D1480638

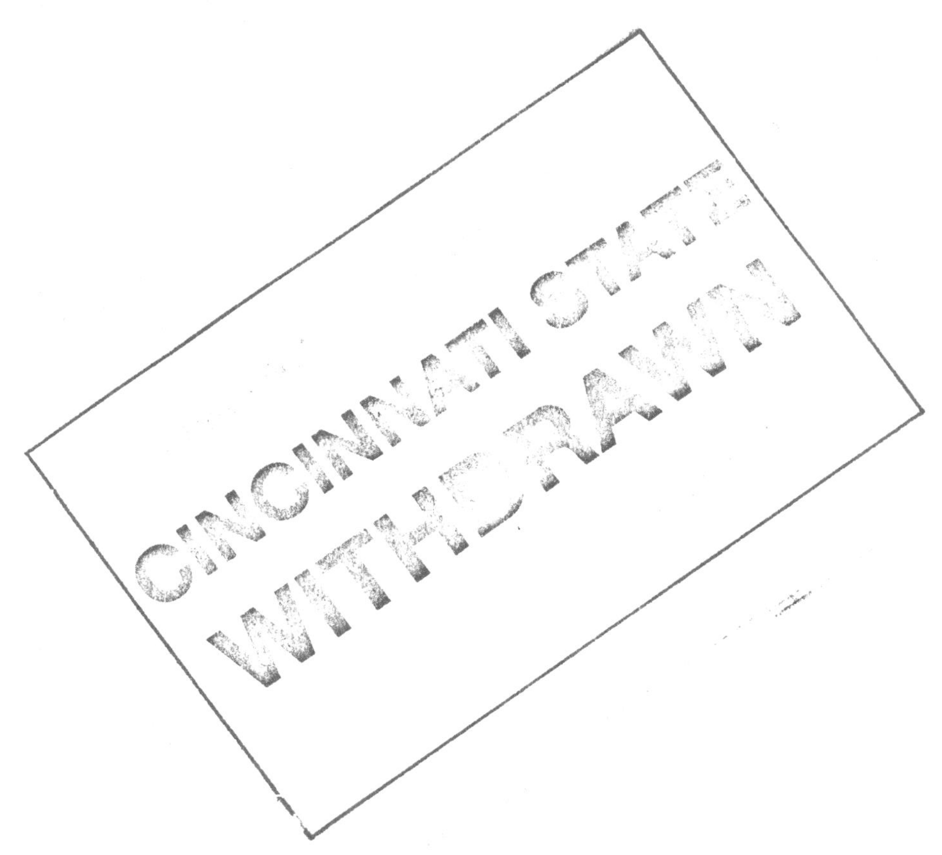
CINCINNATI STATE
WITHDRAWN

Antimicrobial Agents

ANTIBACTERIALS AND ANTIFUNGALS

Antimicrobial Agents

ANTIBACTERIALS AND ANTIFUNGALS

Edited by

André Bryskier, M.D.

Director, Clinical Pharmacology, Anti-infectives
Sanofi-Aventis
Romainville, France

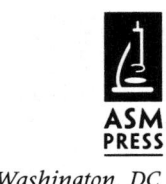

Washington, DC

Cover: *Penicillium* sp., courtesy of Davise H. Larone, MT(ASCP), Ph.D., F(AAM), Weill Medical College and Cornell Medical Center, New York-Presbyterian Hospital

ASM Press
American Society for Microbiology
1752 N Street, N.W.
Washington, DC 20036-2804

Library of Congress Cataloging-in-Publication Data

Antibiotiques, agents antibactériens et antifongiques. English.
Antimicrobial agents : antibacterials and antifungals / edited by André Bryskier.
p. ; cm.
Includes index.
Translation and extensive update of: Antibiotiques, agents antibactériens et antifongiques. 1999.
ISBN-13: 978-1-55581-237-9
ISBN-10: 1-55581-237-6
1. Antibiotics. I. Bryskier, André. II. Title.
[DNLM: 1. Anti-Bacterial Agents—pharmacology. 2. Antifungal Agents —pharmacology. QV 350 A6306 1999a]
RM267.A54313 2005
615'.329—dc22

2005019538

Title of the original French edition: *Antibiotiques, agents antibactériens et antifongiques,* published by Ellipses © 1999 Édition Marketing S.A.

English translation by David Weeks, MA, MèsL, MITI

10 9 8 7 6 5 4 3 2 1

Address editorial correspondence to: ASM Press, 1752 N St., N.W., Washington, DC 20036-2904, U.S.A.

Send orders to: ASM Press, P.O. Box 605, Herndon, VA 20172, U.S.A.
Phone: 800-546-2416; 703-661-1593
Fax: 703-661-1501 Email: Books@asmusa.org Online: Estore.asm.org

I dedicate this work to my wife, Marie Thérèse,
to my two children, Jean-Marie and Marie Isabelle,
and also to my mother for the love they have shown me.

I also wish to dedicate this work to my friend, Jean-François Chantot,
whose constant friendship has been of great support to me.

Contents

Foreword

This book is a tribute to the work of chemists and biologists who have, over the past 50 to 60 years, discovered and developed these "miracle" drugs we call antibiotics and antimicrobials. Antibiotics are natural treasures, essential to the clinician's armamentarium. They control and treat microbes when they cause diseases in people, animals, and plants. One would expect that the cadre of drugs presented in this comprehensive volume would ensure our always having control over microorganisms. In most instances, we can find an effective antibiotic to treat an infection, thanks to the variety we have. Unfortunately, that is not always the case, and too often the drug of first choice fails, leading to prolonged illness, increased costs, and spread of the uncontrolled infectious agent.

Most antibiotics cause minimal harm to the patient, but they are not so specific as to leave no adverse consequence. In the wake of their usage, antibiotics provide strong selective pressure for the propagation of drug-resistant variants among the much larger commensal flora. These so-called "innocent bystanders" surviving antibiotic treatment can subsequently act as reservoirs for resistance traits to be passed on to other neighboring microbes. Moreover, these substances, unlike other therapeutics, are societal drugs. Their use affects a sphere much larger than the individuals who receive them. They impact people at large, broadly affecting the microorganisms associated with the treated patient, as well as others sharing the same environment—hospital room, household, or community.

While the early period following antibiotic development saw the emergence of single drug resistance, today bacteria resistant to more than one drug are more the norm. Some are single resistance determinants that provide cross-resistance to other drugs. Among these, perhaps the most interesting determinants are the multidrug efflux proteins, which can protect the cell from multiple structurally unrelated antibiotics by means of the same mechanism.

We increasingly face organisms whose multiple drug resistance leads to failed treatment and patient death. Modern illnesses and today's technological advances in medicine produce a burgeoning number of patients at risk of infection but immunocompromised due to cancer therapies, transplanted organs, AIDS, and advanced diabetes—conditions where antibiotics are sorely needed. Moreover, as Dr. Bryskier and his colleagues have brought out in this book, there are very few new antibacterials in late-stage development today, and those that have appeared recently already face strains bearing resistance.

Hopefully, new initiatives in research and development will generate a new era of antibiotic discovery which demonstrates rationality in use, and recognition and awareness of the consequences of overuse and misuse. Studies reveal that resistance is not just related to the *amount* used, but also to *how* antibiotics are provided. Chronic low-dose use is optimal for selection of resistance. While we can expect some resistance to emerge with treatment, this sequela does not need to translate to higher frequencies of resistant bacteria and consequent treatment failures. Evidence shows that, with judicious use, we can control such trends and maintain antibiotic efficacy.

This book is unique. I know of none like it, except its original version in French published in 1999. We can thank ASM Press and the authors for pursuing this updated version in English. Now a larger audience of physicians, microbiologists, chemists, pharmacologists, research scientists, and others can benefit from its encyclopedic content. The quality, comprehensive discussion, and illustration of the material are unprecedented. Biologists find themselves lured by chemical structures and chemists are captured by the biology. In one single place, the history, chemical structure, synthesis, mechanisms of action, pharmacology, and efficacy—virtually "all you need to know" about antibiotics—are presented. It is a "bible" in this field, coordinated and largely written by a dedicated clinician, infectious disease expert, colleague, and friend, Dr. André Bryskier. Let's hope that new editions will be needed as new drugs are discovered, to assure us understanding and control of the ever-evolving, ever-responding microbial world.

Stuart B. Levy, M.D.
Boston, Massachusetts
February 2004

Foreword (Revised from the First Edition)

This book, compiled by André Brysker and over twenty-five other experts, is a unique, comprehensive reference on antibiotics. Within these chapters, each antibiotic can be found in the section devoted to the class to which it belongs. Each class is presented by its chemical structure and by means of figures and tables; all the derivatives are then clearly differentiated and classified. The mechanism of action on the bacterial cell and, by consequence, the antibacterial activity is explained, and the relationship between structure and activity is delineated. The pharmacological properties of the compounds and their in vivo distribution underlie the rationale for clinical indication. The potential toxicity to eukaryotic cells and the mechanisms of resistance developed by prokaryotes are considered in each case.

At a time when antibiotics are recognized as a most valuable therapeutic, to be used rationally and prudently, the amount of information given in this book is unprecedented.

Too often the word "antibiotics" is used as one category of therapeutic agents in which many individual agents are comparable. In fact, antibiotics are not so comparable; each agent has different potentials, especially in terms of clinical indications defined by the causal microorganisms and of ecological impact. It is essential to learn the differences between each class, sometimes each subclass or individual agents, to optimize their usage.

Evaluation of an antibiotic may address a diversity of problems: the clinical response and adequate dosage; the status of the patient and his or her defenses against the infection; the causal microorganism, its transmissibility, and its ability to become resistant; and the optimum duration of the treatment and its possible side effects.

In fact, the benefits of anti-infective treatments must be carefully quantified if the cost and the disadvantages are to be evaluated.

The development of new anti-infective agents remains a challenge to all scientific disciplines involved. As in the past, a "good" new product is always difficult to find. The requirements are currently much greater in relation to the increasing knowledge in infectology and the service required by the patient and modern medicine.

This book devotes significant coverage to new acquisitions (molecules under development), which adds to its undisputed usefulness. Descriptions of products used in animals can also be found here.

This book will facilitate the work and enlighten the discussion of all those interested in antibiotics. I express here my best wishes for the success of this fine enterprise.

Jacques F. Acar, M.D.
Paris, June 1999; April 2005

Foreword (Revised from the First Edition)

Foreword to the First Edition

An extraordinary book that is addressed to students, doctors, infectious disease specialists, clinical and basic microbiologists, researchers in the field of infectious diseases, and chemists: it is in this way that we would be tempted to sum up in the simplest form this new treatise on antimicrobial agents. When embarking on such a work, the first question that arises is what its original contribution will be to the wealth of literature already existing in this field. The challenge was therefore a considerable one. However, André Bryskier and the coauthors of these chapters have proved wholly equal to it. There has not previously been a genuine anthology of antimicrobial agents covering the chemical, biochemical, genetic, mechanistic, pharmacokinetic, and toxic aspects of these molecules, not to mention the sophisticated resistance mechanisms developed by the microorganisms against which they are directed.

There are obviously a number of specialist volumes covering specific classes of antibacterial agents and describing some of their fundamental aspects. In practice, however, this type of treatise should serve as a supplement to a larger summary work that acts as a reference source. The need for a reference work reflects the universal dynamic of learning and analysis: from the general summary to the specific case, and not vice versa. The present volume therefore fills an important gap in the vast and fast-moving field of anti-infective agents.

The organization of the book fully obeys this principle of learning. The authors of this work together combine the skills of doctors, microbiologists, and biochemists. From this melting pot has emerged a remarkable synthesis that allows the reader to understand the ins and outs of anti-infective chemotherapy, from its history up to the most recent modern developments. Do not miss the first three chapters at all events. The first recapitulates the principal features of infectious diseases: the leading cause of mortality in humans up until the beginning of the antibiotic era, barely fifty years ago. It highlights the crucial events in the scientific development in this field and the mindset that still underpins our reasoning in the management of infectious diseases and the development of new therapeutic agents. The second chapter is a summary but exhaustive review of the different classes of drugs. It is a synopsis of the contents of the book and an essential reminder of the principal characteristics of the molecules described. Finally, the third chapter reiterates the viewpoint of the bacteria, capable of meeting each of our medical incursions by selecting the most appropriate resistance mutations. This underscores the almost infinite plasticity of the bacterial genome. The epidemiology of resistance is presented in its global universal context and highlights the important and extraordinary ecological changes that antibiotics can inflict on the microbial world if they are not used discerningly. Together, these three chapters provide a prolog to the rest of the book and whet our appetite to discover more.

The following chapters deal systematically with the problem of the development of new anti-infective agents and in particular the details of all the antibacterial and antifungal agents, past, present, and under development. For each class or family of molecules, the presentation is extremely detailed and will satisfy readers of all the levels of competence mentioned earlier. It is difficult to be more precise, and some chapters exceed in detail and novelty many more specialist works already on the market. The chapters dealing with beta-lactams, molecules of the macrolide-lincosamide-streptogramin family, and quinolones in particular are remarkably complete.

Paul Ehrlich, the winner of the Nobel Prize in 1908 for his research into syphilis, advocated the need to discover the "magic bullet" that would destroy the parasite while preserving the host. In less than a century, biomedical research has created not just a bullet, but a whole arsenal. The latter has resulted from exceptional innovative dynamism in academic and industrial research in the second half of this century. However, faced with increasing bacterial resistance, the survival of this therapeutic heritage and the development of new molecules can only be guaranteed by a thorough understanding of the existing inheritance. In this sense, the present work should be found in the library of all doctors specializing in microbiology and infectious diseases. It also belongs in the library of biologists and other specialists interested in these fields. Finally, it belongs in university libraries at the disposal of students. The standard printed version will certainly remain the most convenient source of reference. However, in an area as dynamic as antibiotic resistance and the constant development of new molecules, a computerized version with a regular update would certainly be very welcome. An English translation should also be considered.

We should like here to thank André Bryskier and the coauthors of this work for this remarkable contribution to the field of infectious diseases in general and the pharmacotherapy of bacterial and fungal infections in particular.

Michel Glauser, M.D., and Philippe Moreillon, M.D.
Lausanne University Hospital, Lausanne, Switzerland
Lausanne, 30 June 1999

Preface

Infectious and transmissible diseases have represented one of the great scourges since the dawn of humanity. The awareness of transmissible agents dates back to antiquity in Greece and Egypt. Up to the middle of the 20th century, major epidemics devastated entire populations, sometimes being more murderous than wars. Epidemics of infectious disease have caused profound upheavals in the population and sometimes unexpected sociological and economic changes.

However, despite empirical treatments, it was not until the end of the 19th century that systematic research into anti-infective therapy became established, building on precursors at the beginning of the century such as quinine or emetine. At the same time, scientific advances allowed the parallel development of an improved knowledge of host defense systems and anti-infective chemotherapy. For a long time the two camps were opposed, before being brought together at the end of the 1930s by Gerhard Domagk, who understood that the two systems were complementary and synergistic, an anti-infective agent being merely an aid to the host's defense system by reducing the bacterial burden and thus enabling the host's phagocytes to eliminate any residual bacteria resistant to a given antibacterial agent.

In 1935, Domagk's research culminated in Prontosil, the first of the "sulfa" drugs. Beginning with the great forerunners such as Domagk (sulfonamides, antituberculosis agents), Fleming with Florey and Chain (penicillin), Dubos (thyrothricin), Waksman (streptomycin, neomycin, etc.) and Lehman (para-aminosalicylic acid [PAS]), the field of antibiotic therapy progressed explosively, so that within twenty years the majority of the great families of antibiotics or synthetic antibacterial agents presently used in the treatment of infectious diseases were defined and studied. Some new families for therapeutic use have been discovered since then, but the major innovations have principally involved structural modifications of the molecules within known chemical families.

This enormous progress has coincided with an unprecedented growth in technology and important discoveries in physiology, pathology, and chemistry that have allowed the production of effective therapeutic weapons.

However, thanks to their genetic flexibility, bacteria have adapted to these challenges. The early 21st century is the time of victory for bacteria. The main pathogens in infectious diseases have become progressively resistant to the available antibacterial agents. A long "crusade" will again be necessary to find innovative weapons and original structures with a different mechanism of action to circumvent this adaptation and to overcome this crisis, which will surely be repeated in a few decades' time.

The difficulty is double. Not only have common pathogens acquired resistance, but novel opportunistic microorganisms have emerged among immunosuppressed patients. Furthermore, new pathogens are being discovered, such as *Helicobacter pylori*, against which intensive research is ongoing.

Since the end of the 1980s or the beginning of the 1990s, antibiotic research has begun to change its orientation. Before, the aim of research was to enhance antibacterial activity and enlarge the antibacterial spectrum, to enhance pharmacokinetics, and to improve tolerance and patient comfort (once-a-day administration, lack of bitterness and improved flavor of oral formulations, etc.). Now the goal of anti-infective research is to overcome bacterial resistance.

New antibacterial research is oriented in numerous directions: chemical modification of existing compounds, resulting in analogs with a new mechanism of action (e.g., ketolides, tigecycline, oritavancin, and some new lipopeptides); screening of microorganisms, plants, amphibians, insects, marine stocks, etc., for novel compounds; research into unexploited bacterial targets (peptide deformylase inhibitors) or blockade of resistance mechanisms (efflux pump inhibitors); awareness and adjustment of the use of antibacterials in agriculture (oxazolidinones) and veterinary medicine (mutilins). Current research focuses not only on broad-spectrum derivatives but also on strategies against specific microorganisms (e.g., methicillin-resistant *Staphylococcus aureus* and *H. pylori*).

The increasing variety of families of antibacterial agents and of molecules within them requires classification. It is important to take an interest not only in the molecules that have become drugs, but also in those that have remained unexplored in terms of their therapeutic potential, or those whose development has been stopped prematurely for various reasons: toxicity, difficulty of synthesis, insolubility, high purchase price, or lack of medical need.

This work brings together as much information as possible on the subject of antimicrobial agents. It is intended to provide access for the greatest number of those interested in anti-infective chemotherapy to the information which they require and which is sometimes difficult to find. We hope that we have achieved this aim.

André Bryskier, M.D.
Paris, June 1999; revised July 2005

Contributors

ANTOINE ANDREMONT, Clinical Microbiology, Centre Hospitalier Universitaire Bichat-Claude Bernard, Paris, France

JOSZEF ASZODI, Medicinal Chemistry, Aventis Pharma, Vitry sur Seine, France

EUGÉNIE BERGOGNE-BÉRÉZIN, Clinical Microbiology, Centre Hospitalier Universitaire Bichat-Claude Bernard, Paris, France

ANDRÉ BRYSKIER, Clinical Pharmacology, Anti-infectives, Sanofi-Aventis, Romainville, France (andre.bryskier@wanadoo.fr)

CATHERINE COUTURIER, Microbiology, Sanofi-Aventis, Romainville, France

CHRISTOPHE DINI, Chemical & Physical Sciences, Oroxcell, Romainville, France

LUC DUBREUIL, Clinical Microbiology, Faculty of Pharmaceutical Sciences, Lille, France

CHARLOTTA EDLUND, Department of Microbiology, Pathology and Immunology, Huddinge University Hospital, Karolinska Institutet, and Södertörns Högskola, Stockholm, Sweden

ALAIN FISCH, Emergency Clinics, Centre Hospitalier, Villeneuve Saint Georges, France

RENÉE GRILLOT, Parasitology-Mycology, Centre Hospitalier Universitaire Grenoble, Grenoble, France

JACQUES GROSSET, Clinical Microbiology, Johns Hopkins Hospital, Baltimore, Maryland

JEAN MARC HUSSON, European Academy of Pharmaceutical Medicine, Paris, France

A. JACOLOT, Centre Hospitalier Universitaire Avicenne, Bobigny, France

ANTOINE KAZMIERCZAK, Clinical Microbiology, Centre Hospitalier Universitaire du Bocage, Dijon, France

MICHEL KLICH, Medicinal Chemistry, Hoechst Marion Roussel, Romainville, France

PIERRE LE NOC, Clinical Microbiology, Centre Hospitalier Universitaire Grenoble, Grenoble, France

BERNADETTE LEBEAU, Parasitology-Mycology, Centre Hospitalier Universitaire Grenoble, Grenoble, France

MARC LEBEL, Anapharm, Laval, Québec, Canada

CHUAN LIM, Consultant, Paris, France

JOHN LOWTHER, Clinical Pharmacology, Novexell, Romainville, France

P. NICOLAS, Centre Hospitalier Universitaire Avicenne, Bobigny, France

CARL ERIK NORD, Department of Microbiology, Pathology and Immunology, Huddinge University Hospital, Karolinska Institutet, Stockholm, Sweden

C. PADOIN, Centre Hospitalier Universitaire Avicenne, Bobigny, France

OLIVIER PETITJEAN, Hospital Pharmacy, Centre Hospitalier Universitaire Avicenne, Bobigny, and Clinical Pharmacology, Faculty of Medicine, Paris XIII, France

ÅSA SULLIVAN, Department of Microbiology, Pathology and Immunology, Huddinge University Hospital, Karolinska Institutet, Stockholm, Sweden

MICHEL TOD, Centre Hospitalier Universitaire Avicenne, Bobigny, France

PIERRE VEYSSIER, Internal Medicine, Hôpital de Compiègne, Compiègne, France

Historical Review of Antibacterial Chemotherapy

A. BRYSKIER

1

1. INTRODUCTION

The history of antibacterial agents has been written by a huge number of researchers. Few discoveries in medicine have had so many repercussions as that of penicillin G. All, moreover, have contributed to the success of the new drug: the secret surrounding its birth, the substantial budget invested in its development and industrial production, and finally the fact that it was brought to us by a victorious army. Penicillin G is one of the finest achievements in therapy.

For the first time, medicine had at its disposal a drug in which safety was associated with potent activity. The vicious circle within which anti-infective chemotherapy appeared to be constricted had been broken; activity was no longer inevitably accompanied by toxicity.

Penicillin G is the rallying point for the whole of anti-infective chemotherapy, the history of which can be divided into three periods: the prepenicillin era, the penicillin era, and the postpenicillin era. The history of contemporary anti-infective chemotherapy is more chemical than bacteriological. Purified and therapeutically active substances are obtained by extraction from culture broths or by synthesis or semisynthesis. It is now no longer possible to develop drugs whose chemical structure and pharmacological and toxicological properties are unknown.

1.1. Socioeconomic Consequences of Antibiotic Therapy

In 1935, prophylaxis of infectious diseases was based on studies by Louis Pasteur, Joseph Lister, and Ignaz Semmelweiss. In fact, the control of infections had begun in 1846 with the studies of Semmelweiss, who recommended the use of chlorine, while Lister in 1865 had proposed carbolic acid. The work by Pasteur had stimulated research into vaccines. These studies culminated in the prevention of rabies, diphtheria, tetanus, and, later on, tuberculous meningitis and yellow fever, and also in the recent development of effective vaccines against hepatitis B, typhoid fever, and *Haemophilus influenzae* type b.

In 1935 the treatment of infectious diseases was based principally on serotherapy. Anatoxin vaccines made possible the prevention and treatment of diphtheria and to a lesser extent that of tetanus. Antibacterial sera, on the other hand, possessed more limited activity. Only for cerebrospinal meningitis had mortality initially been spectacularly reduced, but the efficacy of this serotherapy decreased progressively and mortality returned to levels of 70 to 80%.

Apart from a few parasitic diseases, the antibacterial chemotherapy developed by Paul Ehrlich at the end of the 19th century was limited purely to the treatment of syphilis.

Sulfonamide therapy carried great hopes with it, but in fact these were not substantiated until 1945. At that time, penicillin G was a rare and expensive drug, with one vial costing several hundreds of dollars. However, from 1946 onwards, penicillin G was produced in greater quantities and exported worldwide by the United States. It was difficult to handle since it had to be stored at 4°C and few facilities possessed a refrigerator, while the lead time to acquiring the material was 4 to 5 months in Europe. Improvements in chemical and pharmaceutical techniques and in the economic environment gradually made penicillin G more readily accessible.

The advent of anti-infective chemotherapy profoundly altered socioeconomic conditions around the world by prolonging life expectancy, but also by allowing the anarchic growth of the population through a reduction in infant mortality and through the treatment of infectious diseases, such as tuberculosis, leprosy, venereal diseases, lung diseases, and bacterial meningitis, that had been the bane of humanity. Before the introduction of antibacterial agents, the majority of hospitalized patients had been admitted for a disease of infectious origin, a situation that still remains in poor and underdeveloped countries. Hospital departments nowadays, however, chiefly admit patients suffering from neoplasias or cardiovascular diseases. The AIDS epidemic is in the process of completely transforming the reasons for hospitalization.

The introduction of penicillin G and subsequently of streptomycin reduced mortality by 30% in 1947 compared with that in 1938 and prolonged life expectancy, which rose from 42 years in 1960 to more than 70 years in 1967.

A study by the British Ministry of Health showed that the introduction of penicillin G in 1941 reduced infant mortality from congenital syphilis. Rates fell from 1.5 per 1,000 in 1910 to 0.01 per 1,000 in 1954. Mortality and morbidity due to syphilis decreased considerably on all continents, as evidenced in a publication in 1962 from the World Health Organization. A study published in 1962 by the British Ministry of Health showed that important gains had been made in terms of infant mortality since the introduction of antibacterial agents. Infant mortality accounted for 27,000 deaths among children aged 1 to 14 years in 1930, compared with 5,000 in 1960. The introduction of streptomycin and then of other antituberculosis agents exerted a spectacular influence on tuberculosis-related mortality. Scarlet fever, erysipelas, and the other streptococcal skin diseases became curable, and renal and cardiac complications of streptococcal origin declined. The combination of penicillin G and streptomycin provided a treatment for endocarditis of bacterial origin.

However, the changes in the socioeconomic landscape as a result of the new anti-infective therapeutic agents led to the emergence of new infectious diseases. Humanity appeared to have rid itself of the plagues that had altered the economic environment over the centuries and transformed society, such as the great plague and cholera epidemics.

The enrichment of our society and the protection against the social risks associated with disease, as well as the technological progress that has accompanied this prosperity, have resulted in the advent of "high-tech" medicine and surgery, and with them the corollary of the emergence of another form of infectious pathology due to new predators that lie at the basis of the nosocomial or opportunistic infections. The introduction of a new antibacterial agent causes an imbalance in the bacterial ecosystem which, if uncontrolled, results in the emergence in the field of infectious diseases caused by bacteria that until then had been considered laboratory curiosities or that only very rarely affected humans, such as *Mycobacterium avium*. Strains of bacteria considered curable by antibiotics are becoming progressively resistant to these medicines and are at risk of generating new socioeconomic imbalances in the future.

1.2. The Prepenicillin Era

1.2.1. Development of Microbiology

The idea that certain diseases may be due to invisible living beings was proposed by Marcus Terentius Varro in the first century before Christ (116 B.C. to 27 B.C.); in his work *De rerum rusticarum agricultura* (book I, chapter 12), he assumed "the existence of certain animalcules which the eyes cannot see but which, via the air and passing through the mouth and nostrils, enter the body and cause serious diseases there." However, it was not until the end of the 15th century that the first "modern" ideas about infectious diseases were to appear. These related in particular to syphilis.

In 1496 Ulsenius asserted its contagiousness, and then in about 1519 Van Hutten proposed "small winged worms" and Paracelsus "small living organisms" as causative agents. These ideas, although disputed by the majority of doctors, led to prophylactic measures being taken; thus, from 1500 onwards, certain Italian towns instituted health screening of prostitutes.

The first great precursor of bacteriologists was the physician and poet Girolamo Frascator of Verona, Italy. In his treatise on contagious diseases, *De contagione et contagiosis morbis et curatione* (1546), he affirmed the existence of small invisible living organisms that were capable of reproducing and multiplying and which he called contagium vivum or seminaria contagiosis.

He held these responsible for syphilis and tuberculosis. However, these revolutionary ideas in the 16th century found only occasional adherents, such as Montanus in Pavia, Italy.

The first mention of a "direct microbial" observation dates back to 1656 and was made by Athanasius Kircher (1602–1680), who believed he had seen "minute worms" in the blood of patients suffering from plague.

In the middle of the 18th century, the Italian Lazzaro Spallanzani (1729–1799) was the first to succeed in culturing bacteria in bottles containing meat juices, to refute the thesis of spontaneous generation, and to discover bacterial division by fissiparity. He opened the way for experimental research into disinfectants. Spallanzani tested his "animalcules" against various substances, e.g., camphor, terpentine, sulfur, salt water, vinegar, and brandy, and noted that some of them possessed lytic activity. In 1844, Semmelweiss anticipated the infectious origin and method of contagion of the puerperal fever that was decimating new mothers in the hospitals in Vienna, Austria. He blamed its transmission on the hands of the interns and obliged them to disinfect their hands with sodium hypochlorite, which considerably reduced mortality. However, it was not until Pasteur's lecture to the French Academy of Medicine on 18 March 1879 that the causative microorganism was identified: *Streptococcus*.

The last quarter of the 19th century saw the discovery of the principal pathogenic agents thanks to the development of light microscopy, clinical pathology, and culture and identification of bacteria.

The invention of the microscope is attributed to Zacharias Jansen (1588–1628); however, this conventional assumption is currently disputed. It appears that this invention was due to Galileo (1564–1642), who claimed it in the *Saggiatore* (1623). It would seem that Galileo manufactured a microscope in 1610 and that in 1624 he sent a glass to Frederico Cesi which he described precisely in his accompanying letter; the name *microscope* was given to this "glass" in 1625 by Giovanni Faber in his work on Mexican animals. The discovery of the microscope and its use for the study of living beings revolutionized the thinking of scientists; in particular it allowed progress to be made in microbiology, but it also contributed to the acquisition of a basic understanding of the prevention of infectious diseases and the principles of immunity. One of the fathers of protozoology and bacteriology is certainly Antonie van Leeuwenhoek (1632–1723), who constructed a small apparatus in which a biconvex lens was inserted between two copper or silver plates, pierced by a small hole. The object to be studied was held at the focal distance at the top of a rod, the height of which could be adjusted by means of a screw system. The magnifications obtained ranged from ×50 to ×300. Van Leeuwenhoek's descriptions are contained in some 30 letters to Henry Oldenberg, the secretary of the Royal Society of London. Carl von Linné (Carolus Linnaeus), in the 12th edition of *Systema naturae* (1767), aligned himself with the theory of a number of doctors and considered that infectious diseases were due to living beings; Linné's system was adopted by Otto Frederik Müller, who described a genus, *Monas*, that included cocci and bacteria. However, progress in taxonomy was due to Frederich Gmelin, who, in the reedition of *Systema naturae* by C. Linné, added the genus *Bacillaria*. The father of clinical pathology is François-Xavier Bichat (1771 to 1802). He studied the postmortem changes caused by disease in various organs. His studies are reported in several works, including *Anatomie descriptive* (1801 to 1803).

The establishment of the clinical anatomy school by H. Laennec (1781–1826) was to assist in the development of this science, allowing clinicopathological conferences and opening the way to the study of pathophysiology.

Typhoid is one example. In 1813, Petit and Serres described enteromesenteric fever. In 1820, Pierre Bretonneau proposed the name *dothienenteritis*, which his pupil, Armand Trousseau, simplified to *dothienenteria*. In 1829, Pierre Charles Louis applied himself to the description of the clinical and anatomical signs. In 1862, Charles Marchison attributed its origin to poisoning of the drinking water by fecal matter. In 1880, Carl Eberth described the bacillus, which he observed in typhous organs.

It was to Pasteur's credit that not only did he refute definitively the Aristotelian theory of spontaneous generation, but also he showed that fermentation, putrefaction, and certain types of acidification were due to microorganisms; in addition, he was the first to demonstrate that a microorganism was responsible for a specific infection through his study of cholera in chickens. The true father of modern epidemiology is John Snow, who in 1855 explained the mode of transmission of cholera from water contaminated with fecal matter.

In 1887, Anton Weichselbaum, from Vienna, detected a "coffee grain" microorganism in a sample from a patient with purulent meningitis that was negative by Gram staining, a procedure that had recently been developed; it was not until 1903 that he was able to confirm the pathogenicity of this organism by the systematic study of cerebrospinal fluid taken from patients with cerebrospinal meningitis by the lumbar puncture technique developed by H. Quincke in 1890.

Staphylococci were described in 1876 by Pasteur, the gonococcus was described by Albert Neisser in 1879, the diphtheria bacillus was described by Friedrich Loeffler in 1883, the causative agent of whooping cough was described by Jules Bordet and Octave Gengou in 1906, and the causative agent of the plague was described by Alexandre Yersin in 1894.

In 1865, Jean Villemin demonstrated that material from tuberculous lesions on humans, inoculated under the skin of the rabbit or guinea pig, caused the emergence of pulmonary lesions. He thus proved that tuberculosis was an inoculable, contagious, and avoidable disease; in 1882, Robert Koch discovered the pathogenic agent, *Mycobacterium tuberculosis*.

At the same time, the causative agent of malaria was described by Charles Laveran (1880), that of toxoplasmosis was described by Charles Nicolle and L. Manceaux (1908), that of amoebic abscess was described by Robert Koch and G. Gaffky (1886 and 1887), and that of trypanosomiasis was described by J. E. Dutton (1902) and A. Castellani (1903). *Leishmania* was "officially" discovered by W. B. Leishman (1865–1926) in 1900 and C. Donovan in 1903; however, the first observation of the parasite was made in 1885 by D. Cunningham (1843–1914) and Borowski in 1898.

1.3. Empirical Treatments

Infectious diseases had for centuries been treated empirically using plant extracts such as that of "kina-kina," ipecac, qing haosu, and chang san.

Traditional African, Asian, Indian, and Ptolemaic medicines refer to the use of plant extracts.

Molds were probably used in antiquity. A team of anthropologists from the University of Massachusetts (E. J. Basset et al.) observed a fluorescence characteristic of cyclines in the bones of skeletons exhumed from the Sudanese-Nubian civilization (350 B.C.). It is likely that these molds were used by the Greeks, Romans, Carthaginians, Hebrews, and Philistines. It would appear that molds of the *Penicillium* type have been used since ancient times by Egyptians and Hebrews, and they still are in certain regions of the Himalayas, such as Bhutan.

1.4. The First Chemical Agents

The first therapeutic agents that were properly defined chemically were quinine, extracted from the bark of cinchona by Pierre Pelletier and Joseph Caventou (1819), and emetine, which was isolated by Pierre Pelletier and François Magendie in 1817 from ipecac root.

However, the first studies on antibacterial agents began in 1886 with the observation of the antiplasmodial activity of methylene blue by Louis Guttman and Paul Ehrlich.

Felix Mesnil and Charles Nicolle demonstrated the activity of trypan blue against *Trypanosoma brucei*. The first major stage in anti-infective chemotherapy was the introduction by Thomas and Breinl in 1905 of the arsenical derivatives following studies by Ehrlich in the treatment of these infections. For a long time, the treatment of trypanosomiasis was to be based on this type of derivative, such as *p*-aminophenylarsonic acid (Atoxyl).

In 1911, Paul Ehrlich and Sahachiro Hata showed the good activity of arsphenamine in experimental syphilis in the rabbit. Its soluble form, neoarsphenamine, was used in the treatment of syphilis from 1912 until the introduction of penicillin.

Also in 1911, J. Morgenroth and R. Lévy reported good activity by ethylhydrocupreine (Optochine) in the treatment of experimental pneumococcal infections in the mouse. This compound is still used as a laboratory test.

The subsequent stage, following the use and development of the arsenical derivatives, was the development of molecules with a substrate of polyazole dyes. Antimalarial agents were progressively prepared, such as plasmoquine in 1928, mepacrine in 1933, and chloroquine in 1939.

1.5. Sulfonamides

The studies by Ehrlich profoundly affected pharmacological research at the end of the 19th century and beginning of the 20th century. Research was focused on dye substances. Dyes of the sulfonamide type were synthesized in 1908 by P. Gelmo and in 1919 by M. Heidelberger and W. A. Jacobs. The credit for demonstrating the antibacterial activity of sulfamidochrysoidine in vivo in the treatment of experimental streptococcal septicemia, despite the fact that the substance was inactive in vitro, goes to Gerhard Domagk. A few months later, J. Tréfouël and his team showed that sulfamidochrysoidine was metabolized and that only the *para*-aminophenylsulfonamide moiety was active. In 1935, F. M. Mietzch and P. Klave synthesized a series of amino dyes comprising the sulfonamide group, including Prontosil and Rubiazol, which have been used since 1936 in the treatment of infectious diseases. From this observation, more than 5,000 molecules were synthesized and tested between 1935 and 1945.

The sulfonamides were the first broad-spectrum antibacterial medications. They allowed the development of rational methods for the treatment of infectious diseases and were the origin of chemotherapy in clinical microbiology.

The cure of a case of purulent streptococcal meningitis at the Institut Pasteur hospital in Paris, France, represented one of the first clinical success of sulfonamides. Sulfonamides proved effective in the treatment of other streptococcal infections, such as erysipelas and puerperal fever, the mortality of which reached its lowest level prior to the use of penicillin G. The cure of meningococcal meningitis constituted the most spectacular therapeutic success.

Other diseases have been treated with sulfonamides, particularly those due to staphylococci, gonococci, and pneumococci.

The sulfonamides gave rise to the sulfones. Starting from the assumption that the atom of sulfur is the key to the antibacterial activity of the sulfonamides, Tréfouël prepared derivatives in which the sulfur atom was oxidized. The most active derivative was *para*-diaminophenylsulfone, or dapsone. The antibacterial activity of the sulfones was demonstrated in 1937 by two independent teams, those under Ernest F. Fourneau in France and George B. Buttle in the United Kingdom. In 1939, R. Rist demonstrated the antituberculosis activity of the sulfones in vitro and in vivo. However, the results for humans proved disappointing. The relationship between Robert Koch's and Armauer Hansen's bacilli caused Faget in the United States to try sulfones in the treatment of leprosy. The introduction of dapsone by H. Floch and P. Destombes at the Institut Pasteur of Guyana was a decisive stage. The sulfones became one of the cornerstones of the treatment of leprosy.

1.6. Antibiosis

Another route of access to the treatment of infectious diseases was the antagonism of growth between two microorganisms. This effect was called *antibiosis* by Paul Vuillemin in 1889. The first observation of this phenomenon reported in the literature was made by Bartolomeo Bizio, who in 1823 observed the inhibition of the growth of *Serratia marcescens* by molds. The second observation of this phenomenon was made in 1876 by John Tyndall, who demonstrated the activity of *Penicillium*.

In 1877, Louis Pasteur and Jules F. Joubert described the phenomenon of the antagonism existing between *Bacillus anthracis* and other bacteria:

> It is sufficient that the liquid which holds the bacterium in suspension should be combined with other bacteria for the bacterium to perish entirely. These facts justify the greatest possible hope from a therapeutic viewpoint.

Vicenzio Tiberio in 1895 described the inhibitory action of culture filtrates of *Aspergillus flavescens*, *Mucor mucedo*, and *Penicillium glaucum* on different microorganisms, such as the bacilli of anthrax, typhoid fever, cholera, etc. Bartolomeo Gosio, in 1896, was the first to obtain a pure crystalline substance possessing antibiotic activity from *P. glaucum*. In 1897, E. Duchesne confirmed the activity of certain *Penicillium* organisms.

B. anthracis cannot develop in the presence of *Pseudomonas aeruginosa*. In 1899, Rudolf Emmerich and Oscar Low sought to explain this phenomenon. They noted that the filtrate of a 4-week culture of *P. aeruginosa*, evaporated, dialyzed, precipitated with alcohol, and redissolved in water, destroyed certain microorganisms, such as streptococci, staphylococci, and the diphtheria bacillus. They called this substance pyocyanase; it might be considered the first antibiotic from a historical point of view.

Pyocyanase was used by Fortineau in the treatment of anthrax. A number of studies have been devoted to antibiosis. In 1885, A. V. Cornil and Victor Babes postulated that the origin of this antagonism was a substance produced by one microorganism that inhibited the growth of another. This was demonstrated in 1887 by Garré. A number of physicians contributed to these studies: A. de Bary (1879), Catani (1885), E. Freudenreich (1888), Bouchard (1889), Doehle (1889), B. Gosio (1896), and E. Duchesne (1897).

Two pivotal studies should be noted here: the study by Emmerich and Low already mentioned and the 1885 study by Catani, who "insufflated" a bacterium-gelatin mixture into the airways of patients suffering from pulmonary tuberculosis. He obtained satisfactory clinical results. The idea of "bacteriotherapy" postulated in 1881 by Max von Pettenkofer was thus implemented with these two studies.

In 1871, John B. Sanderson demonstrated the impossibility for bacteria to develop in the presence of certain *Penicillium* organisms. Joseph Lister in 1875 reported the same phenomenon, as did Tyndall in 1876 and Roberts in 1874.

Lister, in 1885, reported anecdotally the use of *Penicillium* to treat wounds. In 1886 Gosio isolated a phenolic substance (mycophenolic acid) from *Penicillium brevicompactum* by fermentation, which he crystallized, and demonstrated that it possessed potent "antiseptic" activity against *Bacteridium anthracis*.

In 1897, Duchesne demonstrated antagonism of the growth of *Escherichia coli* in the presence of *P. glaucum*. In 1913, Carl L. Alsberg and Otis F. Black isolated *Penicillium puberulum* from which they obtained "penicillic" acid in crystalline form, which proved to inhibit the growth of *Bacterium coli* (*E. coli*). These in vitro and in vivo studies were not followed up. Almost 40 years were to elapse before these results were to find any echo.

A. Vaudremer, in 1913, showed that filtered extracts obtained from *Aspergillus fumigatus* possessed antistaphylococcal and antituberculosis activity. He attempted to treat tuberculosis with these extracts.

In 1944, Soltys extracted aspergillin; this product was relatively nontoxic and was used in the treatment of staphylococcal skin infections.

The interest aroused by these substances extracted from "molds" or bacteria was considerable, and a methodical search was instituted. Zeller and Schmitz demonstrated the antibacterial activity of a "toxic" substance formed during the metabolism of *Aspergillus niger* and *A. fumigatus*.

1.7. Definition of Antibiotics

In 1941, Selman Waksman christened all of these substances "antibiotics." The term *antibiotic* itself was invented in 1889 by Vuillemin, who also proposed the term *antibiont* for microorganisms that caused antibiosis. An antibiotic is a derivative produced by the metabolism of microorganisms that possesses antibacterial activity at low concentrations and is not toxic to the host. This concept has been extended to molecules obtained by semisynthesis.

The antibacterial agents obtained by total synthesis, such as the quinolones, benzylpyrimidines (co-trimoxazole), nitroheterocycles, and penems, are synthetic antibacterial agents and not antibiotics.

However, usage has meant that any substance possessing antibacterial activity and which is not toxic to the host is referred to as an antibiotic.

1.8. "Antiseptics"

The use of antiseptics for the external treatment of wounds and for asepsis dates back to the middle of the 19th century. Chlorine was isolated as an element in 1809 by Humphry Davy. In 1846, Semmelweiss recommended sodium hypochlorite as an antiseptic. In 1881, Robert Koch demonstrated the antibacterial activity of hypochlorites. Dakin's solution, introduced by Dakin in 1915 as a disinfectant for war wounds, contains 0.45 to 0.50% sodium hypochlorite. Iodine, discovered in 1812 by the Frenchman Courtois, was introduced as a wound disinfectant in 1839 by Davies and was registered in the U.S. Pharmacopeia in 1830 under the name of iodine tincture (tinctura iodini) and iodine liniment. The first studies actually demonstrating the bacterial activity of iodine date back to Casimir Davaine, who worked on the subject between 1874 and 1881.

It was not until the beginning of the 20th century that the different alcohols were used as disinfectants. The use of "systemic disinfectants" came to light in about 1870. In 1871, A. E. Sansom published his treatise *The Antiseptic System: a Treatise on Carbolic Acid and Its Compounds*. In this work, he supported Lister's thesis on antisepsis and proposed the systemic administration of sulfophenolic derivatives. Other phenolic derivatives were tested, such as menthol and thymol. The oils of the phenolic derivatives, such as peppermint, were used by Bradson in 1888 as inhalants in the treatment of pulmonary tuberculosis.

In the 1890s, phenolic derivatives, such as creosote and guaiacol, were administered parenterally.

Bacterial therapy and the use of phenolic derivatives were paralleled by the development of immunotherapy, which gave rise to anatoxic toxinic vaccines.

2. THE PENCILLIN ERA

From 1945, research in the field of antibacterial chemotherapy followed two directions: (i) synthetic antibacterial agents not found in nature and (ii) antibiotics extracted from the fermentation of molds, actinomycetes, and other bacterial genera.

2.1. Antibiotics of Fungal Origin

The prototype of antibiotics of fungal origin is penicillin. The second great family of antibiotics extracted from molds is that of the cephems.

2.1.1. The Discovery of Penicillin

In 1729, Pier Antonio Micheli, in his work *Nova plantarum genera*, described the penicillia, and at the same time it was accepted that Linné's taxon *Mucor crustaceus* (1742) comprised certain penicillia. The genus *Penicillium* established by H. Link in 1809 is a group of molds.

Alexander Fleming (1881–1955) was assigned to a military surgical detachment in Boulogne, France, during the First World War. In treating the wounded, he realized the need for antiseptics more suitable than those available to him. At the end of the war he resumed his work as a microbiologist, and in 1928 he was asked to write a chapter devoted to staphylococci. Because of his professional conscientiousness, he decided to repeat and validate all the experiments described in the literature. The conjunction of Fleming's summer holidays and the presence of C. J. La Touche's mycology laboratory close to Fleming's allowed the greatest discovery of the 20th century: penicillin. On departing on holiday, Fleming left uncovered the petri dishes containing cultures of staphylococci that were to be contaminated by spores of fungal origin. *Penicillium notatum* accidentally contaminated the petri dishes containing cultures of *Staphylococcus aureus*. The era of modern antibiotic therapy thus began obscurely.

In 1929, Fleming published his studies on the potent antibacterial activity of a very active substance known as penicillin, which was capable of inhibiting the growth of *S. aureus* and *Streptococcus pyogenes* and that was also practically devoid of toxicity.

In the first publication, the strain of *Penicillium* had been classified as *Penicillium rubrum* by the mycology team of St. Mary's Hospital in London, England. Raistrick and Tom showed that this was *P. notatum*, a species similar to *Penicillium chrysogenum* described in 1911 by Westling.

The publication by Fleming in 1929 did not attract the attention of the scientific and medical world. Fleming's initial studies were not extended because of the difficulties encountered in isolating and purifying penicillin.

In fact, at the beginning of the 1930s, nothing had changed since the introduction of arsphenamine (Salvarsan) for the treatment of syphilis by Ehrlich. The therapeutic efficacy of the sulfonamides generated new enthusiasm for research into other anti-infective derivatives, allowing the treatment of staphylococcal and pneumococcal infections or tuberculosis. It was in this preantibiotic atmosphere that Howard Florey and Ernst Chain of Oxford University decided to focus their interest on antibacterial agents. Their analysis of the literature led them to rediscover the work by Fleming, and they obtained the strain of *Penicillium* and the Czapek Dox culture medium modified by Raistrick in 1932, which enabled a larger quantity of penicillin to be produced. They then modified the extraction and storage technique.

Florey and Chain published their experimental studies on penicillin in *The Lancet* in 1940. This publication was the starting point of modern antibiotic therapy. The first patients were treated with penicillin in 1941.

The problem of the elucidation of the structure of penicillin and of its industrial production was studied between 1941 and 1944. Its structure was published simultaneously by two independent teams, that of Chain and that of Karl Folkers from Merck Sharp and Dohme. Industrial fermentation was the main work of the chairman of Pfizer Co., John L. Smith. The company specialized in fermentation processes and produced citric acid and vitamin B_2.

The selection of mutants of *P. chrysogenum* produced a better yield. Otto Behrens, from Eli Lilly, observed that *P. chrysogenum* was capable of incorporating various chemical chains and particularly *p*-aminophenylacetic acids. The discovery of the cleavage of the side chain by an enzyme produced by a species of *Streptomyces* or by a strain of *E. coli* yielded the 6-aminopenicillanic nucleus from which a number of semisyntheses were performed, giving rise to the phenoxypenicillins (1959), isoxazolylpenicillins (oxacillin, cloxacillin, and flucloxacillin), ampicillins, α-carboxypenicillins (carbenicillin, and ticarcillin) and *N*-acylpenicillins (azlocillin, mezlocillin, piperacillin, apalcillin, etc.).

2.1.2. The Cephems

The discovery of the antibacterial activity of *Cephalosporium acremonium* extracts occurred as a result of intense research in the area of the antibacterial activity of culture filtrates obtained from the fermentation of actinomycetes.

2.1.2.1. The Discovery Made by Giuseppe Brotzu

In 1945, Giuseppe Brotzu isolated a strain of *C. acremonium* from the sewage discharged into the sea at Cagliari in Sardinia (Italy). This mold produces a substance that inhibits the growth of numerous bacterial species, including staphylococci, salmonellae, pasteurellae, brucellae, vibrios, and shigellae. The culture filtrate and the crude extracts of the fermentation product of *C. acremonium* were injected locally into abscesses, causing them to regress, but pain and fever were noted on injection. As Brotzu did not have the resources necessary to continue the studies in Sardinia, he succeeded in persuading Florey at Oxford University to take an interest in them and in 1948 sent him the strain of *C. acremonium*.

2.1.2.2. The Discovery of Cephalosporin C

Initially two substances were isolated, cephalosporin P, which is active against gram-positive bacteria, and cephalosporin N (penicillin N), which is active against gram-positive and gram-negative bacteria. Penicillin N was one of the substrates that was to give rise to ampicillin.

In 1953, G. G. F. Newton and Edward Abraham discovered a third metabolite, cephalosporin C, that possessed only 10% of the activity of penicillin N. It attracted the attention of researchers at Oxford University because it was much more stable in an acidic medium than penicillin N and because of its greater resistance to hydrolysis by the penicillinase produced by *Bacillus subtilis*. In addition, it was atoxic in mice, and in vivo it protected mice infected with penicillin G-resistant strains of staphylococci and streptococci.

In 1957, E. Felly et al. discovered a mutant strain of *Cephalosporium* producing large quantities of cephalosporin C. Cephalosporin C is a good substrate for chemical modifications.

2.1.2.3. Cephalothin and Cephaloridine

The introduction of penicillin G was rapidly followed by the appearance of clinical strains of penicillin G-resistant *S. aureus*. The need rapidly arose for new antibiotics that could kill these resistant strains. New chemical entities were thus made commercially available with the aim of treating staphylococcal infections due to penicillin G-resistant strains. The example of these in the United States is erythromycin. A number of semisynthetic studies based on penicillin G culminated initially in the phenoxypenicillins and subsequently in the group M penicillins at the beginning of the 1960s. At the same time, research based on cephalosporin C culminated in the semisynthesis of the first cephalosporins.

At the end of 1957, researchers at Glaxo in the United Kingdom succeeded in producing 100 g of cephalosporin C, from which its structure was defined and published in 1961. D. C. Hodgkin and E. N. Maslen confirmed its crystallographic structure.

The third stage was developed from a technique by R. B. Morin at Eli Lilly that allowed hydrolysis of the D-α-aminoadipic chain of the cephem nucleus producing the 7-aminocephalosporanic nucleus (7-ACA).

The first injectable cephalosporin, cephalothin, was prepared by acylation of the 7-ACA nucleus with 2-chlorothienylacetyl. Abraham et al. very rapidly realized that the chain attached to the methylene at position C-3 of the cephem nucleus could be readily displaced by nitrogen chains. When cephalothin sodium is treated with pyridine, the resultant product is cephaloridine.

The success of cephalothin and cephaloridine, which possess good activity against penicillinase-producing strains of *S. aureus*, encouraged research to increase the metabolic stability (because cephalothin is metabolized), enhance the pharmacokinetics, increase the antibacterial activity, and broaden the bacterial spectrum.

Among all the molecules resulting from this first wave of research, cefazolin was semisynthesized by the company Fujisawa. The chain at position C-7 was modified by a tetrazole nucleus and in particular by the introduction at position C-3 of a thiadiazolethiomethylene chain. One of the components of the second and third waves of cephalosporins, a thiomethyl chain to which is attached a heteroatomic nucleus, is seen at position C-3. Cefazolin is less active than cephalothin against penicillin G-resistant strains of *S. aureus*, but its pharmacokinetic profile is characterized by an apparent elimination half-life of more than 3 h. Other molecules from this group have been synthesized, providing only a few marginal advantages over cephalothin.

2.1.2.4. Cefamandole, Cefuroxime, and Other Derivatives

The two main research teams working in the field of cephalosporins produced molecules of an intermediate level in terms of antibacterial innovation but provided the oxyimine chain (cefuroxime) on the one hand and the thiomethyltetrazole nucleus (cefamandole) on the other. The oxyimine chain is the basic structure of all recent molecules; conversely, the thiomethyltetrazole nucleus, which provides good activity against enterobacteria, is present in a number of extended-spectrum (third-generation) cephalosporins, such as cefoperazone, cefmenoxime, latamoxef, cefotetan, and cefminox. These molecules were in some cases abandoned over time because of the antabuse effect they cause and the hypoprothrombinemia associated with disorders of vitamin K metabolism.

Cefamandole and cefuroxime have provided additional activity against enterobacteria producing plasmid-mediated β-lactamases. Cefamandole has the same activity as cephalothin against gram-positive cocci.

2.1.2.5. The New Cephems

In the mid-1970s, the bacterial ecology of hospitals changed and the focus of concerns in anti-infective therapy moved towards *P. aeruginosa* and certain species of Enterobacteriaceae, particularly *Proteus* spp.

Research into β-lactams was conducted simultaneously in the fields of penicillins and cephems. Certain chemical structures developed in the field of penicillins were transposed to cephalosporins; for example, piperacillin and cefoperazone have the same ethyldioxopiperazinyl chain, as do apalcillin and cefpiramide.

The number of cephalosporins increased, and thus the great family of cephems gradually developed. Three routes of research culminated in this family: total synthesis, analysis of the fermentation products, and semisynthesis based on the 7-ACA nucleus.

Total synthesis yielded two classes of cephems: the oxa-1-cephems, of which two molecules were made commercially available, latamoxef and flomoxef, and the carbacephems, one of which has been used therapeutically, loracarbef. Other total syntheses resulted in research molecules such as the isocephems.

The second route was the discovery of the cephamycins from fermentation products. The class of cephamycins comprises cefoxitin, cefotetan, cefminox, cefbuperazone, and cefmetazole. These molecules are less active than cefamandole or cefuroxime, but by virtue of the presence of a methoxy group at position 7α, they have better stability against hydrolysis by certain β-lactamases, such as those produced by *Bacteroides fragilis*.

The third route is the semisynthesis of new derivatives from the 7-ACA nucleus.

2.1.2.6. Cefotaxime and Derivatives

Research into cephalosporins in the mid-1970s was directed towards two poles: *P. aeruginosa* and β-lactamase-producing enterobacteria.

The discovery of the good antipseudomonas activity of sulbenicillin allowed the development of a narrow-spectrum cephalosporin, cefsulodin. This molecule has two points of attraction: a charged nucleus at position 7, pyridinium, and the presence of a negatively charged sulfone group; it possesses two negative charges and a positive charge and subsequently gave rise to ceftazidime through the addition of an oxyimine chain and the 2-amino-5-thiazolyl nucleus. At the same time, cephalosporins derived conceptually from cefamandole with different chains attached at position 7 also came to light: the *N*-acylcephalosporins, such as cefoperazone, cefpiramide, and cefpimizole, possessing moderate activity against *P. aeruginosa* and hydrolyzed to a greater or lesser extent by plasmid-mediated broad-spectrum enterobacterial β-lactamases.

The true innovation in terms of cephalosporins was the discovery of the 2-amino-5-thiazolyl nucleus by researchers from Roussel Uclaf. All of the modern molecules possess this nucleus, which is part of the basic structure. One variant is the 5-amino-2-thiadiazole nucleus, which produces a moderate increase in activity against *P. aeruginosa* but causes a slight reduction in activity against enterobacteria.

The combination of an oxime chain and the 2-amino-5-thiazolyl nucleus gave rise to cefotaxime and its derivatives. The activity associated with the oxime chain was demonstrated by Glaxo in a synthetic intermediate of the α-aminocephalosporins and by researchers from Fujisawa who noted the activity of nocarcidin A, which has a hydroxyimine chain. Only one 2-amino-5-thiazolyl derivative does not possess a methoxyimine chain, which is less stable against hydrolysis by plasmid-mediated β-lactamases.

The various derivatives of this class are characterized by the chain at position C-3. All of them possess a nitrogen heteroatomic nucleus, except for ceftizoxime, which has no chain at position C-3. It is interesting that ceftizoxime has activity identical to that of cefotaxime against penicillin G-sensitive strains of *Streptococcus pneumoniae* but is totally inactive against strains moderately susceptible or resistant to penicillin G, showing that the substituent at position 3 of the cephem nucleus is important in terms of antibacterial activity.

The heteroatomic substituent varies: it can be thiomethyltetrazole (cefmenoxime), triazine (ceftriaxone), or thiazolyl (cefodizime). Depending on their substituents, these nuclei endow these molecules with original profiles, a long apparent elimination half-life (ceftriaxone and cefodizime), and immunomodulatory properties (cefodizime). The thiomethyltetrazole nucleus is the cause of side effects, principally related to the methyl group.

2.1.2.7. Explosion of the Class of β-Lactams

For more than 35 years the penicillins held sway, followed since the 1970s by the cephalosporins. Ongoing research has identified the carbapenems and monocyclic β-lactams during the systematic analysis of fermentation products from mutant strains of known or new species. Several molecules have emerged, such as imipenem, aztreonam, and carumonam. I should also mention β-lactamase inhibitors, such as clavulanic acid.

The second route was the original idea by R. B. Woodward in 1977 of combining the chemical advantages of the penicillins and cephems. This idea gave rise to the penems, molecules obtained by chemical synthesis, some of which are under clinical development, e.g. fropenem (faropenem), ritipenem, and sulopenem.

2.1.2.8. C-3′ Quaternary Ammonium Cephalosporins

Cefotaxime and its derivatives possess excellent activity against the so-called Richmond class I non-β-lactamase-producing enterobacteria (i.e., those producing cephalosporinases) and against streptococci, pneumococci, *H. influenzae*, and *M. catarrhalis*. However, these drugs are moderately active against oxacillin-susceptible strains of *S. aureus* and also against *P. aeruginosa*.

The first molecules to possess activity against *P. aeruginosa* were cefsulodin and, among the 2-amino-5-thiazolyls, ceftazidime, which is moderately active against *S. aureus* and inactive against cephalosporinase-producing strains of enterobacteria.

A new important stage in the history of cephalosporins was the demonstration of the activity of a chain of the quaternary ammonium type, attached at position 3 of the cephem nucleus, against difficult strains of gram-negative bacilli.

The first molecule to be synthesized was cefpirome in 1981, which possesses a cyclopentenopyridinium nucleus, followed some time later by cefepime. Since then, other molecules have joined this group: cefclidin, cefozopran, and, more recently, cefoselis and cefluprenam.

The major characteristic of these molecules is their good activity against cephalosporinase-producing strains of enterobacteria. The mechanism of action has been particularly well studied for *Citrobacter freundii*. These molecules, with their zwitterionic nature, very rapidly penetrate the bacterial wall and reach the periplasmic space that contains the cephalosporinase-like enzymes. They do not have time to be hydrolyzed because they have a twofold characteristic, speed and weak enzymatic affinity, and they bind to penicillin-binding proteins with an affinity similar to that of cefotaxime.

The second characteristic of these compounds is their activity against *P. aeruginosa*. Some of them also have balanced activity between gram-positive cocci and gram-negative bacilli, such as cefpirome and cefozopran, in contrast to cefclidin, which is inactive against *S. aureus*. The good activity against gram-positive cocci is particularly apparent with cefpirome, which possesses good antipneumococcal activity.

2.1.2.9. Cephalosporins of the Year 2000

The story of the cephalosporins is constantly evolving. Three essential chemical features constitute the basic skeleton of future molecules: the 2-amino-5-thiazolyl nucleus, the oxyimine chain at position C-7 of the cephem nucleus, and a quaternary ammonium function at position C-3.

Future molecules will have to resolve the problem posed by the extended-spectrum β-lactamases produced by *Enterobacteriaceae* such as *Klebsiella pneumoniae*, *E. coli*, and *Enterobacter* spp. while at the same time retaining the microbiological properties provided by molecules such as cefpirome and cefepime.

A number of derivatives containing a catechol or pyridone nucleus linked to the oxyimine chain that have not progressed beyond the preclinical stage possess a supplementary and original mechanism of action. In addition to the standard transporin pathway, they employ iron siderophore transporters to penetrate the bacterial wall.

Cephalosporins exhibiting antistaphylococcal activity against strains resistant to methicillin have been produced and are currently under development.

2.1.2.10. Oral Cephalosporins

The search for orally absorbable antibiotics of the β-lactam family that are not destroyed by gastric acidity has resulted in the synthesis of the phenoxypenicillins. The major turning point was the semisynthesis of the α-aminopenicillins, the parent molecule of which is ampicillin. From this basic structure, the semisynthesis of α-aminocephalosporins resulted in cephaloglycin.

Among the α-aminocephalosporins, the most active molecule in vitro is cefprozil, which possesses antibacterial activity and a more advantageous pharmacokinetic profile than that of cefaclor.

Several oral cephalosporins are prodrugs, such as cefotiam hexetil, cefuroxime axetil, cefteram pivoxil, cefetamet pivoxil, cefcamate pivoxil, cefdaloxime penxetil, cefditoren pivoxil and cefpodoxime proxetil. Other molecules are not esterified, such as cefixime and ceftibuten, apart from loracarbef, which is a carbacephem.

All of the new derivatives have a broad antibacterial spectrum and good activity against gram-negative bacilli. The oral cephalosporins are of considerable interest. When the patient's infectious state permits, it is preferable to use the oral rather than the parenteral route. Oral cephalosporins have a number of advantages over other orally administered chemical classes. In contrast to the fluoroquinolones, co-trimoxazole, and cyclines, they may be administered to children, to the elderly, and to pregnant women.

Taking the parenteral cephalosporins as a basis, pharmaceutical studies have been conducted to produce formulations that allow another route of administration. Lipid-type suspensions have been prepared to allow the ingestion of ceftizoxime or ceftriaxone, but this approach appears to have been short-lived. Suppositories constitute another pharmaceutical formulation, ceftizoxime being made commercially available in Japan in this form. The idea is to use this route of administration in young children, for surgical prophylaxis, and in patients for whom the intramuscular route is contraindicated and the intravenous route is not justified.

2.1.3. Antibiotics Extracted from *Bacillus* spp.

In 1907, Nicolle noted that *B. subtilis* was capable of lysing pneumococci. Later, E. Duclaux discovered the same property in other *Bacillus* species. René Dubos in 1939 isolated tyrothricin, a substance possessing antibiotic activity, from a soil organism which he called *Bacillus brevis*. In 1941, René Dubos and Rollin Hotchkiss fractionated the product into two components: gramicidin and tyrocidine. Bacitracin was isolated by A. S. Johnson et al. in 1945 from *Bacillus licheniformis* from the infected wound of a patient. Because of its chemical instability in biological fluids and its poor systemic tolerance, it has been recommended in the treatment of local infections since 1948.

2.1.4. Antibiotics Extracted from *Actinomyces* spp.

After the discovery of penicillin G, the second major advance in antibiotic therapy was the discovery of antibacterial products produced by actinomycetes. All of the major families of antibiotics were progressively discovered: chloramphenicol in 1947, chlortetracycline and oxytetracycline in 1948, erythromycin in 1952, vancomycin in 1955, rifamycin in 1961, gentamicin in 1963, and lincomycin in 1966.

The capacity of a large number of actinomycetes to inhibit bacterial and fungal growth was established at the end of the 19th century. In 1890, G. Gasparini was the first to report these properties for a bacterial species which he called *Streptothrix*. Rudolf Lieske in 1921, Gratia and Dath in 1924, and then Rosenthal in 1925 observed the antibiotic action exerted by Gasparini's *Streptothrix*, which actually is *Streptomyces*. The ubiquitous presence of strains of actinomycetes producing substances possessing antibacterial activity was demonstrated by M. Nakhimovskaia in 1937. Systematic analysis of the fermentation products of different species of actinomycetes began in 1939 in Waksman's laboratory at Rutgers University. In 1939, Waksman and his team showed that 43% of the strains of actinomycetes tested produced substances that possessed antibacterial activity. This production was affected by the composition of the fermentation medium. The first molecule to be isolated was actinomycin in 1940. Between 1939 and 1943, Waksman's team isolated numerous molecules, such as clavacin, fumigacin, chaetomin, micromonosporin, and streptothricin. All of these molecules were too toxic to be developed for human therapy.

2.1.4.1. Aminoglycosides

The objectives that Waksman and his team set themselves were to obtain an antibacterial substance that was active against gram-negative bacilli and the tubercle bacillus. Albert Schatz and S. Waksman demonstrated the antibacterial activity of *Streptomyces griseus* in December 1943 and isolated streptomycin from its fermentation in January 1944. The structure of streptomycin was determined in 1947. The procedures for using streptomycin in the treatment of tuberculosis were defined at a conference devoted to streptomycin in February 1947 in New York. A development program had been set up with the support of the National Research Council and 11 pharmaceutical companies. The synthesis of dihydrostreptomycin was achieved in 1946 by two different teams, those of Q. R. Bartz and R. L. Peck.

However, the appearance of strains resistant to streptomycin and its neuro- and ototoxicity led to the search for other antibacterial agents possessing similar activity. This resulted in the discovery of neomycin in 1949 from the fermentation of *Streptomyces fradiae* and framycetin and hydroxystreptomycin from *Streptomyces griseocarnus*. However, the toxicity of neomycin B and its lack of in vivo activity against the tubercle bacillus restricted its application to local use.

The discovery of kanamycin in 1957 by H. Umezawa and coworkers was the important turning point in the use of aminoglycosides in anti-infective chemotherapy. The other molecules were discovered progressively, such as paromomycin (1959), spectinomycin (1961), gentamicin (1963), ribostamycin (1970), sisomicin (1970), tobramycin (1971), butirosin (1971), lividomycin (1971), apramycin (1973), gentamicin C_{2b} or sagamycin (1974), fortimycin (1976), and seldomycin (1977). Other aminoglycosides have been developed for veterinary use, such as kasugamycin (1965), destomycin (1965), and validamycin (1971).

Following the discovery of kanamycin, a third stage was identified in 1963 in the fermentation medium of *Micromonospora purpurea*, involving the gentamicin complex and sisomicin. These provided a response to the therapeutic challenges posed by infections due to gram-negative bacilli.

In fact, kanamycin possesses a broader antibacterial spectrum than that of streptomycin, but gentamicin and tobramycin (3′-deoxykanamycin B) also include bacterial species such as *P. aeruginosa* in their antibacterial spectra. Gentamicin and kanamycin are pseudotrisaccharides which contain a disubstituted 2-deoxystreptamine nucleus. They differ by the amino sugar attached to the 2-deoxystreptamine: kanosamine for kanamycin and garosamine for gentamicin.

The fourth important event in the terms of the aminoglycosides was the description of the mechanisms conferring resistance to aminoglycosides.

The research focused on molecules that were active against aminoglycoside-resistant strains as a result of enzymatic inactivation and which also were less oto- and nephrotoxic.

On the basis of the biochemical knowledge of the mechanisms of resistance, Umezawa's team carried out the semisynthesis of derivatives resistant to these enzymes. In this way amikacin was prepared from kanamycin A, the former being a molecule that is intrinsically more active than kanamycin and resistant to enzymatic inactivation.

The semisynthetic derivatives of kanamycin B, such as dibekacin (3′,4′-dideoxykanamycin B), are not inactivated by bacterial 3′-phosphotransferases. Habekacin was synthesized from dibekacin. Isepamycin was prepared from gentamicin B and netilmicin was prepared from sisomicin.

The fifth stage was the demonstration of new series of aminoglycosides of the pseudodisaccharide type in the fermentation products of *Micromonospora, Saccharopolyspora, Dactylosporangium*, and *Streptomyces*. These molecules are not inactivated by acetyltransferases, phosphotransferases, or adenyltransferases, except for 3′-acetyltransferase I. Among these derivatives, two have been developed and made commercially available in Japan: fortimicin A (the base compound of astromicin sulfate has been known as fortimicin A) and dactomycin. These two molecules differ in the 2′-aminoformimidoyl group present in the fortimicin A molecule. They are similar in terms of antibacterial activity and possess activity similar to that of gentamicin and amikacin. They are inactive against *P. aeruginosa*.

2.1.4.2. Tetracyclines

The first broad-spectrum antibiotics were the cyclines and chloramphenicol. Chlortetracycline (Aureomycin) was the first molecule of the family of cyclines to be described. On 21 July 1948, at a meeting of the Academy of Sciences of New York, Benjamin J. Duggar, retired professor of botany and mycology at the University of Wisconsin, presented Aureomycin, which had just been extracted from the fermentation of *Streptomyces aureofaciens*. This was an antibiotic in crystallized form, well tolerated and with a broad spectrum, that rapidly occupied an important place in anti-infective therapy. Very shortly afterwards, Kane, Finlay, and Sabin in 1949 from Pfizer reported on oxytetracycline, isolated from *Streptomyces rimosus*. Stephens and coworkers described tetracycline, which they had obtained during studies exploring the chemical structure of the two previous derivatives. They called Terramycin oxytetracycline because of the presence of a hydroxyl group in position 5 and Aureomycin chlortetracycline because of the presence of a chlorine atom in position 7.

Tetracycline is chemically much more stable and is obtained by reduction of chlortetracycline. It was subsequently obtained in the fermentation products of *S. aureofaciens, S. rimosus*, and *Streptomyces viridofaciens*. In 1957, the study of mutant strains of *S. aureofaciens* in order to obtain a tetracycline not contaminated with chlortetracycline resulted in the biosynthesis of an active molecule not possessing the 6α-methyl group: 6-demethyl-7-chlortetracycline, which is chemically much more stable than the other molecules. This derivative produces higher levels in serum, enabling the dosages and dosage intervals to be reduced. It is also an interesting substrate because of the possibility of structural modifications. Chemical modifications have allowed the semisynthesis of more water-soluble products that release tetracycline under physiological conditions. Pyrrolidinomethyltetracycline was made commercially available in 1958, followed shortly afterwards by lysinomethyltetracycline. In 1972, 7-dimethyl-6-deoxytetracycline, or minocycline, was made commercially available.

Two semisynthetic derivatives have been prepared from oxytetracycline and made commercially available: 6-methylene tetracycline (methacycline) in 1965 and 6α-deoxytetracycline (doxycycline) in 1967. Doxycycline was one of the first antibiotics capable of being administered in a single dose.

After intense interest had been aroused in these derivatives, the emergence of resistant strains and the side effects contraindicating their use in pregnant women and children in the growth period resulted in a reduction in their prescription. However, because of their activity against intracellular bacteria, they remained the reference drug in the treatment of chlamydiosis and rickettsiosis. A resurgence of interest occurred as a result of their good activity against strains of chloroquine-resistant *Plasmodium falciparum*. Doxycycline is prescribed in certain regions of the world for the prevention of malaria (Southeast Asia). Recently, minocycline combined with clarithromycin has been proposed for the treatment of certain forms of lepromatous leprosy.

In the treatment of ulcers of duodenal origin and chronic type B gastritis based on the eradication of *Helicobacter pylori*, it has been suggested that cyclines be administered instead of amoxicillin in the triple combination of antiulcer agents, amoxicillin, and 5-nitroimidazoles or macrolides when patients are allergic to amoxicillin.

Recently, the glycine tetracyclines of semisynthetic origin and the dactylocyclines isolated from a strain of *Dactylosporium*, ATCC 53693, have been described. These molecules are active against strains resistant to the other tetracyclines and do not possess cross-resistance with the other cyclines because of a different mechanism of action.

2.1.4.3. Chloramphenicol

In 1947, penicillin G and streptomycin opened a new era in the field of treatment of infectious diseases. Two teams of researchers working in different laboratories in the United States discovered chloramphenicol practically simultaneously. The first team conducted its research in the Osborn Botanical Laboratory of Yale University, where P. R. Burkholder isolated it from a strain of *Streptomyces venezuelae* from a field in Caracas, Venezuela. This discovery was entrusted to Parke-Davis, where Bartz and his team isolated chloramphenicol. The second team, from the University of Illinois, made the same discovery. In fact, H. Carter, David Gottlieb, and L. E. Anderson isolated the same *Streptomyces* strain, strain 8-44, from the compost on a horticultural farm at the Agriculture Botanical Station at Urbana, Ill. This was the first broad-spectrum antibiotic. In 1948 it was synthesized. This antibiotic provided a treatment for typhoid and paratyphoid fevers, as well as for rickettsiosis, ornithosis (psittacosis), brucellosis, and *H. influenzae* infections.

The demonstration of hematotoxicity due to the nitro group encouraged research that gave rise to thiamphenicol, which differs from chloramphenicol through a sulfo group instead of a nitro group.

The development of a pharmaceutical formulation in an oily suspension base yielded a sustained-release drug that could be administered intramuscularly and which is widely used in the treatment of bacterial meningitis in French-speaking black Africa in a dose of two injections at a 24-h interval.

2.1.4.4. Macrolides

Macrolides are antibiotics characterized by a central lactone nucleus of 14 to 16 atoms, to which is attached one (or more) amino or neutral sugars. Erythromycin was described by J. M. McGuire in 1952 and obtained from the fermentation of *Saccharopolyspora erythraeus*. Its structure was elucidated in 1957 by D. F. Wiley et al. The different molecules have gradually been described and extracted by fermentation from various *Streptomyces* spp. or *Micromonospora*.

Among the natural macrolides, the most active molecule is erythromycin A. The main drawback of erythromycin A is its instability in an acidic medium, giving rise to two degradation products through the formation of an oxygenated bridge between the ketone group at position 9 and the hydroxyls at positions 6 and 12. The two resultant compounds are inactive bacteriologically but have the property of stimulating intestinal peristalsis at doses 10 and 3 times less than that of erythromycin A.

Various pharmaceutical and chemical devices have been proposed to circumvent this physicochemical obstacle and thereby increase the quantity of product absorbed.

In pharmaceutical terms, the coating of the active substance with a protective film makes the tablet resistant to gastric juices; a second approach was the film coating of small quantities of active substance in the form of microspheres (pellets), with all the microspheres being contained in a capsule. A second line of approach, combining the pharmaceutical improvements, is the esterification of the hydroxyl group at position 2′ of the desosamine or the preparation of a salt. Several salts of erythromycin have been proposed, such as the lactobionate and the glucoheptonate for intravenous administration and the stearate for oral administration. It is generally accepted that the salt is stable in an acidic medium. Once it crosses the intestinal barrier, the salt releases erythromycin A. This stability in an acidic medium has been questioned by Boggiano and Gleeson (1976).

Several esters of erythromycin A have been developed: the 2′-propionate, the 2′-ethylsuccinate, and, more recently, the 2′-acetate. A third approach is the use of a salt of an ester at position 2′ of erythromycin A. Three derivatives have been developed: erythromycin estolate and RV-11, which are 2′-propionates of erythromycin with a different salt (the lauryl sulfate and the mercaptosuccinate), and erythromycin acistrate, which is a mixture of erythromycin 2′-acetate and erythromycin stearate.

There has been a resurgence of medical interest in erythromycin with the emergence of legionellosis and the identification of the pathogenic potential of *Chlamydia* spp. Research has resumed with the aim of increasing the antibacterial activity and/or absorption of the product.

Blockade of the two anchorage points of the internal ketal, namely, the hydroxyl groups at position 6 (clarithromycin) and at position 12 (davercin), has yielded compounds that are more stable in an acidic medium. Modification of the electron environment of the ketone group at position 9 has been obtained by introducing a fluorine atom at position 8 (flurithromycin).

By blockading the weak point, i.e., the ketone group at position 9, a synthetic intermediate has yielded either roxithromycin by alkylation or dirithromycin by reduction of the oxime or azithromycin by a Beckman reaction. Current research is focused on increasing the antibacterial activity against erythromycin A-resistant strains, and a new subgroup exhibiting such activity has been described, the ketolides.

2.1.4.5. Other Antistaphylococcal Antibiotics

The search for molecules active against penicillinase-producing strains of *S. aureus* has engendered the discovery of several chemical entities, such as the lincosamides, coumarin derivatives (novobiocin, chlorobiocin, and coumermycin), fusidic acid (1960), and vancomycin. The value of the last molecule in treatment will increase as oxacillin-resistant strains of *S. aureus* appear. Mupirocin, a topical antistaphylococcal agent which is derived from a strain of *Pseudomonas fluorescens*, is a separate entity.

2.1.5. Synthetic Antibacterial Agents

Synthetic antibacterial agents other than sulfonamides and sulfones have been synthesized, such as the 5-nitroheterocycles, including 5-nitrofuryl (1944), the 5-nitroimidazoles (metronidazole in 1959), nitroxoline and ethionamide in 1956, trimethoprim in 1957, fosfomycin and the penems in 1977, nalidixic acid in 1962, and the fluoroquinolones at the beginning of the 1980s.

2.1.5.1. Fluoroquinolones

The β-carboxylic pyridones or quinolones are antibacterial or synthetic antibacterial agents first described in 1949 by Price et al.

Barton et al. in 1960 patented about 80 molecules of this family. It was not until 1962 that nalidixic acid was described by Lesher et al. This was isolated from a synthetic intermediate of chloroquine.

Other molecules have been synthesized subsequently: oxolinic acid, which has activity superior to that of nalidixic acid, and two derivatives with substitutions at position 7, either by a piperazine ring (pipemidic acid) or by a pyrrolidine ring (piromidic acid).

Pipemidic acid has a partial cross-resistance reaction with nalidixic acid. Flumequine, a tricyclic molecule, is characterized by the presence of a fluorine atom.

The combination of a fluorine atom and a piperazine or pyrrolidine ring gave rise to a new class of synthetic antibacterial agent: the fluoroquinolones.

Research focused on extending the antibacterial spectrum, obtaining good pharmacokinetics with an absence of metabolization, and achieving better tolerance (central nervous system and light intolerance).

The fluoroquinolones represent a major therapeutic contribution to the treatment of infectious diseases.

2.1.5.2. Benzylpyrimidines

In 1942, G. H. Hitchings' group was interested in purine and pyrimidine base analogs as potential inhibitors of nucleic acid synthesis. The initial studies involved analogs of these bases that could interfere with the metabolism of folic acid in *Lactobacillus casei*. Gradually, however, interest shifted to thymine analogs. It was shown that the 2,4-diaminopyrimidines acted as substituents of thymine but also as inhibitors of the use of folic acid. The first therapeutically usable molecule was pyrimethamine, followed in 1959 by trimethoprim. The cellular target of these molecules, dihydrofolate reductase, was described in 1958 by Osborn and Huennekens. It was shown that the OCH_3 substituents were ideal for activity against *Proteus vulgaris*, an increase in the chain causing a reduction in activity against *P.* but increasing activity against *S. aureus*.

In 1950, Greenberg and Richeson demonstrated the synergistic activity of sulfadiazine and certain 2,4-diamino-5-aryloxypyrimidine derivatives in experimental infections in chickens due to *Plasmodium gallinaceum*. A number of studies by Bushby and G. H. Hitchings resulted in the launch of co-trimoxazole on the market in 1968. The emergence of certain opportunistic infectious agents in the development of AIDS, such as *Pneumocystis carinii*, has revived interest in co-trimoxazole and the search for more active compounds in this field.

3. THE POSTPENICILLIN ERA

Penicillin G remains to date an unrivalled and one of the least expensive antibiotics for a number of infections.

However, it rapidly became clear that penicillin G could not resolve all infectious problems; in particular, it is inactive against gram-negative bacteria, mycobacteria, and intracellular microorganisms. Bacteria reputedly susceptible to penicillin G have progressively become nonsusceptible, such as *S. pneumoniae* and, more recently, *Neisseria meningitidis,* or tolerant, such as viridans group streptococci.

Improvements in medical and surgical techniques have achieved spectacular progress in medicine, but at the same time these have been accompanied by an increase in infectious problems, such as the spread of resistant bacteria and the emergence of opportunistic agents.

The progress in organic chemistry and fermentation methods and the development of microbiological research have allowed the synthesis or semisynthesis of drugs that meet these concerns.

Thus, analysis of the fermentation products of new strains of *Actinomyces, Streptomyces,* or other microorganisms, such as *Nocardia, Flexneria,* or mutants of currently identified strains, has resulted in the isolation of sulfazecin, clavulanic acid, and thienamycin. Likewise, the total synthesis of the derivatives of a known chemical class, such as the quinolones, has given rise to the fluoroquinolones. Semisynthesis starting from the 7-aminocephalosporanic nucleus has yielded the oxyimino-2-amino-5-thiazolyl derivatives, the parent molecule of which is cefotaxime. The emergence of a new infectious agent, *Legionella pneumophila,* has revived interest in the macrolides, giving rise to semisynthetic products such as roxithromycin, and the worldwide spread of macrolide resistance has resulted in intensive modifications of the skeleton of erythomycin A, leading to the discovery of ketolides.

3.1. Future Trends

The directions for future research in anti-infective chemotherapy are difficult to define: will the problems of today be the same as those of tomorrow?

The classical infections remain, but the susceptibilities of bacteria change; opportunistic infections become established, such as the mycobacteriosis that occurs with AIDS; new diseases, such as legionellosis, have appeared, partly as a result of technology (air conditioning); and infectious complications related to antibiotic therapy have arisen, such as pseudomembranous colitis caused by *Clostridium difficile.* New pathogens have emerged, such as *H. pylori* and *Chlamydia pneumoniae.*

Nosocomial infections are to be feared in a hospital environment because of the selection of multiresistant microorganisms, whether extended-spectrum-β-lactamase-producing *Enterobacteriaceae* or cephalosporinase-producing *P. aeruginosa* or other *Pseudomonas* spp., β-lactam-resistant *Acinetobacter,* or other gram-negative bacilli, such as *Stenotrophomonas maltophilia.*

More recently, *Enterococcus faecalis* and *Enterococcus faecium* have become major causes of nosocomial infections in the United States. High-level resistance to aminoglycosides and resistance to glycopeptide antibiotics (in *E. faecium*) are sources of therapeutic problems.

A number of problems still remain to be resolved, such as oxacillin-resistant strains of *S. aureus.* Since penicillin G was first used, penicillinase-producing strains have established themselves. Oxacillin derivatives offered a therapeutic response, but other strains posing substantial therapeutic problems have gradually appeared and spread, such as those resistant to oxacillin, which themselves have become progressively multiresistant, even some of them to vancomycin. Current treatment is based on glycopeptide antibiotics such as vancomycin and teicoplanin, and more recently certain fluoroquinolones, but strains of *S. aureus* of reduced susceptibility to vancomycin were described at the end of the 1900s. The combination cefotaxime-phosphomycin has been proposed by A. Kazmierczak et al. and has been used with considerable success.

Enterobacteriaceae are susceptible to the so-called third-generation cephalosporins, the parent molecule of which is cefotaxime. In the event of resistance to these molecules, the fluoroquinolones may be a therapeutic alternative, albeit with the awareness that they are contraindicated in pregnant women and children, although the benefits should be weighed against the risks. Cefpirome and cefepime can resolve certain therapeutic problems related to AmpC β-lactamase-producing *Enterobacteriaceae.* Cefsulodin, ceftazidime, and cefpirome are active against *P. aeruginosa.* If these molecules are inactive, they may be replaced by certain fluoroquinolones, such as ciprofloxacin, or by carbapenems, such as imipenem and meropenem.

The creativity of the research teams will certainly enable some of these problems to be resolved. There are multiple possibilities: first of all, the analysis of fermentation products of newly isolated bacterial or fungal species or the extraction of new derivatives from mutants of known strains. This approach has allowed the discovery of new compounds, such as dactomycin, fortimicin, sulfazecin, the lankacidins, clavulanic acid, and thienamycin; microorganism "hunters" continue to track down bacteria to discover new compounds resulting from their metabolism that possess antibacterial activity, such as the lipopeptides. Sorangicin A, coloradocin, macquirimycin, arizonins, elfamycins, anthramycins, tiacumycins, etc., metabolites of fungal or bacterial origin that may perhaps become tomorrow's parent molecules, are examples.

The second approach corresponds to the production of semisynthetic new molecules from known structures, such as the cephems, carbapenems, macrolides, ansamycins, cyclines, etc., or the synthesis of new derivatives, such as new quinolones, benzylpyrimidines, and nitroimidazoles.

The third line of approach lies in the hypothetical development or discovery of multipotential molecules. Moreover, these might possess antibacterial activity associated with immunomodulatory properties.

Lastly, just as the pioneers of chemotherapy were interested in the activity of bacterial culture filtrates, so we too must rediscover this enthusiasm and perhaps invest in other "natural" products, such as peptides. Bactericidal activity has been demonstrated in the case of a number of peptides, such as magainins, extracted from the skin of batrachians of the *Xenopus* type; cecropins, defensins extracted from human and rabbit phagocytic cells; and bactenecins, isolated from bovine granulocytes. Likewise, the generation of oxidant stress (tetrachlorodecaxoid) might be a new line of research. The analysis of potential cell targets and genetic research might allow the development of original molecules in the future.

Traditional medicine uses plant extracts which, as in the case of the antimalarial agents, might yield scaffolds that can be chemically altered.

In conclusion, we have a rich therapeutic arsenal for the present and for the near future. In fact, the majority of infections can be treated by the available antibiotic agents, whether third- or "fourth-generation" cephalosporins, fluoroquinolones, new macrolides, or older compounds that have not yet outlived their usefulness.

Certain molecules to come may provide an "oxygen balloon" for the anti-infective therapy of difficult-to-treat microorganisms. Future research into antibacterial chemotherapy should consider not only the potential antibacterial activity of the new derivatives but also their immunological properties. Finally, molecules possessing good oral bioavailability combined with potent bactericidal activity would be very useful in obviating parenteral administration.

REFERENCES

Acar JF, Bryskier A, 1994, Histoire et développement des céphalosporines, Lettre de l'Infectiologue, suppl (maîtrise des infections hospitalières, place de Cefrom®), p 4–7.

Bergogne-Bérézin E, 1993, Le siècle de la microbiologie, Presse Med, 22, 1543–1552.

Boggiano BG, Gleeson M, 1976, Gastric inactivation of erythromycin stearate in solid dosage forms, J Pharm Sci 65, 497–502.

Bryskier A, 1995, L'antibiothérapie au passé, au presént et au futur, Presse Med, 24, 55–65.

Bryskier A, 1996, Historique, classification et perspectives de développement des antibiotiques et des agents antibactériens, Med Ther, suppl, 7–18.

Bryskier A, 1997, Histoire et renouveau des macrolides, Presse Med, 26, 1063–1069.

Bryskier A, 2003, Paul Gehrard Domagk, le découvreur des sulfamides, Chemother J, 12, 97–105, in German.

Bryskier A, Chantot JF, Labro MT, Gasc J-C, 1989, Evolution et tendance moderne de l'antibiothérapie, in Zribi A, Bryskier A, ed, l'Antibiothérapie d'aujourd'hui et de demain, Arnette, Paris, p 11–29.

Fleming A, 1946, Penicillin, Its Practical Application, Butterworth & Co Ltd, London, p 380.

Goldberg HS, Luckey TD, 1955, Introduction, in Goldberg HS, ed, Antibiotics, Their Chemistry and Non-Medical Uses, D. Van Nostrand Co. Inc., Princeton, NJ, p 1–8.

Jukes TH, 1985, Some historical notes on chlortetracyclines, Rev Infect Dis, 5, 702–707.

Lapresle C, 1986, Les sulfamides en médecine, Bull Inst Pasteur, 84, 181–188.

Lepper MH, 1956, Aureomycin (chlortetracycline), monograph 7, p 156, Medical Encyclopedia, New York.

Levaditi C, Vaisman A, Henry-Eveno J, Veillet J, Sandor T, 1952, Le chloramphénicol (chloromycetine) et ses applications therapeutiques, Bailleres JB et fils, Paris, p 171.

Parascandola J, 1980, The history of antibiotics, a symposium, American Institute of the History of Pharmacy, Madison, Wis, 137 p.

Rolison GN, 1988, From Pasteur to penicillin. The history of antibacterial chemotherapy, Zbl Bakt Hyg A 267, 207–315.

Umezawa H, Ueda M, Maeda K, Yagishita K, Kondo S, Okami Y, Utahara R, Osato Y, Nitta K, Takeuchi T, 1957, Production and isolation of a new antibiotic: kanamycin, J Antibiot (Tokyo), 10, 181–188.

Waksman SA, 1949, Streptomycin, Nature and Practical Application, The Williams & Wilkins Co, Baltimore, p 618.

Waksman SA, 1958, Neomycin, Its Nature and Practical Application, The Williams & Wilkins Co, Baltimore, p 412.

Waksman SA, 1968, Actinomycin, Nature, Formation, and Activities, Intersciences Publ, John Wiley & Sons Inc, New York, p 231.

Weinstein L, Ehrenkrantz NJ, 1958, Streptomycin and dihydrostreptomycin, monograph 10, p 116, Medical Encyclopedia, New York.

Woodward TE, Wisseman L, Jr, 1958, Chloromycetin (chloramphenicol), Antibiotics monograph 8, p 159, Medical Encyclopedia, New York.

Antibiotics and Antibacterial Agents: Classifications and Structure-Activity Relationship

A. BRYSKIER

2

1. INTRODUCTION

The modern era of antibacterial chemotherapy began in 1935 with the demonstration of the antibacterial activity of sulfonamides by Gerhard Domagk. This discovery revived research in the area of anti-infective agents. Over the course of the next few years, all of the major families of antibiotics were discovered: penicillins, cephems, aminoglycosides, tetracyclines, macrolides, peptide antibiotics, chloramphenicol, ansamycins, and lincosamides, as well as synthetic antibacterial agents such as the benzylpyrimidines (trimethoprim), fluoroquinolones, fosfomycin, penems (ritipenem and fropenem [faropenem]), and 5-nitroimidazoles (metronidazole and derivatives). The classifications within each family are complex.

2. THE β-LACTAM FAMILY

2.1. Introduction

The β-lactam family comprises four groups of molecules: penams, penems, cephems, and monocyclic β-lactams. To these should be added the β-lactamase inhibitors, some of the structures of which are featured in the four main groups (Fig. 1).

The basic structure of the β-lactams is the azetidinone nucleus, which contains the carbonyl lactam structure essential for the activity of the molecules. To this structure is bound a saturated pentacyclic (penam), unsaturated (penem), or hexacyclic (cephem) ring. The azetidinone nucleus alone (monocyclic β-lactam) can be replaced, and monobactams ($N\text{-}SO_3$, e.g., aztreonam and carumonam), monocarbams, monophosphatams, and other heterocycles (e.g., HR-790) can be distinguished according to the substituents of the nitrogen atom. Because of the complexity of this group, they are currently referred to as monolactams.

All of these molecules are characterized by their route of administration, which may be oral, parenteral, or both. They may be ingested orally with or without esterification (prodrugs) (Table 1). Some compounds have been investigated for use as suppositories, but none have reached clinical use.

2.2. Penicillins

The family of penicillins is complex. The penicillin structure consists of three parts: a thiazolidine nucleus attached to an azetidinone ring and a side chain at the C-6 position by which the penicillins can be distinguished. They are classed as penams, which include the penicillins, oxa-1-penams (e.g., clavulanic acid), and carbapenams.

Within the penicillins, seven groups may be distinguished:

1. Penicillin G
2. Penicillin M
3. Penicillin A
4. α-Substituted penicillins
5. α-Carboxypenicillins and α-sulfopenicillins
6. Amidinopenicillins
7. Oxyiminopenicillins

2.2.1. Penicillin G

Benzylpenicillin (penicillin G) is unstable in an acidic medium. The introduction of a polar group such as an oxygen atom (phenoxypenicillins) or a sulfur atom onto the side chain does not affect the antibacterial activity but increases the stability in an acidic medium. In the case of the phenoxypenicillins, the greater the molecular weight, the better the intestinal absorption. It is for this reason that different groups have been added to the asymmetrical carbon in the α position: methyl (phenethicillin), ethyl (propicillin), and benzene (fenbenicillin).

2.2.2. Group M Pencillins

The emergence of resistant strains of *Staphylococcus aureus* as a result of penicillinase production necessitated the synthesis of molecules stable to hydrolysis by this enzyme. Methicillin differs from penicillin G through the substitution by methoxy groups at positions 2′ and 6′ of the benzene nucleus, causing steric hindrance around the amide bond.

The second type of molecule is characterized by the presence of an isoxazole penta-atomic nucleus in the *ortho* position of the benzene ring, which increases the stability to hydrolysis by *S. aureus* penicillinase. This is augmented by the introduction on the benzene ring of a chlorine atom at position 2′ (cloxacillin) or two chlorine atoms at positions 2′ and 6′ (dicloxacillin) or a chlorine atom at position 2′ and a fluorine atom at position 6′ (floxacillin).

2.2.3. Penicillin A

Penicillin A molecules possess an amino substituent on the α carbon of the chain at position C-6. The essential biological activity is based on the nature and spatial orientation of this side chain. L-Ampicillin is less active against gram-negative

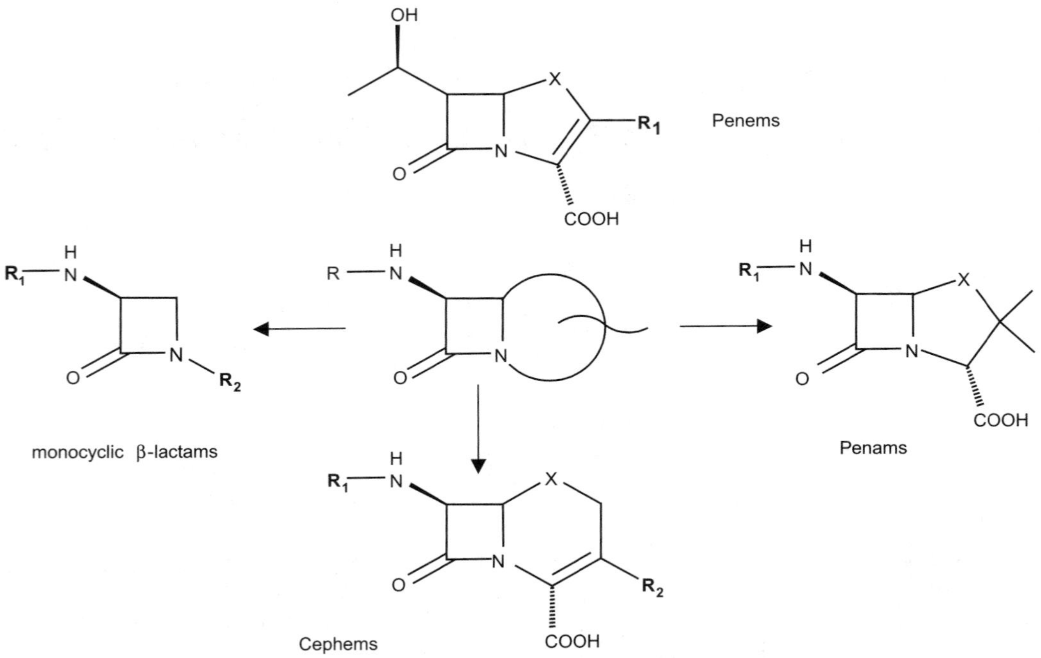

Figure 1 Classification of the β-lactams

Table 1 Oral β-lactams

Drug family	Drug name	Prodrug
Penams	Ampicillin Amoxicillin Penicillin V	Bacampicillin Talampicillin Pivampicillin Lenampicillin
Cephems	Cefadroxil Cefaclor Cephalexin Cefixime Ceftibuten	Cefpodoxime proxetil Cefotiam hexetil Cefuroxime axetil Cefditoren pivoxil Cefetamet pivoxil
Penem	Fropenem	
Carbapenems		Sanfetrinem cilexetil CS-840 DZ 2640 L-084

bacilli than D-ampicillin because of the spatial orientation of the amino group. The introduction of a *para*-hydroxyl group on the benzene nucleus of ampicillin (amoxicillin) increases digestive absorption. Substitution by α-carbamoyl, ureido, acylureido, and carbamoylureido groups gave rise to the N-acylpenicillins. The nature of the chain and its substituents interferes with the antibacterial activity, but not with the pharmacokinetic properties.

2.2.4. α-Carboxy- and α-Sulfopenicillins

The presence of an acid function, such as a carboxylic, sulfamic, or sulfonic group on the carbon in the α position of the side chain in the C-6 position, increases the activity against gram-negative bacilli but decreases the activity against gram-positive cocci. Carbenicillin has a center of asymmetry, but the D and L isomers have identical antibacterial activities.

2.3. Cephems

2.3.1. Classifications

Several thousand compounds have been synthesized since the mid-1960s. There are several classifications: chemical, microbiological, and pharmacokinetic.

Chemically, the cephems may be divided into three groups according to the atom in position 1 of the hexa-atomic ring: cephalosporins (sulfur), carbacephems (methylene), and oxa-1-cephems (oxygen). Each group may be subdivided according to the presence or absence at position 7-α of a methoxy group: cephamycins (e.g., cefoxitin and moxalactam).

Depending on the nature of the α-carbon of the chain at position C-7 of the cephalosporins, they may be subdivided into three groups: CH_2, CH-R, and C=X-Y (Fig. 2).

The cephems may be subdivided into three classes according to their antibacterial spectrum: limited spectrum (groups I and II), broad spectrum (groups III, IV, and V), and narrow spectrum (groups VI and VII) (Fig. 3). Some cephem structures exhibit β-lactamase-inhibitory activity.

2.3.2. Structure-Activity Relationship

It is accepted that the carboxyl group at position 4 must be free and that the presence of a substituent at position 2 of the cephem nucleus is detrimental to the cephalosporins but not to the oxa-1-cephem or carbacephem series. It was gradually realized that the ideal substituent at position 7 is the 2-amino-5-thiazolyl nucleus (cefotaxime and derivatives), which gave rise to the so-called third-generation cephalosporins. One variant is a 5-amino-2-thiadiazolyl nucleus (cefozopran, cefclidin, and cefluprenam) which increases the activity against *Pseudomonas aeruginosa* but slightly decreases that against enterobacteria.

The second stage was the discovery of the activity of a quaternary ammonium chain at position 3 of the cephem nucleus. The first compound was ceftazidime. Further optimization was obtained with cefpirome and cefepime, which

Figure 2 Chemical classification of cephalosporins

are active against certain strains of *Enterobacteriaceae* producing class C β-lactamases (e.g., *Citrobacter freundii*).

In an attempt to increase the activity against *P. aeruginosa* and extended-spectrum-β-lactamase-producing strains of *Enterobacteriaceae*, the oxime chain was replaced by a catechol (RU-59863) or pyridone nucleus, thus adding another mode of action to these molecules. In this type of molecule, the presence of a vinyl chain at position C-3 increases the activity against gram-positive cocci.

The pharmacokinetic properties are located in the chain at position 3. A long apparent elimination half-life has been obtained with ceftriaxone (a triazine nucleus substituted by a hydroxyl) and with cefodizime (bisubstituted thiazolyl nucleus).

Oral absorption of the cephalosporins is complex. There are three types of molecules: α-amino cephems (cefadroxil, cefaclor, and cefprozil), non-α-amino cephems (cefixime and ceftibuten), and prodrugs (cefpodoxime proxetil and cefuroxime axetil).

2.4. Carbapenems

2.4.1. Classification

The carbapenems may be divided into molecules of natural or synthetic origin. Microbiologically, two types of molecule have been synthesized: antibacterials and β-lactamase inhibitors.

Among the compounds of natural origin, more than 50 derivatives have been reported in the literature, grouped into four subclasses according to the side chain at position 6: 5,6-*cis*-hydroxyethyl, 5,6-*trans*-hydroxyethyl (thienamycin), isopropyl, and isopropylidene.

Among the molecules of semisynthetic or synthetic origin, a distinction may be drawn between those with no substituent at position 1 (imipenem) and those with a methyl group at position 1, such as meropenem, panipenem, biapenem, lenapenem, DX-8739, and L-355. Some tricyclic compounds with a closure by a hexa- or pentacycle between C-1 and C-2 have been synthesized.

2.4.2. Structure-Activity Relationship

Carbapenems are complex because they result from an equilibrium between antibacterial activity, chemical stability, and stability against hydrolysis by renal dehydropeptidase I (DHP-I), which is difficult to achieve. To these has been added a fourth parameter, the digestive absorption of carbapenems.

The importance of the following has been demonstrated:

- The stereochemistry at the centers of asymmetry of the molecules
- The role of the chain at position 2 in terms of antibacterial activity, chemical stability, and, to a lesser degree, hydrolysis by DHP-I
- The chain at position C-6, which must be a hydroxyethyl chain, the ethyl group being in the β position (8*R*)
- The substitution at the 1-β position of the carbapenem nucleus, which increases the stability against hydrolysis by DHP-I but reduces the antibacterial activity
- The role played by the chain at position C-2 in terms of antibacterial activity

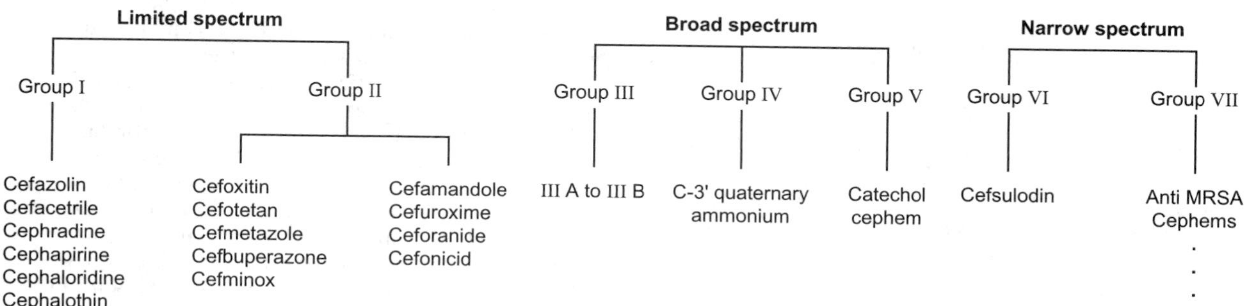

Figure 3 Microbiological classification of the cephems

2-Deoxystreptamine

Streptamine

Streptidine

Figure 4 Aminoglycosides

- The fact that the carbapenem nucleus has antibacterial activity similar to that of ampicillin but is inactive against the β-lactamase-producing bacterial strains

3. AMINOGLYCOSIDES

3.1. Classifications

Several hundred natural molecules or molecules obtained by semisynthesis have been described. The family of aminoglycosides constitutes a complex world whose classification is based on chemical structure. Umezawa (1979) proposed dividing the aminoglycosides into six groups according to a central structure, which is either streptamine, 2-deoxystreptamine, or streptidine (Fig. 4). To these groups should be added a collection of mono-, di-, and trisaccharide molecules which do or do not possess antibacterial activity but which are either precursors of the aminoglycosides obtained by fermentation or molecules that possess activity of the aminoglycoside type but do not have their structures. The classification which I propose derives from that of Umezawa. Group I includes the mono-, di-, and trisaccharide compounds (Fig. 5). Group II contains streptomycin and its derivatives; group III comprises compounds whose 2-deoxystreptamine nucleus is linked to the other sugars by the hydroxyls at positions 4, 5, and 6, thus distinguishing three subgroups: III-A, III-B, and III-C (Fig. 6). Group IV (Fig. 7) consists of a set of compounds whose 2-deoxystreptamine nucleus is attached at positions 4 and 5 to the other sugars. It is possible to distinguish two subgroups in terms of structure: IV-A (pseudotrisaccharide compounds), which contains the ribostamycin derivatives, and subgroup IV-B (pseudotetra- and pentasaccharide molecules), which includes the neomycin B derivatives.

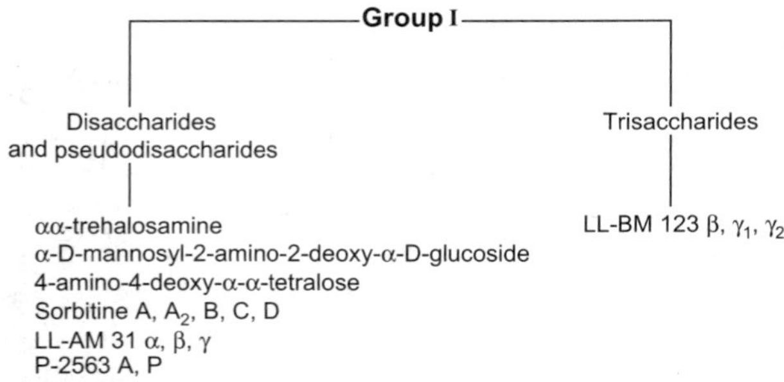

Figure 5 Classification of aminoglycosides (I)

The molecules of ribostamycin derivatives vary in the substituents at position C-1 of the 2-deoxystreptamine and position 3″ of the pentose. For example, butirosins A and B differ through a 5-O-xylose and 5-O-ribose, respectively. In subgroup IV-B, the 2-deoxystreptamine nucleus is identical for all of the compounds; a variable hexose is attached at position C-4. The compounds differ from one another through the substituents on the pentose, to which is attached a hexosamine that varies according to the molecule.

Group V (Fig. 8) consists of derivatives in which the 2-deoxystreptamine is bound to the other sugars by the hydroxyl groups at positions C-4 and C-6. Four subgroups are distinguished within this group: V-A, V-B, V-C, and V-D.

Subgroup V-A is composed of derivatives of kanamycin and of the nebramycin complex and possess kanosamine in common. Several molecules within this subgroup, such as kanamycin, tobramycin, dibekacin, and arbekacin (Habekacin) are used therapeutically. Others, such as butikacin and propikacin, have had their development stopped. These compounds were obtained by semisynthesis and derive either from kanamycin A (such as amikacin, butikacin, BB-K-311) or from kanamycin B (such as tobramycin, dibekacin, arbekacin, and propikacin).

Subgroups V-B, V-C, and V-D have the same amino sugar in common: garosamine. Subgroup V-B comprises the derivatives of gentamicin C, which has yielded the gentamicin complex used therapeutically, sagamicin (gentamicin C_{2b}), isepamicin, and an undeveloped derivative, WIN 42 122-2 (2-hydroxygentamicin C). Subgroup V-C contains compounds that possess a pentose attached at position 6 of the 2-deoxystreptamine. This subgroup is composed of the gentamicin A complex and seldomycins 1, 3, and 5. Subgroup V-D comprises derivatives of sisomicin containing an unsaturated amino sugar, sisosamine, attached at position 4 of the 2-deoxystreptamine. Verdamicin is 6′-C-methylsisomicin. Two semisynthetic derivatives have been developed, netilmicin and 5-episisomicin.

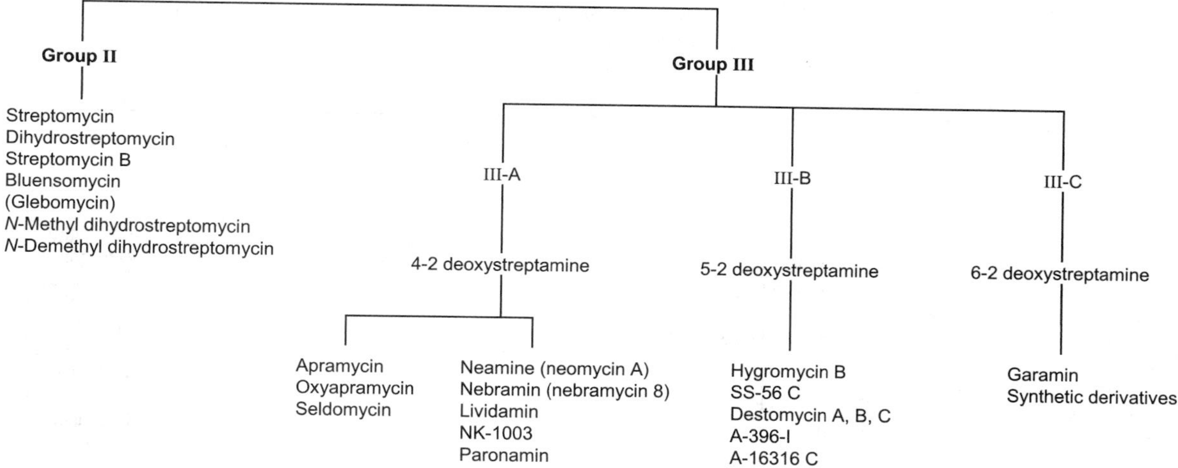

Figure 6 Classification of aminoglycosides (II)

Group VI (Fig. 9) is composed of various molecules that may be divided into three subgroups according to the amino or nonamino nature of the sugars: kasugamycin and myomycin B (neutral sugars), hygromycin A and the validamycin complex (one amino sugar), and derivatives with two amino sugars. Subgroup VI-C consists of a number of derivatives, two of which have yielded drugs, such as the derivatives of spectinomycin and those of fortimicin (astromicin and dactomycin). This group also comprises other molecules, such as the sporaricins and the sannamycin and istamycin complexes.

3.2. Structure-Activity Relationship

Research into aminoglycosides has been geared above all to the identification of new chemical entities obtained from the systematic analysis of the fermentation products of different species of *Streptomyces*, *Micromonospora*, and *Bacillus*. Starting from these parent molecules, either the most active molecule has been purified and developed as a medicinal product, such as streptomycin, neomycin B, tobramycin and kanamycin B, or semisynthetic molecules have been prepared.

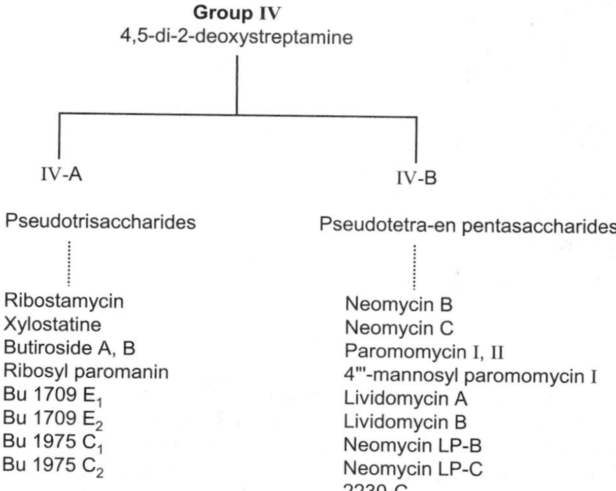

Figure 7 Classification of aminoglycosides (III)

The use of aminoglycosides has been beset by a dual problem: the appearance of resistant strains and a toxicological problem (oto- and nephrotoxicity). The discovery of kanamycin A in 1956 transformed the landscape of the aminoglycosides, but from 1965 onwards about 5% of strains were resistant to kanamycin. Based on studies by Ochiai et al. (1959) and Akiha et al. (1960), who demonstrated the transferability of resistance to certain antibiotics between *Escherichia coli* and *Shigella* spp., Miyamura et al. (1961) were able to demonstrate that shigellae inactivated chloramphenicol. Okamoto et al. (1965) showed that chloramphenicol was inactivated by acetylation through an acetyltransferase. They suggested that kanamycin was inactivated by the same processes. This hypothesis was validated by Umezawa et al., who demonstrated that kanamycin is acetylated at position 6′, yielding 6′-*N*-acetylkanamycin A. This discovery was the cornerstone of all of the research into the aminoglycosides, as the three types of enzymes that inactivate aminoglycosides were progressively discovered: phosphotransferases, acetyltransferases, and nucleotidyltransferases.

The majority of aminoglycosides have similar basic structures and are divided into four groups: streptomycin derivatives, 2-deoxystreptamine derivatives, spectinomycin derivatives, and fortimicin derivatives.

3.2.1. Streptomycin Derivatives

The changes relating to streptomycin centered on the aldehyde function of the L-streptose. The reduction of the aldehyde to a hydroxymethyl derivative (dihydrostreptomycin) did not affect the antibacterial activity, but the reduction to a methyl derivative (compound A) produced a derivative possessing one-tenth of the antibacterial activity of streptomycin. Oxidation of the aldehyde (compound B) yields an inactive derivative.

Modification to the secondary amine of the *N*-methylglucosamine or its methylation (tertiary amine) inactivates the streptomycin molecule (Fig. 10).

Replacement of the guanidino groups on the streptidine by amino or ureido groups substantially reduces the antibacterial activity.

3.2.2. 2-Deoxystreptamine derivatives

The majority of molecules with a 2-deoxystreptamine nucleus have similar structures, making it possible to trace the broad outlines of the structure-activity relationships (Fig. 11).

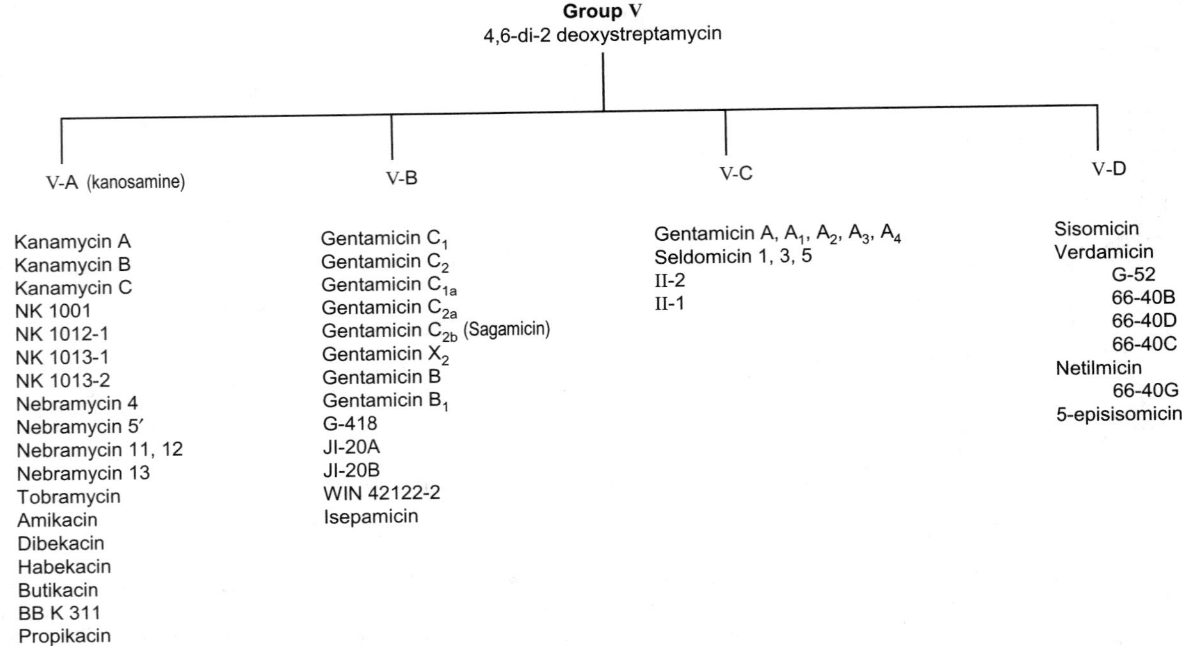

Figure 8 Classification of aminoglycosides (IV)

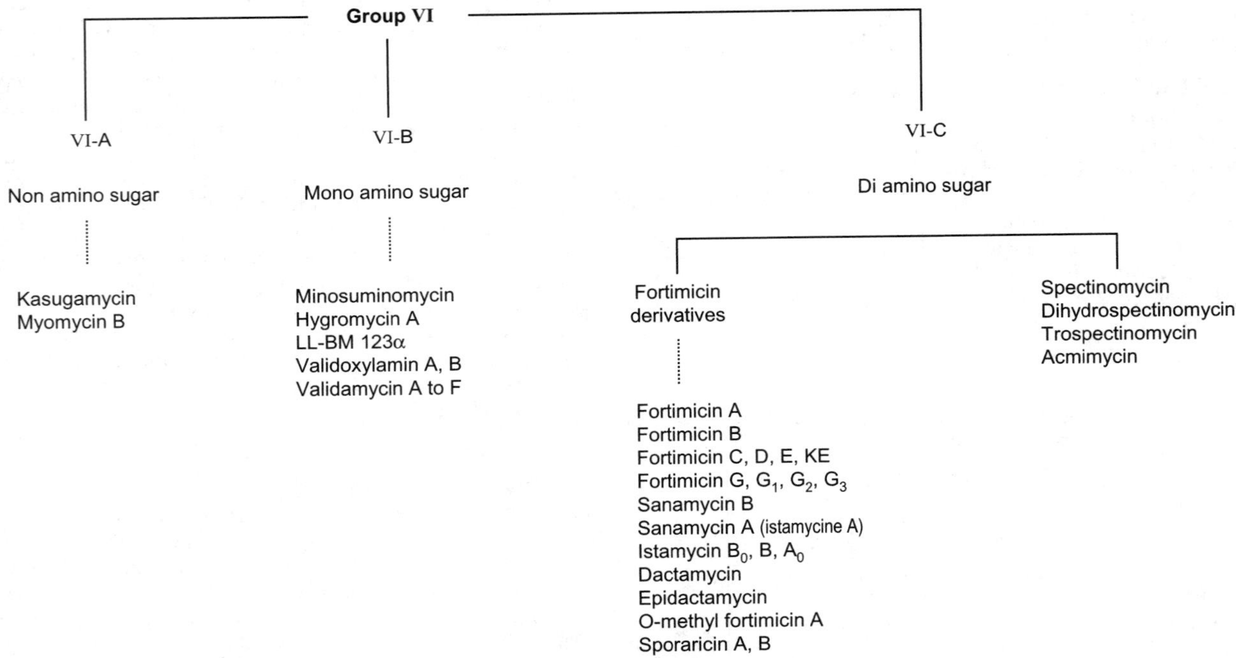

Figure 9 Classification of aminoglycosides (V)

3.2.2.1. Modifications of the A Nucleus

The A nucleus is important in terms of expression of antibacterial activity. It is the target of the enzymes that inactivate the aminoglycosides at the level of the amino groups in positions 6′ and 2′ (acetylation) and the 3′-hydroxyl (phosphorylation). The number and position of the amino groups are important for antibacterial activity. This point has been clearly demonstrated with kanamycins A, B, and C, which differ with respect to their structures in the A nucleus (Fig. 12). Kanamycin B is twice as active as kanamycin A, which is two to four times more active than kanamycin C (Table 2). This demonstrates the importance of the amino groups at

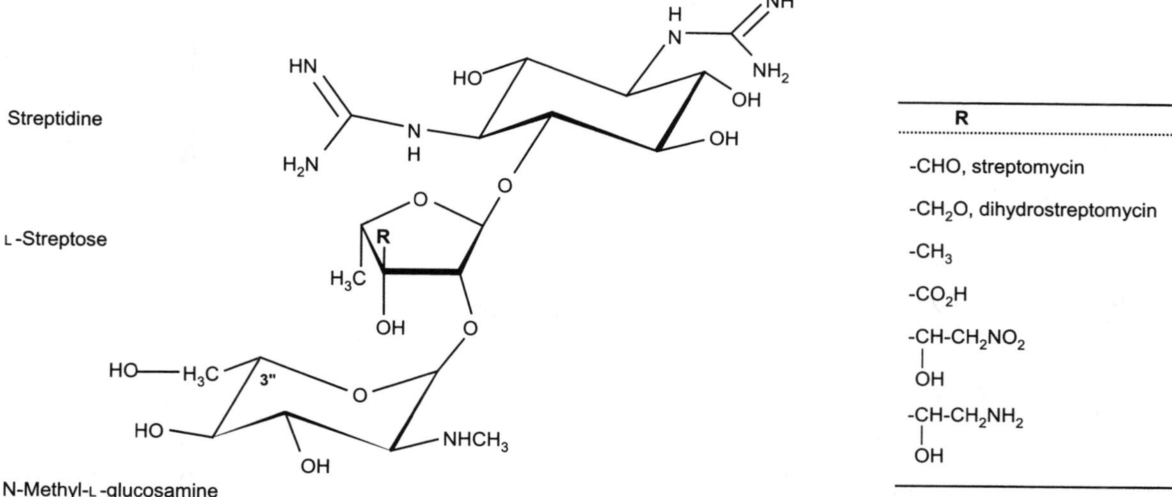

Figure 10 Streptomycin derivatives

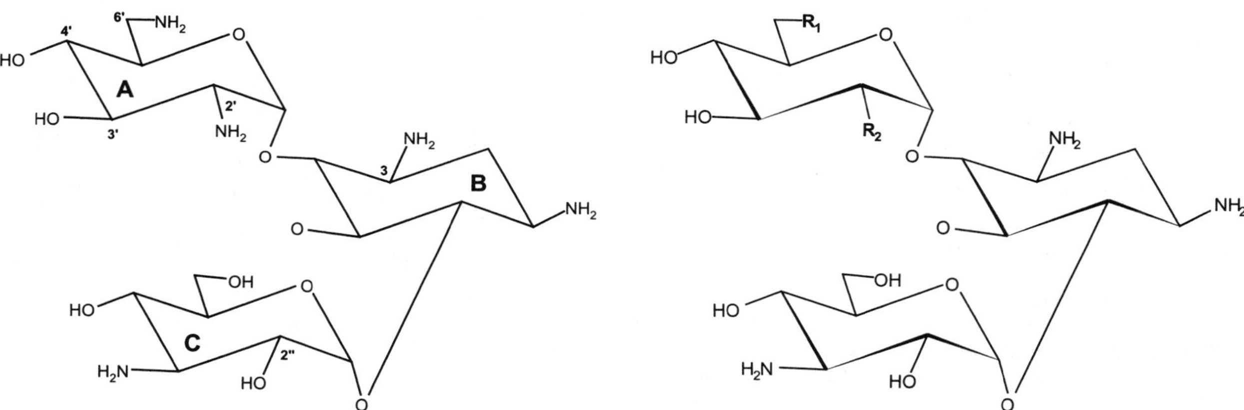

Figure 11 Aminoglycoside A, B, and C nuclei

Figure 12 Kanamycins: structure

Table 2 Antibacterial activities of the kanamycins

Kanamycin	R_1	R_2	MIC (μg/ml)					
			E. coli	*Klebsiella pneumoniae*	*Proteus mirabilis*	*Proteus vulgaris*	*S. aureus*	*P. aeruginosa*
A	NH_2	OH	6.25	3.12	6.25	3.12	6.25	25
B	NH_2	NH_2	1.56	0.78	3.12	1.56	1.56	12.5
C	OH	NH_2	12.5	6.25	1.56	6.25	12.5	>100

positions 2′ and 6′. However, modifications at position 6′, such as C or N methylation, do not modify the activity or may even increase it, as has been demonstrated with gentamicins of the C group (Fig. 13; Table 3). Methylation may be beneficial, as it prevents inactivation by the AAC enzyme (6′). The hydroxyl groups also play an important part in antibacterial activity. Their replacement by a hydrogen causes an increase in activity, whereas other modifications may cause a loss of activity. Conversion of kanamycin B to these derivatives, 3′-deoxykanamycin B (tobramycin), and 3′,4′-dideoxykanamycin B (dibekacin), increases the activity against gram-negative bacilli, particularly *P. aeruginosa*.

The virtually constant presence of a 3′-phosphorylating enzyme in *P. aeruginosa* would explain the lack of activity of aminoglycosides with a 3′-hydroxyl group against this bacterial species. Replacement of the 3′-hydroxyl by a methoxy or

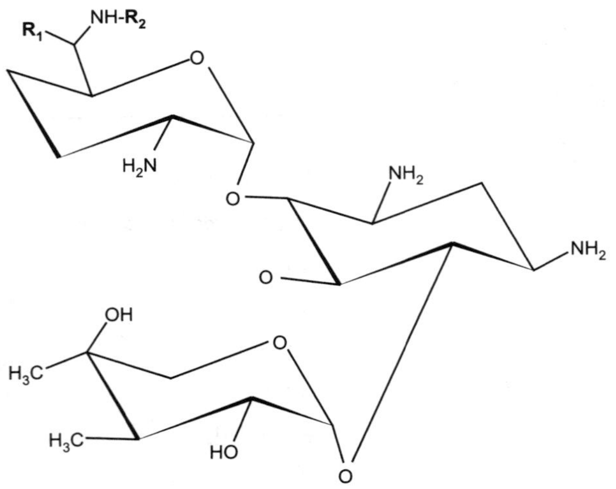

Figure 13 Gentamicins C: structure

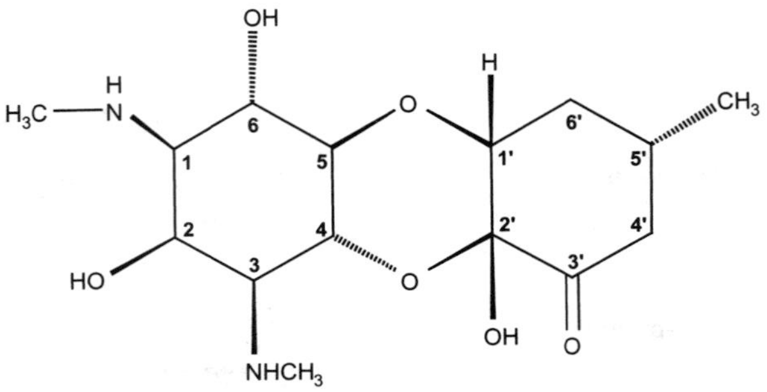

Figure 14 Spectinomycin

amino group causes a loss of activity. The same phenomenon has been demonstrated with other aminoglycosides, such as ribostamycin, butirosin, and neomycin A (neamine).

The presence of double bonds in the A nucleus may alter the activity. In kanamycin B, the replacement of the 3′- and 4′-hydroxyls by a double bond reduces the activity, whereas the introduction of a double bond at positions 4′ and 5′ in gentamicin C_{1a} gives rise to a very active antibiotic, sisomicin. These differences are probably due to a modification in the configuration of the A nucleus.

3.2.2.2. Modifications of the B Nucleus: 2-Deoxystreptamine

The most important structural modification of 2-deoxystreptamine was the acylation of the amino group at position C-1 with 2-hydroxy-4-aminobutyric acid (HABA) to yield amikacin. This modification is the origin of a major increase in activity against *P. aeruginosa* and gentamicin- or tobramycin-resistant strains of enterobacteria. The stereochemistry of the HABA group is important, as the (*S*)-isomer is four times more active than the (*R*)-isomer. In the same way, the attachment of a group in the 1 position of sisomicin increased the activity (1-ethylsisomicin). It is possible to replace the 5-hydroxyl group of sisomicin without reducing the activity.

3.2.2.3. Modifications of the C Nucleus

The nature of the C nucleus varies with the aminoglycoside. If the nucleus is a pyranose, methylation or the absence of the 2″-hydroxyl group (gentamicin C_2) produces a major reduction in activity. Conversely, the activity is not affected by the 2″-NH_2 group (seldomycin). It has recently been reported that arbekacin is inactivated by methicillin-resistant strains of *S. aureus* through the production of a 2″-*O*-phosphorylase. The synthesis of 2″-amino-2″-deoxyarbekacin derivatives has enabled this enzymatic obstacle to be circumvented. The group at position 3″ may be a primary or secondary amine group and may be in an axial or equatorial position. Modifications at position 6″ may be detrimental.

If the nucleus is a furanose, the group at the 3″-hydroxyl may be replaced, as in neomycin, or epimerized as for butirosins A and B. Modifications at position 5″ may be beneficial or deleterious.

3.2.3. Spectinomycin Derivatives

Spectinomycin (formerly known as actinospectacin) (Fig. 14) is an antibiotic isolated from the fermentation products of *Streptomyces flavopersicus* and *Streptomyces spectabilis*. Spectinomycin is a disaccharide antibiotic that possesses a neutral sugar (actinospectose) which is fused to actinamine (*N,N*′-dimethyl-2-*epi*-streptamine) by a β-glycosidic linkage and a hemiacetal type linkage (1,4-dioxane), producing a tricyclic structure. The bond of the B and C structures is in the *cis* position, with a 2′-hydroxyl group in the axial position to the B nucleus. The compound possesses nine centers of asymmetry. Based on the 1,4-dioxane ring, four diastereoisomers may be described.

In an acidic medium, the bonds are hydrolyzed. In an aqueous medium, there is an equilibrium between the form with a 3′-carbonyl and that with a 3′-diol (Fig. 15).

The reduction of the carbonyl at position C-3′ yields the (*S*)- and (*R*)-dihydrospectinomycin derivatives, the antibacterial activities of which range from 0 to 100% of that of spectinomycin according to the bacterial species. The 3′-(*R*)-dihydrospectinomycin isomer is more active than the 3′-(*S*)-dihydrospectinomycin isomer. The 3′-(*R*)-dihydrospectinomycin isomer was detected in the fermentation medium of *S. spectabilis* and would appear to be an intermediate of the biosynthetic pathway of spectinomycin. 3′-(*S*) and 3′-(*R*)-aminospectinomycin derivatives have been synthesized. The 3′-(*R*) derivative has good antibacterial activity, in contrast to the 3′-(*S*)-aminospectinomycin isomer. The difference

Table 3 Antibacterial activities of members of the gentamicin C complex

Gentamicin	R_1	R_2	MIC (μg/ml)			
			E. coli	*Enterobacter* spp.	*Proteus* spp.	*P. aeruginosa*
C_1	CH_3	CH_3	0.3	0.3	0.75	0.75
C_1	H	H	0.3	0.3	0.75	0.75
C_2	CH_3	H	0.3	0.3	0.75	0.75

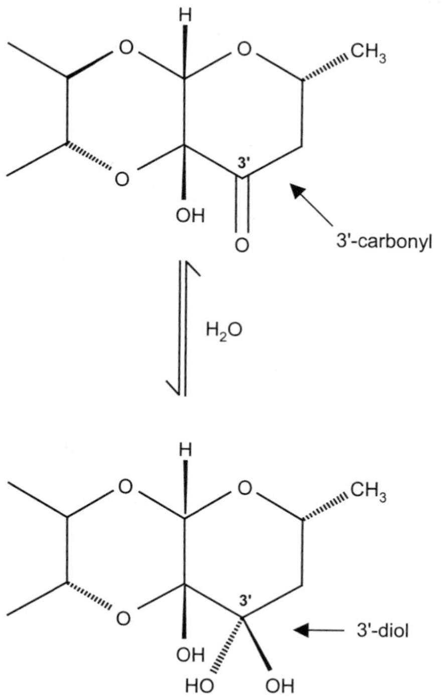

Figure 15 Spectinomycin in an aqueous medium

in activity between the isomers is probably due to the poor binding of the compound at the ribosomal receptor sites, which involves hydrogen bonds. Substitution at the C-3′ position by a halogen (chlorine or bromine) yields relatively inactive compounds. Other modifications have been made at the C-3′ position, such as the 3′-hydroxymethyl derivative which is less active than 3′-(*S*)-dihydrospectinomycin. The attachment of an α-hydroxyl group to this compound occasions weaker antibacterial activity than that of spectinomycin, showing clearly the importance of the hydroxyl groups and their spatial position. The incorporation of an amino function in the chain also restores good antibacterial activity. Alkylation of the amino group reduces the activity in the (*S*) series but increases it in the (*R*) series. The introduction of a second amino function also increases the antibacterial activity. Epimerization of the 2-hydroxyl reduces the activity. Inactivating enzymes may act at this level, as well as on the hydroxyl group at position C-6 (adenylation). Recently, a propyl chain has been attached to the methyl group at position C-3, yielding trospectinomycin, which is 4 to 16 times more active than spectinomycin.

3.2.4. Fortimicin Group

A number of derivatives containing a 1,4-diaminocyclitol were isolated between 1977 and 1979; these constituted the fortimicins. Two molecules have been developed and made commercially available: astromicin sulfate (the base compound of astromicin sulfate has been known as fortimicin A) and dactomycin. These are pseudosaccharide molecules that have in common an amino sugar, fortimine, which is variably replaced according to the molecule. Within the group of fortimicins, a distinction is drawn between two subgroups in terms of the sugar attached at position 6, an unsaturated hexose (sisosamine) or a nonunsaturated hexose, which have variable substitutions at position C-6′ (Fig. 16).

Fortimicin B is less active than fortimicin A, which possesses activity similar to that of kanamycin. It is inactive against *P. aeruginosa*. The structural difference between fortimicins A and B is the presence at position C-4 of a glycine residue. 3-*O*-Methylfortimicin was synthesized to increase the activity against this species, but despite an increase in activity, it still remained weak. Other minor products have been isolated, such as fortimicins C, D, E, KE, KF, and G. Fortimicin C has a hydantoic acid substituting for the glycine of fortimicin A, while fortimicins D and KE are, respectively, 6′-dimethylfortimicins A and B. Fortimicin E is less active and is the epimer at the C-3 or C-4 position of fortimicin B with an equatorial configuration of the cyclitol ring. Fortimicin A is unstable in an alkaline medium and is transformed to fortimicin B by release of the glycyl chain.

Dactomycin is produced by *Dactylosporangium matsuzakiensis*. It differs from fortimicin A in the presence of a *N*-formimidoyl chain on the glycine. A derivative of dactomycin, *epi*-dactomycin, possesses the same antibacterial activity as dactomycin but differs from the latter through the spatial position of the amino group. Sporaricins A and B are produced by *Saccharopolyspora hirsuta* subsp. *kobensis*. The sporaricins are epimers at position C-1 and do not possess 2-hydroxyls. They have antibacterial activity similar to that of the fortimicins.

Sannamycins A and B were isolated from fermentation products of a strain of *Streptomyces*. Sannamycin A (istamycin A) is less active than the derivatives of fortimicin containing a glycine chain. The istamycin complex was isolated from the fermentation of *Streptomyces tenjimariensis*. Four derivatives have been isolated: A_0, A, B_0, and B. The A and B derivatives contain a glycine chain and differ in the C-1 position of the amino group (Fig. 17).

4. MACROLIDES

The macrolides are macrocyclic antibiotics characterized by a central lactone ring containing 12 to 16 members, few double bonds, and no nitrogen atom; one or two amino sugars and/or neutral sugars are attached to the lactone or aglycone ring. The azalides are not included in this definition, as they have an endocyclic nitrogen atom. However, the azalides are not products of natural origin but are obtained by semisynthesis (Beckman rearrangement) using a synthetic intermediate prepared from erythromycin A.

4.1. Classifications

Several classifications have been proposed. The simplest is that combining the central chemical structure (lactone ring) and the natural or synthetic origin of the compound. Among the compounds for therapeutic use, a distinction can be drawn between those that possess 14-, 15-, or 16-membered-ring macrolides (Fig. 18).

4.2. Structure-Activity Relationships

Structural studies of erythromycin A have shown that the orientation of the hydrophilic groups (carbonyl and hydroxyl groups at positions C-6 and C-11) and the hydrophobic groups (methyl groups at positions C-4, C-8, and C-12 and the ethyl chain at position C-13) of the aglycone and D-desosamine plays an important role in the antibacterial activity of erythromycin A.

4.2.1. Chemical Modifications of the Lactone Ring

The chemical modifications of the aglycone may be made directly to the ring or indirectly to the substituents of the aglycone.

		R_1	R_2
Fortimicin	A	CH_3	H
"	C	CH_3	H
"	D	H	H
Sporamicin	A	CH_3	H
Istamycin	A	H	CH_3
Istamycin	B	H	CH_3
Dactamycin		CH_3	H
Fortimicin	B	CH_3	H
	KE	H	H
Sporamicin	B	CH_3	H
Sannamycin	B	H	CH_3

Fortimicin	KF.	H
"	G	CH_3
"	G_1	CH_3
"	G_2	CH_3
"	G_3	CH_3

Figure 16 Group of fortimicins

4.2.1.1. Direct Modifications of the Aglycone

Erythromycin A loses its activity in an acidic medium because of its degradation to a hemiacetal or spiroketal (Fig. 19). The degradation products are bacteriologically inactive and have a weak affinity for the ribosomes. The introduction of a double bond or an epoxy group in erythronolide A causes a loss of antibacterial activity. The introduction of a nitrogen atom at position 10 gives rise to the 14-membered azolides, which are relatively inactive. Cleavage of the L-cladinose yields a product with a 3-hydroxyl which is inactive. Oxidation of this hydroxyl as a 3-keto group has given rise to a new subgroup of macrolides, the ketolides.

The erythronolide nucleus may be extended either by introduction of a nitrogen atom (15-membered azalides) or by enlargement with a 9,12-epoxy (A-69334). These derivatives are more stable in an acidic medium than erythromycin A and more active against gram-negative bacilli.

4.2.1.2. Modifications of the Substituents

The weak point of erythronolide A is the ketone at position 9. The two linking points are the hydroxyls at positions 6 and 11 (Fig. 20).

4.2.1.2.1. Position 6. Clarithromycin is 6-O-methylerythromycin A. It is more active than erythromycin A and more stable in an acidic medium. However, the absence of blockade of the hydroxyl at position 11 means that a degradation product is formed (pseudoclarithromycin) between the 9-keto and the 11-hydroxyl (Fig. 21).

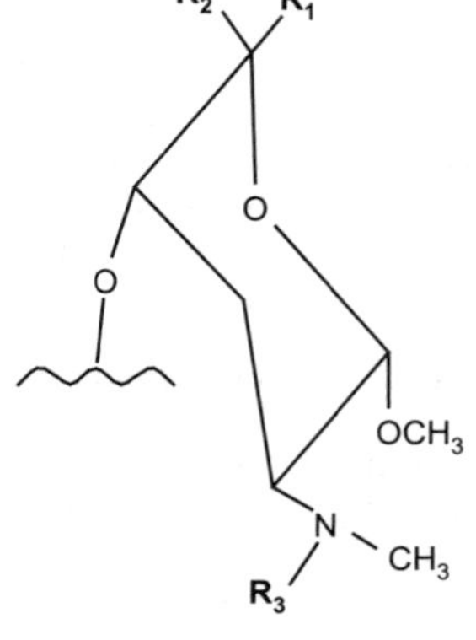

	R_1	R_2	R_3
Istamycin A	NH_2	H	H
Istamycin B	H	NH_2	H
Istamycin A_O	NH_2	NH_2	Glycine
Istamycin B_O	H	H	Glycine

Figure 17 Istamycin derivatives

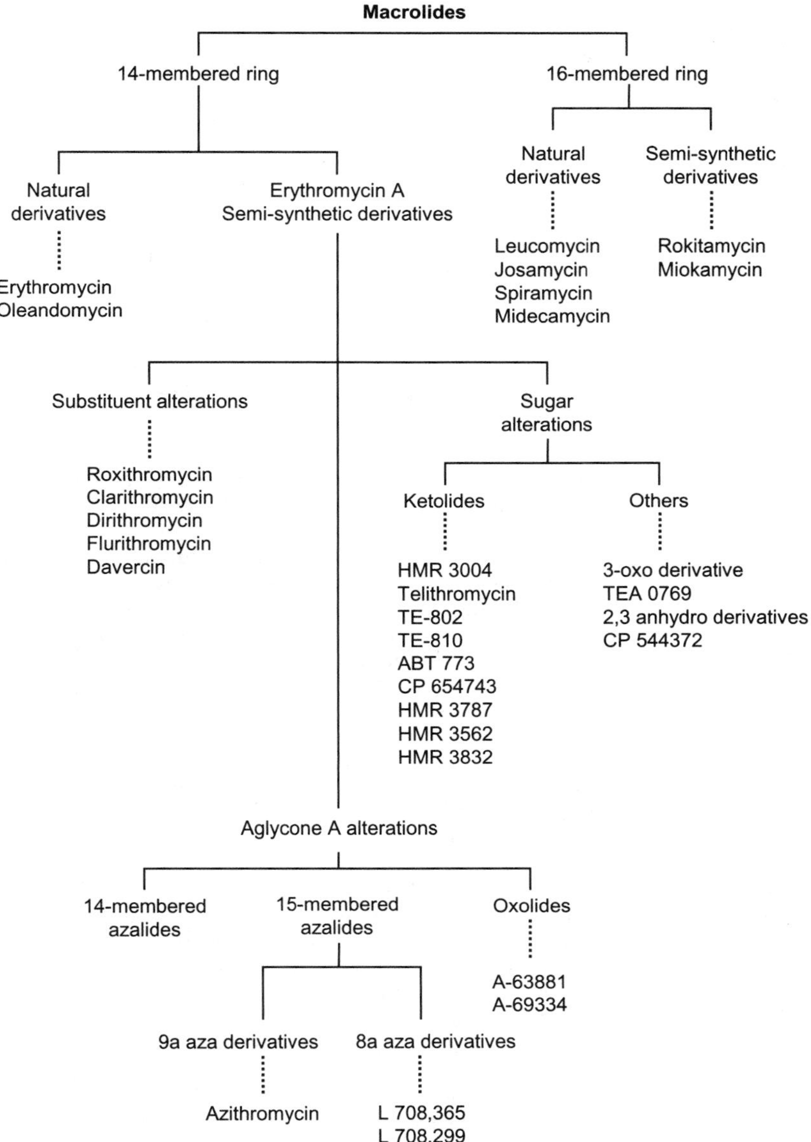

Figure 18 Classification of the macrolides

4.2.1.2.2. Position 8. Erythronolide A has a methyl group at position 8, and its spatial orientation is important for its antibacterial activity.

Replacement of the hydrogen at position 8 by a fluorine atom, which is practically isosteric, in order to increase the stability in an acidic medium yielded flurithromycin (Fig. 22).

4.2.1.2.3. Position 9. A number of modifications have been proposed to prevent inactivation, including the replacement of the ketone by another functional group. Three series of derivatives have been prepared: 9-(S)-erythromycylamine, 9-etheroxime, and the 15-membered azalides (Fig. 23).

4.2.1.2.3.1. ETHEROXIME DERIVATIVES. Different derivatives of the etheroxime type have been synthesized. These vary according to the chain: ether-aliphatic, ether chain containing an amino or sulfo residue, or an oxygen atom. The prototype is roxithromycin, which is stable in an acidic medium and possesses an antibacterial spectrum identical to that of erythromycin A as well as good digestive absorption.

4.2.1.2.3.2. ERYTHROMYCYLAMINE DERIVATIVES. 9-(S)-Erythromycylamine is more active than erythromycin A and 9-(R)-erythromycylamine, but it is weakly absorbed. A number of derivatives have been synthesized to increase the antibacterial activity and to allow absorption of erythromycylamine. The introduction of a supplementary amine group increases hydrophilicity, which affects transparietal penetration of the molecules.

Dirithromycin is a type of prodrug that is active by itself and allows the absorption of erythromycylamine.

4.2.1.2.3.3. AZALIDES. The azalides are not included in Woodward's definition. Two categories of azalides have been described: the 14- and 15-membered azalides. The 15-membered azalides may be divided into two subgroups: the

Figure 19 Degradation of erythromycin A in an acidic medium

9a- and 8a-azalides (Fig. 24). The first series of compounds has increased activity against gram-negative bacilli. Several series of compounds in this group have been prepared. Azithromycin has a methyl group at position 9a, which confers on it the best activity within the first series of synthesized azalides (Table 4). Replacement of the C-4″ hydroxyl of

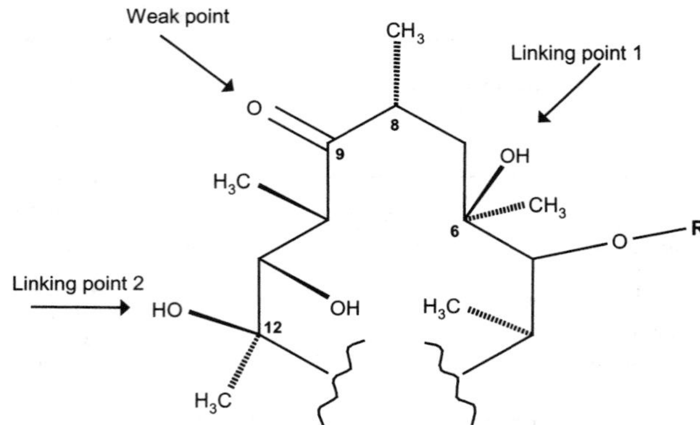

Figure 20 Weak points of erythronolide A

the L-cladinose of azithromycin by an amino group produces increased activity against gram-negative bacilli.

4.2.1.2.4. Positions 11 and 12. Erythromycin A is twice as active as erythromycin B; the compounds differ from one another in the absence of a hydroxyl group at position C-12. Several series of derivatives of erythromycin A have been prepared by modifications at positions 11 and 12. Davercin, which is the cyclic 11,12-carbonate of erythromycin A, is twice as active as erythromycin A.

4.2.1.2.5. Position 14. Clarithromycin is metabolized to 14-hydroxyclarithromycin. The presence of a hydroxyl group at position C-14 does not modify the activity of the erythronolide A nucleus.

4.2.2. Modifications of the D-Desosamine

A number of modifications of the D-desosamine have been published. The *N*-oxide and *N*-dedimethyl derivatives are inactive and have very weak affinity for the ribosomes. The dimethylamino group is important for the antibacterial activity of erythromycin A.

Esters at position 2′ of the hexosamine have been synthesized in order to increase digestive absorption, such as the 2′-ethylsuccinate, 2′-propionate, and 2′-acetyl derivatives, but they are inactive in vitro because they have little affinity for ribosomes. The presence of a 4′-hydroxyl group reduces antibacterial activity, as it is close to the dimethylamino group and may either modify its spatial orientation or cause intramolecular cyclization and thus alter binding to the ribosomes.

4.2.3. Modifications of the L-Cladinose

The absence of L-cladinose on erythromycin A abolishes the antibacterial activity if a hydroxyl is present at position 3, but activity is restored if this hydroxyl is oxidized (3-ketolides).

Erythromycin C, the C-3″ methoxy group of which is replaced by a hydroxyl, is three times weaker than erythromycin A. The 3″-methoxy group is a polar group localized in the proximity of the 3′-dimethylamino group or the 2′-hydroxyl of the desosamine. The 4″-oxime, 4″-amino, and 4″-*O*-sulfonyl derivatives of erythromycin A are two to four times more active than erythromycin A.

5. FLUOROQUINOLONES

The 4-quinolones comprise two types of molecules, those which have substitutions of a fluorine atom at position 6 (fluoroquinolones) and those which do not.

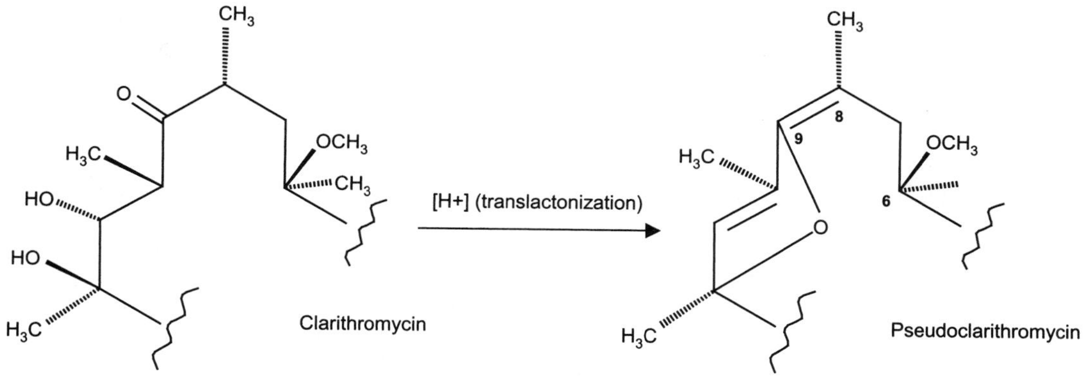

Figure 21 Degradation of clarithromycin in acidic medium

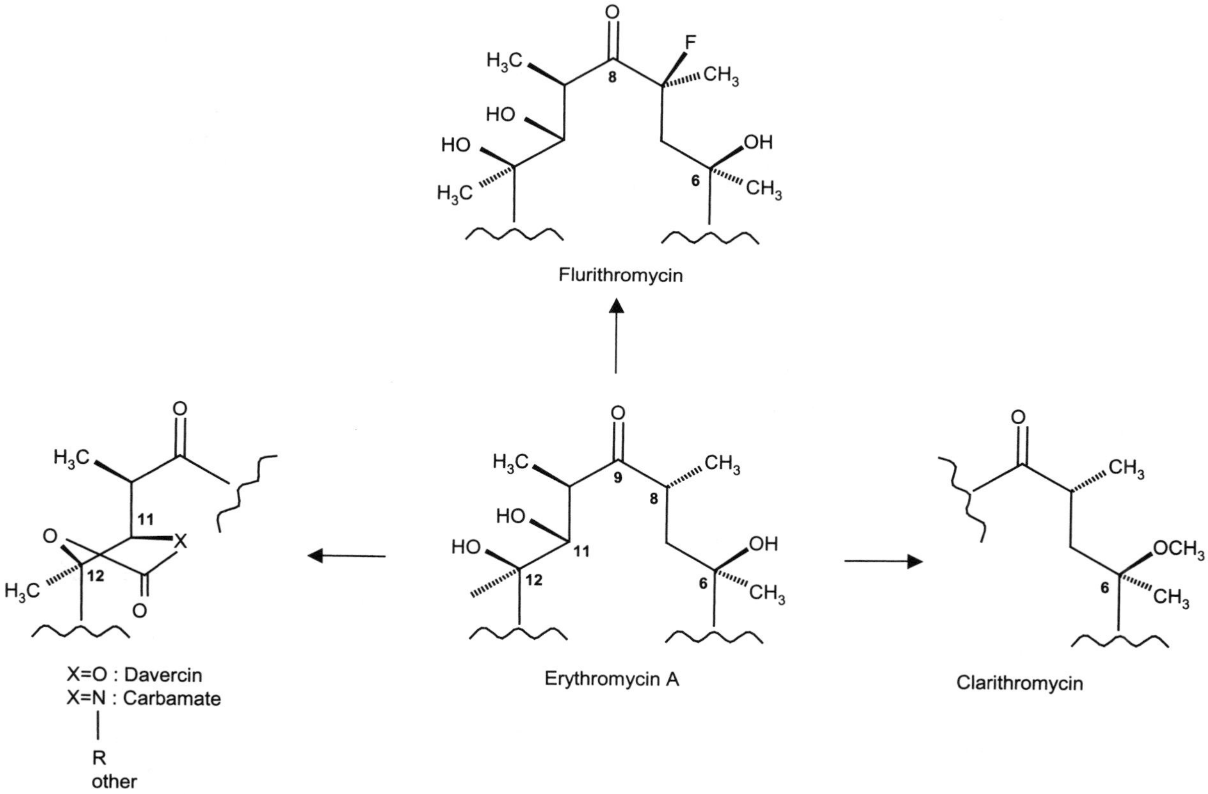

Figure 22 Erythromycin A: modifications of positions C-6, C-8, and C-11 plus C-12

5.1. Classifications

Two classifications have been described: chemical and biological.

5.1.1. Chemical Classification

Four groups may be described according to the structure associated with the pyridone-β-carboxylic ring: mono-, bi-, tri-, and tetracyclic.

The molecules for therapeutic use are pooled in groups II and III. Group II may be divided into two subgroups according to the bicyclic nucleus: quinolene or 1,8-naphthyridone. Group III includes compounds for therapeutic use containing a tricyclic nucleus of the 6,7 type (oxolinic acid), but above all of the 1,8 type (ofloxacin, levofloxacin, rufloxacin, etc.).

5.1.2. Biological Classification

The 4-quinolones may be classified by antibacterial spectrum and metabolization into six subgroups. Groups I and II include compounds whose antibacterial spectrum is limited (to certain species of enterobacteria), groups III and IV comprise derivatives with an extended antibacterial spectrum, and the compounds in groups V and VI have a broad spectrum (Fig. 25).

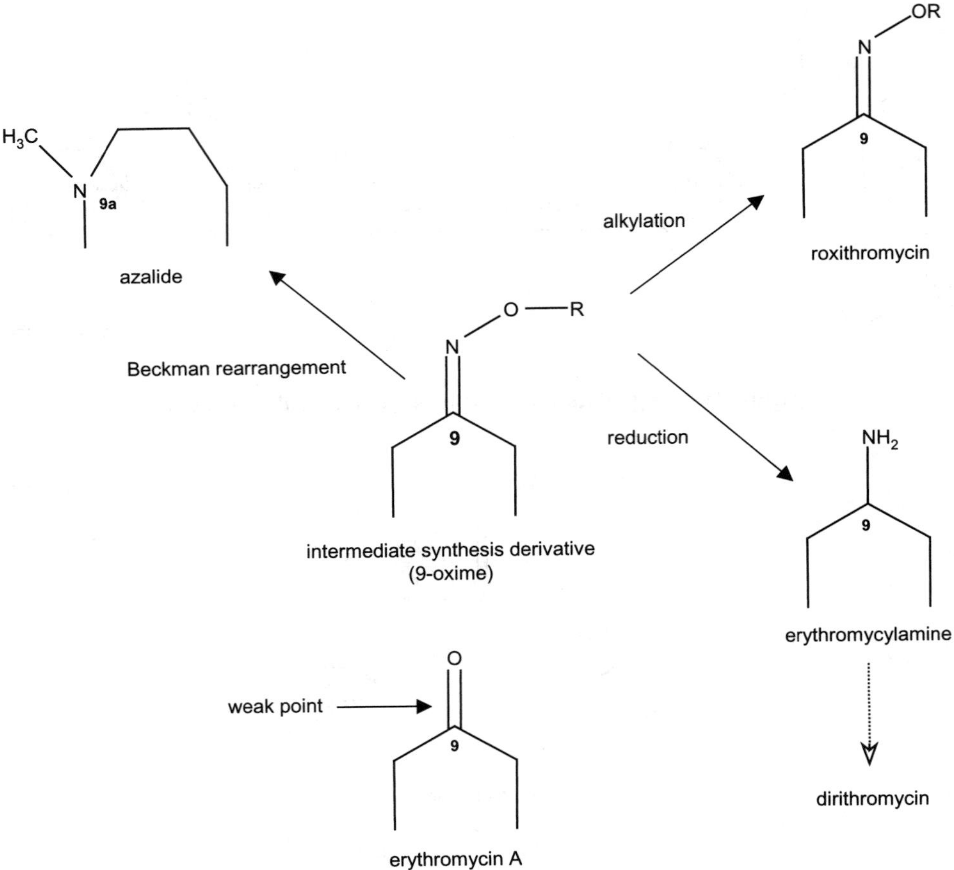

Figure 23 Semisynthesis of 9-erythromycin A derivatives

Figure 24 Azalides Erythromycin A 9a-azalide 8a-azalide

Table 4 Antibacterial activities of the azithromycin derivatives

Drug	MIC (μg/ml)		
	S. aureus	*Enterococcus faecalis*	*E. coli*
Azithromycin	0.39	0.05	0.78
6-O-Methyl azithromycin	0.78	0.05	3.10
11-O-Methyl azithromycin	0.10	0.05	0.78
6,11-Di-O-Methyl azithromycin	0.78	0.78	6.25
6,11,4″-Tert-O-methyl azithromycin	3.10	0.78	6.25

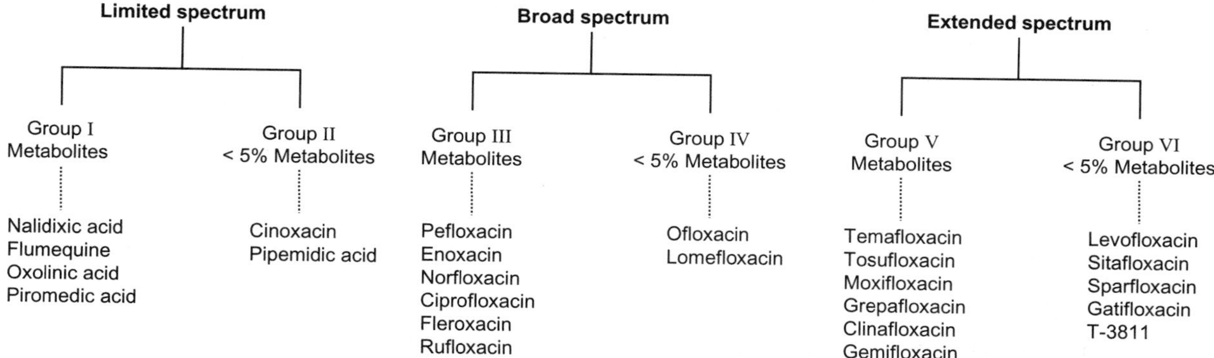

Figure 25 Classification of the 4-quinolones

5.2 Structure-Activity Relationship

5.2.1. Pharmacophore

The pharmacophore unit of the 4-quinolones is composed of a pyridone nucleus and a carboxylic group. This pharmacophore must possess the following minimum structure to be active microbiologically: a double bond at position 2-3 which must not be reduced, a ketone at position 4, which is necessary and which must be free, and the carboxylic group at position 3. All other positions of the quinoline or 1,8-naphthyridone nucleus must or may have substitutions.

5.2.2. Antibacterial Activity

The carboxyl groups at position 3 and the carbonyl groups at position 4 are essential for antibacterial activity as they allow binding of the molecule to the DNA-DNA gyrase complex (Fig. 26). Position 2 must not be replaced, as it is close to the binding site and hindrance at this level would prevent it from binding.

The fluorine atom at position C-6 increases the inhibition of DNA gyrase activity and transparietal penetration.

The presence of a substituent at position 7 increases the antibacterial activity by regulating intrabacterial penetration. A basic group is necessary at position C-7; the nature of the substituents modifies the activity against gram-positive (pyrrolidine > piperazine) or gram-negative (pyrrolidine < piperazine) bacilli. The activity is also affected to a considerable extent by the substituent at the N-1 position. These intervene through steric hindrance and electron interaction. The optimum substituent is the N-1 cyclopropyl (ciprofloxacin) or 1,8-benzoxacin (ofloxacin and levofloxacin). The presence of a methyl group followed by an amino group at position 5 (sparfloxacin) is optimal for antibacterial activity.

5.2.3. Pharmacokinetics

Compounds possessing a 7-*N*-4′-methylpiperazine nucleus are characterized by a long apparent elimination half-life. Substitution at position C-8 by a chlorine or fluorine atom increases oral absorption. The piperazine nucleus is highly metabolized. In order to circumvent this metabolic obstacle, the methyl groups have been attached at position 3′ and/or 5′ of the piperazine (lomefloxacin and sparfloxacin). However, this phenomenon is not avoided with grepafloxacin, which tends to show the importance of the stereochemistry of the compounds.

5.2.4. Safety

The nature of the nucleus at position 7 affects the potentiating effect of nonsteroidal anti-inflammatory drugs on the

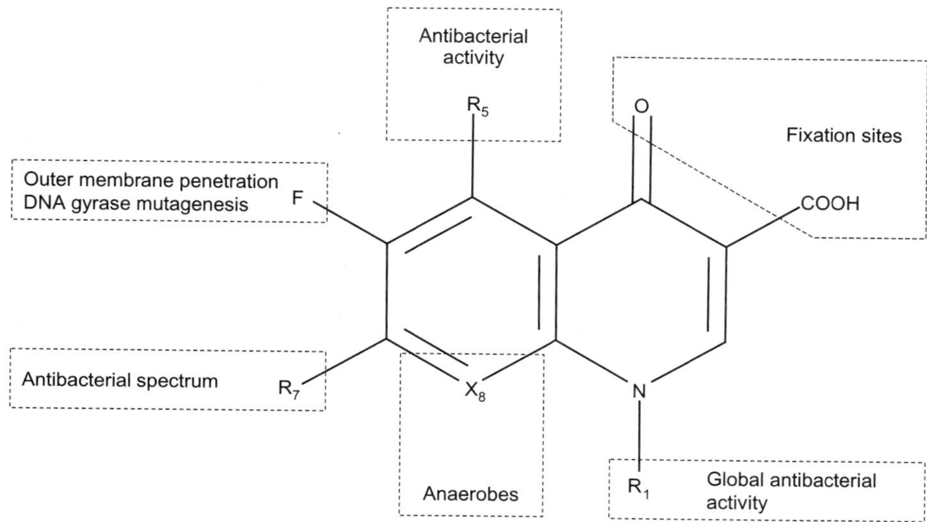

Figure 26 Fluoroquinolones: Antibacterial activity

Table 5 Side effects of fluoroquinolones

Substituent position	Phototoxicity	Solubility	Mutagenicity	Interaction with theophylline	CNS[a]
N-1	–	–	+	+	–
C-5	+	–	+	–	–
C-6	–	–	–	–	–
C-7	–	++	++	+	++
X-8	++	++	++	–	–

[a]CNS, central nervous system.

central nervous system and binding to the γ-aminobutyric acid receptors. Fluoroquinolones with a nonsubstituted piperazine ring (ciprofloxacin, enoxacin, and norfloxacin) exhibit a marked interaction with the nonsteroidal anti-inflammatory drugs, whereas those having an obstructive chain or a pyrrolidine nucleus exert a minimal effect.

The presence of a halogen in C-8 (fluorine or chlorine) increases the risk of phototoxicity of the molecules (Table 5). The genotoxic activity is located in the substituents at positions 1, 7, and 8.

5.2.5. Physicochemical Properties

The majority of fluoroquinolones are zwitterionic molecules that are less soluble at physiological pH. An increase in the solubility in water reduces the risk of crystalluria (tosufloxacin). Substitution at position C-7 by alkyl chains increases solubility in water, as does the presence of a chlorine atom, a methoxy group, or a trimethylfluoro group at position C-8. The presence of an amino acid chain on the pyrrolidine ring increases the hydrosolubility of tosufloxacin and norfloxacin.

6. PEPTIDE ANTIBIOTICS

More than 400 compounds constitute the family of peptide antibiotics. This is an extremely complex class, the borders of which are somewhat vague. The largest family in therapeutic terms are the β-lactams. However, I present here only the other peptides.

6.1. Classification

It is possible to divide the peptides into seven groups (I to VII): linear peptides, cyclic peptides, glycopeptides, glycolipopeptides, lipopeptides, thiazolide polypeptides, and miscellaneous peptides.

Among the cyclic peptides, a few molecules have been made commercially available, such as capreomycin and viomycin (minor antituberculosis agents) and gramicidin S (for topical use). The class of glycopeptides includes numerous compounds, two of which have been made commercially available, vancomycin and ristocetin, although the latter is used only as a laboratory reagent. The glycopeptides may be divided into four groups according to their chemical structures. The classification is based on the structure of the heptapeptide (Fig. 27).

The lipoglycopeptides include numerous compounds and may be divided into two subgroups: glycophospholipid derivatives (teicoplanin and MDL-62873) and the lipoglycodepsipeptide derivatives (ramoplanin).

The lipopeptides are characterized by a peptide chain to which a lipid chain is attached. They may be subdivided into linear and cyclic lipopeptides. The cyclic lipopeptide subgroup contains a very large number of compounds, including the polymyxins and daptomycin.

6.2. Structure-Activity Relationship

6.2.1. Glycopeptides

The antibacterial activity of glycopeptides is based essentially on the peptide part of the molecules. For vancomycin, it is based on amino acids 2, 3, and 4 from the N-terminal acid. The spatial configuration of the amino acids is important in terms of the linkage with D-alanine–D-alanine. The positions requiring the least binding energy are the *R*,*R*,*S*,*R* configuration (amino acids 1, 2, 3, and 4 from the N-terminal acid).

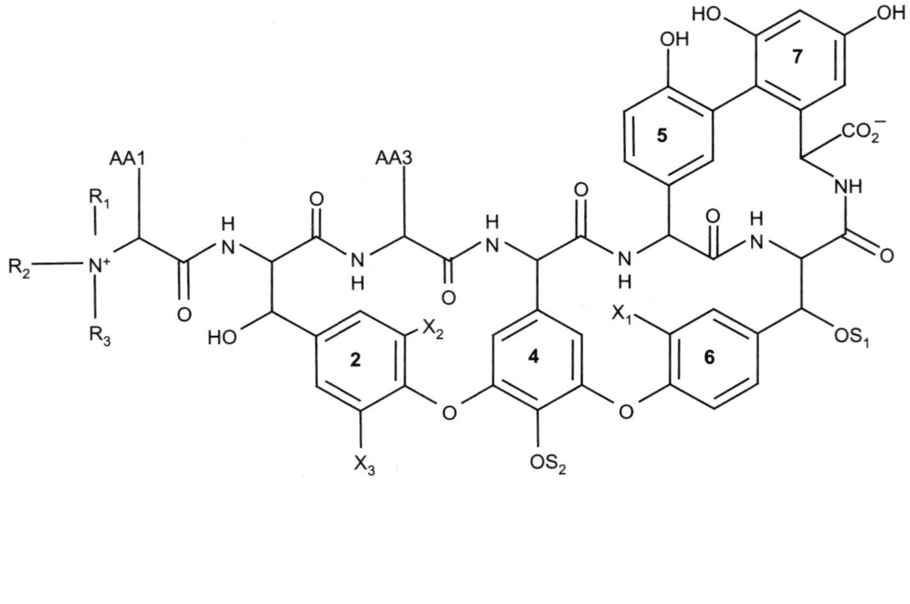

Figure 27 General structure of glycopeptide antibiotics

Vancomycin binds to its substrate via five hydrogen bonds. Sugars such as vancosamine intervene in the binding to the substrate. The NH^{3+}-charged group of vancomycin is important, as it allows binding to the peptide.

6.2.2. Lipoglycopeptides

The teicoplanin complex comprises five major components, A-1 to A-5, and four minor components, RS-1 to RS-4. The lipoglycopeptides are characterized by a glycopeptide ring of the ristocetin type and a lipid chain attached to the amino group of the hexosamine. It has been shown that the two atoms of chlorine at positions 25 and 55 on the aglycone are important for antibacterial activity, as they stabilize the binding of the molecule at the binding site by preventing the mobility of the aromatic rings, in addition to that obtained with the diphenylether group. The chlorine atom at position 55 plays a major role in antistreptococcal activity.

7. ANSAMYCINS

Ansamycin is the name given by Prelog and Oppolzer in 1973 to a series of derivatives possessing a chromophore (aromatic ring) and an aliphatic chain attached on either side of an aromatic ring (ansa). The rifamycins were isolated in 1957 from the fermentation of *Nocardia mediterranei*.

7.1. Classification

It is possible to distinguish two groups of compounds within the family of ansamycins according to the aromatic ring: the naphthalene-type ansamycins and the benzene-type ansamycins. This structural difference is also accompanied by a difference in biological activity. The compounds of the first group are antibacterial or antiviral agents, whereas the second group principally consists of antitumor molecules.

In the first group, apart from the rifamycins (rifamycin S, rifampin, rifapentine, rifabutin, etc.), other compounds have been described, such as halomycins, streptovaricins, tolypomycins, naphthomycins, and awamycin (Fig. 28).

7.2. Structure-Activity Relationship

The rifamycins are characterized by an aliphatic chain which forms a loop between positions 2 and 12 of the naphthalene ring. It is composed of a chain of 17 atoms. The molecules obtained by semisynthesis differ principally through the chain attached at position 3 of the naphthalene nucleus and the presence of a hydroxyl group or its quinone form at position 4.

The chemical modifications of the loop in general cause a reduction in activity. The deacetylation of the acetoxy group at position C-25 and the demethylation at position C-27 represent exceptions. In terms of the naphthalene ring, the hydroxyl groups at positions 1, 2, 9, and 11 should not be modified, as these are essential for antibacterial activity. The most appropriate positions for modification are the carbonyl groups at positions 3 and 4.

8. TETRACYCLINES

Chlortetracycline was described in 1948, followed by oxytetracycline. The molecules were extracted from the fermentation of *Streptomyces aureofaciens* and *Streptomyces rimosus*.

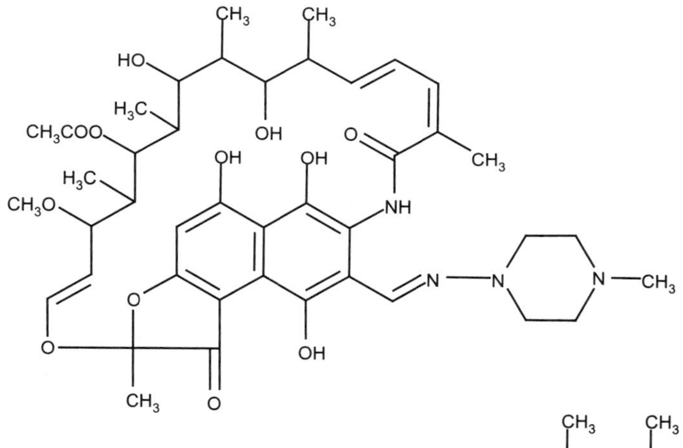

Rifampicin

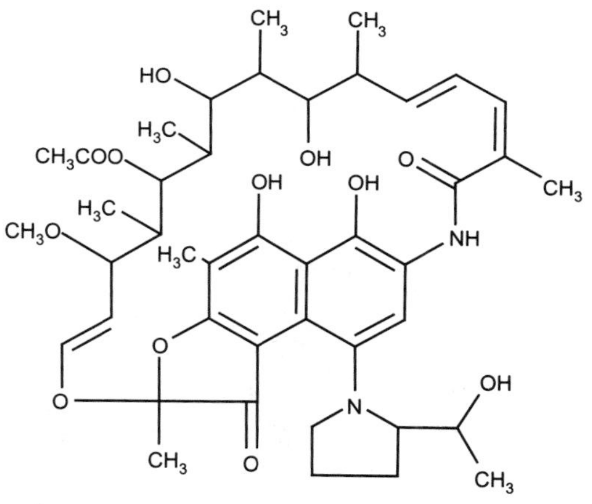

Halomicin

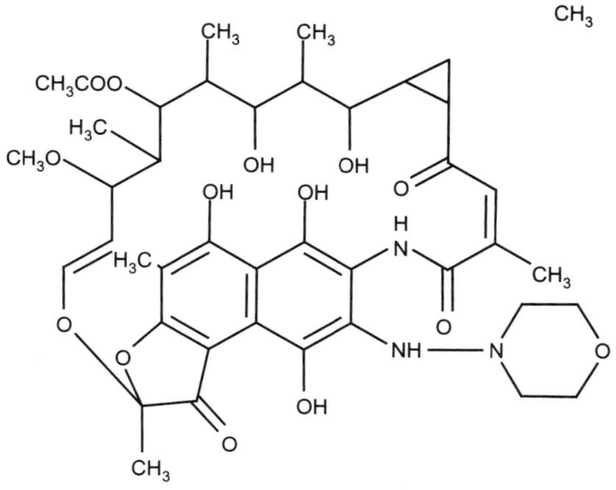

Topylomycin Y

Figure 28 Ansamycins

The description of their chemical structure has allowed the semisynthesis of certain derivatives: tetracycline, doxycycline, minocycline, and other molecules. More recently, molecules of this family have been extracted from *Micromonospora* and *Actinomadura brunea*.

Interest in the cyclines for antibiotic therapy has declined progressively, except in a few indications. Their antiplasmodial activity has long been known, but their use in curative therapy in combination with a fast-acting schizonticide, such as chloroquine, amodiaquine, or quinine, is more recent. This chemical class is enjoying a resurgence of interest in malariology, particularly doxycycline, which is administered as chemoprophylaxis.

8.1. Chemical Structures

The cyclines are polycyclic structures of the perhydronaphthacene carboxamide type. Taking tetracycline as a reference molecule in chemical terms, it is composed of a central skeleton: this tetracyclic structure is an octahydronaphthacene with substitutions in four hydroxyl groups at positions C-3, C-10, C-12, and C-12a, two ketone groups at positions C-1 and C-11, and an *N*-aminodimethyl group at position C-4 and no substituent at position C-9.

The structural variations on this basic skeleton are generally minimal and relate to the C-5, C-6, C-7, and C-8 carbons and the carbamoyl group at position C-2.

Tetracycline has no substituent at position C-5, C-7, or C-8, but a methyl and a hydroxyl are attached at position 6.

Chlortetracycline differs from the basic skeleton in the addition of a chlorine atom at position C-7. This is also found with 6-demethylchlortetracycline and the derivatives Sch-36969, Sch-33256, and Sch-34164, which have variable substituents at position C-8: a methyl or a methoxy for the last two, to which is added in the case of Sch-34164 a hydroxyl at position C-4a; Sch-33256 has a methylcarbamoyl at position C-2.

Oxytetracycline differs from tetracycline through the presence of a supplementary hydroxyl at position C-5 and from 6-deoxytetracycline or doxycycline through demethylation at position C-6; it is structurally very similar to methylene oxytetracycline, which has a methylene at position C-6 without a hydroxyl. Minocycline is a separate entity, possessing no substituents at positions 5 and 6 but a supplementary N-aminodimethylated group at position C-7 (Fig. 29).

Other structures have been studied with the aim of increasing antibacterial activity, such as 6-demethyl-6-deoxytetracycline, 6-thiatetracycline, chelocardin, anhydrotetracycline,

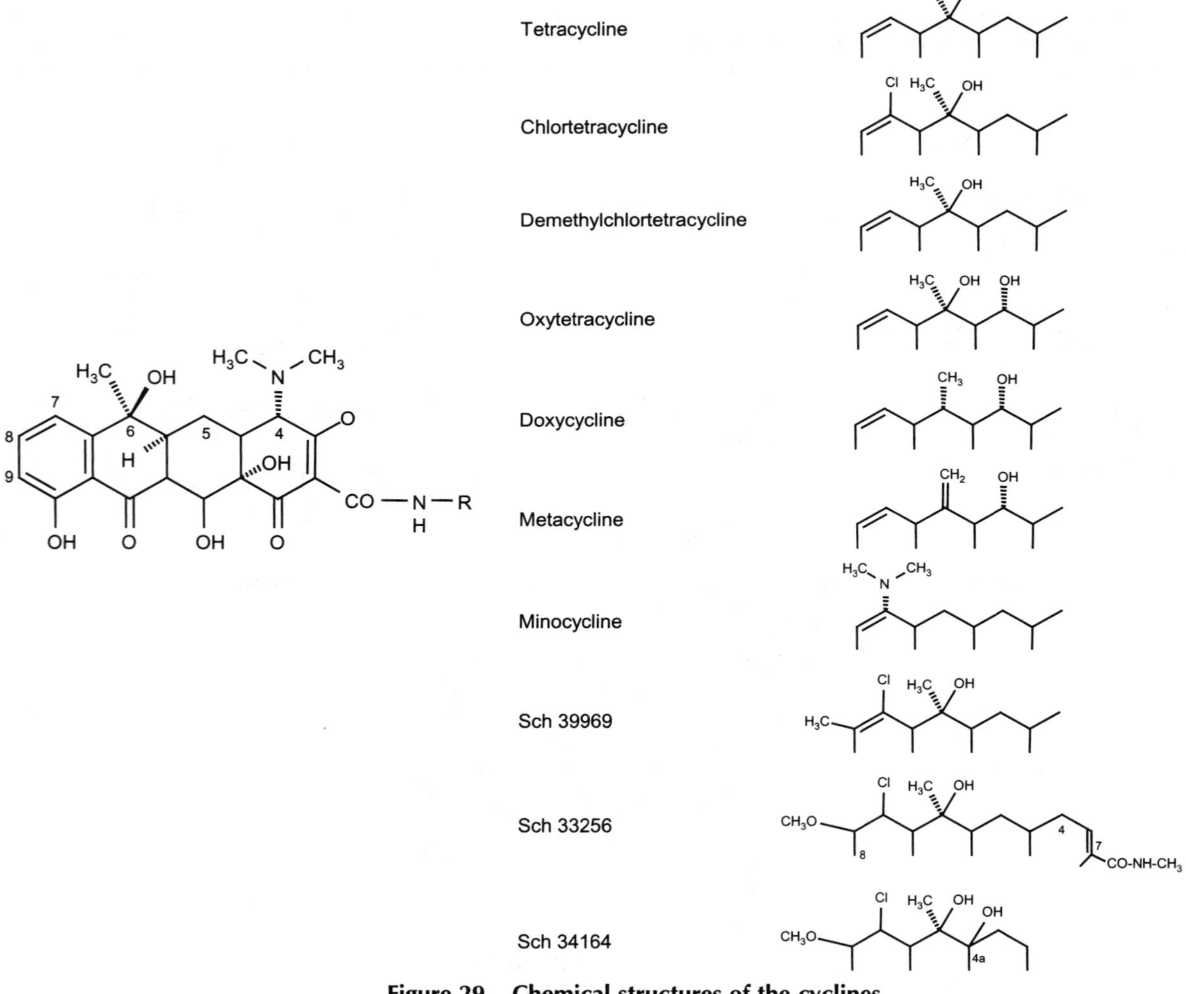

Figure 29 Chemical structures of the cyclines

anhydrochlortetracycline, and 4-*epi*-anhydrochlortetracycline (Fig. 30).

Two new entities have been reported, the glycine tetracyclines and the dactylocyclines, and these are active against tetracycline-resistant bacterial strains (Fig. 31).

8.2. Structure-Activity Relationship

The simplest basic structure possessing in vitro but not in vivo antibacterial activity is 6-demethyl-6-deoxy-4-didemethylaminotetracycline.

All of these cycline derivatives are similar with respect to in vitro antibacterial activity, but perhaps minocycline might be set apart from the other cyclines because of the partial cross-resistance of *S. aureus* to it.

8.2.1. Structural Variations

All of the variations applied to the perhydronaphthacene structure have shown that the presence of the basic *N*-aminodimethyl group at position C-4 is essential for in vivo activity. Structural variations have been made to the nucleus, and various substituents have been proposed.

8.2.1.1. Modification of the Chromophores

Tetracycline possesses two groups of chromophores which separate the hydroxyl at position C-12a: the A ring and the B, C, and D rings.

Modification of these chromophores alters the activity of the cyclines; opening of the B or C ring, extension of the chromophore such as 12a-deoxytetracycline, a substitution of the hydroxyl at position 12a, or aromatization of the A or C ring (5a-,6-anhydrotetracycline, 4a-,12a-anhydrotetracycline) results in loss of all the antibacterial activity.

There is a stereochemical prerequisite, as shown by the activity of the enantiomer of tetracycline, which is half as active as tetracycline.

8.2.1.2. Substituents of the Perhydronaphthacene Ring

Substituents can be found at position C-2. The carbonyl appears to be essential for the activity of the cyclines; conversely, the amide may be replaced.

The reduction in the antibacterial activity of the derivatives with substitutions on the carboxamide group would appear to be related to a modification in lipophilicity rather than a structural modification.

A certain number of cleavable esters have been prepared in order to increase the hydrosolubility of tetracycline: lymecycline, rolitetracycline, pipacycline, etamocycline, and tetrabiguanide. Lymecycline has a cleavable ester of the methylene lysine type. Rolitetracycline is the result of the interaction of tetracycline with formaldehyde and a pyrrolidine ring. This reaction is reversible.

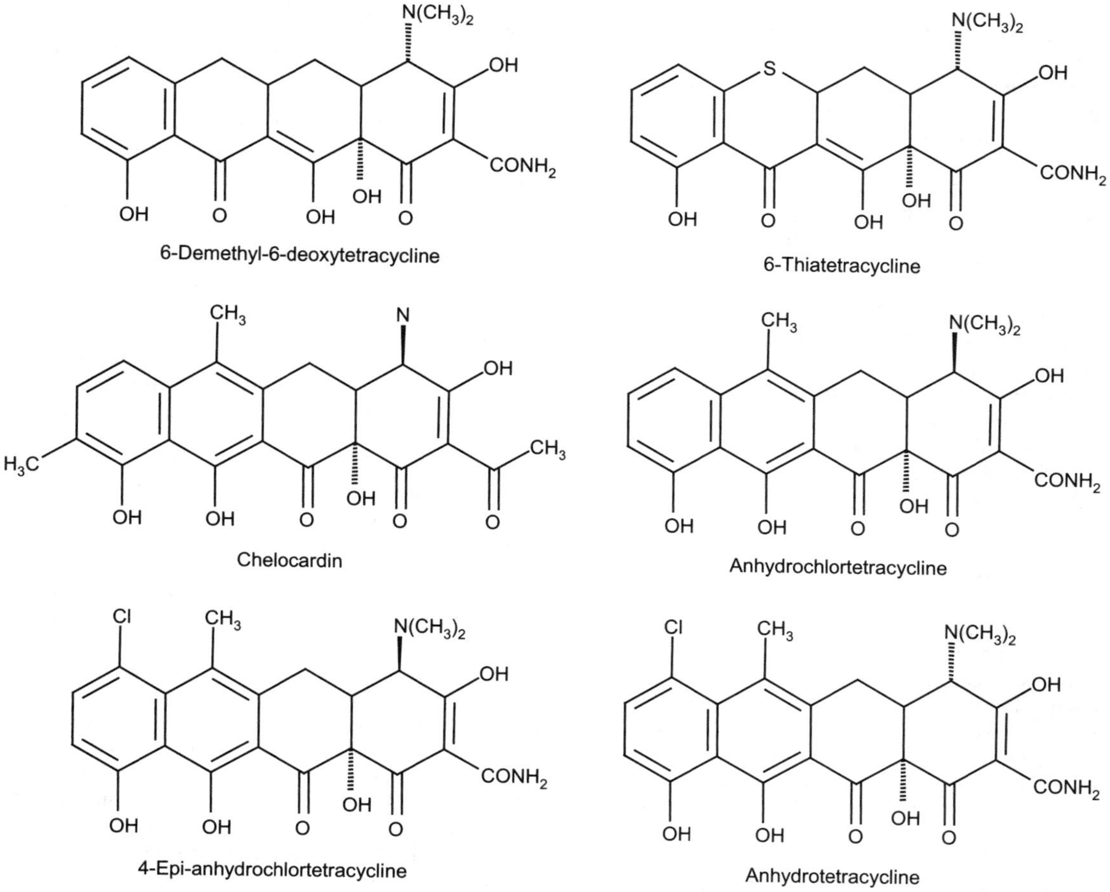

6-Demethyl-6-deoxytetracycline

6-Thiatetracycline

Chelocardin

Anhydrochlortetracycline

4-Epi-anhydrochlortetracycline

Anhydrotetracycline

Figure 30 Other derivatives of the cyclines

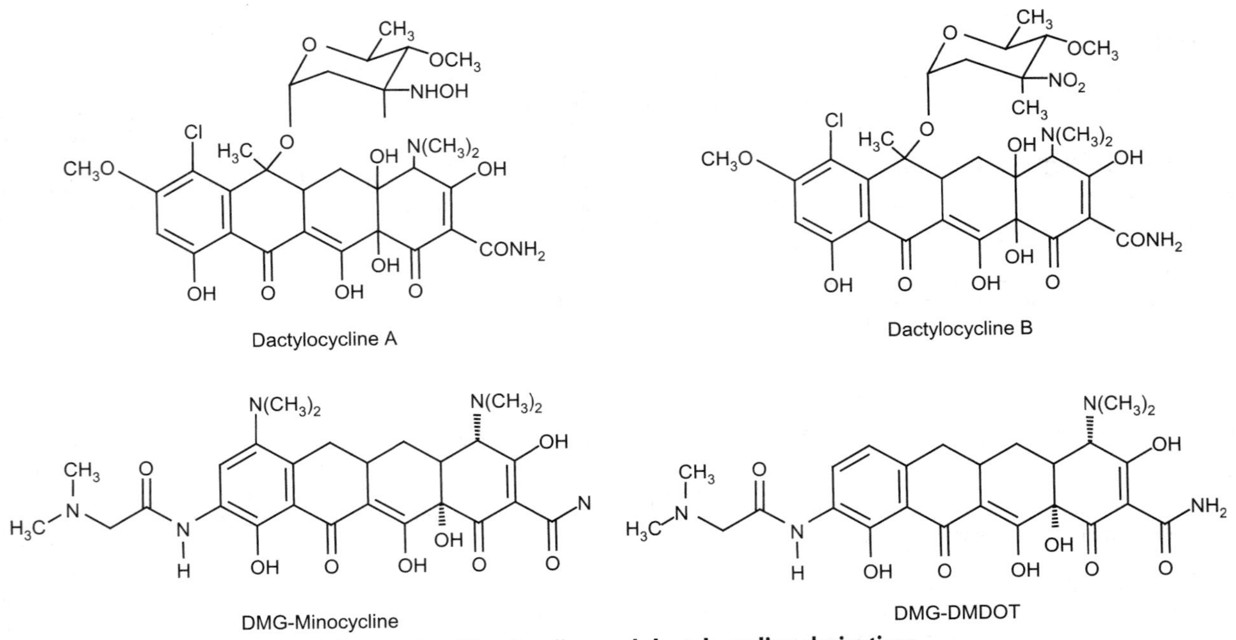

Dactylocycline A

Dactylocycline B

DMG-Minocycline

DMG-DMDOT

Figure 31 Glycylcycline and dactylocycline derivatives

The nonhydrolyzed derivatives possess weaker activity or are devoid of it all together.

8.2.1.2.1. Substituents at position C-4. The tertiary amine function is essential for the in vivo, but not the in vitro, activity. Other derivatives have been proposed, such as 4-methioiodide, 4,6-hemiketal, 4-oxyimino, 4-hydrazino, and 4-hydroxy, but these are devoid of all activity.

8.2.1.2.2. Substituents at position C-6. The most creative approach has been the modifications at position C-6; in fact, these have yielded derivatives that are stable in an acidic medium, allowing substitutions on the aromatic D nucleus. Hydroxylation or methylation at position C-6 is not essential for antibacterial activity. Other substituents also produce appreciable activity. 6-Methylene derivatives are more active than tetracycline. Various substituents of the methylene group have been proposed, particularly thiomethylene, to which are attached phenyl rings or methylphenyl rings, increasing the lipophilia of the molecule.

The position of the substituent interferes with antibacterial activity, with 6-α-deoxytetracycline being more active than 6-β-deoxytetracycline.

8.2.1.2.3. Substituents at position C-7. The electroattractive groups significantly increase in vitro activity. An amino function may be either electroattractive or electrodonating, depending on its protonation.

On the bacterial surface, there would appear to be a microenvironment at a low pH; when the bacterial preparietal zone has an excess of positively charged ions, the amine at position C-7 is protonated and the antibacterial activity increases.

Other groups or heteroatoms have been proposed—chlorine, bromine, and nitro—which also increase the in vitro activity of the cyclines.

8.2.1.2.4. Substituents at position C-9. The electron problems are similar to those with C-7. However, the 9-nitro and 9-chloro derivatives are less active, as is the 9-dimethylamino, because of steric hindrance. The 9-dimethylamino has better in vivo than in vitro antibacterial activity.

Recently, polar methoxy groups have been attached at the C-8 position, giving rise to compounds with variable antibacterial activity: Sch-33256 and Sch-34164.

8.2.2. Physicochemical Properties

The apparently minimal structural variations are capable of modifying the physicochemical properties. The hydrosolubility of a compound depends essentially on certain "polar" groups, such as the hydroxyls. The hydroxyl groups carry electron doublets, explaining their polar nature. This polarity reinforces the hydrosolubility of the compound. For example, oxytetracycline has a supplementary hydroxyl at the C-5 position compared with chlortetracycline and is more hydrosoluble.

Hydrosolubility is also subject to the state of ionization of the compound. The cyclines possess three ionogenic centers. The most hydrosoluble compounds are the most electrically charged compounds. Ionization of the cyclines is a relatively complex phenomenon given the large number of ionogenic centers. The existence of a positive or negative total electric charge (ionized molecules) reduces liposolubility. The tricarbonylmethane system has a high acidity (pK_a1). The second center of activity is the phenolketoenolic system (pK_a2), and the third is the dimethylamine (pK_a3), with minocycline having a fourth dimethylamine center at position C-7 (pK_a4). The values of these different constants are summarized in Table 6.

8.2.2.1. Liposolubility

There is a major variation in the partition coefficient (K_p) (chloroform-water system) according to the molecular structure.

Tetracycline and doxycycline are two isometric molecules whose liposolubilities differ because of the position of the hydroxyls: at β-OH C-6 for tetracycline and at α-OH C-5 for doxycycline. In the tetracycline molecule, the methyl group exerts an influence on the electron density of the hydroxyl group. It repels the binding electrons towards the

Table 6 K_p**s of cyclines**

Drug	$K_p(CHCl_3/H_2O$, pH 7)
Oxytetracycline	0.11
Tetracycline	0.105
Methyleneoxytetracycline	0.117
Demethychlortetracycline	0.148
Doxycycline	0.63
Minocycline	39.4
Chlortetracycline	

oxygen atom by a positive inductive effect. The result is an increase in the electron density and polarity which reinforces the contribution of the hydroxyl at position C-6 to hydrosolubility and reduces the K_p compared to that of the isomer, doxycycline.

9. LINCOSAMIDES

The first lincosamide used therapeutically was lincomycin. Other molecules have been semisynthesized to increase antibacterial activity, such as clindamycin, pirlimycin, and mirincamycin.

Lincomycin is composed of a proline substituted with a 4′-alkyl chain and a thio-octopyranoside, the whole unit being linked by an amide bond (Fig. 32).

9.1. Modifications of the Proline

If the hydrocarbon chain at position C-4′ is increased, optimal activity is obtained with a hexyl group. The isomer in the *cis* position possesses half the activity obtained with the *trans* isomer. The bioavailability increases with the length of the chain, albeit not linearly, whereas the lipophilia increases more regularly.

The *N*-demethyl-4′-alkyl derivatives possess not insignificant antibacterial activity.

9.2. Modifications of the Glucide

The α-thiol group in a β configuration is necessary or even indispensable for the activity of lincomycin. Various substituents of the α-thiol group have been proposed—ethyl, isopropyl, butyl, and methylvinyl—which yield bacteriologically active compounds.

Variations have been made to the substituents at position 7, giving rise to clindamycin, pirlimycin, and mirincamycin. The hydroxyl group at position 7 may be replaced by an *epi*-hydroxy (half the activity of lincomycin) or a 7-keto (2% of the activity of lincomycin); 7-deoxy-(*S*)-chlorolincomycin (clindamycin) possesses four times the activity of lincomycin, and its 7-*epi*-chlorolincomycin isomer is one and a half times more active than lincomycin.

The chain of lincomycin is D-(−)-*threo,* whereas that of clindamycin is L-(+)-*threo*, in an *S* configuration.

9.3. Simultaneous Modifications of the Proline and Glucide

Derivatives possessing modifications at the N-1 and C-4′ positions have been synthesized from clindamycin. It has been shown that the antibacterial activity increases when the length of the chain is extended, reaching an optimum when the substituent at position C-4′ is a pentyl (n-C_5H_{11}).

10. CHLORAMPHENICOL

Chloromycetin was isolated in 1947 by two teams of American researchers from a strain of *Streptomyces venezuelae*, purified in 1948, and crystallized and synthesized in 1949. Subsequently, Japanese researchers isolated other chloromycetin-producing strains: *Streptomyces phaeochromogenes* subsp. *chloromycetine, Streptomyces omiyaensis,* and *Streptosporangium viridogriseum* subsp. *kofuense.*

10.1. Chemical Structure

Chloromycetin is an alcohol whose molecular structure was determined by Rebstock et al. in 1949. It comprises two asymmetrical carbons; it is 2-dichloroacetamido-*para*-nitrophenyl-1,3-propanediol. Chloromycetin is composed of three groups: nitrophenyl, dichloroacetamide, and propanediol. Hydroxylation of carbon 3 of the propanediol is essential for its biological activity (Fig. 33).

Chloramphenicol, a molecule obtained by synthesis, is a levogyrous derivative, D-(−)-*threo*, the physical and biological properties of which are identical to those of chloromycetin. There are four isomers of chloramphenicol, two of the "*erythro*" series and two of the "*threo*" series. The *d* and *l* compounds are distinguished. The difference between the *threo* series and the *erythro* series lies in the position of the hydroxyl attached at position C-1. Only the D-(−)-*threo* has biological activity.

Thiamphenicol is an analog of chloramphenicol with a methylsulfonyl group replacing the nitro group on the phenyl ring.

10.2. Structure-Activity Relationships

The chloramphenicol molecule is composed of three functional units: the nitro group in the *para* position of the phenyl ring, the dichloroacetyl group, and a primary alcohol on carbon 3 of the propanediol chain.

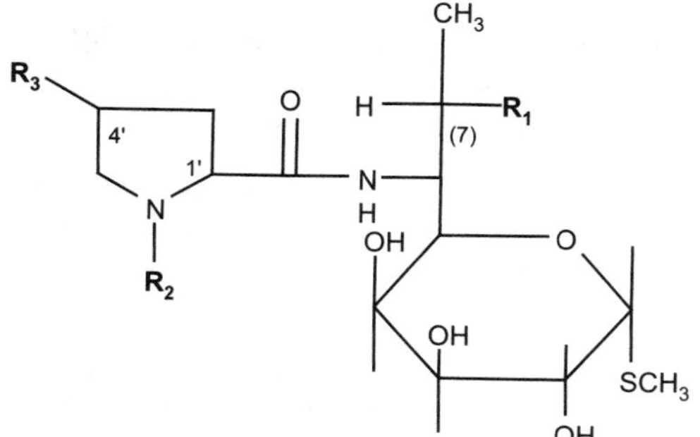

	R_1	R_2	R_3
Lincomycin	-H	$-CH_3$	-n C_3H_7
Clindamycin (U21251 F)	-Cl	$-CH_3$	-n C_3H_7
Mirincamycin (U 24729 A)	-Cl	-H	-n C_3H_{11}
U 26285 A	-Cl	-H	-n C_3H_7

Figure 32 Lincosamide derivatives

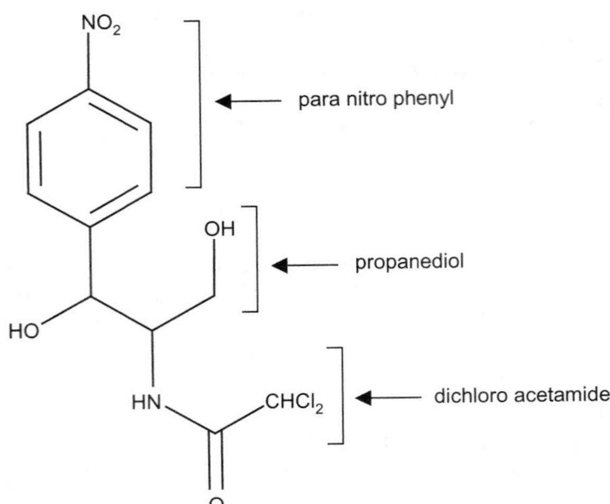

Figure 33 Chloramphenicol

10.2.1. The *p*-Nitrophenyl Group

The presence of a *p*-nitro group in a natural compound is unusual. The three atoms are in the same plane. This group is negatively charged electrically; it can cause mesomerization by electron attraction, enabling the hydroxyl at position C-1 of the propanediol chain to form a hydrogen bond, thus causing a structural modification.

Biotransformation to an amine by reduction of the *p*-nitro group is an important point biologically. By means of a nitroreductase, a nitroso derivative, a hydroxylamine, and an amine are obtained successively. The amine is inactive and is found in the acetylated or nonacetylated form in the urine. It represents 4 to 8% of all the urinary metabolites of chloramphenicol.

Some metabolites possess potential antibacterial activity. Derivatives with an electronegative structure have been synthesized, such as the amine, *R*-methylamine, dimethyl, *R*-sulfonamide, thiomethyl, carbamoyl, carbonitrile, phenyl, benzyl, and hydroxyl groups or the atoms bromine, iodine, fluorine, and chlorine. However, all of these derivatives have weak antibacterial activity.

Only thiamphenicol, in which the *p*-nitro structure has been replaced by *p*-methylsulfonyl, has been developed therapeutically. This group is electronegative and makes the molecule soluble in water, but it is less distributed in the body. It is eliminated in the urine in the nonglucuroconjugated form because of its hydrosolubility.

Replacement of the phenyl nucleus by a thienyl, pyridine, or naphthyl ring yields compounds with interesting antibacterial activity. The steric properties of the aromatic system are not critical for in vitro activity, with the exception of the substituents which must be in the *para* and not the *meta* or *ortho* position.

10.2.2. The Dichloroacetyl Group

Oxidation (cytochrome P450) of the dichloroacetyl side chain gives rise to two derivatives capable of binding covalently to the thiol and amino groups of the proteins. A partially dehalogenated derivative is formed initially, followed by a hydrochloride as the end point of the oxidative process.

On the basis of this knowledge, derivatives have been synthesized in which the chlorine is replaced by a fluorine and the hydrogen is replaced by a halogen, thus preventing the oxidation processes. The steric position of this chain and its size affect antibacterial activity. The activity is inversely proportional to its length.

Substitution of the amine by a methyl group abolishes antibacterial activity.

This chain would appear to intervene principally in the crypticity of chloramphenicol, which penetrates the bacterial wall via a transporter with intrinsic electronic and steric specificity. Because of its electronegative charges and its lipophilia, this chain appears to allow the diffusion of chloramphenicol, since the membrane logP of chloramphenicol is 1.14 (octanol/water).

10.2.3. Primary Alcohol at Position C-3 of the Propanediol Chain

Another series of the second generation of chloramphenicol derivatives is characterized by modifications to the primary alcohol. This plays a major role in the inactivation of chloramphenicol by glucuroconjugation. Substitution by a fluorine derivative increases antibacterial activity, allowing greater resistance to bacterial acetylases. A product has been developed for use in veterinary medicine, florfenicol.

10.2.4. The Propanediol Chain

The propanediol chain includes a primary alcohol and a secondary alcohol. Modifications of this chain have been tried. The presence of a methyl group at position C-2, suppression of the hydroxyls, and an increase in length of the carbon chain abolish antibacterial activity.

The reduction of the hydroxyl group at position C-1 to a ketone has given rise to more than 40 compounds. Two derivatives have 20 to 40 times greater antibacterial activity than chloramphenicol. These are characterized by the presence of an ethylene or a bromine instead of a secondary alcohol.

The antibacterial activity of chloramphenicol may be a function of the spatial position of the three constituents at the ribosomal binding site, but also of the thermodynamics. In fact, the amide bond at position 2 is usually fixed in the *trans* position and the axis of rotation of the hydroxyls is at position 7 or 8, that of the acetamide is at position 1, and that of the aryl is at position 5. The bond between carbons 4 and 5 is 2.7 kcal/mol, whereas the carbon-nitrogen bond at position 3 is 0.6 kcal/mol.

10.3. Other Derivatives

Phenicol derivatives other than chloramphenicol have been described, such as sparsophenicol, which is a chemical combination of chloramphenicol and sparsomycin, and fluorinated derivatives of chloramphenicol and thiamphenicol (Sch-24893, Sch-25298, and Sch-25393), which appear to be more active than the parent molecules.

11. BENZYLPYRIMIDINES

11.1. Introduction

The description of the structure of folic acid in 1946 allowed the development of various compounds inhibiting a constitutive enzyme, dihydrofolate reductase (DHFR). The various research teams worked on these inhibitors in several directions: (i) aminopterin derivatives, e.g., methotrexate; (ii) 2,4-diaminopyrimidines, e.g., antiparasitic and antibacterial agents, like trimethoprim and pyrimethamine; and (iii) the diaminotriazines, particularly the antimalarial agents proguanil and, above all, its metabolite, cycloguanil.

DHFR inhibitors used therapeutically are the result of studies relating to the specificity of this enzyme for bacterial, parasitic, or epithelial cells.

Several hundred molecules have been synthesized. Since the synthesis of trimethoprim, four other molecules possessing antibacterial activity have been used therapeutically or are undergoing clinical development: tetroxoprim, brodimoprim, methoprim, and etioprim (Fig. 34).

Studies of the properties of DHFR initially allowed nonspecific inhibitors to be synthesized, such as methotrexate, followed by specific inhibitors either for bacteria, such as trimethoprim or brodimoprim, or for protozoa, such as pyrimethamine.

The active site of all of the enzymes contains an anionic residue, which is an aspartic acid for bacteria and a glutamic acid for epithelial cells (*E. coli* Asp 27).

The other ionized residue that is markedly involved is arginine 57, which interacts with the α-carboxylic group of the glutamic acid of methotrexate.

The NH atoms of the pyrimidine ring form hydrogen bonds. In *E. coli*, the protons of the nitrogen at position 1 and of the amine group at position 2 also form hydrogen bonds with aspartic acid at position 27. The NH_2 groups also form a bond with tryptophan at position 30 and with the hydroxyl group of the threonine at position 113.

11.2. Classification of DHFR Inhibitors

DHFR inhibitors may be nonspecific or specific, on the basis of which three major classes of therapeutic agents may be distinguished: (i) anticancer agents, e.g., methotrexate; (ii) antiparasitic agents, e.g., pyrimethamine, trimetrexate, and chloroguanidine; and (iii) antibacterial agents, e.g., trimethoprim and derivatives.

The 4′-amino-3′,5′-dimethoxy derivative possesses diuretic activity.

DHFR inhibitors may be divided into three chemical groups: the benzylpyrimidines, the triazinopyrimidines, and the bicyclic derivatives (pteridine, pyrido[2,3]pyrimidines, and quinozalines).

The benzylpyrimidines consist primarily of antiparasitic and antibacterial medications. Only antiparasitic agents are developed from triazinopyrimidines. The anticancer agents belong to a group of bicyclic derivatives.

The antibacterial compounds display good antibacterial activity and a lack of inhibitory activity against epithelial cell DHFR. The most widely used belong to the benzylpyrimidines. These molecules possess three structures that determine the antibacterial activity: a pyrimidine heterocycle, a benzene ring, and a bridge chain.

11.2.1. Pyrimidine Heterocycle

The antibacterial activity of the pyrimidine heterocycle was demonstrated by Russel and Hitchings in 1948. Its activity is based on the presence of amino groups at positions 2 and 4 and the lack of a substituent at position 6.

Roth et al., however, synthesized derivatives of trimethoprim with substitutions at position 6 possessing weaker antibacterial and DHFR-inhibitory activities than trimethoprim.

These authors postulated that the trimethoprim derivatives interact with the enzyme in a given configuration in which the hydrogen at position 6 points towards the center of the benzene ring; another substituent would cause steric hindrance and hence a reduction in affinity. This hypothesis was confirmed by the studies of Baker et al. in 1991.

The second reason for this weak activity is that the substituent at position 6 might reduce the pK_a, except for the alkyls. This would result in a reduction of the proton attraction of the nitrogen at position 1 of the pyrimidine heterocycle by the aspartic acid residue at position 27 of the *E. coli* DHFR. A chlorine atom at position 6 reduces the dissociation constant by 4 units (pK_a3), the compound obtained then being nonionized at physiological pH.

11.2.2. Variations in the Bridge

The nature of the bridge bond undeniably affects the antibacterial activity of the benzylpyrimidines. The best bond is a methylene. The metabolites of trimethoprim with an alcohol or ketone bond are practically inactive. The methylene bond of trimethoprim is inserted in a hydrophobic cleft of the enzyme, explaining the inactivity of alcohols; a hydrophilic substituent alters the angles of torsion between

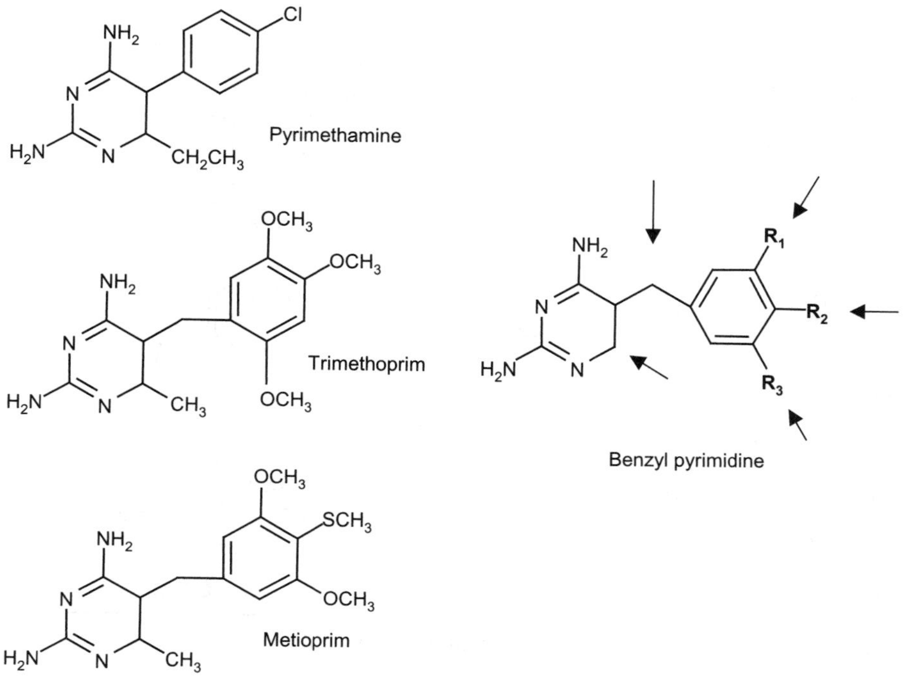

Pyrimethamine

Trimethoprim

Metioprim

Benzyl pyrimidine

Figure 34
2,4-Diaminobenzylpyrimidine

the two rings. In the case of the ketones, electron modification of the substituent at position 5 of the pyrimidine heterocycle reduces the pK_a, which is then on the order of 4.5. Rey-Bellet et al. synthesized compounds with two different bonds. All had weak inhibitory and antibacterial activities.

11.2.3. Benzene Ring

Kompis et al. synthesized a series of trimethoprim analogs in which the benzene ring was replaced by other heterocycles, such as 2′,3′,4′-pyrimidine heterocycles. Their DHFR-inhibitory activities are weak.

Since the studies in 1951 by Falco et al., the best structure has been known to be a benzene ring. It was rapidly apparent that the trisubstituted compounds are more active than the di- or monosubstituted compounds, the lipophilic substituents giving the molecules better activity against gram-positive cocci than against gram-negative bacilli.

11.2.3.1. Substituent at Position 4′ of the Benzene Ring

The substituent at position 4′ of trimethoprim is a methoxy group. Roth et al. in 1980 postulated that one of the factors in the selectivity of trimethoprim might be the presence of the methoxy group outside the plane at position 4′.

Kompis et al. in 1980 reported 38 derivatives differing in the substituent at position 4′. All of the products possessed good affinity for *E. coli* DHFR, with the exception of that with a carboxyl group. However, the amino derivatives were the least active. The presence of an isopropanyl group is responsible for the greater selectivity for bacterial DHFR among the derivatives presented. This chain has the characteristic of being outside the plane bidirectionally relative to the benzene ring. Liebenow et al. synthesized compounds including a hydroxyl. The compounds are active to a greater or lesser extent depending on the nature of the substituents at positions 3′ and 5′. Derivatives comprising a methoxy at position 5′ and a halogen (chlorine or bromine), a hydrogen, or a methyl appear to possess good antibacterial activity.

Roth et al. in 1981 reported 38 derivatives varying in the substituent at position 4′. They suggested that an important function of this substituent, other than a hydrogen, would be to force the two methoxy groups at positions 3′ and 5′ in the *meta* position to move outwards while remaining in the plane of the benzene ring, thus predisposing to an interaction with the enzyme in the inter-*meta* space.

Liebenow et al. synthesized a series of 50 molecules. The compounds possessed methoxy groups at positions 3′ and 5′ varying in terms of their substituents at position 4′; the majority had good antibacterial activity, particularly tetroxoprim (HE-781), for which the group at position 4′ is a dimethoxymethyl chain. However, they noted that the presence of a sulfur atom increased antibacterial activity. The most active would appear to be a 4′-thiomethyl compound.

11.2.3.2. Substituents at Positions 3′ and 5′ of the Benzene Ring

Roth et al. undertook a systematic study of the requirements of the inter-*meta*-benzene space of benzylpyrimidine derivatives that permitted optimal binding to bacterial DHFR by varying the alkyl substituents in the two positions.

Optimal activity was found for *E. coli* DHFR with 3′,5′-diethyl or diethyl-*n*-propyl derivatives occupying the inter-*meta* space, similar to the case with trimethoprim.

These studies strongly suggest that it is the shape of the substituents in the *meta* position rather than their lipophilicity or polarity which plays a preponderant role in their binding to *E. coli* DHFR.

Conversely, the 3′,5′-dialkyl or ether oxygen derivatives exhibit much weaker selectivity for bacterial DHFR.

12. SULFONAMIDES

G. Domagk in 1935 described the curative effect of sulfamidochrysoidine (Prontosil) in a case of streptococcal septicemia. The various studies demonstrated that the active structural unit is *p*-aminobenzenesulfonamide (sulfanilamide).

The sulfonamides are characterized by their capacity for interfering with the synthesis of THF by combining with *para*-aminobenzoic acid, inhibiting the synthesis of dihydrofolates by inhibition of a constitutive enzyme, dihydropteroate synthetase.

12.1. Basis for Activity of the Sulfonamides

Activity of the sulfonamides (Fig. 35 and 36) is based on the following:

- The amino group and the sulfonyl radical must be in the 1,4 position to be active. The amino group at position 4 must not be replaced, or the substituent must be cleaved in vivo.
- Replacement or substitution of the benzene ring abolishes or reduces the antibacterial activity of the resultant compound.
- If SO_2-NH_2 is replaced by SO_2-C_6H_4-*p*-NH_2, the antibacterial activity is similar, but CO-NH_2 or CO-C_6H_4-*p*-NH_2 inactivates the product.
- At position N-1, the compound can only have a monosubstitution, causing a modification in the pharmacokinetic and physicochemical properties; disubstitution reduces antibacterial activity.

According to Moriguchi and Wada, there are two binding sites on the enzyme, which are located about 6.7 to 7 Å from one another; one is specific to the amino group at position 4, and the other is nonspecific.

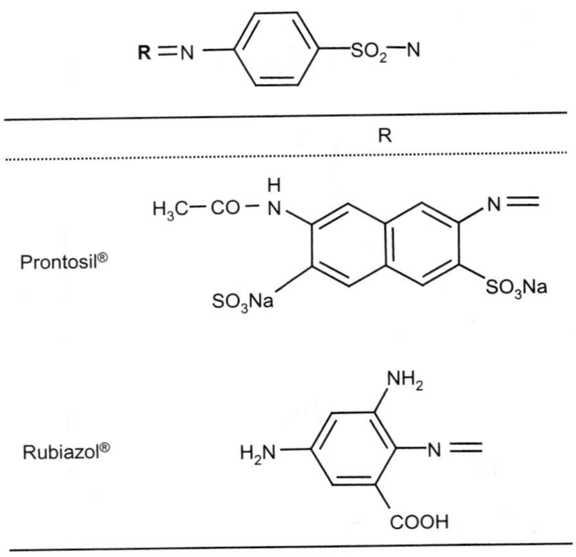

R =N–⟨benzene⟩–SO_2–N

	R
Prontosil®	H_3C–CO–N(H)– naphthalene (SO$_3$Na, SO$_3$Na) –N=
Rubiazol®	H_2N– benzene (NH_2, COOH) –N=

Figure 35 Sulfonamide prodrugs

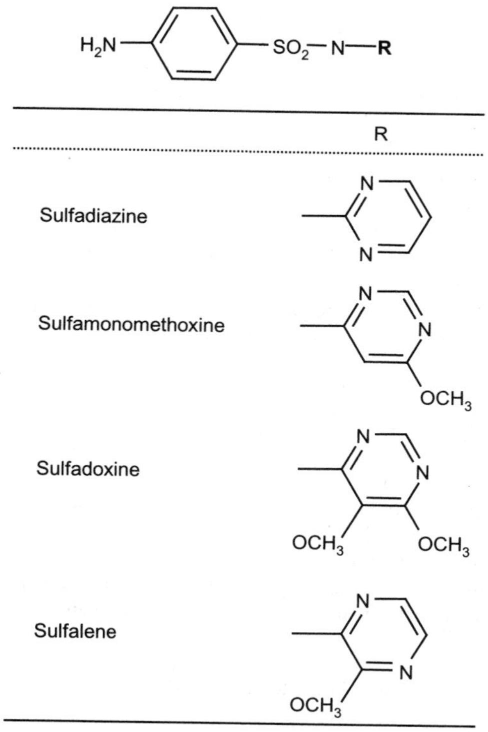

Figure 36 Sulfonamides

The first molecule possessing a heterocycle to be used therapeutically was sulfapyridine in 1938, followed by sulfathiazole. Three compounds possessing a pyrimidine heterocycle have been synthesized; these differ in the absence (sulfadiazine) or presence of one (sulfamerazine) or two (sulfamethazine) methyl groups substituting for the heterocycle at positions 4 and 6.

Two very active and highly hydrosoluble compounds reserved for the treatment of urinary tract infections have come to light: sulfamethizole, which has a thiodiazole heterocycle, and, sulfoxazole, which has an oxazole heterocycle.

Sulfacetamide is a compound possessing an *N*-acyl group substituting for the nitrogen at position 1 which is used in ophthalmology.

The activity of the sulfonamides is dependent on the following:

- The amino group at position 4, which plays a key role in the bacteriostatic activity, which disappears if it is replaced by another group
- The degree of ionization, dependent on the pK_a of the molecules. Compounds with a pK_a of between 6 and 7.4, close to physiological pH, display maximum activity. The pK_a is dependent on the nature of the substituent at the N position.
- The sulfonamides penetrate the cell in a nonionized form but exert their intracellular activity in the ionized form, this being dependent on the electron charge at the N position.

Depending on the substituent at the N-1 position, the sulfonamides possess greater or less antibacterial and even antiparasitic activity.

Sulfamethoxazole has a methyloxazole ring, whereas the oxazole ring of sulfamoxole is dimethylated. These compounds have broad antibacterial spectra, with weak MICs.

Table 7 Half-lives of the sulfonamides

Drug	$t_{1/2}$ (h)
Sulfamethoxypyrazidamine	37
Sulfamethoxydiazine	35
Sulfamethoxypyrazine	65
Sulfadimethoxine	40
Sulfamethoxine	140

12.2. Apparent Elimination Half-Life of the Sulfonamides

The presence of the methyl groups on the pyrimidine hexacycles increases or reduces the apparent elimination half-life according to their position on the ring; the same applies to the methoxy groups, which appear to prolong it still further. The molecule with the longest apparent elimination half-life has methoxy groups at positions 5 and 6 of the ring (sulfamethoxine).

A second phase of development of sulfonamides occurred after 1945, giving rise to two categories of compounds: those having hexacyclic heterocycles with a long apparent elimination half-life and those having pentacycles with a shorter half-life.

Five compounds containing a pyrimidine ring have been synthesized (Table 7).

Three sulfonamides have an apparent elimination half-life on the order of 11 h: sulfamethoxazole, sulfaphenazole, and sulfamoxole.

13. 5-NITROIMIDAZOLES

The chemical class of 5- or 2-nitroheterocycles constitutes a complex family of synthetic antibacterial and antiparasitic agents. They differ from one another through the heterocycle attached to the nitro chain. Thus, 5-nitrofuryl, 5-nitroimidazole, 5-nitrothiazole, and 5-nitrothiophene derivatives have been synthesized. These different derivatives possess antibacterial, antiprotozoal, and anthelmintic activities to various degrees; in 1944, in the course of research undertaken by the Norwich Pharma Co., Dodd and Stilmann demonstrated in a study involving 40 mono- or disubstitution furan derivatives that the introduction of a nitro group at position 5 either caused the appearance of antibacterial activity or increased it. Study of the structure-activity relationships showed the importance of the azomethine group. Exploitation of this fundamental motif resulted in the synthesis of antibacterial and antiprotozoal compounds: nitrofurantoin, furazolidone, and nitrofurazolidone. Other modifications of the chain resulted in the synthesis of derivatives possessing schistosomicidal activity. Based on the concept of isosterism, the furan heterocycle was replaced by other pentagonal heterocycles: nitrothiophene, nitrothiazole, nitroimidazole, nitropyrrole, and nitropyridine. The 5-nitrofuryl derivatives in some cases possess trypanosomicidal activity, such as the nitrofurylthiazoles and nitrofurazones. The first anthelmintics, such as niridazole, were derived from the 5-nitrothiazoles. The therapeutic contribution of the 5-nitroimidazoles has been considerable; in fact, these derivatives, such as metronidazole, possess antibacterial, amoebicidal, and trichomonacidal activities. Metronidazole has recently been proposed for use in the treatment of malaria, but this treatment is disputed.

Green et al. demonstrated that a certain number of nitrofuran derivatives possess not insignificant antimalarial activity.

The molecules have various heterocycles at position 2 of the furyl nucleus, such as triazine (NF-477), pyridazinone (NF-910), and 2-thiazolylamino-2-oxazolidinone (NF-921); nitrofurantoin has moderate antimalarial activity.

Certain 2-aldehyde derivatives of the 5-nitrofuryls would appear to possess antiplasmodial activity.

REFERENCES

Brufani M, 1977, The ansamycins, p 96–212, in Sammes PG, ed, Topics in Antibiotic Chemistry, Horward Ltd.

Bryskier A, 1982, Les inhibiteurs de la dihydrofolate réductase. Classification et relation activité structure, p 19–36, in Modai J, ed, Triméthoprime et sulfamides, Soc Pathol Infect Langue Fr.

Bryskier A, 1983, Classification des céphalosporines et relation activité structure des méthoxy-imino aminothiazolyl céphalosporines, Lyon Pharm, 34, 99–100.

Bryskier A, 1983, Classification des β-lactamines, Pathol Biol, 32, 658–667.

Bryskier A, 1993, Recent advances in fluoroquinolones research, Curr Opin Investig Drugs, 2, 409–415.

Bryskier A, 1993, New pyridone-β-carboxylic acid derivatives, Quinolone Bull, 10(2), 22.

Bryskier A, 1994, Update on fluoroquinolones, Curr Opin Investig Drugs, 3, 41–49.

Bryskier A, Agouridas C, 1993, Azalides: a new medicinal chemical family? Curr Opin Investig Drugs, 2, 687–694.

Bryskier A, Agouridas C, Chantot J-F, 1993, Classification of macrolide antibiotics, in Bryskier A, Butzler J-P, Neu HC, Tulkens PM, ed, Macrolides, Chemistry, Pharmacology and Clinical Uses, Arnette-Blackwell, Paris, p 5–66.

Bryskier A, Agouridas C, Chantot J-F, 1993, Relation structure activity of 14-, and 15-membered ring macrolides, Chemother J, 2, suppl 2, 2–11.

Bryskier A, Agouridas C, Chantot J-F, 1995, New insights into structure-activity relationships of macrolides and azalides, in Neu HC, Acar JF, Young LS, Zinner S, ed, Proc 2nd Int Congr Macrolides Azalides and Streptogramins, Venice, Marcel-Dekker, New York.

Bryskier A, Azsodi J, Chantot J-F, 1993, Parenteral cephalosporin classification, Expert Opin Investig Drugs, 3, 145–171.

Bryskier A, Chantot J-F, 1995, Fluoroquinolones, classification and structure-activity relationships, Drugs suppl—Proc Int Symp New Quinolones Singapore, 1993.

Bryskier A, Labro MT, 1989, Antibiotiques: de nouveaux antipaludéens, in Bryskier A, Labro MT, Paludisme et médicaments, Arnette, Paris, p 133–169.

Chopra I, 1994, Tetracycline analogs whose primary target is not the bacterial ribosome, Antimicrob Agents Chemother, 38, 637–640.

Chopra I, 1994, Glycylcyclines—third generation tetracycline analogues, Expert Opin Investig Drugs, 3, 191–193.

Chu DTW, Fernandes PB, 1991, Recent development in the field of quinolone antibacterial agents, Adv Drug Res, 21, 44–144.

Coulton S, François I, 1994, β-Lactamase: target for drug design, Prog Med Chem, 31, 297–349.

Cox DA, Richardson K, Ross BC, 1977, Aminoglycosides, in Sammes PG, ed, Topics in Antibiotic Chemistry, Horward Ltd, p 5–90.

Della Bella D, 1981, Biological properties of chloramphenicol as related to structural features: from classical knowledge to future developments, in Najean Y, Togoni G, Yunis AA, ed, Safety Problems Related to Chloramphenicol and Thiamphenicol Therapy, Raven Press, New York, p 31–42.

Domagala JM, 1994, Structure-activity and structure-side effect relationships for the quinolone antibacterials, J Antimicrob Chemother, 33, 685–706.

Durckheimer W, Blumbach J, Latrell R, Scheunemann KH, 1985, Recent development in the field of β-lactam antibiotics, Ang Chem, 24, 180–202.

Kirst HA, 1994, Semi-synthetic derivatives of 16-membered macrolide antibiotics, Prog Med Chem, 31, 265–295.

Nagajaran R, 1994, Structure-activity relationships of vancomycin antibiotics, p 195–218, in Nagajaran R, ed, Glycopeptide Antibiotics, Marcel Dekker, New York.

Price KE, 1977, Structure-activity relationships of semi-synthetic penicillins, p 1–86, in Perlman D, ed, Structure-Activity Relationships among Semi-Synthetic Antibiotics, Academic Press.

Price KE, Godfrey JC, Kawaguchi H, 1977, Effect of structural modifications on the biological properties of aminoglycoside antibiotics containing 2-deoxystreptamine, p 299–395, in Perlman D, ed, Structure-Activity Relationships among Semi-Synthetic Antibiotics, Academic Press.

Valcavi U, 1981, Tetracyclines: chemical aspects and some structure-activity relationships, p 502–506, in Gialdroni-Grassi G, Sabath LD, ed, New Trends in Antibiotics: Research and Therapy, Elsevier.

Veyssier P, Bryskier A, 1985, Agents antibactériens de synthèse, Enc Med Chir Thérapeutique, 5-25016 D_{10}.

Epidemiology of Resistance to Antibacterial Agents

A. BRYSKIER

3

1. INTRODUCTION

As each antibacterial is introduced in clinical practice, we hear first of miraculous cures, second of deleterious reactions, and third of the appearance of resistant strains. The goal of antibacterial therapy is to facilitate the eradication of infecting microorganisms from patients in a timely and safe manner while minimizing the emergence and spread of resistance.

Since the introduction of antibiotics into the therapeutic arsenal against infectious diseases, microorganisms have developed means of defense that have protected them against antibacterial agents. The rate of development of this resistance to antibiotic agents at therapeutic doses depends on the chemical complexity of the antibiotics and the genetic material of the bacterium. Currently, whatever the antibiotic used, strains of various bacterial species that are resistant to it preexist. There are a few exceptions, such as a lack of *Streptococcus pyogenes* strains resistant to penicillin G. However, in the laboratory *S. pyogenes* resistant to benzylpenicillin was obtained in 1947 (Gezon, 1948). The mechanism of resistance is carried on a gene which could be plasmid or chromosome mediated. The response of the bacterium is often complex; it may involve preventing the antibiotic from penetrating the bacterial cell wall, inactivating the xenobiotic by enzymes, modifying the site of action of the antibiotic, or synthesizing additional systems that prevent the action of the antibiotic or even actively pump them out (efflux).

All bacterial species and phyla are involved in the phenomenon of resistance to antibacterial agents, sometimes posing genuine therapeutic problems. However, certain antibacterials are responsible for emergence of resistance more frequently than others.

Since 1947, the phenomenon of bacterial resistance has been highlighted by many authors. Resistant and susceptible microorganisms can exist in the same body. As an example, this was demonstrated with two patients with clinical tuberculosus meningitis, for whom streptomycin-susceptible *Mycobacterium tuberculosis* isolates were obtained from cerebrospinal fluid and at the same time streptomycin-resistant organisms were cultured from other lesions (Dowling, 1953).

R. Dubos (1952) wrote that "emergence of resistant strains may be prevented by a rapid termination of the infection. If this occurs soon enough, resistant strains either will have failed to emerge or will have appeared in such small numbers that the host will eradicate them." Dubos was a pioneer in antibiotic therapy and in the exploration of potential consequences of nonprudent use of antibacterials.

Resistance to antibacterial agents is a universal phenomenon that appears to be more acute in some developing countries because of the lack of diversity of the antibiotics available. In industrialized countries, the same phenomenon may be described because of the selective pressure in a given hospital, which has been clearly demonstrated with the intensive use of ceftazidime as single agent therapy or the excessive use of imipenem in intensive care units (ICUs) which has allowed the emergence of resistant *Stenotrophomonas maltophilia*.

Comparison between studies is difficult and could be controversial due to differences in methodology. Only a trend may be drawing. In order to compare data, the sources of samples have to be provided, as well as the nature of the organisms (invasive, chronic, etc.), the ages of the patients (pediatrics, adults, or seniors), and the location (hospital, home care, home, etc.).

2. PROCESS OF BACTERIAL SELECTION

The process of spreading resistance to antibacterials is a complex phenomenon which occurs in three steps. The first step is the acquisition of the resistance trait, which may be due to induction (derepression of efflux genes, β-lactamase induction, etc.) by antibacterials or other drugs (such as salicylic acid) or to acquisition of mobile genes (plasmids, transposons, or integrons) or mutations (on the ribosome, *ropB*, *gyrA* or *-B*, *parC* or *parE*, etc.). Spontaneous mutation is a rare occurrence (about 10^{-7} CFU/ml).

The second step involves selection, mainly antibacterials. Within a standard clone, 10^{-6} to 10^{-7} CFU/ml is already considered less susceptible or resistant to a given antibacterial. However, this level is low and mainly undetectable. The resistant strain will be eradicated by the normal host defense system. When the level of CFU of the resistant strain per ml increases after induction, an antibacterial will kill all susceptible isolates but randomly some susceptible isolates will remain, which permits indirectly the development of resistant strains which could become predominant. All antibacterials are not equal in selecting resistant isolates, for which the MICs will be different from those for wild strains. The number of sequential passages needed to obtain these "mutants" in vitro varies with the antibacterials and with the phenotype and genotype of the strain.

To spread in the host population to create "primary resistance" in patients, resistant pathogens must colonize or infect new hosts. The rate at which this occurs has an important role in determining the timescale on which resistance increases at the level of host population.

Antibacterial resistance substantially impairs the growth rate or virulence of some pathogens, thereby limiting the ability of resistant organisms to spread. The number of organisms present (size of the bacterial population) during transmission from host to host can modify the spread of resistance.

The third step is for the spread of the resistant isolates to become epidemic, and many factors interfere in this phase: cloning of the isolates, the antibacterial involved, and the environment (home care, hospitals, child day care centers, etc.).

3. IN VITRO METHODOLOGY

A large bacterial inoculum size (10^8 CFU/ml) may be a sensitive tool for detecting resistant subpopulations but may cause development of resistance during antibiotic therapy.

A broth microdilution method with a small inoculum size did not allow easy detection of resistant subpopulations.

4. ADAPTATION OF BACTERIA TO AGGRESSION BY ANTIBACTERIAL AGENTS

The adaptation of living beings placed in a hostile environment is quantitative or qualitative. The response to aggression takes the form of a substantial increase in defensive capacities in the first case and the selection of a specific response to the aggression in the second.

4.1. Quantitative Strategy

With the introduction of antibacterial agents, the bacterial world has been confronted with increasing aggression. To counterbalance this aggression, it must adapt to survive. One of the strategies is to increase the production of inactivating enzymes (β-lactamases, dihydrofolate reductase [DHFR], dihydropteroate synthase, etc.).

The dissemination of β-lactamases within bacterial populations occurs through the *bla* gene, interbacterial transmission of which is via transposons or plasmids. The increased production of derepressed cephalosporinases has been one of the responses of gram-negative bacilli to the oxyimino cephalosporins, which are weakly hydrolyzed by broad-spectrum β-lactamases (TEM-1 and -2, SHV-1, and OXA-1 and -2). Resistance to β-lactamase inhibitors may be due to enzymatic hyperproduction through the presence of plasmid multicopies or by reduction of outer membrane penetration by these antibiotics. This hyperproduction of cephalosporinases during treatment poses a major therapeutic problem, as it is one of the causes of failure.

4.2. Qualitative Strategy

The qualitative strategy is based on modification of the cell targets (ribosomes, topoisomerases, penicillin-binding proteins [PBPs], etc.) or modification of the quality of the defensive weapons (β-lactamases).

The strategy of *Enterobacteriaceae* faced with the aggression represented by the oxyimino cephalosporins was the production of conventional enzymes commonly known as extended-broad-spectrum β-lactamases (ESBLs). The substitution of one or more amino acids at the site of action produced greater affinity for these cephems and for aztreonam.

Baquero et al. (1993) showed that mutations could occur at a low level and pass unnoticed in routine use, as the MICs for these molecules are low. A single mutation is probably the starting point. They postulated that the ancestor of TEM-3, which has two mutations at positions 102 (lysine) and 236 (serine), was TEM-18, which only has the mutation at position 102.

The resistance to clavulanic acid and tazobactam is due to a double mutation on the TEM-1 type enzyme. The methionine at position 67 is replaced by an isoleucine, and the methionine at position 180 is replaced by a threonine.

However, the molecular evolution of the β-lactamases is limited by the possible number of mutations that do not cause inactivity of the enzyme.

5. BIOLOGICAL COSTS FOR RESISTANT BACTERIA

The "physiological" modifications in bacteria due to acquired resistance could result in a biological cost for the bacteria, the worst being no survival possibilities.

The biological cost is one of the main determinants of how rapidly and to what extent a resistant mutant will establish itself in an individual or a population.

The cost could be associated either with target alterations in bacteria or with another mechanism of resistance, such as enzyme inactivation.

Chromosomal mutations may be responsible for biological costs to bacteria; however, no such cost has been described. One example is the substitution Lys42 → Arg in *Salmonella enterica* serovar Typhimurium in the streptomycin resistance gene *rpsL*.

Some mutations are associated with low growth rates for organisms in comparison to those of their sensitive counterparts.

The acquisition of plasmids carrying resistance traits requires that bacteria synthesize additional nucleic acids and proteins, thereby increasing the metabolic burden on the organisms. One other main biological cost could be an in vitro or in vivo decrease of virulence.

Infections continue to be a significant cause of morbidity and mortality in both the nosocomial and community settings. The shift in susceptibility greatly affects the ability to successfully treat patients.

6. LOWER RTIs IN THE COMMUNITY

In community-acquired pneumonia, the three most common pathogens collected are *Streptococcus pneumoniae*, *Haemophilus influenzae*, and *Moraxella catarrhalis*. These microorganisms are responsible for community-acquired pneumonia, acute exacerbation of chronic bronchitis, and acute maxillary sinusitis.

They are among the leading causes of primary care physician office visits. Community-acquired pneumonia is the sixth major source of morbidity and mortality in the United States.

The emergence of clinical isolates expressing resistance to one or more standard antibacterials is a significant challenge for patient treatment.

S. pneumoniae, *H. influenzae*, and *M. catarrhalis* belong to the normal oral flora of the upper respiratory tract. Due to the resistance threat, it is imperative to sample and culture respiratory tract infection (RTI) specimens to investigate the susceptibility of pathogens involved in the pathological process.

7. FREQUENCY OF NOSOCOMIAL INFECTIONS

In an important survey (Vincent et al., 1995), the incidence of various infections was assessed, and lower RTI was the main cause of hospital-acquired infections, followed by urinary tract infections and bloodstream infections; other pathologies represented less than one-third of all infections (Table 1).

The prevalence of nosocomial infections varied from 5 to 17% for patients admitted to ICUs in the hospital setting. ICUs are important environments for emergence of bacterial resistance and also for transmission of resistant organisms from patient to patient.

7.1. Risk Factors

Of 116 patients from two different home care facilities, a total of 47 (40.5%) were colonized by gram-negative bacilli that were resistant to ≥1 of the antibacterials tested. Of the resistant microorganisms, 60% were cultured from pharyngeal samples and the 40% remaining were cultured from rectal samples; 36% were obtained from both sites.

Pseudomonas aeruginosa and *S. maltophilia* were commonly isolated from the pharynx, whereas *Klebsiella* spp. and *Escherichia coli* were mostly collected from rectal samples. Approximately two-thirds (30 of 47 [63.8%]) of the organisms showed resistance to ≥2 antibacterials tested.

The major risk factor was tracheostomy: 10 of 11 patients acquired ≥1 antibiotic-resistant microorganism. Nearly equal proportions of colonized and noncolonized patients had been exposed to orally administered antibacterials (Toltzis et al., 1999; Lidsky et al., 2002).

Foreign bodies (tracheostomies, gastrostomy tube, indwelling urinary catheter, etc.) are risk factors because they require considerable manipulations by staff, with the risk of contamination. Decubiti are a significant risk factor for resistant bacillus colonization in elderly patients. Investigations among chronically institutionalized elderly patients have identified oral administration of fluoroquinolones as a risk factor for colonization with resistant bacilli (Lee et al., 1992, 1998; Bonomo, 2000).

In a pan-European collaborative study of ICU, the most frequently isolated organisms were *Enterobacteriaceae*, followed by *P. aeruginosa* (Hanberger et al., 1999) (Table 2).

Table 1 Prevalence of nosocomial infections

Type of infection	% of infections
Pneumonia	46.9
Other lower RTIs	17.8
Urinary tract infections	17.6
Bloodstream infections	12.0
Wounds	6.9
ENT[a] infections	5.1
SSTI[b]	4.8
Gastrointestinal infections	4.5
Cardiovascular infections	2.9
Clinical sepsis	2.0

[a]ENT, ear, nose, and throat.
[b]SSTI, skin and soft tissue infections.

7.2. Nosocomial RTI

The predominant cause of nosocomial pneumonia may be related to the prolonged ventilatory assistance for critically ill patients and the use of mainstream reservoir nebulizers. Both short-term intubation for surgery and longer-term intubation for respiratory failure are associated with the highest reported frequencies of nosocomial pneumonia.

Within hospital-acquired infections, parenchymal lower RTI (pneumonia) ranks second, with about 20% of patients requiring ventilation assistance. Nosocomial pneumonia mortality is high (about 33 to 50%).

S. pneumoniae, H. influenzae, and *Staphylococcus aureus* are leading causes of pneumonias within the early onset of pneumonia (<5 days), and *P. aeruginosa, Acinetobacter baumannii,* and methicillin-resistant *S. aureus* (MRSA) dominate the clinical isolates from later-onset pneumonia (>5 days).

7.3. Urinary Tract Infections

In a collaborative European survey (Dornbusch et al., 1998), 2,512 clinical isolates were collected (Table 3). *P. aeruginosa* was cultured from 4 to 6% of the isolates. *P. aeruginosa* is the third most common cause of urinary tract infection in U.S. hospitals, as well as the second most common cause of lower RTI. *P. aeruginosa* is behind *E. coli* and *Klebsiella pneumoniae*. Another common species is *Proteus mirabilis*.

7.4. Bloodstream Infections

In several European studies, mortality attributed to bacteremia varied from 10 to 50%. Data from Europe and the United States showed an increase in incidence of bacteremia. During the last 20 years, there has been a dramatic change of microbial pathogens within the hospital environment and the wide spread of antibacterial resistance.

Table 3 Main clinical isolates in nosocomial urinary tract infections in Europe (1998)

Organism(s)	Prevalence (%)
Gram-negative bacilli	82
S. aureus	3
Coagulase-negative staphylococci	4
E. faecalis	10
E. faecium	1

Table 2 Prevalence of gram-negative isolates in ICU

Country	Prevalence of gram-negative isolates in ICU (%)			
	P. aeruginosa	*S. maltophilia*	*Acinetobacter*	*Enterobacteriaceae*
Belgium	20	4	2	69
France	25	2	10	59
Portugal	25	2	6	70
Spain	25	2	8	62
Sweden	12	6	3	66

Table 4 Mortality rate versus bacteria in bloodstream infections

Organism	Mortality rate (%)
E. coli	24
K. pneumoniae	27
Enterobacter	28
P. aeruginosa	32
Serratia	26

Table 5 Prevalence of bacteria causing nosocomial bloodstream infections in the Americas in 1997

Organism(s)	Prevalence (%)		
	United States ($n = 6{,}150$)	Canada ($n = 1{,}727$)	Latin America ($n = 1{,}642$)
S. aureus	23.9	20.2	20.5
E. coli	18.6	19.1	12.1
Coagulase-negative staphylococci	12.7	13.1	15.2
Enterococcus spp.	9.6	9.1	2.9
Klebsiella spp.	7.7	7.1	10.3
S. pneumoniae	5.5	4.8	1.9
P. aeruginosa	4.5	4.8	5.6
Enterobacter spp.	3.8	4.1	4.8
Beta-hemolytic streptococci	3.7	3.8	1.5
Acinetobacter	1.6	1.1	5.3

Table 6 Prevalence of bacteria causing nosocomial bloodstream infections in Europe in 1997

Organisms(s)	% of isolated microorganisms
Gram-negative bacilli	52
S. aureus	24
Coagulase-negative staphylococci	15
E. faecalis	7
E. faecium	2

The main organisms isolated from blood cultures associated with mortality in the United States, as determined by the SCOPE study carried out in the early 1990s, are listed in Table 4. Table 5 lists microorganisms that were isolated from the bloodstream in the Americas in a 1997 SENTRY program (Diekema et al., 1999).

Finally, in a European collaborative study, a total of 2,544 blood isolates were consecutively collected (Dornbusch et al., 1998) (Table 6). The figures obtained in that study are close to those obtained by of Diekema et al. in North America and Latin America in the same period. In the Dornbusch study, *P. aeruginosa* represents about 5 to 6% of the isolates (the magnitude observed in the Americas).

7.5. SSTI

Skin and soft tissue infections (SSTI) in hospitals may be consequent to trauma in the community resulting in hospitalization or may occur mainly as a consequence of wound surgery.

In a SENTRY program carried out in 1997 in 20 participating hospitals throughout Europe, approximately 1,000 SSTI isolates were collected. The most frequently isolated organisms are listed in Table 7.

Table 7 Prevalence of bacterial isolates in SSTI in 1997

Organism(s)	Prevalence (%)
Gram-positive bacteria	
S. aureus	39.9
Enterococcus spp.	5.2
Coagulase-negative staphylococci	4.5
Beta-hemolytic streptococci	3.9
Gram-negative bacteria	
P. aeruginosa	12.5
E. coli	7.6
Enterobacter spp.	5.6
P. mirabilis	4.1
K. pneumoniae	3.9
Acinetobacter spp.	4.1

8. GRAM-POSITIVE COCCI

8.1. *S. aureus*

The first strains of penicillin G-resistant *S. aureus* were isolated soon after the introduction of penicillin G into hospitals in London, England. At present, almost 80% of intra- or extrahospital strains are resistant to penicillin G due to a plasmid-mediated penicillinase. Interplasmid transfer occurs by transduction. Four types of extracellular enzymes have been described: A, B, C, and D. These enzymes are distinguished by their amino acid compositions. They hydrolyze group I penicillins, certain *N*-acyl penicillins, cephaloridine, and cefazolin. Strains producing a type A enzyme are more resistant to cefazolin. The production of type D enzyme is often associated with resistance to fusidic acid. Among penicillinase-producing strains, the prevalence of the different enzymes varies. Types A and C are the most common.

8.1.1. Epidemiology of Resistance of *S. aureus* to Methicillin

In the early 1960s, the introduction of methicillin had promised to resolve one of the therapeutic problems associated with infections due to multiresistant, penicillinase-producing *S. aureus*. The first strain was described in the United Kingdom in 1961. The first methicillin- and aminoglycoside-resistant strains were described in Australia in the mid-1970s and shortly afterwards throughout the world. Between 1960 and 1963, a moderate increase in the number of methicillin-resistant strains, on the order of 5%, was noted. Homogeneous populations replaced progressively heterogeneous populations of MRSA.

Between 1965 and 1969 the incidence of methicillin-resistant strains increased from 11 to 28% in Zurich, Switzerland, hospitals. In Denmark in 1967, about a quarter of staphylococcal isolates were methicillin resistant. In France, the incidence of methicillin-resistant strains in nine Parisian hospitals was 12% in 1961, 19% in 1963, and 35% in 1966.

In Greece, between 1978 and 1979, about 50% of strains were methicillin resistant in Athens hospitals.

In the United States, a few strains were isolated in 1963. In fact, no methicillin-resistant strain was isolated in Boston, Mass., hospitals between 1960 and 1967. In 1967, however,

1.4% of isolates were methicillin resistant. From the mid-1970s, the number of resistant isolates has increased progressively, and epidemics have been described in all regions of the United States.

Epidemiological surveillance in Veterans Administration hospitals showed that this type of strain was present in 3 of 137 hospitals in 1975 and 111 of 137 hospitals in 1984. Horan et al. (1986) showed that the distribution of these strains differed according to the type of hospital: 10% in university hospitals, and 4.6 to 6% in nonuniversity hospitals, depending on their size. In 1991, the NNIS survey in the United States showed that 29% of strains of *S. aureus* were methicillin resistant.

In Australia, no resistant strains had been identified as of 1964, but 17% of isolates were methicillin resistant in 1970. In 1993, the frequency of methicillin-resistant strains varied according to geographical location: 25.2% in Queensland and 0.4% in the western region of Australia.

In Hong Kong, Cheng et al. (1988) reported that 25 to 30% of isolates were methicillin resistant. In Korea, in 1989, 46% of strains of *S. aureus* were resistant to methicillin, but 90% were susceptible to ofloxacin.

Likewise, in Ireland the number of methicillin-resistant strains was high, involving about 40% of isolates from septicemic patients.

In Italy, 6% of isolates were resistant in 1981 and 26% were resistant in 1986. From 1968, a further increase in these strains was noted. This study also showed that these strains produced large quantities of penicillinase and were resistant to streptomycin and tetracyclines.

At the beginning of the 1970s, a significant decrease in the number of methicillin-resistant strains was reported. In 1976, methicillin- and gentamicin-resistant strains were described. However, a resurgence of methicillin- and aminoglycoside-resistant strains was noted at the end of the 1970s and the beginning of the 1980s in France, Ireland, Greece, Australia, and South Africa.

Schito et al. (1988) showed that among methicillin-resistant strains, 44, 32, 36, 23, and 21% were also resistant to erythromycin A, cyclines, chloramphenicol, rifampin, and co-trimoxazole, respectively. Resistance associated with aminoglycosides was also noted, differing according to the molecule: 49, 43, 35, and 18% for gentamicin, tobramycin, amikacin, and netilmicin, respectively.

A study undertaken in Japan showed that of 322 strains of MRSA (according to the NCCLS definition), all were susceptible to vancomycin, 20% were susceptible to gentamicin, 90% were susceptible to netilmicin, 100% were susceptible to arbekacin, 10% were susceptible to erythromycin A, 53% were susceptible to minocycline, and 30% were susceptible to ofloxacin.

Lee et al. (1993) reported the incidence of MRSA strains in South Korea. Between 1964 and 1968, no strain was resistant to methicillin. In 1980, 1985, 1990, 1991, and 1992, the percentages of methicillin-resistant strains were, respectively, 14.1, 22, 43.4, 63, and 61%. In 1993, the number of multiresistant strains was high. Clindamycin, erythromycin A, cyclines, and co-trimoxazole were inactive against 88, 97, 86, and 4% of MRSA strains, respectively.

A survey conducted in central Europe in 1991 showed that the incidence of oxacillin-resistant strains of *S. aureus* ranged from 4 to 30.9%, depending on the country.

The number of erythromycin A-resistant strains is high. The proportion of ciprofloxacin-resistant strains ranges from 26 to 47% but is greater than 70% in some countries (Table 8). In this study, all of the strains were susceptible to mupirocin, except in the case of Italy, where 1.5% of MRSA strains were resistant. The majority of methicillin-resistant strains were isolated from pathological specimens from surgical departments.

In a multicenter European study, Voss et al. (1994) collected 7,333 strains of *S. aureus*, 12.8% of which were resistant to methicillin. The proportion varied according to the country or region, from less than 1% in Scandinavia to more than 30% in Italy, Spain, and France. A high level of resistance to ciprofloxacin was noted. More than 60% of these strains came from surgical departments (Table 9).

A study of the prevalence of methicillin-resistant strains of staphylococci was conducted in the Naples region in Italy; rates are listed in Table 10.

In Nigeria, 6.4 and 43% of strains of *S. aureus* in Ibadan and Lagos, respectively, were methicillin resistant. None of these strains was resistant to gentamicin, and 8.5% were resistant to erythromycin A.

In Poland, about 15% of *S. aureus* strains were resistant to methicillin, more than 60% were resistant to cyclines, and 11% were resistant to macrolides and lincosamides; however, these strains remained susceptible to rifampin (92.4%) and aminoglycosides (>90%).

8.1.2. Epidemiology of Resistance to Fluoroquinolones

The number of strains that have become resistant to fluoroquinolones is much greater among the oxacillin-resistant strains than among those which remain susceptible to this antibiotic. In 1984, the number of resistant strains in France was on the order of 5%, with gradual increases in 1985 and 1986 (10 and 15%), reaching a level of 75% in 1987. A plateau on the order of 90% was reached in 1988.

In a Spanish survey conducted in November 1991, Alonso et al. (1993) showed that 15.7% of MRSA strains were resistant to ofloxacin. In a survey undertaken in Sweden by Olsson et al. (1993), 76% of staphylococcal strains were

Table 8 Prevalence of MRSA strains resistant to antibiotics in central Europe[a]

Country	Prevalence of strains resistant to antibiotic (%)				
	Methicillin	Ciprofloxacin	Erythromycin A	Co-trimoxazole	Rifampin
Austria	20.6	83.9	51.6	63.4	22.6
Germany	5.3	91.7	41.7	54.2	20.8
Italy	30.4	89.8	43.8	54	52.6
Czech Republic	4.3	47.1	94.4	17.6	5.9
Hungary	8.6	33.3	85.2	70.4	7.4
Poland	19.7	26.3	36.8	42.1	5.2
Slovenia	30.9	88.2	76.5	38.2	26.5

[a]Data from Voss et al., 1993.

Table 9 Activities of antibiotics against European MRSA strains

Country	Prevalence of strains resistant to antibiotic (%)				
	Oxacillin	Ciprofloxacin	Erythromycin A	Co-trimoxazole	Rifampin
Austria	21.6	82.9	65.0	67.5	17.1
Belgium	25.1	91.7	87.5	75.9	18.6
France	33.6	96.0	83.3	67.2	54.4
Germany	5.5	93.0	38.4	52.3	14
Italy	34.4	83.8	44.6	53.7	57.9
The Netherlands	1.5	55.5	55.5	66.6	44.4
Spain	30.3	84.7	96.8	67.7	39.9
Switzerland	1.8	52.9	58.8	47.1	0
Sweden	0.3	ND[a]	ND	ND	ND
Denmark	0.1	ND	ND	ND	ND

[a]ND, not determined.

Table 10 Susceptibilities of strains of staphylococci resistant to oxacillin and other antibiotics in Italy

Drug	Prevalence of resistance (%)		
	S. aureus	*S. epidermidis*	*S. haemolyticus*
Oxacillin	49	83	85
Vancomycin	0	0	0
Teicoplanin	0	65	75
Ciprofloxacin	100	30	87
Imipenem	100	59	100
Co-trimoxazole	0	60	100
Gentamicin	100	100	100
Netilmicin	75	25	38
Rifampin	100	90	75

resistant to piperacillin and between 4.5 and 15% were resistant to ciprofloxacin, depending on the sampling site.

In Shanghai, China, norfloxacin and ofloxacin were made commercially available in 1986 and 1988, respectively. The resistances to norfloxacin of strains of *S. aureus*, *Staphylococcus epidermidis*, and *Staphylococcus saprophyticus* were multiplied 5-fold (13 to 66%), 1.6-fold (31 to 50%), and 2-fold (20 to 41%), respectively. About 58 to 62% of the strains of *S. aureus* were methicillin resistant.

8.1.3. Resistance to Vancomycin

A reduction in the activity of vancomycin (MIC, 8 to 16 μg/ml) has been demonstrated among strains of coagulase-negative staphylococci, as has a reduction in activity (MIC, 4 μg/ml) against *S. aureus*. A strain (Hu 50) of *S. aureus* exhibiting low-level resistance (MIC, 8 μg/ml) has been described in Japan and in the United States.

8.1.4. Quinupristin-Dalfopristin

Quinupristin-dalfopristin is a combination of streptogramin A (dalfopristin) and streptogramin B (quinupristin). In *S. aureus*, the main mechanism of resistance of quinupristin-dalfopristin is methylation of the 23S rRNA with cross-resistance with macrolides, lincosamides, and streptogramin B.

In the inducible type of resistance, quinupristin remains active because it is not an inducer of methylase; if constitutive, quinuprisitin is inactive and the combination become bacteriostatic due to alteration of quinupristin-dalfopristin activity in vitro and in vivo.

Resistance to dalfopristin is less frequent due to either an efflux or inactivation of streptogramin A.

In 2002, in a worldwide survey, the rates of resistance of quinupristin-dalfopristin were 0.1, 0.3, and 6.5% for *S. aureus* ($n = 3{,}202$), coagulase-negative staphylococci ($n = 838$), and *Enterococcus faecium* ($n = 152$), respectively. No resistant isolates were reported for *S. pneumoniae*, viridans group streptococci, beta-hemolytic streptococci, *Bacillus* spp., *Corynebacterium* spp., or *Listeria* spp. (Streit et al., 2004).

In an epidemiological survey conducted throughout the 15 European Union (EU) countries in 2002 to 2003, no MRSA strains were resistant to quinupristin-dalfopristin, except about 5% in the United Kingdom and Ireland (Felmingham, Aventis Data on file, 2003).

8.1.5. Mupirocin

Mupirocin resistance was detected in *S. aureus* and coagulase-negative staphylococci. Two distinct levels of resistance were differentiated: low (MIC, 8 to 256 μg/ml) due to abnormal isoleucyl-tRNA synthase and high (MIC, >256 μg/ml) due to abnormal isoleucyl-tRNA synthase and an additional abnormal isoleucyl-tRNA synthase encoded by the *ils-2* gene. This additional gene is usually carried by transferable plasmids.

The *mupA* gene was found in organisms with low and high levels of mupirocin resistance (Fujimura et al., 2001; Hodgson et al., 1994).

In a recent epidemiological survey in Korea (2000 to 2001), it was noticed that 16.7% of coagulase-negative staphylococci exhibited low-level mupirocin resistance and 10.3% of the isolates exhibited high-level resistance. These strains were not detected until 1999 (Yun et al., 2003).

In 1997, in a collaborative epidemiological survey carried out in 19 European hospitals, it was found that 1.6 and 5.6% of *S. aureus* and coagulase-negative staphylococci, respectively, showed high-level mupirocin resistance (Schmitz and Jones, 1997).

In Greece in 2001, 2% of *S. aureus* isolates were highly resistant to mupirocin (Maniatis et al., 2001). High-level mupirocin resistance in *S. aureus* has been detected since 1996 in Kuwait (Udo et al., 1999).

8.1.6. Macrolides

In *S. aureus*, erythromycin A resistance is usually due to either ribosomal modifications (23S rRNA methylase mediated by the *ermA*, *ermB*, and *ermC* genes) or an efflux (ATP-dependent pump mediated by the *mrsA* gene).

The *ermA* gene is most often harbored on the transposon Tn*554*, which also encodes resistance for spectinomycin, while the *ermB* gene is often associated with transposon Tn*551* and plasmid pI 258 (penicillinase). The *ermC* gene was infrequently encountered before 1978 and is located on a small plasmid (2.4 to 5 kb).

Since 1997, the potential benefits of macrolide therapy in cystic fibrosis patients have been promoted, and azithromycin is used in a low dose. In this context *S. aureus* isolates, which represent about 20% of the isolates in the sputum of cystic fibrosis patients, began to be highly resistant to 14- and 15-membered-ring macrolides. In one institution, erythromycin A resistance reached 53% among *S. aureus* isolates, compared to 38% in the same geographical area in the general population (Prunier et al., 2003).

The mechanism of resistance was either methylation, efflux, or mutations (23S rRNA—A2058G) or L4 (*rpID* gene) and/or L22 (*rplV* gene) ribosomal protein.

8.1.7. Aminoglycosides

In 1969, the first clinical *S. aureus* isolate resistant to gentamicin was reported (Lacey and Mitchell, 1969). In France, in 1992, the frequency of gentamicin-resistant MRSA was about 7.4%. From 1992 to 1998, this prevalence rate increased progressively to reach between 46.8 and 94.4% in French hospitals. Emergence of MRSA susceptible again to gentamicin was reported in French hospitals. The *aac(6')-aph(2')* gene carried on transposon Tn*400* conferring resistance to all aminoglycosides was lost, and only the *ant(4')* gene remained, which confers resistance to kanamycin, tobramycin, and amikacin.

8.1.8. Small-Colony Variants

It was suggested that small-colony variants of *S. aureus* are associated with persistent and refractory infections which may play a role in clinical resistance. Small-colony variants require menadione, hemin, or thymidine for growth. They also have reduced expression of coagulase and hemolysin. One important subset of small-colony variants has an electron transport deficiency affecting the proton motive force and ATP synthesis and resulting in aminoglycoside resistance.

8.1.9. Community-Acquired MRSA

Recently, true community-acquired MRSA infections (C-MRSA) emerged in many places, such as North America, Europe, Australia, and Japan. They have occurred in 5 to 15% of persons without established risk factors. In the United States, there are at least two different clones. The main risk factor is contact with infected materials, such as pus or other materials through touching wounds or boils, changing someone else's dressing, or sharing personal items.

C-MRSA differs from hospital-acquired MRSA in the following ways:

- C-MRSA tends to be more susceptible to antibacterial classes other than β-lactams.
- Genotypes are different.
- C-MRSA harbors a type IV SSC*mec* (see below) cassette.
- C-MRSA contains a putative virulence factor (Panton-Valentine leukocidin).
- C-MRSA occurs in patients without typical risk factors for MRSA.

8.1.9.1. Genetics

The genetic basis of MRSA is a crucial point (Eady and Cove, 2003). The protein PBP 2a is encoded by the *mecA* gene and a transpeptidase that appears to cooperate with the transglycosidase domain of the native PBP 2 enzyme to restore cell wall biosynthesis in the presence of β-lactams. *mecA* gene expression is controlled by two regulatory proteins encoded by the upstream genes *mecR1* and *mecI* (Hiramatsu et al., 2001). Resistance may be constitutive due to class B complex or inducible (class A). These proteins (class A and class B) are enclosed in a large element named the staphylococcal cassette chromosome (SSC*mec*), which could be transferred with the help of two genes, *ccrA* and *ccrB*, which encode recombinases of the invertase/resolvase family. SSC*mec* is a mobile element which integrates and excises from a specific open reading frame, *orfX*, of the staphylococcal chromosomes; while SSC*mec* carries several genes, only *mecA* is required for methicillin resistance.

There are four type of SSC*mec* described. An additional type of element contains additional DNA including a hypervariable region, one or more integrated plasmids on transposon Tn*554* carrying antibiotic resistance genes.

The product of *mecI* represses *mecA* expression, so that resistance is inducible by exposure to β-lactams. The *mecR1* gene encodes a signal-transducing membrane protein which cleaves MecI due to the protease activity of its cytoplasmic domain.

The *mecA* genes of type I, II, and III SSC*mec* are associated with hospital-acquired infections, and that of type IV is associated with C-MRSA. The *mec* gene may be silent. In a recent epidemiological study, 10% of the European methicillin-susceptible *S. aureus* strains were found to contain the *mecA* gene. The *mecA* gene may have arisen in *Staphylococcus sciuri* or a related commensal of wild animals (Couto et al., 1996).

Hiramatsu et al. identified at least three distinct chromosomal lineages, A, B, and C. Lineage A was found not to harbor type I, II, or III SSC*mec*. Lineages B and C harbored type II. Types I, II, and III are poorly transferable, being too large for bacteriophage transduction, and they lack a sequence that would allow cotransfer by a conjugative plasmid. Type IV, being smaller, is easily transferable by bacteriophages (Stevens, 2003). However, the lack of transposons, integrated plasmids, and other antibiotic resistance genes explains in part the greater susceptibility of C-MRSA (Table 11).

MLST analysis of 369 nosocomial MRSA isolates from 20 countries showed 11 major clones. C-MRSA expressed heterogeneous resistance to methicillin, and almost all strains carried class B *mec* complex within a type IV SSC*mec*. C-MRSA strains which are coresistant to erythromycin A and clindamycin-lincomycin grew significantly faster than C-MRSA susceptible to both compounds (Laurent et al., 2001). This observation implies that erythromycin and clindamycin should not be prescribed as an alternative to β-lactams in patients infected with C-MRSA.

The type IV SSC*mec* element is apparently common among methicillin-resistant coagulase-negative staphylococci from children. It seems that the first coagulase-negative staphylococcus to be colonized with the *mecA* gene was *Staphylococcus haemolyticus*.

8.2. *Streptococcus pneumoniae*

S. pneumoniae continues to be a major cause of mortality and morbidity. It is the leading causative agent of RTIs, the second most common cause of purulent meningitis, and one of the major causes of otitis media.

The sulfonamides were introduced into treatment in about 1936, and the first strains of resistant pneumococci were reported from 1943 onwards. The first cycline-resistant strains were reported in 1962.

Table 11 Characteristics of SSC*mec* types[a]

Element	SSC*mec* type			
	I (34,364 bp)	II (53,017 bp)	III (66,896 bp)	IV (20,920–24,248 bp)
mecA	+	+	+	+
mecR1-mecI	–	+	+	–
ccrAB	+	+	+	+
erm(A)	–	+	+	–
tet(K)	–		+	–
Tn*554*	0	1	2	0
pUB110[b]	–	+	–	–
aad	–	+	–	–

[a]Data from Fridkin and Chambers, 2003.
[b]pUB110 is an integrated plasmid that carries *aad*, the gene for tobramycin and kanamycin resistance.

In 1964, the first strains resistant to erythromycin A were described in a study on the treatment of superinfections during acute exacerbations of chronic bronchitis.

8.2.1. β-Lactams

The number of strains of *S. pneumoniae* resistant to penicillin G has constantly been on the increase for the last 10 years. These strains are found in a number of countries, such as Spain, France, Hungary, Iceland, South Africa, the United States, and various countries in the Middle East, Latin America, and Asia; in other countries (United Kingdom, Belgium, and Germany), the incidence varies (Fig. 1).

More than 80 serotypes or serogroups have been described. There is often confusion in the literature according to whether American or Danish nomenclature is used. The serotypes differ in terms of the site of infection. In parenchymal lower RTIs, serotypes 1, 14, 7, 3, and 4 are the most common, and these are often isolated from healthy carriers. In upper RTIs, serotypes 6, 14, 19, and 23 are most often responsible, and these are isolated with great frequency

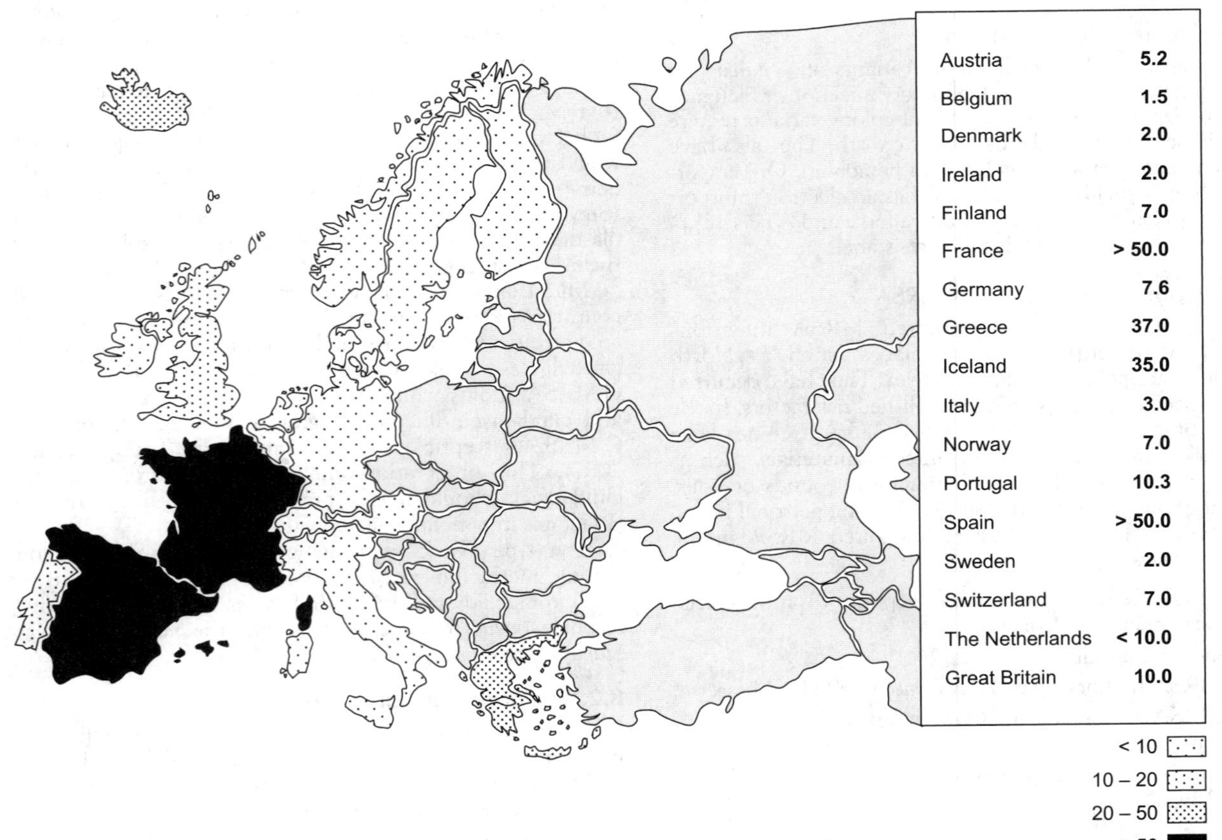

Figure 1 Prevalence of (percent) resistance of *S. pneumoniae* to penicillin G in Europe before 1996

from the nasopharyngeal flora of young children. Since introduction of the vaccine, *S. pneumoniae* isolates with serotypes other than those in the vaccine have emerged at a high frequency and have been found to be resistant to penicillin G or erythromycin A. An exception is serotype 19, for which resistance emerged even under polyvalent vaccination.

A strain of *S. pneumoniae* is described as multiresistant when it is nonsusceptible to at least three antibiotics. The number of strains resistant to erythromycin A is becoming high, and this type of strain has been isolated throughout the world. Erythromycin A resistance usually involves strains that are also of reduced susceptibility or resistant to penicillin G. The first multiresistant strain was described in 1977 in South Africa; this was a strain resistant to penicillin G, erythromycin A, chloramphenicol, tetracycline, and co-trimoxazole. In the region of Durban, South Africa, 15% of the carriage strains were multiresistant in 1978; 56% were multiresistant in the Johannesburg region. An epidemiological study undertaken in Spain between 1978 and 1981 showed that 72% of strains were resistant to tetracycline and 45% were resistant to chloramphenicol, whereas 10% of strains were resistant to penicillin G and 1% were resistant to erythromycin A. In 1989, 10% of strains had become resistant to erythromycin A. In 1976, the first multiresistant strains were reported in the United Kingdom, and the number is increasing. In 1977, 6.8% of strains were resistant to the cyclines. In an epidemiological survey conducted in the United Kingdom in 1990, 3% of strains were of reduced susceptibility to penicillin G, 8.1% were resistant to the cyclines, and 6.5% were resistant to erythromycin A, with a few strains being resistant to amoxicillin. In Northern Ireland in 1988, 12% of strains were resistant to the cyclines, 1% were of reduced susceptibility to penicillin G, and all were susceptible to erythromycin A. In France, the first strains resistant to erythromycin A were described in 1976. Six percent of strains were resistant to erythromycin A in 1978, and the resistance rates were 18.2% in 1983, 26% in 1985, and 29% in 1990. Many strains are resistant to cyclines. Seventy-five percent of strains belonged to serotypes 6, 19, 23, and 24.

Among strains in France, Spain, and Asia resistant to penicillin G, almost 60% were resistant to erythromycin A (Table 12).

Before the late 1990s in Germany and Canada, less than 1% of strains were resistant to erythromycin A. In Hungary, 45 to 60% of strains were multiresistant in 1990.

In Belgium in 1990, rates of resistance to penicillin G, erythromycin A, and the cyclines were, respectively, 1.5, 11.5, and 10.4%. Epidemics of multiresistant strains have been described in the United States.

In Japan, 14% of strains were resistant to minocycline between 1975 and 1977, but no strains were resistant to erythromycin A. In 1987, 7% of the clinical isolates were resistant to erythromycin A and in 1996, 75.2% were resistant.

In 1989, 30% of strains in South Korea possessed reduced susceptibility to penicillin G. In Hong Kong in 1991, 5% of strains were resistant to erythromycin A. The situation has deteriorated dramatically in Southeast Asia (Fig. 2 and 3).

In Turkey, 4% of strains were resistant to erythromycin A in 1977.

In Poland, 90% of strains are susceptible to penicillin G, 7% are of reduced susceptibility, and 3% are resistant to penicillin G and/or chloramphenicol. Strains nonsusceptible to erythromycin A represent about 3%, those nonsusceptible to cyclines represent 44%, and those nonsusceptible to co-trimoxazole represent 5%. The worldwide prevalence of *S. pneumoniae* strains resistant to penicillin G is shown in Table 13; Fig. 4 shows the prevalence of erythromycin A-resistant *S. pneumoniae* strains in Europe in 1997.

Penicillin-resistant strains are infrequent in Russia, except in Siberia (13.5%); two such isolates were reported in Smolensk (Kozlov et al., 2002).

The existence of penicillin G-resistant strains has been known since the experimental studies by Erikson in 1945. However, the first strains of reduced susceptibility to penicillin G (MICs, 0.1 and 0.2 μg/ml) were not isolated until 20 years later by Kislak. In 1967, Hansman et al. in Australia drew attention to the potential therapeutic problem of pneumococcal strains of reduced susceptibility to penicillin G. They had isolated a strain from a hypogammaglobulinemic patient for which penicillin G had a MIC of 0.6 μg/ml. From 1970 onwards, penicillin G-resistant isolates were described in New Guinea and Australia. In New Guinea, the proportion of resistant strains increased progressively, from 12% in 1970 to 33% in 1980.

8.2.2. Cephems

The changes in susceptibility of pneumococci to penicillin G necessitated a revision of the breakpoints for the parenteral cephalosporins active against penicillin G-resistant strains of *S. pneumoniae*. Strains resistant to cefotaxime and ceftriaxone have been isolated in various places. Cefpirome still possesses activity against some of these strains. However, not all the quaternary ammonium-type cephalosporins possess the same activity against strains of pneumococci of reduced susceptibility or resistant to penicillin G (Table 14).

8.2.3. Macrolides

Macrolides are alternatives to β-lactam antibiotics; today there is a huge spread of erythromycin A resistance among *S. pneumoniae* strains worldwide (Table 15).

The mechanism of resistance to erythromycin A is complex and involves at least four mechanisms: methylation [*erm*(B) gene], efflux of the molecule with the *mef*(A) or *mef*(E) gene and the *mel* gene (an ATP-binding cassette) (Gay and Stephen, 2001), mutations (23S rRNA, L4, and

Table 12 Prevalence of penicillin-resistant *S. pneumoniae* with associated resistance to other antibacterial agent

Drug	Breakpoint (μg/ml)	% of isolates		
		Penicillin G, susceptible	Penicillin G, intermediate	Penicillin G, resistant
Erythromycin A	≥8	5.2	39.5	24.6
Clindamycin	≥4	5.2	39	23.7
Tetracycline	≥8	18.9	58.1	64.6
Chloramphenicol	≥8	15.4	49.6	58.7
Co-trimoxazole	≥2/32	24.1	77.5	89.1
Rifampin	≥2	0.6	1.4	2.4
Ciprofloxacin	≥4	0.6	2.3	4.2

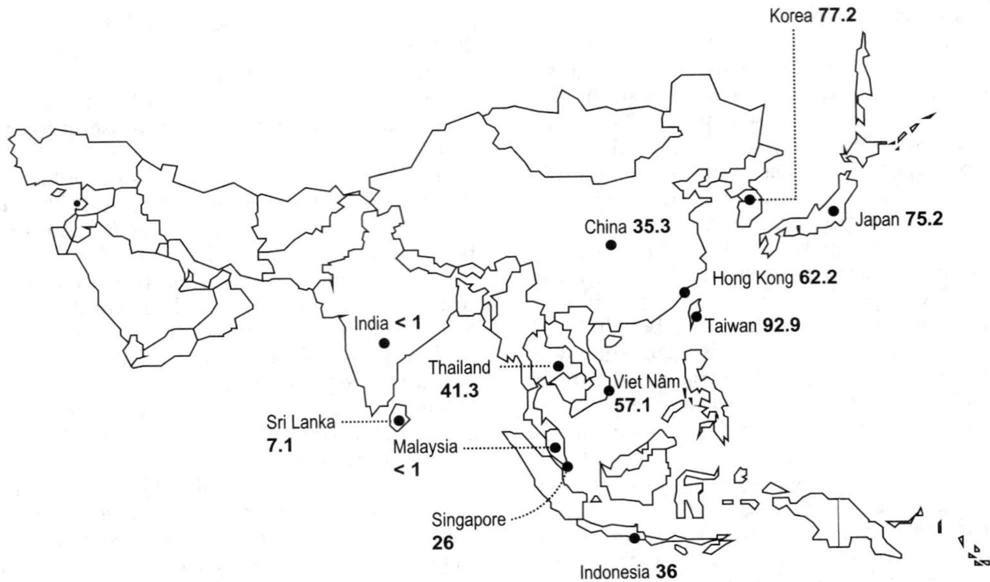

Figure 2 Prevalence of (percent) resistance of *S. pneumoniae* to erythromycin A (1997) in Asia

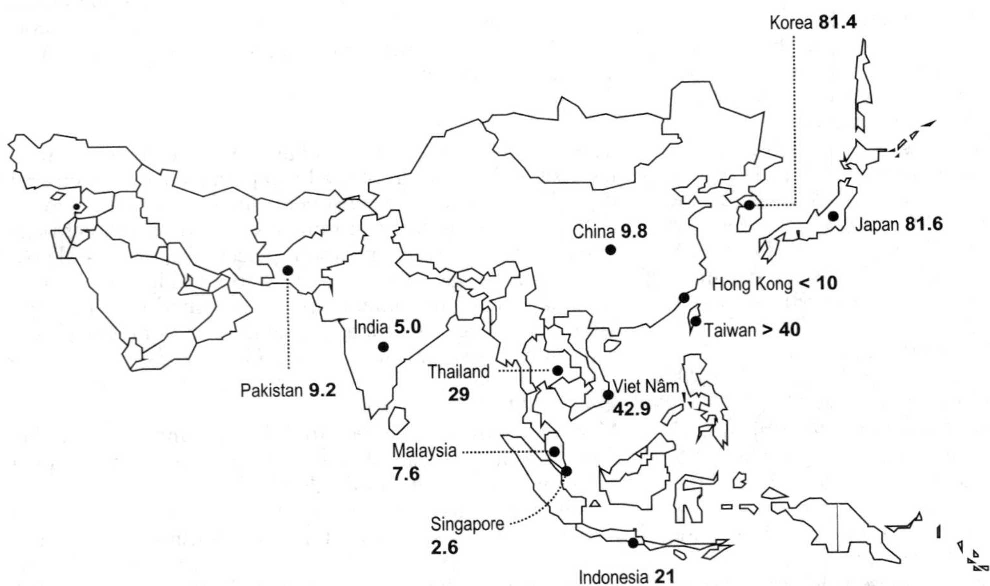

Figure 3 Prevalence of (percent) resistance of *S. pneumoniae* to penicillin G in Asia (1997)

L22 proteins), and inactivations (esterases, phosphotransferases, and glycosidases).

The *mel* gene was found in the Far East, the United States, Mexico, Hungary, and Japan (Farrell et al., 2004). Both the *mef*(A) and -(E) genes and the *mel* gene are located in the macrolide efflux genetic assembly and are cotranscripted.

Since 1974, there have been publications reporting patients suffering from pneumococcal meningitis due to penicillin G-resistant strains. In 1977, the first strains resistant to penicillin G (MIC, 4.0 to 8.0 μg/ml) and chloramphenicol were described in Durban, South Africa. In Europe, there are four main foci of resistance: Spain, Hungary, France, and Iceland.

In Spain, the incidence of penicillin G-resistant strains of *S. pneumoniae* increased from 6% in 1979 to 44% in 1989. An increase of the same amplitude has been found in France. The incidence of resistance was 0.3% from 1980 to 1986, 5.3% from 1987 to 1989, 12.5% in 1990, bordering on 30% from 1992 to 1993, and above 60% in 2002. In Hungary, the incidence of resistance has reached 50%. In Romania, it has attained 25% among clinical isolates in one center. In 1975, an epidemiological study revealed that

Table 13 Epidemiology of resistance of *S. pneumoniae* to penicillin G worldwide[a]

Country	Year(s)	*n*	Prevalence of resistance (%)[b]
Europe			
Austria	1999–2000	178	5.1
Belgium	1999–2000	637	18.8
France	1999–2000	675	>50
Finland	1999–2000	327	39.3
Germany	1997–1998	321	6.9
	1999–2000	330	4.8
Greece	1999–2000	109	51.4
Italy	1999–2000	184	26.1
Ireland	1999–2000	108	27.9
The United Kingdom	1997–1998	663	8.1
	1999–2000	709	9.0
Denmark	1999–2000	376	2.7
Norway	1998–1999	69	3
	1999–2000	192	1.5
The Netherlands	1996–1997	200	8.0
	1999–2000	394	5.1
Luxemburg	1999–2000	184	25
Portugal	1999–2000	344	18
Spain	1999–2000	203	48.3
Sweden	1999–2000	199	10.5
Switzerland	2001–2002	99	5.0
Hungary	1999–2000	46	39.9
Czech Republic	1999–2000	102	33.3
Slovenia	1999–2000	101	34.2
Slovak Republic	1999–2000	100	53.3
Estonia	1999–2000	99	9.0
Lithuania	1999–2000	93	3.3
Latvia	1999–2000	96	10
Poland	1999–2000	97	4.5
Croatia	1999–2000	101	33.3
Romania	1999–2000	99	36.7
Slovenia	2000	NG[c]	18.2
Malta	2000	NG	0
Bulgaria	1999–2000	101	63.3
Russia	2000–2001	468	13.5
Turkey	2001–2002	41	31.7
North America			
The United States	1991–1992		17.8
	1994–1995	1,527	23.6
	1997–1998	1,601	29.5
	1998	195	13.1
	1999–2000	1,531	34.2
	1999–2000	687	31.9
Canada	1999–2000	350	21.2
	1998	1,180	21.3
	1999	1,333	19.6
	2000–2001	1,435	22.9
Latin America			
Mexico	1994–1995	16	38
	1997	285	40.8
Venezuela	1997	73	21.9
Brazil	1997	310	12.9
Argentina	1997	188	19.1
West Indies	1997	84	17.1
Panama	1997	61	23
Chile	1997	99	21.3
Uruguay	1993	NG	7.2
Peru	1993	NG	2.3
Colombia	1993	NG	16

(*Continued on next page*)

Table 13 Epidemiology of resistance of *S. pneumoniae* to penicillin G worldwide[a] (*Continued*)

Country	Year(s)	*n*	Prevalence of resistance (%)[b]
Middle East			
Egypt	1999–2000	51	37
Lebanon	2001	123	73
	2001–2002	47	72.3
Israel	NG	NG	40
Near East			
Saudi Arabia	1996	27	55.5
Kuwait	NG	250	52.8
Africa			
Tunisia	2001–2002	44	40.9
Algeria	2001–2002	39	43.6
South Africa	1996	83	34.9
	2001–2002	196	74.5
Malawi	1997	906	21
Zimbabwe	1994	11	18
	1995	26	19
	1996	10	10
	1997	18	28
	1998	20	45
	1999	41	51
	2000	34	56
Rwanda	1984–1990	383	25.8
Zambia	NG	126	23
Uganda	1993	NG	84
Ghana	2001	NG	17
Kenya	1992–1996	269	27
Togo	1999	114	13.4
Australia	1999–2000	299	9.3
Asia			
Thailand	1996–1997	126	57.9
Singapore	1995	144	13.2
	1996–1997	84	23.1
Malaysia	1996–1997	92	13.1
	1999–2000	100	37
Taiwan	1996–1997	137	38.7
	2001–2002	87	83.9
Korea	1996–1997	177	79.7
	1999–2000	137	81
Hong Kong	1996	44	59.1
	1999–2000	70	58.5
Vietnam	1993–1995	24	8.0
	1996–1997	46	60.8
	1999–2002	36	28
Sri Lanka	1996–1997	41	41.2
Japan	1996–1997	84	65.3
	1999–2000	308	64.3
Indonesia	1997	21	0
	1996–1997	33	21
	1999–2000	NG	42.9
Mainland China	1996–1997	51	9.8
India	1996–1997	183	3.8
	2001–2002	21	0
Bangladesh	1993–1997	361	12.7
Pakistan	1993		9.2
New Guinea	1985	833	60

[a]Data from Felmingham, Aventis data on file, 2002; Silva et al., 1998; Rohani et al., 1999; Gwanzura et al., 2003; Mathai et al., 2001; Kozlov et al., 2002; Inoue et al., 2004; Koh and Lin, 1997; Sangthawan et al., 2003; Turnidge, 2000; Hoban, 1999, 2002; Saha et al., 1999; Parry et al., 2002; Lehmann et al., 1997; Soewignjo et al., 2001; Song et al., 1999; Schito and Marchese, 2004; Denno et al., 2002; El-Kholy et al., 2003; Mokaddas et al., 2001; Bogaerts et al., 1993; Woolfson et al., 1997; Scott et al., 1998, and Uwaydah et al., 2002.

[b]Penicillin-intermediate plus penicillin-resistant strains.

[c]NG, not given.

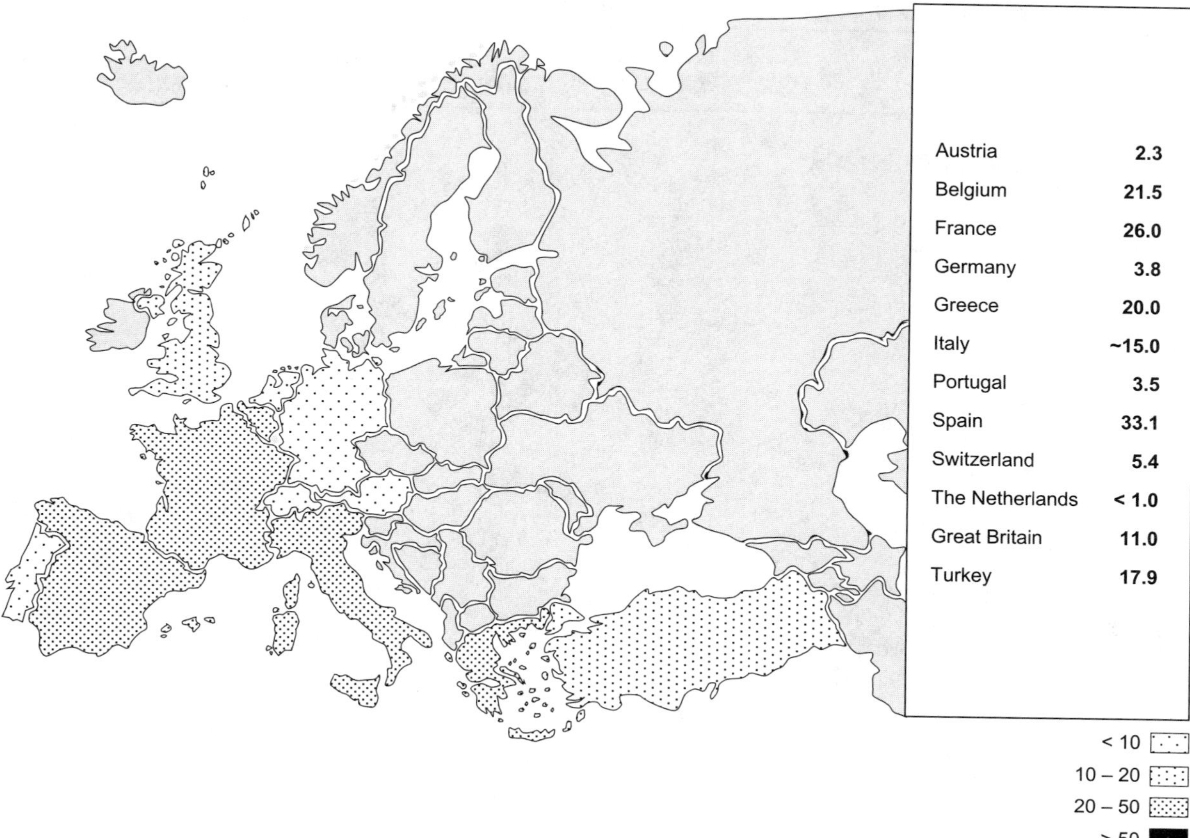

Figure 4 Prevalence of (percent) of resistance of *S. pneumoniae* to erythromycin A in Europe (1997)

almost 27% of strains isolated in Poland were penicillin resistant. In 1988, no strain of *S. pneumoniae* in Iceland was resistant to penicillin. In 1989, 2.3% of isolated strains exhibited reduced susceptibility, and the number of resistant strains has increased progressively since then, with rates of 2.7, 8.4, and 19% in 1990, 1991, and 1992, respectively. In Germany, the incidence of strains of reduced susceptibility was 6% in a recent study. In Belgium, the incidence was 1.5% between 1983 and 1988. In Switzerland, approximately 2.3% of isolates had reduced susceptibility to penicillin G in 1985. In Latin America, the first strains of abnormal susceptibility were isolated in 1987 in Chile and subsequently in Brazil, Argentina, and Venezuela. In Canada and Australia, the incidence of these strains is on the order of 1 to 2%. In the Middle East and Near East, the incidence varies from country to country. It is high in Israel, in some regions affecting 30% of isolates. A recent study in Pakistan showed an incidence of resistance of 6 to 14%, varying according to the disease. In Japan, the incidence of *S. pneumoniae* isolates resistant to penicillin G was less than 1% between 1974 and 1982, but it increased from 5.9 to 27.8% between 1984 and 1991. Strains of abnormal susceptibility have also been described in Malaysia and Bangladesh. The incidence of resistance for the time being is more difficult to assess in the

Table 14 In vitro activities of C3′-quaternary ammonium cephems against *S. pneumoniae*[a]

Drug	MIC (μg/ml) for organism					
	Penicillin susceptible		Penicillin intermediate		Penicillin resistant	
	50%	90%	50%	90%	50%	90%
Cefpirome	0.01	0.03	0.12	0.5	0.5	1.0
Cefepime	0.03	0.03	0.25	1.0	1.0	2.0
Cefclidin	0.25	0.5	1.0	4.0	8.0	8.0
Cefozopran	0.03	0.06	0.25	1.0	2.0	2.0
Cefluprenam	0.03	0.03	0.5	1.0	1.0	1.0
Cefoselis	0.03	0.06	0.125	0.5	0.5	1.0

[a]Data from Geslin et al., 1995, and Appelbaum et al., 1994.

Table 15 Prevalence of erythromycin A-resistant *S. pneumoniae* from 1999 to 2001

Country	n	Year(s)	% Erythromycin A resistant	Prevalence of resistance genes (%)			
				erm(B)	*mef*(A)	*erm*(B) + *mef*(A)	L4
Europe							
Austria	178	1999–2000	6.2	63.6	36.4	0	
Belgium	637		38	NT	NT	NT	
France	675		52.6	97.7	2.3	0	
The Netherlands	394		3.6	25	75	0	
Italy	184		32.4	89.5	10.5	0	
Spain	203		37.4	93.6	5.1	1.3	
Portugal	244		12.4	75	25	0	
Greece	109		43.6	45	55	0	
Finland	327		19.4	32.4	67.6	0	
Sweden	199		4.5	NT	NT	NT	
Denmark	376		2.7	22.2	77.8	0	
Norway	192		3.1	NT	NT	NT	
	69	1998–1999	6				
Iceland	119		8.2	NT	NT	NT	
Germany	330		9.7	NT	NT	NT	
The United Kingdom	709		10.4	32.4	64.9	0	
Ireland	108		9.3	40	60	0	
Luxemburg	184		31	80	20	0	
Czech Republic	102		4.9	80	20	0	
	160	2001	4.3		100	0	
Slovak Republic	100	1999–2000	28	39.3	0	0	60.7
	49	2001	34.7	94.1	0.9		
Hungary	46	2001	39.1	88.8	0.05		Other
Poland	97	1999–2000	27.8	81.5	3.7	11.1	3.7
	108	2001	15.7	88.3	11.7		
Croatia	101	1999–2000	18.2	15.8	3		
	585	2000–2001	18	NT	NT	NT	NT
Slovenia	101	1999–2000	4.9	40	0	40	20
		2000	18.2	ND	ND		
Romania	99	1999–2000	33.3	23.9			16.1
Malta		2000	0				
Switzerland	99	2001	7.1	57	43		
Russia	468	2000–2001	2.5	0.001	0.001	0	0.001
Lithuania	93	1999	5.4	40		40	
Latvia	96	4.2	25		25		50
Estonia	99	2000	13	ND	ND	ND	ND
Bulgaria	101	1999–2000	19.8	30	0	60	10
Turkey	41	2001	7.3	100			
	669	1994–2002	13.6	83.5	16.5		
North America							
The United States	1,527	1994–1995	10.3				
	1,601	1997–1998	19.2				
	195	1998	13.1				
	1,531	1999–2000	26.2				
	687	1999–2000	23.6				
Canada	350	1999–2000	16.6				
Latin America							
Argentina	188	1997	8.5				
Colombia							
Brazil	310	1997	4.8				
Panama	61	1997	14.8				
Venezuela	73	1997	23.3				
Chile	99	1997	9.1				
Mexico	285	1997	25.7				
West Indies	84	1997	1.2				

(Continued on next page)

Table 15 Prevalence of erythromycin A-resistant *S. pneumoniae* from 1999 to 2001 (*Continued*)

Country	*n*	Year(s)	% Erythromycin A resistant	Prevalence of resistance genes (%)			
				erm(B)	*mef*(A)	*erm*(B) + *mef*(A)	L4
Southeast Asia							
Korea	67	1999–2001	85.1	40.4	21.1	38.6	
	137	1999–2000	87.6	43.3	18.3	38.3	0
	31	2001	80.6				
Hong Kong	102	1999–2001	76.5	24.4	66.7	8.9	
	70	1999–2000	71.4	44	56	0	0
	112	2001	76.3				
China	111	2001	73				
Vietnam	60	1999–2001	91.6	45.3	57	49.1	
	63	2001	90.5				
Malaysia	38	1999–2001	44.7	14.3	64.3	21.4	
	44	2001	34.1				
Singapore	17	1999–2001	58.8	44.4	55.6	0	
	32	2001	40				
The Philippines	22	2001	18.2				
	26	1999–2001					
Sri Lanka	39	1999–2001	12.9	75	25	0	
	42	2001	14.3				
Taiwan	47	1999–2001	87.2	70.7	29.3	0	
	86	2001	86				
Thailand	32	1999–2001	50.5	28.6	71.1	0	
	52	2001	36.5				
		2003	34.8	ND	ND		
India	67	1999–2001	1.5	100	0	0	
	77	2001	1.3				
China	86	1999–2001	75.6	76.9	3.1	20	
Japan	308	1999–2001	77.9	52.5	42.5	3.3	0
Africa							
Algeria	39	2001	28.2	100	0	0	
Morocco	13	2001					
Tunisia			44	38.6	82.4	5.8	11.6
Ivory Coast	12	2001	1.0	100			
Togo	114	1999	21				
Senegal	3	2001					
Malawi	906						
South Africa			196	58.2	44.7	15.8	42.1
Middle East							
Lebanon	47	2001	21.3	60	20	20	
Israel	123	2001	36				
Near East							
Saudi Arabia	39	2001	10.3				
Australia	299	1999–2000	13.4	47.5	40	12.5	

[a]Data from Jacobs et al., 2000; Nagai et al., 2002; Felmingham et al., 2003, Felmingham, Aventis data on file, 2002; Song et al., 2004; Doern et al., 2001; Feikin et al., 2003; Hoban et al., 2003; Inoue et al., 2004; Ioannidou et al., 2003; Song et al., 2002; Uwaydah et al., 2002; Leegard et al., 2001; Dagnra et al., 2000; and Sener et al., 2004. NT, not tested; ND, not determined.

other countries in Asia. Outside South Africa and Rwanda (~21%), isolates of abnormal susceptibility have been described in Nigeria, Kenya, Zambia, and certain west African countries. In Tunisia, 11.7% of strains are resistant to penicillin G. However, 25.7, 33.3, and 25.7% of strains were resistant to chloramphenicol, co-trimoxazole, and the cyclines, respectively. In Algeria, the level of resistance is about 12.5%. In Korea, 30% of isolates in 1992 were of reduced susceptibility to penicillin G, but for no strain was the MIC >2 μg/ml.

S. pneumoniae represents about 5.4% of strains isolated from blood cultures in France. It is responsible for about 12 to 18% of cases of purulent meningitis of bacterial origin. Its incidence will increase with the use of anti-*H. influenzae* type B vaccine. It is one of the major pathogenic agents of community-acquired (8 to 75%) or nosocomial (~5 to 7%)

Table 16 Prevalence of resistance to penicillin G and erythromycin A in the United States from 2000 to 2001[a]

Region	*n*	Prevalence of resistance (%)		
		Penicillin G		Erythromycin A resistant
		Intermediate	Resistant	
Southwest	1,349	27	15.4	29.3
South-central	1,455	32.5	13.8	38.9
Southeast	1,063	36.4	14	40.4
Northeast	3,708	27.1	11.5	26.8
North-central	2,106	26.3	11.3	31.8
Northwest	422	17.3	10.4	23.8

[a]Data from Doern and Brown, 2004.

parenchymatous RTIs. The percentage of penicillin G-resistant isolates varies with patient age, sampling period, geographical location, and site of infection. Different epidemiological studies have shown that the number of penicillin G-resistant strains responsible for middle ear infections is increasing regularly, as is the number of such strains responsible for pneumonia. Nasopharyngeal carriage of resistant strains is considerable in certain countries, such as Spain, France, South Africa, Israel, and Hungary. It has reached 34% in Alaska.

In PROTEKT Surveillance Program US 2000-01, the prevalence of *S. pneumoniae* strains resistant to penicillin G and erythromycin A was studied in different geographical areas throughout the United States; rates are shown in Table 16.

The most resistant strains are often those isolated from the middle ear exudate. The percentage of resistant strains isolated from cerebrospinal fluid varies with the surveys.

Resistance of *S. pneumoniae* to telithromycin (Bryskier, 2002) is today a rare occurrence, as it was shown in PROTEKT studies conducted from 1999 to 2004 that for less than 1% of the clinical isolates were the MICs 1 μg/ml (Farrell et al., 2004).

Many extensive and collaborative epidemiological surveys have been performed in Europe, North America, and Asia. In Table 15 data including genotypes and mutation (L4 protein) are reported. In some studies there are discrepancies between azithromycin and erythromycin A susceptibilities. Strains resistant to azithromycin and showing intermediate susceptibility to erythromycin A were found. This phenomenon may be due to the different modes of action of the compounds.

Azithromycin has apparently two binding sites, one in common with erythromycin A and a second linking point in relation to protein ribosomal L4.

1. The nitrogen inserted in the lactone ring does not directly contribute to the binding of azithromycin.
2. The nitrogen is responsible for altering the conformation of the lactone ring, inducing new contacts with Mg^{2+} ions.
3. Binding site 1 of azithromycin interacts with domains IV and V of the 23S rRNA.
4. Binding site 2 of azithromycin interacts with proteins L4 and L22 and domain II of the 23S rRNA through hydrogen bonds between that site and the loop of L4 (Thr64 and Gly60) as well as another putative Mg^{2+} ion.
5. Azithromycin binding sites 1 and 2 are in direct contact through a hydrogen bond between the desosamine sugar and O1 in the lactone ring of azithromycin.

8.2.4. Fluoroquinolones

Many fluoroquinolones, such as levofloxacin, moxifloxacin, and gatifloxacin, are prescribed for treatment of pneumococcal community-acquired pneumonia or pneumococcal exacerbation of chronic bronchitis. In 1996, they were introduced in clinical practice for this purpose. In many surveillance studies (TRUST, PROTEK, LIBRA, SENTRY, and others), the antibacterial activity of levofloxacin as a marker was assessed. The level of resistance is extremely low, under 2%, except in some geriatric institutions in Hong Kong (8%).

An epidemiological survey showed that the prevalence of strains of *S. pneumoniae* resistant to fluoroquinolones was low in France; in 1996 it was 1.2% overall, with regional variations. Rates of sparfloxacin resistance of 6% have been reported in certain geographical areas in France. Table 17 shows the epidemiology of resistance of *S. pneumoniae* to fluoroquinolones in France.

In the United States, the epidemiology of *S. pneumoniae* resistance to levofloxacin was assessed through the TRUST study; results are shown in Table 18.

The prevalence of levofloxacin resistance in Europe was assessed and is reported in chapter 26.

In Asia and Latin America, levofloxacin resistance remains under 2%, except in institutions in Hong Kong.

Table 17 Epidemiology of resistance of *S. pneumoniae* to fluoroquinolones in France[a]

Year	No. of strains	% Resistant
1993	4,054	0.5
1994	4,512	0.6
1995	5,175	0.8
1996	4,804	0.8

[a]Data from Frémaux et al., 1997.

Table 18 Levofloxacin resistance in the United States

Years	*n*	% Resistant[a]
1997–1998	4,140	0.2
1998–1999	4,271	0.6
1999–2000	9,438	0.6
2000–2001	6,307	0.9
2001–2002	7,671	0.9

[a]Levofloxacin intermediate plus levofloxacin resistant.

Table 19 shows fluoroquinolone resistance rates of *S. pneumoniae* around the world.

8.3. *S. pyogenes*

For some years there has been a resurgence of infections due to group A beta-hemolytic streptococci. Very virulent strains have been described in the United States in particular.

Penicillin G has enabled infections due to streptococci of Lancefield group A to be treated successfully. To date, no penicillin G-resistant strain has been reported. In 1954, Lowburry et al. in Great Britain reported the first strain resistant to cyclines; in 1959, the first strain resistant to erythromycin A was reported. In the United States, the first strain resistant to erythromycin A was described in 1959.

Since 1989 the number of erythromycin A-resistant strains has been constantly increasing. In the United Kingdom, Warren et al. reported that in the region of Cambridge only 0.5% of strains were resistant in 1975, whereas the resistance rate in 1987 was 15 to 20%. In Japan, 11.9% of strains were resistant to erythromycin A in 1972, and resistance reached a plateau of 83.1% in 1977 before falling back to 35.4% in 1982. Studies conducted between 1986 and 1987 revealed the existence of three types of bacterial populations in relation to erythromcyin A, one highly susceptible (MIC, ≤0.06 μg/ml), one of intermediate susceptibility (15%) (MIC, 2 to 8 μg/ml), and one highly resistant (MIC, >128 μg/ml) (~25%).

In other countries of Asia, the level of resistance is sometimes poorly known; in 1975, 4.4% of strains were resistant

Table 19 Fluoroquinolone resistance for *S. pneumoniae*

Country	Before 2001		2001–2002		2002–2003		2003–2004[b]	
	n	% R	*n*	% R	*n*	% R	*n*	% R
Latin America								
Argentina			178	0.6				
Brazil			315	0				
Mexico			84	0				
Europe								
France			760	0.9			495	0.21
Germany			1,185	0.2			486	0.21
Italy			813	1.5			230	2.61
United Kingdom			505	0			324	0.31
Spain			649	0.6			301	2.23
Russia			535	0				
Belgium							94	2.13
Denmark							114	0
Finland							44	0
Greece							44	0
Luxemburg							25	8
Norway							49	0
Poland							120	0
Portugal							100	0
Sweden							100	0
The Netherlands							137	0
Northern Ireland							21	0
Canada								
1997–1998	1,179	0.4						
1998–1999	1,333	0.6						
1999–2000	1,593	1.2						
2000–2001	1,421	0.6						
2001–2002			980	1.0				
Asia								
Mainland China			180	1.1	111	0		
Hong Kong			188	8.5	112	8.0		
Taiwan					57	1.8		
Singapore					32	0		
Malaysia					44	0		
Korea			283	2.1	31	0		
Thailand			168	1.2	52	0		
Vietnam					63	0		
Philippines					22	0		
India					77	1.3		
Sri Lanka					42	0		
Africa: South Africa			615	0				
Middle East								
Saudi Arabia					39	0		
Lebanon			123	0				

[a]Data from Sahm et al., 2002; Blosser et al., 2002; Song et al., 2002; Zhanel et al., 2002; Uwaydah et al., 2002; and Kozlov et al., 2002. R, resistant.
[b]2003–2004 data, A. Bryskier, Aventis data on file.

to erythromycin A in Taiwan, whereas 90% were resistant to cyclines. In Australia, the proportion of strains resistant to erythromycin A rose from 1% in 1985 to 9.1% in 1986 and 17.6% in 1987. In Finland, 2% of strains isolated were resistant to erythromycin A in 1989, rising to 27% in certain centers. Also in Finland, the incidence of resistance of *S. pyogenes* to erythromycin A reached 19% in 1993. The reduction in the prescription of erythromycin A resulted in a dramatic fall in the number of resistant strains, with a resistance rate of 8.6% in 1996. In 1990, about 0.7% of isolates in Spain were resistant to erythromycin, and 8% in Turkey were resistant in 1977. In Canada, the percentage of erythromycin A-resistant strains ranged from 0.03 to 2.9%. In Germany, no erythromycin A-resistant strain has been described, but a reduction in the drug's activity has been noted. In France, about 6% of strains are resistant to erythromycin A. In the United States, about 5 to 20% of strains are resistant to erythromycin A. Hryniewicz et al. (1993) have shown that in Poland, all strains of *S. pyogenes* were susceptible to penicillin G, 43% were resistant to cyclines, and 7% were resistant to erythromycin A.

In Italy, the growth in the number of strains of *S. pyogenes* resistant to erythromycin A was spectacular; the incidence rose from 4.6% in 1993 to almost 50% of isolates in 1996, with a marked inflection of the curve in 1995 (37.1%).

In 1990 in New Zealand, the activities of different antibiotics against 434 strains of *S. pyogenes* were tested. All of the strains were susceptible to penicillin G, cefotaxime, and co-trimoxazole. The levels of resistance to erythromycin A, tetracyclines, and chloramphenicol were, respectively, 3.8, 3.5, and 0.3%.

In France, it was noted that the numbers of strains resistant to erythromycin A among streptococci of Lancefield groups C and G were higher than for strains of *S. pyogenes*. Philippon (1994) showed that 8.1 to 22.8% of Lancefield group A and 24.3% of Lancefield group C and G streptococci were resistant to erythromycin A at the Hôpital Saint-Louis in Paris.

The prevalence of resistance to erythromycin A within group A streptococci, as determined by recent surveys, is summarized in Tables 20 and 21.

In PROTEKT 1999-2000, of 382 *S. pyogenes* isolates collected in Canada, 5.2% of them were resistant to erythromycin A (Hoban et al., 2003).

One important bias is that in the recruitment of patients suffering from group A beta-hemolytic streptococci are those for whom the treatment failed due to a resistant strain, increasing artificially the rate of resistance.

8.4. *Enterococcus* spp.

The enterococci are commensals of the human and animal gut, as well as saprophytes of the environment. They are responsible for opportunistic diseases and are naturally resistant to a number of antibiotics.

The genus *Enterococcus* has been separated from the genus *Streptococcus* since 1984. It comprises 14 species, 10 of which have been isolated from pathological specimens from humans. The most commonly encountered species are *Enterococcus faecalis* (80 to 90%) and *E. faecium* (5 to 10%).

Enterococci are essentially the cause of mucocutaneous (surgical wounds, varicose ulcers, and injuries) and abdominal infections, endocarditis, urinary tract infections, and, more rarely, neonatal meningitis.

E. faecalis is the second most common agent responsible for nosocomial infections in the United States. The incidence of enterococcal infections has been constantly on the increase since 1980. *E. faecium* is implicated less commonly than *E. faecalis* in western Europe and in the United States than in Japan.

The enterococci are relatively insensitive to penicillin G (Table 22). They are resistant to the cephalosporins, which often select them in vivo. They are commonly susceptible to vancomycin, except for *Enterococcus gallinarum* and *Enterococcus casseliflavus*.

The activity of aminoglycosides against *E. faecalis* and *E. faecium* is moderate (Table 23).

The first strains of *E. faecalis* resistant to high concentrations of aminoglycosides were isolated in France by Horodniceanu et al. in 1979. Conversely, this type of resistance in *E. faecium* was first described in the United States by

Table 20 Prevalence of *S. pyogenes* resistant to erythromycin A

Country	*n*	No. (%) of resistant strains	Gene(s) (no.)			
			mef(A)	*erm*(B)	*erm*(A)	*erm*(B) + *mef*
Austria	206	20 (9.7)	13	2	5	
Belgium	599	82 (13.7)	33	49		
Denmark	377	11 (2.9)		2	2	7
Finland	133	10 (7.5)	3	3	4	
France	441	38 (8.6)	17	19		
Germany	381	55 (14.4)	12	1	4	
Greece	161	36 (22.4)	23		13	
Iceland	?	? (21.4)	?	?	?	?
Ireland	158	3 (1.9)	1	2		
Italy	269	64 (23.8)	22	22	5	2
Luxemburg	86	9 (10.5)	1	3	2	3
The Netherlands	383	5 (1.3)		2	1	2
Norway	199	2 (1.0)				
Portugal	300	82 (27.3)	16	64	2	
Spain	202	48 (23.8)	40			8
Sweden	199	0 (0.0)				
Switzerland	?	? (2.6)	?	?	?	?
United Kingdom	994	53 (5.3)	16	5	28	1

Table 21 ***S. pyogenes*** **resistance to erythromycin A: prevalence of different genotypes, in central and eastern Europe (including Turkey) and other countries, 1999 to 2000**

Country	*n*	No. (%) of resistant strains	Genes (%)		
			erm(B)	*erm*(A)	*mef*(A)
Bulgaria	106	18 (17.0)		66.7	33.3
Croatia	99	17 (17.2)	28.6	35.7	35.7
Czech Republic	104	8 (7.7)		100	
Estonia	100	13 (13.0)	ND[a]	ND	ND
Hungary	97	5 (5.2)	40	40	20
Latvia	100	9 (9.0)		100	
Lithuania	99	10 (10.1)		100	
Poland	98	16 (16.3)	35.7	64.3	
Romania	103	10 (9.7)	10	10	80
Slovakia	102	16 (15.7)	30.8		69.2
Slovenia	102	13 (12.7)		100	
Russia	600	0 (0.0)			
	100	14 (14.0)	ND	ND	ND
Turkey	92	8 (7.0)	11.1	77.8	11.1
Australia	301	14 (4.7)			57.1[b]
Canada	382	5.2			

[a]ND, not determined.
[b]Remaining strains were nontypeable.

Table 22 **Activities of β-lactams against** ***Enterococcus*** **spp.**

Organism	MIC (μg/ml) of drug							
	PenicillinG		Ampicillin		Piperacillin		Imipenem	
	50%	90%	50%	90%	50%	90%	50%	90%
E. faecalis	1	4	0.5	1	2	4	1	2
E. faecium	8	64	4	32	16	128	4	64
E. gallinarum	0.5	4	0.5	2	8	32	1	4
E. casseliflavus	0.5	0.5	0.25	0.5	4	8	1	4
Enterococcus avium	0.5	2	0.25			16	0.12	2
Enterococcus durans	0.5	2	0.25	0.5	4	8	0.12	1
E. raffinosus	8	64	64					

Table 23 **In vitro activities of aminoglycosides against** ***E. faecalis***

Drug	MIC (μg/ml)
Kanamycin	64–128
Gentamicin	8–16
Tobramycin	8–32
Amikacin	64–256
Netilmicin	4–8
Isepamicin	32–128
Dactocmycin	4–16

Eliopoulos et al. in 1986. Since then a number of resistant strains have been reported in numerous centers in Ireland, the United Kingdom, Austria, Poland, and Singapore.

In a prospective study in the United Kingdom, it was shown that 7.5% of strains of *E. faecalis* were highly resistant to gentamicin, but none were resistant to vancomycin. Of the highly resistant strains, 14% came from urine, 31% came from blood cultures, 20% came from suppuration, and only 4.5% came from feces.

Zervos et al. (1987) demonstrated a relationship between the emergence of strains of *E. faecalis* highly resistant to gentamicin and the prior use of cephalosporins and aminoglycosides. The strains of *E. faecalis* were all resistant to fusidic acid, clindamycin, chloramphenicol, sulfamethoxazole, and amikacin.

The most common mechanism of resistance is the presence of aminoglycoside-inactivating enzymes (phosphotransferases, nucleotidyltransferases, and acetyltransferases). Some enzymes are specific to gram-positive cocci, such as the bifunctional enzyme APH(2′)-AAC(6′). They are plasmid mediated and constitutive.

The first vancomycin-resistant enterococci were isolated in France in 1986 and in the United Kingdom in 1988. Strains of resistant enterococci have been isolated in Italy, but the incidence is low (*E. faecalis*, ~0.9%, and *E. faecium*, ~1.5%). In the hospitals of New York State, the number of vancomycin-resistant strains increased considerably between 1989 and 1991. Table 24 shows the worldwide prevalence of

Table 24 Prevalence of enterococcal isolates resistant to vancomycin or teicoplanin in 1997

Country	*n*	Prevalence % of strains resistant to: Vancomycin	Teicoplanin
Belgium	167	0.6	0.6
France	98	3.1	1.1
Germany	457	2.0	1.3
Italy	323	0.9	0.6
The Netherlands	72	1.4	1.4
Portugal	128	3.9	3.1
Spain	230	3.5	3.5
Switzerland	141	4.2	2.8
The United Kingdom	79	1.3	1.3
The United States		15	ND[a]

[a]ND, not done.

enterococcal isolates resistant to teicoplanin or vancomycin in 1997.

Van den Auwera et al. (1990) showed that oral administration of teicoplanin to volunteers promoted colonization of the digestive tract by strains of *E. faecium* and coagulase-negative staphylococci that were resistant to teicoplanin. Usually this colonization involved strains of *E. faecium*. Overall in *Enterococcus* species at least six resistance phenotypes are reported (Table 25).

In *E. faecalis* and *E. faecium* it has been shown that VanA- or VanB-type resistance to glycopeptides is related to the inducible synthesis of a new precursor of peptidoglycan in which the terminal dipeptide is replaced by a D-Ala–D-lactate depsipeptide, which has a weak affinity for the glycopeptides (Fig. 5). Strains of the VanA phenotype exhibit high-level inducible resistance to vancomycin (MIC, >64 μg/ml) and teicoplanin (MIC, >16 μg/ml). Resistance is crossed with all the derivatives of the glycopeptide family. It is transferable to other gram-positive bacteria, such as *Listeria monocytogenes*, *Lactobacillus*, *Bacillus subtilis*, *S. aureus*, and *Streptococcus* spp., and is transposable through transposon Tn*1546*. This transposon codes for nine proteins. Three genes, *vanH*, *vanA*, and *vanX*, are necessary for the expression of resistance to glycopeptides. The six other genes have transposition functions (*orfI* and *orfII*) or regulation functions (*vanR* and *vanS*) or are accessory genes (*vanY* [D-carboxypeptidase] and *vanZ* [involved in the synthesis of peptidoglycan]).

The VanB phenotype comprises strains of *E. faecalis* and *E. faecium* with variable levels of resistance to vancomycin (MIC, 8 to 1,024 μg/ml) but which remain susceptible to teicoplanin. This is a low-level, inducible, and transferable resistance.

The *vanC-1* and *vanC-2* genes are specific, respectively, for *E. gallinarum* and *E. casseliflavus*. They do not code for a depsipeptide of the D-Ala–D-lactate type and are chromosomally mediated.

The MICs of penicillin G are, respectively, ≤4 and ≥4 μg/ml for *E. faecalis* and *E. faecium*. β-Lactamase production by these organisms was described for the first time in 1991. This type of strain of *E. faecalis* has been detected in the United States, Argentina, and Lebanon. The production of this plasmid-mediated β-lactamase is often associated with the production of a bifunctional enzyme providing low-level resistance to gentamicin. This enzyme is similar to that encoded by the *blaZ* gene of *S. aureus*, but it differs in that it is constitutive and not inducible.

Strains of β-lactam-resistant *Enterococcus raffinosus* and *E. faecium* have been isolated. The MICs of penicillin G for *E. faecium* are usually (22 to 60% of strains) greater than 16 μg/ml, but very resistant strains have been described (MIC, ≥512 μg/ml) in the United States and in certain European countries. This resistance is related to the expression of a low-molecular-weight PBP. The PBP implicated appears to be PBP 5, which is not normally essential but becomes so when all the other PBPs are saturated and inhibited. It is responsible for transpeptidation of the natural precursor and allows the synthesis of the peptidoglycan. In *E. faecium*, the role of PBPs is even more complex because there is additionally a PBP 5′. In the case of *E. raffinosus*, there is also PBP 7 in the resistant strains.

As a general rule, the cephalosporins have a very weak affinity for PBP 5.

Interhuman contamination with *E. faecium* has been shown by numerous studies. Bates et al. (1993) have also isolated these resistant strains from excreta from chickens, pigs, dogs, and horses, but not from sheep or cows. Uncooked food, particularly chicken from supermarkets, was contaminated with *E. faecium*. The authors draw a parallel with contamination with *Salmonella*. They have postulated that these vancomycin-resistant strains would have been selected because antibiotics are used as growth factors (food additives) like avoparcin.

8.5. *Streptococcus agalactiae* (GBS)

Group B streptococci (GBS) are normal commensals of the gastrointestinal and urogenital tracts. GBS are classified in nine serogroups: Ia, Ib, and II to VIII (capsular polysaccharide).

Table 25 Resistance phenotypes of enterococci

Resistance	Acquired					Intrinsic
Phenotype	VanA	VanB	VanD	VanG	VanE	VanC
MIC (μg/ml)						
Vancomycin	64–1,000	4–1,000	64–128	8–16	16	2–32
Teicoplanin	16–512	0.5–1	4–64	0.5	0.5	0.5–1
Expression	Inducible		Constitutive	Inducible		Constitutive Inducible
Location	Plasmid Chromosome		Chromosome	Chromosome		Chromosome
Genetic elements	Tn*1546*	Tn*1547* Tn*1549*				
Modified target	D-Ala–D-Lac			D-Ala–D-Ser		

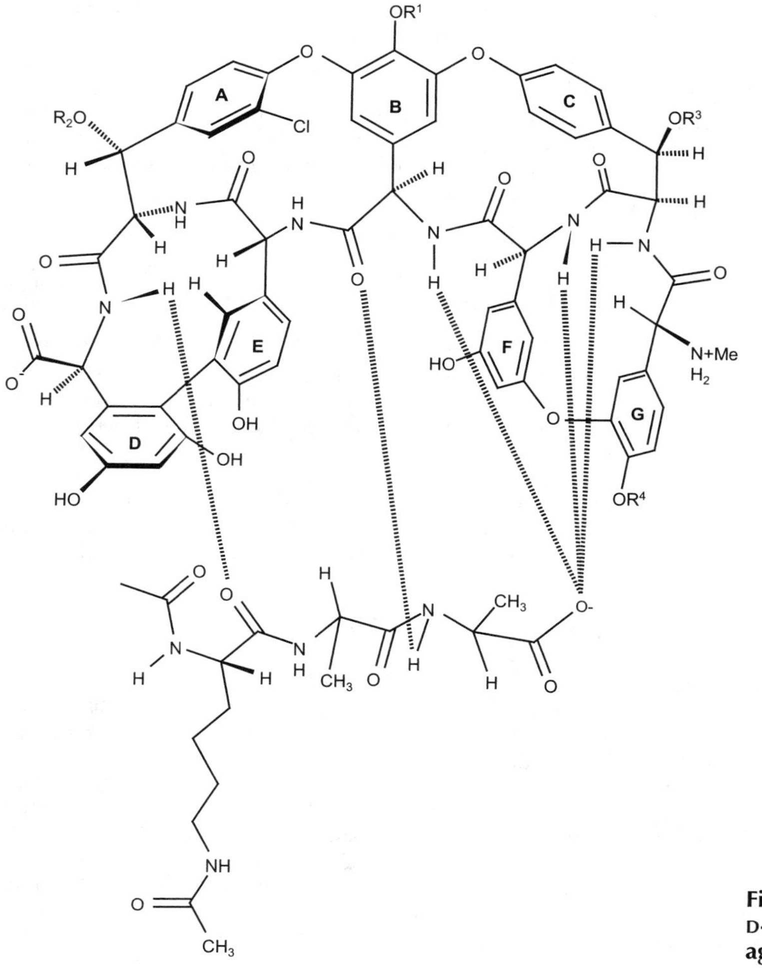

Figure 5 Interaction between D-alanyl–D-alanine and the aglycone of the glycopeptide

GBS are an important cause of neonatal sepsis and of meningitis, infections in pregnant women, and invasive diseases in nonpregnant adults, such as those suffering from diabetes mellitus, malignancy, liver disease, and other immune impairment. GBS infections occur in elderly patients.

Between 15 and 35% of pregnant women were found to be asymptomatic carriers of GBS and in the early onset of the disease (<7 days after delivery), 0.2 to 0.8% of neonates had GBS bacteremia in the United States.

A retrospective study carried out in 2000 by Trijbels-Smeulders et al. reported the incidence for 1,000 live births; data are shown in Table 26.

8.5.1. β-Lactams

In prophylaxis, benzylpenicillin is a drug of choice, and second-line macrolides are recommended.

Resistance to penicillin G is a rare occurrence.

In Canada (Ontario), 196 clinical isolates were collected from 1995 to 1996. One isolate was intermediately susceptible to penicillin G (MIC, 0.5μg/ml).

In the United States, of 574 GBS collected in 1998, 1.8% of the strains were resistant to penicillin G.

Manning et al. (2001) showed that 23 of 150 (15.3%) isolates from healthy carriers were intermediately susceptible to penicillin G.

8.5.2. Aminoglycosides

For serious infections, an aminoglycoside is often administered in combination with a penicillin (benzylpenicillin or amoxicillin) to provide bactericidal synergism.

In the early 1990s, GBS isolates were found to be resistant to streptomycin in France.

In a study carried out in a pediatric hospital in Paris, France (Hôpital Robert Debré), between 1997 and 2002, 2,552 and 3,280 clinical isolates were collected from neonates and mothers, respectively; 5.9 and 0.3% of the strains were highly resistant to kanamycin and/or gentamicin. The rates of kanamycin resistance were 3.7 and 8.5% in 1997 and 2002, respectively. In another study carried out in France, the prevalence rate was 10% (Poyart et al., 2003).

8.5.3. Fluoroquinolones

Up to the year 2000, the MICs of ofloxacin and grepafloxacin for only some strains were slightly increased (Leven et al., 2000).

In 2002, three isolates highly resistant to fluoroquinolones were isolated from Japan (MICs, >32 μg/ml). The resistance mechanism is a mutation at position 81 (Ser81 → Leu) in the *gyrA* gene and another at position 79 in *parC* (Ser79 → Phe) (Kawamura et al., 2003).

Table 26 Incidence of *S. agalactiae* in live births in Europe and in North America

Country	Incidence of GBS/1,000 live births (%)
Austria	2
Belgium	2
France	20.3–0.4
The Netherlands	1.9
The United Kingdom	0.5–2
Finland	0.76
Iceland	0.9
Sweden	1.0
Spain	0.57–2
Italy	0.9
Czech Republic	0.2–1.1
Hungary	1–2
Slovak Republic	1–4
Slovenia	1.8
Norway	1–2
The United States	0.6

8.5.4. Macrolides

GBS resistance to erythromycin A has been reported in many countries: France, Spain, Italy, the United States, Australia, Korea, Taiwan, and many other Asian countries.

In Spain, 18% of the GBS isolates were shown to be resistant to erythromycin A. In North America, in a SENTRY epidemiological program carried out in 2001, of 318 GBS isolates, 69.8, 88.1, and 14.8% were susceptible to erythromycin A, clindamycin, and tetracycline, respectively (Biedenbach et al., 2002).

In another SENTRY program (Andrews et al., 2000) it was revealed that 25 and 14% of neonatal bloodstream isolates in the United States and Canada, respectively, were resistant to erythromycin A and 7% were resistant to clindamycin. In Canada (Ontario), the rate of resistance to erythromycin A increased from 5% in 1995 to 1996 to 13% in 1998 to 1999 (Tyrrell et al., 2000). In Canada, among invasive strains collected in 1996, 7 and 4% were resistant to erythromycin A and clindamycin, respectively (Tyrrell et al., 2000).

In this study, the majority of erythromycin A-resistant isolates possessed an *erm*(TR) gene, an allele of *erm*(A). The *mre*(A) gene is present in all isolates irrespective of the sensitivity to erythromycin A. Resistance to erythromycin A is due to methylation [*erm*(B)] or efflux [*mef*(A)].

Of the Asian countries (Bell et al., 2002), the rate of erythromycin A resistance was found to be high in Taiwan (50%) and Hong Kong (27%); in other countries, the resistance rates were 3, 7, and 5% in Australia, Japan, and Singapore, respectively. No strains in South Africa were resistant to erythromycin A.

8.5.5. Tetracyclines

GBS isolates are often resistant to tetracyclines, even if administration of these drugs is low in patients infected with these organisms.

In the SENTRY program carried out in 2001 in North America, only 14.8% of the GBS isolates were susceptible to tetracycline. Tigecycline MICs range from 0.03 to 0.25 μg/ml irrespective of minocycline MICs (≤0.006 to 16 μg/ml). A similar figure was found in Madrid, Spain, for 115 GBS isolates; only 16.5% of the strains were susceptible to tetracyclines. (Alhambra et al., 2004).

Tetracycline resistance in GBS is mainly due to the presence of the *tet*(M) gene carried on a transposon.

8.5.6. Lincosamides

Usually the resistance pattern for lincosamides followed that for erythromycin A. However, GBS strains resistant to clindamycin and susceptible to erythromycin A due to a *lin*(B) gene have been described.

8.5.7. Chloramphenicol

The rate of resistance to chloramphenicol is usually low, less than 5%.

8.6. *Leuconostoc, Pediococcus,* and *Lactobacillus*

Leuconostoc, Pediococcus, and *Lactobacillus* spp. belong to the saprophytic flora and are naturally resistant to glycopeptides. For some years they have been the source of opportunistic infections in immunodepressed patients. As a general rule, these microorganisms are susceptible to penicillin G. The mechanism of resistance to glycopeptide antibiotics is related to the synthesis of D-Ala–D-lactate, a link in the biosynthesis of peptidoglycan, instead of D-Ala–D-Ala.

9. GRAM-NEGATIVE COCCI

9.1. *Neisseria gonorrhoeae*

In 1999, 360,076 cases of gonorrhea were reported in the United States. Gonorrhea is a major cause of pelvic inflammatory disease.

Up until 1987, *N. gonorrhoeae* was treated with a single dose of penicillin G. *N. gonorrhoeae* was extremely susceptible to benzylpenicillin (MICs, 0.004 to 0.01 μg/ml), but this sensitivity decreased progressively, and by the late 1970s strains emerged that were resistant to penicillin G (MIC, ≥2 μg/ml). Resistance to other antibacterials, including tetracyclines and erythromycin A, also increased during this time.

9.1.1. β-Lactams

Penicillin G resistance arose by two independent mechanisms: plasmid-mediated production of TEM-1 β-lactamase and chromosome-mediated multiple resistance.

Penicillin G has long been the reference drug in the treatment of gonococcal urethritis. Its use was called into question in the mid-1970s with the emergence of resistant strains, particularly in Southeast Asia. The first strains were isolated in the Philippines between 1965 and 1967. Resistance to penicillin G is plasmid mediated.

For some years there has been a decline in the activity of penicillins against *N. gonorrhoeae* due to the production of β-lactamases. The incidence of this resistance varies by country and region. In the Paris region it is on the order of 15%. This enzymatic resistance may be chromosomally or plasmid mediated. In 1983, spectinomycin was recommended in Thailand as the reference treatment because of the marked prevalence of β-lactamase-producing strains resistant to tetracyclines. The first spectinomycin-resistant strain was described in 1981 in California. However, in South Korea and the Philippines, strains resistant to spectinomycin developed rapidly from 1981 onwards, reaching 22.2% in 1988 in the Philippines and 8.9% in 1990 in Thailand. A study undertaken by the World Health Organization in 1988 showed that β-lactamase-producing strains represented 22% in the Fiji Islands, 33.4% in the Emirate of Brunei, 33.2% in Malaysia, 35.7% in Singapore, 40% in Hong Kong, and 44% in the Philippines. In the last country, the prevalence is 73%. In

Korea, the figure for β-lactamase-producing strains was 45% in 1979, reaching 55% in 1987. In Venezuela and Peru, 49% of strains of *N. gonorrhoeae* were β-lactamase producing. In the region of Ibadan in Nigeria, 74.3% of strains were β-lactamase producing. In 1984, Easmon reported that 5% of strains isolated in England were resistant to spectinomycin.

Resistance of chromosomal origin appears to be most widespread and is often accompanied by a reduction in the susceptibility of the strains to spectinomycin, cyclines, sulfonamides, and macrolides. Strains highly resistant to tetracyclines have been described in Australia, probably imported from Southeast Asia.

N. gonorrhoeae has four PBPs, 1, 2, 3, and 4. PBPs 1 and 2 are essential for cell viability. Penicillin G acts mainly on PBP 2. PBP 1 is involved in transformation to high-level penicillin G resistance. The genetic mechanisms include the genes *penA* (encoding PBP 2), *mtr* (erythromycins A to R), and *penB* (efflux for erythromycin A and tetracycline, PBP 1). The *penC* gene was recently described, and if it is present alone, the MICs of penicillin and tetracyclines increase twofold.

In Indonesia, 89% of isolates were resistant to penicillin G (MIC, ≥2 μg/ml), 98% were resistant to cyclines (MIC, ≥2 μg/ml), 18.1% were resistant to spectinomycin (MIC, ≥128 μg/ml), and 97.7% had reduced susceptibility to phenicols (MIC, ~1 to 2 μg/ml).

In Greece, between 1991 and 1998, 575 gonococcal isolates were cultured and tested. Resistances to penicillin G, tetracyclines, erythromycin A, and chloramphenicol were noted.

A high prevalence of plasmid-mediated, high-level resistance to penicillin G and tetracyclines and chloramphenicol has been recognized in Southeast Asia and Africa.

In Japan, the emergence of *N. gonorrhoeae* resistant to 2-amino-5-thiazolyl cephalosporins (cefotaxime and ceftriaxone) and aztreonam was reported in 2001.

In the United States, 29.4% of clinical isolates of *N. gonorrhoeae* were resistant to penicillin, tetracyclines, or both.

In Argentina, 50% of *N. gonorrhoeae* strains showed reduced susceptibility or resistance to penicillin (MIC, ≥0.125 μg/ml).

In Canada, between 1990 and 1994, the MIC at which 50% and 90% of the isolates tested were inhibited (MIC_{50} and MIC_{90}) of ceftriaxone for *N. gonorrhoeae* doubled. In 1994, the MIC distributions for isolates were biphasic for the first time.

In Russia in 2000, 40, 67, 4, and 11% of *N. gonorrhoeae* isolates were resistant to penicillin G, tetracyclines, ciprofloxacin, and spectinomycin, respectively. All strains were susceptible to co-trimoxazole and ceftriaxone (L. Strachounsky, personal communication, 2001).

9.1.2. Fluoroquinolones

N. gonorrhoeae was considered highly susceptible to fluoroquinolones (MIC, ≤0.06 μg/ml). Since 1992, a few strains of reduced susceptibility have been described (MIC, 0.125 to 0.25 μg/ml). Since 1993, resistant strains have been described in Japan, Indonesia, the United States, and Spain. In 1993, 13.7% of strains isolated in Ohio were of reduced susceptibility to ciprofloxacin. Three strains with reduced susceptibility to ciprofloxacin (MIC, 2 μg/ml) have been described in Hawaii. Such strains have also been demonstrated in Australia and Thailand. Ciprofloxacin had a MIC of 16 μg/ml for the Spanish strain, which remained susceptible to tetracyclines and spectinomycin.

In the Philippines, from 1994 to 1997, the proportion of *N. gonorrhoeae* strains highly resistant to ciprofloxacin increased dramatically, from 9 to 49%.

There is a marked prevalence of fluoroquinolone-resistant strains of *N. gonorrhoeae* in Japan. The mechanism of resistance is related to a reduction in intrabacterial accumulation or a double mutation in the *gyrA* and *parC* genes. These resistant strains are less susceptible to ceftriaxone and clarithromycin.

In 1999 in the United States, excluding Hawaii, 0.2% of *N. gonorrhoeae* strains were resistant to fluoroquinolones.

The prevalence of strains with reduced susceptibility to fluoroquinolones has been reported as being over 50% among isolates in Hong Kong, China, the Philippines, Korea, Cambodia, and Thailand.

Resistance may be due to *gyrA* mutations (Ser91 or Asp95) alone or in combination with *parC* mutations (amino acids from 66 to 88 and 91).

9.1.3. Others

The *tet*(M) gene is responsible for high-level tetracycline resistance.

Azithromycin-resistant *N. gonorrhoeae* strains have been reported from the United States and worldwide.

9.2. *Neisseria meningitidis*

Infections caused by *N. meningitidis* are still an important health public problem, because of the severity and highly contagious nature of the disease. *N. meningitidis* can be an etiology of transient fever and bacteremia to meningitis and fulminant septicemia.

Cerebrospinal meningitis was described in the spring of 1805 by Viessieux in Geneva, Switzerland and *N. meningitidis* was initially isolated from cerebrospinal fluid by Weichselbaum in 1887. *N. meningitidis* is classified on the basis of capsular polysaccharide. Capsular polysaccharides are classified into 11 serogroups: A, B, C, X, Y, W 135, Z, 29E, H, I, and K. Serogroups B and C accounted for most of the endemic and sporadic diseases in western countries. Some W 135 and Y isolates have been also reported. In tropical countries, such as the "meningitis belt" of sub-Saharan Africa, the Indian subcontinent, South America, China, and the Middle East, the disease occurs in large spreading epidemics. They are generally due to serogroup A and C strains. Fatality rates associated with these infections are high despite appropriate antibacterial therapy.

The growth medium needs to be adequate, as shown with higher penicillin G MICs observed in Mueller-Hinton broth with lysed blood cells and Haemophilus test medium suggesting that calcium-adjusted MHB is an adequate medium.

Strains of *N. meningitidis* are usually susceptible to penicillin G, β-lactams, chloramphenicol, rifampin, tetracyclines, fluoroquinolones, and macrolides. They have intrinsically low susceptibility to vancomycin. β-Lactams continue to be used for treatment, but in Africa (especially in French-speaking Africa), chloramphenicol is frequently used in epidemic situations.

Chemoprophylatic treatment with rifampin was recommended for nasopharyngeal colonization by *N. meningitidis* for close contacts, to significantly reduce the carriage state.

The first sulfonamide-resistant strains were described at the beginning of the 1960s. Sulfonamides have been administered since 1937 in the treatment of cerebrospinal meningitis. Resistance to sulfonamides may be caused by a mutation in the chromosomal gene for dihydropteroate synthase, with replacement of guanine by thymidine at position 92 resulting in replacement of phenylalanine by a leucine at position 31 and a 6-bp insertion resulting in two extra amino acids (serine 195 and glycine 196). The level of resistance to sulfadiazine was 29% in a 2000 report.

Table 27 Prevalence of resistance to penicillin G in *N. meningitidis*

Country	Year(s)	% Decreased susceptibility
United Kingdom	1985–1999	2.5
Belgium	1990–1995	2.5
The Netherlands	1993–1995	3.3
Greece	1989–1991	48.3
Spain	1994–1997	55.3
France	~2003	30
Scotland	1994–1999	8.3
Sweden	1981–1990	13
Poland	1995–2000	27
Croatia	1994–1999	16
Turkey	~2001	16.7
Cuba	1993–1999	31.5
Argentina	1991–1992	5.6
Israel	1991–1992	9.0
Australia	1994	45
	1999	26
	2002	>66
Canada	1991–1992	5.7
The United States	1998–1999	30.2
Slovenia	1993–1999	1–2
Togo	1999	16.7

In the United States, the first report of decreased susceptibility to penicillin G was in 1945: for 27.8% of the 54 isolates, the penicillin G MICs ranged from 0.1 to 0.5 μg/ml. From 1948 to 1954, 10.4% were shown to have intermediate susceptibility to penicillin G (0.1 to 0.2 μg/ml). From 1983 to 1993 in the Midwest, 15.7% were intermediately susceptible to benzylpenicillin. In two federal surveys conducted in 1991 and 1997, 3.0 and 3.3% of the isolates, respectively, were intermediately susceptible to penicillin G.

In Europe, decreased susceptibility to penicillin G was reported in the early 1970s. Since this period, strains with decreased susceptibility have been described in Greece, Spain, Italy, Portugal, France, Belgium, the United Kingdom, The Netherlands, South Africa, Latin and North America, and Asia (Table 27).

A reduction in the activity of penicillin G (MIC, ≥0.12 μg/ml) has been described in the United Kingdom (England and Wales) and Canada since 1983, in Spain since 1985, and in Greece and South Africa since 1987. In 1999 in Togo, the reduction of susceptibility to penicillin G reached 16.7% (Dagnra et al., 2000), and in Slovenia 1 to 2% of the isolates have been intermediately susceptible to benzylpenicillin since 1993.

The first β-lactamase-producing strain of *N. gonorrhoeae* was described in 1983. This was a plasmid-mediated β-lactamase, the gene for which was carried by an Asiatic-type plasmid of *N. gonorrhoeae* (7.2 kb). However, the strains of reduced susceptibility in Spain were due to a weaker affinity for PBP 2 encoded by the *penA* gene. As for *N. gonorrhoeae*, the modification of PBP 2 appears to be related to the acquisition of certain regions of the gene encoding the PBP 2 of *Neisseria flavescens* and *Neisseria cinerea*. In addition to the decreased affinity for PBP 2, a decreased expression of class 3 porin and PBP 1 may contribute to higher-level resistance of *N. meningitidis* to β-lactams. Class 3 porin and class 2 porin are products of the *porB* gene producing a large channel. Penicillin G and cefotaxime diffuse through the anion-preferred class 3 channel but not easily through the cation-selected class 1 porin channel.

Table 28 Activity of penicillin G against *N. meningitidis* in England between 1985 and 1989

Penicillin G MIC (μg/ml)	No. of strains				
	1985	1986	1987	1988	1989
0.08	579	977	1,155	1,301	1,314
0.16	1	12	28	45	27
0.32	0	0	4	2	12
0.64	0	0	1	2	1
1.28	0	0	1	2	1
≥0.16	0.2	1.2	2.9	3.9	3.1

In a Canadian study from 1979, 827 strains of *N. meningitidis* were isolated and 29 exhibited a reduction in the activity of penicillin G (MIC, 0.25 to 0.5 μg/ml).

In Spain, the number of strains of the penicillin-resistant phenotype rose from 0.8% in 1984 to 8% in 1992.

N. meningitidis comprises 12 serogroups, with serogroups A, B, and C representing 90% of strains responsible for meningitis. In Spain, serogroup B is predominant, but since 1986 the numbers of strains of serogroup C have been increasing, representing 24% in 1990 and 32% in 1991; in 1986, they accounted for fewer than 10% of isolates. Strains of intermediate susceptibility to penicillin G are found three times more often among serogroup C strains. It is possible to divide the strains of *N. meningitidis* of serotypes 1, 2, 3, etc., into subtypes. Strains resistant to penicillin G are usually of serotype 2b, whereas those susceptible to penicillin G are of serotype 2a.

In a Swedish study (1993) conducted over the period from 1981 to 1990, it was shown that 13% of invasive strains were resistant to penicillin G (MIC, ≥0.5 μg/ml). From 1983 to 1984, the isolated strains had reduced susceptibility to the cyclines, and for 82% of strains isolated between 1987 and 1988, the MICs of tetracyclines were greater than 0.5 μg/ml. No strains, even those carrying a plasmid, produced β-lactamases. Reduced susceptibility to sulfadiazine was noted in 45.7% of strains and reduced susceptibility to erythromycin A was noted in 7.5%, compared with 20% for penicillin G and 4 of 188 for rifampin.

In the United Kingdom, the number of strains of *N. meningitidis* isolated is on the increase, with serotypes B and C being isolated with the same frequency. In 1989, penicillin G had a MIC of ≥0.16 μg/ml for about 3.1% of strains (Table 28).

The first strain of *N. meningitidis* of reduced susceptibility to penicillin G (MIC, 0.25 μg/ml) was isolated in North Carolina in 1992. A survey undertaken in 1991 by the Centers for Disease Control and Prevention (CDC) yielded 80 strains, 3 of which were of reduced susceptibility to penicillin G (MIC, 0.125 μg/ml). Chloramphenicol-resistant strains have been described.

In a SENTRY program carried out in the United States from 1998 to 1999, all of the isolates were susceptible to ciprofloxacin and cefotaxime and 54.7% were susceptible to co-trimoxazole. One strain was resistant to rifampin (MIC, >32 μg/ml), and 30.2% were intermediately susceptible to penicillin G.

Resistance to chloramphenicol was reported in Vietnam. In France, resistance was mediated by a chloramphenicol acetyltransferase encoded by the *catP* gene and described first for meningococcal serogroup B isolates.

Rifampin resistance is a rare occurrence. In 1997 in the United States, the rate of rifampin resistance among *N. meningitidis* strains was 3% (MIC, ≥ 8.0 μg/ml). High-level resistance to rifampin is mediated by a mutation in the β-subunit of *ropB*, and a low-level resistance is mediated by a decrease in membrane permeability. Mutations in the *ropB* gene affect two amino acids: Asp542 → Val and His552 → Tyr or Asn.

The *tet*(M) gene confers resistance to tetracyclines.

10. *ENTEROBACTERIACEAE*

10.1. Antibacterial Resistance

10.1.1. β-Lactams

An epidemiological study showed that the resistance rates of gram-negative bacilli are identical in northern and southern Europe. Resistance to ampicillin and piperacillin in northern Europe increased from 8% in 1984 to 26 and 28% in 1987 and 1989, respectively. In central Europe, the resistance rates were 18 and 16% in 1984 and 28 and 26% in 1987 and 1988. In southern Europe, the levels of resistance were 13 and 10% in 1984, compared with 46 and 38% in 1987 and 1988. About 13% of *E. coli* strains and 50% of *P. mirabilis* strains in Korea are susceptible to ampicillin.

The prevalence of resistance to β-lactams among *E. coli* isolates was studied in Porto, Portugal, between 1988 and 1990. A total of 2,036 strains of *E. coli* were collected; the susceptibilities of these strains are summarized in Table 29.

For the 1,126 strains resistant to ampicillin, the production of different β-lactamases was measured: results are shown in Table 30.

Other relatively uncommon enzymes have been identified, such as HMS-1 (0.2%) and OXA-1 (1.5%).

In a survey undertaken by the Hellenic Chemotherapy Society between November 1987 and January 1988 in 19 hospitals in Greece, it was shown that the prevalence of ampicillin-resistant strains of *E. coli* ranged from 42 to 100%, the prevalence of gentamicin-resistant strains was 0 to 35%, and the prevalence of amikacin-resistant strains was 0 to 20% (Table 31).

In an epidemiological study conducted in two university centers in Nigeria between 1987 and 1988, *Enterobacteriaceae* were shown to be very resistant to ampicillin, tetracyclines, chloramphenicol, and co-trimoxazole. The principal species of *Enterobacteriaceae* isolated were *E. coli*, *K. pneumoniae*, and *Proteus* spp. The resistance to gentamicin was high among isolates of *K. pneumoniae* and *Proteus* spp. (Table 32).

Table 29 Susceptibilities to β-lactams of *E. coli* strains isolated in Portugal

Drug	Prevalence of resistance (%)
Ampicillin	55.3
Co-amoxiclav	3.5
Carbenicillin	52.8
Cefoxitin	3.2
Cefotaxime	0.5

Table 30 β-Lactamases isolated from strains of *E. coli* in Portugal

β-Lactamase	Enzymatic prevalence (%)
TEM-1	78.2
SHV-1	7.9
TEM-2	0.5
AmpC	4.7
TEM-6	0.9

Between 1983 and 1989, 520 strains of *E. coli* were isolated from blood cultures in Turku, Finland. The resistance to ampicillin (MIC, ≥16 μg/ml) increased from 33% in 1983 to 66% in 1987 and declined slightly to 44% during the period from 1988 to 1989. This reduction was also found with strains for which the MIC of ampicillin was ≥32 μg/ml.

The isolation of TEM-1-producing strains did not increase proportionally, representing 14% in 1983 and rising to 25% in 1989. Among the β-lactamases produced, TEM-1 was the most frequent, followed by OXA-1 and OXA-2. The majority of TEM-1-producing strains (MIC, ≥32 μg/ml) were also resistant to piperacillin but remained susceptible to cefuroxime. Among these strains, 14 produced chromosomal-type enzymes, including two strains resistant to ceftazidime. Twenty-six strains were resistant to ampicillin through a nonenzymatic mechanism.

The proportion of isolated strains for which the MICs of piperacillin were ≥16 μg/ml increased from 10 to 16% between 1983 and 1986 to 22 to 28% between 1987 and 1989. Two strains were resistant to ceftazidime (MIC, 32 μg/ml) and of reduced susceptibility to cefotaxime (MIC, 1 μg/ml). All of the other strains were susceptible to cefotaxime.

In an epidemiological survey undertaken in Korea in 1991, it was shown that resistance to amikacin was minor, while resistance to gentamicin ranged from 0% (*Citrobacter freundii*) to 62% (*Serratia marcescens*). Species resistant to cefotaxime and its derivatives were uncommon. There was

Table 31 Rates of resistance to antibiotics in Greek hospitals in 1988

Drug	Prevalence of resistance (%)				
	E. coli	*Klebsiella* spp.	*Enterobacter* spp.	*Proteus* spp.	*Serratia* spp.
Ampicillin	52	85	898	59	85
Cefotaxime	5	18	63	7	31
Ceftazidime	5	20	30	5	19
Aztreonam	3	12	19	7	17
Imipenem	0	2	3	2	3
Gentamicin	8	32	35	16	20
Amikacin	7	21	32	8	25
Norfloxacin	2	5	11	3	0

Table 32 Susceptibilities of *Enterobacteriaceae* in Nigeria from 1987 to 1998

Drug	Prevalence of resistance (%)		
	E. coli	*Klebsiella* spp.	*Proteus* spp.
Ampicillin	72–79	85–89	69–79
Co-amoxiclav	0	9	50
Cefotaxime	0–4	14–100	5–25
Chloramphenicol	80–100	76–80	100
Ofloxacin	0	2	0
Co-trimoxazole	76–85	93–99	74–88
Gentamicin	0–12	39–79	38–70
Nalidixic acid	6	3	6
Tetracycline	68–85	76–81	91
Streptomycin	40–55	37–76	20–46

cross-resistance between the cephalosporins, such as cefuzonam, cefotaxime, and ceftazidime. Among strains of *Enterobacter cloacae* resistant to cefotaxime, 7% were also resistant to cefepime. Among strains resistant to gentamicin, 6% were also resistant to cefepime, 63% were resistant to cefotaxime, and 91% were resistant to ceftazidime.

A Spanish epidemiological survey undertaken in November 1991 in 14 centers showed that 5.2% of strains were of reduced susceptibility to ofloxacin (MIC, ≥2 to 8 μg/ml). The proportions of such strains among the different species of *Enterobacteriaceae* were, respectively, 8.3, 1.7, 3.8, 5.3, 22.8, 6.8, and 15.8% for *E. coli, K. pneumoniae, C. freundii, E. cloacae, Enterobacter* spp., *P. mirabilis*, and *S. marcescens*. The activity of ofloxacin against strains of *Providencia* spp. was intermediate.

In the Swedish survey undertaken by Olsson et al. (1993), ciprofloxacin was inactive against 1, 7.5, and 6% of strains of *E. coli, K. pneumoniae*, and *E. cloacae*, respectively.

Alonso et al. (1993) in a Spanish multicenter study (November 1991) reported that among 1,411 strains of *Enterobacteriaceae*, cefotaxime had reduced activity against *Enterobacter* spp. and *S. marcescens* (resistance greater than 8%).

An analysis of the β-lactamases isolated showed that among 60 strains for which the MIC was greater than 1 μg/ml, 34 produced class I enzymes and only 5 had extended-spectrum β-lactamases, principally SHV-5 and TEM-9 (*E. coli*). However, overall, 97.2% of strains of *Enterobacteriaceae* isolated remained susceptible to cefotaxime.

In Poland, 90 and 95% of *Enterobacteriaceae* remained susceptible to the so-called second- and third-generation parenteral cephalosporins, respectively. Fewer than 40% of strains of *E. coli* were susceptible to ampicillin and mezlocillin and 50% were susceptible to cyclines, but 90% were susceptible to gentamicin. Of the strains of *K. pneumoniae*, about 75% were susceptible to ureidopenicillins.

In a survey undertaken in 1991 at the Royal London Hospital, Lin et al. showed that the most common β-lactamase among *Enterobacteriaceae* was TEM-1, followed by TEM-2, SHV-1, and oxacillinase-type enzymes. Their frequency has remained stable since 1982. Among *E. coli* strains, TEM-1 represented 43% of enzymes in 1982 and 46% in 1991. However, enzyme production is increasing for *P. mirabilis*, being 5% in 1982 and 22% in 1991. It is apparently declining for *E. cloacae*, falling from 48 to 17% in 1991. On the other hand, constitutive cephalosporinases have been detected in 13.2% of strains of *E. cloacae, Enterobacter aerogenes, C. freundii, Serratia* spp., and *Morganella morganii* and fewer than 1% of strains of *P. aeruginosa*. Strains of *K. pneumoniae* principally produced enzymes of the SHV-1 type, and TEM-1 and TEM-2 equally. A few strains of *Citrobacter diversus* produced TEM-1 and TEM-2. Eleven out of seventy (15.7%) strains of *K. pneumoniae* produced an ESBL of the TEM-10 type.

The first ESBL was described in 1983 in Germany (SHV-2). The ESBLs have arisen as a result of mutations in the structural genes of the TEM-1 and SHV-1 enzymes. ESBL mutants of TEM or SHV have one to six amino acid substitutions.

All new potent β-lactamases have appeared in all four classes of β-lactamases, such as class D ESBLs (mutants of OXA-2 and -10, plasmid AmpC). In class A enzymes, PER enzymes are another type of new ESBLs. PER-1 was first discovered in *P. aeruginosa* from France. PER-2 was found solely in Argentina.

PER-1 in *P. aeruginosa, Acinetobacter*, and *Salmonella* is spread in Turkey. PER-1 hydrolyzes ceftazidime.

Since their discovery in 1983, numerous ESBLs have been described, deriving via one or two mutations from TEM-1 or -2 or SHV-1. More than 100 enzymes of the TEM type have been described, and above 20 have been described for the SHV type. Some are widely distributed and found in numerous countries, such as SHV-2, SHV-4, SHV-5, and TEM-6, while others are more localized, such as TEM-3 in France, TEM-10 and TEM-12 in the United Kingdom and the United States, and TEM-7 in Greece. These differences are probably due to the antibiotic-prescribing habits in the different countries. They usually involve isolates from small epidemics. The species of *Enterobacteriaceae* most commonly producing these enzymes is *K. pneumoniae*. It would appear that some cephalosporins, such as ceftazidime, are more liable to select these mutants. Genes encoding cephalosporinases are incorporated in the plasmids of certain strains of *Klebsiella* and *E. coli* that have become resistant to cephamycins and to clavulanic acid, tazobactam, and sulbactam (MIR-1 β-lactamase). Other enzymes of this type have also been described for *K. pneumoniae* and *E. coli* from an enzyme found in *C. freundii* (CMY-2), *Klebsiella oxytoca* (MEN-1), and *E. cloacae* (BIL-1). This type of strain has been found in France, Greece, and Pakistan. The TRC-1 enzyme, originating from a TEM, hydrolyzes the β-lactamase inhibitors but not the oxyimino cephems. These strains have been isolated in *E. coli* in France, Spain, and Scotland. The in vitro activities of cefotaxime and ceftazidime against different ESBL-producing strains are summarized in Table 33. The number of β-lactamases in the hospital environment has been increasing since the first report, from 13 in 1970 to above 300 today. The CTX-M enzymes are class A plasmid mediated and are able to hydrolyze cefotaxime. CTX-M2 is widely spread in *E. coli, K. pneumoniae*, and *Salmonella* sp. strains in Paraguay, Uruguay, Chile, and Bolivia.

Enzymes of the TEM type confer variable degrees of resistance depending on the compounds, particularly cefotaxime, ceftazidime, and aztreonam, which are phenotypic markers of resistance. The MICs of cefotaxime are moderately high (MIC, 0.06 to 4 μg/ml), except for TEM-3 and TEM-4 strains (MIC, 32 μg/ml). The values are higher for ceftazidime and aztreonam (MIC, 32 μg/ml), except for TEM-11 and TEM-12 strains (4 and 0.25 μg/ml), whereas the SHV-type enzymes yield high MICs for the three compounds (MIC, ≥32 μg/ml).

It has recently been shown that SHV-1 hyperproduction does not affect the activity of cefotaxime (MIC, 0.01 μg/ml),

Table 33 Activities of cefotaxime and ceftazidime against different ESBL-producing strains

β-Lactamase	MIC (μg/ml) of:	
	Cefotaxime	Ceftazidime
TEM-3	16	32
TEM-4	16	32
TEM-5	64	16
TEM-6	128	1
TEM-7	16	0.06
TEM-9	256	1
TEM-10	64	0.5
CAZ-2	128	2
CAZ-3	32	0.5
CAZ-6	512	8
CAZ-10	4	0.03
SHV-2	4	4
SHV-3	4	4
SHV-4	128	32
SHV-5	128	8
FEC-1	12	200
FUR	2	1
BEL-1	64	16

but it does cause a marked reduction in activities of ceftazidime (MIC, 8 μg/ml) and aztreonam (MIC, 2 μg/ml).

The strains producing these enzymes often have low-level resistance (MIC, 4 to 16 μg/ml) which cannot be detected routinely in the clinical microbiological laboratory. Sirot et al. proposed a simple test of synergy between co-amoxiclav and ceftazidime, cefotaxime, and aztreonam. This test may be compromised if the strains produce a large quantity of cephalosporinases, which can mask the ESBLs. Clavulanic acid is delicate, and false-negative results have been obtained when the disk was too old (more than 7 days outside the protective blister). The prevalence of *K. pneumoniae* isolates producing ESBLs was investigated by Thabaut et al. (1990). In their epidemiological surveys, *K. pneumoniae* accounted for 9% of the strains of *Enterobacteriaceae* isolated from among the 20 hospitals included (one month/year—1,774 strains). In 1985, 0.75% of strains possessed this type of enzyme, whereas in 1987 and 1988, the percentages were 8.4 and 11%, respectively. The enzymes concerned were principally TEM-3, SHV-4, and SHV-5. The resistance of *K. pneumoniae* in France was 15.2% in 1990.

In a survey in 1990, the rates of resistance to ampicillin, ticarcillin, and cephalothin were, respectively, 41, 38, and 25% for strains of *E. coli* and 29, 23, and 13% for strains of *P. mirabilis*. In these species, the rates of resistance to cefotaxime were 1.3 and 0.8%, respectively. In the other species of *Enterobacteriaceae* naturally resistant to ampicillin, the activity of cefotaxime varied with the species. Over a 3-year period, the incidence of resistance to cefotaxime increased from 4.7 to 5.7% and then fell to 5.1%. Significant variations were observed among *Serratia*, *Enterobacter*, and *K. pneumoniae*, with a peak in 1990 for *Serratia* spp. (38.7%) and in 1989 for *Enterobacter* spp. (28.5%) and *K. pneumoniae* (14.3%). The prevalence of resistance in *K. pneumoniae* strains ranges from 0 to 47.6% according to the hospital. In addition, the highest prevalence of resistant strains has been found in ICU (30.6%).

In a study undertaken between January 1988 and August 1989 in the Clermont Ferrand university hospital, 267 strains of ESBL-producing *Enterobacteriaceae* were isolated. The three most common enzymes were TEM-3, CAZ-5, and CAZ-6. The species of *Enterobacteriaceae* involved are listed in Table 34.

Table 34 Distribution of ESBLs according to species of *Enterobacteriaceae*

TEM-3	CAZ-5	CAZ-6
K. pneumoniae	*K. pneumoniae*	*K. pneumoniae*
E. aerogenes		*E. aerogenes*
K. oxytoca		
S. marcescens		*S. marcescens*
E. coli		*E. coli*
E. cloacae		*E. cloacae*
C. freundii		

These strains were found principally in ICU (53.5%), on surgical wards (27.5%), and on medical wards (19%), and chiefly in the urine (43 to 57.4%). Among strains of *K. pneumoniae*, 85% were resistant to all aminoglycosides except for gentamicin and 15% were resistant to all aminoglycosides. The CAZ-6 enzyme was isolated principally from *E. aerogenes*, strains of which were also resistant to aminoglycosides except for gentamicin.

Among the CAZ-5-producing strains, 96% were resistant to all aminoglycosides and 100% were resistant to chloramphenicol, trimethoprim, and fluoroquinolones.

Ciprofloxacin is more slowly bactericidal (18 versus 4 h) against TEM-3-producing strains of *K. pneumoniae*. For these strains, the MIC of cefotaxime is between 2 and 16 μg/ml.

The SHV-4-producing strains of *K. pneumoniae* are resistant to all β-lactams except for cephamycins and imipenem, aminoglycosides except for gentamicin, co-trimoxazole, tetracyclines, and fluoroquinolones.

In Greece, Giammarelou et al. (1993) published a report according to which 46% of strains of *K. pneumoniae* were resistant to ceftazidime (TEM-7), 0.5% were resistant to imipenem, 10% were resistant to ciprofloxacin, and between 36 and 55% were resistant to aminoglycosides. The aminoglycosides are relatively inactive against *Enterobacter* spp., strains of which are resistant to gentamicin (43%), netilmicin (66%), and amikacin (51%). The proportions of strains resistant to ceftazidime, imipenem, and ciprofloxacin are, respectively, 67, 4.2, and 13%.

The proportion of strains of *E. coli* resistant to ampicillin ranges from 60% in the Emirate of Brunei to 96% in Vietnam. In Europe, about 25 to 60% of strains of *E. coli* and 10 to 40% of strains of *P. mirabilis* produce β-lactamases.

In Taiwan in 1999, the antibacterial activities of β-lactams against *Enterobacteriaceae* (i.e., nonfermentative gram-negative bacteria) were assessed. Multiresistant *Aeromonas* and *Acinetobacter* spp. were found to be common. In an epidemiological survey conducted in Japan from 1997 to 1998, *Enterobacteriaceae* were collected from six centers and tested for their susceptibilities to various β-lactams.

Tables 35 and 36 show rates of resistance among gram-negative bacteria in Taiwan in 1999 and in Japan in 1997, respectively.

10.1.2. Fluoroquinolones

An epidemiological survey undertaken in Europe demonstrated that resistance to nalidixic acid taken as a marker remained stable between 1975 and 1986. The incidence of resistant strains has changed little from the introduction of

Table 35 Prevalence of resistance in gram-negative bacteria in Taiwan in 1999 ($N = 60$)

Organism(s)	Prevalence of resistance (%)[a]				
	PIP-TZB	CRO	CAZ	CPO	IMP
E. coli	1.7	16.7	16.7	8.3	0
Klebsiella spp.	3.3	21.7	21.7	67	21.7
Citrobacter spp.	19.3	45	43.3	16.7	1.7
Enterobacter spp.	20	35	38.3	13.3	1.7
Proteus spp.	0	8.3	1.7	0	8.3
Serratia spp.	20	50	8.3	31.7	17
Acinetobacter spp.	53.3	81.7	50	31	33
P. aeruginosa	28.3	28.3	10	30	67

[a]PIP-TZB; piperacillin-tazobactam; CRO, ceftriaxone; CAZ, ceftazidime; CPO, cefpirome; IMP, imipenem.

norfloxacin in 1984 and ofloxacin in 1986. However, the activity of fluoroquinolones varies with the centers. For example, the proportions of resistant strains are less than 1% in Hamburg, Germany, and 8.3% in Innsbruck, Austria. Likewise, there is a difference among the species of *Enterobacteriaceae*, with 1% resistant strains among salmonellae and about 8% resistant strains among *K. pneumoniae* strains. Wiedmann et al. in 1989 showed that the level of resistance to fluoroquinolones remained low, but activity against the different bacterial species was decreasing progressively. For example, the MICs of enoxacin were 2 μg/ml in 1983 and 4 μg/ml in 1986. The percentage of resistant strains (MIC, >4 μg/ml) increased from 1.7 to 6% in 3 years. The same applied to strains of reduced susceptibility (MIC, 2 to 4 μg/ml), which increased from 7.6 to 12.6%. A similar phenomenon has been observed with ofloxacin and ciprofloxacin. Acar et al. observed the same phenomenon with difficult-to-treat *Enterobacteriaceae*, such as *E. cloacae*, *S. marcescens*, and *C. freundii*.

Grüneberg et al. (1993) showed that the activity of ciprofloxacin decreased against bacteria isolated from urinary tract infections, falling from 96.1 to 89.9% for isolates from outpatients between 1987 and 1992 and from 89.8 to 79.8% for inpatients over the same period.

In China, strains of *Enterobacteriaceae* resistant to norfloxacin or ofloxacin were demonstrated in 1992 (Table 37).

Surveys undertaken simultaneously in Canada and the United States showed that strains of *Enterobacteriaceae* resistant to fluoroquinolones (ciprofloxacin and ofloxacin)

Table 37 Activities of fluoroquinolones in China

Organism(s)	*n*	% of strains resistant to:	
		Norfloxacin	Ofloxacin
E. coli	1,901	29	35
K. pneumoniae	788	11	12
E. aerogenes	329	18	22
E. cloacae	379	27	30
P. mirabilis	169	17	17
Proteus vulgaris	49	3	3
Providencia spp.	80	18	18
M. morganii	43	19	8
C. freundii	161	25	21
S. marcescens	124	16	9
Salmonella serovar Typhi	206	1	0
Salmonella spp.	115	1	0

Table 36 Prevalence of resistance among *Enterobacteriaceae* in Japan (1997)

Organism(s)	*n*	Prevalence of resistance (%)[a]		
		CAZ	CPO	IMP
E. coli	210	8.1	0.5	0.5
Klebsiella spp.	219	5.0	0.5	0
Citrobacter spp.	192	23.4	2.6	5.5
Enterobacter spp.	208	25	4.3	0.5
Proteus spp.	200	3.5	0.5	2.5
Serratia spp.	206	6.8	6.8	4.6
Acinetobacter spp.	200	7.0	6.5	4.5
P. aeruginosa	219	15.1	9.6	19.6

[a]CAZ, ceftazidime; CPO, cefpirome; IMP, imipenem.

were infrequent. The most resistant species are *K. pneumoniae* (3 to 11%), *S. marcescens* (7 to 10%), and *Providencia stuartii* (~8%) (Table 38).

Increasing numbers of ciprofloxacin-resistant strains of *E. coli* are being reported.

10.1.3. Carbapenems

A survey conducted in the United States between 1991 and 1992 by C. Thornsberry's team into the activity of imipenem showed that levels of resistance were still low but that among *Proteus* spp., *Providencia* spp., and *M. morganii*, the levels of reduced-susceptibility or resistant strains were not negligible and overall reached 8.7 and 7.1% for *Proteus* spp. and *Providencia* spp., respectively. The activity of imipenem against these bacterial species is summarized in Table 39.

The activity of imipenem overall is good against *E. coli* and *K. pneumoniae*, with a resistance rate of 0.6%. The frequencies of imipenem-resistant strains of *Aeromonas hydrophila*, *Campylobacter jejuni*, and *S. marcescens* were, respectively, 18.6, 9.5, and 4.8%. The mechanisms of resistance are complex.

10.1.4. Aminoglycosides

The resistance of bacteria to aminoglycosides is due either to a modification of the ribosomal target (e.g., streptomycin) or to inactivating enzymes or to a modification of membrane permeability. Modifications of aminoglycosides by inactivating enzymes are one of the principal causes of resistance in *Enterobacteriaceae*. A number of inactivation sites are present on the gentamicin and kanamycin molecules (Fig. 6). There are three types of inactivating enzymes: *O*-acetyltransferases (AAC), *O*-adenyltransferases (ANT), and *O*-phosphotransferases

Table 38 Activities of fluoroquinolones in North America in 1993

Organism	Prevalence of resistance (%) in:	
	The United States[a]	Canada[b]
C. freundii	2	
E. cloacae	2	0
K. pneumoniae	11	3
E. coli	0	0
M. morganii	1	0
P. mirabilis	1	0
P. stuartii	8	4
S. marcescens	7	10

[a]Data from Jones et al., 2002.
[b]Data from Hoban et al., 1997.

Table 39 Activity of imipenem in the United States

Organism(s)	*n*	% with decreased susceptibility	% Resistant
Proteus spp.	11,124	4.5	4.2
P. mirabilis	10,195	4.1	3.8
P. vulgaris	728	8.9	7.2
Proteus penneri	113	8.8	16
Providencia spp.	1,505	2.4	4.7
Providencia alcalifaciens	33	3.0	0
P. rettgeri	403	2.5	2.5
Providencia rustigianii	31	6.5	6.4
M. morganii	1,712	7.2	4.0

(APH) (Table 40). There are two types of acetylases (I and II), but several genes may be involved; for example, nine genes code for AAC(6′)-I and two genes code for AAC(6′)-II. Acetylation of the aminoglycosides occurs on the amino groups at positions 3, 2′, and 6′, whereas adenylation occurs principally at 2″-OH and 4′-OH. Phosphorylation of the 3′-OH groups of kanamycin and neomycin is common. Among *Enterobacteriaceae*, some enzymes are more frequent, such as ANT(2″)-I, AAC(3)-II, AAC(2′)-I, AAC(6′)-II, and APH(3′)-I. Others are much less frequent, such as AAC(6′)-I, AAC(3)-I, AAC(3)-III, AAC(3)-IV, AAC(3)-VI, and ANT(4′)-II, except AAC(6′)-I in Japan.

In an epidemiological survey, it was shown that among *Enterobacteriaceae*, multiple mechanisms of resistance are common in *C. freundii* (32%), *Enterobacter* spp. (44.4%), and *Klebsiella* spp. (53.2%). They are less common in *E. coli* (17%), *Morganella* (15.6%), indole-positive *Proteus* (17.5%), and *Salmonella* and *Shigella* spp. (7.1%).

In *Serratia*, the combination of ANT(2″)-I and AAC(6)-I is carried on a plasmid. In Japan, this combination has been

Table 40 Enzymes inactivating aminoglycosides[a]

Enzyme	Substrate(s)
ANTs	
2″	Gentamicin, tobramycin
3″	Streptomycin
4′	Kanamycin, neomycin
—	Streptomycin
9	Spectinomycin
APHs	
2″	Kanamycin, gentamicin
3′(5″)	Tobramycin
3″	Kanamycin, neomycin
4	Streptomycin
6	Hygromycin, streptomycin
AACs	
1	Apramycin, paromomycin
2′	Gentamicin, tobramycin
3	Kanamycin, gentamicin, tobramycin
6	Kanamycin, gentamicin, tobramycin

[a]Data from Davies.

demonstrated in other species of *Enterobacteriaceae*. Other combinations have been described in Europe and the United States, such as AAC(3)-II and AAC(6′)-I. In Europe, the incidence of combinations in strains of *Enterobacteriaceae* resistant to aminoglycosides was 9.9% from 1984 to 1985, rising to 27% from 1987 to 1988. Combinations are common in Latin America (63 to 85%) and Greece and Turkey (81.8%) and less common in France (34%); South Africa (39.8%); North Africa (16.5%); Italy, Portugal, and Spain (18%); and the Asia-Pacific region (25%).

Among the *Enterobacteriaceae*, *Providencia* and *Serratia* possess four genes of plasmid origin [*aac*(3)-IIa, *aac*(3)-Ib, *ant*(2″)-Ia, and *aac* (3)-Ia] and two genes of chromosomal origin [*aac*(2′)-Ia and *aac*(6′)-Ic], respectively. The *aac*(3)-IIa and *ant*(2″)-IIa genes have long been known and confer resistance to gentamicin, tobramycin, and netilmicin and to

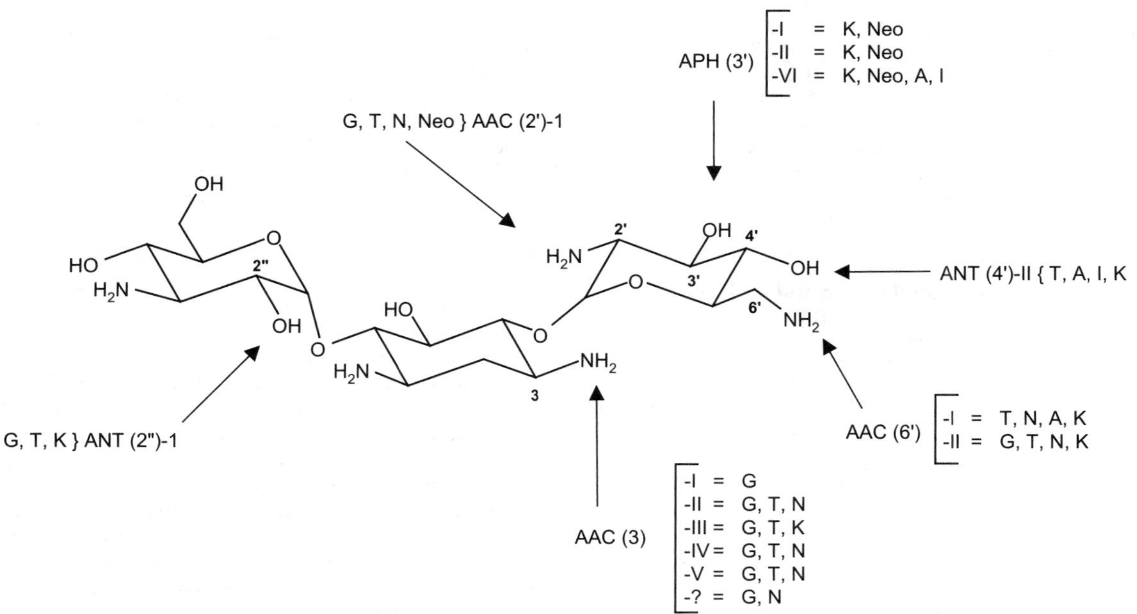

Figure 6 Inactivation sites of aminoglycosides

Table 41 Activities of aminoglycosides in Slovakia

Organism(s)	Prevalence of resistance (%)		
	1990	1991	1992
E. coli	4.5	8.9	8.6
Citrobacter spp.	9.1	15.7	8.3
Klebsiella spp.	0.9	4.0	2.3
Enterobacter spp.	16.1	12.3	6.2
M. morganii		4.8	7.9
P. mirabilis		0.7	0.4
P. rettgeri		2.9	0
S. marcescens		8.7	26.9

gentamicin and tobramycin, respectively. For some years now, an increase has been noted in the presence of the *aac*(6′)-Ib gene, which is responsible for resistance to tobramycin, netilmicin, and amikacin. This gene is rarely alone and is usually associated with other genes that confer resistance to gentamicin. This suggests that this type of resistance appeared in response to pressure of selection. There is a high incidence of the *aac*(6′)-Ib gene in regions in which resistance to aminoglycosides was already high and in which the type of aminoglycosides prescribed changed most, such as Greece, Turkey, Latin America, South Africa, and France.

In Slovakia between 1990 and 1992, the number of strains of *Enterobacteriaceae* resistant to amikacin was stable except for *S. marcescens*, the level of resistance of which increased from 8.7% in 1991 to 26.9% in 1992 (Table 41).

Overall, the rate of resistance to aminoglycosides among *Enterobacteriaceae* is 7% in Slovakia. This is greater than that observed in Germany or Switzerland but is similar to that in Austria, France, Spain, and Portugal.

A survey of the prevalence of strains of gram-negative bacilli and gram-positive cocci resistant to aminoglycosides undertaken by the Paul Ehrlich Society in West Germany, Austria, and Switzerland between 1983 and 1985 showed a low level of resistance to amikacin and an intermediate level of resistance to gentamicin, particularly for *Serratia* spp. (20%) and *Citrobacter* spp. (12%) (Table 42).

A survey conducted in Japan in 1982 showed that 15.3 and 22.4% of strains of *Enterobacteriaceae* were resistant to amikacin and arbekacin, respectively. The proportions of strains of indole-positive *Proteus* resistant to amikacin, arbekacin, and astromicin were, respectively, 16, 5.5, and 4%.

The enzymes most commonly produced by strains of *Enterobacteriaceae* resistant to aminoglycosides are AAC(6′), AAC(2′), and ANT(2″).

Table 42 Resistance to gentamicin and amikacin in 7,500 strains between 1983 and 1985[a]

Organism(s)	Prevalence of resistance (%)	
	Gentamicin	Amikacin
E. coli	1	2
Citrobacter spp.	12	0
Enterobacter spp.	4	1
Klebsiella spp.	3	1
Serratia spp.	21	4
P. mirabilis	4	6
P. aeruginosa	15	2

[a]Data from Naber et al., 1990.

10.1.5. Erythromycin A

The use of erythromycin A in the treatment of traveler's diarrhea or in selective decontamination of the digestive tract allowed the emergence of strains of *E. coli* producing hydrolyzing (esterases) or inactivating (2′-phosphotransferase) enzymes by phosphorylation of the 2′-hydroxyl group of the D-desosamine sugar.

10.2. *Shigella* spp.

Shigellosis represents one of the major causes of dysentery of bacterial origin. Dysentery of bacterial origin is one of the principal causes of morbidity and mortality in the world, mainly in the developing countries. There are about 40 serotypes of *Shigella*, pooled in four serogroups: serogroup A (*Shigella dysenteriae*), serogroup B (*Shigella flexneri*), serogroup C (*Shigella boydii*), and serogroup D (*Shigella sonnei*).

Shigelloses evolve in epidemic cycles. One serotype is dominant for several years and is then replaced by another. For example, in the former Yugoslavia, *S. flexneri* serotype 6 became dominant from 1969, whereas it had been absent before that date. In the 1960s in Kenya, *S. flexneri* serotype 2 was dominant, but it was replaced in 1969 by *S. flexneri* serotype 6. The same applies to the serogroups. At the beginning of the century, *S. dysenteriae* type 1 (*Shigella shigae*) was predominant but was replaced by *S. flexneri,* while for some years now *S. sonnei* has predominated. In the United States, western Europe, and Japan, about 70% of *Shigella* isolates are strains of *S. sonnei* and 30% are strains of *S. flexneri*. This modification has been attributed to better hygiene and socioeconomic conditions. Transmission occurs via food and water, particularly in developing countries (*S. flexneri*) and by interhuman contamination with the highly virulent species (<200 infecting units—*S. sonnei*), which play an important role in industrialized countries with high levels of hygiene. The overall reduction in shigellosis in Japan, Europe, and the United States since the end of the Second World War is due to the improvement in standards of hygiene. Humans are the reservoir, and carriage is about 1 month if no antibiotic therapy is administered to the patient.

Each year, five million to six million deaths occur worldwide among three billion to five billion cases of diarrhea. In developing countries, 45% of cases of diarrhea originate from infection with shigellae or other bacteria.

Oral rehydration is the main symptomatic medication (toxin response), but because of the enteroinvasiveness of shigellae, antibacterial treatment is necessary. Antibiotic treatment reduces the duration of the clinical signs, including diarrhea, and sterilizes the stools, thus breaking the epidemiological chain. In fact, in moderately severe cases of shigellosis, spontaneous resolution of the clinical symptoms occurs in 5 to 7 days.

Retrospective studies in Bangladesh have shown that mortality is higher in *S. sonnei* (10.3%) and *S. dysenteriae* type 1 (6.7%) infections than in the other shigelloses. Shigellosis is a major cause of infant mortality in Bangladesh (9.1%).

Cyclines constituted the first treatment of shigellosis. Local antibiotics such as neomycin are not good medications, as they act only on the intestinal lumen and do not penetrate the intestinal cells.

The recommended treatment currently is co-trimoxazole for 3 days. The emergence of multiresistant strains in Southeast Asia, Africa, and South America has entailed the use, at least in adults, of fluoroquinolones over a period of 3 to 5 days as first-line treatment, in view of the fact that strains resistant to nalidixic acid and, more recently, pefloxacin and enoxacin have been described on the Indian subcontinent. The number of multiresistant strains is increasing regularly. The introduction of a new antibacterial agent is very rapidly followed by the isolation of a clone resistant to the agent.

In North America, strains of *Shigella* resistant to trimethoprim were isolated between 1977 and 1978. Such strains were detected throughout Europe in 1981.

In 1937, *S. sonnei* replaced *S. flexneri* in the United Kingdom. In The Netherlands, following an epidemic of diarrhea due to *S. flexneri* type 2 occurring in December 1983 in a retirement home after the consumption of a salad of deep-frozen prawns from Thailand, the health authorities demanded an inquiry into the prevalence of *Shigella* in their country. Between 1984 and 1989, 3,313 strains of *Shigella* were isolated. The origins of the patients were as follows: indigenous (35%), North African (20%), Middle Eastern (15%), and Southeast Asian (20%). Among the strains isolated, 27.7% were susceptible to all antibiotics. More than half of the strains of *S. flexneri* were multiresistant (ampicillin, chloramphenicol, sulfamethoxazole, and streptomycin). Trimethoprim and co-trimoxazole were inactive against 8 to 25% of strains of *S. flexneri* and 16 to 46% of strains of *S. sonnei*. Four strains of *S. flexneri* were resistant to ampicillin, chloramphenicol, tetracyclines, trimethoprim, sulfamethoxazole, and nalidixic acid. These strains were of reduced susceptibility to norfloxacin.

A study undertaken in Bulgaria between 1973 and 1987 enabled the profiles of susceptibility of 17,126 *S. sonnei* strains to antibacterial agents to be analyzed.

More than 84.3% of the strains were resistant to at least one antibiotic. The strains were most often resistant to, in descending order, tetracyclines, sulfonamides, chloramphenicol, ampicillin, and trimethoprim. From 1973, the number of multiresistant strains increased regularly from 46.8% to reach 72.6% in 1977. After 1981, 79 to 90% of strains were multiresistant. Between 1973 and 1977 there was a predominance of strains with a resistance to tetracyclines only; the percentage of strains resistant to ampicillin was low (1.2%) but increased markedly from 1983, reaching 68.9% in 1987. The level of resistance to chloramphenicol remained stable at 21.6%. Between 1978 and 1982, isolated strains had a combined resistance to tetracyclines, sulfonamides, and streptomycin. The majority of strains became multiresistant from 1983 onwards. The first trimethoprim-resistant strains were isolated from 1980 onwards. Prior to 1987, the proportion of strains resistant to trimethoprim was 20%, rising to 43% in 1987.

In Poland, all strains of *S. sonnei* isolated remain susceptible to chloramphenicol, but more than 50% are resistant to ampicillin and 40% are resistant to co-trimoxazole, whereas 96.8% are susceptible to nalidixic acid.

In Germany, a study conducted between 1989 and 1990 showed that indigenous shigellosis was divided equally between *S. flexneri* and *S. sonnei*. Conversely, imported shigellosis was due predominantly to *S. flexneri* (44%), followed by *S. sonnei* (39.2%), *S. dysenteriae* (10.5%), and *S. boydii* (6.3%). A total of 81.2% of strains were resistant to at least one antibiotic, but the incidence was higher for imported strains (93.5%) than for native strains (62.7%). The majority of strains were multiresistant.

In China, the majority of strains of *S. sonnei* and *S. flexneri* are susceptible to fluoroquinolones, with fewer than 5% of strains being resistant.

In Taiwan, the first strain of multiresistant *S. flexneri* was described in 1976. A modification of the *S. flexneri* serotypes was noted between the study undertaken in 1976 and that conducted between 1982 and 1987. The distribution of serotypes differed; in 1976, serotype 2a was dominant, whereas between 1982 and 1987 the distribution was less homogeneous, with 1a and 1b accounting for 27.3% and serotypes 2a and 2b accounting for 6.23% of *S. flexneri* isolates. In addition, the *S. sonnei* serogroup took over from and gradually replaced the *S. flexneri* serogroup (Table 43).

In the study conducted between 1983 and 1987, the dominant serotypes were *S. sonnei* 1 (29%) and *S. flexneri* 1 (27%). Among these isolates, 80% of strains were resistant to tetracyclines, 87% were resistant to chloramphenicol, 84% were resistant to streptomycin, 52% were resistant to ampicillin, 25% were resistant to nalidixic acid, and 10% were resistant to co-trimoxazole. Among multiresistant strains, the predominant phenotype comprised simultaneous resistance to ampicillin, streptomycin, chloramphenicol, and tetracyclines (28%). These strains possess a transmissible plasmid of 45 to 75 MDa.

The survey undertaken in Malaysia between 1980 and 1981 showed that 80% of strains of *S. flexneri* were resistant to ampicillin, chloramphenicol, tetracyclines, and sulfonamides and 50% were resistant to co-trimoxazole.

In Thailand, two epidemiological surveys showed that *S. flexneri* was the predominant serogroup. The prevalence of shigellosis among diarrheal diseases is on the increase, being 6.1% in 1984 and 17.1% from 1987 to 1988. *Table 44* shows the incidence of *Shigella* serogroups in Thailand from 1984 to 1988.

The number of strains resistant to ampicillin and chloramphenicol is high. The number of strains resistant to co-trimoxazole increased from 25% in 1985 to 81% in 1988 (Table 45).

In the second study, *S. flexneri* was also highly resistant to ampicillin (98%) and co-trimoxazole (88%). *S. boydii* is more susceptible to antibiotics (Table 46).

S. flexneri and *S. sonnei* are nonsusceptible to the action of co-trimoxazole through dual resistance to trimethoprim and sulfamethoxazole. Among these strains, 32% possess a plasmid, the genes of which code for the hyperproduction of type II dihydropteroate synthase (which the majority of strains of

Table 43 Incidence of different *Shigella* species in Taiwan

Organism	% of *Shigella* population	
	1976	1982–1987
S. flexneri	73.1	41
S. dysenteriae	1.6	3
S. sonnei	22.2	47
S. boydii	3.2	9

Table 44 Incidence of different serogroups of *Shigella* spp. in Thailand

Serogroup	% of *Shigella* population	
	1984–1988	1988
S. flexneri	83.5	82.8
S. dysenteriae	15.2	12
S. sonnei	0.9	2.1
S. boydii	0.4	3.0

Table 45 Resistance of *S. flexneri* in Thailand

Drug	Prevalence of resistance (%)				
	1984	1985	1986	1987	1988
Ampicillin	95.7	96.3	92.8	87.5	89.9
Chloramphenicol	96.1	100	90	87.2	91.7
Co-trimoxazole	31	25	57.1	65	80.9
Tetracycline			60		
Nalidixic acid	0	0	0	0	0

Enterobacteriaceae in Thailand possess) and 13% of strains have a gene coding for hyperproduction of type I DHFR.

In Hong Kong and Korea, the *S. flexneri* serogroup is predominant, with a high level of resistance to ampicillin, chloramphenicol, tetracyclines, and co-trimoxazole. In Korea, shigellae account for 1.7% of strains isolated from fecal cultures from diarrheal patients.

In Japan (survey published in 1993), shigellae remained an important cause of diarrhea. Up until 1982, the predominant serogroup was *S. flexneri*. In 1982, *S. flexneri* and *S. sonnei* were equally distributed. In 1988, 40% of isolates were *S. flexneri* and about 60% were *S. sonnei*. The other serogroups represented less than 1% of isolates. About 80% of strains were resistant to tetracyclines, 60% were resistant to co-trimoxazole, 50% were resistant to ampicillin and chloramphenicol, 20% were resistant to nalidixic acid, and a few strains were resistant to norfloxacin.

In Bangladesh two studies showed the predominance of *S. flexneri*, which accounted for between 50 and 60% of isolates, followed by *S. dysenteriae* type 1 (~30%) (Table 47).

The strains of *S. flexneri* and *S. dysenteriae* type 1 are multiresistant, and in the case of the latter species, 69% are resistant to nalidixic acid. The first *S. dysenteriae* strains resistant to nalidixic acid were reported in 1987. Strains of *S. dysenteriae* were particularly resistant to ampicillin (99%), co-trimoxazole (96%), nalidixic acid (69%), and amdinocillin (1%). Chloramphenicol and the cyclines were also relatively inactive.

In India the first epidemic of shigellosis due to multiresistant microorganisms (ampicillin, chloramphenicol, and co-trimoxazole) was described in 1972. Multiresistant strains have been present in India endemically since 1978. A survey undertaken in the region of Vallore between 1989 and 1990 showed that *S. flexneri* was predominant (64.2%), followed by *S. sonnei* (14.8%), *S. boydii* (7.4%), *S. dysenteriae* type 1 (4%), and other serotypes of *S. dysenteriae* (9.7%).

Strains resistant to nalidixic acid have been described since 1987. In the 1989–1990 Vallore study, a strain of *S. dysenteriae* type 1 was resistant to nalidixic acid, pefloxacin, and enoxacin but remained susceptible to the action of ciprofloxacin and ofloxacin. Five strains of *S. flexneri* were resistant to nalidixic acid, and of these, three were resistant to pefloxacin and enoxacin but remained susceptible to ciprofloxacin and ofloxacin. However, the activity of ciprofloxacin was reduced 100-fold (MIC from 0.005 μg/ml to 0.32 μg/ml) and that of ofloxacin was reduced 200-fold (MIC from 0.08 μg/ml to 0.64 μg/ml).

A survey undertaken in Djibouti showed that the incidence of shigellosis in patients with diarrhea was 7.9% and that the *S. flexneri* serogroup was dominant, followed by *S. dysenteriae* type 1 and *S. boydii* equally. In 1989, the rates of resistance to antibiotics were, respectively, 31, 25, 6, and 31% for ampicillin, chloramphenicol, tetracyclines, and co-trimoxazole. All strains were susceptible to nalidixic acid and norfloxacin.

In Saudi Arabia, a retrospective survey between 1985 and 1988 showed that overall, *S. flexneri* and *S. sonnei* accounted for 44 and 43% of isolates, respectively. *S. boydii* represented 10% of isolates and the remainder were *S. dysenteriae*, the serogroup principally imported by workers returning to the country. Among these strains, 80% were resistant to at least two antibiotics. It was found that 54, 72, 77, 53, and 11% of strains were resistant to ampicillin, co-trimoxazole, tetracyclines, chloramphenicol, and piperacillin, respectively.

The serogroup most commonly isolated since 1989 to 1990 is *S. sonnei*.

In Kuwait, the *S. flexneri* serogroup is predominant, followed by *S. sonnei*.

Type 1 *S. dysenteriae* was practically absent from Central America between 1920 and 1969. In 1969, an epidemic with this serogroup was declared in Guatemala. Prior to 1987 all strains of *S. flexneri* 1 and 2 and *S. sonnei* had been susceptible to co-trimoxazole in Guatemala, but the first co-trimoxazole-resistant strain was described in November 1987, and by 1989 29% of strains had become resistant to co-trimoxazole. The strains of *S. flexneri* 6 most commonly isolated were not resistant to co-trimoxazole, and likewise those of *S. sonnei*. These resistant strains were also resistant to chloramphenicol, tetracycline (11 to 13%), and ampicillin (14%). It was found that 3 and 5% of *S. dysenteriae* strains were resistant to tetracyclines and co-trimoxazole, respectively, but susceptible to ampicillin and chloramphenicol. There

Table 46 Resistance of different serogroups of *Shigella* to antibiotics in Thailand

Serogroup	Prevalence of resistance (%)				
	Ampicillin	Chloramphenicol	Cyclines	Co-trimoxazole	Nalidixic acid
S. flexneri	98	99	98	88	0
S. sonnei	44	45	96	72	1
S. boydii	18	42	85	27	0
S. dysenteriae	22	74	91	70	0

Table 47 Incidence of different serogroups of *Shigella* in Bangladesh

Serogroup	Incidence (%)	
	1988	1989
S. flexneri	61.3	53
S. dysenteriae type 1	22.7	31
S. dysenteriae types 2–10	3.8	3
S. boydii	7.6	8
S. sonnei	4.6	5

were few strains of *S. boydii* resistant to co-trimoxazole, ampicillin, and the cyclines—on the order of 2%—and no multiple resistance was noted.

In Brazil, in an epidemiological survey of the prevalence of different pathogenic agents responsible for diarrhea, shigellae were involved in only 5% of cases.

In Nigeria, a survey undertaken between 1984 and 1986 showed that *S. flexneri* was the most common serogroup (68%), followed by *S. sonnei* (23%). A few strains of *S. dysenteriae* were isolated, but no strain of *S. boydii*. Only 48.2% of strains isolated were susceptible to the five antibiotics tested: streptomycin, chloramphenicol, tetracyclines, ampicillin, and sulfonamide. A total of 39.2% were resistant to more than three antibiotics, and 16% of strains were resistant to the five antibiotics.

In Rwanda, cholera has been rife endemically since 1978, with an epidemic episode in 1987. *Vibrio cholerae* represents 34.4% of isolates from fecal cultures, whereas shigellae account for 35.3% and salmonellae account for 7.2%. The strains of *Shigella* are highly resistant to co-trimoxazole, and marked resistance to nalidixic acid has existed since 1985.

In Sudan and Somalia, the strains of *Shigella* are resistant to co-trimoxazole.

10.3. *Salmonella* spp.

In recent years, developed countries have seen significant increases in the occurrence of food-borne pathogens such as *Salmonella* spp., *Campylobacter* spp., and *E. coli* O157 (verocytotoxin-producing *E. coli*). In the same period, these nations have experienced an increase in *Salmonella* isolates with resistance, such as *Salmonella enterica* serotypes Typhimurium and Wien. Table 48 shows the incidence of salmonellae in food.

All *Salmonella* spp. can cause bloodstream infections; the main invasive organisms are *S. enterica* serotypes Typhi, Paratyphi, Choleraesuis, and Dublin.

The mortality associated with bloodstream infections remains high for about 25% of patients. *Salmonella* bacteremia is difficult to treat and may be the initial manifestation of an underlying disease, such as AIDS.

In an epidemiological survey in France, the two most frequent *Salmonella* serovars, in 1994 and 1997, from the hospital network were serovar Typhimurium and *S. enterica* serovar Enteritidis. In 1997, *S. enterica* serovar Hadar appeared to be somewhat more frequent than serovar Enteritidis. It has been the third most frequent serovar in France since 1997.

Emergence of *Salmonella* resistance to antibacterials is a public health concern for humans and animals (e.g., cattle, pigs, and poultry).

Serovar typhimurium DT 104 started to be seen worldwide in 1994.

10.3.1. *S. enterica* Serotype Typhi

Throughout the world some 12 million cases of typhoid fever can be identified annually, corresponding to an incidence of 100 to 1,500 cases per 10^5 inhabitants, depending on the country. Epidemiologically, it is possible to divide the world into three zones. The zones of endemicity are made up of the countries of Southeast Asia, Latin America, Africa, and certain parts of China. The zones of pseudoendemicity include the Middle East and in particular the countries of the Persian Gulf. One-third to one-half of the populations of the Persian Gulf are expatriates originating from the Indian subcontinent. The size of these populations and the flows between the countries and those of the Gulf contribute to the persistence of a stable pseudoendemic state. About 70 to 80% of cases of typhoid fever diagnosed in Bahrain, Kuwait, and Qatar are imported, and 3 to 30% are due to resistant strains. The nonendemicity zones include the industrialized countries. The risks in the United States are associated with travel to the Indian subcontinent, Peru, and Mexico, with an incidence of 58 to 174 cases per 10^6 travelers.

Between 1940 and 1970, the annual incidence of typhoid fever in the United States declined progressively from 75 to 1.7 per 10^6 inhabitants. Between 1970 and 1978, with the exception of one outbreak, the number of annual cases was 350 to 400. A slight increase in incidence in 1978 was noted, with 2.4 per 10^6 inhabitants. By way of example, out of 1,431 cases of typhoid fever between 1977 and 1979, 38% were acquired in the United States and 62% were acquired abroad.

The introduction of chloramphenicol in 1948 had instituted a new era in the treatment of typhoid fever. Treatment with chloramphenicol held sway for more than 50 years and has transformed the prognosis for the disease, which used to be fatal for more than 20% of patients. The emergence of chloramphenicol-resistant strains and the poor bone marrow tolerance, however, required the adoption of a therapeutic alternative. Ampicillin, although less active, and subsequently co-trimoxazole have been widely used.

Table 48 Incidence of salmonellae in food

Source	No. of strains isolated	*S. enterica* serovar	Incidence (%)
Poultry	137	Hadar	40
		Enteritidis	34
Eggs	54	Enteritidis	72
Milk	34	Typhimurium	59
Pork	22	Typhimurium	34
Other	25	Other	Significant

Table 49 Activities of agents against *S. enterica* serovar Typhi in India

Drug	% of organisms with indicated resistance phenotype		
	Susceptible	Intermediate	Resistant
Ampicillin	19.4	31.4	48.3
Chloramphenicol	18.3	3.4	78.3
Trimethoprim	10.8	0	89.1
Sulfamethoxazole	10.8	0	89.1
Ciprofloxacin	100	0	0

The first chloramphenicol-resistant strain was isolated in 1950 in the United Kingdom, 2 years after the first use of chloramphenicol in the treatment of typhoid fever. In rapid succession, chloramphenicol-resistant strains were described on the Indian subcontinent (India, Pakistan, and Bangladesh) and in Nigeria, Greece, Israel, Latin America, and Southeast Asia (Thailand, Vietnam, Indonesia, etc.). In Vietnam, more than 80% of strains have become resistant to chloramphenicol. Several studies show that the nonuse of chloramphenicol could modify the prevalence of chloramphenicol-resistant strains of serovar Typhi. For example, in Thailand more than 80% of strains isolated from pathological specimens in 1977 were resistant. The replacement of chloramphenicol by co-trimoxazole in the therapeutic strategy resulted in a very substantial reduction in the number of chloramphenicol-resistant strains, and in 1982 fewer than 2% were nonsusceptible to the action of chloramphenicol. A study conducted between 1979 and 1985 in the region of Durban, South Africa, showed that the prevalence of chloramphenicol-resistant strains was between 0 and 2% and resistance to ampicillin was less than 0.1%. No strain resistant to chloramphenicol, ampicillin, and co-trimoxazole was detected between 1973 and 1982 in Hong Kong. Between 1978 and 1985, in the United Kingdom, 11 strains out of 2,356 isolated were resistant to chloramphenicol.

Since the Mexico outbreak in 1972, the number of multiresistant strains has been increasing around the world. However, up until the end of the 1980s, the majority of isolates were resistant to a single antibacterial agent. The most common resistance had become that to co-trimoxazole. Strains resistant to trimethoprim were described in France in 1975 and then in the United Kingdom and a very large number of other countries.

Outbreaks of typhoid fever due to strains of serovar Typhi resistant to ampicillin or chloramphenicol have been described throughout the world. The emergence and transmission of multiresistant strains of serovar Typhi poses a major public health problem. Strains of this type have become endemic in numerous countries, and small outbreaks are regularly described. A strain is said to be multiresistant when it is nonsusceptible to at least two antibiotics. Epidemiological multiresistance, in which antibiotics that are not useful therapeutically are tested (a strain may be said to be multiresistant when the antibiotics used in treatment are active), should not be confused with clinical multiresistance, in which two, or all, of the antibiotics used are inactive, such as ampicillin, chloramphenicol, co-trimoxazole, third-generation cephalosporins, and, more exceptionally, fluoroquinolones. In the case of the last group, a few strains resistant to ciprofloxacin have been isolated in India.

In 1967, multiresistant strains (ampicillin, chloramphenicol, and tetracycline) were described almost simultaneously in Aden; Cairo, Egypt; and Pakistan. Two important outbreaks due to strains resistant to chloramphenicol and other antibiotics occurred simultaneously in Mexico and in Kerala, India. Identical outbreaks have since been described in Vietnam (1973 and 1975), Thailand (1974), Korea (1977), and Peru (1979 and 1980). Currently almost 47% of strains in Peru are multiresistant (chloramphenicol, ampicillin, and co-trimoxazole). Epidemiologically, by the end of the 1980s, multiresistant strains had been disseminated across the world, with a marked predominance in Southeast Asia and on the Indian subcontinent.

In the United Kingdom, the number of multiresistant strains increased from 1% in 1986 to 18% in 1991. The majority of patients were contaminated during a stay on the Indian subcontinent or in the Middle East.

Up until 1988, only a few chloramphenicol-resistant strains were occasionally described. The first multiresistant strain was described in 1988. In a study undertaken in 1991, 43% of strains of serovar Typhi were resistant simultaneously to chloramphenicol, ampicillin, and co-trimoxazole, but no strain was resistant to the fluoroquinolones.

In India, about 7 to 13% of strains were resistant to chloramphenicol up until 1988, since then the incidence of resistant strains has increased regularly: 18.6% in 1989, 52% in 1990, and 70.7% in 1991. Since 1989, multiresistant strains have been described in different parts of India (13.2%), reaching about 70% in 1991. Table 49 shows the activities of antibacterial agents, against serovar Typhi in India.

In China, strains of serovar Typhi resistant to norfloxacin were on the order of 2% in 1992 but no ofloxacin-resistant strain was detected as of 1992. Multiresistant strains are on the order of 80% in the Shanghai area. Chloramphenicol, ampicillin, and co-trimoxazole are inactive.

In Senegal, a retrospective study between 1985 and 1991 showed that the serovar most commonly isolated is serovar Typhi (45%), followed by serovar Typhimurium (9%), the remainder being divided among 25 other serovars. More than 50% of strains of serovar Typhi were susceptible to all the antibiotics; only one was multiresistant (<2%). Twenty-nine percent of strains of the other serovars were multiresistant, and 8% of these strains produced an ESBL (serovars Johannesburg, S. Hadar, S. Ordonez, and Tambacounda).

In Bangladesh, the strains of serovar Typhi are often multiresistant but remain susceptible to fluoroquinolones and cefotaxime. Multiresistance in Bangladesh is on the order of 11.9%, but in some regions it may be as high as 44.9%. In a study of these strains, of the 236 collected between 1990 and 1992, 66.5, 72.9, 78.8, 59, and 14%, respectively, were resistant to ampicillin, co-trimoxazole, chloramphenicol, cyclines, and nalidixic acid. The breakpoints used in this study were those of the British Society for Antimicrobial Chemotherapy (1991). The activities of the different antibiotics against serovar Typhi in Bangladesh are summarized in Table 50.

Table 50 **Activities of antibiotics against *S. enterica* serovar Typhi in Bangladesh**

Drug	MIC_{50} (μg/ml)	Break point (μg/ml)	% of resistant strains
Ampicillin	64	8	66.5
Cephalexin	0.12	2	0
Cefotaxime	0.20	1	0
Co-trimoxazole	256	16	72.9
Nalidixic acid	8	8	13.9
Ciprofloxacin	0.01	1	0
Chloramphenicol	128	8	78.1
Tetracycline	16	1	59.5

Typhoid fever is endemic in Pakistan. The first multiresistant strains were described in 1987. The incidence of these strains was 10% in 1987, rising to 60% in 1990. Since 1990, resistance to chloramphenicol has very markedly decreased, and the strains that are currently isolated are resistant to co-trimoxazole and ampicillin. Table 51 shows serovar Typhi resistance in Pakistan from 1986 to 1990.

In a prospective study from 1986 to 1991, Reina et al. (1993) studied the activities of antibiotics against different serovars of *S. enterica* isolated from stools. A total of 2,043 salmonellae were isolated, including serovars Enteritidis (1,213 [59.8%]), Typhimurium (479 [23.4%]), Infantis (128 [6.2%]), Bredeney (34 [1.6%]), and Newport (8 [0.3%]).

In Algeria, resistant strains are infrequent. A few strains were isolated between 1973 and 1978, but between 1979 and 1984 no resistant strain was isolated.

10.3.2. *S. enterica* Serovar Enteritidis

Serovar Enteritidis is the most commonly isolated serovar in Poland and remains highly susceptible to the third-generation parenteral cephalosporins (94%), aminoglycosides (97%), chloramphenicol (99%), co-trimoxazole (88%), and ampicillin (82%). A progressive increase in resistance to ampicillin has appeared, from 12.1% in 1986 to 34% in 1991. Likewise, since 1988 there has been a loss of activity on the part of chloramphenicol and cyclines. No strain resistant to cefotaxime has been described. *S. enterica* serovar Typhimurium var. Copenhagen possesses the highest resistance levels, on the order of 78.8%. The frequencies of resistant strains are summarized in Table 52 according to serotype.

Table 53 **Activities of antibiotics against *Salmonella* spp. isolated in Nigeria**

Drug	Prevalence of resistance (%)
Ampicillin	29–39
Chloramphenicol	2–7
Tetracyclines	18–22
Co-trimoxazole	22–50
Cefotaxime	0
Ofloxacin	0

In Nigeria, strains of *S. enterica* are relatively resistant to ampicillin and co-trimoxazole but remain susceptible to the action of chloramphenicol (Table 53).

In Russia (Moscow and Smolensk), serovar Enteritidis was the main salmonella isolated; susceptibility patterns are reported in Table 54.

10.3.3. *S. enterica* Serotype Typhimurium DT 104

Serotype Typhimurium was first cultured in 1964. Following many animal outbreaks, it was recommended that antibacterials be banned as growth promoters, resulting in a dramatic decrease of the type phage DT 29 (3% of isolation in humans).

Table 51 **Resistance of antibiotics to *S. enterica* serovar Typhi in Pakistan**

Year	No. of strains	Prevalence of resistance (%)				
		Chloramphenicol	Ampicillin	Co-trimoxazole	Multi-drug	Ofloxacin
1986	108	0	0	0	0	0
1987	98	13.3	18.4	13.3	12.2	0
1988	138	10.9	10.9	11.6	10.9	0
1989	132	4.5	3.8	3.8	3.8	0
1990	126	48.4	63.5	66.4	43.6	0

Table 52 **Prevalence of resistance of *S. enterica* serovars other than serovar Typhi to antibiotics**

S. enterica serovar	Prevalence of resistance (%)				
	Ampicillin	Chloramphenicol	Tetracyclines	Co-trimoxazole	Ciprofloxacin
Enteritidis	22.6	1.1	3.5	1.5	0.08
Typhimurium var. Copenhagen	78.8	77.6	76.4	0.8	0.4
Typhimurium	20.6	10.3	32.1	1.7	0
Infantis	7.8	2.3	4.6	3.1	0
Bredeney	5.8	0	14.7	5.8	0
Newport	0	0	12.5	0	0
Others	6.6	2.2	6.6	4.4	0
Total	26.4	11.5	16.1	1.9	0.09

Table 54 *Salmonella* susceptibility to antibacterials in Moscow and Smolensk, Russia, in 1999[a]

Drug	Prevalence of resistance (%)	
	Serovar Enteritidis	*Salmonella* spp.
Ampicillin	2.7	6.3
Cefotaxime	0	0
Co-trimoxazole	0	0
Chloramphenicol	6.7	9.5
Tetracyclines	4.0	10.5
Ciprofloxacin	0	0

[a]Data from L. Stratchounsky, 2001, personal communication.

From 1975 to 1985 an increase was noted in the incidence of multiresistant serovar Typhimurium. The phage type was different from those observed in the 1960s, with the related phage type DTs 204, 193, and 204c predominating. In 1997, 15 and 13% of the isolates showed decreased susceptibility, or resistance, to co-trimoxazole and ciprofloxacin, respectively.

In 1997, the four most common serovars isolated in England and Wales were serovars Enteritidis, Typhimurium, Virchow, and Hadar, comprising 89% of isolates identified. In 1997, serovar Virchow resistant to ciprofloxacin rose from 5 to 14% (1994 to 1997) and resistant serovar Hadar increased from 4 to 50%.

In a 1995 study conducted by the CDC, 20% of serotype Typhimurium DT 104 isolates from human sources were resistant to ampicillin, chloramphenicol, streptomycin, sulfonamides, and tetracyclines.

S. enterica serovar Typhimurium DT 104 isolated since the 1990s represents 15% of salmonella infections in humans, and DT 104 constitutes 43% of all serovar Typhimurium strains.

In Spain, the most common serovars in correlation with food and animals are from pigs (serovar Typhimurium), poultry (serovars Typhimurium and Enteritidis), sheep (serovar Abortus Bovis), and cattle (serovar Typhimurium).

In France, resistance to aminoglycosides except streptomycin or spectinomycin and kanamycin is not commonly observed in serovar Typhimurium. Resistance to apramycin has been found in both veterinary and human strains since 1989 and is plasmid mediated [mainly due to the AAC(3)-IV type].

Quintuple resistance to ampicillin, tetracyclines, chloramphenicol, and streptomycin is chromosomally encoded, and two class 1 intregrons have been characterized.

Serovar Typhimurium DT 104 with resistance to co-trimoxazole and fluoroquinolones has been isolated in many countries, such as the United Kingdom, Germany, France, Spain, and the Czech Republic.

Serovar Typhimurium DT 104 strains producing ESBLs that hydrolyze third-generation cephalosporins and aztreonam have been described.

10.4. Other *Enterobacteriaceae*

In a SENTRY program in North America (1997 to 1998) the susceptibilities of *Enterobacteriaceae* to ceftriaxone and ceftazidime were monitored; rates are presented in Table 55.

In Taiwan, multiresistant *Aeromonas* spp. and *Acinetobacter* spp. are common. Resistance of *Enterobacteriaceae* to antibacterials was assessed in Taiwan; rates are shown in Table 56.

Table 55 Prevalence of resistance in *Enterobacteriaceae* in North America (1997)[a]

Organism	*n*	Prevalence of resistance (%) in Canada		*n*	Prevalence of resistance (%) in the United States	
		CRO	CAZ		CRO	CAZ
Citrobacter	65	16.9	23.1	224	9.9	17
Enterobacter	233	9.5	10.7	939	20	23
S. marcescens	108	0.9	1.9	348	4.3	4.0
E. coli	945	1.8	3.3			
K. pneumoniae	268	2.6	4.5			

[a]CRO, ceftriaxone; CAZ, ceftazidime.

Table 56 Prevalence of resistance to β-lactams in *Enterobacteriaceae* in Taiwan (1996) (*n* = 60)

Organism(s)	Prevalence of resistance (%)[a]				
	PIP-TZB	CRO	CAZ	CPO	IMP
E. coli	1.7	16.7	16.7	8.3	0
Klebsiella spp.	3.3	21.7	21.7	67	21.7
Citrobacter spp.	19.3	45	43.3	16.7	1.7
Enterobacter spp.	20.0	35	38.3	13.3	1.7
Proteus spp.	0	8.3	1.7	0	8.3
Serratia spp.	20	50	8.3	31.7	17
Acinetobacter spp.	53.3	81.7	50	31	3.3
P. aeruginosa	28.3	88.3	10	30	6.7
S. aureus		3.6	16.1	0	0
Coagulase-negative staphylococci		0	0	0	0

[a]PIP-TZB, piperacillin-tazobactam; CRO, ceftriaxone; CAZ, ceftazidime; CPO, cefpirome; IMP, imipenem.

Table 57 Prevalence of resistance to β-lactams in *Enterobacteriaceae* in Japan (1997 to 1998)

Organism(s)	Prevalence of resistance (%)[a]			
	n	CAZ	CPO	IMP
E. coli	210	8.1	0.5	0.5
Klebsiella spp.	219	5.0	0.5	0
Citrobacter spp.	192	23.4	2.6	5.5
Enterobacter spp.	208	25	4.3	0.5
Proteus spp.	200	3.5	0.5	2.5
Serratia spp.	206	6.8	6.8	4.4
Acinetobacter spp.	200	7.0	16.5	4.5
P. aeruginosa	219	15.1	9.6	19.6

[a]CAZ, ceftazidime; CPO, cefpirome; IMP, imipenem.

In Japan a survey was carried out from 1997 to 1998 to determined β-lactam resistance in Enterobacteriaceae; rates are given in Table 57.

10.4.1. *S. marcescens*

S. marcescens has become an important nosocomial pathogen acting as an opportunistic organism. Resistance to β-lactams in *S. marcescens* may be due to the following:

- Elevated class C β-lactamases
- Outer membrane impermeability
- Carbapenemases

Carbapenem resistance may occur via two mechanisms:

- High-level production of class C chromosomal cephalosporinases combined with altered outer membrane permeability. This phenomenon was described for *S. marcescens, E. cloacae, E. aerogenes*, and *Providencia rettgeri* isolates.
- Carbapenemases. In Japan, the prevalence of *S. marcescens* harboring carbapenemases reached 3.8% in certain geographical areas.

10.4.2. *P. mirabilis*

Within *Enterobacteriaceae*, the greatest incidence of ESBLs was found in *K. pneumoniae* and *E. coli*, but other *Enterobacteriaceae*, such as *P. mirabilis*, are able to harbor ESBLs. The prevalence of ESBLs in *P. mirabilis* was assessed in the epidemiological survey conducted by the MYSTIC program; results are given in Table 58 (Mutnick et al., 2002).

Between 1996 and 1998, 1,072 *P. mirabilis* isolates were collected in Clermont-Ferrand hospitals in the center of France; among them, 48.5% were resistant to amoxicillin and 14.2% of all resistant isolates harbored an ESBL (TEM-3 or TEM-66) (Chanal et al., 2000).

10.4.3. *K. pneumoniae*

Klebsiella spp. are opportunisitic pathogens in immunodepressed patients. *Klebsiella* is one of the main *Enterobacteriaceae* harboring ESBLs or plasmid-borne AmpC (*K. oxytoca*).

Table 58 Incidence of ESBLs in *P. mirabilis*

Parameter	1997	1998	1999	2000	2001
No. of strains	61	110	210	196	111
% Producing ESBLs	39.3	9.5	11.3	20.3	18.0

Table 59 Incidence of ESBLs in Europe

Country	No. of strains	ESBL prevalence (%)	
		1994	1997–1998
France	59	19	32
The United Kingdom	23	0	9
Italy	58	15	38
Spain	36	1	5.5
Turkey	44	59	61
Germany	69	17	23
Belgium	59	31	32
The Netherlands	85	16	8

An epidemiological survey conducted in eight countries from 1997 to 1998 showed an increased prevalence of ESBL-producing strains in comparison with a previous survey in 1994 (Table 59).

The prevalences of ESBLs in *K. pneumoniae* show a wide range: 94% in Canada, 87.6% in the United States, 76.1% in the Western Pacific region, 63.3% in Europe, and 49.6% in Latin America. In *K. pneumoniae*, ESBLs were of the TEM, SHV, and CTX-M types. *K. pneumoniae* bacteremia levels were reported to be 3 to 5% and 11.4% in Europe and Canada, respectively, within all cases involving gram-negative bacteria occurring in adults; the mortality rate approached 27 to 34% of patients. It was reported that *K. pneumoniae* causes 1.0% and 5 to 7% of bacteremia cases to in children in the United States and South Africa, respectively. In Canada, 12 of 268 *K. pneumoniae* isolates harbored an ESBL enzyme according to the SENTRY 1997-1998 program. In Chile (1998 to 1999), 8 and 43% of *E. coli* and *K. pneumoniae* isolates, respectively, harbored ESBLs.

10.4.4. *E. coli*

E. coli is among the most important of human pathogens. *E. coli* is responsible for 80 to 90% of cases of uncomplicated urinary tract infection. Treatment of uncomplicated urinary tract infection relies on fluoroquinolones, co-trimoxazole, and fosfomycin trometamol. Resistance to oxyimino cephalosporins (cefotaxime, ceftriaxone, and ceftazidime) is rare in *E. coli* and represents less than 2% of the clinical isolates in most studies. In Poland, there is clearly a high prevalence of *E. coli, K. pneumoniae* and *E. cloacae* resistance to oxyimino cephalosporins due to ESBLs and AmpC enzymes. This resistance is also high in *E. coli* and *K. pneumoniae* cultures from Turkey (26 and 73%, respectively).

In Brazil, ESBL producers were most common among isolates of *E. coli* (19.6%) and *Klebsiella* spp. (39.8%), whereas in the United States and Mexico they were not detected.

In Canada, 31 of 945 *E. coli* isolates were found to harbor an ESBL in the SENTRY 1997-1998 program.

After many years of usage, the level of resistance to fosfomycin remains low (less than 1%). In *E. coli*, fosfomycin is transported into the cell via the GlpT and UhpT transporters. Expression of these genes requires cyclic AMP-cyclic AMP receptor protein complex, and for the *uhpT* gene, the *uhpA*, *uhpB*, and *uhpC* genes are necessary. Resistance may be due to the defect of one or two of these genes by mutations or a plasmid-encoded enzymatic inactivation.

Table 60 Prevalence of difficult-to-treat *Enterobacteriaceae* in nosocomial infections

Type of infection[a]	Prevalence (%)					
	E. cloacae		*S. marcescens*		*Citrobacter*	
	Pediatrics	Adults	Pediatrics	Adults	Pediatrics	Adults
LRTI	12.2					
UTI	10.3	5			4.3	1.0
Pneumonia	9.3	9	4	3.6		
SSTI	8.1					
Bloodstream	6.2	3				

[a]LRTI, lower RTI; UTI, urinary tract infection.

Integrons are genetic elements able to integrate or mobilize gene cassettes by site-specific recombination. Gene cassettes, which often encode antibacterial resistance, are mobile units composed of a gene and an integrase-specific recombination site (59 base elements). Within the four types of integrons, class 1 integrons are the most prevalent among clinical isolates. Today, above 40 cassettes have been identified within class 1 integrons.

For co-trimoxazole, 16 different types of plasmid-borne DHFR have been found in gram-negative bacteria and have been characterized and classified on the basis of their nucleotide sequences and kinetic properties. Family 1, the largest and the most prevalent, is composed of the *dfr1*, *drfIb*, *drfV*, *dfrVI*, *dfrVII*, and *dfr17* genes. All of the proteins encoded by these genes are highly resistant to trimethoprim (MIC, >1,000 μg/ml).

Resistance to streptomycin and spectinomycin can be encoded by the genes *aad1*, *aad2*, *aad3*, and *aad4*, which belong to a cassette-borne aminoglycoside adenyltransferase gene.

10.4.5. *E. cloacae*

The highest prevalence rate of ceftazidime resistance in *Enterobacter* spp. was reported in ICU in Turkey (68%), Russia (56%), and Portugal (48%).

In North America, in the National Nosocomial Infection Surveillance System, the frequency of *E. cloacae* increased significantly in pediatrics patient, from 7 to 12% in the study period. Table 60 shows the prevalence of *Enterobacteriaceae* in nosocomial infections.

10.4.6. *Yersinia pestis*

Y. pestis is the causative agent of plague, a tick-borne infectious disease transmitted to humans through fly bites. Plague is characterized by a bubo or transmitted from human to human, resulting in pneumonia.

The last plague pandemic began in Hong Kong in 1894 and spread throughout the world, establishing many endemic foci (Galimand et al., 1997). Plague reappeared in 1994 in an epidemic form in many countries in Africa (Malawi, Mozambique, and Tanzania), India, Vietnam, and Peru, where plague was silent for at least 30 years. Foci of bubonic plague were reported in many parts of the United States.

Streptomycin, chloramphenicol, and tetracycline alone or in combination are the reference drugs to treat plague, whereas tetracycline or sulfonamides are recommended for prophylaxis. High-level resistance to multiple antibacterials was observed in a clinical isolate of *Y. pestis* in Madagascar (Galimand et al., 1997) as well as a strain harboring plasmid-mediated streptomycin resistance (Guiyoule et al., 2001).

11. NONFERMENTATIVE GRAM-NEGATIVE BACILLI

11.1. *P. aeruginosa*

P. aeruginosa is a nosocomial opportunistic human pathogen in patients requiring intensive care, in immunodepressed patients, in patients suffering from leukemia, in patients with burn wounds, in those with a with long-term indwelling urinary bladder catheter, and in those having specific underlying diseases, such as cystic fibrosis. *P. aeruginosa* is transmitted horizontally. Usually *P. aeruginosa* is associated with single hospitalization unit. It is rarely involved in large hospital outbreaks or interhospital spread. *P. aeruginosa* strains are often multidrug resistant.

The global occurrence of nonfermentative gram-negative bacillus isolates was measured in the SENTRY surveillance program from 1997 to 2001; Table 61 shows the population distribution of 18,569 isolates.

In the SENTRY program carried out in 1997 in Canada, the United States, and Latin America, the rank of various bacterial species was as follows: *Enterobacteriaceae*, gram-positive cocci, and nonfermentative gram-negative bacilli.

During the same period (1997 to 1998) in a survey throughout Europe, about 9,600 clinical isolates were collected from 25 hospitals. Twenty bacterial species represented about 98% of the isolates. The four main pathogens were *E. coli* (20%), *S. aureus* (17.6%), coagulase-negative staphylococci (17.1%), and *P. aeruginosa* (5.3%). The susceptibility profiles of antibacterials are shown in Table 62.

In Russia from 1995 to 1996 and 1997 to 1999, clinical isolates from nosocomial sources were collected, and *P. aeruginosa* represented about 30% of gram-negative bacilli collected (L. Stratchounsky, personal communication, 2001).

Table 61 Incidence of gram-negative bacilli in nosocomial infections

Organism(s)	*n*	% of isolated strains
P. aeruginosa	11,968	64.5
Acinetobacter spp.	3,468	18.7
S. maltophilia	1,488	8.0
Pseudomonas spp.	523	2.8
Aeromonas spp.	258	1.4
Burkholderia spp.	197	1.1
Alcaligenes spp.	184	1.0
Campylobacter spp.	169	0.9
Chryseobacterium	56	0.3
Pasteurella spp.	48	0.2
Other species	210	1.1

Table 62 Susceptibilities of nosocomial pathogens to fluoroquinolones

Drug	% Susceptibility[a]							
	Ec	Pa	Kp	Ac	MRSA	MSSA	MRCoNS	MSCoNS
Ciprofloxacin	91.9	74.9	94.7	50.6	10	89.6	39.9	86
Ofloxacin	92	69.7	94.5	52.7				
Levofloxacin	95.3	71.1	96.5	54.7				
Sparfloxacin					9.7	87.9	37.5	83.5

[a]Ec, *E. coli*; Pa, *P. aeruginosa*; Kp, *K. pneumoniae*; Ac, *Acinetobacter*; MSSA, methicillin-susceptible *S. aurens*: MRCoNS, methicillin-resistant coagulase-negative staphylococci; MSCoNS, methicillin-susceptible coagulase-negactive staphylococci.

Table 63 *P. aeruginosa* susceptibility to antibacterials in Russia[a]

Drug	% Resistance	
	1995–1996	1997–1999
Gentamicin	75	61
Piperacillin	50	45
Piperacillin-tazobactam	41	30
Ciprofloxacin	15	30
Imipenem	7	19
Ceftazidime	11	11
Amikacin	7	6

[a]Data from L. Stratchounsky, 2001, personal communication.

The susceptibility patterns were assessed and are reported in Table 63.

The main mechanisms of resistance to β-lactams are shown in Table 64.

The risks of resistance to antibacterials vary with different antibiotic treatments. A total of 271 patients with pseudomonal infections were treated with various antibacterials. Resistance emerged in 28 patients (10.2%) to the following: ceftazidime (0.8%), ciprofloxacin (9.2%), imipenem (44%), and piperacillin (5.2%). In this study combination therapy with an aminoglycoside did not appear to prevent the emergence of resistance.

In the SENTRY program carried out in North and Latin America in 1997 (Diekema et al., 1999), the susceptibilities of 451 *P. aeruginosa* isolates to various fluoroquinolones were determined; results are shown in Table 65.

In Argentina, 6,343 clinical isolates were collected from nosocomial sources in 27 Argentinean centers. *S. aureus* (22.7%) was the main pathogen isolated, followed by *E. coli* (18.3%), *P. aeruginosa* (13.4%), coagulase-negative staphylococci (9.4%), *K. pneumoniae* (9.2%), *Enterococcus* spp. (7.2%), *Acinetobacter* spp. (5.9%), *E. cloacae* (4.6%), *P. mirabilis* (3.3%), *S. marcescens* (1.3%), and other species (4.7%).

Table 65 Activities of fluoroquinolones against *P. aeruginosa* in the Americas

Drug	% Susceptibility		
	Canada	United States	Latin America
Levofloxacin	83.1	84.8	73.9
Ciprofloxacin	88	88.8	73.9
Gatifloxacin	74.7	81.5	71.7
Sparfloxacin	71.1	96.8	64.0
Trovafloxacin	81.9	79	68.5

Table 66 shows susceptibilities of nosocomial *Acinetobacter* and *P. aeruginosa* isolates in Russia.

11.1.1. β-Lactams

Several mechanisms are implicated in the resistance of *P. aeruginosa* to β-lactams: production of β-lactamases, parietal impermeability, modification of PBPs, and efflux.

P. aeruginosa is resistant to numerous β-lactams. Even the so-called antipseudomonas cephalosporins, such as ceftazidime, are 10 to 100 times less active against *P. aeruginosa* than against *E. cloacae*. This resistance is due in part to weak membrane permeability resulting from porins that are more numerous but less functional.

Imipenem has to cross the outer membrane of *P. aeruginosa* via a specific porin, Opr D2, which has a molecular mass of 48 kDa. This porin is inducible in the presence of glucose.

The second mode of resistance is a modification of the PBPs.

The most common mode of resistance after membrane impermeability is β-lactamase production.

P. aeruginosa produces a chromosomal cephalosporinase (class Id) which, when derepressed, causes resistance to cefsulodin, ceftazidime, and *N*-acylpenicillins, while preserving the activity of imipenem. The actual levels of resistance depend on the quantity of enzymes produced in the absence of induction.

Table 64 Main mechanism of resistance to β-lactams

Strain	% Susceptibility			
	n(%)	Amikacin	Imipenem	Ciprofloxacin
Wild strains	429 (58.1)	77.1	89.3	82.5
PSE-1	48 (6.5)	18.7	79.2	83
Nonenzymatic	116 (15.7)	61.1	82.4	50.9
AmpC	9,212 (5)	33.7	54.3	18.5
AmpC + nonenzymatic	364 (9)	47.2	63.9	16.7

Table 66 Antibacterial susceptibilities of nonfermentative gram-negative bacilli of nosocomial origin in Russia[a]

Drug	% Resistance		
	P. aeruginosa		*Acinetobacter*, ICU
	All wards ($n = 850$)	ICU ($n = 206$)	
Ceftazidime	30	38	83
Cefepime	25	36	83
Imipenem	21	36	9
Piperacillin-tazobactam	35	43	84
Amikacin	36	48	74
Ciprofloxacin	40	53	83

[a]Data from L. Stratchounsky, 2001, personal communication.

Numerous plasmid-mediated β-lactamases have been described: PSE, CARB, TEM, NPS-1, and oxacillinases.

In France and the United Kingdom, about 10 and 2% of strains, respectively, possess enzymes, while the proportion among *Enterobacteriaceae* is greater.

The most common enzymes are PSE-1 (CARB-2) and PSE-4 (CARB-1), which are responsible for resistance to all antipseudomonas penicillins and to cefoperazone and cefsulodin. They do not produce resistance to aztreonam, imipenem, or ceftazidime.

Resistance of *P. aeruginosa* to cephalosporins (cefsulodin, ceftazidime, cefepime, and cefpirome) or aztreonam combined with other antibacterial agents (fluoroquinolones, tetracyclines, and chloramphenicol) is often related to a double porin dysfunction, Opr D and Opr M.

Carbapenems are used as a last resort for treating severe infections attributable to multidrug-resistant gram-negative bacteria such as *P. aeruginosa*. However, *P. aeruginosa* with acquired metallo-β-lactamase IMP-1 emerged. Other enzymes were reported, such as VIM-1 first reported in Italy in 1993, followed by VIM-2 in France and in Greece. Other VIM enzymes were described in Taiwan (VIM-4), in the United States (VIM-4), and in Korea (VIM-2). *P. aeruginosa* clinical isolates producing metallo-β-lactamases were detected in Brazil.

In a collaborative survey within the SENTRY program in North and Latin America in 1997, the susceptibility of *P. aeruginosa* to β-lactams was assessed; results are shown in Table 67.

11.1.2. Fluoroquinolones

P. aeruginosa is one of the bacterial species against which the fluoroquinolones, including ciprofloxacin, possess moderate activity (MIC, 0.5 to 2 μg/ml). The proportion of resistant strains varies by study, not least because the breakpoints are not identical in the different studies.

Table 67 Activities of β-lactams against *P. aeruginosa*

Drug	% Susceptibility		
	Canada	United States	Latin America
Cefepime	90.4	86.6	71.7
Ceftazidime	88	86.6	85.9
Piperacillin-tazobactam	96.4	91.7	85.9
Meropenem	94	94.9	94.6
Imipenem	81.9	88.8	84.8

Table 68 Susceptibility of *P. aeruginosa* to antibacterials in urinary tract infections

Drug	MIC (μg/ml)		% Resistance
	50%	90%	
Ciprofloxacin	0.5	>2.0	37.1
Gatifloxacin	2.0	>4.0	37.6
Levofloxacin	2.0	>4.0	38.1
Cefepime	4.0	16	10
Meropenem	1.0	>8.0	10.5
Piperacillin-tazobactam	8.0	>64	10.5

George et al. showed that the extensive use of ciprofloxacin was associated with a reduction in the susceptibility of strains of *P. aeruginosa*. The proportions of strains for which ciprofloxacin had a MIC of ≤1 μg/ml were 98.6% from 1985 to 1986 and 86.3% in 1989. The proportion of resistant strains (MIC, ≥4 μg/ml) is 3% and remains stable. The number of strains of reduced susceptibility (MIC, 2 to 4 μg/ml) increased from 1% from 1985 to 1986 to 10.8% in 1989. Acar et al. showed that the proportion of strains of *P. aeruginosa* that had become resistant to pefloxacin (MIC, ≥4 μg/ml) increased from 20.1% in 1984 to 33.4% in 1988.

In the Swedish study reported in 1993, 9 to 11% of strains were resistant to ciprofloxacin, 5 to 14% were resistant to imipenem, and 10% were resistant to piperacillin.

In a survey conducted in 1995 in Germany and Switzerland, 11.9% of *P. aeruginosa* isolates were resistant to ciprofloxacin.

In urinary tract infections in 2000, 210 *P. aeruginosa* isolates were tested for their susceptibilities to antibacterials; results are reported in Table 68.

In 2001 surveys performed in Germany, Austria, and Switzerland by the Paul Ehrlich (PEG) Society, 717 *P. aeruginosa* clinical isolates were collected; 76.8 and 79.1% were susceptible to levofloxacin and ciprofloxacin, respectively, whereas in a 1998 survey, 85.6% were susceptible to ciprofloxacin (mode MIC for both studies for ciprofloxacin, 0.25 μg/ml) (M. Kreken, Hafner site PEG).

In an epidemiological study carried out in France, 738 *P. aeruginosa* clinical isolates were collected in 15 hospital centers and the antibacterial susceptibilities were assessed (Table 69) (Cavallo et al., 2001).

Table 69 *P. aeruginosa* susceptibility to antibacterials in cystic fibrosis and non-cystic fibrosis patients in France (2000)

Drug	% Susceptibility of strains from:	
	Non-cystic fibrosis patients ($n = 701$)	Cystic fibrosis patients ($n = 37$)
Ciprofloxacin	60	59
Ticarcillin	58	62
Ceftazidime	76	73
Cefpirome	37	22
Imipenem	82	59
Amikacin	64	27

Table 70 Incidence of resistance of *P. aeruginosa* via a single enzymatic mechanism

Mechanism	Prevalence (%)	Antibacterial(s)
Enzymes		
AAC(2)-1	0	Gentamicin, tobramycin, netilmicin
AAC(6)-1	1.25	Tobramycin, netilmicin, amikacin
AAC(2)-6	18.39	Gentamicin, tobramycin, netilmicin
AAC(3)-1	2.05	Gentamicin
AAC(3)-II	2.2	Gentamicin, tobramycin, netilmicin
AAC(3)-III	0.1	Gentamicin, tobramycin
AAC(3)-IV	0	Gentamicin, tobramycin, netilmicin
AAC(3)-VI	0.15	Gentamicin, tobramycin, netilmicin
AAC(3)-?	0.6	Gentamicin, netilmicin
ANT (2″)-I	11.87	Gentamicin, tobramycin
ANT(4′)-II	0.05	Tobramycin, amikacin, isepamicin
APH(3′)-VI	0.20	Amikacin, isepamicin
Membrane permeability	26.15	Netilmicin, amikacin, isepamicin, gentamicin, tobramycin
All mechanisms	63.01	

In a surveillance epidemiological study carried out in Europe in 1997, 25% of *P. aeruginosa* isolates were resistant to both levofloxacin and ciprofloxacin.

11.1.3. Aminoglycosides

The mechanisms of resistance of *P. aeruginosa* have become extremely complex, and the incidence of resistant strains is increasing. The level of resistance was 37% in 1993, compared with only 15% some 10 years previously. The most common mechanism is modification of transparietal penetration and then inactivation by enzymes of the AAC(6′)-II and ANT(2″)-I types, followed by the combination of several enzymatic mechanisms. In a multicenter, multinational study undertaken from 1992 to 1993, more than 75 different combinations were detected, of which 15 were preponderant. Some of these were present in all regions, and others were specific to certain centers. In this study, 52.3% of strains had an alteration of transparietal penetration. Of 2,284 strains collected, 1,996 presented resistance to at least one aminoglycoside, 37% of which possessed several mechanisms of resistance (two to five). The distribution of enzymatic inactivation of the different aminoglycosides is summarized in Table 70.

11.2. *Acinetobacter* spp.

Acinetobacter spp. are opportunistic gram-negative bacteria responsible for an increasing number of nosocomial infections. Bouvet and Grimont (1986) proposed a new classification: *A. baumannii (Acinetobacter calcoaceticus* subsp. *anitratus*) and non-*A. baumannii*. One of the mechanisms of resistance to β-lactams is the production of a cephalosporinase-type β-lactamase (ACE-1, ACE-2, ACE-3, or ACE-4), enzymes of the TEM-1 type, or carbenicillinases such as CARB-5. This enzyme is present in 9% of isolates of *A. baumannii* at the CHU-Xavier Bichat, Paris, France.

Jolly Guillou et al. have isolated four resistance phenotypes within *Acinetobacter* spp. (Table 71).

The authors demonstrated high resistance to piperacillin (87.5 to 98% piperacillin-resistant strains). Resistance to ticarcillin was on the order of 78.5% (MIC, >256 μg/ml). The addition of clavulanic acid reduced the MIC to 70 μg/ml.

Imipenem is one of the antibiotics active against *Acinetobacter* (MIC, ~0.5 μg/ml). Strains resistant to imipenem (ARI-1 and ARI-2) (~5.5%) have been isolated since 1986.

The proportion of strains of *Acinetobacter* that have become resistant to fluoroquinolones increased from 12.5% to 79.5% between 1984 and 1989.

Amikacin is inactivated by a APH(3′)-VI, which is common in *Acinetobacter* but rare in *Enterobacteriaceae.*

In Greece (Giammarelou et al., 1993), *Acinetobacter* spp. occupied sixth place among nosocomial agents. These strains are resistant to aminoglycosides (>90%). The most common enzymes are APH(3″)-I and APH(3)-VI (21.6%), the latter inactivating amikacin and isepamicin. Three inactivating enzymes were found in 54% of strains, in 46% the combination was AAC(3′)-I, APH(3′)-I, and APH(3′)-VI. In 9.5% of strains, five inactivating enzymes were found. Resistance to aminoglycosides is due to membrane impermeability in 5.4% of strains. A total of 59.6% of these strains are resistant to ciprofloxacin. An ANT(2″)-1 adenylase inactivating gentamicin and tobramycin has been detected in about 30% of species.

Table 71 Antibiotic resistance phenotypes of *Acinetobacter* spp.

Type	Enzyme(s)	% of strains				
		1984	1985	1986	1987	1988
I	Wild	11	11	6	6	2.5
II	Penicillinase	12	4.5	7.5	3	0.5
III	Cephalosporinase	9	12	35	26.5	13
IV	Penicillinase + cephalosporinases	68	72.5	52	64.5	84

In a 1997 SENTRY program, *Acinetobacter* from the bloodstream accounted for 1.6, 1.1, and 5.3% of the isolates in the United States, Canada, and Latin America, respectively (Diekema et al., 1999).

Philippon et al. (1990) described an enzyme of the oxacillinase type in *Alcaligenes denitrificans* subsp. *xylosoxydans*.

12. FASTIDIOUS GRAM-NEGATIVE BACILLI

12.1. *H. influenzae*

H. influenzae represents an important agent in upper and lower RTIs, conjunctivitis, and purulent meningitis. The determination of the in vitro activities of antibacterial agents against *H. influenzae* is complex, as the MIC depends on the culture medium, pH, composition of the incubation atmosphere (CO_2), and size of the inoculum. In addition, this bacterial species requires growth factors, which complicates further still the assessment of the MIC. The lack of standardization is a source of confusion about the published results. At the beginning of the 1960s, ampicillin became the reference antibiotic in the treatment of *H. influenzae* infections. In 1974, the first β-lactamase-producing strains of *H. influenzae* were described. Since then, ampicillin-resistant strains have represented up to 31.7% of clinical isolates in certain centers in the United States.

A European multicenter study showed that the prevalence of ampicillin-resistant strains varied according to the center and country. In Spain it was up to 30%, (non-type b strains), while in Germany it was on the order of 1.6%. In the other European countries it was around 10% (Table 72).

Ampicillin resistance is mainly due to the production of TEM-1 and BRO-1 β-lactamases. ROB-1 is also found in *Pasteurella multocida*. It appears to be of porcine origin, since this enzyme has been demonstrated in *M. pleuropneumoniae*. In an Irish survey, 0.7% of resistant strains were resistant to co-amoxiclav. Another mechanism of resistance has been described: alteration of PBP 1 (β-lactamase-negative antibiotic-resistant strains). For PBP 3, a mutation on the gene *fts* was reported; this gene encodes PBP 3A and PBP 3B, which are involved in peptidoglycan biosynthesis during cell division. Three groups have been described: group I, His 517→Arg, group II, Lys 526→Asn in the conserved motif Lys-Thr-Gly; and group III, Ile377→Met or Thr385→Ser or Phe 389→Leu, which are substituted amino acids in the conserved motif SerSerAsn.

Ampicillin resistance is often accompanied by resistance to chloramphenicol and the cyclines. Resistance to the cyclines was first detected in 1970, and that to chloramphenicol was first detected in 1972. Table 73 shows ampicillin resistance in *H. influenzae* worldwide.

Gould et al. (1994) reported the first strain of *H. influenzae* resistant to ciprofloxacin (MIC, 8 μg/ml) and ofloxacin (MIC, 32 μg/ml). Cefotaxime was active against this nontypeable strain. In the United Kingdom, a multicenter study in 1986 comprising 24 centers showed that of 2,371 strains of nonencapsulated *H. influenzae*, 6% produced β-lactamases, while 4% of ampicillin-resistant strains did not produce any enzyme (MIC, ≥1 μg/ml). The proportions of strains resistant to tetracycline, cefaclor, and cefixime were, respectively, 2.7, 3, and 0.2%. Ampicillin resistance was higher in 1988, at 8.4 and 10%, respectively, for β-lactamase-producing and non-β-lactamases producing strains. Table 74 shows *H. influenzae* resistance to antibiotics in 1990 in the United Kingdom.

The prevalence of β-lactamase-producing strains of *H. influenzae* in Southeast Asia was studied by the World Health Organization in 1988 and varied according to the country: 4.4 to 8% in the Philippines and Vietnam and 17 to 49% in Hong Kong, Malaysia, and China. In 1998 in Japan, the prevalence of β-lactamase-producing strains of *H. influenzae* was 26.8%. In North America from 1999 to 2000, the prevalences were 19.6 and 26.1% for Canada and the United States, respectively. However, there are variations in prevalences of β-lactamase-producing strains among collected *H. influenzae* strains in the United States depending on the survey (Table 75).

In Chile, Argentina, and Venezuela, fewer than 4% of strains of *H. influenzae* were resistant to ampicillin.

In a survey conducted in 1993, 53 and 67% of strains of *H. influenzae* isolated in Canada and the United States, respectively, were susceptible to ampicillin. In 1988, out of 715 strains of *H. influenzae* tested by Dabernat (1989) in France, there were rates of resistance to ampicillin, tetracyclines, and chloramphenicol of 13.98, 8.5, and 1.6%, respectively. Table 76 summarizes the activities of antibiotics against *H. influenzae* in France since 1981.

The strains responsible for otitis are usually nonencapsulated, and fewer than 10% are serotype b. In studies carried out by Gehanno and by Simonet (1988), *H. influenzae* was the principal species responsible for otitis media, isolated from 43% of patients, with *S. pneumoniae* being found in only 23% of patients.

Table 72 Resistance of *H. influenzae* to antibiotics in Europe

Country	Prevalence of resistance (%)							
	Ampicillin		Chloramphenicol		Erythromycin A		Tetracycline	
	b	Non-b	b	Non-b	b	Non-b	b	Non-b
Austria	5	5	2			2	3	6
Belgium	26	17	11	11	2	6	8	18
France	16	9		4	3	17	19	9
Germany	0	2	0	1	6	5	0	3
The United Kingdom	20	8	0	2	0	3	0	2
The Netherlands	12	7	0	1	16	32	4	3
Spain	64	26	41	22	18	20	45	22
Sweden	11	7	9	1	4	10	9	2
Switzerland	6	7	2	2	6	12	2	4

Table 73 Ampicillin resistance among *H. influenzae* isolates[a]

Country	*n*	Year(s)	% Ampicillin resistant
Europe			
Austria	111	1998–2000	5.4
Belgium	224	1998–2000	4.8
France	425	1998–2000	28.2
The Netherlands	228	1998–2000	9.4
Italy	297	1998–2000	5.4
	307	1998–1999	8.1
Spain	292	1998–2000	22.6
	266	2001	29.3
Portugal	369	1998–2000	11.6
Greece	112	1998–2000	13.4
Finland	578	1988–1990	8.0
	297	1995	24.4
Sweden	64	1996	3.0
Denmark	86	1998–9	15.1
Norway	696	1993–1994, 1995	6.7
Germany	345	1998–2000	7.2
The United Kingdom	262	1998–2000	20.2
	152	1998–1999	11.8
	936	1999–2000	24
	152	2001	11.8
Ireland	107	1998–2000	16.8
	936	1999–2000	33
Czech Republic	100	1996	13
		1996	13
		1997	7.9
	276	1998–2000	8.3
Slovak Republic	42	1996	4.8
		1997	5.3
	306	1998–2000	6.5
Hungary	262	1996	3.8
		1997	-
	217	1998–1999	6.5
Poland		1996	3.8
		1997	5.6
Luxemburg	23	2003–2004	13
Switzerland	292	1998–2000	11.3
Russia	143	1998–2000	4.2
Turkey	272	1996–1997	8.8
	12	1999–2000	8.3
North America			
The United States	230	1996	30.4
	2791	1999	32.2
	235	1998–1999	31.9
	2073	1998–2000	30.3
	235	2001	31.9
Canada	637	1995–1996	11.8
	199	1998–1999	26.6
	1407	2000–2001	20.2
Latin America			
Argentina	14	1998	7
	228	1998–1999	21.1
	228	2001	21.1
Colombia	197	2001	10.2
Brazil	23	1998	4
	183	1998–2000	11.5
	163	1998–1999	8.6
Venezuela	13	1996	0
Chile	64	1996	11
Mexico	10	1998	10
	191	1998–2000	24.6
Southeast Asia			
Korea	51	2001	64.7
	55	2002	53.6
	54	2003	53.7
Hong Kong	116	1996	37.1
	379	1998–2000	25.1
Vietnam	78	1999	24
Malaysia	29	1986–1989	10
Singapore	122	1998–2000	27.9
Taiwan	301	1998–1999	18.6
	42	1999–2000	59.5
Thailand	205	1999–2000	45
India	171	1998–1999	17.5
Mainland China	23	1999–2000	4.3
The Philippines	194	1998–1999	28.9
Japan	457	1998–2000	19
Africa			
Tunisia	192	1998–1999	25.9
Kenya	58	1998–1999	8.6
South Africa	303	1998–2000	8.6
	214	1998–1999	18.7
	214	2001	18.7
Kenya	58	1998–2000	8.6
Ethiopia	954	NG[b]	0
Middle East			
Lebanon	167	1998–1999	6
Egypt	89	NG	21
Israel	75	1998–2000	24
	31	1994–1995	24
Near East			
Saudi Arabia	225	1998–2000	20.9
	150	1998–1999	27.3
	86	1996	21.9
	150	2001	23.3
Australia	605	1998–2000	21.2

[a]Data from Acar, 1999; Jacobs et al., 1998, 2003; Bandak et al., 2001; Nishi et al., 2002; Hsueh et al., 2000; Hoban et al., 1997, 2002; Felmingham et al., 2001; 2002; 2003; BSAC Extended Working Party on Respiratory Resistance Surveillance and GR Micro Limited, 2001; Turnidge et al., 2001; Marchese and Schito, 2000; Gür et al., 2002; Kariuki et al., 2003; Youssef et al., 2004; Thabet et al., 2002; Jones et al., 2002; Knudsen et al., 2001; Ringertz et al., 1993; Kristiansen et al., 2001; Manninen et al., 1997; Larson et al., 2000; Critchley et al., 2002; Choo et al., 1990; Bryskier, 2004.

[b]NG, not given.

12.2. *M. catarrhalis*

M. catarrhalis has long been considered a commensal bacterium of the upper airways devoid of pathogenic potential. At the beginning of the 1970s, this bacterial species was susceptible to all the antibiotics used for treatment of the upper respiratory tract, such as penicillin, cyclines, and erythromycin A.

Table 74 Resistance of *H. influenzae* to antibiotics in 1990 in the United Kingdom

Drug[a]	Prevalence of resistance (%)
Ampicillin	
β^+	9.4
β^-	5.2
Co-amoxiclav	5.2
Tetracyclines	4.5
Erythromycin A	86.6
Cefaclor	5.2
Cefixime	0.2

[a]β^+ and β^-, strains did and did not produce, β-lactamase, respectively.

Table 75 Variation of prevalence of β-lactamase-producing *H. influenzae* according to studies

Year(s)	Prevalence (%)	Reference
1999	33	Hoban et al., 1997 (SENTRY)
1996–1997	33.4	Thornsberry (SENTRY)
1997	41.6	Jacobs et al., 1998 (SENTRY)
1997–1998	33	Thornsberry (SENTRY)
1998	33.3	Jones et al., 1999 (SENTRY)
1999–2000	26.1	Hoban et al., 2003 (PROTEKT)

Between 1970 and 1976, no β-lactamase-producing strain of M. *catarrhalis* was detected. In 1981, 56.8% of strains isolated were β-lactamase producing. Since 1977, an increasing number of ampicillin-resistant strains have been isolated from pathological specimens, reaching about 75%.

A French study undertaken in 15 centers determined the prevalence of β-lactamase production among M. *catarrhalis* strains; rates are shown in Table 77.

However, resistance to β-lactams is due not only to β-lactamase production but also to a reduction in membrane permeability.

The majority of β-lactamases produced by M. *catarrhalis* are constitutive and of chromosomal origin. Two enzymes of plasmid origin have recently been detected: BRO-1 and BRO-2.

In the United Kingdom, 6.8% of strains isolated in 1977 were resistant to cyclines, but none were resistant to erythromycin A. In two studies in 1986, 35 and 70% of strains of M. *catarrhalis* were shown to be β-lactamase producing.

In 1991, approximately 4% of strains were resistant to cyclines and erythromycin A but not to co-amoxiclav.

Resistance of M. *catarrhalis* to erythromycin A was reported in 1983 in Sweden (MIC, ≥4 μg/ml), followed by The Netherlands, New Zealand, the United States, Italy, and Japan.

In 1993, only 16 and 13% of strains of M. *catarrhalis* were susceptible to ampicillin in the United States and Canada, respectively.

Other *Moraxella* spp. produce β-lactamases: *Moraxella osloensis, Moraxella lacunata, Moraxella phenylpyruvica,* and *Moraxella urethralis* (*Oligella urethralis*). No β-lactamase activity has been detected in *Moraxella atlantae*.

13. OTHER GRAM-NEGATIVE BACILLI

13.1. *V. cholerae*

V. cholerae O1 is the agent of cholera, an epidemic and strictly human diarrheal disease. Since the beginning of the 19th century, the world has experienced seven cholera

Table 76 Resistance of *H. influenzae* in France (otitis)

Year	Prevalence of resistance (%)		
	Ampicillin	Tetracyclines	Chloramphenicol
1981	5		
1985	16.6	7.6	3.3
1986	10.4	4.7	0.9
1987	18	10.1	0.9
1988	12.8	8.5	ND[a]
1989	23.8	12.3	0.7

[a]ND, not determined.

Table 77 Prevalence of β-lactamase-producing strains of *M. catarrhalis*

Year	No. of β-lactamase-producing strains/total (%)
1987	134/162 (82.7)
1988	185/222 (83.3)
1989	172/221 (77.8)

pandemics, and an eighth of Indian origin began in 1992. The treatment of cholera is based essentially on rehydration of the patients. Antibacterial treatment enables the general status to be improved more rapidly and sterilizes the patient's stools, thus breaking the epidemiological chain. In 1970, treatment with sulfonamides in addition to rehydration was instituted in Iran by Lapeyssonie et al. (1970). In 1961, Rahal et al. (1973) established the transmissibility of plasmid-mediated resistance to antibacterial agents from *Enterobacteriaceae*. Resistance to plasmid-mediated β-lactams took a long time to become established in *V. cholerae*. The first carrier strains were isolated in Algeria in 1973 by Rahal et al. In 1977, plasmid-mediated resistance was described in Asia. The enzymes were of the TEM-1 type.

A new plasmid-mediated β-lactamase, SAR-1, was isolated in 1976 in the fourth cholera epidemic in Tanzania. This involved two strains of *V. cholerae* serotype O1 Inaba.

Resistance to trimethoprim is associated with resistance to the vibriostatic derivative O/129 (2,4-diamino-6,7-diisopropylpteridine). Bougoudogo et al. (1992) studied the susceptibilities to antibiotics of 300 strains collected worldwide between 1982 and 1991. Resistance to vibriostatic compounds appears more common in the Inaba serotype than in the Ogawa serotype. This resistance is associated with that to chloramphenicol, co-trimoxazole, ampicillin, tetracyclines, and, less commonly, nitrofurans.

Outbreaks due to resistant strains have been reported in the Philippines, Tanzania, Malawi, Bangladesh, and Egypt.

The new strain responsible for the eighth pandemic is resistant to furans.

13.2. *Haemophilus ducreyi*

H. ducreyi is a gram-negative coccobacillus responsible for a sexually transmitted disease, chancroid. In South Africa, this is the most common ulcerative genital infection. In Johannesburg, *H. ducreyi* is resistant to sulfonamides (MIC_{90}, >128 μg/ml), tetracyclines, (MIC_{90}, >16 μg/ml), and penicillin G (MIC_{90}, >128 μg/ml), but it remains susceptible to erythromycin A and co-trimoxazole. In 1988, all the strains tested in South Africa were susceptible to erythromycin A and about 10% were moderately resistant to minocycline. By comparison, 50% of strains isolated in

Kenya, the Philippines, and Singapore were resistant to tetracyclines. In 1982, the first strains resistant to erythromycin A were described in Singapore, and strains highly resistant to co-trimoxazole were also reported in 1985 in Africa and Southeast Asia.

13.3. *Campylobacter* spp. and *Helicobacter pylori*

13.3.1. *Campylobacter jejuni* and *Campylobacter coli*

C. jejuni and C. coli constitute one of the etiologies of traveler's diarrhea. Postinfections are rare and consist mainly of neurological immunopathological disorders (Guillain-Barré syndrome). It is transmitted via contamined food and water. The disease is self-limiting, resolving in 3 to 5 days. Campylobacteriosis is considered a zoonotic disease, and animals such as poultry, pigs, and sheep may act as reservoirs for *Campylobacter*. Erythromycin is one of the reference treatments, as are fluoroquinolones. Treatment for *Campylobacter* is often initiated empirically before antibacterial sensitivity tests, and therefore, it is of importance to know the expected susceptibility of *Campylobacter*. This is a prerequisite for appropriate therapy.

In Thailand, 11% of strains of *C. jejuni* and 46% of *C. coli* isolates are resistant to erythromycin A and tetracyclines. In the United States, a survey by the CDC showed that 2.4% of strains were resistant to erythromycin A (MIC, ≥16 μg/ml). Identical results have been reported in Canada. The majority of studies showed that resistance to erythromycin A is associated in particular with *C. coli*.

In studies conducted in France by Mégraud, resistance to erythromycin A has been shown to be minor (1.8 to 3.4%), whereas resistance to cyclines accounts for about 7 to 9% of strains.

In Spain in 1987, fluoroquinolone resistance was practically nonexistent. Rates of resistance to the two antibiotics are 7.4% for *C. jejuni* and 45% for *C. coli*. There is cross-resistance between nalidixic acid and the fluoroquinolones, as demonstrated by Jiménez et al. (1994). From 1997 to 1998, resistance to ciprofloxacin in *C. jejuni* and *C. coli* was higher for strains isolated from broilers (98.7 and 100%) and pigs (100% for *C. coli*) than those isolated from foods (74.4 and 72.7%) or from humans (75 and 70.5%). Regarding erythromycin A resistance, a higher prevalence was found in *C. jejuni* and in *C. coli* cultured from food of chicken origin (17.1 and 50%, respectively) or from pig samples (81.1% for *C. coli*) than in those from human fecal samples (3.2 and 34.5%).

Rautlin et al. showed a progressive reduction in the activity of fluoroquinolones against *C. jejuni* and *C. coli*. Taking 8 μg/ml as the breakpoint (Swedish Committee), the proportion of resistant strains was 4% between 1978 and 1980, increasing to 11% in 1990 and 17% in 1993. The same phenomenon has been observed in The Netherlands and Spain.

In Finland, approximately 3% of *Campylobacter* strains are resistant to erythromycin A and azithromycin.

In Saudi Arabia, a survey was conducted over a period of 12 months between May 1989 and June 1990 in the Jeddah region which showed that the prevalence of *Salmonella* was 6.2%, that of *Campylobacter* spp. was 4.5%, and that of *Shigella* spp. was 4.2%. The isolation of *Campylobacter* peaked between the months of September and November. *C. jejuni* biotype IV represented 69%, and *C. coli* represented 31%. The proportions of erythromycin A- and tetracycline-resistant strains were, respectively, 7.3 and 32.7%. The high prevalence of *C. jejuni* biotype IV had not yet been reported.

A high frequency of isolation of *C. coli* has also been reported in Central Africa, the former Yugoslavia, Hong Kong, and Chile. Resistance of *C. coli* to erythromycin A is also found in Europe and North America.

In Greece from 1998 to 2000, 30.6% of the isolates were resistant to ciprofloxacin and no strains were resistant to erythromycin A.

A low prevalence of chloramphenicol-resistant strains has been shown in many studies.

The emergence of gentamicin resistance in strains isolated from animals could be related to the use of apramycin, which may have selected AAC(3′)-IV-type enzyme. Kanamycin resistance is generally associated with the plasmid-borne *tetO* gene and APH(3′), which had been implicated in kanamycin resistance in *C. coli*.

13.3.2. *H. pylori*

The proportion of metronidazole-resistant *H. pylori* strains is on the order of 25%. In countries with a high macrolide consumption, the primary resistance rate may also attain 15%.

Ampicillin-resistant strains have not been described, but in certain centers a reduction in the drug's activity has been noted. (See chapter 40.)

14. ANAEROBIC BACTERIA

Anaerobic bacteria are potentially pathogenic agents, particularly when the host's defenses are impaired, whether by surgery, neoplasia, malnutrition, or trauma.

The taxonomy of anaerobic bacteria is complex and not definitive. Among gram-negative bacilli, three groups are responsible for infections: *Bacteroides fragilis*, the *Prevotella-Porphyromonas* group, and the *Fusobacterium* group. However, infections in which *Veillonella parvula* is implicated have been described.

The classification of gram-positive bacteria is even more complex: gram-positive cocci (*Peptococcus, Peptostreptococcus*, etc.) and spore-forming (*Clostridium* spp.) or non-spore-forming (*Propionibacterium, Eubacterium*, etc.) bacilli.

Infections caused by *B. fragilis* differ from those due to *Prevotella-Porphyromonas*. The latter are the cause of RTIs both alone and in combination with other microorganisms. *B. fragilis* is responsible for abdominal infections and certain forms of otitis.

14.1. Mechanisms of Resistance

14.1.1. Resistance to β-Lactams

Resistance to gram-negative bacteria is due either to β-lactamase production, the modification of PBPs, or poor transparietal penetration.

The following β-lactamases have been described:

- Cephalosporinases, which hydrolyze cephalosporins, but not cephamycins, and penicillins only weakly
- A penicillinase which also possesses weak cephalosporinase-like activity, produced by *B. fragilis*.
- A large quantity of cephalosporinases which hydrolye cefoxitin, but with a low hydrolysis rate, produced by *B. fragilis*
- β-Lactamases hydrolyzing imipenem and cefoxitin
- Cefoxitinases hydrolyzing cefoxitin but not imipenem, produced by *B. fragilis* (Livermore, 1992) and *Bacteroides distasonis*
- Carbapenamases produced by *B. fragilis* and *B. distasonis* that hydrolyze penicillins and cephalosporins, including

cephamycins. The carbapenamase of *B. distasonis* is inhibited by clavulanic acid, in contrast to that of *B. fragilis*.

- A β-lactamase produced by certain strains of *B. fragilis* group II which have the characteristic of not being inhibited by clavulanic acid, tazobactam, or sulbactam and which have a pI of 5.0

The penicillinases of the *B. fragilis* group are constitutive and have molecular masses of between 26.5 and > 60 kDa. They are periplasmic and associated with the membrane.

The *Prevotella* group produces cephalosporinases or penicillinases. The majority of enzymes produced by this bacterial genus are inhibited by clavulanic acid, tazobactam, sulbactam, moxalactam (latamoxef), and cefoxitin. Likewise, the *Prevotella* enzymes are constitutive and have molecular masses of between 24 and 40 kDa.

Nord et al. have described a penicillinase in *Fusobacterium nucleatum*. This enzyme is constitutive and has a molecular mass of between 21 and 26.5 kDa.

The production of inducible β-lactamases has been described for *Clostridium butyricum*, *Clostridium ramosum*, and *Clostridium clostridioforme*.

A loss of affinity for PBPs 1, 2, and 3 in *B. fragilis* may cause a reduction in the activity of β-lactams. Usually the reduction in activity of cephamycins is related to a reduction in transparietal penetration.

14.1.2. Other Antibiotics

The loss of activity of tetracyclines against anaerobic bacteria is transferable and transposable. It is due to a blockade of intracellular penetration.

The majority of anaerobic bacteria are susceptible to clindamycin, with the exception of *Clostridium difficile*. Clindamycin-resistant strains have been described. Resistance is of the macrolide-lincosamide-streptogramin B type.

With the exception of the spore-forming gram-positive bacteria, the anaerobic bacteria are susceptible to the action of the 5-nitroimidazole derivatives. Resistant strains are uncommon. Resistance is due to one of two mechanisms: either a decrease in parietal penetration or a decrease in nitroreduction.

14.2. Epidemiology of Resistance

For some 15 years, the pressure of selection on the oropharyngeal and fecal floras has resulted in an imbalance in these floras, and we are progressively seeing an increase in the number of resistant strains among anaerobic bacteria. An epidemiological survey undertaken in Spain showed that the proportion of strains of *Peptostreptococcus* of reduced susceptibility to penicillin G (MIC, >0.5 μg/ml) reached 9.5% in 1992. Half of the resistant strains comprised *Peptostreptococcus anaerobius*, followed by *Peptostreptococcus asaccharolyticus*. For 75% of these strains, the MIC of penicillin G was greater than 8 μg/ml. The proportion of strains resistant to cefoxitin (MIC, >2 μg/ml) was 10.5%. There is a correlation between resistance to penicillin G and that to cefoxitin. The level of resistance to metronidazole (MIC, >8 μg/ml) is on the order of 5.5%, while the activity of erythromycin A (MIC, >2 μg/ml) differs according to the species of *Peptostreptococcus*. Overall, 75% of strains isolated are resistant. Clindamycin (MIC, >4 μg/ml) is inactive against 19% of strains. About 1.5% of strains are resistant to co-amoxinclav (MIC, >4/8 μg/ml). Chloramphenicol (MIC, >8 μg/ml) is inactive against only 3% of isolates.

The frequency of resistance of *Clostridium perfringens* to penicillin G is on the order of 12.5%. Resistances to cefoxitin, metronidazole, erythromycin A, and clindamycin are on the orders of 21, 4.5, 37, and 10.5%, respectively.

Rates of resistance to penicillin G are 9, 7, and 18 to 57%, respectively, for the genera *Eubacterium*, *Fusobacterium*, and *Veillonella*. Metronidazole and clindamycin are inactive against 19 and 9% of strains of *Eubacterium*, respectively. Resistance to cefoxitin is on the order of 53.5%. Resistance to metronidazole affects 7.5% of *Veillonella parvula strains*.

Erythromycin A is practically inactive against *Fusobacterium* (75%) and *Veillonella* (66%).

The level of resistance of the *B. fragilis* groups to cefoxitin (MIC, >16 μg/ml) is on the order of 21.5%. There is a difference between the species of this group, the resistance rates being 8 and 67%, respectively, for *B. fragilis* and *Bacteroides thetaiotaomicron*. Levels of resistance to metronidazole and co-amoxiclav are low: 2 and 3.5%, respectively. The global rate of resistance to clindamycin is about 20.5%. In the Swedish survey by Olsson-Olquist, strains of *B. fragilis* resistant to piperacillin, clindamycin, metronidazole, and imipenem represented, respectively, 23, 2, 1, and 0%.

In France, the first strain of imipenen-resistant *B. fragilis* was described in 1987; since then a few strains have been isolated, but they remain infrequent. An epidemiological survey was undertaken between 1988 and 1989 and showed that the activity of the combination of amoxicillin and clavulanic acid had decreased slightly because at a concentration of 2 μg/ml, the growth of 100% of strains was inhibited in 1988 but only 87% of growth was inhibited in 1989. About 15% of strains were resistant to clindamycin (MIC, >4 μg/ml), all were susceptible to chloramphenicol, and 6% were of reduced susceptibility to metronidazole (MIC, 2 to 4 μg/ml).

No metronidazole-resistant strain has been detected among *Prevotella* spp. or *Fusobacterium*. Erythromycin A is inactive against 8% of *Prevotella* spp. The level of resistance of *Fusobacterium* to clindamycin is low, on the order of 3%. Sedaillan et al. (1990) reported the activities of different antibiotics against 475 strains of *Prevotella* (*Prevotella oralis*, 348 strains; *Prevotella melaninogenica*, 107 strains). These strains were isolated from multibacterial flora obtained from gynecological and respiratory infections. Among the strains of *P. oralis*, 40% produced a β-lactamase and clavulanic acid restored the activity of amoxicillin. Table 78 shows activities of antibiotics, against *Prevotella* spp.

In a study conducted on strains of *Prevotella* spp., *Porphyromonas* spp., and *Fusobacterium* spp. collected in the United Kingdom, Appelbaum et al. (1990) showed that 42.3% of the strains of *Prevotella* and *Porphyromonas* and 26.8% of the

Table 78 Activities of antibiotics against *Prevotella* spp.[a]

Drug	MIC (μg/ml)	
	50%	90%
Amoxicillin	2	16
Co-amoxiclav	<0.12	0.25
Piperacillin	1	4
Cefoxitin	1	4
Cefotaxime	0.25	4
Clindamycin	0.12	0.25
Metronidazole	0.25	4

[a]Data from Sedaillan, 1990.

Table 79 Prevalence of β-lactamase-producing strains

Organism(s)	% of β-lactamase-producing isolates
Prevotella bivia	78.6
P. oralis	60
Other species	16.7–45.8
Fusobacterium necrophorum	7.1
Fusobacterium nucleatum	23.5

strains of *Fusobacterium* produced a β-lactamase. This production, however, was species dependent (Table 79).

All of the strains studied were susceptible to metronidazole and imipenem, and depending on the breakpoint adopted, 99.3% (breakpoint, ≥32 μg/ml) and 90.4% (breakpoint, ≤16 μg/ml) were susceptible to cefoxitin.

Bétriu et al. (1993) studied the activities of 11 antibiotics against the *B. fragilis* group. They showed that not all of the cephamycins had the same antibacterial activity against the *B. fragilis* group and that the incidence of resistance to β-lactams varied with the species (Table 80), the most resistant being *B. thetaiotaomicron*, *Bacteroides ovatus*, and *B. distasonis*.

The most active compound was cefoxitin, followed by moxalactam, cefmetazole, and cefotetan. It should be noted that piperacillin and mezlocillin do not have the same activity. Imipenem-resistant strains are infrequent (~1.4%). No strain resistant to metronidazole (MIC, ≥8 μg/ml) or chloramphenicol (MIC, ≥8 μg/ml) has been found. About 20.7% of these strains are resistant to clindamycin (MIC, ≥4 μg/ml).

In a 10-year prospective surveillance study at a Veterans Affairs medical center, only 2% of *C. difficile* isolates were resistant clinically to metronidazole (Johnson et al., 2000). Reports from China, France, and Spain have found clinical *C. difficile* with reduced susceptibility to metronidazole.

High-level resistance to metronidazole in *C. difficile* was reported to occur in horses (Jang et al., 1997).

15. *MYCOBACTERIUM TUBERCULOSIS*

Tuberculosis is one of the oldest diseases of humankind, as evidenced by the lesions found in skeletons of the pre-Columbus era. However, it only became a major public health problem at the time of urbanization and particularly in the industrial era, which fostered the dissemination of the tubercle bacillus. At the beginning of the 19th century, the annual incidence of tuberculosis in the United States was 200 per 10^5 inhabitants.

The introduction of streptomycin into treatment in 1947 produced a spectacular regression in morbidity due to tuberculosis. In 1953, 84,000 new cases were reported in the United States; in 1989, the number of new patients was 23,500.

However, tuberculosis remains a subject of concern throughout the world and has experienced a resurgence of interest in the industrialized countries since 1985 to 1986. About a third of the world's population, i.e. 1,700 million inhabitants, are infected with Koch's bacillus. About eight million new cases are declared annually, and three million deaths are attributed to tuberculosis annually.

In the United States, the incidence of tuberculosis declined by 6% annually up until 1985. From 1986, the number of new patients increased by 16% annually. This recrudescence of the disease is due to several factors, such as the impoverishment of a certain section of the population with an increase in the numbers of homeless, the immigrant populations from countries with highly endemic tuberculosis, overpopulation in poor areas, malnutrition, alcoholism, addictions, lack of medical follow-up, institutionalization of the elderly, and prison overpopulation. A further factor has completely transformed the American scene: AIDS.

In industrial countries, mortality due to tuberculosis is about 3% annually, and a rate of 5.5% has been obtained since 1920 to 1930 through the improvement in socioeconomic conditions and general hygiene. In the developing countries, the incidence of tuberculosis remains very high, as does mortality.

Over the last few years, the incidence of tuberculosis has fallen in Belgium, Finland, and France. It has stabilized in Portugal, the United Kingdom, and Sweden but is on the

Table 80 Resistance to β-lactams among members of the *B. fragilis* group[a]

Drug	Breakpoint (μg/ml)	Prevalence of resistance (%)				
		B. fragilis	*B. thetaiotaomicron*	*B. ovatus*	*B. distasonis*	*B. vulgatus*
Clindamycin	16	12	33	19.2	12.5	50
Cefoxitin	32	6.8	10.2	11.5	25	0
Cefotetan	32	10.3	64.1	34.6	62.5	50
Cefmetazole	32	6.8	12.8	15.3	25	25
Moxalactam	32	8.6	30.7	26.9	62.5	25
Piperacillin	128	8.6	10.2	11.5	25	0
Mezlocillin	128	1.7	5.1	7.6	12.5	0
Imipenem	8	3.4	0	0	0	0
Co-amoxiclav	8	3.4	0	0	0	0
Ampicillin + sulbactam	8	3.4	0	0	0	0
Ticarcillin + clavulanic acid	64	3.4	0	0	0	0

[a]Data from Bétriu et al., 1993.

increase in Austria, Denmark, Ireland, Spain, Germany, The Netherlands, and Switzerland. It is catastrophic in the former Yugoslavia, with an annual incidence of 200 per 10^5 inhabitants in Bosnia.

In western Europe, the highest level is observed in Portugal ($57.7/10^5$) and the lowest level is observed in Denmark ($6.5/10^5$). In the other countries of Europe, the incidence is $\leq 25/10^5$. The population affected is usually elderly. Tuberculosis is affecting human immunodeficiency virus (HIV)-positive patients with increasing frequency, particularly in France, Spain, Italy, and Portugal. In Paris in 1991, tuberculosis was the presenting feature of AIDS in 30% of patients. In France, the decline in tuberculosis was arrested in 1986, when a plateau was reached; a resurgence began in 1992.

Tuberculosis in western countries had become a disease of the poor and deprived. The research programs of the public institutes or public centers no longer counted the tubercle bacillus among their concerns since multiple chemotherapy was very active.

15.1. Multiresistant Strains of the Tubercle Bacilli

Therapy of tuberculosis requires a long treatment. Monotherapy predisposes to the emergence of resistant strains following treatment and results in some therapeutic failures. The frequency of mutation of M. *tuberculosis* varies according to the different antituberculosis agents. It is 10^6 for isoniazid, 10^8 for rifampin, 10^6 for ethambutol, and 10^5 for streptomycin. The probability of a strain of M. *tuberculosis* developing resistance when several antituberculosis agents are combined is therefore low; for the combination of isoniazid and rifampin, for example, it is 10^{14}. Multiple chemotherapy has been recommended since the end of the 1950s. Its application in industrialized countries has produced a reduction in the number of cases of tuberculosis and has had an unexpected consequence, namely, the lack of interest in research in this field. Since the introduction of rifampin in 1960, failures due to secondary resistance are only observed in 20 to 30% of cases, but this is a serious matter since it involves rifampin and isoniazid, which are major antituberculosis agents.

Antibiotic resistance in M. *tuberculosis* has long been known, particularly with streptomycin and isoniazid. Primary resistance of M. *tuberculosis* to isoniazid is greater than 10% in some countries (Table 81).

The appearance of multiresistant strains of M. *tuberculosis,* in other words, nonsusceptible to the two major antituberculosis agents, isoniazid and rifampin, has completely transformed the treatment of tuberculosis.

Table 81 Primary resistance of *M. tuberculosis* to isoniazid

Country	Primary resistance (%)
Bolivia	32.6
Brazil	10.7
Egypt	12.1
India	10.6
Ivory Coast	10.4
Korea	30.6
Mauritania	13.6
Morocco	16.8
South Africa	17.5
Thailand	22.9
Samoa	44.8

In the United States, multiresistant strains have been described in 13 states. Between 1982 and 1986, a survey by the CDC showed that 0.5% of strains isolated were resistant to isoniazid and rifampin. The proportion of such strains reached 3.1% in 1991. Eight outbreaks of nosocomial infection due to multiresistant strains have been described in the United States, affecting about 200 people, including nursing staff. This type of outbreak has also been described in France and Italy.

In a recent survey of the incidence of tuberculosis and the susceptibility of M. *tuberculosis* in the United Kingdom, 46 strains out of 4,099 were multiresistant.

The reason for the emergence of multiresistant strains varies. Poor compliance with treatment and poor prescribing habits are the two main causes.

The risk of an HIV-positive person developing tuberculosis is 10 times greater than in the general population. The annual rate of tuberculosis in this at-risk population is 8%. Because of the marked reduction in cell-mediated immunity, HIV infection reactivates quiescent tuberculosis. It is difficult to treat because of the poor treatment compliance of patients and the side effects associated with the treatment. This results in the selection of resistant strains, which are at risk of dissemination.

In France, almost 10% of strains of M. *tuberculosis* isolated between 1967 and 1970 were resistant to one or more antituberculosis agents. Primary resistance to streptomycin (7.4%) was more common than primary resistance to isoniazid (4.4%). With the use of rifampin in therapy, the rate of primary resistance has declined, falling to 5% between 1980 and 1987. Primary resistance to streptomycin (3.4%) remains more common than primary resistance to isoniazid (2.9%). This might be due to the fact that the streptomycin-resistant strains retain their full virulence, in contrast to isoniazid-resistant strains.

For 80% of streptomycin-resistant strains, the mechanism of resistance is related to mutations in the *rpsL* gene, which encodes the S-12 ribosomal protein, particularly the replacement of the lysine 88 by a glutamine. A second mutation has been shown at the binding site of streptomycin at the 903 and 904 nucleotides which code for 16S rRNA. In the case of low-level resistance, the mechanism involved is a reduction in membrane permeability.

There is no cross-resistance between streptomycin and the other aminoglycosides, such as kanamycin and amikacin.

Since 1988, the frequency of primary resistance has increased, particularly in HIV-positive patients. Primary multiresistance (isoniazid plus rifampin) is on the order of 3%.

A multicenter study conducted in 1992 in the majority of French hospitals showed that 48 strains out of 8,521 were multiresistant. Thirty-one strains out of 48 (65%) were also resistant to another antibiotic, particularly ethambutol and streptomycin.

Fluoroquinolone-resistant strains of M. *tuberculosis* have been described.

The strains of the *Mycobacterium avium* complex that have acquired resistance to 14- and 15-membered-ring macrolides (cross-resistance) have a single point mutation in the V domain of 23S rRNA.

16. *UREAPLASMA UREALYTICUM*

U. urealyticum is an opportunistic and pathogenic agent of the urogenital tract. *U. urealyticum* is sometimes associated with infections of the respiratory tract and central nervous system, which can be life-threatening in neonates. It is one of the etiologies of nongonococcal urethritis and salpingitis.

U. urealyticum is intrinsically resistant to lincomycin and remains susceptible to the action of macrolides. Strains with tetracycline resistance due to the *tet*(M) genes have been isolated. It is, however, difficult to determine the exact prevalence of resistance because of the lack of standardization in the methods for determining susceptibility and the difficulties of isolating strains in routine clinical microbiology laboratories.

17. *CHLAMYDIA* SPP.

The chlamydiae are important pathogens of humans and animals, causing a wide variety of diseases. They have also been reported as pneumonic agents in swine (*Chlamydia suis, Chlamydia pecorum,* and *Chlamydia abortus*).

Emergence of tetracycline-resistant chlamydiae in both humans and animals is of great concern.

There are nine documented cases of human *Chlamydia trachomatis* isolates resistant to tetracyclines. Eight tetracycline-resistant *C. suis* strains were reported on a farm in Nebraska and in Iowa.

18. HOW TO ESTABLISH AN EPIDEMIOLOGICAL SURVEY

To set up a program of postmarketing surveillance of emergence and spread of resistance is a difficult and time-consuming task, but it is compulsory for monitoring the ecological process in front of antibacterials.

The data generated from epidemiological surveys provide physicians with important information to make therapeutic choices on a local scale and to help the scientific community to monitor the prevalence of resistance on a global scale.

The surveillance epidemiological studies have allowed adoption of appropriate measures to control established resistance and limit the emergence of further resistance.

Increasing resistance has limited the options for treating infections.

18.1. Why Epidemiological Studies?

Epidemiological studies are not unequivocal; the aims may be different, and the resulting data may also direct future research.

The best way to extend the life of an antibacterial at the population level is not well understood.

- Resistance makes treatment of patients more complicated.
- Resistance compromises the effectiveness of a disease control program.
- The scale of the problem and the rate at which resistance becomes a problem are highly variable, depending on the antibacterial agent, the pathogen, and the transmission.
- Declines in response to interventions also differ considerably with different pathogen-drug combinations.

18.1.1. Research

In the research field, unfortunately, epidemiological studies are rarely carried out; however, they are an important tool to detect future threats or emergent resistance, and these studies have to be done upstream to investigate the potential medical need. Two distinct studies could be done: a prospective study on a low-level scale in various geographical areas dealing with the pathology (e.g., cystic fibrosis) and an analysis of published data in the literature, but this aspect is less productive and efficient.

18.1.2. Clinical

Epidemiological studies are infection site oriented to investigate two points: main microorganisms involved and their rank in involvement in a given pathology (e.g., otitis media) and the prevalence of resistance of the main pathogens. Clinical studies are the most difficult type of survey to perform.

18.1.3. Microbiology

A microbiology study is the classical survey which involves microorganisms and, indirectly, patients. The clinical isolates may be collected from patients or from carriers.

18.2. Laboratories

For collaborative studies, there are two scenarios to determine MICs: central laboratories and regional laboratories.

18.2.1. Central Laboratories

Central laboratories provide the best situation for testing. All of the facilities have to send the bacteriological sample to the central laboratory for MIC determination, full reidentification, and genetics. The difficult part is the transportation to avoid to loose strains (suitable conditions are needed). The central laboratory will have to use for control reference strains as well as well-identified resistant strains (genetics and enzymatics). Only one methodology is applied.

18.2.2. Regional Laboratories

With regional laboratories, collecting uniform data is more complex. The regional laboratory receives all of the isolates from different local clinical microbiology laboratories in a restricted geographical area. The regional laboratory is in charge of reidentification of all isolates and MIC determinations.

18.2.3. Cross-Validation

The fundamental objective is to obtain reliable data with the same values in all of the regional clinical microbiological facilities participating to the survey. This is accomplished as follows.

18.2.3.1. Material and Methods

The material is composed of well-known and genetic and enzymatic strains as controls; at least 10 of each should be used, and the basic material needs to be the same, for instance, microtiter plates issued from the same manufacturer (dry panel), with the same culture medium. The methodology to perform MIC determinations is the same, such as inoculum size, temperature of incubation, age of subculture, etc.

With each isolate, MICs are determined at least in triplicate and for 3 days.

18.2.3.2. Results

An electronic frame is prepared and given to each regional laboratory to be filled and sent to a central statistical system.

The following should be examined:

- Intralaboratory variations
- Interlaboratory variations

The population distribution versus antibacterials is documented. The interlaboratory variation has to range between -1 and $+1$ dilution from the mean.

An agreement coefficient of $>$85% is considered satisfactory.

When results have less than 85% concordance, the following should be considered:

- The same regional laboratory should always be used; the only other decision would be to eliminate this facility and to find another one in the same geographical area. This is usually of rare occurrence.

- Abnormalities could be found for an antibacterial; it is important to consider that this could be due to chemical instability of the drug substance or to reactivity with the plastic of the wells or other devices.
- The strain to be tested could be unstable, especially resistant isolates.
- The intraclass correlation coefficient is calculated with a confidence interval of 95% (Cuenca-Estrella et al., 2003).

18.3. Methodology

18.3.1. Period for Collecting Strains

The most accurate period for collecting some microorganisms, such as those involved in RTIs, has to be chosen.

18.3.2. Size of Bacterial Sampling

During the recruitment period, all of the given microorganisms are collected, but one organism per patient. To investigate the antibacterial susceptibility, only important bacterial species are collected, such as *S. pneumoniae*. The site of infection needs to be specified (for example, respiratory tract samples, meningitis, blood culture, or wound samples).

18.3.3. Choice of Patients

Ill subjects and carrier subjects must be differentiated. The second criterion is the subject age: neonates, children, adults, and seniors. The third criterion is the physiological status of patients (hepatic or/and renal impairments, burns, obesity, etc.)

18.3.4. Center Selection

It is important to avoid bias via center choice: avoid centers which recruit only patients with failures (such as *Streptococcus pyogenes* in group A beta-hemolytic streptococci) to avoid collection only resistant strains.

Depending on what the epidemiological survey is intended to investigate, patients from ICU (receiving or not receiving ventilatory assistance), hospitalized patients, or patients in the community can be chosen. A differentiation must be made between home care and the community setting.

18.3.5. Strains

All of the collected strains are to be kept in a suitable medium and under proper conditions. The best condition is to test all of the isolates at the same time after reidentification.

When the strain is resistant to a given family of antibiotic, genotyping or sequencing of the major gene involved in resistance, such as the *ropB* gene for rifampin, or a deep analysis of enzyme (β-lactamases, aminoglycoside-inactivating enzymes, etc.) should be done. In the case of an abnormal elevated resistance pattern in a given region in comparison to others, a deep genetic analysis to determine the clone is to be performed (for example, the *eem* gene for *S. pyogenes*).

The genetic and enzymatic evaluations may be performed in a central laboratory. Phenotyping is a minimum to be done; however, discrepancies between genotypes and phenotypes could reach above 10%, as shown for erythromycin A.

Genetic analysis has to be done on strains for which the MICs are equal to or greater than 2 dilutions from the sensitivity breakpoint.

18.3.6. Repetitive Epidemiological Surveys

If the same epidemiological survey is carried out on a 2 to 3-year basis, the strain of the previous year (when it survives) is tested in parallel with the new set of bacteria to really be sure of the trends in resistance; however, the strains need to be collected in the same facilities, from the same type of patients, and from the same site of infection (bronchial secretion, middle ear fluid, etc.) as well as the same location (ICU, urological wards, etc.).

18.3.7. Bactericidal Activity

In some cases, it could be useful to perform kill kinetic curves on random resistant isolates to investigate if some antibacterials have lost their bactericidal activity.

18.4. Results

The most acceptable way to present data is to provide population bacterial distribution, rendering easier the detection of displacement of the mode MICs to the right hand side. The cumulative percentage of sensitivity is related to breakpoints, and comparison has to be done with the same breakpoints to avoid confused results.

19. COMBATING RESISTANCE

Strategies to combat resistance are still a matter of discussion, showing the complexity of the problem that bacteria are able to adapt rapidly as they do in nature to protect themselves against defensive traits of other bacteria.

The following have been proposed:

- Infection control programs to limit the horizontal transmission of multiresistant pathogens
- Control programs to optimize the use of antibiotics
- Restriction of usage: a strategy to limit the use of a specific antibiotic or class. The limitation of this method is that the shift to an alternate class increases prescription and promotes the emergence of resistance.
- Combination therapy; the well-known example is antituberculosis polychemotherapy
- Adapted doses to achieve high levels in serum between doses
- Cycling, which is intended to preserve the activity of antibiotics by scheduled rotation. This technique is highly controversial (Pujol and Gudiol, 2001).
- Prudent use of antibacterials, which has been recommended since the 1950s
- Surveillance studies to adapt therapeutic strategies as well as to detect future problems
- The relationship between volume of prescription and resistance is somewhat difficult to establish. The spread of resistance is a dynamic process; low dosing or noncompliance is often a risk factor. Pharmacokinetics and pharmacodynamics could make it difficult to compare and aggregate consumption of different antibacterials of the same chemical class.

REFERENCES

Acar JF, 1999, Resistance pattern of *Haemophilus influenzae*, J Chemother, 11, 44–50.

Alhambra A, Gomez-Garces JL, Alos JL, 2004, Susceptibility of *Streptococcus agalactiae* isolates from blood and urine to 18 widely used and recently marketed antibiotics, Clin Microbiol Infect, 10, 267–268.

Andrews JI, Diekem DJ, Hunter SK, Rhomberg PR, Pfaller MA, Doern GV, 2000, Group B streptococci causing neonatal bloodstream infection, antimicrobial susceptibility and serotyping results from SENTRY centers in the western hemisphere, Am J Obstet Gynecol, 183, 859–862.

Bandak SI, Allen T, Bolzon DA, Preston DA, Bourchillon SK, Hoban DJ, 2001, Antibiotic susceptibilities among recent clinical isolates of *Haemophilus influenzae* and *Moraxella catarrhalis* from fifteen countries, Eur J Clin Microbiol Infect Dis, 20, 55–60.

Bell JM, Borlace GN, Turnidge JD, SENTRY Asia-Pacific Study Group, 2002, Macrolide resistance in β-hemolytic streptococci from Asia-Pacific region. Results from the SENTRY Asia-Pacific surveillance program 2001, 42nd Intersci Conf Antimicrob Agents Chemother, abstract C2-1986.

Betriu CE, Culebras M, Gomez M, Rodriguez-Avial I, Sanchez BA, Agreda MC, Picazo J, 2003, Erythromycin and clindamycin resistance and telithromycin susceptibility in *Streptococcus agalactiae*, Antimicrob Agents Chemother, 47, 1112–1114.

Betriu CE, Gomez M, Sanchez A, Cruceyra A, Romero J, Picazzo JJ, 1994, Antibiotic resistance and penicillin tolerance in clinical isolates of group B streptococci, Antimicrob Agents Chemother, 38, 2183–2186.

Biedenbach DJ, Stephen JM, Jones RN, 2003, Antimicrobial susceptibility profile among β-haemolytic *Streptococcus* spp. collected in the SENTRY Antimicrobial Surveillance Program—North America, 2001, Diagn Microbiol Infect Dis, 46, 291–294.

Blosser RS, Karginova EA, Karlowsky JA, Critchley IA, Thornsberry C, Sahm DF, Jones ME, 2002, Molecular analysis of *Streptococcus pneumoniae* with elevated MICs to levofloxacin—2001–2002 worldwide surveillance, 42nd Intersci Conf Antimicrob Agents Chemother, abstract C2-1619.

Bogaerts J, Lepage P, Taelman H, Rouvroy D, Batungwanayo J, Kestelyn P, Hitimana DG, van de Perre P, Vandepitte J, Verbist L, et al, 1993, Antimicrobial susceptibility and serotype distribution of *S. pneumoniae* in Rwanda 1984–1990, J Infect, 27, 157–168.

Bonomo RA, 2000, Multiple antibiotic-resistant bacteria in long term care facilities, an emerging problem in the practice of infectious disease, Clin Infect Dis, 31, 1414–1422.

Bryskier A, 2002, Ketolides—telithromycin, an example of a new class of antibacterial agent, Clin Infect Dis, 6, 661–669.

Bryskier A, 2004, Aventis data on file.

BSAC Extended Working Party on Respiratory Resistance Surveillance and GR Micro Limited, 2001, Antimicrobial susceptibility of community-acquired respiratory pathogens in Ireland compared with England, Wales, and Scotland, 41st Intersci Conf Antimicrob Agents Chemother, abstract C2-683.

Cavallo JD, Le Blanc F, Fabre F, Forticq-Esqueönte A, 2001, Surveillance de la sensibilité de *P. aeruginosa* aux antibiotiques en France et distribution des mécanismes de résistances aux bétalactamines, Etude du GERPB en 1999, Pathol Biol, 7, 49–56.

Chanal C, Bonnet R, De Champs C, Sirot D, Labia R, Sirot J, 2000, Prevalence of β-lactamases among 1,072 clinical strains of *Proteus mirabilis*, a 2-year survey in a French hospital, Antimicrob Agents Chemother, 44, 1930–1935.

Choo KE, Ariffi WA, Ahmed T, Lim WL, Gururaj AK, 1990, Pyogenic meningitis in hospitalized children in Kelantan, Malaysia, Ann Trop Paediatr, 10, 80–98.

Cizmann M, Gubina M, Paragi M, Beovic B, Lesnicar G, Slovenian Meningitis Study Group, 2001, Meningococcal disease in Slovenia (1993–1999), serogroups and susceptibility to antibiotics. Int J Antimicrob Agents, 17, 27–31.

Couto I, de Lancastre H, Severinaa E, et al, 1996, Ubiquitous presence of a *mecA* homologue in natural isolates of *Staphylococcus sciuri*, Microb Drug Res, 2, 377–391.

Critchley IA, Blosser-Middleton R, Jones ME, Yamakita J, Aswapokee, Chayakul P, Tharavichitukul P, Vibhagool A, Thornsberry C, Karlowsky IA, Sahm DF, 2002, Antimicrobial resistance among respiratory pathogens collected in Thailand during 1999–2000, J Chemother, 14, 147–154.

Cuenca-Estrella M, Moore CB, Barchiesi F, Bille J, Chryssanthou E, Denning DW, Donnelly JP, Dromer F, Dupont B, Rex JH, Richardson MD, Sancak B, Verweij PE, Rodriguez-Tudela JL, and AFST Subcommittee of the European Committee on Antimicrobial Susceptibility Testing, 2003, Multicenter evaluation of the reproducibility of the proposed antifungal susceptibility testing method for fermentative yeasts, Clin Microbiol Infect, 9, 467–474.

Dagnra Y, Tigossou S, Prince-David M, 2000, Prévalence et sensibilité aux antibiotiques des bactéries isolées des meningitis, Med Mal Infect, 30, 291–294.

Denno DM, Frimpong E, Gregory M, Steele RW, 2002, Nasopharyngeal carriage and susceptibility patterns of *Streptococcus pneumoniae* in Kumasi, Ghana, West Afr J Med, 21, 233–236.

Dermott N, Muscheneim C, Hardley SS, Buan PM, Gorman RV, 1947, Streptomycin in the treatment of tuberculosis in humans. I. Meningitis and generalized hematogeneous tuberculosis, Ann Intern Med, 27, 769.

Diekema DJ, Pfaller MA, Jones RN, Doern GV, Winokur PL, Gales AC, Sader HS, Kugler K, Beach M, the SENTRY Participant Group (America), 1999, Survey of bloodstream infections due to gram-negative bacilli: frequency of occurrence and antimicrobial susceptibility of isolates collected in the United States, Canada, and Latin America for the SENTRY Antimicrobial Surveillance Program, 1997, Clin Infect Dis, 29, 595–607.

Doern GV, Brown SD, 2004, Antimicrobial susceptibility among community-acquired respiratory tract pathogens in the USA, data from Protekt US 2000-01, J Infect, 48, 56–65.

Doern GV, Heilmann KP, Huynh HK, Rhomberg PR, Coffman SL, Brueggemann AB, 2001, Antimicrobial resistance among clinical isolates of *Streptococcus pneumoniae* in the United States during 1999–2000, including a comparison of resistance rates since 1994–1995, Antimicrob Agents Chemother, 45, 1721–1729.

Dornbusch K, King A, Legakis N, the European Study Group on Antibiotic Resistance (ESGAR), 1998, Incidence of antibiotic resistance in blood and urine isolates from hospitalized patients. Report from an European collaborative study, Scand J Infect Dis, 30, 281–288.

Dowling HF, 1953, The effect of the emergence of resistant strains on the future of antibiotic therapy, Antib Annuals 1953–1954, Medicine Encyclopedia Inc., New York.

Dromigny JA, Ndoye B, Macondo EA, Nabeth P, Siby T, Perrier-Gros-Claude JD, 2003, Increasing prevalence of antimicrobial resistance among Enterobacteriaceae uropathogens in Dakar, Senegal, multicenter study, Diagn Microbiol Infect Dis, 47, 595–600.

Eady EA, Cove GH, 2003, Staphylococcal resistance revisited, community-acquired methicillin resistant *Staphylococcus aureus*. An emerging problem for the management of skin and soft tissue infections, Curr Opin Infect Dis, 16, 103–124.

El-Kholy A, Baseem H, Hall GS, Procop GW, Longworth DL, 2003, Antimicrobial resistance in Cairo, Egypt 1999-2000: a survey of five hospitals, J Antimicrob Chemother, 51, 625–630.

Farrell DJ, Morrissey I, Bakker S, Morris L, Buckridge S, Felmingham D, 2004, Molecular epidemiology of multiresistant *Streptococcus pneumoniae* with both *erm*(B)-and *mef*(A)-mediated macrolide resistance, J Clin Microbiol, 42, 764–768.

Feikin DR, Davis M, Nwanyanwu OG, Kazembe PN, Barat LM, Wasas A, Bloland PB, Ziba C, Capper T, Huebner RE, Schwartz B, Klugman KP, Dowell SF, 2003, Antibiotic resistance and serotype distribution of *Streptococcus pneumoniae* colonizing rural Malawian children, Pediatr J Infect Dis, 22, 564–567.

Felmingham D, 2002, Aventis data on file.

Felmingham D, Farrell D, 2001, 2002, 2003, webmaster@grmicro.co.uk.

Felmingham D, Janus C, the e-BASKETT Study Group, 2003, In vitro activity of telithromycin against *Streptococcus pneumoniae* isolated in Europe, Africa, Middle-East and Asia during 2001, ECCMID, Glasgow.

Felmingham D, Reinert RR, Hirakata Y, Rodloff A, 2002, Increasing prevalence of antimicrobial resistance among isolates of *Streptococcus pneumoniae* from the PROTEKT surveillance study, and comparative in vitro activity of the ketolide, telithromycin, J Antimicrob Chemother, 50, suppl 1, 25–37.

Fridkin and Chambers, 2003, UPUA Newsl 21, 2–5.

Fujimura S, Watanabe A, Beighton D, 2001, Characterization of the *mupA* gene in strains of methicillin-resistant *Staphylococcus aureus* with low level of resistance to mupirocin, Antimicrob Agents Chemother, 45, 641–642.

Galimand M, Guiyoule A, Gerbaud G, Rasomanna B, Chanteau S, Carniel E, Courvalin P, 1997, Multidrug resistance in *Yersinia pestis* mediated by a transferable plasmid, N Engl J Med, 337, 677–680.

Gay K, Stephen DS, 2001, Structure and dissemination of a chromosomal insertion element encoding macrolide efflux in *Streptococcus pneumoniae*, J Infect Dis, 184, 56–65.

Gezon HM, 1948, Antibiotic studies on beta-hemolytic streptococci, penicillin-resistance acquired by group A organism, Proc Soc Exp Biol Med, 67, 208.

Giammarelou et al, 1993, 33rd Int Conf Antimicrob Agents, Chemother.

Guiyoule A, Gerbaud G, Buchrieser C, Galimand M, Rahalison L, Chanteau S, Courvalin P, Carniel E, 2001, Transferable plasmid-mediated resistance to streptomycin in a clinical isolate of *Yersinia pestis*, Emerg Infect Dis, 7, 43–48.

Gür D, Özalp M, Sümerkan B, Kaygusuz A, Töreci K, Köksal I, Över U, Söyletir G, 2002, Prevalence of antimicrobial resistance in *Haemophilus influenzae*, *Streptococcus pneumoniae*, *Moraxella catarrhalis* and *Streptococcus pyogenes*, results of a multicenter study in Turkey, Int J Antimicrob Chemother, 19, 207–211.

Gwanzura L, Pasi C, Nathoo KJ, Hakim J, Gangaidzo I, Milke J, Robertson VJ, Heyderman RS, Mason PR, 2003, Rapid emergence of resistance to penicillin and trimethoprim sulfamethoxazole in invasive *Streptococcus pneumoniae* in Zimbabwe, Int J Antimicrob Chemother, 21, 557–561.

Hanberger H, Garcia-Rodriguez JA, Gobernado M, Goossens H, Nilsson LE, Strulens MJ, the French and Portuguese ICU Study Group, 1999, Antibiotic susceptibility among gram-negative bacilli in intensive care units in 5 European countries, JAMA, 281, 67–71.

Hiramatsu K, Cui L, Kuroda M, Ito T, 2001, The emergence and evolution of methicillin-resistant *Staphylococcus aureus*, Trends Microbiol, 9, 486–493.

Hoban D, Waites K, Felmingham D, 2003, Antimicrobial susceptibility of community-acquired respiratory tract pathogens in North America in 1999–2000, finding of the PROTEKT surveillance study, Diagn Microbiol Infect Dis, 45, 251–259.

Hoban DJ, 1999, 2002, Aventis data on file.

Hoban DJ, Balko TV, Kabani AM, Zhanel GG, Karlowsky JA, 1997, Antimicrobial resistance in *Haemophilus influenzae*, a 1996 international surveillance study, 37th Intersci Conf Antimicrob Agents Chemother.

Hodgson JE, Curnock SP, Dyke KGH, Morris D, Sylvester DR, Gross MS, 1994, Molecular characterization of the gene encoding high-level mupirocin resistance in *Staphylococcus aureus* J 2870, Antimicrob Agents Chemother, 38, 1205–1208.

Hsueh PR, Liu YC, Shyr JM, Wu TL, Yan JJ, WU JJ, Leu HS, Chuang YC, Lau YJ, Luh KT, 2000, Multicenter surveillance of antimicrobial resistance of *Streptococcus pneumoniae*, *Haemophilus influenzae*, and *Moraxella catarrhalis* in Taiwan during the 1998–1999 respiratory season, Antimicrob Agents Chemother, 44, 1342–1345.

Inoue M, Lee NY, Hong SW, Lee K, Felmingham D, 2004, Protekt 1999–2000, a multicentre study of the antibiotic susceptibility of respiratory tract pathogens in Hong Kong, Japan and South Korea, Int J Antimicrob Chemother, 23, 44–51.

Ioannidou S, Tassios PT, Zachariadou L, Salem Z, Kanelopoulou M, Kanavaki S, Chronopoulou GC, Petropoulou N, Foustoukou M, Pangalis A, Trikka-Graphakos E, Pappafraggas E, Vatopoulos AC, 2003, In vitro activity of telithromycin (HMR 3647) against Greek *Streptococcus pyogenes* and *Streptococcus pneumoniae* clinical isolates with different macrolide susceptibilities, Clin Microbiol Infect, 9, 704–707.

Jacobs MR, Appelbaum PC, LASER Study Group, 2000, Susceptibility of 1100 *Streptococcus pneumoniae* strains isolated in 1997 from seven Latin American and Caribbean countries, Int J Antimicrob Agents, 16, 17–24.

Jacobs MR, Dagan R, Appelbaum PC, Burch DJ, 1998, Prevalence of antimicrobial-resistant pathogens in middle ear fluid, multinational study of 917 children with acute otitis media, Antimicrob Agents Chemother, 42, 589–595.

Jacobs MR, Felmingham D, Appelbaum PC, Grüneberg RN, the Alexander Project Group, 2003, The Alexander Project 1998–2000 susceptibility of pathogens isolated from community acquired respiratory tract infections to commonly used antimicrobial agents, J Antimicrob Chemother, 52, 229–246.

Jang SS, Hansen LM, Breber JE et al, 1997, Antimicrobial susceptibilities of equine isolates of *Clostridium difficile* and molecular characterization of metronidazole-resistant strains, Clin Infect Dis, 25, suppl 2, S266–S267.

Johnson S, Sanchez JL, Gerding DN, 2000, Metronidazole resistance in *Clostridium difficile*, Clin Infect Dis, 31, 625–626.

Jones ME, Blosser-Middleton RS, Thornsberry C, Karlowsky JA, Sahm DF, 2003, The activity of levofloxacin and other antimicrobials against clinical isolates of *Streptococcus pneumoniae* collected worldwide during 1999-2002, Diagn Microbiol Infect Dis, 47, 579–586.

Jones ME, Karlowsky JA, Blosser-Middleton R, Critchley IA, Thornsberry C, Sahm D, 2002, Apparent plateau in β-lactamase production among clinical isolates of *Haemophilus influenzae* and *Moraxella catarrhalis* in the United States, results from the Libra Surveillance Initiative, Int J Antimicrob Agents, 19, 119–123.

Jones ME, Schmitz FZ, Fruit AC, Acar J, Gupta R, Verhoef J, the SENTRY Participant Group, 1999, Frequency of occurrence and antimicrobial susceptibility of bacterial pathogens associated with skin and soft tissue infections during 1997 from an international surveillance programme, Eur J Clin Microbiol Infect Dis, 18, 403–408.

Kariuki S, Muyodi J, Mirza B, Mwatu W, Daniels J, 2003, Antimicrobial susceptibility in community-acquired bacterial pneumonia in adults, East Afr Med J, 80, 213–217.

Kawamaru Y, Fujiwara H, Mishima N, Tanaka Y, Tanimoto A, Ikawa S, Itoh Y, Ezaki T, 2003, First *Streptococcus agalactiae* isolates highly resistant to quinolones, with point mutations in *gyrA* and *parC*, Antimicrob Agents Chemother, 47, 3605–3609.

Kelly LJ, Thornsberry C, Jones ME, Evangelista AT, Khan J, Karlowsky JA, Sahm DF, 2001, Multidrug-resistant pneumococci isolates in the US, 1997–2001, TRUST surveillance, 41st Intersci Conf Antimicrob Agents Chemother, abstract 2109.

Knudsen AM, Knudsen JD, Jansen ET, Jensen IP, Frimodt-Moller N, 2001, Prevalence of and detection of resistance to ampicillin and other beta-lactam antibiotics in *Haemophilus influenzae* in Denmark, Scand J Infect Dis, 33, 266–271.

Koh TH, Lin RV, 1997, Increasing antimicrobial resistance in clinical isolates of *Streptococcus pneumoniae*, Ann Acad Med Singapore, 26, 604–608.

Kozlov R, Bogdanovitch TM, Appelbaum PC, Ednie L, Stratchounski LS, Jacobs MR, Bozdogan B, 2002, Antistreptococcal activity of telithromycin compared with seven other drugs in relation to macrolide resistance mechanisms in Russia, Antimicrob Agents Chemother, 46, 2963–2968.

Kozlov RS, Appelbaum PC, Kosowska K, Kretchikova OI, Stratchounski LS, 2002, First multicenter study of resistance of nasopharyngeal pneumococci in children from day-care centers in European Russia, 42nd Intersci Conf Antimicrob Agents Chemother, abstract C2-1634.

Kristiansen BE, Sandnes RA, Mortensen L, Tveten Y, Vorland L, 2001, The prevalence of antibiotic resistance in bacterial respiratory pathogens from Norway is low, Clin Microbiol Infect, 7, 682–687.

Lacey RW, Mitchell AAB, 1969, Gentamicin resistant *S. aureus*, Lancet, ii, 1425–1426.

Larson M, Kronwall G, Chuc NT, Karlson I, Lager F, Hanh HD, Tomson G, Falkenberg T, 2000, Antibiotic medication and bacterial resistance to antibiotics, a survey of children in a Vietnamese community, Trop Med Int Health, 5, 711–721.

Laurent F, Lelievre H, Cornu M, et al, 2001, Fitness and competitive growth advantage of new gentamicin-susceptible MRSA clones spreading in French hospitals, J Antimicrob Chemother, 47, 277–283.

Lee YL, Cesario T, Mc Cawley V, et al, 1998, Low level colonization and infection with ciprofloxacin-resistant gram-negative bacilli in a skilled nursing facility, Am J Infect Control, 26, 552–557.

Lee YL, Thrupp LD, Friss RH, et al, 1992, Nosocomial infections and antibiotic utilization in geriatric patients, a pilot prospective surveillance program in skilled nursing facilities, Gerontology, 381, 223–232.

Leegard TM, Bevanger L, Jureen R, Lier T, Melby KK, Caugant DR, Froholm Lo, Hoiby EA, 2001, Antibiotic sensitivity still prevails in Norwegian blood culture isolates, Int J Antimicrob Agents, 18, 99–106.

Lehmann D, Gratten M, Montgomery J, 1997, Susceptibility of pneumococcal carriage isolates to penicillin provides a conservative estimate of susceptibility of invasive pneumococci, Pediatr Infect Dis J, 16, 297–305.

Leven M, Goossens W, De Wit S, Goossens H, 2003, In vitro activity of gemifloxacin compared with other antimicrobial agents against recent clinical isolates of streptococci, J Antimicrob Chemother, 45, suppl S1, 51–53.

Lidsky K, Hoyan C, Salvator A, Rice LB, Toltzis P, 2002, Antibiotic-resistant gram-negative organisms in pediatric chronic care facilities, Clin Infect Dis, 34, 760–766.

Linglof TO, 2002, Aventis data on file.

Maniatis N, Agel A, Legakis NJ, Tzouvelekis LS, 2001, Mupirocin resistance in *Staphylococcus aureus* from Greek hospitals, Int J Antimicrob Agents, 18, 407–408.

Manninen R, Huovinen P, Nissinen A, the Finnish Study Group for Antimicrobial Resistance, 1997, Increasing antimicrobial resistance in *Streptococcus pneumoniae, Haemophilus influenzae* and *Moraxella catarrhalis* in Finland, J Antimicrob Chemother, 40, 387–392.

Marchese A, Schito GC, 2000, Resistance pattern of lower respiratory pathogens in Europe, Int J Antimicrob Agents, 16, S25–S29.

Mathai D, Lewis MT, Kugler KC, Pfaller MA, Jones RN, the SENTRY Antimicrobial Surveillance Program (North America 1998), 2001, Antimicrobial activity of 41 antimicrobials tested against over 2773 bacterial isolates from hospitalized patients with pneumonia. I. Results from the SENTRY antimicrobial surveillance program (North America, 1998), Diagn Microbiol Infect Dis, 39, 105–116.

Mokaddas EM, Wilson S, Sanayal SC, 2001, Prevalence of penicillin-resistant *Streptococcus pneumoniae* in Kuwait, J Chemother, 13, 154–160.

Morton TM, Johnston JL, Patterson J, Archer JL, 1995, Characterization of a conjugative staphylococcal mupirocin resistance plasmid, Antimicrob Agents Chemother, 39, 1272–1280.

Murdoch DR, Reller LB, 2001, Antimicrobial susceptibilities of group B streptococci isolated from patients with invasive disease: 10-year perspective, Antimicrob Agents Chemother, 45, 3623–3624.

Mutnick AH, Turner PJ, Jones RN, 2002, Emerging antimicrobial resistance among *Proteus mirabilis* in Europe, report from MYSTIC program (1997–2001), J Chemother, 14, 253–258.

Nagai K, Appelbaum PC, Davies TA, Kelly LM, Hoellman DB, Andrasevic AT, Drukalska L, Hryniewicz W, Jacobs MR, Kolman J, Miciuleviciene J, Pana M, Setchanova L, Thege MK, Hupkova H, Trupl J, Urbaskova P, 2002, Susceptibilities to telithromycin and six other agents and prevalence of macrolide resistance due to L4 ribosomal protein mutation among 992 pneumococci from 10 central and eastern European countries, Antimicrob Agents Chemother, 46, 371–377.

Nishi J, Yashinaga M, Tokuda K, Masuda K, Masuda R, Kamenosono A, Manayo K, Miyata K, 2002, Oral antimicrobial susceptibilities of *Streptococcus pneumoniae, Haemophilus influenzae*, and *Moraxella catarrhalis* isolated from Japanese children, Int J Antimicrob Agents, 20, 130–135.

Parry CM, Duong NM, Zhen J, Mai NTH, Diep TS, Thinh LQ, Wain J, Chau NVV, Griffiths D, Day NPJ, White NJ, Hien TT, Spratt BG, Farrar JJ, 2002, Emergence in Vietnam of *Streptococcus pneumoniae* resistant to multiple antimicrobial agents as a result of dissemination of the multiresistant 23F-I clone, Antimicrob Agents Chemother, 46, 3512–3517.

Poyart C, Jardy L, Quesne G, Berche P, Trieu-Cuot P, 2003, Genetic basis of antibiotic resistance in *Streptococcus agalactiae* strains isolated in a French hospital, Antimicrob Agents Chemother, 47, 794–797.

Prunier AL, Malbruny B, Laurans M, Brouard J, Duhamel JF, Leclercq R, 2003, High rate of macrolide resistance in *Staphylococcus aureus* strains from patients with cystic fibrosis reveals high proportions of hypermutable strains, J Infect Dis, 187, 1709–1716.

Pujol H, Gudiol F, 2001, Evidence for antibiotic cycling control of resistance, Curr Opin Infect Dis, 14, 711–715.

Ringertz S, Muhe L, Krantz I, Hathaway A, Shamebo D, Freij L, Wall S, Kronwall G, 1993, Prevalence of potential respiratory disease bacteria in children from Ethiopia. Antimicrobial susceptibility of the pathogens and use of antibiotics among the children, Acta Paediatr, 82, 843–848.

Rohani MY, Parasakthi N, Raudzah A, Yasim MY, 1999, In vitro susceptibilities of *Streptococcus pneumoniae* strains isolated in Malaysia to six antibiotics, J Antimicrob Chemother, 44, 852–853.

Saha SK, Rikitomi N, Rutulamina M, Masaki H, Hanif M, Islam M, Watanabe K, Ahmed K, Matsumoto K, Sack RB, Nagatake T, 1999, Antimicrobial resistance and serotype distribution of *Streptococcus pneumoniae* strains causing childhood infections in Bangladesh, 1993 to 1997, J Clin Microbiol, 37, 798–800.

Sahm DF, Thornsberry C, Jones ME, Blosser-Middleton RS, Critchley IA, Evangelista AT, Karlowsky JA, 2002, Correlations of antimicrobial resistance among *Streptococcus pneumoniae* in the US, 2001–2 TRUST surveillance, 42nd Intersci Conf Antimicrob Agents Chemother, abstract C2-1640.

Sangthawan P, Chantaratchada S, Chanthadisai N, Wattanathum A, 2003, Prevalence and clinical significance of community-acquired pneumococcal pneumonia in Thailand, Respirology, 8, 208–212.

Schito GC, Marchese A, 2004, Antibiotic resistance and LRT management, Eur Resp Monography, 9, 135–145.

Schmitz FJ, Jones ME, 1997, Antibiotics for treatment of infections caused by MRSA and elimination of MRSA carriage—what are the choices, Int J Antimicrob Agents, 9, 1–19.

Scott JAG, Hall AJ, Hannington A, Edwards R, Mwarumba S, Lowe B, Griffiths B, Crook D, Marsh K, 1998, Serotype distribution and prevalence of resistance to benzylpenicillin in three representative populations of *Streptococcus pneumoniae* isolates from the coast of Kenya, Clin Infect Dis, 27, 1442–1450.

Sener B, Köseoglu Ö, Gür D, Bryskier A, 2005, Mechanism of macrolide resistance in clinical pneumococcal isolates in a university hospital, Ankara, Turkey, J Chemother, 17, 31–35.

Silva J, Aguilar C, Estrada MA, Echaniz G, Carnalla N, Soto A, Lopez-Antunano FJ, 1998, Susceptibility to new β-lactams of enterobacterial extended-spectrum β-lactamase (ESBL) producers and penicillin-resistant *Streptococcus pneumoniae* in Mexico, J Chemother, 10, 102–107.

Soewignjo S, Gessner BD, Sutanto A, Steinhoff M, Prijanto M, Nelson C, Widjaya A, Arjoso S, 2001, *Streptococcus pneumoniae* nasopharyngeal carriage prevalence, serotype, distribution, and resistance patterns among children on Lombok Island, Indonesia, Clin Infect Dis, 32, 1039–1043.

Song J-H, Chang H-H, Suh JY, Ko KS, Jung S-I, Oh WS, Peck KR, Lee NY, Yang Y, Chongthaleong A, Aswapokee N, Chiu C-H, Lalitha MK, Perera J, Yee TT, Kumararasinghe G, Jamal F, Kamarulazaman A, Parasakthi N, Van PH, So T, Ng TK, on behalf of the ANSORP Study Group, 2004, Macrolide resistance and genotypic characterization of *Streptococcus pneumoniae* in Asian countries: a study of the Asian Network for Surveillance of Resistant Pathogens (ANSORP), J Antimicrob Chemother, 53, 457–463.

Song JH, Jung SI, Oh WS, KIM S, Peck KR, Lee NY, Yang Y, Chiu CH, Lalitha MK, Pererra J, Yee TT, Kamarulzaman A, Parsakthi N, Van PN, Carlos CC, Shibl AM, Ng TK, ANSORP Study Group, 2002, Macrolide and fluoroquinolone resistance among invasive pneumococcal isolates from Asian countries; the Asian Network for Surveillance of Resistant Pathogens (ANSORP) study, 42nd Intersci Conf Antimicrob Agents Chemother, abstract C2-1824.

Song JH, Lee NY, Ichiyama S, Yoshida R, Hirakata Y, Fu W, Chongthaleong A, Asawapokee N, Chiu CH, Lalitha MK, Thomas K, Perrrera J, Yee TT, Jamal F, Warsa UC, Vinh BX, Jacobs MR, Appelbaum PC, Pai CH, 1999, Spread of drug-resistant *Streptococcus pneumoniae* in Asian countries, Asian network for surveillance of resistant pathogens (ANSORP) study, Clin Infect Dis, 28, 1205–1211.

Stevens DL, 2003, Community-acquired *Staphylococcus aureus* infections, increasing virulence and emerging methicillin resistance in the new millennium, Curr Opin Infect Dis, 16, 184–191.

Streit JM, Jones RN, Sader HS, 2004, Daptomycin activity and spectrum, a worldwide sample of 6737 clinical gram-positive organisms, J Antimicrob Chemother, 53, 669–674.

Thabet L, Boutiba I, Kammoun A, Khelif L, Mahjoubi F, Smaoui H, Kechrid A, Ben Redjeb S, Hammani A, 2002, Epidemiologic profile of *Haemophilus influenzae* infection in Tunisia, Tunis Med, 80, 469–472.

Toltzis P, Hoyen C, Spinner-Block S, Salvator AE, Rice LB, 1999, Factors that predict preexisting colonization with antibiotic-resistant gram-negative bacilli in patients admitted to a pediatric intensive care unit, Pediatrics, 103, 719–723.

Trijbels-Smeuders MA, Kollée LA, Adriaase AH, Kimpen JL, Gerards LJ, 2004, Neonatal group B streptococcal infection, incidence and strategies for prevention in Europe, Pediatr J Infect Dis, 23, 172–173.

Turnidge J, 2000, Aventis data on file.

Turnidge JD, Bell JM, the SENTRY Westen Pacific, 2001, Major regional variation in *Haemophilus influenzae* resistance in the Western Pacific, results from SENTRY Western Pacific Plus 1998–2000, 41st Intersci Conf Antimicrob Agents Chemother, abstract C2-687.

Tyrrell GJ, Senzilet LD, Spika JS, Kertesz DA, Alagaratnam M, Lovgren M, Talbot JA, the SENTINEL Health Unit Surveillance System Site Coordinators, 2000, Invasive disease due to group B streptococcal infection in adults, results from a Canadian, population-based, active laboratory surveillance study—1996, J Infect Dis, 182, 168–173.

Udo EE, Farook VS, Mokadas EM, Jacob LE, Sanyal SC, 1999, Molecular fingerprinting of mupirocin-resistant *S. aureus* from a burn unit, Int J Infect Dis, 3, 82–87.

Uwaydah M, Mokhbat JE, Karam-Sarkis D, Barroud-Massif R, Rohban T, 2002, Penicillin-resistant *S. pneumoniae* in Lebanon—the first nationwide study on ambulatory patients, 42nd Intersci Conf Antimicrob Agents Chemother, abstract C2.

Woolfson A, Huebner R, Wasas A, Chola S, Godfrey-Faussett P, Klugman K, 1997, Nasopharyngeal carriage of community-acquired antibiotic-resistant *Streptococcus pneumoniae* in a Zambian pediatric population, Bull W HO, 75, 453–462.

Youssef FG, El-Sakka H, Azab A, Eloun S, Chapman GD, Ismail T, Mansour H, Hallaj Z, Mahoney F, 2004, Etiology, antimicrobial susceptibility profile, and mortality associated with bacterial meningitis among children in Egypt, Ann Epidemiol, 14, 44–48.

Yun HJ, Lee SW, Yoon GM, Kim SY, Choi S, Lee YS, Choi EC, Kim S, 2003, Prevalence and mechanisms of low- and high-level mupirocin resistance in *Staphylococci* isolated from a Korean hospital, J Antimicrob Chemother, 51, 619–623.

Zhanel G, Chan CK, Gin AS, Carrie A, Nichol K, Smith H, Hoban DJ, 2002, Relationship between fluoroquinolone use and fluoroquinolone resistance in *Streptococcus pneumoniae*—analysis of Canadian national data from 1997 to 2002, 42nd Intersci Conf Antimicrob Agents Chemother, abstract C2-1630.

Development of an Antibiotic: Microbiology

A. BRYSKIER

4

1. INTRODUCTION

The life of an antibiotic is the result of a complex series of events that begins with its conception and concludes with its being made commercially available.

Conception is the first major event because it results from the chemist's desire either to create a new chemical entity from a known chemical series or to identify antibacterial activity in a culture filtrate from bacterial or fungal strains, to isolate the active substance or substances, and to modify them structurally. The third eventuality is the total synthesis of a new chemical entity by scientific creativity. Among recent examples, mention might be made of the penems, which were designed in 1977 by Woodward and which are chemical hybrids of the penams and cephems.

Candidates from among the preselected molecules must clear a compulsory hurdle, that of toxicology. If the results obtained prove compatible with clinical development, the second—microbiological—stage involves microbiological studies, which in turn allow phase I and subsequently phase II studies to begin. Thereafter, and in parallel with clinical development, experimental studies enable the so-called specific pharmacology dossier to be compiled, establishing the microbiological identity card of the new molecule. This is then followed by experimental studies to determine the optimal use of the new antibacterial agent, such as adaptation for use on automated devices for determining antibiotic susceptibility. Research into antibacterial activity must not cease with the registration dossier, and considerable energy must be devoted during the lifetime of the drug to epidemiological studies and the search for new indications. A new epidemiological situation might provide new therapeutic indications, as was the case with the identification of the differential activity of the 2-amino-5-thiazolyl cephalosporins against penicillin G-resistant strains of *Streptococcus pneumoniae* (Table 1).

The development of an antibiotic remains a complex matter. An antibiotic is a compound that restores the equilibrium between bacteria and the host's defenses. In contrast to the other therapeutic domains, in the field of infectious diseases drugs are targeted on an external agent, bacteria. For this reason, the preselection of an antibiotic is based on in vitro and in vivo antibacterial performance. Determination of antibacterial activity is the cornerstone of development. Clinical development may be assisted by guidelines (Beam et al., 1993), but with the exception of the specific prerequisites described for the various pathological pictures, there are no guidelines for the development of an antibacterial agent microbiologically.

2. PRESELECTION OF A MOLECULE

Before becoming a drug, the antibacterial agent is only one molecule among a series of compounds prepared by chemists. Preselection is a crucial stage in the life of a new drug. Once a molecule is synthesized, its in vitro activity against a panel of strains belonging to selected bacterial genera and species is determined. The choice of panel is complex. It is the result of a compromise between the specifications laid down in establishing the new research project and systematic analysis of the activity of any new antibacterial chemical entity against common pathogens. The definition of this panel is often difficult, particularly if it is wished to extend the "natural" activity of a chemical family to other bacterial genera. The macrolides are the classic example. At present, the aim of research with respect to new macrolides is to increase the antibacterial activity of the naturally susceptible species, but also to avoid cross-resistance with erythromycin A and to extend it to strains resistant to erythromycin A, such as *S. pneumoniae*. The ketolides are one such example (Agouridas et al., 1994).

It is also a difficult task to establish the panel when testing a new chemical entity. A recent example is daptomycin, a lipopeptide whose antibacterial spectrum principally includes gram-positive cocci and bacteria.

The choice of strains exhibiting different antibiotic resistance phenotypes and that of the molecules that serve for comparison are crucial, because these choices determine the whole way in which the new molecule starts out its life.

The in vitro activity determines the subsequent stage, which involves testing the efficacy of preselected molecules in models of nonspecific experimental infections by administering them parenterally (subcutaneously or intraperitoneally) or orally. Table 2 shows the comparative in vitro and in vivo activities of erythromycin A and roxithromycin against *S. pneumoniae* and *S. aureus*.

The studies conducted during the preselection phase result in the selection of the candidate for clinical development. Selection is based principally on in vitro and in vivo

Table 1 In vitro activities of cephalosporins against *S. pneumoniae*[a]

Drug	MIC (μg/ml)[b]					
	Penicillin S (MIC, <0.12 μg/ml)		Penicillin I (MIC, 0.12–≤1.0 μg/ml)		Penicillin R (MIC, >1.0 μg/ml)	
	50%	90%	50%	90%	50%	90%
Cefotaxime	0.03	0.03	0.25	1.0	1.0	2.0
Ceftriaxone	0.03	0.03	0.25	1.0	1.0	2.0
Cefpirome	0.01	0.03	0.12	0.5	0.5	1.0
Ceftazidime	0.25	0.25	2.0	16	16	16
Cefodizime	0.03	0.03	0.5	2.0	2.0	4.0
Ceftizoxime	0.06	0.06	0.5	8.0	16	16

[a]Data from Frémaux et al., 1992.
[b]S, susceptible; I, intermediate; R, resistant.

Table 2 Comparative in vitro and in vivo activities of erythromycin A and roxithromycin[a]

Organism	Drug	MIC (μg/ml)	PD_{50}[b] (mg/kg)	PD_{50} ratio
S. aureus giorr4	Erythromycin A	0.3	120	3.2
	Roxithromycin	0.6	37	
S. pneumoniae I	Erythromycin A	0.02	375	5.6
	Roxithromycin	0.04	67	

[a]Data from Chantot et al., 1986.
[b]PD_{50}, 50% protective dose.

Table 3 In vivo activities of macrolides[a]

Drug	MIC (μg/ml)	ED_{50}[b] (mg/kg)	
		S. aureus	*Enterococcus* spp.
Roxithromycin	0.296	3.84	2.3
RU-29065	0.126	2.36	20
RU-29702	0.118	1.55	12
Erythromycin	0.151	1.0	1

[a]Data from Gasc et al., 1991.
[b]ED_{50}, 50% effective dose.

activities, but also on the toxicology of the different compounds. Some preselected molecules are sometimes more active than the selected candidate but are not adopted because of their toxicity. The choice is based on the compound that possesses the best balanced antibacterial spectrum and which is best tolerated in animals. Table 3 shows in vivo activities of macrolides against *S. aureus* and *Enterococcus*.

Following selection, the third stage in the process is microbiological; this stage allows the clinical development of the future drug.

3. BASIC DOCUMENTATION

Basic documentation consists of two parts: one involves the acquisition of the essential data for the use of the molecule in microbiological tests, and the second allows the clinical studies to begin.

3.1. Use of the Molecule

The data acquired during this phase are essential to allow experimental studies to begin and to compile the microbiological part of the registration dossier.

The following data are essential:

- The physicochemical properties
- Solubility of the molecule in water and the different solvents used in microbiology
- If the molecule is sparingly soluble or insoluble in water, the method of solubilization must be mentioned in the data sheets given to investigators.
- The interaction with calcium, magnesium, etc.
- The need to add certain factors to the medium

The in vitro activities of cephalosporins containing a catechol nucleus differ according to whether the culture medium contains an excess of iron. The molecules are tested in a medium containing 2,2′-dipyrridyl, which depletes the medium of iron (≤50 μg/liter), and in an iron-rich medium (600 to 2,400 μg/liter instead of 250 to 300 μg/liter). The activity of mupirocin can be modified by the addition of blood when the medium contains isoleucine. The MIC of fosfomycin is determined on Mueller-Hinton medium containing 25 μg of glucose-6-phosphate per ml. The disks for antibiotic sensitivity testing contain 25 μg of glucose-6-phosphate (5 μg of fosfomycin). Sulfonamides and benzylpyrimidines (trimethoprim and brodimoprim) must be tested in a thymidine-depleted medium. It is possible to add thymidine phosphorylase (0.025 to 0.1 U/ml of medium) or, more simply, 5% hemolyzed horse red blood cells to the Mueller-Hinton medium.

The culture medium influences the determination of the MICs. Mueller-Hinton medium from the same manufacturer (lot) or different manufacturers may sometimes produce different bacterial growths and compromise the results, hence the need to observe the M-23 recommendations of the NCCLS (1993). The quality of the Iso-Sensitest medium in determining the activity of aminoglycosides has been called into question because of the lack of standardization (King and Phillips, 1993).

In the macrobroth technique in Iso-Sensitest broth (Oxoid) with an inoculum of 10^4 CFU/ml, the geometric MICs of teicoplanin for *Staphylococcus epidermidis* and *Staphylococcus haemolyticus* were 0.6 and 2.6 μg/ml, respectively (Table 4).

Among the apparently similar Mueller-Hinton media, there are differences in terms of antibacterial activities (Table 5). To differentiate the different Mueller-Hinton media and to be able to propose the use of one of them, the discriminative method is an in vivo murine model of infection with a representative panel of the given bacterial species.

Felmingham et al. (1987) demonstrated that the presence of 10% saponin-lysed horse blood can increase MICs of teicoplanin but not vancomycin for coagulase-negative staphylococci.

There is an "inoculum effect" (increase in MIC with the size of the inoculum) with teicoplanin.

MICs of a given compound using agar and microbroth methods have to be compared by following NCCLS recommendations (NCCLS document M-100). It is a multiparameter study, including different media (Mueller-Hinton, Iso-Sensitest for aerobic bacteria, and Wilkins-Chalgren and Brucella for anaerobes). The in vitro activities are determined in medium without supplementation or with the following additives: whole horse blood, whole sheep blood, and water-lysed horse and sheep blood. Each additive is tested at final concentrations of 2 and 5%. These effects are determined at different inoculum sizes (10^3 to 10^7 CFU/ml). The effect of incubation in ambient air and 5 to 6% CO_2 is also one of the parameters. Depending of the antibacterial spectrum of the new compound, these effects are tested using as test organisms either *Staphylococcus* spp., *Enterococcus* spp., *Haemophilus influenzae*, *S. pneumoniae*, *Streptococcus pyogenes*, *Moraxella catarrhalis*, or anaerobes.

The stability of the molecule in the culture media over time and at different temperatures and pHs is assessed. By way of example, the antibacterial activity of ansamycins against *Mycobacterium tuberculosis* decreases over time in phosphate-buffered saline (PBS) medium or in 7 H9 medium (Table 6).

It is therefore advisable to test the stability of the antibiotic in the culture medium at the same time as determining the antibacterial activity.

The factors influencing bacterial growth should also be determined, although they are not essential in the first phase of development. They are, however, required when submitting the drug dossier for registration. The effect of the size of different inocula on the MIC should be tested. The best examples of this are the cephalosporins (Eng et al., 1985). The increase in the MIC reflects the stability of the different molecules to hydrolysis by β-lactamases (Table 7). Usually, the inoculum is prepared after a 16- to 18-h overnight culture, it is important to check differences between various incubation times (tiny colonies, lysis, etc.).

The content of various ions in the growth medium has to be checked, especially Ca^{2+}, Mg^{2+}, and Mn^{2+}; others, depending on the molecular structure, can also be checked.

The best reading time needs to be determined in various test conditions. It was demonstrated that MICs of telithromycin, azithromycin, and clarithromycin against *H. influenzae* read after 20 h of incubation have a slight tendency to be lower than when read at 16 h and higher than when read at 24 h. Over 99% of MIC results at 16 and 24 h were within plus or minus twofold concentrations of those read at 20 h.

Likewise, some molecules become less bactericidal if the inoculum is increased. The bactericidal activity of the fluoroquinolones decreases above 10^8 CFU/ml, and they become bacteriostatic with an inoculum of more than 10^{10} CFU/ml

Table 4 Medium effect on teicoplanin MICs[a]

Organism	Use of blood in medium	MIC (μg/ml) at indicated inoculum (CFU/ml)					
		ISO agar		DST agar		MH agar	
		10^4	10^6	10^4	10^6	10^4	10^6
S. epidermidis (*n* = 18)	NB	0.6	2.9	2.1	4.5	1.0	2.6
	B	1.3	3.6	1.9	5.0	1.1	3.3
S. haemolyticus (*n* = 14)	NB	2.6	5.4	8.3	17.7	3.8	5.9
	B	7.6	10.2	15.2	22.6	6.2	1.9

[a]Data from Felmingham et al., 1987. ISO, Iso-Sensitest; DST, diagnostic Sensitest; MH, Mueller-Hinton; NB, without blood; B, blood.

Table 5 Effects of Mueller-Hinton medium origin on MICs of teicoplanin and vancomycin

Organism	Medium	$MIC_{50/90}$ (μg/ml)	
		Teicoplanin	Vancomycin
S. aureus (*n* = 37)	Difco Mueller-Hinton agar	4.0/4.0	2.0/2.0
	Bio-Rad Mueller-Hinton agar	8.0/8.0	4.0/4.0
	Difco Mueller-Hinton broth	2.0/4.0	1.0/2.0
S. epidermidis (*n* = 34)	Difco Mueller-Hinton agar	4.0/8.0	2.0/2.0
	Bio-Rad Mueller-Hinton agar	8.0/16	2.0/4.0
	Difco Mueller-Hinton broth	4.0/8.0	2.0/2.0
S. haemolyticus (*n* = 39)	Difco Mueller-Hinton agar	4.0/16	2.0/2.0
	Bio-Rad Mueller-Hinton agar	16/32	2.0/4.0
	Difco Mueller-Hinton broth	4.0/16	1.0/2.0

Table 6 Stability of ansamycins in 7 H9 medium with or without Tween 80[a]

Drug	Medium[b]	Ansamycin concn in medium (μg/ml)		
		Day 0	Day 2	Day 7
Rifampin	Tween 80+	0.8	0.88	0.22
	Tween 80−	0.8	0.70	0.44
	PBS	0.8	0.82	0.42
FCE-22807	Tween 80+	0.68	0.03	0
	Tween 80−	0.69	0.35	0.16
	PBS	0.85	0.34	0.21
FCE-22250	Tween 80+	0.80	0.06	0
	Tween 80−	0.84	0.40	0.18
	PBS	0.94	0.61	0.19
SPA-S-565	Tween 80+	0.70	0	0
	Tween 80−	0.90	0.46	0.13
	PBS	0.80	0.45	0.07

[a]Data from Dickinson and Mitchison, 1990.
[b]Tween 80+, with Tween 80 (0.05% [vol/vol], 37°C, 1μg/ml of solution); Tween 80 −, without Tween 80.

Table 7 In vitro inoculum effect on parenteral cephalosporins[a]

Compound	MIC (μg/ml) for organism at indicated inoculum (CFU/ml):					
	E. coli		*Salmonella* serovar Typhimurium		*K. pneumoniae*	
	5×10^5	5×10^7	5×10^5	5×10^7	5×10^5	5×10^7
Cefotaxime	0.06	0.5	0.06	0.5	0.06	0.5
Ceftriaxone	0.06	1.0	0.5	4.0	0.25	4.0
Ceftazidime	0.12	8.0	0.5	16	0.12	8.0
Cefoperazone	0.25	8.0	1.0	32	0.12	8.0

[a]Data from Eng et al., 1985.

(Smith and Levin, 1988). A certain number of microorganisms require a CO_2-enriched atmosphere to grow, but carbon dioxide causes variations in antibacterial activity by modifying the pH of the culture medium. The best examples of this are the macrolides (Felmingham et al., 1987; Siebor and Kazmierczak, 1993). The pH of the medium may also modify the activity of the molecules. The fluoroquinolones, which possess a piperazine ring at position 7, are less active in an acidic medium than in an alkaline medium. Conversely, compounds which do not have substituents at position 7 are more active in an acidic medium than in an alkaline medium (anionic molecules) (Bryskier et al., 1994).

The presence of horse serum in the culture medium is often necessary for bacterial growth. It is essential to check that MICs do not vary. Klugman and Saunders (1994) showed that the addition of horse serum to Mueller-Hinton medium does not significantly modify the activity of the 2-amino-5-thiazolyl cephalosporins against *S. pneumoniae* (Table 8).

It is possible to use these enriched media to determine the MICs of the different cephalosporins for any strains of *S. pneumoniae*.

The problem of activity in the presence of serum has been studied in detail with daptomycin (Lee et al., 1991). This molecule is very active in vitro against *Enterococcus faecalis*, but therapeutically at the proposed doses it is moderately active because of its strong plasma protein binding.

Testing antibacterial activity in the presence of human serum is not essential for a registration dossier or for a basic understanding of the molecule. In fact, the content of specific proteins (antibodies or complement) or nonspecific proteins (serum albumin, α_1-glycoproteins, etc.) varies from one individual to another. In addition, the reactivity of serum is difficult to standardize, even in a pool, and for this reason the analysis of experimental results is complex.

In the case of the fluoroquinolones, their stability and antibacterial activity must be determined in urine (Table 9) and are generally reduced according to the pH of the urine.

Table 8 Activities of β-lactams in media with and without horse serum[a]

Drug	MIC_{50} (μg/ml)	
	Without serum	With 50% horse serum
Penicillin G	0.015	0.03
Cefpirome	0.03	0.03
Cefotaxime	0.015	0.03
Ceftriaxone	0.015	0.03
Ceftazidime	0.03	0.5
Cefodizime	0.06	0.12
Cefepime	0.03	0.015

[a]Data from Klugman and Saunders, 1994.

Table 9 Effect of urine on the activities of ofloxacin and norfloxacin[a]

Drug	Geometric MIC (μg/ml) in:		
	Urine		Mueller-Hinton broth (pH 7.4)
	pH 5.8	pH 6.8	
Norfloxacin	5.2	3.9	0.083
Ofloxacin	2.9	0.9	0.69

[a]Data from Chantot and Bryskier, 1985.

Table 10 Radius for levofloxacin according to Joan Stokes's method[a]

Resistance phenotype	Radius (mm)	
	S. aureus NCTC 6571	*E. coli* NCTC 10418
Susceptible	≥7	≥9
Intermediate	>3–<7	>3–<9
Resistant	≤3	≤3

[a]Data from Felmingham and Grüneberg, personal communication, 1994.

3.2. Elements of the Dossier Necessary for the Institution of Phases I and II

3.2.1. Microbiological Assays—High-Performance Liquid Chromatography (HPLC)

The choice of culture medium, pH of the medium, and test strain are crucial factors in the fate of the molecule. The method must be sensitive (large, clearly defined, and reproducible zone of inhibition relative to the standard range). The test strain must be taken from referenced and known strains or, in the case of a new strain, be submitted to national collections so as to be readily accessible.

At the same time a clinical assay method, such as high-performance liquid chromatography, must be developed. A good correlation must be obtained between microbiological and chemical methods.

3.2.2. Breakpoints

Before starting phase II clinical studies, it is essential to acquire a reference tool in the clinical microbiology laboratories. The susceptibility to antibacterial agents of a bacterial strain responsible for infection must be known routinely. In the majority of laboratories in hospital centers it is determined by the qualitative method of antibiotic sensitivity testing, which uses the diameter of the zone of inhibition around a disk loaded with a certain quantity of the antibacterial agent. However, the difficulty lies in the fact that the diameter of the paper disk may vary from country to country; in Europe, for example, it is 6 mm, whereas in Japan it is 9 mm. The disk concentration may vary from one country to another. For example, in the majority of European countries and in the United States the disks with oral cephalosporins, such as cefpodoxime, are loaded with 10 μg, whereas in Germany they are loaded with 30 μg. This makes it difficult to compare epidemiological studies of oral cephems with those done in Germany.

The breakpoints can differ in France, Germany (Deutsche Institut für Normung, 1984), Great Britain (British Society for Antimicrobial Chemotherapy, 1991), Sweden (Ericsson and Sherris, 1971; Swedish Reference Group for Antibiotics, 1981), The Netherlands (Werkgroep Richtlijnen Govoeligheidsbepalingen, 1981), the United States (NCCLS, 1997), and Japan (1984). As a general rule, the British Society for Antimicrobial Chemotherapy and Deutsche Institut für Normung systems recommend lower breakpoints for the threshold of sensitivity than those of the Société française de microbiologie and the NCCLS. The Swiss and Dutch breakpoints are similar to those recommended by the European Committee (Baquero, 1990). However, this is not always the case, particularly for the fluoroquinolones, for which the breakpoints of the Société française de microbiologie are 1 to 4 μg/ml and those of the British Society for Antimicrobial Chemotherapy are 2 to 8 μg/ml. There has been an attempt at harmonization in Europe that has produced consensus breakpoints (EUCAST) (Kahlmeter et al., 2003).

In the United Kingdom, microbiologists use the method described by Joan Stokes (1993). This involves comparing the zones of inhibition between the border of the paper disk and the border of the zone of growth of the two strains. The radius is the difference between these two zones, and on the basis of its size it is possible to determine whether an antibiotic is active, moderately active, or inactive (Table 10).

In Europe, harmonization of the methods and breakpoints will be achieved through EUCAST.

3.2.3. Quality Control Strains

It is essential to test the antibiotic against reference strains for quality assurance purposes.

At present it is possible to become lost in the jungle of nomenclatures—ATCC (American) or NCTC (British)—that often cover the same strains. In the United States, quality assurance is well codified. The diameters of the zones of inhibition and the MICs for reference strains are submitted for assessment to the subcommittee for antibacterial susceptibility testing. Once the data are accepted, they are the subject of an official publication by the committee.

The standard strains of *Escherichia coli, Pseudomonas aeruginosa*, and *Staphylococcus aureus* pose no problem; the interpretation for *H. influenzae*, *S. pneumoniae*, and *Neisseria gonorrhoeae*, however, is more difficult. As regards anaerobic bacteria, there is at present no consensus on the part of the NCCLS, merely an ongoing review of the situation.

According to the recommendations of document M-23 of the NCCLS, the activity of the new antibacterial agent must be tested using five lots of culture medium from two manufacturers and a reference batch of Mueller-Hinton medium. The activity against each reference strain must be tested 20 times. Two batches of disks must be tested. Ten laboratories participate in the study.

MICs and zone diameters must be validated during the clinical trials from the local clinical microbiological laboratories. The validation can also be obtained by testing the new compound in 30 different clinical microbiological laboratories.

4. "CORE" DOSSIER

The core dossier involves the compilation of the microbiological dossier that will be incorporated in the pharmacotoxicological expert report of the registration dossier for the new antibacterial agent. It thus enables the antibacterial spectrum and activity to be determined. Whatever the molecule, a knowledge of its intrinsic activity is required in terms of both bacteriostatic activity (MIC) and bactericidal activity. Against common pathogens, the molecule must be tested in a sufficient number of strains (about 100) to determine the MIC at which 50% of the isolates tested are inhibited (MIC_{50}) and the MIC_{90} and to draw the population distribution. Furthermore, testing should be undertaken in several centers distributed in different regions and not just a single center. Three types of strains are used: strains referenced as having or not having a mechanism of resistance, collection strains from a laboratory having served in other studies and providing a point of reference, and freshly isolated clinical strains from patients.

The MIC_{50} represents the intrinsic activity of the compound and must be the basis on which the spectrum and activity of the molecule are established, whereas the MIC_{90} merely reflects the different mechanisms of resistance, which are dependent on the center and the method of collection of the strains.

If the intrinsic value of a compound is to be determined, it is essential to test it against the different bacterial species comprising a bacterial genus, and also against the different strains that possess antibacterial resistance phenotypes.

It is essential to know the antibacterial activity of any metabolite of the antibacterial agent. When the metabolite is active and represents a major component of the kinetics of the drug, the activity of the combination of the parent molecule and its metabolite must be tested to demonstrate the absence of antagonism (Table 11).

4.1. Common Pathogens

The bacterial species and genera are divided into four groups according to morphology and Gram stain.

4.1.1. Gram-Positive Cocci

4.1.1.1. *S. aureus*

It is customary with strains of *S. aureus* to distinguish those which produce penicillinases and those which are resistant to methicillin.

Penicillinase-producing strains account for more than 80% of strains isolated in some regions. If a new antibacterial agent is to be tested against strains of this phenotype, it is important to have a panel of strains possessing the four enzymes A, B, C, and D. Other antistaphylococcal agents must be tested in comparison, such as fusidic acid, which is a good marker of penicillinase type D.

If the activity of a new chemical entity against methicillin-resistant strains is to be demonstrated, it must be tested against strains belonging to the four classes of Tomasz et al. (1991). All of them have to harbor the *mecA* gene.

Jabès et al. (1993) clearly demonstrated the differential activities of the penems and carbapenems in terms of the class to which the staphylococcal strains belonged (Table 12). These molecules are apparently active against classes 1 and 2 but are totally inactive against classes 3 and 4. In addition, it is recommended that the in vitro activity of the molecules

Table 11 In vitro activities of combination of cefotaxime and its main metabolite

Organism(s) tested	No.	No. with:			
		Synergy	Indifference	Antagonism	Additive
Citrobacter spp.	14	13	1	0	0
E. aerogenes	15	10	2	0	3
Enterobacter agglomerans	9	6	1	0	2
E. cloacae	11	11	0	0	0
E. coli	24	21	1	0	2
K. pneumoniae	24	19	4	0	1
M. morganii	9	0	1	8	0
Proteus mirabilis	14	10	0	0	3
Proteus vulgaris	9	4	4	0	1
Providencia spp.	16	5	3	0	3
S. marcescens	16	12	2	0	2
S. aureus	10	9	0	0	1
E. faecalis	9	0	9	0	0
Acinetobacter spp.	4	2	0	0	0
P. aeruginosa	9	0	9	0	0
Pseudomonas spp.	13	8	5	0	0
Total		99	42	8	18

Table 12 In vitro activities of carbapenems against MRSA strains[a]

Drug	MIC (μg/ml)				
	Clinical isolates	Class 1 (CDC-1)	Class 2 (SN-7)	Class 3 (SN-43)	Class 4 (COL)
Methicillin	1.0	3.12	6.25	>100	>100
Ritipenem	0.39	0.19	0.39	100	100
Imipenem	1.56	0.09	0.19	25	25
Meropenem	12.5	0.19	1.56	25	100
Ciprofloxacin	0.19	0.39	0.78	25	6.25

[a]Data from Jabès et al., 1993.

be tested using a Trypticase soy agar medium containing 2% NaCl. The inoculum must be 10^4 CFU/spot, and the incubation temperature must be 30°C. When the inoculum is small, the risk of not detecting hyperresistant heterogeneous strains in classes 1 and 2 is considerable.

It is also necessary to test the compound against multiresistant strains, including resistance to aminoglycosides (gentamicin and amikacin), macrolides, fluoroquinolones, and cyclines.

The macrolides, lincosamides, and streptogramins (MLS_B) must be tested against strains with a known genetic mechanism of resistance (inducible or constitutive). This type of study was conducted in the analysis of the activity of quinupristin-dalfopristin (Table 13) and telithromycin.

Methicillin-resistant *S. aureus* strains (MRSA) with intermediate susceptibility to vancomycin or resistant to vancomycin (due to the *vanA* gene) have been reported. All new compounds for which a putative activity against MRSA is claimed need to tested against MRSA with intermediate susceptibility to vancomycin, and the affinity for PBP 2a needs to be checked (β-lactams).

4.1.1.2. Coagulase-Negative Staphylococci

The coagulase-negative staphylococci comprise numerous species. Here also the antibacterial activity must be tested against methicillin-susceptible or -resistant strains. The species most commonly involved in disease are *Staphylococcus epidermidis, Staphylococcus saprophyticus*, and *Staphylococcus haemolyticus*. In terms of the other species, some 30 strains should provide an idea of the potential activity of the new molecule.

4.1.1.3. *S. pneumoniae*

The emergence of penicillin G-resistant and multiresistant strains requires a number of studies to define the antipneumococcal profile of a new molecule. The simplest test involves determining the in vitro and comparative activities of the molecule against strains that are susceptible (MIC, ≤0.12 μg/ml), intermediate (MIC, 0.12 to 1 μg/ml), or resistant (MIC, >1 μg/ml) to penicillin G. Currently, this panel should also include cefotaxime-resistant strains (MIC, ≥2 μg/ml), as well as those of reduced susceptibility (MIC, 1 μg/ml) and multiresistant, particularly to erythromycin A (MIC, >1 μg/ml), tetracyclines, chloramphenicol, fluoroquinolones, and co-trimoxazole. It is preferable to determine the MIC in an agar medium rather than a broth medium, even in Schaedler's medium, as the results are more arbitrary in a broth medium. However, these tests are not sufficient in themselves, since bactericidal activity must be tested against strains with different β-lactam resistance phenotypes using inocula of different sizes. With the β-lactams and fluoroquinolones, bactericidal activity decreases as the size of the inoculum increases above 10^6 CFU/ml. This modification can be demonstrated by a study of the killing kinetics (F. Baquero, personal communication, 1994). Strains resistant to erythromycin A through an efflux mechanism (erythromycin A-resistant, clindamycin-susceptible, M − phenotype) and having an MLS_B-type mechanism (*erm*-containing strain) and mutation on ribosomal protein L4 or L22 or mutation on the peptidyltransferase loop (e.g., A2058G) must be included, as well as strains resistant to fluoroquinolones. Due to putative dissociation of resistance between erythromycin A and azithromycin, both compounds need to be tested; rare isolates resistant to azithromycin and intermediately susceptible to erythromycin A have been described.

Bactericidal activity against isolates with various resistance patterns are determined from 0 to 6 to 8 h after contact. At 24 h, due to spontaneous lysis, the data are questionable.

S. pneumoniae strains tolerant to vancomycin have been described, but they are apparently of infrequent occurrence. Some isolates are resistant to optochine.

Table 13 In vitro activity of quinupristin-dalfopristin against different antibiotic phenotypes of *S. aureus*[a]

Phenotype[b]	MIC (μg/ml)		
	Quinupristin-dalfopristin	Dalfopristin	Quinupristin
M(S) MLS_B (S)	1	2	0.1
M(R) MLS_B (I)	2	2	0.12
M(R) MLS_B (R)	30	4	0.5

[a]Data from Barrière et al., 1994.
[b]M(S), M(R), macrolide susceptible, resistant; S, susceptible; I, intermediate; R, resistant.

4.1.1.4. *Streptococcus* spp.

Antibacterial activity against streptococci of Lancefield groups A, B, C, G, and F must be determined conventionally. The panel should include strains resistant to erythromycin A, particularly for *S. pyogenes* [*erm(B), erm*(TR/A) and *mef*(A)].

The efflux mechanism of resistance is governed by the *mef*(A) and *mef(E)* genes for streptococci; in *Streptococcus agalactiae*, the gene *mreA* is detected.

This resistance may be due to different mechanisms (MLS_B or efflux). Clindamycin, lincomycin, and, if possible, pristinamycins I and II should always be combined with erythromycin A.

Determination of the activity against viridans group streptococci is more difficult. The bacteriostatic and bactericidal activities must be determined by including strains that are tolerant to penicillin G. Bactericidal activity is determined by killing kinetics.

4.1.1.5. *Enterococcus* spp.

The susceptibilities of the different species of enterococci to antibiotics are established against a panel of strains susceptible or otherwise to vancomycin and gentamicin, in the latter case with strains that have a high level of resistance to aminoglycosides (MIC, >1,000 μg/ml). β-Lactamase-producing strains should certainly be included. Assessment of the bactericidal activity of the compound requires killing kinetics, as has been done with daptomycin.

4.1.2. Gram-Positive Bacilli

Antibacterial activity should be determined against *Listeria monocytogenes, Erysipelothrix rhusiopatihae, Bacillus anthracis* and other *Bacillus* species, *Lactobacillus* spp., *Pediococcus* spp., *Leuconostoc* spp., *Rhodococcus equi*, and *Corynebacterium diphtheriae* and other *Corynebacterium* species (*Corynebacterium jeikeium, Corynebacterium urealyticum*, and other coryneforms).

The activity against *C. jeikeium* must be tested systematically since active antibacterials are few. Activity should also be tested against *Arcanobacterium* (*Corynebacterium*) *haemolyticum* and *Actinomyces* (*Corynebacterium*) *pyogenes*.

There is a resurgence of interest in *C. diphtheriae* because of the epidemic of diphtheria in Russia and Ukraine and recently in Algeria.

4.1.3. Gram-Negative Cocci

Whether in the case of *N. gonorrhoeae* or of *Neisseria meningitidis*, strains exhibiting different antibacterial resistance phenotypes must be tested.

4.1.3.1. *N. meningitidis*

A reduction in the activity of penicillin G (Saez-Nieto et al., 1990) has been demonstrated in many regions, and the mechanism of resistance is similar to that observed with *S. pneumoniae*.

The susceptibilities of isolated strains to penicillin G vary with the region and serogroup. It has recently been shown in Spain that strains belonging to serogroup C have reduced susceptibility to penicillin G. The intensive use of rifampin as prophylaxis is the cause of emergence of strains resistant to this antibiotic. The panel of test strains should therefore include strains susceptible to the antibacterial agents, strains of reduced susceptibility to penicillin G, and strains resistant to rifampin. The strains should be of the serogroups most commonly isolated in diseases, such as B, C, and A. Killing kinetics in the different strains of *N. meningitidis* should be determined. Strains resistant to chloramphenicol have been reported.

4.1.3.2. *N. gonorrhoeae*

The emergence of strains of *N. gonorrhoeae* resistant to penicillin G, tetracyclines, and spectinomycin and, more recently, of reduced susceptibility to fluoroquinolones (Knapp et al., 1994; Putnam et al., 1992) requires the molecule to be tested against strains of different resistance phenotypes. It is probable that strains resistant to the 2-amino-5-thiazolyl cephalosporins (cefotaxime and ceftriaxone) and to the fluoroquinolones will have to be added in the testing panel.

4.1.3.3. *Neisseria* Species

Neisseria species need to be incorporated in a second-line panel to complete the knowledge of the antibacterial spectrum of a new compound.

4.1.4. Gram-Negative Bacilli

4.1.4.1. *Enterobacteriaceae*

The *Enterobacteriaceae* represent a huge world, but a few simple rules will enable the antibacterial profile of a new entity to be determined. It should be borne in mind that the *Enterobacteriaceae* produce enzymes that hydrolyze β-lactams (Philipon et al., 1994), inactivate aminoglycosides to various degrees (Miller and the Aminoglycoside Resistance Study Group, 1994), or become resistant to fluoroquinolones through mechanisms whose genetic basis is chromosomally mediated (Bryskier, 1993).

The new molecule should be tested against the following:

- Isogenic strains, such as *E. coli* 600, which possess the different enzymes hydrolyzing β-lactams or inactivating aminoglycosides
- Strains resistant to the fluoroquinolones, whose mechanism of resistance is known
- Reference strains producing different β-lactamases (class 1, extended spectrum, broad spectrum, etc.) or enzymes which inactivate aminoglycosides (take the strains producing the most common enzymes in each bacterial species)

Initially the scope should be restricted to species with a high frequency of involvement in the various pathological processes. Activity against the less common species should be determined subsequently.

In practice, the activity of the compound must be established against *E. coli*, *Klebsiella pneumoniae*, *Klebsiella oxytoca*, *Citrobacter freundii*, *Serratia marcescens*, *Enterobacter cloacae*, *Enterobacter aerogenes*, *Morganella morganii*, *Providencia* spp., *Proteus* spp., *Shigella* spp., *Salmonella* spp., and *Yersinia enterocolitica*.

For an inhibitor of β-lactamases, the approach is similar to that of standard antibacterials. Often they are inactive against bacteria by themselves, and for a combination to be optimal, it needs to restore activity against bacilli producing class A, C, and D enzymes. Those harboring a metallo enzyme (class B, such as carbapenemases) are different. These combinations are tested in vitro and in vivo against isolates of *Enterobacteriaceae* harboring broad-spectrum β-lactamases, extended-broad-spectrum β-lactamases, class C enzymes (AmpC), and class D enzymes (oxacillinase). Activity against *S. aureus* producing penicillinase is added, as well as that against *P. aeruginosa* (assessment is often difficult due to the complexity of the mechanisms of resistance) and *Acinetobacter*. It must be kept in mind that the compound to restore activity needs to be active by itself against the susceptible targeted bacilli.

In the world of *Enterobacteriaceae*, salmonellae and shigellae occupy a specific place. The new antibacterial agent must be tested against strains resistant to the antibiotics used in the diseases caused by these organisms, namely, ampicillin, chloramphenicol, and co-trimoxazole for salmonellae, plus tetracyclines and nalidixic acid for shigellae. The number of strains resistant to fluoroquinolones is still small, and these strains need not be included in a standard panel.

The following serovars of *Salmonella enterica* at least will have to be tested: Typhi, Enteritidis, and Typhimurium, with strains exhibiting different antibiotic resistance phenotypes; other serovars will have to be tested according to the local epidemiology.

In the case of shigellae, the activity must be tested against the four groups: *Shigella sonnei*, *Shigella flexneri*, *Shigella dysenteriae*, and *Shigella bodii*. The number of strains from clinical isolates is considerable, with the first two species representing the majority of strains responsible for infections. Here, too, a panel of susceptible strains and of those resistant to co-trimoxazole, tetracyclines, and nalidixic acid should be obtained. Strains resistant to fluoroquinolones are rare at present.

4.1.4.2. *P. aeruginosa* and Other Species

The activity of a new antibacterial agent should be determined against wild strains (clinical isolates and collection) and against strains with a known resistance phenotype, whether these are β-lactamase-producing strains (carbenicillinases, oxacillinases, cephalosporinases, etc.) or strains resistant to fluoroquinolones, aminoglycosides (gentamicin, tobramycin, amikacin, and netilmicin), and imipenem (mutant of parietal permeability).

A study of bactericidal activity in combination with other antibacterial agents is essential. This is done by the killing kinetics.

A sufficient number of strains of species other than *P. aeruginosa* must be included in the determination of antibacterial activity and the establishment of the antibacterial spectrum.

4.1.4.3. Other Gram-Negative Bacilli

The following bacterial genera must be included in the characterization of the antibacterial spectrum of the new compound: *Aeromonas hydrophila*, *Stenotrophomonas (Xanthomonas) maltophilia*, *Vibrio cholerae* and other *Vibrio* spp., *Alcaligenes* spp., *Acinetobacter* spp., *Bordetella bronchiseptica*, *Flavobacterium* spp., *Alteromonas* spp., and *Burkholderia* spp.

4.1.4.3.1. *Acinetobacter* spp. The antibacterial activity must be tested against some hundred strains of *Acinetobacter baumannii* with different β-lactam resistance phenotypes (five phenotypes), in particular in response to *N*-acylpenicillins (piperacillin), α-carboxypenicillins (ticarcillin) (singly or combined with a β-lactamase inhibitor [clavulanic acid or tazobactam]), carbapenems, and aminoglycosides.

As *A. baumannii* represents one of the agents of nosocomial pneumonia, it might be important to test a new agent in the model of experimental pneumonia in the immunodepressed mouse.

The other species of *Acinetobacter* should also be included in the panel, but with a very much more limited sample.

4.1.4.3.2. *V. cholerae*. Strains responsible for cholera exhibit profiles of susceptibility to antibiotics which vary according to whether they belong to biovar *V. cholerae* O1, responsible for the seventh pandemic (standard biotype or El Tor), or the new biovar of Indian origin from the region of Bengal, which would appear to be the carrier of the eighth pandemic (*V. cholerae* O139) and which is resistant to co-trimoxazole. Certain non-O1 *V. cholerae* strains have been isolated from patients not exhibiting a choleriform syndrome but with bacteremia often of digestive origin and characterized by nonsusceptibility to colistin.

The new antibacterial agent must be tested against the three types of *V. cholerae* and against strains exhibiting resistance to ampicillin, tetracyclines, and sulfonamides.

4.1.4.4. Fastidious Gram-Negative Bacilli

4.1.4.4.1. *Haemophilus* spp. The susceptibility of *H. influenzae* is studied against a panel of strains including β-lactamase- and non-β-lactamase-producing strains and against strains resistant to ampicillin via a nonenzymatic mechanism. Cephalosporins possess weaker activity against this type of strain, and an oral and a parenteral cephalosporin should be included among the reference compounds.

A difficult and controversial question is the nature of the medium in which the MIC should be determined (Erwin and Jones, 1993; Jones et al., 1994). The strains are distributed between equal numbers of *H. influenzae* type b and non-b strains.

When testing macrolides or ketolides, it is important to use a homemade Haemophilus Test Medium, freshly prepared and with a shelf life of less than 3 to 4 weeks. Variations in MICs according to Haemophilus Test Medium batches produced by different manufacturers have to be investigated. When testing a β-lactam antibiotic with E-test strips, cautions need to be taken when reading the inhibition zones; some erratic colonies could be present in the zone of inhibition due probably to medium osmolarity.

Bactericidal activity has to be determined against strains producing or not producing β-lactamases. For instance, the bactericidal activities determined by killing curve for macrolides against enzyme-producing and non-enzyme-producing strains are different. Macrolides are bacteriostatic mainly against β-lactamase-producing strains. These results were confirmed in animal models.

The other species, such as *Haemophilus parainfluenzae*, *Haemophilus haemolyticus*, *Haemophilus parahaemolyticus*, *Haemophilus paraphrohaemolyticus* and *Haemophilus aegyptius* are included in the panel subsequently. Certain species are responsible for abscesses of the liver, endocarditis, and purulent meningitis.

4.1.4.4.2. *Moraxella* spp. The genus *Moraxella* includes several species, such as *Moraxella lacunata*, *Moraxella bovis*, *Moraxella nonliquefaciens*, *Moraxella phenylpyruvica*, *Moraxella atlantae*, and *Moraxella osloensis*.

M. lacunata and *M. nonliquefaciens* are causative agents of human conjunctivitis and purulent meningitis.

4.1.4.4.3. *M. catarrhalis*. *M. catarrhalis* is a commensal agent of the upper airways responsible for superinfections in chronic bronchitic patients and those with ear, nose, and throat infections, such as otitis media. The strains of *M. catarrhalis* are ROB-1- and ROB-2-type β-lactamase producers and nonproducers, and the three antibiotypes must be included in the test.

The bactericidal activity of a new compound against *M. catarrhalis* needs to be investigated. However, it is somewhat difficult to perform killing curves with this bacterium due to clumping forms, especially with a large inoculum size. This problem has to be overcome.

4.1.4.4.4. *Bordetella pertussis* and other agents of whooping cough. The agent of whooping cough is usually susceptible to macrolides, which are the drugs of choice. The determination of susceptibility is based on strains of *B. pertussis* and *Bordetella parapertussis*. The culture medium and the growth conditions are specific for *B. pertussis*. Recently a new species has been described: *Bordetella holmesii*.

4.1.5. HACCEK

The acronym HACCEK refers to gram-negative bacteria that are uncommon in human pathology but responsible for cases of severe endocarditis. They include *Haemophilus aphrophilus*, *Actinobacillus actinomycetemcomitans*, *Capnocytophaga*, *Cardiobacterium hominis*, *Eikenella corrodens*, and *Kingella*.

The activity of a new compound is determined in the context of the background data required to determine its therapeutic efficacy in the treatment of endocarditis.

4.1.5.1. *Pasteurella* spp.

Pasteurella multocida is responsible for skin infections following bites or scratches by Canidae and Felidae and rarely pneumonia.

Some strains produce ROB-1 β-lactamases, and a number should be included in the panel.

4.1.5.2. *H. ducreyi*

H. ducreyi is a bacterium that is difficult to grow. A special culture medium is prepared at least 3 days before use. The strains tested should exhibit different resistance phenotypes: β-lactamase and non-β-lactamase producing (TEM-1 and ROB-1) and resistant or nonresistant to tetracyclines, sulfonamides, and kanamycin.

Strains resistant to erythromycin A and 2-amino-5-thiazolyl cephalosporins are still uncommon.

4.1.5.3. *Capnocytophaga*

Capnocytophaga species are gram-negative bacilli. *Capnocytophaga ochracea*, *Capnocytophaga sputigena*, and *Capnocytophaga gingivalis* are opportunistic bacteria causing suppurative infections of the oral; ear, nose, and throat; and bone spheres. A few cases of endocarditis have been reported. Strains of *Capnocytophaga* are conventionally resistant to 5-nitroimidazoles and aminoglycosides. The activity of the new antibacterial agent must be determined on the basis of the essential requirements for the treatment of endocarditis.

4.1.5.4. Other Nonfermentative Gram-Negative Bacilli

4.1.5.4.1. *S. maltophilia*. *S. maltophilia* is an opportunistic bacterial agent increasingly involved in nosocomial infections, particularly in intensive care units.

Determination of the susceptibility of *S. maltophilia* to antibacterial agents is not fully standardized. In particular, the disk method has been shown to be unreliable, and the diameters of the zones of inhibition have been shown to depend on the media and their zinc content. *S. maltophilia* produces at least two enzymes: an imipenemase resistant to clavulanic acid and a cephalosporinase susceptible to it. Strains producing little imipenemase are more susceptible to the combination ticarcillin-clavulanic acid than to combinations containing sulbactam or tazobactam (piperacillin-tazobactam). A new molecule should be tested against strains susceptible or resistant to the combination ticarcillin-clavulanic acid.

4.1.5.4.2. *Burkholderia* spp. *Pseudomonas pseudomallei* group II has recently been rechristened *Burkholderia* spp. (Yabuuchi et al., 1992). This group includes *Burkholderia pseudomallei, Burkholderia mallei, Burkholderia cepacia, Pseudomonas gladioli, Burkholderia picketti, Burkholderia caryophylli,* and *Burkholderia solanacearum*. A subspecies of *B. cepacia* was isolated in the bronchial secretions of a cystic fibrosis patient, *Burkholderia cepacia* subsp. *vietnamiensis*, which seems to respond better to available antibacterials. This subspecies need to be tested when a compound is directed against bacteria involved in superinfections in cystic fibrosis patients.

B. cepacia has become a major opportunistic agent but is also found with increasing frequency in patients suffering from cystic fibrosis. The strains isolated are often multiresistant. Conventionally, *B. cepacia* is susceptible to ceftazidime, piperacillin, and co-trimoxazole, but it possesses variable susceptibilities to carbapenems and fluoroquinolones. The strains are usually resistant to aminoglycosides and chloramphenicol.

The antibacterial activity must be tested against strains exhibiting different antibiotic resistance phenotypes. The strains tested must be resistant to one or more of the following antibiotics: imipenem, ceftazidime, co-trimoxazole, piperacillin, and ciprofloxacin. A very high proportion of strains isolated from the bronchial secretions of patients suffering from cystic fibrosis have been found to produce carbapenemases (Simpson et al., 1993).

4.1.6. Anaerobic Bacteria

Determination of the activity of a compound against anaerobic bacteria requires a specialized laboratory. Strains resistant to clindamycin and cephamycins (cefoxitin and cefotetan) must be included for gram-negative bacilli. Strains resistant to 5-nitroimidazoles (metronidazole and derivatives) are infrequent (Dublanchet et al., 1986). This activity should be determined in two different culture media: Wilkins-Chalgren and Brucella. Activity against *Clostridium difficile* is determined separately from that against the other clostridia. Investigation of the in vitro activities of combinations with the new compound and already established antianaerobic compounds have to be done by kill kinetic methods.

4.2. Other Microorganisms

The determination of the activities of new molecules against certain bacterial genera, such as *Treponema pallidum, Borrelia* spp., *H. pylori, Campylobacter* spp., *Mycobacterium* spp., *Mycoplasma* spp., and *Leptospira* spp., is specific.

4.2.1. *H. pylori*

H. pylori is responsible for duodenal ulcers and type B chronic gastritis. The in vitro antibacterial activity is determined at the pH of the gastric environment if the compounds are stable in a highly acidic medium. The antibacterial activity must be determined in combination with Hep-2-type cells, although these tolerate poorly an excessively acidic pH (pH<6). Because of the therapeutic combination with antiulcer drugs such as anti-H_2 or proton pump inhibitors (omeprazole and lansoprazole), the activities of the antibacterial agents must be tested in the presence of these molecules, which may have specific antibacterial activity, such as lansoprazole.

The incidence of resistance of *H. pylori* to metronidazole ranges from 7 to 49% depending on the center. However, there is no standardized method for evaluating susceptibility to metronidazole, which explains the major variability in the assessment of the level of resistance.

De Cross et al. (1993) have developed a method for determining the susceptibility of *H. pylori* to metronidazole by the disk method using the Kirby-Bauer modified technique. This method is moderately reliable, as there is a difference of 10.7% between the agar method and the disk method. Xia et al. (1994) proposed breakpoints for metronidazole against *H. pylori*, and they are shown in Table 14.

There is currently no reference strain that provides quality assurance.

The activity of a new compound is determined against 100 freshly collected strains of *H. pylori* and against strains resistant to metronidazole, clarithromycin, or both of these compounds.

It is essential to have strains of *H. pylori* type 1 in the panel, which are considered to be responsible for ulcerative episodes.

Bactericidal activity should be investigated. In vivo activity at present is more difficult to study, as the murine model of *Helicobacter felis* infection is not truly representative of ulcerative infections in humans. Rodent *H. pylori* models are recommended.

In 2002, the NCCLS introduced quality control strains.

4.2.2. *Campylobacter* spp.

Campylobacter jejuni and *Campylobacter coli* are the *Campylobacter* species most often isolated from pathological products, with *C. jejuni* being more susceptible to

Table 14 Breakpoints of metronidazole against *H. pylori*

Resistance phenotype	Zone diam (mm)	MIC (μg/ml)
Susceptible	≥26	<4
Intermediate	20–26	4–8
Resistant	≤20	>8

antibiotics than *C. coli*. Strains resistant to macrolides and fluoroquinolones should be included in the panel. When exploring the in vitro activities of antibacterials against bacteria involved in gastrointestinal infections, *Campylobacter* strains have to be included in the panel.

4.2.3. *Borrelia* spp.

Borrelia spp. are the causative agents of Lyme disease, which is endemic in the northern hemisphere. Genetic studies have shown that there are several species of *Borrelia*, including *Borrelia burgdorferi*, *Borrelia garinii*, *Borrelia afzelii*, and *Borrelia* strain VS 461 (Péter and Bretz, 1994), associated with different clinical pictures. *B. burgdorferi* is often associated with rheumatological signs and symptoms, and *B. garinii* and *B. afzelii* are associated with neurological and cutaneous syndromes, respectively (acrodermatitis chronica atrophicans).

The panel of strains is chosen from among the different species. BSK II medium is used, and the number of spirochetes is determined using a Petroff-Hausser cell.

Collection strains that have undergone repeated subculturing should be tested, as they grow more rapidly than wild strains. If due care is not taken, it is possible to obtain an incorrect response about the activity of the antibacterial agents tested. In particular, it should not be forgotten that the culture sediment must be subcultured in an antibiotic-free medium to detect the presence of spirochetes, being sure to take a reading after a sufficient number of days so as to allow any regrowth of the bacteria to be detected.

These precautions and the lack of standardization mean that the results obtained may vary from one team to another. The different species of *Borrelia* do not exhibit the same susceptibilities to antibacterial agents (Table 15).

4.2.4. *T. pallidum*

Syphilis is caused by *T. pallidum*, and its treatment is based on benzylpenicillin. However, a therapeutic alternative is necessary when patients have delayed hypersensitivity to penicillin G. There are no in vitro culture models, but there is a model developed by Stamm et al. (1988) which combines bacterial extraction from rabbit testes and a technique of protein synthesis inhibition 4 h after contact of the treponemas with the antibiotic tested. Apart from the susceptible reference Nichols strain, the erythromycin A-resistant strain (due to an A2058G mutation on the peptidyltransferase loop) must be included. The potential activity of the new antibacterial agent in the treatment of syphilis can be quantified by means of a comparative model with penicillin G in the rabbit (Lukehart et al., 1990). These experimental studies must be confirmed by clinical studies (Verdon et al., 1994).

4.2.5. *Mycoplasma* and *Ureaplasma* spp.

There are few compounds that are active against *Mycoplasma* and *Ureaplasma* species, and these principally include macrolides, fluoroquinolones, and cyclines.

The methods are poorly standardized, and interpretation is often difficult. It is difficult to compare the results of different laboratories. For mycoplasmas, the following species should be tested principally: *Mycoplasma pneumoniae*, *Mycoplasma hominis*, and *Mycoplasma genitalium*. The pathogenicity of the other mycoplasmas in human beings is more disputed, so it is not necessary to test the activity of a new molecule in the context of a registration dossier. Strains of *M. pneumoniae* resistant to fluoroquinolones and erythromycin A have been described.

For *Ureaplasma urealyticum*, strains susceptible and resistant to tetracyclines should be tested (Kenny et al., 1986, 1993).

4.2.6. *Nocardia* spp.

Nocardia spp. are bacterial agents that are occasionally responsible for infections, but these are usually associated with immunodepressed states. The genus *Nocardia* includes, among other species, *Nocardia asteroides*, *Nocardia brasiliensis*, and *Nocardia farcinica*. *N. asteroides* is susceptible to aminoglycosides, 2-amino-5-thiazolyl cephalosporins, sulfonamides, oxazolidinones, and tetracyclines (Wallace and Steele, 1988). Fourteen- and fifteen-membered-ring macrolides are ineffective due to enzymatic inactivation on the 2′OH of the D-desosamine.

4.2.7. *Leptospira* spp.

Leptospirosis is an endemic zoonosis due to a bacterial genus, *Leptospira*, that comprises several serogroups and serovars. The serogroups are *Leptospira interrogans* serovars icterohemorrhagiae, Canicola, Grippotyphosa, and Australis.

4.3. Intracellular Bacteria

Few antibiotics have the property of penetrating phagocytic cells. The antibiotics belonging to the following families possibly possess intracellular bioactivity: macrolides, fluoroquinolones, tetracyclines, ansamycins, streptogramins, and lincosamides. The intracellular penetration of peptides should be tested symptomatically (e.g., teicoplanin and oritavancin). For investigational glycopeptides such as dalbavancin and telavancin, there not yet reports on intracellular penetration.

The first stage in the exploration of the intracellular bioactivity of molecules is the determination of their kinetics of penetration and efflux of intracellular accumulation,

Table 15 In vitro activities of different antibiotics against *Borrelia* spp.[a]

Drug	MIC (μg/ml)		
	B. burgdorferi BE 1	*B. garinii* VS 102	*B. afzelii* ACA 1
Doxycycline	0.25	0.125	0.25
Amoxicillin	0.25	0.125	0.25
Roxithromycin	0.062	0.015	0.125
Ceftriaxone	0.031	0.031	0.031
Cefodizime	0.125	0.125	0.25
Cefpirome	0.25	0.25	0.125
Cefpodoxime	4.0	1.0	1.0

[a]Data from Péter and Bretz, 1994.

with the determination of the precise localization of the molecule in the cell. These studies are comparative and are of no value unless they are performed by the same team, since the methodologies vary from one laboratory to another. It is therefore desirable to have results from two different teams.

The second stage consists of testing the intracellular bioactivity of the antibiotic against intracellular species. This type of study is commonly undertaken with *M. tuberculosis* and *Mycobacterium avium* complex. These studies should in the future be generalized to other bacterial genera and intracellular species.

Some intracellular bacteria grow readily on an agar or broth medium, such as *Brucella* spp. The determination of the MIC provides a guideline in terms of activity, but it must be strictly correlated with the intracellular concentrations and the localization of the antibiotic in the cell. The in vitro activity has to be confirmed with a murine brucellosis infection.

The determination of activity against *Chlamydia* spp. varies with the species. The increased knowledge on *Chlamydiaceae* has led to a proposal of a new classification of *Chlamydia*. Three groups have been proposed. Group 1 is divided in subgroups: *Chlamydia* spp. and *Chlamydophila* spp. Groups 2 and 3 are composed of *Simkania* spp. and *Parachlamydia*. *Simkania* spp. are considered to be responsible for bronchitis and pneumonia in humans.

For *Chlamydia pneumoniae*, the bactericidal activities of new compounds have recently been investigated in cell lines with macrolides and ketolides. More experience is needed before conclusions about this method of investigation can be drawn. Animal models of chlamydial infections are not yet validated, but some of them are promising.

For *Chlamydia trachomatis*, the activity of the antibiotic is tested in a cellular medium (McCoy cell or HeLa cell) and in animal models, such as the determination of the fertility rate of mice infected with *C. trachomatis* and treated with the antibiotic, compared to a control.

For *Chlamydia psittaci*, the activity is tested in vitro in a cell line and in a model of experimental pneumonia in the mouse.

In the case of *C. pneumoniae*, only the in vitro determinations are validated, in contrast to the in vivo models. The best type of cell is probably HEp-2, which *C. pneumoniae* penetrates better than McCoy cells.

Activity against *Rickettsia* or related bacteria is determined in a cellular medium. The results obtained vary from one laboratory to another because of different methodologies. Activity should be tested against the main species, such as *Rickettsia conorii*, *Rickettsia rickettsii*, *Rickettsia prowazekii*, *Rickettsia tsutsugamushi*, *Rickettsia typhi*, and *Coxiella burnetii*.

The activity against *Rochalimaea* spp. (*Bartonella* spp.), among which *Rochalimaea henselae* is assuming importance in AIDS patients, should be determined separately in Vero cells, and likewise the activity against different species of *Ehrlichia*, *Afipia felis*, and *Francisella tularensis*.

The in vitro activity against *Legionella* spp. is determined in two culture media with a reference strain. Determination of in vitro activity in charcoal-containing medium (BCYEα) should be avoided, as this type of medium inhibits the activity of macrolides and fluoroquinolones. However, the drug should be tested in macrophages and in vivo in the guinea pig to assess global activity. Combinations with rifampin can be tested by the kill kinetic method.

C. burnetii assays are conducted using human fibroblasts (HEL). Bactericidal activity needs to be investigated. Due to the intracellular location of *C. burnetii* (phagolysosome), only few antibacterials are able to act against this organism. Usually, in vitro activity against this organism is assessed against three strains: the Nine Mile strain (reference strain in the acute phase), strain Q-212, and strain Priscilla (reference strain in the chronic phase).

In vitro activity against *Ehrlichia chaffeensis* is determined in DH 82 cells (canine macrophage cell line) infected with *E. chaffeensis*.

F. tularensis is responsible for tularemia. In vitro activity against this organism is determined in a murine macrophage cell line (P 388D1) in medium supplemented with 10% fetal calf serum and 2 mM glutamine.

Bosea spp. and *Afipia* spp. are α-Proteobacteria. *Afipia* is responsible for cat scratch disease and nosocomial osteitis. *Bosea massiliensis* is associated with nosocomial pneumonia.

Bosea and *Afipia* are associated with amoebae in hospital water supplies. Strains are grown for 72 to 96 h on BCYE agar before being tested in microbroth dilutions (30°C incubation for 72 to 96 h) (La Scola et al., 2004).

4.4. Mycobacteria

A distinction within the mycobacteria should be drawn between *M. tuberculosis*, *Mycobacterium leprae*, and so-called atypical mycobacteria.

4.4.1. *M. tuberculosis*

The new antibacterial agent is tested against reference strain H_{37RV}, which exhibits different antibiotic resistance phenotypes (streptomycin, isoniazid, rifampin, ethambutol, etc.).

If the new antibacterial agent proves active against the H_{37RV} strain, it is tested against a panel of strains from clinical isolates. This panel should include strains of *Mycobacterium africanum*, *Mycobacterium bovis*, and *M. bovis* BCG.

The second stage consists of studying combinations with other antituberculosis agents. Animal models are required.

Conventionally, in vitro antibacterial activity is determined on a Löwenstein-Jensen agar medium impregnated with antibiotic. Currently, however, Middlebrook's agar media are preferred, either the 7 H10 or 7 H11, supplemented with 10% oleic acid-albumin-dextrose-catalase with or without Tween 80 at pH 6.6. The activity of pyrazinamine is tested using the same medium but at pH 5.8. The BACTEC radiometric method may be used at two different pHs (pH 6.8 and pH 7.4).

4.4.2. Atypical Mycobacteria

The new antibacterial agent is tested alone or in combination against different strains of *M. avium* complex. These strains are obtained from human immunodeficiency virus-positive or -negative patients. Combinations with macrophages and with different antibiotics are tested. Depending on the results, a study is conducted in the beige mouse.

Activity is also tested against the other atypical mycobacteria.

4.4.3. *M. leprae*

The search for new antileprosy agents requires that all molecules be tested alone and in combination if they possess a certain potential in this indication. Today, this principally involves the fluoroquinolones and macrolides.

4.5. *Tropheryma whipplei*

T. whipplei is the bacterial agent of Whipple disease, a chronic disease which could be considered when a patient is suffering from an unexplained arthralgia and diarrhea. Part of the bacterial diagnosis relies on duodenal biopsies, but PCR on saliva can orient the diagnosis.

Culture has to be performed on a human fibroblast culture line (HEL). The bacterial growth is long and fastidious for at least 3 months (Raoult et al., 2000).

4.6. Bacteria in Free-Living Amoebae

Hospital-acquired pneumonia occurs in 0.5 to 1% of patients hospitalized, representing 10 to 15% of all nosocomial infections. The etiological agent of pneumonia remains unknown in 20 to 50% of the cases (Marrie et al., 1984).

Aquatic bacteria such as *Legionella* spp., *Pseudomonas* spp., *Stenotrophomonas* spp., *Burkholderia* spp., and *Acinetobacter* spp. may colonize hospital water supplies.

Free-living amoebae have been shown to be a reservoir for *Legionella* spp., *B. pickettii*, *Cryptococcus neoformans*, α-Proteobacteria (*Bosea* and *Afipia*), and *Parachlamydia* spp. (La Scola et al., 2003). Other pathogens may infect free-living amoebae, such as *C. pneumoniae*, *M. avium*, and *L. monocytogenes* (Greub and Raoult, 2002).

5. ANIMAL MODELS

Two types of animal models must be tested: nondiscriminatory models and models of specific experimental infections (Zak and O'Reilly, 1990).

5.1. Nondiscriminatory Models

Nondiscriminatory models are prepared during the preselection phase of a molecule. After determining the in vitro activity, it is essential to determine the in vivo activity parenterally and orally. In fact, the in vitro activity is not necessarily correlated with good in vivo activity (poor absorption, marked metabolization, and toxicity). In these systemic infection models, activity is tested against gram-positive cocci (*S. aureus*, *S. pyogenes*, *S. pneumoniae*, and *E. faecalis*), *Enterobacteriaceae*, and *P. aeruginosa*. The studies are performed comparatively with a molecule of the same class, if one exists.

The selection is made using bacterial strains exhibiting different antibiotic resistance phenotypes, such as *P. aeruginosa* strains exhibiting different susceptibilities to imipenem, ticarcillin, and ceftazidime. However, it is sometimes difficult to test these strains in vivo, as they are not always sufficiently virulent for the mouse, such as with *H. influenzae*.

5.2. Discriminatory Models

Two types of experimental infections may be conducted and serve as a basic requirement for clinical studies.

The first are "organ" infections, such as respiratory tract infections due to *K. pneumoniae* or *S. pneumoniae*, experimental pyelonephritis, endocarditis, experimental abscesses due to *B. fragilis*, experimental *S. aureus* or *P. aeruginosa* osteomyelitis, and experimental diarrhea in the piglet.

In vivo studies are also performed in the immunodepressed mouse with corticosteroids or cyclophosphamide or in the neutropenic mouse if the efficacy of the medicine is to be tested in immunodepressed or neutropenic patients.

The activity of an antibiotic in *H. influenzae* otitis media should be tested in the gerbil or preferably in the chinchilla, although with the knowledge that this model is disputed. *S. pneumoniae* otitis should be tested in the chinchilla, as the gerbil is not a good model since spontaneous resolution occurs too rapidly.

The second type of infection is more specific to a microorganism. These models are used as a basic requirement in respiratory tract infections due to *Legionella pneumophila* (guinea pig) and in infections of the genital tract due to *C. trachomatis* (mouse).

The Syrian hamster model of respiratory tract infections due to *M. pneumoniae* is more controversial.

6. SPECIFIC INDICATIONS

The registration of a specific clinical indication requires detailed pharmacological study. An example of this is pneumococcal infections. The emergence of strains that are resistant or of reduced susceptibility to penicillin G or multiresistant requires the microbiological validation of activity in this indication.

The first stage consists of determining the in vitro activity (MIC) against a panel of strains with variable susceptibilities to penicillin G and cefotaxime. Multiresistant strains (resistance including erythromycin A, clindamycin, tetracyclines, and kanamycin) are also tested. If the activity of a fluoroquinolone is to be tested, strains of various susceptibilities should be included, for example, those for which the MICs of levofloxacin are ≤ 2 and >2 μg/ml. The second stage enables the bactericidal activity to be determined by the killing kinetic technique, testing two inoculum sizes (10^5 and 10^6 CFU/ml). More complex is the third type of study, which attempts to demonstrate the power of selection of the molecule and the frequency and rate of mutation, particularly with fluoroquinolones.

Models of comparative systemic, respiratory (pneumonia and otitis), and meningeal experimental infections demonstrate the potential therapeutic activity of the molecule and help in the choice of doses for phase II.

The same approach is applied for other pathogenic agents, such as *S. aureus* and *P. aeruginosa*.

7. MECHANISMS OF ACTION AND RESISTANCE

Currently, the authorities wish to know the mechanism of action and mechanisms of resistance of antibacterial agents in the current state of scientific knowledge, which is in fact constantly changing because of the ongoing research in this field.

The mechanisms are known to a greater or lesser extent depending on the chemical families. The best known are those of the β-lactams, fluoroquinolones, mupirocin, and fosfomycin.

For β-lactams, studies involve outer membrane passage, action on peptidoglycan synthesis, inhibition of penicillin-binding proteins of different bacterial species, interaction with the different β-lactamases in intact bacterial cells and against enzymes, induction of cephalosporinases, and testing for β-lactamase-inhibitory activity.

For the fluoroquinolones, studies include transparietal passage, affinity for DNA gyrase and DNA gyrase-DNA complex, topoisomerase IV, and the efflux system (e.g., *S. aureus* NorA). The activity of the new fluoroquinolone against the various mutants must be studied.

For macrolides, ketolides, streptogramins, and all antibacterials acting on ribosomes, inhibition of protein synthesis and 30S and 50S and full ribosome assembly has to be investigated. The different mechanisms of resistance are explored, such as methylation (*erm* genes), efflux (*mef* genes), mutation of L4 and L22 ribosomal proteins, and at the 23S rRNA, inactivation by esterases, phosphorylases, and glycosylation. When a mechanism is not clear, a sequence is performed to look for unusual mutations, deletions, etc.

The global evaluation of potentiality of selection is explored through an in vitro model such as sequential passages and in vivo in a murine model.

8. INTERACTION WITH FECAL AND ORAL FLORAS

The study of the impact of a new antibacterial agent on the fecal and oral floras in humans occurs only after phase II once the unit and daily doses have been determined.

The aim of these studies is threefold. The amount of compound and the degradation products or metabolites eliminated in the stools and saliva as well as in sudoriparous glands for fluoroquinolones per 24 h and the duration of this elimination must be assessed after administration of a single dose or repeated doses. The second aim is to quantify the changes in anaerobic flora and *Enterobacteriaceae*, as well as the time necessary for the flora to return to the original level after the end of treatment. The third aim is the assessment of activity against *C. difficile* (Edlund and Nord, 1993). Selection of *Clostridium bolteae* after treatment in children could be of concern.

9. CLINICAL MICROBIOLOGY AND PHASES I AND II: DOSE DETERMINATION

Determination of the dose and rhythm of administration of a new medication is a critical point in development. The in vitro and in vivo studies contribute to the proposal of the doses that might be administered and that will be validated in phase II studies. One example is the determination of the daily oral dose of roxithromycin. Roxithromycin has antibacterial activity similar to that of erythromycin A, but it is 3 to 10 times more active in vivo in models of nondiscriminatory experimental infections, in particular because of its pharmacokinetic profile (Chantot et al., 1986). The preliminary phase II studies were conducted at a third of the dosage of erythromycin A, i.e., 600 mg daily. Dose-finding studies then established the daily dosage as 300 mg (Akoun et al., 1986). Other microbiological studies assist in the choice of the dosage proposed for phase II studies, such as pharmacodynamic models. Subsequently, a certain number of models validate the chosen dosage scientifically, such as the indices proposed by Schentag (1991) and Ellner and Neu (1981) and the bactericidal potency of the serum and cerebrospinal fluid. The concentration of an antibiotic in the cerebrospinal fluid must be at least 10 times the MIC for the pathogenic agent to achieve bactericidal activity (Täuber et al., 1984, 1989). The concentrations in the cerebrospinal fluid are dependent on the phase of meningitis. After a dosage of 200 mg/kg daily of cefotaxime intravenously, the concentrations are higher during the acute phase of the infection (1.7 to 7 μg/ml) and decrease slightly during the phase of attenuation of the disease (1.2 to 4 μg/ml), and during the resolution phase the concentration is 1 μg/ml (0.7 to 1.3 μg/ml) (Periti et al., 1984). When the antibacterial activity decreases, as, for example, with penicillin G or cefotaxime against strains of *S. pneumoniae*, the doses must be increased in order to at least maintain this ratio of 10 so as to obtain bactericidal potency in the cerebrospinal fluid at a minimum of 1:8 (Täuber et al., 1989).

Antibacterial agents may be divided into three categories. The first group is composed of compounds such as the aminoglycosides, fluoroquinolones, and certain macrolides (azithromycin and telithromycin) which possess concentration-dependent activity. The second group comprises β-lactams and macrolides (erythromycin A, roxithromycin, and clarithromycin), glycopeptides whose activity is time dependent. The third group comprises molecules whose activity is principally bacteriostatic, such as the tetracyclines.

The pharmacokinetic parameters and in vitro activity (MIC) enable the therapeutic fate to be evaluated or even predicted.

At present, the following parameters are studied: the area under the curve (AUC)/MIC ratio, the serum peak/MIC ratio, and the length of time for which the concentrations in serum are below the MIC (T>MIC). Another index was proposed by Schentag in 1991, the AUIC, which is equal to the AUC/MIC ratio. This was studied with the injectable cephalosporins, fluoroquinolones, aminoglycosides, metronidazole, and daptomycin. However, this index could be used with other families of antibiotics. The AUIC must be greater than or equal to 125. For the fluoroquinolones which are more rapidly bactericidal, an index of 250 has been proposed by Schentag as the threshold for strong bactericidal activity.

The bactericidal rate of antibiotics is either concentration dependent, as with the aminoglycosides and fluoroquinolones, or concentration independent and time dependent, as with the β-lactams.

The bactericidal rate is higher with the aminoglycosides when the concentrations are very much above the MIC. Optimum activity is achieved when the concentration in plasma is equal to 10 to 12 times the MIC (Moore et al., 1984a, 1984b). Activity depends on the duration and intensity of exposure. A bolus administration achieves an intense early bactericidal effect but a weak late bactericidal effect. This phenomenon may be a source of selection of bacteria with low-level resistance. When the maximum concentration of drug in serum/MIC ratio is greater than or equal to 8, the probability of obtaining antibacterial eradication is high. In animal models, a single dose of an aminoglycoside causes fewer lesions of the Corti organ and renal cells than multiple daily doses.

The bactericidal rate of β-lactams is time dependent and concentration independent. The period during which the concentrations in serum are above the MIC is the best predictive index of therapeutic activity. The bactericidal activity of the β-lactams is saturable in terms of the concentration and is optimal when the concentration in serum is four to eight times the minimal bactericidal concentration against the bacterium studied. Above this concentration, the bactericidal activity does not increase, and in fact a deleterious effect may occur (Eagle-type effect [Eagle et al., 1950]). Because of this saturation phenomenon, the time during which the concentration has a saturating effect should be optimized (T>MIC) rather than the intensity of the exposure (increasing the doses). The efficacy is optimal if T>MIC is 100% for gram-negative bacteria and 50% for gram-positive cocci. This comes down to saying that the concentrations in serum must be greater than the MIC between two drug administrations for gram-negative bacilli but only for 50% of the time in the case of gram-positive cocci because of the absence of a postantibiotic effect (Vogelman and Craig, 1985).

However, these predictive factors may be confuted. For example, ceftriaxone possesses excellent bactericidal activity against *Shigella* spp., with a MIC_{90} of 0.06 μg/ml (Peloux et al., 1994). A single dose of ceftriaxone yields concentrations in plasma that remain above the MIC after 48 h. In a comparative, double-blind efficacy study of ceftriaxone following a single dose in adults suffering from shigellosis, an improvement in clinical status was obtained, but the duration of fecal elimination of shigellae was not modified compared with that obtained with ampicillin or placebo (Kabir et al., 1986; Lolekha et al., 1991).

10. PLACE OF CLINICAL MICROBIOLOGY IN PHASE II AND III CLINICAL STUDIES

A clinical development program for anti-infective agents involves a microbiological component. This program must allow a harmonious clinical development and must be accompanied by a quality assurance program, which at present is purely embryonic or even nonexistent.

Microbiological studies are involved at several levels:

- Sampling of the pathological sample and transport of this specimen
- Isolation and identification of the pathogenic agent
- Determination of the antibacterial activity of the test molecule and that used for comparison
- Phenotype and genotype of the bacterial resistant strain
- Correlation of the in vitro and clinical efficacies to determine the breakpoints

10.1. Pathological Samples

The pathological samples vary: blood, urine, and fecal cultures; bronchial secretions; bronchoalveolar lavage, cerebrospinal, pleural, pericardic, ascites, and joint fluids; pharyngotonsillar specimens; and pus samples of various origins.

The sampling conditions and conditions of transport to the laboratory (transport medium, time, etc.) must be specified and standardized.

Standards for examination must be established: cytological examinations, stained smear examinations with different stains (Gram, May-Grünwald-Giemsa, etc.), and bacterial isolation and identification.

Quantification is necessary for certain pathological specimens, such as urine. This is recommended with other pathological specimens, such as bronchial brushings.

The results of cytobacteriological examinations must be accompanied by biochemical results in certain infections, such as cerebrospinal fluid in meningitis.

Bacterial identification must be complete. For example, the response "*Salmonella* spp." is not acceptable. In fact, the predictable activity of a parenteral cephalosporin differs according to whether *S. enterica* serovar Enteritidis or Typhimurium is involved. The latter has an intracellular development, and β-lactams do not penetrate cells.

The same applies to streptococci, which must be identified in terms of the Lancefield group, and in the event of a therapeutic failure further investigations should be conducted for the purposes of identification. The serogroups and serotypes of pneumococci must be known precisely, with the awareness that these determinations are done in specialized laboratories. In case of failure, identification of *S. pneumoniae* versus *Streptococcus oralis* must be envisaged.

For *H. influenzae*, the determination of the serotypes and biotypes is useful in the event of apparent noneradication of bacteria, enabling the bacterial strains isolated at the beginning of the infection and during treatment to be identified (Kilian, 1976).

When the same bacterial species is isolated from a patient treated with an antibiotic after the discontinuation of treatment or following a presumed clinical and/or microbiological failure, it should be ensured that the identity of the strains at the beginning of the infection is the same as for those isolated subsequently. For some bacterial species, it is possible to undertake a more detailed identification using pulsed-field electrophoresis or other tests. This method of identification yields good results with the majority of *Enterobacteriaceae*, except *Salmonella* spp. and *E. coli*. The method may also be used for *S. pyogenes* and *S. aureus*.

10.2. Determination of Antibacterial Activity

The susceptibility of the bacterial strain considered responsible for the infection is determined in the clinical microbiology laboratory of the center in which the study is being conducted. This involves an antibiotic sensitivity test at the least. The identification of the bacterium, the nature of the sample, the diameters of the zones of inhibition, and the MIC are recorded in the microbiological study book. The MIC and the diameters of the zones of inhibition of the reference strain must be mentioned precisely. In order to facilitate the subsequent analysis of the clinical results, particularly in the event of a therapeutic failure, this test includes other antibiotics so as to enable the antibiotic resistance phenotype of the bacterial strain responsible for the infection to be defined.

The method used for the antibiotic sensitivity test is recorded in the study book, i.e., the Kirby-Bauer method (Bauer et al., 1966), the flooding method (Chabbert, 1982), or the Joan Stokes method in The United Kingdom with specific reference strains (*S. aureus* NCTC 6571, *E. coli* NCTC 10418, *S. pneumoniae* NCTC 12140) (Snell et al., 1988; British Society for Antimicrobial Chemotherapy, 1991). It is essential to know the agar medium used, together with the name of the manufacturer, the batch number, and the expiration date in the case of ready-to-use media. When the media are prepared from a dehydrated powder, a reproducibility test with a reference strain must be included. The use of supplements such as blood (horse, sheep, rabbit, etc.) or growth factors, and the use of 5 to 6% CO_2, etc., should be mentioned.

The origins of the disks (manufacturers), the batch number, quality control strains, and the method of storage must be defined. The method of measuring the zone of inhibition must also be mentioned (calipers, ruler, optical apparatus, etc.).

10.3. Antibiotic Phenotype

Certain tests are performed routinely. For example, in the case of *S. pneumoniae*, the determination of the diameter of the zone of inhibition around a 1-μg oxacillin disk provides an indication of strains resistant to penicillin G. It is advisable to include a ceftizoxime disk because if the diameter is ≤15 mm, there is a high probability that the strain is resistant to cefotaxime and ceftriaxone (MIC, ≥2 μg/ml). This test appears to be less reliable if the strains are of intermediate susceptibility to cefotaxime (MIC, 1 μg/ml). All of these data are confirmed by the determination of the MIC. Another example is the determination of the activity of a new β-lactam against *Enterobacteriaceae*. Cefotaxime, ceftazidime, and, if possible, aztreonam should be tested systemically against co-amoxiclav to detect extended-broad-spectrum β-lactamases using the champagne cork method or the double-disk test (Jarlier et al., 1988).

For the aminoglycosides, it is also possible to determine the enzymatic profile of a bacterial strain against different enzymes and abnormalities of membrane permeability in relation to the diameter of the zone of inhibition (Table 16).

Against *S. aureus* resistant to methicillin, a routine test to detect the gene *mecA* is to use a disk of cefoxitin as recommended by the NCCLS and, if necessary, to confirm with a PCR in case of discrepancies between susceptibility to oxacillin or methicillin and cefoxitin.

Table 16 Zone of inhibition for 50% of clinical isolates resistant to aminoglycosides (1989 to 1991)

Drug[a]	Disk load (μg)	Diam zone (mm)	Zone of inhibition (mm)								
			Gram-negative bacilli							Gram-positive bacteria	
			AAC (3)-IV	AAC (3)-I	AAC (2′)-	AAC (3)-VI	ANT(2″) + AAC(3)-III	ANT (4′)-II	APH (3′)-VI	APH(2″) + AAC(3)	ANT (4′)-I
GEN	10	22	12	13	14	6	8	20	24	6	20
TOB	10	21	6	21	13	17	9	14	26	6	7
NET	30	25	15	25	24	21	22	20	27	18	36
AMI	30	22	23	23	24	21	22	18	8	16	22
ISE	30	24	25	25	24	23	23	18	8	16	21

[a]GEN, gentamicin; TOB, tobramycin; NET, netilmicin; AMI, amikacin; ISE, isepamicin.

10.4. Centralization of Examinations

All of the strains must be stored under good conditions (storage media, temperature, freeze-drying, etc.). A single microbiological laboratory should centralize all of the strains collected during the clinical trial. All strains must be reidentified precisely, including the serogroups or serotypes, and β-lactamase type, the putative mechanisms of resistance (macrolides or ketolides, oxazolidinones, streptogramins, etc.), or aminoglycoside-inactivating enzymes should be detected. The determination of the MIC is repeated systematically by standard methods to provide evaluable results. For fastidious bacterial species that are reputedly difficult to grow, such as *S. pneumoniae*, *S. pyogenes*, *M. catarrhalis*, and *H. influenzae*, it is useful to perform an antibiotic susceptibility test and to determine the MIC of the test antibiotics in parallel. This makes it possible to verify the vitality of the strain tested and avoid assigning it excessively low MICs because of weak bacterial growth. For a given bacterial species, the culture medium and its supplements (except blood) must come from the same batch and same manufacturer. It must be validated systematically using a reference strain.

Other tests might be performed on a given strain if the clinical response is slower than for the majority of strains of a bacterial species, given in terms of bactericidal activities.

Tests should be undertaken in certain bacterial species to detect tolerance phenomena, such as benzylpenicillin for the viridans group streptococci or 2-amino-5-thiazolyl cephalosporins for *H. influenzae*. The simplest test is the determination of the MIC and minimal bactericidal concentration (Allen and Sprunt, 1978).

Determination of the MICs and the diameters of the zones of inhibition (same lot of disks) will establish a correlation between the clinical and microbiological results obtained during the phase II and phase III studies.

10.5. Correlation between Disks and MIC

A correlation between the disk method and the MIC technique is required in certain countries, such as the United States. This involves multicenter studies which allow the collection of clinical isolates over a given period, involving the main bacterial species that grow in an aerobic or aerobic-anaerobic environment and are commonly responsible for infectious conditions.

10.6. Cross-Validation

When two or more central laboratories are involved, a cross-validation of MICs and zone diameters needs to be performed. All clinical isolates collected during the clinical trial

Table 17 Activities of β-lactams against ampicillin-resistant and non-β-lactamase-producing *H. influenzae*

Drug	MIC_{90} (μg/ml)		
	Decreased susceptibility	Susceptible	MIC (μg/ml) for *H. influenzae* NCTC 11931
Ampicillin	5.16	0.52	0.5
Amoxicillin	11.9	0.92	1.0
Co-amoxiclav	6.2	0.64	1.0
Imipenem	6.19	4.14	1.0
Cefazolin	>55.4	30	16
Cefadroxil	>118.7	35.6	16
Cefaclor	>59.1	5.29	4.0
Cefuroxime	5.9	0.69	1.0
Cefotaxime	0.24	<0.06	0.03
Cefepime	1.48	0.11	0.1
Cefpirome	0.7	<0.06	0.06
Cefpodoxime	0.93	0.086	0.1
Cefixime	0.62	0.05	0.06

are exchanged. All of the tests are performed using the same methodology, including culture medium, etc.

If MICs are determined on microtiter trays, a cross-validation between dry and frozen panels is undertaken.

11. EPIDEMIOLOGICAL STUDIES

A difficult exercise is to predict the epidemiology of resistance at the time a new drug is introduced in clinical practice, since between 5 and 10 years will elapse between its synthesis, the initiation of development, and its being made commercially available, and the situation may change rapidly. The first indications heralding changes in the activity of an antibacterial agent against one or more bacterial species must be detected as early as possible. There are always precursor signs. The best example is the reduction in susceptibility of *N. gonorrhoeae* to fluoroquinolones (Knapp et al., 1994; Putnam et al., 1992). Older studies had shown a reduction in the activity of fluoroquinolones against β-lactamase-producing strains.

A reduction in the activity of cefuroxime and other cephalosporins (Table 17) has recently been demonstrated against ampicillin-resistant and non-β-lactamase-producing strains (James et al., 1993).

There is a high risk of emergence of strains resistant to fluoroquinolones among the extended-broad-spectrum-β-lactamase-producing *Enterobacteriaceae* (TEM-3, SHV enzymes, etc.) because a change in killing kinetics has been demonstrated with ciprofloxacin, which occurs after 6 h after contact instead of after 2 h with the non-enzyme-producing strains.

Strains of *S. pneumoniae* resistant to fluoroquinolones have been reported in clinical studies (Garau and Vercken, 1994), but of rare occurrence with a potential risk of dissemination of these strains.

Regular monitoring of the activity of cephalosporins should allow any gradual increase in the MICs to be detected, even if they remain within the therapeutic range. This epidemiological surveillance is difficult to implement and oversee, as it involves a colossal amount of work. In theory, a certain number of laboratory studies should be initiated, but the most realistic surveillance will occur through scientific publications and studies undertaken under the aegis of learned societies, such as those of the European Society of Clinical Microbiology and Infectious Diseases.

12. ADDITIONAL STUDIES

When a new antibacterial agent is introduced in clinical practice, its activity must be tested against strains isolated by clinical microbiology laboratories. The minimum requirement is an antibiotic sensitivity test.

The dissolution process of a new compound needs to be optimized at the beginning of the compound's development to avoid precipitates and false results; as an example, it was shown that glacial acetic acid is one possible and good approach to dissolve macrolides and ketolides (Barry et al., 2004) (Table 18).

However, semiautomatic devices related to the antibiotic sensitivity test are used by some microbiology laboratories. Examples include the Phoenix, MicroScan, and Vitek systems or API strips. The last two methods are unsatisfactory because they are rigid and it is impossible to incorporate a new molecule, in addition to which this choice is made on a discretionary, and not a scientific, basis by the companies manufacturing them.

Other techniques, such as the E-test strips, allow routine determination of MICs in the laboratory. However, their use requires a certain experience, particularly for exigent bacterial species, such as *S. pneumoniae*. It has been noted that for some bacteria and antibacterials the correlation with standard methods is unsatisfactory.

All of these studies should be instituted at the end of development in order for these tests to be ready for the introduction in clinical practice of the new drug.

A correlation between population distribution obtained in clinical trials and those obtained in preclinical studies, as well in epidemiological surveys, has to be done in order to validate the bacterial population collected during these clinical investigations. For example, the level of *H. influenzae* isolates producing β-lactamases or of *S. pneumoniae* isolates resistant to penicillin G and/or erythromycin A has to be of the same magnitude as observed in the epidemiological studies.

Table 18 Performance of telithromycin when microdilution panels were prepared with eight different types of working solutions of telithromycin[a]

Telithromycin solution	Median of 15 MICs (μg/ml)		
	S. pneumoniae ATCC 49619	*S. aureus* ATCC 29213	*H. influenzae* ATCC 49247
Ethanol (9% [vol/vol]) in pH 7.2 buffer			
Water diluent	0.008	0.12	2.0
Buffer diluent	0.008	0.12	1.0
Methanol (9% [vol/vol]) in pH 7.2 buffer			
Water diluent	0.016	0.12	2.0
Buffer diluent	0.016	0.12	1.0
Acetic acid (2.5 ml) in water			
Water diluent	0.008	0.06	1.0
Buffer diluent	0.008	0.06	2.0
DMSO[b] (9% [vol/vol]) in pH 6.5 buffer			
Water diluent	0.008	0.06	1.0
Buffer diluent	0.008	0.06	2.0

[a]Data from Barry et al., 2004.
[b]DMSO, dimethyl sulfoxide.

13. BREAKPOINT DETERMINATIONS

The first step in determining the breakpoints is to determine the load of the test disk and the stability of the drug substance on the paper disk.

Determination of breakpoints is one of the major factors for an antibiotic. A regression analysis is conducted, and the antibacterial is tested against strains for which the MICs are low, medium, and high. The minor and major errors are determined. The second step is to prepare a table which includes for each clinical indication and for each bacterial agent the cure rate (success or failure) as well as microbiological results (eradication); a correlation is made between all MICs and clinical features. Breakpoints are given according the success rate and the MIC.

The mechanism of resistance is an important factor for determining breakpoints for given bacteria. The MIC at which these bacterial species are shown to be resistant is the cutoff and can be considered as the concentration under which the strain is considered susceptible.

14. CONCLUSION

Clinical pharmacology has a multifaceted part to play in the area of anti-infective agents. Its principal role is to determine the intrinsic activity of the new molecule and to establish its antibacterial spectrum. Its second role is to determine the activity of the new antibacterial agent in relation to the molecules used in a given pathological condition. The third aspect is the determination of the activity in a given epidemiological context, such as pneumococcal infections due to penicillin G-resistant strains, ampicillin- and tetracycline-resistant shigellosis, oxacillin-resistant staphylococcal infections, vancomycin-resistant enterococcal strains, extended-spectrum-β-lactamase-producing enterobacteria, and multiresistant tubercle bacilli. Finally, a prospective look at new opportunistic bacterial agents, such as *R. equi*, *Leuconostoc*, and *Pediococcus*, is required.

A key task now is to maintain constant epidemiological surveillance of the changes in resistance so as to monitor constantly the activities of the different antibiotics against problem strains.

REFERENCES

Agouridas C, Bonnefoy A, Chantot JF, 1994, Ketolides, a new distinct semi-synthetic class of macrolides: in vitro and in vivo antibacterial activity, 34th Intersci Conf Antimicrob Agents Chemother, abstract F-168.

Akoun G, Bertrand A, Cambarrère I, Constans P, Dumont R, Guibout P, Kamarec J, Marsac J, Robillard M, Sauvaget J, Thibault P, Voisin C, Safran C, 1986, Clinical evaluation of roxithromycin (RU 28965) in the treatment of hospitalized patients with lower respiratory tract infections, in Butzler JP, Kobayashi H, ed, Macrolides: a Review with an Outlook on Future Development, Excerpta Medica, p 95–99.

Allen JL, Sprunt K, 1978, Discrepancy between minimum inhibitory and minimum bactericidal concentrations of penicillin for group A and group B β-hemolytic streptococci, J Pediatr, 93, 69–71.

Baquero F, 1990, European standards for antibiotic susceptibility testing: towards a theoretical consensus, Eur J Clin Microbiol Infect Dis, 9, 492–495.

Barrière JC, Bouanchaud DH, Desnottes JF, Paris JM, 1994, Streptogramin analogues, Expert Opin Investig Drugs, 32, 115–131.

Barry A, Bryskier A, Traczewski M, Brown S, 2004, Preparation of stock solutions of macrolide and ketolide compounds for antimicrobial susceptibility tests, Clin Microbiol Infect, 10, 78–83.

Bauer AW, Kirby WMM, Sherris JC, Turck M, 1966, Antibiotic susceptibility testing by a standardized single disc method, Am J Clin Pathol, 45, 493–496.

Beam TR Jr, Gilbert DN, Kunin CM, 1993, European guidelines for anti-infective drug products. Introduction, Clin Infect Dis, 17, 787–788.

British Society for Antimicrobial Chemotherapy, 1991, A guide to sensitivity testing, J Antimicrob Chemother, 27, suppl D, 1–47.

Bryskier A, 1993, Fluoroquinolones: mechanisms of action and resistance, Int J Antimicrob Chemother, 2, 151–184.

Bryskier A, Veyssier P, Kazmierczak A, 1994, Fluoroquinolones, propriétés physico chimiques et microbiologiques, Encyclopédie médico-chirurgicales-maladies infectieuses, 8-004-B-10.

Chabbert YA, 1982, Sensibilité bactérienne aux antibiotiques, in Le Minor L, Veron M, ed, Bactériologie médicale, Flammarion, Paris, p 204–212.

Chantot JF, Bryskier A, 1985, Antibacterial activity of ofloxacin and other 4-quinolone derivatives: in vitro and in vivo comparison, J Antimicrob Chemother, 16, 475–484.

Chantot J-F, Bryskier A, Gasc J-C, 1986, Antibacterial activity of roxithromycin: a laboratory evaluation, J Antibiot, 39, 660–668.

Cooper GL, Louie A, Baltch AL, Chu RC, Smith RP, Ritz WJ, Michelsen P, 1993, Influence of zinc on *Pseudomonas aeruginosa* susceptibilities to imipenem, J Clin Microbiol, 31, 2366–2370.

De Cross AJ, Marschall BJ, McCallum RW, Hoffman SR, Barrett LJ, Guerrant RL, 1993, Metronidazole susceptibility testing for *Helicobacter pylori*: comparison of disk, broth, and agar dilution methods and their clinical relevance, J Clin Microbiol, 31, 1971–1974.

Deutsche Institut für Normung, 1984, Methoden zur Empfindlichkeitsprüfung von Bakteriellen Krankenheitseregern (ausser Mycobacterien) gegen Chemotherapeutika, DIN 58940.

Dickinson JM, Mitchison DA, 1990, *In vitro* activities against mycobacteria of two long-acting rifamycins, FCE 22807 and CGP 40/469 A (SPA-S-565), Tubercle, 71, 109–115.

Doern GV, 1992, *In vitro* susceptibility testing of *Haemophilus influenzae*: review of new National Committee for Clinical Laboratory Standards recommendations, J Clin Microbiol, 30, 3035–3038.

Dublanchet A, Caillou J, Emond JP, Chardon H, Drugeon HB, 1986, Isolation of *Bacteroides* strains with reduced susceptibility to 5-nitroimidazole, Eur J Clin Microbiol, 5, 346–347.

Eagle H, Fleishman R, Musselman AD, 1950, Effect of schedule of administration on the therapeutic efficacy of penicillin, Am J Med, 9, 280–289.

Edlund C, Nord CE, 1993, Ecological impact of antimicrobial agents on human intestinal microflora, Alpa Adria Microbiol J, 3, 137–164.

Ellner PD, Neu HC, 1981, The inhibitory quotient: a method for interpreting minimum inhibitory concentration data, J Am Med Assoc, 246, 1575–1578.

Eng RHK, Cherubin C, Smith SM, Buccini F, 1985, Inoculum effect of beta-lactam antibiotics on *Enterobacteriaceae*, Antimicrob Agents Chemother, 28, 601–606.

Ericsson HM, Sherris JC, 1971, Antibiotic sensitivity testing—report of an international collaborative study, Acta Pathol Microbiol Immunol Scand Sect B, 217, suppl 217, 1–90.

Erwin ME, Jones RN, 1993, Roxithromycin in vitro susceptibility testing of *Haemophilus influenzae* by NCCLS methods, J Antimicrob Chemother, 32, 652–654.

Farrell DJ, Felmingham D, 2004, Activities of telithromycin against 13,874 *Streptococcus pneumoniae* isolates collected between 1999 and 2003, Antimicrob Agents Chemother, 48, 1882–1884.

Felmingham D, Robbins MJ, Marais R, Ridgway GL, Grüneberg RN, 1987, The effect of carbon dioxide on the in vitro activity of erythromycin and RU 28965 against anaerobic bacteria, Drugs Exp Clin Res, 13, 195–199.

Felmingham D, Solomonides K, O'Hare MD, Wilson APR, Grüneberg RN, 1987, The effect of medium and inoculum on the activity of vancomycin and teicoplanin against coagulase-negative staphylococci, J Antimicrob Chemother, 20, 609–619.

Forrest A, Nix DE, Ballow CH, Goss TF, Birmingham MC, Schentag JJ, 1993, Pharmacodynamics of intravenous ciprofloxacin in seriously ill patients, Antimicrob Agents Chemother, 37, 1073–1081.

Foster JK, Lentino JR, Strodtman R, DiVincenzo C, 1986, Comparison of in vitro activity of quinolone antibiotics and vancomycin against gentamicin- and methicillin-resistant *Staphylococcus aureus* by time-kill kinetic studies, Antimicrob Agents Chemother, 30, 823–827.

Frémaux A, Sissia G, Rosembaum M, Geslin P, 1992, In vitro activity of cefpirome (HR 810), a new parenteral cephalosporin, against penicillin-susceptible and resistant pnemococci, 32nd Intersci Conf Antimicrob Agents Chemother, abstract 102.

Garau J, Vercken JB, 1994, Efficacy of sparfloxacin in the treatment of 312 cases of pneumococcal community-acquired pneumonia: a pool data analysis, 5th Int Symp New Quinolones.

Gasc J-C, Gouin d'Ambriere S, Lutz A, Chantot J-F, 1991, New ether oxime derivative of erythromycin A. A structure activity relationship study, J Antibiot, 44, 651–668.

Goessens WHF, 1990, Basic mechanisms of bacterial tolerance of antimicrobial agents, Eur J Clin Microbiol Infect Dis, 9, 9–12.

Graig W, 1990, Pharmacodynamics of antimicrobial agents as a basis for determining dosage regimens, Eur J Clin Microbiol Infect Dis, 9, 6–8.

Greub G, Raoult D, 2002, Parachlamydiaceae: potential emerging pathogens, Emerg Infect Dis, 8, 625–630.

Hammerschlag MR, 1994, Antimicrobial susceptibility and therapy of infections caused by *Chlamydia pneumoniae*, Antimicrob Agents Chemother, 38, 1873–1878.

Jabès D, Rossi R, Della Bruna C, Perrone E, Alpegiani M, Andreini BP, Visenti G, Zarini F, Francheschi G, 1993, Activity of new penems against defined MRSA strains, Bioorg Med Chem Lett, 3, 2165–2170.

James PA, Hossain FK, Lewis DA, White DG, 1993, β-Lactam susceptibility of *Haemophilus influenzae* strains showing reduced susceptibility to cefuroxime, J Antimicrob Chemother, 32, 239–246.

Jarlier V, Nicolas MH, Fournier G, Phillipon A, 1988, Extended broad-spectrum β-lactamases conferring transferable resistance to newer β-lactam antibiotics in Enterobacteriaceae: hospital prevalence and susceptibility pattern, Rev Infect Dis, 10, 867–878.

Jones RN, Barry AL, Thornsberry C, 1982, Antimicrobial activity of desacetylcefotaxime alone and in combination with cefotaxime: evidence of synergy, Rev Infect Dis, 4, suppl, S366–S373.

Jones RN, Doern GV, Gerlach HE, Hindler J, Erwin ME, 1994, Validation of NCCLS macrolide (azithromycin, clarithromycin, and erythromycin) interpretive criteria for *Haemophilus influenzae* tested with the Haemophilus Test Medium, Diagn Microbiol Infect Dis, 18, 243–249.

Kabir I, Butler T, Khanam A, 1986, Comparative efficacies of single intravenous doses of ceftriaxone and ampicillin for shigellosis in a placebo-controlled trial, Antimicrob Agents Chemother, 29, 645–648.

Kahlmeter G, Brown D, Goldstein F, MacGowan AP, Mouton JW, Osterlund A, Rodolf A, Steinback M, Urbaskova P, Vatopoulos A, 2003, European harmonization of MIC breakpoints for antimicrobial susceptibility testing of bacteria, J Antimicrob Chemother, 52, 145–148.

Kenny GE, Cartwright FD, 1993, Effect of pH, inoculum size, and incubation time on the susceptibility of *Ureaplasma urealyticum* to erythromycin in vitro, Clin Infect Dis, 17, suppl 1, S215–S218.

Kenny GE, Cartwright FD, Roberts MC, 1986, Agar dilution method for determination of antibiotic susceptibility of *Ureaplasma urealyticum*, Pediatr Infect Dis J, 6, suppl 5, S332–S334.

Kilian M, 1976, A taxonomic study of the genus *Haemophilus* with the proposal of a new species, J Gen Microbiol, 93, 9–62.

King A, Phillips I, 1993, Standardization of Iso-Sensitest agar, J Antimicrob Chemother, 32, 339.

Klugman KP, Saunders J, 1994, *In vitro* susceptibility of penicillin-susceptible and penicillin-resistant pneumococci to parenteral third and fourth generation cephalosporins, 6th Int Congr Infect Dis.

Knapp JS, Washington JA, Doyle LJ, Neul SW, Parekh MC, Rice RJ, 1994, Persistence of *Neisseria gonorrhoeae* strains with decreased susceptibilities to ciprofloxacin and ofloxacin in Cleveland, Ohio, from 1992 through 1993, Antimicrob Agents Chemother, 38, 2194–2196.

La Scola B, Boyadjiev I, Greub G, Khamis A, Martin C, Raoult D, 2003, Amoeba-resisting bacteria and ventilator-associated pneumonia, Emerg Infect Dis, 9, 815–821.

La Scola B, Bryskier A, Raoult D, 2004, Comparison of the in vitro efficacy of telithromycin (HMR 3647) and levofloxacin with 22 antibiotic compounds against Bosea and Afipia species, J Antimicrob Chemother, 53, 683–685.

Lee BL, Sachdeva M, Chambers HF, 1991, Effect of protein binding of daptomycin on MIC and antibacterial activity, Antimicrob Agents Chemother, 35, 2505–2508.

Loleka S, Vibulbandhikit S, Poouyarit P, 1991, Response to antimicrobial therapy for shigellosis in Thailand, Rev Infect Dis, 13, suppl 4, S42–S46.

Lukehart SA, Fohn MJ, Baker-Zander SA, 1990, Efficacy of azithromycin for therapy of active syphilis in the rabbit model, J Antimicrob Chemother, 25, suppl A, 91–99.

Marrie TJ, Durant H, Yates L, 1984, Community-acquired pneumonia requiring hospitalization: 5 years prospective study, Rev Infect Dis, 11, 586–599.

Miller GH, Aminoglycoside Resistance Study Group, 1994, Resistance to aminoglycosides in *Pseudomonas*, Trends Microbiol, 2, 347–352.

Moore RD, Smith CR, Lietman PS, 1984a, The association of aminoglycoside plasma levels with mortality in patients with gram-negative bacteria, J Infect Dis, 149, 443–448.

Moore RD, Smith CR, Lietman PS, 1984b, Association of aminoglycoside plasma levels with therapeutic outcome in gram-negative pneumonia, Am J Med, 77, 657–662.

National Committee for Clinical Laboratory Standards, 1993, Development of *in vitro* susceptibility testing criteria and quality control parameters—tentative guideline, document M23-T, NCCLS, Villanova, Pa.

Nickolai DJ, Lammel CJ, Byford BA, Morris JH, Kaplan EB, Hadley WK, Brooks GF, 1985, Effects of storage temperature and pH on the stability of eleven β-lactam antibiotics in MIC trays, J Clin Microbiol, 21, 366–370.

Peloux I, Le Noc P, Bryskier A, Le Noc D, 1994, In vitro activity of cefpirome and five other cephems against enteric pathogens, 34th Intersci Conf Antimicrob Agents Chemother, abstract E-28.

Periti P, Sueri L, Tosi M, Ciammarughi R, Cadco P, Milanesi B, 1984, Cefotaxime in the cerebral fluid and serum in patients with purulent meningitis, J Antimicrob Chemother, 14, suppl B, 117–123.

Péter O, Bretz AG, 1992, Polymorphism of outer surface proteins of *Borrelia burgdorferi* as a tool for classification, Zentbl Bakteriol, 277, 28–33.

Péter O, Bretz AG, 1994, *In vitro* susceptibility of *Borrelia burgdorferi*, *Borrelia garinii* and *Borrelia afzelii* to 7 antimicrobial agents, in Cevenini R, Sambri V, La Placa M, ed, Advances in Lyme Borreliosis Research, p 167–170.

Philipon A, Arlet G, Lagrange PH, 1994, Origin and impact of plasmid-mediated extended-spectrum beta-lactamases, Eur J Clin Microbiol Infect Dis, 13, suppl 1, 17–29.

Putnam SD, Lavin BS, Stone JR, Oldfield III EC, Hooper DG, 1992, Evaluation of the standardized disk diffusion and agar dilution antibiotic susceptibility test methods by using strains of *Neisseria gonorrhoeae* from the United States and Southeast Asia, J Clin Microbiol, 30, 974–980.

Raoult D, Birg ML, La Scola B, et al, 2000, Cultivation of the bacillus of Whipple disease, N Engl J Med, 342, 620–625.

Saez-Nieto JA, Vasquez JA, Marcos C, 1990, Meningococci moderately resistant to penicillin, Lancet, 336, 54.

Sahm DF, Baker CN, Jones RN, Thornsberry C, 1984, Influence of growth medium on the in vitro activities of second- and third-generation cephalosporins against *Streptococcus faecalis*, Antimicrob Agents Chemother, 20, 561–567.

Schentag J, 1991, Correlation of pharmacokinetic parameters to efficacy of antibiotics: relationships between serum concentrations, MIC values and bacterial eradication in patients with Gram-negative pneumonia, Scand J Infect Dis, suppl 74, 218–234.

Siebor E, Kazmierczak A, 1993, Factors influencing the activity of macrolide antibiotics *in vitro*, in Bryskier AJ, Butzler J-P, Neu HC, Tulkens PM, ed, Macrolides, Chemistry, Pharmacology and Clinical Use, Blackwell-Arnette, Paris, p 197–203.

Simpson IN, Hunter R, Govan JRW, Nelson JW, 1993, Do all *Pseudomonas cepacia* produce carbapenemases? J Antimicrob Chemother, 32, 339–341.

Smith JT, Levin CS, 1988, Chemistry and mechanisms of action of the quinolone antibacterials, in Andriole VT, ed, The Quinolones, Academic Press, p 23–82.

Snell JJS, George RC, Perry SF, Erdman YJ, 1988, Antimicrobial susceptibility testing of *Streptococcus pneumoniae*: quality assessment results, J Clin Pathol, 41, 384–387.

Soussy CJ, Cluzel R, Courvalin P, Comité de l'antibiogramme de la société française de microbiologie, 1984, Definition and determination of *in vitro* antibiotic susceptibility breakpoints for bacteria in France, Eur J Clin Microbiol Infect Dis, 13, 238–246.

Stamm LV, Stapleton JT, Bassford PJ, 1988, In vitro assay to demonstrate high-level erythromycin resistance of a clinical isolate of *Treponema pallidum*, Antimicrob Agents Chemother, 32, 164–169.

Stokes EJ, 1955, Antibacterial drugs, in Clinical Bacteriology, Edward Arnold, London, p 157–192.

Stokes EJ, Ridgway GL, Wren MWD, 1993, Clinical Microbiology, 7th ed, Edward Arnold, London, p 234–278.

Swedish Reference Group for Antibiotics, 1981, A revised system for antibiotic sensitivity testing, Scand J Infect Dis, 13, 148–152.

Täuber MG, Kunz S, Zak O, Sande MA, 1989, Influence of antibiotic dose, dosing interval, and duration of therapy on outcome in experimental pneumococcal meningitis in rabbits, Antimicrob Agents Chemother, 33, 418–423.

Täuber MG, Zak O, Scheld WM, Hengsler B, Sande MA, 1984, The postantibiotic effect in the treatment of experimental meningitis caused by *Streptococcus pneumoniae* in rabbits, J Infect Dis, 149, 575–583.

Tomasz A, Nachman S, Leaf H, 1991, Stable classes of phenotypic expression in methicillin-resistant clinical isolates of staphylococci, Antimicrob Agents Chemother, 35, 124–129.

Verdon MS, Handsfield HH, Johnson RB, 1994, Pilot study of azithromycin for treatment of primary and secondary syphilis, Clin Infect Dis, 19, 486–488.

Vogelman BS, Craig WA, 1985, Postantibiotic effects, J Antimicrob Chemother, 15, suppl A, 37–46.

Wallace RJ, Steele LC, 1988, Susceptibility testing of *Nocardia* species for the clinical laboratory, Diagn Microbiol Infect Dis, 9, 155–166.

Werkgroep Richtlijnen Govoeligheidsbepalingen, 1981, Report, Standaardisatie van govoeligheidsbepalingen, Werkgroep Richtlijnen Govoeligheidsbepalingen, Bilthoven, The Netherlands.

White RL, Kays MB, Friederich LV, Brown EW, Koonce JR, 1991, Pseudoresistance of *Pseudomonas aeruginosa* resulting from degradation of imipenem in an automated susceptibility testing system with predried panels, J Clin Microbiol, 29, 398–400.

Wilkins TD, Chalgren S, 1976, Medium for use in antibiotic susceptibility testing of anaerobic bacteria, Antimicrob Agents Chemother, 10, 926–928.

Williams JD, 1990, Prospects for standardisation of methods and guidelines for disc susceptibility testing, Eur J Clin Microbiol Infect Dis, 9, 496–501.

Xia H, Keane CT, Beattie S, O'Morain CA, 1994, Standardization of disk diffusion and its clinical significance for susceptibility testing of metronidazole against *Helicobacter pylori*, Antimicrob Agents Chemother, 38, 2357–2361.

Yabuuchi E, Kosako Y, Oyaizu H, Yano I, Hotta H, Hashimoto Y, et al, 1992, Proposal of *Burkholderia* gen. nov. and transfer of seven species of the genus *Pseudomonas* homology group II to the new genus with the type species *Burkholderia cepacia* (Palirini and Holmes, 1981) comb. nov. 1992, Microbiol Immunol, 36, 1251–1275.

Zak O, O'Reilly T, 1990, Animal models as predictors of the safety and efficacy of antibiotics, Eur J Clin Microbiol Infect Dis, 9, 472–478.

Penicillins

A. BRYSKIER

1. INTRODUCTION

The discovery by Alexander Fleming in 1928 of the antibacterial activity engendered by *Penicillium notatum* represented an extraordinary event in the study of infectious diseases because it enabled a number of nosocomial and community-acquired infections to be treated, particularly those due to gram-positive cocci. It transformed not only medicine but also the socioeconomic events of the second half of the 20th century.

This discovery passed unnoticed until 1940, when Howard Florey and Ernst Chain started to work on this fungal metabolite.

The second major event in the study of infectious diseases was the identification of metabolites with antibacterial activity in a culture filtrate of *Cephalosporium acremonium*. Among these metabolites, penicillin N (now known as adicillin) was the origin of the group A penicillins. The development of penicillins and cephalosporins occurred in parallel and with the same aim in mind. In 1941, the curative effect of penicillin G was demonstrated in murine experimental infections and very shortly afterwards in humans. The selection of a strain of *Penicillium chryseogenum* and the addition of phenylacetic acid to the culture medium yielded a large quantity of penicillin G.

The instability of penicillin G in an acidic medium was partially circumvented by the preparation of the phenoxypenicillins. The rapid emergence of strains of *Staphylococcus aureus* resistant to penicillin G as a result of the production of penicillinases led to research into molecules that were stable against enzymatic hydrolysis. Research was conducted simultaneously in the areas of penicillins and cephalosporins, culminating in the semisynthesis of the group M penicillins and the first cephalosporins.

Penicillin N, which possesses an α-aminoadipic chain, was the starting point for the production of the α-aminopenicillins, the first molecule of which was ampicillin. New semisyntheses became possible in 1957 with the isolation of the 6-aminopenicillanic nucleus.

The preparation of semisynthetic penicillins yielded molecules that were more active against gram-negative bacilli, particularly *Pseudomonas aeruginosa*, such as the α-carboxypenicillins, the *N*-acylpenicillins, and the α-sulfopenicillins.

2. CLASSIFICATION OF PENICILLINS

Penicillins belong to the family of β-lactams. They are composed of three parts: a thiazolidine nucleus attached to a β-lactam ring and a side chain at position C-6 by which they can be distinguished.

They are grouped within the class of penams, which includes penicillins (dihydrothiazine nucleus), oxa-1-penams, and carbapenams.

The penicillins differ according to the side chain attached at position 6 of the penam nucleus. The following groups are distinguished: penicillin G (group I), penicillin M (group II), penicillin A (group III), 6-α-substituted penicillins (group IV), α-carboxy- and α-sulfopenicillins (group V), amidinopenicillins (group VI), and oxyiminopenicillins (group VII) (Fig. 1).

3. MECHANISM OF ACTION OF PENICILLINS

The penicillins act on peptidoglycan synthesis, causing lysis and cell death. They inhibit one of the stages necessary for the cross-linking of peptidoglycan, transpeptidation, because of the stereochemical similarity between the penicillin molecule and the D-Ala–D-Ala dipeptide. These enzymes are localized in the outer region of the cytoplasmic membrane: penicillin-binding protein (PBP).

The first factor essential to the action of penicillins, particularly in gram-negative bacilli, is their ability to penetrate the walls of these bacteria.

4. RESISTANCE MECHANISMS

Bacteria may become resistant through the production of β-lactamases, enzymes that can be released in the external medium in the case of gram-positive cocci or in the periplasmic space in the case of gram-negative bacteria. Reduction in parietal permeability and a modification in the target (PBP) have been described for various bacterial species or genera (e.g., *S. aureus* and *Streptococcus pneumoniae*).

5. GROUP I: PENICILLIN G AND DERIVATIVES

The original substance known as penicillin was a mixture of several molecules: penicillins F, K, X, and G (Fig. 2). Penicillin

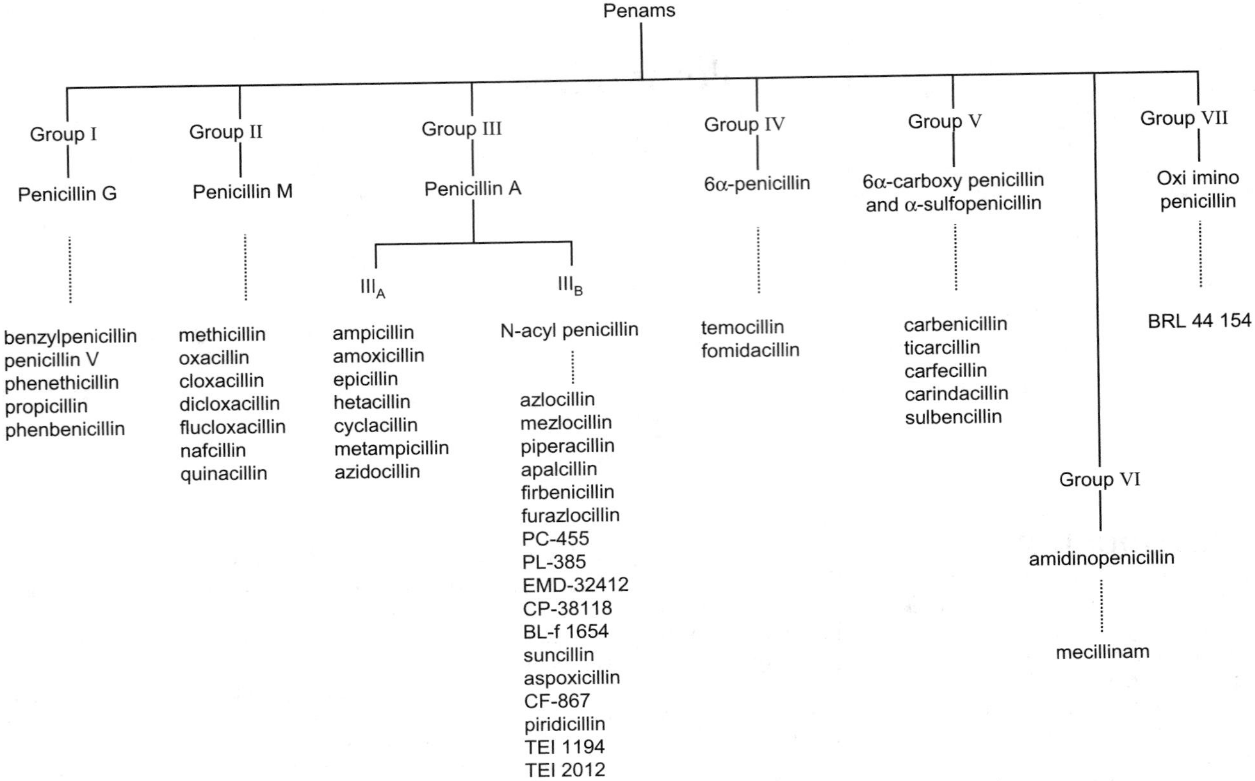

Figure 1 Classification of the penams

G was the most active molecule and has been developed and used therapeutically for more than half a century.

An acetamidobenzyl group is attached to the carbon at position 6 of the azetidinone ring (benzylpenicillin). The instability in an acidic medium means that these molecules are poorly absorbed orally.

The introduction of a polar group on the side chain, such as an oxygen atom (phenoxypenicillin) or a sulfur atom, increases the stability in an acidic medium without altering the antibacterial activity (Table 1). The presence of an electrophilic group in the α position appears to interfere with the electron displacement that inactivates benzylpenicillin. In the case of the phenoxypenicillins, the rule appears to be the higher the molecular weight, the better the intestinal absorption. It is for this reason that different groups have been added to the asymmetrical α carbon: methyl (phenethicillin), ethyl (propicillin), and benzene (fenbenicillin) (Fig. 3).

5.1. Physicochemical Properties

The sodium or potassium salts of penicillin G are soluble in water. One milligram of penicillin G is equivalent to 1,670 U and 1 mg of penicillin V is equal to 1,696 U. Penicillin G and its derivatives are insoluble in chloroform, acetone, and ether. The sodium content of penicillin G is 2.8 mEq/g, and the potassium content 2.6 mEq/g.

The degradation half-life is dependent on the substituent on the carbon in the α position. In an ethanol-water solution (50/50, vol/vol) of pH 1.3 at 35°C, the degradation half-lives are as follows: benzylpenicillin, 3.5 min; α-O-methyl benzylpenicillin, 77 min; phenoxymethylpenicillin, 160 min; α-Cl-benzylpenicillin, 300 min; and α-NH_3^+-benzylpenicillin, 600 min.

The principal physicochemical properties are summarized in Table 1.

5.2. Antibacterial Activity

Penicillin G and its derivatives possess an antibacterial spectrum that includes aerobic and anaerobic gram-positive and gram-negative cocci, gram-positive bacilli, such as *Listeria monocytogenes*, *Corynebacterium diphtheriae*, *Bacillus anthracis*, *Actinomyces* spp., and *Clostridium perfringens;* and the following bacteria: *Pasteurella multocida*, *Streptobacillus moniliformis*, *Spirillum minus*, *Erysipelothrix rhusiopathiae*, *Treponema pallidum*, *Leptospira* interrogans serovar Icterohemorrhagiae, *Borrelia recurrensis*, and *Borrelia burgdorferi*. Activity against *Haemophilus influenzae* is very moderate. They are inactive against *Enterobacteriaceae* and nonfermentative gram-negative bacilli (Table 2).

Penicillin G is a bactericidal antibiotic. A phenomenon of tolerance has been described with penicillin G for *S. pneumoniae*, *Streptococcus pyogenes*, *Streptococcus agalactiae*, streptococci of the viridans group, group C streptococci, certain strains of enterococci, *L. monocytogenes*, and lactobacilli.

5.3. Breakpoints

5.3.1. Breakpoints for Penicillin G

Breakpoints for penicillin G against *S. pneumoniae* are listed in Table 3.

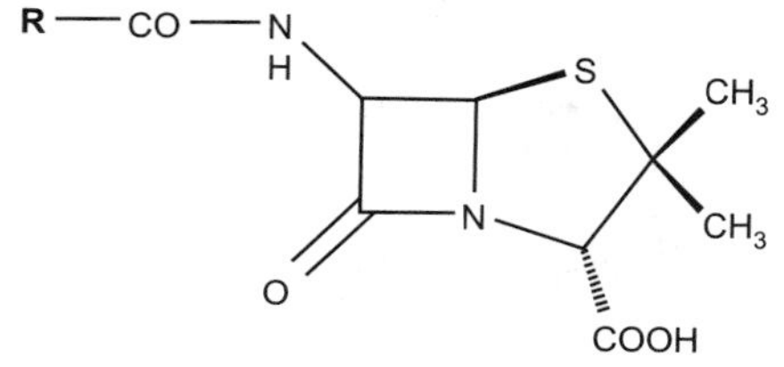

		R
Benzyl	Penicillin G	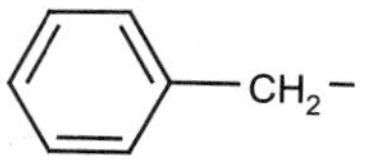 CH_2–
p-hydroxybenzyl	Penicillin X	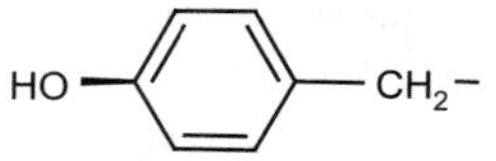 HO CH_2–
2-pentenyl	Penicillin F	CH_3-CH_2-CH=CH-CH_2-
m-amyl	Dihydropenicillin F	CH_3-$(CH_2)_3$-CH_2
n-heptyl	Penicillin K	CH_3-$(CH_2)_5$-CH_2
D-4-amino-4-carboxybutyl	Penicillin N	HOOC-CH(NH_2)-$(CH_2)_2$-

Figure 2 Penicillin produced by *Penicillium*

Table 1 Physicochemical properties of group I penicillins

Drug	Molecular mass (Da)	$t_{1/2}$ degradation (pH 1, 35°C)	pK_a1	$\log_{10} P_u$ n-octanol/water	P_{app} methyl/propanol/water
Penicillin G	334.39	3.5	2.75	1.70	0.501
Penicillin V	350.39	25	2.79	1.95	1.10
Phenethicillin	364.42	16	2.80	2.20	1.55
Propicillin	378.44	13	2.76	2.70	3.02
Fenbenicillin	426.49				
Clometicillin	433.31				

5.3.2. Breakpoints for Cephalosporins

Table 4 shows the breakpoints of cefotaxime and ceftriaxone against *S. pneumoniae* (NCCLS, 1994). The standards listed in the table have been established for strains of *S. pneumoniae* of intermediate susceptibility or resistant to penicillin G.

It is recommended that a 1-μg oxacillin disk be used to detect resistance of a strain of *S. pneumoniae* to penicillin G. A ceftizoxime, cefotetan, or loracarbef disk may be used to detect any reduction in the activity of cefotaxime.

The 1-μg disk is recommended by the NCCLS and the British Society for Antimicrobial Chemotherapy. Since it has become available in France, it has also been recommended there. The 1-μg disk has greater sensitivity, but the use of two disks provides clinical guidance from the outset. Table 5 shows the zones of inhibition of oxacillin.

Attention has recently been drawn to strains classed as resistant to penicillin G in view of the zones of inhibition around the 1-μg oxacillin disk but for which the MIC of penicillin G is in fact ≤0.06 μg/ml. It has been shown that an abnormal gene coding for PBP 2x reduces the susceptibility to oxacillin (MIC, ~1.0 μg/ml). It therefore seems possible to have an oxacillin-resistant and penicillin-susceptible strain. It is recommended that caution be exercised and that the MIC of penicillin G for oxacillin-resistant strains be determined.

5.4. Epidemiology of Resistance to Penicillin G

A number of bacterial species have progressively become resistant to penicillin G, varying in their distribution and incidence according to the center and country.

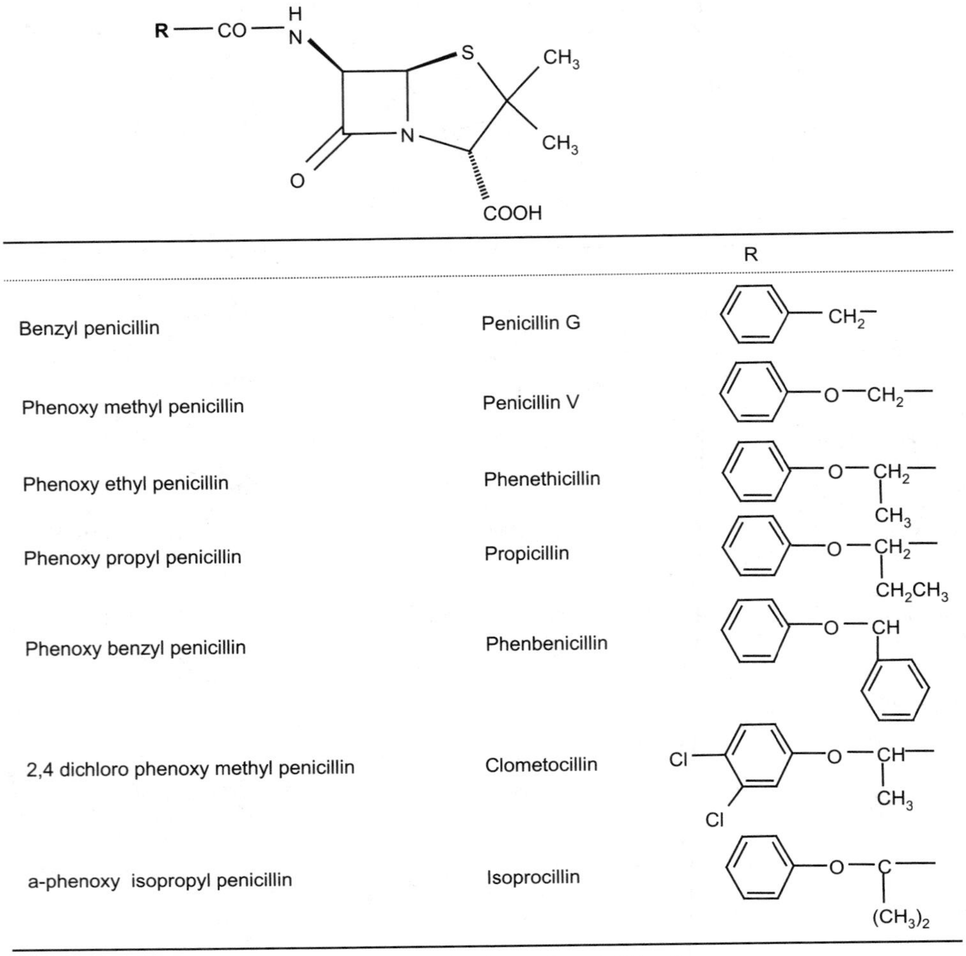

		R
Benzyl penicillin	Penicillin G	C_6H_5—CH_2—
Phenoxy methyl penicillin	Penicillin V	C_6H_5—O—CH_2—
Phenoxy ethyl penicillin	Phenethicillin	C_6H_5—O—CH_2(—CH_3)—
Phenoxy propyl penicillin	Propicillin	C_6H_5—O—CH_2(—CH_2CH_3)—
Phenoxy benzyl penicillin	Phenbenicillin	C_6H_5—O—CH(C_6H_5)—
2,4 dichloro phenoxy methyl penicillin	Clometocillin	$Cl_2C_6H_3$—O—CH(—CH_3)—
a-phenoxy isopropyl penicillin	Isoprocillin	C_6H_5—O—C($(CH_3)_2$)—

Figure 3 Derivatives of penicillin G

Table 2 In vitro activities of the group I penicillins

Organism(s)	MIC (μg/ml)			
	Penicillin G	Penicillin V	Phenethicillin	Propicillin
S. aureus Pen[s]	0.03	0.06	0.06	0.06
S. aureus Pen[r]	>128	>128	>128	>128
S. pyogenes	0.01	0.03	0.06	0.03
S. pneumoniae	0.01	0.03	0.06	0.03
Streptococcus bovis	0.12	0.12		0.5
E. faecalis	2	4	4	4
C. diphtheriae	0.2			
B. anthracis	0.01			
C. perfringens	0.06	0.1	0.1	
N. meningitidis	0.03	0.06	0.12	2
N. gonorrhoeae Pen[s]	0.03	0.12	0.12	0.12
N. gonorrhoeae Pen[r]	>16	>16	>16	>16
H. influenzae Amp[s]	1	4	4	4
E. coli	>128	>128	>128	>128
K. pneumoniae	>128	>128	>128	>128
S. enterica serovar Typhi	8.0	>128	>128	>128
Shigella spp.	64	>128	>128	>128
P. multocida	2	4		8

Table 3 Standards of the French Antibiotic Sensitivity Test Committee (1997)[a]

Organism(s)	Penicillin G (6 μg)					
	MIC (μg/ml)			Zone diam (mm)		
	S	I	R	S	I	R
All bacteria	≤0.25		16	≥29		<8
S. pneumoniae	≤0.12	0.12–1	≥2			

[a]S, susceptible; I, intermediate; R, resistant.

Table 4 Breakpoints of cefotaxime and ceftriaxone against *S. pneumoniae*

Drugs	MIC (μg/ml)		
	Susceptible	Intermediate	Resistant
Cefotaxime and ceftriaxone	≤0.25	0.5–1	≥2

Table 5 Zones of inhibition of oxacillin

Oxacillin disk	Zone diam (mm)	
	Susceptible	Resistant
1 μg	≥19	≤10
5 μg	≥25	≤13

5.4.1. *S. aureus*

The first strains of penicillin G-resistant *S. aureus* were isolated soon after the introduction of penicillin G into London, England, hospitals. At present, almost 80% of intra- and extrahospital strains are resistant to penicillin G, this resistance being due to a plasmid-mediated penicillinase. Interplasmid transfer occurs by transduction. Four types, A, B, C, and D, have been described. These enzymes differ in amino acid composition. These are extracellular enzymes, hydrolyzing group I penicillins, certain *N*-acylpenicillins, cephaloridine, and cefazolin.

5.4.2. *Neisseria gonorrhoeae*

Penicillin G used to be the reference drug in the treatment of gonococcal urethritis. Its use was called into question, however, in the mid-1970s with the emergence of resistant strains, particularly in Southeast Asia. Resistance to penicillin G is mediated via a plasmid carrying the gene coding for production of the broad-spectrum enzyme TEM-1.

5.4.3. *Neisseria meningitidis*

Many publications have reported a reduction in the susceptibility of *N. meningitidis* to penicillin G. This has been described in South Africa, Spain, the United Kingdom, France, and the United States, as well as in other countries.

5.4.4. *S. pneumoniae*

For the last 10 years, the number of strains of *S. pneumoniae* resistant to penicillin G has been constantly on the increase. These strains are found in a number of countries, such as Spain, France, Hungary, Iceland, South Africa, the United States, and numerous countries of the Middle East, Latin America, and Asia; in the other countries, the incidence is variable (United Kingdom, Belgium, and Germany).

5.4.4.1. Definition of Thresholds of Sensitivity

The thresholds of sensitivity are as follows: a strain is said to be susceptible to penicillin G if the MICs are ≤0.1 μg/ml, intermediate if the MICs are between 0.1 and 1.0 μg/ml, and resistant if the MICs are ≥2.0 μg/ml. A strain is said to be multiresistant when three antibiotics are inactive. This principally involves penicillin G, erythromycin A, cyclines, chloramphenicol, and co-trimoxazole. In vitro, penicillin G-resistant strains can be detected using 1-μg oxacillin disks.

5.4.4.2. Epidemiology of Resistance

Penicillin G-resistant strains have been known since the experimental studies by Erikson in 1945. However, the first strains of reduced susceptibility to penicillin G (MICs, 0.1 and 0.2 μg/ml) were not isolated until 20 years later by Kislak. In 1967, Hansman et al. in Australia drew attention to the potential therapeutic problem of pneumococcal strains of reduced susceptibility to penicillin G. They had isolated a strain from a hypogammaglobulinemic patient for which penicillin G had a MIC of 0.6 μg/ml. From 1970 onwards, penicillin G-resistant isolates were described in New Guinea and Australia. In New Guinea, the proportion of resistant strains increased progressively from 12% in 1970 to 33% in 1980.

Since 1974, there have been publications reporting patients suffering from pneumococcal meningitis due to penicillin G-resistant strains. In 1977, the first strains resistant to penicillin G (MICs, 4.0 to 8.0 μg/ml) and chloramphenicol were described in Durban, South Africa. In Europe, there are four main foci of resistance: Spain, Hungary, France, and Iceland.

In Spain, the incidence of penicillin G-resistant strains of *S. pneumoniae* increased from 6% in 1979 to 44% in 1989. An increase of the same amplitude has been found in France. The incidence of resistance was 0.3% from 1980 to 1986 and 5.3% from 1987 to 1989, increasing to 12.5% in 1990 and bordering on 30% from 1992 to 1993. In Hungary, the incidence of resistance has reached 50%. In Romania, it has attained 25% of clinical isolates in one center. In 1975, an epidemiological study revealed that almost 27% of strains isolated in Poland were penicillin resistant. In 1988, no strain of *S. pneumoniae* in Iceland was resistant to penicillin. In 1989, 2.3% of isolated strains exhibited reduced susceptibility, and the proportion of resistant strains has increased progressively since then: 2.7, 8.4, and 19% in 1990, 1991, and 1992, respectively. In Germany, the incidence of strains of reduced susceptibility was 6% at the end of the 1990s. In Belgium, the incidence was 1.5% between 1983 and 1988. In Switzerland, approximately 2.3% of isolates had reduced susceptibility to penicillin G in 1985. In Latin America, the first strains of abnormal susceptibility were isolated in 1987 in Chile and subsequently in Brazil, Argentina, and Venezuela. In Canada and Australia, the incidence on these strains is on the order of 1 to 2%. In the Middle East and Near East, the incidence varies from country to country. It is high in Israel, in some regions affecting 30% of isolates. A recent study in Pakistan showed an incidence of resistance of 6 to 14% according to the disease. In Japan, the incidence of *S. pneumoniae* isolates resistant to penicillin G was less than 1% between 1974 and 1982, but it increased from 5.9 to 27.8% between 1984 and 1991. Strains of abnormal susceptibility have also been described in Malaysia and Bangladesh. The incidence of resistance for the time being is more difficult to assess in the other countries in Asia. Outside South Africa and Rwanda (~21%), isolates of abnormal susceptibility have been described in Nigeria, Kenya, Zambia, and certain west African countries. In Italy, strains of *S. pneumoniae* susceptible to penicillin but resistant to erythromycin A have been described.

5.4.4.3. Resistance and Site of Infection

S. pneumoniae represents about 5.4% of strains isolated from blood cultures in France. It is responsible for about 12 to 18% of cases of purulent meningitis of bacterial origin. Its incidence will increase with the use of anti-*H. influenzae* type B vaccine. It is one of the major pathogenic agents of community-acquired (8 to 75%) or nosocomial (~5 to 7%) parenchymatous respiratory tract infections. The percentage of penicillin G-resistant isolates varies with age, sampling period, geographical location, and site of infection. Different epidemiological studies have shown that the number of penicillin G-resistant strains responsible for middle ear infections is increasing regularly, as are the numbers of strains responsible for pneumonia. Nasopharyngeal carriage of resistant strains is considerable in certain countries, such as Spain, France, South Africa, Israel, and Hungary. It has reached 34% in Alaska.

The most resistant strains are often those isolated from the middle ear exudate. The percentage of resistant strains isolated from the cerebrospinal fluid (CSF) varies with the surveys. Table 6 shows the incidence of penicillin-G resistant pneumococci by sampling site.

In the case of purulent meningitis due to a strain of *S. pneumoniae* resistant or moderately susceptible to penicillin G, treatment is based on the intravenous administration of 300 to 400 mg of cefotaxime per kg of body weight per day or 200 mg of ceftriaxone per kg per day singly or preferably in combination with other antibacterial agents. The objective is to obtain a bactericidal potency in the CSF on the order of 1:8 and in situ concentrations 10 times higher than the MICs or minimum bactericidal concentrations of the antibiotics for the causative strain. When the activity of penicillin G decreases, those of cefotaxime and ceftriaxone decrease also, but not in parallel. Ceftazidime and ceftizoxime are inactive against these strains. When the MIC of cefotaxime is >1.0 μg/ml, the therapeutic alternative is intravenous vancomycin (75 mg/kg/day), with or without intrathecal administration. However, therapeutic failures have been published with vancomycin, probably because of the low concentrations obtained in the CSF.

More than 80 serotypes or serogroups have been described. There is often confusion in the literature according to whether American or Danish nomenclature is used. The serotypes differ in terms of the site of infection. In lower respiratory tract infections of parenchymatous origin, serotypes 1, 14, 7, 3, and 4 are the most common, and they are often isolated from healthy carriers. Serotypes 6, 14, 19, and 23 are most often responsible for upper respiratory tract infections, and they are isolated with great frequency from the nasopharyngeal floras of young children.

5.4.4.4. Mechanism of Resistance

S. pneumoniae possesses six PBPs with molecular masses ranging from 43 to 100 kDa. PBPs 1a and 1b (100 kDa) and 2a, 2b, and 2x (95 to 78 kDa) are the lethal targets of the β-lactams. PBP 1a appears to have a dual enzymatic activity, transglycolase and transpeptidase. PBPs 2a, 2b, and 2x would appear to be transpeptidases.

PBP 3 is a D-D-carboxypeptidase. The mechanism of resistance of pneumococci to the β-lactams involves not β-lactamase production but modification of the cellular targets constituted by PBPs. The affinity of the β-lactams for PBPs is reduced. Abnormal PBPs are not the products of genes that have undergone point mutations but the result of a series of genetic transformations. The DNA comes from other streptococci, such as viridans group streptococci. The activity of penicillin G against viridans group streptococci is also reduced through a modification in PBP 2a (78 kDa). This PBP is identical to PBP 2b of *S. pneumoniae*, suggesting a lateral transfer of the modified gene of PBP 2b from viridans group streptococci to *S. pneumoniae*. The genes coding for PBPs 1a and 2x are localized on the same locus, whereas the genes for PBPs 2b and 3 are localized in different regions on the chromosome. Cefotaxime does not bind to PBP 2b, inhibition of which is considered crucial in induction of the autolytic system.

The genes coding for PBP 2b are divided into two classes, A and B. The changes in the amino acids occur near the active site, preventing access by the β-lactams. These changes do not directly affect the active site of the PBP; for this reason, the bacterial cells have growth comparable to that of susceptible strains.

Resistant strains have major changes in their peptidoglycan. The mono- and oligomeric peptides linked by Ala-Ser bridges (70% of the peptidoglycan of susceptible *S. pneumoniae*) are replaced by peptides essentially linked by means of Ala-Ala dipeptides in the walls of resistant strains. However, in *S. pneumoniae*, the changes in peptidoglycan synthesis do not appear to be correlated with the preferential inhibition of a PBP but are dependent on the relative number of inhibited or free PBPs.

The different types of remodelling may cause resistance to penicillin G and affect the other β-lactams with a different chemical structure in an unpredictable and unequal way.

Table 6 Proportion of penicillin G-resistant pneumococcal strains by sampling site

Country (year)	% Penicillin G-resistant strains					
	Blood culture	Middle ear fluid	Sputum	Nasopharyngeal sample	Pleural fluid	CSF
France (1990)	2.8	47				4
France (1993)	18.7	14	23			33
France (1993)	6	19	17	19		10
Spain (1992)	23.3		42.2		41.7	17
Hungary (1992)	50		48.3	68.7	54.5	50
South Africa (1992)	13.6					31
Pakistan (1993)	11.1			6.8–14.3		
Israel (1993)	39.1	46.3				39.1
Israel (1993)				24		
United States (1993)				24		

Resistance is due to one or more modifications of the affinity for PBPs 1a, 2a, 2x, and 2b (Varon and Gutmann, 1993).

The PBP 1a (100 kDa), 2x (82 kDa), and 2b (78 kDa) genes are mosaics. PBPs, 1a and 2x are also implicated in resistance to cephalosporins, and their genes are transferable in a single stage to a susceptible strain.

The activities of the different β-lactams against strains of *S. pneumoniae* with different resistance phenotypes are summarized in Table 7.

5.4.5. Anaerobes

With the exception of *Fusobacterium*, acquired resistance to penicillin G is rare in strictly anaerobic bacteria.

5.5. Pharmacokinetics

5.5.1. Benzylpenicillins

Benzylpenicillin is unstable in an acidic medium and is destroyed in the stomach.

After intramuscular administration of 600 mg (1 million units), a peak concentration in serum of 12 μg/ml is reached in 30 min.

At the end of an infusion of 2.0 g, the concentration in plasma is between 2.2 and 17 μg/ml. The apparent elimination half-life is on the order of 0.5 h, but there are very substantial interindividual variations.

The apparent volume of distribution is 33 liters. Renal clearance is 350 ml/min (Table 8).

Plasma protein binding is on the order of 50%. Urinary elimination is 50 to 60% from the end of the first hour and principally involves tubular secretion (90%), with glomerular filtration accounting for only 10% of the eliminated dose. Biliary elimination is weak (0.12%), but depending on the MICs for the microorganisms involved in biliary tract infections, penicillin G may have therapeutic activity.

Repeated doses of 3×10^6 U (1.8 g) every 3 h maintain concentrations in plasma on the order of 20 μg/ml.

In neonates, an intramuscular injection of 25 to 50 mg/kg yields mean peak levels in serum of 25 to 35 μg/ml. In infants, the apparent elimination half-life is 3.2 h during the first week of life and 1.4 h from the third week.

Penicillin G is weakly hemodialyzable, with marked variations (5 to 50%).

In patients with renal insufficiency, the apparent elimination half-life may reach 7 to 10 h.

Levels in plasma are lower in diabetic patients.

The addition of procaine prolongs the elimination half-life to 6.0 h and maintains high levels in plasma.

Penicillin G is distributed in all tissues or serous fluids in the body. Concentrations in colostrum and saliva are low. It does not penetrate noninflamed meninges.

In purulent meningitis, the concentrations attain therapeutic levels relative to the MICs for the causative bacteria.

After a dose of 500,000 U/kg in the neonate, peak concentrations in plasma are reached after 4 h and are on the order of 17.1 ± 6.3 μg/ml (mean ± standard deviation), with residual concentrations at 24 h of 2.1 ± 0.98 μg/ml; in CSF, the peak concentration is 0.7 ± 0.35 μg/ml and is attained after 12 h; the residual concentration at 24 h is 0.12 ± 0.05 μg/ml.

Significant levels of penicillin G are found in lung tissue, effusion fluids (pericardial, pleural, synovial, and peritoneal), lymph, muscles, subcutaneous tissues, the tonsils, the middle ear, and abscesses. Certain sites are difficult to access, such as the central nervous system, eye, prostate, and bone.

Penicillin G crosses the fetoplacental barrier. It is present in the fetus and in amniotic fluid.

Biotransformation to benzylpenicilloic acid is on the order of 15 to 20% (Fig. 4).

5.5.2. Phenoxypenicillins

Phenoxypenicillins are more stable in an acidic medium and for this reason can be administered orally.

The peak level in serum is reached in half an hour, and the apparent elimination half-life is on the order of 0.5 h (Table 9). Food reduces the absorption of these drugs.

5.5.2.1. Penicillin V

After intravenous administration of penicillin V, the apparent elimination half-life is on the order of 27 min. Plasma clearance is 800 ml/min, and renal clearance is 400 ml/min. Bioavailability is on the order of 57%.

At concentrations of up to 200 μg/ml, plasma protein binding is between 78.5 and 83.4%.

Table 8 Benzylpenicillin pharmacokinetics (600 mg intravenously)

Parameter	Value
C_{max} (μg/ml)	12
T_{max} (h)	0.5
$t_{1/2\beta}$ (h)	0.5
V (liters/kg)	0.35
CL_P (ml/min)	477
CL_R (ml/min)	350
Urinary elimination (%)	60–90
Protein binding (%)	45–65
Metabolism (%)	15–30

Table 7 Activities of cephalosporins against *S. pneumoniae*[a]

Drug	Pen[s] (MIC, <0.12 μg/ml)		Pen[i] (MIC, 0.12 to ≤1 μg/ml)		Pen[r] (MIC, >1 μg/ml)	
	MIC_{50}	MIC_{90}	MIC_{50}	MIC_{90}	MIC_{50}	MIC_{90}
Cefotaxime	0.03	0.03	0.25	1	1	2
Ceftriaxone	0.03	0.03	0.25	1	1	2
Cefpirome	0.01	0.03	0.12	0.5	0.5	1
Ceftazidime	0.25	0.25	2	16	16	16
Cefodizime	0.03	0.03	0.5	2	2	4
Ceftizoxime	0.06	0.06	0.5	8	16	16

[a] MIC_{50} and MIC_{90}, MIC at which 50 and 90%, respectively, of the isolates tested are inhibited.

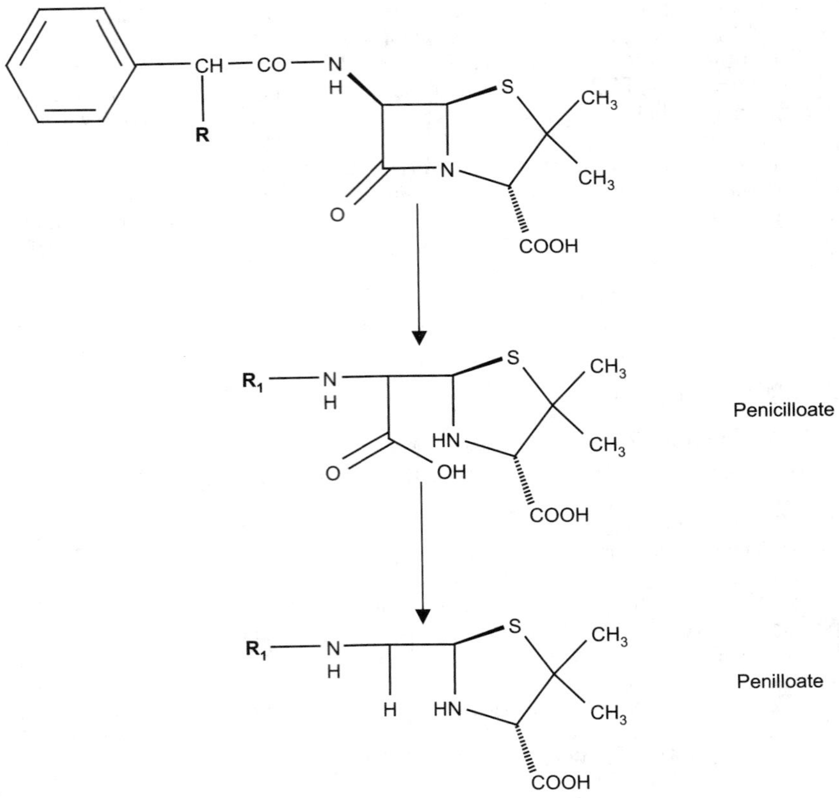

Figure 4 Metabolism of the penams

Table 9 Pharmacokinetics of the phenoxypenicillins

Drug	Dose (mg)	C_{max} (μg/ml)	T_{max} (h)	$t_{1/2}$ (h)	Protein binding (%)	Urinary elimination (%)
Penicillin V	500	3.8	0.75	0.5	60	30–50
Phenethicillin	600	3.4	0.75	0.3	80	20–30
Propicillin	700	7.1	2.5	0.5	85	50

Biotransformation is weak, and two degradation products have been isolated: penicilloic acid and parahydroxypenicillin V. Parahydroxypenicillin V is biologically active.

Penicillin V penetrates the tonsils with a peak concentration on the order of 0.6 mg/kg, compared to a concentration in plasma of 2.6 μg/ml.

5.5.2.2. Penethicillin

Penethicillin is a racemate of which 66% is the *l*-isomer and 34% is the *d*-isomer. The antibacterial activity of the *l*-isomer is slightly greater than that of the *d*-isomer.

The areas under the curve are larger with penethicillin and propicillin than with penicillin V.

After oral administration, 22% of the administered dose is eliminated in the urine in the form of penicilloic acid and a small quantity of 6-aminopenicillanic acid. A polar metabolite possessing antibacterial activity is also found, *para*-hydroxypenethicillin.

The absorption of penethicillin potassium is variable, ranging from 19 to 50% of the administered dose.

Plasma protein binding is between 75 and 82%.

5.5.2.3. Propicillin

Propicillin is a mixture of diastereoisomers. The *l*-isomer is more active than the *d*-isomer or the racemate. Stereospecific absorption and elimination have been described.

For humans, 50 to 53% of the orally administered dose is eliminated in the urine. An unidentified polar metabolite has been detected. Eighty-two percent of the intravenously administered dose is eliminated in the urine. Propicillin is 86 to 89% bound to plasma proteins.

5.5.2.4. Penbenicillin

After oral administration of *dl*-α-phenoxybenzylpenicillin, 20 to 23% of the administered dose is found in the urine. Two metabolites have been detected. Penbenicillin is 97% bound to plasma proteins.

5.5.2.5. Clometocillin

Clometocillin also is a *dl*-α-diastereoisomer. The *d*-isomer is more active than the *l*-isomer. After oral administration, 46% of the administered dose is eliminated renally. Two active metabolites have been identified. Clometocillin is 92% bound to plasma proteins.

5.6. Tolerance

Intolerance reactions are due either to inflammatory phenomena at the injection site or to overdoses. Accidents resulting from overdosage may involve hyperkalemia, encephalopathy, or disorders of hemostasis.

5.6.1. Disorders of Hemostasis

In 1947, Fleming and Fish reported the first hemorrhagic accidents due to penicillin G. Accidents are rare and occur at high doses, often more than 40×10^6 U/day, in patients with renal insufficiency or a predisposing factor: Osler's disease, surgical intervention, or simultaneous administration of aspirin or anti-vitamin K. The platelet changes induced by penicillin G are dose dependent. Penicillin G binds irreversibly to platelets. The number of binding sites is about 4,800. Binding causes a loss of low-affinity receptors for thromboxane A_2 and prostaglandin H_2, inhibition of thromboxane A_2 synthesis, and a modification of intracytoplasmic calcium. Penicillin G modifies the expression of platelet membrane glycoproteins (I_b, I_b-IX, II_b-III_a, and P-selectin).

5.6.2. Encephalopathies

The epileptogenic potency of penicillin G administered intrathecally, intraventricularly, or directly into the cerebral cortex has been known since 1945 (Walker et al., 1945). Encephalopathies subsequent to administration of high intravenous doses have been described since 1964. Even though the frequency is low, on the order of 0.13%, these reactions are severe and can be fatal.

6. GROUP II: GROUP M PENICILLINS

The emergence of penicillinase-producing strains of *S. aureus* necessitated the synthesis of molecules stable against hydrolysis by this enzyme. The first molecule synthesized was methicillin, which differs from benzylpenicillin in the substitution at positions 2′ and 6′ of the benzene ring by methoxy groups, causing steric hindrance around the amide bond.

The second type of molecule is characterized by the presence of an isoxazole pentacycle in the *ortho* position of the benzene ring, the stability of which against hydrolysis by *S. aureus* penicillinases is increased by substitution at position 5′ of a methyl group (oxacillin). The introduction of a chlorine atom at position 2′ (cloxacillin) or two fluorine atoms at positions 2′ and 6′ (dicloxacillin) or a chlorine atom at position 2′ and a fluorine atom at position 6′ (floxacillin) in the benzene ring increases stability against this hydrolysis (Fig. 5).

Molecules similar to methicillin in terms of steric hindrance have been developed: nafcillin, quinacillin, and ancillin (Fig. 6).

6.1. Structure-Activity Relationship

S. aureus penicillinases possess a narrow spectrum and substrate specificity. It is possible to reduce hydrolysis by

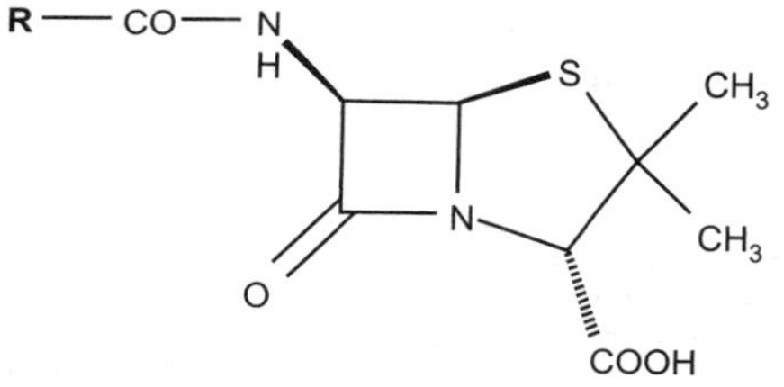

R—CO—NH (penam core: S, CH_3, CH_3, N, O, COOH)

		R
5-methyl-3-phenyl-4-isoxazolyl	oxacillin	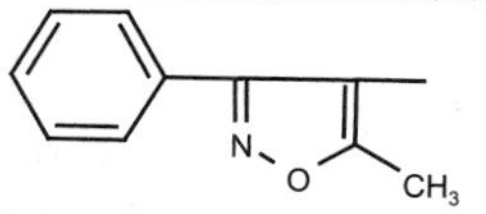 N, O, CH_3
3-(2-chlorophenyl)-5-methyl-4-isoxazolyl	cloxacillin	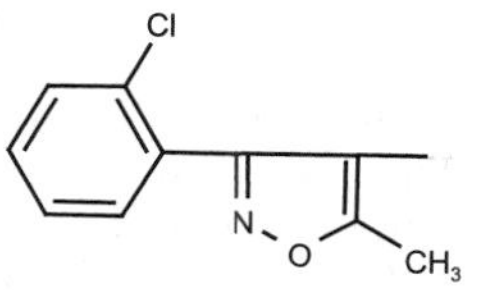 Cl, N, O, CH_3
3-(2,6-dichlorophenyl)-5-methyl-4-isoxazolyl	dicloxacillin	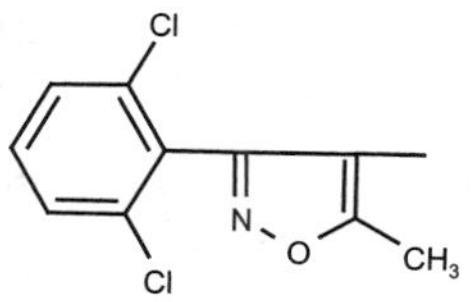 Cl, Cl, N, O, CH_3
3-(2-chloro-6-fluorophenyl)-5-methyl-4-isoxazolyl	flucloxacillin	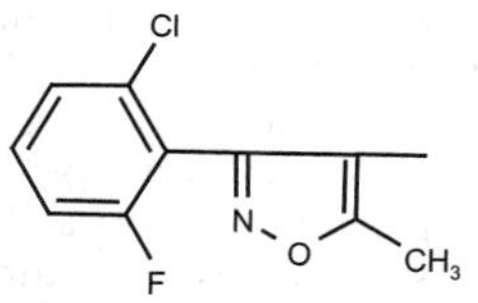 Cl, F, N, O, CH_3

Figure 5 Penicillin M (II) isoxazolylpenicillins

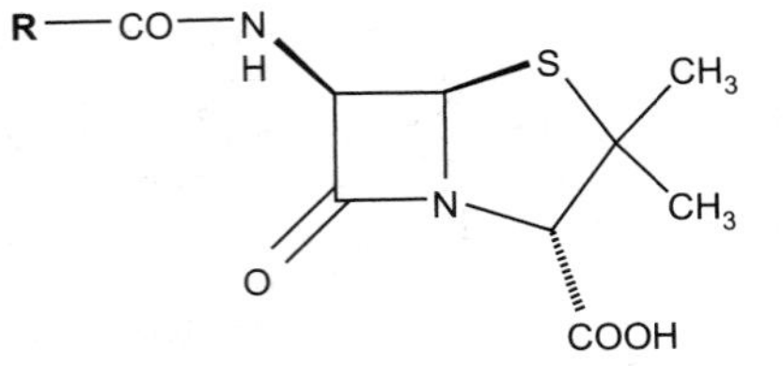

R—CO—NH–(penicillin nucleus: S, CH_3, CH_3, N, O, COOH)

		R
2-ethyl -1-naphthyl	nafcillin	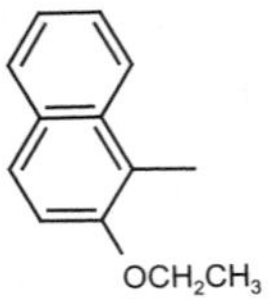 OCH_2CH_3
3-carboxy-2-quinoxalinyl	quinacillin	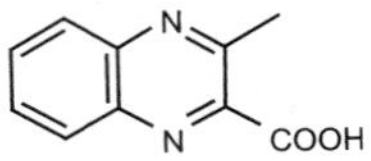 N, N, COOH
2,6-dimethoxy phenyl	methicillin	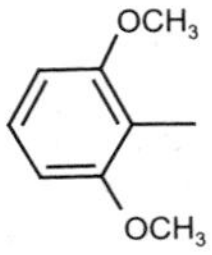 OCH_3, OCH_3
Ortho-biphenyl	Ancillin (diphenycillin)	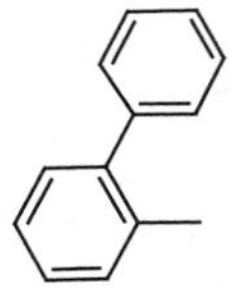
	Prazocillin	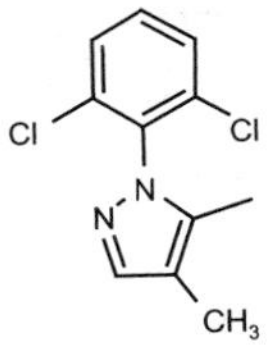 Cl, Cl, N, N, CH_3

Figure 6 Penicillin M group (I)

penicillinases by increasing the steric hindrance around the carbon of the carbonyl-lactam bond, either by increasing the size of the ring attached to the azetidinone nucleus, such as the dihydrothiazine nucleus of the cephalosporins, or by introducing β-lactamase-inhibitory activity (oxacillin). However, these structural modifications often cause a reduction in antibacterial activity.

As a rule, penicillins that are resistant to hydrolysis by penicillinases have an acylated side chain in which the carbon in the α position is quaternary because of the multiple substituents or as a result of incorporation in an aromatic or heterocyclic nucleus. The groups must engender steric hindrance. The introduction of a large hydrophobic group is accompanied by a reduction in activity and antibacterial spectrum. The size of the nucleus plays an important role, but so does the position of the substituents. For example, diphenicillin (ancillin) is *ortho*-biphenylpenicillin, which is stable against hydrolysis by pencillinases; conversely, if the substituents are in the *meta* or *para* position, the molecules are hydrolyzed.

When the nuclei are penta-atomic, hindrance is optimal, with isoxazolylpenicillins substituted by a methyl group and with the presence of a phenyl (oxacillin).

The introduction of another nucleus—furyl or thienyl, or a larger (naphthyl) or more polar (4-pyridine) nucleus—reduces the antibacterial activity. Replacement of the methyl or ethyl group by a larger alkyl, isopropyl, *t*-butyl, or phenyl group maintains the stability against hydrolysis by penicillinases but reduces the antibacterial activity.

Halogenation in the *ortho* position of the phenyl nucleus increases gastrointestinal absorption.

Nafcillin is a 2-ethoxy-1-naphthyl analog that acts by steric hindrance.

6.2. Physicochemical Properties

Methicillin is less stable against acid hydrolysis than the isoxazole penicillins, whose stability is similar to that of the phenoxypenicillins. This stability is probably due to the presence of oxygen and nitrogen atoms in the isoxazole nucleus, these electronegative atoms being protonated more rapidly than those of the carboxyl group.

The physicochemical properties of the different molecules are summarized in Table 10.

Dicloxacillin is relatively unstable at 25°C; plasma samples have to be stored at −70°C. The activity decreases by more than 30% in a month if the samples are stored at −20 or 4°C.

6.3. Antibacterial Properties

The antibacterial spectrum is similar to that of penicillin G. Methicillin is active against gram-positive bacteria and gram-negative cocci such as *N. gonorrhoeae* and *N. meningitidis*. It is, however, 20 to 50 times less active than penicillin G. It is stable against hydrolysis by *S. aureus* β-lactamases and for this reason is active against strains which produce them. Methicillin and nafcillin are both more stable than the isoxazole penicillins, which are, in descending order, dicloxacillin, oxacillin, cloxacillin, and floxacillin.

They are active against *S. pyogenes*, *S. pneumoniae*, and viridans group streptococci but inactive against enterococci.

The metabolites of oxacillin and dicloxacillin are less active than those of cloxacillin and floxacillin against *S. aureus*,

Table 10 Physicochemical properties of group M penicillins

Drug	Mol wt	$t_{1/2}$ degradation (pH 1, 35°C) (min)	pK	Melting point	Na (mmol/g)	Log_{10} P *n*-octanol/water	P_{app} methyl propanol/water
Methicillin	380.42	0.5	2.77	196–197	2.4	1.3	0.363
Oxacillin	401.44	10	2.73	488	2.3	2.31	1.78
Cloxacillin	435.88	15	2.78	170	2.1	2.43	2.4
Dicloxacillin	470.33		2.67	222–225	2	2.91	4.07
Flucoxacillin	453.87		2.76		2	2.61	2.57
Nafcillin	414.48				2.2		

Micrococcus luteus, and *Bacillus subtilis* (Thijssen and Mattie, 1976) (Tables 11 and 12).

In vivo in local experimental infections due to penicillinase-producing *S. aureus*, the isoxazolylpenicillins and methicillin are active if the in situ concentrations are equal to four times the MIC (Table 13). However, such concentrations are rarely attained in endocarditis, osteitis, osteochondritis, and chronic suppurative wounds, in which they are close to the MIC (Renneberg and Forsgren, 1989).

6.4. Breakpoints

The breakpoints of oxacillin recommended by the French Antibiotic Sensitivity Test Committee are listed in Table 14.

6.5. Epidemiology of Resistance

6.5.1. Oxacillinases

Enzymes of the oxacillinase type have been isolated from strains of *Escherichia coli* from Brazil (OXA-4 and OXA-7) and from *P. aeruginosa* (OXA-5 and OXA-6). Oxacillinases have not been described for gram-positive cocci.

These differ from the traditional oxacillinases in their isoelectric point, but they have an identical substrate profile, with one exception, which is that they hydrolyze cefuroxime and cefotaxime. Likewise, an oxacillinase-type enzyme has been described for a strain of *Bacteroides fragilis*. The latter possesses a molecular weight of 41.5 and a pI of 6.9 and hydrolyzes ampicillin more rapidly than cloxacillin. The physicochemical properties are similar to those of the OXA-2, OXA-3, and OXA-6 enzymes, which are dimers. Currently, more than 20 oxacillinases have been described. These are enzymes belonging to Amber's class D. Table 15 summarizes the activities of oxacillinases.

6.5.2. *S. aureus*

6.5.2.1. Epidemiology of resistance of *S. aureus* to methicillin

In the early 1960s, the introduction of methicillin had promised to resolve one of the therapeutic problems associated with infections due to resistant, penicillinase-producing *S. aureus*. The first strain was described in the United Kingdom in 1961 (Barber, 1961; Jevans, 1961). The first methicillin- and aminoglycoside-resistant strains were described in Australia in the mid-1970s and shortly afterwards throughout the world. Between 1960 and 1963, a moderate increase in the number of methicillin-resistant

Table 11 Antibacterial activities of group M penicillins

Organism	MIC (μg/ml)		
	Methicillin	Nafcillin	Isoxazolylpenicillins
S. aureus Pen[s]	1	0.12	0.12
S. aureus Pen[r]	2	0.25	0.25
S. pyogenes	0.25	0.06	0.12
S. pneumoniae	0.25	0.12	0.25
E. faecalis	32	16	32
N. meningitidis	0.25		0.25
N. gonorrhoeae Pen[s]	0.5	2	0.12
N. gonorrhoeae Pen[r]	2	4	>64
E. coli	>128	>128	>128
H. influenzae Amp[s]	2	4	8

Table 12 In vitro activities of group M penicillins against penicillin-susceptible and -resistant *S. aureus*

Drug	MIC (μg/ml)	
	Pen[s]	Pen[r]
Benzylpenicillin	0.05	>128
Methicillin	2	2
Oxacillin	0.5	0.25–1.5
Nafcillin	0.25	0.5
Ancillin	0.25	0.5
Quinacillin	0.5	0.5

Table 13 In vivo activities of group M penicillins

Drug	*S. aureus* producing PC-1[a]	
	1×MIC	4×MIC
Cloxacillin	8	5.2
Floxacillin	7.9	4.2
Dicloxacillin	4.8	4.6
Oxacillin	8	5.3
Methicillin	4.6	4.1
Controls (log_{10} CFU)	9	9

[a]Values are in milligrams per kg.

Table 14 Breakpoints of oxacillin (*S. aureus*)[a]

Drug	Load (μg)	MIC (μg/ml)		Zone diam (mm)	
		S	R	S	R
Oxacillin	5	≤2	>2	≥20	<20

[a]S, susceptible; R, resistant.

Table 15 Activities of oxacillinases

Enzyme	V_{max} with indicated substrate[a]					Cloxacillin inhibition	Molecular weight	pI
	AMP	OXA	CLR	CTX	CFX			
OXA-1	392	197	30			−	23.3	7.4
OXA-2	179	646	37	2	2	−	43.3	7.7
OXA-3	178	336	44			−	41.2	7.1
OXA-4	438	220	194	63	<0.2	+	23	7.5
OXA-5	188	210	89	40	10	−	27	7.62
OXA-6	596	1,048	149	28	<0.2	+	40	7.68
OXA-7	545	702	136	31	41	−	25.3	7.65
OXA-8						−		7.77

[a]AMP, ampicillin; OXA, oxacillin; CLR, clarithromycin; CTX, cefotaxime; CFX, cefoxitin.

strains, on the order of 5%, was noted (Parker and Hewitt, 1970).

Kayser et al. reported that between 1965 and 1969 the incidence of methicillin-resistant strains had increased from 11 to 28% in Zurich, Switzerland, hospitals. In Denmark in 1967, about a quarter of staphylococcal isolates were methicillin resistant (Jessen et al., 1969; Siboni et al., 1968). The incidences of methicillin-resistant strains in nine hospitals in Paris, France, were 12% in 1961, 19% in 1963 (Chabbert et al., 1965), and 35% in 1966 (Soussy and Duval, 1984).

Between 1978 and 1979, about 50% of strains in hospitals in Athens, Greece, were methicillin resistant (Kosmidis et al., 1988).

In the United States, a few strains were isolated in 1963. In fact, no methicillin-resistant strain was isolated in Boston, Mass., hospitals between 1960 and 1967 (Barrett et al., 1968; McGowan, 1988). In 1967, however, 1.4% of isolates were methicillin resistant. From the mid-1970s, the number of resistant isolates has increased progressively, and epidemics have been described in all regions of the United States.

Epidemiological surveillance in Veterans Administration hospitals showed that this type of strain was present in 3 of 137 hospitals in 1975 and 111 of 137 hospitals in 1984 (Preheim et al., 1987). Horan et al. (1986) showed that the distribution of these strains differed according to the type of hospital: 10% in university hospitals and 4.6 to 6% in nonuniversity hospitals depending on their size. In 1991, the National Nosocomial Investigational Surveillance survey in the United States showed that 29% of strains of *S. aureus* were methicillin resistant.

In Australia, no resistant strains had been noted in 1964 (Rountree and Beard, 1968), but 17% of isolates were methicillin resistant in 1970 (Rountree and Vickery, 1973). In 1993, the frequency of methicillin-resistant strains varied according to geographical location: 25.2% in Queensland and 0.4% in the western region of Australia.

In Hong Kong, Cheng and French (1988) reported that 25 to 30% of isolates were methicillin resistant. Likewise, in Ireland the number of methicillin-resistant strains was high (Hone et al., 1981), involving about 40% of isolates from septicemic patients.

In Italy, 6% of isolates were resistant in 1981 and 26% were resistant in 1986 (Schito and Varaldo, 1988).

From 1968, a further increase in these strains was noted. This study also showed that these strains produced large quantities of penicillinase and were resistant to streptomycin and tetracyclines.

At the beginning of the 1970s, a significant decrease in the number of methicillin-resistant strains was reported. In 1976, methicillin- and gentamicin-resistant strains were described (Shanson et al., 1976; Soussy et al., 1976). However, a resurgence of methicillin- and aminoglycoside-resistant strains was noted at the end of the 1970s in France, Ireland, Greece, Australia, and South Africa (Scragg et al., 1978).

Schito and Varaldo (1988) showed that among methicillin-resistant strains, 44, 32, 36, 23, and 21% were also resistant to erythromycin A, cyclines, chloramphenicol, rifampin, and co-trimoxazole, respectively. Resistance associated with aminoglycosides was also noted, differing according to the molecule: 49, 43, 35, and 18% for gentamicin, tobramycin, amikacin, and netilmicin, respectively.

6.5.2.2. Classification of Methicillin-Resistant Strains of *S. aureus*

The phenotypic expression of resistance to methicillin may be heterogeneous or homogeneous. The majority of strains express a heterogeneous resistance phenotype.

However, the distribution of methicillin-resistant strains is much more complex, and three types may be distinguished:

- Borderline resistant *S. aureus*. These strains hyperproduce penicillinases. They were identified in 1986 by Thornsberry et al. These strains produce large quantities of penicillinase and hydrolyze benzylpenicillin rapidly and methicillin and oxacillin partially and slowly; they revert to being susceptible in the presence of a β-lactamase inhibitor, such as clavulanic acid, sulbactam, or tazobactam. They are neither heterogeneous nor multiresistant. These strains do not produce PBP 2a. This group is certainly more complex because a methicillinase has been described, and some of them have modified PBP (Massidda et al., 1992; Varaldo, 1993).
- Modified *S. aureus*. These are strains exhibiting low-level resistance. This resistance is obtained by mutations in several stages, which explains their low incidence. They are characterized by modifications of PBP 2 and PBP 4.
- Methicillin-resistant *S. aureus* (MRSA). This type of resistance is related to the presence of PBP 2a.

Tomasz et al. (1991) proposed dividing the strains into four classes based on the level of methicillin resistance and the degree of heterogeneity of the strains (Table 16).

6.5.2.3. Cell Target

The beginnings of an explanation for the mechanism of resistance to methicillin emerged when PBP 2a was first detected in 1984 (Hartman and Tomasz, 1984).

Table 16 Tomasz's classification

Class	MIC of methicillin (μg/ml) (overall bacteria)	Frequency of highly resistant bacteria	Phenotype
1	3	10^{-7}	Heterogenous stable
2	6–12	10^{-6}	Heterogenous unstable
3	50–200	10^{-3}	Heterogenous stable
4	>400		Heterogenous stable

The first molecular target of the β-lactams is the PBPs. These proteins are bound by a short chain via their N- or C-terminal part to the cytoplasmic membrane, and the greater proportion is oriented towards the bacterial wall. The majority of PBPs constitute an integral part of the terminal synthesis of peptidoglycan.

S. aureus contains five PBPs, 1, 2, 3, 4, and 5, with molecular weights of 85, 80, 75, 70, and 45.

The bactericidal effect of the β-lactams is greatest when PBPs 1, 2, and 3 are inhibited.

In contrast to the PBPs of *E. coli*, which have a dual enzymatic activity (transpeptidase and transglycosylase), in the case of *S. aureus* this activity is supported by other proteins. The first studies showed that PBP 2 and PBP 4 are essential, being responsible for transpeptidation and septation, respectively. PBP 1 is a key target of the β-lactams, albeit not lethal, although its inhibition is a prerequisite for bactericidal activity and bacteriolysis.

Staphylococci may survive with a single PBP. This shows that a single enzyme is capable of bringing about transpeptidation in order to produce a rudimentary peptidoglycan that allows *S. aureus* to survive.

MRSA strains have acquired a supplementary PBP, known as 2a or 2', which binds β-lactams, but with a weak affinity. β-Lactams inhibit the activity of other PBPs, but the presence of PBP 2a is sufficient to allow an adequate quantity of modified peptidoglycan to be synthesized to allow the bacteria to survive. The quality of the peptidoglycan produced is poor, which explains why MRSA strains survive mainly in a hospital environment and are the cause of epidemics of nosocomial infections.

PBP 2a is the product of the *mecA* gene, which is composed of 2,130 bp and localized in the bacterial chromosome on the *mec* determinant. It is found in different species of staphylococci. It possesses an N-terminal domain, which has a transglycosylase function, and a C-terminal domain, which has a transpeptidase function. It has been shown that the *mec* gene is located on a fragment of additional DNA which is absent in isogenic strains susceptible to methicillin. The origin of the *mec* determinant is unknown. Amino acid sequences similar to those of PBP 5 of *Enterococcus hirae* have been identified. However, the nucleotide and amino acid sequences of the product of the *mecA* gene suggest that this gene derives from the fusion of the regulatory region coding for the penicillinases and the PBP structural gene. The *mecA* gene is localized on the chromosome but is regulated from the plasmid-mediated penicillinase genes present in the majority of penicillin-resistant strains of *S. aureus*. The regulatory region is located upstream from the *mecA* gene. There appear to be two regulatory genes, *mecR1* and *mecI*, the proteins of which have a high degree of homology with the products of the staphylococcal *bla* regulatory genes.

The presence of the *mecI* and *mecR1* regulatory genes in some strains of staphylococci is correlated with marked repression of the *mecA* gene, weak induction of transcription of the *mecA* gene in the presence of β-lactams, and a marginal level of resistance to methicillin.

Methicillin-resistant strains possess the *mecA* gene and a deletion of the *mecI* gene.

There is no correlation between the level of methicillin resistance and the quantity of PBP 2a produced.

The *mec* gene is transposable. The Tn*4291* transposon carries the same *mec* gene. The *aadD* gene, which codes for resistance to tobramycin, is similar to the *mec* gene. Likewise, the genes for resistance to mercury, cadmium, and cyclines are associated with the *mec* gene.

The production of the PBP 2a protein is regulated and inducible by β-lactams (class A). In the absence of β-lactamase-producing plasmid, PBP 2a is constitutive (class B). A repressor gene would appear to be common to the penicillinases and to the gene coding for PBP 2a and to be localized upstream from the structural gene of the enzyme. However, non-penicillinase-producing strains may produce β-lactamases by induction of PBP 2a.

MecR1 is a signal-transducing membrane protein which cleaves Mec1, allowing transcription of the gene *mecA*.

The class A-class B complex is located in SCCmec (staphylococcal cassette chromosome), which is a mobile element. SCCmec contains two genes, *ccrA* and *ccrB*, which facilitate SCCmec transfer. These genes encode recombinases of the invertase/resolvase family. Four SCCmec types have been described.

Distinct loci of the *mec* gene and its regulatory genes are probably also important in determining the resistance phenotype.

Berger-Bächi et al. (1992) showed that chromosomal factors independent of PBP 2a are necessary for the expression of high-level resistance to methicillin. These are products of the *fem* (factor essential for methicillin resistance) genes. Currently, four *fem* genes, *femA*, *-B*, *-C*, and *-D*, have been identified, and they are identical to the *aux* (auxiliary) genes described by Tomasz. All strains of *S. aureus*, irrespective of their methicillin susceptibility phenotype, have the *femA* gene. Inactivation of the product of the *femA* gene reduces the level of resistance to methicillin and renders the methicillin-susceptible strains hypersensitive to β-lactams. The same phenomenon has been described with the product of the *femB* gene.

It would appear that isogenic *fem* or *aux* mutant strains have modifications of their autolytic system.

The products of the *femA* and *femB* genes intervene in the synthesis of peptidoglycan and specifically in the formation of the pentaglycine bridge. FemA and FemB are cytoplasmic proteins with molecular weights of 48 and 47, respectively. Their precise biochemical functions in terms of the formation of the interpeptide bond are poorly elucidated. However, the *femA* and *femB* genes intervene in the construction of the peptide pentaglycines, the former after attachment of the first glycine and the latter after attachment of the third glycine. The *femA* and *femB* genes are adjacent. The *femC* gene is localized on *SmaI*IA, and the *femD* gene is localized on *SmaI*I-I. It has been shown that the product of the *femC* gene appears to intervene in the amidation of the carboxyl group of glutamic acid to glutamine during the construction of the peptide (Fig. 7).

Typically MRSA strains are thought to be hospital pathogens. In the community there are at least two distinct types of MRSA: (i) MRSA occurring in the community without hospital contacts and (ii) MRSA following patient discharge from hospital or health care workers carrying MRSA in their nares.

In the community there are at least four different clonal types of MRSA circulating in geographically defined areas having specific virulence factors: exfoliatins (Japan), Panton-Valentine leukocidin (France and the United States), enterotoxins (United States), and α-hemolysin (Australia). β-Lactams appear to upregulate the production of α-toxin in both methicillin-susceptible *S. aureus* (MSSA) and MRSA. Panton-Valentine leukocidin is a cytotoxin that lyses white blood cells and mediates tissue necrosis. These are encoded by the *lukF-PV*, *lukS-PV*, and *lukE-lukD* genes. These isolates possess accessory gene regulator allele type 3 (*agr3*), whereas other MRSA strains possess *agr1* and *agr4*.

Community-acquired MRSA (C-MRSA) strains have been associated with the spread of a single clone. SCCm type IV is mainly found in C-MRSA within EMRSA-15, which is also responsible for MRSA susceptibility to gentamicin as found in France. Some of these isolates are resistant to erythomycin A and clindamycin and less to ciprofloxacin and co-trimoxazole. C-MRSA strains are mainly isolated from patients suffering from skin and skin structure infections.

There are increasing reports of C-MRSA in the United States, France, Japan, Australia, and, to a lesser extent, a few other countries.

It is important to note that in one epidemiological survey in Europe, it was found that about 10% of methicillin-susceptible *S. aureus* isolates harbor a silent *mecA* gene.

6.6. Pharmacokinetics

6.6.1. Methicillin

Methicillin is only used parenterally because it is inactivated in an acidic medium. After administration of 1 g intramuscularly, the peak level in serum is 18 μg/ml and is reached in 0.5 h. The residual concentration at 3 h is 3 to 4 μg/ml (Knudsen and Rolinson, 1960).

After administration of 1 g intravenously (bolus for 5 min), the concentration at the end of infusion is about 60 μg/ml. This concentration is about 120 μg/ml with a dose of 2 g. At the end of the first hour, the concentration in plasma is 7 μg/ml, and at the end of the third hour it is less than 1 μg/ml. Plasma protein binding is between 17 and 43%.

Methicillin is principally eliminated in the urine by glomerular filtration and tubular secretion. About 80% of the administered dose is eliminated renally. Little methicillin is eliminated by hemodialysis. About 2 to 3% of the administered dose is eliminated in the bile.

In the neonate following intramuscular injection of 25 mg/kg, the peak levels in serum are, respectively, 47, 41, 35, and 25 μg/ml for infants aged 4 to 5, 8 to 9, 13 to 15, and 26 to 30 days (McCracken, 1974).

After a dose of 1 g intravenously, the concentration in the CSF is 4.0 μg/ml and the concentration in plasma is 25 μg/ml.

Methicillin penetrates bone better than penicillin G. It penetrates pleural, pericardial, ascites, and osteoarticular fluids well.

6.6.2. Nafcillin

Nafcillin is poorly absorbed, with major interindividual variability. Absorption is affected by the simultaneous ingestion

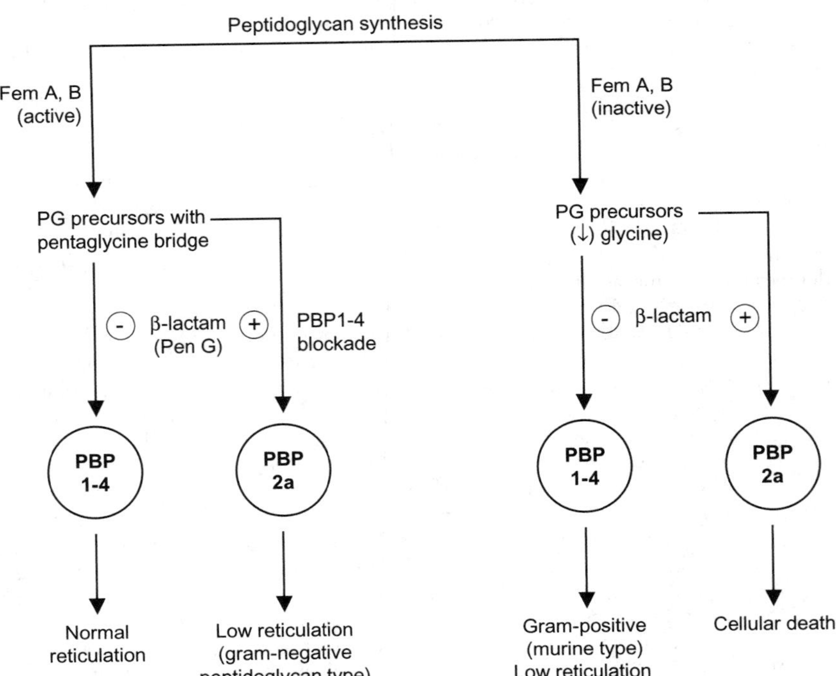

Figure 7 Peptidoglycan (PG) synthesis in MRSA. Pen G, penicillin G.

of food. It is principally administered parenterally (1 g every 4 h or 100 to 200 mg/kg in children).

The concentration in serum at the end of an intravenous infusion of 1 g is 11 μg/ml, and it is 0.5 μg/ml at 6 h (Neu, 1982).

After injection of 1 g intramuscularly, the peak level in serum is 8 μg/ml and is reached in 1 h; the concentration after 6 h is 0.5 μg/ml. After intramuscular administration, the concentrations of nafcillin in plasma are less than those of oxacillin. Nafcillin is 87% plasma protein bound.

Nafcillin is eliminated by glomerular filtration and tubular secretion. After simultaneous administration of probenecid, urinary elimination is 19% rather than 30%. Renal clearance is 160 ml/min, and plasma clearance is 410 ml/min.

Less than 8% of the intramuscularly administered dose is eliminated in the bile. The remainder of the administered dose is inactivated by the liver. Concentrations of nafcillin are higher and elimination is slower in neonates than in infants.

In patients with renal insufficiency, the apparent elimination half-life is not modified. It is also unaffected by hemodialysis. In fact, the loss of renal elimination is partially offset by the hepatobiliary pathway.

The apparent elimination half-life is 1.02 h in healthy volunteers, 1.23 h in cirrhotic patients, and 1.73 h in patients with obstruction of the biliary tract.

High concentrations of nafcillin are obtained in the CSF of patients suffering from purulent meningitis due to *S. aureus*. Concentrations range from 7.5 to 88 μg/ml.

6.6.3. Isoxazolylpenicillins

Isoxazolylpenicillins are administered at a dose of 0.5 g every 6 h in adults and at 50 mg/kg in children. Higher doses are used in the treatment of severe or life-threatening infections.

Oxacillin is the least well-absorbed compound. The peak concentration of cloxacillin in serum is twice that of oxacillin, and those of dicloxacillin and floxacillin are twice that of cloxacillin. The ratio of concentrations in plasma is 1:2:4:4 for oxacillin, cloxacillin, dicloxacillin, and floxacillin.

Food reduces the absorption of isoxazolylpenicillins. This absorption is correlated with the *n*-octanol/water partition coefficient, which increases in the order oxacillin (2.31) < cloxacillin (2.43) < dicloxacillin (2.61) < floxacillin (flucloxacillin) (2.91). The isoxazolylpenicillins are better absorbed orally than are penicillin G, methicillin, and nafcillin, but because of their strong plasma protein binding (>90%), the circulating free fraction is small.

The isoxazolylpenicillins are metabolized to various degrees to three metabolites, two of which are inactive. The active metabolite is obtained by hydroxylation of the methyl group in position 5′ of the isoxazole nucleus, which itself is degraded to a penicilloic acid. The third metabolite is the degradation product, penicilloic acid.

Elimination occurs renally by glomerular filtration and tubular secretion, and probenecid increases the concentrations of these molecules in plasma.

6.6.3.1. Oxacillin

After administration of 500 mg orally, the peak level in serum is 4 μg/ml and is reached in about 1 h. After intramuscular administration, the peak levels in serum are three times those obtained after oral administration (~15 μg/ml).

Oxacillin is highly metabolized. Eight hours after an oral dose of 2 g, the active metabolite 5-hydroxymethyl represents 21% of the administered dose. After a dose of 500 mg orally, 27.4% is eliminated in the urine in the form of oxacillin, 16% in the form of its active metabolite, 22.2% in the form of penicilloic acid, and 22.4% as penicilloic acid of the metabolite.

After a single intramuscular injection of 20 mg of oxacillin per kg to neonates (8 to 15 days), the mean peak level in serum is 51.5 μg/ml, with an apparent elimination half-life of 1.6 h. In infants aged 20 to 21 days, the peak level in serum is 47 μg/ml, with an apparent elimination half-life on the order of 1.2 h. The plasma protein binding of oxacillin is 93%. Diffusion in bone tissue and synovial fluid varies considerably.

6.6.3.2. Cloxacillin

After a single dose of 1 g of cloxacillin intravenously, the area under the curve is 223 μg·h/ml and the apparent elimination half-life is 33 min. Plasma clearance is 155 ml/min. Renal clearance is 113.7 ml/min, and nonrenal clearance is 41.3 ml/min.

After intramuscular administration of 0.5 g, the peak level in serum is 15 μg/ml and is reached in 0.5 h.

After a dose of 0.5 g of cloxacillin orally to volunteers, the peak level in serum is 12.2 ± 6.3 μg/ml and is reached in 45 min. Fifteen minutes after ingestion, the concentration in serum is 4.0 ± 1.0 μg/ml. It then declines slowly and is on the order of 1.35 ± 0.75 μg/ml at 5 h, 0.28 ± 0.18 μg/ml at 12 h, and 0.15 ± 0.14 μg/ml at 24 h (Jamaluddin et al., 1989).

The bioavailability of cloxacillin after a dose of 2 g is 32.9%.

Cloxacillin is eliminated in the urine, accounting for about 56% of the administered dose, together with the active metabolite (12.3%) and the two degradation products (10.6% for penicilloic acid and 2.2% for the other).

After oral or intravenous administration, biliary elimination is 10 to 30% of the administered dose.

After a single dose of 1 g orally, the concentration of cloxacillin in spongy bone is 2.9 mg/kg and that in cortical bone is 1.7 mg/kg. After repeated doses of 1 g every 8 h, the concentrations in bone vary little (2.4 mg/kg in spongy bone and 1.5 mg/kg in cortical bone) (Sirot et al., 1982). Cloxacillin is highly concentrated in synovial fluid. In mandibular bone, the concentration 60 min after administration of 0.5 g is 2.0 ± 0.4 mg/kg (plasma, 3.2 ± 0.5 μg/ml).

The bioavailability is not significantly affected in patients suffering from cystic fibrosis (50% versus 38% in control subjects) after an intravenous dose of 25 mg/kg. Urinary elimination is also similar (64 versus 54.7% in controls). However, the apparent elimination half-life is shorter (46.1 versus 57.1 min) and plasma and renal clearance is more rapid (Table 17).

Table 17 Plasma kinetics of cloxacillin in patients with cystic fibrosis

Patients	AUC (μg·h/ml)	CL_P (ml/min)	CL_R (ml/min)	$t_{1/2\beta}$ (h)	V (mg/kg)	V_{ss} (mg/kg)
Control	187.7	147	94	57.1	71	99
Cystic fibrosis	94	261	123	46.1	91.2	136.5

6.6.3.3. Dicloxacillin

The oral bioavailability of dicloxacillin is 48.8% after a dose of 2 g. The apparent elimination half-life decreases from 43 to 37 min when the dose is increased from 1 to 2 g.

After intravenous administration of a dose of 1 g, the apparent elimination half-life is 42 min, the area under the curve is 307 μg·h/ml, and plasma clearance is 110.8 ml/min. Renal clearance is 67.4 ml/min, and nonrenal clearance is 43.4 ml/min. Urinary elimination is 61% of the administered dose.

Following administration of a single dose of 2 g of dicloxacillin in elderly subjects (Löfgren et al., data on file), the area under the curve is 488 μg·h/ml for young volunteers and 427 μg · h/ml for elderly subjects. The apparent elimination half-lives are, respectively, 1.58 and 1.77 h (Table 18).

In 2-year-old children, concentrations in plasma are between 12 and 40 μg/ml after an oral dose of 25 mg/kg. The peak level in serum is 14.35 ± 6.77 μg/ml and is reached after 1.68 h (0.58 to 3.7 h). The areas under the curve after oral and intravenous administration are, respectively, 70.15 ± 32.2 μg·h/ml and 34.5 ± 18.4 μg·h/ml. Oral bioavailability is about 59.8% ± 24.4%. The apparent elimination half-life is 0.53 ± 0.2 h. Plasma clearance is 156 ml/min/kg. The area under the curve is lower in children aged 6 to 60 months (28.3 ± 13.9 μg·h/ml) than in children over the age of 5 years (58.3 ± 12.9 μg·h/ml). Dicloxacillin is eliminated more slowly than cloxacillin. The elimination rate is 27% lower than that of cloxacillin ($\beta = 0.99$ versus 1.26 h^{-1}).

6.6.3.4. Floxacillin

Paton (1986) demonstrated that the oral bioavailability of 250 mg of floxacillin (flucloxacillin) was similar to that obtained with 500 mg of cloxacillin. The differences are due partly to better digestive absorption but also to slower renal clearance (88 ml/min) than of cloxacillin (102 ml/min) (Table 19).

After intravenous administration of 50 mg/kg in neonates at a gestational age of 33 to 41 weeks, the plasma kinetics are biexponential. The distribution phase is rapid, with a half-life at α phase of 5.7 min. The apparent elimination half-life is 4 h. Nonrenal clearance in the neonate represents 76% of plasma clearance, and renal clearance represents 24%. After oral administration, about 31.6% is absorbed. The apparent elimination half-life is 4.6 h, significantly longer than that in adults (0.76 to 0.88 h) and elderly patients (1.5 h). Plasma clearance is lower than in adults (0.7 versus 1.3 ml/min/kg), due principally to a reduction in renal clearance, which represents 24% of plasma clearance in neonates and 64% in adults. Nonrenal clearance is similar in the neonate, young adult, and elderly subject. The reduction in renal clearance is probably due to the reduction in tubular secretion (Table 20). Oral bioavailablity is lower in the neonate than in the adult. After a dose of 12.5 mg/kg, concentrations in plasma are higher in infants aged 1 to 5 months than in those over 6 months of age. Absorption is greater in children aged over 6 months. The areas under the curve are, respectively, 92 ± 11.5 and 43 ± 9.3 μg·h/ml but are higher in neonates when floxacillin is administered in tablet form (72 ± 10.2 μg·h/ml).

According to Murai et al. (1983), more than 80.9% of the administered dose is eliminated in the urine. Urinary elimination consists of 64.8% floxacillin, 10.5% active metabolite, 3.8% penicilloic acid, and 1% degradation product of the active metabolite.

After doses of 0.5 and 1 g administered intramuscularly, floxacillin concentrations are, respectively, 8.9 μg/ml, 1.3 mg/kg, and 0.9 mg/kg in serum, spongy bone, and cortical bone. After intravenous administration of 2 g at the end of infusion and 12 h afterwards, concentrations in plasma are, respectively, 125.2 and 4.4 μg/ml and those in the cardiac valves are 16.5 and 3.7 mg/kg. In subcutaneous tissue and muscle, the concentrations are 14.7 and 14.2 mg/kg at the end of infusion, with nothing being detectable after 10 h (Frank et al., 1988).

6.7. Tolerance

Methicillin is particularly poorly tolerated. Interstitial nephropathies as well as leukoneutropenia during treatment with methicillin have been described.

The administration of phenylbutazone causes a reduction in cloxacillin and dicloxacillin concentrations in plasma.

Diazepam, phenobarbital, phenytoin, and chlorpromazine interfere to various degrees in the metabolism of the isoxazolylpenicillins.

Table 18 Pharmacokinetics of dicloxacillin in young and elderly subjects[a]

Parameter	Young subjects	Elderly subjects
AUC (μg · h/ml)	488	427
CL_P (liters/h)	4.2	4.75
CL_R (liters/h)	3.18	3.09
CL_{NR} (liters/h)	1.02	1.66
$t_{1/2}$ (h)	1.58	1.77
Urinary elimination (%)	76.5	64.9

[a]Data from Löfgren et al.

Table 20 Pharmacokinetics of floxacillin (flucloxacillin) in neonates of 33 to 42 weeks' gestational age, 50 mg/kg[a]

Parameter	Intravenous	Oral
C_{max} (μg/ml)		69.8 ± 30
$t_{1/2}$ (h)	4.6 ± 1.46	
CL_P (ml/min/kg)	0.74 ± 0.25	
CL_{NR} (ml/min/kg)	0.56 ± 0.18	
CL_R (ml/min/kg)	0.18 ± 0.12	0.19 ± 0.16
F (%)		47.7 ± 12.7
Lag time (h)		0.21 ± 0.14

[a]Values are means ± standard deviations.

Table 19 Comparative oral pharmacokinetics of cloxacillin and floxacillin

Drug	Dose (mg)	C_{max} (μg/ml)	T_{max} (h)	AUC (μg · h/ml)	$t_{1/2}$ (h)[a]	CL_R (ml/min)
Cloxacillin	500	11.9 ± 2.9	0.8	18.6 ± 2.5	0.9 ± 0.1	102
Floxacillin	200	7.7 ± 1.3	0.9	16.8 ± 2.0	1.5 ± 0.2	88

[a]Means ± standard deviations.

The isoxazolylpenicillins may displace bilirubin in premature neonates, whose hepatic function is immature, and be responsible for kernicterus, particularly if the concentrations in plasma are greater than 200 μg/ml (Bratlid, 1976).

7. GROUP III: GROUP A PENICILLINS

In 1960, epidemiological surveys in hospitals showed that the importance of gram-positive cocci had declined markedly in favor of *Enterobacteriaceae* such as *E. coli, Klebsiella pneumoniae*, and *Proteus mirabilis* (Finland, 1970). In a number of cases, the use of ampicillin provided a solution to an acute therapeutic problem. However, epidemics due to ampicillin-resistant *Enterobacteriaceae* were very rapidly described (Finland, 1979).

An increase in the activity of penicillins against gram-negative bacilli was obtained by introducing an ionized group, such as an amino or hydroxyl, in the α position of the side chain at position 6 of the penam nucleus. It was rapidly shown that the introduction of an acid or basic group in the α position increased the activity against gram-negative bacilli. Steric hindrance is partly responsible for this activity, particularly against β-lactamase-producing strains.

7.1. Classification

Group A penicillins may be divided into two subgroups, IIIA and IIIB, according to the presence or absence of a substituent on the amino group. In this way ampicillin and its derivatives can be distinguished from the *N*-acylpenicillins (Fig. 1).

The ampicillin derivatives include two categories of molecules: ampicillin and ampicillin esters; the latter are considered in another chapter.

7.2. Group IIIA: Ampicillin and Its Derivatives

Ampicillin is D-α-aminobenzylpenicillin. It is one of the most widely prescribed antibiotics in the world. The structures of ampicillin and its derivatives are shown in Fig. 8.

7.2.1. Physicochemical Properties

The principal characteristics are summarized in Table 21. The molecules are in the form of the sodium salt for the parenteral route and are soluble in water. The pH of 1% aqueous solutions is between 5 and 8. Ampicillin exhibits acceptable stability in an acidic medium, allowing transit through the gastrointestinal tract.

7.2.2. Structure-Activity Relationship

The penam nucleus is inactive but is essential for the antibacterial activity. Penicillin N (6-D-aminoadipoyl penicillin G) is 100 times less active than penicillin G against gram-positive bacilli but is considerably more active against gram-negative bacteria. Acylation of the amino group increases the activity against gram-negative bacilli. A number of polar groups—amino, hydroxyl, carboxyl, and sulfonyl—increase

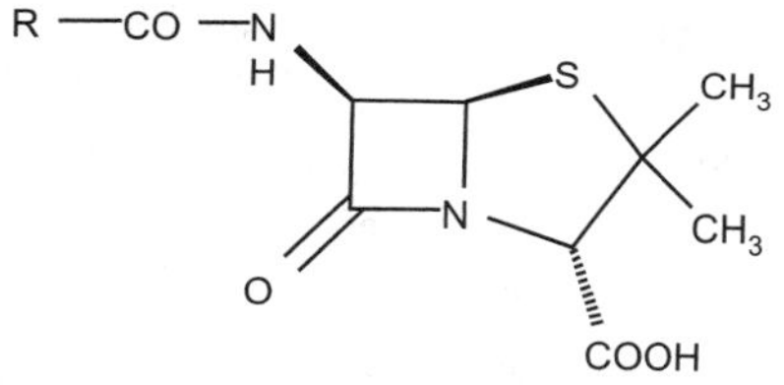

D-α-amino-α-phenyl acetamide	ampicillin	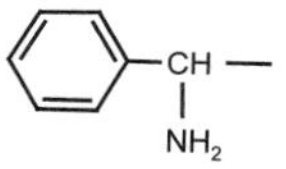 CH — NH2
D-α-amino-α-(p-hydroxy phenyl) acetamide	amoxicillin	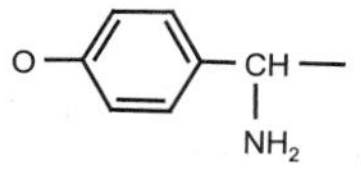 O — CH — NH2
D-α-amino (α-1,4 cyclo hexidien-1-yl) acetamide	epicillin	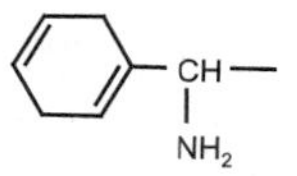 CH — NH2
D-α-azido-α-phenylacetamide	azidocillin	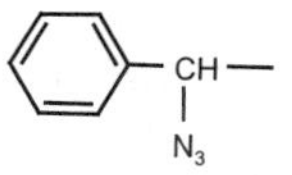 CH — N3
1-aminocyclohexane carboxamide	cyclacillin	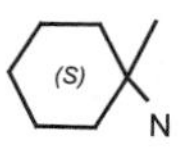 (S) N
2,2-dimethyl-5-oxo-4-phenyl-1-imidazolidinyl	hetacillin	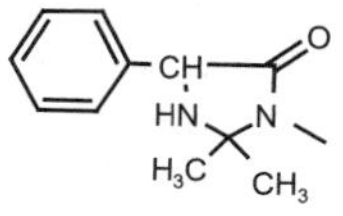 CH O HN N H3C CH3
D-α-Methyl imino-α-phenylacetamide	metampicillin	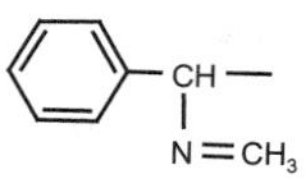 CH — N=CH3

Figure 8 Ampicillin and derivatives

Table 21 Physicochemical properties of the aminopenicillins

Drug	Empirical formula	Mol wt	pK	P_{app} 2-methyl/ propanol/water	Melting point (°C)
Ampicillin	$C_{16}H_{19}N_3O_4S$	349.40	2.53/6.95	0.373	199–203
Amoxicillin	$C_{16}H_{19}N_3O_5S$	365.40	2.67/7.11	0.130	216–218
Epicillin	$C_{16}H_{21}N_3O_4S$	351.42	2.77/7.17	0.438	202
Azidocillin	$C_{16}H_{17}N_5O_4S$	375.42			
Cyclacillin	$C_{15}H_{23}N_3O_4S$	341.42	2.68/7.50	0.866	182–183
Hetacillin	$C_{19}H_{23}N_3O_4S$	398.48			189–191
Metampicillin	$C_{17}H_{19}N_3O_4S$	361.41			
Suncillin	$C_{16}H_{19}N_3O_7S$	429.46			

the activity against gram-negative bacteria. In order to obtain a balance between gram-positive and gram-negative bacteria in terms of activity, the lipophilicity of these molecules must be intermediate.

The biological activity is based essentially on the nature and spatial orientation of the side chain. L-Ampicillin is less active against gram-negative bacilli than D-ampicillin because of the spatial orientation of the amino chain (Table 22).

Structural modifications have yielded epicillin, which is 1,4-cyclohexadienylampicillin, and cyclacillin, which is 1-aminocyclohexylpenicillin.

Amoxicillin is *para*-hydroxyampicillin. The introduction of a substituent on the benzene nucleus reduces the activity against gram-negative bacilli, except for a hydroxyl group in the *para* or *meta* position; these molecules exhibit better bioavailability than ampicillin orally.

The benzene ring may be replaced by a thiophene, isothiazole, or thiazole nucleus; the antibacterial activities of these molecules are similar to that of ampicillin.

Betacin possesses an additional methylene between the α-carbon and the amino group. It exhibits activity against gram-negative bacilli similar to that of ampicillin, but its oral absorption is poor.

Table 22 Antibacterial activities of the isomers of ampicillin

Organism	Ampicillin MIC (μg/ml)	
	D-Isomer	L-Isomer
E. coli	2.5	12.5
K. pneumoniae	1.6	12.5
S. enterica serovar Typhi	1.6	12.5

7.2.3. Antibacterial Activity

Ampicillin is more active than penicillin G against *Enterococcus* spp. and *H. influenzae* but is less active against penicillin-susceptible *S. pneumoniae*, *S. pyogenes*, *Neisseria* spp., and *Clostridium* spp. Conversely, it is active against certain non-β-lactamase-producing species of *Enterobacteriaceae*, such as *E. coli*, *P. mirabilis*, *Salmonella enterica* serovar Typhi and non-serovar Typhi, *Shigella* spp., and *Vibrio* spp. It is active against *L. monocytogenes*, *Bordetella pertussis*, *B. anthracis*, *C. diphtheriae*, *T. pallidum*, and *Yersinia pestis* (Table 23). It is inactive against class I β-lactamase-producing species of *Enterobacteriaceae*, such as *Enterobacter* spp., *Citrobacter* spp., *Serratia marcescens*, and *Morganella morganii*. Likewise, it is inactive against penicillinase-producing strains of *S. aureus* and nonfermenting gram-negative bacilli such as *Pseudomonas*

Table 23 Antibacterial activities of the α-aminopenicillins

Organism(s)	MIC (μg/ml)				
	Ampicillin	Amoxicillin	Epicillin	Cyclacillin	Azidocillin
E. coli	4	4	4	64	64
K. pneumoniae	>128	>128	>128	>128	>128
Enterobacter spp.	>128	>128	>128	>128	>128
Citrobacter spp.	>128	>128	>128	>128	>128
S. marcescens	>128	>128	>128	>128	>128
P. mirabilis	1	1	2	32	32
Proteus indole$^+$	128	128	128	128	128
S.enterica serovar Typhi	1	1	2	32	32
Shigella spp.	2	2	2	32	32
H. influenzae	0.25	0.5	0.25	4	0.25
S. aureus Pen^s	0.1	0.1	0.1	1	0.03
S. aureus Pen^r	>128	>128	>128	>128	>128
S. pneumoniae	0.03	0.03		0.5	0.01
E. faecalis	1	0.5	1	2	1
N. meningitidis	0.06	0.06			
L. monocytogenes	0.25–1	0.25–1			
N. gonorrhoeae Pen^s	0.06	0.12	0.06	0.06	0.01
N. gonorrhoeae Pen^r	>16	>16			2

spp. It is active in vitro and in vivo against *Helicobacter pylori*. On the basis of roundtable held in Dublin, Ireland, in 1991, it is currently recommended that an antiulcer agent (bismuth salt or proton pump inhibitor—omeprazole or lansoprazole) be combined with two antibiotics for a minimum of a fortnight; amoxicillin constitutes the basic antibiotic, combined with a macrolide or 5-nitroimidazole derivative. In the event of hypersensitivity to β-lactams, cyclines may be used. No amoxicillin-resistant strains have as yet been detected, although a reduction in activity has been noted.

Amoxicillin, epicillin, and cyclacillin possess the same antibacterial activity in vitro as ampicillin. Hetacillin and metampicillin are prodrugs of ampicillin. They do not possess antibacterial activity and become active only when ampicillin is released. Azidocillin has the same activity and the same antibacterial spectrum as penicillin G.

7.2.4. Breakpoints

In Table 24, the breakpoints recommended by the French Antibiotic Sensitivity Test Committee are given for ampicillin.

7.2.5. Epidemiology of Resistance to Ampicillin

Anderson and Datta in 1965 isolated a strain of *Salmonella enterica* serovar Typhimurium whose resistance to ampicillin was transferable to *E. coli*. Datta and Kontomichalon (1965) described the first ampicillin-resistant, β-lactamase-producing strain of *E. coli*. This β-lactamase was known as TEM, after the name of a patient, Temoniera. Since the introduction of ampicillin, resistant strains of *E. coli* have been isolated. Of the enzymes of different bacterial species that hydrolyze ampicillin, 75% are TEM-1 (Table 25).

The first strain of *H. influenzae* carrying a plasmid with a resistance gene for ampicillin was isolated in 1974 (Williams and Cavanagh, 1974), followed by a strain of *N. gonorrhoeae* in 1977 and *N. meningitidis* in 1983.

Table 24 Breakpoints of ampicillin[a]

Drug	Load (μg)	MIC (μg/ml)		Zone diam (mm)	
		S	R	S	R
Ampicillin	25	≤4	>16	≥21	<14

[a]S, susceptible; R, resistant.

7.2.5.1. *H. influenzae*

H. influenzae is a pathogenic agent responsible for numerous infectious syndromes: meningitis, epiglottitis, cellulitis, arthritis, and respiratory tract infections, particularly in children under 5 years of age. Ampicillin was the antibiotic of choice in the treatment of *H. influenzae* infections, whether otitis, meningitis, pneumonia, etc. In the United States, ampicillin-resistant strains may represent up to 31.7% of clinical isolates in certain centers (Doern et al., 1988). A European multicenter study showed that the prevalence of ampicillin-resistant strains varied according to the centers and countries, reaching up to 30% in Spain, whereas in Germany it was on the order of 1.6%. In the other European countries it was on the order of 10%. Table 26 shows the susceptibility of *H. influenzae* to various drugs in Europe.

Ampicillin resistance is due principally to the production of a transferable enzyme, TEM-1 (pI 5.4), the gene responsible for which is localized on the TnA transposon. This enzyme is inhibited by clavulanic acid, sulbactam, brobactam, and tazobactam. It may also be chromosomally mediated. It may be related to the production of another enzyme, ROB-1, also found in *P. multocida*. It would appear to be of porcine origin, as this enzyme has been detected in *Actinobacillus pleuropneumoniae*. The modification in affinity for PBP 3A and PBP 3B is responsible for a change in the activity of ampicillin. A nonenzymatic mode of resistance, particularly through modification of PBP, has been described. In an Irish survey, 0.7% of resistant strains were resistant to co-amoxiclav (Augmentin).

Table 25 Frequencies of broad-spectrum β-lactamases

Enzyme(s)	Prevalence (%)
TEM-1	75
TEM-2	3
OXA-1	5
OXA-2	5
OXA-3	3
SHV-1	2
PSE-1	2
PSE-2	NF[a]
PSE-3	NF
PSE-4	NF
Others	3
All enzymes	5

[a]NF, not found.

Table 26 Susceptibilities of *H. influenzae* isolates in Europe

Country	Susceptibility (%) to drug at indicated MIC (μg/ml):			
	Ampicillin, ≤1	Chloramphenicol, ≤2	Tetracycline, ≤2	Co-trimoxazole, ≤10
Germany	97.4	98.5	97.9	92.9
Austria	98.5	98.1	94.7	96.6
Belgium	84.7	94.2	85.1	90.8
Spain	65.9	82.7	79.9	27.2
France	84.0	98.7	87.9	95.7
Italy	96.0	99.5	98.5	79.0
The Netherlands	94.2	97.8	85.9	91.0
The United Kingdom	89.6	98.7	96.0	93.8
Switzerland	93.6	98.7	96.0	93.8

Resistance to ampicillin is due to a TnA transposon and is often accompanied by resistance to chloramphenicol through an acetyltransferase, the gene for which is localized on the TnA transposon insertion site. Resistance to chloramphenicol, which accumulates in the cytoplasmic space through a dual mechanism of diffusion and enzyme-dependent active transport, may be due to a weak intracytoplasmic concentration. Resistance to ampicillin and chloramphenicol is often accompanied by resistance to cyclines.

7.2.5.2. *N. gonorrhoeae*

For some years, there has been a reduction in the activity of penicillins against *N. gonorrhoeae* because of β-lactamase production. The incidence of this resistance varies with the country and region. In the Parisian region, the incidence is on the order of 15%. This enzymatic resistance may be chromosome or plasmid mediated.

Chromosome-mediated resistance appears to be more extensive and is often accompanied by a reduction in the susceptibility of these strains to spectinomycin, cyclines, sulfonamides, and macrolides. The loci of resistance have been reviewed by Dillon et al. (1989) (Table 27).

Regarding plasmid-mediated resistance, five different plasmids have been described:

- African plasmid (5.1 kb) (detected in the United Kingdom). The growth of strains with this plasmid requires arginine. They remain susceptible to cyclines.
- Asian plasmid (7.2 kb) (Far East, United States). Strains with this plasmid are either auxotrophic strains requiring proline to grow or wild strains. They exhibit reduced susceptibility to cyclines. This probably involves a plasmid of the African type that has lost a 2.1 kb fragment. The Asian and African plasmids carry a gene coding for a TEM-1-type β-lactamase and carry 40% of the Tn*2* transposon.
- Toronto plasmid (4.9 kb) was isolated in 1984. The plasmid derives from Asian plasmids with a loss of a 2.3-kb fragment.
- Rio plasmid. This was identified from strains isolated in The Netherlands and Brazil. It involves strains auxotrophic for methionine.
- Nîmes plasmid derived from the African plasmid

Clavulanic acid, sulbactam, and brobactam possess intrinsic in vitro activities against *N. gonorrhoeae* (MIC, 1 to 5 μg/ml) and inhibit the activity of *N. gonorrhoeae* enzymes. The activity of ampicillin (ampicillin-resistant strain, MIC, >10 μg/ml) is restored when the drug is used in combination with a β-lactamase inhibitor (MIC, ≤0.1 μg/ml).

7.2.5.3. *N. meningitidis*

A reduction in the activity of penicillin G has been described in Spain, the United Kingdom, South Africa, and Israel since 1983.

The first β-lactamase-producing strain was described in 1983. This was a β-lactamase of plasmid origin, the gene for which was carried on an Asian-type plasmid of *N. gonorrhoeae* (7.2 kb).

Some publications report strains exhibiting reduced susceptibility to penicillin G (MIC, >0.1 to 0.5 μg/ml) due to reduced affinity for PBP 2. As with *N. gonorrhoeae*, the modification of PBP 2 appears to be related to the acquisition of certain regions of the gene coding for *Neisseria flavescens* PBP 2.

In a Canadian study from 1979, 827 strains of *N. meningitidis* were isolated and 29 exhibited reduced penicillin G activity (MIC, 0.25 to 0.5 μg/ml).

In Spain, the proportion of strains with a penicillin-intermediate phenotype increased from 0.8% in 1984 to 8% in 1992 (Campos et al., 1992).

7.2.5.4. *Moraxella catarrhalis*

M. catarrhalis, formerly *Branhamella* and *Neisseria* (last edition of Bergey's manual), is one of the causative agents of upper (otitis, sinusitis) and lower (superinfection of chronic bronchitis, pneumonia) respiratory tract infections, particularly in patients with an abnormality of the respiratory tract. No β-lactamase-producing strains were detected between 1970 and 1976. In 1981, 56.8% of strains isolated were β-lactamase producing. Since 1977 an increasing number of ampicillin-resistant strains have been isolated from pathological products, reaching a figure of about 75%. In a recent study, Chardon et al. analyzed the susceptibility of *M. catarrhalis* to ampicillin.

Table 28 shows the susceptibilities of strains of *M. catarrhalis* to amoxicillin with and without clavulanic acid.

In a French multicenter study (15 centers), the number of β-lactamase-producing strains was determined; data are shown in Table 29.

However, resistance to the β-lactams was due not only to β-lactamase production but also to a reduction in outer membrane permeability. Table 30 shows the abilities of β-lactams to permeate membranes.

The outer membrane of *M. catarrhalis* is similar to those of the other gram-negative bacilli and comprises 10 to 20 proteins, of which eight are dominant: OmpA to OmpH. These proteins have molecular weights of between 98 and 21. There is a certain interstrain homogeneity.

The majority of β-lactamases produced by *M. catarrhalis* are constitutive and chromosomally mediated. Two plasmid-mediated enzymes have recently been detected: BRO-1 and BRO-2 (BRO = ***BR****anhamella* and ***MO****raxella*).

Table 27 Mechanisms of chromosome-mediated resistance

Genotype	Phenotype	Molecular mechanism
penA	Four to eight times the MIC	Decrease after PBP 2 affinity Decrease peptidoglycan O acetylation New PBP
penB tem	Four times the MIC for penicillin and cycline (*mtr*)	Decrease PBP affinities
ampA ampB	Low-level resistance to ampicillin	
ampC ampD	In combination with *ampA* and *ampB* four times the MIC for ampicillin.	

The two BRO-1 enzymes (pI 5.5, 5.55, and 5.85) and BRO-2 (pI 5.5, 5.9, and 6.25) are very similar; they are attached to the cell and are not produced in large quantities.

BRO-1 is a plasmid-mediated enzyme that has been detected in *M. catarrhalis* and *Moraxella nonliquefaciens*. It hydrolyzes carbenicillin, methicillin, amdinocillin, and cefaclor rapidly and cloxacillin more slowly. The main band has a pI of 5.55. It is found in 90% of β-lactamase-producing strains.

BRO-2 exhibits the same substrate profile. However, strains producing the BRO-2-type enzyme are less resistant to penicillin G than BRO-1-producing ones.

Other moraxellae produce β-lactamases: *Moraxella osloensis, Moraxella lacunata, Moraxella phenylpyruvica,* and *Moraxella urethralis* (*Oligella urethralis*). No β-lactamase enzyme activity has been detected in *Moraxella atlantae*.

Clavulanic acid (geometric MIC, 30.27 μg/ml) and sulbactam (MIC, 5.38 μg/ml) have no intrinsic activity against *M. catarrhalis* but restore the activity of amoxicillin (Table 31).

The relative hydrolysis rates for BRO-1, BRO-2, and TEM-1 are illustrated in Table 32.

Yokota et al. (1986) described a penicillinase-like enzyme produced by *M. catarrhalis* NNBR-8303 with a molecular weight of 33 and a pI of 5.4. It hydrolyzes penicillin G, cefotaxime, and cefmenoxime. It is inhibited by clavulanic acid and sulbactam. This strain produces TEM-1 and two enzymes inactivating aminoglycosides by phosphorylation.

7.2.5.5. *P. multocida*

Pasteurellae are important infectious agents in veterinary infectious diseases (*Mannheimia haemolytica* and *Pasteurella aerogenes*) and in human pathology (*P. multocida*).

The ROB-1 enzyme, similar to TEM, has been isolated in a strain of human *H. influenzae* responsible for purulent meningitis and porcine *A. pleuropneumoniae*. It hydrolyzes carbenicillin more rapidly than penicillin G and cephaloridine more slowly. It is a membrane enzyme. This enzyme has also been isolated in *P. multocida* LNPB9 and LNPB86, *M. haemolytica* LNPB51, and *P. aerogenes* ATCC 27833. These are ampicillin- and carbenicillin-resistant strains. All of these strains possess a 4.4-kb plasmid, except for *P. aerogenes*, for which the ROB-1 resistance gene is chromosomal.

The in vitro activities of different antibacterial agents were tested by Goldstein et al. (1986, 1988) against *P. multocida*; results are shown in Table 33.

Table 28 Susceptibilities of strains of *M. catarrhalis* to amoxicillin with and without clavulanic acid

Drug[b]	MIC (μg/ml)[a]	
	50%	90%
Amoxicillin, β⁻	0.03	0.125
Amoxicillin, β⁺	32	128
Clavulanic acid	16	16
Co-amoxiclav, β⁻	0.015	0.125
Co-amoxiclav, β⁺	0.125	0.25

[a]50% and 90%, MICs at which 50 and 90% of isolates are inhibited, respectively.
[b]β⁻, non-β-lactamase-producing strains; β⁺, β-lactamase-producing strains.

Table 29 β-Lactamase-producing strains in France

Year	% (no./total)	β⁺[a] strains
1987	82.7	(134/162)
1988	83.3	(185/222)
1989	77.8	(172/221)

[a]β⁺, β-lactamase producing.

Table 30 Membrane permeation

Drug	Membrane permeation[a]
Benzylpenicillin	3.4
Amoxicillin	1.3
Carbenicillin	5.5
Cephaloridine	0.93
Cefaclor	1.4
Clavulanic acid	1.1
Sulbactam	1.1
Brobactam	0.9
MM 13902	2.1

[a]IC_{50} for whole cells/IC_{50} for crude extract (enzyme).

Table 31 Activities of β-lactamase inhibitors against β-lactamase-producing strains of *M. catarrhalis*

Drug(s)	MIC (μg/ml) (geometric mean)
Amoxicillin	2.86
Amoxicillin + clavulanic acid (1 μg)	0.14
Amoxicillin + sulbactam	0.15

Table 32 Hydrolysis rates of β-lactamases[a]

Enzyme	Hydrolysis rate (%)				
	PEN	AMP	MET	CEC	CLR
BRO-1	100	75	103	235	17
BRO-2	100	62	112	140	13
TEM-1	100	60	≤1	27	60

[a]PEN, penicillin; AMP, ampicillin; MET, methicillin; CEC, cefaclor; CLR, clarithromycin.

Table 33 MICs for *P. multocida*

Drug	MIC (μg/ml)[a]	
	50%	90%
Penicillin G	<0.06	0.25
Oxacillin	1	8
Ampicillin	0.125	0.25
Co-amoxiclav	0.125	0.125
Cefadroxil	4	8
Cephalexin	4	4
Cefuroxime	0.125	0.25
Tetracycline	0.5	0.5
Ciprofloxacin	<0.03	0.03
Ofloxacin	<0.03	0.06
Erythromycin A	1	4
Roxithromycin	8	32

[a]50% and 90%, MICs at which 50 and 90% of isolates are inhibited, respectively.

7.2.5.6. *Vibrio cholerae*

Plasmid-mediated resistance to β-lactams took a long time to become established in *V. cholerae*. The first carrier strains were isolated in Algeria in 1973 by Rahal et al. In 1977, plasmid-mediated resistance was described in Asia. The enzymes were of the TEM-1 type.

A new plasmid-mediated β-lactamase, SAR-1, was isolated in 1976 during the fourth cholera epidemic in Tanzania. This involved two strains of *V. cholerae* serotype O_1 Inaba, referenced under codes DT 136 and DT 138 (Table 34). The enzyme is carried on plasmids pUK 657 and pUK 658. It has a molecular weight of 33.7 and a pI of 4.9. This enzyme hydrolyzes penicillin G, ampicillin, carbenicillin, cephaloridine, cefamandole, and nitrocefin (Table 35). It does not hydrolyze methicillin, cloxacillin, or cefotaxime.

This enzyme is inhibited by cloxacillin (50% inhibitory dose [ID_{50}], 7 mM) and by clavulanic acid (ID_{50}, 5 mM).

Table 34 MICs for *V. cholerae* DT 136 and DT 138

Drug	MIC (μg/ml)
Ampicillin	>1,000
Carbenicillin	>1,000
Cephaloridine	16
Cephradine	16

Table 35 K_m and V_{max} for *V. cholerae*

Drug	K_m (μM)	V_{max}
Penicillin G	42	100
Ampicillin	68	63
Carbenicillin	190	122
Cephaloridine	93	21
Cefamandole	95	53
Nitrocefin	83	89

The carrier plasmid also possesses the gene for resistance to trimethoprim (dihydrofolate reductase type I).

7.2.6. Pharmacokinetics

The α-aminopenicillins are zwitterionic compounds. They are completely ionized in the gastrointestinal tract and are relatively insoluble. They are absorbed by a saturable transport mechanism and utilize the dipeptide transport system. Their pharmacokinetics are dose dependent, related in part to saturation of the transport system.

Passage of the α-amino-β-lactams occurs via the dipeptide transport system in rodents and in the small intestine in humans. The passage of dipeptides is associated with the penetration of protons via a pH gradient (intraluminal pH < intracellular pH). The gradient is generated and maintained by the Na^+/H^+ exchange system in the enterocyte brush border. The absorption of an Na^+ ion occurs in exchange for a proton. This results in an acidic microenvironment (pH 5.5 to 6.0) in the brush border.

The Na^+/K^+-ATPase system located in the basement membrane of the enterocyte actively eliminates the Na^+ ion from the enterocyte, resulting in the reduction of the intracytoplasmic pool of sodium, causing protons to penetrate the brush border (Fig. 9).

7.2.6.1. Ampicillin

After intravenous administration, the apparent elimination half-life of ampicillin (Fig. 10) is between 1.0 and 1.5 h. The plasma clearance is on the order of 350 ml/min, and 85% of the dose is eliminated in the urine. Biliary elimination represents less than 10% of the administered dose.

Intramuscularly, the bioavailability varies according to the pharmaceutical formulation. The sodium salt of ampicillin trihydrate is 87% absorbed, whereas the benzathine salt is only 37% absorbed.

Oral absorption is moderate, accounting for 32 to 53% of the administered dose. Absorption is dose independent up to a unit dose of 1.0 g. Food delays and reduces the quantity of ampicillin absorbed. It is 18 to 29% plasma protein bound.

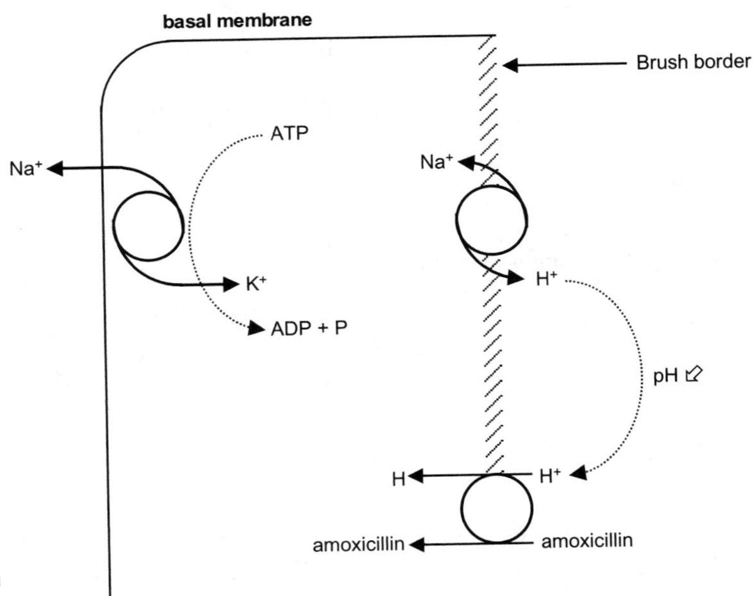

Figure 9 Absorption of amoxicillin by enterocytes

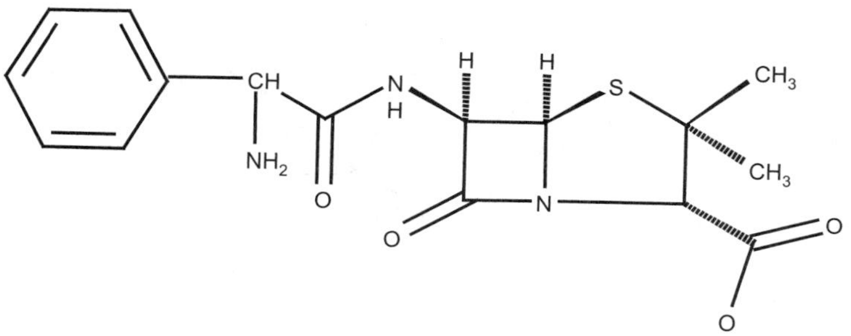

Figure 10 Ampicillin

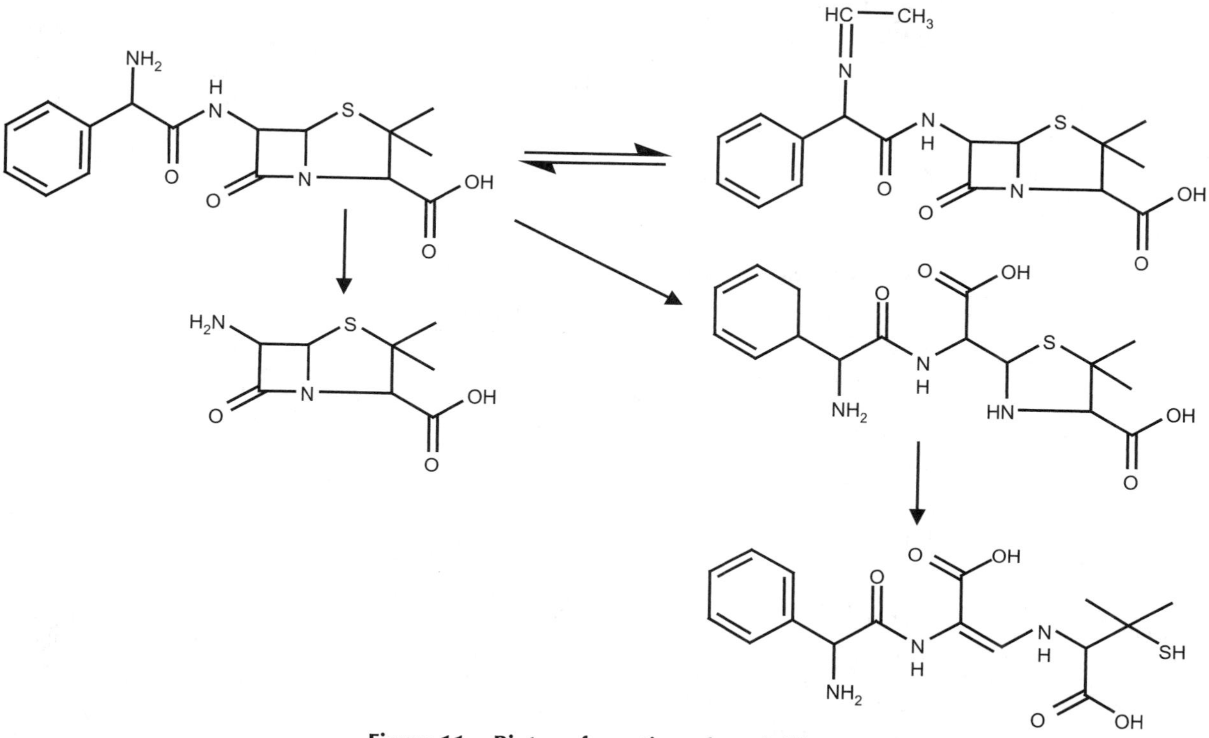

Figure 11 Biotransformation of ampicillin

Ampicillin is biotransformed (Fig. 11). About 10% of the orally administered dose is eliminated in the urine in the form of penicilloic acid. α-Aminobenzylpenamaldic acid has been identified in the urine, as well as traces of 6-aminopenicillanic acid.

Simultaneous administration of probenecid reduces the renal clearance of ampicillin, increasing the concentration in serum by a factor of 2.

Ampicillin readily penetrates interstitial fluid, pleural fluid, synovial fluid, and CSF. The concentrations in bronchial secretions, lung tissue, and renal tissue are high.

Ampicillin is eliminated in colostrum, reaching a concentration 10 to 30% that of serum after 6 h.

7.2.6.1.1. Children. The apparent elimination half-life is 2.2 h in children aged 2 to 5 days, 3.4 h in those 1 day old, and 1.1 h in those over 4 months old.

7.2.6.1.2. Patients with renal insufficiency. When the creatinine clearance is less than 10 ml/min, the plasma clearance is 15% that of subjects with normal renal function, with an apparent elimination half-life of up to 20 h.

7.2.6.1.3. Cirrhotic patients. The concentrations of ampicillin in the ascites fluid are low, and the apparent elimination half-life is increased.

7.2.6.2. Amoxicillin

Amoxicillin (Fig. 12) is *para*-hydroxyampicillin. It is characterized by better oral bioavailability than ampicillin, ranging from 60 to 89% depending on the study (Table 36). This bioavailability varies with the quantity of fluid absorbed, a small volume of fluid being responsible for the poorer dissolution of amoxicillin tablets. It does not appear to be affected by the ingestion of food.

The apparent elimination half-life after intravenous administration is 1.0 to 1.5 h. Renal clearance is 280 ml/min, and plasma clearance is 330 ml/min. The pharmacokinetics of amoxicillin and ampicillin following intravenous administration are superimposable (Table 37). The concentrations of amoxicillin in plasma vary according to the duration of administration; after administration of 250 mg over 3 and 30 min, the concentrations are 63 and 38 μg/ml, respectively. After 500 and 1,000 mg, the concentrations are, respectively, 62.5 and 143 μg/ml. After infusion of 2.0 g of amoxicillin

Figure 12 Amoxicillin

Table 36 Bioavailability of amoxicillin orally[a]

Dose (mg)	Route[b]	C_0 (μg/ml)	C_{max} (μg/ml)	T_{max} (h)	C_{8h} (μg/ml)	AUC (μg · h/ml)	F (%)[c]
1,000	i.v.	77.6		0.08	0.3	53.45	
1,000	p.o.		8.2	1.75	0.3	29.72	56.2 ± 9.4

[a]Data from Westphal et al., 1991.
[b]i.v., intravenous; p.o., per os.
[c]Mean ± standard deviation.

Table 37 Intravenous pharmacokinetics of ampicillin and amoxicillin[a]

Drug	Dose (mg)	Concn in plasma (μg/ml)						
		C_0	0.5 h	1 h	1.5 h	2 h	3 h	6 h
Amoxicillin	500	62.5	14.9	8.4	4.6	3.7	1.9	≤0.5
Ampicillin	500	67.7	16	10	7.1	4.4	2.1	≤0.5
Amoxicillin	1,000	142.7	30.8	19	11.9	8.3	3.9	0.8
Ampicillin	1,000	149.9	31.4	17.9	9.5	6.4	2.9	≤0.5

[a]Data from Brogden et al., 1979.

over 30 min, the concentration at the end of infusion is 133 μg/ml.

Intramuscularly, the bioavailability is on the order of 73.2 to 87.2%. After administration of 250 mg intramuscularly, the peak level in serum is 5.36 μg/ml. The apparent volume of distribution is 0.31 to 0.41 liter/kg at steady state.

Plasma protein binding is 17 to 21%. The plasma kinetics are independent of the dose up to 1.0 g, beyond which they are not linear.

Amoxicillin is eliminated by tubular secretion, as demonstrated by the simultaneous administration of probenecid.

7.2.6.2.1. Children. Because of the physiological immaturity of glomerular filtration and renal tubular secretion in the neonate under 3 weeks of age, amoxicillin is eliminated slowly.

In the normotrophic, hypotrophic, or premature neonate (37 weeks of gestation), the apparent elimination half-life is 5.14 ± 3.43 h, with an apparent volume of distribution of 1.38 liters/kg that is uncorrelated with birth weight (Peskine et al., 1982). The plasma clearance is 0.21 ± 0.3 liter/kg/h. In the premature neonate of 28 weeks' gestation, the apparent elimination half-life is 6.0 h, with a plasma clearance of 0.02 liter/kg/h and an apparent volume of distribution of 0.14 liter/kg. The concentration in plasma is 95 μg/ml at the end of infusion and 19 μg/ml at 8 h.

7.2.6.2.2. Patients with renal insufficiency. It is not necessary to modify the daily dosage in patients with renal insufficiency (Table 38) whose creatinine clearance, is greater than 30 ml/min. Amoxicillin is eliminated by hemodialysis, but only very little by peritoneal dialysis.

7.2.6.2.3. Elderly subjects. In elderly patients, the pharmacokinetics of ampicillin and amoxicillin are identical to those in young adults and dependent on the functional state of the kidney (Table 39).

7.2.6.2.4. Biotransformation. Amoxicillin is transformed to penicilloic acid (Fig. 13). This degradation product represents 35% of the dose eliminated in the urine. Bioautographic assays have not revealed other metabolites.

7.2.6.2.5. Tissue distribution. In patients suffering from meningitis, the concentrations of amoxicillin in the CSF are high, but they vary from patient to patient. After a single intravenous dose of 2.0 g, the concentrations are between 2.9 and 40 μg/ml 1 h after the end of infusion and between 2.6 and 27 μg/ml 1.5 and 4.0 h afterwards. Therapeutic concentrations are reached in other tissues or fluids such as lung tissue, maxillary sinuses, interstitial fluid, etc.

7.2.6.2.6. Interactions with other medicinal products. Prednisolone has no effect on amoxicillin pharmacokinetics.

Table 38 Amoxicillin in patients with renal insufficiency

Creatinine clearance (ml/min)	$t_{1/2}$ (h)
120–80	1.32
80–10	2.77
30–10	6.89
<10	14.5

Table 39 Ampicillin and amoxicillin pharmacokinetics in elderly subjects

Drug	Subjects age (yr)	AUC (μg · h/ml)	$t_{1/2}$ (h)	CL_p (ml/min)	CL_R (ml/min)	Urinary elimination (%)
Ampicillin	>65	39	2.02	205	163	79.7
	<65		1.7	176–239	167	~80
Amoxicillin	>65	42.8	2.17	192	154	81.7
	<65		1.4–2.2	185	136–189	~80

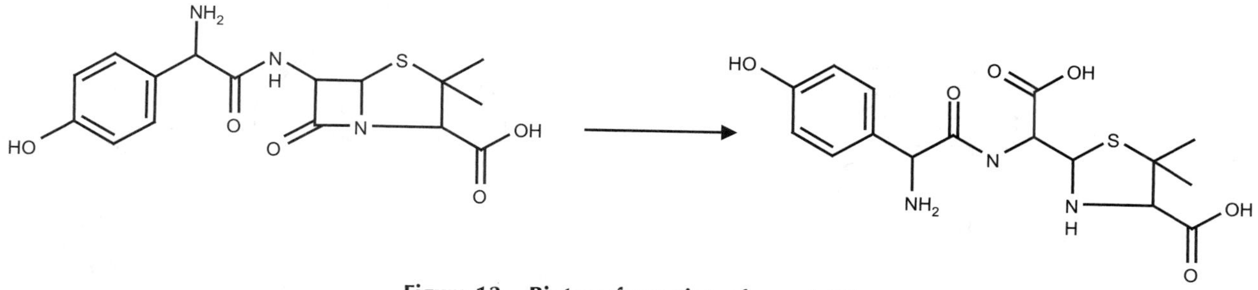

Figure 13 Biotransformation of amoxicillin

Food delays absorption and reduces the maximum concentration of drug in serum but does not significantly affect the bioavailability. Pirenzepine does not affect the pharmacokinetics of amoxicillin. Ranitidine reduces the maximum concentration of the drug and the area under the curve but less than cimetidine, probably because of the better solubility of amoxicillin at a higher pH. Maalox increases the absorption of amoxicillin due to an increase in intestinal motility by $Mg(OH)_2$.

7.2.6.3. Hetacillin

Hetacillin is obtained by condensation of acetone and ampicillin. Hetacillin is rapidly hydrolyzed to ampicillin. The hydrolysis half-life is 20 to 25 min at 37°C and neutral pH. Little hetacillin is detected in the plasma after oral absorption. The peak hetacillin concentration is similar to that obtained with an equivalent dose of ampicillin (Table 40).

The advantage of hetacillin over ampicillin is that it is stable in solution. After intravenous administration of hetacillin, it is detectable in the plasma only for the first hour after infusion. Traces of hetacillin are found in the urine. The plasma half-life of hetacillin is about 11 min, with a plasma clearance of 7.5 liters/min.

Sixty-eight percent of ampicillin is released in the 10 min following intramuscular administration, and 95% is released after 60 min. The plasma peak is reached within 1 h. This suggests that hetacillin is absorbed, reaches the systemic circulation, and is hydrolyzed to ampicillin.

Orally ingested hetacillin is transformed in the gastrointestinal tract, and only ampicillin is detected in the plasma. The bioavailability of ampicillin after absorption of hetacillin is about 30%. It is slightly increased by food.

Sarpicillin is the methoxymethyl ester of hetacillin.

7.2.6.4. Metampicillin

Metampicillin results from the condensation of formaldehyde and ampicillin. The hydrolysis half-life is 1 h in an aqueous medium (37°C, pH 7). Hydrolysis releases ampicillin and formaldehyde (Table 40).

After oral absorption, the pharmacokinetics are those of ampicillin. A small quantity of metampicillin is present in the plasma and urine. Metampicillin is extensively eliminated in the bile (≥10%).

7.2.6.5. Azidocillin

Azidocillin is rapidly transformed to penicillin. Two other metabolites have been detected in the urine: α-azidobenzylpenicilloic acid and α-hydroxybenzylpenicillin (Fig. 14). Azidocillin represents about 5% of the products eliminated in the urine. Urinary levels are dependent on the salt administered: the concentration is 85% after intramuscular administration of the potassium salt, but the concentration is much lower with the dibenzylethylenediamine salt. Azidocillin is eliminated partly via the renal tubules, as demonstrated by simultaneous administration of probenecid.

Table 40 Oral pharmacokinetics of α-aminopenicillins

Drug	Dose (mg)	C_{max} (μg/ml)	$t_{1/2}$ (h)	CL_R (ml/min)	Urinary elimination (%)	Absorption (%)	Protein binding (%)
Ampicillin	500	2.4–6.3	0.6–1.2	210–341	29–60	32–48	15–18
Amoxicillin	500	5.7–10.8	1–1.3	278–297	44–79	≈85	17
Hetacillin	500	2.5–3	1.1–1.3	195–328	28–76	32–42	16
Epicillin	500	2.32–4.7	1–1.2	208	26–35	50	10–30
Metampicillin[a]	500	3	1.8–2		33		

[a]Ampicillin.

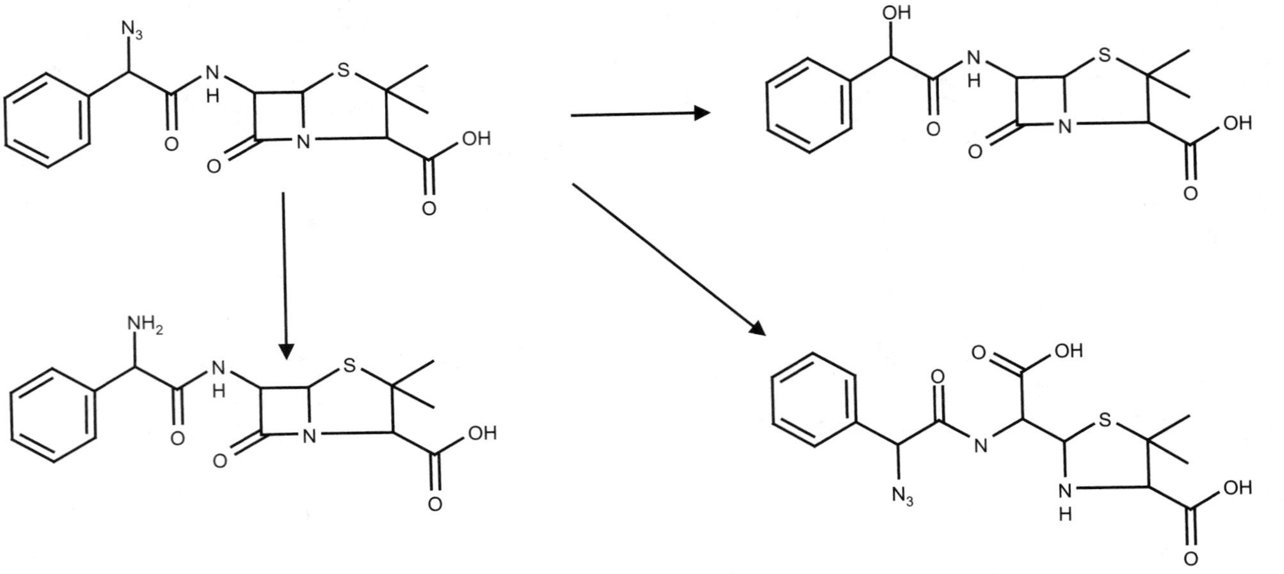

Figure 14 Metabolism of azidocillin

It is 83 to 85% plasma protein bound. It is distributed in the bronchial secretions and amniotic fluid.

7.2.6.6. Epicillin

About 27% of the administered dose is eliminated in the urine in the form of epicillin and of an active metabolite, the structure of which has not been elucidated. Biliary elimination is extensive; peak biliary levels are reached 1 h after ingestion of epicillin.

Plasma protein binding is on the order of 10 to 30% (Table 40).

7.2.6.7. Cyclacillin

After oral administration, 50 to 70% of the dose is eliminated in the urine in the unchanged form, 17% is eliminated in the form of penicilloic acid, and 2% is eliminated in the form of 1-aminocyclohexanecarboxylic acid (Fig. 15).

The absorption and biotransformation of cyclacillin are independent of the administered dose between 250 and 1,000 mg. The apparent elimination half-life is on the order of 15 min and may attain 21 h in patients with renal insufficiency (creatinine clearance, ≤10 ml/min).

It is 18 to 23% plasma protein bound.

7.3. *N*-Acylpenicillins

7.3.1. Physicochemical Properties

The *N*-acylpenicillins (Fig. 16 and 17) are more stable in urine (pH 4.7 to 5.8) than in plasma (pH 7.4) or phosphate buffer (pH 8.8).

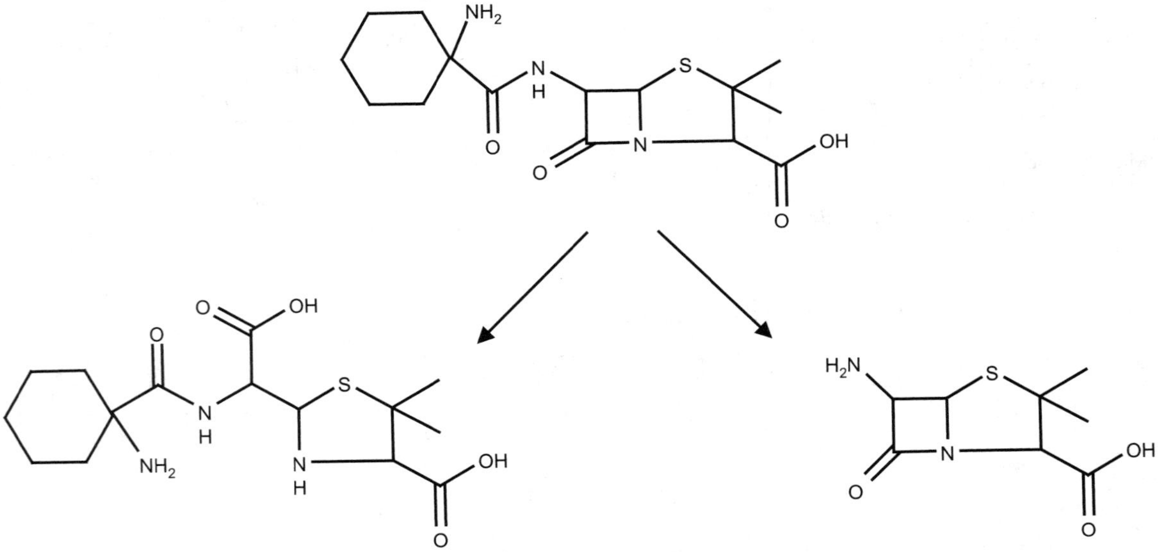

Figure 15 Biotransformation of cyclacillin

	R_1	R_2
Apalcillin	H	
Piperacillin	H	
Furbenicillin	H	
Pirbenicillin	H	
VX-VC 43	OH	
Bay f 5795	H	
Aspoxicillin	OH	$-CHNH_2(CH_2CONHCH_3)$

Figure 16 ***N*-Acylpenicillins (1)**

Maximum stability is obtained at a pH of between 4.0 and 6.0. More acidic pH causes hydrolysis of the carbonyl-lactam bond with the formation of a degradation product, penicilloate, obtained by decarboxylation of penicilloic acid (pH ~3).

At a higher pH (pH 9 to 10), degradation of the β-lactam nucleus occurs with the production of penicilloate. Piperacillin is more stable in an alkaline solution (degradation half-life in an acidic medium, ~4.7 h) than mezlocillin and azlocillin, but at pH 10 piperacillin is entirely degraded within 1 h.

The physicochemical properties of the *N*-acylpenicillins are summarized in Table 41.

7.3.2. Structure-Activity Relationship

Among the *N*-acylpenicillins, four subgroups may be distinguished: the carbamoyls and the ureido-, acylureido-, and carbamoylureidopenicillins (Fig. 18 and 19).

The introduction of a carbamoylpiperazinyl group on the amino residue of ampicillin gave rise to molecules with good activity against *P. aeruginosa*. On the piperazine nucleus, the presence of oxo groups and their position in the ring have little effect on the antibacterial activity of the molecules. The 2′,3′-dioxopiperazine nucleus provides the best antibacterial activity (piperacillin), followed by the 2′-oxopiperazine, piperazine, 3′-oxopiperazine, 3′, 6-dioxopiperazine and 3′,5′-dioxopiperazine nuclei. The length of the alkyl chain on the nitrogen at position 4′ of the piperazine nucleus does not significantly alter the antibacterial activity but does affect the acute toxicity of the molecules and the protein binding and lipophilicity (Table 42). The intravenous median lethal dose varies considerably with the length of the alkyl chain. The greater the length of the chain, the more the toxicity increases.

Numerous molecules have been synthesized by Komatsu et al. (1981), from among which apalcillin (Fig. 20) was selected. Two types of derivatives have been synthesized: molecules with a monocyclic and those with a bicyclic heteroatomic nucleus. Derivatives with a pyridine nucleus are the most active. The presence of a chlorine atom does not affect the activity, whereas a hydroxyl group abolishes it. Identical results have been obtained with pyridazine and pyrimidine nuclei. Among the bicyclic derivatives possessing a quinoline or naphthyridine nucleus, those with a 1,5-naphthyridine nucleus are the most active. Substitution by a hydroxyl group at position 4′ gave rise to apalcillin. Other substituents have been attached at position 6′, such as methylmercapto, dimethylamine, or methoxy. These molecules exhibit weaker

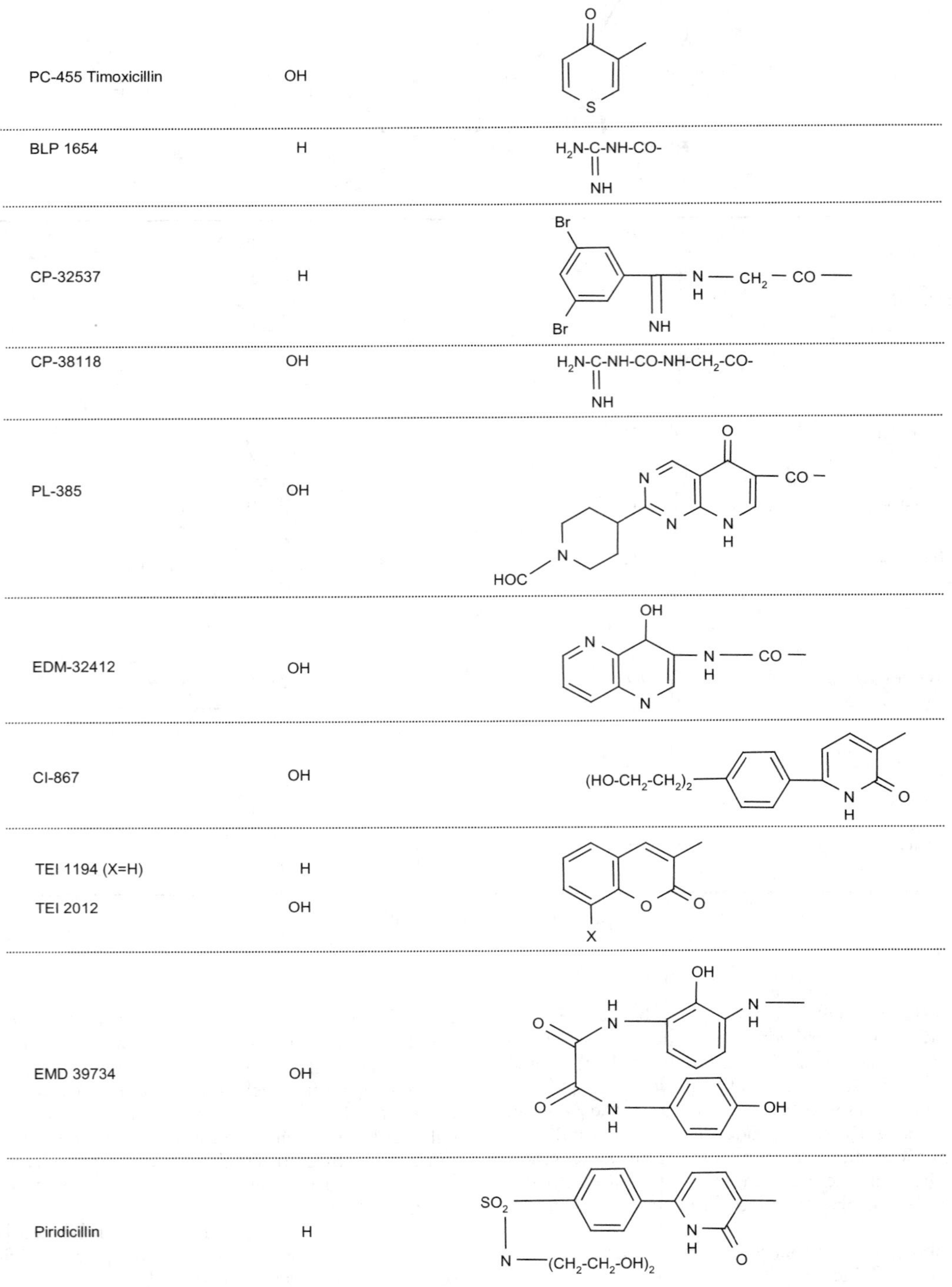

PC-455 Timoxicillin	OH	
BLP 1654	H	H_2N-C(=NH)-NH-CO-
CP-32537	H	
CP-38118	OH	H_2N-C(=NH)-NH-CO-NH-CH_2-CO-
PL-385	OH	
EDM-32412	OH	
CI-867	OH	
TEI 1194 (X=H)	H	
TEI 2012	OH	
EMD 39734	OH	
Piridicillin	H	

Figure 17 *N*-Acylpenicillins (2)

Table 41 Physicochemical properties of *N*-acylpenicillins

Drug	Empirical formular	Molecular weight	pH of solution at 10%	Na (mmol/g)	pK	Melting point (°C)
Azlocillin	$C_{20}H_{22}N_2O_6Sna$	483.5	6.7–7.3	2.17	2.85	
Mezlocillin	$C_{21}H_{24}N_5O_8S_2$	539.6	4.5–8	1.85		200–210
Piperacillin	$C_{23}H_{26}N_5O_7Sna$	539.6	5–7.5	1.98	4.14	180
Ampicillin	$C_{25}H_{22}N_5O_6Sna$	543.5	6.5–8.5	1.84		236–238

activity against *P. aeruginosa*. Replacement of the phenyl nucleus by a cyclohexadienyl, cyclohexenyl, or cyclohexanyl ring reduces the antibacterial activity, as does a benzene ring or an aliphatic chain. The pharmacokinetics in the rat and mouse are little affected by the nature of the substituents on the pyridine, quinoline, and naphthyridine rings. The presence of a cyclohexadienyl, cyclohexenyl, or cyclohexanyl nucleus reduces the concentrations in serum.

7.3.3. In Vitro Antibacterial Activity

The *N*-acylpenicillins are hydrolyzed by *S. aureus* penicillinases and as a rule are less active than penicillin G and ampicillin against gram-positive cocci and bacteria, with the exception of *Enterococcus* spp., against which they possess activity similar to that of ampicillin. They exhibit good activity against anaerobic bacteria. Piperacillin is much more active than ticarcillin against *P. aeruginosa* and *Klebsiella* spp.,

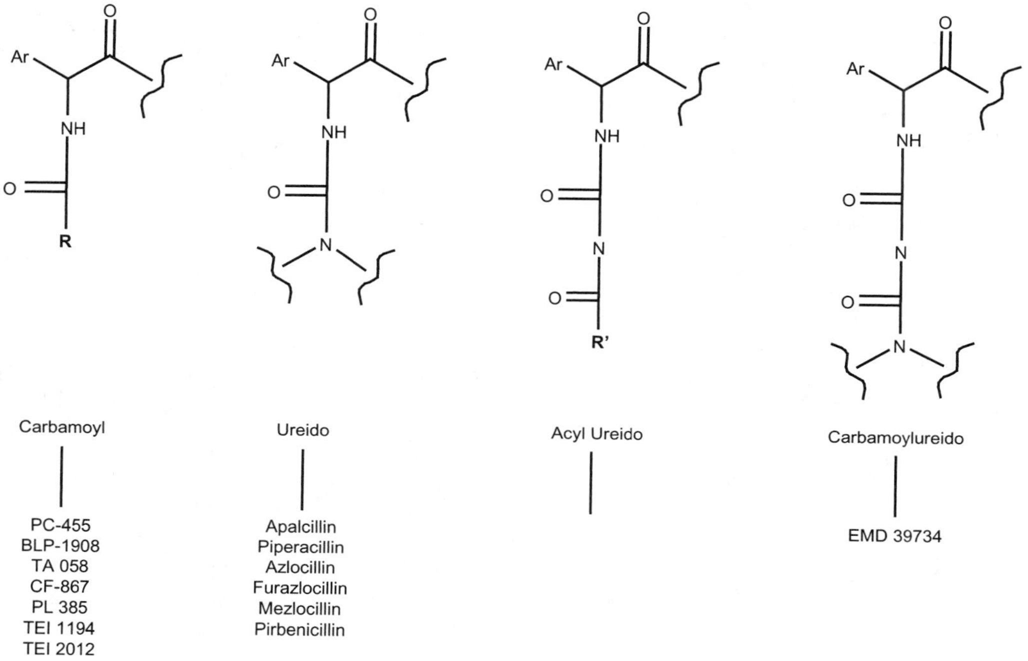

Carbamoyl: PC-455, BLP-1908, TA 058, CF-867, PL 385, TEI 1194, TEI 2012

Ureido: Apalcillin, Piperacillin, Azlocillin, Furazlocillin, Mezlocillin, Pirbenicillin

Acyl Ureido

Carbamoylureido: EMD 39734

Figure 18 ***N*-Acylpenicillins**

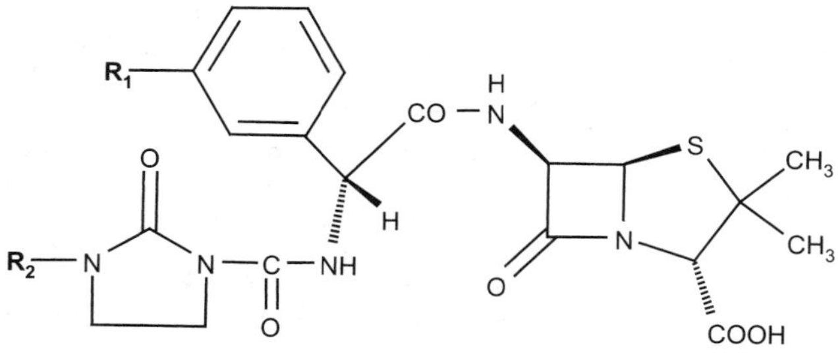

	R_1	R_2
Mezlocillin	H	CH_3SO_2-
Azlocillin	H	H-
Furazlocillin	OH	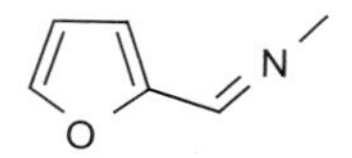 [furfurylideneamino]

Figure 19 ***N*-Acylpenicillin imidazole derivatives**

Table 42 Structure-activity relationship of the piperacillin derivatives

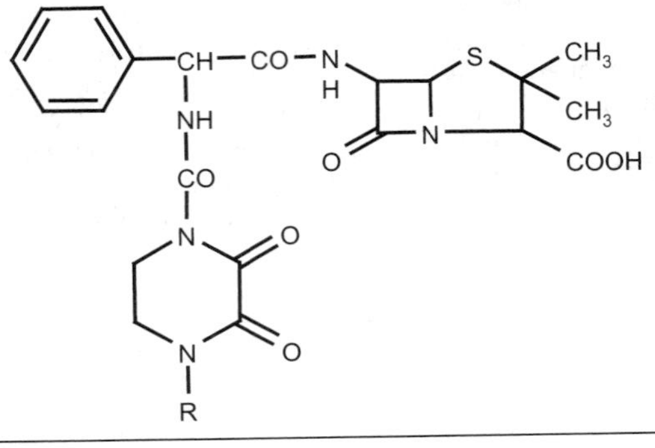

Drug	R	Molecular weight	Protein binding (%)	$CHCl_3$/water-pH 7	50% Lethal dose (mg/kg)
T-1183	$-CH_3$	503.5	15.5	4.3×10^{-3}	4,000
T-1220 (piperacillin)	$-C_2H_5$	517.6	25.3	8.7×10^{-3}	5,000
T-1221	$-C_4H_9$	545.6	35.1	3.9×10^{-2}	1,800
T-1213	$-C_8H_{17}$	601.7	92.0	8.7×10^{0}	300
Ampicillin		349.4	22.9		4,600

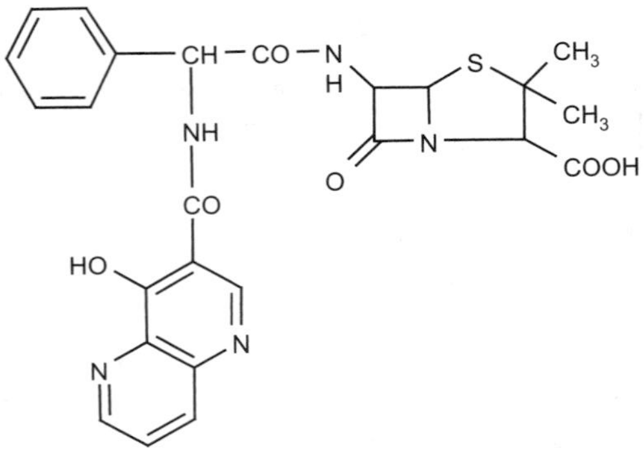

Figure 20 Apalcillin

but its activity against the other gram-negative bacteria is the same. Azlocillin possesses activity similar to that of piperacillin against *P. aeruginosa*, but it is moderately active against *Enterobacteriaceae*. Mezlocillin has the same antibacterial spectrum as ticarcillin but is inactive against *P. aeruginosa* (Tables 43 and 44).

These molecules are hydrolyzed by broad-spectrum β-lactamases, in contrast to the so-called third-generation (expanded-spectrum) cephalosporins.

7.3.4. Breakpoints

The breakpoints for the *N*-acylpenicillins recommended by the French Antibiotic Sensitivity Test Committee are reported in Table 45.

7.3.5. Epidemiology of Resistance

An epidemiological study conducted in Europe showed that resistances of gram-negative bacilli were identical in northern and southern Europe. Resistance to ampicillin and piperacillin increased in northern Europe from 8% in 1984 to 26 and 28% in 1987 and 1988, respectively. In central Europe, the resistances were, respectively, 18 and 16% in 1984 and 28 and 26% in 1987 and 1988. In southern Europe, the levels of resistance in 1984 were, respectively, 13 and 10%, and in 1987 and 1988 they were 46 and 38% (Dornbusch and the European Study Group on Antibiotic Resistance, 1990) (Table 46).

7.3.6. Pharmacokinetics

The pharmacokinetics of *N*-acylpenicillins are shown in Tables 47 and 48.

7.3.6.1. BL-P1654

BL-P1654 (Clarke et al., 1974) is a guanylureidopenicillin. After intravenous infusion of 0.5 and 1.0 g of BL-P1654, the measured concentrations in plasma are, respectively, 41 and 81 μg/ml. At the end of infusion of 0.5 and 1.0 g for 60 min, levels in plasma are, respectively, 22.6 and 47 μg/ml. Six hours after the end of the infusion, the concentrations in plasma are, respectively, 3.4 and 5.4 μg/ml.

The apparent elimination half-life is 2.37 h. Seventy-three percent of the administered dose is found in the urine after 48 h. Plasma protein binding is 20%. Renal clearance is 79 ml/min. Urinary elimination is by glomerular filtration; combination with probenecid does not increase the elimination half-life and does not affect the pharmacokinetic parameters.

Intramuscularly, the bioavailability is excellent. After an intramuscular injection of 1.0 g, the peak concentration in serum of 28.4 μg/ml is reached in 0.75 h.

Renal toxicity led to the development of this molecule being stopped. Administration of 100 to 400 mg/kg to dogs for 4 days caused slowly regressing tubular necrosis.

7.3.6.2. Pirbenicillin

The concentration after infusion of 3.0 g of pirbenicillin in 25 min is 455 μg/ml. The apparent elimination half-life is 78 min, with urinary elimination of 87%.

Table 43 In vitro activities of *N*-acyl- and α-carboxypenicillins

Organism(s)	MIC (μg/ml)						
	Carbenicillin	Ticarcillin	Sulbenicillin	Azlocillin	Mezlocillin	Apalcillin	Piperacillin
S. aureus Pen[s]	1	1	2	1	1	1	0.5
S. aureus Pen[r]	16	16	8	>128	>128	>128	>128
S. pyogenes	0.5	0.25	0.5	0.03	0.06	0.03	0.03
S. pneumoniae	1	0.5	1	0.03	0.03	0.03	0.03
E. faecalis	32	32	32	2	2	4	2
H. influenzae Amp[s]	0.5	0.5		0.06	0.12	0.06	0.03
H. influenzae Amp[r]	>32	>32		4	4	4	4
E. coli	4	4	4	16	4	4	2
K. pneumoniae	>128	>128	>128	64	32	156	16
Enterobacter spp.	16	8		32	4	4	2
Citrobacter spp.	16	8		8	4	4	4
S. marcescens	16	8		16	4	4	2
P. mirabilis	1	1	1	4	1	1	0.5
S. enterica, serovar Typhi	4	4	4	4	4	4	4
Shigella spp.	8	8	8	4	4	4	4
P. aeruginosa	64	32	32	4	32	2	2

Table 44 In vitro activities of *N*-acylpenicillins

Organism	MIC (μg/ml)				
	BLP1654	Pirbenicillin	Furazlocillin	Timoxicillin (PC 455)	Piperacillin
S. aureus Pen[r]	128	32	128		>128
S. pneumoniae	0.5	1	0.25	≤0.1	0.5
H. influenzae Amp[s]/Amp[r]	0.5–16	1–32	0.25–4		0.2–4
E. coli	8	8	1	1.56	2
K. pneumoniae	64	128	2	12.5	8
Morganella morganii	128	32	1	12.5	2
S. marcescens	32	32	2		4
P. aeruginosa	16	16	8	3.13	8

Table 45 Breakpoints for the *N*-acylpenicillins recommended by the French Antibiotic Sensitivity Test Committee[a]

Drug	Load (μg)	MIC (μg/ml)		Zone diam (mm)	
		S	R	S	R
Mezlocillin	76	≤8	>32	≥21	<16
Piperacillin					
Enterococcus	75	≤8	>64	≥20	<12
P. aeruginosa	75	≤16	>64	≥18	<12
Azlocillin	75	≤16	>64	≥19	<13

[a]S, susceptible; R, resistant.

7.3.6.3. Azlocillin

The pharmacokinetics of azlocillin (Singlas and Haegel, 1984) are not linear. Dose independence is evidenced in the lack of proportionality of the concentrations in plasma at the end of infusion. The apparent elimination half-life increases and the plasma clearance decreases when the administered doses are increased. The apparent elimination half-lives are 0.89, 0.98, and 1.5 h and the plasma clearances are 12.2, 9.4, and 6.6 liters/h with doses of 1.0, 2.0, and 5.0 g, respectively, administered in the form of a 5-min bolus (Bergan et al., 1982).

About 60% of the administered dose is eliminated in the urine, the renal clearance being 112 ml/min; extrarenal clearance decreases threefold when the dose is increased from 1 to 5 g, whereas renal clearance decreases by only 30%. The reduction in renal clearance in relation to the dose might be due to the saturation of active tubular secretion. Azlocillin is weakly eliminated in the bile, accounting for between 0.2 and 7.5% of the administered dose.

In patients with renal insufficiency, the apparent elimination half-life is prolonged (Leroy et al., 1980) and the dosage must be adapted accordingly. Azlocillin is eliminated by hemodialysis (30 to 46%). Peritoneal dialysis reduces the elimination half-life from 5 to 6 h to 2.6 h.

The elimination half-life is increased in children under 3 months of age (Table 49).

In premature neonates the apparent elimination half-life is 4.4 h, while in normotrophic neonates it is between 2.6 and 3.4 h; in infants over 3 months of age it is 0.97 h.

Almost 6% of administered azlocillin is eliminated in the form of inactive penicilloate.

Table 46 Epidemiology of resistance of *E. coli* to ampicillin and piperacillin in Europe

Country	% Resistant strains			
	1984		1987–1988	
	Ampicillin	Piperacillin	Ampicillin	Piperacillin
Germany	11	9	25	23
Austria	8	10	23	23
Belgium	48	44	37	33
Denmark			20	20
Spain	8	6	46	42
Finland	11	11	25	25
France	12	10	29	22
Greece	16	14	42	37
Italy	16	8	41	37
The Netherlands	7	4	33	30
Portugal			68	53
The United Kingdom	7	7	50	48
Sweden	6	7	15	12
Switzerland	16	12	20	20

Table 47 Pharmacokinetics of *N*-acylpenicillins

Drug	Dose (g)	C_0 (μg/ml)	C_{1h} (μg/ml)	V (liter/kg)	$AUC_{0-\infty}$ (μg·h/ml)	$t_{1/2\beta}$(h)	CL_P (liters/h)	CL_R (liters/h)	CL_{NR} (liters/h)	Urinary elimination (%)
Azlocillin	1			0.23	89.7	0.89	12.2	7.1	5.1	59.4
	2	368	62	0.20	115.3	0.98	9.4	6.5	2.9	72.5
	5			0.21	164.9	1.53	6.6	4.8	1.8	74.7
Mezlocillin	1			0.55	33.5	0.96	31.2	19.0	12.2	60.8
	2	304	41	0.35	47.2	0.79	21.1	14.2	6.9	67.0
	5			0.38	54.8	1.21	17.0	13.2	3.8	69.0
Piperacillin	1			0.31	57.4	0.83	18.5	9.1	9.5	50.0
	2	41	41	0.30	75.3	1.04	14.0	8.4	5.7	60.9
	5			0.25	76.2	0.92	13.5	9.1	4.3	71.3
Alpacillin	1	30		0.16	82.3	1.05	2.2			18.6
	2	60		0.11	174.9	1.10	2.0			16.5
Furazlocillin	2				5.9	1.01	6.0	6.3	3.7	69.0
	4				7.4	1.01				69.0
BL-P1654	3	30				2.10	1.9	1.4		73.0
Pirbenicillin	1	25			130	1.30				87.0

Table 48 Intravenous pharmacokinetics of *N*-acylpenicillins

Drug	Dose (g)	Infusion time (min)	CL_R (liters/h)	CL_P (ml/min)	Biliary elimination (%)	Protein binding (%)	Urinary elimination (%)	
							Parent compound	Metabolites
Mezlocillin	2	60	122	240	20–30	30	60–70	8–12
Azlocillin	2	60	112	180	5–10	40	50–70	6
Piperacillin	2	60	151	183	10–15	22	50–70	10
Apalcillin	2	60	29	139	20–40	86	18–25	18
Furazlocillin	2	30	72	274	26		69	5–7
Pirbenicillin	3	25					87	NR[a]
BL-P1654	1	30	86	114		20	73	NR

[a]NR, metabolites not identified.

Table 49 Pharmacokinetics of azlocillin in children[a]

Subjects	Dose (mg/kg)	n	k_{el} (h^{-1})	V (liters/kg)	$t_{1/2}$ (h)	CL_P (ml/min)	AUC (μg·h/ml)
Prematures	50	7	0.157	0.34	4.41	1.7	
Neonates	50	7	0.204	0.39	3.40		428
	100	6	0.262	0.29	2.65	4.1	1,020
Infants							
<3 months	100	8	0.368	0.41	1.88	8.1	
>3 months	100	8	0.717	0.26	0.97	22.5	
Children >3 years	75	9	0.745	0.23	0.93	88.9	321

[a]Data from Weingärtner et al., 1982.

Azlocillin crosses the fetoplacental barrier. The levels in serum measured in the umbilical artery and vein 1 to 3 h after intravenous administration of 2.0 g are on the order of 20 μg/ml. In gynecological and colonic tissues, azlocillin levels are between 10 and 50 mg/kg 1 to 2 h after intravenous administration of azlocillin.

Therapeutic concentrations have been detected in bone tissue and bronchial secretions. In burn patients, the kinetics of azlocillin are dependent on the extent of the burnt area. Where the burns are not extensive the pharmacokinetics are identical to those in healthy subjects; in the case of extensive burns, however, extrarenal leakage of azlocillin is substantial (Drugeon et al., 1984).

In children suffering from cystic fibrosis, increases in the volume of distribution of azlocillin (0.8 versus 0.2 liter/kg) and renal clearance (150 versus 80 ml/min) are observed (Bergan and Michalsen, 1979).

Protein binding varies with the concentration, increasing from 30 to 40% as the concentration decreases from 200 to 4.0 μg/ml. It occurs by hydrophobic bonds to albumin (20% ± 2% at 200 μg/ml) and to gamma globulins (17% ± 5% at 200 μg/ml).

7.3.6.4. Mezlocillin

Like azlocillin, mezlocillin is administered intravenously and intramuscularly. There is no consensus on the pharmacokinetics of mezlocillin. Bergan (1978) showed that after administration of 1.0, 2.0, and 5.0 g, the areas under the curve were not proportional to the administered doses. These results contradict those of Lode et al. (1977) and Issell et al. (1978). The apparent half-life is on the order of 1 h. About 60% of the administered dose is found within 24 h in the urine. No active metabolites have been detected in the urine, but 8 to 12% penicilloates are found in the urine.

The apparent elimination half-life is modified in patients with renal insufficiency (Cano et al., 1982) (Table 50).

About 25 to 30% of the dose is eliminated in the bile. In patients with hepatic insufficiency, mezlocillin concentrations in the bile decrease (Bunke et al., 1983) (Table 51).

After intramuscular administration of 1.0 g of mezlocillin, the peak concentration in serum is between 13.2 and 45 μg/ml and is reached in 1.0 to 1.5 h. Mezlocillin does not accumulate after repeated dosing.

Intramuscularly, the bioavailability is 63.4% ± 3.6%.

Simultaneous administration of probenecid reduces the renal clearance of mezlocillin (5.2 versus 10.9 liters/h).

In patients over 70 years of age, the pharmacokinetics of mezlocillin are dependent on the patients' renal function, with an increase in nonrenal clearance and areas under the curve. After a dose of 5.0 g, the area under the curve is 403 ± 95.4 μg·h/ml versus 274.1 ± 31.6 μg·h/ml in young subjects (Table 52) (Meyers et al., 1987).

Table 50 Pharmacokinetics in patients with renal insufficiency

Creatinine clearance (ml/min)	Apparent elimination half-life (h)	
	Azlocillin[a]	Mezlocillin
≥80	1.11 ± 0.17	1.17
80–30	2.03 ± 0.63	1.5–2
30–10	4.01 ± 0.69	2.7–3.2
≤10	5.66 ± 0.07	>6
<5	6.53 ± 1.67	6

[a]Means ± standard deviations.

Table 51 Biliary elimination of mezlocillin

Hepatic behavior	No. of patients	Mean % (range) of the administered dose eliminated in bile (8 h)
Standard	4	20.9 (4.1–26.6)
Moderate	2	12.7 (12.4–13.1)
Severe	8	4.4 (0.05–10.5)

The pharmacokinetics in children are reported in Table 53. In prematures, neonates, or infants aged less than 3 months, the apparent elimination half-life is prolonged.

Plasma protein binding ranges from 28 to 40%.

Mezlocillin readily crosses the fetomaternal barrier but is found only in traces in the colostrum. After administration of 5.0 g, levels of about 10 μg/ml are attained (~35 μg/ml in serum). High concentrations of mezlocillin are measured in the bronchial secretions, peritoneal fluid, bone, the aortic valve, muscle, and cutaneous, hepatic, gynecological, and prostatic tissues.

7.3.6.5. Piperacillin

Piperacillin may be administered intravenously (Table 54) or intramuscularly (Table 55). The pharmacokinetics of piperacillin are not linear. The drug is principally eliminated in the urine. Administration of probenecid increases the area under the curve by 65% and the apparent elimination half-life by 25%, while renal clearance is reduced by 40%. Plasma protein binding is 22% (Tjandramaga et al., 1978).

The apparent elimination half-life is prolonged in patients with renal or hepatic insufficiency (De Schepper et al., 1982; Lange et al., 1982).

Table 52 Pharmacokinetics of mezlocillin in elderly subjects

Subjects	Dose (g)	C_0 (μg/ml)[a]	AUC (μg · h/ml)	$t_{1/2β}$ (h)	CL_P (ml/min)	CL_R (ml/min)	Cl_{NR} (ml/min)
Young	5	383 ± 59.6	274.1	1.21	282	219.3	62.3
Elderly (>70 yr)	5	317 ± 98.2	403	1.13	174	44.98	130.15

[a]Means ± standard deviations.

Table 53 Pediatric pharmacokinetics of mezlocillin[a]

Subjects	Dose (mg/kg)	n	k_{el} (h^1)	V (liters/kg)	$t_{1/2}$ (h)	AUC (μg · h/ml)
Prematures	50	6	0.21	0.26	3.3	929
	75	7	0.195	0.27	3.55	1,415
	100	8	0.302	0.28	2.29	1,182
Neonates	150	6	0.294	0.36	2.38	1,412
	200	7	0.263	0.40	2.45	1,753
Infants						
<3 months	150	7	0.364	0.49	1.93	578
>3 months	150	6	0.782	0.34	0.89	596
Children >3 years	100	6	0.808	0.24	0.86	516

[a]Data from Weingärtner et al., 1982.

Table 54 Pharmacokinetics of ascending intravenous doses of piperacillin[a]

Dose (g)	C_0 (μg/ml)	$t_{1/2β}$ (h)	AUC (μg · h/ml)	CL_P (ml/min)	CL_R (ml/min)	CL_{NR} (ml/min)	Urinary elimination (%)
1	70.7	0.6	36	408.6	303.6	105.1	74.1
2	199.5	0.9	102	301.8	245.7	54.7	81.4
4	330.7	1.02	250	254.2	203.7	53.8	79.8
6	451.8	1.05	437.9	209.6	186.9	24.3	89.1

[a]Data from Tjandramaga et al., 1978.

Table 55 Intramuscular pharmacokinetics of piperacillin[a]

Dose (g)	n	C_{max} (μg/ml)	T_{max} (min)	$t_{1/2β}$ (min)	AUC (μg · h/ml)	CL_P (ml/min)	CL_R (ml/min)	CL_{NR} (ml/min)	Urinary elimination (%)
0.5	8	4.9	33.8	60.2	10.3	584	431.6	152.4	57
1	8	13.3	37.5	68.7	29.2	422.3	314.3	108	57
2	8	30.2	48.8	60.6	85.2	290.8	219.8	71	59
1[b]	8	15.3		65.3	37.8	412.8	264.2		63
1[c]	8	20		84.6	62.3	252.6	157.2		61

[a]Data from Tjandramaga et al., 1978.
[b]With probenecid.
[c]Without probenecid.

In patients undergoing hemodialysis (Francke et al., 1979), the apparent elimination half-life outside the dialysis period is 2.1 h. About 46% of piperacillin is eliminated by hemodialysis (Heim-Duthoy et al., 1986).

The apparent elimination half-life in infants is longer than in adults (Rubio et al., 1982). The half-life is shorter in preadolescents (Thiramoorthi et al., 1983), being 47 min in children aged 1 to 6 months and 29 min in children aged 6 months to 12 years (Wilson et al., 1982) (Table 56).

Piperacillin is metabolized and desethylpiperacillin exhibits good antibacterial activity (Minami et al., 1991) (Tables 57 and 58).

Piperacillin is widely distributed in tissues, including CSF, with concentrations of up to 26 μg/ml.

7.3.6.6. Aspoxicillin

After intravenous administration of 1.0 g (60 min), the concentration at the end of the infusion is 106.4 μg/ml, with an area under the curve of 101.7 μg · h/ml. The apparent elimination half-life is 1.7 h. About 87.9% of the administered dose is eliminated renally.

After intramuscular injection of 1.0 g, the peak concentration in serum is 23.8 μg/ml and is reached in 0.75 h. The area under the curve is 80 μg/ml. Bioavailability is on the

Table 56 Pharmacokinetics of piperacillin in infants (50 mg/kg)[a]

Route	Age (days)	n	k_{el} (h^{-1})	$t_{1/2}$(min)	AUC (μg · h/ml)	CL_P (ml/min)	C_0 (μg/ml)
Intravenous	1–5	17	0.20	217	677	32.3	129
	6–10	12	0.27	162	536	40.5	141
	10	5	0.30	127	505	34.6	154
Intramuscular	1–5	3	0.18	239	606	27.4	
	6–10	4	0.20	244	603	29.2	
	10	3	0.20	211	446	34.6	

[a]Data from Rubio al., 1982.

Table 57 Antibacterial activities of piperacillin and its metabolite[a]

Organism	MIC (μg/ml)	
	Piperacillin	Desethylpiperacillin
S. aureus 209 P	0.78	1.56
S. pyogenes Cook	0.10	0.10
E. coli NIHJ-JC2	1.56	6.25
K. pneumoniae PCI 602	1.56	12.5
E. cloacae 963	1.56	12.5
M. morganii IFO 3848	0.05	0.05
Providencia rettgeri IFO 3850	0.20	0.78
S. marcescens IAM 1184	0.78	12.5
P. aeruginosa NCTC 10490	1.56	6.25

[a]Data from Minami et al., 1991.

Table 58 Pharmacokinetics of YP-14 (desethylpiperacillin) after 2 g of piperacillin intramuscularly

Parameter	Value
C_{max} (μg/ml)	3.1
$AUC_{0-\infty}$ (μg · h/ml)	8.4
T_{max} (h)	1.5
$t_{1/2}$(h)	1.17
Urinary elimination (%)	7.9

order of 80% (Shishido et al., 1982). Plasma protein binding is 24%. Aspoxicillin is metabolized. Simultaneous administration of probenecid does not alter the pharmacokinetic parameters.

In patients with renal insufficiency, the apparent elimination half-life increases when the creatinine clearance is ≤50 ml/min. The apparent elimination half-life between two hemodialysis sessions is 4.1 h.

The pharmacokinetics in children over 3 years of age are similar to those in adults (Table 59).

Penetration of the CSF yields a concentration of between <0.39 and 12.5 μg/ml, depending on the dose (40 to 100 mg/kg). The concentrations in body tissues and fluids are high.

7.3.6.7. Apalcillin

Apalcillin can be administered intravenously. It is 96% bound to plasma proteins. An intravenous pharmacokinetic study (injection over 3 min) at increasing doses showed that the areas under the curve are proportional to the administered doses up to 3.0 g. Plasma clearance is between 108.6 and 157.4 ml/min, and renal clearance is between 20.1 and 34.1 ml/min.

Dose-dependent but relatively high concentrations are detected in the serum 6 h after administration of the product. The apparent elimination half-life is on the order of 1 h. About 18% of the administered dose is eliminated in the urine (Table 60). Two metabolites, which are the enantiomers of penicilloic acid, have been detected in the urine (Borner et al., 1982). Biliary elimination is 20 to 40% of the administered dose (Brogard et al., 1985).

The pharmacokinetics of apalcillin were studied following slow intravenous administration (3 min) of a single dose of 20 to 30 mg/kg in five categories of children. The apparent elimination half-life is long in premature (6.8 h), dysmature (5.4 h), and term neonates (5.0 h). The half-life in neonates and infants over 1 month of age is similar to that in adults. Plasma and renal clearances are also modified in the first category of patients (Table 61).

7.3.6.8. Furazlocillin

The pharmacokinetics are dose dependent. After administration of 1 g of furazlocillin (5 min), the levels in plasma are 214 and 3 μg/ml at the end of infusion and after 4 h, respectively. The apparent elimination half-life is on the order of 1 h. Urinary elimination is 33 to 69%, with the elimination, of a degradation product, furazlocillin penicilloate. Five to 7% of the administered dose is eliminated, with a renal clearance of

Table 59 Pharmacokinetics of aspoxicillin in children

Dose (mg/kg)	n	C_0 (μg/ml)	$t_{1/2\beta}$ (h)	$AUC_{0-\infty}$ (μg · h/ml)	Urinary elimination (%)
10	5	48.3	1.16	50.4	62.7
20	28	229.8	0.9	80.6	67.2
40	12	217.2	1.08	170.5	67.7

Table 60 Pharmacokinetics of ascending doses of apalcillin[a]

Dose (mg)	C_{5min} (μg/ml)	C_{6min} (μg/ml)	AUC (μg · h/ml)	$t_{1/2}$(h)	CL_P (ml/min)	CL_R (ml/min)	Urinary elimination (%)
500	81.7	0.7	63.9	1.06	136.7		22.4
1,000	153.6	1.6	162.3	1.04	109.5		21.2
2,000	228.5	5.3	313.2	1.39	108.6	22.6	14.5
3,000	299.0	5.5	370.7	1.25	144.8	28.6	18.2

[a]Data from Akbaraly et al., 1984.

Table 61 Pediatric pharmacokinetics of apalcillin

Subjects	Dose (mg/kg)	$C_{0.05h}$ (μg/ml)	C_{8h} (μg/ml)	C_{12h} (μg/ml)	AUC (μg · h/ml)	$t_{1/2}$(h)	CL_P (ml/min/kg)	CL_R (ml/min/kg)	Urinary elimination (%)
Premature	20	109.2		15.6	540.2	6.8	0.63	0.17	26.0
Dysmature	20	269.6		17.9	722.4	5.4	0.53	0.17	37.2
Neonates[a]	20	130.0		9.4	674.4	5.0	0.77	0.18	27.0
Neonates[b]	30	344.8		23.4		5.0	0.77	0.18	21.6
Infants[c]	20	210.9	3.4		409.5	2.3	1.14	0.27	20.8
	30	231.3	22			2.3	1.14	0.27	33.4
	30	241.3	0.9		197.7	1.3	2.95	0.48	17.2

[a]Age, <8 days.
[b]Age, 8 days to 1 month.
[c]Age, >1 month

41 ml/min. Plasma clearance is high, on the order of 300 ml/min, with a renal clearance of 80 ml/min and a nonrenal clearance of 221 ml/min. Urinary elimination involves a tubular component. Plasma protein binding is 65%.

The main pharmacokinetic parameters of the *N*-acylpenicillins are recapitulated in Tables 47 and 48.

8. GROUP IV: α-CARBOXY- AND α-SULFOPENICILLINS

The α-aminopenicillins have a broad antibacterial spectrum which includes gram-negative bacilli. However, *P. aeruginosa* is excluded from their spectrum, as well as numerous species of *Enterobacteriaceae* that have progressively become problematical in infectious diseases, such as *Proteus, S. marcescens, Providencia, Citrobacter,* and *Acinetobacter baumannii.*

The synthesis of α-carboxypenicillins has provided a resolution to a certain number of therapeutic problems related to gram-negative bacteria.

8.1. Physicochemical Properties

Carbenicillin is unstable in an acidic medium and is sparingly liposoluble, for which reason it is poorly absorbed by the digestive tract. The physicochemical properties are summarized in Table 62.

8.2. Structure-Activity Relationship

The presence of an acid function such as a carboxyl, sulfamic, or sulfone group on the carbon in the α position of the side chain (Fig. 21) increases the activity against gram-negative bacilli but reduces the activity against gram-positive bacteria. The carbenicillin side chain contains a center of asymmetry. The D- and L-isomers have the same antibacterial activities.

The chemical stability may be improved by esterification of the side chain. Indanyl (carindacillin) and phenyl (carfecillin) esters have been developed. These esters are orally absorbed and rapidly hydrolyzed to carbenicillin.

Replacement of the phenyl nucleus by a thienyl nucleus has yielded ticarcillin, which is twice as active as carbenicillin against the majority of strains of *P. aeruginosa*.

Sulbenicillin was obtained by replacing the carboxyl chain with a sulfone group. This molecule exhibits better chemical stability while retaining antibacterial activity similar to that of the α-carboxypenicillins.

Table 62 Physicochemical properties of α-carboxy/sulfo penicillins

Drug	Mol wt	$t_{1/2}$ (min) degradation, pH 1, 35°C	pK	Log P_u *n*-octanol/water	Na mmol/g	P_{app}	
						pH 5	pH 7
Carfecillin	455.5	25	2.91	2.96	2.1	7.35	0.07
Carindacillin	494.5	25	2.94	3.77	1.9	50.8	0.5
Carbenicillin	378.4	6.3	3.08	1.95	4.8	0.21	0.005
Ticarcillin	384.4				4.7		
Sulbenicillin	414.45	12	2.45	0.59	4.4		

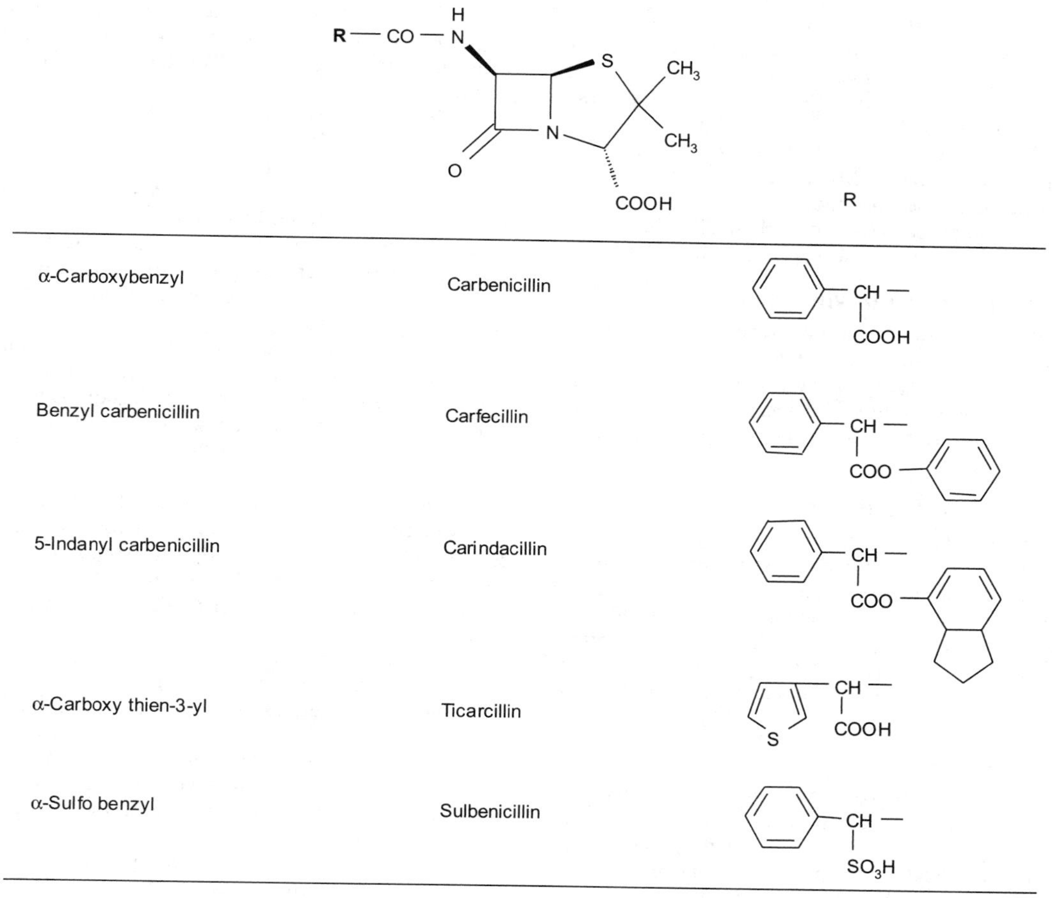

R—CO—N(H)— [penam nucleus: S, CH_3, CH_3, COOH, O]

		R
α-Carboxybenzyl	Carbenicillin	CH— / COOH
Benzyl carbenicillin	Carfecillin	CH— / COO—
5-Indanyl carbenicillin	Carindacillin	CH— / COO—
α-Carboxy thien-3-yl	Ticarcillin	CH— / COOH (S)
α-Sulfo benzyl	Sulbenicillin	CH— / SO_3H

Figure 21 α-Carboxypenicillins and sulfopenicillin

Suncillin (α-sulfoaminobenzylpenicillin) contains a sulfamic acid. This molecule has activity similar to that of carbenicillin against *P. aeruginosa* but is less active against *Enterobacteriaceae*.

Derivatives of benzylpenicillin with an α-5-tetrazole nucleus have antibacterial activities similar to that of carbenicillin in vitro but are less active in vivo.

8.3. In Vitro Antibacterial Properties

8.3.1. Carbenicillin

The spectrum of the α-carboxypenicillins includes gram-negative species susceptible to ampicillin but also other species of *Enterobacteriaceae*, such as *Providencia* spp., *S. marcescens*, *Proteus* spp., *Pseudomonas* spp., *Enterobacter* spp., and even *Bacteroides* spp.; *Klebsiella* spp. are nonsusceptible (Table 43). There is cross-resistance among the different α-carboxypenicillins. Combination with aminoglycosides is synergistic.

8.3.2. Carindacillin

Carindacillin is esterified at the α-carboxyl function, leaving the carboxyl group of the thiazolidine nucleus free. Despite degradation of carindacillin in culture media, it has better activity than carbenicillin against gram-positive cocci, but it is inferior against gram-negative bacilli (Table 63).

Table 63 In vitro activity of carindacillin[a]

Organism(s)	MIC (μg/ml)	
	Carbenicillin	Carindacillin
S. aureus Pen^s	1.56	0.19
S. aureus Pen^r	12.5	12.5
S. pyogenes	0.19	0.003
S. pneumoniae	0.39	0.02
E. faecalis	100	3.12
E. coli	3.12	3.12
K. pneumoniae	>100	50
P. mirabilis	1.56	1.56
P. vulgaris	3.12	3.12
Salmonella spp.	12.5	12.5
S. marcescens	12.5	12.5
Enterobacter aerogenes	6.25	3.12
P. aeruginosa	50	50
H. influenzae	1	1
P. multocida	0.19	0.09

[a]Data from Butler et al., 1973.

8.3.3. Ticarcillin

Ticarcillin is active against gram-positive cocci, but its activity is moderate against penicillinase-producing strains of

S. aureus (MIC, ~8 to 16 μg/ml), and the drug is inactive against *Enterococcus faecalis* (MIC, >32 μg/ml). Likewise, its activity against *L. monocytogenes* is moderate (MIC, ~8.0 μg/ml). Among the *Enterobacteriaceae*, it possesses moderate activity against *S. marcescens* and *Enterobacter* spp. (MIC, ~16.0 μg/ml). Conversely, like carbenicillin it is ineffective against *K. pneumoniae* (MIC, >128 μg/ml). It displays good activity against anaerobic bacteria.

Its spectrum is identical to that of carbenicillin, but it is on average twice as active against susceptible strains (Table 43).

8.4. Factors Influencing In Vitro Activity

The size of the inoculum affects the activity of the α-carboxypenicillins. The culture medium has little influence on the in vitro activity. A pH of between 5.5 and 8.0 yields optimal in vitro activity. The addition of serum to the culture medium does not significantly affect the antibacterial activity.

8.5. Mechanisms of Resistance

The α-carboxypenicillins are hydrolyzed to various degrees by *S. aureus* penicillinases and by certain penicillinase-like enzymes. They are more stable against hydrolysis by class I β-lactamases than the *N*-acylpenicillins. They are unstable to the TEM-type broad-spectrum (TEM-1) or extended-spectrum (TEM-3, etc.; SHV-2, etc.) β-lactamases. More specific enzymes hydrolyze the α-carboxypenicillins: carbenicillinases and PSE.

8.5.1. *Acinetobacter* spp.

Acinetobacter spp. are opportunistic gram-negative bacteria responsible for an increasing number of nosocomial infections. Bouvet and Grimont (1986) have proposed a new classification: *Acinetobacter baumannii* (*Acinetobacter calcoaceticus* subsp. *anitratus*) and non-*A. baumannii*. One of the mechanisms of resistance to β-lactams is the production of β-lactamases, whether these are cephalosporinases (pI 8), TEM-1-type enzymes (pI 5.4), or carbenicillinases such as CARB-5 (pI 6.3). This enzyme is present in 9% of isolates of *A. baumannii* in the Xavier Bichat university hospital (Paris, France). It inactivates carbenicillin and ampicillin but is ineffective against methicillin and oxacillin.

Jolly Guillou et al., isolated five resistance phenotypes among strains of *Acinetobacter* spp: type I, no β-lactamase; type II, presence of a penicillinase; type III, presence of a cephalosporinase; type IV, presence of a penicillinase and a cephalosporinase; and type V, resistance to imipenem.

The changes in these different phenotypes as percentages are given in Table 64.

The authors showed that there was high resistance to piperacillin (87.5 to 98% piperacillin-resistant strains). Resistance to ticarcillin is on the order of 17.5%. (The MIC was >256 μg/ml. The addition of clavulanic acid reduced the MIC to 70 μg/ml.)

Table 64 Resistance phenotypes among *Acinetobacter* strains

Type	Prevalence of phenotype (%)				
	1984	1985	1986	1987	1988
I	11	11	6.0	6.0	2.5
II	12	4.5	7.5	3.0	0.5
III	9.0	12	35	26.5	13
IV	68	72.5	52	64.5	84

Imipenem is one of the antibiotics active against *Acinetobacter* (MIC on the order of 0.5 μg/ml). Imipenem-resistant strains (about 5.5%) have been isolated since 1986.

8.5.2. *P. aeruginosa*

Several mechanisms are involved in the resistance of *P. aeruginosa* to β-lactams: β-lactamase production, parietal impermeability, and modification of PBP.

P. aeruginosa is resistant to numerous β-lactams. Even the antipseudomonal cephalosporins such as ceftazidime are 10 to 100 times less active against *P. aeruginosa* than against *Enterobacter cloacae*.

This resistance is due in part to poor outer-membrane permeability as a result of numerous but less functional porins.

Table 65 shows the MICs of various drugs for a wild-type *P. aeruginosa* strain and one with a mutation in the outer membrane.

Imipenem must pass through the outer membrane of *P. aeruginosa* via a specific porin, Opr D, which has a molecular weight of 48. This porin is inducible in the presence of glucose. The absence of this porin would appear to be the cause of the resistance to imipenem.

The second mode of resistance is a modification in the PBPs.

The most common mechanism of resistance after outer membrane impermeability is β-lactamase production. *P. aeruginosa* produces a chromosomal cephalosporinase (class Id) which, when derepressed, causes resistance to cefsulodin, ceftazidime, and the *N*-acylpenicillins, although the activity of imipenem is preserved. The true levels of resistance depend on the quantity of enzymes produced in the absence of induction.

A number of plasmid-mediated β-lactamases have been described: PSE, CARB, TEM, NPS-1, and OXA.

About 10% of strains in France and 2% of strains in the United Kingdom possess enzymes, while among *Enterobacteriaceae* the proportion is greater.

The most common enzymes are PSE-1 (CARB-2) and PSE-4 (CARB-1), which are responsible for resistance to all antipseudomonal penicillins and to cefoperazone and cefsulodin. They do not cause resistance to aztreonam, imipenem, or ceftazidime.

The activity of these constitutive enzymes is inhibited by clavulanic acid, in contrast to that of cephalosporinase (Sabath and Dalgleish enzyme).

Table 65 Effect of mutation in outer membrane on MICs for *P. aeruginosa*

Drug	MIC (μg/ml)	
	P. aeruginosa K 779/WT	*P. aeruginosa* K 779/61[a]
Carbenicillin	16	0.02
Sulbenicillin	8	0.02
Ticarcillin	4	0.002
Piperacillin	1	0.005
Azlocillin	2	0.005
Cefsulodin	0.2	0.02
Cefotaxime	8	0.01
Cefoperazone	1	0.002
Cefmenoxime	4	0.01

[a]Mutant strain (outer membrane).

Table 66 Carbenicillinases

Enzyme	Other name	Mol wt	pI	Ambler class	Plasmid
CARB-1	PSE-4	32	5.3	A	Dalgleish
CARB-2	PSE-1	26.5	5.7	?	RPL 11
CARB-3	PSE-4		5.75	?	Cilote
CARB-4			4.3		
CARB-5[a]			6.3		
CARB-6[a]			5.7		
AER-1		22	5.9		
PSE-2	OXA-4	12.4	6.1	D	R 151
PSE-3		12	6.9	A	

[a]Data from Jolly-Guillou.
[b]Data from Philippon.

The mechanism of enzyme induction is identical to that of *E. cloacae*.

Philippon et al. (1990) have described an oxacillinase-like enzyme in *Alcaligenes denitrificans* subsp. *xylosoxydans*.

8.5.3. Carbenicillinases and PSE

Enzymes of the carbenicillinase and PSE types belong to Richmond and Sykes class V. PSE-2 strongly hydrolyzes oxacillin, methicillin, and cloxacillin, in contrast to PSE-1, PSE-3, and PSE-4, which weakly hydrolyze 2-amino-5-thiazolyloximino cephalosporins. These enzymes are not specific to *P. aeruginosa,* as they are detected in certain species of *Enterobacteriaceae.*

PSE-1 may be produced by *E. coli, P. mirabilis, Salmonella* spp., and *Shigella sonnei.* PSE-2 has been detected in *E. coli, E. cloacae, K. pneumoniae,* and *Providencia stuartii.*

PSE-3 has been described for *Klebsiella* spp.

The PSE genes are carried by transposons.

These different enzymes differ not only in their physicochemical characteristics (Table 66) but also in their rates of hydrolysis of different substrates (Tables 67 and 68) and their cloxacillin- and pCMB-inhibitory activities.

Morand et al. (1990) showed that the PSE-type enzymes are a heterogeneous class (Tables 67 and 68). The active site of the carbenicillinases contains an alkaline residue of the lysine or arginine type which interacts with the α-carboxy groups of the α-carboxypenicillins.

The carbenicillinases weakly hydrolyze oxacillin and are not inhibited by chlorine ions. CARB-1, CARB-2, CARB-3, and CARB-4 are strongly inhibited by clavulanic acid and the other β-lactamase inhibitors.

8.6. Breakpoints

The breakpoints according to the recommendations of the French Antibiotic Sensitivity Test Committee are given in Table 69.

8.7. Pharmacokinetic Properties

8.7.1. Carbenicillin

Carbenicillin is administered in the form of two diastereoisomers (55% in the D-form). Distribution and elimination are not stereospecific.

After intravenous administration (infusion for 0.25 and 0.5 h), the concentrations at the end of infusion are, respectively, 115 to 140, 127, 300 to 400, and 450 to 750 μg/ml for single doses of 1, 2, 5, and 10 g. At 6 h, residual concentrations are, respectively, <3, 12.5 (4 h), 14.2, and 32 to 45 μg/ml. Renal clearance is ≤100 ml/min. The apparent elimination half-life is between 0.8 and 1.4 h.

Elimination of carbenicillin is urinary and occurs principally by glomerular filtration, the tubular component being minor. In the presence of probenecid, concentrations in serum increase by 25% and renal clearance decreases by 25%. Urinary elimination accounts for about 48% of the administered dose. Biliary elimination is 0.1% of the administered dose. After administration of 1.0 g, peak concentrations in the bile are between 5.7 and 200 μg/ml (39.1 ± 19.7 μg/ml) and are reached within 2 h (concentrations in serum are 48.3 ± 6.1 μg/ml). Carbenicillin is 50% plasma protein bound.

Table 67 Hydrolysis rate of PSE[a]

Enzyme	Hydrolysis rate (%)							
	AMP	CARB	OXA	MET	CLOX	CLA	CMX	CTX
PSE-1	90	97	<2	<2	<2	8	<2	27
PSE-2	267	121	317	803	371	2	—	16
PSE-3	101	253	—	—	3	—	<1	—
PSE-4	88	150	8	16	<2	0	<2	<1

[a]AMP, ampicillin; CARB, carbenicillin; OXA, oxacillin; MET, methicillin; CLOX, cloxacillin; CLA, clarithromycin; CMX, cefuroxime; CTX, cefotaxime.
[b]—, rate of penicillin G is 100%.

Table 68 Enzymatic activities of carbenicillinases and PSE against piperacillin and α-carboxypenicillins

PSE	CARB	Carbenicillin		Ticarcillin		Piperacillin	
		V_{max}	K_m	V_{max}	K_m	V_{max}	K_m
PSE-1	CARB-2	300	70	125	19	21	6
PSE-3		180	22	10	10	19	6
PSE-4	CARB-1	130	120	90	40	22	6.5
	CARB-3	150	100	100	21	38	11

Table 69 Breakpoints of α-carboxypenicillins[a]

Drug	Disk (μg)	MIC (μg/ml)		Diam zone (mm)	
		S	R	S	R
Carbenicillin	100	≤128	>128	≥15	<15
Ticarcillin					
Enterococcus	75	≤16	>64	≥18	<18
P. aeruginosa	75	≤64	>64	≥22	<18

[a]S, susceptible; R, resistant.

After intramuscular administration of 1.0 g of carbenicillin, the peak concentration in serum of 26.3 μg/ml is reached within 1 h. The residual concentration at 6 h is 4.8 μg/ml.

Carbenicillin can be biotransformed into two metabolites, penicilloic acid and benzylpenicillin, by decarboxylation. These two derivatives are quantitatively minor, since 92% of the administered dose is found unchanged in the urine following intravenous administration of carbenicillin.

In the neonate, the plasma clearance is two to four times lower, particularly in 1-day-old or low-birth-weight neonates. After administration of a single dose of 100 mg/kg to a neonate, the peak concentration in serum is between 142 and 217 μg/ml, depending on age. The apparent elimination half-life is 3 to 4 h in the neonate with a birth weight of between 2 and 3 kg and 6 h in the neonate with a birth weight of less than 2 kg.

The apparent elimination half-life of carbenicillin is prolonged in patients with renal insufficiency. It is 15.7 ± 5.2 h in anuric patients. In anuric patients with hepatic insufficiency it is 23.2 ± 9.0 h.

About 30% of carbenicillin is eliminated by hemodialysis. Peritoneal dialysis substantially reduces the elimination half-life of carbenicillin (before dialysis, half-life is ~23 h; during dialysis, half-life is ~7.4 h) despite weak peritoneal clearance (6.8 ml/min). Concentrations in tissue are high (Table 70).

8.7.2. Carfecillin

Carfecillin is a cleavable ester of carbenicillin obtained by esterification of the α-carboxylic function of carbenicillin (Fig. 21).

After a dose of 0.5 g (397 mg of carbenicillin) or 1.0 g (794 mg of carbenicillin), peak concentrations in serum obtained in 2 h are less than 10 μg/ml; the concentration is ≤ 0.1 μg/ml at 6 h. Urinary elimination peaks within the first 4 h (26.5%) (Leigh and Simmons, 1976; Wilkinson et al., 1975). The peak concentration in serum is 1.38 μg/ml and is reached after 2 h, with major interindividual variability.

Table 70 Concentrations of carbenicillin in tissue

Tissue or fluid	Dose	Concn (μg/ml or kg)
CSF	2 g i.v.[a]	8.5
Renal tissue	5 g i.v.	13
Bronchial secretion	2 g i.v.	128–300
Pleural fluid	600 mg/kg	78
Bone tissue	4 g i.v.	152
Synovial fluid	5 g i.v.	20
Peritoneal fluid	4 g i.v.	47
	24 g i.v.	800
	12 g i.v.	525

[a]i.v., intravenous.

The concentrations are higher in patients with renal insufficiency.

Carbenicillin is released after nonspecific hydrolysis intestinally. The phenol nucleus is eliminated in the urine in the form of the glucuronide or sulfate.

8.7.3. Carindacillin

Carindacillin or indanylcarbenicillin is the cleavable ester of carbenicillin (Fig. 21). The 5-indanyl group is attached to the α-carboxylic group of carbenicillin. Carindacillin occurs in the form of a bitter hygroscopic powder. In an acidic medium, the powder becomes coated with a gelatinous film that prevents intestinal absorption. The addition of glycine to the pharmaceutical formulation obviates this physicochemical drawback. Sodium bicarbonate and sodium citrate yield the same effects, but sodium intake is then too high.

Carindacillin is more stable in an acidic medium than carbenicillin, remaining so for at least 24 h.

Carindacillin is markedly more lipophilic than carbenicillin (Table 71) (Butler et al., 1973).

Penicillins with a partition coefficient of more than 2.0 are better absorbed in the gastrointestinal tract.

Because of its high lipophilicity, carindacillin is strongly bound to plasma proteins (~98%).

Hydrolysis of the ester occurs in the intestinal mucosa or liver. In the rat, about 55% of carindacillin is transformed in 1 h to carbenicillin in the intestinal lumen. About 20% of the administered dose is absorbed in the form of carindacillin (Tsuji et al., 1982). In the lumen of the digestive tract, the esters are either absorbed or transformed to carbenicillin, which is only weakly absorbed, or the two products undergo inactivation, being transformed to penicilloic acid. Absorption is increased at pH 5 as the nondissociated forms penetrate the hydrophilic surface of the intestinal mucosa better.

The indole nucleus is 100% eliminated in humans in the form of glucuroconjugated or sulfate derivatives. In dogs, in addition to the previous products, hydroxyl metabolites (1-, 3-, 5-, 6-OH-indanones) are found in the urine.

Carindacillin is rapidly absorbed. The ester is present in the blood circulation for up to 30 min, after which only carbenicillin is detected. After doses of 0.5 and 1.0 g, the peak concentrations in serum are, respectively, 10 and 15 to 17 μg/ml. Urinary elimination is practically complete after 3 h and represents about 30 to 40% of the administered dose.

Simultaneous administration of probenecid increases the concentrations of carbenicillin in plasma.

Above 4.0 g per day, the risk of diarrhea associated with the large quantity of unabsorbed product increases.

Table 71 Lipophilicity of penicillins

Drug	$Log_{10}P$ (*n*-butanol/buffer/phosphate, pH 7.0)
Carbenicillin	0.05
Carindacillin	40–50
Ampicillin	0–26
Benzylpenicillin	2.3
Penicillin V	4.9
Phenoxyethylpenicillin	7.9
Propicillin	15
Oxacillin	9.6
Cloxacillin	12
Dicloxacillin	18–20

Table 72 Pediatric pharmacokinetics of ticarcillin

Age of subjects	No. of children	C_{max} (μg/ml)	C_{min}, 8 h (μg/ml)	$t_{1/2}$ (h)	V (μg/ml)	CL_P (ml/min)
0–7 days, <2 kg	17	167.1	35.1 (12 h)	5.6	663	31
0–7 days, <2 kg	13	135.0	31.5	4.9	715	54
1–8 wk	17	155.2	14.9	2.2	761	118
5–13 yr	7	152.4	37.2	0.9	351	176

8.7.4. Ticarcillin

Mean concentrations after infusion of 1.0, 2.0, and 5.0 g of ticarcillin for 0.5 h are 50, 108, and 250 μg/ml. The apparent elimination half-life is about 70 min. Renal clearance is between 119 and 132 ml/min, and plasma clearance is between 134 and 154 ml/min. Plasma protein binding is 45%.

Elimination is principally renal, involving glomerular filtration and tubular secretion. Simultaneous administration of probenecid reduces the quantity of ticarcillin eliminated in the urine at 6 h (49 versus 72%).

Almost 95% of the administered dose is eliminated in the urine in 12 h.

The kinetics are modified in the neonate and infant under 8 weeks of age (Table 72). The apparent elimination half-life is about 5 to 6 h in the neonate, with a plasma clearance of between 30 and 50 ml/min (>170 ml/min in adults).

In patients with renal insufficiency, the apparent elimination half-life increases with the reduction in creatinine clearance (Table 73).

Following hemodialysis, the clearance of ticarcillin is evaluated as 33 ± 10 ml/min and the apparent elimination half-life is 3.4 ± 0.8 h. Peritoneal dialysis is less effective than hemodialysis. The elimination half-life is 10.6 ± 0.8 h. Peritoneal clearance of ticarcillin is 7.2 ± 1.8 ml/min.

Ticarcillin diffuses readily into the majority of the body's tissues and serous fluids (interstitial, pleural, synovial, and peritoneal). Ticarcillin is distributed in the amniotic fluid. After intravenous administration of 1.0 g, the concentration at the end of the infusion is 1.4 to 3.3 μg/ml.

Biliary elimination of carbenicillin and ticarcillin is high.

8.7.5. Sulbenicillin

Sulbenicillin is a diastereoisomer containing 77% of the D(−) form. After administration of 1.0 g of sulbenicillin intravenously (30-min infusion), the concentration at the end of infusion is about 15.0 μg/ml.

After intravenous administration, the apparent half-life of sulbenicillin is 0.5 to 1.0 h. It is 1.5 to 2.0 h after intramuscular administration.

More than 80% is eliminated in the urine and 6% is eliminated via the hepatobiliary route.

Seventy-five percent of the administered dose is eliminated in the urine with no change in the ratio of stereoisomers. No metabolites have been detected in urine. However, 10 to 20% of the administered dose of sulbenicillin is biotransformed to α-sulfobenzylpenicillin acid. Sulbenicillin is 55% plasma protein bound.

In patients with renal insufficiency, the apparent elimination half-life is prolonged when the creatinine clearance is reduced (Table 74).

8.8. Adverse Effects

The following side effects are reported in the literature for α-carboxypenicillins: phlebitis, hypereosinophilia, hypokalemia, and diarrhea.

Simultaneous administration of cyclosporine and ticarcillin causes an increase in circulating cyclosporine levels (Lambert et al., 1989).

The α-carboxypenicillins are held responsible for agranulocytosis and neurotoxic disorders.

Brown et al. (1975) showed that repeated intravenous administration of ticarcillin in healthy subjects at a dosage of 100 to 300 mg/kg daily affected platelet function. They demonstrated an increase in bleeding time and an anomaly of platelet aggregation. This anomaly occurs very soon after the end of administration and persists for 1 week after the end of administration (Table 75).

9. GROUP V: 6-α-PENICILLINS

Strominger and Tipper (1965) suggested that the 6-α-methylbenzylpenicillins would be better structural analogs of the acyl D-Ala–D-Ala than penicillin G. This hypothesis was tested in 1971 by Böhmer et al., who synthesized some methyl ester derivatives: 6-α- and 6-β-methylbenzylpenicillins. Compared with benzylpenicillin (MIC, 1.0 μg/ml), these two derivatives are inactive against *S. aureus* and *S. pyogenes* (MIC, >500 μg/ml).

Table 73 Elimination half-life of ticarcillin as a function of renal clearance

Creatinine clearance (ml/min)	$t_{1/2}$ (h)[a]
≥60	1.17
60–30	30 ± 0.6
30–10	8.5 ± 2.1
<10	14.8 ± 3.7

[a]Means ± standard deviations.

Table 74 Sulbenicillin in renal insufficiency

Creatinine clearance (ml/min)	$t_{1/2}$ (h)[a]
120	0.45 ± 0.03
50	1.36 ± 0.41
<5	4.59 ± 2.42

[a]Means ± standard deviations.

Table 75 α-Carboxypenicillins and hemostasis[a]

Drug	Dose (mg/kg/day)	No. of subjects	Bleeding time (s)[b]	Quick time (s)[b]	Platelet aggregation[b]
Carbenicillin	300	5	7.9 ± 5.2	20.0 ± 0.06	0.23 ± 0.06
	400	6	6.9 ± 6.4	17.0 ± 3.3	0.27 ± 0.08
Ticarcillin	100	3	4.6 ± 1.6	30.1 ± 3.5	0.47 ± 0.13
	200	6	6.6 ± 1.3	25.5 ± 7.4	0.41 ± 0.13
	300	8	7.3 ± 3.5	14.9 ± 3.8	0.27 ± 0.05
Controls		28	3.7 ± 1.2	24.3 ± 5.5	0.48 ± 5.5

[a]Data from Brown et al., 1974, 1975.
[b]Means ± standard deviations.

Following the publication by Nagarajan et al. (1971), Ho et al. (1972, 1973) synthesized a series of penicillins with substitutions at position 6 and cephems with substitutions at position 7-α. Substitution at position 6-α reduces the antibacterial and transpeptidase inhibitory activity.

The 6-α-methoxypenicillin derivatives are better inhibitors of transpeptidase than the 6-α-methylpenicillin derivatives. The 6-α-methoxypenicillin V derivatives are relatively inactive against *B. subtilis*, as are the 6-α-methoxyampicillin derivatives.

The 6-α-methoxycarbenicillin derivatives possess better activity than carbenicillin against β-lactamase-producing enterobacteria (*Enterobacter* spp., etc.), but they are totally inactive against gram-positive bacteria. The nature of the substituent interferes with the activity.

9.1. Temocillin

Temocillin is 6-α-methoxyticarcillin (Slocombe et al., 1981) (Fig. 22).

9.1.1. Physicochemical Properties

Temocillin ($C_{16}H_{18}N_2O_7S_2$) is a disodium salt with a molecular weight of 414.45. Barton et al. (1986) have shown that penicillins which possess a 6-α-methoxy group are more stable in a weakly acidic or alkaline medium than their analogs without substitutions at position 6. Temocillin is degraded in a highly acidic or highly alkaline pH medium, but by a pathway different from that of the penicillins. There is no formation of penicillanic acid.

9.1.2. Antibacterial Activity

Like the cephamycins, temocillin is less active than its non-6-α-substituted equivalent. The activity is summarized in Table 76.

This molecule has little activity against gram-positive cocci and possesses moderate activity against *Enterobacteriaceae*. Temocillin is less active than cefotaxime or ceftazidime. In vitro, temocillin is active against β-lactamase-producing strains of *H. influenzae*, but in vivo it is inactive in septicemia or meningitis models.

P. aeruginosa, *Pseudomonas* spp., *Campylobacter* spp., and *Acinetobacter* spp. are resistant to temocillin, as are anaerobic gram-negative bacteria such as *B. fragilis*. This resistance would appear to be due to the inability of temocillin to permeate the bacterial outer membrane.

Temocillin is stable to hydrolysis by the majority of β-lactamases, whether plasmid or chromosomally mediated (Richmond class I). In vitro activity is virtually unaffected when the size of the bacterial inoculum increases, but the addition of 50% serum to the culture medium reduces the activity of temocillin two- to fourfold.

The majority of β-lactams bind to PBP in two stages. An initial reversible stage, followed by covalent binding of the antibiotic to PBP, yields a stable complex. It would appear that this weaker activity than that of ticarcillin is related to the method of binding. This molecule binds with a greater or lesser degree of stability to *E. coli* PBP 3 and PBP 5 after an extremely slow recognition phase, as shown by Labia et al. (1984).

9.1.3. Pharmacokinetic Properties

The intravenous pharmacokinetics (3-min bolus) of doses of 3.75, 7.5, and 15 mg/kg were determined by Leroy et al. (1983). The same volunteers also received a single dose of

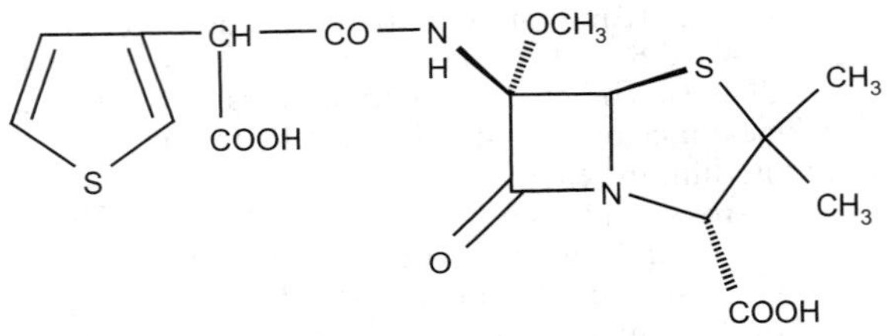

Figure 22 Temocillin

Table 76 In vitro activities of temocillin and fomidacillin

Organism(s)	MIC (μg/ml)	
	Temocillin	Fomidacillin (BRL-36650)
S. aureus	>256	>128
S. pneumoniae	>256	4
E. coli	2.5	0.06
K. pneumoniae	5	0.5
P. mirabilis	2.5	0.12
E. cloacae	5	0.5
S. marcescens	2.5	0.25
M. morganii	2.5	0.25
P. rettgeri	2.5	0.25
Shigella spp.	8	0.25
P. aeruginosa	>256	0.5
H. influenzae	0.5	0.25
M. catarrhalis	0.2	0.06
B. fragilis	256	32
Clostridium difficile	>256	<128

Table 77 Pharmacokinetics of ascending intravenous doses of temocillin

Dose (mg/kg)	C_{max} (μg/ml)	$t_{1/2\beta}$ (h)	CL_P (ml/min)	CL_R (ml/min)	Urinary elimination (%)
3.75	31.3	4.8	47.8	33.1	69.6
7.5	75.1	5.9	40.2	27.4	67.4
15	145.6	5.2	41.5	34.1	71.5

7.5 mg/kg intramuscularly. Levels in serum and urine were measured by a microbiological method using *P. aeruginosa* NCTC 10701 as the test strain. The limit of detection was 1.56 μg/ml. After intravenous administration, the concentrations in serum at the end of the injection were, respectively, 31.3, 75.1, and 145.6 μg/ml. The apparent elimination half-life was between 4.8 and 5.2 h. The plasma clearance was between 40.2 and 47.8 ml/min/1.73 m^2. A total of 67.4 to 71.5% of the administered dose was eliminated unchanged in the 24-h urine (Table 77).

After intramuscular administration of a single dose of 7.5 mg of temocillin per kg, the peak concentration in serum was 26.7 μg/ml and was reached in 1.67 h. The apparent elimination half-life was 5.5 h.

In patients with renal insufficiency, the apparent elimination half-life increases as the creatinine clearance decreases (Table 78).

Hemodialysis causes a reduction of 69.8% in plasma temocillin concentrations. Plasma protein binding is on the order of 85%.

The areas under the curve after intravenous and intramuscular administration are, respectively, 213.97 ± 31.2 and 240.14 ± 25.03 μg · h/ml, and bioavailability is on the order of 100%. Biliary elimination is weak. Metabolization via penicillanic acid is minor.

In common with the other penicillins that have an α-carboxylic group (Hoogmartens et al., 1982), temocillin possesses a center of asymmetry and two diastereoisomers. The ratio between the *R*- and *S*-epimers is 65:35. The pharmacokinetics of the two epimers are summarized in Table 79.

Eight hours after intravenous administration of 1.0 g of temocillin disodium, the ratio between the epimers is modified. The *R*-epimer declines from 61.4 to 42.9%. This change in the *R/S* ratio is due to the apparent elimination half-life, which is shorter for the *R*-epimer (~4.0 h) than for the *S*-epimer (~6.0 h). Plasma clearance is twice as high in the case of the *R*-epimer. The *R*-epimer is less plasma protein bound than the *S*-epimer.

After an injection of 1.0 g of temocillin disodium intravenously, the concentrations measured in the different tissues between 2 and 5 h are 6.6 mg/kg in muscle, 2.5 mg/kg in parotid tissue, 16 mg/kg in sinus mucosa, 9 mg/kg in adipose tissue, and 2 to 16 mg/kg in prostatic tissue.

Table 78 Temocillin in patients with renal insufficiency

Creatinine clearance (ml/min)	$t_{1/2}$ (h)
>80	~5.5
80–30	13.6
30–10	18.9
<10	28.2
Hemodialysis	31.2

Table 79 Plasma pharmacokinetics of temocillin and its diastereoisomers[a]

Parameter (unit)	Temocillin	*R*-Epimer	*S*-Epimer
$t_{1/2\beta}$ (h)	4.8	3.8	6.1
AUC (μg·h/ml)	659	313	360
CL_P (ml/min)	26.1	35.3	17
V (liters)	9.7	10.2	8.3
Urinary elimination, 24 h (%)	70.7		

[a]Data from Guest et al., 1985.

9.2. BRL-20330

BRL-20330 is a prodrug of temocillin obtained by esterification of the α-carboxyl group by an *O*-methylphenyl group (Fig. 23). After absorption, it is converted in the body to temocillin. The plasma pharmacokinetics of oral doses of 400, 600, and 800 mg of BRL-20330 were determined by Basker et al. (1986). The peak levels in serum of 9.8, 12.8, and 15.8 μg/ml were reached within 2 h. The residual concentrations at 12 h were between 3.0 and 6.0 μg/ml.

The areas under the curve increased linearly between 400 and 800 mg (as temocillin base). The apparent elimination half-life was about 6 h. Over a period of 24 h, urinary elimination was about 25% of the administered dose and a small fraction of BRL-20330 (0.2 to 0.5%).

In the presence of food, the peak concentration in serum is reduced (9.0 versus 11.0 μg/ml) and time to maximum concentration of drug in serum is increased, although the bioavailability is unchanged.

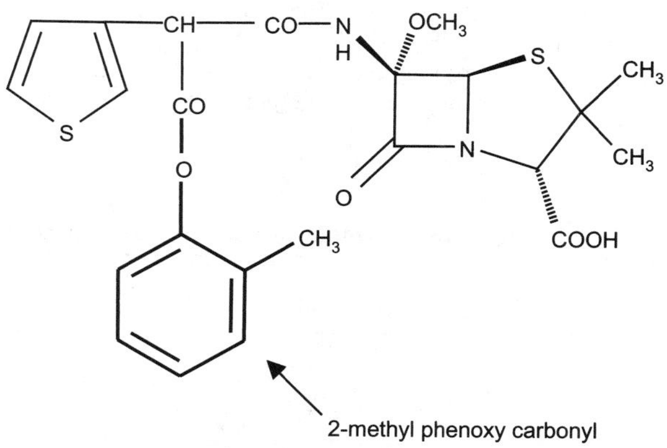

2-methyl phenoxy carbonyl

Figure 23 BRL-20330

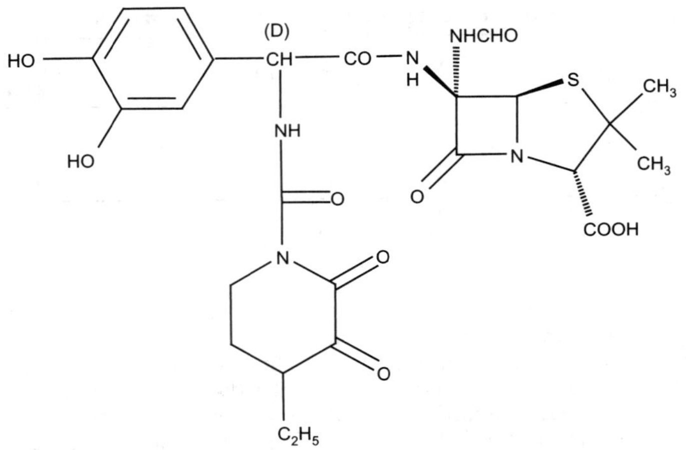

Figure 24 Fomidacillin (BRL-36650)

9.3. Fomidacillin (BRL-36650)

Fomidacillin is a penicillin derived from piperacillin, possessing a dihydroxyphenyl nucleus and a 6-α-foramidine group (Fig. 24).

9.3.1. Antibacterial Activity

Fomidacillin is active against *Enterobacteriaceae* and nonfermenting gram-negative bacilli, but it is inactive against gram-positive bacteria. It is much more active than penicillin and piperacillin (Table 80). It is stable against hydrolysis by the majority of β-lactamases.

9.3.2. Pharmacokinetics

After intravenous doses of 0.5, 1.0, 2.0, and 4.0 g, the peak levels in plasma at the end of infusion (3 min) are, respectively, 57.8, 110.6, 224.7, and 427.0 μg/ml. The areas under the curve are proportional. Plasma clearance is on the order of 150 ml/min, and renal clearance is 83 ml/min. Urinary elimination is 60% of the administered dose. The apparent elimination half-life is between 1.3 and 1.6 h. Plasma protein binding is 30% (Table 81).

After intramuscular administration of 1.0 g, peak levels in serum of 25.5 μg/ml are reached within 1 h; the bioavailability calculated from the area under the curve is on the order of 93%.

Concentrations in the blister fluid after intravenous administration are between 14.7 and 35.8 μg/ml.

In patients with renal insufficiency, the apparent elimination half-life is moderately prolonged in relation to creatinine clearance (Table 82).

In patients undergoing hemodialysis, the apparent elimination half-life during the dialysis period is 3.5 h. About 23.7% of the administered dose is recovered by hemodialysis, with a dialysis clearance of 43.1 ml/min.

Table 80 Comparative activities of fomidacillin, piperacillin, and cefotaxime

Organism(s)	MIC_{50}[a] (μg/ml)		
	Fomidacillin	Piperacillin	Cefotaxime
E. coli	0.06	2	≤0.03
K. pneumoniae	0.25	8	≤0.03
K. oxytoca	0.06	>64	0.5
Enterobacter spp.	0.25	4	0.12
Enterobacter spp.	2	>64	>64
S. marcescens	0.12	16	0.5
Citrobacter spp.	0.25	4	0.12
P. mirabilis	0.12	0.25	≤0.03
Providencia spp.	2	32	0.12
P. aeruginosa	0.25	8	16
Acinetobacter spp.	0.5	32	8
H. influenzae	0.12	≤0.03	≤0.03

[a]MIC_{50}, MIC at which 50% of the isolates tested are inhibited.

10. GROUP VI: AMIDINOPENICILLINS

Amidinopenicillins are molecules having a penam nucleus but which differ from penicillins through an amide bond at position 6. Amdinocillin (mecillinam) is characterized by the presence of an azepine nucleus attached to the amide bond (Fig. 25) (Lund and Tybring, 1972).

Table 81 Intravenous pharmacokinetics for single ascending doses of fomidacillin

Dose (g)	C_{max} (μg/ml)	C_2 (μg/ml)	AUC (μg·h/ml)	$t_{1/2\beta}$ (h)	CL_P (ml/min)	CL_R (ml/min)	CL_{NR} (ml/min)	Urinary elimination (%)
0.5	57.8	8.4	48.6	1.32	157.4	86.6	70.9	56.7
1	110.6	15	103.4	1.42	145.9	83.2	62.8	57.1
2	224.7	30.2	211.3	1.38	144.2	86	58.3	59.4
4	427	61.5	442.4	1.56	135.7	81.5	54.2	60.3

Table 82 Fomidacillin in patients with renal insufficiency

Creatinine clearance (ml/min)	$t_{1/2}$ (h)
130–80	1.96
50–30	2.52
30–15	2.93
15–<10	4.73

10.1. Physicochemical Properties

Physicochemical properties are summarized in Table 83.

10.2. Antibacterial Activity

Amdinocillin is inactive against *S. aureus* and *E. faecalis*, and its activity against *S. pneumoniae* and *S. pyogenes* is moderate. It is inactive against *P. aeruginosa* and nonfermenting gram-negative bacteria, such as *Alcaligenes* and *Flavobacterium* spp. The molecule is also inactive against *H. influenzae*. The activity against *Enterobacteriaceae* varies with the species. The activity is good against *E. coli*, *Citrobacter* spp., *Salmonella* spp., *Shigella* spp., *Yersinia enterocolitica*, and *Enterobacter* spp., but the drug is inactive against *S. marcescens*, *P. mirabilis*, and *Providencia* spp. (Table 84). There is an inoculum effect against broad-spectrum-β-lactamase-producing strains. Amdinocillin would appear to be hydrolyzed in the culture media. The bactericidal activity is dependent on the osmolarity and conductivity of the medium (Neu, 1983). Amdinocillin is capable of rapidly selecting resistant strains, which appear during treatment.

The mechanism of action is different from that of the penicillins and cephalosporins. *E. coli* exposed to amdinocillin produces ovoid forms because it binds to PBP 2 (50% inhibitory concentration [IC_{50}], 0.04 μg/ml) and has no affinity for the other PBPs (IC_{50} > 500 μg/ml). Its activity in combination with other β-lactams is synergistic against β-lactamase-producing strains of *Enterobacteriaceae*, as is its activity in combination with clavulanic acid or sulbactam (Cleeland and Squires, 1983). There is no synergy between amdinocillin and aminoglycosides, chloramphenicol, or cyclines. Amdinocillin is inactive against class I β-lactamase-hyperproducing strains of *Enterobacteriaceae*. It is partially hydrolyzed by TEM-type enzymes and that of *Klebsiella oxytoca* (Richmond and Sykes type IVc).

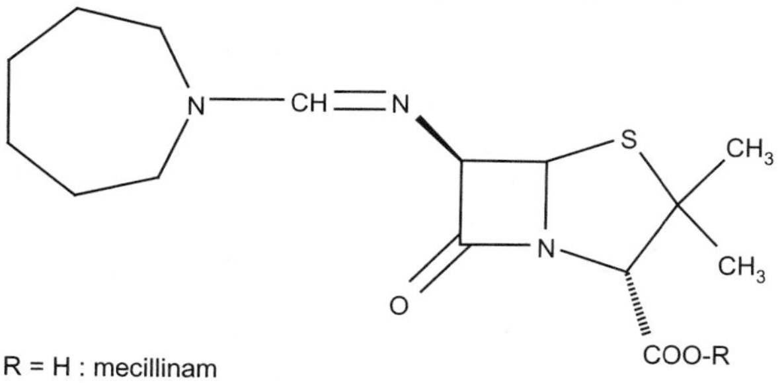

Figure 25 Amdinocillin (mecillinam) and derivatives

Table 83 Physicochemical properties of amidinopenicillins

Drug	Empirical formula	Mol wt	pK
Amdinocillin	$C_{15}H_{23}N_3O_3S$	397.9	7
Pivemecillinam	$C_{21}H_{33}N_3O_5S$	476	8.9
Bacmecillinam	$C_{20}H_{31}N_3O_6S$	478	

10.3. Breakpoints

The breakpoints proposed by the French Antibiotic Sensitivity Test Committee are shown in Table 85.

10.4. Pharmacokinetics

Amdinocillin hydrochloride is not orally absorbed. It is administered intramuscularly and intravenously. Esters of amdinocillin enable it to be absorbed after oral administration.

10.4.1. Amdinocillin

The concentration in plasma at the end of a 15-min infusion of a single dose of 500 mg of amdinocillin hydrochloride is 39.0 ± 7.7 μg/ml. The residual concentration at 6 h is 0.19 μg/ml. The area under the curve is 27.7 ± 4.89 μg·h/ml. The apparent elimination half-life is 0.99 ± 0.31 h. Renal clearance is 3.15 ± 0.92 ml/min/kg, and plasma clearance is 18.7 ± 4.0 liters/h. A total of 88.5% ± 11% of the administered dose is eliminated in the urine in 24 h. Amdinocillin is eliminated by glomerular filtration and tubular secretion.

After intramuscular injection of a dose of 335 mg of amdinocillin dihydrate (~273 mg of anhydrous amdinocillin),

Table 84 In vitro activity of amdinocillin[a]

Organism(s)	MIC_{50} (μg/ml)	MIC_{90} (μg/ml)
S. aureus	>100	>100
S. pneumoniae	1.6	12.5
S. pyogenes	1.6	>100
E. faecalis	>100	>100
L. monocytogenes	>100	>100
E. coli	0.4	12.5
K. pneumoniae	1.6	50
Citrobacter spp.	0.4	100
Salmonella spp.	0.8	1.6
Shigella spp.	0.8	25
Enterobacter spp.	1.6	25
S. marcescens	12.5	>100
P. mirabilis	12.5	12.5
Providencia spp.	50	100
P. aeruginosa	>100	>100
H. influenzae	25	>100
Y. enterocolitica	0.8	1.6
Aeromonas hydrophila	0.4	1.6
Campylobacter jejuni	0.8	1.6

[a]MIC_{50} and MIC_{90}, MIC at which 50 and 90%, respectively, of isolates tested are inhibited.

Table 85 Breakpoints of amdinocillin[a]

Drug	Load (μg)	MIC (μg/ml)		Zone diam (mm)	
		S	R	S	R
Amdinocillin	10	≤2	>2	≥22	<18

[a]S, susceptible; R, resistant.

the peak concentration in serum of 4.5 to 5.0 μg/ml is reached in 30 to 45 min.

Amdinocillin is no longer detectable after 6 h. It is eliminated in the bile (Hares et al., 1982). After administration of 800 mg of amdinocillin, the mean concentration in the gallbladder is 40 μg/ml in nonicteric patients and 12 μg/ml in icteric patients.

Amdinocillin penetrates the CSF only weakly (concentration <1.0 μg/ml).

In patients with a creatinine clearance equal to or less than 10 ml/min, the apparent elimination half-life is 5.5 h (Svarsa and Wessel-Aas, 1980). Plasma protein binding is approximately 10 to 15%.

10.4.2. Amdinocillin Esters

Two esters have been developed, bacmecillinam and pivemecillinam (Fig. 25). Bacmecillinam has an ethoxycarbonyloxyethyl group as the ester, which allows better digestive absorption than the pivaloyloxymethyl group of pivemecillinam. In addition, bacmecillinam tablets dissolve better than those of pivemecillinam.

10.4.2.1. Bacmecillinam

Josefsson et al. (1982) compared the pharmacokinetics of bacmecillinam and pivemecillinam after a single oral dose of 400 mg. The peak concentrations in serum were, respectively, 4.76 and 2.57 μg/ml for bacmecillinam and pivemecillinam. The areas under the curve were greater for bacmecillinam than pivemecillinam.

The pharmacokinetic parameters of doses of 100, 200, and 400 mg of bacmecillinam are summarized in Table 86.

10.4.2.2. Pivemecillinam

After doses of 250 and 500 mg of pivemecillinam (Neu, 1983), the peak concentrations in serum were, respectively, 2.28 and 2.97 μg/ml and were reached in 1.5 h. At 6 h, the concentrations were 0.1 and 0.28 μg/ml, respectively. The areas under the curve were 5.35 and 7.87 μg·h/ml. Absorption was on average 44.5 and 33.1%. Urinary elimination was 29.2 and 24.8%.

After single doses of 200, 400, and 800 mg of pivemecillinam, the peak concentrations in serum were, respectively, 2 to 3, 4 to 5, and 6 to 7 μg/ml. The apparent elimination half-life was less than 1 h. Urinary elimination was 45%.

The apparent elimination half-life can attain 6.0 h in patients with a creatinine clearance of ≤10 ml/min.

The first pharmaceutical formulations of pivemecillinam caused visible changes in the gastric mucosa in the form of hyperemia, bleeding, and erosions.

11. GROUP VII: OXYIMINOPENICILLINS

BRL-44154 is a penicillin which has a 2-amino-5-thiazolyl nucleus on its side chain and an oxime group to which is attached a cyclopentyl nucleus (Fig. 26).

This molecule exhibits good activity against gram-positive cocci and penicillinase-producing or non-penicillinase-producing *S. aureus*, *S. pneumoniae*, and *S. pyogenes*. Its activity is more moderate against viridans group streptococci. It exhibits good activity against β-lactamase-producing and non-β-lactamase-producing strains of *M. catarrhalis* and *H. influenzae*.

It is moderately active against *Enterobacteriaceae* and practically inactive against class I or plasmid-mediated β-lactamase-producing strains. It is inactive against *B. fragilis* and *P. aeruginosa*. It was more active than floxacillin in experimental staphylococcal infections.

It has better affinity for *S. aureus* PBP 2a (IC_{50} > 1,000 μg/ml). BRL-44154 is capable of sterilizing endocarditis vegetations induced by an MRSA strain. In the dog, the apparent elimination half-life is 35 min, with plasma protein binding of 64% and urinary elimination of 64%.

Table 86 Pharmacokinetics of bacmecillinam and pivemecillinam orally[a]

Drug	Dose (mg)	Lag time (h)	C_{max} (μg/ml)	AUC (μg·h/ml)	$t_{1/2}$ (h)	Urinary elimination (%)
Bacmecillinam[b]	100	0.2	1.43	2.21	0.84	47.0
	200	0.24	2.74	3.99	0.95	43.5
	400	0.24	4.76	7.74	1.13	51.4
Pivemecillinam[c]	400	0.27	2.57	5.35	0.73	37.7

[a]Data from Josefsson et al., 1982.
[b]400 mg = 272 mg of mecillinam.
[c]400 mg = 273 mg of mecillinam.

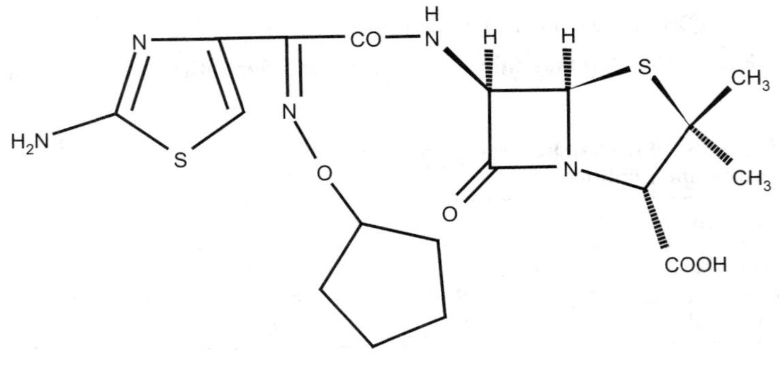

Figure 26 BRL-44154

REFERENCES

Akbaraly JP, Sarlangue J, Santarel M, Heinzel G, Peyraud J, Martin C, 1985, Pharmacokinetics of apalcillin in pediatrics, Pathol Biol, 33, 309–312.

Anderson ES, Datta N, 1965, Resistance to penicillin and its transfer in *Enterobacteriaceae*, Lancet, i, 407–409.

Anderson K, 1951, The aureomycin sensitivity of 100 pathogenic strains of *S. aureus*, J Clin Pathol, 4, 355.

Anonymous, 1984, BRL 20330, *Drugs Future*, 9, 250–251.

Barber M, Methicillin-resistant staphylococci 1965–1975, Lancet, ii, 650–653.

Barrett FF, McGehee RJ Jr, Finland M, 1968, Methicillin-resistant *S. aureus* at Boston City Hospital: bacteriologic and epidemiologic observations, N Engl J Med, 274, 441–448.

Basker MJ, Edmondson RA, Knott SJ, Ponsford RJ, Slocombe B, White SJ, 1984, In vitro antibacterial properties of BRL 36650, a novel 6a-substituted penicillin, Antimicrob Agents Chemother, 26, 734–740.

Basker MJ, Merrikin DJ, Ponsford RJ, Solocombe B, Tasker TCG, 1986, BRL 20330, an oral prodrug of temocillin: bioavailability studies in man, J Antimicrob Chemother, 18, 399–405.

Bengtsson S, Lindholm CE, Osterman K, 1979, Azidocillin levels in tracheobronchial secretions, Scand J Respir Dis, 60, 225–229.

Bergan T, 1983, Review of the pharmacokinetics of mezlocillin, J Antimicrob Chemother, 11, Suppl C, 1–16.

Bergan T, Michalsen H, 1979, Pharmacokinetics of azlocillin in children with cystic fibrosis, Arzneim Forsch, 29, 1955–1957.

Bergan T, Thornsteinsson SB, Steingrimmson I, 1982, Dose-dependent pharmacokinetics of azlocillin compared to mezlocillin, Chemotherapy, 28, 160–170.

Berger-Bächi B, Strassle A, Gustafson JE, Kayser FH, 1992, Mapping and characterization of multiple chromosomal factors involved in methicillin resistance in *Staphylococcus aureus*, Antimicrob Agents Chemother, 36, 1367–1373.

Bodey GP, Horikoshi N, Rodriguez V, 1974, Antimicrob Agents Chemother, 5, 366.

Borner K, Lode H, Elvers A, 1982, Determination of alpalcillin and its metabolites in human body fluids by high-pressure liquid chromatography, Antimicrob Agents Chemother, 22, 949–953.

Brachet-Liermain A, Akbaraly JP, Quentin C, Guyot M, Coux C, Auzerie J, Bebear C, 1983, Etude pharmacocinetique de l'alpacilline apres perfusion, Pathol Biol, 31, 319–322.

Bratlid D, 1976, Pharmacologic aspects of neonatal hyperbilirubinemia, Birth Defects, 12, 184–191.

Brogard JM, Adloff M, Pinget M, Dorner M, Lautier F, 1985, L'élimination biliaire de l'apalcilline: étude experimentale et evaluation chez l'homme, Pathol Biol, 33, 121–128.

Brogard JM, Kopferschmitt J, Dorner M, Lavillaureix J, 1981, Détermination expérimentale et étude clinique de l'élimination biliaire de la mezlocilline, Pathol Biol, 29, 405–410.

Brogden RN, Heel RC, Speight TM, Avery GS, 1979, Amoxycillin injectable: a review of its antibacterial spectrum, pharmacokinetics and therapeutic use, Drugs, 18, 169–184.

Brogden RN, Heel RC, Speight TM, Avery GS, 1980, Ticarcillin: a review of its pharmacological properties and therapeutic efficacy, Drugs, 20, 325–352.

Brown III CH, Natelson E, Bradshaw MJ, Alfrey CP, Williams TW Jr, 1975, Study of the effect of ticarcillin on blood coagulation and platelet function, Antimicrob Agents Chemother, 7, 652–657.

Brown III CH, Natelson E, Bradshaw MJ, Williams TW Jr, Alfrey CP, 1974, The hemostatic defect produced by carbenicillin, N Engl J Med, 291, 265–270.

Brown RM, Wise R, Andrew JM, 1982, Temocillin, in vitro activity and the pharmacokinetics and tissue penetration in healthy volunteers, J Antimicrob Chemother, 10, 295.

Bulger R, Sherris JC, 1968, Decreased incidence of antibiotic resistance among *S. aureus*: a study in a university hospital over a nine year period, Ann Intern Med, 69, 1099–1108.

Bunke CM, Aronoff GR, Brier ME, Sloan RS, Luft FC, 1983, Mezlocillin kinetics in hepatic insufficiency, Clin Pharmacol Ther, 33, 73–76.

Burton G, Dobson CR, Everett JR, 1986, The degradation of temocillin, a 6-α-methoxypenicillin, and identification of the major degradation products, J Pharm Pharmacol, 38, 758–761.

Butler K, English AR, Briggs B, Gralla E, Stebbins RB, Hobbs DC, 1973, Indanylcarbenicillin chemistry and laboratory studies with semisynthetic penicillin, J Infect Dis, 127, suppl, S97–S104.

Campos J, Fuste MC, Trujillo G, Saez-Nieto J, Vaquez J, Loren JG, Vinas M, Spratt BG, 1992, Genetic diversity of penicillin-resistant *N. meningitidis*, J Infect Dis, 166, 173–177.

Cano JP, Rigault JP, Gevaudan MJ, Saingra S, Murisasco A, Charpin J, 1982, Etude pharmacocinétique de la mezlocilline intraveineuse chez les malades à fonction renale normale et chez les insuffisants renaux, Nouv Presse Med, 11, 335–339.

Chabbert YA, Baudins JG, Acar JF, Gerbaud GP, 1965, The natural resistance of staphylococci to methicillin and oxacillin, Rev Fr Etud Clin Biol, 10, 495–506.

Cheng AF, French GL, 1988, Methicillin-resistant *Staphylococcus aureus* bacteremia in Hong Kong, J Hosp Infect, 12, 91–101.

Clarke GP, Libke RD, Ralph ED, Luthy RP, Kirby WMM, 1974, Human pharmacokinetics of BLP 1654 compared with ampicillin, Antimicrob Agents Chemother, 6, 729–733.

Clayton JP, Cole M, Elson SW, Hardy KD, Mizen LW, Sutherland R, 1975, Preparation, hydrolysis and oral absorption of a-carboxy esters of carbenicillin, J Med Chem, 18, 172–177.

Cleeland R, Squires E, 1983, Enhanced activity of beta-lactam antibiotics with amdinocillin in vitro and in vivo, Am J Med, 75(SA), 21–29.

Crowngold T, 1977, Susceptibility of *Yersinia pestis* to trimethoprim and sulfamethoxazole, singly and in combination, as well as to amoxycillin, South Afr J Med Lab Technol, 23, 15.

Datta N, Kontomichalon P, 1965, Pencillinase resistance controlled by infectious R-factors in *Enterobacteriaceae*, Nature, 208, 239–241.

Delgado FA, Stout RL, Whelton A, 1983, Pharmacokinetics of azlocillin in normal renal function: single and repetitive dosing studies, J Antimicrob Chemother, 11, 79–88.

De Schepper PJ, Tjandramaga TB, Mullie A, Verbesselt R, van Hecken A, Verberckmoes R, Verbist L, 1982, Comparative pharmacokinetics of piperacillin in normals and in patients with renal failure, J Antimicrob Chemother, 9 (Suppl B), 49–57.

Doern GV, Jorgensen JH, Thornsberg C, Preston DA, Tubert T, Redding JS, Mahler LA, 1988, National collaborative study of prevalence of antimicrobial resistance among clinical isolates of *Haemophilus influenzae*, Antimicrob Agents Chemother, 32, 180–185.

Dornbusch K, the European Study Group on Antibiotic Resistance, 1990, Resistance to β-lactam antibiotics and ciprofloxacin in Gram-negative bacilli and staphylococci isolated from blood: a European collaborative study, J Antimicrob Chemother, 26, 269–278.

Drugeon HB, Pannier M, Courtieu AL, 1984, Pharmacocinétique de l'azlocilline chez les brûlés, Presse Med, 13, 805–807.

Finland M, 1970, Changing ecology of bacterial infections as related to antibacterial therapy, J Infect Dis, 22, 419–431.

Finland M, 1979, Emergence of antibiotic resistance in hospitals, 1935–1975, Rev Infect Dis, 1, 4–21.

Fleming A, Fish EW, 1947, Influence of penicillin on the coagulation of blood, Br Med J, 2, 243–244.

Francke EL, Appel GB, Neu HC, 1979, Pharmacokinetics of intravenous piperacillin in patients undergoing chronic hemodialysis, Antimicrob Agents Chemother, 16, 788–791.

Frank U, Schmidt-Eisenlohr E, Schlosser V, Spillner G, Schindler M, Daschner FD, 1988, Concentrations of flucloxacillin in heart valves and subcutaneous and muscle tissues of patients undergoing open heart surgery, Antimicrob Agents Chemother, 32, 930–931.

Goerner JR, Massell BF, Jones TD, 1947, Use of penicillin in the treatment of carriers of beta-hemolytic streptococci among patients with rheumatic fever, N Engl J Med, 237, 576–580.

Grose WE, Bodey GP, Hall SW, 1976, Curr Ther Res, 20, 604.

Guest EA, Horton R, Mellows G, Slocombe B, Swaisland AJ, Tasker TCG, 1985, Human pharmacokinetics of temocillin (BRL 17421) side chain epimers, J Antimicrob Chemother, 15, 327–336.

Hansson E, Wahlguist S, 1968, α-Azidobenzylpenicillin. II. Preliminary clinical pharmacology, in Hobby GD, ed, Antimicrobial Agents Chemotherapy, p 568–572. American Society for Microbiology, Washington, D.C.

Hares MM, Hegarthy A, Tomkyns J, Burdon DW, Keighley MRB, 1982, A study of biliary excretion of mecillinam in patients with biliary diseases, J Antimicrob Chemother, 9, 217–222.

Hartman BM, Tomasz A, 1984, Low-affinity penicillin binding protein associated with beta-lactam resistance in *Staphylococcus aureus*, J Bacteriol, 158, 513–520.

Heim-Duthoy KL, Halstenson CE, Abraham PA, Matzke GR, 1986, The effect of hemodialysis on piperacillin pharmacokinetics, Int J Clin Pharmacol Ther Toxicol, 24, 680–684.

Herngren L, Ehrnebo M, Broberger U, 1987, Pharmacokinetics of free and total flucloxacillin in newborn infants, Eur J Clin Pharmacol, 32, 403–409.

Herrell WE, Heilman DG, William HL, 1942, The clinical use of penicillin, Pro Staff Meet Mayo Clinics, 17, 605–616.

Hinderling PH, Gundert-Remy U, Förster D, Gau W, 1983, The pharmacokinetics of furazlocillin in healthy humans, J Pharmacokin Biopharm, 11, 5–30.

Hone R, Cafferkey M, Keane CT, et al, 1981, Bacteremia in Dublin due to gentamicin-resistant *S. aureus*, J Hosp Infect, 2, 119–126.

Hoogmartens J, Roets E, Janssen G, Vanderhaeghe H, 1982, Separation of the side chain diastereoisomers of penicillins by high-performance liquid chromatography, J Chromatogr, 244, 299–309.

Horan TC, White JC, Jarvis WR, Emori TG, Culver DH, Munn VP, et al, 1984, Nosocomial infection surveillance—CDC surveillance summaries, Morb Mortal Wkly Rep, 35, 17SS–29SS.

Issell BF, Bodey GP, Weaver S, 1978, Clinical pharmacology of mezlocillin, Antimicrob Agents Chemother, 13, 180–183.

Jamaluddin ABM, Sarwar G, Rahim MA, Rahman MK, 1989, Assay for cloxacillin in human serum utilising high-performance liquid chromatography with ultraviolet detection, J Chromatogr, 490, 243–246.

Jessen O, Rosendal K, Bulow P, Faber V, Eriksen R, 1969, Changing staphylococci and staphylococcal infections—a ten year study of bacteremia and cases of bacteremia, N Engl J Med, 281, 627–635.

Jevans MP, 1961, Celbenin-resistant staphylococci, Br Med J, i, 124.

Josefsson K, Bergan T, Magni L, Pring BG, Westerlund D, 1982, Pharmacokinetics of bacmecillinam and pivemecillinam in volunteers, Eur J Clin Pharmacol, 23, 249–252.

Kacet N, Russel-Delvallez M, Gremillet C, Dubos JP, Storme L, Lequien P, 1992, Pharmacokinetics study of piperacillin in newborns relating to gestational and postnatal age, Pediatr Infect Dis J, 11, 365–369.

Kayser FH, Morenzoni G, Santanam P, 1990, The second European collaborative study on the frequency of antimicrobial resistance in *Haemophilus influenzae*, Eur J Clin Microbiol Infect Dis, 9, 810–817.

Kees F, Naber KG, Dominiak P, Stockmann P, Meyer GP, Adam D, Grobecker H, 1985, Metaboliten and Umwandlungsprodukte von Penicillinen, Fortschr Antimikr Antineoplast Chemother, band 4-6, 1433–1443.

Knirsch AK, Hobbs DC, Korst JJ, 1973, Pharmacokinetics, toleration, and safety of indanyl carbenicillin in man, J Infect Dis, 127, suppl, 105–110.

Knoiller J, Schonfeld W, Bremm KD, König W, 1988, Degradation of acylaminopenicillins with regard to their pH dependency, Zentbl Bakteriol Hyg A, 267, 531–536.

Knudsen ET, Rolinson GN, 1960, Absorption and excretion of a new antibiotic, BRL 1241, Br Med J, 2, 700–703.

Komatsu T, Noguchi H, Tobiki H, Nakagome T, 1981, Apalcillin (PC 904) and its related compounds, p 87–98, in Mitsuhashi S, ed, Beta-Lactam Antibiotics, Scientific Soc Press, Tokyo.

Kosmidis J, et al, 1988, Staphylococcal infections in hospital: the Greek experience, J Hosp Infect, 11, suppl A, 109–115.

Kwan RH, MacLeod SM, Spino M, Teare FW, 1982, High-pressure liquid chromatographic assays for ticarcillin in serum and urine, J Pharm Sci, 71, 1118–1121.

Labia R, Baron P, Masson JM, Hill G, Cole M, 1984, Affinity of temocillin for *Escherichia coli* K-12 penicillin binding proteins, Antimicrob Agents Chemother, 26, 335–338.

Labinchinski H, 1992, Consequences of interaction of β-lactam antibiotics with penicillin binding proteins from sensitive and resistant *S. aureus* strains, Med Microbiol Immunol, 181, 241–265.

Lambert C, Pointet P, Ducret F, 1989, Interaction ciclosporine-ticarcilline chez un transplante renal, Presse Med, 18, 230.

Lange H, Baler R, Fleishmann N, Frei M, Dapper D, 1982, Elimination of piperacillin in renal impairement, Curr Chemother Immunother, 1, 673–675.

Leigh DA, Simmons K, 1976, The treatment of simple and complicated urinary tract infections with carfecillin, a new oral ester of carbenicillin, J Antimicrob Chemother, 2, 293–298.

Leroy A, Humbert G, Fillastre JP, et al, 1983, Pharmacokinetics of temocillin (BRL 17421) in subjects with normal and impaired renal function, J Antimicrob Chemother, 12, 47–58.

Leroy A, Humbert G, Godin M, Fillastre JP, 1980, Pharmacokinetics of azlocillin in subjects with normal and impaired renal functions, Antimicrob Agents Chemother, 17, 344–349.

Lode H, Niestrath U, Koeppe P, Langmaack H, 1977, Azlocillin und mezlocillin: zwei neue semisynthetische Acylureidopenicilline, Infection, 5, 163–169.

Löfgren S, Bucht G, Hermansson B, Holm SE, Winblad B, Norrby R, Single-dose pharmacokinetics of dicloxacillin in healthy subjects of young and old age, data on file, SmithKline Beecham.

Lund F, Tybring L, 1972, 6-β-Amidinopenicillanic acid—a new group of antibiotics, Nature, 236, 135–137.

Massidda O, Montanari MP, Varaldo PE, 1992, Evidence for a methicillin-hydrolysing β-lactamase in *Staphylococcus aureus* strains with borderline susceptibility to this drug, FEMS Microbiol Lett, 92, 223–227.

McCracken GH Jr, 1974, Pharmacological basis for antimicrobial therapy in newborn infants, Am J Dis Child, 128, 407–419.

McDougal L, Thornsberry C, 1986, The role of β-lactamase in staphylococcal resistance to penicillinase-resistant penicillins and cephalosporins, J Clin Microbiol, 23, 832–839.

McGowan JE Jr, 1988, Gram-positive bacteria: spread and antimicrobial resistance in university and community hospitals in the USA, J Antimicrob Chemother, 21, suppl C, 49–55.

Meyers BR, Mendelson MM, Srulevitch-Chin E, Bradbury K, McMurdo L, Hirschman SZ, 1987, Pharmacokinetic properties of mezlocillin in ambulatory elderly subjects, J Clin Pharmacol, 27, 678–681.

Minami Y, Komuro M, Sakawa K, Ishida N, Shindo T, Matsumoto K, Oishi K, 1991, Human specific metabolite of piperacillin, desethylpiperacillin newly found after 10-year clinical usage, 31st Intersci Conf Antimicrob Agents Chemother.

Murai Y, Nakagawa T, Yamaoka K, Uno T, 1981, High performance liquid chromatographic analysis and pharmacokinetic investigation of oxacillin and its metabolites in man, Chem Pharm Bull, 29, 3290–3297.

Murai Y, Nakagawa T, Yamaoka K, Uno T, 1983, High performance liquid chromatographic determination and moment analysis of urinary excretion of flucloxacillin and its metabolites in man, Int J Pharm, 15, 309–320.

Nauta EH, Mattie H, 1987, Pharmacokinetics of flucloxacillin and cloxacillin in healthy subjects and patients on chronic intermittent haemodialysis, Br J Clin Pharmacol, 2, 111–121.

Neu HC, 1982, Antistaphylococcal penicillin, Med Clin N Am, 66, 51–60.

Neu HC, 1983, Penicillin-binding proteins and role of amdinopenicillin in causing bacterial cell death, Am J Med, 75(2A), 9–20.

Parker MT, Hewitt JH, 1970, Methicillin resistance in S. aureus, Lancet, i, 800–804.

Paton DM, 1986, Comparative bioavailability and half-lives of cloxacillin and flucloxacillin, Int J Clin Pharm Res, 6, 347–349.

Peskine F, Despaux E, Rodiere M, Balmayer B, Kassis J, Fuseau E, Brunei D, 1982, Etude pharmacocinetique et clinique de 1'amoxicilline intraveineuse chez le nouveau-né, Pathol Biol, 30, 476–480.

Phillips I, 1976, β-Lactamase producing penicillin-resistant gonococcus, Lancet, ii, 656–657.

Preheim LC, Rimland D, Bittner MJ, 1987, Methicillin-resistant *S. aureus* in Veterans Administration Medical Centers, Infect Control, 8, 191–194.

Price KE, Chisholm DM, Leitner F, Miesck M, Gourevitch A, 1969, Antipseudomonal activity of α-sulfoaminopenicillins, Appl Microbiol, 17, 881–887.

Price KE, Leitner F, Misiek M, Chisholm DR, Pursiano TA, 1971, BL-P 1654, a new broad-spectrum penicillin with marked antipseudomonal activity, Antimicrob Agents Chemother, 10, 17–29.

Ramsay CH, Bodin NO, Hansson E, 1972, Absorption, distribution, biotransformation, and excretion of azidocillin, a new semisynthetic penicillin, in mice, rats and dogs, Arzneim Forsch, 22, 1962–1970.

Renneberg J, Forsgren A, 1989, The activity of isoxazolyl penicillins in experimental staphylococcal infection, J Infect Dis, 159, 1128–1132.

Rolinson GN, 1981, Ampicillin, p 83–86, in Mitsuhashi S, ed, Beta-Lactam Antibiotics, Springer-Verlag, Berlin.

Rolinson GN, Batchelor FR, 1962–1963, Penicillin metabolites, Antimicrob Agents Chemother, 654–660.

Rountree PM, Beard MA, 1968, Hospital strains of *Staphylococcus aureus* with particular reference to methicillin-resistant strains, Med J Aust, 2, 1163–1168.

Rountree PM, Vickery AM, 1973, Further observations on methicillin-resistant staphylococci, Med J Aust, 1, 1030–1034.

Rubio T, Wirth FH, Karotkin EH, 1982, Pharmacokinetics of piperacillin in newborn infants, Curr Chemother Immunother, 1, 677–678.

Schito GC, Varaldo PE, 1988, Trends in the epidemiology and antibiotic resistance of clinical *Staphylococcus* strains in Italy—a review, J Antimicrob Chemother, 21, suppl C, 67–81.

Scragg JN, Appelbaum PC, Govender DA, 1978, The spectrum of infection and sensitivity of organisms isolated from African and Indian children in a Duban hospital, Trans R Soc Trop Med Hyg, 72, 325–328.

Shanson DC, Kensit JC, Duke R, 1976, Outbreak of hospital infection with a strain of *Staphylococcus aureus* resistant to gentamicin and methicillin, Lancet, ii, 1347–1348.

Shishido H, Matsumoto K, Uzuka Y, Nagatake T, Yamamoto M, Sakuma Y, Yamaguchi T, 1982, Phase I clinical study of TA-058, Curr Chemother Immunother, 1, 329–331.

Siboni K, Poulsen L, Digman E, 1968, The dominance of methicillin-resistant staphylococci in a county hospital, Dan Med Bull, 15, 161–165.

Singlas E, Haegel C, 1984, Pharmacocinetique de l'azlocilline, Presse Med, 13, 788–796.

Sirot J, Lopitaux R, Dumont C, Delisle JJ, Rampon S, Cluzel R, 1982, Diffusion de la cloxacilline dans le tissu osseux apres une administration par voie orale, Pathol Biol, 30, 332–335.

Sjoberg B, Ekstrom B, Forsgren U, 1968, α-Azidobenzylpenicillin I. Chemistry, bacteriology and experimental chemotherapy, p 560–567, in Hobby GD, ed, Antimicrobial Agents Chemotherapy. American Society for Microbiology, Washington, D.C.

Sjövall J, Alvan G, Huitfeldt B, 1986, Intra- and interindividual variation in pharmacokinetics of intravenously infused amoxycillin and ampicillin to elderly volunteers, Br J Clin Pharmacol, 21, 171–181.

Slocombe B, Basker MJ, Bentley PH, Clayton JP, Cole M, Comber KR, Dixon RA, Edmondson RA, Jackson D, Merriken DJ, Sutherland R, 1981, BRL 17421, a novel β-lactam antibiotic highly resistant to β-lactamases, giving high and prolonged serum levels in humans, Antimicrob Agents Chemother, 20, 38–46.

Smith AL, Meeks CA, Koup JR, Opheim KE, Weber A, Vishwanathan CT, 1990, Dicloxacillin absorption and elimination in children, Dev Pharmacol Ther, 14, 35–44.

Soussy CJ, Dublanchet A, Cormier M, Bismuth R, Mison F, Chardon H, Duval J, Fabiani E, 1976, Nouvelles resistances plasmidiques de *S. aureus* aux aminosides (gentamicine, tobramycine, amikacine), Nouv Presse Med, 5, 2599–2601.

Soussy CJ, Duval J, 1984, Evolution de la résistance des staphylocoques aux pénicillines, p 7–25, in Vachon F, Régnier B, ed, Les Infections à staphylocoques meticilline resistants, Arnette, Paris.

Svarsa PL, Wessel-Aas T, 1980, Serum levels of mecillinam in patients with severely impaired renal function, Scand J Infect Dis, 12, 303–305.

Thijssen HHW, Mattie H, 1976, Active metabolites of isoxazolylpenicillins in humans, Antimicrob Agents Chemother, 10, 441–446.

Thiramoorthi MC, Asmar BI, Buckley JA, Bollinger RO, Kauffman RE, Dajam AS, 1983, Pharmacokinetics of intravenously administered piperacillin in preadolescent children, J Pediatr, 102, 941–946.

Tjandramaga T, Mullie A, Verbesselt R, De Schepper PJ, Verbist L, 1978, Piperacillin: human pharmacokinetics after intravenous and intramuscular administration, Antimicrob Agents Chemother, 14, 829–837.

Trunet P, Bouvier AM, Otterbein G, Lepresle E, Lhoste F, Rapin M, 1982, Encéphalopathies dues aux β-lactamines, Nouv Presse Med, 11, 1781–1784.

Tsuji A, Miyamoto E, Terasaki T, Yamana T, 1982, Carbenicillin prodrugs: kinetics of intestinal absorption competing degradation of the α-esters of carbenicillin and prediction of prodrug absorbability from quantitative structure-absorption rate relationship, J Pharm Sci, 17, 403–406.

Varaldo PE, 1993, The "borderline methicillin-susceptible" *Staphylococcus aureus*, J Antimicrob Chemother, 31, 1–4.

Varon E, Gutmann L, 1993, Bases moléculaires de la résistance du pneumocoque aux bêta-lactamines, p 15–24, in Carbon C, Chastang C, Decaze JM, ed, Infections à pneumocoques de sensibilité diminuée aux bêta-lactamines, Springer-Verlag, Paris.

Walker AE, Johnson HC, Case TJ, Kohros JJ, 1946, Convulsive effects of antibiotic agents on cerebral cortex, Science, 103, 116.

Walker AE, Johnson HC, Koliros JJ, 1945, Penicillin convulsions: convulsive effects of penicillin applied to cerebral cortex of monkey and man, Surg Gynecol Obst, 81, 692–701.

Wasz-Hockert O, Nummi S, Vuopala S, Jarvinen PA, 1970, Transplacental passage of azidocillin, ampicillin and penicillin G during early and late pregnancy, Acta Paediatr Scand Suppl, 206, 109–110.

Weingartner L, Sitka V, Patsch R, Thiemann HH, 1982, Azlocillin and mezlocillin: pharmacokinetic studies in children, Curr Chemother Immunother, 1, 642–643.

Westphal JF, Deslandes A, Brogard JM, Carbon C, 1991, Reappraisal of amoxycillin absorption kinetics, J Antimicrob Chemother, 27, 647–654.

Wilkinson PJ, Reeves DS, Wise R, Allen JT, 1975, Volunteer and clinical studies with carfecillin: a new orally administered ester of carbenicillin, Br Med J, ii, 250–253.

Williams JD, Cavanagh P, 1974, Ampicillin-resistant Haemophilus influenzae meningitis, Lancet, i, 864, letter.

Wilson CB, Koup JR, Pheim KE, Adelman LA, Levy J, Still TL, Clausen C, Smith AL, 1982, Piperacillin pharmacokinetics in pediatric patients, Antimicrob Agents Chemother, 22, 442–447.

Cephems for Parenteral Use

A. BRYSKIER AND J. ASZODI

6

1. INTRODUCTION

The modern history of β-lactams began in 1929 with the publication by Alexander Fleming of the antistaphylococcal activity of a culture filtrate of *Penicillium notatum*. Since their introduction into therapeutic use at the beginning of the 1970s, cephalosporins have been among the most potent and most widely used anti-infective agents. They are well tolerated. The development of the cephalosporins has paralleled that of the penicillins.

Table 1 In vitro activities of cephalosporins

Drug	MIC (μg/ml)		
	S. aureus	*E. coli*	*K. pneumoniae*
Cephalosporin C	78	92	27
Cephalothin	0.4	17	2
Cephaloridine	4	5	4
Cefazolin	0.8	2	2

The history of cephalosporins began in 1945 with the discovery of the antibacterial and therapeutic activity of a culture filtrate or crude extract of *Cephalosporium acremonium*. Three substances were isolated by Abraham and Newton's team from the University of Oxford: penicillin N (now known as adicillin), cephalosporin P1, and cephalosporin C. Cephalosporin C possesses modest antibacterial activity (Table 1) but is active against *Staphylococcus aureus* Oxford and is resistant to hydrolysis by *Bacillus subtilis* penicillinase. Penicillin N had not yet been synthesized. The discovery of a mutant strain of *C. acremonium* producing large quantities of cephalosporin C and the development of a chemical process providing a good yield of 7-aminocephalosporanic acid gave rise to the chemistry of the cephalosporins (Fig. 1). The first molecule available was cephalothin, followed by cephaloridine. These have good activity against penicillinase-producing strains of *S. aureus*

HOOC—CH—$(CH_2)_2$—CH_2—CO—N(H) ... NH_2 ... S ... N ... O ... H_2C ... $OCOCH_3$ ... COONa

1) NOCl, HCOOH

2) H_2O

H_3N^+ ... S ... N ... O ... H_2C ... $OCOCH_3$ ... COOH

(yield 40%) **Figure 1 7-Aminocephalosporanic acid (7-ACA)** and also not insignificant activity against certain species of *Enterobacteriaceae*.

At the beginning of the 1970s, the cephamycins (cephems possessing a 7α-methoxy group) were isolated from a culture filtrate of *Streptomyces*. The search for molecules with good activity against gram-negative bacteria passed through several stages: the discoveries of cefsulodin, which is an α-sulfocephalosporin; cefamandole, which was the first molecule to have an *N*-methylthiotetrazole moiety at C-7; and cefuroxime, which represented a major advance with the methoxyimino chain at C-7. The major discovery was that of the 2-amino-5-thiazolyl moiety at position 7 which gave rise to cefotaxime. This discovery was the beginning of the modern era in the use of cephalosporins.

A further small advance was made with ceftazidime with the addition of a C-3′ quaternary ammonium. This molecule is inferior in terms of its activity against gram-positive cocci and *Enterobacteriaceae* but possesses therapeutic activity against *Pseudomonas aeruginosa*.

The chemical picture can consequently be defined: 2-amino-5-thiazolyl and oxyimino chain substituted at position 7 and a quaternary ammonium type chain at C-3′. The difficulty was to synthesize molecules with a balanced antibacterial spectrum. Only cefpirome and cefozopran meet this requirement.

The appearance of enzymes capable of hydrolyzing cefotaxime stimulated research based on the observation by Watanabe et al. of the use of the iron transport route in *Escherichia coli* by a cephalosporin possessing a catechol moiety, E-0702. The new cephalosporins thus also have a catechol or a pyridone group.

2. CLASSIFICATIONS OF CEPHEMS

Because of the importance of the cephems, it is essential to classify them so as to allow their optimal use. Numerous classifications have been proposed: chemical, biological, microbiological, pharmacokinetic, and immunological.

2.1. Chemical Classification

The cephems are characterized by an azetidinone ring, to which is attached an unsaturated hexacycle. Side chains are attached to the two rings. Five classes of cephems may be distinguished in terms of the nature of the moiety: cephalosporins (Fig. 2), cephamycins and cephabacins, oxa-1-cephems, carba-1-cephems, and miscellaneous. The miscellaneous group comprises molecules such as 1-phosphocephems, 2-azacephems, and isocephems (Fig. 3).

The cephalosporins are characterized by an azetidinone ring, to which is attached a dihydrothiazine ring. The cephem

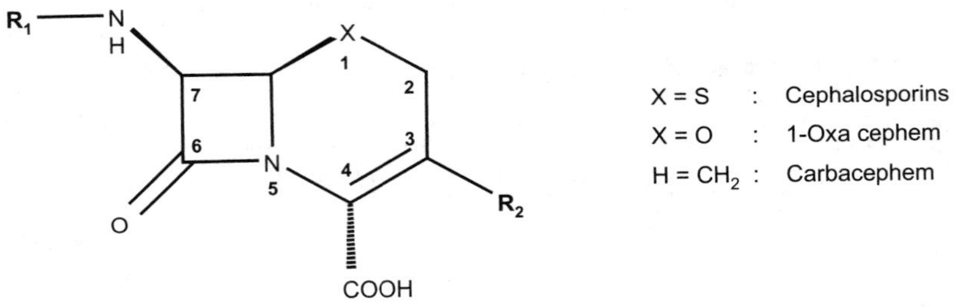

X = S : Cephalosporins
X = O : 1-Oxa cephem
H = CH_2 : Carbacephem

Figure 2 Cephems

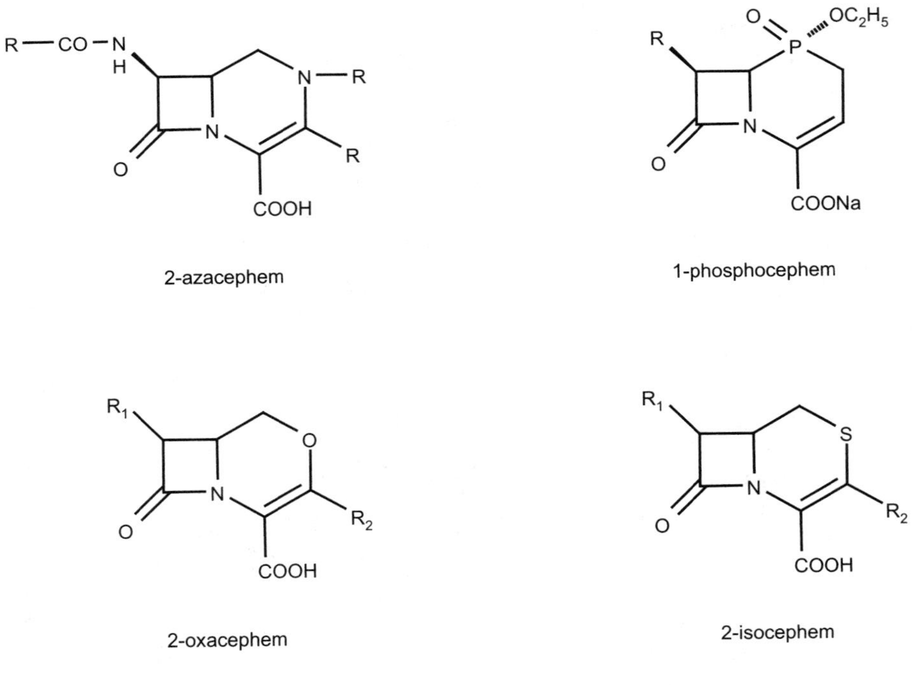

2-azacephem

1-phosphocephem

2-oxacephem

2-isocephem

Figure 3 Other cephems

derivatives are divided according to the nature of the chain on the α carbon at C-7 (CH_2, CH-R, C=X-Y) (Fig. 4).

Three subgroups of cephalosporins may be distinguished according to the side chain at position 7: non-α-substituted cephalosporins, α-substituted cephalosporins, and oxyiminoarylacetyl cephalosporins.

2.1.1. Group 1A: Non-α-Substituted Cephalosporins

Two subgroups may be distinguished: the first category of molecules possesses a metabolizable side chain at C-3 and the second possesses a polyazole heterocycle. Subgroup 1 comprises molecules which may be deacetylated at C-3 by an esterase: cephalothin, cephapirin, and cephacetrile. Subgroup 2 comprises six molecules possessing a heterocycle at C-3: cefotiam, cefazolin, etc. Mention may also be made of cefathiamidine, which has an aminothioisopropyl chain and which appears to be active against *Enterococcus faecalis* and *Enterococcus faecium.*

2.1.2. Group 1B: α-Substituted Cephalosporins

2.1.2.1. α-Amino Cephalosporins

α-Amino cephalosporins have the chemical characteristics of an α-amino group and a phenyl ring replaced by hydroxyl and halogen groups (chlorine). The group at C-3 is a polar or small group which, when combined with the amino group, facilitates oral absorption.

2.1.2.2. Other α-Substituted Cephalosporins

Other α-substituted cephalosporins may be subdivided into three classes:

- The hydroxycephalosporins. Two molecules have currently been developed: cefamandole and cefonicid. They differ in the N-substituent of the tetrazole moiety at C-3: *N*-methyl for cefamandole and *N*-methylsulfone for cefonicid, giving it a long apparent elimination half-life.
- The α-sulfocephalosporins. Currently, only one molecule has been developed: cefsulodin, which has good activity against *P. aeruginosa* (MIC, 1 to 4 μg/ml).

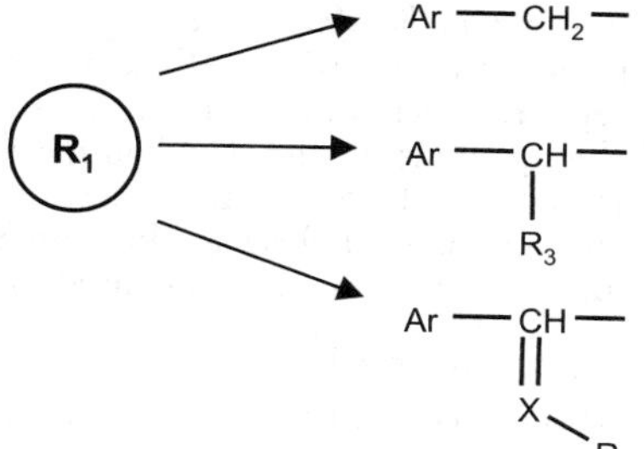

Figure 4 Basic structures of cephalosporins

- *N*-Acylcephalosporins. The asymmetrical carbon in the α position of the chain at C-7 is replaced by a chain comprising a carbamoyl and a variable heterocycle. Several molecules have been described and developed: cefoperazone, cefpiramide, and cefpimizole, which possess *N*-ethyldioxopiperazine, pteridine, and imidazole moieties, respectively. Other molecules of the ureidocephalosporin type have been described, such as KT-180.

2.1.3. Group 1C: Oxyiminoarylacetyl Cephalosporins

With the exception of cefuroxime (furyl moiety), the cephalosporins all comprise a 2-amino-5-thiazolyl or 5-amino-2-thiadiazolyl heterocycle.

The oxyimino group is substituted by an α-hydroxy group or by an alkyl (methyl, isobutyric, etc.), carboxyl, aryl, or phosphonic chain.

Three groups of molecules may be distinguished: derivatives of cefotaxime possessing a 2-amino-5-thiazolyl moiety and a methoxyimino residue with a variable side chain at C-3, C-3′ quaternary ammonium cephalosporins, and derivatives with a catechol moiety at C-3 or C-7.

2.2. Pharmacokinetic Classification

The dosage and dosing frequency of a cephalosporin are the result of a balance between its antibacterial activity and its pharmacokinetic profile.

For the sake of convenience, the cephalosporins may be classified according to their apparent elimination half-life in young subjects with healthy renal function. Three groups may be proposed, I to III (Fig. 5).

Group I comprises molecules with an apparent elimination half-life of less than 1.0 h. Group II is composed of derivatives with a half-life greater than or equal to 1 h and less than 3 h. Molecules in group III have a half-life of more than 3 h but less than or equal to 8 h.

Within these groups, the molecules are divided according to the route of elimination: urinary or biliary ($>$20% of the administered dose). The daily doses in severe but not immediately life-threatening infections in groups II and III are 3 to 4 g and 2 to 3 g, respectively.

This daily dosage has to be modified when the apparent elimination half-lives are greater than 1 h (group I), 3 h (group II), and 8 h (group III).

2.3. Microbiological Classification

The cephalosporins are traditionally divided into first, second, third, and fourth generations. In reality, the cephems may be divided into seven groups on the basis of their antibacterial activities: limited spectrum (groups I and II), broad spectrum (groups III, IV, and V) and narrow spectrum (group VI). A seventh group is made up of molecules that have weak activity but chemical originality, such as 1-phospho- or 1-azacephalosporins (Fig. 6).

2.3.1. Group I Cephalosporins

Group I cephalosporins may be divided into two groups according to their metabolic stability (Fig. 7): the compounds in group IA include molecules metabolized in the liver, i.e., cephalothin, cephacetrile, and cephapirin; those in group IB include nonmetabolized molecules, such as cephaloridine, cefazolin, cephanone, ceftezole, cefazaflur, and cefazedone (Fig. 7). Figure 8 shows the structures of group I cephalosporins. Figure 9 shows the structures of group IB cephalosporins.

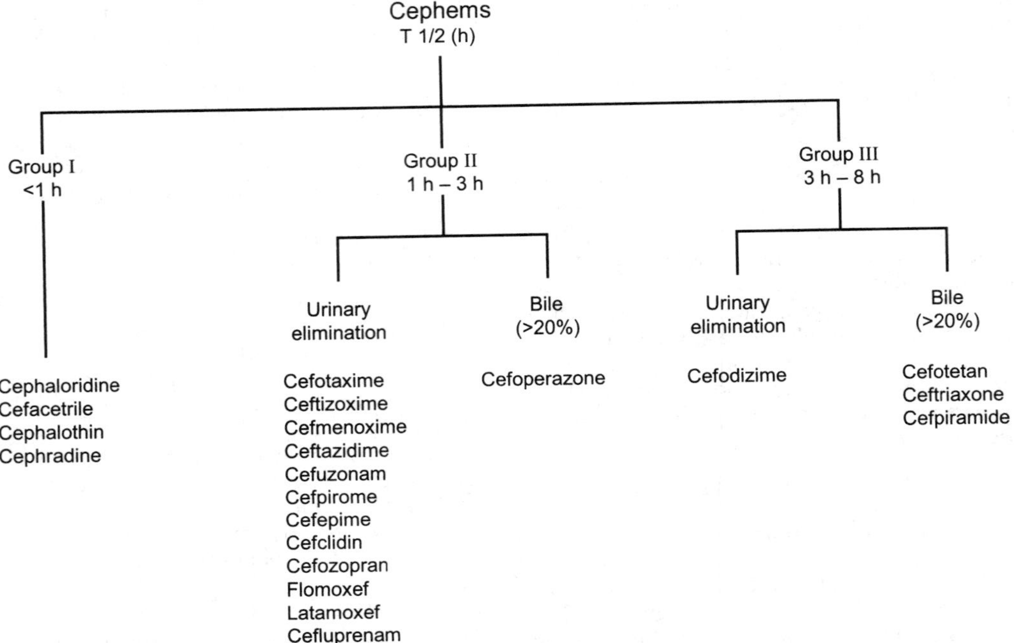

Figure 5 Pharmacokinetic classification of cephems

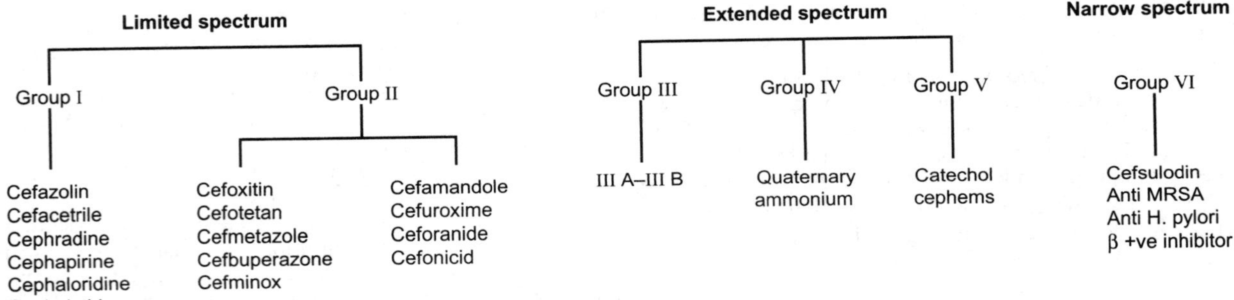

Figure 6 Microbiological classification of cephalosporins

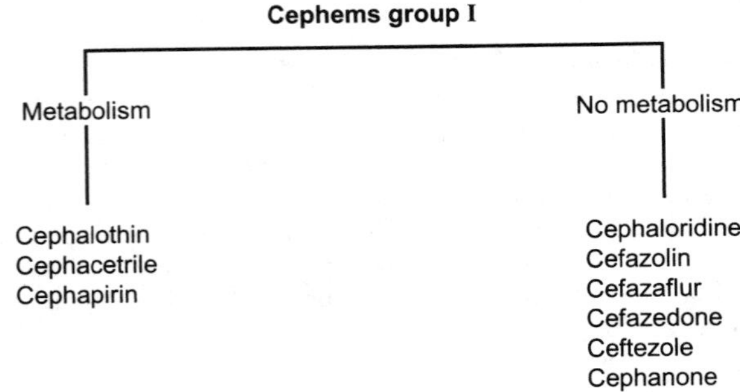

Figure 7 Cephems, group I

2.3.1.1. In Vitro Activity

All of these molecules are characterized by good activity against non-β-lactamase-producing strains of *S. aureus* but weaker activity against penicillinase-producing strains (Table 2), a feature that is particularly apparent with cefazolin and cephaloridine, which are four times less active against penicillin G-resistant strains, whereas this reduction in activity is minor with cephalothin. Cefazolin and cephaloridine are partially hydrolyzed by *S. aureus* penicillinases. These molecules are relatively unstable against hydrolysis by broad-spectrum β-lactamases of *Enterobacteriaceae* and other gram-negative bacilli (TEM-1 and TEM-2, SHV-1, ROB-1, etc.), hence their mediocre activity against strains producing these enzymes, such as *E. coli and Neisseria gonorrhoeae*. They are inactive against type I enzyme-producing species of *Enterobacteriaceae*: *Enterobacter cloacae, Serratia marcescens, Citrobacter freundii, Morganella morganii*, etc. They are also ineffective against *P. aeruginosa* (Table 3).

With the exception of cefazolin, which has a half-life of 3 h, in general the apparent elimination half-life for these molecules is between 0.5 and 1.5 h. In all of these cases more than 70% of the administered dose is eliminated in the urine. Some of them are extensively metabolized (Table 4).

2.3.2. Group II Cephalosporins

Group II comprises cephalosporins whose antibacterial spectrum is limited but whose stability against hydrolysis by broad-spectrum β-lactamases is greater than that of the compounds

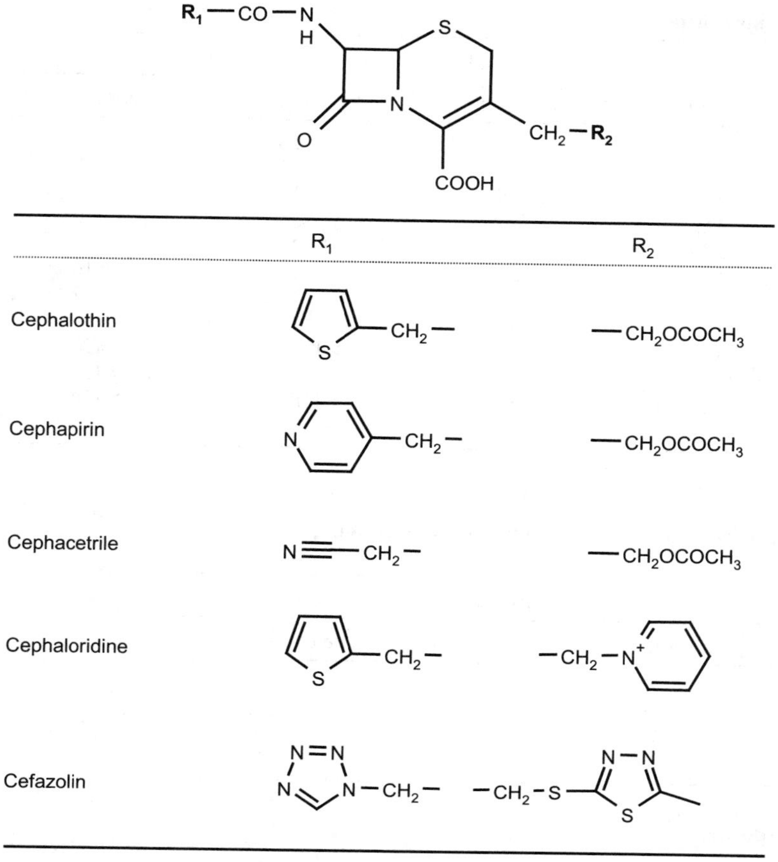

R$_1$—CO—NH … S … N … O … COOH … CH_2—**R**$_2$

	R_1	R_2
Cephalothin	S (ring)—CH_2—	—CH_2OCOCH_3
Cephapirin	N (ring)—CH_2—	—CH_2OCOCH_3
Cephacetrile	N≡—CH_2—	—CH_2OCOCH_3
Cephaloridine	S (ring)—CH_2—	—CH_2—N^+ (ring)
Cefazolin	N=N, N (ring) N—CH_2—	—CH_2—S—(N—N, S ring)—

Figure 8 Group I cephalosporins

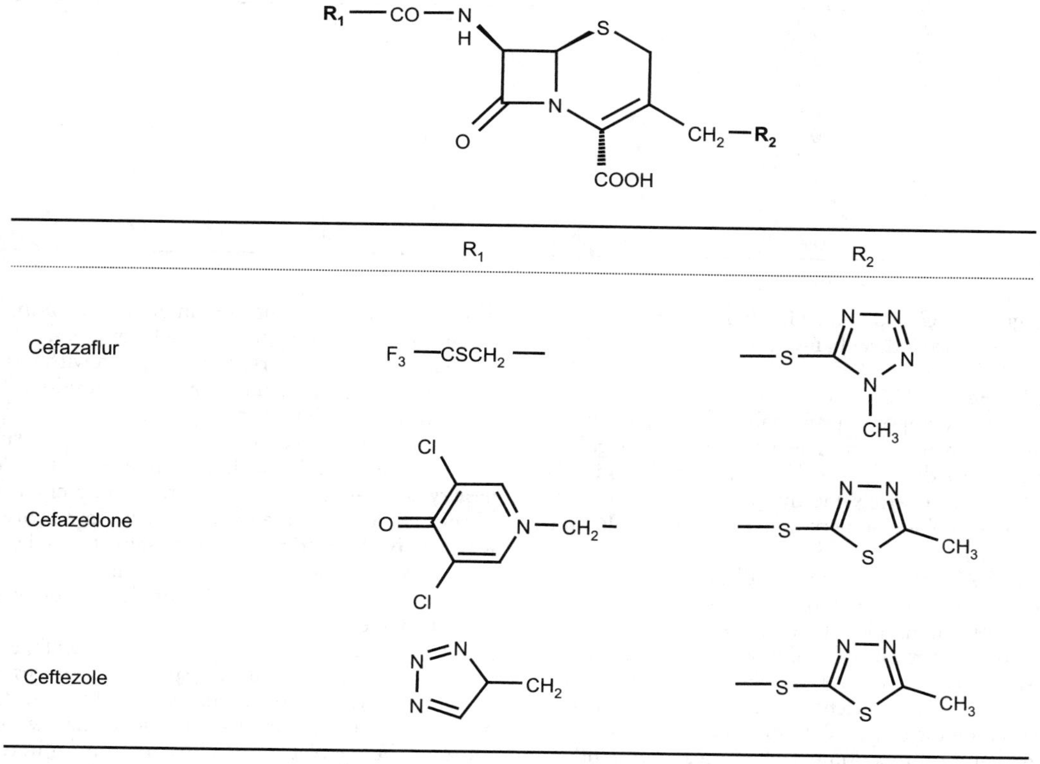

R$_1$—CO—NH … S … N … O … COOH … CH_2—**R**$_2$

	R_1	R_2
Cefazaflur	F_3—$CSCH_2$—	—S—(N—N, N, N ring)—N—CH_3
Cefazedone	Cl, O=(ring)N—CH_2—, Cl	—S—(N—N, S ring)—CH_3
Ceftezole	N=N, N, N (ring)—CH_2	—S—(N—N, S ring)—CH_3

Figure 9 Group IB cephalosporins

Table 2 Antibacterial activities of group I cephalosporins[a]

Organism(s)	MIC (μg/ml)				
	Cephalothin	Cefazolin	Cephacetrile	Cephapirin	Cephaloridine
S. aureus Pen[r]	0.5	1	2	0.5	2
S. aureus Pen[s]	0.25	0.25	1	0.25	0.12
S. pyogenes	0.12	0.12	0.12	0.06	0.03
S. pneumoniae	0.12	0.12	0.25	0.06	0.06
N. meningitidis	0.5	0.25		0.5	0.5
N. gonorrhoeae Pen[r]	0.5	2	8	4	>16
E. coli	4	2	4	4	2
K. pneumoniae	4	2	4	4	4
Enterobacter spp.	>128	>128	>128	>128	>128
S. marcescens	>128	>128	>128	128	>128
Proteus indole+	>128	>128	>128	>128	>128
H. influenzae	4	8		4	4

[a]Data from Rolinson, 1986.

Table 3 Activities of group I cephalosporins against β-lactamase-producing gram-negative bacilli

Drug	MIC (μg/ml)			
	E. cloacae	*P. aeruginosa*	*E. coli*	*Enterobacter aerogenes*
Cephaloridine	100	100	100	100
Cephalothin	294	275	26	112
Cefazolin	50	92	13	93
Cefamandole	1	1	53	106

Table 4 Pharmacokinetics of group I cephalosporins

Drug	C_0 (μg/ml)	$t_{1/2}$ (h)	CL_P (ml/min)	CL_R (ml/min)	Urinary elimination (%)	Protein binding (%)	Metabolism
Cefazolin	140	3	65	65	90	85	–
Cephalothin	70	0.6	470	275	50–70	65	+++
Cephapirin	70	0.1–0.8			50–70	70	+++
Cefazaflur		0.44			73		–
Ceftezole		0.9			87		–
Cefazedone		1.6–1.8			80		–
Cephacetrile	75	1.3			75–98	70	+++
Cephanone		2.1–2.8			88		–
Cephaloridine		1.4	165	125	90	65	20

belonging to group I. Group II may be divided into two subgroups: cephalosporins and cephamycins (Fig. 6).

2.3.2.1. Subgroup IIA

Subgroup IIA is composed principally of four molecules: cefamandole, cefuroxime, ceforanide, and cefonicid (Fig. 10).

Cefamandole was described in 1972 by Ryan. This is the first molecule to have an *N*-methylthiotetrazole chain at position 3 of the cephem moiety. It has a D-mandelamine group at position 7.

Cefamandole sodium is not readily obtainable in a crystalline form. Cefamandole nafate (Fig. 11), which is the *O*-methyl ester of cefamandole base, is used therapeutically. To prevent precipitation of cefamandole base or its *O*-methyl ester, it is essential to add Na_2CO_3 to the bottles for therapeutic use (1.0 g of cefamandole base = 1.11 g of cefamandole nafate for 63 mg [0.28 mol] of Na_2CO_3).

The *O*-methyl ester function is labile in alkaline solution, and cefamandole nafate is 40 to 60% transformed to cefamandole sodium on reconstitution in ampoules for injection. This transformation is very rapid in the body (half-life, ~13 min).

Cefuroxime is the first cephalosporin with a side chain at position 7 to possess an α-oxyimino residue. The moiety attached to this chain is a furyl ring.

Ceforanide and cefonicid possess the same side chain at C-7 as cefamandole, with the difference that the phenyl moiety is substituted by a 5-methylamine chain in the case of ceforanide. The side chain at position 3 is also the same, with an *N*-thiotetrazole moiety substituted by an acetate (ceforanide) or methylsulfonyl (cefonicid).

The antibacterial activities of these four molecules are similar (Table 5).

They possess good activity against penicillinase-producing or non-penicillinase-producing strains of *S. aureus*. Cefonicid is partially inactivated by *S. aureus* penicillinases. They exhibit good activity against streptococci but are inactive against enterococci. These molecules are therefore similar in terms of their activities against gram-positive cocci. They differ essentially

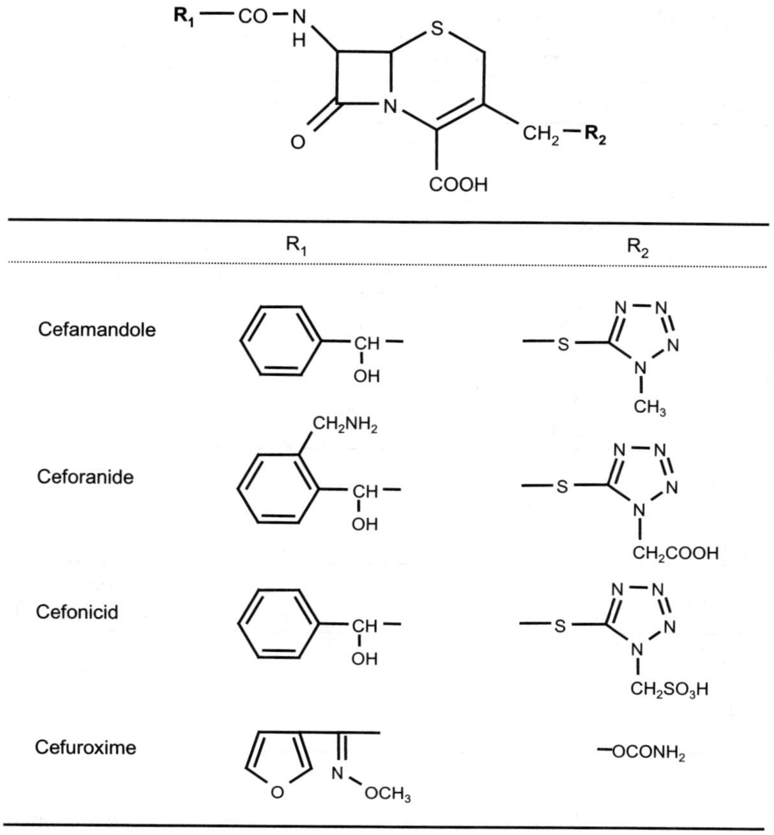

	R_1	R_2
Cefamandole	C_6H_5–CH(OH)–	–S–(1-methyltetrazol-5-yl); N–N, N, N, CH_3
Ceforanide	2-(CH_2NH_2)C_6H_4–CH(OH)–	–S–(tetrazolyl); N–N, N, N, CH_2COOH
Cefonicid	C_6H_5–CH(OH)–	–S–(tetrazolyl); N–N, N, N, CH_2SO_3H
Cefuroxime	2-furyl–C(=N–OCH_3)–	–$OCONH_2$

Figure 10 **Cephems, group IIA**

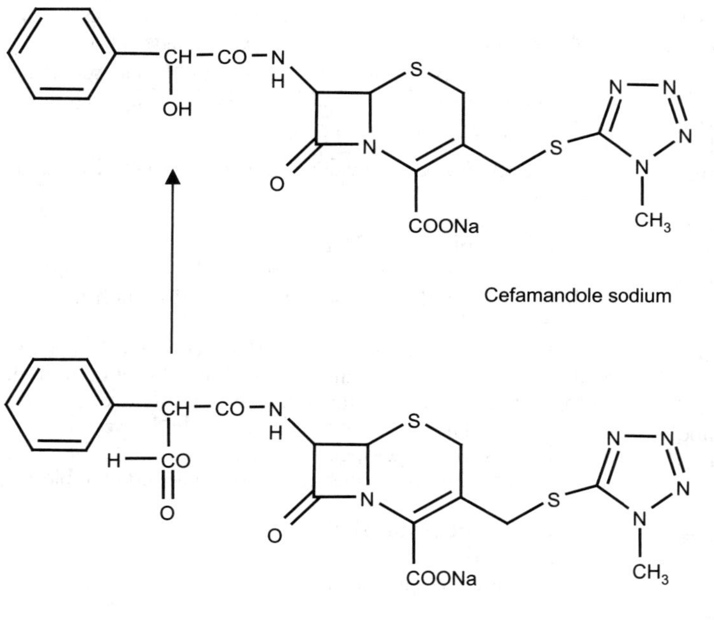

Cefamandole sodium

Cefamandole nafate

Figure 11 **Cefamandole**

through their activities against *Enterobacteriaceae*. They are slightly more active against certain strains of plasmid-mediated β-lactamase-producing *Enterobacteriaceae* and possess better activity against the other strains of *Enterobacteriaceae*.

Pharmacokinetically, only cefonicid has an apparent elimination half-life of more than 3 h. All of these molecules are more than 80% plasma protein bound. They are eliminated principally in the urine (Table 6).

Table 5 In vitro activities of group IIA cephalosporins[a]

Organism	MIC (μg/ml)			
	Cefuroxime	Cefamandole	Ceforanide	Cefonicid
E. coli	1	1	1	1
K. pneumoniae	2	0.5	1	4
Enterobacter sp.	16	32	32	16
Citrobacter	8	8	32	8
S. marcescens	64	>64	>128	64
Proteus indole$^+$	8	8	>32	16
S. enterica serovar Typhi	4	0.5	0.5	
Shigella sp.	2	0.5	0.5	
H. influenzae	0.5	1	8	1
S. aureus Pen^r	1	1	2	4
S. pneumoniae	0.12	0.25	0.12	1
S. pyogenes	0.03	0.06	0.12	0.5

[a]Data from Rolinson, 1986.

Table 6 Pharmacokinetics of group IIA cephalosporins

Drug	Dose (mg)	C_0 (μg/ml)	$t_{1/2}$ (h)	AUC (μg·h/ml)	CL_P (ml/min)	CL_R (ml/min)	Urinary elimination (%)
Cefuroxime	1,000	184.1	1.05	90.8		90.8	>90
Cefamandole	1,000	68	0.7		257	260	90
Ceforanide	1,000	184	2.6	389	33.3	39.2	84.5
Cefonicid	1,000	186.2	5.3	654.2	23	19	83

2.3.2.2. Subgroup IIB: Cephamycins

The cephamycins are characterized by the presence of a 7α-methoxy group on the cephem moiety. The presence of this group gives them greater stability against hydrolysis by plasmid-mediated or chromosomally mediated β-lactamases.

Five molecules are currently available: cefoxitin, cefmetazole, cefotetan, cefbuperazone, and cefminox (Fig. 12).

The cephamycins have the same antibacterial spectrum and the same activity, with a few minor differences (Table 7). They are much less active than the other cephems against gram-positive cocci, and cefotetan and cefbuperazone in particular are inactive against *S. aureus*. They have moderate activity against anaerobic bacteria, including *Bacteroides fragilis*. The plasmid-mediated MIR-1 enzyme hydrolyzes the cephamycins. The pharmacokinetic properties of the cephamycins are summarized in Table 8. Cefotetan has an apparent elimination half-life of more than 3 h. Cefotetan is tautomerized (Fig. 13). There is slight metabolization of cefoxitin, with the formation of descarbamoyl cefoxitin. In patients with renal insufficiency, the dosage must be modified when the creatinine clearance is less than or equal to 30 ml/min (Table 9).

A series of derivatives similar to the cephamycins, the cephabacins, has been described. The molecules are characterized by a 7α-formamide chain instead of a 7α-methoxy group. Figure 14 shows the structures of cephalosporins and cephamycins.

2.3.3. Group III Cephalosporins

Group III comprises molecules that have at least two of the following characteristics:

- The presence of a 2-amino-5-thiazole or 5-amino-2-thiadiazole moiety at position 7 of the cephem moiety
- A broad antibacterial spectrum
- MIC at which 90% of the isolates tested are inhibited (MIC_{90}) less than or equal to 1.0 μg/ml against type I or non-extended-spectrum-β-lactamase-producing Enterobacteriaceae, *Haemophilus influenzae, Neisseria* spp., group A streptococci, and *Streptococus pneumoniae*
- Good stability against hydrolysis by broad-spectrum β-lactamases (TEM-1, TEM-2, SHV-1, ROB-1, etc.)
- Good activity against *P. aeruginosa*

Group III may be subdivided into five subgroups, IIIA to -E (Fig. 15).

2.3.3.1. Subgroup IIIA

Subgroup IIIA consists of cefotiam, a 2-amino-5-thiazolyl cephalosporin, and the *N*-acylcephalosporins such as cefoperazone, cefpimizole, and cefpiramide (Fig. 16).

Cefotiam has better activity than cefotaxime against *S. aureus* and activity similar to that of cefamandole. Cefoperazone and cefpimizole have moderate activity against *P. aeruginosa*. These molecules are hydrolyzed to various degrees by broad-spectrum β-lactamases (Table 10). The pharmacokinetic properties are summarized in Table 11.

2.3.3.2. Subgroup IIIB

All of the derivatives belonging to subgroup IIIB are from the same family chemically as cefotaxime.

2.3.3.2.1. Chemical structures. Chemical structures are shown in Fig. 17. All of these molecules are characterized by a 2-amino-5-thiazolyl moiety and a methoxyimino chain. They differ from one another by the side chain at position 3. Ceftizoxime has no substituent at C-3. Cefotaxime possesses an acetoxymethyl chain. The other molecules have a substituted thioaromatic moiety: ceftriaxone (triazine), cefodizime (thiazole), cefuzonam (thiadiazole), and cefmenoxime

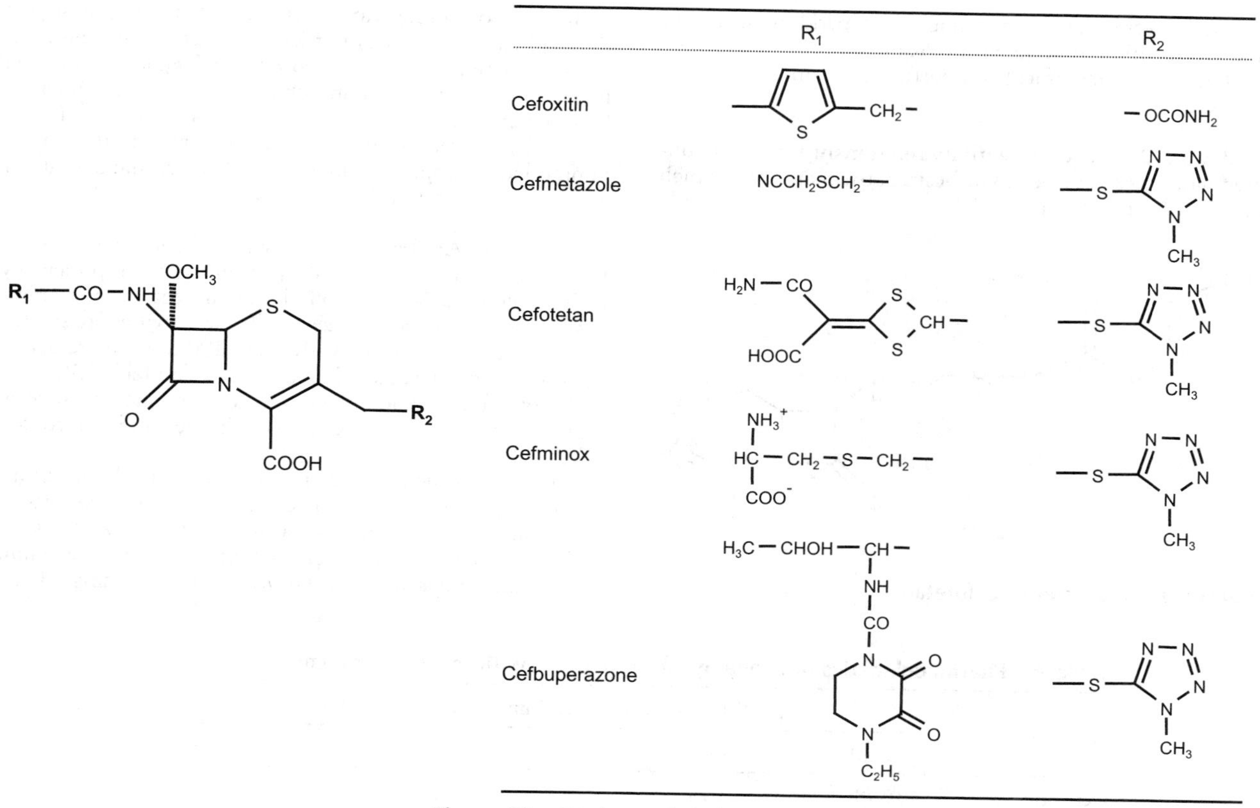

	R_1	R_2
Cefoxitin	(thienyl)–CH_2–	–$OCONH_2$
Cefmetazole	$NCCH_2SCH_2$–	–S–(N-methyltetrazolyl)
Cefotetan	H_2N–CO, HOOC (dithietane) CH–	–S–(N-methyltetrazolyl)
Cefminox	NH_3^+–HC(COO^-)–CH_2–S–CH_2–	–S–(N-methyltetrazolyl)
Cefbuperazone	H_3C–CHOH–CH–NH–CO–(4-ethyl-2,3-dioxopiperazinyl)	–S–(N-methyltetrazolyl)

Figure 12 Cephamycins, group IIB

Table 7 In vitro activities of cephamycins (group IIB)

Organism(s)[a]	MIC_{50} (μg/ml)				
	Cefoxitin	Cefotetan	Cefmetazole	Cefbuperazone	Cefminox
S. aureus	1	8	1	8	12.5
S. pyogenes	1	1	0.5		4
S. pneumoniae	2	2	0.5		1
E. coli (TEM-1)	4	0.5	1	0.25	0.5
E. coli (class I)	8	2	2		
K. pneumoniae CFZ[r]	4	0.5	1	0.5	0.5
Enterobacter CTX[s]	>128	16	>64	1	>128
Enterobacter CTX[s]	>128	>128	>128		>128
Citrobacter spp.	>128	1	>128	8	>32
P. mirabilis	2	0.25	1		0.5
S. marcescens	16	1	16	8	>32
H. influenzae	2	1	4	1	0.5
N. gonorrhoeae	0.5	0.5	2		0.5

[a]CFZ, cefazolin; CTX, cefotaxime.

Table 8 Pharmacokinetics of cephamycins

Drug	Dose (mg)	C_0 (μg/ml)	AUC (μg·h/ml)	$t_{1/2}$ (h)	CL_P (ml/min)	CL_R (ml/min)	Urinary elimination (%)	Protein binding (%)
Cefoxitin	2,000	244	129	1.5	279	221	77	73
Cefmetazole	2,000	290	295	0.8	112	78.7	71	
Cefotetan	100	158	524	4.5	50		61	88
Cefminox	500	68.4	166.8	1.9	180		78	30
	1,000	193.8	335.4	1.9	180		77	30
Cefbuperazone	1,000	83.7		1.7				

(*N*-methyltetrazole). Ceftazidime has a pyridinium moiety and an isobutyric residue on the oxime.

The physicochemical properties are summarized in Table 12.

2.3.3.2.2. Structure-activity relationship. Several hundred molecules have been synthesized, the majority of which have not been developed.

Figure 13 Tautomer of cefotetan

In this group of derivatives, the side chain at position 3 of the cephem moiety does not significantly modify the antibacterial activity. This is based on the 2-amino-5-thiazolyl moiety and on the oxyimino chain (Fig. 18). The chain at C-3 modifies the pharmacokinetic properties (e.g., ceftriaxone and cefodizime) and in some cases invests them with nonantibiotic properties (increase in bactericidal activity of granulocytes by cefodizime).

2.3.3.2.3. Antibacterial activity. These molecules all have the same antibacterial spectrum, which principally includes gram-negative bacilli and gram-negative and gram-positive cocci, except for *S. aureus*. Their activities are similar. Cefotaxime and these derivatives are 100 times more active against *Enterobacteriaceae* than cefamandole (Table 13).

Cefotaxime, cefmenoxime, and ceftizoxime are slightly more active than ceftriaxone, cefodizime, and cefuzonam (Table 14).

These molecules are inactive against methicillin-resistant *S. aureus* (MRSA) strains. They have little activity against *P. aeruginosa* and are inactive against *Listeria monocytogenes* and *Enterococcus* spp. Their activities against penicillin G-resistant strains of *S. pneumoniae* vary according to the

Table 9 Pharmacokinetics of cephamycins in patients with renal insufficiency

Drug	$t_{1/2}$ (h) at indicated creatinine clearance (ml/min):				
	≥80	80–30	30–10	<10	Hemodialysis
Cefoxitin	0.78	1.15	6.31	13.18	21.56
Cefmetazole[a]	0.81 ± 0.08	3.13 ± 0.8	6.9 ± 1.9	14.98 ± 4.7	
Cefotetan	4.2	7.78	9.86	35.1	

[a]Means ± standard deviations.

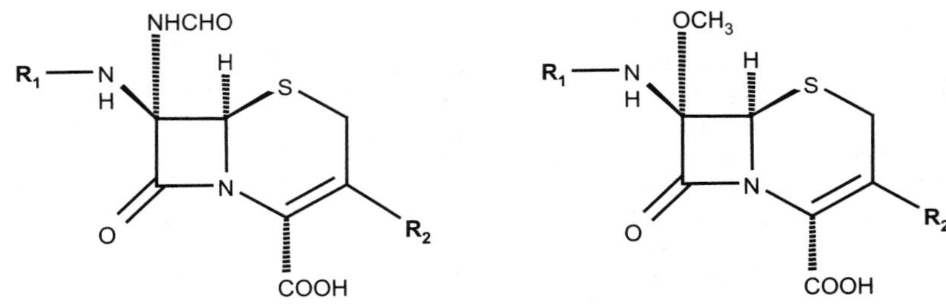

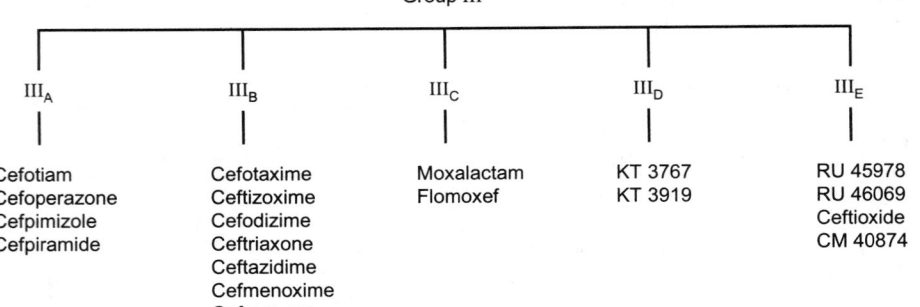

Figure 14 Cephalosporins versus cephamycins

Group III

- III_A: Cefotiam, Cefoperazone, Cefpimizole, Cefpiramide
- III_B: Cefotaxime, Ceftizoxime, Cefodizime, Ceftriaxone, Ceftazidime, Cefmenoxime, Cefuzonam
- III_C: Moxalactam, Flomoxef
- III_D: KT 3767, KT 3919
- III_E: RU 45978, RU 46069, Ceftioxide, CM 40874

Figure 15 Cephems, group III

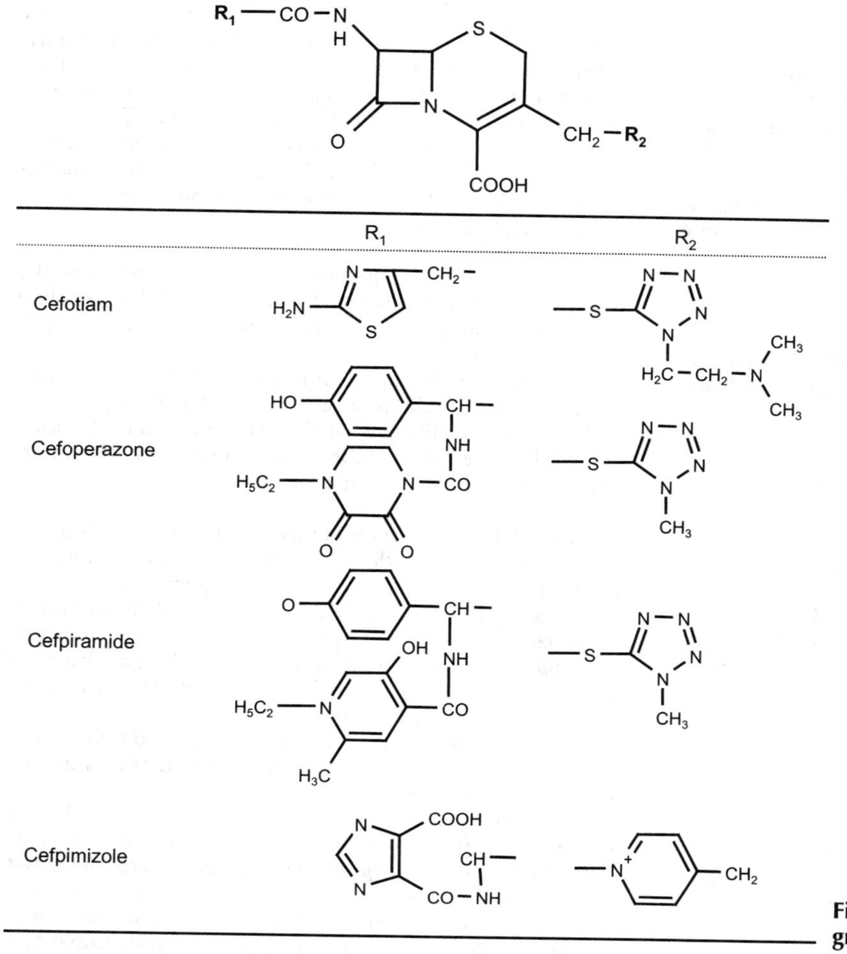

Figure 16 Cephalosporins, group IIIA

Table 10 In vitro activities of *N*-acylcephalosporins (group IIIA)

Organism(s)	MIC (μg/ml)			
	Cefotiam	Cefoperazone	Cefpimizole	Cefpiramide
S. aureus Met[s]	0.5	1	1	1
S. pyogenes	0.06	0.12	1	0.12
S. pneumoniae		0.25	1	0.12
E. coli	0.25	0.12	0.5	0.5
K. pneumoniae	0.25	0.2	4	2
S. marcescens	>128	2	>128	32
Enterobacter spp.	4	1	4	1
Citrobacter spp.	16	4	16	4
P. mirabilis	0.5	1	4	1
S. enterica serovar Typhi	0.25	0.5	4	1
P. aeruginosa	>128	4	8	2
H. influenzae	1	0.25	0.25	0.5

Table 11 Pharmacokinetics of *N*-acylcephalosporins (group IIIA)

Drug	Dose (mg)	AUC (μg·h/ml)	$t_{1/2}$ (h)	CL_P (ml/min)	CL_R (ml/min)	Urinary elimination (%)
Cefpiramide	500	452.9	4.06	20.2	4.7	21.5
Cefpimizole	1,000	120	1.9	118.6	96.2	75
Cefoperazone	1,000	248	2.5	75	20	15–30
Cefotiam	1,000	47.8	1.2	21.1	10.5	59.1

molecule. Cefotaxime and ceftriaxone have good activity against strains that are of intermediate susceptibility or resistant to penicillin G, whereas ceftizoxime is inactive. Strains of reduced susceptibility (MIC, 0.5 to 1 μg/ml) or resistant (MIC, ≥2 μg/ml) to ceftriaxone or cefotaxime have been described (Table 15).

This difference between the molecules in terms of activity against *Enterobacteriaceae* is based on the stability against hydrolysis by β-lactamases as demonstrated by the inoculum size effect and a differential affinity for penicillin-binding proteins (PBP).

The activity of desacetylcefotaxime is similar to that of cefuroxime (Table 16).

The MIC is usually determined in agar or broth medium using an inoculum standardized to 10^5 CFU/ml without serum.

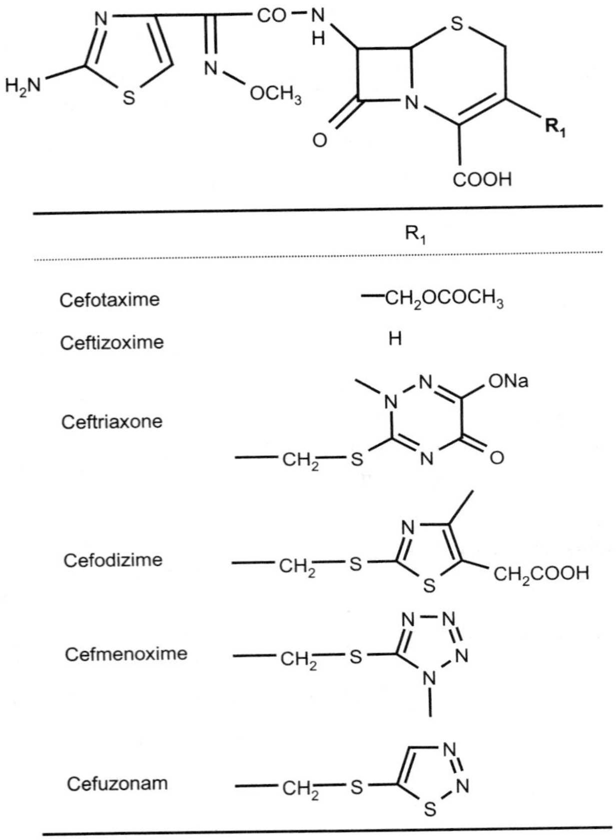

	R_1
Cefotaxime	$—CH_2OCOCH_3$
Ceftizoxime	H
Ceftriaxone	$—CH_2—S$ (N, N, ONa, N, O)
Cefodizime	$—CH_2—S$ (N, S, CH_2COOH)
Cefmenoxime	$—CH_2—S$ (N—N, N, N)
Cefuzonam	$—CH_2—S$ (N, N, S)

Figure 17 Cephems, group IIIB

Eng et al. (1985) studied the effect of inoculum size (at 5×10^5 and 5×10^7 CFU/ml) of four molecules, cefotaxime, ceftriaxone, ceftazidime, and cefoperazone, on activity against a strain each of *E. coli*, *Salmonella enterica* serovar Typhimurium, and *Klebsiella pneumoniae* (Table 17).

If the breakpoints are taken as 1 μg/ml (United Kingdom) and 4 μg/ml (France), the MICs of certain derivatives are greater than the breakpoints when the inoculum size is increased.

When the inoculum size is 5×10^7 CFU/ml, the activities of ceftazidime and ceftriaxone are limited, whereas the activity of cefotaxime is equal to 0.5 μg/ml. The inoculum effect is an indirect reflection of the stability against hydrolysis by β-lactamases.

The addition of human serum reduces the activity of ceftriaxone 8- to 10-fold, reduces that of cefoperazone slightly, and does not modify that of the other molecules. Caution should, however, be exercised when interpreting this information in relation to therapeutic efficacy.

2.3.3.2.4. Pharmacokinetics. With the exception of ceftriaxone and cefodizime, these molecules belong to group II of the pharmacokinetic classification.

For all of these molecules, the bioavailability after intramuscular administration is greater than 90%. The peak concentrations in serum after administration of 1.0 g are between 25.3 μg/ml (cefotaxime) and 76 μg/ml (ceftriaxone) and are reached, on average, within 1 h.

The main parameters after intravenous administration in the form of an intravenous bolus for 3 min or infusion for 0.5 h are presented in Table 18.

Apart from ceftriaxone, which is strongly protein bound and about 40% of the administered dose of which is eliminated in the bile, the majority of the molecules are eliminated in the urine. Ceftriaxone is difficult to use in premature infants or neonates, whose hepatic systems are immature and in whom there is a risk of accumulation of free bilirubin as a result of displacement from the plasma albumin binding sites.

Cefotaxime is metabolized in the liver. Its principal metabolite, deacetylcefotaxime, has antibacterial activity that is greater than or equal to that of cefamandole and pharmacokinetics parallel to those of cefotaxime.

In subjects with an underlying pathological condition (renal insufficiency, hepatic insufficiency, or a combination of the two) and in very young or elderly subjects, it is sometimes necessary to adapt the rhythm of administration or dosage (Tables 19 and 20).

2.3.3.3. Subgroup IIIC: Oxa-1-Cephems

The oxa-1-cephems are synthetic molecules. The observation that oxa-1-cefamandole, oxa-1-cefoxitin, and

Table 12 Physicochemical properties of group IIIB cephalosporins

Drug	Empirical formula	Molecular mass (Da)	Melting point (°C)	pK_a	Na (mmol/g)
Cefotaxime	$C_{16}H_{17}N_5O_7S_2$	455.48	162–163[a]	3.35	4.54
Cefmenoxime	$C_{16}H_{17}N_9O_5S_3$	511.56	171–173	3.4	3.52
Cefodizime	$C_{20}H_{20}N_6O_7S_4$	584.65	—[a]	2.85/3.37/4.18	5.05
Cefuzonam	$C_{16}H_{15}N_7O_5S_4$	513.58			
Ceftriaxone	$C_{18}H_{18}N_8O_7S_3$	554.58	155	3/3.2/4.1	3.3
Ceftizoxime	$C_{15}H_{13}N_5O_5S_2$	383.40	227		2.46
Ceftazidime	$C_{22}H_{22}N_6O_7S_2$	546.57	>170	1.8/2.7/4.1	

[a]Was altered before reaching the melting point.

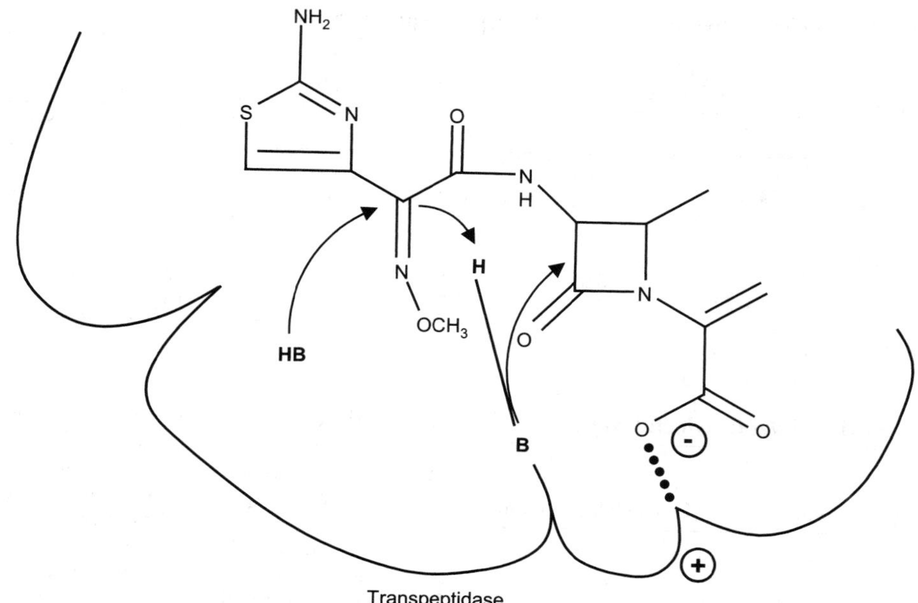

Figure 18 Mechanism of basic intramolecular catalysis of methoxyimino cephalosporins

Table 13 Comparative activities of cefotaxime and cefamandole

Organism(s)[a]	MIC_{50} (μg/ml)	
	Cefamandole	Cefotaxime
E. coli Amp[r]	16	0.12
E. coli Amp[s]	1	0.03
K. pneumoniae CFZ[s]	0.5	0.12
K. pneumoniae CFZ[r]	>128	0.12
Enterobacter spp.	32	0.03
C. freundii	8	0.25
Proteus indole+	8	0.12
S. marcescens	>64	0.12
H. influenzae β−	1	0.03
H. influenzae β+	>8	0.06
S. pneumoniae	0.25	0.12
N. meningitidis	0.06	0.01
N. gonorrhoeae	0.5	<0.01

[a]CFZ, cefazoline; β−, non-β-lactamase producing; β+, β-lactamase producing.

oxa-1-cephalothin had 4 to 16 times the antibacterial activity of their cephalosporin counterparts provided the impetus for intense research.

Several derivatives have been described, such as oxa-1-cefotaxime, oxa-1-E-0702, etc. Two molecules are currently used therapeutically: moxalactam (latamoxef) and flomoxef (Fig. 19).

This class of cephems is characterized by a specific structure. The modifications due to the replacement at position 1 of the sulfur atom by an oxygen atom are substantial. In fact, compared to those in the cephalosporins, the interatomic distance at C-8 and C-9 is shorter and that between N-5 and N-8 is longer. The nitrogen atom at position 5 is outside the C-4–C-6–C-8 plane. The result is a reduction in the amide resonance and increased reactivity of the β-lactam ring.

Acylation of parietal transpeptidases and β-lactamases is greater than with the cephalosporins, the two phenomena being similar. In order to correct this instability against hydrolysis by β-lactamases, a methoxy group has been attached in the α position of C-7, as well as a carboxyl group on the asymmetrical carbon of the side chain at position 7.

Table 14 In vitro activities of group IIIB cephalosporins[a]

Organism	MIC_{50} (μg/ml)				
	Cefotaxime	Ceftizoxime	Cefmenoxime	Ceftriaxone	Ceftazidime
E. coli	0.03	0.03	0.06	0.12	0.12
K. pneumoniae	0.03	0.01	0.03	0.25	0.12
Enterobacter sp.	0.12	0.12	0.12	0.25	0.25
Citrobacter sp.	0.25	0.25	0.25	0.5	0.5
Proteus indole+	0.12	0.06	0.12	0.12	0.12
P. aeruginosa	32	64	32	32	2
H. influenzae	0.03	0.03	0.03	0.03	0.12
S. aureus	2	2	2	4	4
S. pneumoniae	0.12	0.12	0.06	0.25	0.25

[a]Data from Rolinson, 1986.

Table 15 In vitro activities of group IIIB cephalosporins against *S. pneumoniae*[a]

Drug	Pen[s] (MIC, <0.12 μg/ml)		Pen[r] (MIC, 0.12–1 μg/ml)		Pen[r] (MIC, >1 μg/ml)	
	MIC_{50}	MIC_{90}	MIC_{50}	MIC_{90}	MIC_{50}	MIC_{90}
Cefotaxime	0.03	0.03	0.25	1	1	2
Ceftriaxone	0.03	0.03	0.25	1	1	2
Cefpirome	0.01	0.03	0.12	0.5	0.5	1
Ceftazidime	0.25	0.25	2	16	16	16
Cefodizime	0.03	0.03	0.5	2	2	4
Ceftizoxime	0.06	0.06	0.5	8	16	16

[a]Values are in milligrams per liter.

Table 16 In vitro activity of desacetylcefotaxime[a]

Organism	MIC_{50} (μg/ml)	
	Cefotaxime	Desacetylcefotaxime
S. aureus Met[s]	1.6	12.5
S. epidermidis	3.1	25
S. pyogenes	0.025	0.05
S. agalactiae	0.025	0.25
S. pneumoniae	0.05	0.25
H. influenzae	0.01	0.25
N. meningitidis	<0.005	<0.005
E. coli	0.025	0.4
K. pneumoniae	0.05	0.1
S. marcescens	0.1	0.8
C. freundii	0.1	1.6
P. mirabilis	0.001	0.002
Providencia stuartii	3.1	>50
B. cepacia	25	3.1

[a]Data from Neu, 1982.

The carboxyl function provides greater stability against hydrolysis by cephalosporinases, and the 7-methoxy group increases the stability against plasmid-mediated enzymes (extended-broad-spectrum β-lactamases) (Table 21).

The improved activity of moxalactam against gram-negative bacilli is due to better transmembrane penetration and its enhanced activity against the constitutive enzymes of peptidoglycan.

The presence of an N-methylthiotetrazole moiety at position 3 of the cephem moiety is the source of two major side effects: hypoprothrombinemia associated with inhibition of vitamin K epoxide reductase and an antabuse effect through inhibition of aldehyde dehydrogenase.

The presence of an α-carboxylic group on the C-7 chain causes disorders of platelet aggregation (as with the α-carboxypenicillins) (Fig. 20).

Bleeding to various degrees has been described with moxalactam for patients with renal insufficiency.

Changes to the moxalactam molecule have been made to reduce (hypoprothrombinemia) or eliminate (antabuse

Table 17 Effect of inoculum size on activity of cephalosporins[a]

Drug	MIC (μg/ml) at inoculum size (CFU/ml)					
	E. coli		*S. enterica* serovar Typhimurium		*K. pneumoniae*	
	5×10^5	5×10^7	5×10^5	5×10^7	5×10^5	5×10^7
Cefotaxime	0.06	0.5	0.06	0.5	0.06	0.5
Ceftriaxone	0.06	1	0.5	4	0.25	4
Ceftazidime	0.12	8	0.5	16	0.12	8
Cefoperazone	0.25	8	1	32	0.12	8

[a]Data from Eng et al., 1985.

Table 18 Pharmacokinetics of group IIIB and -C cephalosporins

Drug	C_{12h} (μg/ml)	$t_{1/2}$ (h)	$AUC_{0-\infty}$ (μg·h/ml)	CL_P (ml/min)	CL_R (ml/min)	Urinary elimination (%)	Protein binding (%)
Cefotaxime	0.1	1.2	70.4	250	170	50–60	3
Ceftazidime	0.1	2	179	110	85	70–85	10–30
Cefmenoxime	0.1	1.5	90.2	245	170	70–80	40–77
Ceftriaxone	28	6	1006	14	7	45–50	>90
Cefodizime	3.9	3.5	422	21.7	42.9	80	80
Cefuzonam	<0.1	1.2	60.9	279	171	55	
Moxalactam	2.2	2.7	221	92	60	70–80	50
Flomoxef	<0.1	1	82.4	135	60	80	

Table 19 Elimination half-lives of cephalosporins at different physiological ages

Drug	$t_{1/2}$ (h)			
	Neonates	Children	Elderly (>65 yr)	Young
Cefotaxime	3.4	2	1.5	1.2
Cefmenoxime	3.9	1.4	2.4	1.3
Ceftizoxime	3.8	2.1	3.2	1.5
Cefoperazone	6.3	2.4	3.2	2.5
Ceftazidime	4.7	−2	1.9	2
Moxalactam	5.4	4.4	3	2.7
Cefotetan	ND[a]	2.6	3.8	4.2
Ceftriaxone	7.3–18.3	4–6.6	8.9–12.2	6.8–8

[a]ND, not determined.

Table 20 Half-lives of cephalosporins in patients with renal insufficiency

Drug	$t_{1/2}$ (h) at indicated creatinine clearance (ml/min):			
	120–80	80–30	30–10	<10
Cefotaxime	1.2	2.5	2	2
Cefmenoxime	1.3	1.9	7.9	10.1
Ceftazidime	1.5	3.6	9	16.1
Ceftizoxime	1.7	2.7	8.1	34.7
Cefoperazone	2	2.3	2.1	2
Ceftriaxone	8	12.4	11.4	15.7
Cefotetan	3	3.7	4.6	11.1
Moxalactam	2	4.8	8.4	13.6

effect) these side effects and have given rise to flomoxef. The *N*-hydromethylthiotetrazole chain of flomoxef does not inhibit aldehyde dehydrogenase, the disulfiram-like effect of which is absent following simultaneous ingestion of alcohol and administration of flomoxef. In addition, the absence of an α-carboxyl group at C-7 eliminates platelet aggregation.

2.3.3.3.1. Antibacterial activity. Flomoxef possesses a more balanced antibacterial spectrum than moxalactam. In fact, in contrast to moxalactam, it is active against gram-positive cocci; the two molecules possess good activity against *Enterobacteriaceae*, including those producing type I enzymes (Table 22). Against gram-negative bacilli, flomoxef is less active than moxalactam. Cefotaxime is more active than moxalactam against non-enzyme-producing strains.

Moxalactam and flomoxef possess marked activity against gram-negative (*B. fragilis*) and gram-positive anaerobic bacteria (Table 23).

Moxalactam is a racemate. Because of a center of asymmetry, two epimers can be identified. The *R*-(−)-epimer is more active than the *S*-(−)-epimer and the racemate (Table 24).

2.3.3.3.2. 2-Amino-5-thiazolyl methoxyimino derivatives. Shibara et al. have described two β-methyl-1-oxacephem derivatives, OCP-9-176 (L-565575) and OCP-9-231 (Fig. 21). These derivatives possess a broad antibacterial spectrum but are not active against *P. aeruginosa*.

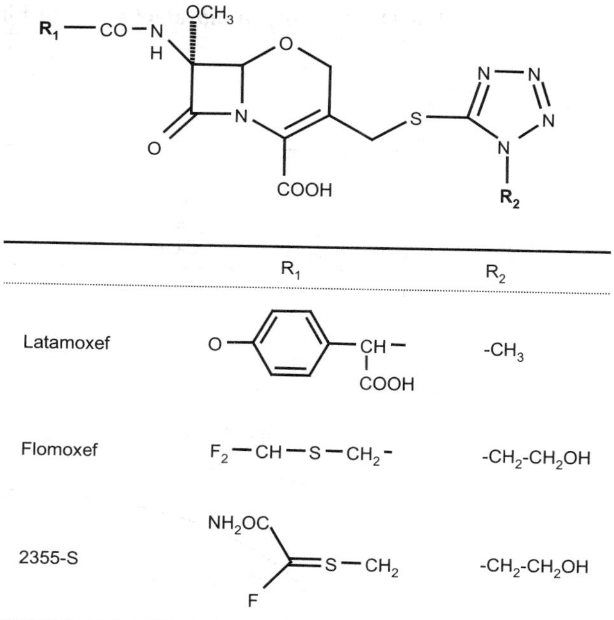

	R_1	R_2
Latamoxef	O–C_6H_4–CH(COOH)–	$-CH_3$
Flomoxef	$F_2-CH-S-CH_2-$	$-CH_2-CH_2OH$
2355-S	NH_2OC(F)C=S–CH_2	$-CH_2-CH_2OH$

Figure 19 1-Oxacephems, group IIIC

The introduction of a carboxyl group on the oxime residue increases the activity against *P. aeruginosa*. OCP-9-176 possesses activity similar to that of ceftazidime (Table 25).

OCP-9-231 possesses a mercaptothiadiazole moiety at position 3 and is two to five times more active against gram-positive and gram-negative bacteria than its 1-oxacephem and 2β-methylcephem analogs. However, this molecule is inactive against type I enzyme-producing *Enterobacteriaceae*.

2.3.3.3.3. Pharmacokinetics. The pharmacokinetics of moxalactam and flomoxef are summarized in Tables 26 to 28.

The pharmacokinetics of flomoxef in children are summarized in Table 29. Probenecid modifies the elimination pharmacokinetics of flomoxef and moxalactam. The molecules are eliminated by glomerular filtration and tubular secretion.

The pharmacokinetics in patients with renal insufficiency are summarized in Table 30. In patients with renal insufficiency, the ratio between the *R*- and *S*-epimers is altered. The *R*-epimer is eliminated preferentially.

Plasma protein binding is 53 and 30% for moxalactam and flomoxef, respectively.

After intramuscular administration, the peak concentration in serum is between 13 and 25 μg/ml and occurs, on average, within 1 h. Bioavailability is close to 100%.

Flomoxef is metabolized. Two metabolites have been detected: flomoxef sulfoxide, which possesses a certain antibacterial activity, and hydroxyethylthiotetrazole (HTT), which is inactive (Fig. 22). The sulfoxide metabolite represents 0.1 to 0.2% of the administered dose eliminated in the urine. HTT is present at high concentrations in plasma and represents 12 to 15% of the product eliminated in the urine (Tables 31 and 32).

2.3.3.4. Subgroup IIID: Carbacephems

Christensen et al. simultaneously synthesized the oxa-1-cephems and 1-carbacephems. They showed that the sulfur heteroatom is not essential for antibacterial activity. Narasida et al. showed that a carbacephamycin derivative possessed good chemical stability.

Table 21 Stability of moxalactam against hydrolysis by β-lactamases[a]

R_1	R_2	Hydrolysis		MIC (μg/ml)		
		P	C	*E. coli* NIJH-JC-2	*E. coli* 73 (P)	*E. cloacae* 233 (C)
H	H	–	–	0.8	>100	>100
COOH	H	–	++	0.2	50	0.4
H	OCH_3	++	±	0.1	0.8	100
COOH (moxalactam)	OCH_3	++	++	0.2	0.4	0.2

[a]Data from Yoshida, 1981. P, penicillinase; C, cephalosporinase.

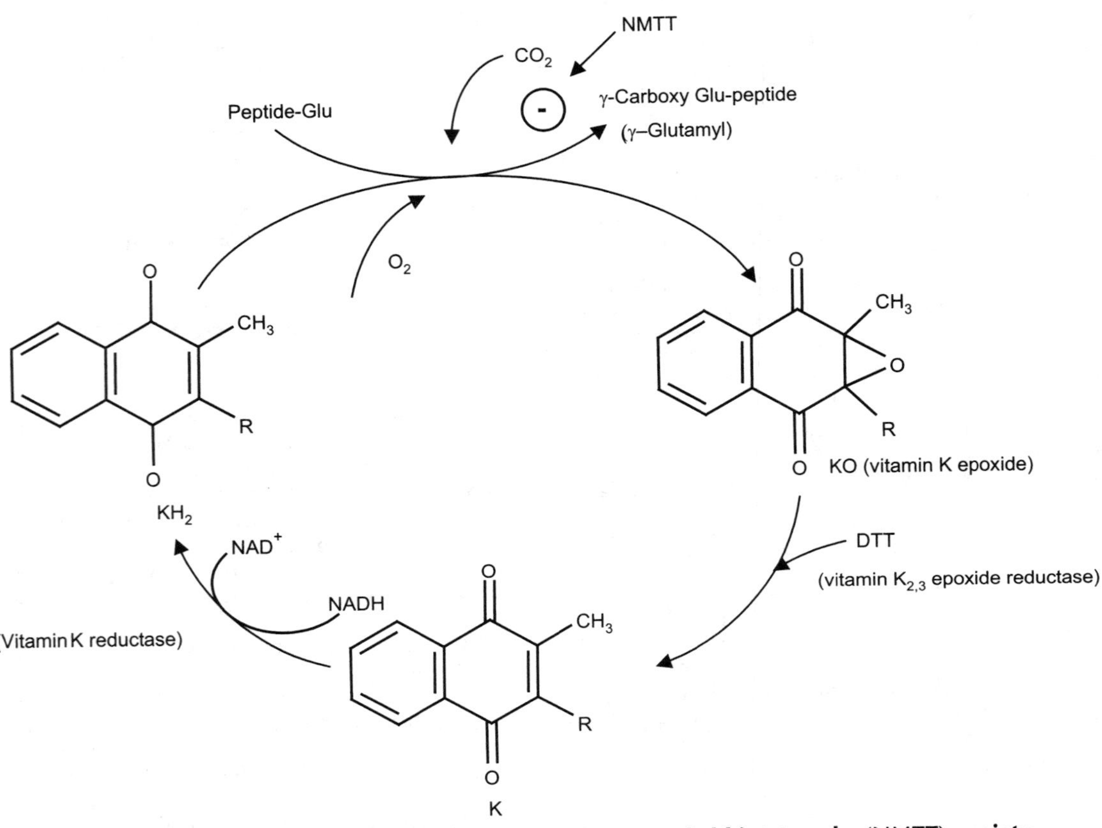

Figure 20 Vitamin K cycle: interference by the *N*-methylthiotetrazole (NMTT) moiety of cephalosporins

The combination of potential antibacterial activity and good chemical stability stimulated research into the 1-carbacephems since it was possible to work on chemically stable molecules, as are cephems, with the hope of being able to synthesize new chemical entities.

Among the carbacephems, two types of molecules have been described: the oral derivatives, of which loracarbef is the prototype, and the parenteral derivatives.

2.3.3.4.1. Derivatives for parenteral use. The first molecule to have been synthesized is carbacephalothin, rapidly followed by carbacefamandole and carbacefoxitin (Firestone et al., 1977). The 1-carbacefoxitin derivative has antibacterial activity, in contrast to carbacefamandole (Table 33). A number of series have been synthesized since then by various research teams.

Doyle et al. (1970) reported the activity of carbacephems with substitutions at position 2 or 3. Uneo et al. (1980) synthesized a series of carbacephems, 1-dethiaceftizoxime (Fig. 23), which is inactive against *S. aureus* but possesses good activity against *Enterobacteriaceae*.

Hirata et al. (1981) synthesized a series of carbacephems. The 2-amino-5-thiazolyl derivatives KT-3767 and KT-3937 (Fig. 24) do and do not possess a 2-hydroxyl group, respectively. The molecules are inactive against *S. aureus* and moderately active (KT-3937) or inactive (KT-3767) against *P. aeruginosa* (Table 34).

Derivatives with a catechol moiety have been synthesized, with or without a C-3′ quaternary ammonium-type chain (Fig. 25). Of these compounds, KT-4788 is the most active molecule, having antistaphylococcal and anti-*P. aeruginosa* activity.

There is a center of asymmetry on the chain at C-7, and the (*S*)-isomer is more active than the (*R*)-isomer against *Enterobacteriaceae*, but the (*R*)-isomer is more active against *S. aureus* and *Staphylococcus epidermidis*.

Table 22 In vitro activities of moxalactam, flomoxef, and cefotaxime[a]

Organism	MIC (μg/ml)		
	Flomoxef	Moxalactam	Cefotaxime
S. aureus 209 P	0.2	6.3	1.6
E. coli NIJHHJC-2	0.1	0.1	0.1
K. pneumoniae	0.05	0.1	0.02
E. cloacae 233	12.5	0.1	0.2
P. aeruginosa ATCC 25619	>100	6.3	1.6

[a]Data from Tsuji et al.

Table 23 Activities of oxa-1-cephamycins against anaerobic bacteria

Organism(s)	MIC (μg/ml)		
	Moxalactam	Flomoxef	Cefoxitin
B. fragilis	0.78	0.78	6.25
Prevotella spp. *Porphyromonas* spp.	0.39	0.1	0.39
Fusobacterium spp.	0.39	0.05	0.2
C. perfringens	3.13	0.39	1.56
C. difficile	12.5	1.56	50
Propionibacterium spp.	0.39	0.05	0.1
Eubacterium spp.	6.25	0.39	0.78
Peptococcus spp.	0.2	0.2	0.2
Peptostreptococcus spp.	3.13	0.78	0.39
Streptococcus spp.	12.5	1.56	6.25
Veillonella spp.	0.39	3.13	0.39

Table 24 In vitro activities of the enantiomers of moxalactam[a]

Organism	Moxalactam *R*(−)-epimer	Moxalactam *S*(−)-epimer	Moxalactam racemate
S. aureus	4	8	4
E. coli TEM-1	0.06	0.12	0.06
K. pneumoniae	0.06	0.12	0.12
P. mirabilis	0.25	0.5	0.25
M. morganii	0.06	0.12	0.06
B. fragilis	0.5	0.5	0.5
H. influenzae β+[b]	0.015	0.03	0.03

[a]Data from Wise et al., 1982.
[b]β+, β-lactamase producing.

A series of derivatives of C-3′ quaternary ammonium have been synthesized (Cook et al., 1989). Two derivatives, LY-214748 and LY-211256 (Fig. 26), possess good activity against gram-negative bacilli, but their activity against *S. aureus* is moderate and they are inactive against *P. aeruginosa* because of a reduction in transmembrane penetration. LY-258360 has better activity against type I β-lactamase-producing strains of *Enterobacteriaceae*. The addition of a pyridinium, imidazole, or catechol moiety does not increase the activity against *P. aeruginosa*, but some of these derivatives have better activity against type I β-lactamase-producing strains of *Enterobacteriaceae* (Table 35). The presence of a methylene between C-3 of the cephem moiety and the quaternary ammonium (C-3′ derivative) increases the antipseudomonal activity, which suggests that the mobility of pyridinium allows better outer membrane penetration. The derivative LY-262290 has a nitroimidazole moiety and is more active against *S. aureus* and streptococci, but its activity against *Enterobacteriaceae* is modest (Cooper, 1992).

A series of derivatives possessing a C-3 sulfonyl has been synthesized by Crowell et al. (1989). In the 2-amino-5-thiazolyl series, irrespective of the substituent in the sulfonyl group, the molecules obtained were inactive against *S. aureus* but did possess antistreptococcal activity. Their activities against *Enterobacteriaceae* varied, but they were devoid of activity against the type I β-lactamase-producing strains of *Enterobacteriaceae* and against *P. aeruginosa*. The most active molecule is LY-214748 (Fig. 26); it possesses a *c*-propyl group attached to the 3-sulfonyl group. Two derivatives possessing a 3-fluoromethyl group have been synthesized. They differ by the presence or absence of a *para*-hydroxyl group attached to the phenyl moiety.

The 3-fluoromethyl group is more electroattractive in the 3-chloro group of cefaclor, suggesting greater antibacterial activity. Like loracarbef, these two molecules are chemically stable. They possess good activity against gram-positive cocci, *H. influenzae*, *E. coli* TEM-1, and *K. pneumoniae*. Only the *p*-hydroxyl derivative is active against cephalosporinase-producing strains of *E. coli* (MIC, ~1 μg/ml). Against gram-positive cocci, their activity is similar to those of the oral cephalosporins, such as cefuroxime. After oral administration, absolute bioavailability is on the order of 88 to 89% in the mouse and 61.5% in the rhesus monkey, with an apparent elimination half-life greater than or equal to that of loracarbef (1.2 and 2 h versus 1 h).

The derivatives of a series possessing a 2-amino-5-thiazolyl cephalosporin ring and a fluoroethyl residue on the oxime exhibited not insignificant activity against the heterogeneously oxacillin-resistant strains of *S. aureus*, having a good correlation with the affinity of these derivatives for PBP 2a (50% inhibitory concentration [IC_{50}] ≤ 10 μg/ml).

Figure 27 shows the structures of LY-264548 and LY-227060.

2.3.3.4.2. Oral derivatives—loracarbef. One molecule is used therapeutically, loracarbef (KT-3777, LY-163892) (Fig. 28).

2.3.3.4.2.1. STRUCTURE ACTIVITY. Structurally, loracarbef is the nonsulfated equivalent of cefaclor. It is derived from a series of carbacephems synthesized by Mochida et al. (1989).

The different molecules are distinguished by the substituent at position 3. The molecule without a substitution at position 3 is inactive. Different azoheterocycles have been attached, thiomethyltetrazole, thiopyridinium, and thiodiazole, both with and without substitutions. Loracarbef, a molecule with a 3-chlorine, belongs to this series. These molecules possess a certain activity against *S. aureus* and *Enterobacteriaceae*, except those producing type I enzymes. Activity against streptococci is variable, but some molecules possess moderate activity against *E. faecalis*.

The molecules are very stable in an aqueous medium compared to their sulfated equivalent (Table 36). The carbacephem-type molecules are asymmetrical, and the substituents on the β-lactam moiety are in the *cis* position; the *cis* stereochemistry of the carbacephems is less stable thermodynamically than the *trans* stereochemistry.

β-Lactams containing a phenylglycine chain have been shown to be less stable under physiological conditions than β-lactams which do not have an amino group. This phenomenon is related to the capacity of the amino group to attack the carbonyl-lactam bond, yielding a diketopiperazine

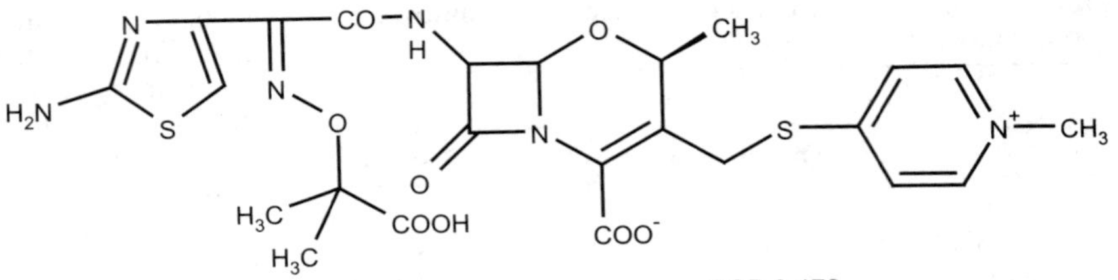

OCP-9-176

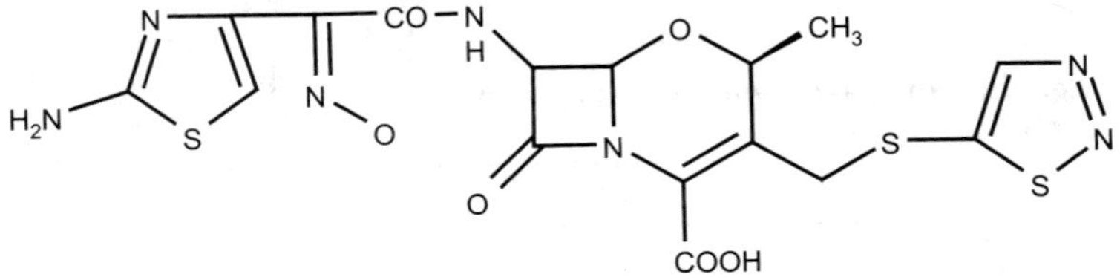

OCP-9-231

Figure 21 2β-Methyl-1-oxacephem derivatives

Table 25 In vitro and in vivo activities of OPC-9-176[a]

Organism	OCP-9-176		Ceftazidime	
	MIC (μg/ml)	ED_{50} (mg/kg)	MIC (μg/ml)	ED_{50} (mg/kg)
S. aureus MB 2865	4	3.1	4	5.2
E. cloacae MB 2646	4	1.6	128	50
K. pneumoniae MB 4005	0.06	3.8	0.03	1.6
P. aeruginosa MB 2835	4	35.7	1	11.8

[a]Data from Gilfillan et al., 1988. ED_{50}, 50% effective dose.

Table 26 Intramuscular pharmacokinetics of 1-oxa-cephamycins

Drug	Dose (mg)	C_{max} (μg/ml)	T_{max} (h)	$AUC_{0-\infty}$ (μg·h/ml)	$t_{1/2}$ (h)	$AUC_{i.v.}/AUC_{i.m.(0.5)}$	F (%)	Urinary elimination (%)
Moxalactam	250	13.4	0.8	59.9	2.5		~100	~90
	500	21.9	1	114.9	2.8	119.6/114.9		
Flomoxef	500	13.5	0.5	32.4	1.3	31.1/32.4	~100	~90
	1,000	24.7	0.5	64.9	1.4			

Table 27 Intravenous pharmacokinetics of flomoxef[a]

Dose (mg)	*n*	$C_{5\,min}$ (ml/min)[b]	C_{6h} (ml/min)	$t_{1/2\beta}$ (h)	$AUC_{0-\infty}$ (μg·h/ml)	Urinary elimination (%)
500	4	39.4 ± 8.4	<0.2	46.2	31.1	80.4
1000	4	102 ± 9.1	0.4	44.2	82.4	70.8

[a]Data from Yasunaga et al., 1987.
[b]Means ± standard deviations.

Table 28 Intravenous pharmacokinetics of moxalactam and flomoxef

Drug	Dose (mg)	*n*	$C_{5\,min}$ (ml/min)	C_{6h} (ml/min)	$t_{1/2\beta}$ (h)	Urinary elimination (%)
Flomoxef	1,000	4	90.8 ± 19.5	0.07	56.3	80.4
Moxalactam	1,000	4	118.8	0.57	110.4	70.8

Table 29 Pediatric pharmacokinetics of flomoxef[a]

Subjects	Age (days)	Dose (mg)	No. of subjects	C_0 (μg/ml)	C_{6h} (μg/ml)	$t_{1/2\beta}$ (h)	$AUC_{0-\infty}$ (μg·h/ml)
Prematures	0–3	10	2	24	8.9	4.1	124
		20	6	54	18.6	4.3	334
		40	6	98.2	39.8	4.7	614
	4–7	10	3	28.6	ND[b]	2.5	108
		20	6	54.6	6.9	2.3	
		40	1	93	20.6	2.9	407
	8	10	1	21.7	4.4	2.6	
		20	7	55.5	10.7	3	167
		40	5	106	14.6	2.1	333
Neonates	0–3	10	8	23.2	6.1	3.4	116
		20	14	54.4	9.6	3	176
		40	3	104	29.7	3.4	486
	4–7	10	3		3.1	1.9	71
		20	14	51.4	6.2	2.3	145
		40	1	95.9	3.4	1.2	196
	8	10	4		1.9	1.6	71
		20	24	51.4	6.2	2.3	145
		40	4	99.2	10.3	1.8	261
Infants	>8	10	3	28.1	0.29	1.1	28
		20	19	50.7	2.3	1.8	108
		40	8	96.8	0.9	0.9	113

[a]Data from Fujii, 1990.
[b]ND, not determined.

Table 30 Apparent elimination half-life of moxalactam in patients with renal insufficiency

Drug	$t_{1/2}$ (h) at indicated creatinine clearance (ml/min)			
	>80	80–30	30–10	<10
Moxalactam	2	4.8	8.4	13.6

by an intramolecular reaction. The β-lactams that contain this phenylglycine chain are in a zwitterionic state at pH 7, as the ammonium group possesses a positive charge and the carboxyl group possesses a negative charge.

For the carbacephems, the ammonium group is strongly attracted by the carboxyl group. A hydrogen-type bond may be created between these two groups. The result is that the ammonium group is located above the plane of the carboxyl group. These compounds have increased chemical stability. For the cephalosporins, the ammonium group is close to the sulfur atom, contributing to greater nucleophilic activity.

Cefaclor differs from cephalexin by the presence of a chlorine atom instead of a methyl group at position 3. The chlorine increases the chemical reactivity of the carbonyl-lactam bond, which in turn increases the binding to PBP. The problem with cefaclor is its instability at 37°C. This problem is resolved with loracarbef, and in fact in plasma at 37°C it is more stable than cefaclor and cephalexin. Loracarbef is stable for more than 120 h, whereas the activity of cephalexin is only 10% of its initial value after 1 h. Derivatives of loracarbef with different substituents on the phenyl moiety have been synthesized.

A total of 94 to 100% of the administered dose of *para*-hydroxyloracarbef is absorbed in the dog, but the renal clearance is more rapid than that of loracarbef. In the baboon, the bioavailability is 35%, with an apparent elimination half-life of 34.6 min (Quay et al., 1987) (Table 37).

The *meta*-methylsulfonamide (LY-228238) and *meta*-ethylsulfonamide (LY-257128) derivatives have poorer bioavailability, whereas their apparent elimination half-lives are longer and their antibacterial activities are similar to that of loracarbef. The *para*-methylsulfonamide derivative (LY-203815) is less active. The derivative of loracarbef with a 3-cyclopropyl group instead of a 3-chlorine is hydrolyzed by β-lactamases (TEM-1, type I, etc.), and its bioavailability in the CD-1 mouse is 78.6%, compared with those of loracarbef and cefaclor, which are 98% (Fig. 29).

Counter et al. (1989) synthesized carbacephem derivatives with a phenylglycyl ring (LY-264548). One of these, LY-227060 (2-amino-5-thiazolyl), has a carboxyethyl side chain at position 3 (Fig. 27).

Different esters have been attached to the carboxyl group at position 4 to enable them to be absorbed. The bioavailability of these derivatives is less than 50%. It is 49% in the mouse and 33% in the monkey.

The derivatives with a substituent at C-2 of the α- or β-methyl type are less active than the derivatives without substitutions at C-2, particularly against gram-negative bacilli.

A series of thiocarbacephems appears to possess not inconsiderable activity against methicillin-resistant strains of *S. aureus* (Fig. 30).

2.3.3.4.2.2. ANTIBACTERIAL ACTIVITY. Loracarbef has the same antibacterial activity as cefaclor (Table 38), with mediocre activity against *S. aureus* and good activity against *Streptococcus pyogenes* and certain species of *Enterobacteriaceae*. The following bacterial species or genera are resistant to loracarbef: *C. freundii*, *E. cloacae*, *S. marcescens*, *Enterobacter* spp., *M. morganii*, *Providencia rettgeri*, *Proteus vulgaris*, *Streptococcus liquefaciens*, *Bordetella pertussis*, *Bordetella parapertussis*, *Enterococcus* spp., and *L. monocytogenes*.

Against anaerobic species, loracarbef inhibits the growth of *Clostridium difficile* (MIC, ~1 μg/ml) but is inactive against *B. fragilis*, other *Clostridium* spp., etc. Loracarbef inhibits the

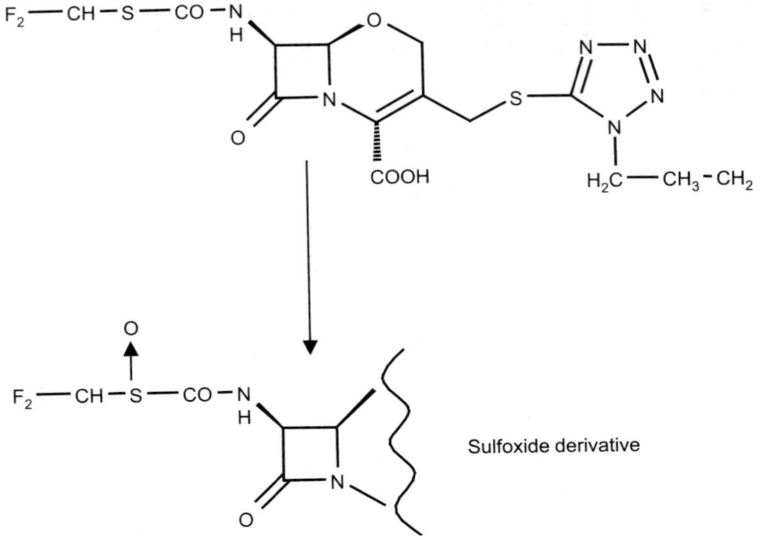

Sulfoxide derivative

Figure 22 Metabolism of flomoxef

Table 31 Metabolism of flomoxef[a]

Dose (mg)	Route[b]	No. of subjects	Plasma concn (μg/ml)[c]		Urinary elimination (%)		
			Flomoxef	HTT	Flomoxef	HTT	Sulfoxide
1,000	i.v.	4	79 ± 5.3	4.3 ± 0.6	84.4	14.5	0.2
1,000	i.m.	4	24.1 ± 6.5	1 ± 0.5	83.4	12.7	0.1

[a]Data from Yasunaga et al., 1987.
[b]i.v., intravenous; i.m., intramuscular.
[c]Means ± standard deviations.

Table 32 Interference of flomoxef with coagulation after repeated doses[a]

Parameter	Day	Bleeding time (s)	Platelet count (mm³, 10³)	ADP	Collagen (% mA)	Epinephrine (% mA)	Arachidonic acid (% mA)	Ristocetin (% mA)
Platelets	0	275	223	50	55.6	11.8	62.5	60.6
	7	217	301	56.2	58.7	16.3	68.8	66.8
		Quick time (s)	APTT (s)	$K_{1,2,3}$ epoxide (AUC_{0-8})	$AUCK_{1,2,3}$ epoxide (AUC K-1)	Vitamin K_1 (ng/ml)		Serum (ng/ml)
Coagulation	0	13.2	29.5					
	7	12.9	28.6	1.3	1.25	0.18		5.3

[a]Data from Andrassy et al., 1991. % mA, mean % of amplitude versus baseline.

Table 33 Comparative activities of cephalosporin and carbacephem derivatives[a]

Organism(s)	MIC (μg/ml)			
	Cefoxitin	Carbacefoxitin	Cefamandole	Carbacefamandole
S. aureus	1.56	6.25	<0.39	1.56
S. pyogenes	0.78	6.25	<0.39	3.12
E. coli	1.56	12.5	<0.39	1.56
K. pneumoniae	3.12	6.25	1.56	1.56
Enterobacter spp.	>100	>100	50	100
Serratia spp.	25	50	>100	>100

[a]Data from Firestone et al., 1977.

in vitro growth of *Helicobacter pylori*, with a MIC on the order of 2 μg/ml. Its activity against *S. pneumoniae* is better than that of cefixime but markedly inferior to those of cefpodoxime and cefuroxime. When the size of the bacterial inoculum is increased, the activity decreases. The molecule is unstable against hydrolysis by β-lactamases.

The breakpoints for loracarbef (NCCLS) are >8 and <32 μg/ml for intermediate strains and ≥32 μg/ml for resistant strains.

It is stable against hydrolysis by the *Moraxella catarrhalis* BRO-1 enzyme but is hydrolyzed by *E. coli* oxacillinases and TEM-2 and by chromosomally mediated type I and IV enzymes. Its stability against hydrolysis is slightly greater than that of cefaclor for enzymes of plasmid origin, such as TEM-1, OXA-1, and OXA-2 (Richmond and Sykes type V). It is hydrolyzed by the Ia enzyme of *E. cloacae* P99 and IVc of *Klebsiella oxytoca* (K1 enzyme).

Overall, its stability against hydrolysis by β-lactamases is less than that of cefadroxil, cephalexin, or cefuroxime.

Loracarbef possesses a certain activity against TEM-6- and TEM-7-producing strains of *E. coli* and against SHV-2-producing strains of *K. pneumoniae*. Loracarbef is inactive against SHV-4-, SHV-5-, and CMY-1-producing strains of *K. pneumoniae*. TEM-3-producing strains are not susceptible to loracarbef (MIC, ~32 μg/ml).

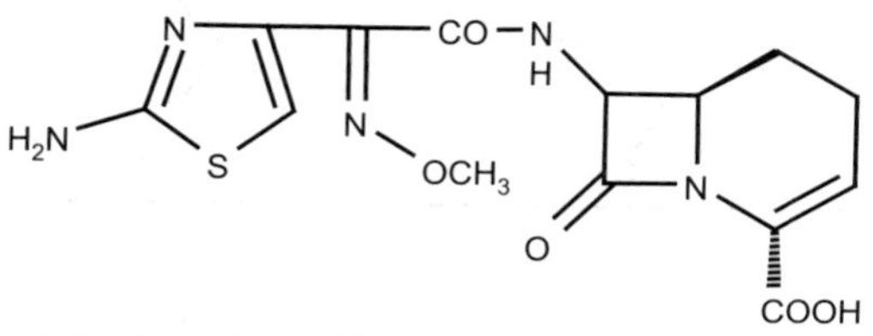

Figure 23 1-Dethiaceftizoxime

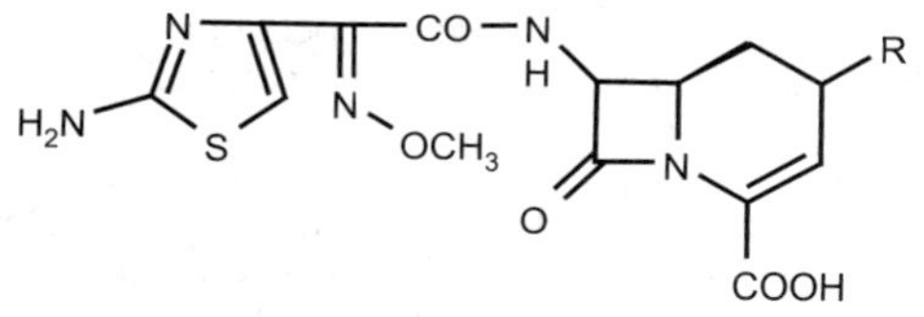

	R
KT 3767	H
KT 3919	α-OH
KT 3933	β-OH
KT 3937	-OH (racemate)

Figure 24 Carbacephems, group IIID

2.3.3.4.2.3. PHARMACOKINETICS. After administration of a single dose of loracarbef, the pharmacokinetics are linear between the studied doses of 50 and 500 mg. The apparent elimination half-life is on the order of 1.2 h. Plasma protein binding of loracarbef is approximately 25%. The product is eliminated renally, and probenecid modifies the kinetics of the product, suggesting tubular elimination. Food modifies the peak concentration in serum and the time to peak, but the area under the curve is similar. There is no plasma accumulation after repeated doses (Table 39).

In children (6 months to 14 years), the kinetics are identical to those in adults (Table 40). In elderly subjects, the pharmacokinetics are correlated with those of creatinine clearance. In patients with renal insufficiency, the pharmacokinetics are modified at less than 50 ml/min, requiring a dosage adjustment. In the effusion liquid from the middle ear, the mean concentrations of loracarbef after doses of 7.5 and 15 mg/kg of body weight are 2.0 and 3.9 μg/ml. In the blister fluid after a single dose of 200 mg, the area under the curve (AUC) is 13.8 μg·h/ml, similar to that in plasma.

After a single dose of 400 mg, the concentration of loracarbef in sinus fluid is 1.1 μg/ml. Likewise, the concentration in tonsillar tissue is on the order of 37 to 58% of that obtained in plasma (1.1 μg/ml). The salivary concentration is on the order of 0.7 μg/ml.

2.3.3.5. Subgroup IIIE: Isocephems

The isocephems are synthetic molecules characterized by the presence of a sulfur, oxygen, or nitrogen heteroatom at position 2 of the cephem moiety. These molecules may be subdivided into subgroups according to the heteroatom present at position 2: 2-isocephems, 2-azacephems, and 2-oxacephems (Fig. 31).

2.3.3.5.1. Isocephems. The first isocephems were synthesized simultaneously by researchers from Roussel-Uclaf and Sumitomo. Two molecules have been presented: RU-45978 and RU-46069 (Fig. 32). These two molecules are characterized by the presence of a 2-amino-5-thiazolyl moiety and either a methyl or a fluoromethyl residue on the oxime. At C-3, the presence of a vinylog chain increases the activity against gram-positive cocci. These are molecules belonging to the C-3′ quaternary ammonium series. A quaternary ammonium-type group is attached to the C-3 position on the propenyl chain. The two molecules possess activity equal to or greater than that of cefpirome against gram-positive cocci, and they are more active than cefpirome against *Enterobacteriaceae*. Their activity against type I

Table 34 Antibacterial activities of carbacephems

Organism	MIC (μg/ml)				
	KT-3767	KT-3937	KT-4380	KT-469	KT-4788
S. aureus 209 P	12.5	25	1.56	25	0.78
E. coli Juhl	0.01	0.01	0.2	0.1	0.1
K. pneumoniae 8045	0.01	0.01	0.1	0.01	0.05
S. marcescens T-26	0.2	0.2	0.78	0.78	6.25
E. cloacae F1510	0.1	0.05	0.05	0.02	0.02
C. freundii F526	0.1	0.02	0.2	0.1	0.1
P. aeruginosa	12.5	3.13	0.78	0.39	0.39

	R_1	R_2
KT 4380	3,4-dihydroxyphenyl	H
KT 4697	5-hydroxy-4-oxopyridyl	H
KT 4788	4,5-dihydroxypyridyl	CH_2–S–(N-methylpyridinium-4-yl)

Figure 25 Catechol-type carbacephems

	R
LY 214748	SO_2-cyclopropyl
LY 258360	3,4-dimethylpyridinium

Figure 26 LY-214748 and LY-258360

enzyme-producing *Enterobacteriaceae* is not bimodal. They are inactive against *P. aeruginosa* (Table 41). In vivo, their activity is slightly superior to that of cefpirome.

2.3.3.5.2. Oxa-2-cephems. Oxa-2-cephem derivatives have been synthesized. In a comparative study (Table 42) (Aszodi et al., 1988), derivatives with an oxygen heteroatom were shown to be less active and less stable against hydrolysis by β-lactamases.

In the isocephem series synthesized by Doyle et al. (1980), oxa-2-cephem derivatives were more active than their cephalosporin equivalents. These molecules possess good activity against gram-positive cocci but variable activity against *Enterobacteriaceae* depending on the side chains at C-7 and C-3.

Matsumoto et al. described a series of derivatives possessing a 2-amino-5-thiazolyl moiety and an oxycyclopentyl residue on the oxime and a pyridiniomethyl chain substituted at C-3. This series, known as OPC-20000, OPC-200011, and their 2-sulfoisocephem equivalent (BDF-12013), possess good antistaphylococcal activity in some cases but are less active than ceftazidime against *Enterobacteriaceae*, while exhibiting activity similar to that against *P. aeruginosa* (Fig. 33).

Tricyclic derivatives, the carboxyl group of which is replaced by a phenol or a pyridinium, have been described (Fig. 34), and likewise derivatives which also have a phosphorus atom at position 3.

Derivatives possessing an oxygen heteroatom at position 3 have been described (Phillips et al., 1983) (Fig. 35) with a methoxy- or thiomethyltetrazole-type substituent at position 2 of the cephem moiety.

2.3.4. Group IV: C-3′ Quaternary Ammonium Cephalosporins

The first optimization of the antibacterial activity of the cephalosporins was the presence of a 2-amino-5-thiazolyl moiety.

The first molecule was cefotaxime. The second optimization was the combination of a 2-amino-5-thiazolyl moiety and a methoxyimino chain which was present in the cefuroxime molecule. The third improvement was the presence of a quaternary ammonium residue. This is present in cephaloridine, cefsulodin, and cefpimizole, but these molecules do not have a

Table 35 In vitro activities of LY-262290 and LY-266941[a]

Organism	MIC (μg/ml)		
	LY (alkyl pyridinium)	LY-262290 (nitroimidazole)	LY-266941 (catechol)
S. aureus	1	0.06	8
S. pyogenes	0.015	0.008	0.06
S. pneumoniae	0.015	0.015	0.125
H. influenzae	0.015	0.015	0.015
E. coli	0.03	1	0.06
K. pneumoniae	0.008	0.015	0.015
E. cloacae	0.12	1	0.25
S. marcescens	0.06	2	0.25
M. morganii	0.06	4	4
P. aeruginosa	128	128	8

[a]Data from Cooper et al., 1992.

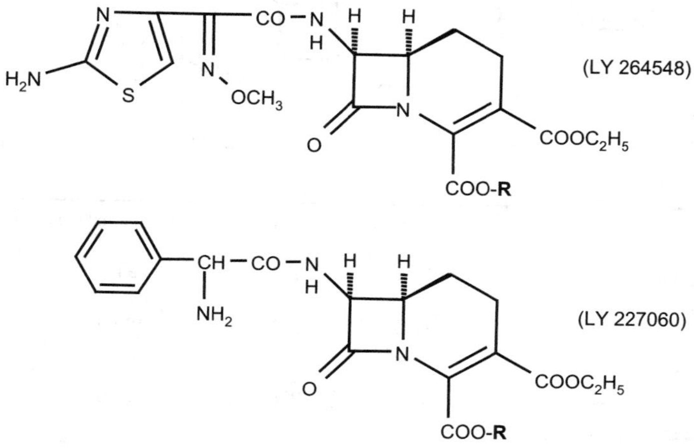

(LY 264548)

(LY 227060)

Figure 27 LY-264548 and LY-227060

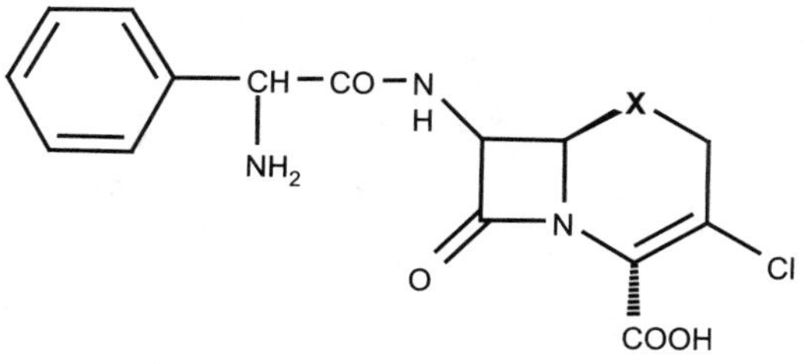

	X
Cefaclor	S
Loracarbef	CH_2

Figure 28 Loracarbef

Table 36 Degradation in an aqueous medium[a]

Drug	$t_{1/2}$ (h) (degradation)
Loracarbef	203
para-Hydroxyloracarbef (LY-213735)	215
Cephalexine	19.4
Cefaclor	1.45

[a]Phosphate buffer, pH 7.4, 35°C.

2-amino-5-thiazolyl moiety. Among the 2-amino-5-thiazolyl derivatives, the first molecule to possess a C-3′ quaternary ammonium moiety was ceftazidime. This was the first molecule of the group to exhibit activity against *P. aeruginosa*. However, its global activity other than against *P. aeruginosa* is inferior to that of cefotaxime or ceftriaxone. Numerous molecules have been synthesized and developed to improve on the basic activity of ceftazidime. Currently, at least six molecules are available or under development for therapeutic use: cefpirome, cefepime, cefclidin, cefozopran, cefluprenam, and cefoselis.

There are two types of molecules: those possessing a quaternary ammonium group at position 7 and those possessing a quaternary ammonium residue at position 3 (Fig. 36).

2.3.4.1. Group IV-1: C-7 Quaternary Ammonium Cephalosporins

Group IV-1 molecules possess a β-(1-benzylpyridinium) chain at position 7. They differ in the chain attached at position 3 of the cephem moiety to the thiomethyl residue. This is either a methyltetrazole (L-640876), methyltriazine (L-652813), or thiadiazine (L-642946) moiety (Fig. 37).

Overall these molecules have moderate antibacterial activity (Table 43). They are inactive against *P. aeruginosa* and moderately active against type I β-lactamase-producing

Table 37 Animal kinetics of loracarbef and *p*-OH-loracarbef (LY-213735)[a]

Animal	Drug	Route[b]	C_{max} (μg·h/ml)	AUC (μg·h/ml)	CL_R (ml/min)	$t_{1/2}$ (h)	Bioavailability (%)
Dog	Loracarbef	i.v.	39.6	7,840	39		
		p.o.	8.9	7,460	31		
	p-OH-loracarbef	i.v.	28.6	2,250	28		
		p.o.	6.7	2,120	24.2		
Baboon	Loracarbef	i.v.	168	3,620		19.6	
		p.o.	12.8	1,720			47
	p-OH-loracarbef	i.v.	212	4,650		34.6	
		p.o.	9.6	1,650			35

[a]Data from Quay et al., 1987.
[b]i.v., intravenous; p.o., per os.

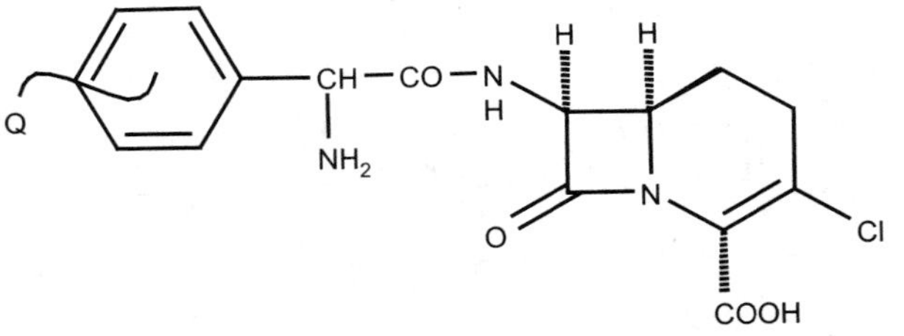

Q — CH—CO—N(H) ; NH_2 ; H H ; O ; N ; Cl ; COOH

	Cmax	T 1/2 (min)	Bioavailability (%)
Cefaclor	25.1	143	91.6
Loracarbef	37.6	673	100.0
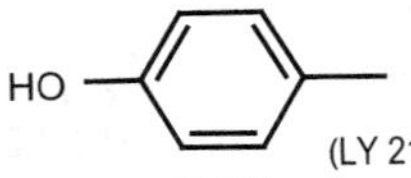 HO— (LY 213735)	31.8	928	100.0
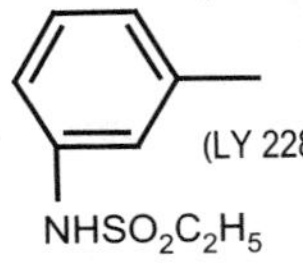 $NHSO_2C_2H_5$ (LY 228138)	42.7	546	66.0
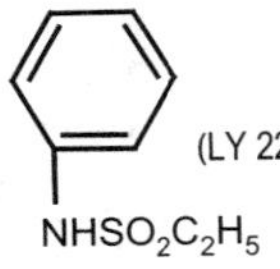 $NHSO_2C_2H_5$ (LY 228238)	38.4	811	75.0

Figure 29 Carbacephem derivatives of the phenylglycine type

strains of *Enterobacteriaceae*. They have the characteristic of preferentially inhibiting *E. coli* PBP 2 activity. Conversely, they have modest activity against anaerobic bacteria. L-652813, like ceftriaxone, possesses a triazine moiety, and its pharmacokinetic profile is similar to that of ceftriaxone in animals (Table 44).

2.3.4.2. Group IV-2: C-3′ Quaternary Ammonium Cephalosporins

Numerous molecules have been described (Fig. 36). They are divided chemically into two subgroups: those possessing a 2-amino-5-thiazolyl moiety and the others, which have a 5-amino-2-thiadiazolyl moiety. The latter increases the antibacterial activity against *P. aeruginosa* by 1 dilution compared with the same molecule with a 2-amino-5-thiazolyl moiety; however, they are slightly less active against *nterobacteriaceae*. Within each subgroup, the molecules have a variable residue on the oxime (methyl or isobutyl). The chain at C-3 differs.

The physicochemical properties of these molecules are summarized in Table 45.

The presence of a quaternary ammonium residue at position 3 of the cephem moiety improves the activity against certain reputedly difficult bacterial species, giving rise to molecules that represent a technological advance.

2.3.4.3. Group IV-2A: 2-Amino-5-Thiazolyl Cephalosporins

The majority of the C-3′ quaternary ammonium type cephalosporins belong to this group IV-2A (Fig. 38).

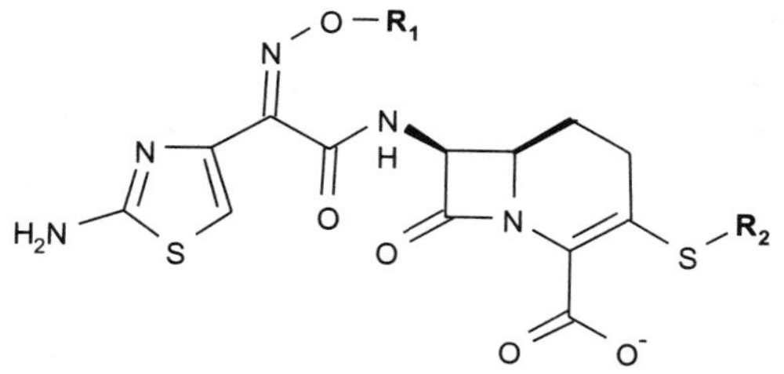

Derivative	R_1	R_2	MIC (μg/ml) *S. aureus* Methi-S	Methi-R
A	CH_2-CH_2F	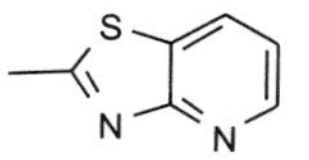	1.0	4.0
B	CH_2-CH_2F	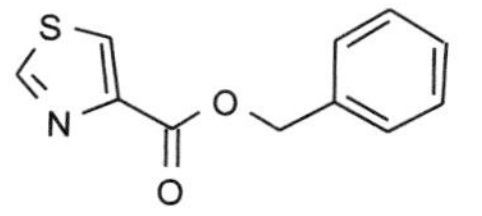	0.5	16.0
C	CH_2-CH_2F	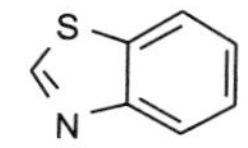	0.5	4.0
D	CH_2-CH_2F	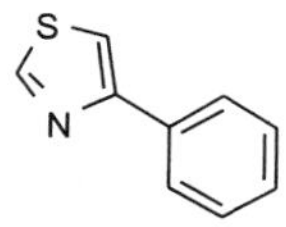	0.5	4.0
E	CH_3	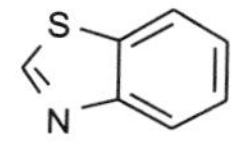	1.0	8.0
F	CH_2-CH_2F	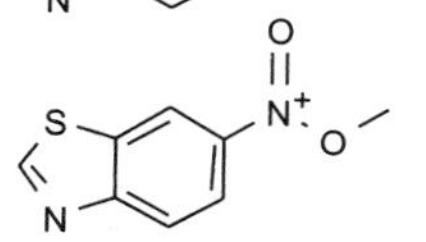	0.5	2.0

Figure 30 Antistaphylococcal activity of thiocarbacephems

Table 38 Comparative in vitro activities of cefaclor and loracarbef[a]

Organism[b]	MIC_{50} (μg/ml) Loracarbef	Cefaclor
S. aureus	4	4
S. pyogenes	0.12	0.12
S. pneumoniae	0.5	0.25
H. influenzae β^-	0.5	1
H. influenzae β^+	0.5	1
M. catarrhalis β^-	0.25	≤0.125
M. catarrhalis β^+	0.5	0.5
E. coli	0.5	1
K. pneumoniae	0.5	2
P. mirabilis	1	2

[a]Data from Doren et al., 1992.
[b]β^-, non-β-lactamase producing; $\beta^{\pm}$, β-lactamase producing.

2.3.4.3.1. Cefpirome. Cefpirome is a 2-amino-5-thiazolyl cephalosporin which possesses a cyclopentenopyridinium moiety at the C-3 position of the cephem moiety. The nature of the chain affects the activity against gram-positive cocci and *Enterobacteriaceae*, particularly those producing cephalosporinases. The moiety at C-3 yields a molecule with a well-balanced antibacterial spectrum (Bryskier and Chantot, 1985). In solution, cefpirome is stable at a pH of between 4 and 7.

2.3.4.3.2. Cefepime. Cefepime is derived from a series of compounds synthesized by Naito et al. (1986). It possesses a 3-(*N*-methylpyrrolidine) moiety at the C-3 position of the cephem moiety. In this series, the alkyl residue on the oxime and the heterocycle at position 3 of the cephem moiety affect stability against hydrolysis by different β-lactamases.

2.3.4.3.3. DQ-2556 and DQ-2522. DQ-2556 possesses a methoxyimino-2-amino-5-thiazolyl chain at position 7 of the cephem moiety and a methylpyridinium chain to which is attached a 3-oxazole moiety at position 4′. DQ-2556 was chosen from a series of molecules synthesized by Ejima et al. (1987). This molecule was selected for its antibacterial activity and its solubility in water. The solubility is dependent on the substituent of the pyridinium moiety. Derivatives with an imidazole, oxazole, or oxadiazole moiety are more soluble in water than those with a pyrazole, triazole, or thiadiazole moiety.

2.3.4.3.4. ME-1228. ME-1228 belongs to the group of C-3′ thiomethylpyridinium cephalosporins with an ethyl group at position 1. It differs from the other molecules by the residue on the oxime group, which is an ethoxy, with the

Table 39 Pharmacokinetics of loracarbef

Dose (mg)	No. of subjects	C_{max} (μg/ml)	T_{max} (h)	$AUC_{0-\infty}$ (μg·h/ml)	$t_{1/2}$ (h)	Urinary elimination (%)
100	9	3.8	1.3	5.6	1.09	79.1
200, fasting	12	9.1	1.3	14.9	1.03	82
200, fed	12	5.1	2.1	13.4	1.1	94.9
200, with probenecid (500 mg)	12	10.4	1.2	26.9	1.52	89.9
400	6	11.4	1.2		1.18	83.4
250	9	10.3	1.1	19.1	1.19	93.2
500	9	15.9	1.3	30.7	1.19	86

Table 40 Pharmacokinetics of loracarbef in children[a]

Dose (mg/kg)	No. of subjects	C_{max} (μg/ml)	T_{max} (h)	$AUC_{0-\infty}$ (μg·h/ml)	$t_{1/2}$ (h)
7.5	9	14.1 ± 4.9	0.67 ± 0.18	23.8 ± 3.6	0.89 ± 0.21
15	10	20.3 ± 3.2	0.9 ± 0.41	40.7 ± 7.6	0.99 ± 0.27

[a]Data from Nelson et al., 1988. Data are means ± standard deviations.

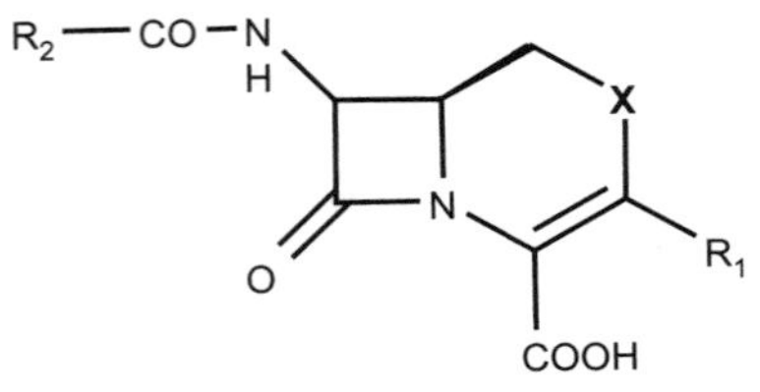

R2—CO—NH, X, N, O, R1, COOH

	X
2-iso cephems	S
2-aza cephems	N-R
2-oxa cephems	O

Figure 31 Isocephems

presence of an asymmetrical center. The isomer (S) is the most active and has been selected. The selection of the molecule was based not only on its antibacterial activity but also on its toxicological profile, which is dependent on the residue on the oxime. The 1-carboxy-1-methylethoxyimino derivatives are more toxic in the mouse (intravenous 50% lethal dose [LD_{50}] < 1 g/kg) than the dimethyl derivative (LD_{50} > 3 g/kg), with the added drawback of a reduction in activity against *P. aeruginosa* (Shibahara et al., 1990).

The stereochemistry of the 1-carboxyethoxyimino chain influences the antibacterial activity, and the (S)-isomers have activity superior to that of the (R)-isomers.

Three derivatives, CP-107, MT-382, and MT-520, possess similar structures.

2.3.4.3.5. CS-461. CS-461 is a 2-amino-5-thiazolyl cephalosporin selected from a series prepared by Nakayama et al. (1991). It possesses a 3-thiazolomethyl chain substituted at position 3′ by a hydroxyethyl chain and at position 4′ by a methyl group. In this series, the molecules with a thiadiazole moiety are less active than those with a thiazole moiety. The substituents on the thiazole moiety interfere markedly with the activity of the molecules.

2.3.4.3.6. Cefoselis (FK-037). Cefoselis is also a methoxyimino-2-amino-5-thiazolyl derivative. It is characterized by a methylpyrazolium chain having a 2′-hydroxyethyl chain and a 3-amino group.

2.3.4.4. Group IV-2B

Members of group IV-2B are shown in Fig. 39.

2.3.4.4.1. Cefclidin (E-1040). A series of derivatives having a 5-amino-2-thiadiazole moiety was synthesized by Sugyama et al. (1992). The derivatives possess a quinuclidine moiety, with or without a substitution at position 3. The dehydroquinuclidine derivatives are less active than the quinuclidine derivative. The derivatives with a 2-amino-5-thiazolyl moiety are less active against *P. aeruginosa*. Derivatives with a 4′-carbamoyl substituent on the quinuclidine moiety are the most active. The residue on the oxime alters the activity. The methoxy group appears to be optimal in relation to an ethoxy, methyl, or cyclopropyl group, particularly against *S. aureus*.

2.3.4.4.2. Cefozopran. Cefozopran (SCE-2787) is a 5-amino-2-thiadiazolyl cephalosporin selected from among a number of derivatives of the bicyclic quaternary ammonium type. It possesses an imidazolepyridazinium moiety at C-3. Replacement of this moiety by a fluorine, methoxy, methyl, chlorine, or thiomethyl has been shown to have an adverse effect on activity against *S. aureus*, *P. aeruginosa*, or both.

2.3.4.4.3. Cefluprenam (E-1077). A series of derivatives has been synthesized by Kamiya et al. Cefluprenam possesses two characteristics: the oxime residue has a fluorine atom, and the chain at the C-3 position is original and has a 5-amino-2-thiadiazolyl moiety.

The originality of the chain at the C-3 position lies in the presence of a double bond. This vinylog produces good activity against gram-positive cocci. A quaternary ammonium-type *N*-α-ethyl-Nα-methylglycinamide chain is attached to this propenyl residue. Cefluprenam has been adopted from among all the derivatives of this series, not only for its

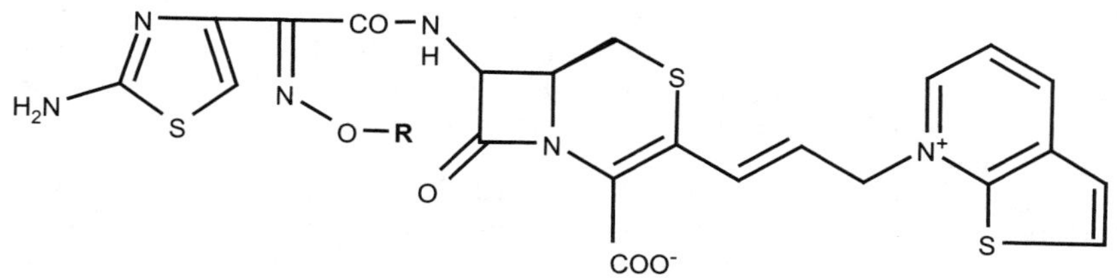

	R
RU 45978	$-CH_3$
RU 46069	$-CHF_2$

Figure 32 Isocephems: RU-45978 and RU-46069

Table 41 In vitro activities of 2-isocephems[a]

Organism	MIC_{50} (μg/ml)		
	RU-45978	RU-46069	Cefpirome
S. aureus Met[s]	0.15	0.015	0.6
S. pyogenes	≤0.0025	≤0.0025	0.005
S. pneumoniae	≤0.0025	≤0.0025	0.005
E. coli	0.005	0.01	0.04
K. pneumoniae		0.01	0.02
C. freundii	0.04	0.02	0.15
P. stuartii	0.04	0.15	0.04
M. morganii	0.005	0.005	0.01
P. aeruginosa	20	20	10

[a]Data from Chantot et al., 1988.

Table 42 Comparative in vitro activities of isocephems with respect to the heteroatom in position 2[a]

Organism	MIC (μg/ml)	
	Sulfur	Oxygen
S. aureus SG 511	1.2	1.2
S. pyogenes A561	≤0.04	≤0.04
P. aeruginosa 1171	5	>40
E. coli TEM	0.3	5
K. oxytoca 1082 E (K1)	10	>40
E. cloacae P99	>40	>40
Serratia strain RG 2532	0.6	5

[a]Data from Azsodi et al., 1988.

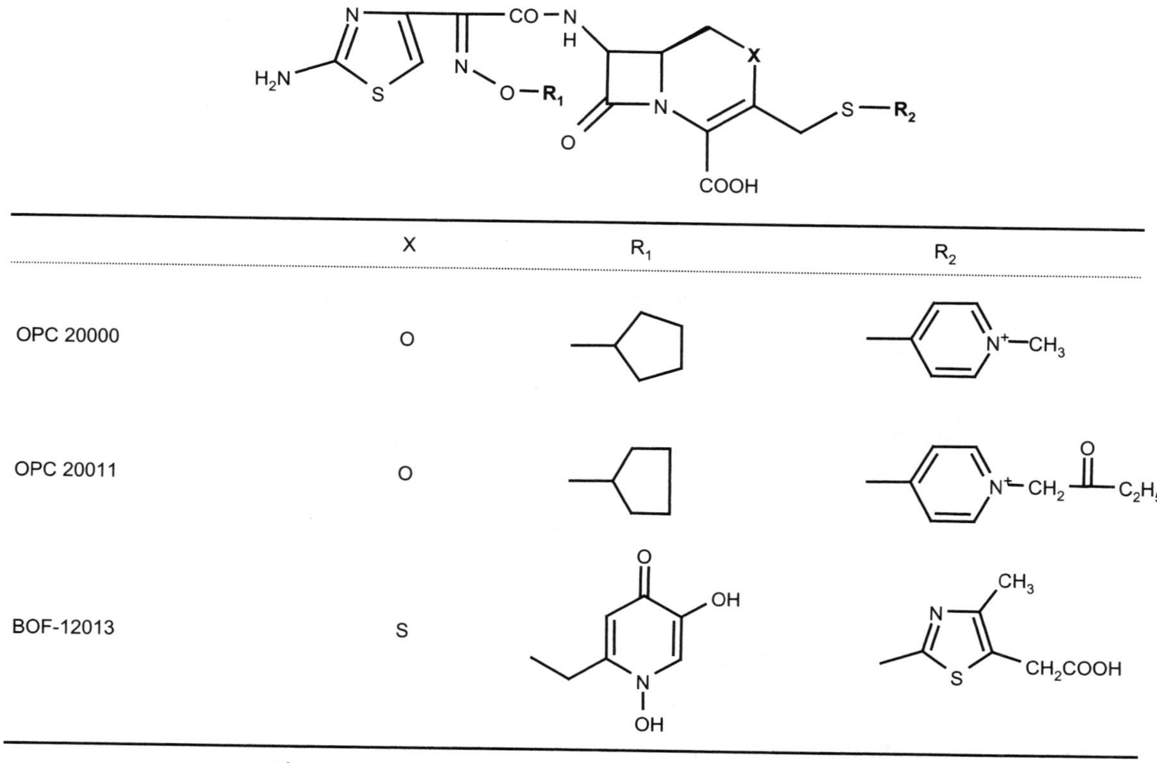

	X	R_1	R_2
OPC 20000	O		
OPC 20011	O		
BOF-12013	S		

Figure 33 Group IIIE 2-isocephems and 2-oxaisocephems

antibacterial activity but also for its physicochemical and toxicological properties.

2.3.4.4.4. FK-518. A series of molecules have been synthesized by Sakane et al. (1990). FK-518 has a 5-amino-2-thiadiazolyl moiety at C-7 and a 3-amino(2-hydroxyethyl)pyrazole chain at C-3. This chain is optimal in this series. In fact, the presence of a methyl group at position 4 of the pyrazole moiety or a different alkyl chain at position 2 reduces the activity against *P. aeruginosa*. This molecule possesses moderate activity against cefoperazone-resistant strains of *P. aeruginosa*.

Figure 34 Oxa-2-cephems: tricyclic derivatives

2.3.4.4.5. YM-40220. YM-40220 is a cephalosporin with a 5-amino-2-thiadiazolyl moiety at C-7. The residue on the oxime is a fluoromethyl group. It has a vinylog chain at C-3 and a 2,2-dimethyl-5-isoxazolidine moiety. Arao et al. (1994) showed that this molecule is twice as active as cefpirome and cefluprenam against oxacillin-susceptible strains of *S. aureus* (MIC_{50}, 0.20 μg/ml) and four times as active against coagulase-negative staphylococci. It possesses activity equivalent to that of cefpirome against streptococci, including penicillin G-resistant *S. pneumoniae*. Against *Enterobacteriaceae*, its activity is similar to that of cefpirome. It is inactive against *Stenotrophomonas maltophilia*, *Burkholderia cepacia*, *Chryseobacterium meningosepticum*, and *P. aeruginosa*, and its activity is similar to that of ceftazidime.

Figure 35 Oxa-3-cephems

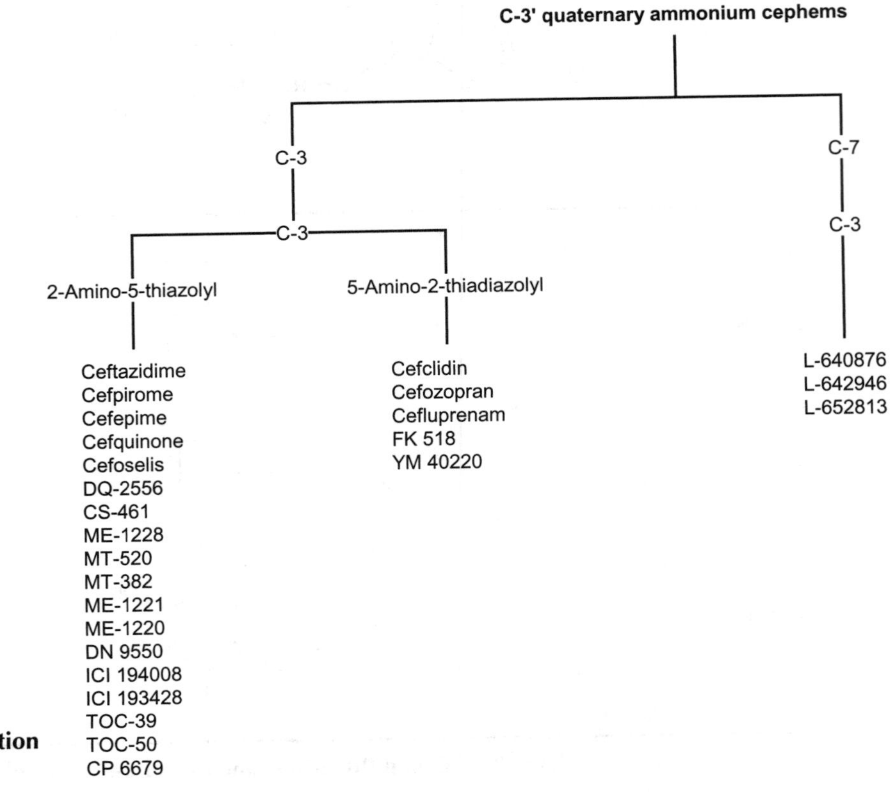

Figure 36 Classification of group IV cephems

2.3.4.5. Antibacterial Activities

Molecules with a C-3′ quaternary ammonium group principally exert activity against cephalosporinase-producing strains because of their speed of penetration and their weak affinity for these periplasmic enzymes. Some of them have better activity than ceftazidime against *P. aeruginosa*, others better activity than cefotaxime against *S. aureus*. Cefpirome and cefozopran have a well-balanced antibacterial spectrum, followed by cefepime. Cefclidin is above all an anti-gram-negative, and in particular antipseudomonal, molecule. Cefoselis possesses good activity against gram-positive cocci and *Enterobacteriaceae* (Tables 46 to 49).

Cefpirome has a well-balanced antibacterial spectrum with good activity against gram-positive cocci, including penicillin G-resistant strains of *S. pneumoniae* (Table 50). It is the most active molecule against penicillin G-resistant strains of *S. pneumoniae*. Its activity against *Enterobacteriaceae*, including type I β-lactamase-producing strains, is good. It possesses good activity against *P. aeruginosa*.

Like the other 2-amino-5-thiazolyl cephalosporins, it is relatively inactive against extended-spectrum-β-lactamase-producing strains.

Cefepime is relatively inactive against *S. aureus* but is more active than cefclidin and ceftazidime, although

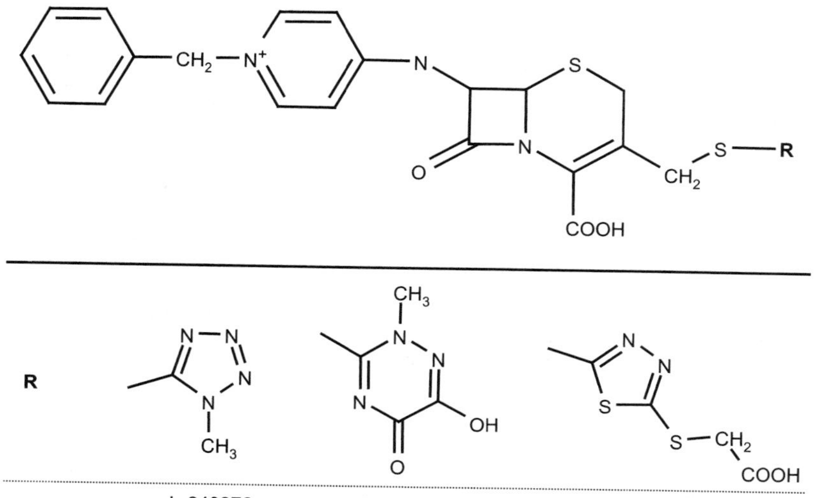

Figure 37 C-7 quaternary ammonium cephalosporins, group IV-1

Table 43 In vitro activities of C-7 quaternary ammonium cephalosporins[a]

Organism	MIC (μg/ml)			
	L-640876	L-652813	L-642946	Cefotaxime
S. aureus	16	1	8	1
E. faecalis	128	>128	>128	32
E. coli	<0.06	≤0.008	0.06	<0.06
Salmonella serovar Typhimurium	0.5	≤0.008	0.03	0.125
E. cloacae (type I)	0.5	0.25	1	128
K. oxytoca (K1)	16	0.5	4	1
K. pneumoniae	8	≤0.008	≤0.008	<0.06
M. morganii	32	≤0.008	0.015	0.5
S. marcescens	128	0.03	0.125	8
P. aeruginosa	>128	>128	>128	64

[a]Data from Koupal, 1983, and Pelak et al., 1987.

Table 44 Pharmacokinetics of L-652813 in animals[a]

Animals	Dose (mg)	Route[b]	L-652813			Ceftriaxone		
			AUC (μg·h/ml)	$t_{1/2}$ (h)	Urinary elimination (%)	AUC (μg·h/ml)	$t_{1/2}$ (h)	Urinary elimination (%)
Mice, CD-1	20	s.c.	73.8	70	53.2	145	63	41
Baboons (rhesus)	10	i.m.	152–190	59–91	40	187–303	89–125	28

[a]Data from Prlak et al., 1987.
[b]s.c., subcutaneous; i.m., intramuscular.

Table 45 Physicochemical properties of C-3′ quaternary ammonium cephalosporins

Drug	Empirical formula	Molecular mass (Da)	Melting point (°C)	pK_a
Cefpirome (sulfate)	$C_{22}H_{24}N_6O_5S_2$	514.6	180	2.51/2.81
Cefepime	$C_{19}H_{24}N_6O_5S_1$	480.6	~150	2.81
Cefclidin	$C_{21}H_{26}N_8O_6S_2$	549.73		
Cefozopran	$C_{19}H_{17}N_9O_5S_2$	551.98		
Cefquinone (sulfate)	$C_{23}H_{24}N_6O_5S_2$	626.7	>200	
Cefluprenam	$C_{20}H_{25}FN_8O_6S_2$	556.59		
DQ-2556	$C_{29}H_{19}N_7O_6S_2$	684.07	145–155	
ME-1228	$C_{23}H_{24}N_6O_7S_3$	586.04	180–183	
CS-461	$C_{20}H_{24}N_6O_{10}S_4$	635.26		
L-640876	$C_{22}H_{21}N_7O_3S_2$	495.57	162–164	
DQ-2522	$C_{22}H_{19}N_7O_6S_2$	540.74	144–155	

markedly less so than cefpirome. Its activity against streptococci is good but is less than that of cefpirome. It possesses the same activity against *Enterobacteriaceae* as cefpirome and better activity than that of cefclidin. Its activities against *P. aeruginosa* and against *H. influenzae* and *M. catarrhalis* are similar to those of cefpirome. It shares with the other molecules of this class mediocre activity against extended-spectrum plasmid-mediated β-lactamase-producing strains of *Enterobacteriaceae*.

The data on the antibacterial activity of CS-461 are fragmentary. Nevertheless, this molecule possesses good activity against methicillin-susceptible *S. aureus* (MSSA) strains and against the strains of *Enterobacteriaceae* tested, and it has moderate activity against *P. aeruginosa*.

The MIC_{50} of cefclidin for *Enterobacteriaceae*, *P. aeruginosa*, *H. influenzae*, and *Neisseria* spp. is 0.25 μg/ml, and the MIC_{90} is between 0.06 and 2.0 μg/ml. Cefclidin is twice as active as ceftazidime and as active as cefpirome and cefepime. It is particularly active against type I enzyme-producing strains of *C. freundii*. It is inactive against *S. aureus*. It is particularly active against *P. aeruginosa*, whether or not the strains are susceptible to ceftazidime or imipenem.

Cefoselis has the same activity as cefpirome against gram-positive cocci and against *P. aeruginosa*. It has the same activity as cefpirome against *Enterobacteriaceae* but possesses weaker activity against type I β-lactamase-producing strains, such as *E. cloacae, S. marcescens, C. freundii, M. morganii*, and *P. rettgeri* with a bimodal bacterial population. It has good activity against strains of penicillin-resistant *S. pneumoniae* (MIC_{50}, ~0.25 μg/ml) (Jones, 1992). Cefoselis is hydrolyzed by extended-spectrum β-lactamases of the CAZ, TEM, and SHV types in a fashion similar to that for cefepime and cefpirome (Table 51). It is also more extensively hydrolyzed by the P99 enzyme than cefepime but to the same extent by the K-1 enzyme of *K. oxytoca*.

Cefluprenam has the same activity as cefepime against gram-positive cocci and activity similar to that of ceftazidime against *P. aeruginosa*. It has good activity against all *Enterobacteriaceae*. The *S. marcescens* population responds bimodally to the action of cefluprenam, while this drug is inactive against ceftazidime-resistant strains of *P. aeruginosa*.

The activity of cefozopran is identical to that of cefpirome against gram-positive cocci and similar to that of ceftazidime against *P. aeruginosa*. It has good activity against *Enterobacteriaceae*, but its activity against *Proteus* spp. is bimodal.

The activity of DN-9550 against gram-positive cocci is similar to that of cefotaxime. DN-9550 possesses moderate activity against *P. aeruginosa* and against *Enterobacteriaceae*. It exhibits bimodal activity against *S. marcescens*, *C. freundii*, *E. cloacae*, and *P. aeruginosa*.

FK-518 possesses moderate activity against gram-positive cocci and is inactive against *S. aureus*. Against *Enterobacteriaceae*, its activity is similar to that of cefclidin. Conversely, it has bimodal activity against type I β-lactamase-producing strains of *Enterobacteriaceae*. It possesses moderate activity against strains of *P. aeruginosa* with variable phenotypes of resistance to β-lactams. Its activity appears to be similar to that of cefclidin (Table 52).

DQ-2556 possesses activity identical to that of cefotaxime against gram-positive cocci, whether streptococci or staphylococci. Against *Enterobacteriaceae*, it is more active than cefotaxime against certain species but has identical activity against others. Against type I β-lactamase-producing strains, it possesses bimodal activity. It is inactive against *P. aeruginosa* (Table 53).

The antistaphylococcal and antistreptococcal activities of ME-1228 are moderate. ME-1228 possesses good activity against *Enterobacteriaceae*. Its activity is bimodal against *C. freundii* ($MIC_{50/90}$, 0.10/25 μg/ml), but minor against *S. marcescens* and *M. morganii*. It has little activity against *P. aeruginosa*.

In the same series, MT-382, MT-520, and CP-107 possess good activity against *Enterobacteriaceae*, but they are inactive against *P. aeruginosa*, while CP-107 possesses activity similar to that of cefpirome against MSSA strains. They are inactive against type I β-lactamase-producing strains of *E. cloacae*, *C. freundii*, and *M. morganii*.

ICI-194008 and ICI-193428 are relatively inactive against *S. aureus* and moderately active against streptococci. They are inactive against penicillin G-resistant strains of *S. pneumoniae* (MIC_{50}, 4 to 32 μg/ml) (Table 54). They are also relatively inactive against *P. aeruginosa*. ICI-193428 is more active against *Enterobacteriaceae* than ICI-194008, with activity similar to that of cefpirome (Table 55).

A series of derivatives with a vinylog type chain at C-3 was synthesized and the molecule TOC-50 was selected (Fig. 40). This molecule is more active than cefpirome against gram-positive cocci, including *S. pneumoniae*. It is active against oxacillin-resistant strains of *S. aureus* (MIC_{50}, ~1.56 μg/ml) and against *E. faecalis* (MIC_{50}, ~0.39 μg/ml). It possesses activity similar to that of cefpirome against *Enterobacteriaceae*, with the exception of *C. freundii* (MIC_{50}, ~6.25 μg/ml) and *S. marcescens* (MIC_{50}, ~12.5 μg/ml). It is inactive against *P. aeruginosa* (MIC, >100 μg/ml). TOC-39 has also been described for this series (Fig. 41).

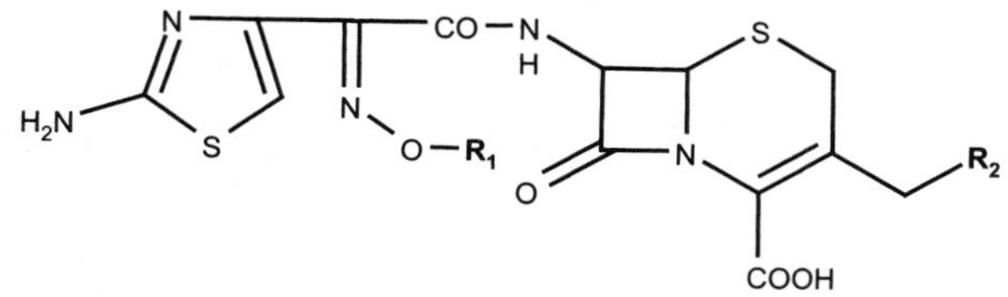

	R_1	R_2
Cefpirome	$-CH_3$	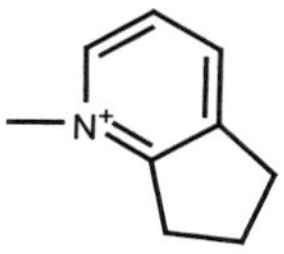 $-N^+$
Cefepime	$-CH_3$	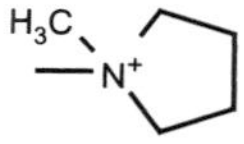 H_3C, $-N^+$
DQ 2556	$-CH_3$	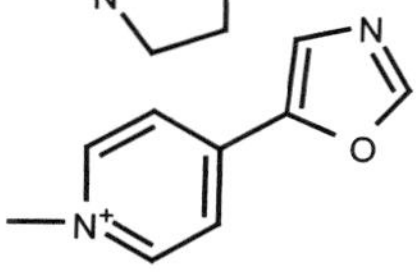 $-N^+$; N, O
Cefoselis	$-CH_3$	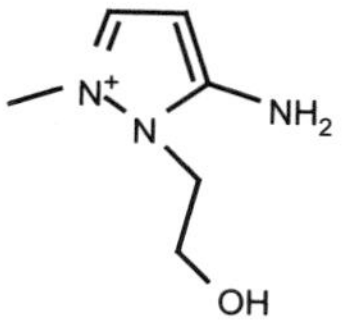 $-N^+$, N, NH_2, OH
ME 1228	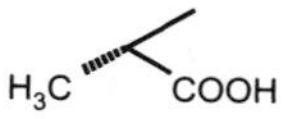 H_3C, COOH	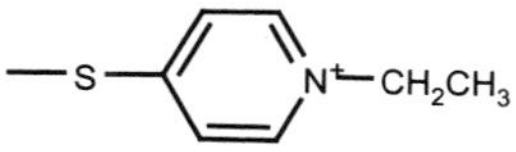 $-S-$, $N^+-CH_2CH_3$
CS-461	$-CH_3$	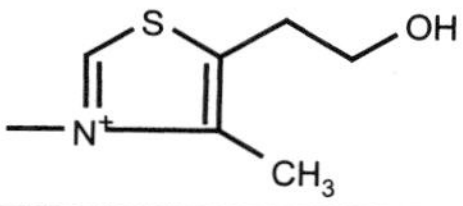 S, OH, $-N^+$, CH_3

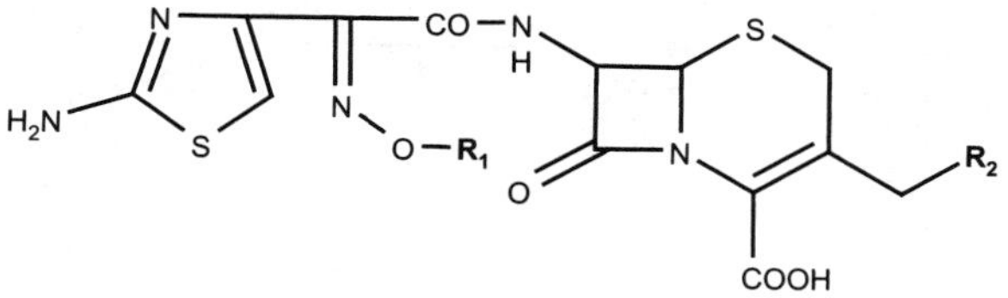

	R_1	R_2
DQ 2522	$-CH_3$	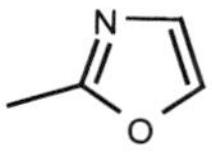 N, O
M-14138	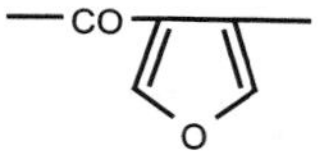 $-CO-$, O	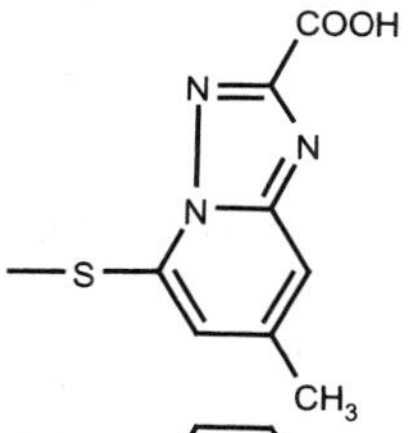 COOH, N, N, N, $-S-$, CH_3
MT 382	$-CH_3$	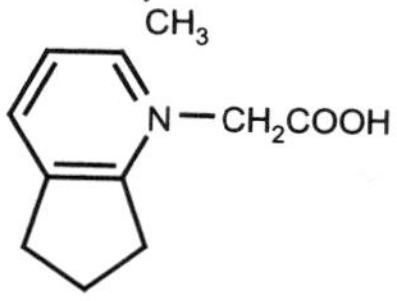 $N-CH_2COOH$
DN 9550	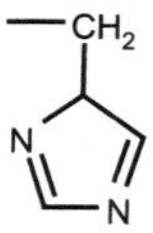 $-CH_2$, N, N	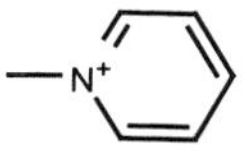 $-N^+$
ME 1220	C_2H_5	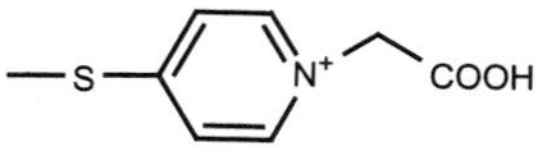 $-S-$, N^+, COOH
ME 1220	CH_2COOH	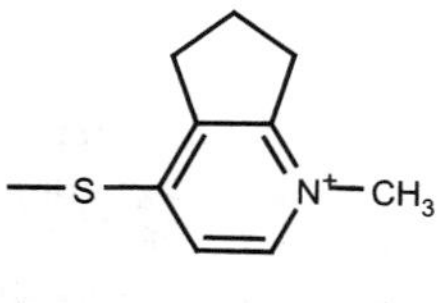 $-S-$, N^+-CH_3

Figure 38 C-3′ quaternary ammonium cephalosporins, group IV-2A

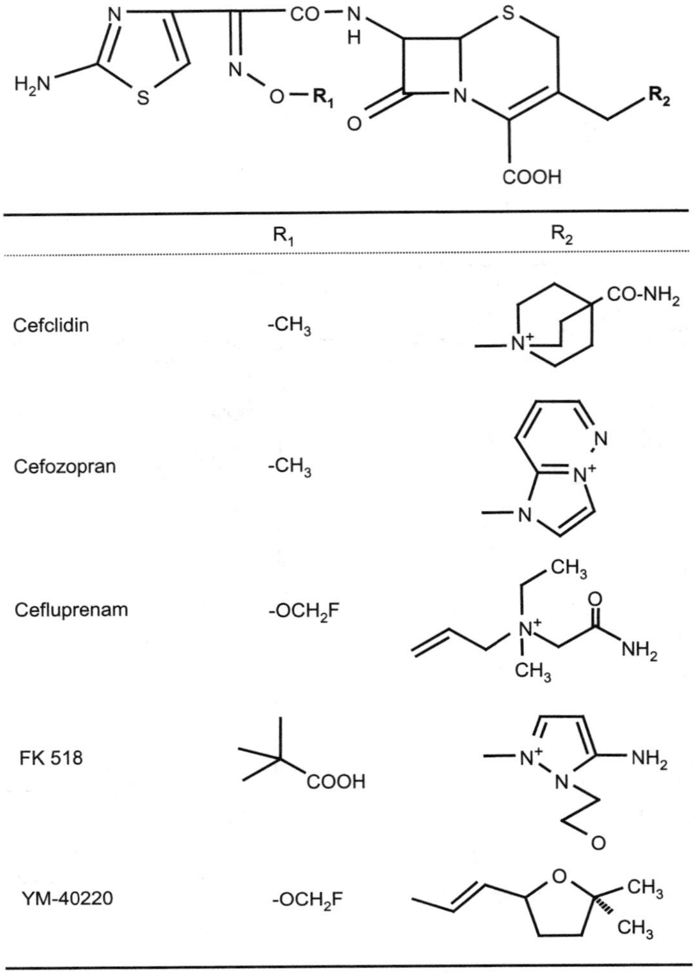

	R_1	R_2
Cefclidin	$-CH_3$	
Cefozopran	$-CH_3$	
Cefluprenam	$-OCH_2F$	
FK 518	COOH	NH_2
YM-40220	$-OCH_2F$	CH_3, CH_3

Figure 39 C-3′ quaternary ammonium cephalosporins, group IV-2B

Table 46 Activities of group IV cephalosporins against gram-positive bacteria

Organism	MIC$_{50}$ (μg/ml)						
	Ceftazidime	Cefclidin	Cefpirome	Cefozopran	Cefluprenam	Cefoselis	Cefepime
S. aureus Met^s	8	16	1	0.78	0.78	0.78	4
Staphylococcus Met^s coagulase negative	8	4	0.5	0.39	0.39	0.78	1
S. pyogenes	0.015	0.015	0.015	0.012	0.012	0.012	0.015
S. agalactiae	0.25	0.12	0.015	0.1	0.05	0.05	0.03
S. pneumoniae	0.25	0.25	0.015	0.05	0.025	0.025	0.03
E. faecalis	>64	>64	4	12.5	1.56	50	32
L. monocytogenes	>64	>64	8				32

MC-02306 is an arylthiocephem which possesses a phenylthio moiety at C-3 replaced by a 2-isothiouronium chain (Fig. 42). This derivative is very soluble in water. It is less active than imipenem against MSSA strains (MIC$_{50}$, 0.25 μg/ml). It is moderately active against methicillin-resistant strains (MIC$_{50}$, 4 μg/ml) and strains of *E. faecalis* (MIC$_{50}$, 2 μg/ml) and *E. faecium* (MIC$_{50}$, 4 μg/ml) but is inactive against vancomycin-resistant strains of *E. faecalis*. It possesses good activity against *S. pneumoniae*, whether or not the strain is resistant to penicillin G (MIC$_{50}$, ~0.125 μg/ml). It possesses good affinity for *S. aureus* PBP 2a (IC$_{50}$, 1.54 μg/ml).

CP-6679 (Fig. 43) has a fluorine atom on the oxime and an imidazothiazolium moiety at C-3. This derivative is moderately active against gram-positive cocci, with the exception of *S. pneumoniae*. In vivo, CP-6679 is four times more active than ceftazidime against *P. aeruginosa*. It is more active than cefpirome against *S. aureus*, *K. pneumoniae*, and *E. cloacae*.

2.3.4.6. Mechanisms of Action and Resistance

The activity of the β-lactams is based on the possibility of penetrating the outer membrane of gram-negative bacilli,

Table 47 Activities of group IV cephalosporins against gram-negative bacilli

Organism(s)	MIC$_{50}$ (µg/ml)				
	Cefoselis[a]	Cefluprenam[b]	Cefpirome	Cefepime	Cefozopran[c]
E. coli	0.05	0.025	0.03	0.03	0.05
K. pneumoniae	0.05	0.025	0.06	0.06	0.05
K. oxytoca	0.5	0.05	0.06	0.06	0.05
E. cloacae	0.1	0.05	0.25	0.25	0.05
C. freundii	0.05	0.05	0.12	0.06	0.05
P. mirabilis	0.05	0.05	0.015	0.03	0.2
M. morganii	0.05	0.025	0.015	0.015	0.2
P. vulgaris	0.2	0.39	0.12	0.03	0.2
P. rettgeri	0.39	0.12	0.25	0.25	0.05
P. stuartii	0.25		0.06	0.06	0.05
S. marcescens	1.56	0.78	0.12	0.12	0.39
P. aeruginosa	6.25	3.13	2	4	0.78
B. cepacia			8	8	0.78
H. influenzae	0.1	0.05	0.06	0.12	0.1
M. catarrhalis	0.78	0.1	0.12	0.2	0.1
N. gonorrhoeae	0.025	0.025	0.06		
Aeromonas spp.		0.06	0.06	0.06	
Acinetobacter spp.	3.13	1.56		0.2	
Y. enterocolitica	0.12		3.13	0.06	
Alcaligenes spp		6.25	50		12.5
Flavobacterium spp.		25	25		12.5

[a]Data from Nishino et al., 1991.
[b]Data from Watanabe et al., 1992.
[c]Data from Iwahi et al., 1992.

Table 48 Comparative activities of C-3′ quaternary ammonium cephalosporins

Organism(s)	MIC$_{50}$ (µg/ml)						
	FK-518[a]	DQ-2556[b]	ME-1228[c]	CS-461[d]	ME-1220	ME-1221[e]	DN-9550[f]
E. coli	0.1	≤0.05	0.05	≤0.01	0.05	0.05	0.1
K. pneumoniae	0.1	≤0.05	0.025	≤0.01	0.05	0.025	0.1
P. mirabilis	0.2	≤0.05	0.025				0.19
M. morganii		0.19	0.025	0.1	0.05	0.013	
C. freundii	0.39	0.78	0.1				0.39
E. cloacae	3.13	0.39	0.2	≤0.01	0.2	0.2	0.39
S. marcescens	1.56	1.56	0.2	≤0.01	0.78	0.2	0.78
Shigella spp.	0.1						
P. aeruginosa	1.56	6.25	3.13	3.1	12.5	6.25	1.56
B. cepacia	1.56		1.56		6.25	6.25	
Alcaligenes xylosoxidans	3.13						
Alcaligenes faecalis	3.13	12.5					3.13
Acinetobacter spp.	-	-	12.5				

[a]Data from Mine et al., 1990.
[b]Data from Fujimoto et al., 1986.
[c]Data from Tamura et al., 1990.
[d]Data from Nakayama et al., 1991.
[e]Data from Okamoto et al., 1991.
[f]Data from Une et al., 1985.

crossing the periplasmic space without being hydrolyzed, and finally inhibiting the activity of PBP.

Using proteoliposomes, Nikaido et al. (1990) showed that cefpirome, cefepime, and cefclidin penetrate the porin channel of *E. coli* and *E. cloacae* more rapidly than ceftazidime. These molecules have also been shown to possess a high degree of resistance to hydrolysis by type I β-lactamases because of their weak affinity. Like the majority of 2-amino-5-thiazolyl cephalosporins, these molecules bind preferentially to *E. coli* or *P. aeruginosa* PBP 3 with inhibitory activity that varies with the molecule. They are also weak cephalosporinase inducers.

As a rule, the effect of the inoculum size is more moderate than for the conventional 2-amino-5-thiazolyls. However, they share the same weakness as cefotaxime and ceftazidime and are less active against strains producing TEM-3 to -26 and SHV-2 to -8.

Table 49 Comparative activities of C-3′ quaternary ammonium cephalosporins

Organism	MIC$_{50}$ (μg/ml)						
	FK-518	DQ-2556	ME-1228	CS-461[a]	ME-1220	ME-1221	DN-9550
S. aureus Met[s]	12.5	1.56	3.13	0.1	1.56	3.13	1.56
S. pyogenes	0.39	0.013	0.2		0.025	0.05	≤0.05
S. pneumoniae	0.39	0.025					≤0.05
N. gonorrhoeae	0.05	0.05					0.1
N. meningitidis	≤0.025						
M. catarrhalis	0.2		0.05				
H. influenzae	0.2	0.05	0.025		0.013	0.013	0.2

[a]For this drug, MIC rather than MIC$_{50}$ is shown.

Table 50 In vitro activities of C-3′ quaternary ammonium cephems against *S. pneumoniae*[a]

Drug	MIC (μg/ml)					
	Pen[s]		Pen[i]		Pen[r]	
	50%	90%	50%	90%	50%	90%
Cefpirome	0.01	0.03	0.12	0.5	0.5	1
Cefepime	0.03	0.03	0.25	1	1	2
Cefclidin	0.25	0.5	1	4	8	8
Cefozopran	0.03	0.06	0.25	1	2	2
Cefluprenam	0.03	0.03	0.5	1	1	1
Cefoselis	0.03	0.06	0.125	0.5	0.5	1

[a]Data from Geslin et al., 1985, and Appelbaum et al., 1994.

Table 51 Hydrolytic activities of β-lactamases against group IV-2 cephalosporins[a]

Enzyme	MIC$_{50}$ (μg/ml)				
	Cefoselis	Cefepime	Cefpirome	Ceftazidime	Cefclidin
E. coli	≤0.06	≤0.06	0.12	0.25	
CAZ-2	8	8	8	>16	16
HMS-1	≤0.06	≤0.06	0.12	0.25	
SHV-1	1	0.5	0.5	2	
SHV-2	32	16	16	>16	32
SHV-3	8	4	>16	>16	16
SHV-4	4	2	16	>16	32
SHV-5	16	16	16	>16	8
TEM-1	≤0.06	≤0.06	0.12	0.25	
TEM-2	0.25	0.5	0.5	0.5	
TEM-3	16	4	8	>16	8
TEM-4	32	8	8	>16	8
TEM-5	4	2	2	>16	4
TEM-6	4	4	4	>16	8
TEM-7	4	8	8	>16	16
TEM-9	8	8	8	>16	16
OmpF$^+$	0.5	>0.06	0.12	0.12	
OmpF$^-$	≤0.06	≤0.06	0.12	0.25	

[a]Data from Jones, 1992.

2.3.4.7. Plasma Pharmacokinetics

The cephalosporins with a C-3′ quaternary ammonium chain all exhibit the same pharmacokinetic profile: an apparent elimination half-life on the order of 2.0 h, preponderant urinary elimination, and the need for adjustment of the dosage for patients with renal insufficiency.

2.3.4.7.1. Cefpirome. After administration of a single intravenous dose of 0.5 to 2.0 g, the apparent elimination half-life is about 2.0 h. Elimination occurs renally, accounting for about 80 to 85% of the administered product (Table 56). After repeated doses there is no plasma accumulation of cefpirome. After intramuscular administration of 1.0 g, the peak

Table 52 Activities of FK-518 and cefclidin against *P. aeruginosa* strains with different resistance phenotypes[a]

P. aeruginosa[b]	MIC_{50} (μg/ml)			
	FK-518	Cefclidin	Ceftazidime	Imipenem
Susceptible		1.56	0.78	3.13
1.56				
CAZ^{s}	6.25	6.25	50	3.13
CFP^{s}	3.13	3.13	12.5	1.56
IMP^{r}	1.56	3.13	6.25	25
GEN^{r}	3.13	6.25	12.5	1.56
CPZ^{r}/GEN^{r}	3.13	6.25	12.5	1.56
CAZ^{r}/CPZ^{r}/GEN^{r}	6.25	12.5	25	3.13
CAZ^{r}/CPZ^{r}/IMP^{r} GEN^{r}	12.5	12.5	100	25

[a]Data from Mine et al., 1990.
[b]CAZ, ceftazidime; CFP, cefpirome; IMP, imipenem; GEN, gentamicin; CPZ, cefoperazone.

Table 53 In vitro activity of DQ-2556

Organism(s)	MIC (μg/ml)	
	DQ-2522	DQ-2556
S. aureus	1.56	1.56
S. pneumoniae	0.05	0.1
E. coli	0.05	0.05
Enterobacter spp.	12.5	12.5
K. pneumoniae	0.39	0.19
P. aeruginosa	50	25

concentration in serum (mean ± standard deviation) of 23.2 ± 6.2 μg/ml is reached in 2.0 h (Table 57). The bioavailability of cefpirome is greater than 95%.

In patients with renal insufficiency, the apparent elimination half-life is more than 3 h when the creatinine clearance is less than or equal to 30 ml/min (Table 58).

Cefpirome is well distributed in body fluids and tissues (Tables 59 and 60).

2.3.4.7.2. Cefepime. The pharmaceutical formulation for intravenous administration contains L-arginine hydrochloride. After administration of a single dose of 1.0 g by infusion for 30 min, the apparent elimination half-life is on the order of 2.3 h, with urinary elimination of 72% (Table 61). In patients with renal insufficiency, the apparent half-life is greater than 3 h when the creatinine clearance is less than 70 to 80 ml/min (Table 58). Probenecid does not significantly alter the pharmacokinetics of cefepime, which suggests that urinary elimination occurs principally by glomerular filtration. Cefepime is eliminated by hemodialysis, and the apparent elimination half-life, which is on the order of 13.5 h before hemodialysis, returns to normal during the hemodialysis session. After administration of 1.0 or 2.0 g intramuscularly, bioavailability is absolute. Peak concentrations in serum of 29.6 ± 4.4 μg/ml and 57.5 ± 9.5 μg/ml are reached on average in 1.5 h with AUCs of 137 ± 11 μg·h/ml and 262 ± 23 μg·h/ml (Table 62). In elderly subjects, the changes in the pharmacokinetics are related to renal function.

2.3.4.7.3. DQ-2556. After administration of single increasing doses of DQ-2556 (250 to 2,000 mg), the pharmacokinetics are linear. The apparent elimination half-life is on the order of 2 h with urinary elimination of 80 to 85% of the administered dose (Table 61). There is no plasma accumulation after repeated doses. Fecal elimination is below the limit of detection (Nakashima et al., 1993).

2.3.4.7.4. Cefluprenam. The pharmacokinetics are linear between 0.25 and 2.0 g as a single intravenous dose in healthy volunteers. The apparent elimination half-life is on the order of 2.0 h, with 80 to 97.5% elimination in the urine. There is no plasma accumulation after repeated doses (Table 61).

2.3.4.7.5. Cefozopran. After a single dose of 1,000 mg by intravenous infusion for 20 min, the apparent elimination half-life is less than 2.0 h (Müller et al.). Urinary elimination is on the order of 90%. After repeated doses, no plasma accumulation was detected. In patients with renal insufficiency, the apparent elimination half-life becomes greater than 3 h when the creatinine clearance is less than 30 ml/min, requiring a dosage adjustment (Table 61).

2.3.4.7.6. Cefclidin. After administration of 1.0 g of cefclidin intravenously, the apparent elimination half-life is 1.9 h, with an AUC of 168.8 μg·h/ml. Eighty-four percent of the administered dose of cefclidin is eliminated in the urine (Table 61).

2.3.5. Group V: Catechol Cephalosporins

2.3.5.1. Introduction

There has been increasing interest over the past few years in β-lactams with a catechol moiety. The catechol cephalosporins represent an advance. In fact, in addition to the conventional activity against enzymes that allow the constitution of peptidoglycan, these molecules penetrate the bacterial outer membrane using the iron transport system.

2.3.5.2. Transport of Iron within the Bacterium

Iron is an essential element for the growth of microorganisms. The extracellular concentrations required are on the order of 0.4 to 4 μm. In humans, iron binds to proteins with an affinity of between 10^{24} and 10^{32} (transferrin and lactoferrin). For their growth, microorganisms must take up the iron bound to these proteins. They do so either via chelators, known as siderophores, which possess a very high affinity for ferric ions (Fe^{3+}) (K_m, ~10^{24} to 10^{52}), or directly.

Iron is an essential element in the cytochrome respiratory chain and in DNA synthesis. At physiological pH, the ferric ion (Fe^{3+}) (10^{-38} M) is insoluble, and therefore bacteria must develop a system that enables them to acquire extracellular iron.

Table 54 In vitro activities of ICI-194008 and ICI-193428 against gram-positive bacteria and cocci

Organism(s)	MIC$_{50}$ (μg/ml)		
	ICI-194008	ICI-193428	Cefpirome
S. aureus	2	4	1
S. epidermidis	4	4	0.5
S. pyogenes	0.125	0.125	≤0.06
S. agalactiae	0.5	0.25	≤0.06
Streptococcus G, C	0.125–0.5	0.125–0.5	≤0.06
Viridans group streptococci Pen^s	0.5	2	0.06
Viridans group streptococci Pen^r	4–32	4–32	0.5–2
S. pneumoniae Pen^r	>64	>64	8
E. faecalis	>64	>64	16
E. faecium	>64	>64	>64
Enterococcus avium	>64	>64	8
L. monocytogenes	64	64	64

Table 55 In vitro activities of ICI-194008 and ICI-193428 against gram-negative bacteria and cocci

Organism(s)^a	MIC$_{50}$ (μg/ml)		
	ICI-194008	ICI-193428	Cefpirome
E. coli	0.125	≤0.06	≤0.06
K. pneumoniae	0.125	≤0.06	≤0.06
E. cloacae	0.25–2	0.125–2	≤0.06–0.5
C. freundii	0.5–4	0.125–4	≤0.06–1
S. marcescens	0.5–0.5	0.25–0.5	0.125–0.25
P. mirabilis	0.125	≤0.06	0.125
M. morganii	0.5–1	0.125–0.5	≤0.06–0.25
P. aeruginosa	4–8	4–8	4–16
B. cepacia	4–16	2–16	4–16
S. maltophilia	4–16	4–16	>128
Aeromonas spp.	0.5	0.25	≤0.06
Acinetobacter spp.	16	32	4
H. influenzae β$^+$/β$^-$	≤0.06	≤0.06	≤0.06
N. gonorrhoeae β$^+$	≤0.06	≤0.06	≤0.06

^{a}β$^+$, β-lactamase producing; β$^-$, non-β-lactamase producing.

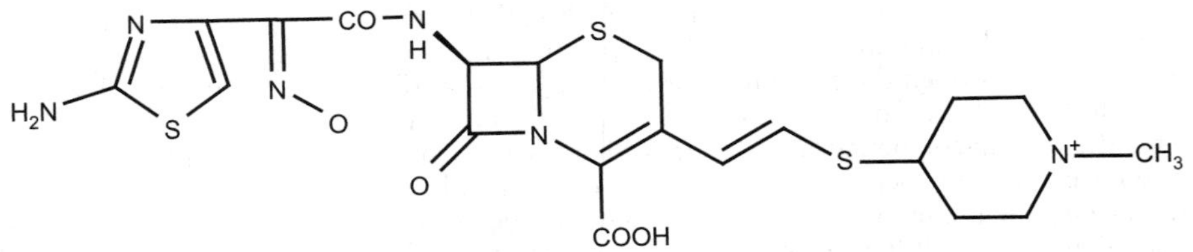

Figure 40 TOC-50

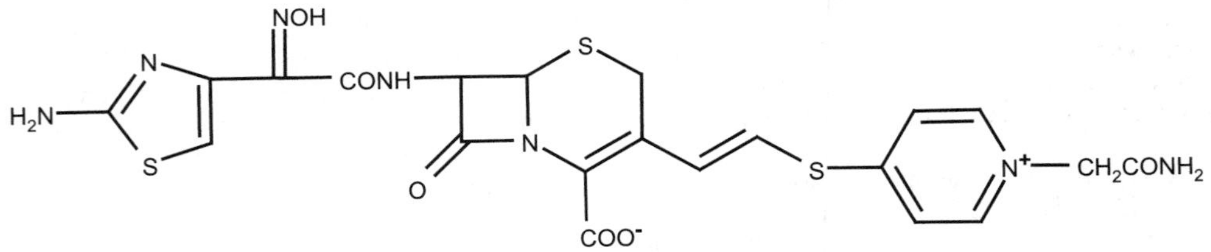

Figure 41 Structure of TOC-39

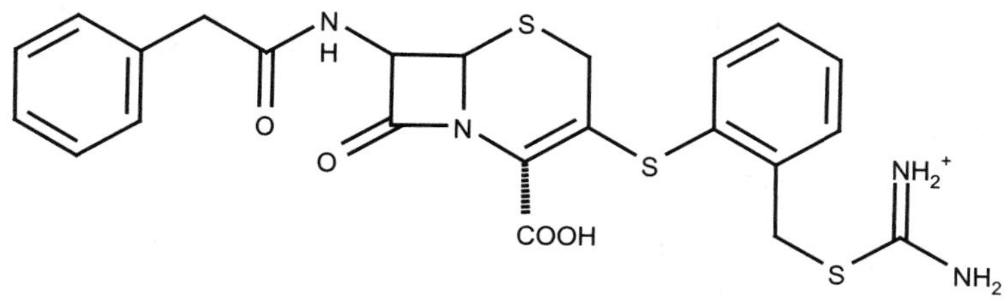

Figure 42 MC-02306

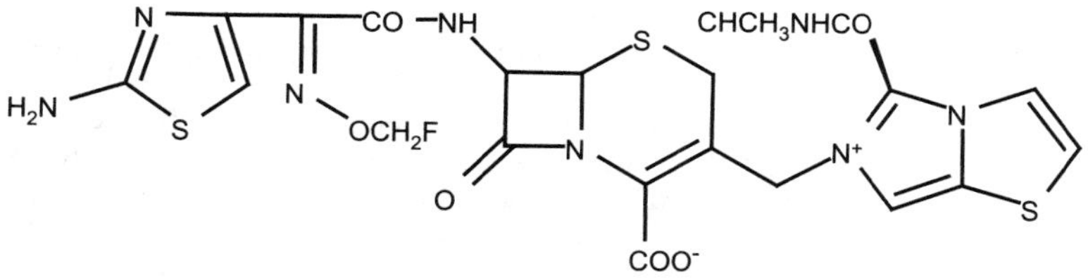

Figure 43 CP-6679

Table 56 Pharmacokinetics in healthy volunteers of cefpirome administered by intravenous route[a]

Dose (mg)	T_{max} (min)	C_{max} (μg/ml)	$t_{1/2\beta}$ (h)	AUC (μg·h/ml)	CL_P (ml/min)	CL_R (ml/min)	Urinary elimination (%)
500	60	57.2 ± 5.6	1.72 ± 0.12	77.8 ± 10.7	109 ± 13	NT[b]	92.3 ± 7.3
1,000	60	86.7 ± 12.9	1.72 ± 0.3	119 ± 20	144 ± 23	NT	80.9 ± 3.4
1,000	5	97.4 ± 28.5	2.3 ± 0.3	156.3 ± 27.8	109.5 ± 20.2	82.1 ± 19.5	75.5 ± 6.9
2,000	60	119 ± 14	1.71 ± 0.14	259 ± 46	133 ± 24	NT	90 ± 5.5
2,000	5	145.7 ± 26.2	2.0 ± 0.3	276 ± 23	121 ± 10	107 ± 10	88

[a]Means ± standard deviations.
[b]NT, not tested.

Table 57 Pharmacokinetics in healthy volunteers of cefpirome administered by intramuscular route[a]

Dose (mg)	C_{max} (μg/ml)	T_{max} (h)	$AUC_{0-\infty}$ (μg·h/ml)	$t_{1/2\beta}$ (h)	Urinary elimination (%)
500	12.2 ± 3.6	1.6 ± 0.6	57 ± 10	2.0 ± 0.2	69
1,000	23.2 ± 11.3	1.9 ± 0.7	116 ± 20	2.0 ± 0.2	75
2,000	43.0 ± 11.3	2.3 ± 1.0	230 ± 33	2.1 ± 0.3	77

[a]Means ± standard deviations.

Table 58 Pharmacokinetics of cefpirome in renally impaired patients

Drug	Dose (g)[a]	$t_{1/2\beta}$ (h) at indicated creatinine clearance (ml/min)[b]			
		>80	30–80	>10–30	<10
Cefpirome	2.0	2.3 ± 0.3	2.6 ± 0.8	9.2 ± 6.6	14.5 ± 5.0
Cefepime	1.0	2.29 ± 0.55	4.89 ± 0.82	10.5 ± 2.96	13.5 ± 2.65
Cefprozan	1.0	115.6 ± 8.8	187.6 ± 45.0	52.3 ± 20.2	109.4 ± 54.3

[a]Given intravenously.
[b]Means ± standard deviations.

A number of studies have shown that the acquisition of iron from the host is a determining factor in the pathogenesis of infection. For example, a large proportion of invasive strains of *E. coli* carry a ColV virulence plasmid on which certain genes enable aerobactin to be synthesized and used. This iron-virulence relationship has also been demonstrated in certain *Vibrio* spp. and in *Neisseria meningitidis*.

In humans, iron is intracellular and complexed to hemoglobin, ferritin, or hemosiderin (storage of intracellular iron) or extracellular, where it is transported by transferrins or lactotransferrins. Bacteria take up iron with or without siderophores.

2.3.5.2.1. Siderophore-independent iron uptake. Certain bacterial species, such as *Neisseria* spp. (*N. meningitidis* and *N. gonorrhoeae*), *H. influenzae*, and *Bordetella* spp., do not produce siderophores; these bacteria chelate iron directly on transport glycoproteins such as transferrin and lactoferrin or from hemin.

2.3.5.2.2. Siderophore-dependent iron uptake. The induction of iron transport in gram-negative bacilli requires the synthesis of siderophores, which are low-molecular-weight iron chelators, and the presence of parietal receptors, which are high-molecular-weight molecules.

2.3.5.3. Siderophores

Bacterial siderophores bind and solubilize iron. They allow iron to be transferred through the bacterial outer membrane. Iron transport is a phenomenon requiring energy (ATP), which is regulated by the *tonB* system. The TonB protein transmits cytoplasmic energy to the parietal receptors, allowing the release of iron from the receptors in the periplasmic region. This *tonB* energy system is regulated by the ExbB and ExbC proteins and probably others also.

The siderophores are of two types: catechols (phenolates) and hydroxamates (Table 63).

Table 59 Cefpirome tissue distribution

Tissue or fluid	Dose (mg)	Mean concn (mg/kg) 2 h	12 h
Prostate	1.0	12.9	1.7
Bronchial mucosa	2.0	33.0	
Blister fluid	1.0	39.2	3.0
Peritoneal fluid	1.0	46.3	10.6
Synovial fluid	1.0	2.8	2.1
Sputum	2.0	2.4	0.5
Myometrium	1.0		
Ovary tissue	1.0		
Fat tissue	1.0		

Table 60 Cefpirome concentrations in cerebral fluid

Fluid	Dose (μg/ml or mg)	Sampling time (h)	Concn in plasma (μg/ml)[a]	Concn in fluid (μg/ml)[a]
Cerebral fluid	2,000	2	61.1 ± 10.5	2.7 ± 0.4
		4	20.5 ± 3.3	4.2 ± 0.8
		8	4.29 ± 0.9	3.6 ± 0.8
		12	3.02 ± 1.0	2.3 ± 1.2
Blister fluid	1,000	2		39.2 ± 7.9

[a]Means ± standard deviations.

Table 61 Pharmacokinetics of C-3′ quaternary ammonium cephalosporins

Product	Dose (μg/ml)	Infusion time (min)	C_o (ml/min)[a,b]	AUC (μg·h/ml)[a]	CL_P (liters/h)[a]	CL_R (liters/h)[a]	$t_{1/2\beta}$ (h)[a]	Urinary elimination (%)[a]	Protein binding (%)
DQ-2556	1,000	5	109 ± 12.4	154 ± 30.5	6.7±1.4	5.7 ± 1.4	1.89 ± 0.42	84.9 ± 3.9	-
	2,000	5	274.2 ± 39.7	285.1 ± 36.1	7.1 ± 0.8	6.1 ± 0.8	1.81 ± 0.19	85.5 ± 1.1	-
Cefluprenam	1,000	60	63.2 ± 4.6	148.3 ± 7.2	6.8 ± 0.3	6.9 ± 0.5	1.87 ± 0.13	90.5 ± 2	
	2,000	60	142.7 ± 5.6	340 ± 39.3	5.9 ± 0.7	5.8 ± 0.7	1.88 ± 0.17	97.5 ± 2	15
Cefclidin	1,000	60	66.1 ± 5.9	168.8 ± 13.3	6 ± 0.5	5 ± 0.4	1.89 ± 0.06	84.3 ± 3.1	≤10
	2,000	60	116.4 ± 21.5	277.1 ± 35	7.3 ± 0.9	6 ± 0.9	1.78 ± 0.11	81.5 ± 5.1	
Cefozopran	1,000	20	176.8 ± 39.9	205.6 ± 20.8	6.8 ± 0.5	5.9 ± 0.5	1.75 ± 0.31	87.7 ± 6	31
Cefepime	1,000	30	63.5 ± 7.8	131 ± 22.8	7.9 ± 0.5	6.6 ± 1.7	2.29 ± 0.55	77.2	16
	2,000	30	132.2 ± 20.8	268 ± 27	7.5 ± 0.7	6.6 ± 0.8	2.07 ± 0.22	85.51	

[a]Means ± standard deviations.
[b]End of infusion.

Table 62 Pharmacokinetics of cefepime administered intramuscularly[a]

Dose (mg)	C_{max} (μg/ml)[b]	T_{max} (h)[b]	$AUC_{0-\infty}$ (μg·h/ml)[b]	$t_{1/2\beta}$ (h)[b]	Urinary elimination (%)[b]
250	7.8 ± 2	1 ± 0.3	33 ± 6	2.35 ± 0.5	65.6
500	13.9 ± 3.4	1.4 ± 0.9	60 ± 8	2.05 ± 0.2	80.8
1,000	29.6 ± 4.4	1.6 ± 0.4	137 ± 11	2.35 ± 0.4	84.6
2,000	57.5 ± 9.5	1.5 ± 0.4	262 ± 23	2.05 ± 0.2	84.6

[a]Data from Barbhaiya et al., 1990.
[b]Means ± standard deviations.

Each microorganism possesses its own system for acquiring iron from the environment.

The transport of iron within the bacterial cell requires the following:

- Receptors on the surface of the bacterial outer membrane
- A control system allowing passage through the outer membrane and the cytoplasmic membrane
- Proteins allowing translocation through the cytoplasmic membrane
- Regulatory proteins found in the periplasmic space
- Export proteins found in the periplasmic space

Different proteins have been identified, together with their functions (Table 64). The nature of the bacterial receptors and the transport mechanism of the siderophores have been studied in particular in *E. coli*.

Enterobactin (Fig. 44) is the prototype siderophore present in the majority of *Enterobacteriaceae*. Enterobactin binds iron through catechol groups and penetrates the bacterial outer membrane in the form of a complex with iron.

The synthesis of enterobactin is governed by numerous chromosomal genes. The penetration of enterobactin is mediated by a transport system under the dependence of the *tonB* gene product, which is bound to the cytoplasmic membrane. The expression of six parietal proteins in *E. coli* K-12, Fiu (83 kDa), FepA, FecA, FhuA, FhiA, and Cir, is coordinated and inversely regulated in response to the body's iron status, as is the production of enterocholine. This regulation is under the dependence of the *fur* locus gene product, with Fe(II) as the aporepressor.

The *fepA* gene codes for a protein parietal receptor, FepA (81 kDa), and *fepB* codes for a permease and four other proteins, FecC, -D, -E, and -G.

The *fes* gene codes for an intracellular esterase which enables ferric iron to be extracted from enterobactin.

Finally, the Fur protein interacts with Fe^{2+} and acts as a repressor of the expression of all of the components of the iron transport system.

Penetration of ferrichrome in *E. coli* requires two genes, *fhuA* and *fhuB*. The FhuA protein is a parietal protein, and FhuB is a cytoplasmic membrane protein.

The products ExbB, FhuC, and FhuD are involved in the use of hydroxamate-type siderophores. FhuE is a parietal receptor for coprogen and ferric rhorodotorulate.

The ferric citrate system is also dependent on the *tonB* and *exbB* genes and on the *fecA* (parietal receptor) and *fecB*, *-C*, *-D*, and *-E* genes, which produce cytoplasmic proteins.

The two parietal proteins Fiu and Cir are also induced in an iron-depleted medium, but their functions have been poorly elucidated.

The *iucABC* genes are responsible for the synthesis of aerobactin, whereas the *iutA* and *iutB* genes code for a parietal receptor and a transport protein. These systems are under the dependence of the *tonB*, *exbB*, and *fhuCDB* genes (Fig. 45).

Table 63 Principal siderophores

Siderophore	Organism
Phenolates (catechols)	
Enterocholin (enterobactin)	*E. coli*
	Salmonella
	Shigella
	Klebsiella
	Enterobacter
Vibriobactin	*Vibrio cholerae*
Agrobactin	*Acinetobacter tumefaciens*
Anguibactin	*Vibrio anguillarum*
Pyochelin	*P. aeruginosa*
Parabactin	*Paracoccus denitrificans*
Hydroxamates	
Aerobactin	*E. coli*
	Klebsiella
	Shigella
	Enterobacter
	Salmonella
	Yersinia intermedia
	Yersinia frederiksenii
	Proteus
	Serratia
	Yersinia kristensenii
Arthrobactin	*Arthrobacter*
Mycobactin	*Mycobacterium*
Pyoverdin	*P. aeruginosa*
Schizokin	*Bacillus megaterium*
Ferrichrome	Yeast

Table 64 Siderophore proteins

Gene	Protein	Molecular mass (kDa)	Transfer/function
fhuA	FhuA	78	Ferrichrome
fhuE	FhuE	76	Coprogen, rhodotorulic acid
iut	Iut		Aerobactin
fecA	FecA	80.5	Dicitrate ferric
fepA	FepA	81	Enterocholin
fui	Fui	83	Dihydroxylbenzoylserine
cir	Cir	74	Dihydrobenzoylserine
feuA	FeuA	74	Enterocholin
feuB	FeuB	81	Colicin B
btuB	BtuB		Vitamin B_{12}—colicin E1
tonB	TonB	36	Regulation
fur	Fur		Regulation

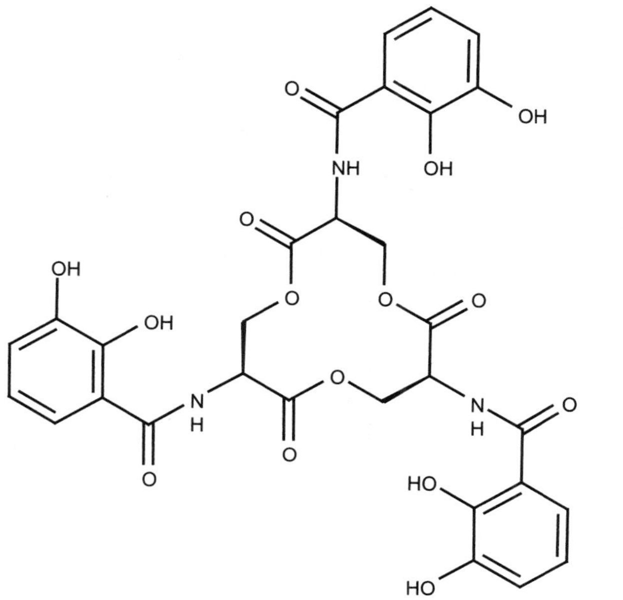

Figure 44 Enterobactin

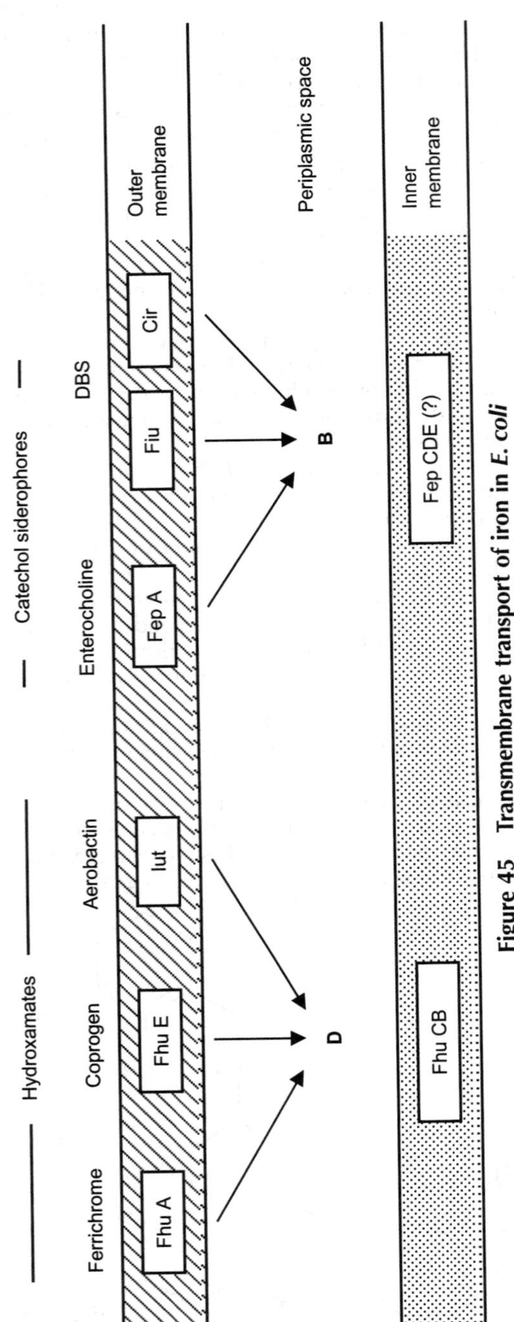

Figure 45 Transmembrane transport of iron in *E. coli*

2.3.5.4. Cephalosporins and Iron Transport

Kaduragamura et al. were among the first to show that subinhibitory concentrations of cefotaxime and ceftriaxone significantly reduce the production of bacterial enterocholine in an iron-depleted medium but do not affect bacterial growth.

The first known anti-infective agents that interacted with the iron transport system were the sulfonamides, which bind covalently to ferrioxamine B, a siderophore similar to ferrichrome.

Watanabe et al. were the first to show that the catechol groups present on a cephalosporin, E-0702, allowed transparietal passage by means of iron transporters dependent on the *tonB* regulation system. This discovery was the origin of a number of studies in this field and the synthesis of numerous molecules with a catechol moiety.

This mechanism of action has been clearly demonstrated using iron transporter mutants. Harris (1993) showed that the presence of a catechol moiety at position 3 or 7 of the cephem moiety did not modify the mode of penetration (Table 65).

The catechol-type cephalosporins mimic the catechol groups present on the siderophores, whether these are in a linear or a cyclic form. Among the catechol-type siderophore transport proteins, the Fiu and Cir proteins were identified by Hantke as being involved in the recognition and transport of the hydroxybenzylserines (such as enterobactin, which is a trimer of 2,3-dihydroxybenzylserine). The catechol-type cephalosporins appear to use this route (Nikaido et al., 1990). In fact, when the two Cir and Fiu proteins are absent, the activity of the molecules decreases by a factor of 1,000. KP-736 is a pyridone-type molecule and uses this route (Tatsumi et al., 1995).

This mechanism of transport of cephems within the bacterial cell increases the periplasmic concentration of the antibiotic. The presence of dipyridyl in the culture medium (iron depletion) does not affect bacterial growth, but in the presence of catechol-type cephalosporins it substantially increases the bactericidal activity of these molecules.

cir fiu mutants have been identified. However, because of the fact that a microorganism possesses several pathways for acquiring iron, the activity of the catechol cephems is slower than in wild-type strains. In addition, this type of mutant is probably nonvirulent and these cephems will continue to use the porin route for their intrabacterial penetration.

2.3.5.5. Antibacterial Activity

A distinction can be drawn between the molecules containing a catechol moiety and those containing a pyridone

Table 65 Activity of GR-69153 against mutant strains (iron transport) of *E. coli*

Genotype	MIC (μg/ml)	
	C-7 catechol GR-69153	Ceftazidime
Wild	<0.008	0.25
ftuA	0.015	0.25
ftuE	0.015	0.25
fecA	<0.008	0.12
fepA	<0.008	0.12
fiu	0.03	0.25
cir	0.015	0.25
cir fiu	0.12	0.25
fur	<0.008	0.12
tonB	0.12	0.12

moiety. Two types of catechol cephalosporin molecules have been synthesized: those possessing a catechol moiety at position 3 and those whose catechol nuclei are at the 7 position of the cephem moiety (Fig. 46).

2.3.5.6. Group V-1A: Cephems with Catechol Moiety at Position 3

Two molecules have been synthesized and studied, BO-1236 (L-658310) and BO-1341 (Fig. 47). The two molecules are intermediates between the C-3′ quaternary ammonium and catechol-type molecules. They have an alkyloxime group at position 7 and a methyl-6,7-dihydroxyisoquinolinium (BO-1341) or *N*-methyl-5-6-dihydroxyisoindolinium (BO-1236) moiety. These two molecules are relatively inactive against gram-positive cocci (Table 66). BO-1236 is more active than BO-1341 against *Enterobacteriaceae*, and in fact the latter possesses bimodal activity against type I β-lactamase-producing strains, such as *E. cloacae* ($MIC_{50/90}$, 0.39/0.25 μg/ml), *C. freundii* ($MIC_{50/90}$, 0.05/25 μg/ml), and *M. morganii* ($MIC_{50/90}$, 0.2/6.25 μg/ml). These two molecules are active in vitro against ceftazidime-resistant strains of *P. aeruginosa* (Table 67). It has been shown that BO-1341 is active against strains of *P. aeruginosa* resistant to ceftazidime (MIC, ~0.8 μg/ml), cefoperazone (MIC, ~0.1 μg/ml), cefsulodin (MIC, ~0.1 μg/ml), imipenem (MIC, ~0.03 μg/ml), and carumonam (MIC, ~0.3 μg/ml).

Another series of derivatives with a catechol moiety at position 3 has also been synthesized (Jung, 1989). These molecules possess good activity against *P. aeruginosa* but weak activity against *S. aureus*.

Imae et al. (1990) synthesized a series of molecules with a broad antibacterial spectrum, including *S. aureus*, and having an unsaturated chain (propenyl) at C-3, the (*E*)-isomer being more active than the (*Z*)-isomer.

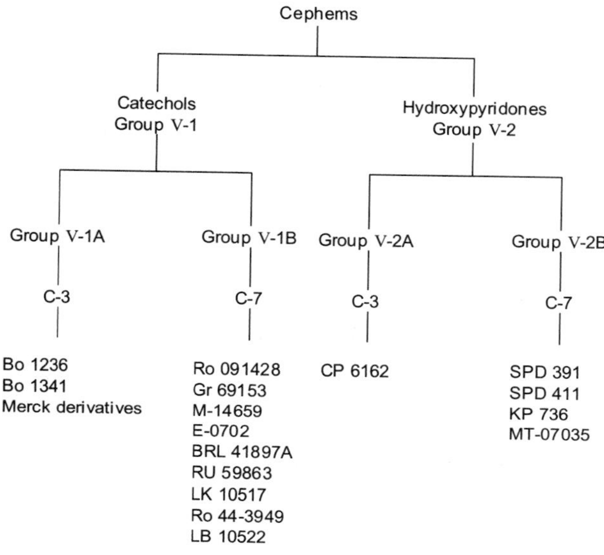

Figure 46 Group V cephalosporins

2.3.5.7. Group V-1B: Cephems with Catechol Moiety at Position 7

The first molecule to have been synthesized was E-0702 (Fig. 48), which exhibits excellent activity against *Enterobacteriaceae*, *P. aeruginosa*, and *Acinetobacter* but weak activity against gram-positive cocci. This molecule possesses a thiocarboxymethyltetrazole at the C-3 position of the cephem moiety. Intermediate molecules have been synthesized and exhibit moderate global activity: M-14648 and M-14646. Several molecules have been synthesized: Ro-09-1227, Ro-09-1428, M-14659, and GR-69153 (cefetecol).

The first three molecules possess a 5-methyltriazolopyrimidine moiety at position 3, substituted by either a carbonyl group (M-14659 and Ro-09-1227) or a hydroxymethyl

Figure 47 Group V-1A cephalosporins

Table 66 In vitro activities of catechol cephems

Organism(s)	MIC$_{50}$ (μg/ml)						
	GR-69153	Ro-09-1428	Ro-09-1227	BO-1236	BO-1341	M-14659	E-0702
S. aureus Met^{s}	4	8	4	25	50	0.78	4
S. aureus Met^{r}	>64	8	>32				
CNS Met[a]	1	2	>32	25	50		8
CNS Met^{r}		16	>32				
S. pyogenes	0.12	0.12	0.25	0.78	1.56		
S. agalactiae	0.5	0.25	0.5		1		
Group C, F, and G streptococci	0.12	0.25	2				
S. pneumoniae Pen^{s}	0.12	0.12	0.25	0.39	1.56		
S. pneumoniae Pen^{r}	1	0.39					
E. faecalis	>32	64	>32	>128	>128	>32	
L. monocytogenes	>32	>64					
E. faecium	>32		>32			>32	
C. jeikeium	>32						
Bacillus cereus			32				
Viridans group streptococci	1						
B. subtilis						12.5	

[a]CNS, coagulase-negative staphylococci.

Table 67 Activity of BO-1236 against nonfermenting gram-negative bacilli

Organism(s)	MIC (μg/ml)			
	BO-1236		Ceftazidime	
	50%	90%	50%	90%
P. aeruginosa CAZ^{s}	0.025	0.2	0.78	1.56
P. aeruginosa CAZ^{r}	0.78	0.78	25	50
B. cepacia	0.1	1.56	1.56	>100
S. maltophilia	0.006	12.5	0.78	>100
Acinetobacter spp.	0.1	0.39	3.12	12.5

[a]CAZ, ceftazidime.

group (Ro-09-1428). GR-69153 does not have a substituent at position 3, like ceftizoxime (Fig. 49).

The molecules possess moderate activity against gram-positive cocci, but this is very inferior to that of cefpirome (Table 68). GR-69153 possesses the same activity as ceftazidime against streptococci. The difference is found in its activity against penicillin G-resistant strains of *S. pneumoniae* (MIC$_{50}$, ~1.0 μg/ml; MIC$_{90}$, ~4.0 μg/ml). The molecules are inactive against *Enterococcus* spp., *L. monocytogenes*, and *Corynebacterium jeikeium*.

GR-69153 exhibits bimodal activity against BRO-1-producing strains of *M. catarrhalis* and *C. freundii*, *E. cloacae*, and *M. morganii*. The same phenomenon was demonstrated with Ro-09-1428 and Ro-09-1227 (Table 69).

The global activity of these molecules against *Enterobacteriaceae* is less good than that of cefpirome or cefotaxime (Table 68).

Likewise, the activity against *H. influenzae* and *M. catarrhalis* is weaker than that of cefotaxime (Table 70).

The activity of GR-69153 against *P. aeruginosa* is better than that of ceftazidime and similar to that of cefclidin. For the other molecules, the activity is practically identical to that of ceftazidime (Table 71).

Recently, a new series of cephalosporins containing a catechol moiety has been described (Aszodi et al., 1993, 1994). One molecule, RU-59863 (Fig. 50), possesses an evenly balanced spectrum of gram-positive cocci, including penicillin G-resistant strains of *S. pneumoniae*, and gram-negative bacilli. In vitro, it is active against numerous strains of extended-spectrum-β-lactamase-producing *Enterobacteriaceae* (of the TEM or SHV type) and against ceftazidime- and imipenem-resistant strains of *P. aeruginosa* (le Noc et al., 1995) (Tables 72 and 73).

A derivative with two catechol nuclei, one at C-3 and the other at C-7, has been described: Ro-44-3949 (Fig. 51). This molecule is moderately active. LB-10522 (Fig. 52) is a new derivative with activity inferior to that of cefpirome.

2.3.5.7.1. Factors affecting in vitro activity. The activity of GR-69153 is not affected by an increase in size of the bacterial inoculum between 10^3 and 10^5 CFU per spot, but above 10^6 CFU/spot it increases moderately against type I or IV β-lactamase-producing *Enterobacteriaceae*, and the MICs increase substantially when the inoculum is 10^6 CFU/spot (Table 74).

The presence of 5% sheep blood in the agar medium increases the activity of GR-69153 twofold. A reduction in pH to below 6 reduces the activity two- to fourfold. An increase in the Mg^{2+} content of the culture medium does not affect the antibacterial activity, nor does incubation in an anaerobic medium. The presence of 2,2′-dipyridyl, which depletes the medium of iron (≤5 μg/dl), does not modify the MIC of GR-69153, but the addition of iron (60 to 240 μg/dl instead of 25 to 30 μg/dl) causes an increase in the MIC.

2.3.5.7.2. Interaction with β-lactamases. These molecules are stable against hydrolysis by TEM-1-, TEM-2-, and SHV-1-type enzymes. They appear to be much less stable against hydrolysis by the *M. catarrhalis* enzyme (BRO-1). They are relatively unstable against enzymes of the SHV-4 and SHV-5 types. Stability against hydrolysis by CAZ-2 varies with the molecule. GR-69153 appears to be less stable than Ro-09-1227. These molecules are slightly hydrolyzed by TEM-3-type enzymes. The currently available molecules

R1—CH—CH—N(H)— ; NH—CO—R2 ; S ; N ; O ; R2 ; R3

Generic	R_1	R_2	R_3
E-0702	HO—	HO, HO, O, O	N—N, N, N, S, N, CH_2COOH
MT 0703	N, H_2N, S	OH, N, OH	—S—, N^+—CH_2CH_2OH

Figure 48 Catechol cephalosporins of the 7-*N*-acyl type: group V-1B

H_2N, N, S, CO—N(H), N, O—R_1, S, N, O, COOH, R_2

	R_1	R_2
Gr 69153	HO, HO, *(S), COOH	H
Ro 09-1428	HO, HO, CO-NH-NH, O	R_3, N, N, N, —S—, N; CH_2OH
Ro 09-1227		R_3=COOH
M 14659	HO, HO, *(S), COOH	COOH, N, N, N, —S—, N, CH_3
LK 10517	HO, HO, (S), COOH	H_2N, NH_2, N^+, N

Figure 49 Group V: cephalosporins containing a catechol moiety

Table 68 **In vitro activities of catechol cephalosporins against *Enterobacteriaceae***

Organism(s)	MIC$_{50}$ (μg/ml)						
	GR-69153	Ro-09-1428	Ro-09-1227	BO-1236	BO-1341	M-14656[a]	E-0702
E. coli	0.12	0.06	0.5	0.01	0.01	0.2	0.01
K. pneumoniae	0.06	0.12	0.5	0.02	<0.06	<0.05	0.02
K. oxytoca	0.06	0.25	0.12	0.25			
E. cloacae	0.5	4	16	0.2	0.39		0.3
C. freundii	0.25	1	16	0.1	0.05	0.78	0.008
P. mirabilis	0.03	0.5	<0.06	0.1	0.01	<0.05	0.05
M. morganii	0.5	2	2	0.2	0.2	0.39	0.1
P. stuartii		0.25	2	0.25			
Salmonella spp.	0.06	<0.03	<0.06	0.06		<0.05	0.001
Shigella spp.	0.06	0.06	1	0.25			
Yersinia enterocolitica	0.25	0.25	0.25				
S. marcescens	0.5	0.5	1	0.39	0.2	0.05	0.06

[a]GR-63116.

Table 69 **Activities of catechol cephalosporins against *Enterobacteriaceae***

Organism	MIC (μg/ml)					
	GR-69153[a]		Ro-09-1227[b]		Ro-09-1428[c]	
	50%	90%	50%	90%	50%	90%
C. freundii	1	>32	0.25	16	1	32
E. cloacae	0.25	>32	1	16	4	32
M. morganii	0.5	8	1	2	2	8

[a]Data from Chin et al., 1991.
[b]Data from Jones et al., 1992.
[c]Data from Chin et al., 1991.

Table 70 **In vitro activities of catechol cephalosporins**

Organism	MIC$_{50}$ (μg/ml)						
	Gr-69153	Ro-09-1428	Ro-09-1227	BO-1236	BO-1341	M-14656[a]	E-0702
H. influenzae	0.12	0.5	0.5	0.39	0.1		
M. catarrhalis	0.5	0.5	0.5	0.02	0.2		
N. gonorrhoeae		<0.06	0.015	<0.06			0.1
N. meningitidis							

[a]GR-63116.

Table 71 **In vitro activities of catechol cephalosporins against nonfermenting gram-negative bacilli**

Organism(s)	MIC$_{50}$ (μg/ml)						
	GR-69153	Ro-09-1428	Ro-09-1227	BO-1236	BO-1341	M-14656[a]	E-0702
P. aeruginosa	0.12	0.25	4	0.02	0.2	1.56	0.1
B. cepacia		8		0.006	0.05		1.26
A. baumannii	4	16		0.1	0.39	6.25	0.3
S. maltophilia	4	>64	2	3.12	1.56		0.39
Aeromonas spp.	0.5	4					
Campylobacter jejuni	0.5						
C. meningosepticum						>128	
Alcaligenes spp.				0.1			

[a]GR-63116.

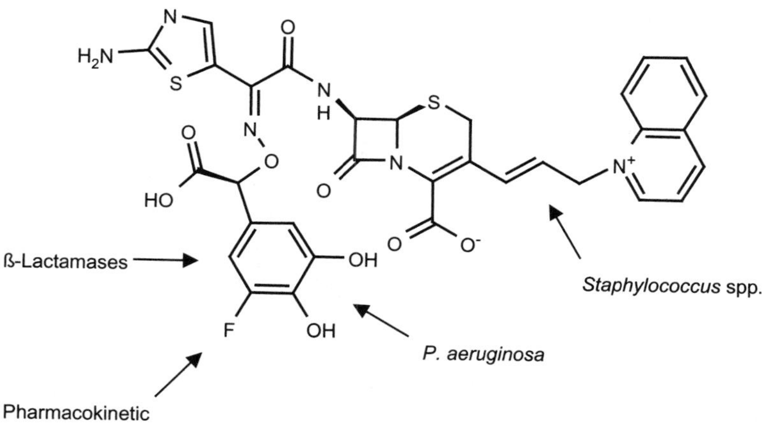

Figure 50 RU-59863 (data from Aszodi et al.)

Table 72 In vitro activity of RU-59863 against gram-negative bacteria[a]

Organism phenotype	MIC$_{50}$ (μg/ml)			
	RU-59863	Ceftazidime	Cefepime	Cefpirome
Enterobacteria				
Susceptible	0.06	0.1	0.06	0.06
Low-level penicillinases	0.06	0.12	0.06	0.06
High-level penicillinase	0.06	0.14	0.08	0.06
High-level cephalosporinases	0.06	0.18	0.06	0.06
Low-level cephalosporinase + high-level penicillinase	0.08	0.4	0.15	0.12
Overexpressed cephalosporinases	0.35	40	0.64	0.84
ESBL[b]	0.23	11	1.2	1.4
P. aeruginosa				
TIC^s CAZ^s IMP[c]	0.58	1.5	2	3.5
TIC^r CAZ^s IMP^s	0.78	2.6	7	8.9
TIC^r CAZ^r IMP^s	0.6	15	10.5	22
TIC^r CAZ^r IMP^r	2.8	23	14	26

[a]Data from Le Noc et al., 1995.
[b]ESBL, extended-spectrum β-lactamase.
[c]TIC, ticarcillin; CAZ, ceftazidime; IMP, imipenem.

Table 73 In vitro activity of RU-59863 against gram-positive cocci

Organism(s)	MIC$_{50}$ (μg/ml)		
	RU-59863	Cefpirome	Cefotaxime
S. aureus Met^s	1.2	1.2	2
S. pneumoniae Pen^s	0.02	0.01	0.03
S. pneumoniae Pen^i	0.3	0.12	0.25
S. pneumoniae Pen^r	0.6	0.5	1
S. pyogenes	0.005	0.015	0.005
S. agalactiae		0.015	0.025
Enterococcus spp.		4	>32

are all hydrolyzed by TEM-9-type enzymes. The TEM-7 enzyme hydrolyzes Ro-09-1428 but the other molecules only very slightly, and likewise the TEM-5 enzyme hydrolyzes Ro-09-1227 and GR-69153 but Ro-09-1428 only slightly (Table 75).

GR-69153 is stable against hydrolysis by TEM-1 produced by *H. influenzae* and *N. gonorrhoeae*, but perhaps slightly less against the BRO-1 enzyme of *M. catarrhalis* (Table 76).

2.3.5.7.3. Pharmacokinetics. The only molecule for which the pharmacokinetics have been studied is GR-69153. This molecule has a long apparent elimination half-life, more than 3 h. It is 70% plasma protein bound (concentrations between 5 and 60 μg/ml). It is eliminated by glomerular filtration and is metabolized hepatically to an active methyl metabolite.

The apparent elimination half-life of the metabolite is on the order of 3.5 h and represents 1 to 2% of the concentration of the parent molecule in plasma. These pharmacokinetic characteristics are summarized in Table 77.

2.3.5.7.3.1. *N*-Acylcephem derivatives. *N*-Acyl-cephalosporin-type molecules or cephamycins have been synthesized with a catechol moiety at position 7 (Ohi et al., 1987).

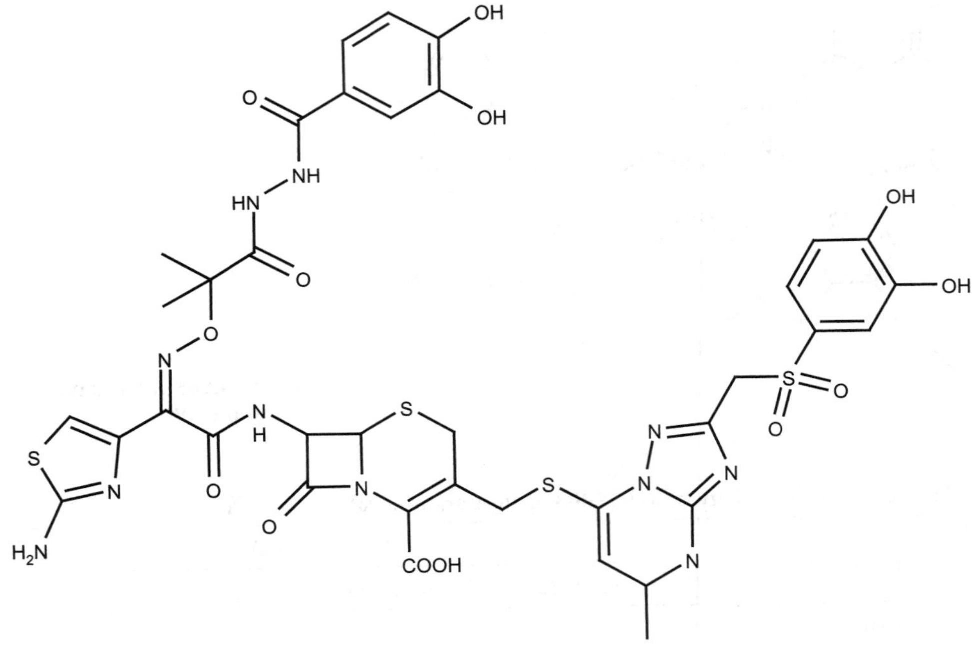

Figure 51 Ro-44-3949

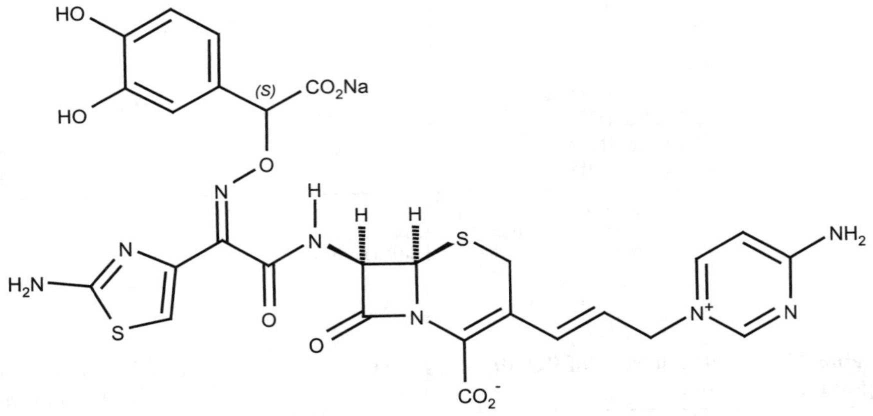

Figure 52 LB-10522

Table 74 Effect of inoculum size on GR-69153 activity[a]

Bacterial species	Enzyme	MIC (μg/ml) with inoculum (CFU/spot)	
		10^5	10^6
E. aerogenes	Ia	8	>8
E. cloacae	Ia (P99)	8	>8
M. morganii	I	0.12	8
P. stuartii	I	0.03	>8
S. liquefaciens	I	0.5	>8
K. oxytoca	IVc (K14)	0.25	8
	IVc (K1)	0.12	>8

[a]Data from Erwin et al., 1991.

Two molecules have good activity against *S. aureus* 209 P JC-I (MIC, ~0.78 μg/ml) and *P. aeruginosa* (MIC, ~0.78 μg/ml), with more moderate activity against *S. marcescens* and *M. morganii* (Fig. 53).

Separate from these, a molecule of the 7α-formamide-cephem type with a catechol and a dioxopiperazine moiety (BRL-41897A ([Fig. 54]) has been described by Basker et al. (1989).

2.3.5.7.3.2. BRL-41897A. It has been shown, by comparison with the derivative BRL-42948A without a catechol moiety, that the iron content of the medium affects the antibacterial activity of the catechol derivative but does not modify β-lactamase production. Likewise, *E. coli* mutants

Table 75 Activities of catechol cephalosporins against *E. coli* 600 containing different enzymes

Enzyme	MIC (μg/ml)			
	Ro-09-1227	Ceftazidime	GR-69153	Ro-09-1428
CAZ-2	2	>16	8	
SHV-1	0.12	1	0.03	0.25
SHV-2	1	>16	0.5	
SHV-3	1	>16	1	
SHV-4	32	>16	32	
SHV-5	>32	>16	4	
TEM-1	<0.06	0.25	0.12	0.015
TEM-2	0.12	0.5	0.3	0.015
TEM-3	1	>16	1	2
TEM-4	1	>16	0.5	
TEM-5	4	>16	16	0.25
TEM-6	8	>16	4	
TEM-7	1	>16	0.5	16
TEM-9	8	>16	8	>64

Table 76 In vitro activity of GR-69153

Organism phenotype	MIC (μg/ml)	
	50%	90%
H. influenzae		
β-lactamase Amp[s]	0.03	0.06
β-lactamase Amp[r]	0.25	0.05
β-lactamase + Amp[r]	0.03	0.03
M. catarrhalis		
β-Lactamase Amp[s]	0.03	0.25
BRO-1	0.12	0.5
BRO-2	0.03	0.06
N. gonorrhoeae		
β-Lactamase$^-$	0.015	0.03
β-Lactamase$^+$	0.03	0.06

have revealed that the route of penetration is subject to the *tonB*, *fiu*, *cir*, and *fluA* (ferrichrome) system (Table 78). This molecule exhibits little activity against gram-positive cocci but appears to be more active against *P aeruginosa*.

2.3.5.8. Group V-2

Other molecules have a pyridone moiety, and preliminary results have been published. These include FK-736, SPD 391, SPD 411, and CP-6162 (Fig. 55).

2.3.5.8.1. Group V-2A: C-7-pyridone derivatives. Several molecules have been described: SPD 391, SPD 411, FK-376, and MT-07035.

A series of derivatives with a 3-isoxazolidinyl moiety at position 3 has been synthesized (Ikeda et al., 1990). These molecules are inactive against MSSA strains and possess activity identical to that of ceftazidime against *Enterobacteriaceae*. Both appear to be more active against *P. aeruginosa* (Table 79).

There is a center of asymmetry at position 3′ of the oxazole moiety. The molecules with an *S* configuration are more active than those with an *R* configuration.

KP-736 is inactive against *S. aureus* and moderately active against streptococci. Its activity against *Enterobacteriaceae* is moderate compared to that of cefotaxime.

MT-07035 is a pyridone derivative which has mediocre activity against MSSA, good activity against *Enterobacteriaceae*, and bimodal activity against *S. marcescens* and *C. freundii*. It is active against ceftazidime-resistant strains of *P. aeruginosa*. The molecule has a center of asymmetry, and only the (*S*)-isomer is active.

2.3.5.8.2. Group V-2B: C-3-pyridone derivatives. A series of derivatives have been synthesized by Shibahara et al. (1989), including CP-6162. This molecule is inactive against MSSA and moderately active against streptococci. Its activity against *Enterobacteriaceae* is identical to that of ceftazidime. The in vitro activity of CP-6162 is not bimodal against strains of *M. morganii*, *E. cloacae*, *C. freundii*, or

Table 77 Pharmacokinetics of cefetecol (GR-69153)[a]

Dose (mg)	*n*	C_{max} (μg/ml)	$AUC_{0-\infty}$ (μg·h/ml)	$t_{1/2}$ (h)	Cl_P (ml/min)	Urinary elimination (%)	
						Cefetecol	Metabolite
125	3	16.9	31		67.2	50.1	3.4
250	6	31.3	56.8	3.7	43.4	51.8	3.3
500	5	71.3	113.7	3.6	43.3	50.6	3
1,000	5	123.9	212.7	2.9	78.3	52.2	3.4
2,000	6	259.5	486.6	3.5	68.6	55.2	4.9

[a]Data from MacKay et al., 1989.

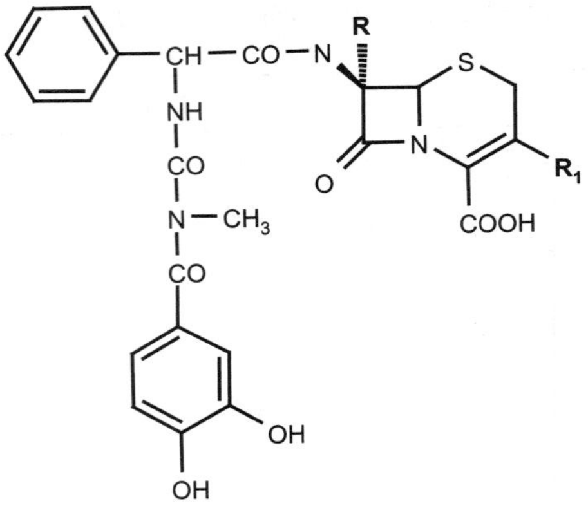

Compound	R	R_1	*S. aureus* 209P	*M. morganii* JU241	*S. marcescens* FU-104	*P. aeruginosa* PS-6
A	H	OAc	0.78	3.13	1.56	0.78
B	OCH_3	MTT*	1.56	0.78	0.39	0.78

MTT*, thiomethyltetrazole

Figure 53 *N*-Acyl cephems

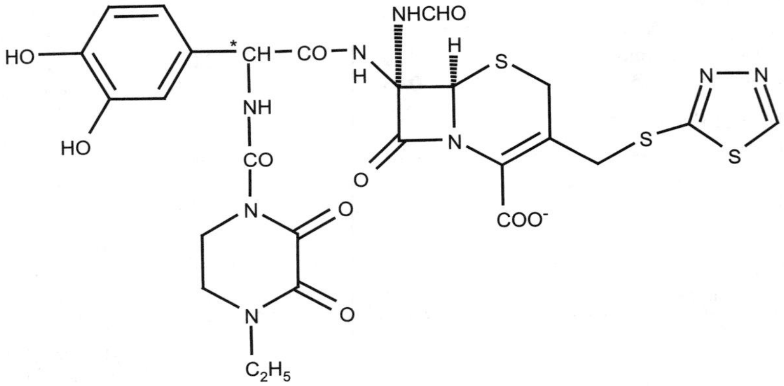

Figure 54 BRL-41897A (C-7-α-formamidinocatechol-cephem)

Table 78 In vitro activity of BRL-4298

Organism	MIC (μg/ml)					
	BRL-41897A		BRL-42948A		Ceftazidime	
	Fe^-	Fe^+	Fe^-	Fe^+	Fe^-	Fe^+
E. coli NCTC 10418	0.008	0.12	0.12	0.12	0.12	0.12
K. pneumoniae T 767	0.015	0.12	0.25	0.12	0.12	0.12
E. cloacae N1	0.06	0.5	0.25	0.5	0.25	0.5
P. mirabilis 977	0.5	0.5	0.5	0.5	0.12	0.12
P. stuartii Agnetti	2	2	2	2	0.5	0.25
S. marcescens US20	0.06	1	0.5	0.5	0.25	0.25
P. aeruginosa NCTC 10662	0.06	2	4	4	2	2
S. aureus Oxford	4	8	4	4	8	8
S. pyogenes CN10	0.5	0.5	0.25	0.5	0.12	0.2

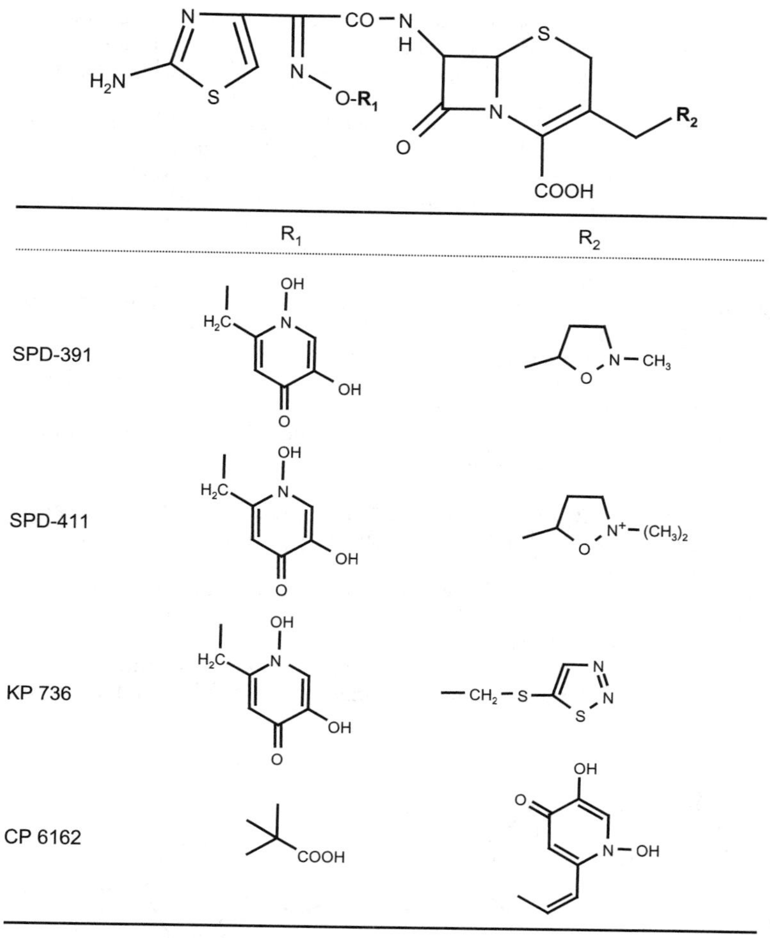

	R_1	R_2
SPD-391		
SPD-411		
KP 736		
CP 6162		

Figure 55 Cephalosporins of the pyridone type, group V2B

Table 79 In vitro activities of pyridone derivatives

Organism(s)	MIC$_{50}$ (μg/ml)				
	KP-736	SPD 391[a]	SPD 411[a]	CP-6162	MT-07035
S. aureus	25	25	12.5	>100	6.25
S. pyogenes	0.2				
S. pneumoniae	0.39			3.13	
E. coli	0.01	0.1	0.2	0.02	0.01
K. pneumoniae	0.01	0.003	0.02	0.01	<0.06
S. marcescens	0.05	0.1	0.1	0.01	0.78
M. morganii	0.01	0.02	0.1	<0.025	
C. freundii	0.02	>100	50	0.025	0.025
E. cloacae	0.39	0.05	0.05	0.39	0.2
P. mirabilis	0.01	0.05	0.2	<0.025	
Salmonella spp.	0.01	0.01	0.01		
P. aeruginosa	0.39	0.1	0.2	0.1	0.1
B. cepacia	0.02			<0.025	
H. influenzae	0.1			0.1	
S. maltophilia	1.56			1.56	
Acinetobacter spp.	0.78			0.39	

[a]For this drug, MIC rather than MIC$_{50}$ is given.

S. marcescens, with good $MIC_{50/90}$ activity (0.20/0.20 μg/ml). CP-6162 is active against ceftazidime-resistant strains of *P. aeruginosa* ($MIC_{50/90}$, 0.20/3.13 μg/ml).

There is a marked inoculum effect at 10^8 CFU/ml against type I β-lactamase-producing strains.

The addition of α-α′-dipyridyl does not modify its activity, as opposed to the addition of $FeCl_3$.

2.3.6. Group VI: Cefsulodin and Anti-MRSA

2.3.6.1. Cefsulodin

There is only one molecule in group VI: cefsulodin. It is original in its antibacterial spectrum, which covers *P. aeruginosa* (Bryskier, 1983), and the fact that chemically it is the only molecule that is substituted by an α-sulfo group at C-7 and by a quaternary ammonium (pyridinium) at C-3 (Fig. 56).

2.3.6.2. Anti-MRSA

At 0.25 to 0.5 μg/ml, a drop in in vitro activity against MRSA ($MIC_{50/90}$, 4.0/4.0 μg/ml), *Staphylococcus haemolyticus* ($MIC_{50/90}$, 8.0/8.0 μg/ml), and *Staphylococcus hominis* (MIC, 1 to 8 μg/ml) was noted. MICs are two- to fourfold higher against *S. aureus* isolates producing β-lactamases. Group VI cephems also include cephems acting against MRSA and *H. pylori* and exhibiting β-lactamase-inhibitory activity (see respective chapters).

In a continuous effort to synthesize new cephem derivatives active against MRSA and vancomycin-resistant enterococci (VRE), new series of compounds have been reported since the last decade, such as RWJ-54428.

The quest for a β-lactam that exhibits MRSA PBP 2a has been conducted for several years. The genetic determinant of MRSA is the gene *mecA*, which is 30 to 50 kb of foreign DNA. The gene *mecA* encodes PBP 2a, which has a low affinity for β-lactam antibiotics (see chapter 5).

In *E. faecium* isolates resistant to vancomycin and ampicillin, the high-level resistance is mediated by overproduction of some PBP and a decrease in the affinity for these enzymes by β-lactam antibiotics. In 1982, penicillinase genes were first reported to be present in *E. faecalis*.

For *S. aureus* β-lactamase which hydrolyzes penicillin G, four immunotypic variants—A, B, C, and D—have been identified and characterized. These β-lactamases are inhibited by clavulanic acid.

2.3.6.2.1. RWJ-54428 (MC-02,479). The antibacterial activity of RWJ-54428 (Fig. 57) is reported in Table 80.

RWJ-54428 was designed to overcome methicillin resistance in MRSA and ampicillin resistance in *E. faecium* by PBP alterations.

MIC_{50}s for MRSA range between 1.0 and 2.0 μg/ml and those for MSSA range between 0.125 and 0.5 μg/ml

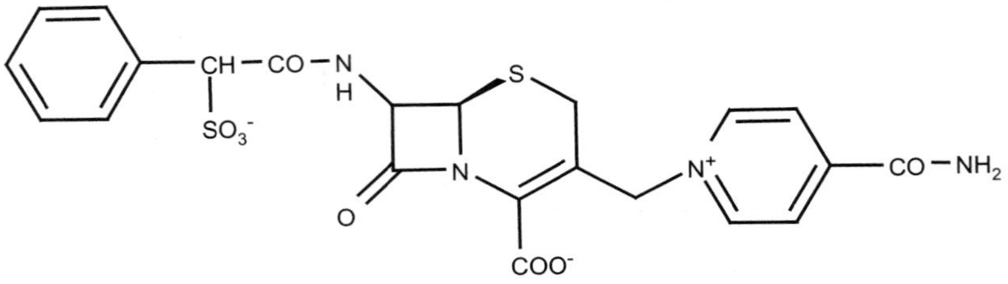

Figure 56 Cefsulodin

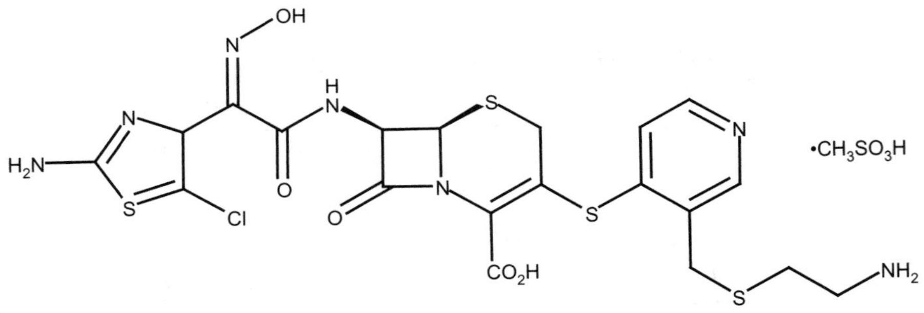

Figure 57 RWJ-54428

Table 80 Activity of RWJ-54428 against *S. aureus* producing β-lactamases

Organism	Enzyme		MIC (μg/ml)		
	Type	Level	RWJ-54428	Cefamandole	Cefaclor
MSSA			0.125	0.25	0.125
	A	0.006	0.25	0.25	0.5
	B	0.024	0.125	2	1
	C	0.034	0.5	2	1
	D	0.030	0.25	1	1
MRSA COL	Negative		1	>8	>8
MRSA 76	Positive	NA[a]	2	>8	>8

[a]NA, not applicable.

irrespective of the immunotypic variants (Table 80) and the susceptibility to vancomycin.

RWJ-54428 inhibits PBP 2a from MRSA and PBP 5 from *Enterococcus hirae* (Table 81).

RWJ-54428 diplays good in vitro activity against *E. faecalis* isolates resistant to ampicillin, with MICs ranging from ≤0.06 to 0.125 μg/ml. RWJ-54428 is poorly active against gram-negative anaerobes, with MIC_{50}s of ≥16 μg/ml, but has better in vitro activity against gram-positive anaerobes, with MIC_{50}s ranging from 0.06 μg/ml (*Peptostreptococcus*) to 0.125 μg/ml (*Propionibacterium*). The compound is weakly active against *Eubacterium* (MIC_{50}, 4.0 μg/ml) and *C. difficile* (MIC_{50}, 8.0 μg/ml).

2.3.6.2.2. RWJ-333441 (MC-04,546). New series have been synthesized, and one compound, RWJ-333441, was selected for further investigation. It differs from RWJ-54528 by the aminothiadiazolyl ring instead of the 2-amino-5-thiazolyl ring at position C-7 of the cephem ring (Fig. 58). RWJ-333441 in vitro is as active as RWJ-54528 against *S. aureus* irrespective of the phenotype of resistance, but it is less active against *E. faecalis* and *E. faecium*. RWJ-333441 is 80-fold more stable in rat serum. The water solubility of RWJ-333441 is 4.4 mg/ml at pH 7.2. RWJ-333441 is more active than RWJ-54528 in staphylococcal mouse disseminated infection, with a 50% effective dose of 0.39 mg/kg (range, 0.3 to 0.5 mg/kg) instead of 1.0 mg/kg (range, 0.7 to 1.6 mg/kg) for RWJ-54528.

RWJ-333441 is stable against hydrolysis by staphylococcal β-lactamase type A (PC-1), type C (V-137), and type D (FAR 19), with a rate of hydrolysis relative to cephaloridine of 7 to 9.

The MIC of RWJ-333441 are not affected by the inoculum size (10^5 to 10^7 CFU/ml). This compound shows a good affinity for PBP 2a of *S. aureus* 67-0, with an IC_{50} of 0.8 μg/ml (MIC, 1.0 μg/ml). The frequency of isolation of resistance to RWJ-333441 in MRSA COL was $<10^{-10}$ at twice the MIC.

The in vitro activity of RWJ-333441 against gram-positive cocci and gram-negative bacilli was investigated.

$MIC_{50/90}$s of RWJ-333441 are ≤0.06/0.06 μg/ml for penicillin G-susceptible, *S. pneumoniae*, viridans group streptococci susceptible to penicillin G, *S. pyogenes*, and *Streptococcus agalactiae*. $MIC_{50/90}$s of RWJ-333441 are 0.5/1.0 μg/ml for MSSA and *E. faecalis*. For *H. influenzae* and *M. catarrhalis*, $MIC_{50/90}$s are 0.5/2.0 μg/ml and ≤0.06/2.0 μg/ml, respectively. For MRSA, *S. epidermidis*, and *S. haemolyticus*, $MIC_{50/90}$s are 2.0/2.0, 1.0/2.0, and 2.0/4.0 μg/ml, respectively. For glycopeptide-intermediate *S. aureus*, MICs are 1.0 and 2.0 μg/ml for *S. aureus* HIP-5836 and HIP-5827; the MICs are 0.125, 0.25, and 2.0 μg/ml for glycopeptide-intermediate *S. epidermidis* strains HIP-4645 and HIP-4680 and *S. haemolyticus* HIP-5979, respectively. RWJ-333441 seems to be poorly active against *E. faecium* strains resistant to ampicillin (MIC_{50}, >32 μg/ml) and resistant to vancomycin (MIC, >32 μg/ml). There is a drop in in vitro activity against *S. pneumoniae* resistant or intermediate to penicillin G (MIC_{50}s, 0.125 and 0.25 μg/ml versus ≥0.06 μg/ml) and against viridans group streptococci resistant to penicillin G (MIC_{50} of 0.5 μg/ml versus MIC of ≤0.06 μg/ml for susceptible strains). RWJ-333441 exhibits activity against *S. pneumoniae* comparable to that of cefotaxime, but RWJ-333441 is more active against viridans group streptococci than is cefotaxime. RWJ-333441 is inactive against *Enterobacteriaceae*, *P. aeruginosa*, and *Acinetobacter* spp. (MIC, >64 μg/ml).

RWJ-333441 is slowly bactericidal against MRSA strain COL (MIC, 2 μg/ml); a decrease of 3.8 log_{10} CFU/ml occurs after 24 h of contact. Against MSSA strain ATCC 29212 (MIC, 0.25 μg/ml) a decrease above 4 log_{10} CFU/ml occurs after 12 h of contact but a regrowth is noted after 12 h. RWJ-333441 exhibits only bacteriostatic activity against *E. faecium* JS26 (ampicillin susceptible) but is bactericidal against *E. faecalis* ATCC 23241 (MIC, 0.125 μg/ml).

Table 81 Affinity for PBP of RWJ-54428

Organism	Drug	MIC (μg/ml) with PBP 1	IC_{50} (μg/ml) with PBP: 1	2	2a	3	4	5
MRSA	RWJ-54428	512			0.7			
	Methicillin	128			587			
	Cefotaxime	0.25			363			
MSSA	RWJ-54428	1	0.2	0.2	NA[a]	0.1		
	Methicillin		0.6	66	NA	<0.03		
E. hirae R40	RWJ-54428	0.5				<0.5	<0.5	0.8
	Imipenem	32				<0.5	<0.5	8.6

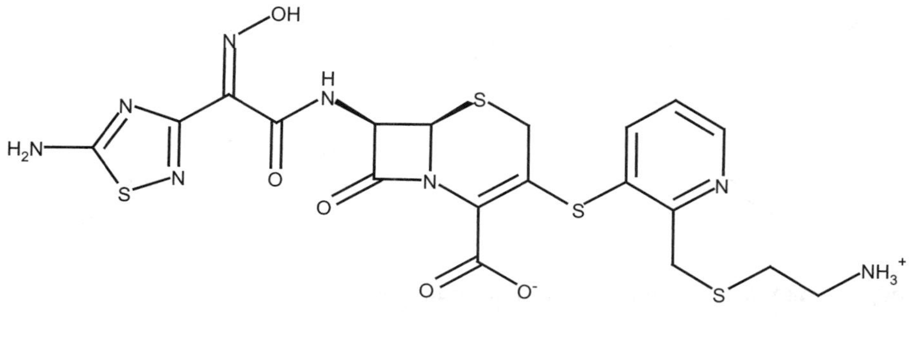

Figure 58 RWJ-333441 (MC 04,546)

Table 82 shows the comparative in vitro activities of RWJ-55428 and RWJ-333441.

2.3.6.2.3. RWJ-333442 (MC-04,699). The aqueous solubility of RWJ-333442 (Fig. 59) improved in comparison with that of RWJ-54428; it was 4.4 mg/ml at pH 7.4. However, an increase in water solubility is desirable for intravenous formulation. A prodrug was synthesized by adding various esters at the C-7 ammonium moiety. Three ester analogs of RWJ-333441 were found to have a water solubility above 20 mg/ml at pH 7.4: the aspartate analog (RWJ-333442), the alanine-alanine analog (RWJ-333443 [MC-04,730]), and the dioxolone analog.

The alanine and alanyl-alanine derivatives were cleared more rapidly (84 and 83% formation in 1 h at 37°C) by human peptidase. The alanyl-alanine was cleared sequentially. The clearance of the aspartyl prodrug occurs more slowly (23% after 1 h at 37°C). The highest bioconversion was observed with aspartate, alanyl-alanine, and dioxolone prodrugs. After 20 min of infusion of 15 mg/kg to rats, a concentration above 35 μg/ml was reached. The aspartate derivative was chosen for further investigations. The pharmacokinetic profile of RWJ-333442 (MC-04,699) was investigated in mice (Swiss Webster), rats (Sprague-Dawley), rabbits (New Zealand White), and monkeys (rhesus macaque) after a single intravenous dose. In all species, total clearance was slower and the apparent elimination half-life was longer than that of RWJ-54428. The elimination rate in urine is about 23%. RWJ-333442 was rapidly converted into RWJ-333441. In less than 3 h, the aspartyl prodrug was not detected.

The antistaphylococcal activities of RWJ-333442 in comparison with RWJ-54428, vancomycin, and quinupristin-dalfopristin against *S. aureus* Smith were investigated in a sepsis model (Swiss-Webster mice) and were also investigated for *S. aureus* 076, a methicillin-resistant strain (male DBA/2 mice). Antibiotics were administered at 0 and 2 h after bacterial challenge (for both MSSA and MRSA, 100 LD_{100}s is 1.0×10^7 CFU/mouse). The ED_{50}s of RWJ-333442, vancomycin, and RWJ-54428 were, respectively, 0.125, 1.0, and 0.125 mg/kg for *S. aureus* Smith and 1.4, 5.6, and 6.5 mg/kg for *S. aureus* 076; the quinupristin-dalfopristin ED_{50} for *S. aureus* 076 (MRSA) was 9.9 mg/kg. In a neutropenic mouse thigh model (male Swiss-Webster mice), the efficacy of RWJ-333442 was tested against various MRSA strains, including glycopeptide-intermediate strains. At a dose of 30 mg/kg, the in vitro postantibiotic effect ranged from 4 to 19 h. Maximum reductions in CFU/per thigh (Δ max log CFU) of 0.97, 1.05, and 1.58 were achieved; these were comparable to those of RWJ-54428. The percentage of a 24-h period that the serum RWJ-333441 concentration exceeded the MIC is the pharmacokinetic-pharmacodynamic parameter that best described the efficacy of RWJ-333441. For non-protein-bound RWJ-333441, the bacteriostatic effect ranged from 12 to 20% for all strains.

Table 82 Comparative in vitro activities of RWJ-55428 and RWJ-333441

Organism	MIC (μg/ml)	
	RWJ-55428	RWJ-333441
S. aureus ATCC 29213	0.25	0.25
S. aureus Col A	0.25	0.25
S. aureus PC-1	0.25	0.25
S. aureus Smith	0.12	0.12
S. aureus Spain 356 (Met[r])	1.0	1.0
S. haemolyticus 05 (Met[r])	2.0	2.0
E. faecalis ATCC 29212	≤0.06	1.0
E. faecium ATCC 35667	0.5	1.0
E. faecium vanA	0.25	2.0
E. faecalis vanB	0.12	0.5
E. faecium A491 (Amp[r])	8.0	>32
Decomposition in water (%/h)	2.4	2.0
Rat serum decomposition (%/h)	56	6
Human serum decomposition	22	1
ED_{50}[a] (mg/kg)	1.0	0.39

[a]ED_{50}, 50% effective dose.

2.3.6.2.4. BMS-247243. Taking a lead compound, BMS-186221 (Fig. 60), which displays good activity against gram-positive cocci, including MRSA, but a poor pharmacokinetic profile due to the metabolism of the C-3 side chain in desacetyl compounds, a series of 1-aminopyridium 4-thiomethyl cephalosporins were synthesized. One compound, BMS-195109, having a sulfonic substituent on the pyridinyl moiety has good water solubility and good in vivo efficacy at a dose of 100 mg/kg per day in rabbit endocarditis due to methicillin-resistant staphylococci.

A second series of derivatives starting from BMS-195109 was synthesized in order to obtain a compound with good antistaphylococcal activity, including MRSA, and good water solubility. This new series bears an acidic moiety at C-7, in order to enhance the water solubility. The target of this series was to obtain C-7 acidic cephalosporins which exhibit a MIC_{50} of ≤4 μg/ml for MRSA, a 50% protective dose (PD_{50}) against MRSA

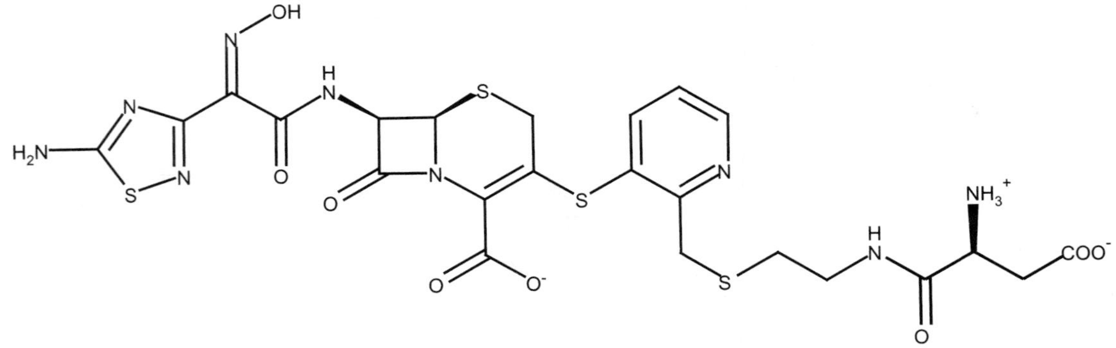

Figure 59 RWJ-333442 (MC 04,699) (L-aspartyl prodrug of RWJ-333441)

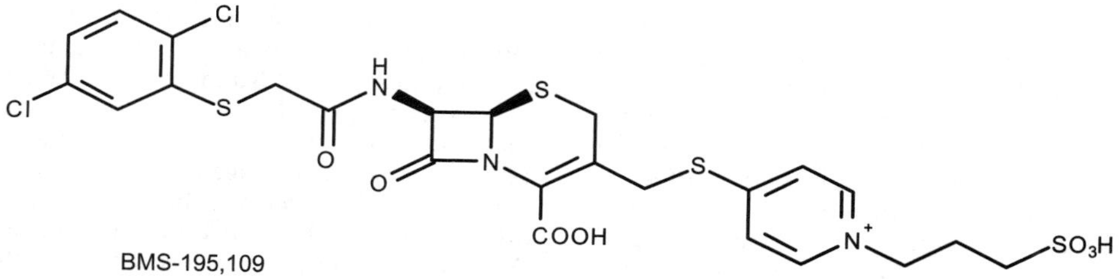

BMS-195,109

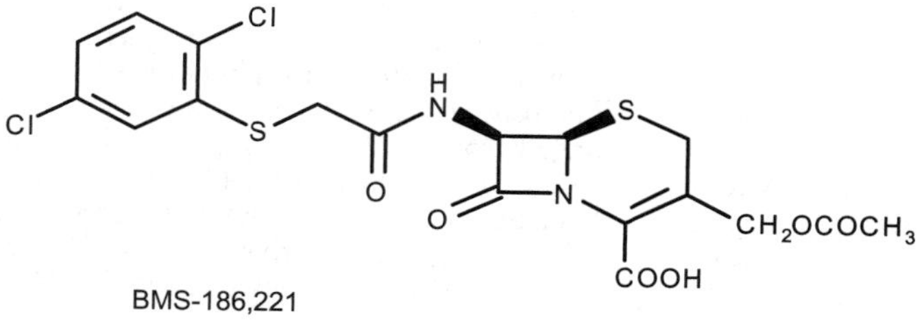

BMS-186,221

Figure 60 BMS-195109 and BMS-186221

mouse disseminated infection of ≤5.0 mg/kg, a water solubility above or equal to 20 mg/ml, and safety in a murine acute-toxicity assay. Numerous leads have been identified. Among the previous series, BMS-196411 (Fig. 61) was chosen as a lead compound for further chemical alterations but was not selected due to unacceptable acute toxicity and water solubility but good anti-MRSA activities, with a MIC of 0.5 μg/ml and a PD_{50} in murine infection of 0.4 to 1.8 mg/kg. BMS-196411 possesses at C-7 a biquaternary moiety. These modification yielded BMS-247243, which is a C-3 biquaternary-C-7 acidic cephalosporin (Fig. 62). BMS-247243 is highly soluble in water at pH 7.0. The activity of BMS-247243 against 250 *Staphylococcus* strains with various phenotypes of resistance was assessed. For fully susceptible *S. aureus*, *S. epidermidis*, *S. haemolyticus*, *Staphylococcus saprophyticus*, *Staphylococcus cohnii*, and

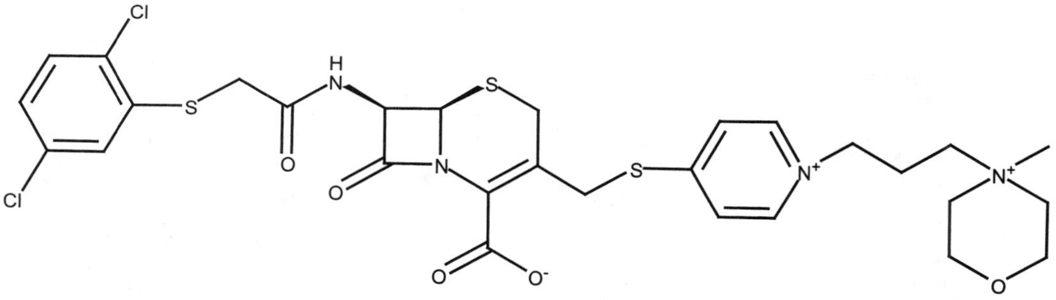

Figure 61 BMS-196411

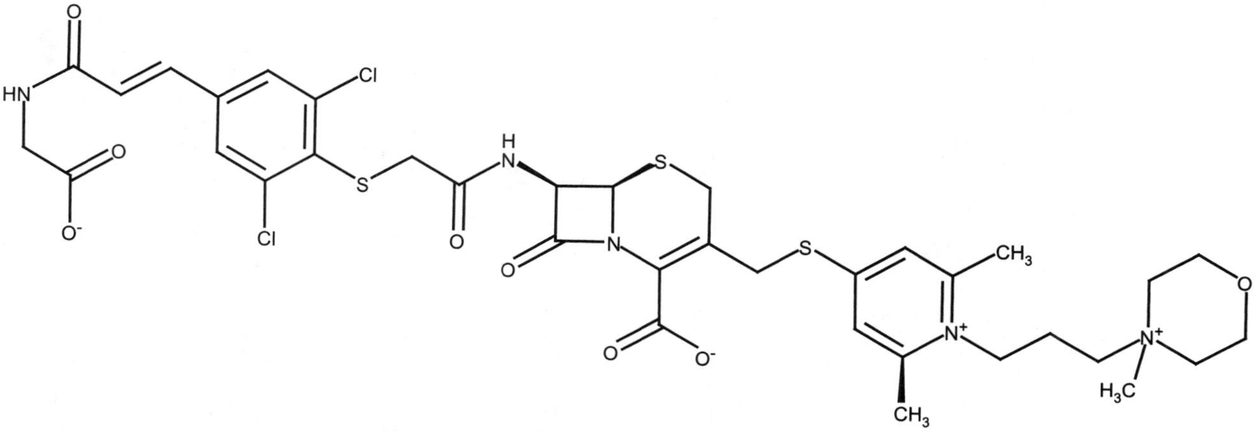

Figure 62 BMS-247243

Staphylococcus capitis strains, the MIC_{50}s ranged from 0.13 to 0.5 μg/ml and the MIC_{50} was 1.0 μg/ml instead of 0.25 μg/ml for non-β-lactamase-producing strains. The rates of hydrolysis by staphylococcal β-lactamase relative to cephaloridine (100%) were 26.2, 4.5, 8.7, and 12.7% for A, B, C, and D enzymes, respectively. The affinity (IC_{50}) of BMS-247243 for PBP 2a of *S. aureus* A-27225 (MRSA) was 0.7 μg/ml, for a MIC of 4.0 μg/ml. The antibacterial spectrum and activity of BMS-247243 were investigated and determined.

Table 83 shows the in vitro activity of BMS-247243. BMS-247243 is highly active against *S. pneumoniae* isolates susceptible to penicillin G ($MIC_{50/90}$ of 0.008/0.06 μg/ml), but a significant drop in activity was noted against *S. pneumoniae* isolates resistant to penicillin G ($MIC_{50/90}$ of 0.5/2.0 μg/ml). For other streptococci, including *S. pyogenes*, *S. agalactiae*, and viridans group streptococci, MIC_{50}s of BMS-247243 ranged from 0.03 to 0.06 μg/ml and MIC_{90}s ranged from 0.03 to 0.5 μg/ml. It is poorly active against *E. faecium* (MIC_{50}, 16 μg/ml), and $MIC_{50/90}$s of 1.0/2.0 μg/ml were noted for *E. faecalis*; however, discriminated data for ampicillin-susceptible and -resistant isolates were not shown. In vitro activity against other gram-positive bacteria was investigated. MICs ranged from 0.06 to 1.0 μg/ml for *Micrococcus* spp., *Leuconostoc* spp., *Pediococcus* spp., *Lactobacillus* spp., *C. jeikeium*, and *L. monocytogenes*. BMS-247243 is inactive against *Enterobacteriaceae* (MIC, >64 μg/ml), *P. aeruginosa* (MIC, >64 μg/ml), *M. catarrhalis* (MIC, ≥16 μg/ml), *H. influenzae* producing a β-lactamase (MIC, ≥16 μg/ml), and *N. meningitidis* (MIC, ≥64 μg/ml). For gram-positive anaerobic bacteria, MIC_{50}s were 2.0, 1.0, and 0.25 μg/ml for *Clostridium perfringens*, *Peptostreptococcus* spp., and *Propionibacterium acnes*, respectively. MICs of 32 μg/ml were shown for two strains of *C. difficile*. BMS-247243 is inactive against *E. faecium* resistant to vancomycin, VanA or VanB phenotype (MIC, >16 μg/ml). For *Enterococcus casseliflavus* VanC, MICs of BMS-247243 ranged from 0.12 to 0.5 μg/ml and for *Enterococcus gallinarum*, MICs of BMS-247243 ranged from 0.12 to 16 μg/ml. At eight times the MIC, BMS-247243, after 6 h of contact, yields a drop of less than 3 $\log_{10}$ CFU/ml for *S. aureus* A-27223 (MIC, 2.0 μg/ml). BMS-247243 exhibits only a

Table 83 BMS-247243 in vitro activity

Organism(s)	*n*	MIC (μg/ml)		
		50%	90%	Range
S. pneumoniae Pen^s	10	0.008	0.06	0.004–0.12
S. pneumoniae Pen^i	10	0.06	0.12	0.016–0.12
S. pneumoniae Pen^r	48	0.5	2.0	0.25–4.0
Streptococcus sanguis	12	0.06	0.5	0.016–2.0
Streptococcus mitis	10	0.03	0.25	0.004–0.5
S. pyogenes	10	0.03	0.03	0.03
S. agalactiae	10	0.06	0.12	0.016–0.12
E. faecalis	18	1.0	2.0	0.5–8.0
E. faecium	11	16	>32	0.06–>64
H. influenzae BLA^{-}[a]	11	2.0	4.0	1.0–8.0
H. influenzae BLA^{+}	12	16	32	2–32
N. meningitidis	18	64	>64	32–>64
C. perfringens	10	2.0	4.0	1.0–8.0
Peptostreptococcus spp.	10	1.0	2.0	0.008–2.0
P. acnes	10	0.25	0.5	0.25–0.5
E. coli	10	>64	>64	>64
S. aureus Met^s	167	0.5	1.0	0.125–2.0
S. aureus Met^r	259	2.0	2.0	0.5–2.0
S. epidermidis Met^s	49	1.0	2.0	0.25–8.0
S. haemolyticus Met^r	33	2.0	4.0	0.125–4.0
S. saprophyticus Met^s	12	0.5	0.5	0.25–0.5
E. faecalis Amp^s	82	0.5	1.0	0.25–0.1
E. faecalis Van^r	11	1.0	1.0	0.25–32
E. faecium Amp^s	22	2.0	4.0	0.25–4.0
E. faecium Amp^r	100	>32	>32	4–>32
E. faecium Van^r	74	>32	>32	1–>32
S. pneumoniae Pen^s	33	≤0.06	≤0.06	≤0.06–0.125
S. pneumoniae Pen^i	30	0.125	0.25	≤0.06–0.5
S. pneumoniae Pen^r	34	0.25	0.5	0.125–0.5
S. pyogenes	13	≤0.06	1.0	≤0.06–1.0
S. agalactiae	9	≤0.06		≤0.06
L. monocytogenes	4			1.0–2.0
Viridans group streptococci Pen^s	9	≤0.06		≤0.06
Viridans group streptococci Pen^i	10	≤0.06	≤0.06	≤0.06
Viridans group streptococci Pen^r	12	0.5	2.0	≤0.015–32
H. influenzae	31	0.5	2.0	≤0.06–4.0
M. catarrhalis	17	≤0.06	2.0	≤0.06–2.0

[a]BLA, β-lactamase.

bacteriostatic effect against *E. faecalis* strain A-27518. A synergistic activity was shown to be species dependent in combination with streptomycin against *E. faecalis*. In murine (female ICR mice, 18 to 23 g) staphylococcal disseminated infections initiated by the intraperitoneal route, treatment started 0 and 2 h after bacterial challenge by the intramuscular route. The PD_{50}s ranged from 0.2 to 3.8 mg/kg for *S. aureus* and from 0.25 to 0.5 mg/kg for coagulase-negative staphylococci. The PD_{50}s were 4.0 and 8.0 mg/kg for *E. faecalis* A-27518 and *E. faecium* A-24885, respectively.

BMS-247243 was administered intravenously to fasted mice at the doses of 5, 40, and 80 mg/kg. The apparent elimination half-lives ranged from 1.3 to 1.7 h, with an AUC from 40 μg·h/ml (5 mg/kg) to 304 μg·h/ml (80 mg/kg). Urine recoveries ranged from 44% (5 mg/kg) to 27% (80 mg/kg) of the administered dose.

In female rabbits (2 to 2.5 kg), staphylococcal (MRSA strain A-27223, MIC, 2 μg/ml) endocarditis was induced with 10^6 CFU of an overnight culture. Therapy started 18 h after bacterial challenge and continued for three consecutive days (10 mg/kg for 8 h). Fifteen hours after the last dose of BMS-247243, cardiac vegetations were removed and bacterial counts were performed. Six of 11 animals treated had vegetation counts below the limit of detection (10^2 CFU/g). For the remaining animals, bacterial counts ranged from 10^4 to 10^9 CFU/g (one animal).

2.3.6.2.5. 3-Dithiocarbamoyl carbacephems and cephalosporins. Series of carbacephems and cephalosporins were synthesized to inhibit PBP 2a of MRSA and PBP 2x of *S. pneumoniae* isolates resistant to cephalosporins.

In a subset of compounds it was shown that the C-3 dithiocarbamates replaced with a 2-isoindanyl moiety are the most active compounds. In this subset of molecule, variations around the oxime residue and the heteroaryl moiety at C-7 position were performed and three compounds were selected for further preclinical investigation: a carbacephem, PGE-9951357 (oxyphenyl at C-7), and cephalosporins PGE-6737410 (2-amino-5-thiazolyl methoxyimino chain at C-7) and PGE-9739390 (2-amino-5-thiazolyl hydroxyimino at C-7 and a substituted isoindanyl moiety) (Fig. 63).

PGE-6737410 is highly soluble in water (>25 mg/ml), but PGE-9739390 is poorly soluble in water (0.015 mg/ml). Both compounds exhibit a good affinity for PBP 2x of *S. pneumoniae*, with IC_{50}s of 0.3 and 0.15 μM, respectively. They also show IC_{50}s of 2.6 and 1.5 μM for PBP 2a of *S. aureus*. Introduction of an amino side chain to the isoindanyl ring reduced the water solubility due to the zwitterionic nature of the compound (PGE-9739390). These two compounds displayed a reasonable chemical stability. The in vitro activities of PGE-9951357, PGE-6737410, and PGE-9739390 against gram-positive and -negative microorganisms were investigated. The most active compound was PGE-9739390, with MIC_{50}s from ≤0.12 to 0.5 μg/ml and MIC_{90}s from 0.12 to 2.0 μg/ml for MRSA and MSSA, *S. pneumoniae* irrespective of the susceptibility to penicillin G, *S. pyogenes*, *S. epidermidis*, viridans group streptococci, and *E. faecalis*. It is inactive against *E. faecium* (MIC_{50}, >32 μg/ml). It is also active against *M. catarrhalis* ($MIC_{50/90}$, ≤0.12/0.25 μg/ml) *H. influenzae* producing or not producing β-lactamase (MIC_{50}, ≤0.12 to 0.25 μg/ml; MIC_{90}, 0.5 to 1.0 μg/ml). It is weakly active against *Enterobacteriaceae*. For

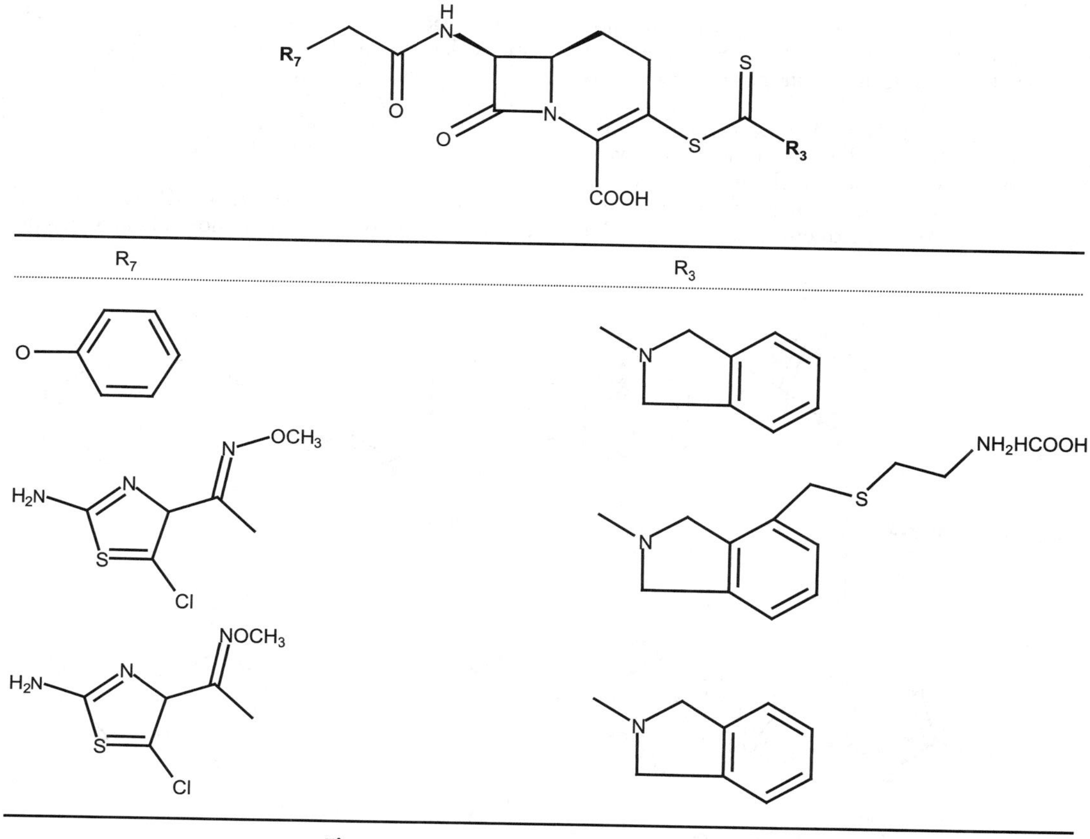

Figure 63 3-Desthiocarbamate cephems

these organisms the most active compound was PGE-6737410, with MIC_{50}s of 0.5, 0.5, and 2.0 μg/ml for *E. coli*, *K. pneumoniae*, and *E. cloacae*, respectively. All of them are inactive against *P. aeruginosa* (MIC, ≥32 μg/ml). PGE-9739390 and PGE-6737410 are stable against hydrolysis by broad-spectrum β-lactamases but not by extended-spectrum β-lactamases tested (TEM-3, TEM-8, TEM-5, and SHV-5).

In disseminated murine (CF-1 male, 18 to 25 g) infections induced by the intraperitoneal route with *S. pneumoniae*, *S. aureus* (methicillin susceptible and resistant), and *E. coli*, and after a therapy which started 1 h and a second administration at 4 h after bacterial challenge by the subcutaneous route, the PD_{50}s were 9.6, 5.6, and 10.98 mg/kg for *S. pneumoniae*, 21.64, 86.75, and 57.06 mg/kg for MSSA, greater than 200 mg/kg for MRSA, and above 100 mg/kg for *E. coli* for PGE-9951357, PGE-6737410, and PGE-9739390, respectively. The pharmacokinetics of the three compounds were investigated in CD rats (270 to 330 g) after a single intravenous dose of 20 mg/kg. The apparent elimination half-lives (means ± standard deviations) ranged from 0.32 ± 0.1 h to 1.4 ± 0.2 h, and the AUCs ranged from 7 ± 1.3 to 58 ± 11 μg·h/ml.

All of these compounds exhibit in vitro activity against gram-positive cocci, except *E. faecium*, but poor in vivo activity.

2.3.6.2.6. HMRZ-4 and HMRZ-62. A series of parenteral cephems were synthesized, TOC-30 and TOC-50, with potential activity against MRSA and enterococci; TOC-50 and TOC-30 are 2-amino-5-thiazolyl cephalosporins having a vinylthio-substituted pyridine at the C-3 position of the cephem moiety. However, due to toxicological features, they were not developed.

It was shown that cephalosporins having a methylthiobenzothiopyran side chain at C-3 of the cephem moiety exhibited enhanced activity against gram-positive organisms (Obi et al., 1995).

In a new series of cephalosporins, having a vinylthio linkage at C-3, various 4-oxo-4*H*-1-benzothiopyrans were attached. In this series, at C-7 the side chain is formed with either thienyl or 2-amino-5-thiazolyl rings with various substituted oxime moieties. All of the thienyl derivatives exhibit good activity against MSSA isolates (MICs, 0.06 to 0.2 μg/ml) and weak activity against MRSA (MICs, 1.56 to 6.25 μg/ml) and VRE (MICs, 0.78 to 12.5 μg/ml); all of them were inactive against *Enterobacteriaceae* and *P. aeruginosa* (MICs, > 100 μg/ml). The 2-amino-5-thiazolyl analogs are poorly active against MRSA and VRE irrespective of the oxime residue but show a higher activity against *E. coli* (MICs, 1.56 to 6.25 μg/ml) than the thienyl derivatives, but they are inactive against *P. aeruginosa* (MICs, 25 to >100 μg/ml). The third subset of analogs are 2-amino-5-thiazolyl hydroxyimino cephems having various heterocycles fixed to the C-3 vinylthio chain. Against MRSA and VRE the most active analogs are a benzothiopyranyls (MICs, 3.13 and 1.56 μg/ml for MRSA and VRE), followed by benzopyranyl analogs (MICs, 6.25 and 25 μg/ml) and benzoxazolyl analogs (MICs, 12.5 and 12.5 μg/ml). The phenyl analog is inactive (MICs, 25 and 50 μg/ml). All of them are inactive against *P. aeruginosa* (MICs, >100 μg/ml) and weakly active against *E. coli* NIHJ-JC2 (MICs, 1.56 to 12.5 μg/ml).

HMRZ-4 (Fig. 64), the compound most active against MRSA and VRE, was selected as a lead compound. A new series of 7-thienylacetamido-3-heterocyclic-fused thiopyran cephalosporins were synthesized. All compounds, having a substituted or not thiophene-fused ring, a furan-fused ring, a pyridine-fused ring, or a pyrazolyl-fused ring, exhibited good activity, with MICs from 0.78 to 3.13 μg/ml and 0.78 to 6.25 μg/ml for MRSA and VRE, respectively. Only one compound was poorly active, having a bulky substituent on the thiopyran ring.

Two subsets of compounds in this new series, having at C-3 a thienothiopyranyl link to the cephem moiety with a thiovinyl chain, were synthesized with various side chains at C-7.

The most active compound has a 2-amino-5-thiazolyl ring replaced with a chlorine atom. MIC_{50} were 0.39, 0.05, 0.78, 0.10, and 3.13 μg/ml for MRSA, *S. aureus* 209P, VRE (NCTC 12201), *E. faecalis* ATCC 21212, and *E. coli* NIHJ-JC2, but the compound is inactive against *P. aeruginosa*. This compound is referred to as HMRZ-62 (Fig. 65).

2.3.6.2.7. BAL 9141 (Ro-63-9141). BAL 9141 (Fig. 66) is a thiadiazolyl hydroxyimino cephem with a pyrrolidone

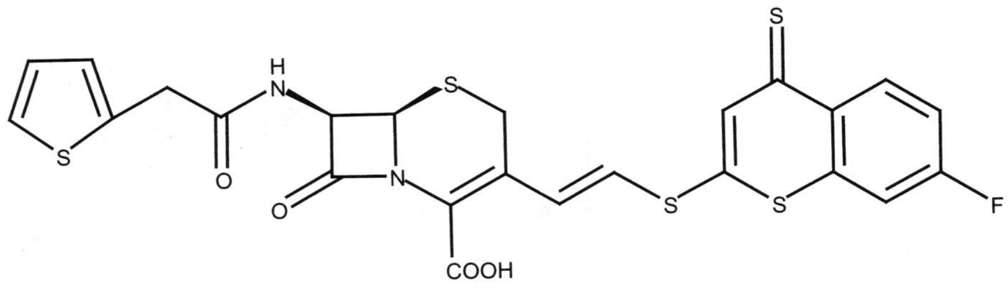

Figure 64 HMRZ-4

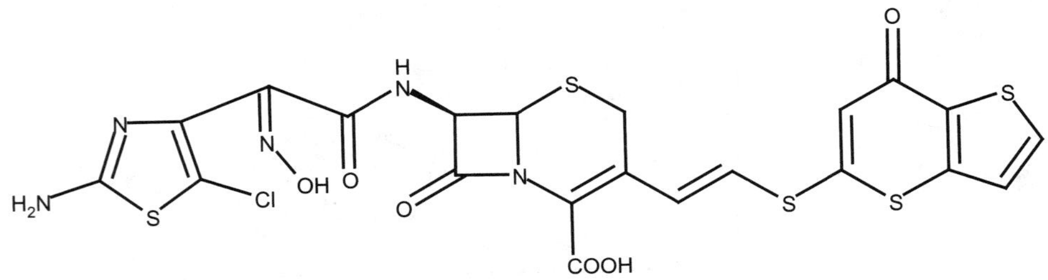

Figure 65 HMRZ-62

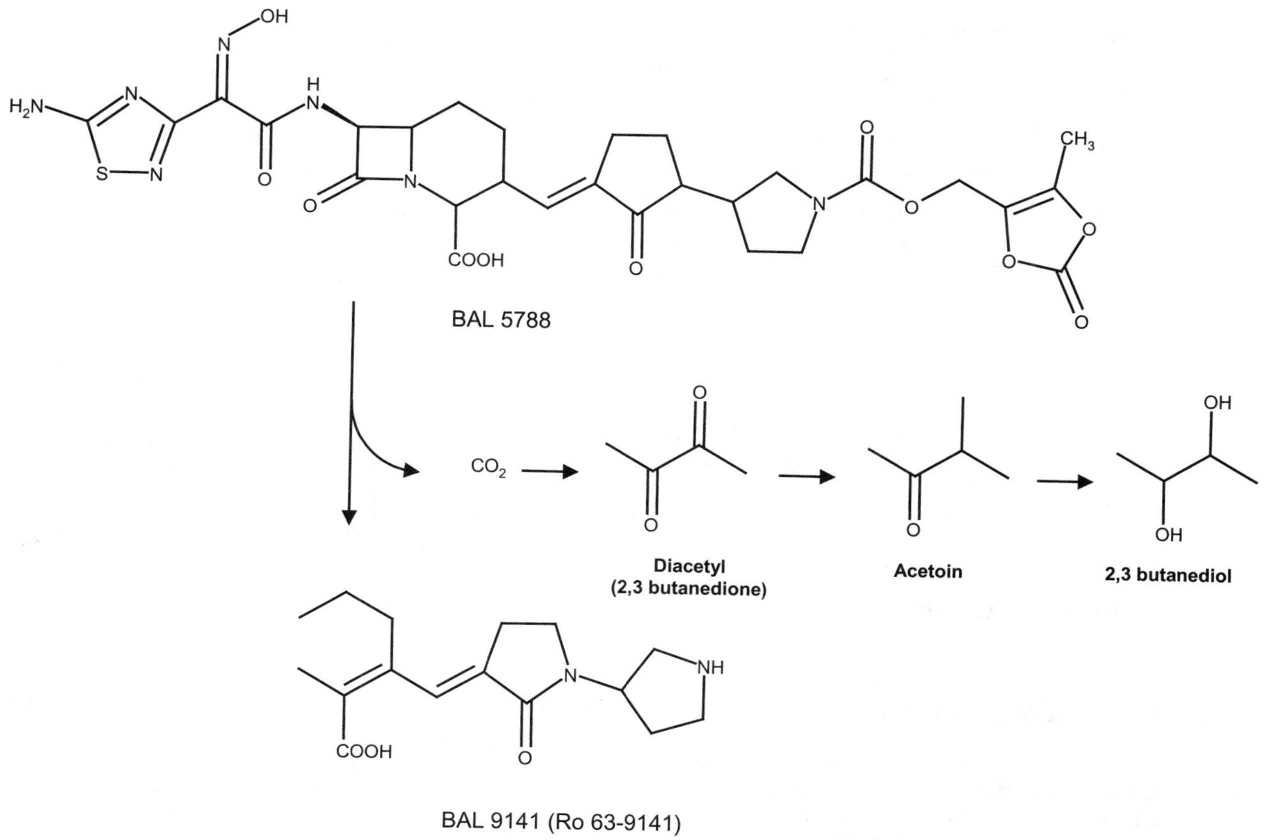

BAL 5788

CO_2

Diacetyl (2,3 butanedione)

Acetoin

2,3 butanediol

BAL 9141 (Ro 63-9141)

Figure 66 BAL-9141

C-3 side chain. BAL 9141 is the prodrug of BAL 5788 (Fig. 66). After absorption, the ester side chain of the prodrug is metabolized in CO_2 and 2,3 butanediol, and the parent compound is released.

BAL 5788 is active in vitro against *S. aureus* isolates irrespective of their susceptibility to methicillin or benzylpenicillin and displays good in vitro activity against *S. pneumoniae* and viridans group streptococci. Against *E. faecalis*, BAL 5788 exhibits a bimodal activity (MIC_{50}, 0.5 μg/ml), but the compound is inactive against *E. faecium* (MIC_{50}, >32 μg/ml) (Table 84).

BAL 5788 exhibits an apparent elimination half-life of 2 to 3 h, being mainly eliminated in urine. The level of the prodrug in plasma is low, representing 0.7 to 3.5% of the maximum concentration of drug in serum of parent compound for less than half the volunteers (15 out of 40) and only for 2 to 4 h sampling intervals (Table 85).

The free drug represents 62% of the compound level in plasma.

2.3.6.2.8. LB-11058. LB-11058 is a 2-amino-5-thiazolyl cephalosporin having a hydroxyimino moiety. The

Table 84 In vitro activity of BAL-9141

Organism(s)	*n*	MIC (μg/ml)		
		50%	90%	Range
MSSA	50	0.5	0.5	0.25–2
MRSA	96	1	2	0.12–2
CoNS[a]	26	0.12	0.25	≤0.015–1
CoNS-Met^r	90	1	2	≤0.015–4
S. pneumoniae Pen^s	261	≤0.015	≤0.015	≤0.015–0.03
S. pneumoniae Pen^i	144	0.06	0.12	≤0.015–0.5
S. pneumoniae Pen^r	114	0.25	0.25	≤0.015–1
Viridans group streptococci Pen^s	38	≤0.015	0.06	≤0.015–0.06
Viridans group streptococci Pen^i	34	0.03	0.25	≤0.015–1
Viridans group streptococci Pen^r	13	0.5	1	0.03–32
E. faecalis	61	0.5	16	0.12–>32
E. faecium	50	>32	>32	0.25–>32

[a]CoNS, coagulase-negative staphylococci.

Table 85 Pharmacokinetics of BAL-9141

Dose (mg)	n	C_{max} (μg/ml)	$t_{1/2}$ (h)	AUC (μg·h/ml)	CL_P (liters/h)	CL_R (liters/h)	Urinary elimination (%)
125	6	9.87	2.84	20.3	6.27	4.6	74.2
250	6	19.5	3.42	43.7	5.81	4.35	76.1
500	6	35.5	3.44	76.6	6.54	5.07	77.5
750	6	59.6	3.47	135	5.74	4.08	71.3
1,000	6	72.2	3.25	151	6.64	4.16	62.5

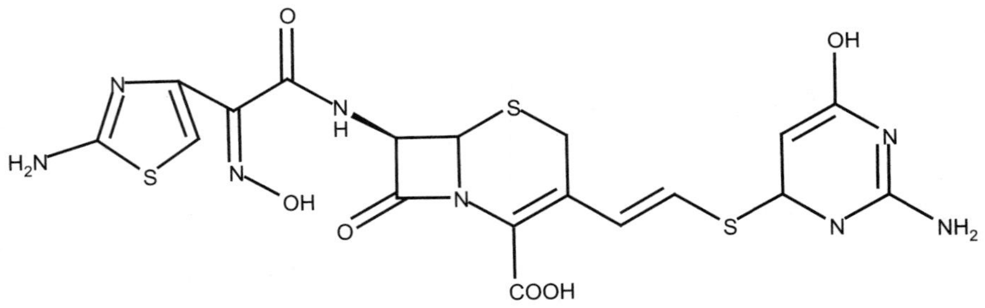

Figure 67 LB-11058

C-3 side chain is a pyrimidyl-substituted vinyl sulfide chain (Fig. 67).

LB-11058 is water soluble (>20 mg/ml) and seems to have a good affinity for PBP 2a (IC_{50}, 0.3 μg/ml).

It is active against *S. aureus, S. pneumoniae*, beta-hemolytic streptococci, and viridans group streptococci but is inactive against *E. faecium*. LB-11058 is active against *S. aureus* isolates producing PC-1 enzyme, whatever the immunotype (Table 86). LB-11058 seems to be bactericidal against MRSA strains (reduction of ≥3 $\log_{10}$ CFU/ml) after 8 h of contact.

2.3.6.2.9. S-3578. S-3578 is an amino-thiadiazolyl cephalosporin with an oxiethyl residue fixed on the oxime. In C-3 a C-3′ quaternary ammonium side chain is fixed (Fig. 68). For MRSA, the MIC is 3.13 μg/ml; for *P. aeruginosa*, the MIC is 1.56 μg/ml.

2.3.7. Group VII: Other Cephems

2.3.7.1. Sulfoxycephems

Various derivatives possessing a sulfoxide or a sulfone at position 1 have been described, such as HR-109 and CM-40876 (Fig. 69). It has been shown that the 1-β-sulfoxide derivatives have good antibacterial activity, particularly against

Table 86 In vitro activity of LB-11058 against *S. aureus* producing β-lactamases

Strains	Type	MIC (μg/ml) at inoculum (CFU/ml): 5×10^5	5×10^6	5×10^7
MSSA	–	0.13	0.13	0.13
ATCC 29213	A	0.13	0.25	0.25
NCTC 9789	A	0.25	0.25	0.5
22260	B	0.25	0.5	0.5
V137	C	0.25	0.25	0.25
FAR 8	D	0.25	0.25	0.25
MRSA	+	0.5	0.5	1
MRSA	–	0.5	0.5	0.5

β-lactamase-producing strains, as they are not a good substrate for these enzymes. The derivative SYN-010 possesses a 1-sulfonyl and is inactive. The original feature of this molecule is that it has a sulfone function. The derivative SYN-012 is identical to SYN-010, but the sulfone in position 1 is not oxidized. This molecule has good activity against *S. aureus* (MIC, ~0.1 μg/ml) but is not active against type I enzyme-producing *Enterobacteriaceae* or against those producing broad-spectrum

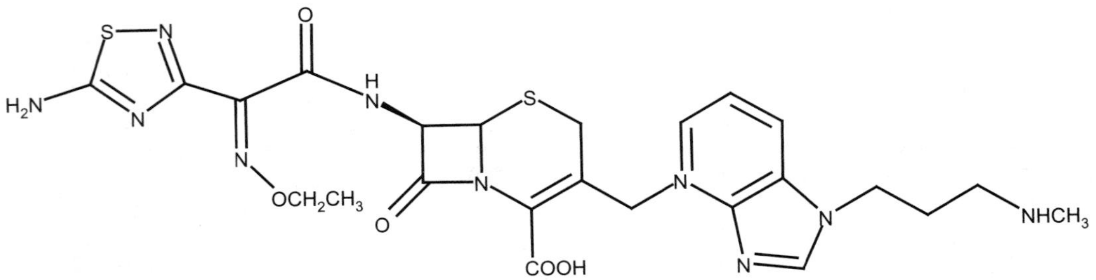

Figure 68 S-3578

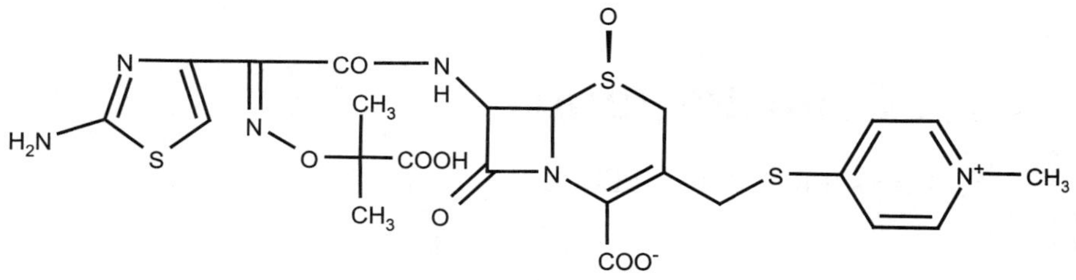

Figure 69 **1-*S*-Sulfoxide cephalosporin, CM-40876**

enzymes (SHV-1, TEM-1 and -2, OXA-1, etc.). However, they open up a new avenue of research.

2.3.7.2. Other Cephems

2.3.7.2.1. Phosphocephems. Satoh et al. replaced the sulfur atom with a phosphorus atom. These molecules do not have antibacterial activity and do not inhibit β-lactamases.

2.3.7.2.2. Azacephems. 1-Azacephem and 2-azacephem derivatives have been described. Their antibacterial activity is unknown.

REFERENCES

The extensive references may be obtained from the author.

Oral Cephalosporins

A. BRYSKIER AND M. LEBEL

7

1. INTRODUCTION

Oral cephalosporins have been in clinical use now for more than 20 years. Those available since the 1970s and 1980s include cephalexin, cephradine, cefadroxil, cefaclor, and, for a decade, cefixime, cefuroxime axetil, cefpodoxime proxetil, cefotiam hexetil, ceftibuten, loracarbef, cefprozil, cefetamet pivoxil, and cefditoren pivoxil. Loracarbef, a carbacephem, is included in this chapter as a cephalosporin.

Few families of oral antibacterials are available in clinics. The most important are penicillins, cephalosporins, macrolides/ketolides, fluoroquinolones, and, to a lesser extent, tetracyclines, lincosamides, and recently oxazolidinones.

Within this category of antibacterials, cephalosporins are considered safe and acid stable, with a broad antibacterial spectrum which covers main common pathogens encountered in everyday physician clinical practice. A diversity of antibacterials are needed to overcome intrinsic or acquired bacterial resistance (e.g., *Haemophilus influenzae* producing β-lactamase).

The first parenteral cephalosporin was issued from the chemical modification of cephalosporin C (especially 7-aminocephalosporanic acid) which was isolated from the fermentation broth of *Cephalosporium acremonium*, now named *Acremonium chrysogenum*. Cephalosporins are acid stable but are poorly absorbed.

The modification of the side chain at the C-7 position of the cephem nucleus, by fixing a D-phenylglycine moiety, yielded cephalexin in 1967 (Wick, 1967). Since then, many series of compounds bearing a 7-D-phenylglycine residue have been synthesized, but only a few have been introduced in clinical practice. The aim of the research within the α-aminocephalosporins was to improve the pharmacokinetic profile, in order to reduce the daily intake. This target was reached with cefadroxil, which differs from cephalexin by a *para*-hydroxyphenyl moiety instead of a phenyl, allowing one or two administrations per day. With the same goal, some esters were prepared, such as cephaloglycin or cephalexin esters. The second target was to enhance the antibacterial activity. This first wave of oral cephalosporins was directed against penicillinase-producing strains of *Staphylococcus aureus*. The second wave was also oriented against gram-negative bacilli. Polar groups were appended at C-3. One compound now in wide use was introduced in clinical practice at this time, cefaclor. With the development of parenteral 2-amino-5-thiazolyl cephalosporins, many efforts were directed to obtain absorbable compounds in this class of cephems.

The first efforts were done within the existing parenteral compounds. Efforts with cefotaxime were unsuccessful. Some results were obtained with ceftizoxime (KY-20, and AS-924) but for KY-20 the absorption rate was too moderate to allow clinical development; for the second molecule, phase III is currently ongoing. Two compounds were esterified and are widely used, cefuroxime axetil and cefotiam-hexetil. An oral formulation of ceftriaxone has been proposed. The α-amino-cephalosporin compounds that been developed include cefprozil and an α-aminocarbacephem, loracarbef, which is close to cefaclor.

Among the 2-amino-5-thiazolyl derivatives, two types of compounds were developed, esterified and nonesterified compounds.

Nonesterified cephems have a hydroxy group (cefdinir and cefmatilen) or an acetoxy residue (cefixime) on the oxime group. Other groups have been appended instead of the oxime ring (ceftibuten).

Many of the new oral cephems are prodrugs, with a cleavable ester at C-4 (carboxylic group). They differ by their C-3 side chains and ester chains. The main compounds are cefpodoxime proxetil, cefetamet pivoxil, cefcamate pivoxil, and cefditoren pivoxil. Research in this field continues, with the goal of extending the antibacterial spectrum and enhancing the antibacterial activity.

2. CLASSIFICATION

Several classifications of the cephalosporins have been proposed. The most commonly used and the most practical is based on the timing of their introduction in clinical practice, which fairly often corresponds to the characteristics of their antibacterial spectrum.

Two classifications can be described: the most reliable one, i.e., the chemical classification, and the vernacular one, i.e., the microbiological classification.

2.1. Microbiological Classification

The microbiological classification can be said to mimic the parenteral cephalosporin classification (Bryskier et al., 1994). Compounds can be divided into three groups according to their antibacterial spectra and in vitro activities. However, it is difficult to insert some compounds which have intermediate antibacterial activity.

The first group (limited spectrum) is divided into two subgroups, I_A and I_B. Group I_A is composed of most of the α-amino cephalosporins, with differences between compounds. All of them display good in vitro activity against gram-positive cocci. They are less active against isolates of *S. aureus* producing penicillinase, and they are inactive against *Enterococcus faecalis*. Against enteric bacilli, cefaclor and to a lesser extent cefatrizine and cefprozil are active (especially against methicillin-susceptible *S. aureus*), but other derivatives exhibit weak antibacterial activity against gram-negative bacilli.

Their antibacterial spectrum includes gram-positive cocci such as *S. aureus*, and *Staphylococcus epidermidis*, and *Streptococcus pneumoniae* and some gram-negative bacilli such as *Escherichia coli*, *Proteus mirabilis*, and *Klebsiella pneumoniae*. A new cephalosporin, cefprozil, in our opinion belongs to this group.

Group II is composed of only one available drug, cefuroxime axetil, and one compound, cefcanel daloxil, which was only developed up to phase III.

These cephalosporins (cefaclor, loracarbef, and cefuroxime axetil) exhibit increased activity against gram-negative bacteria and are more stable against hydrolysis by several types of β-lactamases. The antibacterial spectrum and activity of these cephalosporins include the gram-positive and gram-negative bacteria covered by group I cephalosporins, plus *H. influenzae*, *Moraxella catarrhalis*, and *Neisseria gonorrhoeae* (including β-lactamase-producing strains).

Parenteral cefuroxime belongs to Group II of the parenteral microbiological classification. It is more active than cefaclor, covering gram-negative bacilli and *H. influenzae* as well as gram-positive cocci, but it is less active than compounds of group III.

Group III compounds, which have an extended antibacterial spectrum among the oral cephalosporins, can be divided into two groups, III_A and III_B, according to their in vitro activities against gram-positive cocci, mainly *S. aureus*. Compounds of group III_B are inactive against *S. aureus* and are poorly active against *S. pneumoniae*.

Group III cephalosporins are characterized by a broader coverage of gram-negative bacteria, but sometimes at the expense of good coverage of gram-positive cocci (except for streptococci). In addition, their stability in the presence of β-lactamase hydrolysis is markedly superior to that of group I and II cephalosporins. The microbiological classification in terms of three groups is illustrated in Fig. 1.

2.2. Chemical Classification

On the basis of chemical structure, oral cephalosporins can be divided into six groups.

Groups I and II are composed of α-amino cephalosporins. Group I gathers most common old cephalosporins, which are also subdivided into three subgroups according to the C-3 side chain. In subgroup I_A, only one compound was introduced in clinical practice, cephaloglycin. However, among the compounds with a C-3 aliphatic side chain, four drugs are currently used in clinical practice: cefadroxil, cephalexin, cephradine, and cefprozil. Only two compounds with a polar side chain are available for clinical use, cefaclor and cefroxadines; one compound with an aromatic nucleus is available, cefatrizine. Group III is composed of miscellaneous derivatives, such as ceftibuten.

The more complex group is group IV, composed of oral cephalosporin prodrugs. Group IV is subdivided into four subgroups. The most important one, in terms of clinical use, is group IV_C, with at least four compounds introduced for human clinical use: cefuroxime, cefetamet, cefpodoxime and cefteram (Japan), and cefditoren pivoxil.

Group V, consisting of the aryloxyimino derivative nonesterified compounds, possesses two main drugs: cefixime and cefdinir.

Group VI is composed of carbacephems. Loracarbef is the unique compound of this group.

3. PHYSICOCHEMICAL PROPERTIES

The available chemicophysical data for esterified and non esterified compounds are listed in Tables 1 and 2.

These compounds (ester- and nonester-type compounds) are either colorless (cefaclor and cefuroxime axetil) to slightly yellowish (cefixime, cefprozil, ceftibuten, cefuroxime-axetil, and cefditoren) or brownish (cefpodoxime proxetil) crystalline powder.

Cefprozil is a 9:1 mixture of its *cis*- and *trans*-isomers, and cefuroxime axetil and cefpodoxime proxetil are mixtures of diastereoisomers of almost equal proportions.

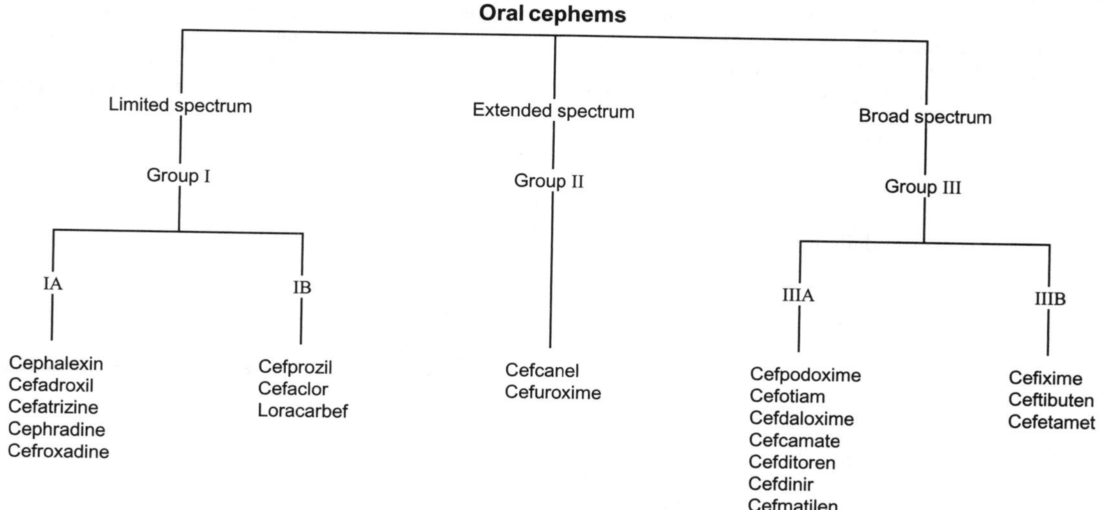

Figure 1 Microbiological classification of oral cephalosporins

Table 1 Chemicophysical properties of α-aminocephalosporins

Generic name	Empirical formula	Molecular mass (Da)	Dissociation constant			Degradation half-life (pH 1, 35°C) (min)	Group (oral)
			pK_a1	pK_a2	pK_a3		
Cephalexin	$C_{16}H_{17}N_3O_4S$	347.40	2.67	6.96		36,000	I
Cefadroxil	$C_{16}H_{17}N_3O_5S$	381.41	2.69	7.22		44,000	I
Cephaloglycin	$C_{18}H_{19}N_3O_6S$	405.44	2.03	6.89		2,100	I
Cephradine	$C_{16}H_{19}N_3O_4S$	349.41	2.63	7.35		38,000	I
Cefaclor	$C_{15}H_{14}ClN_3O_3S$	367.82	1.5	7.17			II
Cefatrizine	$C_{18}H_{18}N_6O_5S_2$	462.50	2.62	6.99		19,000	I
Cefroxadine	$C_{16}H_{19}N_3O_5S$	365.40					II
Loracarbef	$C_{16}H_{16}ClN_3O_4$	349.57					VI
Cefprozil	$C_{18}H_{19}N_3O_5S$	407.5	2.8	7.3	9.7		II

Table 2 Chemicophysical properties of non-α-amino oral cephems

Generic name	Empirical formula	Molecular mass (Da)	Dissociation constant(s) (pK_a1/pK_a2)	Group	
				Oral	Parenteral
Cefpodoxime	$C_{15}H_{17}N_5O_6S_2$	427.5	2.01, 3.17	IVd	
Cefpodoxime proxetil	$C_{21}H_{27}N_5O_9S_2$	557.6	3.2	IVd	
Cefuroxime	$C_{16}H_{16}N_4O_8S$	424.4	2.2		II
Cefuroxime axetil	$C_{20}H_{22}N_4O_{10}S$	510.5		IVd	
Cefetamet	$C_{14}H_{15}N_5O_5S_2$	397.4	2.6, 3.6	IVd	
Cefetamet pivoxil	$C_{20}H_{25}N_5O_7S_2$	511.17	3.1	IVd	
Cefditoren pivoxil	$C_{25}H_{28}N_6O_7S_3$	620.73		IVd	
Cefditoren	$C_{19}H_{18}N_6O_5S_3$	506.59		IVd	
Ceftibuten	$C_{15}H_{14}N_4O_6S_2$	410.43	2.3, 3.2, 4.5	III	
Cefdinir	$C_{14}H_{13}N_5O_5S_2$	395.4		V	
Cefixime	$C_{16}H_{15}N_5O_7S_2$	453.5	2.1, 2.7, 3.7	V	
Cefotiam	$C_{18}H_{23}N_9O_4S_2$	598.5	2.6, 4.6, 7.0		IIIa
Cefmatilen	$C_{15}H_{14}N_8O_5S_4$	569.04	3.2		

Ceftibuten is formulated as the pure active *cis*-isomer but it is partially converted (up to 20%) to the less active *trans*-isomer in serum and liver. In the case of the ester prodrugs, there is no difference in antibacterial activity, since the asymmetric center is located in the ester side chain.

The *cis*- and *trans*-isomers of cefprozil differ in their antibacterial activities. The *trans*-isomer is six- to eight-fold less active against *E. coli, K. pneumoniae, N. gonorrhoeae,* and *H. influenzae.*

Another common characteristic of the cephem prodrug ester is its bitter taste. Cefaclor and loracarbef differ by the substituent in position 1, a sulfur atom (cefaclor) and a methylene (loracarbef). The carbacephem compound is chemically stable compared to its cephalosporin analog (cefaclor).

Ceftizoxime alapivoxilal (AS-924) water solubility is 19.9 mg/ml, and the lipophilicity is estimated at logP 1.15.

4. STRUCTURE-ACTIVITY RELATIONSHIP

The general chemical structure of the cephalosporins is illustrated in Fig. 2. This chemical structure comprises a β-lactam ring, common to the penicillins and cephalosporins, attached to a dihydrothiazolidine ring that characterizes the

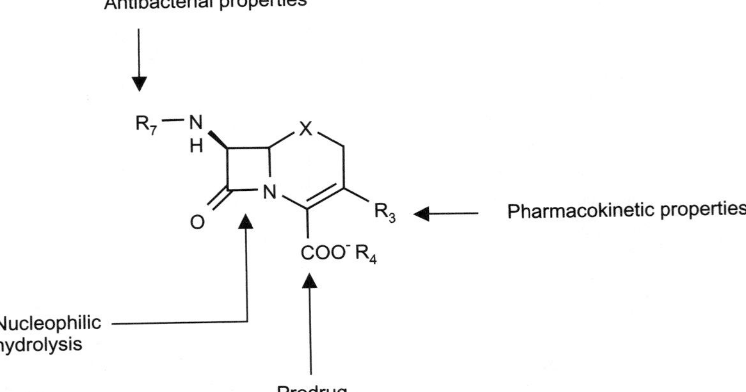

Figure 2 General structure of cephalosporins

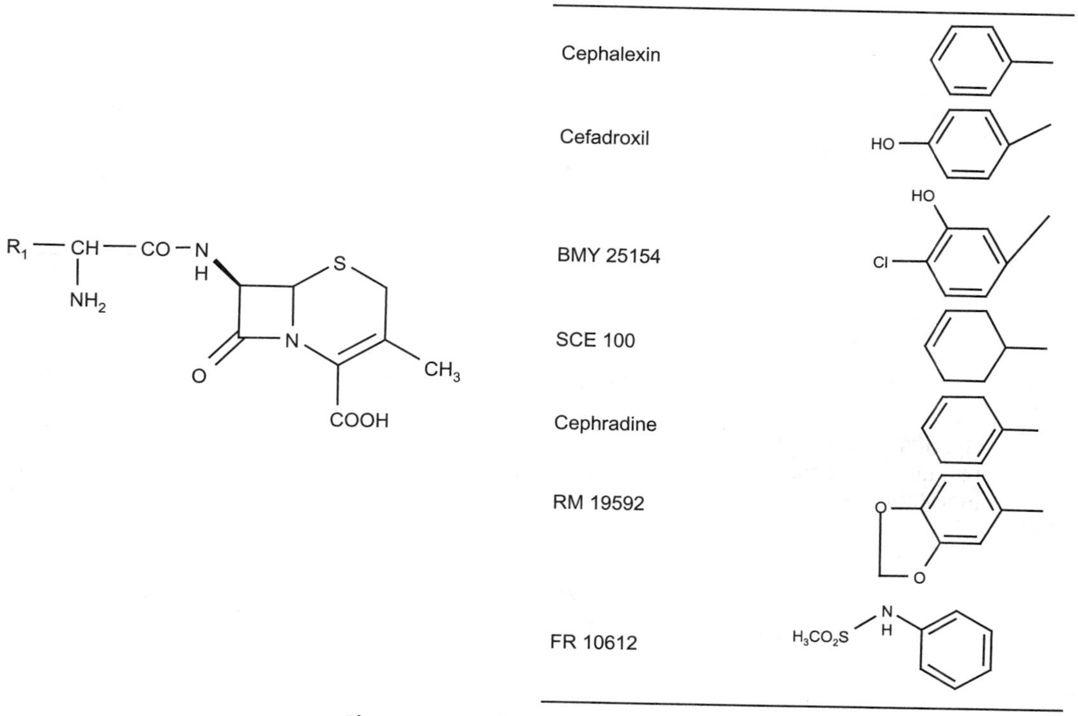

Figure 3 Oral cephems (group IA)

cephalosporins, with its sulfur atom at position 1. In addition, loracarbef possesses a carbon (methylene) at position 1, thus classifying this molecule among the carbacephems.

As a general rule, the substitutions at position 7 affect the antibacterial activity of the cephalosporins as well as their stability against hydrolysis by β-lactamases. Changes at position 3 affect the antibacterial and pharmacokinetic properties, whereas the addition of an ester group to the carboxyl group at position 4 enables the bioavailability of oral cephalosporins to be increased. The chemical structures of all of the oral cephalosporins discussed in this chapter are illustrated in Fig. 3, 4, 5, 6, and 7.

5. ANTIBACTERIAL ACTIVITY

The in vitro activity of oral cephalosporins is well documented. In general, studies of more than 10 isolates and using broth or agar dilution methods with bacterial inocula of 10^4 to 10^6 CFU/ml are considered in this review. The natural antibacterial spectrum of oral cephalosporins covers gram-positive cocci, gram-negative cocci, and some gram-negative bacilli. Numerous studies have been conducted to determine the in vitro activity of oral cephalosporins against common pathogens.

5.1. Factors Affecting In Vitro Activity

It is well known that the inoculum size and the susceptibility test media may affect the activity of β-lactams. The inoculum size effect will be more or less pronounced in all strains producing β-lactamases.

For some bacterial species, MICs of cefpodoxime were determined in different media, at different pHs, with and without human or horse serum and at different inoculum sizes.

Human serum had little effect on MICs and minimum bactericidal concentrations, (Wise et al., 1990) and this was mirrored in the low protein binding, which is 14.3 and 18.3% at 1 and 5 μg/ml, respectively. Horse serum addition also had no effect on MICs (Nishino et al., 1988) (Table 3).

The different culture media did not affect the in vitro activity of cefpodoxime (Chantot et al., 1991; Knothe et al.,

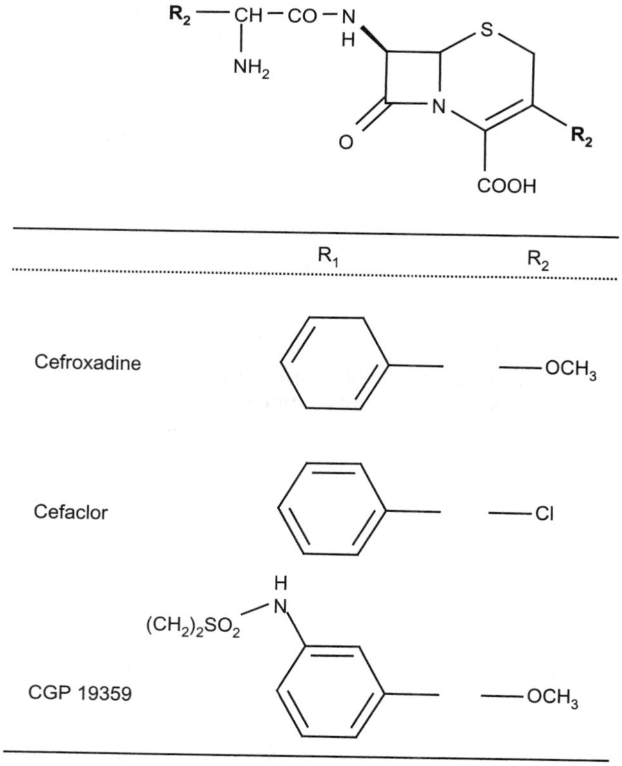

Figure 4 3-Methylcephems (group IB)

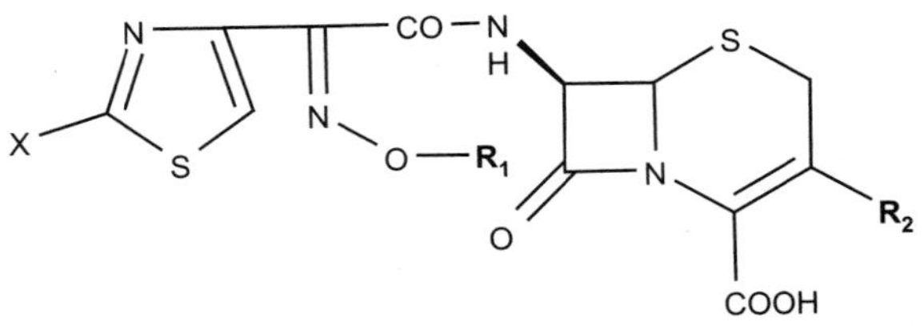

	X	R2	R2
Cefixime	—NH2	—CH2COOH	—CH=CH2
FK 089	—H	—CH2COOH	—H
Cefdinir	—NH2	—OH	—CH=CH2
CGP 33098 A	—NH2	—CH2COOH	S —CH2CH2NH2

Figure 5 Oral cephalosporins (2-amino-5-thiazolyl cephems [unesterified])

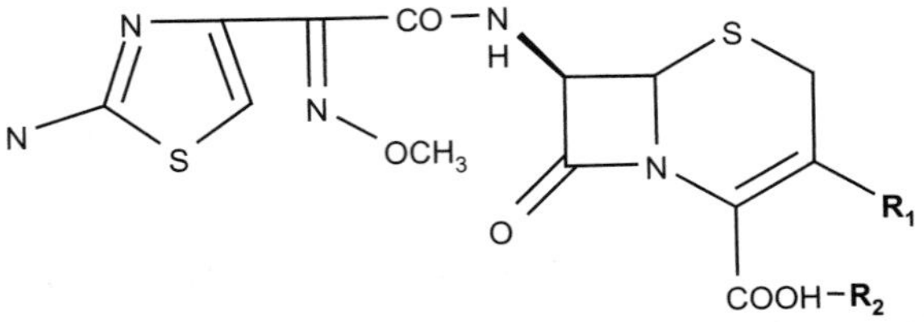

	R1	R2 (ester)
Cefuzonam	—CH2-S— (1,2,3-thiadiazolyl)	—CH(CH3)—O—C(=O)—O—CH2CH3
Cefetamet	—CH3	—CH2-O-CO-C(CH3)3
Cefditoren	—CH=CH— (4-methylthiazolyl, CH3)	—CH2-O-CO-C(CH3)3
Cefpodoxime	—CH2OCH3	—CH(CH3)-O-CO-O-CH(CH3)3
Cefteram	—CH2—N (5-methyltetrazolyl, CH3)	—CH2-O-CO-C(CH3)3

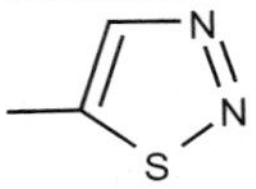

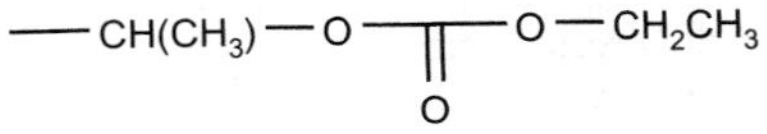

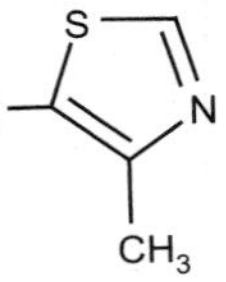

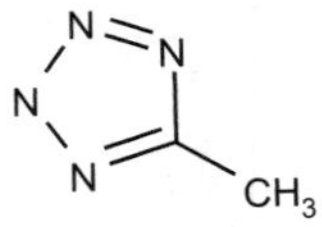

Figure 6 Oral cephalosporins (2-amino-5-thiazolyl cephems [esterified])

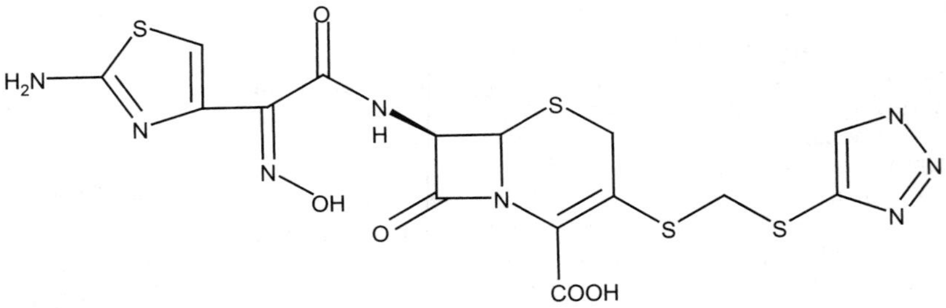

Figure 7 Cefmatilen (S-1090)

Table 3 Effect of horse serum on in vitro activity of cefpodoxime[a]

Strain	MIC (μg/ml) at following % of horse serum:			
	0	10	25	50
S. aureus 209 P-JC	3.13	3.13	3.13	3.13
E. coli NIHJ-JC2	0.39	0.39	0.39	0.39
K. pneumoniae KC-1	0.10	0.10	0.10	0.10
S. marcescens IFO 3736	0.78	0.78	0.78	0.78
P. vulgaris OX-19	0.10	0.10	0.10	0.10

[a]Data from Nishino et al., 1988. Medium H.A (10^6 CFU/ml) was used.

Table 4 Effect of culture medium on in vitro activity of cefpodoxime

Medium	MIC (μg/ml)		
	E. coli 250 HT2	*K. pneumoniae* 238 UC2	*P. mirabilis* 312 UCI
Mueller-Hinton	1.2	0.3	0.04
Nutrient broth 5	0.6	0.15	0.02
AM-3	1.2	0.15	0.04
Trypticase soy broth	0.6	0.15	0.04
Heart-brain broth	0.6	0.15	0.04

1991) (Table 4), nor did the size of the inoculum (Nishino et al., 1988) (Table 5), even against respiratory pathogens (Valentini et al., 1994) (Table 6). The pH of the medium did not significantly affect MICs for gram-negative bacilli (Nishino et al., 1988) (Table 7). At three different temperatures, −4, 22, and 37°C, cefpodoxime at pH 5.0 in distilled water and at pH 7.4 in Mueller-Hinton medium is stable for 168 and 48 h, respectively (Knothe et al., 1991).

The effect of cefpodoxime is modified by large alterations of pH, with a change between pH 5.5 and pH 8.5 causing a 4- to 16-fold variation in MICs. Cefprozil and loracarbef remain unaffected at pH 6 or 8 or in the presence of (inactivated) human serum (Arguedas et al., 1991). However, the in vitro activity drops significantly for both agents at pH 5 and at an inoculum of $>10^5$ CFU/ml.

It is well established that constitutively produced β-lactamases, as well as inducible β-lactamases, contribute to increased MICs. It has been shown that MICs of cefetamet increased to resistant levels for *Enterobacteriaceae* after the inoculum size was raised from 10^5 to 10^7 CFU/ml (Neu et al., 1986).

Increasing the inoculum from 10^5 to 10^7 CFU/ml resulted in a 15- to 50-fold increase in the MIC of cefixime for *E. coli*,

Table 5 Effect of inoculum size on activity of cefpodoxime[a]

Strain	MIC (μg/ml) at following inoculum size (CFU/ml):			
	10^5	10^6	10^7	10^8
S. aureus 209 P-JC	3.13	3.13	3.13	3.13
E. coli NIHJ-JC2	0.39	0.78	0.78	0.78
K. pneumoniae KC-1	0.05	0.10	0.20	0.20
S. marcescens IFO 3736	0.78	0.78	1.56	1.56
P. vulgaris OX-19	0.025	0.05	0.05	0.10

[a]Data from Nishino et al., 1988. Medium HIA (10^6 CFU/ml) was used.

Table 6 Effect of inoculum size on in vitro activity of cefpodoxime against respiratory pathogens[a]

Strain[b]	MIC (μg/ml) at following inoculum size (CFU/ml)			
	10^6	10^7	10^8	10^9
S. pyogenes DB 013SF	0.01	0.01	0.01	0.01
S. pneumoniae DB 038SR	0.01	0.01	0.01	0.01
H. influenzae β^-	0.06	0.06	0.06	0.06
H. influenzae β^+	0.06	0.06	0.06	0.06
M. catarrhalis β^-	0.5	0.5	0.5	0.5
M. catarrhalis β^+	0.25	0.25	0.25	0.25

[a]Data from Valentini et al., 1994.
[b]β^-, non-β-lactamase producing; β^+, β-lactamase producing.

Table 7 Effect of pH on in vitro activity of cefpodoxime

Strain	MIC (μg/ml) at following pH:		
	5.5	7.0	8.5
S. aureus 209 P-JC	0.20	3.13	3.13
E. coli NIHJ-JC2	0.78	0.78	0.39
K. pneumoniae KC-1	0.20	0.10	0.10
S. marcescens IFO 3736	1.56	0.78	0.78
P. vulgaris OX-19	0.05	0.05	0.05

[a]Data from Nishino et al., 1988. Medium H.A (10^6 CFU/ml) was used.

Enterobacter cloacae, *P. mirabilis*, *Serratia marcescens*, *Morganella morganii*, and *K. pneumoniae* (Neu et al., 1984).

5.2. In Vitro Activities

5.2.1. Gram-Positive Bacteria

Like other β-lactams, oral cephalosporins are inactive against *Listeria monocytogenes*. They are inactive against *Corynebacterium jeikeium*.

For staphylococcal species, they are, like all available β-lactamas, inactive against methicillin-resistant isolates. For *S. aureus* isolates susceptible or resistant to penicillin G, two kinds of oral cephems can be described. One subgroup is inactive against *S. aureus*; this subgroup includes cefixime (MIC at which 50% of the isolates tested are inhibited [MIC_{50}], ≥16 μg/ml), cefetamet (MIC, >64 μg/ml), and ceftibuten (MIC_{50}, >64 μg/ml). Loracarbef and cefaclor are less active against penicillin G-resistant isolates, showing a certain degree of susceptibility to hydrolysis by penicillinases produced by *S. aureus*. Among the other cephems, the most active compound is cefdinir ($MIC_{50/90}$, 0.5 μg/ml) whatever the strain, due to its chemical structure (hydroxyimino residue at C-7 position) (Table 8).

Against *S. epidermidis*, ceftibuten, cefetamet, and cefixime are inactive. Other cephalosporins exhibit good activity. However, against penicillin G-resistant isolates of *S. epidermidis*, cefprozil, cefaclor, and loracarbef are less active, with two populations, one susceptible and one resistant. Against coagulase-negative staphylococci, cefetamet, ceftibuten, and cefixime are inactive. The most active compound is cefdinir. Other compounds show the same activity (Table 9).

Table 8 In vitro activities of oral cephems against *S. aureus*[a]

Drug	MIC (μg/ml)			
	S. aureus Pen[s]		*S. aureus* Pen[r]	
	50%	90%	50%	90%
Cefadroxil	2	4	4	8
Cefaclor	2	4	8	16
Loracarbef	1	2	4	16
Cefprozil	0.5	0.5	1	4
Cefuroxime	1	2	2	2
Cefpodoxime	2	4	4	4
Cefixime	16	32	16	32
Cefetamet	>64	>64	>64	>64
Ceftibuten	>64	>64	>64	>64
Cefdinir	0.5	0.5	0.5	0.5
Cefmatilen	0.02	0.05	0.2	0.7

[a]Data from Bauernfeind and Jungwirth, 1991; Felmingham et al., 1994; and Nishino et al., 1997.

All cephalosporins are inactive against *E. faecalis*, *Enterococcus faecium*, and *Enterococcus liquefaciens* (MIC, ≥64 μg/ml).

Against beta-hemolytic streptococci (Lancefield groups A, B, C, and G) (Tables 10, to 13), all compounds show good in vitro activity, except ceftibuten, which is inactive against *Streptococcus agalactiae* (group B streptococci) (Table 10).

Against viridans group streptococci, cefetamet, ceftibuten, cefaclor, and cefadroxil are weakly active or inactive. Cefixime ($MIC_{50/90}$, 0.5/4 μg/ml) and loracarbef ($MIC_{50/90}$, 1/4 μg/ml) are less active than other compounds (MIC_{50}s and MIC_{90}s ranged from 0.03 to 0.25 μg/ml). Against *S. pneumoniae*, Baquero and Loza (1994) have defined three subgroups of cephalosporins against penicillin-susceptible isolates. Cefixime, ceftibuten, and cefetamet are the least active compounds. One of the most active is cefditoren (Table 14).

Table 9 In vitro activities of oral cephalosporins against coagulase-negative staphylococci

Drug	$MIC_{50/90}$ (μg/ml)					
	S. epidermidis	*Staphylococcus haemolyticus*	*Staphylococcus simulans*	*Staphylococcus hominis*	*S. saprophyticus*	*Staphylococcus cohnii*
Cefadroxil	2/2	2/4	2/4	2/4	2/4	8/8
Cefaclor	1/2	1/2	1/2	0.5/4	1/8	4/8
Loracarbef	1/1	1/2	2/2	1/4	2/4	2/8
Cefprozil	0.5/0.5	0.5/2	0.5/0.5	1/2	1/1	2/2
Cefuroxime	0.5/1	1/2	0.5/1	0.25/1	2/4	2/4
Cefpodoxime	1/1	2/4	1/2	1/2	4/8	8/8
Cefixime	4/8	16/32	8/16	4/8	32/64	64/>64
Cefetamet	8/16	16/>64	16/32	8/32	64/>64	>64/>64
Ceftibuten	16/32	64/>64	64/>64	8/>64	>64/>64	>64/>64
Cefdinir	0.06/0.1	0.1/0.5	0.06/0.1	0.06/0.1	0.25/0.25	0.25/1
Cefmatilen	8.0/64	2.0/128			0.39/1.56	

[a]Data from Bauernfeind and Jungwirth, 1991, and Nishino et al., 1997.

Table 10 In vitro activities of oral cephalosporins against group B streptococci (*S. agalactiae*)[a]

Drug	MIC (μg/ml)		
	50%	90%	Range
Cefteram	0.125	0.25	<0.015–2
Cefetamet	1	1	0.5–2
Cephalexin	1	8	0.125–8
Cefaclor	0.5	8	0.125–8
Cefpodoxime	0.06	0.25	0.03–0.25
Cefixime	1.0	2.0	0.5–2
Cefdinir	0.016	0.03	0.008–0.03
Ceftibuten	16	16	16
Cefprozil	0.03	0.06	0.016–0.13
Cefadroxil	0.25	0.25	0.06–0.25
Loracarbef	0.06	0.5	0.06–0.5
Cefdaloxime	0.03	0.06	0.016–0.13
Cefuroxime	0.03	0.06	0.016–0.13
Cefditoren	0.016	0.03	0.016–0.06
Cefcamate	0.03	0.06	0.03–0.03
Cefotiam	0.5	0.25	0.125–0.25
Cefmatilen	0.01	0.03	0.01–0.03

[a]Data from Bauernfeind and Jungwirth, 1991; Knothe et al., 1991; and Neu et al., 1986.

Table 11 In vitro activities of oral cephalosporins against group A streptococci (*S. pyogenes*)[a]

Drug	MIC (μg/ml)		
	50%	90%	Range
Cefteram	≤0.015	0.25	≤0.015–0.25
Cefetamet	0.03	0.5	≤0.15–1
Cephalexin	0.25	4	0.06–4
Cefaclor	≤0.06	2	0.06–4
Cefpodoxime	0.03	0.06	0.016–0.06
Cefixime	0.13	0.25	0.13–0.5
Cefdinir	0.016	0.03	0.008–0.06
Ceftibuten	1	1	0.25–4
Cefprozil	0.03	0.06	0.016–0.13
Cefadroxil	0.13	0.25	0.06–0.25
Loracarbef	0.13	0.13	0.06–0.5
Cefdaloxime	0.016	0.06	0.016–0.06
Cefuroxime	0.03	0.06	0.016–0.25
Cefditoren	≤0.025	≤0.025	≤0.025
Cefcamate	0.008	0.008	0.008–0.016
Cefotiam	0.03	0.06	<0.015–0.06
Cefmatilen	0.006	0.008	0.006–0.008

[a]Data from Bauernfeind and Jungwirth, 1991; Knothe et al., 1991; Neu et al., 1986; and Tamura et al., 1988.

5.2.2. Gram-Negative Bacteria

In terms of activity against *Proteus* and *Providencia* spp., it is possible to divide the oral cephems into two subgroups, those which are poorly active (cefuroxime) and inactive (cefadroxil, loracarbef, cefaclor, and cefprozil) and those which display good in vitro activity, such as cefpodoxime, cefixime, cefetamet, ceftibuten, and cefdinir. However, cefdinir is poorly active against *Proteus vulgaris* (Table 15).

In terms of activity against *Enterobacteriaceae* which are known to produce type 1 β-lactamases, such as *E. cloacae*, *S. marcescens*, *Citrobacter freundii*, and *M. morganii*, oral

Table 12 In vitro activities of oral cephalosporins against group G streptococci[a]

Drug	MIC (μg/ml)		
	50%	90%	Range
Cefteram	0.25	2	≤0.015–4
Cefetamet	0.13	0.5	0.13–0.5
Cephalexin	1	8	0.125–8
Cefaclor	0.06	0.25	0.016–0.25
Cefpodoxime	0.03	0.06	0.016–0.06
Cefixime	0.13	0.25	0.13–0.5
Cefdinir	0.016	0.016	0.008–0.03
Ceftibuten	1.0	1.0	0.5–1
Cefprozil	0.03	0.06	0.016–0.12
Cefadroxil	0.13	0.25	0.06–0.25
Loracarbef	0.13	0.13	0.06–0.25
Cefdaloxime	0.03	0.03	0.016–0.06
Cefuroxime	0.03	0.06	0.016–0.13
Cefotiam	0.03	0.06	<0.015–0.06

[a]Data from Bauernfeind and Jungwirth, 1991; Knothe et al., 1991; and Neu et al., 1986.

Table 13 In vitro activities of oral cephalosporins against group C streptococci[a]

Drug	MIC (μg/ml)		
	50%	90%	Range
Cefteram	0.25	2	≤0.015–4
Cefetamet	0.13	0.5	0.03–0.5
Cephalexin	1	8	0.125–8
Cefaclor	0.03	0.13	0.016–0.13
Cefpodoxime	0.5	0.5	0.03–0.5
Cefixime	0.5	1	0.25–1
Cefdinir	0.008	0.016	0.008–0.016
Ceftibuten	1.0	1.0	0.5–1
Cefprozil	0.016	0.03	0.016–0.03
Cefadroxil	0.06	0.13	0.06–0.13
Loracarbef	0.06	0.13	0.06–0.13
Cefdaloxime	0.016	0.03	0.016–0.03
Cefuroxime	1.0	1.0	0.016–1
Cefotiam			

[a]Data from Bauernfeind and Jungwirth, 1991, and Neu et al., 1986.

cephems can be also divided into two subgroups: (i) compounds totally inactive, e.g., cefadroxil, cefaclor, loracarbef, cefprozil, cefuroxime, and, to a lesser extent, cefdinir, and (ii) those which could display a bimodal activity, such as ceftibuten, cefixime, and cefpodoxime. Cefetamet is inactive against *E. cloacae* and *M. morganii* but remains active against *S. marcescens*. The four latter compounds showed good activity against *C. freundii* (Table 16).

Cefadroxil is poorly active against *E. coli* isolates. Cefaclor and cefprozil are weakly active against *E. coli* resistant to ampicillin. Cefuroxime is also moderately active against *E. coli*, whatever its susceptibility to ampicillin. The 2-amino-5-thiazolyl derivatives cefixime, cefpodoxime, cefetamet, and ceftibuten display identical in vitro activities against *E. coli*.

Table 14 In vitro activities of oral cephalosporins against *S. pneumoniae*[a]

Cephalosporin	MIC (μg/ml)					
	Pen[s]		Pen[i]		Pen[r]	
	50%	90%	50%	90%	50%	90%
Penicillin G	0.015	0.03	0.5	1.0	2.0	4.0
Cefdinir	≤0.06	0.125	0.25	2.0	4.0	8.0
Cefuroxime	0.03	0.03	0.5	4.0	4.0	8.0
Cefpodoxime	0.03	0.06	0.5	2.0	4.0	4.0
Cefaclor	0.5	1.0	4.0	64	64	128
Cefixime	0.25	0.25	4.0	32	32	32
Cefditoren	0.01	0.01	0.25	0.5	1.0	1.0
Cefprozil	0.03	0.125	0.5	4.0	4.0	16.0
Cefetamet	0.25	1.0	4.0	>32.0	4.0	>32.0
Loracarbef	1.0	2.0	4.0	32	≥32	≥32
Cefotiam	0.125	0.25	1.0	4.0	4.0	16

[a]Data from Barry et al., 1997; Frémaux et al., 1993; Linares et al., 1996; Sifaoui et al., 1996; Spangler et al., 1996; and Yee and Thornsberry, 1994.

Table 15 In vitro activities of oral cephems against *Proteus* and *Providencia* spp.

Drug	$MIC_{50/90}$ (μg/ml)			
	P. mirabilis	*P. vulgaris*	*P. rettgeri*	*Providencia stuartii*
Cefadroxil	8/8	>64/>64	>64/>64	32/>64
Cefaclor	4/4	>64/>64	>64/>64	>64/>64
Loracarbef	2/2	>64/>64	64/>64	32/>64
Cefprozil	8/16	>64/>64	16/>64	64/>64
Cefuroxime	4/4	>64/>64	2/8	2/4
Cefpodoxime	0.06/0.1	0.13/1.0	0.06/0.5	0.06/0.5
Cefixime	0.01/0.06	0.01/0.03	0.01/0.1	0.01/0.1
Cefetamet	0.06/0.1	0.12/0.25	0.06/0.25	0.03/0.15
Ceftibuten	0.03/0.03	0.03/0.06	0.008/0.12	0.01/0.06
Cefdinir	0.13/ 0.5	8/32	0.06/0.25	0.06/2
Cefmatilen	0.06/0.12	128/>128	0.5/32	0.1/6.25

Table 16 In vitro activities of oral cephalosporins against *E. cloacae*, *S. marcescens*, *C. freundii*, and *M. morganii*[a]

Drug	$MIC_{50/90}$ (μg/ml)			
	E. cloacae	*S. marcescens*	*C. freundii*	*M. morganii*
Cefadroxil	>64/>64	>64/>64	>64/>64	>64/>64
Cefaclor	>64/>64	>64/>64	32/>64	>64/>64
Loracarbef	32/>64	>64/>64	8/32	32/64
Cefprozil	>64/>64	>64/>64	64/64	>64/>64
Cefuroxime	>64/>64	>64/>64	4/64	>64/>64
Cefpodoxime	0.5/64	4/64	1/8	0.5/64
Cefixime	2/64	1/16	1/8	2/64
Cefetamet	16/64	2/64	1/2	16/64
Ceftibuten	0.25/32	0.25/2	0.5/4	0.25/32
Cefdinir	16/32	8/64	0.5/16	16/32
Cefmatilen	4.0/128	32/128	0.5/4.0	4.0/16

[a]Data from Bauernfeind and Jungwirth, 1991.

Cefadroxil, cefprozil, and, to a lesser extent, cefuroxime are poorly active against *K. pneumoniae* and *Klebsiella oxytoca*; other compounds show good in vitro activity. Cefpodoxime, cefixime, cefetamet, cefdinir, and ceftibuten show a bimodal activity against *Enterobacter aerogenes* and *Serratia liquefaciens*. Other compounds are inactive against these two microorganisms (Table 17). Except ceftibuten ($MIC_{50/90}$, 0.5/8 μg/ml), other compounds are inactive (MIC, >64 μg/ml) or moderately active, with two populations, such as cefpodoxime, cefixime (MIC_{50}, 4 μg/ml), and cefdinir (MIC_{50}, 2 μg/ml), with MIC_{90}s above 32 μg/ml for *Hafnia alvei*.

Except cefixime ($MIC_{50/90}$, 4/8 μg/ml), the 2-amino-5-thiazolyl cephalosporins show good in vitro activity against *Yersinia enterocolitica*. Cefuroxime and cefixime are poorly active. Other compounds are inactive. Cefadroxil and cefuroxime are inactive or poorly active against *Salmonella* spp. and *Shigella* spp. Other compounds show good activity against these microorganisms, except cefixime, which is weakly active against *Shigella* spp. ($MIC_{50/90}$, 2/2 μg/ml) (Table 18).

All available oral cephalosporins are inactive against *Pseudomonas aeruginosa* (MIC, >64 μg/ml), other *Pseudomonas* spp., *Stenotrophomonas maltophilia*, *Burkholderia cepacia*, and *Acinetobacter baumannii*. They are also inactive against *Bordetella pertussis* (MIC, >64 μg/ml).

In terms of activity against *H. influenzae*, two types of oral cephalosporins can be described: compounds which are inactive (cefadroxil, and cephalexin) and those which are poorly active (cefprozil and loracarbef).

In vitro activities of cefpodoxime, cefuroxime, and cephalexin against *Klebsiella rhinoscleromatis* were tested. $MIC_{50/90}$s for cefuroxime and cefpodoxime were 0.06/0.5 and 0.03/0.06 μg/ml, respectively. *K. rhinoscleromatis* is a nonobligate intracellular pathogen (Mikulicz cells) which is responsible for rhinoscleroma, a chronic granulomatous infection of the upper airway (Perkins et al., 1992).

Other compounds display good activity against *H. influenzae* isolates producing or not producing β-lactamases. However, they are slightly less active or poorly active against *H. influenzae* isolates resistant to ampicillin by a nonenzymatic mechanism (Table 19).

New oral cephem derivatives show good activity against *Moraxella* (*Branhamella*) isolates whether or not the strains produce β-lactamases (Table 20).

5.3. Bactericidal Activity

The bactericidal activities of cefpodoxime, cefuroxime, cefixime, cefaclor, cefdinir, and cefditoren were assessed by means of time-kill kinetics against *S. pneumoniae* isolates with different patterns of resistance to penicillin G.

All oral cephalosporins were bactericidal at four times the MIC after 12 h of contact and yielded 90% killing after 6 h. Cefpodoxime and cefdinir were more bactericidal than cefuroxime, cefaclor, and cefixime. Cefditoren was

Table 17 In vitro activities of oral cephalosporins against *Enterobacteriaceae*

Drug	$MIC_{50/90}$ (μg/ml)					
	E. coli Amp[r]	*E. coli* Amp[s]	*K. pneumoniae*	*K. oxytoca*	*E. aerogenes*	*S. liquefaciens*
Cefadroxil	8/8	8/8	8/16	8/8	>64/>64	>64/>64
Cefaclor	4/8	1/2	0.5/8	0.5/1	>64/>64	>64/>64
Loracarbef	0.5/1	0.5/1	0.5/1	0.5/2	32/>64	>64/>64
Cefprozil	2/8	1/2	4/8	4/8	>64/>64	>64/>64
Cefuroxime	2/4	2/4	2/8	2/8	8/64	>64/>64
Cefpodoxime	0.5/0.5	0.25/0.5	0.1/0.5	0.1/1	1/64	2/64
Cefixime	0.25/0.5	0.25/0.25	0.06/0.25	0.03/0.5	1/64	2/32
Cefetamet	0.25/1	0.25/0.5	0.25/0.5	0.1/0.5	0.5/32	0.5/16
Ceftibuten	0.1/0.25	0.1/0.25	0.06/0.1	0.06/0.1	0.5/64	0.25/8
Cefdinir	0.25/0.5	0.25/0.5	0.1/0.5	0.1/0.25	1/>64	4/>64
Cefmatilen		0.12/0.5	0.10/0.25	0.10/1.0	1.56/1.56	

Table 18 In vitro activities of oral cephalosporins against enteric pathogens

Drug	$MIC_{50/90}$ (μg/ml)		
	Salmonella spp.	*Shigella* spp.	*Y. enterocolitica*
Cefadroxil	8/8	4/8	16/32
Cefaclor	2/8	1/1	16/16
Loracarbef	0.5/1	0.5/1	16/64
Cefprozil	0.5/1	2/8	16/32
Cefuroxime	8/16	2/4	4/4
Cefpodoxime	0.25/0.5	0.25/0.25	1/2
Cefixime	0.03/0.1	2/2	4/8
Cefetamet	0.5/1	0.5/0.5	0.25/2
Ceftibuten	0.03/0.06	0.1/0.25	0.1/0.25
Cefdinir	0.1/0.5	0.1/0.25	0.5/1
Cefditoren	0.5/0.5	0.25/4	

Table 19 In vitro activities of oral β-lactams against *H. influenzae*[a]

Drug	MIC (μg/ml)					
	Amp^s		Amp^r β$^+$		Amp^r β$^-$	
	50%	90%	50%	90%	50%	90%
Amoxicillin	0.5	1	8	128	16	32
Co-amoxiclav	0.5	1	0.5	2	8	16
Cefaclor	4	16	4	32	32	64
Cefuroxime	1	2	1	4	2	8
Cefixime	0.12	0.12	0.03	0.12	0.12	1
Cefdinir	0.12	0.25	0.12	0.25	1	1
Cefotiam	0.5	1.0	0.5	1.0		
Cefpodoxime	0.06	0.125	0.06	0.125	0.125	0.125
Cefprozil	2.0	16	16	≥32		
Cefetamet	0.12	0.25	0.25	0.5	0.5	1.0
Loracarbef	2	4	2	8	8	32
Cefditoren	0.015	0.015	0.008	0.015		
Ceftibuten	0.06	0.06	0.06	0.06	2	4
Cefmatilen	0.12	0.5	0.12	0.5		
Sanfetrinem	0.06	0.125	0.06	0.125	0.25	0.50

[a]Data from Briggs et al., 1991; Dabernat et al., 1991; Debbia et al., 1991; Felmingham et al., 1994; Herrington et al., 1996; Sifaoui et al., 1996; and Williams et al., 1992. β$^+$, β-lactamase producing; β$^-$, non-β-lactamase producing.

Table 20 In vitro activities of oral β-lactams against *M. catarrhalis*

Drug	MIC (μg/ml)			
	β-Lactamase$^-$		β-Lactamase$^+$	
	50%	90%	50%	90%
Amoxicillin	0.25	0.5	32	64
Co-amoxiclav	0.06	0.25	0.12	1.0
Cefaclor	0.5	1.0	1.0	4.0
Cefuroxime	0.5	1.0	1.0	2.0
Cefixime	0.06	0.25	0.25	0.5
Cefpodoxime	0.06	0.12	0.25	0.5
Ceftibuten	0.12	2.0	1.0	4.0
Cefetamet	0.5	0.5	1.0	1.0
Cefdinir	0.03	0.06	0.06	0.12
Loracarbef	≤0.25	≤0.25	1.0	2.0
Cefadroxil	2.0	4.0	4.0	4.0
Cephalexin	2.0	4.0	2.0	4.0
Cefroxadine	2.0	2.0	4.0	16
Cefteram	0.03	0.5	0.12	1.0
Cephradine	2.0	2.0	4.0	8.0
Cefditoren	0.03	0.03	0.5	1.0
Cefmatilen			1.0	2.0

[a]Data from Bauernfeind, 1993; Berk et al., 1996; Brenwald et al., 1996; Briggs et al., 1991; Chaïbi et al., 1995; Dabernat et al., 1990; Doern et al., 1991; Laurans and Orfila, 1991; Neu and Chin, 1994; Sarubbi et al., 1989; Sifaoui et al., 1991; and Stobberingh et al., 1987.

the most bactericidal compound (Table 21) (Spangler et al., 1997).

5.4. Breakpoints

5.4.1. French Breakpoints

The breakpoints for oral cephalosporins recommended in France (CA-SFM) are listed in Table 22.

Table 21 Time-kill of oral cephems against *S. pneumoniae*[a]

Drug	No. of strains for which 99% killing is achieved at 4 × MIC after 6 h
Cefditoren	9
Cefpodoxime	6
Cefdinir	6
Cefaclor	6
Cefuroxime	5
Cefixime	4
Amoxicillin	5

[a]Nine strains were tested.

5.4.2. NCCLS Breakpoints

The breakpoints recommended by the NCCLS (1994) are listed in Table 23.

5.4.3. British (BSAC) Breakpoints

The breakpoints recommended by the British Society for Antimicrobial Chemotherapy (BSAC) are listed in Table 24.

6. EPIDEMIOLOGY OF RESISTANCE

Doern et al. (1996) in an epidemiological survey between November 1994 and April 1995 collected 1,527 clinical isolates of *S. pneumoniae* from 30 different U.S. medical centers. Cephalosporins with high intrinsic activity against penicillin G-susceptible isolates (i.e., cefotaxime, ceftriaxone, cefpodoxime, and cefuroxime) were tested, as well as other cephem derivatives. Of these isolates, 216 (14.1%) were intermediately susceptible to penicillin G and 145 (9.5%) were resistant to penicillin G. The percentage of strains not susceptible to penicillin G varied from 2.1 to 52.9% (Miami, Fla.). Among the oral cephalosporins, the rank order of activity is cefpodoxime ≥ cefuroxime > cefprozil ≥ cefixime > cefaclor = loracarbef > cefadroxil = cephalexin.

Table 22 French breakpoints for oral cephems[a]

Generic name	Breakpoint (μg/ml)		Zone diam (mm)		Load (μg)
	S	R	S	R	
Cefadroxil					
Cephalexin	≤8	>32	≥18	<12	30
Cefradine					
Cefotiam (hexetil)	≤1	>2	≥22	<19	
Cefuroxime (proxetil)		>4	≥26	<20	10
Cefixime	≤1	>2	≥25	<22	
Cefpodoxime (axetil)			≥24	<21	10
Cefaclor			≥22	<16	
Loracarbef	≤2	>8	≥22	<15	10
Cefatrizine			≥23	<14	

[a]S, susceptible; R, resistant.

Table 23 NCCLS breakpoints (1994)[a]

Generic name	Breakpoint (μg/ml)		Zone diam (mm)			Load (μg)
	S	R	S	I	R	
Cephalothin, all tested organisms	≤8	≥32	≥18	15–17	≤14	30
Cefpodoxime						10
Haemophilus	≤2		≥21			
N. gonorrhoeae	≤0.5		≥29			
Other organisms	≤2	≤8	≥21	18–20	≤17	
Cefprozil						30
Haemophilus	≤8	≥32	≥18	15–17	≤14	
Other organisms	≤8	≤32	≥18	15–17	≤14	
Cefuroxime						30
Haemophilus	≤4	≥16	≥20	17–19	≤16	30
N. gonorrhoeae	≤1	≥4	≥31	26–30	≤25	
S. pneumoniae	≥0.5	1	≥2			
Other organisms	≤4	≥32	≥23	15–17	≤14	
Cefaclor						
Haemophilus	≤8	≥32	≥20	17–19	≤16	30
Other organisms	≤8	≥32	≥18	15–17	≤14	
Cefixime						
Haemophilus	≤1		≥21			5
N. gonorrhoeae	≤0.25		≥31			
Other organisms	≤1	≥4	≥19	16–18	≤15	
Loracarbef						
Haemophilus	≤8	≥32	≥18	16–18	≤15	30
Other organisms	≤8	≥32	≥18	15–17	≤14	
Cefetamet						10
Haemophilus	≤4	8	≥18	15–17	≤14	
N. gonorrhoeae	≤0.5		≥29			
Other organisms	≤4	≥16	≥18	15–17	≤14	
Ceftibuten						30
Haemophilus	≤2					
Other organisms	≤8	≥32	≥21	18–20	≤17	

[a]S, susceptible; R, resistant; I, intermediate.

MICs of cefpodoxime are summarized in Table 25.

No breakpoints for *S. pneumoniae* have been given for cefpodoxime by the NCCLS. Breakpoints were given only for cefotaxime, ceftriaxone, and cefuroxime (a MIC of ≥2 μg/ml indicates resistance). In this study, about 12% of the isolates were resistant to cefuroxime.

A total of 723 isolates of *M. catarrhalis* were collected from outpatients in 30 U.S. medical centers between November 1994 and May 1995. The overall rate of β-lactamase producing strains was 95.3% ($n = 689$). NCCLS breakpoints for *H. influenzae* were applied in this study. The proportion of isolates susceptible to cefpodoxime was 99%,

Table 24 BSAC breakpoints (1996)

Drug	MIC (μg/ml)	
	Enterobacteriaceae	*S. aureus, M. catarrhalis, H. influenzae*
Cephradine	2–8	2–8
Cephalexin	2–8	2–8
Cefuroxime	1–4	1
Cefpodoxime	1–4	1
Cefixime	1–4	1

Table 25 Activity of cefpodoxime against *S. pneumoniae* (national surveillance, United States)

Penicillin G phenotype	*n*	MIC (μg/ml)		
		50%	90%	Range
Susceptible	1,165	0.03	0.03	≤0.015–4
Intermediate	216	0.5	2	0.06–>16
Resistant	145	4	16	1–>16

Table 26 Susceptibility of *M. catarrhalis* to cefpodoxime

M. catarrhalis phenotype	*n*	MIC (μg/ml)		
		50%	90%	Range
β-Lactamase$^+$	689	1.0	2.0	0.6–8
β-Lactamase$^-$	34	0.12	0.25	0.06–1

compared to 98.5% for cefuroxime and 99.3% for cefixime (Doern et al., 1996). MICs obtained for cefpodoxime are summarized in Table 26.

In a national surveillance study in the United States, 1,537 isolates of *H. influenzae* were recovered. A total of 36.4% of the isolates were found to produce β-lactamases. Thirty-nine strains intermediately resistant or resistant to ampicillin and 17 β-lactamase-producing strains were also resistant to co-amoxiclav (modal MIC, 32 μg/ml). Modal MICs for oral cephems are higher than those for β-lactamase-producing strains (Doern et al., 1997).

Consecutive isolates of *H. influenzae* were collected by the Public Health Laboratory, Bath, United Kingdom, between June 1992 and June 1993. Of 379 isolates, 40 (10.6%) were β-lactamase producers. The overall resistance rate for cefpodoxime was 0.3% (James et al., 1996) (Table 27).

A total of 352 blood culture isolates of viridans group streptococci obtained form 43 U.S. medical centers during 1993 and 1994 were characterized. High levels of penicillin G resistance were noted among 13.4% of the strains; for 42.9% of the strains, penicillin MICS were 0.25 to 2 μg/ml (intermediately susceptible isolates).

Among the cephalosporins tested, the rank order of activity for five cephalosporins against viridans group streptococci was cefpodoxime = ceftriaxone > cefprozil = cefuroxime > cephalexin. The proportions of isolates resistant (MIC, ≥2 μg/ml) were 15, 17, 18, 20, and 96%, respectively. *Streptococcus mitis* was the most resistant organism and *Streptococcus milleri* was the most susceptible (Doern et al., 1996) (Table 28).

The MICs of a broad set of antibacterials, including cefpodoxime, for *Streptococcus pyogenes, S. pneumoniae, H. influenzae, M. catarrhalis, S. aureus, E. coli, K. pneumoniae, P. mirabilis,* and *Staphylococcus saprophyticus* collected during 1992 were determined (Forsgren and Walder, 1994). β-Lactamase production was found in 10% of *H. influenzae* isolates and 80 to 90% of *S. aureus* and *M. catarrhalis* isolates. Among *H. influenzae* isolates, resistance to ampicillin by a nonenzymatic mechanism was recorded in 3%. Decreased susceptibility to penicillin G was detected in 11% of *S. pneumoniae* isolates. Decreased susceptibility to erythromycin A was detected in 9% of *S. pyogenes* isolates in 1992 (Table 29). All isolates of *S. pyogenes*, including those resistant to erythromycin A (9%), were fully susceptible to cefpodoxime. Eleven of the strains showed decreased susceptibility to penicillin G. Six of them were resistant to co-trimoxazole. One strain was resistant to penicillin G (MIC, 2 μg/ml), and the MIC of cefpodoxime for this isolate was 2 μg/ml. Cefpodoxime was stable against hydrolysis by the TEM-1 β-lactamase of *H. influenzae*. MICs reached 4 μg/ml for *H. influenzae* resistant to ampicillin by a nonenzymatic mechanism.

In one survey (Coonan and Kaplan, 1994), 11 oral antibiotics, including oral cephalosporins, were tested against 282 respiratory tract isolates and 431 isolates from severe or invasive diseases involving group A streptococci. Approximately 83% of the 282 pharyngeal isolates could be serologically characterized. Twenty-one different M types were identified. Over half of these isolates were M type 1, 2, 3, 4, or 12. The isolates from severe group A streptococcal infections were predominantly M types 1 and 3. The MIC_{90} of penicillin G was 0.012 μg/ml; for only one isolate was the MIC 0.024 μg/ml. All of 325 isolates were inhibited by a cephalothin concentration of 0.25 μg/ml or less (MIC_{90}, 0.1 μg/ml). At a concentration of 1 μg/ml, cefaclor inhibited 282 isolates (MIC_{90}, 0.5 μg/ml). The MIC_{90} of cefixime was 0.5 μg/ml; however, for 6% of the isolates (16 of 282 strains) the MICs were above the NCCLS breakpoints. The cefpodoxime MIC_{90} was 0.016 μg/ml. For eight (2.8%) of the isolates, the MICs were of 0.5 μg/ml or greater for macrolides (erythromycin A, clarithromycin, and azithromycin). These eight isolates were susceptible to clindamycin. An efflux mechanism of resistance could be involved. A total of 9.8% of the 325 isolates were resistant to tetracycline (MIC, ≥4 μg/ml). The MIC_{90}s of ciprofloxacin were 0.5 μg/ml. For lightly more than 9% of the isolates tested, the MIC of

Table 27 Activity of cefpodoxime against *H. influenzae* (United Kingdom survey)

Organism phenotype	*n*	MIC (μg/ml)			% Resistant
		50%	90%	Range	
β-Lactamase$^-$	399	0.07	0.18	<0.03–6.6	0.3
β-Lactamase$^+$	40	0.07	0.23	<0.03–0.37	0

Table 28 In vitro activities of oral cephems against *H. influenzae* isolates producing β-lactamases and co-amoxiclav resistant[a]

Drug	Modal MIC (μg/ml)			
	Amp[s] (*n* = 977)	Amp[r] β[+] (*n* = 560)	Amp[r] (β[+]) co-amoxiclav[r] (MIC, ≥8 μg/ml) (*n* = 17)	Amp[r] β[−] (*n* = 29)
Amoxicillin	≤1	32	≥128	≥2
Co-amoxiclav	≤1	≤2	≥8	4
Cefpodoxime	0.06–0.12	0.06	0.06–0.12	0.25–0.5
Cefaclor	4	4	4	16–32
Loracarbef	2–4	4	2–4	16
Cefprozil	4	8	4	32
Cefuroxime	1.0	1	1	4–8
Cefixime	0.03		0.03	0.06

[a]Data from Doern et al., 1997. β, β-lactamases.

Table 29 Activity of cefpodoxime in Swedish epidemiological surveillance

Organism(s)	*n*	MIC (μg/ml)			Breakpoint (μg/ml)
		50%	90%	Range	
S. pyogenes	100	0.015	0.015	0.015–0.03	1
S. pneumoniae	100	0.015	0.12	0.015–2	1
H. influenzae	100	0.12	0.12	0.06–4	1
M. catarrhalis	100	1	2	0.25–4	1
E. coli	100	0.5	0.5	0.12–4	1
Klebsiella spp.	100	0.12	0.5	0.06–2	1
E. cloacae	100	1	4	0.12–≥32	1
P. mirabilis	100	0.06	0.12	0.03–0.25	1
S. aureus	100	4	4	2–4	1
S. saprophyticus	100	8	8	4–≥32	1

[a]Data from Forsgren and Walder, 1994.

ciprofloxacin was ≥1 μg/ml. Numerous reports demonstrated an increase in the prevalence of group A streptococci resistant to erythromycin A, an agent long considered the alternative to penicillin G for patients allergic to that drug.

Cephalosporins showed considerable variation in their in vitro activities against group A streptococci. Cefaclor and cefixime are the least active. Cefixime and cefaclor required 30-fold higher concentrations than cefpodoxime.

6.1. β-Lactamase Interactions

6.1.1. Kinetics of Oral Cephem Hydrolysis by β-Lactamases

The rate of hydrolysis is a measure of the ability of an enzyme to hydrolyze a compound that has bound to its active site. It only measures the activity of the enzyme once the compound has bound. The K_m values establish the affinity of the substrate bound to the enzyme; the higher the value, the less affinity there is for the substrate.

Within the α-amino cephalosporins, cefatrizine and cephradine are more stable against β-lactamase hydrolysis than cefaclor. They are poorly hydrolyzed by TEM-1, TEM-2, OXA-2, OXA-3, and SHV-1. Like cefaclor, they are partially hydrolyzed by *S. aureus* penicillinase. Cephradine and cefatrizine are partially hydrolyzed by *M. catarrhalis* enzyme, while cefaclor is totally hydrolyzed. They are partially hydrolyzed by P99 and K-1 enzymes (Neu et al., 1984).

Cefuroxime, cefetamet, cefixime, and cefpodoxime showed poor affinity for TEM-2 and OXA-1 enzymes. Enzyme produced by *K. oxytoca* hydrolyzed cefaclor and cefpodoxime to some extent, whereas breakdown of cefixime and cefetamet was undetectable. All compounds tested exhibited a high affinity for *E. cloacae* chromosomally encoded enzyme. Cefixime, cefetamet, and cefpodoxime were poor substrates for the enzyme of *P. vulgaris* 4917 (Cullmann and Dick, 1990).

It has been shown that ceftibuten is not hydrolyzed by TEM-3, SHV-2, or SHV-3 enzyme, while cefotaxime, ceftazidime, and aztreonam are affected. All of these compounds are good substrates for SHV-4 and SHV-5 enzymes (Thabaut et al., 1994).

Cefdinir is highly hydrolyzed by TEM-3 compared to cefixime and cefuroxime. Cefuroxime and cefdinir are identically hydrolyzed by TEM-5. They display a higher stability against TEM-4 than does cefixime (Thornber et al., 1991). Cefdinir is not hydrolyzed by *S. aureus* PC-1 enzyme. Cefprozil is hydrolyzed more slowly by *S. aureus* penicillinase than is cefaclor. Cefixime is slightly less stable than cefdinir and cefuroxime against TEM-10 enzyme (Payne and Amyes, 1993). In direct enzyme hydrolysis studies, cefpodoxime has been shown to be resistant to hydrolysis by the following β-lactamases: types I and Ia; most I_C (J20) enzymes; and types II, IIa, IV, IVb, IV (Kc), and V (PSE-1) (Ueda et al., 1988). Compared to cefaclor and cefotaxime, it had been shown that cefpodoxime is stable against hydrolysis by type Ia, IIa, IV, and V β-lactamases (Table 30) (Jones and Barry, 1987).

These data were also obtained by Wise et al. (1990). It has been demonstrated that cefpodoxime is not a good substrate for BRO-1 of *M. catarrhalis*.

Table 30 Relative rate of hydrolysis of cefpodoxime versus that of cephaloridin (100%)

Organism	β-Lactamase type	Relative hydrolysis rate		
		Cefpodoxime	Cefaclor	Cefotaxime
E. cloacae	Ia (P99)	4.7	108	<1.0
E. coli	IIIa (TEM-1)	2.9	122	3.2
K. oxytoca	IV (K-1)	3.7	44	3.2
E. coli	V (CARB-2)	2.5	67	<1.0
E. coli	V (OXA-1)	11.7	339	10.5

Table 31 Hydrolysis of oral cephalosporins by β-lactamases of *M. catarrhalis*

Drug	Relative V_{max}	K_m (μM)
Cefpodoxime	19	72
Cephalexin	30	41
Cefadroxil	22	35
Cefaclor	216	76
Cefteram	10	32

β-Lactamase of *M. catarrhalis* belongs to group 2C of the Busch classification. This enzyme hydrolyzes carbenicillin and is inhibited by clavulanic acid. Cefpodoxime is hydrolyzed less by BRO-1 than is cefaclor but slightly more than cefteram. However, the affinity for the enzyme is higher for cefteram (Takenouchi and Nishino, 1991) (Table 31).

6.1.2. In Vitro Activities of Oral Cephems against Isolates Producing β-Lactamases

Kitzis et al. (1990) have tested the in vitro activities of 15 β-lactams against *K. pneumoniae* and isogenic *E. coli* harboring extended-spectrum β-lactamases. All β-lactams were affected by SHV-4 and SHV-5 enzymes as well as TEM-3 and TEM-4 enzymes. α-Aminocephems were less affected by TEM-1 and TEM-7 enzymes. Cefuroxime is not affected by TEM-7 enzyme. It is poorly active against *E. coli* BM684 harboring SHV-4 and SHV-5 enzymes (Table 32).

Of the 2-amino-5-thiazolyl cephalosporins, all are hydrolyzed by TEM-3 and TEM-5 enzymes. The compounds are slightly less active against isolates harboring SHV-1 enzyme, except cefixime. A decrease of activity was noted for SHV-2 and SHV-3. *E. coli* organisms harboring SHV-5 enzymes are less susceptible to oral cephalosporins except for cefetamet.

These results were confirmed in another study. In addition, other compounds were included and other enzymes were inserted in the panel (*E. coli* CF-604, TEM-5, *E. coli* HB 80-251, TEM-6; and *K. pneumoniae* CHO, CMY-1) (Table 33).

Except for cefdinir, ceftibuten, and cefetamet, all of the compounds tested are inactive against *E. coli* CF-604 (TEM-5) and *E. coli* HB 80-251 (TEM-6). Cefetamet and ceftibuten display good activity against *K. pneumoniae* CF-104 (TEM-3) compared to those of other oral cephems. All of the oral cephems tested are inactive against *K. pneumoniae* CHO (CMY-1).

Cefaclor, cefixime, and cefuroxime are less active than cefdinir against *E. coli* 2639E (TEM-9) (Thornber et al., 1991).

6.1.3. Induction of β-Lactamases

Induction of β-lactamases is an important mechanism of antibiotic resistance in species such as *E. cloacae, E. aerogenes, S. marcescens, M. morganii, C. freundii*, and *P. aeruginosa* (Livermore, 1987). The most effective inducers are those that stimulate β-lactamase production at concentrations below the MIC of the inducer for a given strain.

Ceftibuten can be classified as a weak inducer of the class I β-lactamases of *E. cloacae, E. aerogenes*, and *S. marcescens*, such as cefotaxime (Papanicolaou and Medeiros, 1991).

Cefetamet is a poor inducer of β-lactamase from a selected strain of *E. cloacae* (P99 enzyme), *M. morganii* enzyme, the *K. oxytoca* K-1 enzyme, and the inducible β-lactamases of *P. aeruginosa* (Neu et al., 1989).

Ceftibuten was identified as a potent inhibitor of the class Ia β-lactamase (Jones and Barry, 1988). It has been shown

Table 32 In vitro activities of oral cephalosporins against *E. coli* BM684 harboring various β-lactamases

Drug	MIC (μg/ml)										
	E. coli BM684	TEM-1	TEM-2	TEM-3	TEM-4	TEM-7	SHV-1	SHV-2	SHV-3	SHV-4	SHV-5
Cephalexin	4	8	8	16	16	8	8	32	256	32	128
Cephradine	8	16	16	32	16	16	16	32	128	32	128
Cefadroxil	8	8	8	16	16	8	8	32	64	32	128
Cefaclor	1	4	8	32	32	2	64	32	128	32	128
Cefatrizine	1	8	32	64	64	8	64	64	128	64	256
Cefprozil	2	4	64	64	64	4	64	>256	256	64	256
Cefuroxime	4	4	4	64	64	4	16	16	32	8	128
Cefotiam	0.25	0.25	0.5	2	2	0.5	1	8	16	2	8
Cefpodoxime	0.25	0.5	0.5	64	32	1	8	8	32	8	32
Cefixime	0.25	0.25	0.25	4	8	0.25	0.25	1	1	8	32
Cefetamet	0.25	0.25	0.25	4	8	0.25	1	1	2	1	2
Cefotaxime	0.06	0.06	0.06	8	4	0.12	0.06	4	4	1	4
Ceftazidine	0.12	0.25	0.50	16	8	8	4	4	8	16	64
Aztreonam	0.06	0.06	0.2	4	4	0.25	0.12	2	2	32	128

Table 33 Activities of oral cephems against *Enterobacteriaceae* producing extended-spectrum β-lactamases

Drug	MIC (μg/ml)							
	K. pneumoniae CF-104 (TEM-3)	*E. coli* CF-604 (TEM-5)	*E. coli* HB 80-251 (TEM-6)	*E. coli* (TEM-7)	*K. pneumoniae*			
					SH122 (SHV-2)	197 (SHV-4)	160 (SHV-5)	CHO (CMY-1)
Cefadroxil	16	36	16	8	64	>64	>64	>64
Cefaclor	32	32	8	4	16	>64	>64	>64
Cefprozil	64	64	16	16	8	>64	>64	>64
Loracarbef	16	64	4	2	1	>64	>64	>64
Cefuroxime	64	16	16	8	16	64	64	>64
Cefdinir	4	8	1	0.5	8	8	16	64
Cefetamet	0.5	2	4	0.5	0.5	4	8	>64
Cefpodoxime	3.2	16	16	16	64	64	64	>64
Ceftibuten	0.25	1	1	0.12	0.25	8	8	>64
Cefixime	8	32	2	0.5	0.25	>64	>64	>64
Cefotaxime	32	2	2	0.25	32	32	32	128
Ceftazidime	32	128	256	32	16	32	32	4
Cefoxitin	16	16	4	8	8	8	8	512

that ceftibuten is a weak inducer of class Ia enzyme (Papanicolaou and Medeiros, 1991).

It has been shown that cefpodoxime inhibits the hydrolytic action of β-lactamases from certain strains of *C. freundii, E. cloacae, M. morganii,* and *Providencia inconstans* but does not inhibit β-lactamases from other gram-negative bacteria (Todd, 1994).

Induction of synthesis of chromosomal β-lactamases in *E. cloacae, P. aeruginosa,* indole-positive *Proteus, S. marcescens,* and *C. freundii* with cefpodoxime resulted in a 0.8- to 2.3-fold increase in specific enzyme activity. The corresponding figures after induction with cefoxitin ranged from 24- to 270-fold (Stobberingh et al., 1989) (Table 34).

6.2. Outer Membrane Impermeability

Cefetamet demonstrated greater penetration rate across the outer membrane of *P. vulgaris* and *S. marcescens* than did cefixime, cefaclor, and cefuroxime (Mancini et al., 1992). The ability of cefdinir to penetrate the outer membrane of *E. coli* was 1 order of magnitude lower than that of cefaclor and cephalexin but two times higher than that of cefixime (Mine et al., 1989).

The rate of penetration through OmpF porin of *E. coli* is faster for cefixime, than for cefteram and cefditoren. The penetration rates relative to that of cefazolin (=1) are 0.11, 0.31, and 0.36, respectively (Kawaharajo et al., 1992).

Debbia et al. (1991) studied the in vitro activity of ceftibuten against *E. coli* mutants with outer membrane protein alterations. An *ompF* alteration usually increased the ceftibuten MIC eight-fold, compared with no or two-fold changes for *ompA* or *ompC*, respectively (Table 35).

Table 34 Capacity of cefpodoxime to induce β-lactamase[a]

Organism	Cefpodoxime	Cefoxitin
E. cloacae	0.9–1.3	90–272
P. aeruginosa	1.1–1.6	60–260
Indole^{+} *Proteus*	1.0–1.2	25–41
S. marcescens	0.8–1.1	13–140
C. freundii	0.8	24

[a]Each value is the fold increase in specific β-lactamase activity after induction with cefpodoxime or cefoxitin.

6.3. Alterations of PBPs

Resistance due to alteration of penicillin-binding proteins (PBPs) is far more common in gram-positive than in gram-negative bacteria.

S. pneumoniae possesses six PBPs (1a, 1b, 2a, 2b, 2x, and 3). The affinity of β-lactams for PBPs 1a, 2x, 2b, and 2a decreased in penicillin- and cephalosporin-resistant isolates.

Altered forms of PBPs 1a and 2x with low affinity for 2-amino-5-thiazolyl cephalosporins are present in *S. pneumoniae* strains (Munoz et al., 1992). This phenomenon has been observed in *Neisseria meningitidis, N. gonorrhoeae,* and *H. influenzae* (Philpot-Howard, 1984).

7. PHARMACOKINETICS

Table 36 summarizes the pharmacokinetic properties of the different oral cephalosporins.

7.1. Single Oral Doses

Within the α-aminocephalosporins, the highest peak levels in serum (C_{max}) after a single oral dose of 500 mg was achieved for cephalexin (C_{max}, 20.7 μg/ml), and the lowest was achieved for cefroxadin (C_{max}, 4.9 μg/ml). The C_{max} of cefprozil (10.2 μg/ml) is lower than those of cephradine (17.7 μg/ml) and cefaclor (17.3 μg/ml).

Table 35 In vitro activity of ceftibuten against *E. coli omp* mutants

Genotype	MIC (μg/ml)	
	Ceftibuten	Cefaclor
Control	0.125	1.0
ompA	0.125	0.25
ompC	0.25	2.0
ompF	1.0	4.0

Table 36 Pharmacokinetics of oral cephalosporins after a single oral dose to young healthy volunteers

Generic name	Dose (mg)	*n*	C_{max} (μg/ml)	T_{max} (h)	$AUC_{0-\infty}$ (μg·h/ml)	$t_{1/2}$ (h)	Urinary elimination (%)	Protein binding (%)	Reference
Ceftibuten	200	18	9.85	1.75	42.07	2.01			Barr et al., 1991
	400	18	16.99	2.00	79.18	2.29		63	Barr et al., 1991
	800	18	23.34	1.96	117.55	2.25			Barr et al., 1991
Loracarbef	200	10	6.0	1.0	10.6	1.02			Sitar et al., 1994
	400	10	12.0	2.0	27.8	1.02		25	Sitar et al., 1994
Cefpodoxime proxetil	100	12	1.4	2.4	7.03	2.1	40.0		Tremblay et al., 1990
	200	12	2.6	2.4	14.5	2.3	39.2		Tremblay et al., 1990
	400	12	4.5	8.5	26.5	2.4	23.8	21–33	Tremblay et al., 1990
	800	12	6.9	2.9	46.4	2.9	27.9		Tremblay et al., 1990
Cefotiam hexetil	200	12	2.16	1.55	4.16	1.0	34.75		
	400	12	3.43	2.26	8.52	0.9	31.92	40	
Cefixime	200	12	2.5	4.3	21.4	3.9			Faulkner et al., 1987
	400	12	3.6	3.7	25.7	3.1			Faulkner et al., 1987
	800	12	4.9	4.4	37.7	3.7			Faulkner et al., 1987
	1,600	12	7.8	4.3	56.4	3.5		69	Faulkner et al., 1987
	2,000	12	8.9	3.8	67.0	3.4			Faulkner et al., 1987
Cefteram pivoxil	400	6	4.2	1.5	14.2	1.2		74.6	Patel et al., 1986
	800	6	7.0	1.9	24.8	1.2			
	1,200	6	8.3	1.8	27.3	1.2			
Cefditoren pivoxil	100	5	1.7	1.4	3.7	0.8	19.9		Shimada et al., 1989
	200	5	3.4	2.0	10.0	1.1	19.6	91.5	
	300	5	4.4	2.0	13.7	1.1	21.7		
Cephradine	500	12	17.7	0.8	27.5	0.61	~90		Schwinghammer et al., 1990
	1,000	10	27.7	1.1	4	1.1	84	10–20	Pfeffer et al., 1977
	2,000	5	44.9	1.4	102.5	0.86	89.7		Chow et al., 1979
Cefprozil *cis*	500	8	10.2	1.7	29.7	1.33	71		Shyu et al., 1992
Cefprozil *trans*	500	8	1.2	1.6	3.2	1.33	65		Shyu et al., 1992
Cefprozil *cis*	1,000	6	12.3	2.1	45.9	1.7	56.9		Shyu et al., 1991
Cefprozil *trans*	1,000	6	1.1	1.7	4.3	1.9	37.6	36	Shyu et al., 1991
Cefprozil *cis*	250	12	6.1	1.5	16.1	1.4	69.2		Barbhaiya et al., 1990
Cefprozil *trans*	500	12	11.2	1.4	32.0	1.3	62.1		
Cefaclor	250	12	10.6	0.5	8.7	0.5	66.5		Barbhaiya et al., 1990
	500	12	17.3	0.7	17.5	0.6	78.9		Barbhaiya et al., 1990
	1,000	6	34.6	1.1	74.5	0.7	52.7	25	Lode et al., 1979
Cephalexin	250	16	9.3	0.9	14.0	0.5	~80		Pfeffer et al., 1977
	500	12	20.7	0.7	29.0	0.6	~80	18–20	Pfeffer et al., 1977
	ND[a]	9	28.5	1.2	61.8	0.8	89.6		Finkelstein et al., 1978
	2,000	5	50.5	1.4	116.3	0.86	91.9		Chow et al., 1979
Cefadroxil	300	16	9.8	1.2	26.8	1.05	~80		Pfeffer et al., 1977
	500	12	16.2	1.9	47.4	1.3	~80		Pfeffer et al., 1977
	1,000	6	33.0	1.7	108.5	1.6	89.6	18–20	Lode et al., 1979
Cefatrizine	250	10	4.1	1.6	15.9	1.9	63.6	63	Mastrandrea et al., 1985
	500	10	7.1	1.6	27.7	2.9	62.9		Mastrandrea et al., 1985
	500	12	7.37	1.79	24.38	1.5			Couet et al., 1988
Cefroxadin	250		9.7	1.0	13.4	0.7	97.6	10	Yamasaku et al., 1989
	1,000	6	23.0	1.0	70.1	0.9	78.9		Lode et al., 1979
Cefuroxime axetil	250	12	4.8		12		32	50	Harding et al., 1984
	500	12	4.9	2.3	19		32		Finn et al., 1987
	1,000	6	7.3	1.5	23		30		Sommers et al., 1987
	1,000	23	9.9	2.1	36		30		Williams and Harding, 1984
Cefetamet pivoxil	500	16	4.1	4.0	24.6	2.3	51.3	22	Tam et al., 1989
	1,000	16	7.2	4.23	45.3	2.4	47.4		Tam et al., 1989
	1,500	16	9.4	4.6	64.6	2.5	44.6		Tam et al., 1989
	2,000	16	11.4	4.9	88.3	2.8	44.9		Tam et al., 1989
Cefdinir	200	16	1.0	3.31	4.08	1.43	23.0	73	Richer et al., 1995
	300	16	1.55	3.20	6.53	1.46	17.7		Richer et al., 1995
	400	16	2.15	3.0	8.83	1.43	17.3		Richer et al., 1995
	600	16	2.35	3.22	9.84	1.50	12.7		Richer et al., 1995
Cefmatilen	50	12	2.01	3.17	11.37	2.89	20–30	96.6	Nakashima et al., 1993
	75	12	2.58	3.25	15.06	2.99			Nakashima et al., 1993
	100	12	3.10	3.58	19.25	2.84			Nakashima et al., 1993
	2000	12	4.25	3.83	27.52	3.08			Nakashima et al., 1993

[a]ND, not determined.

After a 400-mg dose, the C_{max} of loracarbef is lower than those achieved by cefaclor after a 500-mg dose (12 versus 17.3 μg/ml) but equivalent to that achieved after a 250-mg single dose of cefaclor. After a 400-mg dose of cefpodoxime proxetil, the C_{max} was higher than that of cefotiam hexetil (4.5 versus 3.4 μg/ml) and identical to that achieved after 500 mg of cefetamet pivoxil or cefuroxime axetil.

Among the nonesterified cephalosporins, cefdinir has a lower C_{max} after a 400-mg single oral dose (C_{max}, 2.15 μg/ml) than does ceftibuten (C_{max}, 6.9 μg/ml). Cefixime has a C_{max} (3.6 μg/ml after a 400-mg single dose) close to those of cefpodoxime proxetil, cefuroxime axetil, and cefotiam hexetil.

The times taken to achieve C_{max} (T_{max}) for the new oral cephems range from 1.0 h for loracarbef to above 4.0 h for cefetamet pivoxil and cefixime. The T_{max} of the majority of oral cephems is independent of the dose. For cefixime, the T_{max} lengthens with an increase in dose: for 50 mg the T_{max} is 2.7 h, and for 2,000 mg it is 8.9 h.

Nonlinearity in the relationship between ascending single oral doses and area under the curve from 0 h to infinity ($AUC_{0-\infty}$) has been noted for the majority of nonesterified cephalosporins and prodrug ester cephalosporins.

For cefpodoxime proxetil, the dose-normalized AUC decreased about 25% over the dose range of 100 to 800 mg (Borin et al., 1995). For cefixime, 35% decreases have been noted for the compared AUCs after 50 and 400 mg (Brittain et al., 1985). For cefetamet pivoxil, the dose-normalized AUC decreased 12% with doses between 500 and 2,000 mg (Tam et al., 1989). A linear relationship between AUC and oral doses has been reported for cefprozil (250 to 1000 mg) (Barbhaiya et al., 1990), ceftibuten (25 to 200 mg) (Nakashima et al., 1988), and cefuroxime axetil (125 to 1,000 mg) (Finn et al., 1987).

Among the new oral cephalosporins, the percentage of protein binding of cefpodoxime is the lowest (21 to 33%). Cefditoren displays the highest degree of protein binding, with about 91.5% of the total concentration in serum being protein bound.

Ceftibuten undergoes substantial (about 10%) conversion to the *trans*-isomer. The cefprozil parent compound consists of *cis*- and *trans*-isomers at the propenyl side chain at position 3 of the cephem nucleus in approximately a 90:10 ratio.

These oral β-lactams are eliminated mainly by the renal route. The two carboxymethyl derivatives, ceftibuten and cefixime, are partly eliminated by bile (Westphal et al., 1994). For these two drugs only 40 and 60% of the absorbed drug is recovered in urine.

The renal clearance of the free drug ranges between 150 and 100 ml/min for cefpodoxime proxetil, cefetamet pivoxil, and ceftibuten. Renal clearances are higher for cefuroxime axetil (360 ml/min) and cefprozil (230 ml/min).

The renal elimination mechanisms are primarily glomerular filtration in the first group and glomerular filtration and tubular secretion in the second. Cefixime shows a low renal clearance (80 ml/min) but displays a high hepatic clearance, 60%.

Cefpodoxime proxetil is an equal-part mixture of a pair of diasteroisomers (A and B) that possess optical activity in their ester moieties. Twenty healthy male volunteers received 100 mg of cefpodoxime proxetil of each form, A and B, as a solution in a crossover design. The mean values for the pharmacokinetic parameters are listed in Table 37.

There was no significant difference between the three forms for T_{max}, AUC, and mean retention time. The C_{max} and AUC were higher for compound A than for the racemate (18.7 and 15.7% higher, respectively; $P < 0.05$). There is no significant difference between the racemate and compound B. However, considering the slight difference between compound A and the racemate, the use of the latter is fully justified (Lenfant et al., 1992).

7.2. Multiple Doses

The pharmacokinetics of cefixime were determined after repeated doses of 200 mg twice a day (b.i.d.) ($n = 14$) (group I) or 400 mg once a day ($n = 13$) (group II) for 15 days.

The pharmacokinetics of cefixime after repeated dosing to steady state were similar to the drug profile after single dosing. There was no accumulation of the drug in serum or urine after the multiple-dose regimen (Faulkner et al., 1987) (Table 38).

Given the relatively short apparent elimination half-lives ($t_{1/2}$s) of the oral cephalosporins (1 to 3 h) and dosing intervals, significant accumulations were not recorded, as shown by comparing the $AUC_{0-\infty}$s after the first dose and the last dose of the regimen. The main pharmacokinetic parameters after multiple doses are listed in Table 39.

8. PHARMACOKINETICS IN SPECIFIC POPULATIONS

8.1. Elderly Subjects

Studies on the pharmacokinetics of loracarbef and cefprozil comparing control groups of young subjects with groups of elderly subjects (age ranges of the groups, 20 to 45 and 60 to

Table 37 Bioavailability of diastereoisomers of cefpodoxime proxetil

Form of drug	C_{max} (μg/ml)	T_{max} (h)	$AUC_{0-\infty}$ (μg·h/ml)	CL_R (liters/h)	MRT (h)
Racemate	1.34	2.08	7.0	6.4	4.2
Isomer A	1.59	2.17	8.1	6.1	4.3
Isomer B	1.19	2.38	6.5	6.1	4.3

Table 38 Pharmacokinetics of multiple oral doses of cefixime in healthy volunteers

Parameter (unit)	Day 1		Day 8		Day 15	
	I	II	I	II	I	II
C_{max} (μg/ml)	1.7	2.8	1.8	3.0	1.9	2.7
T_{max} (h)	4.3	4.4	3.1	4.0	3.3	4.0
$AUC_{0-\infty}$ (μg · h/ml)	13.6	24.0	11.9	24.2	12.6	21.6
$t_{1/2}$ (h)	3.4	3.7	3.4	3.7	3.3	4.0
Urinary elimination (%)	14.5	12.4	12.5	11.7	11.9	9.9

Table 39 Pharmacokinetic parameters of oral cephalosporins after multiple doses

Drug	Dose (mg)	Day	C_{max} (μg/ml)	T_{max} (h)	$AUC_{0-\infty}$ (μg·h/ml)	$t_{1/2\beta}$ (h)	Reference
Cefprozil	500	1	11.5	2.3	33.3	0.97	Lode et al., 1992
	500	8	9.3	1.7	27.5	0.91	Lode et al., 1992
Ceftibuten	200	1	10.6		45.7	18.8	Nakashima et al., 1988
	200	14	10.9		49.7	2.2	Nakashima et al., 1988
Cefixime	400	1	2.76		24.6	3.7	Faulkner et al., 1987
	400	15	2.67		19.9	4.0	Faulkner et al., 1987
Cefpodoxime proxetil	200	1	2.2	3.1	11.8	2.7	Tremblay et al., 1990
	200	5	2.3	2.3	11.8	2.3	Tremblay et al., 1990
Cefuroxime axetil	500	1	8.6	2.4	30.3		Sommers et al., 1984
	500	21	9.0	1.8	28.6		Sommers et al., 1984
Cefetamet pivoxil	1,000	1	7.4	4.0	45.7	2.3	Koup et al., 1988
	1,000	10	6.0	4.3	42.5	2.8	Koup et al., 1988
Cefmatilen	200	1	4.86		27.8		Nakashima et al., 1993
	200	15	3.98		24.9		

80 years, respectively) showed that their pharmacokinetics were little affected in the latter population, apart from a slight reduction in total clearance proportional to the decline in glomerular filtration rate observed with age. In fact, the $t_{1/2}$ was slightly prolonged in this age group. However, these differences do not appear to require a dosage adaptation in elderly subjects, subject to the recommendations for use with respect to the greater sensitivity of this population to adverse effects.

In addition, two studies with cefuroxime axetil comparing elderly subjects and middle-aged subjects showed that the $t_{1/2}$, C_{max}, and AUC were slightly increased in elderly subjects. However, the differences observed do not appear to require dosage modifications in this age group.

Some pharmacokinetic studies have shown that for cefixime the AUC, C_{max}, and $t_{1/2}$ were all increased in elderly subjects compared to young adults. The increases were on the order of 20 to 40% depending on the studies. For ceftibuten, the results were similar to those observed with cefixime, with increases of 30 to 50% in the kinetic parameters mentioned above.

Finally, the pharmacokinetic studies conducted with cefetamet pivoxil and cefpodoxime proxetil in elderly subjects showed that there was a slight reduction in total clearance, causing increased $t_{1/2}$s in elderly subjects. However, these changes do not appear to require dosage modifications except in the presence of severe underlying renal insufficiency.

In nonfasting elderly patients, $t_{1/2}$, T_{max}, and AUC increased slightly, while there were no differences in C_{max} and urinary elimination. After a single oral dose of AS-924, the conjugated carnitine increased slightly from 2 to 6 h after dosing.

Several factors influencing pharmacokinetic parameters, such as glomerular filtration, protein concentration, metabolic capacity, and hepatic and renal blood flow, are reduced in the elderly.

Age-related alterations in renal function appear to have the greatest potential influence on the pharmacokinetics of oral cephalosporins. These compounds are not highly protein bound, nor do they undergo significant hepatic metabolism. The glomerular filtration rate decreases by about 35% after the age of 65 years.

Increases in $t_{1/2}$ and AUC have been reported for elderly subjects (Table 40).

The bioavailability values for cefetamet pivoxil and cefpodoxime proxetil in young volunteers were comparable to those in elderly patients. The $t_{1/2}$s for both compounds are significantly prolonged in the elderly as a result of the age-related impairment of renal function. The AUC of cefixime was significantly higher in the elderly than in the young,

Table 40 Pharmacokinetics of oral cephalosporins in the elderly

Drug	Age (yrs)[a]	n	Dose (mg)	C_{max} (μg/ml)	T_{max} (h)	AUC (μg·h/ml)	$t_{1/2\beta}$ (h)	F (%)	Reference
Cefpodoxime proxetil	Y, 31.7 ± 2.2	15	100	1.3	2.7	7.3	2.4		Tremblay et al., 1990
	E, 70.8 ± 1.0	9	100	1.4	3.1	9.0	2.9		Tremblay et al., 1990
Cefetamet pivoxil	Y, 29.5 ± 5	12	1,000	6.2	4.0	39.7	2.2	51.0	Blouin et al., 1989
	E, 69 ± 4	12	1,000	6.8	4.2	47.2	2.8	46.5	Blouin et al., 1989
Cefuroxime axetil	Y	10	500	11.1	1.8	36.4	1.4		Harding et al., 1984
	E, 65–83	10	500	10.3	2.8	59.4	2.4		Veyssier et al., 1988
Cefixime	Y, 20–32	12	400	3.9	3.7	28.6	3.2		Faulkner et al., 1988
	E, 65–74	12	400	4.9	4.2	41.0	3.9		
Cephradine	Y	10	1,000	27.7	1.1		1.1		
	E	9	1,000	35.1	1.1		1.7		
Cefdinir	E, 74–77	3	100	0.85	3.0	4.2	1.8		Shiba et al., 1989
	E, 74–77	2	200	1.15	3.5	6.6	1.9		

[a]Y, young; E, elderly. Means ± standard deviations or ranges are shown.

whereas C_{max} and urinary recovery values did not differ significantly with age.

The pharmacokinetics of cefprozil in young and aged persons (41 to 60 years and 61 to 80 years, respectively) were determined (Wieseman and Benfield, 1993). The $t_{1/2}$s in the elderly were greater than those in younger subjects. After intravenous infusion of cefetamet sodium salt (500 mg) in 12 elderly patients (69 ± 4 years [mean ± standard deviation]) and 12 young volunteers (29 ± 5 years), the total body clearance was on average 22% lower in the elderly (119 versus 155 ml/min), which could be due to reduced renal clearance (88 versus 119 ml/min) in the aged group.

Cefmatilen is metabolized to at least seven metabolites (Fig. 8). The metabolites are a consequence either of a breakdown of the 7-side chain and oxidation or carboxylation of the link moiety (M5 to M7), or opening of the β-lactam ring (carbonyl lactam bound) and cyclization of the obtained compounds (M1 to M4), or movement in space of the hydroxy group on the oxyimino moiety—to an *anti* position instead of a *syn* position (M8).

Cephradine was administered to young and elderly subjects either by the intravenous route (5 min) or orally. After a 1-g administration, the total body clearance was reduced by 45% in elderly patients (4.81 versus 2.64 ml/min/kg), resulting in a corresponding increase in mean AUC by 53% and $t_{1/2}$ by 53%. Renal clearance was reduced (4.11 versus 2.38 ml/min/kg). The relative bioavailability remained unchanged (94 versus 94.8%).

8.2. Children (Excluding Neonates)

According to the available data, it appears that the pharmacokinetics of the following oral cephalosporins are not altered in children: cephalexin, cephradine, cefadroxil, cefaclor, cefprozil, cefixime, and loracarbef. Dosages equivalent to those used in adults per unit of body surface area are therefore recommended.

In the case of cefetamet pivoxil, the pharmacokinetic parameters appear to be similar to those observed in adults after adjustment for body surface area. Thus, doses equivalent to those used in young adults per unit of body surface area are recommended (Table 41).

8.3. Penetration of Oral Cephems in MEF

As highlighted by Bluestone (1992), adequate penetration of new drugs into the middle ear fluid (MEF) of patients with otitis media should be demonstrated.

After administration of 25 mg of oral cephalexin per kg of body weight, the average level in serum achieved at 90 min was 25 μg/ml and levels in MEF were 5 μg/ml (range, 3.1 to 6.5 μg/ml). Concentrations in MEF were lower in younger patients (1 to 24 months) than in older patients (McLin, 1973).

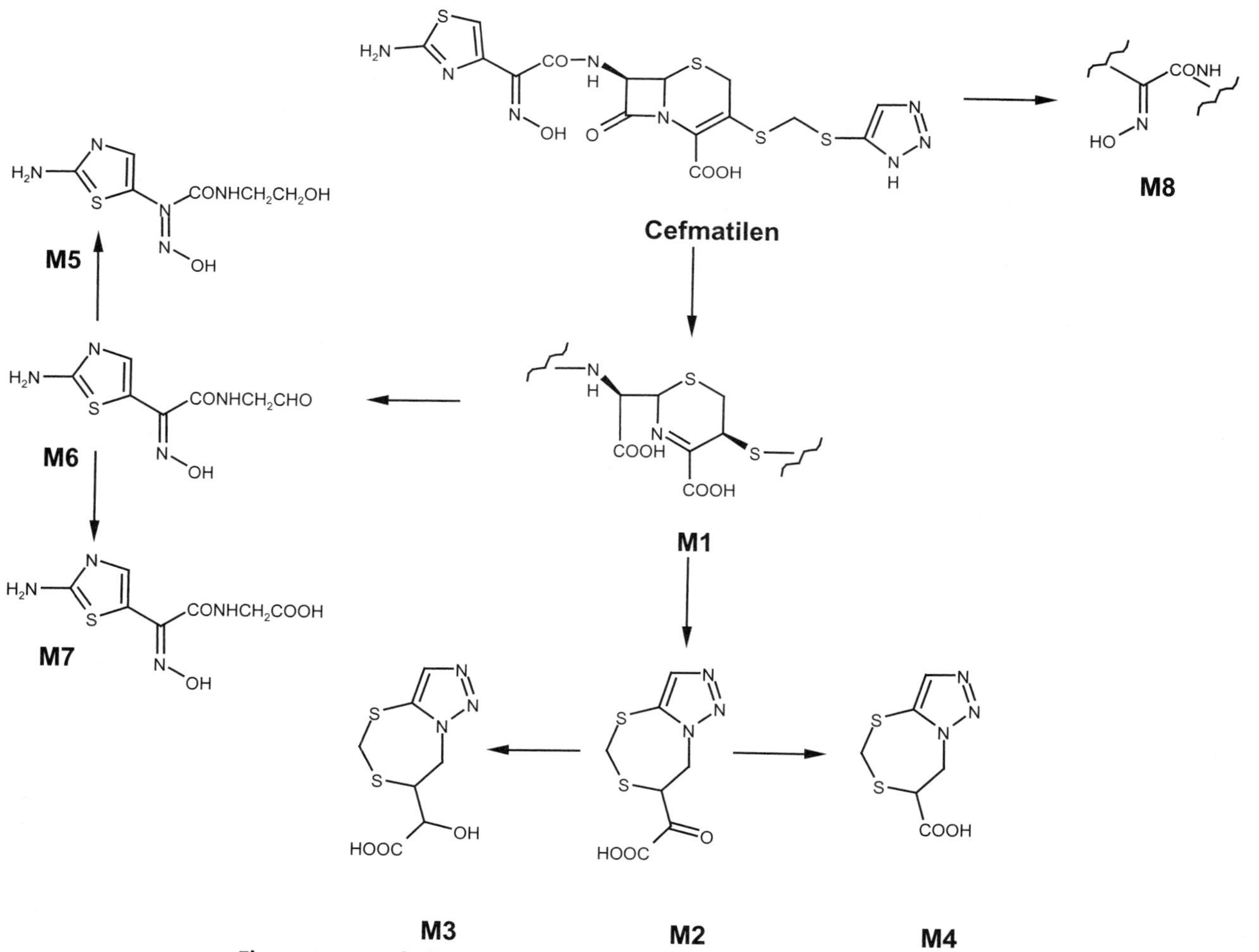

Cefmatilen

M1

M2

M3

M4

M5

M6

M7

M8

Figure 8 Metabolism of cefmatilen (adapted from Nishino et al., 2000)

Table 41 Pharmacokinetics of oral cephalosporins in children[a]

Drug	Age	*n*	Isomer	Dose (mg/kg)	C_{max} (μg/ml)	T_{max} (h)	AUC (μg·h/ml)	Urinary elimination (%)	$t_{1/2\beta}$ (h)	Reference(s)
Loracarbef	4.6–16.7 yr	8		7.5	10.6	0.78	21.4	32–94	1.23	Nahata and Koranyi, 1992
	0.5–16.6 yr	10		15	18.0	0.83	35.6	26–93	1.13	Nahata and Koranyi, 1992
Cefpodoxime proxetil	1.0–17.2 yr	30		2.7–5	2.24	2.55	11.4	1.45	47.1	Kearns et al., 1994; Motohiro et al., 1989
	8–11 yr	3		3	2.0	2.0	10.85	44.7	2.03	Motohiro et al., 1989
		3		6	4.27	2.0	21.80	43.5	2.23	Motohiro et al., 1989
Ceftibuten	0.5–4 yr	20	*cis*	9	16.2	2.2	72.7	2.38		Barr et al., 1993
			trans	9	3.2	2.5	13.9			Barr et al., 1993
			cis	13.5	23.2	2.6	114.8	2.44		Barr et al., 1993
			trans	13.5	3.9	2.6	20.1			Barr et al., 1993
	0.5–3 yr	4	*cis*	4.5	5.3		19.4	1.5	45.7	Barr et al., 1993
	3–5 yr	6	*cis*	4.5	8.3		28.6	1.8	51.3	Barr et al., 1993
	6–11 yr	6	*cis*	4.5	9.1		33.6	2.1	38.6	Barr et al., 1993
	12–17 yr	9	*cis*	4.5	8.1		37.1	2.2	50.3	Barr et al., 1993
	0.5–3 yr	15	*cis*	9.0	9.0		38.7	1.9	45.6	Barr et al., 1993
	3–5 yr	15	*cis*	9.0	9.0		38.7	1.9	45.6	Barr et al., 1993
	6–11 yr	9	*cis*	9.0	16.2		69.1	2.0	54.2	Barr et al., 1993
	12–17 yr	5	*cis*	9.0	16.3		78.4	2.5	56.9	Barr et al., 1993
Cefprozil	8 mo–8 yr	9	*cis*	15	11.6	1.2	28.0	1.8		Saez-Lorens et al., 1990
	8 mo–8 yr	9	*trans*	15	11.6	1.2	2.9	1.7		Saez-Lorens et al., 1990
	8 mo–8 yr	9	*cis*	30	15.1	1.6	44.1	2.1		Saez-Lorens et al., 1990
	8 mo–8 yr	9	*trans*	30	1.6	1.7	4.3	1.6		Saez-Lorens et al., 1990
Cefuroxime axetil	1 mo–11 yr	11		12	3.9		11.3			Ginsburg et al., 1985
	11–68 mo	22		15	4.6		12.6			Ginsburg et al., 1985
				20	5.1		18.5			Ginsburg et al., 1985
Cefixime	2–22 mo	12		8	3.1	4.5	15.1	4.3		Nahata and Koranyi, 1993
	1–13 yr	3		6	2.4	6.0		5.0	26.0	Sunakawa and Iwata, 1986
	5–12 yr	6		7	5.0	4.0		4.8	23.5	Sunakawa and Iwata, 1986
Cefadroxil	1.1–11 yr	16		15	3.7	1.0	0.4	1.3		Ginsburg, 1982
Cephradine	13 mo–8 yr	15		15	21.3	0.5	0.3	0.8		Ginsburg, 1982
Cephalexin	2 mo–6 yr	11		15	23.4	0.5	40	1.0		Ginsburg, 1982
Cefaclor	4 mo–4 yr	10		15	13.1	0.5	20	0.6		Ginsburg, 1982
	34 mo	7		10	10.8	0.5	15	1.0		McCracken et al., 1978
Cefetamet pivoxil	3–17 yr	9		500 mg[b]	5.2	4.8	37.8	2.8	38.1	Hayton et al., 1991
	8–12 yr	4		1,000 mg[c]	6.1	4.7	42.6	2.1	29.9	Hayton et al., 1991
Cefdinir	0.5–2 yr	6		7	2.04	2.0	6.79		1.3	Guttendorf et al., 1992
		6		15	4.11	2.3	13.0		1.2	Guttendorf et al., 1992
	2–12 yr	6		7	2.56	2.3	9.83		1.5	Guttendorf et al., 1992
		6		15	3.60	1.7	13.7		1.5	Guttendorf et al., 1992

[a]Data from Bryskier et al., 1998.
[b]Total of 340 mg of free acid.
[c]Total of 680 mg of free acid.

A single oral dose of cefpodoxime proxetil suspension (4 mg/kg) was administered 2, 3, 4, or 6 h before planned MEF collection. All samples were assayed microbiologically (*Micrococcus luteus*, 0.5 to 16 μg/ml; *Providencia rettgeri*, 0.015 to 0.5 μg/ml). Twenty-four children whose ages ranged from 5 months to 9 years received cefpodoxime proxetil (Table 42) (Van Dyk et al., 1997). From the results obtained by Van Dyk et al. (1997), the concentrations of cefpodoxime reached in the MEF at 6 h exceeded the $MIC_{50/90}$ for penicillin-susceptible *S. pneumoniae* (MIC, ≤0.06 μg/ml) and *H. influenzae* (MIC, ≤0.06 μg/ml) whether or not they produced β-lactamase. In addition, the MIC_{50}s for intermediately susceptible *S. pneumoniae* and *M. catarrhalis* (MIC_{50}, 0.25 μg/ml) are under the levels in MEF at 6 h. However, cefpodoxime levels did not reach the MIC for *S. pneumoniae* isolates resistant to penicillin G (MIC, ≥2 μg/ml). These data were confirmed in an experimental chinchilla model (Bolduc et al., 1996). After 5 and 10 mg of cefpodoxime proxetil per kg, the mean peak levels in MEF were 0.20 and 0.24 μg/ml, respectively (Nelson et al., 1994).

Levels of cefaclor in MEF as determined by different studies are summarized in Table 43.

In one pharmacokinetic study (25 children with serous otitis media) (Krause et al., 1982), it was shown that 2 h after dosing (15 mg/kg), no cefaclor was detected in plasma or MEF (Table 44).

Penetration of cefprozil into the MEF was investigated in patients with chronic otitis media. A total of 89 patients ranging from 7 months to 11 years old were enrolled in this study (Table 45). MEF was removed at times ranging from 0.38 to 5.97 h after oral administration of a single dose of 15 or 20 mg/kg of body weight. Concentrations of cefprozil in plasma were assayed by a high-performance liquid chromatographic method, and those in MEF were assayed by a microbiological assay (*M. luteus* A 24959). The lower limits of quantification were 0.1 and 0.02 μg/ml for plasma and MEF, respectively.

The penetration of cefprozil in MEF was rapid, with levels of 0.17 to 3.0 μg/ml at 0.5 h after dosing. At 5 h after dosing, levels in MEF ranged from 0.18 to 0.59 μg/ml (Shyu et al., 1994). Similar results were obtained by Kafetzis (1994). After 15 mg of cefprozil per kg b.i.d., 2 μg/ml was reached at 2 h in MEF and the trough level at 8 h was 0.1 μg/ml (Table 46).

Two studies were done to evaluate the penetration of ceftibuten into MEF in patients with acute otitis media (Barr et al., 1995). In the first study, 30 pediatric patients received a single oral dose of 9 mg of ceftibuten per kg. Ceftibuten reached a maximum of 4 μg/ml within 4 h of dosing. At 12 h, the ceftibuten concentration was 0.52 μg/ml. In the second study, ceftibuten levels were higher, due mainly to a different methodology. The peak level in MEF was delayed to 2 h from the C_{max} in plasma (Table 47).

MEF cefixime values after the administration of a single oral dose of 8 mg/kg, although varying considerably, average 14% of levels in serum (0.06 to 0.12 μg/ml), which range from 0.76 to 33 μg/ml (Wiedeman and Schwartz, 1992). Levels of cefixime (3 to 5 h after an 8-mg/kg single dose) in MEF from patients with acute otitis media and otitis media with effusion were 1.32 μg/ml (0.35 to 2.86 μg/ml) and 1.51 μg/ml (0.32 to 5.69 μg/ml), respectively, with concentrations in serum of 2.51 and 4.21 μg/ml, respectively (Harrisson et al., 1994).

Loracarbef concentrations in MEF were 2 ± 2.6 μg/ml 2 h after a single oral dose of 7.5 mg/kg and 3.9 ± 2.6 μg/ml after oral administration of 15 mg/kg (Kusmiesz et al., 1990).

At 2 h after administration of a 750-mg dose of cefuroxime, the levels in MEF were 0.73 to 1.7 μg/ml (Martini and Xerri, 1982). At 2 to 5 h after a single 250-mg dose of cefuroxime axetil, the levels of cefuroxime in MEF were 0.20 to 4.85 μg/ml (Haddad et al., 1991).

After a single oral dose of 500 mg of cefatrizine, the levels in MEF were 9.5 and 3.7 μg/ml at 3 and 6 h after dosing, respectively, with concentrations in plasma of 6.2 and 2.9 μg/ml, respectively (Santacroce et al., 1985). Four to six hours after a single oral dose of 200 mg of cefdinir, the concentration in MEF was 0.02 μg/ml and the level in plasma was 0.16 μg/ml (Kawamura et al., 1989).

Table 42 Levels of cefpodoxime in MEF

Time of sampling (h)	Concn (μg/ml) in:	
	Serum	MEF
2	2.64 ± 0.51	0.87 ± 0.67
3	2.48 ± 0.75	0.82 ± 0.61
4	2.01 ± 0.45	0.49 ± 0.25
6	1.01 ± 0.46	0.52 ± 0.24

Table 43 Cefaclor levels in MEF[a]

Dose (mg/kg)	Sampling time (h)	Concn in serum (μg/ml)	Sampling time (h)	Concn in MEF (μg/ml)	Reference
13.3 b.i.d.	2	3.6	2	1.0	Kafetzis, 1994
	4	0.6	4	0.5	Kafetzis, 1994
15	0.5	7	2	1.1	Nelson, 1981
15	1.5–2	6.9	1.5–2	1.3	Krause et al., 1982
20	1.5–2	13	1.5–2	2.8	Eden et al., 1983
20 MD	1.5–2	15.5	1.5–2	4.6	Emston et al., 1985
20	1.5–2	12.3	1.5–2	2.9	Emston et al., 1985
40	1.5–2	33	1.5–2	4.8	Eden et al., 1983
40	1.5–2	31.7	1.5–2	5.9	Emston et al., 1985
40	ND	ND	1.5–2	2.1	Bessaguet et al., 1994
40	2	3.63	2	0.96	Barr et al., 1995
	4	0.69	4	0.49	Barr et al., 1995
	6		6		Barr et al., 1995

[a]MD, multiple doses; ND, not determined.

Table 44 Pharmacokinetics of cefaclor penetration in MEF

Time of sampling (h)	Concn (μg/ml) in:	
	Serum	MEF
0–0.5	12.8 ± 6.7	3.8 ± 2.8
0.5–1	16.8 ± 6.5	2.8 ± 2.1
1–1.5	11.2 ± 3.6	2.3 ± 1.3
1.5–2	6.9 ± 2.6	1.3 ± 0.3
2–3	ND[a]	ND
3–4	ND	ND

[a]ND, not determined.

Table 45 Cefprozil levels in MEF (chronic otitis)

Dose (mg/kg)	Concn (μml) in:	
	Plasma	MEF
15	0.38–15.97	0.06–4.44
20	1.28–21.47	0.17–8.67

8.4. Pharmacodynamics in MEF

The major determinant of efficacy with oral cephalosporins is the time the drug concentrations at the site of infection exceed the MIC for the pathogen. It had been demonstrated with both gram-positive and gram-negative bacteria that bacterial killing occurs when concentrations in serum exceed the MIC for only 40 to 50% of the dosing interval. Maximal killing is found when values exceed the MIC for 60 to 70% of the dosing interval. These results were also found with cefpodoxime proxetil and *S. pneumoniae* (Urban et al., 1995) (Table 48).

Craig and Andes (1996) demonstrated that a MEF/MIC ratio of between 3.2 and 6.3 correlates with 80 to 85% bacterial eradication and that maximal efficacy is seen when the MEF/MIC ratio exceeds 10.

It is difficult to evaluate time above MIC in MEF due to methodology problems in collecting and assaying MEF.

8.5. Oral Cephem Concentrations in Tonsils

Concentrations of the differents oral cephalosporins in tonsils are listed in Table 49.

Table 46 Pharmacokinetics of cefprozil and cefaclor penetration in MEF

Time of sampling (h)	Concn (μg/ml)			
	Cefprozil (15 mg/kg b.i.d.)		Cefaclor (13.3 mg/kg b.i.d.)	
	Serum	MEF	Serum	MEF
2	5.5	2.0	3.6	1.0
4	4.4	1.6	0.6	0.5
6	1.5	1.0		
8	1.0	0.1		

Table 47 Levels of ceftibuten in MEF

Time of sampling (h)	Concn (mg/ml)			
	Study 1		Study 2	
	Serum	MEF	Serum	MEF
2	6.73	0.85	14.48	4.41
4	5.93	4.03	10.02	14.27
6	3.15	1.28	2.72	0.81
8	1.56	0.62		
12	0.8	0.52	1.28	1.29

8.6. Concentrations of Oral Cephems in Sinus Mucosa

Concentrations of oral cephems in sinus mucosa are listed in Table 50.

8.7. Cephem Concentrations in Respiratory Tissues

The concentrations of the different cephalosporins on lung tissue, pleural fluid, and bronchial mucosa have been studied. The existing data are listed in Table 51.

8.8. Concentrations of Cephems in Skin Blisters

Dog, cat, and human bites frequently harbor (*alpha- and beta-hemolytic*) and nonhemolytic streptococci, *S. aureus*, coagulase-negative staphylococci, anaerobes, and *Corynebacterium* spp. *Pasteurella multocida* is a frequent pathogen in dog and cat bites, whereas human bites may become infected with *Eikenella corrodens* as well as a variety of fastidious aerobic and anaerobic veterinary species.

Table 48 Time above MIC for oral cephalosporins against *S. pneumoniae*, *H. influenzae*, and *M. catarrhalis*[a]

Drug	Dose[b]	*S. pneumoniae*						*H. influenzae*		*M. catarrhalis*	
		Pen[s]		Pen[i]		Pen[r]					
		MIC_{90}	T > MIC[c]	MIC_{90}	T > MIC	MIC_{90}	T > MIC	MIC_{90}	T > MIC	MIC_{90}	T > MIC
Cefaclor	13.3 mg/kg t.i.d.	0.5	44	8–16	0	16–32	0	8	0	2	35
Cefuroxime	250 mg b.i.d.	0.12	73	0.5–2	55–33	4–8	23–0	2	33	2	33
Cefixime	8 mg/kg q.d.	0.5	48	4–16	0	32–64	0	0.06	88	0.5	48
Cefpodoxime	5 mg/kg b.i.d.	0.25	62	0.25–2	54–0	2–4	0	0.12	82	1	37
Cefprozil	15 mg/kg b.i.d.	0.25	78	0.5–4	66–28	4–16	28–0	8	16	2	41
Loracarbef	7.5 mg/kg b.i.d.	0.5	42	2–16	26–0	16	0	8	9	2	26

[a]Data from Craig and Andes, 1996. MIC_{90}s are in micrograms per milliliter. T > MICs are in hours.
[b]t.i.d., three times a day; q.d., per day.
[c]T > MIC, time above MIC.

Table 49 Oral cephalosporin concentrations in tonsils

Drug	*n*	Dose (mg)[a]	Sample time (h)	Concn in: Tissue (mg/kg)	Concn in: Plasma (μg/ml)	Reference
Cefpodoxime proxetil	11	100 SD	4	0.24	1.25	Gehanno et al., 1990
			7	0.09	0.39	Gehanno et al., 1990
	12	5.0	3	0.06	1.39	Bairamis et al., 1996
	12		6	0.05	0.66	Bairamis et al., 1996
	12		12	0.05	0.11	Bairamis et al., 1996
Cefuroxime axetil	16	500 SD	1–7	0.5		Dellamonica et al., 1994
	2	15 mg/kg	0–2	0.15	1.42	Jetlund et al., 1991
	5	15 mg/kg	2–3	0.65	1.83	
	3	15 mg/kg	3–4	0.54	2.91	
	3	15 mg/kg	4–5	0.92	3.50	
	6	15 mg/kg	5–6	0.67	2.28	
Cefetamet pivoxil	25	1,000 SD	2	0.82		Blouin and Stoeckel, 1993
			4	1.2		Blouin and Stoeckel, 1993
			6	0.5		Blouin and Stoeckel, 1993
			12	0.3		Blouin and Stoeckel, 1993
Cefprozil	15	7.5 mg/kg	0.7–3.2	0.48–2.42		
Cefaclor	30	500	2	5.2–6	6.1–6.1	Iwasawa, 1979
Cefixime	4	100	3	0.32–0.72	0.9–1.7	Fujimaki et al., 1985
	1	200	3	0.95	2.5	
	21	4 mg/kg MD	5.3	0.5–0.7	1.2	Bégué et al., 1989
Cephalexin	6	1,000	2.5	1.1	24	Adam and Kreutle, 1980
	10	1,000	3.5	0.9	ND[b]	Adam and Kreutle, 1980
	5	1,000	2.0	2.6	23.9	Adam and Kreutle, 1980
	13	1,000	2.0	1.8	11.9	Adam and Kreutle, 1980
	10	1,000	5	0.1	ND	Adam and Kreutle, 1980
	15	1,000 × 4	2	2.0	16.2	Holm and Ekedahl, 1982
			4	2.4	15.9	Holm and Ekedahl, 1982
Cefadroxil	10	1,000	2.5	3.5	20.6	Adam and Kreutle, 1980
	10	1,000	3.5	1.9	ND	Adam and Kreutle, 1980
	10	1,000	5	1.6	ND	Adam and Kreutle, 1980
	10	1,000 × 2	2	2.0	16.2	Holm and Ekedahl, 1982
	5	1,000 × 2	4	2.4	15.9	Holm and Ekedahl, 1982
Cefatrizine	3	500	3	10.7	7.8	Santacroce et al., 1985
	3	500	6	4.2	2.6	Scaglione et al., 1996
Ceftibuten	5	400	2.3	2.3	14.1	Scaglione et al., 1996
	5	400	4.4	5.3	7.4	Scaglione et al., 1996
	5	400	8.3	1.9	2.8	Scaglione et al., 1996
	5	400	12.4	1.0	1.3	Scaglione et al., 1996
	5	400	24.6	0.3	0.15	Scaglione et al., 1996
Cefdinir	2	100	2	0.06–0.3	0.5–1	Kawamura et al., 1989
	2	100	4	0.2	0.7–1	Kawamura et al., 1989
	2	100	5	0.1	0.4	Kawamura et al., 1989
Cefditoren pivoxil	13	200	1.5–4	0.1–0.09	0.5–2	Nishizono et al., 1992
Cefotiam hexetil	6	200	1	0.5	2.2	Mori et al., 1989
	6	200	2	0.3	2.2	Mori et al., 1989
	6	200	2.5	0.1	0.8	Mori et al., 1989
Cefmatilen	15	100	3.0	0.24–1.78	1.79–2.27	Kumazawa et al., 1995

[a]SD, single dose; MD, multiple doses.
[b]ND, not determined.

Cefprozil, loracarbef, and cefpodoxime are more active than cefadroxil, cephalexin, and penicillin G against many aerobic bite wound isolates, including *P. multocida* (except cefpodoxime). In vitro activity against *E. corrodens* remains low except for cefpodoxime. Cefprozil and loracarbef are poorly active against *Peptostreptococcus* spp.

While some clinicians advocate the use of cephalexin and cefadroxil for bite wounds (Callaham, 1980), clinical failures are currently reported. Weber et al. (1984) have noted that cephalexin and cefaclor do not achieve levels in blood that are sufficient to treat *P. multocida* infections.

Some new oral cephalosporins could be alternative treatments according to the origin of the bite wounds. *P. aeruginosa* is a common pathogen in puncture wounds of the foot, e.g., diabetic foot.

Cephalosporins exhibit a time-dependent killing. Thus, the duration for which the drug concentration at its site of action (e.g., skin blister fluid) is above the MIC for a given

Table 50 Concentrations of oral cephalosporins in sinus mucosa

Drug	Dose (mg)	*n*	Time of sampling (h)	Concn in: Plasma (μg/ml)	Concn in: Tissue (mg/kg)	Reference
Cephalexin	500	19	2	19	3.1	Kohonen et al., 1975
Cefpodoxime proxetil	100	3	3		0.34	Shinikawa et al., 1988
	200	2	1	1.79	0.24	
Cefetamet pivoxil	500 MD[a]	13	2	ND[b]	0.8–4.5	Stoeckel et al., 1995
Cefixime	100	4	3	1.4–2.3	<0.01–1.0	Fujimaki et al., 1985
Cefotiam hexetil	100	4	1–5	<0.1–0.7	<0.1–0.5	Furuta et al., 1988
	200	16	1–6.5	<0.1–0.7	<0.1–0.6	Furuta et al., 1988
Cefditoren pivoxil	200	13	2–3.5	0.74–3.19	0.11–0.48	Nishizono et al., 1992
Cefdinir	100	1	4	0.82	0.32	Kawamura et al., 1989
	100	2	4.5	0.76	0.20	Kawamura et al., 1989
	100	1	5	0.92	0.55	Kawamura et al., 1989

[a]MD, multiple doses.
[b]ND, not determined.

Table 51 Oral cephalosporins in respiratory tissues

Drug	Tissue or fluid	No. of subjects	Dose (mg)[a]	Sampling time (h)	Tissue fluid level (mg/kg or μg/ml)	Concn in plasma (μg/ml)	Reference
Cephradine	Lung		500	ND	2.6		
Cefadroxil	Lung	22	500	2–4	7.4 ± 0.7	11.5 ± 1.3	Quintiliani, 1982
	Pleural fluid	4	1,000	3–5	11.4 ± 3.0	9.4 ± 2.5	Quintiliani, 1982
Cefixime	Bronchial mucosa	10	200 MD	3.8	1.5	3.9	Baldwin et al., 1992
		10	400 MD	4.3	2.4	6.6	
	Lung	9	200 MD	4	0.78	2.76	Gallet et al., 1989
				7.8	0.32	1.29	Gallet et al., 1989
		14	400 MD	3.7	1.52	3.76	Gallet et al., 1989
				8.4	1.31	2.76	Gallet et al., 1989
Cefetamet pivoxil	Lung	6	1,000 SD	5	0.96		Blouin and Stoeckel, 1993
				8	1.3		
		6	2,000 SD	5	3.2		
				8	2.0		
Cefaclor	Bronchial mucosa	8	500 MD	0.75–1	4.4		Marlin et al., 1984
		6	1,000 MD	0.75–1	7.7		
	Lung		500	3	0.12	1.68	Imaizumi et al., 1986
		ND[b]	500	5	0.29	0.45	
Cefpodoxime proxetil	Lung	6	200 SD	3	0.63	1.05	Couraud et al., 1990
		6		6	0.52	0.91	
		6		12	0.52	0.36	
	Pleural fluid	18	200 SD	3	0.6	2.7	Dumont et al., 1990
				6	1.9	2.7	
				12	0.78	0.7	
	Bronchial mucosa	13	200 SD	1–5	0.9	1.9	Baldwin et al., 1992
Cefuroxime axetil	Bronchial mucosa	19	500 SD	1–6	1.8	3.9	Baldwin et al., 1992
Cefotiam hexetil	Lung	6	400 MD	3–4	0.25	0.54	Mignot et al., 1994
	Lung	6	800 MD	3–4	0.35	0.69	
	Lung	6	1,600 MD	5–6	0.29	0.58	
Cefatrizine	Lung	4	500 SD	2.0	0.9–1.4	7.5–9.6	Mignini et al., 1985
	Lung	4	500 SD	3.0	1.2–1.6	6.5–7.5	Mignini et al., 1985
	Bronchial mucosa	4	500 SD	3.0	9.4–11.4	7.0–8.0	Mignini et al., 1985
		4	500 SD	6.0	3.4–4.5	2.1–3.1	Mignini et al., 1985

[a]MD, multiple doses; SD, single dose.
[b]ND, not determined.

Table 52 Skin concentrations of oral cephalosporins

Drug	Dose (mg)	n	Time (h)	Concn in: Plasma (μg/ml)	Concn in: Skin tissue (mg/kg)	Reference
Cefpodoxime proxetil	100 MD[a]	14	2–3	2.07	0.43	Zolfino et al., 1992
Cefditoren pivoxil	200	5	0.5	5.42	0.35	Akiyama et al., 1992
	200	5	1.0	14.94	1.06	Akiyama et al., 1992
	200	5	2.0	22.16	1.57	Akiyama et al., 1992
	200	5	4.0	22.94	2.25	Akiyama et al., 1992
	200	5	6.0	17.20	1.41	Akiyama et al., 1992
Cefdinir	100	1	3.0	0.77	0.37	Nogita et al., 1989

[a]MD, multiple doses.

pathogen is most closely correlated with ability to kill and with clinical outcome.

The concentrations of oral cephalosporins in normal skin are summarized in Table 52. Concentrations achieved in skin blisters with different methods are listed in Table 53.

Oral cephalosporins that achieve concentrations above the MIC_{90} for methicillin-susceptible *S. aureus* isolates for 50 to 90% of their dosing interval include cefuroxime (axetil), cephalexin, and cefadroxil. The level of activity against *S. pyogenes* in skin and skin structure infections is reached by most of the oral cephalosporins: cephalexin, cefadroxil, cefaclor, cefprozil, cefuroxime (axetil), loracarbef, and cefpodoxime (proxetil).

Stone et al. (1989) showed that concentrations of cefixime in blister fluid remained above 0.1 μg/ml at 24 h. The $MIC_{50/90}$ for *S. pyogenes* is under ≤0.1 μg/ml, but the $MIC_{50/90}$ is above the peak concentration in blister fluid (3.2 ± 1.0 μg/ml) for methicillin-susceptible *S. aureus*.

Concentrations of cefprozil in blister fluid are above the $MIC_{50/90}$ for *S. pyogenes* for up to 8 h (concentration at 8 h, 0.3 to 1 μg/ml) but remain above $MIC_{50/90}$ for *S. aureus* for up to 3 to 4 h (concentration at 4 h, 3.2 to 6.9 μg/ml) (Nye et al., 1990). After 200- or 400-mg single or multiple doses, levels in skin blister fluid remain above the $MIC_{50/90}$ for *S. pyogenes* for up to 24 h.

8.9. Concentrations in Bone

There are important differences between bone infections in children and adults. The microorganism responsible for bone infections is *S. aureus* in almost 90% of all cases.

Cefadroxil was administered orally in a dose of 1,000 mg at 24, 12, and 2 h prior to the collection of fluid or tissue. The levels in different fluids and tissues are listed in Table 54 (Quintiliani, 1982).

In another study, after a single oral dose of 1,000 mg 4 to 5 h prior to sampling bone ($n = 10$) and muscle ($n = 11$), the concentrations in bone and muscle were 4.2 and 3.0 mg/kg, respectively, while simultaneous levels in serum were 11 to 12 μg/ml (Quintiliani, 1982).

Cefadroxil was given in a dose of 25 mg/kg every 12 h to 28 children, among them 22 who had undergone orthopedic surgery. From all patients, *S. aureus* susceptible to cefadroxil was isolated. Out of the 28 treated children, 23 had good clinical bacteriological and radiological outcomes (Jimenez-Shebab and Barrogan, 1982).

9. RENAL INSUFFICIENCY

Since the majority of oral cephalosporins, apart from cefixime, are principally eliminated via the kidneys, it is not surprising to find that dosage adjustments are recommended in relation to the degree of renal insufficiency. Thus, studies have shown for all the oral cephalosporins mentioned that prolongation of the $t_{1/2}$ is proportional to the degree of renal impairment, which may be explained by reductions in the total clearances of the cephalosporins in the presence of renal insufficiency. The dosages recommended for patients with severe renal insufficiency and a creatinine clearance of less than or equal to 20 ml/min are given in Table 55. In addition, it is important to note that even for cefixime, which is partly eliminated in the bile, a dosage adjustment is suggested in the presence of severe renal insufficiency.

9.1. Renal Dysfunction

For all compounds eliminated mainly by the kidneys, changes in the pharmacokinetic parameters in relation to the degree of renal impairment have been recorded. Peak concentrations, T_{max}, AUC, and $t_{1/2}$ increased and urinary elimination decreased. For all compounds but cefixime and cefetamet, body clearance and renal clearance are closely related to creatinine clearance. For ceftibuten and cefixime, dose adjustments are recommended only for patients with severe renal impairment (creatinine clearance of ≤10 to 20 ml/min). The $t_{1/2}$ of cephalexin increases particularly when the creatinine clearance is below 30 ml/min (Bailey et al., 1970).

9.2. Hemodialysis

Hemodialysis is warranted for patients with end-stage renal failure. This procedure is typically implemented three times a week, and the duration of each dialysis is about 3 h.

Hemodialysis removed about 22% of the administered dose of cefpodoxime proxetil in a study by Borin et al. (1992). Hemodialysis clearance of cefpodoxime was 120 ± 31 ml/min. Cefprozil is removed by hemodialysis. The CI_{HB} is 87 ml/min. Approximately 55% of cefprozil is removed during the 3-h hemodialysis procedure (Shyu et al., 1991). During a 6- to 8-h hemodialysis session, cefadroxil concentrations decreased by 75% (Humbert et al., 1979). Approximately one-third of the administered dose of cefaclor was recovered in the dialysate in a study by Berman et al. (1978). For cephalexin, the mean concentration in serum at end of hemodialysis was 3.3 μg/ml compared to 14.7 μg/ml at the beginning of hemodialysis. The clearance of cephalexin was 25 ml/min (Bailey et al., 1970).

9.3. CAPD

Eight noninfected patients and eight healthy volunteers received a single oral dose of 200 mg of cefpodoxime proxetil (Johnson et al., 1993). Only 5.74% ± 3.1% of the dose was recovered from the dialysate (Table 56). In healthy volunteers,

Table 53 Pharmacokinetics of oral cephems in skin blister fluids[a]

Drug	Subjects (n)	Dose (mg)	C_{max} (μg/ml)		T_{max} (h)		$t_{1/2\beta}$ (h)		Reference
			Plasma	SBF	Plasma	SBF	Plasma	SBF	
Cefpodoxime proxetil									
Cantharidin blister	6	200 SD	2.1	1.7	2.9	3.5	2.6	3.6	
Suction blister	8	200 SD	2.2	1.6	3.1	4.7	2.7	3.0	Borin et al., 1990
	8	200 MD	2.3	1.6	2.3	3.5	2.6	2.3	Borin et al., 1990
	8	400 SD	4.2	2.9	2.9	4.3	2.6	2.7	Borin et al., 1990
	8	400 MD	4.1	2.8	2.4	3.5	2.7	3.2	Borin et al., 1990
Cefetamet pivoxil (cantharidin blister)	9	500 MD	5.1	4.8	2.8	3.9	2.3	3.1	Stoeckel et al., 1995
Cefixime (cantharidin blister)	6	400 SD	3.7	3.2	3.7	6.7	3.8	4.1	Stone et al., 1989
Ceftibuten (canthuridin blister)	6	200 MD	10.9	9.2	1.8	3.7	2.5	1.1	Wise et al., 1990
Cefprozil									
Cantharidin blister	6	500 SD	9.6	4.9	1.9	3.5	1.4	1.4	Nye et al., 1990
Suction blister	12	250 SD	6.1	3.0	1.5	2.4	1.4	2.4	Barbhaiya et al., 1990
	12	500 SD	11.2	5.8	1.4	2.5	1.3	2.2	Barbhaiya et al., 1990
Cefaclor	12	250 SD	10.6	3.6	0.5	1.1	0.5	1.5	Barbhaiya et al., 1990
	12	500 SD	17.3	6.5	0.7	1.0	0.6	1.4	Barbhaiya et al., 1990
Cefuroxime axetil		600 SD	6.4	4.1	2.5	3.3	1.1	1.9	
Cefotiam hexetil									
Cantharidin blister	6	400 SD	2.6	0.9	2.1	3.5	0.8	2.6	Korting et al., 1990
Suction blister	6	400 SD	2.6	0.9	2.1	3.3	0.8	4.6	Korting et al., 1990
Cefdinir		200	1.0	0.5	3.3	4.9	1.4	3.4	Richer et al., 1995
		300	1.6	0.7	3.2	4.9	1.5	3.7	Richer et al., 1995
		400	2.2	0.9	3.0	4.8	1.4	3.9	Richer et al., 1995
		600	2.4	1.1	3.2	4.8	1.5	3.7	Richer et al., 1995

[a]SBF, suction blister fluid, SD, single dose; MD, multiple doses.

Table 54 Bone and synovial levels of cefadroxil

Specimen	n	Concn in: Tissue of fluid (mg/kg or μg/ml)	Serum (μg/ml)
Bone	14	5.0 ± 0.9	21.5 ± 2.8
Muscle	12	6.5 ± 0.9	20.7 ± 2.9
Synovial capsule	21	7.8 ± 1.5	20.5 ± 3.1
Synovial fluid	13	11.0 ± 1.7	25.5 ± 2.0

24.2% ± 13% of the administered dose was recovered from urine, in contrast to only 5.5% ± 6.9% for the five nonanuric patients undergoing continuous ambulatory peritoneal dialysis (CAPD). Peak dialysate cefpodoxime levels occurred on average at 14.8 ± 6 h, with a mean peak level in dialysate of 1.06 ± 0.4 μg/ml. At 6 and 24 h, mean dialysate cefpodoxime levels were 0.6 ± 0.4 and 0.37 ± 0.4 μg/ml, respectively. The cefpodoxime clearance in dialysate was 0.03 ml/min/kg. The main pharmacokinetic parameters of cefpodoxime in CAPD patients are listed in Table 56.

10. HEPATIC INSUFFICIENCY

Very few studies have been undertaken to determine the impact of hepatic insufficiency on the pharmacokinetics of oral cephalosporins since these are principally eliminated renally.

One study that was conducted with cefixime in cirrhotic patients showed that the $t_{1/2}$ was prolonged about twofold (3.5 versus 6.4 h) in these patients. However, two other studies carried out in this patient group with cefprozil and cefetamet pivoxil have shown no significant difference in the plasma pharmacokinetics from those in healthy subjects.

Cefprozil is almost completely absorbed by the gastrointestinal tract. The urinary excretion data show that approximately 40% is cleared through nonrenal mechanisms.

The study conducted by Shyu et al. (1991) showed that the pharmacokinetics of the two isomers of cefprozil are not significantly modified in patients with hepatic impairment.

The bioavailability of cefotiam hexetil is not significantly altered in patients with hepatic impairment. The AUC is about twofold greater than in healthy volunteers, and the $t_{1/2}$ is two times longer than in healthy volunteers.

Cefixime was given in 200-mg oral single doses to volunteers and nine patients with impaired hepatic function (Pugh index range from 7 to 12). The C_{max}s and AUCs are similar for both populations. The $t_{1/2}$ is twice the length of that in the control, as an effect of increased volume of distribution (0.51 ± 0.05 versus 1.05 ± 0.2 liter/kg). However, no change in dosing is required in these patients (Singlas et al., 1989) (Table 57).

11. GASTRECTOMIZED PATIENTS

In gastrointestinal surgery, absorption of a drug may be altered. Gastrectomy may be total (Roux-Y procedure) or subtotal (Billroth I and II) (Table 58).

Table 55 Pharmacokinetics of oral cephalosporins in renally impaired patients after a single oral dose

Generic name	CL_R ml/min	Dose (mg)	*n*	C_{max} (μg/ml)	T_{max} (h)	$AUC_{0-\infty}$ (μg·h/ml)	$t_{1/2\beta}$ (h)	Urinary recovery (%)	Reference
Ceftibuten	≥100	300	6	11.7	2.67	65.6	2.7	67.7	Kelloway et al., 1991
	50–80	300	6	13.9	2.83	94.1	3.85	52.6	
	30–49	300	6	13.0	3.17	167.7	7.07	41.1	
	5–29	300	6	19.5	3.0	472.2	22.28	18.0	
Cefdinir	≥100	100	3	0.49	2.0	2.76	1.66	17.7	
	51–70	100	1	1.49	2.0	10.74	2.41	28.9	Nishitani et al., 1989
	31–50	100	3	0.73	4	7.48	2.92	10.9	
	≤30	100	2	1.59	8	16.94	4.06	14.25	
Cefprozil									
cis	>90	1,000	6	12.3	2.1	45.9	1.7	56.9	
trans	>90	1,000	6	1.1	1.7	4.3	1.9	37.6	Shyu et al., 1991
cis	61–90	1,000	6	16.1	1.8	71.9	2.1	53.4	
trans	61–90	1,000	6	1.4	1.7	5.4	1.9	30.1	
cis	31–60	1,000	6	22.6	2.7	117.0	3.4	46.0	
trans	31–60	1,000	6	1.8	2.9	8.3	1.8	25.1	
cis	≤30	1,000	6	30.4	3.7	260.0	5.2	23.8	
trans	≤30	1,000	6	2.2	3.7	16.1	3.4	10.5	
Cefpodoxime proxetil	>90	200	6	2.34	2.50	14.8	3.55	32.2	
	50–80	200	6	3.53	2.58	26.6	3.53	36.2	St. Peter et al., 1992
	30–49	200	6	3.03	3.67	33.3	5.90	26.2	
	5–29	200	6	3.71	3.75	63.5	9.80	21.7	
Cefixime	>100		6	2.49	2.83	22.0	3.82	27.6	Dhib et al., 1991
	40–80		6	4.65	4.25	71.1	6.60	22.1	Dhib et al., 1991
	20–39		8	5.83	3.68	99.5	8.44	9.2	Dhib et al., 1991
	5–19		6	6.67	4.33	152	13.8	7.1	Dhib et al., 1991
Cefatrizine	>100	500	15	6.9	1.8		1.5		Couet et al., 1991
	10–50	500	15	10.7	2.8		2.6		Couet et al., 1991
Cefetamet pivoxil	>80	1,000	9	5.9	3.9	41.6	2.6	38	Kneer et al., 1989
	40–79	1,000	12	7.8	4.1	77.0	4.4	34	Kneer et al., 1989
	10–39	1,000	15	12.3	4.9	248	10.6	23	Kneer et al., 1989
	<10	1,000	11	41.7	8.4	613	28.8	11	Kneer et al., 1989
Cefuroxime axetil	>85	250	6	5.2	3.0	21.6	1.4	42	Konishi et al., 1993
	50–84	250	6	5.5	3.0	28.5	2.4	33	Konishi et al., 1993
	15–49	250	7	8.6	3.9	89.0	4.6	34	Konishi et al., 1993
	<15	250	9	10.7	6.3	258	16.8	22	Konishi et al., 1993
Loracarbef	>90	400	10	15.4	1.2	32.0	1.29	94.3	Therasse et al., 1993
	75–90	400	5	18.0	1.5	41.8	1.52	76.2	Therasse et al., 1993
	50–75	400	7	21.6	1.4	67.5	2.45	81.7	Therasse et al., 1993
	10–49	400	10	24.7	1.3	168.8	5.62	49.9	Therasse et al., 1993
	<10	400	8	23.0	3.7	1,085.0	31.6		Therasse et al., 1993

Table 56 Pharmacokinetics of cefpodoxime in CAPD patients

Patients	C_{max} (μg/ml)	T_{max} (h)	T_{lag} (h)	$AUC_{0-\infty}$ (μg · h/ml)	$t_{1/2}$ (h)	Urinary recovery (%)
Healthy	1.88	2.44	0.21	10.2	1.98	24.2
CAPD	3.25	12.0	0.56	10.7	24.4	5.5

Table 57 Pharmacokinetics of oral cephalosporins in hepatically impaired patients

Generic name	Patients[a]	Dose (mg)	n	C_{max} (μg/ml)	T_{max} (h)	$AUC_{0-\infty}$ (μ·h/ml)	$t_{1/2\beta}$ (h)	Urinary recovery (%)	Reference
Cefprozil									
cis	H	1,000	12	16.7	1.8	62.7	1.6	65.8	Shyu et al., 1991
trans		1,000	12	1.8	2.0	5.7	1.2	54.0	
Cefprozil									
cis	HP	1,000	12	15.8	1.9	70.7	2.2	61.2	
trans		1,000	12	1.7	2.0	6.7	1.5	50.0	
Cefpodoxime proxetil	H	200	8	2.6	8.4	14.5	2.3	39.2	Tremblay et al., 1990
	HP	200	8	1.7	2.6	10.79	2.68	35.0	Tremblay et al., 1990
Cefotiam hexetil	H	200	12	2.2	1.6	4.2	1.0		
	HP	200	12	2.7	3.0	11.0	2.7		
Cefixime	H	200	ND[b]	3.9	3.6	32.2	3.5	16.0	Singlas et al., 1989
	HP	200	9	3.7	5.2	36.2	6.4	43.0	

[a]H, healthy; HP, hepatically impaired.
[b]ND, not determined.

Table 58 Pharmacokinetics of AS-924 and cefcapene pivoxil in gastrectomized patients

Drug	Procedure	n	C_{max} (μg/ml)	T_{max} (h)	AUC_{0-12} (μg·h/ml)
AS-924	Total gastrectomy	6	2.94 ± 0.73	1.5 ± 0.5	10.32 ± 2.23
	Billroth I	5	2.69 ± 0.41	4.0 ± 0	10.26 ± 2.01
	Billroth II	6	3.33 ± 0.63	2.3 ± 0.8	13.8 ± 2.45
	None (control)	6	2.95 ± 0.39	2.6 ± 0.6	11.36 ± 1.09
Cefcapene pivoxil	Total gastrectomy	9	1.21 ± 0.34	1.8 ± 0.4	4.11 ± 1.21
	Billroth I	7	1.10 ± 0.44	3.7 ± 0.8	3.40 ± 1.65
	Billroth II	3	1.17 ± 0.20	3.3 ± 1.2	3.52 ± 0.90
	None (control)	6	2.62 ± 0.35	2.0 ± 0.3	7.81 ± 0.85

In patients who underwent the Billroth I procedure, the T_{max}s were longer than in healthy volunteers. In patients who underwent the Billroth II procedure, the T_{max}s were not significantly different from those in healthy volunteers. In patients who underwent total gastrectomy, the T_{max}s decreased in comparison with those in healthy volunteers.

In similar studies, it was shown that cefterame pivoxil absorption is modified in gastrectomized patients, due to the Δ^2 conversion. Cefterame pivoxil is inactivated at a weakly acidic pH and alkaline pH due to the Δ^2 conversion.

Cefcapene (cefcamate) pivoxil seems not to undergo Δ^2 conversion in humans. In patients who underwent the Billroth I and II procedures, T_{max}s were longer; T_{max}s decreased in patients who underwent total gastrectomy. Absoption decreased significantly in all cases.

12. METABOLISM

The nonesterified oral cephalosporins are not metabolized, except ceftibuten. The esterified oral cephalosporins are metabolized (isomerization), and the ester side chain is removed by esterases in the intestinal mucosa during enteral absorption and then are metabolized.

12.1. Ceftibuten Metabolism

Formation of metabolites after oral administration of ceftibuten was investigated using high-performance liquid chromatography and thin-layer chromatography. The olefinic isomer of ceftibuten (*trans*-isomer) was recovered in urine and plasma from healthy patients and renally impaired patients.

After a single oral dose of 200 mg of ceftibuten, urine recovery of the *trans*-isomer ranged from 7.3 to 9.8% of the administered dose; up to 12.6% was recovered in the urine after repeated doses (Nakashima et al., 1986) (Table 59).

Wise et al. (1990) found that the peak levels of the *trans*-isomer in plasma were 4.8 to 7% of the peak *cis*-isomer levels. Shiba (1988) found 4.3 to 4.5% of the isomer in plasma and 7.2 to 9.2% in urine, of the total amount of ceftibuten. In renally impaired patients, the renal clearance of the *trans*-isomer decreased and the AUC increased (Kelloway et al., 1991) (Table 60).

Table 59 Urinary recovery of *trans*-ceftibuten

Patient state or dose	n	Dose (mg)[a]	Urinary recovery (%)	
			Ceftibuten	*trans*-Isomer
Fasting	6	200 SD	67.4 ± 7.1	9.8 ± 1.7
Fed	6	200 SD	60.4 ± 4.0	7.3 ± 1.3
1st dose	6	200 MD	72.6 ± 11.0	9.2 ± 2.9
15th dose	6	200 MD	84.0 ± 6.0	10.5 ± 2.5
27th dose	6	200 MD	84.8 ± 4.8	12.6 ± 2.4

[a]SD, single dose; MD, multiple doses.

Table 60 Pharmacokinetics of *trans*-ceftibuten in renally impaired patients

Creatinine clearance (ml/min)	C_{max} (μg/ml)	T_{max} (h)	$AUC_{0-\infty}$ (μg·h/ml)	$t_{1/2\beta}$ (h)	CL_R (ml/min)	Urinary elimination (%)
≥100	2.12	3.5	14.12	2.63	49.89	9.8
50–80	1.18	4.3	19.62	5.37	43.03	15.3
30–49	1.71	6.7	52.20	14.29	15.06	14.7
5–29	2.68	11.3	111.68	19.46	6.51	8.7

trans-Ceftibuten is an active metabolite but it is at least eight times less active than ceftibuten (Nakashima et al., 1989) (Table 61).

12.2 Isomerization of Oral Cephalosporin Esters

The esterified oral cephalosporins undergo reversible isomerization of the Δ^3 double bond to yield a mixture of Δ^3 cephems and Δ^2-unsaturated esters. The cephalosporin free acid does not isomerize under the same conditions. By hydrolysis, Δ^2 cephalosporin esters yield Δ^2 cephalosporins which are bacteriologically inactive.

A proton in the 2 position is abstracted by a base. The resulting ambident carbanion can be reprotonated in the 4 position, giving a Δ^2 ester (Richter et al., 1990).

Δ^2 isomerization has been well studied for cefotiam hexetil. Δ^2 cefotiam represents 1.4% of the administered dose in plasma. The peak concentrations of 0.06 μg/ml (200 mg) and 0.11 μg/ml (400 mg) were achieved 2.5 h after dosing. The $t_{1/2}$ of Δ^2 cefotiam is 1.3 h.

Cefotiam hexetil and cefteram pivoxil are inactivated in the gut due to the conversion of a double bond of the cephem ring (Δ^2 conversion) at a higher pH.

12.3. Metabolism of the Ester Side Chain

Different side chains have been fixed on the C-4 carboxylic group. They are released in the intestinal cell wall by esterase and undergo metabolism.

12.3.1. Acetoxymethyl Side Chain (e.g., Cefuroxime Axetil)

The acetoxymethyl side chain is fixed on the C-4 carboxylic group of cefuroxime axetil and is metabolized in acetaldehyde and acetic acid. The acetaldehyde is rapidly converted into acetic acid.

12.3.2. Isopropyloxycarbonyloxyethyl Group (e.g., Cefpodoxime Proxetil)

The isopropyloxycarbonyloxyethyl side chain is fixed on the C-4 carboxylic group of cefpodoxime; this side chain is mainly metabolized in isopropanol, carbon dioxide, and acetaldehyde.

Table 61 In vitro activity of the *trans*-isomer of ceftibuten

Strain	MIC (μg/ml)	
	cis	*trans*
S. pyogenes C-23	0.2	1.6
S. pneumoniae I	3.1	25
E. coli EC-14	0.05	0.4
K. pneumoniae SR-1	0.012	0.1
P. mirabilis PR-4	0.025	0.2
P. vulgaris CN 329	0.025	0.2
S. marcescens ATCC 13880	0.1	0.78
H. influenzae SR 3508	0.1	0.78

12.3.3. POM

Numerous oral cephalosporins bear the pivaloyloxymethyl (POM) side chain at the C-4 carboxylic group: cefetamet, cefditoren, and cefcamate.

The metabolism of the POM ester side chain has been studied in detail for cefcamate pivoxil (Nakashima et al., 1992; Shimizu et al., 1993; Totsuka et al., 1992).

The metabolism of the POM side chain yielded two components: formaldehyde and pivalic acid.

It has been found that the main metabolite recovered in urine from POM is pivaloylcarnitine (Vickers et al., 1985). Carnitine is an essential cofactor in fatty acid β-oxidation, which takes place mainly in the mitochondrial matrix.

Carnitine acts as a carrier of the acyl groups to transport fatty acids into the mitochodrion inner membrane, which is otherwise impermeable by coenzyme A compounds.

Three subjects received, 0.5 h after a standard meal, 100- or 200-mg tablets of cefcamate pivoxil. Concentrations of cefcamate, pivalic acid, and pivaloylcarnitine in plasma and urine were assayed (Table 62).

Carnitine plays an important role in detoxification of xenobiotics with carboxylic acid in animals and humans.

Other metabolites in humans are glucuronide and glycine conjugates (Melegh et al., 1987).

Conjugation with glycine could be a minor route of excretion of pivalic acid.

After repeated doses, the free carnitine concentrations in plasma were reduced to 65% of the control levels and the plasma pivaloylcarnitine concentration increased, but all returned to normal 3 to 5 days after the completion of the treatment.

The formaldehyde liberated from POM has been hypothesized to be metabolized to carbon dioxide via the C_1 metabolic cycle.

12.3.4. Cyclohexyloxycarbonyl Ethoxy Side Chain (e.g., Cefotiam Hexetil)

The side chain of cefotiam hexetil is metabolized to cyclohexanol and then in three different metabolites, (1,4) cyclohexanediol [(1,4)CH], (1,3)CH, and (1,2)CH, synthesized in the liver.

All of these metabolites are assayed in plasma and urine. However, cyclohexanol levels remain low.

After doses of 400 mg every 8 h for 7 days, cyclohexanol could be detected between 1 and 3 h after dosing. The C_{max} of cyclohexanol is 0.13 μg/ml and is reached 1.7 h after dosing. The $t_{1/2}$ is 1.7 h for an AUC of 0.42 μg · h/ml. Cyclohexanol accounts for less than 1.0% of the administered dose in urine.

(1,2)CH accounts for 36% and (1,3)CH and (1,4)CH account for 18% of the administered dose. The $t_{1/2}$s are long, about 17 h.

In plasma, the peak concentrations of (1,2)CH and (1,3 + 1,4)CH are 0.72 and 0.26 μg/ml and 1.3 and 0.5 μg/ml, respectively, after administration of 200 and 400 mg of cefotiam hexetil. These peaks are reached after an average of 4.5 h for all metabolites. In severe renal impairment, both compounds accumulate (Table 63).

12.4. Gastrointestinal Absorption

12.4.1. Absolute Bioavailability

All of the oral cephalosporin prodrugs exhibit incomplete but comparable bioavailabilities.

The absolute bioavailabilities were reported to be 50% for cefpodoxime proxetil (Tremblay et al., 1990), 55 to 58% for cefetamet pivoxil (Stoeckel et al., 1995), and 52% for cefuroxime axetil (Finn et al., 1987).

The cefuroxime axetil suspension had 10 to 20% lower bioavailability than the tablet form (Donn et al., 1994), while the bioavailability of cefetamet pivoxil syrup is about 30% lower than that of tablets (Ducharme et al., 1993).

The absolute bioavailability of cefprozil is 89% (Shyu et al., 1992). For cefaclor and ceftibuten, absolute bioavailability was not determined. However, recovery of unchanged drug accounts for 90 to 95% of the administered dose for cefaclor (Spyker et al., 1978) and 75 to 90% for ceftibuten (Barr et al., 1991).

The absolute bioavailability of cefixime is less than 50% (Fernandez et al., 1988). Urinary recovery of cefdinir after oral administration is about 36% (Shimada and Soejima, 1987).

The absolute bioavailability of cefotiam hexetil is 45% after oral and intravenous doses of 400 mg.

The absolute bioavailability of cephradine is 94% (Schwinghammer et al., 1990).

The bioavailability of cefpodoxime proxetil tablets relative to the oral solution was 82%, as determined from AUC ratios (Borin et al., 1995).

Based on serum AUCs, the absolute bioavailabilities of cefixime were 52.9, 47.9, and 40.2% after 200-mg oral solution, 200-mg capsule, and 400-mg capsule doses, respectively (Faulkner et al., 1988).

12.4.2. Mechanisms of Gastrointestinal Absorption

12.4.2.1. Nonesterified Cephalosporins

Many studies have been conducted to determine mechanisms involved in the oral absorption of β-lactams.

12.4.2.1.1. Transport system. Oral β-lactams are structural analogs of tripeptides that contain a β-lactam ring, two

Table 62 Pharmacokinetics of pivalic acid and pivaloylcarnitine (plasma)

Drug[a]	Dose (mg)	n	C_{max} (μg/ml)	T_{max} (h)	$t_{1/2\beta}$ (h)	$AUC_{0-\infty}$ (μg·h/ml)	Urinary recovery (%)
Cefcamate	100	3	0.83	4.3	2.24	5.28	93.7
PA	100	3	0.44	3.7	6.07	2.66	92.5
PC	100	3	0.94	4.3	2.64	7.62	89.1
Cefcamate	200	3	2.06	2.3	1.53	10.08	41.3
PA	200	3	1.0	2.3	4.16	5.10	92.5
PC	200	3	2.07	2.3	3.01	13.69	93.8

[a]PA, pivalic acid; PC, pivaloylcarnitine.

Table 63 Pharmacokinetics of cefotiam hexetil metabolites

Parameter (unit)	(1,2) CH		(1,3 + 1,4) CH	
	Normal	Renal impairment	Normal	Renal impairment
C_{max} (μg/ml)	0.72	1.8	0.26	1.1
T_{max} (h)	4.5	6.0	4.4	9.0
$AUC_{0-\infty}$ (μg·h/ml)		33		50
$t_{1/2}$ (h)	15.5	20	16.7	44
Urinary elimination (%)	36	28	18	9.0

peptide bonds, and a free carboxylic acid group. The transporter takes up cephalosporins that exist as zwitterions, such as α-aminocephalosporins, as well as cephalosporins that exist as anions (cefixime and ceftibuten). The cephem molecules are discriminated by the membrane protein, and the structure of the side chain is very important for oral antibiotics to be recognized as tripeptides. The transport of ceftibuten and cephalexin is stereospecific depending on the isomerism of the side chain at the 7 position. The *cis*-isomer of ceftibuten and the D-cephalexin are absorbed, while the *trans*-ceftibuten and L-cephalexin are not taken up.

Muranushi et al. (1995) have shown that there are at least three different transport carriers for oral cephems depending on the N-terminal amino acid of the carrier and the structure of the side chain at the 7 position of molecules.

The first transport system is exemplified by cefaclor (an α-aminocephalosporin) carrier aromatic (hydrophobic) peptides such as Phe-Ala-Ala. The side chains of α-aminocephems are D-phenylglycine. Depending on the orientation of the D-phenyl of cefaclor, it could be taken for L-Phe.

The second one is the relatively hydrophilic concentrative transport system that transports an aliphatic peptide such as Gly-Gly or Glu-Ala-Ala. Ceftibuten could use this carrier system. Ceftibuten has a structure similar to the side chain of glutamic acid, and the nitrogen of the thiazole ring is located at the position of the amino group of glutamic acid.

The third one is a transport system for peptides with a heterocyclic amino acid (tryptophan or histidine) at the N terminus; S-1090 is mainly absorbed through the oligopeptide which recognizes peptides having histidine as the N-terminal amino acid.

12.4.2.1.2. Transport through the basolateral membrane. Once concentrated within the intestinal enterocytes, cephalosporins must leave the cell by the basolateral membrane to enter the bloodstream. A peptide carrier (glycylsarcosine) seems to be located in the basolateral membrane surface and is proton dependent.

It has been shown that cephalexin, cephradine, and loracarbef use a specific basolateral transporter (Hu et al., 1994; Inui et al., 1992).

12.4.2.2. Esterified Cephalosporins

Cefuroxime, cefpodoxime, cefetamet, and cefditoren are not absorbed by the intestinal mucosa. The C-4 ester increases the lipophilicity of the molecule, which diffuses passively through the intestinal mucosa.

Using luminal washing and crude mucosal homogenate, it was observed that hydrolysis of the ester led to the release of free cefpodoxime. The enzyme involved is a choline esterase. It seems that the luminal cefpodoxime proxetil esterase has a broader specificity than the mucosal one (Crauste-Manciet et al., 1997). A carboxylesterase seems to be involved in the release of cefuroxime (Campbell et al., 1987).

The bioavailability of these compounds could be related to the hydrolysis of the ester chain by esterase within the lumen of the intestine.

The esterification of the 2-amino-5-thiazolyl ring may result in increased liphophilicity of the compound but reduced water solubility. To solve the problem of decreased absorption in the gastrointestinal fluid, an amino acid was introduced via the bifunctional prodrug design. Through a series of compounds synthesized, the POM on the C-4 carboxylic group yielded AS-924, an ester of ceftizoxime.

Table 64 shows the pharmacokinetics of esterified oral cephems.

13. ORAL CEPHEMS UNDER INVESTIGATION

13.1. LB-10827

A new class of cephems bearing a 3-pyrimidinyl-substituted sulfonyl, sulfonylmethyl, or sulfonylmethyl-sulfonyl group at the C-3 position of the cephem ring has been synthesized. The targeted bacteria were *S. pneumoniae* isolates resistant to penicillin G.

One compound was selected for further investigation, LB-10827. LB-10827 possesses 2,6-diaminopyrimidinyl-4-thiomethylthio at the C-3 position of the cephem ring and bears a hydroxy residue on the oxime group (Oh et al., 1999).

LB-10827 is more active than cefdinir, cefuroxime, cefprozil, and trovafloxacin against *S. pneumoniae* isolates, irrespective of their susceptibilities to penicillin G.

$MIC_{50/90}$s are ≤0.008/0.016, 0.13/0.13, and 0.5/0.5 μg/ml, respectively, for *S. pneumoniae* isolates susceptible, intermediately susceptible, and resistant to penicillin G. For the last group of microorganisms, trovafloxacin was more active than LB-10827 ($MIC_{50/90}$, 0.25/0.25 μg/ml). LB-10827 also exhibits good in vitro activity against *H. influenzae* isolates producing or not producing β-lactamases ($MIC_{50/90}$, 0.13/0.5 μg/ml) and is 10 times more active than cefuroxime. However, no data were provided for activity against *H. influenzae* harboring a nonenzymatic mechanism of resistance to ampicillin (Paek et al., 1999).

The given antibacterial activity is very difficult to interpret. Data provided for *S. pneumoniae* isolates having a high level of resistance to penicillin G (MIC, 4 μg/ml) showed that LB-10827 activity dropped from 0.008 to 0.5 μg/ml; also, investigation of activity against *H. influenzae* is not well enough documented.

Pneumococcal infections of the lungs were achieved in neutropenic rats induced by cyclophosphamide (Sprague-Dawley rats, 80 to 100 g) by intrabronchial instillation. Tested compounds were administered orally at doses of 2, 10, and 50 mg/kg 18, 26, 42, and 50 h after bacterial challenge with *S. pneumoniae* type III. Bacterial counts were about 4 $\log_{10}$ CFU/lung, whatever the administered doses. Higher burdens were recorded for co-amoxiclav, cefdinir, and trovafloxacin.

In mice (C57 black; six mice, 17 to 19 g), *S. pneumoniae* type III (MIC, 0.008 μg/ml) challenge was performed after intranasal instillation. Tested agents were administered orally 6 h after bacterial challenge and then twice daily for 3 days. With LB-10827 the survival rate was 100% at doses of 50, 17, 5.6, and 1.8 mg/kg. The same survival rate was observed with co-amoxiclav. With cefdinir, a 100% survival rate was recorded after a 50-mg/kg dose, and a 40% survival rate was recorded after a 17-mg/kg dose; for lower doses no survival in mice was recorded (Kim et al., 1999).

LB-10827 may have potential for *S. pneumoniae* isolates resistant to penicillin G. However, data thus for are insufficient, with no use of control rats and no tests with *S. pneumoniae* isolates with different levels of resistance to penicillin G. Other, more convincing studies are warranted.

13.2. Ceftriaxone

Ceftriaxone is only available as a parenteral drug; it is degraded in gastric fluid and also exhibits poor affinity for the peptide transporter PEPT1, and being a hydrophilic compound, it cannot diffuse passively through the enteral membrane.

Table 64 Pharmacokinetics of esterified and nonesterified oral cephems

Drug	Form	n	Dose (mg)	C_{max} (μg/ml)	C_0 (μg/ml)	T_{max} (h)	$AUC_{0-\infty}$ (μg·h/ml)	$t_{1/2}$ (h)	CL_R (ml/min)	CL_P (ml/min)	Urinary elimination (%)	F (%)	Reference
Cephradine	Oral	10	1,000	27.7		1.12		1.12			84	94	Schwinghammer et al., 1990
	i.v.[a]	10	1,000		57.75	0.08		1.12	4.1 (kg)	4.8 (kg)			Schwinghammer et al., 1990
Cefprozil	Oral *cis*	8	500	10.2		1.7	29.7	1.33			71	89	Shyu et al., 1992
	trans	8	500	1.2		1.6	3.2	1.33			65	103	Shyu et al., 1992
	i.v. *cis*	8	500		26	0.5	31.4	1.45	2.4	3.1	76		Shyu et al., 1992
	trans	8	500		2.7	0.5	3.5	1.29	1.9 (kg)	2.8 (kg)	63		
Cefpodoxime proxetil	Oral	12	100	0.96		2.3	4.75	2.4			40.2	50	Tremblay et al., 1990
	i.v.	12	100		2.97	2.0	10.3	2.3	8.1 (kg)	9.9 (liters/h)	80.5		Tremblay et al., 1990
Cefixime	Solution	16	200	3.22		3.1	26.0	3.3			21.3	52.13	Faulkner et al., 1988
	Capsule	16	200	2.92		3.8	23.6	3.4			18.0	41.9	Faulkner et al., 1988
	i.v.	16	200		30.5	0.08	47.0	3.2	29	73	40.8		Faulkner et al., 1988
	Capsule	16	400	4.84		3.8	39.4	3.5			18.0	40.2	Faulkner et al., 1988
Cefotiam hexetil	i.v.	12	400				19.6	1.3	24.6	345	70		
	Oral	12	400	3.3		2.5	8.8	1.0			29	45	

[a]i.v., intravenous.

Bioadhesive polymers that bind to the epithelial cell surface could be useful in drug delivery through the enteric membrane. Three oral formulations of ceftriaxone were prepared using carrageenan as a mucoadhesive polymer and calcium, arginine, and cetylpyridinium chloride as binding agents.

To determine the enteral absorption of those formulations, each formulation was given to male Sprague-Dawley rats through the duodenum at the equivalent of 40 mg of ceftriaxone per kg. The peak concentrations in plasma ranged from 28.8 μg/ml (cetylpyridinium chloride) to 69.1 μg/ml (calcium), with $AUC_{0-\infty s}$ of 136 ± 0.1, 113.5 ± 20.7, and 16.5 ± 56.8 μg·h/ml for the calcium, arginine, and cetylpyridinium formulations, respectively. In comparison with the intravenous administration, the bioavailabilities were 36.2, 30.1, and 43.9%, respectively. However, ceftriaxone alone in this model was absorbed at 13.9%.

13.3. 3-Isoxazolylvinyl Cephalosporins: KST 150,257 and KST 105,290

A series of 3-isoxazolylvinyl cephalosporins has been synthesized. Two compounds, KST 105,257 and KST 150,290 (Fig. 9), esterified at the C-4 position of the cephem ring with a POM chain, showed oral bioavailabilities in mice of 33 and 52%, respectively, values higher than that of cefixime (30%) but lower than that of cefpodoxime proxetil (84%).

They displayed good in vitro activity against gram-positive cocci and *Enterobacteriaceae* not producing β-lactamases. They were inactive against *E. cloacae* P99 and *P. aeruginosa*.

They are claimed to be active against methicillin-resistant *S. aureus*, but no affinity for PBP 2a has been shown, and the in vitro methodology was not clearly stated (Choi et al., 1997; Park et al., 1997).

13.4. AS-924

AS-924 is a prodrug of ceftizoxime, a parenteral cephalosporin. It is a bifunctional prodrug, with a lipophilic group at C-4 (POM group) and a water-soluble group (L-alanyl) fixed on the 2-amino group of the 2-amino-5-thiazolyl moiety at C-7 (Fig. 10).

The ceftizoxime ester is assumed to be stable to isomerization from the Δ^3 to the Δ^2 ester because it has no substituent at the C-3 position. In a rabbit model, the urinary elimination was significantly enhanced by esterification of C-4, from 5.36% to 11.12 to 35.59%. Of the esters, the POM ester showed the highest urinary elimination. Analysis showed a parabolic relationship between logP and urinary elimination values for the monofunctional prodrugs, with an optimum logP of 1.81.

To enhance water solubility, various amino acids were introduced as basic moieties onto the amino group of the thiazole group of ceftizoxime POM. This amino acid increased the water solubility at both pH 4.5 and 6.0.

Urinary elimination in rabbits is increased only by introduction of an L-alanyl moiety.

At the C-4 position the POM is quickly hydrolyzed by intestinal esterase. The hydrolysis of ceftizoxime amide varied according to the amino acids introduced (half-lives from 5.9 to 79.47 min). The L-valine was hydrolyzed most slowly and more than 60% remained after 60 min, while the L-leucine and L-lysine derivatives were almost completely degradated within 30 min. The L-alanine derivative disappeared over 60 min.

Extensive pharmacokinetic studies have been carried out. Ascending dose administration to volunteers (25 to 200 mg) showed a peak concentration ranging from 0.34

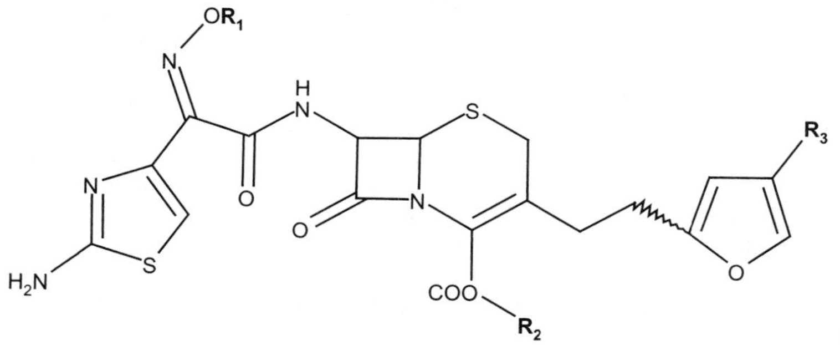

Figure 9 3-Isoxazolylvinyl cephalosporins

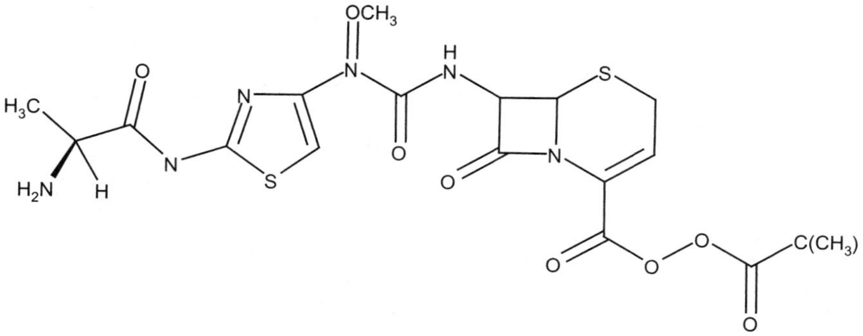

Figure 10 AS-924

to 2.83 μg/ml, which was reached between 1.5 and 2.0 h. The $t_{1/2}$ is 1.3 h, with an AUC_{0-12} ranging from 1.13 to 10.16 μg·h/ml. About 40% of the administered dose is eliminated as ceftizoxime in urine. AS-924 is currently undergoing phase II and III trials in Japan.

13.4.1. Conclusion

This compound has the same antibacterial activity as ceftizoxime, including poor activity against *S. pneumoniae* intermediately susceptible or resistant to penicillin G. However, it is the first compound among the cefotaxime derivatives which is orally absorbed and has reached clinical trials. Previously, cefuzonam prodrug had been described together with a pharmaceutical preparation of ceftizoxime (KY-20), but they never reached clinical trials. The presence of the POM ester chain could be detrimental by decreasing plasma L-carnithine levels by 50% and by producing formaldehyde (data not shown).

14. INTERACTIONS WITH OTHER MEDICINAL PRODUCTS

Two studies conducted with cefaclor and ceftibuten showed that they did not affect the pharmacokinetics of theophylline.

One study showed that simultaneous administration of cefprozil and antacids had few effects on the plasma pharmacokinetics of cefprozil. Similar results were observed with concomitant administration of antacids, anti-H2 (ranitidine), and cefetamet pivoxil, apart from slightly delayed absorption of the last (T_{max}), of about 20%. Conversely, some studies have shown that concomitant ingestion of antacids and/or anti-H2 with cefpodoxime proxetil might significantly reduce absorption of the latter.

The renal elimination of oral cephalosporins often involves two mechanisms, i.e., glomerular filtration and tubular secretion, and it has been shown that concomitant administration of probenecid and oral cephalosporins may delay the excretion of most of them.

15. CLINICAL INDICATIONS

The clinical use of oral cephalosporins depends on a number of factors, including the severity of the infection, the pathogenicity of the bacteria involved, and the pharmacokinetics of the drug. Given their antibacterial spectrum, the oral cephalosporins may be used in a number of infections.

16. ADVERSE EFFECTS

The adverse effects associated with administration of oral cephalosporins are generally benign and infrequent. It is, however, difficult to compare the exact incidence of these reactions among the cephalosporins since the data derive from noncomparative studies with numerous differences in terms of the methodology of recording these adverse effects. Nevertheless, it is possible to compile a general table of adverse effects related to administration of oral cephalosporins.

16.1. Alterations of Microflora

Gastrointestinal disturbances are the most common adverse events reported with oral cephalosporins: nausea, vomiting, and diarrhea.

The composition of microflora can be influenced by antibacterial agents because of incomplete absorption of orally administered drugs, high rate of elimination by bile, and strong activity against microorganisms of the microflora.

Cefuroxime axetil (600 mg/dose every 8 h for 3 days) caused a decrease of *Enterobacteriaceae* in three volunteers who developed diarrhea. *Bacteroides* spp. and anaerobic cocci decreased significantly, but not clostridia (Wise et al., 1984).

Cefixime (200 mg b.i.d. for 7 days) was administered to 10 healthy volunteers. Cefixime was detectable in the feces (237 to 912 mg/kg of feces) from day 1 to day 7. There was a marked decrease in the number of *Enterobacteriaceae* as well as anaerobic flora. *Clostridium difficile* was isolated in five volunteers. Cytotoxin was detected in only one subject. The intestinal microflora normalized within 2 weeks after treatment was stopped (Nord et al., 1988).

Cefpodoxime proxetil was given for 10 days. Cefpodoxime was measured in the feces (0 to 3.65 U of cefpodoxime/g of feces). *C. difficile* was detected (Chachaty et al., 1992). The same results were obtained with cefprozil (500 mg b.i.d. for 8 days) (Lode et al., 1992) and ceftibuten (400 mg g.d. for 10 days) (Brismar et al., 1993). With cefetamet pivoxil in one study (500 mg b.i.d. for 10 days), no *C. difficile* organisms were detected (Novelli et al., 1994).

16.2. Interaction with Absorption

The absorption of oral cephems given concomitantly with other drugs could be affected.

16.2.1. Anti-H2 Receptors and Antacid Drugs

The effect of antacids and anti-H2 receptors on the bioavailability of oral prodrug cephalosporins is of importance, since the solubility of these compounds is pH dependent (Table 65).

Little to no information exists on the potential interaction between cephalexin, cephradine, cefadroxil, cefaclor, and cephaloglycin and antacids or H2 receptor antagonists. Data have been published extensively for cefpodoxime proxetil and to a lesser extent for cefuroxime axetil, cefprozil, and cefixime. Agents which increase gastric pH (e.g., cimetidine, ranitidine, famotidine, and sodium carbonate) could reduce the dissolution of the prodrug cephalosporins, resulting in impaired bioavailability.

Hughes et al. (1989) found that pretreatment with ranitidine and sodium carbonate reduces the bioavailability of cefpodoxime proxetil by 30% (Table 66). Saathoff et al. (1992) showed that the relative bioavailability of cefpodoxime proxetil is reduced by 60% after pretreatment with famotidine and Maalox. After pentagastrin stimulation, the relative bioavailability of cefpodoxime proxetil was greater. These differences could be due partly to a better dissolution of cefpodoxime tablets under acidic conditions, but also to a better solubility of the drug at low pH.

After oral doses of ranitidine (300 mg) and sodium bicarbonate (4 g), the peak concentration in plasma and AUC for cefuroxime axetil are reduced by 19 and 43%, respectively (Sommers et al., 1984).

Antacids seem to have no effect on the relative bioavailabilities of cefixime (Healy et al., 1989), cefprozil (Shyu et al., 1992), ceftibuten (Wiseman et al., 1994), and cefetamet pivoxil (Blouin et al., 1990).

The pharmacokinetic parameters of cefpodoxime were not affected by metoclopramide and anisotropine methylbromide (Uchida et al., 1989). The bioavailabilities of cefetamet pivoxil (Blouin et al., 1990) and cefotiam hexetil have been shown to be slightly affected by ranitidine and Maalox.

16.2.2. Food Interactions

In various studies carried out to investigate the effect of food on the relative bioavailability of oral cephalosporins, it has been shown that there is a delay (T_{max}) of the absorption of the majority of the drugs (Table 67).

Absorption of cefcapene pivoxil was enhanced because de-esterification of the POM moiety of cefcapene pivoxil in the gut was prevented by food intake.

In nonfasting volunteers, the T_{max} of AS-924 was prolonged in the postprandial administration, while C_{max} and AUC increased by 10 to 20%.

16.2.3. Effect of Diet on Absorption

Food produces many complex effects on gastrointestinal function.

Sixteen healthy nonsmoking adults participated in a study of food interaction with cefpodoxime proxetil (200 mg) (Hughes et al., 1989). Six different diets were given: (i) no food (fasting), (ii) a standard diet, (iii) a high-protein diet, (iv) a low-protein diet, (v) a high-fat diet, and (vi) a low-fat diet. The pharmacokinetic parameters are listed in Table 68.

Statistically significant differences in the mean values were determined for the $AUC_{0-\infty}$ among the six diets. Fasted subjects had significantly lower $AUC_{0-\infty}$ relative to the AUC estimates for the subjects receiving any food. Absorption of food increases the overall extent of absorption of cefpodoxime. The composition of the meal does not appear to influence the overall extent of absorption. Food may increase the C_{max} relative to maximum drug concentrations obtained under fasting conditions.

Table 65 Solubilities of oral cephalosporins at various pHs

Drug	pH	Solubility (mg/ml)
Cefpodoxime proxetil	1.5	11.4
	6.8	0.4
Cefuroxime axetil	<1	1.0
Cefetamet pivoxil	1.0	21
	4.0	0.18
	6.8	0.14
Cefixime	2.0	0.34
	4.4	491
Cefprozil	1.8	40
	5 (*cis*)	6.18
	5 (*trans*)	1.0

Table 66 Effects of various drug which modify gastric pH on pharmacokinetics of cefpodoxime (200 mg to 17 volunteers)

Drug	C_{max} (μg/ml)	T_{max} (h)	$AUC_{0-\infty}$ (μg·h/ml)	Urinary elimination (%)
Cefpodoxime proxetil				
Alone (fast)	2.24	2.44	13.40	32.4
+ Ranitidine	1.5	3.65	9.21	23.9
+ Pentagastrin	2.61	2.68	15.30	36.4
+ Sodium bicarbonate	1.31	2.50	8.76	25.8
+ Aluminum hydroxide	1.70	2.50	9.58	27.0

Table 67 Effect of food on oral cephalosporin pharmacokinetic

Drug	Patient state	Dose (mg)	*n*	C_{max} (μg/ml)	T_{max} (h)	$AUC_{0-\infty}$ (μg·h/ml)	Reference
Cefetamet pivoxil	Fasting	1,500	6	7.4	3.0	45.8	Koup et al., 1988
	Fed	1,500	6	9.7	4.8	64.7	
Cefuroxime axetil	Fasting	1,000	6	1.5	7.3	23.4	Sommers et al., 1984
	Fed	1,000	6	1.5	13.6	39.8	Sommers et al., 1984
Cefditoren pivoxil	Fasting	200	6	2.3	1.4	6.28	Shimada et al., 1989
	Fed	200	6	3.4	2.0	10.02	
Cefteram pivoxil	Fasting	400	5	7.4	1.9	24.8	Patel et al., 1986
	Fed	400	5	6.3	2.2	25.3	Patel et al., 1986
Cefixime	Fasting	400		4.24	3.8	32.02	Faulkner et al., 1987
	Fed	400		4.22	4.8	30.78	Faulkner et al., 1987
Cefotiam hexetil	Fasting	400	12	4.8	1.4	9.1	Deppermann et al., 1989
	Fed	400	12	4.4	1.9	10.0	Deppermann et al., 1989
Cefprozil	Fasting	250	12	6.13	1.2	15.0	Barbhaiya et al., 1990
	Fed	250	12	8.70	0.6	8.6	Barbhaiya et al., 1990
Ceftibuten	Fasting	100	6	6.10	2.6	24.2	Nakashima et al., 1986
	Fed	100	6	5.10	3.2	23.2	Nakashima et al., 1986
Loracarbef	Fasting	400	12	19.2	1.1	33.04	Roller et al., 1992
	Fed	400	12	13.64	2.4	35.38	Roller et al., 1992
Cefdinir	Fasting	100	6	1.25	3.5	6.16	Shimada and Soejima, 1987
	Fed	100	6	0.79	4.3	4.04	Shimada and Soejima, 1987
Cefaclor	Fasting	250	12	8.7	0.6	8.60	Barbhaiya et al., 1990
	Fed	250	12	4.29	1.3	7.59	Barbhaiya et al., 1990
Cephalexin	Fasting	1,000	6	38.8	0.9	93	Lode et al., 1979
	Fed	1,000	6	23.1	1.8	70	Lode et al., 1979
Cefadroxil	Fasting	500	16	14.7	0.5	43.3	Pfeffer et al., 1977
	Fed	500	16	16.3	0.6	45.1	Pfeffer et al., 1977
Ceftizoxime alapivoxil	Fasting	100	8	1.52	1.8	5.02	Totsuka et al., 2001
	Fed	100	8	1.72	2.1	6.02	
Cefmatilen	Fasting	100	6	2.79	2.5	20.35	Nakashima et al., 1993
	Fed	100	6	3.78	3.17	25.51	

Table 68 Pharmacokinetics of cefpodoxime proxetil (200 mg) with different diets

Diet	C_{max} (μg/ml)	Lag time (h)	T_{max} (h)	$AUC_{0-\infty}$ (μg·h/ml)	Urinary elimination (%)
Fasting	2.62	0.40	2.75	13.5	41.0
Standard	3.11	0.81	3.25	17.6	51.8
High protein	3.19	0.85	3.78	16.9	64.1
Low protein	3.14	0.82	3.38	17.0	52.2
High fat	3.02	0.62	3.22	16.3	54.0
Low fat	3.25	0.69	3.47	18.0	55.4

16.2.4. Water and Milk Interactions

It was shown that absorption of oral antibiotics such as amoxicillin and erythromycin was significantly reduced when they were taken with a small quantity of water. However, the absorption of ampicillin is less affected than that of amoxicillin by the volume of water (at least 150 ml of water) (Table 69).

For AS-924, there is no difference in absorption after concomitant absorption of water and milk.

16.2.5. Iron Interactions

Cefdinir is a hydroxyiminocephalosporin which complexes with iron ion. When cefdinir (200 mg) and ferrous sulfate (105 mg) are given concomitantly, the bioavailability of cefdinir decreases. When ferrous sulfate is given 3 h after cefdinir intake, the relative bioavailability of cefdinir remains unchanged (Table 70) (Ueno et al., 1993).

16.2.6. Antacid Interactions

Antacids elevate the pH in the stomach, and the water solubility of cephems decreases (Table 71).

After a pretreatment with 150 mg of ranitidine, the plasma parameters of AS-924 were not affected, while those of urine were slightly increased.

16.3. Other Drug Interactions

It has been shown that the administration of an oral dose of 200 mg of ceftibuten every 12 h does not alter the systemic clearance of theophylline given in a single intravenous dose (Bachmann et al., 1990). Ceftibuten, like

Table 69 Effect of volume of water on pharmacokinetics of AS-924 and cefcapene pivoxil

Drug	Quantity of water (ml)	C_{max} (μg/ml)	T_{max} (h)	$t_{1/2}$ (h)	AUC_{0-12h} (μg·h/ml)	Urinary elimination (%)	
						Parent compound	*p*-Carnitine
AS-924	30	2.82	2.3	1.5	10.56	41.6	91
	150	2.94	1.8	1.3	10.36	43.9	90.2
Cefteram pivoxil	30	1.41	2.7	1.2	4.46	20.3	73.7
	150	2.02	1.8	1.1	6.28	27.2	74.3

Table 70 Interaction of cefdinir and ferrous ion

Drug	Dose (mg)	*n*	C_{max} (μg/ml)	T_{max} (h)	$AUC_{0-\infty}$ (μg·h/ml)
Cefdinir					
Alone	200	6	1.71	4.2	10.3
+ Iron	200	6	0.16	1.8	0.78
+ Iron 3 h after	200	6	1.28	3.3	6.55

Table 71 Interactions of ranitidine with AS-924 and cefteram

Drug	*n*	Dose (mg)	C_{max} (μg/ml)	T_{max} (h)	AUC (μg·h/ml)	$t_{1/2}$ (h)	Urinary elimination (%)	
							Parent compound	Δ^2 isomer
AS-924								
Alone	8	100	1.72	2.4	6.22	1.3	47.6	ND[a]
+ Ranitidine	8	150	1.60	2.3	5.74	1.3	46.1	ND
Cefteram								
Alone	8	200	2.32	2.6	7.38	1.0	28.3	0.9
+ Ranitidine	8	150	1.58	2.3	4.56	1.0	17.9	1.4

[a]ND, not determined.

some other β-lactams (ticarcillin, moxalactam [latamoxef], and carbenicillin), possesses a carboxylic group at C-7; its effects on platelet functions and blood coagulation have been tested in humans and animals. Ceftibuten did not affect platelet function or blood coagulation (Nakashima et al., 1988).

The presence of warfarin reduced both the percentage of protein binding and the isomerization rate constant of ceftibuten (Shimada et al., 1993). It is suggested that ceftibuten is isomerized at the warfarin binding site on albumin.

After pretreatment with a single oral dose of either 200 or 400 mg of cefixime, no impairment of the metabolism of vitamin K_1 could be detected in healthy volunteers (Trenk et al., 1990).

The types of unfavorable reactions due to oral cephalosporins might arbitrarily be classified into three categories: gastrointestinal disorders, allergic reactions (cutaneous and systemic), and other adverse effects.

Gastrointestinal disorders comprise diarrhea, nausea, vomiting, dyspepsia, and abdominal cramping. Diarrhea appears to be the most commonly reported adverse effect with cephalosporins. The incidences of gastrointestinal disorders (3 to 10%) appear to be comparable among the oral cephalosporins, apart from cefixime and cefuroxime axetil. In addition, if the last two are excluded, the incidence of diarrhea for the oral cephalosporins appears to be comparable to that for amoxicillin but less than that for amoxicillin-clavulanic acid. In the case of cefixime, the incidence of diarrhea would appear to be 10 to 15%, depending on the study, and more common than with amoxicillin. In addition, the incidence of diarrhea induced by cefuroxime axetil appears to be comparable to that with amoxicillin-clavulanic acid. Finally, there have been only a very few cases of pseudomembranous colitis due to oral cephalosporins, but the few cases reported were for the most part associated with administration of cefixime or cefuroxime axetil.

The incidence of allergic skin reactions (i.e., rash, pruritius, and erythema) appears to be comparable to that due to the other antibiotics of the β-lactam group. A few cases of anaphylaxis have been reported following administration of oral cephalosporins. A few cases of hematological disorders have also been reported, such as hemolytic anemia, neutropenia, and thrombocytopenia.

Lastly, the other adverse reactions reported include fever, headache, transient asymptomatic elevation of hepatic transaminases, and vaginal and oral candidosis.

REFERENCES

Adam D, Kreutle O, 1980, Investigation on the diffusion of cefadroxil and cephalexin into tonsil tissue, Infection, 8, Suppl 5, 580–583.

Adamson I, Edlund C, Sjöstedt S, Nord CE, 1997, Comparative effects of cefadroxil and phenoxypenicillin on the normal oropharyngeal and intestinal microflora, Infection, 25, 154–158.

Adler M, McDonald PJ, Trostmann U, Keyserling C, Tack K, 1997, Cefdinir *versus* amoxicillin/clavulanic acid in the treatment of suppurative acute otitis media in children, Eur J Clin Microbiol Infect Dis, 16, 214–219.

Agger WA, Callister SM, Jobe DA, 1992, In vitro susceptibilities of *Borrelia burgdorferi* to five oral cephalosporins and ceftriaxone, Antimicrob Agents Chemother, 36, 1788–1790.

Akiyama H, Torigoe R, Yamada T, et al., 1992, ME 1207 in the field of dermatology, Chemotherapy, 40, Suppl 2, 619–623.

Almirall J, Morato I, Riera F, Verdaquer A, Priu R, Coll P, Vidal J, Murgai I, Vallas F, Catalan F, 1993, Incidence of community acquired pneumonia and *Chlamydi pneumoniae* infection: a prospective multicenter study, Eur Respir J, 6, 14–18.

Arguedas AG, Arrieta AC, Stutman HR, Akinaro JC, Marks MI, 1991, In vitro activity of cefprozil (BMY 28100) and loracarbef (LY 163892) against pathogens obtained from middle-ear fluid, J Antimicrob Chemother, 27, 311–318.

Aronovitz GH, Doyle CA, Durham SJ, et al, 1992, Cefprozil *vs* amoxicillin-clavulanate in the treatment of otitis media, Infect Med, 9, Suppl C, 19–32.

Ausina V, Coll P, Sambeat M, Puig I, Condom MJ, Luquin M, Ballester F, Prats G, 1988, Prospective study on the etiology of community-acquired pneumonia in children and adults in Spain, Eur J Clin Microbiol Infect Dis, 7, 342–347.

Avril JL, Mesnard R, Donnio PY, 1990, Comparative in vitro activity of cefpodoxime against *Pasteurella multocida*, Int Congr Infect Dis.

Avril JL, Mesnard R, Donnio PY, 1991, In vitro activity of penicillin, amoxycillin and certain cephalosporins, including cefpodoxime, against human isolates of *Pasteurella multocida*, J Antimicrob Chemother, 28, 473–474.

Axelrod JL, Kochman KS, 1980, Cefaclor levels in human aqueous humor, Arch Ophthalmol, 98, 740–742.

Axelrod JL, Kochman KS, 1981, Cephradine levels in human aqueous humor, Arch Ophthalmol, 99, 2034–2036.

Bachmann K, Schwartz J, Jauregui L, Martin M, Nunlee M, 1990, Failure of ceftibuten to alter single dose theophylline clearance, J Clin Pharmacol, 30, 444–448.

Backhaus A, Tinz J, 1990, Cefixim Therapie bei Patienten mit nachgewiesener Gonorrhoe, Infection, 18, Suppl 3, 145–146.

Bailey RR, Gower PEC, Dash CH, 1970, The effect of impairment of renal function and hemodialysis on serum and urine levels of cephalexin, Postgrad Med J, 46, 60–64.

Bairamis TN, Nikolopoulos T, Kafetzis DA, et al, 1996, Concentrations of cefpodoxime in plasma, adenoid and tonsillar tissue after repeated administration of cefpodoxime proxetil in children, J Antimicrob Chemother, 37, 821–824.

Baldwin DR, Andrews JM, Wise R, Honeybourne D, 1992, Broncheoalveolar distribution of cefuroxime axetil and in vitro efficacy of observed concentrations against respiratory pathogens, J Antimicrob Chemother, 30, 377–385.

Baldwin DR, Wise R, Andrews JM, Honeybourne D, 1992, Concentrations of cefpodoxime in serum and bronchial mucosa biopsies, J Antimicrob Chemother, 30, 67–71.

Baquero F, Loza E, 1994, Antibiotic resistance of micro-organisms involved in ear, nose and throat infections, Pediatr Infect Dis J, 13, S9–S14.

Barbhaiya RH, Gleason CR, Shyu WC, Wilber RC, Martin RR, Pittman KA, 1990, Phase I study of single-dose BMY-28100, a new oral cephalosporin, Antimicrob Agents Chemother, 34, 202–205.

Barbhaiya RH, Shukla UA, Gleason CR, Shyu WC, Wilber RB, Pittman KA, 1990, Comparison of cefprozil and cefaclor pharmacokinetics and tissue penetration, Antimicrob Agents Chemother, 34, 1204–1209.

Barbhaiya RH, Shukla UA, Gleason CR, et al, 1990, Comparison of the effects of food on the pharmacokinetics of cefprozil and cefaclor, Antimicrob Agents Chemother, 34, 1210–1213.

Barr WH, Affrime M, Lin CC, Batra V, 1993, Pharmacokinetics of ceftibuten in children, Pediatr Infect Dis J, 12, S55–S63.

Barr WH, Affrime M, Lin CC, Batra V, 1995, Pharmacokinetics of ceftibuten in children, Pediatr Infect Dis J, 14, S93–S101.

Barr W, Lin CC, Radwanski E, Lim J, Symchovicz S, Affrime M, 1991, The pharmacokinetics of ceftibuten in humans, Diagn Microbiol Infect Dis, 14, 93–100.

Barry A, 1997, Antipneumococcal activity of a ketolide (HMR 3647) and seven related drugs in vitro, 37th Intersci Conf Antimicrob Agents Chemother.

Bauernfeind A, 1993, Comparative in-vitro activities of the new quinolone, Bay y 3118, and ciprofloxacin, sparfloxacin, tosufloxacin, CI-960 and CI-990, J Antimicrob Chemother, 31, 505–522.

Bauernfeind A, Jungwirth R, 1991, Antibacterial activity of cefpodoxime in comparison with cefixime, cefdinir, cefetamet, ceftibuten, loracarbef, cefprozil, BAY 3522, cefuroxime, cefaclor and cefadroxil, Infection, 19, 353–362.

Beam TR Jr, Gilbert DN, Kunin CM, 1992, General guidelines for the clinical evaluation of anti-infective drug products, Clin Infect Dis, 15, suppl 1, 5–32.

Bégué P, Garabédian N, Quinet B, Baron S, 1989, Diffusion amygdalienne du cefixime chez l'enfant, Presse Med, 18, 1593–1595.

Berk SL, Kalbfleisch JH, the Alexander Project Group, 1996, Antibiotic susceptibility patterns of community-acquired respiratory isolates of *M. catarrhalis* in Western Europe and in the USA, J Antimicrob Chemother, 38, suppl A, 85–96.

Berman SJ, Boughton WH, Sugihara JG, Wong EGC, Sato MM, Siemsen AW, 1978, Pharmacokinetics of cefaclor in patients with end-stage renal disease and during hemodialysis, Antimicrob Agents Chemother, 14, 281–283.

Bessaguet MF, Champy R, Chassagnac F, Defaye P, Dumont Y, Renaudie P, Servole JP, Denis F, Mounier M, 1994, Concentrations de céfaclor dans l'oreille moyenne chez l'enfant, Med Mal Infect, 24, 719–722.

Blasi F, Cosentini R, Legnani D, Denti F, Allegra L, 1993, Incidence of community acquired pneumonia caused by *Chlamydia pneumoniae* in Italian patients, Eur J Clin Microbiol Infect Dis, 12, 696–699.

Blouin RA, Kneer J, Ambros RJ, Stoeckel K, 1990, Influence of antacid and ranitidine on the pharmacokinetics of oral cefetamet pivoxil, Antimicrob Agents Chemother, 34, 1744–1748.

Blouin RA, Kneer J, Stoeckel K, 1989, Pharmacokinetics of intravenous cefetamet (Ro 15-8074) and oral cefetamet pivoxil (Ro 15-8075) in young and elderly subjects, Antimicrob Agents Chemother, 33, 291–296.

Blouin RA, Stoeckel K, 1993, Cefetamet pivoxil clinical pharmacokinetics, Clin Pharmacokinet, 25, 172–188.

Bluestone CD, 1992, Current therapy for otitis media and criteria for evaluation of new antimicrobial agents, Clin Infect Dis, 14, Suppl 2, S197–S203.

Blummer JL, McLinn SE, Deabate CA, Kafetzis DA, Perrotta RJ, Salgado O, 1995, Multinational multicenter controlled trial comparing ceftibuten with cefaclor for the treatment of acute otitis media, Pediatr Infect Dis J, 14, S115–S120.

Bolduc GR, Tam PG, Pelton S, 1996, Therapeutic approaches to experimental otitis media due to penicillin resistant *Streptococcus pneumoniae*, p 518–519, in Recent Advances in Otitis Media.

Borin MT, Forbes KK, Hughes GS, 1995, The bioavailability of cefpodoxime proxetil tablets relative to an oral solution, Biopharm Drug Disp, 16, 295–302.

Borin MT, Hughes GS, Kelloway JS, Shapiro BE, Halstenson CE, 1992, Disposition of cefpodoxime proxetil in hemodialysis patients, J Clin Pharmacol, 92, 1038–1044.

Borin MT, Hughes GS, Spillers CR, Patel RK, 1990, Pharmacokinetics of cefpodoxime in plasma and skin blister fluid following oral dosing of cefpodoxime proxetil, Antimicrob Agents Chemother, 34, 1094–1099.

Boyle GL, et al, 1970, Intraocular penetration of cephalexin in man, Am J Ophthalmol, 69, 869–872.

Brenwald N, Andrews J, Baswell F, Wise R, 1996, CG 5501 in vitro study against clinical isolates including *Chlamydia* spp and *Mycobacterium tuberculosis*, 36th Intersci Conf Antimicrob Agents Chemother, abstract F54.

Briggs BM, Jones RN, Erwin ME, Barrett MS, Johnson DM, 1991, In vitro activity evaluation of cefdinir (FK 482, CI-983 and PD 1314393)—a novel orally administered cephalosporin, Diagn Microbiol Infect Dis, 14, 424–425.

Brismar B, Edlund C, Nord CE, 1993, Effect of ceftibuten on the normal intestinal microflora, Infection, 21, 373–375.

Brismar B, Edlund C, Nord CE, 1993, Impact of cefpodoxime proxetil and amoxicillin on the normal oral and intestinal microflora, Eur J Clin Microbiol Infect Dis, 12, 714–719.

Brittain DC, Scully BE, Hirose T, Neu HC, 1985, The pharmacokinetic and bactericidal characteristics of oral cefixime, Clin Pharmacol Ther, 38, 590–594.

Brook I, Gober AE, 1997, Monthly changes in the rate of recovery of penicillin-resistant organisms from children, Pediatr Infect Dis J, 16, 255–257.

Brumfitt W, Franklin I, Grady D, Hamilton-Miller JM, 1986, Effect of amoxicillin-clavulanate and cephradine on the fecal flora of healthy volunteers not exposed to a hospital environment, Antimicrob Agents Chemother, 30, 335–337.

Bryskier A, Aszodi J, Chantot JF, 1994, Parenteral cephalosporin classification, Expert Opin Investig Drugs, 3, 145–171.

Callaham M, 1980, Prophylactic antibiotics in common dog bite wounds: a controlled study, Ann Emerg Med, 9, 410–414.

Campbell CJ, Chantrell LJ, Eastmond R, 1987, Purification and partial characterisation of rat intestinal cefuroxime axetil esterase, Biochem Pharmacol, 36, 2317–2324.

Carpentier JL, 1990, Klebsiella pulmonary infections: occurrence at one medical center and review, Rev Infect Dis, 12, 672–682.

Carson JWK, Watters K, Taylor MRH, Keane CT, 1987, Clinical trial of cefuroxime axetil in children, J Antimicrob Chemother, 19, 109–112.

Celin SE, Bluestone CD, Stephenson JY, Imag HM, Collins JF, 1991, Bacteriology of acute otitis media in adults, JAMA, 266, 2249–2252.

Centers for Disease Control, 1993, 1993 sexually transmitted diseases treatment guideline, Morb Mortal Wkly Rep, 42(RR-14), 56–59.

Chachaty E, Depitre C, Mario N, et al, 1992, Presence of *Clostridium difficile* and β-lactamase activities in feces of volunteers treated with oral cefixime, oral cefpodoxime proxetil, or placebo, Antimicrob Agents Chemother, 36, 2009–2013.

Chaïbi EB, Mugnier P, Kitzis MD, Goldstein FW, Acar JF, 1995, β-Lactamases de *Branhamella catarrhalis* et leurs implications phénotypiques, Res Microbiol, 146, 761–771.

Chantot JF, Mauvais P, 1991, RU 51807 (cefpodoxime proxetil), evaluation de l'activité antibactérienne in vitro et in vivo d'une nouvelle céphalosporine active par voie orale, Pathol Biol, 39, 17–27.

Choi KI, Cha JH, Cho YS, et al, 1997, Novel 3-isoxazolylvinyl cephalosporins. I. Synthesis and in vitro antimicrobial susceptibilities, 37th Intersci Conf Antimicrob Agents Chemother, abstract F-182.

Chow M, Quintiliani R, Cunha BA, Thompson M, Finkelstein E, Nightingale CH, 1979, Pharmacokinetics of high-dose oral cephalosporins, J Clin Pharmacol, 19, 185–194.

Cohen R, Roque F, Dort C, et al, 1993, High rates of penicillin-resistant *S. pneumoniae* in otitis media unresponsive to initial antibiotherapy, 33rd Intersci Conf Antimicrob Agents Chemother, 337.

Comité de l'antibiogramme de la Société Française de Microbiologie, 1996, Communiqué 1996, Pathol Biol, 44, 8-I-VIII.

Coonan KM, Kaplan EL, 1994, In vitro susceptibilities of recent North American group A streptococcal isolates to eleven oral antibiotics, Pediatr Infect Dis J, 13, 630–635.

Couet W, Fauvet JP, Laville M, Pozet N, Fourtillan JB, 1991, Pharmacokinetics of oral cefatrizine in patients with impaired renal function, Int J Clin Pharmacol Ther Toxicol, 29, 213–217.

Couet W, Reigner BG, Lefebvre MA, Bizouard J, Fourtillan JB, 1988, Pharmacocinétique de la céfatrizine administrée en doses répétées, Pathol Biolol, 36, 513–516.

Couraud L, Andrews JM, Lecoeur H, Sultan E, Lenfant B, 1990, Concentrations of cefpodoxime in plasma and lung tissue after a single oral dose of cefpodoxime proxetil, J Antimicrob Chemother, 26, suppl E, 35–40.

Cox CE, Graveline JF, Luongo JM, 1991, Review of clinical experience in the United States with cefpodoxime-proxetil in adults with uncomplicated urinary tract infections, Drugs, 42, Suppl 3, 41–50.

Craig W, Andes D, 1996, Pharmacokinetics and pharmacodynamics of antibiotics in otitis media, Pediatr Infect Dis J, 15, 255–259.

Crauste-Manciet S, Huneau JF, Decroix MO, Tomé D, Farinotti R, Chaumeil JC, 1997, Cefpodoxime proxetil esterase activity in rabbit small intestine: a role in the partial cefpodoxime absorption, Int J Pharm, 149, 241–249.

Cullmann W, Dick W, 1990, Cefpodoxime: comparable evaluation with other orally available cephalosporins: with a note on the role of β-lactamases, Int J Med Microbiol, 273, 501–517.

Cullmann W, Then RL, 1991, Cefetamet, its in vitro activity and interaction with β-lactamases and penicillin-binding proteins, Drug Investig, 3, 299–307.

Dabernat H, Avril JL, Boussougant Y, 1990, In vitro activity of cefpodoxime against pathogens responsible for community-acquired respiratory tract infections, J Antimicrob Chemother, 26, suppl E, 1–6.

Dabernat H, Delmas C, Lareng MB, 1991, Infections respiratoires à *Haemophilus influenzae* intérêt du céfuroxime axétil, Med Mal Infect, 21, Hors série, 22–26.

Dagan R, Abramson O, Leibovitz E, Lang R, Gosben S, Greenberg D, Yagupsky P, Liberman A, Fliss DM, 1996, Impaired bacteriologic response to oral cephalosporins in acute otitis media caused by pneumococci with intermediate resistance to penicillin, Pediatr Infect Dis J, 15, 980–985.

Dajani AS, Kessler S, Mandelson R, Uden DL, Todd WM, 1993, Cefpodoxime proxetil *versus* penicillin V in paediatric pharyngitis/tonsillitis, Pediatr Infect Dis J, 12, 275–279.

Debbia EA, Schito GC, Pesce A, 1991, Antibacterial activity of ceftibuten, a new oral third generation cephalosporin, J Chemother, 3, 209–225.

Denny FW, Wannamaker LW, Brink WR, et al, 1950, Prevention of rheumatic fever: treatment of the preceding streptococci infection, JAMA, 142, 151–153.

Deppermann KM, Garbe C, Hasse K, et al, 1989, Comparative pharmacokinetics of cefotiam hexetil, cefuroxime, cefixime, cephalexin and effect of H2 blocker, standard breakfast and antacids on the bioavailability of cefotiam hexetil, 29th Intersci Conf Antimicrob Agents Chemother, abstract 1223.

Dhib M, Moulin B, Leroy A, Hammeau B, Godin M, Johannides R, Fillastre JP, 1991, Relationship between renal function and disposition of oral cefixime, Eur J Clin Pharmacol, 41, 579–583.

Disney FA, Hanfling MJ, Hansinger SA, 1992, Loracarbef *versus* penicillin VK in the treatment of streptococcal pharyngitis and tonsillitis, Pediatr Infect Dis J, 11, S20–S26.

Doern GV, Brueggemann A, Holley HP Jr, Rauch AM, 1996, Antimicrobial resistance of *S. pneumoniae* recovered from outpatients in the United States during the winter months of 1994 to 1995: results of a 30-center national surveillance study, Antimicrob Agents Chemother, 40, 1208–1213.

Doern GV, Brueggemann AB, Pierce G, Holley HP Jr, Rauch A, 1997, Antibiotic resistance among clinical isolates of *H. influenzae* in the United States in 1994 and 1995 and detection of β-lactamase-positive strains resistant to amoxicillin-clavulanate: results of a national multicenter surveillance study, Antimicrob Agents Chemother, 41, 292–297.

Doern GV, Brueggemann AB, Pierce G, Hogan T, Holley HP Jr, Rauch A, 1996, Prevalence of antimicrobial resistance among 723 outpatient clinical isolates of *M. catarrhalis* in the United States in 1994 and 1995: results of a 30-center national surveillance study, Antimicrob Agents Chemother, 40, 2884–2886.

Doern GV, Ferraro MJ, Brueggemann AB, Ruoff KL, 1996, Emergence of high rates of antimicrobial resistance among viridans group streptococci in the United States, Antimicrob Agents Chemother, 40, 891–894.

Doern GV, Vautour R, Parker D, Tubert T, Torres B, 1991, In vitro activity of loracarbef (LY 163892), a new oral carbacephem antibacterial agent, against respiratory isolates of *H. influenzae* and *M. catarrhalis*, Antimicrob Agents Chemother, 35, 1504–1507.

Donn KH, James NC, Powell JR, 1994, Bioavailability of cefuroxime axetil formulations, J Pharm Sci, 83, 842–844.

Doyle CA, Durham JJ, Hamilton HA, et al, 1992, Cefprozil *vs* cefaclor in the treatment of pharyngitis and tonsillitis in adults, Infect Med, 9, suppl E, 66–67.

Ducharme MP, Edwards DJ, McNamara PJ, Stoeckel K, 1993, Bioavailability of syrup and tablet formulations of cefetamet pivoxil, Antimicrob Agents Chemother, 37, 2706–2709.

Dumont R, Andrews JM, Guetat F, Sultan E, Lenfant B, 1990, Concentrations of cefpodoxime in plasma and pleural fluid after a single oral dose of cefpodoxime proxetil, J Antimicrob Chemother, 26, suppl E, 41–46.

Eden T, Amari M, Emston S, et al, 1983, Penetration of cefaclor to adenoid tissue and middle ear fluid in secretory otitis media, Scand J Infect Dis, 39, suppl, 48–52.

Edlund C, Brismar B, Sakamoto H, Nord CE, 1993, Impact of cefuroxime axetil on the normal intestinal microflora, Microb Ecol Health Dis.

Emston S, Amari M, Eden T, et al, 1985, Penetration of cefaclor to adenoid tissue and middle ear fluid effusion in chronic OME, Acta Otolaryngol, 424, 7–12.

Fang GD, Fise M, Orloff J, Arisumi D, Yu VL, Kapoor WA, Grayston JT, Pin Wang S, Kholer R, Muder RR, Yee YC, Rihs JD, Vickers RM, 1990, New and emerging etiologies for community-acquired pneumonia with implications for therapy: a prospective multicenter study of 359 cases, Medicine, 69, 307–315.

Farr BM, Mandell GL, 1994, Gram-positive pneumonia, p 349-367, in Pennington JF, ed, Respiratory Infections—Diagnosis and Management, 3rd ed, Raven Press Ltd, New York.

Faulkner RD, Bohaychuk W, Desjardins RE, et al, 1987, Pharmacokinetics of cefixime after once-a-day and twice-a-day dosing to steady state, J Clin Pharmacol, 27, 807–812.

Faulkner RD, Bohaychuk W, Lanc RA, et al, 1988, Pharmacokinetics of cefixime in the young and elderly, J Antimicrob Chemother, 21, 787–794.

Faulkner RD, Fernandez PB, Laurence G, et al, 1988, Absolute bioavailability of cefixime in man, Clin Pharmacol, 28, 700–705.

Faulkner RD, Yacobi A, Barone JS, Kaplan SA, Silber BM, 1987, Pharmacokinetic profile of cefixime in man, Pediatr Infect Dis J, 6, 963–970.

Felmingham D, Robbins MJ, Ghosh G, Bhogal H, Mehta MD, Leakey A, Clark S, Dencer CA, Ridgway GL, Grüneberg RN, 1994, An in vitro characterization of cefditoren, a new oral cephalosporin, Drugs Exptl Clin Res, 20, 127–147.

Fernandez P, Laurence G, Sia LL, Falkowski AJ, 1988, Absolute bioavailability of cefixime in man, J Clin Pharmacol, 28, 700–706.

File JM Jr, 1996, Aetiology and incidence of community-acquired pneumonia, Infect Dis Clin Pract, 5, Suppl 4, S127–S135.

Finegold SM, Ingram-Drake L, Gee R, et al, 1987, Bowel flora changes in human receiving cefixime (CL 248,635) or cefaclor, Antimicrob Agents Chemother, 31, 443–446.

Finkelstein E, Quintiliani R, Lee R, Bracci A, Nightingale CH, 1978, Pharmacokinetics of oral cephalosporins: cephradine and cephalexin, J Pharm Sci, 67, 1447–1450.

Finn A, Straughn A, Meyer M, Chubb J, 1987, Effect of dose and food on the bioavailability of cefuroxime axetil, Biopharm Drug Dispos, 8, 519–526.

Forsgren A, Walder M, 1994, Antimicrobial susceptibility of bacterial isolates in South Sweden including a 13-year follow-up study of some respiratory pathogens, APMIS, 102, 227–235.

Foy HM, Kenny GE, Cooney MK, Allan ID, 1979, Long-term epidemiology of infection with *Mycoplasma pneumoniae*, J Infect Dis, 139, 681–687.

Frémaux A, Sissia G, Brumpt I, Geslin P, 1993, Cefditoren (ME 1206), a new cephalosporin: in vitro activity against penicillin-susceptible and resistant pneumococci, 18th Int Congr Chemother, abstract 998.

Fujimaki Y, Kawamura S, Watanabe H, Itabashi T, 1985, Clinical and experimental studies of FK027 for otorhinolaryngological infections, 13th Int Congr Chemother.

Furuta S, Tsurumaru H, Fukami S, et al, 1988, Cefotiam hexetil in the field of otorhinolaryngology, Chemotherapy, 36, Suppl 6, 843–857.

Gallet J, Couraud L, Saux MC, Roche G, 1989, Diffusion pulmonaire du cefixime chez l'homme, Presse Med, 18, 1589–1592.

Gehanno P, Andrews JM, Ichou F, Sultan E, Lenfant B, 1990, Concentrations of cefpodoxime in plasma and tonsillar tissue after a single oral dose of cefpodoxime proxetil, J Antimicrob Chemother, 26, Suppl E, 47–51.

Gerber MA, Markowitz M, 1985, Management of streptococcal pharyngitis reconsidered, Pediatr Infect Dis J, 4, 518–526.

Gerber MA, Randolph MF, Chanatry J, Wright LL, DeMeo K, Kaplan EL, 1987, Five *vs* ten days of penicillin V therapy for streptococcal pharyngitis, Am J Dis Child, 141, 224–227.

Geslin P, Frémaux A, Sissia G, Spicq C, Aberrane S, 1996, Rapport du Centre National de référence des pneumocoques années 1994–1995, Créteil.

Ginsburg CM, 1982, Comparative pharmacokinetics of cefadroxil, cefaclor, cephalexin and cephradine in infants and children, J Antimicrob Chemother, 10, suppl B, 27–31.

Ginsburg CM, McCracken GH, Petruska M, Olson K, 1985, Pharmacokinetics and bactericidal activity of cefuroxime axetil, Antimicrob Agents Chemother, 28, 504–507.

Goldstein EJ, 1997, Comparative in vitro activity of HMR 3004, a new ketolide, with azithromycin (AZ), clarithromycin (CL), roxithromycin (RX) and erythromycin (ERY) against 311 aerobic and anaerobic bacteria isolated from human and animal bite wound infections, 37th Intersci Conf Antimicrob Agents Chemother.

Goldstein EJ, Citron DM, 1988, Comparative activities of cefuroxime, amoxicillin-clavulanic acid, ciprofloxacin, enoxacin, and ofloxacin against aerobic and anaerobic bacteria isolated from bite wounds, Antimicrob Agents Chemother, 32, 1143–1148.

Goldstein EJ, Nesbit CA, Citron DM, 1995, Comparative in vitro activities of azithromycin, Bay Y 3118, levofloxacin, sparfloxacin, and 11 other oral antimicrobial agents against 194 aerobic and anaerobic bite wound isolates, Antimicrob Agents Chemother, 39, 1097–1100.

Goldstein F, Kitzis MD, Gutmann L, Acar JF, 1992, Comparative activity of oral cephalosporins against β-lactamase producing pathogens, Med Mal Infect, 22, 535–543.

Gomez J, Branos V, Ruiz-Gomez J, Soto MC, Munoz L, Nunez ML, Canteras M, Valdès M, 1996, Prospective study of epidemiology and prognostic factors in community-acquired pneumonia, Eur J Clin Microbiol Infect Dis, 15, 556–560.

Gooch WM III, McLinn SE, Aronovitz GH, et al, 1993, Efficacy of cefuroxime axetil suspension compared with that of penicillin V suspension in children with group A streptococcal pharyngitis, Antimicrob Agents Chemother, 37, 159–163.

Gooch WM III, Swenson E, Higbee MD, Cocchetto M, Evans EC, 1987, Cefuroxime axetil and penicillin V compared in the treatment of group A beta-hemolytic streptococcal pharyngitis, Clin Ther, 9, 670–677.

Grimm H, 1991, Interpretative criteria of antimicrobial disk susceptibility test with cefpodoxime, Infection, 19, 380–382.

Guay DRP, Meatherall RC, Harding GK, Brown GR, 1986, Pharmacokinetics of cefixime in healthy subjects and patients with renal insufficiency, Antimicrob Agents Chemother, 30, 485–490.

Guttendorf R, Koup I, Misiak P, Hawking P, Olson S, 1992, Pharmacokinetics of cefdinir (CI-983-FK482) in children—NONMEM analysis dose selection and body size factors, 32nd Intersci Conf Antimicrob Agents Chemother, abstract 1227.

Gwaltney JM Jr, 1995, p 585–590, in Mandell GI, Bennett JE, Dolin R, ed, Principles and Practice of Infectious Diseases, 4th ed, Churchill Livingstone, New York.

Gwaltney JM Jr, Hayden FG, 1982, p 399–423, in Proctor DF, Anderson I, ed, The Nose, Upper Airway Physiology and the Atmospheric Environment, Elsevier Biomedical Press, Amsterdam.

Haddad J Jr, Isaacson G, Respler DS, Hart RW, Yilmaz HM, Collins JJ, Bluestone CD, 1991, Concentration of cefuroxime in serum and middle-ear effusion after single dose treatment with cefuroxime axetil, Pediatr Infect Dis J, 10, 294–298.

Hara J, Otani E, Kawamura T, Nagahara F, 1992, Clinical studies of ME 1207 in anterior eye infections and concentrations of ME 1206 in serum and aqueous humor, Chemotherapy, 40, Suppl 2, 660–663.

Harding SM, Williams PE, Ayrton J, 1984, Pharmacology of cefuroxime as the 1-acetoxyethyl ester in volunteers, Antimicrob Agents Chemother, 25, 78–82.

Harrison HR, Magder LS, Boyce WT, 1986, Acute *Chlamydia trachomatis* respiratory tract infections in childhood—serologic evidence, Am J Dis Child, 140, 1067–1071.

Harrisson CJ, Chartrand SA, Rodriguez W, et al, 1994, Middle-ear fluid (MEF) concentrations of cefixime in acute otitis media and otitis media with effusion, in 34th Intersci Conf Antimicrob Agents Chemother, abstract A67.

Hatano K, Nishino T, 1994, Morphological alterations of *Staphylococcus aureus* and *Streptococcus pyogenes* exposed to cefdinir, a new oral broad-spectrum cephalosporin, Chemotherapy, 40, 73–79.

Hayton WL, Walstad RA, Thurmann-Nielsen E, et al, 1991, Pharmacokinetics of intravenous cefetamet and oral cefetamet pivoxil in children, Antimicrob Agents Chemother, 35, 720-725.

Healy DP, Sahai JV, Sterling LP, Racht EM, 1989, Influence of an antacid containing aluminum and magnesium on the pharmacokinetics of cefixime, Antimicrob Agents Chemother, 33, 1994–1997.

Heffron R, 1979, Pneumonia: with Special Reference to Pneumococcus Lobar Pneumonia, p 656–663, Harvard University Press, Cambridge.

Herrington JA, Federici JA, Painter BG, Remy JM, Barbiero ML, Thurberg BE, 1996, In vitro activity of Bay 12-8039, a new 8-methoxy quinolone, 36th Intersci Conf Antimicrob Agents Chemother, abstract F004.

Holm SE, Ekedahl C, 1982, Comparative study of the penetration of penicillin V and cefadroxil into tonsils in man, J Antimicrob Chemother, 10, Suppl B, 121–123.

Holt HA, Bywater MH, Reeves DS, 1990, In vitro activity of cefpodoxime against 1834 isolates from domiciliary infections at 20 UK centers, J Antimicrob Chemother, 26, suppl E, 7–12.

Howie VM, Owen MJ, 1987, Bacteriology and clinical efficacy of cefixime compared with amoxicillin in acute otitis media, Pediatr Infect Dis J, 6, 989–991.

Howie VM, Poussard JH, 1972, Efficacy of fixed combination antibiotics versus separate components in otitis media, Clin Pediatr, 11, 205–214.

Hu M, Chen J, Zhu Y, Dantzig AH, Stratford RE Jr, Kuhfeld MT, 1994, Mechanism and kinetics of transcellular transport of a new β-lactam antibiotic loracarbef across an intestinal epithelial membrane model system (Caco-2), Pharm Res, 11, 1405–1413.

Hughes GS, Heald DL, Barker KB, et al, 1989, The effects of gastric pH and food on the pharmacokinetics of a new oral cephalosporin, cefpodoxime proxetil, Clin Pharmacol Ther, 46, 674–685.

Humbert G, Leroy A, Fillastre JP, Godin M, 1979, Pharmacokinetics of cefadroxil in normal subjects and in patients with renal insufficiency, Chemotherapy, 25, 189–195.

Hyslop D, Bischoff W, 1992, Loracarbef *versus* cefaclor and norfloxacin in the treatment of uncomplicated pyelonephritis, Am J Med, 92, suppl 6A, 86–94.

Imaizumi M, Kajita M, Fujita K, et al, 1986, Clinical studies on the concentration of cefaclor in sera and lung tissues of patients with respiratory diseases, Jpn J Antibiot, 39, 2754–2760.

Inui KI, Yamamoto M, Saito H, 1992, Transepithelial transport of oral cephalosporins by monolayers of intestinal epithelial cell line Caco-2: specific transport systems in apical and basolateral membranes, J Pharmacol Exp Ther, 261, 195–201.

Iravani A, Cox C, Miller D, Schneider R, Sugawara S, Teplitzky B, 1990, A multicenter, dose response study of cefpodoxime proxetil in patients with urinary tract infections, Int Congr Infect Dis.

Iravani A, Richard GA, 1988, A double-blind multicenter comparative study of the safety and efficacy of cefixime *versus* amoxicillin in the treatment of acute urinary tract infections in adult patients, Am J Med, 85, Suppl 3A, 17–23.

Iwasawa T, 1979, Fundamental and clinical studies on cefaclor in the otorhino-laryngologic field, Chemotherapy, 696.

James PA, Lewis DA, Zordens JZ, Gribb J, Dawson SJ, Murray SA, 1996, The incidence and epidemiology of β-lactam resistance in *H. influenzae*, J Antimicrob Chemother, 37, 737–746.

Jetlund O, Walstad RA, Thurmann-Nielsen E, 1991, Comparison of the serum and tissue concentrations of cefuroxime from cefuroxime axetil and phenoxymethylpenicillin in patients undergoing tonsillectomy, Int J Clin Pharmacol Res, 11, 1–6.

Jimenez-Shebab M, Barrogan A, 1982, Oral cefadroxil in the treatment of bone and joint infections in children and adults, J Antimicrob Chemother, 10, suppl B, 149–152.

Johnson CA, Ateshkadi A, Zimmerman SW, et al, 1993, Pharmacokinetics and ex vivo susceptibility of cefpodoxime proxetil in patients receiving continuous ambulatory peritoneal dialysis, Antimicrob Agents Chemother, 37, 2650–2655.

Johnson RC, Kodner CB, Jurkovich PJ, Collins JJ, 1990, Comparative in vitro and in vivo susceptibilities of the Lyme disease spirochete *Borrelia burgdorferi* to cefuroxime and other antimicrobial agents, Antimicrob Agents Chemother, 34, 2131–2136.

Jones RN, 1993, Ceftibuten: a review of antimicrobial activity, spectrum and other microbiologic features, Pediatr Infect Dis J, 12, S37–S44.

Jones RN, Barry AL, 1987, In vitro evaluation of U-76,252 (CS-807): antimicrobial spectrum, beta-lactamase stability and enzyme inhibition, Diagn Microbiol Infect Dis, 8, 245–249.

Jones RN, Barry AL, 1988, Ceftibuten (7432-S, SCH 39720): comparative antimicrobial activity against 4735 clinical isolates, beta-lactamase stability and broth microdilution quality control guidelines, Eur J Clin Microbiol Infect Dis, 7, 802–807.

Jones RN, Barry AL, Pfaller M, Allen SD, Ayers LW, Fuchs PC, 1988, Antimicrobial activity of U-76,252 (CS-807), a new orally administered cephalosporin ester, including recommendations for MIC quality control, Diagn Microbiol Infect Dis, 9, 59–63.

Jones RN, Erwin ME, 1992, Haemophilus test medium interpretative criteria for disk diffusion susceptibility test with cefdinir, cefetamet, cefmetazole, cefpodoxime, cefdaloxine (RU 29246, HR-916 metabolite) and trosectinomycin, Diagn Microbiol Infect Dis, 15, 693–701.

Jousimies-Somer HR, Savolainen S, Ylikoski JS, 1988, Bacteriological findings of acute maxillary sinusitis in young adults, J Clin Microbiol, 26, 1919–1925.

Kafetzis DA, 1994, Multi-investigator evaluation of the efficacy and safety of cefprozil, amoxicillin-clavulanate, cefixime and cefaclor in the treatment of acute otitis media, Eur J Clin Microbiol Infect Dis, 13, 857–865.

Kaplan SL, Mason EO Jr, 1994, Antimicrobial agents: resistance patterns of common pathogens, Pediatr Infect Dis J, 15, 1050–1053.

Kawaharajo K, Miyata A, Kakinuma K, et al, 1992, In vitro and in vivo antibacterial activity of ME1207, a new oral cephalosporin, Chemotherapy, 40, Suppl 2, 51–58.

Kawamura S, Ichikawa GI, Watanabe I, et al, 1989, Fundamental and clinical studies on cefdinir in otorhinolaryngological infection, Chemotherapy, 37, Suppl 2, 1041–1052.

Kayer FH, 1994, In vitro activity of cefpodoxime in comparison with other oral β-lactam antibiotics, Infection, 22, 370–375.

Kearns GL, Darville T, Wells TG, Jacobs RF, Hughes GS, Borin MT, 1994, Single dose pharmacokinetics of cefpodoxime proxetil in infants and children, Drug Investig, 7, 221–233.

Kearns GL, Reed MD, Jacob RF, Ardite M, Yogen RD, Blumer JL, 1991, Single-dose pharmacokinetics of ceftibuten (SCH 39720) in infants and children, Antimicrob Agents Chemother, 35, 2078–2084.

Kelloway JS, Awni WM, Lin CC, et al, 1991, Pharmacokinetics of ceftibuten-*cis* and its *trans* metabolites in healthy volunteers and in patients with chronic renal insufficiency, Antimicrob Agents Chemother, 35, 2267–2274.

Kiani R, Johnson D, Nelson B, 1988, Comparative, multicenter studies of cefixime and amoxicillin in the treatment of respiratory tract infections, Am J Med, 85, Suppl 3A, 6–13.

Kim MY, Kim SH, Yim HJ, Paek KS, Oh SH, Ryu EJ, Lee CS, 1999, In vivo activity of LB 10827, a new oral cephalosporin in pneumonia infection models, 39th Intersci Conf Antimicrob Agents Chemother, abstract F-399.

Kitzis MD, Liassine N, Ferré B, Gutmann L, Acar JF, Goldstein F, 1990, In vitro activities of 15 oral β-lactams against *K. pneumoniae* harboring new extended-spectrum β-lactamases, Antimicrobial Agents Chemother, 34, 1783–1786.

Klein JO, 1994, Selection of oral antimicrobial agents for otitis media and pharyngitis, Infect Dis Clin Pract, 3, 151–157.

Knapp CC, Sierra-Madero J, Washington JA, 1988, Antibacterial activities of cefpodoxime, cefixime, and ceftriaxone, Antimicrob Agents Chemother, 32, 1896–1898.

Kneer J, Tam YK, Blouin RA, Frey FJ, Keller E, Stathakis C, Lunginbuehl B, Stoeckel K, 1989, Pharmacokinetics of intravenous cefetamet and oral cefetamet pivoxil in patients with renal insufficiency, Antimicrob Agents Chemother, 33, 1952–1957.

Knothe H, Shah PM, Eckardt O, 1991, Cefpodoxime: comparative antibacterial activity, influence of growth conditions and bactericidal activity, Infection, 19, 370–376.

Kohonen A, Paavolainen M, Renkonen OV, 1975, Concentration of cephalexin in maxillary sinus mucosa and secretions, Ann Clin Res, 7, 50–53.

Konishi K, Suzuki H, Hayashi M, Saruta T, 1993, Pharmacokinetics of cefuroxime axetil in patients with normal and impaired renal function, J Antimicrob Chemother, 31, 413–420.

Korting HC, Schäfer-Korting M, Kees F, Lukacs A, Grobecker H, 1990, Skin tissue fluid levels of cefotiam in healthy man following oral cefotiam hexetil, Eur J Clin Pharmacol, 39, 33–36.

Korvick JA, Hackett AK, Yu VL, Muder RR, 1991, *Klebsiella pneumoniae* in the modern era: clinicoradiographic correlations, South Med J, 84, 200–204.

Koup JR, Dubach UC, Brandt R, Wyss R, Stoeckel K, 1988, Pharmacokinetics of cefetamet (Ro-15-8076) and cefetamet pivoxil (Ro-15-8075) after intravenous and oral doses in humans, Antimicrob Agents Chemother, 32, 573–579.

Krause PJ, Owens NJ, Nightingale CH, Klimek JJ, Lehmann WB, Quintiliani R, 1982, Penetration of amoxicillin, cefaclor, erythromycin-sulfisoxazole, and trimethoprim-sulfamethoxazole into the middle ear fluid of patients with chronic serous otitis media, J Infect Dis, 145, 815–821.

Kuhlwein A, Nies RA, 1989, Efficacy and safety of a single 400 mg oral dose of cefixime in the treatment of uncomplicated gonorrhoea, Eur J Clin Microbiol Infect Dis, 8, 261–262.

Kusmiesz H, Shelton S, Brown O, Manning S, Nelson JD, 1990, Loracarbef concentrations in middle ear fluid, Antimicrob Agents Chemother, 34, 2030–2031.

Laurans G, Orfila J, 1991, *Moraxella (Branhamella) catarrhalis* dans les infections respiratoires activité in vitro de la cefuroxime, Méd Mal Infect, 21, hors série, 34–40.

Leigh DA, Fraser S, Hannington J, Mason T, 1991, Comparative trial of the efficacy and tolerance of cefpodoxime proxetil and amoxicillin in the treatment of acute and acute-on-chronic bronchitis, Int Congr Chemother.

Lenfant B, Molinier P, Gigliotti G, Coussedière D, Dupront A, Tremblay D, 1992, Bioavailability of the two diastereoisomers of cefpodoxime proxetil in healthy volunteers, Vth World Conf Clin Pharmacol Ther, abstract P 305–05, p 248.

Le Noc P, Croizé J, Bryskier A, Le Noc D, 1990, Activité antibactérienne de quatre céphalosporines à forme orale sur 338 souches de bactéries entéropathogènes, Réunion Interdisc Chemother Anti-infect, 48/P5.

Léophonte P, Rouquet R, Gustin M, et al, 1990, Cefpodoxime proxetil *vs* amoxicillin in the treatment of community-acquired pneumonia in adult patients, Int Congr Infect Dis, abstract 32.

Linares J, Tubau FE, Alcaide F, Ardany C, Garcia A, Martin R, 1996, Antimicrobial resistance of *S. pneumoniae*: comparison of the in vitro activity of 16 antibiotics, Curr Ther Res, 57, suppl A, 57–64.

LiPuma JJ, Daley B, Stull TL, 1990, In vitro activities of cefpodoxime, trospectinomycin and second-generation cephalosporins against *H. influenzae* type b, J Antimicrob Chemother, 25, 535–539.

Livermore DM, 1987, Clinical significance of β-lactamase induction and stable derepression in Gram-negative rods, Eur J Clin Microbiol, 6, 439–445.

Lode H, Müller C, Borner K, Nord CE, Koeppe P, 1992, Multiple-dose pharmacokinetics of cefprozil and its impact on intestinal flora of volunteers, Antimicrob Agents Chemother, 36, 144–149.

Lode H, Schaberg T, Mauch H, 1996, Management of community-acquired pneumonia, Curr Opin Infect Dis, 9, 367–371.

Lode H, Stahlmann R, Koeppe P, 1979, Comparative pharmacokinetics of cephalexin, cefaclor, cefadroxil, and CGP 9000, Antimicrob Agents Chemother, 16, 1–6.

Luger SW, Paparone P, Wormsmer GP, et al, 1995, Comparison of cefuroxime axetil and doxycycline in treatment of patients with early Lyme disease associated with erythema migrans, Antimicrob Agents Chemother, 39, 661–667.

Lundberg C, Carenfelt C, Engquist S, Nord CE, 1979, Anaerobic bacteria in maxillary sinusitis, Scand J Infect Dis, 19, suppl, 74–76.

Mancini R, Massida O, Satta G, 1992, Rate of penetration of cefetamet, cefixime, cefuroxime and cefaclor in different strains of *Enterobacteriaceae*, Med Mal Infect, 22, 544–547.

Mandelman PM, Chaffin DO, 1987, Penicillin binding proteins 4 and 5 of *H. influenzae* are involved in cell wall incorporation, FEMS Microbiol Lett, 239–242.

Marchant CD, Shurin PA, 1982, Antibacterial therapy for acute otitis media: a critical analysis, Rev Infect Dis, 4, 506–510.

Marlin GE, Nicholls AJ, Funnell GR, Bradbury R, 1984, Penetration of cefaclor into bronchial mucosa, Thorax, 39, 813–817.

Marrie TJ, Durant H, Yates L, 1989, Community-acquired pneumonia requiring hospitalization: 5 years prospective study, Rev Infect Dis, 11, 586–599.

Martini A, Xerri L, 1982, Study of diffusion of cefuroxime into middle ear effusions of patients with chronic purulent otitis media, J Antimicrob Chemother, 10, 197–198.

Mastrandrea V, Ripa S, La Rosa F, Ghezzi A, 1985, Pharmacokinetics of cefatrizine after oral administration in human volunteers, Int J Clin Pharm Res, 5, 319–323.

Matsumoto F, Sakurai I, Imai T, 1989, Basic and clinical studies on cefdinir, Chemotherapy, 37, Suppl 2, 426–435.

McCarthy JM, 1994, Comparative efficacy and safety of cefprozil *versus* penicillin, cefaclor and erythromycin in the treatment of streptococcal pharyngitis and tonsillitis, Eur J Clin Microbiol Infect Dis, 13, 846–850.

McCracken GH, Ginsburg CM, Clahsen JC, Thomas ML, 1978, Pharmacokinetics of cefaclor in infants and children, J Antimicrob Chemother, 4, 515–521.

McLin SE, 1973, Serum and middle ear levels of cephalexin, a new cephalosporin in acute otitis media, 8th Int Congr Chemother, 1, 305–310.

McLinn SE, McCarty JM, Perrotta R, Pichichero ME, Reidenberg BE, 1995, Multicenter controlled trial comparing ceftibuten with amoxicillin-clavulanate in the empiric treatment of acute otitis media, Pediatr Infect Dis J, 14, S108–S114.

Melegh B, Kerner J, Bieber LL, 1987, Pivampicillin-promoted excretion of pivaloylcarnitine in humans, Biochem Pharmacol, 20, 3405–3409.

Mendelman PM, Del Beccaco MA, McLin SE, Todd WM, 1992, Cefpodoxime proxetil compared with amoxicillin-clavulanate for the treatment of otitis media, J Pediatr, 12, 459–465.

Mendelman PM, Henzitzy LL, Chaffin DO, et al, 1989, In vitro activities and targets of three cephem antibiotics against *Haemophilus influenzae*, Antimicrob Agents Chemother, 33, 1878–1882.

Mignini F, Magni A, Dainelli D, Patrizi L, 1985, Determinations of tissue levels of cefatrizine in blood, lungs and bronchi, Drugs Exptl Clin Res, 11, 457–460.

Mignot A, Millerioux L, Couraud L, Durgeat S, Joubert M, 1994, Distribution of cefotiam in human lung tissue after multiple oral administration of cefotiam hexetil, Eur J Clin Pharmacol, 46, 383–384.

Milatovic D, 1991, Evaluation of cefadroxil, penicillin and erythromycin in the treatment of streptococcal tonsillopharyngitis, Pediatr Infect Dis J, 10, suppl 10, S61–S63.

Milatovic D, Adam D, Hamilton H, Materman E, 1993, Cefprozil *versus* penicillin V in treatment of streptococcal tonsillopharyngitis, Antimicrob Agents Chemother, 37, 1620–1623.

Miller RA, Brancato F, Holmes KK, 1986, *Corynebacterium hemolyticum* as a cause of pharyngitis and scarlatiniform rash in young adults, Ann Intern Med, 105, 867–872.

Mine Y, Watanabe Y, Matsumoto Y, et al, 1989, Mechanism of action of cefdinir, a new orally active cephalosporin, Chemotherapy, 37, Suppl 2, 122–134.

Mori Y, Baba S, Suzuki K, et al, 1989, Cefotiam hexetil in the otorhinolaryngological field, Chemotherapy, 37, Suppl 2, 810–821.

Motohiro T, Maruoka T, Nagai K, et al, 1989, Pharmacokinetic and clinical studies of cefpodoxime proxetil dry syrup in the field of pediatrics, Jpn J Antibiot, 42, 1629–1666.

Munoz R, et al, 1992, Genetics of resistance to third generation cephalosporins in clinical isolates of *Streptococcus pneumoniae*, Mol Microbiol, 6, 2461–2465.

Muranushi N, Hashimoto N, Hirano K, 1995, Transport characteristics of S-1090, a new oral cephem in rat intestinal brush-border membrane vesicles, Pharm Res, 10, 1488–1492.

Murphy TF, Apicella MA, 1987, Nontypeable *H. influenzae*: a review of clinical aspects, surface antigens and the human response to infection, Rev Infect Dis, 9, 1–15.

Nahata MC, Kolbrenner VM, Barson WJ, 1993, Pharmacokinetics and cerebral fluid concentrations of cefixime in infants and young children, Chemotherapy, 39, 1–5.

Nahata MC, Koranyi KI, 1992, Pharmacokinetics of loracarbef in pediatric patients, Eur J Drug Metabol Pharmacokinet, 17, 201–204.

Nakao H, Ide J, Yanagisawa H, Iwata M, Komai T, Masuda H, Hirasawa T, 1987, Cefpodoxime proxetil (CS 807), a new orally active cephalosporin, Sankyo Kenkyusho Nempo, 39, 1–44.

Nakashima M, Ida M, Yoshida T Kitagawa T, Oguma T, Ishii H, 1986, Pharmacokinetics and safety of 7432-S in healthy volunteers, 26th Intersci Conf Antimicrob Agents Chemother, abstract 591.

Nakashima M, Oguma T, Kimura Y, Sasaki S, Sendo Y, Sendo H, 1996, Phase 1 clinical studies of S-1090: safety and pharmacokinetics, J Infect Chemother, 2, 271–279.

Nakashima M, Uematsu T, Oguma T, et al, 1992, Phase I clinical studies of S-1108: safety and pharmacokinetics in a multiple-administration study with special emphasis on the influence on carnitine body stores, Antimicrob Agents Chemother, 36, 762–768.

Nakashima M, Uematsu T, Takiguchi Y, et al, 1988, Phase I clinical studies of 7432-S, a new oral cephalosporin: safety and pharmacokinetics, J Clin Pharmacol, 28, 246–252.

Nakashima M, Uematsu T, Takiguchi Y, Mizuno A, Uchida K, Matsubara T, 1988, Phase I clinical studies of 7432-S: effect of 7432-S on platelet aggregation and blood coagulation, J Clin Pharmacol, 28, 253–258.

Nakashima M, Uematsu Y, Takiguchi Y, et al, 1989, Phase I studies of 7432-S, a new oral cephem antibiotic, Chemotherapy, 37, Suppl 1, 78–109.

Nelson CT, Mason EO, Kaplan SL, 1994, Activity of oral antibiotics in middle-ear and sinus infections caused by penicillin-resistant *Streptococcus pneumoniae*: implications for treatment, Pediatr Infect Dis J, 13, 585–589.

Nelson JD, Ginsburg CM, MacLeland O, et al, 1981, Concentration of antimicrobial agents in middle ear fluid, saliva and tears, Int J Pediatr Otorhinolaryngol, 3, 327–334.

Nelson JD, Shelton S, Kusmiesz H, 1988, Pharmacokinetics of LY 163892 in infants and children, Antimicrob Agents Chemother, 32, 1738–1739.

Neu HC, Chin NX, 1994, In vitro activity of the new fluoroquinolone CP-99,219, Antimicrob Agents Chemother, 38, 2615–2622.

Neu HC, Chin NX, Labthavikul P, 1984, Comparative in vitro activity and β-lactamase stability of FR 17027, a new orally active cephalosporin, Antimicrob Agents Chemother, 26, 174–180.

Neu HC, Chin NX, Labthavikul P, 1986, In vitro activity and β-lactamase stability of two oral cephalosporins, ceftetrame (Ro 19-5247) and cefetamet (Ro 15-8074), Antimicrob Agents Chemother, 30, 423–428.

Neu HC, Saha G, Chin NX, 1989, Comparative in vitro activity and β-lactamase stability of FK 482, a new oral cephalosporin, Antimicrob Agents Chemother, 33, 1795–1800.

Ng WS, Chau PY, Leung YK, Wong PCL, 1985, In vitro activity of Ro 15-8074, a new oral cephalosporin, against *Neisseria gonorrhoeae*, Antimicrob Agents Chemother, 28, 461–463.

Nishino I, Fujitomo H, Umeda T, 2000, Determination of a new oral cephalosporin, cefmatilen hydrochloride hydrate, and its seven metabolites in human and animal plasma and urine by coupled systems of ion-exchange and reversed phase high-performance liquid chromatography, J Chromat B, 749, 101–110.

Nishino T, Takenouchi T, Ohtsuki M, Tanino T, 1988, In vitro and in vivo antibacterial activity of CS-807, a new oral cephem antibiotic, Chemotherapy, 36, Suppl 1, 72–93.

Nishitani Y, Yamada D, Hayata S, et al, 1989, Basic and clinical studies on cefdinir in urology, Chemotherapy, 37, Suppl 2, 823–840.

Nishizono H, Uchiazono A, Shima T, et al, 1992, Basic and clinical studies on ME 1207 for the infectious disease in the field of otorhinolaryngology, Chemotherapy, 40, Suppl 2, 643–650.

Nogita T, Iozumi K, Shimozuma M, et al, 1989, Skin tissue concentration and clinical evaluation of cefdinir in dermatology, Chemotherapy, 37, Suppl 2, 955–969.

Nord CE, Grahnen A, Eckernäs SA, 1991, Effect of loracarbef on the normal oropharyngeal and intestinal microflora, Scand J Infect Dis, 23, 255–260.

Nord CE, Heimdahl A, Lundberg C, Marklund G, 1987, Impact of cefaclor on the normal human oropharyngeal and intestinal microflora, Scand J Infect Dis, 19, 681–685.

Nord CE, Movin F, Stalberg D, 1988, Impact of cefixime on the normal intestinal microflora, Scand J Infect Dis, 20, 547–552.

Novak E, Paxton LM, Tubbs HJ, Turner LF, Keck CW, Yatsu J, 1992, Orally administered cefpodoxime proxetil for treatment of uncomplicated gonococcal urethritis in males: a dose response study, Antimicrob Agents Chemother, 36, 1764–1765.

Novelli A, Mazzei T, Nicoletti P, et al, 1994, Intestinal flora changes in patients treated with cefetamet pivoxil, cefixime and cefuroxime axetil, J Chemother.

Nye K, O'Neill P, Andrews JM, Wise R, 1990, Pharmacokinetics and tissue penetration of cefprozil, J Antimicrob Chemother, 25, 831–835.

Oh SH, Ryn EJ, Paek KS, Lee SH, Lee CS, 1999, Synthesis and antibacterial activities of LB 10827, a new oral cephalosporin antibiotic, 39th Intersci Conf Antimicrob Agents Chemother, abstract F-397.

Ooishi M, Miyao M, Tuzawa H, et al, 1992, Basic and clinical studies of ME1207 in ophthalmology, Chemotherapy, 40, Suppl 2, 651–659.

Paek KS, Oh SH, Ryu EJ, Lee CS, Kim MY, 1999, In vitro antibacterial activity of LB 10827, a new oral cephalosporin against respiratory pathogens, 39th Intersci Conf Antimicrob Agents Chemother, abstract F-398.

Papanicolaou GA, Medeiros AA, 1991, Ability of ceftibuten to induce the class I beta-lactamases of *E. cloacae*, *S. marcescens* and *E. aerogenes*, Diagn Microbiol Infect Dis, 14, 85–87.

Park SH, Park SY, Kim DY, et al, 1997, Novel 3-isoxazolylvinyl cephalosporins. II. Antibacterial activities against clinical isolates and pharmacokinetics in mice, 37th Intersci Conf Antimicrob Agents Chemother, abstract F-183.

Patel IH, Chang DH, Gustavson L, Reele S, 1986, Dose proportionality and food effect on Ro 19-5248/T2588 absorption in humans, 26th Intersci Conf Antimicrob Agents Chemother, abstract 2027.

Payne DJ, Amyes GB, 1993, Stability of cefdinir (CI-983, FK 482) to extended spectrum plasmid-mediated β-lactamases, J Med Microbiol, 38, 114–117.

Peixoto E, Ramet J, Kissling M, 1993, Cefetamet pivoxil in pharyngotonsillitis due to group A beta-haemolytic streptococci, Curr Ther Res, 53, 694–706.

Perkins BA, Hamill RH, Musher DM, O'Hara C, 1992, In vitro activities of streptomycin and 11 oral antimicrobial agents against clinical isolates of *Klebsiella rhinoscleromatis*, Antimicrob Agents Chemother, 36, 1785–1787.

Perol Y, November 1989, Comparative study of the activity of RU 51746, cefpodoxime sodium salt, against *N. gonorrhoeae*, Roussel Uclaf, data in file.

Péter O, Bretz AG, 1994, In vitro susceptibility of *Borrelia burgdorferi*, *Borrelia garinii* and *Borrelia afzelii* to 7 antimicrobial agents, VI Int Conf Lyme Borreliosis.

Pfeffer M, Jackson A, Ximenes J, Perche de Menezes J, 1977, Comparative human oral clinical pharmacology of cefadroxil, cephalexin, and cephradine, Antimicrob Agents Chemother, 11, 331–338.

Philpot-Howard J, 1984, Antibiotic resistance and *Haemophilus influenzae*, J Antimicrob Chemother, 13, 199–208.

Pichichero ME, 1991, The rising incidence of penicillin treatment failure in group A streptococcal tonsillopharyngitis: an emerging role for the cephalosporins? Pediatr Infect Dis J, 10, S50-S55.

Pichichero ME, Disney FA, Aronovitz GH, Ginsburg C, Stillerman M, 1987, A multicenter randomized, single-blind evaluation of cefuroxime axetil and phenoxymethylpenicillin in the treatment of streptococcal pharyngitis, Clin Pediatr, 26, 453–458.

Pichichero ME, Gooch WM, Rodriguez W, Blumer JL, Aronoff SC, Jacobs RF, Musser JM, 1994, Effective short-course treatment of acute group A β-haemolytic streptococcal tonsillo-pharyngitis, Arch Pediatr Adoles Med, 148, 1053–1060.

Pichichero ME, Margolis PA, 1991, A comparison of cephalosporins and penicillins in the treatment of group A β-hemolytic streptococcal pharyngitis: a meta-analysis supporting the concept of microbial copathogenicity, Pediatr Infect Dis J, 10, 275–281.

Pichichero ME, McLinn SE, Gooch WM III, Rodriguez W, Goldfarb J, Reidenberg BE, 1995, Ceftibuten *vs* penicillin V in group A beta-hemolytic streptococcal pharyngitis, Pediatr Infect Dis J, 14, Suppl, S102-S107.

Poole JM, Rosenberg R, Aronovitz GH, et al, 1992, Cefprozil *vs* cefixime and cefaclor in otitis media in children, Infect Med, 9, suppl C, 21–32.

Portier H, Charvanet P, Gouyon JB, Guetat F, 1990, Five day treatment of pharyngotonsillitis with cefpodoxime proxetil, J Antimicrob Chemother, 26, 79–85.

Pozzi E, Oliva A, 1995, Oral cephalosporins: clinical results in lower respiratory tract infections, Antibiot Chemother, 47, 123–144.

Pugh RNH, Murray LIM, Dawon JL, Pietroni MC, Williams R, 1973, Transection of the oesophagus for bleeding oesophageal varices, Br J Surg, 60, 646–649.

Pukander JS, Paloheim SH, Sipilä MM, 1992, Cefetamet pivoxil in pediatric otitis media, Chemotherapy, 38, Suppl 2, 25–28.

Quintiliani R, 1982, A review of the penetration of cefadroxil into human tissue, J Antimicrob Chemother, 10, suppl B, 33–38.

Ramet J, Pierrard D, Vandenberghe P, De Boecke K, 1992, Comparative study of cefetamet pivoxil and penicillin V in the treatment of group A beta-haemolytic streptococcal pharyngitis, Chemotherapy, 28, Suppl 2, 33–37.

Randolph MF, 1988, Clinical comparison of once-daily cefadroxil and thrice-daily cefaclor in the treatment of streptococcal pharyngitis, Chemotherapy, 34, 512–518.

Reixoto E, Ramet J, Kissling M, 1993, Cefetamet pivoxil in pharyngotonsillitis due to group A beta-hemolytic streptococci, Curr Ther Res, 53, 694–706.

Richer M, Allard S, Manseau L, Vallée F, Pak R, Le Bel M, 1995, Suction-induced blister fluid penetration of cefdinir in healthy volunteers following ascending doses, Antimicrob Agents Chemother, 39, 1082–1086.

Richter WF, Chong YH, Stella VJ, 1990, On the mechanism of isomerization of cephalosporin esters, J Pharm Sci, 79, 185–186.

Rolston KVI, Messer M, Nguyen H, Ho D, Le Blanc B, Bodey GP, 1991, In vitro activity of cefpodoxime against bacterial isolates obtained from patients with cancer, Eur J Clin Microbiol Infect Dis, 10, 581–585.

Rosenfeld RM, Doyle WJ, Swarts DJ, Seroky J, Perez Pinero B, 1992, Third generation cephalosporin in the treatment of acute pneumococcal otitis media—an animal study, Arch Otolaryngol Head Neck Surg, 118, 49–52.

Rotter S, Lode H, Stelzer I, et al, 1992, Pharmacokinetics of loracarbef and interaction with acetylcysteine, Eur J Clin Microbiol Infect Dis, 11, 851–855.

Saathoff N, Lode H, Neider K, Depperman KM, Borner K, Koeppe P, 1992, Pharmacokinetics of cefpodoxime proxetil and interactions with antacid and an H2 receptor antagonist, Antimicrob Agents Chemother, 36, 796–800.

Sader HS, Jones RN, Washington JA, Murray PR, Gerlach EH, Allen SD, Erwin ME, 1993, In vitro activity of cefpodoxime compared with other oral cephalosporins tested against 5556 recent clinical isolates from five medical centers, Diagn Microbiol Infect Dis, 17, 143–150.

Saez-Lorens X, Shyu WC, Shelton S, Kumiesz H, Nelson J, 1990, Pharmacokinetics of cefprozil in infants and children, Antimicrob Agents Chemother, 34, 2152–2155.

Saito A, 1993, Pharmacokinetics and tissue penetrations of cefditoren pivoxil, 18th Int Congr Chemother, abstract P 1122, p. 821.

Santacroce F, Dainelli B, Mignini F, Fasanella L, Marangoni F, Ripa S, 1985, Determination of cefatrizine levels in blood, tonsils, paranasal sinuses and middle-ear fluid, Drugs Expt Clin Res, 11, 453–456.

Sarubbi FA, Verghese A, Caggiano C, Holtsclaw-Berk S, Berk SL, 1989, In vitro activity of cefpodoxime proxetil (U-76,252; CS-807) against clinical isolates of *Branhamella catarrhalis*, Antimicrob Agents Chemother, 33, 113–114.

Scaglione F, Pintucci JP, Demartini G, Dugnani S, 1996, Ceftibuten concentrations in human tonsillar tissue, Eur J Clin Microbiol Infect Dis, 15, 940–943.

Schaadt RD, Yagi BH, Zurenko GE, 1990, In vitro activity of cefpodoxime proxetil (U-76,252; CS-807) against *N. gonorrhoeae*, Antimicrob Agents Chemother, 34, 371–372.

Schatz B, Karavokiros KT, Tauebel MA, Itokazu GS, 1996, Comparison of cefprozil, cefpodoxime proxetil, loracarbef, cefixime and ceftibuten, Ann Pharmacother, 30, 258-268.

Schumacher-Perdreau F, Jansen B, Peters G, 1991, In vitro actvity of cefpodoxime against staphylococci in comparison to other cephalosporins, Eur J Clin Microbiol Infect Dis, 10, 585–588.

Schwartz RH, Freij BJ, Ziai M, Sheridan MJ, 1997, Antimicrobial prescribing for acute purulent rhinitis in children: a survey of pediatricians and family practitioners, Pediatr Infect Dis J, 16, 185–190.

Schwartz RH, Wientzen RI Jr, Pedrera F, et al, 1981, Penicillin V for group A streptococcal pharyngitis: a randomized trial of seven *versus* ten day therapy, JAMA, 246, 1790–1795.

Schwinghammer TL, Norden CW, Gill E, 1990, Pharmacokinetics of cephradine administered intravenously and orally to young and elderly subjects, J Clin Pharmacol, 30, 893–899.

Sheppard M, King A, Phillips I, 1991, In vitro activity of cefpodoxime, a new oral cephalosporin, compared with that of nine other antimicrobial agents, Eur J Clin Microbiol Infect Dis, 10, 573–581.

Shgu WC, Wilber RD, Pittman K, Barbhaiya RH, 1992, Effect of antacid on the bioavailability of cefprozil, Antimicrob Agents Chemother, 36, 962–965.

Shiba K, 1988, Pharmacokinetic evaluation of ceftibuten (7432-S), 28th Intersci Conf Antimicrob Agents Chemother, abstract 452.

Shiba K, Kaji M, Shimada J, Sakai O, 1990, Effects of probenecid on in vivo pharmacokinetics of ME 1207, a new oral cephem antibiotic, 30th Intersci Conf Antimicrob Agents Chemother, abstract 672.

Shiba K, Saito A, Shimada J, et al, 1989, Clinical studies on cefdinir, Chemotherapy, 37, Suppl 2, 345–352.

Shigi Y, Matsumoto Y, Kaizu M, Fujishita Y, Koyo H, 1984, Mechanisms of action of the new orally active cephalosporin FK027, Jpn J Antibiot, 37, 790–796.

Shimada J, Hori S, Oguma T, Yoshikawa T, Yamamoto S, Nishikawa T, Yamada H, 1993, Effects of protein binding on the isomerization of ceftibuten, J Pharm Sci, 82, 461–465.

Shimada K, Kobayashi Y, Shinkai S, Komiya I, Matsumoto T, 1989, Phase I clinical studies on a novel orally active cephem antibiotic, ME1207, 29th Intersci Conf Antimicrob Agents Chemother, abstract 366.

Shimada K, Soejima R, 1987, FK482, a new orally active cephalosporin: pharmacokinetics and tolerance in healthy volunteers, 27th Intersci Conf Antimicrob Agents Chemother, abstract 655.

Shimizu K, Saito A, Shimada J, et al, 1993, Carnitine studies and safety after oral administration of S-1108, a new oral cephem, to patients, Antimicrob Agents Chemother, 37, 1043–1049.

Shinikawa A, Tamura Y, Shimizu K, Miyake H, 1988, CS-807 in otorhinolaryngological infections, Chemotherapy, 36, suppl 1, 1046–1055.

Shyu WC, Haddad J, Reilly J, Khan WN, Campbell DA, Tsai Y, Barbhaiya KH, 1994, Penetration of cefprozil into middle ear fluid of patients with otitis media, Antimicrob Agents Chemother, 38, 2210–2212.

Shyu WC, Pittman KA, Wilber RB, Matzke GR, Barbhaiya RH, 1991, Pharmacokinetics of cefprozil in healthy subjects and patients with renal impairment, J Clin Pharmacol, 31, 362–371.

Shyu WC, Shah WR, Campbell DA, Wilber RB, Pittman KA, Barbhaiya RH, 1992, Oral absolute bioavailability and intravenous dose-proportionality of cefprozil in humans, J Clin Pharmacol, 32, 789–803.

Shyu WC, Wilber RB, Pittman KA, Gorg DC, Barbhaiya RH, 1991, Pharmacokinetics of cefprozil in healthy subjects and patients with hepatic impairment, J Clin Pharmacol, 31, 372-376.

Siebor E, Cordin S, Delpech N, Duez JM, Kasmierczak A, 1990, Etude comparative de l'activité antibactérienne du cefpodoxime sur les entérobactéries productrices de bétalactamases, Pathol Biol, 38, 331–335.

Sifaoui F, Duval F, Boucot I, Leblanc F, Gutmann L, Berche P, 1996, In vitro activity of sanfetrinem (GV 104326) against bacterial isolates from acute otitis media in children, 36th Intersci Conf Antimicrob Agents Chemother, abstract F151.

Sifaoui F, Kitzis MD, Gutmann L, 1996, In vitro selection of one-step mutants of *Streptococcus pneumoniae* resistant to different oral β-lactam antibiotics is associated with alterations of PBP2x, Antimicrob Agents Chemother, 40, 152–156.

Singlas E, Lebrec D, Gaudin C, Montay G, Roche G, Taburet AM, 1989, Influence de l'insuffisance hépatique sur la pharmacocinétique du cefixime, Presse Med, 18, 1587–1588.

Sitar D, Hoban DJ, Aoki FY, 1994, Pharmacokinetic disposition of loracarbef in healthy young men and women at steady state, J Clin Pharmacol, 34, 924–929.

Smith CB, Golden C, Kanner RE, Renzetti AD, 1976, *H. influenzae* and *H. parainfluenzae* in chronic obstructive pulmonary disease, Lancet, i, 1253–1255.

Smith CB, Golden CA, Kanner RE, Renzetti AD, 1980, Association of viral and *Mycoplasma pneumoniae* infections with acute respiratory illness in patients with chronic obstructive pulmonary diseases, Am Rev Respir Dis, 121, 225–232.

Sommers DK, Van Wyk M, Moncrieff J, Schoeman HS, 1984, Influence of food and reduced gastric acidity on the bioavailability of bacampicillin and cefuroxime axetil, Br J Clin Pharmacol, 18, 535–539.

Sommers DK, Van Wyk M, Williams PEO, Harding SM, 1984, Pharmacokinetics and tolerance of cefuroxime axetil in volunteers during repeated dosing, Antimicrob Agents Chemother, 25, 344–347.

Spangler SK, Jacobs MR, Appelbaum PC, 1994, In vitro susceptibility of 185 penicillin-susceptible and -resistant pneumococci to WY-49605 (SUN/SY5555), a new oral penem, compared with those to penicillin G, amoxicillin, amoxicillin-clavulanate, cefixime, cefaclor, cefpodoxime, cefuroxime, and cefdinir, Antimicrob Agents Chemother, 38, 2902–2904.

Spangler SK, Jacobs MR, Appelbaum PC, 1994, Activity of WY-49605 compared with those of amoxicillin, amoxicillin-clavulanate, imipenem, ciprofloxacin, cefaclor, cefpodoxime, cefuroxime, clindamycin, and metronidazole against 384 anaerobic bacteria, Antimicrob Agents Chemother, 38, 2599–2604.

Spangler SK, Jacobs MR, Appelbaum PC, 1996, Activities of RPR 106972 (a new oral streptogramin), cefditoren (a new oral cephalosporin), two new oxazolidinone (U 100592 and U 100766), and other oral and parenteral agents against 203 penicillin-susceptible and -resistant pneumococci, Antimicrob Agents Chemother, 40, 481–484.

Spangler SK, Jacobs MR, Appelbaum PC, 1997, Time-kill studies on susceptibility of nine penicillin-susceptible and -resistant pneumococci to cefditoren compared with nine other B-lactams, J Antimicrob Chemother, 39, 141–148.

Spyker DA, Thomas BL, Sande MA, Bolton WK, 1978, Pharmacokinetics of cefaclor and cephalexin: dosage nomograms for impaired renal function, Antimicrob Agents Chemother, 14, 172–177.

Stillerman M, 1969, Comparison of cephaloglycin and penicillin in streptococcal pharyngitis, Clin Pharmacol Ther, 11, 205–213.

Stillerman M, 1976, Cefatrizine and potassium phenoxymethylpenicillin on group A streptococcal pharyngitis, Antimicrob Agents Chemother, 16, 185.

Stillerman M, 1986, Comparison of oral cephalosporins with penicillin therapy for group A streptococcal pharyngitis, Pediatr Infect Dis J, 5, 649–654.

Stillerman M, Isenberg HD, Moody M, 1972, Streptococcal pharyngitis therapy: comparison of cephalexin, phenoxymethylpenicillin and ampicillin, Am J Dis Child, 123, 457–461.

Stobberingh EE, Houbon AW, Philips JH, 1989, In vitro activity of cefpodoxime, a new oral cephalosporin, Eur J Clin Microbiol Infect Dis, 8, 656–658.

Stobberingh EE, Winderink M, Philips M, Houben A, 1987, *Branhamella catarrhalis*: β-lactamase production and sensitivity to oral antibiotics, including new cephalosporins, J Antimicrob Chemother, 20, 765–766.

Stoeckel K, Hayton WL, Edwards DJ, 1995, Clinical pharmacokinetics of oral cephalosporins, Antibiot Chemother, 47, 34–71.

Stone JW, Linong G, Andrews JM, Wise R, 1989, Cefixime, in-vitro activity, pharmacokinetics and tissue penetration, J Antimicrob Chemother, 23, 221–228.

St Peter J, Borin MT, Hughes G, Kelloway J, Shapiro B, Halstentson C, 1992, Disposition of cefpodoxime proxetil in healthy volunteers and patients with impaired renal function, Antimicrob Agents Chemother, 36, 126–131.

Straffon RA, 1974, Urinary tract infection: problems in diagnosis and management, Med Clin N Am, 58, 545–554.

Sunakawa K, Iwata S, 1986, Clinical evaluation of cefixime in pediatrics, Jpn J Antibiot, 39, 1035–1054.

Swedish Study Group (Christensson et al), 1991, A randomized multicenter trial to compare the influence of cefaclor and amoxycillin on the colonization resistance of the digestive tract in patients with lower respiratory tract infections, Infection, 19, 208–215.

Sydnor A, Gwaltney JM Jr, Cochetto DM, Scheld WM, 1989, Comparative evaluation of cefuroxime axetil and cefaclor for treatment of acute bacterial maxillary sinusitis, Arch Otolaryngol Head Neck Surg, 115, 1430–1433.

Tack K, Keyserling CH, McCarty J, Heddrick JA, 1997, Study of use of cefdinir versus cephalexin for the treatment of skin infections in pediatric patients, Antimicrob Agents Chemother, 41, 739–742.

Takenouchi T, Nishino T, 1991, Antibacterial activity of cefpodoxime against *Branhamella catarrhalis*, Microbiol Immunol, 35, 1059–1071.

Tam YK, Kneer J, Dubach UC, Stoeckel K, 1989, Pharmacokinetics of cefetamet pivoxil (Ro 15-8075) with ascending oral doses in normal healthy volunteers, Antimicrob Agents Chemother, 33, 957–959.

Tamura A, Okamoto R, Yoshida T, Yamamoto H, Kondo S, Inoue M, Mistuhashi S, 1988, In vitro and in vivo antibacterial activity of ME 1207, a new oral cephalosporin, Antimicrob Agents Chemother, 32, 1421–1426.

Tapsall JW, Phillips EA, 1995, The sensitivity of 173 Sydney isolates of *N. gonorrhoeae* to cefpodoxime and other antibiotics used to treat gonorrhea, Pathology, 27, 64–66.

Teele DW, Klein JO, Rosner B, et al., 1989, Epidemiology of otitis media during the first seven years of life in children in Greater Boston: a prospective, cohort study, J Infect Dis, 160, 83–94.

Thabaut A, Meyran M, Sofer L, Morand A, Labia R, 1994, Interactions of ceftibuten with extended beta-lactamases: a bacteriological and enzyme analysis, Drugs Exp Clin Res, 20, 49–54.

Then RL, 1987, Ability of new–β-lactam antibiotics to induce β-lactamase production in *Enterobacter cloacae*, Eur J Clin Microbiol, 6, 451–455.

Therasse DG, Farlow DS, Davidson RL, et al, 1993, Effects of renal dysfunction on the pharmacokinetics of loracarbef, Clin Pharmacol Ther, 54, 311–316.

Thornber D, Wise R, Andrews JM, O'Sullivan N, 1991, The in vitro activity and β-lactamase stability of cefdinir (CI-983, KFK 482): a new oral cephalosporin, 17th Int Congr Chemother.

Thorpe EM Jr, Schwerbke JR, Hook EW III, et al, 1996, Comparison of single-dose cefuroxime axetil with ciprofloxacin in treatment of uncomplicated gonorrhoea caused by penicillinase-producing and non-penicillinase-producing *Neisseria gonorrhoeae* strains, Antimicrob Agents Chemother, 40, 2275–2280.

Tillett WS, Cambier MJ, MacCormack JE, 1944, The treatment of lobar pneumonia and pneumococcal empyema with penicillin, Bull NY Acad Med, 20, 142–178.

Todd JK, Todd N, Damato J, Todd WA, 1984, Bacteriology and treatment of purulent nasopharyngitis, a double-blind, placebo controlled evaluation, Pediatr Infect Dis J, 3, 226–232.

Todd WM, 1994, Cefpodoxime proxetil: a comprehensive review, Int J Antimicrob Agents, 4, 37–67.

Totsuka K, Shimizu K, Konishi M, Yamamoto S, 1992, Metabolism of S-1108, a new oral cephem antibiotic, and metabolic profiles of its metabolites in humans, Antimicrob Agents Chemother, 36, 757–761.

Tremblay D, Dupont A, Ho C, Coussedière D, Lenfant B, 1990, Pharmacokinetics of cefpodoxime in young and elderly volunteers after single doses, J Antimicrob Chemother, 26, Suppl E, 21–28.

Trenk D, Wagner F, Bechtold H, Nier B, Jähnchen E, 1990, Lack of effect of cefixime on the metabolism of vitamin K1, J Clin Pharmacol, 30, 737–742.

Tupasi TE, Calubiran OV, Torres CA, 1982, Single oral dose of cefaclor for the treatment of infections with penicillinase-producing strains of *Neisseria gonorrhoeae*, Br J Vener Dis, 58, 176-179.

Uchida E, Kobayashi S, Kamijo Y, et al, 1989, The effects of ranitidine, metoclopramide and anisotropine methylbromide on the availability of cefpodoxime proxetil in Japanese healthy subjects, IV World Conf Clin Pharmacol Ther 1989, Mannheim-Heidelberg, Eur J Clin Pharmacol, 36, Suppl, 1133, A-266.

Ueda Y, Okubo H, Ida Y, Yanezu S, Sakakibara Y, Yasunaga K, 1988, Laboratory and clinical study on CS-807, Chemotherapy, 36, Suppl 1, 502–511.

Ueno K, Kazahiko T, Tsujimura K, et al, 1993, Impairment of cefdinir absorption by iron ion, Clin Pharmacol Ther, 54, 473–475.

Urban A, Andes D, Craig WA, 1995, In vivo activity of cefpodoxime against penicillin-resistant pneumococci, 19th Int Congr Chemother.

Utsui Y, Inoue M, Mitsuhashi S, 1988, Antibacterial activity of CS-807, a new oral cephalosporin, Chemotherapy, 36, suppl 1, 1–15.

Valentini S, Coratza G, Rossolini GM, Massidda O, Satta G, 1994, In vitro evaluation of cefpodoxime, J Antimicrob Chemother, 33, 495–508.

Van Dyk JC, Terespolsky SA, Meyer CS, Van Niekerk CH, Klugman K, 1997, Penetration of cefpodoxime into middle ear fluid in paediatric patients with acute otitis media, Pediatr Infect Dis J, 16, 79–81.

Venkatesan P, MacFarlane JT, 1991, Epidemiology and pathogenesis of prevention of pneumonia, Curr Opin Infect Dis, 4, 154–159.

Veyssier P, Darchis JP, Devillers A, 1988, Pharmacocinétique du céfuroxime-axétil administré par voie orale chez le sujet âgé, Therapie, 43, 355–359.

Vickers S, Ducan CAH, White SD, et al, 1985, Carnitine and glucuronic acid conjugates of pivalic acid, Xenobiotics, 15, 453–458.

Wald ER, 1985, Epidemiology, pathophysiology and etiology of sinusitis, Pediatr Infect Dis J, 4, S51-S54.

Wald ER, 1991, Purulent nasal discharge, Pediatr Infect Dis J, 10, 329–333.

Wallace RJ Jr, Masher DM, Martin PR, 1978, *Haemophilus influenzae* in adults, Am J Med, 64, 87–93.

Wannamaker LW, Rammelkermp CR Jr, Denny FW, et al, 1951, Prophylaxis of acute rheumatic fever by treatment of the preceding streptococcal infection with various amounts of depot penicillin, Am J Med, 10, 673–695.

Weber DJ, Wolfson JS, Swartz MN, Hooper DC, 1984, *Pasteurella multocida* infections: report of 34 cases and review of the literature, Medicine, 63, 133–154.

Westbloom TU, Gudipati S, Midkiff BR, 1990, In vitro susceptibility of *Helicobacter pylori* to the new oral cephalosporins cefpodoxime, ceftibuten and cefixime, Eur J Clin Microbiol Infect Dis, 9, 691–693.

Westphal JF, Jehl F, Brogard JM, 1994, Cinétique de la clairance biliaire du céfixime chez des patients cholécystectomisés, Therapie 49, 35–39.

Wick WE, 1967, Cephalexin, a new orally absorbed cephalosporin antibiotic, Appl Microbiol, 15, 765–769.

Wiedeman B, Luhmer E, Zühlsdorf MT, 1991, In vitro activity of cefpodoxime and ten other cephalosporins against Gram-positive cocci, *Enterobacteriaceae* and *P. aeruginosa*, including β-lactamase producers, Infection, 19, 365–369.

Wiedeman BL, Schwartz RH, 1992, Effect of blood contamination on the interpretation of antibiotic concentrations in the middle ear fluid, Pediatr Infect Dis J, 11, 244–245.

Wieseman LR, Benfield P, 1993, Cefprozil, a review of its antibacterial activity, pharmacokinetic properties and therapeutic potential, Drugs, 45, 295–317.

Willcox RR, Woodcock KS, 1970, Cephalexin in the oral treatment of gonorrhoea by a double-dose method, Postgrad Med J, 46, suppl, 103–106.

Williams JD, Powell M, Fah Ys, Seymour A, Yuan M, 1992, In vitro susceptibility of *Haemophilus influenzae* to cefaclor, cefixime, cefetamet and loracarbef, Eur J Clin Microbiol Infect Dis, 11, 748–751.

Williams PO, Harding SM, 1984, The absolute bioavailability of oral cefuroxime axetil in male and female volunteers after fasting and after food, J Antimicrob Chemother, 13, 191–196.

Wise R, Andrews JM, Ashby JP, Thornber D, 1990, The in vitro activity of cefpodoxime: a comparison with other oral cephalosporins, J Antimicrob Chemother, 25, 541–550.

Wise R, Bennet SA, Dent J, 1984, The pharmacokinetics of orally absorbed cefuroxime compared with amoxycillin/clavulanic acid, J Antimicrob Chemother, 13, 603–610.

Wise R, Nye K, O'Neill P, Wastenholme M, Andrews JM, 1990, Pharmacokinetics and tissue penetration of ceftibuten, Antimicrob Agents Chemother, 34, 1053–1055.

Wiseman LR, Balfour JA, 1994, Ceftibuten: a review of its antibacterial activity, pharmacokinetic properties and clinical efficacy, Drugs, 47, 784–808.

Yamasaku F, Suzuki Y, Uno K, 1989, Comparative study of pharmacokinetics of cefdinir and cefroxadine in the same healthy volunteers, Chemotherapy, 37, Suppl 2, 441–446.

Yee YC, Thornsberry C, 1994, Penicillin-resistant *Streptococcus pneumoniae* on the rise in the United States: its effect on oral cephalosporins, Antimicrob Infect Dis New Lett, 13, 49–57.

Yourassowsky E, Van den Linden MP, Crokaert F, 1992, Killing rate and growth rate comparison for newer beta-lactamase stable oral beta-lactams against *S. pneumoniae*, *H. influenzae* and *M. catarrhalis*, Chemotherapy, 38, 7–13.

Zolfino I, Senesi S, Campa M, et al, 1992, Human skin disposition of cefpodoxime after oral administration of its proxetil ester, J Antimicrob Chemother, 30, 731–733.

Carbapenems

A. BRYSKIER

8

1. BACKGROUND

Carbapenems belong to the β-lactam family, with a broad antibacterial spectrum that includes gram-positive and gram-negative bacteria. In enzymatic terms they have dual activity: they inhibit the activity of certain β-lactamases and are active against the majority of β-lactamase-producing strains. Some carbapenems are rapidly metabolized in vivo, as evidenced, for instance, by the weak urinary elimination.

Research in the area of carbapenems has involved several stages, starting with the discovery of thienamycin, which is a natural carbapenem. Thienamycin was extracted from the culture filtrate of *Streptomyces cattleya*, which owes its name to the fact that the colonies resembled the orchid of the same name. The extraction, purification, and elucidation of the structure of thienamycin constituted a long and difficult process because of the chemical instability of the molecule. A number of derivatives of thienamycin have an *(S)* configuration at C-8 rather than the *(R)* and have been extracted under the name of epithienamycin S, also known as olivanic acid. Thienamycin is unstable as a result of intermolecular dimerization. A stable compound containing an imidine group instead of the cysteamine chain at position 2 was then semisynthesized and developed: imipenem. The drawback of this molecule, which exhibited an exceptional spectrum and antibacterial activity, is its instability against hydrolysis by renal dehydropeptidase I (DHP-I), a metalloenzyme, and its poor hydrosolubility.

Research into carbapenems has been geared towards increasing the stability against renal DHP-I, and research teams from Merck have shown that the presence of a 1-β-methyl group increases stability against DHP-I. Other groups have been proposed to fill this role. This characteristic is exhibited by some molecules such as meropenem. A number of molecules have been synthesized, but fewer than a dozen of them are undergoing development.

The current research into carbapenems is directed towards the synthesis of molecules that are more stable against hydrolysis by DHP-I, the reduction of neurologic side effects, the improvement of pharmacokinetic characteristics (apparent elimination half-life), oral absorption, and the absence of cross-resistance with imipenem. Another line of research is the combination of a carbapenem and a fluoroquinolone. One major aspect remains the reduction in the cost of synthesis because of the large number of steps required in the synthesis process.

2. CLASSIFICATION

The carbapenems may be divided into molecules of natural origin and those of synthetic origin. Microbiologically, two types of derivatives have been prepared: antibacterial agents and β-lactamase inhibitors.

2.1. Natural Derivatives

More than 50 compounds have been described in the literature, and these may be classified into four subgroups according to the side chain at position 6: 5,6-*cis*-hydroxyethyl, 5,6-*trans*-hydroxyethyl (thienamycin), isopropyl, and isopropylidene (Fig. 1). Their in vitro activities are variable (Table 1).

These molecules possess a carbapen-2-em-3-carboxylic acid nucleus with substituents at positions 2 and 6.

The substituents at position 2 derive from cysteamine, and their chain does or does not have an unsaturated bond, the sulfur atom of which is present in the form of sulfoxide. In the majority of cases, the amino group is acylated, with the exception of thienamycin and its derivatives, in which the amino group is free.

The chain at position 6 may be optically inactive, as in the derivatives carpetimycins A and B; NS-5; PS-5, -6, -7, and -8; northienamycin; and asparenomycin; or optically active, as in the epimers involving C-6 and C-8. All of the isomeric possibilities have been described, with the exception of the 5,6 *cis*, 8*R* diastereoisomer.

2.1.1. Thienamycin and Derivatives

The molecules belonging to the subgroup of thienamycin and derivatives have three characteristics: a 6-α-hydroxylated side chain, a basic chain at position 2, and an unsaturated pentacyclic nucleus.

Thienamycin is a metabolite of *S. cattleya*, but its name derives from the chromophore, β-thioenamine. It is a zwitterionic-type molecule. The stereochemistry of the three asymmetrical centers is 5*R*, 6*S*, 8*R*. A minor fermentation derivative, 9-northienamycin, has a 5*R*, 6*S* configuration.

2.1.2. 5,6-*cis*-Ethyl Carbapenems

There are more than 20 molecules in the 5,6-*cis*-ethyl carbapenem subgroup, the prototypes of which are the epithienamycins, PS-5, OA-6129, and the pluracidomycins.

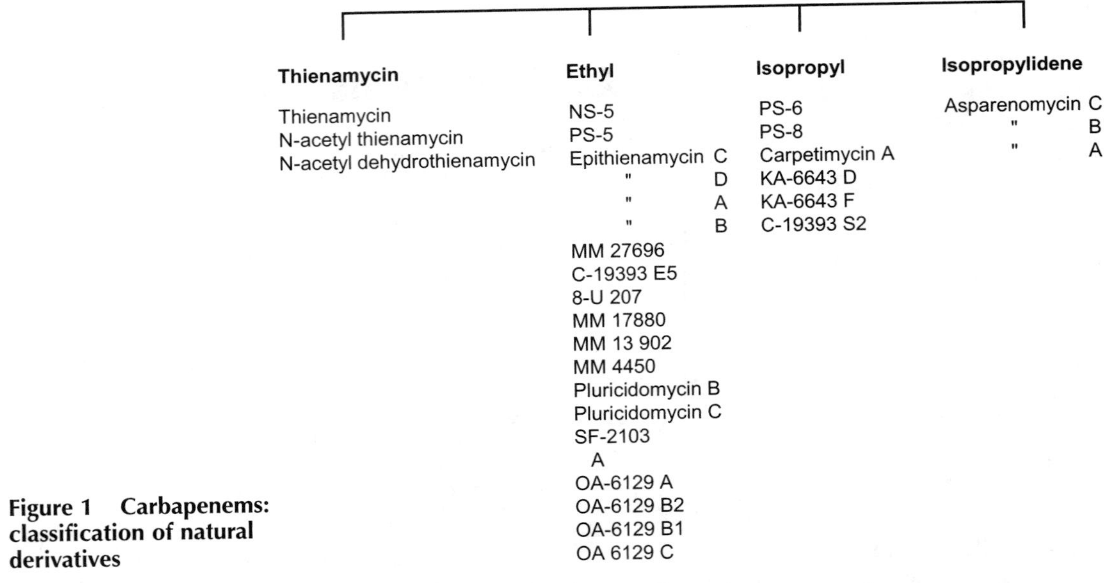

Figure 1 Carbapenems: classification of natural derivatives

Table 1 In vitro activities of the natural carbapenems

Drug	MIC (μg/ml)						
	E. coli TEM+	*P. mirabilis*	*S. marcescens*	*E. cloacae*	*P. aeruginosa*	*B. fragilis*	*S. aureus* Pen^r
Thienamycin	0.32	5	16		2.5	1	0.04
Olivanic acid	1.6	0.2	3.1	12.5	50	0.4	1.6
MM 13902							
Carpetimycin A	0.2	1.6	3.1	3.1	6.25	3.1	0.39
Asparenomycin A	0.4	3.1	12.5	1.6	25		1.6
Pluracidomycin A (SF-2103A)	12.5		100		>100		25
PS-5 (MM 22744)	3.1	12.5	6.3	12.5	25		0.16

All of these molecules are inactive against *Pseudomonas aeruginosa*, except for two diacetylated compounds, and do not have an ion function such as an *O*-sulfate (NS-5 and NA-26978). The compounds without an *N*-acyl group on their side chain are more stable against hydrolysis by DHP-I.

The epithienamycins, or olivanic acids, are produced by *Streptomyces olivaceus* and are composed of two types of molecules: sulfated derivatives (MM 4550 and epithienamycin E) and nonsulfated derivatives (epithienamycins A, C, and D). The derivatives inhibit β-lactamase activity. Some, such as MM-13902, also possess significant antibacterial activity. They are chemically unstable; the most stable of them, MM 13902, has a degradation half-life of 12 h in an aqueous medium at 25°C, but this falls to 4 h at pH 6.

2.1.3. Pluracidomycins

Pluracidomycin A (SF-2103A) was isolated from a strain of *Streptomyces sulfonofaciens*; it has moderate antibacterial activity but also inhibits the activity of numerous β-lactamases.

2.1.4. PS Series

PS-5, -6, -7, and -8 differ by the substituent at the 2′ position of the C-6 chain and the C-2 chain, which may or may not be saturated. They were isolated from *Streptomyces cremeus* subsp. *auratilis*. PS-5 also possesses antibacterial activity.

A large number of derivatives obtained by semisynthesis have been prepared. Those possessing a 4-pyridylthio chain are active against gram-positive bacteria, while those with a D-cysteine-type chain are more active against gram-positive bacteria (Fig. 2).

The OA-6129 series comprises four derivatives: A, B, B_2 and C, characterized by a pantethienyl chain at position 2. They differ in the substituent at C-6, which may be a hydroxyl in the *S* or *R* position, a sulfate, or a hydroxyl in the *S* or *R* position. The antibacterial activity, in descending order, is pantethienyl > sulfomethyl (OA-6129C) > ethyl (OA-6129A) > hydroxyethyl (OA-6129B_2).

2.1.5. Isopropyl Carbapenems

The isopropyl carbapenems comprise 11 molecules. The side chain at position 6 enables two types of molecules to be distinguished: those possessing a hydroxyl group and those possessing a sulfone group.

The side chain at position C-2 may or may not comprise unsaturated groups and sulfoxide groups. Only molecules with a 5,6-*cis* chain have good antibacterial activity.

The presence of a sulfoxide group at C-2 increases the inhibitory activity against penicillinases, but decreases it or is without effect against cephalosporinases, with the exception of that of *Proteus vulgaris* GN 4413.

The number of methylated groups at C-6 interferes to various degrees with the inhibitory activity, depending on whether the compounds possess a hydroxyl or sulfate group at position 8.

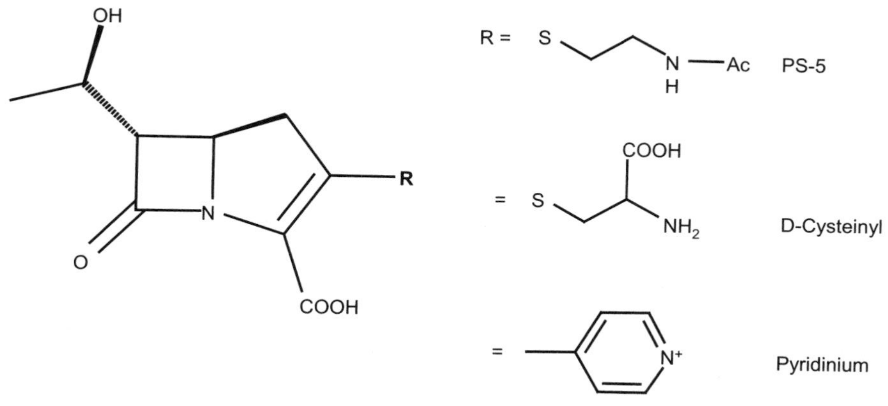

Figure 2 Semisynthetic carbapenems

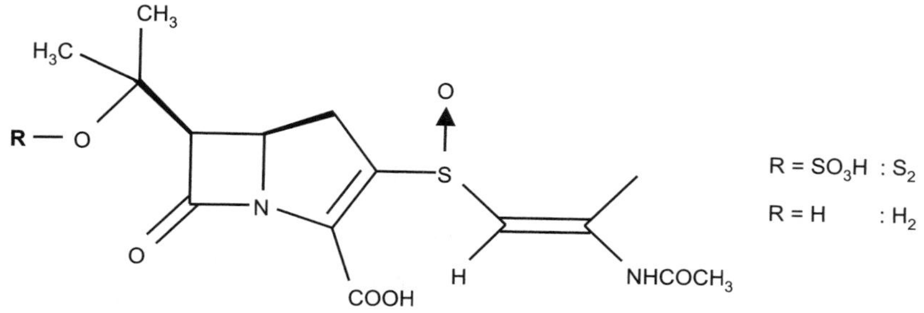

Figure 3 Compounds C-19393 H_2 and S_2

The following molecules belong to this subgroup: carpetimycins A, B, C, and D; C-19393 H_2; and C-19393 S_2 (Fig. 3). The carpetimycins were isolated from *Streptomyces* sp. strain KC-6643 and possess β-lactamase-inhibitory activity similar to that of the olivanic acids (about 10% of that of clavulanic acid). C-19393 H_2 acts in synergy with ampicillin and cefotiam against TEM β-lactamase-producing strains. Carpetimycins A and B are more stable chemically than the epithienamycins, their degradation half-lives at pH 7 in an aqueous medium being, respectively, 187 and 170 h.

2.1.6. Isopropylidene Carbapenems

The isopropylidene carbapenems comprise the asparenomycin series and 6643X. The asparenomycins were isolated from cultures of *Streptomyces tokunonensis* and *Streptomyces argenteolus* and possess an ethylidene chain at C-6. Asparenomycin A has not inconsiderable antibacterial activity and potent β-lactamase inhibitory activity, particularly against β-lactamases of Richmond and Sykes classes Ia, Ib, and Ic.

Asparenomycin A is chemically unstable. At pH 4 and ambient temperature, it is hydrolyzed within 6 h. Oxidation following hydrolysis of asparenomycin A yields aspartic acid.

2.1.7. Other Derivatives

The simplest carbapenem structurally is SQ-27860, which is nonsubstituted. It was isolated from a strain of *Serratia* and *Erwinia* spp. It is chemically unstable.

3. SYNTHETIC MOLECULES

Two groups of molecules are introduced in clinical practice or under development: those nonsubstituted at position 1 and those substituted at position 1 (Fig. 4).

3.1. Molecules Nonsubstituted at Position 1: Imipenem

Only two molecules have been introduced in clinical practice: imipenem and panipenem. Imipenem is a semisynthetic molecule whose basic nucleus is thienamycin. Thienamycin is unstable in an aqueous medium as intermolecular dimerization occurs (Fig. 5). To avoid this phenomenon, the cysteamine residue has to be modified. Imipenem is the imidine derivative of thienamycin or *N'*-formylimidoyl thienamycin.

Biapenem possesses a thiopyrrazolotriazolium chain at position 2. L-695256 belongs to a series of molecules having a heavy chain of the enolyl type at C-2 with an imidazolium nucleus. It is not substituted at position 1 (Fig. 8).

3.2. Molecules Substituted at Position 1

The molecules currently under development have a substituent at position 1, principally a methyl group. Eight molecules for parenteral use (Fig. 6) are currently introduced in clinical practice or undergoing clinical or preclinical development: meropenem, panipenem, ertapenem, DX-8739, lenapenem, doripenem, CL-188624, CL-190294, and CL-191121. They differ in the substituent at position 2, with meropenem possessing a thiopyrrolidinyl nucleus substituted at position 5' by a carbamoyl chain. Panipenem has a thiopyrrolidine nucleus substituted by an acetamidoyl chain. DX-8739 is also a 2-thiopyrrolidine; on the pyrrolidine nucleus a hydroxycarboxypiperazine chain is appended. The pyrrolidine ring is replaced by a 2'-hydroxymethylaminopropyl chain for lenapenem and a sulfamoylcyanomethyl for doripenem (Fig. 7).

The derivative BMS-181189 has an original substituent at 1-β, a guanidoethyl chain, and the substituent at C-2 is a cyanoethylethio chain (Fig. 7).

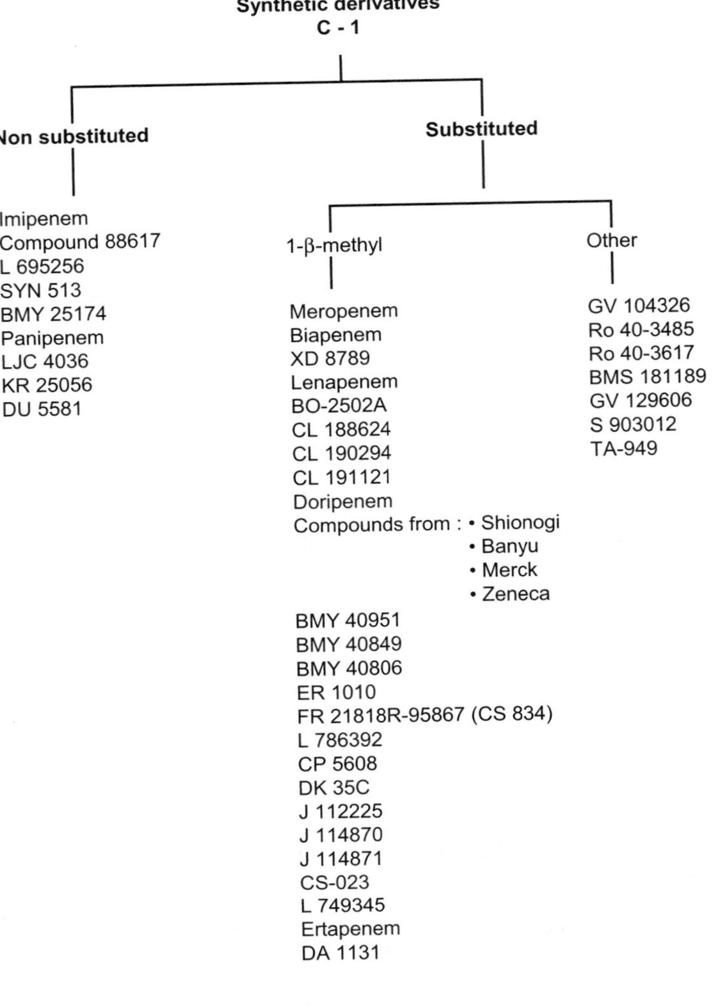

Figure 4 Carbapenems: classification of synthetic derivatives

Figure 5 Dimerization of thienamycin

A series of derivatives possessing a pyrrolidine nucleus at C-2 substituted by an aminohydroxymethyl chain has been synthesized. One molecule has been selected: E-1010 (Fig. 9). It possesses a 3-*(R)*-pyrrolidin-3-yl-*(R)*-hydroxymethyl chain.

FR-21818 is also a 2-thiopyrrolidine carbapenem, the pyrrolyl nucleus of which is substituted at position 4′ by an azabicyclic nucleus (Fig. 10) (Matsumoto et al., 1995).

3.2.1. Tricyclic Molecules

A certain number of molecules have been synthesized with a closure by a pentacyclic or hexacyclic nucleus between C-1 and C-2: these may involve a sanfetrinem carbocyclic nucleus (GV 104326) or a polyheterocyclic nucleus, for example, the presence of a sulfur atom (molecule synthesized by Takeda) (Fig. 11).

A new tricyclic derivative for parenteral use has also been described, GV 129606 (Fig. 12) (di Modugno et al., 1997).

3.2.2. Tetracyclic Molecules

Wollman et al. have synthesized a series of tetracyclic carbapenems (Fig. 13). The presence of two methyl groups at position 1 significantly increases the stability against hydrolysis by DHP-I but significantly reduces the antibacterial activity, particularly against gram-negative bacilli.

The β isomer of the tetracyclic compound (Fig. 14) possesses good activity against gram-positive cocci but is less active than meropenem against gram-negative bacilli. The α isomer is less active against gram-positive cocci and is inactive against gram-negative bacteria. However, these compounds are stable against hydrolysis by porcine DHP-I.

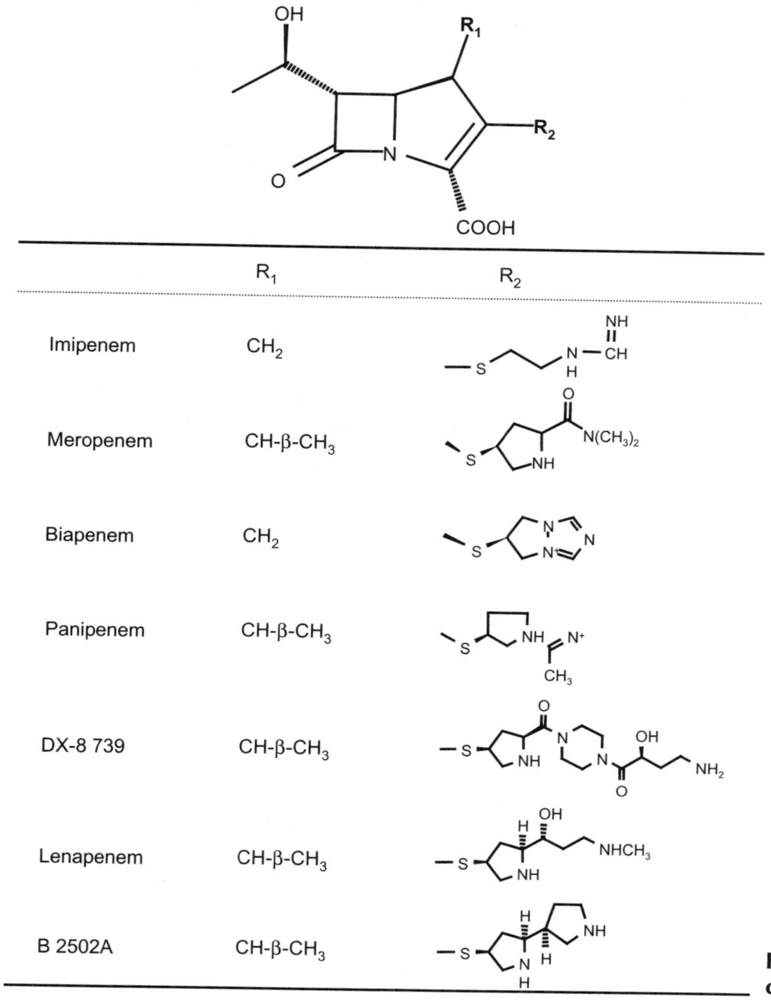

	R_1	R_2
Imipenem	CH_2	
Meropenem	CH-β-CH_3	
Biapenem	CH_2	
Panipenem	CH-β-CH_3	
DX-8 739	CH-β-CH_3	
Lenapenem	CH-β-CH_3	
B 2502A	CH-β-CH_3	

Figure 6 Series of parenteral carbapenems

Substitution of the phenyl nucleus by various groups or fluorine atoms on the β isomer increases the activity against gram-positive cocci, but the molecules are devoid of activity against gram-negative bacilli. Some of them possess excellent stability against hydrolysis by porcine or human DHP-I.

The presence of a piperazine or morpholine nucleus yields molecules that are active against gram-positive cocci but moderately active against gram-negative bacilli.

4. STRUCTURE-ACTIVITY RELATIONSHIPS

The structure-activity relationships of the carbapenems are complex, as they derive from an equilibrium that is difficult to achieve between antibacterial activity, chemical stability, and stability against hydrolysis by renal DHP-I. In addition, research has added the following parameters to these three: the need for good neurologic tolerance compared to that of imipenem, an improvement in the pharmacokinetic profile, and the possibility of oral absorption.

The following have been demonstrated:

- The importance of the stereochemistry with respect to the centers of asymmetry of the molecules.
- The important role of the chain at position 2 in terms of antibacterial activity, chemical stability, and, to a lesser extent, hydrolysis by DHP-I. A hydroxyethyl chain at C-6 yields optimal antibacterial activity, but the ethyl group must be in the β (8*R*) position.
- The substitution at 1-β of the carbapenem nucleus increases stability against hydrolysis by DHP-I but reduces the antibacterial activity, which is dependent on the chain at position 2.
- The chain at position 2 plays an important role in terms of antibacterial activity. The molecules undergoing development have a thiosubstituted chain. The basic substituents increase the activity against gram-negative bacilli, including *P. aeruginosa*.
- Molecules with the carbapenem nucleus, in contrast to the cephem or penam nucleus, possess antibacterial activity similar to that of ampicillin, but they are inactive against β-lactamase-producing strains.
- The zwitterionic carbapenems exhibit good activity against *P. aeruginosa* and good stability against hydrolysis by DHP-I.

4.1. Chain at Position 6

The stability against hydrolysis by β-lactamases is dependent on the chain at C-6. The presence of a hydroxyl group in the β position provides this stability, in contrast to the α-OH epimer, which is unstable. However, this is not involved in stability against hydrolysis by DHP-I. The introduction of a fluorine atom at position 8 has increased stability against DHP-I,

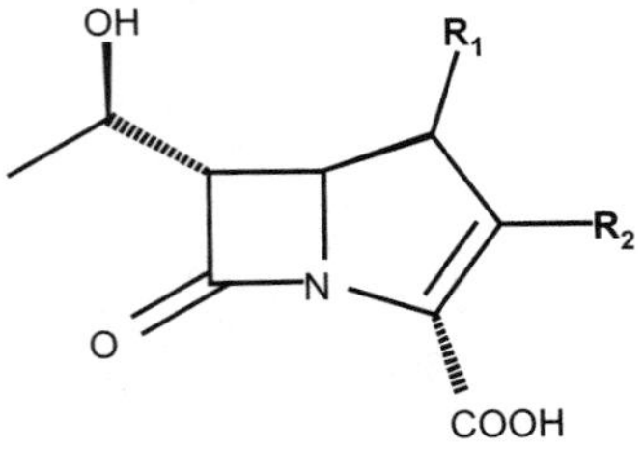

	R_1	R_2
SYN 513	CH_2	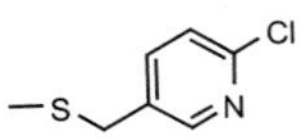
BMY 24 174	CH_2	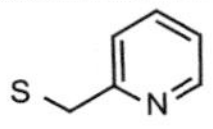
Ro 40-3617	$-CH_2-CH_2-N(H)-C(=NH)-NH_2$	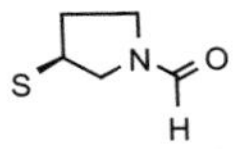
BMS 181189	$-O-CH_2-CH_2-NH_3^+$	$-S-CH_2CH_2CN$
Doripenem	CH-β-CH_3	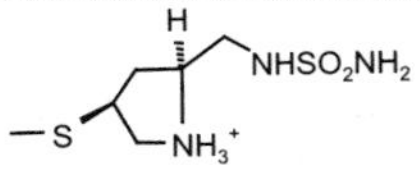
CL 191121	CH-β-CH_3	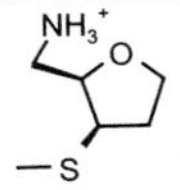
CL 188624	CH-β-CH_3	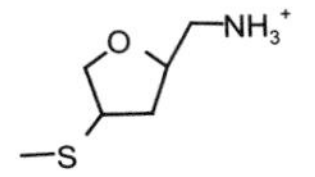
CL 190294	CH-β-CH_3	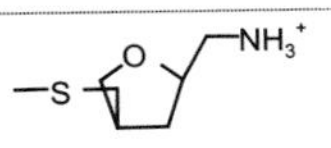
Ertapenem	CH-β-CH_3	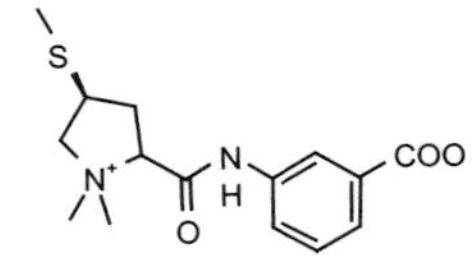

Figure 7 **Series of parenteral carbapenems**

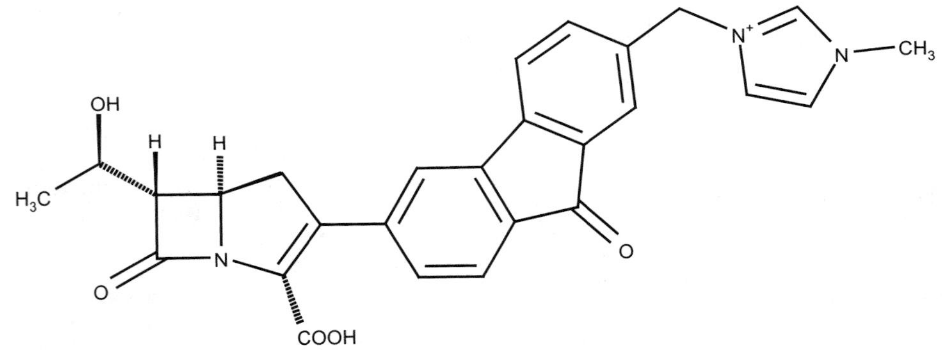

Figure 8 **L-695256**

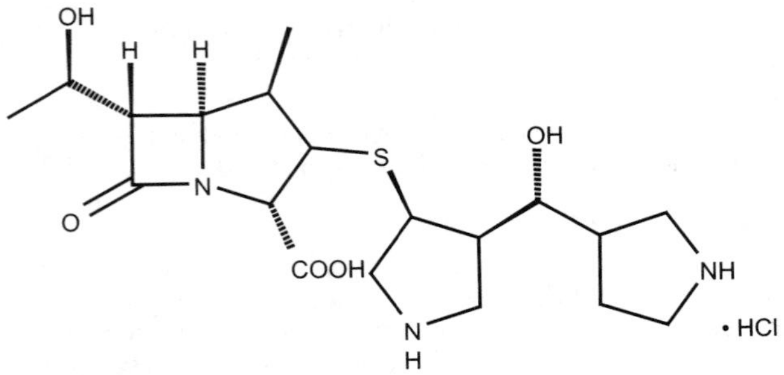

Figure 9 **E-1010 (ER-35786)**

but the antibacterial activity of these derivatives is moderate, and, in particular, they are inactive against *P. aeruginosa*. The fluorine atom must be in the *trans* position (molecule 88-617) (Fig. 15), as it is inactive in the *cis* position. The spatial position of the chain at position 6 is important; thus, if the chain is in the 5,6-*cis* position the derivatives are bacteriologically active, whereas the 5,6-*trans* compounds are inactive (MIC, >128 μg/ml).

The ethyl group of thienamycin and the 7-α-methoxy group of cefoxitin occupy identical spatial positions relative to the lactam carbonyl bond and appear to be responsible for the stability against hydrolysis by β-lactamases for steric reasons. The marked intrinsic activity of the carbapenem

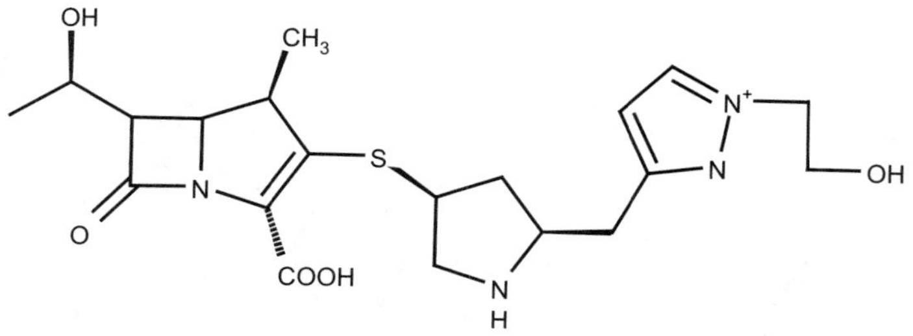

Figure 10 FR-21818

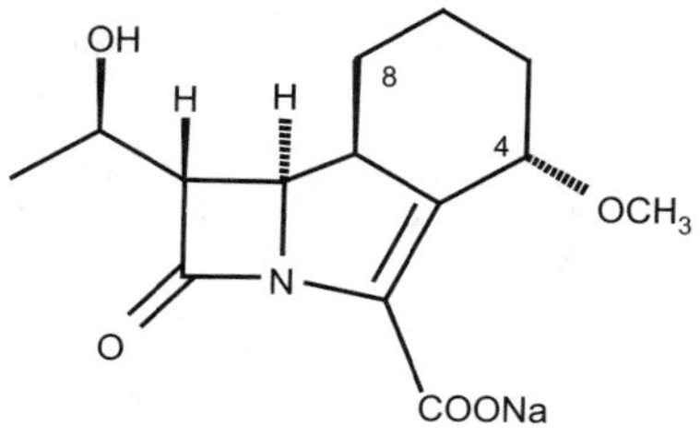

GV 104326

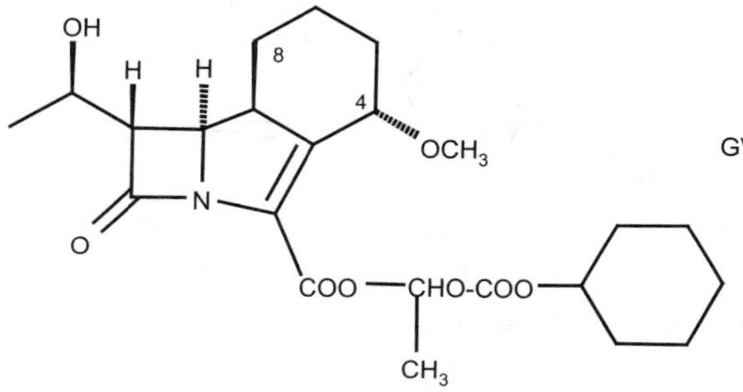

GV 118819 (sanfetrinem cilexetil)

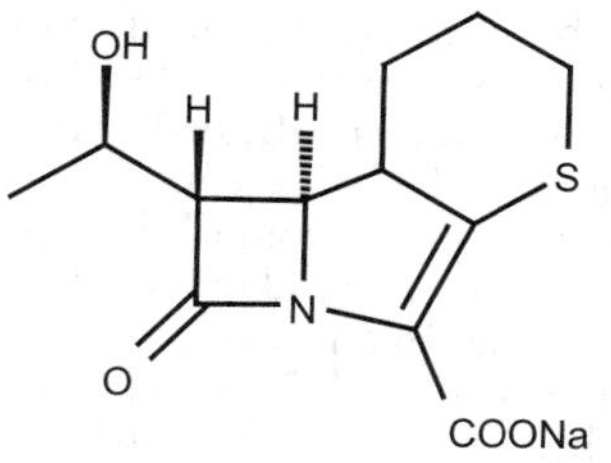

Takeda derivatives

Figure 11 Trinems

Figure 12 GV 129606

nucleus obviates the reduction in antibacterial activity noted with the cephamycins.

The 6-α-hydroxyethyl chain is probably heavily involved in the binding of the molecule at its active site, as shown by the weak activity of the isomer at position 8.

In vitro, the 6-(1-aminoethyl) derivatives are active against gram-negative bacilli but inactive against gram-positive cocci.

It is also possible to increase the stability against hydrolysis by DHP-I by attaching sulfo groups to the 5,6-*cis* carbapenems, but the antibacterial activity of the resultant molecules is weak. The 5,6-*trans* derivatives are more active than the 5,6-*cis* derivatives.

4.2. Chains at Position 2

The chain at position 2 plays an important role in the antibacterial activity but also in the stability against hydrolysis by DHP-I. Hydrophobic or aromatic groups increase the antibacterial activity against gram-positive bacteria; basic groups increase the activity against *P. aeruginosa*.

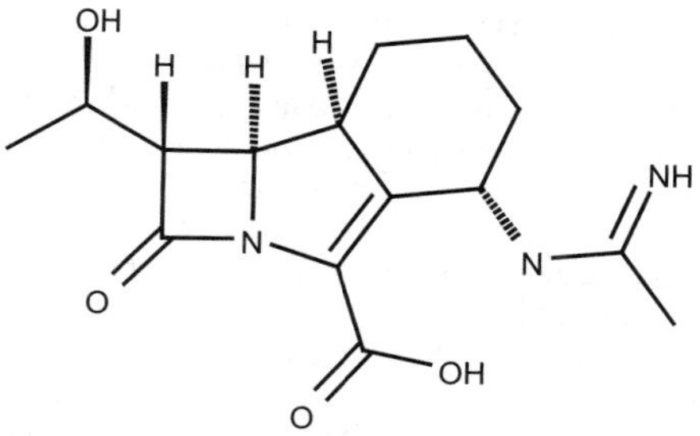

Five molecules undergoing development have a pyrrolidinyl nucleus substituted at position 2. However, the bond

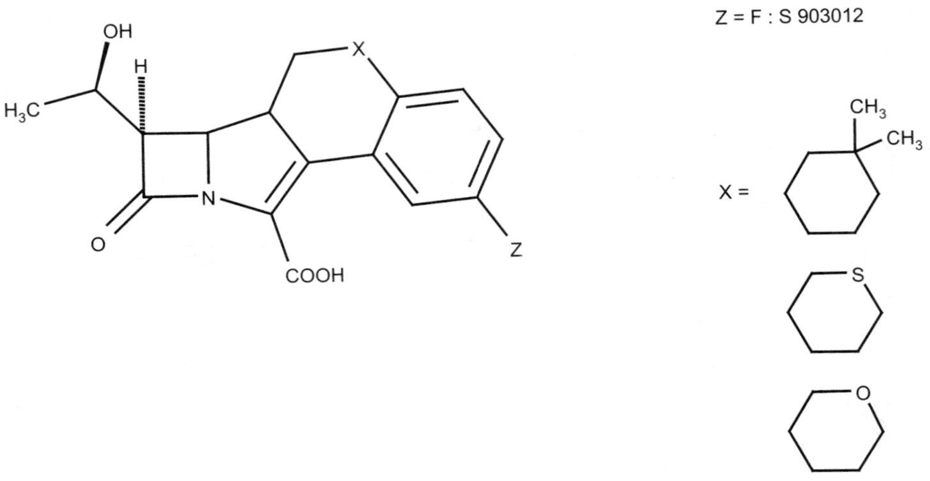

Z = F : S 903012

Figure 13 Tetracyclic carbapenem derivatives

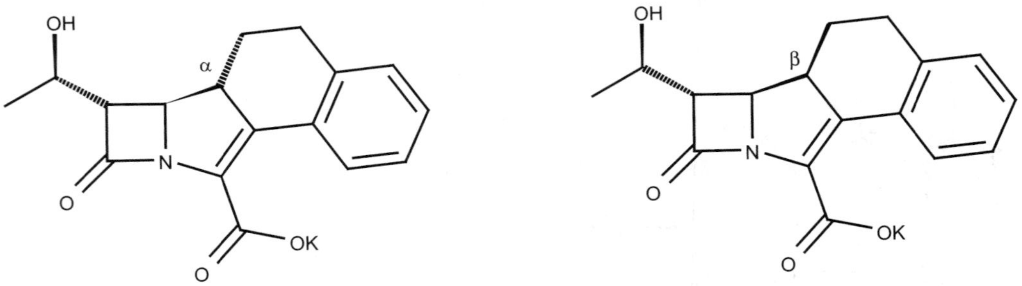

Figure 14 Tetracyclic carbapenems, α and β isomers

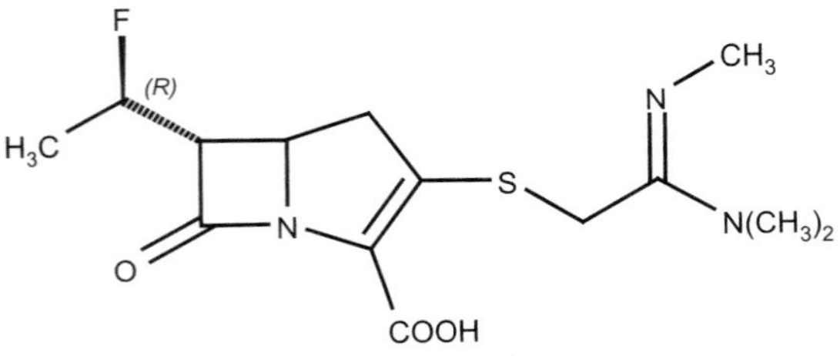

Figure 15 6-Fluorocarbapenem: molecule 88-617 (Mak et al.)

at the thiol residue is important. It has been shown that the two *cis* and *trans* isomers possess similar activities against gram-positive cocci and *Enterobacteriaceae*, but the *cis* isomers are more active against *P. aeruginosa* than the *trans* isomers. The stabilities of the two isomers against hydrolysis by DHP-I are identical. Meropenem is derived from a series of molecules possessing a substituted 5-aminocarbonyl chain attached to the pyrrolidine nucleus. Molecules with substituents at 5′S have the best activity against *P. aeruginosa*.

In the case of DX-8739, the presence of a carboxypiperazine residue increases the antibacterial activity; the presence of a hydroxyl group increases the stability against hydrolysis by DHP-I. The presence of another heterocycle instead of the pyrrolidine nucleus, such as a pyrrole, pyridine, homopiperazine, or azetidine nucleus, reduces the antibacterial activity.

Biapenem has a bicyclic pyrrazolotriazolium nucleus.

Other substituents have been described in patents, such as carbamoylpyrrolidinylthio substituted chains; the substituent of the carbamoyl chain may be a carboxypyridinyl, carboxythiazolyl, carboxyimidazolyl or carboxypyrrolyl (Fig. 16). Derivatives with a 3-amino-1-azetidinylcarboxy-2-pyrrolidinylthio chain have also been described (Fig. 17).

A series of compounds possessing an acetimidoylazetidin-3-4-thiocarbapenem in place of the pyrrolidinyl nucleus have been described by Fujisawa (Fig. 18 and 19).

Shah et al. showed that the presence of a 1-β-methyl group increases the stability against hydrolysis by DHP-I and the chemical stability of the carbapenems. However, the antibacterial activity of the 1-β-methyl derivatives is less good than that of the nonmethylated derivatives. The introduction of an imidine group or a polar heterocycle at C-2 restores this activity against gram-negative bacteria, particularly *P. aeruginosa*.

The methyl group must be in the β position, as the α epimer is less active, less chemically stable, and more strongly hydrolyzed by DHP-I.

A series of carbapenems possessing a 1-β-alkoxy chain has been synthesized by Roche. It has been shown that the size of the substituent at position 1 was less important than the functionality of the chain in terms of antibacterial activity. The increase in the hydrophobicity of the chain at position 1 increases the activity against gram-positive cocci but reduces the activity against gram-negative bacteria. One molecule in this series possesses good antibacterial activity and stability against hydrolysis by DHP-I: Ro-40-3485 (Fig. 20). In this series, the 1-β-alkoxy carbapenems, the presence of an amino group appears to be a prerequisite for good activity against *P. aeruginosa*.

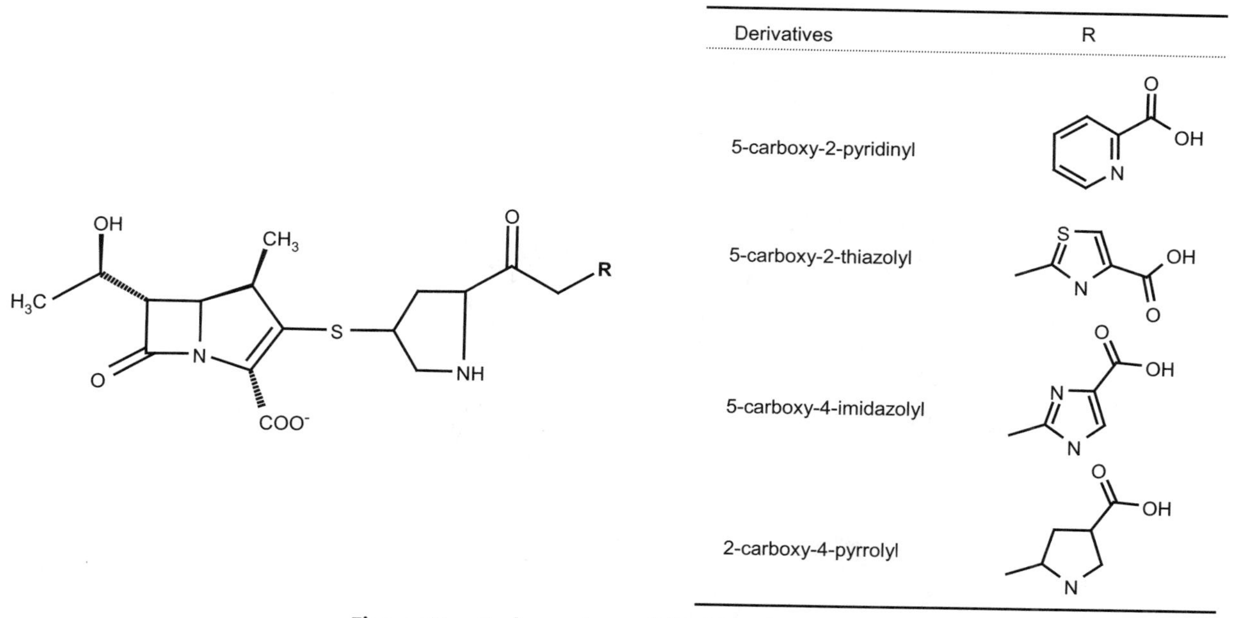

Derivatives	R
5-carboxy-2-pyridinyl	
5-carboxy-2-thiazolyl	
5-carboxy-4-imidazolyl	
2-carboxy-4-pyrrolyl	

Figure 16 Carbamoylpyrrolidinylthio derivatives

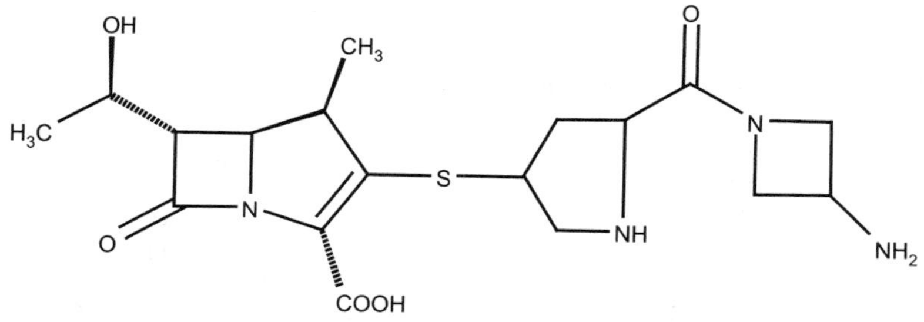

Figure 17 Pyrrolidinyl carbapenem from Sankyo

1-β-Aminoalkyl derivatives have been synthesized. The antibacterial activity is identical when the chain is increased from two to five carbons, and the activity against *P. aeruginosa* is moderately reduced. The introduction of a sulfur atom into the chain or its acylation reduces the activity. Substitution by a guanidine or *N*-formimidoyl group does not modify the antibacterial activity but increases the chemical stability. The presence of an alkyl chain on the amine reduces the antibacterial activity but increases the chemical stability. The 1-β-aminoethyl derivatives are active in vitro but are unstable at high pH, as an intramolecular rearrangement is produced. The attachment of an amino acid or a small peptide prevents this rearrangement. In this series, the chloro-L-alanine derivative (BMY-45465) possesses good in vitro and in vivo activity against *P. aeruginosa* and *Staphylococcus aureus*.

Tricyclic derivatives involving cyclization between positions 1 and 2 have been synthesized. BMY-45301 possesses a heterocycle containing a sulfur; it is weakly active against *P. aeruginosa*. A series of hexacyclic compounds has been synthesized by Takeda.

Penta-, hexa-, hepta-, and octacyclic nuclei have been proposed: one molecule, sanfetrinem (GV 104326), reached the end of phase II and before further development was given up. It possesses a cyclohexyl, the 4′-carbon of which is substituted by an α-methoxy group; the 4′-β-methoxy derivative is less active. The antibacterial activity and stability against hydrolysis by DHP-I are greater when the bond is in the 8-β and not the 8-α position.

Okamoto et al. synthesized three series of carbapenems possessing a 2-thiopyrrolidinyl chain substituted by a hydroxyaminoalkyl group. The first series has an aminoalkyl chain at position 2′ of the pyrrolidine nucleus. The alkyl chains are of variable length and possess a nonsubstituted amino group. The most active molecule is that having an aminopropyl ring. The attachment of an amino group to the 1-hydroxymethyl chain enabled the better antibacterial activity of the aminopropyl derivatives to be demonstrated. The most active molecule is lenapenem. The presence of an amine or a charged group (N^+) significantly reduces the activity against gram-negative bacilli. Likewise, the presence of a 2′-hydroxymethylaminopropyl chain and a methyl substituent at N-1′ or N^+-$(CH_3)_2$ decreases the activity against gram-negative bacilli. Lenapenem is less toxic to mice than the *S*-diastereoisomer.

It was shown that the antipseudomonal activity was enhanced with the introduction of amino groups or quaternized heterocycles to C-2 side chain. The compound containing more basic nitrogen exhibited good antipseudomonal activity. The positive charge in the quaternized heterocyclic

Banyu CH-β-CH_3 1,4 hexa hydrothiazepine

Zeneca CH-β-CH_3

CH-β-CH_3 Carboxythiazolyl

Fujisawa CH-β-CH_3 Azetidinylthio carbapenem

R = Quinolinyl
Quinazolinyl
Isoquinolinyl

Figure 18 Carbamoylpyrrolidinyl carbapenem derivatives

Figure 19 R = methylthio, methoxy, alkyl, carboxyquinoline, quinoxalinyl, quinazolinyl, isoquinolinyl chain at position 1

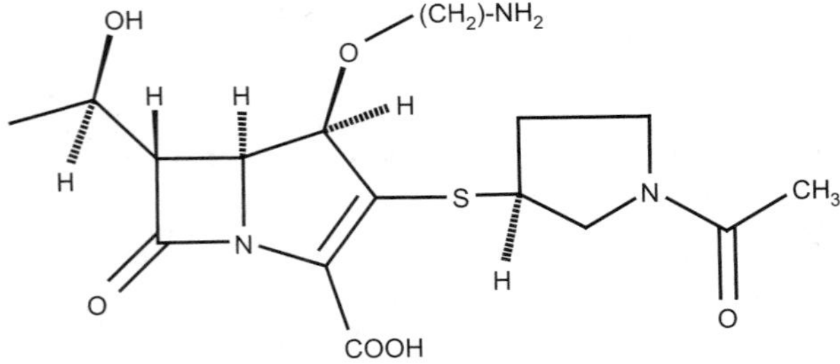

Figure 20 Ro-40-3485

ring imparts a better antipseudomonal activity to these compounds than that of their unquaternized counterparts (Fig. 21).

4.3. β-Lactamase-Inhibitory Activity

The carbapenems with an oxysulfonyl group at position 8 (MM 4550, MM 13902, MM 17880, S_2, S_2M) progressively inhibit β-lactamases. A number of carbapenems have a hydroxyl group, and they inhibit *Escherichia coli* TN 713 or *P. vulgaris* GN 4413 β-lactamases nonprogressively.

E. coli TN 649, *Enterobacter cloacae* TN 1282, and *Serratia marcescens* TN 1281 β-lactamases are progressively inhibited by all carbapenems. The progressive inhibition is irreversible, whereas the nonprogressive inhibition is reversible. C-19393 H_2, PS-5, and clavulanic acid appear to be substrates for the enzymes of *P. vulgaris* GN 4413, which slightly hydrolyzes C-19393 H_2. The inhibitory activity is reversible.

The 5,6-*cis* carbapenems inhibit β-lactamases, even if they are not inhibited by sulbactam or clavulanic acid.

There appears to be a number of structure-activity rules for these products. The presence of a sulfoxide at C-2 increases the inhibitory activity against penicillinases and the cephalosporinase of *P. vulgaris* GN 4413, but it reduces the inhibitory activity against the other cephalosporinases; whether or not the chain at C-2 is saturated, the β-lactamase inhibitory activity of these compounds is unaffected. The carbapenems possessing a single methyl group at position 8 are

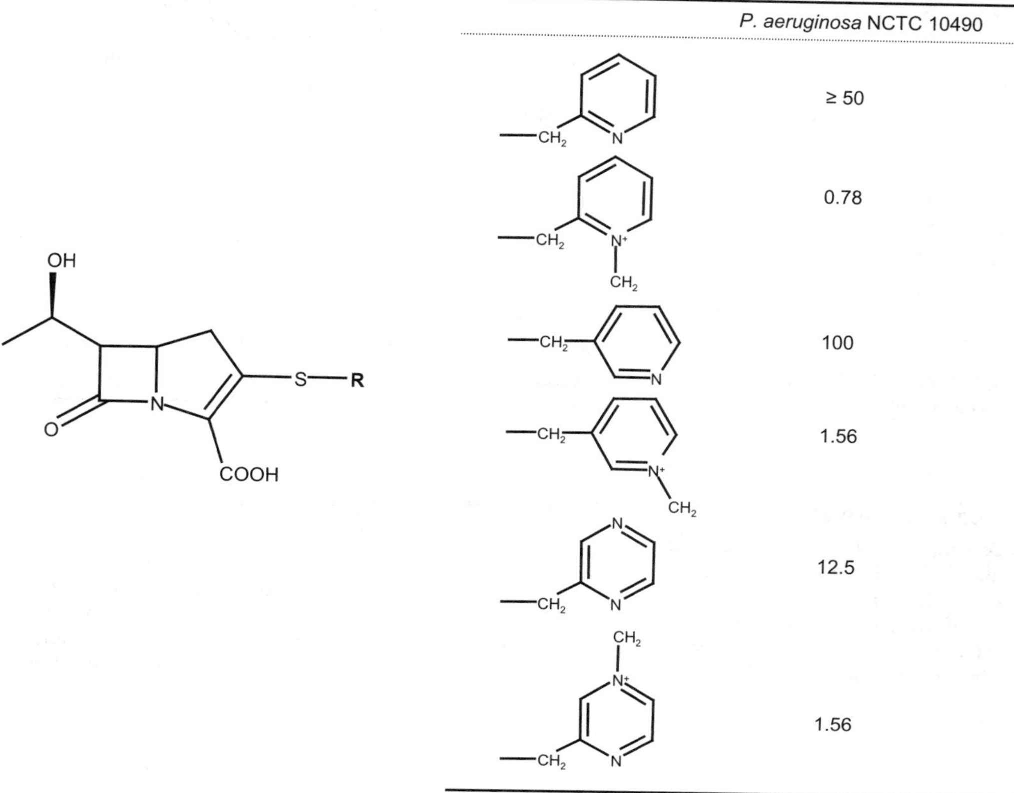

Figure 21 Comparison of unquaternized ring with quaternized ring

more inhibitory than those having two methyl groups in the oxysulfate series.

The chain at position 6 is optically inactive for a certain number of molecules: carpetimycins A and B; NS-5; PS-5, -6, -7, and -8; northienamycin; and the asparenomycins. For the other derivatives, the attachment to the carbapenem nucleus may be in the *cis* or *trans* position (A or B). All of the stereoisomers may be obtained by fermentation, with the exception of the 5,6-*cis*-8*R* diastereoisomer. The 8*S* or 8*R* configuration plays an important role in the profile of the antibiotic. The 5,6-*cis* or -*trans* stereochemistry also affects the antibacterial activity and the stability against hydrolysis by β-lactamases.

Among the 8*S* derivatives, the 5,6-*cis* isomers (MM 22382 and MM 22380) are more active than their *trans* analogs. When the chain is 8*R* (thienamycin and *N*-acetylthienamycin), the activities are similar for the *cis* and *trans* derivatives. The 8*R* and 8*S* derivatives with a 5,6-*trans* attachment at position 6 exhibit strong activity against β-lactamase-producing strains.

The *cis* derivatives have reduced activity because of their instability against hydrolysis by β-lactamases, compared to that of the *trans* isomers.

The good stability of the *trans* isomers against β-lactamases is not surprising, as they have a hindering group (1-hydroxyethyl) on the α side of the carbapenem nucleus, analogous to the α-methoxy substituents of the cephamycins. Thienamycin has the optimal combination (5*R*, 5,6-*trans*, 8*R*).

5. NEW DERIVATIVES

5.1. 2-Biphenyl Carbapenem Derivatives

Di Ninno et al. (1993) showed that derivatives possessing a C-2 quaternary ammonium chain (aminomethylphenyl) have a broad antibacterial spectrum and good stability against hydrolysis by DHP-I. In a new series (1995) they synthesized biphenyl derivatives with the aim of increasing the lipophilia and hence protein binding. They obtained a molecule, the *meta*-biphenyl derivative ($NR_2 = 2'\text{-}NH_2$), which possesses activity similar to that of vancomycin (MIC, ~1 μg/ml) against highly methicillin-resistant strains (MIC, >64 μg/ml).

In another series of carbapenems, the same team also synthesized molecules with some activity against methicillin-resistant *S. aureus* (MRSA) strains (Meurer et al., 1995).

Starting from the preceding series, which possesses a *meta*-biphenyl pharmacophore, they attached a pyridine ring at the 3′-*meta* position of the phenyl nucleus and closed the bridge between the two phenyl nuclei with a heterocyclic nucleus, which yielded a series of molecules. The nitrogen atom was placed in the different positions of the pyridine nucleus, α, β, γ, and δ. Three molecules have good activity against methicillin-resistant strains: the 1,9-dimethyl-α-carbonyl, 2,9-dimethyl-β-carbonyl, and 2-methyl-β-carbonyl carbapenem derivatives (Fig. 22).

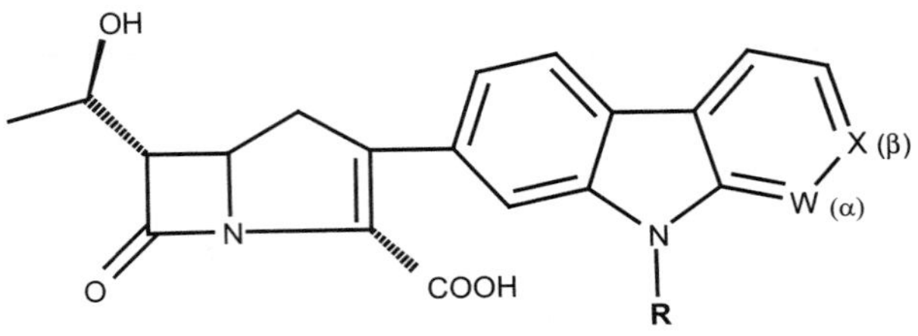

Derivatives	R	W (α)	X (β)
1, 9-dimethyl-a-carbonyl	$-CH_3$	$-N^+-CH_3$	-CH
2, 9 dimethyl-β-carbonyl	$-CH_3$	-CH	$-N^+-CH_3$
2 methyl-β-carbonyl	$-CH_3$	-CH	$-N^+-CH_3$

Figure 22 2-Carbonyl carbapenems

5.2. 2-Hydantoin Carbapenem Derivatives

A series of derivatives possessing a hydantoin chain (Fig. 23) was prepared by Oh et al. (1995). Different heterocycles were attached to this nucleus. All of the molecules obtained possessed good activity against *Streptococcus pneumoniae* and *S. aureus* but moderate activity against *Enterobacteriaceae*, and they were inactive against *P. aeruginosa*.

5.3. Benzothiazolo Carbapenems

See Waddell et al., 1995.

The goal was to obtain a molecule with a good affinity for PBP 2a of MRSA. It was shown that the presence of a benzothiazolyl nucleus attached by a sulfur atom at position 3 of cephalosporins or carbacephems increased the activity against these strains. A thiothiazole nucleus in itself does

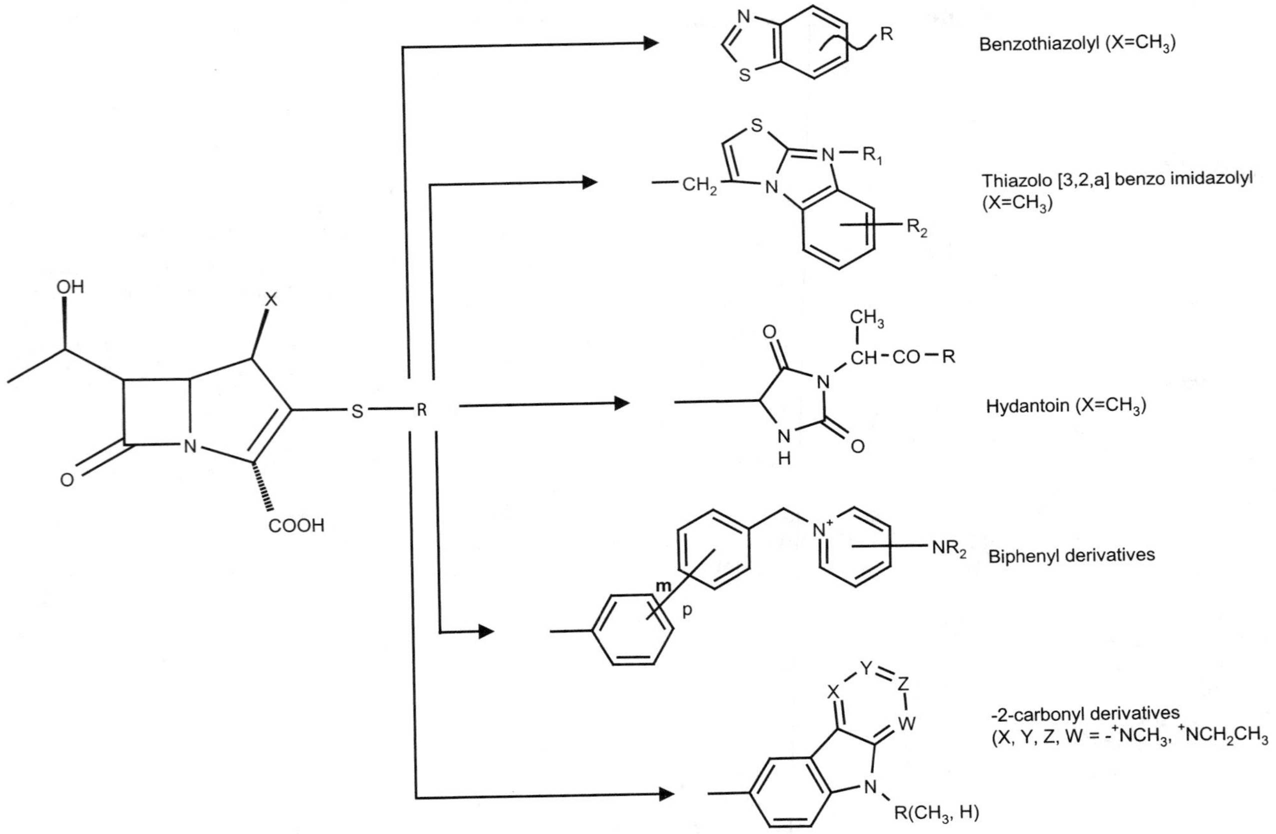

Benzothiazolyl ($X=CH_3$)

Thiazolo [3,2,a] benzo imidazolyl ($X=CH_3$)

Hydantoin ($X=CH_3$)

Biphenyl derivatives

-2-carbonyl derivatives ($X, Y, Z, W = -^+NCH_3, ^+NCH_2CH_3$)

Figure 23 2-Hydantoin carbapenem derivatives

not confer anti-MRSA activity, so it is necessary to have a second ring fused or directly attached at position 4 of the thiazolyl nucleus introduced at position 5. In addition, this second aromatic nucleus must come from a benzene, thiophene, or less active furan nucleus. Replacement of the nitrogen atom in the thiazolyl nucleus by a methylene or the sulfur atom by an oxygen, or by C–N or a C-C double bond, reduces or abolishes the activity compared to that of the benzoimidazole derivative. The electron attractive substituents may be considered to increase the anti-MRSA activity, whereas the electron donor substituents are detrimental to this activity. This activity is correlated with increased affinity for PBP 2a (Fig. 24).

5.4. Thiazolo-[3,2-*a*]-Benzimidazole Carbapenems

Oh et al. (1995) synthesized a series of derivatives with a thiazolo-[3,2-*a*]-benzimidazole chain. The presence of a charged nucleus (quaternary ammonium) slightly increases the activity against *Enterobacteriaceae*. The activity against *P. aeruginosa* is poor.

5.5. Dithiocarbamate Derivatives

A series of 1-β-methyl carbapenems possessing a dithiocarbamate chain has been synthesized with the intention of achieving good activity against MRSA strains.

Several molecules have been selected. One of them in particular has been studied: BO-3482. It is generally less active against gram-positive cocci than imipenem, as well as against *Enterobacteriaceae*. It is inactive against *P. aeruginosa*. It is less hydrolyzed by porcine DHP-I than imipenem, but it exhibits significant epileptogenic potential (Hashizume et al., 1996).

5.6. R-115685 (CS-023)

Within a new series of carbapenems, R-115685 was selected for further investigation. This compound is a 1-β-methyl carbapenem with a complex C-2 side chain: (3*S*, 5*S*)-5[(*S*)-3-[2-3-guanidino)acetylamino]-pyrrolidin-1-ylcarbonyl]-pyrrolidin-3-ylthio group (Fig. 25). R-115685 is a broad-spectrum carbapenem, covering gram-positive and -negative bacteria. Against gram-positive cocci, R-115685 is less than or equally as active as imipenem, with MICs at which 50% of isolates tested were inhibited (MIC_{50}s) ranging from ≤0.03 to 0.12 μg/ml and MIC_{90}s from ≤0.03 to 1.0 μg/ml for *S aureus*, *Staphylococcus epidermidis*, *Staphylococcus haemolyticus*, *Streptococcus pyogenes*, *Streptococcus pneumoniae* with different patterns of resistance to penicillin G, *Streptococcus agalactiae*, *Streptococcus sanguinis*, *Streptococcus oralis*, and *Streptococcus mitis*. It is poorly active against MRSA ($MIC_{50/90}$, 4.0/8.0 μg/ml) and *S. epidermidis* isolates resistant to methicillin. The $MIC_{50/90}$ was 0.5/4.0 μg/ml. For *Enterococcus faecalis* and *Enterococcus faecium*, the MIC_{50}s were 2.0 and >32 μg/ml and the MIC_{90}s were 8.0 and >32 μg/ml, respectively. R-115685 is more active than imipenem against gram-negative bacilli, but its activity is less than or equal to that of meropenem. For *Enterobacteriaceae*, the MIC_{50}s ranged from ≤0.03 to 0.5 μg/ml and the MIC_{90}s ranged from ≤0.03 to 4.0 μg/ml.

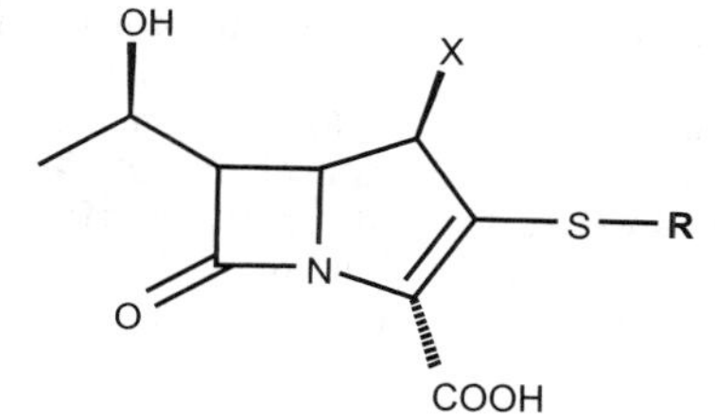

OH X S—R N O COOH

R	MIC (μg/ml) MSSA	MIC (μg/ml) MRSA	IC_{50} (μg/ml) PBP 2a
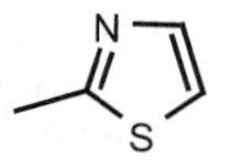 Thiazolyl	0.17	18.2	11.7
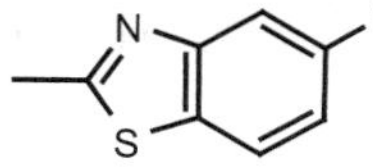 Benzothiazolyl, CF_3 (*)	0.08	1.2	0.9
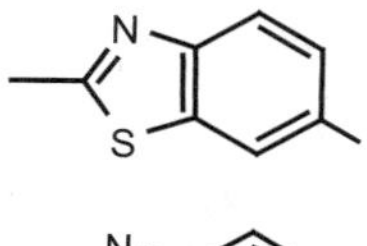 Benzothiazolyl, NO_2 (*)	0.05	1.1	0.6
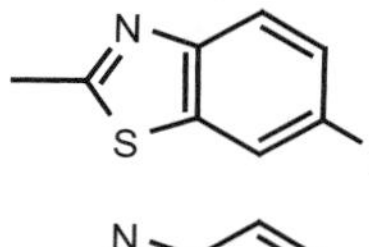 Benzothiazolyl, NH_2 (**)	0.09	9.0	16.8
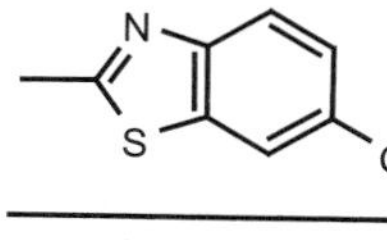 Benzothiazolyl, OC_2H_5 (**)	0.10	4.0	4.7

(*) Electroattractive substituent (**) Electrodonor substituent

Figure 24 Benzothiazolylthio carbapenems

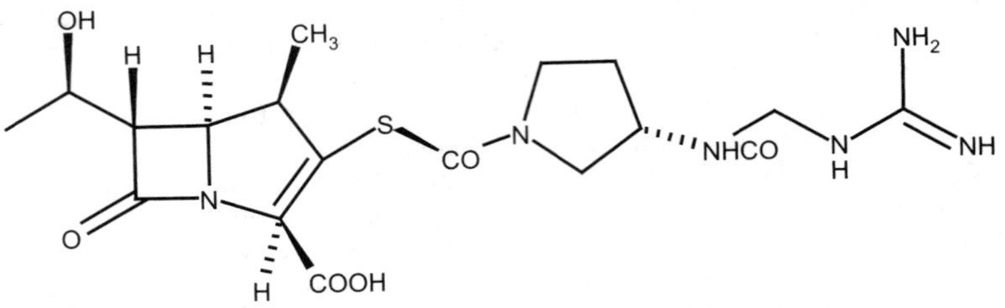

Figure 25 R-115685

R-115685 is as active as meropenem against *P. aeruginosa* ($MIC_{50/90}$, 0.5/4.0 μg/ml), but it is inactive against *Burkholderia cepacia* (MIC_{50}, 32 μg/ml) and *Stenotrophomonas (Xanthomonas) maltophilia* (MIC_{50}, >32 μg/ml). Against *Moraxella catarrhalis* and *Haemophilus influenzae*, R-115685 exhibits good in vitro activity, with MIC_{50}s from ≤0.03 to 0.12 μg/ml and MIC_{90}s from ≤0.03 to 0.25 μg/ml.

R-115685 also displays good activity against anaerobes, comparable to that of imipenem and meropenem against *Bacteroides fragilis* ($MIC_{50/90}$, 0.12/0.5 μg/ml), *Peptostreptococcus* species (MIC_{50}s, ≤0.03 to 0.12 μg/ml; MIC_{90}s, ≤0.03 to 2.0 μg/ml), and *Propionibacterium acnes* ($MIC_{50/90}$, ≤0.03/0.12 μg/ml). R-115685 displays bactericidal activity against *S. pneumoniae* 10 689 after 4 h of contact, but a reduction of about 2.5 $\log_{10}$ CFU/ml was recorded after 4 h of contact with *P. aeruginosa* 10 632. It is impossible to draw any conclusion with such a short time of contact. Like imipenem and meropenem, R-115685 is stable against β-lactamase hydrolysis, including extended-broad-spectrum β-lactamases. It is hydrolyzed by metallo-β-lactamases.

In murine disseminated infections (ddY mice, 4 weeks old) induced by the intraperitoneal route and with treatment administered subcutaneously immediately and 4 h after bacterial challenge, R-115685 was very efficient in gram-positive coccus infection, but less than imipenem and more than meropenem. The 50% effective doses (ED_{50}) were 0.974, 2.63, 7.93, 0.764, 0.122, and 0.552 mg/kg of body weight for *S. aureus* Smith, *S. aureus* 560 (MRSA), *S. aureus* 507 (MRSA; imipenem MIC, >32 μg/ml), *S. epidermidis*, *S. pneumoniae* 2132 (Pen^s), and *S. pneumoniae* 9605 (Pen^r; MIC, 4 μg/ml), respectively. Against gram-negative bacilli, especially *Enterobacteriaceae*, R-115685 is more efficient than imipenem and meropenem, with ED_{50} from 0.308 to 1.12 mg/kg, except for *Enterobacter aerogenes* 100 (ED_{50}, 6.54 mg/kg) and *Proteus mirabilis* 12621 (ED_{50}, 38.7 mg/kg). It is as active as imipenem-cilastatin against *P. aeruginosa* 1008 (ED_{50}, 0.951 mg/kg). After a dose of 20 mg/kg administered subcutaneously to ddY mice, the apparent elimination half-life was 0.19 h, comparable to those of imipenem-cilastatin (0.19 h) and meropenem (0.15 h). In monkeys, after an intravenous dose of 10 mg/kg, the apparent elimination half-lives were 83.4 and 30.9 min for R-115685 and meropenem, respectively. In rabbits, dogs, and rats, the apparent elimination half-lives after 10 mg/kg given intravenously were 42.0, 49.6, and 9.6 min respectively. The recoveries in urine from rats and dogs were 29.6% ± 8.6% and 45.2% ± 4.0% (means ± standard deviations) for the parent compound, respectively, and 31.2% ± 4.8% and 13.1% ± 4.0% for the degradation product obtained by hydrolysis of the β-lactam bound, respectively. With rats, after single and multiple doses of R-115685 of up to 1,000 and 2,000 mg/kg, no animal died. The minimal lethal dose for monkeys is above 800 mg/kg. In male Japanese White rabbits, after a single 200-mg/kg intravenous dose, no degeneration or tubular necrosis was recorded. In Wistar rats (12 weeks old), after a single dose of up to 50 μg/head administered intraventricularly, no electroencephalogram abnormalities were recorded. At 100 μg/head, sharp waves were seen for one out of five animals. At 10 μg/head, seizures occurred with imipenem (two out of five animals), and they occurred for all animals at a dose of 20 μg/head. The hydrolysis rates with DHP-I in human renal microsomes were 0.108 ± 0.023, 0.130 ± 0.189, and 0.931 ± 0.636 nmol/min/mg of protein for R-115685, meropenem, and imipenem, respectively. R-115685 seems to be well tolerated.

5.7. J-114,870

J-114,870 is a 1-β-methyl carbapenem with a C-2 thiopyrrolidinyl-substituted moiety (Fig. 26) which was selected within a series of carbapenem derivatives produced from J-111,347. Using a small inoculum size (10^5 CFU/ml), MIC determinations were done in Mueller-Hinton broth against MRSA. The $MIC_{50/90}$ was 2.0/4.0 μg/ml. Against *P. aeruginosa*, J-114,870 is less active than meropenem, with a $MIC_{50/90}$ of 2.0/4.0 μg/ml.

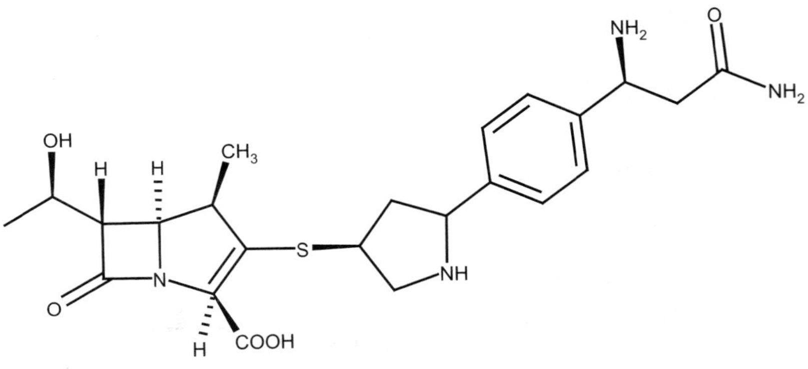

Figure 26 J-114,870

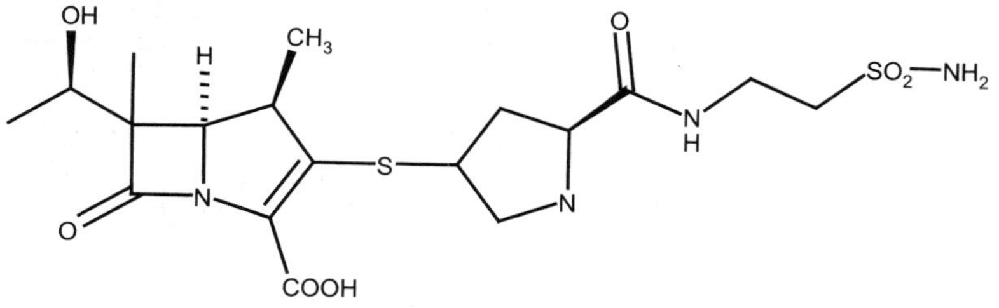

Figure 27 IH-201

In murine (ICR mice) disseminated infections induced by intraperitoneal challenge, treatments started 1 h (one dose) or 1 and 3 h (two doses) postinfection.

After a single dose, the ED_{50} were 0.12 and 6.7 mg/kg for *S. pneumoniae* BB 6230 (Pen[r]) and MRSA BB 6221, respectively. Against MRSA, vancomycin was more effective (ED_{50}, 2.0 mg/kg). After two doses, the ED_{50} of J-114,870 were 3.71 and 2.57 mg/kg against MRSA BB 6221 and MRSA BB 6310, and J-114,870 was more effective than vancomycin, for which the ED_{50} were 4.64 and 3.12 mg/kg, respectively.

5.8. IH-201

IH-201 is a C-2 pyrrolidinyl-substituted 1-β-methyl carbapenem (Fig. 27). IH-201 is less active than meropenem against *Enterobacteriaceae* and gram-positive cocci. The affinities (50% inhibitory concentrations [IC_{50}]) of IH-201, imipenem, meropenem, and cefazolin for [^3H]muscimol binding in cerebral cortical membranes from male Sprague-Dawley rats (5 μM muscimol) were 31.4, 0.9, 27.6, and 1.7 mM, respectively. In mice, after a dose of 40 mg/kg administered subcutaneously, the peak concentration in plasma was 16.0 ± 0.96 μg/ml, with an area under the curve of 11.89 ± 1.13 μg·h/ml and an apparent elimination half-life of 0.32 ± 0.04 h. For meropenem, the peak concentration in plasma was 7.6 ± 0.55 μg/ml, with an area under the curve of 3.29 ± 0.29 μg·h/ml and an apparent elimination half-life of 0.24 ± 0.02 h. The 50% protective doses (PD_{50}) were 2.31, 0.47, and 2.6 mg/kg in murine disseminated infections due to *S. pyogenes* 77A, *E. coli* 078, and *P. aeruginosa* 1771M, respectively.

5.9. CP-5068

CP-6679, a cephalosporin derivative, bears at C-3 position an imidazolo-[5,1-*b*]-thiazolium-6-yl methyl group (Fig. 28). The imidazolium thiazolyl ring was applied to a carbapenem derivative, yielding a lead compound, CP-0697. Chemical alteration of the C-3 moiety side chain yielded CP-5068 (Fig. 28). The rates of human DHP-I hydrolysis relative to that of imipenem (1.0) were 0.06, 0.19, and 0.89 for CP-5068, meropenem, and panipenem, respectively. The IC_{50} were 1.34, 14.61, 0.40, and 1.23 mM for γ-aminobutyric acid A ($GABA_A$) receptor binding for CP-5068, meropenem, imipenem, and panipenem, respectively. At 1,000 mg/kg no proximal tubular necrosis was shown with CP-5068. CP-5068 MIC_{50} and MIC_{90} were 2.0 and 4.0 μg/ml (range, ≤0.063 to 8.0 μg/ml) for 100 MRSA strains. The bactericidal activity against MRSA is strain dependent at four times the MIC. An IC_{50} of 1.7 μg/ml for PBP 2a of *S. aureus* (methicillin resistant)

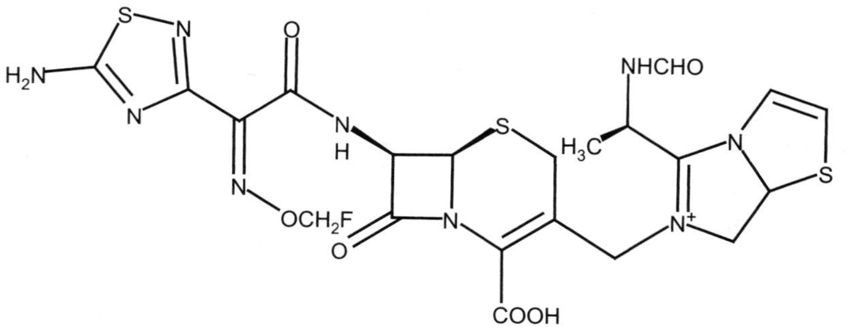

CP-6679 (ME-1209)

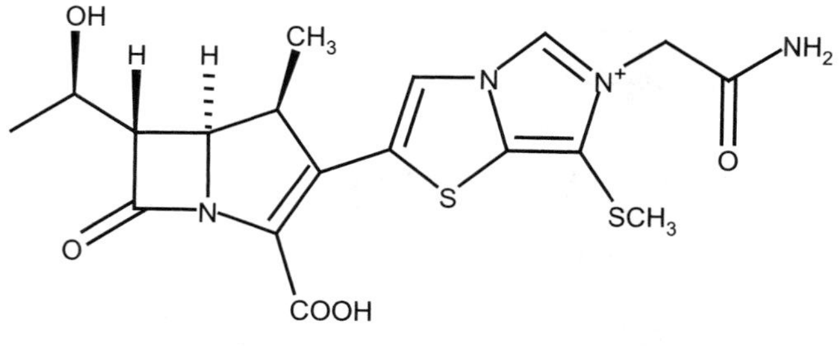

CP-5068

Figure 28 CP-6679 and CP-5068

was noted. No resistant subpopulation was obtained for a concentration of ≥8.0 μg/ml of CP-5068, and the MRSA isolates did not acquire resistance to CP-5608. In disseminated murine staphylococcal infection induced in neutropenic mice (ICR; cyclophosphamide) by intraperitoneal challenge, with treatment started 2 and 4 h after infections, the PD_{50} ranged from 0.087 to 0.10 mg/mouse/day, in comparison with 0.18 to 0.52 mg/mouse/day for vancomycin. For *S. pneumoniae* isolates, the MICs ranged from 0.005 to 0.03 μg/ml. There is no correlation between MIC and alteration of PBP 1a, 2b, or 2x, except for a MIC of 0.03 μg/ml for which all of the isolates exhibited an alteration of the three penicillin-binding proteins (PBPs).

CP-5068 was 16, 32, 4, 16, and 64 times more active than imipenem, meropenem, panipenem, vancomycin, and levofloxacin, respectively, against *S. pneumoniae* resistant to penicillin G. After 8 h of contact at one, two, and four times the MIC, CP-5068 exhibits bactericidal activity, with a reduction of more than 4 $\log_{10}$ CFU/ml. In murine disseminated (male JCI/ICR; 20 to 23 g) infections induced after intraperitoneal administration of an *S. pneumoniae* isolate resistant to penicillin G, with treatment administered 2 and 4 h after bacterial challenge, the PD_{50} for CP-5068 was 0.018 mg/kg/day. Significant bactericidal activity was obtained in pneumococcal lung infections in male CBA/J mice (14 to 19 g).

5.10. CP-5609

Among 200 imidazolthiazolyl carbapenem analogs, CP-5609 was selected for further investigation (Fig. 29). CP-5609 possesses carbamoylmethyl pyridinium as a substituent of the aryl moiety. CP-5609 exhibits good in vitro activity against MRSA, penicillin-resistant *S. pneumoniae* (PRSP), and BLNAR (Table 2).

CP-5609 displays good in vivo activity against MRSA in mice. It also has a high affinity for PBP 2a (IC_{50}, 0.73 g/ml) and a MIC of 1 μg/ml for an MRSA strain (Table 3).

5.11. Isoxazole Carbapenems

A series of 1-β-methyl carbapenems containing a substituted isoxazolopyrrolidinylthio side chain at C-2 was synthesized. All of them exhibit good antistaphylococcal activity and good in vitro activity against *Enterobacteriaceae* and *P. aeruginosa*. Rates of hydrolysis by partially purified porcine renal DHP-I relative to that for meropenem (rate = 1) ranged from 0.80 to 1.66. Compound 1 with a quaternized isoxazolidine exhibits the best stability against DHP-I, and compound 2 and isoxazoline derivative exhibit the highest antibacterial activity (Fig. 30).

Available carbapenems, such as imipenem, meropenem, biapenem, and panipenem, possess an extended broad antibacterial spectrum. However, none of them exerts anti-MRSA activity, and they have a lack of efficacy against penicillin G-resistant enterococci due to a low affinity for the PBPs of these microorganisms.

5.12. DK-35C

DK-35C (Fig. 31) has been known since 1994. The abilities to inhibit [^{3}H]muscimol (5 nM) binding to ($GABA_A$) receptors were assayed using crude synaptic membranes prepared from

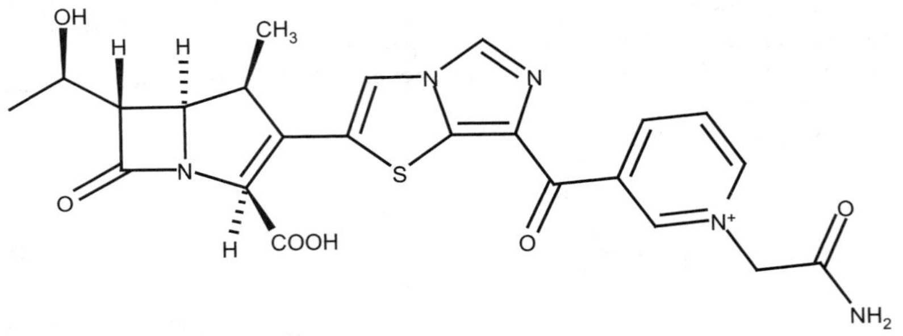

Figure 29 CP-5609

Table 2 In vitro activity of CP-5609

Organism	*n*	MIC$_{90}$ (μg/ml)				
		CP-5609	Vancomycin	Imipenem	Cefotaxime	Levofloxacin
MRSA	100	2	1	64	128	64
PRSP	44	0.031	0.5	0.5	2	1
BLNAR[a]	74	0.25	NT[b]	0.5	1	0.031

[a]NT, not tested.
[b]BLNAR, *H. influenzae*, ampicillin resistant by a nonenzymatic process.

Table 3 Affinity of CP-5609 for PBPs

Compound	MIC (μg/ml) for MSSA	IC$_{50}$ (μg/ml) with PBP					MIC (μg/ml) for MRSA
		1	2	3	4	2a	
CP-5609	0.031	0.01	1.04	0.607	0.047	0.73	1
Imipenem	0.031	0.01	0.76	0.11	0.007	224–229	64

the rat cerebral cortex. The concentrations which inhibit 50% of the specific binding were 0.6, 18, 15.4, and 27.6 mM for imipenem, cefazolin, DK-35C, and meropenem, respectively. After intracerebroventricular injections, the doses which induced convulsions in 50% of rats were 57, 96, 377, and >3,000 nmol/rat for imipenem, cefazolin, DK-35C, and meropenem, respectively. In mice (ICR), pretreatment with 200 to 800 mg of tested β-lactams per kg by intravenous route, followed by intraperitoneal administration of pentylenetetrazole, induced convulsions at 800 mg/kg with cefazolin and 200 mg/kg with imipenem. At 400 mg/kg, no convulsions were recorded with cefazolin, meropenem, or DK-35C. No data have been provided after a dose of 800 mg/kg for DK-35C.

DK-35C possesses a risk of convulsive activities mediated through an interaction with $GABA_A$ receptors.

5.13. C-2 Pyrrolidinylthio Substituted Carbapenems

A new series of 1-β-methyl carbapenems whose C-2 side chains are very close to that of E-1010 has been synthesized. On the C-2 pyrrolidinylthio group, a 3″-, 4″-disubstituted group at 5′ of the pyrrolidine ring was introduced. Among these new analogs (Fig. 32), one compound with unsubstituted diol was the most active compound against gram-positive cocci, except *E. faecium*, and retained good activity against *Enterobacteriaceae* and *P. aeruginosa*. The in vitro activity of this compound ranged between those of imipenem (gram-positive cocci) and meropenem (gram-negative bacilli). It is less stable against porcine DHP-I hydrolysis than meropenem (about 40% reduction of stability) and possesses a pharmacokinetic profile in mice comparable to that of meropenem. The in vivo protective activities in mice are comparable to those of meropenem.

Series of 1-β-methyl carbapenems having at the C-2 position *trans*-3,5-disubstituted 5-aryl pyrrolidinylthio moieties have been synthesized (Fig. 33).

The prototype, J-111,347 (Fig. 33), possesses a benzylamino moiety. It covers gram-positive and gram-negative microorganisms. It was shown that the anti-MRSA and anti-*Pseudomonas* activities were dependent on the stereochemistry on the pyrrolidinyl ring and that the phenyl ring needed to be attached directly to the pyrrolidinyl ring with a *trans* configuration.

J-111,347 was not chosen for further development due to epileptogenic properties, which could be reduced by

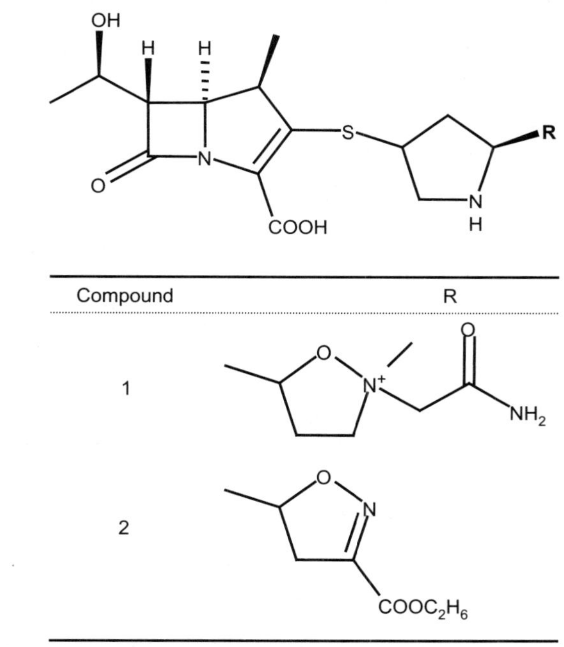

Compound	R
1	
2	$COOC_2H_6$

Figure 30 Isoxazole carbapenems

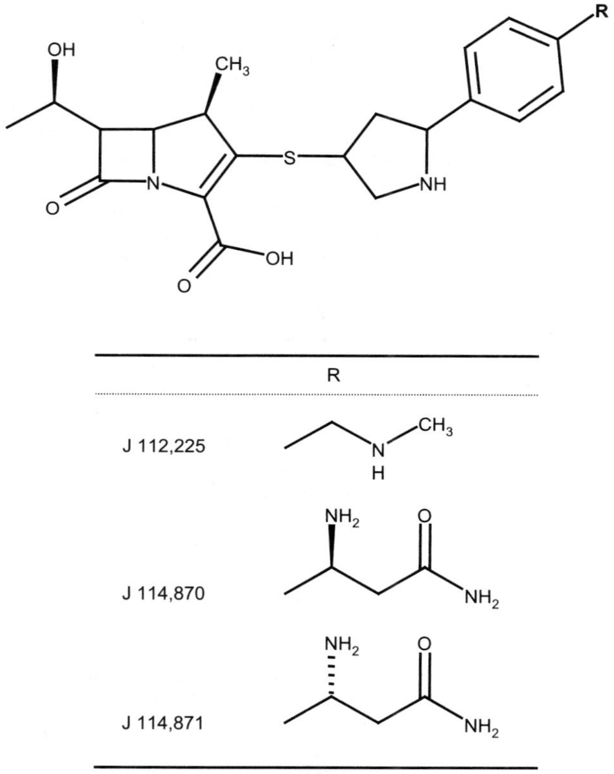

	R
J 112,225	
J 114,870	
J 114,871	

Figure 32 J-111,225 and derivatives

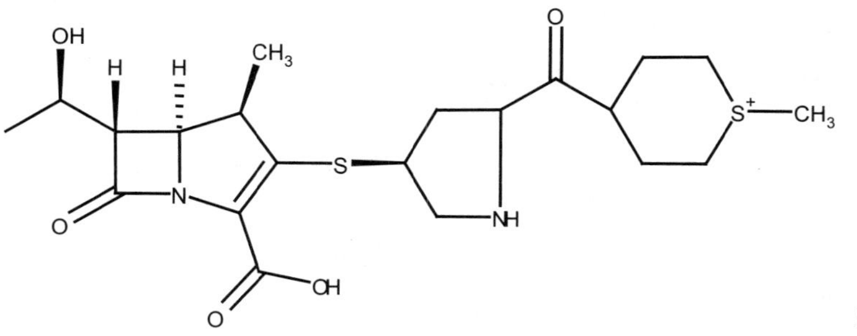

Figure 31 DK-35C

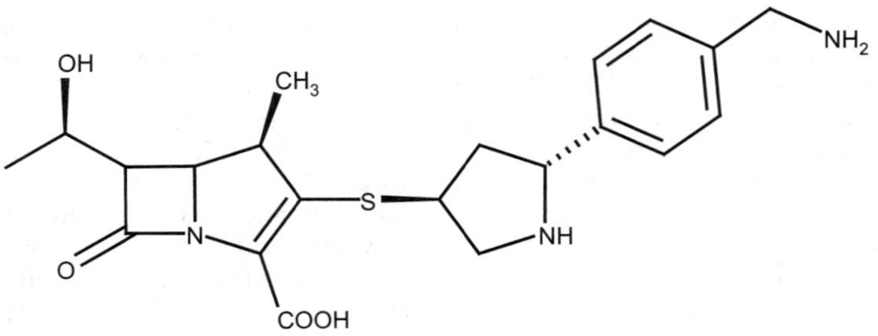

Figure 33 J-111,347

introduction of an α substituent on the benzylamino group or by an *N*-alkyl chain.

Three other compounds have been selected for further investigation: J-111,225, J-114,870, and J-114,871. J-111,225 differs from the prototype analog by an N-methylation of the benzylamino moiety. The stereochemistry is a very important parameter. The *trans* derivative is two to four times more active against gram-positive and gram-negative bacteria than the *cis* analog. Furthermore, the *cis* analog showed epileptogenic properties in mice. This compound is quite stable in solution at pH 5.69 for 8 h at 25°C.

All of these derivatives display good in vitro activity against gram-positive and gram-negative microorganisms.

They are very active against *S. aureus*, *S. pneumoniae*, *S. pyogenes*, and *S. agalactiae*, with MIC_{50}s from ≤0.008 to 0.016 μg/ml. They are poorly active against *E. faecalis* and *E. faecium*, with MIC_{50}s of 2 to 4 μg/ml and above 32 μg/ml. All of them showed good activity against *Enterobacteriaceae*. MIC_{50}s ranged from 0.01 to 0.06 μg/ml, except for *Proteus* species (MIC_{50}, 0.125 to 0.25 μg/ml). In general, they are one to two times less active than meropenem against *Enterobacteriaceae*. They are weakly active against *P. aeruginosa* (MIC_{50}, 2 to 4 μg/ml) compared to meropenem (MIC_{50}, 1 μg/ml). They are also weakly active against *B. cepacia* (MIC_{50}, 8 μg/ml). They showed good activity against *B. fragilis* (MIC_{50}, 0.25 μg/ml) and are weakly active against *Clostridium difficile* (MIC_{50}, 1 to 2 μg/ml).

In vivo, after a single dose in normal mice 1 h after bacterial challenge, the three compounds displayed good activity against methicillin-susceptible *S. aureus* (MSSA) strain Smith, with an ED_{50} from 0.04 to 0.08 mg/kg, compared to 0.5 mg/kg for vancomycin.

The in vivo efficacy against MRSA BB 6221 is less pronounced in normal mice and in immunosuppressed mice (two doses, 1 and 3 h after bacterial challenge). In normal mice, the ED_{50} were 5.26 to 5.42 mg/kg for carbapenems and 2.56 mg/kg for vancomycin. In immunosuppressed mice, the ED_{50} were comparable to that of vancomycin (7.75 to 8.53 mg/kg, versus 8.83 mg/kg for vancomycin) except for J-114,871 (ED_{50}, 5.99 mg/kg). J-111,225 showed a better activity in a disseminated pneumococcal murine infection (ED_{50}, 0.29 mg/kg) than penicillin G (MIC, 2 μg/ml; ED_{50}, 4.36 mg/kg) but less than imipenem (MIC, 0.5 μg/ml; ED_{50}, 0.16 mg/kg). Against *E. coli*, *Klebsiella pneumoniae*, and *P. aeruginosa*, J-111,225 is less active than meropenem.

For MRSA, MIC_{50}s were 2.0 μg/ml; however the methodology to determine MICs was not clearly defined, which is also the case for MICs of methicillin and the type of MRSA strain (homogeneous or heterogeneous). It seems that these analogs showed bactericidal activity at four times the MIC (J-111,225 and J-111,347), with a reduction of 3 $\log_{10}$ CFU/ml at 6 h, or at the MIC (J-114,870 and J-114,871) after 2 h of contact.

The affinity for PBP 2a is high compared to that of imipenem. The IC_{50} (^{14}C benzylpenicillin) were 2.6 and 2.5 μg/ml for J-111,347 and J-111,225, respectively.

For J-110,441, the relative hydrolysis rate with IMP-1 of *P. aeruginosa* is very low (1 to 8%).

A potentiation of activity has been obtained with J-110,441 in combination with imipenem against *S. marcescens* (IMP-1), *P. aeruginosa* (IMP-1), *S. maltophilia* (L-1), and *B. fragilis* (CcrA).

The relative rate of hydrolysis of imipenem by DHP-I is comparable to that of meropenem in humans, but the rates of hydrolysis of J-111,225, J-114,870, and J-114,871 are almost 3, 4, and 2.5 times the imipenem rate, respectively, in rhesus monkeys. In rhesus monkeys, the urinary recovery is higher when J-111,225 is administered with cilastatin (65%) than when given alone (10 mg/kg intravenously) (~14%). The same figures apply for J-114,870 (73.9 versus 9.5%) and J-114,871 (59.3 versus 21.1%). The protein binding in humans ranges from 21.5% (J-111,871) to 38.8% (J-111,225). The apparent elimination half-lives are around 1 h, like for imipenem-cilastatin.

No nephrotoxicity has been found in rabbits. Repeated doses of 50 mg/kg daily for 29 days have been well tolerated in monkeys.

5.14. DA-1131

DA-1131 is a C-2 pyrrolidinyl substituted 1-β-methyl carbapenem. The side chain replacing this ring is 3-methanesulfonylamino-1-propenyl (Fig. 34).

DA-1131 is more stable than imipenem and meropenem against DHP-I in animals and humans (Table 4).

5.15. Carbapenems with Anti-MRSA Activity

Intensive research on new carbapenem derivatives exhibiting anti-MRSA activity is currently ongoing.

In the field of carbapenems, few compounds have been claimed to be effective against MRSA by having a high affinity for PBP 2a. Among these are, L-695256, SM-17466 and derivatives, BO-3483, BO-3411, BO-3482, and L-786392.

Among a series of 2-naphthylcarbapenem analogs having an appropriate positioning of a cationic moiety, one compound had been found to have enhanced activity against MRSA (MIC range, 0.25 to 8 μg/ml) and retained some activity against *Enterobacteriaceae* but not against *P. aeruginosa*.

Merck researchers have synthesized previous carbapenems with anti-MRSA activity. Two series of compounds have yielded 1-aryl derivatives, L-695256 and L-742728, and a 2-benzothiazolylthio analog, L-763863. The side chains of these derivatives have been replaced by cationic groups. The lipophilic core of the side chain provided for binding to PBP 2a of MRSA, whereas the cationic substituent attenuates serum protein binding and improves the pharmacokinetics.

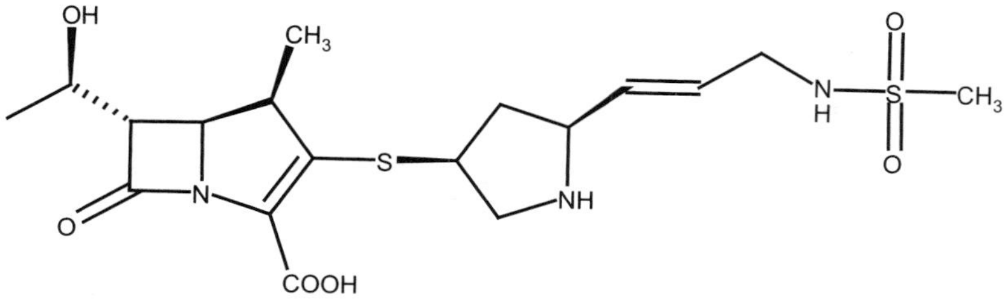

Figure 34 DA-1131

Table 4 Interactions of DHP-I with DA-1131 and comparators

Animal	V_{max}/K_m ratio		
	Imipenem	Meropenem	DA-1131
Mouse	13.7	21.1	6.2
Rat	22.5	13.5	6.0
Rabbit	8.2	23.4	5.5
Dog	39	16.5	12.6
Pig	19.8	0.95	0.74
Human	6.2	2.41	1.39

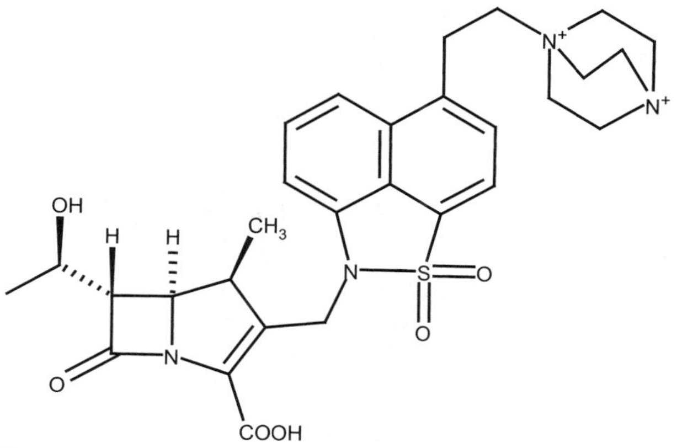

Due to an immune toxicity in rhesus monkeys, all of these compounds have not been developed. The immunotoxicity was believed to result from nonspecific acylation of the cell surface lysine residue by these compounds, followed by recognition and response to the appended hapten. It was hypothesized that the main component of the hapten was the lipophilic residue of these compounds. To avoid the release of the anti-MRSA pharmacophore during the opening of the β-lactam ring, a series of compounds have been prepared with a more stable link between the pharmacophore and the carbapenem ring. It was shown that a 2-tricyclic sulfamido residue could be a useful analog. L-784113, the unsubstituted (naphthosultamyl) methyl carbapenem was found to possess good anti-MRSA activity. A cationic side chain was fixed on the naphthosultamyl moiety, yielding L-786392 (Fig. 35).

L-786392 is moderately active against *Enterobacteriaceae*, with MIC_{50}s of about 2 μg/ml, and inactive against nonfermentative gram-negative bacilli. It is very active against anaerobic gram-positive bacteria, including *C. difficile* (MIC_{50}, 0.125 μg/ml). It is 1 or 2 dilutions (in tube tests) less active than imipenem against *S. pyogenes* (MIC_{50}, 0.016 μg/ml) and *S. pneumoniae*.

L-786392 displays moderate in vitro activity against *E. faecalis* (MIC_{50}, 2 μg/ml) and *E. faecium* (MIC_{50}, 4 μg/ml). It is more active against *Enterococcus gallinarum* (MIC_{50}, ≤0.03 μg/ml). However, irrespective of the profile of resistance to vancomycin, L-786392 showed bactericidal activity against *E. faecalis* CL 5244 (Van^r isolate), but it seems only bacteriostatic against *E. faecium* CL 5272. The antistaphylococcal activity has been tested by the microdilution method in Mueller-Hinton medium supplemented with 2% NaCl at 35°C for 20 h (MSSA) or 22 to 46 h (MRSA). The inoculum size was 10^7 to 10^8 CFU/ml. For a set of MRSA clinical isolates, the $MIC_{50/90}$ of L-786392 was 2/4 μg/ml (MIC of methicillin, >512 μg/ml). Against coagulase-negative staphylococci resistant to methicillin, the $MIC_{50/90}$ was 2/4 μg/ml.

Against MSSA and methicillin-susceptible coagulase-negative staphylococci, the $MIC_{50/90}$s were 0.03/0.03 and 0.008/0.015 μg/ml, respectively.

Figure 35 L-786392

The affinities of L-786392 for PBP 2a of *S. aureus* COL and PBP 5 of *E. hirae* ATCC 9790 were determined; the IC_{50} were 1.7 and 0.2 μg/ml, respectively.

Immunosuppressed outbred CD-1 mice (cyclophosphamide) were challenged with a VanA-resistant *E. faecium* CL 5053 in a localized thigh model. The MIC of L-786392 was 8 μg/ml. At 20 mg/kg, a 2.3-$\log_{10}$ CFU/ml reduction was obtained after multiple doses over a 5-day period.

In staphylococcal murine systemic infections, the ED_{50} were 0.02 and 3.90 mg/kg against MSSA (strain MB 2985) and MRSA (7-6 virginale), respectively. In thigh infections at 40, 20, 10, and 5 mg/kg, the reductions of MRSA by L-786392 were 4.78, 5.57, 5.17, and 2.9 $\log_{10}$ CFU/ml, respectively. At low doses, the reductions were 2.9, 1.4, and 0.5 $\log_{10}$ CFU/ml, at 5, 2.5, and 1.25 mg/kg, respectively. After intranasal infection of mice with a penicillin G-resistant *S. pneumoniae* strain, L-786392 sterilized mouse lung tissue at doses of 50 and 5 mg/kg when administered 1 and 4 h after bacterial challenge.

As for all β-lactams, the pharmacodynamic parameter for efficacy of L-786392 is time above the MIC.

In the carbapenem class, it was shown that the pharmacokinetic behavior in chimpanzees could predict human pharmacokinetics, as has been demonstrated with ertapenem.

The intravenous pharmacokinetics of L-786392 have been evaluated after a 10-mg/kg dose in chimpanzees compared to imipenem with and without cilastatin. Both compounds were assayed by a high-performance liquid chromatography (HPLC) method. The apparent elimination half-lives in chimpanzees were 1.79, 2.46, and 0.94 h, and the urinary eliminations were 8, 56, and 13% for L-786392 alone, for L-786392 with addition of cilastatin, and for imipenem-cilastatin, respectively. Protein binding levels were 75 and 65% for chimpanzees and humans, respectively.

The preliminary toxicological tests, including a 4-week tolerability test in rhesus macaques, did not detect any abnormalities. No histological nephrotoxicity in rabbits with up to 225 mg/kg, as well as no convulsive effects after a dose above 200 μg intracisternally in rats, was found; these effects were found at a dose of 20 μg for imipenem. No immunogenicity, which is due in previous series to the release of the side chain, have been identified in rhesus monkeys.

5.16. J-111,225

J-111,225 is not active against *S. marcescens* or *P. aeruginosa* harboring an IMP-1 enzyme or against *S. maltophilia* (L-1) or *B. fragilis* (CcrA). However, the hydrolysis rate relative to that of imipenem is low for IMP-1 of *P. aeruginosa* but not for the three other species. Another derivative, J-110,441 (Fig. 33), is a good inhibitor of class C enzyme of *E. cloacae* and of TEM-1. However, no data have been presented concerning extended-broad-spectrum β-lactamases.

Previous data have been published on the in vitro and in vivo activities of J-111,225, but no data have been reported concerning the correlation between the chemical structure and anti-MRSA activities and epileptogenicity due to the C-5 stereochemistry of the side chain. J-111,225 is characterized by an unusual C-5 stereochemistry of the side chain in comparison with known carbapenems having a *cis*-substituted 3-pyrrolidinylthio side chain, such as meropenem. The four diastereoisomer analogs of J-111,225 were synthesized to investigate their in vitro activities and epileptogenicities.

In terms of the C-3 configuration, the (3-*S*) isomers were significantly more active than the corresponding (3-*R*) isomers. Of the two (3-*S*) isomers, the *trans*-(5-*R*) isomer was four times more active than the corresponding *cis*-(5-*S*) isomers against MRSA and *P. aeruginosa*. In addition, no epileptogenicity was recorded after intracerebroventricular injection (200 μg/rat head) of the 5-*trans* isomer analog, whereas the 5-*cis* isomer analog produced severe adverse effects at the same dose.

5.17. C-2 Thiazolyl Carbapenems

A series of C-2 thiazolylthio derivatives has been synthesized. Three compounds were selected for further investigation: SM-197438, SM-232721, and SM-232724 (Fig. 36). They display moderate in vitro activity against gram-positive cocci, especially against MRSA (Table 5).

SM-216601, having a 4-dihydropyrrolydinyl thiazolyl side chain at position C-2, was selected for further investigation against MRSA (physicochemical properties: pK, 8.54; logP, 0.343). SM-216601 displayed good in vitro ($MIC_{50/90}$, 1.0/2.0 μg/ml) and in vivo (ED_{50}, 2.89 mg/kg) activities against MRSA. The affinity for PBP 2a is high (IC_{50}, 0.99 μg/ml). It displayed poor activity against gram-negative enteric bacilli and it is inactive against *P. aeruginosa* (Ueda et al., 2004).

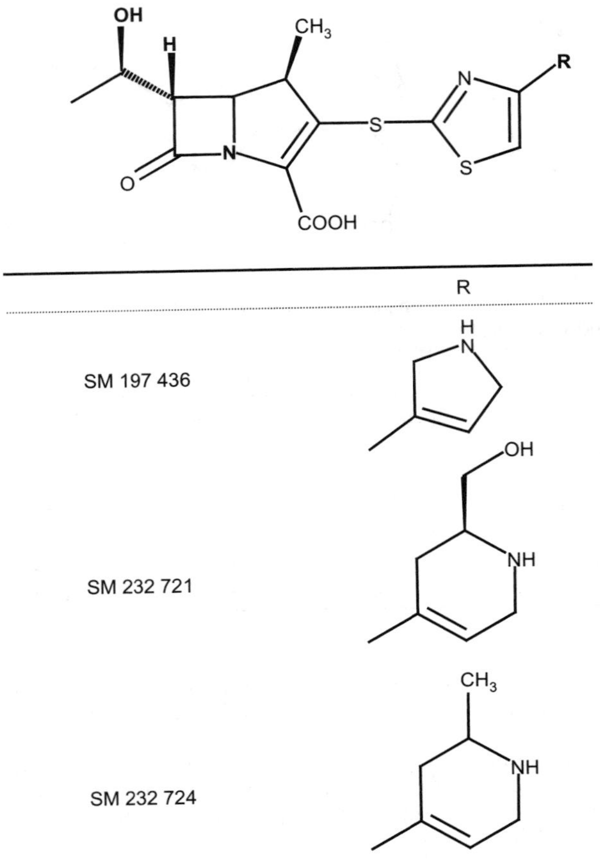

Figure 36 C-2-thiothiazol substituted carbapenems SM-197438, SM-232721, and SM-232724

Table 5 In vitro activities of thiazolylthio carbapenem derivatives

Microorganism[a]	MIC_{50} (μg/ml)		
	SM-197438	SM-232721	SM-232724
MRSA	2	1	1
MRSE	2	2	1
PRSP	0.25	0.125	0.06
E. faecalis	1	1	0.5
E. faecium	0.5	<0.25	<0.25
E. faecium (VRE)	4	2	2
S. pyogenes	≤0.008	≤0.008	≤0.008
S. agalactiae	≤0.008	≤0.008	≤0.008
B. subtilis	≤0.008	≤0.008	≤0.008
L. monocytogenes	≤0.008	0.16	0.016
E. coli	0.25	0.5	0.5
K. pneumoniae	0.031	0.125	0.031

[a]MRSE, methicillin-resistant *S. epidermidis*; VRE, vancomycin-resistant enterococcus.

5.18 C-2 Pyrrolydinyl Isoxazoloethenyl Moiety Carbapenems

A series of 1-β-methyl carbapenems with a substituted pyrrolidinyl moiety at C-2, having an isoxazolothienyl chain at 5′, were synthesized. A derivative, P 91022, was selected for further investigation. This analog is more active than imipenem against gram-positive cocci (one dilution). Against gram-negative enteric bacilli it exhibited in vitro activity similar to meropenem. In murine disseminated infections, whatever the bacteria involved, this compound is more active than meropenem (ED_{50}, 0.05 to 1.12 versus 0.26 to 4.11 mg/kg) (Yoo et al., 2004).

5.19 C-2 Pyrrolydinyl-5′-Substituted Thiourea Cyclic Carbapenems

A series of 1-β-methyl carbapenems having a pyrrolidinyl at C-2 position and substituted at 5′ with a thiourea cyclic side chain were synthesized. Among them one compound was selected for further investigation: IIId (Hawon Pharma nomenclature). This compound is more active than meropenem against gram-positive cocci, but less so than imipenem. It is as active as, or more than, meropenem against gram-negative enteric bacilli, with good activity against *P. aeruginosa* (Han et al., 2004).

Table 6 In vitro activities of carbapenems

Microorganism(s)	MIC$_{50}$ (μg/ml)							
	Imipenem	Meropenem	Panipenem	Biapenem	DX-8739	Lenapenem	Doripenem	BMS-18139
MSSA	0.025	0.25	0.05	0.1	0.2	0.1	0.03	0.32
MRSA	0.78	0.1	0.78	0.39	25	12.5	64	14.54
S. epidermidis Met[s]	0.1	0.2	0.2	0.1		0.05	0.03	0.23
S. epidermidis Met[r]	0.25	4					1	1.28
S. pyogenes	<0.0006	<0.0006	<0.0006	<0.0006		<0.006	0.003	0.02
S. agalactiae	0.012	0.06	<0.006	0.12		<0.006	0.03	0.04
S. pneumoniae	<0.006	<0.006	<0.006	<0.006		0.025	0.008	
PRSP	0.12	0.25					0.12	
E. faecalis	0.78	3.13	0.78	1.56		1.56	4	3.46
E. faecium	>128	>128	128	ND[a]		4	>64	11.95
Enterococcus avium	0.78	1	1	0.25		2		
Enterococcus liquefaciens		8						
L. monocytogenes	0.05	4	0.05	0.05		0.06		
Corynebacterium diphtheriae	0.012		0.025	<0.019				
C. jeikeium	1	0.25		8			>32	
B. anthracis	0.12		<0.06					
B. subtilis ATCC 6633	<0.01		<0.006	0.01				
Erysipelothrix rhusopathiae	<0.02	0.01						
Rhodococcus equi	<0.3	<0.3						
N. asteroides	1							
P. aeruginosa	1.56	0.78	6.25	0.78	0.39	0.39	0.39	
B. cepacia	2	0.5	25	12.5		8		0.95
S. maltophilia	>128	>128	>128	>128		>128	>128	
A. faecalis	0.1	0.06	0.1					
A. baumannii	0.2	0.2	0.1	0.1		0.2	0.25	
C. coli/jejuni	0.07	0.03					0.004	
C. meningosepticum	25		2.5			0.2		
Eikenella corrodens	0.1							
B. bronchiseptica	0.5							
A. hydrophila	0.05	0.01						
Vibrio cholerae	1.56		0.78				0.25	
Helicobacter pylori	0.13	0.06						
A. xylosoxidans	0.78		0.39					
Burkholderia pseudomallei	1							
H. influenzae	1.5–<6	0.05		0.78	ND	0.5	0.25	0.4
M. catarrhalis	0.015	0.008	0.013	0.06		0.01	0.015	0.02
Moraxella spp.	<0.08							
N. gonorrhoeae	0.12	0.008	0.1	0.06			0.015	
N. meningitidis	0.05	0.01			0.06		0.015	
P. multocida	0.5							
Gardnerella vaginalis		0.03						
B. pertussis	0.1		0.2					
M. lacunata	<0.19			<0.19				
H. aegyptius	0.78			0.78				

[a]ND, not determined.

6. IN VITRO ANTIBACTERIAL ACTIVITY

Analysis of the in vitro activity is complex. In fact, due account must be taken of the antibacterial spectrum, which includes gram-positive and gram-negative cocci, gram-positive and gram-negative bacilli, and anaerobic species. The carbapenems have a postantibiotic effect on gram-negative bacilli.

6.1. Gram-Positive Cocci

See Tables 6, 7, and 8.

The carbapenems possess good activity against gram-positive cocci, such as staphylococci, streptococci, and certain species of enterococci. They are inactive against *E. faecium* (MIC$_{50}$, >128 μg/ml) and against MRSA strains and methicillin-resistant *S. epidermidis*. They possess good activity against viridans group streptococci: *S. sanguinis*, *Streptococcus milleri*, *S. mitis*, *Streptococcus salivarius*, and *Streptococcus mutans* (MIC$_{50}$ of imipenem, ~0.01 μg/ml). Likewise, their activity against all coagulase-negative staphylococci is good (MIC$_{50}$, ~0.1 μg/ml) (Table 8).

Imipenem and panipenem are the most active molecules, followed by lenapenem and then meropenem and biapenem.

Table 7 In vitro activities of the new carbapenems CL-188624, CL-190294, and CL-191121

Microorganism(s)[a]	CL-188624	CL-190294	CL-191121	Biapenem	Imipenem	Meropenem	GV 129606
MSSA	0.25	0.12	0.03	0.06	≤0.015	0.12	>8
MRSA	16	8	>16	>16	>16	>16	>8
CoNS Met[r]	>16	16	>16	>16	>16	>16	>8
E. faecalis	2	1	0.5	2	1	4	8
E. faecium	8	8	8	32	8	32	
S. pneumoniae Pen[s]	≤0.015	≤0.015	≤0.015	≤0.015	≤0.015	≤0.015	≤0.015
S. pneumoniae Pen[i]	0.12	0.12	0.12	0.06	0.03	0.12	
PRSP	1	1	0.5	0.5	0.3	0.5	0.25
S. pyogenes	≤0.06	≤0.06	≤0.015	≤0.015	≤0.015	≤0.015	≤0.015
S. agalactiae	0.03	0.06	≤0.015	≤0.015	≤0.015	0.06	
E. coli	0.06	0.06	0.03*	0.06	0.12	0.03	0.03
E. coli CAZ[r]	0.06	0.12	0.03	0.03	0.12	0.03	
K. pneumoniae	0.06	0.12	0.12	0.12	0.12	0.06	0.25
K. pneumoniae CAZ[r]	0.12	0.25	0.12	0.12	0.25	0.06	
Klebsiella oxytoca	0.12	0.12	0.06	0.12	0.25	0.03	0.12
S. marcescens	0.25	0.25	1	1	1	0.12	1
E. cloacae	0.06	0.06	0.06	0.06	1	0.06	0.12
E. aerogenes	0.25	0.25	0.5	0.25	1	0.06	0.25
C. freundii	0.12	0.06	0.06	0.06	1	0.03	0.06
Citrobacter diversus	0.03	0.03	≤0.015	0.03	0.12	≤0.015	0.03
Salmonella spp.	0.06	0.06	0.03	0.03	0.12	0.03	
Shigella spp.	0.25	0.25	0.25	0.25	0.25	0.03	
M. morganii	1	1	1	1	4	0.25	1
P. mirabilis	1	1	2	2	2	2	0.25
Providencia spp.	0.5	0.5	1	1	1	0.06	
M. catarrhalis	0.03	0.03	≤0.015	≤0.015	≤0.015	≤0.015	
H. influenzae	0.5	0.5	0.25	0.5	0.5	0.06	
B. fragilis	0.5	0.5	0.25	0.25	0.12	0.25	0.25
P. aeruginosa	8	8	4	0.25	1	0.5	4
B. cepacia	8	8	8	2	8	2	
S. maltophilia	>256			>256	>256	>256	

[a]CoNS, coagulase-negative staphylococci; CAZ, ceftazidime.

Table 8 In vitro activities against coagulase-negative staphylococci

Microorganism	MIC$_{50}$ (μg/ml)				
	Imipenem	Meropenem	Biapenem	Lenapenem	Doripenem
S. epidermidis Met[s]	0.1	0.2	0.12	0.12	0.02
S. epidermidis Met[r]	0.25	4	4		
Staphylococcus saprophyticus	0.03	0.25	0.03	0.05	0.1
Staphylococcus simulans	0.06	0.13			
Staphylococcus hominis	0.03	0.13			
Staphylococcus warneri	0.13	0.13			
S. haemolyticus	0.03	0.13		1.56	0.39
Staphylococcus capitis				6.25	

6.2. Gram-Positive Bacilli

Overall, the carbapenems possess good activity against gram-positive bacilli, particularly *Listeria monocytogenes* (except for meropenem) and *Corynebacterium jeikeium*. The activity against *Nocardia asteroides* is more limited. The most active molecules are imipenem and panipenem, followed by meropenem and biapenem (Table 6).

6.3. Gram-Negative Cocci

The carbapenems exhibit good activity against *Neisseria gonorrhoeae* and *Neisseria meningitidis* (Table 6).

6.4. *Enterobacteriaceae*

See Tables 9 and 10.

The carbapenems possess remarkable activity against *Enterobacteriaceae*; in particular, they are active against strains producing plasmid-mediated broad-spectrum (TEM-1, SHV-1, etc.) and extended-spectrum (TEM-3 to TEM-26, SHV-2 to 5, CAZ, etc.) enzymes and chromosomally mediated enzymes (class I). The most active molecule is meropenem, and the least active is imipenem. The other molecules, such as lenapenem, biapenem, panipenem, doripenem, and the new derivatives (E-1010 and FR-21818), have intermediate

Table 9 In vitro activities of carbapenems against *Enterobacteriaceae*

Microorganism(s)	MIC$_{50}$ (μg/ml)							
	Imipenem	Meropenem	Panipenem	Biapenem	DX-8739	Lenapenem	Doripenem	GV 129606
E. coli	0.1	0.01	0.1	0.02	0.05	0.06	0.02	0.03
K. pneumoniae	0.78	0.05	0.1	0.39	0.05	0.12	0.05	0.25
P. mirabilis	1.56	0.1	0.78	1.56	0.1	2	0.1	0.25
Salmonella spp.	0.25	0.03	0.05			0.2	0.03	
Shigella spp.	0.2	0.03	0.1			0.2	0.03	
M. morganii	3.13	0.1	0.78	0.78		1	0.2	1
E. cloacae	0.39	0.05	0.2	0.1	0.2	0.12	0.03	0.06
S. marcescens	0.78	0.39	0.39	0.78	0.1	0.25	0.12	1
P. vulgaris	1.56	0.1	0.78	1.56	0.2	1	0.12	0.25
C. freundii	0.39	0.05	0.2	0.1		0.12	0.02	0.06
Yersinia enterocolitica	0.25	0.03	0.2			1.12	0.06	
Hafnia alvei	<0.1	0.03	0.2					

Table 10 In vitro activity of E-1010[a]

Microorganism	MIC$_{50}$ (μg/ml)				
	E-1010	MER	IMP	CAZ	Cefclidin
S. aureus Met^s	0.1	0.2	0.25	12.5	25
E. faecalis	12.5	25	6.25	>100	>100
E. coli	0.05	0.025	0.2	0.2	0.1
C. freundii	0.2	0.2	0.78	50	3.13
S. marcescens	0.78	0.29	0.78	3.13	3.13
H. influenzae	1.56	0.39	12.5	0.78	0.2
P. aeruginosa	3.13	6.25	12.5	50	6.25
P. aeruginosa IMP^r	6.25	25	25	50	6.25
P. aeruginosa MER^r	6.25	25	25	50	12.5
P. aeruginosa CAZ^r	6.25	25	25	100	25
P. aeruginosa CEF^r	6.25	25	25	100	25

[a]IMP, imipenem; MER, meropenem; CAZ, ceftazidime; CEF, cefpirome.

activity. Among *Enterobacteriaceae*, the carbapenems possess weaker activity against *Proteus* spp. and *Providencia* spp. than do the cephalosporins.

6.5. Other Gram-Negative Bacteria

The carbapenems are active against ceftazidime-susceptible and -resistant strains of *P. aeruginosa*. The activity against the other species of *Pseudomonas* is variable, being good against *P. stutzeri* (MIC$_{50}$ of meropenem, ~0.06 μg/ml) and *P. acidovorans*, variable against *P. pickettii*, and weak against *P. putida*, and *P. fluorescens*. They are inactive against *B. cepacia* (Table 11). The carbapenems are inactive against *S. maltophilia* and *Chryseobacterium* (*Flavobacterium*) *meningosepticum*. They

Table 11 In vitro activities of carbapenems against *Pseudomonas* spp. and *Burkholderia* spp.

Microorganism	MIC$_{50}$ (μg/ml)		
	Imipenem	Meropenem	BMS-181139
B. cepacia	>32	8	0.95
P. pickettii	>4	>4	
P. putida	1	2	0.42
P. acidovorans	1	0.25	
P. stutzeri	0.25	0.06	0.25
B. pseudomallei	1		

possess good activity against *Alcaligenes faecalis*, *Acinetobacter* spp., *Aeromonas hydrophila*, *Bordetella bronchiseptica*, *Alcaligenes xylosoxidans*, *Campylobacter jejuni*, and *Campylobacter coli*. Against *P. aeruginosa*, the most active molecule is lenapenem. This molecule has cross-resistance with the other carbapenems, and its activity against imipenem- and meropenem-resistant strains is markedly reduced. Only lenapenem and biapenem remain active against ceftazidime-resistant strains. The activity of meropenem and imipenem is reduced by 2 dilutions in comparison with activity against wild strains. Among the carbapenems, panipenem is inactive against *P. aeruginosa* (MIC, ~6.25 μg/ml). Meropenem possesses activity similar to that of lenapenem against imipenem-susceptible strains, but against the other phenotypes it is half as active and the organisms become resistant or their susceptibility is intermediate. Biapenem is only active against imipenem- and ceftazidime-susceptible strains and is inactive against the other phenotypes (Table 12).

The activity against *H. influenzae*, *Haemophilus ducreyi*, *Haemophilus aegyptius*, *M. catarrhalis*, *Pasteurella multocida*, *Bordetella pertussis*, and *Moraxella lacunata* is good. Meropenem exhibits better activity than imipenem.

6.6. Anaerobic Microorganisms

See Table 13.

The activities of all the carbapenems against anaerobic gram-negative bacteria, *B. fragilis*, *Prevotella* spp.,

Table 12 In vitro activities of carbapenems against *P. aeruginosa*

P. aeruginosa (no. of isolates)	MIC$_{50}$ (μg/ml)						
	Imipenem	Meropenem	Biapenem	Panipenem	Lenapenem	Ceftazidime	Doripenem
Imipenem^s (128)	1.56	0.39	0.78	6.25	0.39	3.13	0.25
Imipenem^r (22)	12.5	6.25	12.5	25	3.13	12.5	4
Meropenem^r (13)	12.5	12.5	12.5	25	6.25	25	
Ceftazidime^r (39)	3.13	3.13	1.56	12.5	1.56	25	
Imipenem + meropenem^r (10)	12.5	12.5	25	25	6.25	25	
Imipenem + ceftazidime^s (12)	12.5	12.5	25	25	6.25	25	

Table 13 In vitro activities of carbapenems against anaerobic bacteria

Microorganism(s)	MIC$_{50}$ (μg/ml)							
	Imipenem	Meropenem	Panipenem	Biapenem	DX-8739	Lenapenem	Doripenem	GV 129606
B. fragilis	0.1	0.2	0.1	0.3	0.39	0.03	0.25	0.25
Fusobacterium spp.	0.2	0.008	0.1	0.1		0.25	0.06	
Veillonella parvula	0.39	≤0.025	0.1	0.2	≤0.05	0.2		
Peptostreptococcus spp.	≤0.025	0.2	≤0.025	0.39		0.01	0.12	
Peptococcus spp.	0.1	0.2	0.1	0.1				
P. acnes	0.05	0.39	0.1	0.39		0.06		
Eubacterium spp.	1.56	0.78	0.78	0.78				
Mobiluncus spp.	≤0.025	≤0.025		≤0.025				
Bifidobacterium spp.	0.05	0.05		0.2				
C. perfringens	0.05	0.025	0.1	≤0.025		0.016	0.03	0.06
C. difficile	3.13	3.13	6.25	6.25		0.5	2	
G. vaginalis	0.39	≤0.025		0.39				
Prevotella spp.	≤0.25	0.05	≤0.05	0.1		0.03	0.06	
Porphyromonas gingivalis	≤0.025	≤0.025	≤0.05	≤0.025			0.06	

Porphyromonas spp., and *Fusobacterium* are good, as are the activities against gram-positive cocci, gram-negative cocci, and gram-positive bacilli, with the exception of *C. difficile*; however, there are differences in the activities. The MIC$_{50}$ is 6.25 μg/ml for lenapenem and meropenem and greater than or equal to 50 μg/ml for imipenem and biapenem. The most active molecule is meropenem, while the other molecules are similar in terms of activity.

6.7. Factors Affecting In Vitro Activity

When the size of the bacterial inoculum is increased from 10^3 to 10^6 CFU/ml, the MICs of imipenem remain unchanged. Above 10^8 CFU/ml, the MICs of imipenem for *Klebsiella*, *Citrobacter*, *Enterobacter*, *Proteus*, and *P. aeruginosa* increase 4- to 16-fold.

Imipenem is inactivated in thioglycolate-containing media and agar media; it is less stable at 35°C than at 4°C. In solution, imipenem is relatively stable when frozen at −70°C; at 4°C it is unstable. Imipenem is rapidly inactivated when the pH of the agar medium increases to 7 to 8 and is more stable in an acidic medium. The presence of CO_2 increases the MICs fourfold.

6.8. Postantibiotic Effect

The postantibiotic effect is defined as the time during which antibacterial activity persists in the absence of the antibiotic.

Like the penicillins or cephems, the β-lactams exert a postantibiotic effect against gram-positive cocci but not gram-negative bacilli. Imipenem exerts a postantibiotic effect of 1 to 3 h, depending on the bacterial species studied, which is concentration and contact time related.

In contrast to the case with the cephalosporins, a postantibiotic effect has been described with carbapenems against *Enterobacteriaceae*. After short-term exposure to 8 μg of imipenem per ml, a postantibiotic effect against *E. cloacae*, *E. coli*, *K. pneumoniae*, *P. aeruginosa*, and *S. marcescens* was found.

6.9. Combinations with Other Antibiotics

The combination imipenem-amikacin or imipenem-gentamicin is synergistic or additive against *P. aeruginosa*.

The combination of imipenem and a fluoroquinolone is synergistic against *Enterobacter* and *P. aeruginosa*. Combinations of imipenem with tetracyclines or erythromycin A are antagonistic to *E. faecalis* and *S. aureus*.

6.10. Breakpoints

The breakpoints proposed by Weiss et al. (1992) for biapenem are as follows: susceptible, ≤4 μg/ml and ≥16 mm; resistant, ≥16 μg/ml and ≤13 mm. Those of imipenem are as follows: susceptible, ≤4 μg/ml and ≥22 mm; resistant, >8 μg/ml and <18 mm.

7. MECHANISMS OF ACTION

Carbapenems are low-molecular-weight molecules of a zwitterionic nature which readily penetrate the outer membrane of gram-negative bacilli through porins. Their chemical nature enables them to cross the periplasmic space rapidly and reach their target, the PBPs.

When *Enterobacteriaceae* are placed in contact with imipenem, ovoid or spherical but not filamentous bacterial forms occur. The bacteria end by lysing.

Table 14 Affinities of carbapenems for *E. coli* NIHJ-JC2 PBPs

PBP	IC_{50} (μg/ml)		
	Imipenem	Meropenem	Doripenem
1a	0.3	0.86	>6.3
1b	1.3	1.1	2.1
2	0.038	<0.013	0.017
3	>12.5	0.32	4
4	>12.5	>6.3	>6.3
5	0.27	1	>6.3
6	0.9	>6.3	>6.3
MIC (μg/ml)	0.1	0.01	0.025

Table 15 Affinities of carbapenems for *P. aeruginosa* PAO1 PBP

PBP	IC_{50} (μg/ml)		
	Imipenem	Meropenem	Doripenem
1a	0.2	0.27	0.29
1b	0.27	0.15	0.28
2	<0.1	<0.1	<0.1
3	0.64	<0.05	0.07
4	<0.05	<0.05	<0.05
5	0.58	15	>25
MIC (μg/ml)	1.56	0.78	0.78

Table 16 Affinities of carbapenems for *S. aureus* 209 FDA PBP

PBP	IC_{50} (μg/ml)		
	Imipenem	Meropenem	Doripenem
1	<0.2	<0.1	<0.1
2	0.4	0.071	0.47
2a[a]	260	>400	160
3	>6.3	0.076	>6.3
4	<0.1	<0.05	<0.1

[a]From strain SRM 710 (MRSA).

Carbapenems bind to the bacterial peptidases, PBPs which are responsible for the synthesis of peptidoglycan.

The affinity of the carbapenems for *E. coli* PBP is strong in the case of PBPs 2, 1, and 1b and variable for PBP 3, which, when inhibited, is responsible for filamentation. In contrast to meropenem, imipenem has very weak affinity for PBP 3 (Table 14). Likewise, meropenem has greater affinity for *P. aeruginosa* PAO1 PBP 3 than does imipenem (Table 15). Imipenem and meropenem have a strong affinity for *S. aureus* 209P FDA PBPs 2 and 4, while there is a strong affinity for PBP 3 in the case of imipenem. There is no affinity for MRSA PBP 2a, which is also the case with meropenem (Table 16).

The carbapenems are capable of exerting bactericidal activity against strains in the stationary phase. This activity is concentration and structure dependent. Imipenem is capable of bactericidal activity against *E. coli* in the stationary phase in cerebrospinal fluid. It appears to bind to one PBP in particular, PBP 7, which appears only during this phase.

Ohya et al. (1991) have shown that the antipseudomonal activity of panipenem is maximal in a medium deprived of basic amino acids (L-lysine, L-histidine, and L-arginine). This increase in activity would appear to be due to a reduction in competition at the OprD porin, facilitating the transport of basic amino acids, such as histidine, or small peptides containing basic amino acids.

The new molecules CL-191121, CL-188624, and CL-190294 do not, like imipenem, employ the OprD porin of *P. aeruginosa* to cross the outer membrane (Table 17).

8. MECHANISMS OF RESISTANCE

There are a number of mechanisms of resistance to carbapenems. These are based on single or multiple phenomena: crossing of the bacterial wall, modification of the target (PBP), and hydrolysis by β-lactamases.

8.1. β-Lactamases

The carbapenems are stable against hydrolysis by staphylococcal penicillinases and plasmid-mediated enzymes of gram-negative bacilli, and likewise they are resistant to hydrolysis by extended-spectrum β-lactamases, which hydrolyze cefotaxime, ceftazidime, or aztreonam (TEM-3, etc., SHV-2 to -8, CAZ, MIR-1, CEP-1, etc.) (Table 18). The carbapenems are not hydrolyzed by cephalosporinases of *Enterobacteriaceae* or *P. aeruginosa* (Table 19).

Imipenem is a potent inducer of chromosomally mediated β-lactamases of *E. cloacae*, *Citrobacter freundii*, and *P. aeruginosa* but is not hydrolyzed by these enzymes.

The imipenemases are chromosomal metalloenzymes (Amber class B) capable of hydrolyzing the carbapenems. The cofactor of this enzyme is Zn^{2+}, which is located at the active site.

These enzymes have been described to occur in various bacterial species: *S. maltophilia*, *Bacillus cereus*, *Legionella gormanii*, *A. hydrophila*, *Aeromonas sobria*, and *Flavobacterium odoratum*. More recently, they have been detected in *E. cloacae*, *S. marcescens*, and *B. fragilis*. In *S. marcescens*, the activities of imipenem (MIC, 16 to 32 μg/ml, versus 0.25 to 0.5 μg/ml for the susceptible strain) and meropenem (MIC, 0.25 μg/ml, versus 0.03 μg/ml) differ since the rates of hydrolysis by this enzyme, Sme-1, are different. Likewise, biapenem is less hydrolyzed by this enzyme than meropenem (V_{max}, 4.3 versus 52). Biapenem is less hydrolyzed by *S. maltophilia* L1 carbapenemase than is imipenem (2.9 versus 290).

Table 17 Activities of different carbapenems against *P. aeruginosa* wall mutant strains

Strain	MIC (μg/ml)				
	Imipenem	Biapenem	CL-188624	CL-190294	CL-191121
27853a	2	0.5	32	32	16
D2 mutant	32	8	32	32	16
D2 mutant Quinn	16	16	64	64	16

Table 18 In vitro activities of carbapenems against β-lactamase-producing *Enterobacteriaceae*

Strain	Enzyme(s)	MIC (μg/ml)				
		Imipenem	Biapenem	Cefotaxime	Ceftazidime	Aztreonam
E. coli	TEM-1, TEM-2	0.25	<0.12	<0.12	<0.12	<0.12
	TEM-3	0.25	<0.12	256	32	16
	TEM-7	0.25	0.25	0.5	128	4
	TEM-12	<0.12	<0.12	<0.12	8	1
K. pneumoniae	SHV-1	<0.12	<0.12	8	32	64
E. coli	SHV-2	<0.12	<0.12	16	4	2
K. pneumoniae	SHV-5	<0.12	<0.12	8	256	>256
	CEP-1	0.25	<0.12	8	32	64
	MIR-1	0.5	0.5	>256	>256	128

Table 19 Activities of carbapenems against class I β-lactamase-producing strains

Microorganism	MIC_{50} (μg/ml)				
	Biapenem	Imipenem	Ceftazidime	Cefotaxime	Aztreonam
E. cloacae	<0.12	1	128	32	64
C. freundii	0.25	1	128	32	32
S. marcescens	0.25	0.5	0.5	128	2
M. morganii	1	2	16	16	1
P. vulgaris	0.25	0.5	0.25	256	256
P. aeruginosa	0.25	0.5	32	>256	32

8.2. Bacterial Outer Membrane

The loss of activity of imipenem is often associated with a modification of the bacterial outer membrane, preventing its passage. In *P. aeruginosa*, the reduction in the parietal protein OprD and the loss of the 47-kDa protein prevents penetration by imipenem or meropenem. A reduction in the penetration by fluoroquinolones is also observed.

In *E. aerogenes*, the outer membrane penetration of imipenem appears to be dependent on a 40-kDa outer membrane protein.

Imipenem, meropenem, biapenem, and lenapenem contain positively charged basic groups at position 2 which allow the molecules to penetrate the wall of *P. aeruginosa* via the canal of the parietal protein OprD, which allows through molecules of 350 to 400 Da. BMS-181139 exhibits only partial cross-resistance with imipenem and meropenem since it does not use the OprD pathway. The basic amino acids that use this pathway inhibit the penetration of imipenem and panipenem, but not that of BMS-181139.

The carbapenems possessing a basic group at position 1 or 6 do not penetrate the outer membrane of *P. aeruginosa* via OprD. The same applies if the molecule has an amino group at position 1 or 6.

For example, meropenem (1-β-methyl) and its derivative, BMY-45047 (1-ethylguanidine), cross the outer membrane of *P. aeruginosa* by different routes. Carbapenems that contain a basic substituent are much more active against *P. aeruginosa* than those that do not.

A mutation on the *nalB* gene of the *P. aeruginosa* chromosome (*cfxB*, *nfxB*, and *nfxC*) causes a cross-resistance reaction with fluoroquinolones, chloramphenicol, cyclines, and erythromycin A, with hyperproduction of the parietal protein OprM (49 kDa). A mutation of the *nfxB* or *nfxC* type causes cross-resistance with the fluoroquinolones and chloramphenicol, with hyperproduction of the proteins OprJ (54 kDa) and OprN (50 kDa), respectively. *nfxC* resistance associated with the efflux system OprM (50 kDa)-MexC (46 kDa)-MexD (100 kDa) is localized in the cytoplasmic membrane of *P. aeruginosa*. This complex is associated with multiresistance, including to β-lactams.

It has been shown that the resistance of *P. aeruginosa* to carbapenems is due principally to the loss of the OprD protein, but also to the slow but significant hydrolysis by chromosomally mediated β-lactamases. The degree of hydrolysis by these enzymes differs according to the molecule. Imipenem, biapenem, and panipenem are hydrolyzed and their activity is restored by a high concentration of sulbactam, but not by clavulanic acid. The activities of meropenem and lenapenem are little affected by the presence of sulbactam (Hazumi et al., 1995).

8.3. PBPs

About 12% of strains of *Acinetobacter baumannii* are resistant to imipenem. *A. baumannii* has seven PBPs, five of which are major proteins (24, 40, 49, 61, 65, 84, and 95 kDa). In imipenem-resistant strains, PBPs are difficult to visualize, except those of 24 kDa, as imipenem has weak affinity for this protein.

8.4. Epidemiology of Resistance

The emergence of resistant strains of *P. aeruginosa* was observed with the use of imipenem monotherapy in patients suffering from cystic fibrosis. It is possible to select this type of strain in vitro. However, this parietal type of resistance is unstable and reversible. In Boston, Mass., the number of resistant strains has increased from 10% in 1984 to about 30% at present.

The intensive use of imipenem as monotherapy has allowed the emergence of opportunistic microorganisms such as *S. maltophilia*, particularly in intensive care units.

A retrospective study undertaken by Philips et al. (1989) showed the activity of imipenem to be stable in the Netherlands. Over a period from 1986 to 1988, Nösner et al. (1988) noted no increase in the number of resistant strains of *Enterobacteriaceae*.

Table 20 Physicochemical properties of carbapenems

Drug	Empirical formula	Molecular weight	International code	pK1	pK2	pK3
Imipenem	$C_{12}H_{17}N_3O_4S$	317.36	MK-0787	3.2	9.9	
Meropenem	$C_{17}H_{25}N_3O_5S$	383.46	SM-7388			
Panipenem	$C_{15}H_{21}N_3O_4S$	339.42	CS-533			
Biapenem	$C_{15}H_{18}N_4O_4S$	350.39	L-J10627			
Doripenem	$C_{15}H_{24}N_4O_6S_2$	420.51	S-4661			
Lenapenem	$C_{18}H_{29}N_3O_5S$	453.98	BO-2727			
	$C_{19}H_{29}N_3O_5S$	447.98	E-1010			
Ertapenem	$C_{22}H_{24}N_3O_7S$	474.52	MK-0826			
Cilastatin	$C_{16}H_{25}N_2O_5S$	380.43	MK-0791	2	9.2	4.4
Betamipron	$C_{10}H_{11}NO_3$	193.2	CS-443			
	$C_7H_9NO_7$	222	WS-1358 A_1			
	$C_6H_7NO_7$	208	WS-1358 B_1			

In surveys conducted in 1999 and 2000 in 10 and 15 centers, respectively, in the United States, it was shown that mainly all isolates of *Enterobacteriaceae* remain susceptible to meropenem and that meropenem was not active against around 16 to 20% of *P. aeruginosa* and *A. baumannii* isolates.

For *P. aeruginosa*, a few class B carbapenem-hydrolyzing β-lactamases have been characterized, such as IMP-1, IMP-3, VIM-1, and VIM-3.

In Japan, IMP-1 enzymes were found in 1.3% of *P. aeruginosa* isolates in a survey conducted from 1976 to 1977. In the northern part of Italy and in Greece, *P. aeruginosa* isolates have been shown to harbor VIM-1.

In 1985 in Scotland, the first known *A. baumannii* isolate with a carbapenemase known as ARI-1 (OXA-23) was isolated.

9. PHYSICOCHEMICAL PROPERTIES

Table 20 summarizes the physicochemical properties of the main carbapenems already introduced in clinical practice or under development. The major problem with the carbapenems is their chemical instability in solution.

A solution of imipenem is stable at −70°C for 1 year but deteriorates rapidly in a ready-to-use medium supplemented with cations of the Mueller-Hinton type. The solution degrades rapidly at −20°C. The degradation half-lives are 13.9 h for thienamycin, 19.5 h with imipenem, and 36.3 h for the 1-β-methyl imipenem derivative in a 1-mg/ml solution. In a 250-μg/ml solution, the degradation half-lives are 0.3, 0.7, and 36.3 h, respectively.

Bigley et al. (1986) studied the stability of imipenem at 40, 25, and −20°C in 17 different infusion solutions. The stability of imipenem was dependent on its concentration in the solution. A 2.5-μg/ml solution is more stable than a 5.0-mg/ml solution. Imipenem is more stable when the solutions are maintained at 4°C than when they are kept at 25°C; the stabilities are identical at 4, −10, and −20°C. The best stability is obtained in 0.9% sodium chloride. Imipenem-cilastatin should not be reconstituted with a solution containing lactate. Smith et al. (1990) showed that imipenem is degraded in a weakly acidic (pH 4) or alkaline (pH 9) medium. In an acidic medium (pH 4), a reaction occurs between the β-lactam bond and the protonated carboxyl group, with the formation of a diketopiperazine (Fig. 37). At pH 9, imipenem is degraded by three parallel reactions: hydrolysis of the lactam carbonyl bond, hydrolysis of the formimidoyl group to an amino group, and an intermolecular reaction between the β-lactam and the formimidoyl group. Cilastatin is degraded in solution to cilastatin sulfoxide.

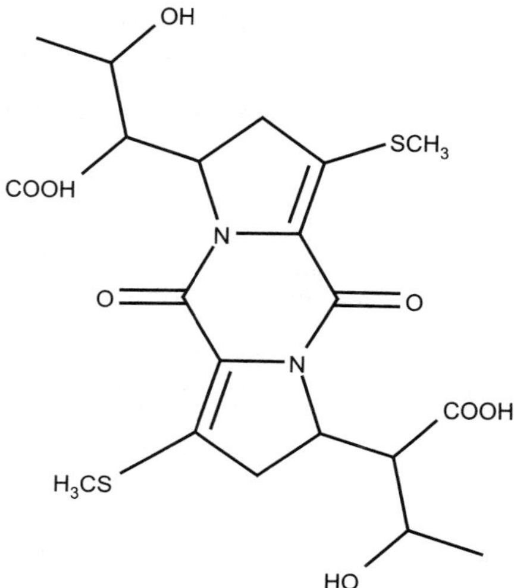

Figure 37 Diketopiperazine: Degradation product of imipenem in solution at pH 7.4

In the meropenem series, the introduction of a 1-β-methyl group increases the hydrolysis half-life compared to that of the 1-α-methyl series (310 versus 27 min).

The stability of panipenem is at least 5 days at −20°C and 28 days at −80°C in plasma. In urine, the stabilities at −20 and −80°C are at least 7 and 42 days. Betamipron is stable for at least 42 days at −20 and −80°C.

In the natural carbapenem series, the C-19393 series has been particularly studied for its chemical stability.

C-19393 H_2 and S_2 differ in terms of the side chain at position 2. The S_2 molecule has a chain attached to the thiol residue, [1-sulfoxy-1-methylethyl], and the chain of the H_2 molecule is 6-[1-hydroxy-1-methylethyl]. These products are stable in 0.05 M phosphate buffer at 60°C at a pH of between 6 and 7. When the pHs are equal to 5 and 8, the degradation half-lives are, respectively, 1.8 and 2.8 h, whereas for a pH of 6 to 7 it is 7.4 h. The presence of a sulfoxide residue increases the chemical stability in an acidic medium, but to a lesser degree in an alkaline medium.

Lenapenem hydrochloride crystallizes. The crystal is stable at room temperature at 40°C. It is soluble in water. The solution is stable at room temperature for several hours (8 h for 5 to 10 mg/ml at 25°C). Lenapenem is relatively stable in an acidic medium.

10. ASSAY METHODS

10.1. Imipenem

As imipenem is unstable, biological specimens should be taken in iced tubes and stored on ice. Blood samples must be centrifuged as rapidly as possible using a refrigerated centrifuge. Plasma or urine should be mixed equally with a morpholinopropanesulfonate glycol buffer (pH 6.8) and frozen immediately at −70°C or preferably in liquid nitrogen. The microbiological method uses *Bacillus subtilis* ATCC 6633 as a test strain (medium 1; Oxoid), with a threshold of susceptibility of 0.1 μg/ml. The HPLC method enables imipenem to be detected with a sensitivity on the order of 0.3 μg/ml and cilastatin with limits of 0.75 μg/ml for plasma and 2.5 μg/ml for urine.

10.2. Meropenem

The plasma and urinary assays of meropenem by a microbiological method involve *E. coli* NIHJ-JC2 as the test strain. Using the chromatographic method, the limits of detection of meropenem are 0.06 μg/ml in plasma and 1.0 μg/ml in urine. The metabolite ICI-213689 is detected at a level of 10 μg/ml in urine. For the plasma assays, a radioimmunological method may be used.

10.3. Panipenem-Betamipron

The microbiological assay method uses *B. subtilis* SANK 76959 in brain-heart medium as the test strain. The limits of detection are 0.02 μg/ml for plasma and urine and 0.08 μg/ml for tissue.

For assays by an HPLC method, the limits of detection for panipenem are 0.3 μg/ml in plasma and 1.0 μg/ml in urine. Those of the metabolite are 1.0 and 5.0 μg/ml in urine and plasma, respectively. For betamipron, the limits of detection are, respectively, 0.2, 0.5, and 0.4 μg/ml in plasma, urine, and tissue.

10.4. Biapenem

Biapenem is assayed by a microbiological method using *S. aureus* IFO 14607 or *B. subtilis* ATCC 11778 (antibiotic medium 1) as the test strain. An HPLC method has been described by Weiss et al. (1992), but the limit of sensitivity is not known.

11. PHARMACOKINETICS

11.1. Plasma Pharmacokinetics in Healthy Volunteers

The plasma pharmacokinetics of the carbapenems are complex because of their hydrolysis by renal DHP-I to various degrees, depending on the molecule, with major interindividual variability. In addition, the data published in the literature are fragmentary, even for well-established molecules such as imipenem, and for this reason they are sometimes difficult to interpret.

11.1.1. Imipenem

At the end of a 30-min infusion of imipenem-cilastatin at 1.0 g each, the concentrations in plasma are 52.1 and 65.0 μg/ml. Imipenem is weakly bound to plasma proteins (13 to 20%).

The apparent elimination half-life is on the order of 1.0 h and does not vary with the administered dose. The plasma clearance is between 165 and 200 ml/min/1.73 m^2. That of cilastatin is between 207 and 218 ml/min (Table 21).

Imipenem is eliminated renally. It is hydrolyzed by renal DHP-I. The addition of cilastatin increases the renal clearance (56 versus 157 ml/min) and the quantity of unchanged product eliminated in the urine (22 versus 70%). The quantity recovered in the feces is on the order of 0.6% of the administered dose.

Simultaneous administration of imipenem-cilastatin and probenecid causes a reduction in plasma (218 versus 89 ml/min) and renal (173 versus 70 ml/min) clearance and an increase in the apparent elimination half-life (0.8 h versus 1.7 h), but the quantity of imipenem collected in the urine is identical (about 75%). According to Reeves et al. (1983), the renal clearance is due to glomerular filtration of 86 ml/min and tubular secretion of 44 ml/min. Biliary elimination is weak, but the concentrations obtained in the bile are greater than the MICs for the main microorganisms involved in hepatobiliary infections. The peak concentration in the bile is obtained 10 min after the end of infusion: 10 μg/ml (1.5 to 16.7 μg/ml). One hour after the end of the infusion, it is between 8 and 9 μg/ml. The apparent elimination half-life in the bile is 1.24 h.

11.1.2. Meropenem

An ascending-dose study (Bax et al., 1989) was undertaken with doses of 0.25, 0.5, and 1.0 g in a volume of 60 ml (30-min infusion).

The results are summarized in Tables 22 and 23. The concentrations obtained at the end of the infusion and the areas under the curve are proportional to the administered dose. About 79% of the administered dose is recovered unchanged in the urine. The apparent elimination half-life is about 1 h, with a plasma clearance of 250 to 300 ml/min and high renal clearance (about 200 to 226 ml/min).

In the presence of probenecid, the apparent elimination half-life of meropenem is increased (0.98 versus 1.30 h), as is the area under the curve (61.5 versus 95.4 μg·h/ml). Plasma and renal clearances are reduced.

The hydrolysis product, ICI-213689, represents about 20% of the administered product. Plasma protein binding is weak and represents less than 10%.

Table 21 Pharmacokinetics of imipenem

Dose (mg)	Drug	C_0 (μg/ml)	AUC (μg·h/ml)	$t_{1/2\beta}$ (h)	CL_P (ml/min)
250	Imipenem		22	0.85	189
	Cilastatin		2.1	0.83	190
500	Imipenem		38.8	0.92	224
	Cilastatin		40	0.90	212
1,000	Imipenem	52.1	74.1	0.93	165–200
	Cilastatin	65	73.1	0.84	207–218

Table 22 Comparative pharmacokinetics of imipenem and meropenem

Drug	Dose (mg)	C_{max} (μg/ml)	$AUC_{0-\infty}$ (μg·h/ml)	$t_{1/2}$(h)	CL_R (ml/min)	CL_P (ml/min)	Urinary elimination (%)
Meropenem	1,000	61.6	77.5	1	188	139	75
Imipenem-cilastatin	1,000	69.9	94.38	1.1	183	135	74

11.1.3. Panipenem-Betamipron

Panipenem is hydrolyzed by DHP-I. Betamipron prevents this hydrolysis indirectly by inhibiting the transport of panipenem into the proximal tubule cells. In the absence of betamipron, panipenem is hydrolyzed by DHP-I to a degradation product, SM-1. In the phase I study conducted by Nakashima et al. (1990), the combination panipenem-betamipron was administered to volunteers in ascending doses (0.125, 0.250, 0.5, and 1.0 g) in the form of an infusion of 100 ml in 60 min. The results are summarized in Table 23.

There is linearity between the concentrations obtained at the end of the infusion and the areas under the curve of panipenem and betamipron. The apparent elimination half-lives are on the order of 1.0 h for panipenem and 0.6 h for betamipron. The plasma clearance of betamipron is very high, on the order of 400 ml/min, while that of panipenem is lower, being on the order of 180 to 190 ml/min. The urinary elimination of betamipron is on the order of 95 to 99% of the administered dose. That of panipenem is 30%, and that of the degradation product, SM-1, is about 50%.

No accumulation of panipenem or betamipron has been found following repeated doses. The two products have not been detected in the feces (<10%). Plasma protein binding is 3.9% for panipenem and 74.9% for betamipron.

11.1.4. Biapenem

A phase I study was conducted by Nakashima et al. (1991) with ascending doses of biapenem (150, 300, and 600 mg) in the form of an infusion for 1.0 h. The concentrations obtained at the end of the infusion were linear among the three doses, as were the areas under the curve. The apparent elimination half-life was about 1 h. There was no accumulation after repeated dosing. Urinary elimination was about 60% of the administered dose (Table 23). The fecal concentration was less than 1.0 μg/g.

11.1.5. Lenapenem

Nakashima et al. (1993) administered single and ascending doses of lenapenem hydrochloride to 30 volunteers: 25, 50, 125, 250, 500, and 1,000 mg. After infusion for 30 min, the concentrations were linear over the range of doses from 250 to 1,000 mg, as were the areas under the curve. Plasma clearance was 131.5 ml/min, and renal clearance was 123 ml/min. No product was detected in the feces. The apparent elimination half-life was 1.5 h. Urinary elimination was about 70% (Table 23). After a dose of 1.0 g, the salivary concentration was on the order of 0.72 μg/ml. Plasma protein binding was weak.

11.1.6. Doripenem

Nakashima et al. (1994) administered an intravenous infusion (0.5 h) of ascending doses of doripenem to 40 volunteers. The apparent elimination half-life was less than 1 h, but more than 75% of the product was eliminated unchanged in the urine (Table 24).

11.1.7. Ertapenem

Ertapenem (L-749345 or MK 0826) is a 1-β-methyl carbapenem characterized by a carboxyphenylaminocarbonyl chain attached to a pyrrolidinylthio nucleus.

In terms of its antibacterial activity, this molecule is inferior to imipenem and meropenem. The major innovation is its pharmacokinetic profile, as it has a long apparent elimination

Table 23 Pharmacokinetics of carbapenems

Drug	Dose (mg)	No. of subjects	Infusion (min)[a]	C_{max} (μg/ml)	AUC_{0-8} (μg·h/ml)	$t_{1/2\beta}$ (h)	CL_P (ml/min)	Urinary elimination (%)	
								Drug	Metabolite
Panipenem	125	2	60 (P)	6.8	11.72	1.13	181.2	30.4	
			(B)	4.47	5.31	0.65	415.8	106.3	
	250	5	60 (P)	14.26	23.2	1.14	182.8	31	53.8
			7.25 (B)	8.9	0.65	484.5	99.7		
	500	5	60 (P)	27.51	45.21	1.19	188.5	28.5	48.6
			15.59 (B)	19.7	0.67	445.2	93.2		
	100	5	60 (P)	49.27	84.8	1.23	194.3	28.3	45.1
			(B)	23.68	31.3	0.76	536.6	95.4	
Biapenem	150	5	60	8.8	14.7	0.97		62.1	<1
	300	5	60	17.3	29.2	1.03		62.1	<1
	600	5	60	32.4	55.4	10.4		64	<1
Meropenem	250	6	30	12.1	14.4	1.01	300	76	<1
	500	5	30	25.6	30.1	0.97	283	83	<1
	1,000	6	30	55.4	66.9	0.96	254	79	<1
Lenapenem	250	6	30	17.6	32	1.54	133	77	
	500	6	30	38.8	66.3	1.50	128	71	
	1,000	6	30	71.9	120.2	1.41	140	71	

[a]P, panipenem; B, betamipron.

Table 24 More pharmacokinetics of carbapenems

Dose	Drug (mg)	n	C (μg/ml) 0.5h	12h	24h	AUC (μg·h/ml)	$t_{1/2}$ (h)	CL_P (ml/min)	CL_R (ml/min)	Urinary elimination (%)
Ertapenem	500	6	78.2	5.5	0.8	298	4.1	10.9	28.3	37.5
	1,000	6	144.2	10.3	1.5	575	4.2	10.1	29.5	35.2
	2,000	6	268.2	17.5	2.5	986	4.0	12.2	34.4	34.8
	3,000	6	253.0	26.9	3.8	1,376.1	3.9	13.6	31.0	35.8
CS-023	50	6	3.62			6.26	1.55			64.4
	100	6	6.18			12.2	1.56			74.1
	200	6	13.4			23.5	1.48			51.6
	350	6	24.9			47.9	1.64			54.9
	700	6	44.2			87.3	1.76			59.4
	1,400	6	102			170	1.88			68.9
	2,100	6	135			272	2.06			69.6
E-1010	250	6	9.9			1.69		151.8	235	66.6
	500	6	21.2			1.69		112	221.6	59.9
	1,000	7	41.4			1.5		151.9	237.6	61.9
Doripenem	125	6	8.1			8.7	0.85			75
	250	6	18.1			20.2	0.90			75
	500	6	33.1			34.4	0.86			75
	1,000	0	63			75.6	0.96			75

Table 25 Pharmacokinetics of imipenem (single dose) in cystic fibrosis patients[a]

Dose (mg/kg)	n	Drug	$t_{1/2}$ (h)	V_{ss} (liters)	CL_p (ml/min/1.73 m²)	AUC (μg·h/ml)	CL_R (ml/min/1.73 m²)	Urinary elimination (%)
30	7	Imipenem	0.8	0.34	262.4	25.4	122.7	49.8
60	5	Cilastatin	0.9	0.30	252.9	24.4	195.2	78.4
		Imipenem	1.0	0.25	181.0	76.1		
		Cilastatin	0.7	0.23	221.2	65.5		
90	4	Imipenem	0.8	0.27	220.0	81.5		
		Cilastatin	0.7	0.25	267.0	79.7		

[a]Data from Reed et al., 1985.

half-life (half-life at β phase ~4.5 h) and high residual concentrations in plasma at 12 h (~3.8 μg/ml for 250 mg), and the urinary elimination is between 30 and 45% of the administered dose (Majundar et al., 1996).

In healthy young volunteers, L-749345 was administered in the form of a slow infusion for 30 min. Blood samples were taken at 5°C, and the plasma recovered after centrifugation in a refrigerated centrifuge was stabilized and stored at −70°C.

The principal pharmacokinetic parameters are summarized in Table 24.

Plasma protein binding was 97.1% for a concentration of 25 μg/ml.

12. PHARMACOKINETICS IN SPECIFIC POPULATIONS

12.1. Burn Patients

Twelve patients suffering from second-degree and/or third-degree burns over 13 to 82% of their bodies received imipenem-cilastatin intravenously at a dose of 500 mg every 6 h. The concentrations in plasma obtained at the end of infusion (60 min) were between 13.5 and 28.5 μg/ml. The steady-state concentrations were between 16.6 and 37.1 μg/ml. No significant differences were found between the plasma clearance (208.5 ml/min) and apparent elimination half-lives (1.12 h) in burn patients and healthy volunteers. There is, however, major interindividual variability.

12.2. Cystic Fibrosis Patients

The pharmacokinetics of the combination imipenem-cilastatin were studied in 17 pediatric patients over 12 years of age suffering from cystic fibrosis. Three doses were administered, 7.5, 15, and 22.5 mg/kg, every 6 h for 3 days. The pharmacokinetic parameters after the first dose and at steady state are summarized in Table 25. The pharmacokinetics are identical to those in healthy adults. A daily dose of 90 to 100 mg/kg is recommended for the treatment of *P. aeruginosa* infections.

12.3. Elderly Subjects

A pharmacokinetic study of imipenem-cilastatin was conducted in subjects aged 65 to 75 years. The pharmacokinetic parameters are superimposable on those of young adults (Table 26), and there is no need to modify the dosage.

Table 26 Pharmacokinetics of imipenem-cilastatin in 65- to 75-year-old subjects (500 and 500 mg by infusion)

Parameter (unit)	Imipenem	Cilastatin
k_{el} (min^{-1})	0.74	0.61
$t_{1/2}$ (h)	0.97	1.26
V (liters)	0.24	0.2
AUC (μg·h/ml)	46.1	72.2
CL_P (ml/min)	175	119
CL_R (ml/min)	94.8	64.3
Fe (%)	0.56	0.54

13. PHARMACOKINETICS OF CARBAPENEMS IN PEDIATRIC PATIENTS

13.1. Imipenem

There is dose dependence and an increase in the apparent elimination half-life of imipenem (2.5 h) and cilastatin (9.1 h) in neonates and premature infants (<37 weeks) compared with the kinetic parameters obtained in adults, associated with a reduction in the plasma clearance (0.15 liter/h/kg for imipenem and 0.03 liter/h/kg for cilastatin). Cilastatin accumulates in the plasma after repeated doses, in contrast to imipenem. The proportions attributable to renal and nonrenal clearance are 16 and 8% in premature infants, compared to 52 and 44% in adults.

13.2. Meropenem

Numerous studies have been conducted with meropenem at intravenous doses of 10, 20, and 40 mg/kg.

In pediatric patients over the age of 6 months, the pharmacokinetics are identical to those in adults, with an apparent elimination half-life of between 0.8 and 1.0 h. The area under the curve is 60 μg·h/ml after a dose of 20 mg/kg, and the concentration in plasma at the end of the infusion (30 min) is between 30 and 70 μg/ml. The urinary elimination of meropenem ranges from 40 to 80%, depending on the patient (Table 27).

13.3. Panipenem-Betamipron

In the incremental-dose kinetic study of the combination at equal doses of panipenem and betamipron (10, 20, and 30 mg/kg), no dose dependence was demonstrated. The concentrations obtained at the end of the infusion (30 min) were, respectively, 26.7 and 18.3, 64.8 and 38.7, and 91.7 and 50.8 μg/ml after 10, 20, and 30 mg/kg. The apparent elimination half-lives were on the order of 1.0 and 0.5 h for panipenem and betamipron, respectively. About 30% of the administered dose of panipenem is eliminated in the urine; the figure is 70% for betamipron. The area under the curve is proportional to the administered dose (Table 28).

14. PHARMACOKINETICS IN PATIENTS WITH RENAL INSUFFICIENCY

14.1. Imipenem

Several studies have been undertaken. The study conducted by Verpoolen et al. (1984) is summarized in Table 29.

The apparent elimination half-life increases when the creatinine clearance decreases. When the creatinine clearance is less than 15 ml/min, the daily dosage must be reduced from 4 to 2.0 g. The apparent elimination half-life of cilastatin increases more than that of imipenem between dialysis sessions.

Imipenem and cilastatin are eliminated by hemofiltration and hemodialysis, but only 3.2% of imipenem and 5.4% of cilastatin are eliminated by peritoneal dialysis over a period of 6 h.

Imipenem penetrates the peritoneal dialysis fluid when administered parenterally. The peak concentration is reached at 8 h and represents about 20 to 30% of the peak concentration in plasma (2 μg/ml for 500 mg intravenously and 14 μg/ml for 1,000 mg intravenously).

14.2. Meropenem

Christensson et al. (1992) studied the pharmacokinetics of meropenem in patients with renal insufficiency (Table 30). The authors recommended an adaptation of the daily dosage. In subjects with healthy renal function, a dose of 0.5 to 1.0 g must be administered every 6 to 8 h; when the creatinine clearance is between 50 and 29 ml/min the same dose must be administered every 12 h, when it is between 30 and 10 ml/min a dose of 0.25 to 0.50 g must be administered every 12 h, and below 10 ml/min the dosage is 0.25 to 0.5 g every 24 h.

14.3. Panipenem-Betamipron

Koda et al. (1989) reported the pharmacokinetics of panipenem and betamipron in patients with renal insufficiency. The apparent elimination half-life increases in patients with a creatinine clearance of less than 30 ml/min, as does the area under the curve. A modification of the dosage is therefore necessary. As with the combination imipenem-cilastatin, betamipron, which undergoes extensive renal elimination, accumulates more than panipenem (Table 31).

14.4. Ertapenem

The impact of altered renal function caused by 1 g of ertapenem given intravenously was investigated in 24 patients with various renal dysfunctions versus healthy volunteers. The concentration of ertapenem in plasma was modified for mild dysfunction for the unbound fraction. The apparent elimination half-life was prolonged for both total and unbound ertapenem concentrations. The area under the curve from 0 h to infinity increased more for unbound than total ertapenem with increasing renal impairment. The renal clearance declined more than five-fold for total drug and eight-fold for unbound drug (Table 32).

Table 28 Pharmacokinetics of panipenem-betamipron in pediatric patients

Dose (mg/liter)	C_{max} (μg/ml)	$t_{1/2\beta}$ (h)	Urinary elimination (%)
10/10	26.7	0.99	25
20/20	64.8	0.82	25
30/30	91.7	1.02	25

Table 27 Pharmacokinetics of meropenem in pediatric patients

Patient group	Dose (mg/kg)	C_0 (μg/ml)	$AUC_{0-\infty}$ (μg·h/ml)	$t_{1/2}$ (h)	CL_P (ml/min)	CL_R (ml/min)	Urinary elimination (%)
Premature infants	10	20.45	86.3	3.22	3.61	1.4	32.1
	20	44.4	181	2.78	3.58	1.37	43.6
	40	79.5	330	2.76	4.57	2.41	43.1
Neonates	10	21.7	68.3	2.46	8.88	3.09	33.0
	20	40.6	134	1.95	9.72	3.46	32.0
	40	79.7	200	1.72	11.4	3.53	31.6

Table 29 Pharmacokinetics of imipenem in patients with renal insufficiency[a]

Group	Creatinine clearance (ml/min)	Drug	k_{el} (min^{-1})	$t_{1/2\beta}$ (h)	CL_P (ml/min)	CL_R (ml/min)	Urinary elimination (%)
I	>80	Imipenem	0.013	52	0.39	788	13.4
		Imipenem-cilastatin	0.012	55	0.31	1,073	43.4
		Cilastatin	0.012	54	0.25	1,015	59.1
II	80–30	Imipenem	0.01	69	0.24	1,551	19.5
		Imipenem-cilastatin	0.009	75	0.26	1,548	43.7
		Cilastatin	0.008	80	0.18	1,980	65.8
III	30–20	Imipenem	0.005	118	0.35	2,404	18.2
		Imipenem-cilastatin	0.005	127	0.28	2,991	33.9
		Cilastatin	0.004	149	0.18	4,855	58.8
IV	<10	Imipenem	0.004	155	0.24	3,594	9
		Imipenem-cilastatin	0.004	159	0.23	3,932	13.5
		Cilastatin	0.004	417	0.27	11,843	39.2

[a]Data from Verpoolen et al., 1984.

Table 30 Pharmacokinetics of meropenem in patients with renal insufficiency[a]

Creatinine clearance and drug	Volunteers (no.)	C_{max} (μg/ml)	T_{max} (h)	AUC (μg·h/ml)	$t_{1/2}$ (h)	CL_P (ml/min)	CL_R (ml/min)	Urinary elimination (%)
>80 ml/min								
Meropenem	5	30.3		36	0.93	186	142	77
Metabolite		1.51	0.58	4.63	2.31			22
80–30 ml/min								
Meropenem	5	31.7		89.8	2.34	74	41	53
Metabolite		1.89	3.6	31	9.11			13
30–5 ml/min								
Meropenem	7	33.1		156	3.82	53	23	38
Metabolite		3.46	7.44	163	23.6			6
<5ml/min								
Meropenem	5	53.1	53.1	393	6.81	19		
Metabolite		11.7	11.7	405				

[a]Data from Christensson et al., 1992.

Table 31 Pharmacokinetics of the combination panipenem-betamipron in patients with renal insufficiency[a]

Group	Creatinine clearance (ml/min)	Drug	C_0 (μg/ml)	k_{el} (liters h^{-1})	AUC (μg·h/ml)	$t_{1/2\beta}$ (h)	Urinary elimination (%)
I	>60	Panipenem	30.8	0.49	53.5	1.42	35.5
		Betamipron	18.1	1.02	20.4	0.71	98.5
II	60–30	Panipenem	27.8	0.41	61.5	1.78	28
		Betamipron	20.5	0.63	37.6	1.31	73
III	<30	Panipenem	25.9	0.19	126.1	3.94	11.9
		Betamipron	25.8	0.14	194.7	5.77	82.5

[a]Data from Koda et al., 1989.

Table 32 Pharmacokinetics of ertapenem in patients with renal insufficiency[a]

Creatinine clearance (ml/min)	n	C_0 (μg/ml) (30-min infusion)	$AUC_{0-\infty}$ (μg·h/ml)	$t_{1/2}$ (h)	CL_P (ml/min)	Urinary elimination up to 36 h (%)
>90	16	154.9	572	3.9	29.5	43.1
60–90	6	181.7	800	5	21.8	39.8
59–31	7	166.2	1,036	6.9	17	38.3
30–5	6	124.8	1,747	12.9	10	22.5
<10	7	148	2,038	12.9	9	NA[b]
Hemodialysis	5	120.4	1,622	17.4	11.6	NA

[a]Data from Christensson et al., 1992.
[b]NA, not available.

15. TISSUE DISTRIBUTION

15.1. Imipenem-Cilastatin

Imipenem reaches therapeutic levels in cerebrospinal fluid and in peritoneal, pleural, pancreatic, and biliary fluids. The concentrations vary with the individual, and the sampling time after the end of the infusion and in relative terms as a function of the dose.

After a dose of 1.0 g, the concentrations of imipenem and cilastatin in the cerebrospinal fluid are not insignificant when the meninges are not inflamed, with little variation according to the sampling time (0 to 8 h): 0.4 to 0.75 μg/ml for imipenem and 0.08 to 0.9 μg/ml for cilastatin. In bacterial meningitis, the concentrations of imipenem range from 0.5 to 11.0 μg/ml and those of cilastatin range from 0.25 to 1.4 μg/ml.

In pancreatic fluid after a dose of 500 mg, the mean peak concentration of 1.7 μg/ml is reached 1.5 h after the end of the infusion.

In inflammatory blister fluid (induction by cantharidin), the concentration is 6.2 μg/ml 30 min after the end of the infusion and then decreases slowly to reach 0.5 μg/ml at 6 h.

Penetration of peritoneal fluid measured during abdominal surgical procedures is on the order of 30 μg/ml 15 min after the end of the infusion of 1.0 g, and it is 5 to 7 μg/ml 3 to 4 h later.

Concentrations in pleural fluid after an infusion of 250 or 500 mg range from 1.2 to 31.0 μg/ml between the end of the infusion and 4 h afterwards, irrespective of the dose; cilastatin concentrations are between 1.6 and 4.9 μg/ml. In synovial fluid after a dose of 1.0 g, concentrations are between 7.9 and 20.4 μg/ml, depending on the sampling period.

Less than 1% of the administered dose is eliminated in the bile. However, the fecal concentration of imipenem ranges from 0.7 to 22.2 mg/kg.

The concentrations in the different tissues are presented in Table 33.

Concentrations in bronchial tissue are on the order of 1.1 to 3.2 mg/kg after an infusion of 1.0 g; in lung tissue the concentrations vary time dependently from 2.1 mg/kg (2.0 h) to 12.1 mg/kg (0.5 h). In bronchial secretions, a mean peak concentration of 2.0 μg/ml was obtained at 2 h. In tonsillar tissue, the mean concentration after a dose of 500 mg was 2.2 mg/kg.

In uterine and ovarian tissues and in the fallopian tubes, the concentrations were between 2.2 and 3.8 mg/kg after a dose of 1.0 g. Concentrations in the tissues of the digestive apparatus, colon, ileum-jejunum, peritoneum, abdominal

Table 33 Tissue and fluid concentrations of imipenem

Tissue or fluid	Dose (g)	Concn (μg/ml or mg/kg)	Sampling time (h)
Aqueous humor	1	2.9	2
Peritoneal fluid	1	35.3	0.5
		18.5	2.5–3 h
Blister fluid (cantharides)	1	6.5	0.5
		0.8	6
Bronchial secretion	1	0.85	0.5
		1.96	1
		2.1	2
		1.26	4
		0.64	6
Lung: parenchyma	1	12.1	0.25
		6.6	0.5
		5.6	1
		2.1	2
Skin	0.5	15.45	0.25
Subcutaneous tissue	0.5	2.18	0.25
Fascia	0.5	13.52	0.25
Muscle	0.5	6.6	0.25
Colon tissue	0.5	2.07	0.25
Peritoneal tissue	0.5	8.24	0.25
Noninflamed tissue	1	0.4–0.9	
Inflamed tissue		0.25–11	
Pancreatic fluid	0.5	1.7	1.5
Pleural fluid	0.25	1.2–31	0–4
	0.5	14.7	0–4
Renal tissue			
Cortex	1	16–79	ND[a]
Medulla	1	14–102	ND
Prostatic tissue	0.5	2.3–13.8	0.5
		1.6–12.7	1
		<0.5–8.6	2
		0.5–2	3.5
Synovial fluid	1	20.4	1
		13	2
		7.9	3

[a]ND, not determined.

muscles, fascia, subcutaneous tissue and fat were between 2.18 and 15.45 mg/kg 45 min after the end of the infusion.

In prostatic tissue, the mean concentration was 5.3 mg/kg after a dose of 500 mg of imipenem-cilastatin. In the renal cortex and medulla the concentrations were 16 to 79 and 14 to 102 mg/kg, respectively.

15.2. Meropenem

After an infusion of 500 mg of meropenem, concentrations were 4 mg/kg in the submaxillary glands and 1.0 mg/kg in the tonsils 45 min after the end of the infusion, and concentrations were 0.35 to 6.0 mg/kg in the mucosae of the maxillary and ethmoidal sinuses and in the auricular epithelium. In the uterine and ovarian tissues and in the fallopian tubes, the concentrations ranged from 7.65 to 13.0 mg/kg, with levels of 2.10 to 7.34 μg/ml in the retroperitoneal fluid.

In burn patients, the concentrations of meropenem were 11.65 mg/kg in necrotic skin and 9.28 mg/kg in healthy skin.

Levels of 0.20 to 1.05 μg/ml were measured in the tear fluid between 0 and 4 h after the end of the infusion, with a peak of 1.25 μg/ml. In the aqueous humor, the meropenem concentration was 0.52 μg/ml (plasma, 18.6 μg/ml) 20 min after the end of the infusion.

15.3. Panipenem-Betamipron

Tissue distribution studies were conducted following administration of a single dose of 0.5 or 1.0 g of panipenem-betamipron.

After a dose of 1.0 g, the concentrations of panipenem were 1.74 to 8.74 μg/ml in sputum; 4.91 μg/ml in pancreatic fluid; 5.85 mg/kg in uterine, ovarian, and tubal tissues; and about 3.0 mg/kg in the ileojejunal wall. After a dose of 0.5 g, the concentrations of panipenem were 1.6 to 12.5 mg/kg in the bladder wall, 0.1 to 0.5 μg/ml in pancreatic tissue, 0.72 μg/ml in the lymph nodes, 2.63 mg/kg in the submaxillary glands, 7.8 μg/ml in the maxillary sinus, 0.25 mg/kg in the mandibular bone, 1.15 μg/ml in the aqueous humor, 0.2 to 1 mg/kg in the stomach wall, 0.5 mg/kg in the colonic wall, 1.0 mg/kg in the subcutaneous fat, and 0.2 to 1 mg/kg in the peritoneal tissue.

In the renal tissue, panipenem and betamipron had the following concentrations, respectively, after an infusion of 0.5 g: renal medulla, 7.0 to 14.4 and 29 to 113.7 mg/kg; cortex, 2.1 to 18.9 and 25.7 to 208.5 mg/kg; and uterine, ovarian, and tubal tissues, 1.5 to 3.21 and 3.21 to 5.74 mg/kg.

After doses of 0.5 g every 12 h for 3 days, the mean concentration in the peritoneal fluid was 1 to 2 μg/ml.

Concentrations in the cerebrospinal fluid in pediatric patients with purulent bacterial meningitis range from 0.40 to 6.84 μg/ml for panipenem and 0.77 to 0.95 μg/ml for betamipron at doses of 20 to 40 mg/kg.

15.4. Biapenem

Few studies relating to tissue distribution have been published. After a dose of 600 mg by infusion, a concentration of 0.9 μg/ml has been measured in the pancreatic fluid, 2.6 mg/kg has been measured in the gastric wall, and 0.6, 1.8, and 1.5 mg/kg have been measured in the subcutaneous fat, peritoneal tissue, and abdominal muscles, respectively.

16. TOLERANCE OF CARBAPENEMS

16.1. Renal Tolerance

16.1.1. Renal DHP-I

Renal DHP-I is a peptidase-type metalloenzyme described by Greenstein.

It is capable of hydrolyzing the lactam carbonyl bond of carbapenems and penems. Mitsuhashi et al. (1988) purified renal DHP-I of human origin. It is a protein with a molecular weight of 135 and an isoelectric point of 4.75. Campbell et al. characterized renal DHP-I as an enzyme that acts on unsaturated dipeptides, such as glycyldehydrophenylalanine (Gdp). The dipeptidases act selectively on dipeptides with free amino and carboxyl groups. For this reason, it seems unlikely that carbapenems without a free amino group would be susceptible to the action of DHP-I. Penicillin G, cephaloridine, and aztreonam are not hydrolyzed by DHP-I. It appears that this action is specific to the carbapenem skeleton (Table 34).

DHP-I extracted from rat lung has a molecular weight of 150 and comprises two 80-kDa subunits. Its activity is inhibited by cilastatin, *ortho*-phenantholine, which is a chelator of metal ions, and ATP. Rat kidney and lung are important organs for the metabolism of glutathione and its derivatives. The derivatives of glutathione are hydrolyzed to glutamate and cysteinylglycine by γ-aminoglutamyltransferase localized in the brush border (microvilli) of the proximal tubules. DHP-I hydrolyzes cysteinylglycine to cysteine. It also enables D_4 leukotrienes to be converted to E_4.

Tanimura et al. (1991) studied the dehydropeptidase activity in different human and animal organs. They showed that the activity differs with the organ and the animal species.

DHP-I activity is strong in renal tissue in the monkey, dog, mouse, rat, and rabbit. It is weaker in the kidney and lung, except in the rat, where the activity is strong (Table 35).

In humans, dehydropeptidase activity is marked in renal tissue, being maximal in the renal cortex (2,795 ± 549 mU/g of tissue), followed by the medulla (1,546 ± 539 mU/g of tissue). Extensive activity has been detected in the appendicular wall (832 ± 761 mU/g of tissue). Elsewhere, the activity is less than 200 mU/g of tissue in the following order: lung, colon, esophagus, ileum-jejunum, liver, gallbladder, pancreas, and spleen.

Histochemical studies in rat renal tissue have shown that the enzyme is localized in particular in the brush border of

Table 34 Penems hydrolysis by DHP-I[a]

Drug	K_m (mM)	V^b_{max}
Gdp	0.133	100
Imipenem	1.020	0.86
Sch-29482	0.476	0.65
Carpetimycin A	0.167	0.64
Carpetimycin B	1.110	0.38
Cilastatin	0.096	

[a]Data from Mitsuhashi et al., 1988.
[b]Percent of Gdp hydrolysis rate.

Table 35 DHP-I activity in various tissues[a]

Animal	mU/g of tissue		
	Liver	Kidney	Lung
Human		1,638	42
Baboon	53.1	1,647	143
Dog	29.4	2,914	92
Rabbit	24	597	137
Rat	48.9	312	702
Mouse	76.3	942	133

[a]DHP-I activity was tested using Gdp as a substrate.

the proximal tubules and the basement membrane, and in the juxtaglomerular region. The enzyme is not localized in the distal tubules.

16.1.2. Stability of Carbapenems against Hydrolysis by DHP-I

Carbapenems are hydrolyzed at the lactam carbonyl bond by DHP-I. Their relative stabilities are dependent on the chain at C-3 and C-6.

Studies by Sukamoto et al. (1991) in the PS-5 series showed that the stability against hydrolysis by DHP-I varies according to the origin of the enzyme tested and that the activity is not necessarily of the Michaelis-Menten type. The in vitro activity does not necessarily reflect the in vivo activity, so both tests are required.

DHP-I hydrolyzes all carbapenems or penems to various degrees, whether of natural origin, such as thienamycin, carpetimycins A and B, PS-5, and epithienamycins, or of synthetic origin, such as imipenem. The stability of the natural molecules against hydrolysis by DHP-I is dependent on the nature of the side chain at position 2.

The penems and carbapenems have an ene-lactam-type structure which is homologous with that of the dehydropeptides. However, the cephalosporins that also possess this structure are not susceptible to hydrolysis by DHP-I.

The weak urinary elimination of thienamycin or imipenem in the different animal species (mice, rats, dogs, pigs, and monkeys) is due to the extensive metabolization of the molecules in the renal tissue. DHP-I is a metalloenzyme that contains zinc and acts as a class B β-lactamase. Norrby et al. (1983) have shown that there is major interindividual variability with respect to hydrolysis by DHP-I by analyzing the quantity of imipenem eliminated in the urine of volunteers. They defined a group of weak metabolizers (urinary elimination of imipenem >16%) and strong metabolizers (urinary elimination of imipenem <16%).

The presence of a 1-β-methyl group increases stability against DHP-I (Table 36).

The resistance to hydrolysis varies with the animal species. Meropenem is more strongly hydrolyzed by mouse, rabbit, and monkey DHP-I than is imipenem, but meropenem is more stable against hydrolysis by guinea pig and dog enzymes (Table 37). Meropenem is four times more stable than imipenem against DHP-I of human origin (Table 38).

Porcine and murine DHP-I differ in terms of their biochemical properties. The pig enzyme is inactivated by EDTA and 1,10-phenanthroline, in contrast to that of the mouse. Gdp is hydrolyzed more rapidly by porcine DHP-I than are the carbapenems, in contrast to the enzyme of murine origin. The interpretation of the results in experimental murine infections must take into account this phenomenon.

Takahagi et al. (1991) showed that the hydrolysis of panipenem differs according to the animal species and the tissues. Panipenem is extensively hydrolyzed in the liver in animals and humans, and also in the lung tissue in the rat (Table 39).

The stability of the carbapenems under development or already introduced in clinical practice was tested by Hikida et al. (1992) using DHP-I of porcine and human origin.

Biapenem is the most stable molecule, relative to meropenem, panipenem, and meropenem (Table 40).

The introduction of a hydroxyl group into the carboxypiperazine chain in the molecule DX-8739 increases the stability against DHP-I. At doses of 200, 400, and 800 mg/kg in the rat, no tubular necrosis is observed. This derivative has stability against human DHP-I similar to that of meropenem and is hydrolyzed more by monkey and dog DHP-I than is meropenem.

Lenapenem is more stable against hydrolysis by DHP-I than imipenem and meropenem in vivo, as demonstrated by the lack of effect of cilastatin in experimental murine *P. aeruginosa* infections (Table 40).

Table 36 Stability against hydrolysis by DHP-I and affinity of carbapenems

Drug	Mouse DHP-I		Pig DHP-I	
	K_m (mM)	V_{max} (mmol/g)	K_m (mM)	V_{max} (mmol/g)
Gdp	0.28	100	0.92	100
Imipenem	3.6	74	7	59
1-β-Methyl imipenem	2.7	16	4.9	5.2
Meropenem	5.7	250	11	2.3
Desmethyl meropenem	8.4	1,800	5.8	65
Meropenem analog	1.8	190	53	44

Table 37 Activity of DHP-I against imipenem and meropenem[a]

Animal	Meropenem		Imipenem	
	K_m (mM)	V_{max} (mmol/g)	K_m (mM)	V_{max} (mmol/g)
Mouse	5	5	3	1.6
Rat	3.2	2.8	8.3	8.3
Guinea pig	8.3	0.91	13	14
Rabbit	1.9	5.7	2.8	2.5
Pig	8.3	1	11	11
Dog (beagle)	14	2	17	14
Monkey (rhesus)	10	56	4.8	2.9
Human	2	0.09	6.3	1

[a]Data from Fukasawa et al., 1992.

Table 38 Residual activity of four carbapenems after contact with DHP-I

Drug	% Activity after contact with:			
	Pig DHP-I		Human DHP-I	
	0.25 h	4 h	0.5 h	4 h
Imipenem	0	0	45	0.1
Meropenem	55	0.2	84.8	28.7
Panipenem	13.7	0	66.4	4.3
Biapenem	96.8	73.7	100	95.6

[a]Data from Hikida et al., 1992.

Table 39 Hydrolysis of panipenem by DHP-I[a]

Animal	nmol of panipenem/min/g of tissue		
	Liver	Kidney	Lung
Human		130	10.9
Monkey	348	496	ND[b]
Dog	128	791	35.7
Rabbit	116	854	38.7
Rat	166	569	715
Mouse	20	448	ND

[a]Data from Takahagi et al., 1991.
[b]ND, not determined.

Table 40 In vivo activity (mouse) of carbapenems in the presence of cilastatin in systemic infections due to *P. aeruginosa* BB 5746[a]

Drug	Combination with cilastatin	MIC (μg/ml)	ED_{50} (mg/kg)
Lenapenem	–	0.12	0.27
	+		0.29
Meropenem	–	0.39	6.72
	+		1.42
Imipenem	–	0.39	6.13
	+		0.92

[a]Mice (n = 8) were infected with 2.9×10^5 CFU each (315 50% lethal doses).

Doripenem (Table 41) is much more stable against this hydrolysis than are imipenem and meropenem.

16.1.3. Cilastatin (L-Cysteinylthiohexenoate)

Imipenem is hydrolyzed in the renal tubular cells and causes tubular necrosis in the rabbit and monkey.

DHP-I and the other peptidases of the brush border serve to cleave natural peptides. Research into inhibitors of this enzyme has been directed towards molecules containing the dehydropeptide bond, which have little if any effect on the peptidases acting on the L-L-peptidases.

Among the numerous inhibitors synthesized, the acylamino-(S+)-dimethylcyclopropylamide series has proved the most interesting. Because of the presence of an L-cysteine, the molecule is of a zwitterionic type, which provides maximum inhibitory activity.

The first inhibitor to be selected and used in humans is MK-0789 (Fig. 38); because of the local irritant phenomena found in animals receiving high doses of MK-0789 during toxicity studies, another inhibitor, cilastatin (MK-0791), was selected to be combined with imipenem. MK-0789 has a better affinity for human and porcine DHP-I (IC_{50}, 0.08 and 0.08 μM) than does cilastatin (IC_{50}, 0.11 and 0.13 μM).

In combination with imipenem, cilastatin penetrates the basal membrane of proximal tubule epithelial cells via an anion transporter which is inhibited by probenecid (Fig. 39).

Cilastatin has no antibacterial activity. Combination with imipenem prevents tubular necrosis.

Table 41 Ratio of hydrolysis rate to affinity for DHP-I of doripenem

Animal	V_{max}/K_m ratio		
	Doripenem	Meropenem	Imipenem
Mouse	0.12	0.45	1
Rat	0.18	0.41	1
Guinea pig	0.039	0.08	1
Dog	0.06	0.17	1
Monkey	1.5	4.8	1
Human	0.05	0.12	1

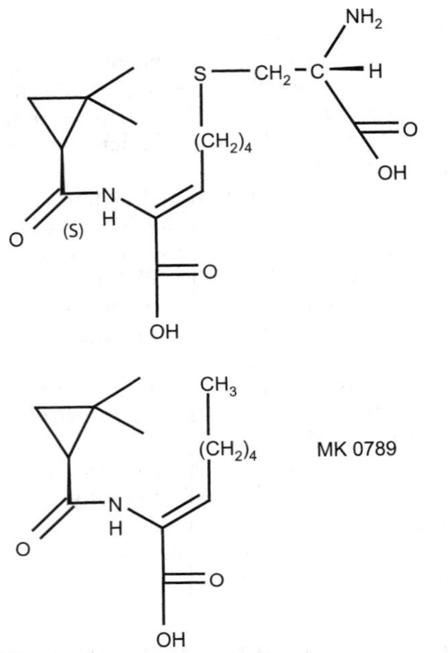

Figure 38 DHP-I inhibitors

16.1.4. Betamipron

Betamipron is *N*-benzyl-β-alanine (Fig. 40). It does not inhibit DHP-I. In vivo, administered simultaneously with panipenem, imipenem, or cephaloridine to albino male rabbits, it prevents necrosis of the proximal tubules (Fig. 41).

Betamipron is secreted by the anion transport system. It protects the renal tubules by inhibiting the transport of panipenem into renal tubular cells (Fig. 42 and 43).

The activities of cilastatin and betamipron are illustrated in Fig. 42.

16.1.5. WS-1358 A_1 and WS-1358 B_1

Two inhibitors of renal DHP-I have been identified in culture filtrates of *Streptomyces parvulus* subsp. *tochigiensis* (Hashimoto

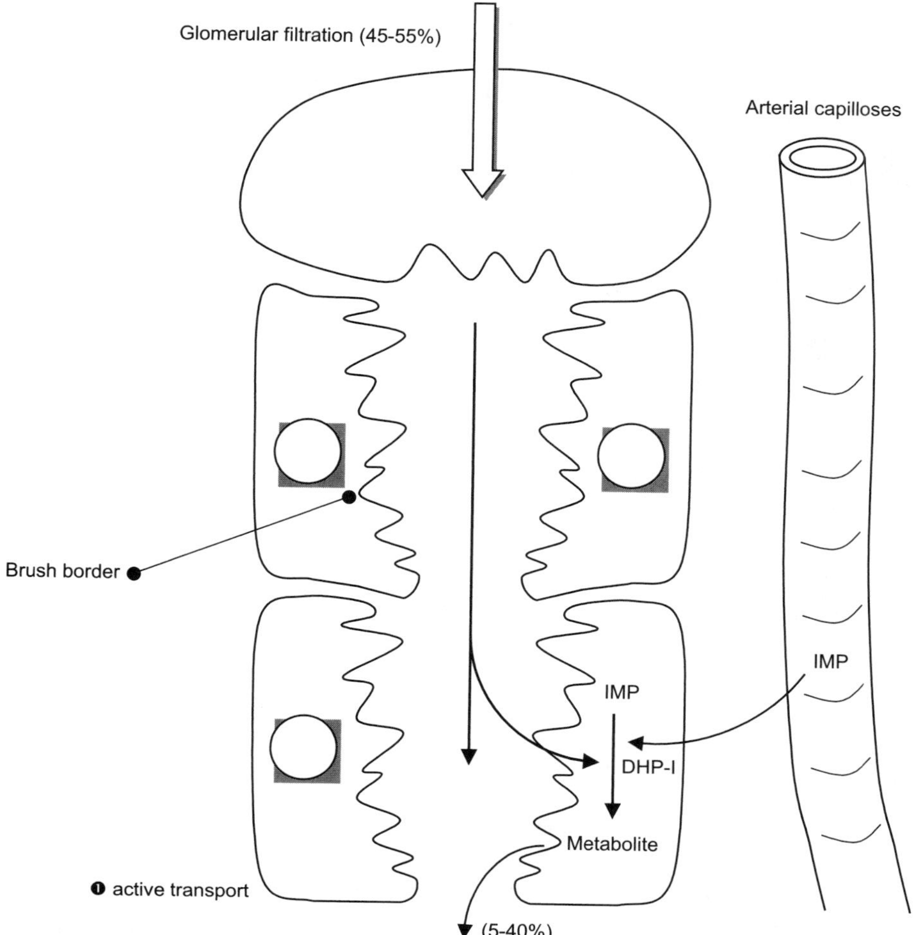

Figure 39 Urinary elimination of imipenem

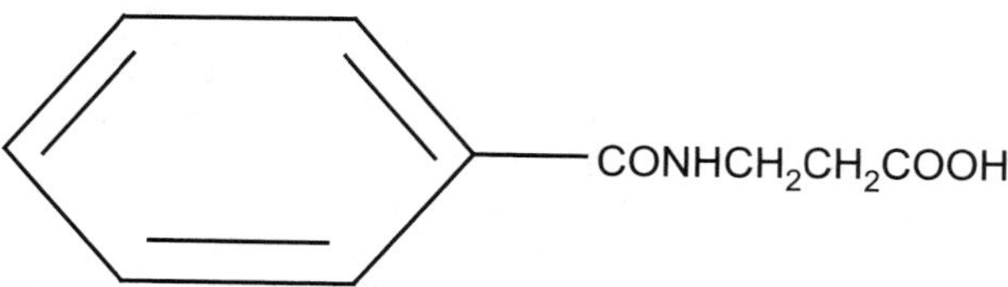

Figure 40 Betamipron

et al., 1990): WS-1358 A_1 (FR-104007) and WS-1358 B_1 (FR-104008). WS-1358 A_1 is 2-hydroxy-2-hydroxyaminocarbonyl-3-methyl glutamic acid, and WS-1358 B_1 is the dimethyl derivative (Fig. 44).

The two derivatives are soluble in water, sparingly soluble in methanol, and insoluble in acetone, chloroform, and *n*-hexane.

WS-1358 A_1 and B_1 inhibit the DHP-I activity of the pig renal cortex. The IC_{50} are 3 and 600 nM, respectively, compared to 130 nM for cilastatin. They are inactive bacteriologically, the intravenous ED_{50} in the mouse being greater than 1,000 mg/kg.

16.2. Neurologic Tolerance of Carbapenems

β-Lactams are known to have proconvulsive activity, particularly penicillins and cephalosporins. For patients with renal insufficiency, convulsive seizures have been reported following administration of imipenem-cilastatin. The development of a penem or a carbapenem must take into account this information. Pharmacological evaluation is difficult. Several methods have been proposed, including that of Schliamser et al. (1988) and that of Rotiroti et al. (1983).

The first method is based on the identification of the neurotoxicity of β-lactams in terms of the epileptogenic threshold in the New Zealand White rabbit. The epileptogenic threshold for imipenem is 86 mg/kg, compared to 486 mg/kg for benzylpenicillin. The concentration of imipenem alone in rabbit cerebrospinal fluid is low, but the concentration in cerebral tissue is high (4.7 ± 9.2 mg/kg) (Table 42).

Williams et al. (1988) showed that imipenem alone or in combination with cilastatin potentiates the convulsive effect of pentylenetetrazole (metrazole) in the Swiss-Webster mouse. This has been confirmed by other authors, who have shown a potentiating effect of doses of 150 mg each of imipenem and cilastatin per kg intravenously (Patel and Giles, 1989; Hikida et al., 1990). At a dose of 150 mg/kg, imipenem causes clonic seizures; the drug becomes fatal above 300 mg/kg. Meropenem and biapenem do not potentiate metrazole, even at doses of 400 and 600 mg/kg intravenously.

The cerebral concentrations of imipenem and biapenem after administration of 50 mg/kg to rats are identical (Table 43).

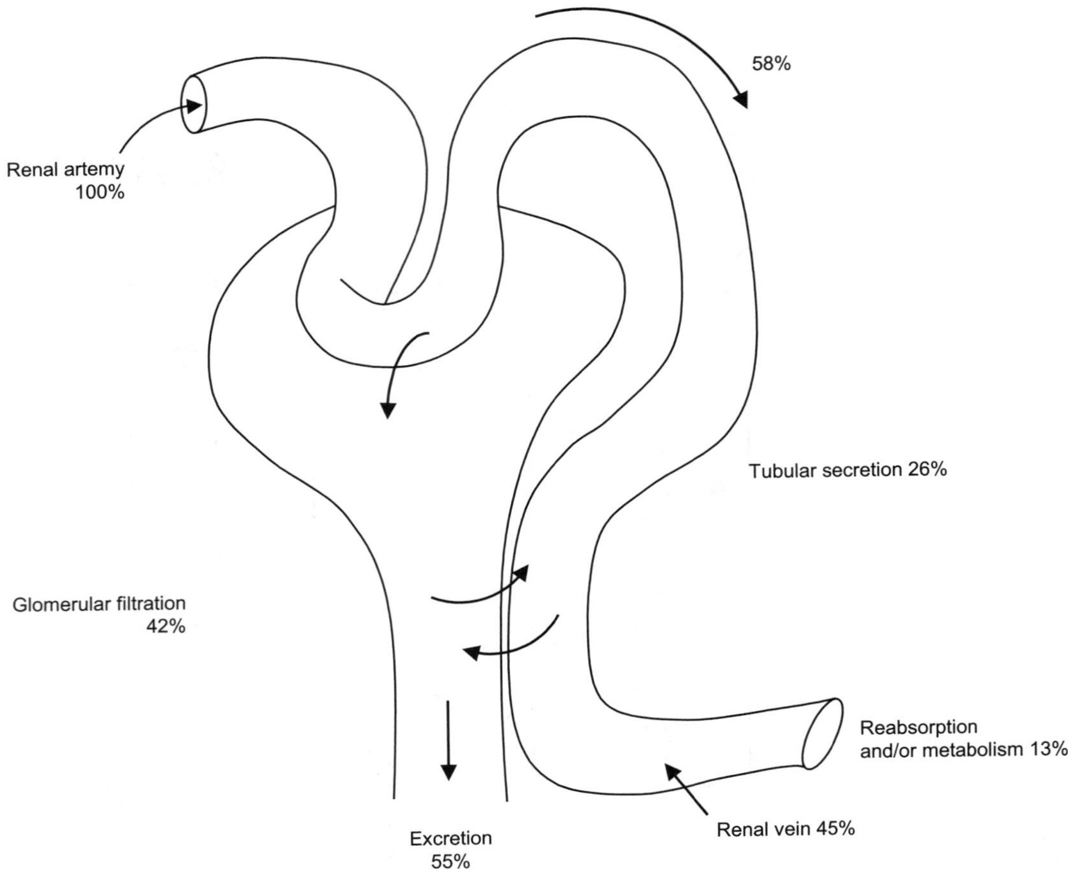

Figure 41 Urinary elimination of panipenem in the rabbit

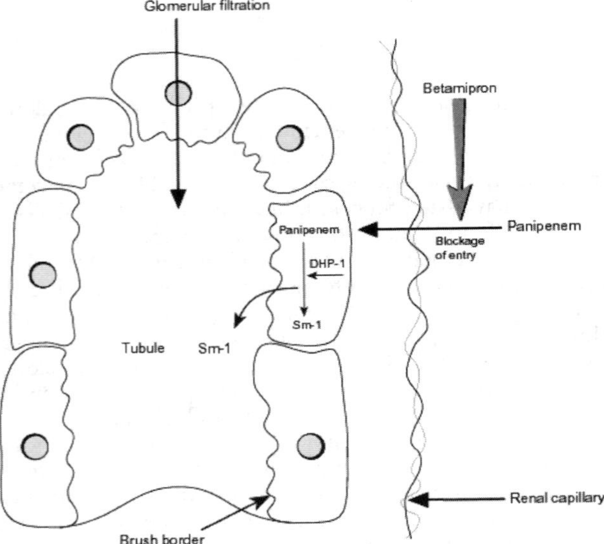

Figure 42 Inhibition of the transport of panipenem by betamipron in the brush cells of the proximal tubules

Imipenem and cefazoline inhibit the binding of [^{3}H]γ-aminobutyric acid to synaptic membranes in the rat brain. Biapenem exhibits only weak inhibitory activity, as does lenapenem.

Sunagawa et al. (1991) have shown that the convulsive properties of carbapenems are dependent on the structure at C-2 but that substituents at C-1 are also involved.

By comparison with meropenem and imipenem at the intracisternal dose of 50 μg per mouse (SIC: ddy), DX-8739 does not cause convulsions, in contrast to imipenem, with which 100% of mice were observed to convulse. At a dose of 150 μg dose per mouse, 45% of the mice had clonic convulsions and 25% had clonic extensions.

Imipenen, panipenem, and cefazoline induce dose-dependent convulsions in mice after intraventricular administration. Five hundred nanomoles of lenapenem caused convulsions in 20% of the mice, compared to doses of 14, 20, and 16 nmol for imipenem, panipenem, and cefazolin, respectively.

17. INDICATIONS FOR CARBAPENEMS

The studies currently available concern imipenem-cilastatin (Tienam) and meropenem (Meronem).

The therapeutic indications are dependent on the antibacterial spectrum and the tissue diffusion of these antibiotics.

Other factors are involved:

- The monomicrobial or polymicrobial features
- The severity of the infection
- The underlying predisposition of the host, particularly immunodepression
- Community or nosocomial acquisition

Carbapenems may be used as monotherapy or in combination, usually with aminoglycosides, to avoid the emergence

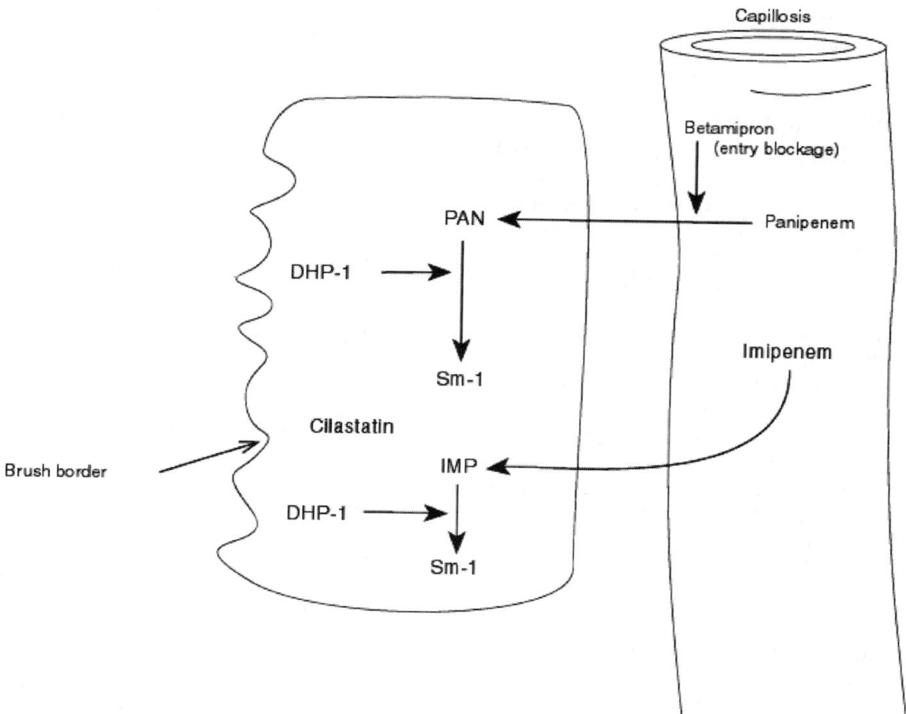

Figure 43 Metabolism of panipenem and imipenem by DHP-I

of resistant strains, increase the killing rate, and/or extend the antibacterial spectrum.

An empirical (probabilist, first-line) procedure is often used in severe life-threatening infections before the bacteria responsible for the infections are identified.

The dosages of imipenem-cilastatin are dependent on the severity of the infection: 1 g every 12 h in infections of moderate severity and up to 4 g daily in severe infections.

R
OH
COOH
COOH
CONHOH

R = CH_3 : WS 1358 A_1 (FR 104007)
R = H : WS 1358 B_1 (FR 104008)

Figure 44 DHP-I inhibitors

Table 42 Pharmacokinetics of carbapenems (dose, 100 mg/kg intravenously) in rabbit cerebrospinal fluid in experimental meningitis due to *S. aureus* 209P[a]

Drug	Concn (μg/ml)			AUC (μg·h/ml)			$t_{1/2}$ (h)
	C_{max}	1 h	2 h	1 h	2 h	3 h	
Imipenem	13.3	11.8	4.55	9.2	14.1	17.7	85.8
Meropenem	4.42	1.9	0.57	10.4	13.9	15.7	50.9
Panipenem	16.2	14.9	3.75	10.9	15.9	19	62.9

[a]Data from Hasuta et al., 1991.

Table 43 Concentrations of carbapenems in rat cerebral tissue

Drug	Dose (mg)[a]	Concn (μg/g)			
		Brain, 5 min	Plasma		
			15 min	5 min	15 min
Imipenem-cilastatin	50/50	0.83	0.64	147.5	87.5
Biapenem	50	0.95	0.65	153.4	94.15
Cefazolin	50	1.32	0.88	200.9	118.2

[a]Given intravenously.

The dosages must be reduced in the case of renal insufficiency. In pediatric patients, the dosages range from 15 to 25 mg/kg every 6 h.

17.1. Mixed Polymicrobial Infections

In intra-abdominal infections (essentially peritonitis), obstetrical or gynecological infections, infections of the cutaneous and subcutaneous tissue, bone and joint infections, and parenchymatous respiratory infections (for which an inhalational mechanism is postulated), the causative bacteria are usually gram-positive cocci, *Enterobacteriaceae*, or anaerobic bacteria (streptococci or *Bacteroides* spp.). The antibacterial spectrum of the carbapenems predicates their use in this type of indication.

During mixed infections, the bacterial flora may be modified by factors related to the host (essentially immunodepression with the risks of colonization by *P. aeruginosa*, etc.), by prior antibiotic therapy, and by the acquisition of resistant strains through cross-transmission during hospitalization. In mixed infections, the carbapenems are preferentially included in the proposed therapeutic regimens.

17.2. Other Infections

Because of the risk of septic shock, bacteremia requires rapid and appropriate empirical treatment. Carbapenems in combination with aminoglycosides are recommended, particularly if these infections are of nosocomial origin.

During febrile episodes in neutropenic patients, carbapenems may be used from the outset or secondarily when another so-called first-line antibiotic therapy has failed to demonstrate efficacy. Use of imipenem-cilastatin as monotherapy has been compared with combinations of cephalosporins and aminoglycosides, with identical results, but the frequency of convulsions in the imipenem-cilastatin group (up to 6%) reduces their use in these indications.

Where severe and of nosocomial origin, pyelonephritis is amenable to treatment by carbapenems.

Despite good diffusion through the blood-brain barrier and its intrinsic activity against the majority of bacteria responsible for meningitis, imipenem-cilastatin is not used in purulent meningitis of bacterial origin because of the adverse neurologic effects (convulsive episodes). Meropenem is currently undergoing evaluation in the treatment of meningitis. Carbapenems are also effective against penicillin G-resistant strains of *S. pneumoniae*.

During the evolution of cystic fibrosis, acute episodes with parenchymatous involvement are due to *P. aeruginosa*, which produces a biofilm, and carbapenems are a therapeutic alternative. However, the risk of selecting a resistant strain is considerable. Their activity against *B. cepacia* is moderate.

17.3. Nosocomial Infections

Nosocomial infections are usually due to resistant bacterial strains. The gram-negative bacteria responsible for this type of infection are usually *Serratia* spp., *Enterobacter* spp., indole-positive *Proteus* spp., *Citrobacter* spp., *P. aeruginosa*, and, more recently, *K. pneumoniae*, the strains of which produce extended-spectrum β-lactamases, and *A. baumannii*, responsible for epidemics. These nosocomial infections have major consequences for hospital morbidity and mortality. Carbapenems are indicated during these infections and are sometimes the only therapeutic resort. Coadministration with aminoglycosides restricts the emergence of resistant strains. Carbapenems are inactive against MRSA or methicillin-resistant strains of coagulase-negative staphylococci and against enterococci responsible for nosocomial infections.

Investigation of new carbapenem derivatives exhibiting anti-MRSA activity is ongoing.

Numerous compounds are at different stages of development; some are already licensed, such as ertapenem (L-749345, MK-0826), or at an exploratory stage. Few of them have reached phase I, or the preclinical stage.

18. ORAL CARBAPENEMS

See Fig. 45.

18.1. Sanfetrinem (GV 104326)

GV 104326 (Fig. 46) from Glaxo belongs to the trinem subclass of carbapenems. Trinems are characterized by a tricyclic system. The third ring could be a five-, six-, or seven-membered-ring carbocycle or heterocycle.

Many compounds have been synthesized with various endocyclic atoms (sulfur, oxygen, and nitrogen) and side chain fixed at the C-4′ position (Fig. 47). For instance, within this subclass of derivatives a series with 4′-amino moiety had been synthesized. Many derivatives with a C-4′ amino tertiary function display good in vitro activity, including enhanced antipseudomonal activity (MIC, 4 μg/ml) for the amino group (NH_2) and the monomethylamino group ($NH\text{-}CH_3$). For other moieties the antipseudomonal activity was weak, such as NH-cyclopropyl or $N\text{-}(CH_3)_2$. Hydrophilic substituents such as amino or ammonium in the C-4′ position improve penetration of the outer membranes of gram-negative bacteria. (Fig. 48).

Trinems with aryl substituents at the C-4′ position have been synthesized by Merck and Sankyo (Fig. 48). These trinems were substituted with all known aryl spacers possessing cationic groups, including naphthosultam (Merck product), benzothiazolylthiomethyl, and pyrrolidinylthiomethyl derivatives. The two latter compounds exhibited MICs of 0.001 to 0.05 μg/ml and 1.5 μg/ml for MSSA and MRSA, respectively.

The relative configuration 4α, 8β represents one of the best compromises in terms of activity and biological stability within trinems.

Sanfetrinem (GV 104326) is esterified to yield the orally available form sanfetrinem cilexetil (GV 118819). The development of this molecule was stopped after phase II.

GV 104326 possesses an α-OCH_3 at position 4′ on the hexyl ring, which gives an enhanced chemical stability against DHP-I in comparison with that of imipenem (seven times).

The 8β position allowed a better stability than the 8α position against DHP-I hydrolysis.

GV 104326 is highly active in vitro and in vivo against gram-positive cocci (Table 44), except MRSA (MIC_{50}, ≥12.5 μg/ml), and moderately active against *Enterococcus* spp. (MIC_{50}, ≥1.56 μg/ml). It displays good activity against *Enterobacteriaceae*, but less against those potentially producing class C β-lactamases (*S. marcescens*, *E. aerogenes*, and *E. cloacae*). It is inactive against *P. aeruginosa* (MIC_{50}, ≥25 μg/ml) and *C. difficile* (MIC_{50}, ≥4.0 μg/ml) (Table 44).

In murine infections, sanfetrinem-cilexetil is more active than imipenem-cilastatin against infections induced by *Enterobacteriaceae* but exhibits activity similar to that of imipenem-cilastatin against gram-positive coccus infections (Table 45).

GV 104326 is stable against hydrolysis by broad-spectrum and PSE β-lactamases, but it is more or less hydrolyzed by TEM-10, an extended-broad-spectrum β-lactamase. GV 104326 lost activity against strains producing zinc-containing

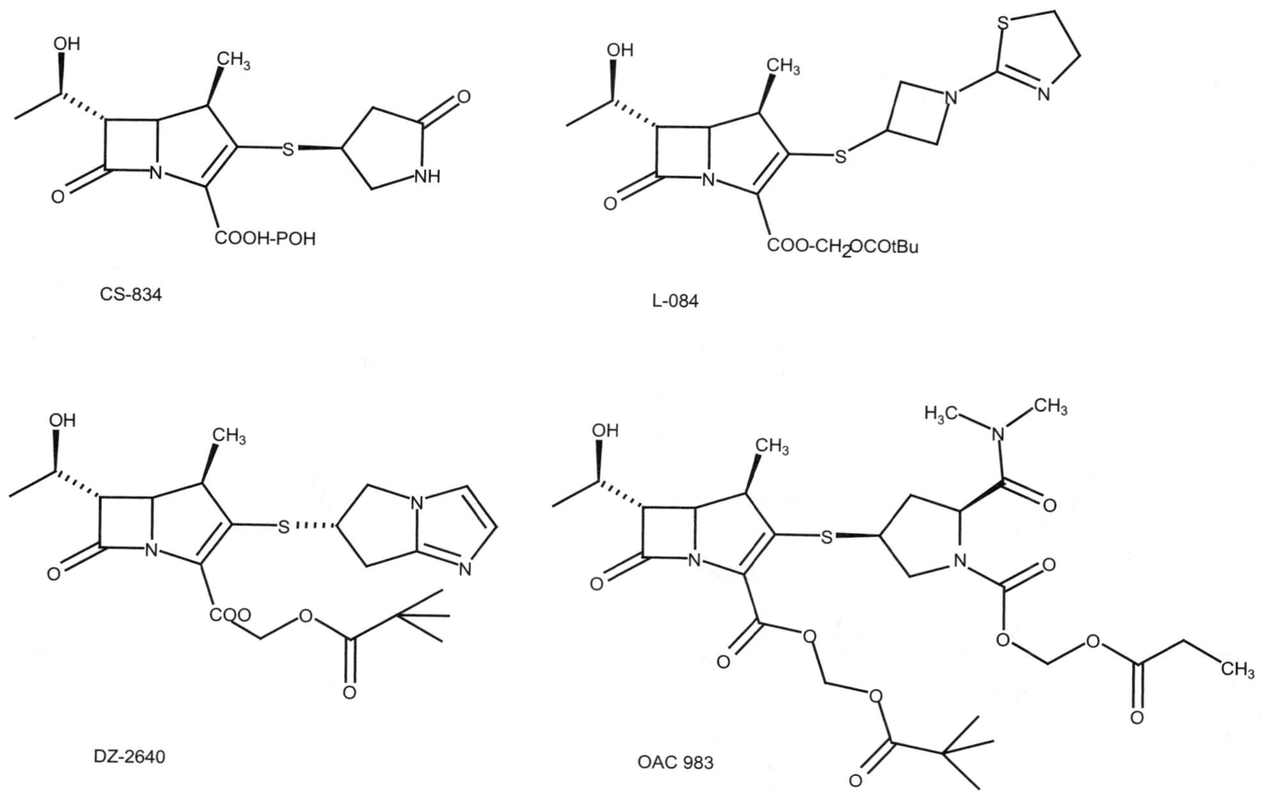

CS-834

L-084

DZ-2640

OAC 983

Figure 45 New oral carbapenems

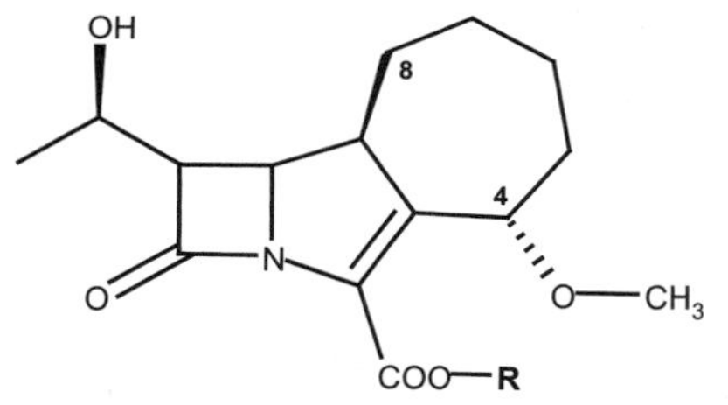

	R
GV 104326 (sanfetrinem sodium)	Na
GV 118819 (sanfetrinem cilexetil)	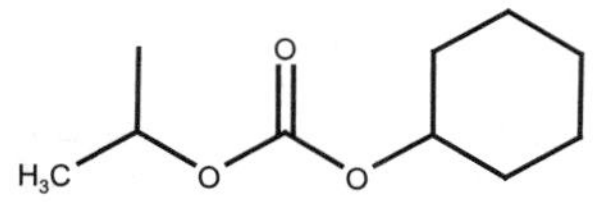

Figure 46 Oral trinems GV 104326 and GV 118819

enzymes (class B). It is hydrolyzed by class A (Sme-1) and class B (IMP-1) carbapenemases.

18.2. DZ 2640 and DU-6681

DZ 2640 is an oral carbapenem obtained by esterification of the carboxyl group with a pivaloyloxymethyl (POM) chain (Fig. 49) (Kawamoto et al., 1996).

DZ 2640 is a prodrug of DU-6681. The C-2 side chain is composed of a bicyclic imidazolyl ring. The position of the two nitrogen atoms influences the in vitro activity of these derivatives, as well as the stereochemistry due to the chiral center. However, all of them display good in vitro activity (Fig. 50).

DU-6681 is the (*S*)-isomer, which exhibits a two-fold-higher potency than the (*R*)-isomer against both gram-positive and gram-negative bacteria. The nonsubstituted bicyclic ring (imidazolyl) is more active than the substituted ring, whatever the substituent fixes on the nitrogen or the carbon atoms.

The pharmacokinetics are also influenced by the nitrogen location in the ring as well as the stereochemistry. In rats, the (*S*)-isomer shows phamacokinetics different from those of the (*R*)-isomer (Fig. 51).

In this series it was shown that the POM ester and the isopoxycarboxylethyl ester showed good bioavailability among the various proposed esters (Fig. 50).

The in vitro activity of DU-6681 is not affected by various culture media, namely, Mueller-Hinton agar, nutrient agar, heart infusion agar, brain-heart infusion agar, and Trypticase soy agar. The alteration of pH, the size of the inoculum (10^4 to 10^7 CFU/ml), and human serum do not affect MICs.

The frequencies of spontaneous mutants are summarized in Table 46.

The in vitro activity in comparison with those of fropenem (faropenem) and R-95867 is listed in Table 47.

Time-kill studies showed a rapid bactericidal effect against *S. aureus*, *S. pneumoniae*, and *E. coli*.

DU-6681 is not hydrolyzed by class A enzymes but is hydrolyzed by class B enzymes such as L1 of *S. maltophilia*. DU-6681 is not stable against class C hydrolysis.

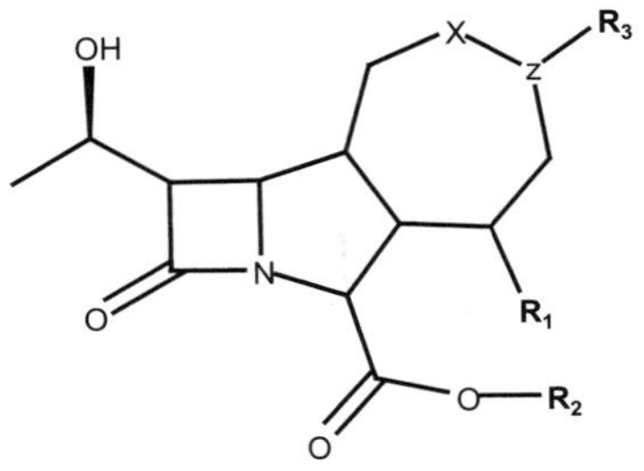

Compounds from	R_2	R_1	R_3	X	Z
Sanfetrinem sodium	Na	OCH_3	H	CH_2	CH_2
Glaxo-Wellcome (1)	Na	$O(CH_2)_2$-$N(CH_3)_3$	H	CH_2	CH_2
Glaxo-Wellcome (2)	Na	-S-CH_3	H	CH_2	CH_2
Glaxo-Wellcome (3)	Na	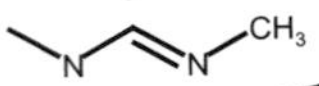 N N CH_3	H	CH_2	CH_2
Glaxo-Wellcome (4)	Na	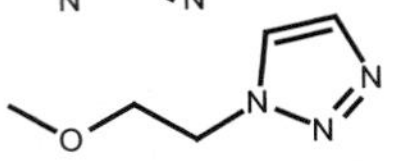 O N N N	H	CH_2	CH_2
Glaxo-Wellcome (5)	Na	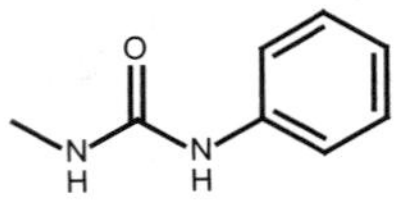 O N H N H	H	CH_2	CH_2
Glaxo-Wellcome (6)	Na	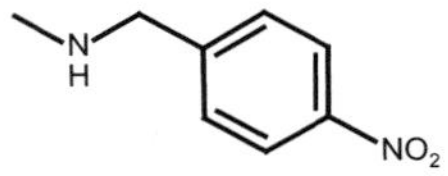 N H NO_2	H	CH_2	CH_2
Montreal University	Na	H	-OCH_3	CH_2	CH_2
Takeda (1)	Na	H	H	O	CH_2
Takeda (2)	Na	OH	H	O	CH_2
Takeda (3)	Na	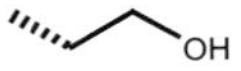 OH	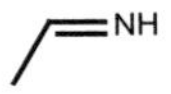 NH	O	CH_2
Takeda (4)	Na	OCH_3	H	CH_2	S

Figure 47 Tricyclic trinems

18.3. CS-834

CS-834 is the prodrug of R-95867 by esterification of the carboxylic moiety. This is a 1-β-methyl carbapenem with an (*R*)-5-oxopyrrolidinylthio chain at position 2. The ester at position 3 is a POM chain (Fig. 52).

The chemical instability was a major obstacle for the development of oral carbapenems. The 1-β-methyl substitution of carbapenem compounds improving this stability allowed the development of such derivatives.

Miyauguchi et al. (1997) have synthesized series of 1-β-methyl carbapenems with a variety of C-2 side chains. They discovered that a C-2 amide group resulted in compounds with high antibacterial activity and stability against DHP-I.

Among them, CS-834, with a POM ester at C-4, was selected for further development.

It was shown that compounds with only a phenyl moiety are active only against gram-positive bacteria. Compounds with a carboxamide group display better in vitro activities against gram-negative organisms but are poorly active against *Enterobacteriaceae* which produce class C β-lactamases. Compounds having an alkylcarboxamide are more potent against gram-negative bacteria but less against gram-positive bacteria.

The best antibacterial activity, excluding against *P. aeruginosa*, was achieved when a five-membered cyclic amide system was introduced at the C-2 position depending on the pyrrolidinyl position of the oxo function. When the five-membered cyclic amide system is present at the C-2 position, the resulting compound is weakly active; when the system is present at the C-5′ position of the pyrrolidinyl ring, the resulting compound exhibits potent activity against gram-positive and gram-negative bacteria. The (*R*)-isomer is slightly more active than the (*S*)-isomer. The 1-H counterpart of the (*R*)-isomer of the 5-oxo analog exerts the same antibacterial activity. This compound seems to be slightly more potent in vitro than GV 104326.

A stereoselective effect of the chiral center in the C-2 side chain was observed in urinary recovery. The urinary recovery of the (*R*)-isomer was only 46%. Simultaneous administration of cilastatin with the (*S*)-isomer resulted in enhanced urinary recovery, equal to that of the (*R*)-isomer.

The degradation rate by mouse DHP-I was lower for the (*R*)-isomer than for the (*S*)-isomer. The urinary recovery of the 1-H carbapenem analog was only 8% (Table 48).

In order to optimize the oral absorption of the (*R*)-isomer, several ester derivatives were prepared. The oral absorption of these prodrugs was evaluated using urinary elimination as a parameter in mice.

Among them, the POM urinary recovery was 47% and the 1-methylcyclohexylcarbamoyloxymethyl analog had a 55% urinary recovery.

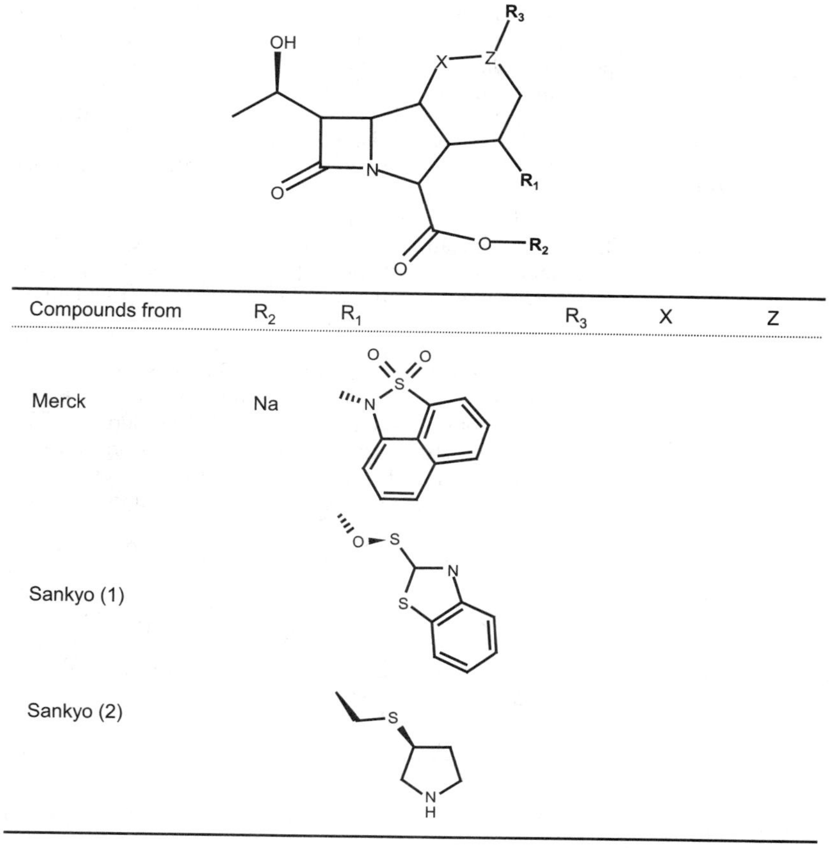

Compounds from	R_2	R_1	R_3	X	Z
Merck	Na				
Sankyo (1)					
Sankyo (2)					

Figure 48 Tricyclic trinems

The most promising compounds were selected for pharmacokinetic analysis, which was conducted in dogs; the best profile was obtained with POM.

18.4. TA-949

TA-949 is a 1-substituted carbapenem (Fig. 53) having at the C-2 position an (*R*)-pyrrolidine-2-thion-4ylthio group and an isobutyryloxy methyl ester on the C-3 carboxylic group. No data on the antibacterial activity are available. It would be of interest to have these data due to the original substituent in position 1.

18.5. KR 21,056

A series of 1-β-methyl carbapenems with another C-2 side chain has been synthesized. One compound was selected for further development, KR 21,056 (Fig. 54).

KR 21,012 possesses in C-2α an (*R*)-isopropyl chain (Fig. 54). It seems highly stable against porcine DHP-I hydrolysis, and the apparent half-life of degradation is above 5 h, as for sanfetrinem (for imipenem, the half-life is 0.55 h). A POM prodrug (KR 21,056) has been prepared to allow oral absorption.

KR 21,012 is a broad-spectrum oral carbapenem. It covers gram-positive cocci and *Enterobacteriaceae*. It is inactive against *P. aeruginosa*. It is as active as fropenem (also known as faropenem), an oral penem, against gram-positive cocci, but it is two to three times more active than fropenem against *Enterobacteriaceae*. It is active against *E. coli* producing class A β-lactamases (not specified) and class C enzymes produced by *E. cloacae* P99 and 1194E, like fropenem and sanfetrinem. In disseminated mouse (ICR mice) infections, KR 21,012 is more active than sanfetrinem and fropenem against *S. aureus* Y-80-1953 and *E. coli* 078 and equally as active as sanfetrinem, but KR 21,012 is more active than fropenem, against *S. pyogenes* A-77 and *E. cloacae* M501.

In mice after a 40-mg/kg single dose, administered subcutaneously, the apparent elimination half-lives are 0.69, 0.55, and 0.27 h for KR 21,012, sanfetrinem, and fropenem, respectively, with areas under the curve of 20.9, 27.39, and 10.01 μg·h/ml, respectively. Urinary recoveries at 24 h were 25.1, 20.5, and 12.2%, respectively.

Preliminary toxicological data showed good tolerance in mice and rabbits.

18.6. L-084

A series of 1-β-methyl carbapenems has been synthesized at Lederle (Japan) in order to obtain an orally absorbed compound. It had been shown that compounds having lipophilic and less basic C-2 side chains have an enhanced oral absorption but are less active.

LJC-11036 is a new esterified 1-β-methyl carbapenem which exhibits excellent in vitro activity, superior or equal to that of imipenem, and could be of interest as an oral β-lactam antibiotic.

LJC-11036 is stable against DHP-I hydrolysis. After incubation at 30°C for 4 h, the residual amount of LJC-11036 decreased only about 11% from the initial amount, while imipenem decreased by 50% after 1 h of incubation.

LJC-11036 has a 1-(1,3-thiazol-2-yl) azetidin-3-ylthio group at the C-2 position and an esterified POM group

(L-084). It is more active than imipenem against gram-positive cocci, but it is weakly active against enterococci. It is more active than imipenem against *Enterobacteriaceae* and *H. influenzae*, but it is poorly active against *P. aeruginosa*.

Table 44 In vitro activity of sanfetrinem (GV 104326)

Organism[a]	*n*	MIC (μg/ml) 50%	MIC (μg/ml) 90%
MSSA	32	0.05	0.05
MRSA	33	0.125	100
MSSE	38	0.05	0.39
MRSE	32	3.13	50
S. pyogenes	32	≤0.006	0.012
S. pneumoniae Pen[s]	28	≤0.006	0.012
S. pneumoniae Pen[r]	21	0.1	0.2
S. agalactiae	24	0.025	0.05
E. faecalis	30	1.56	1.56
E. faecium	28	1.56	3.13
E. avium	30	1.56	25
E. coli	41	0.39	0.78
K. pneumoniae	40	0.2	1.56
C. freundii	64	0.78	3.13
E. cloacae	38	1.56	6.25
E. aerogenes	40	1.56	6.25
S. marcescens	50	3.13	12.5
P. mirabilis	40	0.2	0.39
P. vulgaris	40	0.2	0.39
Providencia rettgeri	37	0.78	3.13
M. morganii	38	0.78	6.25
P. aeruginosa	40	25	100
Acinetobacter calcoaceticus	41	0.78	1.56
H. influenzae	52	0.1	0.78
M. catarrhalis	45	0.025	0.1
N. gonorrhoeae	18	0.05	0.1
C. difficile	13	4	8
B. fragilis	34	0.06	0.25
C. perfringens	20	≤0.0015	0.03

[a]MSSE, methicillin-susceptible *S. epidermidis*; MRSE, methicillin-resistant *S. epidermidis*.

LJC-11036 exhibits good in vitro activity against *E. coli* producing class A or C β-lactamases, including extended-spectrum β-lactamases. It is two to four times more active than imipenem. It is poorly active against *E. coli* producing class B enzyme (IMP-1). LJC-11036 showed no inducibility capacity for a class C β-lactamase (*E. cloacae* KU69).

LJC-11036 is more active than imipenem against *Peptostreptococcus* spp., *C. difficile* (MIC_{50}, 2 μg/ml), *Clostridium perfringens*, *Veillonella* spp., *B. fragilis*, and other *Bacteroides* spp. and shows activity comparable to that of imipenem against *Prevotella* spp., *Porphyromonas* spp., and *Fusobacterium nucleatum*. LJC-11036 inhibits β-lactamase activity produced by *B. fragilis*.

L-084 issued from research of compounds having less basic side chains and esterification of the C-3 carboxylic group. L-084 is the prodrug of LJC-11036, by esterification of the 4-carboxylic group of the penem ring with a POM group (Fig. 55).

In a phase I study, after a single ascending oral dose of 25 to 200 mg, a linear dose response was observed between 25 and 150 mg. The mean peak concentrations in plasma ranged from 1.27 ± 0.62 μg/ml (25 mg) to 5.93 ± 2.16 μg/ml (200 mg), with areas under the curve of 0.90 ± 0.12 μg·h/ml

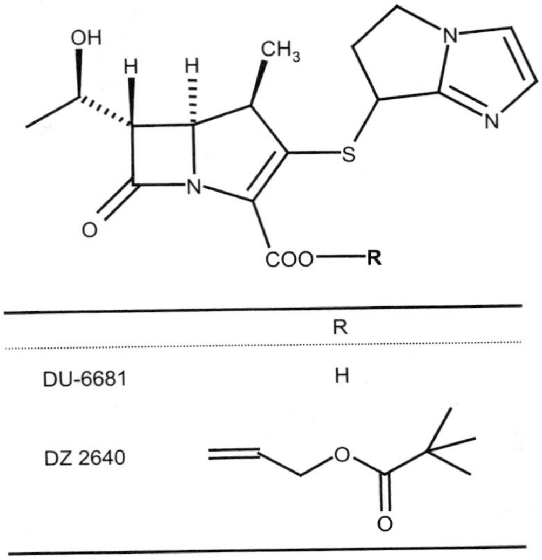

	R
DU-6681	H
DZ 2640	

Figure 49 DU-6681 and DZ 2640

Table 45 In vivo activity of sanfetrinem (GV 104326)

Challenge strain	Dose/mouse (CFU)	Antibiotic	ED_{50} (mg/kg)	MIC (μg/ml)
S. aureus 663E	2×10^4	Sanfetrinem	0.2	0.2
		Imipenem	0.1	0.1
S. aureus 853 E	3.6×10^7, β^+	Sanfetrinem	0.3	0.2
		Imipenem	0.1	0.1
S. pneumoniae 157E	1.2×10^6	Sanfetrinem	0.02	<0.01
		Imipenem	0.02	<0.01
E. coli 851E	1.2×10^4	Sanfetrinem	0.2	0.5
		Imipenem	0.4	0.5
K. pneumoniae 1977E	2.1×10^5	Sanfetrinem	0.5	1.0
		Imipenem	0.7	2.0
P. mirabilis 1315 E	9×10^5	Sanfetrinem	0.5	1.0
		Imipenem	6.2	4.0
M. morganii 1375 E	6×10^5	Sanfetrinem	0.2	2.0
		Imipenem	1.2	4.0
C. freundii 3374	3.6×10^7	Sanfetrinem	1.6	4.0
		Imipenem	1.6	2.0

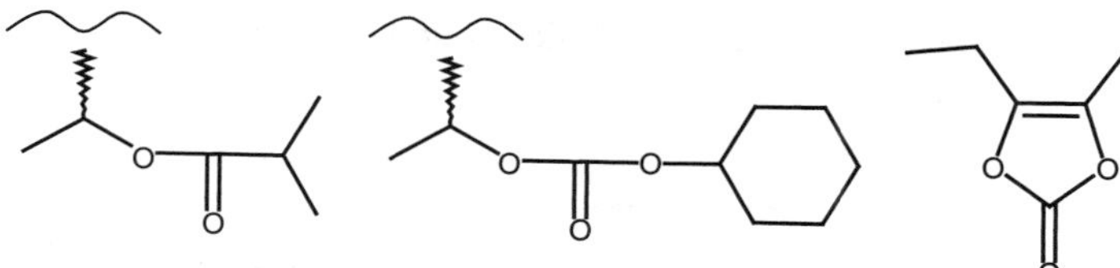

	DZ 2640	DZ 2640 + HCl salt	HCl salt	HCl salt	HCl salt
Cmax (µg/ml)	5.23	7.27	7.66	3.39	0.59
AUC (µg.h/ml)	4.94	5.04	5.06	3.41	0.22
Urinary elimination (%)	24.6	30.40	22.20	17.30	2.80

Figure 50 Esters of DU-6681

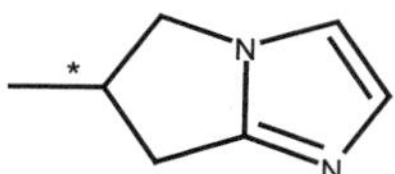
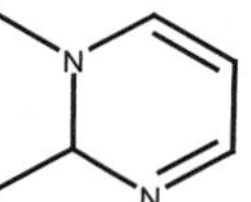
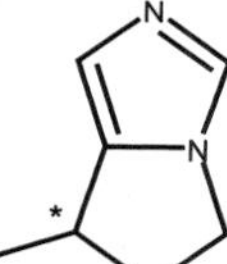

	DZ 2640	R-isomer	S-isomer	R-isomer	S-isomer	R-isomer
Cmax (µg/ml)	5.23	3.48	3.83	2.20	19.88	7.00
AUC (µg.h/ml)	4.84	2.77	2.98	1.89	17.44	4.09
Urinary elimination (%)	24.6	11.2	15.8	12.2	18.5	14.90
DHP-I **	6.0	12.0	0.3	1.0	1.0	2.00

* Chiral center
** Hydrolysis relative to imipenem (100)

Figure 51 Pharmacokinetics of DZ 2640 and derivatives in the rat

Table 46 Spontaneous mutants

Drug	Frequency of mutants
DU-6681	3.2×10^{-7}
Cefdinir	1.1×10^{-6}
Cefpodoxime	7×10^{-6}

(25 mg) to 7.03 ± 1.14 µg·h/ml (200 mg). The apparent elimination half-lives ranged from 0.28 to 0.43 h. The urinary elimination is predominant, with 63 to 73% of the administered doses recovered in urine. A metabolite was identified in urine that represents 10% of the eliminated compound.

The ester side chain is metabolized in pivalic acid, leading to a net decrease of L-carnitine. This is a well-known adverse effect due to the POM side chain. Usually the metabolism of this side chain yields pivalic acid and formylaldehyde; the level of the latter metabolite was not given in this presentation.

In murine (CBA/JNCrj mice) pneumococcal pneumonia, L-084 is more active than fropenem, oral cephalosporins, and amoxicillin, with ED_{50} of 1.96 mg/kg, versus 20 mg/kg.

18.7. OCA-983

A novel series of aminomethyl tetrahydrofuranylthio (THF) 1-β-methyl carbapenem peptide prodrugs has been synthesized to enhance oral absorption relative to that of the parent compounds. Several different amino acids have been appended to the aminomethyl THF residue. Prodrugs with amino acids showed improved oral absorption, while the D-forms were poorly active. Prodrugs with alanine, valine, isoleucine, and phenylalanine substituents have the best oral efficacy in murine infections.

A series of 1-β-methylcarbapenems containing a 2-aminomethylene-substituted THF side chain was synthesized and reported in 1994 (Fig. 56). The aim of this series of 1-β-methylcarbapenem analogs was to obtain derivatives with enhanced activity against gram-negative bacilli and with oral activity, both mediated through the use of the peptide transport system. A double ester prodrug has been prepared, and it is transported through the phospholipid bilayer.

An effort was initiated to produce synthetic peptidic prodrugs of these carbapenem derivatives by addition of amino acids at the aminomethyl group of each selected carbapenem molecule in an attempt to improve oral absorption and efficacy through the di- and tripeptide transport system. The pure diastereoisomer CL-191121 was extensively esterified with different amino acids: alanine, valine, isoleucine, and phenylalanine.

The efficacies of CL-191121 and the four prodrug analogs were evaluated in a murine (female CD-1 mice, 20 ± 2 g) model of disseminated infections induced by *Enterobacteriaceae* (including strains producing broad- and extended-broad-spectrum β-lactamases) *S. aureus* Smith, and *S. pneumoniae* isolates susceptible or resistant to penicillin G.

Table 47 In vitro activities of oral carbapenems

Organism(s)[a]	*n*	MIC$_{50}$ (μg/ml)			
		DU-6681	R-95867	LJC-11036	Fropenem
S. pneumoniae Pen^s	33	≤0.008	≤0.008	≤0.006	≤0.008
PRSP	19	0.03	0.06	0.05	0.06
H. influenzae β$^-$	12	0.015	0.03	0.05	0.12
H. influenzae β$^+$	28	0.03	0.06		0.25
M. catarrhalis	25	0.03	0.06	0.025	0.25
MSSA	39	0.03	0.12	0.025	0.12
MRSA	58	8	64	6.25	>128
MSSE	33	0.015	0.06	0.1	0.06
MRSE	28	1	32		32
S. pyogenes	29	≤0.008	0.015	≤0.006	0.015
E. avium	13	8	32		8
E. faecalis	28	4	16		2
E. faecium	26	128	>128		>128
Enterococcus raffinosus	13	64	128		128
E. coli	31	≤0.008	0.015	≤0.025	1
K. pneumoniae	28	0.015	0.015	≤0.025	0.5
S. marcescens	23	0.12	0.5	0.39	8
E. cloacae	22	0.03	0.25	0.05	4
E. aerogenes	23	0.03	0.25		2
C. freundii	22	0.03	0.12		2
P. vulgaris	21	0.12	0.12		2
P. mirabilis	22	0.06	0.12	0.39	2
M. morganii	22	0.25	0.5		2
P. rettgeri	21	0.12	0.12		2
A. baumannii	10	2	0.5		8
P. aeruginosa	31	16	32	6.25	>32
V. cholerae	25	0.12	0.12		1
Vibrio parahaemolyticus	25	≤0.008	≤0.008		0.06
Salmonella spp.	9	≤0.008	0.015		
Shigella spp.	5	≤0.008	0.015		
S. maltophilia	23	>100			>100

[a]β$^-$, non-β-lactamase producing; β$^+$, β-lactamase producing; MSSE, methicillin-susceptible *S. epidermidis*; MRSE, methicillin-resistant *S. epidermidis*.

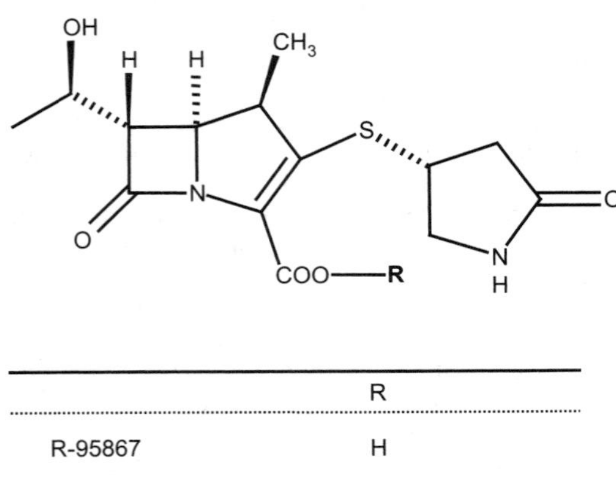

Figure 52 CS-834

The parent compound, CL-191121, nonesterified, possesses good in vivo efficacy when administered subcutaneously, but a modest efficacy after oral administration due to poor enteral absorption. Peptidic derivatives (alanine and valine) were strongly active against all challenging strains, including those producing extended-broad-spectrum β-lactamases. These increasing oral efficiencies can be attributed to an increasing level of circulating parent compound in serum.

CL-191121 is less active in vitro than meropenem against *Enterobacteriaceae*, especially against *Enterobacter* spp., *Morganella morganii*, *P. mirabilis*, *Providencia* spp., and *S. marcescens* (MIC$_{90}$, ≥2.0 μg/ml). It is as active as imipenem against gram-positive cocci, including *S. pneumoniae* isolates, irrespective to their susceptibility to penicillin G. CL-191121 is hydrolyzed by metallo-β-lactamases. It has the same stability as imipenem against hydrolysis by serine β-lactamases, but CL-191121 has an enhanced stability to Sme-1 and Imi-1 in comparison with that of imipenem.

CL-191121 is highly stable against hydrolysis by human renal dehydropeptidase, with a relative rate of hydrolysis of 4.4, versus 100 for imipenem. However, the relative hydrolysis rate is comparable to that of meropenem (4.4, versus 5.3 for meropenem) and higher than that observed with biapenem (4.4, versus 1.7 for biapenem).

CL-191121 esterified with a valine residue (Fig. 57), OCA-983, was selected for further investigation.

In preliminary pharmacokinetic analysis (ascending dose) of OCA-983, after administration of 100- to 800-mg oral doses to volunteers, peak concentrations in plasma ranged from 0.8 μg/ml (100 mg) to 3.5 μg/ml (800 mg), with areas

Table 48 Urinary recovery of R-95867 in mice

1-β-Methyl carbapenem	Urinary recovery (%)		DHP-I degradation rate
	Without cilastatin	With cilastatin	
(*R*)-Isomer (R-83201)	75	84	1.0
(*S*)-Isomer	46	78	3.3
1-H carbapenem	8	64	14.2

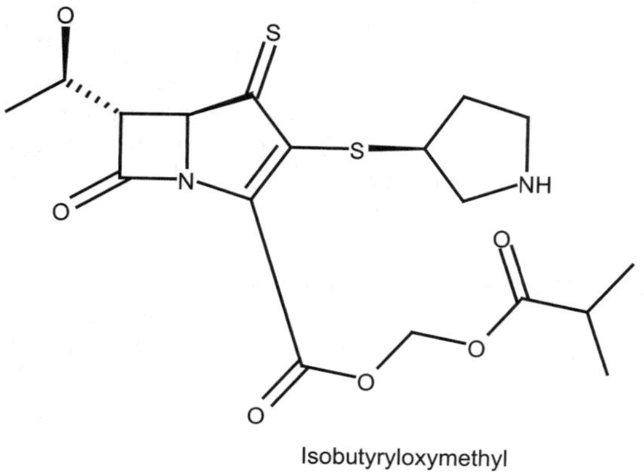

Isobutyryloxymethyl

Figure 53 TA-949

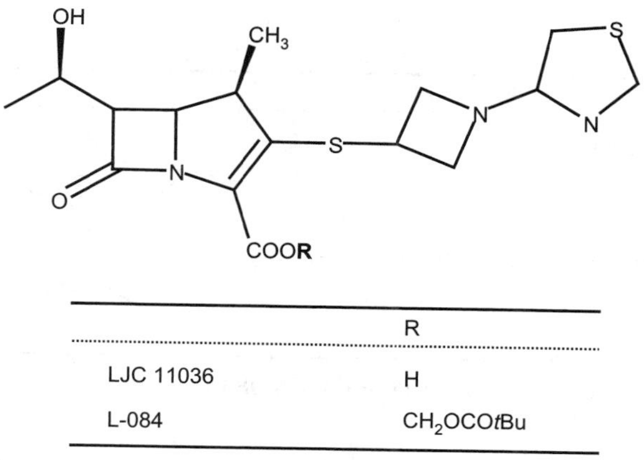

	R
KR 21012	H
KR 21056	

Figure 54 KR 21,056

	R
LJC 11036	H
L-084	$CH_2OCOtBu$

Figure 55 L-084 and LJC-11036

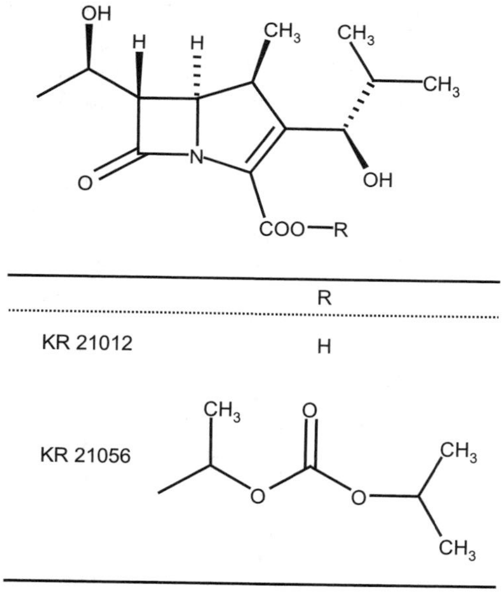

	R
CL 188 624	
CL 190 294	
CL 191 121	

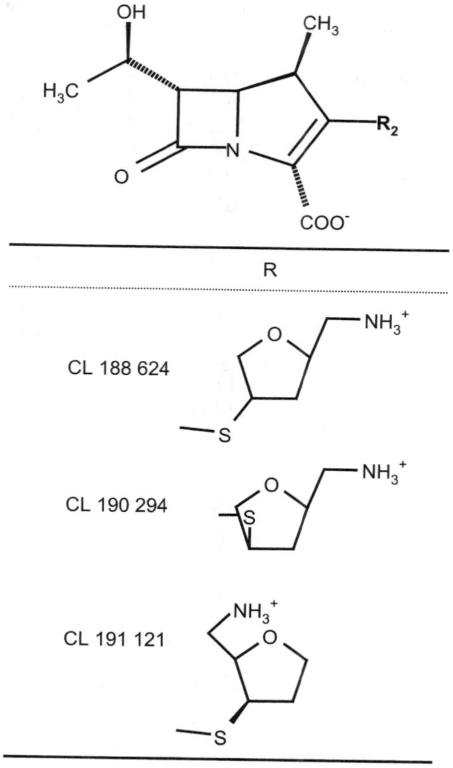

Figure 56 THF carbapenems

under the curve of 2.34 (100 mg) to 13.5 μg·h/ml (800 mg). The apparent elimination half-life was 1.4 h.

18.8. Pharmacokinetics of Oral Carbapenems

Today all of the oral carbapenems are prodrugs, and for a 100-mg oral dose the maximum concentration of the parent compound in serum (C_{max}) ranged from 0.97 μg/ml (CS-834) to 4.06 μg/ml (L-084), with an apparent elimination half-life of ≤1 h. The parent compound is eliminated mainly in urine (Table 49).

The urinary elimination of DU-6681 is extremely rapid and is almost completed after 4.0 h.

Plasma protein binding rates 2 and 4 h after oral administration of a single dose of 200 mg were 25.6 and 23.3%, respectively.

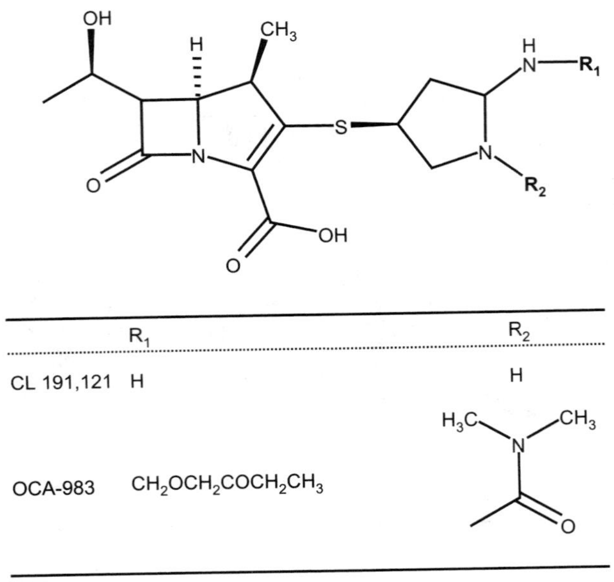

	R_1	R_2
CL 191,121	H	H
OCA-983	$CH_2OCH_2COCH_2CH_3$	

Figure 57 CL-191121 and OCA-983

After intravenous dosing with GV 104326 (infusion over 30 min), the plasma clearance ranged from 359 to 1,000 ml/min and the renal clearance ranged from 237 to 345 ml/min. The intact ester form is not detected in plasma and is rapidly eliminated, explaining the short elimination half-life (0.68 to 1.67 h for a 4-g single dose).

The oral absorption of DZ 2640 is slightly delayed by food (Table 50).

The pharmacokinetics of sanfetrinem-cilexetil were assessed in a pediatric population of patients, as were concentration of the compound in the middle ear fluid (MEF) of patients suffering from otitis media. The mean C_{max} is 0.3 μg/ml (0.1 to 4.6 μg/ml), which is reached 1.0 h after a 10-mg/kg dose of sanfetrinem-cilexetil. In MEF after 1 h the mean concentration was 0.9 μg/ml (0.09 to 2.56 μg/ml). The sanfetrinem level in MEF was assayed after 6 h for only one patient and was 0.1 μg/ml.

18.9. Other Oral Carbapenems

A series of double ester 2-pyrrolidinyl 1-β-methylcarbapenems for oral use has been produced (Fig. 58). CL-191121 demonstrated some oral activity, with an ED_{50} of 2 to 4 g/kg against *E. coli* infection in mice.

Table 49 Pharmacokinetics of ascending doses of oral carbapenems

Compound	Dose (mg)	*n*	C_{max} (μg/ml)	T_{max} (h)	AUC (μg·h/ml)	$t_{1/2}$ (h)	Urinary elimination (%)
GV 104326/GV 118819 (sanfetrinem)	250	4	1.16	0.68	2.55	1.0	31.95
	500	12	3.53	0.75	6.68	1.29	26.35
	1,000	12	4.21	0.75	11.16	2.34	21.83
	2,000	8	6.91	0.63	14.48	2.31	16.49
CS-834 (R-95867)	50	6	0.51	1.08	0.94	0.76	30
	100	6	0.97	1.25	1.91	0.73	32.5
	200	6	1.59	1.38	3.30	0.77	27.2
	400	6	2.51	1.67	6.61	0.66	33.5
L-084 (LJC-11036)	25		1.27	0.51	0.90	0.28	67.8
	50		2.13	0.61	1.83	0.42	69.1
	75		2.75	0.54	2.18	0.38	54
	100		4.06	0.50	3.47	0.41	72
	150		5.85	0.58	5.57	0.50	73.4
	200		5.93	0.72	7.03	0.43	63
OCA-983 (CL-191121)	25	6		0.9		0.28	63
	100	6	0.8	1.42	2.34	1.4	
	200	6	1.6	1.58	4.37	1.3	73
	400	6	2.7	1.58	8.5	1.3	
	800	6	3.5	2.2	13.5	1.4	
DZ 2640 (DU-6681)	25	6	0.26	1.0	0.302	0.47	34.9
	50	6	0.68	1.08	0.779	0.59	44.9
	100	6	1.0	1.38	1.534	0.69	37.5
	200	6	2.0	1.13	3.128	0.89	38.9
	400	6	2.5	1.42	5.093	0.71	31.9

Table 50 Influence of food on pharmacokinetics

Drug	Dose (mg)	Status	C_{max} (μg/ml)	T_{max} (h)	AUC (μg·h/ml)	Urinary elimination (%)
DZ 2640	100	Fasting	1.09	1.05	1.713	72
	100	Fed	0.93	1.5	1.565	73
L-084	100	Fasting	0.82	1.56	1.65	34.1
	100	Fed	0.95	1.50	2.00	32.0

Compound	C log P	R_1	R_2	SOD	SCD	Ratio SOD/SSC
				ED$_{50}$ (mg/kg) *E. coli* 311		
A 1	1.28	CH_2OCOPr	$CH_2OCOOEt$	0.56	0.40	1.40
2	2.04	CH_2OCOPr	CH_2OCOBu	1.60	1.90	0.84
3	1.89	CH_2OCOPr	CH(Me)OCOOPr	1.40	2.10	0.67
4	3.09	CH_2OCOPr	$CH_2OCOOC_6H_{10}$	1.50	1.90	0.78
5	0.75	CH(Me)OAc	$CH_2OCOOEt$	0.83	0.59	1.40
6	1.50	CH_2OCOPr	$CH_2OCOOEt$	1.30	0.49	2.60
7	1.58	CH(Me)OCOPr	$CH_2OCOOEt$	0.72	0.45	1.60
8	1.67	CH_2OCOBu	$CH_2OCOOEt$	0.96	0.73	1.30
9	1.98	CH(Me)OCOBu	$CH_2OCOOEt$	0.42	0.48	0.91
10	2.08	$CH_2OCOC_6H_5$	$CH_2OCOOEt$	0.76	0.54	1.40

SOD : Single oral dose
SCD : Subcutaneous dose

Figure 58 ED$_{50}$ (mg/kg) for THF carbapenems against acute lethal *E. coli* infection in mice. SOD, single oral dose; SCD, subcutaneous dose.

However, the ED$_{50}$ by the subcutaneous route are 11 to 14 times lower than those obtained with the oral route. Ideally the ratio of ED$_{50}$ after a single oral or subcutaneous dose should approach 1.

It was investigated whether a double ester would improve the oral absorption. The double ester prodrug will be directed in order to facilitate absorption through the phospholipid membrane by eliminating the ionic nature and increasing the lipophilicity of the parent compound CL-191121 (pK 3.1, 9.1; logP, −3.02).

The bis double esters are inactive, and all of them exhibited a higher stability than imipenem against DHP-I hydrolysis. In the mouse model the bis double ester exhibited a higher bioavailability than the monoester. This fact is correlated with the logP (Fig. 58).

Double esterification of meropenem yielded KL-3744 and KL-3758 with a bioavailability after oral absorption in cats of 23.37 and 18.20%, respectively (Kunishiro et al., 2004).

REFERENCES

Albers-Schonberg G, Arison BH, Hensens OD, et al, 1976, Structure and absolute configuration of thienamycin, J Am Chem Soc, 100, 6491–6499.

Bax RP, Bastain W, Featherstone A, Wilkinson DM, Hutchinson M, Haworth SJ, 1989, The pharmacokinetics of meropenem in volunteers, J Antimicrob Chemother, 24, suppl A, 311–320.

Calandra GB, Brown BK, Grad LC, Ahonkhai V, Wang C, Aziz MA, 1978, Review of adverse experiences and tolerability in the first 2516 patients treated with imipenem-cilastatin, Am J Med, 78, 73–78.

Calandra GB, Wang C, Azizi M, Brown KR, 1986, The safety profile of imipenem/cilastatin: worldwide clinical experience based on 3470 patients, J Antimicrob Chemother, 18, suppl E, 193–202.

Campbell BJ, 1970, Renal dipeptidase, Methods Enzymol, 19, 722–729.

Campbell BJ, Lin YC, Davis RV, Ballew E, 1966, The purification and properties of a particulate renal dipeptidase, Biochim Biophys Acta, 118, 371–386.

Christensson BA, Nilson-Ehle I, Hutchison M, Haworth SJ, Oqvist B, Norrby SR, 1992, Pharmacokinetics of meropenem in subjects with various degrees of renal impairment, Antimicrob Agents Chemother, 36, 1532–1537.

di Modugno E, Broggio R, Erbetti I, Lowther J, 1997, In vitro and in vivo antibacterial activities of GV 129606, a new broad-spectrum trinem, Antimicrob Agents Chemother, 41, 2742–2748.

Di Ninno F, Muthard DA, Salzmann T, 1995, The discovery and synthesis of 2-biphenylcarbapenems active against methicillin resistant staphylococci, Bioorg Med Chem Lett, 5, 945–948.

Fujii R, Nishimura T, 1992, Pharmacokinetics and efficacy of panipenem/betamipron in pediatrics, 32nd Intersci Conf Antimicrob Agents Chemother.

Fukasawa M, Sumita Y, Harabe ET, Tanio T, Nouda H, Kohzuki T, Okuda T, Matsumura H, Sunagawa M, 1992, Stability of meropenem and effect of 1 β-methyl substitution on its stability in the presence of renal dehydropeptidase I, Antimicrob Agents Chemother, 36, 1577–1579.

Greenstein JP, 1948, Dehydropeptidases, p 117–169, in FF Nord, ed, Advances in Enzymology and Related Subjects of Biochemistry, Interscience, New York.

Han TH, Cho HY, Cho JH, Oh CH, 2004, Synthesis and biological activity of 1β-methyl carbapenems having cyclic thiourea moieties, 44th Intersci Conf Antimicrob Agents Chemother, abstract F-328.

Hashizume T, Shibata K, Nagano R, et al, 1996, In vitro and in vivo evaluation of Bo-3482, a novel dithiocarbamate carbapenem, 36th Intersci Conf Antimicrob Agents Chemother, abstract F-118.

Hazumi N, Kato Y, Hashizume T, Matsuda K, 1995, Effects of a β-lactamase inhibitor, sulbactam, on the activity of carbapenems against *Pseudomonas aeruginosa*, J Antibiot, 48, 1364–1367.

Hikida M, Kawashima K, Yoshida M, Mitsuhashi S, 1992, Inactivation of new carbapenem antibiotics by dehydropeptidase-I from porcine and human renal cortex, J Antimicrob Chemother, 30, 129–134.

Hikida M, Masukawa Y, Kitazumi K, Kavashima K, Naruki T, Nishiki K, Furukauwa Y, Kamei C, Tasaka T, 1990, Benign neurotoxicity of LJC 10627, a novel 1-p-methyl carbapenem antibiotic, 30th Intersci Conf Antimicrob Agents Chemother, abstract 901.

Kahan JS, Kahan FM, Goegelman R, Currie SA, Jackson M, Stapley EO, Miller TW, Miller AK, et al, 1979, Thienamycin, a new β-lactams antibiotic. 1. Discovery, taxonomy, isolation and physical properties, J Antibiot, 32, 1–12.

Kawamoto I, Miyauchi M, Endo R, Hisaoka M, Yasuda H, Kuwahara S, 1996, CS-834, a new oral carbapenem. 1. Structure-activity relationships of 2-substituted 1β-methyl carbapenems, 36th Intersci Conf Antimicrob Agents Chemother, abstract F-105.

Kropp H, Sundelof JG, Hajdu R, Kahan FM, 1982, Metabolism of thienamycin and related carbapenem antibiotics by the renal dipeptidase, dehydropeptidase, Antimicrob Agents Chemother, 22, 62–70.

Kunishiro K, Shirahase H, Matsui H, Kitagawa M, et al, 2004, Novel orally active prodrugs of meropenem, KL-3744 and KL-3758: synthesis and pharmacokinetics, 44th Intersci Conf Antimicrob Agents Chemother, abstract F-534.

Kusube K, Taniguchi S, Nakamura M, Watanabe N, Ohba F, Horie T, 1995, ER-35786, a new antipseudomonal carbapenem. IV. Pharmacokinetics in laboratory animals, 35th Intersci Conf Antimicrob Agents Chemother, abstract F-154.

Le Anza WJ, Wildonger KJ, Miller TW, Christensen BG, 1979, *N*-Acetimidoyl and *N*-formimidoylthienamycin derivatives, antipseudomonal β-lactam antibiotics, J Med Chem, 22, 1435–1436.

Leroy A, Fillastre JP, Borsa-Lebas F, Etienne I, Humbert G, 1992, Pharmacokinetics of meropenem (ICI 194,660) and its metabolite (ICI 213,689) in healthy subjects and in patients with renal impairment, Antimicrob Agents Chemother, 36, 2794–2798.

Leroy A, Fillastre JP, Etienne I, Borsa-Lebas F, Humbert G, 1992, Pharmacokinetics of meropenem in subjects with renal insufficiency, Eur J Clin Pharmacol, 42, 535–538.

Majundar A, Birk K, Blum RA, Cairns AM, et al, 1996, Pharmacokinetics of L-749345, a carbapenem antibiotic, in healthy male and female volunteers, 36th Intersci Conf Antimicrob Agents Chemother, abstract F-130.

Matsumoto Y, Matsumoto S, Morinaga C, Tawara S, Tanaka A, Barret D, Matsuda K, Chiba T, Sakane K, 1995, FR-21818, a new parenteral carbapenem. Preclinical evaluation of in vitro antibacterial activity, 35th Intersci Conf Antimicrob Agents Chemother, abstract F-146.

Meurer LC, GuthiKonda RN, Huber JL, Di Ninno F, 1995, The synthesis and antibacterial activity of 2-carbolinyl carbapenems, potent anti-MRSA/MRCNS agents, Bioorg Med Chem Lett, 5, 767–772.

Mitsuhashi S, Fuse A, Mikami H, Saino Y, Inoue M, 1988, Purification and characterization of human renal dehydropeptidase I, Antimicrob Agents Chemother, 32, 587–588.

Miyadera T, Sugimura Y, Hashimoto T, Tanaka T, Iiono K, Shibata T, Sugawara S, 1983, Synthesis and in vitro activity of a new carbapenem, RS-533, J Antibiot, 36, 1034–1039.

Nakamura M, Watanabe N, 1995, ER-35768, a new antipseudomonal carbapenem. II. In vitro antibacterial activity, 35th Intersci Conf Antimicrob Agents Chemother, abstract F-152.

Nakashima M, Uematsu T, Kanamaru M, 1990, Phase I study of CS-976 (CS 533/CS-443), a new injectable carbapenem antibiotic agent, 30th Intersci Conf Antimicrob Agents Chemother, abstract 897.

Nakashima M, Uematsu T, Ueno K, 1991, Pharmacokinetics and safety of L-627, a new parenteral carbapenem, in healthy volunteers, 31st Intersci Conf Antimicrob Agents Chemother, abstract 819.

Oh CH, Ham YN, Hong SY, Cho JH, 1995, Synthesis and antibacterial activity of new 1β-methyl-carbapenem having a thiazolo [3, 2-a] benzimidazole moiety, Arch Pharmacol, 328, 289–291.

Ohya S, Fukuoka T, Masuda N, Iijima M, Yasuda H, Kuwahara S, 1991, Panipenem shows strange antipseudomonal activity in low-amino-acid media and biological fluids than in standard susceptibility test media, 31st Intersci Conf Antimicrob Agents Chemother, abstract 832.

Patel JB, Giles RE, 1989, Meropenem, evidence of lack of proconvulsive tendency in mice, J Antimicrob Chemother, 24, suppl A, 307–309.

Reed MD, Stern RC, O'Brien CA, Yamashita TS, Myers CM, Blumer JL, 1985, Pharmacokinetics of imipenem and cilastatin in patients with cystic fibrosis, Antimicrob Agents Chemother, 27, 583–588.

Rotiroti D, de Sarro GB, Musolino R, Nistico G, 1983, A new model of experimental epilepsy: the cefazolin-induced epilepsy, Prog Clin Biol Res, 124, 129–144.

Sato N, Sasho M, Kamada A, Suzuki T, Ashizawa K, Sugiyama L, 1995, ER 35786, a new antipseudomonal carbapenem. I. Synthesis and structure-activity relationships of 2-substituted 1b-methyl carbapenems, 35th Intersci Conf Antimicrob Agents Chemother, abstract F-151.

Shibamoto N, Sakamoto M, Fukagawa Y, Ishikura I, 1982, Pharmacological studies on carbapenem antibiotics. Isolation of a PS-5 inactivating factor from the rat kidney, J Antibiot, 6, 729–735.

Sigura M, Ito Y, Hirana K, Sawaki S, 1978, Purification and properties of human kidney dipeptidase, Biochim Biophys Acta, 522, 544–550.

Sunagawa M, Matsumura H, Ohno Y, Nakamura M, Fukasawa M, 1991, Meropenem, a 1-β-methyl carbapenem with low neurotoxic side effects: structure-activity relationship for convulsive liability, 31st Intersci Conf Antimicrob Agents Chemother, abstract 167.

Takahagi H, Hirota T, Matsushita Y, Maramatsu S, Tanaka M, Matsuo E, 1991, In vitro dehydropeptidase-I activity and its hydrolytic activity of panipenem in several tissues in animal species and their influence on the disposition of panipenem in vivo, Chemotherapy, 39, suppl 3, 236–241.

Tanimura H, Ochai M, Takahaji H, Hirota T, 1990, Localization of dehydropeptidase-I (enzyme hydrolyzing carbapenems) in human tissues, 30th Intersci Conf Antimicrob Agents Chemother, abstract 898.

Ueda Y, Kanazawa K, Takemoto K, Eriguchi, Sunigawa M, 2004, SM-216601, a novel parenteral 1β-methyl carbapenem: in vitro and in vivo antimicrobial activity, 44th Intersci Conf Antimicrob Agents Chemother, abstract F-330.

Waddell SY, Ratdiffe RW, Szumiloski SP, Wildonger KJ, Wilkening RR, Blizzard T, et al, 1995, Benzothiazolylthio carbapenems, potent anti-MRSA agents, Bioorg Med Chem Lett, 5, 1427–1432.

Welch CL, Campbell BJ, 1978, Fed Proc, 37, 1533.

Williams PD, Bennet DB, Comereski CR, 1988, Animal model for evaluating the convulsive liability of β-lactam antibiotics, Antimicrob Agents Chemother, 32, 758–760.

Wise R, 1986, In vitro and pharmacokinetic properties of the carbapenems, Antimicrob Agents Chemother, 30, 343–349.

Wollmann T, Gerlach U, Hörlein R, Krass N, Lattrell R, Limbert M, Markus A, 1993, Novel tetracyclic carbapenems, synthesis and biological activity, in Bentley PH, Ponsford R, ed, Recent Advances in the Chemistry of Anti-Infective Agents, Royal Society of Chemistry, p 50–65.

Yoo KH, Lee KS, Kang YK, Lee K, et al, 2004, Novel 1β-methyl carbapenem with sodium 5-(3- and 5-carboxylic acid) isoxazoloethenyl moieties, 44th Intersci Conf Antimicrob Agents Chemother, abstract F-327.

Penems

A. BRYSKIER

9

1. INTRODUCTION

Penems are synthetic molecules belonging to the β-lactam family. The original synthesis of the penems resulted from scientific curiosity on the part of Woodward (1977), who was interested in the combination of a penam-type pentacycle and a cephalosporin-like double bond. The first molecule to be synthesized was the 7-phenyl-2-methyl penem derivative (Fig. 1). This is a hybrid between the penam nucleus and the "ene-lactam" of the cephems. Since the description of the first penem by Woodward in 1976, a number of molecules have been synthesized. Despite attempts at development with Sch-29482 and Sch-33433, no medicinal product has yet been introduced in clinical practice. Currently fropenem (faropenem), ritipenem, and sulopenem are in phase II or III or in preregistration in Japan, Europe, and the United States.

2. CLASSIFICATIONS

Penems are characterized by the presence of an unsaturated pentaatomic ring attached to the azetidinone ring. Three groups may be distinguished in terms of the heteroatom attached at position 1 (Fig. 2 and 3): the penems (1-sulfur), the carbapenems (5-CH_2), and the oxa-1-penems.

Within the penems, five subgroups (A to E) may be distinguished according to the side chain attached at position 2: thiopenems (Sch-29482, Sch-33443, and sulopenem), oxypenems (HR-664), aminopenems, alkylpenems (ritipenem), and arylpenems (fropenem and TMA 3176) (Fig. 4).

3. PHYSICOCHEMICAL PROPERTIES

Penems are low-molecular-weight molecules (Table 1). Sch-33443 is stable for 24 h in phosphate buffer at 37°C and in culture media when stored at 4°C. Its activity decreases to 87% in the presence of 50% serum.

Ritipenem is stable in medium with a pH of between 4.4 and 7.0, in which case the degradation half-life is greater than 100 h. When the pH is very acidic (pH 1.7), the half-life is 1.7 h, and at alkaline pH (pH 9.0), it is 5.85 h.

4. STRUCTURE-ACTIVITY RELATIONSHIP

Penems are β-lactams with an unsaturated nucleus at position 2,3 and a sulfur atom at position 1 (thiazolidine nucleus). Various studies have shown that the chain that produces optimum activity at C-6 is a 1-(*R*)-hydroxyethyl group oriented in the α position, as for the carbapenems. This group is responsible for the stability against hydrolysis by β-lactamases. The pharmacokinetic properties, antibacterial activity, and toxicological properties are based on the C-2 side chain.

Several series of molecules have been synthesized in order to extend the antibacterial spectrum, increase the activity against *Enterobacteriaceae*, obtain better chemical stability and better stability against hydrolysis by renal dehydropeptidase, and reduce lipophilicity.

4.1. Modifications at Positions 5, 6, and 8

The absence of substituents at position 6 does not abolish the antibacterial activity of the penems, but the molecules are only moderately active against gram-positive cocci and *Enterobacteriaceae* (Table 2). They are inactive against β-lactamase-producing *Enterobacteriaceae*. The introduction of an ethyl group at position 6 either reduces the activity (*trans*) or abolishes it (*cis*). The 6-methoxypenem derivatives are relatively inactive and chemically unstable.

The introduction of a 6-(1-hydroxyethyl) group increases the antibacterial activity and stability against hydrolysis by β-lactamases. However, these properties are dependent on the stereochemistry. Only the 5*R*,6*S*,8*R* isomer is active, whereas the other three isomers, 5*R*,6*S*,8*S*, 5*R*,6*R*,8*R*, and 5*R*,6*R*,8*S*, are inactive. The 6-hydroxyethyl derivatives are less active than the 6-(1-hydroxyethyl) derivatives against β-lactamase-producing strains (Table 3). The addition of a methyl group at position 8 does not increase the antibacterial activity. Among the isomers, the 5*R* isomers are responsible for the antibacterial activity of the penems.

4.2. Modifications at Position 2

4.2.1. Thiopenems

Among the 2-thiopenem derivatives, the most active are those with a 2-thioethyl group (Sch-29482) (Alfonso et al., 1984). The presence of a larger, lipophilic residue of the 2(2-phenylthioethylthio) type reduces the activity against gram-negative bacteria but not that against gram-positive bacteria. This is a general tendency, the increase in size and lipophilicity of the chain reducing the antibacterial activity. The introduction of small polar groups (F, Cl, and OH) does not significantly alter the spectrum or antibacterial activity (Kawamoto et al., 1986).

Figure 1 7-Phenyl-2-methyl penem (Woodward, 1976)

A series of 2-alkylthiopenem derivatives has been synthesized, including in particular alcohols and carbamates. In the carbamate series, the addition of an oxygen atom or a supplementary amino group reduces the antibacterial activity. A derivative, Sch-33443, has been developed up to the beginning of phase III and possesses a 2(2-carbamoyloxyethylthio) chain at C-2 (Fig. 5). Other carbamate derivatives have good antibacterial activity: nitrile and cyanoamidine derivatives. The presence of a carboxyl group at C-2 reduces the activity against gram-positive bacteria.

Among a series of 2-thiopenems, CP-65207 (sulopenem) has a 1-oxotetrahydrothiophene chain.

Nishi et al. (1993) have shown that the presence of a quaternary ammonium at C-2 (pyridinium) increases the stability against hydrolysis by dehydropeptidase I (DHP-1). Some derivatives exhibit good antibacterial activity, as has already been demonstrated with a series of carbapenems (Kim et al., 1987). These derivatives possess good activity against gram-negative bacilli. However, although they are 15 to 50 times more stable against hydrolysis by porcine DHP-I than imipenem and Sch-34343, the penems are more resistant than the carbapenems with identical side chains at position 2 (Sunagawa et al., 1992). This increase in stability is due to the presence of a pyridinium nucleus, but also the

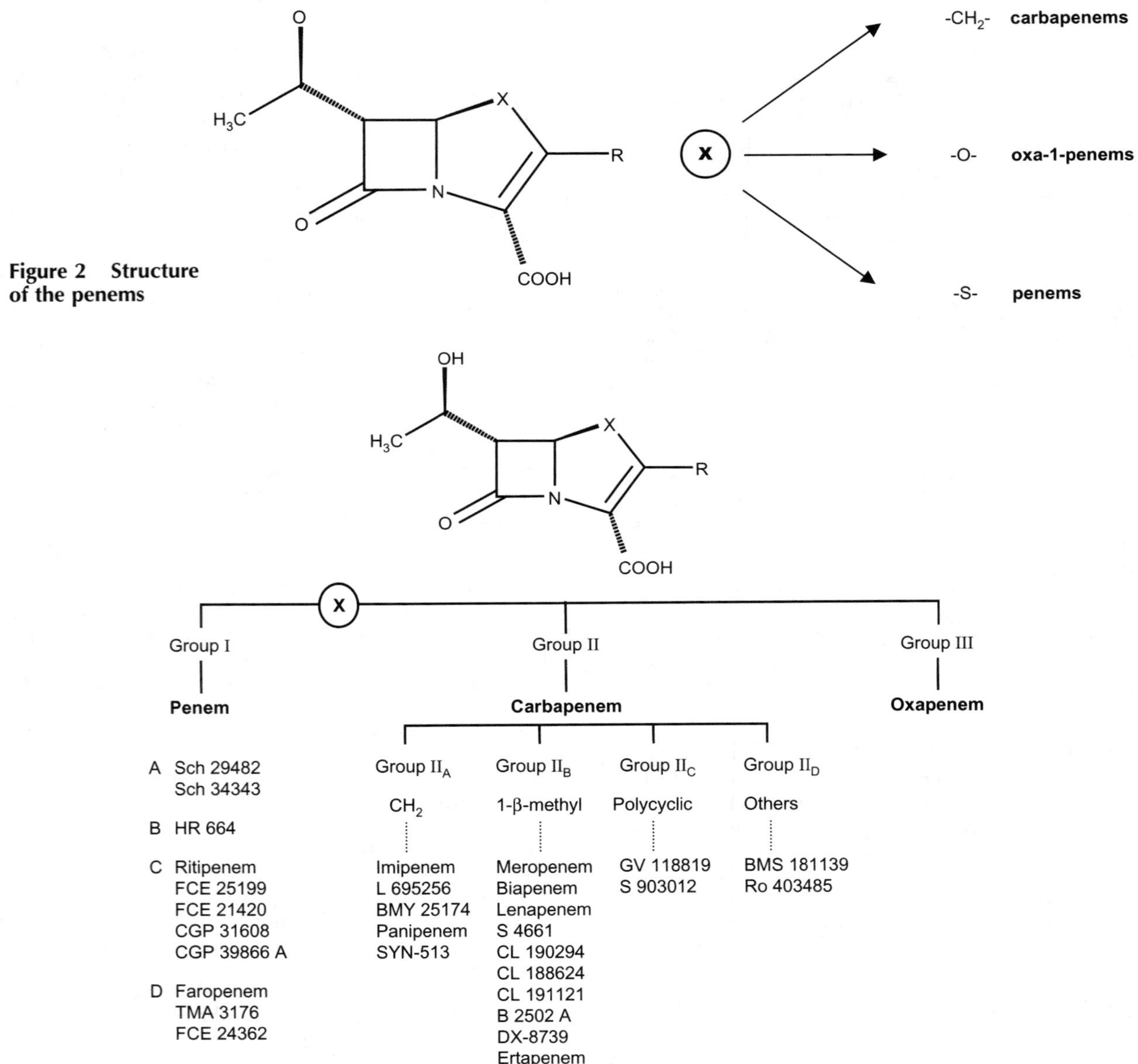

Figure 2 Structure of the penems

Figure 3 Classification of the penems

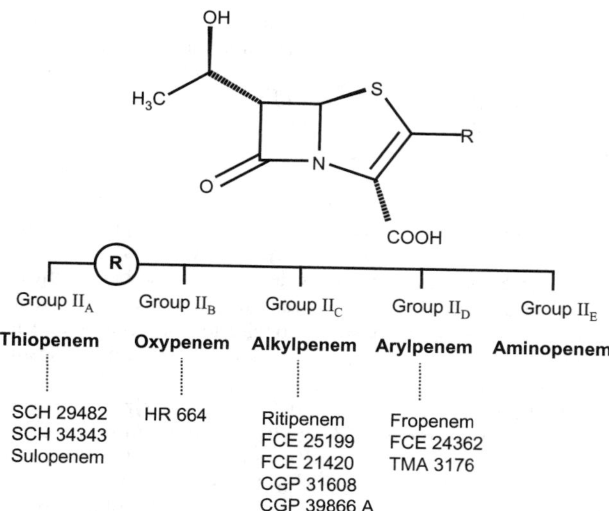

Figure 4 Classification of the penems

Table 1 Physicochemical properties of penems

Drug	Empirical formula	Mol wt	pK
Sch-29482	$C_{10}H_{13}NO_4S$	275.22	
Sch-34343	$C_{11}H_{13}N_2O_6S_2$	356.34	
Ritipenem	$C_{10}H_{12}N_2O_6S$	288.28	
Fropenem	$C_{12}H_{15}NO_5S$	285.32	3.44
CGP-31608	$C_9H_{12}N_2O_4S$	244.26	
Sulopenem	$C_{11}H_{14}NO_5S_3$	336.24	
HR-664	$C_{15}H_{13}N_2O_6S$	349.15	
FCE-25199	$C_{15}H_{17}NO_8S$	371.36	
FCE-21420	$C_{11}H_{13}NO_6S$	287.29	

bicyclic structure. The position of the nitrogen atom in the pyridinium ring plays an important role in the biological activity of the molecules. Some derivatives (Fig. 6) have good activity against *Pseudomonas aeruginosa* (MIC, ~3.13 μg/ml, versus 1.56 μg/ml for imipenem). The bicyclic derivatives of a zwitterionic nature have good activity against gram-negative bacilli, which is dependent on the nature of the ring. Compounds with an imidazole nucleus are less active (Nishi et al., 1994). Molecules with a pentacyclic nucleus attached to the quaternary ammonium are less active than those which have a hexacyclic nucleus. Moreover, here again the spatial orientation of the bicyclic nucleus determines the antibacterial activity.

4.2.2. 2-Alkylpenems

Farmitalia Carlo Erba has synthesized several series of 2-alkylpenems. The first series yielded ritipenem (FCE-22101), which has a 2-CH_2-X functional group. Several series have been prepared with the aim of extending the antibacterial spectrum so as to obtain good stability against hydrolysis by renal dehydropeptidase and reduce the lipophilicity of the molecules. A second series of the alkylaminopenem type has been synthesized involving the presence of a quaternary ammonium group, amino substituted groups, N-heterocycles, and *N*-imidazole. One of these derivatives exhibited good antibacterial activity but was chemically unstable. To obviate this chemical instability, a third series was prepared by attachment of a substituted or nonsubstituted 2-phenyl residue. These molecules possess good bioavailability and good stability against hydrolysis by renal dehydropeptidase, but their activity against *Enterobacteriaceae* remains moderate, while plasma protein binding is strong. A fourth series of compounds was prepared by attaching a *p*-phenylene at C-2.

A fifth series of derivatives with a 2-pyridinium nucleus was proposed. The isosteric substitution CH→N in the C-2 arylpenem class produced an increase in antibacterial activity while retaining good stability against hydrolysis by DHP-I (Bedeschi et al., 1990). Excellent in vivo activity was demonstrated in this series among the 2-(3-pyridyl) derivatives, as well as good oral absorption of the acetoxymethyl ester, with bioavailability on the order of 67%. The molecules have good stability against hydrolysis by porcine DHP-I. FCE-24362 (Fig. 5) is a derivative which has a (pyridiniomethyl)phenyl chain at C-2, and in vivo the 50% effective dose for gram-positive cocci and gram-negative bacilli is ≤1 mg/kg of body weight.

Table 2 In vitro activities of penems not substituted at position 6

Organism	MIC (μg/ml)			
	Methyl	Ethyl	S-CH_2-phenyl	Ampicillin
S. aureus 209P	2	1	0.5	0.06
Bacillus subtilis ATCC 6633	2	0.5	0.5	0.06
E. coli 10536	32	1	8	1
K. pneumoniae 815502	8	4	>64	64

Table 3 Antibacterial activity and isomerism in positions 5, 6, and 8

Organism	MIC (μg/ml)			
	5*R*,6*S*,8*R*	5*R*,6*S*,8*S*	5*R*,6*R*,8*R*	5*R*,6*R*,8*S*
S. aureus 209P	0.125	16	16	0.5
B. subtilis ATCC 6633	0.03	16	8	0.125
E. coli 10536	0.5	>16	4	0.25
K. pneumoniae 815502	0.5	>16	16	16
Providencia strain Hewitt 104	0.5	>16	16	>16

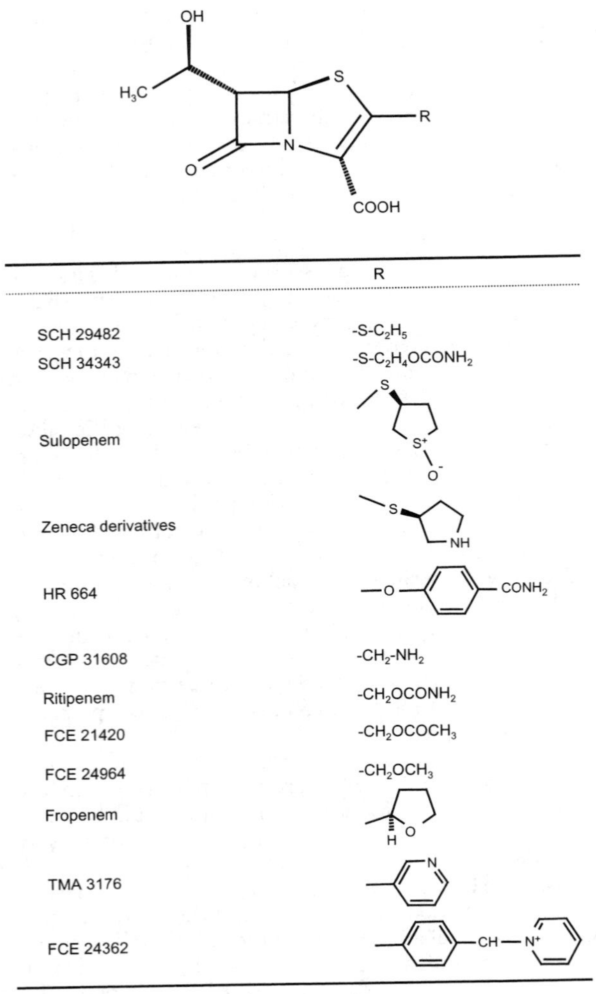

	R
SCH 29482	$-S-C_2H_5$
SCH 34343	$-S-C_2H_4OCONH_2$
Sulopenem	
Zeneca derivatives	
HR 664	$-O-C_6H_4-CONH_2$
CGP 31608	$-CH_2-NH_2$
Ritipenem	$-CH_2OCONH_2$
FCE 21420	$-CH_2OCOCH_3$
FCE 24964	$-CH_2OCH_3$
Fropenem	
TMA 3176	
FCE 24362	

Figure 5 Thiopenem derivatives

An alkyl-lactone or alkylamine series has been synthesized. The lactonyl derivatives are more active than the lactamyl derivatives, and within each subgroup the *S*-isomer is more active than the *R*-isomer (Table 4).

A series of derivatives with a quaternary ammonium has been synthesized (Perrone et al., 1987) (Fig. 7). A number of molecules possessed chains similar to that of the cephalosporins of this class. The derivative with a methylpyrrolydinium at C-2 (Fig. 7) is very active against gram-positive cocci and gram-negative bacilli but is chemically very unstable.

A series of 2-phenoxyalkyl derivatives has been synthesized. The molecules possess a narrow antibacterial spectrum which includes gram-positive cocci and anaerobic bacteria. They are inactive against gram-negative bacteria. Plasma protein binding is greater than 90%.

In the series of 2-*N*-pyrimidylalkylpenem-type molecules, some derivatives have good activity against gram-positive and gram-negative bacteria and against anaerobic bacteria. Plasma protein binding varies, and one of the characteristics is that of having a long apparent elimination half-life in mice. One molecule, CGP-39866A, possesses good pharmacokinetics, but it has weaker activity than does its isomer (Fig. 8 and Table 5). Prodrugs have been prepared to increase the bioavailability.

Table 4 Antibacterial activities of the 2-alkyl-lactone and 2-alkyl-lactam derivatives

Organism	MIC (μg/ml) of isomer				
	S	R	S	R	S
S. aureus 10B	0.02	0.02	0.02	0.02	0.02
Streptococcus pyogenes Aronson	0.02	0.05	0.01	0.05	0.02
H. influenzae NCTC 4560	1	2	1	2	1
E. coli 205	0.1	1	0.05	0.5	0.1
S. marcescens 344	1	4	1	2	1
E. cloacae P99	0.5	2	0.5	2	0.5

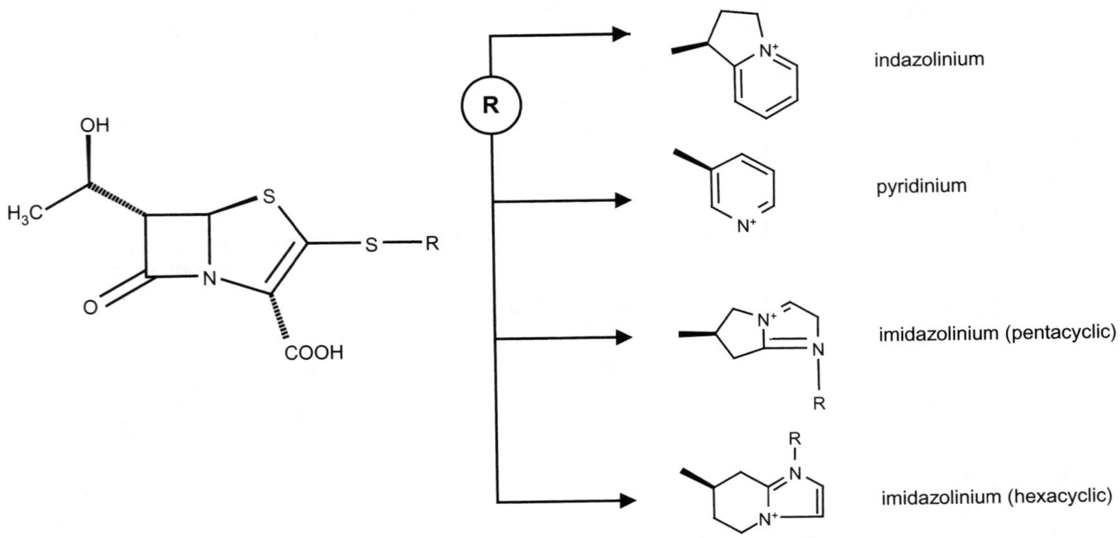

indazolinium

pyridinium

imidazolinium (pentacyclic)

imidazolinium (hexacyclic)

Figure 6 Penems/quaternary ammonium derivatives

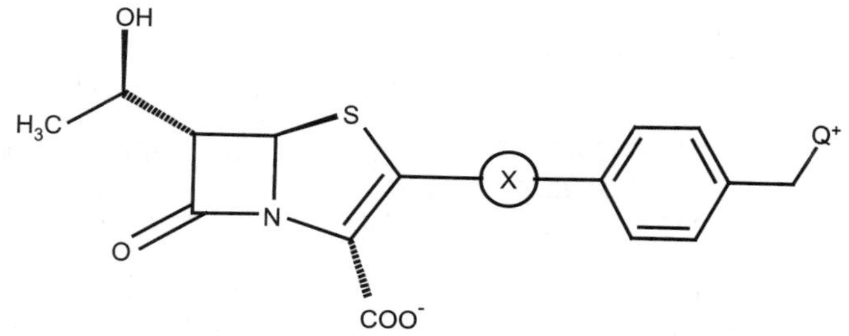

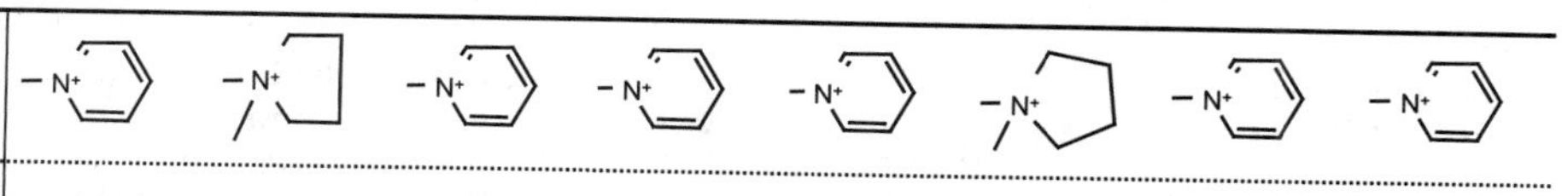

Q+ / X	=	=	O	S	CH_2O	CH_2O	CH_2OCO	CH_2OCONH
S. aureus	0.01	0.04	0.04	0.01	0.01	0.02	0.01	0.04
S. pyogenes	0.01	0.005	0.01	0.01	0.005	0.01	0.005	0.01
E. faecalis	1.56	6.25	6.25	6.25	1.56	3.12	0.78	0.39
K. aerogenes 1082 E	0.39	0.78	0.56	0.78	1.56	1.56	1.56	0.78
E. coli B (β-lactamase)	0.54	2.20	1.09	1.56	0.78	1.09	1.09	1.09
E. cloacae	0.38	0.78	1.56	1.56	1.56	1.56	1.56	0.78
E. cloacae P-99	1.56	6.25	1.56	3.12	3.12	6.25	3.12	3.12
Proteus indole+	0.54	1.09	6.25	2.20	1.56	3.51	1.09	1.56
C. freundii ATCC 8090	0.19	0.78	1.56	1.56	0.78	0.78	1.56	1.56

Figure 7 Quaternary ammonium—pyridinio(methyl)phenyl penem (from Perrone et al., 1987)

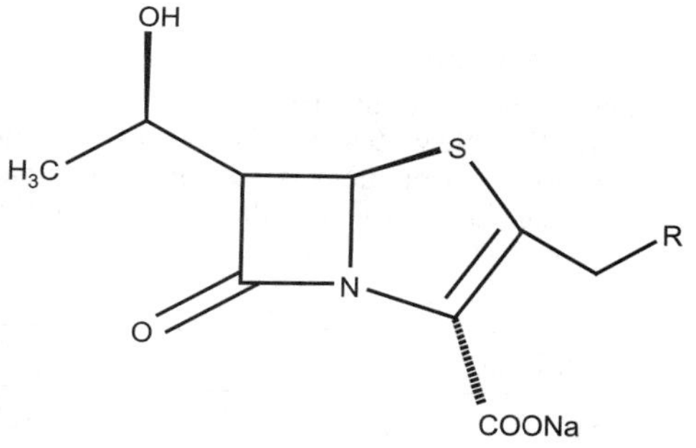

	R
CGP 39866 A	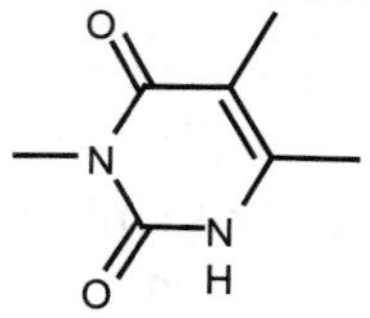
Isomer	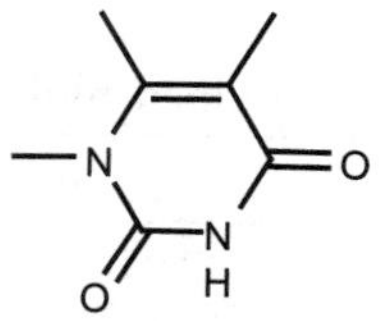

Figure 8 CGP-39866A and its isomer

Table 5 In vitro activities of CGP-39866A and its isomer

Organism	MIC (μg/ml)	
	CGP-39866A	Isomer
S. aureus 10B	0.05	0.5
S. aureus A331 Met[r]	0.2	2
S. pneumoniae Q13	0.05	0.05
H. influenzae P23	0.1	1
E. coli 205	1	0.5
K. pneumoniae 327	1	16
C. difficile RX2	4	1
B. fragilis L01	0.5	

4.2.3. 2-Oxypenems

See Cooke et al., 1984.

Among the derivatives of the oxypenem series, the presence of a carbamoyl group at position 4′ yields antibacterial activity greater than that of molecules with substitutions at position 2′ or 3′ (Table 6).

The increase of the alkyl chain on the carbamoyl group reduces the activity against gram-negative bacilli. The most active molecule, HR-664, possesses a carbamoyl group (Seibert et al., 1987). The 2-phenoxy derivatives are more active than the 2-alkoxy derivatives.

4.2.4. 2-Arylpenems

A series of 19 2-arylpenem derivatives has been synthesized (Ishiguro et al., 1988). The derivatives possess penta- or

Table 6 Activities of oxypenems

Organism	MIC (μg/ml) with indicated position on the phenyl ring[a]		
	2	3	4
S. aureus SG 511	0.19	0.1	0.05
S. pyogenes 77A	0.1	0.1	0.05
E. coli 205	1.56	0.39	0.19
E. coli TEM+	6.25	0.78	0.39
E. cloacae P99	12.5	3.13	3.13
Salmonella enterica serovar typhimurium MZ II	3.13	0.78	0.78

[a]In all cases there was an H at R.

hexacyclic nuclei or acyclic chains. There is substantial isomerism at position 2 because of the presence of an asymmetrical carbon (Table 7). The pentacyclic series is more active than the hexacyclic series. Within the pentacyclic series, derivatives that have a cycle with an oxygen and that are not unsaturated are more active than those with an unsaturated nucleus of the furyl type. The position of the oxygen heteroatom relative to the bond to the penem nucleus determines the antibacterial activity. Derivatives with an alycyclic chain are inactive against *Enterobacteriaceae* and have variable activity against gram-positive cocci.

The presence of a catechol nucleus at C-2 increases the activity against gram-negative bacilli.

4.2.5. 2-Dithiocarbamate Penems

A series of 2-dithiocarbamate penems has led to the isolation of a few molecules with good activity against gram-positive cocci, but the activity against gram-negative bacilli is weak, including that of a derivative with a catechol nucleus (Altamura et al., 1993) (Fig. 9).

4.2.6. 2-Aminomethyl Penem Derivatives

The presence of a 2-aminomethyl chain at position 2 increases the stability of the molecules against hydrolysis by DHP-I. The attachment of chains to the aminomethyl group reduces the activity against gram-negative bacteria. However, the unsaturated N-heterocyclic derivatives (e.g., imidazole) may exhibit good antibacterial activity (Girijavallabhan et al., 1986) (Fig. 10).

4.3. Isomers

4.3.1. Fropenem (Faropenem)

There is a center of asymmetry at C-2 on the tetrahydrofuryl nucleus of fropenem. The *R*-isomer (SUN-5555) is more active than the *S*-isomer (SUN-4434). The *S*-isomer is more active against gram-positive bacteria but is inactive against *Enterobacteriaceae*. This phenomenon has been demonstrated in the whole series of synthesized derivatives (Table 8).

4.3.2. Sulopenem

The sulopenem molecule possesses two centers of asymmetry, one on the thiol of the thiotetrahydrothiophene nucleus at C-2. The *R*-isomer (CP-70429) and the *S*-isomer (CP-81054) have the same in vitro activity (Table 9 and Fig. 11).

5. NEUROLOGIC AND RENAL TOLERANCE

5.1. Neurologic Tolerance

5.1.1. Fropenem

At doses of up to 100 mg/kg, fropenem does not cause convulsions or death in mice, in contrast to imipenem-cilastatin, which induces convulsions at a dose of 300 mg/kg, accompanied by death in the murine model. Fropenem has a weak affinity for the γ-aminobutyric acid receptors (Hori et al., 1992).

5.1.2. Ritipenem

See Schliamser et al., 1988.

In the New Zealand White rabbit, the epileptogenic threshold of ritipenem is 102 mg/kg, compared to 486 and 86 mg/kg for benzylpenicillin and imipenem, respectively.

Table 7 Activities of 2-arylpenem derivatives

Organism	MIC (μg/ml)							
	SUN-5555 (*R*)	SUN-4434 (*S*)	SUN-4194	SUN-4196	SUN-5262	SUN-4771 (*R*)	SUN-4770 (*S*)	SUN-3519
S. aureus 209P	0.05	0.05	0.39	0.2	0.03	0.1	0.1	0.2
E. coli NIHJ-JC2	0.78	6.25	25	12.5	50	6.25	50	0.78
K. pneumoniae PCI 602	0.39	1.56	3.13	3.13	0.2	0.1	3.13	1.56
S. marcescens IAM 1136	1.56	25	25	25	25	25	>50	12.5
B. fragilis GM 7000	<0.025	0.1	0.39	0.39		0.1	0.78	0.1

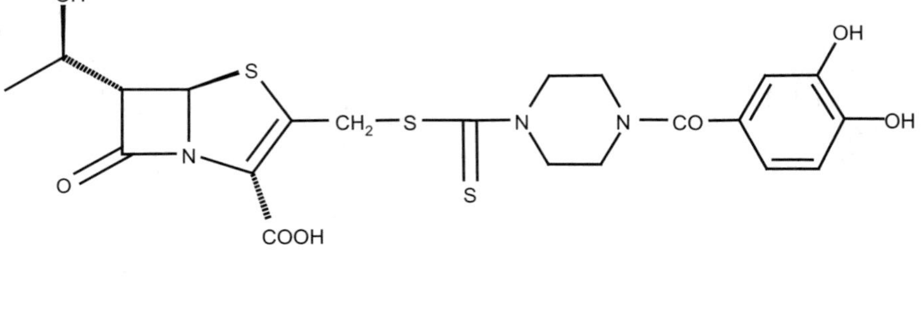

Figure 9 Penems/dithiocarbamate (catechol derivative)

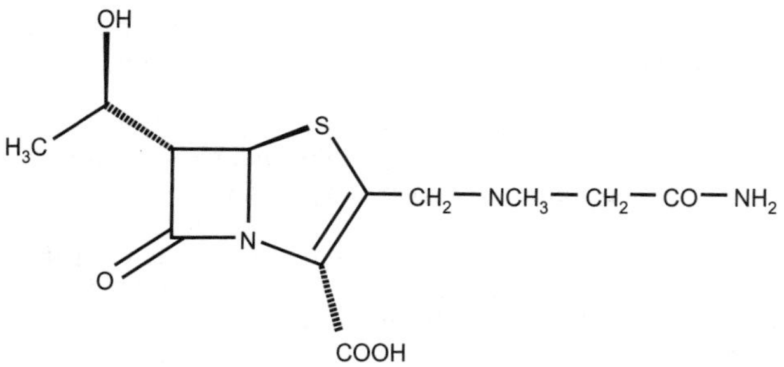

Figure 10 Men 1070

Table 8 Antibacterial activities of the isomers SUN-5555 and SUN-4434

Organism	MIC (μg/ml)	
	SUN-5555	SUN-4434
S. aureus 209P	0.05	0.05
E. coli NIHJ-JC2	0.78	6.25
K. pneumoniae	0.39	1.56
S. marcescens	1.56	25
P. mirabilis	1.56	6.25
Citrobacter freundii	25	>50
B. fragilis	<0.025	0.1

The concentrations of imipenem and ritipenem in cerebrospinal fluid are low, but the concentrations in cerebral tissue are high, 4.7 ± 9.2 and 5.5 ± 1.3 mg/kg (mean ± standard deviation) for imipenem and ritipenem, respectively.

It has been shown that the toxic effect on the central nervous system is due to the zwitterionic and lipophilic nature of the molecules and that it might be suppressed by the insertion of a second anionic center. Other derivatives in this series, such as FCE-24362, have been synthesized and have displayed excellent antibacterial activity, but they have not been developed because of their neurotoxicity (Perrone, 1988).

Table 9 Antibacterial activities of the *S*- and *R*-isomers of sulopenem

Organism	MIC (μg/ml)	
	CP-70429 (CP-65207 *R*)	CP-81054 (CP-65207 *S*)
S. aureus	0.1	0.1
S. epidermidis	0.1	0.1
E. faecalis	1.56	3.12
S. pyogenes	≤0.025	≤0.025
E. coli Amp^r	0.05	0.05
K. pneumoniae	0.1	0.1
E. cloacae	0.78	1.56
Morganella morganii	0.78	1.56
S. marcescens	0.2	0.2

5.2. Renal Dehydropeptidase

In the presence of cilastatin, the plasma pharmacokinetic parameters of ritipenem are unaffected. Conversely, the elimination of the degradation products P-1 and P-2 is reduced, with an increase in the urinary elimination of ritipenem (37 to 80%) with a high interindividual coefficient of variation (~36%).

The two stereoisomers of CP-65207 are more stable against hydrolysis by porcine and human DHP-I than imipenem (Table 10).

In the dog, intravenous administration of CP-65207 and a DHP-I inhibitor revealed that urinary elimination is not increased (~40%) for CP-65207, whereas it is increased from 1 to 14% for imipenem. It is therefore likely that CP-65207 is markedly less metabolized than imipenem in the dog proximal tubules.

In humans, the urinary elimination of the *S*-isomer (CP-70429) is twice that of the *R*-isomer (CP-81054) (46 versus 26%).

The urine of volunteers receiving the racemate has an odor of sulfur, in contrast to that of volunteers receiving the *S*-isomer. The odor is probably due to the *R*-isomer, which is less polar than the *S*-isomer.

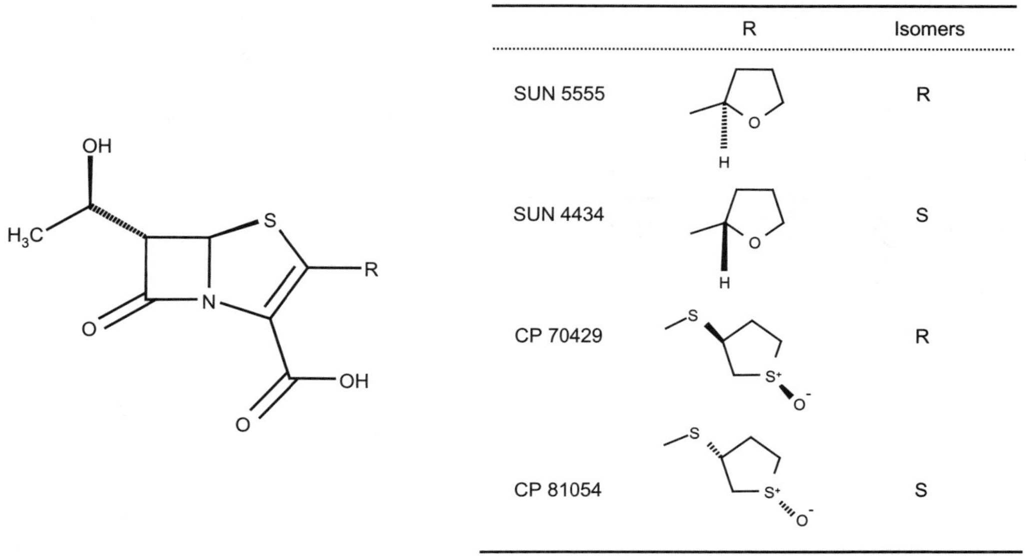

	R	Isomers
SUN 5555		R
SUN 4434		S
CP 70429		R
CP 81054		S

Figure 11 Isomers of fropenem and sulopenem

Table 10 Hydrolysis of the isomers of CP-65207 by DHP-I

Drug	% Hydrolysis in 20 min	
	Human DHP-I DPH	Pig DHP-I
CP-81054	2.25	4.01
CP-70429	1.43	3.09
Imipenem	2.96	23.29

Coadministration of cilastatin and fropenem (10 mg/kg intravenously) to rats causes a 28% reduction in plasma clearance of the molecule. Study of the metabolism by DHP-I in the different tissues showed that fropenem is degraded in the lung and renal tissues (Fig. 12). In renal tissue, 30% activity remains after 1 h, but 80% remains when fropenem is used in combination with cilastatin. In the presence of pure human DHP-I, the apparent degradation half-life of fropenem is 1.8 h, compared to 3 h for imipenem.

6. ANTIBACTERIAL ACTIVITY

6.1. Antibacterial Spectrum and Activity

The penems possess good activity against gram-positive cocci, particularly methicillin-susceptible strains. Against ofloxacin-resistant strains of *Staphylococcus aureus* (MIC, ≥6.25 μg/ml), fropenem has bimodal activity, with a MIC at which 50% of isolates tested are inhibited (MIC_{50}) of 0.2 μg/ml but a MIC_{90} of >100 μg/ml. The same applies for *Staphylococcus epidermidis*.

However, these molecules are not bactericidal against such strains. The penems are inactive against *Enterococcus faecium* (MIC, ≥128 μg/ml), and they have moderate activity against *Enterococcus faecalis* (MIC, ~4 μg/ml) (Table 11). For vancomycin-resistant strains of *E. faecalis* fropenem has a MIC_{50} of 8 μg/ml.

The molecules possess good activity against streptococci, including penicillin G-resistant strains of *Streptococcus pneumoniae*. The penems have good activity against strains of the viridans group streptococci.

Ritipenem possesses good bacteriostatic activity against *Streptococcus sanguinis* (MIC, 0.25 μg/ml), *Streptococcus mutans* (MIC, 0.125 μg/ml), and *Streptococcus milleri* (MIC, 0.25 μg/ml) but does not exert any bactericidal activity against the same species, with minimum bactericidal concentrations (MBCs) of 32, >32, and 32 μg/ml, respectively. The activity of ritipenem against *Streptococcus salivarius* is moderate (MIC and MBC, 2 and 4 μg/ml, respectively). This phenomenon has also been demonstrated with FCE-24362. In the case of fropenem, bactericidal activity has been demonstrated against streptococci of the viridans group, including strains tolerant to penicillin G. The penems possess good activity against *Listeria monocytogenes* (MIC, ~0.25 μg/ml), *Erysipelothrix rhusiopathiae, Corynebacterium diphtheriae* (MIC, ~0.1 μg/ml), and *Bacillus anthracis*. Conversely, they are inactive against *Corynebacterium jeikeium* (MIC, >128 μg/ml) (Table 12). Fropenem possesses moderate activity against *Leuconostoc* and *Lactobacillus* spp. (MIC_{50}, 4 μg/ml). Fropenem and imipenem have the same activity against *Gemella morbillorum* (MIC_{50}, ≤0.025 μg/ml).

The activity of the penems against *Enterobacteriaceae* is inferior to that of the parenteral cephems, particularly against *Enterobacter cloacae* and *Serratia marcescens*. They are inactive against nonfermentative gram-negative bacilli, such as *Pseudomonas* spp., *Acinetobacter* spp., and *Stenotrophomonas (Xanthomonas) maltophilia*, but against *Alcaligenes* the activity is variable (Table 13).

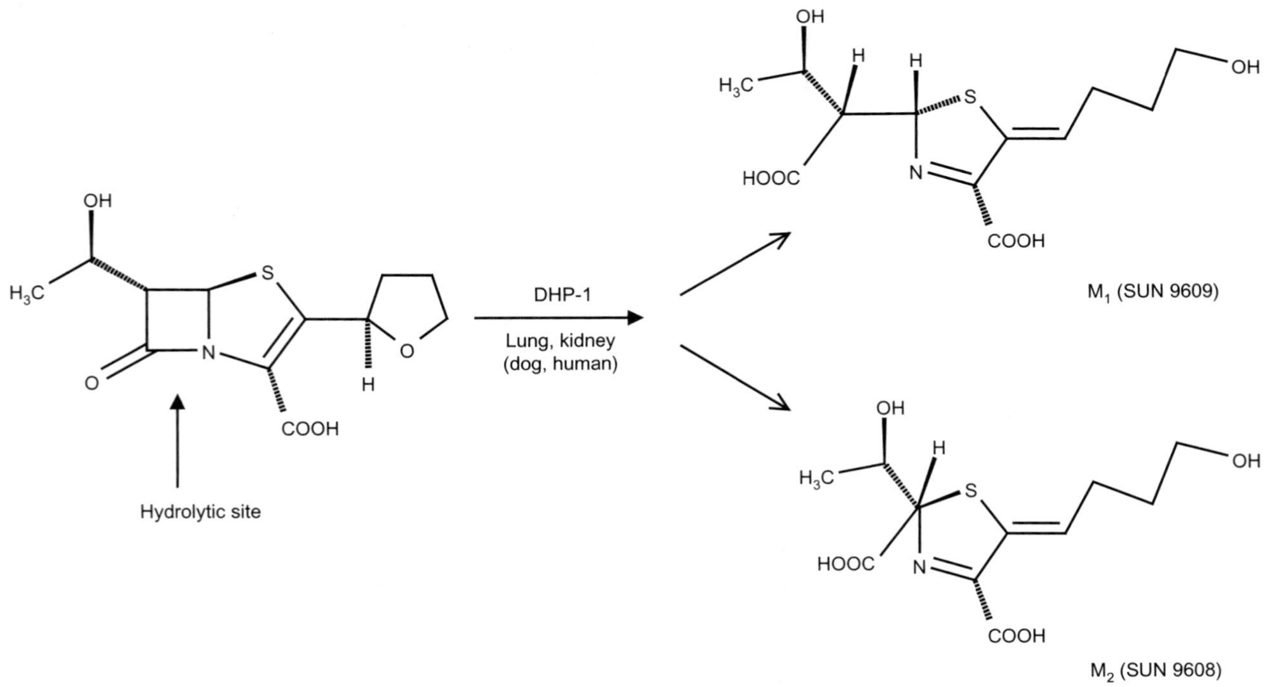

Figure 12 Hydrolysis of fropenem by DHP-I

Table 11 Activities of penems against gram-positive cocci

Organism(s)	MIC$_{50}$ (μg/ml)								
	Sch-29482	Sch-34343	Ritipenem	Fropenem	Sulopenem	HR-664	CGP-31608	TMA-3176	Men 1070
S. aureus	0.06	≤0.12	0.03	0.12	0.1	0.03	0.05	0.1	0.06
S. pyogenes	0.06	0.03	0.007	≤0.02	0.06	0.01	0.5	0.01	0.03
Streptococcus agalactiae	0.06	0.06	0.03	0.06	≤0.03	0.06	0.5		0.13
S. pneumoniae	0.01	0.03	0.03	≤0.02	0.008	≤0.01	0.25	0.01	0.03
E. faecalis	4	4	4	0.78	4	2	16	0.78	8
E. faecium	≥128	≥128	8	>128		6.25			
Enterococcus avium				3.13					
Viridans group streptococci	6.3	0.03		0.03		0.5	25	0.05	
Streptococcus bovis	0.2	≤0.015	0.5			0.25			
S. milleri	0.06		0.005					0.05	
Staphylococcus saprophyticus		0.25		0.5		0.5	3.2		
S. epidermidis	0.4	0.12	0.12	0.06	<0.03	0.03	0.12	0.1	
Staphylococcus warneri		0.25		0.12					
Staphylococcus hominis		0.12		0.25					

Table 12 In vitro activities of penems against gram-positive bacilli

Organism	MIC$_{50}$ (μg/ml)							
	Sch-29482	Sch-34343	Ritipenem	Fropenem	Sulopenem	HR-664	CGP-31608	TMA-3176
L. monocytogenes	0.25	0.25	0.4	0.12	NT[a]	0.25	0.5	
C. diphtheriae		1		0.78	NT		0.05	0.5
C. jeikeium		>128	>128		NT	>16	>25	
E. rhusiopathiae	0.25				NT	0.08		
B. anthracis				<0.02	NT	0.01	0.19	
B. subtilis ATCC 6633	0.02			<0.02	NT		0.19	

[a]NT, not tested.

Table 13 Activities of penems against gram-negative bacilli

Organism(s)	MIC$_{50}$ (μg/ml)								
	Sch-29482	Sch-34343	Ritipenem	Fropenem	Sulopenem	HR-664	CGP-31608	TMA-3176	Men 1070
E. coli	0.5	0.5	0.5	0.78	≤0.03	0.5	4	0.39	0.5
E. coli Amp^r			0.5		≤0.03		4		
K. pneumoniae	0.5	0.25	0.5	0.78	0.12	1	4	0.39	1
Salmonella spp.	0.5	0.25	1	0.1	0.06	0.5	2		
Shigella spp.	0.25	0.25	0.5	0.78	≤0.03	0.5	4		
E. cloacae	1.6	1	0.39	0.2	0.2	2	4	1.56	2
C. freundii	0.8	1	0.6	0.78	0.06	2	4	1.56	1
S. marcescens	6.3	2	3.12	1.56	0.25	4	8	25	2
M. morganii	1.6	1	2	0.78		2	4	0.78	2
P. mirabilis	0.5	0.5	1	1.56	0.25	1	2	0.39	8
K. oxytoca	0.4	0.25	0.5	0.39	0.06	1		0.39	
Providencia stuartii	0.8	0.5	1	0.78		1	6.2	0.39	8
Yersinia enterocolitica	2	0.25	0.5	1	0.06	8			
Yersinia pseudotuberculosis			0.5–4				12.5		
Aeromonas spp.	0.4	4	3.1			2	1		
P. aeruginosa	>128	128	128	128	32	128	64	64	
Acinetobacter	8	4	4	6.25	0.5	16		12.5	2
S. maltophilia	>128	>64	>128	<128		>128	128		
Alcaligenes faecalis	3.1	0.5		0.78					
Flavobacterium		128							
Burkholderia cepacia		8							

The penems exhibit good activity against β-lactamase-producing and non-β-lactamase-producing strains of *Haemophilus influenzae, Moraxella catarrhalis*, and *Neisseria gonorrhoeae*. The activity against *Pasteurella multocida, Haemophilus ducreyi, Gardneralla vaginalis*, and *Neisseria meningitidis* appears to be good. By contrast, the activity against *Bordetella pertussis* is moderate for ritipenem (MIC, ~4 μg/ml), although it appears to be better for fropenem (MIC, ~1 μg/ml) (Table 14).

The activity against anaerobic bacteria, whether gram positive or gram negative, is excellent, except against *Clostridium difficile* (MIC, >2 μg/ml) (Table 15).

The activity of Sch-29483 and ritipenem against *Mycobacterium tuberculosis* $H37_{RV}$ is not insignificant. Conversely, Sch-29483 is inactive against atypical mycobacteria (Table 16).

6.2. Mechanism of Action of Penems

After crossing the outer membrane, the penems penetrate the periplasmic space, in which the β-lactamases are found, and finally reach their target, the penicillin-binding proteins (PBP), which are enzymes responsible for the synthesis of peptidoglycan.

6.2.1. β-Lactamases

The penems are stable against hydrolysis by β-lactamases and may also inhibit the activity of some of them.

Ritipenem inactivates the enzymatic activity of *E. cloacae* class Ia, *Proteus vulgaris* class Ic, and *Escherichia coli* CS2/RE45 type V β-lactamases. It does not inactive the *Proteus mirabilis* IIb, *E. coli* CS/RE45 type III (TEM-1), or *Klebsiella oxytoca* type IVb enzyme.

Table 14 In vitro activities of penems

Organism(s)	MIC$_{50}$ (μg/ml)								
	Sch-29482	Sch-34343	Ritipenem	Fropenem	Sulopenem	HR-664	CGP-31608	TMA-3176	Men 1070
H. influenzae β$^-$	≤0.1	≤0.1	0.5	0.25		0.5	0.5	1	2
H. influenzae β$^+$	≤0.1	≤0.1	0.5	0.25	0.12	0.5	0.5		2
M. catarrhalis β$^-$		≤0.1	0.12	0.03	≤0.03		0.25	1	
M. catarrhalis β$^+$		≤0.1	0.12	0.06	≤0.03		0.25		0.25
B. pertussis		4		0.78			4		
P. multocida	≤0.01	0.5					0.25		
G. vaginalis		0.125		0.2					
H. ducreyi			0.5						
N. gonorrhoeae β$^-$	0.03	0.06	0.06	≤0.03	0.06		0.5		
N. gonorrhoeae β$^+$	<0.1	0.06	0.06	0.06			0.5		
Campylobacter jejuni	0.1		3.1						
N. meningitidis	0.1	≤0.1	≤0.06	≤0.03			0.78	0.05	
Helicobacter pylori			0.004						
Vibrio parahaemolyticus	0.006								
Vibrio cholerae	1								

[a]β$^-$, non-β-lactamase producing; β$^+$, β-lactamase producing.

Table 15 In vitro activities of penems against anaerobic bacteria

Organism(s)	MIC$_{50}$ (μg/ml)								
	Sch-29482	Sch-34343	Ritipenem	Fropenem	Sulopenem	HR-664	CGP-31608	TMA-3176	Men 1070
B. fragilis	0.25	0.06	0.06	0.13	0.1	0.125	1	3.13	0.25
Prevotella spp.	0.03	0.125	0.06	0.1		0.6			
Porphyromonas spp.		0.25	0.03	≤0.025					
Fusobacterium spp.	0.01	0.03	0.03	0.13		0.3	0.5	0.1	
Veillonella spp.	0.125	0.25		0.2					
Mobiluncus		0.06		0.2					
Propionibacterium		0.5	0.03	0.6		0.01	2	0.1	
Eubacterium		0.125	1	0.78					
Bifidobacterium		0.25		0.1			2		
Peptostreptococcus	0.25	0.125	0.06	0.39	0.1	0.01			0.25
Peptococcus	0.03	0.125	0.06	0.05	3.12	0.01			
C. difficile	6.25	4	4	4	2		2		
Clostridium perfringens	0.5	0.6		0.5	0.02	0.3			
Clostridium tetani		0.015				0.25			
Actinomyces spp.		≤0.06		0.2					

Table 16 Activities of penems against mycobacteria

Organism	MIC (μg/ml)	
	Sch-29482	FCE-22101
Mycobacterium tuberculosis H37$_{RV}$	6.2	0.06–0.5
Mycobacterium kansasii	1.6	
Mycobacterium scrofulaceum	6.2	
Mycobacterium intracellulare	12.5	
Mycobacterium fortuitum	>100	3.1–12.5
Mycobacterium chelonae	>100	
Mycobacterium bovis		0.06–0.5

The affinity (K_i) for the β-lactamases varies according to the class of enzyme. Table 17 shows the comparative affinities of ritipenem, imipenem, and ceftazidime for certain β-lactamases.

Ritipenem is stable against hydrolysis by class I β-lactamases. Like the other derivatives, it is stable against hydrolysis by plasmid-mediated extended-spectrum β-lactamases (Table 18). In fact, ritipenem, fropenem, and pseudopenem possess good activity against extended-spectrum-β-lactamase-producing *Klebsiella pneumoniae* strains of the SHV-2, SHV-3, and TEM-3 types (Table 19). HR-664 is stable against hydrolysis by enzymes of the TEM-3, TEM-5, and TEM-7 types.

6.2.2. PBP

Ritipenem possesses greater affinity for *S. aureus* PBP 2 and 3 than does imipenem. However, it has weaker affinity for PBP 2a of methicillin-resistant strains of *S. aureus* and greater affinity for PBP 2a than does imipenem.

Ritipenem possesses higher affinity for *S. pneumoniae* PBP 3, 1a, and 1b. Affinity for PBP 2b is a characteristic of the penems. This phenomenon would partly explain the good activity of this molecule against strains of *S. pneumoniae* for which the MIC of penicillin G is greater than 1 μg/ml.

In *E. coli*, the penems have a strong affinity for PBP 2, followed by PBP 1a and 1b (Table 20). Sch-34343 strongly inhibits *Bacteroides fragilis* PBP 1c.

6.2.3. PAE

At a concentration of 30 μg/ml, ritipenem possesses postantibiotic effects (PAE) of 3 h against *E. coli* and 6 h against *S. aureus*. After 2 h of exposure, a reduction of 4 $\log_{10}$ CFU is obtained for *E. coli*; by contrast, the activity against *S. aureus* is slower, where exposure of 4 h is required to obtain a reduction of 2 $\log_{10}$ CFU.

Table 17 Affinity of ritipenem for β-lactamases

Organism	β-Lactamase class[a]	K_i (μM)		
		Ritipenem	Imipenem	Ceftazidime
E. cloacae Ne K39	Ia	0.12	0.14	2.17
P. vulgaris 33	Ic	8.11	0.16	8,200
P. mirabilis JY 10	IIb	8	8.47	831
E. coli CS2 RK1	II (TEM-1)	212	2.38	20,900
K. pneumoniae 42	IVb	167	1.38	20,900
E. coli CS2/RE45	V	0.48	4.13	11,300

[a]Richmond and Sykes classification.

Table 18 Hydrolysis of penems by β-lactamases

Organism	Enzyme type	Richmond classification	% Hydrolysis					
			Ritipenem	Imipenem	Cefotaxime	Sch-34343	Sch-29482	HR-664
E. coli	TEM-1	III	<1	0	<1	0	0	<0.1
	TEM-2	III	<1	0	<1	0	0	<0.1
Klebsiella	SHV-1	III	0	0	0	0	0	<0.1
E. coli	OXA-2	V	0	0	0	0	0	
P. aeruginosa	PSE-1	V	4	0	0	1.6	0	<0.1
	PSE-2	V	5	0	2	0	0	
	PSE-3	V	0	0	0	33	0	
	PSE-4	V	3	0	2	0	0	<0.1
	OXA-3	V	0	0	0			
	P99	Ia	<1	0	0			<0.1
E. cloacae	K-1	IV	1	0	0	0	0	<0.1
K. oxytoca		Ic	1	0	10	0		<0.1
P. vulgaris		Ic	0	0	0	0	0	<0.1
M. morganii		Ic	0	0	0	<1	0	<0.1
P. aeruginosa		Id	0	0	0	0	0	<0.1
S. aureus			0	0	0	<1	0	0.3
M. catarrhalis			0	0	0	0	0	<0.1
S. maltophilia								5.3

Table 19 Activity of ritipenem against extended-spectrum-β-lactamase-producing strains of *K. pneumoniae*

Compound	MIC (μg/ml) for *K. pneumoniae* strain			
	Wild type	SHV-2	SHV-3	TEM-3
Ritipenem	0.8	1	0.7	0.8
Imipenem	0.1	0.2	0.12	0.25
Aztreonam	0.05	1.4	6.5	4.5
Cefotaxime	0.05	14	20	10
Moxolactam	0.05	0.2	0.9	0.3

Fropenem has a PAE identical to that of imipenem. After contact for 2 h at four times the MBC, the PAE are 1.45 h for *E. coli* and 2.13 h for *S. aureus*.

6.2.4. Factors Affecting In Vitro Activity

The bacterial inoculum has little effect on the in vitro activity of penems. Conversely, the pH of the medium affects the MIC. The activity of fropenem is modified if the pH of the medium is between 5.5 and 8.5, but this varies according to the bacterial species. This phenomenon has also been found with other penems, such as HR-664, particularly against gram-positive cocci (Table 21).

Among gram-positive cocci, there is no effect of the bacterial inoculum (10^3 to 10^8 CFU/ml) on the MIC, but in the case of *Enterobacteriaceae* the MIC increases by 1 dilution between 10^7 and 10^8 CFU/ml. The addition of horse serum modifies the MIC, which increases by 1 dilution (concentrations of 10, 25, and 50% horse serum). The MIC of fropenem is ≤0.025 μg/ml for *S. aureus* at acidic pH and 0.1 μg/ml at neutral or basic pH. For gram-negative bacteria, the MICs are higher at acidic pH (pH 5) than at neutral pH. The nature of the culture medium does not interfere with the MIC (Nishino et al., 1994).

6.2.5. Activity against Bacteria in the Stationary Phase

It has been shown that ritipenem, fropenem, FCE-25199, and CGP-31608 are bactericidal against strains of *E. coli* in the stationary phase.

6.2.6. Critical Concentrations

Barry et al. proposed the following critical concentrations for ritipenem: sensitivity ≤4 μg/ml (≥17 mm), and resistance, >8 μg/ml (≤13 mm), for a disk content of 10 μg.

The Swedish group has proposed different critical concentrations. The definitions of sensitivity and resistance were established with a disk content of 10 μg: sensitivity, ≤4 μg/ml (≥18 mm), and resistance, 16 μg/ml (<10 mm).

For fropenem, Fuchs et al. (1994) proposed using a disk content of 5 μg with a concentration limit of ≤2 μg/ml. The diameters of the zones of inhibition were, respectively, ≤12 and ≥16 mm for resistant and susceptible strains, respectively.

7. PHARMACOKINETICS

The currently available penems are administered parenterally, principally intravenously; in the case of ritipenem, the intramuscular route appears to be possible. The oral route is possible for fropenem, but for the other medicinal products esterification of the molecules is necessary.

The penems have certain pharmacokinetic characteristics in common, including an apparent elimination half-life on the order of 1 h, a certain stability against hydrolysis by renal DHP-I, and preponderant urinary elimination. Gootz et al. have shown that, as with penicillins, plasma protein binding increases with the hydrophobic nature of the C-2 side chain. The penems that possess a C-2 polar group (polar aliphatic chains of charged nuclei) are weakly or moderately plasma protein bound. Penems with nonpolar side chains are strongly protein bound. The size of the C-2 chain does not affect the bond.

7.1. Parenteral Pharmacokinetics

7.1.1. Ritipenem

After infusion of 0.5 to 2 g, the pharmacokinetics are linear at the end of the infusion, with a concentration of between 30 and 161 μg/ml. The apparent elimination half-life is 0.5 h, with urinary elimination on the order of 30%. Plasma clearance is extensive and greater than 500 ml/min. The two degradation products, P_1 and P_2, represent 36 and 6%, respectively, of the product eliminated in the urine. The renal clearance of ritipenem is on the order of 170 ml/min.

Table 20 Affinity for *E. coli* PBP

E. coli strain	Compound	MIC (mg/liter)	IC_{50}[a] (μg/ml) for PBP:					
			1a	1b	2	3	4	5/6
NIHJ-JC2	Ritipenem		0.025	0.03	0.016	0.5	0.069	0.12
K-12DCO	Sch-34343		1	1	0.25	32	16	1
NIHJ-JC2	Fropenem	0.78	0.3	7.5	<0.1	17.8	0.2	2.3
W7	Sulopenem		0.2	1.1	0.02	<4.2	2.1	>2.1
K-12	HR-664		>1	>1	0.1	0.1	>1	0.1

[a] IC_{50}, 50% inhibitory concentration.

Table 21 In vitro activity of HR-664 at different pHs

Strain	MIC (μg/ml) at pH:							
	5.5	6	6.5	7	7.5	8	8.5	9
S. aureus Met[s]	<0.002	<0.002	0.008	0.015	0.062	0.125	0.25	0.25
S. aureus Met[r]	0.015	0.015	0.015	0.062	0.062	0.125	0.25	1
S. pyogenes	0.008	0.008	0.015	0.015	0.031	0.062	0.125	0.125

After intramuscular administration of 500 mg, the peak concentration in serum of 8.27 ± 0.7 μg/ml is reached in 0.5 h, with an area under the curve of 12.39 μg·h/ml. The residual concentration at 4 h is 0.28 μg/ml. Urinary elimination is 25%.

7.1.2. Sulopenem

Following an infusion of sulopenem, the concentrations in plasma 5 min after the end of infusion are 33 μg/ml for the *R*-isomer and 29 μg/ml for the *S*-isomer. After a rapid distribution phase (half-life at alpha phase, ~13 min), the apparent elimination half-lives are respectively, 53 and 55 min for the *R*- and *S*-isomers. The concentration of sulopenem is 1 μg/ml at 3.5 h. Urinary elimination is 46% of the administered dose for the *S*-isomer and 26% in the case of the *R*-isomer.

Administration of 1 g of the *S*-isomer yields a concentration in plasma of 70 μg/ml. After an α distribution phase, the concentration of the *S*-isomer declines rapidly. The parameters of the *S*-isomer are identical to those obtained with the racemate (Table 22). Urinary elimination is 36%.

7.1.3. Fropenem

After a 30-min infusion of 250 mg, 500 mg, 1 g, and 2 g, the concentrations at the end of the infusion are, respectively, 22.9, 37.5, 66.3, and 126 μg/ml. The residual concentrations at 8 h are on the order of 0.1 μg/ml for the first two doses and are on this order at 12 h for the 1- and 2-g doses. The areas under the curve are, respectively, 36, 55.4, 99.7, and 204.4 μg·h/ml. The apparent elimination half-life is on the order of 0.90 h. The plasma clearance is between 110 and 144 ml/min. After administration of 1 g, the peak concentrations of the degradation products M-1 and M-2 in serum are 2.66 and 1.35 μg/ml and occur after about 30 min, with half-lives on the order of 1.37 and 2.27 h, respectively (Table 22).

7.1.4. CGP-31608

After administration of a 5-min infusion of 0.25 to 2.0 g of CGP-31608, the distribution phase is rapid, with a half-life at α phase of between 0.04 and 0.26 h and an apparent elimination half-life of between 0.12 and 1 h. About 71 to 84% of the administered dose is eliminated in the urine.

7.1.5. Sch-34343

At the end of the infusion of 1 g of ^{14}C-labeled Sch-34343, the concentration is on the order of 39 μg/ml. The distribution half-life is 0.16 h, and the apparent elimination half-life is 0.8 h. Plasma clearance is 7.52 ml/min/kg, and the apparent volume of distribution is 525 ml/kg. Urinary elimination is 23.6%, whereas the radioactivity accounts for 87.9% of the administered dose. In the feces the radioactivity is 0.8%. There are about six metabolites in the urine. Plasma protein binding is 56.6%.

7.2. Oral Pharmacokinetics

Table 23 shows the oral kinetics of penems.

7.2.1. Esters

See Fig. 13.

With the exception of fropenem, which, like the cephalosporins, is absorbed orally via the dipeptide pathway, the penems are esterified. In order to increase the proportion of thiopenem absorbed, the molecule has been esterified (Fig. 13).

In the β-lactam family, the choice of a prodrug is limited to labile esters attached to the carboxyl group, which must be free because it is partly responsible for the antibacterial activity and the hydrophilicity of the molecules.

Several types of esters have been attached to the penems: substituted or nonsubstituted acyloxymethyl, acyloxyallyl, and dioxolone. The first type of ester is metabolized, yielding formaldehyde and pivalic acid which is attached to the carnithine (Table 24). The acyloxymethyl chains are cleaved in two stages: an initial nonsteric cleavage on the terminal part of the ester, followed by spontaneous degradation of the intermediate part of the ester, which is unstable, to hydroxymethyl and formaldehyde, and then release of the β-lactam molecule. The production of formaldehyde may cause various adverse effects.

An isopropoxycarbonyloxyethy-type (cefpodoxime proxetil) or oxycarbonyloxyethyl (bacmecillinam) esterified chain is decomposed to isopropanol, CO_2, and acetaldehyde. Isopropanol is metabolized to acetone and CO_2. The dioxolone residue is metabolized to butanedione (Fig. 14).

7.2.2. Ritipenem Acoxil (FCE-22891)

Ritipenem acoxil is the prodrug of FCE-22101. Escalating-dose pharmacokinetics are linear up to 2 g. Residual levels in plasma at 4 h are on the order of 1 μg/ml. The bioavailability is on the order of 42% (Table 23).

Following administration of 1 g of ritipenem acoxil orally (0.8 g of ritipenem) to elderly subjects, the peak concentration in serum is 7.1 μg/ml and is reached in 1.4 h with an area under the curve of 18 μg·h/ml. The apparent elimination half-life is 1.2 h. Renal clearance is 132.6 ml/min, with urinary elimination on the order of 14%. The degradation product P-1 is present in the circulation and urine, but the P-2 product is present only in the urine (Table 25).

Food does not appear to affect the pharmacokinetics of ritipenem acoxil significantly (Table 26).

Table 22 Parenteral kinetics of the penems

Drug	Dose (mg)	Infusion time (h)	C_0 (μg/ml)	AUC (μg·h/ml)	V (liters)	$t_{1/2}$ (h)	CL_R (ml/min)	Protein binding (%)	Urinary elimination (%)
Sch-34343	1,000	0.5	39	29.2		0.8		57	23.6
CP-65207-S	1,000	0.03	69.8	54.1	24	1	35.5	10	31.5
CP-65207-R	1,000	0.03	36.4	23.4	27.6	1	56.9		26.8
CP-65207-S			37.2	23.3	31.1	1	38		46
Fropenem	250	0.5	30.9	36		0.95		95	29.5
	500	0.5	56.5	56.1		0.87			23
	1,000	0.5	92.6	99.6		0.87			27.4
	2,000	0.5	174.3	204.3		0.83			28.4

Table 23 Oral kinetics of penems

Drug	Dose (mg)	C_{max} (μg/ml)	T_{max} (h)	AUC (μg·h/ml)	$t_{1/2}$ (h)	Urinary elimination (%)	Absorption (%)	Protein binding (%)
Sch-29482	125	2.8	1	6	0.95			94
	250	5.1	1.1	12.4	1.1	2		
	500	12.8	0.7	31	1.3			
	750	18.7	1.1	48.3	1.4			
	1,000	16.3	1.2	68.1	1.3			
Ritipenem acoxil	750	6	0.5	8	0.4	14		42
	1,000	9	0.5	14	0.8	12	42	
	1,000	8.3	<1	11	0.9	14		
	1,500	12	0.5	13	0.5	13		
	2,000	14	0.5	23	0.5	11		
Sulopenem pivoxil	500(*S*)	1.18		2.26		23.5	35.8	10
	500(*R*)	1.07		2.18		12.2	31.6	
	1,000(*S*)	1.79		4.19		20.3	29.8	
	1,000(*R*)	1.57		3.74		8.3	23.8	
Fropenem	150	2.36	0.96	3.95	0.76	3.12	20	95
	300	6.24	1.04	11.72	0.79	6.78		
	600	7.37	1.42	19.59	0.82	5.25		
Fropenem ester	75	3.58	1.5	7.19	0.87	14.3		
	150	5.38	2.17	12.33	0.89	14.1		
	300	12.7	1.42	28.87	0.89	20.4		

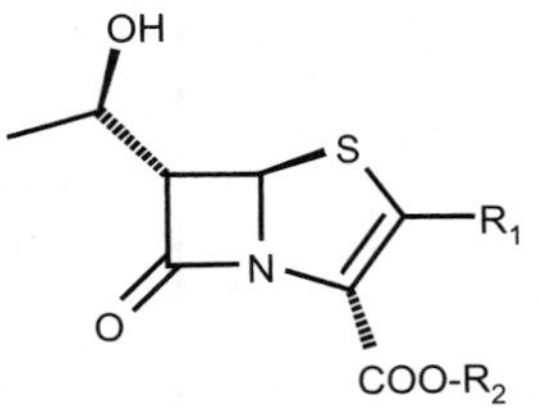

OH
S
R_1
N
O
COO-R_2

	Ester (R_2)	Parent compound
FCE 25199	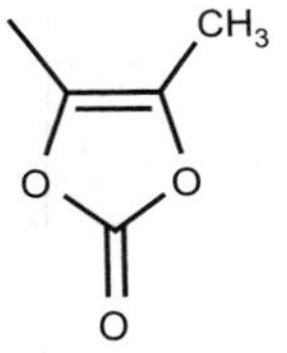 CH_3, O, O, O	FCE 24964
SUN A 0026		Fropenem
CP 65207	$-CO-C(CH_3)_3$	Sulopenem
Ritipenem-acoxil	$-CH_2OCOCH_3$	Ritipenem
TMA-230	$-CH_2OCOCH_3$	TMA-3176

Figure 13 Penem esters

7.2.3. Sulopenem (CP-65207)

Oral administration of the pivaloyloxymethyl ester of sulopenem yields high concentrations of the two isomers in plasma (Table 23). The *S*-isomer is better absorbed than the *R*-isomer. It has been postulated that administration of 1 g of the ester of the *S*-isomer would yield peak concentrations of 4.3 μg/ml, with residual concentrations of more than 1 mg/liter at 3.5 h. The ester is hydrolyzed in the gastrointestinal tract and is not detected in the peripheral blood.

Table 24 Production of formaldehyde by esters

Drug	Formaldehyde (%)	Ester
Penamicillin	7.4	Acetoxymethyl
Pivampicillin	6.5	Pivaloyloxymethyl
Pivemecillinam	6.8	Pivaloyloxymethyl
Sultamicillin	5	Pivaloyloxymethyl
Cefteram pivoxil	5	Pivaloyloxymethyl
Pivecephalexin	6.5	Pivaloyloxymethyl
Ritipenem acoxil	8.3	Acetoxymethyl

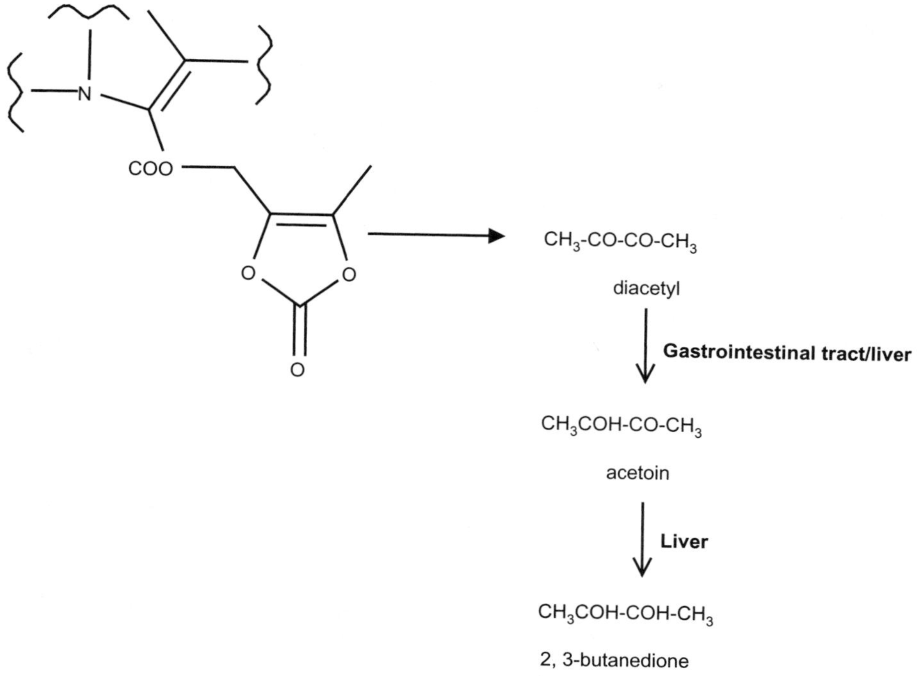

Figure 14 Metabolism of the dioxolenone ester

7.2.4. Sch-29482

Volunteers ingested single doses of 125, 250, 500, 750, and 1,000 mg of Sch-29482. The peak concentrations in serum were between 2.8 and 26.3 μg/ml and were reached in about 1 h. The apparent elimination half-life was 1 h. The areas under the curve were proportional to the ingested dose and were between 6 and 68.1 μg·h/ml. Urinary elimination was on the order of 2%.

7.2.5. Fropenem

Doses of 150, 300, and 600 mg of fropenem have been administered to volunteers. The peak concentrations are between 2.36 and 7.37 μg/ml and are reached in 1 h. The apparent elimination half-life is on the order of 1 h. Urinary elimination is 5 to 6% of the administered dose.

After a dose of 600 mg, the peak concentration of the M-1 metabolite in serum is 0.2 μg/ml, with urinary elimination corresponding to 11% of the administered dose. The M-2 product is not detected in the blood, but 4.4% is eliminated in the urine. In the case of fropenem, 25% of the administered dose is absorbed. Food does not significantly affect the pharmacokinetics of fropenem. The apparent elimination half-life is longer in elderly patients than in young adults, about 1.61 ± 0.53 h, and likewise the area under the curve is higher, 16.49 μg·h/ml for an oral dose of 300 mg.

Fropenem has been esterified by an ester of the dioxolenone type to increase its gastrointestinal absorption. After doses of 75, 150, and 300 mg of the ester, the peak concentrations in serum are between 3.6 and 12.7 μg/ml and are reached in 1.4 to 2.2 h. The apparent elimination half-life is about 0.89 h. The areas under the curve are between 7.19 and 28.87 μg·h/ml. Residual concentrations at 12 h are on the order of 0.1 to 0.2 μg/ml. Urinary elimination is between 14 and 20% of the administered dose. Food does not significantly affect the peak concentration in serum or the area under the curve, but it does cause a reduction in urinary elimination (Table 27).

Table 25 Pharmacokinetics of ritipenem acoxil and fropenem in elderly subjects

Drug	Dose (mg)	C_{max} (μg/ml)	T_{max} (h)	AUC (μg·h/ml)	$t_{1/2}$ (h)	CL_R (ml/min)	Urinary elimination (%)
Ritipenem	500	7.1	1.4	18	1.2	132	14.3
Metabolite P-1		2.1	2.6	9.8			11
Metabolite P-2							2.6
Fropenem	500	3.5	3.2	3.2	1.6		

Table 26 Effect of food (500 mg) on pharmacokinetics of ritipenem acoxil

Drug	Status of subjects	C_{max} (μg/ml)	T_{max} (h)	AUC (μg·h/ml)	$t_{1/2}$ (h)
Ritipenem	Fasting	4.98	0.72	6.61	0.63
	Fed	3.53	1.59	7.41	0.93
Metabolite P-1	Fasting	0.96	1.43	2.28	5.89
	Fed	0.95	2.57	2.86	3.33

Table 27 Effect of food on pharmacokinetics of fropenem

Status of subjects	Dose (mg)	C_{max} (μg/ml)	T_{max} (h)	AUC (μg·h/ml)	$t_{1/2}$ (h)
Fasting	300	6.24 ± 2.9	1.04 ± 0.4	1.01 ± 0.4	11.7 ± 8.3
Fed	300	4.25 ± 1.6	2.8 ± 0.5	0.96 ± 0.2	9.8 ± 4.6

Table 28 Pharmacokinetics of fropenem in children

Dose (mg/kg)	n	C_{max} (μg/ml)	AUC (μg·h/ml)	$t_{1/2}$ (h)	Urinary elimination (%)
3 (fed)	1	0.33	0.84	0.95	1.71
5 (fasting)	10	2.09	4.35	1.2	4.13
5 (fed)	24	1.21	3.36	1.33	4.17
10 (fasting)	4	2.96	8.28	0.89	6.02
10 (fed)	21	2.45	6.66	1.17	4.64
15 (fed)	3	4.3	12.05	0.82	7.97

The pharmacokinetics of fropenem in children have been investigated at different doses using a syrup. At doses of 3, 5, 10, and 15 mg/kg, the peak concentrations are 0.33, 2.09, 2.96, and 4.3 mg/liter, respectively. The apparent elimination half-life is about 1 h. Urinary elimination is between 4 and 8% of the administered dose (Table 28). In elderly subjects, the apparent elimination half-life is slightly longer (1.61 ± 0.53 h), depending on the creatinine clearance. After a single dose of 300 mg orally, the peak concentration in serum is 3.49 ± 2.62 mg/liter and is reached in 3.17 ± 1.27 h, with an area under the curve of 16.49 ± 16.42 mg·h/liter (Table 28).

REFERENCES

Alfonso A, Ganguly AK, Girijavallabhan V, McCombie S, 1984, A synthesis of penem antibiotics, p 266–279, in Brow AG, Roberts SM, ed, Recent Advances in the Chemistry of β-Lactam Antibiotics, The Royal Society for Chemistry.

Altamura M, Giannotti D, Perrotta E, Sbraci P, Pestellini V, Arcamone M, 1993, Synthesis of new penem dithiocarbamates, Bioorg Med Chem Lett, 3, 2159–2164.

Bedeschi A, Visentin G, Perrone E, Giudici F, Zarini F, Franceschi G, Meinardi G, Castellani P, Jabes D, Rossi R, Delia Bruna C, 1990, Synthesis and structure-activity relations in the class of 2-(pyridyl) penems, J Antibiot, 43, 306–313.

Bryskier A, 1995, Penems: new oral β-lactam drugs, Expt Opin Investig Drugs, 4, 705–724.

Cooke MB, Moore KW, Ross BC, Turner SE, 1984, Synthesis and some antibacterial properties of 2-oxypenems, p 100–115, in Brow AG, Roberts SM, ed, Recent Advances in the Chemistry of β-Lactam Antibiotics, The Royal Society for Chemistry.

Edwards DMF, Pellizzoni C, Strolin Benedetti M, Bizien A, Molinari M, Lebeaut A, Sassella D, 1993, FCE 22891, pharmacokinetics in the elderly, 6th Eur Congr Clin Microbiol Infect Dis.

Foulds G, Knirsch AK, Lazar JD, Tensfeldt TG, Gerber N, 1991, Pharmacokinetics of the penem CP-65207 and its separate stereoisomers in humans, Antimicrob Agents Chemother, 35, 665–671.

Franceschi G, Foglio M, Alpegiani M, Battistini C, Bedeschi A, Perrone E, Zarini F, Arcamone F, 1983, Synthesis and biological properties of sodium (5R,6S,8R)-6-a-hydroxyethyl-2-carbamoyloxymethyl-2-penem-3-carboxylate (FCE 22101) and its orally absorbed esters FCE 22553 and FCE 22891, J Antibiot, 36, 938–941.

Fuchs PC, Barry AL, Sewell DL, 1994, Antibacterial activity of WY-49605 (SUN 5555) and six other oral agents and selection of disk content, 34th Intersci Conf Antimicrob Agents Chemother.

Fujii R, Nishimura T, 1994, Pharmacokinetic and clinical studies of fropenem dry syrup in the pediatric field, 9th Mediter Congr Chemother.

Girijavallabhan V, Ganguly AK, Liu Y-T, Pinto PA, Patel N, Hare RH, Miller GH, 1986, A new class of penems—C-2-N-substituted compounds—synthesis and antibacterial activity, J Antibiot, 39, 1187–1190.

Gootz T, Girard D, Schelkley W, Tensfeldt T, Foulds G, Kellogg M, Stam J, Campbell B, Jasys J, Kelbaugh P, Volkmann R, Hamanaka E, 1990, Pharmacokinetic studies in animals of a new parenteral penem CP-65207 and its oral prodrug ester, J Antibiot, 43, 422–432.

Gootz T, Retsma J, Girard A, Hamanaka E, Anderson M, Sokolowski S, 1989, In vitro activity of CP-65207, a new penem antimicrobial agent, in comparison with those of other agents, Antimicrob Agents Chemother, 33, 1160–1166.

Hori S, Shimida J, Hirotsu I, Inomata N, Hayashi Y, Nishimura M, Ohno T, Ishihara T, 1992, Lesser epileptogenic activity of SY 5555, a novel penem antibiotic, 32nd Intersci Conf Antimicrob Agents Chemother, abstract 393.

Inoue E, Mitsuhashi M, 1994, In vitro antibacterial activity and β-lactamase stability of SY-5555, a new oral penem antibiotic, Antimicrob Agents Chemother, 38, 1974–1979.

Ishiguro M, Iwata H, Nakatsuka T, Tanaka R, Maeda Y, Nishihara T, Noguchi T, Nishino T, 1988, Synthesis and in vitro activity of novel 2-chiral substituted penems, J Antibiot, 41, 1685–1693.

Kawamoto I, Endo R, Sugawara S, 1986, Synthesis and antimicrobial activity of a new penem, sodium (5R,6S)-2-(2-fluoroethylthio)-6-[(1R)-1-hydroxyethyl]penem-3-carboxylate, J Antibiot, 39, 1551–1556.

Kim CU, Misco PF, Luh BY, Hitchcock JM, 1987, Synthesis and in vitro activity of C-2 quaternary heterocyclic alkylthiocarbapenems, J Antibiot, 40, 1707–1715.

Lode H, Saathoff A, Hampel B, Deppermann KM, Borner K, Koeppe P, Rau M, Carella G, 1988, Pharmacokinetics of FCE 22891, a new oral penem, 28th Intersci Conf Antimicrob Agents Chemother, abstract 160.

Mitsuhashi M, Franceshi G, 1991, Penem Antibiotics, Japan Scientific Society Press and Springer Verlag, p 130.

Nakashima M, 1994, Pharmacokinetics and safety investigation of fropenem in healthy male volunteers, 9th Mediter Congr Chemother.

Nishi T, Higashi K, Soga T, Takemura M, Sato M, 1994, Synthesis and antibacterial activity of new 2-substituted penems II. J Antibiot, 47, 357–369.

Nishi T, Higashi K, Takemura M, Sato M, 1993, Synthesis and antibacterial activity of new 2-substituted penems. I. J Antibiot, 46, 1740–1751.

Nishino T, Maeda Y, Ohtsu E, Kolzuka S, et al, 1989, Studies on penem antibiotics. II. In vitro activity of SUN 5555, a new oral penem, J Antibiot, 42, 977–988.

Nishino T, Okamoto K, Iwao K, Otsuki M, 1994, In vitro and in vivo antibacterial activities of SY 5555, a novel oral penem antibiotic, Chemotherapy, 42, suppl 1, 51–71.

Okonogi K, Iwahi T, Nakao M, Noji Y, 1993, Antibacterial activities of a new oral penem, TMA-230, and its active form, AMA-3176, 33rd Intersci Conf Antimicrob Agents Chemother, abstract 927.

Perrone E, 1988, Penems: conception and evolution of a new class of β-lactam antibiotics, Il Farmaco, suppl 12, 1075–1095.

Perrone E, Alpegiani M, Bedeschi A, Giudici F, Zarini F, Franceschi G, 1986, 2-(Quaternary ammonio)-methyl penems, J Antibiot, 39, 1351–1355.

Perrone E, Alpegiani M, Bedeschi A, Giudici F, Zarini F, Franceschi G, Della Bruna C, Jabes D, Meinardi G, 1987, Novel quaternary ammonium penems: the [(pyridinio)methyl]-phenyl derivatives, J Antibiot, 40, 1636–1639.

Phillips I, Wise R, Neu HC, 1982, An oral penem antibiotic: Sch 29482, J Antimicrob Chemother, 9, suppl C.

Reeves D, Speller D, Spencer R, Daly PJ, 1989, FCE 22101, a new penem antibacterial, and its oral prodrug FCE 22891, J Antimicrob Chemother, 23, suppl C.

Schliamser SE, Broholm K-A, Liljedahl A-L, Norby RS, 1988, Comparative neurotoxicity of benzylpenicillin, imipenem/cilastatin and FCE 22101, a new injectable penem, J Antimicrob Chemother, 22, 687–695.

Seibert G, Isert D, Klesel N, Limbert M, Pries A, Schrinner E, Cooke M, Walmsley J, Bentley PH, 1987, HRE 664, a new parenteral penem. I. Antibacterial activity in vitro, J Antibiot, 40, 660–667.

Sunagawa MH, Matsumura H, Inoue T, Fukasawa M, 1992, New penem compounds with 5′-substituted pyrrolidinylthio group at a C-2 side chain. Comparison of their biological properties with those of carbapenem compounds, J Antibiot, 45, 500–504.

Takamoto M, Ishibashi T, 1994, Pharmacokinetic profile of fropenem in elderly patients with respiratory infections, 9th Mediter Congr Chemother.

Wise R, Andrews JM, Piddock LJV, 1987, In vitro activity of CGP 31608, a new penem, Antimicrob Agents Chemother, 31, 267–273.

Wise R, Phillips I, 1985, Sch 34343—a new parenteral penem, J Antimicrob Chemother, 15, suppl C.

Woodward RB, 1977, Recent advances in the chemistry of β-lactam antibiotics, p 167–180, in Elks J, ed, Recent Advances in the Chemistry of β-Lactam Antibiotics, Special Publication N-23, The Chemical Society, London.

Monocyclic β-Lactams

P. LE NOC

10

1. INTRODUCTION

The systematic search for bacterial production of metabolites resulted in the discovery of a new family of β-lactams, the monocyclic β-lactams, characterized by a monocyclic structure (azetidinone heterocycle) differing from the double ring encountered in penicillins, cephalosporins, penems, and carbapenems. These compounds are produced by certain bacterial species found in the environment (water, soil, and plants) and belonging to different genera: *Gluconobacter*, *Acetobacter*, *Pseudomonas*, *Chromobacterium*, and *Agrobacterium*. The natural monocyclic β-lactams are weak antibacterial agents but are characterized by good stability against hydrolysis by β-lactamases.

The first monocyclic β-lactam to be developed and then used therapeutically was SQ-26776, or aztreonam. It is derived from a natural monocyclic β-lactam isolated from *Chromobacterium violaceum*, SQ-26180 (Fig. 1). This compound was demethoxylated at C-3 and substituted with a 2-amino-5-thiazolyl oxime moiety on the acyl side chain at position 3 of the β-lactam ring and an α-methyl group at position 4 (Fig. 2). A number of molecules have been synthesized subsequently; all retain the 2-amino-5-thiazolyl oxime group but differ in the substitutions at positions 1 and 4 of the β-lactam ring or at the oxime side chain.

Among these compounds, two are currently introduced in clinical practice: one internationally, aztreonam (SQ-26776); the other locally in Japan, carumonam (Ro-17-2301, AMA-1080).

2. CLASSIFICATION

The monocyclic β-lactams may be divided into several groups depending on the moiety attached to the nitrogen of the β-lactam ring:

- The sulfomonolactams or monobactams ($-SO_3-$), comprising aztreonam (SQ-26776), carumonam (Ro-17-2301) (Fig. 3), and BO-1165 (Fig. 4)
- The monosulfactams ($-OSO_3-$), comprising, among others, SQ-30213 (tigemonam) (Fig. 5) and SQ-83831 (Fig. 6)
- The monocarbams (sulfonylaminocarbonyl group), including U 78 608 (Fig. 7), SQ-83360 (pirazmonam) (Fig. 8), and SQ 83 691 (Fig. 9)

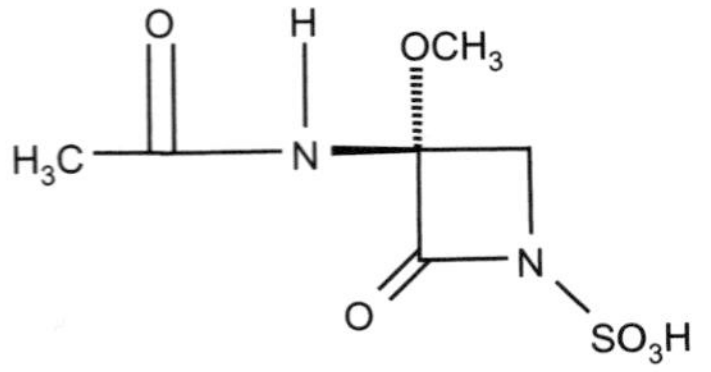

Figure 1 SQ-26180

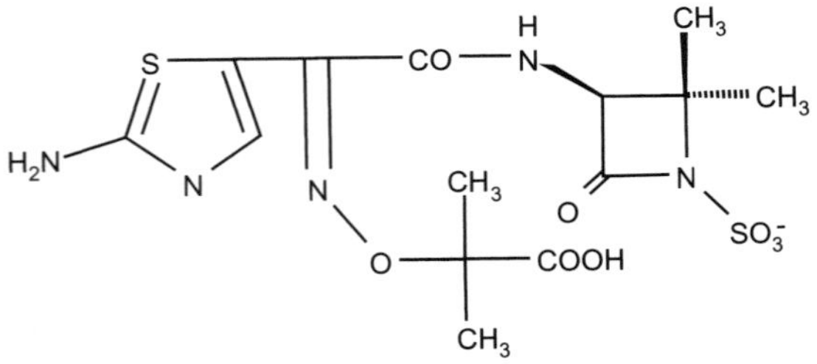

Figure 2 Aztreonam (SQ-26776)

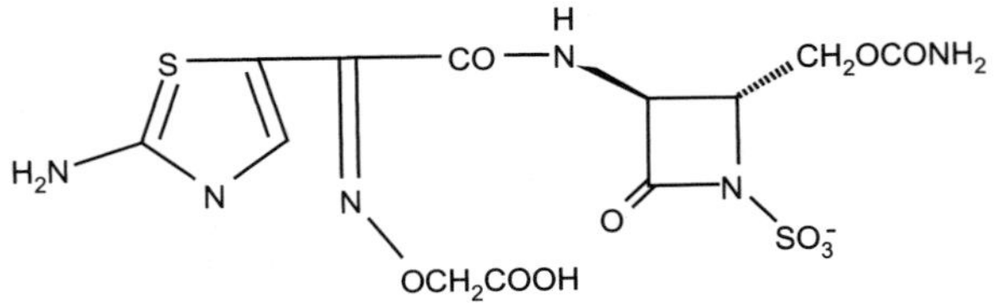

Figure 3 Carumonam (Ro-17-2301, AMA-1080)

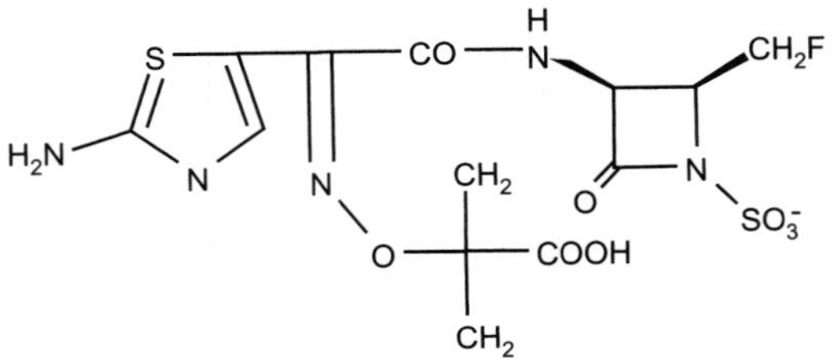

Figure 4 BO-1165

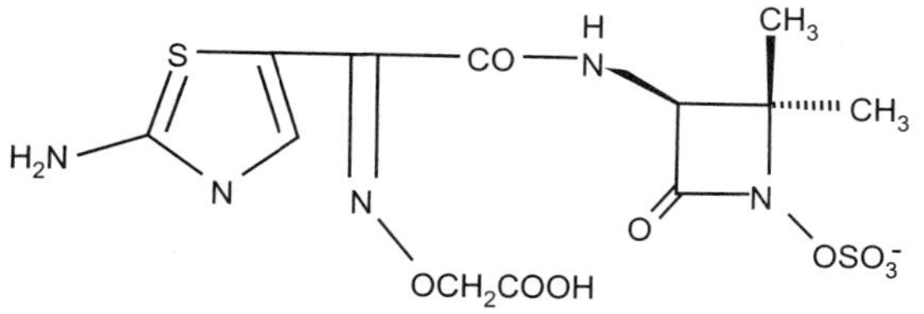

Figure 5 Tigemonam (SQ-30213)

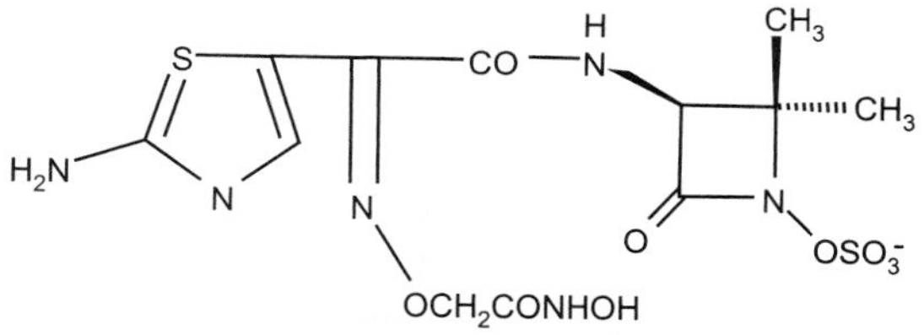

Figure 6 SQ-83831

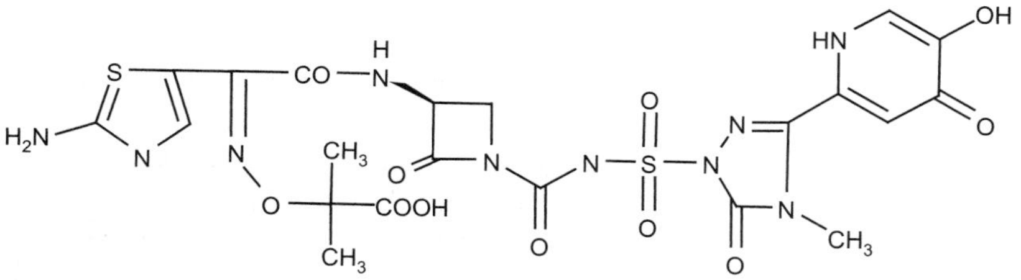

Figure 7 U-78608

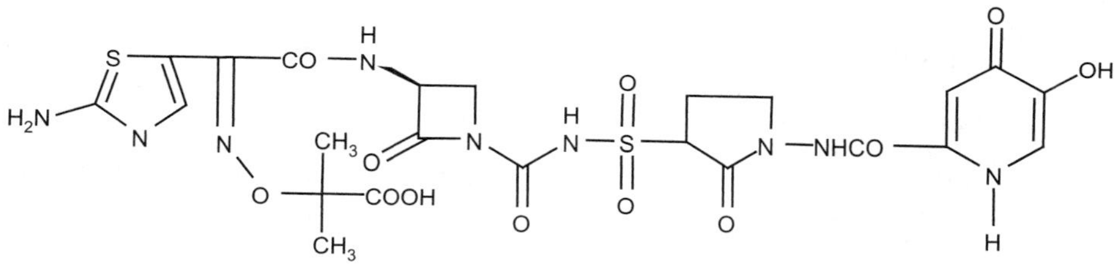

Figure 8 Pirazmonam (SQ-83360)

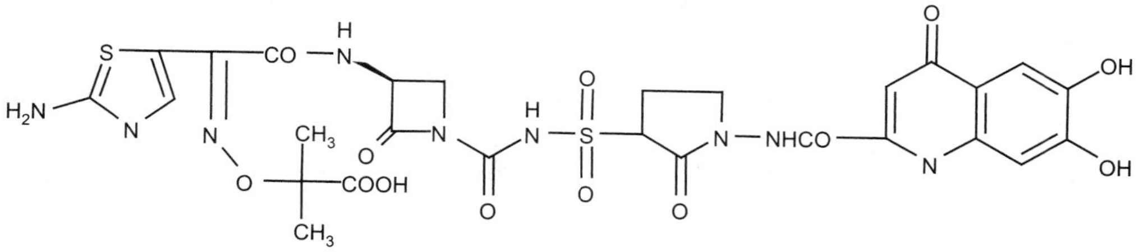

Figure 9 SQ-83691

- The monophosphams (phosphonate group), the most active of which is SQ-30590 (Fig. 10)
- The monocyclic β-lactams with a tetrazole group, such as HR-790 (formerly designated RU-44790) (Fig. 11).

3. STRUCTURE-ACTIVITY RELATIONSHIPS

This chapter is confined to a few models of monocyclic β-lactams in which the structural changes are accompanied by changes to their antibacterial properties. Table 1 compares for each molecule the groups attached at N-1 or C-4 of the azetidinone ring in the α or β position and those substituting for the oxime group.

3.1. Groups Attached at N-1

Groups attached at N-1 primarily act in the first place as activators of the β-lactam ring, but they may also exhibit intrinsic antibacterial activity (phosphonate moiety with anti-*Pseudomonas aeruginosa* activity). They also allow rings to be attached, thereby increasing the antibacterial activity.

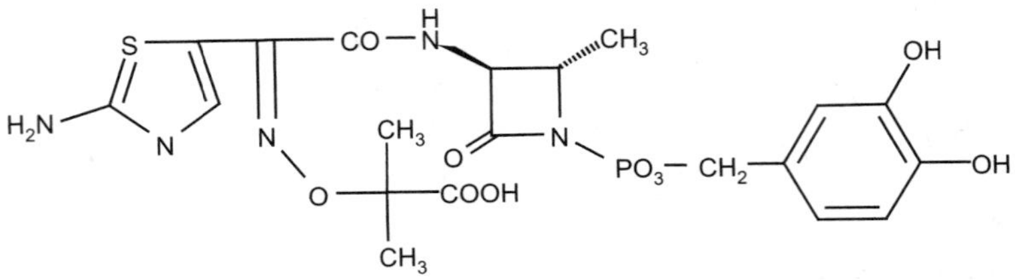

Figure 10 SQ-30590

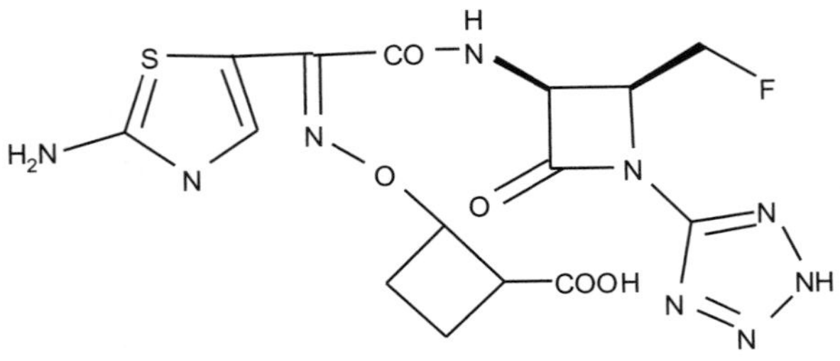

Figure 11 HR-790

Thus, the 5-hydroxy-4-pyridone (U-78608 and pirazmonam), catechol (SQ-30590), and bicyclic catechol (SQ-83691) derivatives increase the activity of the molecule against nonfermentative gram-negative bacilli, particularly *Pseudomonas* spp. In addition, the combination of a phosphonate group and a catechol nucleus (SQ-30590) may cause the compound to be resistant to certain cephalosporinases, such as the E2 and P99 enzymes of *Enterobacter cloacae*. The same applies to the tetrazole group of HR-790: this is involved in the increased activity of the compound against bacteria producing cephalosporinases or certain extended-spectrum β-lactamases.

3.2. Substitutions at C-3

The thiazole heterocycle carrying an amino group (2-amino-5-thiazolyl) present in all monocyclic β-lactams is responsible for the marked activity of these compounds against gram-negative bacilli through the increase in affinity of the molecule for the penicillin-binding proteins (PBP), particularly PBP 3. The aminothiazolyl ring, however, does not in itself ensure good stability against hydrolysis by the most common β-lactamases. The addition of an oxyimino group, also common to all the molecules, guarantees the desired stability.

3.3. Groups at C-4

Groups at C-4 involve either (i) a methyl group in the α position or a carbamoyloxymethyl group in the β position (carumonam) or (ii) a fluoromethyl group in the α (BO-1165) or β (HR-790) position. The aim of all of these groups is to increase the stability against β-lactamases. Thus, the carbamoyloxymethyls and fluoromethyls increase the activity of the analog derivatives possessing them against the K-1 enzyme (Richmond and Sykes group IV) of *Klebsiella oxytoca*.

3.4. Substitutions at the Oxime

Substitutions at the oxime moiety generally extend the antibacterial spectrum to include other gram-negative bacilli due to the thiazole heterocycle (confined to *Enterobacteriaceae*). The $C(CH_3)_2$ COOH groups present in a certain number of molecules increase their antipseudomonal activity. The same applies to the CH_2 CONHOH group of SQ-83831 and the carboxylcyclobutyl group of HR-790, which produce an interesting change in the antibacterial activity by improving the efficacy of these compounds against certain species of beta-hemolytic streptococci. This activity, however, remains inadequate for therapeutic use.

Table 1 Monocyclic β-lactams: nature of substituents at positions 1 and 4 of the azetidinone heterocycle and at the oxime side chain

Substituent(s)				Code no. (generic name)
N-1	Oxime	C-4 (α)	C-4 (β)	
$-SO_3-$(sulfomonolactams)	$C(CH_3)_2COOH$	CH_3	CH_3	SQ-26776 (aztreonam)
	CH_2COOH	H	CH_2OCONH_2[a]	Ro-17-2301 (carumonam)
	Carboxycyclopropyl	CH_2F[b]	H	BO-1165
$-OSO_3-$(monosulfactams)	CH_2COOH	CH_3	CH_3	SQ-30213 (tigemonam)
	$CH_2CONHOH$	CH_3	CH_3	SQ-83831
Sulfonyl-amino-carboxyl groups (monocarbamates)				
+5-Hydroxy-4-pyridones[c]	$C(CH_3)_2COOH$	H	H	U-78608
+5-Hydroxy-4-pyridones[c]	$C(CH_3)_2COOH$	H	H	SQ-83660 (pirazmonam)
+Catechol dicyclic	$C(CH_3)_2COOH$	H	H	SQ-83691
Tetrazole group	Carboxycyclobutyl	H	CH_2F	HR-790
Phosphonate group (monophosphams + catechol)	$C(CH_3)_2COOH$	CH_3	H	SQ-30590

[a]Carbomoyloxymethyl.
[b]Fluoromethyl.
[c]The two molecules differ by the bridge between the sulfonylcarboxyl and 5-hydroxy-4-pyridase moieties.

4. PHYSICOCHEMICAL PROPERTIES

The monocyclic β-lactams are soluble in water in the form of sodium salts.

5. IN VITRO ANTIBACTERIAL PROPERTIES

5.1. Bacteriostatic Activity

Table 2 lists the MICs at which 50% of the isolates tested are inhibited (MIC_{50}s) and MIC_{90}s of the monocyclic β-lactams for the principal bacterial species. The two figures noted for certain compounds (aztreonam, carumonam, tigemonam, and BO-1165) indicate the range of MIC_{50}s or MIC_{90}s reported in different studies. (Chantot et al., 1986; Chin and Neu, 1988; Deforges et al., 1983; Fuchs et al., 1988; Le Noc et al., 1987; Matsuda et al., 1986; Nelet et al., 1989; Neu and Labthavikul, 1981; Neu et al., 1986; Neu and Chin, 1987; Soussy et al., 1986; Thanbaut et al., 1985; Wise et al., 1981; Zurenko et al., 1990).

This table defines the spectrum of activity of the monocyclic β-lactams: activity of all molecules against gram-negative cocci (*Neisseria* spp. and *Moraxella catarrhalis*), *Haemophilus influenzae*, and *Enterobacteriaceae;* variable activity against *Pseudomonas* spp. and *Acinetobacter baumannii* depending on the compound; and lack of activity against gram-positive cocci and anaerobic bacteria.

5.1.1. *Enterobacteriaceae*

The global activities of aztreonam, carumonam, and tigemonam are on the same order: 90 to 95% of isolates are inhibited by concentrations equal to or less than 4 μg/ml.

A low incidence of strains for which the MIC is ≤8 μg/ml was found in the various studies, often involving derepressed cephalosporinase-producing strains (*E. cloacae, Serratia marcescens, and Citrobacter freundii*).

A few differences in activity are observed according to bacterial species: tigemonam and carumonam are more active against *K. oxytoca* than aztreonam (maximum MIC_{90}s, 0.25 and 2 μg/ml, respectively, versus 32 μg/ml). Tigemonam is more active against *E. cloacae* and *C. freundii* than aztreonam (maximum MIC_{90}s, 16 and 8 μg/ml, respectively, versus 64 μg/ml).

Among the more recently developed monocyclic β-lactams, U-78608, SQ-83360, and HR-790 have better global activity than the previous compounds, inhibiting 95% of isolates at concentrations equal to or less than 1 μg/ml. The difference in activity is particularly marked with respect to certain chromosomally mediated cephalosporinase-producing species (*E. cloacae, S. marcescens*, and *C. freundii*), and the MIC_{90}s of these three compounds for these species are two to eight times lower than those of aztreonam and carumonam. For *E. cloacae*, the maximum MIC_{90}s of these three monocyclic β-lactams are 0.6 to 0.25 μg/ml, versus 16 to 64 μg/ml for aztreonam and carumonam; for *C. freundii*, the same values are 0.12 to 1.2 μg/ml, versus 8 to 64 μg/ml. The activity of BO-1165 is intermediate between those of these two groups of compounds.

5.1.2. *P. aeruginosa*

Aztreonam, carumonam, BO-1165, and HR-790 have similar activities against *P. aeruginosa*. Depending on the study, 50 to 60% of strains are inhibited by 4 μg/ml and 70 to 90% are inhibited by 8 μg/ml. Tigemonam is markedly less active than the previous two monocyclic β-lactams in terms both of the MIC_{50} (64 to 128 μg/ml versus 2 to 4 μg/ml) and of the number of strains inhibited (11% of strains affected at 8 μg/ml). Two compounds (U-78608 and SQ-83360) are more effective than the previous ones against this species: their MIC_{90}s are 1 μg/ml, compared with 8 μg/ml for aztreonam, and 4 μg/ml, as opposed to 32 μg/ml, for ciprofloxacin-resistant strains.

5.1.3. Other Pseudomonas Species

All of the molecules have limited activity against strains of *Burkholderia cepacia* (MIC_{50}s, 2 to 32 μg/ml). Aztreonam, carumonam, tigemonam, and BO-1165 are inactive against *Stenotrophomonas maltophilia*; U-78608 and SQ-83360 may be active against this species (MICs of 2 to 8 μg/ml).

5.1.4. *A. baumannii*

The only two monocyclic β-lactams that are active against *A. baumannii* are SQ-83360 and U-78608, with MICs of 0.25 to 8 μg/ml.

5.1.5. *Neisseria* spp., *M. catarrhalis,* and *H. influenzae*

All of the monocyclic β-lactams inhibit *Neisseria* spp., *M. catarrhalis*, and *H. influenzae* at concentrations equal to or less than 0.25 μg/ml. The MICs for β-lactamase-producing and non-β-lactamase-producing strains of *M. catarrhalis* and *H. influenzae* do not vary.

5.1.6. Gram-Positive Cocci

The monocyclic β-lactams are inactive against *Staphylococcus aureus* (MIC_{50}s from 32 to >128 μg/ml), *Streptococcus pneumoniae*, and *Enterococcus faecalis* (MIC_{50}s, greater than 64 μg/ml). Lancefield group A, C, and G streptococci are slightly less resistant than staphylococci. Against the latter, tigemonam and HR-790 have the best relative activities (MIC_{50}s from 1 to 8 μg/ml, compared with 16 to 32 μg/ml for the other compounds), but these activities are usually insufficient for the two compounds to be considered for therapeutic use.

5.1.7. Anaerobes

The monocyclic β-lactams are ineffective against anaerobic species. The MIC_{50}s vary with the study, from 8 to 128 μg/ml for *Bacteroides fragilis* and from 64 to >128 μg/ml for *Clostridium* spp. These compounds therefore do not affect the natural anaerobic flora.

5.2. Variations in Bacteriostatic Activity According to Nature of the Medium and Size of the Inoculum

See Chantot et al., 1986; Chin and Neu, 1988; Fuchs et al., 1988; Neu and Labthavikul, 1981; Neu et al., 1986; Neu and Chin, 1987; and Wise et al., 1981, 1985.

The nature of the medium used to determine the MIC (Mueller-Hinton, heart-brain, Trypticase soy, or nutrient agar) always has a limited influence on MICs, i.e., of not more than 1 or 2 dilutions.

Variations in the pH of the culture medium from 5.5 to 7.5 only affect the MICs within the limits of 1 dilution.

The addition of 50% serum to the medium is without effect.

The inoculum size effect is very limited (difference of 1 dilution) for all of the compounds between 10^3 and 10^6 CFU per ml. The only variation observed in this case concerned the K-1 enzyme-producing strains of *K. oxytoca*, where the variation in inoculum size caused an increase in the MIC of aztreonam, associated with an increase in the hydrolysis of the compound.

Table 2 Activities of monocyclic β-lactams against different bacterial species

Species	Monocyclic β-lactam	MIC (μg/ml)	
		50%	90%
E. coli	Aztreonam	0.03–0.25	0.06–4
	Carumonam	0.03–0.12	0.06–2
	Tigemonam	0.12–0.5	0.25–0.5
	BO-1165	0.015–0.12	0.06–0.25
	U-78608	0.015	0.06
	SQ-83360	0.008	0.12
	HR-790	0.08	0.15
K. pneumoniae	Aztreonam	0.03–0.25	0.06–8
	Carumonam	0.03–0.12	0.06–4
	Tigemonam	0.12–0.5	0.25–1
	BO-1165	0.015–0.06	0.03–0.5
	U-78608	0.015	0.12
	SQ-83360	0.008	0.12
	HR-790	0.08	0.15
K. oxytoca	Aztreonam	0.03–2	0.03–32
	Carumonam	0.03–0.06	0.06–0.25
	Tigemonam	0.12–0.5	0.25–2
	BO-1165	0.015–0.06	0.06–0.12
	HR-790	0.08	0.15
E. cloacae	Aztreonam	0.03–4	0.25–64
	Carumonam	0.06–1	0.12–32
	Tigemonam	0.25–2	0.25–16
	BO-1165	0.12–0.5	0.25–8
	U-78608	0.06	0.25
	SQ-83360	0.12	0.5
	HR-790	0.15	0.6
Enterobacter aerogenes	Aztreonam	0.06–0.5	0.25–4
	Carumonam	0.03–0.25	0.06–1
	Tigemonam	0.25–0.5	0.25–2
	BO-1165	0.06	0.5–1
	U-78608	0.03	0.06
	SQ-83360	0.06	0.12
	HR-790	0.15	0.3
S. marcescens	Aztreonam	0.06–0.5	0.25–4
	Carumonam	0.03–0.25	0.06–1
	Tigemonam	0.25–0.5	0.25–2
	BO-1165	0.06	0.5–1
	U-78608	0.03	0.06
	SQ-83360	0.06	0.12
	HR-790	0.15	0.3
A. baumannii	Aztreonam	2–32	16–128
	Carumonam	4–16	8–128
	Tigemonam	32–>128	64–>128
	BO-1165	16–32	32–64
	U-78608	1	>40
	SQ-83360	0.5	2
	HR-790	40	>40
P. aeruginosa	Aztreonam	2–8	4–64
	Carumonam	2–8	2–64
	Tigemonam	64–128	>128
	BO-1165	4–8	16–32
	U-78608	0.12	1
		0.12[a]	4
	SQ-83360	0.12	1
		0.006[a]	8
	HR-790	5	10
B. cepacia	Aztreonam	4–32	16–128
	Carumonam	4–32	8–64
	Tigemonam	2–16	8–64
	BO-1165	2–8	4–64
	U-78608	4	>64
	SQ-83360	4	>64
	HR-790[b]	ND[c]	ND
S. maltophilia	Aztreonam	≥128	>128
	Carumonam	8–64	16–128
	Tigemonam	64–>128	≥128
	BO-1165	32–64	64–>128
	U-78608	2	8
	SQ-83360	4	8
	HR-790	40	40
Neisseria gonorrhoeae	Aztreonam	0.04–0.06	0.06–0.12
	Carumonam	0.06–1	0.06–2
	Tigemonam	0.03–0.06	0.06–0.25
	BO-1165	0.015	0.06
M. catarrhalis	Aztreonam	≤0.12	≤0.12
	Carumonam	≤0.12	≤0.132
	Tigemonam	0.06–0.12	0.12–0.25
H. influenzae	Aztreonam	0.03–0.12	0.03–0.12
	Carumonam	0.04–0.12	0.06–0.25
	Tigemonam	0.06–0.12	0.12–0.25
	BO-1165	0.03	0.06
	U-78608[d]	0.12	0.25
	SQ-83360[d]	0.12	0.25
	HR-790	≤0.0025	0.02
S. aureus	Aztreonam	32–128	>128
	Carumonam	32–128	>128
	Tigemonam	>128	>128
	BO-1165	32–128	>128
	HR-790	>40	>40
P. vulgaris	Aztreonam	0.03–0.12	0.03–1
	Carumonam	0.015–0.12	0.015–1
	Tigemonam	0.03–0.5	0.03–0.5
	BO-1165	0.015–0.06	0.03–0.12
	U-78608	0.015	0.03
	SQ-83360	0.03	0.06
	HR-790	0.02	0.04
P. mirabilis	Aztreonam	0.015–0.12	0.015–0.5
	Carumonam	0.015–0.12	0.015–0.25
	Tigemonam	0.015–0.5	0.03–0.5
	BO-1165	0.015–0.06	0.015–0.06
	U-78608	0.015	0.03
	SQ-83360	0.015	0.06
	HR-790	0.02	0.04
M. morganii	Aztreonam	0.015–0.25	0.03–1
	Carumonam	0.015–0.12	0.06–2
	Tigemonam	0.03–0.5	0.06–1
	BO-1165	0.015–0.06	0.06–0.5
	U-78608	0.12	
	SQ-83360	0.12	
	HR-790	0.01	0.3
Providencia stuartii	Aztreonam	0.015–0.25	0.03–0.5
	Carumonam	0.015–0.12	0.03–0.25
	Tigemonam	0.015–0.5	0.06–1
	BO-1165	0.015–0.06	0.06–0.5
	U-78608	0.008	0.25
	SQ-83360	0.008	0.25
	HR-790	0.2	0.15
	U-78608	0.03	0.12

(Continued on next page)

Table 2 Activities of monocyclic β-lactams against different bacterial species *(Continued)*

Species	Monocyclic β-lactam	MIC (μg/ml)	
		50%	90%
	SQ-83360	0.06	0.25
	HR-790	0.08	1.2
Salmonella sp.	Aztreonam	0.015–0.25	0.03–0.5
	Carumonam	0.015–0.12	0.03–0.25
	Tigemonam	0.12–0.5	0.12–1
	BO-1165	0.03–0.06	0.03–0.12
	U-78608	≤0.008	≤0.008
	SQ-83360	≤0.008	≤0.008
	HR-790	0.008	0.15
Shigella sp.	Aztreonam	0.015–0.25	0.03–0.25
	Carumonam	0.015–0.12	0.03–0.12
	Tigemonam	0.25	1
	BO-1165	0.03–0.06	0.06
	U-78608	0.03	0.06
	SQ-83360	0.06	0.25
	HR-790	0.04	0.08
Streptococcus pyogenes	Aztreonam	16–32	≥128
	Carumonam	16–32	≥128
	Tigemonam	1–8	8
	BO-1165	16–32	≥128
	HR-790	2.5	20
E. faecalis	Aztreonam	>64	>64
	Carumonam	>64	>128
	Tigemonam	>128	>128
	BO-1165	>64	>64
B. fragilis	Aztreonam	32–128	≥128
	Carumonam	8–32	16–128
	Tigemonam	16	16
	BO-1165	32–128	≥128
Clostridium sp.	Aztreonam	64	≥128
	Carumonam	>128	>128
	Tigemonam	>128	>128
	BO-1165	64	≥128

[a]*P. aeruginosa* strains ciprofloxacin resistant
[b]MIC range (0.6 to 0.5 μg/ml).
[c]ND, not determined.
[d]Identical MIC for susceptibility to ampicillin.

The inoculum effect is clearly more marked at 10^7 to 10^8CFU per ml. The MIC of the monocyclic β-lactams may increase four-fold or more for certain species, particularly for *Klebsiella* spp., *Enterobacter* spp., *Serratia* spp., and *Citrobacter* spp. This inoculum effect appears to be less consistent with tigemonam than with aztreonam and carumonam.

5.3. Bactericidal Activity

5.3.1. Minimum Bactericidal Concentrations (MBC)

See Chin and Neu, 1988; Fuchs et al., 1988; Neu and Labthavikul, 1981; Neu et al., 1986; Neu and Chin, 1987; and Wise et al., 1981, 1985.

As with the other β-lactams, the MBC of the monocyclic β-lactams are equal to one or two times the MICs for the majority of species. The exceptions observed are with *E. cloacae* (aztreonam) and *P. aeruginosa* (aztreonam and carumonam), the MBC for which may be equal to four times the MIC or more.

The MIC-MBC difference may also increase with the addition of serum to the medium or in the case of a large inoculum (10^7 to 10^8CFU/ml). This is observed in the first case with aztreonam against *Proteus mirabilis* and *P. aeruginosa* and in the second case with aztreonam against *Morganella morganii*, *Proteus* spp., and *Providencia* spp.

5.3.2. Killing Kinetics

See Chantot et al., 1986; Matsuda et al., 1985; and Shah et al., 1981.

The monocyclic β-lactams that have been the subject of killing kinetics studies (aztreonam, carumonam, and HR-790) have killing kinetics similar to those of the other β-lactams. A reduction of 99.9% of the bacterial inoculum is usually obtained in 2 to 6 h for *Escherichia coli* and 4 to 8 h for *Klebsiella pneumoniae*, *S. marcescens*, and *P. mirabilis*. The bactericidal activity becomes dose independent once the antibiotic concentrations exceed the MIC.

The monocyclic β-lactams, however, have weak bactericidal activity against *P. aeruginosa*.

5.4. In Vitro Antibiotic Combinations

In vitro antibiotic combinations have been studied in particular with aztreonam and to a lesser extent with carumonam (Neu et al., 1986; Wise et al., 1981).

The combination of a monocyclic β-lactam with an antibiotic active against gram-positive bacteria (macrolides and related substances and glycopeptides) is usually neutral. The combination of a monocyclic β-lactam with an antibiotic active against anaerobes (clindamycin or metronidazole) is additive or neutral.

The effect of the combination of a monocyclic β-lactam with another antibiotic active against gram-negative bacteria varies according to the nature of the latter: synergistic or additive in the case of an aminoglycoside, neutral or rarely additive in the case of a fluoroquinolone, and neutral or, very rarely, synergistic when another β-lactam is combined with a monocyclic β-lactam (piperacillin, cefoperazone, or ceftazidime). Rare cases of antagonism have been observed for combinations with fluoroquinolones.

6. MECHANISMS OF ACTION

All of the monocyclic β-lactams bind to PBP 3 of gram-negative bacteria, for which they have a high affinity (Chantot et al., 1986; Thabaut et al., 1985; Wise et al., 1985; Zurenko et al., 1990). Aztreonam also binds to PBP 1a, but to a lesser extent. PBP 3 exhibits transpeptidase activity and is involved in the formation of the bacterial division septum. Inhibition of this enzyme causes filamentation of the bacteria and the arrest of bacterial multiplication (initial bacteriostatic activity). Filamentation is usually followed by lysis of the bacteria (bactericidal activity). For some species, this filamentation may not be followed by lysis, but even then there is still a loss of viability.

7. STABILITY OF MONOCYCLIC β-LACTAMS AGAINST β-LACTAMASES

7.1. Plasmid-Mediated β-Lactamases

See Chantot et al., 1986; Chin and Neu, 1988; Fuchs et al., 1988; Gutmann et al., 1989; Kitzis et al., 1990; Matsuda et al., 1986; Neu and Labthavikul, 1981; Neu et al., 1986; Neu and Chin, 1987; Nelet et al., 1989; Thabault et al., 1985; Wise et al., 1981, 1985; and Zurenko et al., 1990.

The monocyclic β-lactams represent very weak substrates for the standard β-lactamases of gram-negative bacilli and for this reason are very stable against the hydrolytic activity of these enzymes, whether TEM, OXA, HMS-1, PSE, etc. In particular, they are highly stable against the TEM-1, OXA-2, and SHV-1 enzymes, the most common plasmid-mediated β-lactamases among the *Enterobacteriaceae*. Aztreonam, however, is slightly hydrolyzed by the PSE-2 enzyme produced by *P. aeruginosa*, which causes a limited increase in the MIC (8 μg/ml). This enzyme, however, is of little clinical importance.

The behaviors of the monocyclic β-lactams in response to extended-spectrum β-lactamases are dependent on the molecule and bacterial species (Table 3).

Aztreonam and tigemonam are the most susceptible compounds and are hydrolyzed by a number of these enzymes: TEM-3, TEM-7, SHV-2, SHV-3, SHV-4, and SHV-5. The MIC may be increased 8- to 512-fold. The lowest figures relate to SHV-2 (2 to 4 μg/ml) and TEM-7 (1 to 8 μg/ml), and the highest relate to SHV-4 and SHV-5 (32 to >128 μg/ml).

Carumonam in particular is hydrolyzed by SHV-4 and SHV-5 (MIC from 8 to 16 μg/ml). It is little affected by SHV-2 (MIC, 0.25 μg/ml), TEM-3 (MIC, 0.25 μg/ml) and TEM-7 (MIC, 0.12 μg/ml).

HR-790 is stable against TEM-3 (MIC, 0.6 μg/ml), SHV-2 (MIC, 0.15 μg/ml), and SHV-4 (MIC, 0.3 to 1.2 μg/ml). The MICs here are 30 to 60 times lower than for aztreonam. BO-1165 is also presented as being more stable than aztreonam against these enzymes.

7.2. Chromosomal β-Lactamases

See Chantot et al., 1986; Chin and Neu, 1988; Fuchs et al., 1988; Kitziz et al., 1990; Matsuda et al., 1986; Neu and Labthavikul, 1981; Neu et al., 1986; Neu and Chin, 1987; Nelet et al., 1989; Thabault et al., 1985; Wise et al., 1981, 1985; and Zerenko et al., 1990.

7.2.1. Natural Cephalosporinases

Chromosomal cephalosporinases are produced naturally by certain gram-negative bacilli (*Klebsiella* spp., *Enterobacter* spp., *S. marcescens, Citrobacter* spp., *M. morganii*, and *Pseudomonas* spp.). The enzymes most widely studied for their activity against monocyclic β-lactams are the K-1 enzyme (Richmond and Sykes group IV) produced by certain strains of *K. oxytoca* and the Ia and Id enzymes (Richmond and Sykes) produced, respectively, by *E. cloacae* P99 and *P. aeruginosa*. The activity of these enzymes varies with the compound.

Aztreonam is hydrolyzed by K-1 and is also unstable against Ia and Id. Carumonam is stable against K-1 but is affected by the Ia enzyme of *E. cloacae* P99 (MIC, ~4 μg/ml). BO-1165 is stable with respect to the previous enzymes but very slightly hydrolyzed by the Ic enzyme of *Proteus vulgaris*. U-78680, SQ-83360, and HR-790 are stable against the hydrolytic activity of K-1 and relatively nonsusceptible to all Richmond and Sykes group I enzymes.

Table 3 Behavior of monocyclic β-lactams against the new plasmid-mediated extended-spectrum β-lactamases[a]

Enzyme	Aztreonam	Carumonam	Tigemonam	HR-790
TEM-3	+	(+)	+	–
TEM-7	(+)	(+)	(+)	ND
SHV-2	(+)	(+)	(+)	–
SHV-3	+	+	+	ND
SHV-4	+	+	+	(+)
SHV-5	+	+	+	ND

[a]+, high MICs due to β-lactamase hydrolysis; (+), MICs-below breakpoints due to low hydrolysis rate; –, no hydrolysis; ND, not determined.

7.2.2. Derepressed Cephalosporinases

Aztreonam, carumonam, and tigemonam have reduced activities against derepressed mutants of gram-negative bacilli producing high cephalosporinase levels. The observed elevations of the MIC, however, vary with the species: the highest figures relate to *E. cloacae* and *C. freundii* (4 to 32 μg/ml); the increase in MICs remains moderate for *P. vulgaris* and *M. morganii* (1 to 2 μg/ml) and *S. marcescens* (1 to 4 μg/ml) and are often still compatible with therapeutic use of the product. The MICs observed with tigemonam as a rule are 1 or 2 dilutions lower than those observed with aztreonam and carumonam. The activity of Bo-1165 is also reduced with respect to these strains. HR-790 appears to exhibit the greatest efficacy against these mutants, with MICs 20 times lower than those exhibited by aztreonam.

7.3. Permeability Mutants

A study concerning the activities of aztreonam, carumonam, and tigemonam showed that permeability mutants affected the activity of tigemonam (fourfold elevation of the MIC) more than those of the other two compounds (Nelet et al., 1989).

8. INHIBITION OF β-LACTAMASES

The monocyclic β-lactams may behave like β-lactamase inhibitors (Chantot et al., 1986; Chin and Neu, 1988; Neu and Labthavikul, 1981; Neu et al., 1986; Neu and Chin, 1987; Zurenko et al., 1990). This property only applies to the chromosomally mediated β-lactamases, as the monocyclic β-lactams are all poor inhibitors of plasmid-mediated β-lactamases (TEM-1, OXA, SHV-1, etc.). Aztreonam is thus a strong inhibitor of the Ia (*E. cloacae* P99), Id (*P. aeruginosa*), and K-1 (*K. oxytoca*) enzymes.

Carumonam, tigemonam, and BO-1165 are also strong inhibitors of Ia and Id enzymes, but they are inactive against K-1. The compounds U-78608 and SQ-38360 are weak inhibitors of Ia, while SQ-83360 exhibits no inhibitory activity.

9. INDUCTION OF β-LACTAMASES

None of the monocyclic β-lactams are β-lactamase inducers (Chin and Neu, 1988; Neu et al., 1986; Neu and Chin, 1987).

10. INTERFERENCE BY MONOCYCLIC β-LACTAMS WITH HOST DEFENSE SYSTEMS

10.1. Interference with Phagocytic Cells

Cooperation between monocyclic β-lactams and phagocytic cells has been demonstrated in two studies (Adinolfi et al., 1989; Iida-Tanaka et al., 1986).

At subinhibitory concentrations, aztreonam and carumonam significantly increase the phagocytic activity and bactericidal activity of murine macrophage lines against different species of *Enterobacteriaceae* and *P. aeruginosa*. The changes in the bacterial cell wall caused by these monocyclic β-lactams appear to facilitate phagocytosis and render the bacteria more susceptible to the bactericidal substances released by the macrophages, hydrogen peroxide and superoxide anion.

In a study conducted on mouse macrophages, aztreonam exhibited greater intracellular antibacterial activity than extracellular activity. This activity is increased still further in the presence of immunoserum. This would appear to be related to an interaction of the monocyclic β-lactam with the macrophage O_2-independent bactericidal system, since this was still found in macrophages with impaired oxidative metabolism.

10.2. Interference with the Immune System

The monocyclic β-lactams rarely cause the synthesis of specific immunoglobulin G or E. Cross-reactivity with the other β-lactams is absent or very weak, and the monocyclic structure of these compounds might be the cause of this phenomenon.

11. PHARMACOKINETICS OF MONOCYCLIC β-LACTAMS

11.1. Pharmacokinetics in Healthy Volunteers

Table 4 lists the pharmacokinetic parameters of aztreonam and carumonam observed in healthy adult volunteers after parenteral administration of 1 g as an example. The figures shown represent the ranges of values reported in the different studies (Horber et al., 1986; Stutman et al., 1984; Swabb, 1985; WeideKamm et al., 1984).

The monocyclic β-lactams exhibit the general pharmacokinetic behavior of β-lactams, with similar parameters for the two types of compounds.

11.1.1. Pharmacokinetics after Intravenous Administration of a Single Dose

The pharmacokinetics observed are satisfactorily described by an open, linear, two-compartment pharmacokinetic model. The levels in serum and the areas under the curve are proportional to the administered doses: thus, the mean concentrations in serum obtained at the end of intravenous administration of 1 and 2 g are, respectively, 125 and 242 μg/ml for aztreonam and 77 and 150 μg/ml for carumonam. The elimination half-lives of the two compounds are on the order of 1.3 to 1.8 h, comparable to that of ceftazidime. Their apparent volumes of distribution are moderate, 0.15 to 0.20 liter per kg; the plasma clearance values are also very similar, between 1.3 and 2 ml/min/kg. Two parameters, however, distinguish the two monocyclic β-lactams: protein binding, which is higher for aztreonam (56%) than for carumonam (18 to 20%), and the higher renal clearance for carumonam (75 to 125 ml/min) than for aztreonam (50 to 56 ml/min).

Table 4 Pharmacokinetic parameters of aztreonam and carumonam in healthy adults after administration of a single dose of 1 g[a]

Parameter	Aztreonam	Carumonam
C_{max} (μg/ml)		
Intravenous (bolus)	99.5–176.33	77.7–125.6
Intramuscular	36.1–66	
T_{max} (h), intramuscular	0.6–1	
Residual concn at 12 h (μg/ml)		
Intravenous	0.57	0.7–1.4
Intramuscular	0.65	
AUC (μg·h/ml)		
Intravenous	148–232	113.4–170
Intramuscular	152–230	
Urinary elimination (% at 24 h)		
Intravenous	57–74	74–85
Intramuscular	63–81	
$t_{1/2\beta}$	1.5–1.8	1.3–1.7
V (liter/kg)	0.15–0.21	0.15–0.23
Protein binding (%)	56	18–20
CL_P (ml/min)	1.3–1.67	1.4–2
CL_R (ml/min)	50–56	75–125
Biliary elimination (μg/ml)	39–43	13.3
Fecal excretion (%) (active form)	1–1.3	2.2–3.5

[a]Data from Swabb, 1985, and Weidekamm et al., 1984.

Renal excretion is predominant (60 to 80% of the administrated dose in 24 h) and occurs by tubular secretion and glomerular filtration for aztreonam and almost exclusively by glomerular filtration for carumonam. The monocyclic β-lactams are excreted in the active form (90% of the administered dose for aztreonam). The urinary levels observed 16 to 24 h after intravenous administration of 1 g are between 2 and 2.8 μg/ml.

Biliary excretion is weak and is greater for aztreonam than for carumonam; fecal excretion accounts for 1 to 3% of the administered dose, sufficient to alter the susceptible aerobic flora (*Enterobacteriaceae*) from the third day of treatment.

11.1.2. Pharmacokinetics after Intramuscular Administration of a Single Dose

The pharmacokinetics observed here can best be described by a linear one-compartment pharmacokinetic model (absorption-elimination). The time to reach the peak concentration in serum is about 1 h, and the bioavailability evaluated from the area under the curve is approximately 100%. Levels in serum are also proportional to the administered doses, with peaks lower than those obtained intravenously (mean peak concentrations in serum of 22 and 46 μg/ml after administration of 1 and 2 g, respectively).

The other parameters are identical to those observed following intravenous administration.

11.1.3. Pharmacokinetics after Administration of Repeated Doses

Repeated dosing does not affect the pharmacokinetic parameters of the two monocyclic β-lactams: the apparent elimination half-life, apparent volume of distribution, and plasma clearance remain dose independent.

The peak concentrations in serum obtained after a single administration of 1 or 2 g of monocyclic β-lactam are greater than the MIC_{90}s for the most common species of *Enterobacteriaceae* and the majority of strains of *P. aeruginosa*. Residual levels observed after 12 h (0.5 to 1.4 μg/ml after administration of 1 g) are still effective against the most susceptible species of *Enterobacteriaceae*. Urinary levels observed 16 to 24 h after administration of 1 g are also greater than the MIC_{90}s for the most common species of enterobacteria.

11.2. Pharmacokinetics in Patients with Renal Insufficiency

Table 5 shows the variations in four pharmacokinetic parameters—apparent volume of distribution, elimination half-life, plasma clearance, and urinary excretion—in patients with renal insufficiency after intravenous administration of 1 g of aztreonam or carumonam (Horber et al., 1986).

Table 5 Pharmacokinetic parameters of aztreonam and carumonam in patients with renal insufficiency after intravenous injection of 1 g[a]

Parameter	Creatinine clearance (mg/min)			
	>80	80–30	29–10	<10
Apparent volume of distribution (liter/kg)				
Aztreonam	0.22	0.17	0.18	0.19
Carumonam	0.18	0.18	0.18	0.18
$t_{1/2\beta}$ (h)				
Aztreonam	2	3.4	4.8	6
Carumonam	1.7	4.5	6.6	11.3
CL_P (ml/min)				
Aztreonam	107	46	34	29
Carumonam	98.8	39.1	24.6	13.6
Urinary elimination (%)				
Aztreonam	58	40	58	1.4
Carumonam	78.2	54.6	42.6	12.2

[a]Data from Swabb, 1985, and Horber et al., 1986.

The plasma clearance of the two compounds is linearly related to creatinine clearance: it parallels that of renal function. The urinary excretion decreases in an identical way.

The elimination half-life increases proportionally to the degree of renal insufficiency. Serum protein binding decreases slightly as renal insufficiency increases.

Only the apparent volume of distribution remains unchanged, irrespective of the creatinine clearance.

The variations observed imply that the dosage of these monocyclic β-lactams should be adapted for the degree of renal insufficiency.

11.3. Pharmacokinetics in Children

Table 6 shows the variation in the main pharmacokinetic parameters in children after intravenous administration of 30 mg of aztreonam per kg of body weight (Stutman et al., 1984).

The concentrations in serum (100 μg/ml on average) and the apparent volume of distribution (0.30 liter/kg) exhibit no significant variations with age. Conversely, the apparent elimination half-life and the bioavailability, evaluated in terms of the area under the curve, are inversely proportional to age. The half-life is thus 5.7 h in premature infants and 1.7 h in children in the age range from 1 month to 2 years.

The lowest plasma clearance is observed in premature babies (0.94 ml/min). This rate then increases, with similar values in term neonates, infants, and children up to 2 years (1.41 to 1.87 ml/min). The elimination rate becomes identical to that of adults from 2 years (2.5 ml/min). Urinary concentrations of aztreonam remain high for a prolonged period (76 to 111 μg/ml after 24 h). Serum and urinary concentrations obtained after administration of a dose of 30 mg per kg remain higher than the MIC_{90}s for the majority of species of enterobacteria or strains of *P. aeruginosa*, and aztreonam can therefore be used therapeutically.

11.4. Pharmacokinetic Constants in Elderly Subjects

Two parameters are affected: the elimination half-life is increased and the plasma clearance is decreased in parallel with the creatinine clearance, thus necessitating an adjustment of the dosage.

11.5. Pharmacokinetic Constants in Patients with Hepatic Insufficiency

Pharmacokinetic constants were studied in subjects suffering from hepatic cirrhosis. The elimination half-life was increased (2.2 h in the case of biliary cirrhosis and 3.2 h in the case of alcoholic cirrhosis); the plasma clearance was also decreased, likewise justifying a dosage adjustment.

12. TISSUE DISTRIBUTION

Table 7 shows the concentrations of aztreonam obtained in the extravascular fluids and in a few tissues. Aztreonam diffuses into the bile, various effusion fluids, the renal parenchyma, the pulmonary parenchyma (the levels obtained after a single or repeated administration of 2 g attain 15 to 22 μg/g), the skin, and the female genital organs at useful concentrations. The concentrations obtained are considerably above the MIC_{90}s for the majority of species of gram-negative bacilli covered by the spectrum of activity of this monolactam.

The behavior of aztreonam, however, must be interpreted for a few sites where antibiotics diffuse poorly, such as the bronchial mucus, cerebrospinal fluid, prostate, and aqueous humor.

12.1. Bronchial Secretions

The concentrations observed vary from one study to another, but the mean levels obtained are usually low, from 1 to 5 μg/ml (Morel et al., 1985). These levels are sufficient to inhibit the growth of *Haemophilus* spp. or *M. catarrhalis* but are insufficient to inhibit that of some strains of *P. aeruginosa* (superinfection of cystic fibrosis).

12.2. Cerebrospinal Fluid

The concentrations obtained are up to 3.2 μg/ml in adults with inflamed meninges and may exceed this figure in children (Modai et al., 1986). These concentrations are sufficient to inhibit the gram-negative bacteria responsible for

Table 6 Pharmacokinetic parameters of aztreonam in children after intravenous injection of 30 mg/kg[a]

Subjects	C_{max} (μg/ml)	AUC (μg·h/ml)	$t_{1/2\beta}$ (h)	V (liter/kg)	CL_s (ml/min)
Prematures	83	325.2	5.71	0.36	0.94
Neonates					
<7 days	97.8	306.7	2.56	0.26	1.41
7 days–1 mo	97.4	256.8	2.43	0.30	1.68
1 mo–2 yr	118.7	228.9	1.70	0.20	1.87
>2–12 yr	96.9	189.4	1.67	0.29	2.50

[a]Data from Stutman et al., 1984.

Table 7 Tissue distribution of aztreonam

Tissue or fluid	Concn obtained	
	μg/ml	%
Extravascular fluid		
Bile (1 g intravenous)	39–43	0.2–0.5
Bronchial secretions		
1 g intravenous, 2 days	0.4–1.15 (days 1 and 3)	0.8–4.6
2 g intravenous	4.8–18.7 (at 2 h)	
CSF[a]		
Adult (2 g intravenous)		
Noninflamed meninges	0.5 and 1 (1 and 4 h after injection)	
Inflamed meninges	1.9 and 3.2 (1 and 4 h after injection)	
Child (30 g/kg intravenous), inflamed meninges	2.4–20.8	3.1–24.1
Pleural fluid (2 g intravenous)	51	
Pericardial fluid (2 g intravenous)	33	
Peritoneal fluid (1 g intravenous)	16	
Synovial fluid (2 g intravenous)	83	
Aqueous humor		
1–2 g intravenous	2.1–12.5	
2 g intravenous	1.2–2.2	
Tissue		
Kidney (2 g intravenous)	67	
Prostate (1 g intravenous)	2.9–7.8	
Lung (1g intravenous)	≥2 (30–90 min after injection)	10–22
Bone (1 g intravenous)	16	
Skin (2 g intravenous)	25	
Endometrium (1 g intravenous)	11–25 (1–2 h after injection)	33–100
Myometrium	18–30 (1–2 h after injection)	
Fetus—maternal transfer	27–33	

[a]CSF, cerebrospinal fluid.

meningitis: *Neisseria meningitidis*, *H. influenzae*, and enterobacteria (*E. coli* and *Salmonella* spp.). They may, however, be inactive against enterobacteria and *Pseudomonas* spp. involved in nosocomial meningitis.

12.3. Prostate

The concentrations reported range from 2.9 to 7.8 μg/g. These are higher than the MIC_{90}s for the species of *Enterobacteriaceae* that may be implicated in prostatitis, but they may be less than the MIC_{90}s for certain strains of *P. aeruginosa* (postoperative infections).

12.4. Aqueous Humor

The concentrations observed are on the order of 2 μg/ml, comparable to those obtained with ceftazidime and ceftriaxone. These are active against *Haemophilus* spp. and the *Enterobacteriaceae* responsible for endophthalmitis but ineffective against *P. aeruginosa*, which is also involved in these infections following ocular surgery.

13. DRUG INTERACTIONS

13.1. Interaction with Probenecid

Combined with aztreonam, probenecid causes a significant reduction in the plasma clearance of the compound by reducing its tubular secretion by half. Glomerular filtration, however, is unaffected. Probenecid also slightly increases the elimination half-life and the apparent volume of distribution of the product.

Combined with carumonam, it does not cause any change in the elimination half-life or plasma clearance since the compound is virtually not eliminated at all by tubular secretion. The apparent volume of distribution, however, is slightly increased, although this might be due to displacement of the serum protein-bound fraction of the antibiotic.

13.2. Interaction with Furosemide

Combined with aztreonam, furosemide causes a slight reduction in the renal clearance of the compound, from 0.88 to 0.77 ml/min/kg.

13.3. Interaction with Other Antibiotics

No laboratory or clinical interaction has been reported, irrespective of the antibacterial activity of the combinations.

14. TOLERANCE

14.1. Allergic Reactions

The absence of or very weak cross-reactivity between monocyclic β-lactams and the other β-lactams limits these reactions, none of which have been reported.

14.2. Clinical or Laboratory Reactions

Clinical or laboratory reactions remain exceptional and may be divided into the following:

- General clinical reactions: transient, moderate headache subsequent to administration of monocyclic β-lactam;

sensation of tiredness; abnormal sensation of taste; erythematous and pruriginous rash; and moderate diarrhea

- Local clinical reactions: pain at the intramuscular injection site and irritation of the interior of the vein
- Laboratory reactions: hypereosinophilia; moderate thrombocytopenia; moderate increases in transaminases (5% of cases), γ-glutamyltransferase, and alkaline phosphatase. These reactions are reported with aztreonam in particular.

14.3. Changes in Intestinal Flora

On the basis of their spectrum of activity, the monocyclic β-lactam spare anaerobic bacteria, gram-positive bacteria, and yeasts. They are, however, active against gram-negative aerobic floras, which they destroy and which disappear from the third day of treatment. Selection of resistant bacteria then becomes possible, and rare cases of enterocolitis due to *S. aureus* and urinary tract infections due to *E. faecalis* or *E. cloacae* have been reported.

15. CLINICAL INDICATIONS

The activity of the monocyclic β-lactams against gram-negative bacilli is comparable to that of the aminoglycosides, and a number of authors have proposed substituting the former for the latter in therapeutic regimens to avoid the risks of nephrotoxicity.

15.1. In Monotherapy

Monotherapy is confined to documented infections due to susceptible gram-negative bacteria, particularly severe upper urinary tract infections, septicemia, and soft tissue infections.

15.2. In Bitherapy

Monocyclic β-lactams are used as first-line treatments for infections in which a mixed flora is suspected. This is the case with severe intra-abdominal infections, gyneco-obstetric infections, and pneumonia in intensive care units. Monocyclic β-lactams may be combined with an antibiotic that is active against gram-positive bacteria and/or a compound active against anaerobes. Monocyclic β-lactam–aminoglycoside combinations are also recommended.

The use of parenteral monocyclic β-lactams orally for digestive tract decontamination prior to intestinal surgery should not be recommended, as this practice has caused a number of episodes of diarrhea and a few cases of pseudomembranous colitis.

REFERENCES

Adinolfi LE, Utili R, Dilillo M, Tripodi MF, Attanassio V, and Ruggiero G, 1989, Intracellular activity of cefamandole and aztreonam against phagocytosed *E. coli* and *S. aureus*, J Antimicrob Chemother, 24, 927–935.

Chantot JF, Seibert G, Klich M, and Teutsch G, 1986, RU 44 790: in-vitro and in-vivo antibacterial activity of a new N-tetrazolyl monocyclic β-lactam, 26th Intersci Conf Antimicrob Agents Chemother, abstract 844.

Chin NX, and Neu HC, 1988, Tigemonam, an oral monobactam, Antimicrob Agents Chemother, 32, 84–91.

Deforges L, Le Van Thoi J, Soussy CJ, Duval J, Thabaut A, Meyran M, Acar JF, Kitzis MD, Chanal M, Cluzel M, Morel C, 1983, Activité in vitro de l'aztreonam sur les bacilles gram negatif hospitaliers. Resultats d'une étude multicentrique, Pathol Biol, 31, 488–491.

Fuchs PC, Jones RN, Barry AL, the Collaborative Antimicrobial Susceptibility Testing Group, 1988, In vitro antimicrobial activity of tigemonam, a new orally administered monobactam, Antimicrob Agents Chemother, 32, 346–349.

Gutmann L, Ferre B, Goldstein FW, Rizk N, Pinto-Schuster E, Acar JF, and Collatz E, 1989, SHV-5, a novel SHV-type β-lactamase that hydrolyzes broad-spectrum cephalosporins and monobactams, Antimicrob Agents Chemother, 33, 951–956.

Horber F, Egger HJ, Weidekamm E, Dubach UC, Frey FJ, Probst PJ, and Stoeckel K, 1986, Pharmacokinetics of carumonam in patients with renal insufficiency, Antimicrob Agents Chemother, 29, 116–121.

Iida-Tanaka K, Tanaka T, Irino S, Nagayama A, 1986, Enhanced bactericidal action of mouse macrophages by subinhibitory concentrations of monobactams, J Antimicrob Chemother, 18, 239–250.

Kitzis MD, Liassine N, Ferre B, Gutmann L, Acar JF, Goldstein F, 1990, In vitro activities of 15 oral β-lactams against *Klebsiella pneumoniae* harboring new extended-spectrum β-lactamases, Antimicrob Agents Chemother, 34, 1783–1786.

Le Noc P, Croize J, Le Noc D, 1987, Activité antibactérienne comparée d'un nouveau monobactam, le carumonam (RO 17-2301, AMA 1080) sur des bactéries hospitalières résistantes aux bêtalactamines, Pathol Biol, 35, 451–456.

Matsuda H, Nagashima M, Nakagawa S, Inoue M, Mitsuhashi S, 1986, In vitro antibacterial activity of BO 1165, a new monobactam antibiotic, J Antimicrob Chemother, 17, 747–753.

Matsuda K, Hamana Y, Inoue M, Mitsuhashi S, 1985, In vitro antibacterial activity of AMA-1080, J Antimicrob Chemother, 16, 539–547.

Modai J, Vittecoq D, Decazes M, Wolff M, Meulemans A, 1986, Penetration of aztreonam into cerebrospinal fluid of patients with bacterial meningitis, Antimicrob Agents Chemother, 29, 281–283.

Morel C, Vergnaud M, Malbruny B, Meulemans A, Morocq N, 1985, Aztreonam: diffusion dans le mucus bronchique, Pathol Biol, 33, 533–537.

Nelet F, Gutmann L, Kitzis MD, Acar JF, 1989, Tigemonam activity against clinical isolates of Enterobacteriaceae and Enterobacteriaceae with known mechanisms of resistance to β-lactam antibiotics, J Antimicrob Chemother, 24, 173–181.

Neu HC, Chin NX, 1987, In vitro activity and β-lactamase stability of a new monobactam, BO-1165, Antimicrob Agents Chemother, 31, 505–511.

Neu HC, Chin NX, Labthavikul P, 1986, The in vitro activity and β-lactamase stability of carumonam, J Antimicrob Chemother, 18, 35–44.

Neu HC, Labthavikul P, 1981, Antibacterial activity of a monocyclic betalactam, SQ 26 776, J Antimicrob Chemother, 8(suppl E), 111–121.

Shah PM, Losert-Bruggner B, Stille W, 1981, Bactericidal activity of SQ 26 776, J Antimicrob Chemother, 8(suppl E), 77–80.

Soussy CJ, Le Van Thoi J, Duval JR, 1986, Activité in vitro du carumonam (RO 17-2301) sur les bactéries hospitalières, Pathol Biol, 34, 573–576.

Stutman HR, Marks MI, Swabb EA, 1984, Single-dose pharmacokinetics of aztreonam in pediatric patients, Antimicrob Agents Chemother, 26, 196–199.

Swabb EA, 1985, Review of the clinical pharmacology of the monobactam antibiotic aztreonam, Am J Med, 78(suppl 2A), 11–18.

Thabaut A, Meyran M, Huerre M, 1985, Activité comparée in vitro de deux monobactams: le RO 172 301 (AMA 1 080) et l'aztréonam, de la ceftazidime et du cefotaxime sur les bacilles à gram négatif, Pathol Biol, 33, 404–407.

Weidekamm E, Stoeckel K, Egger HJ, Ziegler WH, 1984, Single-dose pharmacokinetics of Ro 17-2301 (AMA-1080), a monocyclic β-lactam, in humans, Antimicrob Agents Chemother, 26, 898–902.

Wise R, Andrews JM, Hancox J, 1981, SQ 26,776 a novel β-lactam; an in vitro comparison with other antimicrobial agents, J Antimicrob Chemother, 8(suppl E), 39–47.

Wise R, Andrews JM, Piddock LJV, 1985, The in vitro activity of RO 17-2301, a new monobactam, compared with other antimicrobial agents, J Antimicrob Chemother, 15, 193–200.

Zurenko GE, Truesdell SC, Mannonyagi B, Mourey RJ, Laborde AC, 1990, In vitro antibacterial activity and interaction with β-lactamases and penicillin-binding proteins of the new monocarbam antibiotic U 78 608, Antimicrob Agents Chemother, 34, 884–888.

β-Lactam Prodrugs

A. BRYSKIER

11

1. DEFINITION OF A PRODRUG

1.1. Definition

A prodrug is a provisional chemical entity that enables the undesirable properties of a drug to be masked or eliminated. In fact, the use of a medicinal product may be restricted by its physicochemical properties, such as poor membrane permeation.

A prodrug is pharmacologically inactive, and its spontaneous or enzymatic transformation is necessary to obtain the release of the parent molecule. This release may occur prior to absorption, in the digestive tract, during absorption, or at a specific site.

A prodrug consists of the parent molecule and a nucleus that enables it to cross a physiological barrier and then be cleaved enzymatically or otherwise with the release of the parent molecule and nucleus, which follows its own course through the metabolic pathways of the body (Fig. 1) (Ferres, 1983).

1.2. Applications of Prodrugs

Prodrugs have the following applications:

- Increase in bioavailability and crossing of various physiological barriers
- Increase in duration of pharmacological action
- Increase in quantity of product at the specific active site
- Reduction in side effects
- Improvement in organoleptic properties
- Increase in chemical stability and hydrosolubility

1.3. Different Prodrugs

1.3.1. Development of Prodrugs

The most commonly prepared prodrugs are those requiring enzymatic cleavage. The body is rich in hydrolases. Esterases are ubiquitous and of different kinds and are present in the liver, kidney, and blood and in certain organs.

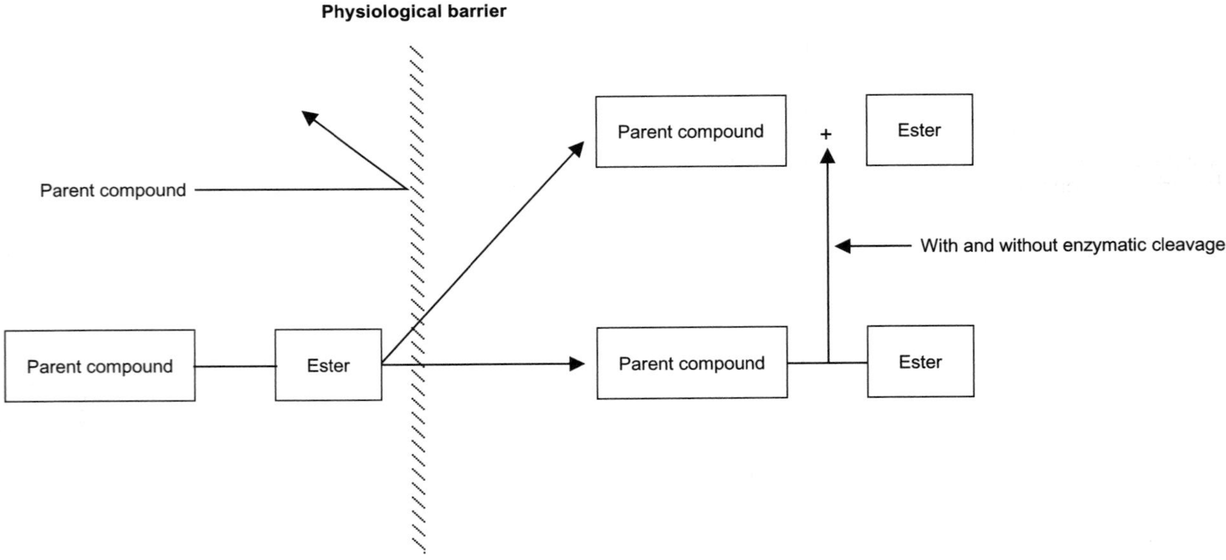

Figure 1 Mechanism of a prodrug

Esters are the most common prodrugs, while amides have been tried but are chemically unstable.

In 1945, Richardson et al. reported that simple esters at the C-3 position of the penicillins were inactive in vitro but could exhibit good in vivo activity depending on the animal species. The esters were hydrolyzed in the mouse and rat but not in the monkey, dog, or rabbit. Two years later, Ungar showed that rabbit and human sera do not contain the same esterases as those present in the rat, mouse, and guinea pig. They concluded from this study that only esterified penicillins that are chemically unstable can be effective in humans. In 1952, Ungar and Muggleton described the first ester of penicillin G: penicillin penethemate. In 1965, Jansen and Russell described the first labile ester, 3-acetoxymethylpenicillin or penamecillin, which is rapidly hydrolyzed by esterases to penicillin G. The same year Bunn et al. described hetacillin, a prodrug of ampicillin.

The studies by Jansen and Russell had a major impact on research into prodrugs. In 1970, Daehne et al. described a series of acetoxymethyl-type esters of ampicillin, including pivampicillin (C-3 pivaloyloxymethyl ampicillin). Pivampicillin is completely hydrolyzed enzymatically in rats, dogs, and humans.

One year later the Leo Research Center reported a substantial increase in the absorption of cephaloglycin when it is esterified by an acetoxymethyl group.

Fabre et al. in 1972 reported the good oral absorption of carindacillin, which is the α-indanyl ester of carbenicillin. In 1974, Clayton et al. and Shiobara et al. described the 3-phthalidyl ester of ampicillin (talampicillin). In 1975, Clayton et al. described another ester of carbenicillin, carfecillin, which is the α-phenyl ester.

A fourth type of ester, the acyloxyallyls, has been reported by the Kanebo Research Center; lenampicillin has a 2-oxo-1,3-dioxolone-5′-methyl nucleus.

1.3.2. Concept of the Double Ester

See Bundgaard, 1991.

A prodrug which is intended to improve digestive absorption must fulfill at least two criteria: be orally absorbed and be capable of releasing the parent molecule. The latter is usually difficult to achieve.

A simple ester at C-3 is often too stable. Additionally, the carboxyl group at C-3 (penicillin) or C-4 (cephems) is essential for the expression of antibacterial activity, and the esters are inactive bacteriologically. Research culminated in the most ingenious of ideas in terms of prodrugs: the concept of the double ester.

The solution was found and described in 1965 by Jansen and Russell from the Wyeth Research Centre. An esterifiable carboxyl group was attached to the second hydroxyl group of the gemediols. The simplest of the double esters is acetoxymethyl. The ester is hydrolyzed by specific esterases and the resultant product is unstable (hydroxymethyl), so penicillin is rapidly released, together with formaldehyde. Acetic acid is also released during the first stage.

Ferres (1983) (Table 1) showed that certain esters are rapidly hydrolyzed, whereas substitution of the methylene residue at the CO-CH bond by relatively sterically nonhindering groups (V) does not modify the hydrolysis rate. Sterically hindering groups, on the other hand, reduce it significantly (VI).

The thioesters (VII) are more stable, as are the carbamate-type esters (VIII). The group IX esters are totally stable.

Bodor (1977) proposed replacing the carboxyl groups by tertiary amines. These quaternary ammonium-type compounds are unstable and might improve the pharmacokinetic properties.

1.3.3. Mutual Prodrugs

Mutual prodrugs are prodrugs that combine two pharmacologically active compounds and in which each of the compounds acts as a prodrug for the other.

These prodrugs must be well absorbed. After their absorption, the two parts must be released simultaneously and in large quantities. Maximum pharmacological activity must be obtained with a 1:1 ratio. The distribution and mode of elimination must be identical.

The combination of ampicillin and probenecid (Fig. 2) has been described. Probenecid blocks the active tubular secretion of ampicillin. This derivative was administered to monkeys and dogs. Plasma ampicillin levels were below those obtained with other esters of ampicillin.

The second example is the combination ampicillin-mecillinam.

The third example is sultamicillin (Fig. 3), which is the combination of ampicillin and sulbactam. Sulbactam is absorbed in this form since on its own it is poorly absorbed, in contrast to clavulanic acid.

After administration of 500 mg of sultamicillin, the mean peak concentrations in serum are, respectively, 5.1 and 8.7 μg/ml for sulbactam and ampicillin. Digestive absorption is 60 and 70% of the administered dose. In addition, there is no food effect for sulbactam (Table 2) (Foulds et al., 1982).

1.3.4. Bifunctional Prodrugs

1.3.4.1. Cefcanel Daloxate

Cefcanel (Fig. 4) is not absorbed by the gastrointestinal tract. Esterification at C-4 of the carboxyl group increases the lipophilicity and absorption but consequently reduces

Table 1 Hydrolysis rate of esters

Hydrolysis	Compound	-R
rapid	I	$-CH_2OCOCH_3$
	II	$-CH_2OCO-R$
	III	$-CH_2OCOOCH_3$ (carbamate)
	IV	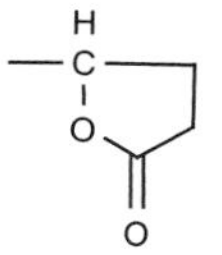 —CH(H)–O– lactone ring with C=O (lactonyl)
moderate	V	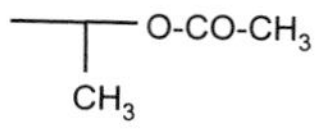 —CH(CH_3)—O-CO-CH_3
	VI	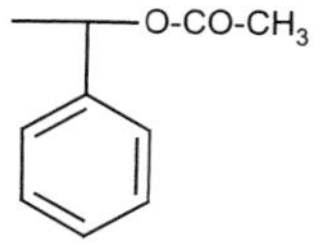 —CH(C_6H_5)—O-CO-CH_3
	VII	$-CH_2-S-CO-CH_3$
slow	VIII	$-CH_2OCON(CH_3)_2$
lack	IX	$-CH_2COOCH_3$

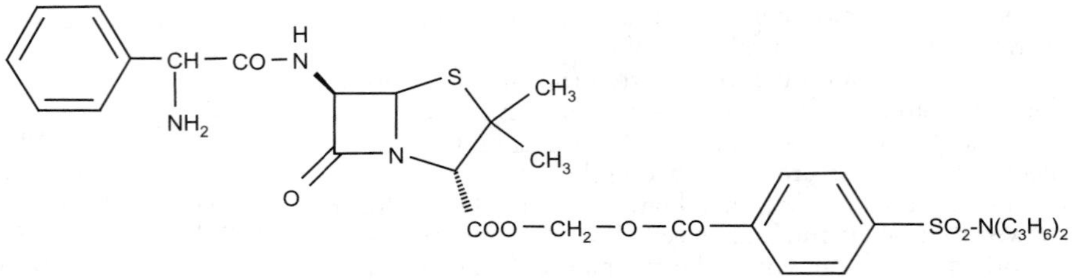

Figure 2 Ampicillin-probenecid

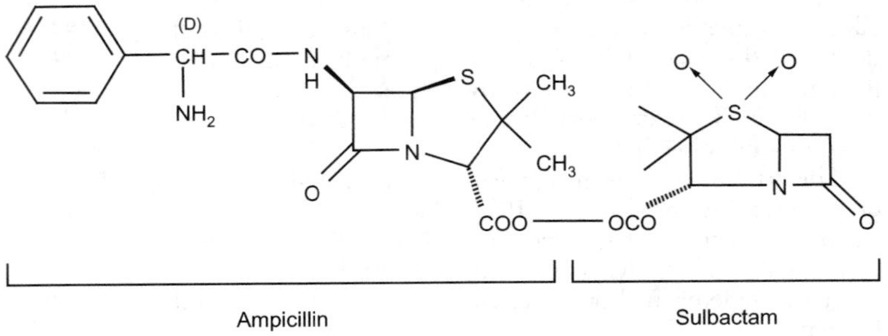

Figure 3 Sultamicillin

the solubility in water. In order to circumvent this obstacle, an L-alanine was attached at C-7 to the α-hydroxyl group (Table 3). Cefcanel daloxate is stable in the stomach. It is hydrolyzed in the small intestine, colon, and cecum. In the intestine, cefcanel monoester (KY-106) is released in the intestinal mucosa and only cefcanel is found in the portal vein (Fig. 5) (Nishimura et al., 1988).

Several amino acids have been tested, such as isoleucine, valine, methionine, leucine, lysine, proline, and glutamic acid. In mice, the best bioavailability is obtained with an L-alanine, L-proline, or L-lysine. L-Isoleucine and valine yield the worst scores (Table 4).

After administration of 150, 300, and 600 mg of cefcanel daloxate, peak concentrations in serum of 8, 5, and

Table 2 Pharmacokinetics of ampicillin and sulbactam

Form	Dose (mg)	C_{max} (μg/ml)		$t_{1/2}$ (h)		Urinary elimination (%)	
		Ampicillin	Sulbactam	Ampicillin	Sulbactam	Ampicillin	Sulbactam
Tablet	100	8.7	5.1	0.74	0.70	72	52
Tablet	750	11	8.3	0.79	0.79	62	49
Tablet	250	2.6	3.6	1.24	1.24	69	50
Tablet	250	2.5	2.8	1.37	1.37	82	52

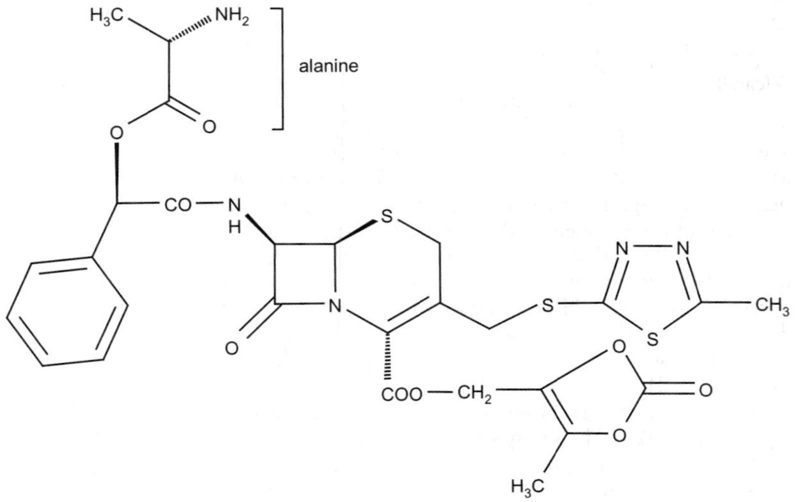

Figure 4 Cefcanel daloxate

Table 3 Physicochemical properties of cefcanel daloxate

Drug	Water solubility (μg/ml)	Lipophilicity (1 *n*-octanol/water pH 6.5)	Hydrolysis (min)	
			Rat serum (1%)	Intestine, homogeneous (1%)
Cefcanel	>500	0.0098		
Cefcanel monoester	0.02	39	NT[a]	NT
Cefcanel daloxate	>500	7.8	3.7	2.2

[a]NT, not tested.

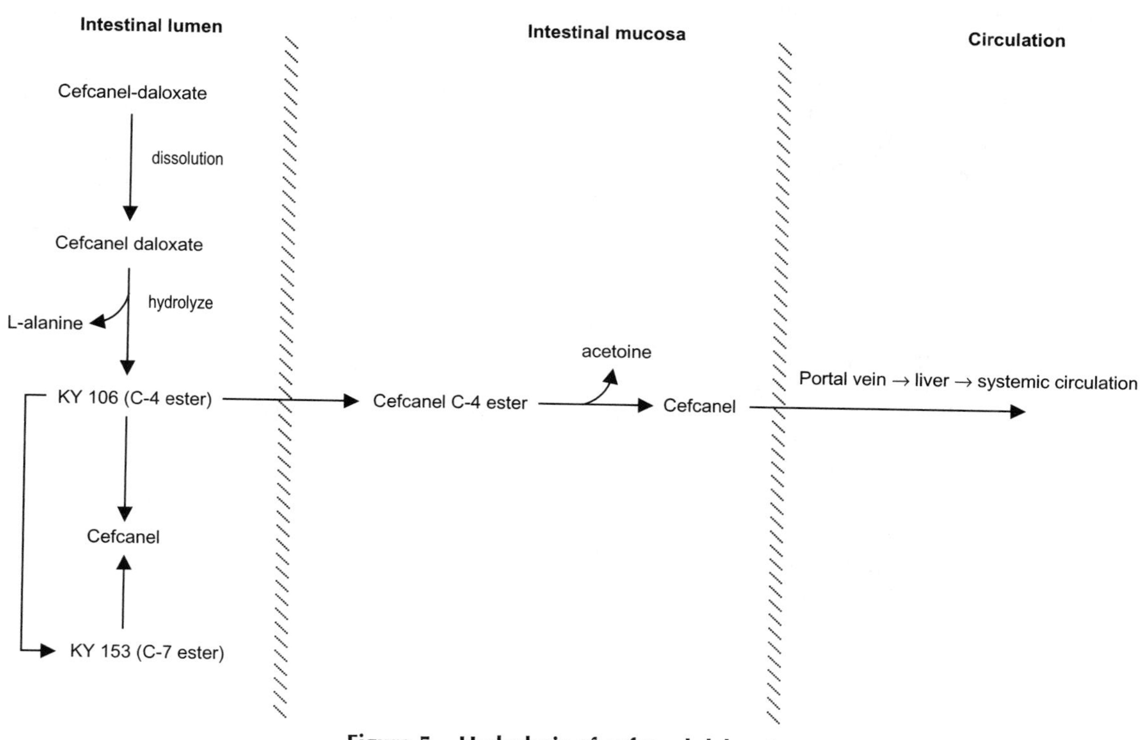

Figure 5 Hydrolysis of cefcanel daloxate

Table 4 Role of amino acids at C-7α-OH in the absorption of cefcanel

Drug or amino acid	AUC (μg·h/ml)	Bioavailability (%)
Cefcanel	0.33	1.5
Cefcanel monoester (C-4)	0.43	2
L-Alanyl	5.91	27.4
L-Valyl	1.35	6.3
L-Leucyl	4.53	21
L-Isoleucyl	1.68	7.8
L-Methionyl	2.83	13.1
L-Lysyl	7.03	32.6
L-Glutamyl	4.17	19.3
L-Propyl	5.76	26.7

4.7 μg/ml are reached at 0.5, 0.6, and 0.75 h, respectively. Between 150 and 300 mg, the areas under the curve are proportional, but above 300 mg the pharmacokinetics are no longer linear. The apparent elimination half-life is 1 h. Urinary elimination rates are, respectively, 41, 38, and 30%.

1.3.4.2. FK-020

Ceftizoxime is not absorbed orally. Ueda et al. (1983) attempted to combine different vehicles to obtain the absorption of ceftizoxime. The presence of ethyl cellulose achieves this. With a suspension of 10% ceftizoxime (500 mg) containing ethyl cellulose and 4% triglycerides, a peak concentration in serum of 3.6 μg/ml is reached in 3.3 h. The area under the curve is 17.3 μg·h/ml, and urinary elimination is 9.6% in 24 h.

A bifunctional prodrug of ceftizoxime was synthesized by Nishimura et al. (1990). A pivaloyloxymethyl chain was attached to the carboxyl group at C-4 and an amino acid, L-alanine, was attached to the amino group of the 2-amino-5-thiazolyl nucleus (Fig. 6).

The oral bioavailability is between 8 and 20%, depending on the animal species (Table 5).

The organoleptic properties of the C-4 esters of ceftizoxime (Table 6) have shown that greater sweetness is

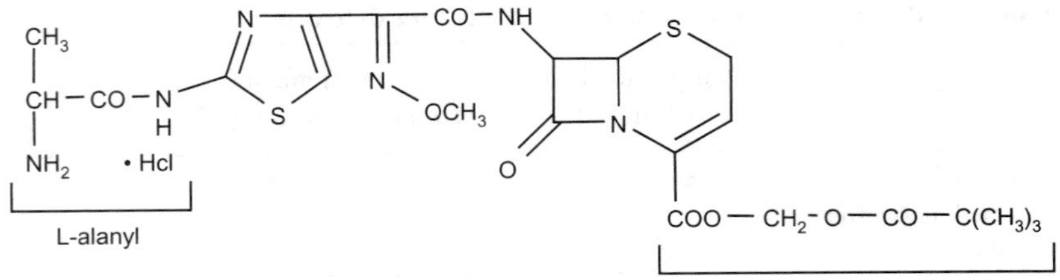

Figure 6 FK-020 (AS-924)

Table 5 Bioavailability of KY-20 in animals

Drug	Route of administration[a]	Dog AUC (µg·h/ml)	Dog Urinary elimination (%)	Rabbit AUC (µg·h/ml)	Rabbit Urinary elimination (%)	Rat AUC (µg·h/ml)	Rat Urinary elimination (%)	Mouse AUC (µg·h/ml)	Mouse Urinary elimination (%)
KY-20	p.o.	14.4	19.1	10.4	33.8	1.4	7.8	2.8	6.5
Ceftizoxime	i.v.	87.8	98.7	32.5	86	18.7	76.6	19.9	61.4
Bioavailability (%)	p.o./i.v.	16.8	19.4	31.9	39.3	7.6	10.2	14	10.6

[a]p.o., per os; i.v., intravenously.

Table 6 Organoleptic properties of the esters of ceftizoxime

Compound	-R	Sweetness (Saccharose = 1)	Bitterness	Urinary elimination (%) [rat]
I	$-CH_2OCOC(CH_3)_3$	333	±	8.0
II	$-CH_2OCOCH(CH_3)_3$	120	+	4.0
III	$-CH_2OCOCH_2(CH_3)_3$	8	+	6.5
IV	$-CH_2OCOCH_2CH(CH_3)_3$	13	++	5.7
V	$-CH(CH_3)O-CO-CH(CH_3)_2$	67	+	8.9
VI	$-CH(CH_3)O-CO-CH(CH_3)_2$	27	+	4.9
VII	$-CH(CH_3)O-CO-CH(CH_3)_2$–cyclohexyl 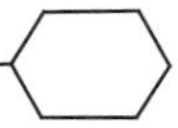	0	++	7.1

obtained with the pivaloyloxymethyl chain, but a slight bitterness still persists.

2. INTESTINAL ABSORPTION

The factors affecting intestinal absorption are of two kinds: physiological and pharmaceutical. The physiological factors are summarized in Table 7 (Bechgaard, 1982).

Physicochemical properties play a major role, particularly pK, solubility in water, and lipophilicity. The pharmaceutical form is important, as the bioavailability may be correlated with the dissolution time of the tablet and the release of the active substances. For the same active substance, the pharmaceutical formulation can increase the resistance to the environmental medium as well as the bioavailability.

Gastric emptying is regulated by the neuroendocrine system, as well as factors such as the degree of gastric distention, the composition and viscosity of the food bolus, the pH, and the temperature.

Table 7 Factors influencing digestive absorption

Gastrointestinal transit	Gastric release
Intestinal fluid	pH: bile
Absorption site	Surface; specific transporters
Metabolism	Hepatic; extrahepatic
Physiological state	Neonates; elderly
Pathological state	
Drug pharmacological effects	

Liquids and small particles are eliminated more rapidly from the stomach than solids. The gastric emptying time is between 10 and 50 min depending on the volume and temperature of the liquids. The higher the temperature, the lower the gastric emptying rate. Intraindividual variations are minor compared to interindividual variations.

Gastric pH in humans is normally between 1 and 3. The pH increases with food and may reach 6 to 7. Bile increases the duodenal pH, which may reach 5 to 6. In the distal part of the small intestine and in the colon, the pH is 7 to 8 and is unaffected by the food bolus.

2.1. Neonates

Absorption, distribution, and elimination of numerous medications in neonates differ from those in children and adults because of the biochemical, functional, and enzymatic immaturity of a number of organs. Some drugs undergo little if any absorption in adults, such as sulfaguanidine, cefazolin, and cefamandole, but are absorbed in neonates (Morita et al., 1992).

Morita et al. (1992) studied the absorption of cefazolin and cephradine in neonatal and 1-, 2-, and 3-week-old rats. Cefazolin is a polar derivative that is absorbed during the first 2 weeks of life of the rat (Table 8). The rats are weaned from the third week, and anatomical changes in the intestinal loops appear: elongation and narrowing of the microvilli. The intestine no longer allows the passage of proteins, and enzymatic activity increases. It is possible to induce these changes early in the jejunum, but not the ileum, using cortisone. There is a linear relationship between intestinal absorption of cefazolin and the intraluminal concentration in 1-week-old rats. This absorption is not modified by carnosine or glycylglycine. Conversely, with cephradine, absorption is a saturable phenomenon in rats of the same age, and absorption is inhibited by carnosine and glycylglycine.

3. ABSORPTION OF β-LACTAMS

3.1. General Remarks

The small intestine plays a major role in homeostasis. Biopolymers, like proteins, carbohydrates, and lipids, are digested in the form of small fragments by the action of digestive enzymes. The proteins are hydrolyzed to oligopeptides by pancreatic and gastric enzymes. The oligopeptides are then degraded to di- or tripeptides by peptidases localized in the enterocyte membranes.

Different experimental models have been proposed to study the absorption of the α-amino-β-lactams. Currently, the model most commonly used in vitro is the Caco 2 cell, which comes from a colonic cell line of carcinomatous origin. The following enzymatic activities have been detected in the membrane of this cell: dipeptidylpeptidase IV, aminopeptidase N, and phenolsulfotransferase. Conversely, there is no UDP-glycuronyltransferase activity (Artusson and Karlsson, 1991). A dipeptide transporter is present. It is generally accepted that absorption of amino acids occurs via a series of transporters localized in the membrane of the basolateral and apical poles of the enterocytes, which are Na^+ dependent or independent.

By contrast, absorption of tripeptides occurs via a proton gradient localized in the membranes of the basolateral and apical poles of the enterocytes (Thwaites et al., 1993).

3.2. β-Lactams

The β-lactams may be considered tripeptide analogs (Fig. 7). It has been shown in the rat that there are different transporters and that the α-aminopenicillins and α-aminocephems are absorbed differently according to the pH gradient.

When the pH gradient is markedly increased, an increase occurs in the absorption of the α-aminocephems, in contrast to the α-aminopenicillins, whose absorption is not affected by the proton gradient (internal pH = external pH = pH 7.5).

3.2.1. Chemical Structure

The α-aminocephems are amphoteric molecules which have a negatively charged group (COO^-) and a positively charged group (NH^{3+}). They are not hydrolyzed by intestinal hydrolases.

The chemical structure interferes with intestinal absorption. The presence of a hydroxyl group on the phenyl nucleus in the *para* position of ampicillin (amoxicillin) or cephalexin (cefadroxil) increases intestinal absorption.

The cephalosporins that have a 7-phenylglycine chain are orally absorbed. However, certain non-α-amino molecules are absorbed, such as cefixime, cefdinir, FK-089, and ceftibuten, and they also use the dipeptide transport route.

Stereospecificity of the transporter has been demonstrated for cephalexin. The *l*-isomer is less well absorbed in the rat than the *d*-isomer.

Ceftibuten is a dianionic molecule which has a center of asymmetry on the side chain in position 7 of the cephem nucleus (Fig. 8). The *cis* isomer of ceftibuten is

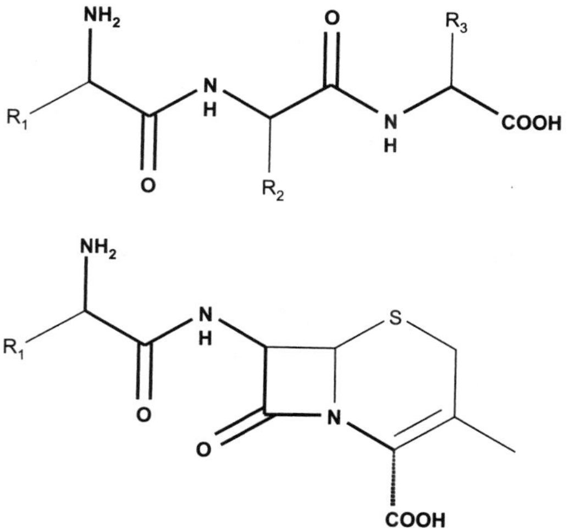

Figure 7 Structural analogies between tripeptides and cephems

Table 8 Oral kinetics of cefazolin in the neonatal rat (20 mg/kg)

Age of rats	Cefazolin			Cephradine		
	C_{max} (μg/ml)	T_{max} (h)	AUC (μg·h/ml)	C_{max} (μg/ml)	T_{max} (h)	AUC (μg·h/ml)
1 wk	3.48	6.36	51.86	7.42	2.83	111.44
2 wk	4.13	2.2	22.69	5.32	2.23	64.6
3 wk	ND[a]	ND	ND	4.33	1.97	18.54
Adult	ND	ND	ND	4.47	0.67	12.3

[a]ND, not determined.

well absorbed, whereas the *trans* isomer is not absorbed (Yoshikawa et al., 1989). In addition, this molecule has three ionizable groups (two carboxyl groups, pK 2.3 and 3.2, and an amino group on the 2-amino-5-thiazolyl nucleus, pK 4.5).

3.2.2. Physicochemical Properties

The absorption of the molecules depends on the liposolubility and the degree of ionization, which is dependent on the pH of the environment and the pK of the molecule (Irwin et al., 1987) (Table 9).

The surface of the intestine is a lipid barrier. Schanker et al. proposed the "pH-partition" model for the absorption of drugs, by which the degree of absorption of bases and weak acids depends on their liposolubility and their degree of ionization. This hypothesis predicts that molecules with a pK of less than 3 will be weakly absorbed. Penicillins and cephalosporins are antibiotics in which the pK of the carboxyl group is between 2 and 3 (Fig. 9).

Figure 8 Ceftibuten

Table 9 Lipophilicity of cephalosporins[a]

Drug	LogP *n*-octanol/water, 37°C, pH 7.4
Cefazolin	−4.92
Cephalothin	−4.3
Cefazaflur	−3.98
Cephaloridine	−1.52
Cephradine	−1.15
Cephalexin	−1.1
Cephaloglycin	−1.05

[a]Data from Irwin et al., 1987.

The lipophilicity of the antibiotics varies according to the nature of the side chains and the pH in the intestinal lumen. At intestinal pH (pH 6 to 7), all β-lactams are weakly liposoluble.

3.3. Transport Systems

The α-amino-β-lactams use the saturable dipeptide transport system in the intestine, but also in the renal tubules (Fig. 10).

One of the systems has a weak affinity and a strong transport capacity, and the second has a strong affinity but a weak transport capacity.

Studies with cefixime and ceftibuten have shown that there are two pH-dependent types of transporters. Type I functions at neutral pH, and type II functions at acid pH. There is a third type of passage, but this is still poorly defined and probably involves passive diffusion of the antibiotic.

Type II is used by non-α-aminocephalosporins such as ceftibuten, cefixime, and cefdinir, whereas the α-aminocephalosporins use type I and type II transporters (Table 10). The interior of the enterocytes is normally negatively charged relative to the intestinal lumen, where there is an acidic microenvironment on the surface of the epithelium. This is maintained by the Na^+/H^+ antiport system of the brush border and the Na^+/K^+ ATPase pump of the basolateral border (Lucas et al., 1976; Westphal et al., 1995) (Fig. 11).

3.3.1. Penicillins

With the exception of the 7-phenylglycine penicillins, the absorption of penicillins is dependent on their lipophilicity and their stability in an acidic medium.

The lipophilic penicillins and the phenoxy (penicillin V and derivatives) or isoxazolyl (oxacillin and derivatives) analogs cross the brush border membrane by a saturable phenomenon.

3.3.2. Cephalosporins

3.3.2.1. α-Amino Cephalosporins

Quay and Forster (1970) were the first to show that absorption of cephalexin in the jejunum is inhibited by a dipeptide, L-phenylalanylglycine. α-Aminocephalosporins are effectively absorbed in the small intestine, even if they are ionized at physiological pH, and are poorly liposoluble.

Using an in vitro model, Lowther et al. (1990) showed that penetration inside the enterocytes is a saturable phenomenon, as demonstrated by the non-dose dependency (Table 11).

Figure 9 pK values of penams and cephems

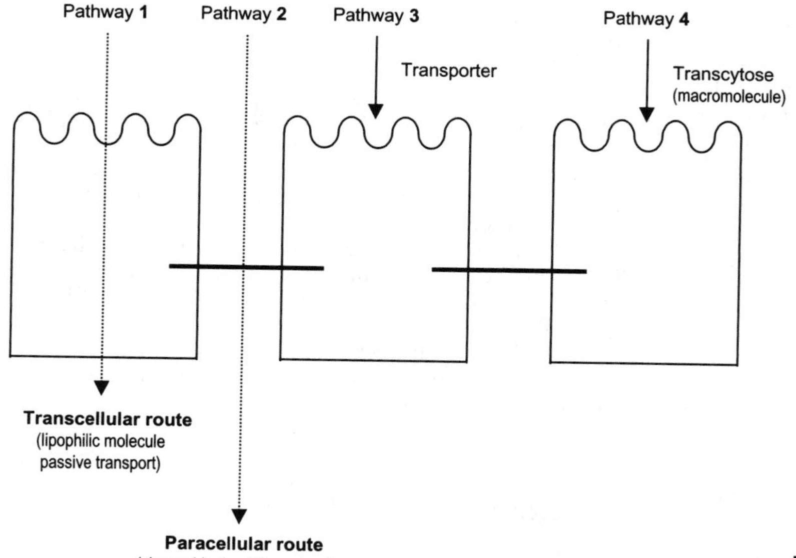

Figure 10 Transepithelial transport of xenobiotics

Table 10 Transport systems used by different cephalosporins

Class A, type I/II	Class B, type II
Cefaclor	Cefixime
Cephalexin	Ceftibuten
Cefadroxil	FK-089
Cephradine	Cefdinir

3.3.2.2. Ceftibuten, Cefixime, FK-089, and Cefdinir

Ceftibuten is transported into the enterocyte by means of a pH gradient. The initial penetration, like that of cefaclor, is concentration dependent and a function of the pH gradient. Transport is electrogenic and associated with a transfer of positive charges across the membrane (Yoshikawa et al., 1989).

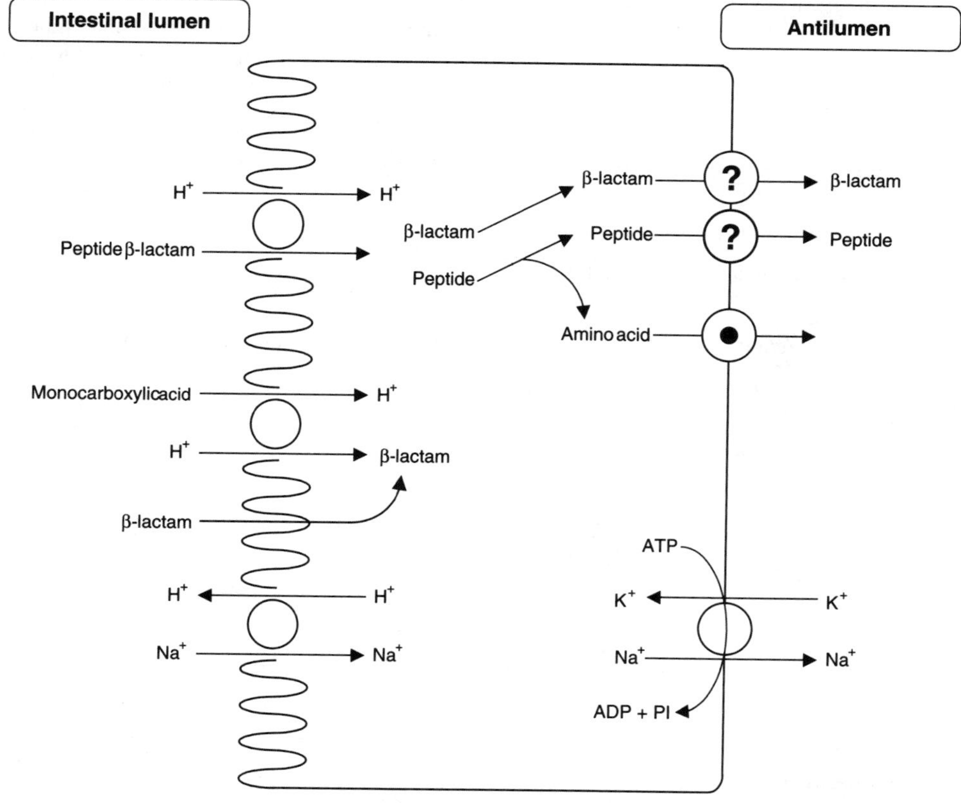

Figure 11 Intestinal absorption of β-lactams

Table 11 Relationship between enterocytes and bioavailability[a]

Drug	Penetration in enterocytes (oral) (nmol/mg of proteins/30 s)	Bioavailability per os (%) in humans
Cefadroxil	4.4	85
Cephradine	3.1	95
Cephalexin	2.9	90
Cefaclor	3	50
Cefixime	2.1	30
Cefoxitin	<0.6	0
Cefazolin	<0.4	0.0
Cefuroxime	<0.4	1
Cephalothin	<1	0

[a]Data from Lowther et al., 1990.

The absorption of ceftibuten increases as the pH decreases, as opposed to what is observed with cefaclor, cephradine, and cefixime. Ceftibuten is cotransported with a proton in exchange for an OH^-. The transport process is affected by the membrane potential.

The absorption of cefixime and FK-089 also requires an acidic medium (pH, ~4.5 to 5) compared to cephradine (pH 6.0).

It has been shown with FK-089 that the lipophilicity of the molecule increases when the pH decreases (Table 12).

The pharmacokinetics of FK-089 are summarized in Table 13.

Table 12 Lipophilicity of FK-089 as a function of pH[a]

pH	P_{app} (2-methyl/propanol/water, 27°C)
2	1.535
3	0.454
3.5	0.064
4	0.017
4.5	0.004

[a]Data from Tsuji et al., 1986.

For ceftibuten, cefaclor, and cephradine, penetration is $[H^+]$ dependent (Fig. 12).

Cefdinir utilizes the dipeptide transport pathway, but also that of the monocarboxyl acids, such as acetic acid and lactic acid. These two pathways are saturable. The dipeptide pathway accounts for 35% of absorption, that of the monocarboxyl acids accounts for 30%, and a passive diffusion pathway accounts for 25%, while 10% of cefdinir is transferred by an unknown mechanism.

Other derivatives whose mechanism of absorption has not been described are currently in the preclinical development stage, such as S-1090, FK-312, CP-0467, and BK-218 (Fig. 13).

Overall, the different oral cephalosporins may be classified into two subgroups, A and B, on the basis of the importance of pH in their penetration into the enterocyte (Table 10).

4. PENICILLIN PRODRUGS

4.1. Penicillin G

Penicillin G is a weak acid (pK, ~2.7) and is weakly lipophilic ($\log_{10} P = 1.76$). It is unstable in an acidic medium and for this reason is weakly absorbed orally. Esters have been synthesized to increase its lipophilicity. The first esters were single esters of the alkyl or aryl type, which did not provide good release of penicillin G. Blood penicillin G levels were subject to major interspecies and intraspecies variations.

4.1.1. Penethamate Hydroiodide

See Fig. 14.

The first esters synthesized were diakylaminoethyls, and the prototype was *N,N*-diethylaminoethyl penicillin G. The half-life of cleavage to penicillin G is about 30 min at pH 7.4 and 37°C. This molecule is more lipophilic and more stable in an acidic medium (pK 8.5) than penicillin G. This type of ester is hydrolyzed slowly in tissues and blood. This is probably related to the degree of protein binding, which is extensive for this ester and prevents the esterases from acting on the amino group. The mechanism of hydrolysis is summarized in Fig. 15.

Table 13 Pharmacokinetics of FK-089[a]

Dose (mg)	C_{max} (μg/ml)	T_{max} (h)	$t_{1/2}$ (h)	AUC (μg·h/ml)	CL_R (ml/min)	Urinary elimination (%)
125	1.59	2.3	1.96	8.1	118.1	43.7
250	2.44	2.9	2.15	12.8	146.5	33.6

[a]Data from Suematsu, 1985.

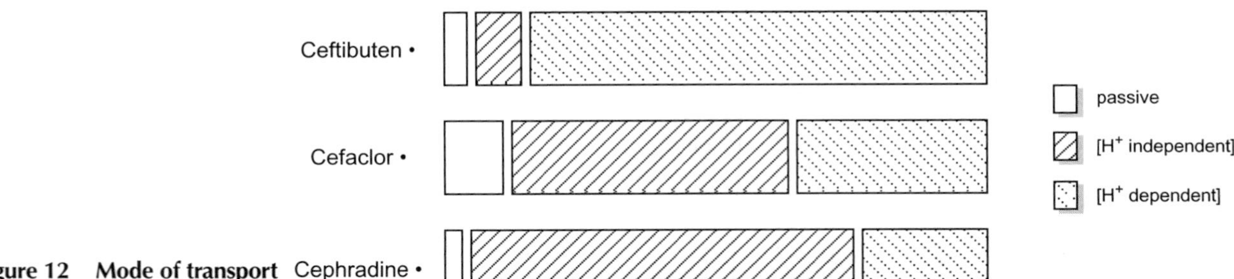

Figure 12 Mode of transport of cephems

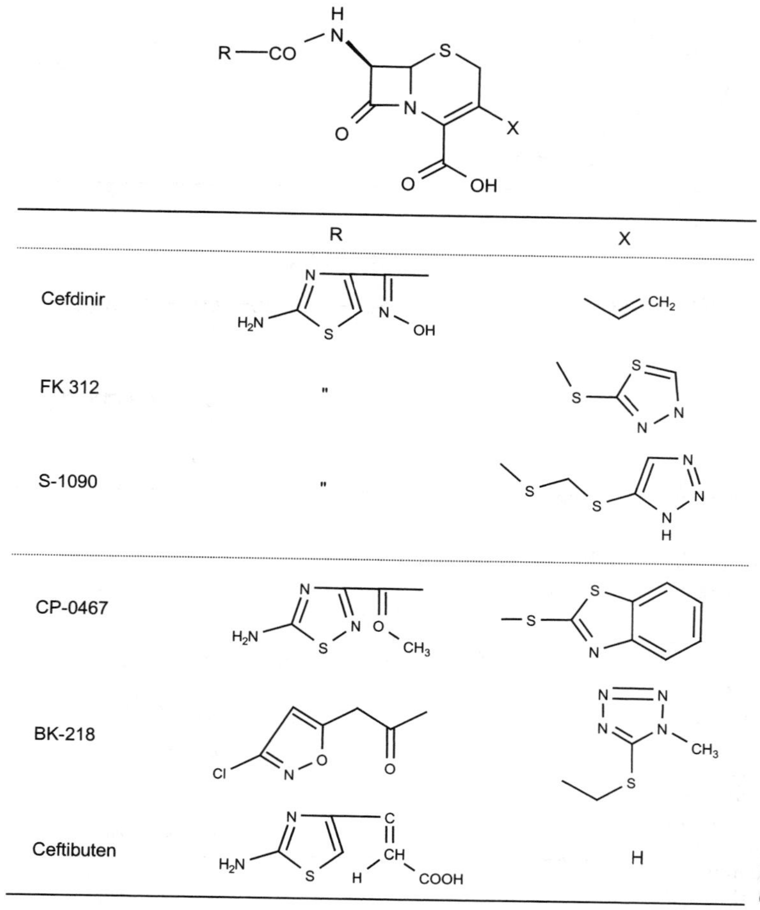

Figure 13 S-1090, FK-312, CP-0467, and BK-218

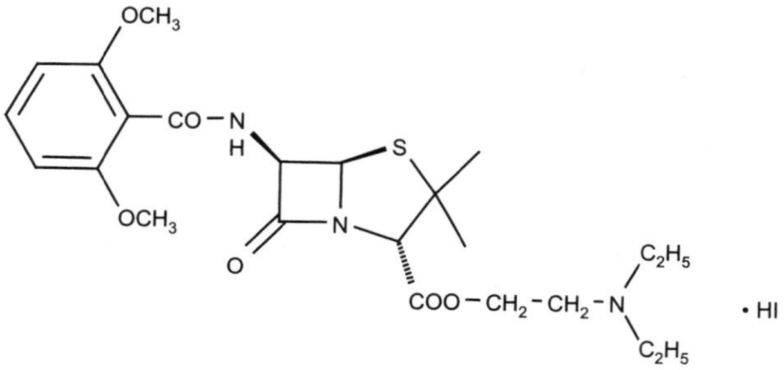

Figure 14 Penicillin penethamate

Penethamate was the first prodrug to exhibit apparent selectivity. After intramuscular administration, the concentrations in the lung are higher with penethamate than with penicillin G. However, this compound is poorly absorbed orally, and intramuscular administration is painful.

4.1.2. Penamecillin and the Aminoacyloxymethyl Esters

See Fig. 16.

Penamecillin was the first double ester by virtue of the presence of an acetoxymethyl chain. Penamecillin is more lipophilic and more stable in an acidic medium than penicillin G. The ester is sparingly soluble in water. To circumvent this obstacle, an amino group was incorporated into the acetoxymethyl chain. The pharmacokinetics of two of these

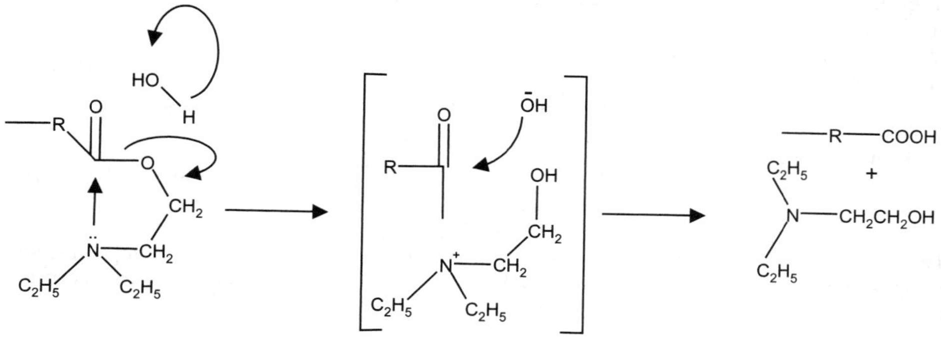

Figure 15 Mechanism of hydrolysis of penicillin G penethamate

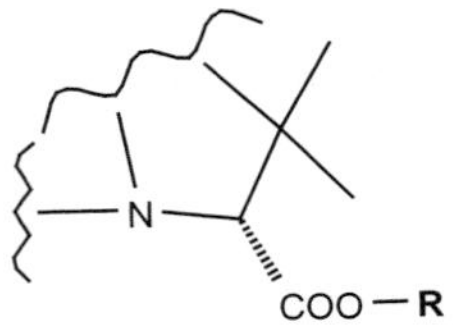

	R
Penamecillin	CH_2OCOCH_3
Amino acyl oxymethyl penicillins	$CH_2—O—CO—CH(NH_2)—CH(CH_3)_2$
" "	$CH_2—O—CO—CH(NH_2)—CH_2COOCH_3$

Figure 16 Penamecillin

esters have been studied in humans, and a three- to fourfold increase in the levels of penicillin G in plasma has been demonstrated.

4.2. Methicillin

Methicillin was esterified using *N,N*-aminoalkyl-disubstituted chains in order to try to increase its stability in an acidic medium and its digestive absorption. Normally methicillin is weakly orally absorbed in humans and animals. *N,N*-Diethylaminoethyl methicillin hydroiodide is well absorbed orally in mice and monkeys. This ester is more rapidly hydrolyzed in the mouse than in the monkey, but little is detected in the blood of the mouse in contrast to the monkey.

A structure-activity relationship study showed that the aminoalkyl esters with a tertiary amino group are weakly hydrolyzed to methicillin because of extensive plasma protein binding (Table 14).

4.3. Ampicillin and Derivatives

Ampicillin is an α-aminopenicillin of semisynthetic origin. It is stable in an acidic medium, and 30 to 40% of the administered dose is absorbed. Daehne et al. (1970) showed that it was possible to increase the quantity of orally absorbed ampicillin by esterifying the molecule using an acetoxymethyl chain. The presence of an amino group was considered to be responsible for better dissolution in the digestive tract. Several esters have been developed and are used therapeutically (Fig. 17).

4.3.1. Pivampicillin

Pivampicillin is pivaloyloxymethylampicillin, which was developed by the Leo Research Center and introduced in clinical practice in 1972. Shindo et al. (1975) studied the site of pivampicillin hydrolysis in different animal species. In the dog, pivampicillin is found in the portal vein, but this is not the case in the rat, mouse, or monkey. Because of the quantitative importance of esterases in the human intestine, pivampicillin is rapidly hydrolyzed to ampicillin, pivalic acid, and formaldehyde and is not found in the systemic circulation.

4.3.2. Talampicillin

Talampicillin, the second ester of ampicillin to be introduced in clinical practice, was marketed by Beecham in 1972. It is phthalidylampicillin.

Table 14 Methicillin esters

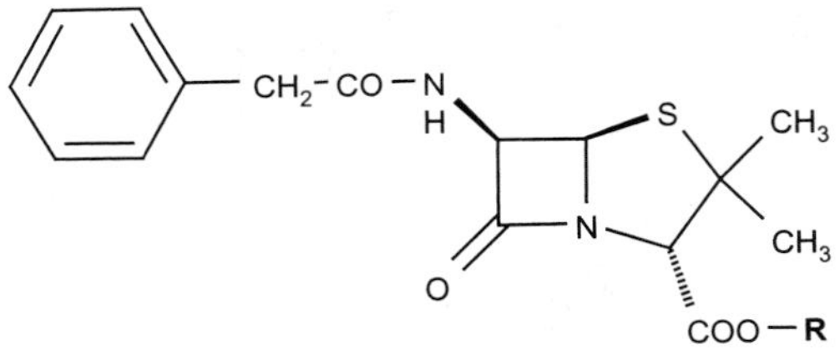

R	% hydrolysis 15 min: Buffer pH 7.4	% hydrolysis 15 min: Blood
$—CH_2CH_2N(CH_3)_2$	68	59
$—CH_2\text{-}CH_2N(C_2H_5)_2$	68	58
$—CH\text{-}[CH_2\text{-}N(C_2H_5)2]_2$	94	68
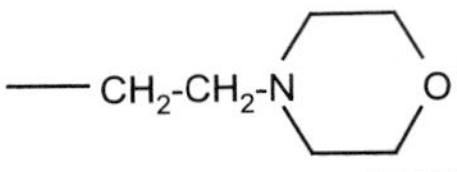 $—CH_2\text{-}CH_2\text{-}N$ (morpholino)	24	23
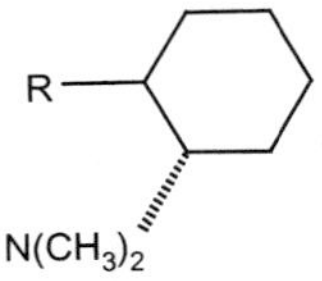 R-cyclohexyl-$N(CH_3)_2$	47	8
$—CH_2\text{-}CH_2\text{-}N^+(CH_3)_2$	< 25	< 25

Talampicillin may be detected in the portal vein of the dog, but not in the rat.

4.3.3. Bacampicillin

Bacampicillin is the third ester of ampicillin to have been introduced in clinical practice by Astra in 1977. It is ethoxycarbonyloxyethylampicillin.

The lactone and carbonate present in talampicillin and bacampicillin may be regarded as structural variants of the aryloxymethyl chains.

	R	Metabolites (prodrugs)
Ampicillin	H	
Pivampicillin	$-H_2C-OCO-C(CH_3)_3$	$H\text{-}CHO + (CH_3)_3\text{-}C\text{-}COOH$
Bacampicillin	$-CH(CH_3)\text{-}O\text{-}CO\text{-}O\text{-}C_2H_5$	CH_3CHO, C_2H_5OH, CO_2
Talampicillin	—CH—O—C(=O)—(benzene ring)	(benzene ring)—COOH, —CHO
Lenampicillin	$-H_2C-$ (dioxolone ring, C=O) $-CH_3$	$CH_3\text{-}COCHOHCH_3$, CO_2

Figure 17 Ampicillin esters

The plasma ampicillin levels obtained after oral administration of the three esters are two to three times greater than those obtained with ampicillin alone. The difference between these three chains lies in their metabolism.

Talampicillin and bacampicillin contain a center of asymmetry, but only the racemates are therapeutically available. The pharmacokinetics of the two epimers of talampicillin have revealed no difference in terms of levels in plasma and urinary elimination of ampicillin (Table 15). In addition, hydrolysis of the two isomers of the ester is identical (Table 16).

The bioavailabilities of ampicillin after absorption of pivampicillin, talampicillin, and bacampicillin are reported in Table 17.

The peak concentration in serum is reached much more rapidly after absorption of the esters than with ampicillin, and the bioavailability of the esters is less sensitive to inter- and intraindividual variations than is the bioavailability of ampicillin itself. Food interferes with the kinetics of ampicillin. After administration of pivampicillin with food, the peak concentration in serum and the area under the curve are lower than those of ampicillin administered alone. For talampicillin and bacampicillin the effect of food would appear to be negligible (Table 18).

Two studies have been undertaken in children, one with pivampicillin and the other with bacampicillin. The study conducted by Eriksson and Bolme (1981) in 38 children aged from 6 months to 6 years showed that pivampicillin was better absorbed in children than ampicillin and that absorption was better with tablets than with suspension.

Table 16 Hydrolysis of the ester of talampicillin

Medium or site of hydrolysis	Value	$t_{1/2}$ (min)	
		Isomer a	Isomer b
Phosphate buffer	pH 7.4	>25	>25
Human blood	90%	<2	<2
	10%	3	<2
	2%	10	4
Intestine	10%	2	<2
Human liver	0.02%	25	20

Table 15 Pharmacokinetics of the epimers of talampicillin

Talampicillin	n	Concn in plasma (μg/ml) at min: 20	40	60	90	120	240	360	Urinary elimination (%)
Racemate	10	1.8	5.8	6.5	4.7	3.6	0.8	0.3	73
Epimer A	9	1.5	5.8	5.6	5.4	3.1	0.6	0.2	72
Epimer B	9	1.5	5.5	5.3	4.1	2.5	0.5	0.1	68
Ampicillin (250 mg)	10	0.3	1.7	2.4	2.3	2.2	0.9	0.2	43

Table 17 Bioavailability of the esters of ampicillin

Drug	n	Dose (mg)	C_{max} (μg/ml)	AUC (μg·h/ml)	Urinary elimination (%)
Bacampicillin	9	400	7.4	15	80
Ampicillin	10	278	2.6	9	56
Bacampicillin	5	200	4.4		72
	5	400	6.8		74
	5	800	12		85
Ampicillin	5	500	2.6		30
Bacampicillin	13	800	8.3	17	
	4	800	11.3	20	
	4	1,600	14.5	32	
Bacampicillin	11	900	6	11	
	11	1,600	17.3	36	
Ampicillin	11	2,000	7.5	18	
Talampicillin	10	371	6.2		69
Ampicillin	10	250	2.6		43
Talampicillin	10	742	7.4	16	66
Ampicillin	10	1,000	6.2	18	42
Talampicillin	32	250	4.8		70
Ampicillin	32	250	2.6		43
Talampicillin	10	250	3.2	7	66
Ampicillin	10	500	4	14	38
Bacampicillin	11	400	8.3	16	72
Pivampicillin	11	398	7.1	15	65
Ampicillin	11	178	3.7	10	45
Bacampicillin	10	400	6	16	54
Pivampicillin	10	350	4.9	13	43
Ampicillin	10	500	3.6	16	30

Table 18 Food effects on pharmacokinetics of ampicillin and ampicillin esters

Drug	n	Dose (mg per os)	Food	C_{max} (μg/ml)	T_{max} (h)	AUC (μg·h/ml)	Urinary elimination (%)
Pivampicillin	15	350	+	3.3	2	8	55
Pivampicillin	15	350	−	5.1	1	15	62
Ampicillin	15	350	−	4.5	2	15	35
Talampicillin	32	250	+	3.3	1		62
Talampicillin	32	250	−	4.7	0.7		64
Ampicillin	32	250	+	1.5	2		23
Ampicillin	32	250	−	2.5	1.5		39
Bacampicillin	12	400	+	6.6	1		
Bacampicillin	12	400	−	6.1	1		
Bacampicillin	12	800	+	12.7	1	26	75
Bacampicillin	12	800	−	11.1	1	28	75

Ginsburg et al. (1981) compared the pharmacokinetics of two preparations of bacampicillin (Veegum and microcapsules) in 24 children. Although the ampicillin content was 25% lower (equimolar base), the bioavailability with bacampicillin was twice that obtained with ampicillin. Bacampicillin is bitter, and these two preparations were also intended to improve the organoleptic properties. It appears that microcapsules are more acceptable than the Veegum formulation and yield higher plasma ampicillin levels (Table 19).

In patients suffering from celiac disease localized in the proximal part of the small intestine, absorption of ampicillin is unaffected, but that of pivampicillin is reduced (Table 20).

4.3.4. Lenampicillin

Sakamoto et al. (1984) developed a fourth type of ester with an acyloxyallyl nucleus. They prepared 3-phthalidylene and 2-oxo-1,3-dioxolone esters with substitutions at position 5′. Several substituents were proposed: methyl, butyl, phenyl, etc. The highest ampicillin levels were obtained with nuclei with a methyl group (Table 21). Derivatives possessing a 5′-methyl and 5′-phenyl group are well absorbed, and levels in plasma are high in the mouse. They are moderately stable in an acidic medium. The nonsubstituted derivative is too labile in the digestive tract. The 5′-*ter*-butyl derivative is 10 times more stable than the 5′-methyl or 5′-phenyl derivatives in mouse blood, yielding low ampicillin levels. Lenampicillin has been developed.

Lenampicillin is more rapidly hydrolyzed than talampicillin and bacampicillin in serum (Table 22). From 53 to 59% of the compound administered is eliminated in the urine in the form of ampicillin, and about 20% is eliminated in the form of the *S*-isomer of ampicillin.

Table 19 Pharmacokinetics of bacampicillin according to pharmaceutical formulation

Drug	Vehicle	n	Dose per os (mg/kg)	C_{max} (μg/ml)	T_{max} (h)	AUC (μg·h/ml)	$t_{1/2}$ (h)
Bacampicillin	Veegum	13	27.8	7.6	1	20	1.4
	Microcapsules	7	27.8	14.4	1	29	1.8
Ampicillin	Trihydrate suspension	13	25	4.8	1	13	1.7

Table 20 Pharmacokinetics of ampicillin in patients suffering from celiac disease

Drug	n	Patient status	Dose (mg)	C_{max} (μg/ml)	T_{max} (h)	Urinary elimination (%)
Pivampicillin	8	Healthy	350	4.2	1	28
	10	Celiac	350	4.4	1	44
Ampicillin	11	Healthy	500	4.4	2	34
	8	Celiac	500	3.2	2	26

4.3.5. Other Ampicillin-Ester Derivatives

The main line of research in terms of prodrugs has involved esterification of the carboxyl group at C-3 of the thiazolidine nucleus. Other research has been conducted into modifying the amino group of the C-6 side chain of ampicillin.

4.3.5.1. Hetacillin

Hetacillin is the result of the action of acetone on ampicillin, producing 6-(2,2-dimethyl-5-oxo-4-phenyl-1-imidazolidinyl)penicillanic acid (Fig. 18).

The conversion of hetacillin to ampicillin in vivo is rapid (half-life, ~11 min) and occurs by chemical conversion without enzymatic intervention. Following intramuscular administration, 68 and 90% of the compound assayed 10 and 60 min, respectively, after the injection is ampicillin. The peak serum ampicillin concentration is reached in 1 h. This suggests that the majority of the injected compound is absorbed in the form of hetacillin. Orally, hetacillin is hydrolyzed in the digestive tract in the form of ampicillin. The bioavailability of ampicillin is 38%, and its absorption is increased with food.

Table 22 Hydrolysis of lenampicillin (KBT-1585)

Plasma source	$t_{1/2}$ (min) of ester release		
	KBT-1585	Talampicillin	Bacampicillin
Human	4	7.4	138.6
Dog	5.4	15.4	231
Rat	4.6	3.7	3.5

The different pharmacokinetics of hetacillin and ampicillin failed to show any marked superiority of hetacillin over ampicillin.

4.3.5.2. Sarpicillin

Hetacillin was esterified by a C-3 methoxymethyl chain (Fig. 18), and this double prodrug is known as sarpicillin.

Sarpicillin is partially hydrolyzed in the digestive tract, and part of it is found in the circulation. The conversion half-life of sarpicillin to ampicillin in plasma is about 20 min, whereas that of pivampicillin, bacampicillin, and talampicillin is less

Table 21 Derivatives of lenampicillin (pharmacokinetics in the mouse)

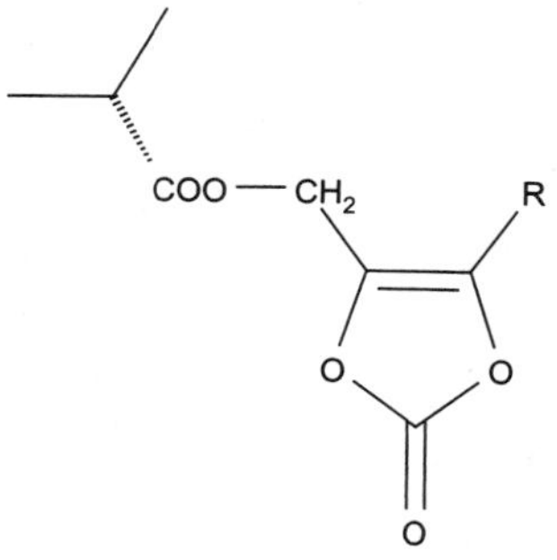

COO — CH_2, R, O, O, O

R	(C) ampicillin (μg/ml) 15	30	60	120	Gastric	Intestine	Blood (%)
H	31.0	22.5	11.9	5.6	6.0	1.60	> 2
CH_3	43.1	33.1	21.3	3.1	12.6	2.70	> 2
$(CH_3)_3$	18.5	10.5	8.2	3.3	> 20	> 20	20
Phenyl	35.2	26.3	19.4	5.0	9.0	2.50	> 2
Ampicillin trihydrate	11.3	14.4	10.6	3.1	-	-	-

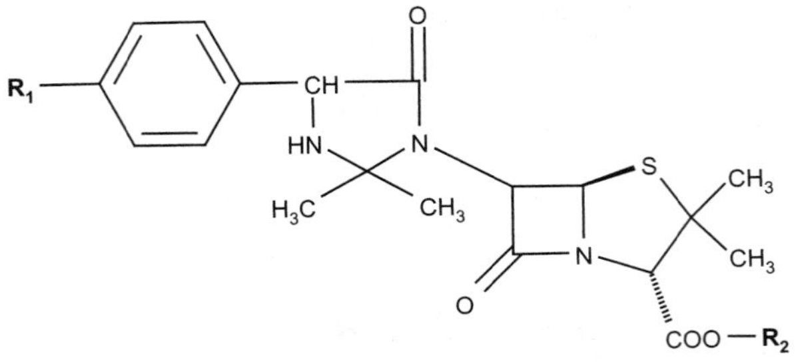

	R_1	R_2
Hetacillin	-H	-H
Sarpicillin	-H	$-CH_2OCH_3$
Hetamoxicillin	-OH	-H
Sarmoxicillin	-OH	$-CH_2OCH_3$

Figure 18 α-Aminopenams

than 1 min. Sarpicillin is more lipophilic than ampicillin and for this reason is absorbed and is detectable in the systemic circulation. It is likely that the tissue concentrations are much higher than those of ampicillin, but they have not been measured in humans. In fact, ampicillin concentrations in the dog (prostatic fluid) and rabbit (cerebrospinal fluid) after administration of sarpicillin are much higher.

4.3.5.3. Hetamoxicillin and Sarmoxicillin

Amoxicillin is the *para*-hydroxyphenyl derivative of ampicillin. Smyth et al. studied the plasma pharmacokinetics of amoxicillin after administration of 500 mg of sarmoxicillin orally (Table 23). Sarmoxicillin is a cationic molecule and is 30 to 600 times more lipophilic than amoxicillin, which is an amphoteric molecule. High salivary amoxicillin levels are detected after administration of sarmoxicillin, but not after administration of amoxicillin. About 10 to 20% of the prodrug is present in the systemic circulation after ingestion of sarmoxicillin.

4.4. Derivatives of Carbenicillin

The simple alkyl or aryl esters at C-3 of the thiazolidine nucleus are usually resistant to enzymatic hydrolysis in humans, but such esters are hydrolyzed if they are attached to the side chain.

Two derivatives of carbenicillin have been used therapeutically and exhibit this type of ester.

Carfecillin and carindacillin are the α-indanyl and α-phenyl esters of carbenicillin. Absorption is due probably to an increase in the lipophilicity and stability of carbenicillin in an acidic medium. The release of carbenicillin from the esters (aryls) occurs rapidly in vivo and in plasma and tissues (Hobs, 1972). The effect of the ester structure on the bioavailability of carbenicillin in humans and the characteristics of hydrolysis have been studied by Clayton et al. (1975). The aryl derivatives are more rapidly hydrolyzed than the alkyl derivatives.

4.5. Derivative of Temocillin: BRL-20330

BRL-20330 is a prodrug of temocillin obtained by esterification of the α-carboxyl group by an *O*-methylphenyl group (Fig. 19). After absorption it is converted in the body to temocillin. The peak levels in serum of 9.8, 12.8, and 15.8 μg/ml are reached 2 h after oral administration of 400, 600, and 800 mg of BRL-20330. The residual concentrations at 12 h are between 3.0 and 6.0 μg/ml. The areas under the curve increase linearly between 400 and 800 mg (in temocillin base equivalent). The apparent elimination half-life is about 6 h. Over a 24-h period, urinary elimination accounts for about 25% of the administered dose and a small fraction of BRL-20330 (0.2 to 0.5%).

In the presence of food, the peak concentration in serum is reduced (9.0 versus 11.0 μg/ml) and time to maximum concentration in serum is increased, but the bioavailability is unchanged.

5. CEPHALOSPORINS

Parenteral cephalosporins are not absorbed by the gastrointestinal tract, as they are present in the digestive tract in the ionic form and are poorly liposoluble because of the pK of the carboxyl group at position 4 of the cephem nucleus, which is detrimental to the passage of molecules across lipid membranes. Esterification of the carboxyl groups increases the lipophilicity (Yoshimura et al., 1985). However, even with the esters, it has been shown that the substituent at the C-3 position of the cephem nucleus plays an important role in the gastrointestinal absorption of non-α-aminocephalosporins.

5.1. Cephaloglycin

Acyloxymethyl derivatives of cephaloglycin have been developed by Binderup et al. (Fig. 20). These esters are better absorbed than cephaloglycin, with urinary elimination on

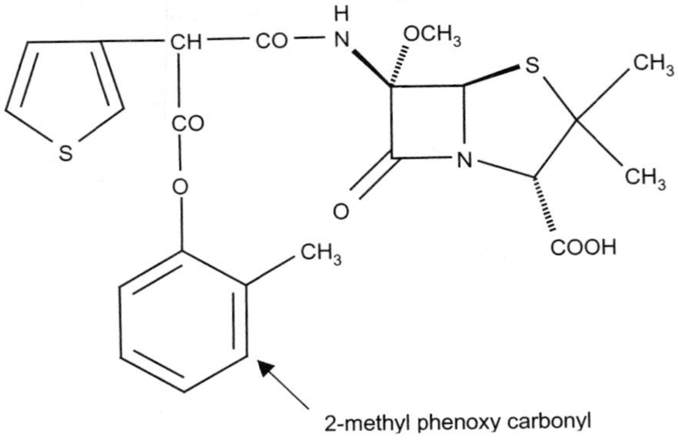

2-methyl phenoxy carbonyl

Figure 19 BRL-20330

Table 23 Pharmacokinetics of sarmoxicillin after 500 mg of amoxicillin base

Drug administered	Drug detected	C_{max} (μg/ml)	T_{max} (h)	$t_{1/2}$ (h)	AUC (μg·h/ml)
Amoxicillin		6.4	1.8	1.1	17.3
Sarmoxicillin	Amoxicillin	3.7	1.4	1.7	10.9
	Sarmoxicillin	1.2	0.5	0.3	1

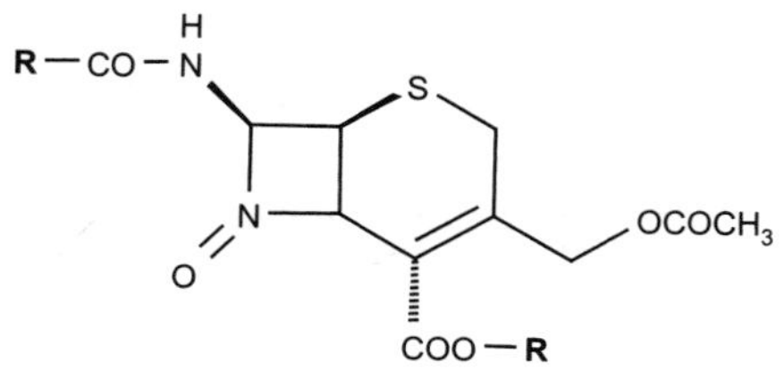

R = H	cephaloglycin
R = $CH_2OCO(CH_3)_3$	cephaloglycin CPE
R = CH_2OCOCH_3	cephaloglycin CPA

Figure 20 Cephaloglycin prodrug

the order of 60%, as opposed to 20% for nonesterified cephaloglycin. Peak levels in serum are higher, but after 4 h the concentrations in plasma are identical (Table 24).

5.2. Cephalexin

Esterification at C-4 of the carboxyl group of cephalexin by a pivaloyloxymethyl or phthalidyl chain increases the bioavailability of cephalexin (Foresta et al., 1977).

5.3. Cefamandole

Wheeler et al. (1979) showed that acetoxymethylcefamandole is weakly absorbed orally and that the presence of different glycyloxymethyl chains does not increase its absorption. This is probably due to poor hydrolysis gastrointestinally.

Cefamandole esterified by a pivaloyloxymethyl or phthalidyl chain is better absorbed. Cefamandole is isomerized at Δ^2-Δ^3. The Δ^2 isomer is inactive.

5.4. Cefuroxime Axetil

Cefuroxime is esterified at C-4 by a 1-acetoxyethyl chain. The bioavailability of cefuroxime axetil varies according to the authors and study conditions (Singlas). With the commercially available pharmaceutical formulation, the bioavailability is between 55 and 65%. It decreases as the pH increases, as with the changes induced by ranitidine or sodium bicarbonate. The apparent elimination half-life is on the order of 1 to 1.5 h. The principal pharmacokinetic parameters are given in Table 25.

5.5. YM-22561

YM-22561 is a 2-amino-5-thiazolyl cephalosporin with a 1,3-dithiolane nucleus at C-3. The molecule is esterified at C-4 by an acetoxyethyl chain (Fig. 21). This molecule

Table 24 Pharmacokinetics of the esters of cephaloglycin

Drug	Concn (μg/ml)					Urinary elimination (%)
	0.5 h	1 h	2 h	4 h	6 h	
Cephaloglycin	0.6	1	0.8	0.3	<0.1	18
Cephaloglycin CPE[a]	5.8	3.7	1.1	0.2	<0.1	61
Cephaloglycin CAE[a]	7.7	4.1	1.6	0.4	<0.1	68

[a]See Fig. 20.

Table 25 Pharmacokinetics of esterified oral cephalosporins

Drug	Dose (mg)	C_{max} (μg/ml)	T_{max} (h)	AUC (μg·h/ml)	$t_{1/2}$ (h)	Urinary elimination (%)
Cefpodoxime proxetil	100	1.55	3.2	7.54	1.7	41.8
	200	3.02	3.4	15.81	1.9	46.4
Cefuroxime axetil	250	4.8	2.5	12.2	1.2	32
	500	6.4	2.5	27	1.2	30
	1,000	7.3	1.5	23	1.2	30
Cefotiam hexetil	200	2.16	1.55	4.16	1	34.7
	400	3.43	2.26	8.52	0.87	31.9
Cefetamet pivoxil	500	4.1		24.6	2.3	51.3
Cefteram pivoxil	100	0.85	1.18	2.01	0.78	33.2
	200	1.7	1.6	5.52	0.9	18.7
	400	4.2	1.5	14.2	1.2	
	800	7	1.9	24.8	1.2	
	1,200	8.3	1.8	27.3	1.2	
Cefdaloxime penxetil	200	3.95	3.15	21.4	2.16	62
Cefcapene pivoxil	50	0.58	1.1	1.37	1.17	28.1
	100	0.79	1.4	2.27	1.03	23.3
	150	1.55	1.6	4.34	0.99	26.5
	200	1.49	1.7	4.36	1.1	22.4
Cefditoren pivoxil	200	1.99	1	5.12	1.09	11.6
AS-924 (ceftizoxime)	25	0.34	1.5	1.13	1.2	39.1
	50	0.79	1.8	2.7	1.3	43.9
	100	1.38	2	5.01	1.3	41.8
	200	2.83	2	10.16	1.3	40.5

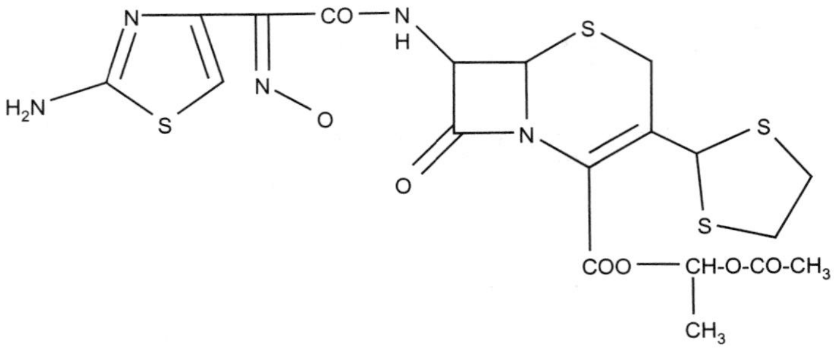

Figure 21 YM-22561 (YM-22508)

exhibits weaker activity against gram-positive cocci than does cefdinir and moderate activity against *Enterobacteriaceae*. In the mouse, rat, and monkey, the apparent elimination half-life is on the order of 1.9 h, with urinary elimination of 4 to 15% depending on the animal species. Bioavailability is on the order of 16.4% in the mouse. Plasma protein binding is on the order of 87.8% in humans.

5.6. Cefpodoxime Proxetil

Cefpodoxime proxetil is a 2-amino-5-thiazolyl cephalosporin. Several esters have been attached at C-4 to the cefpodoxime molecule. Only the 1-(isopropoxycarbonyl-oxyethyl) yields high levels in plasma in the mouse compared to the 1,3-dioxolene-5-methyl derivative, for which the urinary elimination is 22%, as opposed to 76% for cefpodoxime proxetil. The principal pharmacokinetic parameters are listed in Table 25.

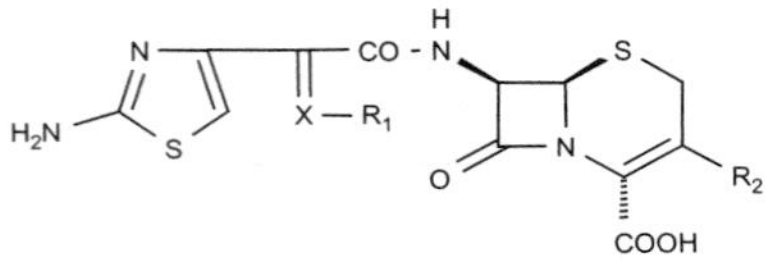

	X-R_1	R_2
Cefpodoxime	-$NOCH_3$	-CH_2OCH_3
Cefetamet	-$NOCH_3$	-CH_3
Cefteram	-$NOCH_3$	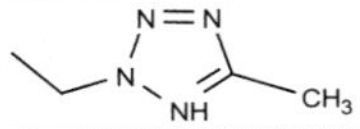
Cefditoren	-$NOCH_3$	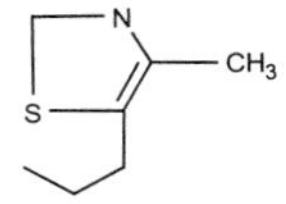
Ceftrazonal	-$NOCH_3$	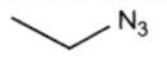
Cefcamate	-CH_2-CH_2-CH_3	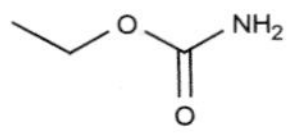
Cefdaloxime	-N-OH	-CH_2OCH_3
SC-002	-N-OH	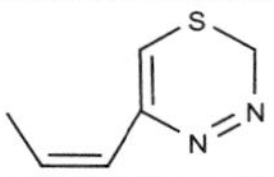
S-1090	-N-OH	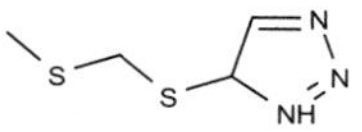
E-1100	-N-OH	-$CH_2OCON(CH_3)_2$
YM-22508	-N-OH	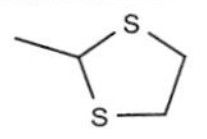

Figure 22 Oral cephalosporins (esterified)

5.7. Pivaloyloxymethyl Cephalosporins

Certain cephalosporins have been developed with a pivaloyloxymethyl chain as the ester at C-4, such as cefetamet pivoxil, cefteram pivoxil, cefditoren pivoxil, cefcamate pivoxil, and SC-004 (SC-004 is SC-002 esterified). (Fig. 22).

The plasma pharmacokinetics in healthy adult volunteers are summarized in Table 25.

5.8. Cefdaloxime Penxetil

Cefdaloxime penxetil is a 2-amino-5-thiazolyl cephalosporin (Fig. 22) belonging to the subgroup of C-7α-OH cephems. It is esterified at C-4 by a pivaloyloxyethyl group. Like all the chains with a 1-hydroxyethyl group, the ester possesses a center of asymmetry (Fig. 23). It has been shown that the pharmacokinetics (absorption) differ according to the isomer. The *S*(−) isomer (HR-916K) is better absorbed in dogs (Table 26) and humans than the *R*(−) isomer (HR-916J) and the racemate (HR-916B) (Klesel et al., 1992).

In humans, after a dose of cefdaloxime penxetil tosylate equivalent to 200 mg of active substance, the peak concentration in serum is 3.95 μg/ml and is reached in 3.15 h, with an apparent elimination half-life of 2.16 h. Urinary elimination is 62% of the administered dose (Table 25).

5.9. Cefotiam Hexetil

Nishimura et al. demonstrated that the 1-acyloxyalkyl esters occasioned good absorption of cefotiam. They showed that the combination of an alkyl group of the methyl, ethyl, or propyl type and a cycloalkyl on the acyloxy residue increased the bioavailability. Another series was prepared which showed that the oxa, aza, and thia chains incorporated in a 1-(cyclohexylacetoxy)alkyl chain produced better absorption of cefotiam than the 1-(ethoxycarbonyloxyethyl) chain. *N*-Cyclohexylcarbamoyloxymethyl precludes the absorption of cefotiam. 1-Cyclohexyloxycarbonyloxyethyl has two diastereoisomers. In the mouse, the levels in plasma, bioavailability, and absorption are identical (Table 27). The solubility in water is greater than 1 mg/ml at pH 4.5.

Cefotiam is esterified at C-4 by a cyclohexanol chain. From 30 to 35% of the administered dose of cefotiam is eliminated via the urine by glomerular filtration and tubular secretion, with renal clearance of 250 to 300 ml/min. The apparent elimination half-life is about 1 h. The oral bioavailability of cefotiam hexetil is 43% ± 4% (mean ± standard deviation) for a dose of 400 mg.

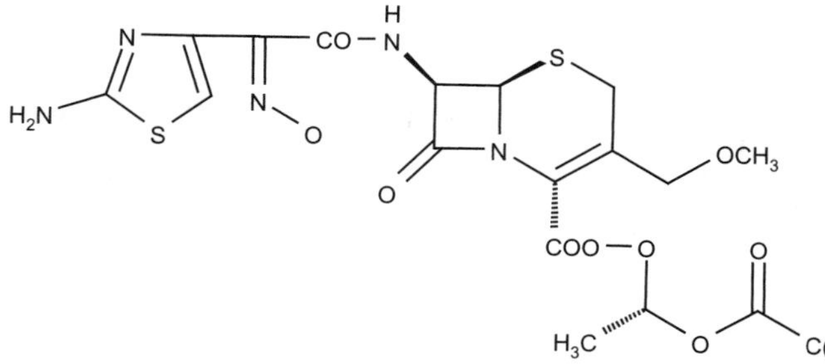

(Chain 1 *(S)* pivaloyloxy ethyl) **Figure 23 Cefdaloxime penxetil**

Table 26 Pharmacokinetics of cefdaloxime penxetil in the dog

Cefdaloxime penxetil	Route[a]	C_{max}/C_0 (μg/ml)	T_{max} (h)	$t_{1/2}$ (h)	AUC_{0-7} (μg·h/ml)	Urinary elimination (%)
Racemate	p.o.	15.9 ± 6.9	4.6 ± 2.2		68.7 ± 29.1	39.2 ± 8.2
Isomer *R*(−)	p.o.	7.7 ± 2.1	5.1 ± 2.7		33 ± 11.7	19.7 ± 3.6
Isomer *S*(−)	p.o.	26.7 ± 3	6 ± 2.3		83.4 ± 32	677 ± 4.5
Cefdaloxime	i.v.	226 ± 37		2.1 ± 0.2	117 ± 31.7	86 ± 9.7

[a]p.o., per os; i.v., intravenously.

Table 27 Cefotiam hexetil: pharmacokinetics of the isomers in the mouse (100 mg/kg orally)

Isomer	C_0 (μg/ml)	C_1 (μg/ml)	C_2 (μg/ml)	AUC (μg·h/ml)	Bioavailability (%)
α	28.5	6.05	0.39	24.8	63.9
β	19.6	7.41	0.57	23.7	61.1

5.10. Ceftrazonal Bopentil (Ro-41-3399/Ro-41-6890)

Ceftrazonal bopentil is a cephalosporin with a 3′-azidomethyl group at C-3 (Fig. 24). A whole series of esters has been synthesized: 2-(alkyloxycarbonyl)-2-alkylidene ethyl. Replacement of the carbonyl group by another electrodonor group (ketone, sulfone, or nitrile) abolishes absorption and saturation of the double bond. Ro-41-3399 has a 2-isobutoxycarbonyl-2-propylidene ethyl chain. The molecule is isomerized at Δ^2-Δ^3.

5.11. Baccefuzonam

Curran et al. prepared a series of esters of cefuzonam. They attached several chains: ethoxycarbonyloxyethyl, adamantadylcarbonyloxymethyl, acetoxymethyl, phthalidyl, and miristoyloxymethyl. The CL-118673 derivative is the ethoxycarbonyloxyethyl ester of cefuzonam. This compound is well absorbed in the mouse, as demonstrated by its oral pharmacokinetics and activity in experimental infections.

5.12. AS-924

Esterification of ceftizoxime increases its lipophilicity. To enhance oral absorption and water solubility, amino acids as basic moieties have been introduced into the weak basic amino group on the aminothiazolyl ring.

AS-924 is a bifunctional prodrug.

In a series of experiments, it was shown that increasing lipophilicity was an important factor to enhance oral absorption. The most useful moiety was pivaloyloxymethyl. However, it was accompanied by a high decrease of water solubility. To enhance oral absorption and water solubility, amino acids as basic moieties have been introduced onto the weak basic amino group on the aminothiazolyl ring. When an L-alanine is added to the pivaloyloxymethyl ceftizoxime, urinary recovery in animals increases from 32 to 43%.

The partition coefficient of AS-924 is logP 1.2, and water solubility is 19.9 mg/ml (pH 4.5) and 4.32 mg/ml (pH 6.0). In comparison, for ceftizoxime sodium the logP is −3.29 and water solubility is >25 mg/ml with a urine recovery in animals of 5.36% ± 1.62%.

Ceftizoxime ester is thought to be stable and not prone to isomerize from Δ^3 ester to Δ^2 ester.

About 90% of pivaloylcarnitine is eliminated in urine. The concentrations of Δ^2 ceftizoxime in plasma and urine were below the detection limit after a single oral dose of AS-924.

Pharmacokinetics have been investigated in various physiopathological situations (Table 28).

5.13. Cefditoren Pivoxil

Cefditoren exhibits good in vitro activity against gram-positive cocci (Table 29).

6. PENEMS

With the exception of fropenem (faropenem), 20% of the orally administered dose of which is absorbed by using the dipeptide pathway like the oral cephems, the penems must

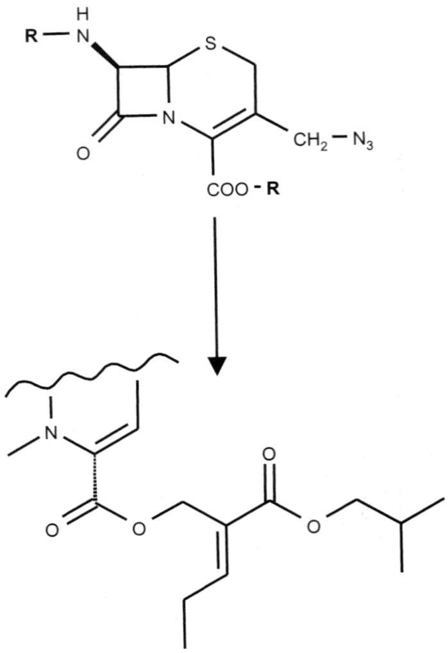

Ro 41-6890

Ro 41-3399 (ceftrazonal bopentil)
Chain 2-isobutoxy carbonyl-2-propylidene

Figure 24 Ceftrazonal bopentil (Ro-41-3399/Ro-41-6890), a cephalosporin with a 3′-azidomethyl group at C-3

Table 28 Pharmacokinetics of AS-924 in various physiological situations

Condition	Dose (mg)	*n*	C_{max} (μg/ml)	T_{max} (h)	$AUC_{0–12}$ (μg·h/ml)	$t_{1/2β}$ (h)	Urinary elimination (%)
Fasting	100	8	1.52	1.8	5.02	1.3	43.4
Fed	100	8	1.72	2.1	6.02	1.4	49.7
Ranitidine	100	8	1.6	2.3	5.74	1.3	
Elderly	100	8	1.67	2.6	7.41	1.7	45.2
Young	100	8	1.72	2.1	6.02	1.4	49.7
Water, 30 ml	200	5	2.82	2.3	10.56	1.5	
Water, 150 ml	200	5	2.94	1.8	10.36	1.3	49.3
Milk	200	5	2.13	1.8	10.63	1.3	44.1

be esterified to be absorbed (Fig. 25). Several types of esters have been attached to the carboxyl group: substituted or nonsubstituted acyloxymethyl, acyloxyallyl, and dioxolone. Ritipenem acoxil, sulopenem pivoxil, and SUN-A-026 (fropenem ester) are under development.

7. CARBAPENEM

7.1. GV 104326

A series of tricyclic derivatives that can be esterified and orally absorbed has been described by Perboni et al. (1993). GV 104326 (a trinem) reached only phase II clinical development. The molecule is esterified (GV 118819) (Fig. 26). The ester is a (cyclohexyloxy)carbonyloxyethyl (or hexetil) chain. The activity of the molecule is dependent on the substitution of the hexyl ring and the disposition of this substituent at position 4. The methoxy group must be in the α position. The location of the bond at position 8 is very important. When the bond is in the β position, the molecule is much more stable against hydrolysis by renal dehydropeptidase than if it is in the α position.

GV 104326 has activity different from that of imipenem against gram-positive cocci. Imipenem is more active against *Staphylococcus aureus* and coagulase-negative

Table 29 In vitro activity of cefditoren against gram-positive cocci

Organism(s)[a]	*n*	MIC (μg/ml)[b]		
		50%	90%	Range
S. pneumoniae Pen[s]	189	0.016	0.03	≤0.004–0.12
S. pneumoniae Pen[i]	145	0.12	0.5	0.016–2.0
S. pneumoniae Pen[r]	76	0.5	2.0	0.25–4.0
S. pyogenes	89	0.008	0.016	0.04–0.016
Streptococcus agalactiae	53	0.03	0.06	0.016–0.06
Group C streptococci	65	0.016	0.12	0.008–0.12
Group G streptococci	82	0.016	0.12	≤0.001–0.25
Group F streptococci	15	0.12	0.12	≤0.001–0.25
Enterococcus spp.	40	>64	>64	32–>64
MSSA	21	0.5	1.0	0.25–1.0
MSSE	100	0.25	0.5	0.03–0.5
Clostridium perfringens	100	4	16	0.25–16
Haemophilus influenzae	214	≤0.01	0.03	≤0.01–0.4
Viridans group streptococci	241	0.12	0.5	0.008–4.0

[a]MSSA, methicillin-susceptible *S. aureus*; MSSE, methicillin-susceptible *S. epidermidis*.

[b]50% and 90%, MICs at which 50 and 90% of isolates tested are inhibited, respectively.

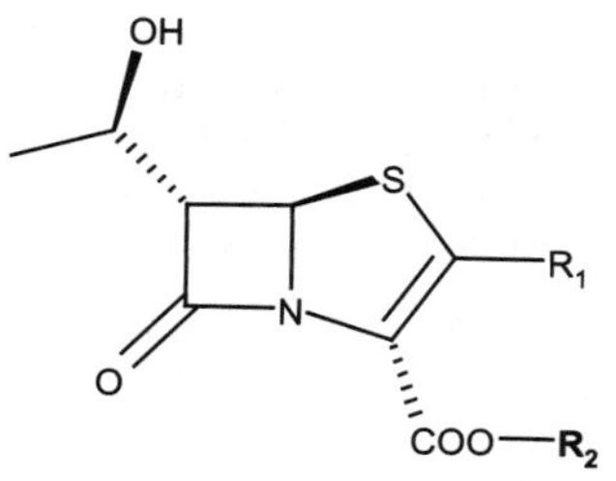

	Ester (R_2)	Parent compound
FCE 25199	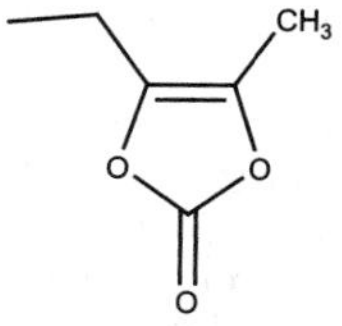 (5-methyl-2-oxo-1,3-dioxol-4-yl)methyl	FCE 24964
SUN A 0026		Fropenem
CP 65207	$-CO-C(CH_3)_3$	Sulopenem
Ritipenem-acoxil	$-CH_2OCOCH_3$	Ritipenem
TMA-230	$-CH_2OCOCH_3$	TMA-3176

Figure 25 Penem esters

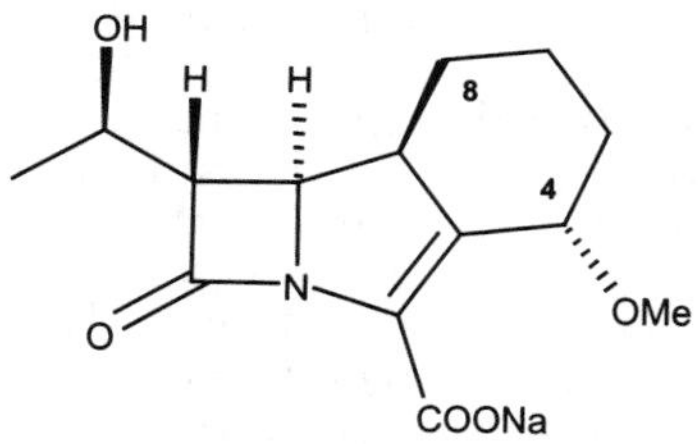

GV 104326

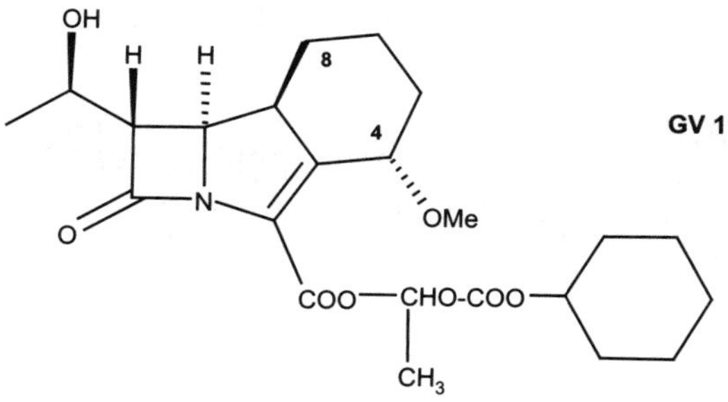

GV 118819 (Sanfetrinem-cilexetil)

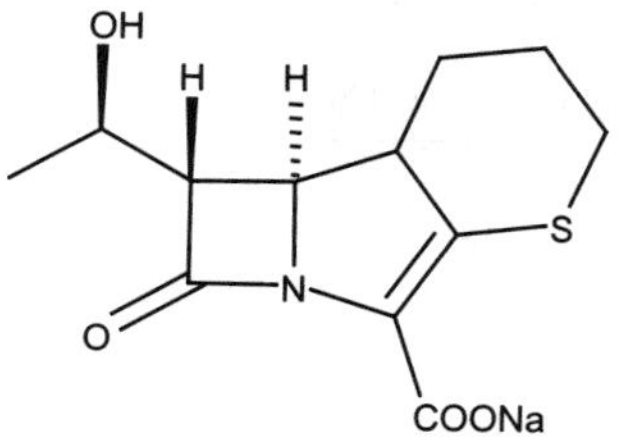

Takeda derivatives

Figure 26 Trinems

Table 30 In vitro activity of sanfetrinem (GV 104326)

Organism(s)	MIC_{50}[a] (μg/ml)	
	GV 104326	Imipenem
S. aureus Met[s]	0.06	<0.015
Coagulase-negative staphylococci	0.03	≤0.015
S. pneumoniae	0.003	0.003
S. pyogenes	0.007	0.003
Enterococcus faecalis	2	1
Enterococcus faecium	1	2
S. agalactiae	0.03	≤0.015
E. coli	0.5	0.25
Klebsiella pneumoniae	1	0.25
Klebsiella oxytoca	0.5	0.5
Enterobacter aerogenes	2	1
Enterobacter cloacae	1	0.5
Citrobacter freundii	1	0.5
Proteus mirabilis	0.5	4
Proteus vulgaris	1	8
Morganella morganii	2	2
Serratia marcescens	8	1
H. influenzae	0.06	0.5
Moraxella catarrhalis	0.12	0.12

[a]MIC_{50}, MIC at which 50% of isolates tested are inhibited.

Table 31 Stability against hydrolysis by β-lactamases

Organism	MIC (μg/ml)		
	GV 104326	Cefpodoxime	Imipenem
E. coli J-53-2	0.5	0.5	0.1
TEM-1	0.5	0.5	0.1
TEM-2	0.2	0.5	0.06
TEM-3	0.2	32	0.06
TEM-5	0.5	16	0.1
TEM-6	2	32	0.1
TEM-7	1	8	0.1
TEM-9	2	>32	0.1
K. pneumoniae TEM-10	0.5	8	0.1
E. coli J-53 SHV-1	0.2	1	0.1
E. coli J-53 SHV-3	1	32	0.06
K. pneumoniae K-1 (−)	0.5	0.1	0.1
K. pneumoniae K-1	1	8	0.1
E. cloacae P99 (−)	0.5	0.5	0.1
E. cloacae P99	2	>32	0.1
E. coli ES-2 PSE (−)	0.5	0.5	0.1
E. coli ES-2 PSE 1	0.5	1	0.1
E. coli ES-2 PSE 2	0.5	0.2	0.1
E. coli ES-2 PSE 3	0.5	0.5	0.1
E. coli ES-2 PSE 4	0.5	0.2	0.1

staphylococci. GV 104326 is much more active against *Streptococcus pneumoniae* in vitro and in vivo than amoxicillin or cefpodoxime (Di Modugno et al., 1994). Its activities against *Streptococcus pyogenes* and enterococci are similar. Against *Enterobacteriaceae*, GV 104326 is more active than imipenem (Table 30). It is inactive against *Pseudomonas aeruginosa* (MIC, >32 μg/ml). Against *Bacteroides fragilis* it is more active (MIC at which 50% of isolates tested are inhibited, 0.06 μg/ml) than cefoxitin, piperacillin, and metronidazole. GV 104326 is relatively inactive against *Clostridium difficile* (MIC, 1 to 8 μg/ml). It is less stable against hydrolysis by β-lactamases than imipenem (Table 31) (Di Modugno et al., 1993). The rate of hydrolysis by dehydropeptidase I is greater for GV 104326 than for imipenem. GV 104326 binds to *Escherichia coli* penicillin-binding proteins 1a and 2.

After administration of single doses of 0.25 to 4 g of GV 104326 intravenously in the form of an infusion over 0.5 h, the peak concentrations at the end of the infusion are between 9.86 and 174 μg/ml. The apparent elimination half-life is between 0.68 and 1.67 h. GV 104326 is principally eliminated renally, representing about 60% of the administered dose (Table 32). After administration of a single dose (0.25 to 2 g) of the ester (GV 118819X) in the form of a suspension in hydroxypropyl methylcellulose (Methocel), the peak concentrations of GV 104326 in serum are between 1.16 and 6.91 μg/ml and are reached in less than 1 h, and 17 to 32% of the administered dose is eliminated in the urine (Table 33). After oral elimination in the form of a suspension, the absolute bioavailability is on the order of 40% (Ethymiopoulos et al., 1994). Plasma protein binding is on the order of 8%.

7.2. DZ 2640

DZ 2640 is the prodrug of DU-6681a, which is esterified by a pivaloyloxymethyl group on the carboxyl group at position 4 (Fig. 27). DU-6681a is a 1-β-methylcarbapenem with a bicyclic nucleus (imidazolyl) at position 2. This is the (S)-enantiomer. DZ 2640 was selected on the basis of the pharmacokinetic parameters obtained in rats following administration of an oral dose of 20 mg/kg. In vitro, DU-6681a is more active than fropenem and cefpodoxime against gram-positive and gram-negative bacteria. It is inactive against *P. aeruginosa* and *Stenotrophomonas maltophilia*. DZ 2640 is rapidly absorbed in the rat, mouse, and monkey. On the basis of the area under the curve, the product is 33.1% absorbed in the rat (Nishi et al., 1995; Aoki et al., 1995).

8. METABOLISM

The different types of esters attached to the carboxyl group at C-4 are summarized in Fig. 28. They are metabolized, and various metabolites have been detected (Fig. 29).

Table 32 Intravenous pharmacokinetics of GV 104326

Dose (g)	C_0 (μg/ml)	AUC (μg·h/ml)	$t_{1/2}$ (h)	CL_P (liters/h)	CL_R (liters/h)	Urinary elimination (%)
0.25	9.86	7.6	0.68	33.92	17.45	59.7
0.5	19.3	15.34	0.74	32.63	20.71	58.3
1	13.2	35.04	1.13	28.55	19.67	62.5
2	95.1	83.67	1.17	23.92	14.23	62.5
4	174	186	1.67	21.51	14.21	65.4

Table 33 Pharmacokinetics of GV 118819X (orally)

Dose (g)	C_{max} (μg/ml)	T_{max} (h)	AUC (μg·h/ml)	$t_{1/2}$ (h)	CL_R (liters/h)	Urinary elimination (%)
0.25	0.16	0.88	2.55	1	22.02	31.95
0.5	3.53	0.75	6.68	1.29	20.18	26.35
1	4.21	0.75	11.16	2.34	19.51	21.83
2	6.91	0.63	14.48	2.31	17.94	16.49

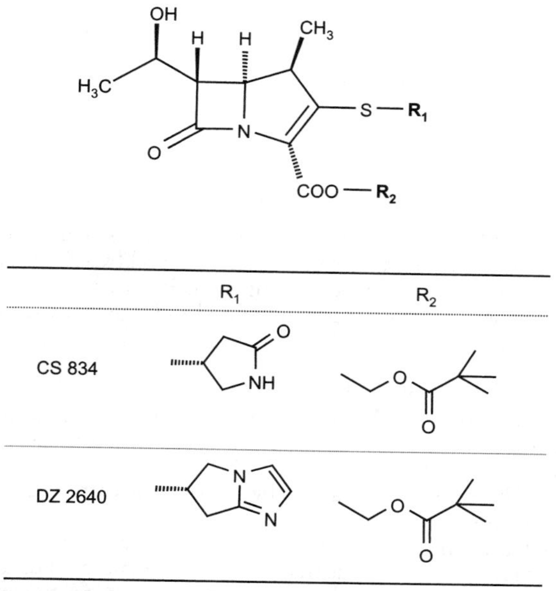

Figure 27 DZ 2640 and CS-834

8.1. Δ^{3-2} Isomerism

Miyauchi et al. (1989) and Saab et al. (1988) showed that in a phosphate buffer (0.5 M, pH 6.86, 37°C) a number of molecules are isomerized at Δ^2. This isomerism is reversible in an alkaline medium but not in an acidic medium. In the digestive tract, the pH may reach 8 as a result of pancreatic secretions. The ionized forms are due to gastric secretions. The pH affects the degradation of the pivalyloxymethyl esters. An increase in pH increases the degradation constants. If the concentration in the buffer is increased, only the isomerization increases, whereas degradation does not increase. When serum albumin is added, the isomerization constants are increased. This derives from a catalytic phenomenon due to the amino acids or to a change of configuration, occasioning a structural change that enhances isomerization by increasing the ionic form (Fig. 30).

The electrodonor nature of the substituent at C-3 modifies the degree of degradation and isomerization. The mechanism of isomerization between Δ^3 and Δ^2 is related to the deprotonation at C-2 (Fig. 31).

Studies conducted to optimize the geometry of the double bond between C-3 and C-4 and the substituent at C-3 have shown that the energy level of the least occupied orbital is correlated with log $k_{1.2}$.

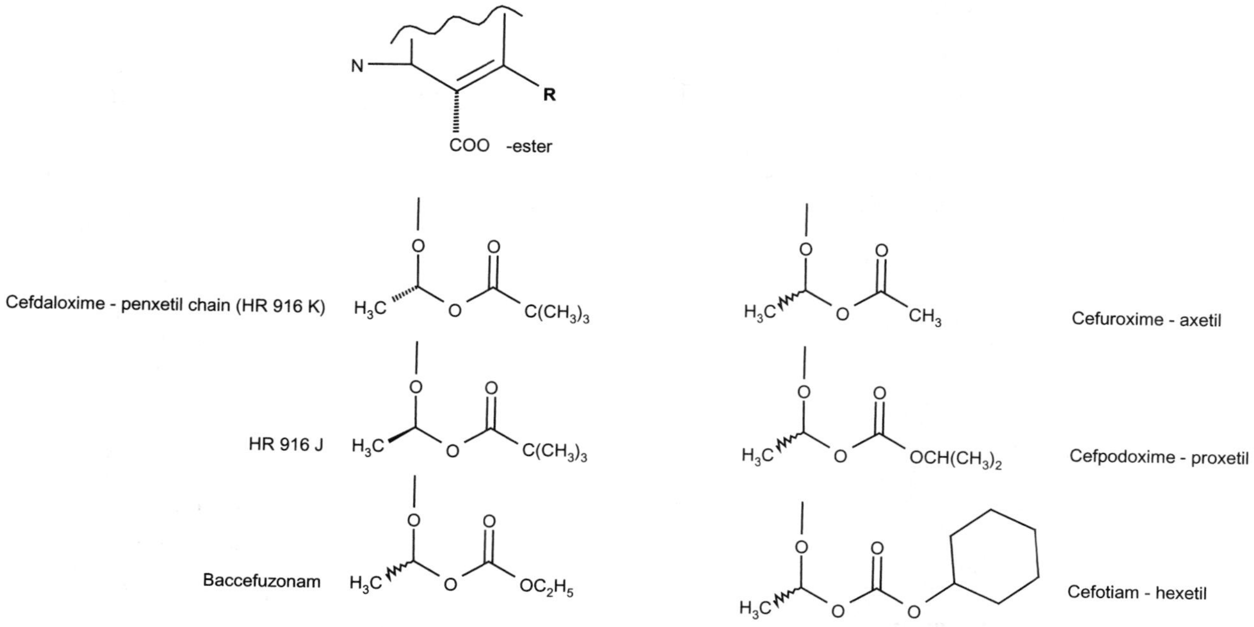

Figure 28 Various esters of oral cephalosporins

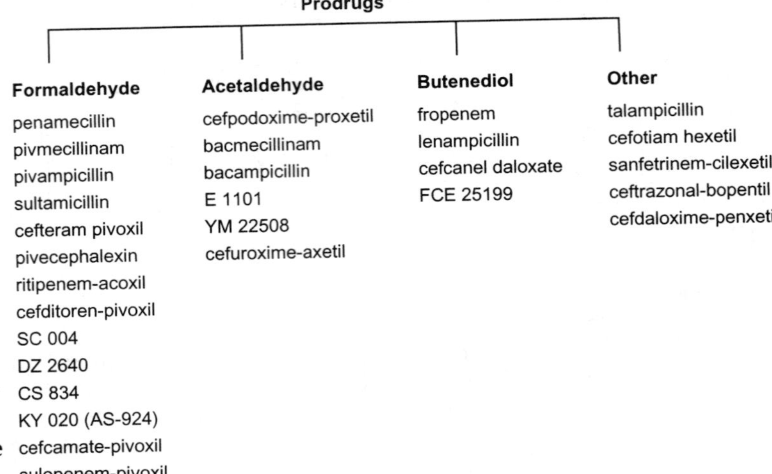

Figure 29 Metabolites of the ester chain

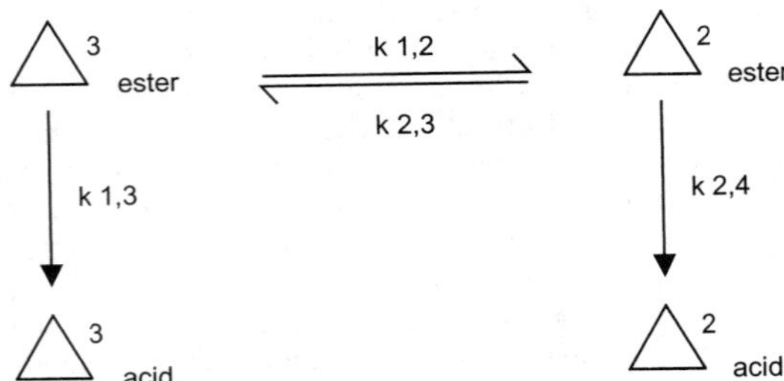

Figure 30 Cephalosporin metabolism ($\Delta^3 \rightarrow \Delta^2$ isomerization)

8.2. Pivaloyloxymethyl

A number of β-lactams have a pivaloyloxymethyl type of ester. Among the penicillins, pivampicillin and pivmecillinam may be mentioned here. A number of oral cephalosporins possess this ester, such as cefetamet, cefteram, cefditoren, cefcamate, KY-020, and SC-004 (Fujii, 1993). Among the penems, ritipenem has this ester. The pivaloyloxymethyl ester is metabolized to formaldehyde and pivalic acid.

8.2.1. Pivalic Acid (Trimethylacetic Acid)

Pivalate is converted in vivo to its coenzyme A ester, which, because of its structure, cannot be metabolized unless the acyl group is transferred to an acyl acceptor of the carnitine type. This transfer is catalyzed by one or more carnitine acyltransferases.

L-Carnitine is an essential factor involved in the β-oxidation of fatty acids that occurs in the mitochondria. It acts as a transporter of the acyl groups that transfer the fatty acids through the mitochondrial cytoplasmic membrane, which is normally impermeable to coenzyme A (Fig. 32). About 100 mmols of carnitine is present in the body of a 70-kg adult. It is localized in bone and cardiac tissue (~98%).

Figure 31 $\Delta^3 \rightarrow \Delta^2$ isomerization

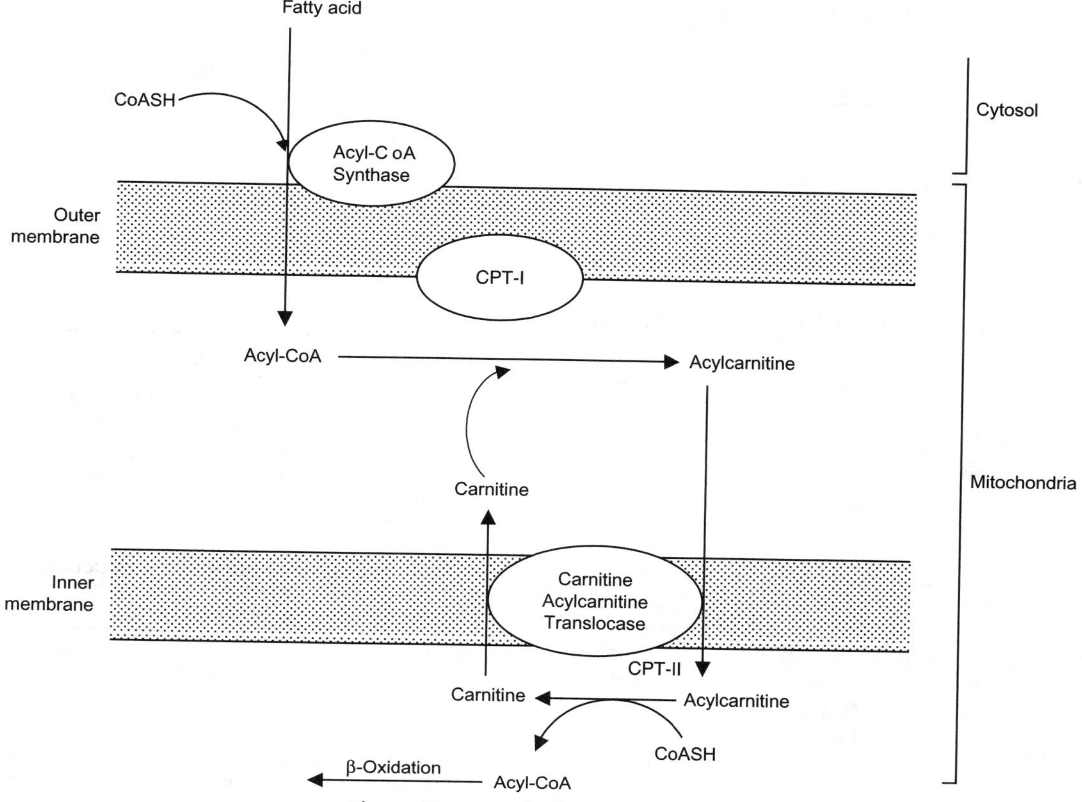

Figure 32 Metabolism of carnitine

Overconsumption of carnitine may be the cause of metabolic dysfunction.

The production of pivaloylcarnitine has been described, with the depletion of carnitine after the use of pivampicillin, cefcamate pivoxil, and cefditoren pivoxil (Fig. 33).

8.2.1.1. Cefcamate Pivoxil (S-1008, Cefcapene)

After administration of repeated doses of cefcamate pivoxil, the concentrations of carnitine plasma decrease, whereas those of pivaloylcarnitine increase (Table 34). After administration of 200 mg every 8 h for 7 days, the concentration of carnitine

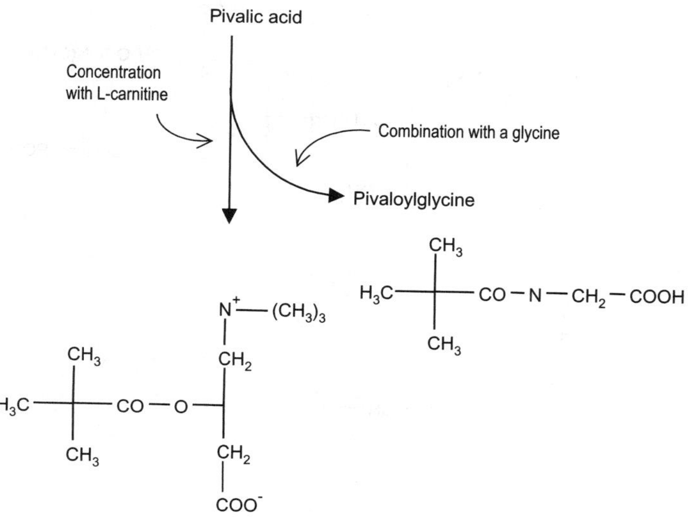

Figure 33 Metabolism of pivalic acid

Table 34 Metabolism of cefcamate

Drug	Dose (mg)	C_{max} (μg/ml)	T_{max} (h)	$t_{1/2}$ (h)	AUC (μg·h/ml)	Urinary elimination (%)
Cefcapene	100	0.83	4.33	2.24	5.28	35
	200	2.06	2.33	1.53	10.08	41
Pivalic acid	100	0.44	3.67	6.07	2.66	92.5
	200	0.99	2.33	4.16	5.1	
Pivaloylcarnitine	100	2.07		3.01	13.7	93.8

Table 35 Effect of the ester of cefcamate on metabolism[a]

Time	Glucose (mM)	3-HB (μM)	FFA (μM)	TG (mM)	Urea (mM)
Before treatment	5.24 ± 0.11	271.8 ± 62.3	408.6 ± 54.4	1.24 ± 0.21	4.61 ± 0.25
After treatment	6.76 ± 0.3	41.9 ± 18.5	263.5 ± 29.4	1.41 ± 0.12	3.74 ± 0.18
Significance	NS	$P < 0.05$	$P < 0.5$	NS	$P < 0.05$

[a]3-HB, 3-hydroxybutyrate; FFA, free fatty acids; TG, triglycerides; NS, not significant.

in plasma is 20 nmol/ml from the fifth day of treatment. Four to five days after the end of treatment, plasma carnitine levels return to normal (40 to 50 nmol/ml). There is also a marked increase in urinary elimination of pivaloylcarnitine.

Cefcamate pivoxil is also isomerized to Δ^2-cefcamate pivoxil and Δ^2-cefcamate (<2%) (Totsuka et al., 1992).

The same phenomenon has been described with pivampicillin and cefditoren pivoxil. The same metabolism products would probably be found with cefetamet pivoxil, cefteram pivoxil, and ritipenem acoxil.

After repeated administration of pivampicillin, a reduction in 7-β-hydroxybutyrates and triglycerides has been found on the seventh day, but no change in blood glucose levels has been noted (Table 35).

8.2.2. Formaldehyde

Variable quantities of formaldehyde are released, depending on the molecule (Table 36). The true impact of the formation of formaldehyde remains unclear. Numerous studies undertaken at the request of the Food and Drug Administration have shown that formaldehyde added to the drinking water of rats at doses of up to 125 mg/kg of body weight/day for 2 years caused no tumors. In addition, formaldehyde is not teratogenic at doses of up to 185 mg/kg/day.

Table 36 Prodrugs and aldehyde production

Drug	% HCHO	Ester
Penamecillin	7.4	Acetoxymethyl
Pivmecillinam	6.5	Pivaloyloxymethyl
Pivampicillin	6.8	Pivaloyloxymethyl
Sultamicillin	5	Aldehyde linker
Cefteram pivoxil	5	Pivaloyloxymethyl
Pivecephalexin	6.5	Pivaloyloxymethyl
Ritipenem acoxil	8.3	Pivaloyloxymethyl

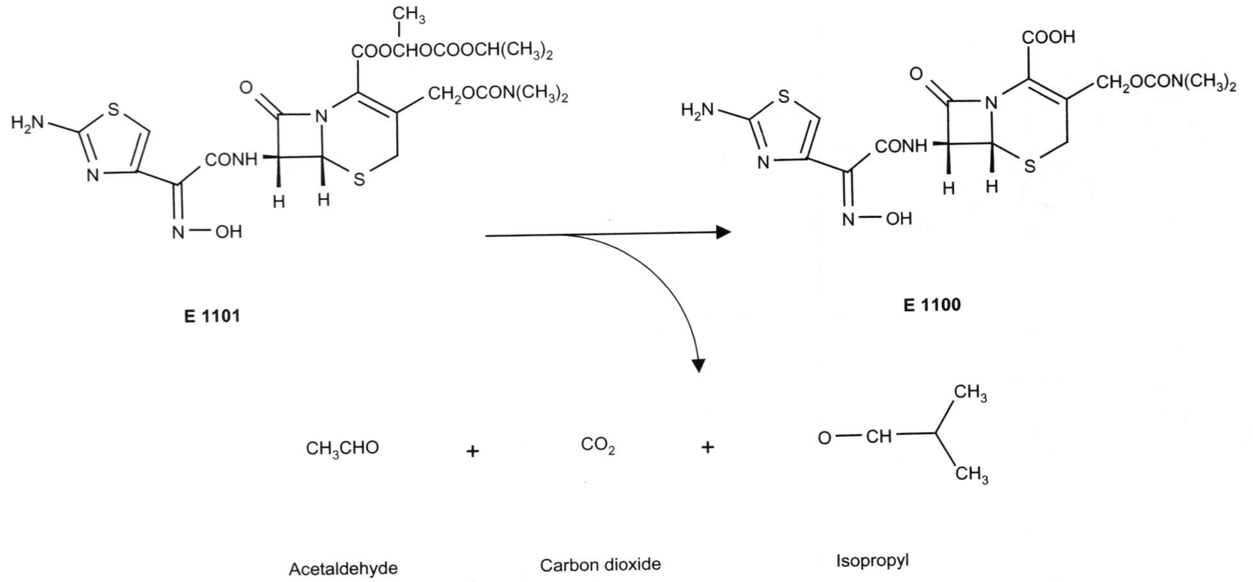

Figure 34 Acetaldehyde, carbon monoxide, and isopropyl (from Watanabe et al., 1994)

However, a genotoxic activity has been demonstrated with some molecules in in vitro tests, and these effects have been attributed to formaldehyde.

Abnormalities of the gastric mucosa in the form of hyperhemia and bleeding have been detected by fiberoptic endoscopy after ingestion of pivampicillin (Hey et al., 1982).

8.3. Isopropoxycarbonyloxyethyl Chain

Cefpodoxime proxetil (Fig. 22) is metabolized to cefpodoxime and its ester is metabolized to isopropanol and acetaldehyde. Isopropanol is then degraded. Cefpodoxime is also isomerized at Δ^3-Δ^2. This metabolism has also been demonstrated with E-1101, which is transformed to E-1100 (Fig. 34).

8.4. Acyloxyallyl Nucleus

The 3-phthalidylene-type esters of ampicillin are rapidly hydrolyzed, and the prodrug enables ampicillin to be well absorbed. The mechanism of hydrolysis involves an initial attack on the terminal lactone part followed by electron transfer and cleavage of the ester, releasing ampicillin and a vinylketone (Fig. 35).

The esters of the 2-oxo-1,3-dioxolone type are hydrolyzed by electron transfer after cleavage of the cyclic carbonate (Fig. 36). The hydrolysis products are ampicillin, CO_2, and an α-carbonyl derivative such as acetoin (lenampicillin), which is transformed to 2,4-butenediol (Fig. 37). Acetoin is used as a food additive.

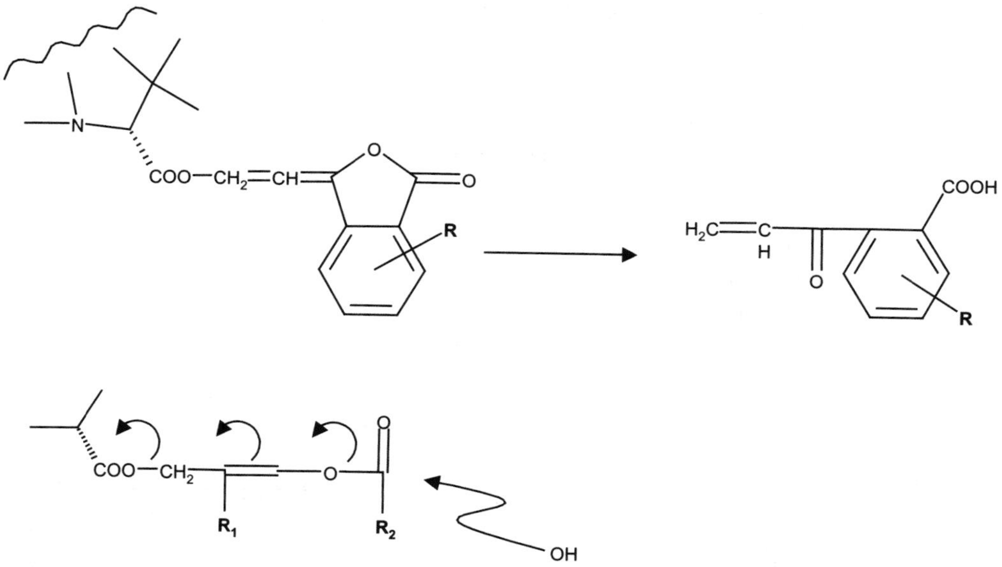

Figure 35 Degradation of the 3-phthalidylene ampicillins

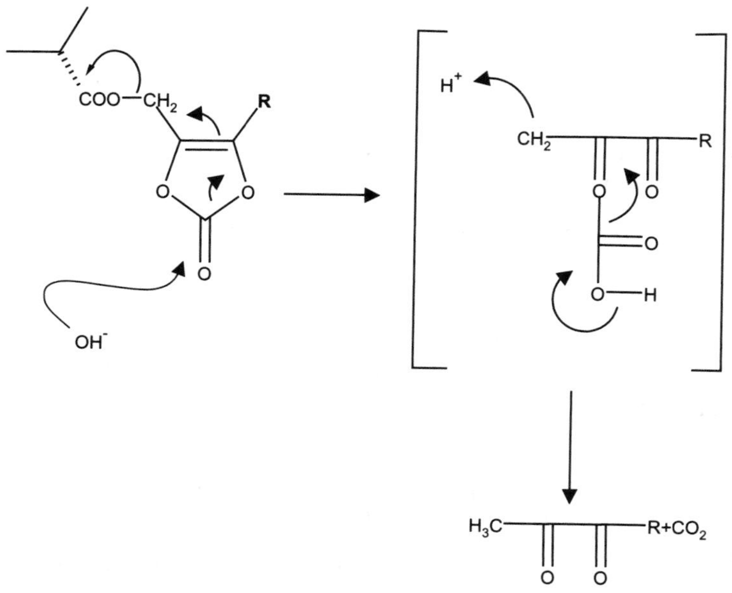

Figure 36 Degradation of the 1,3-dioxolene nucleus

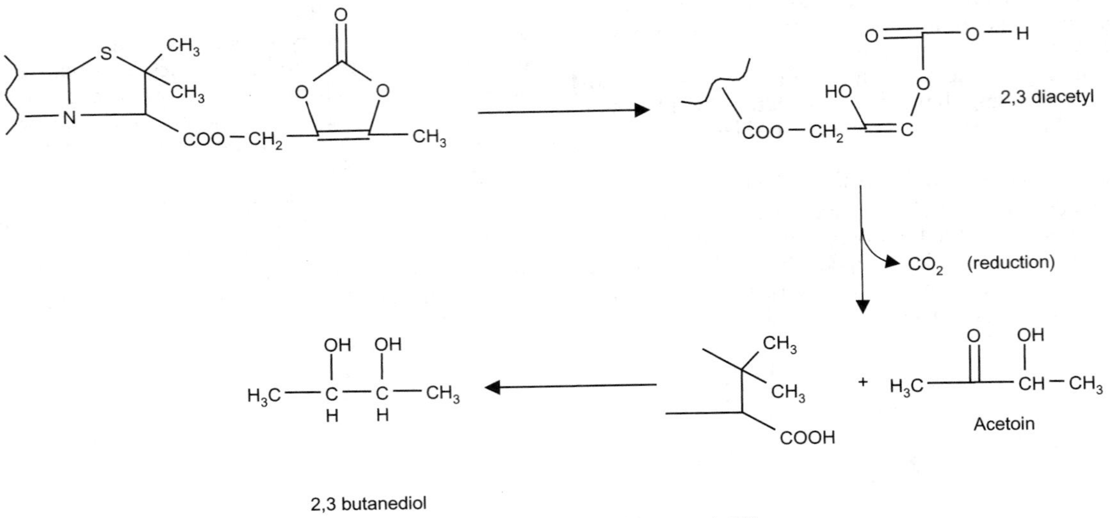

2,3 diacetyl

CO_2 (reduction)

Acetoin

2,3 butanediol

Figure 37 Metabolism of lenampicillin

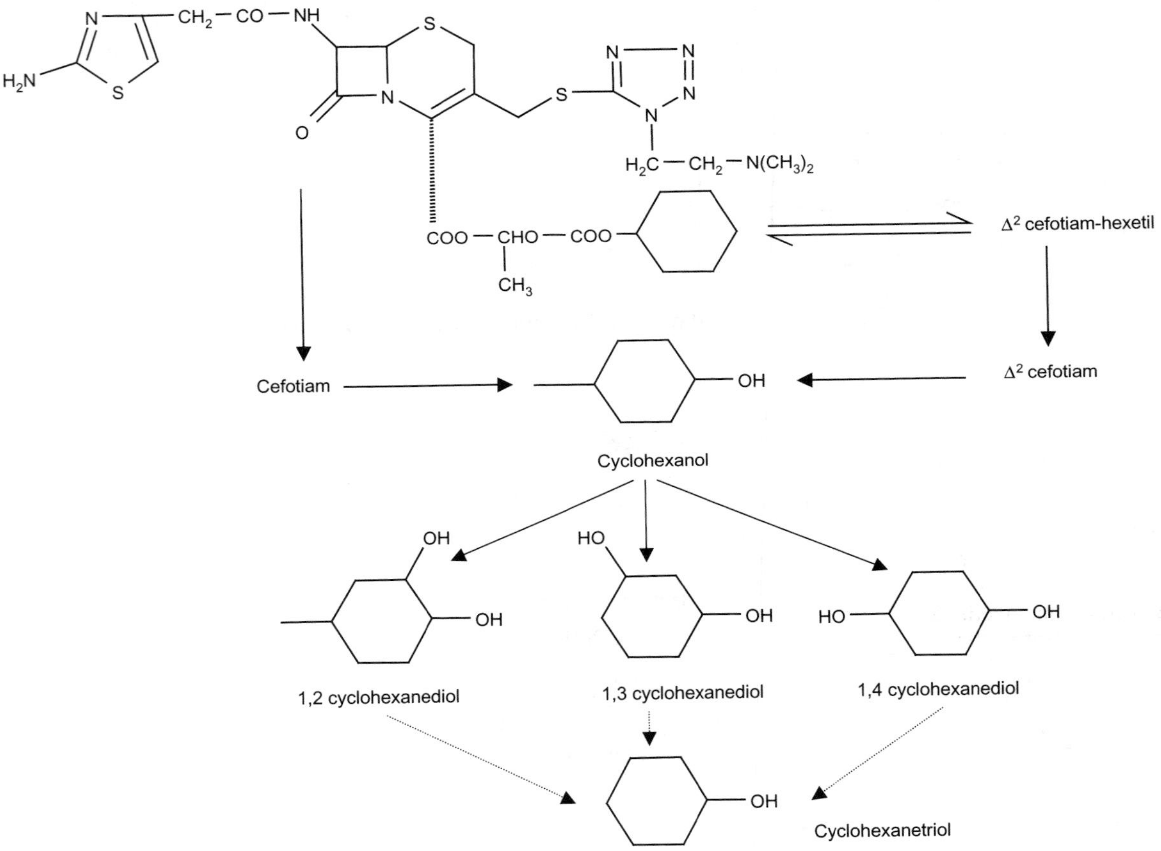

Δ² cefotiam-hexetil

Δ² cefotiam

Cefotiam

Cyclohexanol

1,2 cyclohexanediol

1,3 cyclohexanediol

1,4 cyclohexanediol

Cyclohexanetriol

Figure 38 Chemical metabolism of ester of cefotiam hexetil

8.5. Cyclohexanol (Cefotiam Hexetil)

Cefotiam is released after hydrolysis of the ester chain of cefotiam hexetil in the intestinal parietal cells. A small fraction is isomerized to Δ²-cefotiam (Fig. 38).

The lipophilic side chain of cefotiam is transformed to cyclohexanol, which is not found in the plasma, and its urinary elimination represents less than 1% of the administered dose. It is metabolized in the liver to cyclohexanediols and

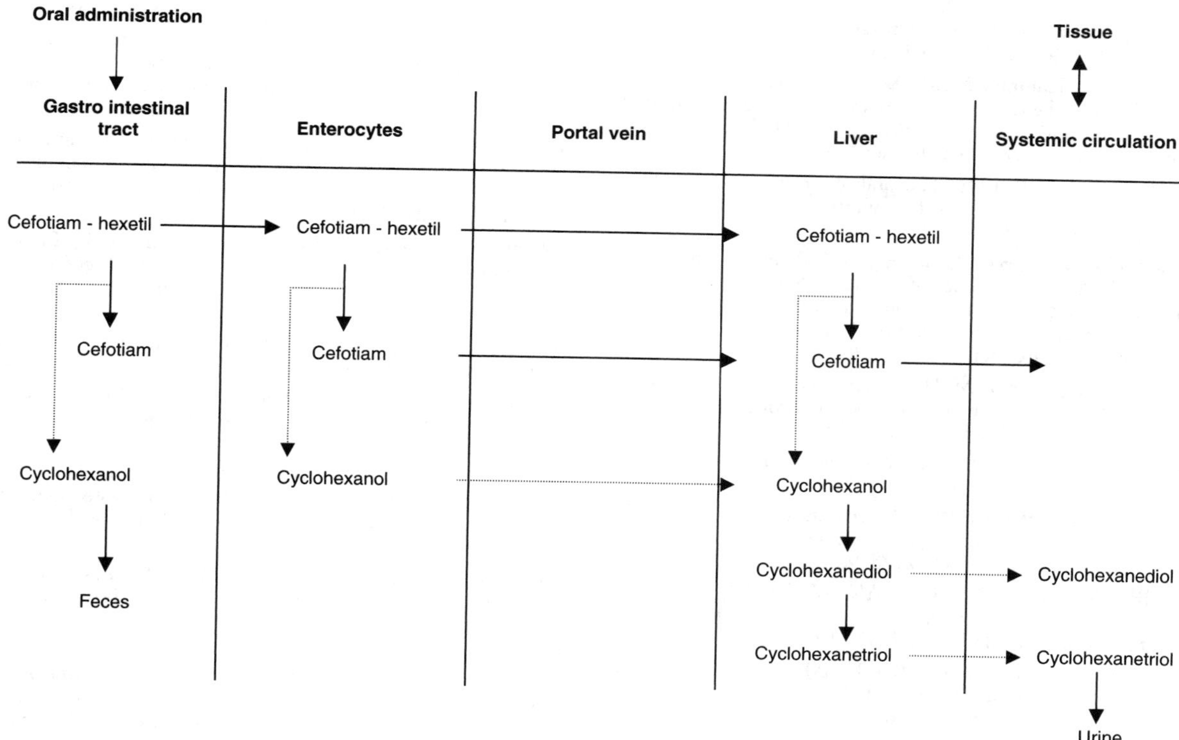

Figure 39 Metabolism of cefotiam hexetil (from Tanayama et al., 1988)

cyclohexatriols, traces of which are found in the systemic circulation (Fig. 39). The concentrations of cyclohexanediols in plasma are proportional to the doses of cefotiam hexetil ingested. Their formation is slow, requiring about 4 to 5 h. Their elimination in the urine is on the order of 35 to 40% (1,2-cyclohexanediol) and 18 to 20% (1,3 and 1,4-cyclohexanediols) of the administered dose. These products are eliminated slowly, with an apparent elimination half-life on the order of 15 to 17 h. After repeated doses of cefotiam hexetil (400 mg three times) the metabolites accumulate, reaching steady-state levels of 4 to 5 μg/ml for 1,2-cyclohexanediol and 2.0 to 2.5 μg/ml for the 1,3- and 1,4-cyclohexanediols (Table 37).

8.6. Cefuroxime Axetil

Cefuroxime is esterified by a 1-acetoxyethyl chain. Following its absorption, cefuroxime axetil is hydrolyzed to cefuroxime and Δ^2-cefuroxime axetil. Δ^2-Cefuroxime is released in the liver and is present in the portal vein. The ester released in the intestinal mucosa is metabolized to acetic acid and acetaldehyde.

Table 37 Elimination of the metabolites of cefotiam hexetil

Drug	Administered dose (%)	$t_{1/2}$ (h)
Cefotiam	35	1
Δ^2-Cefotiam	1.4	1.3
Cyclohexanediol	0.5	1.7
1,2-Cyclohexanediol	36	15.5
1,2- + 1,4-Cyclohexanediol	18	16.7

REFERENCES

Aoki H, Sekiguchi M, Akahane K, Tsutmi Y, Korenaga H, Hayano T, Hayakawa I, 1995, DZ2640, a new oral carbapenem antibiotic. 3. Pharmacokinetics and safety in laboratory animals, 35th Intersci Conf Antimicrob Agents Chemother, abstract F-135.

Artusson P, Karlsson J, 1991, Correlation between oral absorption in humans and apparent drug permeability coefficients in human intestinal epithelial (CaCo2) cell culture, Biochem Biophys Res Commun, 175, 880–885.

Bechgaard H, 1982, Critical factors influencing gastrointestinal absorption—what is the role of pellets? Acta Pharm Technol, 2, 149–157.

Binderup E, Godtfredsen WO, Roholt K, 1971, Orally active cephalosporin esters, J Antibiot, 24, 767–773.

Bodor N, 1977, Chapter 7, in Roche EB, ed, Design of Biopharmaceutical Properties through Prodrugs and Analogs, American Pharmacology Association and Academy of Pharmaceutical Sciences.

Bundgaard H, 1991, Novel chemical approaches in prodrug design, Drugs Fut, 16, 443–448.

Bunn PA, Milicich S, Lunn JS, 1965, Pharmacological properties of hetacillin in the human, Antimicrob Agents Chemother, 947–950.

Clayton JP, Cole M, Elson SW, Ferres H, 1974, BRL 8988 (talampicillin), a well-absorbed oral form of ampicillin, Antimicrob Agents Chemother, 5, 670–671.

Clayton JP, Cole M, Elson SW, Hardy KD, Mizen LW, Sutherland R, 1975, Preparation, hydrolysis, and oral absorption of α-carboxy esters of carbenicillin, J Med Chem, 18, 172–177.

Daehne WV, Frederiksen E, Gundersen E, Lund F, Morch P, Petersen HJ, Roholt K, Tybring L, Godtfredsen WO, 1970, Acyloxymethyl esters of ampicillin, J Med Chem, 13, 607–612.

Di Modugno E, Erbetti I, Hammond SM, Lowther J, Piccoli L, Zampicinni L, 1994, Activity of the tribactam GV 118819 against penicillin resistant experimental *Streptococcus pneumoniae*, 34th Intersci Conf Antimicrob Agents Chemother, abstract F 80.

Di Modugno E, Hammond SM, Xerri L, Gaviraghi G, 1993, In vitro activity of the tribactam GV 104326 against gram-positive, gram-negative, and anaerobic bacteria, 33rd Intersci Conf Antimicrob Agents Chemother, abstract 128.

Eriksson M, Bolme P, 1981, The oral absorption of ampicillin, pivampicillin and amoxycillin in infants and children, Acta Pharmacol Toxicol, 49, 38–42.

Ethymiopoulos C, Capriati A, Barrington P, Patel J, Sheny EVB, Bye A, 1994, Pharmacokinetics of GV 104326, a novel tribactam antibiotic, following single intravenous and oral (as its prodrug GV 188819X) administration in man, 34th Intersci Conf Antimicrob Agents Chemother, abstract F 82.

Fabre J, Burgy C, Rudhart M, Herrera A, 1972, The behaviour in man of CP 15464, a carbenicillin absorbed following oral administration, Chemotherapy, 17, 334–343.

Ferres H, 1983, Prodrugs of β-lactam antibiotics, Drugs Today, 19, 499–538.

Foresta P, Ramacci MT, De Witt P, Capatani N, Faneli O, 1977, A new cephalosporin derivative (ST-21) orally administered in laboratory animals, Arzneim Forsch, 27, 819–823.

Foulds JP, Stankewich JP, Knirsch AK, Weidler DJ, 1982, The pharmacokinetics of sultamicillin in man, 22nd Intersci Conf Antimicrob Agents Chemother, abstract 519.

Fujii, 1993, Cefditoren-pivoxil (CDTR-PI): pharmacokinetics. Influence on carnitine metabolism and clinical evaluation in pediatric patients, 33rd Intersci Conf Antimicrob Agents Chemother, abstract 897.

Ginsburg CM, McCracken GH Jr, Clahsen J, Zweighaft T, 1981, Comparative pharmacokinetics of bacampicillin and ampicillin suspensions in infants and children, Rev Infect Dis, 3, 117–120.

Hey H, Frederiksen HJ, Thoup Andersen J, 1982, Gastroscopic and pharmacokinetic evaluation of a new pivmecillinam tablet, Eur J Clin Pharmacol, 22, 63–69.

Hobs DC, 1972, Metabolism of indanyl carbenicillin in dogs, rats, and humans, Antimicrob Agents Chemother, 2, 272–275.

Irwin VP, Quigley JM, Timoney RF, 1987, Quantitative relationships between in vitro antibacterial activities of cephalosporins and their n-octanol/water partition coefficients, Int J Pharm, 34, 241–246.

Jansen ABA, Russell TJ, 1965, Some novel penicillin derivatives, J Chem Soc, 65, 2127–2132.

Klesel N, Adam F, Isert D, Limbert M, Markus A, Schrinner E, Seibert G, 1992, RU 29246, the active compound of the cephalosporin prodrug ester HR 916. III. Pharmacokinetic properties and antibacterial activity in vivo, J Antibiot, 45, 922–931.

Lowther J, Hammond SM, Russell K, Fairclough PD, 1990, Uptake of cephalosporins by human intestinal brush-border membrane vesicles, J Antimicrob Chemother, 25, 183–185.

Lucas ML, et al, 1976, Relationship of the acid micro-climate in rat and human intestine to malabsorption, Biochem Soc Trans, 4, 154–156.

Miyauchi, M, et al, 1989, Studies on orally active cephalosporin esters. II. Chemical stability of pivaloyloxymethyl esters in phosphate buffer solution, Chem Pharm Bull, 37, 2369–2374.

Morita E, Mizuno N, Nishikata M, Takahashi K, 1992, Effect of gastrointestinal maturation on absorption of β-lactam antibiotics, J Pharm Sci, 81, 337–340.

Nishi T, Ishida Y, Sugita K, Ohtsuka M, Takemura M, Hayakawa I, Hayano I, 1995, DZ-2640, a new oral carbapenem antibiotic. 1. Structure activity relationships and in vitro activity, 35th Intersci Conf Antimicrob Agents Chemother, abstract F-133.

Nishimura K, Yoshimi A, Kitagawara M, Hashizumo H, Muro H, Kasai M, Hatano S, Kakeya N, 1990, KY-20, a new sweet tasting and orally absorbed prodrug of ceftizoxime; oral absorption and efficacy in animals, 30th Intersci Conf Antimicrob Agents Chemother, abstract 674.

Nishimura K-I, Nishizawa S, Yoshimi A, Nakamura M, Nishimura M, Kakeya N, 1988, KY-109, a new bifunctional prodrug of cephalosporin. II. Mechanism of oral absorption, Chem Pharm Bull, 36, 2128–2134.

Perboni A, Donati D, Rossi T, Tamburini B, Tarzia G, Gaviraghi G, 1993, Tricyclic β-lactams (tribactams); potent DHP-1 and β-lactamase stable antibiotics, 33rd Intersci Conf Antimicrob Agents Chemother, abstract I27.

Quay JF, Forster L, 1970, Cephalexin penetration of the surviving rat intestine, Physiologist, 13, 287.

Richardson AP, Walker HA, Loeb P, Miller I, 1945, Metabolism of methyl and benzyl esters of penicillin by different species, Proc Exp Biol Med, 60, 272–276.

Saab AN, Dittert LW, Hussain AA, 1988, Isomerization of cephalosporin esters: implications for the prodrug ester approach to enhancing the oral bioavailabilities of cephalosporins, J Pharm Sci, 77, 906–907.

Sakamoto F, Ikeda S, Tsukamoto G, 1984, Studies on prodrugs. II. Preparation and characterization of (5-substituted 2-oxo-l,3-dioxolen-4-yl)methyl esters of ampicillin, Chem Pharm Bull, 32, 2241–2248.

Shindo H, Kawai K, Fukuda K, Muyazaki K, Arita T, 1975, Absorption and metabolism of pivampicillin—site of ester hydrolysis and the species difference, Annu Rep Sankyo Res Gab, 27, 150–151.

Shiobara Y, Tachibana A, Sasaki H, Watatanabe T, Sado T, 1974, Phthalidyl D-α-aminobenzylpenicillate hydrochloride (PC-183), a new orally active ampicillin ester, J Antibiot, 27, 665–673.

Thwaites DT, Hirst BH, Simmons NL, 1993, Direct assessment of dipeptide/H + symport in intact human intestinal (CaCo2) epithelium: a novel method utilising continuous intracellular pH measurement, Biochem Biophys Res Commun, 194, 432–438.

Totsuka K, Shimizu K, Konishi M, Yamamoto S, 1992, Metabolism of S-1108, a new oral cephem antibiotic, and metabolic profiles of its metabolites in humans, Antimicrob Agents Chemother, 36, 757–761.

Ueda I, Shimojo F, Kozatani J, 1983, Effect of ethylcellulose in a medium chain triglyceride on the bioavailability of ceftizoxime, J Pharm Sci, 72, 454–458.

Ungar J, Muggleton PW, 1952, Accumulation of diethylaminoethanol ester of penicillin in inflamed lung tissue, Br Med J, 1, 1211–1213.

Westphal J-F, Jehl F, Brogard J-M, Carbon C, 1995, Amoxicillin intestinal absorption reduction by amiloride: possible role of the Na+/H+exchanger, Clin Pharmacol Ther, 57, 257–264.

Wheeler WJ, Preston DA, Wright WE, Huffman GW, Osborne HE, Howard DP, 1979, Orally active esters of cephalosporin antibiotics. 3. Synthesis and biological properties of aminoacyloxymethyl esters of 7-[O-(−)-mandelamido]-3-[[(1-methyl-H-tetrazol-5yl)thio]methyl]-3-cephem-4-carboxylic acid, J Med Chem, 22, 657–661.

Yoshikawa T, Muranuoshi N, Yoshida M, Oguma T, Hirano K, Yamada H, 1989, Transport characteristics of ceftibuten (7432 S), a new oral cephem, in rat intestinal brush-border membrane vesicles: proton-coupled and stereoselective transport of ceftibuten, Pharm Res, 6, 302–307.

Yoshimura Y, Hamaguchi N, Yashiki T, 1985, Synthesis and relationship between physicochemical properties and oral absorption of pivaloyloxymethyl esters of parenteral cephalosporins, Int J Pharm, 23, 117–129.

Peptidoglycan Synthesis Inhibitors

A. BRYSKIER AND C. DINI

12

1. INTRODUCTION

Bacterial peptidoglycans were first identified in the 1940s. The nucleotide precursors were isolated and characterized in 1949. Peptidoglycan biosynthesis has been investigated in many bacterial species. It was found that penicillin-binding proteins (PBPs) can be bifunctional enzymes. Several antibacterials inhibit peptidoglycan synthesis, such as fosfomycin, β-lactams, glycopeptides, lipoglycopeptides, bacitracin, and moenomycin.

2. PEPTIDOGLYCAN

Peptidoglycan (murein) is a continuous covalent macromolecular structure located outside of the cytoplasmic (inner) membrane of almost all eubacteria; it is found exclusively in microorganisms.

2.1. Peptidoglycan Function

The main function of peptidoglycan is to withstand the internal osmotic pressure and to maintain a defined cell shape.

Peptidoglycan also participates in the cell division process. Most gram-positive bacteria, such as *Bacillus subtilis* and *Staphylococcus aureus*, have a thick cell wall composed of peptidoglycan, while gram-negative bacteria have an additional outer membrane. In mycobacteria the outer leaflet consists of mycolic acid, an unusual lipid containing more than 70 carbon chains with only a few double bonds.

2.2. Peptidoglycan Structure

Peptidoglycan is a giant molecule composed of linear glycan chains linked by short peptides. The glycan chains are small and repeated units composed of *N*-acetylglucosamine (GlcNAc) and *N*-acetylmuramic acid (MurNAc). The sugars are linked by β-1,4-glycoside bridges.

Position 3− of muramic acid bears a pentapeptide side chain of the general structure L-Ala–γ-D-Glu–X–D-Ala–D-Ala, in which X can be either L-lysine or a *meso*-diaminopimelic acid.

2.3. Peptidoglycan Biosynthesis

Peptidoglycan biosynthesis is a complex process involving at least three stages, namely, intracytoplasmic monomer formation, monomer transfer through the inner membrane with specific steps, and polymerization at the cell surface. Each step involves several enzymes which all are potential targets for novel antibacterial agents.

2.3.1. UDP-GlcNAc Formation

The peptidoglycan monomer consists of two sugars, namely, GlcNAc and MurNac-pentapeptide, which also derives from GlcNAc.

Glucosamine-6-phosphate is synthesized from fructose-6-phosphate in a reaction catalyzed by glucosamine-6-synthase. Glucosamine-6-phosphate is converted into glucosamine-1-phosphate by phosphoglucosamine mutase (GlmM). Glucosamine-1-phosphate is converted into UDP-GlcNac by glucosamine-1-phosphate acetyltransferase and GlcNAc-1-phosphate uridyltransferase (GlmU). The *glmU* gene product is bifunctional, and the C-terminal domain catalyzes acetylation of glucosamine-1-phosphate to yield GlcNAc-1-phosphate, while the N-terminal part catalyzes uridylation of GlcNAc-1-phosphate to provide UDP-GlcNAc (Fig. 1). Thereafter, UDP-GlcNAc is used for the assembly of both peptidoglycan and the lipid A component of bacterial lipopolysaccharide (Fig. 2) and for chitin assembly in fungi.

2.3.1.1. GlmS

D-Glutamine:D-fructose-6-phosphate amidotransferase (GlmS) catalyzes the conversion of D-fructose-6-phosphate into glucosamine-6-phosphate. This enzyme is encoded in *Escherichia coli* by the *glmS* gene (Wu and Wu, 1971).

The amide functionality of glutamine is used as an ammonia source. It is a bienzyme complex with two structurally and functionally distinct domains. The N-terminal glutaminase domain catalyzes hydrolysis of glutamine to glutamate, while

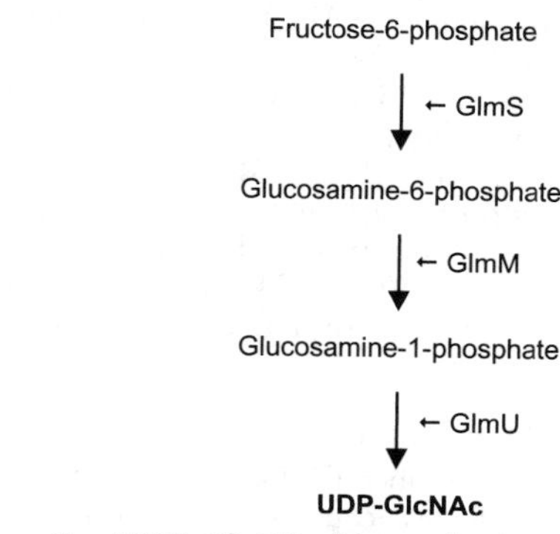

Figure 1 UDP-GlcNAc biosynthesis

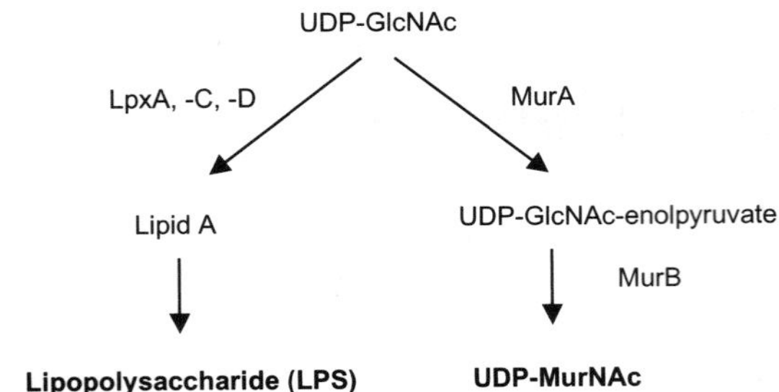

Figure 2 Lipopolysaccharide (LPS) or UDP-MurNac biosynthesis

releasing an equivalent of ammonia. The C-terminal corresponds to the domain for conversion of fructose-6-phosphate to glucosamine-6-phosphate. Each domain was overproduced and crystallized and their three-dimensional structure was determined at high resolution (Isupov et al., 1996; Teplyakov et al., 1998).

The glutamine and fructose-6-phosphate binding sites were studied using substrate analogs, and the residues involved in their binding were identified (Bearne, 1996; Leriche et al., 1997; Bearne and Blouin, 2000).

Naturally occurring and synthetic inhibitors of the GlmS synthase have been described. Recently, novel electrophilic glutamine analogs based on 6-diazo-5-oxonorleucine were reported as very potent inhibitors (Walker et al., 2000).

2.3.1.2. GlmM

In the second step, GlmM catalyzes the interconversion of glucosamine-6-phosphate to glucosamine-1-phosphate (Fig. 1). It is the product of the *glmM* gene in *E. coli*. The *glmM* gene was shown to be essential in *E. coli*, but genetic data recently suggested that in *S. aureus* there could be an alternative pathway for glucosamine-1-phosphate biosynthesis (Glanzmann et al., 1999).

Purified *E. coli* GlmM was shown to be active only in a phosphorylated form containing one bound phosphate and separable from the unphosphorylated form (Mengin-Lecreulx and van Heijenoort, 1996; Jolly et al., 1999).

2.3.1.3. GlmU

The last two steps for the preparation of UDP-GlcNAc are acetylation and uridylation (Fig. 1). They are catalyzed by the product of the *glmU* gene in *E. coli*. The corresponding gene has been identified in several other bacterial species. The GlmU protein from *E. coli* is a bifunctional enzyme. Its C-terminal domain catalyzes acetylation of glucosamine-1-phosphate into GlcNAc-1-phosphate, whereas its N-terminal domain catalyzes uridylation to yield UDP-GlcNAc (Mengin-Lecreulx and van Heijenoort, 1994).

The two domains are functionally independent, and each one is essential for cell viability (Gehring et al., 1996; Pompeo et al., 2001).

The crystal structures of *Streptococcus pneumoniae* GlmU and its complex with UDP-GlcNAc and Mg^{2+} were determined (Kostrewa et al., 2001). When UDP-GlcNAc and Mg^{2+} are bound at the uridyltransferase active site, the protein structure is in a closed form.

2.3.2. UDP-MurNAc Formation

UDP-MurNAc formation from UDP-GlcNAc is a two-step process: (i) MurA transferase catalyzes the transfer of an enolpyruvate from phosphoenolpyruvate to position 3− of GlcNAc, yielding UDP-GlcNAc-enolpyruvate, and (ii) the enolpyruvate moiety is reduced into D-lactoyl by MurB reductase to yield UDP-MurNAc. MurA is inhibited by fosfomycin.

2.3.2.1. MurA

UDP-GlcNAc enolpyruvyl transferase (MurA) is a 44-kDa protein which is the enzyme responsible for the first committed step in bacterial cell wall biosynthesis. It catalyzes the transfer of an enolpyruvate from phosphoenolpyruvate to UDP-GlcNAc (Marquardt et al., 1992; Brown et al., 1995). Although only one gene exists in gram-negative bacteria for MurA, two genes are present in gram-positive bacteria (Du et al., 2000).

A free open MurA form was observed from the *Enterobacter cloacae* X-ray structure with 1.8-Å resolution (Eschenburg and Schonbrunn, 2000). The substrate, UDP-GlcNAc, and fosfomycin have been cocrystallized with *E. coli* MurA at 1.8-Å resolution. Fosfomycin is a naturally occurring inhibitor of MurA, which behaves like a phosphoenolpyruvate analog (Brown et al., 1994). This compound is clinically used as an antibiotic.

2.3.2.2. MurB

UDP-*N*-acetylenolpyruvylglucosamine reductase (MurB) is a 38-kDa protein that reduces the enolpyruvyl group of UDP-*N*-acetylenolpyruvylglucosamine. MurB is a flavine-dependent reductase (FAD). Reduction of the enolpyruvate group of UDP-GlcNAc-enolpyruvate to UDP-MurNAc by MurB flavoprotein occurs in a two-step process: first, bound FAD is reduced by (NADPH + H^+), and then $FADH_2$ reduces the enolpyruvyl group at position C-3 to yield UDP-MurNAc.

The *S. aureus* MurB (326 amino acids) crystal structure in a free form at 2.3 Å was recently published (Benson et al., 2001).

2.3.3. UDP-MurNAc-Pentapeptide Formation

L-Alanine, D-glutamic acid, and *meso*-diaminopimelic acid (or L-lysine) are sequentially added onto the lactyl side chain of UDP-MurNAc by their respective ligases (MurC, MurD, and MurE [see below]) to yield UDP-MurNAc-tripeptide. Finally, the dipeptide D-Ala–D-Ala is added by MurF (see below) to yield UDP-MurNAc-pentapeptide (Fig. 3).

L-Alanine, D-glutamic acid, and *meso*-diaminopimetic acid induce carboxy activation of a C-terminal amino acid residue of the nucleotide substrate into an acyl-phosphate intermediate.

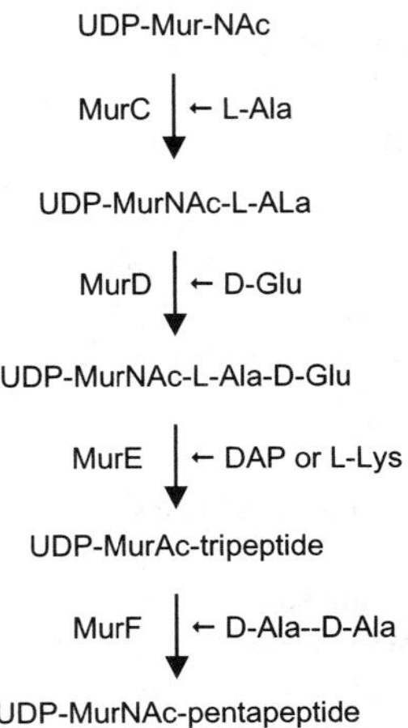

Figure 3 Pentapeptide biosynthesis

After nucleophilic attack and elimination of a phosphate, a peptide bond is formed. This mechanism is similar to that of the ATP-dependent amide-forming enzymes, such as glutamine synthase and glutathione synthase (Fig. 4).

The *mur*C to *mur*F genes are all essential in bacteria. In addition, according to available genomic sequences, the corresponding Mur proteins are highly conserved among bacterial species. Consequently, a potential inhibitor of these enzymes would be expected to be antibacterial and to have a broad spectrum.

2.3.3.1. MurC

UDP-*N*-acetylmuramate L-alanine ligase (MurC) is a 50-kDa protein which adds an L-alanine to the growing amino acid side chain (Liger et al., 1995b). A free-form X-ray crystal structure of *E. coli* MurC at 3.5-Å resolution has been reported (Emanuele et al., 1996). The specificities of various MurC synthetases for D-alanine and UDP-MurNAc were investigated with closely structurally related analogs accepted as substrates or functioning as competitive inhibitors (Hammes et al., 1973; Mizuno et al., 1973; Ishiguro 1982; Michaud et al., 1987; Liger et al., 1991; Liger et al., 1995b; Emanuele et al., 1996; Gubler et al., 1996).

2.3.3.2. MurD

UDP-*N*-acetylmuramoyl-L-alanine D-glutamate ligase (MurD) is a 47-kDa protein which adds a D-glutamic acid to UDP-*N*-acetylmuramoyl-L-alanine. An X-ray structure (free form) of *E. coli* MurD at 2.4 Å has been reported. Moreover, an X-ray cocrystal MurD with the substrate (UDP-*N*-acetylmuramoyl-L-alanine) has been reported at 1.95-Å resolution (Bertrand et al., 1997, 1999; Bertrand et al., 2000). The high specificity of MurD for D-glutamate was confirmed by studying structurally related analogs as substrates or inhibitors (Michaud et al., 1987; Pratviel-Sosa et al., 1994; Auger et al., 1995; Tanner et al., 1996; Gegnas et al., 1998; Gobec et al., 2001).

2.3.3.3. MurE

UDP-*N*-acetylmuramoyl-L-alanyl-D-glutamate-*meso*-diaminopimelate ligase (MurE) is a 52-kDa protein which adds an L-lysine in gram-positive bacteria and *meso*-diaminopimelic acid in gram-negative bacteria to the growing cell wall chain (Michaud et al., 1990; Mengin-Lecreulx et al., 1996; Mengin-Lecreulx et al., 1999).

An X-ray cocrystal of *E. coli* MurE with the product of the enzymatic reaction UDP-*N*-acetylmuramoyl-L-alanyl-ε-D-glutamyl-*meso*-diaminopimelate has been reported at 2.0-Å resolution (Gordon et al., 2001). It shares a three-domain topology comparable to that of the other Mur ligases. By its ε-amino group, *meso*-diaminopimelate or lysine is involved in the cross-linking between the peptide subunits of the glycan chains and thus plays a key role in the integrity of peptidoglycan. In a given organism *meso*-diaminopimelic acid and D-lysine are both present as cell metabolites, but its MurE synthetase generally efficiently discriminates between the two amino acids by catalyzing the addition of only one of them to the UDP-MurNAc–L-Ala–D-Glu precursor.

The search of related analogs as substrates or inhibitors led to active compounds with 50% inhibitory concentrations (IC_{50}) up to 1 μM (Abo-Ghalia et al., 1988; Zeng et al., 1998).

2.3.3.4. MurF

UDP-*N*-acetylmuramoyl-L-alanyl-D-glutamyl-*meso*-diaminopimelate-D-alanyl-D-alanine ligase (MurF) is a 46-kDa protein which adds a D-alanyl–D-alanine peptide onto the growing cell wall chain (Anderson et al., 1996).

An X-ray crystal structure of *E. coli* MurF at 2.3-Å resolution has been reported (Yan et al., 1999, 2000). The specificity profile for the D-alanyl–D-alanine peptide substrate has been studied with D-Ala–D-Ala analogs accepted as substrates or functioning as inhibitors (Neuhaus and Struve, 1965; Hammes et al., 1973; Schleifer et al., 1976; Duncan et al., 1990; Bugg et al., 1991; Billot-Klein et al., 1994; Reynolds et al., 1994; Arthur et al., 1996).

2.3.4. Transmembrane Transfer (Translocation Steps)

Final peptidoglycan assembly takes place on the outer side of the inner membrane, in the periplasmic space. To reach this site, the monomer-pentapeptide has to cross the hydrophobic inner membrane.

The phospho-MurNAc-pentapeptide unit crosses the cytoplasmic membrane with the help of an undecaprenyl phosphate lipid carrier. There is a series of membrane reactions involving MraY, a phospho-MurNAc-pentapeptide translocase I encoded by the *mraY* gene in *E. coli*, and yielding lipid I (undecaprenol-diphospho-MurNAc-pentapeptide. Translocase II (or glycosyltransferase) then attaches a GlcNAc residue from UDP-GlcNAc to lipid I, yielding lipid II (encoded by *murG* in *E. coli*). The next step is the migration of these dimeric units to the outside of the cell membrane. The mechanism of translocation remains unknown. The final step of peptidoglycan biosynthesis is the assembly of the various monomeric-pentapeptide–lipid II intermediates on the outside of the inner membrane (Fig. 5).

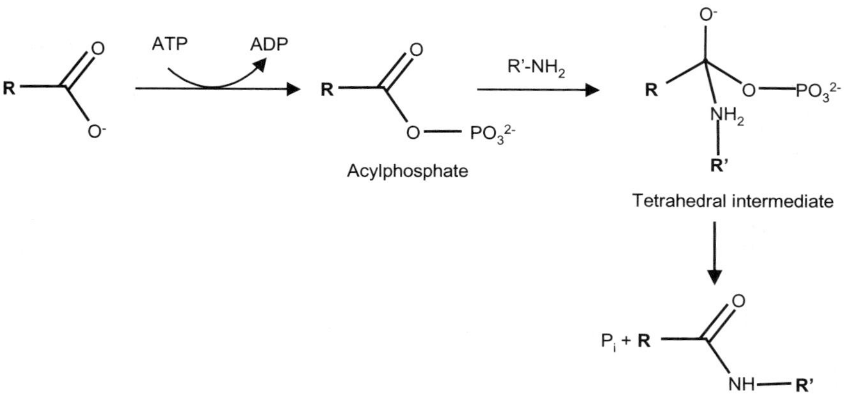

Figure 4 Mechanism of reaction catalyzed by ATP-dependent amide-forming enzymes (MurC to MurF)

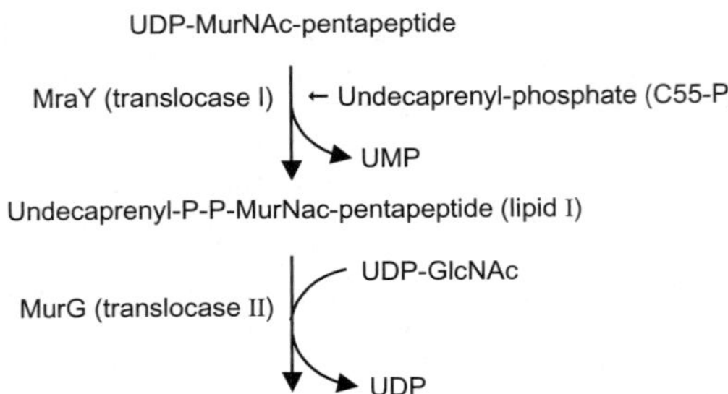

Figure 5 Lipid II biosynthesis

The *mur*G and *mraY* genes are essential in bacteria and have been identified in many bacterial genomes. Consequently, a potential inhibitor of their respective products would be expected to be antibacterial and to display a broad spectrum.

2.3.4.1. MraY

The two-dimensional membrane topology of the *E. coli* and *S. aureus* MraY transferases, which catalyze the formation of the first lipid intermediate (lipid I) of peptidoglycan synthesis, was established using the β-lactamase fusion system. This study led to a topological model possessing 10 transmembrane segments, five cytoplasmic domains, and six periplasmic domains including the N- and C-terminal ends. The agreement between the topologies of *E. coli* and *S. aureus*, their agreement to a fair extent with predicted models, and a number of features arising from the comparative analysis of 25 ortholog sequences strongly suggested the validity of the model for all eubacterial MraY transferases. The primary structures of the 10 transmembrane segments diverged among orthologs, but they retained their hydrophobicity, number, and size. The similarity of the sequences and distribution of the five cytoplasmic domains in both models, as well as their conservation among the MraY orthologs, clearly suggested their possible involvement in substrate recognition and in the catalytic process.

Comparison of the amino acids sequences of MraY from six microorganisms showed that hydrophobic and hydrophilic domains are regularly alternated. The predictive topology of the protein allows the proposal that the active site is located on the inner side of the bacterial cell wall. Mg^{2+} is essential to catalyze the transfer of undecaprenyl phosphate to 1-phospho-MurNac-pentapeptide, yielding lipid II.

Many inhibitors have been described for this essential enzyme (see section 3.6.), but none is clinically used as an antibiotic yet.

2.3.4.2. MurG

MurG is a glycosyltransferase located on the inner side of the cytoplasmic membrane. MurG fixes a GlcNAc residue on lipid I. The final resulting lipid intermediate is transferred by an unknown mechanism through the hydrophobic environment of the membrane to external sites where monomer units are added to the growing peptidoglycan chain.

2.3.5. Peptidoglycan Maturation: PBPs

All eubacterial outer membranes possess a set of PBPs involved in the late steps of peptidoglycan biosynthesis. High-molecular-weight PBPs (class A or B) are essentially two-domain proteins. In class B PBPs, the N-terminal chain is probably involved in interactions with other membrane proteins.

More than 30 class A high-molecular-weight PBPs have been identified in gram-positive and gram-negative bacteria.

E. coli PBP 1a is the most intensively investigated class A PBP.

PBP 1b contains a 65-amino-acid N-terminal cytoplasmic tail followed by a 24-amino-acid transmembrane domain and a 757-amino-acid periplasmic region with transglycosylation and transpeptidation domains clearly separated by an inert linker. Part of the transglycosylase (corresponding to the first 163 amino acids) is located in the periplasmic space. This is also the case in *S. pneumoniae*.

Glycosyltransferase activity has only been studied with *E. coli* PBPs 1a, 1b, and 1c.

Monofunctional enzymes with solely transpeptidase or glycosyltransferase activity have been identified. A number of membrane-bound non-PBP monofunctional glycosyltransferases (Mgt) capable only of catalyzing the formation of non-cross-linked peptidoglycan have been found in *E. coli*, *Micrococcus luteus*, *S. aureus*, and *S. pneumoniae*. The corresponding genes were detected in *E. coli*, *Haemophilus influenzae*, *Klebsiella pneumoniae*, *Neisseria gonorrhoeae*, and *Ralstonia eutropha* and other gram-negative bacteria.

In a given microorganism, there are several peptidoglycan glycosyltransferases. For instance, in *E. coli*, there are four enzymes catalyzing transglycosylation reactions (PBPs 1a, 1b, and 1c and Mgt), and there are four in *S. pneumoniae* (PBPs 1a, 1b, and 2a and Mgt).

The final step in peptidoglycan biosynthesis is transpeptidation between the amino terminus of *meso*-diaminopimelic acid (in most gram-negative bacteria) or a peptide cross-link (most gram-positive bacteria) and the carbonyl group of D-alanine at position 4 of a second peptide side chain (Fig. 6).

2.3.5.1. Transglycosylation

The mature peptidoglycan is assembled on the cell surface by transglycosylation and transpeptidation reactions catalyzed by PBPs. Transglycosylation of lipid II consists of a glycosyl transfer reaction involving displacement of the α-diphospho-undecaprenyl group by the C-4 hydroxy group of GlcNAc resulting in an inversion of the configuration of the anomeric center, leading to mostly β-1,4 linkages between sugar residues.

The precise mechanism of transglycosylation is not yet known. In the periplasmic space, linear assembly of glycan chains presumably proceeds by sequential addition of disaccharide-pentapeptide units at either the reducing end or the nonreducing end (Fig. 7).

Lipid II is an acceptor substrate in the first case and a donor substrate in the second case. In the first hypothesis, the growing glycan chain to undecaprenyl pyrophosphate is the glycosyl donor substrate, which is transferred to the 4-hydroxy group of the GlcNAc unit of lipid II, which itself serves as the glycosyl acceptor substrate. This mechanism has been established in a few gram-positive microorganisms.

In the second hypothesis, lipid II functions as the donor, and its disaccharide-peptide is transferred to the 4-hydroxyl group of the GlcNAc of the growing chain, which serves as the acceptor.

2.3.5.2. Transpeptidation

Peptidoglycan is cross-linked by amide links between the ε-amino side chain of lysine or *meso*-diaminopimelic acid and

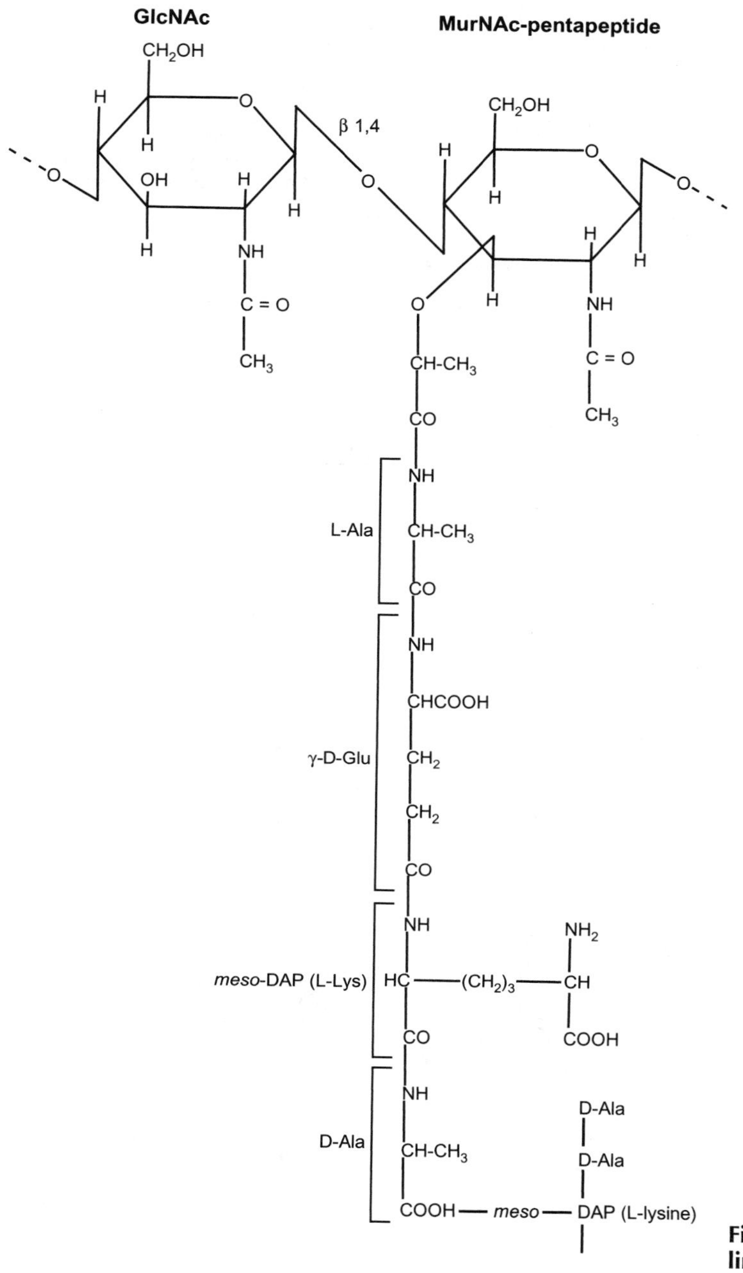

GlcNAc

MurNAc-pentapeptide

CH_2OH H H OH H H H NH C = O CH_3 β 1,4 O CH_2OH H H H H H NH C = O CH_3 O CH-CH_3 CO

L-Ala: NH, CH-CH_3, CO

γ-D-Glu: NH, CHCOOH, CH_2, CH_2, CO

meso-DAP (L-Lys): NH, HC—$(CH_2)_3$—CH (NH_2, COOH), CO

D-Ala: NH, CH-CH_3, COOH— *meso* — DAP (L-lysine) — D-Ala — D-Ala

Figure 6 Peptide cross-linking

position 4 of a second side chain. The nature of the diamino acid residues of the peptide bridge and the extent of peptidoglycan cross-linking vary according to the bacterial species. The nascent peptidoglycan loses one D-alanine. This step can be inhibited by vancomycin, teicoplanin, and derivatives. Replacement of D-alanine by a D-lactic acid blocks the action of vancomycin. Each peptide chain is linked to another peptide chain by a short peptide bridge (cross-linking), resulting in a complex network. Free endogenous *meso*-diaminopimelic acid is either irreversibly decarboxylated into L-lysine or used to form a cross-linking peptide. Newly polymerized peptidoglycan can be used either for elongation or for septation.

3. PEPTIDOGLYCAN BIOSYNTHESIS INHIBITORS

3.1. MurA Inhibitors

The best-known inhibitor of MurA is fosfomycin (Fig. 8), which is a phosphoenolpyruvate analog. The inactivation of MurA by fosfomycin results from its covalent linkage to the active-site cysteine residue (Cys115). The nucleophilic attack by Cys115 occurs at the C-2 position of fosfomycin, opening the epoxide ring and resulting in a covalent bond between C-2 and Cys115 (Kahan et al., 1974; Skarzynski et al., 1996).

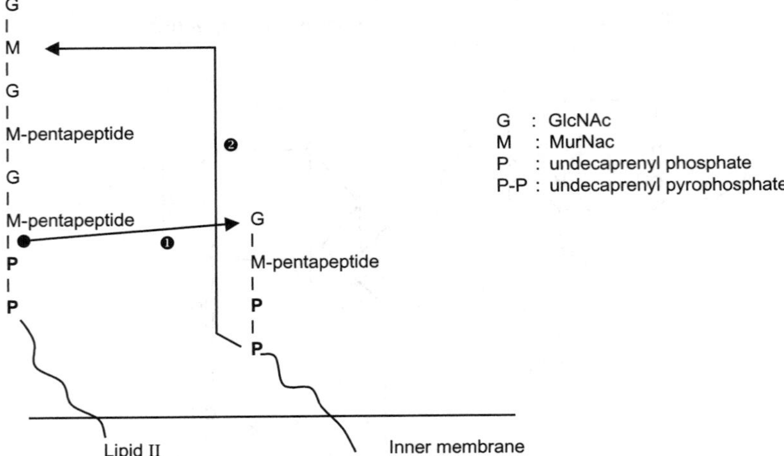

Figure 7 Transglycosylation

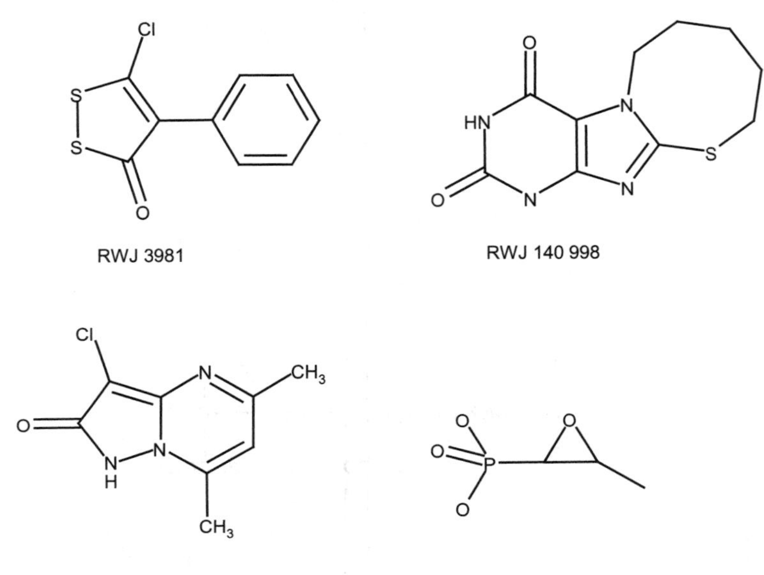

Figure 8 MurA inhibitors

Fosfomycin enters bacteria by active transport by both the L-α-glycerophosphate and glucose-6-phosphate uptake systems. Fosfomycin is clinically used as an antibiotic.

Other *E. coli* MurA inhibitors have been described, including a cyclic disulfide (RWJ-3981), a purine analog (RWJ-140998), and a pyrazolopyrimidine (RWJ-110192). They were discovered by screening the chemical library of Johnson and Johnson (Fig. 8). Their IC_{50} (0.02 to 0.9 μM) are lower than that of fosfomycin. Fosfomycin has irreversible inhibitory activity, as do RWJ-3981 and RWJ-140998. These three compounds inhibit not only MurA enzyme but also DNA, RNA, and protein synthesis. Their MICs are similar to those of fosfomycin for gram-positive cocci (*S. aureus* and *Enterococcus* spp.), ranging from 8 to >32 μg/ml (fosfomycin MIC, 1 to >32 μg/ml).

The predicted binding of these three compounds is as follows:

- RWJ-3981 binds 7.1 Å from the sulfur of the catalytic Cys115. The carbonyl oxygen of the inhibitor may form strong hydrogen bonds with Arg120 and Arg 397. The sulfur atoms can make hydrophobic contacts with the side chain carbon atoms of Met90 and Arg91.
- The pyrazolone ring of RWJ-110192 binds Cys115, and the carbonyl oxygen can form a strong hydrogen bond with Arg91 (guanidium ring).
- RWJ-140198 binds approximately 8.7 Å from the sulfur of Cys115. The dioxopyrimidine nucleus of RWJ-140198 may bind as follows: the amino group (NH) of the pyrimidone ring forms a strong hydrogen bond with Asp305,

while the carbonyl oxygen may form a hydrogen bond to Asn23; Arg120 may form a hydrogen bond with one of the nitrogen atoms of the imidazole ring. Phe3328 can form hydrophobic contacts with the methylene carbons of the imidazole ring.

Synthesis of structural analogs of these three compounds showed that the disulfur and chlorine atom are essential for RWJ-3981 activity.

3.2. MurB Inhibitors

MurB is responsible for reducing enoylpyruvyl UDP-MurNAc. MurB involves two half-reactions. Enzyme-bound FAD serves as a redox intermediate. The first half-reaction is the reduction of FAD to $FADH_2$ by NADPH. The second half-reaction is the reduction of UDP-GlcNAc enolpyruvate to UDP-MurNAc. Inhibitors of MurB (4-thiazolidinones) have been synthezised (Fig. 9).

Thiazolidinones that contain an *n*-butyl group (synthesized from norleucine) are the most active compound so far prepared. Their stereochemistry seems to play a significant role in their potency. Diastereoisomers are synthesized from D-norleucine. These molecules were intended to mimic key diphosphate enzyme interactions and to be able to orient the resulting side chains in such a way that they would occupy space in a way similar to that of the glucosamine and uridine moieties of the substrate.

3.3. MurC Inhibitors

The specificities of various MurC synthetases for D-alanine and UDP-MurNAc were investigated with closely structurally related analogs accepted as substrates or functioning as competitive inhibitors. A series of phosphinate transition state analogs was synthesized (Hammes et al., 1973; Mizuno et al., 1973; Ishiguro, 1982; Michaud et al., 1987; Liger et al., 1991; Liger et al., 1995b; Emanuele et al., 1996; Gubler et al., 1996). Among them, a phosphinate derivative mimicking the transition state of the MurC reaction (Fig. 10) showed an IC_{50} of 49 μM.

3.4. MurD Inhibitors

As MurD enzyme adds a D-glutamic acid, various transition state analogs of the nucleotide substrate have been prepared (Auger et al., 1995; Tanner et al., 1996; Gegnas et al., 1998; Gobec et al., 2001). They are phosphinate-based inhibitors. The best IC_{50} (<1 nM) was obtained with a phosphinate compound mimicking very closely the transition state (Fig. 11).

Based on a computer-based molecular design strategy, a series of macrocyclic derivatives has been prepared (Fig. 12). They showed good activity against MurD, with IC_{50} ranging from 0.7 to 9 μM, depending on their substitution pattern (Horton et al., 2003).

3.5. MurE Inhibitors

The best inhibitors were phosphinate analogs. Phosphinates act as slow-binding inhibitors by mimicking the tetrahedral intermediate formed in the reaction (Abo-Ghalia et al., 1988; Le Roux et al., 1992; Zeng et al., 1998). Two major compounds were prepared displaying IC_{50} of 1.1 and 700 μM (Fig. 13). According to their respective chemical structures, it becomes clear that the UDP moiety is necessary for good inhibition.

3.6. MurF Inhibitors

Measuring the concomitant release of radiolabeled inorganic phosphate from ATP can monitor the D-alanyl–D-alanine-adding activity of MurF. Pseudo-tri- and -tetrapeptide aminoalkylphosphinic acids have been prepared as transition state analogs of MurF. These inhibitors were poorly active (200 to 700 μM) (Miller et al., 1998).

Series of MurF inhibitors have been recently synthesized (Fig. 14); the IC_{50} were 8.0 and 1.0 μM for compounds 1 and 2, respectively. The cyano group of compound 1 is essential for MurF-inhibitory potency. The replacement of the cyano group with amides, amine, or ethyl ester resulted in significant or complete loss of activity. Both cyano and amide NH may be involved in hydrogen bonding interactions with the enzyme (Gu et al., 2004).

3.7. MraY Inhibitors

MraY is a suitable antibacterial target even if no antibacterials were introduced in clinical practice, despite the number of inhibitors found to be active against this enzyme. These inhibitors can be classified in different families (Fig. 15): nucleoside antibiotics, lipopeptide antibiotic (amphomycin), and peptide inhibitor (protein E). Nucleoside antibiotics can

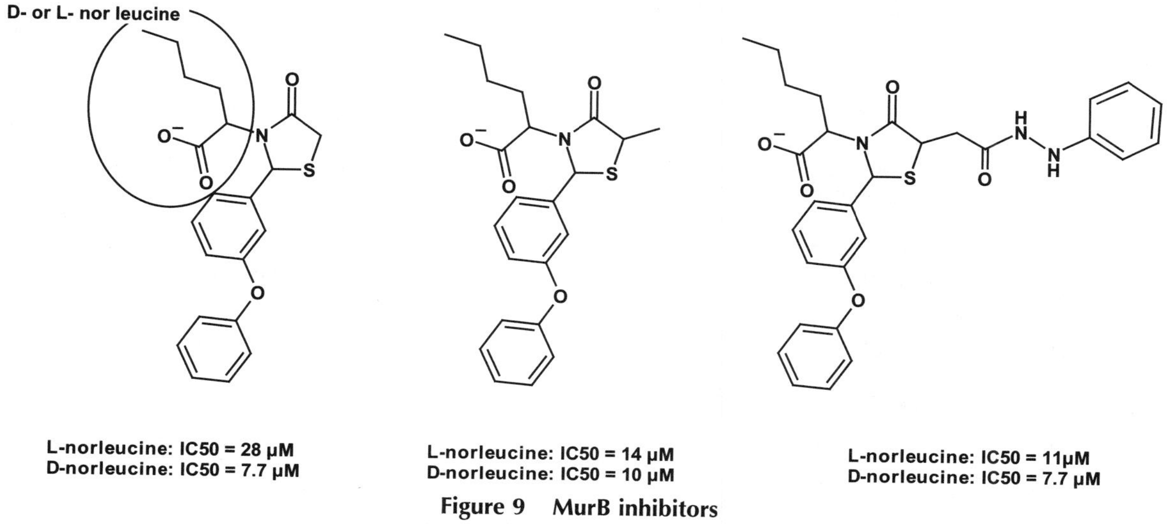

D- or L- nor leucine

L-norleucine: IC50 = 28 μM
D-norleucine: IC50 = 7.7 μM

L-norleucine: IC50 = 14 μM
D-norleucine: IC50 = 10 μM

L-norleucine: IC50 = 11μM
D-norleucine: IC50 = 7.7 μM

Figure 9 MurB inhibitors

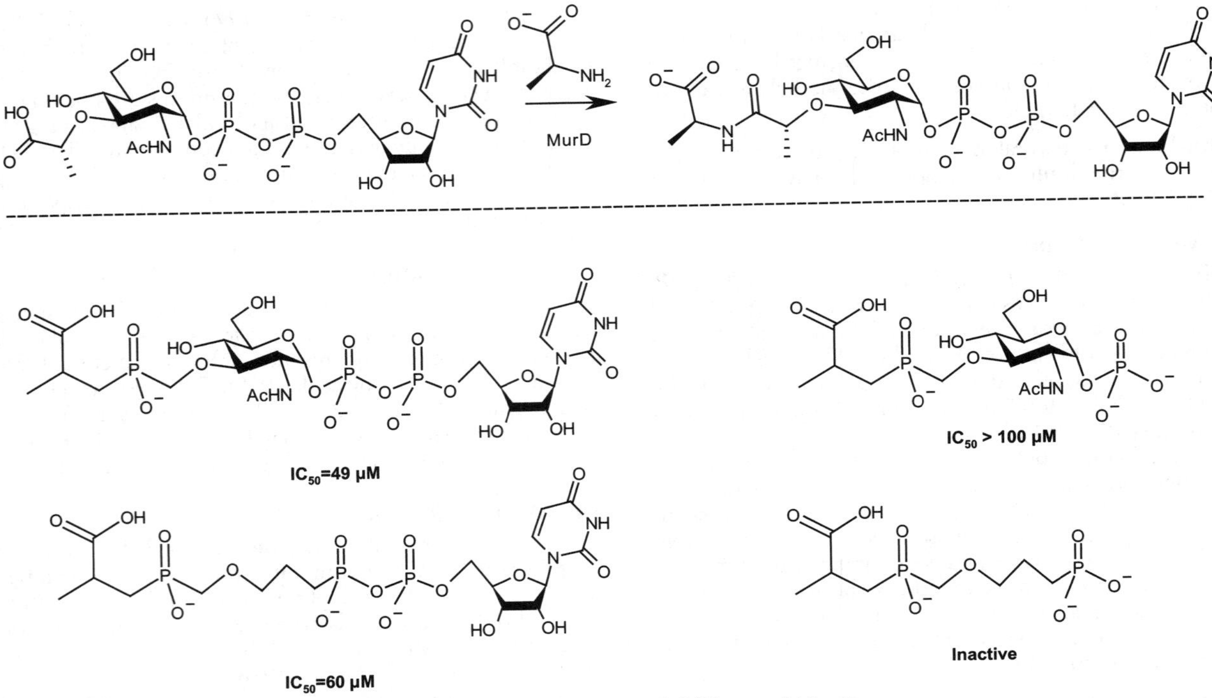

MurD

IC_{50}=49 μM

IC_{50} > 100 μM

IC_{50}=60 μM

Inactive

Figure 10 Phosphinate inhibitors of MurC

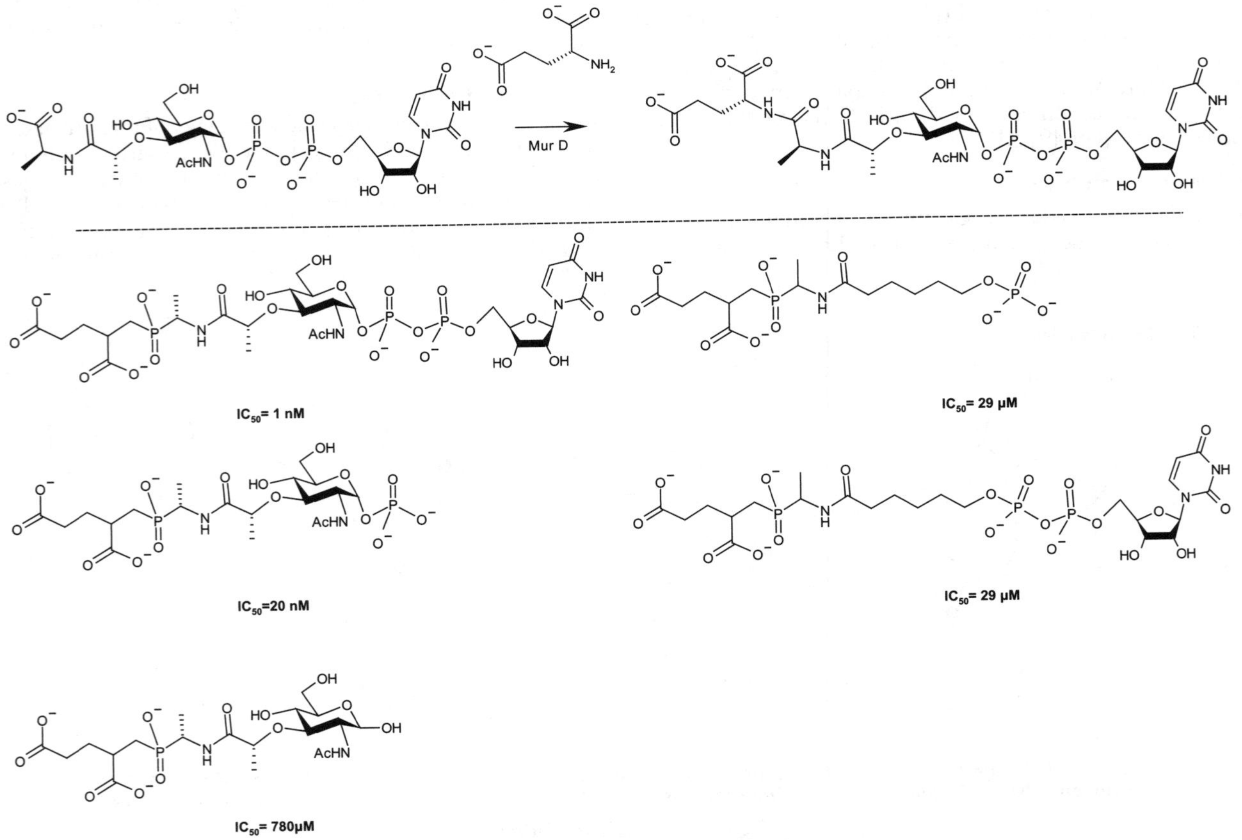

Mur D

IC_{50}= 1 nM

IC_{50}= 29 μM

IC_{50}=20 nM

IC_{50}= 29 μM

IC_{50}= 780μM

Figure 11 Phosphinate inhibitors of MurD

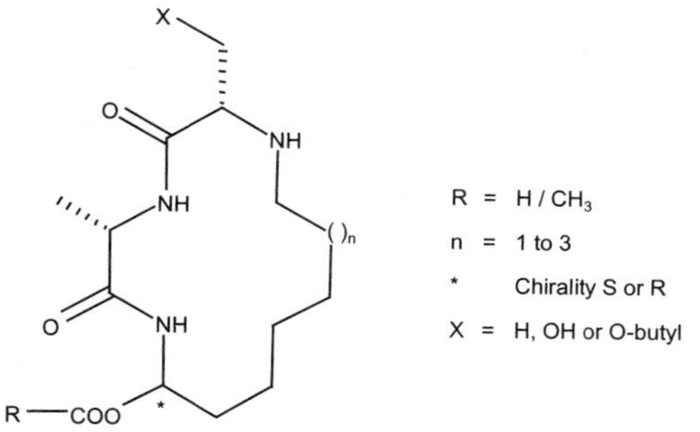

Figure 12 Macrocyclic derivatives

be subdivided into different classes according to their chemical structures and/or their respective modes of action against MraY: the tunicamycin group (which also contains streptovirudins and corynetoxins), the ribosamino-uridine group (with liposidomycins, riburamycins, caprazamycins, muraymycin, and FR-900493), and finally the capuramycin group.

Some of them possess activities against gram-positive bacteria (e.g., tunicamycins, riburamycins, and amphomycin), against *Mycobacterium* spp. (liposidomycins and capuramycins), and against *Pseudomonas* spp. (mureidomycins and related compounds). When known, the mechanisms of inhibition appear to be different for all of the classes aforementioned.

The tunicamycin group is known to be highly toxic. Amphomycin, liposidomycins, mureidomycins, and capuramycins showed acceptable 50% lethal doses (LD_{50}) when administered in mice.

Moreover, target selectivity towards MraY versus other glycosyltransferases seems to be the determinant factor for toxicity discrimination (Schwartz and Datema, 1980).

These compounds inhibit the biosynthesis of the lipid I, which is the product of the MraY enzymatic reaction (Fig. 16).

3.7.1. Nucleoside Antibacterials

Not all nucleoside antibacterials act as translocase inhibitors. Some of them exhibit antimycobacterial and anti-*Candida albicans* activities (toyocamycin MICs of 2.0 and 1.0 μg/ml for eukaryotic cells, which they killed by inhibiting phosphatidylinositol kinase of the A-431 cell membrane, with IC_{50} of 3.3 μg/ml [e.g., tubercidin and sangivamycin] [Fig. 17]).

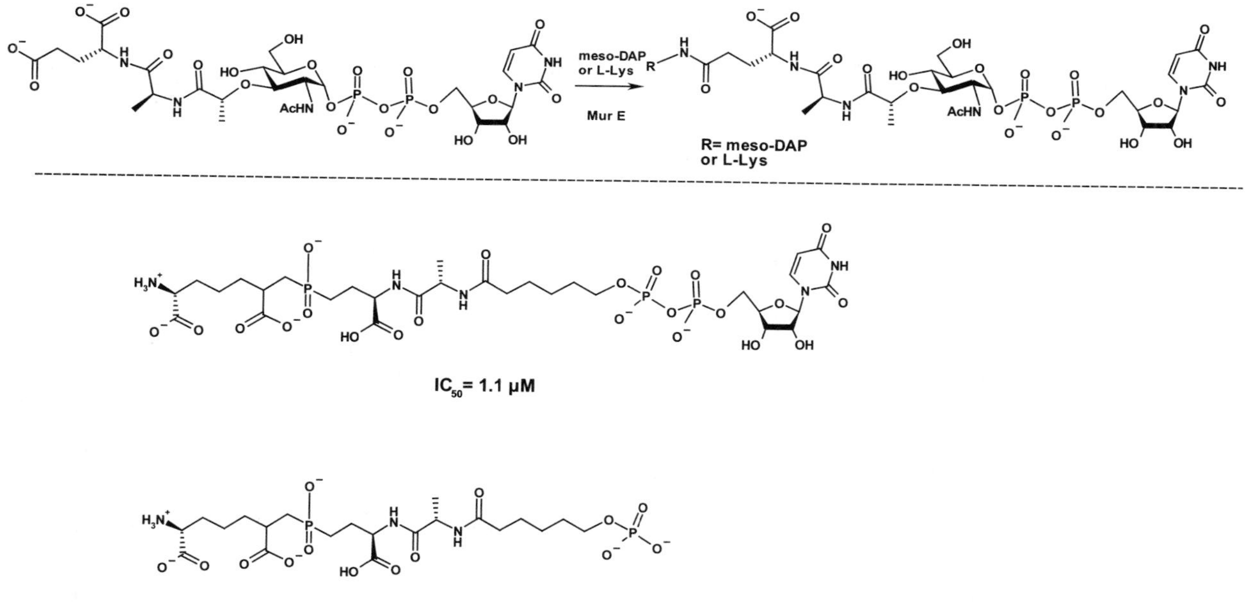

Figure 13 Phosphinate inhibitors of MurE

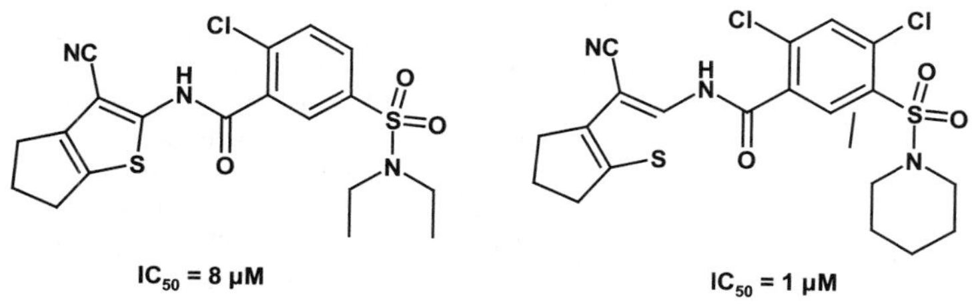

Figure 14 MurF inhibitors (Gu et al., 2004)

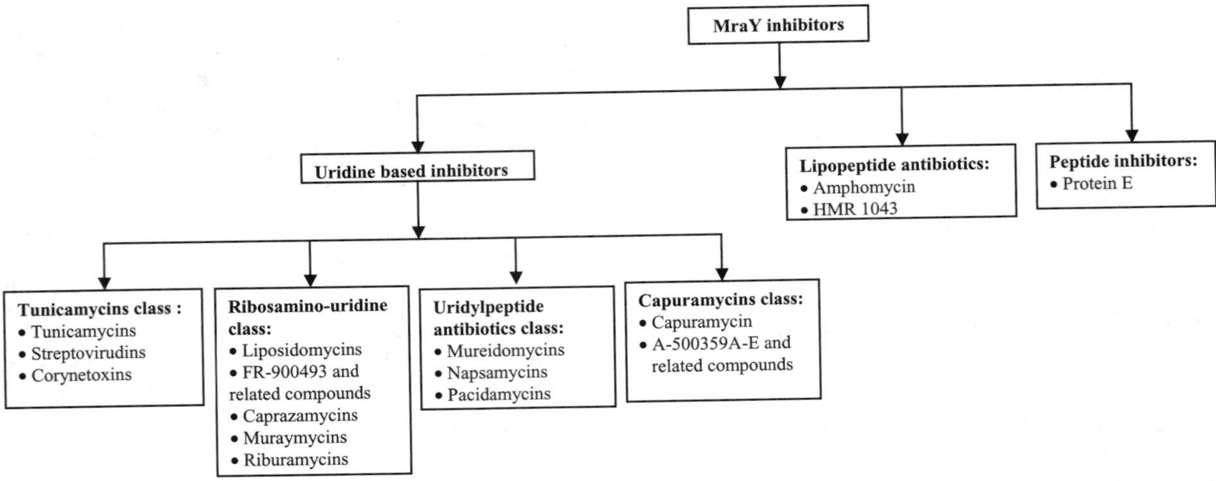

Figure 15 Classification of MraY inhibitors

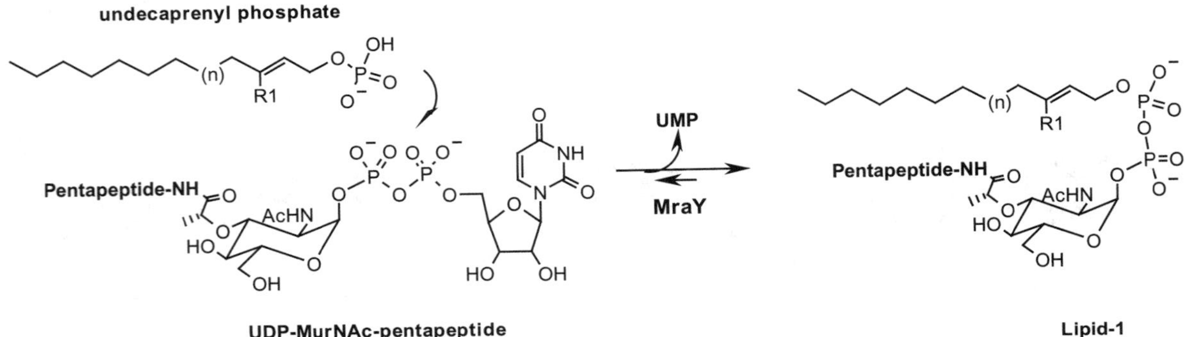

Figure 16 MraY enzymatic reaction

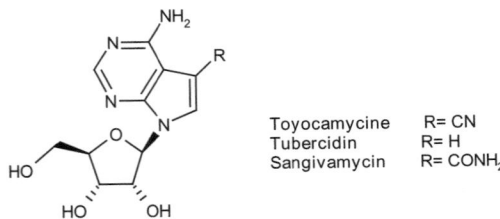

Toyocamycine R= CN
Tubercidin R= H
Sangivamycin R= $CONH_2$

Figure 17 Nucleoside antibiotics that are non-MraY inhibitors

3.7.1.1. Class 1: Tunicamycin Group (Tunicamycins, Streptovirudins, and Corynetoxins)

Tunicamycins were the first inhibitors discovered in class 1. They were isolated from the fermentation broth of *Streptomyces lysosuperficus* in 1971 through their antiviral properties (Takatsuki and Tamura, 1971). Thereafter, streptovirudins and corynetoxins were respectively isolated from the fermentation broth of *Streptomyces griseoflavus* (Eckardt et al., 1980) and *Corynebacterium rathayi* (Vogel et al., 1981).

The chemical structures of these compounds are very close to each other. Actually, overlaps exist between these families, which differ stricto sensus by the lipid side chains they carry (Table 1). The scaffold of this class is made of a dialdo undecose residue (tunicamine). This unusual sugar is involved at each reducing end in glycosylic bonds:

- With a GlcNAc residue, through a 11′-β,1″-α-*O*-glycosidic bond
- With uracil or dihydrouracil through a 1′-β-*N*-glycosidic bond

3.7.1.1.1. Tunicamycins. From the antibacterial point of view, tunicamycin (Table 1) exhibited especially anti-gram-positive-organism activities (e.g., against *Bacillus* spp., with MICs from 0.3 to 10 μg/ml). However, they also showed additional in vitro cellular activities against viruses and fungi, as well as antitumoral properties. However, their in vivo antibacterial activity was compromised by acute toxicity. As an example, corynetoxins were identified as the causative agents of annual ryegrass intoxication of cattle in New Zealand (Edgar et al., 1982). The LD_{50} was estimated at 4.5 mg/kg of body weight. This toxicity is explained by their high inhibitory activity upon glycoconjugate biosyntheses, such as of techoic acids, glycosaminoglycans, and glycoproteins. They inhibit GlcNAc-1-phosphate transferase rather than MraY. Their lack of specificity (as antibacterial, antiviral, antitumoral, and antifungal) is certainly

Table 1 Tunicamycins, streptovirudins, and corynetoxins

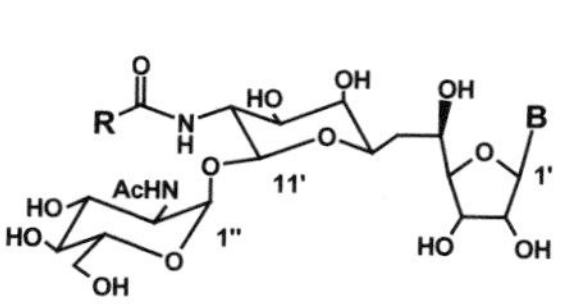

	Code	Fatty chain (R)	Base (B)
Tunicamycins	I		Uracil
	II	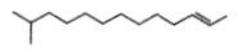	Uracil
	III	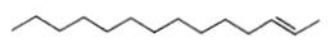	Uracil
	IV	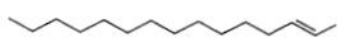	Uracil
	V	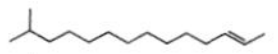	Uracil
	VI	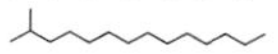	Uracil
	VII	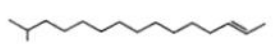	Uracil
	VIII	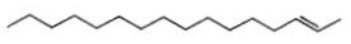	Uracil
	IX	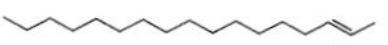	Uracil
	X	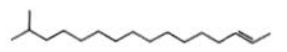	Uracil
Streptovirudins	A1	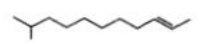	Dihydrouracil
	B1	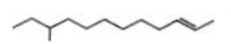	Dihydrouracil
	B1a	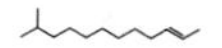	Dihydrouracil
	C1	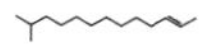	Dihydrouracil
	D1	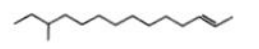	Dihydrouracil
	A2	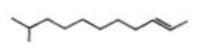	Uracil
	B2	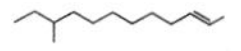	Uracil
	B2a	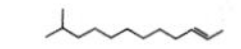	Uracil
	C2	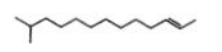	Uracil
	D2		Uracil
Corynetoxins	S15a	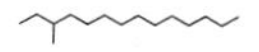	Uracil
	H16i	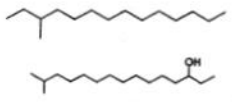	Uracil
	U16i	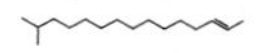	Uracil
	H17a	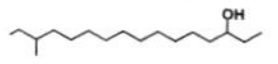	Uracil
	S16i	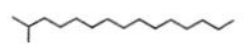	Uracil
	U17a	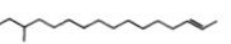	Uracil
	U17i	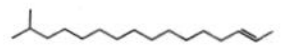	Uracil
	S17a	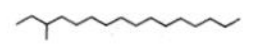	Uracil
	H18i	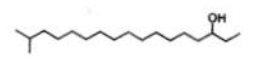	Uracil
	U18i	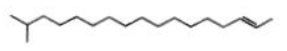	Uracil
	H19a	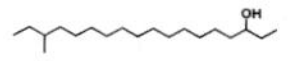	Uracil
	S18i	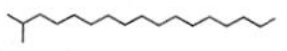	Uracil
	U19a	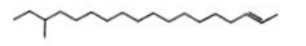	Uracil
	S19a	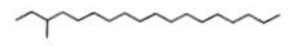	Uracil

the consequence of their lack of selectivity against various glyscosyltransferases (Schwartz and Datema, 1980).

The mode of action of tunicamycin against *E. coli* MraY was established throughout enzymatic inhibition studies. It turns out that tunicamycin is competitive to UDP-MurNAc-(Nε-Dns) pentapeptide (K_i=550 nM) and not competitive to undecaprenyl phosphate substrate.

3.7.1.1.2. Streptovirudins. Streptovirudins have 10 components which varied on the fatty acid side chain (Table 1). Streptovirudins were isolated in 1975 from the fermentation broth of *Streptomyces griseoflavus* subsp. *thuringiensis*. In some compounds (A_1, B_1, B_{1a}, C_1, and D_1) the uracil moiety is replaced by a dihydrouracil (Table 1). These compounds are active against enveloped viruses. They also exhibit activity against gram-positive bacteria and especially *Bacillus* spp. (MICs, 0.3 to 10 μg/ml).

3.7.1.1.3. Corynetoxins. Fourteen components have been isolated from the fermentation broth of *C. rathayi*, and all exhibit ryegrass-like toxicity (Table 1).

3.7.1.2. Class 2: Ribosamino-Uridine Class of Antibacterials

All inhibitors exhibiting a ribosamino-uridine (Fig. 18) subunit in their chemical structures have been gathered in the same class. This particular disaccharide unit was demonstrated as the minimal structural element from the liposidomycin structure required for preserving anti-MraY activity (Dini et al., 2000). As a consequence, this can be extrapolated to all ribosamino-uridine-containing compounds. This includes liposidomycins, muraymycins, caprazamycins, FR-900493 series, and riburamycins, from which this crucial motif has been deduced.

3.7.1.2.1. Liposidomycins. Liposidomycins, like tunicamycins, are fatty acyl nucleoside antibacterials; however, they are not toxic and are specific inhibitors of MraY. Liposidomycins were extracted from the fermentation broth of *Streptomyces griseosporum* in 1985 (Isono et al., 1985). There are 12 known natural liposidomycins. These natural compounds contain a ribosamino-uridine subunit, a diazepanone ring, and a fatty acid side chain. Their classification depends

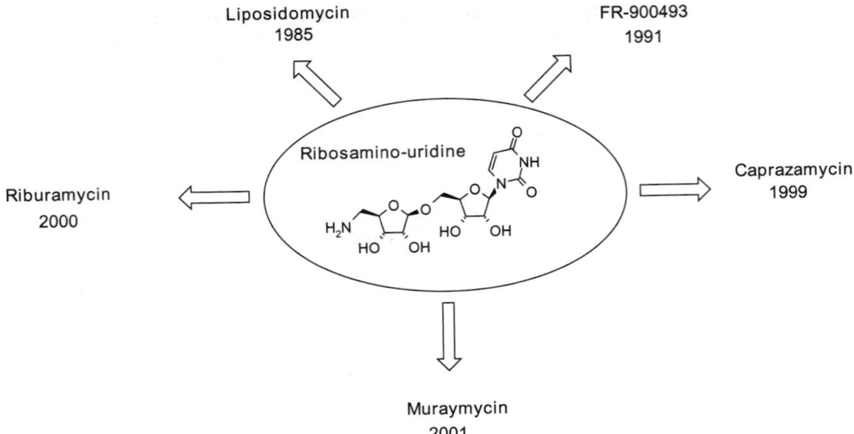

Figure 18 Ribosamino-uridine is the minimal structural requirement in this class to inhibit MraY

on the nature of the fatty side chain, the presence or absence of a sulfate group, and the presence or absence of a 3-methylglutaric residue (Table 2).

In the case of liposidomycin A, the order for peptidoglycan inhibition activity is A-(I) > A-(III) > A-(IV) > A-(II). Additionally, it is worth noting that types III and IV display better antibacterial activities than types I and II. This difference might be attributed to the absence of sulfate group for types III and IV, allowing a better cell membrane penetration (Kimura et al., 1998).

Liposidomycin B is a slow-binding inhibitor of MraY ($K_i = 550$ and 80 nM). It is competitive to undecaprenyl phosphate but not to UDP-MurNAc-(Nε-Dns) pentapeptide (Brandish et al., 1996b).

In contrast to tunicamycins, liposidomycins do not inhibit glycoconjugate biosynthesis at low concentrations (e.g., liposidomycin B does not inhibit glycoprotein biosynthesis in mammals; $IC_{50} > 400$ μg/ml). Moreover, the four types of liposidomycin A showed no cytotoxic activity against BALB/3T3 cells at up to 25 μg/ml, whereas tunicamycin was potently cytotoxic ($IC_{50} = 0.05$ μg/ml) in the same assay system. This absence of cytoxicity translates well in vivo: liposidomycins were administered intravenously up to 500 mg/kg in mice without evidence of acute toxicity (Kimura et al., 1998).

They are active against gram-positive bacteria and also against *Mycobacterium phlei* (MIC, 1.6 μg/ml). Their global antibacterial activity remains low, probably in part because of their high hydrophilicity (membrane penetration).

3.7.1.2.2. Caprazamycins. Seven components designated A to G have been reported (Table 3). These compounds were extracted from a culture of a *Streptomyces* sp. (Takeuchi et al., 1999, 2001).

Table 2 Liposidomycin classification

3-methylglutaric residue

LPM-	R1	R2 = Type I	R2 = Type III	R2 = Type II	R2 = Type IV
A		SO3H	H	SO3H	H
B		SO3H	H	-	-
C		SO3H	H	SO3H	H
G		SO3H	H	-	-
H		SO3H	H	-	-
K		SO3H	H	-	-
L		SO3H	H	-	-
M		SO3H	H	-	-
N		SO3H	H	-	-
X		-	H	-	-
Y		-	H	-	-
Z		SO3H	H	-	-

Table 3 Caprazamycin chemical structure

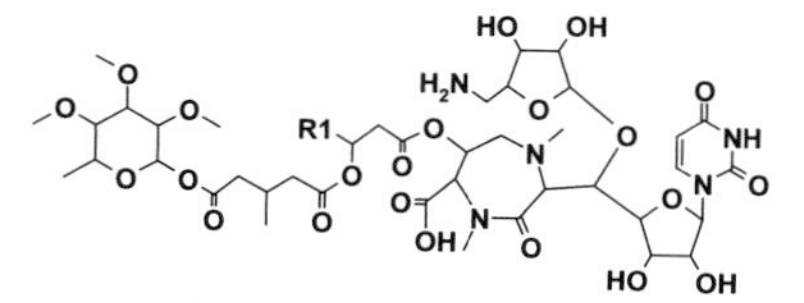

Caprazamycins	R1=
A	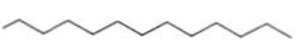
B	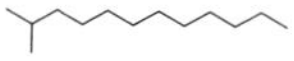
C	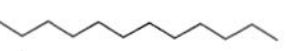
D	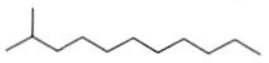
E	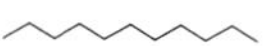
F	
G	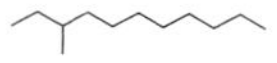

The major difference in caprazamycin chemical structures compared with liposidomycins resides in the presence of a monosaccharide unit fixed to the 3-methylglutaric acid residue, with fatty acid side chains of different lengths.

The major component, caprazamycin B, exhibits anti-*Mycobacterium tuberculosis* activity (MIC, 3.13 μg/ml for the $H37_{RV}$ strain) and excellent activity against *Mycobacterium avium* complex (MICs, 0.05 to 0.78 μg/ml). Caprazamycin B has therapeutic efficacy at 1.5 mg/kg·day in a pulmonary tuberculosis infection model in mice, when administered intranasally (Igarashi et al., 2002).

3.7.1.2.3. FR-900493 and derivatives. FR-900493 was extracted from the fermentation broth of *Bacillus cereus* (Ochi et al., 1989).

The major chemical difference observed between liposidomycins and FR-900493 resides in the presence of an N-functionalized amino acid residue in the FR-900493 structure (Fig. 19), instead of the diazepanone ring of liposidomycins.

FR-900493 displays antistaphylococcal activity in vitro (MIC, 3.13 μg/ml) and in vivo in a murine staphylococcal infection model. The LD_{50} in mice after intravenous administration is above 500 mg/kg.

Series of semisynthetic compounds have been prepared. One of them, compound 77 (Fig. 19), exhibited MICs of 6.25 μg/ml for *S. aureus* 2550 and 12.5 μg/ml for *E. coli* 29 (Yoshida et al., 1993).

3.7.1.2.4. Muraymycins. Muraymycins (Fig. 20) were extracted from the fermentation broth of a *Streptomyces* sp. Nineteen components have been identified (McDonald et al., 2002). Among them are muraymycins A1 and C1 (Fig. 20).

Like FR-900493, muraymycins present an N-functionalized amino acid residue instead of diazepanone (in the case of liposidomycins). However, the substituents are more complex.

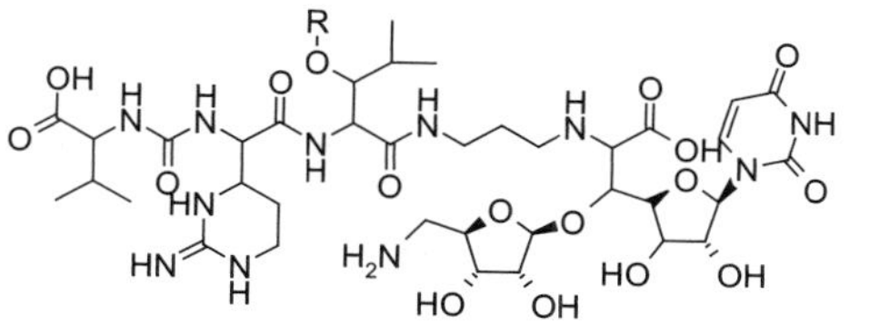

Muramycin A1 ; R= COC11H22N(HO)C(NH2)=NH
Muramycin C1 ; R= H

Figure 20 Muraymycins

Muraymycins inhibit lipid I formation. One component, muraymycin 1, demonstrated activity against gram-positive bacteria, with MICs of 2 to 8 μg/ml for methicillin-resistant and susceptible *S. aureus* (MRSA and MSSA, respectively), MICs of 2 to 64 μg/ml for a *Streptococcus* sp., and MICs of 16 to 64 μg/ml for an *Enterococcus* sp. The compound was also very active against a permeable *E. coli* organism, with a MIC of <0.5 μg/ml. However, the compound showed much weaker or no activity against rough (8 μg/ml) and wild-type (>128 μg/ml) *E. coli* strains. Animal efficacy studies indicated that muraymycin 1 was active when dosed intravenously in an *S. aureus* lethal-infection model, with a 50% effective dose of 1.1 mg/kg (McDonald et al., 2002).

3.7.1.2.5. Riburamycins. Riburamycins are synthetic and simplified analogs of liposidomycins. They have been designed on the basis of molecular-modelling assumptions throughout superimposition studies of liposidomycins, tunicamycins, and the nucleotide substrate of MraY, UDP-MurNAc-pentapeptide (Dini et al., 2000).

Such studies highlighted the minimal and essential part of the liposidomycin structure necessary to preserve significant enzyme-inhibitory activity ($IC_{50} = 50\,\mu M$): it consists of a ribosamine residue linked to uridine through a $\beta(1 \rightarrow 5)$ glycosidic bond, hence the given name of "ribosamino-uridine class" (Fig. 21).

Regarding the functional groups of riburamycin, the following statements apply:

- Only the 3′ OH group is essential for antibacterial activity (Dini et al., 2001).
- Basic groups such as secondary amines or amidine and guanidine are tolerated at position 5″−. However, any other substituents led to inactive compounds.
- Uracil is crucial for binding to MraY (Dini et al., 2001a).

Furthermore, addition of a chiral center at position 5′− corresponding to the L-tallofuranose series led to an improved inhibitor (5 μM), whereas the other isomer (D-allofuranose series) was almost inactive (Fig. 21).

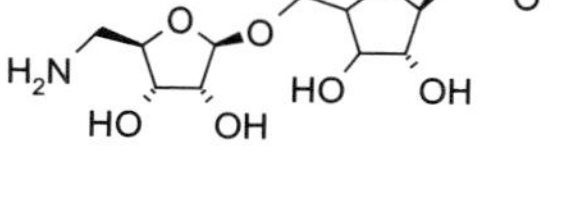

FR900493

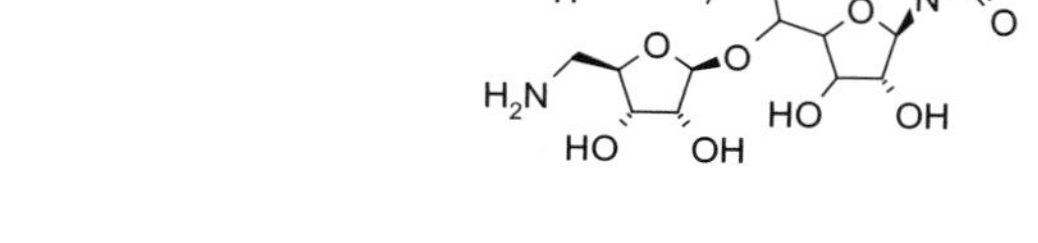

77

Figure 19 FR-900493 and compound 77 described in a Fujisawa patent

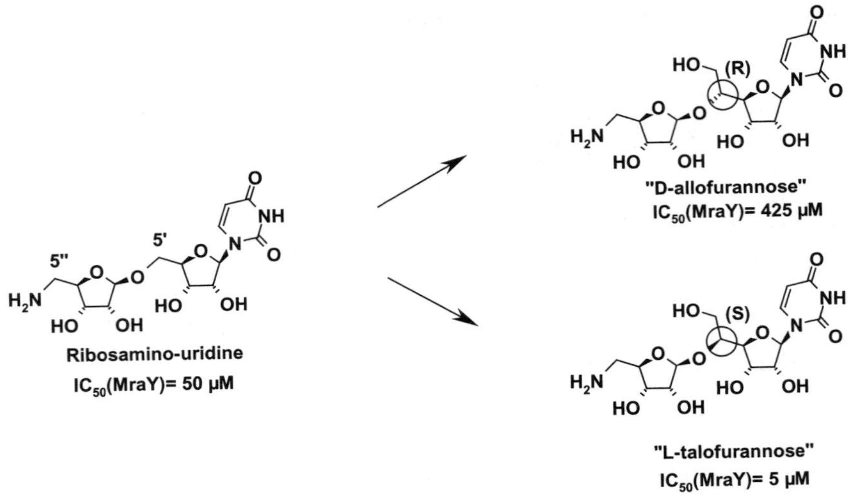

Figure 21 Ribosamino-uridine is the template of the riburamycin series

Extensive functionalization at position 6′− of riburamycins compounds led to antibacterial compounds. The antibacterial activity was correlated with the presence of lipophilic substituents (Dini et al., 2002). For instance, RU-75411, which carries a long fatty acid chain at position 6′− (Fig. 22), demonstrated activity against sensitive and multiresistant gram-positive strains (Table 4). In parallel, this compound showed powerful inhibitory activity against MraY (IC_{50}=0.08 µM) (Biton et al., 2002).

3.7.1.3. Class 3: Uridylpeptide Antibiotics

Class 3 comprises naturally occurring inhibitors of MraY: mureidomycins, pacidamycins, and napsamycins, which were isolated from the fermentation broth of *Streptomyces flavidovirens*, *Streptomyces coeruleorubidus*, and *Streptomyces candidus*, respectively. This class also includes semisynthetic derivatives: the dihydropacidamycins.

Uridylpeptide antibiotics share the same chemical template: a 3′-deoxyuridine sugar attached via an enamide linkage to a peptide chain and linked via an N-glycosidic bond to uracil or dihydrouracil (Fig. 23). Major differences come from the nature of the amino acids composing the polypeptide side chain (Table 5).

The pharmacological characteristics of these compounds are the following: good inhibitory activity on MraY from both *Pseudomonas aeruginosa* and *E. coli*, and low toxicity. However, the narrow spectrum and the high frequency of resistance for this class are weaknesses.

3.7.1.3.1. Mureidomycins. Mureidomycins were first isolated in 1989 from the fermentation broth of *S. flavidovirens* SANK 60486 (Inukai et al., 1989). Mureidomycins A to F (Table 5) are active against *P. aeruginosa*. Among them, mureidomycin C was the most active component, with MICs of 0.1 to 3.13 µg/ml for many strains of the target organism. Its activity was comparable to that of cefoperazone, ceftazidime, and cefsulodin (Isono et al., 1989). Mureidomycin C-resistant mutants of *P. aeruginosa* appeared spontaneously at a high frequency when cultured in the presence of the antibiotic (10^{-5} to 10^{-6} CFU/ml). No cross-resistance was observed with β-lactam antibiotics. A rapid decrease of turbidity along with spheroplast formation and cell lysis was observed when cells of *P. aeruginosa* were grown in the presence of mureidomycin C. Mureidomycins exhibited low toxicity (no acute deleterious effects were observed at doses up to 400 mg/kg) and protected mice from experimental infection with *P. aeruginosa* (50% effective dose=50 to 69 mg/kg for components A, B, and C and above 100 mg/kg for component C). They are inhibitors of peptidoglycan synthesis, and their specific target is MraY (Inukai et al., 1993).

The mode of action of mureidomycin A on *E. coli* MraY has been established throughout enzymatic inhibition studies. Mureidomycin A exhibited slow-binding-type inhibition (K_is of 36 and 2 nM, respectively) and was competitive with respect to both UDP-MurNAc-(Nε-Dns) pentapeptide and undecaprenyl phosphate (Brandish et al., 1996a; Brandish et al., 1996b).

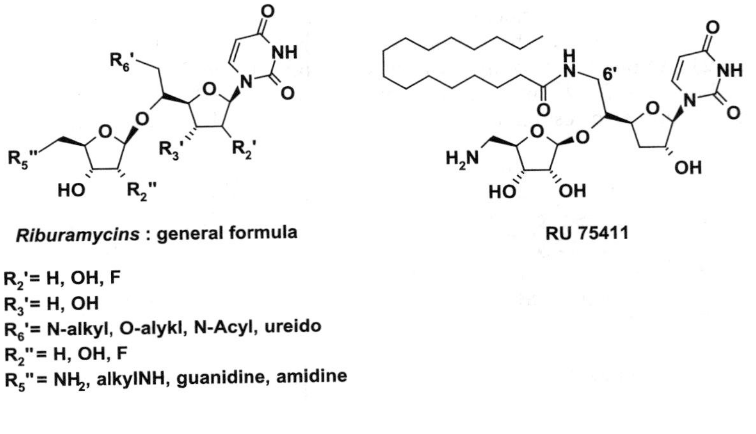

R_2'= H, OH, F
R_3'= H, OH
R_6'= N-alkyl, O-alykl, N-Acyl, ureido
R_2"= H, OH, F
R_5"= NH_2, alkylNH, guanidine, amidine

Figure 22 Riburamycins

Table 4 Riburamycin activity against gram-positive bacteria, including multiresistant strains

Microorganism	Phenotype	MIC (μg/ml)	
		Teicoplanin	RU 75411
S. aureus 011HT3	*oxaS eryS*	≤0.04	5
S. aureus 011HT18	ATCC 13709 Smith	0.6	2.5
S. aureus 011HT1	*novR*	≤0.04	2.5
S. aureus 011DU5	*novR tetR*	≤0.04	20
S. aureus 011CB20	*oxaR eryRc tetR*	≤0.04	10
S. aureus 011GO71	*oxaR eryS tetR*	0.3	40
S. aureus 011GO64	*oflR oxaR eryRc tetR*	0.6	40
S. aureus 011GR91	*priR oxaR eryR novR*	0.08	5
S. epidermidis 012GO20	*oxaS eryS tetR*	0.3	5
S. epidermidis 012GO42	*oxaR*	5	5
Coagulase-neg staph 012HT5	*oflR oxaR tetR*	2.5	5
S. pyogenes 02A1SJ1	*vanS eryRc*	≤0.04	2.5
S. pyogenes 02A1UC1	*vanS eryS*	≤0.04	2.5
S. pyogenes 02A1FI6	*eryR*	≤0.04	2.5
Group G strep 02GOCB2	*tetR rifR novR*	≤0.04	5
S. pneumoniae 030BI2	*eryR*	≤0.04	5
S. milleri 02milGR12	*eryS vanS*	≤0.04	2.5
E. faecium 02D3AP9	*vanR teiR*	>40	5
E. faecium 02D3HT12	*teiR vanR eryR tetR*	>40	5
E. faecium 02D3IP2	*teiR vanR eryR tetR*	5	5
E. faecium 02D3HM3	*vanA eryR tetR*	>40	5

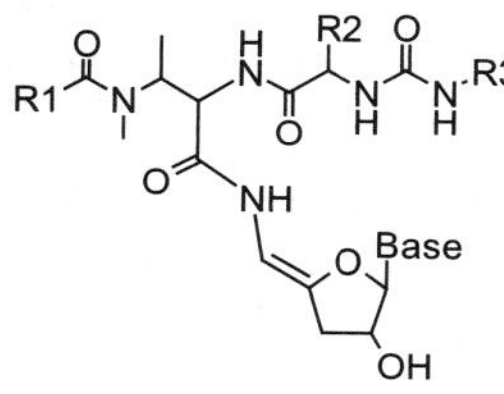

Base= uracil or dihydrouracil

Figure 23 Uridylpeptide antibiotic template

3.7.1.3.2. Pacidamycins. Pacidamycins (Table 5) were isolated in 1989 from a culture of *S. coeruleorubidus* AB 1183-64 (Chen et al., 1989; Karwowski et al., 1989). Their antibacterial activity is limited to *P. aeruginosa* (MICs, 8 to 64 μg/ml). Their MICs for other organisms, such as *Enterobacteriaceae*, *S. aureus*, most streptococci, and other *Pseudomonas* species, are higher than 100 μg/ml. The activity of these compounds was one- to twofold less in serum than in broth. Time-kill curves were performed using four

Table 5 Mureidomycin, pacidamycin, and napsamycin chemical structures

Pacidamycins (PCDs)	Napsamycins (NAPs)	Mureidomycins (MRDs)
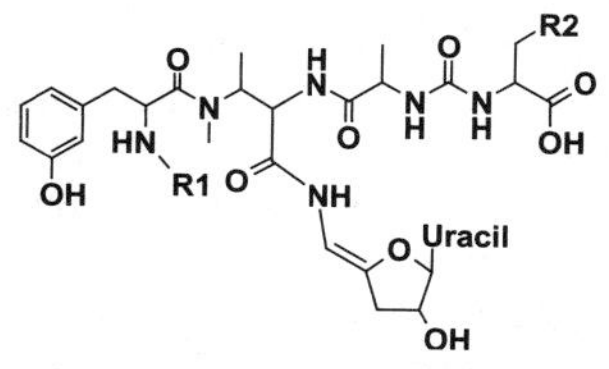	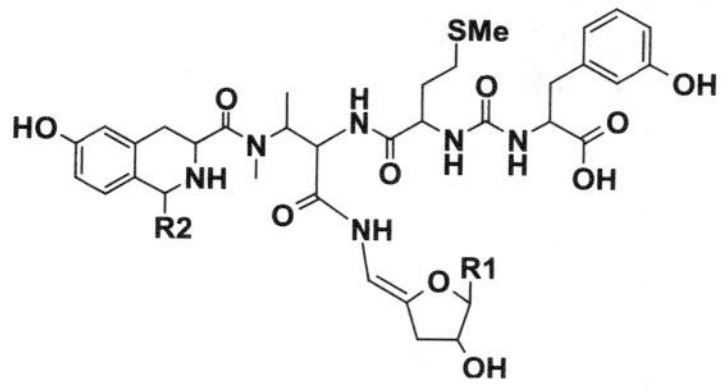	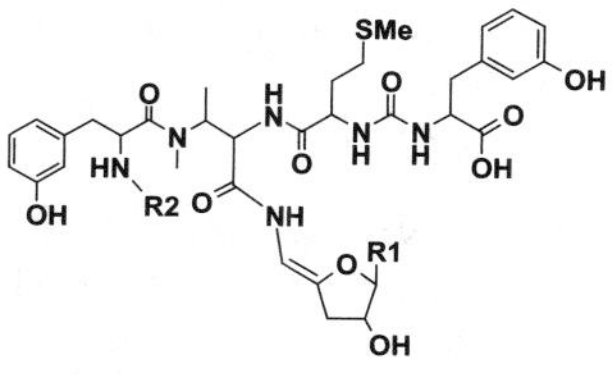
PCD-1; R1 = alanyl, R2 = 3-indolyl PCD -2; R1 = alanyl, R2 = phenyl PCD -3; R1 = alanyl, R2 = m-HOC_6H_4 PCD -4; R1 = H, R2 = 3-indolyl PCD -5; R1 = H, R2 = phenyl PCD -6; R1 = glycyl, R2 = 3-indolyl PCD -7; R1 = glycyl, R2 = phenyl	NAP-A; R1 = uracil, R2 = H NAP-B; R1 = uracil, R2 = CH_3 NAP-C; R1 = dihydrouracil, R2 = H NAP-D; R1 = dihydrouracil, R2 = CH_3	MRD-A; R1 = uracil, R2 = H MRD-B; R1 = dihydrouracil, R2 = H MRD-C; R1 = uracil, R2 = glycyl MRD-D; R1 = dihydrouracil, R2 = glycyl MRD-E; see below MRD-F = Napsamycin-A
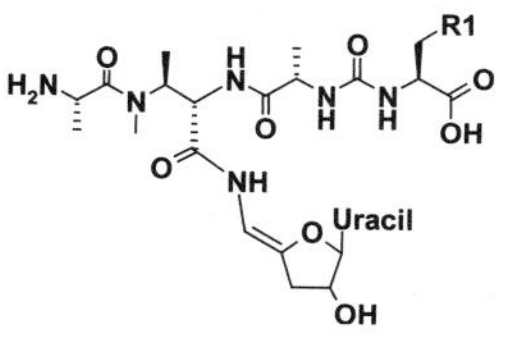		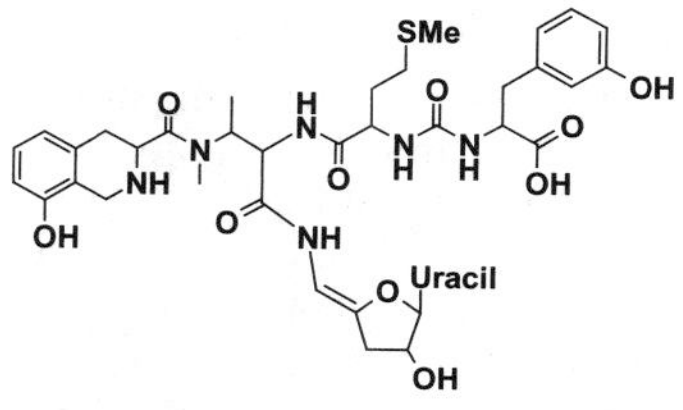
PCD -D; R1 = 3-indolyl		MRD-E

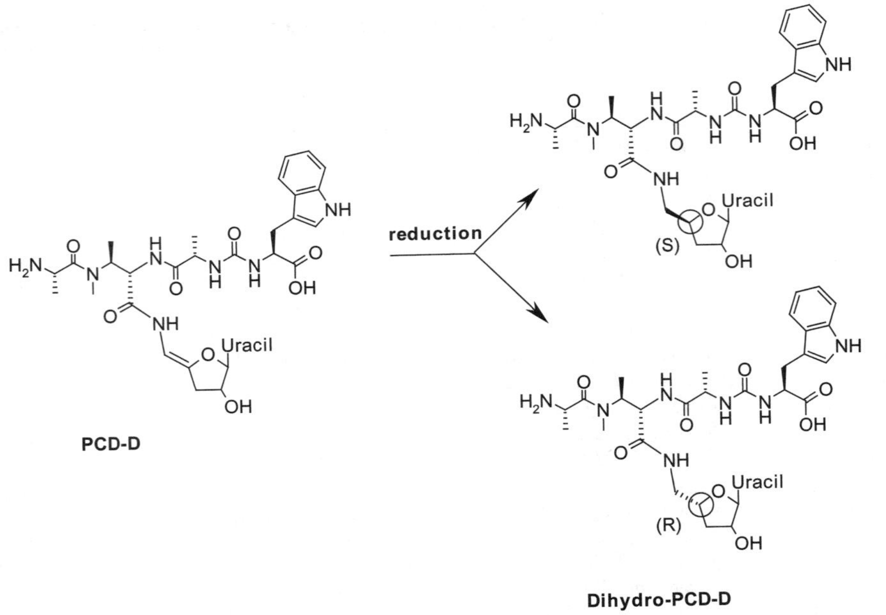

Figure 24 Dihydropacidamycin D isomers are reduction products of pacidamycin D

and eight times the MIC of pacidamycin 1. It was bactericidal against *P. aeruginosa* (3-$\log_{10}$ CFU/ml decrease in 4 to 6 h). At 24 h, resistant mutants were found in the cultures. The frequency of resistance to these compounds was $<3.5 \times 10^{-6}$. The pacidamycins were inactive against *P. aeruginosa* in mouse protection tests. After a single subcutaneous injection of 25 mg of pacidamycin 1 per kg, the maximum concentration in serum was approximately 50 μg/ml and the serum half-life was 0.5 h (Fernandes et al., 1989).

Some chemical modifications were performed on this series, either through semisynthetic or combinatorial approaches (Lee and Hecker, 1999; Boojamra et al., 2001). Interestingly, it was shown that the enamide bond of UPAs is not mandatory for preserving good MraY inhibition. Reduction of this chemical group led to two isomers of dihydropacidamycin D (Fig. 24). The (*R*)-isomer showed better antipseudomonal activity (MIC, 32 μg/ml) than the (S)-isomer (MIC, 512 μg/ml), and its antipseudomonal activity was similar to that of pacidamycin D (MIC, 64 μg/ml).

3.7.1.3.3. Napsamycins. Four napsamycins (Table 5) were discovered in 1994 in a culture of *Streptomyces* sp. strain HIL Y-82,11372. They are specific for *Pseudomonas* sp. inhibition, with MICs from 6.25 to 50 μg/ml (Chatterjee et al., 1994). But only weak activity was shown against other gram-negative and -positive bacteria (MIC, >100 μg/ml).

3.7.1.4. Capuramycin and Derivatives

The chemical template of the series comprises a uracil-containing nucleoside, an unsaturated uronic acid (Fig. 25).

Capuramycins were isolated from a culture filtrate of *Streptomyces griseus* in 1986 (Yamaguchi et al., 1986). Depending of their substitution pattern, they exhibit various degrees of MraY inhibition (Table 6), with IC_{50} of 0.01 to 0.3 μg/ml (Kimura and Bugg, 2003).

A-500359A exhibited reversible inhibition, which was mixed type and noncompetitive with respect to UDP-MurNAc-(Nε-Dns) pentapeptide ($K_i = 0.0079$ μM) and undecaprenyl phosphate, respectively. They are active against *Mycobacterium* species, with MICs ranging from 8 to 12.5 μg/ml (Hotoda et al., 2003a; Hotoda et al., 2003b). A single intravenous administration of A-500359A at a dose of 500 mg/kg showed no toxicity in mice.

Even though capuramycins' name was given because of the presence of a caprolactam ring in the first component isolated, this residue is not compulsory for good MraY inhibition: as an example, A-500350E is as active as capuramycin itself. Moreover, about 70 semisynthetic derivatives were synthesized from A-500350E (Hotoda et al., 2003b). These compounds were tested against MraY and against *Mycobacterium smegmatis* (Table 7).

Some of them were further evaluated against M. *avium*, *Mycobacterium intracellulare*, and *Mycobacterium kansasii*; compound 65 had MICs similar to those of isoniazid (Table 8).

3.7.2. Lipopeptide Antibiotic: Amphomycin

Amphomycin is a lipopeptide antibiotic (Fig. 26). It was isolated from the fermentation broth of *Streptomyces canus* in 1953. It is an undecapeptide containing 3-isododecanoic acid fixed to the N-terminal aspartic residue by an amide linkage. Amphomycin forms a complex with dolichyl phosphate in the presence of Ca^{2+}, preventing the MraY reaction from occurring. It is active against gram-positive cocci, with MICs at which 50% of isolates tested are inhibited of 2 to 4 μg/ml for MSSA and MRSA and of 0.5 to 1 μg/ml for streptococci and enterococci. They are essentially active when Ca^{2+} is present in the culture medium. The LD_{50} was determined at 120 mg/kg administered intravenously in mice. It is currently used as a topical antibacterial in veterinary medicine.

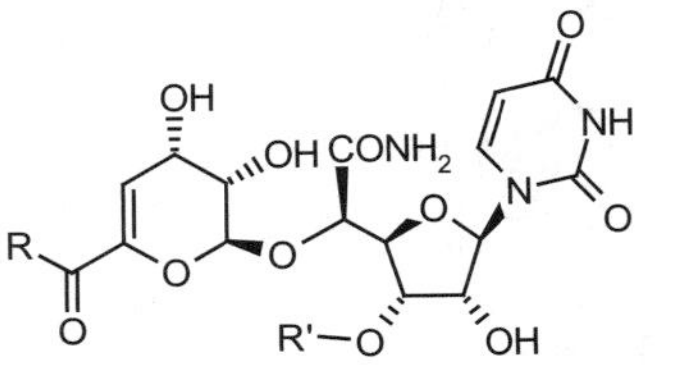

Figure 25 Capuramycin template

Table 6 Inhibitory activity of capuramycin and closely related compounds against MraY

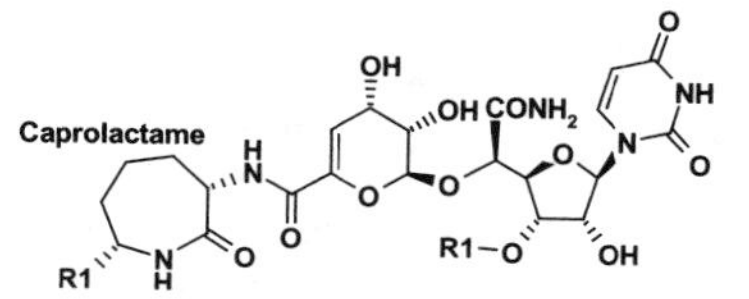

	R1	R2	R3	IC_{50}*(μg/ml)
Capuramycin	Me	OH	Me	0.01
A-500359A	H	OH	Me	0.01
A-500359B	Me	OH	H	0.07
A-500359C	Me	H	Me	0.3
A-500359D	H	OH	H	0.08

*against translocase I

Table 7 Evaluation of capuramycin and related compounds against MraY and *M. smegmatis*

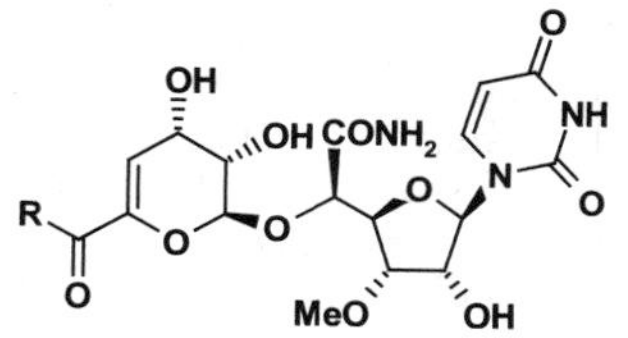

Compound	R	Translocase I IC_{50} (ng/ml)	*M. smegmatis* MIC (μg/ml)
Capuramycin	see. Table	10(18 nM)	12.5
A-500359A	see. Table	10	6.25
A-500359E	MeO–	27	>100
9*	Cyclohexyl-NH–	30	12.5
19*	Ph(CH2)2NH–	21	12.5
34*	PhCH2NH–	120	50
47*	PhNH–	6.5	6.25
65*	3,4-diF–PhNH–	9	6.25

*given name from the publication (Hotoda et al., 2003b)

Table 8 Evaluation of capuramycin and related compounds against *M. avium*, *M. intracellulare*, and *M. kansasii* and comparison with rifampin and isoniazid

Compound	MIC (μg/ml)		
	M. avium	*M. intracellulare*	*M. kansasii*
Capuramycin	8	8	8
A-500359A	8	4	16
47[a]	16	4	8
65[b]	2	0.5	1
Rifampin	0.125	0.125	0.25
Isoniazid	1	8	2

[a]Given name in (Hotoda et al., 2003b).

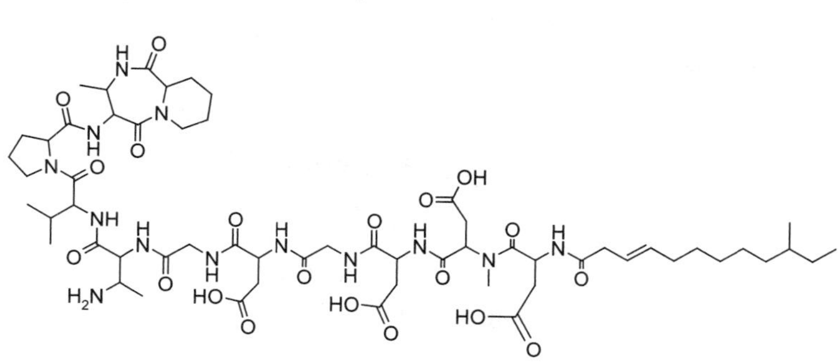

Figure 26 Amphomycin

3.7.2.1. HMR 1043, HMR 1082

HMR 1043 (Fig. 27) and HMR 1082 are, respectively, the calcium and disodium salts of a semisynthetic cyclic lipopeptide. HMR 1043 exhibits good activity against gram-positive cocci (Table 9) (Bemer et al., 2003).

Translocase I (MraY) inhibits protein E. This polypeptide is composed of 93 amino acids and contains a transmembrane helix. Protein E is produced by the bacteriophage ΦX174. Protein E is synthesized in the cytoplasm and then transferred to the inner membrane. It is suspected to tightly interact with the 10 transmembrane segments of MraY protein, resulting in MraY inhibition.

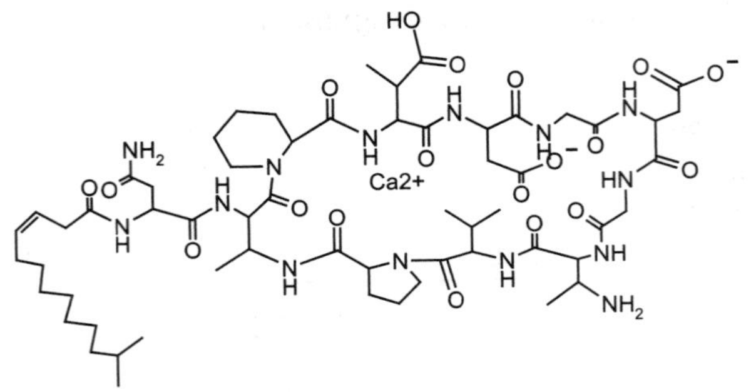

Figure 27 HMR 1043 (friulimicin)

3.8. MurG Inhibitors

MurG (translocase II) catalyzes the passage from lipid I to lipid II (Fig. 28). It is a membrane-associated protein. MurG was described in 1965, and its gene was identified in the 1980s.

Ramoplanin (Fig. 29), which is an antibiotic under development (see chapter 30), was found to inhibit peptidoglycan biosynthesis and preferentially lipid II formation, whereas lipid I synthesis was not affected (Somner and Reynolds, 1990; Crouvoisier et al., 1999). However, its mode of action was reconsidered, and it appears that ramoplanin tends to complex with most peptidoglycan intermediates (Cudic et al., 2002), as it does for lipid II.

3.9. Lipid Pyrophosphorylase Inhibitors: Bacitracin

Bacitracin was isolated in 1943 from *Bacillus* spp. Bacitracin is active against gram-positive cocci and bacilli and also some archaeobacteria, such as *Methanobacterium*, *Methanococcus*, and *Perkinsus marinus* (agent of oyster infection). Bacitracin binds several divalent metal ions to form 1:1 complexes: $Ca^{2+} > Ni^{2+} > Co^{2+} > Zn^{2+} > Mn^{2+}$. Bacitracin binds to metal via its imidazolyl ε-nitrogen. The involvement of the histidine-imidazolyl ring and the carboxylate groups of Asp and Glu is also proposed. The thiazolyl ring may bind Mn^{2+} at pH 6.6. Zinc binds to bacitracin through the δ-N imidazolyl ring of histidine, the sulfur atom of the thiazole ring, and the Glu carboxylate. The tight binding of bacitracin with undecaprenyl pyrophosphate prevents recycling of the sugar carrier, thereby inhibiting cell wall synthesis. Metallobacitracin binds very tightly to undecaprenyl pyrophosphate, preventing the hydrolysis into undecaprenyl phosphate. Hydrolysis is an essential step in peptidoglycan biosynthesis (Fig. 30).

It was found that exposure to bacitracin led to the synthesis of the lactate-containing UDP-MurNAC-pentapeptide precursor that is required for vancomycin resistance. An ABC

Table 9 In vitro activity of HMR 1043

Organism[a]	*n*	MIC (μg/ml)		
		HMR 1043	Daptomycin	TEC[b]
MSSA	7	0.5–2.0	0.25	1.0
MRSA	4	2.0	0.5	16
VISA	5	4.0	1.0	16
MSSE	7	0.5–4.0	0.25	1.0
MRSE	8	1.0–4.0	2.0	2.0
Staphylococcus haemolyticus TEC[s]	10	0.5	0.25	4.0
S. haemolyticus TEC[s]	11	8.0	0.5	16
Enterococcus faecalis	12	4.0	1.0	0.25
E. faecalis VanA	13	1.0	2.0	16
E. faecalis VanB	17	4.0	1.0	0.25
Enterococcus faecium	15	2.0	2.0	0.5
E. faecium VanA	16	2.0	2.0	16
E. faecium VanB	17	4.0	0.5	0.5
Listeria monocytogenes	18	8.0	4.0	0.5
S. pneumoniae	20	0.5–4.0	0.125	0.125
Streptococcus pyogenes	23	1.0	1.0	0.125
Streptococcus agalactiae	26	1.0	0.25	0.25

[a]VISA, vancomycin-intermediate *S. aureus*; MSSE, methicillin-susceptible *Staphylococcus epidermidis*; MRSE, methicillin-resistant *S. epidermidis*.
[b]TEC, teicoplanin.

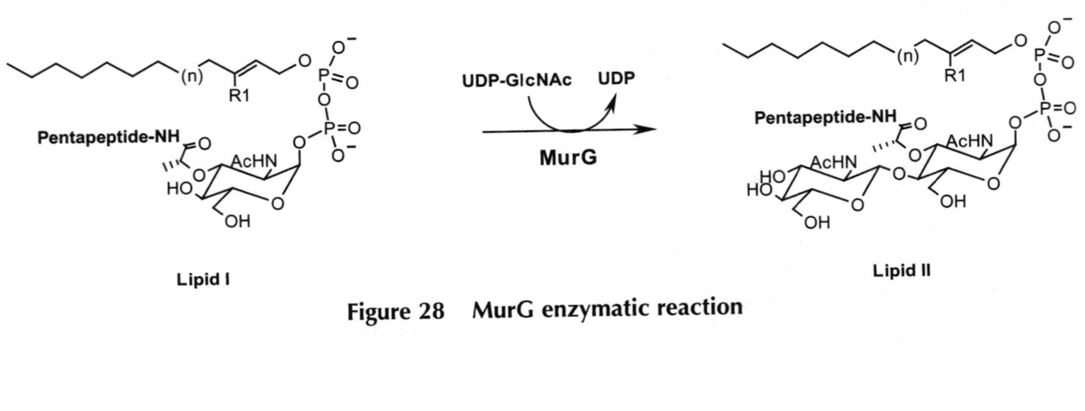

Figure 28 MurG enzymatic reaction

Figure 29 Ramoplanin

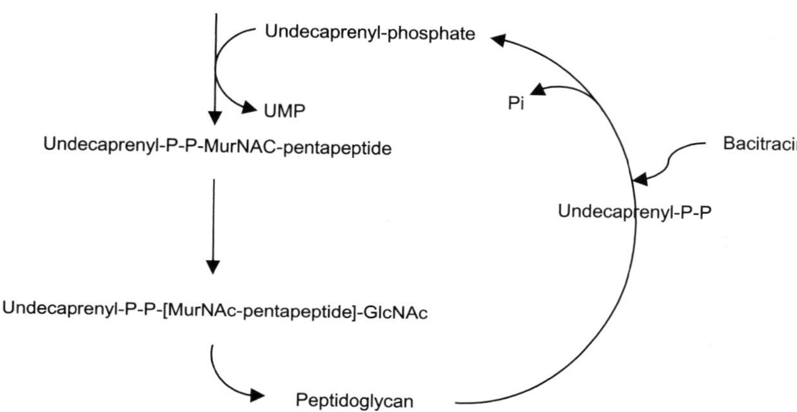

Figure 30 Mode of action of bacitracin

transporter system (efflux) has been shown to be involved in bacitracin resistance.

3.10. Peptidoglycan Maturation Inhibition

3.10.1. Transglycolase Inhibitors

Only a few compounds have been found to inhibit the transglycosylation step of peptidoglycan synthesis.

3.10.1.1. Moenomycin

The moenomycin group of antibiotics are phosphoglycolipid compounds (Fig. 31) produced by various species of *Streptomyces*. Moenomycin A is the main component and is produced by *Streptomyces bambergiensis*. Moenomycin is a polysaccharide chain linked to a C-25 hydrophobic tail moenocinol via a phosphoric acid diester and a glycerol acid unit.

This natural product is an inhibitor of the essential transglycosylase reaction that polymerizes GlcNAc-β-1,4-MurNAc-pentapeptide-pyrophosphoryl-undecaprenol (lipid II) into bacterial peptidoglycan (El-Abadla et al., 1999). Moenomycin inhibits enzyme interaction with the normal lipid II substrate and/or nascent lipid-linked peptidoglycan. Based on structural similarities between moenomycin and lipid II, it has been proposed that moenomycin might compete with the substrate at the enzyme binding site (Ritzeler et al., 1997).

Monofunctional glycosyltransferases (Mgt) from *S. aureus* and *S. pneumoniae* are sensitive to moenomycin A, contrary to those from *E. coli* and *M. luteus*. The oligosaccharide motif of moenomycin is selectively recognized. There are two recognition sites for moenomycin-type transglycosylation inhibitors on the enzyme: one on the donor site and the other on the acceptor site. Moenomycin A presumably binds to the donor site.

Even though most studies evaluating the biochemical mechanism of antibacterial activity have been performed with the gram-negative bacterium *E. coli*, moenomycin is mostly active against gram-positive bacteria. This lack of efficiency against gram-negative bacteria is attributed to the presence of the outer membrane, which prevents access to the biochemical target. TS0510, the hydrogenated form of moenomycin, is as active as moenomycin itself (Fig. 31). Moreover, degradation of TS0510 yielding tetra-, tri-, and disaccharides (TS0511, TS0512, and TS0514, respectively) did not drastically compromise the antibacterial efficiency of the series (Goldman et al., 2000; Goldman and Gange, 2000).

3.10.1.2. Vancomycin-Like Inhibitors

Even though vancomycin resistance is mainly due to acquisition of D-lactate instead of a D-alanine in the terminus of the pentapeptide side chain, semisynthetic derivatives of vancomycin bearing a disaccharide fixed to the nitrogen of vancosamine sugar were shown to interact with the transglycosylation complex (Chen et al., 2003).

This confirms that vancomycin analogs with a biaryl substituent on the vancosamine moiety possess a second mechanism of action (Ge et al., 1999).

Figure 32 shows the structure of chlorobiphenyl vancomycin.

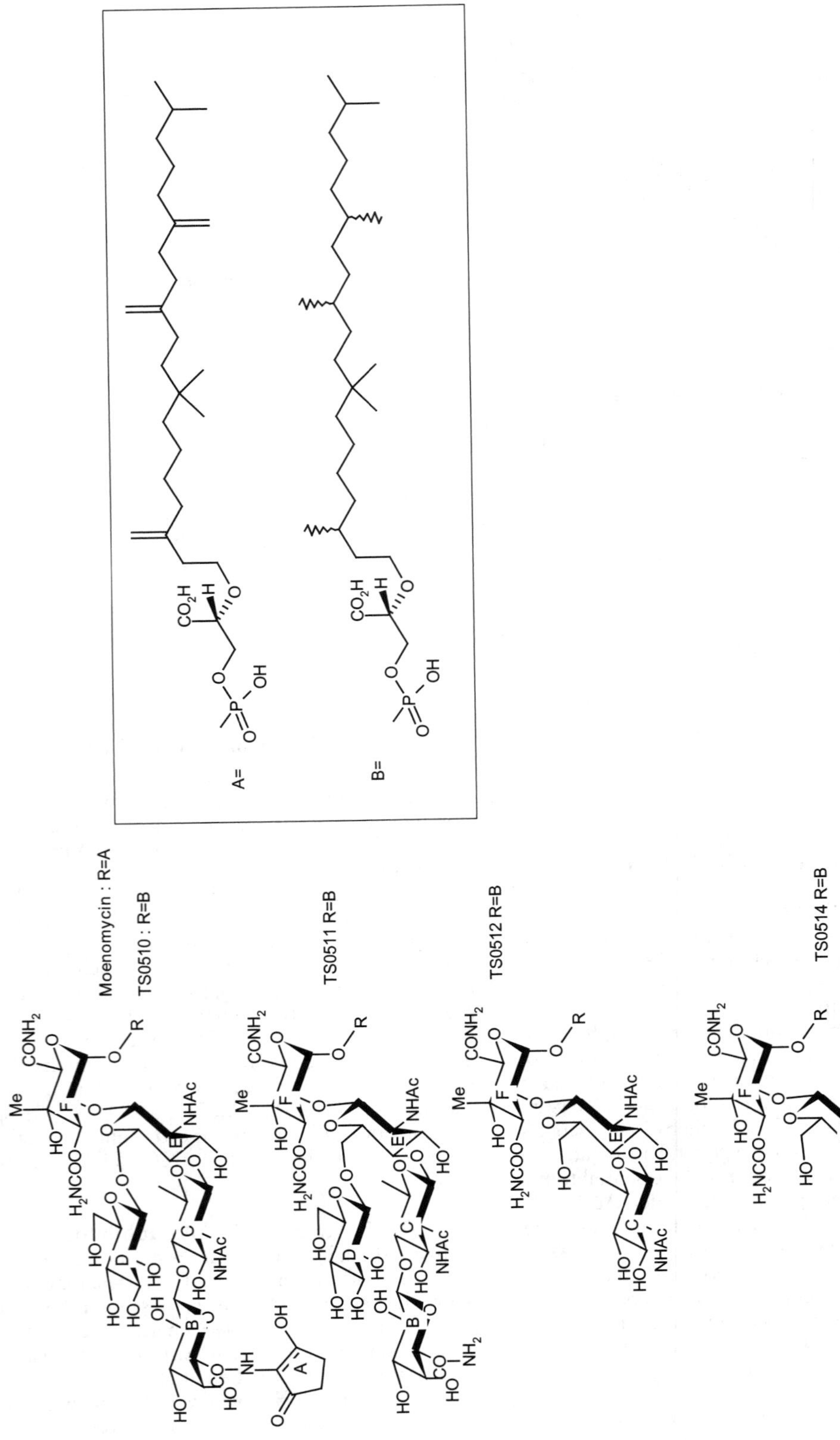

Moenomycin : R=A
TS0510 : R=B

TS0511 R=B

TS0512 R=B

TS0514 R=B

Figure 31 Moenomycin A

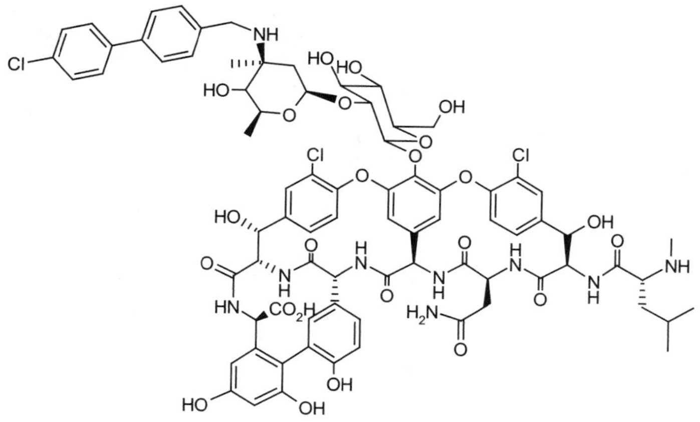

Figure 32 Chlorobiphenyl vancomycin

3.10.2. Transpeptidase Inhibitors

Glycopeptide antibiotics (see chapter 32) and β-lactam antibiotics (see chapters 5 to 7) are transpeptidase inhibitors.

4. MERSACIDIN

Mersacidin (Chatterjee et al., 1992) is a lantibiotic. Lantibiotics are gene-encoded peptides that contain unusual thioether amino acids and/or 3-methyllanthionine. Lantibiotics are classified into two groups: A and B. Group A is composed of nisin, subtilin, epidermin, Pep5, and epilancin K7. Lantibiotic group B contains mersacidin, cinnamycin, phosphatidylethanolamine, duramycin, and actagardin.

Mersacin is produced by fermentation of *Bacillus* sp. strain HIL Y-85,54728. Mersacidin is composed of 20 amino acids, including 4-thioether amino acids (3-methyllanthionine and 2-aminovinyl-2-methylcysteine). This leads to the formation of four intramolecular heterocycle rings. In addition, mersacidin possesses the uncommon amino acid αβ-didehydroalanine.

Mersacidin is active against gram-positive cocci, including MRSA, and inhibits cell wall formation by forming a complex with lipid II.

REFERENCES

Abo-Ghalia M, Flegel M, Blanot D, Van Heijenoort J, 1988, Synthesis of inhibitors of the meso-diaminopimelate-adding enzyme from Escherichia coli, Int J Pept Protein Res, 32, 208–222.

Anderson MS, Eveland SS, Onishi HR, Pompliano DL, 1996, Kinetic mechanism of the Escherichia coli UDPMurNAc-tripeptide D-alanyl-D-alanine-adding enzyme, use of a glutathione S-transferase fusion, Biochemistry, 35, 16264–16269.

Arthur M, Reynolds P, Courvalin P, 1996, Glycopeptide resistance in enterococci, Trends Microbiol, 4, 401–407.

Auger G, van Heijenoort J, et al, 1995, J Prakt Chem, 337, 351.

Bearne SL, 1996, Active site-directed inactivation of Escherichia coli glucosamine-6-phosphate synthase, determination of the fructose 6-phosphate binding constant using a carbohydrate-based inactivator, J Biol Chem, 271, 3052–3057.

Bearne SL, Blouin C, 2000, Inhibition of Escherichia coli glucosamine-6-phosphate synthase by reactive intermediate analogues, the role of the 2-amino function in catalysis, J Biol Chem, 275, 135–140.

Bemer P, Juvin M-E, Bryskier A, Drugeon H, 2003, In vitro activities of a new lipopeptide, HMR 1043, against susceptible and resistant gram-positive isolates, Antimicrob Agents Chemother, 47, 3025–3029.

Benson TE, Harris MS, Choi GH, Cialdella JI, Herberg JT, Martin JP Jr, Baldwin ET, 2001, A structural variation for MurB, X-ray crystal structure of Staphylococcus aureus UDP-N-acetylenolpyruvylglucosamine reductase (MurB), Biochemistry, 40, 2340–2350.

Bertrand JA, Auger G, Fanchon E, Martin L, Blanot D, van Heijenoort J, Dideberg O, 1997, Crystal structure of UDP-N-acetylmuramoyl-L-alanine D-glutamate ligase from Escherichia coli, EMBO J, 16, 3416–3125.

Bertrand JA, Auger G, Martin L, Fanchon E, Blanot D, Le Beller D, van Heijenoort J, Dideberg O, 1999, Determination of the MurD mechanism through crystallographic analysis of enzyme complexes, J Mol Biol, 289, 579–590.

Bertrand JA, Fanchon E, Martin L, Chantalat L, Auger G, Blanot D, van Heijenoort J, Dideberg O, 2000, Open structures of MurD, domain movements and structural similarities with folylpolyglutamate synthetase, J Mol Biol, 301, 1257–1266.

Billot-Klein D, Gutmann L, Sable S, Guittet E, van Heijenoort J, 1994, Modification of peptidoglycan precursors is a common feature of the low-level vancomycin-resistant VANB-type Enterococcus D366 and of the naturally glycopeptide-resistant species Lactobacillus casei, Pediococcus pentosaceus, Leuconostoc mesenteroides, and Enterococcus gallinarum, J Bacteriol, 176, 2398–2405.

Biton J, Braham K, et al, 2002, Synthesis and in vitro evaluation of riburamycin (Ru75411), activity against MraY, antibacterial profile, and mechanism of action (MOA) on whole cells, 42nd Intersci Conf Antimicrob Agents Chemother.

Boojamra CG, Lemoine RC, et al, 2001, Stereochemical elucidation and total synthesis of dihydropacidamycin D, a semisynthetic pacidamycin, J Am Chem Soc, 123, 870–874.

Brandish PE, Burnham MK, et al, 1996, Slow binding inhibition of phospho-N-acetylmuramyl-pentapeptide-translocase (Escherichia coli) by mureidomycin A, J Biol Chem, 271, 760.

Brandish PE, Kimura K, et al, 1996, Modes of action of tunicamycin, liposidomycin B, and mureidomycin A, inhibition of phospho-N-acetylmuramyl-pentapeptide translocase from Escherichia coli, Antimicrob Agents Chemother, 40, 1640–1644.

Brown ED, Marquardt JL, Lee JP, Walsh CT, Anderson KS, 1994, Detection and characterization of a phospholactoyl-enzyme adduct in the reaction catalyzed by UDP-N-acetylglucosamine enolpyruvoyl transferase, MurZ, Biochemistry, 33, 10638–10645.

Brown ED, Vivas EI, Walsh CT, Kolter R, 1995, MurA (MurZ), the enzyme that catalyzes the first committed step in peptidoglycan biosynthesis, is essential in Escherichia coli, J Bacteriol, 177, 4194–4197.

Bugg TD, Wright GD, Dutka-Malen S, Arthur M, Courvalin P, Walsh CT, 1991, Molecular basis for vancomycin resistance in Enterococcus faecium BM4147, biosynthesis of a depsipeptide peptidoglycan precursor by vancomycin resistance proteins VanH and VanA, Biochemistry, 30, 10408–10415.

Chatterjee S, Chatterjee DK, et al, 1992, Mersacidin, a new antibiotic from Bacillus, in vitro and in vivo antibacterial activity, J Antibiotics, 45, 839–845.

Chatterjee S, Nadkarni SR, et al, 1994, Napsamycins, new Pseudomonas active antibiotics of the mureidomycin family from Streptomyces sp HIL Y-82, 11372, J Antibiot, 47, 595–598.

Chen L, Walker D, et al, 2003, Vancomycin analogues active against vanA-resistant strains inhibit bacterial transglycosylase without binding substrate, Proc Natl Acad Sci USA, 100, 5658–5663.

Chen RH, Buko AM, et al, 1989, Pacidamycins, a novel series of antibiotics with anti-Pseudomonas aeruginosa activity. II. Isolation and structural elucidation, J Antibiot, 42, 512–20.

Crouvoisier M, Mengin-Lecreulx D, et al, 1999, UDP-N-acetylglucosamine, N-acetylmuramoyl-(pentapeptide) pyrophosphoryl undecaprenol N-acetylglucosamine transferase from Escherichia coli, overproduction, solubilization, and purification, FEBS Lett, 449, 289–292.

Cudic P, Kranz JK, et al, 2002, Complexation of peptidoglycan intermediates by the lipoglycodepsipeptide antibiotic ramoplanin, minimal structural requirements for intermolecular complexation and fibril formation, Proc Natl Acad Sci USA, 99, 7384–7389.

Dini C, Collette P, et al, 2000, Synthesis of the nucleoside moiety of liposidomycins, elucidation of the pharmacophore of this family of MraY inhibitors, Bioorg Med Chem Lett, 10, 1839–1843.

Dini C, Drochon N, et al, 2001a, Synthesis of analogues of the O-beta-d-ribofuranosyl nucleoside moiety of liposidomycins. Part 1. Contribution of the amino group and the uracil moiety upon the inhibition of MraY, Bioorg Med Chem Lett, 11, 529–531.

Dini C, Drochon N, et al, 2001b, Synthesis of analogues of the O-beta-d-ribofuranosyl nucleoside moiety of liposidomycins. Part 2. Role of the hydroxyl groups upon the inhibition of MraY, Bioorg Med Chem Lett, 11, 533–536.

Dini C, Didier-Laurent S, et al, 2002, Synthesis of sub-micromolar inhibitors of MraY by exploring the region originally occupied by the diazepanone ring in the liposidomycin structure, Bioorg Med Chem Lett, 12, 1209–1213.

Du W, Brown JR, Sylvester DR, Huang J, Chalker AF, So CY, Holmes DJ, Payne DJ, Wallis NG, 2000, Two active forms of UDP-N-acetylglucosamine enolpyruvyl transferase in gram-positive bacteria, J Bacteriol, 182, 4146–4152.

Duncan K, van Heijenoort J, Walsh CT, 1990, Purification and characterization of the D-alanyl-D-alanine-adding enzyme from Escherichia coli, Biochemistry, 29, 2379–2386.

Eckardt K, Wetzstein H, et al, 1980, Streptovirudin and tunicamycin, two inhibitors of glycolipid synthesis, differentiation by use of gel chromatography, HPLC and hydrolysis, J Antibiot (Tokyo), 33, 908–910.

Edgar JA, Frahn JL, et al, 1982, Corynetoxins, causative agents of annual ryegrass toxicity; their identification as tunicamycin group antibiotics, J Chem Soc, 4, 222–224.

El-Abadla N, Lampilas M, et al, 1999, Moenomycin A, the role of the methyl group in the moenuronamide unit and a general discussion of structure-activity relationships, Tetrahedron, 55, 699–722.

Emanuele JJ Jr, Jin H, Jacobson BL, Chang CY, Einspahr HM, Villafranca JJ, 1996, Kinetic and crystallographic studies of Escherichia coli UDP-N-acetylmuramate, L-alanine ligase, Protein Sci, 5, 2566–2574.

Fernandes PB, Swanson RN, et al, 1989, Pacidamycins, a novel series of antibiotics with anti-Pseudomonas aeruginosa activity. III. Microbiologic profile, J Antibiot, 42, 521–526.

Ge M, Chen Z, Onishi HR, Kohler J, Silver LL, Kerns R, Fukuzawa S, Thompson C, Kahne D, 1999, Vancomycin derivatives that inhibit peptidoglycan biosynthesis without binding D-Ala-D-Ala, Science, 284, 442–443.

Gegnas LD, Waddell ST, Chabin RM, Reddy S, Wong KK, 1998, Inhibitors of the bacterial cell wall biosynthesis enzyme MurD, Bioorg Med Chem Lett, 8, 1643–1648.

Gehring AM, Lees WJ, Mindiola DJ, Walsh CT, Brown ED, 1996, Acetyltransfer precedes uridylyltransfer in the formation of UDP-N-acetylglucosamine in separable active sites of the bifunctional GlmU protein of Escherichia coli, Biochemistry, 35, 579–585.

Glanzmann P, Gustafson J, Komatsuzawa H, Ohta K, Berger-Bachi B, 1999, glmM operon and methicillin-resistant glmM suppressor mutants in Staphylococcus aureus, Antimicrob Agents Chemother, 43, 240–245.

Gobec S, Urleb U, Auger G, Blanot D, 2001, Synthesis and biochemical evaluation of some novel N-acyl phosphono- and phosphinoalanine derivatives as potential inhibitors of the D-glutamic acid-adding enzyme, Pharmazie, 56, 295–257.

Goldman RC, Baizman ER, et al, 2000, Differential antibacterial activity of moenomycin analogues on gram-positive bacteria, Bioorg Med Chem Lett, 10, 2251–2254.

Goldman RC, Gange D, 2000, Inhibition of transglycosylation involved in bacterial peptidoglycan synthesis, Curr Med Chem, 7, 801–820.

Gordon E, Flouret B, Chantalat L, van Heijenoort J, Mengin-Lecreulx D, Dideberg O, 2001, Crystal structure of UDP-N-acetylmuramoyl-L-alanyl-D-glutamate, meso-diaminopimelate ligase from Escherichia coli, J Biol Chem, 276, 10999–11006.

Gu YG, Florjancic AS, et al, 2004, Structure-activity realationship of novel potent MurF inhibitors, Bioorg Med Chem Lett, 14, 267–270.

Gubler M, Appoldt Y, Keck W, 1996, Overexpression, purification, and characterization of UDP-N-acetylmuramyl, L-alanine ligase from Escherichia coli, J Bacteriol, 178, 906–910.

Hammes W, Schleifer KH, Kandler O, 1973, Mode of action of glycine on the biosynthesis of peptidoglycan, J Bacteriol, 116, 1029–1053.

Horton JR, Bostock JM, et al, 2003, Macrocyclic inhibitors of the bacterial cell wall biosynthesis enzyme MurD, Bioorg Med Chem Lett, 13, 1557–1560.

Hotoda H, Daigo M, et al, 2003, Synthesis and antimycobacterial activity of capuramycin analogues. Part 2. Acylated derivatives of capuramycin-related compounds, Bioorg Med Chem Lett, 13, 2833–2836.

Hotoda H, Miyuki F, et al, 2003, Synthesis and antimycobacterial activity of capuramycin analogues. Part 1. Substitution of the azepan-2-one moiety of capuramycin, Bioorg Med Chem Lett, 13, 2829–2832.

Igarashi M, Nakagawa S, et al, 2002, 42nd Intersci Conf Antimicrob Agents Chemother, abstract F-2031, p 232.

Inukai M, Isono F, et al, 1989, Mureidomycins A-D, novel peptidyl nucleoside antibiotics with spheroplast forming activity. I. Taxonomy, fermentation, isolation and physicochemical properties, J Antibiot, 42, 662–666.

Inukai M, Isono F, et al, 1993, Selective inhibition of the bacterial translocase reaction in peptidoglycan synthesis by mureidomycins, Antimicrob Agents Chemother, 37, 980–983.

Ishiguro EE, 1982, Inhibition of uridine 5'-diphosphate-N-acetylmuramyl-L-alanine synthetase by beta-chloro-L-alanine in Escherichia coli, Can J Microbiol, 28, 654–659.

Isono K, Uramoto M, et al, 1985, Liposidomycins, novel nucleoside antibiotics which inhibit bacterial peptidoglycan synthesis, J Antibiot, 38, 1617–1621.

Isono F, Katayama T, et al, 1989, Mureidomycins A-D, novel peptidylnucleoside antibiotics with spheroplast forming activity. III. Biological properties, J Antibiot, 42, 674–679.

Isupov MN, Obmolova G, Butterworth S, Badet-Denisot MA, Badet B, Polikarpov I, Littlechild JA, Teplyakov A, 1996, Substrate binding is required for assembly of the active conformation of the catalytic site in Ntn amidotransferases, evidence from the 18 A crystal structure of the glutaminase domain of glucosamine 6-phosphate synthase, Structure, 4, 801–810.

Jolly L, Ferrari P, Blanot D, Van Heijenoort J, Fassy F, Mengin-Lecreulx D, 1999, Reaction mechanism of phosphoglucosamine mutase from Escherichia coli, Eur J Biochem, 262, 202–210.

Kahan FM, Kahan JS, Cassidy PJ, Kropp H, 1974, The mechanism of action of fosfomycin (phosphonomycin), Ann NY Acad Sci, 235, 364–386.

Karwowski JP, Jackson M, Theriault RJ, Chen RH, Barlow GJ, Maus ML, 1989, Pacidamycins, a novel series of antibiotics with anti-Pseudomonas aeruginosa activity. I. Taxonomy of the producing organism and fermentation, J Antibiot 42, 506–511.

Kimura K, Ikeda Y, et al, 1998, Selective inhibition of the bacterial peptidoglycan biosynthesis by the new types of liposidomycins, J Antibiot, 51, 1099–1104.

Kimura K, Bugg TDH, 2003, Recent advances in antimicrobial nucleoside antibiotics targetting cell wall biosynthesis, Nat Prod Rep, 20, 252–273.

Kostrewa D, D'Arcy A, Takacs B, Kamber M, 2001, Crystal structures of Streptococcus pneumoniae N-acetylglucosamine-1-phosphate uridyltransferase, GlmU, in apo form at 233 A resolution and in complex with UDP-N-acetylglucosamine and Mg(2+) at 196 A resolution, J Mol Biol, 305, 279–289.

Le Roux P, Auger G, et al, 1992, Synthesis of new peptide inhibitors of the meso-diaminopimelate-adding enzyme, Eur J Med Chem, 27, 899–907.

Lee VJ, Hecker SJ, 1999, Antibiotic resistance versus small molecules, the chemical evolution, Med Res Rev, 19, 521–542.

Leriche C, Badet-Denisot MA, Badet B, 1997, Affinity labeling of Escherichia coli glucosamine-6-phosphate synthase with a fructose 6-phosphate analog—evidence for proximity between the N-terminal cysteine and the fructose-6-phosphate-binding site, Eur J Biochem, 245, 418–422.

Liger D, Blanot D, van Heijenoort J, 1991, Effect of various alanine analogues on the L-alanine-adding enzyme from Escherichia coli, FEMS Microbiol Lett, 64, 111–115.

Liger D, Masson A, Blanot D, van Heijenoort J, Parquet C, 1995, Over-production, purification and properties of the uridine-diphosphate-N-acetylmuramate, L-alanine ligase from Escherichia coli, Eur J Biochem, 230, 80–87.

Liger D, Masson A, Blanot D, van Heijenoort J, Parquet C, 1996, Study of the overproduced uridine-diphosphate-N-acetylmuramate, L-alanine ligase from Escherichia colim Microb Drug Resist, 2, 25–27.

Marquardt JL, Siegele DA, Kolter R, Walsh CT, 1992, Cloning and sequencing of Escherichia coli murZ and purification of its product, a UDP-N-acetylglucosamine enolpyruvyl transferase, J Bacteriol, 174, 5748–5752.

McDonald LA, Barbieri LR, Carter GT, Lenoy E, Lotvin J, Petersen PJ, Siegel MM, Singh G, Williamson RT, 2002, Structures of the muraymycins, novel peptidoglycan biosynthesis inhibitors, J Am Chem Soc, 124, 10260–10261.

Mengin-Lecreulx D, van Heijenoort J, 1994, Copurification of glucosamine-1-phosphate acetyltransferase and N-acetylglucosamine-1-phosphate uridyltransferase activities of Escherichia coli, characterization of the glmU gene product as a bifunctional enzyme catalyzing two subsequent steps in the pathway for UDP-N-acetylglucosamine synthesis, J Bacteriol, 176, 5788–5795.

Mengin-Lecreulx D, van Heijenoort J, Park JT, 1996, Identification of the mpl gene encoding UDP-N-acetylmuramate, L-alanyl-gamma-D-glutamyl-meso-diaminopimelate ligase in Escherichia coli and its role in recycling of cell wall peptidoglycan, J Bacteriol, 178, 5347–5352.

Mengin-Lecreulx D, Falla T, Blanot D, van Heijenoort J, Adams DJ, Chopra I, 1999, Expression of the Staphylococcus aureus UDP-N-acetylmuramoyl- L-alanyl-D-glutamate, L-lysine ligase in Escherichia coli and effects on peptidoglycan biosynthesis and cell growth, J Bacteriol, 181, 5909–5914.

Michaud C, Blanot D, Flouret B, Van Heijenoort J, 1987, Partial purification and specificity studies of the D-glutamate-adding and D-alanyl-D-alanine-adding enzymes from Escherichia coli K12, Eur J Biochem,166, 631–637.

Michaud C, Parquet C, Flouret B, Blanot D, van Heijenoort J, 1990, Revised interpretation of the sequence containing the murE gene encoding the UDP-N-acetylmuramyl-tripeptide synthetase of Escherichia coli, Biochem J, 269, 277–278.

Miller DJ, Hammond SM, Anderluzzi D, Bugg TDH, 1998, Aminoalkylphosphinate inhibitors of D-Ala-D-Ala adding enzyme, J Chem Soc Perkin Trans, 1, 131–142.

Mizuno Y, Yaegashi M, Ito E, 1973, Purification and properties of uridine diphosphate N-acetylmuramate, L-alanine ligase, J Biochem (Tokyo), 74, 525–538.

Neuhaus FC, Struve WG, 1965, Enzymatic synthesis of analogs of the cell-wall precursor - I - kinetics and specificity of uridine diphospho-N-acetylmuramyl-L-alanyl-D-glutamyl-L-lysine, D-alanyl-D-alanine ligase (adenosine diphosphate) from Streptococcus faecalis R, Biochemistry, 10, 120–131.

Ochi K, Ezaki M, et al, 1989, Antibiotic FR-900493 manufacture with Bacillus EP-333177, Fujisawa Pharmaceutical Co, Ltd, Japan.

Pompeo F, Bourne Y, van Heijenoort J, Fassy F, Mengin-Lecreulx D, 2001, Dissection of the bifunctional Escherichia coli N-acetylglucosamine-1-phosphate uridyltransferase enzyme into autonomously functional domains and evidence that trimerization is absolutely required for glucosamine-1-phosphate acetyltransferase activity and cell growth, J Biol Chem, 276, 3833–3839.

Pratviel-Sosa F, Acher F, Trigalo F, Blanot D, Azerad R, van Heijenoort J, 1994, Effect of various analogues of D-glutamic acid on the D-glutamate-adding enzyme from Escherichia coli, FEMS Microbiol Lett, 115, 223–228.

Reynolds PE, Snaith HA, Maguire AJ, Dutka-Malen S, Courvalin P, 1994, Analysis of peptidoglycan precursors in vancomycin-resistant Enterococcus gallinarum BM4174, Biochem J, 301, 5–8.

Ritzeler O, Hennig L, et al, 1997, Synthesis of a trisaccharide analogue of moenomycin A-12, implications of new moenomycin structure-activity relationships, Tetrahedron, 53, 1675–1694.

Schleifer KH, Hammes WP, Kandler O, 1976, Effect of endogenous and exogenous factors on the primary structures of bacterial peptidoglycan, Adv Microb Physiol, 13, 245–292.

Schonbrunn E, Eschenburg S, Krekel F, Luger K, Amrhein N, 2000, Role of the loop containing residue 115 in the induced-fit mechanism of the bacterial cell wall biosynthetic enzyme MurA, Biochemistry, 39, 2164–2173.

Schwartz R, Datema R, 1980, Inhibitors of protein glycosylation, Trends Biochem Sci, 65–67.

Skarzynski T, Mistry A, Wonacott A, Hutchinson SE, Kelly VA, Duncan K, 1996, Structure of UDP-N-acetylglucosamine enolpyruvyl transferase, an enzyme essential for the synthesis of bacterial peptidoglycan, complexed with substrate UDP-N-acetylglucosamine and the drug fosfomycin, Structure, 4, 1465–1474.

Somner EA, Reynolds PE, 1990, Inhibition of peptidoglycan biosynthesis by ramoplanin, Antimicrob Agents Chemother, 34, 423–429.

Takatsuki A, Tamura G, 1971, Tunicamycin, a new antibiotic. III. Reversal of the antiviral activity of tunicamycin by aminosugars and their derivatives, J Antibiot (Tokyo), 24, 232–238.

Takeuchi T, Igarashi M, et al, 1999, Antibiotic caprazamycins and process for producing the same, WO 2001012643-A1, Zaidan Hojin Biseibutsu Kagaku Kenkyu Kai, Japan.

Takeuchi T, Igarashi M, et al, 2001, Caprazamycin manufacture with Streptomyces for control of acid-fast bacteria, JP 2003012687, Meiji Seika Kaisha, Ltd, Japan.

Tanner ME, Vaganay S, van Heijenoort J, Blanot D, 1996, Phosphinate inhibitors of the D-glutamic acid-adding enzyme of peptidoglycan biosynthesis, J Org Chem, 61, 1756–1760.

Teplyakov A, Obmolova G, Badet-Denisot MA, Badet B, Polikarpov I, 1998, Involvement of the C terminus in intramolecular nitrogen channeling in glucosamine 6-phosphate synthase, evidence from a 16 A crystal structure of the isomerase domain, Structure, 6, 1047–1055.

Vogel P, Petterson DS, et al, 1981, Isolation of a group of glycolipid toxins from seedheads of annual ryegrass (Lolium rigidum

Gaud) infected by Corynebacterium rathayi, Aust J Exp Biol Med Sci, 59, 455–467.

Walker B, Brown MF, Lynas JF, Martin SL, McDowell A, Badet B, Hill AJ, 2000, Inhibition of Escherichia coli glucosamine synthetase by novel electrophilic analogues of glutamine—comparison with 6-diazo-5-oxo-norleucine, Bioorg Med Chem Lett, 10, 2795–2798.

Wu HC, Wu TC, 1971, Isolation and characterization of a glucosamine-requiring mutant of Escherichia coli K-12 defective in glucosamine-6-phosphate synthetase, J Bacteriol, 105, 455–466.

Yamaguchi H, Sato S, et al, 1986, Capuramycin, a new nucleoside antibiotic: taxonomy, fermentation, isolation and characterization, J Antibiotics, 39, 1047–1053.

Yan Y, Munshi S, Li Y, Pryor KA, Marsilio F, Leiting B, 1999, Crystallization and preliminary X-ray analysis of the Escherichia coli UDP-MurNAc-tripeptide D-alanyl-D-alanine-adding enzyme (MurF), Acta Crystallogr D Biol Crystallogr, 55 (Pt 12), 2033–2034.

Yan Y, Munshi S, Leiting B, Anderson MS, Chrzas J, Chen Z, 2000, Crystal structure of Escherichia coli UDPMurNAc-tripeptide D-alanyl-D-alanine-adding enzyme (MurF) at 23 A resolution, J Mol Biol, 304, 435–445.

Yoshida Y, Yamanaka H, et al, 1993, Preparation of uronic acid (FR-900493) derivatives as antibacterial agents, JP05078385, Fujisawa, Pharma.

Zeng B, Wong KK, Pompliano DL, Reddy S, Tanner ME, 1998, A phosphinate inhibitor of the meso-diaminopimelic acid-adding enzyme (MurE) of peptidoglycan biosynthesis, J Org Chem, 63, 10081–10085.

β-Lactamase Inhibitors

A. KAZMIERCZAK

13

1. INTRODUCTION

The most widespread mechanism of bacterial resistance to β-lactams is the biosynthesis of chromosomal or plasmid-mediated β-lactamases. It is therefore understandable that the main aim of pharmaceutical companies is to find new β-lactams that are not hydrolyzed by these enzymes. Over the past 30 years a new approach to this problem of bacterial resistance of enzymatic origin has involved the discovery of β-lactamase inhibitors which, when combined with a β-lactam, protect the latter from enzymatic inactivation and thus preserve its activity against β-lactamase-producing bacteria. At present there are three β-lactamase inhibitors that are already in therapeutic use: clavulanic acid, sulbactam, and tazobactam. These are β-lactams that possess antibacterial activity but at concentrations that are incompatible with therapeutic use, except for *Neisseria* and *Acinetobacter*, against which only sulbactam is active. Sulbactam and tazobactam are sulfones of penicillanic acid, and brobactam is a bromine derivative of penicillanic acid, while in the case of clavulanic acid the sulfur of the thiazolidine ring is replaced by an oxygen, thus making it a clavam (Fig. 1).

2. β-LACTAMASES AND HYDROLYSIS REACTIONS

β-Lactamases hydrolyze the β-lactam–carbonyl bond of the β-lactams, thus inactivating the antibiotic by the following kinetic pathway:

$$E + S \underset{k-1}{\overset{k\,1}{\Longleftrightarrow}} E \cdot S \xrightarrow{k\,2} E - S \xrightarrow{k\,3} E + P$$

The enzyme (E) and the substrate (S) form a noncovalent, and hence reversible, complex, known as a Michaelis-Menten complex ($E \cdot S$). The substrate then induces a

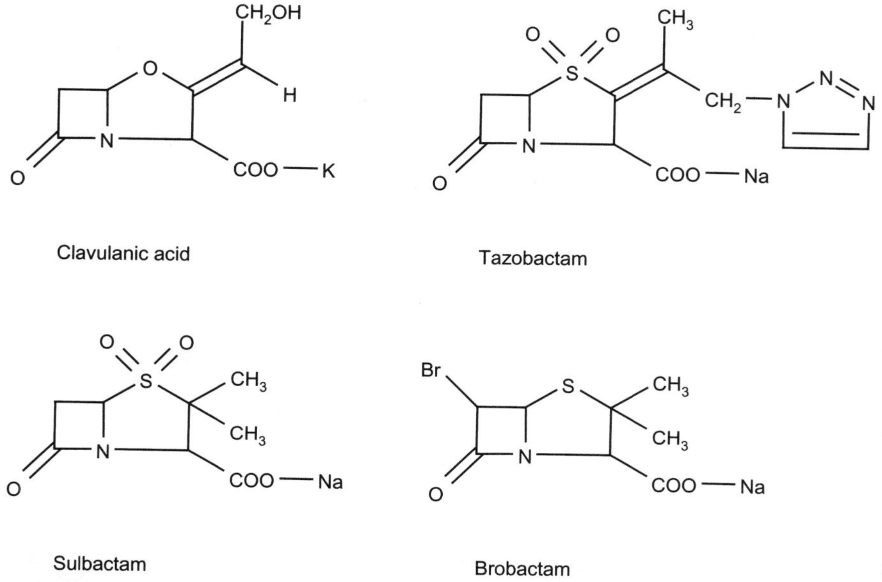

Figure 1 Chemical formulae of β-lactamase inhibitors

change in the configuration of the enzyme, allowing hydrolysis of the β-lactam ring by the hydroxyl function of the serine residue localized at the active site of the enzyme, culminating in the formation of a covalent acylenzyme intermediate ($E - S$). This intermediate is then deacylated, releasing the inactive product (P) and regenerating the enzyme (E).

The rate (v) of the enzymatic reaction increases with the concentration of substrate (S) to reach a maximum rate (V_{max}) which no longer varies with an excess of substrate. It is calculated by the Michaelis-Menten equation $v = V_{max} \cdot S/(K_m + S)$, where K_m is the quantity of substrate for which the hydrolysis rate is equal to half the maximum rate. This equation can be converted to the Lineweaver-Burk linear plot $1/v$ as a function of 1/S, which facilitates the calculation of the Michaelis-Menten constants K_m and V_{max} (Fig. 2). K_m (expressed as a micromolar concentration) is independent of the substrate concentration and defines the affinity of the enzyme; the more it increases, the more the affinity of the enzyme for the substrate decreases. V_{max} is generally reported as a percentage of the V_{max} of penicillin G as the reference β-lactam. The V_{max}s of different β-lactams (substrate profile) thus serve to characterize a β-lactamase.

It should be realized that the characterization of a β-lactamase on the basis of the substrate profile is not always suitable for predicting the activity of a β-lactam against a bacterial strain that produces this β-lactamase. Thus, the V_{max}s of carbenicillin (10.0) and cephalothin (10.6) are identical for the penicillinase TEM-1, so the two antibiotics might be expected to have similar activities. In fact, only cephalothin remains active against strains producing this type of penicillinase. This may be explained by the fact that TEM-1 has very different affinities for these two antibiotics, since the K_m of cephalothin (230 μM) is 23 times weaker than that of carbenicillin (10 μM).

In practice, therefore, both K_m and V_{max} must be taken into account in predicting the activity of a β-lactam. To this end, Pollock (1965) proposed the concept of enzymatic efficiency which corresponds to the ratio V_{max}/K_m, while Labia (1974) proposed the concept of enzymatic stability for the ratio K_m/V_{max}. This is also a relative value expressed as a percentage of that for the reference antibiotic; the larger it is, the less the antibiotic is hydrolyzed.

3. β-LACTAMASES AND INHIBITION REACTIONS

The β-lactamase-inhibitory properties of a given molecule are studied in the presence of a reference β-lactam (penicillin G for penicillinases and cephalothin for cephalosporinases). Thus, some β-lactams prove to be competitive inhibitors that enter into competition with the reference substrate at the active site of the β-lactamases, thus modifying the kinetics of hydrolysis of the latter: either they are delayed, but still run their course, or they are stopped more or less rapidly (Fig. 3).

In the first eventuality, the inhibitor reacts like a substrate with the enzyme, culminating in its hydrolysis and regeneration of the enzyme, which can then participate in new reactions. This is then a reversible competitive inhibitor, which is the case with penicillin M and the third-generation (broad-spectrum) cephalosporins for cephalosporinases.

In the second eventuality, the stage involving formation of the covalent acylenzyme intermediate ($E - I$) is followed by the fragmentation of the molecule into compounds that bind covalently to sites on the enzyme other than the active site. The resultant inactivated enzyme is unable to exert catalytic activity (Fig. 4). There is then irreversible competitive inhibition, and the inhibitor is known as a suicide inhibitor. This is the case with clavulanic acid, sulbactam, and tazobactam against penicillinases and extended-spectrum β-lactamases, and also with sulbactam, tazobactam, moxolactam, and aztreonam against cephalosporinases.

During the hydrolytic reaction of the reference substrate in the presence of the inhibitor, the K_m of the reference

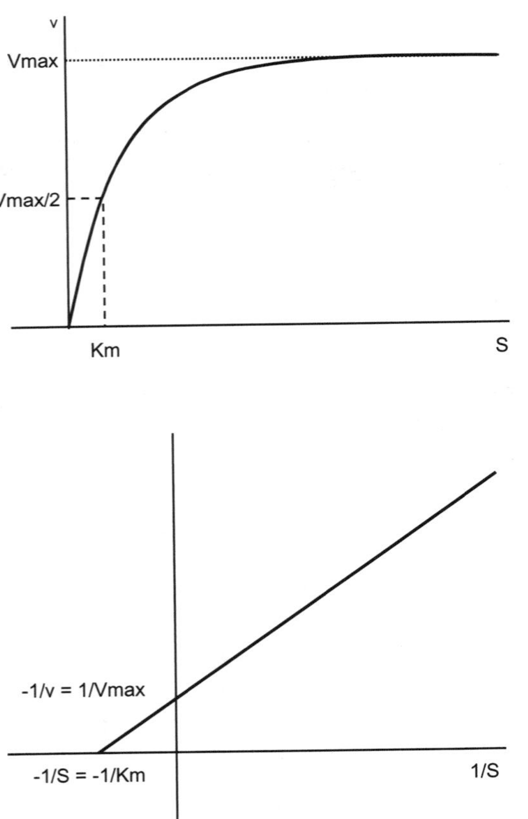

Figure 2 Enzymatic reaction rate as a function of substrate concentration and Lineweaver-Burk linear plot

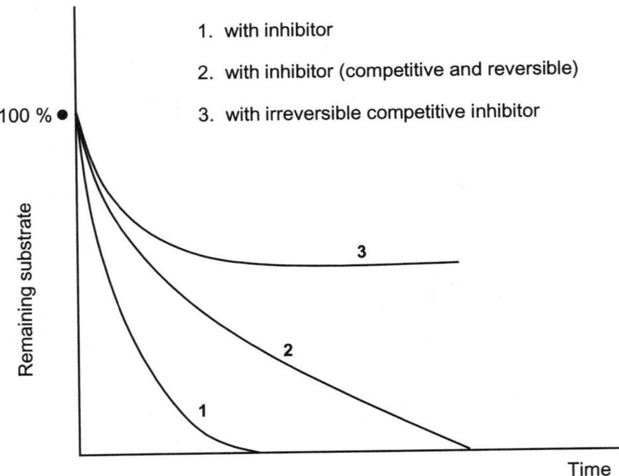

Figure 3 Kinetics of enzymatic hydrolysis (disappearance of substrate) according to the type of enzyme inhibitor

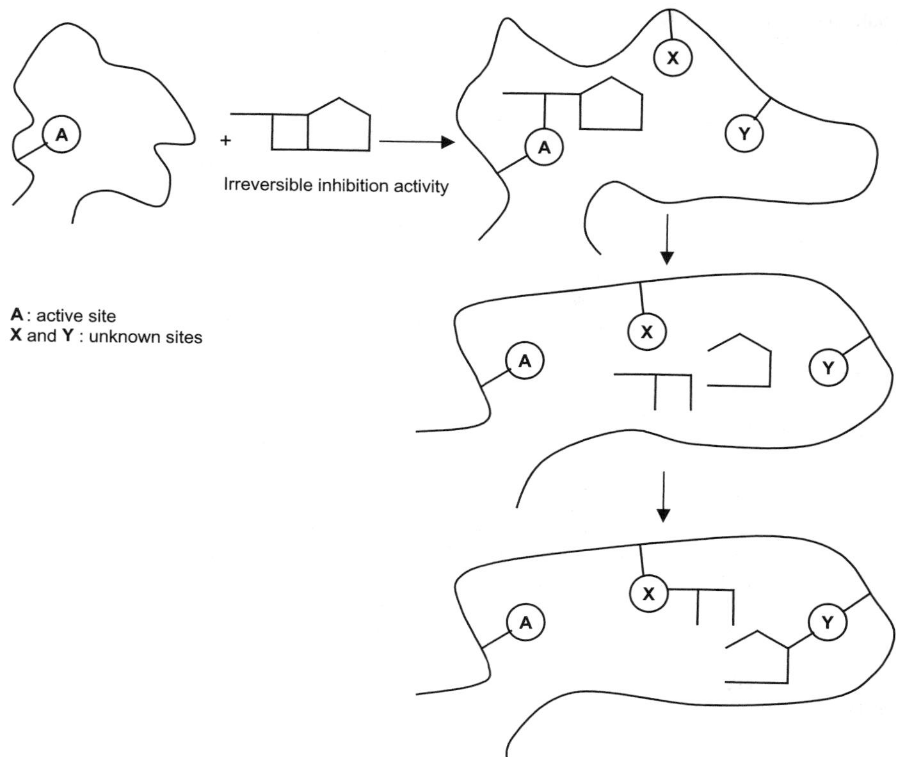

Figure 4 Graphical representation of irreversible enzymatic inhibition of β-lactamases (R. Labia)

substrate increases as a function of the affinity (K_i) of the inhibitor for the enzyme and its concentration (I). K_m becomes the following: $K'_m = K_m(1 + I/K_i)$. The kinetics of hydrolysis obtained in the presence of different concentrations of inhibitor enable $K'm$ to be determined from the Lineweaver-Burk plot, from which the constant of inhibition may be deduced: $K_i = K_m \cdot I/(K'_m - K_m)$ (Fig. 5). Like K_m, the constant of inhibition (K_i) is independent of the concentration of inhibitor; the lower the K_i is, the higher the affinity of the enzyme for the inhibitor.

As the K_i is not easy to determine, it is generally preferred to determine the concentration of inhibitor that reduces the V_{max} of the hydrolysis of a reference substrate by 50% (I_{50}). This involves placing a given concentration of enzyme and reference substrate in contact simultaneously with variable concentrations of inhibitor and observing the change in the hydrolysis reaction. Since the I_{50} is equal to the $K_i(1 + S/K_m)$, where S is the concentration of reference substrate and K_m is its constant of affinity for the β-lactamase, comparison of the results between studies must be performed under the same experimental conditions for one or more inhibitors; it may also be noted that the I_{50} can never be equal to the K_i (Tables 1 and 2) but may approximate it as the ratio S/K_m tends towards zero.

For any new β-lactam with β-lactamase-inhibitory properties, it is important to establish the mechanism of inhibition on the basis of the determination of the I_{50}, which must be undertaken not only in simultaneous competition with the reference substrate, but also following preincubation of the enzyme with the inhibitor, using a standard preincubation period of 10 min to assess whether this inhibition is time dependent. Comparison of the I_{50}s obtained with and without preincubation therefore provides information about the mode of action of the inhibitor. If they are the same, it is a reversible inhibitor. If they decrease after incubation, it is an irreversible inhibitor.

In general, the term β-lactamase inhibitor is reserved for β-lactams whose spectrum of inhibition covers all the β-lactamases to various degrees. Clavulanic acid, sulbactam,

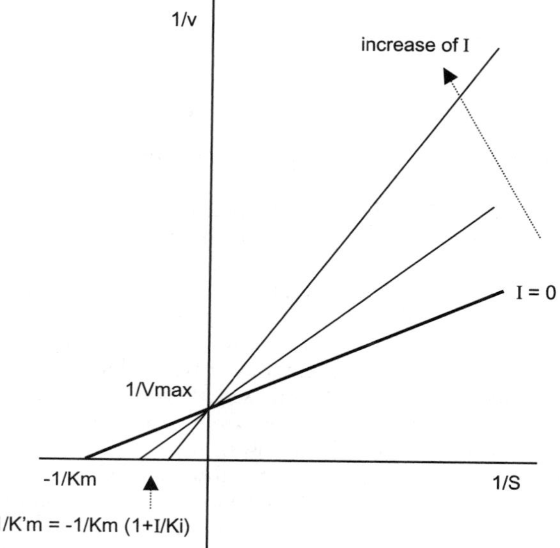

Figure 5 Lineweaver-Burk plot showing the variation in K_m as a function of the concentration of competitive inhibitor

Table 1 Inhibition constants for different β-lactamases

Strain	β-Lactamase	K_i (μM)		
		Clavulanic acid	Sulbactam	Tazobactam
E. coli BM694	TEM -1	0.73	1.1	0.038
	SHV-1	0.19	1.7	0.057
	SHV-2	0.11	0.17	0.04
	TEM-3	0.44	0.12	0.043
	SHV-5	0.11	0.18	0.036
M. morganii 86	C	180	34	2.3
Citrobacter freundii 79	C	250	64	13
Enterobacter cloacae 82	C	>1,000	380	48
Serratia marcescens 89	C	>1,000	120	229

Table 2 I_{50}s for different β-lactamases

Strain	β-Lactamase	I_{50} (μM)		
		Clavulanic acid	Sulbactam	Tazobactam
E. coli BM694	TEM-1	0.06	1.69	0.07
E. coli	TEM-2	0.08	1.3	
E. coli 1527E	OXA-1	1.5	4.7	
E. coli 1573E	OXA-2	1.3	0.3	
E. coli 1894E	OXA-3	55	12	
E. coli BM694	SHV-1	0.057	7.5	0.15
Pseudomonas aeruginosa 1973E	PSE-1	1.0	30	
	PSE-2	0.04	3.4	
P. aeruginosa 1920E	PSE-3	0.02	5.5	
P. aeruginosa 1959E	PSE-4	0.07	3.2	
E. coli BM694	SHV-2	0.017	0.46	0.065
	TEM-3	0.026	0.05	0.02
	SHV-5	0.0045	0.40	0.022
M. morganii 86	C	150	0.40	0.08
C. freundii 79	C	40	3.1	0.35
E. cloacae 82	C	45	6.5	1
S. marcescens 89	C	200	9	13
P. vulgaris 1028	C	0.03	0.1	
P. rettgeri 401H	C	188	0.2	
Providencia stuartii 45C	C	>500	5.3	
S. aureus 88	PC-1	0.1	3.6	

and tazobactam are currently the only ones to meet this criterion.

On the basis of the K_i and I_{50} (Tables 1 and 2), which are weight values expressed in micromolar concentrations, clavulanic acid generally proves to be the best inhibitor of penicillinases (TEM-1 and -2, SHV-1, OXA, PSE, and *S. aureus* penicillinases); conversely, it is inactive against cephalosporinases except for those of *Proteus vulgaris* and *Bacteroides fragilis*. Tazobactam is a better inhibitor of penicillinases and cephalosporinases than sulbactam. The three inhibitors exhibit comparable activities against extended-spectrum β-lactamases. It should be stressed that the inhibitory activity of sulbactam and tazobactam against cephalosporinases is considerably weaker than that against penicillinases and, particularly, extended-spectrum β-lactamases. Nevertheless, from a therapeutic point of view these inhibitors are still of some use against *Pr. vulgaris*, *Providencia rettgeri*, *Morganella morganii*, and *B. fragilis* cephalosporinases.

4. IN VITRO ACTIVITY OF β-LACTAMASE INHIBITORS

Like all β-lactams, the inhibitors bind to penicillin-binding proteins (PBP). Clavulanic acid has a strong affinity for *Escherichia coli* PBP 2, and sulbactam and tazobactam have strong affinities for PBP 1a.

Despite this binding to PBP, inhibitors are generally relatively inactive in themselves (MIC greater than 8 μg/ml) because of their weak ability to penetrate the bacteria. Usually the intrinsic activity of clavulanic acid is greater than that of sulbactam, which is itself greater than that of tazobactam. It should be noted that sulbactam has the specific feature of being active against *Acinetobacter*, with MICs of less than 2 mg/liter for carbenicillin-susceptible strains and equal to 8 to 16 mg/liter for resistant strains. It is also highly active against *Neisseria* (Table 3).

Synergy of antibacterial activity of a β-lactam in combination with a β-lactamase inhibitor can be evaluated in various ways. Standard agar diffusion methods may be used

Table 3 MICs of β-lactamase inhibitors for different bacterial species

Organism(s)	MIC (μg/ml)		
	Clavulanic acid	Sulbactam	Tazobactam
Enterobacteriaceae	16–128	32–>128	128–4,096
P. aeruginosa	256	>512	>512
S. aureus	16	32–>256	32
Acinetobacter	4–16	0.5–2	4–32
Haemophilus	32	128	64
Neisseria	0.03–8	0.03–2	

routinely with the following commercially available disks: Augmentin (amoxicillin plus clavulanic acid: 20 μg + 10 μg), Claventin (ticarcillin plus clavulanic acid: 75 μg + 10 μg), Unasyn (ampicillin plus sulbactam: 10 μg + 10 μg), and Tazocilline (piperacillin plus tazobactam: 75 μg + 10 μg). Thus, comparison of the diameters of the zones of inhibition of the antibiotics alone and in combination with the inhibitor can be used to assess synergy, although this is best quantified by studies of the MIC in a liquid or solid medium.

The checkerboard technique, which is undertaken using a micromethod in a broth medium, is certainly the best for evaluating this synergy, as each of the antibiotic concentrations is tested in the presence of each of the concentrations of inhibitor. After the MICs of the antibiotic (A) and the inhibitor (I) are recorded, the lowest active concentrations in combination (IC) are noted. The synergy is then defined by the FIC index, which is equal to IC of A/MIC of A + IC of I/MIC of I. This index must be ≤0.5, corresponding to a reduction in MIC of at least a factor of 4 for the two compounds combined. It should be noted that a FIC index of very much less than 0.50 may be obtained with a very high MIC and a very low IC without there being any therapeutic application for the combination insofar as the IC are above the levels in serum and, in particular, those of the infectious focus. In practice, this implies that antibacterial activity is restored to the β-lactam in the presence of the inhibitor at a concentration equivalent to one-fourth of the peak concentration in serum, i.e., 4 μg/ml for clavulanic acid, 8 μg/ml for tazobactam, and 16 μg/ml for sulbactam.

Although the checkerboard technique is the reference method, comparisons of the antibacterial activities of combinations of β-lactams with each of the three inhibitors have essentially been effected in the presence of 8 mg of inhibitor per liter (Tables 4 and 5).

It is thus apparent that the combinations of ampicillin, amoxicillin, and carbenicillin with clavulanic acid are, with a few exceptions (*Staphylococcus aureus*, and *Haemophilus influenzae*), more effective than those with tazobactam and particularly sulbactam, not only against penicillinase-producing bacterial species, as predicted by the K_i and I_{50}, but also against species producing extended-broad-spectrum β-lactamases even though the three inhibitors have similar K_is and/or I_{50}s for this type of β-lactamase (Tables 1 and 2).

Thus, determination of the parameters of enzymatic inhibition (K_i and I_{50}) is not sufficient to estimate the activity of the inhibitors against *Enterobacteriaceae*. Allowance should also be made for the penetration of the inhibitor into the bacterium (assessed indirectly by its MIC), the susceptibility of the β-lactamase to the inhibitor, and the quantity of β-lactamase biosynthesized. For example (Table 6), the chromosomally mediated penicillinase SHV-1 is produced at a low level in *Klebsiella pneumoniae*, which confers low-level resistance to amoxicillin (MIC, 128 μg/ml). Although sulbactam is a weaker inhibitor of the β-lactamase SHV-1 than tazobactam and clavulanic acid (K_i = 1.7, 0.057, and

Table 4 MICs of β-lactams alone or in combination with 8 mg of inhibitor per liter against strains producing a single β-lactamase

Strain	β-Lactamase	Antibiotic	MIC (μg/ml)			
			Alone	+Clavulanic acid	+Sulbactam	+Tazobactam
S. aureus 5353	PC-1	Amoxicillin	16	<0.5	<0.5	<0.5
H. influenzae 31	TEM-1	Amoxicillin	64	<0.5	<0.5	<0.5
E. coli C1a	TEM-1	Amoxicillin	>2,048	1	512	4
	TEM-2	Amoxicillin	>2,048	2	>2,048	32
	OXA-1	Amoxicillin	256	2	32	32
	OXA-2	Amoxicillin	256	1	1	2
	OXA-3	Amoxicillin	64	0.5	0.5	1
	SHV-1	Amoxicillin	>2,048	0.5	1,024	8
K. pneumoniae 2222	SHV-1	Ampicillin	128	1	2	2
E. coli C600	TEM-3	Ampicillin	1,000	8	8	8
	TEM-4	Ampicillin	1,000	8	8	8
	TEM-5	Ampicillin	1,000	8	32	16
	SHV-2	Ampicillin	>16,000	16	≥256	128
	SHV-3	Ampicillin	>16,000	16	≥256	64
	SHV-4	Ampicillin	>16,000	8	≥256	32
	SHV-5	Ampicillin	500	8	8	8
E. cloacae 82	C	Ampicillin	256	128	64	8
M. morganii 86	C	Ampicillin	256	256	8	1
C. freundii 79	C	Ampicillin	128	64	4	2
S. marcescens 89	C	Ampicillin	128	128	128	128
P. vulgaris 486	C	Amoxicillin	256	4	4	2
B. fragilis 42	C	Amoxicillin	32	≤0.5	≤0.5	≤0.5
P. aeruginosa 38	C	Carbenicillin	8	32	8	8

Table 5 MICs of β-lactams alone and in combination with 8 mg of inhibitor per liter against strains producing one or two β-lactamases

Strain	β-Lactamase(s)	Antibiotic	MIC (μg/ml)			
			Alone	+Clavulanic acid	+Sulbactam	+Tazobactam
E. cloacae 82	C	Carbenicillin	4	4	4	4
	C + TEM-1	Carbenicillin	>2,048	16	>2,048	32
M. morganii 86	C	Carbenicillin	≤0.5	≤0.5	≤0.5	≤0.5
	C + TEM-1	Carbenicillin	128	<0.5	1	<0.5
C. freundii 79	C	Carbenicillin	4	4	4	4
	C + TEM-1	Carbenicillin	>2,048	16	2,048	16
S. marcescens 89	C	Ampicillin	128	128	128	128
	C + TEM-1	Carbenicillin	>2,048	16	128	8
P. aeruginosa 38	C	Carbenicillin	8	32	8	8
	C + PSE-1	Carbenicillin	>2,048	128	1,024	1,024
	C + PSE-2	Carbenicillin	128	32	128	128
	C + PSE-3	Carbenicillin	>2,048	32	32	32
	C + PSE-4	Carbenicillin	>2,048	16	32	32
K. pneumoniae 2222	SHV-1	Amoxicillin	128	1	2	2
	SHV-1 + TEM-1	Amoxicillin	>2,048	16	>2,048	32

Table 6 MICs in the presence of 8 mg of inhibitor per liter as a function of the quality of β-lactamase biosynthesized

Strain	β-Lactamase	Antibiotic	MIC (μg/ml)			
			Alone	+Clavulanic acid	+Sulbactam	+Tazobactam
K. pneumoniae 2222	SHV-1	Amoxicillin	128	1	2	2
E. coli C1a	SHV-1	Amoxicillin	>2,048	0.5	1,024	8
E. coli C600	SHV-1[a]	Ampicillin	≥16,000	16	≥256	≥256
E. coli C1a	TEM-2	Amoxicillin	>2,048	2	>2,048	32
E. coli C600	TEM-2[b]	Ampicillin	≥16,000	64	≥256	128

[a]Specific activity, 9,000 mU/mg of protein.
[b]Specific activity, 24,000 mU/mg of protein.

0.19 μM and I_{50} = 7.5, 0.15, and 0.057 μM, respectively; cf. Tables 2 and 3), it restores the activity of amoxicillin at concentrations similar (2 mg/liter) to those of the other two inhibitors when the three are tested at 8 mg/liter. Conversely, in *E. coli*, which is a high-level producer of the plasmid-mediated β-lactamase SHV-1, depending on the β-lactamase production levels and for the same concentration of inhibitor (8 mg/liter), the activity of amoxicillin is not restored in the presence of sulbactam (1,024 mg/liter), but is restored in the presence of clavulanic acid (0.5 mg/liter) and incompletely so with tazobactam (8 mg/liter); when this β-lactamase is produced at a very high level (MIC of ampicillin, ≥ 16,000 mg/liter), the activity of the β-lactam is not restored by sulbactam or tazobactam (MIC, ≥ 256 mg/liter) and is incompletely restored by clavulanic acid (MIC, 16 mg/liter). Similar results (MIC of amoxicillin, ≥ 2048 mg/liter) are observed with TEM-2-producing *E. coli* (Table 6).

The antibacterial activity of a β-lactam–inhibitor combination is a function not only of the level of bacterial β-lactamase production and the quality of the inhibitor but also of the capacity of the β-lactam to be less susceptible to the hydrolytic activity of the β-lactamase. Thus, compared with ampicillin and ticarcillin, piperacillin and, in particular, cefoperazone are less hydrolyzed by the penicillinases TEM-1 and TEM-2 and by the TEM-type extended-spectrum β-lactamases. Although tazobactam and, in particular, sulbactam are less inhibitory than clavulanic acid against TEM-1 and TEM-2 and the three inhibitors have similar activities against extended-spectrum β-lactamases of the TEM type, the combinations piperacillin-tazobactam and, particularly, cefoperazone-sulbactam are markedly more active than the combination of ampicillin or ticarcillin plus clavulanic acid (Table 7). It can therefore be understood that the ideal combination would comprise the best inhibitor with the least hydrolyzed β-lactam.

In 1993, clavulanic acid was solely available as a fixed combination with amoxicillin or ticarcillin, and tazobactam was available only in combination with piperacillin. While proposed in a fixed combination with ampicillin, only sulbactam was also available for extemporaneous combination with the most appropriate β-lactam for the β-lactamase-producing bacterial species concerned. By way of example, the results presented in Fig. 6, 7, and 8 are significant in this respect. It can be seen that for three TEM-3-producing species, the combinations of sulbactam plus cefotaxime, ceftazidime, and aztreonam are more effective than the fixed combinations clavulanic acid-ticarcillin and tazobactam-piperacillin.

5. PHARMACOKINETICS OF INHIBITORS

The main pharmacokinetic characteristics of the three inhibitors currently used therapeutically are presented in Table 8.

With 70% bioavailability following oral administration, clavulanic acid has proved to be well absorbed by the intestinal

Table 7 Activity of the β-lactam–β-lactamase inhibitor combinations (8 mg/liter) against *E. coli* C600 transconjugants producing a plasmid-mediated β-lactamase

β-Lactamase	MIC (μg/ml)[a]			
	AMP + CLA	TICAR + CLA	CFP + SUL	PIP + TZB
TEM-1	8	16	≤0.25	2
TEM-2	64	256	16	256
TEM-3	8	32	≤0.25	2
TEM-4	8	32	≤0.25	2
TEM-5	8	16	≤0.25	2
TEM-6	16	64	≤0.25	8
TEM-7	16	32	≤0.25	4
TEM-9	8	64	≤0.25	2

[a]AMP, ampicillin; CLA, clavulanic acid; TIC, ticarcillin; CFP, cefoperazone; SUL, sulbactam; PIP, piperacillin; TZB, tazobactam.

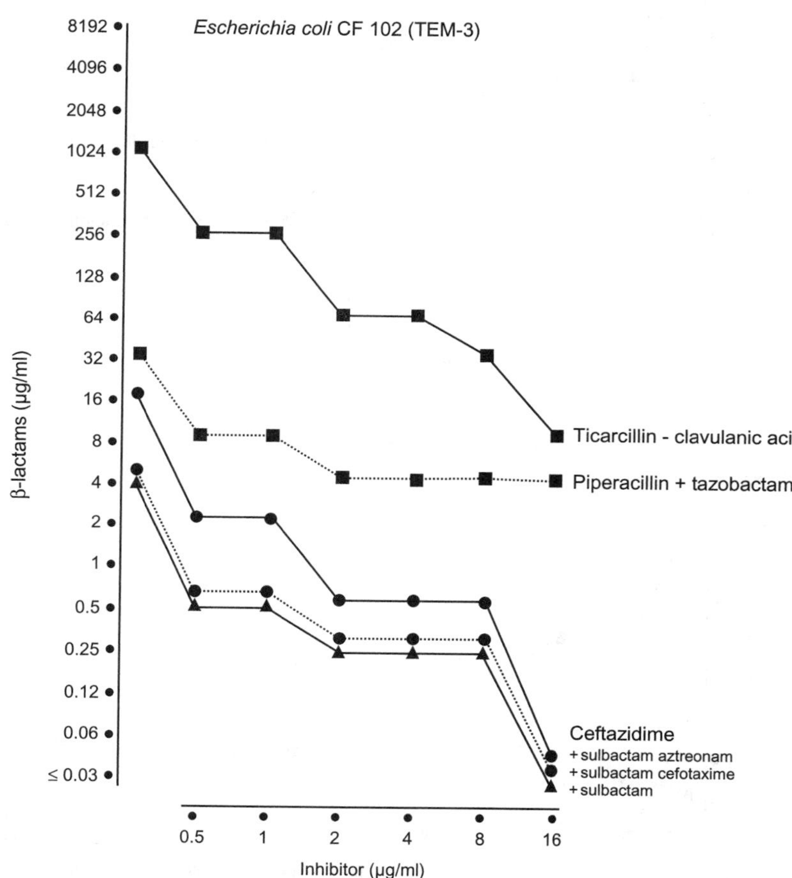

Figure 6 MICs of β-lactams in the presence of different concentrations of inhibitors against *E. coli* CF 102 synthesizing the extended-broad-spectrum β-lactamase TEM-3

mucosa; as the same applies to amoxicillin (80% bioavailability), the combination of the two products is suggested for oral administration. Conversely, sulbactam is weakly absorbed, since its bioavailability is less than 10%. Nevertheless, to allow it to be administered orally in combination with ampicillin, which is itself less well absorbed than amoxicillin (50% bioavailability), the two products are linked by a double esterification producing a single molecule or prodrug: sultamicillin. This double prodrug is well absorbed by the intestinal mucosa. It undergoes hydrolysis by enterocyte esterases, resulting in the release of sulbactam and ampicillin into the general circulation, with 80% bioavailability for the two products. Tazobactam, for its part, probably has the same characteristics of absorption as sulbactam, but as it is proposed in combination with piperacillin, it can only be used parenterally.

Clavulanic acid is to a large extent eliminated hepatically, since about 50% of the administered dose is not found in the urine after intravenous injection. Conversely, elimination of sulbactam and tazobactam is essentially renal,

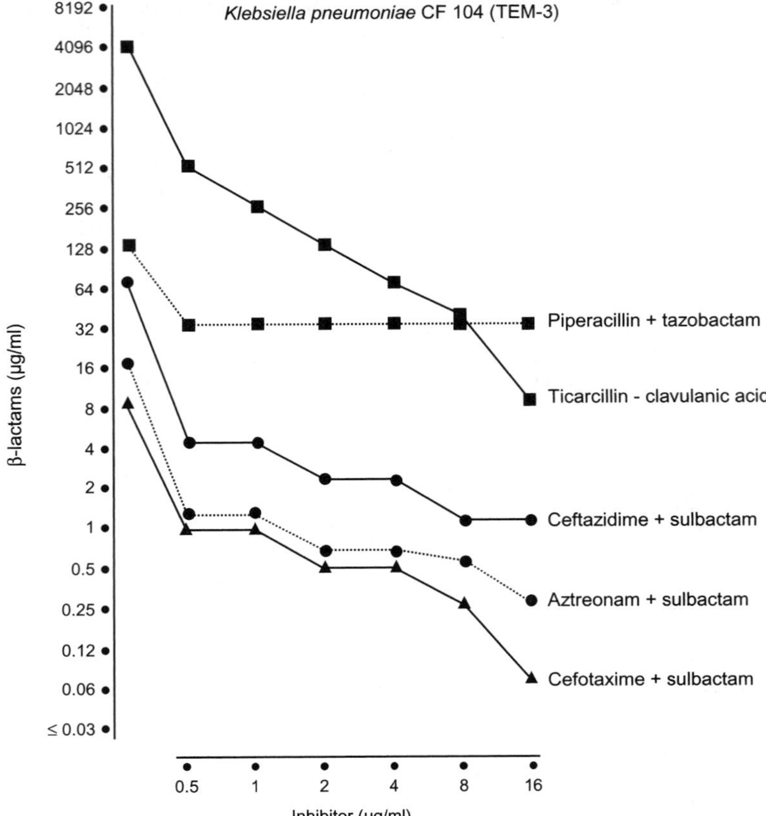

Figure 7 MICs of β-lactams in the presence of different concentrations of inhibitors against *K. pneumoniae* CF 104 synthesizing the extended-broad-spectrum β-lactamase TEM-3

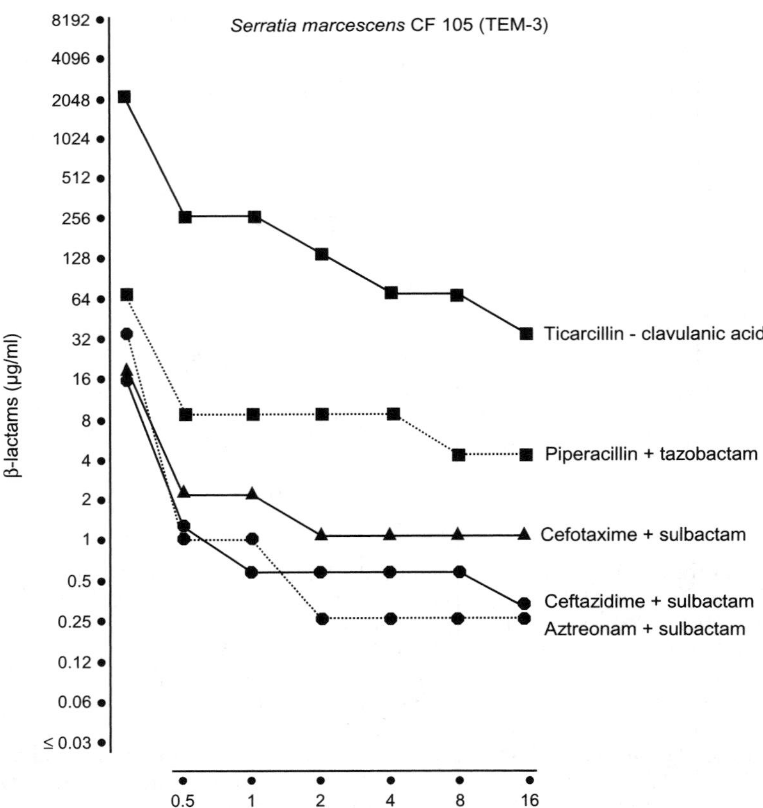

Figure 8 MICs of β-lactams in the presence of different concentrations of inhibitors against *S. marcescens* CF 105 synthesizing the extended-broad-spectrum β-lactamase TEM-3

Table 8 Pharmacokinetic parameters of β-lactamase inhibitors[a]

Parameter	Clavulanic acid[b]		Sulbactam[c]		Tazobactam,[d] i.v.
	p.o.	i.v.	p.o.	i.v.	
Protein binding (%)	20–25		35–40		23
C_{max} (mg/liter)	2.8	13.8	8.9	55	34.4
T_{max} (h)	1.3		1.0		
$t_{1/2}$ (h)	0.8	0.8	0.9	1.1	0.8–0.9
CL_P (ml/min)		215		262	197–202
CL_R (ml/min)		105	150	204	104
AUC (mg·h/liter)	7	17	16.7	62	41.4–43.4
Urinary elimination (%)	43	49	66	77	55.4
Metabolites in urine (%)					20

[a]p.o., per os; i.v., intravenously.
[b]Amoxicillin + clavulanic acid: 125/500 mg and 0.2/1 g.
[c]Sulbactam-ampicillin: 294/440 mg and 1/2 g.
[d]Tazobactam-piperacillin: 0.5/4 g.

involving tubular secretion, which is not found with clavulanic acid. In addition, it should be stressed that 20% of injected tazobactam is eliminated in the form of the urinary metabolite M1.

The following inhibitor–β-lactam fixed combinations are proposed for therapeutic use:

- Orally
  - Clavulanic acid-amoxicillin (Augmentin: 31.25/125 mg, 62.5/250 mg, and 125/500 mg)
  - Sulbactam-ampicillin (Unasyn: 147/220 mg in the form of sultamicillin tosylate dihydrate)
- Intravenously or intramuscularly
  - Clavulanic acid-amoxicillin (Augmentin: 50/500 mg and 0.2/1 or 2 g)
  - Clavulanic acid-ticarcillin (Timentin: 0.1/1.5 g, 0.2/3 g, and 0.2/5 g)
  - Sulbactam-ampicillin (Unasyn: 0.125/0.25 g, 0.25/0.5 g, 0.5/1g, and 1/2 g)
  - Tazobactam-piperacillin (Tazocilline: 0.25/2 g and 0.5/4 g)

Where there is an appreciable difference in renal elimination (clavulanic acid and amoxicillin or ticarcillin; tazobactam and piperacillin), the other pharmacokinetic parameters of the two components of the inhibitor–β-lactam combination are comparable in healthy subjects, particularly their plasma kinetics, which are parallel. The same is not the case in patients with renal insufficiency. Thus, for a creatinine clearance ranging from 130 to 5 ml/min, the elimination half-lives of clavulanic acid, amoxicillin, and ticarcillin increase by factors of 3, 18, and 8.6, respectively, those of sulbactam and ampicillin increase by a factor of 20, and those of tazobactam and piperacillin increase by factors of 8 and 2, respectively. Thus, hepatic elimination compensates for a deficiency of renal elimination for clavulanic acid and piperacillin. In patients with hepatic insufficiency, there is no appreciable modification of the pharmacokinetics of tazobactam and piperacillin; it may validly be assumed that the same applies to the combination of clavulanic acid plus amoxicillin or ticarcillin, and it is clear that this does not affect the combination sulbactam-ampicillin.

6. CONCLUSION

The inhibitor and the β-lactam present in the bacterium compete for binding to the active site of the β-lactamase. As the inhibitors generally have a better affinity for the enzyme, the β-lactam may escape the hydrolytic activity of the β-lactamase if the concentration of inhibitor combined with it is sufficient to inactivate all of the β-lactamase molecules. If that is not the case, the free enzyme molecules will bind to the same number of β-lactam molecules, the remainder being allowed to exert antibacterial activity as long as the hydrolysis rate is low. It can thus be seen that the ideal combination is that of the best inhibitor with the β-lactam most resistant to the hydrolytic activity of the β-lactamases. The fixed combinations that are currently available therapeutically do not always fulfill this criterion because of the type of enzyme produced and/or the level of enzyme production. To offset this, sulbactam is proposed on its own for use in a flexible combination with the β-lactams most resistant to β-lactamases. The results obtained therapeutically suggest that clavulanic acid and tazobactam might also be proposed alone. This would then allow the prescription of the most suitable combination of inhibitor and β-lactam for the bacterial species responsible for the infection.

REFERENCES

Arisawa M, Then RL, 1982, 6-Acetylmethylenepenicillanic acid (Ro 15-1903), a potent β-lactamase inhibitor. I. Inhibition of chromosomally and R-factor-mediated β-lactamases, J Antibiot, 35, 1578–1583.

Gutmann L, Kitzis MD, Yamabe S, Acar JF, 1986, Comparative evaluation of a new β-lactamase inhibitor, YTR 830, combined with different β-lactam antibiotics against bacteria harboring known β-lactamases, Antimicrob Agents Chemother, 29, 955–957.

Jacoby GA, Carreras I, 1990, Activities of β-lactam antibiotics against *Escherichia coli* strains producing extended-spectrum β-lactamases, Antimicrob Agents Chemother, 34, 858–862.

Kitzis MD, Billot-Klein D, Goldstein FW, Williamson R, Tran Van Nhieu G, Carlet J, Acar JF, Gutmann L, 1988, Dissemination of the novel plasmid-mediated β-lactamase CTX-1, which confers resistance to broad-spectrum cephalosporins, and its inhibition by β-lactamase inhibitors, Antimicrob Agents Chemother, 32, 9–14.

β-Lactamase Inhibitors Under Research

ANDRÉ BRYSKIER, CATHERINE COUTURIER, AND JOHN LOWTHER

14

1. INTRODUCTION

β-Lactams belong to a huge family of antibiotics. The main modes of resistance to β-lactams are modification of cell targets (penicillin-binding proteins), impermeability of the cell wall, efflux, and production of inactivating enzymes, the β-lactamases.

β-Lactamases are a complex family of enzymes, and currently more than 300 unique β-lactamases have been reported for gram-positive and gram-negative bacteria.

The discovery of β-lactam resistance occurred in 1940, when Abraham and Chain reported that an extract from a crushed strain of *Escherichia coli* inactivated benzylpenicillin. In 1944, Kirby emphasized the clinical significant of β-lactamase of *Staphylococcus aureus*. Rapidly it became apparent that a large variety of β-lactamases are produced by gram-negative bacteria. For instance, the first β-lactamase-producing strain of *Haemophilus influenzae* was reported in 1974 (Laufs et al., 1981).

The first clinical isolates of *Enterobacteriaceae* resistant to cefotaxime emerged in 1985 in France and Germany simultaneously, and then these isolates spread worldwide. In 1945, an anti-β-lactamase serum to fight against penicillin G inactivation was investigated, but the results were disappointing. In 1946, Reid described various organic compounds as β-lactamase inhibitors. In 1950, Behrens and Garrisson suggested that small molecules structurally related to benzylpenicillin might behave as substrate analogs and act as competitive β-lactamase inhibitors.

In 1956, Abraham and Newton validated this hypothesis by showing that cephalosporin C is able to inhibit β-lactamase from *Bacillus cereus*. In early 1960, methicillin and oxacillin were introduced in clinical practice. It was demonstrated that they are active as competitive inhibitors of β-lactamases produced by gram-negative bacteria. In 1960, the concept of combining a useful β-lactamase-susceptible antibiotic with a β-lactamase inhibitor was used in combining ampicillin with oxacillin in the treatment of urinary tract infection. This approach fell with the availability of cephems.

The discovery resulted in intensive research to find new β-lactamase inhibitors even if they were not useful in clinics due to the high level of inhibitor required.

In 1972, Cole et al. reported that more than 1,000 penicillin analogs had been tested as β-lactamase inhibitors and only a few molecules exhibited inhibitory activity; from these one was selected for further investigation, BRL-1437 (Fig. 1).

BRL-1437 is a potent inhibitor of cell free β-lactamases but unfortunately was ineffective as a synergistic antibacterial due to its poor bacterial cell wall penetration. In 1979, Brown et al. reported that olivanic acid compounds produced by *Streptomyces olivaceus* exhibited β-lactamase-inhibitory activities, but none were developed due to their poor ability to penetrate the bacterial cell wall.

In 1977, Reading and Cole reported the isolation of clavulanic acid from the fermentation broth of *Streptomyces clavuligerus*. The discovery of the first clinically useful compound was the starting point of intensive research resulting in the discovery of other compounds, such as sulbactam and tazobactam.

In 1980, a β-lactamase inhibitor with a non-β-lactam structure was isolated from a *Micromonospora* strain: izumenolide (Fig. 2).

Research on β-lactamases led to different classifications, one of which is the Ambler classification describing four classes: A, C, D (serine β-lactamases), and B (metalloprotease β-lactamases).

Currently the research in this field is mainly oriented towards broad-spectrum β-lactamase inhibitors covering all serine active-site β-lactamases (class A, class C, and class D), especially AmpC—enzymes, which have started to become a real problem in terms of resistance resulting in therapeutic failure. However, with the emergence of metallo-enzymes (CcrA, IMP-1, and class B), specific research is also directed in this field.

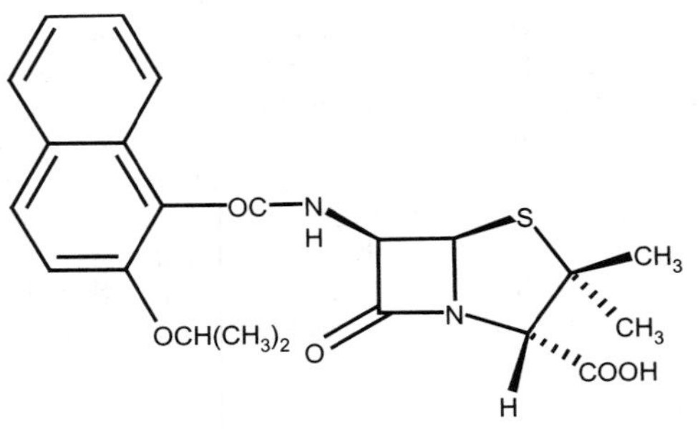

Figure 1 BRL-1437

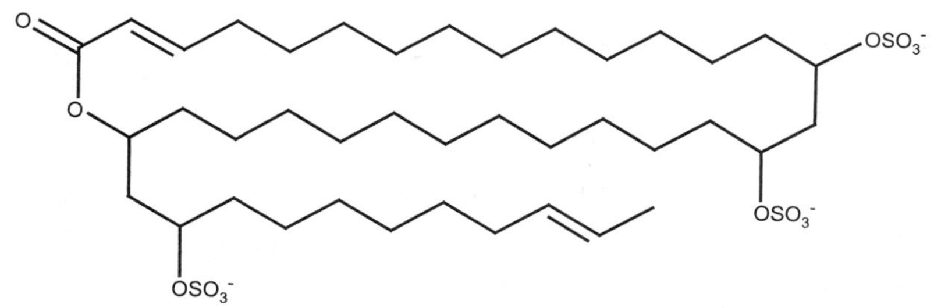

Figure 2 Izumenolide

2. ROLE OF β-LACTAMASES

In gram-positive bacteria, β-lactamases are secreted into the external medium and have been described for *S. aureus* and *Enterococcus faecium*. In gram-negative bacteria they are located in the periplasmic space.

β-Lactamases efficiently catalyze the irreversible hydrolysis of the amide bond of the β-lactam ring, yielding biologically inactive products.

Since the beginning of the β-lactam era, β-lactamases have played a double role: (i) as a source of β-lactam resistance and (ii) as an incentive for the development of new β-lactams.

There is not only emergence of new enzymes from class A β-lactamases but also an emergence of bacteria producing chromosomal or plasmid-mediated AmpC-type β-lactamases which result in resistance to all known cephems. These enzymes are especially prevalent in nosocomial gram-negative pathogens. The intensive use of carbapenems has resulted in spread of class B enzymes in *Pseudomonas aeruginosa*, *Stenotrophomonas maltophilia*, *Serratia* spp., etc.

Unfortunately, a new challenge is the emergence of a novel TEM-derived, plasmid-encoded β-lactamase resistant to inhibition by clavulanic acid.

3. RATIONALE FOR RESEARCH ON β-LACTAMASE INHIBITORS

The elimination of the problem of β-lactamase production or activity is essential to ensure the continuing clinical utility of β-lactams as antibacterial agents. The challenge is particularly important and difficult, since the plasmid- and transposon-mediated spread of β-lactamase genes both within and among bacterial species is a facile process. Unfortunately, there has been little advance in this field even if in recent years intensive research has been conducted. But none of the studies has resulted in the introduction of a suitable drug in the clinic.

To circumvent β-lactamase activity, two strategies have been commonly used:

- Chemical alteration of β-lactams leading to methicillin, oxacillin, or the 2-amino-5-thiazolyl cephems, and the C-3′ quaternary ammonium cephems (cefpirome and cefepime), cephamycins, and carbapenems
- Introduction of a β-lactamase inhibitor in combination with a partner such as amoxicillin, ampicillin, ticarcillin, piperacillin, and cefoperazone

Interest in combining relatively inert β-lactam derivatives in synergy with β-lactams was high because of the idea that the inert compound would bind competitively to the β-lactamase, thereby protecting the active substrate from hydrolysis.

4. CLASSIFICATIONS OF β-LACTAMASES AND RELATED INHIBITORS

β-Lactamase classification is complex, and many schemes have been published over half a century, making classification a little confusing for the nonspecialist. The first classification was based on biological activities: penicillinases and cephalosporinases. A more complex classification was subsequently proposed by Richmond and Sykes (1973), which was completed by a classification for gram-negative organisms by Sykes et al. A specific classification proposed by Mitsuhashi et al. (1981) is used in Japan.

Currently two classifications are used: that of Ambler and that of Bush et al.

Four classes have been described according to the Ambler classification: classes A, C, and D (serine β-lactamase) and B (metallo-β-lactamase). In Table 1 the two classifications are put in correspondence.

4.1. Class A Serine β-Lactamases

The most prevalent β-lactamases are those belonging to class A, such as PC from *S. aureus*, TEM-1 and -2 from *E. coli*, and TEM-1 and -2 and SHV-1 from *Klebsiella pneumoniae*. In class A (group 2be) a common feature is the spread of extended-spectrum β-lactamases (ESBL) such as CTX-M (Table 2).

The first β-lactamase inhibitors introduced in clinical practice are directed against class A β-lactamases such as TEM-1 or TEM-2 and SHV-1, found mainly in *K. pneumoniae* but also in other microorganisms, such as *E. coli*, *H. influenzae*, and *Moraxella catarrhalis*. These inhibitors are clavulanic acid and two penicillanic acid sulfones: sulbactam and tazobactam.

However, many other compounds have been described but for various reasons were not developed:

- Biphenyl tetrazole
- Thiols (SB 264218)
- Thiolesters (thiomandelic acid)

Class A β-lactamase inhibitors (e.g., co-amoxiclav) are active against ESBL, which are able to hydrolyze cefotaxime, ceftazidime, and aztreonam.

Table 1 Correspondence between classifications of Ambler and Bush et al.

Classification of Ambler	Classification of Bush et al.
Class A (TEM, SHV, PC, CTX-M)	Groups 2a, 2b, 2be, 2br, 2c, 2d, 2e, 2f
Class B (metalloenzymes)	Groups 3a, 3b, 3c
Class C (cephalosporinases)	Group 1
Class D (oxacillinases)	Group 4

Table 2 β-Lactamases of class A (classification of Bush et al.)

Classification	Preferred substrates	Enzyme(s)
2a	Penicillins	Penicillinases from gram-positive cocci
2b	Penicillins and cephems	TEM-1 (R-TEM), TEM-2, SHV-1
2be	Penicillins, narrow- and extended-spectrum cephems, monocyclic β-lactams	TEM-3 (CTX-1), TEM-4, TEM-5 (CAZ-1) to TEM-26, SHV-2 to SHV-6, CTX-M, *K. oxytoca* K1
2br	Penicillins	TEM-30 (IRT-2), TEM-31 (IRT-1) to TEM-37 (IRT-7), TRC-1
2c	Penicillins, carbenicillin	PSE-1, PSE-3, PSE-4
2e	Cephems	Inducible cephalosporinase from *P. vulgaris*
2f	Penicillins, cephems, carbapenems	NMCA (*Enterobacteriaceae*), Sme-1 (*S. marcescens*)

In 1993 in France, *E. coli* resistant to co-amoxiclav or sulbactam-ampicillin was reported. One explanation is the presence of an inhibitor-resistant enzyme of type TEM (IRT) or SHV. Since then, IRT has been described for *E. coli*, *Citrobacter freundii*, *K. pneumoniae*, *Klebsiella oxytoca*, *Proteus mirabilis*, *Enterobacter cloacae*, and *Shigella sonnei*. IRT-containing isolates remain susceptible to first-generation (narrow-spectrum) cephalosporins, cephamycins, and carbapenems.

4.2. Class B Metallo-β-Lactamases

Class B β-lactamases belong to group 1 of the family of zinc metallohydrolases, which is composed of 16 groups.

In class B, three subgroups have been described, B1, B2, and B3 (Table 3).

Many metallo-β-lactamases play a role in intrinsic resistance to β-lactams, and additionally some IMP or VIM β-lactamases are emerging worldwide as a source of acquired resistance to carbapenem in gram-negative bacteria.

IMP enzymes were first isolated in clinical isolates of *Serratia marcescens* and *P. aeruginosa*, but they have been also found in *K. pneumoniae*, *Alcaligenes* spp., *Acinetobacter* spp., and *Shigella* spp.

There are not yet available class B inhibitors in clinical usage, explaining partly the intensive research in this field. The first metalloenzyme inhibitor was directed against *B. cereus* BCII. It was a cyclic phosphonate.

A number of metalloenzyme inhibitors have been described:

- Biphenyl tetrazole
- Thiols (SB 264218)
- Thiolesters (thiomandelic acid)
- Trifluoromethyl alcohol
- α-Ketones
- Hydroxamates
- Penems
- Succinic acids
- Phosphates
- Phenazines

The discovery of broad class B inhibitors is difficult due to the functional architecture of the active site, which differs from one enzyme to another. Most of the research currently is directed against IMP-1 enzyme.

IMP-1 enzyme is a zinc β-lactamase that hydrolyzes all β-lactams except aztreonam. It is scattered in Enterobacteriaceae and *P. aeruginosa* isolates from Asia, Europe, and Canada.

Zinc-containing β-lactamases hydrolyze nearly all β-lactams, including clavulanic acid.

Sites of metallo-β-lactamases give to the enzyme the potential to bind two zinc(II) ions, although their affinities

Table 3 Class B β-lactamase classification

Subgroup	Active site	Microorganism	Enzyme
B1 (broad substrate profile)	Site 1: His116, His118, His196 Site 2: Asp120, Cys221, His263	*Chryseobacterium meningosepticum*	BLAB
		Chryseobacterium indologenes	IND-1, -2, -3
		B. cereus	BCII
		B. fragilis	CcrA (cfiA)
		P. aeruginosa	IMP-1 to VIM-1 to -3
		Chryseobacterium gleum	CGB1
		Empedobacter brevis	EBR-1
		Flavobacterium johnsoniae	John-1
B2 (efficiently hydolyze only carbapenems)	Site 1: Asn116, His118, His196 Site 2: Asp120, Cys221, His263	*A. hydrophila*	CphA, Cph2
		Aeromonas sobria	Imi S
		Serratia fonticola	Sfh1
B3 (broad spectrum, mainly directed against cephems)	Site 1: His116, His118, His196 Site 2: His121, Ser221, His263	*S. maltophilia*	L1
		C. meningosepticum	GOB1
		Janthinobacterium lividum	THIN1
		Flueribacter gormanii	FEZ 1

for the zinc could be quite different. *B. cereus* has two binding sites for zinc(II), of low and a high affinities, whereas *Bacteroides fragilis* and *S. maltophilia* present two high-affinity binding sites for zinc(II).

4.3. Class C Serine β-Lactamases

Class C enzymes are either chromosomally or plasmid encoded. Under normal conditions class C enzymes produced by gram-negative bacteria are repressed. The chromosomally encoded enzymes are produced mainly by *C. freundii*, *E. cloacae*, *Enterobacter aerogenes*, *Morganella morganii*, *S. marcescens*, and *P. aeruginosa* and to some extent by *E. coli*. Plasmids encoding class C β-lactamases have been discovered worldwide, mainly in *K. pneumoniae* (MIR-1, CMY-1, FOX-1, and MOX-1) and to a lesser extent in *E. coli* and other *Enterobacteriaceae*. A dendrogram of chromosomal and plasmid-encoded class C enzymes shows the diversity of genes and relationship of some plasmid-mediated enzymes to some chromosomal enzymes. The dendrogram of group C β-lactamases can be divided into at least five or six clusters (Table 4).

Chromosomally encoded class C β-lactamases rapidly degrade cephalosporins, and available β-lactamase inhibitors do not inhibit them. Ceftazidime and other cephems are stable against AmpC enzyme hydrolysis due to their bulky R_1 side chain, making unfavorable interactions with the enzyme, especially with the Val211 and Tyr221 residues. To relieve their interactions these β-lactams rotate into a conformation that blocks formation of the deacylation high-energy intermediate. Class C enzymes achieve their activity by increasing the size of the active site, allowing cephems to relax into a catalytically competent conformation. Numerous compounds are active against class C enzymes, while some are active against both class A and class C enzymes.

A nonrestrictive list of potential molecules against class C enzymes follows:

- BRL-42715
- Rhodamines
- Penicillanic acid sulfones
- Boronic acid
- α-Keto heterocycles

4.4. Class D Serine β-Lactamases

The OXA-type enzymes have been reported for *Enterobacteriaceae* and *P. aeruginosa*. OXA-type β-lactamases hydrolyze benzylpenicillin, oxacillin, methicillin, and, in some cases, 2-amino-5-thiazolyl cephems, C-3′ quaternary ammonium cephems, and carbapenems (OXA-23, -24, -25, -26, and -27). They are resistant to inhibition by P-CMB and susceptible to chlorine anion.

The OXA-10 β-lactamase X-ray structure became available recently. This enzyme has an uncommon lysine carbamate (carboxylate lysine) in its active site (lysine carbamate 70). The carboxylated lysine should be the residue that promotes acylation of the active-site serine by the substrate. These β-lactamases are weakly inhibited by clavulanic acid.

Table 4 Class C β-lactamase clusters[a]

Cluster and/or source	Enzyme(s)
C. freundii	AmpC chromosomal β-lactamase of *C. freundii*; BIL-1, CMY-2 to -7, LAT-1, LAT-2
Enterobacter	P99, MIR-1, ACT-1
M. morganii	DHA-1, DHA-2
Aeromonas	CMY-1-8-9, FOX-1 to -5, MOX-1 and -2
P. aeruginosa	Chromosomal β-lactamase
Hafnia alvei	ACC-1

[a]Data from Philippon et al., 2002.

5. β-LACTAMASE INHIBITORS

In the clinical setting there are only three drugs available: clavulanic acid, sulbactam, and tazobactam. In contrast, in research hundreds of molecules have been tested. β-Lactamase inhibitors can be divided globally into two groups: β-lactams and non-β-lactams (Fig. 3).

5.1. Inhibitors with β-Lactam Structures

The first natural inhibitor was reported in 1948 and named notalysine by Hatter and colleagues. This compound was produced by *Penicillium* spp., including *Penicillium notatum*.

Many compounds have been obtained either by screening of natural products or by semisynthesis. A nonexhaustive list of compounds follows:

- Clavulanic acid
- Penicillanic acid (brobactam)
- Penicillanic acid sulfones (sulbactam and tazobactam)
- Cephem sulfones
- Alkylidene cephems
- Penems and carbapenems
- Oxa-1-penem (AM-112)
- Monocyclic β-lactams
- Bridged β-lactams
- Codrugs

5.2. Clavulanic Acid and Derivatives

Clavulanic acid and four analogs possessing the oxa-1-penam ring have been isolated from fermentation of *S. clavuligerus* ATCC 27064. Only clavulanic acid has been shown to inhibit β-lactamases.

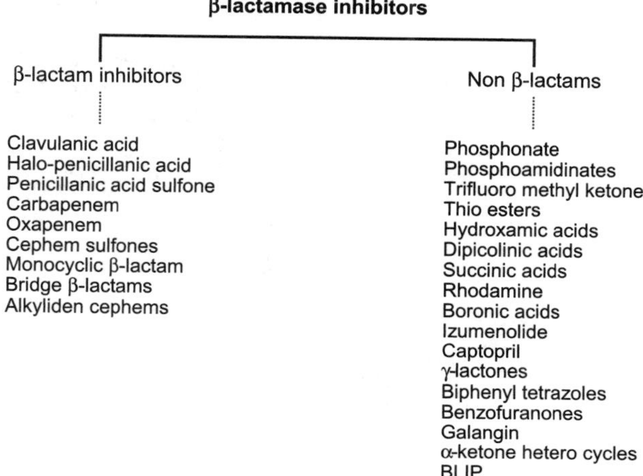

Figure 3 Classification of β-lactamase inhibitors

Since the extraction in 1976 of clavulanic acid (Fig. 4), many compounds have been obtained from natural sources. Derivatives of clavulanic acid have been obtained from the fermentation broth of *Streptomyces antibioticus* subsp. *antibioticus* Tü 1718 (Fig. 5).

Unfortunately, not all of these derivatives exhibit anti-β-lactamase activities; for instance, Ro-22-5417 acts as an inhibitor of methionine synthesis.

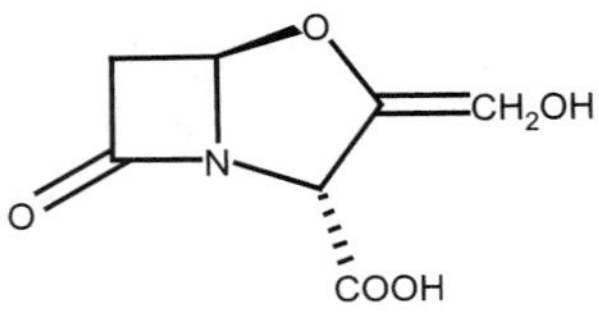

Figure 4 Clavulanic acid

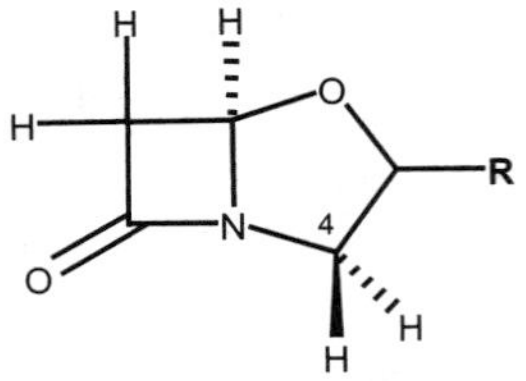

	R	C_4
Clavam-2 carboxylic acid	–COOH	H
2-hydroxy methyl clavam	$-CH_2OH$	H
2-formyl oxymethyl clavam	$CH_2O{-}C(=O){-}H$	H
β-hydroxy-propionyl clavulanic acid	$CH_2O{-}C(=O){-}CH_2CH_2OH$	COOH

Figure 5 Clavam derivatives

A number of compounds of this medicinal chemical class have been prepared to explore the structure-activity relationship. It was shown that (i) the lack of the C-4 carboxylic group does not eliminate the β-lactamase inhibitory activity and (ii) a catalytic group at position 2 enhances the inhibitory activity 4 to 10 times.

Alterations of clavulanic acid were performed by replacing the C-2 hydroxyl group with a variety of triazolyl-substituted rings. Some of them show a slight improvement in activity over clavulanic acid (Fig. 6).

A number of substituted amidoethenylthio derivatives and their corresponding sulfoxides have been synthesized.

Clavulanic acid acts as a suicide substrate and efficiently acylates most class A β-lactamases. The compound fails to inactivate the DD-peptidases. The guanidinium moiety of clavulanic acid anchors a molecule of water, which serves as the source of a critical proton.

The resistance to clavulanic acid may be due to the alteration of Asp244. Class C β-lactamases are not inhibited by clavulanic acid, due probably to a poor recognition resulting in an inefficient acylation.

Clavulanic acid and few analogs possessing the oxa-1-penam ring have been isolated from the fermentation of *S. clavuligerus* ATCC 27064. Only clavulanic acid has been shown to inhibit β-lactamases.

The conversion of clavulanic acid into endocyclic double-bond isomers yields high activity against class C β-lactamases, such as P99 (Fig. 7 and Table 5), whereas clavulanic acid has low activity against these β-lactamases.

5.3. Penicillanic Acid Derivatives

Since the beginning of the penicillin era, penicillanic acids were shown to have β-lactamase-inhibitory activity. It was shown by Cole et al. that analogs having a phenyl, naphthyl, and quinolyl moiety at C-6 position especially substituted with an alkoxy side chain were potent β-lactamase inhibitors. One of them was selected for further investigation: BRL-1437 (Fig. 8).

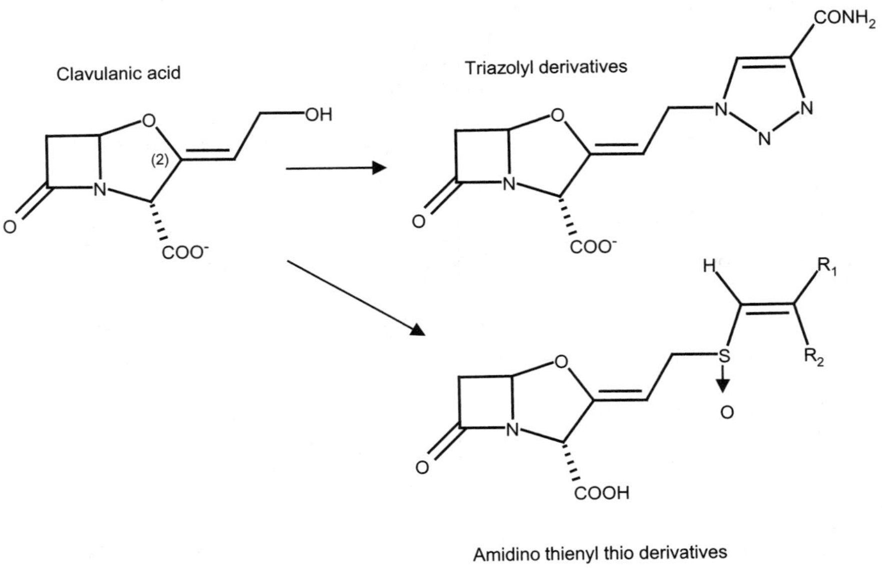

Clavulanic acid

Triazolyl derivatives

Amidino thienyl thio derivatives

Figure 6 Clavulanic derivatives

BRL 20780

BRL 19378

Figure 7 Analogs of clavulanic acid

5.3.1. BRL-1437

BRL-1437 (2-isopropoxy-1-naphthyl) penicillanic acid is a semisynthetic penicillanic derivative. It was found that the ketone functionality was important after the initial acylation reaction. A nucleophilic imine residue in the active site of the enzyme can further react with the keto group to yield a cross-linked iminium acyl-enzyme, which is a stable inactivated enzyme.

Similar properties were found when the acetyl group was replaced by a CN. However, the compound was poorly active or devoid of activity when tested against the whole bacterial cell due to its chemical instability. The chemical stability was improved by reducing the 6-exocyclic double bond, but the inhibitory activity was lost. This activity may be regained by converting the sulfide into a sulfone. The therapeutic use of BRL-1437 was limited due to poor oral absorption (Greenwood and O'Grady, 1975).

5.3.2. Halo Penicillanic Acids

Semisynthetic penicillanic derivatives such as halo penicillanic acid sulfones were designed to mimic the mechanism of enzyme inactivation observed with clavulanic acid.

In this chemical class, halo penicillanic acids were extensively explored. All of them exhibit weak antibacterial activity, but some have potential as β-lactamase inhibitors. The 6α and 6β mono- and bisubstituted compounds have been prepared bearing either a chlorine, a bromine (brobactam), or an iodine atom.

The sulfur state was changed by oxidation of a sulfide to a sulfoxide or a sulfone. The 6α-chloro penicillanic acid sulfone was the most active derivative, but unfortunately it was less active than sulbactam.

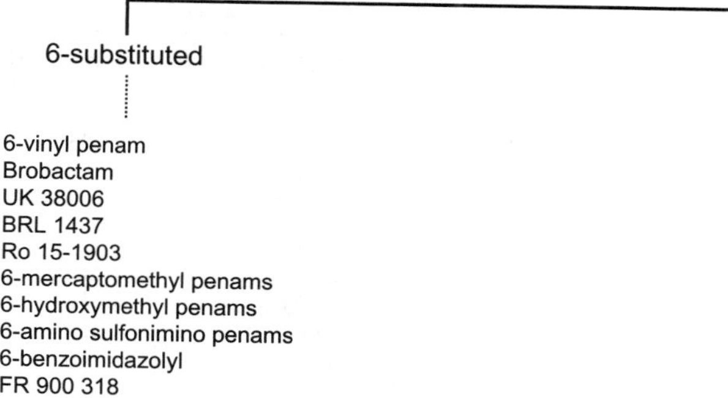

Figure 8 Penicillanic acid derivatives

The 6β-iodo derivatives display activity almost similar to that of sulbactam.

The stereochemistry at position 6 is an important factor. Usually the 6β halo analogs are more potent inhibitors of β-lactamases than the 6α derivative counterparts.

The 6-halo penams exhibit low antibacterial activity, with the exception of activity against *Neisseria* spp.

5.3.2.1. Brobactam

Brobactam (Fig. 9) is a 6-bromo penam partly developed in combination with pivampicillin (2085P) (Neu, 1983).

Brobactam was more active than clavulanic acid (Table 6) against various enzymes, including those of class C.

The combination 2085P is efficiently absorbed from the gastrointestinal tract, and after enzymatic hydrolysis of the pivaloyloxymethyl ester group, 2085P is released in the blood as ampicillin and brobactam in an approximate ratio of 3:1. The main parameters in healthy adult volunteers are shown in Table 7.

In murine infections (intraperitoneal), 2085P was more active than co-amoxiclav (Table 8).

5.3.2.2. UK-38006

UK-38006 is the 6β-iodo penicillanic acid. UK-38006 (Fig. 10) has no antibacterial activity. This compound is able to inactivate class C as well as class A and class D enzymes.

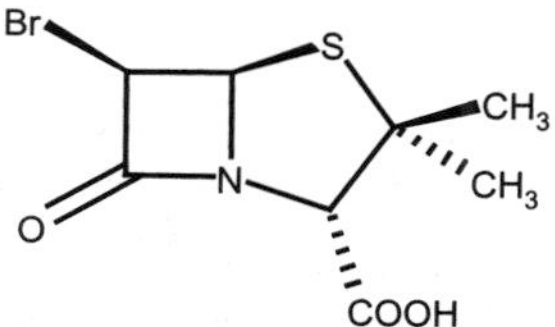

Figure 9 Brobactam

Table 5 Inhibitory activities of clavulanic acid derivatives

Compound	IC$_{50}$ (μg/ml)					
	E. coli JT4	*E. aerogenes* E70	*P. mirabilis* C889	*E. cloacae* P99	*P. aeruginosa*	*S. aureus* Russel
Clavulanic acid	0.07	0.015	0.03	115	>40	0.06
BRL-20780	0.2	3.6	<0.08	>40	>40	<0.08
BRL-19378	0.18	6.5	4.0	0.16	0.18	0.11

Table 6 Inhibitory activity of brobactam

Organism	Enzyme	IC_{50} (μM)	
		Brobactam	Clavulanic acid
E. coli	TEM-1	0.008	0.01
	SHV-1	0.008	0.005
	OXA-1	0.25	0.1
	OXA-2	0.005	10
	OXA-3	0.63	1.6
	HMS	0.32	0.013
	TEM-2	0.005	0.016
E. cloacae	C	0.59	6.6
	C	0.68	11
	C	0.32	7.9
	C	0.45	3.5
C. freundii	C	0.25	13
P. vulgaris	C	0.008	0.05
M. morganii	C	0.028	6

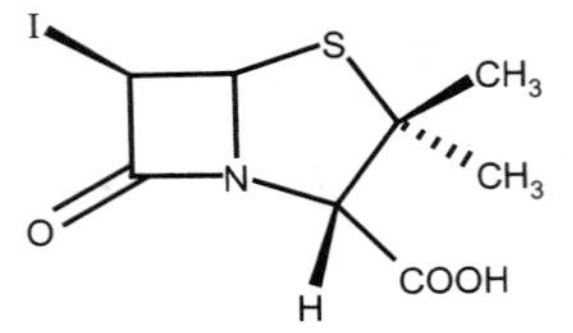

Figure 10 UK-38006

Table 9 Inhibitory activity of UK-38006

Organism	Class	Enzyme	IC_{50} (μg/ml)[a]	
			No preincubation	Incubation
E. coli	C		11.4	0.88
K. aerogenes	A	K1	15.7	0.14
E. coli	A	TEM	0.31	0.013
E. coli	D	OXA-1	0.88	0.013
S. aureus	A	PC-1	>160	0.39

[a]Nitrocefin.

However, it is less active than clavulanic acid (Table 9) (Moore and Brammer, 1981).

Combinations with ampicillin significantly decreased MICs for *H. influenzae*, *S. aureus*, *Neisseria gonorrhoeae*, and methicillin-resistant *S. aureus* (MRSA) but were ineffective against *P. aeruginosa*.

UK-38006 synergized effectively with piperacillin and mezlocillin and less with cephalothin. UK-38006 potentialized ampicillin in vivo.

5.3.3. Other Derivatives

Recently a new series of derivatives having a mercaptomethyl side chain or a hydroxymethyl moiety at positions C-6 has been reported (Fig. 11). All of them are inactive, with MICs above 128 μg/ml, but all of the 6-mercaptomethyl analogs exhibit good inhibitory activity against metallo-β-lactamases L1 and BCII. In contrast, the C-6 hydroxymethyl analogs have no activity against class B enzymes.

The oxidation (sulfone) of the sulfur atom does not affect the anti-class B activities of these analogs.

The mercaptomethyl penicillanic acid sulfones inhibit both class A and class B enzymes.

A series of benzoimidazolyl hydroxy derivatives has been prepared, and many of them are potent β-lactamase inhibitors (Fig. 12).

A series of S-aminosulfenimines at position C-6 has been reported (Fig. 13) which exhibits moderate inhibitory activity. The *N*-carboethoxy-*S*-aminosulfenimine penam sulfone is a strong inhibitor of *B. cereus* BCI. It is more active than sulbactam.

Table 7 2085P pharmacokinetics[a]

Dose (mg)[a]	C_{max} (μg/ml)		T_{max} (min)		AUC (μg·h/ml)		Urinary elimination (%)	
	AMP	BPA	AMP	BPA	AMP	BPA	AMP	BPA
250, Fasting	4.11	1.38	44	51	7.41	2.4	62.5	50.2
500, Fasting	6.83	2.67	58	66	14.35	4.9	57.2	49
500, Fed	6.73	2.51	55	65	16.13	5.62	61.1	51.8
1,000	10.65	3.56	67	75	30.56	10.44	60.3	48.3

[a]AMP, ampicillin; BPA, brobactam.

Table 8 In vivo activity of 2085P in comparison with co-amoxiclav

Microorganism	MIC (μg/ml)		PD_{50}[a] (mg/kg)	
	2085P	Co-amoxiclav	2085P	Co-amoxiclav
S. aureus CJ8	2.1	20	18	32
E. coli HA 159	66	63	112	186
K. pneumoniae HE 34	4.2	4.0	39	52
M. morganii H352	33	>250	148	>313
P. mirabilis HJ34	8.3	16	83	274

[a]PD_{50}, 50% protective dose.

Figure 11 6-Hydroxymethyl penems

Figure 12 Benzoimidazolyl penams

Table 10 Inhibitory activity of benzoimidazolyl hydroxy penam

Compound	R_1	Enzyme inhibition (%)	
		S. aureus	*E. coli*
A	H	95	57
B	CH_3	96	72
C	C_2H_5	93	33
D	Propionyl	88	58
G	$CH=CH_2$	100	86
K	CH_2CH_2OH	85	43
L	CH_2CH_2F	82	51
M	$CH_2CH_2OCH_3$	93	61
N	Δ	78	23
S	CH_2COOH	62	24
T	CH_2OCHBu	92	40
W	Phenyl	93	95
Clavulanic acid		85	81
Sulbactam		46	40

Figure 13 *N*-Carboxy-*S*-aminosulfenimino penicillinate

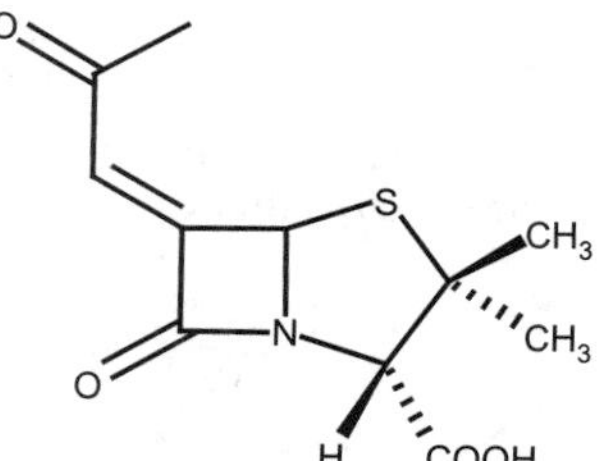

Figure 14 Ro-15-1903

A series of benzoimidazolyl hydroxy penams showing potent inhibitory activity against β-lactamases (Table 10) has been reported.

5.3.4. Ro-15-903

Ro-15-903 (Fig. 14 and 15) (Adam et al., 1986) is the 6-acethylmethylene penicillanic acid. It is active against AmpC enzymes.

5.4. Penicillanic Acid Sulfones

Since the discovery of sulbactam, various penicillanic acid sulfones with different functionalities at positions C-2α, C-2β, and C-6 have been designed and studied extensively as potential β-lactamase inhibitors (Fig. 16 and 17).

5.4.1. Sulbactam Analogs

Sulbactam has low oral bioavailability. For this reason extensive research was undertaken to enhance the oral absorption by fixing on the C-4 carboxylic group a lipophilic double ester, such as pivoxil.

Sultamicillin (combination of sulbactam and ampicillin) partially solved the pharmacokinetic problems.

Another ester was proposed but was not developed: KB-2585 (Fig. 18).

5.4.2. Tazobactam Derivatives

Tazobactam is the 2-β-substituted sulbactam (Fig. 19) with a tetrazolyl moiety.

The 2α-isomer of tazobactam was prepared (Fig. 20). In cell extracts the inhibitory activity was comparable to that of tazobactam against TEM-2.

Ro 15-1903

Figure 15 Reactivity of Ro-15-1903

Penicillanic acid sulfones

- C-6-substituted
  - Triazolyl penams
  - CL 186 195
  - CL 186 369
  - Nitrile oxidomethyl penams
  - Sulfoamido penams
  - S-aminosulfenimino penams
  - GD-40
  - 6-spirocyclopropyl derivatives
- C-6 and C-2 substituted
  - 6-halo-2-halo penams
- C-2 substituted
  - 2α
    - Tazobactam derivatives
    - Methylene penam
  - 2β
    - Sulbactam
    - Tazobactam
    - Ro 48-1220
    - Methylene penam
    - Acrylonitrile penam

Figure 16 Classification of penicillanic acid sulfones

Figure 17 Chemical modifications of penicillanic acid sulfones

Figure 19 Tazobactam

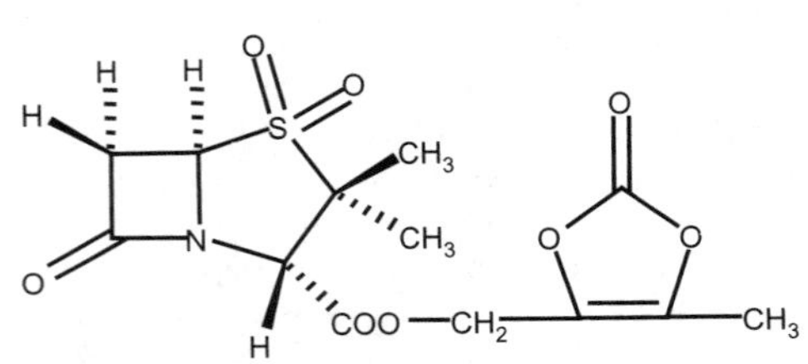

Figure 18 KB-2585

5.4.3. Other Penicillanic Sulfone Derivatives

The chemical structures of penicillanic acid sulfones under research are very complex. Three subgroups of compounds can be identified (Fig. 21).

Those having a substituent at the C-6α or C-6β position compose the first group, those having a substituent at the C-2α or C-2β position compose the second group, and the third group is composed of compounds having a substitution

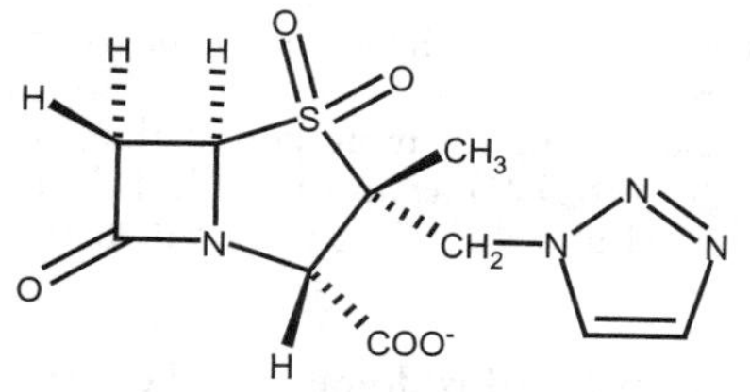

Figure 20 2α-Isomer of tazobactam

at both sides of the molecule core. Some compounds are able to inhibit class A and class C β-lactamases.

5.4.3.1. C-6 Substituted Penicillanic Acid Sulfone Derivatives

5.4.3.1.1. Ro-48-1220. Ro-48-1220 is a (Z)-2-β-acrylonitrile penam sulfone (Fig. 22) (Tzouvelekis et al., 1997). It is a potent inhibitor of group 2b (TEM-1 and -2 and SHV-1) and group 2be (extended-spectrum) β-lactamases. It is as active as clavulanic acid but exerts a higher activity than tazobactam (Table 11).

Against ESBL, Ro-48-1220 (4 μg) restored activity of ceftriaxone and to a lesser extent that of ceftazidime. In combination with both cephems, Ro-48-1220 restored activity for class C enzymes (Table 12).

Ro-48-1220 is more potent than sulbactam and clavulanic acid.

5.4.3.1.2. CL-186195. Novel isoxazolinyl penam sulfones exhibited good inhibitory activity against P99 and class B (CcrA) enzymes. They are activated by phosphate buffer, unlike penam sulfones that have been described previously (Yamaguchi et al., 1985).

Compounds CL-186195 and CL-186659 (Fig. 23) were able to inactivate the metallo-β-lactamases from *B. fragilis*, although the sulfones were shown to behave like poor substrates at low concentrations. Both act synergistically with piperacillin against *E. cloacae* P99 and *E. coli* CcrA but not against *E. coli* TEM-1.

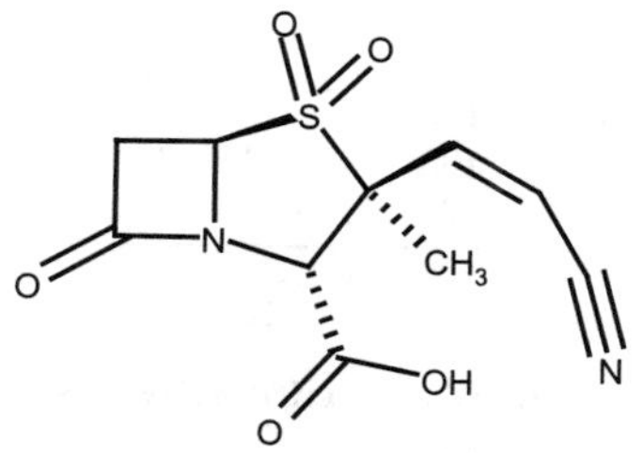

Figure 22 Ro-48-1220

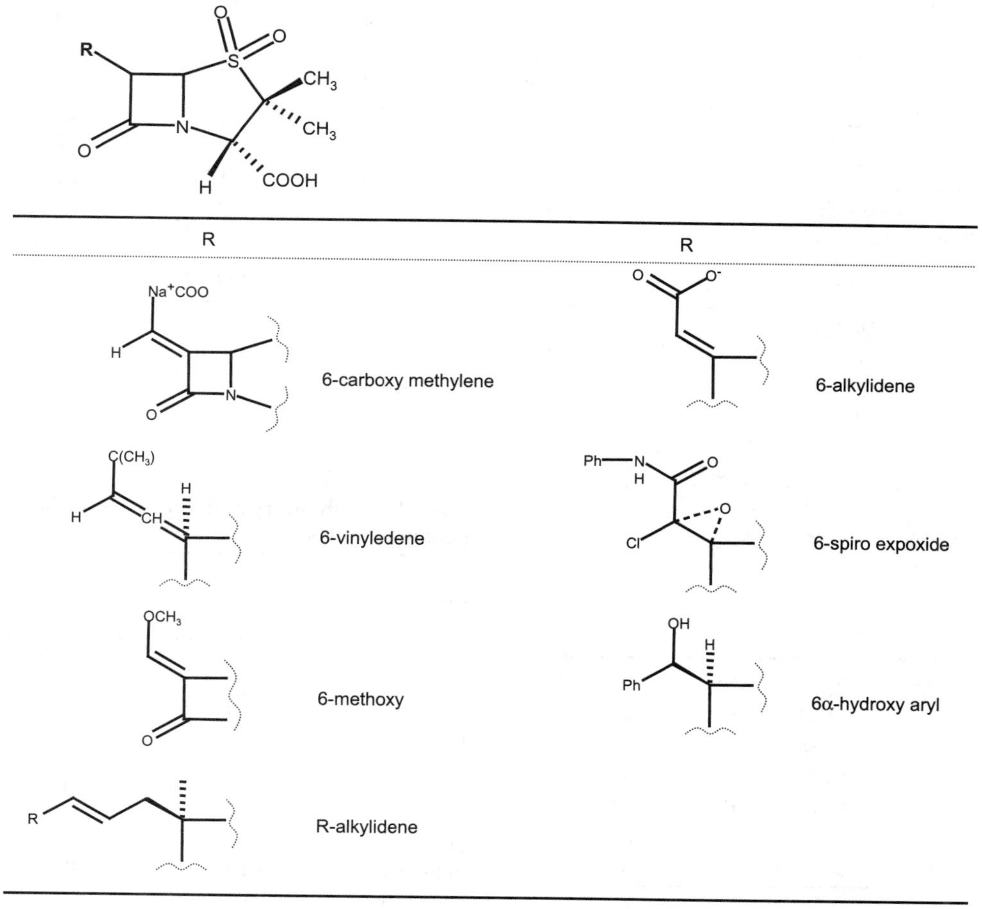

Figure 21 C-6-substituted penam sulfones

Table 11 IC_{50}s of Ro-48-1220 for various β-lactamases

Enzyme	IC_{50} (μM)		
	Clavulanic acid	Tazobactam	Ro-48-1220
TEM-1	0.01	0.05	0.08
TEM-2	0.2	0.09	0.08
TEM-3	0.04	0.04	0.04
TEM-10	0.02	0.02	0.06
TEM-26	0.03	0.03	0.03
TEM-28	0.04	0.02	0.08
SHV-1	0.05	0.24	0.27
SHV-2	0.05	0.18	0.40
SHV-5	0.02	0.10	0.16
MIR-1	>100	9	0.5
LAT-1	>100	13	0.8
C. freundii C	>100	12	0.7
E. cloacae C	>100	10	0.6
E. aerogenes C	>100	12	1.2
S. marcescens C	>100	26	1.7
P. aeruginosa C	>100	10	0.5

It has been shown that the stereochemistry at position 5′ of the isoxazolinyl moiety is important. In the case of CL-186195 the *S*-isomer is more potent than the *R*-isomer counterpart (CL-186194) against metallo-β-lactamases.

The 3-thienyl and 4-tolyl contributed to the inhibitory activity.

5.4.3.1.3. 6-Nitriloxidomethyl Penam Sulfones. Molecular-modelling studies with several β-lactamase structures revealed that there is ample space in the active site to accommodate larger substituents at the C-6 position. A suitable side chain may slow the hydrolysis of the β-lactam nucleus and thereby increase the inhibitory activity.

Several research groups have introduced an isoxazolyl ring via a methylene bridge.

Substitution at the level of the isoxazole ring may increase the inhibitory activity against CcrA enzyme (class B). It was also shown that the β isomer is more active than the α isomer (compound C versus compound D) (Table 13 and Fig. 24).

5.4.3.1.4. 6-Sulfoamido penicillanic sulfone derivatives. It was suggested that the introduction of an

Table 12 In vitro activities of Ro-48-1220 in combination with cephems against class C enzymes

Strain[a]	Enzyme	MIC (μg/ml)[b]			
		CRO	CRO + Ro	CAZ	CAZ + Ro
E. coli C600	LAT-1	16	0.5	32	0.5
C. freundii 56 I	C	1.0	<0.5	1.0	<0.5
C. freundii 56 D	C	64	4.0	128	4.0
E. cloacae 473 I	C	1.0	<0.5	2.0	<0.5
E. cloacae 473 D	C	128	4.0	64	4.0
E. aerogenes 27 I	C	2.0	1.0	2.0	0.5
E. aerogenes 27 D	C	32	2.0	64	4.0
S. marcescens 40 I	C	1.0	<0.5	1.0	0.5
S. marcescens 40 D	C	16	1.0	16	1.0
P. aeruginosa 160 I	C			2.0	1.0
P. aeruginosa 160 D	C			128	2.0
P. aeruginosa R43 D	C			128	8.0

[a]I, inducible; D, derepressed.
[b]CRO, ceftriaxone; Ro, Ro-48-1220; CAZ, ceftazidime.

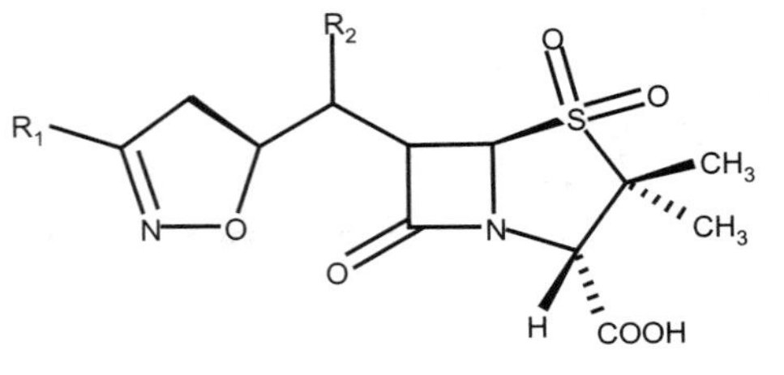

Compound	CL	R_1	R_2	IC_{50} (μM)
186 194		4-tolyl	H	2.0
186 195		4-tolyl	H	1.7
186 659		4-tolyl	OAc	3.9
186 325		C_2H_5	H	7.7
186 395		Br	H	2.4
186 369		3-thienyl	H	3.5

Figure 23 Isoxazoline sulfones (metalloenzymes)

Table 13 Inhibitory activities of 6-nitriloxidomethyl penam sulfones

Compound	IC_{50} (μM)		
	TEM-1	CcrA	AmpC
A	3.8	4.3	7.1
B	2.3	25	53
C	0.31	1.4	6.3
D	0.003	6.3	4.8
E	1.0	6.0	0.86
F	20	0.37	9.8
G	0.66	2.2	2.5
H	27	0.33	5.1
Sulbactam	1.4	>400	66
Tazobactam	0.06	>400	48

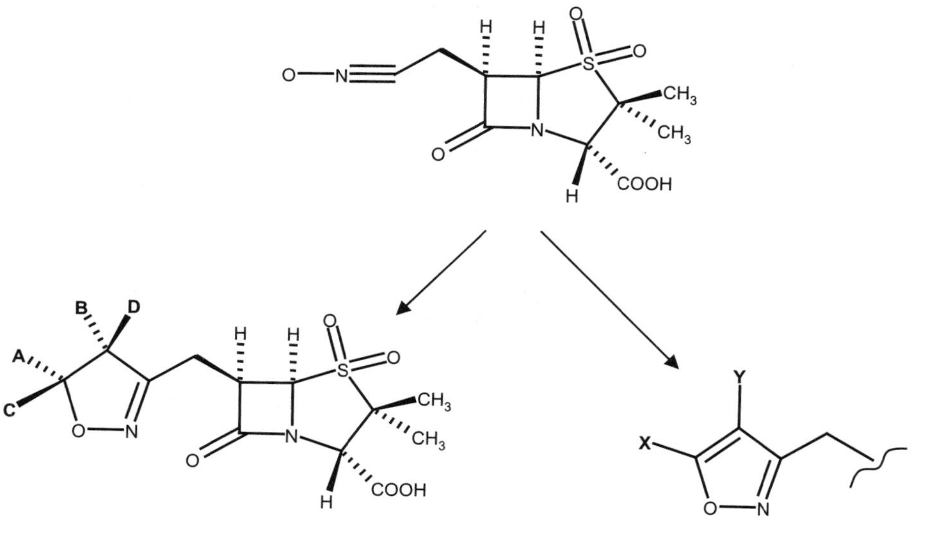

	A	B	C	D
Compound A	$COOCH_3$	H	H	H
Compound B	H	H	$COOCH_3$	H
Compound C	SO_2Ph	H	H	H
Compound D	S-Ph	H	H	H

	X	Y
Compound E	$COOCH_3$	H
Compound F	H	SO_2Tol
Compound G	COPh	H

Figure 24 6-Nitriloxido-methyl penam sulfones

electron-withdrawing group in the amino group of 6β-amino penicillanic acid would increase the acidity of the 6α-hydrogen atom, leading to a faster formation of a β-amino acrylate system. Several series of compounds have been synthesized, and the most promising derivative was the 6β-trifluoromethylene sulfamido penicillanic acid sulfone, which inhibits the *B. cereus* BCII (569/H) β-lactamase. Several similar compounds were prepared which also exhibited good inhibitory properties (Fig. 25).

5.4.3.1.4.1. FR-900318. FR-900318 (Fig. 26) is a 6-sulfoamino penicillanic acid sulfone which was isolated from the fermentation broth of *Aspergillus candidus*. This compound is inactive against gram-positive cocci and bacilli (MICs, ≥250 μg/ml) and gram-negative bacilli (MICs, ≥1,000 μg/ml). FR-900318 exhibits weak inhibitory activity against class 2b β-lactamases, less than sulbactam (Yamashita et al., 1983).

5.4.3.1.4.2. 6β-Cysteine sulfamido penam sulfones. The β amino acrylate is a common intermediate through which proceeds inhibition of β-lactamases by sulbactam and related compounds.

In a series of 6β-aryl or alkyl sulfamido penam sulfones (Fig. 27), it was shown that some analogs exhibited inhibitory activity against β-lactamases and a synergy of action with ampicillin.

5.4.3.1.4.3. 6β Hydroxyalkyl penicillinoic sulfones. A new 6β-hydroxyalkyl penicillanic acid sulfone was disclosed (Cohen et al., 2004). This compound in combination with amoxicillin is more active than tazobactam against broad-spectrum β-lactamases of respiratory pathogens. In vivo, in murine disseminated infections, the combination of penicillin-sulfone and amoxicillin restored in vivo efficacy

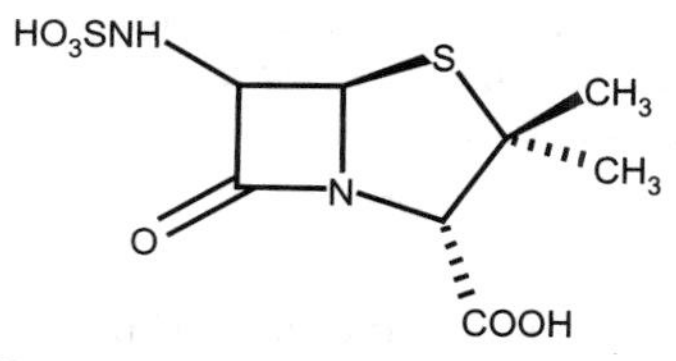

Figure 26 FR-900318

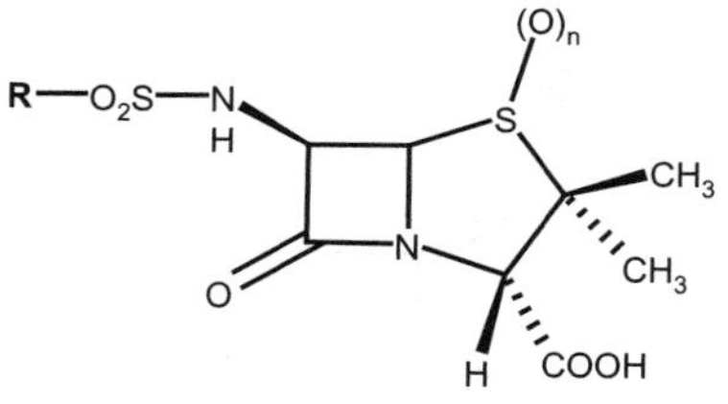

Figure 25 6β-Sulfamido penicillanic acid sulfones

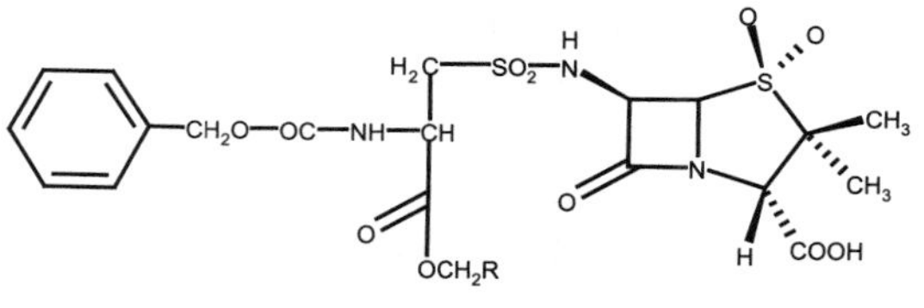

Figure 27 6β-Cysteine sulfonamido penicillanic acid sulfones

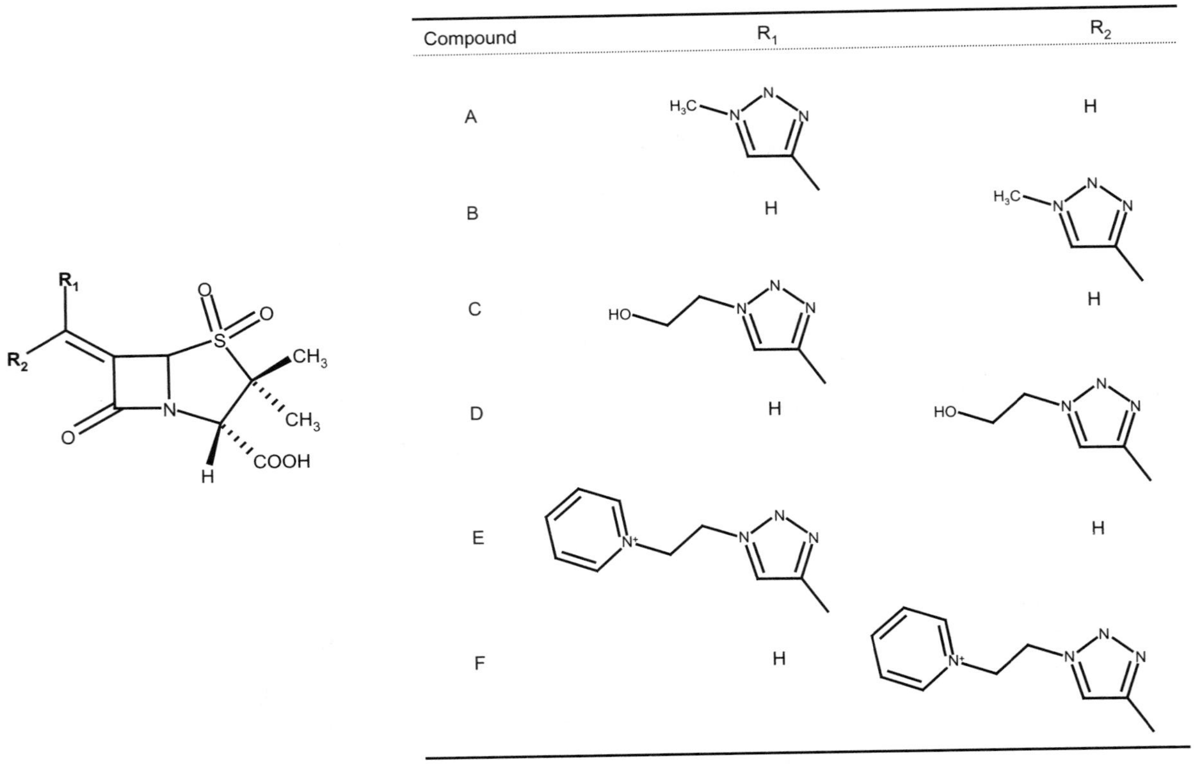

Figure 28 Triazolyl penam sulfones

against *H. influenzae* and *M. catarrhalis* producing broad-spectrum β-lactamases.

5.4.3.1.5. 6-Heterocyclic derivatives. A number of 6-heteroaryl substituted methylene penams have been reported in the literature or in patents as potent inhibitors of β-lactamases. Many of them are ineffective in synergism tests due to impermeability problems.

A series of triazolyl penam sulfones (Fig. 28) has been synthesized. They differ in the N_1 substituent. Six analogs with various groups have been tested, as well as two isomeric types for each of them. They are devoid of both antibacterial activity and inhibitory activity against *B. cereus* BCI. Only a few of them displayed inhibitory activity against R-TEM of *E. coli* (class 2b, TEM-1) as well as against *E. cloacae* class C enzyme. This is reported for compounds A, C, and E in Table 14.

Table 14 Inhibitory activities of 6-triazolyl penam sulfones

Compound	IC$_{50}$ (μM)		
	BCI	R-TEM	C
A	>20	0.2	0.7
B	>20	>20	>20
C	>20	0.34	0.4
D	>100	>200	>20
E	20	0.11	21
F	>100	>100	1.5
Tazobactam	0.31	0.076	2.4
Sulbactam	23	4.9	20

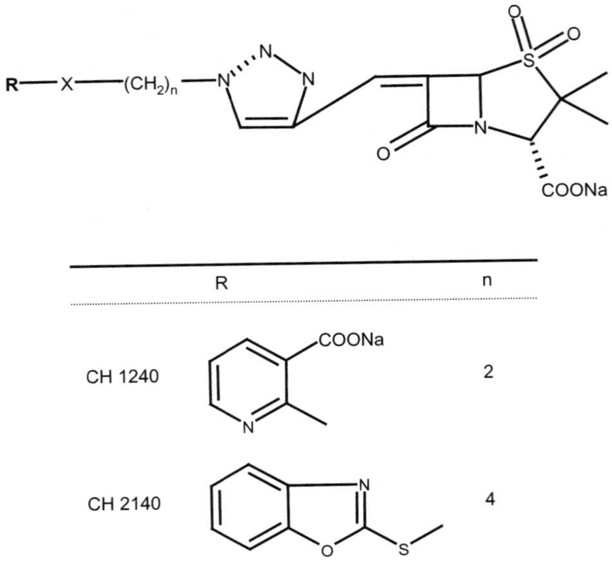

Against R-TEM they are less active than tazobactam but more active than sulbactam. In combination with ampicillin these compounds are less active than tazobactam.

These exomethyl derivatives, such as CH-1240 and CH-2140 (Fig. 29), were tested in vivo in experimental infections due to *P. aeruginosa* in mice. The combination of CH-1240 and cefoperazone did not provide protection. Protection was better in infection due to *E. coli* 3457E and *Citrobacter diversus* 2046E in mice when CH-1240 was used

Figure 29 CH-1240 and CH-2140

in combination with either ampicillin or amoxicillin (Park et al., 1998).

5.4.3.1.6. Other 6-side chains of penam sulfones. A variety of residues have been fixed at the C-6 position (Fig. 30).

The 6-carboxymethylene derivatives exhibited a broad spectrum of inhibitory activity, including partially irreversible inhibitory activity against β-lactamase of *E. cloacae* P99.

The 6-vinylidene analogs, especially the *tert*-butyl derivative, were found to be potent inhibitors of class C enzyme, especially for P99 of *E. cloacae*.

The 6-methoxymethylene derivative was only active on the cell free enzyme, and development was stopped for this reason.

Introduction of an αβ unsaturated system via a methylene bridge at position C-6 gave rise to compounds having inhibitory activity against TEM-1 and AmpC. For some molecules possessing a side chain with a $COCH_3$ or $COOCH_3$, potent inhibition of metalloenzyme (CcrA, with a 50% inhibitory concentration [IC_{50}] of 3.0 or 1.4 μM, respectively) was seen.

The 6α-alkylidene series (Fig. 31) gave rise to some compounds having IC_{50}s of 45 nM against P99 enzymes and 120 nM against TEM-2 β-lactamases.

Following an initial intramolecular attack of the carboxylic group on the imine, the double bond is isomerized, leading to the formation of a stabilized β-amino-β-acyloxiacrylate-enzyme complex.

The 6-spiro epoxide analog has been shown to be a good β-lactamase inhibitor. The chlorine atom is crucial for inhibitory activity. Replacement with a hydrogen yielded a less active analog. A 6-spirocyclopropyl penam sulfones series demonstrated good inhibitory activity (Fig. 32).

Introduction of 6-hydroxyarylalkyl substituents led to effective class C β-lactamase inhibitors. The 6α-hydroxymethyl analog exhibits IC_{50}s of 8 and 160 nM against TEM-1 and AmpC, respectively.

Figure 30 6-Mercapto or 6-hydroxy methyl penam sulfones

Figure 31 6-Alkenyl penicillanic acid sulfone

The 6αβ-hydroxyisopropyl derivatives are inhibitors of class D enzyme (OXA-10).

In order to investigate whether the 6β-acyl amido group could be replaced by substituents of similar steric shape, the amido group was replaced by an olifenic bond. A series of vinyl derivatives was obtained. Some derivatives displayed weak antibacterial activity.

5.4.3.1.6.1. GD-40. GD-40 is the 6α-2β-chloromethyl penam sulfone (Fig. 33), and it has good inhibitory activity against class A β-lactamases such as TEM-1 or SHV-2 (Table 15) (Danelon et al., 1998).

5.4.3.2. C-2 Substituents

Substituents may be fixed at position C-2α or C-2β of the penam ring. Various substituents have been proposed and tested (Fig. 34).

It was shown that the 2,3-β-methylene analogs of sulbactam exhibited anti-β-lactamase activities, and this resulted in the discovery of tazobactam.

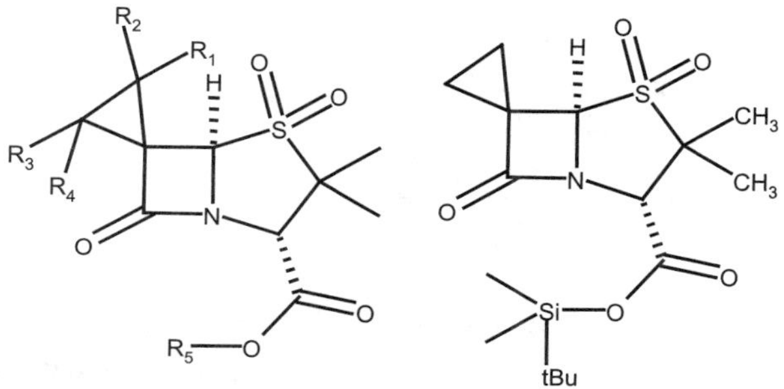

Figure 32 6-Spirocyclopropyl penam sulfones

Figure 33 GD-40

Table 15 In vitro activity of GD-40 against class A enzymes in comparison with other inhibitors

Inhibitor	Enzyme	IC_{50} (μM)	
		No preincubation	Preincubation
Brobactam	TEM-1	0.484	0.0139
	SHV-2	0.0520	0.0003
Tazobactam	TEM-1	0.0456	0.0333
	SHV-2	0.0265	0.0075
Sulbactam	TEM-1	0.826	1.074
	SHV-2	0.0676	0.419
Clavulanic acid	TEM-1	0.419	0.2499
	SHV-2	0.3502	0.072
GD-40	TEM-1	0.4910	0.6510
	SHV-2	0.0008	0.6500

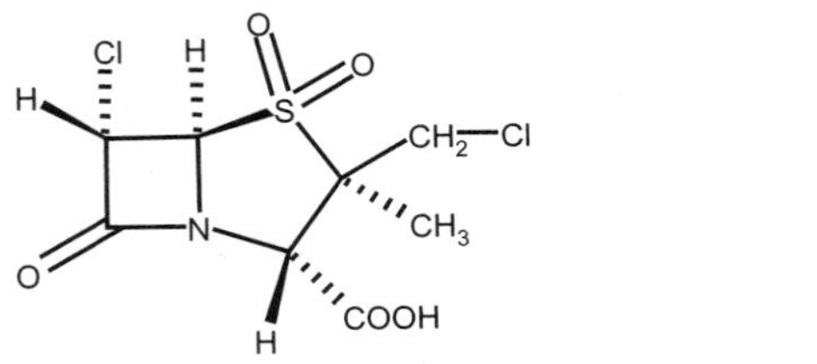

6α-halo (chloro) 2β-chloro methyl penam sulfone

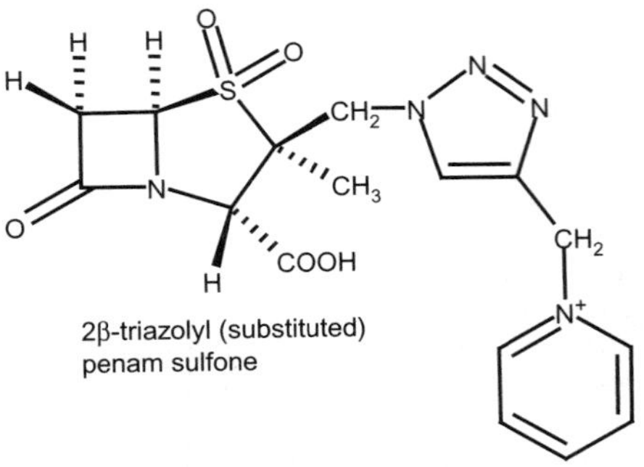

2β-triazolyl (substituted) penam sulfone

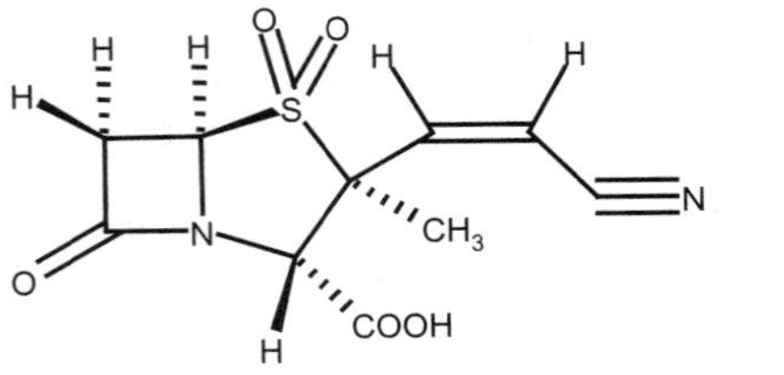

2β-acrylonitrile penam sulfone (Ro 48-1220)

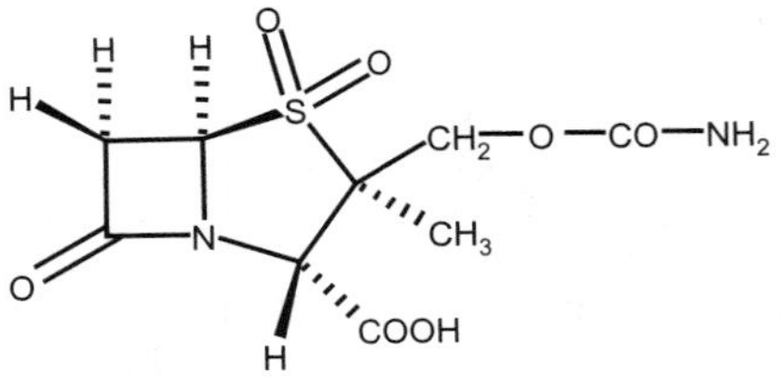

2β-carbamoyl methyl penam sulfone

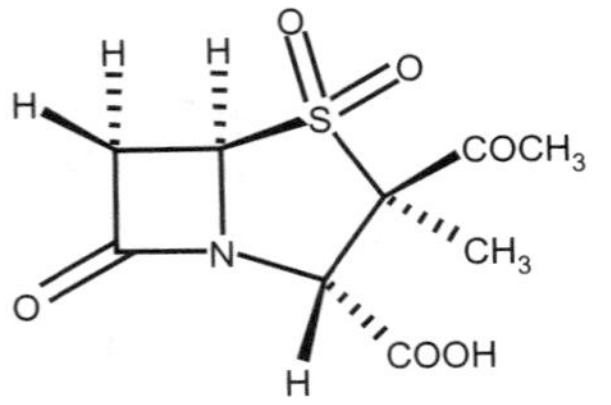

2β-acetyl penam sulfone

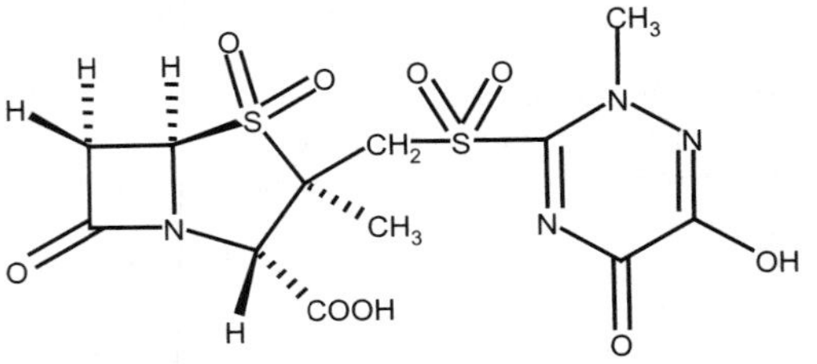

2β-triazolyl sulfonyl penam sulfone

Figure 34 C-2β-substituted penam sulfones

The 2,3α-methylene analog displayed better inhibitory activity against *E. cloacae* P99 than sulbactam (IC_{50}, 12 versus 20 μM) (Fig. 35).

In general, it is thought that the β-lactamases recognize β-methylene as a cephem.

The triazolylo sulfonyl methyl analog displayed high inhibitory activity against class C enzymes. In the series of 2β-triazolyl-substituted compounds, one possessing a methylpyridinium group exhibited good inhibitory activity against class C enzymes in combination with piperacillin, as well as against TEM and SHV enzymes. When substituted with a 2β-carbamoyl side chain, however, the compounds were less active than sulbactam.

A series of 2β-acetyl penam sulfones exhibited good inhibitory activity and in combination a synergistic activity with piperacillin and ceftazidime against chromosomally mediated class 1 enzymes and also against isolates producing TEM, SHV, or OXA-type β-lactamases.

Series of 2β-alkoxy carbonyl penam sulfones (Fig. 36) have been prepared. Many various substituents have been fixed on the carbonyl moiety, such as sodium, methyl, ethyl, trifluoromethyl, pyridinium, and tetrazolyl rings. Most of them have inhibitory properties similar to that of tazobactam against *E. coli* TEM-1 and *K. pneumoniae* and *P. aeruginosa* class C enzymes.

When combined with piperacillin, none of them displayed synergistic activity compared to the combination tazobactam-piperacillin against class A- or class D-producing strains.

Some derivatives with a 2β-halo (chlorine) atom seem very active against class A- β-lactamases.

5.4.3.3. C-2 and C-6 Substituents

Various penam sulfones with double substitutions have been reported, such as those with a 6α-hydroxy methyl side chain and a 2β-iminomethyl residue.

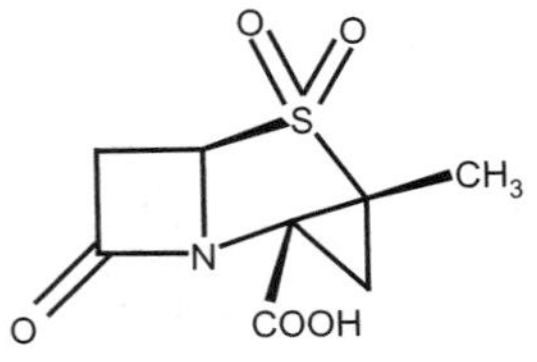

Figure 35 2,3α-Methylene penam

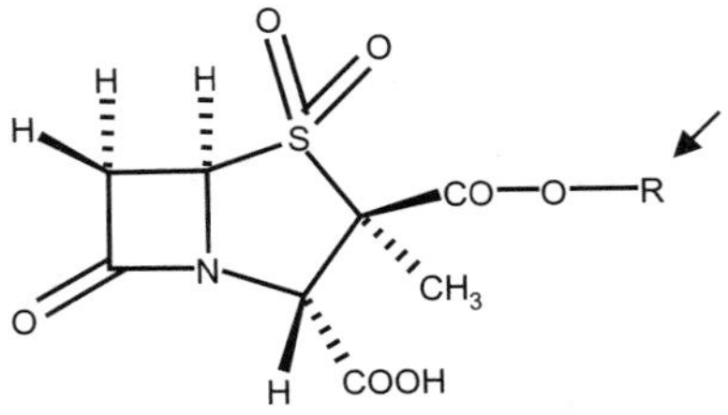

Figure 36 2β-Alkoxycarbonyl penam sulfones

In this series of 6α-hydroxy methyl analogs, some displayed potent inhibitory activity against class C enzymes, including those of *P. aeruginosa*.

Double substitution at C-2β and C-6 with a chlorine atom yielded compounds very active against class A β-lactamases.

A series having a 6-carbamoylmethyl and a C-2β-methyl/chlorine has been prepared; unfortunately they exerted poor activities (Fig. 37).

5.5. Penem Derivatives

The discovery of carbapenems from natural sources and penem synthesis by Woodward in the mid-1970s were key steps in the β-lactam field.

Very early on it was shown that carbapenems have dual potencies—antibacterial activity and β-lactamase inhibition.

Penems in general as β-lactamase inhibitors can be divided into three classes: penems, carbapenems, and oxa-1-penems (Fig. 38).

5.5.1. Carbapenems

Carbapenems may be obtained either by natural sources or by synthetic pathways.

5.5.1.1. Natural Carbapenems

At least 30 carbapenems from natural sources have been isolated. The nomenclature is extremely confusing; sometimes two generic names have been given for the same molecule.

6α-hydroxy benzyl-2β-methoxy imino methyl penam sulfones

6α-carbamoyl methyl-2β-chloro methyl penam sulfones

6α-halo-2β-halo methyl penam sulfones

Figure 37 C-6- and C-2β-substituted penam sulfones

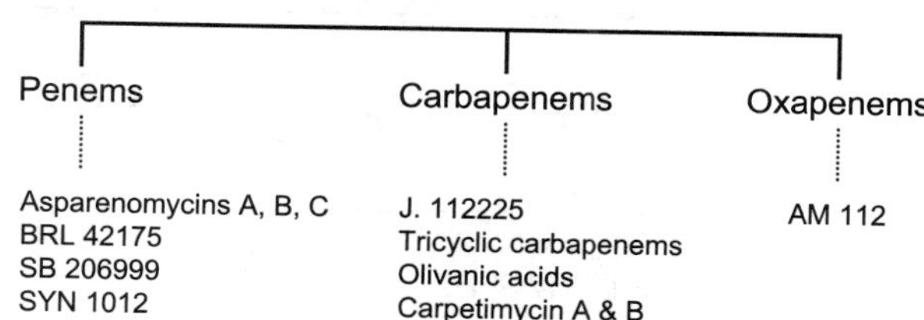

Figure 38 Classification of penems as β-lactamase inhibitors

5.5.1.1.1. Olivanic acids. Various strains of *Streptomyces* have been found to produce a complex of structurally related carbapenems which exhibit broad-spectrum antibacterial activity and exert β-lactamase-inhibitory activities. The broth complex includes at least seven distinct components designed with the prefix "MM."

The different names of compounds which were isolated from *S. olivaceus* ATCC 21379 are listed in Table 16.

All olivanic acids differ from thienamycin in the following ways:

- They have a C-2 aminothio side chain saturated or not.
- The chiral center of the C-6 hydroxy group has an *S* configuration.

All of them exhibited good inhibitory activity against class A and class C enzymes (Table 17).

Derivatization of the olivanic acids has been studied mainly through the esterification of the carboxylic group; modification of the hydroxyl moiety by acylation, elimination, reduction, and replacement; and halogenation or isomerization of the *trans*-acetamidol thio side chain.

MM 4550 (Fig. 39) is particularly active against penicillinases, whereas MM 13902 and MM 17880 are mainly active against class C enzymes, such as those of *E. coli* and *E. cloacae*. The β-lactamase inhibition was found to be progressive and irreversible.

5.5.1.1.2. PS-5. PS-5 (Fig. 40) is a natural carbapenem antibiotic isolated from the fermentation broth of *Streptomyces cremeus* subsp. *auratilis* ATCC 31358 or *Streptomyces fluvoviridis*. PS-5 is active against some gram-positive and gram-negative bacteria and exhibits inhibitory

Table 16 Corresponding components between Merck and Beecham classifications

Merck classification	Beecham classification	Other classification
MM 17880	Epithienamycin F	
MM 13902	Epithienamycin E	
MM 4550	696-SY2-A	
MM 22380	Epithienamycin A	Sankyo 17927 A_1
MM 22282	Epithienamycin B	Sankyo 17927 A_2
MM 22381	Epithienamycin C	
MM 22383	Epithienamycin D	

Table 17 Affinities of MM 4550 for β-lactamases[a]

Strain	IC_{50} (μg/ml)			
	MM 4550[b]		Clavulanic acid[c]	
	Incubation	Preincubation	Incubation	Preincubation
S. aureus MB9	0.016	0.0037	0.84	0.02
E. coli K-12 R-TEM	0.0014	0.00046	0.56	0.08
K. aerogenes A	0.002	0.0008	0.11	0.01
P. mirabilis C889	0.0006	0.00035	0.69	0.01

[a]Data from Basker et al., 1980.
[b]Benzylpenicillin was used as substrate.
[c]Amoxicillin was used as substrate.

Figure 39 MM 4550

Figure 40 PS-5

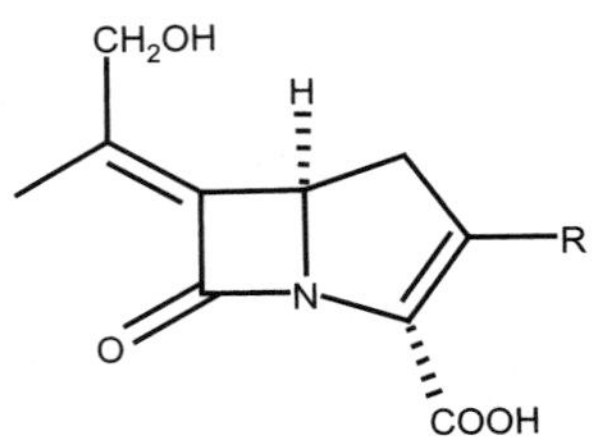

Asparenomycin	R
A	$-S(O)-CH=CH-NH-CO-CH_3$
B	$-S(O)-CH_2-CH_2-NH-CO-CH_3$
C	$-S-CH=CH-NH-CO-CH_3$

Figure 41 Asparenomycins

activity against β-lactamases. It differs from olivanic derivatives by the lack of an oxygen functionality in the C-6 ethyl side chain. Derivatization of PS-5 by modifications of the carboxyl group and the acetamido thio side chain has been reported (Sakamoto et al., 1984).

PS-5 is a potent inhibitor of *Bacillus licheniformis*. PS-5 is hydrolyzed by β-lactamases of *B. cereus*, *Proteus vulgaris*, *C. freundii*, and *Streptomyces* spp. With this exception, PS-5 behaves like clavulanic acid.

5.5.1.1.3. Asparenomycins. MC-690 SY A2 has been reported as a metabolite of *S. fulvoridis* in 1977. However, as an unknown structure it was reported as early as 1973 to be a β-lactamase inhibitor.

Three components have been described (Fig. 41), A, B, and C, which differ by the C-2 side chain. The C-6 side chain is through a double bond (Murakami et al., 1982).

5.5.1.1.4. Carpetimycins. Carpetimycins are produced by *Streptomyces* and are closely related to olivanic acids. They exhibit a broad antibacterial spectrum including *P. aeruginosa* but with a moderate in vitro activity (MIC, 6.25 μg/ml for *P. aeruginosa*), as well as potent inhibitory effects on β-lactamases (Nakayama et al., 1980).

The nomenclature is also a little confusing: carpetimycin A is also known as C-19393 H_2, and carpetimycin B is also known as C-19393-S_2 (Fig. 42).

Carpetimycins A and B exhibit good inhibitory activity against β-lactamases of *E. coli* and *P. vulgaris* 69 (class C) (Table 18).

The IC_{50}s of these carbapenems for 10 types of β-lactamases are less than 0.04 μg/ml for carpetimycin A and under 0.2 μg/ml for carpetimycin B.

	R_1	R_2	n
MM 22382	H	H	0
MM 13902	SO_3H	H	0
MM 4550	SO_3H	H	1
Carpetimycin A	H	CH_3	1
Carpetimycin B	SO_3H	CH_3	1

Figure 42 Carpetimycins

Table 18 Inhibitory activities of carpetimycins

Drug	IC_{50} (nM)	
	E. coli[a]	*P. vulgaris* 69[b]
Carpetimycin A	0.64	0.52
Carpetimycin B	0.21	0.74

[a]Benzylpenicillin (penicillin G) was used as substrate.
[b]Cephaloridine was used as substrate.

5.5.1.2. Tricyclic Carbapenems

A series of tricyclic carbapenems (Fig. 43) has been reported. Two of them were selected for further investigations: LEK 156 and LEK 157, having inhibitory activity against class C enzymes such as ACT-1, CMY-1, and MIR-1.

It was highlighted that some tricyclic derivatives exhibit inhibitory activity against class C enzymes (IC_{50}, 1.8 to 5.0 μM (Vilar et al., 2001).

5.5.1.3. Synthetic Carbapenems

Numerous compounds have been synthesized, and one was partially developed: BRL-42175.

5.5.1.3.1. BRL-42715. BRL-42175 exhibits good synergistic activity with cefazolin and piperacillin. This compound has no intrinsic antibacterial activity (Tables 19 and 20).

The mechanism of action of BRL-42715 is summarized in Fig. 44. The acyl-enzyme intermediate formed initially can undergo both hydrolysis and rapid rearrangement to the more stable dihydrothiazepine derivative (Woodnutt et al., 1992).

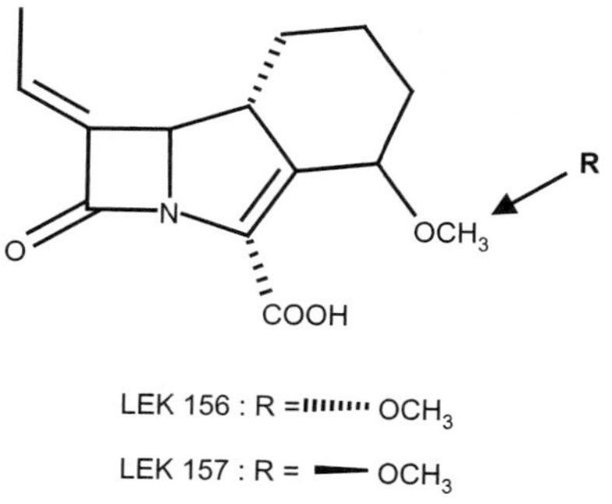

Figure 43 LEK 156 and LEK 157

BRL-42175 penetrates strongly into the periplasmic space of gram-negative bacilli (Table 21).

The development of BRL-42715 was given up mainly due to its chemical instability.

5.5.1.3.2. SYN-1012. SYN-1012 is chemically close to BRL-42715 (Fig. 45), having a propylidene side chain on the triazolyl ring (Phillips et al., 1997).

This derivative was also chemically unstable, and development was stopped.

5.5.1.3.3. SB 206999. Figure 46 shows the structure of SB 206999, while Table 22 shows its inhibitory activity.

5.5.1.3.4. J-111,225. J-111,225 (Fig. 47) has no antibacterial activity but exerts an inhibitory activity against β-lactamases of classes A, B, and C (Table 23) (Nagano et al., 2000).

The main weaknesses of penems are hydrolysis by the dehydropeptidase I (DHP-I) renal enzyme and seizures.

The relative rate of hydrolysis compared to imipenem by porcine renal DHP-I is 0.25, and there was no epileptogenicity detected in five rats (200 μg/rat head).

5.5.1.3.5. Other derivatives. For the carbapenem series, intensive research has shown the following:

- The 6-ethylidene penems are potent inhibitors of β-lactamases, reducing the MICs of ampicillin and cephalexin.
- The alkylidene series resulted in one compound, BRL-42175.

In the 6-ethylidene penem series the replacement of the methyl group at C-8 by a thienyl or a furyl ring enhanced the synergistic activity against β-lactamases.

Table 20 Synergistic activity of piperacillin and BRL-42175

Strains	MIC (μg/ml)		
	Piperacillin	BRL-42175	Piperacillin + BRL-42175
E. coli E 96	64	16	1
E. coli 41548	512	8	≤0.25
P. mirabilis R 238	256	32	8
E. cloacae 812/13	128	64	16
B. fragilis VP 18708	128	64	4

Table 19 Synergistic activity of BRL-42175 and cefazolin

Strain	MIC (μg/ml)		
	Cefazolin	BRL-42175	Cefazolin + BRL-42175
E. coli T4 1507	64	32	2
E. cloacae T626	512	>64	64
S. marcescens OG4	512	64	2
C. freundii W114	256	32	0.25
Providencia rettgeri WM 16	512	64	1
B. fragilis UP 18708	256	32	2
M. morganii Stockpart	128	64	4

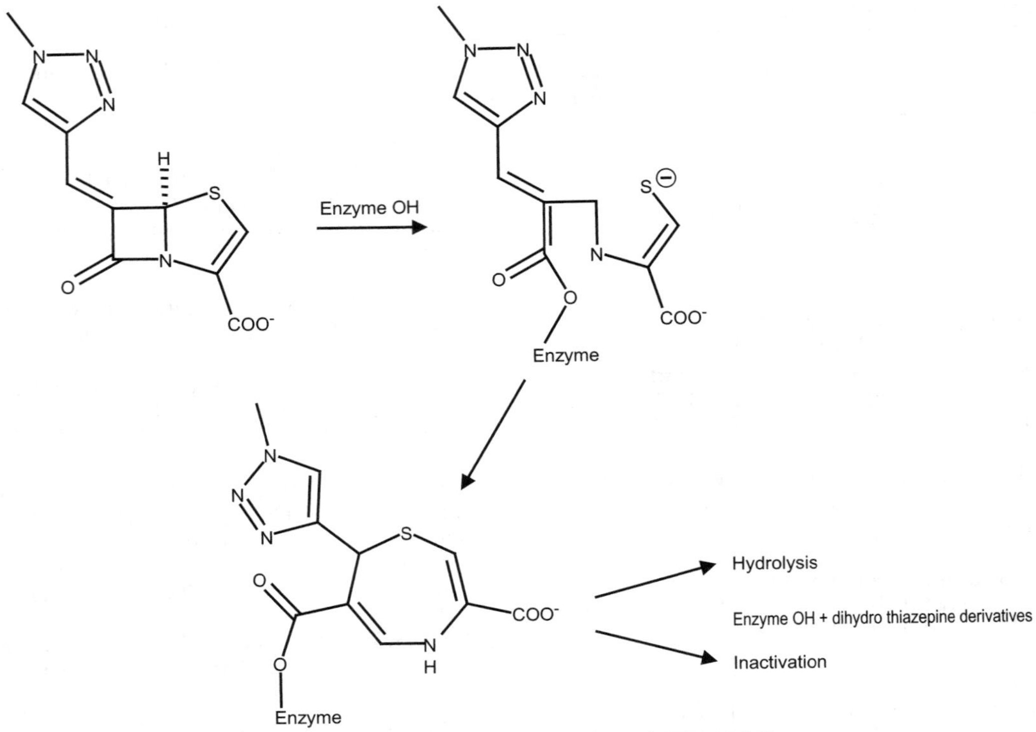

Figure 44 Mechanism of action of BRL-42175

Table 21 Penetration of β-lactamase inhibitors into the periplasmic space

Microorganism	Enzyme	Compound	Whole cell	Sonicate
E. coli NCTC 11560	TEM-1	Clavulanic acid	0.8	0.244
		Sulbactam	35.3	1.18
		Tazobactam	1.18	0.02
		BRL-42175	0.09	0.007
K. pneumoniae 1082E	K1	Clavulanic acid	0.069	0.0109
		Sulbactam	32.8	2.31
		Tazobactam	196	54.9
		BRL-42175	131	0.732
E. cloacae	P99	Clavulanic acid	1,429	2,311
		Sulbactam	3,020	510
		Tazobactam	601	997
		BRL-42175	2.8	0.0592

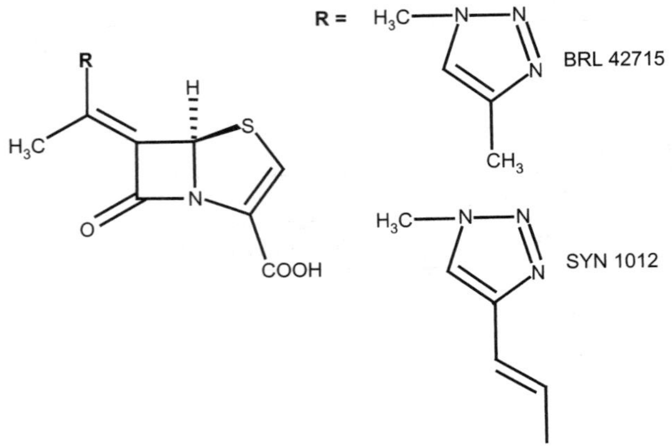

Figure 45 SYN-1012 and BRL-42175

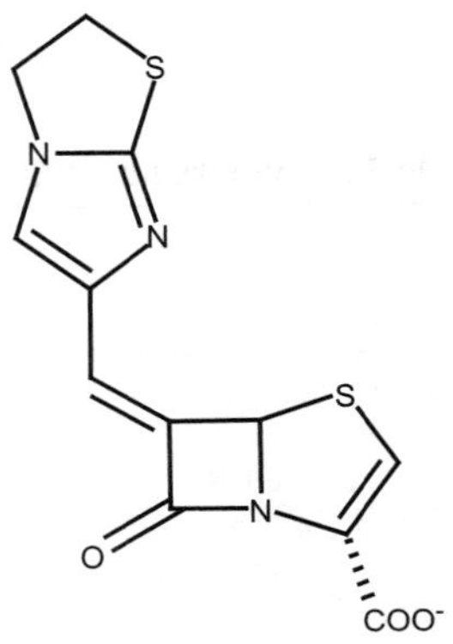

Figure 46 SB 206999

Table 22 Inhibitory activity of SB 206999

Enzyme	Class	IC_{50} (μM)	
		Clavulanic acid	SB 206999
PC-1	A	0.063	0.01
TEM-1	A	0.06	<0.005
CcrA	B	>500	NT[a]
P99	C	>50	<0.005
OXA-1	D	0.71	0.01

[a]NT, not tested.

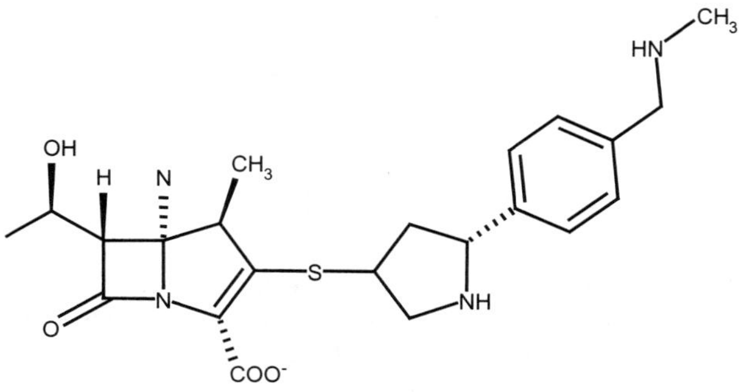

Figure 47 J-111,225

5.5.1.4. Tribactams

Some derivatives exhibit high affinity for class C enzymes of *E. cloacae* 908R (IC_{50}, 1.8 to 5.0 μmol/liter) and low affinity for class A enzymes (IC_{50}, 32 to 120 μmol/liter) (Copar et al., 2002).

5.5.2. Oxa-1-Penem

In the oxa-1-penem subclass, only one compound is currently under evaluation: AM-112 (Jamieson et al., 2003). Three series of oxa-1-penems were developed. In the first two, developed in 1978 and 1993, the compounds were potent inhibitors of β-lactamases but had poor chemical stability. In the third one, AM-112 represents a compound selected for further development.

5.5.2.1. AM-112

AM-112 (Fig. 48) contains a quaternary substituent at position C-2 which greatly improves the molecular stability. This molecule is zwitterionic. At C-6 the hydroxyethyl group has the *R* configuration. AM-112 is prepared by a seven-step synthesis. AM-112 exhibits DHP-I stability similar to that of meropenem. The best potential partner seems to be ceftazidime, cefepime, or aztreonam.

AM-112 does not possess antibacterial activity (MIC, ≥32 μg/ml). A concentration of 4 μg/ml restores activity of ceftazidime against strains producing class A enzymes, including ESBL, and class C enzymes. It is also active against class D β-lactamases (OXA-1 to -7) (Table 24).

In a molecular-modelling study it was shown for TEM-1 that the nitrogen of the heterocyclic ring of AM-112 was hydrogen bonded to water-323, which H bonds in the main chain amino and carboxylic group and has a hydrogen bond interaction with Arg244. The terminal amino group of the C-2 side chain forms H bonds with the side chain hydroxyl group of Ser235 and also with Arg244 via a water molecule (water-402).

AM-112 displays pharmacokinetics in rodents similar to those of ceftazidime (Table 25).

5.5.3. Methylidene Penem Derivatives

In a series of derivatives, three compounds were selected for investigation in combination with piperacillin. They were active against class C enzymes (IC_{50}, 1.5 to 6.2 nM) and broad-spectrum β-lactamase (TEM-1) and weakly active against class B enzymes. In vivo in murine disseminated

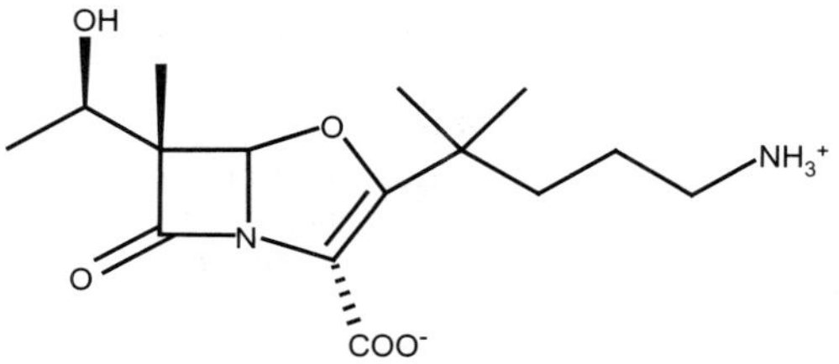

Figure 48 AM-112

Table 24 Inhibitory activity of AM-112 in comparison with clavulanic acid

Enzyme	Class	IC_{50} (μM)	
		Clavulanic acid	AM-112
TEM-1	A	0.12	2.26
TEM-10	A	0.03	0.224
SHV-5	A	0.008	0.16
P99	C	11.4	0.002
S2	C	327	0.07
StA	C	449	0.002
OXA-1	D	99	0.005
OXA-5	D	202	0.0007

Table 23 Inhibitory activity of J-111,225

Organism	Enzyme	Class	Hydrolysis (%)	K_i (μM)	MIC (μg/ml)
P. aeruginosa	IMP-1	B	4	0.17	32
B. fragilis	CcrA	B	59	15	>128
S. maltophilia	L-1	B	43	10	32
B. cereus	BCII	B	59	12	NT[a]
E. coli	Penicillinase	A	<1	2.82	NT
E. cloacae		C	<1	>1	NT

[a]NT, not tested.

Table 25 Pharmacokinetics of AM-112 in rodents when coadministered with ceftazidime

Animal	Dose of AM-112 (CAZ[a]) (mg/kg)	$t_{1/2}$ (min)		AUC (μg·min/ml)	
		AM-112	CAZ	AM-112	CAZ
Mouse	10 (0)	5.8		327.2	
	10 (20)	6.2	7.6	765.8	410.2
	50 (0)	8.9		1,330.5	
	50 (100)	12.9	13.5	1,178.6	2,586.4
	100 (0)	9.0		2,513.8	
	100 (200)	6.4	10.0	2,339.3	3,757.4
Rat	10 (0)	9.8		181.8	
	10 (20)	6.9	13.6	199.4	546.9
	50 (0)	9.0		1,546.4	
	50 (100)	9.3	15.1	846.4	2,634
	100 (0)	11.5		2,963.5	
	100 (200)	6.8	19.6	2018	6,413.2

[a]CAZ, ceftazidime.

infections, all three compounds exerted 50% effective doses ranging from 22 to 97 mg/kg of body weight.

The mode of action of these derivatives is the formation of 1,4-thiazepine ring (Venkatesan et al., 2004).

5.6. Monocyclic β-Lactams

Many monocyclic β-lactams from natural sources have high affinity for class A and class C β-lactamases (e.g., the IC_{50} for *E. cloacae* P99 is ~0.0007 nM), but they seem to have less affinity for class A enzymes.

It was shown that nocarcidin A (Fig. 49) and desthiobenzylpenicillin are substrates of β-lactamases of *B. cereus* 569/H/9, *E. coli* W3310, and *S. aureus* PC-1.

Nocarcidin is a complex of seven components, A through G, isolated from *Nocardia uniformis* subsp. *tsuyamanensis* ATCC 21806 (Pratt et al., 1980).

Few compounds have been prepared in this subclass of β-lactamase inhibitors.

5.6.1. SYN-2190

SYN-2190 (Fig. 50) is a monocyclic β-lactamase inhibitor which possesses a 1,5-dihydroxy-4-pyridone side chain at position C-3 (Nishida et al., 1999). It is a potent inhibitor of class C β-lactamases but not those of other types.

SYN-2190 has no intrinsic antibacterial activity. It uses the TonB pathway, a ferric uptake pathway, as do catecholic cephalosporins. It was shown that SYN-2190 restores the in vitro activity of ceftazidime and cefpirome against β-lactamase-derepressed *P. aeruginosa* (Table 26).

Tazobactam exhibited moderate inhibitory activity against class C β-lactamases. SYN-2190 has strong inhibitory activity against class C. The synergy with cephems is concentration dependent. The α-methyl group at position C-4 of aztreonam (Fig. 51) increases the antibacterial activity and the stability against β-lactamases. A 4-phenyl monobactam (Fig. 52) has been synthesized with the aim of obtaining a scaffold of β-lactamase inhibitors.

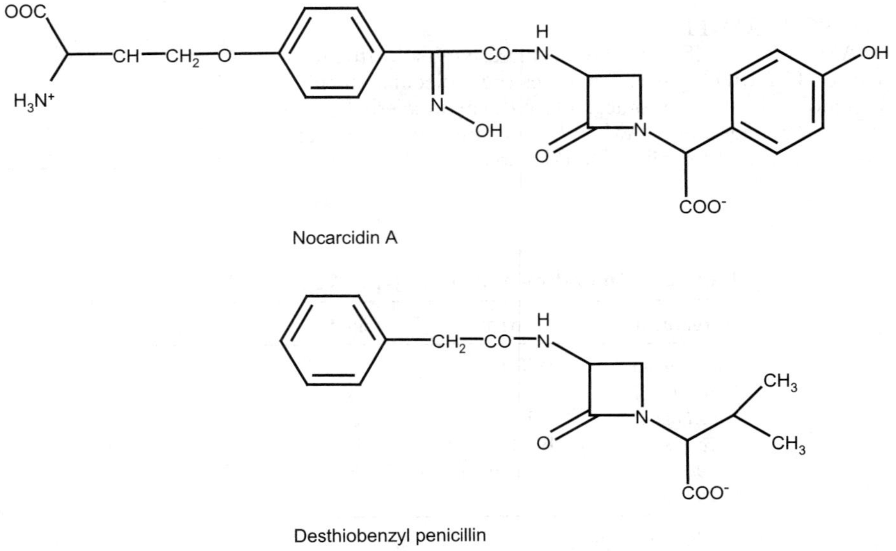

Figure 49 Nocarcidin A and desthiobenzyl penicillin

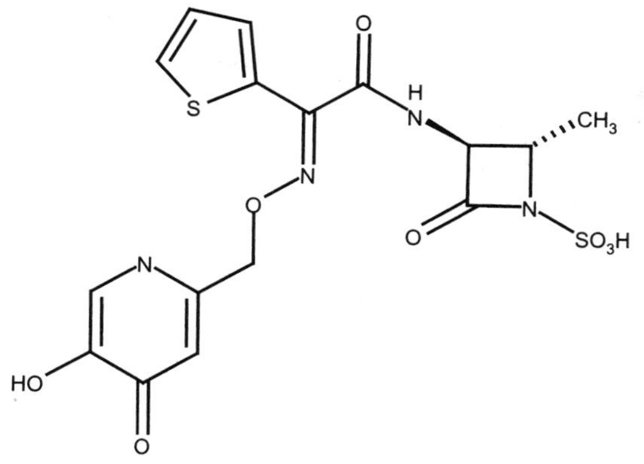

Figure 50 SYN-2190

Figure 51 Aztreonam

Table 26 Inhibitory activity of SYN-2190

Bush group	Microorganism	IC_{50} (μM)	
		SYN-2190	Tazobactam
1	*P. aeruginosa* 46012	0.01	2.264
	E. cloacae P99	0.006	4.995
	M. morganii	0.002	0.433
	C. freundii	0.002	1.931
2b	*E. coli* TEM-1	>20	0.007
2be	*K. pneumoniae* TEM-3	7.894	0.008
2e	*P. vulgaris*	>20	0.002

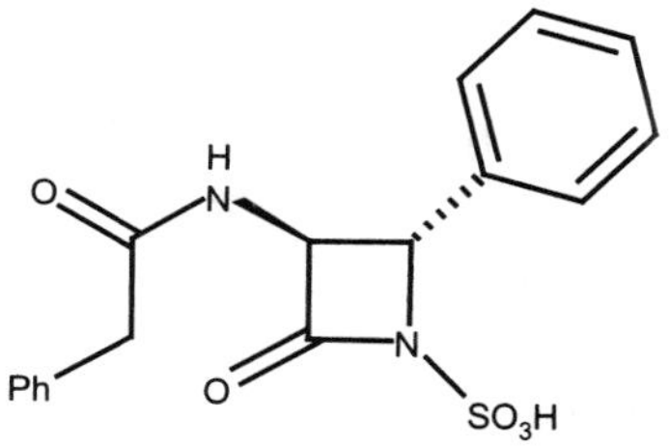

Figure 52 Phenyl acetamidino phenyl monobactam

5.6.2. Thienamonobactam

New racemic thienamonobactams (Fig. 53 and 54) have been designed as hybrids between thienamycin and aztreonam. One compound exhibits significant inhibitory activity against *C. freundii* class C β-lactamases (Nagano et al., 1997).

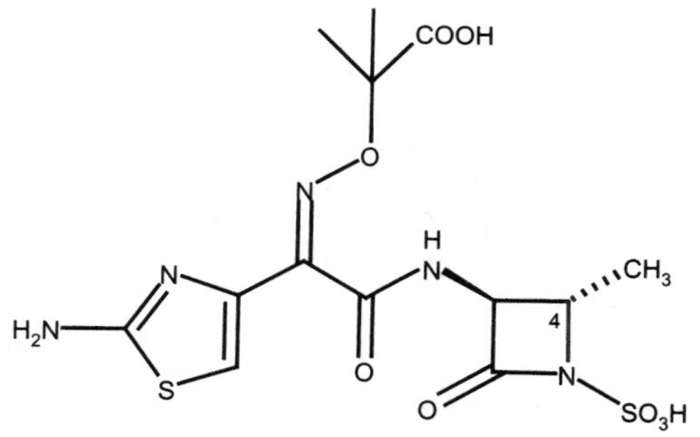

5.7. Cephem Derivatives

In 1972, O'Callaghan and Morris showed that cefoxazole (Fig. 55) with a cloxacillin side chain (isoxazole nucleus) is a potent inhibitor of β-lactamases produced by *E. cloacae*. However, high concentrations of cefoxazole are needed to obtain synergistic activity.

The same year, from a series of cephem derivatives, one compound was selected for further studies due to its inhibitory activity toward β-lactamases: 443/1. This compound exerts activity against TEM-1 of *E. coli* (IC_{50},

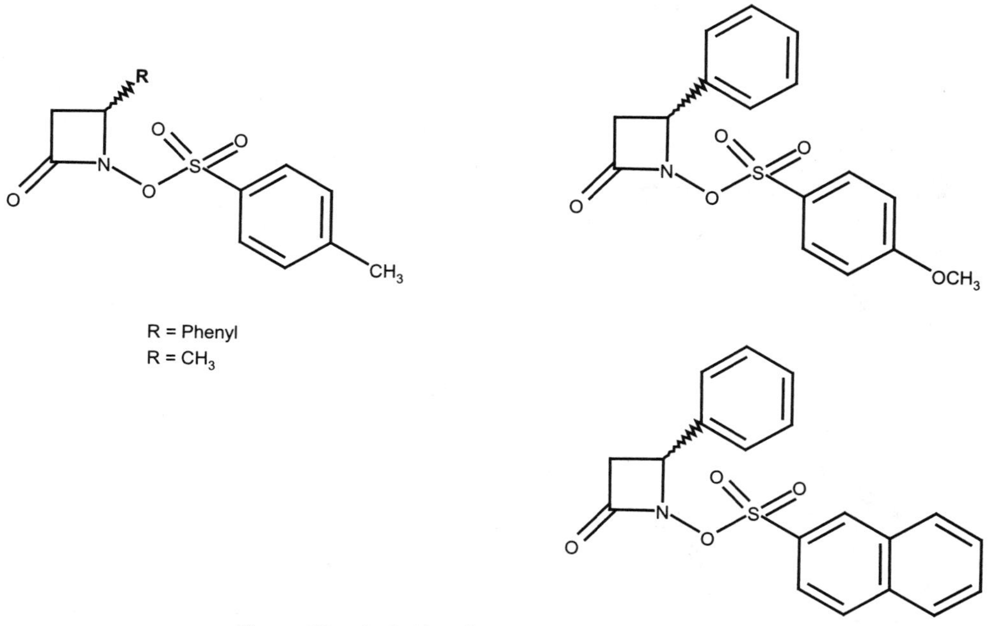

R = Phenyl
R = CH_3

Figure 53 *N*-Sulfonyloxy monocyclic β-lactams

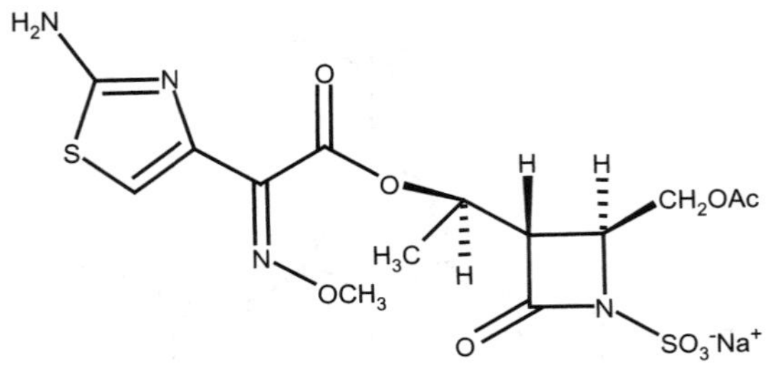

Figure 54 Thienamonobactam

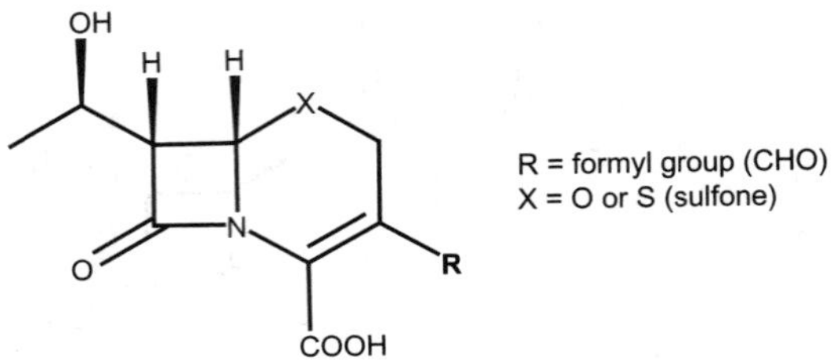

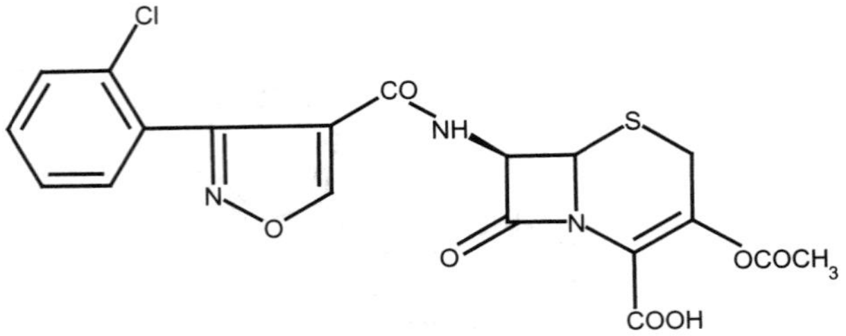

Figure 55 Cefoxazole

0.01 nM) and against class C enzyme of *E. cloacae* P99 (IC_{50}, 0.01 nM), as well as against *S. aureus* PC-1 (IC_{50}, 0.72 nM).

In 1980, thioxime cephems (Fig. 56) were shown to be potent inhibitors of class C enzymes. However, inhibition diminishes with time and is fully reversible upon dialysis. It seems likely that these compounds are poor substrates for class C enzymes.

In 1990, it was shown by Nishimura et al. that 7α-hydroxyethyl sulfone cephems (Fig. 57) and sulfoxide having a C-3 formyl side chain exhibited potent anti-β-lactamase activities.

R = formyl group (CHO)
X = O or S (sulfone)

Figure 57 Cephem sulfones

In 1994, the 7-vinyl cephem sulfones (Fig. 58), showing β-lactamase-inhibitory activity, were reported. The 7-(α-*tert*-butyl vinylidene) cephem was found to be a potent inhibitor of class C (P99) enzymes. Recently the 7α-alkylidene cephems were shown to be inhibitors of β-lactamases (class A and class B) (Fig. 59).

In 1996, Farina et al. prepared a cephem with the potential to be a β-lactamase inhibitor. The idea was to follow a concept for the generation of an allylic sulfoxide at the active site which is in rapid equilibrium with the corresponding sulfonates via a [2,3] double bond rearrangement.

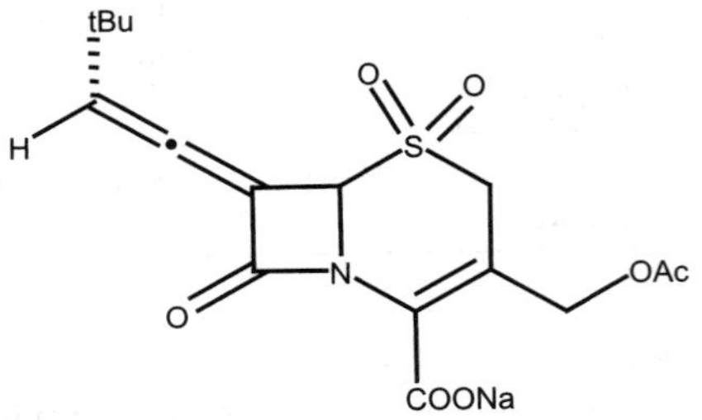

Figure 58 7-Vinyl cephems

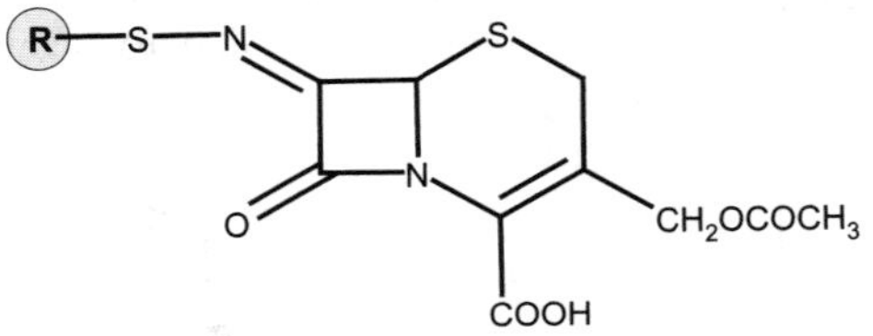

Compound	R	IC_{50} (mg/L) I_a	II_b	III_a	Iv_c*
A	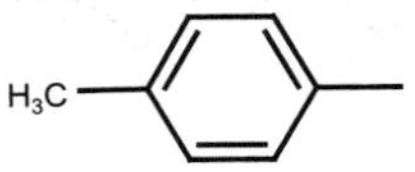 H_3C–	0.125	0.02	> 300	> 300
B	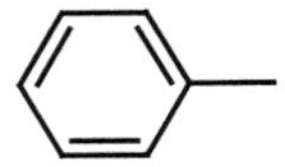	0.003	0.09	113	> 125
C	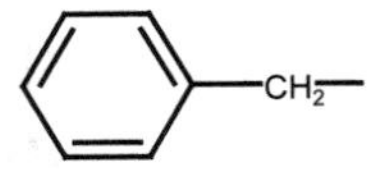 –CH_2–	0.88	0.88	> 125	> 125
D	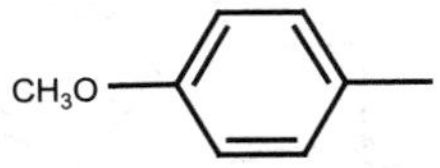 CH_3O–	0.48	0.31	> 125	> 125
E	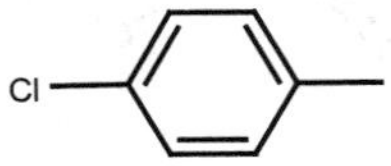 Cl–	0.38	0.44	63	> 125

Figure 56 Thioxime cephems (IV_c, Richmond and Sykes classification)

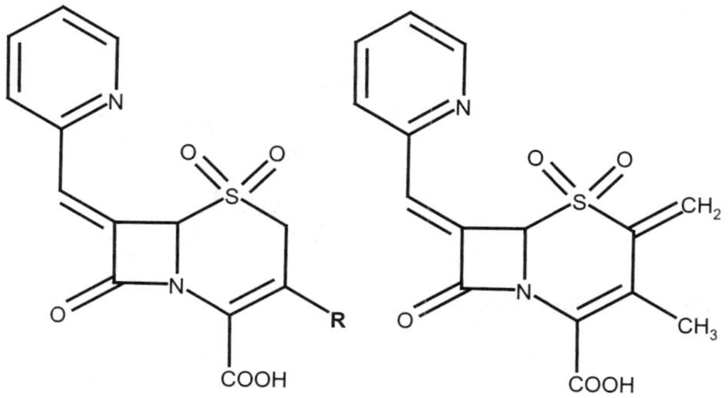

Figure 59 7α-Alkylidene cephems

In this series, none was found to be an inhibitor, but they were good substrates. The lack of inhibition is probably related to rapid hydrolysis of the acyl-enzyme intermediate by the β-lactamase (Fig. 60).

Some benzocarbacephems with inhibitory activity have been synthesized (Fig. 61).

5.8. Bridged β-Lactams

The design of bridged β-lactams originated from the study of class C β-lactamase interactions and the structure and kinetics of a β-lactamase from *C. freundii* 1203.

The idea was to delay the deacylation reaction of the acyl-enzyme complex by blocking the water molecule involved in hydrolysis.

Molecular modelling suggested that penams, cephems, and monocyclic β-lactams possessing *cis* C3-C4 substituents could rotate without steric hindrance due to protein side chains. This rotation allows access by a molecule of water,

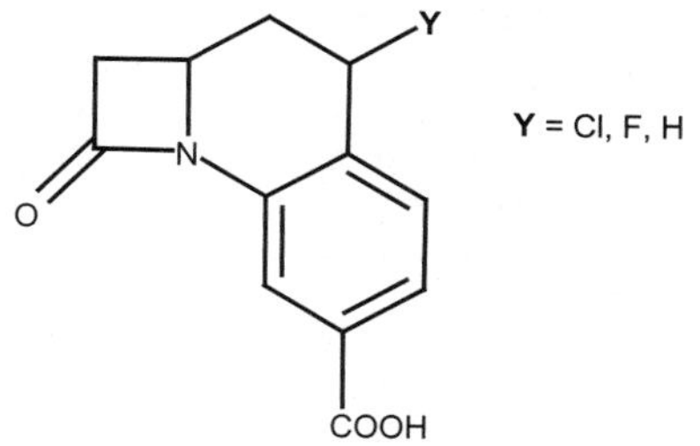

Y = Cl, F, H

Figure 61 Benzocarbacephems

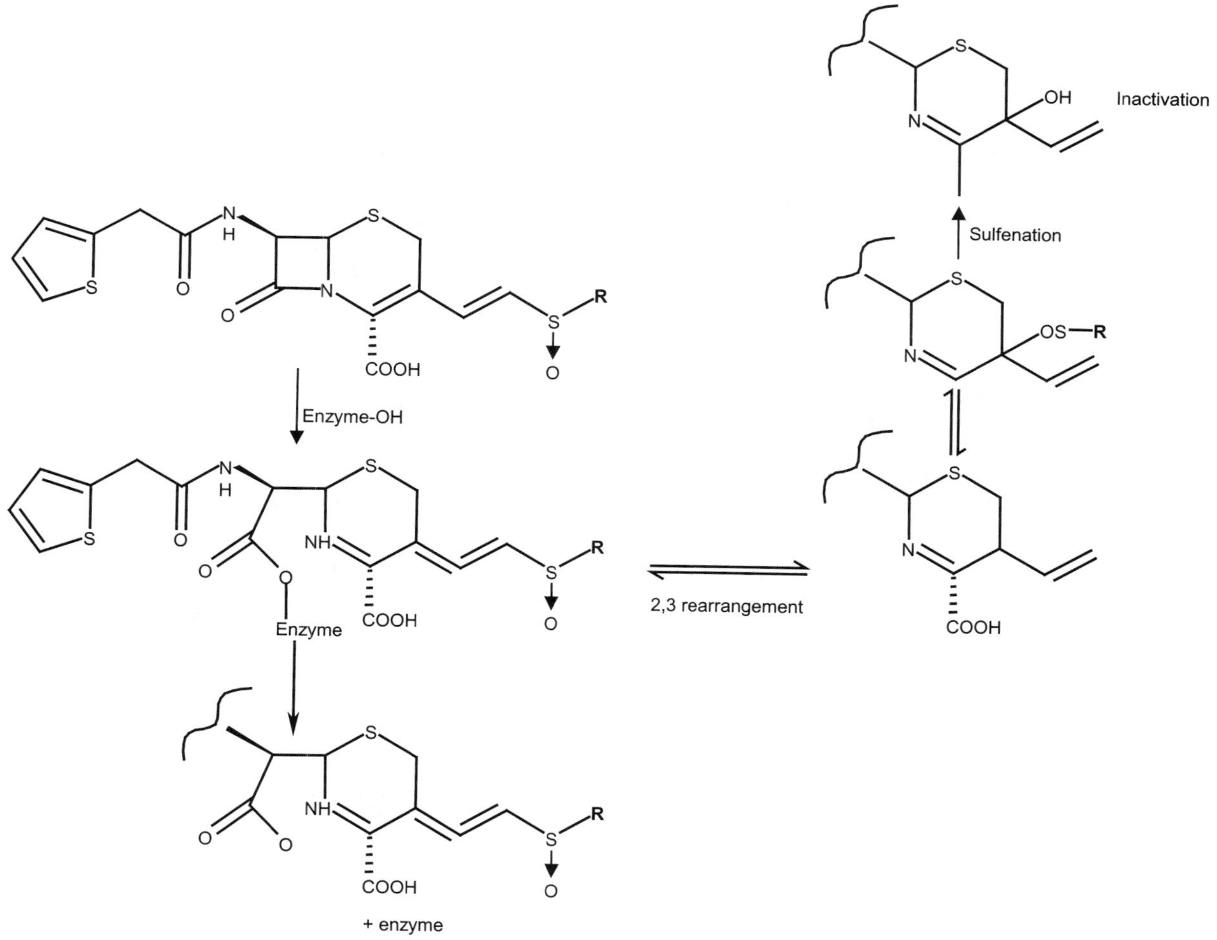

Enzyme-OH

2,3 rearrangement

Sulfenation

Inactivation

+ enzyme

Figure 60 Allylcephem plus sulfenation

which could lead to hydrolysis of the ester by class C enzymes.

To stabilize the acyl-enzyme complex, a rearrangement in a suitable system blocking the access of a molecule of water is required. During the initial process, the counterclockwise rotation about the C3-C4 bond relaxes the eclipsed conformation of the intact β-lactam. The NSO_3 group blocks the accessible face of the ester group so that the molecule of water cannot reach the ester functionality. Clockwise rotation due to a left conformation is less favorable because it allows the steric interaction between the C-4 methyl substituent and Tyr150 and Leu119.

In 1998 the first bridge monobactam was reported; it exhibited potent inhibitory activity against class C enzymes (IC_{50}, <10 nM). These molecules are less effective against class A and class B (IC_{50}, >100 nM), due to the different mechanism of hydrolysis than those of class C.

A good synergy was observed between some of the molecules and ceftriaxone, with MICs from 64 to 0.25 μg/ml (Livermore and Chen, 1997).

A third series was reported which showed various substituents on the nitrogen atom of the β-lactam ring of the monocyclic β-lactam (-OSO_3H-sulfactam, or OCH_2COOH- oxamazine) (Fig. 62).

The oxamazine derivatives are ineffective as β-lactamase inhibitors, but the sulfactams exhibited lower inhibitory potency than the bridge monobactam analogs.

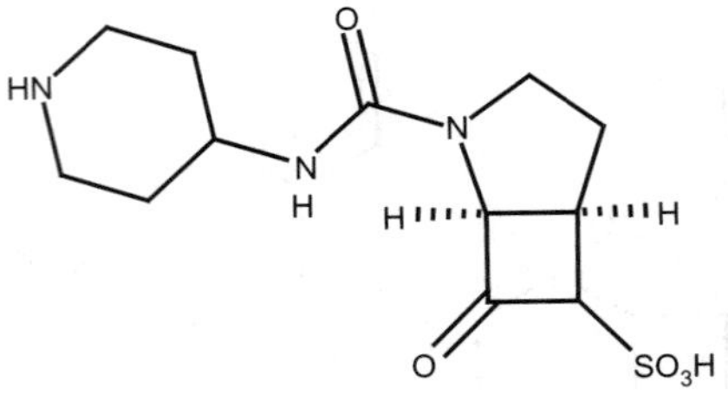

Figure 63 Ro-48-1256

One derivative, Ro-48-1256 (Fig. 63), was tested in combination with imipenem, meropenem, piperacillin, and ceftazidime against *P. aeruginosa* isolates. The combination of Ro-48-1256 and imipenem was always synergistic against isolates producing inducible or derepressed class C β-lactamases, leading to a drop in MIC from 2 to 4 μg/ml to 0.25 to 0.5 μg/ml or from 8 to 16 μg/ml to 1 to 2 μg/ml for those lacking of OprD protein (D_2 porin). Ceftazidime and piperacillin were also potentiated against derepressed organisms but not against those for which the enzymes remained inducible.

5.9. Codrugs

A series of codrugs combining clavulanic acid and penams with a phenyl bridge has been synthesized; they have moderate inhibitory activity (Fig. 64) (Hakimelahi et al., 2002).

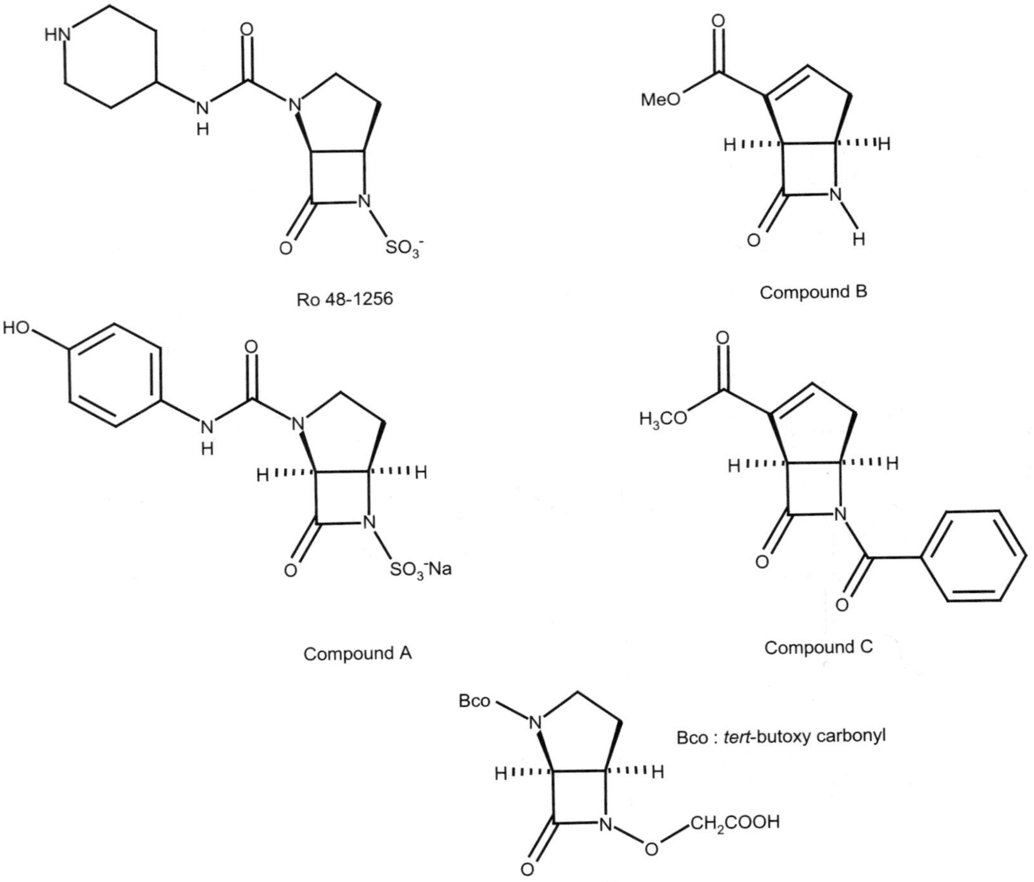

Ro 48-1256

Compound B

Compound A

Compound C

Bco : *tert*-butoxy carbonyl

Figure 62 Bridged monobactams

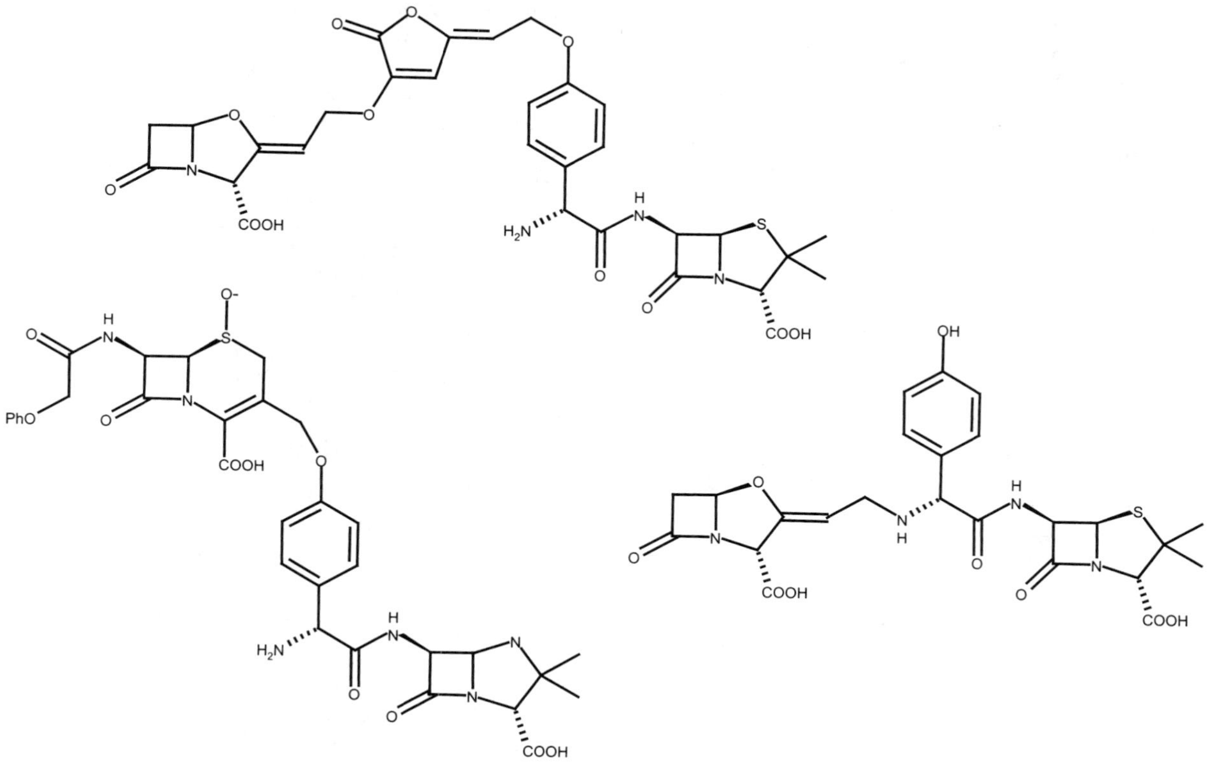

Figure 64 Codrugs as β-lactamase inhibitors

6. NON-β-LACTAMS AS β-LACTAMASE INHIBITORS

Numerous compounds have been reported as having potential as β-lactamase inhibitors. To circumvent β-lactamase inactivation, combinations of β-lactams and β-lactamase inhibitors have been introduced in clinical practice. However, all of the drugs are β-lactams, and when exposed to the molecules, bacteria acquire resistance. To escape from this vicious circle, non-β-lactam inhibitors may be an alternative.

6.1. Succinic Acid Derivatives

The 2,3-(*SS*) disubstituted succinic acids (Fig. 65) are potent inhibitors of IMP-1 enzyme (IC_{50}, 0.009 μM). These compounds were found by screening in the Merck Chemical Library. Succinic acid itself is poorly active, with an IC_{50} of 6.3 μM (Toney et al., 2001).

The addition of an (*R*)-methyl group at one of the benzylic positions led to an approximatively fivefold increase of activity (IC_{50}, 0.013 μM), whereas the addition of an (*S*)-methyl group resulted in a drastic loss of activity (IC_{50}, ≥2.7 μM).

6.2. Rhodamine

By screening of their chemical library, researchers at Johnson & Johnson identified rhodamine as a promising lead for an inhibitor of β-lactamases (Fig. 66) (Jin et al., 1999; Grant et al., 1999).

Rhodamine inhibits class C (P99) and class A (TEM-1) β-lactamases (IC_{50} of 2.6 and 8.7 μM, respectively).

A series was synthesized. It was shown that the most selective compounds are those lacking a substituent at the ring nitrogen and those having a nitro group on the benzylidene phenyl ring (IC_{50} for P99 enzyme, 43 μM).

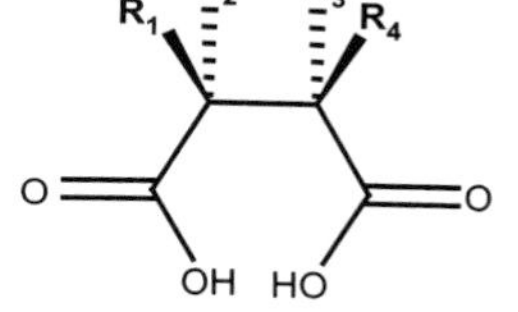

Compound	R_1	R_2	R_3	R_4	Configuration	IC_{50} (μM) for IMP-1
1	$ArCH_2$	H	$ArCH_2$	H	*S*, *S*	*S*, *S*
2	$PhCH_2$	H	$PhCH_2$	H	*S*, *S*	*S*, *S*

Figure 65 Succinic acid derivatives

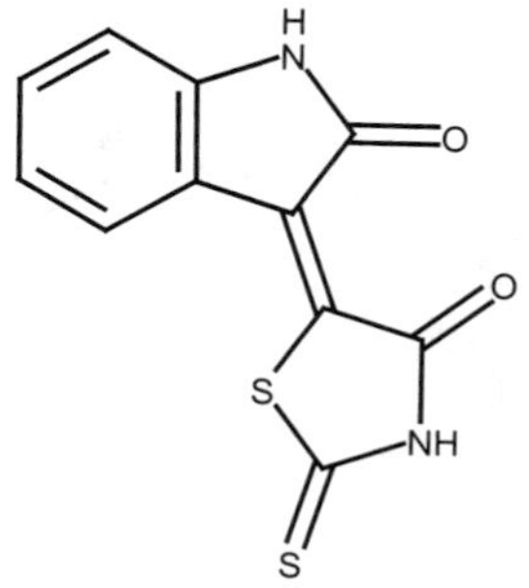

Figure 66 Rhodamine

The addition of a two-carbon spacer to mimic the cephalosporin substrate of class C β-lactamases improved the inhibitory activity.

Some compounds of the second series exhibited inhibitory activity against P99 enzyme and a synergistic activity with piperacillin against resistant isolates. However, some of them have antibacterial activity (Fig. 67).

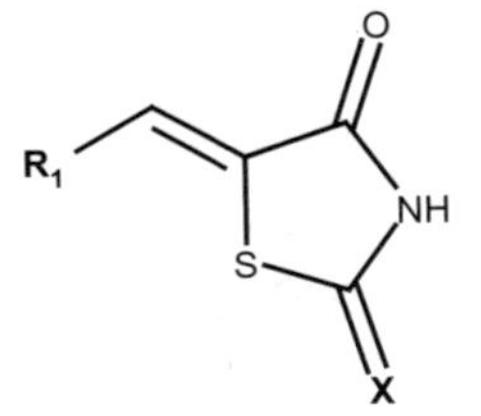

X	R_1	IC_{50}(μM) P99	MIC(mg/liter)
S	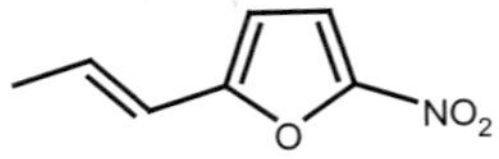	0.41	2.0
O		> 50	0.5

Figure 67 Rhodamine analogs

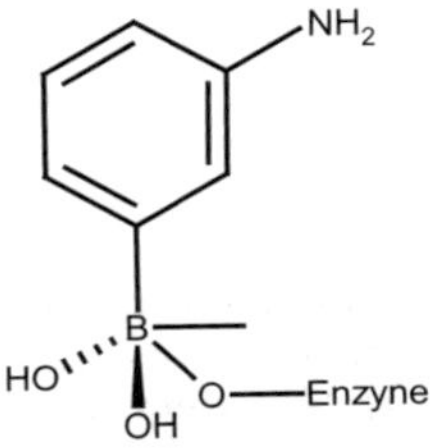

Figure 68 Arylboronic acid

6.3. Boronic Acid Analogs

Boronic acid analogs are serine β-lactamase inhibitors. They act as competitors, forming reversible adducts with the catalytic serine of enzymes and adopting a tetrahedral geometry thought to ressemble to that of a high-energy intermediate.

The original lead has modest affinity for β-lactamases. The arylboronic acids (Fig. 68) have variable affinities for class C enzymes (Weston et al., 1998).

Substitution with different NH-R groups leads to some compounds with higher affinity than that of the parent compound (K_i = 7.3 μM). Some of them have K_is equal to 0.08 to 1.6 μM. However, none of them has antibacterial activity.

Some compounds inhibit the activity of class C enzymes as well as those of *S. aureus* (PC-1: K_i, 2 to 6 μM) and TEM-1 (K_i, 2.5 to 7.3 μM) (Fig. 69).

6.4. Phosphonate Derivatives

Among non-β-lactam inhibitors, the phosphonates have shown particularly interesting activity against class C β-lactamases (Fig. 70 to 72) (Li et al., 1997).

These molecules have been shown to both acylate and phosphorylate the active-site serine residue.

The cyclic phosphonates are reversible covalent inhibitors of P99 β-lactamase but are not substrates. One compound bearing a phenyl ring was shown to inhibit both class A and class C enzymes. Even though it was a cyclic compound, the reaction was not irreversible because the 4-phenylcyclic phosphate with the TEM-β-lactamases was slowly reversible.

6.5. Galangin

Flavonoids are a group of hydroxylated benzyl-γ-pyrone derivatives widely distributed in plants. More than 4,000 flavonoids have been reported. Flavonoids can inhibit the activity of zinc-containing metallopeptidases due to radical scavenging or metal chelation. Galangin (Fig. 73) is a 3,5,7-trihydroxyflavone, which inhibits L-1 metalloprotease of *S. maltophilia*. It was assumed that the 4-keto and 5-hydroxy

Ki (μM)		
PC-I	TEM-I	P99
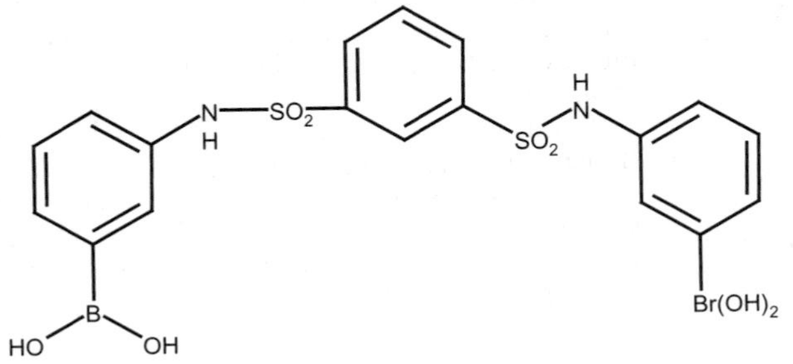 3.2	7.3	0.45
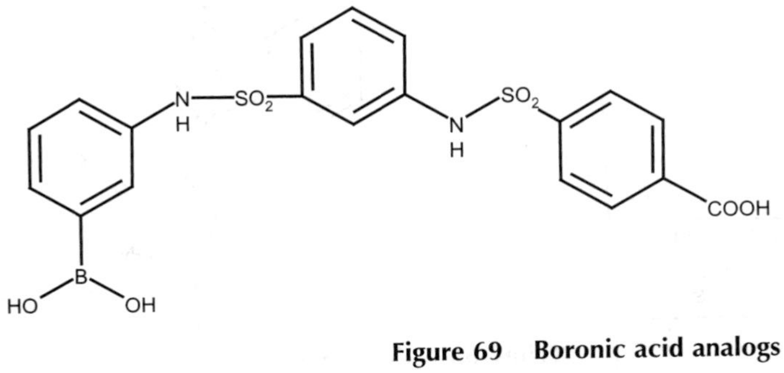 2.0	2.5	0.17

Figure 69 Boronic acid analogs

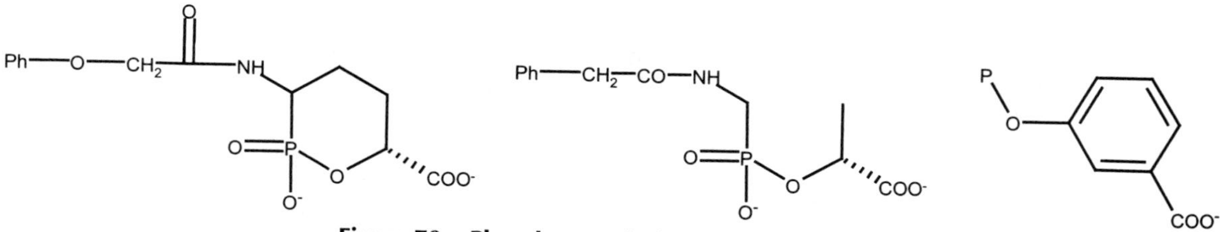

Ph—O—CH$_2$—C(=O)—NH ... O=P ... O ... COO$^-$ ... O$^-$

Figure 70 **Phosphonate derivatives (anti-class B enzymes)**

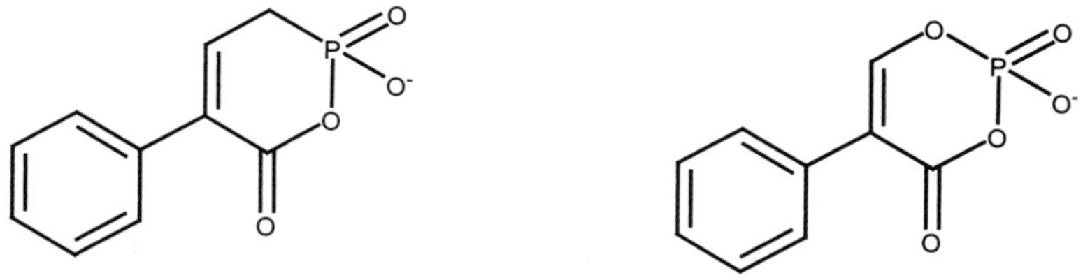

Cyclic phosphonate β-lactamase inhibitors

Phosphate β-lactamase inhibitors

Figure 71 **Cyclic phosphonates**

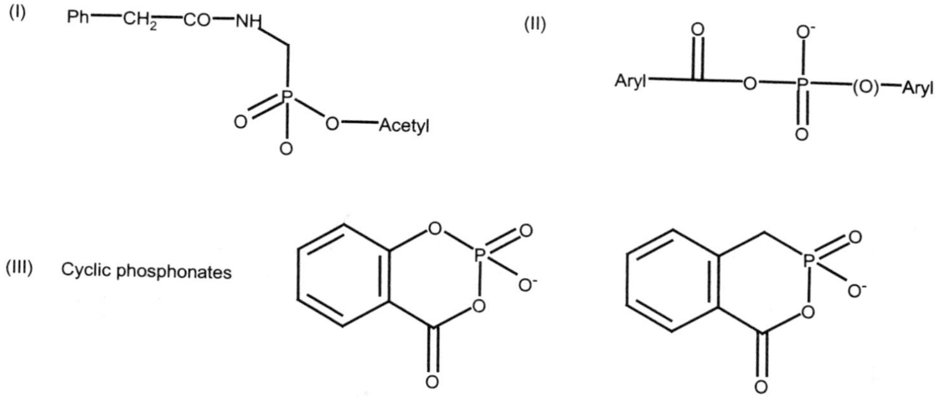

(I) Ph—CH$_2$—CO—NH ... O—Acetyl

(II) Aryl—C(=O)—O—P(O$^-$)(=O)—(O)—Aryl

(III) Cyclic phosphonates

Figure 72 **Phosphonate β-lactamase inhibitors**

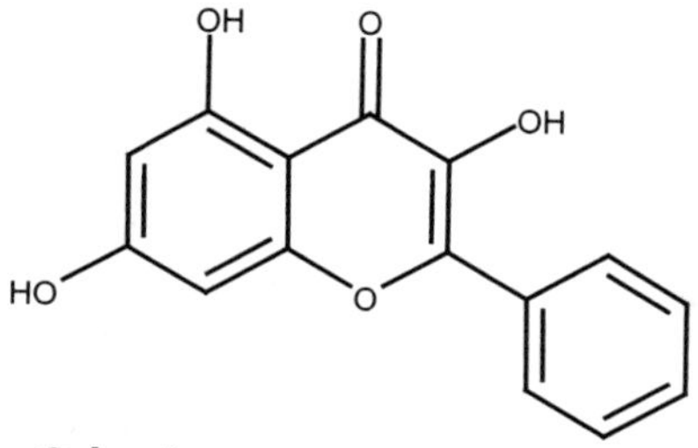

Figure 73 **Galangin**

groups from galangin bond to the zinc ion in the protein (Denny et al., 2002).

6.6. Epigallocatechin Gallate

Epigallocatechin gallate is a main constituent of catechins. This molecule enhances the in vitro activity of β-lactams against MRSA.

Epigallocatechin gallate inhibits penicillinase activity, restoring the activity of penicillin G against penicillinase-producing *S. aureus*.

6.7. Thiol Derivatives

Thiols are known inhibitors of metalloproteases because of their ability to coordinate the active-site zinc.

It was shown that cysteinyl dipeptidases are inhibitors of *B. cereus* 563/H/9 class B metallo-β-lactamase. *N*-Carbobenzoxy-D-phenylalanine has a K_i of 3.0 μM against *B. cereus* β-lactamase (Payne et al., 1997) (Fig. 74).

6.8. Captopril

Captopril (Fig. 75) and enalapril are potent inhibitors of the zinc-dependent angiotensin-converting enzyme.

Captopril was found to inhibit the *B. cereus* zinc β-lactamase, with a K_i of 41 μM, whereas enalapril, which does not contain a thiol group, is practically ineffective against β-lactamases. Captopril is a mercaptocarboxamide inhibitor of several metalloenzymes.

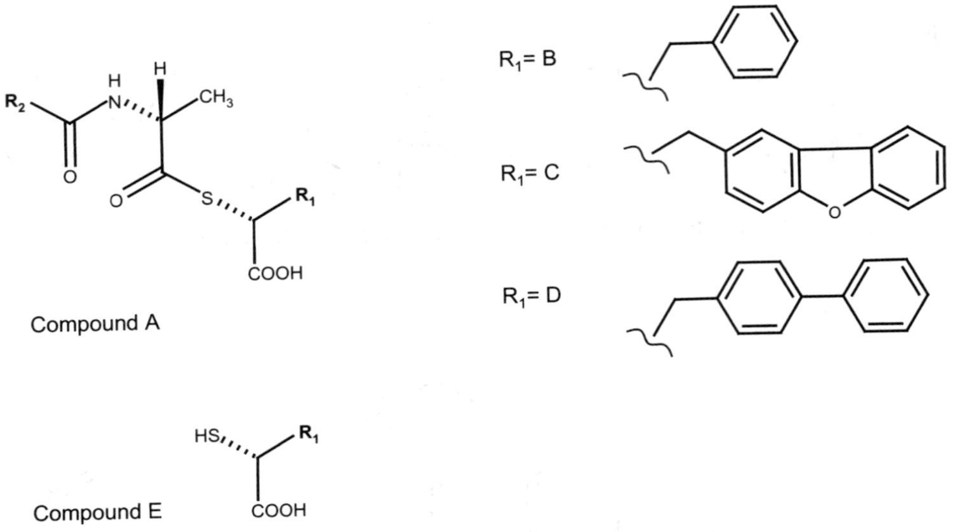

Compound A

Compound E

R_1= B

R_1= C

R_1= D

Figure 74 Thiol esters and thiol β-lactamase inhibitors

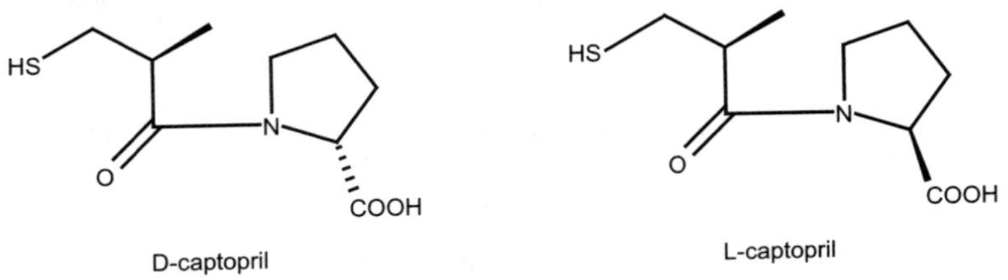

D-captopril

L-captopril

Figure 75 Captopril derivatives

Captopril may serve as a starting point for drug design by enabling the identification of protein inhibitors. D-Captopril has a higher affinity than L-captopril for β-lactamases of class B (*B. fragilis*). Diastereoisomers of captopril contain a D- and an L-proline.

6.9. *N*-Aryl Sulfonyl Hydrazones

A series of *N*-aryl sulfonyl hydrazones has been synthesized (Fig. 76). Some of them exhibit potent inhibitory activity, with IC_{50}s of 1.6 to 6.3 μM for IMP-1 metallo-β-lactamase. They seem to be poor inhibitors of *B. cereus* BCII enzyme (Siemann et al., 2002).

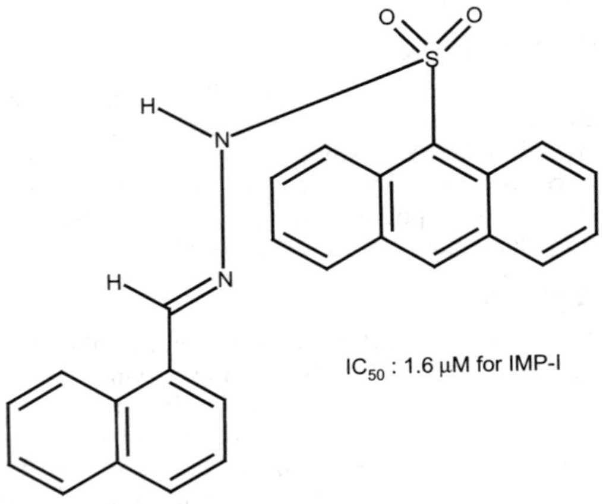

IC_{50} : 1.6 μM for IMP-I

Figure 76 *N*-Aryl sulfonyl hydrazones

6.10. α-Keto heterocycles

A series of α-keto heterocycle has been prepared. The benzoxazole derivatives were ineffective as β-lactamase inhibitors. The tetrazolyl derivative was the best β-lactamase inhibitor of the series against P99 β-lactamase (Kumar et al., 2001) (Fig. 77).

6.11. Benzofuranones

It has been shown that acyclic (thio)depsipeptides are substrates of both β-lactamases and D-D-peptidases (Adediran et al., 2001) (Fig. 78).

6.12. Dipicolinic Acids

Metalloenzymes (class B) are usually inhibited not by β-lactamase inhibitors but by uncommon chemical entities such as EDTA. By screening of the chemical library of Lederle, more than 70,000 natural products were tested against the CcrA metallo-β-lactamase. An *Actinomyces* strain, LL-10G 568, produces two dipicolinic acid derivatives. These compounds have been known since the early 1980s, but their inhibitory properties were not identified. They were isolated from a culture of *Pseudomonas putida* (Yang et al., 1994).

Both compounds are pyridine-2-carboxylic acid (Fig. 79) substituted with a side chain at position 6: monothiocarboxylic acid.

The natural products LL-10G 568α and LL-10G 568β are potent inhibitors of class B enzymes, but it was shown that LL-10G 568 lacking a free sulfhydryl group had weak inhibitory activity against metallo-β-lactamases (Table 27).

Figure 77 **α-Keto heterocycles as β-lactamase inhibitors**

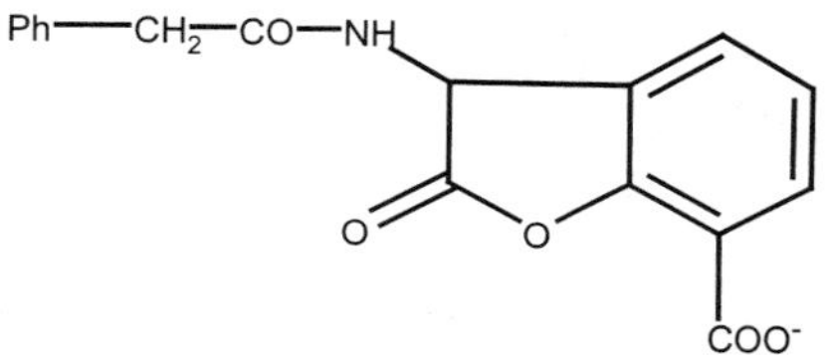

Figure 78 **Benzofuranones**

	R_1	R_2
Dipicolinic acid	OH	OH
Dipicolinic dimethyl ester	OCH_3	OCH_3
LL-10G568α	ONa	SH
LL-10G568a-mono-S methyl ester	ONa	SCH_3
LL- 10G568β	SH	SH
LL- 10G568β-di-S-methyl ester	SCH_3	SCH_3

Figure 79 **Dipicolinic acid derivatives**

They are poorly effective against *S. aureus* PC-1 (IC_{50}, >250 μM) or TEM-2 (IC_{50}, >250 μM), SHV-1, TEM-26, P99 (IC_{50}, >250 μM), and Sme-1 (IC_{50}, >44 μM).

6.13. SB 236049, SB236050, and SB238569

Extracts from *Chaetomium funicola* exhibit inhibitory activity against class B β-lactamase of *B. cereus* BCII.

Three extracts, SB 236049, SB 236050, and SB 238569 (Fig. 80), with K_is of 79, 17, and 3.4 μM for the BCII, *P. aeruginosa* IMP-1, and *B. fragilis* CfiA metalloenzymes, respectively, were investigated.

None of them display an efficacy against *S. maltophilia* L-1 enzyme (IC_{50}, >1,000 μM).

SB 236050 exhibits key polar interactions with Lys184, Asn193, and His162 and a stacking interaction with the indole ring of Trp49.

The three extracts have good synergistic activity with meropenem (Payne et al., 2002).

Table 27 **Inhibitory activities of dipicolinic derivatives against class B enzymes**

Microorganism	Enzyme	IC_{50} (μM)			
		LL-10G 568α	LL-10G 568β	Dipicolinic acid	LL-10G 568 di-*S*-methyl ester
B. fragilis	CcrA	0.29	0.14	4.2	250
S. maltophilia	L-1	1.2	0.6	7.6	340

SB 236 050

SB 236 569

SB 236 049

Figure 80 SB 236050, SB 238569, and SB 236049

6.14. Biphenyl tetrazoles

Biphenyl tetrazoles (Fig. 81) have been found to be inhibitors of metallo-β-lactamases. Some of them also display antagonism with angiotensin II.

In a series of biphenyl tetrazoles containing a 3-*n*-butylphenylpyrazole-5-carboxylate, it was shown that a single 2-chlorine is crucial for recognition of *B. fragilis* enzyme.

One derivative was found to be a modest inhibitor of IMP-1 (Toney et al., 1999).

6.15. Trifluoromethyl

Trifluoromethyl ketones (Fig. 82) are known inhibitors of serine proteases and carboxypeptidase A (zinc enzyme). It was shown that simple trifluoromethyl ketones were inhibitors of *B. cereus* BCII (Cook et al., 1998).

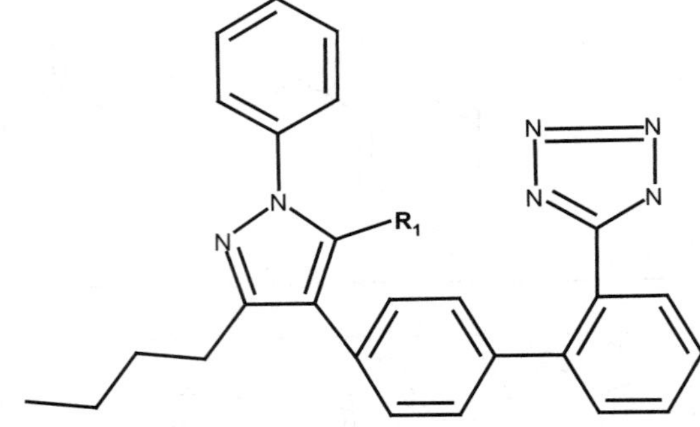

Figure 81 Biphenyl tetrazole β-lactamase inhibitors

R = CH_3 or $PhCH_2$

Figure 82 Trifluoromethyl ketones

In a series, *N*-phenoxyacetyl substituted trifluoromethyl ketones and alcohols were tested as inhibitors of β-lactamases from *S. maltophilia*, *Aeromonas hydrophila*, *B. cereus*, and *P. aeruginosa*. It was demonstrated that trifluoromethyl ketones and alcohols derived from D-alanine, L-alanine, L-phenylalanine, and D-phenylalanine exhibited significant inhibition of the metallo-β-lactamases of *S. maltophilia* and *A. hydrophila* but were less active against the enzymes from *B. cereus* and *P. aeruginosa* (Table 28 and Fig. 83).

In another series, it was demonstrated that some trifluoromethyl ketone derivatives display in vitro activity against gram-positive bacteria but not against gram-negative bacilli, except compound E, which exerted weak activity against *E. coli* (MIC, 3.9 to 7.8 μg/ml) and also against yeasts.

The combination of compound E (Fig. 84) with promethazine was significantly synergistic against *E. coli* isolates, especially the proton pump-deficient mutant.

Compound E is a 2-trifluoromethyl benzoxazole analog. Removal of the methylene resulted in a loss of potency, and replacement of benzoxazole with an another aromatic ring resulted in a significant reduction of potency.

Table 28 Activities of trifluoromethyl analogs against class B enzymes

Compound	Configuration	K_i (μM)		
		S. maltophilia	*B. cereus*	*P. aeruginosa*
A	*S*	>5,000	300	400
A′	*R*	35	700	400
B	*S*	>5,000	11,000	500
B′	*R*	>5,000	30	60
C	*S*	1.5	300	300
C′	*R*	3.0	700	500
D	*S*	15	500	539
D′	*R*	NT[a]	1,000	NT

[a]NT, not tested.

R = CH_3 A or A'
R = $PhCH_2$ B or B'

R = CH_3 C or C'
R = $PhCH_2$ D or D'

Figure 83 Trifluoromethyl ketones and alcohols

Compound E

Figure 84 Trifluoromethyl ketone analogs

Some trifluoromethyl ketones (compounds F to K) have anti-*Helicobacter pylori* activities similar to that of metronidazole and close to that of clarithromycin (Fig. 85).

6.16. BLIP

A culture filtrate of *S. clavuligerus* yielded a protein, BLIP, which was a inhibitor of β-lactamase.

BLIP inhibits class A and certain class C β-lactamases (e.g., *E. coli*) but has no effect against class C produced by *E. cloacae*. This enzyme is encoded by a chromosomal gene. The protein contains 165 amino acids for a molecular mass of 17,523 Da. The gene seems also to encode a 36-amino-acid signal sequence.

Several, but not all, β-lactamases are inhibited by BLIP (Thai et al., 2001). BLIP inhibits the plasmid pUC and chromosomally mediated β-lactamase of *E. coli* and inhibits *B. cereus* type I β-lactamase. BLIP showed no inhibitory activity against *E. cloacae* β-lactamase or *B. cereus* BCII.

Few peptides with inhibitory effects against β-lactamases have been described. One preliminary description of a peptide isolated from *Streptomyces gedanensis* which acted as an inhibitor of *S. aureus* penicillinase was published in 1972. No further investigation was carried out on this peptide.

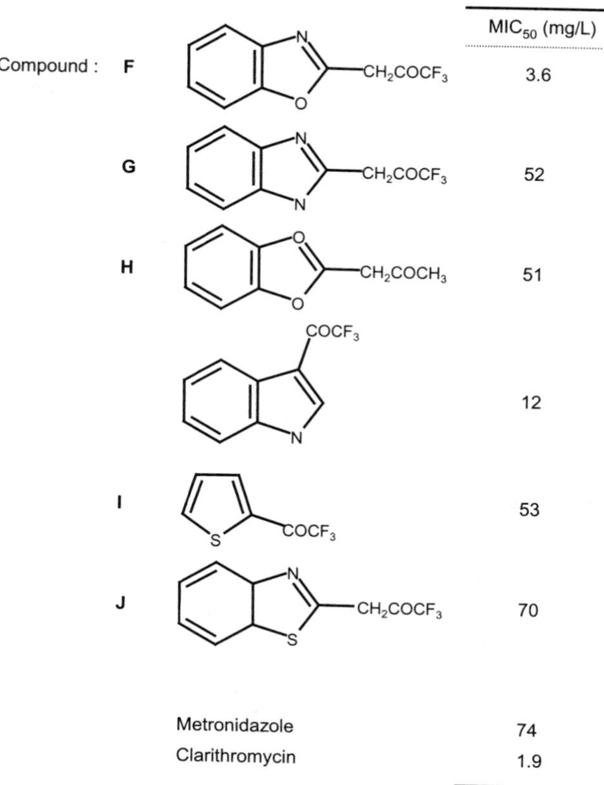

Figure 85 Anti-*H. pylori* activity of trifluoromethyl ketones

6.17. NB 2001

NB 2001 is a cephem with a 2-thienylacetamido side chain at C-7 (Fig. 86). In addition, NB 2001 contains a prodrug form with triclosan which is converted to its active form by a β-lactamase (Li et al., 2002).

Triclosan has a broad antibacterial spectrum, and it acts via inhibition of enoyl acyl carrier protein reductase (FabI).

NB 2001B exhibits good activity against gram-positive cocci through triclosan and moderate activity against gram-negative organisms through cephalothin. It is active against TEM-1, for which it is a good substrate (Table 29).

6.18. Thioesters

Simple thiodepsipeptides (compound A) has been reported to inhibit several metalloenzymes, with widely varying potencies. Introduction of hydrophobic C-terminal substituents enhanced the activity (compounds B, C, and D) (Fig. 87).

Figure 86 NB 2001

Table 29 Activity of NB 2001

Microorganism	*n*	MIC (μg/ml)[a]	
		50%	90%
S. aureus	20	0.12	0.25
Staphylococcus epidermidis	15	0.06	0.06
MRSA	20	0.12	0.5
MRSE[b]	15	0.06	0.25
S. pneumoniae Pen[s]	4	0.12	
S. pneumoniae Pen[r]	6	2.0	
Enterococcus faecalis	10	4.0	8.0
E. faecalis Van[r]	5	4.0	
M. catarrhalis	20	≤0.004	≤0.004
H. influenzae	20	0.5	1.0
E. aerogenes	30	4.0	8.0
E. cloacae	30	20	8.0
E. coli	30	4.0	8.0
K. pneumoniae	30	8.0	16
P. aeruginosa	10	>32	>32

[a]50% and 90%, MICs at which 50 and 90% of isolates are inhibited, respectively.
[b]MRSE, methicillin-resistant *S. epidermidis*.

They are substrates for IMP-1 enzyme and are hydrolyzed to thiols (compound E), which themselves are potent inhibitors of IMP-1.

The (*R*)-stereochemistry of the α-mercapto acid center is important for the inhibitory activity of these compounds (Fig. 88).

They are poorly active against *B. fragilis* CcrA enzyme. These thioesters are reversible competitive inhibitors. They increased the sensitivity of an IMP-1-producing laboratory strain of *E. coli* to the carbapenem L-742728 (Table 30).

Compound F, on which R = Ph CH (NH)CO, was found to be a good inhibitor of several metallo-β-lactamases (Table 31).

It has been hypothesized that the mercaptoacetic thiol ester derivatives are hydrolyzed by the enzyme; this hydrolysis releases the mercaptoacetic component, which irreversibly binds to the enzyme, forming a disulfide with the cysteine active site.

6.19. Thiomandelic Acid

Thiol compounds as simple as mercaptoacetic acid can be a potent inhibitor of class B enzymes either as free thiols or in the protected form of a thioester. Thiomandelic acid has good affinity for class B enzymes (Table 32).

Comparison of thiomandelic acid and *para*-substituted analogs with compounds lacking SH and COOH shows that the third group is essential for inhibition but the carboxylate group is not. Replacement of the third group by hydroxyl, bromo, or amidoxime moieties abolishes inhibitory activity.

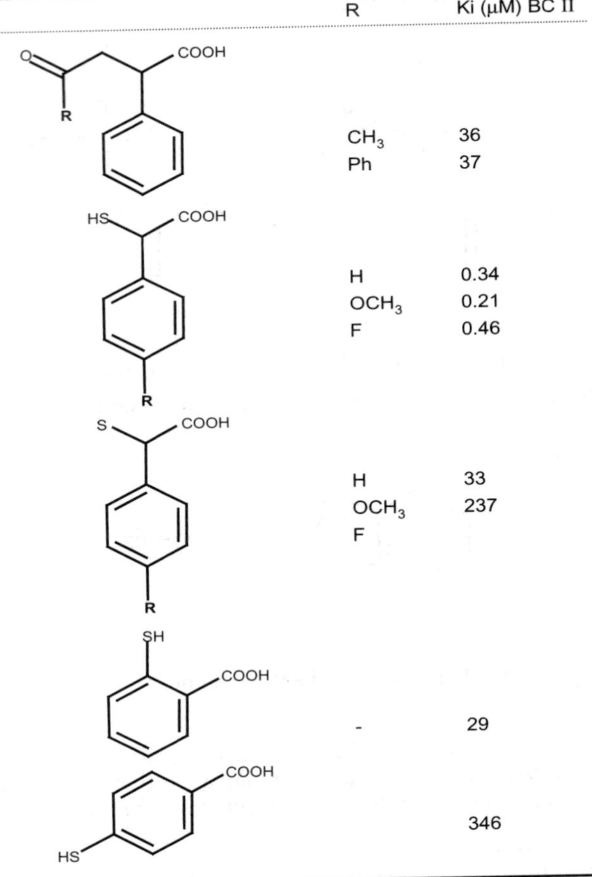

R
Ki (μM) BC II
COOH
R
CH3 36
Ph 37
HS
COOH
H 0.34
OCH3 0.21
F 0.46
R
S
COOH
H 33
OCH3 237
F
R
SH
COOH
- 29
COOH
HS
346

Figure 87 Thioester β-lactamase inhibitors

6.20. γ-Lactones

A natural γ-lactone, A-factor (2-isocapryloilhydroxymethyl-γ-butyro lactone), stimulates sporulation in *Streptomyces griseus*. Other γ-lactones possess inhibitory activity against β-lactamases.

Within a series, two derivatives (Gal et al., 2000) (Fig. 89) were tested (compounds A and B) (Table 33).

In this series, non-γ-lactones exhibited antibacterial activity (MIC, >1,000 μg/ml). The overall activity against various β-lactamases was weak and less than that of sulbactam.

6.21. Izumenolide

Izumenolide was isolated in 1980 from the fermentation broth of *Micromonospora chalcea* subsp. *izumensis*. It is a

Compound F

Thiomandelic acid

R = H/OCH$_3$/F

Figure 88 Thioester β-lactamase inhibitors: compound F and thiomandelic acid

Table 30 Activities of thioesters

Compound	IC_{50} (μM)	
	IMP-1	CcrA
A	240	>1,000
B	20	>1,000
C	12	>1,500
D	3.6	1,000

Table 31 Activity of compound F against class B

Microorganism	Enzyme	IC_{50} (μM)
B. cereus	BCII	38
S. maltophilia	L-1	3
A. hydrophila	CphA	3.5

Table 32 Affinity of thiomandelic acid for class B enzymes

Microorganism	Enzyme	K_i (μM)
B. cereus	BCI	0.34
B. fragilis	CfiA	0.80
S. maltophilia	L-1	0.081
P. aeruginosa	IMP-1	0.029
Acinetobacter baumannii	IMP-2	0.059
P. aeruginosa	VIM-1	0.23
C. meningosepticum	BlaB	0.56
Legionella gormanii	FEZ-1	0.27
A. hydrophila	CphA	144

macrocyclic compound which contains three sulfate esters. It is a potent inhibitor of β-lactamases from gram-negative bacteria, such as R-TEM β-lactamase, which is irreversibly inhibited. The synergistic activity with ampicillin is weak due to permeability problems. The mode of action was not well explored (Liu et al., 1980).

The IC_{50}s of izumenolide for different β-lactamases are reported in Table 34.

The specificity of izumenolide may be related to the anion sulfates. This hypothesis is strengthened by the fact that sodium dodecyl sulfate (SDS) and panosialin (Fig. 90) and some other alkylbenzene sulfates also inhibit β-lactamases (Bush et al., 1980).

Panosialin is distributed in *Streptomyces* strains and is a mixture of different components.

SDS is recognized as a general inhibitor of enzymes, including β-lactamases (Table 35).

The IC_{50}s for several long fatty acids are shown in Table 36.

TEM enzymes are also inhibited in a nonprogressive manner by the relatively nonspecific inhibitor panosialin (*n*-alkylbenzene disulfite).

Table 34 Inhibitory activity of izumenolide

Microorganism	Enzyme	IC_{50} (μg/ml)
B. cereus	BCI	280
B. cereus	BCII	660
S. aureus	PC-1	>1,000
E. cloacae	P99	0.1
E. coli	TEM-1	0.4
E. coli	TEM-2	0.01
K. aerogenes	K1	0.2

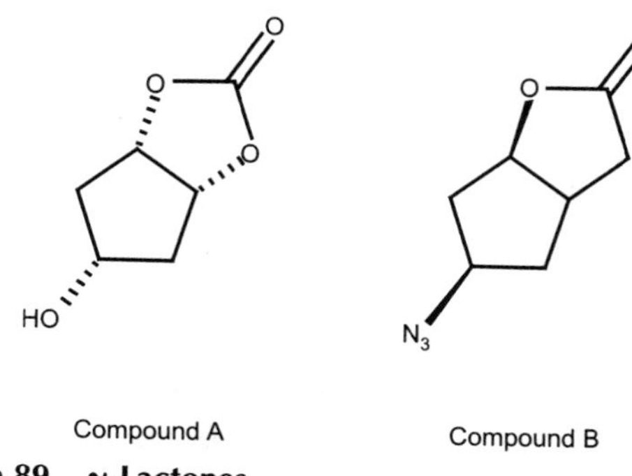

Figure 89 γ-Lactones

$OSO_3^-Na^+$
$(CH_2)_{14}CH_3$
$OSO_3^-Na^+$
$CH_3(CH_2)_{10}CH_2OS_3^-Na^+$
Sodium dodecyl sulfate

Figure 90 Panosialin

Table 33 Activities of γ-lactones against different enzymes

Microorganism	Enzyme	Group	IC_{50} (μg/ml)		
			Compound A	Compound B	Sulbactam
S. aureus	PC-1	2a	>1,000	100	3.5
B. cereus		2a	770	100	2.4
P. vulgaris		1	460	75	0.12
E. cloacae	P99	1	330	60	5.0
E. coli	R-TEM	2b	605	65	12.2
K. oxytoca	K1	2bc	15	100	3.5
K. oxytoca		2be	20	100	2.5
E. coli		2d	385	57	0.2
P. aeruginosa		2c	390	88	0.24

Table 35 Inhibitory characteristics for sulfate-containing inhibitors of TEM-2

Compound	IC_{50} (μg/ml) for TEM-2 enzyme
SDS	54
Panosialin	0.23
Izumenolide	0.01

Table 36 β-Lactamase-inhibitory activities of long fatty acids

Compound	Empiric formula	IC_{50} (nM)
Decanoic acid	$CH_3(CH_2)_8COOH$	>1.0
Lauric acid	$CH_3(CH_2)_{10}COOH$	0.4
Myristic acid	$CH_3(CH_2)_{12}COOH$	0.09
Palmitic acid	$CH_3(CH_2)_{14}COOH$	>0.5
SDS		0.01

6.22. AVE 1330A

AVE 1330A is a novel β-lactamase inhibitor (Fig. 91). It does not exhibit any antibacterial activity. It is a *trans* isomer, showing two structural features: a carbonyl-lactam bond and a structure which mimics monobactam. AVE 1330A restores activities of ceftazidime against gram-negative bacilli harboring ESBL and AmpC enzymes. It is inactive against class B enzymes. These activities was confirmed in disseminated murine infections due to ESBL-containing bacilli (Bonnefoy et al., 2004).

Figure 91 AVE 1330A

AVE 1330A has a pharmacokinetic profile similar to that of ceftazidime (half-life, ~1.0 h) in mice and protein binding of 15% (ceftazidime, 17% in humans) (Aventis, data in file, 2004).

7. CONCLUSION

The emergence of bacteria in hospitals and in the community producing new ESBL and chromosomal or plasmid-mediated class C enzymes is responsible for new medical threats, and therefore there is a need for broad-spectrum β-lactamase inhibitors.

Intensive research on β-lactamase inhibitors is needed for the following:

- To enlarge the inhibitory spectrum to cover class C and class B enzymes
- To overcome the rapid spread of ESBL
- To be prepared for an eventual reduction of activity of existing compounds, such as clavulanic acid

The most important families of inhibitors are listed in Fig. 92.

REFERENCES

Abraham EP, Chain E, 1940, An enzyme from bacteria able to destroy penicillin, Nature, 146, 837–841.

Abraham EP, Newton CG, 1956, A comparison of the action of penicillinase on benzylpenicillin and cephalosporin N and the competitive inhibition of penicillinase by cephalosporin C, Biochem J, 63, 628–634.

Adam S, Then R, Angehrn P, 1986, Potential prodrugs of 6-acetylmethylenepenicillanic acid (Ro 15-1903), J Antibiot, 39, 833–838.

Adediran SA, Cabaret D, Drouillat B, Pratt RF, Wakselman M, 2001, The synthesis and evaluation of benzofuran-e-nones as β-lactamase substrates, Biorg Med Chem Lett, 9, 1175–1183.

Ambler RP, 1980, The structure of β-lactamases, Phil Trans R Soc (London), 289B, 321–331.

Basker MJ, Boon RJ, Hunter PA, 1980, Comparative antibacterial properties in vitro of seven olivanic acid derivatives, MM 4550, MM 13902, MM 17880, MM 22380, MM 22381, MM 22382 and MM 22383, J Antibiot, 33, 878–884.

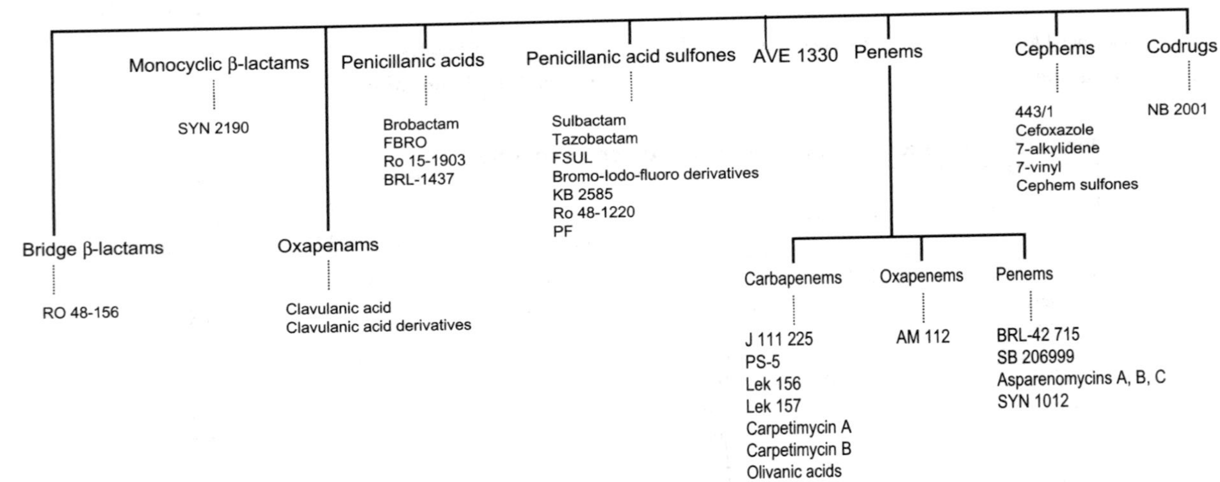

Figure 92 β-Lactamase inhibitors

Behrens OK, Garrisson L, 1950, Inhibitors for penicillinase, Arch Biochem, 27, 94–98.

Bonnefoy A, Dupuis-Hamelin C, Steier U, Delachaume C, Seyes C, Stachyra T, Guitton M, Lampilas M, 2004, In vitro activity of AVE 1330A, an innovative broad-spectrum new β-lactamase inhibitor, J Antimicrob Chemother, 54, 410–417.

Brown AG, Corbett DF, Eglington AJ, Howarth TT, 1979, Structures of olivanic acid derivatives MM 22380, MM 22381, MM 22382 and MM 22383; four new antibiotics isolated from Streptomyces olivaceus, J Antibiot, 32, 961–963.

Bush K, 1986, Evaluation of enzyme inhibition data in screening for new drugs, Drugs Exp Clin Res, 12, 565–576.

Bush K, Freudenberger J, Sykes RB, 1980, Inhibition of Escherichia coli TEM-2 β-lactamase by the sulfated compounds izumenolide, panosialin and sodium dodecyl sulfate, J Antibiot, 33, 1560–1562.

Bush K, Jacoby GA, Mederos AA, 1995, A functional classification scheme for β-lactamases and its correlation with molecular structures, Antimicrob Agents Chemother, 39, 121–133.

Buynak JD, Doppalapudi VR, Rao S, Nidamarthy CD, Grey A, 2000, The synthesis and evaluation of 2-substituted 7(alkylidene) cephalosporin sulfones as β-lactamase inhibitors, Biorg Med Chem Lett, 10, 847–851.

Buynak JD, Vogeti L, Doppalapudi R, Solomon GM, Chen H, 2002, Cephalosporin-derived β-lactamase inhibitors, part 4—the C-3 substituents, Biorg Med Chem Lett, 12, 1663–1666.

Chen YL, Hedberg K, Guarino K, Retsema JA, Anderson M, Manousos M, Barrett J, 1991, (6R, 8S)-(2-benzimidazolyl)hydroxymethyl penicillanic acids as potent antibacterial agents and β-lactamase inhibitors, J Antibiot, 44, 870–884.

Cohen MA, Huband MD, Gootz TD, 2004, In vitro activity of 6β-hydroxyalkyl penicillanic acid sulfone, an inhibitor of β-lactamases in combination with amoxicillin and ceftazidime evaluated versus contemporary clinical isolates, 44th Intersci Conf Antimicrob Agents Chemother, abstract F 321, p 194.

Cole M, 1979, Inhibition of β-lactamases, in Hamilton-Miller JMT, Smith JT, ed, β-Lactamases, Academic Press, London.

Cole M, Elson S, Fullbrook PD, 1972, Inhibition of the β-lactamases of Escherichia coli and Klebsiella aerogenes by semisynthetic penicillin, Biochem J, 127, 295–308.

Cook GK, Hornback WJ, McDonald JH III, Munroe JE, Snyder NJ, 1998, 3-Trifluoromethylcarbacephems, synthesis of broad spectrum antibacterial compounds, Bioorg Med Chem Lett, 8, 1261–1266.

Copar A, Prevec T, Anzic B, Mesar T, Selic L, Vilar M, Solmajer T, 2002, Design, synthesis and bioactivity evaluation of tribactam β-lactamase inhibitors, Bioorg Med Chem Lett, 12, 971–975.

Danelon G, Mascaretti O, Radice M, Power P, Calcagno ML, Mata EG, Gutkind G, 1998, Comparative in-vitro activities of GD-40 and other β-lactamase inhibitors against TEM-1 and SHV-2 β-lactamases, J Antimicrob Chemother, 41, 313–315.

Denny BJ, Lambert PA, West PW, 2002, The flavonoid galangin inhibits the L1 metallo-beta-lactamase from Stenotrophomonas maltophilia, FEMS Microbiol Lett, 208, 21–24.

Gal ZS, Koncz A, Szabo I, Deak E, Benko I, Baradas GY, Hernadi F, Kovacs P, 2000, A synthetic gamma-lactone group with beta-lactamase inhibitory and sporulation initiation effects, J Chemother, 12, 274–279.

Grant EB, Guiadeen D, Bush K, Baum EZ, Foleno B, Jin H, Montenegro DA, Hlasta DJ, 1999, The synthesis and SAR of the rhodamines as novel class C β-lactamase inhibitors, 39th Intersci Conf Antimicrob Agents Chemother, abstract 404, p 299.

Greenwood D, O'Grady F, 1975, Potent combinations of beta-lactam antibiotics using the beta-lactamase inhibition principle, Chemotherapy, 21, 330–341.

Hakimelahi GH, Shia KS, Xue C, Hakimelahi S, Moosavi-Movahedi AA, Saboury AA, Khalafi-Nezhad A, et al, 2002, Design, synthesis, and biological evaluation of a series of β-lactam-based prodrugs, Bioorg Med Chem, 10, 3489–3498.

Jamieson CE, Lambert PA, Simpson IN, 2003, In vitro and in vivo activities of AM-112, a novel oxapenem, Antimicrob Agents Chemother, 47, 1652–1657.

Jin H, Montenegro DA, Melton J, Hlasta DJ, Guiadeen D, Grant EB, Foleno B, Fernandez J, Baum EZ, Bush K, 1999, Novel rhodamine as class C β-lactamase inhibitors, 39th Intersci Conf Antimicrob Agents Chemother, abstract F-405, p 300.

Kumar S, Pearson AL, Pratt RF, 2001, Design, synthesis, and evaluation of α-ketoheterocycles as class C β-lactamase inhibitors, Bioorg Med Chem, 9, 2035–2044.

Laufs R, Riess F, Jahn G, Fock R, Kaulfer Z, 1981, Origin of *Haemophilus influenzae* R-factor, J Bacteriol, 147, 563–568.

Li N, Rahil J, Wright ME, Pratt RF, 1997, Structure-activity studies of the inhibition of serine beta-lactamases by phosphonate monoesters, Bioorg Med Chem, 5, 1783–1788.

Li Q, Lee JY, Castillo R, Hixon MS, Pujol C, Doppalapudi VR, Shepard HM, Wahl GM, Lobl TJ, Chan MF, 2002, NB2001, a novel antibacterial agent with broad-spectrum activity and enhanced potency against beta-lactamase-producing strains, Antimicrob Agents Chemother, 46, 1262–1268.

Liu WC, Astle G, Wells JS Jr, Trejo WN, Principe PA, Rathnium ML, Parker WL, Kocy OR, Sykes RB, 1980, Izumenolide—a novel β-lactamase inhibitor produced by Micromonospora. I. Detection, isolation and characterization, J Antibiot, 33, 1256–1261.

Livermore DM, Chen HY, 1997, Potentiation of β-lactams against Pseudomonas aeruginosa strains by Ro-48-1256, a bridged monobactam inhibitor of AmpC β-lactamases, J Antimicrob Chemother, 40, 335–343.

Mitsuhashi S, Inoue M, 1981, Mechanism of resistance to β-lactam antibiotics, p 41–56, in Mitsuhashi S, ed, Beta-Lactam Antibiotics, Japan Scientific Press, Tokyo.

Mollard C, Moali C, Papamicael C, Damblon C, Vessilier S, Amicosante G, Schofield CJ, Galleni M, Frere JM, Roberts GC, 2001, Thiomandelic acid, a broad spectrum inhibitor of zinc beta-lactamases, kinetic and spectroscopic studies, J Biol Chem, 276, 4515–4523.

Moore BA, Brammer KW, 1981, 6β-Iodo penicillanic acid (UK-38006), a β-lactamase inhibitor that extends the antibacterial spectrum of β-lactam compounds, initial bacteriological characterization, Antimicrob Agents Chemother, 20, 327–331.

Murakami K, Doi M, Yoshida T, 1982, Asparenomycins A, B and C, new carbapenem antibiotics. V. Inhibition of beta-lactamases, J Antibiot, 35, 39–45.

Nagano R, Adachi Y, Hashizume T, Morishima H, 2000, In vitro antibacterial activity and mechanism of action of J 111225, a novel 1β-methyl carbapenem against transferable IMP-1 metallo-β-lactamase producers, J Antimicrob Chemother, 45, 271–276.

Nagano Y, Kumagai T, Kobayashi S, Tamai S, Ohta K-I, Inoue Y, Kishi K, 1997, Synthetic approach toward the development of new β-lactamase inhibitors, Heterocycles, 46, 193–198.

Nakayama M, Iwasaki A, Kimura S, Mizoguchi T, et al, 1980, Carpetimycins A and B, new β-lactam antibiotics, J Antibiot, 33, 1388–1390.

Neu, HC, 1983, β-Lactamase inhibitory activity of iodopenicillanate and bromopenicillanate, Antimicrob Agents Chemother, 23, 63–66.

Nishida K, Kunugita C, Uji T, Higashitani F, Hyodo A, et al, 1999, In vitro and in vivo activities of Syn 2190, a novel β-lactamase inhibitor, Antimicrob Agents Chemother, 43, 1885–1890.

O'Callaghan C, Morris A, 1972, Inhibition of beta-lactamases by beta-lactam antibiotics, Antimicrob Agents Chemother, 2, 442–448.

Park KW, Yim CB, Kim KH, 1998, Comparative activity of novel β-lactamase inhibitors, 6-exomethylene penam sulfones (CH 1240, CH 2140), in experimental mouse infection model, Arch Pharm Res, 21, 527–530.

Payne DJ, Bateson JH, Gasson BC, Proctor D, Khushi T, Farmer TH, Tolson DA, Bell D, Skett PW, Marshall AC, Reid R, Ghosez L, Combret Y, Marchand-Brynaert J, 1997, Inhibition of metallo-beta-lactamases by a series of mercaptoacetic acid thiol ester derivatives, Antimicrob Agents Chemother, 41, 135–140.

Payne DJ, Hueso-Rodriguez JA, Boyd H, Concha NO, Janson CA, Gilpin M, Bateson JH, Cheever C, Niconovich NL, Pearson S, Rittenhouse S, Tew D, Diez E, Perez P, De La Fuente J, Rees M, Rivera-Sagredo A, 2002, Identification of a series of tricyclic natural products as potent broad-spectrum inhibitors of metallo-beta-lactamases, Antimicrob Agents Chemother, 46, 1880–1886.

Philippon A, Arlet G, Jacoby G, 2002, Plasmid-determined AmpC-type β-lactamases, Antimicrob Agents Chemother, 46, 1–11.

Phillips OA, Czajkowski DP, Spevak P, Singh MP, Hanehara C, Kunugita A, Hyodo A, Micetich RG, Maiti SN, 1997, SYN 1012—a new β-lactamase inhibitor of penem skeleton, J Antibiot, 50, 350–356.

Pratt RF, Anderson EG, Odeh I, 1980, Certain monocyclic β-lactams are β-lactamase substrates: nocarcidin and desthiobenzyl penicillin, Biochem Biophys Res Commun, 93, 1266–1273.

Reading C, Cole M, 1977, Clavulanic acid, a beta-lactamase-inhibiting beta-lactam from *Streptomyces clavuligerus*, Antimicrob Agents Chemother, 11, 852–857.

Richmond MH, Sykes R, 1973, The beta-lactamases of gram-negative bacteria and their possible physiological role, Adv Microb Physiol, 9, 31–88.

Sakamoto M, Ishikura T, Fukagawa Y, 1984, Synergism of PS-5 with penicillins and cephalosporins in antimicrobial activity against beta-lactam-resistant gram-negative microorganisms, J Antibiot, 37, 1414–1422.

Siemann S, Evanoff DP, Marrone L, Clarke AJ, Viswanatha T, Dmitrienko GI, 2002, N-Arylsulfonyl hydrazones as inhibitors of IMP-1 metallo-beta-lactamase, Antimicrob Agents Chemother, 46, 2450–2457.

Singh R, Cooper RDG, 1994, Synthesis and biological evaluation of 6-azabicyclo [320] hept-2-ene derivatives as potential antibacterial agents and β-lactamase inhibitors, Tetrahedron, 50, 12049–12064.

Tanizawa K, Santoh K, Kanaoka Y, 1989, Diketene analogs as β-lactamase inhibitors, Chem Pharm Bull, 37, 824–825.

Thai W, Paradkar AS, Jensen SE, 2001, Construction and analysis of β-lactamase-inhibitory protein (BLIP) non-producer mutants of Streptomyces clavuligerus, Microbiology, 147, 325–335.

Toney JH, Cleary KA, Hammond GG, Yuan X, May WJ, Hutchins SM, Ashton WT, Vanderwall DE, 1999, Structure-activity relationships of biphenyl tetrazoles as metallo-beta-lactamase inhibitors, Bioorg Med Chem Lett, 20, 2741–2746.

Toney JH, Hammond GG, Fitzgerald PM, Sharma N, Balkovec JM, Rouen GP, Olson SH, Hammond ML, Greenlee ML, Gao YD, 2001, Succinic acids as potent inhibitors of plasmid-borne IMP-1 metallo-beta-lactamase, J Biol Chem, 276, 31913–31918.

Tzouvelekis LS, Gazouli M, Prinarakis EE, Tzelepi E, Legakis NJ, 1997, Comparative evaluation of the inhibitory activities of the novel penicillanic acid sulfone Ro 48-1220 against beta-lactamases that belong to groups 1, 2b, and 2be, Antimicrob Agents Chemother, 41, 475–477.

Venkatesan AM, Mansour TS, Dos Santos O, Agarwal A, Petersen PJ, Weiss WJ, Yang Y, Shlaes DM, Abe T, Ushirogochi H, Yamamura I, Kumagai T, 2004, Novel penems bearing a bicyclic heterocycle on methylidene linkage as broad spectrum β-lactamase inhibitors and their mechanism of inactivation, 44th Intersci Conf Antimicrob Agents Chemother, abstract F-320.

Vilar M, Galleni M, Solmajer T, Turk B, Frere JM, Matagne A, 2001, Kinetic study of two novel enantiomeric tricyclic beta-lactams which efficiently inactivate class C beta-lactamases, Antimicrob Agents Chemother, 45, 2215–2223.

Weston GS, Blaquez J, Baquero F, Shoidez BK, 1998, Structure-based enhancement of boronic acid-based inhibitors of AmpC β-lactamases, J Med Chem, 41, 4577–4586.

Woodnutt G, Berry V, Mizen L, 1992, Simulation of human serum pharmacokinetics of cefazolin, piperacillin, and BRL 42715 in rats and efficacy against experimental intraperitoneal infections, Antimicrob Agents Chemother, 36, 1427–1431.

Yamaguchi A, Adachi A, Hirata T, Adachi H, Sawai T, 1985, Conversion of cloxacillin into a progressive inhibitor of beta-lactamases by sulfonation and its activity against various types of these enzymes, J Antibiot, 38, 83–93.

Yamashita M, Hashimoto S, Ezaki M, Iwami M, Komori T, Kohsaka M, Imanaka HJ, 1983, FR-900318, a novel penicillin with beta-lactamase inhibitory activity, J Antibiot, 36, 1774–1776.

Yang Y, Roll DM, Wildey MJ, Lee MD, Greenstein M, Maiese WM, Bush K, 1994, Inhibition of metallo-β-lactamases by LL-10G568α and LL-10G568β, 34th Intersci Conf Antimicrob Agents Chemother, abstract C-56.

γ-Lactams and Derivatives

A. BRYSKIER

15

1. INTRODUCTION

The β-lactams represent the largest clinical class of antibiotics. However, the activity of the β-lactams is declining, as a result either of their enzymatic inactivation by chromosomally or plasmid-mediated β-lactamases, of the reduction in their ability to cross the bacterial outer membrane, or of a modification of their affinity for their bacterial target, the penicillin-binding proteins (PBP), which are in fact enzymes involved in peptidoglycan synthesis. Several solutions have been proposed to overcome this reduction in activity. The first involves the search for natural molecules in hypersensitive mutants, and a number of new molecules have been discovered: sulfazecins, cephabecins, formacidins, and lactivicins.

The second solution that has been proposed is the replacement of the azetidinone ring by other rings: cyclobutanone, β-sulfam, and thionolactam. However, these structures have failed to yield prototypes with active molecules.

Interest has since turned to the pentacycles, which possess certain affinities for PBP, such as the γ-lactams, pyrazolidinones, and isoxazolidinones (lactivicin). The general structure is shown in Fig. 1.

2. γ-LACTAMS

Derivatives of the γ-lactam-type penicillin had been synthesized since 1949. However, research in this area did not really start until the beginning of the 1980s.

Baldwin et al. (1983) took as their hypothesis the idea that the azetidinone ring was not necessary for antibacterial activity and that only the amide bond was essential. They synthesized two γ-lactam analogs of carbapenicillanic acid (Fig. 2). These molecules were devoid of antibacterial activity and β-lactamase-inhibitory activity. The same authors synthesized molecules with an azetidinone ring (Fig. 3) that were devoid of antibacterial activity and inhibitory activity against *Bacillus cereus* class I β-lactamases. A similar amino derivative appears to possess a certain antibacterial activity (Fig. 4). The first γ-lactam molecules to exhibit antibacterial activity (Fig. 5) were described by Baldwin et al. (1986) and Boyd et al. (1986). It appeared that greater activity could be obtained with penem-like derivatives because of the possibility of electronic modifications at the nitrogen (Fig. 6). A γ-lactam analog of ceftizoxime was synthesized, but it did not possess antibacterial activity (Fig. 7). It was shown that bicyclic γ-lactams with a side chain at C-7 rather than at C-6 and in the β position have a configuration identical to that of the β-lactams. It was postulated that this

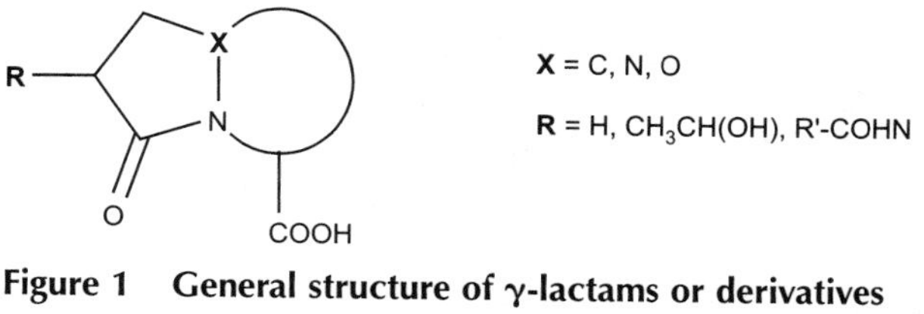

X = C, N, O

R = H, $CH_3CH(OH)$, R'-COHN

Figure 1 General structure of γ-lactams or derivatives

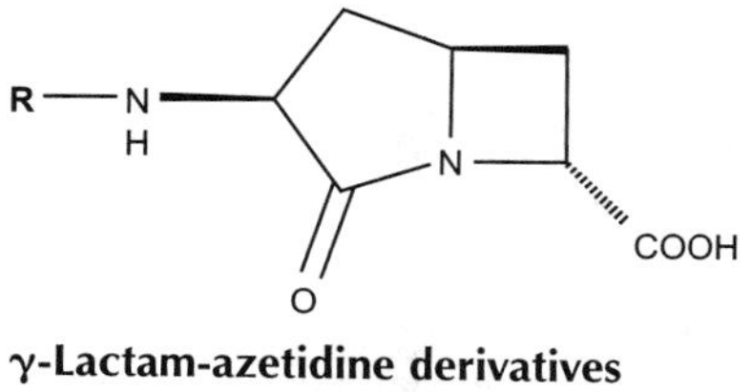

Figure 3 γ-Lactam-azetidine derivatives

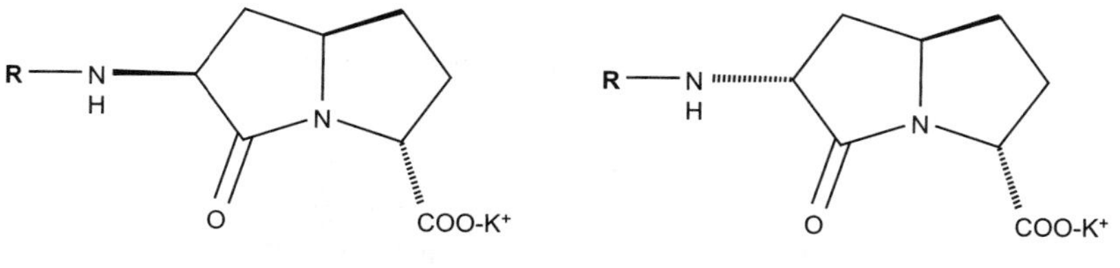

Figure 2 γ-Lactam derivatives of carbapenicillanic acid

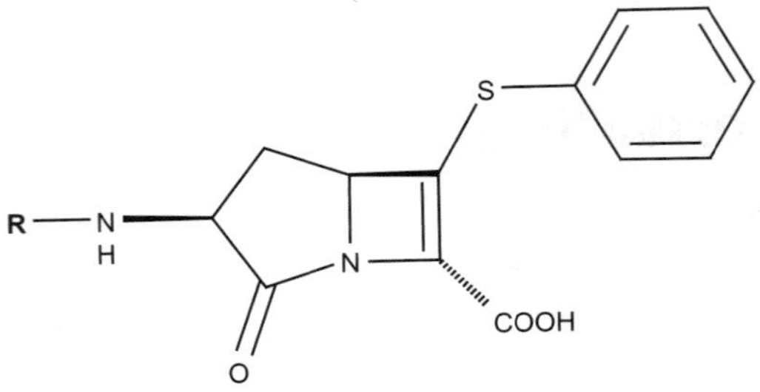

Figure 4 β-Lactam-azete derivatives

side chain was important for the antibacterial activity of the β-lactams. There is a center of asymmetry at C-7, and the *S*-isomer is more active than the *R*-isomer against gram-positive cocci (Table 1).

Among the carbapenem analogs, there is a sulfoxide derivative with moderate antibacterial activity (Fig. 8), as well as the derivative with a 2-amino-5-thiazolyl methoxyimine chain at C-7 (Fig. 9). Hahiguchi et al. (1982) synthesized a series of γ-lactam derivatives which are carbapenem analogs and have a cysteamine chain. They differ in the chain at C-7 and the substituents of the cysteamine residue (Fig. 10). All of these compounds possess weak activity against gram-negative bacilli. The sulfone derivative is more active than the sulfide derivative. The *trans* isomer is more active, with MICs of 25, 6.25, and 25 μg/ml for *Escherichia coli*, *Proteus mirabilis* 21100, and *Klebsiella pneumoniae* IFO 3317, than is the *cis* isomer, with MICs of 100, 25, and 100 μg/ml for the same microorganisms.

γ-Oxapenam- and γ-oxapenem-type derivatives have been synthesized, as well as monocyclic β-lactam analogs (Fig. 11), but these are devoid of activity.

3. PYRAZOLIDINONES

Researchers from Eli Lilly studied the activity of the pyrazolidinone nuclei in the γ-lactam family. The first derivative, derivative A (Fig. 12), is active against *Staphylococcus aureus*.

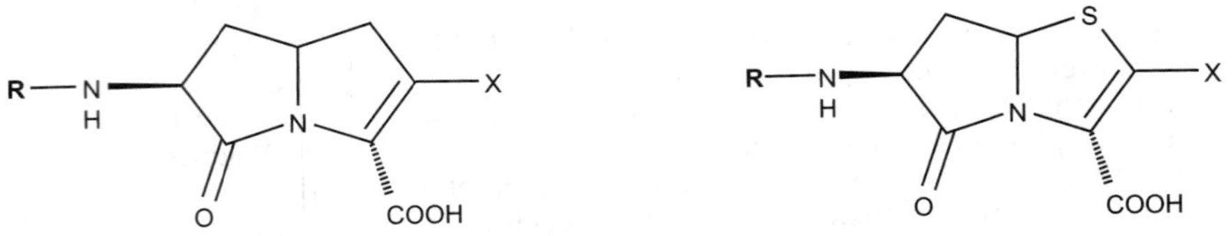

Figure 5 γ-Lactam-penem derivatives

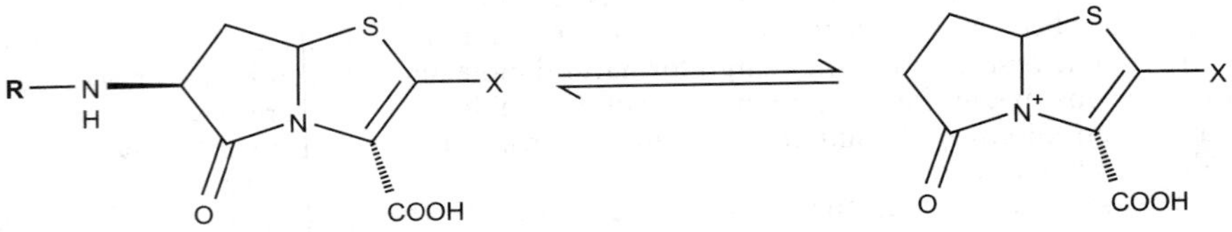

Figure 6 γ-Lactam-penem electronic alterations

Table 1 In vitro activities of the γ-lactam isomers

Strain	MIC (μg/ml)	
	S-Isomer	*R*-Isomer
Streptococcus pneumoniae Park	128	4.0
S. pyogenes C-203	64	8.0

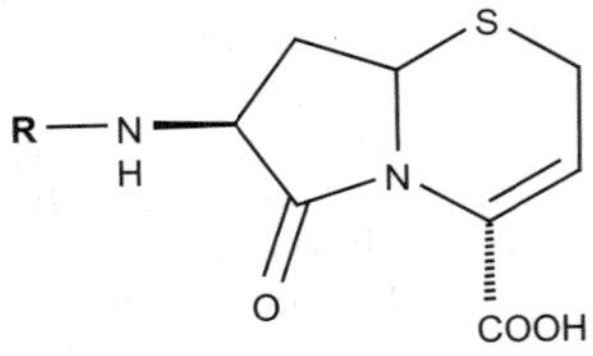

Figure 7 γ-Lactam analog of ceftizoxime

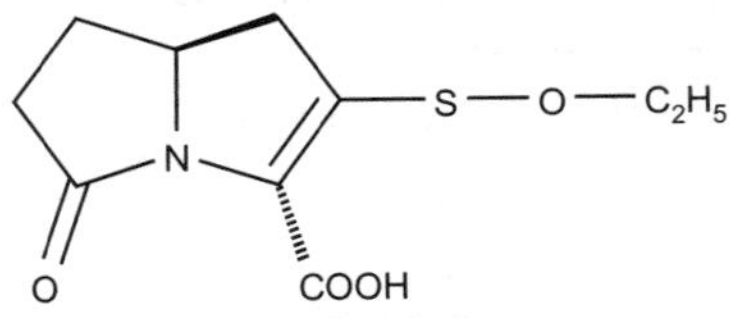

Figure 8 γ-Lactam sulfoxide derivative

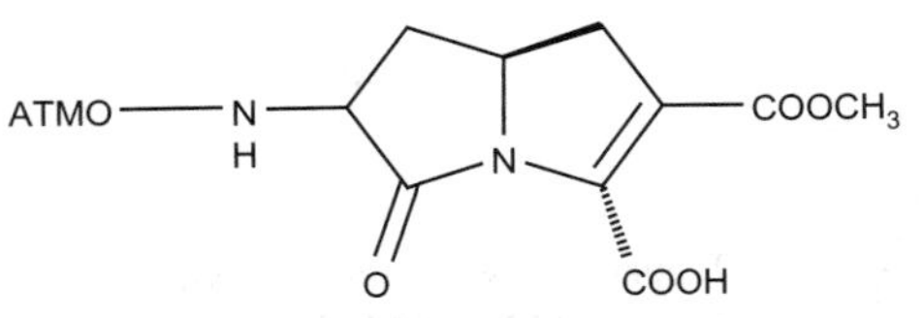

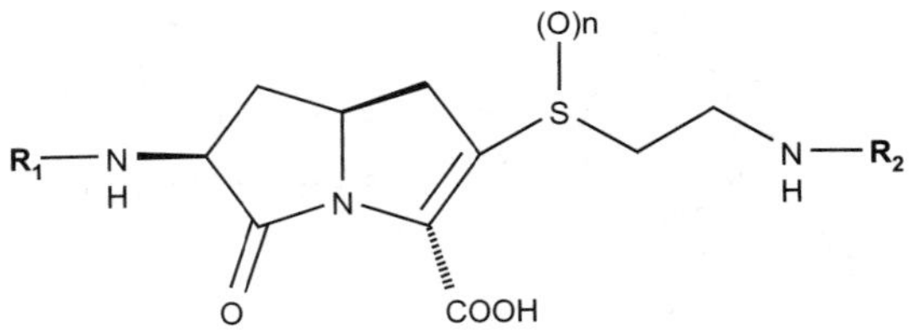

R_1	R_2	N
Phenylglycine	Ac	0
Amino thiazolyl methoxyimine	Ac	0
Phenylglycine	H	0
Phenylglycine	H	2

Figure 9 γ-Lactam methoxiimine derivative

Figure 10 γ-Lactam carbapenem derivatives

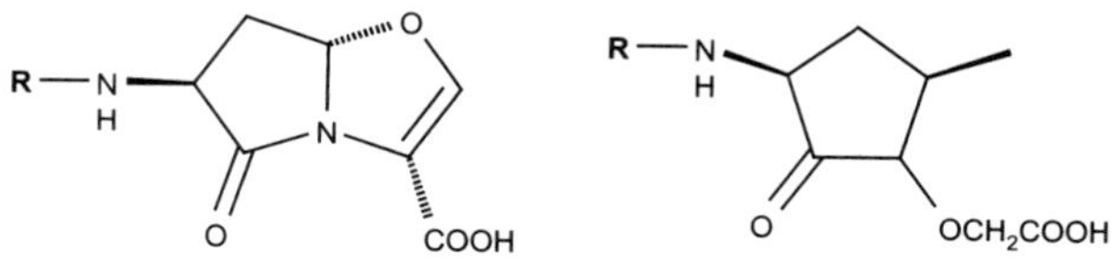

Figure 11 γ-Lactam monolactam derivatives

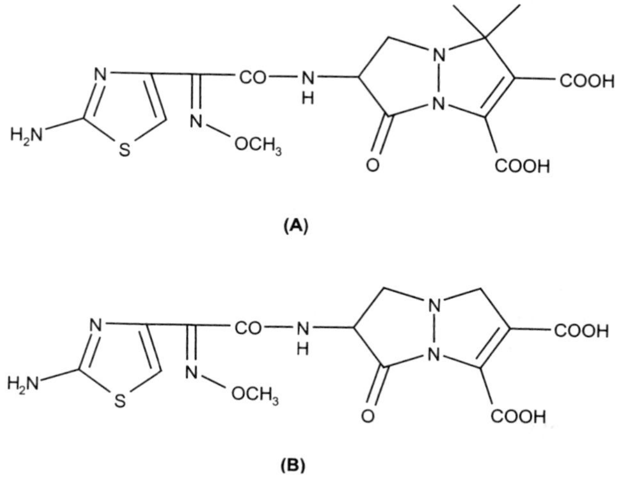

(A)

(B)

Figure 12 γ-Lactam from Eli Lilly

A new series was synthesized, and 3-methyl ester and 3-acetyl derivatives exhibited good antibacterial activity. The opening of the γ-lactam ring is dependent on the substituent at C-3. The cyano (LY-255262) and sulfone (LY-193239) derivatives are more active against gram-negative than against gram-positive bacteria. However, they are inactive against *Pseudomonas aeruginosa* and *S. aureus* (MIC, ≥32 μg/ml) (Table 2).

The replacement of the carbon at position 3 by a sulfur atom failed to produce more active molecules.

The increase in lipophilicity of the substituent at C-3 or on the oxime residue enhanced the activity against gram-positive bacteria but decreased that against gram-negative bacteria.

The *S*-isomer has been shown to be more active than the racemate against gram-negative bacteria. The *S*-isomer in the chain at C-7 has a configuration similar to that of the cephems and penems.

The LY-221124 derivative has a C-7 chain of the imipenem type and is devoid of antibacterial activity.

4. LACTIVICINS

4.1. Lactivicin

Lactivicin is an antibacterial agent isolated from the fermentation of *Empedobacter lactamgenus* YK-258 and *Lysobacter albus* YK-422.

This is a molecular entity comprising an isoxazolidinone (*S*-cycloserine) and γ-lactam nucleus connected by a simple C-N bond. Lactivicin is a mixture of two epimers, A and B, in a ratio of 53:47 (Fig. 13).

Lactivicin is an acidic antibiotic that is soluble in water. The physicochemical properties of lactivicin and the methylated esters of the carboxyl group are summarized in Table 3.

Lactivicin is a non-β-lactam antibiotic that shares the microbiological properties of the β-lactams:

- Binding to PBP
- Susceptibility to hydrolysis by cephalosporinases and pencillinases
- Induction of β-lactamase
- Activity against certain anaerobic bacterial species
- Inactivity against mycoplasmas

In addition, it possesses weak inhibitory activity against certain β-lactamases. The antibacterial activity of lactivicin

Table 2 Comparative activities of C-3-substituted pyrazolidinone derivatives

Substitution	MIC (μg/ml)		
	S. pyogenes C-203	*K. pneumoniae* X68	*Providencia rettgeri* C24
SO_2CH_3	0.25	0.25	0.06
CN	0.5	0.50	0.25
$COCH_3$	0.5	2.0	0.25
CO_2CH_3	4.0	8.0	1.0
$CONHC_2H_5$	1.0	32	8.0
COOH	8.0	64	8.0
2-Thiophene	>128	>128	>128
Benzyl	>128	>128	>128

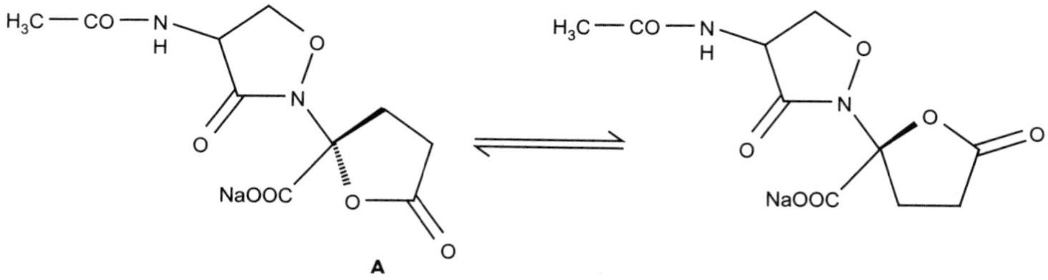

A

Figure 13 Lactivicins

Table 3 Physicochemical properties of lactivicin

Property[a]	Lactivicin (A)	Methyl esters (B)	Methyl esters
Appearance	White powder	Colorless crystals	Colorless crystals
Melting point (°C)		163–166	180–181
Specific rotation	−24.1°	76.7°	−112°
C=	0.5, H_2O	0.62, $CHCL_3$	0.51, $CHCL_3$
MW	295	287	287
Empirical formula	$C_{10}H_{11}N_2O_7Na$	$C_{11}H_{14}N_2O_7$	$C_{11}H_{14}N_2O_7$
UV λ_{max} (E)	216 (4,050)	216 (3,720)	217 (4,000)
Solvent	H_2O	CH_3OH	CH_3OH
IR $S_{max}^{(KBr)}$ (cm^{-1})	1,780, 1,730, 1,660	1,800, 1,750, 1,760, 1,650	1,815, 1,805, 1,760, 1,740, 1,665

[a]MW, molecular weight; E, absorbance; IR S_{max}, infrared spectra.

Table 4 Antibacterial activity of lactivicin

Strain	MIC (μg/ml)
S. aureus 209P	6.25
S. pyogenes E-14	1.56
S. pneumoniae 1	6.25
Corynebacterium diphtheriae Tront	0.78
E. coli NIHJ-JC2	100
Citrobacter freundii IFO 12681	100
K. pneumoniae DT	100
Sernatia marcescens IFO 12648	100
P. aeruginosa IFO 3455	100
Acinetobacter calcoaceticus IFO 13006	50

is summarized in Table 4. Lactivicin is active against gram-positive bacteria and inactive against gram-negative bacteria. In vivo, lactivicin has moderate activity (Table 5).

Table 5 Activity of lactivicin after intraperitoneal infection in the mouse (subcutaneous administration)

Strain	MIC (μg/ml)	ED_{50}[a] (mg/kg)
S. aureus 308 A-1	25	25.4
S. pyogenes E-14	1.56	2.05
E. coli O-111	50	7.10

[a]ED_{50}, 50% effective dose.

It has a dual mechanism of action: (i) inhibition of peptidoglycan synthesis and (ii) inhibition of the activity of membrane proteins with a thiol group.

The mechanism of action of lactivicin is similar to that of the β-lactams. They act by irreversible acylation of PBP by opening of the γ-lactam nucleus. The resultant oxime is then degraded (Fig. 14).

4.2. Synthetic Derivatives

Synthetic derivatives have been prepared to reduce the parenteral toxicity and to increase the activity and antibacterial spectrum. The acute toxicity is 400 mg/kg of body weight subcutaneously and more than 400 mg/kg orally.

The lack of the γ-lactam nucleus suppresses the antibacterial activity (Fig. 15). Derivatives with a D-phenylglycyl group are inactive because they are unstable in a neutral or

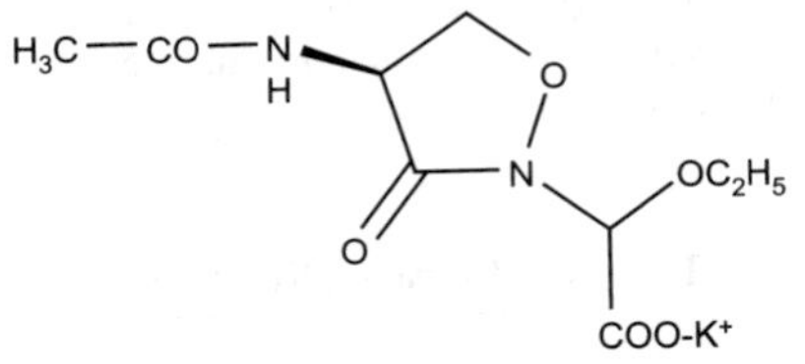

Figure 15 Lactivicin: lack of γ-lactam ring

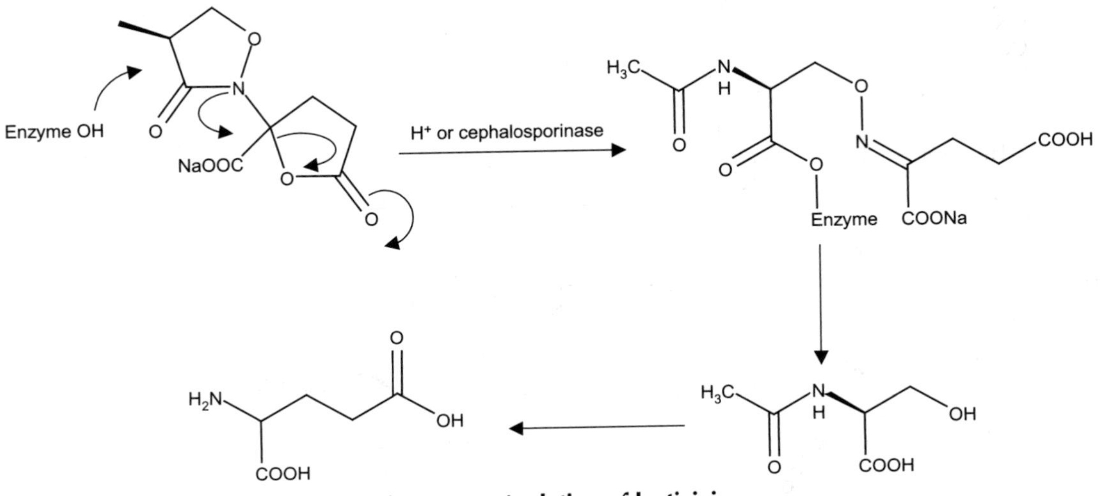

Figure 14 Acylation of lactivicin

basic medium. The methoxyimino-2-amino-5-thiazolyl derivatives are the most active (Fig. 16). The molecules bind to *E. coli* PBP 3 (Table 6).

Monolactam analog derivatives have yielded orally absorbed molecules (Table 7).

Monolactam analog derivatives have been synthesized, as well as azalactivicins. Among the latter, the non-N-substituted derivatives are weakly active, while the N-acetylated and N-methylated derivatives are inactive against *E. coli* O-111 and *Streptococcus pyogenes* E-14 (Fig. 17).

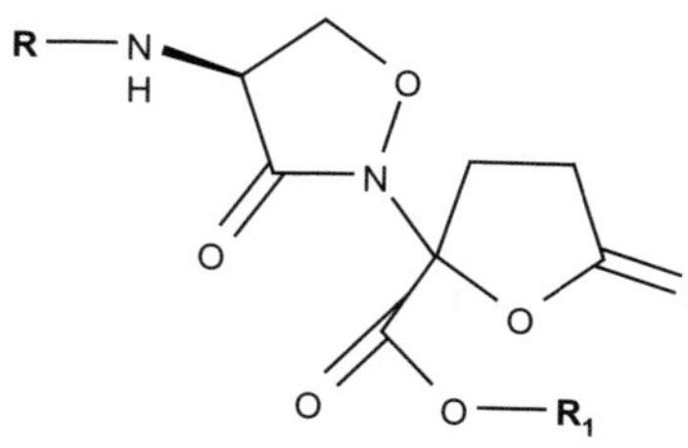

	R	R_1
Lactivicin	Acetyl	Na
Phenylglycine	Ph-CH_2-CO-	Na
Phenylglycine esterified	Ph-CH_2-CO-	-CH_2O-CO-C$(CH_3)_2$
Thiadiazolyl	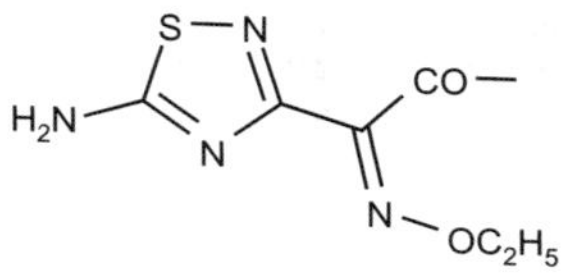 H_2N-thiadiazolyl-C(=N-OC_2H_5)-CO-	

Figure 16 Methoxyimino-2-amino-5-thiazolyl derivatives

Table 6 In vitro activities of derivatives of lactivicin

Strain	MIC (μg/ml)[a]						
	Lactivicin	D-Cycloserine	MAT	HAT	BAT	Th	Pyr
S. aureus 209P	3.13	12.5	12.5	1.56	>100	0.39	<0.1
E. coli NIHJ-JC2	100	25	0.39	3.13	0.78	6.25	12.5
C. freundii IFO 12681	100	50	3.13	1.56	0.78	12.5	100
K. pneumoniae DT	100		0.78	3.13	0.2	6.25	12.5
S. marcescens IFO 12648	100	>100	3.13	6.25	0.39	>100	>100
Proteus vulgaris IFO 3988	100	100	0.78	3.13	<0.1	6.25	100

[a]MAT, methoxyimino amino-2-thiazolyl; HAT, hydroxyiminothiazolyl; BAT, isobutyliminothiazolyl; Th, 2-methylthienyl; Pyr, 2′-chloro-4′-thiomethylpyridone.

Table 7 In vivo activities of lactivicin derivatives

Compound	Strain	MIC (μg/ml)	ED_{50} (mg/kg)[a]
Lactivicin	*S. aureus* 308 A-1	25	25.4 s.c.
	S. pyogenes E-14	1.56	2.05 s.c.
	E. coli O-111	50	71.0 s.c.
Phenylglycine derivative	*S. aureus* 308 A-1	0.78	21.1 s.c.
	S. pyogenes E-14	<0.1	0.65 s.c.
	E. coli O-111	3.13	17.7 s.c.
Phenylglycine derivative ester	*S. aureus* 308 A-1		17.7 p.o.
	S. pyogenes E-14		1.39 p.o.
	E. coli O-111		40.4 p.o.
Thiadiazyl derivative	*S. aureus* 308 A-1	12.5	25 s.c.
	E. coli O-111	0.39	0.44 s.c.

[a]ED_{50}, 50% effective dose; s.c., subcutaneous; p.o., per os.

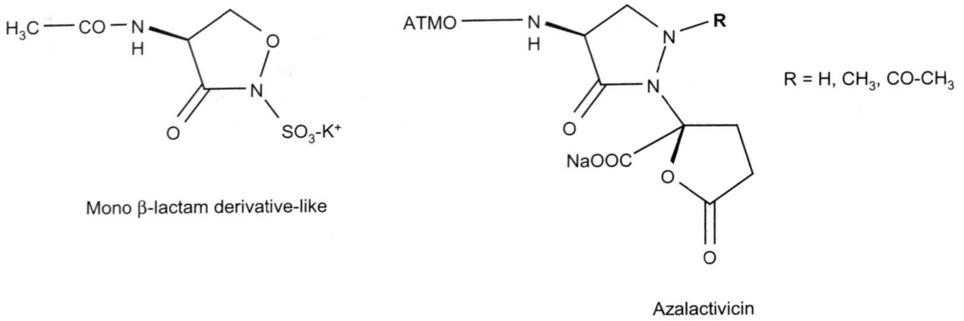

Mono β-lactam derivative-like

$R = H, CH_3, CO\text{-}CH_3$

Azalactivicin

Figure 17 Monolactam and azalactavicins

REFERENCES

Billot-Klein D, Gutimann L, Collatz E, Van Heijenoort J, 1992, Analysis of peptidoglycan precursors of vancomycin-resistant enterococci, Antimicrob Agents Chemother, 36, 1487–1490.

Courvalin P, 1990, Resistance of enterococci to glycopeptides, Antimicrob Agents Chemother, 34, 2291–2296.

Duncan K, van Heijenoort J, Walsh CT, 1990, Purification and characterization of the D-alanyl-D-alanine-adding enzyme from Escherichia coli, Biochemistry, 29, 2379–2386.

Gardner AD, 1940, Morphological effects of penicillin on bacteria, Nature, 3713, 837–838.

Labischinski H, Barnickel G, Naumann D, Ronspeck W, Bradaczek H, 1985, Conformational studies on the bacterial cell wall peptide analog phenylacetyl D-alanyl D-alanine: comparison between conformations of cell wall peptide analog and those of penicillin G, Biopolymers, 24, 2087–2112.

Malhotra KT, Nicholas RA, 1992, Substitution of lysine 213 with arginine in penicillin binding protein 5 of Escherichia coli abolishes D-alanine carboxypeptidase activity without affecting penicillin binding, J Biol Chem, 267, 11386–11391.

Waxman DJ, Strominger JL, 1982, β-Lactam antibiotics: biochemical modes of action, in Morin RB, Gorman M, ed, Chemistry and Biology of β-Lactam Antibiotics, vol 3, Academic Press, New York.

Wright GD, Molinas C, Arthur M, Courvalin P, Walsh CT, 1992, Characterization of VanY, a DD-carboxypeptidase from vancomycin-resistant *Enterococcus faecium* BM4147, Antimicrob Agents Chemother, 36, 1514–1518.

Aminocyclitol Aminoglycosides

P. VEYSSIER AND A. BRYSKIER

16

1. INTRODUCTION

The aminoglycosides are amino sugars that may be divided in terms of their chemical structures into two main groups: streptomycin and its derivatives on the one hand and the 2-deoxystreptamine group on the other (Table 1). They are hydrosoluble, basic, organic compounds with a molecular weight of 500 to 800. Their optimal antibacterial activity occurs at pH 7.5 to 8.5.

Aminoglycosides are rapidly bactericidal antibiotics, acting in particular on aerobic gram-negative bacilli, staphylococci, and gram-positive bacilli. They are weakly active or inactive against anaerobes, streptococci, and pneumococci. Their combination with β-lactams, fluoroquinolones, and polypeptide antibiotics is synergistic. Their bactericidal activity is usually concentration dependent, and there is a postantibiotic effect. These two properties, combined with a reduction in toxicity, account for the reduction in the number of injections for the same daily dosage.

They act essentially on the bacterial ribosome by interfering with the reading of the genetic code and inhibiting all stages of protein synthesis. Acquired resistance is usually plasmid mediated and transferable and is related to inactivating enzymes. The pharmacokinetics are comparable among the different products: no digestive absorption, weak or nonexistent protein binding, similar elimination half-lives (2 to 3 h), poor tissue diffusion, and essentially renal elimination in the active, nonmetabolized form by glomerular filtration associated with tubular reabsorption, engendering accumulation in the renal parenchyma with accompanying toxic risks.

Aminoglycosides are nephro- and ototoxic to various degrees, hence the need to monitor renal function and to use serum assays to adapt the dosages. Short-term treatments and administration in two divided doses or even once daily reduce the risk of toxicity.

Therapeutic indications include, in particular, severe hospital-acquired infections due to aerobic gram-negative bacilli or staphylococci, and the aminoglycosides are almost always used in combination. Their indications in the community are limited. In terms of prophylaxis, there are few indications apart from the prevention of infectious endocarditis or infection in orthopedics.

2. CHEMICAL STRUCTURE AND CLASSIFICATION

The aminoglycosides may be divided into three groups (Table 1).

- Streptomycin and its derivatives, combining streptidine with a pentose and a glucosamine (Fig. 1)
- The deoxystreptamines, divided into two groups according to whether the substitutions occur at 4,5 or 4,6

Table 1 Different classes of antibiotics: aminocyclitol aminoglycosides

Deoxystreptamines		Other
4,5-Bisubstituted	4,6-Bisubstituted	
Neomycin Ribostamycin Lividomycin Paromomycin Butiromycin	Kanamycins A, B, C Dideoxykanamycin[a] Tobramycin Gentamicins Sisomicin Netilmicin[a] Amikacin[a] Sagamicin Dibekacin[a] Arbekacin[a] Isepamicin	Streptomycin Spectinomycin Apramycin (deoxystreptamine) Fortimicin Kasugamicin Istamicin Dactomycin

[a]Semisynthetic.

(Fig. 2 and 3). The group of 4,5-substituted deoxystreptamines includes the neomycins, paromomycin, butirosins, ribostamycin, and lividomycin. These products also all include a ribose molecule in their formulas. The group of 4,6-substituted deoxystreptamines comprises the kanamycins and derivatives, dibekacin, amikacin and arbekacin (Habekacin), tobramycin, sisomicin and *N*-acetylsisomicin, and netilmicin (Fig. 4 and 5).

- The structure of the fortimicins includes an aminocyclitol, fortamine, instead of the deoxystreptamine (Fig. 6). Spectinomycin is an aminocyclitol with a structure similar to that of streptomycin.

In the compounds that represent the "true aminoglycosides," the deoxystreptamines, the substituents on the 2-deoxystreptamine ring are numbered 1,6, the substituents on the amino sugar linked by a glycoside bond at position 4 are numbered 1′,6′, and the substituents at position 5 or 6 of the 2-deoxystreptamine ring are numbered 1″,6″, etc. In the

Streptidine

L-streptose

N-methyl-L-glucosamine

R
-CHO, streptomycin
$-CH_2OH$, dihydrostreptomycin
$-CH_3$
$-CO_2H$
$-CH(OH)-CH_2NO_2$
$-CH(OH)-CH_2NH_2$

Figure 1 Streptomycin derivatives

	R_1	R_2	R_3	R_4
Ribostamycin	NH_2	OH	H	H
Butirosin A	NH_2	H	H	$COCH(OH)(CH_2)_2NH_2$
Butirosin B	NH_2	OH	H	$COCH(OH)(CH_2)_2NH_2$

Figure 3 4,5-Deoxystreptamines: ribostamycin and butirosins

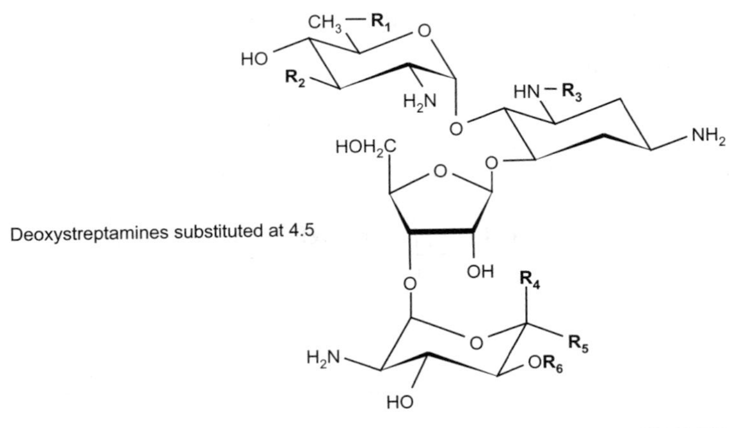

	R_1	R_2	R_3	R_4	R_5	R_6
Neomycin B	NH_2	OH	H	CH_2NH_2	H	H
Neomycin C	NH_2	OH	H	H	H	H
Lividomycin A	OH	H	H	CH_2NH_2	H	α-D-Mannose pyranosyl
Lividomycin B	OH	H	H	CH_2NH_2	H	H
Paromomycin I	OH	OH	H	CH_2NH_2	H	H
Paromomycin II	OH	OH	H	H	CH_2NH_2	CH_2NH_2

Figure 2 Structures of neomycins, lividomycins, and paromomycins

	R_1	R_2	R_3	R_4	R_5
Kanamycin A	NH_2	OH	H	OH	OH
Kanamycin B	NH_2	NH_2	H	OH	OH
Kanamycin C	OH	NH_2	H	OH	OH
Amikacin	NH_2	OH	$COCHOH(CH_2)_2NH_2$	OH	OH
Dibekacin	NH_2	H	H	H	H
Habekacin	NH_2	NH_2	NH_2	H	H
Tobramycin	NH_2	NH_2	NH_2	OH	OH

Figure 4 Derivatives of kanamycin

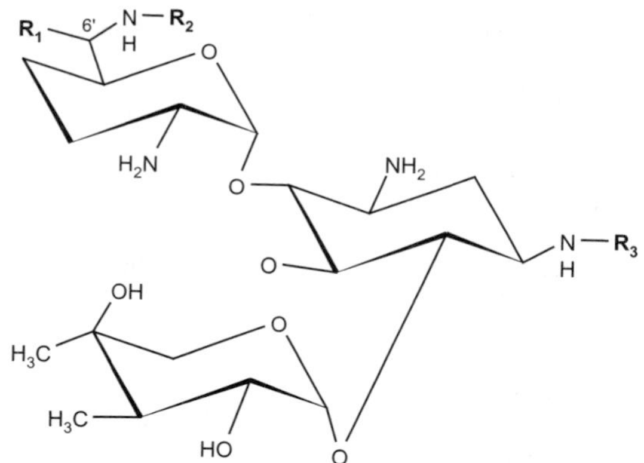

Gentamicin	R_1	R_2	R_3
" C1	CH_3	CH_3	H
" C1A	H	H	H
" C2	CH_3	H	H
Sisomicin	NH_2	H	H
Netilmicin	NH_2	H	C_2H_5

Figure 5 Derivatives of gentamicin

case of streptomycin and its derivatives which contain a substituted streptamine, the carbon atoms of this ring are numbered 1,6 and the other rings are numbered sequentially 1′,6′, etc.

		R_1	R_2
Fortimicin	A	CH_3	H
"	C	CH_3	H
"	D	H	H
Sporamicin	A	CH_3	H
Istamycin	A	H	CH_3
Istamycin	B	H	CH_3
Dactinomycin		CH_3	H
Fortimicin	B	CH_3	H
	KE	H	H
Sporamicin	B	CH_3	H
Sannamycin	B	H	CH_3

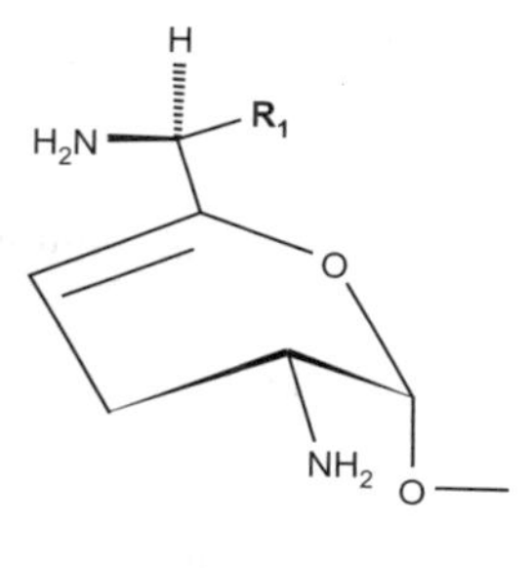

Fortimicin	KF	H
"	G	CH_3
"	G_1	CH_3
"	G_2	CH_3
"	G_3	CH_3

Figure 6 Fortimicin group

3. PHYSICOCHEMICAL PROPERTIES

See Tables 2 and 3.

The aminoglycosides are basic organic compounds with a pK_a of between 7.5 and 8. Their molecular weight is low (500 to 800), which renders them dialyzable. These antibiotics are used in the form of the sulfate. They are presented as a white powder (or yellowish [sisomicin]). This powder is amorphous, odorless, hydrosoluble, and slightly bitter. Aminoglycoside solutions are stable for several months at room temperature and at neutral pH. They are heat stable (and can therefore be incorporated in the cements used in orthopedics). However, these antibiotics are susceptible to variations in pH and have optimal activity at a pH of between 7.5 and 8.5. Gentamicin is composed of three fractions: C_1, 28.3%; C_{1a}, 37.1%; and C_2, 37.1%. Neomycin consists of neomycins B (85%), C (14%), and D, E, and F (1%).

Table 2 Physicochemical properties of aminoglycosides

Generic name	Empirical formula	Mol wt	Melting point (°C)	Identification	Optical rotation	pK_a
Streptomycin	$C_{21}H_{39}N_7O_{12}$	581.58	190–200	White powder No odor Hygroscopic	$(\alpha)^{25}{}_D$ 84	7.7
Kanamycin	$C_{18}H_{36}N_4O_{11}$	484.5	ND[a]	White powder Crystalline powder No odor or light	Kanamycin A, $(\alpha)^{24}{}_D + 146°$; kanamycin B, $(\alpha)^{21}{}_D + 114°$	7.2
Gentamicins	$C_{19-21}H_{39}N_5O_7$	449.56–477.61	94–100 (C_1) 107–123 (C_2)	White to yellowish powder	Gentamicin C_1, $(\alpha)^{25}{}_D + 158°$; gentamycin C_2 $(\alpha)^{25}{}_D + 160°$	8.2
Tobramycin	$C_{18}H_{37}N_5O_9$	497	168	White powder No odor	$(\alpha)_D + 128°$	7.4 cy 1 6.2/7 cy 2 7.6/6.8 cy 8
Sisomicin	$C_{18}H_{37}N_5O_7$	447.5	198–201	White powder Yellow-brownish	$(\alpha)^{26}{}_D + 189°$	
Netilmicin	$C_{21}H_{41}N_5O_7$	475.55	ND	White powder Yellow	$(\alpha)^{25}{}_D + 88°$ to $96°$	8.1
Amikacin	$C_{22}H_{43}N_5O_{13}$	585.6	203–204	Yellow, white powder	$(\alpha)^{20}{}_D + 99°$	
Dibekacin	$C_{18}H_{37}N_5O_8$	451.54	240–241	Yellow, white powder No odor, bitter	$(\alpha)^{20}{}_D + 132°$	
Isepamicin	$C_{22}H_{43}N_5O_{12}$	569.61			$(\alpha)^{26}{}_D + 110.9°$	

[a]ND, not determined.

Table 3 More physicochemical properties of aminoglycosides

Generic name	Water solubility	Solubility in organic solvent	pH	Expiration time (yrs)	Atmosphere
Streptomycin	Highly soluble (200–500 mg/ml)	Sparingly soluble to insoluble (0.30 mg/ml)	4.5–7 (water, 25%)	4	Ambient
Kanamycin	20%	Insoluble	6.5–8 (water, 1%)	3	Ambient
Gentamicins	Highly soluble (1 g/ml)	Insoluble	3.5–5.5 (water, 4%)	3	Ambient
Tobramycin	Highly soluble (538 mg/ml)	Sparingly insoluble to insoluble (10–20 mg/ml)	9–11 (solution, 10%) base 3.5–7 sulfate (water solution, 1 and 5%)	2	Ambient
Sisomicin	Highly soluble	Insoluble	3.5–5.5 (water solution, 4%)	3	Ambient
Netilmicin	Highly soluble	Insoluble	3.5–5.5 (water solution, 4%)	3	Ambient
Amikacin	20% in distilled water	Insoluble	9–11 (base in water solution to 1%)	3	Ambient (reconstituted) 12 h to ambience (10 days at 4°C)
Dibekacin	Highly soluble (1 g/ml)	Insoluble	10 (base solution, 50 mg/ml) 6–8 (sulfate solution, 50 mg/ml)	3	Ambient 24 h (reconstituted solution)

4. ANTIBACTERIAL SPECTRUM AND ACTIVITY

See Table 4.

The aminoglycosides are broad-spectrum antibiotics essentially active against gram-negative bacteria (cocci, coccobacilli, and bacilli) and against staphylococci. They are also active against gram-positive bacilli such as *Listeria monocytogenes*, *Corynebacterium diphtheriae*, and *Bacillus anthracis*. However, they are inactive against obligate anaerobic bacteria and against streptococci and pneumococci.

Table 4 Antibacterial spectra of aminoglycosides

Susceptible	Naturally resistant
Enterobacteriaceae	*Burkholderia cepacia*
P. aeruginosa	*Stenotrophomonas maltophilia*
Acinetobacter	*Flavobacterium*
S. aureus	*Streptococcus* spp.
Staphylococcus epidermidis	*Bacteroides* spp.
Haemophilus influenzae	*Clostridium* spp.
Neisseria gonorrhoeae	*Legionella* spp.
Neisseria meningitidis	*Mycoplasma* spp.
Mycobacteria	
Alcaligenes spp.	

A penicillin-aminoglycoside combination, on the other hand, exerts synergistic and bactericidal activity on streptococci with low-level resistance to streptomycin (MIC, <1,000 mg/liter). This synergistic effect may be due to better penetration of the bacterial cell by the aminoglycoside as a result of the inhibition of peptidoglycan synthesis by penicillin G.

Bacteria affected by nontoxic concentrations in the serum, 4 to 8 mg/liter for the majority of products and 8 to 16 mg/liter for amikacin, are considered susceptible. The concentration of divalent cations in the culture media for antibiotic sensitivity testing may affect the MIC for certain species, particularly *Pseudomonas aeruginosa*. A high Ca^{2+} or Mg^{2+} concentration may increase the MIC for the majority of strains by a factor of 8 or 16. It has therefore been agreed to standardize the media (for example, Mueller-Hinton) with concentrations similar to physiological conditions (20 to 30 mg of Mg per liter and 50 to 100 mg of Ca per liter). To assess the efficacy of aminoglycosides, it is not sufficient to compare the mean MICs; the concentration in serum/MIC ratio in particular must also be established. Against *Enterobacteriaceae*, the activities of gentamicin, tobramycin, sisomicin, isepamicin, and netilmicin are comparable: the MICs of these aminoglycosides for all bacteria do not differ significantly (0.15 to 4 mg/liter), although amikacin is less active in terms of MIC. However, taking into account the concentrations in serum obtained with a standard unit dosage, 20 mg/liter for amikacin and 4 to 8 mg/liter for gentamicin, the index of antibiotic activity (concentration in serum/MIC) of amikacin is comparable to that of the other aminoglycosides.

Although the antibacterial activities are similar from one product to another, studies have shown particular molecules to be more interesting with regard to certain bacteria. Tobramycin thus appears to be the product that is usually most active against *P. aeruginosa*. Some products (streptomycin and kanamycin) are more active against *Mycobacterium tuberculosis*, while amikacin is more active against atypical mycobacteria and is the only one that is active against *Nocardia*.

Paromomycin is active against certain protozoa. Dactomycin, which is a pseudodisaccharide (2″-*N*-formimidoylfortimicin A), is active against *P. aeruginosa* but, like all aminoglycosides, inactive against streptococci. It is moderately active against staphylococci. Compared to gentamicin and amikacin, dactomycin has good activity against numerous gram-negative bacteria and is highly active against *Proteus* and *Serratia*. The activity of dactomycin tested against strains producing the majority of the most common inactivating enzymes in clinical practice [except AAC(6′) and APH(2″)] persists, but activity is decreased against AAC(3′)-I-producing strains, although to a lesser extent than is observed with fortimicin A (the base compound of astromicin sulfate has been known as fortimicin A). The rate of acetylation by this enzyme is half that observed with fortimicin A. The in vivo activity is correlated with the in vitro observations. The activities of O-demethylfortimicin, hapagentamicin B, and 5-episisomicin were compared with the activities of the aminoglycosides used clinically. Hapagentamicin B is the most active compound against staphylococci and indole-positive *Proteus*. 5-Episisomicin is very active against *Pseudomonas*.

Arbekacin (Habekacin; 1-NHABA-dibekacin) was studied for its antibacterial spectrum. This product is relatively nonsusceptible to inactivating enzymes [except for AAC(2′) and AAC(6′)-IV]. There is no cross-resistance to this molecule in the case of gram-negative bacilli such as aminoglycoside-resistant *Serratia* and *Pseudomonas*, particularly those resistant to amikacin. In a study of the susceptibility of *P. aeruginosa* to aminoglycosides, arbekacin was shown to be slightly more effective than amikacin, whereas there was no difference in the incidence of resistance to these two products. Arbekacin appears to have a potent effect against strains of *Staphylococcus aureus* and *Staphylococcus epidermidis*, even when the strains are highly resistant to gentamicin and amikacin [AAC(3)] (Collatz et al., 1988).

The aminoglycosides are bactericidal antibiotics. Their minimum bactericidal concentrations are very close to the MICs, and an in vivo bactericidal effect is readily achieved. The bactericidal effect is obtained rapidly in vitro, within 4 to 6 h. It is concentration dependent for the majority of bacterial species. There is a postantibiotic effect.

A study of antibiotic combinations has shown that there is frequent synergy between β-lactams and fluoroquinolones. There may be antagonism (more rare in vivo) with bacteriostatic antibiotics. Synergistic combinations are usually prescribed in severe infectious states, but the superiority of such combinations over monotherapy has only rarely been demonstrated, other than in neutropenic subjects.

5. MODE OF ACTION OF AMINOGLYCOSIDES

The antibiotics of the aminoglycoside family are bactericidal. The majority of studies relating to their mode of action have been undertaken with streptomycin.

The ribosome has been identified as the prime target of all the aminoglycosides tested. There are in fact alterations of the ribosomes in the mutants observed, and the ribosomal proteins affected by mutation have been identified and characterized.

Despite the fact that the ribosome has been identified as the primary target of the action of aminoglycosides, studies relating to the exact mode of action are complicated by the fact that these products (kanamycin and gentamicin have the same action as streptomycin) have different and apparently unrelated effects on cultured bacteria. Thus, membrane changes, inhibition of protein synthesis, modifications of RNA synthesis, and morphological changes are observed. Inhibition of protein synthesis at the ribosomal level constitutes the most likely mechanism of the mode of action of aminoglycosides. The concomitant effects contribute to the bactericidal activity, the aminoglycosides concentrated in the cell being capable of producing lethal effects because of the role of the membrane changes in particular.

The action of streptomycin at the ribosomal level is exerted essentially on the S12 protein. There is in fact a spontaneous emergence of highly streptomycin-resistant

Escherichia coli mutants in a single step, and these strains have a modification in their S12 protein which controls the overall efficacy of the translation of RNA to protein.

In contrast to streptomycin, spectinomycin, and kasugamycin, the neomycins, kanamycin, and gentamicin act at a number of ribosomal sites. This explains the possibility of obtaining single-step resistant mutants possessing high-level resistance to these products from the outset. These antibiotics also act as inhibitors of protein synthesis by disrupting RNA translation.

The lethal action of the majority of aminoglycosides is therefore probably due to an irreversible combination with certain ribosomal proteins and additional effects of the product on the cell membrane function (Davies). The irreversible nature of the binding to ribosomal proteins distinguishes the bactericidal activity of the aminoglycosides from the bacteriostatic action of other protein synthesis inhibitors, such as chloramphenicol.

The mode of penetration of the aminoglycosides into the bacterial cell is an important process. These molecules must first cross the outer membrane and the cytoplasmic membrane before penetrating the cytoplasm. The differences in activity of streptomycin, gentamicin, and amikacin against *E. coli* and *P. aeruginosa* are partly due to the capacity of the antibiotic for penetration and not to differences in affinity or susceptibility of the ribosomal proteins.

There are three stages in the penetration of an aminoglycoside into a bacterium. The first stage is adsorption to the cell surface as a result of ionic interactions. The second stage requires metabolic energy provided by a gradient between the inside and outside of the cell, and this stage may be blocked by mutation. It may also be disrupted if the conditions required by the production of oxidative energy for the transport of aminoglycosides are not strictly observed. This explains the reduced susceptibility of anaerobes to aminoglycosides and the reduction in the activity of aminoglycosides against facultative anaerobes (*Enterobacteriaceae*) in the case of a relatively anaerobic infection (deep focus). The third and final stage is rapid and is associated with the binding of the compound to the ribosome. In some mutants with an alteration in the ribosome, there may be a reduction in ribosomal binding. These mutants are rare in the clinical situation. There are mutations affecting the cell penetration phase with a reduction in binding to the ribosomal proteins, but the increase in extracellular concentrations with a secondary increase in penetration may offset these abnormalities.

6. STRUCTURE-ACTIVITY RELATIONSHIP OF AMINOGLYCOSIDES

A number of studies have been conducted on the structure-activity relationships of aminoglycosides. Early studies with streptomycin suggested that the number of amino groups determined the efficacy of the compound. However, other groups are equally important. Thus, streptamine replaces deoxystreptamine without affecting the efficacy of neomycin. Fortimicin contains neither streptamine nor deoxystreptamine, but its structure contains groups whose arrangement engenders identical behavior towards ribosomal receptors. Compounds containing an epistreptamine group are less active, but other changes to the deoxystreptamine ring do not necessarily alter the activity of the product. This ring is very important, but it is not the sole factor in the activity (Nagabushan et al., 1982).

Other structural modifications are known. The loss of a hydroxyl group does not alter the activity against the ribosome but affects the antibacterial spectrum of the aminoglycoside. The superior activity of gentamicin and tobramycin against *P. aeruginosa* appears to be related to differences in the transport properties of the 3′-OH and 3′-deoxy compounds. The antipseudomonal activity of amikacin is enhanced by protection against enzymatic inactivation through substitution on the 1 amino group. Other structural modifications may cause changes in the spectrum of the aminoglycosides. For example, against resistant strains, changes in structure may restrict the activity of the inactivating enzymes. The number of amino groups affects the activity of the compounds, and some of these groups are more important than others. This is the case with 6′, which is more important than 2′. Thus, kanamycin B with a 2′,6-diamino sugar is more active than kanamycin A with a 2′-amino sugar. The amino groups on the deoxystreptamine ring also vary in importance. The 3-amino group is the most important. It cannot be modified. The 1-amino group may be modified without altering the activity of the antibiotic by acetylation or alkylation. Netilmicin and amikacin, modified on the 1-amino group, are the most effective by virtue of the protection afforded against the activity of inactivating enzymes. The role of the amidino groups on the streptamine ring of streptomycin has also been studied. Modified analogs have been synthesized, yielding activity against strains harboring plasmids conferring resistance to streptomycin.

The capacity of aminoglycosides to penetrate the bacterial cell also constitutes a major chapter in the structure-activity relationships. The passive and active transport of the antibiotic and its binding to ribosomal proteins can be affected by structural changes in the aminoglycosides, but they are particularly affected by changes in bacterial structure, represented essentially by mutations causing alterations in the ribosomal proteins but also abnormalities of transfer in the cell membrane.

7. MECHANISMS OF BACTERIAL RESISTANCE TO AMINOGLYCOSIDES

Certain bacteria may be naturally and consistently resistant to aminoglycosides, particularly obligate anaerobes such as *Bacteroides* and *Clostridium*, or certain aerobes and anaerobes such as *Streptococcus pyogenes*, *Streptococcus pneumoniae*, and *Enterococcus faecalis*. For the streptococci as a whole, the resistance is low level, between 16 to 256 mg/liter for streptomycin and between 4 and 128 mg/liter for gentamicin, and this low level may be explained by ineffective active transport through the bacterial membrane. *Treponema*, *Leptospira*, and *Actinomycetes* spp. are naturally resistant to aminoglycosides.

The bacteria may acquire resistance to aminoglycosides, and this phenomenon was exacerbated in the years from 1985 to 1990. Resistance may by acquired by four different mechanisms: alteration of the target, interference with transport of the antibiotic, enzymatic inhibition of the antibiotic, and substitution of the target. The first three mechanisms are secondary to chromosomal or plasmid-mediated mutations. The fourth is only observed after acquisition of a resistance plasmid or a transposon. Aminoglycoside resistance may occur after mutation (alteration-interference) or after the acquisition of a plasmid (enzymatic action).

Alteration of the ribosomal target is related to a mutation, the substitution of a single amino acid causing a reduction in the affinity of the ribosome for the aminoglycoside. This often causes high-level resistance from the outset. This resistance is not crossed between aminoglycosides, given the multiplicity of the binding sites of the different aminoglycosides. It is a rare event in clinical practice and has been observed in particular with streptomycin. For the majority of aminoglycosides, multiple mutations are needed to obtain high levels of resistance. A defect of cellular permeability (interference with transport of the antibiotic) is involved more often than ribosomal resistance. Penetration is related to passive diffusion through the porins of the outer membrane and active transport requiring energy across the cytoplasmic membrane. Mutations affecting the active transport system cause decreased accumulation of the antibiotic in the cell. These resistant mutants grow in dwarf colonies and are more often found when aminoglycosides are used extensively or as monotherapy (staphylococci, and *P. aeruginosa*). They are nonsusceptible to all aminoglycosides, which raises major therapeutic problems. The mechanism is poorly elucidated but appears to involve a lack of membrane oxidative energy.

Enzymatic inactivation of the aminoglycosides is the type of resistance most commonly observed in clinical practice. The enzymes are divided into three classes according to the reactions that they catalyze (phosphorylation or nucleotidylation of a hydroxyl group and acetylation of an amino group) and into subclasses depending on the sites that they modify. Some only modify compounds that are structurally similar, whereas others modify molecules of a very different structure. Thus, APH(2″) of gram-positive cocci only modifies the 4,5-bisubstituted deoxystreptamines, whereas APH(3′5″) modifies the 4,5- and 4,6-bisubstituted deoxystreptamines. Given the overlap of the enzyme substrate profiles, a compound may be modified by several enzymes (seven in the case of kanamycin B). It is for this reason that an aminoglycoside may select various inactivating enzymes, particularly as some (gentamicin, for example) are molecular complexes. The problem of in vivo selection and dissemination of the resistance mechanisms is exacerbated by the fact that the majority of aminoglycoside-resistant strains harbor plasmids that code for several enzymes (Shannon and Phillips, 1982) or combine several resistance factors.

The enzymes are necessary and sufficient to confer resistance on the host bacterium, but only phosphotransferases confer very high levels of resistance. The enzymes are synthesized constitutively: they are detected in cells cultured in the absence of antibiotic. There is no inactivation of the antibiotic in the culture media. The enzyme confers on the host the capacity to multiply and increase in the presence of higher concentrations of unmodified antibiotic. Resistance is due to the equilibrium between ineffective aminoglycoside transport in the bacterium and enzymatic inactivation of these molecules. The resistance phenotype depends both qualitatively and quantitatively on the host. An enzyme may produce low-level resistance in a *Staphylococcus* and very high-level resistance in a *Streptococcus*. This confirms that a resistance mechanism does not have a level in itself. It acts by amplifying the resistance level of the host.

The inactivating enzymes are of three types (Fig. 7):

- Phosphotransferases (APH) have five subtypes, phosphorylating a hydroxyl group by O phosphorylation
- Nucleotidyltransferases (ANT) have five subtypes, binding an adenyl or other nucleotides to an OH (O adenylation)
- Acetyltransferases (AAC) have three subtypes, binding an acetyl to an NH_2 (N-acetylation)

Kanamycin may be inactivated by seven enzymes: APH(3′), APH(2″), ANT(4′), ANT(2″), AAC(3′), AAC(2′), and AAC(6′).

Gentamicin may be inactivated by APH(2″) and ANT(2″) and, depending on these constituents, by three types of acetyltransferases. Unlike tobramycin, it is not susceptible to ANT(4′).

Dibekacin has no hydroxyl groups at 3′ and 4′. As the phosphotransferases APH(3′)-I and APH(3′)-II and the nucleotidyltransferase ANT(4′) have their site of action at this point, they cannot therefore inactivate this molecule. However, it is inactivated by the same enzymes as kanamycin.

Netilmicin escapes the action of phosphotransferases and nucleotidyltransferases, particularly ANT(4′), but it is inactivated by numerous acetyltransferases [variable action in the case of AAC(3′)-I and AAC(3′)-III but consistent for AAC(3′)-II, AAC(2′), and AAC(6′)].

Amikacin is the most active aminoglycoside in vitro. This product is only susceptible to certain acetyltransferases [AAC(6′)] and to APH(3′) (staphylococci and enterococci) and ANT(4′) found in rare strains of enterococci.

Dactomycin is acetylated by AAC(3′)-I on the amino group at position 4.

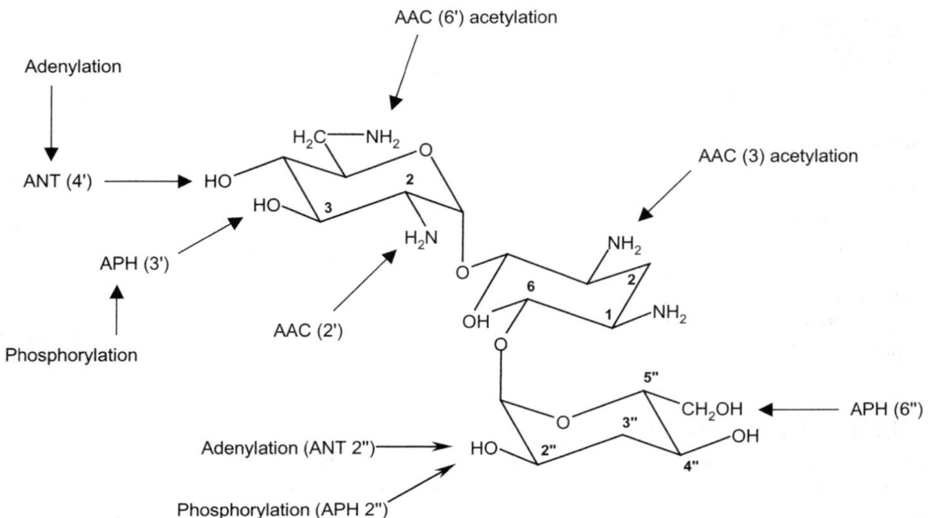

Figure 7 Sites of enzymatic inactivation(s) of aminoglycosides

Arbekacin is stable against inactivating enzymes, except AAC(2′) and AAC(6′)-IV, and has good activity against certain strains of *S. aureus* and *S. epidermidis*, even those resistant to amikacin.

The frequencies of resistance of gram-negative bacilli to aminoglycosides are about 2% for amikacin, 10% for netilmicin, and 12 to 13% for gentamicin and tobramycin. The frequency of inactivating enzymes in the gram-negative bacteria isolated in North America, South America, Asia, and Europe has been studied. There appears to be a correlation between the use of aminoglycosides and the type of enzymes observed. The AAC(6′) enzymes are the most commonly found in Asia (one-third are responsible for resistance to amikacin), while AAC(3′) enzymes are predominant in Chile and the Netherlands (95 and 70%). In the United States, 42% of resistant strains produce AAC(2″), 25% produce AAC(6″), and 17% produce AAC(3′). The dissemination of resistance to amikacin has been described and appears to be related to the preferential use of this medicine in certain hospitals. Plasmids carrying genes coding for the AAC(6′) type of inactivating enzymes are disseminated among the *Enterobacteriaceae*. The genes responsible are carried by IncC plasmids in France.

The role of the use of antibiotics in the development and/or selection of resistant strains has been studied, particularly for amikacin. Over 10 years of use, the incidence of resistance to amikacin has increased only moderately. It has not been clearly shown that there is a relationship between the selection of amikacin-resistant bacteria and heavy prescription. The expression of resistance is constitutive, whether the antibiotic is present or not. The use of aminoglycosides primarily provides a favorable environment for the selection of resistant strains. The study of genes coding for certain types of enzymatic resistance has shown a possible link with the regulatory elements of a TEM-1-type β-lactamase gene carried by a transposable element. This suggests the possibility of increased selection of amikacin-resistant strains in treatment with β-lactams susceptible to TEM-1, whereas a combination with cefotaxime would not have this effect (Acar et al., 1986).

However, it seems reasonable to think that the more the aminoglycosides are used, the higher the probability of selecting aminoglycoside-resistant strains.

8. PHARMACOLOGY OF AMINOGLYCOSIDES

The aminoglycosides can only be used parenterally, except for intestinal infections or indications for decontamination. Absorption is complete following intramuscular administration. Protein binding is weak or nonexistent. The apparent elimination half-life is about 2 h, and elimination is predominantly renal with glomerular filtration and tubular reabsorption. The pharmacokinetics of elimination are independent of the dose and route of administration. Tissue diffusion is poor, but renal accumulation occurs, particularly in the cortex. Renal insufficiency causes a marked increase in the elimination half-life and requires a dosage adaptation.

9. PHARMACOLOGY IN HUMANS

The pharmacokinetics of the aminoglycosides were initially considered to be very simple. It was assumed that the molecules were located in extracellular compartments, as the aminoglycosides were considered not to be present in the majority of tissues. A one-compartment model was therefore considered appropriate. Their nephrotoxicity was considered dose dependent and infrequent. Ototoxicity did occur, but only, it was believed, if the prescription was continued despite a renal toxic effect. After 1970, arguments against the one-compartment model began to surface: the incomplete recovery of aminoglycosides in the urine, the possible accumulation in the renal parenchyma, and the elevation of the peak and trough concentrations after repeated doses; although impairment of renal function might explain this increase in concentrations, it could not be confirmed. Likewise, even imperceptible modifications of renal function could not account for the biphasic reduction in concentrations noted by different authors after repeated doses. There was a persistence of aminoglycosides in all subjects after the last dose and a biphasic elimination with a second phase half-life of about 100 h (Kahlmeter et al., 1978). Since then a two-compartment model has appeared to be best suited to describe these data. The first distribution phase is very rapid. The second phase of apparent elimination is slower. The apparent half-life is about 2 h for all aminoglycosides. The accumulation of aminoglycosides in the renal cortex explains the existence of a third deep compartment with a half-life of between 50 and 100 h.

Plasma protein binding is negligible at therapeutic doses (0 to 30%). There is no competition between bilirubin and the aminoglycoside at the binding sites.

The aminoglycosides do not cross the intestinal barrier after oral or rectal administration of neomycin or paromomycin, and less than 5% is found in the urine. Ophthalmic administration is possible. The intrathecal or intraventricular route may be used in certain infections of the central nervous system. In fact, only the parenteral route is used for systemic infections. After an intramuscular injection, absorption is rapid and complete. The peak concentrations in serum are usually obtained 1 to 2 h after the injection and are dose dependent. Bioavailability is close to 100%, as shown by comparative studies following intramuscular or intravenous administration. The pharmacokinetic parameters are summarized in Table 5.

Gentamicin, tobramycin, sisomicin, netilmicin, and dibekacin are administered clinically at a unit dose of 1 to 2 mg/kg of body weight. The peak concentrations in serum obtained after intramuscular injection are between 4 and 7 mg/liter. Streptomycin, kanamycin, and amikacin are prescribed clinically at unit doses of about 7.5 mg/kg (~500 mg). The peak concentrations in serum obtained are between 15 and 25 mg/liter. The same unit doses administered by intravenous infusion (30 to 60 min) yield higher peak levels in serum, but the elimination pharmacokinetics are unchanged and are independent of the route of administration (half-life, 2 h). The serum distribution half-life is between 0.20 and 0.40 h for all aminoglycosides.

Pharmacokinetic studies conducted with the same subjects at different doses showed that the pharmacokinetics are dose independent. The concentration and area under the curve are proportional to the dose and are not affected by the dosage regimen, nor is the elimination half-life. This, combined with studies on the efficacy and toxicity, is an argument for single daily administration.

10. METABOLISM AND EXCRETION

The biotransformation of aminoglycosides is negligible (<10%). They are found almost entirely in the unchanged, biologically active form in the urine.

Table 5 Principal pharmacokinetic parameters of aminoglycosides in subjects with normal renal function

Compound	Dose, i.m.[a]	C_{max} (μg/ml)	T_{max} (h)	$t_{1/2\beta}$ (h) concn	V (liter/kg)	Mean urinary (μg/ml)	Urinary elimination (% at 24 h)	Clearance (ml/min)	
								Renal	Total
Streptomycin	500 mg	15–20	1	2.5–3	0.2–0.3	300–500	70	70–80	
Kanamycin	500 mg	20–25	1	2.2–2.5	0.23	200–600	80–85	70–80	
Gentamicin	1 mg/kg	4–5	1	2–2.5	0.24–0.32	40–100	75–85	75	90–120
Tobramycin	1.5 mg/kg	5–7	1	2–2.5	0.28–0.32	50–200	75–90	80–90	100–120
Sisomicin	1 mg/kg	4–5	0.6–0.9	2–2.4	0.20–0.26	10–100	75–95	50–85	65–110
Netilmicin	2 mg/kg	5–7	0.7–1.1	2–2.4	0.1–0.32	100–200	70–90	65–100	70–100
Amikacin	500 mg	15–25	0.6–1.4	1.5–2.1	0.24–0.35	200–600	70–90	80–120	140–160
Dibekacin	1 mg/kg	4–5	0.4–0.8	2–2.5	0.16–0.3	50–100	80–90	50–120	55–140
Lividomycin	500 mg	20–25	0.5–1.5	1.2–2.6	0.25–0.35	300–600	75–95	60–120	90–150
Fortimicin	5 mg/kg	23.8 ± 8[b]		1.8 ± 0.5	0.14 ± 0.08	270–600	85 ± 18	115 ± 23	
Isepamicin	15 mg/kg	42	1.33	2.6	0.27 ± 0.05		97.3	101 ± 25.2	100

[a]i.m., intramuscular.
[b]Mean ± standard deviation.

10.1. Biliary Excretion

The biliary route constitutes only a very accessory route of elimination of aminoglycosides (0.5 to 2% of the administered dose) with no enterohepatic cycle. Hepatobiliary disorders for this reason have little effect on elimination.

Effective biliary concentrations of kanamycin, gentamicin, and tobramycin have been found in patients not exhibiting biliary obstruction. Conversely, penetration of the bile tract is poor in the presence of biliary calculi or severe hepatic insufficiency.

10.2. Renal Elimination

The renal pathway is the essential route of elimination of the aminoglycosides. Urinary concentrations are very high, and elimination is rapid. Eighty to 90% of the administered dose is found in the urine at 24 h (Table 5). Administration of probenecid does not affect the elimination, which tends to prove the absence of tubular secretion. Aminoglycosides are eliminated by glomerular filtration and are partly reabsorbed in the proximal tubule. For this reason, the renal clearance is less than the creatinine clearance (CL_{CR}) (Table 5).

Total serum clearance is similar to renal clearance, thus confirming the absence of metabolism.

11. RENAL BEHAVIOR OF AMINOGLYCOSIDES AND ITS EFFECTS

11.1. Normal Behavior

There are a number of arguments to demonstrate that glomerular filtration is the only route of elimination of aminoglycosides and that there is no tubular excretion in humans. There remains some uncertainty about tubular reabsorption. There is tubular reabsorption from the urinary filtrate and also from the peritubular capillaries, although this is weak. Tubular reabsorption involves two stages which differ in rapidity, level, and order of magnitude.

There is initial binding to the peritubular cells in the membrane brush border, after which the product is transported into the cell. This stage is slower and more rapidly saturated than the first (between 5 and 25 mg/liter). It is related to a membrane effect that requires energy: pinocytosis and the combination of active and passive transport may also be involved. After reabsorption by the proximal tubule, a small amount of antibiotic diffuses into the peritubular fluids, but the greater part remains within the cells. This process of accumulation persists throughout the whole of the treatment.

11.2. Toxic Behavior

There is also a debate about the intracellular site of injury when toxic concentrations are reached. The slowness of the renal lesion suggests a lysosomal lesion with an impairment of protein synthesis, whereas an early lesion of the VIIIth cranial nerve and the loss of enzymes from the border membrane indicate more a disorder of energy production and use. Markers of the effects of aminoglycosides on the kidney are β_2-microglobulin, renal enzymes (which are of much greater interest), the formation of casts, and, more straightforwardly, variations in CL_{CR}.

12. DISTRIBUTION IN BODY TISSUES AND FLUIDS

Diffusion of the aminoglycosides is rapid. The apparent volume of distribution corresponds to 20 to 30% of body weight, a volume equivalent to that of the extracellular fluids (Table 5).

12.1. Cerebrospinal Fluid

After parenteral administration, the aminoglycosides diffuse weakly into the cerebrospinal fluid (CSF). When the meninges are healthy, the ratio of the levels in CSF and serum is less than 10%. In meningeal inflammation, penetration is slightly increased but the CSF concentrations usually remain below the MICs for the bacteria responsible for infection, except in neonates.

Intrathecal or intraventricular administration combined with parenteral treatment yields effective levels in the CSF for periods of 12 to 18 h.

12.2. Bronchial Secretions

The concentrations reached in the bronchi are usually below the MICs for the majority of bacteria responsible for bronchopulmonary infections. The peak concentrations measured in purulent sputum range from 1 to 6 mg/liter for gentamicin and 3 to 4 mg/liter for amikacin. It is very difficult to predict the efficacy of aminoglycoside treatment in bronchial infections. Some authors recommend their use in aerosols or instillations, but the indications remain disputed (Guillaume et al., 1992).

12.3. Renal Parenchyma

Aminoglycosides accumulate in the renal cortex, where the concentrations are 2 to 3 times higher than those measured in the medulla and 20 to 30 times higher than the peak concentrations in serum. They are released only very slowly from the renal tissue compartment. This binding is responsible for the increase in peak levels in serum and residual levels and for the persistence of not insignificant concentrations in serum several weeks after the discontinuation of treatment, particularly if this has been prolonged. It may be accompanied by damage to the tubular epithelium, with an increase in the elimination half-lives.

12.4. Transplacental Passage

The aminoglycosides diffuse fairly well into the placenta and fetus. However, fetal penetration is limited by their polar nature. The ratios of the concentrations in maternal blood and cord blood range from 1.2 for streptomycin to 6.7 for tobramycin.

12.5. Other Tissues and Serous Fluids

Finally, aminoglycosides, which are not liposoluble, diffuse very poorly into adipose tissue. Their diffusion into bone is weak and variable. By contrast, they diffuse fairly well into ascites fluid and pleural, pericardial, and synovial effusions, where their concentrations attain 25 to 50% of levels in serum.

13. PHARMACOKINETICS AS A FUNCTION OF DIATHESIS

13.1. Patients with Renal Insufficiency

The pharmacokinetics of elimination of the aminoglycosides are dependent almost exclusively on renal function. Renal insufficiency produces major changes in the pharmacokinetics. It increases the peak concentrations in serum variably according to the compound. In the case of amikacin and lividomycin, this increase may be as much as 50% in patients with severe renal insufficiency, and there is a risk that the ototoxic threshold will be reached if the unit dosage is not adjusted.

The elimination half-life increases proportionally to renal insufficiency as the CL_{CR} decreases (Table 6), to the extent that half-lives 20 to 30 times greater than those observed in healthy subjects are obtained. This prolongation is particularly marked once the CL_{CR} falls below 30 ml/min.

The apparent volume of distribution is not affected. Extrarenal clearance increases but remains weak.

Correlations have been established for each aminoglycoside between the elimination half-lives or constants and serum creatinine levels or CL_{CR} (Table 7).

These correlations enable the elimination half-life to be calculated in relation to the degree of renal insufficiency and the dosage to be adapted accordingly.

It should be noted that urinary elimination, however much reduced, enables effective antibacterial concentrations to be obtained as long as the CL_{CR} is greater than 30 ml/min.

13.1.1. Hemodialysis

The aminoglycosides are weakly bound, if at all, to plasma proteins and are readily dialyzable. About 50% of the quantity of antibiotic present in the body is eliminated during a hemodialysis session of 4 to 6 h. The dialysis of gentamicin is 24 ml/min, and that of tobramycin is 49 ml/min. The dialysis depends more on the nature of the dialyzer than on blood and dialysate flows.

13.1.2. Peritoneal Dialysis

Peritoneal dialysis is much less effective than hemodialysis in eliminating aminoglycosides. The elimination half-lives of amikacin are about 20 h during peritoneal dialysis and about 5 h during hemodialysis. Peritoneal clearance of gentamicin is weak (5 to 10 ml/min). During peritoneal dialysis, the introduction of aminoglycosides into the dialysate results in stable levels in serum within 24 h.

13.2. In Elderly, Obese, Dehydrated, and Febrile Patients and Those with Major Burns

The elimination half-lives of aminoglycosides vary considerably in elderly subjects, from 0.3 to 32.7 h for gentamicin, which requires that treatment be monitored.

Table 7 Correlations between half-life or elimination rate constant and serum creatinine levels or CL_{CR} for some aminoglycosides

Compound	Correlation
Amikacin	$t_{1/2} = 0.25$ creat.[a] + 0.12; $K_e = 0.003\ CL_{CR} + 0.008$
Sisomicin	$t_{1/2} = 0.29$ creat. + 2.38; $K_e = 0.002\ CL_{CR} + 0.002$
Netilmicin	$t_{1/2} = 0.23$ creat. + 2.87; $K_e = 0.002\ CL_{CR} + 0.017$
Dibekacin	$t_{1/2} = 0.28$ creat. + 1.14; $K_e = 0.003\ CL_{CR} + 0.006$

[a]creat., serum creatinine level.

Table 6 Apparent elimination half-lives of aminoglycosides in patients with renal insufficiency

Compound	$t_{1/2}$ (h)				
	CL_{CR} (ml/min)			Hemodialysis	
	30–80	10–30	<10	Before-after	During
Gentamicin	3–5	5–15	15–40	48–72	10
Tobramycin	4–12	12–20	20–24	56–60	10
Sisomicin	5–10	15–25	30–70	40–70	6–13
Netilmicin	5–6.5	15–25	20–30	30–35	5–6
Amikacin	7	10–25	35–60	45–60	4–7
Dibekacin	5–7	8–20	25–30	40–70	2.5–4
Lividomycin	6–10	10–22	30–100	35–50	5–10
Isepamicin	2–5	5–19	11–26	41.5	3.05

In obese subjects, the apparent volume of distribution in relation to total body weight is reduced. It is therefore preferable to refer to lean body weight in calculating dosages.

Dehydration reduces urinary elimination of aminoglycosides.

In patients with major burns, the frequent increase in glomerular filtration reduces the elimination half-lives of aminoglycosides (0.7 to 1.5 h).

Hyperthermia does not affect the elimination half-lives of aminoglycosides. However, levels in serum are reduced, and 3 h after intramuscular injection of gentamicin, concentrations in serum are 40% lower than those observed in apyretic subjects.

13.3. In Children and in the Perinatal Period

In neonates, absorption after intramuscular administration is more rapid, the apparent volume of distribution is higher (40 to 60% of body weight), peak levels in serum are lower, and renal elimination is slower than in adults. In children with normal renal function, the elimination half-lives are slightly lower than those in adults (1 to 1.5 h). They may reach 14 h in cases of severe renal insufficiency. The immaturity of renal function is responsible for delayed elimination during the first stage of life. The apparent elimination half-life of aminoglycosides is then 5 to 6 h. In the full-term neonate, it is higher in the first 4 days of life and when the body weight is less than 2 kg. In premature infants, the situation is further exacerbated, particularly if the gestational period is less than 28 to 30 weeks, body weight is less than 1 kg, and age is less than 1 week, when the elimination half-life may exceed 16 h and thus expose the child to the risk of toxicity.

In the neonate and premature infant, elimination half-lives are inversely correlated with the duration of gestation, birth weight, age, and CL_{CR}. Conversely, accumulation in the renal parenchyma is weaker in the neonate. In addition, hypoxemia is responsible for a reduction in glomerular filtration, which increases the elimination half-lives of aminoglycosides.

Various formulas have been proposed according to gestational age and birth weight, such as the proposed dosage intervals for gentamicin during the first week of life (Collatz et al., 1987) (Table 8).

However, the value of these therapeutic modalities in terms of efficacy and toxicity remains to be established.

In patients with cystic fibrosis, there is an increase in total clearance compared to that in healthy adults, but with no increase in renal clearance. There may therefore be an extrarenal elimination pathway, which would explain the weaker efficacy of the aminoglycosides in these patients and the benefit of increasing the dosages.

13.3.1.General Considerations

There is no effect of circadian rhythm on the pharmacokinetics of aminoglycosides. In patients receiving a protein-rich diet, there is a reduction in the elimination half-life and an increase in total clearance compared with those in fasting subjects. This fact might account for certain interindividual variations and should be borne in mind when setting up pharmacokinetic studies.

Several studies have demonstrated that the monitoring of levels in serum is necessary for patients aged between 6 months and 18 years if treatment exceeds 10 days or if there is an abnormality of renal function.

A number of authors have stressed the importance of the risks of drug interference, which are liable to exacerbate the toxic effects specific to aminoglycosides.

Table 8 Dosage frequency of gentamicin according to gestational age

For a 2.5-mg/kg dose	
Gestation period (wks)	Frequency of administration (h)
<28	24
29–30	18
>36	12

14. DRUG INTERACTIONS — PHYSICOCHEMICAL INCOMPATIBILITIES

14.1. Drug Interactions

The drug interactions observed with aminoglycosides are particularly detrimental when they are liable to exacerbate the specific toxic effects of these antibiotics: ototoxicity, nephrotoxicity, and curarizing effect. Their prescription should be avoided for anesthetized patients receiving curare agents. However, the curarizing effect of aminoglycosides may be avoided by administering calcium chloride and/or anticholinesterases. Their nephrotoxicity may be potentiated by the concomitant prescription of other medications that are themselves nephrotoxic, particularly amphotericin B, vancomycin, methoxyflurane, cisplatin, and daunorubicin. Combination with cephalosporins is possible on the condition that renal function and concentrations in serum are monitored, particularly for at-risk patients. Furosemide and ethacrynic acid markedly potentiate the risk of ototoxicity, but also that of nephrotoxicity.

Prolonged oral administration of neomycin has been held responsible for an intestinal malabsorption syndrome. This antibiotic may inhibit the gastrointestinal absorption of digoxin and vitamin B_{12}.

Particular emphasis should be placed on the partial inactivation of aminoglycosides by certain antibiotics and heparin.

14.1.1. Aminoglycoside-β-Lactam Interaction

Aminoglycosides may be inactivated in the presence of high concentrations of penicillins or cephalosporins. This inactivation may be explained by the formation of a complex between aminoglycosides with four or five free amino groups and certain penicillins, such as carbenicillin and ticarcillin, that possess two carboxyl groups. The formation of this complex depends on the concentration of the aminoglycoside and the penicillin or cephalosporin, the temperature, and the contact time. Amikacin is the least sensitive to this inactivation, while tobramycin is the most sensitive.

The in vivo inactivation of aminoglycosides is greater in patients suffering from severe renal insufficiency and may require dosage adjustments; in fact, the elimination half-life of aminoglycosides may be substantially prolonged, from 50 to 60 h to 20 to 30 h in these patients.

14.1.2. Aminoglycoside-Heparin Interaction

Inactivation of aminoglycosides by high concentrations of heparin (>10 to 100 U/ml) occurs essentially in vitro when blood samples are taken in heparinized tubes: in this case a slight reduction in the antibacterial activity of aminoglycosides may be observed.

Heparin does not inactivate aminoglycosides in vivo. In fact, the heparin concentrations found in patients treated with anticoagulants are very much lower than the inhibitory concentrations (<5 U/ml): in vivo inactivation of aminoglycosides by heparin is therefore negligible. However, sufficiently high levels of heparin (>100 U/ml) may be observed when aminoglycosides and heparin are injected simultaneously in the same infusion set. Thus, in the event of coadministration of heparin and an aminoglycoside, the following apply:

- A heparin infusion must be discontinued during an infusion of an aminoglycoside if the same infusion route is used, particularly if this involves a peripheral vein and the use of a small-diameter catheter.
- It is, however, possible to infuse heparin and an aminoglycoside jointly by two different approaches.
- In addition, blood samples for the assay of aminoglycosides should on no account be taken in heparinized tubes.

The main drug interactions or interferences of aminoglycosides are summarized in Table 9.

14.2. Physicochemical Incompatibilities of Aminoglycosides

The main physicochemical incompatibilities of several aminoglycosides are given in Table 10.

14.3. Risk of Interference with Laboratory Tests

As aminoglycosides have a nephrotoxic potential, they can cause proteinuria. At therapeutic doses they can also cause various degrees of hypomagnesemia, the mechanism of which is disputed: either by a reduction of digestive absorption of Mg^{2+} or, following intramuscular administration, by disruption of tubular reabsorption of magnesium.

More specifically, neomycin and kanamycin may cause a reduction in blood ammonium levels by an action on the producing bacteria, neomycin and kanamycin may cause a reduction in cholesterol (formation of salts with bile acids), and gentamicin may cause a reduction in blood uric acid.

15. INCIDENTS AND ACCIDENTS ASSOCIATED WITH AMINOGLYCOSIDES

Aminoglycosides have both renal and cochleovestibular toxicity. This constant toxicity risk, associated with variable interindividual susceptibility, is acceptable and controllable in

Table 9 Drug interactions or interference

Drug(s) used in combination with aminoglycosides	Interaction	Follow-up
Ethacrynic acid or furosemide	Enhancement of nephro- and/or ototoxicity effects	Combination to be banned, check regular kidney function
Penicillin V	Oral neomycin may diminish oral absorption of penicillin V	Avoid combining, or use parenteral penicillin
Broad-spectrum penicillins (carbenicillin, ticarcillin)	Partial inactivation	Not combined; monitoring of plasma aminoglycoside levels
Cephems	Partial inactivation; enhancement or decrease of nephrotoxicity	Kidney functions
Clindamycin	Enhancement of nephrotoxicity (?)	Kidney function
Amphotericin B	Enhancement of nephrotoxicity	Kidney function
Polymyxins	Enhancement of nephrotoxicity	Combination to be banned
Oral anticoagulants	Orally administered aminoglycosides may reduce vitamin K production, yielding enhancement of anticoagulant effect	Decrease the daily dose of anticoagulants and check regular coagulation tests
Methoxyflurane	Aminoglycosides enhance nephrotoxicity effects	Combination to be banned; kidney function
Heparin	Heparin partially inactivates aminoglycosides	No simultaneous infusion of the two drugs and no use of heparin-containing tubes for aminoglycoside assays
5-Fluorouracil	Neomycin may decrease oral absorption of 5-fluorouracil	Combination to be banned; kidney function
Cisplatin	Accumulation of nephrotoxic effects	Kidney function
Daunorubicin	Orally administered aminoglycosides may reduce methotrexate absorption	
Methotrexate		
Digoxin	Neomycin and other aminoglycosides may reduce gastrointestinal digoxin absorption	
Succinylcholine, tubocurarine	Risk of neuromuscular blockage	Check the level of curare at the end of anesthesiology; combination of calcium and a cholinesterasic drug to be administered before and after the curare administration
Colchicin	Alterations of vitamin B_{12} gastrointestinal absorption; colchicin enhances this dysabsorption	Neomycin decreases vitamin B_{12} absorption
Diltiazem	Glomerular filtration is improved and renal toxicity is decreased	Protective combination

Table 10 Physicochemical incompatibilities of aminoglycosides

Drug(s)	Incompatibility with:			Notes
	Injectable solutions	Other antibacterial agents	Other drugs	
Streptomycin sulfate	Sodium bicarbonate, electrolytes	Amphotericin B, carbenicillin, chloramphenicol (hemisuccinate), erythromycin (glucoheptonate), isoniazid, lincomycin, nitrofurantoin, novobiocin, oxytetracycline, sulfadiazine, sulfafurazole (diethanolamine)	Barbiturates, calcium (gluconate), chlorothiazide, heparin, phenytoin, riboflavin, triamcinolone	
Kanamycin	Sodium bicarbonate, proteolysates	Amphotericin B, cephalosporins, chloramphenicol, erythromycin, lincomycin, nitrofurantoin, penicillins, polymyxin B	Aminophylline, chlorpromazine, vitamin B complex and hydrosol multivitamin, heparin, hydrocortisone, hydroxydione, methylprednisolone, pentobarbital + phenobarbital, thiopental, phenytoin	
Gentamicin and sisomicin		Amphotericin B, cephalosporins, penicillins	Dopamine, heparin, hydrocortisone	It is recommended that other drugs not be used in combination with these antibiotics.
Tobramycin sulfate	Appears to be compatible with a large number of solutions, except those containing ethanol	Cephalosporins, penicillins		
Amikacin sulfate		Amphotericin B, cephalosporins, erythromycin, nitrofurantoin, penicillins, tetracyclines, sulfadiazine	Chlorothiazide, dexamethasone, heparin, phenytoin, group B vitamins with vitamin C, warfarin	It is recommended that amikacin not be mixed with other drugs in the same syringe or same infusion bottle. Recommended solutions: 0.9% isotonic NaCl solution, 5% isotonic glucose solution, 10% glucose solution
Netilmicin		Penicillins, cephalosporins	Heparin, vitamin B	
Dibekacin			Heparin, group B vitamins	

severe infections but unacceptable in minor infections. The mechanism is complex. The risk must be limited by a knowledge of the risk associated with interactions and age and by compliance with the rules governing prescriptions: short-term treatment and application of new treatment modalities (once or twice daily), possibly with the monitoring of peak and trough levels in serum.

15.1. Nephrotoxicity

Aminoglycosides are antibiotics that are known for their narrow therapeutic index and high risk of tubulointerstitial nephropathy as a result of the potential accumulation of the compound and the fact that the toxic concentrations are fairly close to effective concentrations. The risk is increased with drug combinations, particularly in debilitated patients and during treatments lasting longer than 10 days. The frequency of renal impairment is estimated at 3 to 25% depending on the drug, adopting an increase of 5 or 10 mg/liter, for creatinine levels of less than or more than 30 mg/liter, respectively, as a marker of nephrotoxicity.

Renal impairment is often confined to the appearance of proteinuria and/or extensive leukocyturia, with the occasional occurrence of acute renal failure in which diuresis is maintained. An increase in urinary elimination of certain enzymes (alanine aminopeptidase in particular) and β_2-microglobulin is found, although it cannot be claimed that this is a true sign of toxicity. Renal impairment is clinically very difficult to detect: no fever and no lower back pain, hematuria or oliguria. The warning signs can only be detected by monitoring the laboratory parameters, but these are in any case difficult to interpret for patients with functional instability. This is to emphasize the value of monitoring concentrations in serum in order to adjust the dosages. Sometimes, however, a hypokalemic and hypocalcemic syndrome may be noted, although no other proximal or distal tubular disorders have been reported.

Renal histology reveals acute tubular nephropathy with interstitial edema without cellular infiltration. The basal enzymes are not destroyed, even when there is tubular necrosis. Regression is therefore possible with tubular regeneration and functional and histological restoration.

The aminoglycosides have differing nephrotoxicities, with gentamicin appearing to be the most toxic. The nephrotoxicities of the other aminoglycosides vary with the species, sex, dose, and treatment duration. Other factors are involved (age, hemodynamic status, and concomitant medications). Netilmicin would appear to be the least potentially nephrotoxic compound; amikacin and tobramycin are apparently the best tolerated. However, comparative studies are insufficient and are no longer ethically acceptable, so short-term treatments are the rule.

In animals it is possible to obtain the clinical and laboratory effects observed in humans. Histologically, a proximal lesion is observed with rarefaction of the brush border. The subsequent intracellular lesions are dominated by lysosomal changes. The accumulation of aminoglycosides has been demonstrated by autoradiography with accumulation of the radioactive compound at the lysosomal level. At the intrarenal biochemical level, inhibition of glycolysis, mitochondrial oxidative phosphorylation, and mitochondrial electron transport have been demonstrated.

Four stages in the formation of aminoglycoside-associated renal lesions may be described. First of all is a functional phase lasting 24 to 48 h after the beginning of treatment, reflected essentially in an increase in the excretion of β_2-microglobulins. There then follows a phase (3 to 5 days) of microscopic cellular damage in the proximal tubule. The nephrons with proximal tubular lesions cannot fulfill their function of reabsorbing water, electrolytes, and proteins. The mechanism of protection associating glomerular filtration with a satisfactory tubular reabsorption function must be activated. This activation marks the beginning of the third phase, with a sharp fall in glomerular filtration. Elevation of serum creatinine is the marker event in the monitoring of treatment. It occurs 2 to 10 days after the onset of the first changes in the urinary sediment. The reduction in glomerular filtration is progressive. The juxtaglomerular apparatus plays a role in controlling this event, but tubuloglomerular feedback appears to function independently of any hormonal or nervous influence, and this process can only be monitored by studying the changes in CL_{CR}. Treatment remains symptomatic pending histological restitution and functional restoration. During the third phase, elements of regeneration of the tubular cells appear. This does not prevent the appearance of new tubular lesions if exposure to the aminoglycoside continues. The third stage may be exacerbated by other drugs, with increasing creatinine levels. These are essentially loop diuretics, one of the effects of which is to block the feedback-induced reduction in glomerular filtration. Although their effect is beneficial in that they increase diuresis, at the same time they increase the urinary concentration of the aminoglycoside and enhance the risk of tissue injury associated with accumulation.

The fourth phase is one of cellular regeneration. CL_{CR} normalizes and is evidence of the return to normal of glomerular function and tubular reabsorption. It is interesting that the regenerated tubular cells are temporarily less susceptible to injury by an aminoglycoside or any other substrate toxic for the tubule. The functional recovery time depends on a number of factors, e.g., nutritional status and exposure to other toxic agents. An improved knowledge of the "refractory" state to the toxicity of aminoglycosides during recovery is important in order to be able to establish the optimum dosage intervals if treatment is resumed (Schentag, 1982).

The nephrotoxicity of aminoglycosides depends on a number of parameters. It may be dependent on intrarenal accumulation rate; changes in membrane permeability, particularly of the lysosomal membrane; and degree of intracellular biochemical changes. It may also depend on the pharmacokinetics of the aminoglycoside.

After administration of the product, the reduction in concentration in serum occurs by two independent pathways with interindividual variations: tissue binding and renal elimination. Different patients may therefore have similar tissue concentrations and clinical effects but differing degrees to which the drug is toxic in them. In about 5% of patients there is marked tissue accumulation and a rapid increase in concentration in serum, with a major risk of nephrotoxicity, whereas in the majority of individuals there is normal tissue binding and urinary elimination, with a minor toxicity risk. However, the reaction is unpredictable, and during treatment the peak and trough concentrations in serum should be monitored so as to adapt the unit dosage and/or the dosage intervals. The ideal is to treat the patient for a short period, selecting the best method of administration.

Certain factors predispose to the onset of nephrotoxicity:

- Age, because of the physiological reduction in renal function which predisposes to overdoses and frequent drug combinations
- The administered dose (total dose more than unit dose)
- Above all, the rhythm of administration. A single daily injection appears to be less nephrotoxic than the same dose administered three times.

The nephrotoxicity of aminoglycosides is increased by salt depletion (salt-free diet or use of furosemide). Metabolic acidosis exacerbates this effect. A calcium-rich diet reduces nephrotoxicity. Alkalosis has no effect.

The nephrotoxicity of aminoglycosides may be affected by combination with other drugs, some of which have an intrinsic nephrotoxic effect, such as amphotericin B, vancomycin, cisplatin, and certain antimitotic agents. Combination with cephalosporins or ureidopenicillins would appear to exert a more protective effect. Diltiazem also has a favorable effect (Lortholary et al., 1992).

To prevent nephrotoxicity, the use of aminoglycosides should therefore be reserved for serious infections, the daily dosage should be restricted (particularly in subjects over the age of 60 years), treatments should be short (8 to 10 days), combinations should be effected with products that, if possible, are nontoxic or weakly toxic, renal concentration should be monitored, concentrations in serum should be tested to adapt the dosages and/or rhythm of administration, and a single daily dosage is preferred (De Broe et al., 1991; Tulkens, 1991).

15.1.1. Conclusion

Despite problems related to interindividual susceptibility, the nephrotoxicity of aminoglycosides remains a risk associated with the total dose, tissue accumulation, and a number of other factors. Rational use of these drugs starts with the choice of dosage regimens adapted to the CL_{CR} (calculated and then measured). Patients should be monitored at steady state by determining the CL_{CR} and possibly by serum assays so as to be able to analyze any situation of therapeutic failure.

Conversely, in high-risk patients in whom it is more difficult to monitor renal function, monitoring of concentrations in serum is used to maintain effective therapeutic levels. The residual concentrations are important parameters for detecting excessive tissue uptake on days 4 to 6 of treatment.

If nephrotoxicity occurs, the drug should be discontinued where possible, or its dosage should be reduced. Patients must be correctly hydrated and compensated electrolytically. Loop diuretics should always be avoided (except in an emergency related to a fluid overload).

An indication for elimination by hemodialysis is rare (trough levels of 4 mg/liter and creatinine increasing rapidly). Following dialysis, levels in serum rapidly return to their previous values in high-risk patients because of release from the tissues, whereas redistribution is less rapid in patients with tissue accumulation and a lower risk. Measurement of concentrations 6 to 8 h after the end of dialysis enables the type of tissue storage to be assessed. Peritoneal dialysis is perhaps more useful, as the equilibration time is longer, thus allowing more product accumulated in tissue to be extracted.

Obviously the ideal is to prevent nephrotoxicity.

15.2. Cochleovestibular Toxicity

Aminoglycosides have both a cochlear and a vestibular toxic potential. Vestibular lesions in general precede cochlear lesions. This is evidenced in dizziness, ataxia, and nystagmus, which usually regress and/or are compensated to a greater or lesser extent. Cochlear injury, which is more serious, may occur during treatment or several days or even several months after discontinuation of the aminoglycoside. Sometimes preceded by tinnitus, it is usually revealed by a sudden loss, at least apparently, of unilateral or bilateral auditory acuity which is irreversible and not amenable to instrumentation. The studies performed, both with animals and with humans, yield divergent results and do not allow a precise hierarchy of the different aminoglycosides to be established in terms of ototoxicity. Overall, streptomycin, gentamicin, and tobramycin have a predominantly vestibular toxicity, whereas kanamycin and amikacin have an essentially cochlear tropism. The frequencies of vestibular lesions are on average estimated at 3.5% for gentamicin, tobramycin, and amikacin and 1.4% for netilmicin (Kahlmeter and Dahlager, 1984). The incidence of these side effects may attain 10% or even 20% in the presence of these risk factors:

- High daily doses
- Treatment prolonged for more than 10 days
- Previous administration of aminoglycosides
- Simultaneous administration of other ototoxic medications, such as furosemide or ethacrynic acid
- Renal insufficiency
- Advanced age
- Previous auditory lesion

The toxicity of the aminoglycosides to the cochleovestibular apparatus may be explained by their rapid distribution into the internal ear fluids (peri- and endolymph), culminating in high concentrations over prolonged periods. The elimination half-lives in the perilymph are about 12 h.

The histological lesions are currently well known: destruction of the ciliated sensory cells of the internal ear, maximal in the basal spiral of the cochlea and the ciliated cells of the ampullar and vestibular crests. The mechanism remains poorly understood. Current research suggests reversible binding of aminoglycosides to the membrane surfaces of the sensory cells and then irreversible incorporation into these membranes, with a disorder of permeability predisposing to intracellular penetration. Aminoglycosides bind to polyphosphoinositol-rich membranes by competition with calcium on the phosphate groups. They thus affect the mitochondria and endoplasmic reticulum and disrupt cellular metabolism. Finally, their action on ribosomal metabolism is comparable to that observed on bacterial ribosomes.

Pharmacokinetic studies have shown the importance of the peak concentrations in serum in these accidents. Concentrations of more than 10 to 12 mg/liter for gentamicin, sisomicin, tobramycin, netilmicin, and dibekacin and greater than 30 to 40 mg/liter for amikacin would appear to be potentially ototoxic. More recently, greater significance has been attributed to the area under the concentration in serum time curve, which would appear to be a more reliable reflection of the accumulation of aminoglycosides in the body. In fact, no criterion provides a definite prediction of ototoxicity.

Thus, the best guarantee is to follow the rules governing prescription. The following should be avoided:

- Excessively high unit doses, exposing the patient to potentially ototoxic concentrations
- Treatment durations exceeding 10 days
- Combination with other ototoxic drugs: particularly in high-risk patients. Monitoring of the audiogram, with in particular a fall in acute frequencies being a warning signal, must be systematic in these patients.

Currently, it would seem that netilmicin is the least ototoxic compound. A number of studies appear to confirm a reduction in the risk of ototoxicity in short-term treatments and when amikacin or netilmicin is administered in one or two injections in adults (Tulkens, 1991) or children (Viscoli et al., 1991).

15.3. Curarizing Action

The curarizing action, involving neuromuscular blockade, is manifested in a flaccid paralysis with possible respiratory impairment. This reaction has been observed after intraperitoneal administration of neomycin or streptomycin during general anesthesia involving curare agents. This effect has not been observed for other aminoglycosides at the usual dosages.

The principal mechanism of the neuromuscular depression of aminoglycosides is competitive antagonism with the calcium ions at the presynaptic level. This phenomenon has been studied in particular for neomycin and streptomycin, with which it is observed at moderate concentrations. At high concentrations, these antibiotics also have a postsynaptic action on the acetylcholine receptors. Tobramycin has in particular a presynaptic action, and netilmicin has a postsynaptic action. Kanamycin has weaker effects.

This curarizing action of aminoglycosides is inhibited by calcium ions. In practice, therefore, it is advisable to prohibit intraperitoneal instillations of aminoglycosides and to refrain from prescribing these antibiotics to anesthetized patients receiving curare agents and to myasthenic patients, in the knowledge that "curare-like" effects are reversible with calcium chloride and neostigmine.

15.4. Other Adverse Effects

Central and/or peripheral neurologic lesions have been observed following lumbar intrathecal or intracisternal administration at dosages greater than the recommended doses.

Allergic reactions have been reported in exceptional cases, but local tolerance otherwise is excellent.

16. DOSAGE AND ROUTE OF ADMINISTRATION

Therapeutic levels of aminoglycosides are close to toxic levels. Any circumstance altering elimination exposes the patient to a risk of overdosage and toxicity.

16.1. Route of Administration

Aminoglycosides are commonly administered intramuscularly. The intravenous route is reserved for contraindications to the intramuscular route (anticoagulants). In this case, in order to avoid excessively high peak levels in serum, a bolus intravenous administration is prescribed and a unit dose is administered by infusion over 30 min or preferably using a constant-flow-rate syringe, not combined with any other substance. Subcutaneous administration is possible, but absorption is slow. The local route may also be used, but lumbar intrathecal or intraventricular administration in certain cases of bacterial meningitis has caused it to lose much of its theoretical and practical value. Oral administration is reserved for certain gastrointestinal infections and for oral decontamination.

16.2. Dosage

16.2.1. In Subjects with Normal Renal Function

In the treatment of systemic infections, the unit dose should be given every 8 or 12 h. Studies have shown that urinary concentrations obtained at 24 h are always greater than the MIC at which 50% of the isolates tested are inhibited for the majority of susceptible bacteria, irrespective of the frequency of administration.

Recent data have shown the value of a single daily dose in reducing the risk of toxicity. Animal models (Collatz et al., 1986) and studies with humans (Tulkens, 1991; Van der Auwera, 1991) have demonstrated the value of this rhythm of administration in terms of antibacterial activity in severe infections (Table 11). The use of aminoglycosides in a single daily injection is currently validated for amikacin and netilmicin (Beaucaire et al., 1991). Supplementary studies will be necessary (Levison, 1992) to confirm these results.

Table 11 Dosages of aminoglycosides in subjects with normal renal function

Compound	Dosage (mg/kg/day)	
	Adults	Children
Gentamicin	3	3
Tobramycin	3–5	3–5
Sisomicin	3–4.5	
Netilmicin	6–7.5	4–6
Amikacin	15	15
Isepamicin	15	

16.2.2. In Patients with Renal Insufficiency

In patients with renal insufficiency (Table 12), the dosages must be adapted. It is possible to reduce the doses or increase the interval between doses. If the interval between doses is increased, the elimination half-life should be calculated and the dose should be administered every three half-lives. In patients with very severe renal insufficiency, half the dose may be administered every half-life. Tables are available for the prescriber.

If the interval between doses is not modified, it is possible, after a normal initial dose, to administer a maintenance dose adapted according to the normograms. In practice, a simplified treatment may suffice. Levels in serum should be systematically monitored and the dosage adapted accordingly.

In the case of peritoneal dialysis, following a loading dose, 10 mg of gentamicin, tobramycin, or netilmicin per liter or 20 mg of amikacin per liter may be added to the dialysis solution to maintain effective concentrations in serum.

Table 12 Dosage of aminoglycosides in patients with renal insufficiency

Compound	Dosage at indicated CL_{CR}[a]		
	30–80 (mg/kg/day)	10–30 (mg/kg/36 h)	<10 (mg/kg)
Gentamicin	1	1	1 (48–72 h)
Tobramycin	1	1	1 (48–72 h)
Sisomicin	1	1	1 (48–72 h)
Netilmicin	2	2	2 (72 h)
Dibekacin	1	1	1 (72 h)
Amikacin	7.5	7.5	7.5 (72 h)
Isepamicin	8	8 (72 h)	8 (96 h)

[a]The units given apply to the dosages.

16.2.3. Specific Cases

In elderly subjects, the dosage should be adapted for CL_{CR}.

For obese patients, reference should be made to the ideal weight plus 40% and not the actual weight.

In burn patients, the dosages should be increased but the concentrations in serum should be monitored. The dosages for children are identical to those for adults. Finally, for neonates, several factors need to be taken into account.

17. CURRENT CLINICAL INDICATIONS OF AMINOGLYCOSIDES

17.1. In a Hospital Setting

With the exception of certain upper urinary tract infections, aminoglycosides are used in combination with β-lactams and/or glycopeptides (vancomycin), lipoglycopeptides (teicoplanin), or fluoroquinolones.

The essential indications are as follows:

- Systemic staphylococcal infections, in combination with a penicillin M or a "first-generation" (limited-spectrum) cephalosporin. If the strain is resistant to gentamicin, aminoglycosides must be avoided.

- Severe infections due to focalized aerobic gram-negative bacilli, with or without positive blood cultures
- *P. aeruginosa* infections, in combination with a β-lactam (cephalosporin or carbapenem)
- *Listeria* infections
- Septicemia with or without enterococcal endocarditis, particularly in cases involving streptomycin-resistant strains
- Meningitis due to gram-negative bacilli resistant to conventional β-lactams. However, the use of fluoroquinolones, third-generation cephalosporins, and carbapenems has reduced the indications for local treatments.
- Infections in neutropenic patients, subject to combination with a β-lactam. Amikacin is used extensively here without any obvious increase in resistance as a result of this intensive use.
- Postoperative infections following abdominal surgery, in combination with antibiotics effective against *Bacteroides*
- Infections in patients undergoing ambulatory peritoneal dialysis where the use of gentamicin in the injected solutions may be an effective alternative
- Infections due to *Nocardia* or atypical mycobacteria may also be considered, as may cystic fibrosis.

Prophylactically, aminoglycosides may be used in oral digestive decontamination or parenterally in combination with amoxicillin in high-risk patients.

The interest in new derivatives resistant to inactivating enzymes and with weaker toxicity is considerable.

17.2. In the Community

In monotherapy, the only indication is certain forms of pyelonephritis in young patients. Treatment is limited to 8 days. It is also possible to treat uncomplicated lower urinary tract infections in young women with a single injection (netilmicin, 4.5 mg/kg).

In view of the large number of penicillin G-resistant strains, gonococcal infection may be treated by spectinomycin at 2 g/day intramuscularly in simple forms and at 4 g/day in two injections for 3 days in disseminated forms.

A combination is the rule in other situations (when pregnancy requires the prescription of an aminoglycoside). This may involve severe exacerbations of chronic bronchitis (the addition of an aminoglycoside may sometimes avoid hospitalization), complicated urinary tract infections, or subacute osteoarticular infections (combination and then switch to prolonged oral treatment with a β-lactam or fluoroquinolone).

The main progress in the prescription of aminoglycosides, both in the community and in the hospital, has been represented by the rhythm of administration of the daily dose: one or two injections daily with a reduction in the total duration of treatment.

18. CONCLUSION

Despite the development of cephalosporins and fluoroquinolones, aminoglycosides remain valuable antibiotics in the treatment of severe infections. Substantial progress has been made in terms of understanding the mechanisms of resistance and toxicity. Pharmacodynamic studies with animals and humans have allowed the validation of new rules governing prescriptions: short-term treatment and daily administration, providing the same efficacy and considerably reducing the risks of oto- and nephrotoxicity.

REFERENCES

Acar JF, Goldstein FW, Menard R, Bleriot JP, 1986, Strategies in aminoglycoside use and impact on resistance, Am J Med, 80, 6B, 82–90.

Beaucaire G, Leroy O, Beuscart C, Karp P, et al, 1991, Clinical and bacteriological efficacy and practical aspects of amikacin given once daily for severe infections, J Antimicrob Chemother, 27, suppl C, 91–103.

Collatz E, Carbon C, Humbert G, 1986, Aminoglycosides (aminocyclitols), in Peterson PK, Verhoef I, ed, Antimicrobial Agents Annual 1986, p 1–16, Elsevier Science Publishers.

Collatz E, Carbon C, Humbert G, 1987, Aminoglycosides (aminocyclitols), in Peterson PK, Verhoef I, ed, Antimicrobial Agents Annual 1987, p 1–13, Elsevier Science Publishers.

Collatz E, Carbon C, Humbert G, 1988, Aminoglycosides (aminocyclitols), in Peterson PK, Verhoef I, ed, Antimicrobial Agents Annual 1988, p 1–13, Elsevier Science Publishers.

Davies JE, Aminoglycoside aminocyclitol antibiotics and their modifying enzymes, p 790, in Antibiotics in Laboratory Medicine.

De Broe ME, Verbist L, Verpooten GA, 1991, Influence of dosage schedule on renal cortical accumulation of amikacin and tobramycin in man, J Antimicrob Chemother, 27, suppl C, 41–47.

Guillaume C, Faurisson F, Peytavin G, 1992, Pharmacokinetics of nebulized tobramycin in mechanically ventilated patients with bacterial pneumonia, 32nd Intersci Conf Antimicrob Agents Chemother, poster 207.

Kahlmeter G, Dahlager JI, 1984, Aminoglycoside toxicity. A review of clinical studies published between 1975 and 1982, J Antimicrob Chemother, 13, suppl A, 9–22.

Kahlmeter G, Jonsson S, Kamme C, 1978, Multiple compartment pharmacokinetics of tobramycin, J Antimicrob Chemother, 4, suppl, 5-11.

Levison ME, 1992, New dosing regimens for aminoglycoside antibiotics, Ann Intern Med, 117, 693–694.

Lortholary O, Nochy D, Heudes C, Carbon C, 1992, Glomerular alterations due to netilmicin in rabbits, functional and morphological approach. Prevention with diltiazem in rabbits, 32nd Intersci Conf Antimicrob Agents Chemother, poster 292.

Nagabushan TL, Miller GH, Weinstein MJ, 1982, Structure activity relationships in aminoglycoside aminocyclitol antibiotics, p 3–27, in Whelton A, Neu HC, ed, The Aminoglycosides, Marcel Dekker Inc, New York.

Schentag JJ, 1982, Aminoglycoside pharmacokinetics as a guide to therapy and toxicology, p 143–167, in Whelton A, Neu HC, ed, The Aminoglycosides, Marcel Dekker Inc, New York.

Shannon K, Phillips I, 1982, Mechanism of resistance to aminoglycosides in clinical isolates, J Antimicrob Chemother, 9, 91–102.

Tulkens P, 1991, Pharmacokinetics and toxicological evaluation of a once daily regimen versus conventional schedules of netilmicin and amikacin, J Antimicrob Chemother, 27, suppl C, 49–61.

Van der Auwera P, 1991, Pharmacokinetic evaluation of single daily dose amikacin, J Antimicrob Chemother, 27, suppl C, 63–71.

Viscoli C, Dudley M, Ferrea G, Boni L, Castagnola E, et al., 1991, Serum concentrations and safety of single daily dosing of amikacin in children undergoing bone marrow transplantation, J Antimicrob Chemother, 27, suppl C, 113–120.

Spectinomycin

A. BRYSKIER

17

1. STRUCTURE AND STRUCTURE-ACTIVITY OF SPECTINOMYCIN

Spectinomycin (formerly known as actinospectacin) (Fig. 1) is an aminocyclitol antibiotic isolated from the fermentation broths of *Streptomyces flavopersicus* and *Streptomyces spectabilis*. Spectinomycin is a disaccharide antibiotic with a neutral sugar (actinospectose) fused to actinamine (*N,N'*-dimethyl-2-*epi*-streptamine) by a β-glycoside bond and a hemiacetal type of bond (1,4-dioxane), producing a tricyclic structure (Wiley et al., 1963). The bond of the B/C structure is in the *cis* position with a 2′-hydroxyl group axial to the B nucleus. The molecule has nine centers of asymmetry. Starting from the 1,4-dioxane nucleus, four diastereoisomers may be described (Cochran et al., 1972).

In an acidic medium, the bonds are hydrolyzed. In an aqueous medium, there is an equilibrium between the form with a 3′-carbonyl and that with a 3′-diol (Fig. 2).

Reduction of the carbonyl at C-3′ yields the (*S*)- and (*R*)-dihydrospectinomycin derivatives, the antibacterial activities of which range from 0 to 100% of that of spectinomycin depending on the bacterial species. The 3′-(*R*)-dihydrospectinomycin isomer is more active than the 3′-(*S*)-isomer. The 3′-(*R*)-dihydrospectinomycin isomer was detected in the fermentation broth of *S. spectabilis* and would appear to be an intermediate of the biosynthesis pathway of spectinomycin. 3′-(*S*)- and 3′-(*R*)-aminospectinomycin derivatives have been synthesized. The 3′-(*R*)-isomer has good antibacterial activity, in contrast to the 3′-(*S*)-aminospectinomycin isomer. The difference in activity between the isomers is probably due to the poor binding of the molecule at the ribosomal receptor sites, which occurs through hydrogen bonds. Substitution at C-3′ by a halogen (chlorine or bromine) produces molecules that are relatively inactive. Other changes have been made at C-3′, such as the 3′-hydroxymethyl derivative, which is less active than 3′-(*S*)-dihydrospectinomycin. The attachment of an α-hydroxyl group to this molecule reintroduces antibacterial activity weaker than that of spectinomycin, showing clearly the importance of the hydroxyl groups and their spatial positions. Incorporation of an amino function in the chain also restores good antibacterial activity. Alkylation of the amino group reduces the activity in the (*S*) series but increases it in the (*R*) series. The introduction of a second amino function also increases antibacterial activity. Epimerization of the 2-hydroxyl reduces the activity. Inactivating enzymes may intervene at this point, as well as on the hydroxyl group at C-6 (adenylation). Trospectomycin results from the attachment of a propyl chain to the methyl

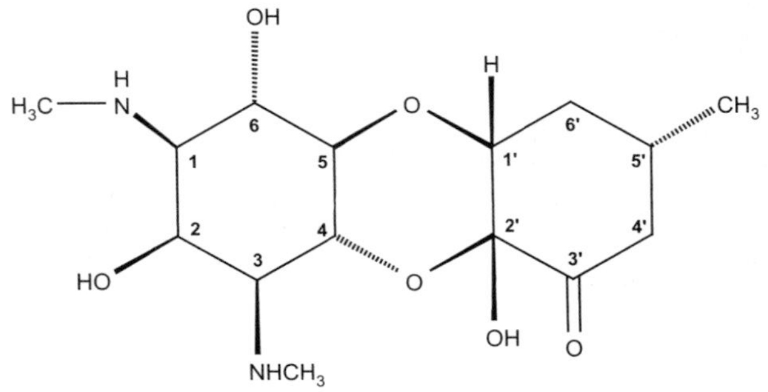

OH H H H_3C—N O CH_3 6 6′ 1 5 1′ 5′ 2 4 2′ 4′ 3 3′ HO O OH O $NHCH_3$

Figure 1 Spectinomycin

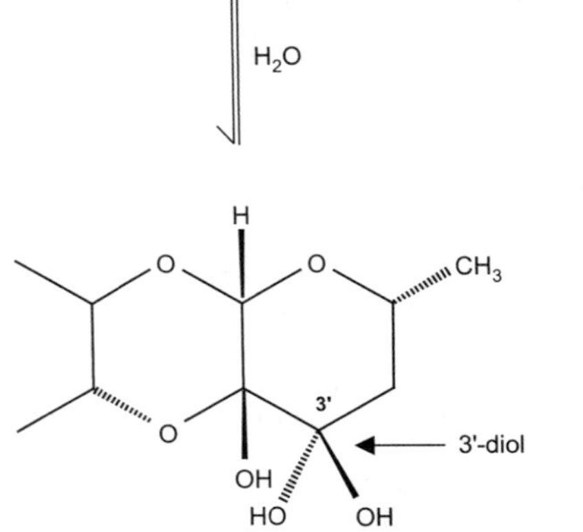

H O O CH_3 3′ O OH O 3′-carbonyl

H_2O

H O O CH_3 3′ O 3′-diol OH HO OH

Figure 2 Spectinomycin in an aqueous medium

group at C-3. It is 4 to 16 times more active in vitro than spectinomycin (Fig. 3).

2. PHYSICOCHEMICAL PROPERTIES

Spectinomycin pentahydrate dihydrochloride is a white crystalline powder which is freely soluble in water. The pH of a 1% aqueous solution is between 3.8 and 5.6. Spectinomycin is a dibasic antibiotic with pKs of 6.95 and 8.70. The physicochemical properties are summarized in Table 1.

3. ANTIBACTERIAL ACTIVITY

Spectinomycin and trospectomycin are inactive or weakly active against methicillin-susceptible and -resistant strains of *Staphylococcus aureus* and coagulase-negative staphylococci. Likewise, they are inactive against *Streptococcus pyogenes, Streptococcus agalactiae*, streptococci of Lancefield groups C and G, and enterococci. Trospectomycin exhibits good activity (MIC at which 50% of isolates tested are inhibited [MIC_{50}], ~2 μg/ml) against penicillin G-susceptible and -resistant strains of *Streptococcus pneumoniae*, whereas spectinomycin is inactive (MIC_{50}, ~16 μg/ml). Against gram-positive bacilli, trospectomycin is more active than spectinomycin (MIC_{50}, ~8 μg/ml) (Table 2).

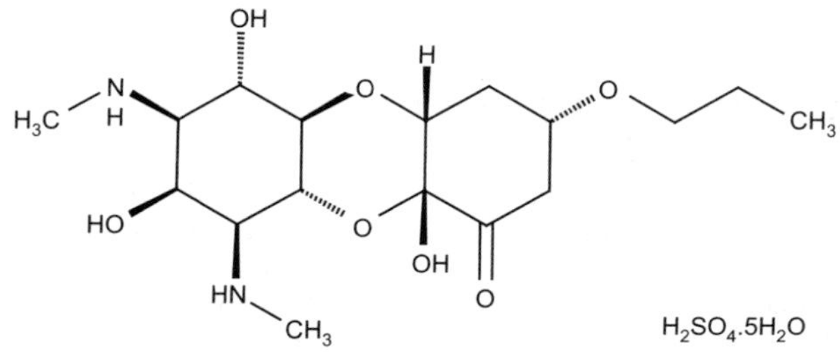

$H_2SO_4.5H_2O$

Figure 3 Trospectomycin sulfate

Both molecules have good activity against *Moraxella catarrhalis*. Only trospectomycin is active against *Haemophilus influenzae* (MIC_{50}, ~1 μg/ml); spectinomycin is inactive (MIC_{50}, ~16 μg/ml). They are inactive against *Acinetobacter* spp. and *Pseudomonas aeruginosa*. Against *Enterobacteriaceae* they are moderately active. Spectinomycin is more active than trospectomycin, with the exception of *Salmonella* spp. and *Shigella* spp. (Zurenko et al., 1988) (Table 3).

Spectinomycin is inactive against anaerobic bacteria, while trospectomycin possesses activity weaker than that of clindamycin (Gismondo et al., 1991; Jacobus and Tally, 1988) (Table 4).

A single dose of more than 40 mg of trospectomycin per kg of body weight eliminated *Treponema pallidum* in experimental syphilitic lesions in the rabbit (Rice et al., 1988). Spectinomycin is inactive against *T. pallidum*.

Trospectomycin and spectinomycin possess good activity against *Haemophilus ducreyi* ($MIC_{50/90}$, 0.12/0.25 versus 4/4 μg/ml) (Sanson-Lepors et al., 1986).

Trospectomycin has activity similar to that of the cyclines against *Mycoplasma pneumoniae* (MIC_{90}, ~1 μg/ml). It is inactive against *Mycoplasma hominis* (MIC_{50}, >128 μg/ml). Activity against *Ureaplasma urealyticum* is moderate (MIC_{50}, ~16 μg/ml) (Yancey and Klein, 1988) (Table 5).

Chlamydia trachomatis is susceptible in vitro to the activity of trospectomycin, 99.9% of its growth being inhibited by this drug at a dose of 12.5 μg/ml (Zurenko et al., 1988). Trospectomycin inhibits the growth of *Chlamydia pneumoniae* at concentrations of between 5 and 40 μg/ml (Kuo and Grayston, 1988). Trospectomycin appears to be active against *Chlamydia psittaci*.

Table 1 Physicochemical properties of spectinomycin and trospectomycin

Drug	Empirical formula	Mol wt	CAS no.[a]	Melting point (°C)	pK
Spectinomycin	$C_{14}H_{24}N_2O_7$	332.25	1695-77-8	184–194	6.95/8.7
Trospectomycin	$C_{17}H_{30}N_2O_7$	562.58	088851-61-0		

[a]CAS no., *Chemical Abstracts* number.

Table 2 Activity of spectinomycin against gram-positive bacteria

Organism(s)	MIC_{50} (μg/ml)	
	Spectinomycin	Trospectomycin
S. aureus	128	16
S. aureus OXA[r a]	>128	32
Coagulase-negative staphylococci	64	8
Enterococcus faecalis	128	16
Enterococcus spp.	128	16
S. agalactiae	>128	32
S. pyogenes	128	4
Group C and G streptococci	32	4
S. pneumoniae Pen[s]	16	2
S. pneumoniae Pen[r]	16	2
Listeria monocytogenes	32	8
Corynebacterium jeikeium	16	8
Bacillus spp.	64	16

[a]OXA, oxacillin.

Table 3 In vitro activity of spectinomycin against gram-negative bacilli

Organism(s)[a]	MIC_{50} (μg/ml)	
	Spectinomycin	Trospectomycin
H. influenzae β^-	16	1
H. influenzae β^+	8	0.5
M. catarrhalis	8	4
E. coli	16	32
Citrobacter freundii	32	32
Citrobacter diversus	16	16
Enterobacter spp.	16	32
K. pneumoniae	16	32
Morganella morganii	32	8
Proteus mirabilis	32	32
Providencia stuartii	>1,024	32
Serratia marcescens	32	128
Acinetobacter	32	16
P. aeruginosa	128	256

[a]β^-, non-β-lactamase producing; β^+, -lactamase producing.

Table 4 In vitro activity of spectinomycin and trospectomycin against anaerobes

Organism(s)	MIC_{50} (μg/ml)	
	Spectinomycin	Trospectomycin
Bacteroides fragilis	4	1
Bacteroides thetaiotaomicron	8	4
Bacteroides ovatus	8	2
Bacteroides distasonis	2	0.5
Bacteroides vulgatus	4	1
Bacteroides bivius	2	≤0.12
Bacteroides oralis	2	≤0.12
Eikenella corrodens	1	
Clostridium difficile	16	1
Clostridium spp.	4	0.5

Trospectomycin is much more active than spectinomycin against spectinomycin-susceptible strains of *Neisseria gonorrhoeae*, including strains resistant to ampicillin through a plasmid-mediated (PPNG) or chromosomal (CMRNG) mechanism, with or without resistance to tetracyclines. Spectinomycin is inactive against *Neisseria meningitidis*, whereas trospectomycin has moderate activity (MIC_{50}, ~4 μg/ml) (Peeters et al., 1984; Zurenko et al., 1988). Trospectomycin has good activity against *Helicobacter pylori* (MIC_{50} between 0.2 and 0.7 μg/ml, depending on the pH) (Debets-Ossenkopp et al., 1995). Against *Mycoplasma agalactiae*, $MIC_{50/90}$s were 0.52/0.938 μg/ml, with the drug being less active than tylosin and enrofloxacin ($MIC_{50/90}$, 0.12 μg/ml) (Loria et al., 2003).

4. MECHANISMS OF ACTION AND RESISTANCE

Spectinomycin and trospectomycin inhibit protein synthesis. They act by binding to the 30S ribosomal subunit with different affinities, which might explain the difference in terms of their antibacterial activities (50% inhibitory concentration, 4.4 versus 10 μM) (Laborde and Mourey, 1987). They inhibit the initiation process of the peptide chain (Reusser, 1976). They act on the 16S rRNA. Like aminoglycosides, they act by inhibiting translocation (they cause translational errors). They bind on the A site. Their target sites include ribosomal domains in which the accuracy of the codon-anticodon is assessed. In particular, they bind to a highly conserved motif of 16S rRNA, which leads to alterations in the ribosome function.

Spectinomycin binds at position N-7 of 16S rRNA residue G1064. Probably this binding occurs on helix 34 of the 16S rRNA. Binding of spectinomycin is thought to stabilize helix 34, inhibiting the binding of elongation factor G, thereby blocking translocation of peptidyl tRNA from the ribosome A site to the P site.

Plasmid-mediated enzymatic inactivation of spectinomycin occurs by adenylation of the hydroxyl group at position 6. A second mechanism involving mutation in protein ribosomal L2, S5, and S12 causing high-level resistance in *Escherichia coli* and *N. gonorrhoeae* has been described. A change occurs in the ribosome, preventing spectinomycin from binding. A methylase has been described for a strain of *Klebsiella pneumoniae*. This methylase, ArmA, is encoded by the *armA* gene. In ring II, the amino groups at positions 1 and 3 are essential for the binding to the decoding site of 16S rRNA of prokaryotic cells. Most aminoglycosides bind to a loop where bases A1408, A1493, and A1492 are located. Methylation can be plasmid mediated.

Trospectomycin exhibits cross-resistance with spectinomycin.

5. EPIDEMIOLOGY OF RESISTANCE OF *N. GONORRHOEAE*

Penicillin G used to be the reference drug in the treatment of gonococcal urethritis. Its use was called into question in the mid-1970s with the emergence of resistant strains, particularly in Southeast Asia. The first strains were isolated in the Philippines between 1965 and 1967.

In Thailand, in 1983, spectinomycin was recommended as the reference treatment because of the marked prevalence of β-lactamase-producing and tetracycline-resistant strains. The first spectinomycin-resistant strain was described in 1981 in California. However, from 1981 spectinomycin-resistant strains developed rapidly in South Korea and the Philippines, reaching 22.2% in 1988 in the Philippines and 8.9% in 1990 in Thailand. Easmon reported in 1984 that 5% of strains isolated in England were resistant to spectinomycin.

Chromosomally mediated resistance appears the most widespread form and is often accompanied by a reduction in the susceptibility of the involved strains to spectinomycin, cyclines, sulfonamides, and erythromycin A.

In Indonesia, 89% of isolates were resistant to penicillin G (MIC, ≥2 μg/ml), 98% were resistant to cyclines (MIC,

Table 5 In vitro activity of spectinomycin against bacteria responsible for genital infections

Organism	MIC_{50} (μg/ml)			
	SPT[a]	Trospectomycin	Tetracycline	Ampicillin
M. pneumoniae	0.5	0.5	0.5	
M. hominis	1	16	4	
U. urealyticum	32	16	4	
N. gonorrhoeae SPT^s, Amp^s	16	1	0.25	≤0.125
N. gonorrhoeae SPT^s, Amp^r	16	2	2	16
N. gonorrhoeae SPT^r, Amp^s	>256	>256	2	0.125
N. gonorrhoeae SPT^r, Amp^r	>256	256	2	16
N. gonorrhoeae CMRNG, SPT^s	16	2	1	0.25

[a]SPT, spectinomycin.

≥2 μg/ml), 18.1% were resistant to spectinomycin (MIC, ≥128 μg/ml), and 97.7% were of reduced susceptibility to phenicols (MIC, ~1 to 2 μg/ml).

In Durban, South Africa, from 1999 to 2000, the rate of resistance to spectinomycin for *N. gonorrhoeae* reached 32%. In Nigeria, the resistance rate reached 62.3%.

In Trinidad and Tobago no isolates resistant to spectinomycin had been detected. All isolates studied recently in Sweden (1999) were susceptible to spectinomycin.

For a Spanish strain for which the MIC of ciprofloxacin was 16 μg/ml, the activities of the tetracyclines and spectinomycin remained unchanged.

6. BREAKPOINTS

The breakpoints of spectinomycin recommended by the French Antibiotic Sensitivity Test Committee are ≥64 μg/ml for *N. gonorrhoeae*.

7. PHARMACOKINETICS

7.1. Spectinomycin

After an intravenous dose of 500 mg, the apparent volume of distribution is 8.6 liters and the plasma clearance is 4.73 liters/h, with an apparent elimination half-life of 1.66 h (Wagner, 1977).

Spectinomycin is rapidly absorbed intramuscularly. The peak concentration in serum of 103 μg/ml is reached after 1 h with a dose of 2 g, and the peak is 160 μg/ml after 2 h following a dose of 4 g; at the end of the first hour the concentration in plasma is 127 μg/ml. At 8 h, the residual concentrations are, respectively, 15 and 31 μg/ml for doses of 2 and 4 g. Renal and plasma clearances are, respectively, 2.21 to 3.74 liters/h and 3.9 to 5.2 liters/h. After single doses of 500 mg intravenously and intramuscularly, the area under the curve is 111 mg·h/liter (Wagner et al., 1968) and the renal and plasma clearances are, respectively, 3.22 and 4.52 liters/h, with residual concentrations after 8 h of 1.9 and 2.2 μg/ml, respectively.

Urinary elimination after 48 h is 77% of the administered dose (Brogden et al., 1972).

Probenecid does not retard the urinary elimination of spectinomycin. Protein binding is weak.

After a dose of 40 mg/kg in children, peak levels in serum of 64.3 μg/ml are reached at 1 h (Rettig et al., 1980). Urinary elimination accounts for 70% of the administered dose.

In patients with renal insufficiency, the apparent elimination half-life increases as the creatinine clearance decreases (Table 6). Fifty percent of the administered dose of spectinomycin is eliminated by hemodialysis (Kusumi et al., 1981).

After administration of 2 g intramuscularly, the concentrations (means ± standard deviations) obtained between 65 and 130 min are 23.2 ± 11.7 mg/kg and 12.1 ± 6.3 mg/kg in the uterine cervix and fallopian tubes, respectively. After a dose of 4 g, the concentrations obtained between 95 and 130 min are, respectively, 21.9 ± 6.3 mg/kg and 11.9 ± 4.6 mg/kg (Elder et al., 1977).

Table 6 Half-life of spectinomycin in patients with renal insufficiency

Creatinine clearance (ml/min)	$t_{1/2}$ (h)
120–80	1.5
80–40	4.7–4.9
40–5	10.4–17.9
<5	18.5–29.3

7.2. Trospectomycin

The intravenous and intramuscular pharmacokinetics were determined at doses of 75 to 1,000 mg. Intravenously, trospectomycin was administered in the form of an infusion over 20 min. The assays were performed by a microbiological method (*S. epidermidis*) and by high-performance liquid chromatography. The limits of detection were, respectively, 0.6 μg/ml and 25 ng/ml.

The concentrations at the end of the infusion were proportional to the administered dose, as were the areas under the curve (Table 7) (Novak et al., 1987).

The same applies after intramuscular administration (Table 8); after repeated doses (every 12 h for 7.5 days) there is no accumulation (Novak et al., 1988). At low doses, 70% of the administered dose is eliminated in the urine, but at high doses (1,000 mg), about 25% is eliminated in the feces. This would suggest saturation of urinary elimination and

Table 7 Intravenous pharmacokinetics of ascending doses of trospectomycin

Dose (mg)	C_{max} (μg/ml)	AUC (μg·h/ml)	k_{el} (h^{-1})	$t_{1/2}$ (h)
75	5.2	7.1		
150	9.9	15.5		
300	28.9	41.9	0.4	1.7
450	42	63.4	0.4	1.9
600	45.3	84.1	0.3	2.2
750	52.9	109.4	0.3	2.6
900	78.3	127.4	0.3	2.1
1,000	82.4	157	0.3	2.2

Table 8 Intramuscular pharmacokinetics of ascending doses of trospectomycin

Dose (mg)	C_{max} (μg/ml)	AUC (μg·h/ml)	k_{el} (h^{-1})	$t_{1/2}$ (h)	Urinary elimination (%)
300	11.1	34.7	0.51	1.4	23–42
600	18.5	80.9	0.36	2	41.50
1,000	30.3	131	0.35	2	27–72

Table 9 Comparative intravenous and intramuscular pharmacokinetics (1 g) of trospectomycin

Parameter (unit)	Intravenous	Intramuscular
C_{max} (μg/ml)	81.2	28.7
AUC_{0-18h} (μg·h/ml)	156.2	116.2
T_{max} (h)		1.25
$t_{1/2}$ (h)	49	47.8
Urinary elimination (%)	21.8	21.8

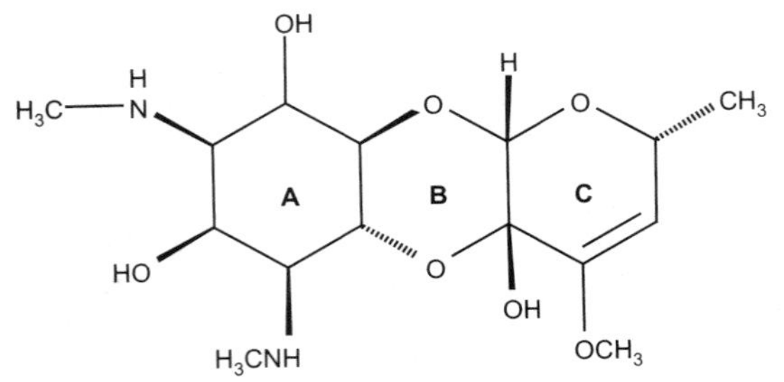

Figure 4 Acmimycin

Table 10 In vitro activity of acmimycin

Organism	MIC (μg/ml)	
	Acmimycin	Spectinomycin
S. aureus ATCC 6538P	100	100
S. epidermidis sp-a1-1	50	50
S. pyogenes NY5	3.1	12.5
Bacillus subtilis ATCC 6633	25	25
E. coli NIHJ-JC2	50	25
P. aeruginosa IAM 1095	100	1,000

compensation by the biliary route (Bye and Dring, 1987). Following intramuscular administration, about 80% of the dose is absorbed (Table 9) (Zurenko et al., 1988).

8. ACMIMYCIN

Acmimycin was isolated from the fermentation broth of *Streptomyces* sp. strain AC 4559 (FERM P-6645) in 1984 (Awata et al., 1986). It is distinguished structurally by a modification of the C ring (Fig. 4). This molecule is soluble in water, sparingly soluble in methanol, and insoluble in acetone and ethyl acetate. Its antibacterial activity is very similar to that of spectinomycin (Table 10).

REFERENCES

Awata M, Hayashi M, Muto N, Sakakibara H, 1986, Acmimycin, a new aminoglycoside antibiotic, Agric Biol Chem, 50, 239–241.

Brogden RN, Avery GS, 1972, New antibiotics: epicillin, minocycline and spectinomycin—a summary of their antibacterial activity, pharmacokinetic properties and therapeutic efficacy, Drugs, 3, 314–330.

Bye A, Dring LG, 1987, The pharmacokinetics of trospectomycin, 27th Intersci Conf Antimicrob Agents Chemother, abstract 272.

Cochran TG, Abraham DJ, Martin LL, 1972, Stereochemistry and absolute configuration of the antibiotic spectinomycin: an X-ray study, JCS Chem Comm, 494–495.

Debets-Ossenkopp YJ, Namavar F, MacLaren DM, 1995, Effect of an acidic environment on the susceptibility of Helicobacter pylori to trospectomycin and other antimicrobial agents, Eur J Clin Microb Infect Dis, 14, 353–355.

Elder MG, Bywater MJ, Reeves DS, 1977, Pelvic tissue and serum concentrations of various antibiotics given as pre-operative medication, Br J Obst Gynecol, 64, 887–893.

Gismondo MR, Chisari G, Lo Bue AM, 1991, In vitro activity against aerobes and anaerobes of trospectomycin versus spectinomycin, Drugs Exp Clin Res, 17, 101–104.

Jacobus NV, Tally FP, 1988, Activity of trospectomycin against Bacteroides fragilis and other Bacteroides species, Antimicrob Agents Chemother, 32, 584–586.

Kuo CC, Grayston JT, 1988, In vitro susceptibility of Chlamydia sp. strain TWAR, Antimicrob Agents Chemother, 32, 257–258.

Kusumi R, Metzler G, Fass R, 1981, Pharmacokinetics of spectinomycin in volunteers with renal insufficiency, Chemotherapy, 37, 95–98.

Laborde AL, Mourey RJ, 1987, Mechanism of action of trospectomycin, a novel spectinomycin analog, 27th Intersci Conf Antimicrob Agents Chemother, New York, abstract 266.

Loria GR, Sammartino C, Nicholas RA, Ayling RD, 2003, In vitro susceptibilities of field isolates of Mycoplasma agalactiae to oxytetracycline, tylosin, enrofloxacin, spiramycin and lincomycin-spectinomycin, Res Vet Sci, 75, 3–7.

Novak E, Griffith DL, Paxton LM, Metzler CM, Francom SF, 1988, Human safety and pharmacokinetics of multiple intramuscular doses of trospectomycin sulfate (U-63366F)—a novel spectinomycin analogue, 28th Intersci Conf Antimicrob Agents Chemother, abstract 97.

Novak E, Zurenko GE, Paxton LM, Francom SF, Oliver LK, 1987, Trospectomycin sulfate [6′-N-propylspecinomycin (U-63366F)]: safety and pharmacokinetics in man after single-dose iv administration, 27th Intersci Conf Antimicrob Agents Chemother, abstract 271.

Peeters M, Van Dyck E, Piot P, 1984, In vitro activities of the spectinomycin analog U-63366 and four quinolone derivatives against Neisseria gonorrhoeae, Antimicrob Agents Chemother, 26, 608–609.

Rettig JP, Nelson JD, Kusmies H, 1980, Spectinomycin therapy for gonorrhoea in prepubertal children, Am J Dis Child, 134, 359.

Reusser F, 1976, Effect of spectinomycin on peptide chain initiation, J Antibiot, 29, 1328–1333.

Rice RJ, Thompson SE, Arko RJ, Hunter EF, Burleigh PM, Craig BT, Larsen AF, 1988, Tissue fluid penetration and antitreponemal activity of trospectomycin (a new spectinomycin analog) in the rabbit syphilis model, Sex Transm Dis, 15, 152–155.

Sanson-Lepors MJ, Casin IM, Thebault M-C, Arlet G, Perol Y, 1986, In vitro activities of U-63366, a spectinomycin analog; roxithromycin (RU 28965), a new macrolide antibiotic; and five quinolone derivatives against Haemophilus ducreyi, Antimicrob Agents Chemother, 30, 512–513.

Wagner JC, 1977, Pharmacokinetic parameters estimated from intravenous data by uniform methods and some of their uses, J Pharmacokinet Biopharm, 5, 161–182.

Wagner JC, Novack E, Leslie LG, Metzler CM, 1968, Absorption, distribution and elimination of spectinomycin dihydrochloride in man, Int J Clin Pharmacol, 1, 261–285.

Wiley PF, Argoudelis AD, Hoeskema H, 1963, The chemistry of actinospectacin. IV. The determination of the structure of actinospectacin, J Am Chem Soc, 85, 2652–2659.

Yancey RJ Jr, Klein LK, 1988, In vitro activity of trospectomycin sulphate against Mycoplasma and Ureaplasma species isolated from humans, J Antimicrob Chemother, 21, 731–736.

Zurenko GE, Ford CW, Novak E, 1988, Trospectomycin, a novel spectinomycin analogue: antibacterial activity and preliminary human pharmacokinetics, Drugs Exp Clin Res, 14, 403–409.

Zurenko GE, Yagi BH, Vavra JJ, Wentworth BB, 1988, In vitro antibacterial activity of trospectomycin (U-63366F), a novel spectinomycin analog, Antimicrob Agents Chemother, 32, 216–223.

Macrolides

A. BRYSKIER AND E. BERGOGNE-BÉRÉZIN

18

1. DEFINITION OF MACROLIDES

The name "macrolide" comes from macro (large) and olide (lactone).

The macrolides are hydrophobic molecules having a central 12- to 16-membered-ring lactone with few or no double bonds and no nitrogen atom. Several amino or neutral sugars may be attached to the lactone nucleus.

The azalides are not included in Woodward's definition, as they have an endolactone nitrogen atom. Nevertheless, because of their chemical origin they are semisynthetic derivatives of erythromycin A, and due to their antibacterial spectrum they belong to the macrolide family.

2. CLASSIFICATIONS

There are several classifications of macrolides: a chemical classification and a simplified classification that considers the lactone structure and the natural or semisynthetic origin of the molecule, on the basis of which the macrolides can be classified into four groups. The natural macrolides of importance in human pathology are the 14- and 16-membered-ring macrolides; the semisynthetic derivatives of importance in human pathology are the 15-membered-ring macrolides (azalides).

The 14-membered-ring macrolides are divided into two groups: those of natural origin, such as erythromycin A (Fig. 1) and oleandomycin, and those obtained by semisynthesis from erythromycin A. The latter may be separated into three subgroups: those with a modified substituent of the lactone nucleus, such as roxithromycin, clarithromycin, dirithromycin, flurithromycin, and davercin (group II_A); those whose lactone nucleus has undergone modification, involving two subgroups, azalides (azithromycin) and oxolides (group II_{B1} and II_{B2}); and a third subgroup with a modification of the neutral sugar: ketolides and derivatives (group II_C) (Fig. 2).

Groups III and IV comprise, respectively, the 16-membered-ring natural molecules, such as josamycin, spiramycin, and midecamycin, and the molecules obtained by semisynthesis, such as miokamycin and rokitamycin.

3. ERYTHROMYCIN A

The introduction of sulfamidochrysoidine (Prontosil) and sulfachrysoidine (Rubiazol) into therapy in 1936 and the structural modifications of sulfonamides by Tréfouël's team from the Institut Pasteur in Paris, France, stimulated research into new anti-infective compounds. The presence of antibacterial substances produced by microorganisms had been known and used therapeutically since the end of the 19th century. The rediscovery of Alexander Fleming's work by Florey and Chain's team from the University of Oxford culminated in the use of penicillin F and subsequently penicillin G of American origin, and the studies by Dubos on thyrothricin caused a "broad wave" of isolation of compounds of natural origin. The discovery of streptomycin and neomycin by S. Waksman represented a new historical turning point, with the interest of the pharmaceutical industry then focusing on these new drugs. Two broad-spectrum antibiotics were very rapidly isolated, oxytetracycline (Pfizer) and chloromycetin (Parke-Davis).

The anti-infective arsenal of the end of the 1940s appeared to meet the requirements for gram-positive cocci (penicillin G) and gram-negative bacilli (*Salmonella*, *Shigella*, and *Vibrio cholerae*), with chloramphenicol, oxytetracycline,

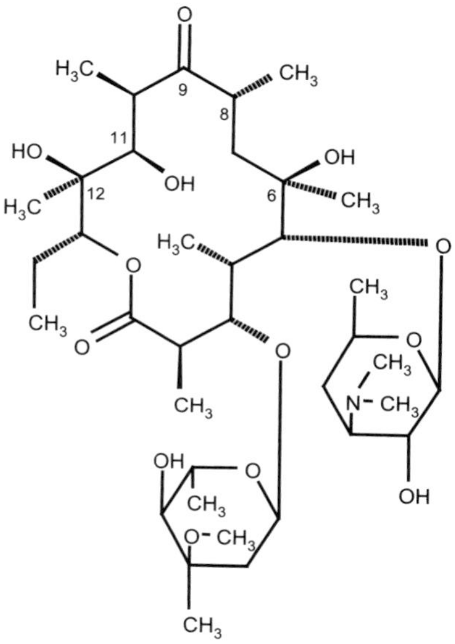

Figure 1 Erythromycin A

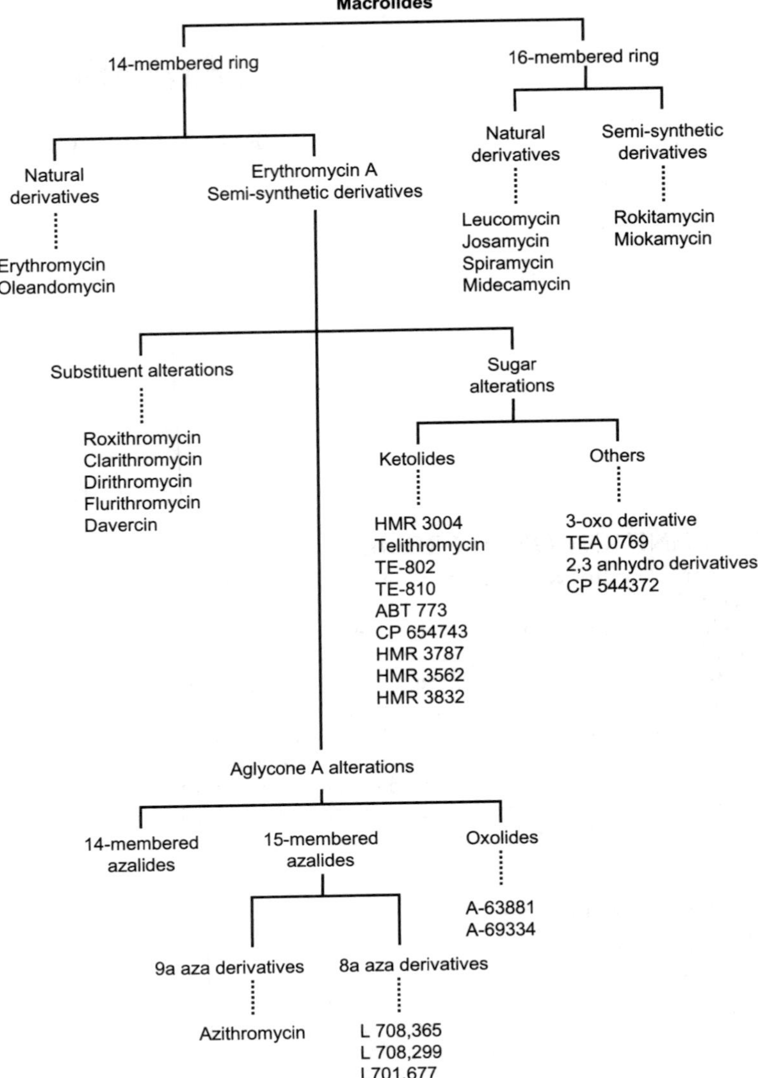

Figure 2 Classification of macrolides

and streptomycin; antituberculosis agents (streptomycin); and antirickettsial agents (chloramphenicol).

However, it rapidly became apparent that the bacterial world is complex, plastic, adaptive, and not homogeneous. Whereas initially low doses of antibiotics were sufficient to cure an infection, the bacteria rapidly became less receptive and new pathogenic agents emerged.

The introduction of benzylpenicillin, more stable than penicillin F and produced in larger quantities, allowed staphylococcal infections to be treated. However, the first therapeutic failures were reported at the beginning of the 1950s, and other drugs had to be found.

3.1. Discovery of Erythromycin and the Other Macrolides

Against this epidemiological background, which had taken the medical profession of the time by surprise, and in the euphoria created by the analyses of fermentation metabolites, a systematic search was performed to discover antistaphylococcal compounds.

Among these compounds, erythromycin was discovered by researchers at Eli Lilly in 1952.

This molecule lived up to expectation: it was active against penicillinase-producing strains of *Staphylococcus aureus*. This characteristic allowed it to be rapidly introduced into clinical practice in the United States.

During the same period, other macrolides were discovered from fermentation broths of microorganisms, such as oleandomycin, the leucomycin complex, tylosin, and the spiramycin complex (Table 1).

Table 1 Discoveries of macrolides

Drug	Organism	Yr
Erythromycin A	*Saccharopolyspora erythraea*	1952
Oleandomycin	*Streptomyces antibioticus*	1954
Spiramycin(s)	*Streptomyces ambofaciens*	1954
Josamycin	*Streptomyces narbonensis* subsp. *josamyceticus* sp. nov.	1957
Midecamycin	*Streptomyces mycarofaciens*	1971
Tylosin	*Streptomyces fradiae*	1961

3.2. Erythromycin A and Its Problems

Erythromycin produced in a fermentation broth is a molecular complex comprising at least six different components, A to F. Only erythromycin A has sufficient antibacterial activity to be used therapeutically.

Only a few companies are capable of extracting a compound with a high purity of erythromycin A content.

For various chemical reasons, erythromycin A, like penicillin G, is unstable in an acidic medium.

The chemical structure of erythromycin A causes it to degrade in an acidic medium. The two degradation products, the hemiketal and spiroketal derivatives of erythromycin A, are bacteriologically inactive, although the hemiketal derivative has the biological property of stimulating intestinal peristalsis. It is partly responsible for the gastrointestinal disorders attributable to erythromycin A.

Erythromycin A is the most active molecule among the natural derivatives, but it has the drawback of being bacteriostatic or slowly bactericidal.

Erythromycin A is insoluble in water, and a pediatric form is difficult to obtain because of its bitterness.

3.3. Erythromycin A: Pharmaceutical and Chemical Solutions

The various problems associated with erythromycin A fostered a search for answers.

In the 1950s and 1960s, the in vitro activity of erythromycin A against common pathogens was on the same order as that of the molecules available at that time. The problems involved preparing a solution for parenteral use, masking the bitterness, and improving acid stability.

Various salts of erythromycin A, such as erythromycin A glucoheptonate and lactobionate, which are still used therapeutically despite the poor venous tolerance of these products, were prepared in order to obtain a formulation for intravenous use.

The search for an intramuscular form resulted in the preparation of erythromycin A ester. An increase in the bioavailability of erythromycin A was then found.

Esterification of the hydroxyl group at position 2′ of the D-desosamine masked the bitterness of erythromycin. This type of approach was also adopted for oral chloramphenicol with a stoichiometric mixture with palmitic acid and repeated with erythromycin A with a stoichiometric mixture with a fatty acid. Erythromycin A stearate was selected.

Once the bitterness had been masked, either by esterification or by means of a mixture with a fatty acid, the idea was then conceived that, since erythromycin A is only partially degraded in an acidic medium, unlike penicillin G, it would be possible to preserve it either by means of pharmaceutical protection, such as a film coating of the tablet, or by manufacturing micropellets included in capsules (e.g., Eryc).

The hypothesis that esterification, a stoichiometric mixture with a fatty acid or a combination of the two active substances, would increase the stability and absorption of erythromycin A resulted in the production of numerous derivatives: erythromycin stearate, erythromycin 2′-ethyl succinate, erythromycin 2′-propionate, erythromycin estolate (combination of ethyl succinate and lauryl sulfate), erythromycin acistrate (2′-acetate and stearate), and RV-11 (2′-propionate mercaptosuccinate) (Fig. 3).

3.4. Failures and Disappointments with Erythromycin A Esters

The improvement of the assay techniques very rapidly showed that the pharmacokinetics of the 2′-esters and salts of erythromycin A were erratic (Table 2). In addition, gastrointestinal disorders were not controlled, particularly with erythromycin stearate.

New preparations of erythromycin have recently been proposed as a result of technological improvements in pharmaceutical formulation.

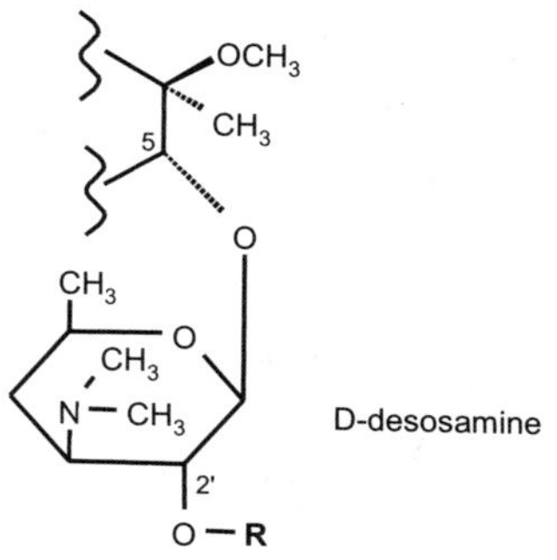

D-desosamine

2'-ester	R	Salt
Acistrate	$COCH_3$	$CH_3(CH_2)_{16}COOH$
Ethylsuccinate	C_2H_5-OOC-$(CH_2)_2$-COOH	-
Estolate	$OCCH_2CH_3$	$C_{12}H_{25}OSO_3H$
Propionate	$OCCH_2CH_3$	-
RV-11	$OCCH_2CH_3$	HS — CH - COOH H_2C — COOH

Figure 3 Erythromycin A 2′-esters

3.5. Limit of Erythromycin A Stearate

The mixture of erythromycin stearate is unstable in an acidic medium, as has been demonstrated by several teams. A pharmacokinetic study undertaken with the 250-mg tablet has clearly demonstrated that erythromycin A is degraded in an acidic medium to a hemiketal derivative, and similar proportions of erythromycin A and its degradation product have been detected in the sera of volunteers (Table 3).

In addition, the plasma pharmacokinetics vary according to the origin of the tablets. A 50% lower relative bioavailability than that of the reference drug has been found.

3.6. Limit of the 2′-Ester Derivatives

In order to be active, erythromycin A must be released very rapidly, and only the free form possesses antibacterial activity.

A study has shown that the rate of release of erythromycin A from its ester varies with the nature of the ester. The apparent half-life of release for a concentration in plasma of 5 μg/ml is longest for the 2′-propionate (247 min) and shortest for the 2′-ethyl succinate (60 min) (Table 4).

The second difficult point is the metabolism of the ester in some cases, particularly the ethyl succinate, which may not be totally "detached" from the 2′-hydroxyl group of the D-desosamine and may produce a bacteriologically inactive erythromycin A hemisuccinate.

3.7. Other Macrolides

Other 16-membered-ring macrolides, such as the spiramycin complex, have been introduced in clinical practice although principally in France, as have the derivatives of leucomycin (josamycin) in Japan and Europe. Midecamycin A_1 has also

Table 2 Plasma pharmacokinetics of erythromycin A

Erythromycin[a]	Dose (g)	C_{max} (μg/ml)	T_{max} (h)	AUC (μg·h/ml)	$t_{1/2}$ (h)
Base	0.25	1.3	3.4	1.6	1.6
	0.50	2	3.7	2	2
Stearate	0.25	0.9	2.2	3	1.6
	0.50	2.4	1.8	8.8	1.9
2′-Ethyl succinate	0.50	1.2	1.1	4.5	1.7
	1	3	1	9.1	1.7
Acistrate	0.4	2.2	2.6	12.3	3
E-base (pellets)	0.25	1.9	1.4	5.4	2
	0.50	3.8	1.4	13.2	2.5
	1	6.5	1.3	28.6	3
2′-Propionate	0.50	4.4	2	16.5	6.1
	1	5.6	1.5	31.9	4
Estolate	0.50	4.2	3.5		
	0.25	0.4	3.6	1.9	
12′-Propionate mercaptosuccinate	1	5.6	1.6	52.8	5.1

[a]Concentrations in erythromycin base.

Table 3 Plasma pharmacokinetics of erythromycin A stearate (250 mg orally)

Parameter	Erythromycin A	Anhydroerythromycin A
C_{max} (μg/ml)	0.9 ± 0.2	0.3 ± 0.1
T_{max} (h)	2.6 ± 0.4	2 ± 0
$t_{1/2}$ (h)	1.5 ± 0.1	3.3 ± 2.4
$AUC_{0-\infty}$ (μg·h/ml)	4.5 ± 1	4.1 ± 2.4

Table 4 Hydrolysis half-life of the 2′-esters of erythromycin A (37°C)

2′-Ester of erythromycin A	Half-life at concn (plasma)	
	100 μg/ml	5 μg/ml
2′-Propionyl	69	247
2′-Ethylsuccinyl	39	60
2′-Acetyl	39	170
2′-Butyryl	188	353
2′-Valeryl	492	478

been introduced in clinical practice in Japan and in some European countries.

Their in vitro activity is less than that of erythromycin A, and they are either extensively metabolized, as in the case of josamycin, or not, as with spiramycin. As the latter is a mixture of three components, a single compound has been developed in Japan, acetylspiramycin 1. These molecules are much more stable in an acidic medium.

A 14-membered-ring derivative possessing antibacterial activity similar to that of erythromycin A but stable in an acidic medium has been introduced in clinical practice, oleandomycin, in the form of oleandomycin triacetate, but unfortunately it has major adverse effects as a result of drug interactions (cytochrome P450) (Fig. 4).

3.8. Revival of the Macrolides

Erythromycin A was intended above all to provide a response to the emergence of penicillinase-producing strains of *S. aureus*. The discovery of vancomycin did not supplant the use of erythromycin because of its poor tolerance, but the semisynthesis of penicillin M (methicillin and oxacillin) and the first parenteral cephalosporins (cephalothin and cephaloridine) led to a decline in the use of erythromycin A, to their advantage.

Two circumstances were to cause a revival of interest in the macrolides: an improvement in microbiological techniques, providing a better understanding of the pathophysiology of certain infections, and the demonstration of the pathogenic potential of *Chlamydia trachomatis*.

In addition, the epidemic of Legionnaire's disease respiratory tract infections demonstrated the superiority of erythromycin A over the β-lactams. This activity is related to the fact that *Legionella pneumophila* is an intracellular pathogen and the fact that the β-lactams do not accumulate in phagocytic cells, in contrast to the macrolides, tetracyclines, fluoroquinolones, and ansamycins.

The interest devoted to these new microbiological entities and the discovery of their importance in the pathogenesis of community-acquired respiratory diseases caused a resurgence of research into the macrolides.

3.9. The Search for New Macrolides

The period of the revival of interest in the macrolide family occurred at a time of great ferment in anti-infective medicinal

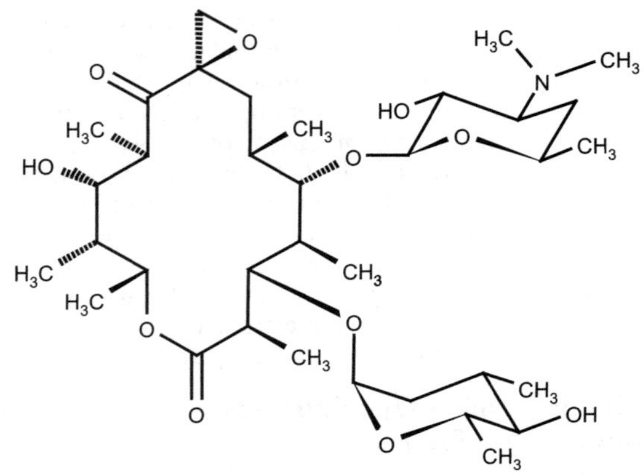

Figure 4 Oleandomycin

chemistry, with three major discoveries that were to totally transform the panorama of anti-infective chemotherapy: the discoveries of cefotaxime and its derivatives, the fluoroquinolones, and the carbapenems. This period also corresponds to the end of the great era of discoveries in terms of aminoglycosides.

Although a few attempts have been made to produce semisynthetic derivatives in the 16-membered-ring macrolide group with miokamycin (a derivative of midecamycin) and rokitamycin (a derivative of leucomycin A_5), the focus of efforts has been principally on the derivatives of erythromycin A.

Why erythromycin A? It is the most widespread molecule, it is the most active in terms of in vitro antibacterial activity, and it is a good substrate for chemical modifications.

A number of studies have shown that it is possible to modify the structure of erythronolide A without losing the antibacterial activity.

3.10. Modifications of Erythronolide A

The aims of the structural modifications of erythronolide A were to increase the acid stability of the molecule, to allow better oral bioavailability, to increase the activity against intracellular bacteria, and to increase the intraphagocytic concentration. No increase in activity against common pathogens was sought, nor was an increase in activity against bacterial strains resistant to erythromycin A, which were infrequent at the end of the 1970s and beginning of the 1980s, sought.

3.11. How To Increase Acid Stability

An understanding of the role of the weak point of erythronolide A, namely, the keto group at position 9, and the two anchor points, i.e., the hydroxyl groups at position 6 and 12, in the inactivation process enabled molecules to be prepared in which these sites were blocked. The presumption of the possibility of increasing the stability in an acidic medium was enhanced by the stability at a low pH of oleandomycin and erythromycin B, which have no hydroxyl groups at C-12.

Schematically, three pathways were to be used: blockade of the weak point at position 9, noncleavable esterification of the hydroxyl at C-6 (clarithromycin) or attachment of a carbonate or carbamate residue at C-11 and C-12 (davercin), or an attempt to increase the electronic stability of the 9-keto group by isosteric replacement of the hydrogen at C-8 by a fluorine atom (flurithromycin) (Fig. 5).

The attachment of an oxime group at position 9 gave rise to a synthetic intermediate which when alkylated yielded roxithromycin, when reduced yielded erythromycylamine (and subsequently dirithromycin), and when subjected to a chemical reaction allowing the endocyclic inclusion of the nitrogen atom, yielded azithromycin (Fig. 6).

3.12. Characteristics of the New Molecules

The aim pursued was an increase in the acid stability of the macrolides. This was fully achieved with roxithromycin and azithromycin. The degradation product that can be obtained after a long period of contact at very acidic pH is a molecule without an L-cladinose and one which is bacteriologically inactive. It has a hydroxyl group at position 3. Clarithromycin is slightly less stable, as the hydroxyl group at position 12 may react with the 9-keto group to yield an inactive derivative, pseudoclarithromycin.

The second characteristic is the pharmacokinetic profile. The molecules are divided into two categories, those with

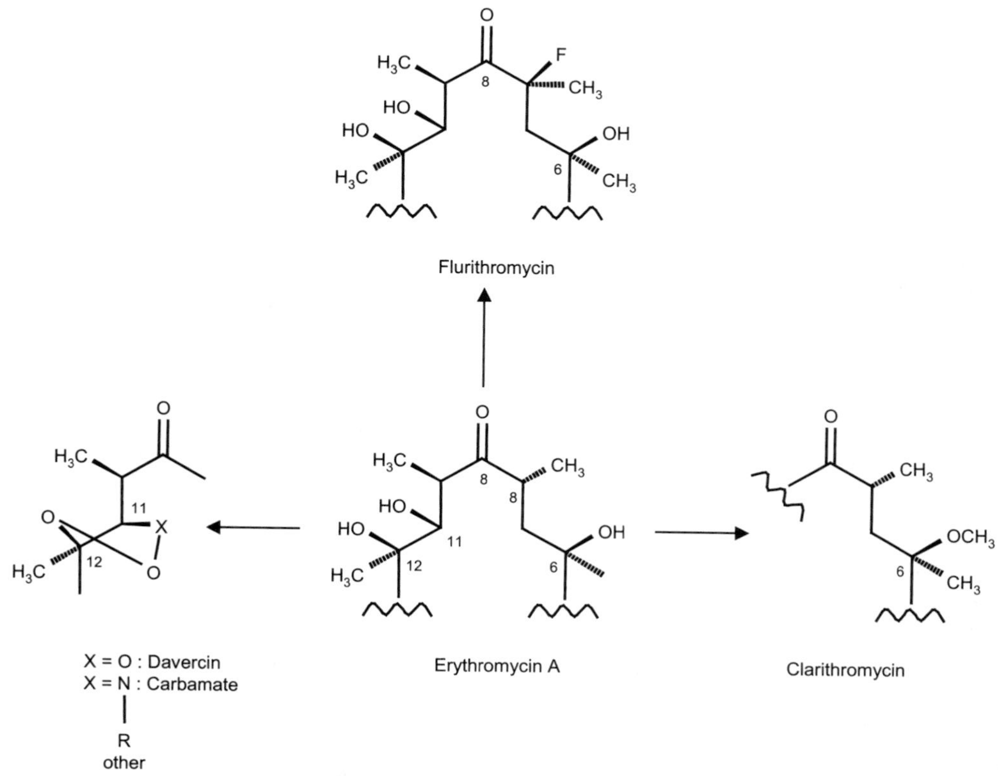

Figure 5 Modification of the substituent at position 8

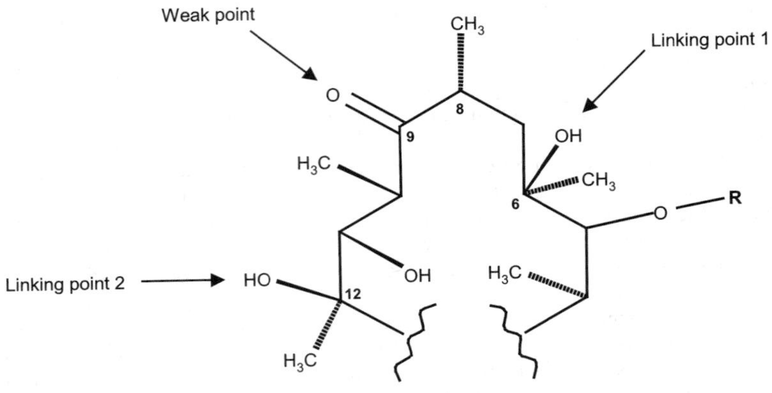

Figure 6 Sites of modification of erythromycin A

extensive plasma pharmacokinetics (roxithromycin and clarithromycin) and those in which cellular pharmacokinetics are predominant, such as azithromycin and dirithromycin, a phenomenon related to the greater basicity of these molecules. This difference in pharmacokinetics is also associated with different pharmacodynamics; the activity of molecules in the first group is said to be time dependent, while that of the second group is concentration dependent. The first group includes erythromycin, roxithromycin, and clarithromycin, and the second group is composed of azithromycin.

In terms of antibacterial activity, the different molecules are very similar to erythromycin A, with which they share the mechanisms of resistance, whether of the macrolide-lincosamide-streptogramin B (MLS_B) type, by efflux (*Streptococcus pneumoniae* and *Streptococcus pyogenes*), by enzymatic inactivation (2′-phosphotransferase), or by hydrolysis of the aglycone by an esterase (detected mainly in *Escherichia coli*).

In terms of activity against atypical and intracellular bacteria, these new molecules are more active in vitro and in vivo than erythromycin A and accumulate to a much greater extent in phagocytic cells.

3.13. Contributions of the New Macrolides

In therapeutic terms, the new molecules provide access to infections due not only to common pathogens but also, above all, to intracellular and atypical bacteria. Some of them are part of the treatment of specific infections, such as those due to *Helicobacter pylori*, *Mycobacterium avium*, and *Mycobacterium leprae*.

3.14. The Search Continues

Erythromycin A has been one of the responses to the therapeutic requirements of staphylococcal infections due to penicillinase-producing strains. By virtue of their physicochemical, pharmacokinetic, and bacteriological properties, roxithromycin and the other derivatives have been incorporated in the therapeutic arsenal against respiratory tract infections and have been the pivotal medications for certain infectious entities.

The resurgence of diphtheria and the noneradication of whooping cough have made them the antibiotics of first choice.

However, the emergence of strains resistant not only to erythromycin A (such as *S. pyogenes*) but also to penicillin G (*S. pneumoniae*) among the bacteria responsible for respiratory tract infections has necessitated a renewal of our portfolio of antibacterial agents and the discovery of new derivatives that do not exhibit total cross-resistance with erythromycin A. One of the responses to this medical need in this medicinal chemical class is the ketolides (see chapter 19).

4. STRUCTURE-ACTIVITY RELATIONSHIPS

4.1. Chemical Modifications of Erythromycin A

The first studies involving erythromycin A as a substrate were directed towards increasing its acid stability, eliminating its bitterness, and improving its solubility in an aqueous medium.

The conformational study of the erythromycins revealed the importance of the spatial orientation of the hydrophilic groups (carbonyl-lactone, carbonyl-ketone, and hydroxyls at C-6 and C-11) and the hydrophobic groups (methyl groups at C-4, C-8, and C-12 and the ethyl chain at C-13) of the aglycone and the D-desosamine, which play an important role in the attachment to ribosomal nucleotides via the hydroxyl at C-2′ and the dimethylamine group at C-3′. This bonding occurs via hydrogen bonds between the hydrogen and the nitrogen of the nucleotide bases and erythromycin.

Further hydrogen bonds are formed between the ribosomal nucleotides and the hydroxyl groups at C-11 and C-12, the carbonyl at position 9, the methoxy group at position 3″, and probably the hydroxyl at C-6.

4.1.1. Modifications of the Aglycone

Erythromycin A rapidly loses its antibacterial activity in an acidic medium because of its degradation. The degradation products are bacteriologically inactive and bind only weakly to ribosomes.

The introduction of a double bond or an epoxy group into erythromycin A reduces the antibacterial activity. The introduction of a nitrogen atom at position 10 yields a 14-membered-ring N-10 azalide.

Enlarging the aglycone is another route of modification. Two examples of this are the 15-membered-ring azalides (azithromycin) with the introduction of a nitrogen atom at position 8a or 9a and 9,12-epoxy erythromycin A (A-69334) (oxolide). These derivatives are more stable in an acidic medium, and some of them also possess activity against gram-negative bacilli.

4.1.2. Modifications and Substituents of the Aglycone

Substituents of the aglycone may be modified; the various derivatives are more stable in an acidic medium and have better gastrointestinal absorption or increased antibacterial activity.

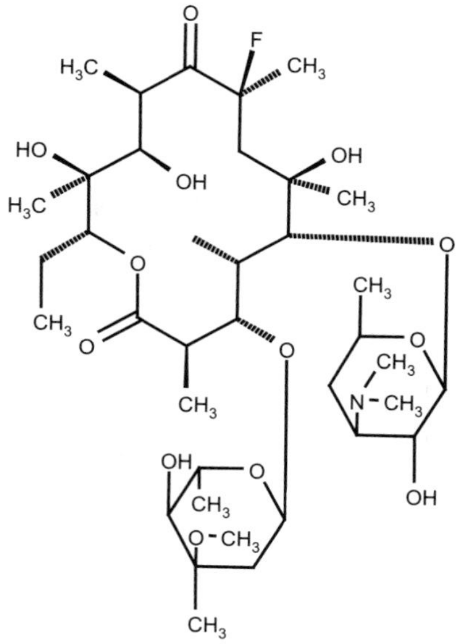

Figure 7 Flurithromycin

4.1.2.1. Modifications at Position 6

The hydroxyl at position 6 is the anchor point of the enolether between the 9-keto and the hydroxyl at position 6. Blockade of the hydroxyl group at position 6 by a noncleavable ester has yielded 6-*O*-methylerythromycin A or clarithromycin. This molecule is more active than erythromycin A and more stable in an acidic medium. However, because of the nonblockade of the hydroxyl at position 12 and of the 9-keto, this product is degraded in an acidic medium and yields pseudoclarithromycin.

4.1.2.2. Modifications at Position 8

The spatial position of the methyl group at position 8 has a major influence on the antibacterial activity. Replacement of the hydrogen at position 8 by a fluorine atom, which is isosteric (flurithromycin), indirectly increases the acid stability. In vitro, flurithromycin is less active than erythromycin A, but in vivo it is two to four times more active (Fig. 7).

4.1.2.3. Modifications at Position 9

A number of chemical modifications have been proposed to prevent the inactivation of the erythronolide A nucleus, including blockade of the 9-keto group. Three series of derivatives have been prepared: 9(S)-erythromycylamine, the ether-oxime derivatives, and the 15-membered-ring azalides.

9(S)-Erythromycylamine has antibacterial activity similar to that of erythromycin A, but it is poorly absorbed. The introduction of a 9-*N*-1-oxazine chain has yielded a prodrug, dirithromycin (Fig. 8).

Five ether-oxime series have been prepared. Among these 80 molecules, roxithromycin was selected for its pharmacokinetic, microbiological, and toxicological profiles. It is stable in an acidic medium and has excellent oral bioavailability, on the order of 50% of the administered dose, and an apparent elimination half-life on the order of 12 h (Fig. 9).

4.1.2.4. Modifications at Position 11,12

Erythromycin A is twice as active as erythromycin B. It differs from the latter by the absence of a hydroxyl group at position 12. A number of derivatives with an 11,12-carbonate have been synthesized and are twice as active as erythromycin A.

4.1.3. Modifications of the D-Desosamine

Numerous modifications of the D-desosamine have been proposed, but all entail a reduction in antibacterial activity. This is an essential group for the antibacterial activity of erythromycin A; its absence abolishes any antibacterial activity.

The hydroxyl group at position 2′ of the D-desosamine is the support for the cleavable esters of erythromycin A.

The presence of a hydroxyl at 4′ reduces the antibacterial activity. The hypothesis has been postulated that the slightest modification of the spatial orientation of the D-desosamine or the dimethylamine group prevents proper binding to the ribosome.

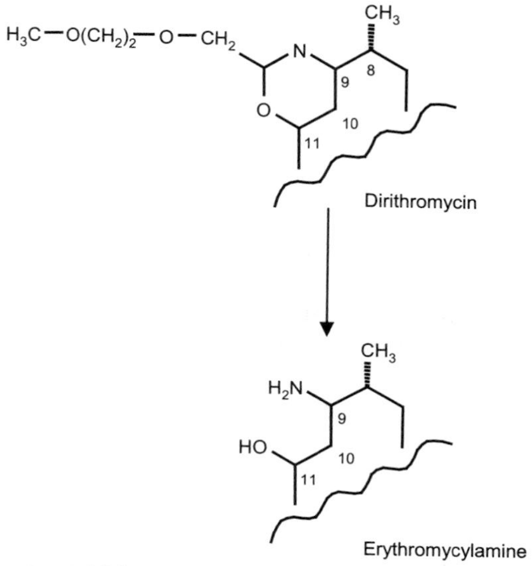

Figure 8 Dirithromycin

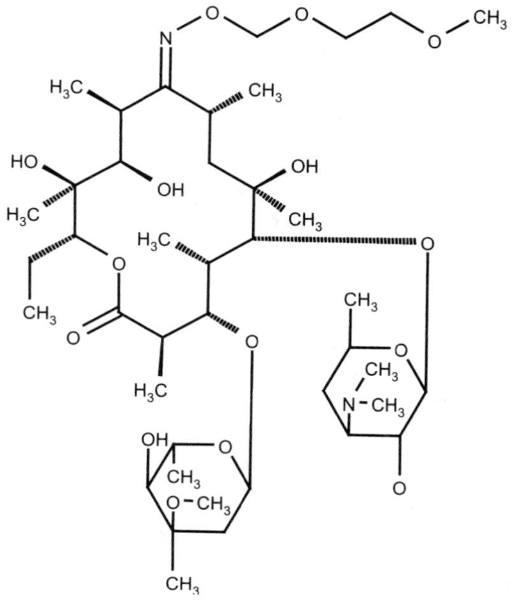

Figure 9 Roxithromycin

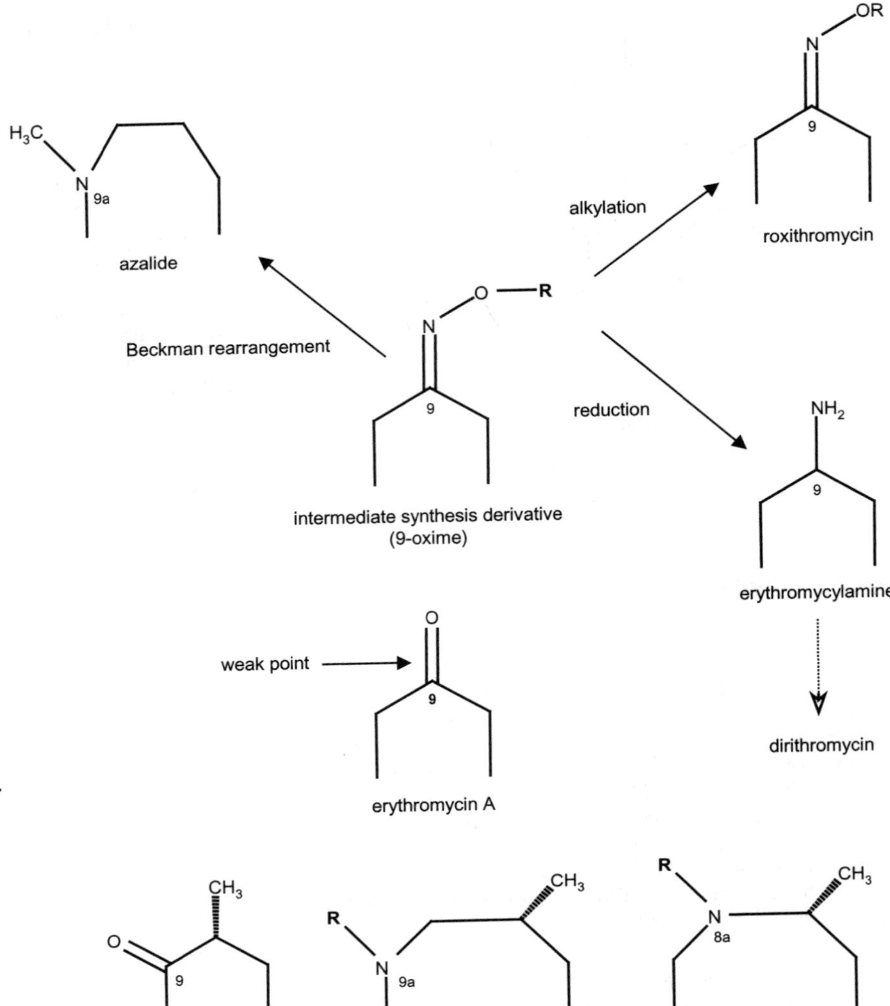

Figure 10 Chemical modifications of 9-*N*-oxime erythromycin A

Figure 11 8a- and 9a-azalides

4.1.4. Modifications of the L-Cladinose

The antibacterial activity of erythromycin C, which differs from erythromycin A by the presence of a hydroxyl group at 3″ instead of a methoxy, is a third of that of erythromycin A, and at the same time its binding to the ribosome is reduced.

The absence of the L-cladinose does not prevent antibacterial activity, as has been demonstrated with the ketolides. The important factor is the reduction of the hydroxyl group at position 3 of erythronolide A.

4.2. Azalides

The azalides are obtained from a synthetic intermediate, erythromycin A 9-oxime, by a Beckman reaction (Fig. 10). Two categories have been described, the 14- and 15-membered-ring azalides.

4.2.1. 15-Membered-Ring Azalides

The 15-membered-ring azalides can be subdivided into two subgroups according to the position of the endocyclic nitrogen in the lactone nucleus: 9a- and 8a-azalides (Fig. 11).

The first molecule used therapeutically was azithromycin, which is characterized by a nitrogen atom substituted by a methyl group at position 9a (Fig. 12). A molecule for veterinary use, tulathromycin, was recently introduced in clinical veterinary practice.

Numerous derivatives of azithromycin have been synthesized. A characteristic of azithromycin and its derivatives is that they have good activity against certain gram-negative

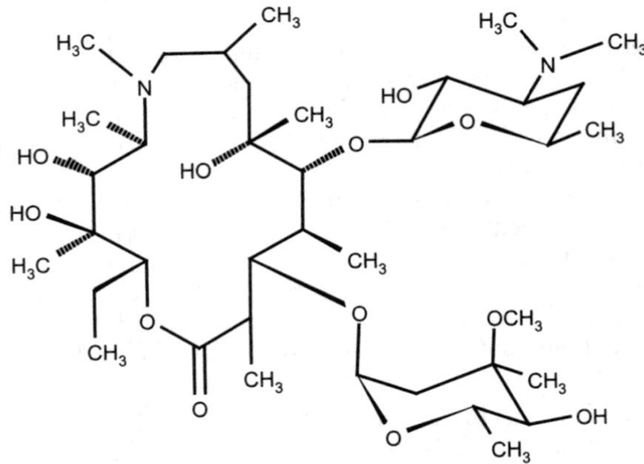

Figure 12 Azithromycin

Table 5 In vitro activities of azalides against *E. coli*

Drug	MIC (μg/ml) for *E. coli*
Azithromycin	0.78
6-*O*-Methylazithromycin	3.1
11-*O*-Methylazithromycin	0.78
6,11-Di-*O*-methylazithromycin	6.25
6,11,4″-2-Tri-*O*-methylazithromycin	6.25

bacilli, but to the detriment of activity against gram-positive cocci (Table 5).

A series of derivatives possessing an endocyclic nitrogen atom at position 8a has been synthesized (Fig. 13). A number of 8a-azalide derivatives have in vitro activity comparable to that of azithromycin.

Figure 13 8a-Aza-8a-homeoerythromycin

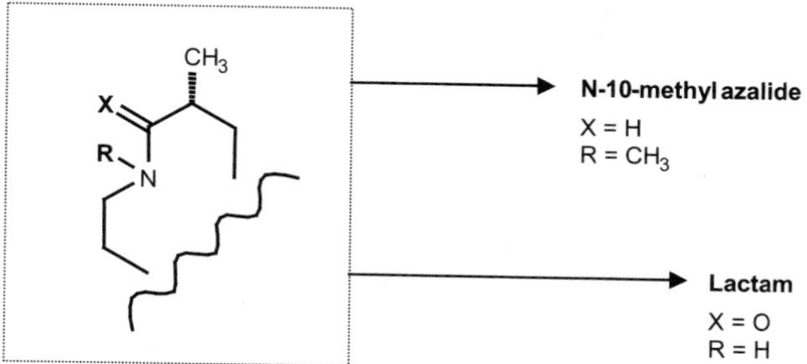

Figure 14 14-Membered-ring azalides

4.2.2. 14-Membered-Ring Azalides

A series of 14-membered-ring azalides has been described. The 10-aza derivative (Fig. 14) is half as active as azithromycin against gram-positive bacilli and four times less active against gram-negative bacilli (Table 6).

5. PHYSICOCHEMICAL PROPERTIES

5.1. Principal Properties

The principal physicochemical properties of the macrolides are presented in Table 7.

5.2. Stability Acidic Medium

Erythromycin A and, to a lesser extent, spiramycin and josamycin are unstable in an acidic medium.

Erythromycin A is degraded by the formation of a hemiketal or a spiroketal form of erythronolide A (Fig. 15).

Josamycin (leucomycin A_3) may be converted in an acidic medium to isojosamycin, which has a hydroxyl group at C-13 because of the rearrangement of the dienole system of josamycin.

Spiramycin is a complex formed by three major components (I to III), which differ in the substituent at position 3 of the lactone nucleus: 3-OH (spiramycin I), 3-*O*-acetyl (spiramycin II), and 3-*O*-propionyl (spiramycin III) (Fig. 16).

The spiramycins are much more stable than erythromycin A in an acidic medium. Rupture of the L-mycarose occurs under very acidic conditions, and the neospiramycins, which are the desmycarosyl derivatives, are more active in vitro than the parent molecule but are inactive in vivo.

The macrolides of group II_A, comprising roxithromycin and clarithromycin, and group II_{B1} are much more stable in an acidic medium than erythromycin A.

Roxithromycin is highly stable at pH 4.2 compared to erythromycin base and erythromycin 2′-propionate. After

Table 7 Physicochemical properties of macrolides

Drug	pK	Mol wt
Erythromycin A	8.6	733.94
Oleandomycin	8.5	687.89
Clarithromycin	8.3	747.96
Roxithromycin	9.2	837.04
Dirithromycin	9.2	835
Erythromycylamine	8.9	734
Flurithromycin		751.95
Azithromycin	8.9–9.1	748.9
Josamycin	7.1	828.02
Midecamycin	6.9	813.99
Spiramycin I	7.7	843.06
Miokamycin	6.5	898.05
Rokitamycin	6.3	828

Table 6 In vitro activities of the 14-membered azalides

Drug	MIC (μg/ml)			
	S. aureus	*S. pyogenes*	*H. influenzae*	*E. coli*
Erythromycin A	0.25	0.015	2	32
Azithromycin	0.5–1	0.03	0.25–1	1–2
10-*N*-Methylazalide	2–4	0.125	2–8	4–8
10-*N*-Azalidelactam	>128	>128	>128	>128
10-*N*-Methyl-4″-aminoazalide	4	0.125	1	4

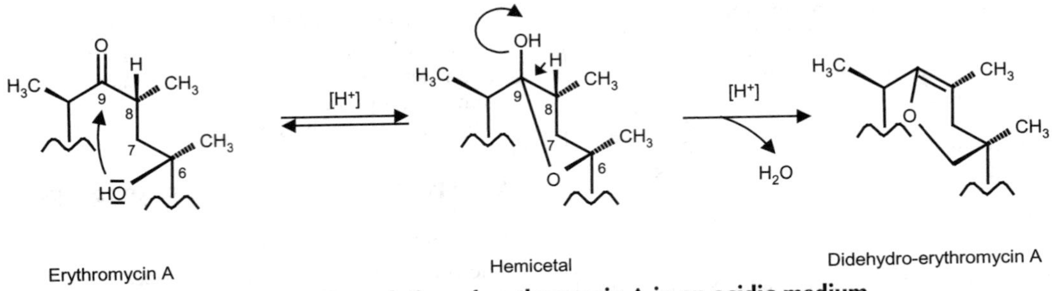

Erythromycin A

Hemicetal

Didehydro-erythromycin A

Figure 15 Degradation of erythromycin A in an acidic medium

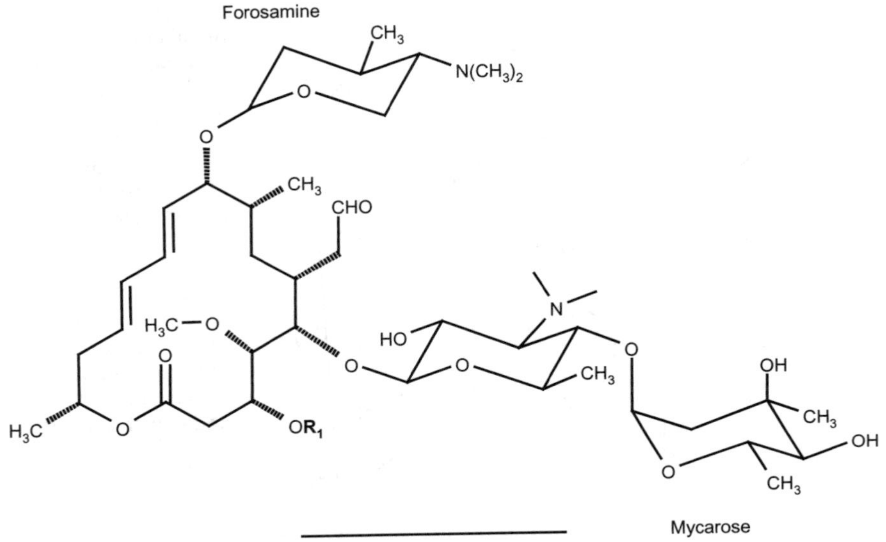

Forosamine

Mycarose

	R_1
Spiramycin I	-H
Spiramycin II	$-COCH_3$
Spiramycin III	$-COCH_2CH_3$

Figure 16 Spiramycins

1 h of contact, more than 90% of the activity still remains. At pH 1.2, erythromycin A is inactivated within 10 min, while 30% of the activity of roxithromycin remains (Fig. 17).

Clarithromycin is 6-O-methylerythromycin A (Fig. 18), and for this reason one of the anchor points, the hydroxyl at position 11, remains free. A degradation product that is bacteriologically inactive occurs under conditions of extreme acidity: pseudoclarithromycin (Fig. 19).

After a sufficiently long contact time and under highly acidic conditions (pH ~1.2), a bacteriologically inactive degradation product is formed, but one which is very stable in an acidic medium as a result of the detachment of the L-cladinose attached at position 3 of the aglycone nucleus (Fig. 20).

6. INTRACELLULAR ACCUMULATION OF MACROLIDES

The macrolides penetrate phagocytic cells, thereby allowing the treatment of infections due to intracellular bacteria, such as *Chlamydia* spp. and *Legionella* spp.

The macrolides may be divided into two groups (Table 8).

The mean ratios of cell concentrations to those present in the extracellular medium are presented in Table 9.

The concentration in other cells, such as epithelial cells, is rarely studied.

7. IN VITRO ACTIVITY OF MACROLIDES

7.1. Natural Antibacterial Spectrum

The natural antibacterial spectrum of the macrolides, irrespective of their structure, includes gram-positive bacteria; gram-negative cocci; fastidious gram-negative bacilli, such as *Haemophilus influenzae, Moraxella catarrhalis, Pasteurella* spp., and *Bordetella* spp.; anaerobic bacteria; intracellular bacteria; mycoplasmas and related species; spirochetes; bacteria responsible for gastrointestinal infections (*V. cholerae* and other *Vibrio* spp. and *Campylobacter* spp.); and *H. pylori*.

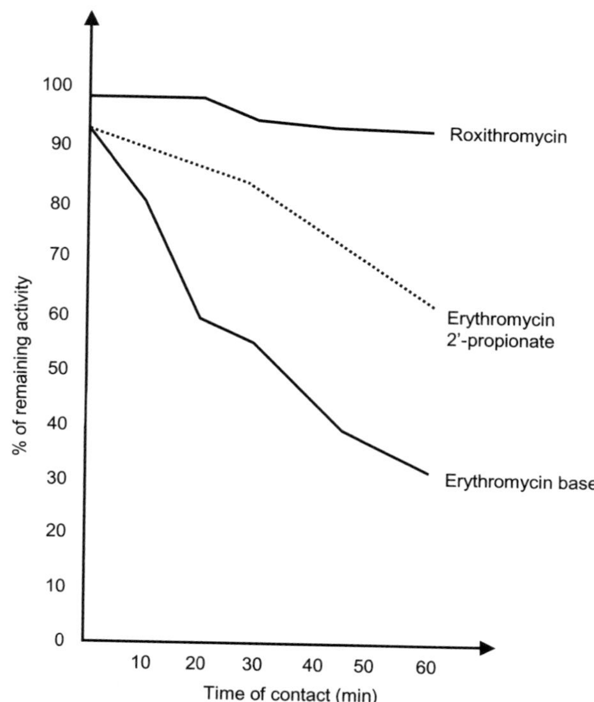

Figure 17 Stability of roxithromycin at pH 4.2

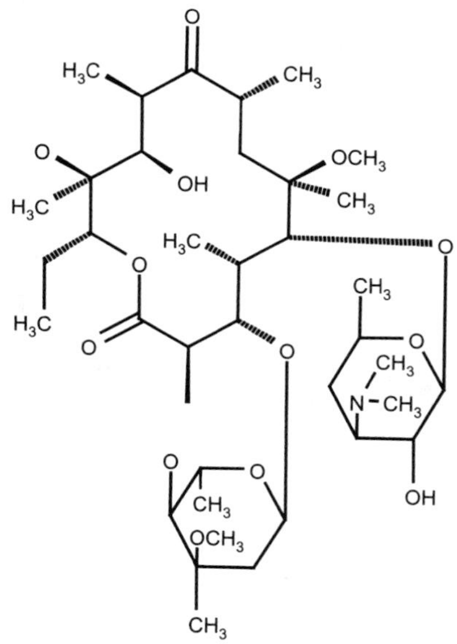

Figure 18 Clarithromycin

Clarithromycin

[H^+] (translactonization)

Pseudoclarithromycin

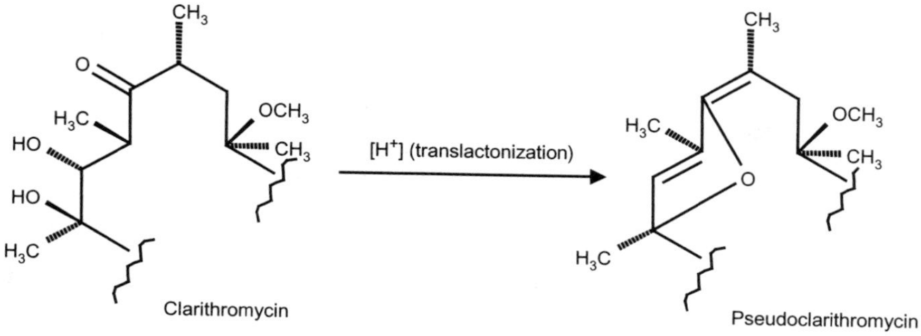

Figure 19 Pseudoclarithromycin

7.2. Activity of Natural Macrolides against Common Pathogens

Erythromycin A is the reference macrolide among the macrolides of natural origin, such as oleandomycin, josamycin, spiramycin, and midecamycin. It is 10 times more active than oleandomycin, 2 to 10 times more active than josamycin, 2 to 12 times more active than spiramycin, and up to 10 times more active than midecamycin (Table 10).

Spiramycin is the least active molecule, relative to josamycin and erythromycin A. Its activity is similar to that of oleandomycin.

7.3. In Vitro Activity of Group II_A and II_{B1} Macrolides against Common Pathogens

The macrolides have the same antibacterial spectrum as erythromycin A.

Azithromycin, which is a more basic molecule, has better in vitro activity against gram-negative bacilli.

7.3.1. Gram-Positive Cocci

Erythromycin A overall is less active than clarithromycin but more active than azithromycin, roxithromycin, and dirithromycin (Table 11). These molecules are weakly active against enterococci (*Enterococcus faecalis* and *Enterococcus faecium*) and have moderate activity against viridans group streptococci.

7.3.2. Gram-Positive Bacilli

Group II_A and II_{B1} macrolides have good activity against *Corynebacterium diphtheriae* and remain the reference molecules against this bacterial species. Erythromycin A-resistant strains have been described. The molecules have not insignificant activity against the group of lactic bacilli (*Lactobacillus* spp., *Pediococcus* spp., and *Leuconostoc* spp.). Conversely, they are inactive against *Corynebacterium jeikeium*, *Corynebacterium urealyticum*, and *Nocardia* spp. The least active molecule is azithromycin. There are no data on the activity of dirithromycin against many of these bacterial species (Table 12).

7.3.3. Gram-Negative Bacteria

The activity is moderate against *Neisseria gonorrhoeae* and *Pasteurella multocida*. However, it is good against *Bordetella pertussis*. The macrolides are the reference treatment for whooping cough. Some erythromycin A-resistant strains have been described. The activity against *H. influenzae* is disputed because of the difficulties of determining the MIC, the most active molecule being azithromycin, which is effective against some gram-negative bacteria.

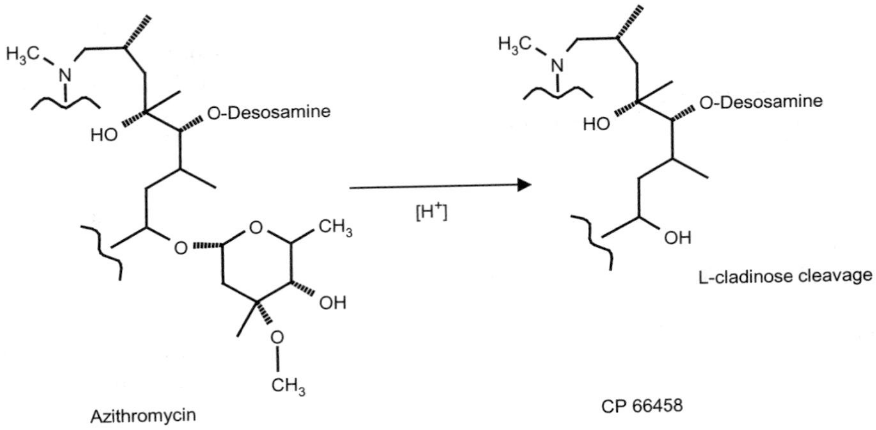

Figure 20 Azithromycin: degradation in an acidic medium

Table 8 Classification of macrolides according to their intracellular properties

Group	Drug	Properties
I	Azithromycin Dirithromycin Erythromycylamine	Bibasic compound Nonsaturable accumulation Intragranular site; $\Delta G > 100$ kJ/mol; slight efflux
II	Erythromycin A Roxithromycin	Monobasic compound Quick accumulation and plateau
	Clarithromycin	Granular and cytoplasmic location; $\Delta G = 60–70$ kJ/mol; quick efflux

The activities against bacteria responsible for gastrointestinal diseases, such as *Campylobacter jejuni* and *V. cholerae*, appear to be moderate, but a high concentration in the lumen of the digestive tract eradicates these bacteria. Activity against *H. pylori* is good, and clinical studies with clarithromycin (MIC at which 50% of isolates tested are inhibited [MIC_{50}], 0.015 μg/ml) have demonstrated good activity (Table 13).

The activity of the macrolides against *H. pylori* varies with the pH of the medium. As a general rule, as with the other bacterial species, the in vitro activity decreases in an acidic medium (Table 14).

The incidence of clarithromycin-resistant strains of *H. pylori* varies from country to country, ranging from 3% (Germany) to 16% (Poland) (Table 15).

In the industrial countries, the macrolides continue to be the drugs of first choice in the treatment of diarrhea due to *C. jejuni* because the incidence of macrolide-resistant strains is low (2 to 5%) and is remaining stable, in contrast to the fluoroquinolones. The macrolides are active against fluoroquinolone-resistant strains of *C. jejuni*. Azithromycin is the most active molecule (MIC_{50} and MIC_{90}, 0.6 and 0.12 μg/ml), and midecamycin is the least active (MIC_{50} and MIC_{90}, 2.0 and 4.0 μg/ml) (Table 16).

7.3.4. Anaerobic Bacteria

The activity of erythromycin A against anaerobic gram-negative bacilli is weak, in contrast to that of the other macrolides (Table 17). Conversely, its activity against gram-positive anaerobic bacteria is good. The results, however, are difficult to interpret, as the presence of an incubation atmosphere containing 6% CO_2 increases the MICs.

7.3.5. Intracellular and Atypical Bacteria

Erythromycin A was the source of the initial therapeutic successes against *L. pneumophila* pneumonia. However, the semisynthetic macrolides of groups II_A and II_B are more active. They are very active against *C. trachomatis*, an agent responsible for nongonococcal urethritis and trachoma; conversely, their activity, while still good, is weaker against *Chlamydia (Chlamydophila) pneumoniae*. They are very active against *Mycoplasma pneumoniae* and *Ureaplasma urealyticum*. They are inactive against *Mycoplasma hominis*, which is responsible for pelvic inflammatory disease in women (Table 18).

Chlamydia psittaci is responsible for pneumonia of avian origin. The activities of the different macrolides tested are summarized in Table 19.

The activity against *M. avium* is difficult to interpret, and the results vary according to the author. Good in vivo activity in the beige mouse and therapeutically has been demonstrated with the semisynthetic macrolides.

They also exhibit a certain activity against *M. leprae* in the mouse footpad model, and the combination clarithromycin-minocycline has been tested successfully in the treatment of lepromatous leprosy.

In the current state of knowledge, it is impossible to obtain *M. leprae* from a culture on agar media or in broth. Its growth is obtained by using the mouse footpad model or from certain in vitro metabolic inhibition systems demonstrating therapeutic activity of a compound.

In an in vitro model of reduction of the oxidation of [^{14}C]palmitic acid, erythromycin A (concentration, ≥2 μg/ml), and M-119-31 caused a reduction in oxidation. Roxithromycin is more active. Azithromycin is the least active in this model, while clarithromycin causes a reduction at a concentration of 0.125 μg/ml. Comparable results have been obtained by measuring the concentration of bacillary ATP after incubation for 3 weeks in the presence of antibiotics.

In vivo, in control BALB/c mice, bacterial growth plateaus 3 to 4 months after inoculation. In mice treated with erythromycin A, growth is comparable to that obtained

Table 9 Accumulation ratios (cellular/extracellular) of the main macrolides (in vitro)[a]

Macrolide	Cells	Cellular/extracellular ratio (time)	Method
Erythromycin A	PN 1 (h)	4.4–18 (30 min)	RA
		1–10 (30 min)	B
	MP alveolar (H)	18–38 (46)[b] (30 min)	RA
	MP (H)	1.5–7 (24 h)	RA
	Mo (H)	4.2	
	Fibroblasts (H)	25 (1 h)–97 (72 h)	
	M4	4 (15 min)	RA
	MP (cell line S)	3.6–6 (24 h)	RA
	Hepatocytes (R)	11 (60 min)	RA
	McCoy, HEp-2	4–5 (20 min)	RA
Roxithromycin	PN (H)	14–100 (30–60 min)	RA
	MP alveolar (H)	61 (190)[b]–2 (30 min)	RA
	MP (H)	2–6 (24 h)	RA
		25 (15 min)	RA
	Hepatocytes (R)	19–31 (60 min)	RA
Clarithromycin	PN (H)	9–16–100 (30 min)	RA
Dirithromycin	PN (H)	7 (15 min)–36 (120 min)	RA
	PN (H)	5 (5 min)–20 (120 min)	RA
	PN (H)	60 (30 min)–140 (120 min)	RA
		3–5 (180 min)	B
		15–60 (5 min)–128–300 (120 min)	HPLC
	Mo (H)	200 (40 min)	RA
		5–6 (180 min)	B
	MP alveolar (H)	668 (40 min)	RA
		300 (120 min)	HPLC
	Fibroblasts (H)	174 (60 min)–3738 (72 h)	RA
	MP peritoneal(s)	20 (60 min)–100 (24 h)	RA
	MP (cell line S)	38–99 (24 h)	RA
	J774	10 (5 min)–41.5 (24 h)	RA
	NRK Cells	40 (10 min)–312 (24 h)	RA
	Fibroblasts	19 (5 min)–93 (24 h)	RA
Spiramycin	MP alveolar (H)	20–35 (120 min)	HPLC
	MP (guinea pig)	25 (120 min)	HPLC
Josamycin	PN (H)	16 (15 min)–21 (45 min)	RA
	MP (rabbit)	40 (15 min)	RA
Rokitamycin	PN (H)	30 (15 min)	RA
	MP alveolar (H)	120 (30 min)	RA

[a]PN, neutrophils; MP, macrophages; MO, monocytes; H, human; S, mice; R, rats; RA, radiolabelling; B, microbiology; HPLC, high-performance liquid chromatography.
[b]Cells from smoking subjects (data from Labro, 1997).

Table 10 In vitro activities of natural macrolides against common pathogens

Organism	MIC (μg/ml)[a]				
	ERY A	OLEA	JOSA	SPIR	MID
S. aureus 209 P-JC	0.1	0.78	0.2	0.78	0.1
S. epidermidis spal 1	0.1	0.78	0.39	0.78	0.78
S. pyogenes NY-5	0.012	0.2	0.05	0.39	0.1
S. agalactiae 1020	0.025	0.39	0.2	0.2	0.39
E. faecalis 1501	0.39	3.13	1.56	0.78	1.56
C. diphtheriae PW8	≤0.006	0.05	0.05	0.1	0.05
Bacillus subtilis ATCC 6683	0.5	0.78	0.2	0.78	0.2

[a]ERY A, erythromycin A; OLEA, oleandomycin; JOSA, josamycin; MID, midecamycin.

in untreated mice. Of mice treated with roxithromycin, four of six were positive in the fourth month postinoculation and all were positive in the fifth month postinoculation.

It was not possible to detect *M. leprae* in mice administered clarithromycin (minimum level of 1.6×10^4 CFU/g), even 5 months postinoculation.

The activity against *Rickettsia* or related species is more difficult to interpret. The macrolides have good activity (Table 20).

The macrolides possess good activity against *Bartonella* spp. (Table 21).

7.3.6. Spirochetes

Roxithromycin and azithromycin are very effective in experimental infection in the rabbit with *Treponema pallidum* strain Nichols, whereas these molecules have cross-resistance

Table 11 In vitro activities of group II_A and group II_B macrolides against gram-positive cocci

Organism(s)	MIC$_{50}$ (μg/ml)[a]					
	ERY A	CLA	AZI	ROX	DIR	MIO
S. aureus Met^{s} Ery^{s}	0.25	0.25	1	0.5	0.5	1
S. epidermidis Met^{s} Ery^{s}	0.25	0.12	0.5	0.5	0.25	0.1
S. pyogenes (group A)	0.06	0.015	0.06	0.12	0.12	0.1
S. agalactiae (group B)	0.06	0.015	0.06	0.12	0.25	0.5
Streptococcus (groups C and G)	0.06	0.03	0.12	0.12	0.12	0.2
S. pneumoniae Pen^{s}	0.06	0.015	0.06	0.06	0.12	0.06
S. pneumoniae Pen^{i}	0.12	0.015	0.06	0.06	0.12	0.2
S. pneumoniae Pen^{r}	0.12	0.015	0.06	0.06	0.25	0.2
E. faecalis	4	4	8	8	16	2
E. faecium	>64	>64	>64	>64	>64	8
Viridans group streptococci	2	1	4	4		0.1

[a]ERY A, erythromycin A; CLA, clarithromycin; AZI, azithromycin; ROX, roxithromycin; DIR, dirithromycin; MIO, miokamycin.

Table 12 In vitro activities of group II_A and group II_B macrolides against gram-positive bacilli

Organism(s)	MIC$_{50}$ (μg/ml)[a]					
	ERY A	CLA	AZI	ROX	DIR	MIO
Listeria monocytogenes	0.25	0.06	0.5	0.25	2	1
Erysipelothrix rhusiopathiae	0.25	0.12		0.5		
C. diphtheriae	0.008	0.004	0.015	0.008	0.015	
Nocardia spp.	16	16	≥128	64		4
Pediococcus spp.	0.125	0.06	0.125	0.06		
Lactobacillus spp.	0.06	0.015	0.06	0.06		
Leuconostoc spp.	0.06	0.03	0.125	0.125		
C. jeikeium	>128	>128	>128	>128	>128	>32
C. urealyticum	>64	>64	>64	>64	>64	>128
G. vaginalis	0.06	0.008	0.06	0.03		0.01

[a]ERY A, erythromycin A; CLA, clarithromycin; AZI, azithromycin; ROX, roxithromycin; DIR, dirithromycin; MIO, miokamycin.

Table 13 In vitro activities of group II_A and II_B macrolides against gram-negative bacilli

Organism	MIC$_{50}$ (μg/ml)[a]					
	ERY A	CLA	AZI	ROX	DIR	MIO
Neisseria meningitidis	0.12	0.015	0.015	0.06		0.01
N. gonorrhoeae	0.25	0.25	0.12	0.5	1	
M. catarrhalis	0.12	0.06	0.03	0.12	0.12	
H. influenzae	4	4	1	8	16	16
P. multocida	4	2	1	4		
B. pertussis	0.06	0.015	0.03	0.12		
V. cholerae	4	4	0.5	8		
C. jejuni	1	1	0.12	4	1	4
H. ducreyi	0.06	0.008	0.015	0.03		
Vibrio parahaemolyticus	4	8	0.5	16		
H. pylori	0.25	0.015	0.25	0.12		
Eikenella corrodens	4	4	1	8		
G. vaginalis	0.01	0.01	0.01	0.01		0.01
B. melitensis	4	2		8		8

[a]ERY A, erythromycin A; CLA, clarithromycin; AZI, azithromycin; ROX, roxithromycin; DIR, dirithromycin; MIO, miokamycin.

Table 14 In vitro activities of macrolides against *H. pylori* as a function of pH of the culture medium

Drug	MIC_{50} (μg/ml)		
	pH 7.5	pH 6.5	pH 5.5
Erythromycin A	0.2	2	16
Azithromycin	0.12	1	8
Clarithromycin	0.03	0.06	0.25
Dirithromycin	1	4	16
Roxithromycin	0.25	1	4
Spiramycin	1	8	32
Midecamycin	1	2	4

Table 15 Resistance of *H. pylori* to clarithromycin

Country	% resistant strains (1996)
Germany	3
Belgium	10.5
Canada	1.3
Spain	12
United States	9
France	10
Greece	1.2
Hungary	7
Ireland	6
Italy	5
The Netherlands	1
United Kingdom	7
Switzerland	5.8
Poland	16

with erythromycin A, as has been demonstrated with an erythromycin A-resistant strain of *T. pallidum*.

Erythromycin A and azithromycin are active against *Leptospira* spp. Azithromycin is active in vivo in hamsters infected with *Leptospira interrogans* serovar Canicola (Table 22).

Table 16 In vitro activities of macrolides against *C. jejuni*

Drug	MIC (μg/ml)	
	50%	90%
Erythromycin A	0.12	1
Azithromycin	0.06	0.12
Clarithromycin	0.25	2
Dirithromycin	0.25	0.25
Erythromycylamine	0.5	1
Flurithromycin	0.5	0.5
Roxithromycin	1	4
Miokamycin	0.25	1
Spiramycin	2	4
Rokitamycin	0.5	2
Midecamycin	1	2

7.3.6.1. *Borrelia burgdorferi*

Lyme disease is an endemic disease localized in the northern hemisphere and transmitted by ticks.

B. burgdorferi sensu lato is divided into three subspecies: *B. burgdorferi* sensu lato, *Borrelia garinii*, and *Borrelia afzelii*. The three species are responsible for different syndromes: rheumatological, neurologic, and dermatological.

The activities of roxithromycin differ with the species: roxithromycin is most active against *B. garinii* (MIC_{50}, 0.01 μg/ml, 10 strains), followed by *B. burgdorferi* sensu lato (MIC_{50}, 0.06 μg/ml, 5 strains) and *B. afzelii* (MIC_{50}, 0.125 μg/ml, 10 strains).

This activity is comparable to that of ceftriaxone, the MIC_{50} of which is 0.03 μg/ml for the three species. Roxithromycin is bactericidal against *B. garinii* VSBM (MIC and minimum bactericidal concentration [MBC], 0.06 μg/ml) and *B. afzelii* (MIC and MBC, 0.03 and 0.06 μg/ml); it is slightly less bactericidal against *B. burgdorferi* sensu lato MAC 3EMCNY (MIC and MBC, 0.03 and 0.125 μg/ml).

7.3.7. Other Bacterial Genera

Macrolides are inactive in vitro and in vivo against *Enterobacteriaceae*, with a few minor exceptions. Azithromycin has a certain activity against *E. coli*, *Salmonella*

Table 17 Activities of macrolides against anaerobic bacteria[a]

Organism(s)	MIC_{50} (μg/ml)[b]					
	ERY A	CLA	AZI	ROX	DIR	MIO
B. fragilis	16	2	8	32		2
Bacteroides thetaiotaomicron	8	4	8	32		16
Prevotella melaninogenica	0.5	0.06	0.125	0.25		
Porphyromonas spp.	0.06	≤0.06	0.125	≤0.06		
Propionibacterium spp.	0.016	≤0.008	0.03	0.03		
Peptostreptococcus spp.	2	0.25	1.0	4.0		
Peptococcus spp.	2	1	1	4		0.5
Veillonella spp.[c]	8–32	0.12–16	0.5–16	8–64		
Clostridium spp.	64	32	>64	>64		
Clostridium difficile	32	>64	8.0	64		
Fusobacterium spp.	0.25	≤0.06	0.25	0.5	2	2

[a]Data from Dubreuil, 1997, personal communication.

[b]ERY A, erythromycin A; CLA, clarithromycin; AZI, azithromycin; ROX, roxithromycin; DIR, dirithromycin; MIO, miokamycin.

[c]MIC range, in micrograms per milliter.

Table 18 In vitro activities of macrolides against intracellular and atypical bacteria

Organism	MIC$_{50}$ (μg/ml)[a]					
	ERY A	CLA	AZI	ROX	DIR	MIO
L. pneumophila	0.25	0.03	0.12	0.12		0.06
C. pneumoniae	0.125	0.06	0.125	0.125		
C. trachomatis	0.03	0.004	0.03	0.03		
M. pneumoniae	0.015	0.004	0.03	0.03		0.5
M. hominis	>64	>64	>64	>64	>64	
U. urealyticum	0.5	0.03	1	0.5		0.5

[a]ERY A, erythromycin A; CLA, clarithromycin; AZI, azithromycin; ROX, roxithromycin; DIR, dirithromycin; MIO, miokamycin.

Table 19 Activities of macrolides against *C. psittaci* LOTH[a]

Drug	% Intracellular inclusions							
	0.05		0.5		5		50	
	24 h	48 h	24 h	48 h	24 h	48 h	24 h	48 h
Erythromycin A	70	8.3	0	0	0	0	0	0
Josamycin	69	8.3	7.1	0.6	5.4	1.2	3.8	0.2
Spiramycin			7.4	2.5	7.4	6.5	8.6	7
Roxithromycin	76.2	0.26	0	0	0	0	0	0

[a]Data from Orfila et al., 1995.

Table 20 Activities of macrolides against *Rickettsia* spp.[a]

Organism	MIC$_{50}$ (μg/ml)[b]				
	ERY A	CLA	AZI	ROX	DIR
R. akari	16	2	0.25	8	16
R. conorii	8	4	16	16	16
R. prowazekii	2	0.125	0.25	1	16
R. rickettsii	16	8	8	16	16

[a]Data from Ives et al., 1997.
[b]ERY A, erythromycin A; CLA, clarithromycin; AZI, azithromycin; ROX, roxithromycin; DIR, dirithromycin.

Table 21 Activities of macrolides against *Bartonella* spp.[a]

Organism	MIC$_{50}$ (μg/ml)[b]				
	ERY A	CLA	AZI	ROX	DIR
B. henselae	0.125	0.03	0.015	0.125	0.125
B. quintana	0.25	0.06	0.03	0.25	1
B. elizabethae	0.75	0.06	0.02	0.06	0.1

[a]Data from Ives et al., 1997.
[b]ERY A, erythromycin A; CLA, clarithromycin; AZI, azithromycin; ROX, roxithromycin; DIR, dirithromycin.

spp., and *Shigella* spp., but therapeutic activity still remains to be demonstrated.

They are inactive against *Acinetobacter* spp., *Pseudomonas* spp., and other nonfermenting gram-negative bacteria.

They may exhibit a certain in vitro activity against *Brucella* spp., but they are inactive in vivo because of the lack of similarity in terms of intracellular localization.

They are also inactive against *Coxiella* spp.

Table 22 In vitro activities of antibiotics against *L. interrogans* serovars[a]

L. interrogans serovars	MIC (μg/ml)[b]				
	ERY A	AZI	DOX	AMO	PEN G
Canicola	0.02	0.02	0.78	0.01	0.19
Icterohemorrhagiae	0.02	0.02	1.6	0.01	0.03
Grippotyphosa	0.02	0.02	1.6	0.01	0.19
Hardjo	0.01	0.01	0.78	0.004	0.06
Pomona	0.01	0.03	0.78	0.01	0.13

[a]Data from Johnson et al., 1992.
[b]ERY A, erythromycin A; AZI, azithromycin; DOX, doxycycline; AMO, amoxicillin; PEN G, penicillin G.

7.4. In Vitro Activity of 16-Membered-Ring Macrolides (Groups III and IV)

Erythromycin A is more active than miokamycin, the derivative obtained by semisynthesis from midecamycin. It possesses activity comparable to that of josamycin (Fig. 21), irrespective of the bacterial species (Tables 23 and 24).

7.5. Breakpoints

The breakpoints of the macrolides vary according to the committee, and not all macrolides have been referenced by the committees, hence a certain difficulty in interpreting epidemiological results.

The breakpoints adopted by the French Antibiotic Sensitivity Test Committee are given in Table 25.

The breakpoints of erythromycin A used by the other committees are given in Table 26.

The breakpoints are different in the United States (NCCLS) (Tables 27 and 28). The values for *S. pneumoniae* are different from those for staphylococci.

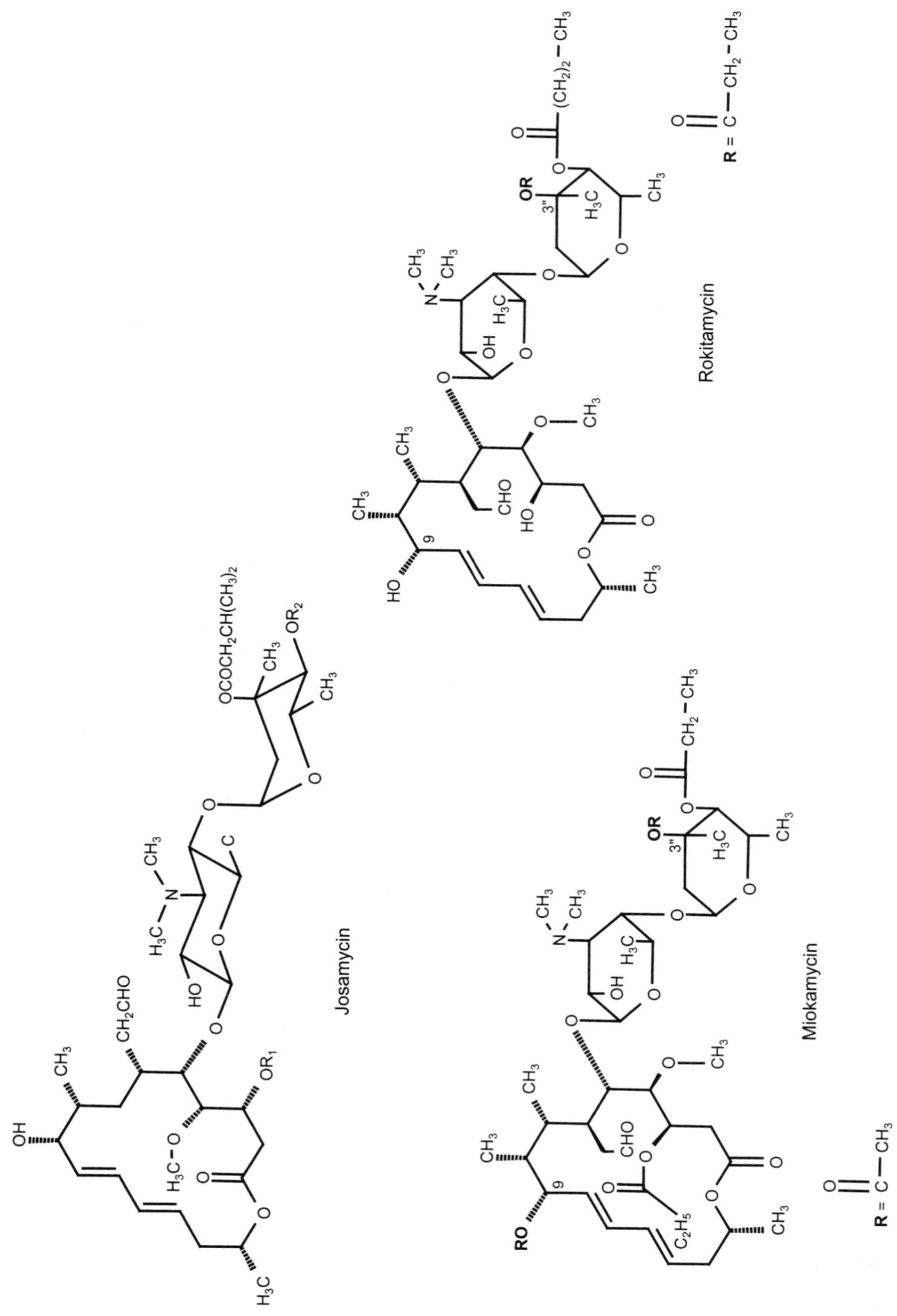

Josamycin

Rokitamycin

Miokamycin

Figure 21 16-Membered-ring macrolides

Table 23 In vitro activities of 16-membered-ring macrolides

Organism(s)	MIC$_{50}$ (μg/ml)[a]		
	ERY A	MIO	JOS
S. aureus Met[s], Ery[s]	0.25	2	2
Coagulase-negative staphylococci, Met[s]	0.25	1	1
S. pyogenes (group A)	0.06	0.12	0.12
S. agalactiae (group B)	0.06	0.25	0.25
Streptococcus groups C and G	0.06	0.12	0.12
Viridans group streptococci	2	0.12	0.25
S. pneumoniae Pen[s]	0.06	0.25	0.12
S. pneumoniae Pen[i]	0.12	0.25	0.12
S. pneumoniae Pen[r]	0.12	0.12	0.12
E. faecalis	4	4	8
E. faecium	>64	>64	>64
C. diphtheriae	0.008	0.06	0.06
C. jeikeium	>128	>128	>128
L. monocytogenes	0.25	1	1
Nocardia spp.	16	16	32
G. vaginalis	0.06	0.03	0.03
N. meningitidis	0.12	0.12	0.12
N. gonorrhoeae	0.25	0.12	0.25
M. catarrhalis	0.12	0.5	0.5
H. influenzae	4	32	32
H. ducreyi	0.06	0.06	0.12
B. pertussis	0.06	0.06	0.12
V. cholerae	4	32	16
V. parahaemolyticus	4	64	32
C. jejuni	1	1	0.5
H. pylori	0.25	0.03	1
L. pneumophila	0.25	0.12	0.5
C. trachomatis	0.03	0.25	0.06
C. pneumoniae	0.5	0.5	0.5
M. pneumoniae	0.015	0.03	0.015
M. hominis	>64	0.12	0.12
U. urealyticum	0.5	0.12	0.5
B. fragilis	4	1	1
P. melaninogenica	0.5	0.06	0.12
Fusobacterium spp.	2	4	8
Peptostreptococcus spp.	4	1	0.5
Clostridium perfringens	2	1	2
Clostridium spp.	0.5	0.25	0.25
C. difficile	1	0.5	0.25
M. avium complex	64	64	128

[a]Ery A, erythromycin A; MIO, miokamycin; JOS, josamycin.

Table 24 In vitro activities of 16-membered-ring macrolides[a]

Organism(s)	MIC$_{50}$ (μg/ml)[b]		
	JOS	SPI	ROK
S. aureus Met[s]	1	1	0.5
S. epidermidis	1	0.5	0.25
S. pyogenes	0.12	0.12	0.25
S. pneumoniae	0.12	0.03	0.12
S. agalactiae	0.25	0.12	0.25
Viridans group streptococci	0.25	0.03	0.12
L. monocytogenes	1.0	4	1
M. catarrhalis	0.5	2	0.25
H. influenzae	32	8	8
C. jejuni	0.5	0.5	1
L. pneumophila	0.5	16	0.25
B. pertussis	0.12	0.12	0.03

[a]Data from Hardy et al., 1988.
[b]JOS, josamycin; SPI, spiramycin; ROK, rokitamycin.

8. MECHANISM(S) OF ACTION OF MACROLIDES

8.1. Ribosomes and Macrolides

The most widely studied mechanism of action is that of erythromycin A. The available data, however, are fragmentary, and the puzzle is far from being solved.

The target of the macrolides is intrabacterial, the ribosome. Before reaching it, the molecule has to cross one (in gram-positive organisms) or two (in gram-negative organisms) barriers. A number of studies have shown that intrabacterial accumulation is not blocked by metabolic inhibitors.

Erythromycin A and its derivatives penetrate gram-positive bacteria and also *H. influenzae* passively. The relative susceptibility of *H. influenzae* to the macrolides appears to be due to the absence of an O antigen chain and also the presence of large pores allowing the passage of molecules with a molecular weight of more than 1,400.

The macrolides inhibit protein synthesis by binding to the 50S subunit of the bacterial ribosomes.

The 50S ribosomal subunit of *E. coli* comprises 32 proteins (4,228 amino acids, with a molecular weight of 460) and two rRNAs, 23S and 5S. 23S rRNA is composed of 2,904 nucleotides, and 14 proteins of the 50S subunit are associated with the 23S rRNA (L1, L2, L3, L4, L6, L7, L10, L11, L12, L13, L16, L20, L23, and L24).

Table 25 Breakpoints of macrolides of the French Antibiotic Sensitivity Test Committee (1997)

Drug	Disk load (μg)	MIC (μg/ml)		Zone diam (mm)	
		Susceptible	Resistant	Susceptible	Resistant
Erythromycin A	15	≤1	>4	≥22	<17
Dirithromycin	15	≤0.12	>4	≥28	<16
Clarithromycin	15	≤1	>4	≥22	<17
Roxithromycin	15	≤1	>4	≥22	<17
Azithromycin	15	≤0.12	>4	≥32	≤19
Spiramycin	100	≤1	>4	≥24	<19
Josamycin	15	≤1	>4	≥24	<19
Midecamycin	15	≤1	>4	≥24	<19

Table 26 Breakpoints of erythromycin A (15-μg disks)

Committee or country[a]	Concn (μg/ml)	
	Susceptible	Resistant
BSAC (United Kingdom)	≤0.5	
DIN (Germany)	≤2	≥8
SRGA (Sweden)	≤1	≥4
Norway	≤1	≥4
CFA (France)	≤1	≥4

[a]BSAC, British Society for Antimicrobial Chemotherapy; DIN, German Institute for Standardization; SRGA, Swedish Reference Group for Antibiotics; CFA, Comité Français Antibiogramme.

Table 27 NCCLS breakpoints for *S. pneumoniae* (1997)[a]

Drug	MIC (μg/ml)		
	Susceptible	Intermediate	Resistant
Erythromycin A	≤0.25	0.5	≥1
Azithromycin	≤0.50	1	≥2
Clarithromycin	≤0.25	0.5	≥1
Dirithromycin	≤0.50	1	≥2

[a]Data from Table 2G and 2H of the January 1998 edition (NCCLS).

Table 28 NCCLS breakpoints for staphylococci (1997)

Drug	MIC (μg/ml)		
	Susceptible	Intermediate	Resistant
Erythromycin A	≤0.5	1–4	≥8
Azithromycin	≤2.0	4	≥8
Clarithromycin	≤2.0	4	≥8
Dirithromycin	≤2.0	4	≥8

It has been shown that erythromycin A binds to a single site of the ribosomal subunit.

In 1987, Cundliffe et al. showed that erythromycin A bound to the site from 2058 to 2062 of domain V of the 23S rRNA of *E. coli*.

In the presence of macrolides, peptidyl-tRNA accumulates in the bacterial cell, causing depletion of the free tRNA necessary for activation of the α-amino acids. The presence of erythromycin A causes the release of a basic amino acid-rich peptide chain by transient inhibition of transpeptidation.

Translocation is impaired by the nascent peptide, which adheres to the surface of the ribosome, generating friction forces. This phenomenon is optimal with effect from a certain chain length, when it becomes a floating strip.

What appears certain is that erythromycin A modifies the interaction between peptidyl-tRNA and the peptidyltransferase donor site (Fig. 22).

Menninger's theory is consistent with the hypothesis that erythromycin A binds to the L4 and L22 proteins near the exit channel of the nascent peptides, causing destabilization of peptidyl-tRNA during translocation and inducing dissociation of peptidyl-tRNA from the ribosomes during the elongation phase of protein synthesis.

8.2. Peptidyltransferase Center

The recent emergence of high-resolution crystal structures and research on ribosomes and ribosome-targeted antibacterials have made a significant step forward.

8.2.1. Macrolide Action

It has been shown that lincosamides and 16-membered-ring macrolides which possess an L-mycarose sugar inhibit the peptidyltransferase enzymatic activity.

Fourteen- and 15-membered-ring macrolides as well as streptogramin B analogs block the entrance of the exit channel of the 50S ribosomal subunit.

By blocking the exit channel, the 14- and 15-membered-ring macrolides induce premature dissociation of peptidyl-tRNA from the ribosome. This "drop-off" event occurs just after initiation of protein synthesis.

8.2.2. Nascent Peptide

All nascent peptides have different chemical properties. For instance, synthesis of polyphenylalanine is poorly inhibited by erythromycin A and by streptogramin B, while these compounds are strong inhibitors of incorporation of basic amino acids.

The translation reaction contains a hydrolase: peptidyl-tRNA hydrolase. Peptidyl-tRNAs that dissociate from the ribosome by drop-off are hydrolyzed by this enzyme, but not those remaining bound to the ribosome.

The length of the drop-off nascent peptide is compound dependent.

Spiramycin, josamycin, and clindamycin, which bind close to the peptidyltransferase center, induce dissociation of peptidyl-tRNA of 2 to 4 amino acid residues.

Erythromycin A and streptogramin B are responsible for a drop-off of 6 to 8 amino acid residues. These molecules do not reach the peptidyltransferase center.

The ketolides telithromycin and cethromycin, which are smaller, allow polymerization of 9 to 12 amino acid residues.

On the basis of the second amino acid of the peptidyl chain, the length will differ in methylated (*erm*) and nonmethylated ribosomes. With josamycin, in methylated ribosomes, the second amino acid may be a glycine and the drop-off peptide will induce a di- or tripeptide -tRNA, and in nonmethylated (valine) ribosomes only a dipeptide will be induced. For spiramycin, only a tetrapeptide is removed in methylated ribomes (*erm*) and a dipeptide is removed in nonmethylated ribosomes. For erythromycin A, the length of the drop-off of the peptidyl chain is the same whatever the status of the ribosome. Telithromycin causes a drop-off of a chain containing 9 to 12 amino acid residues in nonmethylated ribosomes but fails to inhibit synthesis of full-length *erm* peptide with 9 amino acids.

8.2.3. Residues

The binding site of MLS antibacterials is located in the entrance of the exit tunnel before it is constricted by the ribosomal proteins L4 and L22.

Fourteen- and 15-membered-ring macrolides reduce the diameter of the tunnel entrance from 18 to 19 Å to less than 10 Å. In the remaining space, part is occupied by a hydrated Mg^{2+} ion, leaving a passage for the nascent peptide of 6 to 7 Å. These compounds block the progression of the nascent peptide by steric hindrance. Telithromycin and cethromycin due to the lack of L-cladinose leave more space for the growing peptide than erythromycin A, explaining why the drop-off of peptidyl-tRNA is of a

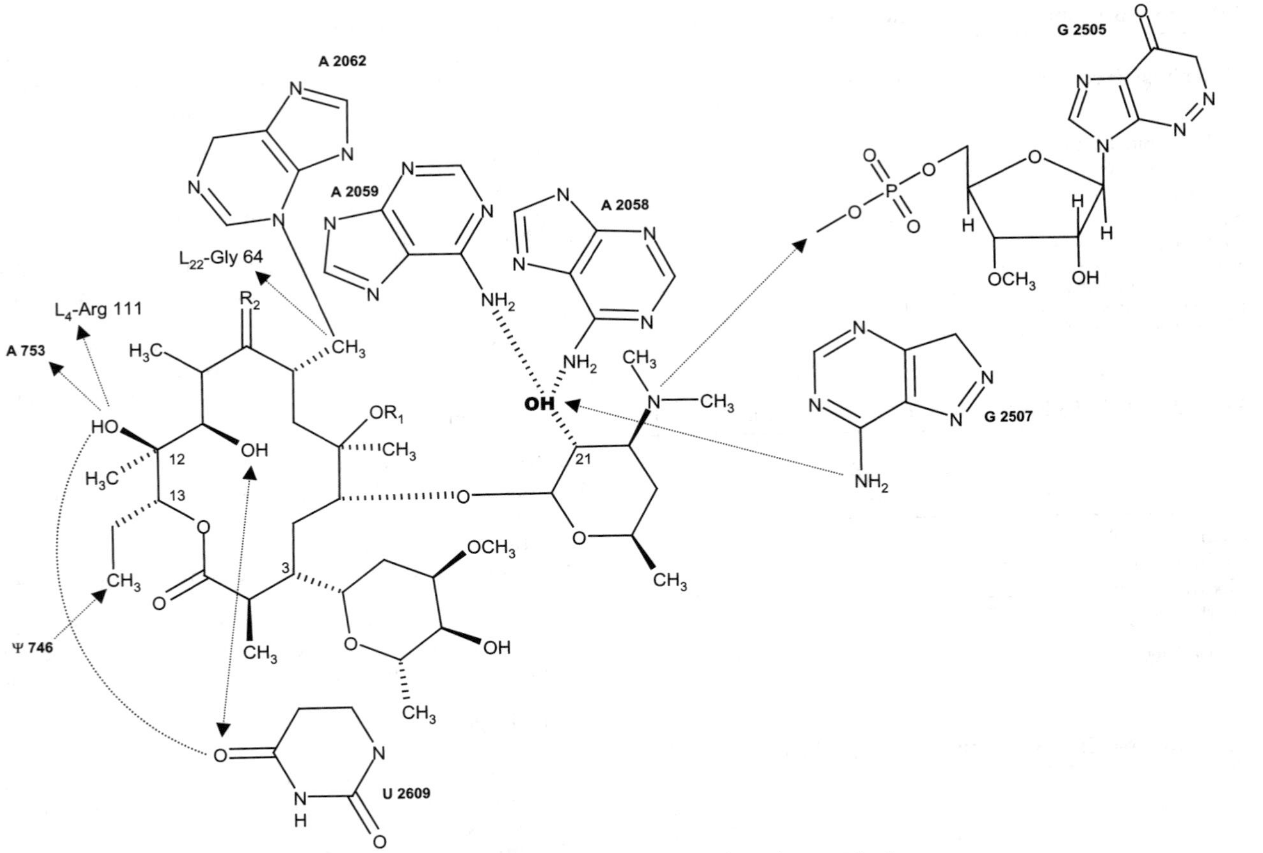

Figure 22 Electronic interactions of erythromycin A

magnitude of 9 to 12 amino acid residues instead of 6 to 8 amino acid residues for erythromycin A.

Erythromycin A and streptogramin B lose their ability to inhibit protein synthesis beyond a critical peptide length due to a stronger affinity for ribosomes of long peptide chains for the ending ribosomal sites.

8.2.4. Macrolide Binding to the 50S Ribosomal Subunit

The 23S rRNA of the 50S ribosomal subunit is essential for the binding of the MLS_B antibacterials. This includes A2058, A2059, and A2062. A2062 forms a covalent bond with the ethylaldehyde side chain of the 16-membered-ring macrolides.

The distances between compounds and the peptidyltransferase center vary with the antibacterials:

- Josamycin, 4.2 Å
- Clindamycin, 4.6 Å
- Spiramycin, 6 Å
- Erythromycin A, 10.6 Å
- Telithromycin, 12.9 Å

The interaction of erythromycin A and domain V of the 23S rRNA is shown in Fig. 22.

Erythromycin A and related analogs are composed of three structural components: the lactone ring and the D-desosamine and L-cladinose sugars.

D-Desosamine is a key element of erythromycin A antibacterial activity. Two moieties are involved in its attachment: 2′-OH and the dimethylamino group.

The 2′-OH group forms three hydrogen bonds: N^6 and N^4 of adenine 2058 and N^6 of adenine 2059. The methylation of the N^6 of adenine 2058 causes steric hindrance for the binding of erythromycin A by preventing the formation of hydrogen bonds to the 2′-OH group. This also occurs with A2058G mutation by disruption of the hydrogen bond.

The dimethylamino group when protonated (>96%) interacts through ionic interactions (pH dependent) with the oxygen of G2505.

Three hydroxyl groups of the lactone ring are within hydrogen-binding distance of the 23S rRNA: 6-OH, 11-OH, and 12-OH.

The 6-OH moiety may form a hydrogen bond with the N^6 atom of adenine 2062. Even with a 6-methoxy group (clarithromycin), the oxygen atom is still at hydrogen-bonding distances to N^6 of adenine 2062.

The 11-OH and 12-OH groups could each form a hydrogen bond with the O^4 atom of uracil 2609.

The active groups of the L-cladinose sugar are not involved in hydrogen bond interactions with the 23S rRNA. The etheroxime side chain of roxithromycin does not have interactions with the 23S RNA or ribosomal proteins, but enters in the exit tunnel. Erythromycin A does not interact with helix 35 of domain II. The distance between 11-OH of the lactone ring and N^4 of adenine 752 is 8.5 Å, and the methyl group at position 13 of the lactone ring is 4.5 Å from O^2 of guanine 745 of helix 35.

Ribosomal proteins L4 and L22, implicated in erythromycin A resistance, are at different distances: L4 is 8 Å away from 12-OH and L22 is 9 Å away from 8-CH_3. Probably mutations at these levels have indirect effects on the 23S rRNA.

8.3. Inhibition of Ribosomal Subunit Synthesis

Another mode of action has been shown, the process of bacterial ribosomal formation.

In the absence of erythromycin A, 50S formation in cells proceeds through two intermediate precursor particles (particles 32S and 43S). The final 50S subunits contain a macrolide-binding site.

In the presence of erythromycin A, the growth results in drug binding to a second target site formed on a 50S precursor particle. Antibiotic binding at this site inhibits further subunit formation, and the incomplete particle is degraded by cellular ribonuclease activities, leading to the accumulation of RNA oligonucleotides in cells and ribosomal depletion (Fig. 23).

In the presence of erythromycin A, azithromycin, and clarithromycin, the 50S ribosomal subunit synthesis was reduced by 40% or more. This effect was shown in methicillin-susceptible and -resistant *S. aureus*, MLS_B-resistant *S. aureus*, and *H. influenzae*. Flurithromycin, roxithromycin, and 14-OH clarithromycin have equivalent inhibitory activities on 50S synthesis and display similar protein-inhibitory activities. Oleandomycin and spiramycin have poor effects on 50S subunit synthesis.

9. EPIDEMIOLOGY OF RESISTANCE TO ERYTHROMYCIN A

An analysis of the literature relating to resistance to erythromycin A is complex. In fact, the breakpoints used to define a resistant strain vary from 0.5 to 8 μg/ml depending on the study. It is rare for the bacterial populations to be distributed in such a way that the results can be harmonized. This difficulty is compounded by the method of determining the activity of erythromycin A (MIC in broth or agar media, antibiotic susceptibility test, presence of 5 to 6% CO_2, and inoculum size), hence the care required to interpret the data, which provide a semiquantitative insight into the phenomenon of resistance.

Lancefield group A streptococci are etiological agents of common infections, such as tonsillitis or impetigo, but also of severe and life-threatening infections. These infections are also the seedbed for secondary incapacitating conditions, such as acute rheumatic fever and acute glomerular nephritis.

No penicillin G-resistant strains of *S. pyogenes* have been described to date. Conversely, the number of erythromycin A-resistant strains is on the increase.

In Finland, Italy, and the United States, the incidence of resistance is high, exceeding 40%. A spectacular reduction in the level of resistance in Finland should be noted, which had fallen to less than 20% in 1996. This involves the replacement by an erythromycin A-susceptible serotype, since there is no reversal of resistance.

Higher levels have been reported for other beta-hemolytic streptococci in France, 22.8 and 24.3%, respectively for Lancefield group C and G streptococci.

Table 29 shows rates of resistance of Lancefield group A streptococci to erythromycin A.

H. Seppälä in Finland has described a new, noninducible resistance phenotype that does not appear to involve a methylase and that affects the activity of streptogramin B, clindamycin, and 16-membered-ring macrolides.

Erythromycin A-resistant strains of *Streptococcus agalactiae* have been described, and they possess different mechanisms of resistance.

Erythromycin A-resistant strains have been described among the following species: *M. avium, H. pylori, M. pneumoniae,* and *T. pallidum*. These are isolated cases. The combination of resistances to penicillin G and to erythromycin A among clinically isolated strains of *S. pneumoniae* is much

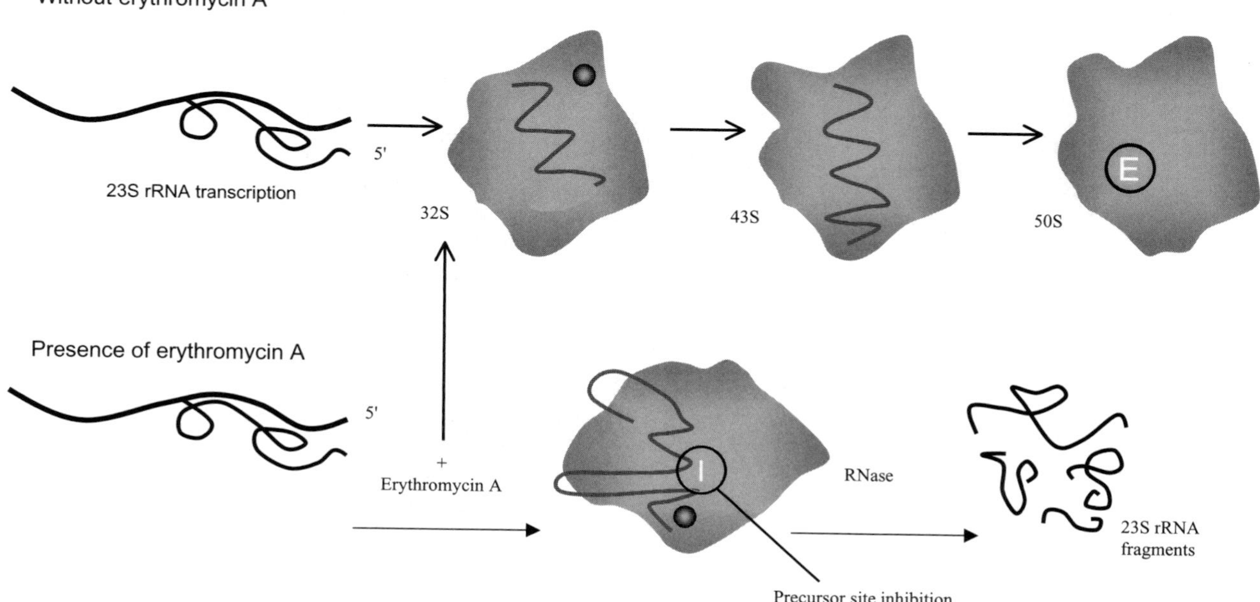

Figure 23 Inhibition of 50S ribosomal subunit biosynthesis

Table 29 Resistance of Lancefield group A streptococci to erythromycin A

Country	Resistance (%)	Yr
France	8	1994
Italy	54	1997
Spain	40	1997
United States	16	1994
Taiwan	22	1995
Finland	16.2	1997
Australia	17.6	1996
Japan	>30	1997
Germany	<1	1993
Norway	17	1990
United Kingdom	23	1990
Slovenia	4.1	1995

more concerning. Likewise, numerous strains of enterococci and staphylococci have become resistant to erythromycin A.

Clarithromycin is beginning to be widely used in *H. pylori* infections, and the incidence of resistance ranges from 1 to 16%.

The acquisition of resistance to azithromycin appears to be possible in the species *C. pneumoniae*, as has been demonstrated by M. Hammerschlag's team (1998).

9.1. *S. pneumoniae*

Erythromycin A-resistant strains may be classified into three categories:

- Strains resistant to erythromycin A but remaining susceptible to penicillin G, which are a common occurrence in Italy
- Multiresistant strains with a high incidence
- Strains resistant to erythromycin A but susceptible to clindamycin and streptogramin B (efflux)

Alarming levels of erythromycin A-resistant strains have been recorded in Asia, but lower levels have been recorded in the Indian subcontinent (Fig. 24).

In North America, levels of resistance to erythromycin A are high and have reached 20%.

In Europe, there is a large variation between countries. The highest levels of resistance have been reported in Spain and France, and low levels, often correlated with resistance to penicillin G, have been reported in Germany and the United Kingdom (Fig. 25).

It should, however, be noted that the level of resistance to erythromycin A is often higher than that to penicillin G. What affect the actual level of resistance still more are the breakpoints used, which range from 0.5 μg/ml (United States) to 8 μg/ml (certain European countries).

A recent study showed that there was a large number of erythromycin A-resistant strains among gram-positive cocci in the United States (Table 30).

The intensive use of clarithromycin in the treatment of gastroduodenal infections due to *H. pylori* has led to the substantial emergence of resistant strains (Fig. 26).

10. RESISTANCE MECHANISMS

There are currently four recognized mechanisms of resistance to erythromycin A: modifications in the ribosomal target, inactivation of the molecule, efflux, and mutations in the 23S rRNA and ribosomal proteins L4 and L22.

10.1. Modification of the Ribosomal Target

10.1.1. Resistance by Methylation

Resistance of the MLS_B type has been described since 1956 for certain strains of staphylococci. It has subsequently been described for streptococci and enterococci. This resistance is due to dimethylation of *E. coli* adenosine 2058 or 2059 via a transferase the cofactor of which is an S-adenosylmethionine, allowing the binding of one or two methyl groups on adenine 2058 or 2059 of the 23S rRNA located at domain V (peptidyltransferase transfer center). The methyltransferases are under the control of at least eight *erm* (erythromycin resistance methylase) genes (Table 31).

The result is a reduction in the affinity between erythromycin A and the ribosome, causing the incapacity of the antibiotic to inhibit protein synthesis. The genes responsible for these methyltransferases are carried by a plasmid or

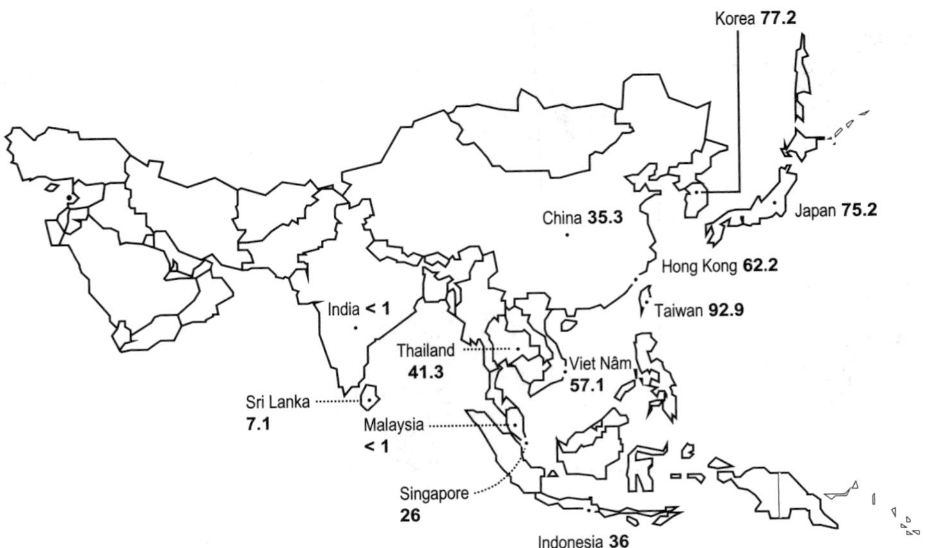

Figure 24 ***S. pneumoniae*: resistance to erythromycin A in Asia**

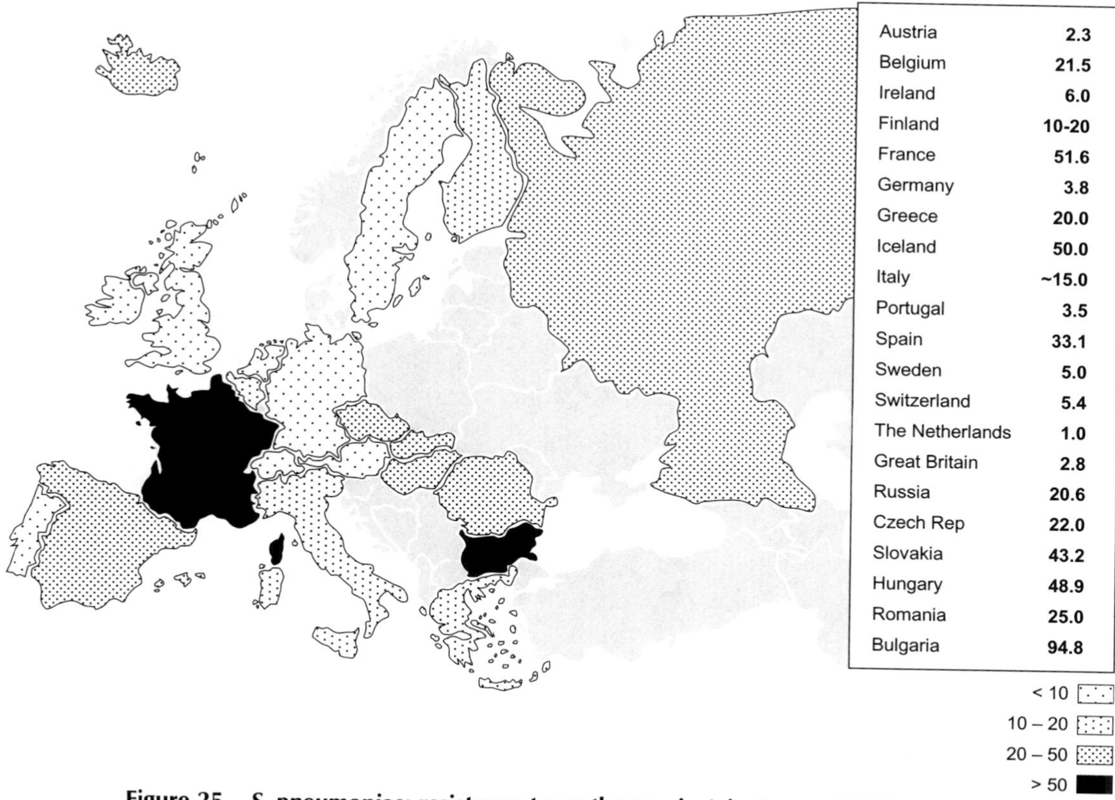

Figure 25 ***S. pneumoniae*: resistance to erythromycin A in Europe (1999 to 2000)**

Table 30 Epidemiology of resistance among gram-positive cocci in the United States

Organism(s)	*n*	Resistance (%)
Enterococcus spp.	649	88
S. aureus	1,410	39
Staphylococcus, coagulase negative	457	62
S. pyogenes	115	16
Viridans group streptococci	53	43

located on the chromosome. The mode of expression of this resistance may be inducible or constitutive.

10.1.1.1. *ermC* Gene (Plasmid pE194)

The regulation of the methyltransferase produced by the *ermC* gene of staphylococci and carried by the plasmid pE194 has been the most widely studied.

Its expression depends on the regulatory region coding for the synthesis of a small regulatory peptide, located upstream from the structural gene coding for the methylase. At the 5′ terminus of the regulatory region of the mRNA there are four complementary inverse sequences that can pair with one another and that surround the site of ribosomal binding and the initiation codons for the synthesis of methyltransferase.

The gene of the regulatory peptide and that of the methylase are transcribed simultaneously in the 5′→3′ direction by a single mRNA. This mRNA thus comprises two coding regions.

The ribosomes are bound to another RNA sequence known as the Shine-Dalgarno (SD) sequence or ribosome binding site located a few bases before the initiation codon.

Translation of the mRNA occurs in the 5′→3′ direction. It starts with that of the open reading frame of the regulatory peptide and should continue with that of the methylase. However, in the case of the *ermC* mRNA, the 5′ terminus exhibits a series of inverse repetitions that form loops on pairing (conformation I).

The SD-1 ribosome binding site and the codon initiating the synthesis of the regulatory peptide are accessible to the ribosomes and are normally translated via loop 1, which does not constitute an obstacle. In the absence of erythromycin A, these loops sequester the SD-2 ribosome binding site and the subsequent translation initiation codon, thus preventing synthesis of methylase because of their inaccessibility to the ribosomes.

Erythromycin A causes inhibition by binding to the 50S fraction of the ribosome. It is this inhibition which probably produces a conformational rearrangement of the mRNA with a modification of the loop (Fig. 27). Having remained free, the SD-2 site and the initiation sequences may be recognized by the ribosomes and allow synthesis of the enzyme (conformation II). The gene coding for the methylase will be translated by the ribosomes that have remained free or are weakly methylated naturally. When all the ribosomes are methylated, inhibition can no longer occur and the mRNA molecules return to a resting configuration. There is a self-regulating system of methyltransferase synthesis.

A comparable but more complex mechanism has been demonstrated with the *ermA* determinant of *S. aureus* and

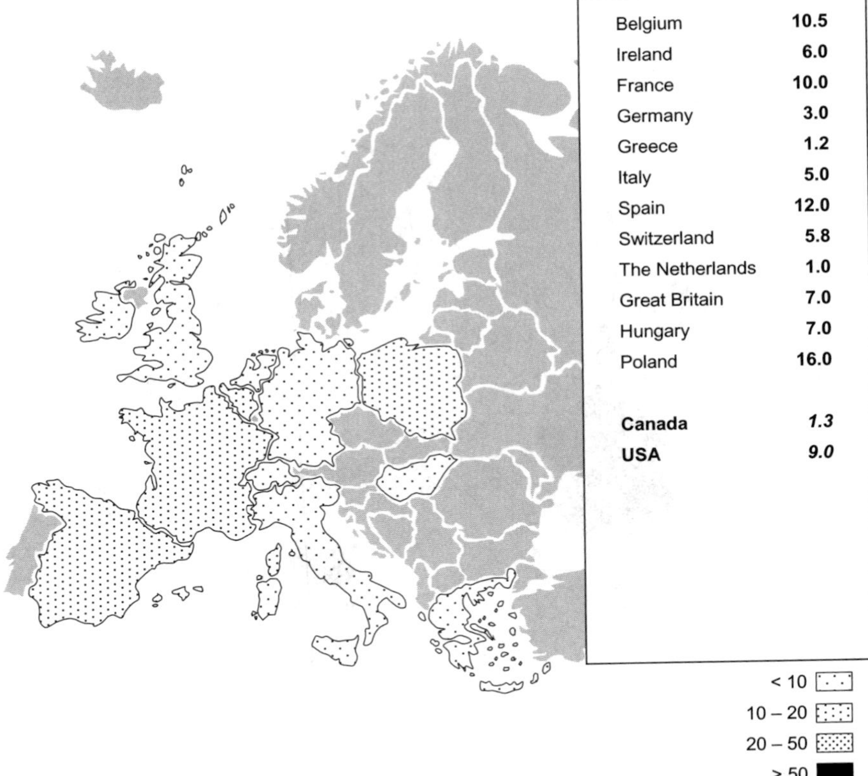

Figure 26 ***H. pylori*: resistance to erythromycin A in Europe (1999)**

Table 31 ***erm* genes and bacteria**

Gene	Bacterial species	Location
ermA	*S. aureus* and coagulase-negative staphylococci	Tn*554*
ermA′	*Arthrobacter*	Chromosome
ermAM	Streptococci (groups A and B), *Streptococcus sanguinis, S. pneumoniae, E. faecalis, Pediococcus acidilactici, K. pneumoniae*	Tn*1545*
ermB	*S. aureus*	(Tn*1551*)[a]
ermBC	*E. coli*	Tn*917*
ermC	*Staphylococcus* spp., *B. subtilis*	pE194
ermD	*Bacillus licheniformis*	Chromosome
ermE	*Saccharopolyspora erythraea*	Chromosome
ermF	*B. fragilis, Bacteroides ovatus*	pBF41 (Tn*4351*)
ermG	*B. sphaericus*	Chromosome
ermP	*C. perfringens*	Chromosome

[a]Parentheses indicate possible location.

the *ermG* determinant of *Bacillus sphaericus*, expression of which is inducible. There are two regulatory peptides here, and induction assumes a series of detachments-reattachments of the regions of inverse repetition in a cascade.

The regulation of resistance is posttranscriptional; it does not occur at the time of the transcription of DNA to mRNA but on the translation of RNA.

The first *Bacteroides fragilis* strain exhibiting MLS_B resistance of a constitutive type was reported in 1976. The determinants are of either plasmid or chromosomal origin. The *ermF* gene is located on a transposon, Tn*4351*, itself carried by a 41-kb plasmid, pBF4.

MLS_B-type resistance has also been demonstrated in *Campylobacter* spp.

10.1.1.2. Inducible and Constitutive Phenotypes

The difference between the 14- and 16-membered-ring macrolides in terms of inductive potency appears to be related to the amino acid composition and the length of the regulatory peptide.

The variants isolated carry mutations, deletion(s), substitution(s), or duplications of the regulatory region of the methylase so that the ribosome binding sites and the initiation codon of the methylase are permanently accessible.

The constitutive or inducible nature appears to be related not to the class of the *erm* determinant but to the nature of the regulatory region related to the structural gene.

In *S. pneumoniae* resistant to erythromycin A (constitutive type), it was shown by sequence analysis that 187 bp of

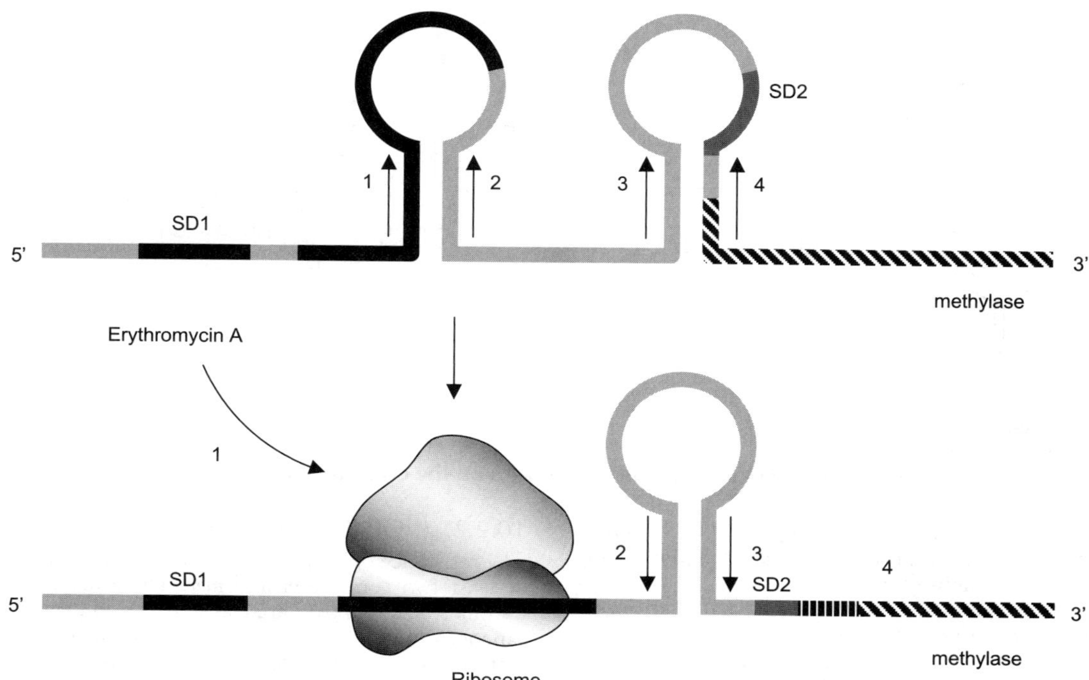

Figure 27 The *ermC* gene: schematic representation of the conformational rearrangement following inhibition by erythromycin A

tandem repeats which includes the ribosome binding site for the *erm*(B) gene was inserted in the attenuator of the *erm*(B) gene in *S. pneumoniae*. This alteration prevents the formation of the mRNA stem-loop structure in the translational attenuator of the *erm*(B) gene.

10.1.2. Resistance to Macrolides by Ribosomal Mutation

Resistance to erythromycin A is due to a mutation in domain V of the 23S rRNA. The acquisition of resistance by *M. pneumoniae* is due not to methylation on its 23-rRNA but to a single nucleoside mutation at 2063 (A→G) or 2064 (A→G). Nucleotide 2064 corresponds to nucleotide 2059 of *E. coli*. There is inducible resistance to 16-membered-ring macrolides in which activity is preserved but at a very reduced level, or a constitutive form involving total resistance (Table 32).

In *M. avium*, a mutation (a single operon) occurs in domain V, causing a nucleotide substitution at position 2274 (A→G or G→T) (position 2058 in *E. coli*).

Table 32 Resistance of *M. pneumoniae* to erythromycin A[a]

Drug	MIC (μg/ml) for *M. pneumoniae* 129[b]		
	ERY^s	ERY^r (inducible)	ERY^r (constitutive)
Erythromycin A	0.004–0.01	>100	125
Spiramycin	0.16–0.63	20	>160
Midecamycin	0.08	5	>100
Clindamycin	1.6–3.1	>1,000	50
Miokamycin A	0.16–1.25	0.31	0.31

[a]Data from Lacier et al., 1995.
[b]ERY, erythromycin.

Clarithromycin-resistant mutant strains of *H. pylori* are readily obtained in vitro. The mutation sites (two operons) are at positions 2143 (A→C) and 2144 (A→G) (2058 and 2059 in *E. coli*). *erm*-type genes have not been detected in *H. pylori*.

A mutation designated as *ery*A exhibits a modification of the L4 protein, preventing erythromycin A from binding to the ribosomes. The *ery*B mutation causes a modification of the L22 protein, and the *ery*C mutation affects the maturation of rRNA and the 30S ribosomal subunit. These last two mutations do not have a clear expression in terms of resistance to erythromycin A in the current state of our knowledge.

10.2. Mechanism(s) of Resistance by Inactivation

Resistance by inactivation has been described for *S. aureus*, *Staphylococcus haemolyticus*, and *E. coli* but has not been described to date for streptococci. Macrolide-inactivating enzymes have been demonstrated, consisting of those that phosphorylate or glycosylate the 2′-OH group of the D-desosamine and those that hydrolyze the lactone ring (esterases).

10.2.1. Esterases

Courvalin et al. have described two esterases (I and II), isolated from gram-negative bacilli, which hydrolyze the lactone nucleus of erythromycin A and oleandomycin (Fig. 28).

The hydrolysis rate varies with the substituents at C-9, C-6, and C-11. Compared to erythromycin A (hydrolysis rate [V] [100%], 0.2 to 0.6 μg/ml/min), clarithromycin is more rapidly hydrolyzed (V = 26.2) than roxithromycin (V = 15.7), although less so than erythromycin A. Compounds with a C-9 oxime and a C-11 carbamate chain are hydrolyzed 30 times more slowly than erythromycin A (V = 3.6).

Genetic studies have shown that the genes producing these enzymes have a plasmid as a support. Esterase I is the

R : α-L cladinose
R : D-desosamine

Figure 28 Mode of action of esterases on the erythronolide A ring

product of the *ercA* gene and is composed of 349 amino acids, whereas esterase II is the product of the *ercB* gene and is composed of 419 amino acids.

The enzymes produced by the *ercA* and *ercB* genes have been isolated principally from *E. coli*, but also from certain strains of *Klebsiella pneumoniae*. It has recently been shown that the *S. aureus* strain 01A1032 produces an esterase similar to that encoded by *ercB*. This enzyme is not capable of hydrolyzing azithromycin but principally hydrolyzes 14- and 16-membered-ring macrolides, while the *ercA* and *ercB* enzymes only hydrolyze the 14-membered-ring macrolides.

The esterase of this *S. aureus* strain inactivates erythromycins A, B, and C, 11,12-carbonate erythromycin A, clarithromycin, 11,12-carbonate clarithromycin, 11,12-carbonate azithromycin, and oleandomycin. It does not inactivate 4″-epiazithromycin, in contrast to the *E. coli* esterases.

It should be noted that 8a-*N*-azithromycin is not a good substrate for the three enzymes (Figure 29).

10.2.2. 2′-OH Glycosyltransferase

The resistance of *Streptomyces lividans* to macrolides involves at least two genes: *erm* and *mgt*. These are bound to the chromosome, and they are transcribed and expressed simultaneously. The *erm* gene product is a methyltransferase that introduces a methyl group into A2058 of 23S rRNA. The *mgt* gene of *S. lividans* produces a glycosyltransferase that inactivates macrolides by using UDP glucose or UDP galactose as a cofactor.

This inactivation is selective for the 16-membered-ring macrolides with D-mycaminose as an amino sugar (tylosin, desmycosin, etc.). In fact, angolamycin, in which the sugar is angolosamine (2-deoxymycaminose), is not a good substrate. Inhibition by binding to the 2′-OH-desmycaminose group is maximal when the molecule is monosaccharidic at C-5 of the lactone nucleus.

This enzyme, 2′-O-glycosyltransferase, has also been described for *Streptomyces vendargensis*.

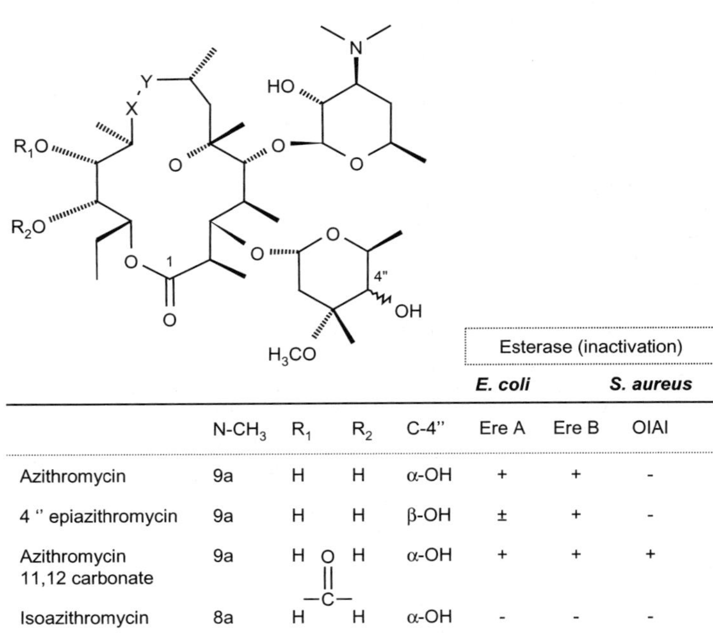

	N-CH_3	R_1	R_2	C-4"	Esterase (inactivation) *E. coli* Ere A	*E. coli* Ere B	*S. aureus* OIAI
Azithromycin	9a	H	H	α-OH	+	+	-
4 " epiazithromycin	9a	H	H	β-OH	±	+	-
Azithromycin 11,12 carbonate	9a	H $\overset{O}{\overset{\|}{-C-}}$	H	α-OH	+	+	+
Isoazithromycin	8a	H	H	α-OH	-	-	-

Figure 29 Structure of miokamycin and its principal metabolites

10.2.3. 2′-O-Phosphotransferases

Macrolide 2′-O-phosphotransferases have been described for *E. coli* and *Streptomyces coelicolor*.

These are inducible intracytoplasmic enzymes that inactivate 14- or 15-membered-ring macrolides by binding to a phosphate on the 2′-OH group of the D-desosamine (Fig. 30).

The enzymes of *E. coli* are relatively inactive against 16-membered-ring macrolides, but *S. coelicolor* 2′-phosphotransferase inactivates spiramycin and tylosin.

2′-O-Phosphotransferase (MPH-2′) was first described in Japan, followed by MPH-2′I (oleandomycin 2′-phosphotransferase) and then, in Europe, MPH-2′II.

O'Hara et al. (1996) showed that not all 14-membered-ring macrolides had the same substrate specificities for these enzymes (Table 33).

The inactivation of oleandomycin is 16, 20.5, and 20.6 nmol per mg of protein for the Tf481A, L441D, and BM2506 enzymes, respectively. It is 860 nmol of oleandomycin per mg per cell/h. MPH-2′I does not inactivate kanamycin A, B, or C; gentamicin C_1, C_{1a}, or C_2; or the other aminoglycosides containing amino sugars of the desosamine type (Fig. 31).

Compared to erythromycin A and oleandomycin, clarithromycin and roxithromycin are less hydrolyzed by the *ercA* product.

The difference is marked with respect to inactivation by 2′-O-phosphotransferases. Roxithromycin is relatively insensitive to inactivation by MPH-2′II compared to clarithromycin, and likewise there is a difference in reaction towards MPH-2′I between the two compounds, suggesting that the C-9 chain exerts a favorable action with respect to inhibition by MPH-2′. The presence of Mg^{2+} is essential for the activity of MPH-2′, and the active site of the enzyme must comprise a phenylalanine, a tyrosine, a tryptophan, or a histidine.

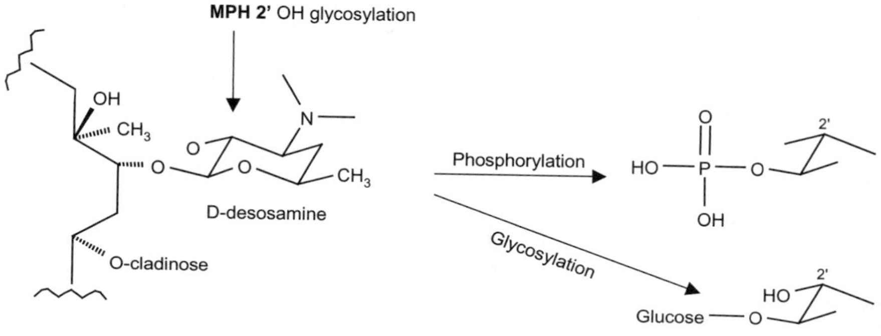

Figure 30 Inactivation of erythromycin A

Table 33 Inactivation of macrolides by MPH-2′[a]

Enzyme	*E. coli* strain	% Inactivation[b]				
		OL	EM	CAM	RXM	LM
MPH2″I	Tf-481 A	100	87	64	37	1
	L 441 D	100	82	73	47	1
MPH2″II	BM 2506	100	23	17	0	61
EM (*ercA*) esterase	BM 694/pAT 63	100	15	8	7	0

[a]Data from O'Hara et al., 1996.
[b]OL, oleandomycin; EM, erythromycin A; CAM, clarithromycin; RXM, roxithromycin; LM, leucomycin.

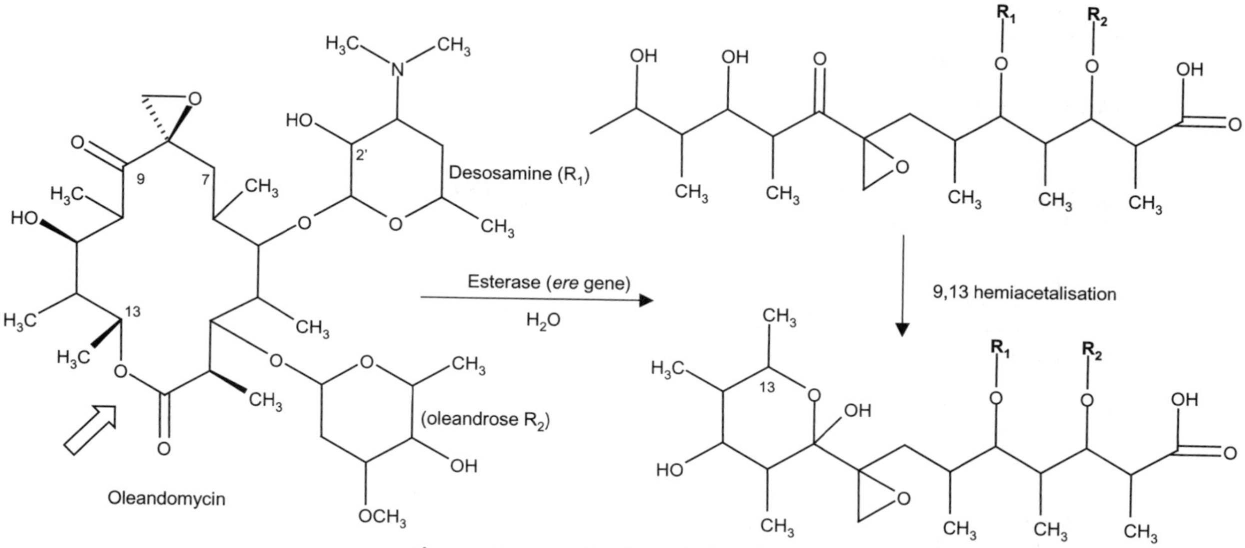

Figure 31 Inactivation of oleandomycin

10.3. Mechanism of Resistance by Efflux

A number of transport systems have been held responsible for resistance to drugs, whether the efflux system via P-glycoprotein (*mdrL* gene) for anticancer agents or other efflux systems for antibacterial agents such as the macrolides, tetracyclines, or fluoroquinolones.

In a staphylococcal outbreak in Hungary in 1977, strains of *S. aureus* were collected that were resistant to erythromycin A, oleandomycin, and streptogramin B but susceptible to 16-membered-ring macrolides and lincosamides. They were resistant to mycinamycins I and II (16-membered-ring macrolides).

These were the first resistant strains of the MS type described epidemically.

In 1993, Eady et al. showed that a third of erythromycin A-resistant strains of coagulase-negative staphylococci (*Staphylococcus epidermidis*) possessed dual resistance, to erythromycin A and streptogramin B but not to lincosamides.

The gene responsible for this resistance is *mrsA*. The product of this gene is a protein composed of 488 amino acids containing two hydrophobic intracytoplasmic domains that bind to the ATP of a transporter superprotein of the ABC transporters.

Other genes are involved in the extensive efflux in *S. aureus*: *smp* and/or *stp*. The *stp* gene encodes a protein that binds the ATP of a transporter protein, and the *smp* gene codes for a hydrophobic transmembrane protein, that appears to be the efflux pump. These are plasmid-mediated genes.

In a recent study, it was shown that in five species of coagulase-negative staphylococci, the *ermC* gene (50.6%) was the most common, alone or in combination with a second *erm* gene. The *ermA* and *ermB* genes were only present in 5.9 and 7.2% of strains, respectively, and 33% of strains possessed the *mrsA* gene.

In Hungary, it has been shown that 25.6% of erythromycin A-resistant strains from 27 regions collected over a period of 12 months possessed the MS phenotype (efflux). In the United States, this phenotype was demonstrated in a New Jersey hospital in 7.3% of erythromycin A-resistant strains of coagulase-negative staphylococci.

In Denmark, the study of 428 erythromycin A-resistant strains of *S. aureus* collected between 1959 and 1988 showed that such strains carried the *ermA* gene until 1971, and then the *ermC* gene became dominant between 1984 and 1988. Only six strains do not carry the *ermA* or *ermC* gene; four of these carry the *mrsA* gene.

Energy-dependent efflux resistance under the control of the *mtr* gene has been described for *N. gonorrhoeae*. This efflux system is nonspecific to macrolides, as it is similar to that described for *Pseudomonas aeruginosa* (*mexAB-oprKI*) and *E. coli* (*acrAB* and *acrEF*).

Streptococcal strains with an M phenotype have an efflux system different from that described for staphylococci.

The strains of *S. pneumoniae* and *S. pyogenes* with an M phenotype are resistant to erythromycin A but remain susceptible to clindamycin and streptogramin B. The MICs of erythromycin A, however, are moderately increased (Table 34). The activity of erythromycin A is less affected than in the case of resistance of the MLS_B type.

This system is under the control of the *mef* gene (for macrolide efflux), which is the *mefA* gene for *S. pyogenes* and *mefE* for *S. pneumoniae*.

An *mreA* gene (macrolide resistance efflux), different from the *mef* gene, has been demonstrated in *S. agalactiae*; strains with this gene are resistant to the 14-, 15-, and 16-membered-ring macrolides.

10.4. Other Mechanisms

Resistance to erythromycin A, but not to lincosamides or streptogramin B, has been described for a strain of *S. epidermidis* carrying a 26.5-kb pNE24 plasmid. This resistance is constitutive under the control of the *erpA* gene, which causes a modification of the membrane permeability, evidenced by a low intrabacterial concentration of [^{14}-C]erythromycin A. It does not affect the 16-membered-ring macrolides.

The activities of antibiotics of the MLS group are summarized in Table 35.

10.5. Combinations of Resistance Mechanisms

Combinations of several resistance mechanisms have been found, such as the *erm-mef* combination in *S. pneumoniae* (Table 36).

10.6. Pentapeptides

It was shown that overexpression of a short segment of *E. coli* 23S rRNA (positions 1235 to 1268) renders all *S. pneumoniae* resistant to erythromycin A.

A nascent pentapeptide can interact directly with erythromycin A and displace the antibacterials from the ribosome. These peptides act as "bottle brushes," cleaning the ribosome from the bound erythromycin A.

This E-peptide is translated by the ribosome. The rRNA-encoded E-peptide is not normally expressed because the SD region of the peptide open reading frame is sequestered in the 23S rRNA secondary structure. E-peptide affects only the ribosome on which it has been translated. Sequence analysis revealed a consensus sequence, MXLXV, which could be recognized in the majority of E-peptides. Different pentapeptides confer resistance to different macrolides. The pentapeptide for ketolides, the K-peptide, is MRFFY. The

Table 34 Activities of 14-membered-ring macrolides against streptococci resistant to erythromycin A by efflux[a]

Drug	Susceptibility[b]		MIC (μg/ml)	
	Erythromycin A	Clindamycin	50%	90%
Erythromycin A	S	S	≤0.06	≤0.06
	R	R	>32	>32
	R	R	4	8
Clarithromycin	S	S	≤0.06	≤0.06
	R	R	>32	>32
	R	S	2	4

[a]Data from Barry et al., 1997.
[b]S, susceptible; R, resistant.

Table 35 Activities of antibiotics of the MLS group against different strains of *S. aureus*[a]

Mechanism	Genotype	ERY	16-membered	LIN	CLIN	Strep B	Strep A	Strept
Target alteration	*erm* inducible	R	S	S	S	S	S	S
Inactivation	*erm* constitutive	R	R	R	R	R	S	S
	linA	S	S	R	(S)	S	S	S
	isa	S	S	I	I	S	R	I
Efflux	*saa-sbh (vgb)*	S	S	S/I	S/I	R	R	R
	mrsA	R	S	S	S	S	S	S
	eprA							

[a]ERY, erythromycin A; LIN, lincomycin; CLIN, clindamycin; Strep B, Strep A, and Strept, streptogramins; R, resistant; S, susceptible.

Table 36 Combination of mechanisms of resistance to erythromycin A in *S. pneumoniae*[a]

Mechanism	% with mechanism of resistance		
	Europe ($n = 77$)	United States ($n = 114$)	Japan ($n = 80$)
mefE$^+$	21	61	43
ermAM$^+$	73	32	56
mef/erm$^+$	3	5	1
mef/unknown	4	2	

[a]Data from Acar, 1998.

size of the peptide, 3 to 6 amino acids, and its amino acid sequence are essential for its functions (Fig. 32).

11. PLASMA PHARMACOKINETICS OF MACROLIDES

11.1. Oral Pharmacokinetics in Healthy Young Subjects

The absorption and bioavailability vary according to the molecule, partly explaining the difference in unit and dosage rhythm of the different macrolides.

Absorption is rapid, with a lag time often on the order of 0.25 h (roxithromycin and clarithromycin). The peak concentration in serum varies from 0.4 μg/ml (azithromycin, 500 mg) to 11 μg/ml (roxithromycin, 300 mg), is reached after a period of between 0.6 h (rokitamycin) and 4.0 h (dirithromycin), and is dependent on the dose absorbed. The relative bioavailability ranges from 3.7 μg·h/ml (rokitamycin) to 132 μg·h/ml (roxithromycin, 300 mg) and is dependent on the administered dose, but it is not proportional to the dose for certain molecules with nonlinear pharmacokinetics. The apparent elimination half-life ranges from 0.1 h (miokamycin) to 44 h (dirithromycin). The absolute bioavailability of the different molecules ranges from 10% (dirithromycin) to about 50 to 60% (roxithromycin and clarithromycin). It is on the order of 37% for azithromycin and 14-hydroxyclarithromycin, the main metabolite of clarithromycin (Table 37).

Plasma protein binding is mainly to the α_1-glycoproteins for the erythromycin A derivatives and ranges from 15% (josamycin) to more than 90% (roxithromycin).

Elimination occurs mainly by the hepatobiliary route, and only with clarithromycin is about 30% of the administered dose eliminated in the urine (Table 38).

For miokamycin, a reduction in the apparent elimination is noted as the unit dose increases, particularly for the Mb-9a and Mb-6 metabolites. Conversely, the pharmacokinetics of

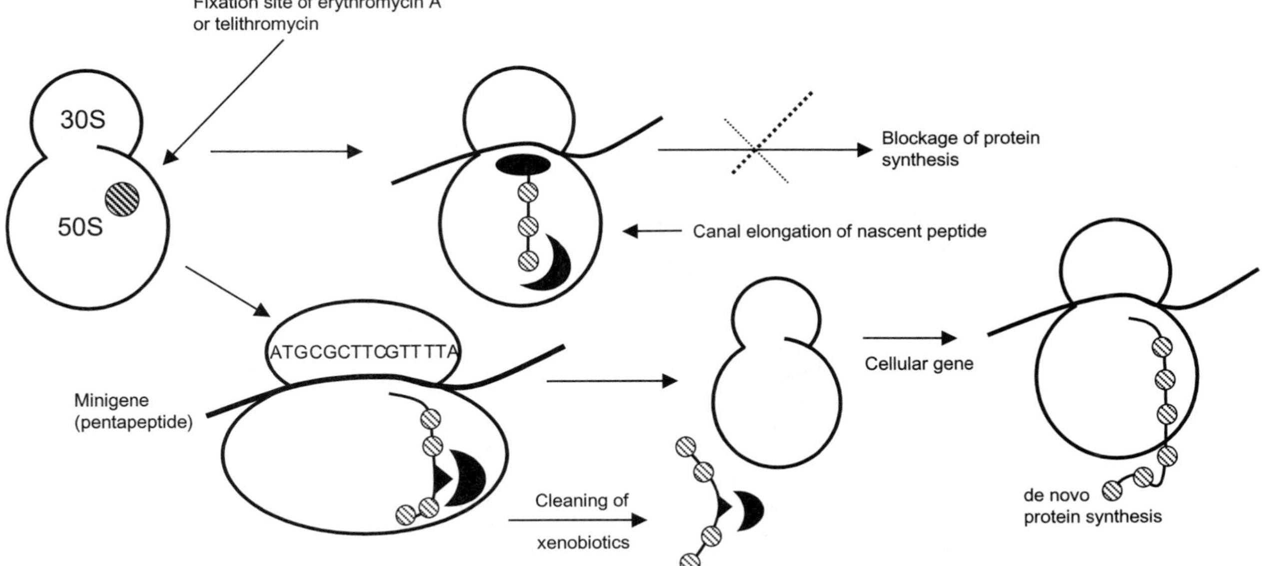

Figure 32 Bottle brush mechanism of resistance

Table 37 Plasma pharmacokinetics of macrolides

Drug	*n*	Dose (mg)	Metabolites	C_{max} (μg/ml)	T_{max} (h)	AUC/F (μg·h/ml)	$t_{1/2\beta}$ (h)
Azithromycin		500		0.35 ± 0.1	0.9 ± 0.9	3.58 ± 1.2	NA[a]
	1	500		0.59 ± 0.2	2.2 ± 0.02	3.35 ± 0.4	41.2 ± 4.3
	2						
Clarithromycin	6	100	C	0.35	1.46	1.67	2.27
	6		DH-C[b]	0.35	2.09	3.06	2.4
	8	200	C	0.6	1.56	2.99	2.3
	8		OH-C	0.41	2.29	3.4	3.37
	6	400	C	0.13	1.86	8.55	3.6
	6		OH-C	0.78	2.11	7.52	3.89
		600	C	2.03	1.83	15.44	3.64
	8		OH-C	1.06	2.45	9.95	3.84
	8	800	C	2.63	2.67	24.73	4.25
	7		OH-C	1.02	2.72	10.72	5.09
	8	1,200	C	3.97	2.2	44.6	5.98
	6		OH	1.54	2.61	23.9	9.19
		250	C	0.7–0.8	1.7 ± 1.9	4–4.2	2.6–2.8
			OH	0.6–0.7	2.2–2.3	4.6–4.9	3.9–5.1
		500	C	1.77–1.89	2.3	11.1–11.7	3.3–3.5
			OH	0.7–0.8	2.3–2.8	6.1–6.9	6.4–6.6
Dirithromycin	1	250		ND[c]			
	2						
	1	500		0.29 ± 0.2	4	0.86 ± 0.6	32.5
	2						
	1	750		0.64 ± 0.4	4	1.84 ± 1.2	30.6
	2						
	1	1,000		0.41 ± 0.2	4	1.61 ± 1.1	31.9
	2						
Roxithromycin		150		7.9 ± 0.6	1.9	81 ± 10	10.5 ± 1.4
		300		10.8 ± 0.6	1.5	132 ± 17	11.9 ± 0.5
		450		12.2 ± 0.7	1.3	170 ± 20	13.8 ± 0.9
Flurithromycin	1	500		1 ± 0.7	0.92	0.4	3.54
	2						
	1	750		1.58 ± 0.3	0.72	3.52	2.8
	2						
	1	375		1.41 ± 0.5	1	4.41	3.94
	2						
Oleandomycin	1	1,000		2.8	2.6	10.8	3.4
	2						
Spiramycin		1,000		0.96	3	5.43	5.37
		1,500		1.53	3	9.8	5.52
		2,000		1.65	4	11.26	6.23
		500		2.14		6.19	4.51
Josamycin		1,000		2.74	0.75	4.2	1.5
	1	400		0.33	0.77	0.91	1.51
	2						
	5	1,000		2.41	0.75	4.9	2
Oleandomycin		1,000		4	1	14	4.2
Midecamycin		400		0.25	0.5	0.34	1
	5	600		0.8	1		
		1,200		1.9	2		
Rokitamycin		600		1.9	0.6	3.7	2
Miokamycin[d]		600		3.01	2	3	1
		400	Mb-12	0.6	0.48	0.73	1.24
			Mb-6	0.17	0.6	0.28	1.47
			Mb-9a	0.16	0.73	0.27	1.45
		800	Mb-12	1.37	0.52	1.72	1.32
			Mb-6	0.44	0.65	0.76	1.71
			Mb-9a	0.4	0.83	1.46	2.34
		800	Mb-12	1.73	0.79	2.59	1.31
			Mb-6	0.66	0.83	1.46	2.34
			Mb-9a	0.57	1.06	1.33	2.09

[a]NA, not available.
[b]14-hydroxyclarithromycin
[c]ND, not determined.
[d]Microbiological assay.

Table 38 Urinary elimination of macrolides

Drug	Dose (mg)	Urinary elimination (%)
Erythromycin A		
Lactobionate	125–900	5.6–17.1
Base	250	6.4
Base (pellet)	250–1,000	5–9
Stearate	1,000	2–7.5
2′-Propionate	1,000	5.5
2′-Acistrate	400	5
Troleandomycin	1,000	15–20
Josamycin	1,000	4.4
Spiramycin	2,000	4.4
Midecamycin	600	3.3
Miokamycin	400–1,200	0.9–4.5
Roxithromycin	300	5–10
Azithromycin	500	~10
Clarithromycin	200–1,200	~30
Flurithromycin	750	3.3
Dirithromycin	500	1–3

the Mb-12 metabolite are linear over the range of doses studied (400 to 1,200 mg). Miokamycin is not found in the circulation after oral administration in humans, but the principal metabolites, such as Mb-12, Mb-9a, and Mb-6, can be assayed. A major interindividual variability is noted.

Erythromycin is released slowly from erythromycin A ethyl succinate after being absorbed. A peak concentration in plasma one-tenth that of the ester appears 4.0 h after absorption of the medication, whereas the ester appears 1.5 h after ingestion (Table 39).

After administration of a single dose of erythromycin A estolate, the plasma circulation consists of 80% 2′-propionate and 20% erythromycin base. After repeated doses of 250 mg of erythromycin A estolate (erythromycin A 2′-propionate dodecyl sulfate), the proportions are the same (Table 40).

Food does not affect the plasma pharmacokinetics of erythromycin A estolate, although this effect is dependent on the pharmaceutical formulation.

Table 39 Pharmacokinetics of erythromycin A ethyl succinate[a]

Drug	C_{max} (μg/ml)	T_{max} (h)	$AUC_{0-\infty}$ (μg·h/ml)
Total erythromycin A ester	0.48	1.5	1.22
Total erythromycin A	0.03	4	0.04

[a]Data from Yakatan et al., 1985. A single dose of 400 mg was used.

Table 40 Pharmacokinetics of erythromycin A estolate[a]

No. of doses (250 mg)	n	Form of drug	C_{max} (μg/ml)	T_{max} (h)	$AUC_{0-\infty}$ (μg·h/ml)
1	8	Base	0.39 ± 0.22	3.6	1.85 ± 1.06
		Estolate	1.66 ± 1.12	2.5	
5	24	Base	1.13 ± 0.37	3	7.37
		Estolate	4.35 ± 1.12	2	

[a]Data from Yakatan et al., 1985.

Using a high-performance liquid chromatographic method with electrochemical detection (limit of detection, 5 ng/ml), the residual concentrations of azithromycin (500 mg on day 1 and 250 mg on the following 4 days) were measured up to 120 h after the last dose (216 h after the first dose).

Residual levels at the limit of quantitation (5.7 ± 1.7 ng/ml [mean ± standard deviation]) were measured 216 h after the first dose. Results are shown in Table 41.

11.2. Intravenous Pharmacokinetics of Macrolides

Few of the macrolides introduced into clinical human practice have pharmaceutical formulations that allow intravenous administration for therapeutic use. They have often been studied in terms of their absolute bioavailability by means of a formulation prepared for this purpose, such as dirithromycin and roxithromycin. There is no parenteral formulation for josamycin, rokitamycin, miokamycin, or midecamycin.

11.2.1. Erythromycin Base

Two salts of erythromycin have been used, the lactobionate and the glucoheptonate.

11.2.1.1. Erythromycin A Lactobionate

Erythromycin A lactobionate is the most widely used parenteral formulation but is poorly tolerated. The mean bioavailability is 35.2% (10.5 to 79.3%) (Table 42).

11.2.1.2. Erythromycin A Glucoheptonate

After intravenous administration to 20 volunteers of 300 mg of erythromycin glucoheptonate dissolved in 10 ml of water for injections for 4 min, the apparent elimination half-life was about 2 h. The concentration at the end of the injection was 40 μg/ml. The concentrations at 2 and 6 h were, respectively, 2.56 and 0.32 μg/ml. Urinary elimination was about 15% (Table 42).

11.2.2. Spiramycin Adipate

The pharmaceutical formulation is spiramycin adipate. Following slow administration of 500 mg of spiramycin adipate, the mean concentration in plasma at the end of the infusion was 2.14 μg/ml, with an area under the curve of 6.19 μg·h/ml and plasma clearance of 84 liters/h. The absolute bioavailability was between 33 and 39%.

11.2.3. Azithromycin

After administration of 500 mg of azithromycin intravenously, the area under the curve was about 10 μg·h/ml, the apparent elimination half-life was 35 to 40 h, and urinary

Table 41 Residual concentrations of azithromycin in plasma after repeated doses[a]

Time after last dose (h)	Global time (h)	Concn in plasma (ng/ml)
0	96	34 ± 3
24	120	40.5 ± 3.4
48	144	26.5 ± 1.1
72	168	18.1 ± 2.5
96	192	10.3 ± 2.3
120	216	5.7 ± 1.7

[a]Data from Fourtillan et al., 1990.

Table 42 Pharmacokinetics of macrolides administered intravenously

Drug	*n*	Dose (mg)	C_0 (μg/ml)	AUC (μg·h/ml)	$t_{1/2\beta}$ (h)	CL_P(liters/h)	CL_R (liters/h)	Urinary elimination (%)
Erythromycin lactobionate	5	125	~10	4.6	1.3	28.1	1.5	5.6
	5	250	10	10.5	1.3	28.9	1.3	4.8
Erythromycin glucoheptonate	4	500	40	19.4	2.4	25.3	2.7	16.3
	3	900	40	41	2.4	26.3	4.4	17.1
								13
Spiramycin adipate	20	300	40					
Dirithromycin							8.6	7.6
Azithromycin	12	500	2.28	8.49	5.54	66.2		
	4	100	1.5	1.4–5.7	16–65	13–64		1.1–2.8
Clarithromycin	12	500	3.87	10.1	52.2	51.2	4	7.9
C 14-OH[a]	20	250	2.8	8.4	2.8	32.1		
			0.8	4.4	5.1	50.8		

[a]C 14-OH, 14-hydroxyclarithromycin.

elimination was 12.2%. The concentration at the end of the infusion was 10 μg/ml, and the bioavailability about 37%. After administration of 1, 2, and 4 g of intravenous azithromycin, the concentrations in plasma at the end of the 2 h of infusion were 3.1, 6.8, and 9.9 μg/ml, with (areas under the curve) of 23.4, 45.6, 82.1 μg·h/ml, respectively.

11.2.4. Dirithromycin

Dirithromycin was administered intravenously in the form of a slow infusion (100 mg). The concentrations in serum at the end of the infusion were between 1.3 and 1.7 μg/ml, with an area under the curve of 1.4 to 5.7 μg·h/ml and a plasma clearance of 13 to 64 liters/h. Urinary elimination was 1.1 to 2.8%. The absolute bioavailability was about 10%.

11.2.5. Clarithromycin

The published results are more sparse and difficult to interpret. Increasing-dose pharmacokinetics have been determined with administration of 75 to 100 mg by infusion. The main metabolite, 14-hydroxyclarithromycin, has a long elimination half-life (5.3 to 9.3 h) compared to that of the parent molecule (2.1 to 4.5 h); conversely, the concentrations in plasma of the metabolite at the end of infusion are one-tenth those obtained with the parent molecule.

Increasing doses have been administered intravenously to healthy volunteers in the form of a slow infusion; results are shown in Table 43.

11.2.6. Roxithromycin

After an infusion of 50 mg over a period of 2 h to 12 healthy subjects, the concentration in plasma was 8.06 μg/ml, with concentrations at 12 h of 1.3 μg/ml and at 48 h of 0.246 μg/ml. The pharmacokinetic parameters were as follows: area under the curve, 53.8 μg·h/ml; half-life, 12.87 h; plasma clearance, 0.97 liter/h; and urinary elimination, 8.3% of the administered dose. For infusion of 100 and 150 mg of roxithromycin, the concentrations in plasma at the end of the 2-h infusion were 7.76 and 10 μg/ml, respectively, with areas under the curve of 81.8 and 125 μg·h/ml, respectively. The total clearance was 1.28 liters/h after a 100-mg infusion.

11.2.7. Bioavailability of Macrolides

The bioavailability of the macrolides is summarized in Table 44.

11.3. Repeated Doses

The administration of repeated doses of macrolides simulates treatment and enables any accumulation of the drug to be studied.

Table 44 Absolute bioavailability of macrolides

Drug	Bioavailability (%)
Erythromycin stearate/lactobionate	35
Spiramycin adipate	36 ± 14
Clarithromycin	47
Azithromycin	37
Dirithromycin	50–60
Roxithromycin	50–60

Table 43 Clarithromycin concentrations in plasma at the end of infusion of increasing doses

Dose (mg)	C_0 (μg/ml)		$t_{1/2}$ (h)	
	Clarithromycin	14-OH[a]	Clarithromycin	14-OH
75	1.25		2.1	
125	1.87	0.21	2.3	7.2
250	4.75	0.47	2.6	5.1
500	6.95	0.83	3.2	7
1,000	9.4	1.06	4.5	9.3

[a]14-OH, 14-hydroxyclarithromycin.

The parameters that best enable the extent of this accumulation to be assessed are the ratio of the residual concentration after the last dose to that obtained after the first dose and the ratio of the areas under the curve after the last and first administrations. In the event of accumulation, elimination is delayed and the apparent elimination half-life is prolonged.

Analysis of the pharmacokinetic parameters after repeated dosing enables the time at which steady state is reached to be determined. The concentrations in plasma at the peak level in serum increase as a function of the multiplication coefficient obtained with the different ratios.

The most frequently published coefficient of accumulation is obtained from the ratio of the areas under the curve and ranges from 1.1 (roxithromycin, 300 mg, repeated doses) to 11.1 (josamycin, repeated doses). The apparent elimination half-life may be prolonged to various degrees. It is prolonged almost sixfold for josamycin, but only by 30% for roxithromycin or 1.5 times for flurithromycin. Steady state is reached with the fourth dose for roxithromycin and the fifth dose for clarithromycin (Table 45).

11.4. Clarithromycin Slow-Release Formulation

After 500 or 1,000 mg of the slow-release formulation of clarithromycin, all of the pharmacokinetic parameters were the same except the time to reach the peak concentration in plasma, which was longer (about 6 h).

The main advantage of these formulations is to have the possibility to administer clarithromycin once a day instead of twice a day with similar clinical efficacy.

11.5. Effect of Food

Food may affect the absorption of macrolides. The changes may be minor, with the maintenance of the relative bioavailability but a delay in the time to the peak concentration in serum and a reduction in its size. Another example is the reduction in relative bioavailability. These changes will govern the dosage regimen of the medication to obtain the optimal effect.

These modifications may be due to physiological changes in the gastrointestinal tract or physical or chemical interactions between the food and the drugs.

The bioavailability of erythromycin A is not significantly affected after administration of food when the drug is administered in the form of the ethyl succinate (area under the curve from 0 h to infinity, 7.48 ± 3.98 μg·versus 4.86 ± 3.28 μg·h/ml [800-mg single dose]) or acistrate. Conversely, it is reduced after ingestion of erythromycin A stearate or erythromycin base in pellet form (Eryc). The bioavailability is not significantly modified after ingestion of clarithromycin, azithromycin, flurithromycin, or miokamycin (Mb-12) (Table 46).

12. PHARMACOKINETICS AT DIFFERENT STAGES OF LIFE

The pharmacokinetics of the drugs may vary with age, particularly in relation to hepatic metabolism (immaturity), digestive absorption, and the state of the renal system.

12.1. Pharmacokinetics in the Elderly Patient

In theory, the category of elderly is reached at the age of 65 years. However, this limit is artificial. The pharmacokinetics may allow the dosage to be modified if the drug is accumulated at a level that might entail a risk of toxicity.

12.1.1. Erythromycin A

One gram of erythromycin A stearate was administered twice daily for 7 days to eight young subjects (26 to 34 years) and to eight elderly subjects (65 to 82 years). The concentrations in plasma were measured by a microbiological method using *Sarcina lutea* ATCC 9341 as the test strain.

The results are reported in Table 47. After seven doses an accumulation of 1.43 (area under the curve) and 1.64 (peak plasma concentration) was noted in the elderly subjects, but not in the young volunteers.

This accumulation is nonlinear and might be due to saturation or inhibition of the enzymatic metabolism of erythromycin A.

The increase in peak concentrations in serum and area under the curve in elderly patients should highlight the potential risk of adverse effects associated with marked accumulation of erythromycin A.

12.1.2. Spiramycin

After slow intravenous administration of 500 mg of spiramycin adipate, the areas under the curve are 2.5 times

Table 45 Macrolides: repeated dose pharmacokinetics

Drug	*n*	Dose (mg)	Administration[a]	Dose no.	C_{min}	RAUC	$t_{1/2}$ first dose (h)	$t_{1/2}$ last dose (h)
Josamycin	6	1,000	8h × 3d	7	12.2 ± 3	11.1 ± 3.9	1	5.8 ± 0.8
Spiramycin		500	8h × 6d	18	2.05	1.6	4.51 ± 0.6	6.25 ± 1.3
Erythromycin base	10	500	8h × 4d	12		2.57		
Azithromycin	14	500	24h × 3d	3		1.99		
	14	500	500 + 250 × 4d	5		2.49		
Clarithromycin	17	250	12h × 3d	5	1.9(1.6)	1.5(1.1)		
	17	250	12h × 5d	7	2.2(1.9)	1.6(1.2)		
Roxithromycin	20	150	12 × 11d	22		1.4	8.3 ± 4.3	12.4
	20	300	24h × 11d	11			10.9 ± 6.5	13.05 ± 6.8
Flurithromycin	12	750	12h × 5d	9		1.41	2.8	4.2
Miokamycin	12	800	12 × 8d	16		1.2(Mb12)	1.24(Mb12)	1.34
						2.1(Mb6)	1.73(Mb6)	
Erythromycin RV-11	19	1,000						2.23
						1.4	5.1	5.2

[a]8h × 3d, every 8h for 3 days; the other expressions for administration follow this model.
[b]R, ratio.

Table 46 Macrolide pharmacokinetics after food

Drug	n	Dose (mg)	Status[a]	C_{max} (μg/ml)	T_{max} (h)	$AUC_{0-\infty}$ (μg·h/ml)
Erythromycin A						
Base (Eryc)		500	Fasting	2.0	3.53	7.08
			Fed	1.65	4.89	5.23
Base (Eryc)	2	333	Fasting	1.36	3.25	4.99
	7		Fed	0.49	5.05	1.87
Stearate			Fasting	3.57	1.28	9.46
		500	Fed	1.65	2.36	4.12
Stearate	1		Fasting	2.09	3.34	4.99
	6	500	Fed	0.3	1.04	1.04
Acistrate	1	400	Fasting	2.23	2.6	12.7
	0	400	Fed	2.7	3.5	12.3
Ethyl succinate	1	800	Fasting	2.71	1.28	7.48
	8	800	Fed	1.54	2.39	4.86
Azithromycin	1	500	Fasting	0.31	2.6	1.4
	0	500	Fed	0.15	3.4	0.8
Dirithromycin		500	Fed	0.24	5.7	1.29
		500	Fasting	0.36	6	1.86
Roxithromycin		150	Fasting	6.6	2.5	76.3
		150	Fed	2.9	7.1	55.2
Clarithromycin	2	500	Fasting	2.51	2	16.18
	6	500	Fasting, 14-OH	0.97	2.1	11.69
			Fed, C	1.65	2.8	13.67
			Fasting, 14-OH	0.88	3	11.18
Flurithromycin	8	500	Fasting	1.51	2.5	5.58
		500	Fed	1.61	1.5	4.86
Miokamycin	1	800	Fasting, Mb-12	1.57	0.54	1.9
	2	800	Fed, Mb-12	1.24	0.29	1.55

[a]C, clarithromycin; Mb-12, main metabolite of miokamycin; 14-OH, 14-OH clarithromycin.

Table 47 Pharmacokinetics of erythromycin A stearate in elderly patients after repeated doses

Dose	Subject group	C_{max} (μg/ml)	T_{max} (h)	$AUC_{0-\infty}$ (μg·h/ml)	$t_{1/2\beta}$ (h)	CL_P/F (liters/h/kg)
1st	Young	8	1.5	2.6	29.1	0.64
	Elderly	13	1.7	4.1	60.9	0.31
7th	Young	6.8	2.0	2.3	25.1	0.69
	Elderly	14.8	2.7	4.8	78.8	0.22

higher than in young subjects, with a prolongation of the apparent elimination half-life from 4.5 to 9.8 h.

After administration of 500 mg three times daily, spiramycin is accumulated in elderly patients in a ratio of 2.9, whereas after the first dose it is 3.2 times higher than in young subjects (Table 48).

Table 48 Pharmacokinetics of spiramycin in elderly subjects after repeated intravenous doses of 500 mg every 8 h for 6 days

Parameter	n	Young	Elderly
C_{max} (μg/ml)	18	2.14 ± 0.32	2.58 ± 0.82
	18	3.10 ± 0.70	4.66 ± 0.79
C_{min} (μg/ml)	18	0.18 ± 0.05	0.57 ± 0.12
	18	0.37 ± 0.12	1.66 ± 0.47
CL_P/F (liters/min)	18	1.42 ± 0.30	0.53 ± 0.14
	18	1.18 ± 0.30	0.44 ± 0.10
$t_{1/2\beta}$ (h)	18	4.3 ± 0.7	9.8 ± 3.2
	18	6.2 ± 1.3	13.5 ± 8.7

12.1.3. Josamycin

There is no change in the bioavailability of josamycin in elderly patients, but the published data are sparse and poorly documented.

12.1.4. Clarithromycin

Comparative pharmacokinetics in 12 young healthy subjects (<30 years) and elderly subjects (>65 years) ingesting 500 mg of clarithromycin every 12 h for 5 days showed that clarithromycin was rapidly absorbed, with absorption coefficients of 1.04 ± 0.41 h^{-1} and 0.80 ± 0.43 h^{-1} in the young and elderly subjects, respectively. The peak concentrations in serum of the parent molecule and the metabolite and the residual concentrations at 12 h (1.69 ± 0.69 μg/ml versus 0.73 ± 0.27 μg/ml) were significantly increased. The area under the curve was significantly increased in elderly patients, but the plasma clearance was reduced (300 ± 97 ml/min versus 476 ± 112 ml/min), as was the renal clearance (84 ± 31 ml/min versus 168 ± 35 ml/min). Rates of

Table 49 Pharmacokinetics of macrolides in elderly patients

Drug	Subject group	Dose (mg)	Route[a]	C_{max} (μg/ml)	T_{max} (h)	$AUC_{0-\infty}$ (μg·h/ml)	$t_{1/2}$ (h)	CL_P (liters/h)
Spiramycin	Young	500	i.v.	2.14		6.7	4.5	32
	Elderly	500	i.v.	2.51		16.7	9.8	84
Josamycin	Young	1,000	p.o.			6.25	1.69	
	Elderly	1,000	p.o.			6.25	3.4	
Miokamycin (Mb-12)	Young	800	p.o.	1.34	0.67	1.92	1.24	
	Elderly	800	p.o.	1.15	0.58	2.52	2.36	
Roxithromycin	Young	300	p.o.	9.7	1.6	122.6	11.2	
	Elderly	300	p.o.	10.8	2.06	197.3	15.5	
Dirithromycin	Young	500	p.o.	0.34	3.90	0.91		
	Elderly	500	p.o.	0.52	4.80	2.42		
Clarithromycin	Young	500	p.o.	2.41		18.9	4.9	
	Elderly	500	p.o.	3.28		30.8	7.7	
14-OH clarithromycin	Young	500	p.o.	0.66			7.2	
	Elderly	500	p.o.	1.33			14.0	
Azithromycin	Young	500	p.o.	0.41	2.5	2.5		
	Elderly	500	p.o.	0.38	3.8	3.0		

[a]i.v., intravenously; p.o., per os.

Table 50 Pharmacokinetics of dirithromycin in elderly patients (dose of 500 mg once a day)

Day	Parameter	Pharmacokinetics by age ($n = 5$):				
		19–50 yr	65–69 yr	70–74 yr	74–80 yr	>80 yr
1	C_{max} (μg/ml)	0.34	0.59	0.45	0.18	0.52
	T_{max} (h)	3.9	3.0	5.25	3.0	4.8
	AUC (μg·h/ml)	0.91	1.82	1.29	0.4	2.42
10	C_{max} (μg/ml)	0.36	0.43	0.48	0.27	0.85
	T_{max} (h)	4.1	3.6	5	3.8	4.8
	AUC (μg·h/ml)	1.83	2.57	1.81	1.12	4.3

urinary elimination of the parent molecule were similar in the two groups (30.4% ± 12.8% versus 36.2% ± 7%). The pharmacokinetics of the principal metabolite were parallel to those of the parent molecule (Table 49).

12.1.5. Azithromycin

The pharmacokinetics of azithromycin were studied in 12 young subjects (22 to 39 years) and 12 elderly subjects (67 to 80 years). Following repeated oral administration of 500 mg on the first day and 250 mg daily for 4 days, the pharmacokinetics of azithromycin were little altered in the elderly subjects (Table 49).

12.1.6. Dirithromycin

The pharmacokinetics of dirithromycin after a single dose or repeated doses (10 days) of 500 mg daily were studied in a population of elderly subjects. They were divided into four groups according to their age range (Table 50). There were no major differences between the four groups. However, marked interindividual variability was observed.

12.1.7. Roxithromycin

A single dose of 300 mg was administered orally to elderly and young subjects as well as dose of 150 mg every 12 h for 6 days. The apparent elimination half-life was unaffected. The area under the curve was increased, but it remained within the limits of those found at steady state in young subjects (Table 51).

12.2. Pharmacokinetics in Children

Specific pharmacokinetic studies are required in children because of the continuous change in body weight and the distribution of extravascular water, the hepatic immaturity, the lower protein binding levels, and even the immaturity of the kidneys.

12.2.1. Erythromycin A

Various pharmacokinetic studies have been undertaken with erythromycin base, erythromycin ethyl succinate, and erythromycin estolate in children during fasting or after a meal; results are shown in Table 52.

12.2.2. Oleandomycin

Oleandomycin has been used therapeutically in the form of triacetyloleandomycin. Begué et al. (1981) administered a single dose of 50 mg of triacetyloleandomycin per kg of body

Table 51 Pharmacokinetics of roxithromycin in elderly subjects

Parameter	Single dose (300 mg)	Multiple doses (150 mg every 12 h for 6 days)
$t_{1/2}$ (h)	26.7 ± 3.0	27.2 ± 3.5
AUC (mg·h/ml)	148 ± 27(0–60 h)	83 ± 10(0–12 h)
CL_R (0–8 h) (liters/h)	0.06 ± 0.01	0.26 ± 0.07

Table 52 Pharmacokinetics of erythromycin in children

Erythromycin form or patient status	n	Age	Dose (mg/kg)	C_{max} (μg/ml)	T_{max} (h)	AUC (μg·h/ml)	$t_{1/2}$ (h)
Base	ND[a]		15	3.4	2–3		
Ethyl succinate	6	Neonate	10	1.1 ± 0.5	1.8	6.32 ± 0.63	2.26 ± 0.4
After food	11	19 mo	15	1.4 ± 0.6	1.0	4.8	1.7
Fasting	18	19 mo	15	0.82 ± 0.7	1.0	2.4	1.4
	26	1.5 days	10	1.5	1.0	15.1	4.2
	ND	15 days	10	2.0	3.0	18.3	4.5
Estolate	6	1 mo	10	1.6 ± 0.6	2.7 ± 0.4	17.2 ± 4.9	4.0
Fed	20	19 mo	10	4.8 ± 2.5	2.0	40	5.1
Fasting	1	19 mo	10	4.7 ± 2.9	2.0	45	3.5

[a]ND, not disclosed.

weight to 28 children suffering from respiratory tract infections and 1 suffering from pyoderma.

The levels in plasma were measured in 20 children and were, respectively, 2.13 ± 1.44 μg/ml, 1.04 ± 0.95 μg/ml, and 0.32 ± 0.44 μg/ml at 2, 4, and 8 h, with an apparent elimination half-life of 2.35 h.

12.2.3. Roxithromycin

Several pharmacokinetic studies have been conducted with children and are summarized in Table 53.

12.2.4. Sixteen-Membered-Ring Macrolides

Apparently no report had been issued on the pharmacokinetics of spiramycin or midecamycin in children.

The pharmacokinetics of josamycin propionate were determined by Del Mastro (1984). Those of rokitamycin were established in neonates (Table 54).

12.2.5. Clarithromycin

Twenty-four children aged 0.5 to 10 years received a single dose or repeated doses (every 12 h for 4 to 5 days) of 7.5 mg of clarithromycin per kg in the form of a suspension prepared from granules for reconstitution (125 ml/5 ml). The single dose was administered before or after food.

After a single dose, the pharmacokinetics were similar to those observed in adults with the same pharmaceutical formulation. After multiple doses, the ratio of the areas under the curve after the last and first administrations were 1.6 for clarithromycin and 1.8 for 14-hydroxyclarithromycin.

Food (potato purée) did not significantly affect the bioavailability of clarithromycin or its principal metabolite. There was a major interindividual variation in the concentrations in plasma. The lag time was longer than in adults (Table 55).

Thirteen low-body-weight neonates received 15 or 30 mg of clarithromycin per kg. The neonates included in this study were born after 27 ± 1 week of gestation and had been delivered between 11 and 36 days previously.

The apparent elimination half-life was higher than in adults. The results are summarized in Table 56. A marked interindividual variation may be noted.

Thirty-one children aged 2 to 12 years received clarithromycin in the form of a suspension of 7.5 mg/kg every 12 h for 7 days. These children suffered from chronic otitis necessitating the insertion of grommets.

It was possible to obtain plasma and middle ear effusion fluid from 24 children on day 5 and 2.5 h after drug administration. The results are listed in Table 57.

Table 53 Pharmacokinetics of roxithromycin in children

Study	Patient age	n	Dose (mg/kg)	C_{max} (μg/ml)	T_{max} (h)	AUC (μg·h/ml)	$t_{1/2}$ (h)
Bégué et al.	1–12 mo	8	2.5	4.77 ± 0.5	1.8	43.5 ± 7.7	14.6 ± 4.8
	1–12 mo	9	5	14.9 ± 2.9	2.6	97.9 ± 17.4	10.4 ± 2.4
	1–8 yr	7	2.5	5.9 ± 1.5	2.0	49 ± 11	9.0 ± 1.5
Demotes-Mainard et al.	1–18 mo	5	2.5	10.1 ± 3.0	1.3	61.5 ± 22.5	19.8 ± 9.7
	1.5–5 yr	7	2.5	8.7 ± 4.9	1.6	57.6 ± 31.8	21 ± 1.4
	5–13 yr	6	2.5	8.9 ± 7.0	1.6	62.9 ± 51.7	20.8 ± 6.9
Boccazi et al.	10 mo–13 yr	8	5	9.1 ± 1.1	1.0	60.9 ± 19	15.7 ± 2.1
	1–12 yr	16	10	14.5 ± 2.9	1.5	100.6 ± 20.8	14.6 ± 1.7

Table 54 Pharmacokinetics of 16-membered-ring macrolides in children

Drug	n	Patient age	Dose (mg/kg)	C_{max} (μg/ml)	T_{max} (h)	AUC (μg·h/ml)	$t_{1/2}$ (h)
Josamycin propionate			14.3	0.86 ± 0.3	2.0	2.88	1.03
			14.3 every 12 h for 4 days	2.14 ± 0.6	2.0	1.7	1.24
Rokitamycin	8	<1 mo	10	0.78	0.5	1.21	1.0
Miokamycin (Mb-12)	3		5	0.09			0.8
	3		10	0.33			0.7

Table 55 Pharmacokinetics of clarithromycin in children

Patient status and dosing	n	Drug[a]	C_{max} (μg/ml)	T_{max} (h)	$AUC_{0-\infty}$ (μg·h/ml)
Fasting, single dose	10	C	3.59 ± 1.47	3.1 ± 1.0	10 ± 5.49
	10	M	1.19 ± 0.37	3.2 ± 1.0	3.66 ± 1.49
Fed, single dose	10	C	4.58 ± 2.76	2.8 ± 0.7	14.2 ± 9.39
	10	M	1.26 ± 0.46	4.0 ± 1.0	4.37 ± 1.79
Fasting, multiple doses	10	C	4.60 ± 2.08	2.8 ± 1.0	15.7 ± 6.72
	10	M	1.64 ± 0.75	2.7 ± 1.7	6.69 ± 2.97

[a]C, clarithromycin; M, metabolite.

Table 56 Pharmacokinetics of clarithromycin in low-body-weight neonates

n	Length of pregnancy (wks)	Wt of neonates (mg)	No. of days after birth	Dose (mg/kg)	C_{max} (μg/ml)	AUC (μg·h/ml)	T_{max} (h)	$t_{1/2}$ (h)	k_{el} (h^{-1})
8	27 ± 2	995 ± 266	19 ± 9	15	0.6 ± 0.51	3.66 ± 3.2	3.2 ± 1.8	11.4 ± 10.9	0.1
5	27 ± 1	1,077 ± 233	25 ± 11	30	1.6 ± 0.6	8.95 ± 4.3	3.1 ± 1.9	6.3 ± 4.4	0.1

Table 57 Concentrations of clarithromycin in plasma and middle ear fluid

Drug	Concn (μg/ml) in:	
	Plasma	MEF[a]
Clarithromycin	1.73 ± 1.21	2.53 ± 2.31
14-OH clarithromycin	0.82 ± 0.32	1.27 ± 0.99

[a]MEF, middle ear fluid.

The concentrations of clarithromycin and 14(*R*)-hydroxyclarithromycin were measured in the middle ear pus of 32 children aged 0.5 to 12 years suffering from otitis media after administration of 7.5 mg of a suspension of clarithromycin per kg every 12 h for 3 days (steady state, 3 days).

The concentrations in plasma and middle ear pus were determined 2, 4, and 24 h after administration of the last dose.

In 60% of patients (19 of 32), the middle ear pus had dried up by the sixth administration.

At 2 h, the concentrations in plasma of clarithromycin and those in the middle ear fluid were similar, but the concentrations were greater at 4, 8, and 12 h, reaching a plateau at 4 h in the middle ear fluid. Those of the metabolite were from the outset higher at 2 h (2.32 versus 1.34 μg/ml) (Table 58).

12.2.6. Azithromycin

Azithromycin suspension was administered in the form of a single dose of 12 mg/kg to 13 children and in repeated doses for 5 days to 8 children; results are shown in Table 59.

Azithromycin was administered to 14 children in the form of a suspension in repeated doses for 5 days with the following dosage regimen: one loading dose on the first day (10 mg/kg) followed by 5 mg/kg for 4 days.

After the last dose, the peak concentration in serum was 0.38 ± 0.14 μg/ml and was reached in 2.5 ± 1.1 h. The area under the curve was 3.11 ± 1.03 μg·h/ml.

Table 59 Repeated-dose pharmacokinetics of azithromycin in children

Dose	n	C_{max} (μg/ml)	T_{max} (h)	$t_{1/2}$ (h)	CL/F (liters/kg/h)
1	13	3.5	2.4	49.7	4.2
5	8	3.6	2.4	69.8	5.8

Table 58 Pharmacokinetics of clarithromycin in middle ear fluid

Drug	Sampling time (h)	n	Concn in plasma (μg/ml)	n	Concn in MEF[a] (μg/ml)
Clarithromycin	2	7	2.93 ± 2.76	2	3.02
	4	1	3.42 ± 1.44	5	8.3 ± 2.48
	8	4	1.11 ± 0.66	0	
	12	7	0.68 ± 0.44	4	7.38 ± 3.81
14-OH clarithromycin	2	7	1.34 ± 1.14	1	2.52
	4	1	1.77 ± 0.5	4	2.89 ± 0.78
	8	4	0.83 ± 0.19	1	1.49
	12	7	0.85 ± 0.43	4	3.77 ± 1.28

[a]MEF, middle ear fluid.

The residual concentrations 24, 48, and 72 h after the last dose were, respectively, 0.07 ± 0.03 μg/ml, 0.06 ± 0.02 μg/ml, and 0.03 ± 0.01 μg/ml.

12.2.7. Distributions in the Middle Ear Fluid (Effusion)

The concentrations in plasma of other macrolides and those in the effusion fluids of patients with serous otitis or in pus from patients with acute otitis are presented in Table 60.

12.2.8 Distribution of Macrolides in Tonsils and Saliva

12.2.8.1. Concentrations in Tonsils

Table 61 shows concentrations of macrolides and ketolides in tonsils.

12.2.8.2. Concentrations in Saliva

Therapeutic concentrations of antibiotics maintained throughout the day would be considered beneficial for treatment of pharyngitis. However, as it was noted for penicillin V eliminated in saliva at concentrations well in excess of the MIC for viridans group streptococci, maintaining these concentrations could contribute to the disturbance of the oral flora, which is a potential factor of selection of resistant mutants.

Table 62 shows concentrations of macrolides and ketolides in saliva. In volunteers receiving telithromycin, the mean peak concentrations in plasma and saliva were 2.35 μg/ml (range, 1.46 to 3.74 μg/ml) and 3.05 μg/ml (range, 1.49 to 5.39 μg/ml), respectively, 24 h after the first administration. The residual concentrations at 24 h were 0.01 and 0.07 μg/ml in plasma and saliva, respectively. The areas under the curve at 24 h were 9.27 and 15.6 μg·h/ml in plasma and saliva, respectively. The ratio of the areas under the curve in saliva and plasma was 1.7. On day 10 the ratio was 1.6. In volunteers receiving clarithromycin, the mean peak concentrations in plasma and saliva were 2.98 μg/ml (range, 1.74 to 4.94 μg/ml) and 2.38 μg/ml (range, 0.78 to 4.58 μg/ml), respectively, 24 h after the first administration. At 24 h, clarithromycin was not detected in plasma and saliva. The areas under the curve at 10 h were 18.1 and 13.3 μg·h/ml in plasma and saliva, respectively. The ratio between the areas under the curve in saliva and plasma was 0.7. On day 10 the ratio was 1.0. In the clarithromycin group the concentrations in plasma and saliva were similar on days 1 and 10. After administration of 500 mg of azithromycin once daily for three consecutive days, important concentrations of azithromycin could be detected for up to 6.5 days in saliva.

The plasma/saliva concentration ratio ranged from 0.21 to 0.30 after administration of erythromycin acistrate (400 mg three times a day). The degree of hydrolysis of 2′-acetyl erythromycin was higher in saliva (61 to 78%) than in plasma (27 to 41%). In plasma, the percentage of hydrolysis was inversely correlated with the concentration of acid α_1-glycoprotein. The antibiotic concentration was clearly higher in plasma than in saliva.

For dirithromycin, the concentrations achieved after repeated doses of 500 mg are low, 0 to 1.4 μg/ml and 0 to 0.088 μg/ml in plasma and saliva, respectively, and individual variations are important.

13. PHARMACOKINETICS IN PATHOLOGICAL PREDISPOSITIONS

13.1. Hepatic Insufficiency

With the exception of clarithromycin, macrolides are eliminated mainly by the hepatobiliary route. They are also dependent on the concentration in plasma of α_1-glycoproteins, to which they are bound (Table 63).

The pharmacokinetics of these drugs may be altered, particularly in patients with hepatic insufficiency (grade C of the Child-Pugh classification).

13.1.1. Erythromycin A

Barré et al. (1987) studied the pharmacokinetic parameters of erythromycin A lactobionate in five cirrhotic patients (Child-Pugh grades B and C) and six healthy volunteers. These subjects received 500 mg of erythromycin base by infusion for 30 min. The levels in plasma were measured by a microbiological method using *S. lutea* as the test strain (limit of detection, 0.07 μg/ml).

The mean apparent elimination half-life was prolonged in the cirrhotic patients (2.24 ± 0.89 h versus 1.36 ± 0.43 h). The free fraction was greater in the cirrhotic patients (58.3% ± 17.7%) than in the healthy volunteers (30.5 ± 2.8%),

Table 60 Distribution of macrolides in the middle ear fluid (or effusion)

Drug	Doses (mg/kg)	Concn (μg/ml) in: Plasma	Concn (μg/ml) in: MEF[a]
Erythromycin			
Ethyl succinate	12.5 (4 doses)	0.45–2.0	0.24–1.02
	15–20 (3 doses)	0.5–4.2	0.1–11
	15	1.55	0.6
Estolate	12.5 (4 doses)	4.15–12.3	1.68–>8.0
	15	1.0	0.6–1.0
	10		0.6–5.2
Josamycin	25[b]	0.55 ± 0.3	1.2 ± 1.8
	25[c]	1.9 ± 1.6	0.9 ± 0.7
	25[d]	0.4 ± 0.3	1.8 ± 3.4
Roxithromycin	2.5 every 12 h (2 doses)	0.58 ± 0.06	0.9 ± 0.2

[a]MEF, middle ear fluid.
[b]Acute otitis.
[c]Chronic otitis.
[d]Serous otitis.

Table 61 Macrolide and ketolide concentrations in tonsils[a]

Compound	Dose	*n*	Sampling time (h)	Concn (mg/kg or μg/ml) in:	
				Plasma	Tissue
Erythromycin					
Estolate	125 mg SD	5	4–6	0.28–5.10	0.16–2.6
	125 mg MD	5	4–6	0.48–3.8	0.34–1.2
Ethyl succinate	100 mg MD	20	2	2.8 ± 0.13	3.39 ± 0.28
		20	3	2.4 ± 0.12	2.72 ± 0.23
		20	4	1.44 ± 0.13	1.98 ± 0.12
Stearate	500 mg t.i.d. MD	12	3.5	1.32 ± 0.95	0.72 ± 0.58
Base	30 mg/kg MD	10	3	2.46–7.9	0.91–7.10
	500 mg t.i.d. MD	12	4	1.78 ± 1.41	0.86 ± 1.06
Acistrate	500 mg MD, EA	14	3–8	5.79 ± 2.08	2.87 ± 2.11
	500 mg MD, E		3–8	2.16 ± 0.89	1.36 ± 0.91
Oleandomycin triacetylate	1,000 mg MD	12	2.5–3.5	1.41	4.09
	50 mg/kg	35	2–3	2.27	12.2
Roxithromycin	5 mg/kg + 2.5 mg/kg MD	17	6	2.23 ± 0.32	R 2.91 ± 0.29
		17	6	2.23 ± 0.32	L 2.87 ± 0.64
	5 mg/kg SD	18	1	4.9 ± 1.1	6.0 ± 1.0
		18	2	6.6 ± 1.55	6.0 ± 1.0
		18	4	4.71 ± 1.36	6.0 ± 1.0
	5 mg/kg SD	18	6	2.71 ± 0.41	6.0 ± 1.0
		18	12	1.60 ± 0.22	6.0 ± 1.0
	5 mg/kg MD	10	4	5.6 ± 1.9	4.63 ± 0.97
Clarithromycin	250 mg MD	60	1	1.36 ± 0.48	1.88 ± 0.35
			2	1.82 ± 0.46	3.76 ± 1.98
			4	1.14 ± 0.32	6.74 ± 3.83
			6	0.70 ± 0.21	5.48 ± 2.5
			8	0.26 ± 0.11	4.16 ± 1.51
			12	0.12 ± 0.04	2.6 ± 0.65
Flurithromycin	500 mg MD	11	4	0.67 ± 0.13	L 1.32 ± 0.21
		11	4	0.67 ± 0.13	R 1.43 ± 0.20
Dirithromycin	500 mg MD	11	4	0.18	3.6
		11	15	0.08	1.8
		15	24	NS	1.37 ± 0.55
	500 mg MD, 5 days	8	13	0.20 ± 0.07	4.62 ± 0.97
	500 mg MD, 10 days	4	14	0.17 ± 0.10	3.47 ± 2.84
Azithromycin	10 mg/kg MD		12–204	0.13 ± 0.027	12.1 ± 4.5
	20 mg/kg MD		12–204	0.13 ± 0.027	12.1 ± 4.5
	250 mg (2 doses)	5	13	0.03	4.5
		5	23	0.01	3.9
		8	59	0.01	4.3
	250 mg (2 doses)	3	83	0.006	2.5
		3	178	0.006	0.93
	10 mg/kg SD	4	24	0.047 ± 0.001	10.33 ± 3.9
		5	48	0.014 ± 0.0008	7.21 ± 4.04
		6	96	0.008 ± 0.002	9.3 ± 3.74
		5	192	0.004	1.49 ± 0.48
Spiramycin	50, 75, and 100 mg/kg MD	9	12–84	NS	8–78
	3,000 mg MD	4	12	NS	21.5–40
Josamycin	500 mg SD	30	4	0.76 ± 0.22	21.24 ± 6.5
		20	4	1.81 ± 0.06	13.62 ± 2.7
		10	3	0.4 ± 0.1	3.1 ± 0.7
		23	1	2.8 ± 0.29	14.7 ± 5.05
Miokamycin	600 mg SD	36	1–6	NS	3.9 ± 0.8
	600 mg MD	20	2	1.3 ± 0.33	3.2 ± 0.82
			4	0.5 ± 0.14	1.75 ± 0.31
			6	0.35 ± 0.13	0.52 ± 0.19
			8	0.13 ± 0.06	0.3 ± 0.08
			12	ND	0.12 ± 0.05

(Continued on next page)

Table 61 Macrolide and ketolide concentrations in tonsils[a] *(Continued)*

Compound	Dose	*n*	Sampling time (h)	Concn (mg/kg or μg/ml) in:	
				Plasma	Tissue
Rokitamycin	600 mg SD	2	0.5	0.5	≤0.04
		2	0.75	0.5	≤0.04
		2	1.0	1.24	0.86
		2	1.5	0.71	0.55
		2	2	0.67	0.43
		1	4	0.14	0.13
Telithromycin	800 mg SD	6	3	1.24 ± 0.29	3.95 ± 0.5
			12	0.23 ± 0.32	0.88 ± 0.5
		8	24	0.06 ± 0.01	0.72 ± 0.29

[a]NS, nonspecified; SD, single dose; MD, multiple doses; ND, nondetectable; EA, erythromycin acistrate; E, erythromycin; t.i.d., three times a day.

Table 62 Concentrations of macrolides and ketolides in saliva

Compound	Dose and patient status	*n*	Sampling time (h)	Concn (μg/ml) in:	
				Plasma	Saliva
Erythromycin					
Estolate	10 mg/kg, fed, NS	18	2–4	4.7 ± 2.0	≥0.1
	10 mg/kg, fasting, NS	20	2–4	4.8 ± 2.5	≥0.1
Ethyl succinate	15 mg/kg, fed, NS	18	2–4	0.82 ± 0.66	0.1–1.0
	15 mg/kg, fasting, NS	11	2–4	1.4 ± 0.64	0.1–1.0
Propionate	7.5 mg/kg SD	8	2	4.07 ± 0.29	0.84 ± 0.09
Stearate	7.5 mg/kg SD	8	2	2.15 ± 0.14	0.57 ± 0.08
Base	200 mg SD, i.m.	20	1	1.11	1.11
			2	1.19	1.01
			3	0.96	1.29
Roxithromycin	300 mg + 150 mg (3 doses)	24	1–12	6.12 ± 1.94	0.67 ± 0.12
Clarithromycin	300 mg SD	3	2.5	1.49	1.93
	500 mg b.i.d., 1 day	10	24	2.98	2.38
	500 mg b.i.d., 10 days	10	24	3.87	4.29
Dirithromycin	500 mg o.d., 2 days	20	24	0.10 ± 0.20	0.09 ± 0.16
	500 mg o.d., 3 days		24	0.14 ± 0.07	0.16 ± 0.13
	500 mg o.d., 4 days		24	0.20 ± 0.30	0.23 ± 0.25
	500 mg o.d., 5 days		24	0.27 ± 0.32	0.18 ± 0.20
	500 mg o.d., 7 days		24	0.27 ± 0.34	0.26 ± 0.26
Azithromycin	500 mg MD	28	12	NS	2.14 ± 0.3
Josamycin	1,500 mg + 500 mg MD	4	NS	2.61	1.03 ± 0.43
Spiramycin	1,000 mg (2 doses) MD	6	3	1.6 ± 0.5	1.4 ± 0.5
	1,500 mg MD	3	NS	2.4–4.3	3.1–6.9
	2,000 mg MD	3	NS	2.1–4.0	5.1–13
	3,000 mg MD	3	NS	2.3–4.0	9.6–14
Rokitamycin	400 mg NS	5	1	3.14 ± 1.04	0.3
Telithromycin	800 mg, 1 day	10	24	2.35	3.04
	800 mg, 10 days	10	24	2.03	3.06

[a]SD, single dose; MD, multiple doses; NS, nonspecified; i.m., intramuscular; o.d., every day.

probably because of the marked reduction in the level of circulating α_1-glycoproteins.

Plasma clearance was reduced in these patients (24.2 ± 8.3 liters/h versus 34.2 ± 12.1 liters/h). Clearance of the free fraction was reduced still further (42.2 ± 10.1 liters/h versus 113.2 ± 44.2 liters/h), as was nonrenal clearance of the free fraction (31.6 ± 7.5 liters/h versus 98.6 ± 41.5 liters/h), but renal clearance of the free fraction was unchanged (11.2 ± 5.5 liters/h versus 14.5 ± 4.1 liters/h).

13.1.2. Clarithromycin

The pharmacokinetics of clarithromycin and its principal metabolite, 14-hydroxyclarithromycin, were studied with alcoholic patients suffering from various degrees of hepatic insufficiency (Child-Pugh grades B and C). In grade B and C patients, there was a significant modification of the pharmacokinetic parameters of the parent molecule and its principal metabolite. The apparent elimination half-life increased, whereas the ratios of the peak concentrations in serum and the areas under the curve of the parent molecule and the metabolite decreased significantly.

13.1.3. Azithromycin

The pharmacokinetics of azithromycin were investigated after administration of a single dose of 500 mg orally to 6 healthy volunteers, 10 patients with grade A hepatic insufficiency, and

6 patients with Child-Pugh grade B. Results are shown in Table 64. The pharmacokinetic parameters were not significantly modified.

13.1.4. Roxithromycin

The pharmacokinetics of roxithromycin were studied in 12 healthy volunteers and 10 cirrhotic patients (Pugh grades 9 to 11) after a single dose of 150 mg orally.

Table 63 Protein binding of macrolides

Drug	Protein binding (%)
Erythromycin	60–90
Roxithromycin	73–96
Clarithromycin	42–70
Azithromycin	37
Dirithromycin	19
Josamycin	15
Spiramycin	73–95
Midecamycin	40–48
Miokamycin	47
Mb-12	13
Mb-9a	3
Mb-6	7
Mb-1	29
Mb-5	9
Mb-2	25
Rokitamycin	74

The apparent elimination half-life was prolonged (10.5 ± 1.4 h versus 25.2 ± 1.9 h), as was the renal clearance (Table 65).

13.1.5. Dirithromycin

Sixteen patients suffering from chronic hepatitis or a hepatobiliary condition (Child-Pugh grade A) received 500 mg of dirithromycin orally once daily for 10 days.

The apparent elimination half-life was prolonged to 51.8 and 74.7 h, respectively, in patients with parenchymatous and hepatobiliary lesions, compared to 42 h in healthy volunteers. The peak levels in serum and the areas under the curve were reduced compared to those in healthy volunteers.

In 11 cirrhotic patients (Child-Pugh grades A and B), Mazzei et al. (1993) showed that the apparent half-life was prolonged, the peak concentration in serum was increased, and the plasma clearance was decreased (Table 66).

13.1.6. Josamycin

The pharmacokinetics of a single oral dose of 1,250 mg of josamycin in 5 patients with hepatic insufficiency were studied in comparison with those of 14 healthy volunteers.

The peak concentration in serum was higher in the healthy volunteers than in the subjects with hepatic insufficiency (6.87 versus 1.66 μg/ml), but the apparent elimination half-lives were identical. In two patients with obstruction of the biliary tract, the elimination of josamycin was reduced.

The pharmacokinetics of josamycin were modified in severely cirrhotic patients, with a prolongation of the apparent elimination half-life (5.36 versus 1.05 h) after single and repeated doses of 1.0 g.

Table 64 Pharmacokinetics of azithromycin in patients with hepatic insufficiency

Subjects	n	C_{max} (μg/ml)	T_{max} (h)	AUC (μg·h/ml)	$t_{1/2}$ (h)	Urinary elimination (%)
Healthy volunteers	6	0.29	3.0	4.9	53	11
Hepatic impairment grade A	10	0.39	2.8	4.8	61	12
Hepatic impairment grade B	6	0.51	2.2	4.0	68	16

Table 65 Pharmacokinetics of roxithromycin in patients with hepatic insufficiency

Subjects	n	C_{max} (μg/ml)	T_{max} (h)	AUC_{0-72} (μg·h/ml)	$t_{1/2}$ (h)	U_{0-72h}[a] (mg)	CL_R (ml/min)
Healthy volunteers	12	7.9 ± 0.7	1.9	81 ± 10	10.5 ± 1.4	17.4	3.63 ± 0.4
Hepatically impaired patients	10	5.8 ± 1.4	2.1	118 ± 29	25.2 ± 1.9	28.1	7.0 ± 2.0

[a]U, urinary elimination.

Table 66 Pharmacokinetics of dirithromycin in patients with hepatic insufficiency

Subjects	n	Day	C_{max} (μg/ml)	T_{max} (h)	$t_{1/2}$ (h)	AUC_{0-24} (μg·h/ml)	CL_P (liters/kg)	CL_R (liters/kg)	CL_{NR} (liters/kg)
Healthy volunteers	5	1	0.39	5.0	10	1.56	5.51	0.06	5.45
	5	10	0.69	4.8	42	6.45	1.91	0.04	1.87
Patients with hepatic insufficiency									
Parenchymatous	8	1	0.48	6.3	14.4	3.11	5.11	0.05	2.86
	8	10	0.34	5.3	51.8	4.05	2.10	0.04	2.05
Hepatobiliary diseases	8	1	0.83	3.8	14.4	4.48	3.41	0.02	1.13
	8	10	0.78	3.5	74.7	6.60	1.17	0.03	1.4

13.1.7. Miokamycin

Miokamycin was administered at a dose of 900 mg to six healthy volunteers and six cirrhotic patients. The plasma assays were performed by a microbiological method using a test strain, *S. lutea* ATCC 9341. The peak concentration in serum was increased, as was the area under the curve. However, these results are difficult to interpret, as the relationships between the severity of the hepatic insufficiency and the metabolites were unknown (Table 67).

13.2. Patients with Renal Insufficiency

The macrolides are eliminated by the hepatobiliary route, and only clarithromycin is significantly eliminated via the kidneys.

In patients with a creatinine clearance of less than 30 ml/min, the pharmacokinetic parameters of clarithromycin are modified and necessitate a dosage adjustment. A loading dose of 500 mg is followed by a maintenance dose of 250 mg every 12 h.

It has been shown that renal clearance of dirithromycin is modified in patients with a creatinine clearance of less than 20 ml/min; dirithromycin is not hemodialyzable.

The concentrations in plasma are higher in patients with renal insufficiency (15.7 ± 1.4 μg/ml) than in healthy volunteers after a dose of 150 mg of roxithromycin.

This elevation might be due to the sharp reduction in α_1-glycoprotein levels in this category of subjects. The lack of correlation between total clearance and creatinine clearance and the major interindividual variations of the pharmacokinetics in these patients mean that no dosage modification is recommended.

13.3 Ileostomy

Twelve patients having an ileostomy for more than a month were given either a 1-h infusion of 500 mg or a 500-mg capsule. The percentages of recovery in the ileostomy bag were 15.2% (including degradation products) and 62% (including 15.1% degradation products) after intravenous and oral administration, respectively. The azithromycin clearance in the ileostomy bag was 9.5 liters/h (plasma clearance, 46.6 liters/h).

14. RECTAL PHARMACOKINETICS

A pharmacokinetic study comparing erythromycin base (250 mg) administered orally and rectally was conducted by Pozzi et al. (1982).

The peak concentration in serum was lower (0.9 μg/ml) and appeared more rapidly after rectal administration than after administration by the oral route, with a 30% smaller area under the curve (Table 68).

When erythromycin base was administered rectally in the form of a solution (12.5 ml of a 40-mg/ml solution) for 5 min to six healthy volunteers, the mean bioavailability of a dose of 500 mg was about 3.2% (0.2% to 19.4%). The peak concentration in serum was 0.111 μg/ml, and the area under the curve was 0.319 μg·h/ml, compared to a concentration of 3.993 μg/ml at the end of a 60-min infusion and an area under the curve of 10 μg·h/ml.

Azithromycin was administered intravenously, orally, duodenally, or ileocecally to 11 volunteers (dose, 500 mg). The mean bioavailability when azithromycin was given orally was 0.438 ± 0.107, as opposed to 0.499 ± 0.09 and 0.367 ± 0.123 when the drug was given duodenally and ileocecally, respectively (Table 69).

15. METABOLISM

The macrolides are metabolized to various degrees in the liver. The metabolites may or may not have antibacterial activity. The most extensively metabolized molecule is miokamycin, with 13 metabolites, and the least metabolized are roxithromycin and azithromycin.

15.1. Metabolism of Erythromycin A Derivatives

It is important to stress one point: the products of hepatic metabolism and the degradation products due to instability in an acidic medium should not be confused.

The degradation products in an acidic medium are the hemiketal and spiroketal derivatives of erythromycin A, products having lost the L-cladinose (descladinose roxithromycin,

Table 67 Pharmacokinetics of miokamycin in cirrhotic patients

Subjects	*n*	Dose (mg)	C_{max} (μg/ml)	T_{max} (h)	AUC (μg·h/ml)	$t_{1/2}$ (h)
Healthy volunteers	6	900	0.28	0.83	0.48	1.18
Cirrhotic patients	6	900	0.93	0.75	1.75	1.78

Table 68 Rectal pharmacokinetics of erythromycin base

Form	Dose (mg)	C_{max} (μg/ml)	C_{6h} (μg/ml)	C_{8h} (μg/ml)	T_{max} (h)	$AUC_{0-\infty}$ (μg·h/ml)
Oral	250	1.06	0.59	0.26	3.50	4.14
Suppository	250	0.9	0.2	ND[a]	2.17	3.29

[a]ND, not determined.

Table 69 Gastrointestinal bioavailability of azithromycin

Route	C_{max} (μg/ml)	T_{max} (h)	AUC (μg·h/ml)	F
Intravenous	2.82 ± 0.51	0.8	8.14 ± 1.77	
Oral	0.347 ± 0.095	1.9	3.58 ± 1.22	0.438 ± 0.107
Duodenal	0.842 ± 0.328	1.2	4.02 ± 0.96	0.499 ± 0.091
Ileocecal	0.407 ± 0.426	0.7	3.04 ± 1.46	0.367 ± 0.123

clarithromycin, or azithromycin), or pseudoclarithromycin, which has no antibacterial activity.

Roxithromycin is only weakly metabolized, with less than 5% being found in the urine, involving the mono- and amino-didemethyldesosamine.

Among the derivatives of erythromycin A, the most extensively metabolized molecule is clarithromycin. Eight metabolites have been described (M-1 to M-8) (Fig. 33).

The principal metabolite is the M-5 metabolite, which is 14-hydroxyclarithromycin. It possesses activity comparable to that of the parent molecule. 14-Hydroxyclarithromycin may be eliminated in the form of two epimers, (*R*) and (*S*). The (*R*) epimer has activity comparable to that of clarithromycin, whereas the (*S*) epimer is four to eight times less active than the parent molecule (Table 70).

The M-1 metabolite (N-demethyl) accounts for 1.9% of the metabolites eliminated in the urine.

The M-4 metabolite is a degradation product: descladinose clarithromycin.

Azithromycin is metabolized in the liver, but few metabolites are found in the urine. The principal metabolites are 3′-*N*-demethylazithromycin and 9a-*N*-demethylazithromycin (Table 71).

The distribution of the main identified metabolites of azithromycin is given in Table 72. There are 10 biliary metabolites (B to K).

The most extensively metabolized molecule is miokamycin. More than 13 metabolites have been described (Fig. 34 and Fig. 35).

Miokamycin is not found in the blood circulation. The metabolites Mb-12, Mb-6, and Mb-9a are the most important quantitatively. Mb-12, Mb-6, and Mb-9a exert 84, 38, and 21% of the antibacterial activity of the parent molecule.

Josamycin is metabolized in the liver. Three metabolites have been isolated from the plasma and urine. These are 4″-deisovaleryljosamycin (leucomycin U) and products resulting from hydroxylation of carbon 14 of the aglycone nucleus (15-hydroxyjosamycin) or the β carbon of the 4″-isovaleryl chain (β-hydroxyjosamycin). The MICs for *S. aureus* 209 P are, respectively, 0.78, 1.56, 1.56, and 12.5 μg/ml for josamycin, 15-hydroxyjosamycin, β-hydroxyjosamycin, and deisovaleryljosamycin.

Rokitamycin is metabolized to three principal compounds: leucomycin A_7, leucomycin V, and 4″-*O*-(β-hydroxy butyrylrokitamycin). The concentrations in serum of these three metabolites and of rokitamycin, 30 min after a single dose of 1,200 mg of rokitamycin, represent, respectively, 9, 33, 40, and 18% of the levels in plasma. Leucomycin V is then metabolized to 14-hydroxyleucomycin V (Fig. 36).

No studies of spiramycin metabolism in humans have been published. Studies with rat hepatocytes have shown minimal metabolism.

16. TISSUE DISTRIBUTION

The pharmacokinetic properties of the macrolides and their physicochemical characteristics indicate extensive tissue distribution; a number of experimental studies have confirmed the presence of high concentrations of macrolides in the tissues and biological fluids of the main potential sites of infection corresponding to the indications of the macrolides (Table 73).

16.1. Respiratory Tract

The macrolides are extensively distributed in all respiratory tissues. The peak concentrations in lung tissue and bronchial mucosa are between 3 mg/kg for erythromycin and 20 mg/kg for spiramycin, with mean values of 4 to 6 mg/kg for the majority of molecules. In the lung, high levels of azithromycin have been measured at 96 h; the presence of continuing high concentrations in lung tissue at 8 h (3.80 ± 1.05 mg/kg) has been noted for clarithromycin. There is extensive distribution in the pleural fluid, on the order of 4 to 6 μg/ml, for erythromycin and roxithromycin. Penetration of macrolides in tissues of the ear, nose, and throat sphere is excellent. All the macrolides attain tissue levels two to three times higher than the levels obtained in plasma. In tonsillar and sinus tissues, the concentrations are generally between 1 and 6 mg/kg. The concentrations of erythromycin, roxithromycin, and clarithromycin in the inflammatory fluid of the middle ear are between 0.8 and 2.5 μg/ml. In tear fluid, the concentrations are about 1 to 2 μg/ml for erythromycin and may reach 4.80 μg/ml for roxithromycin.

16.2. Genital Tract

The concentrations of the different macrolides have been determined in uterovaginal and ovarian tissues and in the cervical mucus. Tissue concentrations are between 1 and 3 mg/kg. The concentrations in the cervical mucus are between 0.45 and 2.07 μg/ml. Transplacental passage has only been studied for erythromycin and roxithromycin. Concentrations in amniotic fluid and fetal tissues are between 0.35 and 1.20 μg/ml. The concentrations of josamycin, miokamycin, roxithromycin, and dirithromycin in prostate tissue are between 2.5 and 6 mg/kg.

16.3. Other Distribution Sites

In the skin, the concentrations are dependent on the administered dose and are similar to those in plasma. In suction blister fluid, reflecting the concentrations in the extravascular (interstitial) medium (study models in cantharide-induced suction blisters), the measured concentrations range from 1.5 μg/ml for erythromycin to 5 μg/ml for roxithromycin. Roxithromycin concentrations in cerebral tissue (45 to 200 μg/g) are high. In gastric tissue, concentrations of the different macrolides (azithromycin, clarithromycin, and roxithromycin) are between 0.6 and 18 mg/kg. In the gums and alveolar bone and in synovial fluid, the macrolides attain levels ranging from 0.5 to 4 mg/kg. They do not reach detectable concentrations in cerebrospinal fluid.

17. PHARMACODYNAMICS

The thigh infection models in immunosuppressed and normal mice have shown that macrolides can be separated into two categories: those which are time dependent, such as erythromycin, roxithromycin, and clarithromycin, and those which are concentration dependent, like azithromycin and dirithromycin.

18. DRUG INTERACTIONS

18.1. List of Drugs

Macrolides have the capacity to interfere with the metabolism and pharmacokinetics of other drugs (Table 74).

18.2. Hepatic Metabolism

A number of macrolides have the capacity to interfere with the hepatic metabolism of certain drugs metabolized in the liver. Erythromycin A is metabolized by the cytochrome P450 oxidizing system in a number of animal species and in humans.

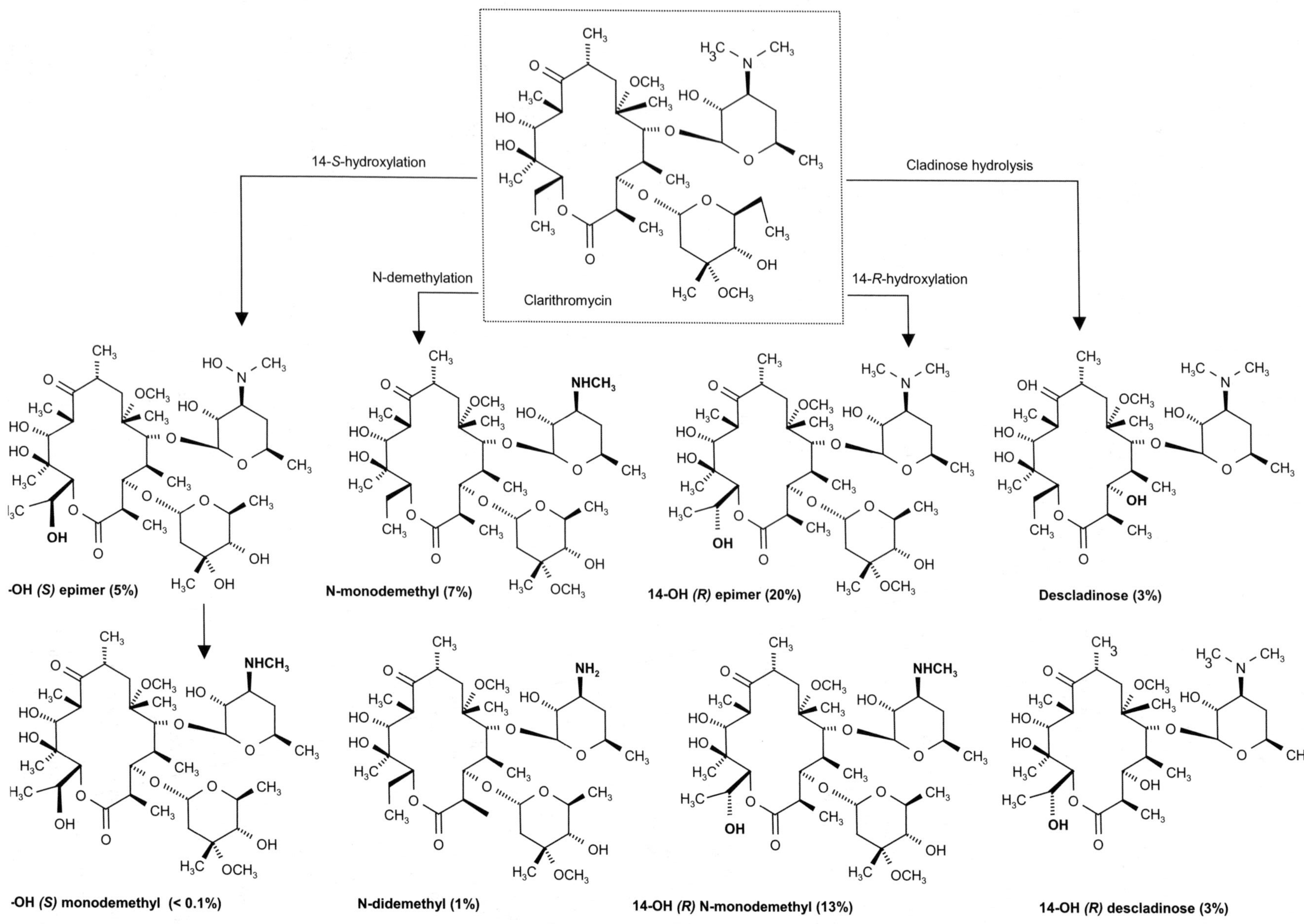

Figure 33 Metabolism of clarithromycin

Table 70 In vitro activities of clarithromycin metabolites

Microorganism	MIC (μg/ml)								
	Clarithromycin	M-1	M-2	M-3	M-4	M-5	M-6	M-7	M-8
S. aureus 209-P	0.05	0.78	3.13	12.5	12.5	0.10	0.78	25	12.5
S. aureus Smith	0.10	1.56	6.25	25	25	0.20			
S. epidermidis 1D 552	0.05	0.78	3.13	12.5	12.5	0.20			
S. pneumoniae 11D 553	≤0.012	0.05	1.56	0.10	0.78	0.025			
S. pyogenes 11ID 689	≤0.012	0.20	0.78	0.20	3.13	0.025			
B. subtilis ATCC 6633	0.05	0.78	6.25	12.5	12.5	0.1			
S. lutea ATCC 9341	0.025	0.10	0.39	1.56	3.13	0.025			
E. faecalis ATCC 8043	0.025	0.10	0.39	3.13	3.13	0.05			
M. *catarrhalis* NNBr-1	0.05	0.78	12.5	12.5	6.25	0.05	0.39	12.5	12.5
H. influenzae J-48	3.13	100	>100	>100	>100	3.13			
N. gonorrhoeae TCC-2	≤0.012	0.20	1.56	0.10	0.78				

Table 71 Distribution of azithromycin products after repeated oral administration (total of 1.5 g over 5 days)

Excreta	Fraction of distribution (%)			
	Azithromycin	3′-*N*-Demethylazithromycin	9a-*N*-Demethylazithromycin	Descladinose azithromycin
Bile	67	18	8	5.7
Urine	91	1	1.3	6.6

Table 72 Metabolites of azithromycin

Metabolite	Structure	Mol wt	Elimination	
			Bile	Urine
B	3′-*N*-Demethyl	735	+	+
C	9a-*N*-Demethyl	735	+	+
D	3′-*N*,3′-*N*,*N*-Demethyl	721	+	−
E	3′-*N*-Demethyl, 9a-*N*-demethyl	721	+	−
F	3′-*N*-Demethyl, 3″-*O*-demethyl	721	+	−
G	Hydroxydesosamine	765	+	−
H	Descladinose	591	+	+
I	3′-*N*-Demethyldescladinose	577	+	−
J	9a-*N*-Demethyldescladinose	577	+	−
K	Hydroxyaglycone	765	+	−

18.2.1. Cytochrome P450 System

The human liver comprises the following families of isoenzymes: CYP1A, CYP2A, CYP2B, CYP2C, CYP2E, CYP3A, and CYP4A.

The largest family in quantitative terms is CYP3A, which represents 30 to 50% of all isoenzymes. The CYP3A family is itself subdivided into several subgroups: CYP3A4, CYP3A5, and CYP3A7.

CYP3A4 is one of the most important groups in adults. Conversely, CYP3A5 is the largest subfamily of isoenzymes in the fetus but is present in only 10 to 30% of adult livers. CYP3A7 is present in fetal livers and in 54 to 89% of adult livers.

There is a major interindividual variability in the activities of the isoenzymes, which can vary up to 10- to 20-fold. This partly explains why some subjects react differently to drug combinations.

18.2.2. Cytochrome CYP3A4

The macrolides are a good substrate for cytochrome CYP3A4. The macrolides may be divided into three groups.

Molecules in group I do not form complexes in vitro and in vivo, even with the microsomes of rats pretreated with oleandomycin or dexamethasone. Josamycin, midecamycin, and spiramycin belong to group I.

Molecules in group II induce CYP3A4 isoenzymes but do not form complexes with the isoenzymes, although they can form complexes with other isoenzymes induced by glucocorticoids (in vitro and in vivo). Clarithromycin, roxithromycin, flurithromycin, dirithromycin, and azithromycin belong to this group.

Molecules in group III induce isoenzymes and form complexes in vitro and in vivo following single or repeated doses and after pretreatment with dexamethasone. Erythromycin A, oleandomycin, and troleandomycin belong to this group.

D-Desosamine is the amino sugar of erythromycin and oleandomycin. It possesses an R-N $(CH_3)_2$ tertiary amine function. This tertiary amine is demethylated and preoxidized by cytochrome CYP3A4 to a (R-N=O) nitroso metabolite which forms an inactive and stable complex with ferrous iron (Fe^{2+}).

The compound binds initially to Fe^{3+}-oxidized cytochrome and is reduced via an $NADPH_2$ oxidase reductase to ferrous iron (Fe^{2+}).

In the oxidized center, the unit is attached to the four nitrogen atoms of the tetrapyrrole nuclei of the heme. The fifth bond is attached to the cysteine of the apoprotein. The six sites that remain free can bind molecular oxygen or other substrates (Fig. 37).

18.2.3. Drug Interference

Certain drugs may be oxidized by CYP3A4. The macrolide-CYP3A4 complex prevents the metabolism of these drugs and may cause iatrogenic intoxication, as has been demonstrated with theophylline, carbamazepine, terfenadine, midazolam, cyclosporine, cisapride, etc.

Compound	R_1	R_2	R_3	R_4	R_5	Relative antibacterial activity
Miokamycin	$COCH_3$	H	H	$COCH_3$	COC_2H_5	2.62
Mb1	$COCH_3$	H	H	H	$COCH_3$	2.33
Mb2	$COCH_3$	H	H	H	H	1.30
Mb3	$COCH_3$	OH	H	H	H	0.73
Mb5	$COCH_3$	H	OH	H	H	0.78
Mb6	H	H	H	H	H	1.00
Mb9a	H	OH	H	H	H	0.54
Mb9b	H	H	OH	H	H	0.58
Mb12	H	H	H	H	$COCH_3$	2.21
Mb13	H	OH	H	H	$COCH_3$	1.35
Midecamycin	H	H	H	H	H	ND

Figure 34 Structure of miokamycin and its principal metabolites

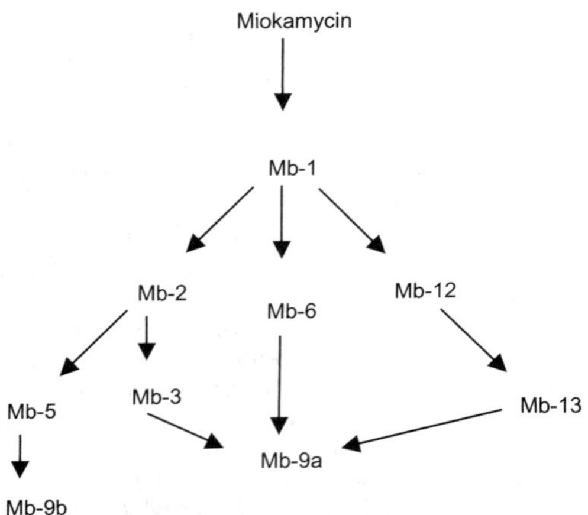

Figure 35 Metabolism of miokamycin (from Shomura et al., 1981)

18.2.3.1. Carbamazepine

Coadministration of carbamazepine with erythromycin A may prolong the apparent elimination half-life of carbamazepine and reduce the concentration in plasma of the 10,11-epoxide metabolite. The risk is principally neurologic.

18.2.3.2. Cyclosporine

The biotransformation of cyclosporine is very sensitive to variations in hepatic monooxygenases. In animal or human hepatic microsomal fractions, oleandomycin, erythromycin A, josamycin, rokitamycin, midecamycin, roxithromycin, and clarithromycin are competitive inhibitors of the metabolism of cyclosporine, whereas spiramycin has no effect.

18.2.3.3. Midazolam

Midazolam is a 1,4-benzodiazepine which is extensively used as a hypnotic agent and in anesthesia induction.

After administration of erythromycin base (500 mg every 8 h) for 1 week to 12 volunteers, administration of 15 mg of midazolam altered the pharmacokinetics of midazolam by increasing the peak concentration in serum 8-fold and the area under the curve 12-fold. The elimination of midazolam was delayed (Table 75).

18.2.3.4. Terfenadine

Terfenadine is an antihistamine which is rapidly metabolized. The lack of metabolism causes accumulation of the parent molecule, which is cardiotoxic above a certain level.

Three groups of six volunteers received 60 mg of terfenadine every 12 h for 1 week. After 1 week, one group simultaneously received 400 mg of erythromycin base every 8 h for 7 days, another group received 500 mg of clarithromycin every 12 h for 7 days, and the third group a daily dose of 250 mg of azithromycin for 5 days. A significant increase in the area under the curve was found with erythromycin base and clarithromycin, but not with azithromycin (Table 76).

No modification of the pharmacokinetics of terfenadine was noted when it was administered with dirithromycin.

18.2.3.5. Theophylline

Theophylline is N-demethylated by CYP1A2, against which erythromycin is inactive. However, it is also 8-hydroxylated, probably by CYP3A4.

18.2.4. Rare Interactions

18.2.4.1. Phenytoin

Phenytoin is an antiepileptic drug. Simultaneous administration of erythromycin base reduces its activity. Phenytoin is a weak inducer of CYP3A4 in humans.

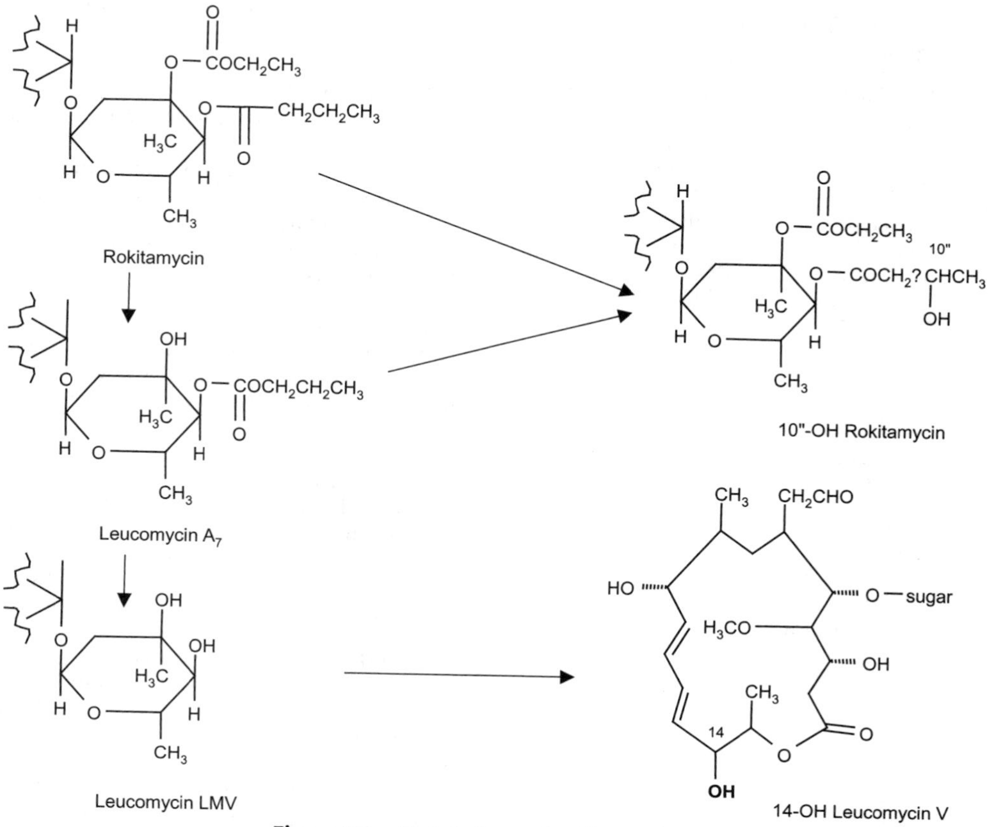

Figure 36 Metabolism of rokitamycin

Table 73 Tissue distribution of macrolides

Compound	Dose (mg)	Concn in serum (μg/ml)	Peak concn (mg/kg or μg/ml): Respiratory tract			Genital tract		
			Bronchial mucosa	Bronchial secretions	Sinus	Prostate	Uterus	Amniotic fluid/fetus
Erythromycin	500[a]	3.08	7.20	1.05	0.9–1.8	0.14–1.05	0.8–6.5	0.06–3.6
Oleandomycin	200[b]	6.26		3.77	2.68		2.24–2.10	
Roxithromycin	150[a]	2.51		3.10	4.15	2.81	1.8	0.58
Clarithromycin	500[a]	2.4			2.18			
Spiramycin	2,000[a]	0.39	13–36	7.3	2–8.8		4.2–23.5	0.63
Josamycin	1,000[a]	2.3		1.6	2.8	5.9		
Miokamycin	600[a]			5.16		4.9		
Azithromycin	500[b]		3.89	0.23	1.34			
Dirithromycin	500[a]	0.22	1.9	1.3		6.52		

[a]Multiple doses.
[b]Single dose.

18.2.4.2. Sodium Valproate

Valproic acid is a very widely used antiepileptic agent. The metabolism of valproic acid is partially inhibited by erythromycin via CYP3A4. The increase in concentrations in serum of valproic acid causes signs of intoxication (anorexia, nausea, vomiting, and ataxia).

Other drugs may produce side effects when administered with macrolides (Table 77). An overview that summarized this subject was published by Rosental and Adam (1995).

19. OTHER EFFECTS OF MACROLIDES

A number of publications have shown that macrolides have nonantibiotic pharmacological effects. Some of these effects have been studied for their therapeutic potential (motilide) or are the subject of important basic research: anti-inflammatory or cardiological effects. The therapeutic application of the antiparasitic activity of macrolides is a separate aspect (Bryskier and Labro, 1993).

Table 74 Nonexhaustive list of drugs whose metabolism may interfere with that of macrolides

Alfentanil, sufentanil	Dialtazem	Methylprednisolone
Antipyrine	Digoxin	Phenytoin
Astemizole	Disopyramide	Rifampin, rifabutin
Bromocriptine	Ergotamine	Sodium valproate
Carmabazepine	Ethyl estradiol	Theophylline
Cyclosporine	Felodipine	Triazolam, midazolam
Cimetidine	Glybenclamide	Verapamil
Cisapride	Levodopa, carbidopa	Warfarin
Clozapine	Lovastatin	Zidovudine

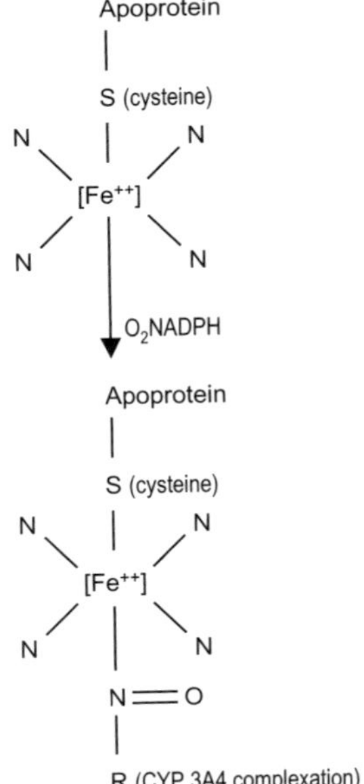

Figure 37 Cytochrome P450 interactions

19.1. Antiparasitic Activity of Macrolides

The macrolides possess antiparasitic properties that have been demonstrated since their first use. They are active against protozoa and are used therapeutically in the treatment of toxoplasmosis or malaria. However, they have not insignificant activity against certain intestinal protozoa, such as *Entamoeba histolytica* and *Giardia intestinalis*.

19.1.1. Intestinal Parasites

19.1.1.1. *E. histolytica*

E. histolytica is an enteric pathogenic agent responsible for dysentry but also for an invasive disease (amoebic hepatitis). In 1954, MacGoven et al. demonstrated that erythromycin A possessed amoebicidal activity in vitro and in vivo (in Wistar rats). This activity was confirmed in humans in 1956 by Nor Eldin. Azithromycin was shown in vitro and in vivo (gerbil model) to possess not inconsiderable activity against *E. histolytica*.

19.1.1.2. *G. intestinalis*

Giardiasis is a common intestinal infection due to *G. intestinalis*.

In 1956, Nor Eldin demonstrated the therapeutic activity of erythromycin in giardiasis. In vitro, azithromycin exhibited good activity, comparable to that of metronidazole. However, it was relatively inactive in vivo in a murine model (neonatal mouse).

19.1.1.3. *Blastocystis hominis*

B. hominis is a pathogenic agent responsible for moderate, recurrent diarrhea. A single study with erythromycin in human immunodeficiency virus patients revealed no activity either by metronidazole or by erythromycin A.

19.1.1.4. *Isospora belli*

I. belli is responsible for short-lasting, spontaneously resolving diarrhea. However, in certain patients, it is responsible for chronic infections. The standard treatment is co-trimoxazole. One patient was treated successfully for 15 days with 2.5 mg of roxithromycin per kg every 12 h.

19.1.1.5. Cryptosporidiosis

Cryptosporidium parvum is a ubiquitous coccidium responsible for spontaneously resolving diarrhea, but also for chronic diarrhea in immunodepressed patients, such as AIDS patients.

The potential activity of macrolides was studied in vivo in an experimental infection in dexamethasone-immunodepressed rats (Sprague-Dawley). It was shown schematically that spiramycin and oleandomycin were inactive and that azithromycin, erythromycin, and clarithromycin reduced the parasite burden, with azithromycin appearing to be the most active.

Two clinical studies with AIDS patients have clearly shown that roxithromycin significantly reduces the parasite burden and causes a marked improvement in the patients' general status.

19.1.2. Toxoplasmosis

Following an acute infection, *Toxoplasma gondii* forms cysts that can persist throughout life in certain tissues, including the brain. This phenomenon is the origin of acute toxoplasmic episodes, particularly in AIDS patients, producing major

Table 76 Bioavailability of terfenadine in combination with macrolides

Drug	AUC (ng·h/ml)		
	Erythromycin	Clarithromycin	Azithromycin
Terfenadine	1,312	1,053	1,712
Terfenadine + macrolide	2,747	2,699	1,749

Table 75 Pharmacokinetics of the combination of midazolam and erythromycin base

Drug	C_{max} (μg/ml)	T_{max} (h)	$AUC_{0-\infty}$ (μg·h/ml)	$t_{1/2}$ (h)	F (%)
Midazolam	70 ± 9.0	80 ± 13	12 ± 1.0	2.4 ± 0.4	0.33
Midazolam-erythromycin	189 ± 16	53 ± 8.0	53 ± 7.0	5.7 ± 0.5	0.82

Table 77 Drug interference by macrolides

Drug	Theophylline	Carbamazepine	Cyclosporine	Midazolam	Terfenadine
Erythromycin	+	+	+	+	+
Oleandomycin	+	+	+	+	NT
Azithromycin	–	–	NT	–	–
Clarithromycin	(+)	+	+	+	+
Dirithromycin	(+)	NT	+	NT	
Roxithromycin	(+)	–	(+)	+	+
Josamycin	+	–	+	NT	NT
Spiramycin	–	NT	–	NT	NT
Rokitamycin	(+)	NT	+	NT	NT
Midecamycin	–	NT	NT	NT	NT
Miokamycin	–	+	+	NT	NT
Flurithromycin	NT	+	NT	NT	NT

neurologic disorders. The macrolides inhibit the in vitro multiplication of tachyzoites, albeit at high concentrations.

The results must be interpreted with reference to other macrolides and for the same author, since the methodology varies from one team to another. The in vitro activity is reported in Table 78.

Roxithromycin, clarithromycin, and azithromycin allow survival in peritoneally induced acute murine toxoplasmosis. High doses, however, are necessary (300 to 50 mg/kg). It would appear that only azithromycin is able to protect mice infected with the virulent RH strain of *T. gondii* from toxoplasmic encephalitis.

The combination of pyrimethamine with macrolides is synergistic.

19.1.3. *Pneumocystis carinii*

In vitro, macrolides have no activity against *P. carinii*. In combination with a sulfonamide, macrolides have synergistic activity in immunodepressed Sprague-Dawley rats infected with a strain of *P. carinii*.

19.1.4. Malaria

Plasmodium falciparum malaria remains one of the major causes of morbidity and mortality in the world. The progressive increase in the number and incidence of chloroquine-resistant strains of *P. falciparum* has necessitated the search for therapeutic alternatives.

Erythromycin, roxithromycin, and azithromycin have been shown to possess slow schizonticidal activity. The combination of these macrolides with a major antimalarial agent (quinine or 4-aminoquinoline) suppresses acute malarial episodes.

19.2. Prokinetic Activity of Erythromycin A

The gastrointestinal side effects of erythromycin are not serious and are expressed principally in the form of abdominal cramps, nausea, and sometimes diarrhea.

It has been shown that these effects are due principally to the hemiketal inactivation product of erythromycin A, which interferes with the motilin receptor. This phenomenon has been demonstrated in humans, rabbits, and dogs, but not in rats or guinea pigs.

Various studies have shown that phase 3 of intestinal contractions is stimulated by weak doses of erythromycin.

The site of action of erythromycin, however, is dose dependent. It has been shown that erythromycin stimulates intestinal smooth muscle through dihydroxypyridine- and nickel-sensitive calcium channels.

Table 78 In vitro activity of macrolides against *T. gondii* (MRC_5 fibroblasts)[a]

Drug	First effective dose (μg/ml)	IC_{50}[b] (μg/ml)
Erythromycin	0.2	3.0
Oleandomycin	4.0	6.5
Midecamycin	1.0	12
Spiramycin	1.0	12
Josamycin	0.10	1.7
Azithromycin	0.10	1.2
Clarithromycin	0.05	0.8
Roxithromycin	1.0	2.0

[a]Data from Derouin et al., 1987, 1990.
[b]IC_{50}, 50% inhibitory concentration.

In 1990, Urbain et al. and Janssens et al. showed the usefulness of low doses of erythromycin in diabetic patients suffering from gastroparesis. Doses of 40 mg accelerated gastric emptying. Likewise, in the opossum, erythromycin stimulated the emptying of Oddi's sphincter, which was confirmed in patients.

This phenomenon has been demonstrated with the 14- and 15-membered-ring derivatives, but not with the 16-membered-ring derivatives (midecamycin, leucomycin, josamycin, and acetylspiramycin).

A number of agents derived from erythromycin A, motilides without antibacterial activity, have been synthesized as prokinetic agents.

These derivatives are erythromycin A enolethers, in which the amino group of the desosamine is substituted by an ethyl group instead of a methyl group, or even with other groups preventing binding to bacterial ribosomes (Fig. 38).

19.3. Cardiovascular Effects

Erythromycin A has electrophysiological properties similar to those of class 1A antiarrhythmic agents; these properties cause an increase in the atrial and ventricular refractory period.

In predisposed subjects, erythromycin A may engender fatal arrhythmias or syncopes.

Rubart et al. showed that erythromycin A modifies potassium fluxes in canine myocardial tissue, which might be responsible for QT interval prolongation and arrhythmias.

In vitro and in vivo studies have shown that this pharmacological effect of erythomycin A is dose dependent and that there is a correlation between the infusion rate and the increase in the QT interval.

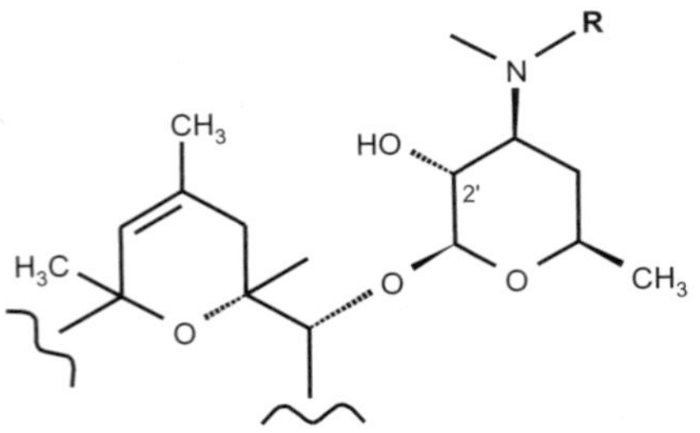

	R
EM 523	$—C_2H_5$
EM 536	$—CH_2≡N—Br$
GM-611	—Isopropyl

Figure 38 Prokinetic agents

Recent studies have led to the cloning of a set of genes that code for proteins involved in the potassium fluxes, such as the K_V 1.5 protein. In myocardial tissue, potassium fluxes through the potassium channels play an important role in terms of repolarization phenomena.

Erythromycin A blocks the K_V 1.5 channel at therapeutic concentrations. This blockade is time, frequency, and voltage dependent.

Erythromycin A acts on the activation phase of the K_V 1.5 potassium channel by acting on the intracellular aspect of the channel.

19.4. Anti-Inflammatory Effects

The macrolides possess anti-inflammatory properties in humans and animals.

Erythromycin has antioxidant properties. The properties may be beneficial. They have been demonstrated with the 14- and 15-membered-ring macrolides and are based on the presence of the neutral sugar L-cladinose.

20. THERAPEUTIC INDICATIONS

Among antibacterial agents, the macrolides are the best tolerated. In contrast to other antibiotics, it is theoretically possible to administer them to all age groups irrespective of the underlying pathophysiological status.

20.1. Standard Clinical Indications

The standard indications for macrolides are infections of the ear, nose, and throat sphere, but extreme caution must be exercised in otitis media due to *H. influenzae*, irrespective of the macrolide. In lower respiratory tract infections, the macrolides are the drugs of choice in pneumonia due to intracellular bacteria or *M. pneumoniae*. Macrolides are a good alternative to replace β-lactams in parenchymatous and nonparenchymatous lower respiratory tract infections. Some cutaneous and subcutaneous infections may be treated successfully with macrolides. Macrolides are the anti-infective agents of choice in the treatment of nongonococcal urethritis due particularly to *C. trachomatis* or *U. urealyticum*. Despite good in vitro activity, macrolides are not recommended in the treatment of gonococcal urethritis. Likewise, the treatment of vaginitis due to *Gardnerella vaginalis* is based not on macrolides, despite their good in vitro activity, but on metronidazole. Syphilis is treated with β-lactams, although macrolides may be a therapeutic alternative. Pelvic inflammatory disease due to *C. trachomatis* or *Mycoplasma* spp. is also a good therapeutic indication for macrolides, except for *M. hominis*, which is naturally resistant to the 14- and 15-membered-ring macrolides.

Whooping cough is due to *B. pertussis*. Despite vaccination, this disease is always present, although usually in deceptive clinical forms. Macrolides represent the treatment of choice. Some are used in combination with metronidazole in orodental infections. In the current state of knowledge, there is insufficient experience with the new macrolides in the prevention of streptococcal or enterococcal endocarditis following tooth extraction in certain susceptible patients. Macrolides represent one of the treatments of choice of intestinal infections due to *Campylobacter jejuni* or *Campylobacter coli*. Erythromycin used to be administered in pharyngeal diphtheria, and the resurgence of this infection in certain eastern European countries might allow the new molecules to be used in this indication.

20.2. Unconventional Clinical Indications

20.2.1. Bacterial Infections

Macrolides might be another therapeutic option in certain pathological situations. However, they should be administered in combination with another antibacterial agent and never as single-agent therapy. A number of pharmacological and clinical studies are currently underway to explore their potential place in the therapeutic arsenal.

Macrolides have found a place in the eradication of *H. pylori*. They are an alternative to the 5-nitroimidazoles in the combination of an antiulcer agent (omeprazole or lansoprazole) with amoxicillin.

B. burgdorferi is highly susceptible to macrolides. The clinical results are very variable. It appears that combination with another antibacterial agent, like co-trimoxazole, yields good results.

In vitro results indicate potential activity for certain macrolides against *Brucella melitensis* in combination with other antibacterial agents.

Macrolides are used in *M. avium-Mycobacterium intracellulare* complex infections. Clarithromycin, roxithromycin, and azithromycin have good in vitro activity against this complex. Clinical results have shown good efficacy for clarithromycin.

Clarithromycin possesses good therapeutic activity against *M. leprae*, particularly in combination with minocycline.

20.2.2. Parasitic Infections

It has been shown since the mid-1950s that erythromycin has good antiparasitic activity.

Spiramycin has been recommended in the treatment of acute toxoplasmosis in France for more than 30 years.

Pharmacological studies have shown the good activity of certain macrolides against *E. histolytica* and *G. intestinalis*. A patient suffering from an infection due to *I. belli* was treated successfully with roxithromycin. The therapeutic activity of macrolides in *C. parvum* diarrhea in AIDS patients is disputed. Macrolides do not eradicate the parasite but sometimes reduce the parasite burden. There is a high incidence of cerebral toxoplasmosis in AIDS patients. Activity against tachyzoites is variable in vitro and in animals, but activity against cerebral cysts is disappointing. Clarithromycin-pyrimethamine or azithromycin-pyrimethamine combinations have produced interesting results in the treatment of cerebral toxoplasmosis. In *P. carinii* pneumonia, the activity of macrolides in combination with other antibacterial agents is under study.

Table 79 Preventive activity of roxithromycin in ischemic events in patients suffering from unstable angina

Event	% of patients with event		P
	Placebo ($n = 93$)	Roxithromycin ($n = 93$)	
Relapse	5.40	1.1	0.63
Myocardial infarction	2.2	0	0.9
Death	2.2	0	0.9
Infarction + death	4.3	0	0.242
Relapses + infarction + death	10	1.1	0.036

Erythromycin in combination with quinine or a 4-aminoquinoline has good activity against chloroquine-resistant or -susceptible strains of *P. falciparum*.

20.3. Clinical Research

The fact that *H. pylori* is the etiological agent of duodenal ulcers and chronic gastritis has revived interest in etiopathogenic research into the bacterial or viral origin of certain nosologic entities such as coronary diseases. Recent studies have shown the potential for cytomegalovirus and *C. pneumoniae* to be involved in coronary atheromatous disease.

It has been shown that high levels of chlamydial antigen and antichlamydia antibody of the immunoglobulin A type and immune complexes containing lipopolysaccharide from *C. pneumoniae* (a gram-negative bacterium) are more frequent in patients suffering a myocardial infarct.

A number of studies have shown the presence of *Chlamydia* in arterial tissue at different stages of atheromatous disease.

C. pneumoniae is an obligate intracellular bacterium which lives principally in monocytes (present in atheromatous plaques) and perhaps in epithelial cells. The (lipopolysacchride-induced) procoagulant and inflammatory activity of *C. pneumoniae* is poorly understood.

A recent study has reported the efficacy of roxithromycin in the prevention of ischemic events in patients suffering from unstable angina but without a precise microbiological status.

This study has the merit of opening up a new line of research in cardiological therapy (Table 79).

Another study has shown the potential role of azithromycin.

REFERENCES

Bryskier A, 1992, Newer macrolides and their potential target organisms, Curr Opin Infect Dis, 5, 764–772.

Bryskier A, 1997, Novelties in the field of macrolides, Expert Opin Investig Drug, 6, 1697–1709.

Bryskier A, 1998, Roxithromycin: a review of its antimicrobial activity, J Antimicrob Chemother, 41, suppl B, 1–21.

Bryskier A, 1998, New research in macrolides and ketolides since 1997, Expert Opin Investig Drug, 8, 1171–1194.

Bryskier A, Agouridas C, 1993, Azalides: a new medicinal chemical family, Curr Opin Investig Drugs, 2, 687–694.

Bryskier A, Agouridas C, Chantot JF, 1992, Acid stability of macrolides, Chemotherapia, suppl, 156–158.

Bryskier A, Agouridas C, Chantot JF, 1993, New insights into the structure activity relationship of macrolides and azalides, p 3–29, in Neu HC, Young LS, Zinner SH, Acer JF, ed, New Macrolides, Azalides and Streptogramins in Clinical Practice, Marcel Dekker, New York.

Bryskier A, Agouridas C, Chantot JF, 1994, New medicinal targets for macrolides, Expert Opin Investig Drug, 3, 405–410.

Bryskier A, Agouridas C, Gasc JC, 1993, Classification of macrolide antibiotics, p 5–66, in Bryskier AJ, Butzler JP, Neu HC, Tulkens PM, ed, Macrolides, Chemistry, Pharmacology and Clinical Use, Arnette-Blackwell, Paris.

Bryskier A, Butzler JP, Tulkens PM, 1996, Les nouveaux macrolides de la chimie à la thérapeutique, Medisearch, 92, 9–29.

Bryskier A, Chantot JF, Gasc JC, 1986, Antibacterial activity of roxithromycin: laboratory evaluation, J Antibiot, 39, 660–668.

Bryskier A, Chantot JF, Gasc JC, Chretien P, 1990, Roxithromycin, a new potent and well-absorbed macrolide, Fortsc Antimikrob Antineopl Chemother Bans, 9–1, 1–17.

Bryskier A, Cornaglia G, 2004, What is the current role of macrolides and ketolides in the treatment of group A streptococcal pharyngitis, p 124–142, in Péchère JC, Kaplan EL, ed, Streptococcal Pharyngitis, vol 3, Karger, Basel.

Bryskier A, Labro MT, 1993, Antiparasitic activity of macrolide antibiotics, p 307–320, in Bryskier AJ, Butzler JP, Neu HC, Tulkens PM, ed, Macrolides, Chemistry, Pharmacology and Clinical Use, Arnette-Blackwell, Paris.

Bryskier A, Labro MT, 1994, Macrolides: nouvelles perspectives thérapeutiques, Presse Med, 23, 1762–1766.

Champney WS, 1998, Inhibition of translation and 50 S ribosomal subunit formation in S. aureus by 11 different ketolide antibiotics, Curr Microbiol, 37, 418–425.

Chu SY, Deaton R, Cavanaugh D, 1992, Absolute bioavailability of clarithromycin after oral administration in humans, Antimicrob Agents Chemother, 36, 1147–1150.

Depootere I, Peters TL, Matthij G, Cachet T, Hoogmartens J, Vantrappen G, 1989, Structure-activity relationship of erythromycin-related macrolides in inducing contractions and displacing bound motilin in rabbit duodenum, J Gastroenterol Mol, 1, 150–159.

Djockic S, Kobrehel G, Lazarewski G, 1987, Antibacterial in vitro evaluation of 10-dihydro-10-deoxo-11-azaerythromycin A: synthesis and structure activity relationship of its acyl derivatives, J Antibiot, 40, 1006–1015.

Fiese EF, Steffen SH, 1990, Comparison of acid-stability of azithromycin and erythromycin A, J Antimicrob Chemother, 25, suppl A, 39–47.

Foulds G, Stepard EM, Johnson RB, 1990, The pharmacokinetics of azithromycin in human serum and tissue, J Antimicrob Chemother, 25, suppl A, 173–182.

Gasc JC, Gouin d'Ambrières S, Lutz A, Chantot JF, 1991, New ether oxime derivatives of erythromycin A. Structure activity relationship, J Antibiot, 44, 313–330.

Godfried MH, 2003, Clarithromycin (Biaxin) extended-release tablet: a therapeutic review, Expert Rev Anti-infect Ther, 1, 9–20.

Hardy DJ, Hensey DM, Beyer JM, Vojkko C, McDonald EJ, Fernandes PB, 1988, Comparative in vitro activity of new 14-, 15, and 16-membered macrolides, Antimicrob Agents Chemother, 32, 1710–1719.

Itoh Z, Ohmura S, 1987, Motilides, a new family of macrolide compounds mimicking motilin, Dig Dis Sci, 32, 915.

Kirst HA, 1993, Expanding the therapeutic potential of macrolide compounds, p 143–151, in Krohn K, Kirst HA, Maag H, ed, Antibiotics and Antiviral Compounds, Chemical Synthesis and Modifications, VCH, New York.

Labro MT, 1998, Immunological effects of macrolides, Curr Opin Infect Dis, 11, 681–688.

Labro MT, 2000, Interference of antibacterial agents with phagocyte functions: immunomodulation or "immuno-fairy tales," Clin Microbiol Rev, 13, 615–650.

Labro MT, 2002, Cellular accumulation of macrolide antibiotics, intracellular activity, p 37–52, in Schönfeld W, Kirst HA, eds, Macrolide Antibiotics, Burhaüser Verlag, Basel.

Moritomo S, Takashi Y, Watanabe Y, Omura S, 1984, Chemical modifications of erythromycin. I. Synthesis and antibacterial activity of 6-O-methyl erythromycin A, J Antibiot, 37, 187–189.

Omura S, Nakagawa A, 1981, Biosynthesis of 16-membered macrolide antibiotics, Antibiotics (New York), 4, 175–192.

Roden BA, Chemburka S, Freiberg I, Ku YY, Pariza B, 1995, Synthesis of the macrolide antibiotic, oxolide, Bioorg Med Chem Lett, 5, 1307–1310.

Shiomura T, Someya S, Unemura K, Nishio M, Murata S, 1982, Metabolism of 9,3″-diacatyl midecamycin. I. The metabolic fate of 9,3″-diacatyl midecamycin, Yakugakuzasshi (Japan), 102, 781–795.

Weisblum B, 1995, Erythromycin resistance by ribosomal modification, Antimicrob Agents Chemother, 39, 577–585.

Ketolides

A. BRYSKIER

19

1. INTRODUCTION

Each new wave of macrolides always coincides with a medical need. The ketolides belong to the third wave of macrolides.

Erythromycin A was discovered at a time when a medication was required that was active against penicillinase-producing strains of *Staphylococcus aureus*. Very shortly after the introduction of penicillin G into clinical practice, penicillin G-resistant strains of *S. aureus* emerged and spread in hospitals in London, England. These strains then spread around the world. This situation required a response, and this came from the pharmaceutical industry with intensive research that was to result in the semisynthesis of methicillin, the isoxazolylpenicillins (oxacillin and floxacillin), and the first parenteral cephalosporins, such as cephalothin and cephaloridine. Other antibiotic families came into existence, such as the macrolide family, several natural derivatives of which were isolated from the fermentation broth of different microorganisms.

Among the macrolides of natural origin, erythromycin A was the most active molecule in vitro. However, the use of erythromycin A was rapidly limited by the use of other antibacterials that were active against *S. aureus* and because of its bacteriostatic activity. The other weak point was its erratic pharmacokinetics, since it is instable in an acidic medium. Despite attempts to overcome this physicochemical obstacle, such as esterification of the hydroxyl group at position 2′ of the D-desosamine, the stoichiometric mixture with the stearate or the mixture of a salt and a 2′-ester such as erythromycin A estolate (erythromycin A lauryl sulfate and 2′-propionate), the pharmacokinetics are unsatisfactory.

These combined problems resulted in erythromycin A and the other macrolides falling into disuse, with a few clinical exceptions. Although used in the treatment of respiratory tract diseases in the same way as β-lactams or tetracyclines, erythromycin A was reserved above all for the treatment of certain bacterial infections such as diphtheria, whooping cough, chancroid, or intestinal infections due to *Campylobacter jejuni* (Bryskier, 1992).

The semisynthetic macrolides of the second wave, such as roxithromycin, clarithromycin, azithromycin, and dirithromycin (Bryskier et al., 1995), are the result of the revival of interest in macrolides with the discovery of *Legionella pneumophila* (Blackman et al., 1978) or the medical interest in intracellular bacteria such as *Chlamydia* spp. These new molecules had to exhibit better antibacterial activity than erythromycin A against *Legionella*, *Chlamydia*, and *Mycoplasma* spp., good stability in an acidic medium, and good gastrointestinal absorption. Activity similar to that of erythromycin A against common pathogens was acceptable. These aims were generally achieved. The principal objective was to improve the pharmacokinetic qualities of the macrolides.

The pharmacokinetic problem was resolved with these new molecules, but the problem of the pharmacokinetics of the macrolides is a complex one. Two types of pharmacokinetics may be described for these molecules: those with simple plasma pharmacokinetics, such as roxithromycin and clarithromycin, and those whose plasma pharmacokinetics are more complex, such as azithromycin and dirithromycin, for which "tissue-directed pharmacokinetics" have been proposed. The first group of molecules has "time-dependent" pharmacokinetics, and the second group has "concentration-dependent" pharmacokinetics.

A new therapeutic era was introduced with the use of these drugs, but this coincided with the postpenicillin era, which is characterized by the emergence of strains resistant to a number of antibiotics, including macrolides. The second wave of macrolides established the therapeutic value of this medicinal chemical class through the extension of these therapeutic indications in response to a new therapeutic requirement: gastrointestinal infections due to *Helicobacter pylori*, infections from opportunistic bacteria in AIDS patients (such as disseminated infections due to *Mycobacterium avium* complex or *Bartonella* spp.), and lepromatous leprosy (in combination with minocycline). The new macrolides are also among the therapeutic combinations proposed for the treatment of parasitic diseases (cerebral toxoplasmosis, cryptosporidiosis, etc.) in AIDS patients (Bryskier, 1992).

Considerable research into the use of roxithromycin and azithromycin for the potential antibacterial treatment of atheromatous disease and asthma is under way.

The third wave of macrolides must respond to this new epidemiological environment, including the emergence of erythromycin A-resistant strains among gram-positive cocci, *Campylobacter* spp., *H. pylori*, *M. avium* complex, etc.

In addition, new medical expectations have arisen as a result of the emergence of penicillin G-resistant strains of *Streptococcus pneumoniae*, since these strains are capable of becoming multiresistant. Several drugs from different chemical classes will be required in therapy to be able to combat these new predators.

Research has been directed towards a third wave of molecules: compounds retaining the pharmacokinetic advances of the second wave of drugs and the antibacterial advances against atypical and intracellular bacteria, but active against erythromycin A-resistant bacterial strains. The requirements did not necessitate the extension of the antibacterial spectrum to include gram-negative bacteria. This research has resulted in the discovery of a new chemical entity: the ketolides.

2. EPIDEMIOLOGY OF RESISTANCE TO MACROLIDES

Over the past 10 years we have experienced a rapid extension of resistance to erythromycin A. The bacterial species most affected are the streptococci, including *S. pneumoniae*, *Streptococcus pyogenes*, streptococci of Lancefield groups C and G, viridans group streptococci, and *Streptococcus agalactiae*. Staphylococcal resistance to erythromycin A is particularly marked among oxacillin-resistant strains. It is much less obvious if there are erythromycin A-resistant strains among intracellular bacteria, particularly *Chlamydia pneumoniae*. However, failures have been reported, with the isolation of a strain for which the MIC of azithromycin had been multiplied 10-fold (MIC of 2 μg/ml) at the end of treatment with erythromycin. There do not appear to be strains of *Haemophilus influenzae* that are resistant to erythromycin A, but this molecule is already relatively inactive by nature.

The rapid and worrying emergence relates particularly to *S. pyogenes*, of which more than 40% of strains are resistant to erythromycin A in certain regions of Italy. This phenomenon used to be even greater in Japan, with an average of 80% of strains resistant, but the current incidence would appear to be less than 20%.

S. pneumoniae is the second species whose susceptibility to erythromycin A has decreased considerably. In France, more than 50% of penicillin G-resistant strains of *S. pneumoniae* are resistant to erythromycin A. There is a similar phenomenon in Spain. An epidemiological survey of resistance to erythromycin A has been taken in Southeast Asia, showing a loss of activity of erythromycin A against *S. pneumoniae* in alarming proportions, particularly in Japan, Taiwan, Hong Kong, and Korea.

2.1. Mechanism of Resistance

The mode of resistance to macrolides is complex. Several mechanisms have been described. The MLS_B mechanism is common to macrolides, lincosamides, and streptogramin B. A second mechanism, of efflux, involves the 14- and 15-membered-ring macrolides, but not clindamycin.

Enzymatic inactivation mechanisms have been described for *Escherichia coli* (esterase) or involving 2′-phosphotransferase or glycosylation (inactivation of the 2′-hydroxyl group of D-desosamine).

3. CLASSIFICATION

The semisynthesis of new macrolides requires a revision of the classification proposed in 1996 (Bryskier et al., 1997).

In fact, among the 14-membered-ring macrolides, a distinction must continue to be drawn between natural molecules, such as erythromycin (A to G) and oleandomycin, and molecules obtained by chemical modification of erythromycin A.

The second group of 14-membered-ring macrolides is subdivided according to the type of chemical modifications: those relating to the substituents (group II_A), those relating to the aglycone or erythronolide A (neutral group II_B), and those which involve a modification of the sugars by the addition (3′-oxomacrolides) or removal (ketolides) of one such sugar (Fig. 1).

At present, three subgroups may be described among the macrolides obtained by semisynthesis from erythromycin A. The first contains roxithromycin, clarithromycin, flurithromycin, and davercin.

The second subgroup is slightly more complex and may be subdivided into two. Two types of modification of the aglycone may be considered: enlargement of the aglycone by insertion of a nitrogen atom (15-membered-ring azalides) or oxygen (oxolides), or insertion of a nitrogen atom without alteration of the size of the aglycone (14-membered-ring azalide).

The third subgroup is related to the removal of the neutral sugar. The 3-OH group obtained was oxidized, yielding a 3-carbonyl group which characterized ketolides (Fig. 2).

4. KETOLIDES

The ketolides belong to group II_C of the classification of macrolides. They have the following characteristic: they have a 3-keto group instead of α-L-cladinose at position 3 of erythromycin A (Fig. 3) (Bryskier et al., 1997).

4.1. Precursors of the Ketolides

There are natural derivatives of the 14-membered-ring macrolides which do not have an L-cladinose at position 3 of the aglycone nucleus: picromycin and narbomycin (Fig. 4).

In 1951, Brockman and Henkel described a bitter substance which they named picromycin. It is produced by fermentation from *Streptomyces felleus*, but also from *Streptomyces flavochromogenes* under the name of amaromycin.

In 1955, Corbaz et al. described narbomycin, which they isolated from the fermentation of *Streptomyces narbonensis* strain ETH7346. Muxfelt et al. (1968) showed that narbomycin is 12-deoxypicromycin.

Both molecules are characterized by a 14-membered aglycone ring, which is the picronolide. These derivatives have only the amino sugar, D-desosamine, at position 5 of the aglycone ring. Another important feature is the absence of a hydroxyl group at position 6, in contrast to erythromycin A. Picromycin and narbomycin have good activity against *S. aureus*, *S. pyogenes* (MIC between 0.1 and 1.0 μg/ml), and *Corynebacterium diphtheriae* and are inactive against gram-negative bacilli. Narbomycin is active against erythromycin A-resistant strains of gram-positive cocci (Fig. 5). In vivo, narbomycin is inactive even at high doses.

Le Mahieu et al. (1974) prepared certain derivatives from erythromycin A without the L-cladinose, having an oxime function instead of a 9-keto at position 9. They showed that the 3-hydroxyl and 3-O-benzyl derivatives are inactive (antibacterial activity of <1% compared to that of erythromycin A), with the 3-keto derivative also being only weakly active (Fig. 6).

The lack of antibacterial activity of the 3-O-benzyl derivatives was also demonstrated by Asaka et al. (1997). The MICs are greater than 100 μg/ml for all gram-positive cocci.

4.2. Structure of Ketolides

All ketolides are characterized structurally by the absence of an α-L-cladinose at position 3 of the erythronolide A and the presence of a 3-keto group.

Three types of ketolides have been synthesized. The first two are those obtained by modifications of the keto group at

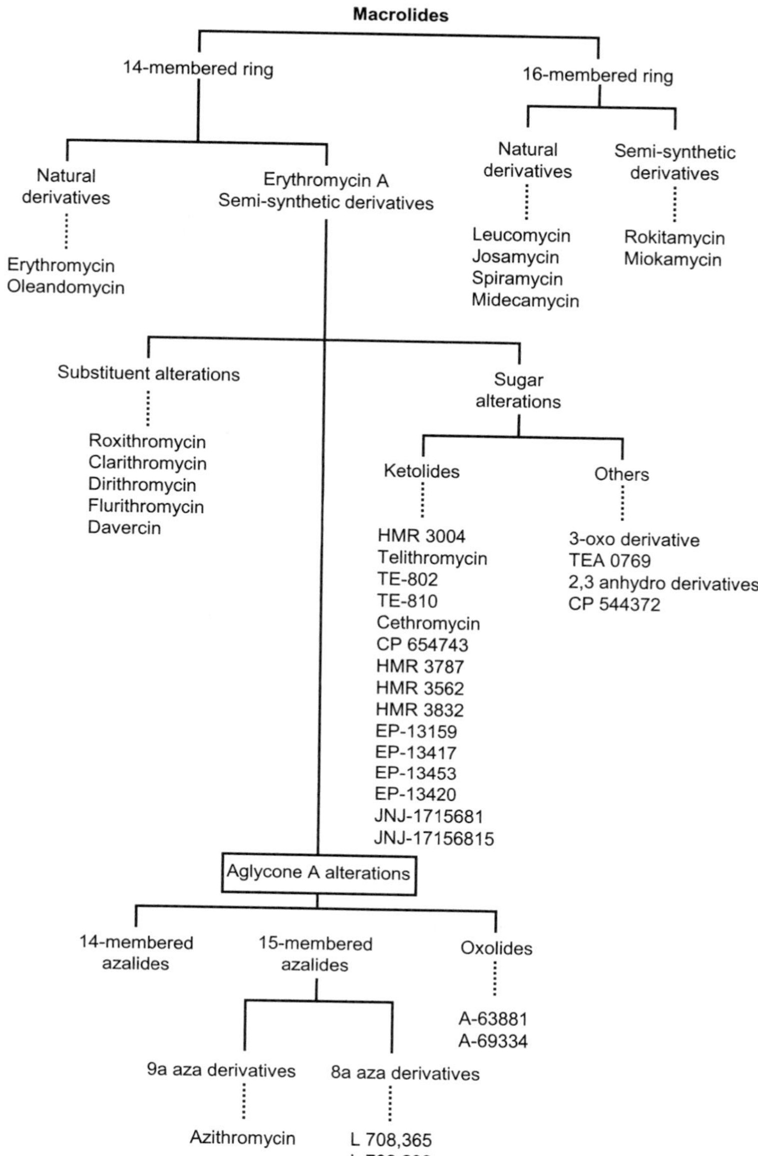

Figure 1 Classification of 14- and 15-membered-ring macrolides

position 9 of erythromycin A and those possessing a side chain at C-11 and C-12. In order to avoid hemiketalization between the hydroxyl group at position 6 and the keto group at position 3, a methyl group has been fixed to the hydroxyl group at position 6 (Fig. 7). The third group is composed of molecules with a carbamate at C-11 and C-12 and a side chain at C-6.

Several types of side chains have been attached at C-11 and C-12: a carbamate chain or a carbazate chain. Different aromatic rings have been attached to these chains, such as quinoline (HMR 3004), pyridinyl and imidazolyl (telithromycin), or a tricyclic system (TE-802).

4.3. Characteristics of Ketolides

Ketolides have the following main characteristic: high acid stability. Compounds without an α-L-cladinose obtained in an acidic medium have been shown to be stable (e.g., azithromycin and roxithromycin) (Fig. 8).

The derivatives are weakly inductive of resistance because of the absence of L-cladinose, as has been demonstrated with compounds that differ only by the presence of an L-cladinose.

4.4. Structure-Activity Relationship of Ketolides

Ketolides are prepared from erythromycin A. They differ from it by the presence of a methyl group at position 6, the lack of L-cladinose, and a side chain attached on the carbamate residue at C-11 and C-12 with or without an *O*-allyl chain at C-6 (Fig. 9), or even at C-9 of the erythronolide A nucleus, such as RU-504 (Fig. 10).

4.4.1. 6-*O*-Methyl Group

In contrast to clarithromycin, in which the 6-O-methyl group prevents hemiketalization between the 9-keto group and the 6-OH, causing inactivation of the molecule, in the ketolides it prevents ketalization between the hydroxyl group at position 6 and the keto group at position 3 (Fig. 10).

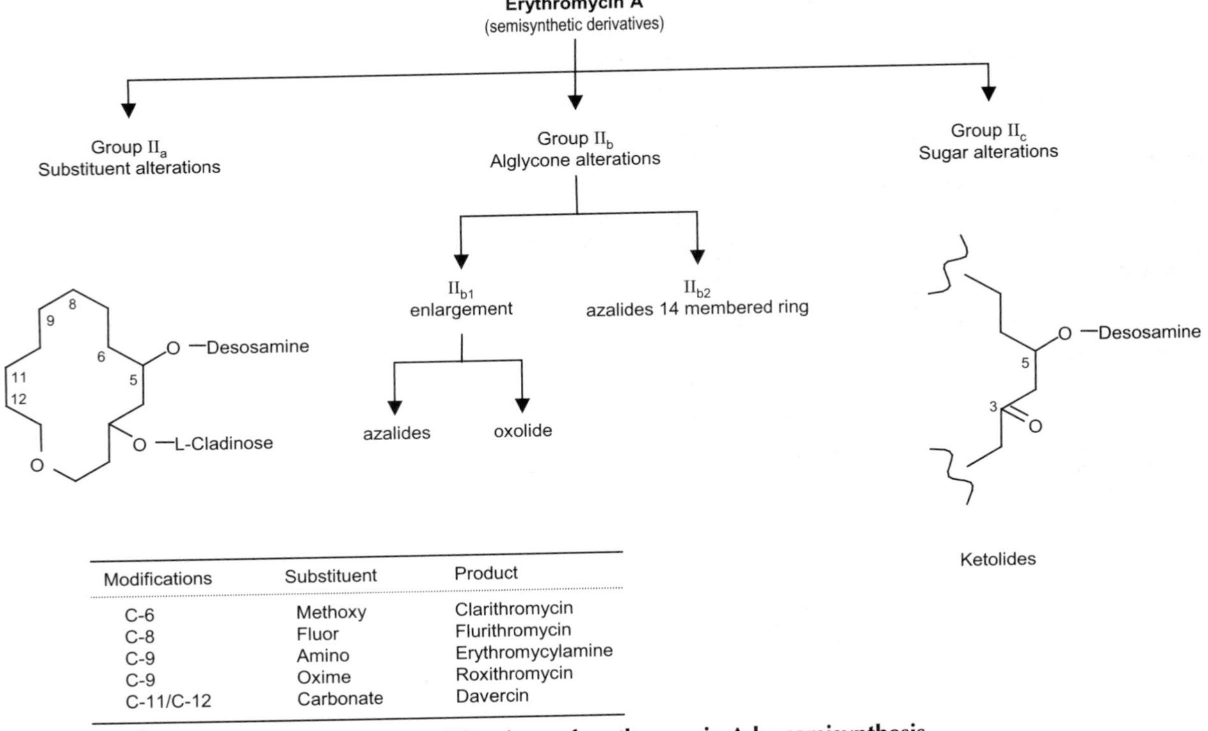

Modifications	Substituent	Product
C-6	Methoxy	Clarithromycin
C-8	Fluor	Flurithromycin
C-9	Amino	Erythromycylamine
C-9	Oxime	Roxithromycin
C-11/C-12	Carbonate	Davercin

Figure 2 Modifications of erythromycin A by semisynthesis

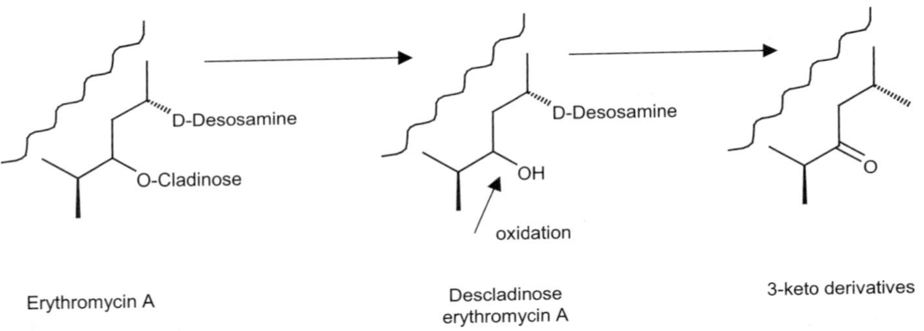

Figure 3 Definition of a ketolide

4.4.2. L-Cladinose

The lack of L-cladinose reduces the activity against clarithromycin-susceptible strains, even with the addition of an oxime at position 9 instead of a 9-keto. However, the lack of L-cladinose makes it possible to overcome resistance to erythromycin A for an isolate harboring an inducible MLS_B mechanism of resistance. This has been clearly demonstrated in reference strains of *S. aureus*. Conversely, the available ketolides are inactive against strains with constitutive MLS_B mechanisms of resistance to erythromycin A (Table 1). This allows increased stability in an acidic medium.

4.4.3. Carbamate Residue at C-11 and C-12 of Erythronolide A

4.4.3.1. Carbamate Residues

The carbamate or carbazate residue is responsible for the antibacterial activities of the different compounds and their pharmacokinetic profiles.

In order to increase the stability of erythromycin A in an acidic medium, the various weak points have been blocked chemically. The hydroxyl group at position 12 was first masked by a cyclic 11,12-carbonate residue. This derivative is four times more active than erythromycin A and has a long apparent elimination half-life. However, one of the drawbacks of such derivatives could be their hepatotoxicity (Kingsley et al., 1983).

Baker et al. (1988) synthesized a series of derivatives of erythromycin A with a cyclic carbamate between positions C-11 and C-12 of erythromycin A.

A series of derivatives of clarithromycin with a carbamate chain has been synthesized (Fig. 11). These derivatives have better antibacterial activity than clarithromycin against *S. pyogenes* strains resistant to erythromycin A by an MLS_B mechanism, but this antibacterial activity is not within the therapeutic margin (Table 2) (Fernandes et al., 1989).

Substitution of carbons 11 and 12 of the aglycone ring increases the activity against clarithromycin-susceptible strains, even in the absence of L-cladinose. The activity is also found against erythromycin A-resistant strains and is double that of the nonsubstituted compound.

The antibacterial activity of erythromycin A is increased when a carbonate (davercin) or carbamate (A-62514) residue is attached at C-11 and C-12.

RU-57708, which is the ketolide derivative of A-66321, has good activity against erythromycin A-resistant strains harboring an inducible MLS_B mechanism (Table 3).

The ketolide derivative is more active than its L-cladinose counterpart against erythromycin A-susceptible strains. Conversely, the in vitro activities against strains of *S. pyogenes* that are resistant by an efflux mechanism are comparable for the two derivatives.

The lack of L-cladinose increases the activity of the carbamate derivatives against *S. pneumoniae* and *S. pyogenes*, but the activity against strains that are resistant through an

Picromycin

Narbomycin

Figure 4 Picromycin and narbomycin

Figure 6 9-Oxime-3-keto-erythromycin A derivative (Le Mahieu et al., 1974)

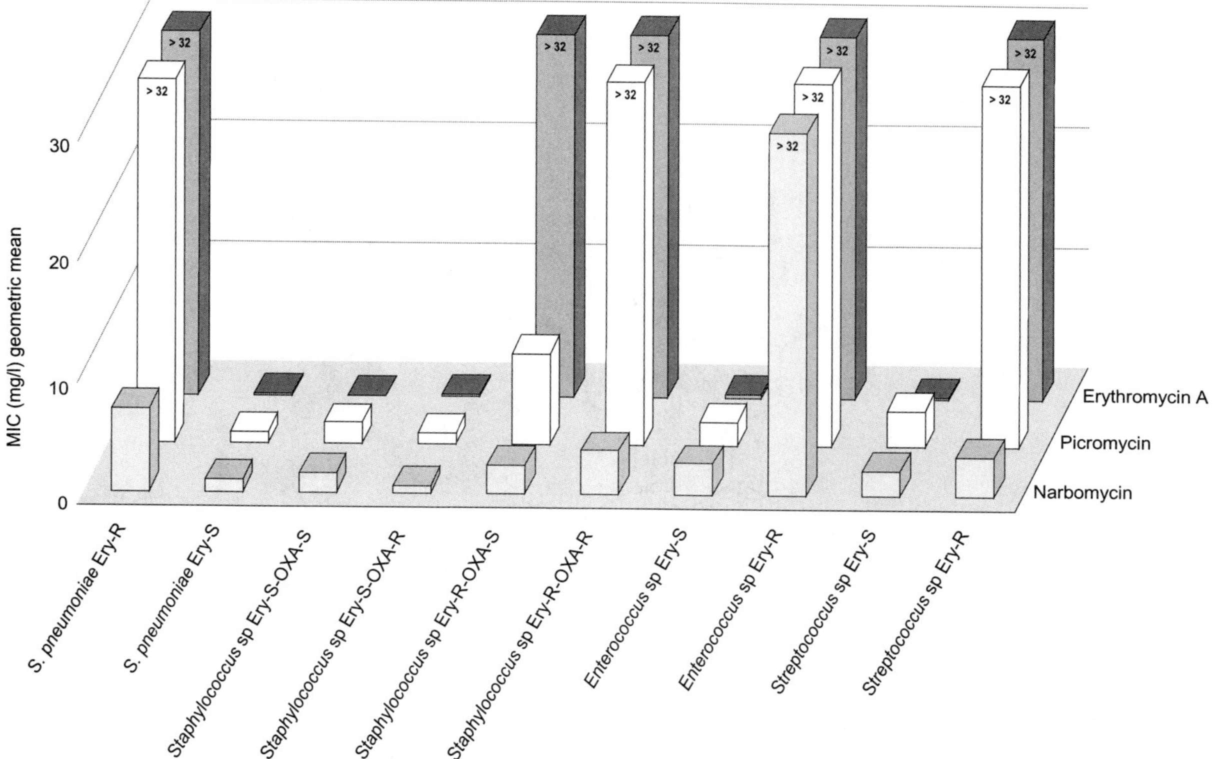

Figure 5 In vitro activity of narbomycin

Interaction

Internal ketalization

Stable derivative

Figure 7 **Hemiketalization between C-6 hydroxyl and 3-keto**

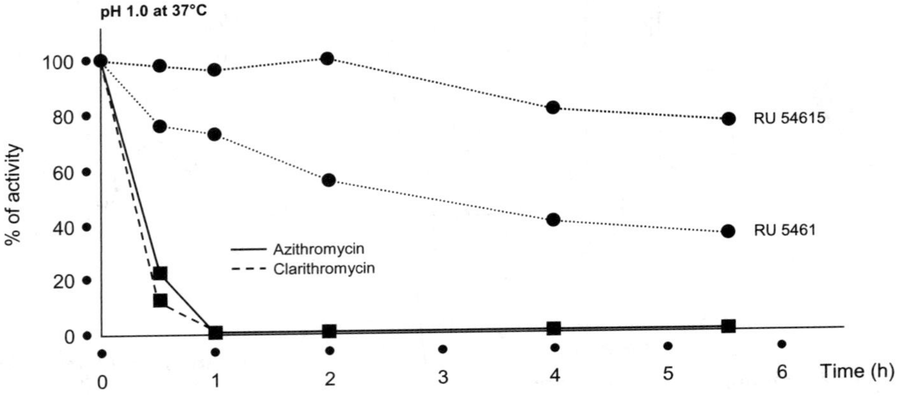

Figure 8 **Acid stability of ketolides**

I, X = COOMe
X = NH_2, OH, OMe, NO_2, $CONH_2$, F

Figure 9 **11,12-Carbamate and C-6-*O*-alkyl derivative**

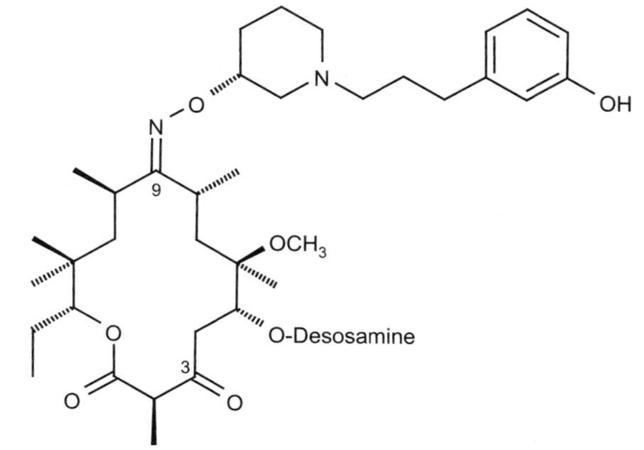

Figure 10 RU-504 (9-oxime ketolide)

Table 1 In vitro activity of descladinose clarithromycin

Organism (no. of isolates)	$MIC_{50/90}$ (μg/ml)	
	Descladinose clarithromycin	Clarithromycin
S. aureus (25)	1.56/3.13	0.39/0.39
S. pyogenes (23)	0.20/0.39	0.05/0.05
S. pneumoniae (13)	0.20/0.39	0.05/0.78
E. faecalis (17)	1.56/2.13	0.39/3.13
H. influenzae (20)	25/25	6.25/6.25
S. aureus Ery[r] (MLS_B)	0.78/1.56	>100
S. pneumoniae Ery[r]	0.20/0.39	1.56

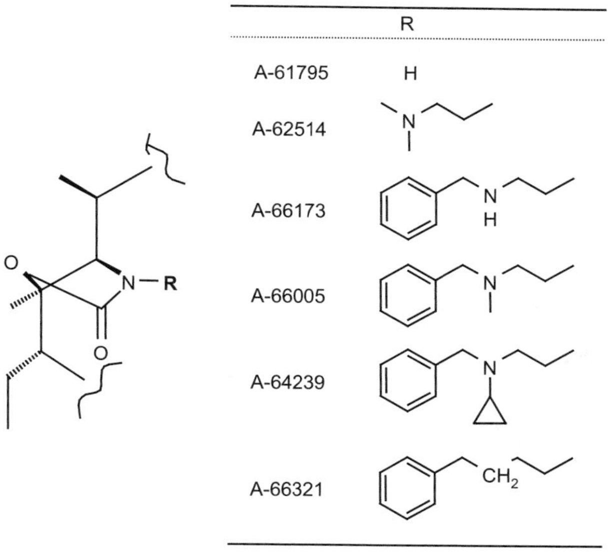

Figure 11 Carbamate derivatives of clarithromycin

efflux mechanism appears to be related to the nature of the chain attached to the carbamate (Table 4).

The nature of the carbamate chain exerts a major influence on the antibacterial activity of the different compounds. The key points in terms of activity are the length of the chain and the presence or absence of a heteroatom (oxygen, sulfur, or nitrogen). The incorporation of a heteroatom

Table 2 In vitro activities of the carbamate derivatives of clarithromycin

Drug	MIC (μg/ml) for *S. pyogenes* strain			
	EES61	2548[a]	2707	930[b]
A-61795	0.12	1	0.06	64
A-62514	0.12	4	0.25	64
A-66173	0.06	0.25	0.03	4
A-66005	0.03	0.25	0.03	4
A-64239	0.12	0.50	0.12	4
A-66321	0.12	0.50	0.06	8
Clarithromycin	0.06	2	0.06	>128

[a]Strain 2548 is erythromycin resistant (efflux).
[b]Strain 930 has constitutive MLS_B-type resistance.

Table 3 In vitro activity of RU-57708 versus A-66321[a]

Organism	MIC (μg/ml)		
	Phenotype[b]	A-66321	RU-57708
S. aureus 6538 P	Ery[s]		0.39
S. aureus A-5177	Ery[r] (I)		0.20
S. aureus A-5278	Ery[r] (C)		100
S. pyogenes EES 61	Ery[s]	0.06	0.02
S. pyogenes 2548	Ery[r] efflux	0.5	0.39
S. pyogenes 930	Ery[r] (C)	>128	50

[a]Data from Griesgraber et al., 1996.
[b]I, inducible; C, constitutive.

Table 4 Activities of carbamate ketolides against *S. pyogenes* and *S. pneumoniae* resistant to erythromycin A by efflux

Drug	MIC (μg/ml)	
	S. pyogenes PIU 3548	*S. pneumoniae* S 646
Erythromycin A	6.2	16
A-223322	1.56	4
A-223324	1.56	4
A-223321	3.1	4
A-223323	0.39	2

plays a major role in terms of activity against *H. influenzae* (Phan et al., 1998).

However, it should be realized that it is difficult to obtain a compound with very marked activity against both gram-positive cocci and *H. influenzae*. The best compromise must be made in order to obtain optimal activity, as has been obtained with telithromycin.

4.4.3.2. Carbamate-Cyclic Imine Chain

The combination of substitution at C-11 and C-12 of erythromycin A and modification of the keto at position 9 was obtained by cyclization between the carbamate and a cyclic imine from C-9, giving rise to several series of derivatives, the prototype of which is TE-802. Compounds substituted at C-11 and C-12 have good activity against *Enterococcus faecalis*.

Certain derivatives with a cyclic imine chain substituted on the 11,12-carbamate have been prepared. They have the general characteristic of ketolides, namely, that of being active against strains resistant to erythromycin A by an inducible MLS_B mechanism. It is the level of this activity which varies depending on the nature and spatial position of the substituent on the cyclic imine ring.

Dimethylation (TE-806) and the presence of a β-methyl (TE-935) do not substantially modify the activity against *S. pneumoniae, S. pyogenes,* or *S. aureus*. The in vitro activity of TE-943 (α-methyl) against *E. faecalis* is half of those of other molecules (Fig. 12).

Numerous variants with an additional ring on the cyclic amine have been prepared, yielding tetracyclic ketolides. Tetrahydrofuran, cyclopentyl, or pyrrolidine rings have been attached. None of these derivatives is more active than TE-802 (Phan et al., 1998).

4.4.3.3. Carbazate Chain

In order to increase the antibacterial activity and to try to overcome the obstacle of the lack of activity against strains of *S. aureus* resistant to erythromycin A by a constitutive MLS_B mechanism, a carbazate chain has been proposed (Fig. 13).

Several series of derivatives with a cyclic carbazate between positions C-11 and C-12 of the aglycone have been synthesized (Griesgraber et al., 1996).

It has been shown that the nonsubstituted carbazate ketolide derivative has good activity against erythromycin A-susceptible strains and those resistant by an inducible but not a constitutive MLS_B mechanism and likewise against *S. pyogenes*. However, the stereochemistry of the derivative is important, the 10-(*R*)-carbazate being 10 to 30 times more active than the 10-(*S*)-carbazate (a methyl is attached at position 10). Different alkyl or oxyalkyl chains have been attached, but the compounds obtained are less active against *S. aureus* than the nonsubstituted derivative. Likewise, the presence of an alicyclic chain does not increase the antibacterial activity compared to that of the initial 10-(*R*)-carbazate derivative.

N-Alkyl or imino derivatives are more active. The best derivatives are those with a substituted phenyl (chlorine or methoxy) or a phenylpropyl.

HMR 3004 has a quinoline nucleus attached to the carbazate by a propyl chain (Fig. 14). This molecule is more active than the previous molecules. Numerous investigations have been performed with this prototype molecule.

Like the other ketolides, this molecule is active against gram-positive cocci strains resistant to erythromycin A by an inducible MLS_B mechanism. It has excellent in vitro activity against gram-positive cocci, intracellular bacteria, and mycoplasmas, including *Mycoplasma hominis*, which is atypical for a 14-membered-ring macrolide. Its antibacterial activity is summarized in Table 5.

4.4.4. 9-Oxime Substituent

In a new series of ketolide derivatives, it was shown that (E)-9-oxime derivative with a piperidyl moiety and a 11,12-carbamate gained in vitro activity against *S. pyogenes* constitutively resistant to erythromycin A (MIC, 0.6 μg/ml for constitutively resistant *S. pyogenes*, instead of >4.0 μg/ml) (Denis et al., 2003) (Fig. 15).

	R_1	R_2
TE-802	H	H
TE-935	CH_3	H
TE-943	H	CH_3
TE-806	CH_3	CH_3

Figure 12 Derivatives of the 11,12, cyclic 9-amine ketolide type

C_{11}-C_{12} carbamate derivatives (HMR 3647, TE-810)

C_{11}-C_{12} carbazate derivatives (HMR 3004)

Figure 13 Carbamate and carbazate ketolides

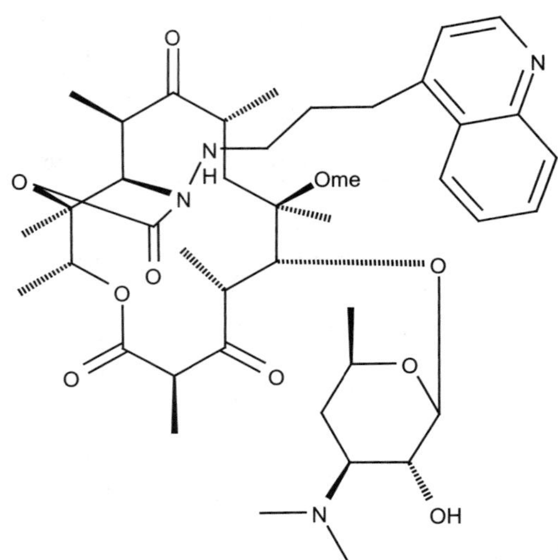

Figure 14 HMR 3004

Table 5 In vitro activity of HMR 3004[a]

Organism(s)	MIC (μg/ml) 50%	MIC (μg/ml) 90%
S. aureus Oxa[s] or Oxa[r] Ery[s]	0.03	0.06
S. aureus Oxa[s] or Oxa[r] Ery[r] (I[b])	0.06	0.128
S. pyogenes	0.008	0.015
Viridans group streptococci	0.015	0.03
S. agalactiae	0.015	0.015
S. pneumoniae	0.008	0.008
M. hominis	0.12	0.5
M. pneumoniae	0.0002	0.001
L. pneumophila	0.008	0.03
E. faecalis	0.015	0.03

[a]Data from Felmingham, 1996.
[b]I, inducible.

4.4.5. Activity against Strains Resistant by an MLS_B-Type Mechanism

The lack of L-cladinose does not abolish the activity of the erythromycin A derivative. The presence of a 3-keto or 3-O-substituted group increases the activity against strains of gram-positive cocci resistant to erythromycin A by an inducible but not a constitutive type of MLS_B mechanism.

4.5. Stability in an Acidic Medium

It has been clearly demonstrated that the different ketolides studied are very stable in an acidic medium, even if the pH is 1.2, depending on the substituent fixed on the aglycone. This stability is different from that obtained with clarithromycin, azithromycin, or roxithromycin.

Roxithromycin is stable in an acidic medium when the pH is 4.2. More than 90% of the antibacterial activity remains after exposure for more than 1 h (Fig. 16); the same applies to azithromycin.

Figure 15 9-Oxime piperidyl carbamate ketolide

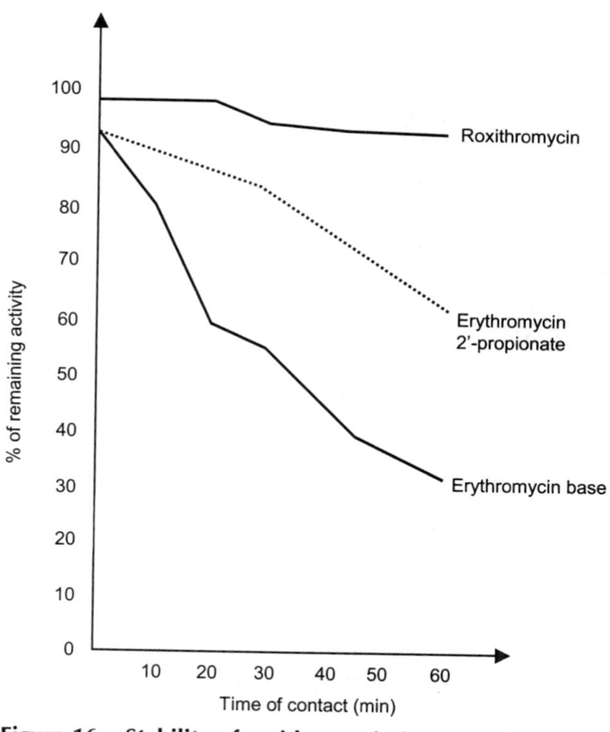

Figure 16 Stability of roxithromycin in an acidic medium (pH 4.2) (Bryskier et al., 1993)

The ketolides HMR 3004, telithromycin, TE-810, and TE-802 are not destroyed at pH 1.2 after more than 6 h of contact (Fig. 17).

It has been shown that azithromycin and roxithromycin are hydrolyzed at the β-O-glycoside bond at position 3 in an acidic medium (pH 1.2). The resultant descladinose product has a 3-hydroxyl on the lactone nucleus. These compounds are highly stable in an acidic medium (Fiese and Steffen, 1990; Bryskier et al., 1993a).

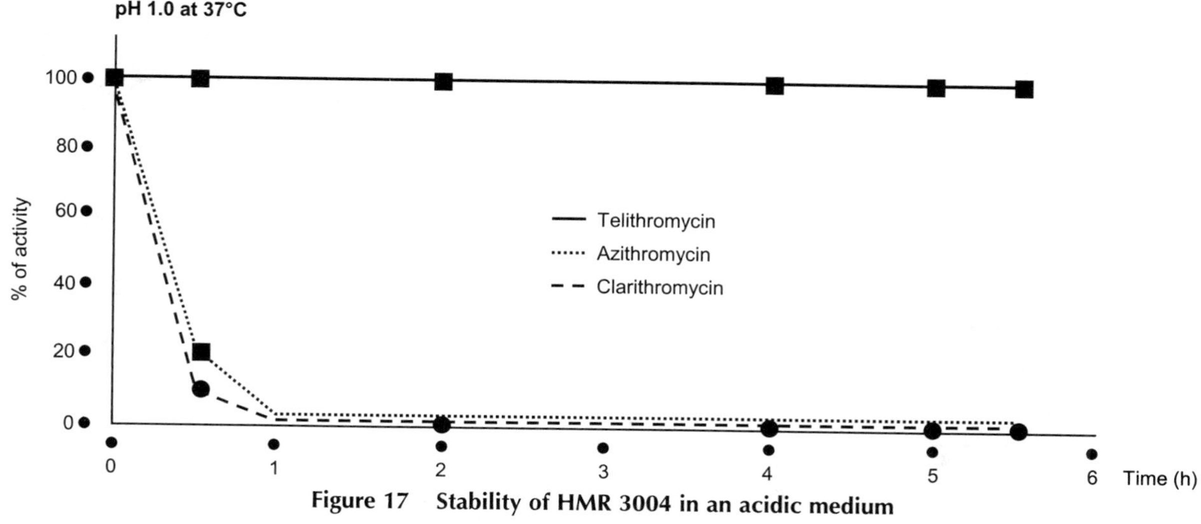

Figure 17 Stability of HMR 3004 in an acidic medium

5. TELITHROMYCIN (HMR 3647)

Telithromycin is a ketolide characterized by an alkyl chain containing two heterocycles, imidazolyl and pyridinyl, which are attached to the carbamate residue at C-11 and C-12 of the erythronolide A nucleus by a propyl chain (Fig. 18).

5.1. Physicochemical Properties

The physicochemical properties are summarized in Table 6. Telithromycin is very stable in an acidic medium. More than 90% of its activity remained after contact for 6 h or more (24 h) in an acidic medium at pH 1.2.

5.2. In Vitro Antibacterial Activity

The antibacterial spectrum of telithromycin encompasses that of the macrolides but also includes the majority of gram-positive bacteria.

Telithromycin is more active in vitro than clarithromycin against gram-positive and gram-negative cocci, and also against erythromycin A-susceptible strains of gram-positive bacilli. It is active against strains of gram-positive cocci resistant to erythromycin A by an efflux or (inducible) MLS_B mechanism of resistance.

5.2.1. Staphylococci

The strains of *S. aureus* are divided into oxacillin-susceptible and -resistant strains. However, the activity of telithromycin against these strains is dependent on their susceptibility to erythromycin A and the mechanism of resistance to erythromycin A: inducible or constitutive MLS_B.

Against strains susceptible to erythromycin A or resistant by an inducible mechanism, telithromycin has excellent activity (oxacillin-susceptible or -resistant strain), with MICs at which 50 and 90% of isolates tested are inhibited (MIC_{50} and MIC_{90}, respectively) of 0.06 and 0.12 μg/ml. However, against strains resistant to erythromycin A by a constitutive MLS_B mechanism, telithromycin is inactive (Table 7).

Clarithromycin is inactive against erythromycin A-resistant strains, irrespective of the mechanism of resistance. The activity of telithromycin against the different species of coagulase-negative staphylococci is good, with MIC_{50}s and MIC_{90}s of 0.03 and 0.25 μg/ml (Kitzis et al., 1997; Felmingham et al., 1998).

5.2.2. Streptococci

Telithromycin is very active against beta-hemolytic streptococci of Lancefield groups A, B, C, and G when the strains are susceptible to erythromycin A, with MIC_{50}s and MIC_{90}s of 0.008 and 0.015 μg/ml. The in vitro activity remains excellent against erythromycin A-resistant strains, particularly where an efflux mechanism is involved, whereas that of clarithromycin is markedly decreased (Table 8).

5.2.3. *S. pneumoniae*

Strains of *S. pneumoniae* that are susceptible or resistant to penicillin G, erythromycin A, ofloxacin, co-trimoxazole, or tetracyclines are highly susceptible to telithromycin.

The antibacterial activity persists whether the strain is resistant by an MLS_B mechanism or by efflux (erythromycin-resistant, clindamycin-susceptible strain: M-phenotype).

Against strains resistant to erythromycin A by an MLS_B mechanism, clarithromycin is inactive (MIC, >32 μg/ml).

The MIC_{50}s and MIC_{90}s of telithromycin are ≤0.008 and 0.25 μg/ml (Table 9) (Barry et al., 1997; Visalli et al., 1997).

5.2.4. Viridans Group Streptococci

The activity of telithromycin is good against viridans group streptococci, irrespective of the resistance phenotype (erythromycin A-resistant, penicillin G-resistant) (Table 10).

5.2.5. Gram-Positive Bacilli

The gram-positive bacilli comprise several bacterial genera and species, including *Listeria* spp., *Bacillus* spp., *Erysipelothrix rhusiopathiae*, coryneforms, and lactic bacilli.

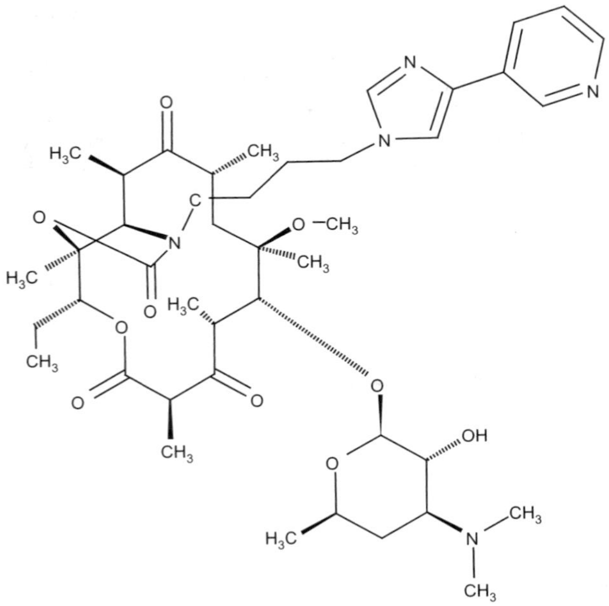

Figure 18 Telithromycin

Table 7 Telithromycin: in vitro activity against *S. aureus*

S. aureus phenotype[a]	MIC (μg/ml) Telithromycin 50%	Telithromycin 90%	Clarithromycin 50%	Clarithromycin 90%
Oxa^s Ery^s	0.04	0.08	0.5	0.5
Oxa^s Ery^r (I)	0.08	0.3	>40	>40
Oxa^s Ery^r (C)	>40	>40	>40	>40
Oxa^r Ery^s	0.12	0.25	0.5	0.5
Oxa^r Ery^r (I)	0.12	0.13	>40	>40
Oxa^r Ery^r (I)	>128	>128	>128	>128

[a]I, inducible; C, constitutive.

Table 6 Telithromycin and HMR 3004: physicochemical properties

Drug	Empirical formula	Mol wt	pK_a	LogP	Melting point (°C)
HMR 3004	$C_{43}H_{64}N_4O_{10}$	797.01	5.5; 8.7	4.1	183
Telithromycin	$C_{43}H_{54}N_5O_{10}$	812	5.1; 3; 8.7	3.5	177

Table 8 Telithromycin: activity against *S. pyogenes*[a]

Drug	MIC$_{50}$ (μg/ml)			
	MLS$_B$ constitutive	MLS$_B$ inducible	Efflux	Susceptible
Telithromycin	4	1	≤0.06	0.06
Erythromycin A	>128	>128	8	0.06
Clarithromycin	>128	>128	4	0.03
Roxithromycin	>128	>128	16	0.12
Josamycin	>128	>128	8	0.12
Rokitamycin	2	≤0.06	≤0.06	0.12
Clindamycin	>128	≤0.06	0.25	0.12
Amoxicillin	0.01	0.01	0.007	0.007

[a]Data from Coccuza et al., 1998.

Table 9 Telithromycin: in vitro activity against *S. pneumoniae*

S. pneumoniae phenotype[a]	MIC (μg/ml)			
	Telithromycin		Clarithromycin	
	50%	90%	50%	90%
Pen^s	0.03	0.06	0.2	0.25
Pen^i	0.03	0.06	0.25	0.5
Pen^r	0.03	0.25	0.5	>64
Ery^s clindamycin susceptible	0.03	0.03	0.03	0.03
Ery^r clindamycin resistant	0.03	0.03	>32	>32
Ery^r clindamycin susceptible	0.25	0.5	2	4
Tetracycline resistant	0.01	0.01	0.06	0.06
Co-trimoxazole resistant	0.03	0.06	0.06	0.08
Ofloxacin resistant	0.03	0.03	0.25	0.25

Table 10 Activity of telithromycin against viridans group streptococci

Viridans group streptococcus phenotype	MIC (μg/ml)			
	Telithromycin		Clarithromycin	
	50%	90%	50%	90%
Pen^s Ery^s	0.005	0.02	0.01	>32
Pen^r	0.06	0.12	1	64
Ery^r	0.03			

Diphtheria is again emerging as a public health problem in certain European countries such as Russia and the Ukraine, and even in Caucasian republics such as Georgia. Antibiotic treatment is based on penicillin G or erythromycin A. Erythromycin A-resistant strains have been described.

Telithromycin is very active against *C. diphtheriae*, whether or not the strain is toxigenic, with MIC$_{50}$s and MIC$_{90}$s of 0.004 and 0.008 μg/ml (Engler et al., 1997).

The activity against *Listeria monocytogenes* is excellent, with MIC$_{50}$s and MIC$_{90}$s of 0.03 and 0.25 μg/ml, and also against *E. rhusiopathiae* (MICs, ≤0.015 and 0.06 μg/ml).

The lactic bacilli form a complex group that includes the following bacterial genera: *Lactobacillus*, *Leuconostoc*, *Pediococcus*, and *Lactococcus*. Medical interest has recently focused on these bacterial genera because of the increasingly common description of infections due to these opportunistic bacteria in immunodepressed patients such as AIDS patients (Table 11) (Torres et al., 1997).

The in vitro activity of telithromycin against the various species that make up the group of coryneforms is excellent.

The world of coryneforms has evolved considerably as a result of the taxonomic classifications. A number of species are involved in nosocomial infections, such as *Corynebacterium jeikeium* and *Corynebacterium urealyticum*.

Telithromycin is very active against the majority of corynebacteria. The distribution of the strains of *C. jeikeium* with regard to the antibacterial activity of telithromycin is bimodal. Likewise, because of difficulties of taxonomic positioning, there is a difference among authors with respect to the activity of *C. urealyticum*.

Telithromycin has been shown to have good activity against erythromycin A-resistant strains of corynebacteria (MIC, ≥0.5 μg/ml) (Table 12).

Table 11 Telithromycin: in vitro activity against gram-positive bacilli

Organism(s)	MIC (μg/ml)		
	50%	90%	Range
C. diphtheriae	0.004	0.008	0.004–0.015
L. monocytogenes	0.03	0.03	0.03–0.06
Bacillus spp.			0.06–0.12
E. rhusiopathiae			≤0.015–0.06
Rhodococcus spp.	0.25	0.25	≤0.015–0.25
Leuconostoc spp.	0.007	0.25	≤0.007–0.25
Pediococcus spp.	≤0.03	≤0.03	≤0.03
Lactobacillus spp.	0.007	0.125	≤0.007–0.25
Lactococcus spp.			≤0.03–2

Table 12 In vitro activity of telithromycin against erythromycin A-resistant coryneforms (MIC, >0.5 μg/ml)

Organism	*n*	MIC (μg/ml)	
		50%	90%
C. urealyticum	16	0.5	2
C. jeikeium	25	0.25	>128
Corynebacterium amycolatum	36	0.12	0.5
Corynebacterium pseudodiphtheriticum	10	0.06	0.12
Corynebacterium striatum	21	16	32
Corynebacterium minutissimum	6	0.03	0.06

5.2.6. *Enterococcus* spp.

Telithromycin has good activity against *E. faecalis* compared to clarithromycin. Telithromycin is active against gentamicin-resistant, β-lactamase-producing, erythromycin A-resistant, and vancomycin-teicoplanin-resistant (VanA) strains. Clarithromycin is inactive (Table 13).

Telithromycin is also active, albeit moderately, against *Enterococcus faecium*, with little variation according to the resistance phenotype (Table 14).

5.2.7. *Neisseria meningitidis*

N. meningitidis strains of reduced susceptibility to penicillin G have been described in certain regions of the world, particularly in Spain, South Africa, the United States, Israel, and, to a lesser extent, France.

Rifampin-resistant strains are increasingly common; conversely, some erythromycin A- or spiramycin-resistant strains have been observed which harbor an efflux mechanism of resistance mediated by Mtr (encoded by the *mtr* gene).

The activity of telithromycin is excellent, with MIC_{50}s and MIC_{90}s of 0.015 and 0.125 μg/ml.

5.2.8. Bacteria Responsible for Lower Respiratory Tract Infections

Lower respiratory tract infections, whether parenchymatous (pneumonia) or nonparenchymatous (superinfection of acute exacerbation of chronic bronchitis), are due to common pathogens or to intracellular or atypical bacteria.

The common pathogens most commonly involved in lower respiratory tract infections are *S. pneumoniae*, *H. influenzae*, and, more marginally, *Moraxella catarrhalis*.

5.2.8.1. *H. influenzae*

The determination of the in vitro activity of an antibacterial agent against *H. influenzae* is always difficult, as it is poorly standardized. The media used vary: Haemophilus test medium (HTM), Mueller-Hinton medium supplemented with red blood cell extract, 3% Fildes, IsoVitaleX, and laked horse blood plus NAD.

HTM is the medium currently recommended by the NCCLS Subcommittee for Antibiotic Sensitivity Testing. However, it is prepared in each laboratory and must be used within 3 weeks of its preparation.

This is further compounded by the complexity of the culture medium and the addition of 5 to 6% CO_2 to the incubation atmosphere, which in the case of macrolides markedly affects the in vitro activity.

Telithromycin has in vitro activity similar to that of azithromycin against *H. influenzae* and greater than that of clarithromycin and roxithromycin. Telithromycin exerts bactericidal activity at two to four times the MIC after 12 h of contact with the antibiotic. In vivo, telithromycin has better activity than azithromycin in lung bacterial clearance of murine pneumococcal pneumonia.

5.2.8.2. *Bordetella pertussis*

B. pertussis is responsible for whooping cough. Macrolides remain the reference antibiotic treatment. Erythromycin A-resistant strains are rare.

The activities of telithromycin and other macrolides are presented in Table 15.

5.2.8.3. Intracellular Bacteria

The intracellular bacteria responsible for pneumonia are mainly *C. pneumoniae* and *L. pneumophila*.

5.2.8.3.1. C. *pneumoniae*. The determination of the activity of an antibacterial agent against *C. pneumoniae* can be difficult, as it depends on the number of strains available, which are few, and the cell lines.

The latter point is crucial, as it has been well demonstrated that certain cell lines allow better growth of *C. pneumoniae*, such as the HEp-2 line, as opposed to the McCoy line. Penetration of the antibiotic into the cells is dependent on the pH of the culture broth, its calcium content, and probably other poorly established parameters.

The activities of different macrolides, including telithromycin, are summarized in Table 16.

C. pneumoniae is an intracellular agent of relatively recent discovery (Graystone et al., 1989) that appears to be implicated in numerous pathological processes, such as lower respiratory tract infections and perhaps asthma, and atheromatous diseases.

In some clinical studies it had been shown that roxithromycin (Gurfinkel et al., 1997; Gurfinkel, 1998) and

Table 13 Activity of telithromycin against *E. faecalis*[a]

Organism	*n*	MIC (μg/ml)			
		Telithromycin		Clarithromycin	
		50%	90%	50%	90%
E. faecalis	20	0.12	2	4	>128
E. faecalis HLGR	20	1	4	>128	>128
E. faecalis BLA+	10	0.12	4	>128	>128
E. faecalis VanA	10	0.5	0.5	>128	>128
E. faecalis VanB	21	8	16	>128	>128
E. faecalis Ery[r]	12	2	2	>128	>128

[a]Data from Schülin et al., 1997, and Hoban et al., 1997.

Table 14 Activity of telithromycin against *E. faecium*[a]

E. faecium phenotype	MIC (μg/ml)			
	Telithromycin		Clarithromycin	
	50%	90%	50%	90%
Wild	2	8	>128	>128
HLGR	8	8	>128	>128
VanA	4	4	>128	>128
VanB	4	16	>128	>128
Ery[r]	2	2	>128	>128

[a]Data from Schülin et al., 1997.

Table 15 Activities of telithromycin and 14- and 15-membered-ring macrolides against *B. pertussis*[a]

Drug	MIC (μg/ml)	
	50%	90%
Telithromycin	0.03	0.03
Erythromycin A	0.06	0.06
Clarithromycin	0.015	0.03
Roxithromycin	0.12	0.5
Azithromycin	0.03	0.03

[a]Data from Hoppe et al., 1998.

Table 16 **Activities of macrolides against *C. pneumoniae*[a]**

Drug	MIC (μg/ml)	MCC[b] (μg/ml)
Telithromycin	0.125	0.125
Roxithromycin	0.125	0.125
Azithromycin	0.125	0.125
Erythromycin A	0.03	0.03

[a]Data from Roblin et al., 1997.
[b]MCC, minimal chlamydial concentration.

azithromycin (Gupta et al., 1997) significantly improve the prognosis for coronary diseases when added to the underlying symptomatic treatment.

5.2.8.3.2. *L. pneumophila*. Erythromycin A and its derivatives and rifampin represent the reference antibacterial agents for the treatment of *L. pneumophila* pneumonia.

The in vitro activity may be biased if it is determined on a charcoal-containing medium (buffered charcoal-yeast extract). In the case of macrolides, it must always be determined on a charcoal-free medium (buffered yeast extract). The activity of telithromycin is excellent. The activities of different macrolides are presented in Table 17.

5.2.8.3.3. *Parachlamydia* and *Simkania*. Trophozoites of *Acanthamoeba* hosting chlamydia-like bacteria have been isolated from patients with fever associated with use of humidifiers in Vermont (Hall's coccus strain) and from nasal mucosa (strain Bn9). The use of antibiotics directed against *Parachlamydia* has been reported for 8 of 376 patients suffering from community-acquired pneumonia. *Parachlamydia* does not grow on an acellular medium. An in vitro infection model of amoebae (*Acanthamoeba polyphaga*) had been developed to test antibacterials. *Parachlamydia* spontaneously causes lysis of amoebae after culture for 3 to 5 days. The inhibitory effect of antibacterials on cell lysis was investigated to determine MICs (Table 18).

5.2.8.3.4. *Tropheryma whipplei*. *T. whipplei* is responsible for a chronic disease, Whipple's disease, which is characterized by arthralgia and diarrhea.

MCR5 cells were infected with *T. whipplei*. The growth of *T. whipplei* was inhibited according to the method of quantification of the copies of DNA (Table 19).

5.2.8.3.5. *Afipia* and *Bosea* Species. Nosocomial pneumonia, a frequent complication associated with morbidity, and mortality, is one of the leading cause of morbidity from nosocomial infections. Community-acquired pneumonia is associated with a case fatality rate of up to 8.8%. In about 47 to 55% of cases of community-acquired pneumonia no bacterial agents are identified.

Table 17 **Activities of macrolides against *L. pneumophila*[a]**

Drug	MIC (μg/ml)	
	50%	90%
Telithromycin	0.03	0.12
Erythromycin A	0.25	0.5
Clarithromycin	0.03	0.03
Azithromycin	0.12	1
Roxithromycin	0.12	0.12
Josamycin	0.25	0.25
Miokamycin	0.12	0.12

[a]Data from Felmingham et al., 1997.

Table 18 **In vitro activities of antibacterials against *Parachlamydia***

Drug	MIC (μg/ml)	
	BN9	Hall's coccus
Telithromycin	0.25	0.5
Erythromycin A	0.5	0.5
Penicillin G	>32	>32
Amoxicillin	>32	>32
Ceftriaxone	2	1
Gentamicin	0.5	1
Thiamphenicol	>32	>32
Doxycycline	0.25	1
Co-trimoxazole	0.25/2.5	2/10
Rifampin	0.25	0.25
Ciprofloxacin	>16	>16
Vancomycin	>16	>16

Table 19 **Activities of antibacterials against *T. whipplei***

Drug	Concn (μg/ml) inhibiting growth
Penicillin G	100
Streptomycin	10
Rifampin	4
Doxycycline	4
Co-trimoxazole	1.6/8.0
Ciprofloxacin	2.0
Levofloxacin	0.25
Telithromycin	0.25

By means of amoebic coculture procedures, many fastidious amoebic resistant bacteria have been isolated from the environment (water), such as *Legionella* spp., *Afipia*, *Bosea*, *Parachlamydia* spp., and *Rhodobacter* spp.

Afipia species belong to the α-Proteobacteria (*Bradyrhizobiaceae* family). The genus *Afipia* is composed of at least six species: *A. felis*, *A. clevelandensis*, *A. broomeae*, *A. massiliensis*, *A. birgiae*, and *Afipia* genospecies 1, 2, and 3. For the genus *Bosea* the following species have been reported: *B. massiliensis*, *B. minatitlanensis*, *B. thiooxidans*, *B. eneae*, and *B. vestrisii*.

MICs of various antibacterials were determined for both *Afipia* and *Bosea* species. The microtiter plates were used for MIC determinations after a 72- to 96-h subculture on buffered charcoal-yeast extract agar (Table 20).

In general, both *Afipia* spp. and *Bosea* spp. are poorly susceptible to β-lactams, colistin, and vancomycin. The antibacterial activities of other antibacterial agents vary according to bacterial species. Apparently *Afipia* genospecies 1, 2, and 3 are the least susceptible pathogens.

It was demonstrated that *A. felis* is able to grow intracellularly. The mechanism of intracellular survival of *A. felis* was shown to be a phagosome-lysosome inhibiting factor. Uptake by macrophages directly into a nonendocyctic compartment is induced.

5.2.9. Bacteria Involved in Sexually Transmitted Diseases

The sexually transmitted diseases are mainly due to *Neisseria gonorrhoeae*, *Chlamydia trachomatis*, *Haemophilus ducreyi*, and *Gardnerella vaginalis*. Syphilis is due to *Treponema pallidum*

Table 20 In vitro activities of antibacterials against *Afipia* and *Bosea*

Drug	MIC (μg/ml)	
	Afipia spp.	*Bosea* spp.
Telithromycin	2–16	≤0.25–128
Erythromycin A	16–128	0.5–128
Ciprofloxacin	≤0.25–32	1.0–128
Levofloxacin	≤0.25–>256	≤0.25–64
Penicillin G	8.0–256	2.0–256
Amoxicillin	4.06–>256	1.0–>256
Ticarcillin	0.5–128	≤0.25–256
Piperacillin	≤0.25–64	4.0–>256
Cefoxitin	≤0.25–>256	2.0–>256
Cephalothin	2.0–>256	1.0–>256
Ceftriaxone	≤0.25–>256	≤0.25–>256
Ceftazidime	2.0–>256	≤0.25–>256
Cefepime	≤0.25–>256	≤0.25–>256
Imipenem	≤0.25–32	0.5–64
Amikacin	≤0.25–>256	0.5–256
Netilmicin	≤0.25–>256	0.5–6.0
Tobramycin	≤0.25–128	1.0–64
Gentamicin	≤0.25–32	1.0–128
Doxycycline	4.0–>256	≤0.25–4.0
Rifampin	4.0–>256	0.5–16
Colimycin	>256	16–>256
Vancomycin	>256	2.0–>256

Table 21 Telithromycin: activity against bacteria responsible for sexually transmitted diseases[a]

Organism	MIC (μg/ml)	
	50%	90%
N. gonorrhoeae	0.12	0.12
H. ducreyi	0.004	0.008
G. vaginalis	≤0.002	≤0.002
U. urealyticum	0.06	0.06
M. hominis	2	4
C. trachomatis	0.008	0.008

[a]Data from Felmingham et al., 1997.

Table 22 Telithromycin: in vitro activity against anaerobic bacteria

Organism(s)	MIC (μg/ml)	
	50%	90%
B. fragilis	8	8
B. thetaiotaomicron	4	8
Prevotella melaninogenica	0.125	0.25
Porphyromonas spp.	0.06	0.5
Peptostreptococcus spp.	0.03	0.03
Propionibacterium spp.	≤0.008	≤0.008
C. perfringens	0.125	0.125
C. difficile	0.25	>64

and appears to be experiencing a resurgence of epidemic proportions in certain regions of Great Britain and eastern Europe.

Macrolides are highly active against *N. gonorrhoeae*, irrespective of the resistance profile of the strain isolated (resistance to penicillin G, spectinomycin, tetracyclines, etc.), but the therapeutic activity is often disappointing.

Chancroid is a sexually transmitted disease due to *H. ducreyi* and is widespread; macrolides represent the standard treatment. Telithromycin is highly active against this bacterial species (Table 21).

C. trachomatis is the causative agent of trachoma in regions of endemicity, especially desert regions such as the Sahara and sub-Saharan regions, but in particular of nongonococcal urethritis in nondesert regions, and is also responsible for pelvic inflammatory disease resulting in tubular sterility.

Determination of the activity of the new antibacterial agents against *C. trachomatis* is based not only on the in vitro activity in a cellular medium but also on the preventive activity of tubular infertility in the mouse.

The activity of telithromycin is good, with MICs on the order of 0.008 μg/ml. Those of azithromycin ranged from 0.03 to 0.06 μg/ml.

Ureaplasma urealyticum is often implicated in or associated with nongonococcal urethritis. The activity of telithromycin is good, with a MIC_{50} and MIC_{90} of 0.06 μg/ml.

5.2.10. Anaerobic Bacteria

Telithromycin in vitro possesses moderate activity against gram-negative bacilli of the *Bacteroides* sp. type but good activity against *Porphyromonas* and *Prevotella* spp. and variable activity against *Fusobacterium* spp., particularly *F. mortiferum* and *F. varium*. It has excellent activity against gram-positive bacteria (Ednie et al., 1997) (Table 22).

In a murine model of abdominal abscess induced by *Bacteroides fragilis*, the activity of telithromycin was shown to be comparable to that of clindamycin at a dose of 1.25 mg/mouse twice a day (Table 23).

5.2.11. Bacteria Implicated in Infections following Animal Bites

Animal bites or scratches are common and result in several thousand medical consultations annually.

They are the cause of an important morbidity. In addition, human bites are more common than is reported. Certain bacterial species are responsible for infections following human bites, such as *Eikenella corrodens*.

The activity of telithromycin is reported in Table 24.

5.2.12. *Toxoplasma gondii*

Telithromycin inhibits the growth of *T. gondii* tachyzoites at a concentration of 0.5 μg/ml. Following experimental infection with tachyzoites of the virulent RH strain (intraperitoneal injection) or cysts of the C-56 strain, telithromycin exhibited good activity.

At a dose of 30 mg/kg of body weight, telithromycin provides protection against infection by cysts of the C-56 strain.

At a dose of 50 mg/kg for 10 days, telithromycin enabled 30% of mice to survive, while 100% survived at doses of 100 or 200 mg/kg/day.

In previous studies using the same model, spiramycin had been shown to provide no protection. The doses necessary to prevent the death of mice in acute toxoplasmosis are summarized in Table 25.

6. MECHANISMS OF ACTION

The mechanism of action of HMR 3004, telithromycin, cethromycin, and other derivatives (RU-57708) has been

Table 23 Telithromycin: in vivo activity against *B. fragilis*[a]

Drug	Dose (mg, b.i.d.[b])	No. of mice with intra-abdominal abcess/total	Cure rate (%)	*B. fragilis* CFU/mg
None (control)		10/13	23	1.4×10^6
Telithromycin	1.25	4/13	69	1.4×10^7
Clindamycin	2.5	3/13	77	1.4×10^4
Metronidazole	2.5	5/13	61	1.2×10^4
Cefotetan	2.5	5/12	58	2.9×10^4

[a]Data from Thadepalli et al., 1998.
[b]b.i.d., twice a day.

Table 24 Telithromycin activity against bacteria responsible for infections due to animal bites[a]

Organism(s)	MIC (μg/ml) 50%	90%	Range
Staphylococcus intermedius	0.03	0.12	0.015–0.03
Streptococcus canis	0.03	0.06	0.03–0.06
Actinomyces spp.			≤0.015–8
Ef-4b	0.25	0.25	0.125–1
E. corrodens	0.25	0.25	≤0.015–1
Pasteurella multocida	1	1	0.25–1
Neisseria weaveri	0.125	0.25	≤0.015–1
Weeksella zoohelcum	0.5	0.5	0.25–1

[a]Data from Goldstein, 1997.

Table 25 ED_{100} in the prevention of acute toxoplasmosis[a]

Drug	ED_{100} (mg/kg/day)
Telithromycin	100
Clarithromycin	300
Azithromycin	200
Roxithromycin	500
Spiramycin	>500

[a]Data from Araujo et al., 1997.

explored. The results obtained are not definitive. In fact, the mechanism of action of macrolides and ketolides in general is not completely elucidated.

Mechanisms of action are complex, but those of macrolides, tetracyclines, lincosamides, streptogramins, oxazolidinones, chloramphenicol, and pleuromutilins share the same target: they inhibit protein synthesis of bacteria.

Table 26 Affinity of ketolides for ribosomes

Drug	K_{diss} (M)
Erythromycin A	$(1.4 \pm 0.2) \times 10^{-8}$
HMR 3004	$(1.6 \pm 0.3) \times 10^{-9}$
Telithromycin	$(1.3 \pm 0.3) \times 10^{-9}$
RU-66252[a]	$(2.9 \pm 0.2) \times 10^{-9}$
RU-56006	$(1.8 \pm 1) \times 10^{-7}$

[a]L-Cladinose counterpart of HMR 3004.

Macrolides and ketolides penetrate in the cell via passive diffusion.

The affinity for ribosomes is higher for ketolides than for erythromycin A. The dissociation constants are summarized in Table 26.

Cethromycin binds tightly to ribosomes in comparison to erythromycin A (Table 27).

Ketolides have at least a dual mode of action, acting on the exit tunnel of the 50S ribosomal subunit and blocking the ribosomal subunit assembly.

6.1. Exit Tunnel

The exit tunnel passes through the middle of the 50S ribosomal subunit and is paved by the RNA loop mainly. The tunnel is about 100 Å in length, with a diameter up to 25 Å, and spans the 50S ribosomal subunit. The tunnel accommodates a peptide of 25 to 40 amino acids of any sequence and any conformation. The tunnel is formed with proteins L22 and L4. L22 protein is the largest contributor to the surface of the tunnel and with L4 protein forms the narrow part of the tunnel. L22 protein consists of a single domain with three α-helices packed against a three-stranded anti-parallel β-sheet which forms a hydrophobic core.

Three amino acid deletions from the side of the β-hairpin are responsible for erythromycin A resistance (Met82, Arg84, and Lys83).

Table 27 Dissociation constants

Drug	*S. pneumoniae* K_1 (M^{-1} min^{-1})[a]	K_{-1} (min^{-1})[b]	K_{diss} (M)[c]	*S. aureus* K_1 (M^{-1} min^{-1})	K_{-1} (min^{-1})	K_{diss} (M)
Erythromycin A	5.28×10^5	0.0215	4.1×10^{-8}			
Roxithromycin	4.3×10^5	6.1×10^{-3}	1.4×10^{-8}	4.3×10^5	6.1×10^{-3}	1.4×10^{-8}
Cethromycin	2.62×10^6	0.0016	6.1×10^{-10}			
HMR 3004	1.0×10^7	1.5×10^{-3}	1.5×10^{-10}	1.4×10^6	8.4×10^{-8}	6.0×10^{-10}

[a]K_1, rate constant.
[b]K_{-1}, reverse rate constant.
[c]K_{diss}, dissociation constant (K_1/K_{-1}).

L4 protein mutation prevents erythromycin A binding, and L22 protein mutation neutralizes the effect of binding.

In L4 protein mutation, one of the major changes was substantial narrowing of the tunnel entrance, which does not bind erythromycin A, making the opening smaller than an erythromycin A molecule. Presumably, telithromycin being smaller than erythromycin A, telithromycin remains active in L4 mutation.

The growing polypeptide is protected by the ribosome from enzymatic digestion until the nascent protein is large enough to fold rigidly and protect itself. Only if the growing chain finds its way into the tunnel does the process of protein biosynthesis continue, because during the initial step, the first four amino acids of the newly formed peptide may not be fixed in the space.

Partly, the functionality of ketolides is related to those of 14- and 15-membered-ring macrolides. Ketolides do not inhibit peptidyltransferase enzyme; they block the entrance to the tunnel in the large ribosomal subunit, through which the nascent peptide exits. Blockade of the exit tunnel by ketolides induces premature dissociation of peptidyl-tRNAs from the ribosome. Such a "drop-off"occurs just after initiation of protein synthesis, when the nascent polypeptide chain is short. The released peptide is composed of 9 to 12 amino acid residues irrespective of the methylation status of the ribosome.

6.2. Peptidyltransferase Center

At the ribosomal level, interactions between cethromycin (ABT-773) and the 23S rRNA have been investigated. It was shown that the L-cladinose sugar does not interact with the peptidyltransferase center.

The peptidyltransferase center consists of domains II and V, which form a pocket with 5S rRNA. Ketolides are fixed on domain V (A2058 and A2059) and domain II (A752 and A790). The 5S rRNA plays an important role in the ribosome. The putative binding of 5S rRNA with ribosomal protein L18 and L5 was mapped within the 23S rRNA segment from 2250 to 2410, near the central loop of domain V. There is a cross-linker between U89 of 5S rRNA and C2475 of 23S rRNA. At the same time, U89 can be cross-linked to several positions in domain II of 23S rRNA (U958, G1022, and G1138). 5S rRNA forms a functional link between two 23S rRNA domains. In particular, 5S rRNA could help to properly juxtaposition domains II and V in the ribosomal tertiary structure.

Cethromycin and telithromycin interact, like erythromycin A, with domain V through desoamine sugar and aglycone.

Ketolides are composed of two additional parts: a carbamate residue and a long side chain either on the carbamate, such as for telithromycin, or through the 6-hydroxyl group, as for cethromycin. The aryl group is believed to form an additional interaction with the ribosome, compensating for the free-energy loss due to the adenine dimethylation.

The carbamate of cethromycin forms a network of hydrophobic interactions with bases 2606 to 2611 and uracil 2609 of domain V. The hydrogen bond between O^4 of U2609 and N^2 of the carbamate residue may be responsible for enhancement of cethromycin affinity for ribosomes compared with that of erythromycin A. The flexibility of the side chain of both ketolides allows the moiety to occupy spatial positions. The N^3 of the quinolylallyl chain of cethromycin forms a hydrogen bond with $O^{2'}$ of U790 of domain II, which is located at the junction of helices 32 and 35a. Telithromycin forms hydrogen bonds with A752 of domain II (hairpin 35).

By comparing cethromycin and roxithromycin (which possesses a long etheroxime side chain at position 9 of the aglycone), it was demonstrated that domain IV of 23S rRNA contributes to the positioning of the long side chain of cethromycin through hydrophobic interactions with U1782.

A group of five ribosomal proteins is essential: L16, L2, L3, L4, and L5. L2 has been shown to interact with Met-tRNA and AcPhe-tRNA and to enhance the rate of spontaneous hydrolysis of the aminoacyl moieties from tRNAs.

6.3. Blockade of Ribosome Assembly

The 30S subunit has a 21S subunit intermediate, and the 50S subunit has two intermediates, 32S and 43S. The inhibition of ribosomal subunit assembly yields to the accumulation of precursor particles in the bacterial cell which are destroyed by an RNase. The inhibitory activity of the 11,12-carbonate is higher than those of carbamate derivatives; however, the carbonate seems to induce liver toxicity.

The available ketolides inhibit the assembly of 50S subunits of *S. aureus* and *S. pneumoniae*. It is less clear if for gram-positive cocci they partly inhibit the assembly of the 30S subunit.

For *H. influenzae*, telithromycin and cethromycin have equivalent inhibitory activities against the assembly of 30S and 50S ribosomal subunits, having in fact only one target 23S rRNA as the difference for gram-positive cocci.

7. MECHANISM OF RESISTANCE OF KETOLIDES

The two main mechanims of resistance are methylation and efflux. Mutations accounted for less than 5% in various epidemiological surveys of macrolides.

7.1. Induction of Resistance

Various ketolides have been shown not to be capable of inducing resistance to other macrolides. This phenomenon has been explored with strains of *S. aureus, S. pneumoniae*, and *S. pyogenes* (Bonnefoy et al., 1997) in the presence of ketolides and their counterpart with an L-cladinose and with clarithromycin, erythromycin A, and azithromycin.

Only the ketolides do not induce resistance to macrolides (Fig. 19 and 20). It was originally shown that the lack of L-cladinose in narbomycin and picromycin (natural ketolides) resulted in the lack of inducibility of methylase.

7.2. Efflux

Gram-positive cocci remain susceptible to the activity of HMR 3004, telithromycin, and cefthromycin. Activity of the other macrolides depends on the extent of the efflux (Table 28).

For obvious reasons, ketolides are able to overcome the efflux mechanism of resistance due to Mef, MreA, and MsrA in *S. pneumoniae, S. pyogenes, S. aureus*, and *S. agalactiae*.

Macrolide and ketolide transport into the bacterial cell is a passive process, independent of energy and facilitated by the intracellular binding site, the ribosome.

Protonation of the desosamine may enhance the intracellular uptake through porins, especially if they are large enough; however, it remains a minor way of intracellular penetration.

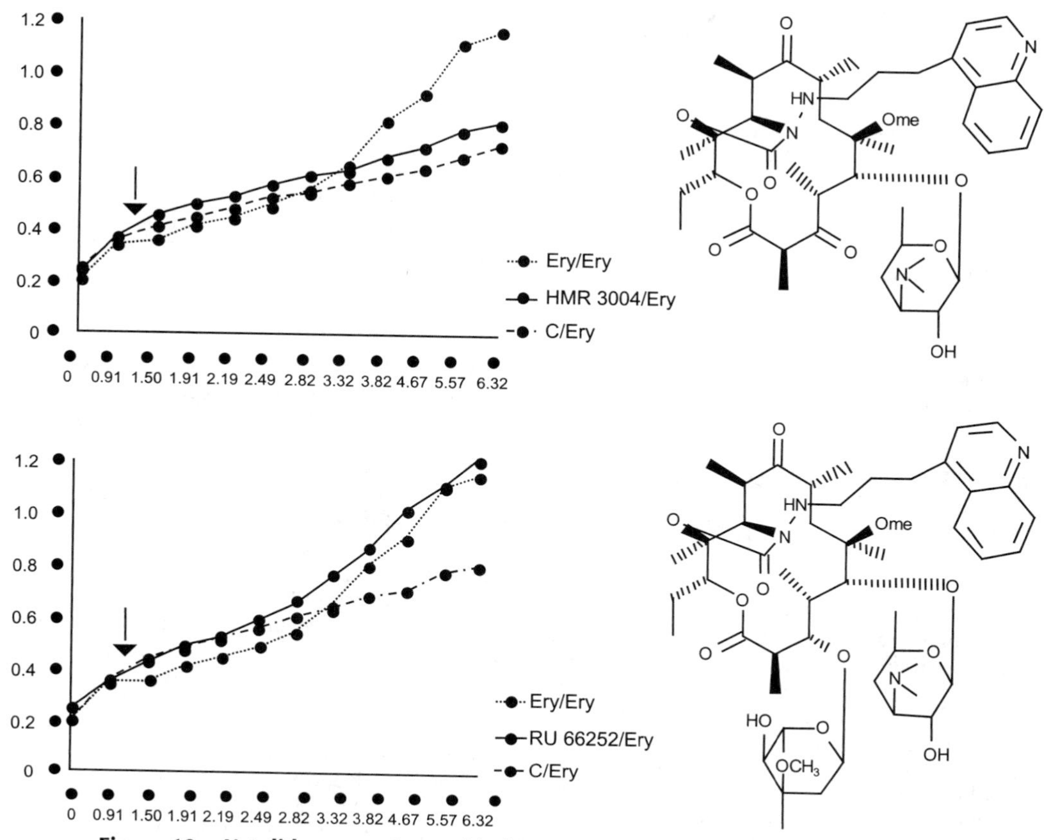

Figure 19 Ketolides: experimental induction (*S. aureus*) (Bonnefoy et al., 1997)

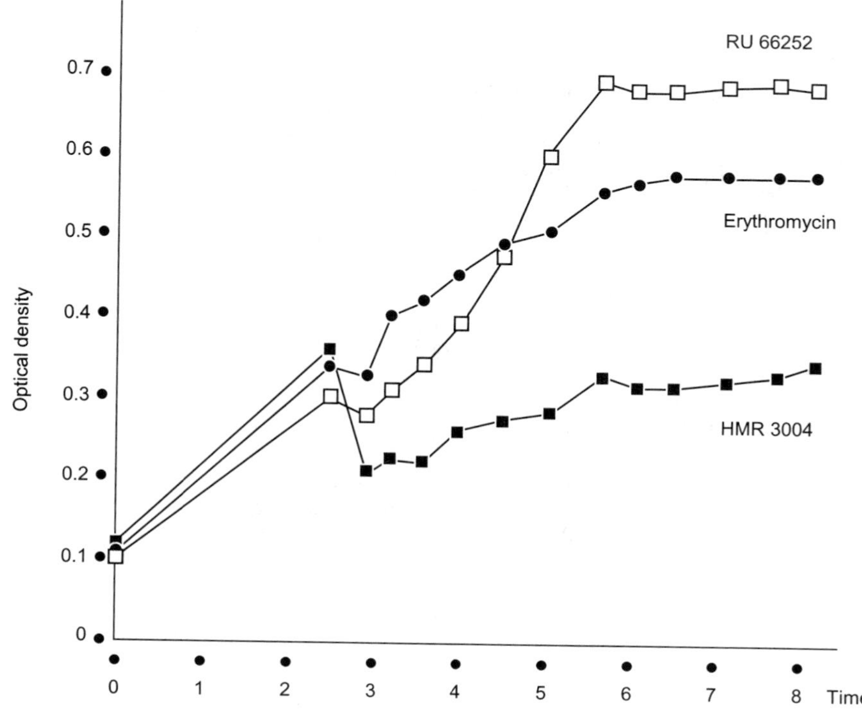

Figure 20 Ketolides: experimental induction (*S. pyogenes*) (Bonnefoy et al., 1997)

Table 28 HMR 3004: resistance by efflux

Organism	Resistance mechanism or strain	Gene or phenotype	MIC (μg/ml)[a]			
			HMR 3004	Ery A	Cla	Josa
S. aureus	Efflux	*mrsA*	0.01	0.1	0.1	0.25
	Efflux	*mrsA* (multicopies)	0.12	32	32	0.25
S. pneumoniae	UA978	*mef*	0.06	0.5	0.5	0.3
		Sensitive	0.002	0.02	0.04	0.5

[a]Ery A, erythromycin A; Cla, clarithromycin; Josa, josamycin.

Methylation of ribosomes induces only minor changes in the membrane properties, and the interference with ketolide uptake is minimal.

Erythromycin A accumulation dropped about 70 to 80% after *erm* induction. Ketolides could accumulate in the bacterial cell to preinduction level, and the concentration remains high enough to interfere with the ribosome.

7.2.1. Mef Pumps

The efflux mechanism of resistance of *S. pneumoniae* involves a Mef protein, which binds to macrolides and ketolides and extrudes them from the bacterial cell, resulting in reduced intracellular drug concentrations. In *mef*-containing strains, there is competition between the ribosome and the Mef binding sites for the intracellular compound. Ketolides, which possess tight ribosome binding kinetics, may not bind tightly to the efflux pump, yielding in a net influx which exceeds the capacity of the pump.

7.2.2. MsrA Pumps

The resistance gene found in *Staphylococcus epidermidis* encodes MS resistance. The resistance gene is carried by plasmid pUL 5050. This plasmid expressed erythromycin A resistance constitutively, but streptogramin B resistance remains inducible. This transporter belongs to the ATP cassette. Telithromycin remains active against these isolates, with MICs of 0.05 to 2.0 μg/ml.

7.2.3. MreA Pumps

MreA pumps have been described for *S. agalactiae*. Telithromycin remains active against isolates with MreA pumps, with MICs of ≤0.015 to 0.06 μg/ml. For these isolates, erythromycin A MICs were 1.0 to 8.0 μg/ml, azithromycin MICs were 8.0 to 64 μg/ml, and clarithromycin MICs were 0.5 to 2.0 μg/ml.

7.2.4. AcrAB-TolC Pump

In gram-negative bacilli, the AcrAB-TolC efflux pump is responsible for erythromycin A resistance. It was demonstrated that telithromycin has a transport system other than that used by erythromycin A. Telithromycin seems not to be a good substrate for the TolC channel.

7.2.5. Gene *mat*(A)

An additional gene involved in efflux of erythromycin A has been recently reported for streptococci. The transport system is ATP dependent (Iannelli et al., 2004).

7.3. Methylation

Two types of methylated resistance have been described: inducible and constitutive.

Originally, constitutive macrolide resistance was applied to strains of gram-positive bacteria that are resistant to erythromycin A, clindamycin, and streptogramin B (MIC, >128 μg/ml).

MLS_B inducible resistance results in lower MICs for erythromycin A (MICs of 1 to 16 μg/ml), and lincosamides (clindamycin) remain active.

Erythromycin A acts as an inducer, resulting in an increase in methylase production, causing resistance. Ketolides are not inducers of resistance to macrolides.

Both ketolides remain susceptible to an isolate harboring an inducible MLS_B mechanism of resistance.

It was demonstrated that if A2058 is mono- or bimethylated, erythromycin A becomes inactive. If A2058 is monomethylated telithromycin remains active, but if this base is bimethylated telithromycin becomes inactive.

The dimethylation of the N^6 atom would not add a bulky substituent causing steric hindrance for the binding but would prevent the formation of hydrogen bonds to the 2′-OH group of D-desosamine.

A2058 is one of the few nucleotides of the peptidyltransferase center that is not conserved among phylogenetic domains. Mitochondrial and cytoplasmic RNAs of higher eukaryotes have a guanine instead of an adenine. The G-C base pair seems to maintain the proper conformation of A2058. In many eubacteria the base pair is an A-U.

All available ketolides are inactive against isolates harboring a constitutive methylase. In an isolate of *S. pneumoniae* showing an MLS_B constitutive type of resistance to both erythromycin A and telithromycin, sequence analysis showed that a 187-bp tandem repeat was inserted, including the ribosome binding site (SD-2) for the *erm*(B) gene, resulting in a new ribosome binding site, SD-2′, in the attenuator of the *erm*(B) gene of this mutant.

In the constitutive *erm*(A) gene of *S. aureus*, it was shown that deletions and duplications of different sizes account for constitutive gene expression (deletion of 26 to 141 bp, tandem duplication of 12 bp, and a point of mutation).

7.4. Mutations

Mutations in domain V and in proteins L4 and L22 have been reported.

In L4 mutation there is a 3-amino-acid substitution: $_{69}GTG_{71} \rightarrow {}_{69}TPS_{71}$. This occurs in a highly conserved region ($_{63}$KPWRQK**GTG**RAR$_{74}$). Telithromycin remains active against *S. pneumoniae* isolates harboring this mutation. The MIC_{50} and MIC_{90} are 0.12 and 0.25 μg/ml. For 14- and 15-membered-ring macrolides the MICs were 32 to >64 μg/ml. MICs for pristinamycin were 0.5 to 1.0 μg/ml, and those for clindamycin were 0.06 to 0.12 μg/ml.

In L22, an 18-bp insertion resulted in the addition of 6 amino acids: $_{69}$GTG**REKGTG**RAR$_{74}$. This strain is resistant to all macrolides, with an increase in the MIC of telithromycin (MIC, 3.12 μg/ml).

23S rRNA mutations in domain V were reported for many bacterial species, including *S. pneumoniae, S. pyogenes, S. aureus, Mycoplasma pneumoniae, Helicobacter pylori, Propionibacterium acnes, T. pallidum*, and *Borrelia burgdorferi*. Mutation occurs mainly on A2058→G, rendering all of these isolates resistant to erythromycin A and, to a lesser extent, to ketolides.

Other mutations have been reported to render telithromycin less active, such as U2609→C, which confers resistance to telithromycin but increases bacterial cell susceptibility to erythromycin A. This mutation appears to be located within the compound binding site and may directly affect interaction of the telithromycin molecule with the ribosome. One mutant selected by clarithromycin (MIC, >32 μg/ml) that showed decreased susceptibility to telithromycin (MIC, 4 μg/ml) had a single base deletion (A752) in domain II. The C2611→U mutation confers mild resistance to macrolides and telithromycin; this was obtained in laboratory experiments. In laboratory studies, mutations at A2058 or A2059 of domain V of 23S rRNA yielded three different mutations: A2058→T, A2059→G, and A2058→G; telithromycin activity dropped in comparison with that for a wild type. Mutation in hairpin 35 at U754→A renders bacterial cells resistant to low concentrations of erythromycin A and telithromycin.

7.5. "Bottle Brush"

It was discovered that overexpression of a short segment of *E. coli* 23S rRNA (positions 1235 to 1268) rendered cells resistant to erythromycin A.

Translation of a minigene sequence within 23S rRNA produces pentapeptide binding to the ribosome, but the resistance mechanism is unknown.

The rRNA-encoded pentapeptide is not normally expressed because the Shine-Dalgarno region of the peptide open reading frame is sequestered in the 23S rRNA secondary structure. This pentapeptide, K-peptide, is specific to ketolides (Table 29).

Table 29 Pentapeptide sequences from K-peptides

Peptide	Pentapeptide sequence	Ketolide MIC (μM)
Wild type	None	10
K1	MLYKP	80
K2	MKDTS	60
K3	MRFFV	100
K15	MSWKI	80

7.6. Inactivations

The bacteria usually covered by the antibacterial spectrum of the macrolides do not inactivate the molecules. However, a few strains of *E. coli* produce esterases that can hydrolyze the erythronolide A ring. Telithromycin is less hydrolyzed than erythromycin A, even in the presence of high concentrations of esterases, and remains within the therapeutic range (MIC, 0.50 μg/ml) (Table 30).

HMR 3004, telithromycin, and others, however, are inactivated by the binding of a phosphate to the hydroxyl group at position 2′ of the D-desosamine sugar (P. Courvalin, 1996, personal communication). *Nocardia* spp. are resistant to macrolides and ketolides due to the production of inactivating enzymes (phosphorylases and glycosylases).

7.7. Selection of Mutants

The ability of sequential subcultures in subinhibitory concentrations of telithromycin, azithromycin, roxithromycin, clindamycin, and pristinamycin to select for resistance was investigated. The study was performed with five erythromycin A-susceptible and six erythromycin A-resistant *S. pneumoniae* strains, the latter group including three examples of each containing *mef*(E) or *erm*(B) gene. Overall, 54 mutants were derived for which the MIC of at least one of the antibiotics was increased. Of these, only for three were the telithromycin MICs >1 μg/ml. In contrast, for 34 and 28 mutants the MICs of azithromycin and clarithromycin, respectively, were >1 μg/ml. While exposure to telithromycin did select for pneumococcal mutants for which the MICs were increased, the MICs nevertheless remained within the susceptibility range.

8. PHARMACODYNAMICS

The pharmacodynamics of telithromycin have been studied in the neutropenic (ICR) and nonneutropenic (Swiss) mice infected with *S. pneumoniae* (different antibiotic resistance phenotypes) and *S. aureus*. An experimental infection was induced in a thigh (localized infection), and treatment was administered 2 h after the infection with different doses and at different dosage frequencies. The static dose was determined from the residual bacterial count in the thigh abscess. At the same time, the plasma pharmacokinetics were determined. All of these data indicate the dosage frequency and the type of pharmacodynamics (time or concentration dependent).

It has been shown with telithromycin that the response is independent of the rhythm of administration. The bacteriostatic dose is comparable, irrespective of the rhythm of administration, suggesting that a single daily dose is sufficient (Table 31).

Table 30 Mechanisms of inactivation of macrolides[a]

E. coli enzyme(s)	Gene	MIC (μg/ml)[b]					
		Telithromycin	Ery A	Cla	Josa	Lin	Prist
Esterases		0.03	10	4	8	8	4
	ercA	0.5	>128	>128	8	8	4
	ercB	0.5	64	ND	8	8	4
2′-Phosphotransferase	*mphA*	64	>128	>128	ND	ND	128

[a]Data from Courvalin, 1996, personal communication.
[b]Ery A, erythromycin A; Cla, clarithromycin; Josa, josamycin; Lin, lincomycin; Prist, pristinamycin; ND, not determined.

Table 31 Telithromycin: dosage frequency[a]

Rhythm of administration (h)	Static dose (mg/kg)
3	21.0 ± 3.2
8	18.5 ± 2.8
12	18.0 ± 1.7
24	29.1 ± 4.8

[a]Data from Vesga et al., 1997.

The second point that has been demonstrated is that there is a good correlation between efficacy and concentration, particularly the area under the curve (Fig. 21).

9. INTRACELLULAR CONCENTRATIONS

Telithromycin gradually accumulates in polymorphonuclear leukocytes, like azithromycin, but without any saturation phenomenon at 180 min (Fig. 22). The activation energy is high (128 kJ/mol). It accumulates strongly in the granules (60%) and is eliminated progressively from the cell (efflux) (Fig. 23). Telithromycin uses a transport system to penetrate the phagocytic cell.

10. PHARMACOKINETICS OF TELITHROMYCIN

10.1. Pharmacokinetics in Healthy Volunteers

The pharmacokinetics of telithromycin administered orally as a single dose or in repeated doses of 800 mg once daily show that the peak concentration in serum of 1.99 μg/ml occurs within 1 or 2 h. The area under the curve after a single oral dose is 7.25 μg·h/ml and after repeated doses for 10 days is 8.4 μg·h/ml. The accumulation ratio is 1.2. The apparent elimination half-life is between 10.6 and 13.4 h. Telithromycin is eliminated mainly nonrenally, urinary elimination being less than 15% of the administered dose (Table 32).

From a comparison of the areas under the curve of the plasma and the inflammatory fluid obtained after a cantharide-induced suction blister, the ratio is 1.38. After a dose of 600 mg, the peak concentration (0.44 μg/ml) in the suction blister fluid occurs 9 h after administration and the concentration at 24 h is 0.08 μg/ml, with a median residence time of 11.06 h.

In open single-dose or multiple-dose studies, telithromycin was given orally to 12 healthy volunteers at the dose of 800 mg once a day. Telithromycin was assayed in plasma by using a validated high-performance liquid chromatography method with detection by fluorimetry. The limits of quantification were 0.005 μg/ml in plasma and 0.5 μg/ml in urine.

Following multiple doses of 800 mg once a day, steady-state was reached after 2 days of dosing. The overall accumulation ratio after multiple dosing is about 1.42.

The rate and extent of absorption of telithromycin are unaffected by food intake.

In vitro binding to human serum albumin is 45 to 49% at concentrations up to 2.44 μg/ml. The percent binding to α_1-acid glycoprotein is about 30% for a concentration of 0.07 μg/ml. The total level of binding to plasma protein is about 70% at concentrations up to 1.02 μg/ml.

The absolute bioavailability after 800 mg of telithromycin was 57%.

Telithromycin distribution in lung tissue has been assessed after a single oral dose of 800 mg. Results are summarized in Table 33.

10.2. Pharmacokinetics in the Elderly

In elderly volunteers after oral single or repeated doses of 800 mg of telithromycin once a day, the accumulation ratio is about 1.17, in comparison to 1.45 in young volunteers. Steady state was reached after 2 days of dosing. At steady state the maximum concentration in serum and area under the curve were two times higher in elderly subjects than in young volunteers. Renal clearance decreased with age. However, it was recommended not to change the daily dose or the rhythm of administration of telithromycin in elderly patients (Table 34) (Perret et al., 2002).

10.3. Pharmacokinetics in Renally and Hepatically Impaired Patients

Twelve patients with hepatic impairment with a Child-Pugh score of ≥6 and ≤13 (A, B, and C) were enrolled in a pharmacokinetic study in comparison with 20 healthy volunteers. After a single oral dose of 800 mg of telithromycin,

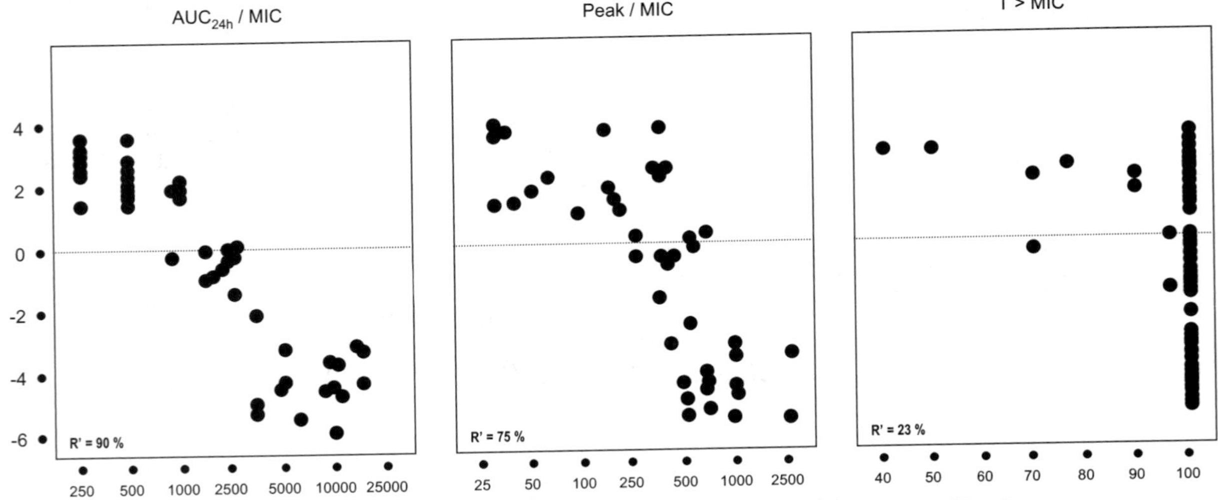

Figure 21 Telithromycin: correlation between efficacy and pharmacokinetic or pharmacodynamic parameters (Vesga et al., 1997)

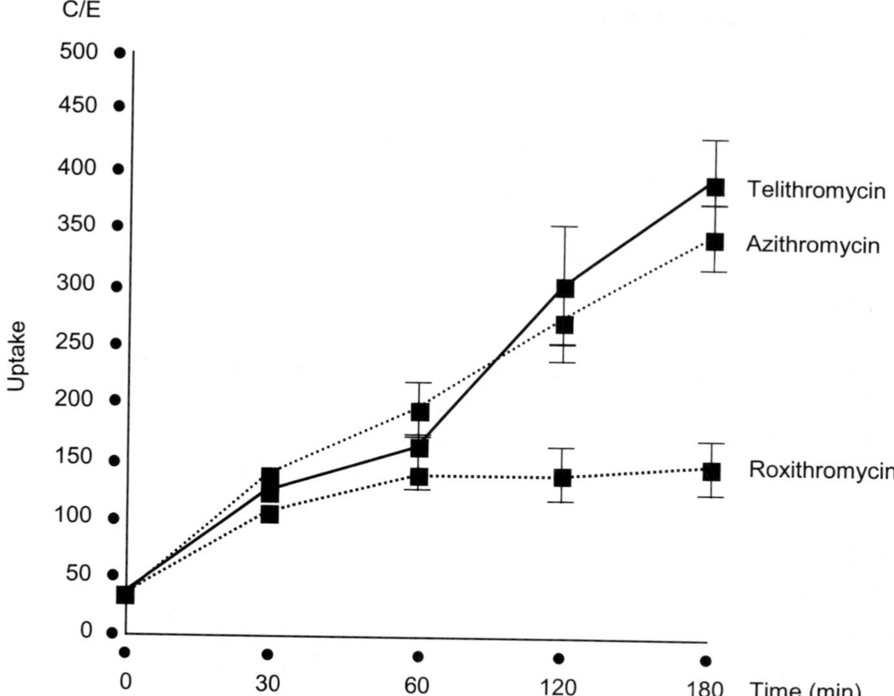

Figure 22 Cellular/extracellular ratio of telithromycin in human granulocytes (Labro et al., 1997, 1998)

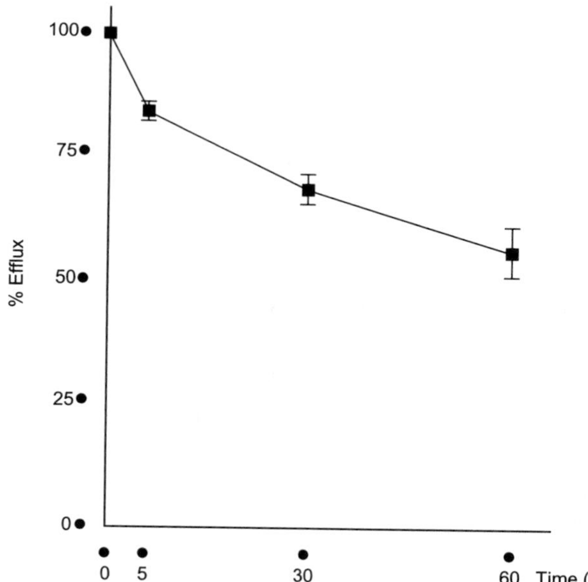

Figure 23 Telithromycin efflux (Labro et al., 1998)

the pharmacokinetic behavior of telithromycin was moderately altered in patients with impaired liver function (Tables 35 and 36). The decrease of telithromycin metabolic clearance is partially compensated for by a 50% increase in renal clearance.

Telithromycin pharmacokinetics were investigated after a single oral dose of 800 mg of telithromycin in 40 patients with various degrees of renal impairment (Table 37). Peak

Table 32 Pharmacokinetics of telithromycin administered orally (repeated doses)

Parameter	Day 1 ($n^a = 18$)	Day 11 ($n^a = 18$)
C_{max} (μg/ml)	1.90 ± 0.8	2.27 ± 0.71
T_{max} (h)	1.0 (1–2)	2.0 (0.5–3.0)
C_{24} (μg/ml)	0.029 ± 0.013	0.07 ± 0.05
AUC_{0-24} (μg·h/ml)	8 ± 2.6	12.5 ± 5.4
$t_{1/2\gamma}$ (h)	7.16 ± 1.3	12.5 ± 5.4
Urinary elimination (%) (0–72 h)	12.66 ± 4.2	17.7 ± 4.7
CL_R (liters/h)	12.32 ± 2.1	12.5 ± 4.3

[a]n, number of volunteers.

concentrations in plasma and areas under the curve increased 1.4- to 1.5-fold, respectively, in renally impaired patients in comparison with healthy volunteers. The apparent elimination half-life increased slightly in renally impaired patients in comparison with healthy volunteers.

10.4. Metabolism

Telithromycin metabolism is mediated by CYP3A4 and CYP2D6. Four metabolites have been described (Fig. 24). Three of them retained antibacterial activity, and one is considered inactive (Tables 38 and 39).

One of the metabolites, RU-78849, is totally inactive, whereas RU-72365 exhibits good antipneumococcal activity (Table 38).

Fifty-seven percent of the dose reaches the systemic circulation as unchanged compound and is eliminated by multiple pathways as follows:

- Seven percent is excreted unchanged in feces by the biliary route and/or intestinal secretions.

Table 33 Lung distribution of telithromycin

Time of sampling (h)	n	Concn of telithromycin			
		Plasma (μg/ml)	Bronchial mucosa (mg/kg)	ELF[a] (μg/ml)	Alveolar macrophages (μg/ml)
1–3	5	1.07	0.68	5.4	65
6–8	6	0.61	2.2	4.2	100
24	6	0.07	3.5	1.17	41
48	6	LOQ[b]	LOQ	0.30	2.15

[a]ELF, epithelial lining fluid.
[b]LOQ, limit of quantification.

Table 34 Telithromycin pharmacokinetics in elderly subjects

Parameter	Elderly		Young	
	Day 1	Day 10	Day 1	Day 10
C_{max} (μg/ml)	3.0	3.6	1.99	1.84
T_{max} (h)	0.5	0.75	1	2.0
C_{24} (μg/ml)	0.057	0.142	0.025	0.046
AUC_{0-24} (μg·h/ml)	11.56	17.2	7.25	8.49
$t_{1/2\gamma}$ (h)	11.46	14.23	10.64	13.4
Urinary elimination (%) (0–72 h)	10.9	18	12.0	14.5
CL_R (liters/h)	7.35	7.83	13.07	12.98

Table 35 Telithromycin pharmacokinetics in hepatically impaired patients after a single oral dose of 800 mg

Parameter	Hepatically impaired patients ($n = 12$)	Healthy volunteers ($n = 20$)
C_{max} (μg/ml)	1.99	2.32
T_{max} (h)	0.75	1.0
C_{24} (μg/ml)	0.087	0.039
$AUC_{0-\infty}$ (μg·h/ml)	11.1	10.1
Urinary elimination (%) (0–72 h)	22.4	13.1
CL_R (liters/h)	17.3	10.78

Table 36 Pharmacokinetics of telithromycin in hepatically impaired patients after repeated 800-mg doses[a]

Parameter	Hepatically impaired patients		Healthy volunteers	
	Day 1	Day 7	Day 1	Day 7
C_{max} (μg/ml)	1.54	1.8	1.73	1.92
T_{max} (h)	3.0	2.0	1.5	3.0
AUC_{0-24} (μg·h/ml)	9.11	12.4	8.74	13.3
$t_{1/2}$ (h)		11.9		11.0

[a]Data from Cantalloube et al., 2003.

- Thirteen percent is excreted unchanged in the urine.
- Thirty-seven percent is metabolized by the liver.

The elimination of the metabolites is summarized in Table 39.

10.5. Ascending Doses

After repeated doses the steady state was achieved on the second or third day. A slight accumulation was observed with multiple doses after 7 days, with a ratio for the areas under the curve from 0 to 24 h of 1.3 to 1.49. After the final dose (in multiple doses), telithromycin was quantifiable in plasma after the 400- and 800-mg regimen. Telithromycin was still quantifiable in 14 of 16 subjects after the final dose in the 7-day multiple-dose phase in the 1,600-mg group (Table 40).

RU-76363, an alcohol analog (metabolite) resulting from the loss of the aryl ring, is the main hepatic metabolite of telithromycin. Its pharmacokinetics are summarized in Table 41.

Table 37 Telithromycin pharmacokinetics in renally impaired patients after a single oral dose of 800 mg

Parameter	Value at indicated creatinine clearance (ml/min)[a]			
	>80	80–41	40–11	≤10
C_{max} (mg/liter)	2.25	3.0	3.25	2.13
T_{max} (h)	1.15	1.30	1.10	1.35
C_{24} (mg/liter)	0.029	0.055	0.066	0.05
$AUC_{0-\infty}$ (mg·h/liter)	10.09	14.31	16.0	10.79
$t_{1/2\beta}$ (h)	10.66	11.41	12.58	14.64
CL_R (liters/h)	9.34	5.71	2.63	0.36[b]
Urinary elimination (%)	10.96	9.57	5.51	0.46[b]

[a]Unless otherwise indicated, 10 patients were studied.
[b]Two patients were studied.

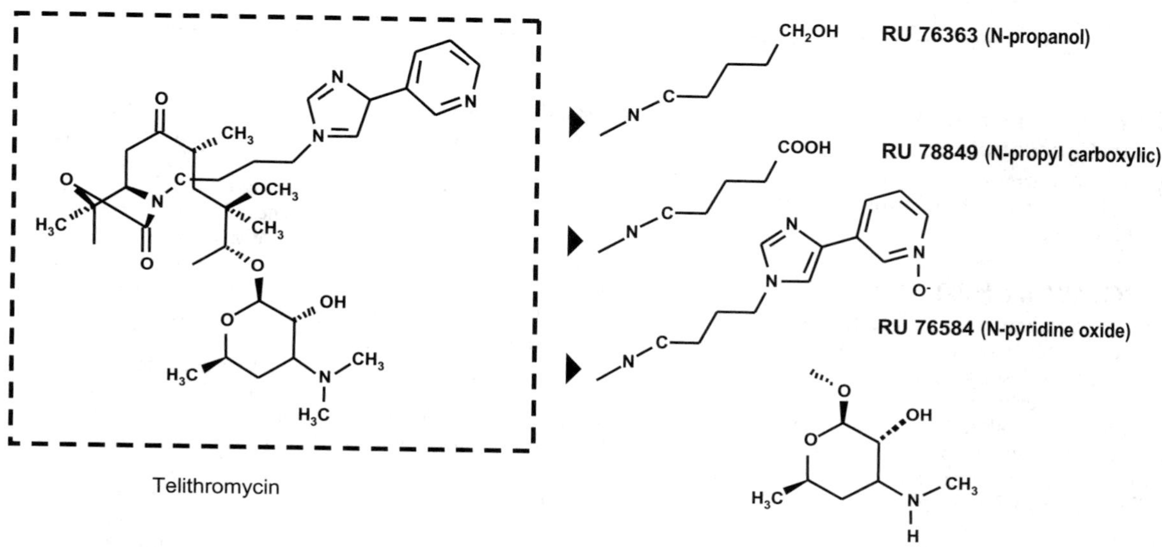

Figure 24 Metabolites from telithromycin

Table 38 In vitro activities of telithromycin metabolites

Organism[a]	n	MIC (μg/ml)				
		Telithromycin	RU-78849	RU-76584	RU-76363	RU-72365
MSSA Ery[s]	10	0.06	>16	10–20	10	0.5–1.0
MRSA Ery[r]	10	>32	>16	>16	>16	>16
S. pneumoniae Ery[s]	10	0.015	10–20	0.06	0.03	≤0.008–0.015
S. pneumoniae Ery[r]	10	0.015	>16	0.06–0.12	>16	0.03

[a]MSSA, methicillin-susceptible *S. aureus*; MRSA, methicillin-resistant *S. aureus*.

Table 39 Elimination of telithromycin and its main metabolites

Waste product	HMR 3647	RU-76363	RU-72365	RU-78849	RU-76584	Total
Feces	20.2	2.71	1.97	11.5	0.71	37.1
Urine	11.8	1.23	0.07	0.29	0.10	13.8

Table 40 Pharmacokinetics of telithromycin after ascending doses[a]

Dosing regimen	Dose (mg)	C_{max} (μg/ml)	T_{max} (h)	$AUC_{0-\infty}$ (μg·h/ml)	$t_{1/2}$ (h)	C_{24} (μg/ml)
Single dose	400	0.8	1.0	2.57	6.68	0.006
	800	1.9	1.0	8.25	7.16	0.03
	1,600	4.07	1.0	23.1	10.13	0.10
Multiple doses (day 7)	400	0.83	1.0	4.01	7.70	0.02
	800	2.3	1.0	12.59	9.8	0.07
	1,600	4.5	1.0	35.9	18.7	0.30

[a]Data from Namour et al., 2001.

Table 41 Pharmacokinetics of RU-76363

Dose (mg)	C_{max} (μg/ml)	T_{max} (h)	$AUC_{0-\infty}$ (μg·h/ml)	$t_{1/2}$ (h)	C_{24} (μg/ml)
400	0.05	1.5	0.277	2.96	0.0008
800	0.13	2.0	0.974	3.45	0.005
1,600	0.24	3.0	2.37	4.00	0.02

10.6. Pediatric Patients and Middle Ear Fluid Telithromycin Concentrations

Telithromycin concentrations in middle ear fluid were assessed in children suffering from otitis media (Cantalloube et al., 2004) (Table 42).

11. CETHROMYCIN (ABT 773)

Cethromycin is a carbamate ketolide having a propylene quinolyl side chain fixed on the hydroxyl at position C-6 (Fig. 25). It seems to be less bactericidal against *S. pneumoniae* than telithromycin. Cethromycin exhibits a slow bactericidal activity which occurs after 12 h of contact for strains susceptible to erythromycin A, but it is weakly bactericidal against *erm*(B)-containing strains, with a reduction of $\leq$2.0 $\log_{10}$ CFU/ml for two and eight times the MIC after 6 h of contact. Against *S. pneumoniae,* the bactericidal activity is strain dependent irrespective of the susceptibility to erythromycin A. Cethromycin seems to be more active than telithromycin against *mef*(E)-containing *S. pneumoniae.* Thirty percent of the *S. pneumoniae* isolates were inhibited by concentrations of 0.008 and 0.03 μg/ml for cethromycin and telithromycin, respectively. On the other hand, telithromycin is more active against *erm*(B)-containing *S. pneumoniae*. The population distribution for telithromycin is larger, with MICs of 0.008 to 0.5 μg/ml for *erm*(B)-containing *S. pneumoniae* and 0.008 to 1.0 μg/ml for *mef*(E)-containing *S. pneumoniae,* versus 0.008 to 0.125 μg/ml for both *erm*(B)- and *mef*(E)-containing *S. pneumoniae* for cethromycin. The in vivo efficacy in rodent infections was assessed by mouse protection tests and rat lung infection models. In the mouse protection tests, the mice were challenged intravenously with a 100-fold 50% lethal dose (LD_{50}) of the infecting bacteria. Treatment started 1 and 5 h postinfection. The 50% effective doses (ED_{50}) were 10.47, 12.5, and 2.5 mg/kg for *S. aureus* 10649, *S. pneumoniae* 6303, and *S. pyogenes* C-203 (all are susceptible to erythromycin A), respectively. Rats were inoculated intratracheally with a pneumococcal suspension (10^6 to 10^8 CFU). Treatment with cethromycin started 18 h after bacterial challenge (oral route) for 3 days. To yield a 2-$\log_{10}$ CFU/liter reduction in the lungs in comparison with the control required ED_{50} of <0.63, 7.0, and 1.6 mg/kg/day for *S. pneumoniae* 6307, *S. pneumoniae* 5649 (M-phenotype), and *S. pneumoniae* 6396 (MLS_B phenotype), respectively.

Cethromycin exhibits good in vitro activity against erythromycin-A susceptible *S. pyogenes* (MIC, 0.008 μg/ml), but a drop in activity was observed when the isolate harbored an underlying mechanism of resistance to erythromycin A (MIC, 1.0 μg/ml). Cethromycin is weakly active against *H. influenzae* (MIC_{50} and MIC_{90}, 2.0 and 4.0 μg/ml). Cethromycin exerted a slow bactericidal activity which occurred after 12 to 24 h of contact and (at twice the MIC) for 9 out of 10 strains tested. Cethromycin exhibited good in vitro activity against gram-positive anaerobic bacteria, with MIC_{50}s of $\leq$0.015 μg/ml and MIC_{90}s of $\leq$0.015 to 0.03 μg/ml. Cethromycin displayed good in vitro activity against *Porphyromonas* and *Prevotella* spp. (MIC_{50}s ranged from $\leq$0.015 to 0.06 μg/ml, and MIC_{90}s ranged from $\leq$0.015 to 0.125 μg/ml). It is poorly active against *Fusobacterium nucleatum* (MIC_{50} and MIC_{90}, 4 and 8 μg/ml). Against other aerobic microorganisms involved in bite wound infections, cethromycin exhibited good in vitro activity, except against *Pasteurella* spp. (MIC_{50}, 0.5 to 1.0 μg/ml).

Table 42 Telithromycin concentration in middle ear fluid

Fluid and dosing regimen[a]	*n*	Dose (mg/kg)	Mean concn in MEF (μg/ml)				
			3 h	12 h	24 h	36 h	48 h
MEF, SD	22	20	1.32	0.45	0.82	3.19	0.17
MEF, SD	25	30	2.21	1.71	3.29		
MEF, MD	60	20	1.82	6.24	1.61	0.37	1.41
Extracellular MEF, SD	22	20	1.16	1.51	0.80		

[a]MEF, middle ear fluid; SD, single dose; MD, multiple doses.

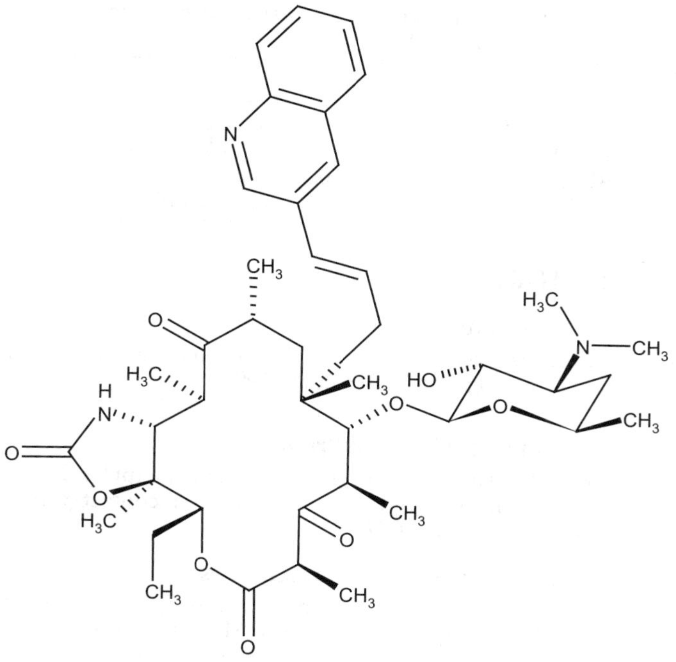

Figure 25 Cethromycin (ABT-773)

The 24-h area under the curve and MIC are the pharmacokinetic and pharmacodynamic parameters that best predict the in vitro activity of cethromycin.

In a phase I, single-center, randomized, placebo-controlled, double-blind, parallel-group, fasting study, five or six volunteers per group received orally 100 to 1,200 mg of cethromycin. Peak concentrations in plasma ranged (mean ± standard deviation) from 0.14 ± 0.06 μg/ml (100 mg) to 1.17 ± 0.36 μg/ml (1,200 mg) and were reached between 0.9 h (100 mg) and 5.1 h (1,200 mg). The areas under the curve from 0 h to infinity ranged from 0.63 ± 0.25 μg·h/ml (100 mg) to 10.95 ± 0.4 μg·h/ml (1,200 mg). The total clearance ranged from 124 ± 113 liters/h to 254 ± 92 liters/h. The apparent elimination half-lives ranged from 3.6 ± 0.5 h (100 mg) to 6.6 ± 1.0 h (1,200 mg). Fifteen healthy volunteers received 400 mg of cethromycin in fasting and fed conditions. The peak concentrations in plasma were 0.47 ± 0.21 μg/ml and 0.45 ± 0.15 μg/ml in fasting and fed conditions, respectively. The areas under the curve from 0 h to infinity were comparable (3.47 ± 1.66 μg·h/ml versus 3.55 ± 1.42 μg·h/ml), as were the times to reach the peak concentration in plasma: 2.7 ± 0.8 h and 3.4 ± 1.5 h in fasting and fed conditions, respectively. However, there is an important interindividual variation in peak concentration in plasma and area under the curve.

12. HMR 3004

HMR 3004 is a ketolide bearing a cyclic hydrazano carbamate at the C-11 and C-12 positions of the erythronolide A ring, on which a quinoline moiety is linked by a propyl side chain (Fig. 14). HMR 3004 was more active than clarithromycin against erythromycin A-susceptible isolates (MIC_{50}, 0.01 μg/ml) and retained activity against inducible (MLS_B) resistant *S. aureus* (MIC_{50}, 0.04 μg/ml), but it is inactive against constitutively MLS_B erythromycin A-resistant strains. Against enterococci HMR 3004 is highly active irrespective of their susceptibility to vancomycin (MIC_{50}, 0.01 to 0.06 μg/ml). HMR 3004 exhibited good activity against beta-hemolytic streptococci, including *S. pyogenes* (MIC_{50}, 0.06 μg/ml) isolates resistant to erythromycin A.

It also shows high activity against viridans group streptococci (MIC_{50}, ~0.001 μg/ml). Against *S. pneumoniae* isolates susceptible (MIC_{50}, 0.016 μg/ml) or resistant (MIC_{50}, 0.06 μg/ml) to erythromycin A, HMR 3004 displays good activity. It exerts a strong and identical in vitro activity against *S. pneumoniae* isolates susceptible or intermediately susceptible to penicillin G (MIC_{50}, 0.016 μg/ml), but slightly lower activity has been noted against penicillin G-resistant strains (MIC_{50}, 0.06 μg/ml); clarithromycin can be considered inactive (MIC_{50}, 2 μg/ml). The available macrolides are poorly active or inactive against anaerobes as a whole. Compared to metronidazole, HMR 3004 shows enhanced activity against *B. fragilis* (MIC_{50}, ~0.5 μg/ml). It is four times more active than metronidazole against *Bacteroides thetaiotaomicron* (MIC_{50}, 0.15 μg/ml). It is, respectively, two and eight times more active than clarithromycin and azithromycin against *Fusobacterium* spp. (MIC_{50}, 0.06 μg/ml).

It is highly active against *Clostridium* and *Peptostreptococcus* spp. It is more active than clarithromycin against *H. influenzae* (MIC_{50}, ~1 μg/ml) and shows identical activity against *M. catarrhalis* (MIC_{50}, 0.12 μg/ml). Unusual among the macrolides is the strong activity against *N. meningitidis* (MIC_{50}, 0.007 μg/ml). Preliminary results show that HMR 3004 is effective against *Chlamydia* and *Legionella* spp. One interesting characteristic is the good in vitro activity of HMR 3004 against *M. hominis* (MIC, ~0.2 μg/ml) and *Mycoplasma fermentans* (MIC, 0.2 μg/ml), which are usually resistant to 14-membered-ring macrolides. It is effective against *M. pneumoniae* (MIC, 0.01 μg/ml) and 5 to 100 times more active than comparators against *U. urealyticum*, whatever the resistance to tetracycline (MIC, 0.01 μg/ml).

The in vivo antibacterial activity of HMR 3004 was explored compared to those of erythromycin, clarithromycin, azithromycin, and pristinamycin. In murine septicemia due to erythromycin-susceptible *S. aureus*, HMR 3004 and clarithromycin show comparable activity (50% protective dose

[PD_{50}], 20 mg/kg; MIC, 0.01 μg/ml). However, it shows good in vivo activity against *S. aureus* resistant to erythromycin A by an inducible mechanism (PD_{50}, 13 mg/kg), whereas clarithromycin was totally inactive (PD_{50}, >100 mg/kg). It is also more active (PD_{50}, 17 mg/kg) than clarithromycin (PD_{50}, 30 mg/kg) against *S. aureus* resistant to erythromycin A by an inducible mechanism and to oxacillin.

Against *S. pneumoniae*, whatever the susceptibility of the isolate to erythromycin A, HMR 3004 shows good activity. PD_{50}s range between 15.8 mg/kg (erythromycin-susceptible strain) and 42 mg/kg (erythromycin-resistant isolate [constitutive mechanism]). Against erythromycin-resistant isolates, whatever the mechanism of resistance, other tested macrolides were inactive (PD_{50}, >50 mg/kg). HMR 3004 displays good in vivo activity against *S. pyogenes* (PD_{50}, 16 mg/kg) and *S. agalactiae* (PD_{50}, 36 mg/kg). It is more active than pristinamycin against enterococci, with PD_{50}s between 11 mg/kg (erythromycin- and vancomycin-resistant *E. faecium*) and 22 mg/kg (erythromycin-resistant *E. faecium*).

In experimental murine septicemia induced by *H. influenzae*, HMR 3004 showed in vivo activity close to that of azithromycin. PD_{50}s ranged between 142 mg/kg (ampicillin susceptible) and 410 mg/kg (ampicillin resistant, β-lactamase negative).

Experimental pneumonia was induced in Swiss mice by intratracheal inoculation of virulent *S. pneumoniae* isolates either susceptible to erythromycin A (*S. pneumoniae* 4241) or constitutively erythromycin resistant (*S. pneumoniae* 6254). The drug administration started at 6 and 18 h after challenge. Two regimens were given intraperitoneally: 50 and 100 mg/kg. MICs for HMR 3004 were 0.01 and 0.5 μg/ml for erythromycin A-susceptible and erythromycin-resistant isolates, respectively. When administered every 6 or 24 h, survival rates were 92 and 54%, respectively. Comparatively, there was no survival with erythromycin. C5 + BV6 mice were intratracheally infected with *H. influenzae* type b (10^8 CFU). Bacterial lung clearance was assayed after a single oral dose of 100 mg of HMR 3004 per kg or 50 mg of azithromycin per kg, administered 16 h after challenge. The compounds exhibited identical activities, with a 2.5-log CFU reduction in burden compared to the control. Initial clearance (at 6 h) was more efficient with HMR 3004 than with azithromycin.

HMR 3004 is highly accumulated in polymorphonuclear neutrophils, with an extracellular/intracellular ratio above 400. HMR 3004 uptake occurs rapidly, and in approximately 5 min intracellular concentrations reach a plateau. Uptake is different from that of telithromycin and similar to that of HMR 3562 and HMR 3787, which rapidly concentrate but to a lower level than HMR 3004.

The pharmacokinetics of HMR 3004 after a single oral dose of 600 mg are summarized in Table 43.

The pharmacokinetics of HMR 3004 after ascending doses (oral route) are listed in Table 44.

Table 43 Pharmacokinetics of HMR 3004 and telithromycin in humans after 600 mg (oral)

Parameter	HMR 3004	Telithromycin
C_{max} (μg/ml)	0.16 ± 0.30	0.90 ± 0.13
C_{24} (μg/ml)	ND[a]	0.01 ± 0.01
T_{max} (h)	1.75	1.5
$AUC_{0-\infty}$ (μg·h/ml)	0.59 ± 0.11	4.09 ± 0.55
$t_{1/2}$ (h)	2.25 ± 0.16	11.0 ± 1.90

[a]ND, not determined.

Table 44 Pharmacokinetics after ascending oral doses of HMR 3004

Parameter	300 mg	600 mg	900 mg
C_{max} (μg/ml)	0.056 ± 0.011	0.164 ± 0.29	0.28 ± 0.044
T_{max} (h)	1.0	1.75	3.0
$AUC_{0-\infty}$ (μg·h/ml)	0.120 ± 0.02	0.59 ± 0.11	1.45 ± 0.26
$t_{1/2}$ (h)	1.73 ± 0.14	2.25 ± 0.16	3.26 ± 0.35

13. TE-810

13.1. Structure

TE-810 is a ketolide with a cyclic carbamate group at C-11 and C-12 (Fig. 26) (Asaka et al., 1995a).

13.2. Physicochemical Properties

TE-810 is very stable in an acidic medium (pH 1.2). No degradation product is observed 2 h after contact with a solution at pH 1.2 at 37°C.

13.3. In Vitro and In Vivo Activities

TE-810 has good activity against strains of *S. aureus* resistant to erythromycin A by an inducible MLS_B mechanism but is inactive against strains of the constitutive MLS_B type, which is confirmed by good activity in disseminated staphylococcal infections (ED_{50} for *S. aureus* Smith, 0.047 mg/mouse). It is more active than clarithromycin (ED_{50}, 0.34 mg/mouse). It is four times more active than clarithromycin in disseminated pneumococcal infections (ED_{50} for *S. pneumoniae* IID 553, 0.3 versus 0.12 mg/mouse).

In murine respiratory infections due to *H. influenzae* J-48, lung bacterial clearance is greater than that obtained with clarithromycin but comparable to that obtained with azithromycin.

13.4. Animal Pharmacokinetics

In the mouse and monkey after an oral dose of 5 mg/kg, 34.2 and 24.6%, respectively, of TE-810 is eliminated in the urine.

The peak concentrations in serum and areas under the curve are higher than those obtained after administration of clarithromycin or azithromycin, but the apparent elimination half-lives are shorter (Table 45).

14. TE-802

TE-802 is a ketolide belonging to the derivatives with a cyclic carbamate at C-11 and C-12. It possesses a cyclic amine between C-9 and C-11 (Fig. 27) (Asaka et al., 1995b).

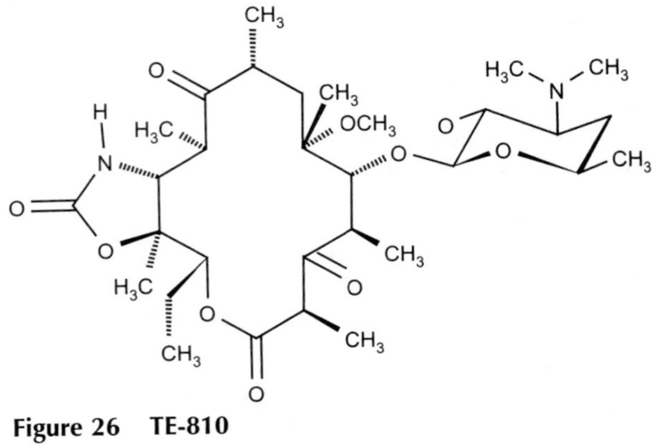

Figure 26 TE-810

Table 45 Pharmacokinetics of TE-810 in animals after a dose of 5 mg/kg orally

Day	C_{max} (μg/ml)	T_{max} (h)	C_{12} (μg/ml)	C_{24} (μg/ml)	$AUC_{0-\infty}$ (μg·h/ml)	$t_{1/2}$ (h)
1	1.99	1	0.1	0.03	7.25	10.6
10	1.84	2	0.2	0.05	8.4	13.4

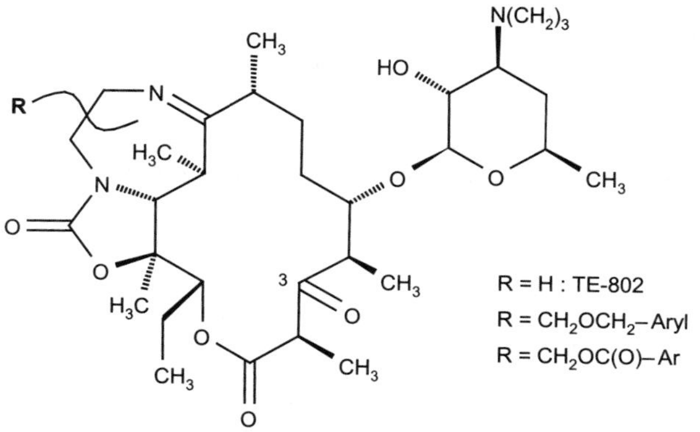

Figure 27 Tricyclic ketolides: monosubstitution on the imine nucleus

14.1. Physicochemical Properties

TE-802 is highly stable in an acidic medium at pH 1.2.

14.2. Structure-Activity Relationship and Antibacterial Activities

As stated above, TE-802 belongs to the cyclic carbamate C-11 and C-12 derivatives. It differs from TE-810 by the presence of a cyclic imine between C-9 and C-11.

Several derivatives have been synthesized, distinguished by the substituents of the cyclic imine group. Five derivatives have been studied: TE-802, TE-935, TE-942, TE-943 and TE-806.

The five compounds are more active than clarithromycin and azithromycin against *E. faecalis* but are weakly active against *H. influenzae* and have activity similar to that of clarithromycin against the other gram-positive cocci.

They are active to various degrees against strains of *S. aureus* resistant to erythromycin A by an inducible MLS_B mechanism, whereas clarithromycin is inactive. By contrast, they are inactive against strains of *S. aureus* resistant by a constitutive MLS_B mechanism (Fig. 28).

TE-802 is less active than clarithromycin against *L. pneumophila* ATCC 33152 (MIC, 0.78 versus 0.10 μg/ml), *H. pylori* ATCC 43504 (MIC, 0.10 versus 0.05 μg/ml), and *C. trachomatis* F/UW-6/CX (MIC, 0.125 versus 0.004 μg/ml).

In disseminated murine infections, TE-802 is 2 to 10 times more active than clarithromycin or azithromycin. Pulmonary bacterial clearance of *S. pneumoniae* J-4 is greater after treatment with TE-802.

After a dose of 5 mg/kg orally in the rat, the peak concentration in serum of 0.09 μg/ml is reached after 2 h, with an area under the curve of 0.43 mg·h/liter and an apparent half-life of 4.8 h, equivalent to that observed with azithromycin (4.6 h).

15. 11,12-CARBAMATE, 6-ARYLALKYL MACROLIDES

A series of ketolide-type compounds has been described recently by Abbott. They possess a nonsubstituted carbamate at C-11 and C-12 and a variable arylalkyl chain attached at C-6 (Fig. 29).

A derivative possessing a quinoline nucleus substituted at position 5′ by a methoxycarbonyl group has good activity against gram-positive cocci, including strains resistant to erythromycin A by an efflux mechanism or an inducible MLS_B mechanism (Table 46).

16. 2-FLUOROKETOLIDES

16.1. Haloketolides

Using TE-802 as a lead compound, new chemical modifications at position C-2 of the erythronolide A ring have been explored to improve the in vivo efficacy of TE-802.

The C-2 hydrogen has been replaced by either a fluorine atom, a chlorine atom, or a bromine atom.

A-229339 (with a C-2 chlorine) is inactive or poorly active against *S. aureus*, *S. pneumoniae*, *S. pyogenes*, and *H. influenzae*. A-216599 (C-2 bromine) is four times less active than TE-802 against *S. aureus* and *S. pneumoniae* strains susceptible to erythromycin A. It is weakly active against *S. pneumoniae* resistant to erythromycin A by an efflux mechanism (MIC, 4 μg/ml) and poorly active against *H. influenzae* (MIC, 8 μg/ml). A-241550 (2-fluorine) is two times more active than TE-802, except against *S. pyogenes* PI02548 harboring an efflux mechanism of resistance (MIC, 0.5 versus 0.2 μg/ml). The 2-fluorine substituent improved slightly the in vivo efficacy and enhanced the potency in *H. influenzae* infections.

16.2. HMR 3562 and HMR 3787

Introduction of halogen at the C-2 position of the erythronolide A ring leads to the synthesis of HMR 3562 and HMR 3787. Both compounds are 2-fluoroketolides. They differ by the side chain substituting the 11,12-carbamate residue. HMR 3562 is the 2-fluoro counterpart of telithromycin, and HMR 3787 has a bicyclic moiety (imidazolo pyridyl) links to the 11,12-carbamate residue through a butyl side chain.

The relative importance of position 2 of erythronolide A of ketolides has been studied by introduction of various electrophiles (halogen atoms or a methyl group) as well as new 2,3-enol ether derivatives.

Position 2 of ketolides needs to remain tetrahedral and tolerates only very small substituents such as fluorine; planar analogs such as the 2,3-enol ether result in a loss of antibacterial activities. It was shown that the 2-chloro and 2-methyl analogs were less active than clarithromycin or the parent ketolide, especially against *S. aureus* harboring inducible MLS_B resistance. The most active compounds are HMR 3562 and HMR 3787. HMR 3562 differs from the structural point of view from telithromycin by having a 2-fluorine, and HMR 3787 differs by having a bicyclic ring on the carbamate side chain. Previous series of 2-fluoroketolides were described (Denis et al., 1999). A fluorine atom, a chlorine atom, or a bromine atom replaced the C-2 hydrogen. The C-2 bromine and C-2 chlorine analogs were poorly active, and the 2-fluoro TE-802 exhibited only a slight improvement in vivo.

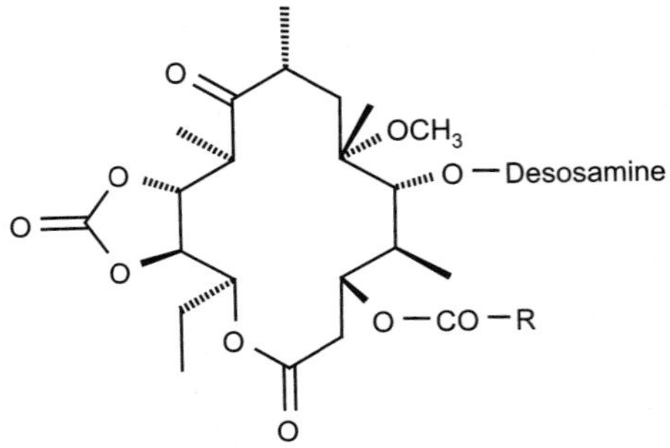

		S. aureus 209P	*S. aureus* (inducible)	*S. aureus* (constitutive)
3(O-methoxybenzyl)	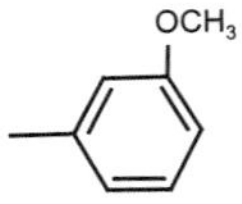 OCH_3	3,13	3,13	100
3-O(4-nitrobenzyl)	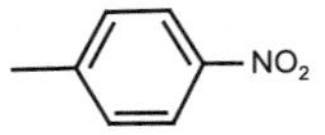 NO_2	3,13	6,25	100
3-O(4-nitrophenylacetyl) (TEA-0769)	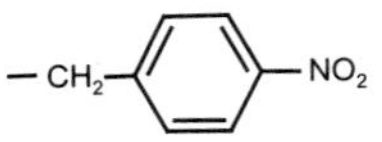 $— CH_2$ NO_2	0,10	0,20	>100
Clarithromycin	L-cladinose	0,10	>100	>100

Figure 28 3-Acyl erythromycin A

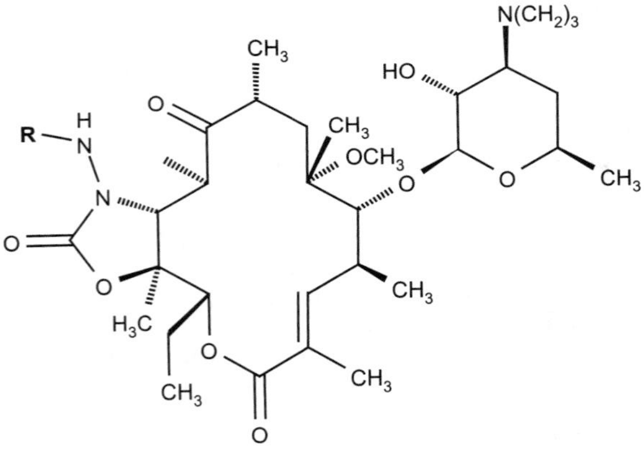

Figure 29 Carbamate macrolides

HMR 3562 and HMR 3787 were tested for their in vitro activities against gram-positive and gram-negative cocci and some gram-negative bacilli as well as against *M. pneumoniae*, *L. pneumophila*, *Chlamydia* spp., and *Mycobacterium tuberculosis* (Felmingham et al., 1999).

16.2.1. HMR 3787

HMR 3787 (Fig. 30) seems to be more active against gram-positive cocci than HMR 3562, except against *S. pneumoniae* isolates resistant to erythromycin A, against which HMR 3562 is one tube test dilution more active (MIC_{50} and MIC_{90}, 0.015 and 0.12 μg/ml), and HMR 3787 exhibits activity against *S. pneumoniae* isolates susceptible to erythromycin A comparable to that of telithromycin, with a MIC_{50} and MIC_{90} of 0.008 and 0.015 μg/ml. HMR 3787 also retains activity against *S. pneumoniae* isolates harboring an underlying mechanism of resistance to erythromycin A, such

Table 46 In vitro activity of compound I

Animals	Compound[a]	C_{max} (μg/ml)	T_{max} (h)	$t_{1/2}$ (h)	$AUC_{0-\infty}$ (μg·h/ml)	Urinary elimination (%)
Mice	TE-810	1.16	0.5	1.54	2.73	34.2
	Cla	0.30	0.5	1.66	0.52	3.8
	Azi	0.38	1.0	2.30	1.11	9.4
Rats	TE-810	0.40	1.0	1.40	1.26	NT[b]
	Cla	0.16	2.0	1.73	0.46	NT
	Azi	0.25	2.0	4.61	0.53	NT
Monkeys	TE-810	1.15	1.0	1.99	3.70	24.6
	Cla	0.72	1.0	1.74	2.49	7.1
	Azi	0.25	0.5	2.63	0.60	2.1

[a]Cla, clarithromycin; Azi, azithromycin.
[b]NT, not tested.

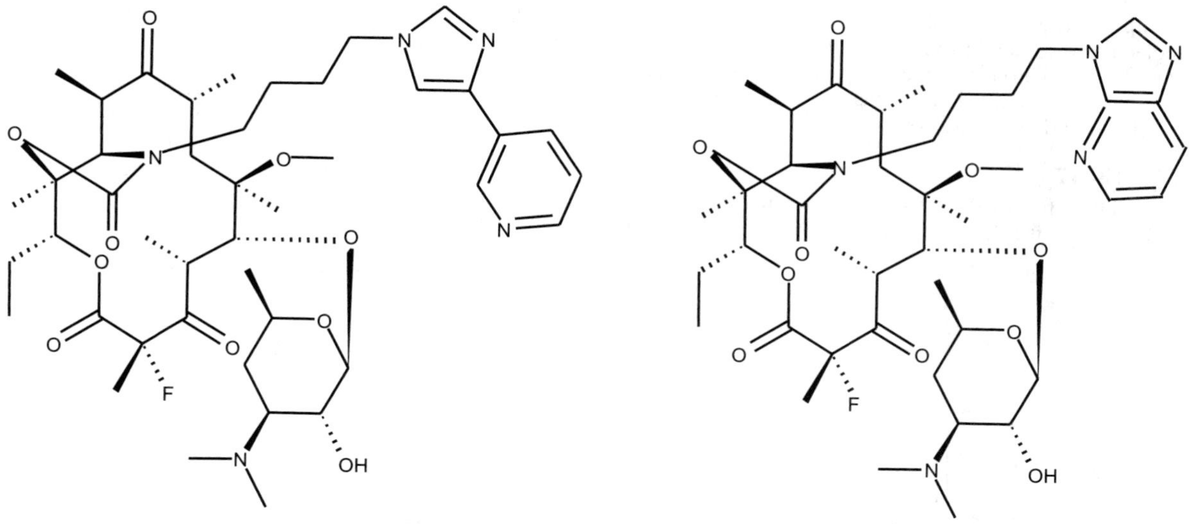

Figure 30 HMR 3787 and HMR 3562

as MLS_B [*erm*(B)], efflux [*mef*(E)], and ribosomal protein mutation (proteins L4 and L22).

For *E. faecium* strains resistant to erythromycin A, the MIC_{50} and MIC_{90} were 0.5 and 0.5 μg/ml. Both compounds are active against *C. diphtheriae, L. monocytogenes, N. gonorrhoeae, N. meningitidis, M. catarrhalis*, and *B. pertussis*. For *H. influenzae*, the MIC_{50} and MIC_{90} were 1.0 and 2.0 μg/ml and 1.0 and 1.0 μg/ml for HMR 3562 and HMR 3787, respectively. They exhibit good activity against *H. pylori, L. pneumophila, C. trachomatis, C. pneumoniae, M. pneumoniae*, and *U. urealyticum*. Only HMR 3787 exhibits significant activity against *M. hominis* (MIC_{50} and MIC_{90}, 0.5 and 1.0 μg/ml). They are inactive against *M. tuberculosis* (MIC, ≥64 μg/ml).

In murine disseminated infections, both compounds are more active than clarithromycin against *S. aureus, S. pyogenes, S. pneumoniae*, and *S. agalactiae* infections irrespective of the susceptibility of the bacterial isolates to erythromycin A. The difference in in vivo activity between the compounds is strain dependent.

Female Swiss (OF-1) mice (20 to 23 g) were infected intratracheally with around 10^5 CFU of *S. pneumoniae* (erythromycin A-susceptible and erythromycin A-resistant isolates; MIC, >128 μg/ml). Treatment was initiated subcutaneously 18 h after bacterial challenge and given every 8 h for 3 days. After 50 or 100 mg/kg, the survival rate for mice challenged with the susceptible *S. pneumoniae* strain was 80 to 100%; with the *S. pneumoniae* strain resistant to erythromycin A the survival rates were around 90% for HMR 3562 and 45 to 60% for HMR 3787. The bacterial lung clearance was higher.

It was shown that both compounds are strongly accumulated by human neutrophils, with an intracellular/extracellular ratio greater than 100 within the first 5 min. Both are mainly located in the granular compartment of neutrophils, and they are moderately released from loaded polymorphonuclear leukocytes. For both compounds, against *S. pneumoniae* susceptible to erythromycin A a strong bactericidal activity was recorded; the same was the case with *mef*(A)-containing *S. pneumoniae*. For both compounds the bactericidal activity against *erm*(B)-containing *S. pneumoniae* occurred more slowly.

After 6 and 12 h of contact irrespective of the mechanism of resistance to erythromycin A, HMR 3787 exhibits bactericidal activity, with a reduction above 3 $\log_{10}$ CFU/ml at low concentrations (MIC or twice the MIC). HMR 3787 is highly active against *S. pyogenes* susceptible to erythromycin A (modal MIC, 0.015 μg/ml). Against *S. pyogenes* harboring the *erm*(TR) or *mef*(A) gene as a mechanism of resistance to erythromycin A, HMR 3787 is two times more active than telithromycin. Only isolates for which erythromycin A exhibits a MIC of >64 μg/ml were chosen to investigate the potential of HMR 3787 against *erm*(B)-containing strains. Half of the isolates range in the intermediate zone of susceptibility to HMR 3787 using the resistance breakpoint for telithromycin (MIC, >2 μg/ml). The HMR 3787 MIC_{50} and MIC_{90} are 2.0 and 2.0 μg/ml for *H. influenzae*.

HMR 3787 exhibits comparable activity against *S. aureus* susceptible to erythromycin A, or slightly higher (MIC_{50}, 0.06 μg/ml, versus 0.12 μg/ml for telithromycin). HMR 3787 seems to be the most active ketolide against *C. pneumoniae* and *L. pneumophila*, with MIC ranges of 0.06 to 0.12 μg/ml and 0.004 to 0.004 μg/ml, respectively. This excellent activity is correlated with the intracellular concentration of HMR 3787. HMR 3787 is extremely active against *M. pneumoniae*, with a MIC_{50} and MIC_{90} of 0.0005 to 0.0005 μg/ml.

16.2.2. HMR 3562

HMR 3562 (Fig. 30) exhibited activity comparable to that of HMR 3787 against *S. aureus* strains susceptible to erythromycin A (MIC_{50} and MIC_{90}, 0.06 and 0.06 μg/ml). Against erythromycin A-resistant isolates, as for HMR 3787 and telithromycin, the antistaphylococcal activity is delineated in inducible MLS_B and constitutive MLS_B strains, being only active against inducible MLS_B strains.

HMR 3562 retained good antipneumococcal activity against erythromycin A-resistant isolates (MIC_{50} and MIC_{90}, 0.03 and 0.06 μg/ml) and against all streptococci. HMR 3562 also exhibits good activity against gram-positive bacilli. It is bactericidal against *S. pneumoniae*.

16.3. EP-13159

A series of 2-fluoroketolides was synthesized. These compounds are 6,11-*O*-bridged ketolides. The aim of this bridge was to improve the stability of the compound by preventing intramolecular hemiketal formation and to enhance rigidity. They are 9-oxime ketolides. One compound was selected for further investigation: EP-13159 (Fig. 31). This derivative seems to be as active as telithromycin (Table 47).

16.4. EP-13417

EP-13417 differs from EP-13159 by the heteroaryl moieties (Fig. 31). In vitro, it is less active than telithromycin against *H. influenzae* (the MIC_{50} and MIC_{90} of EP-13417 were 4 and 16 μg/ml, versus 1.0 and 8.0 μg/ml for telithromycin) and *S. aureus*.

EP-13417 exerts good in vivo activity, similar to that of telithromycin, against pneumococcal *mef*-containing strains (ED_{50}, 14.9 versus 18 mg/kg) and against staphylococcal infection (ED_{50}, 17.4 versus 18 mg/kg). In mice, EP-13417 possesses a long apparent elimination half-life (Table 48).

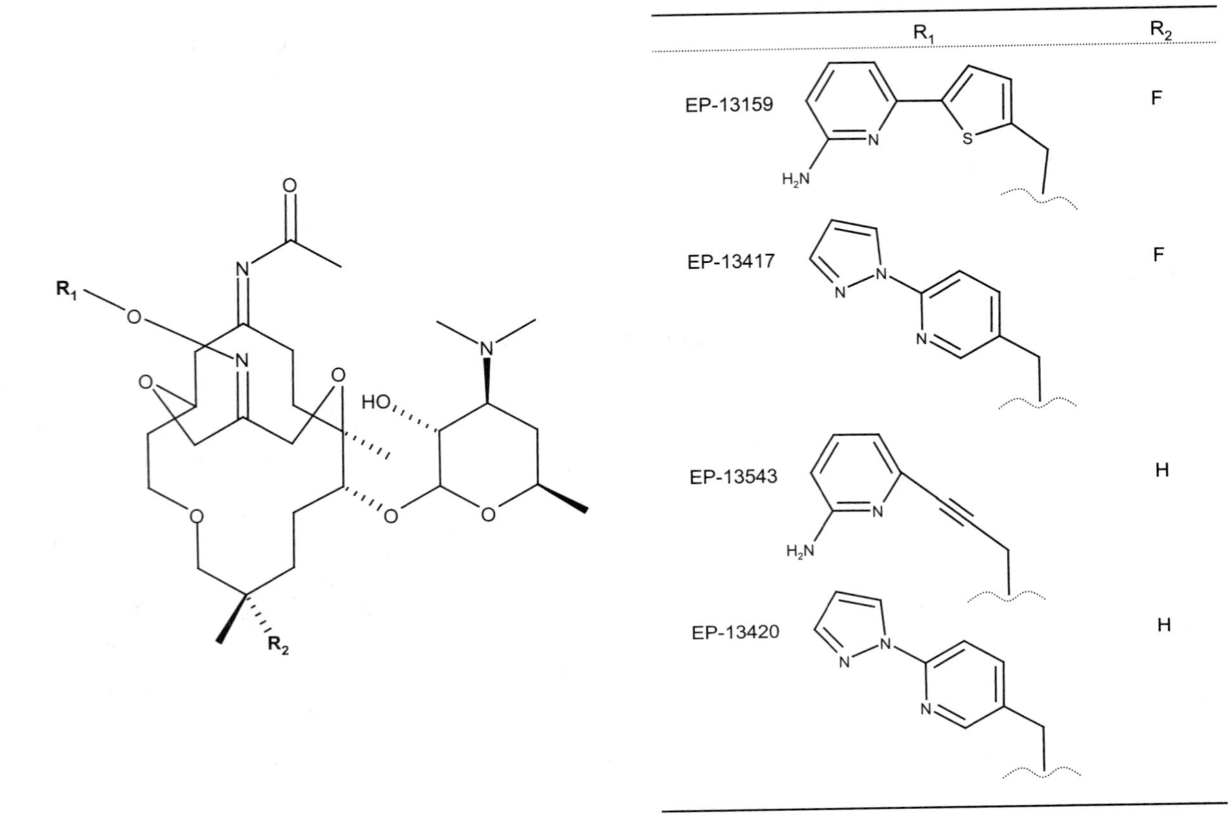

	R_1	R_2
EP-13159		F
EP-13417		F
EP-13543		H
EP-13420		H

Figure 31 Bridged bicyclic ketolides

Table 47 In vitro activity of EP-13159

Organism(s)	Drug	MIC (μg/ml) 50%	90%	Range
S. aureus	EP-13159	0.125	4.0	
	Telithromycin	0.125	>64	
VRE[a]				
E. faecalis ATCC 29212	EP-13159			0.06
	Telithromycin			0.03
E. faecalis ATCC 19434	EP-13159			0.06
	Telithromycin			0.03
E. faecium ATCC 51575	EP-13159			1.0
	Telithromycin			8.0
E. faecium ATCC 900221	EP-13159			1.0
	Telithromycin			8.0
S. epidermidis ATCC 12228	EP-13159			0.125
	Telithromycin			0.125
S. epidermidis ATCC 12228 (multidrug-resistant)	EP-13159			0.125
	Telithromycin			0.125

[a]VRE, vancomycin-resistant enterococci.

Table 48 Pharmacokinetics of ketolides in mice after administration of 25 mg/kg (oral doses)

Drug	C_{max} (μg/ml)	T_{max} (h)	AUC_{0-24} (μg·h/ml)	$t_{1/2}$ (h)	Oral bioavailability (%)
EP-13417	1.7	1.0	16.6	3	84
EP-13159	0.9	3.0	8.2	2.6	54
EP-13420	2.5	1.5	17	3.3	89
EP-13543	1.6	1.0	4.4	2.1	40
Telithromycin	5.5	1.0	16	1.5	73
Clarithromycin	0.8	0.5	1.8	1	49

16.5. 6-*O*-Arylpropargyl 9-Oxime-2-Fluoro-Carbamate Ketolide

It was reported that 9-oxime derivatives of macrolides and ketolides exhibited improved antibacterial activity against streptococci and staphylococci. The 2-fluoro ketolides have been shown to be effective against erythromycin A-resistant strains, with improved pharmacokinetic properties.

In a new series of 6-arylpropargyl-carbamate analogs (Fig. 32), it was shown that the 2-fluoro analogs did not exert any improved antibacterial activity compared to the H-counterpart, with the exception of *S. pyogenes* (MIC of 8 versus 32 μg/ml) (Beebe et al., 2004).

16.6. JNJ 17155528 and JNJ 17155437

Following the synthesis of a series of 15-methyl ketolides (Abbanat et al., 2001), a series derived from this analog was synthesized with a naphthyridone moiety: JNJ 17155528 and JNJ 17155437. They exhibited good antipneumococcal activity (MICs, ≤0.0015 to 0.03 μg/ml) and moderate activity against *H. influenzae* (MIC, 2 μg/ml). They are active against *erm*(B)- and *mef*(A)-containing *S. pneumoniae.* (MICs, 0.06 to 0.12 μg/ml). They have activity similar to that of telithromycin (Macielag et al., 2003).

16.7. JNJ 17156581 and JNJ 17156815

In a series of 2-fluoroketolides, two derivatives were selected for further investigation: JNJ 17156581 and JNJ 17156815. They are composed of a 6-O-biheteroaryl-2-propenyl side chain. They differ by the heteroaryl moiety (Fig. 33).

They were obtained from a genetically modified strain of *Streptomyces erythraeus* and cloned in *Streptomyces coelicolor.* The 15-methyl-deoxy-erythromycin B obtained was synthetically modified, yielding these two derivatives. In vitro they had antibacterial activity similar to that of telithromycin (Table 49).

17. OTHER KETOLIDE DERIVATIVES

17.1. HMR 3832

HMR 3832 is a new ketolide derivative having an amino phenyl moiety on the carbamate side chain, instead of a pyrridinyl ring for telithromycin (Fig. 34). It exhibits good activity against gram-positive cocci, including beta-hemolytic streptococci (Lancefield groups A, B, C, and G), with a MIC_{50} and MIC_{90} of 0.03 and 0.06 μg/ml. For *S. pneumoniae*, the MIC_{50}s and MIC_{90}s of HMR 3832 were 0.03 to 0.06 μg/ml and 0.06 to 0.25 μg/ml, respectively. HMR 3832 exhibits good activity against *E. faecalis* (MIC_{50} and MIC_{90}, 0.06 and 0.06 μg/ml), *C. diphtheriae* (MIC_{50} and MIC_{90}, 0.008 and 0.015 μg/ml), *C. jeikeium* (MIC_{50} and MIC_{90}, 0.06 and 0.25 μg/ml), and *L. monocytogenes* (MIC_{50} and MIC_{90}, 0.06 and 0.06 μg/ml). HMR 3832 is inactive against *Nocardia* spp. (MIC_{50}, 32 μg/ml). HMR 3832 exhibited activity comparable to that of clarithromycin against erythromycin A-susceptible gram-positive cocci, but it retained activity against gram-positive cocci isolates harboring a mechanism of resistance to erythromycin A.

HMR 3832 exhibited better in vitro activity than clarithromycin against *H. influenzae* (MIC_{50} and MIC_{90}, 2.0 and 4.0 μg/ml), but the MICs increased twofold when the organism was incubated in 5 to 6% CO_2. HMR 3832 shows good activity against *N. gonorrhoeae* (MIC_{90}, 0.12 μg/ml),

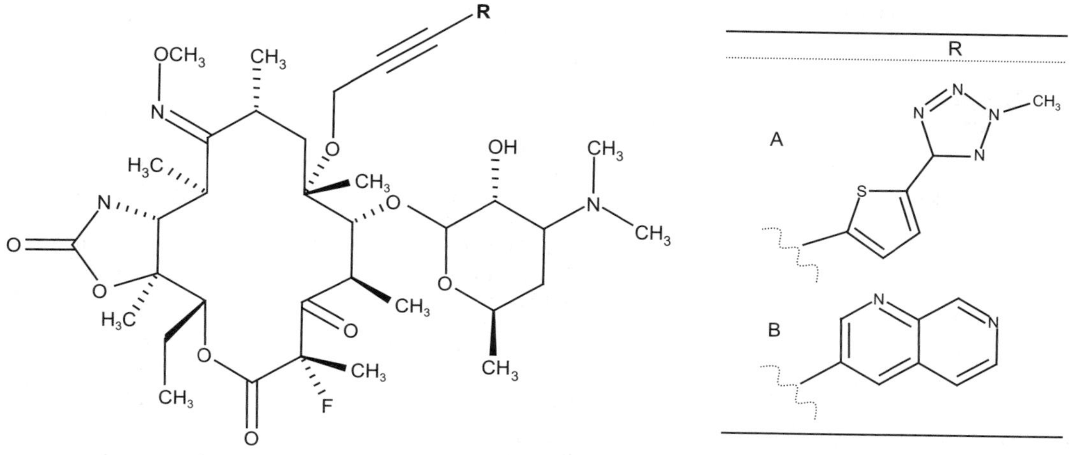

Figure 32 *O*-Arylpropargyl-9-oxime-2-fluoro-carbamate ketolide

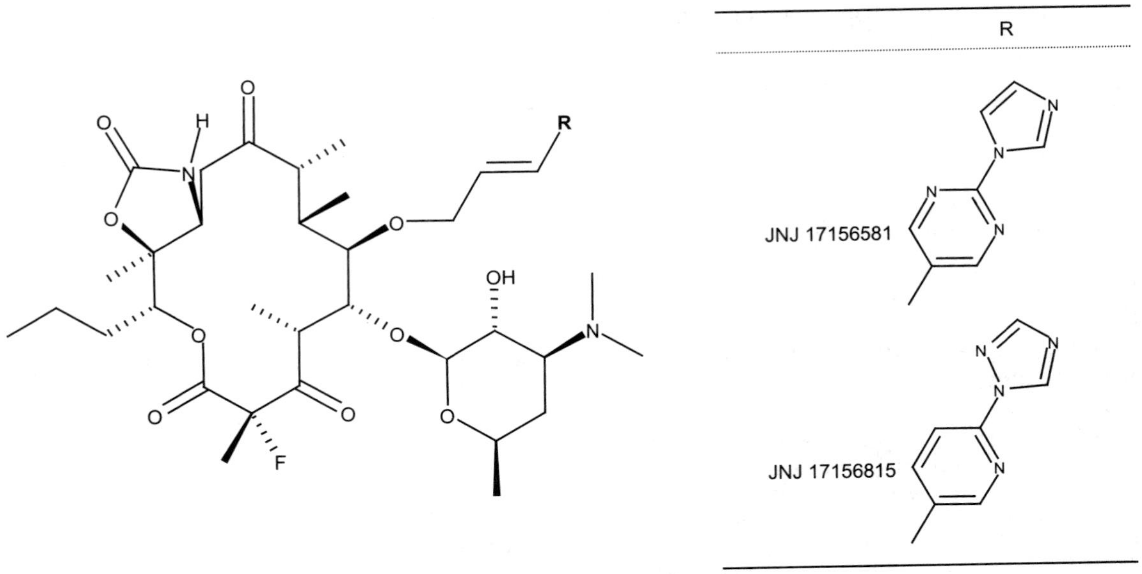

Figure 33 6-*O*-Heteroaryl propenyl ketolides

Table 49 In vitro activities of JNJ 17156581 and JNJ 17156815

Microorganism	*n*	Compound	MIC (µg/ml) 90%	MIC (µg/ml) Range
S. pneumoniae				
Ery[s]	7	Telithromycin		≤0.015
		JNJ 17156581		≤0.015
		JNJ 17156815		≤0.015
erm(B)	10	Telithromycin	0.06	≤0.015–0.12
		JNJ 17156581	0.06	≤0.015–0.5
		JNJ 17156815	0.06	≤0.015–0.06
mef(A)	10	Telithromycin	0.25	0.03–0.25
		JNJ 17156581	0.12	≤0.015–0.12
		JNJ 17156815	0.12	≤0.015–0.12
mef(A) + *erm*(B)	2	Telithromycin		0.5
		JNJ 17156581		0.06–0.12
		JNJ 17156815		0.12–0.25
L4 mutation	1	Telithromycin		0.06
		JNJ 17156581		0.06
		JNJ 17156815		0.06
23S rRNA mutation	1	Telithromycin		0.03
		JNJ 17156581		0.03
		JNJ 17156815		0.03
S. pyogenes				
Ery[s]	1	Telithromycin		0.015
		JNJ 17156581		0.015
		JNJ 17156815		0.015
erm(TR)	23	Telithromycin	0.06	0.015–0.06
		JNJ 17156581	0.06	0.015–0.06
		JNJ 17156815	0.03	0.015–0.06
erm(B)	3	Telithromycin		8–>8
		JNJ 17156581		1–2
		JNJ 17156815		1–4
mef(A)	7	Telithromycin		0.5–1
		JNJ 17156581		0.12–0.25
		JNJ 17156815		0.12–0.25
H. influenzae	12	Telithromycin	4	0.5–4
		JNJ 17156581	8	1–8

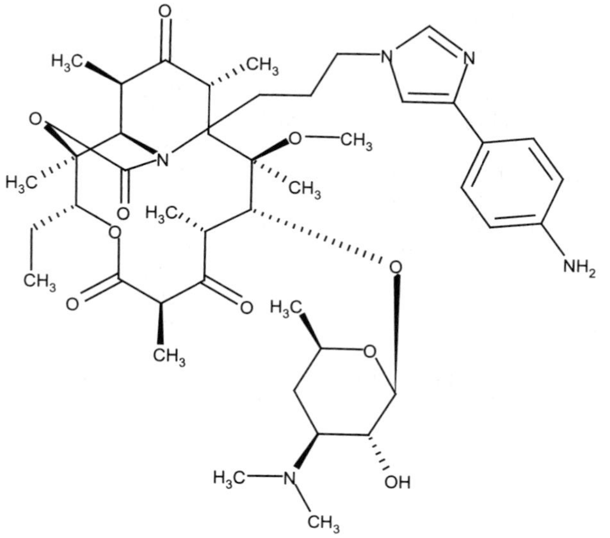

Figure 34 HMR 3832

N. meningitidis (MIC_{50} and MIC_{90}, 0.06 and 0.12 μg/ml), *M. catarrhalis* (MIC_{50} and MIC_{90}, 0.06 and 0.12 μg/ml), and *B. pertussis* (MIC_{90}, 0.12 μg/ml). It is inactive against *Enterobacteriaceae* and *Pseudomonas aeruginosa* (MIC, ≥32 μg/ml). HMR 3832 displays good in vitro activity against anaerobes: *Peptostreptococcus* spp., *Clostridium perfringens*, and *Clostridium difficile* (MIC_{50}s, 0.03 to 0.12 μg/ml; MIC_{90}s, 0.12 to 0.5 μg/ml). In the case of gram-negative anaerobic bacilli, HMR 3832 exhibits good in vitro activity against *Prevotella* (MIC_{50}, 0.25 μg/ml), and *Porphyromonas* spp. but weak activity against the *B. fragilis* group (MIC_{50} and MIC_{90}, 8 and 64 μg/ml).

For *H. pylori* the MIC_{90}s were 0.25 and 0.03 μg/ml for HMR 3832 and clarithromycin, respectively. HMR 3832 was inactive against *M. tuberculosis* (MIC, >64 μg/ml).

For gram-positive bacteria, the in vitro activity of HMR 3832 in comparison to that of clarithromycin is summarized in Table 50.

17.2. 11-*O*-Substituted Ketolides

Few series of 11-*O*-substituted ketolides have been synthesized, with and without an allyloxy moiety at position 12. The C-12 allyloxy derivatives were shown to be less active than erythromycin A. The length of the linker at position C-11 demonstrated that those having a three-carbon chain are less potent than those with a four- or five-carbon chain. However, they are less active than erythromycin A.

17.3. EP-13543

EP-13543 (Fig. 31) differs from EP-13417 by the lack of a 2-fluorine atom. In vitro, it is as active against pneumococci and staphylococci but less active against *H. influenzae* than telithromycin A, but it is more active in vivo in pneumococcal infection (ED_{50}, 11 versus 18 mg/kg) and staphylococcal infections (ED_{50}, 11 versus 18 mg/kg).

EP-13543 differs from EP-13420 by the aryl substituent on the side chain (Fig. 31). It has the same activity as telithromycin against pneumococci and staphylococci, but it is less active against *H. influenzae*. In vivo, EP-13543 is more active against pneumococcal infections (ED_{50}, 7.7 mg/kg) but less active against staphylococcal infections (ED_{50}, 20.3 mg/kg) than telithromycin.

17.4. EP-13420

EP-13420 is a bridged ketolide (Fig. 35). Its activity was tested against *M. avium* complex. It is not active against clarithromycin-resistant strains. In vivo in murine infections (beige mouse), it is more active against *M. avium* complex than clarithromycin at a daily dose of 100 mg/kg (Bermudez et al., 2004).

The pharmacodynamic model of infection in ICR mice challenged with *S. pneumoniae* demonstrated a concentration-dependent activity (Maglio et al., 2004).

17.5. 9-Keto Bridged Ketolides

The 11,12-carbamate group is essential for overall antibacterial activity because it increases the rigidity of the ketolide conformation (Baker et al., 1988).

The purpose of this series of compounds of bridged bicyclic ketolides was to improve the stability by preventing intramolecular hemiketal formation, increasing the rigidity of the ketolide conformation and providing a point for aryl group attachment. These ketolides are active against *S. pneumoniae* (MIC, 0.13 μg/ml) and inactive against *H. influenzae* (MIC, >64 μg/ml) (Wang et al., 2004).

17.6. CP-654,743

A novel series of ketolide derivatives has been synthesized. All compounds are characterized by a 11, 12-carbamate residue on which a butyl imidazolyl pyridyl chain is fixed like for telithromycin. The molecules differ by the substituents at C-2 (Fig. 36). All of them possess a C-9 methyloxime group. Among all of these derivatives, the C-2F analogs displayed

Table 50 In vitro activity of HMR 3832 against gram-positive bacteria

Organism(s)	*n*	MIC (μg/ml)			
		HMR 3832		Clarithromycin	
S. aureus Ery[s]	22	0.12	0.12	0.12	0.12
Coagulase-negative staphylococci	22	0.12	0.12	0.12	0.12
S. pyogenes	23	0.03	1.0	0.01	8.0
S. agalactiae	23	0.03	0.03	0.01	0.03
Lancefield group C and G streptococci	44	0.03	0.03	0.03	0.03
Viridans group streptococci	35	0.06	0.25	1.0	>64
S. pneumoniae	21	0.03	0.06	0.01	0.01
S. pneumoniae Ery[r]	20	0.06	0.25	>64	>64
E. faecalis	21	0.06	0.06	0.25	0.25
C. diphtheriae	20	0.008	0.01	0.004	0.004
L. monocytogenes	26	0.06	0.06	0.12	0.12

the highest antibacterial activity. CP-654,743, the C-2 unsubstituted analog, exhibited a higher antibacterial activity than other analogs. CP-654,743 was selected for further preclinical investigation.

CP-654,743 exhibits good antipneumococcal activity against isolates susceptible to erythromycin A (MIC_{90}, 0.004 μg/ml), but a drop of activity was noted for *S. pneumoniae* isolates harboring an underlying mechanism of resistance to erythromycin A, with MIC_{90}s of 0.125 and 0.25 μg/ml for *erm*(B^+) and *mef*(E^+)-containing *S. pneumoniae*. CP-654,743 is highly active against *S. pyogenes* susceptible to erythromycin A, but an important drop of activity was shown when an *erm*(B^+)/*erm*(A^+) gene or a *mef*(A^+) gene is present: the MIC_{90} of CP-654,743 was 2.0 μg/ml.

In a model of pneumococcal peritonitis in mice (female Swiss, CF-1; 18 to 20 g) induced intraperitoneally with an LD_{100} of *S. pneumoniae* with various patterns of resistance to erythromycin A, and treated orally at 0.5 and 4.0 h after bacterial challenge, the PD_{50}s were 25.4, 22.7, and 42.5 mg/kg for MLS-resistant and penicillin G-susceptible, MLS_B- and penicillin G-resistant, and M-phenotype and penicillin G-susceptible *S. pneumoniae* isolates, respectively. Female C3H/HeN mice (18 to 20 g) were infected intranasally with an LD_{100} of a log-phase pneumococcal culture (~10^4 to 10^6 CFU per mouse). Oral therapy was initiated 18 h following bacterial challenge and administered twice a day for 2 days. Of mice infected with erythromycin A- with and penicillin G-susceptible *S. pneumoniae* isolates, 100% survived after an oral dose of 25 mg/kg and 80% survived after a dose of 6.25 mg/kg. About 20% of the mice survived after an oral dose of 1.56 mg/kg. Of mice infected with penicillin-susceptible but erythromycin A-resistant *S. pneumoniae*, the survival rates

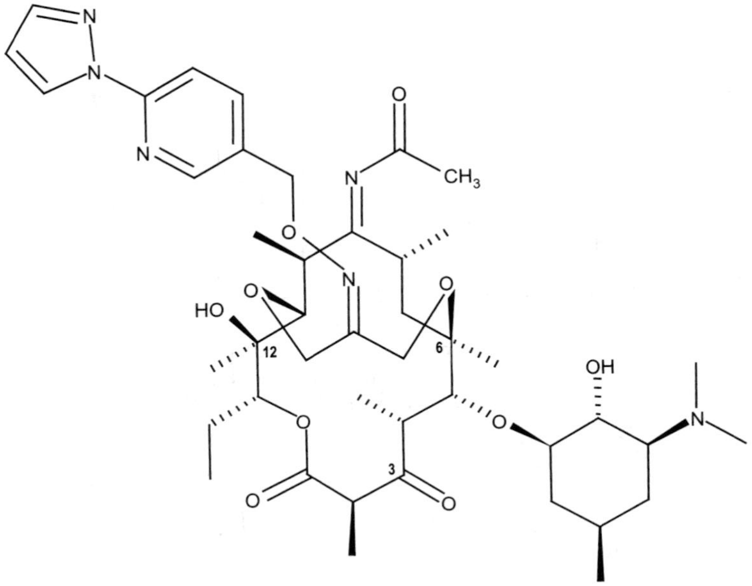

Figure 35 EP-13420

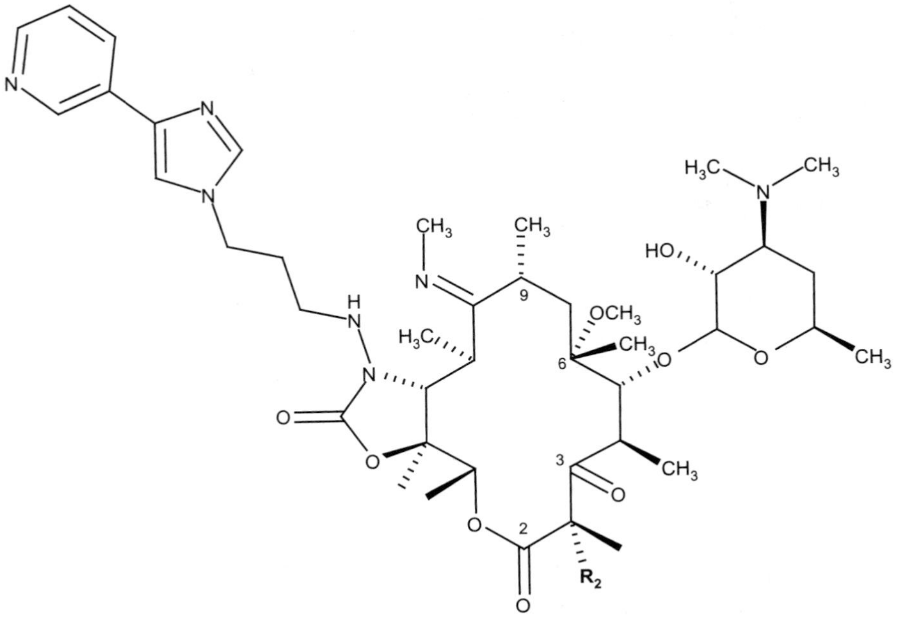

	R_2
CP 654734	F
CP 654745	CH_3
CP 659931	OH
CP 605006	H
CP 660035	C(C)OCH_3

Figure 36 9-Oxime-2 substituted ketolides

were 100, 80, and 10% after 100, 25, and 6.25 mg/kg. These results correlate well with the ED_{50}, which were 4.5, 18.0, 28.0, and 22.7 mg/kg for penicillin G-resistant and M-phenotype penicillin G-susceptible *S. pneumoniae* isolates.

Female Mongolian gerbils (6 to 7 weeks, 18 to 20 g) were challenged with 10^3 CFU of *H. influenzae* via intrabulla instillation. Oral therapy was initiated 18 h after bacterial challenge and given three times per day for 2 days at 100, 50, 25, and 12.5 mg/kg. The ED_{50} were 23 and 22.4 mg/kg for CP-654,743 and telithromycin, respectively. Bacterial clearance was obtained with a dose of 100 mg/kg/day for both compounds. At 12.5 mg/kg/day no clearance was obtained with CP-654,743; at this dose of telithromycin, bacterial clearance was obtained in 20% of the gerbils.

After intravenous administration of 10 mg of CP-654,743 and telithromycin per kg to rats and monkeys, the areas under the curve for the compounds were comparable in rats (3.8 versus 3.3 μg·h/ml) and were higher for telithromycin in monkeys (8.6 versus 5.5 μg·h/ml). In monkeys the apparent elimination half-lives were 3.0 and 9.7 h for CP-654,743 and telithromycin, respectively. The solubility of CP-654,743 in water is comparable to that of telithromycin at pH 7.0 (>65 μg/ml), and the lipophilicity is higher for CP-654,743 than for telithromycin (C-logP, 6.64 versus 3.54).

17.7. C-13 Modified Ketolides

A series of ketolide derivatives was produced from erythromycin A templates produced in a genetically engineered *S. coelicolor* strain, allowing evaluation of structure-activity relationships of C-13 substitutions. This strain was fermented with an appropriate diketide thioester precursor to yield 6-deoxyerythronolide B analogs with C-13 methyl or vinyl groups in place of the ethyl group. A second series was prepared from picromycin, a natural ketolide which does not possess a C-6 methoxy group or C-10 methyl functionalities in comparison with erythromycin A (Fig. 37).

Two compounds having the 11, 12-carbamate residue on which a butyl imidazolyl pyridyl chain was fixed and having either an ethyl or a vinyl group at C-13 (Fig. 37) are poorly active in vitro, especially against gram-positive cocci harboring an underlying mechanism of resistance to erythromycin A (*mef* or *erm*). However, in vitro activity is retained against *erm*-containing *S. pneumoniae* (MICs, 2.0 to 4.0 μg/ml, versus >16.0 μg/ml for erythromycin A) and *mef*-containing *S. pneumoniae* (MIC, 0.5 μg/ml, versus 2.0 μg/ml for erythromycin A).

Replacement of the C-13 ethyl group on telithromycin with a methyl or vinyl group yielded two- to four-fold or two- to eight-fold increases, respectively, in the MIC, and the resulting analogs were inactive against *S. aureus* strains containing an inducible *erm* gene (MICs, 16 μg/ml).

Only 40% of the Swiss Webster mice were protected with the two picromycin analogs after being challenged with *S. aureus* strain Smith and treated by the subcutaneous route with a dose of 20 mg/kg, 1 h after bacterial challenge.

17.8. GW 581506 (PL1023)

GW 581506 (PL1023) is a 3-keto azalide. This compound exhibits moderate in vitro activity against *S. pneumoniae* isolates susceptible to erythromycin A (MIC_{50} and MIC_{90}, 0.5 and 0.5 μg/ml), and it is inactive against isolates resistant to erythromycin A [*mef*(E)-containing strain] (MIC_{50} and

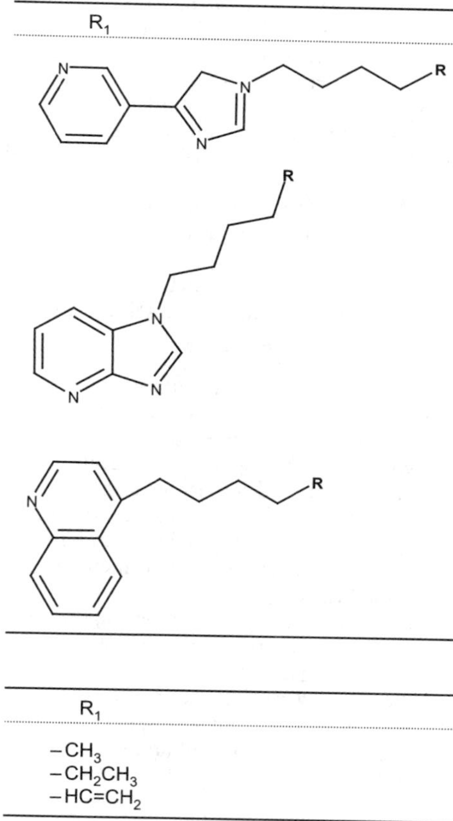

Figure 37 **13-Modified substituted ketolides**

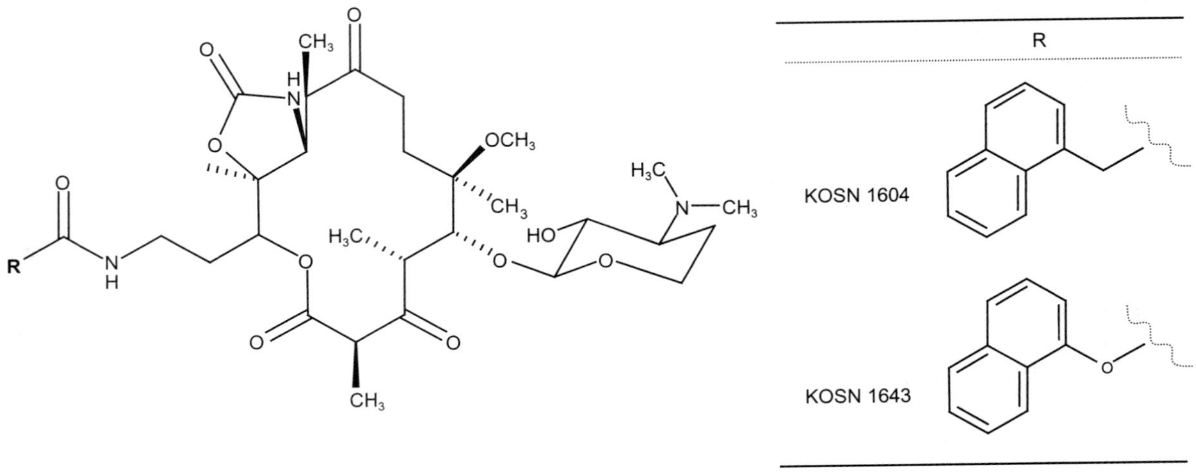

	R
KOSN 1604	
KOSN 1643	

Figure 38 15-Amido ketolides

MIC_{90}, 8.0 and 8.0 μg/ml) and against *erm*(B)-containing strains (MIC, >128 μg/ml). It is weakly active against *S. aureus* and *H. influenzae*. Other keto-8aN-azalides have been prepared and exhibited moderate activity or were considered inactive.

17.9. 15-Amido Ketolides

A series of 15-amido ketolides has been synthesized (Fig. 38). They are less active in vitro than telithromycin, with MICs ranging from 0.025 to 6.25, 0.25 to 12.5, and 3.12 to 6.25 μg/ml for *S. pneumoniae*, *S. aureus*, and *H. influenzae*, respectively. For KOSN 1643 the oral bioavailabity in mice is about 37%. For KOSN the bioavailability is less than 15% in mice. For both the apparent elimination half-lives ranged from 0.8 to 1.9 h, with peak concentrations in plasma of 100 and 156 μg/ml after oral administration and 766 and 798 μg/ml after intravenous administration for KOSN 1604 and KOSN 1643, respectively (Ashley et al., 2004).

17.10. GW 773546 and GW 708408

A new series of ketolide derivatives (Fig. 39) has been synthesized and tested against *S. pneumoniae* and *H. influenzae*. Against these microorganisms they had similar in vitro activities (Table 51) (Appelbaum et al., 2004; Pankuch et al., 2004).

17.11. Lactone Ketolides

A series of ketolides bearing a five-membered lactone ring fused to positions 11 and 12 was prepared (Fig. 40) (Hunziker et al., 2004). Some derivatives exhibited good in vitro activity against *S. pneumoniae* resistant to erythromycin A (MIC, 0.25 μg/ml) and activity against *H. influenzae* (MICs, 0.25 to 4.0 μg/ml) similar to that of telithromycin. Activity against *S. pneumoniae* was strongly dependent on the nature of the side chain attached to the five-membered lactone ring via the sulfide bridge.

In vivo in disseminated pneumococcal murine infections they exerted good activity irrespective of the susceptibility to erythromycin A. Against *S. pyogenes* disseminated infections in mice the ED_{50} were 7.1 and <1.5 mg/kg after oral and subcutaneous administrations, respectively (telithromycin ED_{50}, 5.0 and 1.2 mg/kg for oral and subcutaneous administrations, respectively).

	R
GW 773546	
GW 708408	

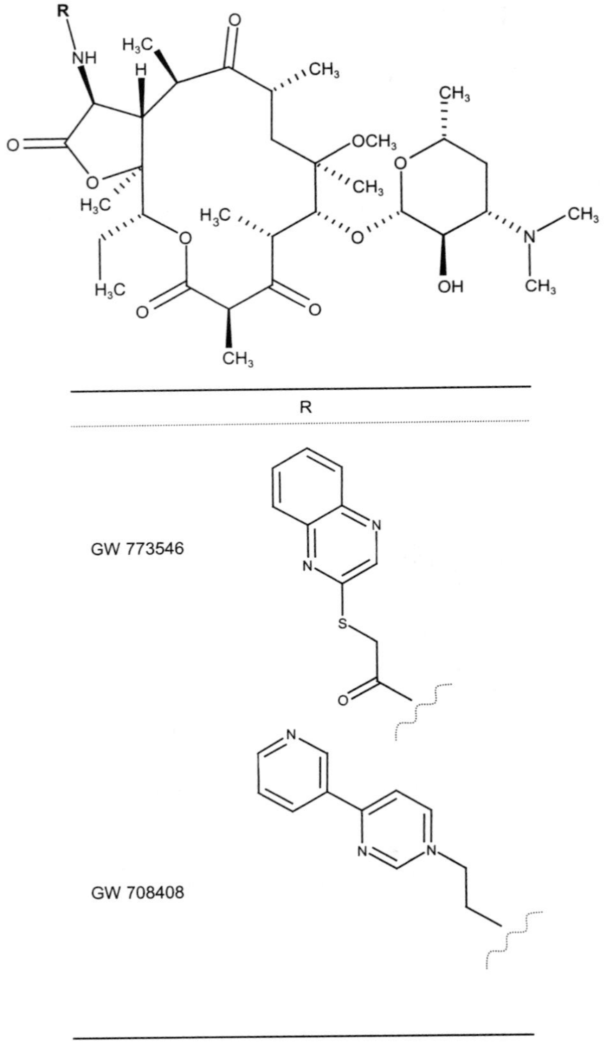

Figure 39 GW 773546 and GW 708408

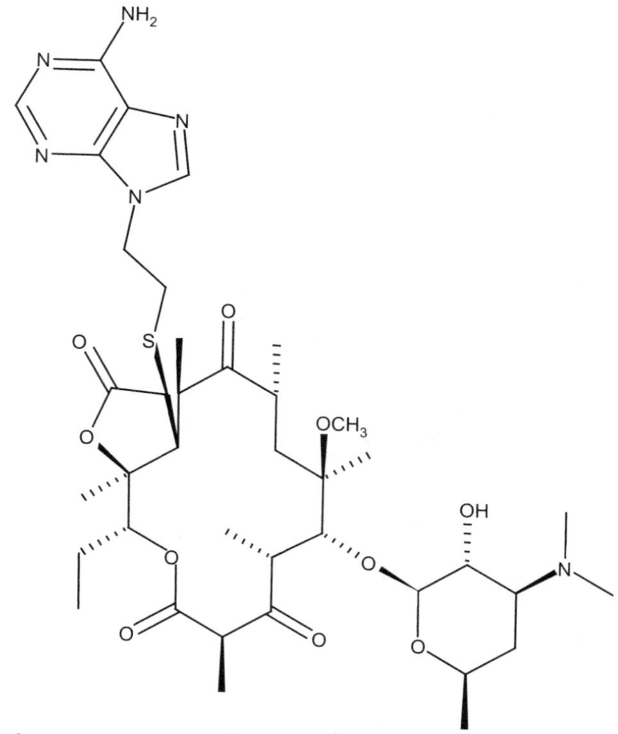

Figure 40 Lactone ketolides

The oral bioavailability in mice is around 60%, with an apparent elimination half-life of 1.1 to 1.2 h.

17.12. JNJ 17069546

A series of C-6 carbamates was prepared, and among the molecules one was further investigated, JNJ 17069546. This pyrimidinyl phenyl-propenyl carbamate ketolide (Fig. 41) is active against *S. pneumoniae* irrespective of the susceptibility to erythromycin A of the isolate (MICs, 0.03 to 0.06 μg/ml) and weakly active against *H. influenzae* (MIC, 4.0 μg/ml). In murine disseminated pneumococcal infections the ED_{50} were 1.8 and 4.4 mg/kg after oral (20 mg/kg) and subcutaneous (10 mg/kg) administrations, respectively (telithromycin ED_{50}, 15 and 15 mg/kg after oral and subcutaneous administrations, respectively (Henninger et al., 2004).

17.13. Oleandomycin Derivatives

New series of oleandomycin derivatives have been prepared (GW 580483X [PL1329]) which are 9-oxime derivatives exhibiting moderate activity against *S. pneumoniae*, *S. pyogenes*, and *S. aureus* susceptible to erythromycin A and are inactive against *erm*(B)-containing isolates and *H. influenzae*.

It seems that oleandomycin with a lack of L-cladinose is totally inactive.

17.14. A-217213

A-217213 is an 11,12-carbamate ketolide bearing a 6-O-propargyl-3-quinoline side chain (Fig. 42). In vitro and in vivo in disseminated pneumococcal infections in mice (ED_{50}, 11.1 mg/kg, versus 12.5 mg/kg for telithromycin), A-217213 exhibited similar antibacterial activities (Table 52).

17.15. Bifunctional Ketolides

A series of bifunctional ketolides has been synthesized in order to be used as probes for ribosome interaction (Fig. 43). RU-64004 and ABT-773 bear a quinolyl group which moves freely and allows the formation of a suitable conformation for effective binding. The C-3 cladinose moiety is placed above the macrolide ring and blocks one of the two pathways leading to the anchor-left isomer. Removing the C-3 cladinose allows the formation of the anchor-right isomerother descladinosyl derivatives. Both are inactive against erythromycin A-resistant *S. pneumoniae* isolates (Ma et al., 2002).

17.16. TEA 0769 and TEA 0777

Le Mahieu et al. (1975) showed that the 3-O-benzylerythromycin A derivative was inactive, as has been confirmed by various teams.

Several series of compounds with different chains substituting for the 3-OH group have been prepared (Asaka et al., 1997), and two compounds have been selected: TEA 0769 and TEA 0777 (Fig. 29).

Three different series have been prepared, comprising 6-O-methyl, 6-OH derivatives with an 11,12-carbonate, and 9-oxime, with three different types of chains attached to the 3-O-carbonyl: 3-methoxybenzoyl, 4-nitrobenzoyl, and 4-nitrophenylacetyl.

The most encouraging series is that involving an 11,12-carbonate and 6-OCH_3 (TEA 0769) and the derivative

Table 51 Antipneumococcal and anti-*H. influenzae* activities of GW 773546 and GW 708408

Organism[a]	*n*	MIC (μg/ml)			
		GW 773546		GW 708408	
		50%	90%	50%	90%
H. influenzae β$^+$	89	1.0	2.0	2.0	4.0
H. influenzae β$^-$	115	1.0	2.0	2.0	4.0
H. influenzae BLNAR	19	0.5	2.0	1.0	4.0
S. pneumoniae Ery^s	164	0.008	2.0	0.016	0.016
S. pneumoniae erm(B)	78	0.03	0.016	0.03	0.5
S. pneumoniae mef(E)	57	0.06	0.5	0.125	0.25
S. pneumoniae L4 mutation	19	0.06	0.125	0.06	0.125

[a]β$^+$, β-lactamase producing; β$^-$, non-β-lactamase producing.

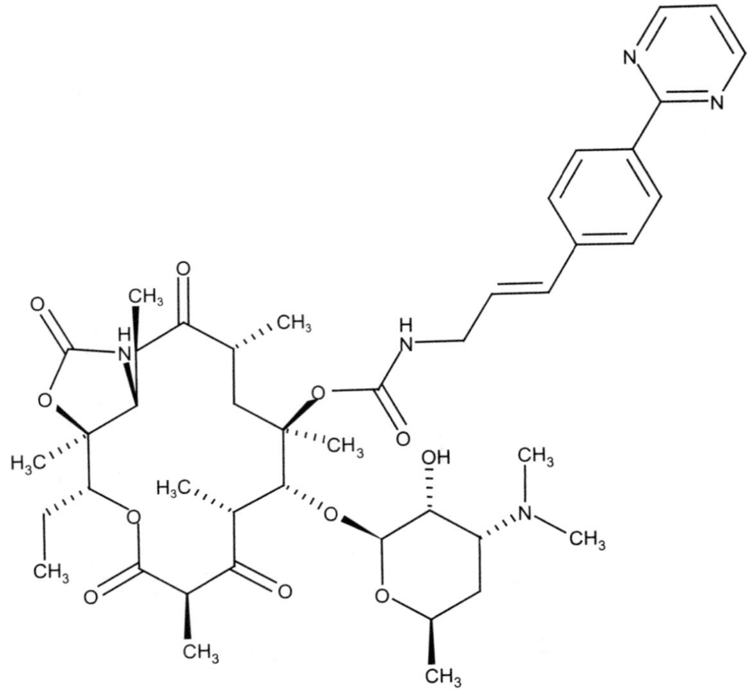

Figure 41 JNJ 17069546

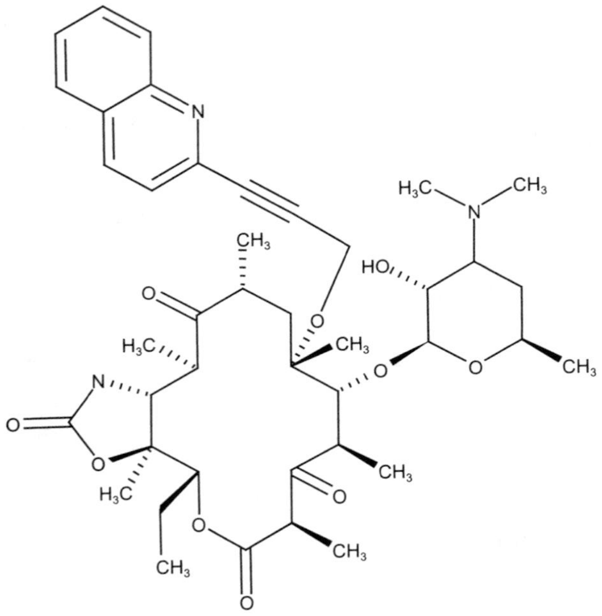

Figure 42 A-217213

without the carbonate (TE 0777). They possess good in vitro activity against erythromycin A-resistant (induced) *S. aureus* 209 P (MIC, 0.20 μg/ml) and *S. aureus* B12 (MIC, 0.30 μg/ml), but they are inactive against erythromycin A-resistant (constitutive) *S. aureus* 138 (MIC, >100 μg/ml).

The in vivo activity of TEA 0769 and TEA 0777 is weaker than that of clarithromycin, despite a threefold-higher concentration than that of clarithromycin in the mouse lung.

17.17. FMA 0713

FMA 0713 is an α-methoxyimino acylide (Fig. 44). It is less active in vitro than telithromycin against gram-positive cocci (Table 53) (Sugiyama et al., 2004).

17.18. 2,3-Anhydroerythromycin A Derivatives

A series of 2,3-anhydroerythromycin A derivatives with a 6-methoxy group and a cyclic carbamate between C-11 and C-12 has been synthesized (Elliott et al., 1997a, 1998) (Fig. 29). These derivatives have good antibacterial activity against erythromycin A-susceptible strains of gram-positive cocci or those resistant as a result of an inducible, but not a constitutive, MLS_B type of mechanism. The molecules

Table 52 In vitro activity of A-217213[a]

Organism	*n*	MIC (μg/ml) A-217213 50%	A-217213 90%	Telithromycin 50%	Telithromycin 90%
S. aureus	16	0.03	0.03	0.06	0.12
S. pneumoniae Ery[s]	30	0.004	0.004	0.015	0.015
S. pneumoniae mef(A)	23	0.03	0.06	0.12	0.25
S. pneumoniae erm(B)	31	0.008	0.12	0.004	0.06
H. influenzae	21	1.0	2.0	2.0	2.0

[a]Data from Nilius et al., 2001.

Table 53 In vitro activity of FMA 0713

Organism	n	MIC (μg/ml) 50%	90%
S. pneumoniae Ery[s]	24	0.06	0.06
S. pneumoniae Ery[r] *mef*(A)	24	0.12	0.25
S. pneumoniae Ery[r] *erm*(B)	25	0.12	0.12
S. pneumoniae Ery[r] *erm*(B)+*mef*(A)	14	0.5	1.0
S. pyogenes Ery[s]	24	0.25	0.5
S. pyogenes Ery[r] *mef*(A)[a]	8	0.25	
S. pyogenes Ery[r] *erm*(B)	13	0.25	
S. pyogenes Ery[r] *erm*(TR)[a]	3	0.25	0.5
S. aureus Ery[r] (inducible)	23	0.5	0.5

[a]MIC range, in micrograms per milliliter, is shown.

Tetracycle left (Abbott)

Tetracycle right (Abbott)

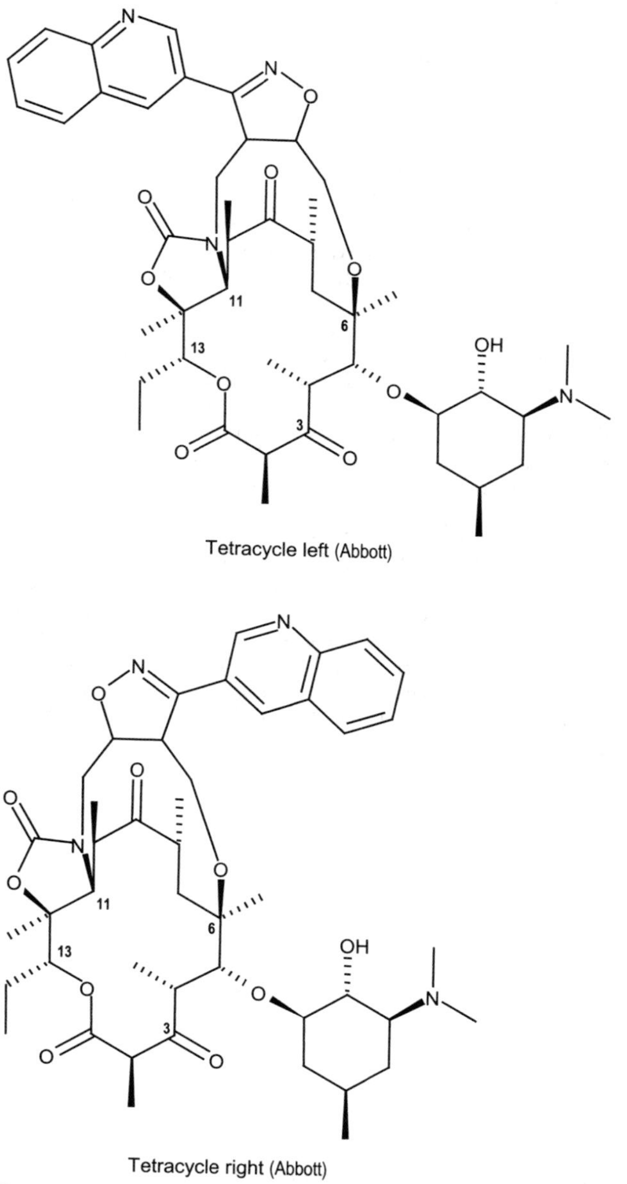

Figure 43 Bifunctional ketolides

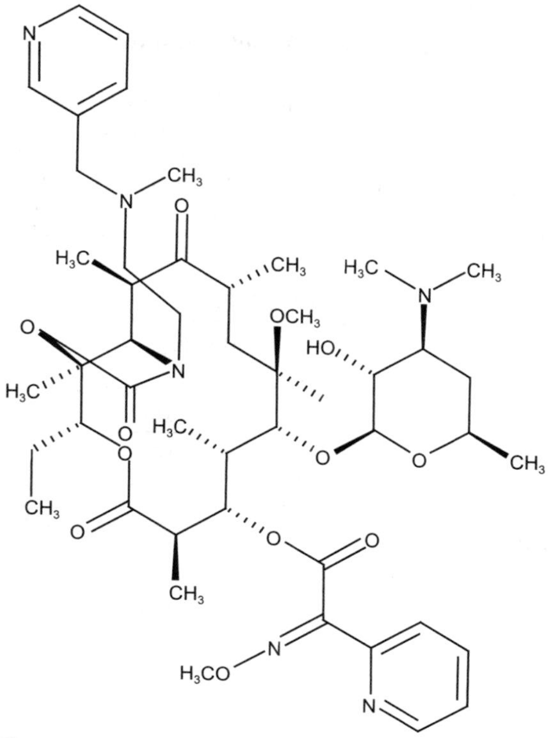

presented are inactive against *H. influenzae*. However, the activity varies with the chain attached to the carbamate residue. The length of the chain between the carbamate and the ring is important. A chain comprising two or four carbons yields greater activity than that with one or three carbons. The presence of electrodonor groups on the phenyl nucleus increases the activity. The sterically hindering nuclei (e.g., quinolinyl) reduce the activity of the molecules. However, there is no in vivo activity in murine models of septicemia due to *S. aureus* NCTC 10649 M and *S. pneumoniae* ATCC 6303.

A second series with a carbazate residue between C-11 and C-12 of the aglycone nucleus has been synthesized with the aim of obtaining in vivo activity with the 2,3-anhydroerythromycin A derivatives (Griesgraber et al., 1998). The in vitro activity depends on the stereochemistry and particularly the epimer at position 10. The 10-(*R*)-carbazate derivatives are active compared to the 10-(*S*)-carbazate derivatives. The A-179364 derivative is inactive (Fig. 45). The most active molecule is A-179796, which has good activity against erythromycin A-susceptible strains of *S. aureus*, *S. pyogenes*, and *S. pneumoniae* or those resistant to erythromycin A by an inducible, but not a constitutive, type of MLS_B mechanism (Table 54).

Certain derivatives have moderate activity against *H. influenzae* (MIC between 2 and 16 μg/ml).

A number of other derivatives have in vivo activity. However, it is less than that of clarithromycin against *S. aureus* NCTC 10649 M, but three selected derivatives have better activity in a murine pneumococcal infection model (*S. pneumoniae* ATCC 6303).

Figure 44 FMA 0713

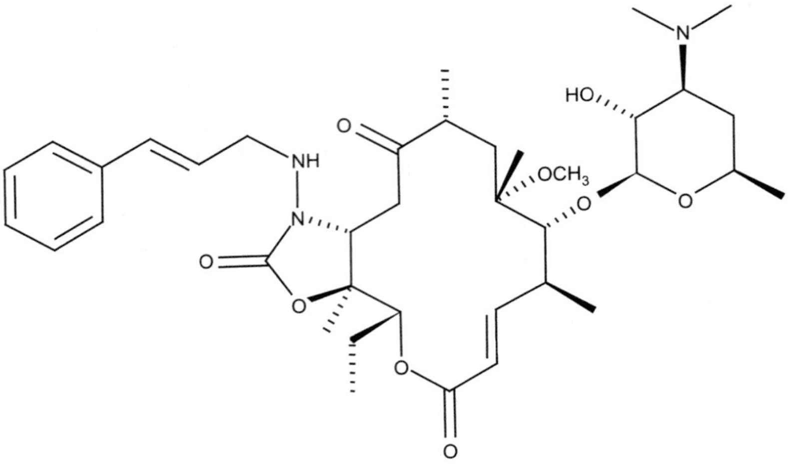

		R
A-179796	10 *(R)*	—
A-179797	10 *(S)*	'''''''''''

Figure 45 A-179796 and A-179797

The derivatives comprising a nonsubstituted (A-168903) or substituted hydropyrazole residue are inactive in vitro (Griesgraber et al., 1997).

17.19. 3-Deoxyclarithromycin

A 3-deoxy-3-descladinosyl erythromycin A series has been synthesized (Elliott et al., 1997b) (Fig. 46). The 3-deoxyclarithromycin derivative has been transformed to other derivatives, 9-oxime, 9-*O*-alkyloxime, 11,12-carbonate, and 11,12-carbamate. These derivatives are weakly active against *S. aureus, S. pneumoniae*, and *S. pyogenes*.

17.20. Derivatives from 16-Membered-Ring Macrolides

It was demonstrated that josamycin, kitasamycin, tylosin, and other leucomycin derivatives can be converted in new 14-membered-ring macrolides. The josamycin derivative, EP-263 (Fig. 47), is less active than josamycin against *S. pneumoniae* and *S. pyogenes* harboring a *mef* gene, but it is more active than erythromycin A against these isolates

Table 54 In vitro activity of A-179796

Organism	Phenotype[a]	MIC (μg/ml) A-179796, 10-(R)	MIC (μg/ml) A 179797, 10-(S)
S. aureus 6538 P	Ery^s	0.07	12.5
S. aureus A-5177	Ery^r(I)	0.1	6.2
S. aureus A-5278	Ery^r(C)	100	50
S. pyogenes EES61	Ery^s	0.06	4
S. pyogenes PIU 2548	Ery^r (efflux)	0.5	8
S. pyogenes 930	Ery^r (C)	32	16
S. pneumoniae ATCC 6303	Ery^s	0.03	1
S. pneumoniae 5649	Ery^r (efflux)	1	4
S. pneumoniae 2979	Ery^r (C)	32	16
H. influenzae DILL	Amp^r	8	>64

[a]I, inducible; C, constitutive.

(*S. pneumoniae*, EP-263 MIC, 0.25 versus 8.0 μg/ml; *S. pyogenes*, EP-263 MIC, 0.5 versus 16 μg/ml). The derivative from kitasamycin, EP-1126, is poorly active (MIC, 16 μg/ml). In the josamycin series, compounds with a 9-amino group were synthesized, EP-935 and EP-263. EP-935 has the same antibacterial activity as EP-263; both are more active against erythromycin A-susceptible strains of *S. pneumoniae* (MIC, 0.06 versus 0.25 μg/ml) than they are against resistant strains. To enhance the antibacterial activity of 16-membered-ring macrolides, chemical alterations of the 4′-hydroxyl of tylosin have been done, as well as C-23 carbamates or esters. Some of them displayed improved activity against isolates harboring the *mef* gene (Fig. 48).

17.21. GW 587726 (PL1441)

GW 587726 (PL1441) is an 8aN-azalide with a 3-acetophenyl (nitrophenyl) derivative. At the position the 6-hydroxy group of the aglycone is substituted with a methyl group. This compound is active against *S. pneumoniae* resistant to erythromycin A (MIC_{50} and MIC_{90}, 0.06 and 0.12 μg/ml), but it is inactive against isolates harboring an *erm*(B) gene (MIC_{50} and MIC_{90}, >128 μg/ml) and exhibits reduced activity against *S. pneumoniae* isolates expressing a *mef*(E) gene

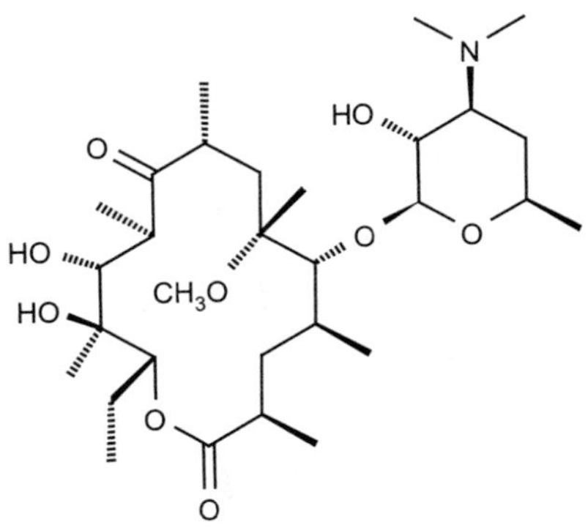

Figure 46 3-Deoxyclarithromycin

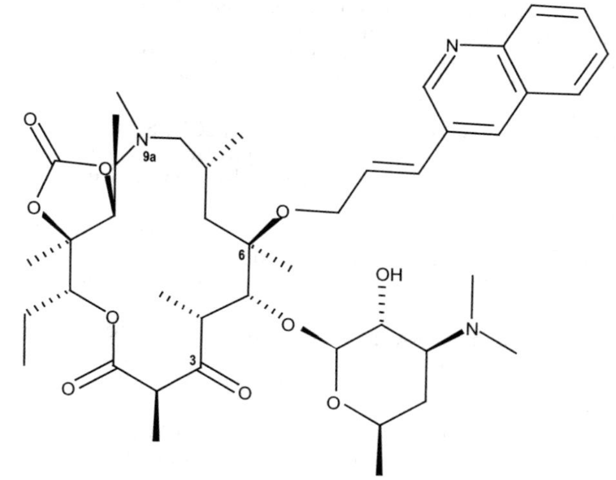

Aza-ketolide (Abbott)

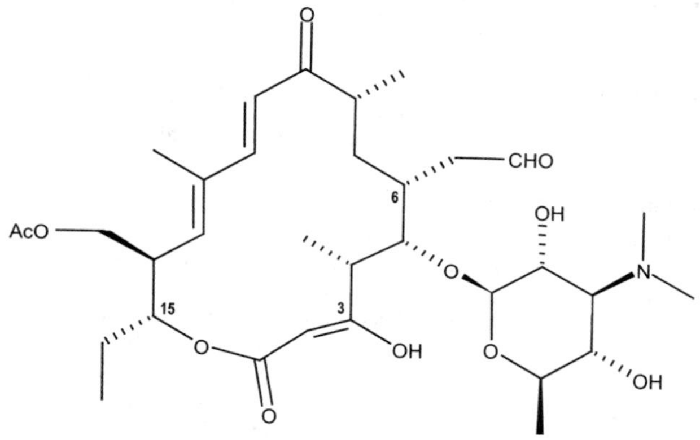

Ketolide derived from tylosin (Elanco)

Figure 47 Tylosin and aza-ketolide analogs

(MIC_{50} and MIC_{90}, ≤0.25 μg/ml). It is moderately active against *S. pyogenes* susceptible to erythromycin A (MIC_{50} and MIC_{90}, 1.0 and 2.0 μg/ml), and it is inactive against isolates resistant to erythromycin A by a constitutive MLS_B mechanism (MIC, >128 μg/ml). It is poorly active against *H. influenzae* (MIC_{50} and MIC_{90}, 4.0 and 6.0 μg/ml).

This compound exhibits a lower affinity for ribosomes of *Bacillus subtilis* and *S. aureus* than does azithromycin, for 50% inhibitory concentrations of 2.8 and 1.0 μg/ml respectively. The affinity for the ribosome of *S. aureus* resistant to erythromycin A is poor (50% inhibitory concentration, >256 μg/ml).

REFERENCES

Abbanat D, Ashley G, Carney J, Fardis M, Foleno B, Hilliard J, Li Y, Licari P, Loeloff M, Macielag M, Melton J, Stryker S, Wira E, Bush K, 2001, In vitro and in vivo activities of 15-methyl ketolide derivatives of erythromycin A, 41st Intersci Conf Antimicrob Agents Chemother, abstract F-1173.

Appelbaum PC, Ednie L, Kelly L, Matic Y, 2004, Anti-pneumococcal activity of two novel macrolides, GW 773546 and GW 708408, compared with 5 other agents by MIC, 44th Intersci Conf Antimicrob Agents Chemother, abstract F-1400.

Asaka T, Kashimura M, Ishi T, et al, 1997, New macrolide antibiotics, acylides (3-O-acyl-S-O desosaminyl erythronolides), synthesis and biological properties, 37th Intersci Conf Antimicrob Agents Chemother, abstract F-262, p 190.

Asaka T, Kashimura M, Misawa Y, et al, 1995a, A new macrolide antibiotic, TE-810. Synthesis and biological properties, 35th Intersci Conf Antimicrob Agents Chemother, abstract F-177, p 144.

Asaka T, Kashimura M, Misawa Y, et al, 1995b, A new macrolide antibiotic, TE-802. Synthesis and biological properties, 35th Intersci Conf Antimicrob Agents Chemother, abstract E-176, p 143.

Ashley GW, Li Y, Liu G, Ma W, Myles D, Shaw S, Zhang D, Zheng H, 2004, 15-Amido ketolides, a new class of ketolide antibacterial agents, 44th Intersci Conf Antimicrob Agents Chemother, abstract F-1409.

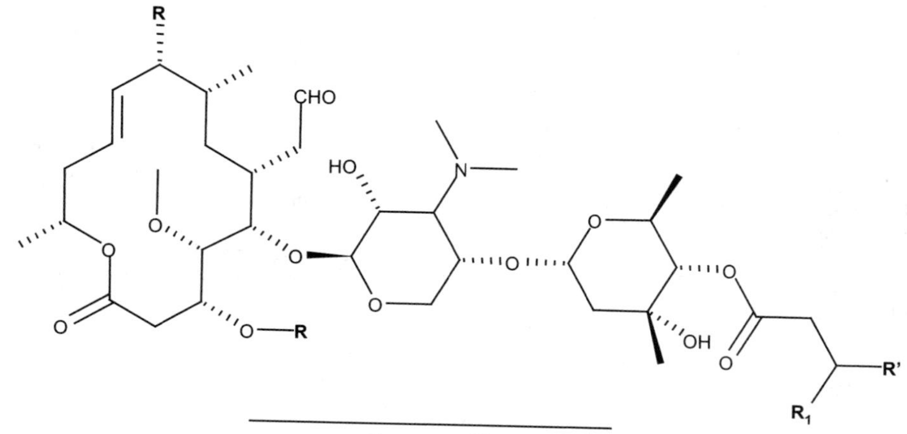

	R	R'	R_1
EP-263	OH	CH_3	$COCH_3$
EP-935	$N(CH_3)_2$	CH_3	$COCH_3$
EP-1126	OH	H	H

Figure 48 EP-263, EP-935, and EP-1126

Baker WR, Clark JD, Stephens RL, Kim KH, 1988, Modification of macrolide antibiotics. Synthesis of 11-deoxy-11-(carboxyamino)-6-O-methyl erythromycin A 11,12-(cyclic esters) via an intramolecular Michael reaction of O-carbamate with an α,β-unsaturated ketone, J Org Chem, 53, 2340–2345.

Barry AL, Brown SD, Fuchs PC, 1997, Antipneumococcal activity of a ketolide (HMR 3647) and seven related drugs *in vitro*, 37th Intersci Conf Antimicrob Agents Chemother, abstract F-107, p 164.

Beebe X, Yang F, Bui MH, Mitten MJ, Ma Z, Nilius AM, Djuric SW, 2004, Synthesis and antibacterial activity of 6-O-arylpropargyl-9-oxime-11,12-carbamate ketolides, Bioorg Med Chem Lett, 14, 2417–2421.

Bermudez LE, Inderlied CB, Kolonoski P, Aralat P, Petrosky M, Wu M, Wang G, Niu D, Young LS, 2004, In vitro and in vivo activity of 6-11 bridged-bicyclic ketolides (including EP 013420) against *Mycobacterium avium* complex (MAC), 44th Intersci Conf Antimicrob Agents Chemother, abstract F-1408.

Blackman J, Hicklin MD, Chandler F, 1978, Legionnaires' diseases, pathological and historical aspect of a new disease, Arch Pathol Lab Med, 102, 337–343.

Bonnefoy A, Denis A, Bretin F, Fromentin C, 1999, In vivo antibacterial activity of two ketolides, HMR 3562 and HMR 3787, highly active against respiratory pathogens, 39th Intersci Conf Antimicrob Agents Chemother, abstract 2156, p 352.

Bonnefoy A, Girard AM, Agouridas C, Chantot JF, 1997, Ketolides lack inducibility properties of MLS(B) resistance phenotype, J Antimicrob Chemother, 40, 85–90.

Bryskier A, 1992, Newer macrolides and their potential target organisms, Curr Opin Infect Dis, 5, 764–772.

Bryskier A, 1997, Novelties in the field of macrolides, Exp Opin Investig Drugs, 6, 1697–1709.

Bryskier A, Agouridas C, Chantot JF, 1993a, Acid stability of new macrolides, J Chemother, 5, suppl 1, 158–159.

Bryskier A, Agouridas C, Chantot JF, 1995, New insights into the structure-activity relationship of macrolides and azalides, p 330, in Neu HC, Young LS, Zinner SH, Acar JF, ed, New Macrolides, Azalides and Streptogramins in Clinical Practice, Marcel Dekker, New York.

Bryskier A, Agouridas C, Chantot JF, 1997, Ketolides, new semisynthetic 14-membered-ring macrolides, p 39–50, in Zinner SH, Young LS, Acar JF, Neu HC, ed, Expanding Indications for the New Macrolides, Azalides and Streptogramins, Marcel Dekker, New York.

Bryskier A, Agouridas C, Gasc JC, 1993b, Classification of macrolide antibiotics, p 5–66, in Bryskier AJ, Butzler JP, Neu HC, Tulkens PM, ed, Macrolides: Chemistry, Pharmacology and Clinical Use, Arnette-Blackwell, Paris.

Bryskier A, Labro MT, 1994, Macrolides, nouvelles perspectives thérapeutiques, Presse Med, 223, 1762–1766.

Cantalloube C, Scaglione F, Pukander J, Van Dyk K, Pascual MH, Montay G, Leroy B, 2004, Telithromycin concentration in middle-ear fluid in children with acute otitis media or otitis media with effusion, 44th Intersci Conf Antimicrob Agents Chemother, abstract A7.

Cantalloube C, Vargayava V, Sultan E, Vacheron F, Batista I, Montay G, 2003, Pharmacokinetics of the ketolide telithromycin after single and repeated dose in patients with hepatic impairement, Int J Antimicrob Agents, 22, 112–121.

Cocuzza CE, Tomasini A, Reuzetti D, et al, 1998. Ketolide (HMR 3647) in vitro activity on 4000 strains of *S. pyogenes* isolated in northern Italy, 4th Int Conf Macrolides, Azalides, Streptogramins, Ketolides, abstract 1.06, p 21.

Collette P, Douthwaite S, Monkin A, Mauvais P, 1998, Similarities and differences in ketolides and macrolide interaction within two distinct domains of 23 ribosomal RNA, 4th Int Conf Macrolides, Azalides, Streptogramins, Ketolides, abstract 1.2, p 25.

Corbaz R, Ettlinger L, Gaumann E, et al, 1955, Stoffwechselprodukte von Actinomyceten, Helv Chim Acta, 38, 935–942.

Denis A, Agouridas C, Bonnefoy A, Bretin F, Fromentin C, Bonnet A, 1999, Synthesis and antibacterial activity of 2-halogeno, 2-methyl, and 2,3 enol-ether ketolides using β-keto-ester chemistry, 39th Intersci Conf Antimicrob Agents Chemother, abstract 2152, p 351.

Denis A, Pejac JM, Bretin F, Bonnefoy A, 2003, Synthesis of 9-oxime-11,12 carbamate ketolides through a novel diamineation reaction of 11,12-hydrazinocarbamate ketolide, Bioorg Med Chem, 11, 2389–2394.

Ednie LM, Jacobs MR, Appelbaum PC, 1997, Comparative anti-anaerobic activities of the ketolides HMR 3647 (RU 66647) and HMR 3004 (RU 64004), Antimicrob Agents Chemother, 41, 2019–2022.

Elliott RL, Pireh D, Griesgraber G, et al, 1997a, Synthesis and in vitro activity of novel 2,3-anhydro 6-O-methyl-11,12-carbamate erythromycin analogues, 37th Intersci Conf Antimicrob Agents Chemother, abstract F-265, p 191.

Elliott RL, Pireh D, Griesgraber G, et al, 1998, Anhydrolide macrolides. I. Synthesis and antibacterial activity of 2,3 anhydro-6-O-methyl 11,12 carbamate erythromycin analogues, J Med Chem, 41, 1651–1652.

Elliott RL, Pireh D, Nilius AM, et al, 1997b, Novel 3-deoxy-3-descladinosyl-6-O-methyl erythromycin A analogues. Synthesis and in vitro activity, Bioorg Med Chem Lett, 7, 641–647.

Engler KH, Warner M, George RC, 1997, In vitro susceptibility of *Corynebacterium diphtheriae* to a new macrolide, HMR 3647, 37th Intersci Conf Antimicrob Agents Chemother, abstract F-124, p 167.

Felmingham D, 1996, HMR data in file.

Felmingham D, 1997, HMR data in file.

Felmingham D, Robbins MJ, Clark S, Mathias I, Bryskier A, 1998, The comparative *in vitro* activity of HMR 3647 against speciated coagulase-negative *Staphylococcus* spp., 4th Int Conf Macrolides, Azalides, Streptogramins, Ketolides, abstract 1.07, p 21.

Felmingham D, Robbins MJ, Leakey A, et al, 1997, The comparative in vitro activity of HMR 3647, a ketolide antimicrobial, against clinical bacterial isolates, 37th Intersci Conf Antimicrob Agents Chemother, abstract F-116, p 166.

Felmingham D, Robbins MJ, Mathias I, Bryskier A, 1999, In vitro activity of two ketolides, HMR 3562 and HMR 3787, against clinical bacterial isolates, 39th Intersci Conf Antimicrob Agents Chemother, abstract 2154, p 351.

Fernandes PB, Baker WR, Freiberg LA, Hardy DJ, McDonald EJ, 1989, New macrolides active against *Streptococcus pyogenes* with inducible or constitutive type of macrolide-lincosamide-streptogramin B resistance, Antimicrob Agents Chemother, 33, 78–81.

Fiese EP, Steffen SH, 1990, Comparison of the acid stability of azithromycin and erythromycin A, J Antimicrob Chemother, 25, suppl A, 39–47.

Goldstein E, 1997, HMR data on file.

Graystone JT, Wang SP, Kuo CC, Campbell LA, 1989, Current knowledge on *C. pneumoniae* strain TWAR, an important cause of pneumonia and other acute respiratory diseases, Eur J Clin Microbiol, 8, 191–202.

Griesgraber G, Elliott RL, Kramer MJ, et al, 1997, Synthesis and in vitro activity of novel 2,3-anhydro-11-hydrazo-6-O-methyl-11,12-carbamate erythromycin derivative, 37th Intersci Conf Antimicrob Agents Chemother, abstract F-267, p 191.

Griesgraber G, Kramer MJ, Elliott RL, et al, 1998, Anhydrolide macrolides. 2. Synthesis and antibacterial activity of 2,3-anhydro-6-O-methyl-11,12-carbazate erythromycin A analogues, J Med Chem, 41, 1660–1670.

Griesgraber G, Or YS, Chu DTW, Nilius AM, Johnson PM, Flamm RK, Henry RE, Plattner JJ, 1996, 3-Keto-11,12-carbazate derivative of 6-O-methyl erythromycin A. Synthesis and in vitro activity, J Antibiot, 49, 465–477.

Gupta S, Leatham E, Carrington D, Mendall M, Kaski JC, Camm J, 1997, Elevated *Chlamydia pneumoniae* antibodies, cardiovascular events, and azithromycin in male survivors of myocardiac infarctus, Circulation, 96, 404–407.

Gurfinkel E, 1998, Is there a role for macrolides in atherosclerosis? 4th Int Conf Macrolides, Azalides, Streptogramins, Ketolides, abstract 8, p 19.

Gurfinkel E, Bozovich G, Daroca A, Beek E, Mautuer B, 1997, Randomised trial of roxithromycin in non-Q-wave coronary syndromes, ROXIS pilot study, Lancet, 350, 404–407.

Henninger TC, Xu X, Abbanat D, Baum EZ, Foleno BD, Hilliard JJ, Burh K, Hlaska DJ, Macielag MJ, 2004, Synthesis and antibacterial activity of C-6 carbamate ketolides, a novel series of orally active ketolide antibiotics, Bioorg Med Chem Lett, 14, 4495–4499.

Hoban D, Karlowsky J, Weshnoweski B, Kabani A, Zhanel G, 1997, In vitro activity of a new ketolide, HMR 3647, against geographically diverse Canadian isolates of *Enterococcus* spp., 37th Intersci Conf Antimicrob Agents Chemother, abstract F-119, p 166.

Hoppe JE, Bryskier A, 1998, *In vitro* susceptibility of *B. pertussis* and *B. parapertussis* to the ketolides HMR 3004 and HMR 3647, to the macrolides azithromycin, clarithromycin, erythromycin A and roxithromycin and to the ansamycins, rifampicin and rifapentine, 4th Int Conf Macrolides, Azalides, Streptogramins, Ketolides, abstract 1.13, p 23.

Hunziker D, Wyss PC, Angehrn P, Mueller A, Marty HP, Holm R, Kellenberger L, Bitsch V, Biringer G, Wolf A, Stämpfi A, Schmitt-Hofmann A, Cousot D, 2004, Novel ketolide antibiotics with a fused five-membered lactone ring. Synthesis, physicochemical and antimicrobial properties, Bioorg Med Chem, 12, 3503–3519.

Iannelli F, Santagi M, Doquier JD, Cassone M, Oggioni MR, Rossolini G, Stefani S, Pozzi G, 2004, Type M resistance to macrolides in streptococci is not due to the mef(A) gene but to mat(A) encoding an ATP-dependent efflux pump, 44th Intersci Conf Antimicrob Agents Chemother, abstract C1-1188.

Kingsley E, Gray P, Tolman KC, Tweedale R, 1983, The toxicity of metabolites of sodium valproate in culture hepatocytes, J Clin Pharmacol, 23, 178–185.

Kitzis MD, Goldstein FW, Bismuth R, Meigi M, Acar JF, 1997, Comparative in vitro activity of HMR 3647, a new ketolide antibiotic, against *S. aureus* (SA) and coagulase negative staphylococci (CNS), 37th Intersci Conf Antimicrob Agents Chemother, abstract F-111, p 165.

Ma Z, Li L, Rupp M, Zhang S, Zhang X, 2002, Regio selective synthesis of bifunctional macrolides, for probing ribosomal binding, Org Lett, 4, 987–990.

Macielag M, Abbanat D, Ashley G, Foleno B, Fu H, Li Y, Wira E, Bush K, 2003, Structure-activity studies of 15-methyl ketolides, optimization of the heterocyclic substituent, 43rd Intersci Conf Antimicrob Agents Chemother, abstract F-1662.

Maglio D, Sun HK, Patel T, Banevicius MA, Nightingale CH, Nicolau DP, Araya A, Wang G, Chen Z, Phan LT, 2004, Pharmacodynamics of a new bridged bicyclic ketolide EP 013420 in a murine *Streptococcus pneumoniae* pneumonia model, 44th Intersci Conf Antimicrob Agents Chemother, abstract F-1407.

Namour F, Wessels DH, Pascual MH, Reynolds D, Sultan E, Lenfant B, 2001, Pharmacokinetics of the new ketolide telithromycin (HMR 3647) administered in ascending single and multiple doses, Antimicrob Agents Chemother, 45, 170–175.

Nilius AM, Mitten M, Bui MH, Hensey-Rudloff D, Clark R, Ma Z, Meulbroek J, Flam RK, 2001, In vitro and in vivo activities of A-217213, a new ketolide antibiotic against respiratory pathogens, 41st Intersci Conf Antimicrob Agents Chemother, abstract F-1172.

Pankuch G, Jacobs MR, Appelbaum PC, 2004, In vitro activity of GW 773546 and GW 708408, telithromycin, erythromycin, azithromycin and clarithromycin against 223 *Haemophilus influenzae* by MIC, 44th Intersci Conf Antimicrob Agents Chemother, abstract F-1398.

Perret C, Lenfant B, Weinling E, Wessels DH, Scholtz HE, Montay G, Sultan E, 2002, Pharmacokinetics and absolute bioavailability of an 800-mg oral dose of telithromycin in healthy young and elderly volunteers, Chemotherapy, 48, 217–223.

Phan LT, Or YS, Chen Y, Chu DTW, Ewing P, Nilius AM, Bui MH, Raney PM, Hensey-Rudloff D, Mitten M, Henry RF, Plattner JJ, 1998, 2-Substituted tricyclic ketolides, new antibacterial macrolides. Synthesis and biological activity, 38th Intersci Conf Antimicrob Agents Chemother, abstract F-127, p 264.

Sugiyama H, Suzuki K, Oyauchi R, Yamasaki Y, Nanaumi K, Kaneda Y, Kawauchi H, Akashi T, Manaka A, Asaka T, Nakaike S, 2004, FMA 0713, α-methoxyimino acylide, antibacterial activity against *Streptococcus pneumoniae, Streptococcus pyogenes*, and *Staphylococcus aureus*, 44th Intersci Conf Antimicrob Agents Chemother, abstract F-1397.

Torres C, Zarazaga M, Tenorio C, Saenz Y, Portillo A, Baquero F, 1997, Susceptibility of *Lactobacillus, Leuconostoc* and *Pediococcus* to ketolide HMR 3647 and other antibiotics, 37th Intersci Conf Antimicrob Agents Chemother, abstract F-247, p 188.

Vesga O, Andes D, Craig WA, 1997, Comparative in vivo activity of HMR 3647, azithromycin (AZI), clarithromycin (CLA) and roxithromycin (ROX) against *S. pneumoniae* (SP) and *S. aureus* (SA), 37th Intersci Conf Antimicrob Agents Chemother, abstract F-258, p 189.

Vesga O, Craig WA, 1997, Impact of macrolide resistance on the in vivo activity of a new ketolide, HMR 3647, against *S. pneumoniae* (SP) and *S. aureus* (SA), 37th Intersci Conf Antimicrob Agents Chemother, abstract F-259, p 189.

Vesga O, Craig WA, Bonnat C, 1997, In vivo pharmacodynamic activity of HMR 3647, a new ketolide, 37th Intersci Conf Antimicrob Agents Chemother, abstract F-255, p 189.

Visalli MA, Jacobs MR, Appelbaum PC, 1997, Antipneumococcal activity of HMR 3647 (RU 6647), a new ketolide, compared to other drugs, by time-kill, 37th Intersci Conf Antimicrob Agents Chemother, abstract F-109, p 164.

Wang G, Niu D, Qiu YL, Phan LT, Chen Z, Polemeropoulos A, Or YS, 2004, Synthesis of novel 6,11-O-bridged bicyclic ketolides via palladium-catalyzed bis-allylation, Org Lett, 6, 4455–4458.

Streptogramins

A. BRYSKIER

20

1. INTRODUCTION

The streptogramins form a complex group of unique antibacterial agents. Several literature reviews have summarized the natural streptogramins (Cocito, 1979; Paris et al., 1990; Vaquez, 1967, 1975). This family has experienced a resurgence of interest because of the therapeutic difficulties associated with staphylococcal and enterococcal infections and the semisynthesis of a hydrosoluble and injectable derivative of pristinamycin, dalfopristin-quinupristin (RP-59500), and two antibacterial agents for oral use (RPR 106972 and XRP 2868).

2. CLASSIFICATIONS AND PHYSICOCHEMICAL PROPERTIES OF NATURAL STREPTOGRAMINS

The streptogramins are composed of a mixture of two types of molecules: group A streptogramins and group B streptogramins. Each molecular complex contains both structures, but several compounds of each of the two groups may belong to the complex. These two structures act synergistically at the microbiological level. The two components are macrocyclic lactones and peptides.

2.1. Molecular Complex

About a dozen molecular complexes have been isolated from the fermentation of different species of *Streptomyces*. Only two of them have been introduced in clinical practice: pristinamycin (Pyostacine) and virginiamycin (Staphylomycine) (Table 1). One semisynthetic derivative was also introduced in clinical practice, dalfopristin-quinupristin (Synercid).

2.2. Group A Streptogramins

The structure is that of macrocyclic peptolides (Fig. 1).

Four structures have been described for group A, which is also known as pristinamycin II. The synonyms of pristinamycin II are listed in Table 2; they possess the same empirical formula, $C_{28}H_{35}N_3O_7$, and the same molecular weight of 525.

Table 1 Streptogramins of natural origin

Antibacterial(s)	Code no.	Drug	A component	B component	Microorganism
Pristinamycin	RP-7293	Pyostacine	Pristinamycins II_A and II_B	Pristinamycins I_A, I_B, and I_C	*Streptomyces pristinaspiralis*
Virginiamycin		Staphylomycin	Virginiamycins M and M_2	Virginiamycins S_1, S_2, S_3, and S_4	*Streptomyces virginiae*
Streptogramin			Streptogramin A	Streptogramin B	*Streptomyces diastaticus*
Madumycin	A 2315A		Madumycin II	Madumycin I	
Mikamycin			Mikamycin A	Mikamycin B	*Streptomyces mikaensis*
Ostreogrycins	E 129		Ostreogrycins A, C, D, R, and Q	Ostreogrycins B_1, B_2, and B_3	*Streptomyces ostreogriseus*
Partricin			Partricins A and B		
Plauracin	A 2315A		Plauracin II	Plauracin I	*Streptomyces diastaticus*
Synergistins	PA 114		Synergistin A	Synergistins B_1 and B_3	*Streptomyces olivaceus*
Vernamycin			Vernamycin A	Vernamycin B (α, β, and δ)	*Streptomyces liodensis*
Etamycin					*Streptomyces griseus* NRRL 2426

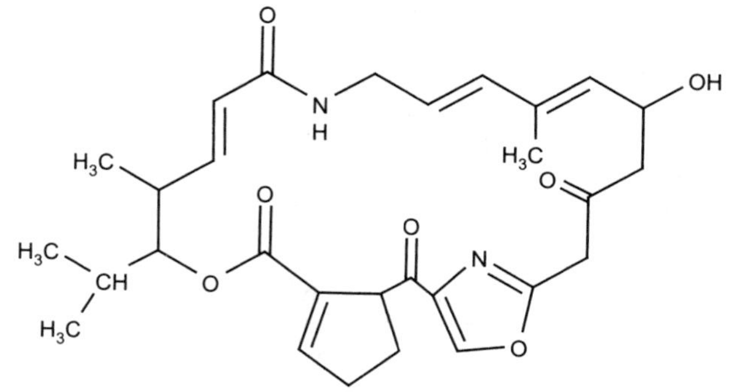

Synonyms :

Streptogramin A	Ostreogrycin G
Mikamycin A	Virginiamycin M2
PA 114 A	Pristinamycin IIB
Pristinamycin IIA	
Vernamycin A	
Virginiamycin M1	
Staphylomycin M	

Figure 1 Streptogramin A

Pristinamycin II (Fig. 1) is divided into two subgroups, II_A and II_B. All of the derivatives in these subgroups contain an aminodecanoic acid and an oxazole nucleus. The other components of group II are griseoviridin and madumycin I.

2.3. Group B Streptogramins

The derivatives belonging to group B are cyclic depsipeptides with a molecular weight of about 800. Nine different types of molecules have been described, including the large group comprising pristinamycin I and other derivatives (Table 3).

Two derivatives are structurally similar to pristinamycin I_A (Fig. 2): virginiamycin S_1 and vernamycin C (doricin). However, 12 different molecules have been described, distinguished by minor modifications involving substitution by an alkyl or methylamide group. The majority of these molecules contain a pipecolic acid or a derivative, except for vernamycin C, which contains an aspartic acid, and partricin A, which contains a proline (Table 4). This variety of substituents is understandable, as pipecolic acid is synthesized from aspartic or pyruvic acid. Etamycin (Fig. 3) and plauracin differ from these molecules, as they are composed of other amino acids.

2.4. Physicochemical Properties of Streptogramins

The compounds in group A and those in group B differ in terms of their solubilities in water and organic solvents.

Table 2 Group A streptogramins

Pristinamycin II_A	Pristinamycin II_B
Virginiamycin M_1	
Streptogramin A	
Synergistin A	
Mikamycin A	
Ostreogrycin A	Ostreogrycin G
Vernamycin A	

Table 3 Group B streptogramins

Pristinamycin I_A	Pristinamycin I_B	Pristinamycin I_C
Streptogramin B		
Mikamycin B		
Ostreogrycin B	Ostreogrycin B_2	Ostreogrycin B_1
Vernamycin B	Vernamycin B_2	Vernamycin B_1
Synergistin B		

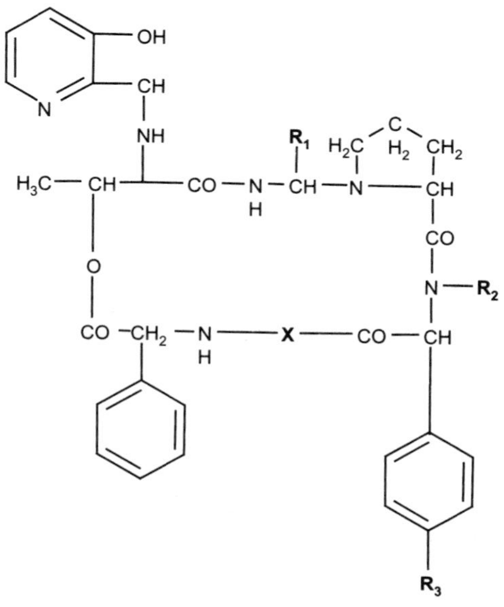

	R_1	R_2	R_3	X
Streptogramin B	$-CH_2CH_3$	$-CH_3$	$-N(CH_3)_2$	-4-oxopipecolic acid
Vernamycin Bβ	$-CH_2CH_3$	$-CH_3$	$-NH-CH_3$	-4-oxopipecolic acid
Vernamycin Bγ	$-CH_3$	$-CH_3$	$-N(CH_3)_2$	-4-oxopipecolic acid
Vernamycin Bδ	$-CH_3$	$-CH_3$	$-N(CH_3)_2$	-4-oxopipecolic acid
Vernamycin C	$-CH_2CH_3$	$-CH_3$	$-NH-CH_3$	-3-hydroxy-4-oxopipecolic acid
Patricin A	$-CH_2CH_3$	$-CH_3$	$-N(CH_3)_2$	proline
Patricine B	$-CH_2CH_3$	$-CH_3$	-H	pipecolic acid
Virginiamycin S1	$-CH_2CH_3$	$-CH_3$	-H	-4-oxopipecolic acid
Virginiamycin S2	$-CH_2CH_3$	-H	-H	-4-hydroxy-4-oxopipecolic acid
Virginiamycin S3	$-CH_2CH_3$	$-CH_3$	-H	-3-hydroxy-4-oxopipecolic acid
Virginiamycin S4	$-CH_3$	$-CH_3$	-H	-4-oxopipecolic acid

Figure 2 Streptogramin B derivatives

Table 4 Group B streptogramin derivatives

Drug	R_1	R_2	R_3	X
Partricin B	C_2H_5	CH_3	H	Picolic acid
Virginiamycin S_1	C_2H_5	CH_3	H	4-Oxopicolic acid
Virginiamycin S_4	CH_3	CH_3	H	4-Oxopicolic acid
Virginiamycin S_2	C_2H_5	H	H	4-Hydroxypicolic acid
Virginiamycin S_3	C_2H_5	CH_3	H	4-Oxopicolic acid
Pristinamycin I_A	C_2H_5	CH_3	$N(CH_3)_2$	4-Oxopicolic acid
Pristinamycin I_B	C_2H_5	CH_3	$NHCH_3$	4-Oxopicolic acid
Pristinamycin I_C	CH_3	CH_3	$N(CH_3)_2$	4-Oxopicolic acid
Vernamycin B_δ	CH_3	CH_3	$NHCH_3$	4-Oxopicolic acid
Ostreogrycin B_3	C_2H_5	CH_3	$N(CH_3)_2$	3-Hydroxy-4-oxopicolic acid
Vernamycin C (doricin)	C_2H_5	CH_3	$N(CH_3)_2$	Aspartic acid
Partricin A	C_2H_5	CH_3	H	Proline

Group A and B molecules are soluble in chloroform and dimethyl sulfoxide. They are moderately soluble in ethanol; factor B is freely soluble in acetone. Groups A and B differ in their solubilities in ether and ethyl acetate, group A molecules being insoluble. The molecules of both groups are insoluble in water (Table 5).

2.5. Antibacterial Activities

These molecules possess different antibacterial activities (Table 6), but their antibacterial spectra include gram-positive cocci and bacilli, gram-negative cocci, *Haemophilus*, *Moraxella*,

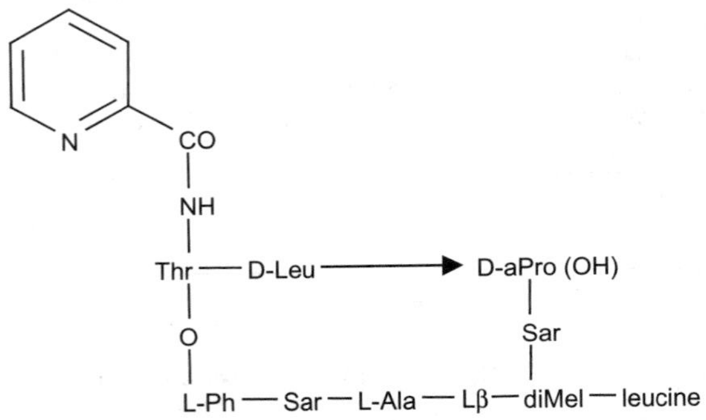

Figure 3 Etamycin (viridogriseine)

Table 5 Solubility of streptogramins (μg/ml)

Substance	Group A streptogramins	Group B streptogramins
Highly soluble		
Dimethylformamide	100	100
Dimethyl sulfoxide	100	
Chloroform	50	100
Dioxane	50	80
Soluble		
Ethanol	20	50
Methanol	20	5
Acetone	20	170
Isopropanol	40	
Butanol	40	
Methylethylacetone	40	
Butyl acetate	40	
Weakly soluble		
Ethyl acetate	5	250
Amyl acetate	4	
Benzene	3	80
Toluene	1	10
Ether		
Nonsoluble		
Hexane	10^{-1}	10^{-1}
Water	10^{-4}	10^{-4}

Table 6 Comparative activities of natural streptogramins

Organism	MIC (μg/ml)					
	Pristinamycin	Streptogramin	Synergistin	Mikamycin	Etamycin	Virginiamycin
S. aureus	0.70	0.60	0.19	32	0.31	1.0
S. pyogenes	0.10	0.05	0.08		0.63	0.07
S. pneumoniae	0.15	0.25	3.12	6.0		0.07
E. faecalis	0.20	1.49	0.39			0.50
Corynebacterium diphtheriae	0.02	0.04	0.39	1.0		
Bacillus subtilis	0.70		0.78	32	2.50	1.0
Neisseria gonorrhoeae	0.20		3.12			
H. influenzae						
Bordetella pertussis		0.04	3.12		5.0	
M. tuberculosis		5.0		200		20

Bordetella, certain intracellular bacteria (*Chlamydia* and *Rickettsia*), and *Mycobacterium tuberculosis*.

3. PRISTINAMYCINS

Pristinamycin (RP-7293) is a streptogramin of natural origin comprising two components, pristinamycin I and pristinamycin II.

The ratios between the two groups of compounds are 30 to 40% for component I (group B) and 60 to 70% for component II (group A).

3.1. Pristinamycin I

Pristinamycin I is a mixture of three macrolactone peptides, pristinamycins I_A (RP-12535), I_B (RP-13919), and I_C (RP-17899), accounting for, respectively, 80 to 95%, 3 to 5%, and 2 to 5% of the mixture of pristinamycin I. Components I_B and I_C differ from I_A in the absence of a methyl group.

The macrolactone ring of compound I_A is composed of six amino acids: (*S*)-threonine, (*R*)-α-aminobutyric acid, (*S*)-proline, (*S*)-*N*-methyl-4-dimethylaminophenylalanine, (*S*)-4-oxopipecolic acid, and (*S*)-phenylglycine. The amino function of the (*S*)-threonine is acylated by 3-hydroxypicolinic acid. Compound I_B possesses an (*S*)-*N*-methyl-4-methylaminophenylalanine instead of the 4-dimethylaminophenylalanine residue. In compound I_C, an (*R*)-alanine replaces the (*R*)-α-aminobutyric acid (Fig. 4).

In aqueous solution, the dimethylaminophenylalanine function is protonated (pK 4.1) and the hydroxyl group of picolinic acid is deprotonated (pK 7.3). Pristinamycin I_A is sparingly soluble in water but is soluble in organic solvents (Table 5). In an aqueous acidic medium (pH 1), pristinamycin I_A is stable for at least 24 h at room temperature. The macrocycle is degraded in an alkaline medium (pH > 9). The total synthesis of pristinamycin I_A has not been performed.

3.2. Pristinamycin II

Pristinamycin II of natural origin is a mixture of two compounds, II_A and II_B. They belong to group A of the streptogramins. These two unsaturated macrocyclic derivatives differ in the degree of oxidation of the proline residue: the II_A derivative is quantitatively the most important and has a hydroxyproline nucleus that replaces the (*R*)-proline residue of the II_B derivative.

The ratio of II_A to II_B in the natural compound extracted from *Streptomyces* is between 90:10 and 90:3, depending on the fermentation conditions.

Pristinamycin II contains an endolactone oxazole nucleus. In an aqueous solution, pristinamycin II does not have acidic and/or basic properties. In phosphate buffer (50 mM sodium phosphate, pH 7.5) and at 20°C, the solubility of the crystalline form of pristinamycin II_A is 50 μg/ml and that of the amorphous form is 250 μg/ml. Pristinamycin II_A is less soluble in organic solvents than pristinamycin I_A, except for methanol (Table 5).

In an acidic medium (pH < 3), the molecule is decomposed to six unidentified degradation products. At a pH of >6, pristinamycin II is decomposed to two degradation products differing from those obtained in a more acidic medium. The stability is thus pH dependent.

The biosynthesis of virginiamycin M (*Streptomyces virginiae*) is identical to that of pristinamycin II_A and is obtained from the following residues: acetic acid, valine, glycine, proline, and serine. The oxazole nucleus has a serine as its origin. Total synthesis has not been performed.

3.3. Structure-Activity Relationship of Pristinamycin

The group A and B compounds themselves possess variable bacteriostatic activities against gram-positive bacteria. Their combination is synergistic, and against certain bacterial species they exert bactericidal activity.

Structural modifications have been effected, but these are relatively few because of the chemical instability and structural complexity of these compounds. The structure-activity relationships of pristinamycin have been summarized in a review (Le Goffic, 1985).

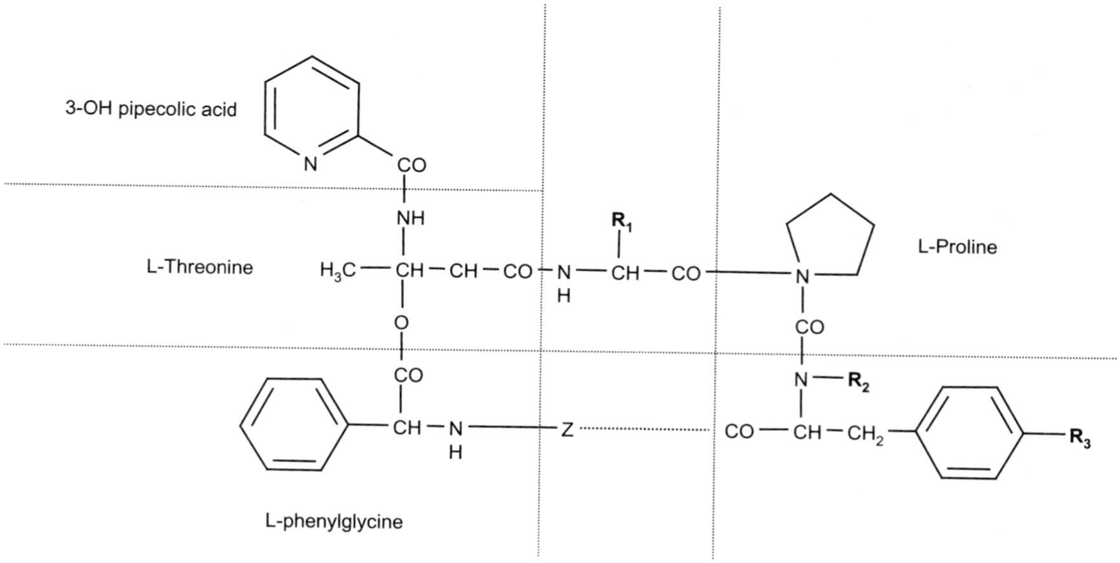

R_1 = D-alanine or D-α-aminobutyric acid

Figure 4 Pristinamycin I

3.3.1. Group A Compounds (Pristinamycin II)

Chemical modifications and the acquisition of plasmid-mediated resistance have shown that the hydroxyl group at position 13 is important for the activity of the molecule, since its acetylation (resistance mechanism) or its oxidation prevents the creation of a hydrogen bond between the carbonyl group at position 6 and the hydroxyl at position 13; the molecule then becomes inactive.

Reduction of the ketone at position 15, as well as the α or β position of the 15-hydroxyl, has little effect on the antibacterial activity. The reduction of the ethylene functions causes a loss of activity in pristinamycin II_A, except for the pyrrole nucleus, which may be modified and in particular may undergo reduction without losing its antibacterial activity (Gale et al., 1981).

3.3.2. Group B Compounds (Pristinamycin I)

Pipecolic acid may be replaced by aspartic acid (vernamycin) or 4-hydroxyl derivatives.

Chemically, the carbonyl function of pipecolic acid may be reduced to two isomers with the same antibacterial activity as pristinamycin I_A.

The phenol function of the pipecolic nucleus may be modified. Acetylation does not affect the antibacterial activity, but esterification by an allyl group causes a loss of activity.

3.4. Antibacterial Activity of Pristinamycin

The antibacterial activity has been reviewed by Kernbaum (1985), and various microbiological studies have established its activity against *Chlamydia* spp. (Orfila and Haider, 1984), *Mycoplasma* spp. (Bébéar et al., 1988), *Rickettsia* spp. (Raoult and Drancourt, 1988), *Legionella pneumophila* (Dournon and Rajagopalan, 1988), and *Haemophilus influenzae* (Dabernat and Delmas, 1988).

Pristinamycin is particularly active against gram-positive cocci. It has good activity against methicillin-resistant or -susceptible strains and constitutive or inducible erythromycin A-resistant strains of *Staphylococcus aureus* (Pechère, 1992) and against methicillin-resistant or -susceptible strains of *Staphylococcus epidermidis*. Activities against common pathogens are given in Table 7, and those against other microorganisms are given in Tables 8 and 9. However, it is inactive against *Treponema pallidum* and *Brucella* spp.

3.4.1. Synergy Between Factors A and B

The combination of the two components is synergistic in terms of activity against erythromycin-susceptible or -resistant strains of *S. aureus*. This synergy is independent of the respective percentages of the two constituents within a large range of (20 to 80%) for each factor. However, in vivo, a higher quantity of pristinamycin II than pristinamycin I must be administered for this synergy to manifest itself in experimental *S. aureus* infections in the mouse because of the poor absorption of pristinamycin II_A. Nguyen (1988) studied 43 strains of *Streptococcus pneumoniae*, 22 of which were susceptible to erythromycin A and 21 of which were resistant. The MICs of pristinamycin and the two constituents are given in Table 10. Erythromycin A-resistant and -susceptible strains were susceptible to pristinamycin. Factors I and II act synergistically.

3.4.2. Postantibiotic Effect

Videau (1965) described the phenomenon of postantibiotic effect. Following brief contact, the bacteria are no longer capable of multiplying until a period of 15 to 20 h has elapsed. This phenomenon has been detected in vitro and in vivo in mice.

3.4.3. Breakpoints

The French Antibiotic Sensitivity Test Committee has adopted a breakpoint of 2 μg/ml for pristinamycin and virginiamycin. This corresponds to a diameter of greater than or equal to 19 mm for a 15-μg disk.

3.4.4. Antibiotic Combinations

The combinations of streptogramins plus aminoglycosides, rifampin, or β-lactams are synergistic.

Table 7 Antibacterial activity of pristinamycin

Organism(s)[a]	MIC (μg/ml)	MIC_{50} (μg/ml)	Mode MIC (μg/ml)
MSSA Ery^s		≤0.12	
MRSA Ery^s		1.0	
MRSA Ery^r		0.5	
MSSE		0.25	
MRSE Ery^r		0.25	
S. pyogenes	0.06–0.1	≤0.06	
Streptococcus agalactiae		≤0.06	
S. pneumoniae	0.25		
E. faecalis	0.20–15	2.0	
H. influenzae			0.5–1.0
S. pneumoniae Ery^s	0.12		
S. pneumoniae Ery^r	0.25		
Neisseria meningitidis	0.20		0.06
N. gonorrhoeae	0.05–0.3		
M. catarrhalis	0.05		
B. pertussis	0.2–1.0		
Pasteurella spp.	0.3–15		
Bacillus anthracis	0.25–0.5		
C. diphtheriae	0.02–0.06		
Listeria monocytogenes	1.5		
Leptospira spp.	0.02–0.03		

[a]MSSE, methicillin-susceptible *S. epidermidis*; MRSE, methicillin-resistant *S. epidermidis*.

Table 8 Activities of streptogramins against anaerobes

Organism(s) (no. of strains)	MIC (μg/ml)		
	Pristinamycin	Pristinamycin I_A	Pristinamycin II_A
B. fragilis (30)	0.5	32	64
Fusobacterium spp. (14)	0.25	16	0.5
Clostridium spp. (40)	0.06	1.0	4.0
Propionibacterium spp. (30)	0.03	2.0	0.06
Peptostreptococcus spp. (21)	0.03	0.25	0.5
Veillonella parvula (5)	2–16	8–64	8–16
Actinomyces spp. (5)	2–16	1.0–8.0	0.25–2
Bifidobacterium spp. (5)	0.03–0.06	8–64	0.12–0.25
Eubacterium spp. (3)	0.03–4	1–64	0.12–32

Table 9 Activity of pristinamycin against intracellular and atypical bacteria

Organism	Mode MIC (μg/ml)
Mycoplasma pneumoniae	0.02
Mycoplasma hominis	0.2
Ureaplasma urealyticum	0.5
L. pneumophila	0.25
Rickettsia conorii	2.0
Rickettsia rickettsii	2.0
Coxiella burnetii	NT[a]

[a]NT, not tested.

For streptococci, the combination pristinamycin-streptomycin was bactericidal against 60% of 220 strains tested by Christol et al. (1971). This bactericidal activity was manifested against 18% of the 82 enterococcal strains, 94% of the 21 strains of group H streptococci, 81% of the 52 viridans streptococci strains, and 86% of the 64 strains of other groups.

The combination pristinamycin-gentamicin proved bactericidal to 40% of the 17 strains of group D streptococci responsible for endocarditis.

Combinations with penicillin G or ampicillin may be additive or synergistic, and likewise the combination pristinamycin-rifampin is additive.

For staphylococci, pristinamycin combined with rifampin was bactericidal against 69% of the 16 tested strains responsible for septicemia; combination with an aminoglycoside induced bactericidal activity against 50% of the same strains.

Combination with fusidic acid or co-trimoxazole is synergistic, while the combination pristinamycin-chloramphenicol is antagonistic.

3.5. Mechanism of Action of Pristinamycin

Streptogramins act through the inhibition of bacterial protein synthesis by binding sequentially to bacterial ribosomes. Pristinamycin II_A appears to bind irreversibly, thus releasing a receptor site for pristinamycin I_A. Components A and B bind to the 50S subunit, which explains their bacteriostatic activity. Pristinamycins II_A and I_B (group A and B) inhibit protein synthesis at different steps of the process.

Protein synthesis is a complex phenomenon which occurs by combination with ribosomal and cytoplasmic factors. This process can be divided into three steps: (i) the initiation phase, involving initiation factors, 1, 2, and 3; (ii) the elongation phase, with elongation factors Tu (EF-Tu), EF-Ts, and EF-G; and (iii) the termination phase, with release factors 1, 2, and 3.

The two ribosomal subunits (30S and 50S) join at the initiation phase to form the 70S ribosome and separate at the termination phase.

The elongation phase involves the positioning of two RNA derivatives at the two sites of the 50S subunit: the A-site for an aminoacyl-tRNA and the P-site for a peptidyl-tRNA precursors.

The positioning of the aminoacyl-tRNA is promoted by EF-Tu. A peptide bond is formed between the carboxyl terminus of the peptide chain and the P-site and the NH_2 of the amino terminus of the aminoacyl-tRNA at the A-site. The third step in the elongation process (EF-G dependent) and

Table 10 Antibacterial activity of pristinamycin

Organism	MIC (μg/ml)		
	Pristinamycin	Pristinamycin I_A	Pristinamycin II_A
H. influenzae	0.5	64	0.5
S. pneumoniae Ery[s]	0.2–1.0	0.5–8	1.0–>8.0
S. pneumoniae Ery[r]	0.12–1.0	4–16	1.0–>8.0
S. aureus Ery[s]	0.12	2–4	2.0
S. aureus Ery[r]	0.25	8	2.0
Campylobacter jejuni Ery[s]	4–8	128–512	8.0–16
C. jejuni Ery[r]	6–>64	>256	>64

GTP hydrolysis for energy involves the translocation of the peptidyl-tRNA from the A-site to the P-site.

Aumercier and Le Goffic (1992) have proposed the following mechanism of action (Fig. 5). The L24 protein belongs to the exit channel of the nascent peptides synthesized in the ribosomes, and proteins L10 and L11 are close to one another and essential for peptidyltransferase activity.

Pristinamycin II_A or its semisynthetic derivative RP-54476 binds strongly to the bacterial ribosome and modifies the conformation of the L10 and L11 proteins. This conformational change increases the affinity for pristinamycin I_A or its semisynthetic derivative (RP-57669), and the presence of L24 causes the formation of a stable stoichiometric ternary complex (1:1).

Most nascent peptides exit the ribosome through a tunnel in the 50S subunit. The binding sites for the macrolide-lincosamide-streptogramin B (MLS_B) antibiotics are located in the beginning of the tunnel, which is constricted by the ribosomal proteins L4 and L22. Streptogramin B prevents nascent peptides from entering the tunnel. There is a strong correlation between the space available between the compound and the peptidyltransferase center and the length of peptides in the peptidyl-tRNAs that dissociate from the ribosome under the influence of the compound.

Streptogramin B causes dissociation of hexapeptidyl-tRNA from the ribosome.

The nascent peptide releases will grow to a point where further peptidyl transfer is inhibited by steric hindrance and this inhibition leads to dissociation of the peptidyl-tRNA from the ribosome.

Streptogramin A loses its ability to inhibit protein synthesis on ribosomes with peptides that have grown beyond a critical length. This results in a reduction in the diameter of the peptide exit channel. If this channel is too narrow, peptides accumulate at the peptidyltransferase site. This causes ribosomal dysfunction, which can block the activity of peptidyl-tRNA synthetase, causing a marked reduction in the concentration of free tRNA in the cell. As this tRNA is essential for activation of the amino acids prior to their incorporation in the peptide chains, this can result in cell death.

Both streptogramins A and B penetrate the bacterial cell by passive diffusion.

Group A streptogramins act on the early stage of the protein synthesis, especially on the elongation phase of translation. Group B streptogramins exert inhibitory activity at the end of the process during extension of the peptide chain, causing premature detachment of the incomplete chain.

Type A components inactivate the donor and acceptor sites of peptidyltransferase, thus interfering with corresponding functions of the enzyme.

They block two of the peptide chain elongation steps: aminoacyl-tRNA binding to the A-site of the ribosome and peptide bond formation with peptidyl-tRNA at the P-site.

A tight linkage of these derivatives with the two ribosomal sites requires a stable interaction of their aminoacyl components with peptidyltransferase. Such interaction is prevented by group A streptogramins.

Group B streptogramins inhibit the peptide bond formation and release an incomplete peptide chain.

The binding site is located at the base of the central protuberance of 50S subunits.

In the presence of type A streptogramin, ribosomal initiation complexes are assembled apparently in the normal fashion but are functionally inactive. Group A streptogramins block substrate attachment to both the acceptor site and the donor site at the peptidyltransferase catalytic center. Group A streptogramins do not bind to ribosomes engaged in protein synthesis.

Group B streptogramins inhibit the two first steps of the elongation phase (aminoacyl-tRNA binding to the A-site and peptidyltransferase from the P-site) and do not affect translocation, the third step (A-site to P-site). Group B streptogramins interact with the ribosome engaged in protein synthesis.

3.6. Resistance to Streptogramins

3.6.1. Epidemiology of Resistance

Until 1975, resistance to streptogramins was infrequent, on the order of 1 to 3%. In 1975 the first strain of *S. aureus* with a pristinamycin I_A and II_A resistance plasmid not associated with the conventional mechanism of macrolide resistance was isolated in France. A hospital epidemic associated with this plasmid has been described in various hospital centers and represents 4 to 5% of strains isolated. However, the level of resistance has remained low and affects about 1% of methicillin-susceptible strains of *S. aureus* (MSSA) and 10% of methicillin-resistant strains (MRSA).

A new mechanism of resistance was described in 1984: isolated resistance to factor A (pristinamycin II_A) and lincosamides (LSA phenotype) conferring low-level resistance to streptogramins. This mechanism is found in about 0.5% of MSSA strains. *Enterococcus faecalis* and *Enterococcus faecium* are naturally resistant to pristinamycin II_A. Factor B (pristinamycin I_A) acts alone.

In an epidemiological survey carried out from 2001 to 2002 in 16 European countries, 454 *E. faecium* isolates and 585 MRSA strains were collected. The overall rates of resistance to dalfopristin-quinupristin were 20.9 and 0.2%, respectively, for a breakpoint of $\geq$4 μg/ml for *E. faecium* and MRSA.

The prevalence rates for the individual countries are reported in Table 11.

In Taiwan an epidemiological survey was conducted between January 1996 and December 1999 for susceptibility of gram-positive cocci to dalfopristin-quinupristin. A total of 1,287 clinical isolates were collected.

All MSSA strains were susceptible to dalfopristin-quinupristin (MIC, $\geq$2 μg/ml). The prevalence rates for dalfopristin-quinupristin resistance are reported in Table 12.

Among coagulase-negative staphylococci, the most resistant were *Staphylococcus cohnii* (48%), *Staphylococcus capitis* (39%), and *Staphylococcus saprophyticus* (36%).

In studies carried out in the United States and Canada from 1996 to 1997, the rates of resistance were reported to be 0.3, 1, 2.3, and 3% for MSSA, MRSA, *S. pneumoniae*, and other gram-positive cocci, respectively. Thirteen percent of *E. faecium* isolates were resistant to dalfopristin-quinupristin.

In Taiwan in 2001, 419 *Streptococcus pyogenes* isolates were collected, and about 2% were resistant to dalfopristin-quinupristin and 6% showed an intermediate susceptibility. Between 2001 and 2002, 936 *S. pneumoniae* isolates were collected in Taiwan, and of them 6% were resistant to dalfopristin-quinupristin and 23% exhibited an intermediate susceptibility.

In a survey conducted in the United Kingdom over a 2.5-year period (January 1997 to June 1999), vancomycin-resistant enterococci (VRE) were collected from 858 patients in 136 hospitals.

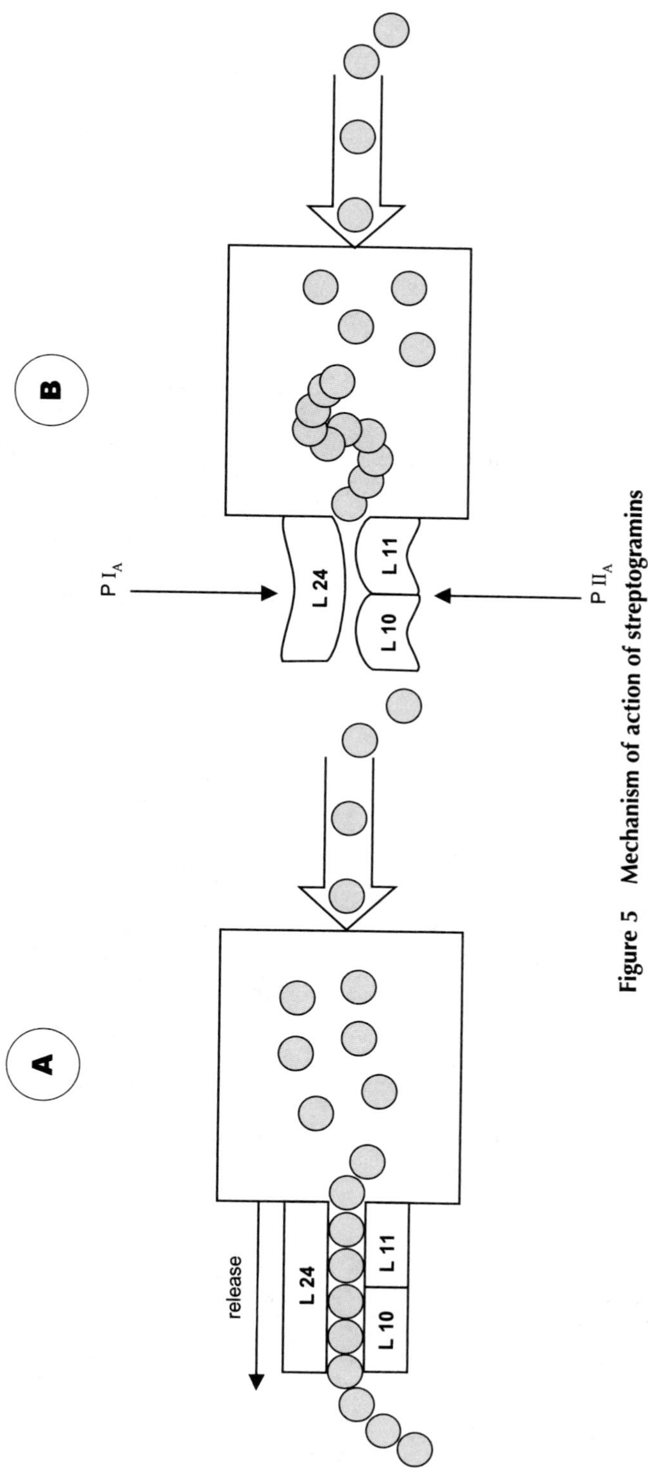

Figure 5 **Mechanism of action of streptogramins**

Table 11 Prevalence of dalfopristin-quinupristin resistance in Europe

Country or region	*E. faecium*		MRSA	
	n	% Resistant	*n*	% Resistant
Scandinavia	23	8.7	48	<1
The Netherlands	25	12	42	<1
Belgium	46	26.1	48	<1
Luxembourg	6	50	14	<1
Italy	64	25	62	<1
Spain	63	33.3	32	<1
Portugal	33	24.2	64	<1
France	56	25	47	<1
Greece	12	25	82	<1
Germany	84	10.7	82	<1
United Kingdom/Ireland	42	9.5		1.2

Table 12 Prevalence of dalfopristin-quinupristin resistance in Taiwan

Organism(s)[a]	Prevalence of resistance (%)
MSSA	0
MRSA	31
CoNS	16
S. pneumoniae	8
Viridans group streptococci	51
VSE	85
VREF	66
Leuconostoc	100
Lactobacillus	50
Pediococcus	87

[a]CoNS, coagulase-negative staphylococci; VSE, vancomycin-susceptible enterococci.

MICs were determined on DST agar containing 5% lysed horse blood; of the 657 *E. faecium* isolates, 77.8% were susceptible to dalfopristin-quinupristin at MICs of ≤ 2 μg/ml. MICs of dalfopristin-quinupristin may be influenced by blood. In the same study, comparison of dalfopristin-quinupristin activities with and without horse blood showed about fourfold-lower MICs without blood than with 5% blood.

Dalfopristin-quinupristin was shown to be less active against *Enterococcus casseliflavus*, *Enterococcus gallinarum*, and *Enterococcus raffinosus* (MICs, 4 to ≥16 μg/ml).

Because dalfopristin-quinupristin is inactive against *E. faecalis*, it is important to correctly identify *E. faecium*.

In the Protek study conducted from 2000 to 2001, it was shown that less than 0.02% of *S. pneumoniae* strains are resistant to dalfopristin-quinupristin. Each isolate had a 5-amino-acid tandem duplication in the L22 ribosomal protein gene (*rplV*), preventing synergistic ribosomal binding of the streptogramin combination. Similar gene duplication has been reported for dalfopristin-quinupristin resistant *S. aureus*.

For *S. aureus* resistant to linezolid (MIC, >128 μg/ml), the MIC of dalfopristin-quinupristin is ≤0.25 μg/ml. For *E. faecium* resistant to linezolid, the MIC at which 50 and 90% of isolates are inhibited ($MIC_{50/90}$) for dalfopristin-quinupristin is ≤0.5/1 μg/ml.

3.6.2. Mechanism of Resistance

See Leclercq et al., 1992.

The antibacterial spectrum of the MLS_B group does not include the gram-negative bacilli. *Enterobacteriaceae*, *Pseudomonas* spp., and *Acinetobacter* are resistant through their outer membrane impermeability to these hydrophobic molecules.

Acquired resistance of the MLS_B type is due to four mechanisms: modification of the antibiotic target, inactivation of the antibiotics, reduction of outer membrane permeability, and efflux.

The resistance phenotypes corresponding to the various mechanisms are summarized in Table 13.

3.6.2.1. Genes Involved in Resistance

Many genes encode streptogramin resistance, a complex phenomenon which could be specific for each component. The genes are listed in Table 14.

Table 13 Staphylococcal resistance phenotypes[a]

Mechanism of resistance	Gene	Erythromycin A	Lincomycin	Pristinamycin I	Pristinamycin II	Pristinamycin
Target alteration	*ermI*	R	S	S	S	S
	ermC	R	R	R	S	(S)
Inactivation	*eri*	R	S	S	S	S
	linA	S	R	S	S	S
	lsa	S	I	S	R	(S)
	saa-sbh	S	S/I	R	R	R
Permeability alteration	*erpA*	R	S	S	S	S

[a]R, resistant; S, susceptible; I, intermediate; (S), apparently susceptible.

Table 14 Genes involved in streptogramin resistance

Microorganism(s)	Mechanism	Gene(s)	Targeted streptogramin	Notes
Staphylococcus spp.	Factor A inactivation	*vat*	A	
	Efflux	*vga*	A	
	LSA	Unknown	A	
	Mutation of L22	*rplV*	B	
	Mutation of L4	*rplD*	B	
	Mutation of 23S RNA (constitutive)	*erm*	B	
	Mutation of 23S RNA (inducible)	*erm*	B	After induction by erythromycin A
	Efflux	*mrs*(A)	B	After induction by erythromycin A
	Factor B inactivation	*vgb*	B	
E. faecium	Factor A inactivation	*vat*	A	
	LSA	Unknown	A	
	Ribosome methylation (constitutive)	*erm*	B	
	Ribosome methylation (inducible)	*erm*	B	After induction by erythromycin A
	Factor B inactivation	*vgb*	B	
S. pneumoniae	Ribosomal methylation (constitutive)	*erm*	B	
	Ribosomal methylation (inducible)	*erm*	B	After induction by erythromycin A
	Mutations to 23S RNA and L22 and L4 proteins	*rrl, rplD, rplV*	B	

The gene *vga* is plasmid borne but nonconjugative. The *vga*, gene encodes an ATP binding protein that mediates efflux of group A streptogramins.

The VgA protein is a 522-amino-acid protein (molecular mass, 60,115 Da). This protein is mainly found in coagulase-negative staphylococci.

Other *vga* genes have been reported, such as *vga*(B), which encodes a 552-amino-acid protein (molecular weight, 61,327), or the *vga*(A) gene in *S. aureus*.

Low-level resistance may be due to LSA chromosomal resistance (MIC of dalfopristin-quinupristin, ≤ 4 μg/ml). Less frequently, streptogramin B is responsible for resistance. The *vgb* or *erm* genes are involved.

3.6.2.1.1. *E. faecium*. Mainly inactivating enzymes are responsible for streptogramin resistance in *E. faecium*. Group B resistance is mainly due to domain V (23S rRNA) methylation by the *erm* gene or mutation on domain V or ribosomal protein L22 or L4. Group B streptogramin is not sufficient to confer full resistance to dalfopristin-quinupristin, conversely, group A streptogramin generally confers resistance to dalfopristin-quinupristin.

Group A streptogramin resistance is due either to an inactivating enzyme such as acetyltransferase (*vat* genes) or to an efflux pump (*vga* or *mstA* genes). The *vat(B)* gene is plasmid borne and encodes an inactivating enzyme.

3.6.2.2. Modification of the Bacterial Target

Modification of the bacterial target, an MLS_B type of resistance, is based on a specific and unique modification of the bacterial ribosome. Resistant strains produce a methylase responsible for the methylation of adenine 2058 of the 23S rRNA of the *Escherichia coli* 50S subunit. There is cross-resistance between macrolides, lincosamides, and streptogramin B (pristinamycin I).

The phenotype may be constitutive, and the strains are resistant to all macrolides and lincosamides and susceptible to streptogramins because of the activity of compound A (pristinamycin II) and the existence of synergistic activity between the A and B components of pristinamycin.

The phenotype may be inducible, and the strains are resistant to 14- and 15-membered-ring macrolides and susceptible to 16-membered-ring macrolides, lincosamides, and streptogramins. Strains of *S. aureus* are resistant only to 14- and 15-membered-ring macrolides (erythromycin A and derivatives and azalide) through the production of a methylase.

The phenotypes are related not to the *erm* gene but to the nature of the regulatory region associated with the structural gene of the methylase.

MLS_B resistance in streptococci may be of the constitutive or inducible type. Enterococci, pneumococci, and viridans group streptococci have constitutive MLS_B resistance. Inducible expression occurs above all in group A, C, G, and B streptococci and in certain viridans group streptococcal strains.

3.6.2.3. Inactivation of Streptogramins

Enzymatic inactivation of pristinamycin or virginiamycin was described in 1975. Some strains of *S. aureus* are capable of acetylating the hydroxyl group at position 13 of pristinamycin II_A through a plasmid-mediated *O*-acetyltransferase and producing an inactive derivative since it has no ribosomal affinity (de Meester and Rondelet, 1977; Le Goffic et al., 1977).

S. aureus possesses a hydrolase on the same plasmid that opens the macrolactone ring of pristinamycin I_A and causes it to lose its antibacterial activity despite good ribosomal binding.

The majority of these *S. aureus* strains have reduced susceptibility to lincosamides.

Inactivation of factor A (pristinamycin II) has been described for staphylococci and *E. faecium*.

3.7. Pharmacokinetics of Pristinamycin

3.7.1. Assay Methods

The assay of pristinamycin is complex because pristinamycin II is destroyed by intraerythrocytic enzymes. To try to reduce the effect of hemolysis of the erythrocytes, blood must be collected in an acetone-rich medium (3 or 4 volumes of acetone to 1 volume of blood).

3.7.2. Pharmacokinetics in Adults

There are no published pharmacokinetic data for children, elderly subjects, or patients with renal or hepatic insufficiency. The pharmacokinetics in adults were reviewed by

Table 15 Pharmacokinetics of pristinamycin components after administration of 2 g orally

Component	C_{max} (μg/ml)	T_{max} (h)	$t_{1/2\beta}$ (h)	AUC (μg·h/ml)	Lag time (min)
pI_A	0.8	3.03	4.03	2.2	23.3
pII_A	0.6	3.01	2.8	1.2	18.3

Table 16 Pharmacokinetics of pristinamycin and virginiamycin[a]

Parameter (unit)	Pristinamycin	Virginiamycin
C_{max} (μg/ml)	1.0	1.0
T_{max} (h)	1.0–2.0	2.0–4.0
$t_{1/2}$ (h)	5.0 (PI)	5.0 (M)
	2.8–8.0 (PII)	8.0 (S)
Protein binding (%)	40–45 (PI)	40–45 (M)
	80–90 (PII)	80–90 (S)
Hepatic elimination	+ + + (<10% metabolites)	+ + + (<10% metabolites)
Renal elimination (%)	10 (PI)	10 (M)
	~2 (PII)	2 (S)

[a]PI, pristinamycin I; PII, pristinamycin II; M, virginiamycin M; S, virginiamycin S.

Kernbaum (1985). In adults, pristinamycin and virginiamycin are not inactivated by gastric fluid. About 15 to 18% of pristinamcyin II_A and virginiamycin M is absorbed in the ileojejunal section. There is also weak absorption of the I_A fraction.

After administration of 500 mg of pristinamycin or virginiamycin, the concentration in plasma is about 1 μg/ml at 2 h. Concentrations in plasma are minimal or nonexistent from 4 to 6 h, depending on the subject (Videau, 1965).

The apparent elimination half-lives are 4 to 5 h for pristinamycin I_A and virginiamycin M and 2.8 to 8 h for pristinamycin II_A and virginiamycin S. After administration of 2 g orally, the maximum concentrations of drug in serum for pristinamycins I_A and II_A are, respectively, 0.8 and 0.6 μg/ml and are attained in about 3 h. The apparent elimination half-lives are, respectively, 4 and 2.8 h. Initial levels in plasma are detectable from about 20 min. The areas under the curve are 2.2 and 1.2 mg.h/liter. The global peak concentration in serum (pristinamycins I_A and II_A) is 1.34 ± 0.7 μg/ml (mean ± standard deviation) and is reached in 3 h (Koechlin et al., 1990) (Table 15). Plasma protein binding is 40 to 50% for pristinamycin I and 80 to 90% for pristinamycin II. Synergistins are metabolized in the liver, but this metabolism has not been studied. Elimination occurs principally in the bile and urinary elimination is weak, on the order of 10% for pristinamycin I and 2% for pristinamycin II (Table 16).

The pharmacokinetic parameters of the I_A and II_A components were determined after repeated doses of 2 g of pristinamycin for 7 days. Sixteen volunteers were included in this study. The ratio of pristinamycin I to pristinamycin II was 30:70. Pristinamycin I is composed principally of a mixture of three components, I_A (80 to 95%), I_B (3 to 15%), and I_C (2 to 5%); pristinamycin II is composed of a mixture of two main constituents, II_A (90 to 97%) and II_B (3 to 10%). Blood samples were taken in a dry tube and acidified immediately (5 ml of blood in 0.5 ml of 0.129 M sodium citrate and 1.25 ml of 0.25 N HCl). The assays were performed using a radioimmunological method. The limits of sensitivity were, respectively, 1 and 2 μg/ml for pristinamycins I and II. The concentrations of the two components in plasma may also be determined by high-performance liquid chromatography. There is a good correlation between the two methods.

After a single dose of 2 g in fasting subjects, the peak concentrations in serum of 915 ± 538 ng/ml (I_A) and 123 ± 63 ng/ml (II_A) were reached in 2 and 2.75 h, respectively. The areas under the curve were 3,029 ± 2,541 ng·h/ml (I_A) and 373 ± 287 ng·h/ml (II_A). Repeated doses were administered with food, and the components of pristinamycin were rapidly absorbed. After the first dose, the peak concentrations of pristinamycins I and II in serum were, respectively, 875 ± 325 ng/ml and 1,497 ± 417 ng/ml and were reached between 0.5 and 2 h. The peak concentrations of pristinamycin I_A, determined by high-performance liquid chromatography, were 2.6 times greater than those of pristinamycin II_A on the first day (898 versus 361 ng/ml), and the areas under the curve were 3.8 times greater than those of pristinamycin II_A (2,709 versus 689 ng.h/ml).

The apparent elimination half-lives of pristinamycins I and II were, respectively, 1.6 ± 0.6 h and 4.7 ± 1.3 h, whereas those of pristinamycins I_A and II_A were similar and short (1.9 ± 0.7 h and 1.3 ± 0.7 h, respectively).

On day 8, the pharmacokinetic parameters were relatively unchanged (Table 17).

Pristinamycin II_A is metabolized to derivatives similar to those of pristinamycin I_A, as these metabolites are recognized by the antibodies in radioimmunological assay.

The tissue distribution of pristinamycin has not been studied in humans. Benazet and Bourat (1965) studied the tissue distribution in animals of pristinamycin I_A and virginiamycin M_1, which are distributed uniformly in all of the organs.

Aumercier et al. (1985) studied the distribution of radiolabeled pristinamycin II_A in female mice (Charles River) by autoradiography. They demonstrated rapid absorption of II_A and a marked concentration in the digestive and urinary tracts. Concentrations in the skin and bone marrow are high. Pristinamycin does not cross the meningeal barrier.

3.8. Drug Interference

Pristinamycin does not interfere with cytochrome P450. There is the possibility of a metabolic interaction between pristinamycin and cyclosporin, which may be responsible for acute nephrotoxicity (Gagnadoux et al., 1987). It interferes with the metabolism of methotrexate (Thyss et al., 1993).

Table 17 Pharmacokinetics of pristinamycins I and II after repeated doses (2 g/day)[a]

Parameter (unit)	Day 1				Day 8			
	RIA		HPLC		RIA		HPLC	
	PI	PII	PI_A	PII_A	PI	PII	PI_A	PII_A
Repeated doses (fed)								
C_{max} (ng/ml)	875	1,497	898	361	809	1,492	814	335
T_{max} (h)	1	1	1	0.75	1	1	1	0.5
AUC_{0-t} (ng·h/ml)	2,563	5,190	2,709	689	1,998	5,174	2,139	513
$t_{1/2}$ (h)	1.6	4.1	1.9	1.3	2.3		1.5	0.8
Single dose (fast)								
C_{max} (ng/ml)			915	123				
T_{max} (h)			2	2.75				
AUC_{0-t} (ng·h/ml)			3,029	373				

[a]RIA, radioimmunoassay; HPLC, high-performance liquid chromatography; PI, PII, PI_A, and PII_A, pristinamycins I, II, I_A, and II_A, respectively.

4. DALFOPRISTIN-QUINUPRISTIN (RP-59500)

Pristinamycin remains an antibacterial complex with good antistaphylococcal activity, particularly against methicillin- and erythromycin A-resistant strains. Its use in the hospital environment has been restricted by the absence of a parenteral form due to the poor solubility of pristinamycin in water. The objective has been to prepare derivatives with the same antibacterial activity as pristinamycin but with greater hydrosolubility. One compound has been developed: dalfopristin-quinupristin (RP-59500).

4.1. Structure-Activity Relationship

Semisynthesis from the isolated I_A and II_A constituents has yielded hydrosoluble derivatives (Fig. 6).

4.1.1. Pristinamycin I_A Derivatives: RP-57669

Paris et al. (1985) have released the chemical structures of more than 80 derivatives obtained by semisynthesis from pristinamycin I_A. They introduced an amino function at the 5δ position in 5δ-thiomethylene or at the 5γ position.

Some 15 5γ-amino pristinamycin I_A derivatives have been prepared; these have good antibacterial activity, and some have 3.7 to 10% solubility in water. Thirty derivatives of the 5δ-aminoethylene pristinamycin I_A type have better activity than pristinamycin I_A and moderate solubility in water, between 1 and 10%. More than 20 derivatives of the 5δ-alcoylthiomethylene type have been prepared with activity similar to that of pristinamycin I_A, but they are sparingly soluble (1%). The best solubility is that obtained with the 5δ-alcoylthiomethyl derivatives, which is greater than 5%. That of pristinamycin I_A is on the order of 0.1% (Fig. 7).

In addition, Aumercier et al. (1985) showed that the presence of substituents at the 5α and 5δ positions might alter the affinity of pristinamycin I_A for ribosomes. The presence of substituents at the 5δ position and the presence of a sulfur atom confer more pronounced antibacterial properties than the 5γ substituents.

The acid salts of the thiomethyl derivatives are the most soluble in water. They have good antibacterial activity, whether the strains of *S. aureus* are susceptible or resistant to erythromycin A, and act synergistically with pristinamycin II_A. The (*SR*)(3*S*)-thiomethylquinuclidine derivative has been selected (RP-57669) (Fig. 8).

4.1.2. Pristinamycin II Derivatives

The semisynthetic derivatives of pristinamycin II_A with an amino substituent at position 26 are soluble in water. About 120 derivatives have been synthesized in three pristinamycin II_B series: 26-thio, 26-sulfinyl, and 26-sulfonyl pristinamycin II_B. The solubility of these derivatives is between 1 and 5%.

The level of oxidation of the sulfur atom attached to the proline residue plays an important role in the biological activity of the derivatives obtained by semisynthesis. The thioether derivatives are less active than pristinamycin II_A and are not synergistic in vitro with pristinamycin I_A, but they possess good synergistic activity with the I_A compound in vivo in the mouse; it is possible that they are transformed in vivo to sulfinyl or sulfonyl derivatives which are active in vitro against susceptible strains not resistant to erythromycin A.

The length of the chain between the sulfur atom and the nitrogen atom has a marked effect on the activity: compounds with two methylenes between the sulfur and the nitrogen are more active than those with three or four methylenes.

The (26*S*)-diethylaminoethylsulfonyl pristinamycin B derivative (RP-54476) has been selected.

Dalfopristin-quinupristin is composed of a combination of the two components RP-57669 and RP-54476 in a ratio of 30:70 (wt/wt) (Fig. 9).

4.2. Antibacterial Activity

RP-59500 has the same antibacterial spectrum as pristinamycin and similar in vitro activity (Tables 18, 19, and 20).

The ratios of cellular and extracellular concentrations of the RP-54476 and RP-57669 components in the macrophage line J774 are, respectively, 30:1 and 60:1. Efflux is rapid (Barrière et al., 1994).

The approved NCCLS breakpoint is ≤1 μg/ml (diameter of zone of inhibition, ≥18 mm) for a disk load at 7.5 μg (ratio, 30:70).

Dalfopristin-quinupristin MICs for GISA strains (glycopeptide-intermediate *S. aureus*) are 0.5 to 1.0 μg/ml.

A left-side endocarditis was induced in male New Zealand White rabbits (2 to 5 kg) with 10^8 CFU of vancomycin-resistant *E. faecium* (VREF) (MIC, 0.5 μg/ml) and GISA (MIC, 0.25 μg/ml) strains per ml. They were treated with either dalfopristin-quinupristin (75 mg/kg of body weight) every 8 hours (q8h) or linezolid (50 mg/kg q12h), with or

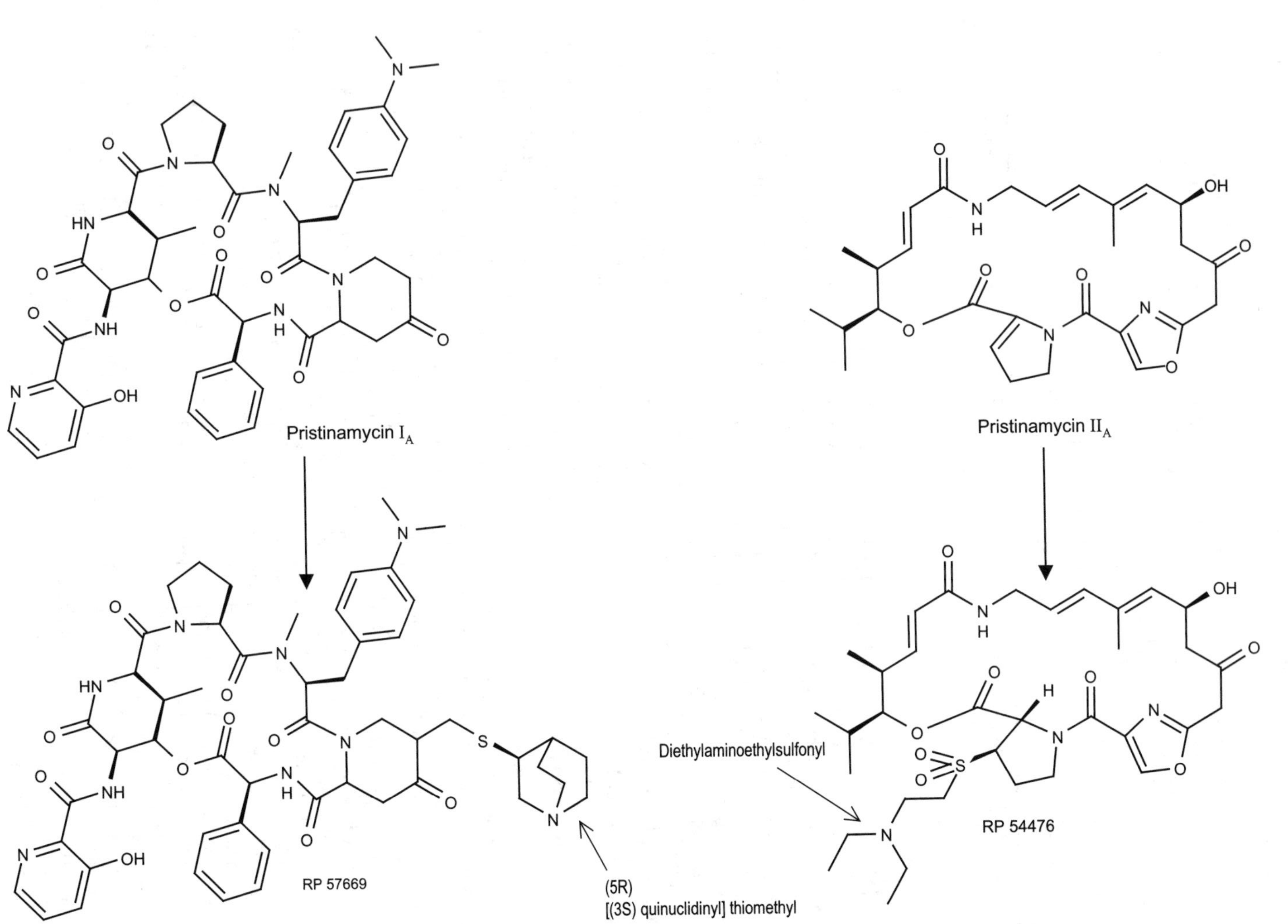

Figure 6 **Pristinamycin I_A and II_A derivatives**

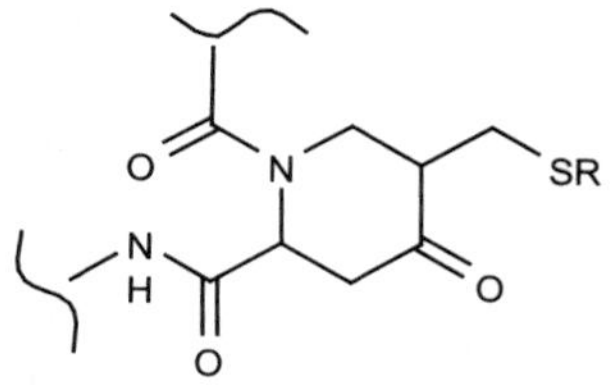

-S-R	Derivative alone Ery-S	Derivative alone Ery-R	In combination withPII Ery-S	In combination withPII Ery-R	Synergy	Water solubility (%)
—S—$(CH_2)_3$—$N(CH_3)_2$	2	2	0.12	0.25	+	10
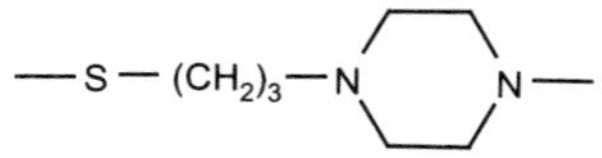 —S—$(CH_2)_3$—N(piperazine)N—	1	2	0.12	0.25	+	5
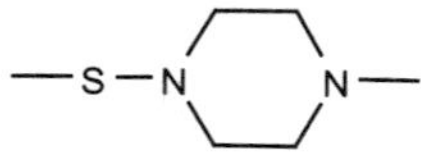 —S—N(piperazine)N—	1	1	0.12	0.25	+	5
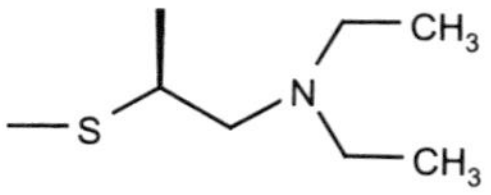 —S—CH(CH3)CH2—N(CH_3)(CH_3)	1	2	0.12	0.50	+	7-5
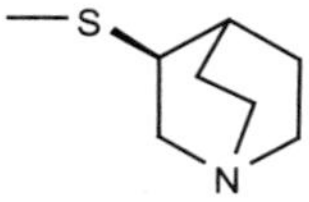 —S—(quinuclidinyl)	1	1	0.25	0.25	+	
Pristinamycin I_A	2-4	8	0.12	0.25	+	0.10

Figure 7 Comparative activity of the 5δ-thiomethyl pristinamycin I_A derivatives against *S. aureus* (adapted from Barrière et al.)

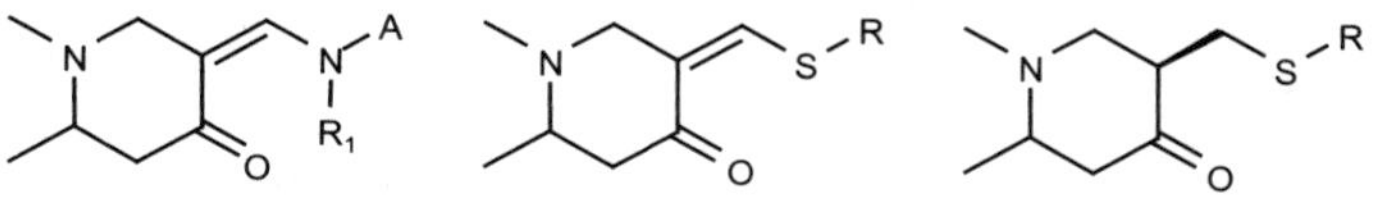

		5-aminomethylene	5-thiomethylene	5-thiomethyl	Pristinamycin I_A
Alone	Erythromycin A-S	8	4	1	2-4
	Erythromycin A-R	30	8	1	8
In combination with	Erythromycin A-S	1	0.25	0.25	0.12
	Erythromycin A-R	0.5	0.50	0.25	0.25
	Synergy	0	+	+	+

Figure 8 Pristinamycin I_A derivatives

without ampicillin and ampicillin-sulbactam (intramuscularly, 100 mg/kg q8h) for 5 days. Blood cultures were obtained and animals were sacrificed 12 h following the last dose of the study drug. Vegetations were removed and quantitative bacterial counts were expressed as $\log_{10}$ CFU per gram of vegetations (Table 21).

4.3. Pharmacokinetics

In a phase I study (Etienne et al., 1992), dalfopristin-quinupristin was assayed by a microbiological method using *Micrococcus luteus* ATCC 9341 as the test strain. The limit of detection in plasma was 0.1 μg/ml. The plasma assays of the two components RP-57669 and RP-54476 and that of the active metabolite RP-12536 (the metabolite of RP-54476) were performed by means of a high-performance chromatographic method. The limits of sensitivity were 0.1 μg/ml for RP-57669, 0.125 μg/ml for RP-54476, and 0.04 μg/ml for RP-12536.

The samples were taken in an acidic medium (tubes containing 0.05 N HCl for high-performance liquid chromatography and 0.25 N for the microbiological assays).

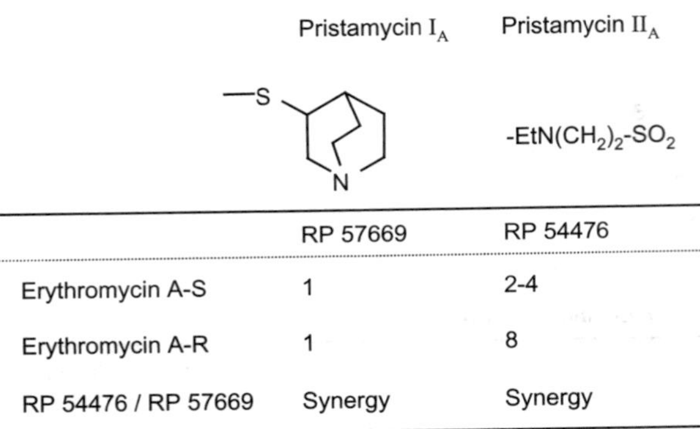

Pristamycin I_A
Pristamycin II_A
—S
N
$-EtN(CH_2)_2-SO_2$
RP 57669
RP 54476
Erythromycin A-S
1
2-4
Erythromycin A-R
1
8
RP 54476 / RP 57669
Synergy
Synergy

Figure 9 Dalfopristin-quinupristin

Table 18 In vitro activity of dalfopristin-quinupristin (I)

Organism(s)	MIC (μg/ml)	
	50%	90%
S. aureus Met[s]	≤0.12	0.5
S. aureus Met[r], Ery[s]	0.5	0.5
S. aureus Ery[r]	0.5	1.0
S. epidermidis Met[s]	0.25	0.25
S. epidermidis Met[r]	0.25	1.0
S. saprophyticus	1.0	8.0
Staphylococcus hominis	0.25	1.0
Staphylococcus haemolyticus	1.0	1.0
Group C and G streptococci	0.25	0.5
S. pyogenes	0.25	0.5
S. agalactiae	0.5	0.5
Viridans group streptococci	1.0	1.0
S. pneumoniae Ery[s]	0.25	0.25
S. pneumoniae Ery[r]	0.5	1.0
S. pneumoniae Pen[s]	0.5	1.0
S. pneumoniae Pen[i]	0.5	0.5
S. pneumoniae Pen[r]	0.5	1.0
E. faecalis Ery[s]	4.0	8.0
E. faecalis Ery[r]	4.0	8.0
E. faecium	1.0	4.0
Enterococcus avium	2.0	8.0
Corynebacterium spp.	0.12	0.5
Listeria spp.	1.0	1.0
Micrococcus spp.	0.06	0.12
Stomatococcus spp.	0.12	
Bacillus spp.	1.0	1.0

The three derivatives were stable for at least 6 months in an acidic medium at −20°C. In the absence of HCl, the components degraded within 24 h.

After repeated administrations to 10 young male volunteers of a dose of 7.5 mg of dalfopristin-quinupristin per kg for 5 days (q12h) and 4 days (q8h), there was no significant accumulation of either component (Table 22). The accumulation ratio ranged between 1.16 and 1.43.

The pharmacokinetic parameters are summarized in Tables 23 and 24. RP-59500 was administered in the form of an infusion over 1 h. Peak concentrations of RP-59500 were between 0.95 ± 0.22 μg/ml (dose, 1.4 mg/kg) and 24.20 ± 8.82 (dose, 29.4 mg/kg). These concentrations increased dose dependently, except for RP-54476, which was rapidly converted to its active metabolite RP-12536. The activity of RP-59500 was detectable 6 h after the end of the infusion.

Table 19 In vitro activity of dalfopristin-quinupristin (II)

Organism(s)[a]	MIC (μg/ml)	
	50%	90%
N. meningitidis	0.25	0.25
N. gonorrhoeae β⁻	0.5	1.0
N. gonorrhoeae β⁺	0.5	0.5
M. catarrhalis	1.0	1.0
H. influenzae β⁻	2.0	4.0
H. influenzae β⁺	2.0	2.0
L. monocytogenes	2.0	2.0
L. pneumophila	0.12–0.5	0.25–0.5
Legionella dumoffii	0.05	1.0
Legionella micdadei	1.0	2.0
Legionella longbeachae	0.25	1.0
Gardnerella vaginalis	0.01	0.06
Bacillus fragilis	4.0	4.0
Clostridium perfringens	≤0.12	0.25
Clostridium difficile	0.12	0.12
Propionibacterium acnes	0.03	0.12
Fusobacterium ssp.	0.06	0.12
Peptostreptococcus spp.	0.03	0.12
Actinomyces israeli	0.12	0.25
Clostridium clostridioforme	0.5	0.5
Clostridium innocuum	0.5	1.0
Clostridium ramosum	0.5	4.0
Eubacterium spp.	2.0	4.0
Corynebacterium amycolatum	0.25	0.25
Corynebacterium jeikeium	0.25	0.5

[a]β⁻, non-β-lactamase producing; β⁺, β-lactamase producing.

Six volunteers received an infusion of a single dose of 12 mg of dalfopristin-quinupristin per kg (ratio, 30:70 for RP-57769 and RP-54476) for 60 min. The assays in suction blister and plasma fluids were performed by a microbiological method for which the test strain was *Sarcina lutea* (limits of detection, 0.125 μg/ml of plasma and 0.25 μg/ml of suction blister fluid).

The peak concentrations in serum and suction blisters were, respectively, 8.65 ± 0.92 μg/ml and 2.41 ± 0.75 μg/ml. The areas under the curve were, respectively, 11.2 ± 1.45 μg·h/ml and 9.19 ± 2.02 μg · h/ml. The penetration was 84.49% ± 11.36%. The apparent elimination half-life of RP-59500 was 1.48 ± 0.64 h (Bernard et al., 1994) (Table 25).

The interindividual variabilities are 20 to 29% and 25 to 32% for quinupristin and dalfopristin, respectively.

Two other metabolites occur through a nonenzymatic process, like pristinamycin II_A: gluthatione-quinupristin and cysteine-quinupristin.

The hepatic clearance and the fecal elimination are 74.7 and 77.5% for quinupristin and dalfopristin, respectively. Protein binding rates are 55 to 78% and 11 to 26% for quinupristin and dalfopristin, respectively.

For a 44-year-old man suffering from VREF ventriculitis, the level of dalfopristin-quinupristin was assessed after 1, 2, and 4 mg of dalfopristin-quinupristin once a day administered by the intrathecal route, knowing that it had been shown that quinupristin and dalfopristin penetrate poorly into the cerebral fluid of infected rabbits.

The patient received quinupristin and dalfopristin locally and intravenously (7.5 mg/kg) in association with chloramphenicol. Data are summarized in Table 26.

Table 20 In vitro activities of dalfopristin-quinupristin and the two components

Organism(s)	MIC$_{50}$ (μg/ml)		
	Dalfopristin-quinupristin	RP-57669	RP-54476
S. aureus Ery^s	0.5	1.0	2.0
S. aureus Ery^r	0.5	4.0	4.0
S. aureus Ery^r Met^r	0.5	4.0	4.0
S. epidermidis Ery^s	0.25	2.0	1.0
S. epidermidis Ery^r	0.25	2.0	0.5
S. epidermidis Ery^r Met^r	0.12	4.0	0.5
S. pyogenes	0.25	1.0	0.5
S. agalactiae Ery^s	0.5	8.0	2.0
Group C and G streptococci	0.25	8.0	0.5
S. pneumoniae	0.5	2.0	1.0
Viridans group streptococci	1.0	16	>16
E. faecalis Ery^s	4.0	32	0.5
E. faecalis Ery^r	8.0	>64	>32
L. monocytogenes	2.0	>16	>16
H. influenzae	2.0	>16	4.0
M. catarrhalis	0.5	4.0	1.0
N. gonorrhoeae	0.5	>16	>16
N. meningitidis	0.25	0.5	0.5
B. fragilis	4.0	32	>32

Table 21 Endocarditis in rabbits

Survival (no. survivors/ no. infected)		Compound	Log$_{10}$ CFU/g of vegetations			
VREF	GISA		n[a]	VREF	n	GISA
		None (control)	6	5.89 ± 1.13	8	8.55 ± 0.65
5/9	7/9	Dalfopristin-quinupristin	9	5.95 ± 1.6	9	8.58 ± 0.9
8/8	7/11	Linezolid	8	3.58 ± 1.4	11	6.91 ± 1.84
4/8		Ampicillin	6	8.45 ± 0.85	10	<3.54 ± 2.85
5/12		Ampicillin + Q-D	10	2.95 ± 0.08		NT[b]
8/9		Ampicillin + linezolid	7	3.71 ± 1.71	8	<1.85 ± 0.76

[a]n, number of rabbits.
[b]NT, not tested.

Table 22 Pharmacokinetics of dalfopristin-quinupristin after repeated doses

Dosing interval	Day	C_{max} (μg/ml)	C_{min} (μg/ml)	AUC (μg·h/ml)	$t_{1/2}$ (h)	CL_p (liters/kg)
q12h						
Quinupristin	1	2.31	BLQ[a]	2.44	0.82	0.93
	5	2.53	BLQ	2.96	0.87	0.77
Dalfopristin	1	5.92	BLQ	6.24	0.61	0.83
	5	6.81	BLQ	7.78	0.79	0.91
Pristinamycin II_A	1	0.84	BLQ	1.39	1.28	
	5	1.11	BLQ	2.09	1.57	
Glu-Q	1	0.3	BLQ	0.5	1.70	
	5	0.38	BLQ	0.78	1.85	
Cys-Q	1	0.25	BLQ	0.58	1.96	
	5	0.49	BLQ	1.11	2.06	
q8h						
Quinupristin	1	2.39	BLQ	2.60	0.75	0.90
	4	2.79	BLQ	3.22	0.85	0.73
Dalfopristin	1	6.20	BLQ	6.44	0.45	0.87
	4	7.22	BLQ	7.81	0.70	0.73
Pristinamycin II_A	1	0.82	BLQ	1.39	1.26	
	4	1.10	BLQ	2.01	1.97	
Glu-Q	1	0.31	BLQ	0.53	2.11	
	4	0.42	BLQ	0.88	1.81	
Cys-Q	1	0.25	BLQ	0.56	1.81	
	4	0.59	BLQ	1.26	2.65	

[a]BLQ, below limit of quantification.

Table 23 Pharmacokinetics of dalfopristin-quinupristin (RP-59500)

Compound	Dose (mg/kg)	C_{max} (μg/ml)	AUC_{0-8h} (μg·h/ml)	$t_{1/2}$ (h)
RP-59500	12.6	10.7	15.94	1.39
RP-57669		8.54		0.56
RP-54476		7.15		
RP-12536		1.27		0.84
RP-59500	16.8	12.82	19.74	1.27
RP-57669		10.93		0.56
RP-54476		4.82		
RP-12536		1.47		0.93
RP-59500	22.4	14.05	22.93	1.53
RP-57669		13.53		NT[a]
RP-54476		4.36		
RP-12536		1.68		0.95
RP-59500	29.4	24.2	37.7	1.32
RP-57669		19.93		0.61
RP-54476		6.90		
RP-12536		2.44		0.75

[a]NT, not tested.

Table 24 Intravenous pharmacokinetics of dalfopristin and quinupristin[a]

Compound	Dose (mg/kg)	C_0 (μg/ml)	AUC (μg·h/ml)	$t_{1/2}$ (h)	Cl_P (liters/h/kg)	V (liters/kg)
Quinupristin	5	1.2	1.41	0.87	1.13	1.37
	10	2.3	2.98	1.02	1.04	1.35
	15	3.58	4.69	0.96	0.99	1.37
Dalfopristin	5	4.55	4.5–7	0.4	0.99	0.55
	10	6.38	7.18	0.52	1.2	0.88
	15	8.17	9.04	1.05	1.4	1.93

[a]Data from Montay et al., 1994.

Table 25 Pharmacokinetics of dalfopristin-quinupristin in suction blister fluid

Sample	C_{max} (μg/ml)	t_{max} (h)	AUC_{0-6h} (μg·h/ml)	$t_{1/2}$ (h)	Cl_P (liters/h)
Plasma	8.6 ± 0.92		11.21 ± 1.45	1.48 ± 0.61	74 ± 10.2
Blister fluid	2.41 ± 0.55	1.66 ± 0.51	9.19 ± 2.02		

Table 26 Levels of dalfopristin and quinupristin in cerebrospinal fluid

Sample	Dose (mg)	Sampling time	Concn in cerebrospinal fluid (μg/ml)[a]				
			Q	Glu-Q (RPR 100391)	Cyst-Q (RP-64012)	D	PII_A (RP-12536)
1	1	Baseline	BLQ	0.021	0.046	BLQ	0.06
2	1	1.7	2.75	0.1	0.38	0.64	3.9
3	1	3.0	0.53	0.07	0.23	0.09	1.14
4	1	3.9	0.32	0.07	0.23	0.05	0.85
5	1	7.0	0.21	0.06	0.17	BLQ	0.28
6	2	Baseline	0.28	0.02	0.03	BLQ	1.13
7	2	1.2	27.2	0.2	0.51	22	BLQ
8	2	2.2	4.0	0.2	0.55	1.7	10.2
9	2	3.2	0.99	0.2	0.52	0.08	2.72
10	2	8.2	0.21	0.13	0.30	BLQ	0.69

[a]Q, quinupristin; D, dalfopristin; PII_A, pristinamycin II_A; BLQ, below limit of quantification.

4.3.1. Tolerability

Dalfopristin-quinupristin appears to have been well tolerated during phase II and III clinical studies, except in the vein. Muscular pain has been reported. Phase II and III clinical trials were performed as a recommended regimen of 7.5 mg/kg q12h and q8h for more severe infections.

Like pristinamycin, this combination does not interfere with cytochrome P450 (Martinet et al., 1992).

5. RPR 106972

RPR 106972 (Fig. 10) is an oral pristinamycin derivative comprising two derivatives, one from pristinamycin I_B (RPR 112808) and the other from pristinamycin II_B (RPR 106950).

5.1. Antibacterial Activity

In vitro, RPR 106972 is less active than dalfopristin-quinupristin against staphylococci, whether or not these are susceptible to methicillin or erythromycin A. It is on average twice as active against streptococci, enterococci, *H. influenzae*, and *Moraxella catarrhalis* (Table 27) (Berthaud et al., 1995).

The pristinamycin I_B (RPR 112808) and II_B (RPR 106950) constituents themselves are less active against staphylococci than the RP-59500 constituents.

For penicillin G-resistant strains of *S. pneumoniae*, the MIC_{50}s are increased by 5 dilutions compared with those for susceptible strains (MIC_{50}s, 0.015 to 2 μg/ml) (Spangler et al., 1995).

This molecule has in vivo bactericidal activity in a murine model of *S. pneumoniae* experimental infection (Berthaud et al., 1995).

5.2. Pharmacokinetics

The 200-mg tablets and later the 500-mg tablets were used for most of the phase I trials. The 250-mg tablets were used in Japan.

The maximum concentrations of drug in serum ranged from 35 to 1,000 ng/ml for pristinamycin I_B and from 86 to 1,100 ng/ml for pristinamycin II_B. The areas under the curve reached 3,200 ng·h/ml for pristinamysin I_B and up to 2,600 ng·h/ml for pristinamycin II_B. A high interindividual variability was observed in all studies. Concentrations in

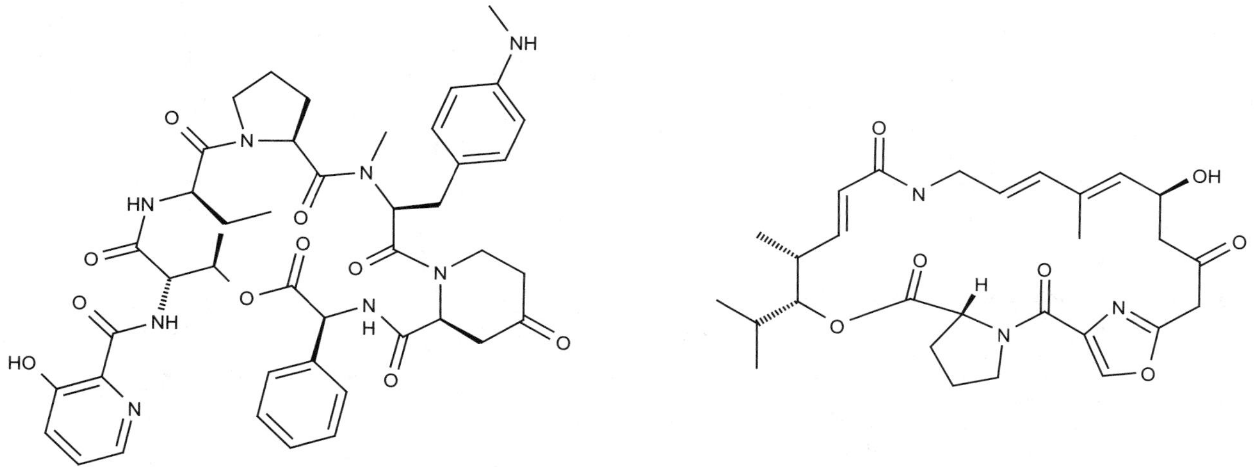

Pristinamycin I_B

Pristinamycin II_B

Figure 10 Oral streptogramin

Table 27 In vitro activity of RPR 106972 and its components

Organism(s)	MIC_{50} (μg/ml)		
	RPR 106972	RPR 12808	RPR 106950
S. aureus	0.5	>4.0	16
S. epidermidis	0.12		
Coagulase-negative staphylococci	0.25	2.0	16
Group A, B, C, and G streptococci	0.06		
S. pneumoniae Pen^s	0.03	0.25	0.125
S. pneumoniae Pen^i	0.125	0.25	1.0
S. pneumoniae Pen^r	0.25	1.0	8.0
Enterococcus spp.	2.0		
Neisseria spp.	0.12		
M. catarrhalis	0.25		
H. influenzae	1.0		
Legionella spp.	0.25		

plasma were higher for pristinamycin II_B than for pristinamycin I_B (ratio, 1.1 to 1.4). The bioavailability after administration of the 500-mg tablet was about 60%. The half-lives of pristinamycins I_B and II_B are 1.0 to 1.5 h. Pharmacokinetics are not modified by gender or age.

When the compound was given with food, the improvement was more pronounced for pristinamycin II_B than for pristinamycin I_B. A delay in time to peak concentration of drug in serum was also noted in association with high-fat meals and with milk. In Japanese volunteers, the bioavailability increased with food; however, the times of administration differed between both studies. In the Caucasian study, the compound was administered 0.5 h before food, and in the Japanese study, the compound was administered with food (Table 28).

Grapefruit juice increases the overall bioavailability but delays the time to peak concentration of drug in serum without influencing the peak concentration of drug in serum. Grapefruit inhibits the premetabolism of CYP 450 3A4. Pristinamycins I_B and II_B are metabolized through CYP 450 3A4.

In blister fluid, the peak concentration of pristinamycin I_B was 25% of the concentrations in plasma; the peak concentration of pristinamycin II_B in blister fluid was 6%.

The main parameters are reported in Table 29.

The protein binding of pristinamycin I_B in plasma was 25 to 40% at 1.0 to 2.0 h postdose, while the binding of pristinamycin II_B varied between 71 and 84% at 1.0 to 2.0 h postdose.

Unchanged compounds were 40 to 60% and 10% of the radioactivity in plasma for pristinamycins I_B and II_B, respectively.

In excreta radioactivity contains mainly pristinamycin I_B and RP-73430 (N-desmethyl derivative). Up to 24 metabolites of pristinamycin I_B have been detected. In feces, unchanged pristinamycin I_B represented 73% of the dose. Pristinamycin II_B was also one of the main compounds. Up to 34 metabolites

Table 28 Pharmacokinetics of RP-106972 after food

Dose (mg)	n	Status	Pristinamycin I_B			Pristinamycin II_B		
			C_{max} (μg/ml)	T_{max} (h)	AUC (μg·h/ml)	C_{max} (μg/ml)	T_{max} (h)	AUC (μg·h/ml)
1,000	16	Fasting	0.30	0.75	0.61	0.48	0.5	0.72
	16	Milk	0.38	2.25	0.91	0.57	1.75	1.23
500	16	Meal	0.35	1.75	1.14	0.63	1.0	1.59
	20	Water	0.16	0.5	0.27	0.26	0.5	0.35
	20	Grapefruit	0.17	2.0	0.33	0.30	1.0	0.53

Table 29 Pharmacokinetics of RP-106972

Administration	Doses (mg)[a]	Pristinamycin I_B			Pristinamycin II_B			n
		C_{max} (μg/ml)	T_{max} (h)	AUC (μg·h/ml)	C_{max} (μg/ml)	T_{max} (h)	AUC (μg·h/ml)	
Single	200	0.034	0.5	0.161	0.096	0.5	0.226	8
	400	0.12	0.8	0.279	0.21	0.8	0.321	8
	800	0.30	1.0	0.615	0.59	0.5	0.865	8
	1,200	0.32	1.3	0.706	0.57	0.5	0.956	8
	2,400	0.71	2.0	1.770	0.90	1.5	1.83	6
	3,600	0.60	1.5	1.450	0.85	0.75	1.64	6
	4,000	1.0	1.5	3.220	1.14	1.0	2.61	6
	250	0.08	1.3	0.18				6
	500	0.15	1.0	0.28				6
	1,000	0.56	0.8					6
	2,000	0.65	0.9					6
	3,000	0.82	1.4					6
Multiple								
Day 1	600	0.18	0.5	0.210	0.45	0.5	0.47	6
	1,200	0.39	0.5	0.530	0.80	0.5	0.94	6
	1,800	0.48	0.75	1.190	0.79	0.5	1.77	6
	500 b.i.d.	0.15	1.0	0.37	0.44	0.5	0.65	6
	1,000 b.i.d.	0.37	0.5	0.80	0.66	0.5	1.07	6
	1,000 t.i.d.	0.33	0.75	1.05	0.62	0.5	1.49	6
Day 10	600	0.17	0.75	0.370	0.40	0.5	0.71	6
	1,200	0.40	0.5	0.620	0.74	0.5	1.08	6
	1,800	0.34	2.0	0.850	0.89	0.5	1.73	6
Day 7	500 b.i.d.	0.11	0.75	0.25	0.39	0.75	0.61	6
	1,000 b.i.d.	0.37	1.5	0.91	0.41	1.0	0.97	6
	1,000 t.i.d.	0.19	0.75	0.48	0.44	0.5	0.81	6

[a]b.i.d., twice a day; t.i.d., three times a day.

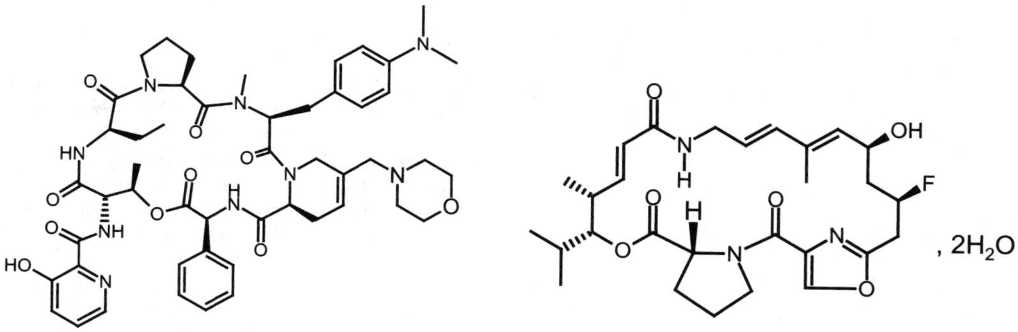

RPR202868 RPR132552A , $2H_2O$

Figure 11 XRP 2868

Table 30 In vitro activity of XRP 2868

Organism(s)[a]	*n*	MIC (μg/ml)					
		XRP 2868		Pristinamycin		Dalfopristin-quinupristin	
		50	90	50	90	50	90
MSSA	16	0.12	0.12	0.25	0.50	0.25	0.50
MRSA	25	0.12	0.25	0.25	1.0	0.25	0.50
GISA[b]	3	0.12		0.25		0.12	
S. aureus Lin[ra]	1	0.25		0.5		0.25	
S. pyogenes	27	≤0.06	≤0.06	0.12	0.12	0.25	0.25
S. agalactiae	15	0.06	0.06	025	0.25	1.0	1.0
Group C and G streptococci	15	0.12	0.25	0.25	0.25	1.0	1.0
Viridans group streptococci	20	0.12	0.25	0.5	0.5	1.0	1.0
S. pneumoniae Ery[s]	141	0.12	0.25	0.25	0.25	0.5	0.5
S. pneumoniae Ery[r]	120	0.25	0.5	0.25	0.5	0.5	1.0
S. epidermidis	14	0.06	0.5	0.12	1.0	0.12	0.25
E. faecalis	21	1.0	2.0	2.0	8.0	8.0	16
E. faecalis Van[r]	16	1.0	2.0	4.0	8.0	8.0	32
E. faecium	11	≤0.06	0.5	0.25	0.5	0.5	2.0
E. faecium VanA	12	0.12	0.25	0.25	0.5	0.5	1.0
E. faecium Lin[rb]	12	0.12	0.25	0.25	0.5	1.0	
E. faecium Q/D[rb]	3	1.0		2.0		4.0	
E. casseliflavus	15	0.5	0.5	1.0	1.0	2.0	4.0
E. gallinarum	15	0.25	0.5	0.5	0.5	2.0	2.0
E. avium	10	0.5	1.0	0.5	2.0	2.0	4.0
E. raffinosus[b]	3	0.5		1.0		2.0	
C. jeikeium	10	≤0.03	0.25	0.12	0.5	0.25	0.5
H. influenzae β⁻	50	0.25	0.5	1.0	2.0	2.0	4.0
H. influenzae β⁺	79	0.25	1.0	1.0	2.0	4.0	4.0
H. influenzae BLNAR	21	0.25	0.5	1.0	1.0	2.0	4.0

[a]β⁻, non-β-lactamase producing; β⁺, β-lactamase producing; BLNAR, non-β-lactamase-producing strains.
[b]MIC (in micrograms per milliliter).

Table 31 Activity of XRP 2868 against well-defined *S. pneumoniae* (genotypes)

Mechanism	No. of strains for which the MIC is (in μg/ml):					Total
	0.06	0.12	0.25	0.5	1.0	
23S rRNA		1	1			2
ermB	3	17	6	2		26
L4			2	15		17
mef	3	16	4	1		24
Total	6	34	13	18		69

were distinguished, among them RP-60389 (*trans*-diol dervative) and RP-60388 (*cis*-diol derivative). In feces, unchanged pristinamycin II_B accounted for 36% of the dose.

The main route of elimination of both components was via bile, with less than 5% of the administered dose being recovered in urine.

6. XRP 2868

XRP 2868, a new semisynthetic oral streptogramin, consists of a 30:70 combination of RPR 202868 (a pristinamycin I_A derivative and RPR 132552A (a pristinamycin II_B derivative) (Fig. 11).

XRP 2868 is more active in vitro and in vivo than pristinamycin and dalfopristin-quinupristin (Table 30). Irrespective of the mechanism of resistance to erythromycin A, XRP 2868 remains active (Table 31), except for a L4 mutation.

XRP 2868 is rapidly bactericidal (less than 2 h) against *S. pneumoniae* and *H. influenzae*. Against isolates resistant to erythromycin A, XRP 2868 remains bactericidal, but slowly; this was also shown with telithromycin-resistant pneumococci, which today are rarely isolated.

REFERENCES

Aujard Y, Bingen E, 1988, Synergistines et infections sévères à staphylocoques de l'enfant, p 125–130, in Pocidalo JJ, Vachon F, Coulaud JP, Vildé J, ed, Macrolides et synergistines, Arnette.

Aumercier M, Capman ML, Marlard M, Le Goffic F, 1985, Autoradiography of tissue distribution of the IIA constituent of the pristinamycin, J Antimicrob Chemother, 16, suppl A, 201–204.

Aumercier M, Lacroix P, Capman MI, Le Goftic F, 1985, Dérivés hydrosolubles du facteur IA des pristinamycines: interactions avec le ribosome bactérien, Pathol Biol, 33, 497–501.

Barrière JC, Bouanchaud DH, Desnottes JF, Paris JM, 1994, Streptogramin analogues, Expert Opin Investig Drugs, 3, 115–131.

Barrière JC, Bouanchaud DH, Paris JH, Tollen O, Harris NV, Smith C, 1992, Antimicrobial activity against Staphylococcus aureus of semisynthetic injectable streptogramins, RP 59500 and related compounds, J Antimicrob Chemother, 30, suppl A, 1–8.

Bébéar C, Renaudin H, Texier-Maugein J, de Barbeyrac B, 1988, Activité in vitro des macrolides et de la pristinamycine sur les mycoplasmes, p 155–161, in Pocidalo JJ, Vachon F, Coulaud JP, Vildé J, ed, Macrolides et synergistines, Arnette.

Benazet F, Bourat G, 1965, Etude radiographique de la répartition du constituant IA de la pristinamycine (7293 RP), C R Acad Sci, 260, 2522–2525.

Benazet F, Dubost M, 1968, Etude biologique de la pristinamycine, activité in vitro, activité chez l'animal de laboratoire, circulation, métabolisme, Rev Med, 9, 6–23.

Bernard E, Bensoussan M, Bensoussan F, Etienne S, Cazenave I, Carsenti-Etesse E, Le Roux Y, Montay G, Dellamonica P, 1994, Pharmacokinetics and suction blister fluid penetration of a semisynthesis injectable streptogramin RP 59500 (RP 57669/RP 54476), Eur J Clin Microbiol Infect Dis, 13, 768–771.

Berthanol N, Charles Y, Gouin AM, Hereau B, Rousseau J, Desnottes JF, 1995, RPR 106972, a new oral streptogramin: in vitro antibacterial activity, 35th Intersci Conf Antimicrob Agents Chemother, abstract F-112.

Berthaud N, Huet Y, Bourgues A, Bussiere JC, Santeole M, Selingue M, Desnottes JF, 1995, In vivo bactericidal activity of RPR 106972, a new oral streptogramin in S. pneumoniae mouse septicemia, 35th Intersci Conf Antimicrob Agents Chemother, abstract F-116.

Boon B, Gilbert M, Lamy F, 1973, Etude des taux plasmatiques et urinaires de la virginiamycine chez l'homme, Thérapie, 28, 367–377.

Burridge R, Warren C, Phillipps L, 1986, Macrolide, lincosamide and streptogramin resistance in Campylobacter jejuni/coli, J Antimicrob Chemother, 17, 315–321.

Chevalier P, Paccaly A, Bourriot JP, Le Roux Y, Montay G, Thebault JJ, Chassard D, Pichard E, 1995, Etude de la pharmacocinétique des pristinamycines chez des volontaires en bonne santé, Med Mal Infect, 25, 1153–1160.

Christol D, Boussougant Y, Buré A, Witchitz J, Zribi A, Dupuis M, 1971, A propos de 220 souches de streptocoques isolées d'hémoculture en milieu hospitalier: étude de l'action bactéricide des antibiotiques et leurs associations, Lyon Med, 225, 99–108.

Cocito C, 1979, Antibiotics of the virginiamycin family, inhibitors which contain synergistic components, Microbiol Rev, 43, 145–192.

Dabernat H, Delmas C, 1988, Activité in vitro des macrolides et des pristinamycines sur Haemophilus influenzae, p 163–173, in Pocidalo JJ, Vachon F, Coulaud JP, Vildé J, ed, Macrolides et synergistines, Arnette.

de Meester C, Rondelet J, 1977, Résistance à la viriginiamycine chez le staphylocoque, Pathol Biol, 25, 685–689.

Dournon E, Rajagopalan P, 1988, Effets de la pristinamycine sur la légionellose expérimentale du cobaye, p 165–182, in Pocidalo JJ, Vachon F, Coulaud JP, Vildé J, ed, Macrolides et synergistines, Arnette.

Dubost M, Pascal C, 1965, Méthodes de dosages des constituants de la pristinamycine dans les liquides biologiques, Ann Inst Pasteur, 109, 490–504.

Etienne SD, Montay G, Le Liboux A, Frydman A, Garaud JJ, 1992, A phase 1, double-blind, placebo-controlled study of the tolerance and pharmacokinetic behaviour of RP 59500, J Antimicrob Chemother, 30, suppl 1, 123–131.

Gagnadoux MF, Loirat C, Pillion G, Bertheleme JP, Pouliquen M, Guest G, Broyer M, 1987, Néphrotoxicité due à l'interaction pristinamycine-ciclosporine chez le patient transplanté rénal, Presse Med, 16, 1781.

Gale EF, Cundliffe E, Reynolds PE, Richmard MA, Wasing MJ, 1981, Antibiotic inhibition of ribosome function, p 502–547, in The Molecular Basis of Antibiotic Action, 2nd Inter et Wilson.

Koechlin C, Kempf JF, Jehl F, Monteil H, 1990, Single oral dose pharmacokinetics of the two main components of pristinamycin in humans, J Antimicrob Chemother, 25, 651–656.

Lafaix C, Bouvet E, Dublanchet A, Dubernat H, Carrere C, Picq JJ, Etienne J, 1985, The in vitro activity of pristinamycin against Haemophilus influenzae and Neisseria meningitidis, J Antimicrob Chemother, 16, suppl A, 221–223.

Latorest H, Fourgesud M, Richet H, Lagrange PH, 1988, Comparative in vitro activities of pristinamycin, its components, and other antimicrobial agents against anaerobic bacteria, Antimicrob Agents Chemother, 32, 1094–1096.

Leclercq R, Nantas L, Soussy CJ, Duval J, 1992, Activity of RP 59500, a new parenteral semisynthetic streptogramin, against staphylococci with various mechanisms of resistance to macrolide-lincosamide-streptogramin antibiotics, J Antimicrob Chemother, 30, suppl A, 67–76.

Le Goffic F, 1985, Structure activity relationship in lincosamide and streptogramin antibiotics, J Antimicrob Chemother, 16, suppl 1, 13–21.

Le Goffic F, Capmau ML, Bonnet D, Cerceau C, Soussy C, Dublanchet A, Duval J, 1977, Plasmid-mediated pristinamycin resistance PAC IIA, a new enzyme which modifies pristinamycin IIA, J Antibiot (Tokyo), 30, 665–669.

Maillard M, Pellerat J, 1965, Comportement de la pristinamycine dans le sang humain, Ann Inst Pasteur, 109, 314–316.

Martinet MR, Vedrine Y, Piquet V, Frydman A, 1992, Lack of effect of streptogramins on hepatic drug metabolism enzyme in the rat, Drug Metab Disp, 20, 490–495.

Nguyen J, 1988, Activité in vitro antipneumococcique des streptogramines, p 115–118, in Pocidalo JJ, Vachon F, Coulaud JP, Vildé J, ed, Macrolides et synergistines, Arnette.

Orfila J, Haider F, 1984, Action de la pristinamycine sur les Chlamydia, Pathol Biol, 32, 443–445.

Paris JM, Barrière JC, Smith C, Bost PE, 1990, The chemistry of pristinamycins, p 182–248, in Lukacs G, Ohno M, ed, Recent Progress in the Chemical Synthesis of Antibiotics, Springer-Verlag.

Paris JM, Rolin O, Corbet JP, Cotrel C, Bouanchaud DH, 1985, Relation structure-activité des dérivés semi-synthétiques du constituant PIA de la pristinamycine, Pathol Biol, 33, 493–496.

Pechère JC, 1992, In vitro activity of RP 59500, a semisynthetic streptogramin against staphylococci and streptococci, J Antimicrob Chemother, 30, suppl A, 15–18.

Preud'homme J, Belloc A, Charpentié Y, Tarridec P, 1965, Un antibiotique formé de deux groupes de composants à synergie d'action: la pristinamycine, C R Acad Sci 260, 1309–1312.

Raoult D, Drancourt M, 1988, Macrolides et rickettsioses, p 163–166, in Pocidalo JJ, Vachon F, Coulaud JP, Vildé J, ed, Macrolides et synergistines, Arnette.

Roberfroid M, Dumont P, 1972, Absorption and metabolism of tritionlabelled factor M1 of virginiamycin by oral and parenteral administration, J Antibiot (Tokyo), 25, 30–38.

Rolin O, Bouanchaud DH, 1988, Activité antipneumococcique de la pristinamycine dans deux modèles expériementaux de la souris, p 120–124, in Pocidalo JJ, Vachon F, Coulaud JP, Vildé J, ed, Macrolides et synergistines, Arnette.

Spangler S, Jacobs M, Appelbaum P, 1995, Antipneumococcal activity of RPR 106972 (a new oral streptogramin) and oral β-lactams, 35th Intersci Conf Antimicrob Agents Chemother, abstract F-113.

Tamaka N, 1975, Mikamycin, in Corcoran JN, Hahn FE, ed, Antibiotics, vol 3, Springer-Verlag.

Tenover FC, Baker CN, 1995, RP 59500 (quinupristin/dalfopristin): development of peritoneal disk diffusion break point for testing RP 59500 (quinupristin/dalfopristin), an injectable streptogramin, 35th Intersci Conf Antimicrob Agents Chemother, abstract D-30.

Thyss A, Milano G, Renée N, Cassulo-Viguier E, Jambon P, Soler C, 1993, Severe interaction between methotrexate and a macrolide-like antibiotic, J Natl Cancer Inst, 85, 582–583.

Vaquez D, 1967, The streptogramin family of antibiotics, p 387–403, in Gottlieb D, Shaw PD, ed, Antibiotics, vol 1, Springer-Verlag.

Vaquez D, 1975, The streptogramin family of antibiotics, p 521–534, in Corcoran JN, Hahn PE, Antibiotics, vol 3, Springer-Verlag.

Videau D, 1965, La pristinamycine et le phénomène de bactériospause, Ann Inst Pasteur, 108, 602–622.

Videau D, Roiron V, 1965, Titrages et taux sanguins de la pristinamycine chez l'homme, Presse Med, 73, 2101–2103.

Lincosamines

A. BRYSKIER

21

1. INTRODUCTION

Lincomycin was isolated in 1962 from the fermentation of *Streptomyces lincolnensis* subsp. *lincolnensis*. The fermentation medium also contained other components of lincomycin: lincomycin B (4′-depropyl-4′-ethyllincomycin), lincomycin C (1-demethyl-1-ethylthiolincomycin), lincomycin D (1-demethyllincomycin), and lincomycin S (1′-demethyl-1-ethylthiolincomycin). With the exception of lincomycin D, the different molecules exhibit good antibacterial activity against gram-positive cocci, apart from *Enterococcus faecalis*.

Within this family, one molecule—celesticetin—was isolated in 1955 by Deboer et al. from the fermentation broth of *Streptomyces caelestis*, the structure of which was elucidated in 1968 by Hoeksema. It differs from lincomycin by the presence of a methoxy group instead of a hydroxyl group at position 7. A derivative of celesticetin has been described which, in contrast to celesticetin, is inactive, while the latter has weaker antibacterial activity than that of lincomycin.

Numerous derivatives have been prepared from lincomycin by semisynthesis to enlarge the antibacterial spectrum and enhance the antibacterial activity. A series of 7-chlorolincomycin derivatives has been synthesized, yielding clindamycin. Two human medicinal drugs have been in clinical practice, lincomycin and clindamycin; pirlimycin has been used in veterinary medicine. Mirincamycin has only undergone clinical development. These molecules, particularly clindamycin, possess antibacterial, and to a certain extent antiprotozoal, activity.

1.1. Chemical Structures

The lincosamides consist of three components: an amino acid, a sugar, and an amide bond connecting these two moieties to one another.

The amino acid residue is an L-proline substituted by a 4′-alkyl-(*trans*-1-methyl-4-*n*-propyl-L-proline) chain. The sugar is lincosamine.

Lincosamine is a thiooctopyranoside.

Clindamycin is the 7(S)-chlorodeoxylincomycin derivative (Fig. 1). Pirlimycin (U-57930E) is the 4-*cis*-ethyl-L-pipecolic derivative of clindamycin.

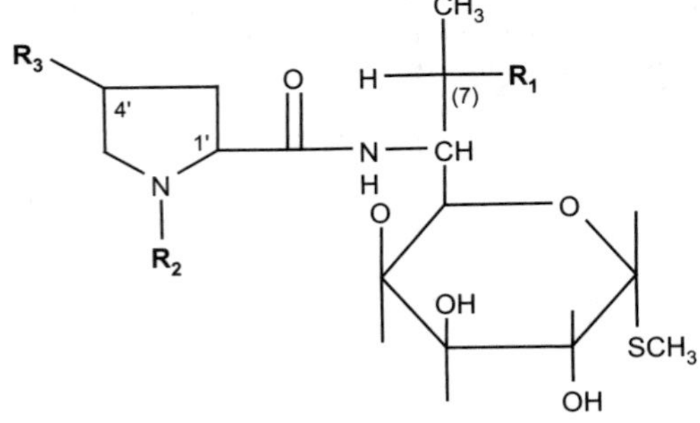

	R_1	R_2	R_3
Lincomycin	-H	$-CH_3$	-n C_3H_7
Clindamycin (U 21251 F)	-Cl	$-CH_3$	-n C_3H_7
Mirincamycin (U 24729A)	-Cl	-H	-n C_5H_{11}
U 26285 A	-Cl	-H	-n C_3H_7

Figure 1 Lincosamides

1.2. Physicochemical Properties

1.2.1. Lincomycin

Lincomycin is a weak base. Lincomycin hydrochloride is soluble in water, methanol, and ethanol and poorly soluble in organic solvents such as acetone, ether, and chloroform.

1.2.2. Clindamycin

Clindamycin hydrochloride (1,090 mg of clindamycin hydrochloride is equivalent to 1,000 mg of clindamycin base) is soluble in water but is less soluble in ethanol, chloroform, and ether than is lincomycin hydrochloride.

There is also a palmitate salt of clindamycin hydrochloride for oral use.

Clindamycin phosphate (1,200 mg is equivalent to 1,000 mg of clindamycin base) is soluble in water.

The principal physicochemical characteristics are summarized in Table 1.

Table 1 Physicochemical properties of lincosamides

Drug	Form	Empirical formula	Mol wt	pK	Lipophilicity (n-octanol/water)	Water solubility (mg/ml)
Lincomycin	Base	$C_{18}H_{34}N_2O_6S$	406.56	7.6		400–600
	Chlorhydrate	$C_{18}H_{34}N_2O_6S,HCl\text{-}H_2O$	461.01		15	500–1,000
Clindamycin	Base	$C_{18}H_{33}ClN_2O_2S$	424.98	6.2		
	Chlorhydrate	$C_{18}H_{33}ClN_2O_5S, HCl\text{-}H_2O$	461.44	7.45/7.6	1.85	5–10
	Phosphate	$C_{18}H_{34}ClN_2O_8S$	504.98	5.75/8.05	166.1	200–300
	Palmitate HCl	$C_{34}H_{63}ClN_2O_6S$, HCl	699.86	7.6		<1

Physiological solutions of lincomycin are stable for 24 h at room temperature. A number of compounds with which lincomycin is incompatible have been reported: β-lactams (penicillin G, cloxacillin, methicillin, ampicillin, ticarcillin, and cephalothin), novobiocin, hydrocortisone, streptomycin, vitamin B, and potassium canrenoate.

The following compounds have been reported to be incompatible with clindamycin phosphate: ampicillin, calcium gluconate, magnesium sulfate, phenytoin, group B vitamins, and barbiturates.

Solutions containing tobramycin sulfate and clindamycin phosphate are unstable.

1.3. Structure-Activity Relationship

1.3.1. Modifications of the Nucleus

Various substituents have been introduced at N-1′ and C-4′. Optimal antibacterial activity is obtained by increasing the length of the hydrocarbon chain at position C-4′ in the presence of a hexyl group. The isomer in the *cis* position has half the antibacterial activity of the *trans* isomer.

However, the enhanced in vitro activity does not parallel the in vivo activity. The optimum is achieved when the hydrocarbon chain reaches six carbons. The bioavailability increases with the length of the chain, but nonlinearly, whereas the lipophilicity increases more regularly. 5′-Propyl, 4′-ethoxy (*cis* and *trans*), 4′-carboethoxy, and 4′-tosyloxy derivatives have been synthesized, but their activities are weaker than that of lincomycin.

1.3.2. Variations at N′-1

The *N*-demethyl-4′-alkyl derivatives have not insignificant antibacterial activity. *N*-Demethyllincomycin is weakly active, but increasing the length of the chain at C-4′ enhances its activity.

The introduction of different alkyl groups yields various results. As a general rule, *N*-demethyl-*N*-ethyllincomycin is active and the *N*-ethyl derivatives are more active than the *N*-methyl derivatives. However, the increase in the alkyl chain at this point first reduces and then abolishes the activity.

Among the *N*-demethyl-*N*-ethyl-4′-alkyl molecules, the derivative with five carbon atoms is the most active, with double the activity for the *trans* derivatives as opposed to the *cis* derivatives.

1.3.3. Modification of the Carbohydrate

The α-thiol group in the β configuration is necessary for the activity of lincomycin. Various substituents of the α-thiol group have been proposed—ethyl, isopropyl, butyl, and methylvinyl—and have yielded bacteriologically active molecules. The absence of the α-thiol group results in a molecule which is weakly active, if at all.

Variations have been made to the substituents at position 7, giving rise to clindamycin, pirlimycin, and mirincamycin.

The hydroxyl group at position 7 may be replaced by an *epi*-hydroxy (half the activity of lincomycin) or a 7-keto (2% of the activity of lincomycin); 7-deoxy-7(*S*)-chlorolincomycin has four times the activity of lincomycin, and its 7-*epi*-chlorolincomycin isomer is one and a half times more active than lincomycin.

The 7(*S*)-bromolincomycin derivative is eight times more active, but replacement of the hydroxyl group by a hydrogen yields a derivative with one-tenth the activity of clindamycin.

Pirlimycin has been described by Karim et al. This is a derivative of 7(*S*)-chloroclindamycin. It differs in that the amine residue is a 4-*cis*-ethyl-L-pipecolic acid. Several bacteriological studies have shown that this molecule is less active than clindamycin against *Staphylococcus aureus* but is three to four times more active against anaerobic bacteria. It appears to possess antimalarial activity.

The chain of lincomycin is in the D(−) *threo* position, whereas that of clindamycin is in the L(+) *threo* position, in the *S* configuration.

1.3.4. Simultaneous Modifications of the Proline and the Carbohydrate Residue

Margerlein and Kajan synthesized derivatives from clindamycin with variable substituents at N-1 and C-4′ of the proline.

While the *N*-demethyllincomycin derivative possesses only 2% of the activity of lincomycin against *S. aureus*, this is not the case with the derivatives of clindamycin. Some molecules exhibit greater activity.

Some authors have shown that the antibacterial activity increases with the length of the 4′-alkyl chain, reaching a maximum when the substituent at C-4′ is a pentyl (n-C_5H_{11}). These results are obtained in vitro with lincomycin. However, in vivo the results are different, with the activity following a parallel course.

1.3.5. Antibacterial Activity

Lincosamides are antibiotics whose antibacterial spectrum includes gram-positive cocci, anaerobic bacteria, and certain so-called atypical bacteria. Enterobacteria, *Pseudomonas* spp., and *Acinetobacter* spp. are excluded from the antibacterial spectrum of the lincosamides (Tables 2, 3, and 4).

The lincosamides possess good antistaphylococcal activity. They are active against methicillin-susceptible *S. aureus* strains but not against methicillin-resistant strains (MIC, >64 μg/ml). They are active against coagulase-negative staphylococci, with the exception of *Staphylococcus cohnii*, *Staphylococcus sciuri*, and *Staphylococcus xylosus*, which have low-level resistance to lincomycin and to streptogramin type B. The MICs of lincomycin are 4 to 8 μg/ml, as opposed to

Table 2 In vitro activity of lincomycin

Organism(s)	MIC (μg/ml)
S. aureus	0.2–3.1
S. aureus Met^r	>64
S. epidermidis	0.8–1.5
S. pyogenes	0.04–0.5
S. pneumoniae	0.01–0.5
E. faecalis	6–100
Enterococcus faecium	0.4–100
N. gonorrhoeae	16
N. meningitidis	>5
B. pertussis	3.12–50
H. influenzae	16–128
C. diphtheriae	0.4
M. pneumoniae	4.0
M. hominis	0.6
Pasteurella multocida	1.6
H. pylori	3.2–12
U. urealyticum	>64
C. jejuni	1.6–>50
C. trachomatis	256
Nocardia spp.	3.1–>100
Actinomyces spp.	0.03–1.0
B. fragilis	>0.1–2.5
Peptostreptococcus spp.	>0.1–1.6
C. perfringens	>0.1–1.6
C. difficile	>64
Veillonella spp.	>0.1–6.2
Prevotella melaninogenica	>0.1–0.4
Fusobacterium spp.	>0.1–6.2
Eubacterium spp.	>0.1–3.1
Propionibacterium spp.	>0.1–1.6
Eikenella corrodens	<0.02–10
Bifidobacterium spp.	0.1–1.6
Porphyromonas spp.	0.1

Table 3 In vitro activity of clindamycin

Microorganism(s)	MIC (μg/ml)		
	50%	90%	Range
S. aureus Met^s	0.12	0.125	
S. aureus Met^r	1.0	>16	
Coagulase-negative staphylococci	0.25	>16	
S. pyogenes	0.03	0.06	
Streptococcus agalactiae	0.06	0.5	
S. pneumoniae Pen^s	0.125	0.25	
S. pneumoniae Pen^r	1.0	16	
Enterococcus spp.	>16	>16	
Viridans group streptococci	0.5	0.5	
N. meningitidis			>5
N. gonorrhoeae			2.0
B. pertussis			0.25–>8
B. bronchiseptica			≤32
H. influenzae			8.0
M. pneumoniae			1.0
M. hominis			0.03
U. urealyticum			2.0
C. trachomatis			1.0
C. jejuni	0.4	0.8	0.1–>50
H. pylori	0.5	2.0	0.25–2.0
G. vaginalis	0.003	0.06	0.2–2.0
Nocardia spp.			0.78–0.25
Actinomyces spp.			0.03–0.25
L. pneumophila			12.5
C. diphtheriae			≤0.2

Table 4 In vitro activity of clindamycin against anaerobes

Organism(s)	MIC (μg/ml)
Peptostreptococcus spp.	0.05
Eubacterium limosum	0.2
Propionibacterium acnes	0.01
Bifidobacterium spp.	0.01
Clostridium ramosum	0.78
C. perfringens	0.025
C. tetani	≤0.006
C. difficile	6.25
Clostridium novyi	0.01
Clostridium sporogenes	6.25
Veillonella parvula	0.025
B. fragilis	0.1
B. thetaiotaomicron	1.56
P. melaninogenica	0.025
Prevotella spp.	≤0.006
Porphyromonas spp.	≤0.006
Fusobacterium spp.	≤0.01

0.5 to 1 μg/ml for susceptible strains. They are inactive against enterococci. They possess good activity against group A and B streptococci, viridans group streptococci, and *Streptococcus pneumoniae*. These strains appear to be inhibited by concentrations of about 0.4 μg/ml. The lincosamides are active against *Corynebacterium diphtheriae*, *Nocardia* spp., and *Bacillus anthracis* but are inactive against *Listeria monocytogenes*. Clindamycin is active against *Erysipelothrix rhusiopathiae*. They are inactive or weakly active against *Neisseria meningitidis* and *Neisseria gonorrhoeae*, *Haemophilus influenzae*, *Moraxella catarrhalis*, and *Pasteurella* spp. Clindamycin is active against *Bordetella pertussis*, but lincomycin is inactive. Clindamycin is inactive against *Bordetella bronchiseptica*. Against *Campylobacter jejuni*, clindamycin possesses good activity (MIC at which 50% of isolates tested are inhibited [MIC_{50}], ~0.4 μg/ml), whereas lincomycin is inactive. The activity of clindamycin against *Helicobacter pylori* is good (MIC, ~1 μg/ml).

The lincosamides are inactive against *Legionella pneumophila*. Clindamycin has activity against *Chlamydia trachomatis*, with a MIC on the order of 1.0 μg/ml, whereas lincomycin is inactive (MIC, ~ 256 μg/ml). In contrast to the 14-membered-ring macrolides, apart from certain ketolides, clindamycin is active against *Mycoplasma hominis* but is weakly inactive against *Mycoplasma pneumoniae* and *Ureaplasma urealyticum*. Clindamycin is active against *Gardnerella vaginalis* (Table 3). Lincomycin is active against *Leptospira* spp. Clindamycin has good activity against anaerobes.

Among gram-positive anaerobes, clindamycin has good activity against *Clostridium perfringens*, *Clostridium tetani*, and *Clostridium difficile*. Its activity against *Bifidobacterium*, *Peptococcus*, *Peptostreptococcus*, and *Propionibacterium* spp. is moderate. It exhibits good activity against *Eubacterium*.

Among gram-negative anaerobes, clindamycin displays good activity against the *Bacteroides fragilis* group, with the exception of *Bacteroides thetaiotaomicron*, *Porphyromonas* spp., and *Prevotella* spp. The activity against *Veillonella* spp. is good (MIC, ~0.05 μg/ml).

1.3.5.1. Breakpoints

The breakpoints recommended by the French Committee for Antibiotic Susceptibility Testing, which belongs to the French Microbiology Society, are summarized in Table 5.

For quality control, reference strain *S. aureus* ATCC 25923 was used; its zone of inhibition is 24 to 30 mm.

1.3.5.2. Mechanisms of Action

The lincosamides act on the 50S subunit of the bacterial ribosome. The binding sites are similar to those for erythromycin A. The lincosamides prevent transpeptidation during the formation of the peptide chain by inhibiting peptidyltransferase.

1.4. Resistance Mechanisms

The antibacterial spectrum of the lincosamides does not include gram-negative bacilli. The "natural" resistance of Enterobacteriaceae, *Pseudomonas* spp., and *Acinetobacter* spp. may be explained by the relative impermeability of the bacteria cell wall to these hydrophobic molecules. In gram-positive cocci, penetration is a passive phenomenon. The enterococci have natural resistance to the lincosamides. Acquired resistance to lincosamides is of the macrolide-lincosamide-streptogramin B (MLS_B) type and may be due to three mechanisms: modification of the bacterial target, modification of the antibiotics, and reduction of parietal permeability (Table 6).

The modification of the target is due to methylation of an adenine residue on the 23S RNA of the 50S subunit by a bacterial methylase.

In *S. aureus*, when the phenotypical expression is of a constitutive type, the resistance encompasses all macrolides, lincosamides, and streptogramin B; conversely, when it is of an inducible type, there is a dissociation between the three molecular groups and the lincosamides remain active, even if the activity is reduced. In streptococci, in contrast to *S. aureus*, the lincosamides can induce resistance.

A plasmid-mediated 3-lincomycin- or 4-clindamycin-*O*-nucleotyltransferase has been detected in *S. aureus*. There is high-level resistance to lincomycin, and a reduction in susceptibility to clindamycin has been noted (Fig. 2).

In coagulase-negative staphylococci, the essential mechanism of resistance is of the MLS_B type and is identical to that of *S. aureus*. These species possess more specific resistance mechanisms, such as a reduction in permeability to 14-membered-ring macrolides as has been described for *Staphylococcus epidermidis*. The 14-membered-ring macrolides may also be inactivated enzymatically; this resistance phenotype has been described for *Staphylococcus hominis*, *Staphylococcus haemolyticus*, and *Staphylococcus saprophyticus*.

Like *S. aureus*, certain species may inactivate lincomycin or clindamycin by a plasmid-mediated enzyme: *O*-nucleotidyltransferase.

It has been shown that strains of *B. fragilis* are divided into three groups:

- Those which are very susceptible to clindamycin (MIC, ≤0.25 μg/ml)
- Those which are moderately susceptible (MIC, 0.25 to 8 μg/ml)
- Those which are resistant (MIC, ≥16 μg/ml)

Strains of *S. pneumoniae* and *Streptococcus pyogenes* susceptible to clindamycin and resistant to erythromycin A derivatives have been described. This dissociation is due to an efflux resistance mechanism.

Table 5 Critical concentrations of lincosamides (CFA-SFM-France, 2002)

Drug	Disk load	MIC (μg/ml)	Zone diam (mm)
Lincomycin	15 μg	2–8	>21–<17
Clindamycin	2 IU	2	>15

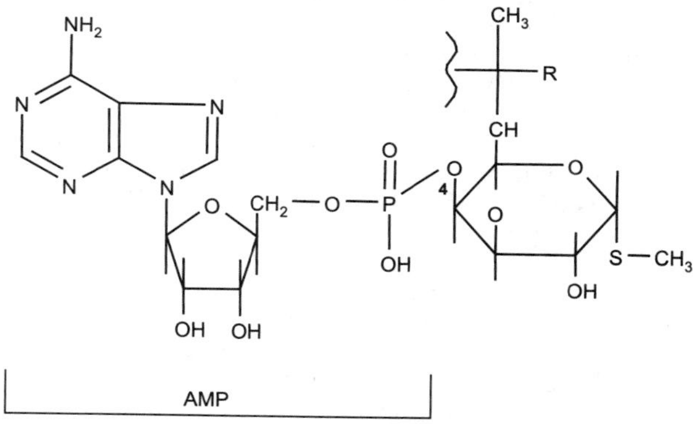

NH2 N N N N O CH2 O P O OH OH OH O 4 O CH3 R CH O O S—CH3 OH AMP

Figure 2 Inactivation of lincosamides by nucleotidylation at position 4

Table 6 Resistance phenotypes

Mechanism of resistance	Genotype[a]	Phenotype[b]		
		Erythromycin A	Lincomycin	Clindamycin
Methylation	*erm* (I)	R	S	S
	erm (C)	R	R	R
Inactivation	*eri*	R	S	S
	linA	S	R	S
	lsa	S	I	S
	saa-sbh	S	S/I	S/I
Permeability	*erpA*	R	S	S

[a]I, inducible; C, constitutive.
[b]R, resistant; S, susceptible; I, intermediate.

1.5. Epidemiology of Resistance

In 1981, an epidemiological survey showed that about 5% of strains belonging to the *B. fragilis* group, 10% of strains of *Clostridium* other than *C. perfringens*, 10% of strains of *Peptostreptococcus*, and about 90% of strains of *Fusobacterium* were resistant to clindamycin.

In France, about 16 to 20% of strains of *B. fragilis* are resistant to clindamycin (MIC, >4 μg/ml).

In Spain, the rate of resistance to clindamycin for the *B. fragilis* group was about 1% in 1975, increasing to 7 to 8% in 1987. A study in 1992 showed that 19% of strains of *Peptostreptococcus*, 10.5% of strains of *C. perfringens*, 19.5% of all clostridia, 9% of *Eubacterium* isolates, and 20.5% of strains of the *B. fragilis* group were resistant to clindamycin. In the *B. fragilis* group, resistance varied according to the bacterial species, being about 20% for *B. fragilis*, 29% for *B. thetaiotaomicron*, 34% for *Bacteroides distasonis*, and 36.9% for *Bacteroides ovatus*. A high rate of resistance to erythromycin A (94%) was noted for *Fusobacterium*, but the rate of resistance to clindamycin was 3%, suggesting a mechanism other than MLS_B.

The prevalence of clindamycin resistance in *S. pneumoniae* and *S. pyogenes* is reported in chapter 18.

1.6. Antiparasitic Activity

Clindamycin exhibits antiplasmodial and antitoxoplasmic activities and might represent secondary treatment or a therapeutic alternative.

1.6.1. Antiplasmodial Activity

In 1967, Lewis et al. showed that clindamycin and its derivatives possessed good antiplasmodial activity, in contrast to lincomycin, which is devoid of it. The most active molecule was *N*-demethyl-7(*S*)-chloro-4′-pentyllincomycin, or mirincamycin (Table 7) (see also below).

The antibacterial and antimalarial activities of the *trans* and *cis* isomers have been shown not to vary significantly.

Lewis et al. showed that lincomycin possessed no activity against *Plasmodium berghei* in murine infection. By contrast, its 7-chlorolincomycin derivative, or clindamycin, has antiplasmodial activity. The activity of the 1′-demethyl-7(*S*)-clindamycin derivatives is similar to, or greater than, that of clindamycin, chloroquine, or diphenyl sulfone. Among these derivatives, 4′-depropyl-4′(*S,R*)-pentylclindamycin (U-24729A), or mirincamycin, has the best antiplasmodial activity and is active against chloroquine- and/or diphenyl sulfone-resistant strains.

Hill reported that clindamycin at high doses (greater than 62.5 mg/kg of body weight) possessed tissue activity following a single administration 3 h after intravenous challenge with sporozoites of *P. berghei*, and Peters reported tissue activity in a study with *Plasmodium yoelii nigeriensis* after a single administration of 10 to 30 mg of clindamycin per kg.

Table 7 Curative activity in mice infected with *P. berghei*

Drug	50% Protective dose (mg/kg)	
	Subcutaneous route	Oral route
Lincomycin	<160	<400
Clindamycin	19	39
Mirincamycin	4.7	12
U–26285A	16	28
Chloroquine	8.1	14
Dapsone	25	38

Jacob and Powers demonstrated a lack of activity of these molecules against gametocytes.

1.6.2. Mode of Action

Powers et al. studied the morphological changes induced by clindamycin and its metabolite *N*-demethyl clindamycin.

Clindamycin has three main metabolites: *N*-demethyl clindamycin, *N*-demethyl clindamycin sulfoxide, and clindamycin sulfoxide. *N*-Demethyl clindamycin is bacteriologically more active than clindamycin.

In clinical terms, these molecules have weak activity during the first 2 or 3 days, which explains the need to combine them with a fast-acting schizonticide such as quinine or amodiaquine.

The first ribosomal modifications appear after 24 h; more marked morphological changes occur during the following two parasitic cycles, particularly in the nuclear and mitochondrial apparatuses.

Seaberg et al. demonstrated that clindamycin reduces protein and nucleic acid synthesis in *Plasmodium falciparum*. This determination was performed by measuring uptake of tritiated isoleucine and hypoxanthine.

The activity of clindamycin and its main metabolites is time dependent.

1.6.3. Resistance to Clindamycin

Jacobs and Koonts succeeded in selecting a clindamycin-resistant strain after 42 passages over a period of 300 days. This strain remained stable after 51 passages over 1 year. This study was also conducted with minocycline, for which partial resistance was obtained after 86 passages over 600 days, with instability and a return to susceptibility after 16 passages. The rate of occurrence of resistance with clindamycin and minocycline is lower than with chloroquine, quinine, or pyrimethamine; in the case of pyrimethamine a resistant strain was obtained after 9 to 12 passages over 60 or 85 days. There is no cross-resistance between these various anti-infectives.

Koontz et al. studied the penetration of clindamycin and the main metabolites into the erythrocytes of mice infected with a clindamycin-susceptible and a clindamycin-resistant strain of *P. berghei*.

They showed that the mechanism of resistance to clindamycin was not related to a phenomenon of intraerythrocytic penetration. The concentrations of clindamycin in erythrocytes infected or not infected with a susceptible or resistant strain are similar. The molecules are rapidly extruded.

1.6.4. Clinical Use

Several clinical studies have been conducted with clindamycin.

Clyde et al. administered clindamycin at a dose of 450 mg every 6 h for 14 days to four patients to treat a *Plasmodium vivax* infection. A relapse occurred between 41 and 51 days after the end of treatment.

Millers et al. treated 13 nonimmune subjects with chloroquine-susceptible or chloroquine-resistant *P. falciparum* infections with a combination of clindamycin at a dosage of 450 mg every 6 h for 3 days and quinine, the latter not having satisfactory activity alone. A curative effect was obtained with the combination, but major gastrointestinal disorders were noted. Hall et al. noted the same signs of intolerance and reduced the doses of clindamycin.

Peirera et al. treated 52 patients orally or intravenously at a dosage of 20 mg/kg for 5 to 7 days, with good results. Other studies have also been undertaken in Brazil by various teams.

No studies on mirincamycin have been published, although the drug appears to be better tolerated in monkeys than clindamycin. At dosages of 80 and 160 mg/kg orally for 28 days, no abnormalities were observed in monkeys.

If clindamycin has to be used, Rieckmann recommends that a fast-acting schizonticide, such as quinine or amodiaquine, be administered first, followed by clindamycin, to avoid problems of gastrointestinal intolerance.

1.6.4.1. Activity against *Toxoplasma gondii*

Clindamycin has been proposed as replacement therapy in the treatment of encephalic toxoplasmosis in patients intolerant to sulfonamides.

There are contradictory studies on the in vitro activity of clindamycin. Derouin et al. showed that lincomycin partially inhibits the growth of toxoplasmas at concentrations greater than 0.3 μg/ml. Clindamycin exerts an inhibitory effect at 0.5 ng/ml and above, but the 90% inhibitory concentration is 100 μg/ml. The discrepancy in the results between the different studies is probably due to slow inhibition of the growth of the parasite, which occurs after 24 h.

It has been shown that clindamycin alone or in combination with pyrimethamine possesses curative activity in acute murine toxoplasmosis. Clindamycin exhibits protective activity against murine cerebral toxoplasmosis. The mechanism of action of clindamycin against *T. gondii* is unknown.

There are articles reporting good activity of the combination clindamycin-pyrimethamine (50 mg/day) in the treatment of acute cerebral toxoplasmosis, with maintenance treatment of 25 mg of pyrimethamine per day and 1.2 g of clindamycin twice weekly.

Multicenter studies have shown the potential interest of clindamycin combined with pyrimethamine in the treatment of acute cerebral toxoplasmosis.

Clindamycin has been proposed as treatment for toxoplasmic chorioretinitis.

1.6.4.2. Activity against *Pneumocystis carinii*

The combination primaquine-chloroquine exerts good activity in vitro and in vivo in experimental pneumonia in the rat (Queener et al., 1988).

Ruf and Potile (1989) tested the combination of clindamycin (900 mg every 6 h intravenously) and primaquine (30 mg daily orally) in eight patients. A marked clinical improvement was observed from the fifth day of treatment onwards.

2. PHARMACOKINETICS

2.1. Plasma Pharmacokinetics

2.1.1. Lincomycin

Lincomycin is presented in several pharmaceutical forms: oral, intravenous, intramuscular, and rectal. *Micrococcus luteus* is used in the microbiological assay, and chromatographic methods have been described.

2.1.1.1. Oral Form

After administration of 500 and 1,000 mg, peak concentrations in serum are reached in 2 to 4 h and are 1.8 to 5.3 μg/ml and 2.5 to 6.7 μg/ml, respectively. The consumption of food affects the bioavailability. Concentrations in plasma are detectable for about 12 h. Absorption of lincomycin represents about 20 to 35% of the administered dose.

Fecal elimination is 30 to 40% of the administered dose over a period of 72 h.

The bioavailability of lincomycin after oral administration is not affected by celiac disease or colonic diverticulosis, but a reduction in the concentrations in plasma has been demonstrated in patients with Crohn's disease.

2.1.1.2. Intravenous Form

After an infusion over 1 h, the concentrations obtained range from 9.1 μg/ml (300 mg) to 36.2 μg/ml (500 mg). The areas under the curve are proportional to the administered doses (300 to 1,500 mg). The mean apparent elimination half-life is 5 h, and about 40% of the administered dose is eliminated in the urine.

Plasma protein binding, principally to albumin, is dose dependent and ranges from 28 to 86%, depending on the dose and the method of determination. On average it is 75% (Table 8).

The volume of distribution is dose dependent, due to protein saturation. The volumes of distribution at steady state (mean ± standard deviation) are, respectively, 63.7 ± 23.8 liters, 78.8 ± 11.0 liters, and 10.5 ± 43.1 liters after infusion of 600, 1,200, and 2,400 mg of lincomycin for 1 h. The apparent volume of distribution is between 26.0 and 32.7 liters.

Plasma clearance is dose dependent because of protein saturation and is 13.32 ± 2.26 liters/h. The clearance of the free fraction is between 28.6 liters/h for 2,400 mg intravenously and 36.4 liters/h for 1,200 mg intravenously. Renal clearance is weak, on the order of 43 ml/min (2.6 liters/h). Urinary elimination is on the order of 30 to 40% (Tables 9 and 10).

Table 8 Protein binding of lincomycin (albumin) by ultrafiltration

Concn in plasma (μg/ml)	Protein bound (%)
2	84.6 ± 2.2
4	78.6 ± 1.6
8	75.6 ± 1.4
16	64.1 ± 2.1

Table 9 Intravenous pharmacokinetics of lincomycin

Dose (mg)	Infusion time (min)	n	C_0 (μg/ml)	AUC (μg·h/ml)	$t_{1/2}$ (h)	CL_P (liters/h)	CL_R (liters/h)	Urinary elimination (%)
300	60	6	9.1	35.5	4.57			32.8
600	60	6	16.8	61.6	4.63			37.1
900	60	6	26.1	92.5	5.18	13.32	5.1	46.0
1,200	60	6	34.1	122.3	5.62			37.9
1,500	60	6	36.2	126.2	5.23			37.3

Table 10 Intravenous pharmacokinetics of lincomycin

Dose (mg)	V_{ss} (liters)	CL_P (liters/h)	CL_P (liters/h) of free fraction	$t_{1/2}$ (h)
600	63.7 ± 232.8	9.94 ± 2.52	32.81 ± 5.78	5.12 ± 1.48
1,200	78.8 ± 11.0	10.04 ± 2.04	36.38 ± 5.95	5.45 ± 0.97
2,400	105.1 ± 43.1	11.79 ± 2.43	28.61 ± 8.62	6.41 ± 1.03

After an intravenous dose of 500 mg, fecal elimination of lincomycin is about 14% over 96 h.

2.1.1.3. Intramuscular Form

After a single intramuscular administration of 600 mg, the peak concentration in serum is between 7.2 and 18.5 μg/ml and is reached after between 0.5 and 5 h. After repeated doses of 600 mg, the residual concentration (8 h) is 6.4 μg/ml. After a daily dose of 500 mg, the residual concentration at 24 h is 1.1 μg/ml. The apparent elimination half-life range is 4 to 5 h. The plasma clearance is dose dependent and is between 0.098 and 0.139 liter/kg.

Urinary elimination is between 10 and 47%, depending on the study. Fecal elimination after a dose of 500 mg is 4 to 6% over a period of 48 to 72 h.

The bioavailability after intramuscular administration appears to be absolute.

2.1.1.4. Rectal Form

After administration of a 500-mg suppository of lincomycin, the peak concentration in serum of 1.1 μg/ml is reached in 1.5 h, with an area under the curve of 8.9 μg·h/ml, compared to a peak of 2.8 μg/ml and an area under the curve of 25.7 μg·h/ml after administration of a rectal solution of lincomycin.

2.1.1.5. Specific Underlying Diseases

2.1.1.5.1. Patients with renal insufficiency. After intramuscular administration of 600 mg of lincomycin, the apparent elimination half-life, the peak concentration in serum, and the area under the curve are increased. Lincomycin is not dialyzable.

2.1.1.5.2. Patients with hepatic insufficiency. After a single dose of 600 mg intramuscularly to patients with hepatic insufficiency, the apparent elimination half-life is increased (8.90 versus 4.85 h) and the peak concentration in serum is decreased (9.2 versus 12.8 μg/ml).

2.1.1.5.3. Children. After an intramuscularly administered dose of lincomycin of 3.33 mg/kg, the peak concentration in serum of 9.6 μg/ml (5.7 to 15.9 μg/ml) is reached in 1 h. After repeated doses of 3.33 mg/kg every 8 h for 3 days, the peak concentration in serum is 9.2 μg/ml and the residual concentration is 2.2 μg/ml.

Lincomycin was administered in the form of capsules to a small number of children. After a dose of 250 mg (39.3 mg/kg/day) every 8 h for 7 days, the peak concentration in serum was 7.8 μg/ml and the residual concentration was 2.7 μg/ml (Table 11).

2.1.1.6. Metabolism

A small amount of lincomycin is inactivated in the liver. The metabolites have not fully been characterized and are devoid of antibacterial activity.

Table 11 Pharmacokinetics of oral lincomycin (capsule) after repeated doses

Dose (mg/kg/day)	Regimen	n	C_{max} (μg/ml)	C_{min} (μg/ml)
22.2–26.2	64 × 6–10 days	3	1.5	0.8
39.3	84 × 7 days	1	7.8	2.7
44.0	64 × 8 days	1	8.1	0.8
51.0	64 × 7 days	1	16.9	2.8

2.1.1.7. Tissue Distribution

Biliary elimination is extensive, ranging from 30 to 40% of the administered dose.

The concentrations obtained in bone range from 0.7 to 9.4 mg/kg, depending on the method of administration but not the dose.

Concentrations in the bronchial mucosa, lung tissue, and pleural fluid are moderate.

The concentrations obtained in the cerebrospinal fluid are weak and exhibit major interindividual variations. The concentrations obtained in cerebral tissue range from 0.5 to 1.92 mg/kg after intravenous infusion of 40 to 50 mg/kg.

Concentrations in the ascites fluid are high. Concentrations in the ocular apparatus are high for the aqueous humor (1.3 to 156.2 μg/ml) and vitreous (19.5 μg/ml).

Transplacental passage is not insignificant, since after intramuscular administration of 600 mg the concentration in the amniotic fluid is 1 to 3 μg/ml.

2.1.2. Clindamycin

Clindamycin is presented in the form of clindamycin phosphate for parenteral use and in the form of clindamycin hydrochloride for oral use. The assays are performed by a high-performance liquid chromatographic method or by a microbiological method using *M. luteus* as the test strain.

2.1.2.1. Intravenous Form

See Table 12.

Clindamycin phosphate is soluble in water. This solubility is pH dependent: at pH 7 the solubility is between 200 and 300 mg/ml, whereas at pH 4 it is 25 mg/ml. Clindamycin phosphate is administered in the form of an infusion over 10 to 45 min, depending on the dose to be administered. Clindamycin phosphate is slowly hydrolyzed to clindamycin, with a hydrolysis half-life of between 3 min (1,200 mg) and 1 min (300 mg). About 10% of the drug is present in the serum after 8 h in the form of clindamycin phosphate. The peak concentration in serum of clindamycin appears about 3 h after the end of the infusion and is between 5.4 μg/ml (300 mg) and 15.87 μg/ml (1,200 mg). The apparent elimination half-life of clindamycin is 2 to 3 h, whereas that of clindamycin phosphate is 0.04 to 0.16 h. The apparent volume of distribution is between 43 and 75 liters. Plasma clearance is on the order of 0.18 liters/h/kg for clindamycin and

Table 12 Pharmacokinetics of clindamycin intravenously and intramuscularly

Dose (mg)[a]	n	T_{max}	C_0 (μg/ml)[b]		Vit[c]	CL_P (liters/h/kg)		$t_{1/2}$ (h)	C_{max} (μg/ml)	Lag time (h)	k (h^{-1})
			Clin PO_4	Clin		Clin PO_4	Clin				
300 i.v.	6	10 min	14.66	5.4	5.08	0.18	0.32	1.98			
600 i.v.	6	20 min	26.98	8.42	8.86	0.19	0.39	4.19			
900 i.v.	6	30 min	31.20	10.37	14.9			3.80			
1,200 i.v.	6	45 min	49.75	15.87	10.32	0.21	0.48	2.50			
300 i.m.	6	2.6 h							5.61	0.31	11.72
450 i.m.	6	3.03 h							5.20	0.34	
600 i.m.	6	3.19 h							5.28	0.22	13.03

[a]i.v., intravenously; i.m., intramuscularly.
[b]Clin, clindamycin.
[c]Vit, hydrolysis rate of clindamycin PO_4 in serum per hour.

0.40 liters/h/kg for clindamycin phosphate. Binding to α_1-glycoprotein is on the order of 92 to 93%.

Clindamycin is mainly eliminated by the hepatobiliary route. The metabolites of clindamycin are found in the urine and stools, but about 28% of the parent compound is found in the urine.

2.1.2.2. Intramuscular Form

After administration of single doses of 300, 450, or 600 mg of clindamycin phosphate, the peak concentrations in serum are between 3.17 and 6.56 μg/ml and are reached in 1.5 to 3.0 h. It is possible to detect clindamycin in the serum after 20 min. About 75% of the drug reaches the plasma in the form of clindamycin.

2.1.2.3. Oral Form

See Table 13.

After absorption, clindamycin palmitate (hydrochloride) is rapidly hydrolyzed in the intestinal lumen before being absorbed in the form of the hydrochloride, and the palmitate is no longer detectable in the serum. The bioavailability is on the order of 80%. The degrees of absorption are identical after single and repeated doses. The bioavailability of clindamycin does not appear to be affected by the ingestion of food, although the absorption is delayed by food consumption.

Clindamycin hydrochloride is poorly soluble in water, and the solubility is pH dependent; when the pH is less than 6, the solubility is greater than 160 mg/ml, whereas between 7 and 8 the solubility is weak, on the order of 2.7 ± 1.0 μg/ml.

After administration of a single dose of 150, 300, or 450 mg of clindamycin hydrochloride, the peak concentrations in serum are between 2.56 and 5.58 μg/ml and appear within 1 h.

According to studies, the dose eliminated in the urine ranges from 8 to 26%. A number of metabolites are eliminated in the urine. Traces of clindamycin hydrochloride are found there, in contrast to clindamycin phosphate, for which 1 to 2% of the administered dose is eliminated in this form.

Six adult volunteers received 300 mg of radiolabeled clindamycin hydrochloride. The radioactivity in the stools was 61% ± 5.2% over a period of 168 h, and the radioactivity in the urine was 29.8% ± 2.9%.

2.1.2.4. Metabolism

Clindamycin is hydrolyzed in the liver. The majority of results have been obtained with clindamycin hydrochloride, but the metabolism involves the free form of clindamycin.

Seven metabolites have been described (Fig. 3): *N*-demethyl clindamycin, clindamycin sulfoxide, hydroxy-clindamycin, clindamycin-*N*-demethyl sulfoxide, clindamycose, 5′-oxoclindamycin, and 5′-oxoclindamycin sulfoxide.

Apart from *N*-demethyl clindamycin, which has antibacterial activity similar to that of clindamycin, the derivatives are devoid of activity (Table 14).

Fecal elemination and urinary elimination of the metabolites differ. In the feces, there is a greater proportion of 5′-oxidated or 5′-hydroxylated metabolite, and about 35 to 40% of fecal radioactivity after oral administration of clindamycin hydrochloride consists of unidentified polar metabolites.

After a single dose of 300 mg of clindamycin hydrochloride, the compounds eliminated in the urine are distributed as follows: clindamycin, 27%; clindamycin sulfoxide, 37%; *N*-demethyl clindamycin, 6%; and clindamycin-*N*-demethyl sulfoxide, 2%. A hydroxyl derivative and a carboxyl derivative, both incompletely identified, have been detected, and each accounts for about 15% of the compounds eliminated in the urine.

2.1.2.5. Pharmacokinetics in Patients with Renal Insufficiency

Clindamycin is mainly eliminated by the hepatobiliary route and metabolized in the liver. It is not significantly eliminated after hemodialysis or peritoneal dialysis.

It has been recommended that when the creatinine clearance is less than 10 ml/min the daily dosage be reduced by a half, as the apparent elimination half-life increases, with major interindividual variability (mean half-life of 5.28 h compared to 2 h). Lode and Kelley expressed an opinion authorizing the use of clindamycin irrespective of the degree of renal insufficiency, but they suggested that the drug not be administered for more than 3 weeks. Craig et al. (1981) showed that α_1-glycoprotein levels increased substantially in patients with renal insufficiency (up to 3,000 μg/ml, compared to 400 to 800 μg/ml). Clindamycin binds extensively to α_1-glycoprotein

Table 13 Pharmacokinetics of clindamycin orally

Dose (mg)	n	k_a	Lag time (h)	$t_{1/2\alpha}$ (h)	T_{max} (h)	C_{max} (μg/ml)
150	12	9.68 ± 5.75	0.28 ± 0.14	0.103 ± 0.07	0.77 ± 0.34	2.56 ± 0.68
300	8	6.41 ± 3.55	0.22 ± 0.05	0.16 ± 0.11	0.91 ± 0.38	3.44 ± 0.87
450	8	8.20 ± 4.65	0.17 ± 0.09	0.13 ± 0.09	0.76 ± 0.31	5.58 ± 1.26

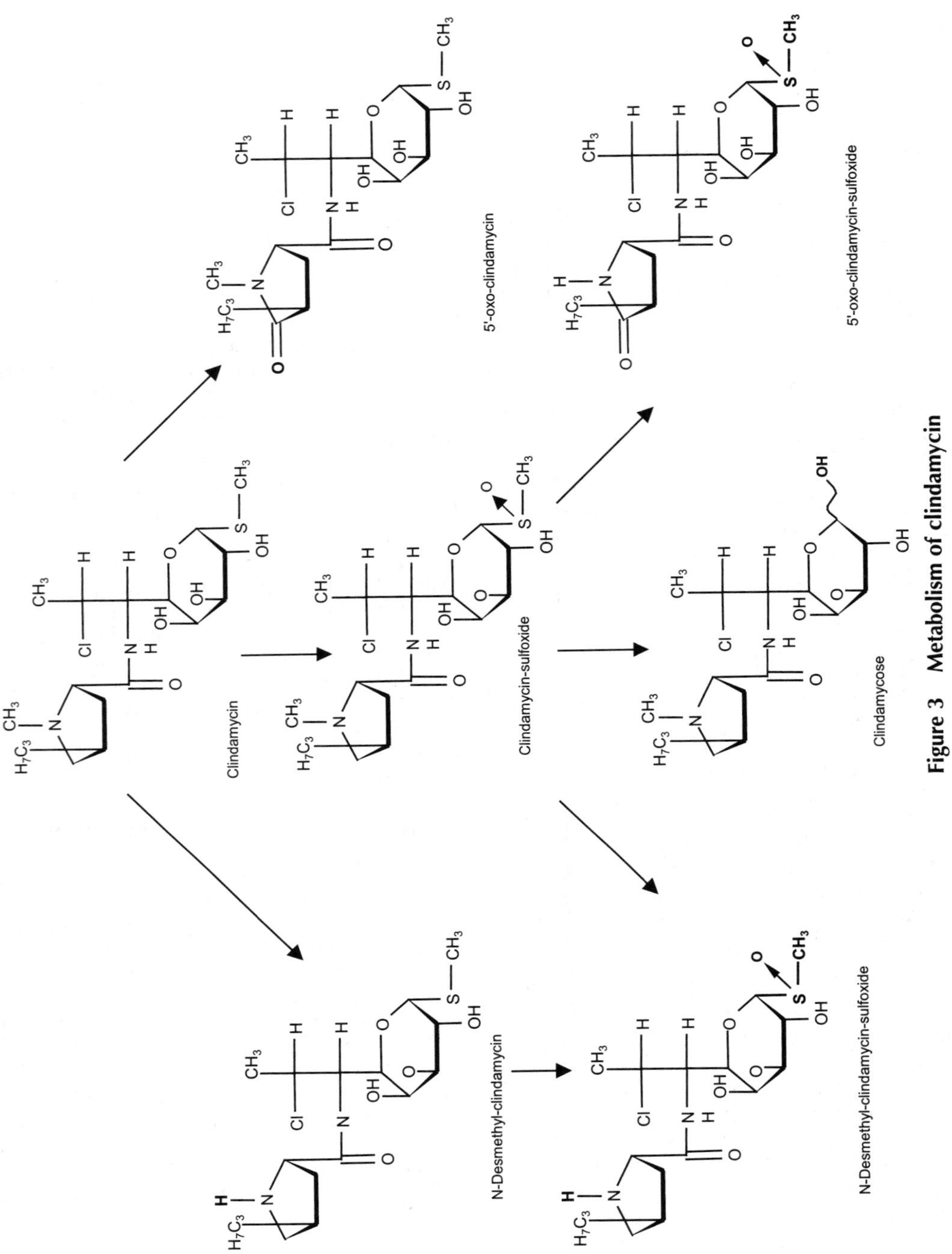

Figure 3 Metabolism of clindamycin

Table 14 Antibacterial activities of clindamycin metabolites

Metabolite	Antibacterial activity relative to that of clindamycin	Urinary elimination (%)
Clindamycin	1	27
N-Demethyl clindamycin	1.4	6
Clindamycin sulfoxide	0.15	35
Hydroxyclindamycin	0.13	15
Clindamycin-*N*-demethyl sulfoxide	0.03	2
Clindamycose	0.03	
5′-Oxoclindamycin	<0.002	Feces
5′-Oxoclindamycin sulfoxide	<0.02	Feces

(about 93%). This yields higher levels in plasma in patients with renal insufficiency, in whom the free fraction is ≤8.5%; in patients with normal kidneys it is <6.5%. Clindamycin also binds to plasma albumin (4%).

In peritoneal fluid, about 3% of the dose of clindamycin phosphate is hydrolyzed to clindamycin in 2 to 4 h. The peritoneal dialysis fluid must contain a concentration of 167 μg of clindamycin phosphate per ml to be certain of exerting therapeutic activity.

2.1.2.6. Pediatrics Subjects

Bell et al. studied the pharmacokinetics of clindamycin in children under the age of 1 year. The apparent elimination half-life is longer in premature neonates (8 to 68 h) than in term neonates (3 to 6 h) during the first 4 weeks. It remains unchanged during the first year of life. As plasma clearance is lower in neonates, after the fourth week the plasma clearance increases (1.6 versus 0.29 to 0.68 liters/h). It is also higher in children weighing more than 3 kg (1.9 versus 0.310 liters/h). The rates of urinary elimination of clindamycin are 16% in premature neonates, 14.4% in neonates under 4 weeks of age, and 22.8% in neonates over 4 weeks of age. Against the background of these differences in the clearance of clindamycin, the authors recommend a dosage of clindamycin phosphate of 30 mg/kg/day in four daily doses for children weighing less than 3.5 kg; in premature infants it should be reduced to 15 mg/kg/day in three daily doses.

In premature children at a dosage of 15 mg/kg/day, the peak concentration in serum is between 5.2 and 13.7 μg/ml, with residual concentrations at 8 h of between <0.1 and 3.8 μg/ml.

In children over 2 months of age, the apparent elimination half-life is the same as that in adults.

After a single dose of 75 mg of clindamycin hydrochloride to children, clindamycin is detectable in the plasma after 0.15 ± 0.12 h, and the peak concentration in serum of 2.26 ± 0.77 μg/ml is reached in about 1 h. The apparent elimination half-life is 2 h. Plasma clearance is similar to that in adults (Table 15).

The concentrations in plasma after a dose of 20 mg/kg in four divided doses (30-min infusion) to three groups of children (group I, premature neonates <28 days old; group II, term neonates <28 days old; and group III, neonates >28 days old) did not vary significantly; they were, respectively, 10.92, 10.45, and 12.69 μg/ml. Likewise, the residual concentrations were not significantly different at 6 h: 5.52, 2.80, and 3.03 μg/ml (Table 16).

Table 15 Pharmacokinetics of clindamycin hydrochloride in children

Parameter	Value
k_a (h^{-1})	8.64 ± 3.36
Lag time (h)	0.15 ± 0.12
$t_{1/2\alpha}$ (h)	0.09 ± 0.03
T_{max} (h)	0.56 ± 0.25
C_{max} (μg/ml)	2.26 ± 0.77
V (liters/kg)	0.86
$t_{1/2}$ (h)	2.0
Dose	75-mg single dose
n	11

A dosage of 20 mg/kg in four divided doses is therefore proposed for children aged over 4 weeks and weighing more than 3.5 kg or in term neonates aged more than 1 week. For premature infants and up to the fourth week of life, a dosage of 15 mg/kg/day in three divided doses is recommended.

2.1.2.7. Elderly Patients

A pharmacokinetic study was undertaken with elderly subjects versus young subjects after a single dose of 300 mg orally and intravenously. The fractions absorbed were similar in the young and elderly subjects (0.92 versus 0.85). The apparent elimination half-life, apparent volume of distribution, and plasma clearance after intravenous administration did not differ significantly: 2.46 versus 2.79 h, 0.71 versus 0.75 liter/kg, and 3.36 versus 3.11 ml/min/kg, respectively. The dosage need not be modified in elderly subjects.

2.1.2.8. Patients with Hepatic Insufficiency

In patients with hepatic insufficiency, the apparent elimination half-life is prolonged. It is 5 to 15 h, compared to 2.5

Table 16 Pharmacokinetics of clindamycin in neonates

Group	n	Dose (mg/kg/day)	C_{max} (μg/ml)	C_{min} (μg/ml), 6 h	$t_{1/2}$ (h)	CL_P (ml/h)	Urinary elimination (%)
Premature, <28 days old	16	15–20	10.92	5.52	8.68	2.94	16
Full term, <28 days old	5	20	10.45	2.80	3.60	0.678	14.4
>4 wks old	19	20	12.69	3.03	3.01	1.589	22.8

to 3.6 h in healthy volunteers. A reduction in the plasma clearance in cirrhotic patients has been demonstrated, with a reduction in protein binding to 79% (versus 93%). However, the apparent volume of distribution at steady state does not vary significantly (0.583 ± 0.18 liter/kg versus 0.693 ± 0.25 liter/kg).

Sattler et al. showed that the clearance of clindamycin phosphate can be correlated with the prothrombin time and antipyrine clearance.

2.1.2.9. Pregnancy

Clindamycin rapidly crosses the fetoplacental barrier. High concentrations of clindamycin have been detected in the liver, kidney, and lungs, and low levels have been detected in cerebral tissue, bone, or muscles of fetuses from spontaneous abortions occurring between the 10th and 22nd weeks of gestation (Table 17).

Four hours after a single oral dose of 150 mg of clindamycin hydrochloride, the mean concentration in colostrum is 1.3 μg/ml (0.7 to 3.8 μg/ml). After intravenous administration of 150 mg of clindamycin phosphate, mean concentrations in colostrum between 1 and 6 h after the end of infusion are 0.3 μg/ml (1.0 h) to 0.8 μg/ml (6.0 h); concentrations in plasma are higher still, 2.6 μg/ml (1.0 h) and 0.9 μg/ml (6.0 h).

In 54 patients undergoing cesarean section and receiving 600 mg of clindamycin phosphate prophylactically, the mean peak concentration in serum was between 6 and 7 μg/ml. Twenty minutes after the end of drug administration, the concentration in serum in the umbilical cord was about 3 μg/ml. Clindamycin was not detected in the amniotic fluid 30 and 60 min after the end of the infusion.

Concentrations in serum in neonates for the first 6 h of life were at least 2 μg/ml.

Concentrations in plasma in pregnant women are the same as those in nonpregnant women.

2.1.2.10. Tissue Concentrations

2.1.2.10.1. Intraphagocytic concentrations. The intracellular/extracellular concentration ratio in neutrophils is between 11 and 15, while in macrophages and monocytes it is 23. Inside the cell clindamycin is localized in the cytoplasm and granules. The ratio of intracellular/extracellular concentrations is on the order of 1.7 to 4 for lincomycin.

2.1.2.10.2. Concentrations in tissue. Clindamycin exhibits good penetration of saliva, bronchial secretions, lung tissues, pleural fluid, the prostate, seminal fluid, bones, and joints. Conversely, concentrations in the eye and cerebrospinal fluid are relatively low.

2.1.2.10.3. Biliary elimination. Brown et al. have shown that the concentration obtained in the bile in patients with a Kehr drain after cholecystectomy was 2.5 to 3 times that detected in plasma.

2.2. Safety

The main side effect of clindamycin is pseudomembranous colitis due to *C. difficile*. The incidence of this colitis varies from one center to another and ranges from 0.1 to 10%.

Hypotension and even cardiorespiratory arrest have been reported at high intravenous doses of lincomycin, particularly after rapid administration.

3. THERAPEUTIC INDICATION

3.1. Lincomycin

The clinical indications of lincomycin are limited. Lincomycin is used in infections due to gram-positive bacteria, such as staphylococci and streptococci, particularly bone, skin and skin structure infections.

3.2. Clindamycin

The principal indications of clindamycin are infections caused by anaerobic bacteria, particularly infections of intestinal or vaginal origin. In polymicrobial and mixed infections, clindamycin must be combined with another antibacterial agent, such as an aminoglycoside.

4. VIC-105555

It was shown that 7-methyl 4′-pentyl prolamide lincosamides (Fig. 4) exhibited higher antibacterial activity

Table 17 Concentrations of clindamycin in fetal tissue (after oral administration)

Tissue	Concn (μg/ml or mg/kg)	
	Single dose ($n = 7$)	Multiple doses ($n = 9$)
Plasma	0.32	0.70
Liver	0.90	2.10
Kidneys	0.90	1.80
Spleen	0.09	1.20
Lung	0.70	1.20
Brain	0.08	0.50
Muscle	0.30	1.10
Bone	ND[a]	0.8

[a]ND, not determined.

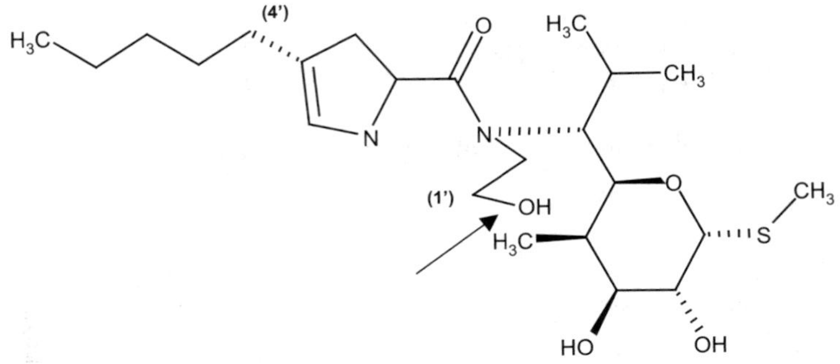

Figure 4 VRC-105555 (7-methyl lincosamine)

against gram-positive organisms than clindamycin (Lewis et al., 2004) both in vitro and in vivo (Park et al. 2004). For methicillin-resistant *S. aureus* the MIC_{50} and MIC_{90} were 0.25 and 0.25 μg/ml, and in vivo the 50% effective doses were 0.13 and 0.32 mg/kg, respectively. VCR 105555 exhibits a longer elimination half-life.

REFERENCES

Cachural G, Tally FP, 1982, Factors affecting the choice of antimicrobial therapy for anaerobic infection, J Antimicrob Chemother, 10, suppl A, 11–22.

Derouin F, Nalpas J, Chastang C, 1988, Mesure in vitro de l'effet inhibiteur de macrolides, lincosamides et synergistines sur la croissance de Toxoplasma gondii, Pathol Biol, 36, 1204–1210.

Hofflin JM, Remington JS, 1987, Clindamycin in a murine model of toxoplasmic encephalitis, Antimicrob Agents Chemother, 31, 492–496.

Lewis JG, Atuegbu AE, Chen T, Kumar SA, Patel DV, Hackbarth CJ, Asano R, Wu C, Wang W, Yuan Z, Trias J, White RJ, Gordeev MF, 2004, Novel antimicrobial 7-methyl lincosamine: prolamide analogs, 44th Intersci Conf Antimicrob Agents Chemother, abstract F-1388.

Lewis JG, Gu S, Kumar SA, Chen T, O'Dowd H, Patel DV, Hackbarth CJ, Asano R, Park C, Blais J, Wu C, Wang W, Yuan Z, Trias J, White RJ, Gordeev MF, 2004, Novel antimicrobial 7-methyl lincosamine: prolamide analogs, 44th Intersci Conf Antimicrob Agents Chemother, abstract F-1389.

Park C, Blais J, Candioni G, Jabes D, Kubo A, Maniar M, Margolis P, Hackbarth C, Lewis J, Gordeev M, White R, Trias J, 2004, VIC 105555, a new lincosamide with improved in vitro efficacy and good in vivo activity, 44th Intersci Conf Antimicrob Agents Chemother, abstract F-1392.

Queener SF, Bartlett MS, Richardson JD, Durkin MM, Jay MA, Smith JW, 1988, Activity of clindamycin with primaquine against *Pneumocystis carinii* in vitro and in vivo, Antimicrob Agents Chemother, 32, 807–813.

Ruf B, Potile HD, 1989, Clindamycin/primaquine for Pneumocystis carinii pneumonia, Lancet, ii, 625–626.

Oxazolidinones

A. BRYSKIER

22

1. INTRODUCTION

The aryl-oxazolidinones constitute a huge family composed of different chemical entities: antibacterials, agriculture derivatives, monoamine oxidase inhibitors, and antihistaminics.

The first compounds were synthesized in 1982, and three of them were introduced in clinical practice: toloxatone, almoxatone, and cimoxatone. All of these derivatives are devoted to use for the central nervous system. Some of them were used as antihistaminics in the therapy of hypersensitivity.

The first antibacterial derivatives were prepared for agricultural use as pesticides for the treatment of tomato infections (*Agrobacterium tumefaciens* and *Xanthomonas vesicatoria*).

These derivatives possessed a 4′-methyl sulfonyl and were used at 200 ppm.

In 1984, the first analog for human therapy was reported: S-6123 (Fig. 1), which is a *para*-benzenyl oxazolidinone with either a 5-methoxymethyl or a 5-hydroxy group. This compound exhibited moderate antistaphylococcal and antistreptococcal activities and was inactive against *Enterobacteriaceae*.

In 1987, optimization of S-6123 yielded two compounds from Dupont de Nemours research (Fig. 2). Both compounds exerted good activity against gram-positive bacteria, and in addition some analogs exhibited antituberculosis activity. DuP 721 development was given up due to lethal toxicity in rats after oral repeated doses (100 mg/kg) every 12 h for 15 days. This toxicity was supposed to result from bone marrow toxicity. This adverse effect was also observed with other analogs, such as U-92300.

After the successful introduction in clinical practice of linezolid, many pharmaceutical companies have undertaken intensive research to enhance antibacterial activity against gram-positive bacteria, to expand the antibacterial spectrum to fastidious gram-negative bacteria, to overcome linezolid resistance among *Staphylococcus aureus* strains and *Enterococcus* spp., and to demonstrate better water solubility.

The oxazolidinones belong to a new chemical class of synthetic antibacterial agents. Only linezolid was introduced into clinical practice; for some analogs development was given up for obvious reasons, while other analogs are still in the exploratory or development phase.

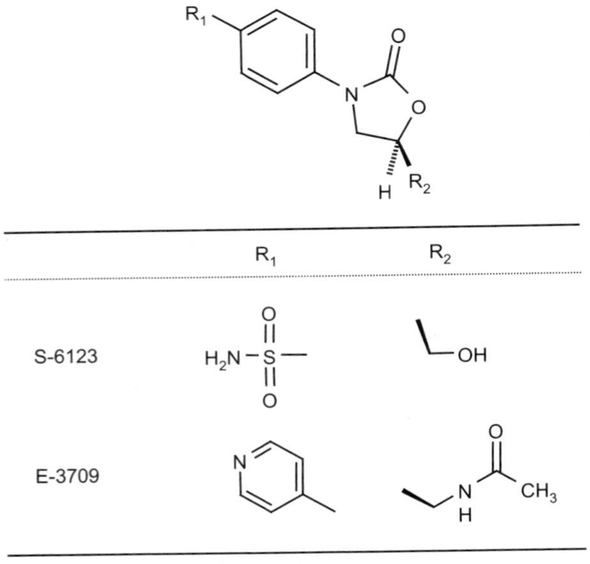

	R_1	R_2
S-6123	H_2N-SO_2-	$-CH_2OH$
E-3709	4-pyridyl	$-CH_2-NH-CO-CH_3$

Figure 1 S-6123 and E-3709

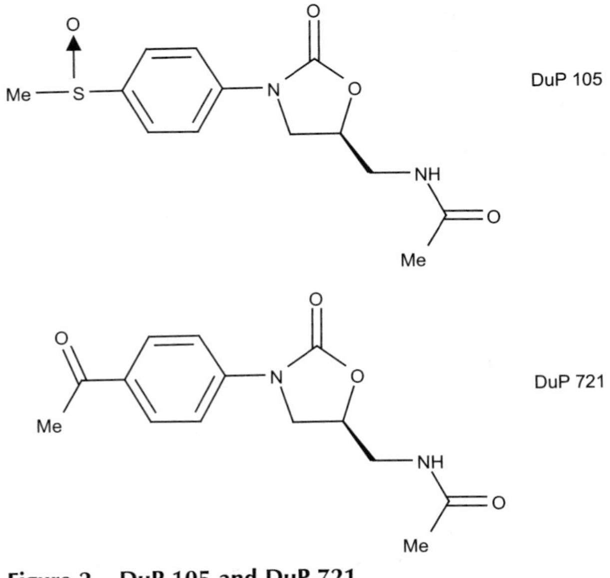

DuP 105

DuP 721

Figure 2 DuP 105 and DuP 721

These compounds are characterized by their activity against gram-positive cocci and bacilli and against *Mycobacterium tuberculosis*.

Certain tricyclic derivatives appear to be active against *Mycobacterium avium*.

2. CHEMICAL STRUCTURES

Numerous series of analogs have been synthesized by many pharmaceutical companies, such as DuPont, Merck, Pharmacia-Upjohn, Bayer, Johnson and Johnson, Ranbaxy, Dr Reddy, and Dong A (Table 1); these analogs have in common a pharmacophore composed of a 2-oxazenecaolidinyl nucleus substituted at position 5 by at least an acetamido methyl side chain and a substituted phenyl nucleus appended at position 3 of the 2-oxazolidinone nucleus. The first molecule in this series, S-6123, was relatively inactive in vitro (Fig. 1).

DuP 721 and DuP 105 differ from one another in the chain in the *para* position of the phenyl nucleus: *p*-acetyl (DuP 721) and *p*-methylsulfinyl (DuP 105) (Fig. 2).

A series of molecules has been synthesized by Pharmacia-Upjohn. They have the same pharmacophore as the previous molecules, but a fluorine atom is appended instead of a phenyl, and they have variable azolyl moieties, such as piperazinyl (U-100592), thiomorphonyl (U-100480), morphonyl (U-100766), and pyridinium (E-3709) (Fig. 3).

Other derivatives with 5-methylvinyl or cyanomethylvinyl chains or different aryl substituents at position 3 of the

Table 1 Pharmaceutical companies involved in oxazolidinone research

Pharmaceutical company	Compound
Roussel-Uclaf	*N*-Glycoxylo oxazolidinones
Marion Merrel-Dow	Oxazolidinone-like derivatives
Dupont de Nemours	DuP 105, DuP 721
Pharmacia-Upjohn	Linezolid, eperezolid, and numerous analogs
Pharmacia-Upjohn-Vicuron	VRC-3599, VRC-3406, VRC-322, VRC-3839, VRC-3054, VRC-3055, VRC-3816, and numerous analogs
Astra-Zeneca	AZD 2563 and numerous analogs
Ranbaxy	Ranbezolid
Dr Reddy	ABX 96, DRF 8417, and numerous analogs
Johnson and Johnson	RWJ-302397, RWJ-306490, and numerous analogs
Bayer Pharma	Numerous analogs
Dong-A	DA-786, DA-7867, DA-70157, DA-70218
Kuwait University	PH-027
Orchid Chemical & Pharmaceutical	OCID 0050

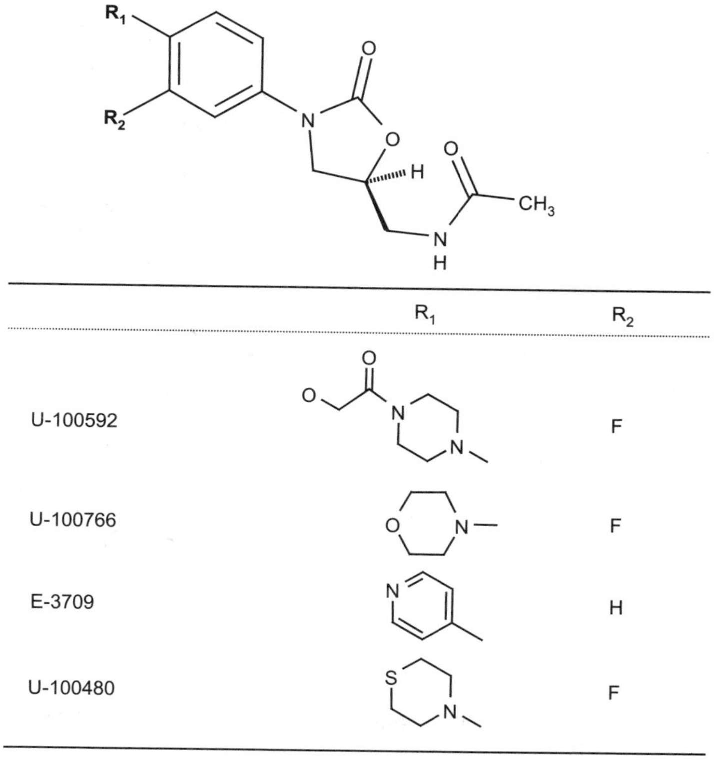

	R_1	R_2
U-100592	[structure]	F
U-100766	[structure]	F
E-3709	[structure]	H
U-100480	[structure]	F

Figure 3 Aryl phenyl-substituted oxazolidinones

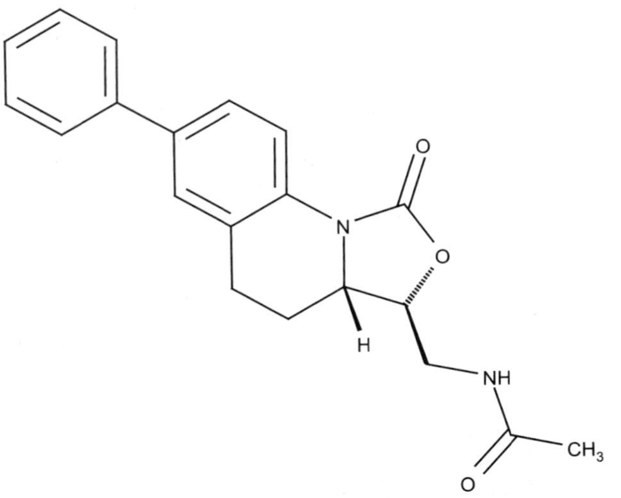

Figure 4 Tricyclic oxazolidinone derivatives

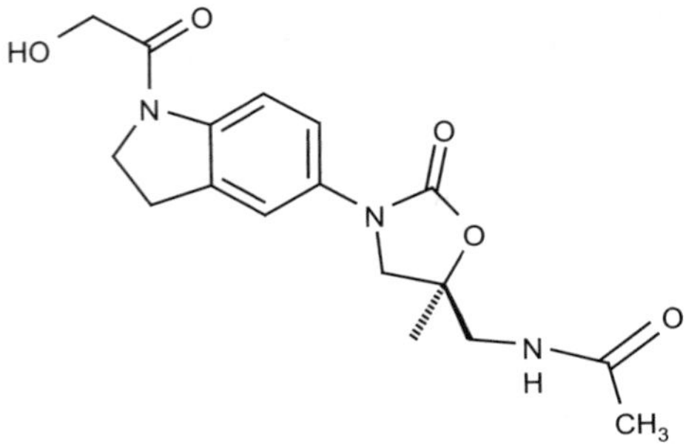

Figure 5 U-97456

cycloalkylbenzene type have been described. A series of derivatives possessing a tricyclic ring with the oxazolidinone core has been synthesized (Fig. 4), and one of the derivatives seems to be active against *M. tuberculosis*. A previous series with an indolinyl nucleus led to the preselection of U-97456 (Fig. 5). Series of phenylazepinyl analogs have been synthesized (Fig. 6), as well as a series with different aryl substituents by Bayer (Fig. 7).

3. STRUCTURE-ACTIVITY RELATIONSHIP

Modifications of all parts of the pharmacophore have been done. The biological properties are dependent on the side chain at the C-5 position and the aryl or alkyl moiety at position 4′ of the phenyl ring.

3.1. C-5 Position

Structure-activity relationship studies have shown that the *l* isomer (center of asymmetry at position 5) is active, whereas the *d* isomer is inactive.

In a series in which certain derivatives possess as a substituent at position 5 a chlorine atom or a hydroxyl group, the most active derivative is that with a *para*-sulfophenyl moiety at position 3. None of the analogs with an amino group is active.

Overall, the presence of a halogen group or a carbon, sulfone, phosphate, or carboxyl chain reduces the antibacterial activity. In the series of compounds with an acetamido methyl side chain at position 5, two derivatives were found to be active: DuP 721 and a 5-nitro derivative.

Some compounds have a fluorine atom instead of a methyl group and remain active (VRC-3816 and VRC-3839).

A sulfur atom instead of an oxygen atom (carbonyl) leading to a thioacetamido methyl side chain resulted in more active analogs.

Replacement of the methyl group by an aryl substituent did not alter the antibacterial activity, as shown by AZD 2563.

In AZD 2563 derivatives the oxygen atom was replaced with a nitrogen atom in order to improve the pharmacokinetic profile. In general the N-linked heterocycles exhibit higher in vivo activity (*S. aureus*) and those with weak efficacy have a high clearance.

Replacement of the (thio)acetamido methyl side chain by another moiety resulted in inactive derivatives.

It was believed that the acetamidomethyl side chain at C-5 of the oxazolidinone was the optimal moiety with a limited bulk on the terminus. However, it was shown that closely related moieties such as carbamate or amide analogs possess good in vitro activity and improved pharmacokinetic properties.

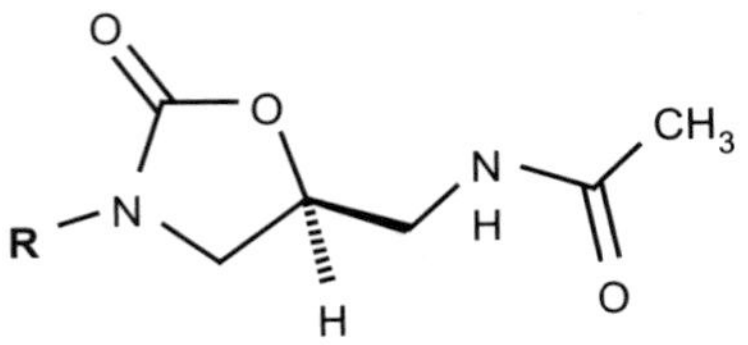

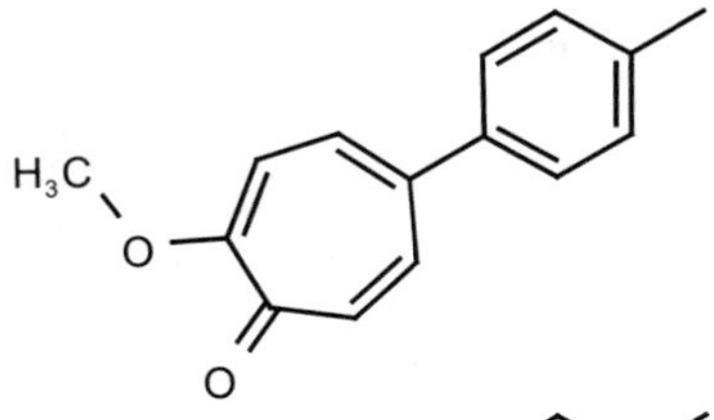

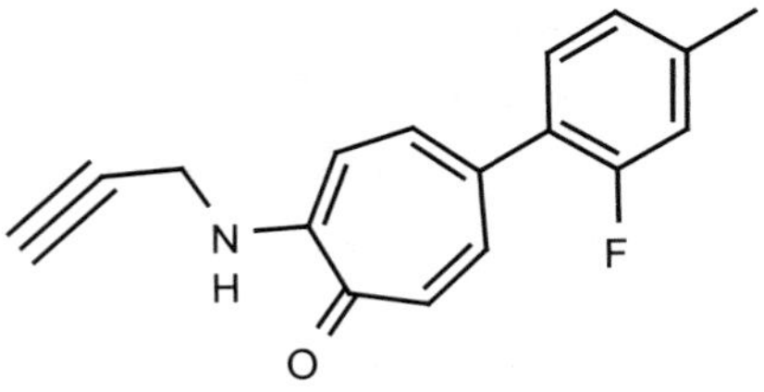

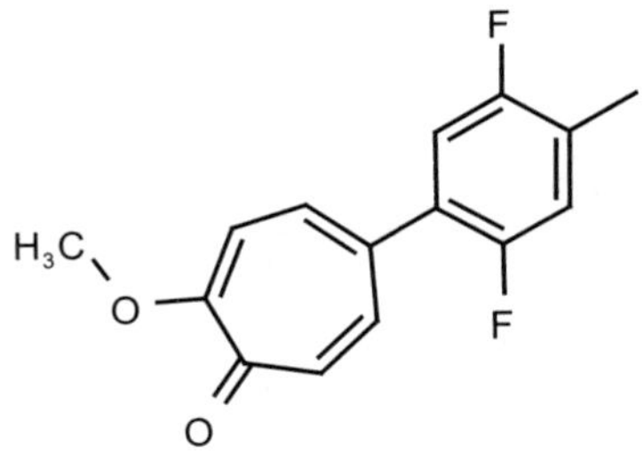

Figure 6 Phenylazepinyl oxazolidinones (Pharmacia-Upjohn)

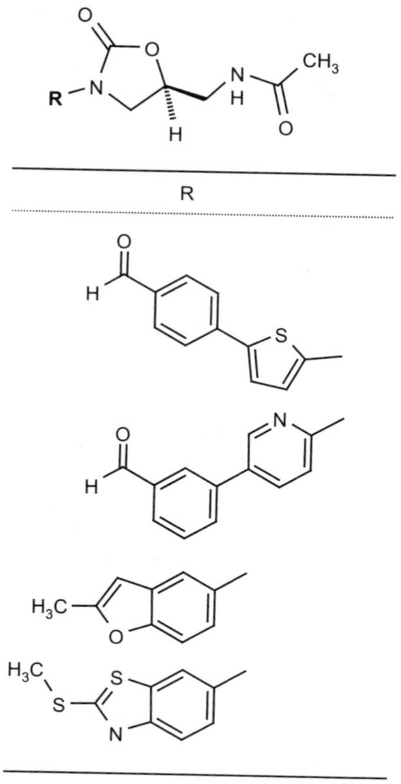

Figure 7 **Aryl oxazolidinone derivatives (Bayer)**

In a new series, optimization of the acetamido group at the C-5 position of the central core was undertaken. Series with six-membered heterocycles, isoxazole, and other five-membered heterocycles were synthesized. All of these analogs have a dihydropyranyl moiety attached on the fluorophenyl ring. In the six-membered series, the 2′-pyridyloxy analogs exhibited activity comparable to that of linezolid, but moving the pyridinyl nitrogen to the 3′-4′ position yielded analogs with decreased in vitro activity in comparison with that of linezolid.

The phenyl and the methyl pyridyl analogs were inactive (MIC, >128 μg/ml). Five-membered-ring analogs were more active than the six-membered-ring derivatives. Isoxazole analogs were more active than the 2′-pyridinyl analogs. But all of them are poorly active in vivo due to poor water solubility. It was shown in a previous study that 5′-thioacetamidomethyl analogs have increased activity compared to their desthio counterpart. Incorporation of a thio ether residue yielded very active compounds in the oxidized form.

The most active compounds in the five-membered-ring series were obtained with sulfur-containing heterocycles. The combination of side chain thioheterocycles and methylsulfono substituents yielded highly active compounds exhibiting high in vitro activity, with MICs of 0.13 μg/ml for *S. aureus*, but poor in vivo activity. In a new series, the endocyclic oxygen in heterocycles was replaced by a nitrogen. The best compound was the 1,2,5-thiadiazole analog. The amino-linked compounds were more potent than the oxygen-linked series (twofold increase in activity). However, in vivo activity, probably due to metabolism, was not correlated with in vitro activity; the 1,2,5-thiadiazole analogs were less potent than the isoxazole derivatives.

In a new series with the two subsets of molecules, those having an oxymethyl and those having an amino-linked five-membered ring at C-5 of the core ring, were combined with various heterocycles at C-4 and hexa- and pentaheterocycles. Cyanopyrrolyl analogs and imidazolyl analogs were highly active in vitro but poorly active in vivo, mainly due to water solubility problems.

VRC-322 (Fig. 8) belongs to a new series which was synthesized to improve the activity against gram-positive cocci, including *S. aureus* isolates resistant to linezolid, and to enlarge the antibacterial spectrum to fastidious gram-negative bacilli involved in respiratory tract infections, such as *Haemophilus influenzae* and *Moraxella catarrhalis*.

The strategy was to keep the morphonyl ring of linezolid but to alter the carbamoyl side chain at C-5 by replacing the methyl group by alkyl and aryl moieties. No compounds in this series were able to overcome the linezolid resistance in *S. aureus*.

VRC-322, the cinnamide fluorophenyl analog, was equipotent to linezolid, demonstrating that certain C-5 bulky groups could be tolerated.

3.2. N-3 Substituents

The antibacterial activity is the result of an equilibrium between the chains at positions C-5 and N-3 of the oxazolidinone ring.

The group attached at position 3 alters the lipophilicity of the molecules. The most hydrophilic derivatives have a sulfonamide, methylsulfone, or methylsulfonide group. In the presence of an acetyl group, the molecule is moderately hydrophilic. The most lipophilic molecules have a thiomethyl- or isopropyl-type chain. In the series produced by Brickner et al. (1996), the

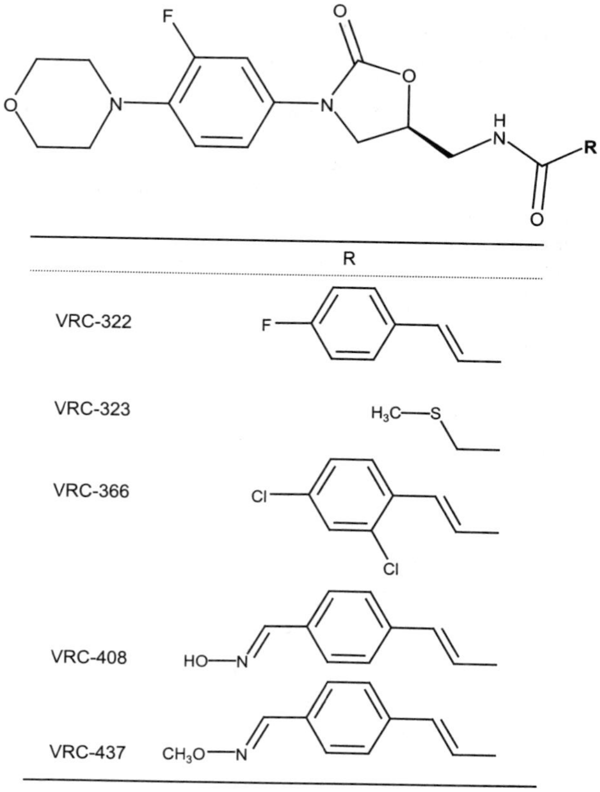

Figure 8 **VRC-322**

presence of a hydroxyacetyl chain and a fluorine atom optimizes the in vitro activity.

3.2.1. Link between N-3 and the Phenyl Ring

The link between N-3 of the oxazolidinone ring and C-1 of the phenyl ring is essential for the antibacterial activity. Addition of various alkyl groups, such as carbonyl, nitro, sulfonyl, or methyl, significantly reduced the antibacterial activity.

3.2.2. Phenyl Ring

The phenyl ring, the N-3–C-1 bond, and the oxozolidinone ring compose the core of the molecule; bulky substituents reduce the antibacterial activities.

The phenyl ring could be substituted. However, the location of the appended substituent is responsible for the antibacterial activity. The most active compounds are those for which the substituents are appended in the *para* position.

The phenyl ring may be substituted by a fluorine atom or two (positions 3′ and 5′). A substitution in the *meta* position (positions 2′ and 6′) significantly reduced the antibacterial activity.

It has been shown that a 3′-fluorine compound is more active than the unsubstituted counterpart.

At position 4′ of the phenyl ring (*para* position) numerous groups have been appended; these may be alkyl groups, such as amino-alkyl groups or non-amino moieties (sulfonyl, sufide, or sulfoxide), or aryl groups (azolyl); the azolyl groups may be mono-, bi-, or tricyclic.

Three type of molecules have been reported: those having a C-N, C-C, or S-C link between the phenyl ring and the C-4′ substituent.

The first compound with such an aryl group, a pyridine, was E-3709.

3.3. Oxazolidinone Ring

Efforts have been focused on the identification of bioisosteric replacements of the oxazolidinone ring. In previous series, the oxazolidinone ring was replaced by dihydrofuran-2-one or pyrrolidin-2-one rings (i.e., ZM 302061) (Fig. 9).

In a new series of bioisosteres of oxazolidinone, the isoxazoline ring system was identified for replacement of the oxazolidinone ring. Like for oxazolidinone, the absolute configuration at the C-5 position is essential for antibacterial activities. The (*R*)-isomer is active, whereas the (S)-isomer is inactive. Two compounds, PNU-173954 and PNU-171832 (Fig. 10), exhibited comparable in vivo efficacies in staphylococcal murine disseminated infections.

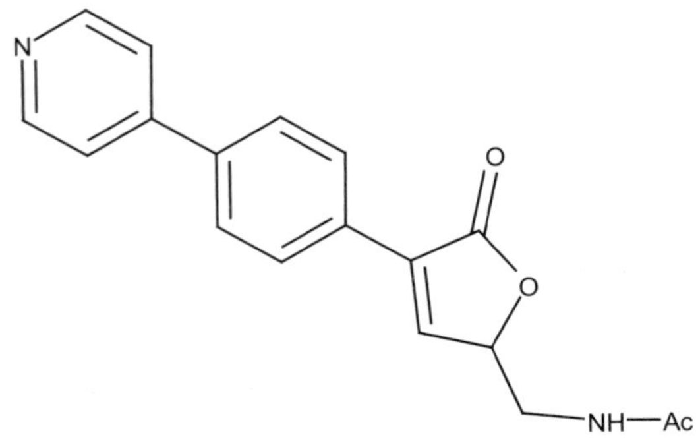

N O O NH—Ac

Figure 9 ZM 302061

4. PHYSICOCHEMICAL PROPERTIES

Oxazolidinones are molecules which are obtained by total synthesis. Six stages are necessary to obtain the active (S)-isomer of DuP 721, with a yield of about 60%.

The physical and chemical properties of DuP 721 and linezolid are summarized in Tables 2 and 3.

5. DuP 105 AND DuP 721

5.1. Antibacterial Activities

The antibacterial spectrum of DuP 105 and DuP 721 includes gram-positive cocci, gram-positive bacilli, anaerobic bacteria, and M. *tuberculosis*. They are inactive against gram-negative bacilli (Table 3). They do not possess antifungal activity.

DuP 721 is more active than DuP 105. It possesses activity equivalent to that of vancomycin (Table 4). It is particularly active against methicillin- or gentamicin-resistant strains of S. *aureus* and coagulase-negative staphylococci.

The pH of the medium (pH 6 to 8) and the addition of up to 50% serum to the culture medium do not affect the antibacterial activity of DuP 721 or DuP 105. Conversely, as with vancomycin, there is a very extensive inoculum effect (Table 5). An increase in the size of the inoculum from 10^3 to 10^5CFU/ml causes a two- to four-fold increase in the MIC. When the inoculum is 10^7 CFU/ml, the in vitro activity is markedly reduced. DuP 105, DuP 721, and vancomycin possess bacteriostatic activity. No mutants have been detected among the strains of staphylococci tested at inocula of up to 10^9 CFU/ml.

Under anaerobic conditions, the MIC increases only two-fold at most. The addition of 3% NaCl, 3 mM Ca^{2+}, 3 mM Mg^{2+}, 9 mM Mg^{2+}, or glucose-6-phosphate (25 μg/ml) to the culture medium (Mueller-Hinton) does not significantly modify the antibacterial activity.

Barry (1988) proposed a MIC of ≤4.0 μg/ml as the breakpoint for DuP 721. At this concentration, 87% of the strains of gram-positive cocci are susceptible, 13% of them possess intermediate activity (MIC, ~8.0 μg/ml), and none are resistant (MIC, ≥16.0 μg/ml).

The combination of DuP 721 and ciprofloxacin or norfloxacin may be synergistic, additive, or antagonistic, depending on the strains tested.

Irrespective of the resistance phenotype, DuP 721 would appear to possess good activity against M. *tuberculosis*, with a MIC of between 0.3 and 1.25 μg/ml and a minimum bactericidal concentration of 2.5 μg/ml (Table 6). DuP 721 is bactericidal for a 10^5-CFU/ml inoculum of the H_{37RV} strain of M. *tuberculosis* in 4 days. Stottmeier (1987) failed to detect any mutants among a population of 10^9 CFU/ml in 7 H10 medium. DuP 721 is inactive against M. *avium* and other species of atypical mycobacteria (Table 7). The in vitro activity of two derivatives against *Legionella pneumophila* is moderate.

DuP 721 and DuP 105 are weakly active against anaerobes (Table 8). These molecules have bacteriostatic activity.

5.2. In Vivo Activity

In acute murine infections (female CF-1 mice) due to S. *aureus* or *Enterococcus faecalis* STCO 19, DuP 721 possesses the same activity as vancomycin subcutaneously and is more active than DuP 105. Its oral activity is good (Table 9).

DuP 721 and DuP 105 are active in S. *aureus* experimental infections in cyclophosphamide-immunodepressed mice, but the 50% effective doses (ED_{50}s) are two to four times higher than those necessary in immunocompetent mice (Table 10).

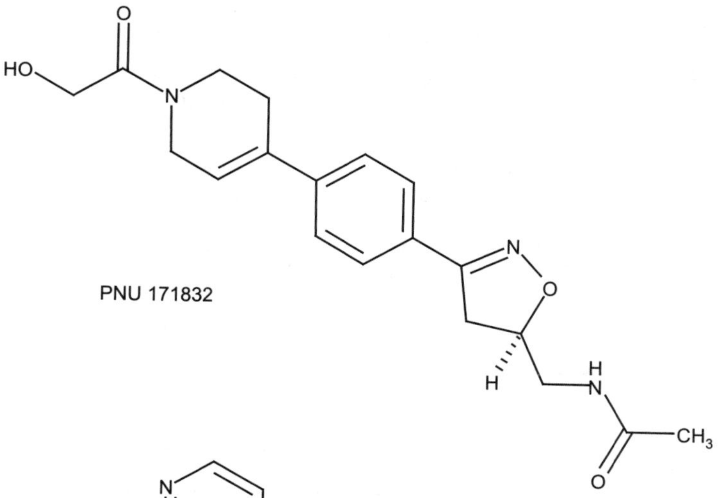

PNU 171832

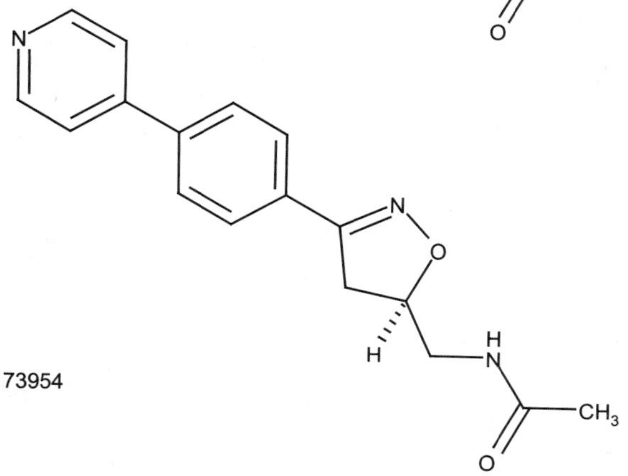

PNU 173954

Figure 10 Aryl (substituted) phenyl oxazolidinones

Table 2 Physicochemical properties of DuP 721

Parameter	Value
Empirical formula	$C_{14}H_{16}N_2O_4$
Mol wt	274.1
Melting point (°C)	190.5
$[\alpha]_D^{20}$	−51° (c=1, DMF)

Table 3 Physicochemical properties of linezolid

Parameter	Value
Empirical formula	$C_{16}H_{20}FN_3O_4$
Mol wt.	337.35
Melting point (°C)	179
$[\alpha]_D^{20}$	−9° (c = 0.919 $CHCl_3$)
Water solubility	3.2 mg/ml (pH 6.8)
Log P	0.55 *n*-octanol/water (amphiphilic compound)
pK	1.8
CAS number	165 800-03-3

In experimental murine renal infections, administration of DuP 721, DuP 105, or vancomycin causes a reduction in the number of bacteria present in renal tissue. The doses required are high.

Table 4 In vitro activities of DuP 105 and DuP 721 against gram-negative and gram-positive bacteria

Microorganism(s)	MIC (μg/ml)	
	DuP 721	DuP 105
MSSA	0.25	2.0
MRSA	0.25	2.0
S. epidermidis Met[s]	0.5	2.0
S. epidermidis Met[r]	0.25	4.0
Staphylococcus haemolyticus	2.0	8.0
Staphylococcus hominis	2.0	8.0
S. pneumoniae	1.0	4.0
S. pyogenes	0.5	2.0
Streptococcus agalactiae	1.0	2.0
Streptococcus group C	0.5	2.0
Streptococcus group F	0.5	2.0
Viridans group streptococci	1.0	4.0
Streptococcus group G	0.5	2.0
Listeria monocytogenes	4.0	16
E. faecalis	1.0	8.0
Corynebacterium jeikeium	0.25	2.0
Bacillus subtilis	0.25	
H. influenzae	32	64
M. catarrhalis	8.0	32
E. coli	>128	>128
Klebsiella spp.	>128	>128
Proteus spp.	>128	>128
Serratia spp.	>128	>128

Table 5 Effect of inoculum size on DuP 721

Organism	Inoculum size (CFU/ml)	MIC (μg/ml)		
		DuP 721	DuP 105	Vancomycin
S. aureus ATCC 29213	10^3	2.0	8.0	1.0
	10^5	4.0	32	1.0
	10^7	>64	>64	64
S. epidermidis Met[r]	10^3	1.0	2.0	1.0
	10^5	4.0	16	1.0
	10^7	>64	>64	64
E. faecalis	10^3	2.0	8.0	1.0
	10^5	4.0	16	2.0
	10^7	>64	>64	>64

Table 6 Activity of DuP 721 against *M. tuberculosis*[a]

Compound	H_{37RV}				*M. tuberculosis*			
	Susceptible (*n* = 1)	INH[r] (*n* = 2)	RIF[r] (*n* = 2)	STR[r] (*n* = 1)	Susceptible (*n* = 10)	INH[r] + RIF[r] + STR[r] (*n* = 3)	INH[r] + RIF[r] (*n* = 15)	ETM[r] (*n* = 1)
DuP 721	1.25	0.97	0.97	0.97	1.5	1.97	1.5–4	
RIF	0.04		>250		0.06			
INH	0.04	30			0.06–0.48		>250	
Rifabutin	0.03		250		0.1–0.4			
ETM	0.2		259					50
STR			0.08	100				

[a]INH, isoniazid; RIF, rifampin; STR, streptomycin; ETM, ethambutol.

Table 7 Activity of DuP 721 against atypical mycobacteria

Microorganism	MIC (μg/ml)
M. avium	>250
Mycobacterium gordonae	3.9
Mycobacterium intracellulare	>250
Mycobacterium fortuitum	3.9
Mycobacterium kansasii	1.95
Mycobacterium scrofulaceum	15.6

Table 8 In vitro activities of DuP 721 and DuP 105 against anaerobes

Microorganism(s)	MIC (μg/ml)	
	DuP 721	DuP 105
Peptococcus spp.	0.5	4.0
Clostridium spp.	2.0	8.0
Peptostreptococcus spp.	0.5	4.0
Propionibacterium spp.	0.25	1.0
B. fragilis	8.0	32
Prevotella spp.	4.0	16
Fusobacterium spp.	0.5	8.0

In a murine implant model with 10^7 CFU of *Bacteroides fragilis*, good activity was demonstrated for DuP 721, but not for DuP 105 (50 mg/kg of body weight subcutaneously). Metronidazole is much more effective.

5.3. Assay Methods

Microbiological and chromatographic methods have been described for DuP 721 and DuP 105. The microbiological method uses *Sarcina lutea* ATCC 9341 in saline BBL medium as a test strain. The limit of detection is 4.0 μg/ml. The chromatographic method allows detection at up to 0.5 μg/ml. There is a good correlation between the two assay methods.

Table 9 In vivo activities of DuP 721 and DuP 105 in CF-1 mice

Microorganism	ED$_{50}$ (mg/kg)[a]				
	DuP 721		DuP 105		Vancomycin, s.c.
	s.c.	p.o.	s.c.	p.o.	
S. aureus 1A	3.8	5.1	9.0	16.6	3.3
MRSA	2.2	2.8	11.9	12.7	4.9
S. aureus Smith	6.1	6.6	16.3	15.1	1.2
E. faecalis STCO 19	2.5	3.1	6.3	14.1	11.8

[a]s.c., subcutaneously; p.o., per os.

Table 10 Experimental infections in immunocompetent and immunosuppressed mice

Compound	ED$_{50}$ (mg/kg)	
	Immunocompetent mice	Immunosuppressed mice
DuP 721	3.5	17.0
DuP 105	9.0	37.5
Vancomycin	3.3	3.1

5.4. Animal Pharmacokinetics

Oral and intravenous pharmacokinetics have been determined in the dog, rat, and mouse for DuP 721 (Table 11). Urinary elimination is more extensive in the rat (~40%) and

Table 11 Animal pharmacokinetics of DuP 721

Animal	Dose (mg/kg)	Route[a]	n	C_{max} (μg/ml)	T_{max} (min)	$t_{1/2}$ (min)	CL (ml/min/kg)	V (liters/kg)	F (%)	Urinary elimination (%)
Mice	20	p.o.	3	1.57	10	52			1.1	11.9
	20	i.v.	3			62	21.3	1.6		12.5
Rats	20	p.o.	2	14.7	30	121			0.9	36.1
	20	i.v.	2			111	5.7	0.9		44.1
Dogs	10	p.o.	1	6.4	30	120			1.3	3.2
	10	i.v.	1			74	13.4	1.9		1.4

[a]p.o., per os; i.v., intravenously.

weaker in the dog (~4%). The apparent elimination half-life is between 1 h (mice) and 2 h (rats, and dogs).

The mouse pharmacokinetics of DuP 105 have been investigated. The peak concentration in serum at 0.5 h is equivalent to that obtained with DuP 721, with an apparent elimination half-life of 0.5 h, compared to 1 h for DuP 721.

6. LINEZOLID AND EPEREZOLID

6.1. Antibacterial Activities

Linezolid (PNU-100766) is mainly active against gram-positive bacteria, including methicillin-resistant *S. aureus* (MRSA) (Table 12). Vancomycin and teicoplanin are more active than linezolid; the MICs at which 50% of isolates tested are inhibited MIC_{50}s for linezolid range from 1.0 to 2.0 μg/ml, and those of vancomycin and teicoplanin range from ≤0.5 to 1.0 μg/ml. Linezolid and levofloxacin exhibit the same antipneumococcal activities (MIC_{50}, 1.0 μg/ml).

Azithromycin and clarithromycin are two to four times more active than linezolid against *Pasteurella* (MIC_{50}, 2 to 4 μg/ml).

Eperezolid (U-100592) is twice as active in vitro as linezolid. Both molecules are active against strains of *S. aureus* (MIC_{50}, ~4 μg/ml) and *Staphylococcus epidermidis* (MIC_{50}, 1 to 2 μg/ml) irrespective of the activity of methicillin, but they are less active than vancomycin. They are very active against *Streptococcus pneumoniae*, whatever the susceptibility

Table 12 In vitro activity of linezolid

Organism(s)	n	MIC (μg/ml) 50%	MIC (μg/ml) 90%
MSSA	102	2.0	2.0
MRSA	53	2.0	2.0
S. epidermidis Met[s]	22	2.0	2.0
S. epidermidis Met[r]	28	1.0	2.0
Staphylococcus saprophyticus	30	1.0	1.0
S. agalactiae	50	1.0	1.0
Streptococcus milleri	28	2.0	2.0
S. pyogenes	20	1.0	1.0
Group C, G, and F streptococci	15	2.0	2.0
S. pneumoniae Pen[s]	177	0.5	1.0
S. pneumoniae Pen[i]	162	0.5	1.0
S. pneumoniae Pen[r]	68	1.0	1.0
S. pneumoniae Ery[r]	16	0.5	1.0
E. faecalis Van[s]	29	2.0	2.0
E. faecalis Van[r]	31	2.0	4.0
E. faecium Van[s]	36	2.0	2.0
E. faecium VanA	23	2.0	2.0
E. faecium VanB	22	2.0	4.0
Enterococcus avium	10	2.0	4.0
Enterococcus raffinosus	10	2.0	4.0
Enterococcus gallinarum	9	2.0	
Enterococcus casseliflavus	10	4.0	4.0
Bacillus cereus	10	1.0	1.0
L. monocytogenes	10	2.0	2.0
C. jeikeium	10	2.0	2.0
Pasteurella multocida	30	2.0	2.0
Other *Pasteurella* spp.[a]	17	2.0	32
Pasteurella multocida subsp. *septica*	43	2.0	2.0
Pasteurella canis	21	2.0	2.0
Pasteurella dagmatis	19	4.0	4.0
P. stomatis	19	4.0	8.0

Organism(s)	n	MIC (μg/ml) 50%	MIC (μg/ml) 90%
Mannheimia haemolytica	7	>32	
Actinobacillus	9	4.0	
Neisseria weaveri	13	8.0	16.0
EF-4b	13	8.0	80
Weeksella zoohelcum	10	1.0	2.0
Eikenella corrodens	20	8.0	16.0
Bordetella pertussis	21	4.0	4.0
Bordetella parapertussis	34	16	16
Neisseria gonorrhoeae	14	8.0	16
H. influenzae	10	16	16
M. catarrhalis			
Helicobacter pylori	14	16	>16
M. pneumoniae	8	8.0	
M. hominis	11	8.0	16
Borrelia burgdorferi		>2	
Legionella spp.	30	4.0	8.0
Clostridium spp.	20	2.0	2.0
Clostridium perfringens	50	2.0	2.0
Clostridium difficile	79	1.0	2.0
Peptostreptococcus spp.	17	1.0	2.0
Prevotella spp.	27	2.0	2.0
Porphyromonas spp.	25	1.0	2.0
Prevotella heparinolytica	13	2.0	2.0
Fusobacterium spp.	28	0.5	0.5
Propionibacterium acnes	30	0.5	0.5
B. fragilis	100	4.0	4.0
Mobiluncus	7	0.25	
Eubacterium	4	4.0	
Lactobacillus	3	2.0	
Actinomyces	3	1.0	
Nocardia spp.	62	2.0–4.0	

[a]*Pasteurella multocida* subsp. *gallicida* and *Pasteurella pneumotropica*.

to penicillin G (MIC_{50}s, 0.25 and 0.5 to 1 μg/ml, respectively). These molecules inhibit the growth of enterococci, including strains resistant to vancomycin, ampicillin, and minocycline, at concentrations of between 1 and 4 μg/ml. Bactericidal activity has been found against anaerobes such as *B. fragilis* (MIC_{50}, 1 to 2 μg/ml), *Clostridium* spp. (MIC_{50}, 2 μg/ml) and *Peptostreptococcus*, but the molecules are less active against *Prevotella* (MIC_{50}, 2 to 4 μg/ml). The in vitro activities of the two compounds against *Mycoplasma pneumoniae* (MIC, ~4 μg/ml) and *Mycoplasma hominis* (MIC, 4 to 32 μg/ml) are weak.

Two derivatives of U-100480 have been modified by oxidation, U-101603 (sulfoxide, X = SO) and U-101244 (sulfone, X = SO_2). They are more active than isoniazid (MIC, 2 μg/ml) against *M. tuberculosis* H_{37RV} (MIC, 0.125 μg/ml). They are active against multiresistant strains.

The MIC_{50} and MIC_{90} of eperezolid are 1 and 2 μg/ml, while those of linezolid are and 4 and 8 μg/ml, respectively. The activity against anaerobic bacteria is presented in Table 12. MICs for *Nocardia* spp. were determined by the E-test method, with which values are 4- to 16-fold lower than MICs obtained by the broth method. NCCLS breakpoints for linezolid are given in Table 13.

In vivo in murine systemic infections, eperezolid is more active against *S. aureus* and *Enterococcus faecium* than vancomycin, but eperezolid is less active than vancomycin against *E. faecalis*.

Linezolid is bacteriostatic against staphylococci and enterococci.

A weak in vitro postantibiotic effect (PAE) was shown for staphylococci at four times the MIC (0.6 to 1.4 h), but not for *E. faecalis*.

During clinical trials and therapy, development of resistant isolates of *Enterococcus* spp. and *S. aureus* occurred. In vitro resistance to linezolid occurs at a frequency of 10^{-9} to 10^{-11}.

Table 13 Linezolid breakpoints (NCCLS)[a]

Pathogen(s)	MIC (μg/ml)			Zone diam (mm)		
	S	I	R	S	I	R
Staphylococcus spp.	≤4			≥21		
Enterococcus spp.	≤2	4	≥8	≥23		
S. pneumoniae	≤2			≥21		
Streptococcus spp.	≤2			≥21		

[a]S, susceptible; I, intermediate; R, resistant.

6.2. Pharmacology and Toxicology

After oral administration, the lethal dose for dogs and rats is 500 mg/kg/day. After repeated dosing for a month, the no-effect dose for both species is 20 mg/kg/day. No adverse events have been shown for a concentration in plasma of less than 8 μg/ml.

For a dose of 40 to 50 mg/kg, a bone marrow atrophy had been shown, yielding to a clear drop in neutrophils, platelets, and erythrocytes.

Linezolid is not a substrate, inhibitor, or inducer of cytochrome P450.

6.3. Pharmacodynamics

The pharmacodynamics of linezolid have been studied in immunocompetent and in neutropenic mice, using the thigh pneumococcal infection model (*S. pneumoniae* Pen^s or Pen^r).

The pharmacodynamics of linezolid seem to be time dependent. The time above the MIC (T>MIC) for *S. pneumoniae* and *S. aureus* is about 40%.

In vivo the PAEs range from 3.6 to 3.8 h and from 3.1 to 3.9 h for *S. pneumoniae* and *S. aureus*, respectively, at doses of 20 and 80 mg/kg.

6.4. Human Pharmacokinetics

The intravenous pharmacokinetics have been determined. After a single dose of 1,500 mg, the apparent elimination half-life is 2.5 h and the concentrations in plasma are dose dependent.

Ascending-dose pharmacokinetics have been determined with eperezolid after administration of a single oral dose. The areas under the curve (0.83 to 40.1 μg·h/ml) and the peak concentrations in serum (0.15 to 9.78 μg/ml) increase linearly between 50 and 2,000 mg (capsules).

The apparent elimination half-life is between 2.4 h (50-mg capsule) and 6.9 h (2,000-mg capsules). Plasma and renal clearance is independent of the administered dose. Urinary elimination is about 50% (Table 14).

Twelve volunteers aged 25 to 53 years received a single dose of 375 mg of linezolid orally, either during fasting or after a rich meal, and then an infusion of 375 mg of linezolid (2-mg/ml solution) for 30 min after a wash-out period of 7 days. This was a randomized, open, crossover study.

The peak concentration in serum of 7.6 μg/ml was reached in 1.52 h, and the mean apparent elimination half-life was 5.0 h. About 30% of the parent molecule was eliminated in the urine. From a comparison of the areas under the plasma curve after intravenous and oral administrations, the absolute

Table 14 Pharmacokinetics of eperezolid (U-100592)

Form	Dose (mg)	C_{max} (μg/ml)	T_{max} (h)	AUC (μg·h/ml)	$t_{1/2}$ (h)	CL/F (liters/h)	CL_R (ml/min)	Fe (%)
Capsules	50	0.153	1.58	0.829	2.41	65.6	400	40.4
	100	0.332	1.90	1.51	2.32	75.1	610	52.5
	200	0.852	2.0	3.27	5.5	63.9	477	46.4
	400	1.75	2.0	8.17	8.06	52.4	435	52.3
	1,500	7.02	1.33	30.3	6.90	52.1		
	2,000	9.78	1.5	40.1	6.90	51.5		
Suspension	200	1.72	0.75	4.63	3.40	46.5	391	51.3
	400	3.26	0.66	9.09	4.56	45.9	505	63.4
	700	2.90	1.0	12.3	12.2	58.3	516	48.6
	1,000	5.73	0.7	20.0	12.2	54.5	454	50.6

bioavailability is on the order of 100%. The principal pharmacokinetic parameters are summarized in Tables 15 and 16.

Food does not alter the pharmacokinetics of linezolid. It delays absorption and slightly reduces the peak concentration in serum (Table 17).

After five doses of 600 mg of linezolid given every 12 h to each of six volunteers, no accumulation was reported. There are no significant differences between pharmacokinetics in young and elderly subjects (Table 18).

In patients suffering from a renal impairment with a creatinine clearance under 40 ml/min, an increase of plasma clearance was observed (Table 19).

Approximately 30% of a dose of linezolid is eliminated during a 3-h hemodialysis session begun 3 h after dosing. Hemodialysis removes the main metabolites.

Table 15 Linezolid: oral pharmacokinetics

Dose (mg)	C_{max} (μg/ml)	T_{max} (h)	$AUC_{0-\infty}$ (μg·h/ml)	$t_{1/2}$ (h)
375	8.21	1.67	65.5	4.98
500	10.4	1.38	74.3	4.59
625	12.7	1.33	102	4.87

Linezolid is primarily metabolized by nonenzymatic chemical oxidation of the morpholine ring into two inactive ring-opened carboxylic acid metabolites: an aminoethoxy acetic acid metabolite (A, or PNU-142585) and a hydroethyl glycine metabolite (B, or PNU-142300) (Fig. 11). They represent approximately 40 and 10% of the administered dose eliminated in urine and 6 and 3% of the administered dose eliminated in feces.

Study of the metabolism of eperezolid in the rat and dog and in vitro in human hepatocyte preparations showed that more than 90% of the radioactivity was eliminated in the urine in the unchanged form. In the rat, a sulfoconjugated metabolite of biliary origin was isolated. In dog urine and hepatic preparations a deacetylated derivative was isolated. Radioactivity was detected in all organs in the rat, except the central nervous system.

A study of U-100480 metabolism in the rat using the radiolabeled product revealed two metabolites in the urine but not in the feces, U-101603 (sulfoxide) and U-101244 (sulfone), which possess good antibacterial activity against *M. tuberculosis*.

The pharmacokinetics of linezolid are not altered in patients with mild to moderate hepatic impairment (Child-Pugh classes A and B) (Table 20).

Table 16 Linezolid: intravenous pharmacokinetics (single dose)

Dose (mg)	C_0 (μg/ml)	$AUC_{0-\infty}$ (μg·h/ml)	$t_{1/2}$ (h)	CL_P (ml/min)	CL_R (ml/min)	Urinary elimination (%)
250	6.4	27.1	5.4	58.5	43.1	27.8
500	11.2	82.9	5.9	107.24	34.9	33.3
750	14.4	104.9	4.9	125	40.8	33.9

Table 17 Linezolid pharmacokinetics after a single oral dose of 375 mg (fasting and food effects)

Subject status	C_{max}/C_0 (μg/ml)	T_{max} (h)	$AUC_{0-\infty}$ (μg·h/ml)	$t_{1/2}$ (h)	CL_P (ml/min)	CL_R (ml/min)	Urinary elimination (%)
Fasting	7.6	1.52	51.7	5.2			29.5
Fed	6.2	2.17	50.0	5.0			33.7
Intravenous	10.8	0.5	50.3	5.2	146	45.5	34.7

Table 18 Pharmacokinetics of linezolid in elderly subjects after a single oral dose of 600 mg

Subject age	n	C_{max} (μg/ml)	T_{max} (h)	$t_{1/2}$ (h)	CL_P (ml/min/kg)	CL_R (ml/min/kg)
Young	8	11.7 ± 2.3	1.0	5.3 ± 1.7	1.67 ± 0.27	0.44 ± 0.07
Elderly (≥65 yrs)	7	11.9 ± 2.9	1.2	4.6 ± 1.3	1.63 ± 0.44	0.31 ± 0.06

Table 19 Linezolid: pharmacokinetics in renally impaired patients

Group	Creatinine clearance (ml/min)	n	Plasma clearance (liters/h)	Elimination constant (liters/h)
1	>80	6	5.8 ± 1.3	0.12 ± 0.03
2	40–79	5	5.3 ± 2.5	0.13 ± 0.04
3	10–39	4	8.4 ± 4.8	0.17 ± 0.09
4	Hemodialysis (after)	4	4.9 ± 1.5	0.09 ± 0.04
	Hemodialysis (before)	4	8.8 ± 2.5	0.12 ± 0.05

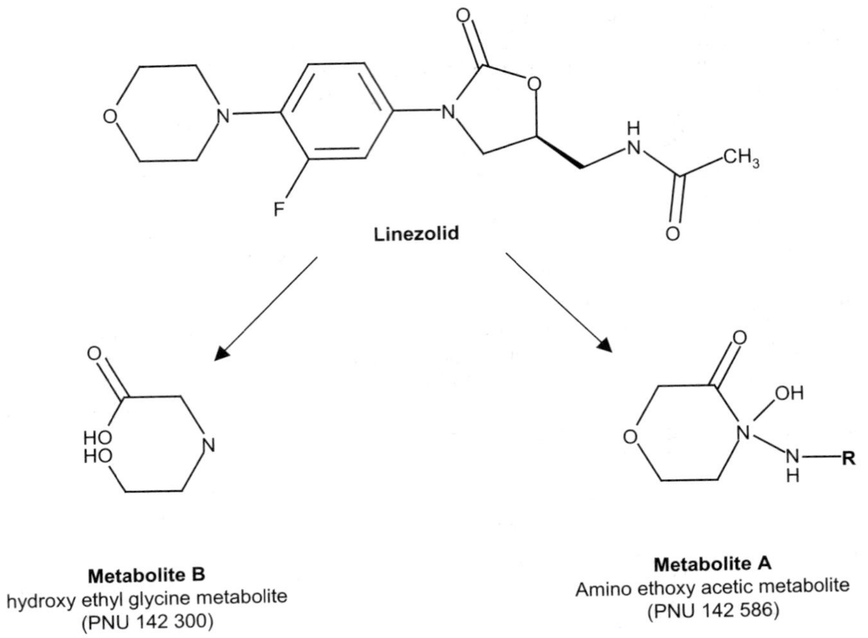

Figure 11 Linezolid metabolism

Table 20 Linezolid in hepatically impaired patients

Parameter	Liver-impaired patients, class A	Healthy volunteers
n	7	8
C_{max} (μg/ml)	11.5 ± 2.0	11.9 ± 1.8
T_{max} (h)	1.43 ± 0.93	1.44 ± 0.90
AUC (μg·h/ml)	128 ± 60	97 ± 31
$t_{1/2}$ (h)	6.77 ± 3.11	5.43 ± 1.58

There is no significant difference in pharmacokinetics according to gender or race.

Protein binding of linezolid is about 31% and is independent of the dose. Linezolid is eliminated in saliva and in sweat. In epithelial lining fluid the level 4 h postdose is 64.2 μg/ml (plasma, 15.5 μg/ml) and in alveolar macrophages it is 2.2 μg/ml; in skin blister fluid the concentration reaches a peak of 16.4 μg/ml 3 h postdose, with a half-life of 5.7 h and an area under the curve of 155.3 μg·h/ml. In cerebral fluid (shunt) the linezolid level ranged from 7.5 to 12.6 μg/ml.

Twelve patients undergoing total hip replacement were given 600 mg of linezolid as a 20-min infusion. The penetration in bone, fat, and muscle were assessed, and results are shown in Table 21.

In children the pharmacokinetic properties of two regimens were assessed; results are shown in Table 22.

Table 21 Linezolid tissue distribution

Sampling time (min)	Concn (μg/ml)		
	Bone	Fat	Muscle
10	9.1	4.5	10.4
20		5.2	13.4
30	6.3	4.1	12.0

Table 22 Pharmacokinetics of linezolid in children (intravenous route)

Parameter	Value at dose:	
	1.5 mg/kg	10 mg/kg
C_{max} (μg/ml)	2.5 ± 0.8	15.3 ± 4.7
T_{max} (h)	0.56 ± 0.1	0.54 ± 0.07
$AUC_{0-\infty}$ (μg·h/ml)	5.22 ± 3.1	44.2 ± 17.0
$t_{1/2}$ (h)	3.1 ± 1.1	2.7 ± 0.9
CL_P (liters/h/kg)	0.36 ± 0.16	0.26 ± 0.11
C_{12} (μg/ml)	0.04 ± 0.08	0.33 ± 0.51
C_{24} (μg/ml)	0.008 ± 0.016	0.07 ± 0.14

7. AZD 2563

AZD 2563 (Fig. 12) possesses a C-5 side chain substituted by an aryl moiety and a piperidinyl ring substituted by an *N*-dihydropropionyl substituent.

In a series, a replacement of the oxygen in the C-5 side chain by another linker to the isoxazole ring, such as NH, was investigated for effectiveness against gram-positive bacteria. In many cases the replacement by NH of the oxygen linkage yielded more potent compounds.

7.1. Antibacterial Activity

AZD 2563 is more active than linezolid. The MIC_{50} and MIC_{90} for *S. pneumoniae* are 0.5 and 1.0 μg/ml and 1.0 and 2.0 μg/ml for AZD 2563 and linezolid, respectively, irrespective of the susceptibility to penicillin G. Against other gram-positive bacteria the two compounds display the same antibacterial activities (Table 23).

Linezolid is more active against gram-negative anaerobes than is AZD 2563. Against gram-positive organisms the two compounds exhibit the same antibacterial activities. For *Aerococcus*, *Leuconostoc*, and *Rhodococcus* the MICs are 2.0 μg/ml, for *Dermabacter hominis* the MICs are 0.5 μg/ml, and for *Lactobacillus* the MICs are 0.5 and 1.0 μg/ml, respectively.

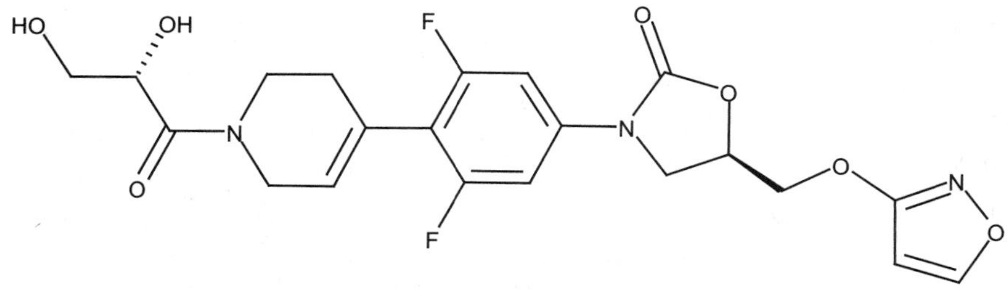

Figure 12 AZD 2563

Table 23 In vitro activity of AZD 2563

Microorganism(s)[a]	n	MIC (μg/ml)			
		AZD 2563		Linezolid	
		50%	90%	50%	90%
MSSA	70	0.5	1.0	2.0	2.0
MRSA	40	1.0	1.0	2.0	2.0
MSSE	70	1.0	2.0	1.0	2.0
MRSE	45	0.5	1.0	1.0	2.0
S. haemolyticus	51	0.5	1.0	1.0	2.0
S. pyogenes	42	0.5	1.0	1.0	1.0
S. agalactiae	66	1.0	2.0	1.0	1.0
S. pneumoniae	385	0.5	1.0	1.0	2.0
Viridans group streptococci		0.5	1.0	1.0	1.0
E. faecalis	53	1.0	2.0	2.0	2.0
E. avium	10	1.0	1.0	1.0	2.0
E. faecium	42	1.0	2.0	2.0	2.0
E. casseliflavus	15	1.0	1.0	2.0	2.0
E. gallinarum	18	2.0	2.0	2.0	4.0
E. raffinosus	10	1.0	2.0	2.0	2.0
Corynebacterium spp.	48	0.25	0.25	0.25	0.5
Listeria spp.	27	2.0	2.0	2.0	2.0
Micrococcus spp.	11	0.5	1.0	1.0	1.0
Stomatococcus spp.	6	0.5		1.0	
Bacillus spp.	23	0.5	1.0	1.0	1.0
C. jeikeium		0.25	2.0	0.5	4.0
H. influenzae	40	>128		16	32
M. catarrhalis	28	16	32	4.0	4.0
Peptostreptococcus spp.	75	1.0	2.0	1.0	2.0
P. acnes	16	0.5	0.5	0.5	0.5
C. perfringens	20	2.0	2.0	2.0	2.0
C. difficile	12	1.0	2.0	2.0	2.0
B. fragilis	10	>16		4.0	4.0
Prevotella/ Porphyromonas spp.	27	4.0	16	1.0	2.0
Fusobacterium spp.	24	2.0	>16	0.5	2.0

[a]MSSE, methicillin-susceptible *S. epidermidis*; MRSE, methicillin-resistant *S. epidermidis*.

It was proposed that breakpoints may be the following: susceptible, ≤2 μg/ml (≥20 mm), and resistant, ≥8 μg/ml (≤16 mm).

There were no marked effects of media (agar or broth), pH of the medium (pH 5, 6, 7, or 8), inoculum size, or addition of serum up to 25%.

AZD 2563, like linezolid, exerts only bacterioststic activity.

After serial passages the frequency of mutants was 10^{-8}.

In a neutropenic-mouse model of thigh infection due to *S. pneumoniae* (6 weeks, 23 to 27 g), at doses of 20 and 80 mg/kg, the in vivo PAEs were 2.8 and 8.1 h, respectively, and in immunocompetent mice the PAE is above 24 h.

The pharmacodynamics for AZD 2563 are concentration dependent (area under the curve/MIC).

In order to improve the pharmacokinetic behavior, series of AZD 2563 analogs have been synthesized by modifying the side chain fixes on the tetrahydropyridine ring. In vivo some of them are more efficient than the parent compound (two to three times).

8. RANBEZOLID

Ranbezolid (RBx 7644) (Fig. 13) is a piperazinyl phenyl oxazolidinone, the piperazine ring being substituted by a nitrofuryl ring.

8.1. Antibacterial Activity

Against common pathogens, including MRSA, ranbezolid displays in vitro activity similar to that of linezolid. Ranbezolid is active against gram-negative anaerobes (Mathur et al., 2004), while linezolid is poorly active (Table 24).

Ranbezolid displays bacteriostatic activity.

In vitro the PAE against MRSA at 562 and 8 times the MIC are 3.0 and 5.0 h after exposures of 1 and 2 h, respectively (linezolid, 2.0 and 2.0 h).

8.2. In Vivo Efficacy

Ranbezolid is more efficient than linezolid in murine infections (Table 25).

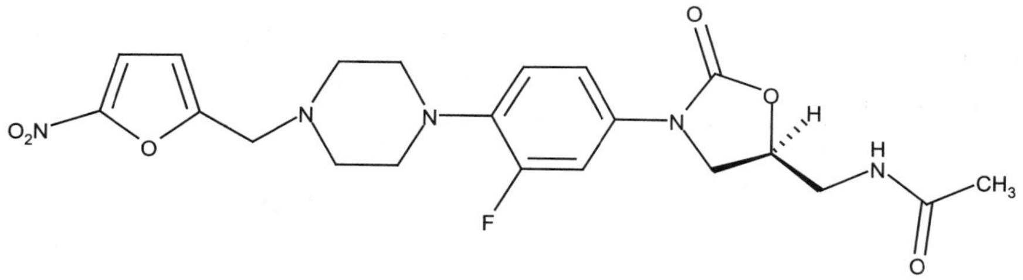

Figure 13 Ranbezolid

Table 24 In vitro activity of ranbezolid

Microorganism(s)[a]	*n*	MIC (μg/ml)			
		Ranbezolid		Linezolid	
		50%	90%	50%	90%
MSSA	50	1.0	2.0	2.0	2.0
MRSA	154	2.0	2.0	2.0	2.0
MSSE	23	0.5	2.0	1.0	2.0
MRSE	31	0.5	2.0	1.0	1.0
E. faecalis	31	10	2.0	2.0	2.0
E. faecium	35	2.0	2.0	2.0	2.0
Bacillus spp.	4	0.06		1.0	
S. pneumoniae	196	0.5	1.0	1.0	2.0
H. influenzae	10	16	32	8.0	16
M. catarrhalis	3	0.5		4.0	
N. gonorrhoeae	17	2.0	16	8.0	16
M. tuberculosis	30	2.0	8.0	1.0	64
M. avium	14	4.0	16	16	32
B. fragilis	26	0.06	0.125	4.0	4.0
Bacteroides thetaiotaomicron	12	0.06	0.125	4.0	4.0
Bacteroides distasonis	12	0.06	0.25	4.0	4.0
Fusobacterium nucleatum	11	0.06	0.03	0.5	1.0
Prevotella/Porphyromonas	57	0.06	0.25	2.0	2.0
Prevotella bivia	11	0.25	0.5	2.0	4.0
Peptostreptococcus spp.	52	≤0.008	0.01	1.0	2.0
P. acnes	11	1.0	2.0	0.5	0.5
C. perfringens	20	0.06	0.06	2.0	8.0
C. difficile	10	0.03	0.03	2.0	2.0

[a]MSSE, methicillin-susceptible *S. epidermidis*; MRSE, methicillin-resistant *S. epidermidis*.

8.3. Animal Pharmacokinetics

The pharmacokinetic profile of ranbezolid was determined in rats and mice after intravenous and oral administrations (Table 26).

9. MECHANISMS OF ACTION AND RESISTANCE

The oxazolidinones cannot cross the outer membrane of gram-negative bacilli, which explains their lack of activity against *Enterobacteriaceae*. It was shown for linezolid that the affinity for ribosomes of gram-positive bacteria is higher than that for ribosomes of gram-negative bacilli. Probably linezolid is less active against gram-negative bacilli due to an important efflux system through the AcrAB-TolC efflux pump.

DuP 721, eperezolid, linezolid, and other oxazolidinone derivatives are potent protein synthesis inhibitors. They block this synthesis before the initiation phase, an event that occurs before the interaction between f-Met-tRNA and the 30S ribosomal subunit. Inhibition occurs only after a cycle of synthesis. DuP 721 must inhibit the recognition site at position 3′ of the binding site of mRNA. In an acellular system, it does not inhibit elongation and does not inhibit the end of synthesis of the polypeptide chain. Likewise, it does not inhibit the initiation of the polypeptide chain. To exert an inhibitory effect, DuP 721 must act in a cellular medium (Fig. 14), where there is inhibition of the elongation factors. In summary, they block the initiation process. They bind the 50S rRNA through domain V of the 23S rRNA (U2113, A2114, A2119, U2118, and C2153). It was also shown that linezolid interacts with the 16S rRNA (site A864) of the 30S ribosomal subunit. At the level of the 50S subunit linezolid also interacts with protein L1. Linezolid does not inhibit the peptidyltransferase activity.

Even if it seems that mutants are difficult to obtain after 20 sequential passages, only a single step is needed. The frequency is above 10^{-9}.

A mutation in the 23S rRNA gene has been detected in linezolid- or eperezolid-resistant *S. aureus* and *E. faecalis* strains. In *E. faecalis* this involves a mutation of the uridine to a guanine (base 2528), and in *S. aureus* it involves a mutation of a uridine to a guanine at base 2447. For *E. faecium* a mutation on domain V of 23S rRNA has been reported (G2576U).

10. NEW INVESTIGATIONAL MOLECULES

New series of oxazolidinones have been synthesized with the intention of increasing the solubility in water so as to be able to prepare a pharmaceutical formulation for intravenous use, enlarge the antibacterial spectrum or enhance the antibacterial activity, or overcome linezolid resistance.

New chemical alterations have been directed to the C-4′ position of the phenyl ring or to both the C-5 side chain of the oxazolidinone ring and the phenyl ring.

10.1. Morphonyl and Piperazinyl Rings and Esters

Oxidation of the piperazinyl or morphonyl nucleus of linezolid or eperezolid increases the solubility in water 100-fold (linezolid, 2.9 mg/ml, versus 470 mg/ml for *N*-oxide linezolid).

Efforts have been centered around the morpholine ring (linezolid) in incorporating a novel thiomorpholine C-ring in place of the morpholine residue.

10.1.1. PNU-288034

Sulfoxide, sulfones, and thiomorpholine analogs, such as PNU-288034 (Fig. 15), have emerged as promising candidates.

Table 25 In vivo activity of ranbezolid

Organism	Ranbezolid			Linezolid		
	MIC (μg/ml)	ED_{50} (mg/kg)[a]		MIC (μg/ml)	ED_{50} (mg/kg)	
		i.v.	p.o.		i.v.	p.o.
MRSA	1.0	1.56	5.2	2.0	4.42	5.6
MRSE[b]	0.125		2.79	2.0		9.12
E. faecalis	1.0	6.25	10.51	2.0	3.12	8.83

[a]i.v., intravenously; p.o., per os.
[b]MRSE, methicillin-resistant *S. epidermidis*.

Table 26 Rodent pharmacokinetics of ranbezolid

Animal	Dose (mg/kg)	Route[a]	C_{max} (μg/ml)	T_{max} (h)	AUC (μg·h/ml)	$t_{1/2}$ (h)	Bioavailability (%)
Mouse	6.25	p.o.	4.54	0.5	6.8	1.2	107.9
	12.5	p.o.	5.73	0.25	9.27	1.4	
	25	p.o.	16.58	0.25	30.7	1.1	
	75	p.o.	19.56	0.5	60.44	2	
	125	p.o.	45.93	0.5	136.7	2	
	6.25	i.v.	12.29		6.3	1.7	
Rat	5.0	p.o.	3.47	0.25	7.55	1.2	114
	15	p.o.	7.06	0.75	22	2.3	94
	50	p.o.	11.07	2.0	73	2.9	114
	5.0	i.v.	5.54		6.61	1.3	
	15	i.v.	24.24		23.17	1.6	
	50	i.v.	47.5		63.97	1.3	

[a]p.o., per os; i.v., intravenously.

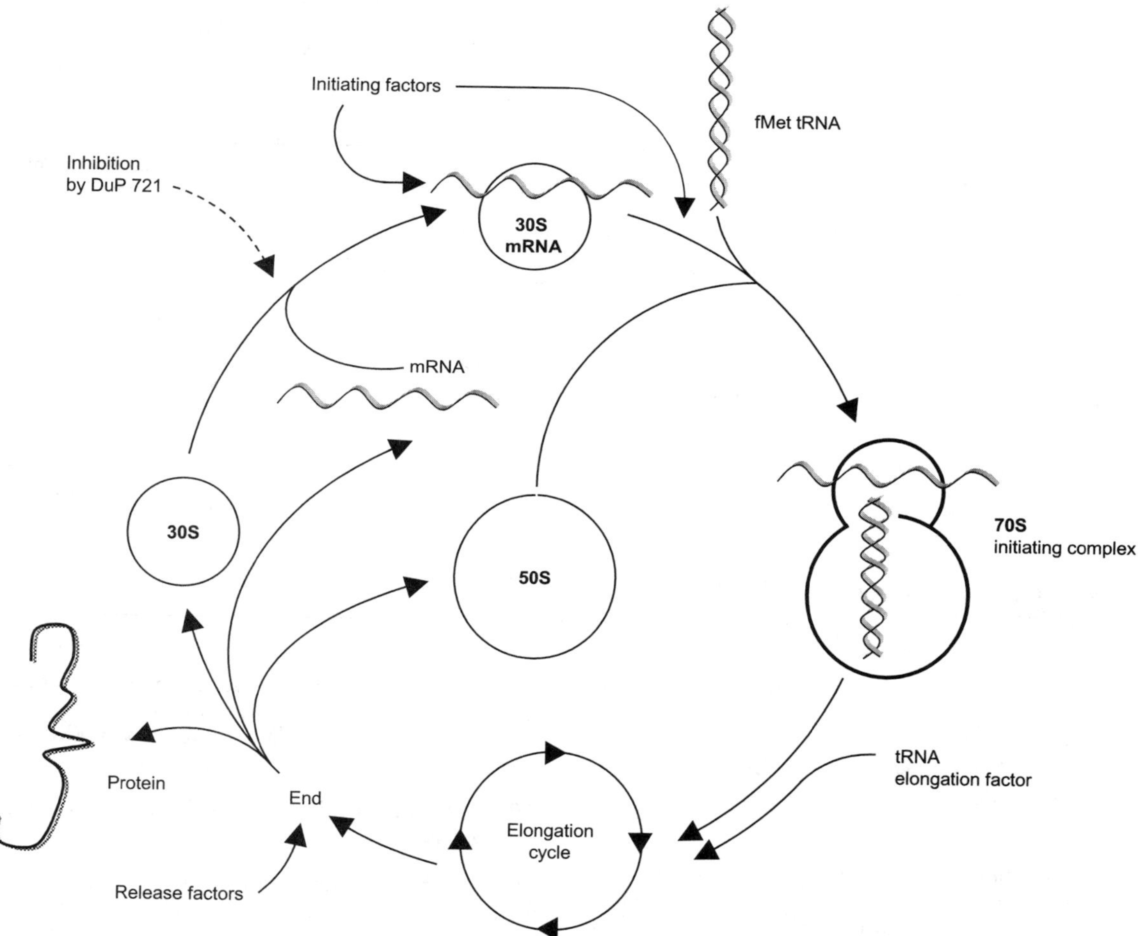

Figure 14 Mechanism of action of DuP 721

10.1.2. Oxazolidinone Derivative Esters

A series of esters of eperezolid has been synthesized in order to increase its solubility in water, which is 4.2 mg/ml in a phosphate buffer at pH 7. The prodrugs with an ionizable chain (succinate or phosphate) are soluble in water. A certain number of these esters possess antibacterial activity, such as eperezolid glycinate (PNU 101099) and eperezolid phosphate (PNU-101850) (Fig. 16).

These two derivatives have intravenous pharmacokinetics in animals comparable to those of eperezolid, but orally they are inferior. It is possible to obtain analogs of linezolid with activity similar to that of the parent molecule by modifications

Figure 15 PNU-288034

	R		Water solubility (mg/ml)
PNU 101 099		Glycinate	150.0
PNU 101 850		Phosphate	25.7
Eperezolid	H	-	4.2
Linezolid	H		2.9

Figure 16 Oxazolidinone derivative esters

at C-5. However, when the size of the N substituent increases, the antibacterial activity decreases. It is possible to replace the morphonyl and piperazinyl nuclei by 4-piperidinyl, pyranyl, or thiopyranyl nuclei while still preserving antibacterial activity.

10.1.3. PH-027

PH-027 is a morphonyl oxazolidinone with a triazole ring at C-5 position (Fig. 17). PH-027 belongs to a series of analogs for which an aryl moiety, substituted or not, was appended at the C-5 position. PH-027 exhibits good antibacterial activity in vitro against gram-positive cocci, with a MIC range from 0.5 to 2.0 μg/ml. Against gram-positive and -negative anaerobes, PH-027 displays good activity (MICs, 0.5 to 2.0 μg/ml).

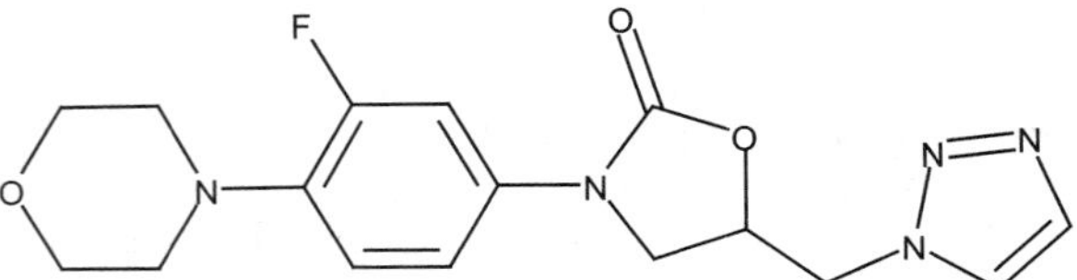

Figure 17 PH-027

10.2. Monocyclic Rings: Five-Membered-Ring Derivatives

10.2.1. Thienyl and Pyridyl Rings

Two series of derivatives with either an *N*-thienyl or *N*-pyridyl nucleus have been synthesized (Fig. 18). However, a second ring attached to the *N*-thienyl or *N*-pyridyl is essential for good antibacterial activity. Two protagonists have been obtained, a 4-(4-pyridinyl-2-pyridyloxazolidinone) and the equivalent in the *N*-thienyl series.

10.2.2. Azolylphenyl Oxazolidinones

The azolylphenyl oxazolidinones, a new series, are composed of novel derivatives having as a third ring a pyrrolyl, pyrazolyl, imidazolyl, triazolyl, thidiazol, imidazolyl (Fig. 19), or

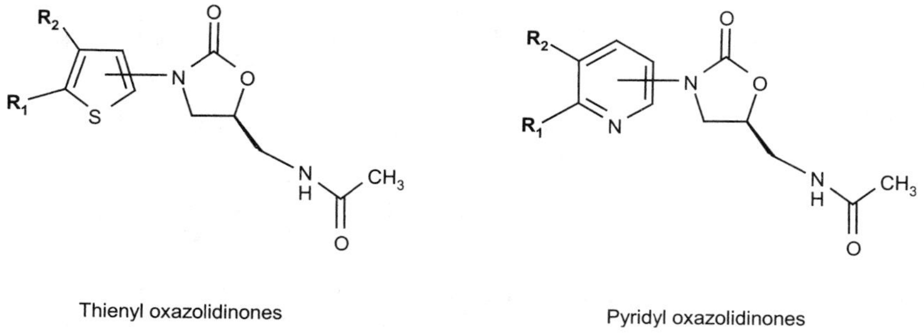

Thienyl oxazolidinones

Pyridyl oxazolidinones

Figure 18 Pyridyl and thienyl oxazolidinones

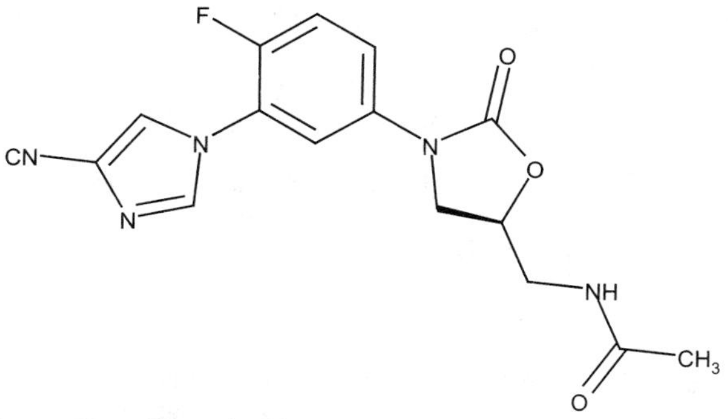

Figure 19 Cyano imidazolyl oxazolidinones

tetrazolyl moiety. Compounds bearing an imidazolyl or a 1H-1,2,4-triazolyl ring show better water solubility (3.2 or 2.6 mg/ml, respectively). Some analogs having a pyrrolyl or a 1H-1,2,3-triazolyl ring display increased activity against gram-negative bacteria, such as PNU-140457 (Fig. 20). Compounds having a 3-cyanopyrrolyl (PNU-171933) and 4-cyanopyrazolyl (PNU-172576) had a MICs of ≤0.5 μg/ml for *S. aureus* and of 2 to 4 ug/ml for *H. influenzae* and

	R
PNU 140,457	
PNU 176,798	

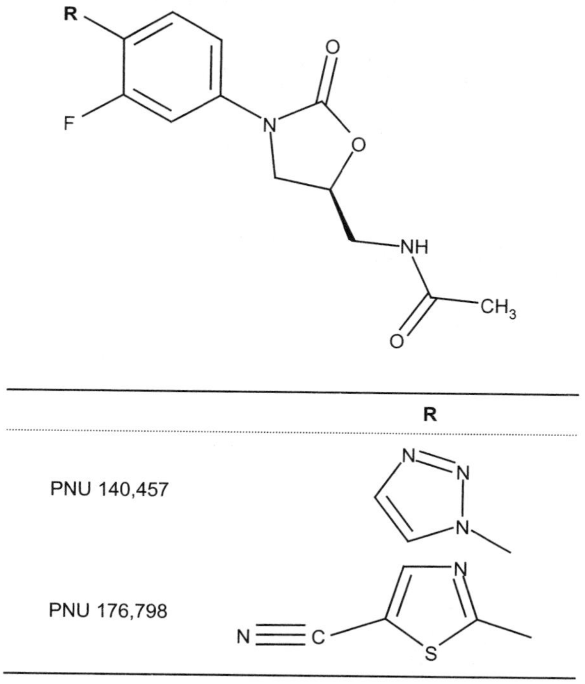

Figure 20 Azolylphenyl oxazolidinones

M. catarrhalis. These analogs have good pharmacokinetic behavior in Sprague-Dawley rats, with apparent elimination half-lives of 5.1 and 5.3 h, respectively (9.9 mg/kg intravenously and 42.9 mg/kg orally).

10.2.2.1. 1,3-Thiazolylphenyloxazolidinone

A series of 1,3-thiazolylphenyloxazolidinone analogs having a C-C linkage has been synthesized. Only one derivative showed moderate activity against *H. influenzae* AI30063 and *M. catarrhalis* MC 30,607, with MICs of 2 and 0.5 μg/ml, respectively. This compound is a 5-cyano-1,3-thiazolyl analog (PNU-176798). However, it is poorly soluble in water (0.016 mg/ml).

10.2.2.2. PNU-182347

A series of 2-substituted 1,3,4-thiadiazolylphenyloxazolidinone thioamides was synthesized. The aim of the continuous investigation of oxazolidinone was to expand the antibacterial spectrum of linezolid to fastidious gram-negative bacilli such as *H. influenzae*. In a previous report, it had been demonstrated that oxazolidinone analogs having a 1,3,4-thiadiazolyl moiety fixed on the fluorophenyl of the oxazolidinone core possessed good in vitro activity against gram-positive and -negative bacteria. In this new series of oxazolidinone analogs having a thioamide side chain, one compound, PNU-182347 (Fig. 21), was selected for further preclinical investigation. This compound is poorly soluble in water: 0.033 mg/ml at pH 7.0. PNU-182347 exhibited good in vitro activity against MRSA and *S. aureus* susceptible to methicillin (MSSA), *S. epidermidis* resistant to methicillin, *S. pneumoniae*, *E. faecalis* susceptible to vancomycin, *H. influenzae*, and *M. catarrhalis*, with MICs of <0.5 μg/ml. In murine staphylococcal disseminated infections, after an oral administration of PNU-182347, the ED_{50} was >20 mg/kg; in comparison, the linezolid ED_{50} was 8.0 mg/kg.

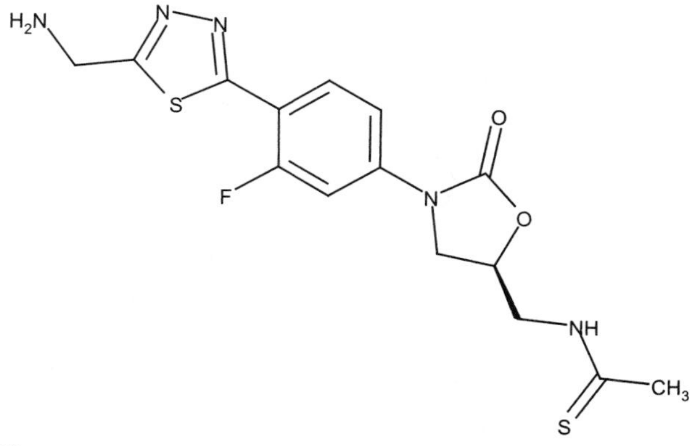

Figure 21 PNU-182347

10.2.2.3. RWJ-302377 and RWJ-306490

A series of piperidinylfluorophenyl oxazolidinone derivatives was synthesized. Variations were made on substituents of the piperidinyl nitrogen. Two compounds were selected for further investigation: RWJ-302377 and RWJ-306490 (Fig. 22). Neither of them was more active than linezolid. RWJ-306490 exhibited antistaphylococcal activity in disseminated murine (Swiss-Webster) infection induced intraperitoneally with 10^5 CFU of *S. aureus* Smith per ml. After administration of RWJ-306490 subcutaneously at 1.0 and 3.0 h after bacterial challenge, the ED_{50} was 13.2 mg/kg/day (versus 2.7 mg/kg/day for linezolid).

10.2.2.4. Pyrrolopyrimidine Oxazolidinones

A series of pyrrolopyrimidine analogs has been reported, and three compounds have been selected for further investigation: JNJ 1026217, JNJ 10391849, and JNJ 10283104 (Fig. 23).

In vitro they are more active than linezolid, with MICs from 0.5 to 2.0 μg/ml for MRSA, MSSA, *E. faecalis*, and *E. faecium* (linezolid MICs, 1.0 to 2.0 μg/ml).

In vivo they exert similar efficacies in murine infections induced with MRSA, with ED_{50}s of 11 to 17 mg/kg (subcutaneous route of administration) (linezolid ED_{50}, 11 mg/kg).

10.2.2.5. DA-7686

DA-7686 is a pyridine-containing oxazolidinone derivative. Most of the pyridine derivatives exhibited a MIC_{90} of 0.39 μg/ml for MRSA isolates; the MIC_{90}s ranged from 0.78 to 1.56 μg/ml for *S. pneumoniae* isolates resistant to penicillin G and for *M. catarrhalis*. In murine staphylococcal disseminated infections, DA-7686 was claimed to be twofold more active than linezolid, with ED_{50}s of 8.6 and 3.6 mg/kg after an oral administration for MRSA and MSSA, respectively.

10.2.2.6. DA-7867

DA-7867 is a substituted pyridylphenoxy oxazolidinone (Fig. 24). The water solubility and the lipophilicity (logP) are pH dependent.

Many aryl substituents have been appended to the fluorophenyl ring. Some of analogs exhibit a higher in vitro activity than linezolid against *H. influenzae*, with MICs of 1.56 μg/ml, such as DA-7880, DA-7888, DA-7894, DA-8997, and DA-7898, with good antistaphylococcal activity (MICs from 0.39 to 0.78 μg/ml) and activity against vancomycin-resistant enterococci (VRE) (MICs from 0.39 to 0.78 μg/ml).

The compounds with isoxazole and pyrrazol moieties showed high in vitro activity but low in vivo efficacies.

10.2.2.6.1. Antibacterial activity. The antibacterial activity of DA-7867 is summarized in Table 27.

10.2.2.6.2. In vivo activity. DA-7867 is two to six times more active in vivo than is linezolid (Table 28).

In male ICR mice (18 to 20 g), after intranasal inoculation of 40 μl of penicillin-resistant *S. pneumoniae*, the ED_{50}s were 0.9 and 46.8 mg/kg for DA-7867 and linezolid, respectively.

The PAEs for VRE and MRSA for 1 h of contact and at four times the MICs ranged from 1.0 h up to 1.63 h.

10.2.2.6.3. Animal pharmacokinetics. The pharmacokinetics in mice and rats were assessed for oral and intravenous administrations (Table 29).

10.2.2.7. VRC-3406

In a series of 3′-fluoro-4′-thioether 3-phenyloxazolidinones, VRC-3406 (Fig. 25) was chosen for further investigation. This compound possesses a 2′-nitrothiazolyl thio ring attached to the 3′-fluorophenyl moiety. The compound was the most active of this series, but no activity was demonstrated against *S. aureus* isolates resistant to linezolid, *H. influenzae*, or *M. catarrhalis*.

10.2.2.8. VRC-3054 and VRC-3055

A series of 4′-amido-3′fluoro-phenyloxazolidinones, was synthesized with various five- and six-membered heterocycles attached on the 4′-amino group. None of them were active against *S. aureus* isolates resistant to linezolid (MIC, >64 μg/ml), and the most active compounds, VRC-3054 and VRC-3055 (Fig. 26), possess on the 4′-amido group thiazole and 2′-chloropyridinyl moieties, respectively. They exhibit in vitro activity similar to that of linezolid, and in murine disseminated infections induced with *S. aureus*

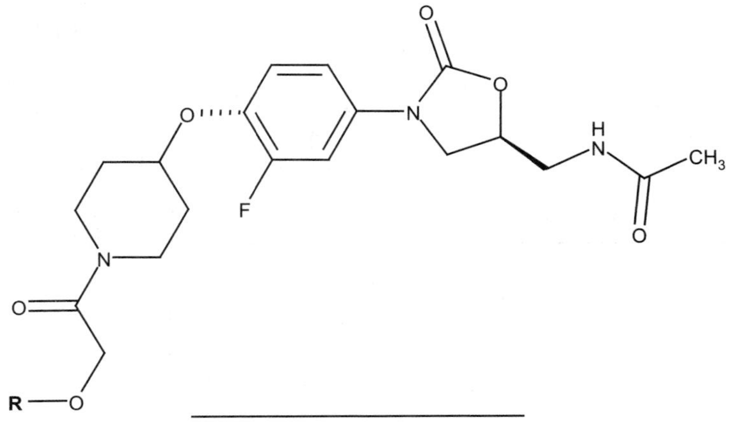

	R
RWJ 302 377	pH CH_2O
RWJ 306 490	H

Figure 22 Pyridinyloxy-substituted oxozolidinones

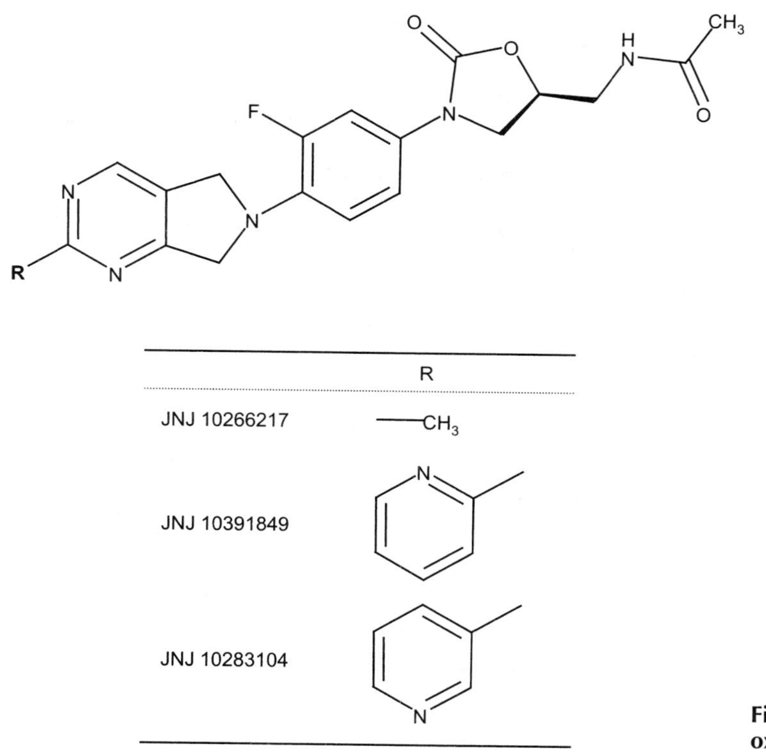

	R
JNJ 10266217	CH_3
JNJ 10391849	
JNJ 10283104	

Figure 23 Pyrrolopyrimidine oxazolidinones

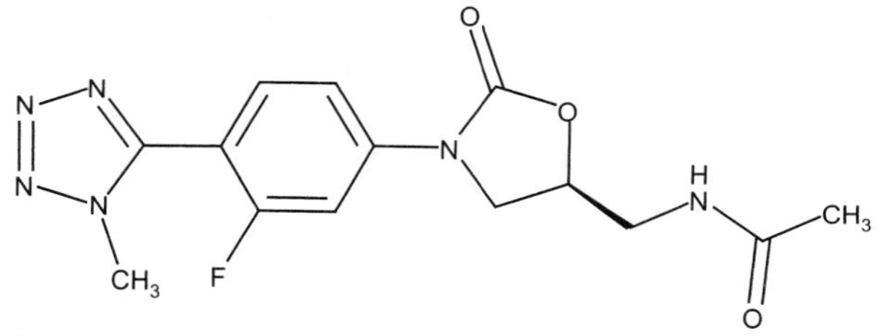

Figure 24 DA-7867

Smith, the ED_{50}s were 8.5, 7.5, and 5.5 mg/kg for VRC-3054, VRC-3055, and linezolid, respectively.

10.2.2.9. VRC-3816 and VRC-3839

A new series of tetrahydro-4-(2*H*)-thiopyran oxazolidinones exemplified by PNU-176723 and PNU-141659 was produced by modifying the C-5 side chain. Two compounds, VRC-3816 and 3839 (Fig. 26), exhibit activity in vitro comparable to that of linezolid, with a slight enhancement of in vitro activity against *H. influenzae* (MICs, 4 and 8 μg/ml, instead of 8 to 16 μg/ml for linezolid). The monofluoro (VRC-3816) and the difluoro thiopyran analogs were tested in a disseminated staphylococcal (*S. aureus* UC 9213 Met^r) murine infections; the ED_{50}s after oral administration were 3.75, 6.52, and 5.0 mg/kg for VRC-3816, VRC-3839, and linezolid, respectively.

10.2.2.10. VRC-3599

In a new series of 4′-acyl amino-3′-fluoro-phenyloxazolidinones, new six- and five-membered heterocycles were attached to 4′-amino group. The nitrofuran analog (VRC-3599) (Fig. 27) exhibits enhanced activity against *S. aureus* resistant to linezolid (MIC, 8 μg/ml, versus >64 μg/ml for linezolid) and against *H. influenzae* (MIC, 2 to 8 μg/ml, versus 8 to 16 μg/ml for linezolid).

VRC-3599 is more efficient in murine infections (Alderley Park mice) than linezolid and is devoid of toxicological effects.

Table 27 In vitro activity of DA-7867

Microorganism(s)	*n*	MIC (μg/ml)			
		DA-7867		Linezolid	
		50%	90%	50%	90%
MSSA	33	0.25	0.25	2.0	2.0
MRSA	30	0.12	0.25	2.0	2.0
MSCoNS	22	0.1	0.12	1.0	1.0
MRCoNS	29	0.12	0.25	1.0	2.0
VRE	10	0.12	0.12	2.0	2.0
S. pneumoniae	22	0.03	0.03	4.0	2.0
S. pyogenes	15	0.06	0.12	0.5	1.0
S. agalactiae	15	0.06	0.12	0.5	1.0
H. influenzae	24	3.13	3.13	8.0	8.0
M. catarrhalis	24	0.5	0.5	4.0	4.0
Peptostreptococcus spp.	56	≤0.06	0.12	1.0	2.0
C. perfringens	17	0.12	0.12	2.0	2.0
C. difficile	15	0.12	0.25	2.0	2.0
B. fragilis	34	1.0	2.0	4.0	4.0
B. thetaiotaomicron	15	2.0	4.0	4.0	8.0

[a]MSCoNS, methicillin-susceptible coagulase-negative staphylococci; MRCoNS, methicillin-resistant coagulase-negative staphylococci.

Table 28 In vivo efficacy of DA-7867

Microorganism(s)	Compound	MIC (μg/ml)	ED_{50} (mg/kg)
MSSA	DA-7867	0.78	3.4
	Linezolid	3.13	8.0
MRSA	DA-7867	0.78	2.6
	Linezolid	3.13	8.3
S. pneumoniae III	DA-7867	0.39	11.6
	Linezolid	6.25	66
S. pneumoniae Pen^r	DA-7867	0.39	2.4
	Linezolid	6.25	5.9
VRE	DA-7867	0.20	4.5
	Linezolid	1.56	28.4

10.2.2.11. PNU-288034

Two fluorine atoms are attached on the phenyl ring, as is a thiomorphonyl moiety (Fig. 15).

In this series it was shown that at the C-5 position a thioamide moiety leads to more active derivatives than a carboxamide residue.

The selected analog, PNU-288034, exhibits in vitro activity similar to that of linezolid against both gram-positive cocci and fastidious gram-negative bacilli. For gram-positive cocci the MIC_{50} and MIC_{90} range from 0.5 to 1.0 μg/ml and 1.0 to 2.0 μg/ml, respectively. For *H. influenzae* the MIC_{50} and MIC_{90} are 8.0 and 16 μg/ml.

Table 29 Pharmacokinetics of DA-7867 in rodents

Animals	Compound	Dose (mg/kg)	Route[a]	C_{max} (μg/ml)	T_{max} (h)	AUC (μg·h/ml)	$t_{1/2}$ (h)	*F* (%)
Mice	DA-7867	5	i.v.	9.76	0.0016	35.8	7.37	
		5	p.o.	4.24	1.0	32.5	5.56	90.8
	Linezolid	5	p.o.	5.19	0.08	4.43	0.63	
Rats	DA-7867	5	p.o.	5.75	1.25	139	12.4	54.1
		5	i.v.	39.3	0.016	257	15.8	
	Linezolid	5	p.o.	6.5	0.139	9.2	0.94	

[a]i.v., intravenously; p.o., per os.

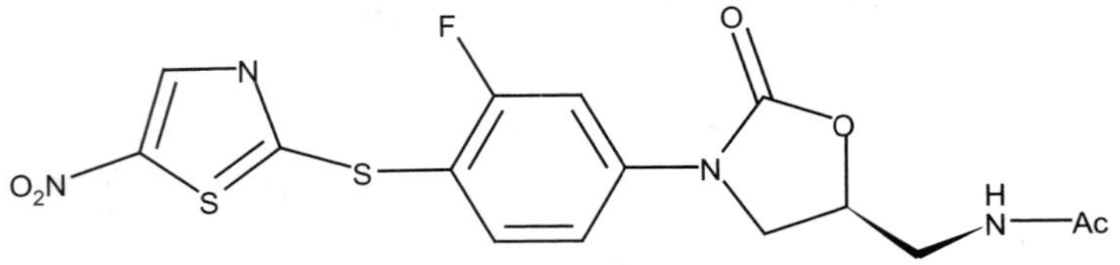

Figure 25 VRC-3406

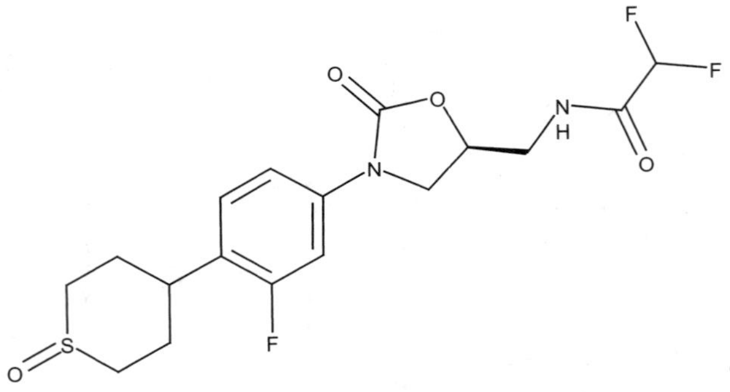

VRC-3839

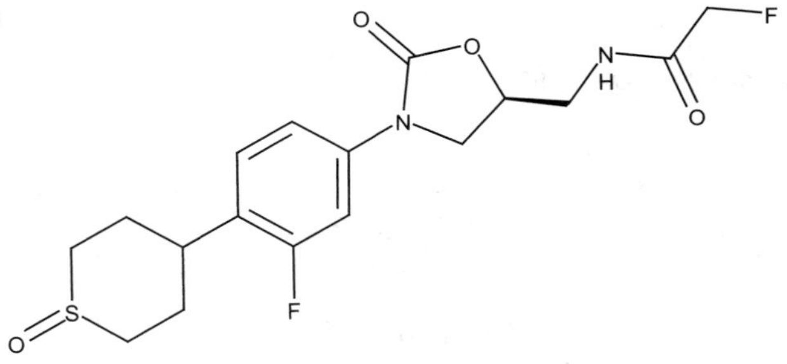

VRC-3816

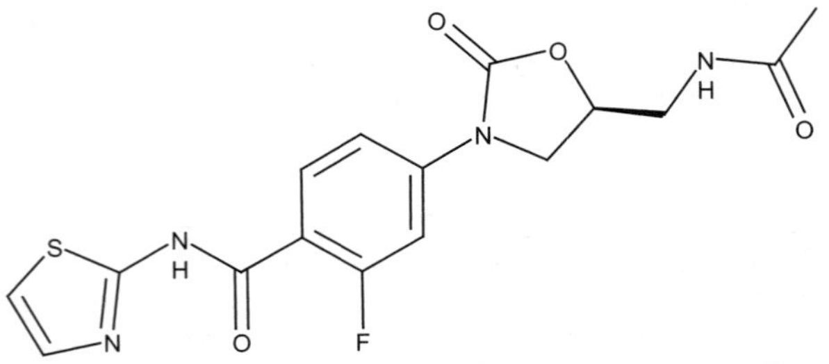

VRC-3054

Figure 26 VRC-3054, VRC-3816, and VRC-3839

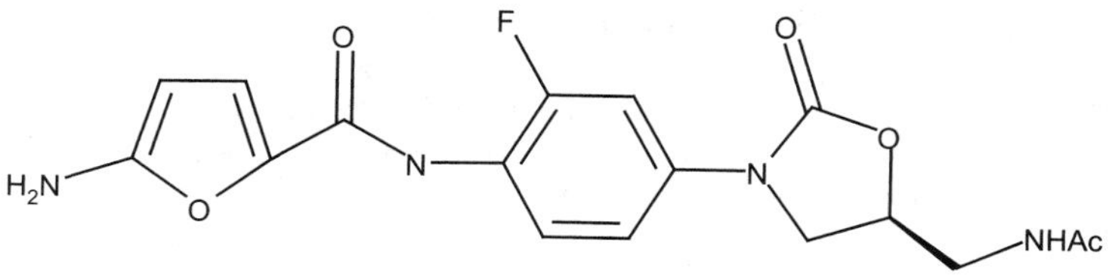

Figure 27 VRC-3599

In a model of endocarditis induced with an MRSA isolate in male New Zealand White rabbits, negative cultures were obtained (50 mg/kg), like for vancomycin (25 mg/kg intravenously).

10.2.3. Tetrahydrothiopyranyl Phenyloxazolidinone Sulfoxides and Sulfones

The morpholine ring of linezolid could be modified while retaining antibacterial activity, especially when the replacement was done with a 3,6-dihydro-4-(2*H*)-thiopyran ring.

A new series of thiopyranyl sulfoxide and sulfone analogs has been synthesized with various side chains replacing the acetamido group. Some analogs in this series exhibited enhanced in vitro activities, including against fastidious gram-negative bacilli such as *H. influenzae* and *M. catarrhalis*. Some analogs showed higher water solubility, up to 20.2 mg/ml, such as compound B.

Biotransformation of PNU-176723 (Fig. 28), a *cis* isomer of the tetrahydro-4-(2*H*)-thiopyranyl phenyloxazolidinone sulfoxide, to the corresponding *trans* isomer was investigated in rats (Sprague-Dawley). The *cis* isomer was biotransformed to the *trans* isomer, and an additional metabolite, a sulfone metabolite, was obtained. It seems that the bioconversion occurs via reduction of the sulfoxide to the sulfide by bacteria in the gastrointestinal tract, followed by the preferential presystemic oxidative metabolism of the sulfoxide to the *trans* sulfoxide.

10.2.4. Carbon-Carbon-Linked Five- or Six-Membered Heteroaryl Phenyloxazolidinones

The link between the phenyl ring and the heterocycle appended on this moiety may be either a carbon-carbon bond, a sulfur-carbon bond, or a nitrogen-carbon bond.

The morpholine ring of linezolid was replaced with various five- or six-membered-ring moieties such as pyrazole, thiophene, oxazole, thiazole, 2,4-oxadiazole, 2,4-thiadiazole, and 2,4-thiomorpholine phenyl rings.

Two cyanothiophene analogs exhibited good in vitro activity against gram-positive cocci, and one of them had good activity against *M. catarrhalis* (MIC, ≤0.5 μg/ml) but was devoid of activity against *H. influenzae* (MIC, >64 μg/ml). A cyanothiophene analog also exhibited good activity against gram-positive cocci (MIC, ≤0.12 to 0.25 μg/ml) and against *M. catarrhalis* (MIC, 0.25 μg/ml) and *H. influenzae* (MIC, 2 μg/ml, versus 16 μg/ml for linezolid). A methyloxazole derivative and thiazole analog also displayed good activity against gram-positive organisms but

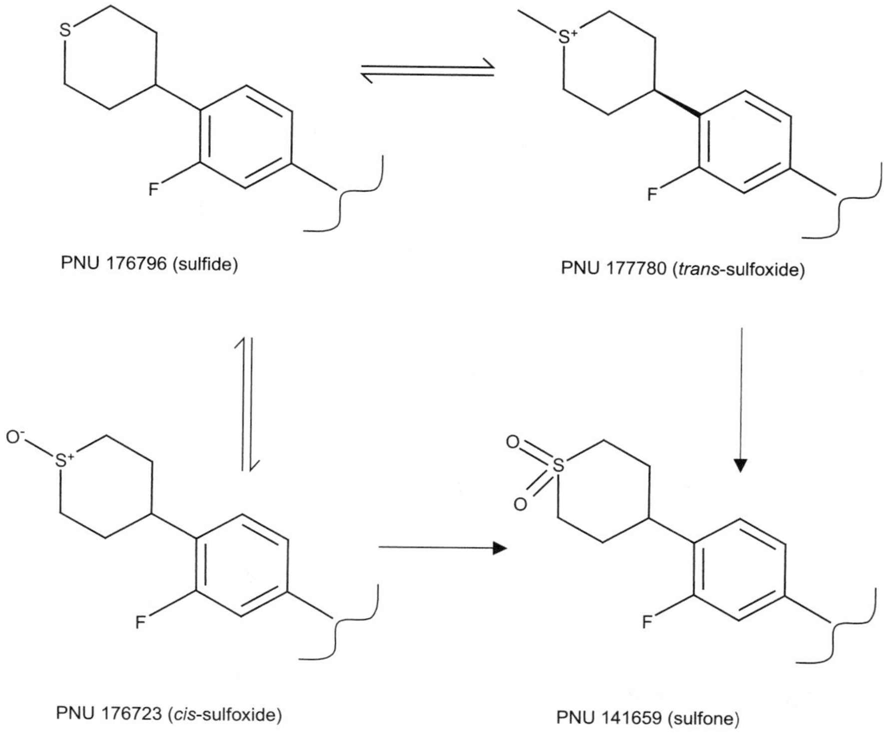

Figure 28 *cis-trans* conversion of tetrahydro-4(H)-thiopyranyl oxazolidinone analogs (adapted from Frils et al., 1999)

were less active against fastidious gram-negative bacilli than was the cyanothiophene analog.

10.2.5. DRF 6991 and DRF 8129

A seris of chalcone oxazolidinones has been synthesized (Fig. 29). The two compounds differ by fluorine atom fixes on the phenyl ring. They are weakly active; the in vitro activity was greatly enhanced by modification of the C-5 side chain to a thioacetamide (DRF 12035) instead of an acetamide. For the latter compound the MICs were 0.25, 2, and 2 μg/ml for *S. aureus*, *E. faecalis*, and *E. faecium*, respectively; for the counterpart the MICs were 4, 8, and 16 μg/ml, respectively.

10.3. Bicylic Ring Derivatives

New series of oxazolidinones having benzothiazolyl, benzoxazolone, or bispyridyl moieties have been synthesized (Figs. 30 and 31). Within these three series, compounds having various N-acetyl side chains have been produced.

10.3.1. Benzothiazolone

Benzothiazolone analogs showed higher activity than linezolid against *S. aureus* and *S. pneumoniae*. The in vitro activities of these analogs are comparable to those of linezolid against *S. pyogenes*, *E. faecium*, and *E. faecalis*. The bis-pyrridyl analogs are two to four times less active than linezolid.

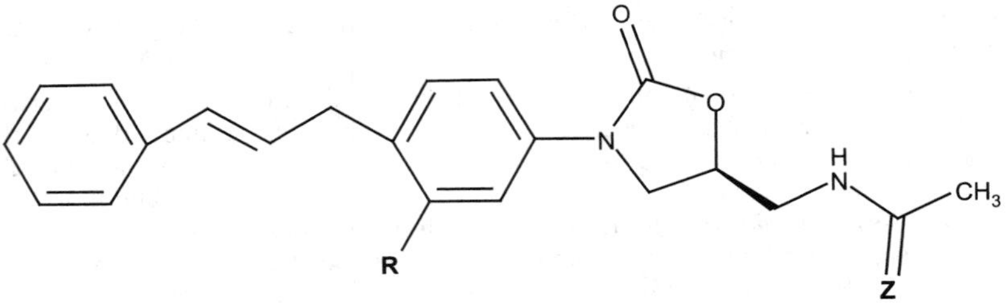

	R	Z
DRF 8129	F	O
DRF 6991	H	O
DFR 12035	F	S

Figure 29 Chalcone oxazolidinones

R—N O O H N R O

Benzoxazolidinone

Benzothiazolone

Bis pyridyl

Figure 30 Bicyclic oxazolidinones

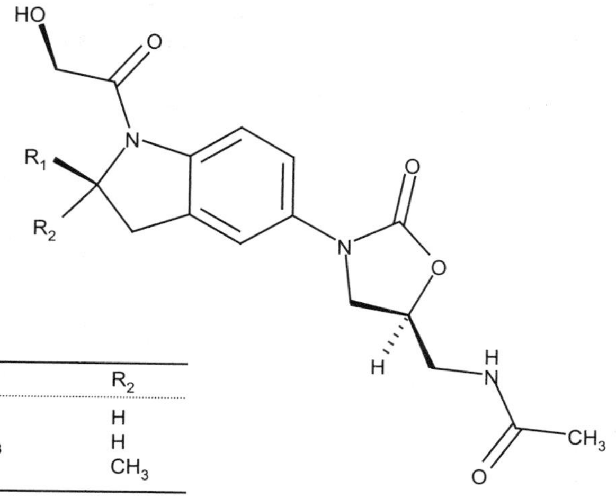

	R_1	R_2
PNN 97 456	H	H
PNU 180 164	CH_3	H
PNU 180 157	H	CH_3

Figure 31 Indanyl oxazolidinones

In mice (CFW-1), concentrations in serum after administration of 50 mg/kg by the intravenous or subcutaneous route (benzothiazolone) were two times higher than those reached with linezolid.

In cyclophosphamide-treated mice (CFW-1) challenged with *E. faecium* L4001, the benzothiazolone analog was more effective than the bis-pyrridyl analog, linezolid, and vancomycin after a dose of 25 mg/kg administered subcutaneously. At 25 mg/kg, all mice challenged with *S. aureus* 48N were cured, compared to 80% with linezolid. A high cure rate (90%) was obtained at 50 mg/kg with both heteroaryl compounds, compared to 50% with linezolid.

It was possible to modify the benzothiazolone derivatives. However, some of them were devoid of antibacterial activity. The *N*-acetyl side chain influences the levels in serum in CFW-1 mice. After an oral dose of 50 mg/kg, the peak concentrations in serum were about 35, 25, and 25 μg/ml for propionamide, methylcarbamate, and acetamide chains, respectively.

It has been shown that benzothiazolone analogs displayed higher in vitro activity against *S. aureus* 133 than benzoxazolone analogs. Within the wide range of the substituents in position 3 of the heterocycle, small and nonpolar substituents are preferable. Only small substituents like fluorine are tolerated on the benzoheterocycles.

10.3.2. Pyrazinoindole and Oxazinoindole Oxazolidinones

Within a series of pyrazinoindole and oxazinoindole analogs of oxazolidinone, two compounds exhibited higher activity against gram-positive cocci than linezolid, especially the oxazinoindole analog. MICs ranged from ≤0.12 to 0.25 μg/ml for *Staphylococcus* spp., *Streptococcus pyogenes*, and *S. pneumoniae* (linezolid MICs, 1 to 2 μg/ml). Enhanced in vitro activity was shown against *H. influenzae* 28 (MIC, 0.5 μg/ml). However, the pharmacokinetics after oral absorption are unfavorable (bioavailability, ~16%).

10.3.3. Benzoxazinone and Benzothiazinone Oxazolidinones

In a series of benzoxazinone and benzothiazinone oxazolidinones, the most active analog exhibited in vitro activity comparable to that of linezolid. In mice (female CFW-1), the pharmacokinetic profile after 1 mg/kg intravenously was better with the selected compound than with linezolid. An apparent elimination half-life of 1.5 h, versus 0.5 h for linezolid, was recorded (Haebich et al., 1999).

10.4. Tricyclic Rings

10.4.1. Imidazo-Benzoxazinyl Oxazolidinone

The aim of the imidazo benzoxazingl-oxazolidinone series was to optimize the antibacterial activity of linezolid by expanding the antibacterial spectrum to fastidious gram-negative bacilli and to increase the activity against gram-positive cocci. It was shown that imidazo-benzoxazinyl analogs of oxazolidinone exhibit good in vitro activity against gram-positive cocci, and some of them exhibit good activity against *H. influenzae, M. catarrhalis*, and *M. pneumoniae*. A broad range of structure variations on the tricyclic ring system was tolerated. Variations on the acetamido side chain yielded highly active analogs. A discriminative test of cytotoxicity on J-774 macrophages and the 3T3-A31 (mouse fibroblasts, BALB/c) cell line showed that most analogs active against *H. influenzae* are also cytotoxic. One compound (Fig. 32) was selected for further preclinical investigation.

The new imidazo-benzoxazinyl oxazolidinone analog is four- to eightfold more active than linezolid against *S. aureus*, coagulase-negative staphylococci, *S. pyogenes*, *E. faecium*, and *S. pneumoniae* (MICs ranged from 0.125 to

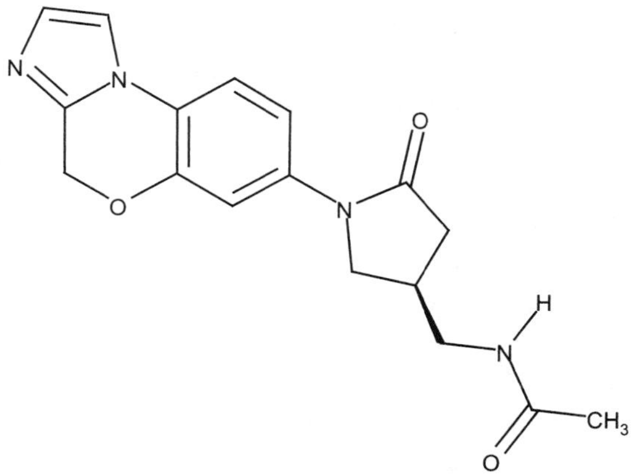

Figure 32 Imidazo-benzoxazinyl oxazolidinones

1.0 μg/ml, versus 0.5 to 2.0 μg/ml for linezolid). It is four to eight times more active than linezolid against *M. catarrhalis* (MICs ranged from 0.5 to 1.0 μg/ml, versus 4.0 to 8.0 μg/ml for linezolid) and two to eight times more active than linezolid against *H. influenzae* (MICs ranged from 2.0 to 4.0 μg/ml, versus 8 to 16 μg/ml for linezolid). In vitro activity was shown against *Proteus vulgaris* 1017 and *Proteus mirabilis* 1235 (MICs, 4.0 μg/ml) and *Escherichia coli* 455/7 (MIC, 2.0 μg/ml). Female CFW-1 mice were infected by intraperitoneal administration of 4×10^8 CFU of *S. aureus* 133 per ml and were treated orally once 0.5 h after bacterial challenge. The survival rates were 60 and 20% for the imidazo-benzoxazinyl oxazolidinone and linezolid, respectively, after a dose of 25 mg/kg. Female CFW-1 mice were infected by the intranasal route with 10^5 to 10^6 CFU of *S. pneumoniae* 1707/4 per ml and treated 2 and 5 h after challenge with 5 and 25 mg/kg. The imidazo-benzoxazinyl oxazolidinone analog was more effective in reducing the lung burden than linezolid after a dose of 25 mg/kg (reduction of ≥3 $\log_{10}$ CFU/lung in 24 h). Female NMRI mice were infected intranasally with 10^6 to 10 CFU of *H. influenzae* strain 9 per ml and treated 2, 6, and 24 h postinfection. A slight reduction of bacterial burden (~1 $\log_{10}$ CFU/lung) versus control was noted after a high dose, 200 mg/kg.

In CFW-1 mice after a single oral dose of 25 mg of the imidazo-benzoxazinyl oxazolidinone per kg, the peak concentration of 0.4 μg/ml was reached in 0.3 h, with an area under the curve of 0.3 kg·h/liter. These pharmacokinetics compared unfavorably with those of linezolid (area under the curve, 1.4 kg·h/liter).

10.4.2. ABX 96

ABX 96 is a tricyclic oxazolidinone having an azolobenxozapenyl moiety (Fig. 33). It displays good in vitro activity similar to that of linezolid, with MICs of 2.0 μg/ml for *S. aureus*, *E. faecalis*, and *E. faecium*. The in vivo activity of ABX 96 is lower than that of linezolid in murine staphylococcal infection, with ED_{50}s of 10.10 and 12.5 mg/kg for the subcutaneous and the oral routes, respectively (linezolid, 2.18 and 5.38 mg/kg, respectively).

The pharmacokinetic parameters in Swiss mice are shown in Table 30.

Table 30 Pharmacokinetics of ABX 96 in mice after oral and subcutaneous administrations

Parameter	ABX 96	Linezolid
C_{max} (μg/ml)	12.9	27.09
T_{max} (h)	1.5	0.5
AUC (μg·h/ml)	52.9	83.45
K_{el} (h^{-1})	0.58	0.61
$t_{1/2}$ (h)	1–3	1.15
ED_{50} (mg/kg)[a]		
s.c.	10.10	2.18
p.o.	12.5	5.38

[a]s.c., subcutaneously; p.o., per os.

10.4.3. DRF 8417

DRF 8417 is a tricyclic derivative characterized by a thioacetamide side chain at the C-5 position and a fused ring at the C-3 position (Fig. 34).

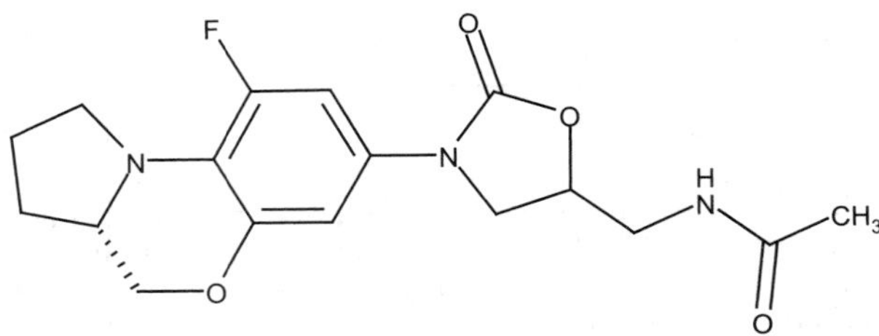

Figure 34 DRF 8417

10.4.3.1. Antibacterial Activity

DRF 8417 is twice as active in vitro as linezolid (Table 31).

Table 31 In vivo activity of DRF 8417

Microorganism	MIC (μg/ml)	
	DRF 8417	Linezolid
S. aureus	0.5	1.0
E. faecalis	1.0	1.0
S. pneumoniae	0.125	2.0
H. influenzae	8.0	16
M. catarrhalis	0.5	8.0

In staphylococcal infection in mice (*S. aureus* ATCC 29213), DRF 8417 is also two times more active (ED_{50}s, 2.26 and 1.2 mg/kg orally and subcutaneously, respectively) than linezolid (ED_{50}s, 5.38 and 2.18 mg/kg orally and subcutaneously, respectively).

Figure 33 ABX 96

The pharmacokinetics orally and intravenously for mice and rats are summarized in Table 32.

A single metabolite has been identified, a C-5 carbamate of DRF 8417 (Fig. 35). This metabolite is moderately active, with MICs from 4 to 8 μg/ml.

10.5. C-4′ Alkyl Phenyl Derivatives

A series of 4′-sulfide and 4′-sulfoxide oxazolidinone derivatives has been reported.

Electron-withdrawing acyclic 4′-substituents may confer enhanced antibacterial activity. The sulfoxide functionality can impart improved water solubility.

The thionamide analogs are more potent than their carboxamide counterparts. They are equipotent to linezolid.

10.6. PNU-29195

A series of oxazolidinones has been synthesized with the aim of enhancing the activity against *H. influenzae* and *M. catarrhalis*. These analogs have fixed on the phenyl ring C-oxatane thietane substituents. They are substituted or not.

Among the disclosed analogs, none of them exhibits better activity against *H. influenzae* (MIC, 8.0 μg/ml) than

Table 32 Pharmacokinetics of DRF 8417 in rodents

Animals and parameter	Oral			Intravenous (10 doses)
	1 dose	3 doses	10 doses	
Mice				
C_{max} (μg/ml)	0.65	1.39	5.17	16.4
T_{max} (h)	1.0	0.25	1.0	
AUC (μg·h/ml)	1.54	3.35	14.74	33.44
$t_{1/2}$ (h)	0.93	1.06	1.18	1.2
F (%)	46.1	33.1	44.2	
Rats				
C_{max} (μg/ml)	1.19	4.25	11.35	13.94
T_{max} (h)	1.63	1.25	1.0	
AUC (μg·h/ml)	7.43	22.68	75.46	71.47
$t_{1/2}$ (h)	2.57	2.46	2.63	3.18
F (%)	104	105	103	

R–C(=S)–OCH_3 → R–C(=O)–OCH_3

R–C(=S)–OCH_3

Sulfine intermediate

Figure 35 Metabolism of DRF 8417

linezolid. However, most of them display better antistaphylococcal activity (MIC, 1.0 μg/ml) than linezolid, and many of them display higher in vitro activity against *E. faecalis* (MICs, 0.5 to 2.0 μg/ml) and antipneumococcal activity (MICs, 0.25 to 1.0 μg/ml). However, in vivo against staphylococcal infections they are less active than linezolid.

10.7. VRC-3408

A series of oxazolidinone has been synthesized having a thioester at position 4′ of the phenyl ring. It was previously shown that small fixed 4′-aliphatic groups seem to be preferable to polar hydrophilic functionalities.

This series has incorporated 4′-sulfoxide and 4′-sulfones with the idea that 4′-acyclic electron-withdrawing functionalities will improve water solubility.

It was shown that replacement of a thioester group for a sulfoxide functionality can enhance activity against fastidious gram-negative bacilli.

4′-Sulfone analogs are generally less active than thioester or sulfoxide counterparts.

Small heterocyclic thioester groups are tolerated, e.g., the nitro thiazole analog VRC-3408. The fluoroalkyl-substituted sulfoxide, VRC-3962, is equipotent to linezolid.

Incorporation of a thioacetamido methyl side chain at C-4 instead of an amino group yields enhanced antibacterial activity (Fig. 36).

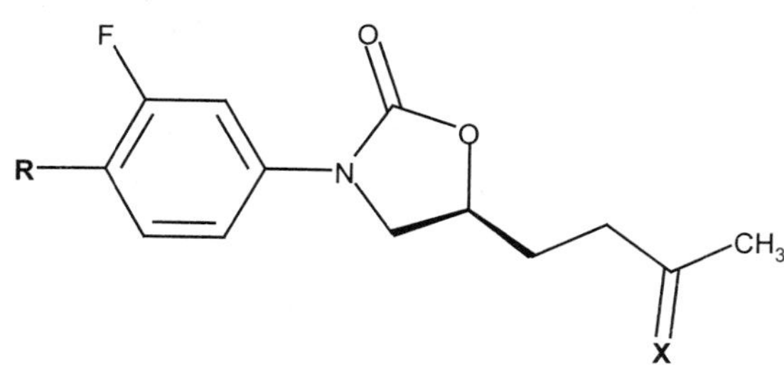

VRC	R	X	MIC (μg/ml) *S. aureus*	VRE	*S. pneumoniae*	*H. influenzae*
3116	H_3C–S–	O	4.0	8.0	1.0 - 2.0	32 -> 64
3803	H_3C–S–	S	1.0 - 4.0	2.0	0.5	32 - 64
3804	H_3C–S(=O)–	O	4.0	4.0	1.0	8 - 64
3909	H_3C–S(=O)–	S	1.0 - 2.0	1.0	0.25 - 0.5	16 - 32

Figure 36 VRC-3408

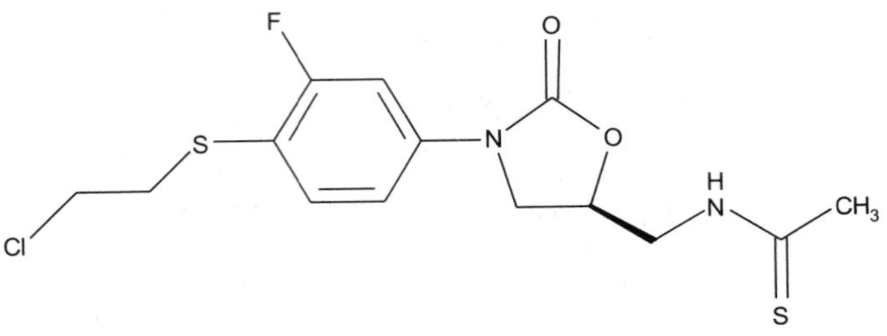

Figure 37 4′-Sulfide and 4′-sulfoxide oxazolidinones

In the sulfoxide series, less lipophilic aliphatic groups are generally preferred: chloroethyl thioether (VRC-3408) (Fig. 37) versus the hydroxy ethyl counterpart (VRC-3343).

10.8. 4′-Acylamino, 4′-Urea, and 4′-Thiourea-Phenyl Oxazolidinones

Early studies on structure-activity relationship have shown a good tolerance towards 4′ substitutions on the phenyl ring. Several functionalities have been appended on the phenyloxazolidinone pharmacophore (Fig. 38).

Acylurea or acylthiourea 4′ groups have been selected based on their potential for hydrogen bonding and for base pair-type interactions.

4′-Acylthioureas are more active than acylurea (e.g., thiourea) counterparts (VRC-4003 and VRC-4020).

Some of them, such as VRC-3807 and VRC-3808, are very active against fastidious gram-negative bacilli.

10.9. RBx 8700

RBx 8700 (Fig. 39) is a new oxazolidinone showing in vitro activity against *Enterococcus* spp. resistant to linezolid (Upadhyay et al., 2004). RBx 8700 is a piperazinyl oxazolidinone on which a nitro thienyl is appended. Its in vitro activity against *Enterococcus* spp. is listed in Table 33.

10.10. Triazolyl Methyl Oxazolidinone

One of the concerns of the available oxazolidinones is the inhibition of monoamineoxidase (MAO), especially type A due to a structural similarity to MAO inhibitors such as toloxatone. This inhibition could be a cause of severe hypertension as a result of ingestion of tyramine-containing food.

It has been shown that the 1,2,3-triazolyl moiety is a good alternative for the acetamide moiety (Fig. 40) (Reck et al., 2004).

10.11. OCID 0050

OCID 0050 is an investigational oxazolidinone (Fig. 41) tested only against streptococci (Solanski et al., 2004). It is a piperazinyl analog on which a pyrazinyl thioacetamide side chain was fixed.

Modal MICs for streptococci are 0.5 to 1.0 μg/ml (linezolid modal MIC, 2.0 μg/ml; ranbezolid modal MICs, 0.5 to 4.0 μg/ml).

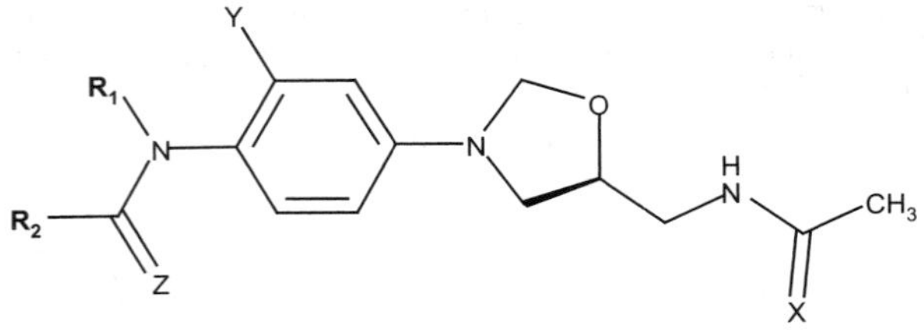

Figure 38 4′-Acylaminophenyl oxazolidinones

Table 33 Antienteroccocal activity of RBx 8700

Microorganism	*n*	MIC (μg/ml)		
		RBx 8700	Linezolid	Vancomycin
E. faecalis	16	0.5–8	4–64	2–>16
E. faecium	6	1–4	8–16	2–>16

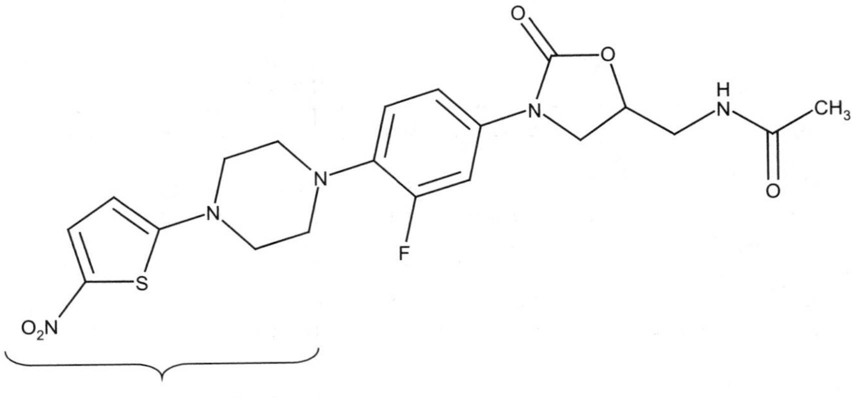

5-nitro-thienyl piperazinyl moiety

Figure 39 RBx 8700

Compound	R	R'	MIC (μg/ml) S.a	Spn	Hi	MAO (μM)
1	$C(=O)CH_3$	-	1.0	0.25	1.0	5.9
2	triazolyl–R'	H	1.0	0.50	2.0	3.4
3	triazolyl–R'	CH_3	1.0	0.50	2.0	25
4	triazolyl–R'	CCH	2.0	0.50	2.0	> 200

S.a : *S. aureus*, **Spn** : *S. pneumoniae*, **Hi** : *H. influenzae*, **MAO** : monoamine oxidase

Figure 40 5-Triazolyl oxazolidinones

Figure 41 OCID 0050

REFERENCES

Ashtekar DR, Costa-Periera R, Shrinivasan T, Lyyer R, Vishvanathan N, Rittel W, 1991, Oxazolidinone, a new class of synthetic antituberculosis agent, in vitro and in vivo activities of DO 721 against Mycobacterium tuberculosis, Diagn Microb Infect Dis, 14, 465–471.

Ashtekar DR, Costa-Perira R, Nagrajan K, Vishvanathan N, Bhatt AD, Rittel W, 1993, In vitro and in vivo activities of nitroimidazole CGI 17341 against Mycobacterium tuberculosis, Antimicrob Agents Chemother, 37, 183–186.

Barbachyn MR, Hutchinson DK, Brickner SJ, et al, 1996, Identification of a novel oxazolidinone (U-100480) with potent antimycobacterial activity, J Med Chem, 39, 680–685.

Barry AL, 1988, In vitro evaluation of DO 105 and DO 721, two new oxazolidinone antimicrobial agents, Antimicrob Agents Chemother, 32, 150–152.

Brickner SJ, 1991, Tricyclic [6,6,5]/[6,6,5]-fused oxazolidinone antibacterial agents, Antimicrobial Patent Fast Alert, (June) p AM 16.

Brickner SJ, Hutchinson DK, Barbachyn MR, et al, 1996, Synthesis and antibacterial activity of U100592 and U-100766, two oxazolidinone antibacterial agents for potential treatment of multidrug-resistant Gram-positive bacterial infections, J Med Chem, 39, 673–679.

Britteli DR, Gregory WA, Corless PF, Park CH, 1988, Aminomethyloxazolidinylethylenylbenzene derivatives useful as antibacterial agents, European Patent 31 6594.

Brumfitt W, Hamilton-Miller JMT, Gargen RA, 1989, Variation in response of Gram-positive cocci to the combination DO 721 and ciprofloxacin, J Antimicrob Chemother, 24, 465–467.

Daly JS, Eliopoulos GM, Reiszner E, Moellering R Jr, 1988, Activity and mechanism of action of DO 105 and DO 721, new oxazolidinone compounds, J Antimicrob Chemother, 21, 721–730.

Daly JS, Eliopoulos GM, Willey S, Moellering RC, 1988, Mechanism of action in vitro and in vivo activities of S-6123, a new oxazolidinone compound, Antimicrob Agents Chemother, 32, 1341–1346.

Eustice DC, Feldman PA, Slee AM, 1988, The mechanism of action of DuP 721, a new antibacterial agent: effects in macromolecular synthesis, Biochem Biophys Res Commun, 150, 965–971.

Eustice DC, Feldman PA, Zajac I, Slee AM, 1988, Mechanism of action of DO 721: inhibition of an early event during initiation of protein synthesis, Antimicrob Agents Chemother, 32, 1218–1222.

Eustice DC, Britteli DR, Feldman PA, Brown LJ, Borkowski JJ, 1990, An automated pulse labelling method for structure-activity relationship studies with antibacterial oxazolidinones, Drugs Exptl Clin Res, 16, 149–155.

Gregory WA, Britteli DR, Wang CLJ, Wuonala MA, McRipley RJ, Eustice DC, Eberly VS, Slee AM, Forbes M, 1989, Antibacterials, synthesis and structure-activity studies of 3-aryl-2oxooxazolidinones. 1. The "B" group, J Med Chem, 32, 1673–1681.

Haebich D, Bartel S, Endermann R, Guarnieri W, Haerter M, Kroll HP, Raddatz S, Riedl B, Rosentreter U, Ruppelt M, Stolle A, Wild H, 1999, Synthesis and antibacterial activity of novel heteroaryl oxazolidinones. II. Benzoxazinone- and benzthiazinone-oxazolidinones, 39th Intersci Conf Antimicrob Agents Chemother, abstract 566, p 310.

Lizondo J, Rabasseda X, Castaner J, 1996, Linezolid, Drugs of the Future, 21, 1116–1123.

Mathur T, Singhal S, Khan S, Upadhyay D, Yadav A, Rubra S, Das B, Rattan A, 2004, Ranbezolid (Rbx 7644) has concentration dependent bactericidal activity against anaerobes, 44th Intersci Conf Antimicrob Agents Chemother, abstract F-1416.

Neu HC, Novelli A, Saba G, Chin NX, 1988, In vitro activities of two oxazolidone antimicrobial agents, DO 721 and DO 105, Antimicrob Agents Chemother, 32, 580–583.

Reck F, Zhen F, Girardot M, Kern G, Eyermann J, Hales NJ, Ramsey Rr, Gravenstock MB, 2004, Novel (5R)-1,2,3-triazolyl methyl oxazolidinone as antibacterial agents with reduced activity aginst monoamine oxidase A, 44th Intersci Conf Antimicrob Agents Chemother, abstract F-1423.

Slee AM, Wuonola MA, McRipley RJ, Zajac I, Zawada MJ, Bartholomew PT, et al, 1987, Oxazolidinones, a new class of synthetic antibacterial agents: in vitro and in vivo activities of DuP 105 and DO 721, Antimicrob Agents Chemother, 37, 1791–1797.

Solanski SS, Kumar DS, Velmurujan R, Samuel MM, Mathiyazhagan K, Singh G, Pandey S, Srinivas ASSV, Argawal SK, Guha MK, 2004. In vitro activity of investigational pyrazinyl thioacetamide oxazolidinine OCID 0050 and ten other standard agents against streptococci, 44th Intersci Conf Antimicrob Agents Chemother, abstract F-1412.

Stottmeier KD, 1987, DO 721, in vitro antituberculosis activity of oxazolidinones, a novel family of antimicrobics, 27th Intersci Conf Antimicrob Agents Chemother, abstract 240.

Upadhyay D, Shinghal S, Mathur P, Khan S, Kalia V, Rao M, Bhadauriya T, Malhota S, Rudra S, Das B, Rattan A, 2004, Rbx 8700: a second generation oxazolidinone showing activity against linezolid resistant enterococci, 44th Intersci Conf Antimicrob Agents Chemother, abstract F-1413.

Wang CL, Wuonola MA, 1990, Aminomethyl oxazolidinylcycloalkyl benzene derivatives useful as antibacterial agents, US Patent 4985429.

Wang CLJ, Gregory WA, Wuonola MA, 1989, Chiral synthesis of DO 721, a new antibacterial agent, Tetrahedron, 45, 1323–1326.

Zajac I, Lam GN, Hoffman HE, Slee AM, 1987, Pharmacokinetics of DO 721, a new synthetic oxazolidinone antibacterial, 27th Intersci Conf Antimicrob Agents Chemother, abstract 247.

Fusidic Acid

A. BRYSKIER

23

1. INTRODUCTION

Fusidic acid is a steroidal antibiotic isolated in 1960 by Godtfredsen et al. from a culture filtrate of *Fusidium coccineum*, a fungal species isolated by fecal culture from a monkey. Fusidic acid has steroid primary structure but without corticosteroid activity.

This was a chance discovery during the systematic search among *Fusarium* spp. for an enzyme necessary for the manufacture of 6-aminopenicillanic acid (penicillin amidase). The demonstration of antistaphylococcal activity resulted in the purification of a compound known as fusidic acid. The first clinical trials in 1962 confirmed its antistaphylococcal activity. Fusidic acid is used in the treatment of both topical and systemic infections due to staphylococci.

2. CLASSIFICATIONS

Fusidic acid belongs to a family of naturally occurring antibiotics, the fusidanes, having in common a tetracyclic ring system with the unique chair-boat-chair conformation separating them from steroids. These compounds have in common the same carboxylate side chain links to the tetracyclic ring at C-17 via a double bond and an acetate group at C-16.

The steroidal antibiotics are divided into four classes: fusidic acid and its derivatives, helvolic acid and its derivatives, cephalosporin P_1 and its derivatives (Fig. 1), and viridomic acids A, B, and C.

2.1. Fusicidic Acid

A certain number of components of fusidic acid have been isolated from the culture filtrate of *F. coccineum*. Nine of them have been identified, seven of which (A to G) are very similar to fusidic acid. They are obtained from the main biosynthetic pathway of fusidic acid (Fig. 2). Two other similar derivatives of fusidic acid have been described: fusilactidic acid and 7,8-dehydropseudofusidic acid (Fig. 3). Fusilactidic acid has weaker antibacterial activity than fusidic acid.

2.2. Helvolic Acid

Helvolic acid was discovered in 1943 from a culture filtrate of *Aspergillus fumigatus*. It has the same chemical skeleton as fusidic acid, but the substituents of the A, B, and C rings are different. Its antibacterial spectrum is identical to that of fusidic acid, but it is less active. Helvolic acid may be obtained from the fermentation of *Cephalosporium caerulens*. Other derivatives have been extracted from this species: helvolinic acid, 6-deacetoxyhevolic acid, and 1-dehydro-3-keto-2-deoxyfusidic acid (Fig. 4).

2.3. Cephalosporin P_1

Cephalosporin P_1 was isolated from the culture supernatant of *Cephalosporium acremonium*, which also produces penicillin N and cephalosporin C.

C. acremonium likewise produces small quantities of antibiotics designated under the names of cephalosporins P_2 to P_5. In 1972, a Japanese group described a strain of *Cladosporium* whose fermentation yields small quantities of cephalosporin P_1 and viridomic acids A, B, and C (Fig. 5).

Cephalosporin P_1 exhibits good antistaphylococcal activity (Table 1).

There is cross-resistance between cephalosporin P_1 and fusidic acid in *Staphylococcus aureus*. The mutation frequencies (means ± standard deviations) are $1.6 \times 10^{-6} \pm 0.4 \times 10^{-6}$ and $7.6 \times 10^{-7} \pm 1.3 \times 10^{-7}$ for cephalosporin P_1 and fusidic acid, respectively.

3. PRODUCTION

Fusidic acid is extracted from the fermentation broth of *F. coccineum*, *Mucor ramannianus*, *Cephalosporium lamellaecula*, *Paecilomyces fusidioides*, and *Epidermophyton floccosum* 8051.

4. STRUCTURE AND PHYSICOCHEMICAL PROPERTIES

4.1. Structure

Fusidic acid has a tetracyclic structure of the triterpene type (fusidane or protostane nucleus). The *trans-cis-trans* stereochemical configuration of the A, B, and C nuclei is unusual. A cyclophenanthrene chain is attached to this tetracyclic nucleus at position 17.

Fusidic acid possesses 10 asymmetrical carbons and a double bond, giving rise to *cis-trans* isomerism between C-7 and C-20.

Fusidanes differ from the nonsteroidal anti-inflammatory drugs by the presence of a methyl group at position C-13 instead of C-14 and C-8 and by the presence of an unsaturated side chain with eight carbon atoms.

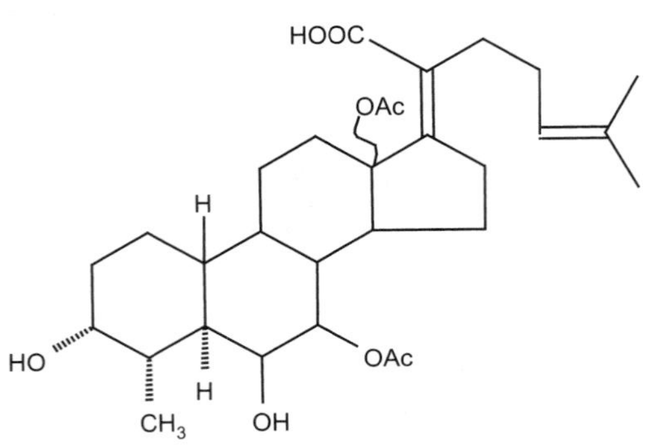

Cephalosporin P_1

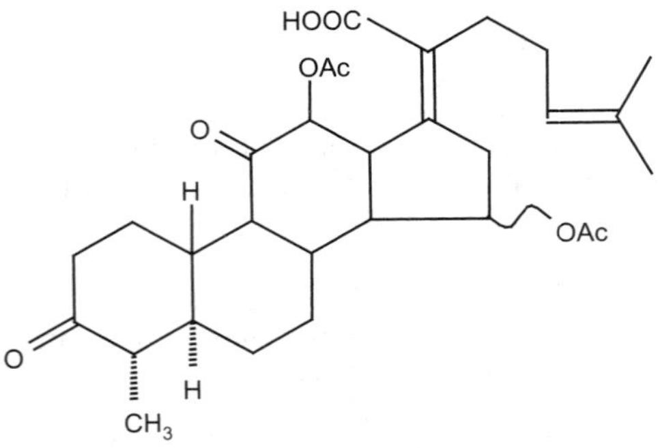

Helvolic acid

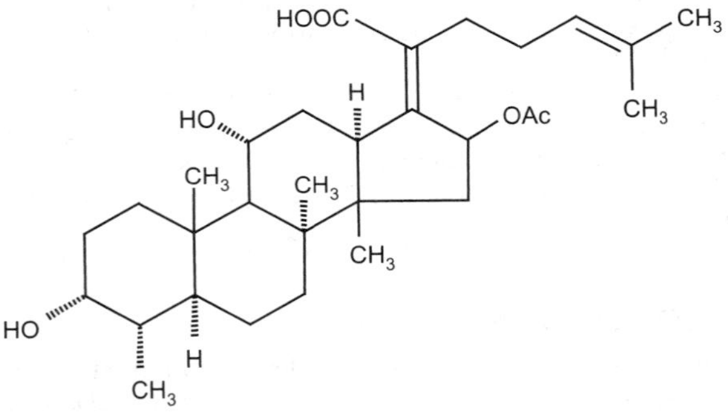

Fusidic acid

Figure 1 Fusidanes

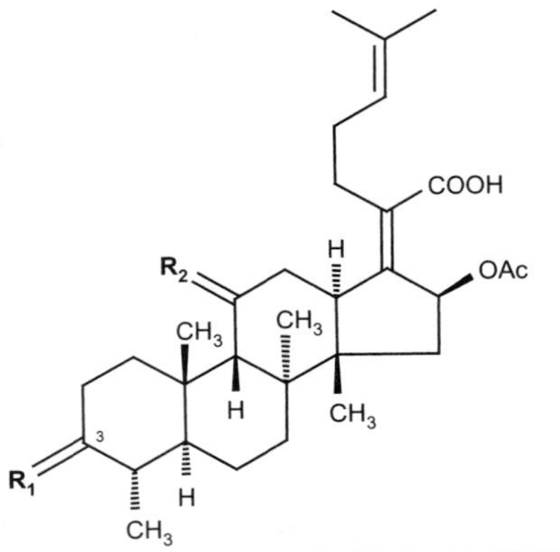

		R_1	R_2
Derivatives	A	O	α-OH
"	B	H, α-OH	O
"	C	H, β-OH	H, α-OH
"	D	H, α-OH	H, β-OH

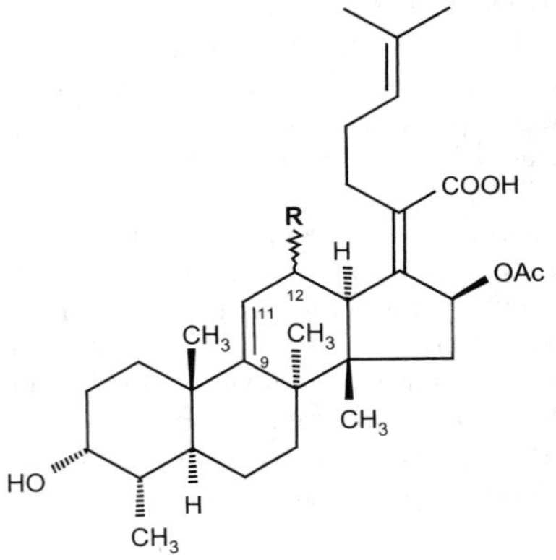

	R
E	H
F	OH

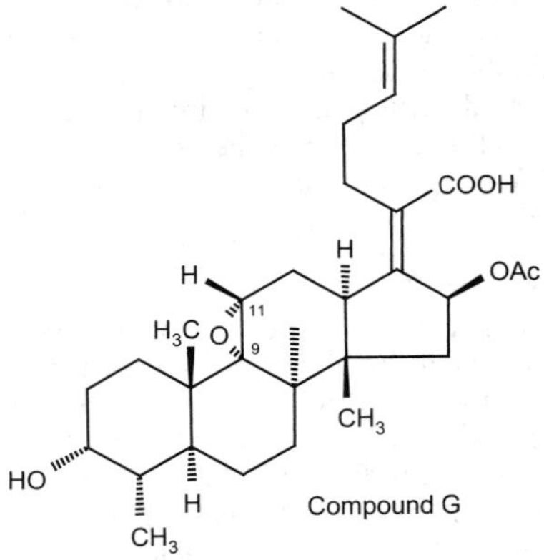

Compound G

Figure 2 Fusidic acid derivatives

4.2. Physicochemical Properties

The pharmaceutical forms used clinically are sodium fusidate for the oral route and the diethanolamine salt for the injectable route (580 mg of diethanolamine salt is equivalent to 500 mg of fusidic acid base). The pediatric suspension is fusidic acid hemihydrate. Sodium fusidate is a crystalline substance with a melting point of 220°C.

Sodium fusidate is soluble in water and ethanol. It is insoluble in chloroform, hexane, dioxane, acetone, and pyridine.

With a molecular weight of 516.9 and an empirical formula of $C_{31}H_{48}O_6$, fusidic acid has a pK of 5.35 (weak acid). It is a lipophilic molecule.

The physicochemical properties are summarized in Table 2.

The partial synthesis of fusidic acid was undertaken in 1977.

5. STRUCTURE-ACTIVITY RELATIONSHIP

A number of fusidic acid derivatives have been synthesized, and some features of the structure-activity relationship have

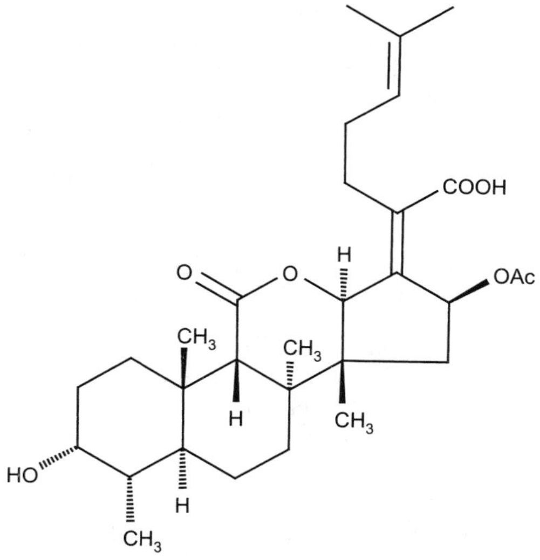

Fusilactidic acid

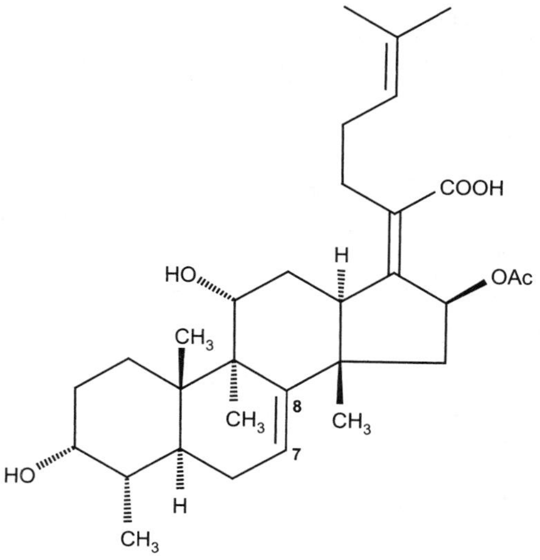

7, 8 dehydropseudofusidic acid

Figure 3 Fusidic acid derivatives

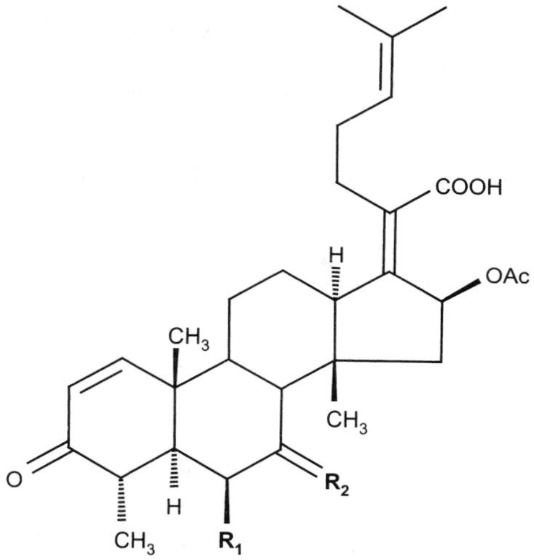

	R_1	R_2
Helvolic acid	O-Ac	O
Helvolic acid	OH	O
6-Deoxyhelvolic acid	H	O
1-Dehydro-3-keto 11-deoxy fusidic acid	H	H_2

Figure 4 Helvolic acid derivatives

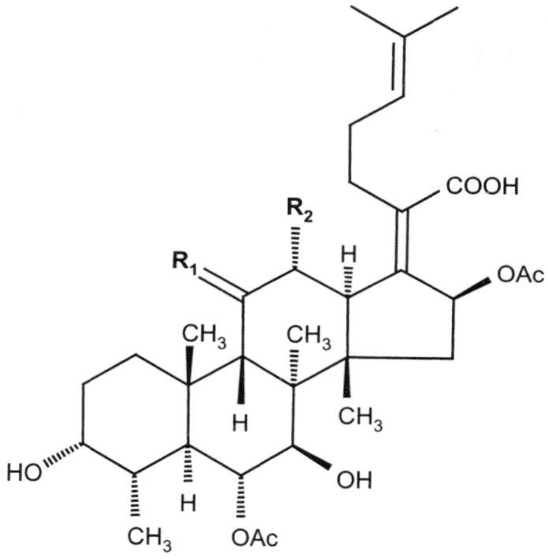

	R_1	R_2
Cephalosporin P_1	H_2	H
Viridomic acid A	O	H
Viridomic acid B	O	OH
Viridomic acid C	H, β-OH	H

Figure 5 Cephalosporin P_1 derivatives

been established. Modifications have been made to the eight regions of the molecule (Fig. 6), A to H.

- The double bond of the side chain may be reduced at C-24–C-25. The resultant derivative, 24,25-dihydrofusidic acid, has activity similar to that of fusidic acid against *S. aureus*. It therefore appears that this double bond is not necessary for the antibacterial activity (modification A).
- The 17,20 bond must be present and geometrically correct; derivatives such as tetrahydrofusidic acid, lumifusidic acid, 24,25-dihydrolumifusidic acid, and tetrahydrolumifusidic acid are inactive (modification B).

Table 1 In vitro antistaphylococcal activity of cephalosporin P_1

Organism[a]	n	MIC (μg/ml)[b]	
		50%	90%
MSSA	37	0.06–8.0	0.25–0.5
MRSA	28	0.12–>256	0.25–4.0
GISA	7	0.125	

[a]MSSA, methicillin-susceptible *S. aureus*; GISA, glycopeptide-intermediate *S. aureus*.

[b]50% and 90%, MICs at which 50 and 90% of isolates are inhibited, respectively.

Table 2 Physicochemical properties of fusidic acid

Parameter	Fusidic acid	Fusidate
Empirical formula	$C_{31}H_{48}O_6$	$C_{31}H_{48}O_6Na$
Molecular weight	516.6	538.7
pK	5.35	
Specific rotation	$[\alpha]_D^{20} = -9°$	$[\alpha]_D^{20} = +5°$ -8°
Sodium content		7.26 mg/ml (0.32 mEq/ml)
Log$_P$ (*n*-octanol/water)		
Solubility		
Water	(+)	+++
Ethanol	+++	++
Ether	(+)	(+)
Benzene	+++	(+)
Acetone	+++	–
Chloroform	+++	–
Pyridine	+++	–
Melting point (°C)	192–193	220

- Modification of the carboxyl group (modification C) at C-21, i.e., esterification, gives rise to molecules with variable activities. The methyl ester derivatives are inactive, while the β-diethylaminoethyl has weak activity against fusidic acid-susceptible and -resistant *S. aureus* strains. The amino, hydrazine, and hydroxylamine derivatives are weakly active, while derivatives of the secondary and tertiary amine types are inactive. The carboxyl group is essential for antibacterial activity.
- The modifications of the methyl group (modification D) at C-27 yield derivatives with 10% of the activity of fusidic acid.
- The modifications at position 16 (modification E) are very numerous; the 16α derivatives are less active than the 16β derivatives, which emphasizes the importance of the stereochemistry at position 16.
- The axial orientation of the hydroxyl group at C-11 (modification F) is very important for antibacterial activity. The group at the 11α position is responsible for greater activity than 11β, but its oxidation (11-keto) or the formation of an 11,32 ether or the presence of a 12,13 double bond yields molecules with antibacterial activity equivalent to 5% of that of fusidic acid.

5.1. Modification of the B Ring (Modification G)

Three molecules have been prepared: 7α-hydroxyfusidic acid, 7-oxofusidic acid, and 6β-hydroxy-7-oxofusidic acid. The 7α-hydroxyfusidic derivative has weak antistaphylococcal activity (10% of that of fusidic acid) but is twice as active against streptococci.

5.2. Modification of the A Ring (Modification H)

Numerous modifications have been made to the A ring. In the natural form, the metabolite, 3-keto-fusidic acid, is eliminated in animals and humans. A number of compounds have also been prepared by semisynthesis.

Oxidation of the 3α-hydroxyl group to a ketone reduces the antibacterial activity by about 15 to 20%, whereas epimerization at C-4 yields derivatives with 10% of the activity of fusidic acid.

Other derivatives possessing variable antibacterial activities have been prepared. In the various series produced, the most active derivative is 3α-azido-3-deoxyfusidic acid, which has activity equal to 30% of that of fusidic acid. The

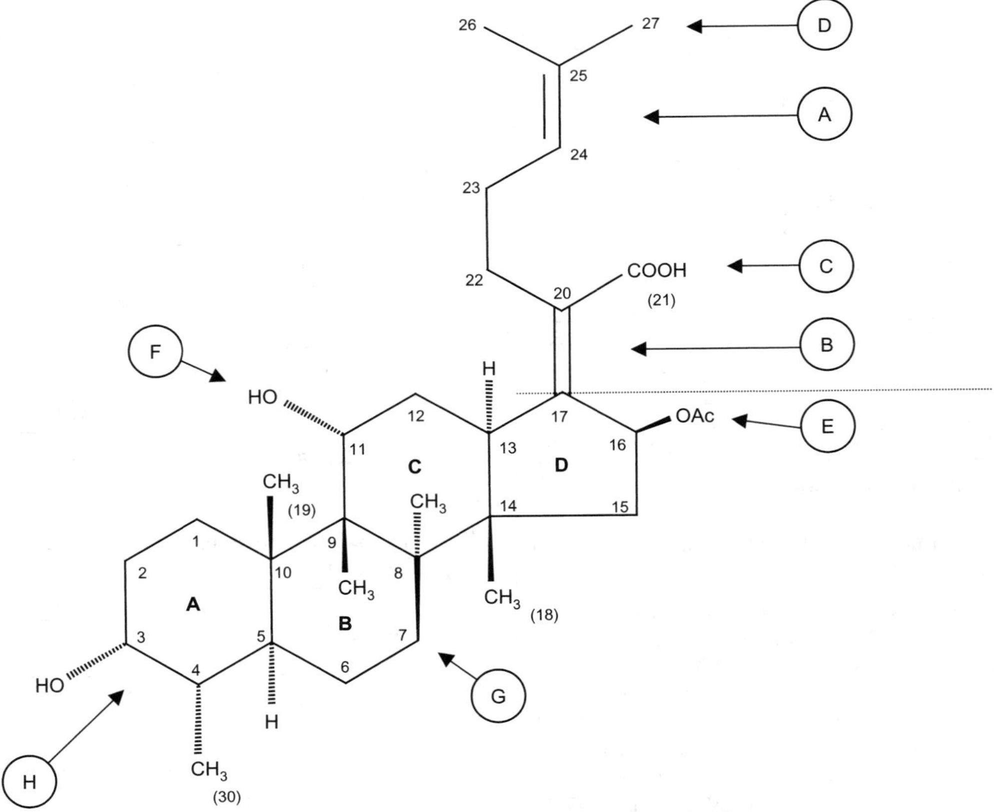

Figure 6 Structure-activity relationship in fusidanes

3α-nitro and 3α-chloro derivatives have 10 and 3% of the activity of fusidic acid, respectively; all other derivatives are inactive. The 3β derivatives are less active; only 3β-bromo- and 3β-iodo-3-deoxyfusidic acids have antibacterial activity equal to 10% of that of fusidic acid.

5.3. 17*S*-20*S* Methanefusidic Acid

As part of the new interest in improving the antibacterial and pharmacokinetic properties of fusidic acid, the role of Δ17(20) double bond in the side chain was investigated.

It was demonstrated that the flexible side chain between C-17 and C-20 yields a compound with a potency similar to that of fusidic acid. Structure-activity relationship studies showed the importance of the orientation of the fusidic acid side chain in a limited bioactive space above the ring plane.

5.4. Conclusion

The double bond at position 24,25, the stereochemistry of the 17,20 bond, and the carboxyl group are important.

The derivatives with hydroxyl groups at 3α and 11α are more active than their isomers.

It is possible to change the substituents at position 16,3, and conversion of the 11α-hydroxyl group to a ketone is possible.

Modification at C-17–C-21 is possible in a certain configuration.

6. TOXICOLOGICAL AND PHARMACOLOGICAL PROPERTIES

The acute toxicity, expressed as the 50% lethal dose in the mouse, rat, and dog, is summarized in Table 3.

Irrespective of the animal species considered, an infusion of sodium fusidate causes local intolerance, evidenced in hardening of the veins and perivenous tissues. Fusidic acid has no teratogenic or embryotoxic effect in animals.

7. ANTIBACTERIAL PROPERTIES

Fusidic acid has a narrow antibacterial spectrum that incorporates gram-positive cocci, gram-positive bacilli, gram-negative cocci, and fastidious gram-negative bacilli such as *Moraxella catarrhalis*, *Haemophilus influenzae*, and *Bordetella pertussis*. It has good in vitro activity against *Mycobacterium tuberculosis* (MIC at which 50% of isolates tested are inhibited, 1.0 μg/ml). The MIC for *M. tuberculosis* by either the proportion method or the BACTEC system is 1.0 μg/ml. It is inactive against *Enterobacteriaceae* and nonfermentative gram-negative bacilli. It also encompasses anaerobic gram-positive cocci and bacilli. Its activity is exerted mainly against methicillin-susceptible or -resistant strains of *S. aureus* and against coagulase-negative staphylococci. It is a bacteriostatic antibiotic. Fusidic acid exhibits weak activity against streptococci, enterococci, and pneumococci. It is active against *Corynebacterium diphtheriae*, *Neisseria meningitidis*, and *Neisseria gonorrhoeae* (Tables 4, 5, and 6).

Bacteriostatic activity against *Mycobacterium leprae* in a murine model has been described.

The MICs increase with the size of the bacterial inoculum (10^4 to 10^6 CFU/ml) and are also pH dependent. They are inversely proportional to the pH of the medium; the MICs for *S. aureus* are, respectively, 0.02, 0.05, and 0.16 μg/ml at pHs of 6, 7, and 8.5. The MICs increase in the presence of serum.

The breakpoints recommended by the French Antibiotic Sensitivity Test Committee are summarized in Table 7.

The intracellular concentrations are between 40 and 100% of the extracellular concentration (HeLa cells, human fibroblasts, human neutrophils, and murine macrophages).

Table 4 In vitro activity of fusidic acid

Organism(s)	MIC (μg/ml)[a]		
	50%	90%	Range
S. aureus Met[s]	0.03	0.06	
S. aureus Met[r]	0.04	0.08	
S. epidermidis	0.03	0.06	
Staphylococcus saprophyticus	3.12	3.12	
S. pyogenes	8.0	16	
Streptococcus agalactiae	>16	>16	
Streptococcus F	4.0	4.0	
Streptococcus G	4.0	16	
Streptococcus pneumoniae			8.0
Enterococcus faecalis			3.12
C. diphtheriae	0.004	0.04	
Corynebacterium jeikeium			<0.06
Corynebacterium pseudodiphthericum			<0.2
Nocardia asteroides	1.56	3.12	
N. gonorrhoeae	0.6		
N. meningitidis	0.03	0.12	
M. catarrhalis			1.0
H. influenzae			5.0–10
B. pertussis	0.08	0.2	
Legionella pneumophila	0.125	0.125	
Listeria monocytogenes			>25
Bacillus anthracis			0.06–1.5
Brevibacterium casei			0.06–0.5
Dermatobacter hominis			0.06–1.0
Turicella otitidis			0.06–0.5
Pleisiomonas spp.			0.01–32
Escherichia coli			>128
Serratia spp.			0.01–32
Yersinia spp.			>16
Lactobacillus plantarum			4.0–≥256
Lactobacillus paracasei/ L. rhamnosus			≥256
Lactobacillus acidophilus			≥256
Lactobacillus sakei/curvatus			32–≥256

[a]50% and 90%, MIC at which 50 and 90% of isolates are inhibited, respectively.

Table 3 Acute toxicity of fusidic acid

Species	LD_{50}[a] (mg/kg) with route:			
	Oral	Intramuscular	Intravenous	Intraperitoneal
Mouse	860	125	180	170
Rat	300	203	140	

[a]LD_{50}, 50% lethal dose.

Table 5 In vitro activity of fusidic acid against anaerobes

Organism(s)	MIC (μg/ml)[a]	
	50%	90%
Clostridium perfringens	0.12	0.5
Clostridium difficile	0.01	2.0
Clostridium tetani	0.01	
Peptococcus spp.	0.25	0.5
Peptostreptococcus spp.	0.25	0.5
Propionibacterium acnes	0.25	1.0
Veillonella parvula	2.0	4.0
Fusobacterium necrophorum	16	32
Bacteroides fragilis	2.0	16
Eikenella corrodens	0.25	0.5
Prevotella melaninogenica	0.25	1.0

[a]50% and 90%, MIC at which 50 and 90% of isolates are inhibited, respectively.

Table 6 In vitro activity against atypical and intracellular pathogens

Organism	MIC (μg/ml)
M. tuberculosis	1.0
Mycoplasma pneumoniae	1.6
Mycoplasma hominis	0.8
Mycoplasma fermentans	0.4
Ureaplasma urealyticum	1.6
Chlamydia trachomatis	4.0
Borrelia burgdorferi	>4

Table 7 Breakpoints of the French Antibiotic Sensitivity Test Committee (2003)

Phenotype	MIC (μg/ml)	Zone diam (mm)
Susceptible	<2	≥22
Resistant	>16	<15

8. MECHANISMS OF ACTION

See Fig. 7.

8.1. Protein Synthesis

The process of protein synthesis by the ribosome includes three main phases: initiation, elongation, and termination.

Protein synthesis is a complex process during which the ribosome and various translation factors interact in a precisely coordinated and regulated fashion. Several of those factors are members of the GTPase superfamily of proteins, and their function on the ribosome is facilitated or accompanied by hydrolysis of GTP to generate GDP and an inorganic phosphate. Elongation factor Tu (EF-Tu) and EF-G are involved in the elongation process.

- Initiation factor 2GTP promotes the binding of initiator tRNA to the ribosomal P-site and recruits the 50S subunit to the 30S initiation complex
- EF-Tu is responsible for delivery of the incoming aminoacyl-tRNA (aa-tRNA)
- EF-G promotes translocation of the ribosome along mRNA by one codon. EF-G is a large GTPase, consisting of five domains, that promotes the directional movement of mRNA and tRNA on the ribosome in a GTP-dependent manner.
    - Domain 1 comprises two subdomains, the GTP binding G domain and the G domain. The catalytic arginine is probably located in the G domain in which there are at least eight arginine residues, of which two, R29 and R59, are located in the vicinity of β-phosphate of GDP. R29 is involved in GTP hydrolysis, and R59 influences ribosome binding and translocation.
    - Domain 2 is a β-stranded barrel.
    - The structure of domain 3 is not known completely.
    - Domain 4 is elongated and possesses an unusual field where two parallel β-strands are connected by an α-helix, forming a left-handed structure similar to a fold observed in ribosomal protein 5S, one domain of DNA gyrase B, and the ribosomal P protein. The tip of domain 4 interacts with the decoding region of the 30S subunit.
    - Domain 5 has a doublly split β-α-β fold. Domains 2 and 5 have interfaces with domain 1; domains 4 and 5 and probably 3 are believed to form a structural unit allowing a lever-like movement of domain 4 relative to domain 1. Domains 3, 4, and 5 mimic the tRNA structure in the EF-Tu ternary complex, whereas domain 4 can be related to the tRNA anticodon arm.
- Release factor 3 promotes the release of release factors 1 and 2 from the ribosome following tRNA hydrolysis at termination.
- EF-2 represents the eukaryotic and archaeal counterpart of EF-G.
- Ribosome recycling factor (RRF) has two domains, I and II, corresponding to the anticodon and acceptor arms of tRNA, respectively.
- GTPase: all of the translational GTPase factors bind to a single or overlapping site on the ribosome. The GTPase activity of EF-G is stimulated by isolated ribosomal proteins L7 and L12. The recent determination of the crystal structure of the 70S ribosome has revealed that all of the regions that have been implicated in factor binding, namely, the α-ricin sarcin loop (nucleotide 2660), the L11 binding region of the 23S rRNA (1060 region), and the L7 and L12 stalk, are located in sufficiently close proximity to form a single factor-binding site.
- Proteins L7 and L12: the stalk of the 50S ribosomal subunit is comprised of two dimers of the 12-kDa proteins L7 and L12 (L7 differs from L12 by an acetylated N terminus). There is a contribution of L7 and L12 to GTPase activation of EF-G on the ribosome.
- Proteins L10 and L11: both proteins are bound to the 1060 region of 23S RNA. These proteins have a number of conserved arginine residues which could act as arginine fingers. L10 does not contribute to the GTPase activation of EF-G.

The elongation phase of protein synthesis starts with the insertion of an aa-tRNA into the A-site by EF-Tu. It begins with the ribosome having a peptidyl-tRNA in the P-site and a free codon in the A-site. During the first step, a complex of aa-tRNA and EF-Tu binds to the A-site, and following codon recognition and GTP hydrolysis, aa-tRNA is released from EF-Tu and is accommodated in the P-site. Once the aa-tRNA is accommodated, the peptide is formed, resulting in deacylated tRNA in the P-site and peptidyl-tRNA in the A-site.

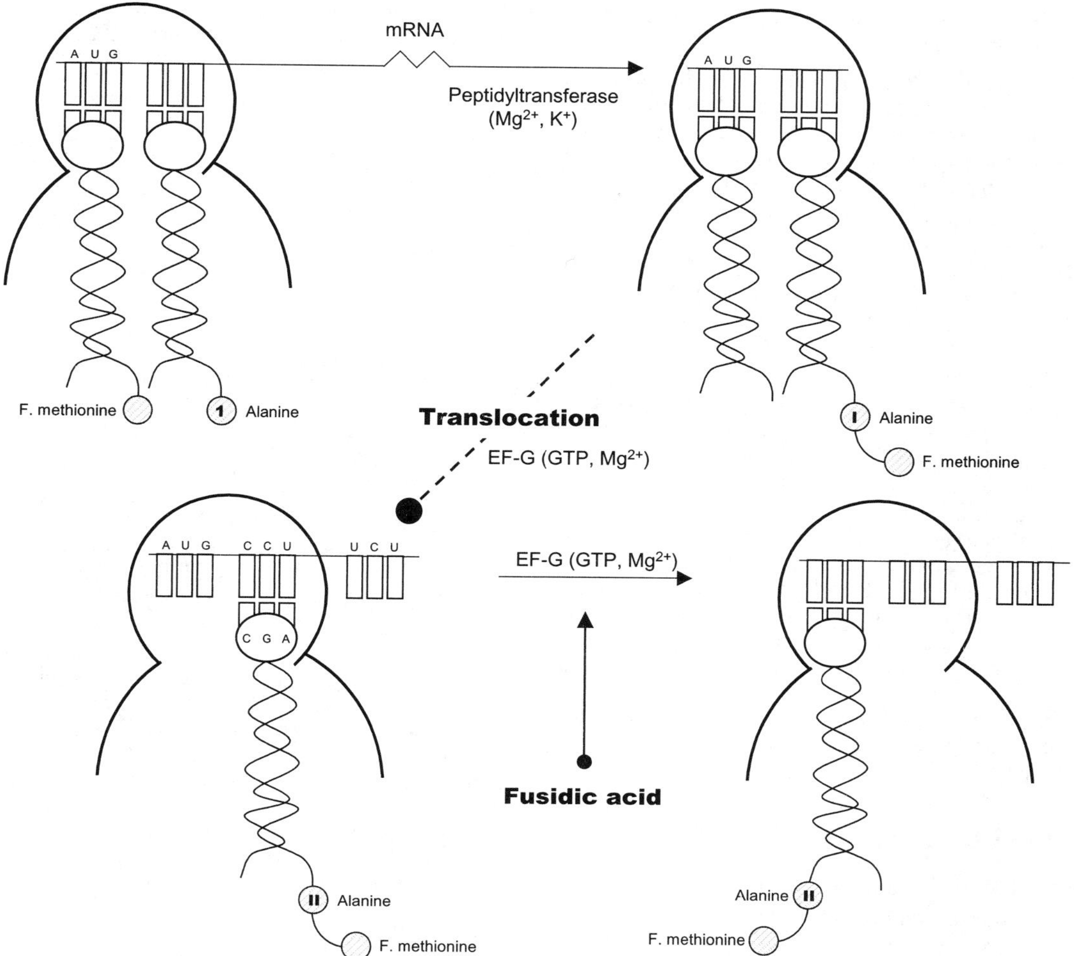

Figure 7 **Translocation**

The next step is translocation. Subsequent binding of EF-G to the ribosome triggers the movement of tRNA from the A-site to the P-site in a process known as translocation. EF-G binding to the ribosome is labile but can be trapped by an antibacterial agent.

During the translocation step of the elongation cycle, two tRNAs together with the mRNA move synchronously and rapidly on the ribosome. The movement is catalyzed by the binding of EF-G and GTP hydrolysis, which affect both translocation and turnover of EF-G.

A functional cycle for the ribosome was first suggested by Mangiarotti et al. In this cycle, 30S and 50S ribosomal subunits periodically are coupled with mRNA, direct synthesis of a protein chain, and dissociate during the release of a complete chain.

After the translocation termination step, RRF and EF-G disassemble the posttermination ribosomal complex, deacylated tRNA and mRNA. The disassembly requires GTP hydrolysis.

RRF binds to the A-site and goes through a "translocation like" motion to occupy the P-site with the help of EF-G, resulting in the release of deacylated tRNA bound to the P- and E-sites; however, the A-site is empty. The A-site is prevented from being occupied by aa-tRNA of EF-G. At the end there is a release of mRNA by the action of both the EF-G–GDP complex and RRF; this release may be inhibited by blockade due to fusidic acid, and the EF-G–GTP complex is released by the ribosome first, followed by the mRNA and, at the end, RRF. The interaction of the prokaryotic translocation factor EF-G with the ribosome has been shown to involve the transient formation of a ternary complex involving the ribosome, G-factor, and GDP. The release of tRNA is a prerequesite for mRNA release.

8.2. Fusidic Acid

A number of antibacterials that inhibit bacterial protein synthesis are thought to act by stabilizing particular conformation of the ribosome, effectively preventing structural changes that occur during translocation.

Fusidic acid does not penetrate the outer membrane of gram-negative bacilli. Fusidic acid inhibits protein synthesis at the translation stage (reading of mRNA). It acts on EF-G.

Fusidic acid and kirromycin prevent the dissociation of factors from the ribosome when the GTP is hydrolyzed. Fusidic acid binds with high affinity to EF-G on the ribosome after GTP hydrolysis.

Fusidic acid acts by stabilizing the EF-G–GTP complex, with the following consequences:

- Blockade of peptidyl-tRNA at the P-site on the ribosome. In fact, after the binding of an aa-tRNA to the A-site on the ribosome, followed by normal translocation, the A-site remains occupied by an EF-G–GTP–fusidic acid complex, which prevents any further binding of aa-tRNA.
- Blockade of translocation. Fusidic acid allows translocation and GTP cleavage but prevents the release of EF-G from the ribosome and traps the ribosome in the post-translocational state. After hydrolysis and translocation, the release of EF-G is inhibited by fusidic acid. Therefore, it allows a single round of tRNA translocation but prevents multiple rounds.

Fusidic acid inhibits the release of mRNA from the ribosome. One possible binding site for fusidic acid can be between domain 5 and GTPase. Other fusidic acid binding sites were also proposed near the GTP binding site and the area of the effector loop (residues 40 to 65).

Other antibacterials, such as thiostrepton and viomycin, are known to block the previous step, the release of tRNA.

Thiostrepton inhibits GTP hydrolysis by preventing the binding of EF-G–GTP to the ribosome. However, it seems that it allows EF-G binding and GTP hydrolysis but inhibits the release of produced inorganic phosphate and hence the translocation.

Viomycin prevents translocation of tRNA but does not inhibit GTP hydrolysis. Viomycin inhibits the release of tRNA by RRF and EF-G.

9. RESISTANCE MECHANISMS

9.1. Prevalence of Resistance

The number of fusidic acid-resistant strains of *S. aureus* has not been explored worldwide, only in some geographical areas. Whether methicillin susceptible or resistant, the percentage of strains that have become resistant to fusidic acid is on the order of 1%. This percentage is slightly higher for *Staphylococcus epidermidis*, on the order of 2.5% in France, 8.8% in the United Kingdom, and 8% in Italy.

In 2002, in the United Kingdom up to 34% of the *S. aureus* isolates in dermatology were shown to be resistant to fusidic acid. For bacteremic patients, the rate of resistance to fusidic acid among staphylococcal isolates overall was 2% in 1990 and reached 6.8% in 2000.

Brown and Wise reported an increase from 8.1% in 1995 to 17.3% in 2001 in the rate of resistance to fusidic acid among community methicillin-susceptible *S. aureus* isolates from 28 centers.

An increased incidence of fusidic acid-resistant *S. aureus* strains in dermatology has been noted in Sweden since the mid-1990s due to a clonal spread among Swedish children of an *S. aureus* strain.

From 1996 to 1997, the antibacterial susceptibility of methicillin-resistant *S. aureus* (MRSA) in sub-Saharan countries, including Malta, was investigated; the results are summarized in Table 8.

Two main mechanisms of resistance to fusidic acid can be described: mutation and efflux. In clinical isolates resistant to fusidic acid, a mutation in the *fusA* gene, which encodes EF-G, had been reported. Resistance in natural isolates may also result from acquisition of *fusB*, a poorly characterized plasmid-mediated resistance mechanism.

Table 8 Prevalence of fusidic acid and rifampin resistance among MRSA isolates in sub-Saharan countries

Country	*n*	% of isolates resistant to:	
		Fusidic acid	Rifampin
Nigeria	42	71.4	69.4
Kenya	38	42.9	23.1
Cameroon	27		88.9
Ivory Coast	26		61.5
Morocco	21	47.6	
Senegal	21	66.7	81
Tunisia	15	0	46.7
Malta	10	80	100

In a study comparing cephalosporin P_1 and fusidic acid mutants, it was shown that mutations arose in the *fusA* gene; these are identified in clusters I and II, corresponding to amino acid residues 418, 404, 408, 436, 452, 478, 656, and 666.

Some sites are important for resistance development, such as residues 451 to 464 and in particular histidine 457, which is thought to interact directly with fusidic acid.

The replacement of histidine 457 occurs quite often in two steps. A mutation (C$\underline{A}$C$\rightarrow$C$\underline{T}$A) yielding H-457$\rightarrow$Q (leucine) occurs first; a second silent nucleotide substitution would need to arise subsequently in the same codon (H$\rightarrow$N).

It is hypothetized that mutation Q-457, despite conferring resistance to fusidic acid (MIC, 64 μg/ml), has unsatisfactory translocase activity, resulting in selection of the compensatory mutation Q$\rightarrow$L (MIC, 256 μg/ml).

These mutations influence the conformational dynamics of the elongation factors.

Many mutations are found in domain III of EF-G.

The AcrAB system belonging to the RND family confers resistance to fusidic acid by an efflux mechanism.

There is no cross-resistance with other molecules active against gram-positive cocci.

9.2. Selection of Mutant Strains In Vitro

It has been shown with MRSA that the frequency of selection of mutant strains is on the order of 10^{-8} for concentrations of between 1.25 and 12.5 μg of fusidic acid per ml.

With strains of *S. epidermidis* at fusidic acid concentrations of between 1 and 5 μg/ml, the frequency of isolation of mutant strains is between 0.5×10^{-7} and 2.5×10^{-8}. When fusidic acid is used in combination with other antibacterials, the time to appearance of mutant strains is longer.

The frequency of mutation is $<10^{-11}$ for a combination of 30 μg of fusidic acid per ml with 16 μg of rifampin per ml.

9.3. Extrinsic Resistance

Gram-negative bacilli are resistant to fusidic acid. This resistance is related to outer membrane impermeability and efflux.

9.4. Acquired Resistance

Acquired resistance may be plasmid or chromosomally mediated. Chromosomal resistance is the result of modification of EF-G. This modification causes a reduction in the affinity of fusidic acid for the factor. This effect has been demonstrated in a spontaneous mutant strain of *S. aureus*.

Plasmid-mediated resistance has been demonstrated in *S. aureus*. The mode of resistance is related to a modification of membrane permeability associated with a modification of the phospholipid levels in the outer membrane, and not to enzymatic inactivation or a modification of the cell target.

10. ANTIBIOTIC COMBINATIONS

The treatment of staphylococcal infections usually requires a combination of antibiotics. There is synergistic, additive, and indifferent, but rarely antagonistic, activity with aminoglycosides, cyclines, co-trimoxazole, chloramphenicol, novobiocin, rifampin, macrolides, and related substances. Combinations with β-lactams, vancomycin, and fosfomycin produce variable results, some of which are antagonistic. Combination with fluoroquinolones is antagonistic.

11. PAE

The postantibiotic effect (PAE) for *S. aureus* was 3.3 h but occurred at concentrations of 1,000 times the MIC (44 to 125 μg/ml). At 100 times the MIC (4.4 to 12.5 μg/ml), the PAE ranged between 0.8 and 1.75 h. The maximum PAE for *Streptococcus pyogenes* was 3.5 h at five times the MIC (10 to 20 μg/ml).

12. ANTIPARASITIC ACTIVITY

Farthing and Inge in 1986 showed that fusidic acid inhibits the growth of *Giardia lamblia* in vitro. Likewise, fusidic acid inhibits the growth of *Plasmodium falciparum* (50% inhibitory concentrations 50 μg/ml). Fusidic acid acts synergistically or additively with chloroquine against *P. falciparum*.

13. PLASMA PHARMACOKINETICS

Fusidic acid in the form of the sodium salt is administered orally, and sodium fusidate in the form of the diethanolamine salt is administrated intravenously (580 mg is equivalent to 500 mg of sodium fusidate).

13.1. Assay Methods

Microbiological and high-performance liquid chromatographic methods have been published.

The microbiological methods use the following test strains: *Corynebacterium xerosis* NCTC 9755 and *S. aureus* NCTC 6571. Different chromatographic methods for assays in pharmaceutical forms and for biological fluids have been published.

13.2. Oral Pharmacokinetics

After oral administration of incremental doses of fusidic acid (250 to 1,000 mg), the pharmacokinetics are not linear. The apparent elimination half-life is about 10 h. It has been shown that there is major interindividual variability, with a mean peak concentration in serum of 20 μg/ml. There is variable accumulation after administration of repeated doses of fusidic acid and its main metabolite, 3-keto-fusidate. Steady state is reached on day 4, and the peak concentration is 80 μg/ml.

The main parameters are summarized in Table 9.

Comparison between the areas under the curve of fusidic acid (500 mg) in the fasted state and after food shows a reduction of about 15% in relative bioavailability. The peak concentrations in serum are similar, and the time to reach the peak is delayed by about 1.0 h.

Table 9 Intravenous pharmacokinetics of sodium fusidate[a]

Parameter (unit)	Single dose	Repeated doses
C_0 (μg/ml)	52.4 ± 4.7	123.1 ± 11.6
$t_{1/2}$ (h)	9.8 ± 0.7	14.2 ± 1.9
AUC (μg·h/ml)	411 ± 44	894 ± 77
Cl_P (ml/min)	21.8	11.1 ± 1.2
V (liters/kg)	0.3 ± 0.04	0.21 ± 0.02

[a]Values are means ± standard deviations.

13.3. Intravenous Pharmacokinetics

After infusion of a single dose of 500 mg of sodium fusidate for 120 min, the concentration in plasma at the end of infusion is 52.4 ± 4.7 μg/ml, with an apparent elimination half-life on the order of 10 h and a plasma clearance of 22 ml/min. The volume of distribution is small, on the order of 0.3 l/kg.

After repeated doses, the apparent half-life increases nonsignificantly.

13.4. Elimination

Fusidic acid is eliminated via the bile. About 2% of the parent compound is eliminated, and the remainder is composed of metabolites.

Urinary elimination is negligible, about 1%. Fecal elimination accounts for 2% of the administered dose.

13.5. Metabolism

See Fig. 8.

The metabolism of sodium fusidate has been studied in the bile of patients with a drain following cholecystectomy. Seven metabolites have been identified, three of which are important in quantitative terms (A, D, and G).

Metabolite G is the glucuronic derivative and accounts for about 15% of the administered dose. Metabolite C is the dicarboxylic acid derivative and accounts for 10% of the dose. Metabolite E is the hydroxyl derivative of dicarboxylic acid and accounts for 3% of the dose.

3-Keto-fusidate (metabolite A) is found in traces in the bile but is the only metabolite identified in plasma. After administration of repeated doses, it accumulates in parallel with the fusidate and reaches a plateau of 10 to 15 μg/ml, equivalent to 15% of the steady-state levels of sodium fusidate.

Only metabolites A, C, E, and G have been identified, together with the 3-keto derivative.

Metabolites C, G, and E are weakly active. 3-Keto-fusidate is four times less active than fusidic acid.

13.6. Underlying Diseases

The pharmacokinetic parameters are unchanged in patients with renal insufficiency, as fusidic acid is eliminated in the bile. Hemodialysis and peritoneal dialysis do not affect the pharmacokinetics of fusidic acid.

In patients with hepatic impairment, administration of fusidic acid must be avoided because of the possibility of (reversible) jaundice. It has recently been shown that the pharmacokinetics of fusidic acid in certain patients with hepatic insufficiency are unchanged.

However, in these patients the potential modifications of the metabolism of fusidic acid are unknown; it would seem that the concentrations of 3-keto-fusidic acid are not modified in patients with cholestasis.

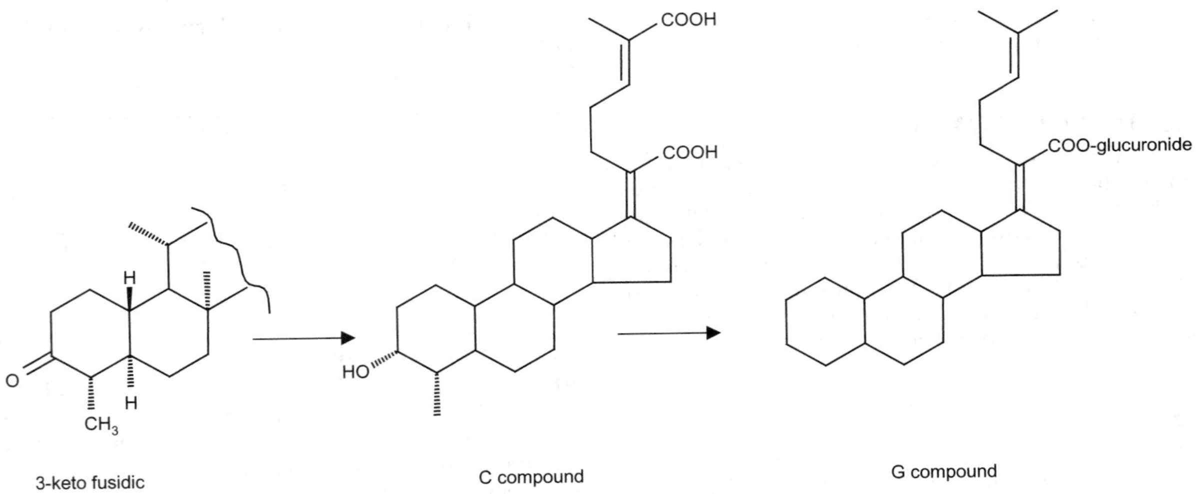

3-keto fusidic — C compound — G compound

Figure 8 Metabolism of fusidic acid

In hemodialysis patients, the mean maximum concentration of drug in serum for the first dose was 13 μg/ml (2.0 to 25.5 μg/ml) and that for the sixth dose was 40.5 (10.1 to 69 μg/ml). Concentrations in serum were not reduced by hemodialysis (Table 10).

Fusidic acid concentrations of 1.0 to 2.3 μg/ml were detected in peritoneal fluid from six of the seven CAPD patients.

13.7. New Oral Formulation

After a 250-mg dose of a new oral formulation (single administration) the fusidic acid concentration was measured; results are shown in Table 11.

The bioavailability for the new film-coated tablet is approximately 91%.

14. TISSUE DISTRIBUTION

Fusidic acid is highly albumin bound, on the order of 97 to 98%. There are three binding sites with a high constant of affinity.

Fusidic acid concentrates well in the liver, skin, subcutaneous fat, muscle, lungs, renal tissue, bone, pleural tissue, and tears, but it does not cross the meningeal barrier. Table 12 summarizes the main tissue distribution results.

The concentrations of fusidic acid in the synovial fluid of patients suffering from rheumatoid arthritis or osteoarthritis are 40 to 80% of the concentrations detected in plasma.

The concentrations in cortical bone are on the order of 0.2 to 1.7 μg/ml after doses of 500 mg (every 8 h for 4 to 31 days). Bone concentrations increase with the duration of treatment.

The concentration in cardiac tissue is 30% of that in plasma. Fusidic acid attains therapeutic concentrations in skin, suction blister fluid, and necrotic tissue.

Table 10 Fusidic acid concentrations in patients undergoing hemodialysis and CAPD

Patient group	Concn (range), mg/liter, after:	
	1st dose	6th dose
Hemodialysis	13 (2.0–25.5)	40.5 (10.1–69.9)
CAPD	16 (4.8–33.8)	33.9 (23.4–61.9)

In the bronchial secretions of children suffering from cystic fibrosis, the concentrations are on the order of 0.1 to 1.6 μg/ml, whereas those in serum are greater than 10 μg/ml.

Fusidic acid does not penetrate the cerebrospinal fluid and only weakly penetrates the aqueous humor.

Local instillation of fusidic acid in the form of eyedrops yields a concentration of 1.4 μg/ml at 12 h, with an apparent elimination half-life of 19 h (1% microcrystalline suspension or carbomer).

15. EYEDROPS

After instillation of 1% viscous eyedrops in healthy volunteers, the concentrations of fusidic acid were measured; results are shown in Table 13.

The apparent elimination half-life is about 7.3 h.

16. OTHER PROPERTIES

Fusidic acid acts on mononuclear cells by reversibly reducing the amounts of interleukin 1 (IL-1) and tumor necrosis factor alpha (TNF-α) released by activated cells. The production of T-cell-derived IL-2 and interferon is also suppressed, as are costimulatory activities of IL-1 and IL-6 on T cells. Fusidic acid also prevents the inhibitory effect of IL-1β and the stimulatory effect of IL-6 on glucose-induced insulin production in vitro.

Both IL-1 and IL-6 are thought to be of pathogenic importance for the development of diabetes. There is apparently a positive effect of fusidic acid on the course of diabetic patients with newly diagnosed disease.

Table 11 Concentrations of fusidic acid after administration in a new oral formulation (single 250-mg dose)

Parameter	Value (μg/ml)
C_{max}	11.6
C_{max}, unbound	0.58
C_{8h}	4.2
C_{8h}, unbound	0.21
C_{12h}	1.5
C_{12h}, unbound	0.75

Table 12 Tissue distribution of fusidic acid

Site	Patient characteristic	Dose[a]	Tissue level (mg/kg)	Concn in serum (μg/ml)	Ratio of levels in tissues and serum
Synovial fluid		1.5 × 3 d	47	71	68
		1.5 × 7 d	48.7	61	81
		1.5 × 7 d	16	34	40
Infected bone	Osteomyelitis	1.5 × 5 d	7.3	24.3	31
			4.6 (cortical)	25.8	23
			2.3	25.8	11
			9.7	25.8	52
Noninfected bone	Surgery	1.5 × 5 d	12.3	26.7	46
		1.5 × 7 d	21.3	44.7	47
		1.5 × 13 d	25.4	27.1	93
		1.5 × 7 d	17.9	39.9	45
			31.9	39.9	80
Myocardium	Surgery	500 mg i.v.	10.7	32.4	33
Sputum	Cystic fibrosis	1,000 mg × 2 × 7 d	0.6–0.4	10–50	5–10
	Pus	1.5 g	17.2	20.7	17
Fat	Surgery	1.5 × 3 d	12.4	72.1	17
Eye	Cataract	1.5 × 1 d	0.33	23.3	
		1.5 × 2 d	1.12	52.3	
		1.5 × 3 d	1.25	63.2	
Burn wounds		1.5 × 3 d	97.7	23.7	412
		1.5 × 15 d	41.1	24	171
		1.5 × 14 d	30.1	7.6	500
Blister fluid	Healthy volunteers	500 mg		24.4	42 (1 h)
					46 (2 h)
					28 (3 h)

[a]d, days; i.v., intravenous.

Table 13 Concentrations measured after instillation of 1% viscous eyedrops in healthy volunteers

Sampling time (h)	Concn (μg/ml)
1	15.7
3	15.2
6	10.5
12	7.3

Fusidic acid has been used successfully in various rodent models and some human autoimmune diseases, such as endogenous uveitis, Guillain-Barré syndrome, T-cell-dependent hepatitis lesions, Crohn's disease, Behcet's colitis, and multiple sclerosis.

Seven patients undergoing continuous ambulatory peritoneal dialysis (CAPD) were given 500 mg per day for 7 days. An accumulation was seen, and in 12 out of 15 patients, steady-state pharmacokinetics had not been achieved by the third day.

17. CLINICAL INDICATIONS

Fusidic acid is an antistaphylococcal antibiotic that does not exhibit cross-resistance with the β-lactams or rifampin. It must be used in combination with other antibacterial agents because of the rapid emergence of resistant strains.

The effect of local therapy of nostrils with fusidic acid cream (20 mg of sodium fusidate per liter) was investigated in 30 untreated patients with lepromatous leprosy. The cream was applied twice a day for 4 weeks. This cream was effective in reducing the morphological index in 2 weeks.

REFERENCES

Godtfredsen WO, Von Daehne W, Tybring L, Vangedal S, 1966, Fusidic acid derivatives - I - Relationship between structure and antibacterial activity, J Med Chem, 9, 15–22.

Okuda S, Iwasaki S, Sair MI, Machida Y, Inoue A, Tsuda K, 1967, Stereochemistry of helvolic acid, Tetrahedron Lett, 24, 2295–2302.

Taburet AM, Guibert J, Kitzis MD, Sorensen H, Acar JF, Singlas E, 1990, Pharmacokinetics of sodium fusidate after single and repeated infusions and oral administration of a new formulation, J Antimicrob Chemother, 25, suppl B, 23–31.

Verbist L, 1990, The antimicrobial activity of fusidic acid, J Antimicrob Chemother, 25, suppl B, 1–5.

von Daehne W, Lorch H, Godtfredsen WO, 1968, Microbiological transformations of fusidane-type antibiotics. A correlation between fusidic acid and helvolic acid, Tetrahedron Lett, 47, 4843–4846.

Yamaki H, 1965, Inhibition of protein synthesis by fusidic and helvolinic acids, steroidal antibiotics, J Antibiot, 18, 228–232.

Tetracyclines

ANDRÉ BRYSKIER

24

1. INTRODUCTION

The tetracyclines were the first group of broad-spectrum antibacterial antibiotics to be described. The first cycline, chlortetracycline, was isolated in 1944 from *Streptomyces aureofaciens* by B.M. Duggar and introduced into clinical practice in 1948. Oxytetracycline, isolated from *Streptomyces rimosus*, was described in 1950, while the prototype, tetracycline, produced by catalytic dehalogenation of chlortetracycline, was described in 1953. The semisynthetic analogs doxycycline and minocycline were discovered in 1966 and 1972, respectively.

The use of tetracyclines is less widespread now than in the past due to the emergence of antibacterial resistance to these antibiotics and the discovery of more effective and selective molecules. Other factors affecting their use and efficacy include their not insignificant toxicity, weak absorption, and molecular instability. They remain, however, fairly extensively used in nonhospital environments for the treatment of respiratory tract infections and infections due to microorganisms not currently susceptible to other intracellularly concentrated antibiotics, such as *Chlamydia, Mycoplasma,* and *Rickettsia.*

2. CHEMICAL STRUCTURES

At pH 7 the tetracyclines are present in the form of crystalline bases. They are only slightly soluble in water and rapidly form sodium salts and hydrochlorides. They are stable in the form of the drug substance and the hydrochloride, but they rapidly lose their activity in solution.

The tetracyclines are complex polycyclic structures of the perhydronaphthacene carboxamide type. The carboxamide group is normally at position 2. The structural variations from the reference molecule, tetracycline, among the tetracyclines are minimal. These structural variations affect the C-5, C-6, and C-7 carbons, which constitute the specific sequence of each cycline. Certain tetracyclines also have variations at C-8 and a carbamoyl group at C-2. Tetracycline has no substituent at position 7 but possesses a methyl and a hydroxyl at position 6. Chlortetracycline has a chlorine atom at position 7. Oxytetracycline has a hydroxyl substituent at position 5. Doxycycline, or deoxyoxytetracycline, has lost a hydroxyl group in the 6β position. Finally, minocycline does not have substituents at positions 5 and 6, but it has an additional dimethylamino group at position 7.

The chemical structures of the main tetracyclines are depicted in Fig. 1.

3. CLASSIFICATION

According to the most recent studies of their mode of action, the tetracyclines may be divided into two classes: (i) so-called "typical" tetracyclines, such as tetracycline, chlortetracycline, minocycline, and doxycycline, which act on bacteria by inhibiting protein synthesis in the ribosome, and (ii) so-called "atypical" tetracyclines, such as chelocardin, anhydrotetracycline, 6-thiatetracycline, anhydrochlortetracycline, and 4-*epi*-anhydrochlortetracycline, which act on bacteria by interfering with the electrochemical gradient of the bacterial membrane and thus promoting lysis and cell death by stimulating autolytic enzyme activity.

Tetracyclines may be classified in terms of their pharmacokinetic properties into (i) short-acting tetracyclines, such as oxytetracycline, tetracycline, and chlortetracycline; (ii) intermediately acting tetracyclines, such as demeclocycline and metacycline; and (iii) long-acting tetracyclines, such as doxycycline and minocycline. They are also divided in terms of their date of discovery and their plasma half-life into (i) first-generation natural tetracyclines with an intermediate half-life, such as chlortetracycline, oxytetracycline, tetracycline, lymecycline, demeclocycline, and rolitetracycline; (ii) second-generation semisynthetic tetracyclines with a long apparent elimination half-life, such as methacycline, doxycycline, and minocycline; and now (iii) third-generation tetracyclines with 9-substituted analogs overcoming tetracycline resistance.

4. PHYSICOCHEMICAL PROPERTIES

The physicochemical properties of the tetracyclines may be modified by minimal structural variations. The hydrosolubility of a molecule is dependent on certain polar groups, such as the hydroxyls, which are frequently found in the tetracyclines at C-5 and C-6, and the state of ionization of the molecule. Thus, oxytetracycline, which has an additional hydroxyl at position 5, is more hydrosoluble than chlortetracycline. Similarly, the most hydrosoluble molecules are those that are the most electrically charged. It should, however, be mentioned that ionization of the tetracyclines is a complex phenomenon, given the presence of three ionogenic centers in these molecules. Each of these ionogenic centers becomes

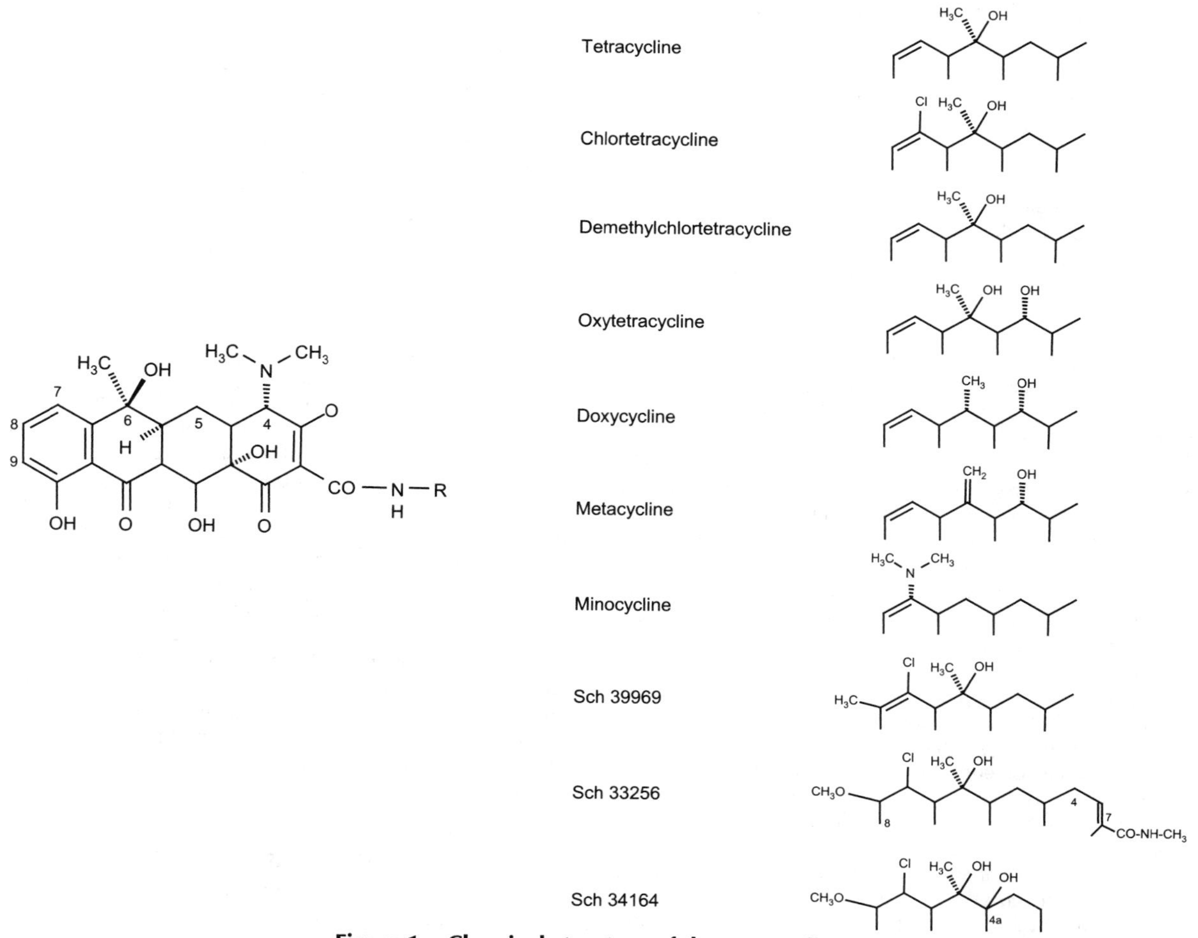

Figure 1 Chemical structure of the tetracyclines

ionized at a certain critical pH value (pK_a); when the pH is equal to the pK_a, there is a change in the state of ionization of the ionogenic center. By looking at these characteristics, it is possible to study and determine the degree of ionization of the tetracyclines as a function of the pH.

Liposolubility increases the rate of penetration of the antibiotic into the cytoplasmic membrane, which is composed principally of phospholipids. At isoelectric pH (about 5.5), the positive charges offset the negative charges and hence the total charge is equal to 0. This pH corresponds to the maximum liposolubility, which can be evaluated by the maximum partition coefficient between oil and water. When the antibiotic is at the interface of the aqueous and lipid media, it divides between the two phases according to a coefficient based on its lipophilicity and hydrophilicity. This coefficient (K_p) expresses the liposolubility as a value relative to the hydrosolubility. The partition coefficients of different tetracyclines have been determined experimentally in a chloroform ($CHCl_3$)-water system or an *n*-octanol–water system. In this system, the value of the solubility in chloroform or in *n*-octanol is a measurement of liposolubility. The coefficients of partition vary with the pH and the molecular structure. Table 1 presents certain characteristics of the tetracyclines.

Chelate formation between the tetracyclines and the Mg^{2+} cation is due to the keto and hydroxyl groups at positions C-11 and C-12. At physiological pH only an Mg^{2+} cation is chelated, whereas at very basic pH a second cation may also be complexed at C-1 or C-10.

Several adverse events due to tetracyclines seem to be related to the degradation products, such as Fanconi-type syndrome, due to the presence of anhydrotetracycline and 4-*epi*-anhydrotetracycline, the major toxic degradation product of the parent compound.

5. IN VITRO PROPERTIES

The tetracyclines are markedly more active in vitro in an acidic medium than in an alkaline medium. The antibacterial spectra are almost similar for all tetracyclines. However, major differences are observed in the degrees of activity against microorganisms. In general, lipophilic substances are more active than hydrophilic substances. Minocycline is thus the most active of the molecules, followed by doxycycline. As oxytetracycline and tetracycline are more hydrophilic, the MICs are two to four times higher than for minocycline and they are therefore the least active tetracyclines. It should, however, be noted that in gram-negative bacteria the opposite applies. In clinical microbiological laboratories the susceptibility tests are performed by means of an antibiogram using a disk loaded with 30 μg.

The tetracyclines are bacteriostatic antibiotics, the ratio of minimum bactericidal concentration to MIC being on

Table 1 Physicochemical properties of cyclines

Tetracycline	Empirical formula	Mol wt	pK	log *P*
Oxytetracycline	$C_{22}H_{24}N_2O_9$	460.4	3.3, 7.3, 9.1	−4.9
Tetracycline	$C_{22}H_{24}N_2O_8$	444.45	3.3, 7.7, 9.7	−2.56
Chlortetracycline	$C_{22}H_{23}ClN_2O_8$	478.89	3.3, 7.44, 9.27	−0.89 (pH 7.5)
Demeclocycline	$C_{21}H_{21}N_2O_8$	469.86	3.3, 7.2, 9.3	−2.46, −0.60 (pH 6.6)
Methacycline	$C_{22}H_{24}N_2O_8$	442.43	3.1, 7.6, 9.5	−3.6, −0.37 (pH 7.5)
Minocycline	$C_{23}H_{27}N_3O_7$	457.49	2.8, 5.0, 7.8, 9.5	−1.37
Doxycycline	$C_{22}H_{24}N_2O_8$	444.45	3.5, 7.7, 9.5	−0.22 (pH 7.4)

average 4. They may possibly have a bactericidal effect on bacterial strains for which the MICs are very low when levels in serum and tissue are greater than the minimum bactericidal concentration.

The antibacterial spectrum and activity of the tetracyclines include numerous gram-positive and gram-negative bacteria, anaerobes, rickettsiae, mycoplasmas, chlamydiae, *Helicobacter pylori*, and spirochetes. Certain tetracyclines are also active against a number of mycobacteria (*Mycobacterium marinum* and *Mycobacterium leprae*) and protozoa, such as *Plasmodium* spp., *Entamoeba histolytica, Balantidium coli, Giardia lamblia*, and *Toxoplasma gondii*.

The postantibiotic effect is used to describe the period of persistent suppression of bacterial growth following short-term exposure to the antibiotic. This result derives from exposure of the microorganisms to the antibiotic and not from the presence of subinhibitory concentrations of the antibiotic. A postantibiotic effect of tetracycline has been demonstrated with *Escherichia coli* in vitro, but only at antibiotic concentrations equal to or greater than the MIC. The effect is greatest at a concentration 8 to 16 times the MIC. The dose-response curves illustrating the antibiotic effect suggest a tetracycline-receptor type of interaction. As the tetracyclines normally bind to specific units of the ribosomes of susceptible bacteria, the postantibiotic effect might represent the time they take to diffuse from the ribosomes.

The appearance of numerous forms of bacterial resistance considerably restricts the indication for tetracyclines nowadays. About half the strains of streptococci and staphylococci are now resistant. The situation is similar with gram-negative bacteria, and resistance is often observed in *E. coli, Klebsiella* spp., *Neisseria gonorrhoeae, Moraxella (Branhamella) catarrhalis, Haemophilus influenzae, Shigella* spp., *Salmonella* spp., *Pseudomonas aeruginosa*, and *Proteus mirabilis*, which are not susceptible to tetracyclines, and *Burkholderia pseudomallei*. Some anaerobic bacteria are susceptible to tetracyclines.

The MIC at which 50% of isolates tested are inhibited (MIC_{50}) and MIC_{90} of tetracycline, doxycycline, and minocycline for certain aerobic, facultatively anaerobic, and strictly anaerobic bacteria are listed in Tables 2 and 3.

The MIC of doxycycline for *Chlamydia psittaci* is 0.12 μg/ml.

6. MECHANISMS OF ACTION

The efficacy of an antibiotic against a microorganism depends both on its affinity for a given target structure and its ability to cross the various structural barriers that bar access to it.

Table 2 MICs of tetracycline, doxycycline, and minocycline for facultative aerobic and anaerobic bacteria

Microorganism(s)	MIC (μg/ml)					
	Tetracycline		Doxycycline		Minocycline	
	50%	90%	50%	90%	50%	90%
Gram positive						
S. aureus	3.1	100	1.6	25	0.5	3.1–6.3
S. pyogenes	0.8	3.1	0.5	1.6		0.8
S. pneumoniae	0.5	2	0.04	0.2	0.04	0.2
Gram negative						
N. gonorrhoeae	0.06	8	<0.5	1.6	<0.05	1.6
Neisseria meningitidis	0.8	3.1	1.6	3.1	1.6	3.1
H. influenzae	3.1	6.25	1.6	3.1	1.6	3.1
Haemophilus ducreyi	16	28	1	4	1	2
E. coli	2	64	2	64	2	64
Klebsiella pneumoniae	1	128	4	32		
Enterobacter cloacae	2	4	2	4		
M. catarrhalis	0.5	1	0.25	0.25	0.12	0.25
Bordetella pertussis	2	4	0.25	2	0.03	1.25
Brucella spp.	0.5	1	0.25	1	0.25	1
B. pseudomallei	6.25	12.5	1.6	3.1	1.6	3.1
C. jejuni	0.8	25	<0.5	6.3		
H. pylori	0.5	1			0.06	0.125

Table 3 In vitro activities of tetracycline, doxycycline, and minocycline against anaerobic bacteria and other pathogens

Microorganism(s)	MIC (μg/ml)					
	Tetracycline		Doxycycline		Minocycline	
	50%	90%	50%	90%	50%	90%
Gram positive						
Streptococcus spp.	0.5	4.0	0.2	1.0		
Clostridium perfringens	2	64	0.06	0.12	0.03	0.06
Actinomyces spp.	0.5	2.0	0.5	2.0		
Gram negative						
Fusobacterium spp.	0.125	2.0	0.125	0.5	0.125	0.5
Bacteroides fragilis	8		0.2	8.0	8.0	16.0
Others						
M. pneumoniae	1.0	2.0	0.5	0.5	0.5	1.0
M. hominis	1.0	2.0	0.12	0.5	0.12	0.12
Legionella pneumophila	2.0	4.0		4.0		4.0
C. trachomatis	0.003	0.125	0.06	0.125	0.06	0.06
Nocardia asteroides	32	32	4.0	32	2.0	8.0
B. burgdorferi	<0.25	2.0	<0.25	2.0	<0.12	
G. lamblia	36	130	6.4	22	5.2	18
U. urealyticum	1.0	40	0.5	1.0	0.25	0.5

In the case of gram-negative bacteria, the first obstacle to be overcome is the bacterial outer membrane. The tetracyclines probably penetrate the periplasmic space via transmembrane proteins forming hydrophilic channels, known as porins. In *E. coli*, it is via the major porin OmpF that the tetracyclines cross the bacterial outer membrane. Since the outer membrane is relatively impermeable to hydrophobic compounds because of the presence of lipopolysaccharide in its outer layer, the activity of the tetracyclines is correlated with the degree of liposolubility of the molecules. Thus, compared to doxycycline and minocycline, oxytetracycline and tetracycline, which are more hydrophilic, have markedly lower MICs for *E. coli* K-12 in proportion to their respective partition coefficients.

6.1. Outer Membrane of Gram-Negative Bacteria

Passage through the outer membrane in *E. coli* and *Staphylococcus aureus* occurs both by passive diffusion and by active transport through the porins OmpC and OmpF as positively charged cations. The latter mechanism allows the tetracyclines to accumulate in the cytoplasm at concentrations up to 100 times greater than the external concentrations.

The cationic metal ion-antibiotic complex is attracted by the Donnan potential across the outer membrane.

6.2. Periplasmic Space

In the periplasm the complex dissociates to liberate uncharged tetracycline, which could diffuse through the lipid bilayer of the inner membrane.

6.3. Inner Membrane

To cross the cytoplasmic membrane, tetracyclines need an energy-dependent proton motive force (ΔpH).

6.4. Cytoplasm

After crossing the cytoplasmic membrane, the cycline molecules diffuse into the cytoplasm, form a complex with Mg^{2+}, and reach their target structure, the ribosomes.

The ensuing inhibition of protein synthesis is due to the binding of the tetracycline molecule to a single site, localized on the 30S ribosomal subunit (Fig. 2). The codon-anticodon interaction between tRNA and mRNA is interrupted, blocking the elongation phase, i.e., the attachment of the aminoacyl-tRNA complex at site A of the ribosome. The cycline binding site on the 30S ribosomal subunit is modeled by proteins S3, S7, S14, and S19 of the main domain. The binding of the tetracyclines to their target is reversible, which would explain their purely bacteriostatic nature.

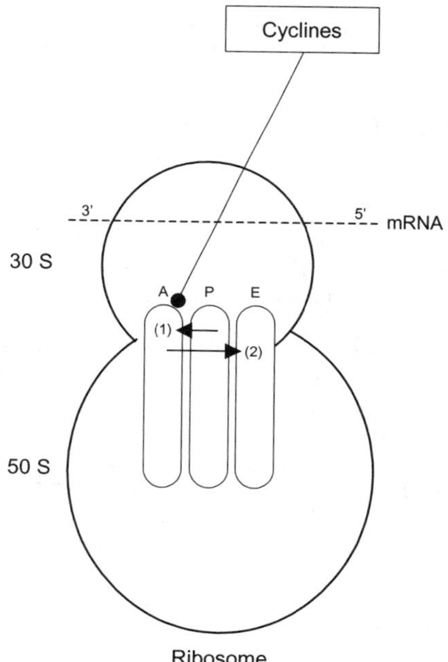

Figure 2 Sequence of protein synthesis and site of action of the tetracyclines. (1) Binding of aminoacyl-tRNA to the A-site in the form of a complex with GTP and elongation factor Tu (EF-Tu). (2) Translocation in the presence of EF-Tu and EF-G. The tetracyclines inhibit the attachment of the aminoacyl-tRNA complex to the ribosomal site (1).

The binding pocket of tetracyclines seems to be composed of protein S7 and the following bases of 16S rRNA: G693, U1052, C1054, G1300, and G1338.

It has been suggested that tetracycline positions C-10 to C-2 are involved in hydrogen binding with the ribosome and are therefore unavailable for chemical alterations.

Tetracyclines interact indirectly with the 16S rRNA through primary distortion of the ribosome.

The divalent Mg^{2+} cation forms a bifurcated ionic pairing with the oxygen atom at the C-11 and C-12 positions.

In vitro, the tetracyclines have an inhibitory effect not only on prokaryotic ribosomes but also on the mitochondrial ribosomes of eukaryotic cells. This would explain the antiplasmodial activity (slow-acting schizonticides) of the tetracyclines. Mammalian cell ribosomes, for their part, have very little affinity for these antibiotics.

In vivo, however, only prokaryotic cells are affected by tetracyclines. This selective action would appear to be due less to structural differences between ribosomes of different origin than to the incapacity of eukaryotic cells, as opposed to bacterial cells, to accumulate tetracycline molecules actively in the cytoplasm.

Certain derivatives similar to tetracyclines, such as chelocardin and 6-thiatetracycline, are bactericidal rather than bacteriostatic agents. This particular feature appears to be due to an original mechanism of action. In fact, these derivatives act not on protein synthesis but rather by causing extensive damage to the bacterial cytoplasmic membrane.

7. RESISTANCE MECHANISMS

The therapeutic use of tetracyclines is increasingly undermined by the frequent emergence of resistance. It indiscriminately affects all species theoretically belonging to the antibacterial spectrum of activity of the tetracyclines. In the great majority of cases this development is due to the acquisition of genetic resistance determinants by a previously susceptible bacterial population.

The spread of resistance within the same bacterial population or between species is facilitated by the fact that these determinants are carried by plasmids and transposons (e.g., Tn*10*). A recent example of this phenomenon is the propagation of the *tet*(M) resistance determinant among numerous strains of *N. gonorrhoeae*, *Ureaplasma urealyticum*, and *Mycoplasma hominis*. Isolated originally on a transposon of the *Streptococus* genus, *tet*(M) is now carried on a conjugation plasmid in a number of species (Table 4).

7.1. Mechanisms

7.1.1. Efflux

Active efflux of tetracycline is a resistance mechanism found in both gram-positive and gram-negative bacteria. The nomenclature for tetracycline resistance determinants has been recently revised (Table 4).

Most of the efflux proteins confer resistance to tetracycline but not to minocycline or glycylcycline in gram-positive cocci. In contrast, the *tet*(B) gene in gram-negative bacteria encodes an efflux protein which confers resistance to both tetracycline and minocycline, but not to glycylcyclines. Each of the efflux genes encodes an about 44-kDa membrane-bound protein. At least 16 groups of proteins have been reported. The multiplicity of these genetic resistance determinants has necessitated the adoption of a complex nomenclature based on the cross hybridization technique. There are at present 16 classes of determinants of resistance to tetracyclines, designated *tet*(A) to *tet*(Z). Each class thus comprises only genes exhibiting a relatively high degree of homology (Table 4).

Table 4 Tetracycline resistance determinants

Tet determinant or gene	GenBank Accession no.
Tet A	X00006
Tet B	J01830
Tet C	J01749
Tet D	X65876
Tet E	L06940
Tet F (?)	Unsequenced
Tet G	S52437
Tet H	U00792
Tet I (?)	Unsequenced
Tet J	AF038993
Tet K	M16217
Tet L (plasmid)	M11036
Tet L (chromosomal)	X08034
Tet P	L20800
Tet V	AF030344
Tet Y	AF070999
Tet Z	AF121000
otrB	AF079900
otr-3 (*tcrC*)	D38215
Tet30	AF090987

The *tet* genes, in gram-negative organisms, first described in *Enterobacteriaceae* and *Pseudomonas*, are now found in *Neisseria* spp., *Vibrio* spp., *Haemophilus* spp., *Mannheimia*, and *Treponema*.

Tetracycline resistance genes are not expressed in the absence of compounds. In gram-negative bacteria, a repressor protein blocks transcription in the absence of tetracyclines by binding to an operator site near the transcription initiation site upstream of the structural genes encoding efflux protein.

The Tet proteins consist of two interdependent domains, Tetα (amino-terminal half) and Tetβ (carboxy-terminal half), both of which are required for the full tetracycline resistance phenotype.

Induction occurs when tetracyclines enter the bacterial cell and bind to the repressor, resulting in repressor release from the operator sequence and allowing for transcription and translation of tetracycline efflux protein.

7.2. Ribosomal Protection

Tetracycline resistance due to ribosome protection is encoded by the *tet*(M) gene and its homologs, the *tet* genes O, Q, PC(B), S and T. The resistance mechanism is also linked to its location on a transposon: Tn*916*, Tn*1721* (class A), or Tn*10* (class B).

Ribosomal protection proteins are inducible without a repressor protein which regulates gene expression. These genes apparently use ribosome stalling mechanisms which prevent the nascent mRNA from prematurely terminating.

The genes involved in ribosomal protection are *tet*(M), *tet*(Q), *tet*(S), *tet*(W), *tet*(O), *tet*(T), *otr*(A), and *tet*(P)(B).

It is believed that *tet*(M) binds to the ribosome adjacent to the tetracycline-binding site on the 30S ribosomal subunit. Upon binding, a GTP hydrolysis-dependent process causes a local conformational change of the tetracycline-binding site to the ribosome.

This mechanism has been reported for *Streptococcus* spp., *Campylobacter* spp., *Eikenella*, *Veillonella*, *Gardnerella*, *Fusobacterium*, *Clostridium*, and *Mycoplasma*.

The *tet*(Q) gene is often associated with a large conjugative transposon which carries the *ermF* gene, which encodes an rRNA methylase, upstream from the *tet*(Q) gene.

Many gram-negative and gram-positive bacteria, including anaerobes, carry both the *tet*(Q)I and *ermF* genes.

In addition, two genes, *rteA* and *rteB*, which are believed to play a role in the transfer of conjugative elements in *Bacteroides*, *Clostridium*, *Actinobacillus*, *Prevotella*, *Selenomonas*, and *Veillonella*, are carried on a transposon.

7.3. Mutations

Mutations in the 30S ribosomal subunit have been reported for *H. pylori* and *Propionibacterium acnes*. These mutations occur in the vicinity of the putative tetracycline-binding site.

In *P. acnes* a point mutation occurs at C1058→G in tRNA.

Other mutations decrease tetracycline resistance:

- The *rpsL* gene, which encodes the S12 ribosomal protein, decreases tetracycline resistance in the presence of *tet*(M) protein.
- The *E. coli miaA* gene encodes an enzyme that catalyzes the first step in the modification of A37 on tRNA that reads codons starting with U. This is located near the anticodon and with modification decreases the rate of elongation and increases the number of errors at the first position of the codon. Mutations in *miaA* in the presence of *tet*(M) reduced the level of tetracycline resistance in *E. coli*.

7.4. Enzymatic Inactivation

The *tet*(X) gene encodes an enzymatic alteration of tetracyclines which was found on a transposon in *Bacteroides*. The *tet*(X) gene is linked to the *ermF* gene. The *tet*(X) gene encodes 44-kDa cytoplasmic protein in the presence of both oxygen and NADPH, which renders tetracyclines inactive.

7.5. Unknown Mechanism(s)

The *tet*(U) gene encodes an 11.8-kDa protein, and the *ort*(C) gene codes for unknown protein. The functions of both proteins are unknown.

7.6. Epidemiology of Resistance

Prior the mid-1950s, the majority of commensal and pathogenic bacteria were susceptible to tetracyclines. Among 433 isolates of *Enterobacteriaceae* collected between 1917 and 1954, 2% were resistant to tetracyclines.

In 1953, the first tetracycline-resistant bacterium was isolated: a *Shigella dysenteriae* strain. In 1955, a multidrug-resistant *S. dysenteriae* strain was isolated (resistant to tetracycline, chloramphenicol, and streptomycin) and represented 0.02% of the total isolates tested.

By 1960, multidrug-resistant *S. dysenteriae* represented 10% of the isolates in Japan.

Recently *Salmonella enterica* serovar Typhimurium DT04 isolates were found to carry a class 1 integron containing a variety of antibiotic resistance genes, including for tetracyclines.

In an epidemiological survey carried out in 1994, it was shown that 90% of methicillin-resistant *S. aureus* strains, 70% of *Streptococcus agalactiae* strains, 70% of multidrug-resistant *Enterococcus faecalis* strains, and 60% of multidrug-resistant *S. pneumoniae* strains were resistant to tetracycline.

It was reported in the mid-1980s that *H. influenzae* can be resistant to both chloramphenicol and tetracycline; the two resistance genes are on the same transposon.

The commensal flora consists of microorganisms which are present in and on surface of a host and not thought to cause disease. The organisms are often beneficial for the host, providing nutrients and inhibiting the growth of potential pathogens by preventing them from becoming established. These bacteria possess the same *tet* genes, plasmids, transposons, conjugative transposons, and integrons as the potential pathogens.

Many oral viridans group streptococci have acquired *tet*(M), *tet*(O), *tet*(L), and *tet*(K) genes, as have *S. pneumoniae*, and *Streptococcus pyogenes*. Most people today carry tetracycline-resistant viridans group streptococci in their mouths regardless of the use of tetracycline therapy.

7.6.1. *S. pneumoniae*

There is an increased prevalence of *S. pneumoniae* isolates resistant to tetracycline, as reported in Table 5.

Tetracycline resistance is frequently associated with penicillin G resistance, as shown in the Alexander Project from 1992 to 1996 (Table 6).

The same kind of resistance profile has been demonstrated in North America in the Protekt study from 1999 to 2000 (Table 7).

The pattern of *S. pneumoniae* resistance to tetracycline was assessed in the Alexander Project from 1992 to 1996; this study showed an established resistance to tetracycline in many countries (Table 8).

In Thailand, 11 and 78.9% of penicillin G-susceptible and -resistant *S. pneumoniae* isolates, respectively, are resistant to tetracycline.

Table 5 Prevalence of tetracycline-resistant *S. pneumoniae* strains in Protekt studies

Country	Protekt 1999–2000		Protekt 2001–2002	
	n	% Resistance	*n*	% Resistance
Argentina	55	18.2	29	27.6
Australia	114	9.6	118	9.3
Austria	57	17.5	92	5.4
Belgium	28	14.3	73	24.7
Brazil	260	14.2	215	14
Canada	350	10.9	514	8.0
Ireland	53	30.2	57	10.5
France	184	44.0	191	47.1
Germany	325	11.7	693	14
Hong Kong	70	74.3	58	87.9
Hungary	54	63	60	40
Indonesia	7	71.4	NT[a]	NT
Italy	119	25.2	284	21.5
Japan	308	78.6	627	79.9
Mexico	203	32.6	80	43.8
The Netherlands	51	5.9	NT	NT
Poland	68	45.6	77	18.2
Portugal	106	19.8	93	14
Korea	137	90.5	110	87.3
Spain	133	36.1	442	37.6
Sweden	64	3.1	72	1.3
Switzerland	111	9.0	NT	NT
Turkey	77	24.7	101	19.8
United Kingdom	91	9.9	91	6.6
United States	337	16.6	174	21.3

[a]NT, not tested.

Table 6 Combined resistance of penicillin G and tetracycline within *S. pneumoniae*

Penicillin G resistance phenotype	% Resistance[a]				
	1992	1993	1994	1995	1996
Susceptible	5.5	4.0	10.4	9.0	10.8
Intermediate	37.5	28	53.4	44	37.7
Resistant	50	35.1	61.9	47.4	50.7

[a]breakpoints, ≥4μg/ml.

Table 7 Combined resistance of penicillin G and tetracycline within *S. pneumoniae* in North America

Penicillin G resistance phenotype	United States		Canada	
	n	% Resistance	n	% Resistance
Susceptible	192	1.6	276	2.9
Intermediate	35	25.7	37	37.8
Resistant	110	40.9	37	100

Table 8 Prevalence of *S. pneumoniae* isolates resistant to tetracycline (1992–1996)

Country	% Resistance				
	1992	1993	1994	1995	1996
United Kingdom	2.3	1.9	6.4	5.3	6.8
Northern Ireland	2.6	0	0	0	2.9
France	22.7	21.1	40.8	32.5	27.9
Spain	26.6	11.8	37.3	33.1	29.4
Germany	10	7.1	18.8	7.8	5.3
Italy	12.9	5.2	20.3	18.5	22.8
The Netherlands					6.2
Belgium					17.8
Switzerland					6.4
Austria					3.7
Poland					37.2
Hungary					22
The Czech Republic					1.3
Slovakia					8.9
Saudi Arabia					11.1
South Africa					7.2
Mexico					27.5
Brazil					10.5
Hong Kong					81.8

7.6.2. *H. influenzae* and *M. catarrhalis*

In Canada, irrespective of the susceptibility to ampicillin, the prevalence of doxycycline resistance is 1.4% (BLNR) to 1.9% (β-lactamase producers). Only 0.2% of *M. catarrhalis* clinical isolates were resistant to doxycycline.

7.6.3. Gram-Positive Cocci

The Sentry Antimicrobial Surveillance Programme in North America in 1997 reported on the prevalence of clinical isolates resistant to antibacterials, including tetracycline, among pathogens involved in skin and skin structure infections (Table 9).

Table 9 Prevalence of gram-positive cocci resistant to tetracycline in North America in 1997

Microorganism(s)[a]	*n*	MIC (μg/ml)		% Resistance
		50%	90%	
MRSA	89	>8	>8	75.3
MSSA	315	≤4	>8	15.9
MRCoNS	20	≤4	>8	30
MSCoNS	26	≤4	>8	11.5
Enterococcus spp.	53	>8	>8	60.3
Beta-hemolytic streptococci	39	≤2	16	47.8

[a]MRSA, methicillin-resistant *S. aureus*; MSSA, methicillin-susceptible *S. aureus*; MRCoNS, methicillin-resistant coagulase-negative staphylococci; MSCoNS, methicillin-susceptible coagulase-negative staphylococci.

7.6.4. UTI

The antibacterial activity of tetracycline is frequently assessed in urinary tract infections (UTI). In two studies conducted in Latin America in 1998 and North America in 1997, it was shown that tetracycline is weakly active against *P. aeruginosa* and *P. mirabilis* (Table 10).

In Lebanon in 1997, tetracycline resistance was assessed among gram-negative bacteria. The following species were fully resistant to tetracycline: *Proteus* spp., *M. morganii*, and *Serratia* spp. For *E. coli*, and *Klebsiella* spp., the prevalence ranged between 60.9 and 66.5%. Fifty percent and 80% of *Citrobacter* and *Enterobacter* spp. were resistant to tetracycline, respectively.

7.6.5. *Salmonella* spp.

A survey was conducted in Poland from 1998 to 1999 on the pattern of *Salmonella* resistance to tetracyclines. All *Salmonella* isolates were weakly susceptible to tetracycline, with differences among serovars (78 to 100% resistance).

7.6.6. *Chlamydia*

A number of *Chlamydia trachomatis*-like isolates, such as *Chlamydia suis*, *Chlamydia percorum*, and *Chlamydophila abortus*, have been isolated from cases of porcine pneumonia.

Recently, numerous *C. sus scofa* isolates resistant to tetracycline (MIC, >4 μg/ml) have been recovered from swine.

7.6.7. *Campylobacter* spp.

From 1997 to 1998, about 40 and 100% of *Campylobacter jejuni* isolates from broilers and other foods respectively, were resistant to tetracyclines. From pigs and food, 97 and 91% of *Campylobacter coli* isolates were resistant to tetracyclines.

Table 10 Prevalence of tetracycline resistance in UTI

Organism(s)	Year	*n*	% Resistance
E. coli	1998	262	56.5
	1997	643	28
K. pneumoniae	1998	48	36.2
	1998	156	17.9
P. aeruginosa	1997	36	97.2
	1998	76	96.1
P. mirabilis	1998	20	95
Enterobacter spp.	1998	14	57.1
	1997	52	13.5
Enterococcus spp.	1997	165	50.3

7.6.8. N. gonorrhoeae

It is well known that tetracyclines are less efficient against gonococci. For instance, in a survey in Argentina from 1985 to 1999, about 82 to 95% of the isolates were resistant to tetracyclines.

8. PHARMACOKINETICS

The main pharmacokinetic data are summarized in Table 11. The tetracyclines are well absorbed orally and reach excellent levels in serum, the best molecules being tetracycline, minocycline, and doxycycline. The last also has the advantage of a very long elimination half-life (19 h) and a maximum concentration in serum of 5 to 6 μg/ml, allowing it to be administered once daily (200 mg) after a double loading dose (400 mg). The bioavailability is improved when the antibiotic is taken in the fasted state or at least 1 to 2 h before a meal.

The tetracyclines are eliminated to differing degrees in the urine and stools. Urinary elimination depends on glomerular filtration, with urinary elimination rates of 60% for tetracycline, 35% for minocycline, and 10% for doxycycline. Tetracyclines must not be used in patients suffering from renal insufficiency, except for doxycycline. In fact, doxycycline possesses an extrarenal (gastrointestinal) route of elimination. Once the antibiotic is eliminated by this route, it binds to magnesium or calcium in the intestinal lumen and cannot be absorbed. The tetracyclines cross the fetoplacental barrier and are distributed in the fetus, where, because of their avidity for calcium, they interfere with bone and tooth development. The tetracyclines are also secreted in breast milk, and their use during lactation in the postpartum period should be prohibited.

Hepatic insufficiency does not appear to affect serum cycline levels. However, because of their potential hepatotoxicity, the administration of tetracyclines to patients with hepatic insufficiency is not recommended.

9. TISSUE DISTRIBUTION

The majority of antibacterial agents rarely attain sufficient intracellular concentrations to treat bacterial intracellular infections effectively. The tetracyclines accumulate in phagocytic cells.

After oral administration, the tetracyclines follow an enterohepatic cycle, with hepatic concentrations 5 to 10 times higher than the levels reached in serum. They can be detected in small quantities in the lung, spleen, brain, and saliva. In the case of tetracycline, the concentrations in the cerebrospinal fluid are approximately 90 to 70% lower than the levels in serum, whereas in the synovial fluid and mucous membrane of the maxillary sinuses the concentrations are equal to those in serum. Minocycline is the most lipophilic of the tetracyclines at physiological pH, followed by doxycycline, which explains their great capacity for diffusion in cerebral tissue, the eyes, and the prostate. Minocycline can penetrate respiratory secretions, saliva, and tears. The tetracyclines are secreted by the sebaceous glands, enabling them to be used in the treatment of acne.

10. DRUG INTERACTIONS

10.1. Reduced Absorption

Food can cause a reduction in the absorption of tetracyclines. This is particularly evident with tetracycline, chlortetracycline, methacycline, and demeclocycline. All of the tetracyclines (although to a lesser extent in the case of doxycycline) form complexes with divalent or trivalent cations, complexes which are not absorbable. Thus, their absorption is markedly reduced when they are administered simultaneously with calcium, magnesium, and aluminum found in antacid agents, milk, iron, or syrups containing iron. Sodium bicarbonate also reduces their absorption. Cimetidine has also been reported to reduce the absorption of tetracycline.

10.2. Hepatic Metabolism

The antiepileptic agents, particularly carbamazepine, phenytoin, and barbiturates, reduce the apparent elimination half-life of doxycycline by almost 50% while increasing its hepatic metabolism. Chronic ingestion of alcohol has also been reported to cause a reduction in the elimination half-life of doxycycline (but not that of tetracycline), probably through the induction of hepatic microsomal enzymes.

10.3. Increased Nephrotoxicity

The administration of anesthetics such as methoxyfluranes with tetracyclines can cause nephrotoxicity. It would appear that this interaction also occurs with fluorinated anesthetic agents, which in principle are less nephrotoxic. Administration of diuretic substances with tetracyclines causes an increase in serum urea levels by a mechanism that remains to be elucidated.

10.4. Interaction with Other Antibiotics

The administration of bacteriostatic agents such as tetracyclines in combination with bactericidal agents can cause antagonism. This subject, however, remains a matter of dispute.

10.5. Interaction with Contraceptives

There have been reports of women treated with tetracyclines and receiving oral contraception who have become pregnant. Reduction of bacterial hydrolysis of conjugated estrogen in the intestine may be the origin of this.

Table 11 Pharmacokinetic parameters of tetracyclines

Tetracycline	Dose (mg)	Oral absorption (%)	T_{max} (h)	C_{max} (μg/ml)	$t_{1/2}$ (h)	Protein binding (%)	Urinary elimination (%)
Oxytetracycline	500	58	2.2	1.4	9	35	70
Tetracycline	500	80	3.6	1.4	8	65	60
Chlortetracycline	500	28		5.5	6	47	18
Demeclocycline	300	66	4.0	1.8	12	91	40
Methacycline	300	60	4.0	2.5	14	90	60
Minocycline	200	95	2.6	2.6	15	76	10
Doxycycline	200	93	2.6	5.2	19	93	38

11. SAFETY

11.1. Hypersensitivity

Hypersensitivity reactions to tetracyclines are rare but may include anaphylactic shock, urticaria, periorbicular edema, rashes, and morbilliform rashes. When a patient is allergic to a given cycline, he or she must be considered allergic to all tetracyclines.

11.2. Photosensitivity

Photosensitivity reactions consist of a reddish rash on regions of skin exposed to sunlight, commonly accompanied by onycholysis. They are more common with demeclocycline but have been described with all tetracyclines. This reaction is currently considered a toxic reaction due to the accumulation of antibiotic in the skin, rather than an allergic type of reaction.

11.3. Hyperpigmentation

There have been reports of increased pigmentation of the skin and nails and asymptomatic pigmentation of the thyroid gland following prolonged administration of minocycline.

11.4. Effect on Bones and Teeth

Discoloration of the teeth ranging from greyish-brown to yellow has been reported for 80% of children treated with tetracyclines in certain populations. This effect is permanent and may be associated with hypoplasia of the dental enamel and a reduction of skeletal growth in premature infants. The discoloration effect due to the tetracyclines is strictly related to the dose of antibiotic administered. The effects on teeth, and to a lesser extent on bone growth, may last for up to 8 years after administration of the antibiotic. This is why some authors do not recommend the use of tetracyclines in children before the age of 12 years. Exceptions to this rule might be represented by children suffering from Rocky Mountain spotted fever who tolerate oral medication. Nevertheless, therapy with more than a single dose must be avoided at all costs in view of the dental and bone problems. Of all the tetracyclines, doxycycline appears to be the least often responsible for dental problems in children because of its reduced capacity for chelating calcium.

11.5. Gastrointestinal Effects

The tetracyclines are irritant substances and frequently cause disorders during oral administration. Esophageal ulcerations have been reported, particularly for patients taking their medication with little or no fluid. Administration of food does not affect the absorption of minocycline, doxycycline, or oxytetracycline, but the other tetracyclines are much less well absorbed under these conditions. Because of the modification of the intestinal flora, diarrhea is a complication commonly associated with the administration of poorly absorbed tetracyclines.

11.6. Oral and Genital Mucosae

Overgrowth of *Candida* spp. may be a problem. Glossitis probably represents a hypersensitivity reaction.

11.7. Hepatic Function

The hepatotoxicity of the tetracyclines, first described with chlortetracycline, is now known for all tetracyclines. It appears on histopathological examination as a microvesicular lipid change and is accompanied by high mortality. These cases are usually observed in pregnant women with renal insufficiency receiving more than 2 g of tetracycline daily.

11.8. Renal Function

The administration of tetracyclines exacerbates preexisting renal insufficiency by inhibiting protein synthesis, giving rise to uremia as a result of the metabolism of amino acids. Demeclocycline may cause renal tubular lesions associated with diabetes insipidus. Demeclocycline has been used in patients with chronic inappropriate secretion of antidiuretic hormone in order to correct this defect. This approach may produce a state of renal insufficiency in cirrhotic patients. Administration of expired tetracycline may cause reversible Fanconi-like syndromes with renal tubular acidosis as a result of the degradation of tetracycline to its *epi*-anhydro form. Fortunately, nowadays the formulations have been modified to avoid this problem.

11.9. Teratogenic Effect

With the exception of two isolated cases of skeletal malformation (of different kinds) reported for humans receiving treatment with tetracyclines during pregnancy, it would appear that the tetracyclines do not have a proven teratogenic risk. The results of experimental studies in animals are contradictory with respect to the teratogenicity of tetracyclines: some authors have reported inhibited growth and skeletal deformities in the rat and chicken, whereas according to other authors this risk is nonexistent. Several authors have reported yellow or brown discoloration of the milk teeth in children born to mothers treated with tetracyclines (tetracycline and oxytetracycline) during the second and particularly the third trimesters of pregnancy.

11.10. Nervous and Sensory Systems

Minocycline is the only cycline that causes dizziness, tinnitus, and ataxia at therapeutic doses. These effects generally occur on the second and third days of treatment and are more commonly observed in women than men. These side effects resolve a few days after the discontinuation of treatment. The majority of tetracyclines can cause a cerebral pseudotumor syndrome, characterized by a benign increase in intracranial pressure in children and adults.

11.11. Hemorrhagic Syndrome

A hemorrhagic diathesis may develop with the use of tetracyclines as a result of interference with endogenous vitamin K production.

11.12. Superinfection

Intestinal colonization by cycline-resistant microorganisms is commonly observed following treatment with tetracyclines, but in general these episodes are not clinically significant. More rarely, fulminant diarrhea can be observed as a result of staphylococcal enteritis. Conversely, oral or vaginal candidiasis may complicate therapy with tetracyclines and often requires specific treatment.

12. CLINICAL INDICATIONS

Tetracyclines are the drugs of choice for a number of infections, particularly for several sexually transmitted diseases, and for the treatment of acute pelvic inflammatory syndromes. Their use should be avoided in children (under the age of 12 years), pregnant women, and people suffering from liver or kidney disease (with the exception of doxycycline). Unless indicated otherwise, the drug of choice is tetracycline hydrochloride orally. Doxycycline is the preferred molecule when intravenous administration is necessary. Because of its very favorable pharmacokinetics, doxycycline is tending to become the most widely prescribed cycline in outpatient medicine.

12.1. Treatment of Choice

The tetracyclines are currently considered the drugs of choice in the early stages of Lyme disease (*Borrelia burgdorferi*) with a predominance of cutaneous manifestations (erythema chronicum migrans), while penicillin is preferred for cases of refractory arthritis and in meningeal involvement. Tetracycline is used in the treatment of relapsing fever (*Borrelia recurrentis*). Doxycycline is effective in the prophylaxis and treatment of leptospirosis. The tetracyclines are used in the treatment of several sexually transmitted diseases (urethritis, rectitis, epididymitis, cervicitis, endometritis, adnexitis, perihepatitis, and venereal lymphogranuloma) and conjunctivitis associated with *C. trachomatis*. The tetracyclines are the drugs of choice for infections due to *C. psittaci* (ornithosis), *Vibrio cholerae* (cholera), *Vibrio vulnificus*, *M. marinum* (minocycline only), and *Mycoplasma pneumoniae* (macrolides can also be used). Combined with chloramphenicol, tetracyclines are used for the treatment of severe forms of melioidosis (*B. pseudomallei*). They are combined with streptomycin and rifampin for the treatment of severe forms of brucellosis and with streptomycin for the treatment of *Yersinia pestis* infections. Doxycycline in combination with amikacin is used for the treatment of *Mycobacterium fortuitum* and *Mycobacterium chelonae* infections. Tetracyclines are used in cases of nonspecific urethritis and urethral syndrome. Following a large number of cases of infertility observed in patients treated inadequately for acute pelvic inflammatory disease, current treatment involves the administration of tetracyclines combined with other antibiotics. Rickettsial infections are treated with tetracyclines, with chloramphenicol generally being used in severe forms: Rocky Mountain spotted fever (*Rickettsia rickettsii*), different types of typhus (*Rickettsia mooseri*, *Rickettsia prowazekii*, and *Rickettsia tsutsugamushi*), boutonneuse fever (*Rickettsia conorii*), Q fever, and ehrlichiosis.

12.2. Effective Therapy

Tetracyclines are considered as alternative therapy in infections due to *Campylobacter fetus* and *C. jejuni*, *Pasteurella multocida*, *Burkholderia mallei*, *Yersinia enterocolitica*, *Treponema pallidum*, *P. acnes* (acne), *Francisella tularensis* (tularemia), and *Spirillum minus* and *Streptobacillus moniliformis* (rat-bite fever). Tetracyclines are also considered as possible therapy in chronic bronchitis (acute episodes), infections due to *N. gonorrhoeae* (particularly when an infection associated with *C. trachomatis* is not excluded but resistance is a problem), actinomycoses, yaws (oropharyngeal), necrotizing ulcerative gingivitis, Whipple's disease, anthrax, and certain types of prostatitis.

12.3. Alternative and Effective Prophylaxis

Doxycycline alone and tetracycline combined with neomycin have been used as alternative and effective prophylaxis for preoperative preparation in colonic surgery, although better antianaerobic agents are now available. Minocycline is used for the prophylaxis of meningococcal meningitis, but rifampin remains the first choice. Doxycycline has been used for the prophylaxis of traveler's diarrhea, but co-trimoxazole is now preferred.

The usual dosages (for adults) of tetracyclines are as follows: oxytetracycline, orally, 500 mg four times a day; tetracycline hydrochloride, orally, 250 to 500 mg four times a day; methacycline, orally, 300 mg twice a day; demeclocycline hydrochloride, orally, 300 mg twice a day; doxycycline (calcium or monohydrate), 200 mg (or 100 mg/12 h) once on the first day and then 100 mg/day (in sexually transmitted diseases, 100 mg/12 h); and minocycline, orally, 200 mg once on the first day and then 100 mg/12 h.

ADDITIONAL BIBLIOGRAPHY

Duggar BM, 1948, Aureomycin, a product of the continuing search for new antibiotics, Ann N Y Acad Sci, 51, 177–181.

Fourtillan JB, Lefebvre MA, 1980, Correlations structure-activité dans la famille des tetracyclines, Nouv Presse Med, 9, 64–70.

Hlavka JJ, Boothe JH, ed, 1985, The tetracyclines, Springer-Verlag, Berlin, Handb Exp Pharmacol, 78, 1–451.

Igarashi K, Kaji A, 1970, Relationship between sites 1,2 and acceptor donor sites for the binding of aminoacyl tRNA to ribosomes, Eur J Biochem, 14, 41–46.

Neu HC, 1978, A symposium on tetracyclines, a major appraisal: introduction, Bull N Y Acad Med, 54, 141–155.

Oliva B, Gordon G, McNicholas P, Ellestad G, Chopra I, 1992, Evidence that tetracycline analogs whose primary target is not the bacterial ribosome cause lysis of *Escherichia coli*, Antimicrob Agents Chemother, 36, 913–919.

Rasmussen B, Noller HF, Daubresse G, Oliva B, Misulovin Z, Rothstein DM, Ellestad GA, Gluzman Y, Tally FP, Chopra I, 1991, Molecular basis of tetracycline action: identification of analogs whose primary target is not the bacterial ribosome, Antimicrob Agents Chemother, 35, 2306–2311.

Siegel D, 1978, Tetracyclines, new look at old antibiotic. I. Clinical pharmacology, mechanism of action, and untoward effects, N Y State J Med, 78, 950–956.

Siegel D, 1978, Tetracyclines, new look at old antibiotic. II. Clinical use, N Y State J Med, 78, 1115–1120.

Tetracyclines Under Investigation

A. BRYSKIER

25

1. INTRODUCTION

The tetracyclines are antibacterial agents whose biological spectrum covers gram-positive and -negative bacteria, intracellular bacteria, mycoplasmas, and protozoa such as *Plasmodium falciparum* (Gialdroni-Grassi, 1993). Since the discovery of chlortetracycline in 1945 (Duggar, 1948), the tetracyclines have been used for almost 60 years as anti-infective agents, but also as food additives and in veterinary medicine. The price of the success of this therapeutic class has been the emergence of cycline-resistant strains, which has resulted in the progressive reduction of their use. Research in the past few years has enabled semisynthetic derivatives to be prepared or isolated from fermentation products of molecules active against cycline-resistant bacterial strains.

2. CLASSIFICATION OF CYCLINES

The tetracycline structure comprises the perhydronaphthacene core and various substituents attached to this skeleton at positions 5, 6, and 7 (Fig. 1) (Blackwood and English, 1970). They differ in their physicochemical properties and their pharmacokinetics. However, their antibacterial spectra are identical and they exhibit cross-resistance, with the exception of minocycline. Tetracycline analogs have been synthesized, such as chelocardin (cetocycline or cetotrin), which is bactericidal. The cyclines may be divided into two groups (Fig. 2): the bacteriostatic molecules, which act on the ribosome only, and the bactericidal molecules, which act on the cytoplasmic membrane (Chopra et al., 1992) (Table 1).

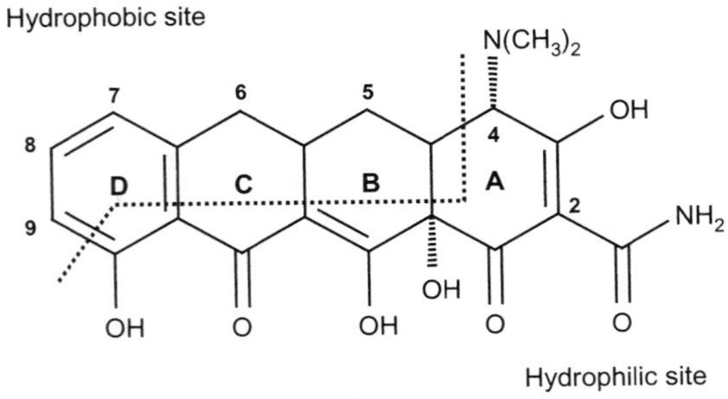

Figure 1 Structure of tetracyclines

2.1. Group 1

The group 1 cyclines are bacteriostatic and inhibit protein synthesis in the ribosome. They interact at the codon-anticodon level (between tRNA and mRNA) by preventing acyl-tRNA from binding to the A-site of the 30S fraction of the ribosome, but the molecular mechanism is poorly elucidated. Binding to the 30S ribosome is reversible, which explains the bacteriostatic activity of these molecules. The S3, S7, and S19 ribosomal proteins are present at the binding site. Tetracycline appears to bind directly to the S7 protein and to the region of 16S RNA from bases 892 to 1054. The hydroxyl group of tetracycline binds to the A892 base.

2.2. Group 2

The cyclines of group 2 do not act directly on protein synthesis (Chopra, 1994; Rasmussen et al., 1991). Their activity appears to be related to the substitution at C-4 by substituents in a β configuration. They may, however, bind to 16S rRNA, although their affinity is insufficient to induce inhibition of protein synthesis. They act on the cytoplasmic membrane. At physiological pH, the tetracyclines exist as a mixture of two forms (Rogalski, 1985): (i) a low-energy, nonionized, lipophilic form and (ii) a high-energy zwitterionic form (Hughes et al., 1979). The nonionized form allows transmembrane penetration, and the zwitterionic form allows ribosomal binding.

3. TETRACYCLINE RESISTANCE MECHANISMS

Resistance to the action of tetracyclines is due principally to the acquisition of the Tet determinant and not to a chromosomally mediated mutation. The mechanisms of resistance of *Neisseria gonorrhoeae* are an exception. Resistance is based on a sequence of genetic modifications in the chromosome: *tet*, *mpr*, and *penB*. In *Escherichia coli*, a combination of mutations at the *mar* locus has been demonstrated.

The resistance mechanisms were first studied for gram-negative bacilli. Sixteen determinants of resistance to tetracycline (Tet) and three to oxytetracycline (Otr) have been described. Among the 16 determinants, 13 are associated with plasmids or transposons and are involved in the efflux resistance mechanisms and 3 are associated with the chromosome and play a role in the mechanisms of ribosomal modification (Tables 2 and 3) (Roberts, 1994).

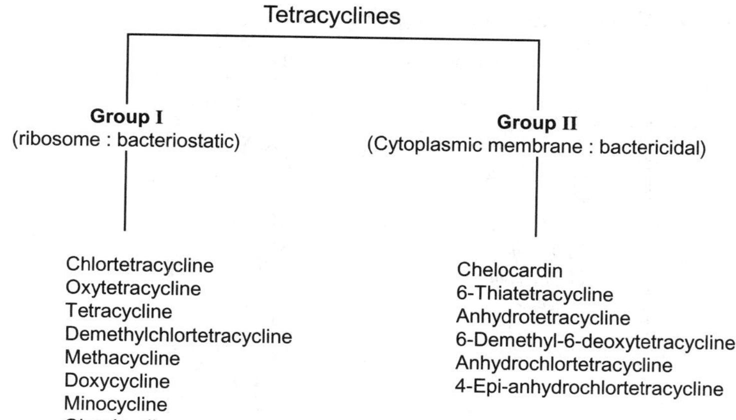

Figure 2 Tetracycline classification

Table 1 Comparative activities of cyclines against *E. coli* K-12[a]

Compound	MIC (μg/ml)	Activity		
		Bacteriostatic	Bactericidal	Ribosome
Tetracycline	0.25	+		+
Chlortetracycline	1.0	+		+
Minocycline	0.25	+		+
Doxycycline	1.0	+		+
Anhydrochlortetracycline	2.0		+	–
6-Thiatetracycline	8.0		+	–
Chelocardin	0.5		+	–
4-*epi*-Anhydrochlortetracycline	0.25		+	–
Glycylcyclines	8.0		+	+

[a]Data from Chopra et al., 1992.

Table 2 Localization of Tet determinants[a]

Plasmid	Chromosome
Tet A–E	Tet B (rare)
Tet X	
Tet G, H	
Tet K	Tet K
Tet L	Tet L (rare)
Tet M (rare)	Tet M
Tet O	Tet O
Tet P	
	Tet Q
Tet S	
	OtrA–OtrC

[a]Data from Roberts, 1994.

Table 3 Resistance mechanisms and determinants

Efflux	Ribosome	Enzymatic	Unknown
A–E	M	X	OtrC
G, H	O		
K	S		
L	Q		
A(P)	B(P)		
OtrB	OtrA		

In outline, three resistance mechanisms may be described:

- An energy-dependent efflux pump based on proteins introduced into the cytoplasmic membrane (Levy, 1992)
- Alterations of the ribosomal target
- Enyzmatic modifications and inactivation of tetracycline

3.1. Efflux

Various gram-negative (Table 4) and gram-positive (Table 5) bacilli have Tet determinants, conferring resistance to tetracyclines by an energy-dependent efflux system. This resistance is mediated by a 37-kDa protein consisting of 12 hydrophobic membrane regions, separated from one another by hydrophilic regions. This efflux system with a protein support allows one proton to be exchanged for a tetracycline-cation complex (Fig. 3) and acts as an antiport system (Yamaguchi et al., 1991). The tetracyclines are exported by the antiport system (of the metal-tetracycline/H^+ type) in the form of a chelation complex with divalent cations such as Mg^{2+}, Mn^{2+}, and Ca^{2+} (Fig. 3 and 4).

The tetracycline molecule penetrates the bacterial cell in the neutral TH^2 form and then dissociates into H^+ and TH^-. TH^- binds to Mg^{2+} and forms a TH-Mg^{2+} complex that is unable to cross the inner membrane spontaneously. Tetracycline accumulates in the cytoplasm of the bacterial cell through a ΔpH due to the high Mg^{2+} ion concentration. The presence of the TetA protein allows the TH-Mg^{2+} complex to be exported as a substrate in a ratio of 1:1 with a proton (antiport system) (Fig. 5).

Table 4 Distribution of Tet resistance determinants among gram-negative bacilli[a]

Efflux		Ribosomal and/or efflux	
Microorganism	Tet determinant(s)	Microorganism	Tet determinant(s)
Actinobacillus	B	*Bacteroides*	MQX
Aeromonas	ABDE	*Campylobacter*	O
Citrobacter	ABCD	*Eikenella*	M
Edwardsiella	AD	*Fusobacterium*	M
Enterobacter	BCD	*Veillonella*	M
Escherichia	ABCDE	*Haemophilus*	BM
Klebsiella	AD	*Kingella*	M
Moraxella	B	*Neisseria*	M
Pasteurella	BDH	*Prevotella*	Q
Pleisiomonas	ABD		
Proteus	ABC		
Pseudomonas	AC		
Salmonella	ABCDE		
Serratia	ABC		
Shigella	ABCD		
Yersinia	B		
Vibrio	ABCDEG		

[a]Data from Roberts, 1994.

Table 5 Tet determinants of gram-positive bacilli[a]

Microorganism	Tet determinant(s)
Actinomyces	L
Streptomyces	KL, OtrA–OtrC
Bacillus	KL
Lactobacillus	O
Corynebacterium	M
Listeria	KLMS
Gardnerella	M
Eubacterium	KM
Mobiluncus	O
Peptostreptococcus	KLMO
Clostridium	KLMP
Mycobacterium	KL, OtrA, OtrB
Mycoplasma	M
Ureaplasma	M
Gemella	KLMO
Staphylococcus	KLMO
Enterococcus	KLMO
Aerococcus	MO

[a]Data from Roberts, 1994

Resistance involving an efflux system is usually inducible. TetA to -E and Tet-G and H contain structural and repressor genes that allow the expression of this transport system. The *tet*(A) and *tet*(R) gene repressor and the TetA export molecule recognize the tetracyclines in the form of the chelation complex. The efflux proteins possess sequences of amino acids similar to those of other efflux systems involved in multiresistance to quaternary ammoniums, chloramphenicol, and fluoroquinolones (Nikaido, 1994). In gram-positive bacteria, the *tet*(K) and *tet*(L) genes produce proteins that are regulated by an mRNA, such as those described for the *erm* genes, which code for an rRNA methylase, and the *cat* genes, which code for a chloramphenicol acetyltransferase. The Tet P determinants of *Clostridium* correspond to two genes: *tetA*(P), which produces an efflux protein, and *tetB*(P), which codes for a modified ribosomal protein.

3.2. Ribosome

The proteins responsible for resistance to tetracycline through a modification of the ribosomal target are Tet(M), Tet(O), Tet(S), Tet(B)(P), Tet(Q), and Otr(A). They are a 72.5-kDa cytoplasmic protein. They possess an amino acid sequence similar to that of elongation factor Tu (EF-Tu) and EF-G.

Tet(M) and Tet(O) are 70% homologous in terms of their amino acid sequence, and likewise Otr(A), Tet(B)(P), and Tet(Q) are 45% homologous and form a third group.

They appear to prevent the binding of tetracyclines to the ribosomes. Tet(M) exhibits GDPase activity. Expression of these genes requires a modification of tRNA.

3.3. Modification of Tetracycline

The only example of enzymatic inactivation has been demonstrated in *Bacteroides fragilis* with the presence of a *tet*(X) determinant. The enzyme requires oxygen to be expressed (Speer and Salyers, 1988).

4. STRUCTURAL MODIFICATIONS OF TETRACYCLINES

It has been shown that structural modifications in the hydrophobic zone of the molecule (Fig. 1) may cause an increase in antibacterial activity, whereas modifications in the hydrophilic zone cause a reduction in activity. Certain derivatives in which the D nucleus has been modified have antibacterial activity.

5. BACTERICIDAL CYCLINES

The group 2 cyclines, the principal molecules of which are chelocardin (Oliver et al., 1963) and 6-thiatetracycline (Fig. 6), are bactericidal by acting on the bacterial cytoplasmic membrane (Chopra et al., 1992).

Replacement of the carbon atom at position 6 of the C ring by a sulfur atom or an oxygen atom yields the heterotetracyclines. This modification is the origin of molecules

Figure 3 Tetracycline interaction with magnesium ion

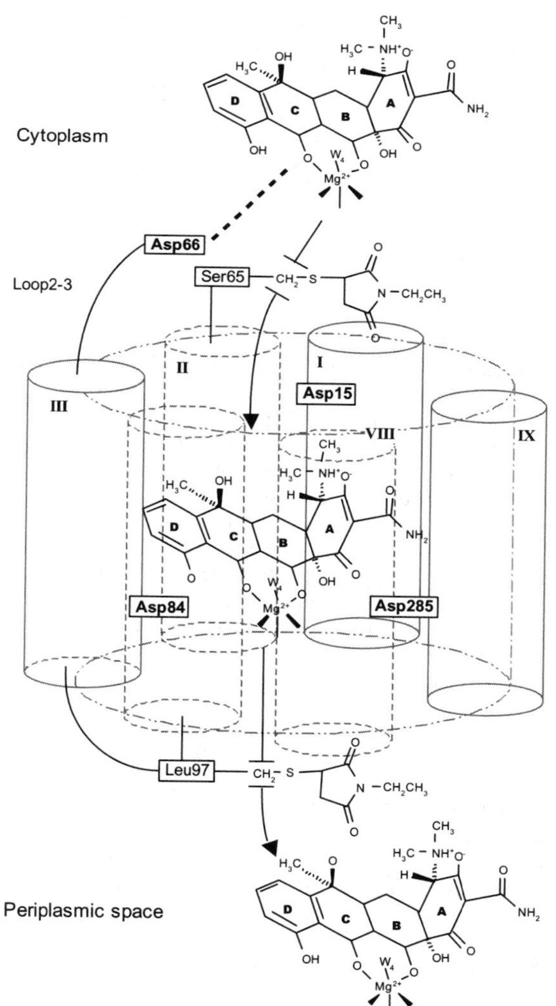

Figure 4 Translocation of tetracycline-Mg complex

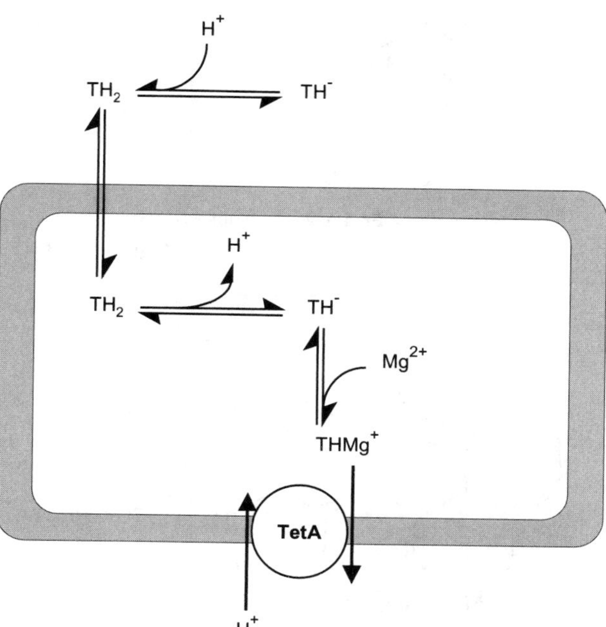

Figure 5 Tetracycline transport systems: tetracycline-Mg^{2+} complex

that are active against tetracycline-resistant bacterial strains. Thiatetracyclines have undergone preliminary development, but this was stopped due to neurologic toxicity. Among the thiatetracyclines, three molecules have been partially developed, including thiacycline, or EMD-33330 (Fig. 7). Thiacycline is active against strains of *E. coli* carrying plasmids for resistance to tetracycline (Russell and Ahon-Khai, 1982). Thiacycline is bactericidal against gram-negative bacilli, in contrast to doxycycline. Resistance takes longer to develop with thiacycline than with tetracycline or doxycycline.

6-Demethyl-6-deoxytetracycline

6-Thiatetracycline

Chelocardin A

Anhydrochlortetracycline

4-Epi-anhydrochlortetracycline

Anhydrotetracycline

Figure 6 Bactericidal tetracyclines

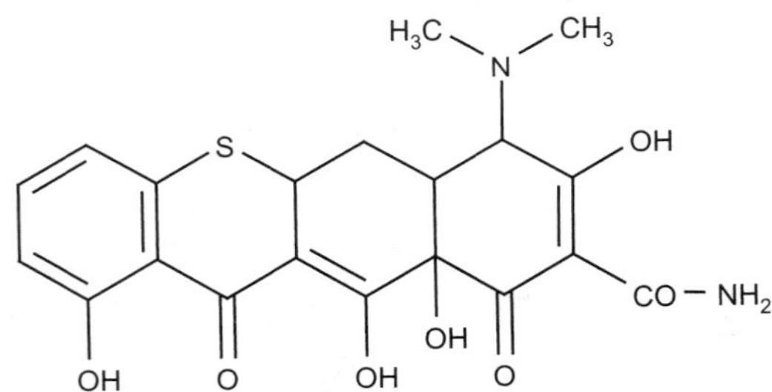

Figure 7 Thiacycline (EMD-33330)

The pharmacokinetics of thiacycline were determined versus those of doxycycline by Dingeldein and Ungethüm (1979) in 17 volunteers. Single doses of 100 and 200 mg of thiacycline and 200 mg of doxycycline were administered orally. The assays were performed by a microbiological method using *Bacillus cereus* ATCC 1178 as the test strain.

The apparent elimination half-life was very long, on the order of 22 h, compared to that of doxycycline, which is 15 h. In contrast to doxycycline, thiacycline is not eliminated renally (~4 versus 41%). After a dose of 200 mg, the peak concentration in serum was 4.18 μg/ml and was reached in 3.3 h (Table 6). Plasma protein binding was greater than 95%. After a single dose of 200 mg of thiacycline, the residual concentrations at 24 and 72 h were, respectively, 2.85 and 0.86 μg/ml.

6. DACTYLOCYCLINES

The dactylocyclines were isolated from *Dactylosporangium* (ATCC 53693) (Wells et al., 1992). Two major and four minor components have been isolated. Dactylocycline A is the dominant product in the fermentation broth. The sugar is identical to that described for evernimicin and viriplanin. It is a pyranose linked by a glycoside bond at position 6 of the C ring (Tymiak et al., 1992; Devasthale et al., 1992) (Fig. 8). The aglycone, dactylocyclinone or Sch-34164 (Fig. 9) (Patel et al., 1987a, 1987b), possesses cross-resistance with the tetracyclines and is active against gram-negative bacteria. The dactylocyclines are active in vitro against tetracycline-resistant and -susceptible bacteria. They are less active against gram-positive bacteria (Tymiak et al., 1993) (Table 7).

7. GLYCYLCYCLINES

7.1. Structural Modifications

Chemical modifications have been made to the D ring. Several series of molecules have been semisynthesized by attachment of different substituents at positions C-7 and C-9 of the D ring of 6-demethyl-6-deoxytetracycline (Sum et al., 1994).

Four types of molecules have thus been synthesized (Fig. 10).

In the first series, the molecules have an amino group at position 9. They are active against strains of *Staphylococcus*

Table 6 Pharmacokinetics of thiacycline[a]

Compound	Dose (mg)	C_{max} (μg/ml)	T_{max} (h)	$AUC_{0-\infty}$ (μg·h/ml)	$t_{1/2}$ (h)	CL_P (liters/h)	CL_R (liters/h)	Urinary elimination (%)
Thiacycline	100	2.5	2.8	87.7	21.9	1.2	0.05	4.2
	200	4.2	3.3	163.4	27.3	1.3	0.04	3.2
Doxycycline	200	3.4	2.0	57.2	15.3	3.6	1.5	41

[a]Data from Dingeldein et al., 1979.

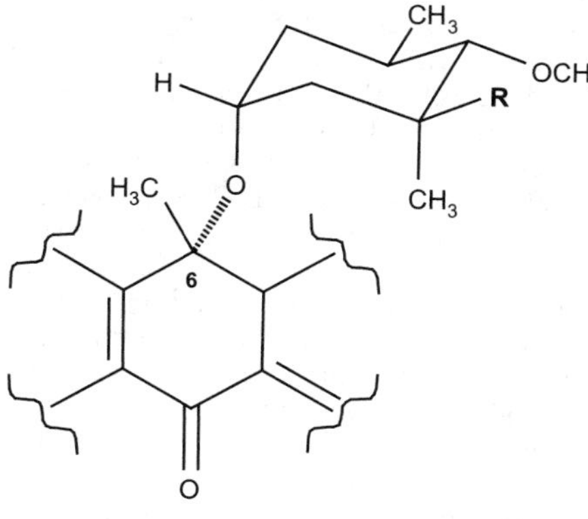

Dactylocycline	R
A	-NHOH
B	$-NO_2$
C	$-NO_2$+O
D	-NHOAc
E	-OH
F	unknown

Figure 8 Dactylocyclines

	R_1	R_2	R_3
Chlortetracycline	-H	-H	-H
Sch 36969	$-OCH_3$	-H	-H
Sch 33256	$-OCH_3$	$-CH_3$	-H
Sch 34164	$-OCH_3$	-H	-OH

Figure 9 8-Methoxychlortetracyclines

aureus with a *tet*(M) (ribosome) and *tet*(K) (efflux) determinant, but they are weakly active against tetracycline-resistant strains of gram-negative bacilli. They are also chemically unstable.

In the second series, the substituent at position 9 is an aminoforamido group. These derivatives are active against strains of *S. aureus* possessing a *tet*(M) determinant but are devoid of activity against gram-negative bacilli.

In the third series, the compounds of the 9-aminoacetamido type are markedly less active than the foramido derivatives.

Table 7 In vitro activities of dactylocyclines

Microorganism	Tetracycline sensitivity[a]	MIC (μg/ml)			
		Tetracycline	Dactylocycline A	Dactylocycline B	Sch-34164
S. aureus	S	0.4	1.6	6.3	6.3
	R	100	6.3	3.1	>100
Staphylococcus epidermidis	S	0.8	6.3	3.1	12.5
	R	50	3.1	3.1	>100
E. faecalis	S	1.6	25	6.3	25
	R	>100	25	6.3	>100
Enterobacter cloacae	S	3.1	>100	>100	100
	R	3.1	>100	>100	>100
E. coli	S	1.6	6.3	25	3.1
	R	>100	>100	>100	>100
K. pneumoniae	S	0.8	100	100	12.5
	R	>100	>100	>100	>100

[a]S, susceptible; R, resistant.

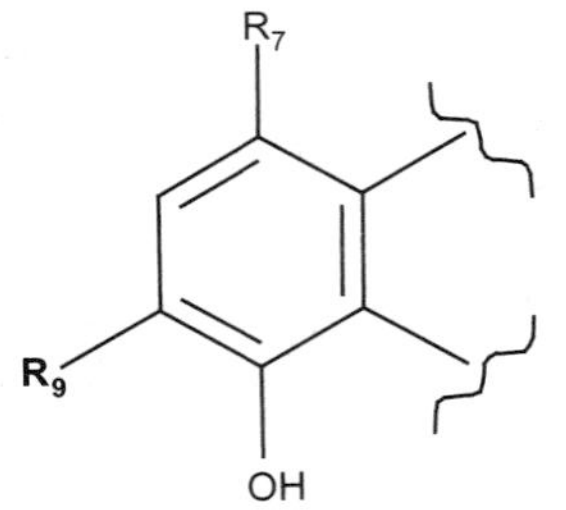

	R_9
9-amino derivatives	$-NH_2$
9-foramido derivatives	-NH-CHO
9-acetamido derivatives	$-NH-CO-CH_3$
9-N-glycine derivatives	$-NH-CO-CH_2N(CH_3)_2$

Figure 10 Cyclines: 9-substituted derivatives

In the fourth series, the amino group has been substituted by a glycyl and another basic group, a dimethylamino. These derivatives have antibacterial activity different from that of tetracycline or minocycline. They are active against gram-positive tetracycline- or minocycline-resistant strains. They are active against *E. coli* and *S. aureus* strains with the *tet*(M) determinant (ribosome) and against *E. coli tet*(A), -(B), -(C), and -(D) (efflux). They are active against methicillin-resistant strains of *S. aureus* and against certain vancomycin-resistant strains of enterococci.

7.2. Resistance Mechanisms

The good activity of glycylcyclines against strains resistant to tetracycline via an efflux mechanism is not due to their inability to induce resistance. The glycyl group prevents the binding of glycylcycline to the *tet*A protein, preventing its membrane translocation (Someya et al., 1995). CL-331928 inhibits the binding of acyl-tRNA to the A-site of the ribosome more markedly than tetracycline or minocycline (Yamamoto et al., 1994; Ishii et al., 1994).

7.3. Antibacterial Activity

Compared to minocycline, the two derivatives DMG-minocycline and CL-331928 are less active against gram-positive cocci, except for *Enterococcus faecalis* and *Streptococcus agalactiae*, against which the two compounds are inactive. The most active molecule is minocycline (Table 8) (Testa et al., 1993; Goldstein et al., 1994; Eliopoulos et al., 1994). Against penicillin G-susceptible strains of *Streptococcus pneumoniae*, CL-331928 is more active than minocycline. Conversely, minocycline is inactive in vitro (MIC at which 50% of isolates tested are inhibited [MIC_{50}], ~4 μg/ml) and in vivo (50% effective dose [ED_{50}], ~40 mg/kg of body weight) against strains of penicillin G-resistant *S. pneumoniae*, whereas CL-331928 is active in vitro (MIC_{50}, ~0.12 μg/ml) and in vivo (ED_{50}, ~0.53 mg/kg) (Petersen et al., 1994a, 1994b). Minocycline is inactive (MIC, ~4 μg/ml) against tetracycline- and methicillin-resistant strains of *S. aureus* [*tet*(M)] and moderately active in vivo (ED_{50}, ~1.6 mg/kg), whereas CL-331928 has good in vitro activity (MIC, ~0.25 μg/ml). CL-331928 has good activity against methicillin- and fluoroquinolone-resistant strains (Kondo and Hiramatsu, 1994). Against strains with *tet*(M) and *tet*(K) determinants and multiresistant to antibiotics, minocycline is inactive in vitro (MIC, ~4 μg/ml) and in vivo (ED_{50}, ~16 mg/kg); CL-331928 has only moderate activity (MIC, ~2 μg/ml; ED_{50}, ~3 mg/kg). In experimental respiratory tract infections with a penicillin G-susceptible strain of *S. pneumoniae*, CL-331928 and minocycline have the same activity as ampicillin. Although the strain of *S. pneumoniae* is penicillin G resistant, CL-331928 is the most active molecule. It produces reductions of 3 $\log_{10}$ CFU/ml compared to the control and 2 $\log_{10}$ CFU/ml compared to minocycline and ampicillin.

Against *Enterobacteriaceae* the glycylcyclines are more active than minocycline, which itself is markedly more active than tetracycline except against *Morganella morganii*. CL-331928 and DMG-minocycline have equivalent activities, except against *Proteus* spp., *M. morganii*, and *Providencia* spp., against which CL-331928 has good activity, in contrast to DMG-minocycline (MIC_{50}, ~2 to 4 μg/ml) (Table 9). They are inactive against *Pseudomonas aeruginosa*. Tetracycline and CL-331928 are inactive against *Stenotrophomonas maltophilia*, in contrast to minocycline and DMG-minocycline, which display good activity, the MIC_{50}s being, respectively, 0.25 and 1 μg/ml. They have moderate activity against *Burkholderia cepacia*. Their activity against

Table 8 In vitro activities of glycylcyclines

Microorganism(s)	MIC_{50} (μg/ml)			
	DMG-minocycline	CL-33928	Minocycline	Tetracycline
S. aureus Met^s	0.25	0.25	0.06	0.25
S. aureus Met^r	0.25	0.25	0.06	0.25
CoNS^s Met^s	0.5	1.0	0.25	1.0
CoNS Met^r	0.25	0.25	0.12	0.5
E. faecalis	0.12	0.12	8.0	32
E. faecium	0.06	0.06	0.03	0.25
Enterococcus Van^r	0.03	0.06	0.03	0.5
S. agalactiae	0.12	0.25	16	32
S. pneumoniae	0.25	0.5	0.25	0.05
S. pyogenes	0.25	0.5	0.25	0.5
Listeria monocytogenes	0.12	0.12	0.01	0.25

[a]CoNS, coagulase-negative staphylococci.

Table 9 In vitro activities of glycylcyclines against *Enterobacteriaceae* and gram-negative bacilli

Microorganism	MIC$_{50}$ (μg/ml)			
	DMG-minocycline	CL-331928	Minocycline	Tetracycline
E. coli	0.25	0.5	0.5	1.0
K. pneumoniae	1.0	1.0	2.0	1.0
Klebsiella oxytoca	0.5	0.5	1.0	0.5
Citrobacter freundii	1.0	1.0	2.0	1.0
Citrobacter diversus	0.5	0.5	0.5	1.0
Serratia marcescens	2.0	2.0	1.0	8.0
E. cloacae	1.0	1.0	2.0	1.0
Enterobacter aerogenes	1.0	0.5	2.0	1.0
Shigella	0.25	0.25	1.0	0.5
Salmonella	0.5	0.5	1.0	1.0
Proteus mirabilis	4.0	0.5	8.0	32
Proteus vulgaris	2.0	0.5	2.0	8.0
Providencia	4.0	2.0	16	64
M. morganii	2.0	1.0	2.0	0.5
P. aeruginosa	16	16	16	32
B. cepacia	4.0	4.0	1.0	4.0
S. maltophillia	1.0	4.0	0.25	8.0
M. catarrhalis	0.06	0.12	0.06	0.25
N. gonorrhoeae	0.5	0.5	0.5	2.0
H. influenzae	0.25	0.5	0.12	0.25

N. gonorrhoeae, *Haemophilus influenzae*, and *Moraxella catarrhalis* is good (Table 9).

Minocycline and tetracycline are inactive against anaerobic gram-negative bacilli; by contrast, the two glycylcycline derivatives have good activity, with MIC$_{50}$s on the order of 0.25 μg/ml (Nord et al., 1993; Watanabe et al., 1994). They all have good activity against anaerobic gram-positive bacteria (Table 10).

The *Mycoplasma pneumoniae* strains are two to four times more susceptible to the glycylcyclines than to tetracycline. They are active against tetracycline-resistant strains of *Ureaplasma urealyticum* carrying the *tet*(M) determinant. This is responsible for the resistance of *Mycoplasma hominis* and *U. urealyticum* to tetracyclines (Table 11) (Kenny and Cartwright, 1994).

Tetracycline is inactive against *E. coli*, *S. aureus*, and *E. faecalis* strains with a *tet* determinant (efflux or ribosome), with MICs of ≥32 μg/ml. The MICs of minocycline are lower and dependent on the nature of the *tet* determinant. The MICs of DGM-minocycline and CL-331928 for *S. aureus* and *E. faecalis* are increased compared to those of a strain without the determinant, but they remain within the range of potential therapeutic activity. The MICs of the two compounds for *E. coli tet*(A) or *tet*(C) are high (MIC, ~2 μg/ml) compared to the control (MIC, ~0.25 μg/ml), but for strains of *E. coli tet*(B), -(D), and -(M), the MICs are identical to those of the control (Table 12).

In vivo, CL-331928 is 2 to 10 times more active than minocycline (Nishino et al., 1994).

7.4. Tigecycline

Tigecycline (GAR-936) is the *t*-butylglycylamido derivative of minocycline (Fig. 11).

7.4.1. In Vitro Activity

The in vitro activity of tigecycline is reported in Table 13. Tigecycline is highly effective against *Chlamydia* spp. (Table 14). It also has good in vitro activity against microorganisms involved in pelvic inflammatory disease, such as *M. hominis*, but it has weaker activity against *U. urealyticum*.

Table 10 In vitro activities of glycylcyclines against anaerobes

Microorganism(s)	MIC$_{50}$ (μg/ml)			
	DMG-minocycline	CL-331928	Minocycline	Tetracycline
B. fragilis	0.25	0.5	4.0	16
B. fragilis group	0.25	0.5	1.0	2.0
Prevotella	0.25	0.5	8.0	32
Clostridium difficile	0.03	0.06	0.03	0.25
Clostridium perfringens	0.12	0.12	0.06	4.0
Clostridium spp.	0.03	0.06	0.01	0.06
Gram-positive cocci	0.06	0.12	4.0	32
Propionibacterium acnes	0.03	0.06	0.12	
Fusobacterium	0.01	0.03	0.03	

Table 11 In vitro activities of glycylcyclines against *Mycoplasma* spp.

Microorganism	MIC_{50} (μg/ml)				
	DMG-minocycline	CL-331928	Minocycline	Tetracycline	Doxycycline
M. pneumoniae	0.5	0.25	0.5	1.0	0.5
M. hominis Tet^s	0.25	0.12	0.12	1.0	0.12
M. hominis Tet^r	0.25	0.25	>64	64	32
U. urealyticum Tet^s	1.0	2.0	0.25	1.0	0.5
U. urealyticum Tet^r	8.0	4.0	32	>64	64

Table 12 In vitro activities of glycylcyclines against tetracycline-resistant bacteria

Microorganism	Determinant	MIC (μg/ml)			
		DMG-minocycline	CL-331928	Minocycline	Tetracycline
E. coli	*tet*(B)	0.25	0.25	16	>64
	tet(A)	2.0	2.0	4.0	32
	tet(C)	2.0	2.0	4.0	64
	tet(D)	0.12	0.25	8.0	>64
	tet(M)	0.25	0.25	64	32
	None	0.25	0.5	0.5	1.0
S. aureus	*tet*(K)	1.0	1.0	0.12	64
	tet(M)	0.25	0.25	8.0	64
	None	0.25	0.12	0.06	0.25
E. faecalis	*tet*(M)	0.25	1.0	16	>64
	None	0.06	0.12	2.0	16

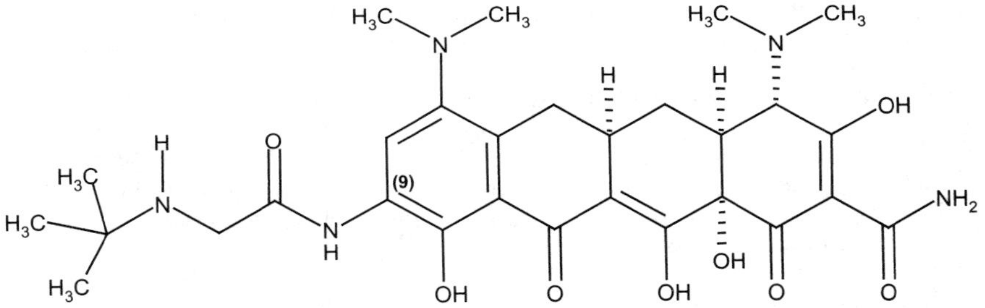

Figure 11 Tigecycline

Tigecycline is active against *M. pneumoniae* (MIC_{90}, 0.25 μg/ml). It is less active than doxycycline against *Bacillus anthracis* (MIC_{50} and MIC_{90}, 0.12 and 0.5 μg/ml, versus 0.06 and 012 μg/ml for doxycycline). It is moderately active against *Legionella pneumophila* (MIC_{50} and MIC_{90}, 4.0 and 8.0 μg/ml).

Tigecycline exhibits similar in vitro activities against *S. pneumoniae* (MICs, 0.06 to 0.5 μg/ml) irrespective of the susceptibility of the isolates to tetracycline. Resistance to tetracycline is common within viridans group streptococci. However, this resistance is not homogeneous among viridans group streptococci; *Streptococcus bovis* is the most resistant, and *Streptococcus salivarius* is the only one for which no resistant strain has been detected. Tigecycline exhibits good in vitro activity against *Streptococcus mitis*, *Streptococcus anginosus*, *Streptococcus sanguinis*, *S. bovis*, and *S. salivarius*, with MICs under 0.25 μg/ml.

Tigecycline remains active against *S. aureus* susceptible or resistant to tetracycline (MICs, 0.25 to 1.0 μg/ml). It displays relatively good in vitro activity against rapidly growing mycobacteria but weak activity against slowly growing mycobacteria (Table 15). For *Nocardia* spp., the MIC_{50} and MIC_{90} were 2.0 and 4.0 μg/ml, respectively.

7.4.2. In Vivo Activity

In a murine infection due to *S. aureus* Smith, the ED_{50}s were 0.6 and 36 mg/kg after intravenous and oral therapy, respectively (minocycline ED_{50}s, 0.52 and 0.53 mg/kg, respectively).

The in vivo efficacies of tigecycline and minocycline against isolates resistant to tetracycline were assessed (Table 16).

7.4.3. Pharmacodynamics

Time above an MIC range of 0.5 to 4.0 μg/ml was a better predictor of the in vivo efficacy than maximum concentration in serum and area under the curve. The level of tigecycline should be maintained at least 50% of the time of the unbound compound to achieve 80% of maximum efficacy.

Table 13 In vitro activity of tigecycline

Microorganism(s)[a]	*n*	MIC (μg/ml)					
		Tigecycline		Minocycline		Tetracycline	
		50%	90%	50%	90%	50%	90%
MRSA Tet^{s}	52	0.25	0.5	0.12	0.25	0.5	2.0
MRSA Tet^{r}	54	0.12	1.0	16	32	>32	>32
cMRSA	32	0.25	0.5	0.12	0.12	0.5	4.0
MRSE	44	≤0.06	1.0	0.5	1.0	2.0	>32
MSSE	10	0.25	0.5	0.25	0.25	0.5	32
E. faecalis	11	0.25	0.5	8.0	8.0	32	32
E. faecium Van^{s}	81	0.06	0.125	0.06	4.0	0.25	32
Enterococci, VanA	42	≤0.06	≤0.06	≤0.06	16	0.5	>32
Enterococci, VanB	20	≤0.06	0.12	0.5	8.0	2.0	>32
Enterococci, VanC	19	≤0.06	≤0.06	≤0.06	16	0.5	>32
S. pneumoniae Pen^{s}	7	≤0.06	0.12	4.0	16	0.25	>32
S. pneumoniae Pen^{r}	47	≤0.06	≤0.06	0.06	16	>32	>32
S. pyogenes	10	0.12	0.25	16	0.12	0.25	0.25
S. agalactiae	10	0.25	0.25	0.06	16	32	32
E. coli (MIC, 1.0 μg/ml)	32	0.5	0.5	8.0	16	>32	>32
E. coli (MIC, 0.5 μg/ml)	14	0.5	0.5	0.5	0.5	1.0	2.0
Shigella spp.	26	0.25	0.5	2.0	4.0	>32	>32
K. pneumoniae	10	1.0	2.0	2.0	4.0	2.0	2.0
K. oxytoca	10	1.0	1.0	2.0	2.0	2.0	2.0
C. freundii	10	1.0	2.0	4.0	4.0	2.0	2.0
C. diversus	10	1.0	1.0	2.0	4.0	2.0	4.0
Salmonella spp.	14	1.0	1.0	2.0	16	2.0	>32
Shigella spp.	188	0.12	0.25	ND[b]	ND	ND	ND
Yersinia enterocolitica	18	0.25	0.25	ND	ND	ND	ND
S. marcescens	10	4.0	4.0	8.0	8.0	32	>32
E. cloacae	10	1.0	2.0	4.0	4.0	4.0	4.0
E. aerogenes	10	1.0	1.0	2.0	2.0	2.0	2.0
Providencia spp.	10	4.0	8.0	16	>32	>32	>32
P. mirabilis	15	4.0	8.0	8.0	16	16	32
P. vulgaris	15	4.0	4.0	2.0	4.0	8.0	32
M. morganii	10	4.0	4.0	4.0	4.0	2.0	2.0
P. aeruginosa	10	16	16	8.0	8.0	16	>32
B. cepacia	10	2.0	4.0	0.5	2.0	2.0	4.0
Acinetobacter baumannii	443	0.5	2.0	≤0.12	2.0	4.0	>32
S. maltophilia	10	2.0	4.0	0.12	0.25	16	16
M. catarrhalis	14	0.12	0.25	0.03	0.06	0.12	0.25
N. gonorrhoeae	22	0.5	1.0	0.5	32	1.0	>32
H. influenzae	15	0.5	1.0	0.12	0.25	0.25	0.5
B. fragilis group	12	0.5	2.0	2.0	4.0		
B. fragilis	14	2.0	2.0	8.0	8.0		
Prevotella spp.	11	0.5	1.0	8.0	16		
C. difficile	10	0.12	0.12	0.03	4.0		
C. perfringens	10	0.5	1.0	≤0.06	4.0		
Campylobacter jejuni	166	≤0.06	0.12	ND	ND	ND	ND
Anaerobic gram positive	15	0.12	0.25	4.0	16		
B. fragilis	272	1.0	8.0	ND	ND	ND	ND
B. thetaiotaomicron	40	1.0	8.0	ND	ND	ND	ND
Bacteroides uniformis	27	2.0	8.0	ND	ND	ND	ND
Bacteroides ovatus	40	2.0	16	ND	ND	ND	ND
Bacteroides caccae	15	4.0	16	ND	ND	ND	ND
Bacteroides vulgatus	16	0.5	8.0	ND	ND	ND	ND

[a]MRSA, methicillin-resistant *S. aureus*; cMRSA, community-acquired MRSA; MRSE, methicillin-resistant *S. epidermidis*; MSSE, methicillin-susceptible *S. epidermidis*.
[b]ND, not determined.

7.4.4. Pharmacokinetics

Ascending doses were administered to eight volunteers in each group and showed a long elimination half-life (Table 17). A single-dose 100-mg infusion (over 1 h) was administered to male and female healthy volunteers; pharmacokinetics are shown in Table 18. The pharmacokinetics are not influenced by age or gender. This compound exhibits a long apparent elimination half-life. After food intake, the area under the curve is moderately altered, as is the concentration at the end of infusion (Table 19).

Table 14 Antichlamydial activity of tigecycline

Organism	Compound	*n*	MIC (μg/ml)	MBC[a] (μg/ml)
Chlamydia trachomatis	Tigecycline	5	0.03–0.125	0.03–0.125
	Doxycycline	5	0.25	0.25
	Ofloxacin	5	0.25–0.5	0.25–0.5
	Clarithromycin	5	0.06	0.06
Chlamydia pneumoniae	Tigecycline	10	0.125–0.25	0.125–0.25
	Doxycycline	10	0.125–0.5	0.125–0.5
	Ofloxacin	10	0.25–0.5	0.25–0.5
	Clarithromycin	10	0.015–0.125	0.15–0.125

[a]MBC, minimum bactericidal concentration.

Table 15 In vitro activity of tigecycline against mycobacteria

Microorganism	*n*	MIC (μg/ml)							
		Tigecycline		Tetracycline		Minocycline		Doxycycline	
		50%	90%	50%	90%	50%	90%	50%	90%
Mycobacterium avium	11	>32	>32	>128	>128	>64	>64	>32	>32
Mycobacterium kansasii	5	32		128		8.0		16	
Mycobacterium xenopi[a]	1	16		128		32		32	
Mycobacterium marinum	5	16		8.0		4.0		16	
Mycobacterium simiae[a]	1	>32		>128		>64		>128	
Mycobacterium fortuitum	10	≤0.06	≤0.12	16	32	32	32	64	128
Mycobacterium abscessus	18	≤0.12	0.25	128	>128	>64	>64	>64	>128
Mycobacterium chelonae	22	≤0.06	≤0.12	32	>128	16	>64	>64	>128

[a]MIC, in micrograms per milliliter.

Table 16 In vivo activity of tigecycline in comparison with minocycline

Microorganism	Gene(s)	Compound	ED_{50} (mg/kg)	MIC (μg/ml)
S. aureus UBMS 90-2	*tet*(U)	Tigecycline	1.0	0.12
		Minocycline	1.8	2.0
S. aureus UBMS 88-7	*tet*(K)	Tigecycline	2.1	0.5
		Minocycline	2.0	0.25
MRSA[a]		Tigecycline	0.79	0.5
		Minocycline	0.31	0.12
	tet(M)	Tigecycline	0.84	0.5
		Minocycline	1.6	4.0
	tet(M) + *tet*(K)	Tigecycline	2.3	1.0
		Minocycline	16	4.0
S. pneumoniae ATCC 6301		Tigecycline	1.3	0.12
		Minocycline	3.9	0.12
S. pneumoniae Pen[r]		Tigecycline	0.61	0.12
		Minocycline	20	4.0
E. coli 311		Tigecycline	1.7	0.5
		Minocycline	3.2	1.0
E. coli	*tet*(A)	Tigecycline	1.6	0.5
		Minocycline	16	4.0
	tet(C)	Tigecycline	1.5	0.25
		Minocycline	14	4.0
	tet(M)	Tigecycline	3.5	0.25
		Minocycline	>32	>32
E. coli minocycline resistant		Tigecycline	1.6	0.5
		Minocycline	32	32
E. coli	*tet*(B)	Tigecycline	3.9	0.5
		Minocycline	>32	32

[a]MRSA, methicillin-resistant *S. aureus*.

Table 17 Pharmacokinetics of tigecycline in healthy volunteers (ascending doses)

Dose (mg)	C_0 (ng/ml)	AUC (ng·h/ml)	$t_{1/2}$ (h)	CL (liters/h/kg)	CL_R (liters/h/kg)
12.5	108.5	753	11	0.29	
25	252	2,255	32	0.20	
50	383	2,558	18	0.28	
75	566	3,658	21	0.29	1.0
100	911	6,396	38	0.20	2.6
200	1,643	12,426	42	0.25	3.0
300 (fed)	2,817	17,856	46	0.25	2.7

Table 18 Pharmacokinetics of tigecycline according to gender

Subjects	*n*	C_{max} (μg/ml)	AUC (μg·h/ml)	CL_P (liters/h/kg)	$t_{1/2}$ (h)
Young males	9	0.9	4.2	0.3	22
Young females	8	1.0	5.1	0.3	17
Elderly males (65–75 yr)	8	0.9	4.3	0.3	19
Elderly females (65–75 yr)	7	1.0	5.1	0.3	16
Elderly males (>75 yr)	8	1.0	5.5	0.3	19
Elderly females (>75 yr)	8	1.1	5.3	0.3	21

Table 19 Pharmacokinetics of tigecycline after food intake

Parameter	*n*	200 mg, fasting	200 mg, fed
C_0 (μg/ml)	8	2.189	1.528
AUC (μg·h/ml)	8	14.462	11.719
$t_{1/2}$ (h)	8	53	54
CL (liters/h/kg)	8	0.20	0.22
CL_R (liters/h/kg)	8	1.8	2.2

Tigecycline is well concentrated in cells with a rapid intake (18.10% ± 3.79% after 0.08 h) (mean ± standard deviation), reaching a plateau at 2.0 h, with a cellular/extracellular ratio of 21.11 ± 5.20. At 2.0 h, 66.53% ± 2.98% is extruded from the cell (efflux).

8. 8-METHOXYCHLORTETRACYCLINE DERIVATIVES

Three 8-methoxychlortetracycline derivatives have been described. They are characterized by the presence of a methoxy group at position 8 of the D ring. These compounds have been isolated from fermentation of *Actinomadura brunea* (Sch-33256) (Patel et al., 1987a), *Dactylosporangium vescum* ATCC 39499 (Sch-34164) (Patel et al., 1987b), and a mutant of *A. brunea* (Sch-36969) (Smith et al., 1987). Structurally (Fig. 9), these molecules differ from one another by the substituent at 2′ or 4a. Sch-34164 is 4a-OH-Sch-36969, and Sch-33256 is 2′-CH_3-Sch-36969.

8.1. Antibacterial Activity

See Cacciapuoti et al., 1987.

Against tetracycline-susceptible strains (MIC, ≤4 μg/ml), Sch-36969 is the most active molecule among the three 8-methoxychlortetracycline derivatives, with a MIC_{GM} (GM is geometric mean) of 4.2 μg/ml, followed by Sch-34164 (MIC_{GM}, ~7.8 μg/ml) and Sch-33256 (MIC_{MG}, ~33 μg/ml). However, they are less active than tetracycline (MIC_{GM}, 2.3 μg/ml) and doxycycline (MIC_{GM}, 3.4 μg/ml) and slightly more active than minocycline (MIC_{GM}, 5.2 μg/ml). They are inactive against tetracycline-resistant strains (MIC, >4 μg/ml) and exhibit cross-resistance.

Against methicillin-susceptible and -resistant *S. aureus* strains the most active molecule is Sch-36969, with MIC_{GM}s of 0.14 and 0.21 μg/ml against methicillin-susceptible and -resistant strains, respectively (Table 20).

Against the streptococci, including *S. pneumoniae* and *E. faecalis*, Sch-36969 has good in vitro activity, with MIC_{GM}s of between 0.04 and 0.12 μg/ml. The least active molecule is minocycline, with MIC_{GM}s of between 1.4 and 2.5 μg/ml. Among the new compounds, Sch-34164 is the least active, particularly against *E. faecalis* (MIC_{GM}, 5.7 μg/ml). Sch-36969 also has good activity against gram-negative and gram-positive anaerobic bacteria, with the exception of *Fusobacterium* spp. (MIC_{GM}, 2.5 μg/ml). The activity is less good against *H. influenzae* (MIC_{GM}, 2.5 μg/ml).

The difference among these three molecules in terms of their in vitro activity is related to the chemical structure. The presence of a methyl group at the N-2′ position of the A ring reduces the activity against gram-negative bacilli (Sch-33256). This fact has already been demonstrated with other tetracycline derivatives (Valcavi, 1981).

Table 20 Antistaphylococcal activities of 8-methoxychlortetracyclines

Compound	MIC (μg/ml)	
	S. aureus Met^s	*S. aureus* Met^r
Sch-36969	0.14	0.21
Sch-33256	0.48	0.86
Sch-34164	2.8	5.4
Tetracycline	0.48	0.79
Doxycycline	0.36	0.43
Minocycline	1.6	12

In vivo in the murine model of infections versus chlortetracycline and tetracycline, Sch-36969 was less efficient against *S. aureus* (50% protective dose [PD_{50}], 0.8 to 10.5 mg/kg) than chlortetracycline (PD_{50}, 0.2 to 7.5 mg/kg). With *E. coli* the PD_{50} was 15 mg/kg, versus 3 mg/kg for chlortetracycline. The values for *Klebsiella pneumoniae* were 225 and 75 mg/kg for Sch-36969 and chlortetracycline, respectively.

8.2. Pharmacokinetics in the Monkey

Two hours after oral administration of 20 mg of Sch-36969 and chlortetracycline per kg, the peak concentrations in serum were, respectively, 0.8 and 3 μg/ml, with areas under the curve of 4.5 and 16.1 mg·h/liter, respectively. These poor pharmacokinetic performances explain the mediocre in vivo activity.

8.3. Other 8-Methoxy Derivatives

Several antitumor tetracycline natural products with weak activity against gram-positive cocci have been reported, such as SF 2575 and TAN 1518 A and B (Fig. 12).

SF 2575 was isolated from a culture of *Streptomyces* sp. strain 2575. This structure contains a salicyloxy group at C′ and a glycoside acylated with an angelic acid at C-9. TAN 1518 was isolated from a culture of *Streptomyces* sp. strain 16012. They exhibit inhibitory activity against DNA topoisomerase I of mammalian cells.

9. PTK 0796 (BAY 73-6944)

PTK 0796 is an aminoethylcycline: 7-dimethylamino,9-(2,2-dimethylpropyl)-aminoethylcycline (Fig. 13). The physicochemical properties of PTK 0796 are the following: molecular weight, 556.65; logP, 0.79 ± 0.750; pK_1, 4.50 ± 1.0; pK_2, 9.74 ± 0.5; and melting point, 224°C. The in vitro activity of PTK 0796 is shown in Table 21.

PTK 0796 exhibits activity against isolates harboring *tet* genes (Table 22). Its in vivo activity is shown in Table 23, and its pharmacokinetics in animals are illustrated in Table 24.

10. OTHER TETRACYCLINES

10.1. Efflux Pump Inhibitor

The 13-(alkylthio)-5-deoxytetracyclines (Fig. 14) are efficient inhibitors of tetracycline efflux in everted vesicles of *E. coli* D1-209. Compound B was shown to have synergistic activity when tested in combination with doxycycline

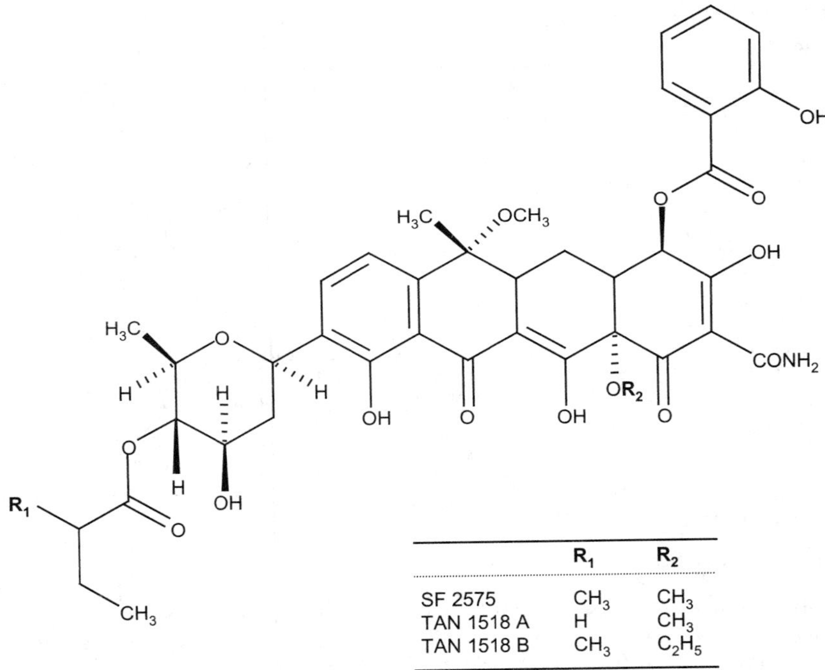

	R_1	R_2
SF 2575	CH_3	CH_3
TAN 1518 A	H	CH_3
TAN 1518 B	CH_3	C_2H_5

Figure 12 8-Methoxytetracyclines

H_3C N CH_3 H H H_3C N CH_3 CH_3 OH CH_3 H_3C N H CH_3 OH OH O OH O O

Figure 13 PTK 0796 (Bay 73-6944)

Table 21 In vitro activity of PTK 0796

Microorganism(s)[a]	n	MIC (μg/ml)							
		PTK 0796		Tetracycline		Minocycline		Doxycycline	
		50%	90%	50%	90%	50%	90%	50%	90%
MSSA	16	0.125	0.215	≤0.06	0.125	≤0.06	0.125	≤0.06	≤0.06
MRSA	39	0.25	0.5	0.25	64	0.25	8.0	0.125	8.0
MRSA, multiresistant	10	0.5	0.5	>64	>64	8.0	8.0	8.0	8.0
E. faecium	14	0.25	0.5	32	64	8.0	16	2.0	8.0
E. faecium Van[r]	19	0.25	0.5	32	64	8.0	16	2.0	4.0
E. faecium, multiresistant	12	0.25	0.5	32	64	8.0	16	2.0	4.0
E. faecalis	31	0.25	0.5	32	64	8.0	16	4.0	16
E. faecalis, multiresistant	3	0.25		32		8.0		4.0	
S. pneumoniae	41	≤0.06	0.125	32	32	2.0	8.0	2.0	4.0
S. pneumoniae Pen[r]	23	≤0.06	≤0.06	32	32	8.0	8.0	4.0	4.0
S. pneumoniae, multiresistant	18	≤0.06	≤0.06	32	32	8.0	8.0	4.0	4.0
S. pyogenes	30	0.125	0.25	64	64	0.25	8.0	≤0.06	64
S. agalactiae	18	0.125	0.125	64	64	16	16	8.0	8.0
E. coli	23	1.0	2.0	>64	64	≤0.06	0.25	1.0	64
K. pneumoniae	14	2.0	4.0	>64	>64	≤0.06	32	2.0	32
H. influenzae	53	1.0	2.0	32	32			0.5	4.0
E. aerogenes	10	2.0	2.0			1.0	2.0		
E. cloacae	10	4.0	4.0			4.0	4.0		
M. morganii	10	32	64			32	32		
P. mirabilis	10	16	16			32	>32		
Providencia rettgeri	5	16				32			
Providencia stuartii	5	16				>32			
P. vulgaris	10	8.0	16			4.0	16		
S. marcescens	10	4.0	4.0			4.0	4.0		
Salmonella spp.	10	2.0	4.0			2.0	4.0		
Shigella spp.	10	0.5	1.0			16	32		
A. baumannii	21	2.0	8.0			1.0	32		
B. cepacia	11	4.0	16			8.0	>32		
P. aeruginosa	10	32	32			16	16		
S. maltophilia	11	4.0	4.0			1.0	2.0		
M. catarrhalis	10	0.25	0.25			0.25	0.25		

[a]MSSA, methicillin-susceptible *S. aureus*; MRSA, methicillin-resistant *S. aureus*.

Table 22 In vitro activity of PTK 0796 against strains resistant to tetracycline

Microorganism	Gene(s)	n	MIC (μg/ml)		
			PTK 0796	Tetracycline	Doxycycline
S. aureus	*tet*M	19	0.125–1.0	32–>64	2.0–16
	*tet*A	5	0.125–0.25	16–32	1.0–4.0
E. faecalis	*tet*M	13	0.125–0.5	32–64	2.0–8.0
	*tet*M or *tet*L	2	0.25	2–>64	8.0–16
	*tet*K	1	0.12	32	4.0
	*tet*O	1	0.12	32	4.0
S. pneumoniae	*tet*M	22	≤0.06	4.0–64	2.0–4.0
S. pyogenes	*tet*M	17	≤0.06–0.5	4.0–64	2.0–16
	*tet*O	4	≤0.06–0.25	32–64	8.0
H. influenzae	*tet*B	20	0.5–2.0	8.0–64	0.5–8.0
	*tet*B and *tet*M	2	1.0–2.0	16	2.0
E. coli	*tet*A	4	2.0	64–>64	16

against *E. coli* resistant to tetracycline harboring the *tet*(A) or *tet*(B) determinant and *S. aureus* bearing the *tet*(K) determinant. Compound A exhibits synergistic activity against *E. coli* harboring the *tet*(A) determinant and additive activity against other tetracycline-resistant organisms.

10.2. Other 9-Substituted Glycyl Deoxytetracyclines

A series of 9-substituted glycyl derivatives has been disclosed, exhibiting in vitro activity against Tet(M) resistant *S. aureus* and *E. coli* or isolates carrying other Tet determinants.

Table 23 In vivo activity of PTK 0796

Microorganism	Compound	MIC (μg/ml)	ED_{50} (mg/kg)
S. aureus ATCC 29213	PTK 0796	0.5	0.4
	Minocycline	0.5	1.0
MRSA strain A5	PTK 0796	0.5	5.9
	Minocycline	2.0	35.2
E. faecalis 29212	PTK 0796	0.5	4.5
	Minocycline	2.0	71.0
E. coli C 189P4	PTK 0796	0.5	4.3
	Minocycline	0.5	4.5

Table 24 Pharmacokinetics of PTK 0796 in animals

Animals	Dose (mg/kg)	C_{max} (μg/ml)	AUC (μg·h/ml)	$t_{1/2}$ (h)	CL_P (ml/h/kg)
Mice (CD-1)	10	2.43	6.23	5.56	1,506
Rats (Sprague-Dawley)	5	0.83	2.97	3.24	1,241
	10	1.71	5.62	3.61	1,343
	20	3.11	12.53	4.25	1,189
	40	3.39	16.07	NC[a]	1,939
Monkeys (cynomolgus)	25	79.73	72.83	11.27	268.4

[a]NC, not calculated.

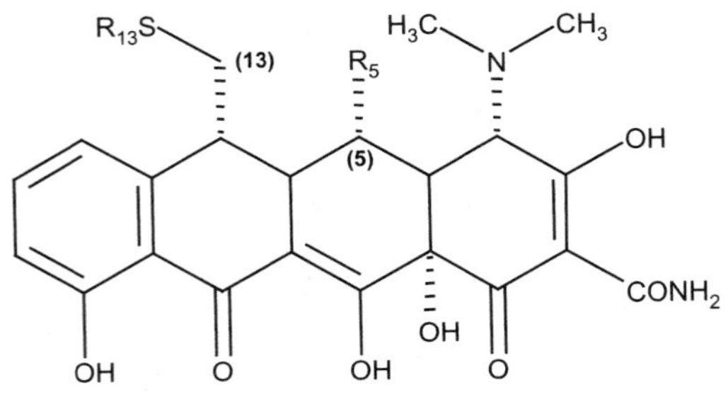

Compound	R_5	R_{13}	IC_{50} (μM)
A	OH	$CH_2S(CH_2)_2Cl$	0.7
B	OH	$CH_2S(CH_2)_3Cl$	0.6
C	H	$CH_2S(CH_2)_3COOH$	43.2
D	H	$CH_2SOC_6H_5$	0.7
E	H	CH_2-cyclopentyl	0.4
F	OH	CH_2-cyclohexyl	0.6
G	OH	$(CH_2)_5CH_3$	4.7
H	OH	$CH_2CH(CH_3)_2$	0.4
Tetracycline			13.2

Figure 14 13-Alkylthio tetracycline

Some are also substituted at the 7 position with a dimethyl amino group or at position 8 with a chlorine atom.

10.3. 7-Substituted Tetracyclines

Series of 7-phenyl substituted analogs have been prepared. It was claimed that they are active against *E. coli*, *S. aureus*, and *E. faecalis*. Other 7-substituted derivatives have been synthesized, such as 7-nitro, 7-carbamoyl, 7-carbonyl, 7-keto, and 7-urea as well as 7-alkenyl and 7-alkyl analogs.

10.4. 8-Bromo Derivatives

Series of 8-bromo or 8-alkenyl derivatives were claimed in patents and seem to exhibit activity against *S. aureus* and *E. coli*.

REFERENCES

Blackwood RK, English AR, 1970, Structure-activity relationships in the tetracycline series, Adv Appl Microbiol, 13, 237–266.

Cacciapuoti A, Moss EL, Menzel F Jr, Cramer CA, Weiss W, Loebenberg D, Hare RS, Miller GH, 1987, In vitro and in vivo characterization of novel 8-methoxy derivatives of chlortetracycline, J Antibiot, 40, 1426–1430.

Chopra I, 1985, Mode of action of the tetracyclines and the nature of bacterial resistance to them, p 317–392, in Hlavka JJ, Boothe IH, ed, Handbook of Experimental Pharmacology, vol 78, Springer-Verlag, Berlin.

Chopra I, 1994, Tetracycline analogs whose primary target is not the bacterial ribosome, Antimicrob Agents Chemother, 38, 637–640.

Chopra I, Hawkey PM, Hinton M, 1992, Tetracyclines, molecular and clinical aspects, J Antimicrob Chemother, 29, 245–277.

Chopra I, Howe TGB, Linton AH, Linton KB, Richmond MH, Speller DCE, 1981, The tetracyclines: prospects at the beginning of the 1980s, J Antimicrob Chemother, 8, 5–21.

Devasthale PV, Mitscher LA, Telikepalli H, Vander Velde D, Zou J-Y, Ax HA, Tymiak AA, 1992, Dactylocyclines, novel tetracycline derivatives produced by a Dactylosporangium sp. III. Absolute stereochemistry of the dactylocyclines, J Antibiot, 45, 1907–1913.

Dingeldein E, Ungethüm W, 1979, Pharmacokinetics of EMD 33 330, a totally synthetic tetracycline, 19th Intersci Conf Antimicrob Agents Chemother, abstract 510.

Duggar BM, 1948, Aureomycin: a product of the continuing search for new antibiotics, Ann N Y Acad Sci, 51, 177–181.

Eliopoulos GM, Wennersten CB, Cole G, Moellering RC Jr, 1994, In vitro activities of two glycylcyclines against gram-positive bacteria, Antimicrob Agents Chemother, 38, 534–541.

Gialdroni-Grassi G, 1993, Tetracyclines—extending the atypical spectrum, Int J Antimicrob Chemother, 3, suppl, S31–S46.

Goldstein FW, Kitzis MD, Acar JF, 1994, *N,N*-Dimethylglycylamido derivative of minocycline and 6-demethyl-6-deoxytetracycline, two new glycylcyclines highly effective against tetracycline-resistant gram-positive cocci, Antimicrob Agents Chemother, 38, 2218–2220.

Hughes LJ, Stezowski JJ, Hughes RE, 1979, Chemical structural properties of tetracycline derivatives. 7. Evidence for the coexistence of the zwitterionic and nonionized forms of the free base in solution, J Am Chem Soc, 101, 7655–7657.

Ishii Y, Ohno A, Miyazaki S, Tateda K, Matsumoto T, Yamaguchi K, 1994, A study on antimicrobial activity of CL 331928 (DMG-DMOT) and mino to S. aureus, 34th Intersci Conf Antimicrob Agents Chemother, abstract F-88.

Kenny GE, Cartwright FD, 1994, Susceptibilities of *Mycoplasma hominis, Mycoplasma pneumoniae,* and *Ureaplasma urealyticum* to new glycylcyclines in comparison with those to older tetracyclines, Antimicrob Agents Chemother, 38, 2628–2632.

Kondo N, Hiramatsu K, 1994, In vitro antimicrobial activity of CL 331928 (DMG-DMOT), a new glycylcycline to methicillin-resistant Staphylococcus aureus (MRSA) clinical strains, 34th Intersci Conf Antimicrob Agents Chemother, abstract F-90.

Levy SB, 1992, Active efflux mechanism for antimicrobial resistance, Antimicrob Agents Chemother, 36, 695–703.

Nikaido H, 1994, Prevention of drug access to bacterial targets: permeability barriers and active efflux, Science, 264, 382–388.

Nishino T, Yoshida M, Otsuki M, 1994, In vitro and in vivo activities of CL 331928 (DMG-DMDOT), a new glycylcycline compound, 34th Intersci Conf Antimicrob Agents Chemother, abstract F-104.

Nord CE, Lindmark A, Persson I, 1993, In vitro activity of DMG-Mino and DMG-DM Dot, two new glycylcyclines, against anaerobic bacteria, Eur J Clin Microbiol Infect Dis, 12, 784–786.

Oliver TJ, Prokop R, Bower R, Otto RB, 1963, Chelocardin, a new broad-spectrum antibiotic. I. Discovery and biological properties, Antimicrob Agents Chemother, 1962, 583–591.

Patel M, Gullo VP, Hegde VR, Horan AC, Gentile F, Marquez JA, Miller GH, Puar MS, Waitz JA, 1987a, A novel tetracycline from Actinomadura brunnea. Fermentation, isolation and structure elucidation, J Antibiot, 40, 1408–1413.

Patel M, Gullo VP, Hegde VR, Horan AC, Marquez JA, Vaughan R, Puar MS, Miller GH, 1987b, A new tetracycline antibiotic from a Dactylosporangium species. Fermentation, isolation and structure elucidation, J Antibiot, 40, 1414–1418.

Petersen PJ, Jacobus NV, Shelofsky AG, Sum P-E, Testa RT, Tally FP, 1994a, In vitro activity of a novel glylcylcycline compound TGB-mino, 34th Intersci Conf Antimicrob Agents Chemother, abstract F98.

Petersen PJ, Jacobus NV, Testa RT, Tally FP, 1994b, In vivo efficacy of a glycylcycline, DMG-DMDOT, 34th Intersci Conf Antimicrob Agents Chemother, abstract F-98.

Rasmussen B, Noller HF, Daubresse G, Oliva B, Misulovin Z, Rothstein DM, Ellestad GA, Gluzman Y, Tally FP, Chopra I, 1991, Molecular basis of tetracycline action: identification of analogs whose primary target is not the bacterial ribosome, Antimicrob Agents Chemother, 35, 2306–2311.

Roberts MC, 1994, Epidemiology of tetracycline-resistance determinants, Trends Microbiol, 2, 353–357.

Rogalski W, 1985, Chemical modification of the tetracyclines, p 179–316, in Hlavka JJ, Boothe IH, ed, Handbook of Experimental Pharmacology, vol 78, Springer-Verlag, Berlin.

Russell AD, Ahonkhai I, 1982, Antibacterial activity of a new thiatetracycline antibiotic, thiacycline, in comparison with tetracycline, doxycycline and minocycline, J Antimicrob Chemother, 9, 445–449.

Smith EB, Munayyer HK, Ryan MJ, Mayles BA, Hegde VR, Miller GH, 1987, Direct selection of a specifically blocked mutant of Actinomadura brunnea—isolation of a third 8-methoxy substituted chlortetracycline, J Antibiot, 40, 1419–1425.

Someya Y, Yamaguhi A, Sawai T, 1995, A novel glycylcycline, 9-(*N,N*-dimethylglycylamido)-6-demethyl-6-deoxytetracycline, is neither transported nor recognized by the transposon Tn*10*-encoded metal-tetracycline/H^+ antiporter, Antimicrob Agents Chemother, 39, 247–249.

Speer BS, Salyers AA, 1988, Characterization of novel tetracycline resistance that functions only in aerobically grown *Escherichia coli,* J Bacteriol, 170, 1423–1429.

Sum P-E, Lee VJ, Testa RT, Hlavka JJ, Ellestad GA, Bloom JD, Gluzman Y, Tally FP, 1994, Glycylcyclines. 1. A new generation of potent antibacterial agents through modification of 9-aminotetracyclines, J Med Chem, 37, 184–188.

Testa RT, Petersen PJ, Jacobus NV, Sum P-E, Lee VJ, Tally FP, 1993, In vitro and in vivo antibacterial activities of the glycylcyclines, a new class of semisynthetic tetracyclines, Antimicrob Agents Chemother, 37, 2270–2277.

Tymiak AA, Aklonis C, Bolgar MS, Kahle AD, Kirsch DR, O'Sullivan J, Porubcan MA, Principe P, Trejo WH, Ax HA, Wells JS, Andersen NH, Devasthale PV, Telikepalli H, Vander Velde D, Zou J-Y, Mitscher LA, 1993, Dactyloglycines: novel tetracycline glycosides against tetracycline-resistant bacteria, J Org Chem, 58, 535–537.

Tymiak AA, Ax HA, Bolgar MS, Kahle AD, Porubcan MA, Andersen NH, 1992, Dactylocyclines, novel tetracycline derivatives produced by Dactylosporangium sp. II. Structure elucidation, J Antibiot, 45, 1899–1906.

Valcavi V, 1981, Tetracyclines: chemical aspects and some structure-activity relationships, p 3–25, in Gialdroni-Grassi G, Sabath LD, ed, New Trends in Antibiotics: Research and Therapy, Elsevier/North Holland.

Watanabe K, Tanaka-Bandoh K, Kato N, Kato H, Ueno K, 1994, In vitro and in vivo activity of CL 331928 (DMG-DMDOT), a new glycylcycline against anaerobic bacteria, 34th Intersci Conf Antimicrob Agents Chemother, abstract F-106.

Wells JS, O'Sullivan J, Aklonis C, Ax HA, Tymiak AA, Kirsch DR, Trejo WH, Principe P, 1992, Dactylocyclines, novel tetracycline derivatives produced by Dactylosporangium sp. I. Taxonomy, production, isolation and biological activity, J Antibiot, 45, 1892–1898.

Yamaguchi A, Ono N, Akasaka T, Noumi T, Sawai T, 1991, Stoichiometry of metal-tetracycline:H+antiport mediated by transposon Tn10-encoded tetracycline resistance protein in Escherichia coli, FEBS Lett, 282, 416–418.

Yamamoto T, Hiramatsu K, Kaji A, 1994, Mode of action of CL 331,928 (DMG-DMDOT), a new glycylcycline, 34th Intersci Conf Antimicrob Agents Chemother.

Fluoroquinolones

A. BRYSKIER

26

1. INTRODUCTION

The pyridone-β-carboxylic acids, or 4-quinolones, are synthetic antibacterial agents first described in 1949. Barton et al. patented about 80 molecules of this chemical family.

Nalidixic acid was described in 1962 (by Lesher et al.). The first chemical studies were undertaken on a contaminant of a synthetic intermediate of chloroquine, which is a 4-aminoquinoline. Nalidixic acid (1,8-naphthyridone) is the first molecule in the series. The replacement of the nitrogen atom at position 8 by a carbon atom gave rise to the quinolone-type derivatives, the first molecule of which to be used therapeutically was oxolinic acid.

Nalidixic acid is active against certain species of the family *Enterobacteriaceae*; at the time of its introduction into clinical practice in 1963, nalidixic acid was restricted to the treatment of urinary tract infections. Despite an attempt at intravenous administration, its use in the treatment of severe infections remains limited because of its moderate activity (MIC, 4 to 16 μg/ml), marked plasma protein binding (92 to 97%), and poor tolerance.

The development of the 4-quinolones progressed slowly. An increase in antibacterial activity was achieved with the synthesis of oxolinic acid, which is four times more active than nalidixic acid. A moderate extension of the antibacterial spectrum, but not of the activity, was obtained with the synthesis of pipemidic acid (*Pseudomonas aeruginosa*), piromidic acid (*Staphylococcus aureus*), and flumequine.

Pipemidic acid exhibits partial cross-resistance with nalidixic acid. The chemical originality of pipemidic acid and piromidic acid is that they have an aromatic nucleus at position 7 of the pyrido[2,3-*b*]pyrimidine ring. Flumequine has a fluorine atom.

The fluoroquinolones arose from the idea of combining an aromatic nucleus at position 7—7-piperazinyl—and a fluorine atom at position 6 of the quinoline nucleus (pefloxacin, norfloxacin, etc.) or the 1,8-naphthyridone nucleus (enoxacin). Norfloxacin represented a microbiological revolution among the 4-quinolones, as it is 10 to 100 times more active than nalidixic acid and possesses a broad antibacterial spectrum. However, it has the drawback of poor bioavailability, which prevents it from being used in systemic infections. The introduction of a methyl group at position 4′ of the piperazinyl ring resolved the pharmacokinetic problem while moderately reducing the antibacterial activity (pefloxacin).

On the basis of these initial studies, it appeared essential to optimize the 7-piperazinyl and 6-fluorine combination. This optimization was obtained by substituting the nitrogen at position 1 of the quinoline nucleus with a cyclopropyl group (ciprofloxacin) instead of an ethyl group. Other substituents were attached at position 1: benzoxazine (ofloxacin), 2′,4′-difluorophenyl (temafloxacin), methylamino (amifloxacin), oxetane (WQ-1197), and difluoroaminophenyl (ABT-492).

The resultant molecules have a broad antibacterial spectrum and bactericidal activity, enabling severe infections to be treated orally or parenterally.

A number of pharmaceutical companies have undertaken research into the fluoroquinolones. Several hundred molecules have thus been synthesized with the aim of finding unpatented chemical structures or synthetic pathways. This amount of compounds has provided a better understanding of the structure-activity relationships of this chemical class. In the search for new chemical entities, it has proved necessary to remedy the shortcomings of the available 7-piperazinyl derivatives: correcting the lack of activity against streptococci, pneumococci, and anaerobes; reducing the side effects; obtaining low-level (<5%) metabolism of molecules; and, finally, reducing or eliminating the interaction between the quinolones and the metabolism of theophylline and other drugs.

These studies have shown that almost all of the positions of the central core can be substituted, including the 5 position of the quinoline nucleus (sparfloxacin), but that the 4-keto and 3-carbonyl groups are not substitutable, except in the latter case by cleavable esters (norfloxacin). Other heterocycles have been attached at position 7, giving rise to molecules that are active against pneumococci and streptococci, particularly those possessing a 3-aminopyrrolidinyl (clinafloxacin) or a bicyclic ring (trovafloxacin and moxifloxacin), or new 7-piperazinyl derivatives (levofloxacin and grepafloxacin) and azetidinyl (ABT-492), etc.

Current research is directed towards molecules with good in vitro and in vivo activities against gram-positive cocci of the *Streptococcus* genus (*Streptococcus pneumoniae*), with good neurologic and cardiological tolerance, and lacking a phototoxic effect. Ideally these drugs should be administered in a single daily oral or parenteral regimen.

One of the main problems at present, as with all antibacterial agents, is the emergence of resistant strains among

Enterobact eriaceae (*Escherichia coli, Salmonella enterica* serovar Typhi), *Staphylococcus* spp., *Neisseria gonorrhoeae, P. aeruginosa*, and *Campylobacter*.

2. CHEMICAL STRUCTURES

All of the molecules belonging to the fluoroquinolones have in common a pyridone-β-carboxylic acid nucleus. The nitrogen at position 1 is substituted by a variable group (Fig. 1). The optimal substituent is a cyclopropyl (ciprofloxacin), followed by the benzoxazine (ofloxacin and levofloxacin), 2′,4′-difluorophenyl (temafloxacin and tosufloxacin), methylamino (amifloxacin), and fluoroethyl (fleroxacin). The minimum essential group is the ethyl chain (pefloxacin, norfloxacin, enoxacin, and lomefloxacin). Other substituents have been proposed at position 1 (Fig. 2), but no molecules have been developed as medicinal products. The majority of 4-quinolones are bicyclic derivatives. Tricyclic molecules have been synthesized and used therapeutically, such as flumequine, ofloxacin, levofloxacin, rufloxacin, and pazufloxacin, and marbofloxacin in veterinary medicine.

In terms of the research and development of antibacterial agents, this is one of the most dynamic therapeutic classes.

Different substituents have been proposed at positions 7, 8, and 5 (Fig. 3, 4, 5, and 6).

Recent molecules such as trovafloxacin, moxifloxacin, garenoxacin, and ecenofloxacin have a bicyclic nucleus at C-7 (Fig. 7).

1,8 naphthyridine derivatives

Quinoline derivatives

Figure 1 Pyridone-β-carboxylic derivatives

Substituents at C-5

NH_2	CH_3	OCH_3
Sparfloxacin	Grepafloxacin	SYN 1193
WQ 0175	BMY 43748	SYN 1253
PD 124816		
SYN 987		
FD 501		
FD 103		
KRQ 10196		

Figure 3 Fluoroquinolones: C-5 substituents

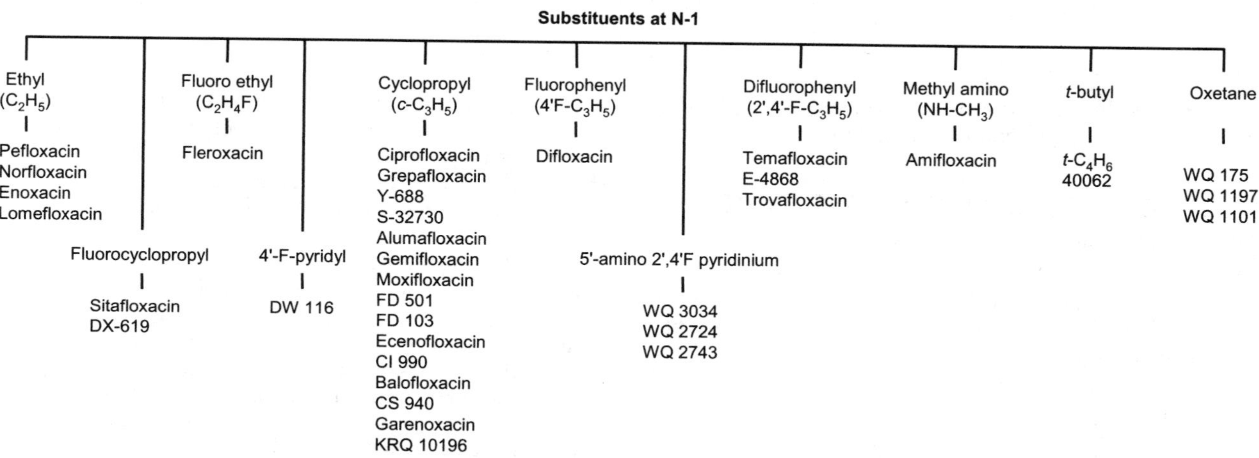

Figure 2 Fluoroquinolones: N-1 substituents

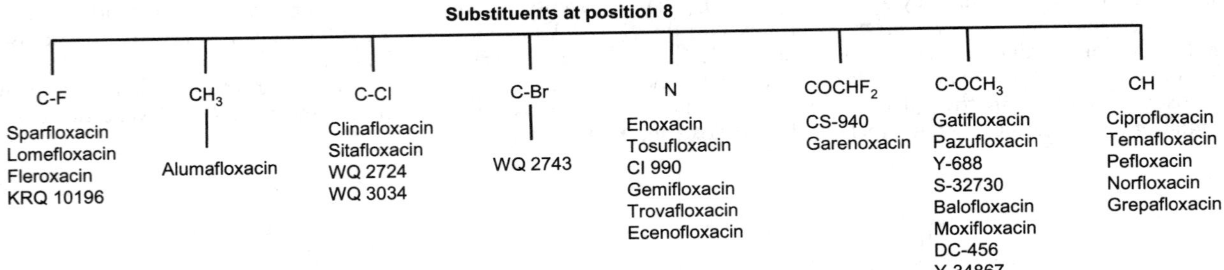

Figure 4 Fluoroquinolones: C-8 substituents

	R_1	R_5	R_8	R_3'	R_4'	R_5'
Ciprofloxacin	c-C_3H_5	H	H	H	H	H
Pefloxacin	C_3H_5	H	H	H	CH_3	H
Norfloxacin	C_3H_5	H	H	H	H	H
Enoxacin	C_3H_5	H	N	H	H	H
Lomefloxacin	C_3H_5	H	C-F	CH_3	H	CH_3
Sparfloxacin	c-C_3H_5	NH_2	C-F	CH_3	H	CH_3
Fleroxacin	C_2H_4F	H	C-F	H	CH_3	H
Gatifloxacin	c-C_3H_5	H	C-OCH_3	CH_3	H	H
Grepafloxacin	c-C_3H_5	CH_3	H	CH_3	H	H
DW 116	5'-pyridyl	H	H	H	CH_3	H

Figure 5 7-Piperazinyl derivatives

Quinoline derivatives with a heptacycle, such as FD501 and FD103, have been reported in the literature (Fig. 8).

3. STRUCTURE-ACTIVITY RELATIONSHIP

All of the molecules currently under development have the following characteristics:

- A fluorine atom at position 6, except garenoxacin, T-3912, PG 9262932, and analogs (Procter and Gamble derivatives)
- A nitrogen substituent at position 1
- No substituent of the 4-keto group
- No substituent of the 3-carbonyl group
- An aromatic nucleus at position 7

The exceptions are the new molecule garenoxacin, Procter and Gamble derivatives, which do not have a fluorine atom at position 6 (Fig. 9), the molecule MF5137 (Fig. 10), which possesses an amino group at position 6 in place of a fluorine atom, and 6-nitro analogs.

3.1. Pharmacophore

The pharmacophore unit of the pyridone-β-carboxylic acids consists of a pyridone nucleus and a carboxyl group. The minimum chemical structure necessary for a derivative to possess antibacterial activity is the presence of an irreducible double bond at 2-3 and a free keto function at position 7. The carboxyl group at position 3 might be replaced by a bioisoster of the thiazolidinone type.

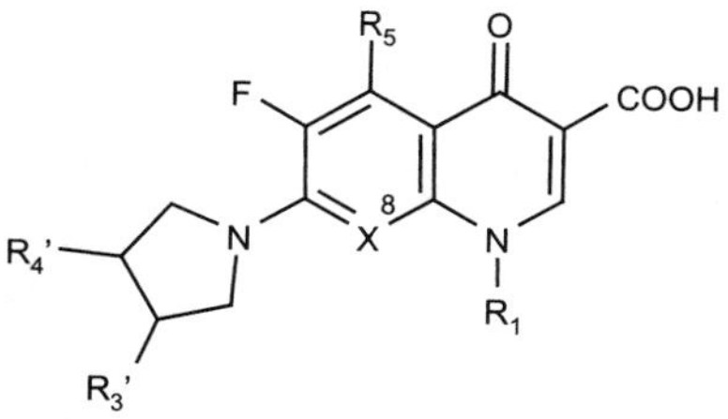

	R_1	R_5	R_8	R_3'	R_4'
Clinafloxacin	c-C_3H_5	H	Cl	NH_2	H
Sitafloxacin	c-F- C_3H_5	H	Cl	NH_2	c-C3H5
CI 990	c-F- C_3H_5	H	N	NH_2	H
Tosufloxacin	2',4' diF-phenyl	H	N	NH_2	H
Alumafloxacin	c-C_3H_5	NH_2	CH_3	NH_2	c-C_3H_5
Gemifloxacin	c-C_3H_5	H	N	-CH_2-NH_2	=$NOCH_3$
S-32730	c-C_3H_5	H	OCH_3	CH_2	-CH_2-NH_2
Y-688	c-C_3H_5	H	OCH_3	CH_2F	-CH_2-NH_2
DC-756	c-C_3H_5	H	CH	NH_2	CH_2F

Figure 6 7-Pyrrolidinyl derivatives

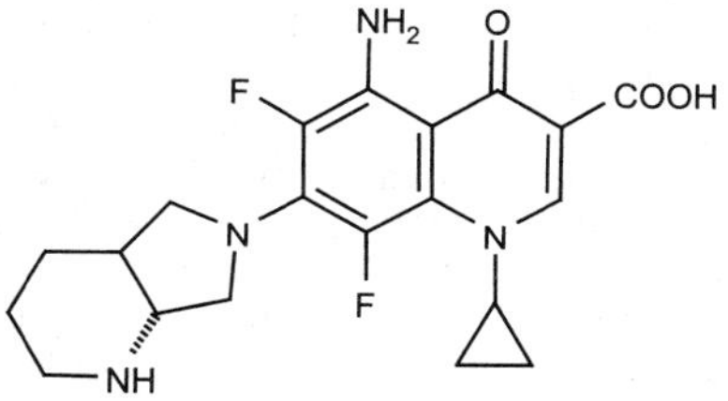

KRQ 10196

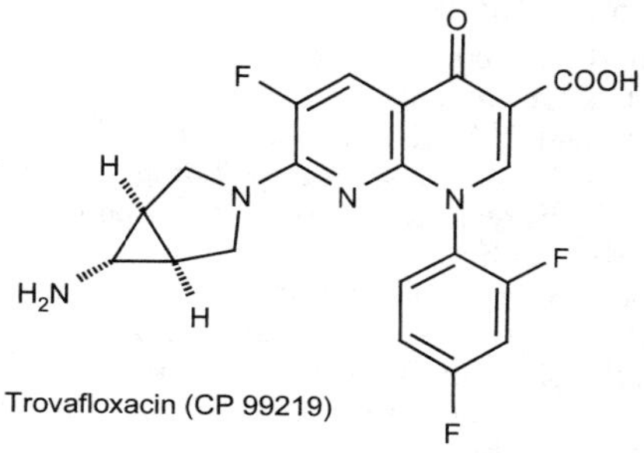

Trovafloxacin (CP 99219)

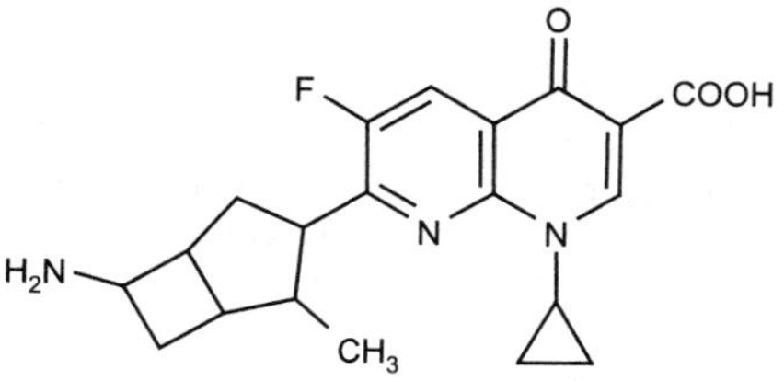

Ecenofloxacin (CFC-222)

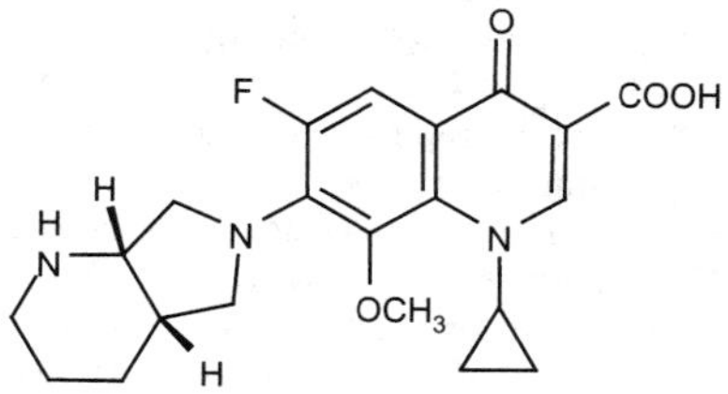

Moxifloxacin (BAY 12-8039)

Figure 7 7-Bicyclic derivatives

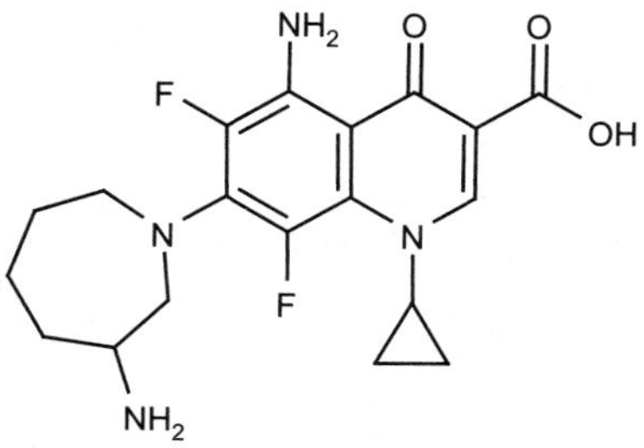

FD 501

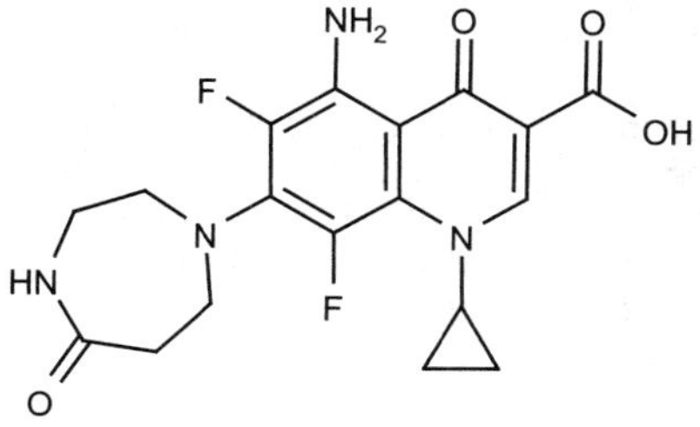

FD 103

Figure 8 FD501 and FD103

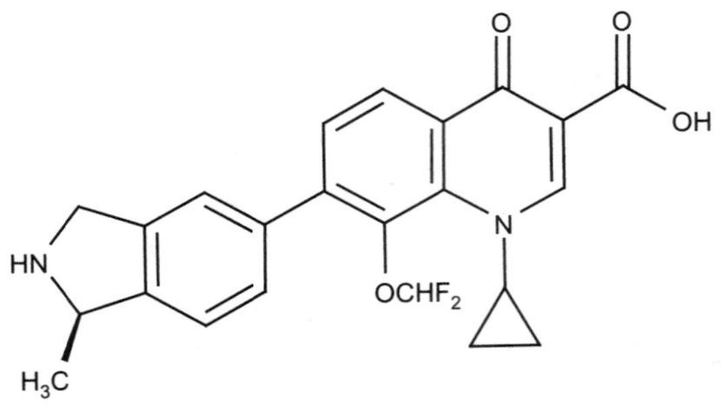

Figure 9 Garenoxacin

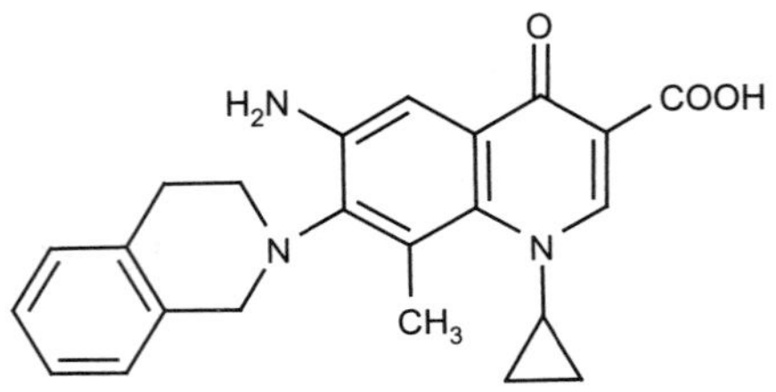

Figure 10 MF5137

3.2. Antibacterial Activity

See Fig. 11.

The antibacterial activity depends on several factors: the aromatic system associated with the pyridone-β-carboxylic acid nucleus, the substituents, and their spatial disposition. These substituents produce greater affinity for the target enzymes (DNA gyrase and topoisomerase IV) but also allow penetration of the bacterial outer membrane.

3.2.1. Effect of Substituents

The 3-carboxyl and 4-carbonyl groups are essential for the expression of antibacterial activity, as they allow the molecule to bind to the bacterial DNA-DNA gyrase complex. Position 2 must remain free, as it is too close to the binding site on the enzyme. Inhibition of the gyrase and intrabacterial penetration are increased by the fluorine atom at position 6. The substituent at position 7 is responsible for an increase in antibacterial activity. The substituents at position 7 play a very important role in the phase of intrabacterial penetration. The presence of a basic group increases the antibacterial activity. They appear to improve binding at the enzyme sites. It has been shown in a series of derivatives that the activity against gram-negative bacteria increases in the following order: 3′-hydroxypyrrolidinyl < 4′-methylpiperazinyl ≤ 3′-methylpiperazinyl < piperazinyl < 3′-aminopyrrolidinyl. The activity against gram-positive bacteria is as follows: piperazinyl < 3′-methylpiperazinyl ≤ 4′-methylpiperazinyl < 3′-hydroxypyrrolidinyl < 3′-aminopyrrolidinyl.

The antibacterial activity is markedly affected by the steric hindrance of the substituent at position 1. Compounds with a methyl group are more active than those with a shorter or longer alkyl chain. When the steric hindrance of a substituent at position 1 is comparable to that of the ethyl group, the antibacterial activity is similar (fluoroethyl-fleroxacin). Ciprofloxacin has a cyclopropyl at N-1 that is larger than the ethyl group, which contradicts the previous theory. The same applies to the *t*-butyl substituent (BMY-40062). This molecule exhibits good activity against gram-positive bacteria. Apart from the steric hindrance, there are other factors that play a role, such as spatial position and electronic interaction.

The contribution of the substituent at position C-5 may increase the antibacterial activity, irrespective of the nature of the substituent at C-7, in the following order: OH ≤ F ≤ OCH_3 ≤ NH_2 < CH_3. However, the important factor in the activity of the compounds with a substituent at C-5 is the steric hindrance.

3.3. Optical Isomers

The majority of available fluoroquinolones do not have a center of asymmetry. A number of them are racemates or isomers.

3.3.1. Isomers of Ofloxacin

Ofloxacin is a fluoroquinolone with a tricyclic structure, characterized by a center of asymmetry at the methyl attached to the oxazine (Fig. 12). Levofloxacin is twice as active as ofloxacin (racemate) and 128 times more active than the *d* isomer (DR-3554). This characteristic is due not to a greater affinity for the DNA-DNA gyrase complex in the case of the *l* isomer but to the possibility of a larger number of molecules of levofloxacin binding to this site: four molecules of *S* isomer (levofloxacin) versus one molecule of *R* isomer (DR-3554).

3.3.2. Isomers of Temafloxacin

Temafloxacin has a center of asymmetry at C-3′ of the piperazinyl nucleus. The in vitro activities of the two isomers against gram-positive and gram-negative bacteria are identical (Table 1).

However, the *S*(−) enantiomer is more active in vivo than the *R*(+) enantiomer. The two enantiomers have the same inhibitory activities towards DNA gyrase in the supercoiling of *E. coli* H 560 DNA, with 50% inhibitory concentrations (IC_{50}s) of 0.52 and 0.78 μg/ml for the *S*(−) enantiomer and *R*(+) enantiomer, respectively.

3.3.3. Tosufloxacin

The *R*(+) enantiomer is 1 to 2 $\log_2$ more active than the *S*(−) enantiomer against aerobic and anaerobic gram-positive and gram-negative bacteria. However, the pharmacokinetic properties are comparable (Table 2).

3.3.4. Sitafloxacin

Sitafloxacin has two centers of asymmetry, one located at the 3′-amino substituent of the 7-pyrrolidinyl nucleus and the other located at the fluorine attached to the cyclopropyl ring in the N-1 position.

Four stereoisomers have been described (Fig. 13). The four stereoisomers have excellent antibacterial activity. Sitafloxacin is the most active molecule (Table 3).

The inhibitory activities of the four molecules against *E. coli* KL-16 DNA gyrase are similar, with DU-6857 and DU-6858 having less affinity. Sitafloxacin has the greatest affinity for *S. aureus* 209 P topoisomerase IV (IC_{50}, 0.39 ± 0.15 μg/ml) (mean ± standard deviation), with DU-6857 (IC_{50}, 1.44 ± 0.07 μg/ml) and DU-6858 (IC_{50}, 0.21 ± 0.06 μg/ml) having a weaker affinity.

3.3.5. Trovafloxacin

Trovafloxacin has a center of asymmetry in the amino group attached to the bicyclic ring at position 7.

The pharmacokinetics differ according to the position of the NH_2 group (Fig. 14).

3.3.6. Gatifloxacin

Gatifloxacin has two enantiomers with identical pharmacokinetics, which are linear between 200 and 800 mg orally (Table 4).

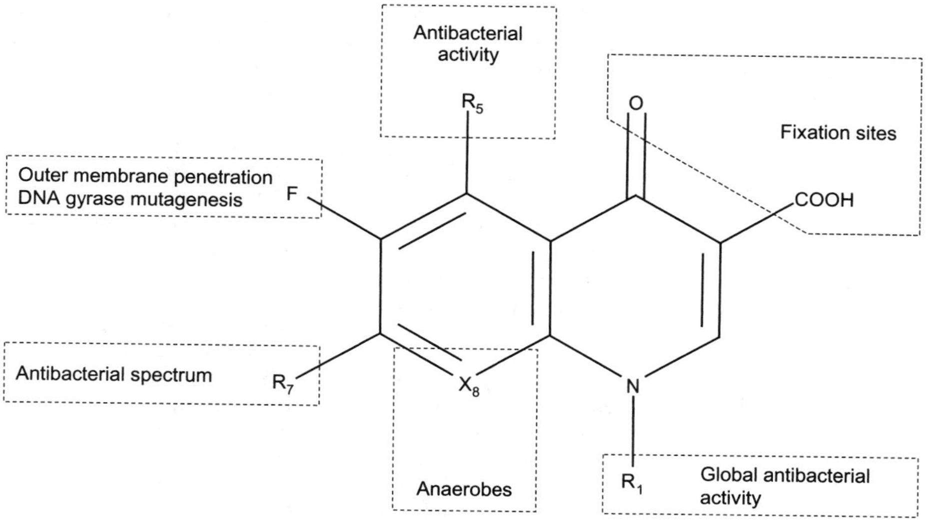

Antibacterial activity
Fixation sites
Outer membrane penetration
DNA gyrase mutagenesis
Antibacterial spectrum
Anaerobes
Global antibacterial activity

Figure 11 Antibacterial activities of the fluoroquinolones in terms of the substituents

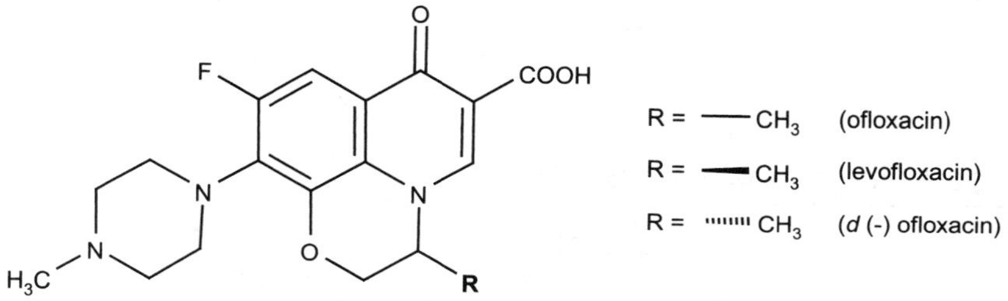

R = CH_3 (ofloxacin)
R = CH_3 (levofloxacin)
R = CH_3 (*d* (-) ofloxacin)

Figure 12 Levofloxacin (4-quinolone/*l*-isomer of ofloxacin)

Table 1 In vitro and in vivo activities of the enantiomers of temafloxacin

Activity	Organism	S(−) temafloxacin	R(+) temafloxacin	Temafloxacin racemate
In vitro (MIC, μg/ml)	*S. aureus* 6338P	0.1	0.1	0.1
	E. faecalis ATCC 8043	0.78	0.78	0.78
	S. pyogenes EES 61	0.39	0.39	0.39
	E. coli Juhl	0.05	0.05	0.05
	P. aeruginosa K799/WT	0.39	0.39	0.39
	S. pneumoniae 6303	4.7	17.2	6.2
In vivo (ED_{50}, mg/kg s.c.[a])	*E. coli* Juhl	0.3	1.2	0.5
	P. aeruginosa A 5007	10.3	10.7	10.3

[a]s.c., subcutaneously.

Table 2 Tosufloxacin: pharmacokinetics of the enantiomers

Isomer	C_{max} (μg/ml)	T_{max} (h)	$t_{1/2\beta}$ (h)	AUC (μg·h/ml)	Urinary elimination (%)
R(+) Isomer	0.40	2.6	3.60	2.78	35.4
S(−) Isomer	0.44	2.4	3.49	2.87	32.4

3.3.7. WCK 919

Two isomers of WCK 919 have been described, WCK 1152 and WCK 1153. The asymmetric center is located on the amino group appended on the 7-pyrrolidyl moiety. One of them is twice as active than the other. The asymmetric center is responsible for the tolerance of this derivative.

3.4. Antimycobacterial Activity

Several series of derivatives have been synthesized to establish the relationships between the structures and the activity against *Mycobacterium tuberculosis* and *Mycobacterium avium* complex (MAC).

3.4.1. *M. tuberculosis*

Derivatives with a 7-piperazinyl nucleus are slightly less active than derivatives with a 7-pyrrolidinyl nucleus. In addition, if the substituent at N-1 is a cyclopropyl, the substituent at C-8 producing the optimal molecule is, in the following order, methoxy > bromine > chlorine, nonsubstituted = fluorine = ethoxy > nitrogen (1,8-naphthyridine nucleus) > trifluoromethyl. Conversely, if the substituent at N-1 is the 2′,4′-difluorophenyl, the substituent at C-8 yields a different

Sitafloxacin (DU-6859a) DU-6856

DU-6857 DU-6858

Figure 13 Enantiomeric derivatives of sitafloxacin

optimal antituberculous activity (Fig. 15). The 1,8-naphthyridone derivatives seem to be inactive against *M. tuberculosis* (see chapter 44).

3.4.2. MAC

The fluorinated quinolones show good in vitro activity against *Mycobacterium kansasii*, *Mycobacterium xenopi*, and *Mycobacterium fortuitum*. The in vitro activity against MAC is method and strain dependent. One compound, WIN 57273, has good activity against gram-positive organisms, with MICs for 90% of isolates, tested (MIC_{90}s) ranging between 1.0 and 4.0 μg/ml.

Among 88 derivatives synthesized and tested, the following substituents have been shown to be important in terms of activity against MAC: a cyclopropyl nucleus at N-1, a fluorine atom at C-6 and C-8, and a heterocycle at C-7. The presence of a piperazinyl nucleus produces the best results against MAC (Klopman et al., 1993).

It has been hypothesized that the mechanism of resistance is associated with bacterial cytochrome P450 activity. Resistant strains may have enhanced P450 activity in the periplasm, resulting in an increased rate of quinolone metabolism, which leads to the breakpoint required to be effective not being reached. Quinolones with an N-1 cyclopropyl

Table 3 In vitro activities of the diastereoisomers of sitafloxacin

Organism	MIC (μg/ml)			
	Sitafloxacin	DU-6856	DU-6857	DU-6858
S. aureus PDA 209 P	0.008	0.016	0.063	0.063
S. pyogenes G 36	0.063	0.125	0.5	0.5
S. pneumoniae J 24	0.031	0.063	0.5	0.25
E. faecalis ATCC 19433	0.25	0.25	1	1
E. coli KL-16	0.008	0.016	0.031	0.063
K. pneumoniae type 1	0.031	0.031	0.063	0.425
P. aeruginosa PAO 1	0.125	0.25	0.25	0.54

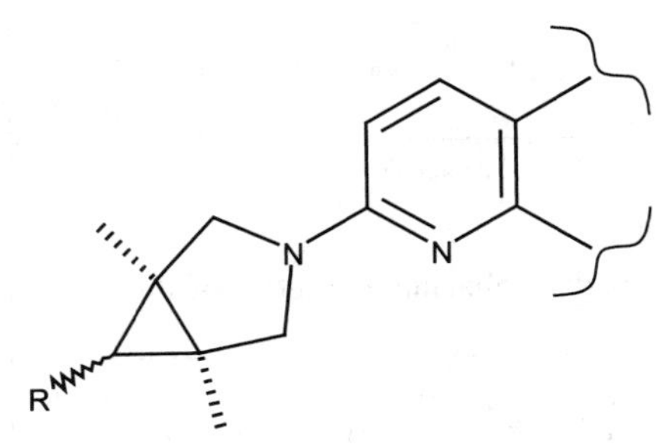

	In vitro activity	In vivo activity	Pharmacokinetics (animal)
H_2N	+++	+++	+++
H_2N	+++	+	+

Figure 14 Enantiomers of trovafloxacin

Table 4 Pharmacokinetics of the enantiomers of gatifloxacin

Dose (mg)	Enantiomer	C_{max} (μg/ml)	T_{max} (h)	AUC (μg·h/ml)	$t_{1/2}$ (h)	CL_R (liters/h)	Urinary elimination (%)
200	*R*	0.99	1	6.99	6.9	10.89	36.9
	S	0.98	1	7.2	7.1	10.53	36.9
400	*R*	1.92	1.25	16.71	7.15	10.83	44.9
	S	1.88	1.25	17.07	7.41	10.65	45.24
600	*R*	2.68	2	26.73	7.46	9.2	40
	S	2.59	2	27.18	7.87	9.1	40.2
800	*R*	3.54	2	37.61	7.25	9.1	41.4
	S	3.50	2.3	38.57	7.58	8.9	41.6

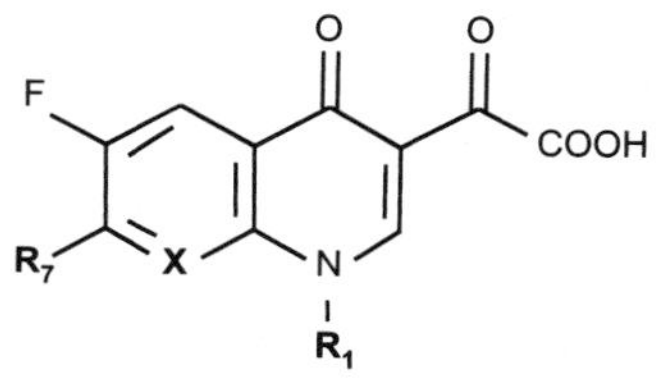

	R_1	X	R_7	MIC (μg/ml) *M. fortuitum*	MIC (μg/ml) *M. tuberculosis*
PD 163753	Cyclopropyl	C-Br	3'-methyl piperazinyl	≤ 0.03	0.76
PD 161144	Cyclopropyl	C-OCH_3	4'-ethyl	≤ 0.03	0.39
PD 163048	*tert*–butyl	N	3'-methyl piperazinyl	0.03	0.78
PD 163049	*tert*–butyl	N	3', 5' dimethyl piperazinyl	0.03	0.78
PD 161148	Cyclopropyl	C-OCH_3	3'-ethyl piperazinyl	0.03	0.10
Ciprofloxacin	Cyclopropyl	CH_2	piperazine	0.06	0.25
Sparfloxacin	Cyclopropyl	C-F	3', 5' dimethyl piperazinyl	0.06	0.06

Figure 15 Fluoroquinolones: structure-activity relationships and mycobacteria

might initiate suicidal inactivation of the metabolizing enzyme via the cyclopropylamine (Fig. 16).

3.4.3. *Mycobacterium ulcerans*

The subcutaneous tropical infection called Buruli ulcer is due to *M. ulcerans*. *M. ulcerans* is resistant to many antibacterials, and the main treatment today is surgery. Some fluoroquinolones have been tested (Table 5) (Dhople and Namba, 2002; Thangaraj et al., 2000). There is a synergy between sitafloxacin and rifampin.

3.5. Esterified Quinolones

Because of their poor solubility, a number of fluoroquinolones have been esterified by attachment of an amino acid to the amino group of the bicyclic nucleus, such as trovafloxacin, yielding alatrofloxacin, which can be used intravenously (Fig. 17).

Prulifloxacin, a thiazetoquinoline fluoroquinolone substituted by an ester chain (prulifloxacin dioxil), has been introduced into clinical practice in Japan (Fig. 18) and some other European countries (e.g., Italy).

Innumerable other esters have been synthesized, such as ofloxacin *N*-succinimyl (Fig. 19) and derivatives of tosufloxacin and norfloxacin (Fig. 20 and 21).

3.6. Natural Quinolones

The quinolones of natural origin differ from the synthetic derivatives by the presence of a 3-β-methyl group instead of a 3-β-carboxyl group (Fig. 22) and the presence of a substituent at position 2.

Several derivatives have been extracted by fermentation of various organisms.

3.6.1. Aurachins

Aurachins A to D are molecular complexes extracted by fermentation of the *Myxobacterium* genus. *Stigmatella aurantiaca* Sga15 produces structurally different antibiotics: stigmatellin, a mixture of myxalamides, and aurachins (Fig. 23). These four molecules have good in vitro activity against gram-positive cocci and gram-positive bacilli (coryneforms).

3.6.2. G1499-2

G1499-2 is a quinolone extracted by fermentation from *Cytophaga johnsonae* ATCC 21123. It is specific because it has a side chain at C-3 containing a cyclopropylidene group (Fig. 24). It inhibits the growth of *S. aureus* Oxford VI and *Bacillus subtilis*, but it is inactive against the other gram-positive and gram-negative bacteria.

3.6.3. Pyo III to XII Derivatives

A number of antibacterial agents obtained by fermentation from strains of marine *Pseudomonas* (VI) or from plants (VII to XII) have a quinoline-type structure, substituted at C-2 by different aliphatic chains and at C-3 by a β-methyl group (Fig. 25).

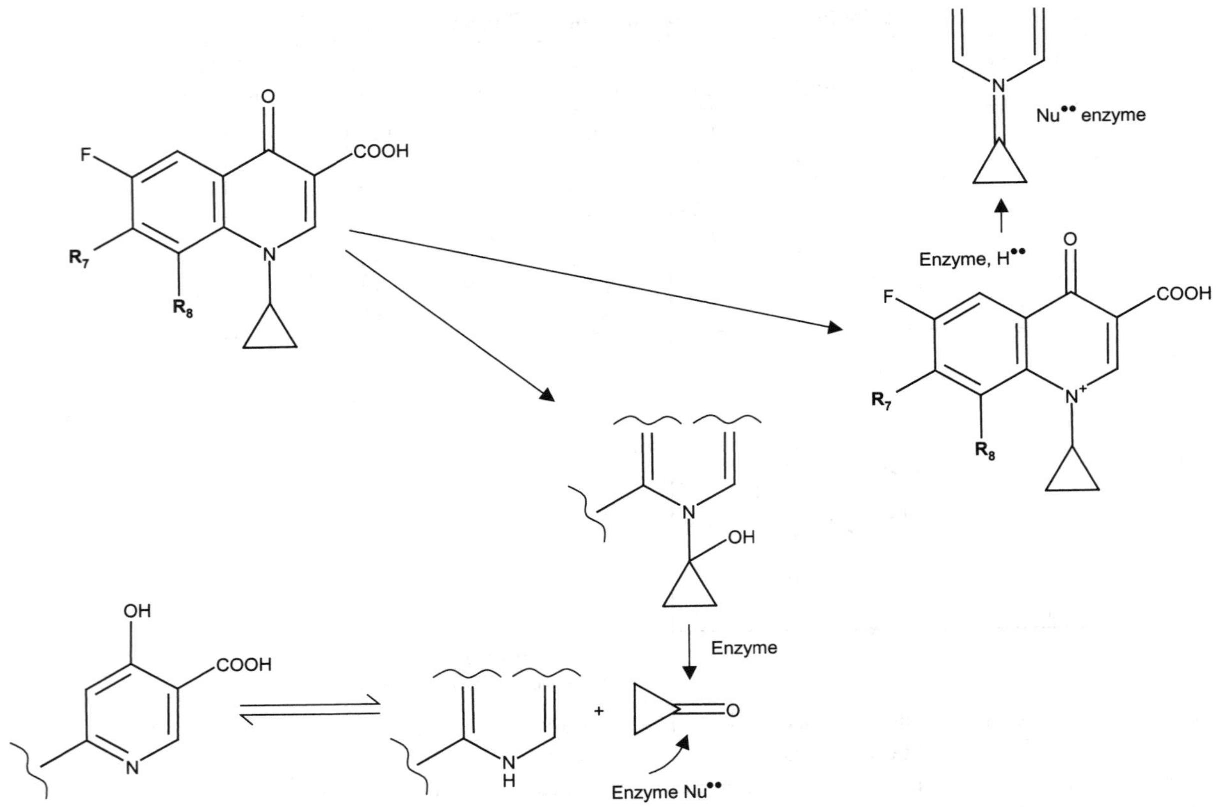

Figure 16 Cytochrome P450 methylamine dehydrogenase inactivation with N-1 cyclopropyl quinolones

Table 5 In vitro activities of some fluoroquinolones against *M. ulcerans*

Drug	MIC (μg/ml)
Sitafloxacin	0.125–2.0
Ofloxacin	0.5–2.0
Levofloxacin	0.25–1.0
Ciprofloxacin	0.5–2.0
Sparfloxacin	0.12–0.5
Rifampin	0.25–0.5

3.6.4. Quinolinol Derivatives

Several metabolites have been isolated from *Burkholderia cepacia* strain Burkh: pyrrolnitrin, isopyrrolnitrin, oxypyrrolnitrin, and a quinoline derivative, 2-(2-heptenyl)-3-methyl-4-quinolinol (Fig. 26).

3.6.5. CL-38489

Eight natural molecules of CL-38489 possess specific activity against *Helicobacter pylori* (Fig. 27). These have been extracted from *Pseudonocardia* sp. strain CL 38489.

3.6.6. YM-30059

YM-30059 (Fig. 28) is a 3-β-methylquinolone derivative extracted by fermentation from *Arthrobacter* sp. strain YL 027295. It is very active against *S. aureus*, including methicillin-resistant strains (MIC, 6.25 μg/ml), in contrast to tosufloxacin. It is inactive against gram-negative bacilli (MIC, >100 μg/ml) and *Mycobacterium smegmatis* ATCC 607 (MIC, 12.5 μg/ml).

3.6.7. *Evodia rutaecarpa*

The fruit of *E. rutaecarpa* (Rutaceae), which is a traditional chinese drug (wu-chu-yu), has long been used in the treatment of abdominal pain, dysentery, amenorrhea, migraine, and nausea. Gosyuyu, a crude extract of the fruit of *E. rutaecarpa*, exhibits marked anti-*H. pylori* activity. Purification yielded the active components, which are composed of two compounds. They are two quinolone derivatives (Fig. 29) which are characterized by an N-1 methyl and no substituent at position 3 (no methyl group such as for natural quinolone, or β-carboxylic group for synthetic derivatives) and a C-2 long alkyl chain: a 8-tridecenyl and 7-tridecenyl for compound A (evocarpin) and compound B, respectively, in a ratio of 10:1, and they cannot be separated from each other.

MICs obtained by the agar dilution method ranged from 0.02 to 0.05 μg/ml (albumin agar after 3 days under microaerobic conditions), and MICs of 2 μg/ml were recorded for *H. pylori* strains NCTC 11916, NCTC 11637, and ATCC 43504. These compounds are poorly active against *Campylobacter jejuni, Vibrio parahaemolyticus, Salmonella enterica* serovar Enteritidis, *E. coli*, and *P. aeruginosa*. In a clinical trial, the combination of omeprazole, amoxicillin, and gosyuyu (gosyuyu, jujube, ginger, and ginseng) yielded in 31 patients an 87% rate of eradication of *H. pylori*.

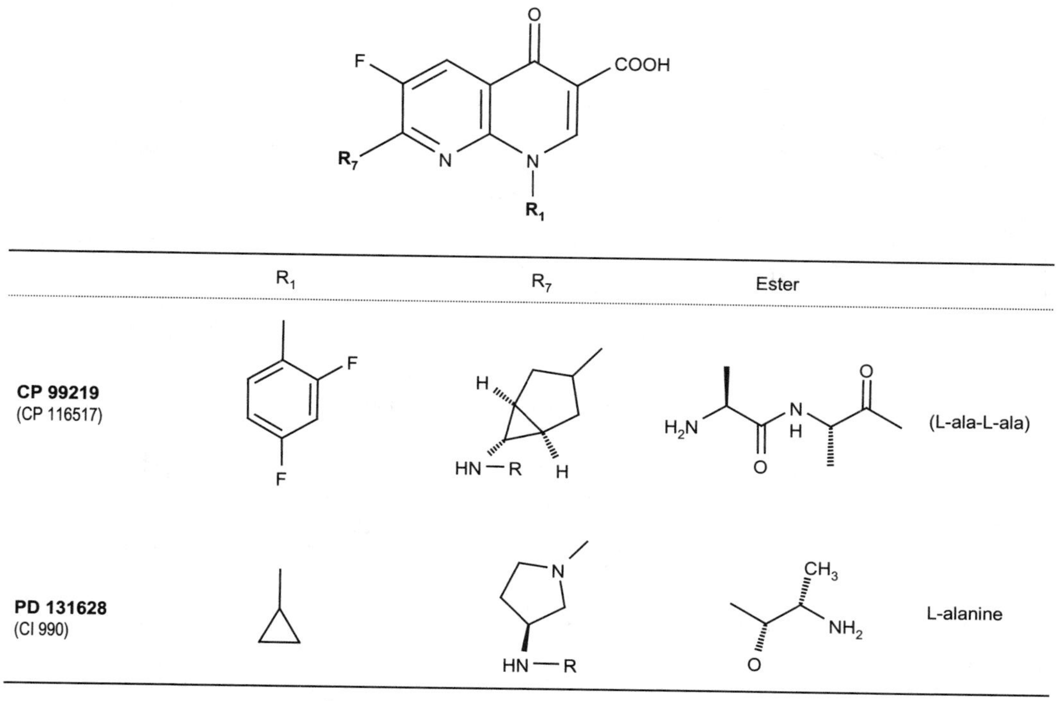

	R_1	R_7	Ester	
CP 99219 (CP 116517)		HN—R	H_2N	(L-ala-L-ala)
PD 131628 (CI 990)		HN—R	CH_3, NH_2	L-alanine

Figure 17 Trovafloxacin (esterification)

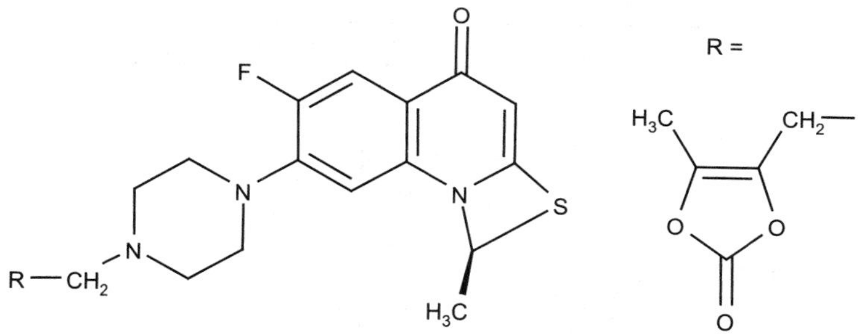

Figure 18 Prulifloxacin dioxil (NAD 394)/(NAD 441A)

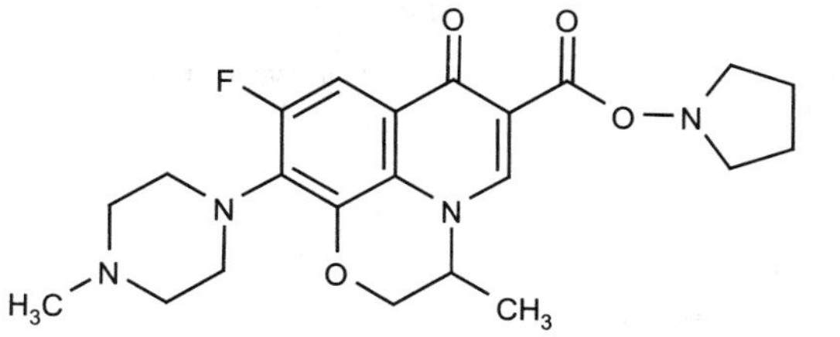

Figure 19 Ofloxacin: *N*-succinimyl ester

4. CLASSIFICATIONS

The pyridone-β-carboxylic acids may be classified according to their chemical structure or their biological properties. They can also be distinguished in terms of their physicochemical properties. The natural quinolones are distinct.

4.1. Chemical Classification

See Fig. 30.

The central nucleus—and the essential minimum in order to belong to the fluoroquinolones—is the pyridone-β-carboxylic acid nucleus. Four chemical groups of 4-quinolones may be described in terms of the number of rings associated with this nucleus.

Group I comprises monocyclic derivatives, such as Ro-13-5478 (Fig. 31).

Group II is composed of bicyclic derivatives, the second ring of which may be pentaatomic (T-14097) (Fig. 32), hexaatomic, or heptaatomic. Within group II, four subgroups have been described: those possessing a 1,8-naphthyridone nucleus (IIA_1) (nalidixic acid and enoxacin), a quinoline nucleus (IIA_2) (the majority of fluoroquinolones), a pyrido[2,3-*b*]pyrimidine nucleus (IIA_3) (pipemidic acid and piromidic acid), and a cinnoline nucleus (IIA_4) (cinoxacin). The molecules may be fluorinated or not, or aminated (MF5137) at position 6. Within the fluorinated subgroups IIA_1 and IIA_2, the molecules are divided according to the nucleus attached at position 7 (piperazinyl, pyrrolidinyl, pyrryl, azetidinyl, bicyclic, or others) (Fig. 33 and 34).

Subgroup IIA_2 (quinolines) can also be subdivided according to the substituent attached at position 8 of the quinoline nucleus (CH_2, F, Cl, CH_3, OCH_3, or CHF_2).

R	Water solubility (mg/ml)	Hydrolysis rate (human plasma) (min)
H (tosufloxacin tosylate)	0.65	-
H (tosufloxacin HCl)	0.10	-
Ala-Ala	23.00	3.0
Gly-Phe	98.00	6.9
Nval-Nval	44.00	2.1
Ala-Nval	26.00	1.3

Figure 20 Ester of tosufloxacin

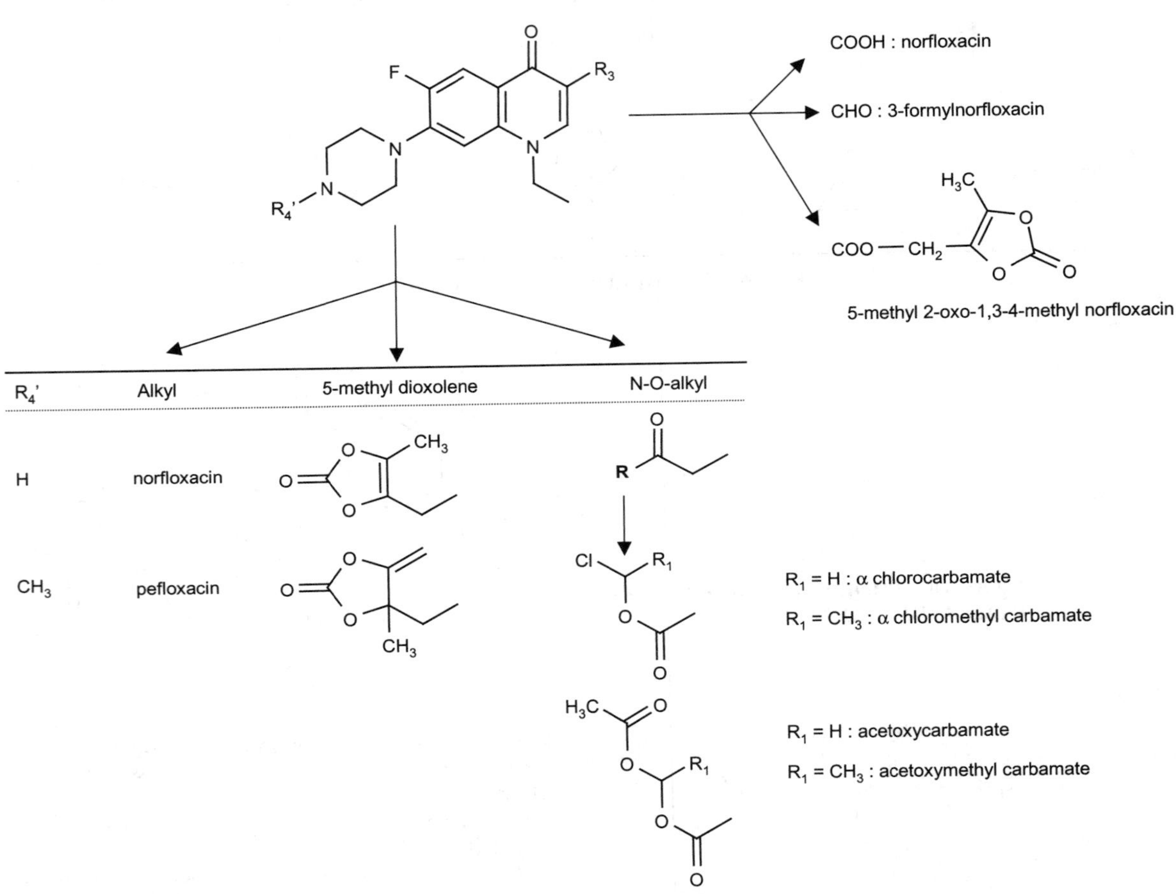

Figure 21 Prodrugs of norfloxacin

Pyridone β-carboxylic

Pyridone β-methyl

Figure 22 3β-Methyl quinolones

Group III is composed of tricyclic molecules, divided into nonfluorinated (oxolinic acid and miloxacin) and fluorinated (ofloxacin, abufloxacin, rufloxacin, ibafloxacin, levofloxacin, prulifloxacin, etc.).

Group IIIB can be subdivided according to the position of the third ring. The majority of molecules are classed together in subgroup $IIIB_1$, in which the third ring is located between N-1 and C-8. Subgroup $IIIB_2$ comprises the other molecules, including prulifloxacin. Subgroup IIIB is highly diverse, with numerous molecules under development or already introduced into clinical pratice: ofloxacin and levofloxacin

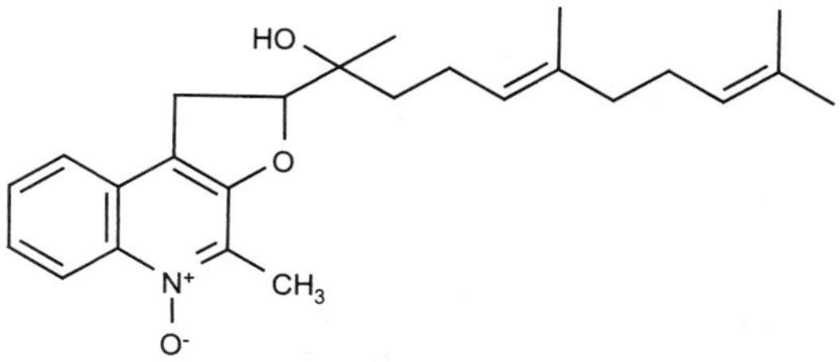

Aurachin A

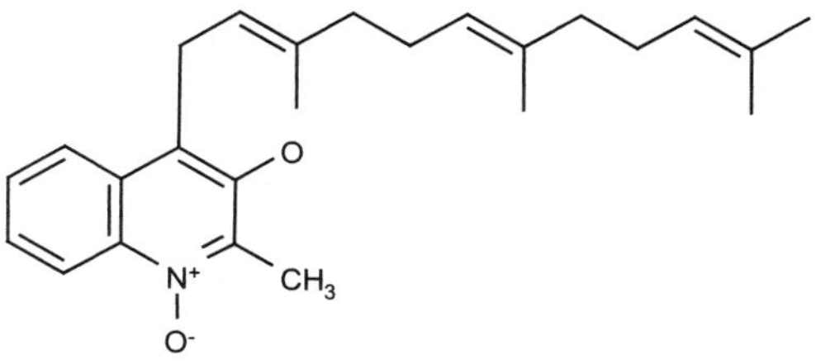

Aurachin B

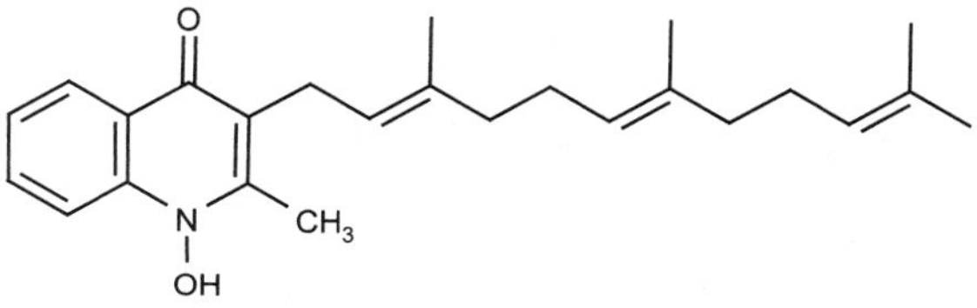

Aurachin C

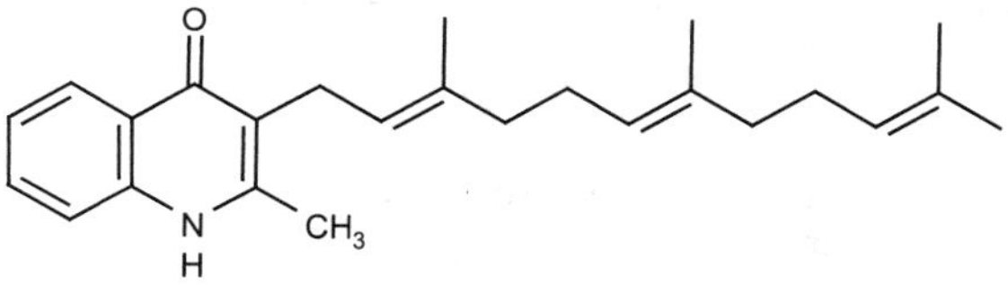

Aurachin D

Figure 23 Aurachins

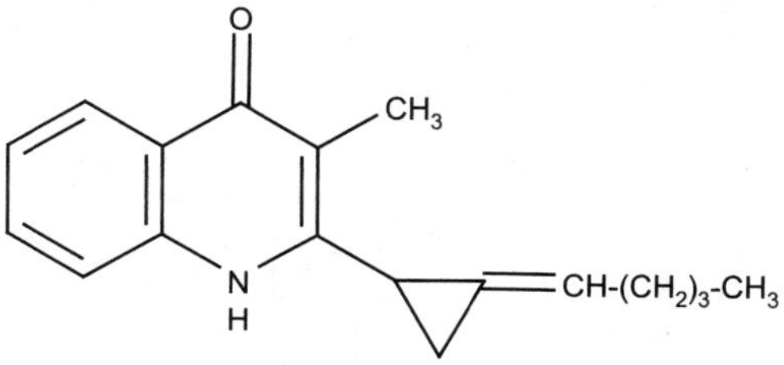

$CH-(CH_2)_3-CH_3$

Figure 24 G1499-2

(oxazine), marbofloxacin (benzodiazine), and rufloxacin (benzothiazine) (Fig. 35).

Group IV contains few molecules and includes quadricyclic molecules such as KB-5246 (Fig. 36).

More recently, esters of existing molecules have been synthesized in order to increase their bioavailability or hydrosolubility, such as norfloxacin and tosufloxacin. The binding of a small peptide to trovafloxacin has allowed the

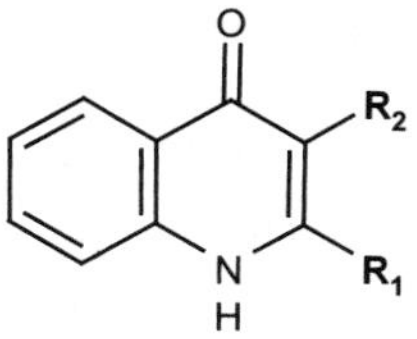

	R_1	R_2
III	$(CH_2)_6$-CH_3	H
IV	$(CH_2)_8$-CH_3	H
V	$CH=CH(CH)_4CH_3$	H
VI	$(CH_2)_4$-CH_3	H
VII	CH_2-$CH=CH$-$(CH_2)_3$-CH_3	CH_3
VIII	$(CH_2)_2(CH=CHCH_2)_2$-CH_3	H
IV	$(CH_2)_8CH_2OH$	H
X	$(CH_2)_9COCH_3$	H
XI	$(CH_2)_3$-$CH=CH$-CH_2CH_3	H
XII	$(CH_2)_{10}$-CH_3	H

Figure 25 Quinolones of natural origin (Pyo III to XII)

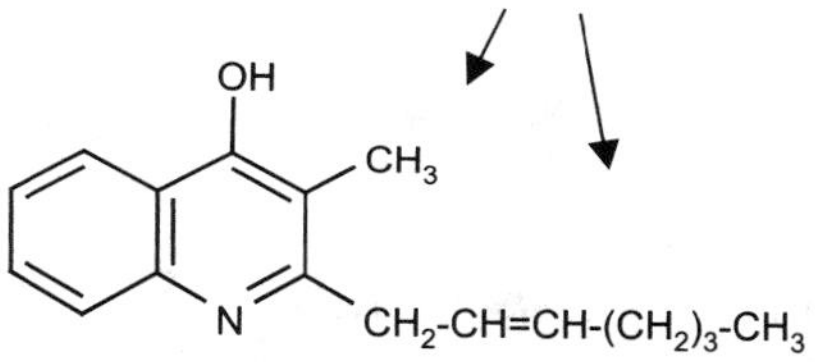

CH_2-$CH=CH$-$(CH_2)_3$-CH_3

2(2-heptenyl)-3-methyl-4-quinolinol

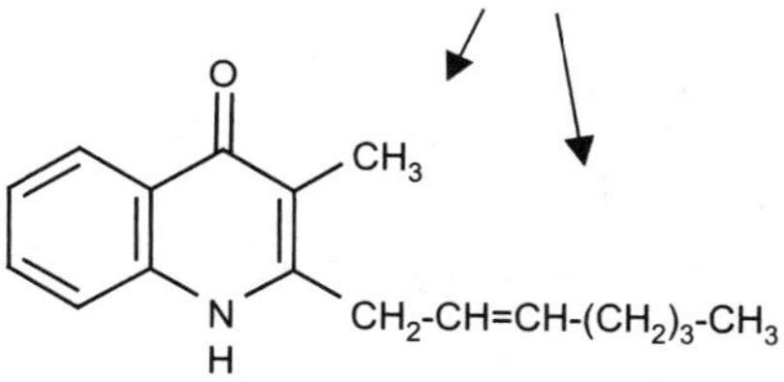

CH_2-$CH=CH$-$(CH_2)_3$-CH_3

Natural quinolones (I)

Figure 26 Quinolinol derivatives

preparation of a parenteral formulation possessing the same activity as the parent molecule.

4.2. Biological Classification

See Fig. 37.

The 4-quinolones may be divided in terms of their antibacterial spectra and their metabolism. Three groups may be described. Each group is in turn subdivided according to the metabolism (>15%) of the molecule.

Group I is composed of molecules with an antibacterial spectrum confined to the *Enterobacteriaceae*. Group IA comprises metabolized molecules such as nalidixic acid, oxolinic acid, piromidic acid, flumequine, and miloxacin. Group IB is composed of nonmetabolized molecules (<5%) such as pipemidic acid and cinoxacin.

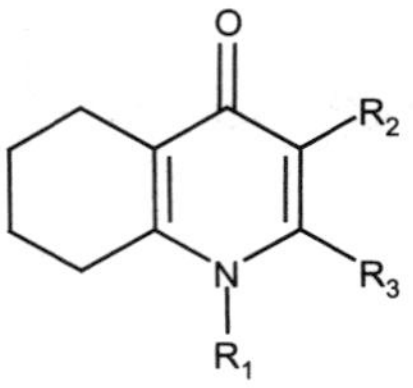

	R_1	R_2	R_3	Diameter of inhibition zone (mm) – (0.5-μg disk)
CJ 13136	H	CH_3	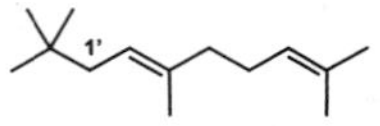 [structure, 1']	23
CJ 13217	CH_3	CH_3	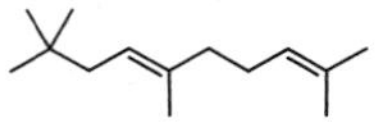 [structure]	24
CJ 13536	CH_2-S-CH_3	CH_3	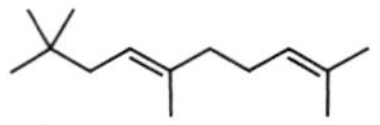 [structure]	12
CJ 13564	CH_3	CH_3	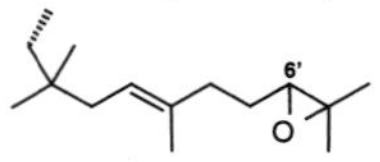 [structure, 6', O]	29
CJ 13565	H	H	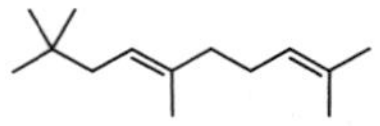 [structure]	17
CJ 13566	CH_3	H	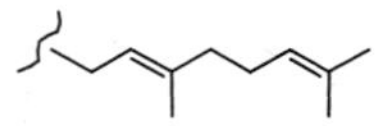 [structure]	16
CJ 13567	CH_3	H	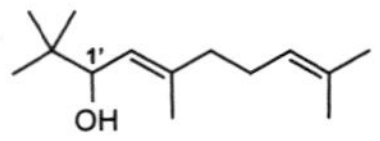 [structure, 1', OH]	8
CJ 13568	CH_3	H	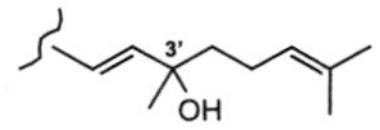 [structure, 3', OH]	20

Figure 27 CL-38489 derivatives

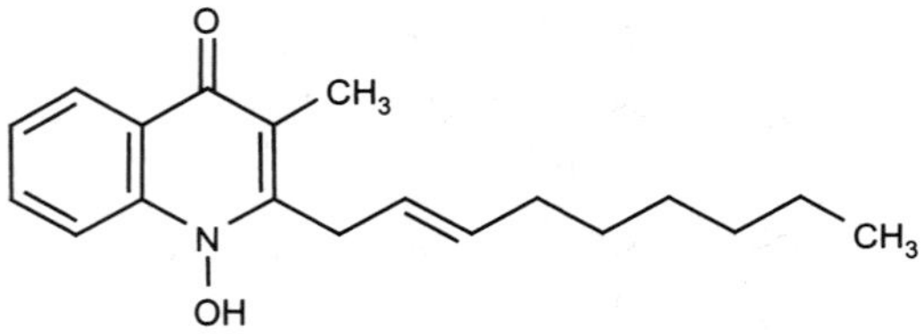

Figure 28 YM-30059

Molecules with an extended antibacterial spectrum are classed in groups IIA and IIB. Their antibacterial activity does not include strict anaerobic or aerotolerant bacteria (streptococci, including *S. pneumoniae*) (Fig. 38).

The number of molecules in this group is large, particularly in group IIA, which contains the metabolized molecules. It may be subdivided into four subgroups according to the heterocycle attached at position 7 of the quinoline or 1,8-naphthyridone nucleus: IIA_1, 7-piperazinyl derivatives (ciprofloxacin, norfloxacin, pefloxacin, and fleroxacin); IIA_2, 7-pyrrolyl; IIA_3, 7-pyrryl; and IIA_4, 7-miscellaneous, which includes derivatives of the type of 7-morpholine, 7-piperidinyl (balofloxacin), 7-azetidinyl, etc.

Group III comprises molecules whose antibacterial spectrum and activity incorporate streptococci and *S. pneumoniae* and, to various degrees, strict anaerobic bacteria. It is also subdivided into groups IIIA and IIIB according to the metabolism of the molecules (Fig. 37).

4.3. Classification by Physicochemical Properties

The majority of new fluoroquinolones have two ionizable functions: the 3-carboxyl group and a protonizable site at position 7, such as a 7-piperazinyl heterocycle. The pK of the carboxyl group is about 6.0 ± 0.3, which is independent of the substituent at position 7. The pK of the basic function at position 7 is, on average, 8.8 and is dependent on the chemical nature of the substituent.

It is possible to distinguish two types of molecules (Table 6): acid compounds and zwitterionic derivatives. In the case of the latter, at neutral pH 90% is in the zwitterionic form and the remainder is in the nondissociated acidic form, thus promoting their membrane permeation.

The capacity of the molecules to cross the bacterial outer membrane is also dependent on the lipophilicity of the derivatives. The molecular mass of the fluoroquinolones as a general rule is less than or equal to 400 Da and plays a certain part in transporin passage, the limit of which is 650 Da for *Enterobacteriaceae* and 342 Da for *P. aeruginosa*. In the case of the last species, the three-dimensional configuration of the molecules plays a predominant role.

Three groups of molecules may be distinguished in terms of the *n*-octanol/water or phosphate partition coefficient: less than 0.1, between 0.1 and 2.0, and greater than 2.0 (Table 7).

1-methyl-2 [(Z)-8-tridecenyl-4 (*1H*)]-quinolone (evocarpin)

1-methyl-2 [(Z)-7-tridecenyl-4 (*1H*)]-quinolone

Figure 29 ***E. rutaecarpa* extract products**

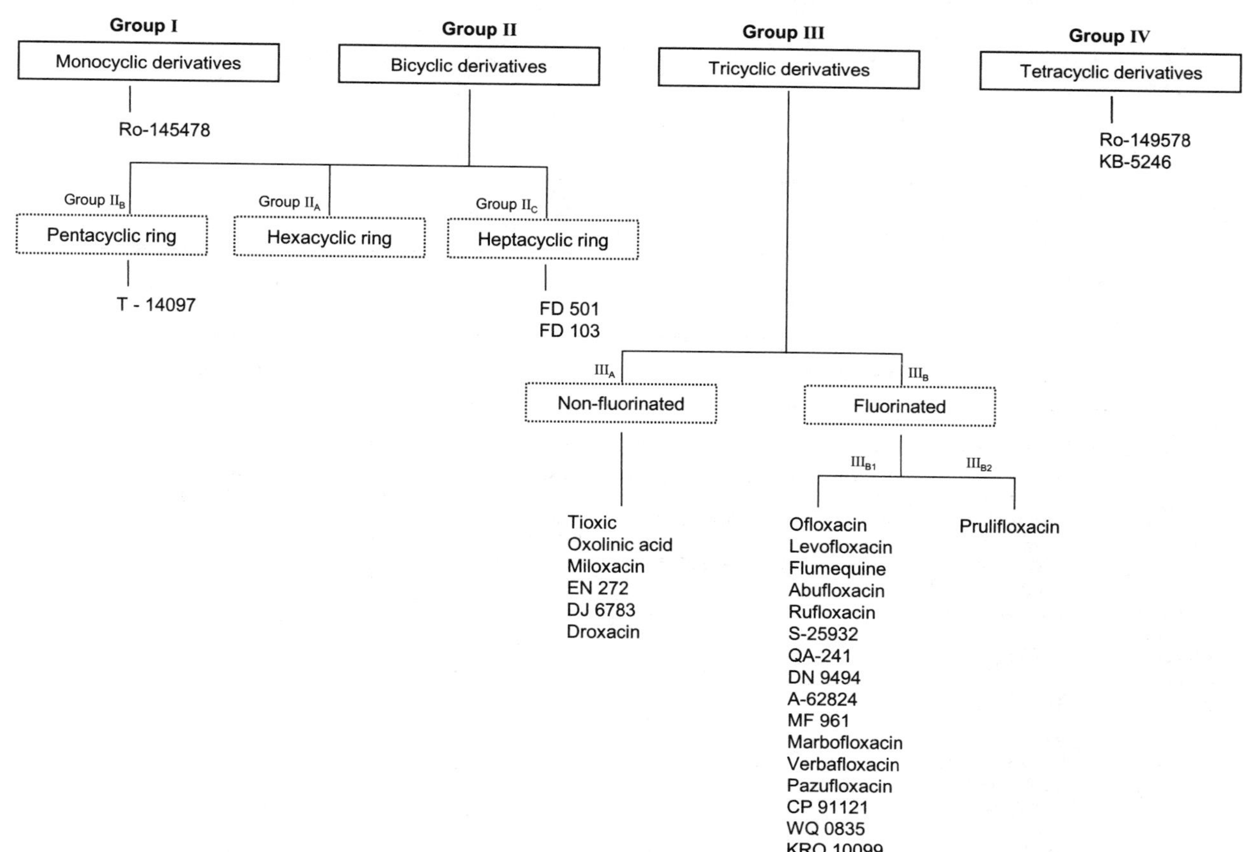

Figure 30 Chemical classification of fluoroquinolones

Figure 31 Pyridone β-carboxylic acid, monocyclic derivative: Ro-13-5478

5. ANTIBACTERIAL ACTIVITY OF FLUOROQUINOLONES

5.1. Factors Affecting the In Vitro Activity of Fluoroquinolones

5.1.1. Effect of pH

The fluoroquinolones are amphoteric molecules. Their charge is dependent on the pH of the medium. Quinolones with a piperazinyl ring at position 7 are less active in an acidic medium than in an alkaline medium. Conversely, molecules with no aromatic substituent at position 7 are more active in an acidic medium than in an alkaline medium (ionic type of molecules) (Fig. 39).

At acidic pH the 7-piperazinyl derivatives are positively charged, and at alkaline pH they are negatively charged.

	R_2	R_1
c :	C_2H_5	H
d :	C_2H_5	CH_3
e :	C_2H_5	H

Pyrazolo [3,4-*b*] pyridines

T 14097

a : R=$COOC_2H_5$

b : R=NO_2

Furo [2,3-*b*] pyridine

Figure 32 Quinolones: bicyclic derivatives with a pentacycle

Nonsubstituted molecules are neutral. Some molecules have a 7-piperazinyl nucleus and represent an exception to this, such as difloxacin, which appears to be relatively insensitive

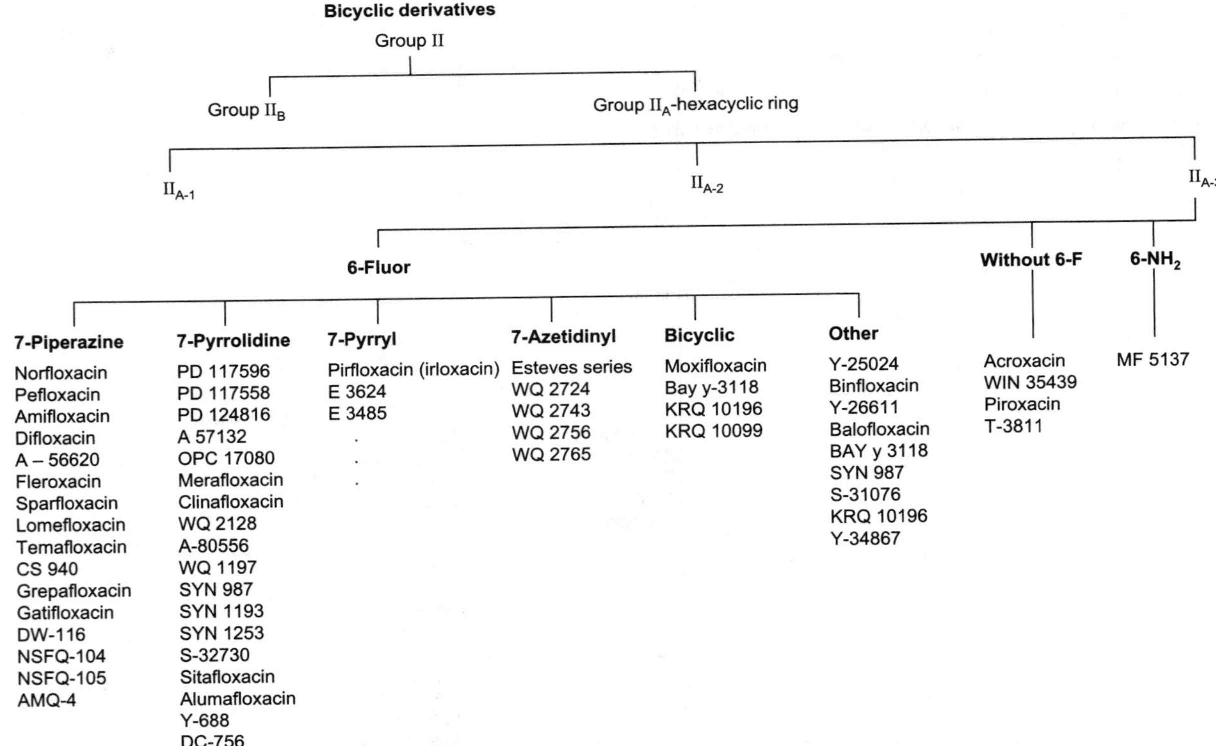

Figure 33 Chemical classification of fluoroquinolones (group II_A)

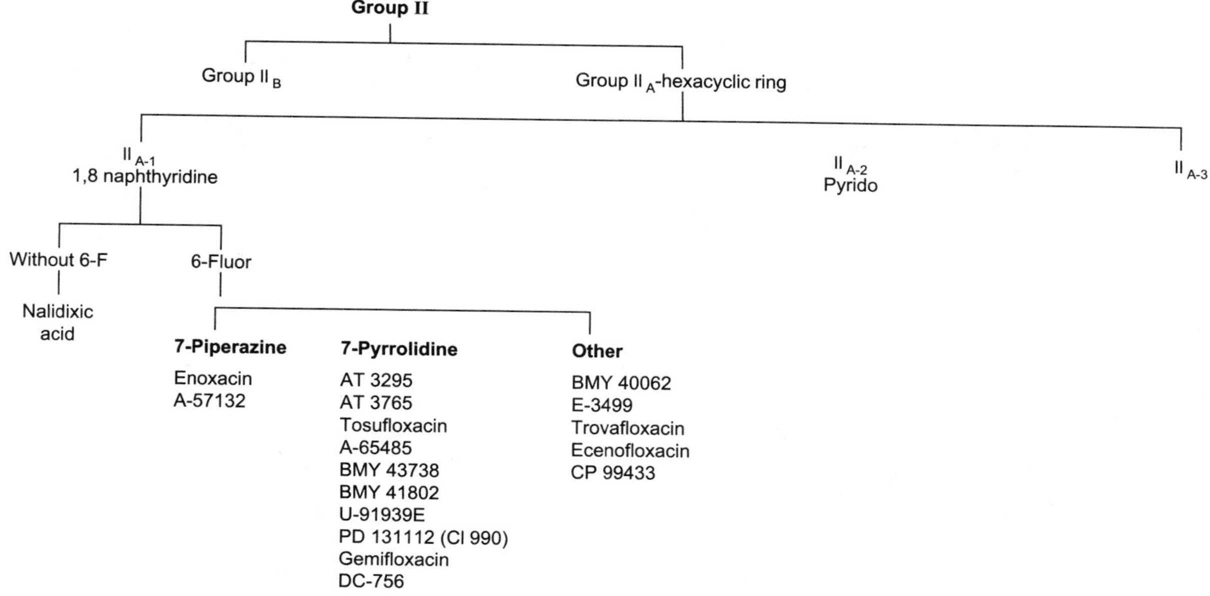

Figure 34 Chemical classification of fluoroquinolones (group II_A)

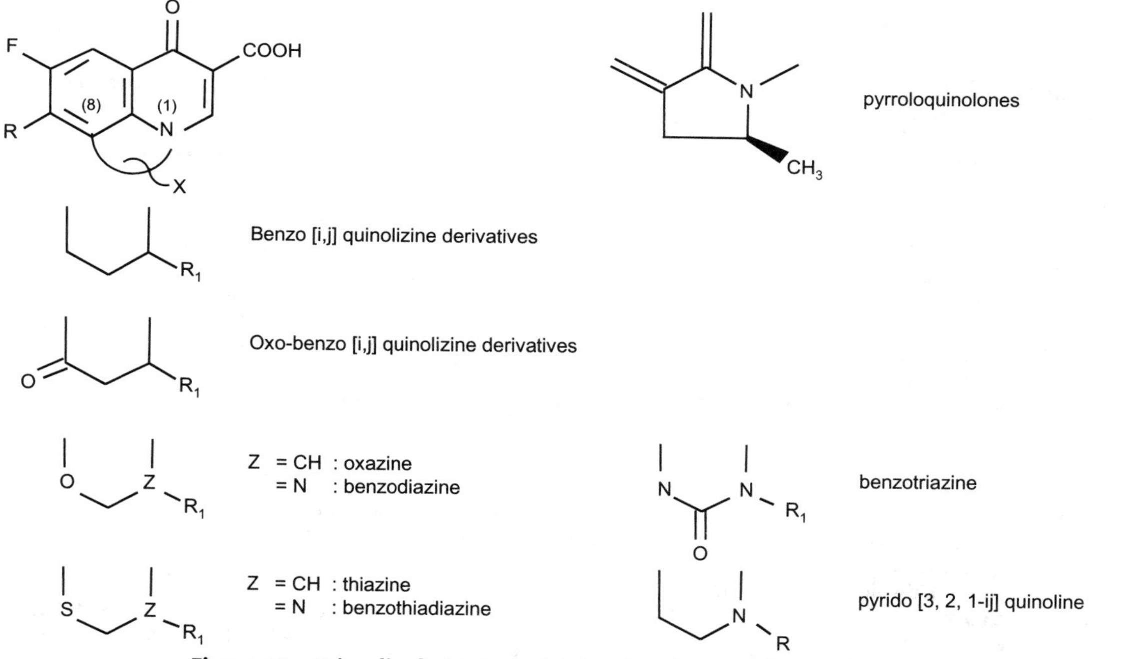

Figure 35 Tricyclic derivatives: 1,8 bond at the quinoline nucleus

to the action of pH. The clinical significance of these phenomena remains to be determined.

5.1.2. Effect of Urine

The standard use of 4-quinolones is in the treatment of complicated and noncomplicated upper or lower urinary tract infections. Tests to determine the in vitro activity of these molecules have been conducted in culture media supplemented with urine.

The fluoroquinolones are less active in urine than in standard culture media, with the MICs being increased 8- to 64-fold. For a number of molecules this reduction in activity may be partly explained by their reduced activity at acidic pH. This is true with all molecules: ciprofloxacin, ofloxacin, enoxacin, and pefloxacin. However, pH alone

Figure 36 Tetracyclic derivatives

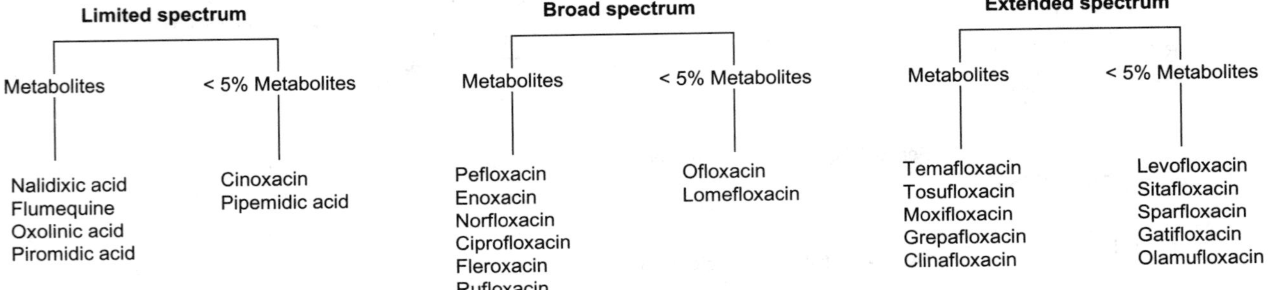

Figure 37 Biological classification of fluoroquinolones

is not sufficient to explain these modifications of activity. The presence of a high concentration of magnesium ions in the urine is one of the main causes of the increase in MIC; the usual level of divalent ions in the urine is 8 to 10 mM, whereas in a standard Mueller-Hinton medium it is 0.3 mM. However, therapeutically the MICs are always lower than the concentrations obtained on elimination of these drugs.

5.1.3. Other Tissues and Fluids

The pH also varies in the bronchial secretions of infected patients. The same applies to bone tissue in patients with osteomyelitis. The pH is usually acidic, and this environment may affect the activity of the fluoroquinolones.

The effect of the pH of the peritoneal dialysis fluid on the activity of ciprofloxacin against *S. aureus* and coagulase-negative staphylococci has been studied. The activity against coagulase-negative staphylococci is slightly reduced. In the dialysate at pH 5.5, the activity of ciprofloxacin against *E. coli* and *P. aeruginosa* is reduced, although it still remains at therapeutic levels.

5.1.4. Effect of Cations

The content of the culture media in terms of magnesium and calcium ions substantially affects the MICs and minimum bactericidal concentrations (MBCs). An excessive presence of magnesium ions causes a reduction in antibacterial activity. This antagonism is less important with molecules that do not have a 7-piperazinyl nucleus.

This effect is more marked in terms of the MICs for *P. aeruginosa*, in a fashion similar to that of the aminoglycosides. The MICs for *Enterobacteriaceae*, *P. aeruginosa*, and *S. aureus* increase eightfold in the presence of 10 mM magnesium ions in Mueller-Hinton medium. The same applies in the presence of 2.4 mM calcium ions. It is impossible to increase the calcium content further, since beyond this limit it forms a precipitate in Mueller-Hinton medium (Table 8).

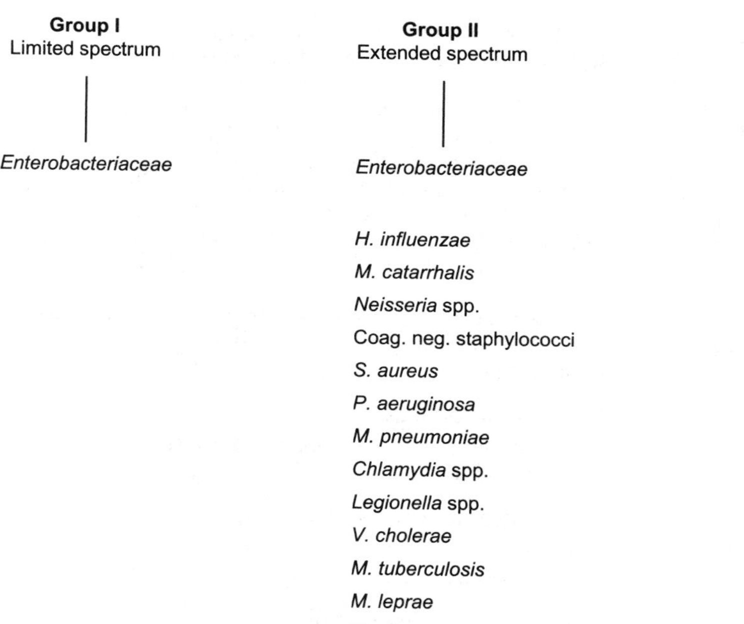

Figure 38 Microbiological classification of fluoroquinolones

Table 6 Physicochemical properties of quinolones

Drug	Mol wt	pK 1	pK 2	pI	Ionic type
Ofloxacin	360.4	5.7	7.9	7.14	Amphoteric
Ciprofloxacin	331.4	6	8.8	7.42	Amphoteric
Norfloxacin	319.3	6.3	8.7	7.34	Amphoteric
Pefloxacin	333.4	6.3	7.6	6.9	Amphoteric
Lomefloxacin	351.3	5.99	9.01	7.56	Amphoteric
Fleroxacin	369.34	5.5	8.1	6.78	Amphoteric
Sparfloxacin	392.4	6.25	9.3		Amphoteric
Temafloxacin	417.4	5.75	8.7	7.18	Amphoteric
Tosufloxacin	404.3	5.8	8.7		Amphoteric
Rufloxacin	363.4	5.6	8.75		Amphoteric
Difloxacin	399.4	6.06	7.63	6.85	Amphoteric
Enoxacin	320.3	6.31	8.69	7.5	Amphoteric
Amifloxacin	334.35	6.28	7.39	6.84	Amphoteric
Levofloxacin	361.3	5.3	8	6.8	Amphoteric
Sitafloxacin	409.82				Amphoteric
Moxifloxacin	437.9	6.4	9.5		Amphoteric
Grepafloxacin	359.4	7.1	7.8	7.95	Amphoteric
Gatifloxacin	402.42				Amphoteric
Trovafloxacin	416.36	5.87	8.09	6.98	Amphoteric
Clinafloxacin	332.33				Amphoteric
Ecenofloxacin	408.86				Amphoteric
Prulifloxacin	349.39				Amphoteric
Prulifloxacin ester	461.46				Amphoteric
Pazufloxacin					Amphoteric
Nalidixic acid	232.2	0.86	5.99		Acid
Pipemidic acid	303.3	5.8	8.7		Amphoteric
Oxolonic acid	261.2		6.9		Acid
Flumequine	261.26	6.2			Acid
Piromidic acid	288.3	5.78			Amphoteric
Cinoxacin	262.2		4.7		Acid
Miloxacin	263.2				Acid
Rosoxacin	312.3				Acid

Table 7 Physicochemical properties of quinolones

Hydrophilic derivatives (logP < 0.01)	Weakly hydrophilic derivatives (logP = 0.1–2)	Hydrophobic derivatives (logP > 2)
Ciprofloxacin	Miloxacin	Nalidixic acid
Norfloxacin	Ofloxacin	Oxolonic acid
Enrofloxacin	Tosufloxacin	Piromidic acid
Pipemidic acid	Pefloxacin	Difloxacin
E-4695	Sparfloxacin	Rosoxacin
E-4868	Rufloxacin	Clinafloxacin
Lomefloxacin	Temafloxacin	Sitafloxacin
	Grepafloxacin	DU-6688
	Fleroxacin	Trovafloxacin
	Gatifloxacin	
	Levofloxacin	
	Tosufloxacin	
	AM-1174	
	BMY-43748	
	Moxifloxacin	

5.1.5. Effect of Inoculum Size

If the size of the bacterial inoculum is increased, the MICs are changed little, if at all, whereas the bactericidal activity is altered. The bactericidal activity decreases beyond 10^8 CFU/ml, and the 4-quinolones become bacteriostatic beyond 10^{10} CFU/ml (Fig. 40). It has been shown that the bactericidal activity of the fluoroquinolones against *S. pneumoniae* decreases when the size of the bacterial inoculum increases.

5.2. Gram-Positive Cocci and Bacilli

5.2.1. *Staphylococcus* spp.

The majority of fluoroquinolones have good antistaphylococcal activity (Table 9).

The activity of some fluoroquinolones has been tested against strains of *S. aureus* of reduced susceptibility to vancomycin in vitro and in vivo. Their activity is reduced against the ATCC 29213 strain of *S. aureus*, which is susceptible to vancomycin and the fluoroquinolones (Table 10).

In an experimental abscess model in CD-1 mice, the Michigan strain proved nonvirulent. The median protective doses (PD_{50}) for clinafloxacin were 14 ± 9.0 mg/kg of body weight and 15.0 ± 4.6 mg/kg for the Mu 50 and New Jersey strains, respectively, and the PD_{50} were >100 mg/kg with ciprofloxacin.

Clinafloxacin appears to possess the best activity against these strains, albeit very reduced compared to that against normal strains.

5.2.2. *Streptococcus* spp.

The activity of fluoroquinolones against streptococci is shown in Table 11.

5.2.3. *Enterococcus* spp.

The in vitro activity of fluoroquinolones against *Enterococcus* spp. is demonstrated in Table 12.

5.3. Gram-Positive Bacilli

The in vitro activity of some fluoroquinolones against gram-positive bacteria is reported in Table 13.

The fluoroquinolones have moderate activity against *Listeria monocytogenes* (MIC, ≥2.0 μg/ml) Table 14.

Against *Corynebacterium diphtheriae* (MIC_{50}, 0.03 to 0.25 μg/ml), the activity is variable. For *Corynebacterium jeikeium* the MICs are ~0.50 μg/ml for ciprofloxacin, ofloxacin, and temafloxacin and >1.0 μg/ml for pefloxacin and lomefloxacin.

For *Rhodococcus equi* the MICs are between 0.25 and 0.5 μg/ml for ciprofloxacin and ≥2.0 μg/ml for the other 4-quinolones. MICs of 1.0 μg/ml were reported for moxifloxacin, trovafloxacin, and ciprofloxacin.

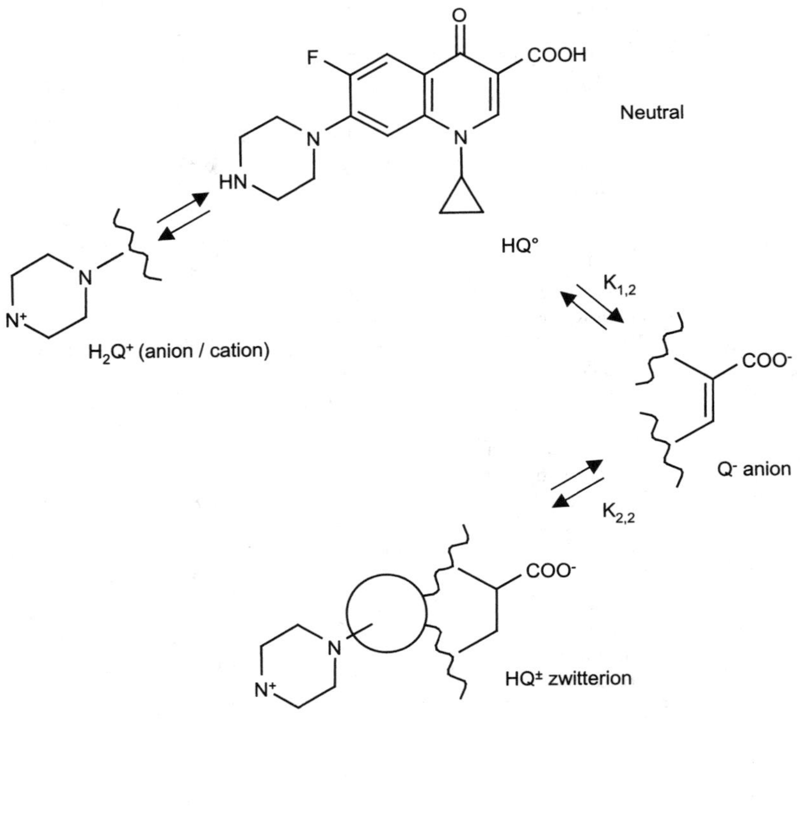

Figure 39 Ionization of quinolones: pH effect

Table 8 Effects of cations on the activity of ofloxacin and levofloxacin in Mueller-Hinton broth[a]

Microorganism	Drug	MIC (μg/ml)		
		Alone	+4.5 mM Ca^{2+}	+9 mM Mg^{2+}
E. coli 5800	Ofloxacin	0.03	0.06	0.25
	Levofloxacin	0.03	0.03	0.12
K. pneumoniae 8708	Ofloxacin	0.03	0.12	0.5
	Levofloxacin	0.03	0.06	0.25
E. cloacae 80	Ofloxacin	0.5	0.5	1
	Levofloxacin	0.25	0.12	0.5
S. marcescens 86	Ofloxacin	0.12	0.25	1
	Levofloxacin	0.12	0.12	0.5
P. aeruginosa 158	Ofloxacin	1	1	4
	Levofloxacin	0.5	0.5	2

[a]Data from Neu et al., 1989.

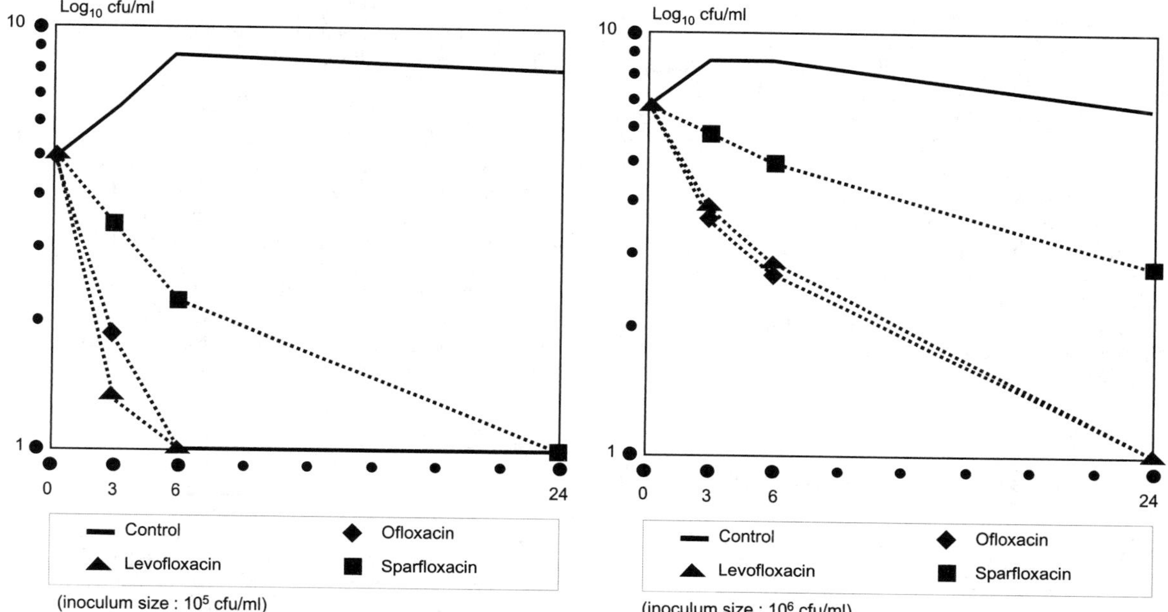

Figure 40 ***S. pneumoniae*** **2816 (cefotaxime resistant) (killing pharmacokinetics) (adapted from Baquero et al., 1996; HMR data on file)**

Table 9 In vitro activities of fluoroquinolones against *Staphylococcus* spp.

Microorganism	MIC$_{50}$ (μg/ml)[a]										
	OFX	LVX	CIP	PEF	TEM	MXF	CLX	GRX	SPX	SIT	GAT
MSSA	0.5	0.25	0.25	0.5	0.01	0.06	0.5	0.12	0.06	0.03	0.12
S. epidermidis Met[s]	0.5	0.25	0.5	0.5	0.03	0.06	0.06	0.12	0.12		2
Staphylococcus haemolyticus	0.25	0.12	0.12		1	0.06	0.06	0.06	0.12		2
S. saprophyticus	1	0.5	0.25		0.12	0.12	0.03	0.12	0.12		0.25
Staphylococcus capitis	0.5	0.25	0.25		0.12	0.03			0.12		0.12
S. warneri	0.5	0.25	0.25		0.03	0.03	0.06		0.06		0.12
Staphylococcus hominis	0.5	0.12	0.25		0.03	0.06	0.06	0.03	0.06		0.12
Staphylococcus lugdunensis	0.5	0.25	0.25						0.06		
Staphylococcus simulans	0.25	0.12	0.12		0.06	0.03	0.03		0.06		0.06

[a]OFX, ofloxacin; LVX, levofloxacin; CIP, ciprofloxacin; PEF, pefloxacin; TEM, temafloxacin; MXF, moxifloxacin; CLX, clinafloxacin; GRX, grepafloxacin; SPX, sparfloxacin; SIT, sitafloxacin; GAT, gatifloxacin.

Table 10 Activities of fluoroquinolones against strains of *S. aureus* of reduced susceptibility to vancomycin

Drug	MIC (μg/ml)			
	Japan Mu50	Michigan 97 A1: 963 sm	New Jersey 992	ATCC 29213
Ciprofloxacin	32	64	32	0.25
Ofloxacin	16	64	32	0.5
Sparfloxacin	16	16	8	0.06
Levofloxacin	8	32	16	0.25
Grepafloxacin	16	16	8	0.03
Trovafloxacin	2	1	2	0.01
Clinafloxacin	0.5	1	0.5	0.01

Ciprofloxacin has proved to be active in the treatment of *Erysipelothrix rhusiopathiae* endocarditis (MIC, 0.03 μg/ml).

Against the genus *Nocardia*, the activity of the fluoroquinolones varies with the species, but the activity is moderate for *Nocardia asteroides* (MIC, ≥2.0 μg/ml). They are inactive against *Nocardia brasiliensis* (MIC, ≥4.0 μg/ml), *Nocardia otiditiscaviarum* (MIC, ≥8.0 μg/ml), and *Nocardia nova* (MIC, ≥16.0 μg/ml). The activity is moderate against *Nocardia farcinica* (MICs, ≥0.39 to 1.56 μg/ml for tosufloxacin, ciprofloxacin, and ofloxacin and >16.0 μg/ml for norfloxacin and enoxacin).

The activity of ciprofloxacin against *Leuconostoc citreum* is 2.0 μg/ml, but the MICs of sparfloxacin, trovafloxacin, and gatifloxacin are between 0.12 and 0.5 μg/ml. The activity against *Pediococcus* spp. is moderate (Table 13). For *Lactobacillus*, the MICs of moxifloxacin, trovafloxacin and ciprofloxacin were 0.125, 05, and 0.125 to 16 μg/ml, respectively.

5.3.1. *Bacillus anthracis*

The in vitro activities of fluoroquinolones and other antibacterials are reported in Tables 15 and 16. MICs are against the vegetative form (Bryskier, 2002).

5.4. *Enterobacteriaceae*

The fluoroquinolones are active against *Enterobacteriaceae*, including strains resistant to third-generation (extended-spectrum) cephalosporins by β-lactamase production, but not those that are resistant as a result of an abnormality of membrane permeability. The activity of the fluoroquinolones against nalidixic acid-resistant strains is reduced but may remain within the range of therapeutic efficacy. In fact, it has been shown that the activity differs according to the susceptibility to nalidixic acid. When the MICs of nalidixic acid are greater than 128 μg/ml, the (geometric) MICs are greater than 2 μg/ml for ciprofloxacin and greater than 15 μg/ml for lomefloxacin. For the majority of strains of *Enterobacteriaceae*, the fluoroquinolones have MICs of ≤0.5 μg/ml. The modal MICs are 0.016 μg/ml for ciprofloxacin, 0.06 μg/ml for ofloxacin and norfloxacin, and 0.12 μg/ml for amifloxacin, difloxacin, enoxacin, fleroxacin, pefloxacin, and lomefloxacin (Table 17). It is 4.0 μg/ml for nalidixic acid.

5.5. Other Gram-Negative Bacilli

The fluoroquinolones have limited activity against the majority of strains of *P. aeruginosa* (MICs between 0.25 and 2.0 μg/ml). The activity against *Pseudomonas fluorescens* (MIC, ~0.5 μg/ml) and *Brevundimonas putida* (MIC, ~0.5 μg/ml) is good, except for fleroxacin (MIC, ~2.0 μg/ml). They are inactive against *Burkholderia pseudomallei* (MIC, ≥4.0 μg/ml). Against *Acinetobacter* spp. the activity is variable, the MICs being 0.25 μg/ml for ciprofloxacin and ofloxacin and 2.0 and 4.0 μg/ml for pefloxacin and norfloxacin, respectively. They are inactive against *Stenotrophomonas maltophilia* (MIC,

Table 11 Activities of fluoroquinolones against streptococci

Organism(s)	MIC_{50} (μg/ml)[a]												
	OFX	LVX	CIP	PEF	LOM	TEM	MXF	GRE	SIT	SPX	CLX	GAT	FLE
S. pyogenes	1	0.5	0.5	4	4	0.12	0.12	0.5	0.03	0.25	0.12	0.25	4
Streptococcus agalactiae	2	1	1		8	0.12	0.25	0.25	0.06	0.5	0.12	0.25	8
Group C and G streptococci	1	0.5		4	4	0.12	0.12	0.5	0.01	2	0.12	0.2	4
Viridans group streptococci	4	1	0.5		4	0.12	0.25	0.5	0.03	0.25	0.12	0.25	4

[a]LOM, lomefloxacin; FLE, fleroxacin; for other abbreviations, see Table 9, footnote *a*.

Table 12 In vitro activities of fluoroquinolones against *Enterococcus* spp.

Organism	MIC_{50} (μg/ml)												
	OFX	LVX	CIP	PEF	LOM	TEM	MXF	GRE	SIT	SPX	CLX	GAT	FLE
E. faecalis	2	1	1	4	4	0.25	0.5	0.5	0.06	0.5	0.008	0.5	4
E. faecalis Van[r]	2	1	1			1			0.25	0.5	0.12	0.25	
E. faecium	8	2	2		8	0.5	2	4	1	1	0.12	2	8
E. faecium VanA	>128	64	64			8	2			64	2	16	
Enterococcus casseliflavus	4	2	1							0.5	2	0.25	
Enterococcus avium	4	2	1					0.25		1	2		
Enterococcus gallinarum	4	2	2				0.5			0.5	0.5	1	
Enterococcus raffinosus	2	1	1						2	0.5	2		

[a]See Table 11, footnote *a*.

Table 13 In vitro activities of fluoroquinolones against gram-positive bacilli

Organism(s)	MIC (μg/ml)[a]									
	OFX	LVX	CIP	SPX	TEM	MXF	GRE	CLX	SIT	GAT
C. diphtheriae	0.25	0.12	0.06		0.03	0.03				
Lactobacillus spp.	2	1	1	0.25	0.5	0.5				16
Pediococcus spp.	16	8	16	4	2	2				4
Leuconostoc spp.	2	2	2	0.5	0.25	0.12				0.25
E. rhusiopathiae	0.25	0.12	0.06	0.03						
Nocardia spp.	8	4								
L. monocytogenes	2	1	0.5	1	0.12	0.25	1	0.25	0.5	1
Bacillus spp.	0.12	0.12	0.12	0.06	0.03					
C. jeikeium	1	0.25	2	0.12	2	2		0.12	0.03	
Stomatococcus spp.	2	1	0.25	0.01				0.03		
Corynebacterium minutissimum	0.25	0.12	0.03	2				0.01		
Corynebacterium striatum	4	2	4	2				0.12		
Corynebacterium xerosis	2	4	2	1				0.06		
Corynebacterium urealyticum	8	4	4					0.06		
R. equi	2	2	0.5	0.25	0.5	8				
Micrococcus spp.	2	1	2							

[a]For abbreviations, see Table 9, footnote *a*.

Table 14 Fluoroquinolones and *L. monocytogenes*[a]

Compound	*n*	MIC (μg/ml)	
		50%	90%
Trovafloxacin	15	0.25	0.25
Levofloxacin	15	1.0	1.0
Ciprofloxacin	15	1.0	1.0
ABT-492	15	0.12	0.12
Gatifloxacin	26	0.5	0.5
Garenoxacin	17	0.5	0.5
Moxifloxacin	17	0.5	0.5
Ofloxacin	17	2.0	2.0
Ciprofloxacin	17	1.0	1.0

[a]Data from Fung-Tomc et al., 2000.

Table 15 In vitro activities of quinolones against *B. anthracis*

Fluoroquinolone	*n*	MIC (μg/ml)	
		50%	90%
Ciprofloxacin	74	0.06	0.06
	28	0.03	0.03
	96	0.06	0.06
	22	0.06	0.06
	18	0.25	2.0
	96	0.125	0.25
	18	0.25	1.0
Gatifloxacin	1		
	20	0.12	0.12
Trovafloxacin	1		
Pefloxacin	96	0.125	0.5
Nalidixic acid	96	4.0	8.0
Ofloxacin	96	0.25	0.25
	22	0.06	0.06
	18	1.0	2.0
Sparfloxacin	18	0.5	0.5

Table 16 In vitro activities of quinolones and other antibacterials against *B. anthracis*[a]

Antibacterial	MIC (μg/ml)
Erythromycin A	0.20
Roxithromycin	0.39
Azithromycin	0.39
Clarithromycin	0.10
Josamycin	0.20
Midecamycin	0.39
Miokamycin	0.78
Rokitamycin	0.20
Leucomycin	0.39
Dalfopristin-quinupristin	0.20
Teicoplanin	0.20
Vancomycin	1.56
Minocycline	0.10
Nalidixic acid	6.25
Pipemidic acid	1.56
Miloxacin	3.13
Norfloxacin	0.39
Ofloxacin	0.10
D-Ofloxacin	0.10
Levofloxacin	0.05
Sparfloxacin	0.05
Tosufloxacin	0.01
Pazufloxacin	0.05
Balofloxacin	0.05
Lomefloxacin	0.20
Enoxacin	0.39
Fleroxacin	0.39
Grepafloxacin	0.025

[a]Data from Bryskier, 2002.

~4.0 μg/ml), except clinafloxacin and moxifloxacin (MIC_{50}, ~0.5 μg/ml), and against *B. cepacia*, *Alcaligenes odorans*, and *Alcaligenes faecalis* (Table 18). They are active against *Agrobacter* spp. (MIC_{50}, ~0.25 μg/ml).

Table 17 In vitro activities of fluoroquinolones against *Enterobacteriaceae*

Organism	MIC$_{50}$ (μg/ml)[a]												
	OFX	LVX	CIP	PEF	SPX	TEM	MXF	GRE	CLX	GAT	LOM	SIT	FLE
E. coli	0.06	0.03	0.01	0.12	0.03	0.03	0.06	0.06	≤0.008	0.03	0.12	0.008	0.03
K. pneumoniae	0.25	0.12	0.03	0.12	0.06	0.06	0.12	0.03	0.01	0.06	0.25	0.03	0.12
Klebsiella oxytoca	0.06	0.03	0.01	0.12		0.03	0.12	0.12	≤0.008	0.03	0.25	0.03	0.12
C. freundii	0.25	0.25	0.03	0.5	0.06	0.06	0.12	0.12	0.01	0.06	0.25	0.03	0.12
S. marcescens	0.25	0.12	0.12	0.5	0.25	0.25	0.25	0.25	0.03	0.25	0.25	0.06	0.25
M. morganii	0.06	0.03	0.03	0.12	0.12	0.25	0.25	0.12	≤0.008	0.06	0.5	0.008	0.03
E. cloacae	0.12	0.06	0.01	0.12	0.03	0.01	0.06	0.03	0.01	0.06	0.12	0.03	0.12
Enterobacter aerogenes	0.25	0.06	0.03	0.12	0.03	0.06	0.12	0.06	0.01	0.06	0.25	0.06	0.12
P. stuartii	1	0.25	2	0.5	0.25	8	4	0.12	0.25	0.12	0.25	0.06	0.12
Providencia rettgeri	0.06	0.5	0.06		0.25	0.25	0.12	0.25	0.03	0.12	1	0.008	0.5
Protens mirabilis	0.12	0.06	0.03	0.25	0.25	0.06	0.25	0.25	0.01	0.12	2		0.12
Y. enterocolitica	0.12	0.06	0.03	0.12	0.06	0.03	0.12	0.03	0.008	0.03	0.25	0.06	0.12
Hafnia alvei	0.06	0.03	0.03		0.06	0.03	0.12		0.03	0.03			0.06

[a]See Table 11, footnote *a*.

Table 18 In vitro activities of fluoroquinolones against nonfermentative gram-negative bacilli

Organism(s)	MIC (μg/ml)[a]									
	OFX	CIP	LVX	SPX	TEM	CLX	CAZ	IMP	GAT	MXF
P. aeruginosa	2	0.25	0.5	1	0.5	0.12	2	1	2	4
Pseudomonas fluorescens/putida	2	0.25	1	1	1	0.25	4	2	0.5	1
B. cepacia	16	8	8	4	8	2	8	16	4	4
S. maltophilia	4	4	2	1	1	0.25	64	256	1	0.5
A. faecalis/odorans	4	4	2	2	4	0.5	8	1	0.5	
Alcaligenes xylosoxidans	16	8	8	8	32	2	16	1	8	4
Moraxella/Oligella	0.25	0.06	0.06	0.06	0.12	0.01	2	0.12		
Acinetobacter spp.	0.5	0.25	0.25	0.06	0.03	0.06	4	2	0.12	0.06
Pseudomonas stutzeri	0.5	0.06	0.12	0.12	4	0.01	1	0.5	0.12	0.25
Brevundimonas diminuta	16	16	8	1	0.25	2	128	1		
Mycoides odoratus	4	4	2	0.5	1	1	>128	16		
Chryseobacterium meningosepticum	4	2	2	0.5	0.12	1	128	8	0.12	
C. indologenes/gleum	2	1	1	0.25	0.25	0.5	16	32		
Other GNB[b]	2	0.5	1	0.25	0.25	0.25	16	0.5		
Ralstonia pickettii	1	0.25	0.5		0.12	0.25			0.25	0.12

[a]CAZ, ceftazidime; IMP, imipenem; for other abbreviations, see Table 9, footnote *a*.
[b]GNB, gram-negative bacilli: *Shewanella putrefaciens, Sphingomonas paucimobilis, Pseudomonas alcaligenes, R. pickettii, Pseudomonas mendocina, Brevundimonas vesicularis, Flavimonas oryzihabitans, Chromobacterium violaceum, Methylobacterium* spp., *Comamonas acidovorans, Comamonas testosteroni, Sphingobacterium multivorum, Agrobacterium radiobacter, Moraxella osloensis, Moraxella phenylpyruvica, Moraxella nonliquefaciens*, and *Oligella urethralis*.

5.5.1. Gram-Negative Bacilli Responsible for Gastrointestinal Infections

The activity of the fluoroquinolones against gram-negative bacilli responsible for intestinal infections is good: *Vibrio cholerae* (MICs, 0.002 to 0.05 μg/ml), *Plesiomonas shigelloides* and *V. parahaemolyticus* (MIC, ~0.06 μg/ml), *Aeromonas hydrophila* (MIC, ~0.015 μg/ml), and *Aeromonas caviae* (MIC, ~0.125 μg/ml). The activity against *C. jejuni* and *Campylobacter coli* is good (MIC, ~0.25 μg/ml), as is the activity against *Yersinia enterocolitica* (MIC$_{50}$, ≤0.12 μg/ml).

5.5.2. *H. pylori*

The in vitro activity of the different fluoroquinolones is moderate (MIC$_{50}$ of ciprofloxacin, 0.25 μg/ml; MIC$_{50}$ of ofloxacin, 1.0 μg/ml). The concentrations of ciprofloxacin, ofloxacin, and enoxacin in the gastric mucosa have been determined. The mean concentration of ofloxacin is 5.0 mg/kg. In therapeutic terms, monotherapy is disappointing, and a combination with an antiulcer agent (omeprazole or lansoprazole) might be interesting.

Y-34867 is a 7-morpholine derivative with in vitro activity comparable to that of amoxicillin and clarithromycin against *H. pylori* ATCC 43504. The MIC is 0.025 μg/ml for these three derivatives, whereas the MIC of sparfloxacin, levofloxacin, and tosufloxacin is 0.3 μg/ml.

In vivo in a murine model (ICR mouse), the activity of Y-34867 was 30 times greater than that of clarithromycin. Bacterial eradication (*H. pylori* 1907) was obtained with a dose of 3 mg/kg every 12 h for 7 days, whereas there was only 80% eradication with 100 mg of clarithromycin per kg. No bacterial eradication was obtained with 100 mg of amoxicillin per kg (Fig. 41).

For garenoxacin, moxifloxacin, levofloxacin, and trovafloxacin, MICs ranged from 0.03 to 0.25 μg/ml.

5.5.3. Other Gram-Negative Bacilli

The mean MIC for *Moraxella lacunata*, responsible for ocular infections, is 0.25 μg/ml. The activity against *Bordetella pertussis* (MIC, ~0.12 μg/ml) and *Bordetella parapertussis* (MIC, ~0.50 μg/ml) is good, whereas against *Bordetella bronchiseptica* (MIC, ~4.0 μg/ml) it is variable. *Chryseobacterium* spp. and *Mycoides* (formerly classified as *Flavobacterium*) in the family of *Cytophagaceae* is a heterogeneous group of nonfermentative gram-negative bacilli. They are responsible for neonatal meningitis and severe infections in immunosuppressed patients. MIC_{50}s of 1.0, 0.25, 0.25, and 2.0 μg/ml were reported for levofloxacin, sparfloxacin, clinafloxacin, and ciprofloxacin, respectively (Tables 18 to 20).

The in vitro activity of the fluoroquinolones against *Pasteurella multocida* is good (MIC_{50}s, 0.01 to 0.12 μg/ml), which is also the case in clinical use. Ofloxacin, ciprofloxacin, and pefloxacin have good activity against *Francisella tularensis* (MICs, 0.12 to 2.0 μg/ml). Ciprofloxacin has good activity against *Haemophilus aphrophilus* (MIC, 0.3 μg/ml). Against *Eikenella corrodens*, which is responsible for infections

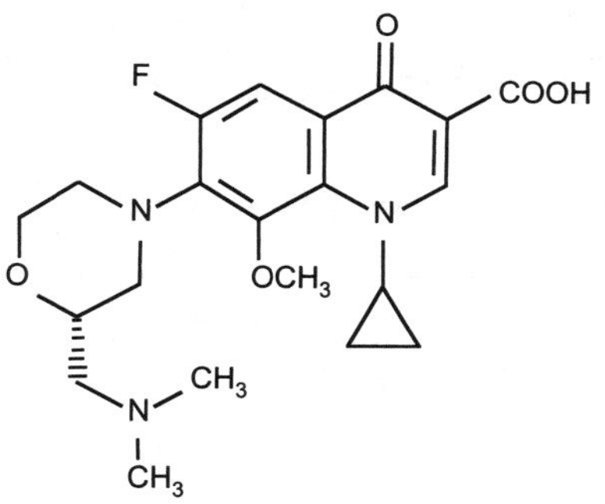

Y-34867

In vitro* activity - *H. pylori

	MIC_{50} (μg/ml)
Y-34867	0.025
Levofloxacin	0.39
Sparfloxacin	0.20
Amoxicillin	0.012
Clarithromycin	0.025

***In vivo* (murine infection - *H. pylori* 1907)**

	MIC (μg/ml)	Dose (mg/kg bid day 7)	Clearance (%)
Control	-	-	0
Y-34867	0.025	3	100
		10	100
Amoxicillin	0.39	30	100
		100	100
Clarithromycin	0.05	30	0
		100	80

Figure 41 Activity of Y-34867 against *H. pylori*

Table 19 In vitro activities of fluoroquinolones against nonfermentative gram-negative rods[a]

Organism(s)	*n*	MIC_{50} (μg/ml)[b]					
		TVA	CIP	OFX	LVX	SPX	CLX
P. aeruginosa	89	0.5	0.25	2.0	1.0	1.0	0.25
P. putida/fluorescens	13	1.0	0.25	2.0	1.0	1.0	0.25
B. cepacia	49	8.0	8.0	16	8.0	4.0	2.0
S. maltophilia	82	1.0	4.0	4.0	2.0	1.0	0.5
Acinetobacter spp.	52	0.06	0.5	0.5	0.5	0.06	0.125
A. faecalis	27	4.0	4.0	4.0	2.0	2.0	0.5
A. xylosoxidans	40	32	8.0	16	8.0	8.0	2.0
Moraxella/Oligella	9	0.125	0.06	0.25	0.06	0.06	0.016
P. stutzeri	10	0.125	0.06	0.5	0.125	0.125	0.016
B. diminuta	11	4.0	16	16	8.0	1.0	2.0
M. odoratus	12	0.25	4.0	4.0	2.0	0.5	1.0
C. meningosepticum	10	1.0	2.0	4.0	2.0	0.5	1.0
C. indologenes/gleum	9	0.125	1.0	2.0	1.0	0.25	0.5

[a]Data from Visalli et al., 1997.
[b]TVA, trovafloxacin; for other abbreviations, see Table 9, footnote *a*.

following human bites or endocarditis, the activity of the fluoroquinolones is good (MIC_{50}, ~0.03 μg/ml). The in vitro activity of fluoroquinolones against *B. pertussis* has been determined and is reported in Table 20.

5.6. Other Pathogenic Agents

5.6.1. *Rickettsia* spp.

The standard treatment of rickettsiosis is based on the administration of cyclines. However, these are slow acting, and an alternative with more bactericidal drugs would seem beneficial. For *Rickettsia conorii*, which is localized and proliferates in the cytoplasm of the phagocytes, ciprofloxacin and sparfloxacin have a MIC of 0.25 μg/ml, pefloxacin has a MIC of 0.50 μg/ml, and ofloxacin has a MIC of 1.0 μg/ml. For *Rickettsia rickettsii*, the MIC of ciprofloxacin and pefloxacin is 1.0 μg/ml and that of sparfloxacin is 0.25 μg/ml. Ciprofloxacin, ofloxacin, and sparfloxacin have good in vitro activity against *Coxiella burnetii* (see below). Ciprofloxacin has also been used successfully in the treatment of murine typhus (*Rickettsia typhi* or *Rickettsia tsutsugamushi*). For *R. conorii* and *R. rickettsii* the MIC_{50}s are 0.25, 0.5, 0.5, and 1.0 μg/ml for clinafloxacin, pefloxacin, sparfloxacin, and ciprofloxacin, respectively. The studies undertaken by Ives et al. (1997) are summarized in Table 21.

The differences in the activities of the fluoroquinolones according to different authors are due to different methods of determination.

5.6.2. *Bartonella* spp.

Table 22 shows the in vitro activity of fluoroquinolones against *Bartonella* spp.

Table 20 In vitro activities of fluoroquinolones against *B. pertussis*[a]

Compound	No. of strains	MIC_{90} (μg/ml)
Ofloxacin	34	0.12
Ciprofloxacin	34	0.06
Fleroxacin	33	0.12
Enoxacin	33	0.5
Tosufloxacin	6	0.01
Levofloxacin	34	0.06
Sparfloxacin	53	0.03
Clinafloxacin	6	0.03
Trovafloxacin	34	0.06
Moxifloxacin	34	0.03
Grepafloxacin	34	0.03
Gatifloxacin	11	0.03

[a]Data from Hoppe, 1998, and Bauernfeind et al., 1998.

Table 21 In vitro activities of fluoroquinolones against *Rickettsia* spp.[a]

Organism	MIC_{50} (μg/ml)[b]				
	CIP	LVX	OFX	SPX	TVA
Rickettsia akari	5.6	28.8	10.4	23.2	>32
R. conorii	14.7	6	1.4	0.85	>32
Rickettsia prowazekii	3	8	9.4	1.05	>32
R. rickettsii	8	24	32	>32	>32

[a]Data from Ives et al., 1997.
[b]See Table 19, footnote *b*.

Table 22 In vitro activities of fluoroquinolones against *Bartonella*[a]

Organism	MIC_{50} (μg/ml)[b]				
	CIP	LVX	OFX	SPX	TVA
B. elizabethae	20.8	19.2	0.004	>32	>32
B. henselae	15.2	6	0.0078	8	>32
B. quintana	19.2	9.2	16.8	>32	>32

[a]Data from Ives et al., 1997.
[b]See Table 21, footnote *b*.

5.6.3. *C. burnetii*

C. burnetii is the causative agent of Q fever, a zoonosis that may be responsible for atypical pneumonia and hepatitis in humans. Coxiellae, like the rickettsiae, are strictly intracellular bacteria. Coxiellae are localized in the phagolysosome and develop at acidic pH.

The fluoroquinolones possess bacteriostatic activity against the three strains of *C. burnetii* tested in cell culture (Table 23).

5.6.4. *Brucella* spp.

The activity of the fluoroquinolones against *Brucella melitensis* is moderate (MIC_{50}s, 0.25 to 4.0 μg/ml) (Table 24) and not bactericidal.

Table 23 Activities of fluoroquinolones against *C. burnetii*[a]

Compound	Concn (μg/ml)	Strain susceptibility[b]		
		Nine Mile[c]	Q 212[d]	Priscilla[d]
Pefloxacin	1	S	I	R
Ciprofloxacin	1	S	I	I
Ofloxacin	1	S	S	S
	0.125	R	R	R
	0.25	R	R	R
	0.5	I	R	R
	2	S	S	S
Levofloxacin	0.125	R	R	R
	0.25	I	R	R
	0.5	S	R	I
	1	S	I	R
	2	S	S	S

[a]Data from Maurin et al., 1998.
[b]S, susceptible; R, resistant; I, intermediate.
[c]Clinical isolate from acute infection.
[d]Clinical isolate from chronic infection.

Table 24 In vitro activities of fluoroquinolones against *B. melitensis*[a]

Compound	MIC (μg/ml)	
	50%	90%
Ciprofloxacin	1.0	1.0
Ofloxacin	2.0	2.0
Levofloxacin	0.5	0.5
Trovafloxacin	1.0	1.0
Sitafloxacin	0.06	0.06
Moxifloxacin	1.0	1.0
Grepafloxacin	1.0	2.0
Rifampin	1.0	1.0
Doxycycline	0.25	0.25

[a]Data from Trujillano-Martin et al., 1999.

The activity is pH dependent. Clinically the fluoroquinolones are inactive, which is probably explained by the intraphagolysosomal localization of the brucellae and the intracytoplasmic localization of the 4-quinolones. They are totally inactive in vitro against *Brucella abortus* (MIC, ~4.0 μg/ml).

Ofloxacin was administered for 4 weeks or longer at a daily dose of 400 mg to 21 patients suffering from an infection due to *B. melitensis*. The immediate therapeutic results were good, but 15% of patients relapsed within 4 to 5 months of the end of treatment.

5.6.5. *Borrelia* spp.

The fluoroquinolones tested in BSK II medium are inactive in vitro. For *Borrelia burgdorferi*, the MIC_{50}s of ciprofloxacin and ofloxacin are greater than 2.0 μg/ml. Those of nalidixic acid and oxolinic acid are, respectively, 300 and 100 μg/ml. For *Borrelia hermsii*, the MIC of ofloxacin is 2.0 μg/ml. The MICs of moxifloxacin, levofloxacin, and trovafloxacin may reach 4.0 μg/ml, and that of garenoxacin may reach 0.25 μg/ml (Table 25).

5.6.6. *Afipia felis*

A. felis is one of the agents responsible for cat scratch diseases, together with *Bartonella henselae*. It is a gram-negative bacillus that develops in macrophages after inhibition of phagolysosomal fusion. The MIC of ciprofloxacin is on the order of 8.0 μg/ml.

5.6.7. *Yersinia pestis*

Plague is an infectious disease which remains endemic in Southeast Asia, Africa, and Asia; a few sporadic cases are reported each year in the United States. Streptomycin, chloramphenicol, and tetracycline are the reference drugs. Resistant strains have been reported in Madagascar.

The in vitro and in vivo activities of the fluoroquinolones have been demonstrated by several teams. In vitro the fluoroquinolones are more active than the reference molecules (Table 26).

In vivo, Butler (1983) showed that, despite its good activity, the efficacy of ampicillin is inferior to that of streptomycin. Goto et al. (1998) tested the activities of different antibacterial agents against a strain of *Y. pestis* (strain 2) that is very virulent in the mouse (Table 27).

They showed there was no correlation between the in vitro and in vivo activities of the fluoroquinolones in the DDY mouse. Grepafloxacin was the most active molecule in vitro (MIC, 0.008 μg/ml) but the least active in vivo (100% effective dose [ED_{100}], 2 mg/mouse). The most active molecule in vivo was levofloxacin (ED_{100}, 0.08 mg/mouse). In vivo, tetracycline was not active at doses of up to 10 mg/mouse, whereas minocycline was more active in vitro (MIC, 0.5 μg/ml) and in vivo (ED_{100}, 10 mg/mouse). β-Lactams were inactive in vivo. The activity of the aminoglycosides was variable. Gentamicin was more active than arbekacin and isepamicin, the latter resulting in survival of 16.6% of mice at high doses (Table 27).

Table 25 In vitro activities of quinolones against *Borrelia* spp.

Compound	MIC (μg/ml)	
	50%	90%
Nalidixic acid	256	256
Norfloxacin	4.0	8.0
Pefloxacin	16	32
Fleroxacin	>16	>16
Ofloxacin	4.0	8.0
Ciprofloxacin	1.0	2.0
Levofloxacin	2.0	4.0
Grepafloxacin	0.5	0.25
Gatifloxacin	0.25	1.0
Trovafloxacin	0.5	1.0
Moxifloxacin	1.0	2.0
Clinafloxacin	0.5	1.0
Sitafloxacin	0.25	0.5
Gemifloxacin	0.06	0.5
Sparfloxacin	0.5	1.0
Garenofloxacin	0.5	1.0
Ceftriaxone	0.03	0.03

Table 26 In vitro activities of antibiotics against *Y. pestis*[a]

Compound	MIC (μg/ml)	
	50%	90%
Ciprofloxacin	0.03	0.06
Ofloxacin	0.12	0.25
Levofloxacin	<0.03	<0.03
Doxycycline	0.5	1
Tetracycline	2	4
Gentamicin	0.5	1
Streptomycin	4	4
Chloramphenicol	2	4
Rifampin	4	8
Sulfamethoxazole	8	16
Trimethoprim	0.5	1
Penicillin G	1	2
Ampicillin	0.25	0.5
Ceftriaxone	0.01	0.03

[a]Data from Smith et al., 1995, and Klugman et al., 1996.

Table 27 In vivo activities of fluoroquinolones against *Y. pestis*

Compound	MIC (μg/ml)	ED_{100} (mg/mouse)
Oral		
Ofloxacin	0.06	0.4
Ciprofloxacin	0.01	2
Sparfloxacin	0.01	0.4
Grepafloxacin	0.008	2
Prulifloxacin	0.03	2
Pazufloxacin	0.01	2
Levofloxacin	0.03	0.08
Chloramphenicol	8	>10
Ampicillin	0.25	>10
Cefdinir	0.25	>10
Tetracycline	2	>10
Minocycline	0.5	10
Fosfomycin	128	>10
Subcutaneous		
Cefotaxime	0.12	>10
Imipenem-cilastatin	0.25	>10
Panipenem-betamicron	0.25	>10
Gentamicin	1	0.4
Isepamicin	0.5	>10
Arbekacin	0.5	2

A virulent, fluoroquinolone-resistant strain of *Y. pestis* induced following exposure to nalidixic acid has been reported in Russia (mutation rate, 10^{-10} to 10^{-8}). The high intraphagocytic concentrations of the fluoroquinolones and the low MIC might be of considerable interest in the treatment of plague.

5.6.8. *Neisseria meningitidis*

The activity against *N. meningitidis* is excellent (MIC, ~0.015 μg/ml); it has been suggested that fluoroquinolones be used in the chemoprevention of cerebrospinal meningitis (Table 28).

5.6.9. Microaerophilic and Fastidious Organisms

Microaerophilic and fastidious microorganisms might be involved in severe infections in humans. In vitro data for some of them are reported in Table 29.

5.7. Anaerobic Bacteria

The taxonomy of the anaerobic bacteria is constantly changing, and for this reason it is difficult to follow the literature in this field. In addition, the reference media for determining the activities of the antibacterial agents vary with the country and the time; for instance, the medium recommended by the NCCLS in the United States changed in 1998. Previous studies were carried out on Wilkins-Chalgren medium, but since 1998 Brucella medium has been used, the composition of which differs among manufacturers so that it is difficult to standardize the methods for determining the activities of the different molecules.

Among the clinically most important anaerobic bacteria, the following two groups may be identified. The first is gram-negative bacteria such as *Bacteroides* (which contains at least 10 species), *Prevotella* spp., *Porphyromonas* spp., *Fusobacterium* spp., and other species less commonly found in patients, such as *Bilophila* spp., *Sutterella* spp., and *Veillonella* spp. The second is gram-positive bacteria; a distinction can be drawn between gram-positive cocci (*Peptostreptococcus* spp.) and sporulating (*Clostridium* spp.) and nonsporulating (*Propionibacterium*, *Eubacterium*, and *Actinomyces* spp.) gram-positive bacilli.

The activities of the fluoroquinolones vary and depend on the structure of the molecules. However, it appears that the activity is greater when it is determined in heart-brain broth supplemented with 5% laked sheep blood and 1 μg of vitamin K_1 per ml than when obtained in Brucella medium with laked sheep blood or in Wilkins-Chalgren medium. This effect is particularly marked when the molecules have weak activity.

As a general rule, the fluoroquinolones are relatively inactive against strict anaerobic bacterial species or genera.

Ciprofloxacin, ofloxacin, lomefloxacin, pefloxacin, and fleroxacin are inactive against gram-negative bacilli, and the MIC_{50}s are ≥4.0 μg/ml for the *Bacteroides fragilis* group, with the exception perhaps of tosufloxacin (MIC_{50}, ~1.0 μg/ml). The MIC_{50}s are also on the order of 2.0 μg/ml for *Prevotella melaninogenica*, other *Prevotella* spp., and *Fusobacterium* spp. Among the new molecules, grepafloxacin and gatifloxacin may also be considered inactive (MIC_{50}, ≥2 μg/ml). Trovafloxacin, clinafloxacin, and sitafloxacin have good in vitro activity against anaerobic gram-negative bacilli (Table 30).

Against *Mobiluncus* spp., the most active molecules are clinafloxacin and sitafloxacin (MIC_{50} and MIC_{90}, 0.05 and 0.05 μg/ml), as well as sparfloxacin (MIC_{50} and MIC_{90}, 0.10 and 0.10 μg/ml). The activity of levofloxacin (MIC_{50} and MIC_{90}, 0.78 and 0.78 μg/ml) and ciprofloxacin (MIC_{50} and MIC_{90}, 0.39 and 0.39 μg/ml) is moderate.

Table 28 In vitro activities of fluoroquinolones against *N. meningitidis*

Compound	MIC (μg/ml)	
	50%	90%
Ofloxacin	0.01	0.01
Ciprofloxacin	0.004	0.004
Sparfloxacin	0.008	0.008
Flerofloxacin	0.03	0.03
Levofloxacin	0.008	0.008
Trovafloxacin	0.004	0.004
Sitafloxacin	0.002	0.002
Moxifloxacin	0.008	0.015

Table 29 In vitro activities of ABT-492 and comparators against microaerophilic microorganisms

Organism(s)	*n*	MIC (μg/ml)					
		ABT-492		Gatifloxacin		Moxifloxacin	
		50%	90%	50%	90%	50%	90%
Desulfomonas	8	0.12–4		0.25–8		0.12–32	
Desulfovibrio	16	0.12	0.12	0.12	0.5	0.12	1.0
Mitsuokella	1	0.12		0.25		0.5	
Selenomonas	6	0.12		0.25–1.0		0.25–1.0	
Captocytophaga	21	0.12	0.12	0.12	32	0.12	64
Campylobacter gracilis	11	0.12	0.12	0.12	16	0.12	32
Campylobacter rectus	32	0.12	0.5	0.12	32	0.12	64
Actinomyces spp.	14	0.12	0.25	0.2	2.0	1.0	4.0
Actinobacillus actinomycetemcomitans	25	2.0	4.0	0.12	0.12	0.12	0.12
Propionibacterium spp.	5	0.12		0.25–1.0		0.25–0.5	
Gemella morbillorum	30	0.12	0.12	0.25	0.5	0.5	0.5
Streptococcus constellatus	19	0.12	0.12	0.5	1.0	0.25	0.5
Staphylococcus intermedius	41	0.12	0.12	0.5	0.5	0.25	0.5
Streptococcus milleri group	27	0.12	0.12	0.5	1.0	0.25	0.5

Table 30 In vitro activities of fluoroquinolones against anaerobic gram-negative bacteria

Compound	MIC_{50} (μg/ml)				
	B. fragilis	*Bacteroides* spp.	*Prevotella* spp.	*Fusobacterium* spp.	*Porphyromonas* spp.
Ofloxacin	4	8	4	2	4
Ciprofloxacin	4	8	1	1	1
Fleroxacin	16	16		32	8
Lomefloxacin	8	16	4	4	4
Levofloxacin	2	2	2	1	2
Sparfloxacin	2	2	2	1	2
Trovafloxacin	0.12	0.25	2	0.5	2
Grepafloxacin	2	4	2	0.12	2
Moxifloxacin	0.25	0.25	0.25	0.06	0.25
Gatifloxacin	1	1	1	0.05	0.05
Clinafloxacin	0.12	0.12	0.06	0.06	0.06
Sitafloxacin	0.06	0.5	0.12	0.06	0.12

Against gram-positive bacteria, ofloxacin, tosufloxacin, temafloxacin, and ciprofloxacin have good activity against *Peptostreptococcus* spp. (MIC_{50}, ~0.5 μg/ml), with grepafloxacin (MIC_{50}, ~1.0 μg/ml) being the least active molecule. Pefloxacin, norfloxacin, and enoxacin are inactive (MIC, ≥2.0 μg/ml).

They also possess good activity against *Clostridium perfringens* (MIC_{50} between 0.06 μg/ml for clinafloxacin and 0.5 μg/ml for the oldest molecules). Against *Clostridium difficile* the majority of molecules are inactive (MIC_{50}, ≥4.0 μg/ml); pseudomembranous colitis has been described after administration of ciprofloxacin and ofloxacin. Clinafloxacin, sitafloxacin, and trovafloxacin have good in vitro activity against *C. difficile*.

Among fluoroquinolones, it is possible to distinguish molecules with good global in vitro activity against anaerobic bacteria, such as trovafloxacin, clinafloxacin, and sitafloxacin and some under investigation (Tables 30 and 31).

5.7.1. *B. fragilis* Group

The *B. fragilis* group is composed at least of 10 species. Few quinolones have been tested against them (Table 32).

5.8. Agents of Respiratory Tract Infections

The pathogenic agents responsible for lower respiratory tract infections are divided into common pathogens and atypical intracellular agents.

5.8.1. Common Pathogens

See Table 33.

The causative agent of parenchymatous or nonparenchymatous lower respiratory tract infections is principally *S. pneumoniae*, a species against which the fluoroquinolones were reputedly inactive clinically. The other pathogenic agents are *Haemophilus influenzae* (8 to 20%) and, more rarely, *Moraxella catarrhalis* (~1%).

5.8.1.1. *S. pneumoniae*

Two types of fluoroquinolones are currently described: derivatives that cannot be used therapeutically for community-acquired pneumonia, such as ofloxacin, ciprofloxacin, pefloxacin, fleroxacin, lomefloxacin, and enoxacin, and those that are clinically active against pneumococci, whether or not the strains are resistant to penicillin G or erythromycin A. The first molecule to exhibit good antipneumococcal activity was temafloxacin, followed by sparfloxacin. Currently a number of molecules are available for the treatment of pneumococcal infections, such as levofloxacin, trovafloxacin, grepafloxacin, moxifloxacin, gatifloxacin, sitafloxacin, gemifloxacin, and clinafloxacin. Other molecules at the development stage also have good antipneumococcal activity, such as garenoxacin and alumafloxacin (Fig. 6 and 9). The activities of the fluoroquinolones are the

Table 31 In vitro activities of fluoroquinolones against anaerobic gram-positive bacteria

Compound	MIC_{50} (μg/ml)			
	C. perfringens	*C. difficile*	*Peptostreptococcus*	*P. acnes*
Ofloxacin	0.5	8	0.5	0.5
Ciprofloxacin	0.5	8	1	0.5
Fleroxacin	1	16	2	
Levofloxacin	0.25	4	0.25	0.5
Trovafloxacin	0.12	1	0.06	
Grepafloxacin	0.5		1	
Moxifloxacin	0.25	2	0.06	0.25
Gatifloxacin	0.5	2	0.5	0.5
Sparfloxacin	1	8	0.5	0.5
Sitafloxacin	0.12	0.06	0.06	≤0.02
Clinafloxacin	0.06		0.06	
Tosufloxacin	0.25	2	2	2

Table 32 In vitro activities of quinolones against the *B. fragilis* group

Bacteroides species	*n*	MIC50 (µg/ml)		
		Garenoxacin	Trovafloxacin	Moxifloxacin
B. fragilis	289	0.5	0.5	1.0
B. thetaiotaomicron	185	1.0	1.0	2.0
B. distasonis	98	1.0	2.0	1.0
B. ovatus	90	1.0	2.0	4.0
B. vulgatus	86	2.0	2.0	4.0
B. uniformis	26	1.0	2.0	2.0
B. caccae	53	1.0	1.0	1.0
B. eggerthii	1	1.0[a]	1.0[a]	1.0[a]
B. merdae	1	1.0[a]	1.0[a]	1.0[a]
B. stercoris	1	1.0[a]	1.0[a]	1.0[a]

[a]MIC, in micrograms per milliliter.

Table 33 In vitro activities of fluoroquinolones against common pathogens responsible for lower respiratory tract infections

Compound	MIC50 (µg/ml)			
	S. pneumoniae	*H. influenzae*	*M. catarrhalis*	*Haemophilus parainfluenzae*
Ofloxacin	2	0.025	0.12	0.02
Ciprofloxacin	2	0.012	0.03	0.008
Fleroxacin	8	0.03		
Sparfloxacin	0.25	0.012	0.01	0.01
Levofloxacin	1	0.012	0.06	0.01
Grepafloxacin	0.25	≥0.006	0.03	0.01
Tosufloxacin	0.25	≥0.006	0.01	
Gatifloxacin	0.25	0.008	0.03	≤0.03
Moxifloxacin	0.25	0.03	0.12	0.01
Trovafloxacin	0.12	0.01	0.03	0.01
Clinafloxacin	0.12	0.008	0.008	0.008
Gemifloxacin	0.03	≤0.004	0.01	0.01
Sitafloxacin	0.03	≤0.015	≤0.015	

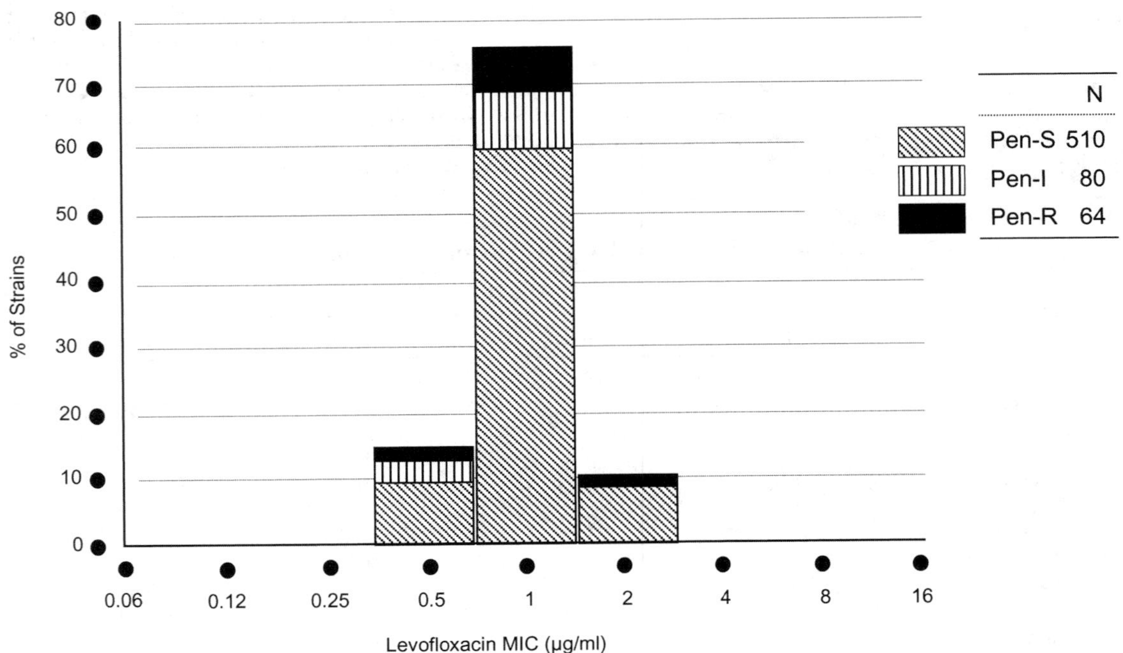

Figure 42 Distribution of the bacterial population of *S. pneumoniae* (654 strains)

same against all strains of *S. pneumoniae*, irrespective of their susceptibility to penicillin G or erythromycin A. These molecules would appear to be more bactericidal against penicillin G-resistant strains but not those resistant to cefotaxime or ceftriaxone (MIC, ≥2 μg/ml). The population distribution of levofloxacin is shown as an example in Fig. 42 (Barry et al., 1996, HMR data on file).

In vitro activity, based on the MIC, does not necessarily reflect clinical activity. Potential activity is assessed on the basis of other parameters, such as the killing kinetics and animal models (pneumonia and meningitis).

The other species conventionally involved are as follow:

- *H. influenzae*, whether the strains are β-lactamase producing or not or resistant to β-lactams through a nonenzymatic mechanism; the fluoroquinolones have excellent activity (MIC, ~0.03 μg/ml). Fluoroquinolone-resistant strains are rare but have been described in Spain for cystic fibrosis patients and in France.
- *M. catarrhalis*, whether the strains are β-lactamase producing or not.

The MICs are between 0.01 and 0.12 μg/ml.

5.8.2. Atypical and Intracellular Microorganisms

Lower respiratory tract infections may be due to obligate or nonobligate (*Lagionella pneumophila*) intracellular agents, or to *Mycobacterium pneumoniae*. Table 34 shows the in vitro activity of fluoroquinolones against these organisms.

5.8.2.1. C. *pneumoniae*

The in vitro activity varies from one molecule to another; however, as with the macrolides, it is difficult to draw a definitive conclusion, as the study methods vary with the authors and as the use of cell media more favorable for bacterial growth may alter the results. The in vitro activity of fluoroquinolones is shown in Table 35.

5.8.2.2. *Chlamydia psittaci*

See Table 36.

The activities of the different molecules must be assessed in in vitro cell lines and in experimental murine pneumonia.

Table 34 In vitro activities of fluoroquinolones against atypical and intracellular bacteria responsible for respiratory tract infections

Compound	MIC_{50} (μg/ml)		
	M. pneumoniae	*C. pneumoniae*	*L. pneumophila*
Ofloxacin	1	0.5	0.015
Ciprofloxacin	2	0.25–4	0.008
Fleroxacin	4	2–8	
Pefloxacin	2	2	0.15
Lomefloxacin	2	0.25	
Levofloxacin	0.5	0.12–0.5	0.008
Sparfloxacin	0.25	0.006–0.5	0.002
Grepafloxacin	0.12	0.006–0.5	≤0.016
Trovafloxacin	0.25	1	≤0.004
Moxifloxacin	0.12	0.06	0.015
Sitafloxacin	0.03	0.06	≤0.03
Enrofloxacin	0.5		
Gatifloxacin	0.06	0.25	0.01
Temafloxacin	1		

Table 35 In vitro activities of fluoroquinolones against *C. pneumoniae*[a]

Compound	MIC (μg/ml)
Garenoxacin	0.015–0.03
Levofloxacin	0.5–1.0
Moxifloxacin	0.125–1.0
Clarithromycin	0.015–0.06
Trovafloxacin[b]	0.5
Ofloxacin[b]	0.5–1.0
Ciprofloxacin[b]	0.5
Gemifloxacin[b]	0.25
Grepafloxacin[c]	0.12
Gatifloxacin[b]	0.12
Trovafloxacin	0.06–0.125
Sparfloxacin	0.06
Olamufloxacin	0.016–0.03
Sitafloxacin	0.03–0.125
Temafloxacin	0.125
WCK 919	0.03–0.06
Norfloxacin	16

[a]Data from Roblin et al., 1999; Kimura et al., 1997; Miyashita et al., 1997; Miyashita et al., 2001; and Niki et al., 1997.
[b]MIC_{50}, in micrograms per milliliter.
[c]MIC_{90}, in micrograms per milliliter.

Table 36 In vitro activities of fluoroquinolones against *C. psittaci*[a]

Compound	MIC (μg/ml)	
	Range	50%
Sitafloxacin	0.03–0.06	0.06
Sparfloxacin	0.03–0.06	0.06
Tosufloxacin	0.125	0.125
Ofloxacin	0.5–1.0	0.5
Ciprofloxacin	1.0–2.0	1.0
Moxifloxacin	0.03–0.125	
Gatifloxacin	0.06	0.06
Levofloxacin	0.125	0.125
Olamufloxacin	0.03	0.03
Temafloxacin	0.06–0.125	
Grepafloxacin	0.06	
Norfloxacin	16	
Doxycycline	0.03	

[a]Data from Miyashita et al., 1997, 2001, 2002; Kimura et al., 1993; and Niki et al., 1997.

Ofloxacin has proved to be clinically active in *C. psittaci* infections at a dose of 600 mg daily for a mean period of 14 days.

Certain fluoroquinolones are more active than erythromycin A, but markedly less than doxycycline or minocycline. Ciprofloxacin and ofloxacin have respective MICs of 0.5 and 1.0 μg/ml, and tosufloxacin has a MIC of 0.06 μg/ml.

The activities of different fluoroquinolones have been determined in experimental murine pneumonia due to the MP strain of *C. psittaci*. After a dose of 10 mg/kg administered 24 h following infection, 100% of mice survived with temafloxacin, sparfloxacin, and minocycline; the figures after ofloxacin and ciprofloxacin were 80 and 75%, respectively. At a dose of 5 mg/kg, mortality rates were 100% with ciprofloxacin and 70% with ofloxacin. There was 100% survival with the other fluoroquinolones.

5.8.2.3. *L. pneumophila*

The activity of ciprofloxacin and ofloxacin against *L. pneumophila* is good (MIC, ≤0.06 μg/ml), while that of pefloxacin is moderate (MIC_{50}, 1.0 μg/ml). The recent molecules are very active against *L. pneumophila* (Table 37).

In pneumonia due to *L. pneumophila* serogroup 1 in guinea pigs, fluoroquinolones have been tested; results are shown in Table 38.

5.8.2.4. *F. tularensis*

In 12 patients, the MICs of ciprofloxacin for *F. tularensis* isolates were 0.0015 to 0.03 μg/ml.

5.8.2.5. *M. pneumoniae* and Other Species

Standardization of MICs is difficult, as *M. pneumoniae* is a pathogenic agent that grows slowly and requires 20% serum for its growth.

The activities of the different fluoroquinolones are variable. For *M. pneumoniae*, ciprofloxacin, lomefloxacin, and pefloxacin have MIC_{50}s of ≥2.0 μg/ml. Enoxacin, ofloxacin, and levofloxacin have MIC_{50}s of ~0.5 μg/ml. Sparfloxacin, trovafloxacin, and grepafloxacin are more active (MIC_{50}s, 0.12 to 0.25 μg/ml) (Table 39).

5.9. Agents of Sexually Transmitted Diseases

The activity of the fluoroquinolones against *N. gonorrhoeae* is excellent, whether the strain is β-lactamase producing or not (penicillinases and cephalosporinases) and whether it is resistant or susceptible to tetracyclines and spectinomycin. The MICs for susceptible strains are ≤0.008 μg/ml. It has been shown with the fluoroquinolones that strains resistant to other antibiotics are slightly less susceptible and vice versa. In the United Kingdom, the incidence of ciprofloxacin-resistant isolates has increased since 1998 depending on the geographical area. This phenomenon is also of concern in Baltic countries and Russia and the European countries of the former Soviet Union.

Table 40 shows the in vitro activity of fluroquinolones against different resistance phenotypes of N. gonorrhoeae.

The clinical activity of fluoroquinolones in chancroid is good, and in fact the MICs for *Haemophilus ducreyi* are on the order of 0.03 μg/ml.

Against the agents responsible for vaginosis, *Gardnerella vaginalis* (MIC, ≥0.5 μg/ml, except for sitafloxacin [MIC_{50} and MIC_{90}, 0.10 and 0.10 μg/ml]) and *Mobiluncus* spp. (MIC_{50} and MIC_{90}, 0.05 to ≥4.0 μg/ml), the activity is variable (Tables 41 and 42).

Prevotella bivia is one of the causative agents of vaginosis. This anaerobic species is relatively nonsusceptible to the action of fluoroquinolones. The molecule that appears to be the most active is trovafloxacin (Table 43).

Chlamydia trachomatis is one of the causes of uterine cervicitis and pelvic inflammatory disease, sequentially related to infertility and ectopic pregnancy in women. The activities of the different molecules against *C. trachomatis*, responsible for nongonococcal urethritis, cervicitis, and certain types of salpingitis, are variable (Table 44).

Ofloxacin has good activity (MIC_{50}, ~0.5 μg/ml), followed by levofloxacin (MIC_{50}, ~1.0 μg/ml). Molecules such as ciprofloxacin (MIC_{50}, 4.0 μg/ml), enoxacin (MIC_{50}, ~16 μg/ml), and norfloxacin (MIC_{50}, ~8.0 μg/ml) are inactive, or weakly active like pefloxacin (MIC, ~2.0 μg/ml). Sitafloxacin, moxifloxacin, gatifloxacin, trovafloxacin, and gemifloxacin have excellent activity (MIC_{50}, 0.06 μg/ml), while for grepafloxacin and gatifloxacin, the MIC_{50}s are, respectively, 0.125 and 0.25 μg/ml. Garenoxacin and levofloxacin MICs are 0.015 and 0.5 μg/ml, respectively. Against *Chlamydia* strain Iol, moxifloxacin has good activity (MIC and minimum chlamydial concentration, 0.06 μg/ml).

Against *Mycoplasma hominis* and *Ureaplasma urealyticum*, the in vitro activities also are variable (Table 45).

The determination of the in vitro activity of antibiotics against *Mycoplasma* spp. is poorly codified. For this reason there are extremely wide interlaboratory variations, hence the need for caution in interpreting the results. Several factors can interfere with the MIC. The use of a broth medium with a pH indicator yields MICs that as a rule are twice as high as when the in vitro activity is determined in a solid medium. The pHs of the media differ for *M. hominis*

Table 37 In vitro activities of fluoroquinolones against *L. pneumophila*[a]

Compound	MIC (μg/ml) 50%	MIC (μg/ml) 90%
Erythromycin A	0.25	2.0
Olamufloxacin	0.008	0.032
Levofloxacin	0.032	0.063
Ciprofloxacin	0.032	0.032
Sparfloxacin	0.008	0.032
Gatifloxacin	0.008–0.03	0.016–0.03
Garenoxacin	0.016	0.06
Moxifloxacin	0.12[b]	
WCK 919	0.06[b]	
Grepafloxacin	0.06[b]	
Trovafloxacin	0.25	0.25
ABT-492	0.12	0.25

[a]Data from Higa et al., 2003.
[b]MIC range, in micrograms per milliliter.

Table 38 In vivo efficacies of fluoroquinolones in pneumonia of guinea pigs due to *L. pneumophila*[a]

Compound	Dose (mg/kg)	Log_{10} CFU/ml/lung 24 h	48 h	72 h	96 h	144 h	192 h
Control		6.4	6.6	6.0	100% mortality		
WCK 1153	10	4	2.3	1.5	1.5	0.36	<1
	30	1.9	1.8	0.4	0.4	0.4	<1
Moxifloxacin	10	4.3	2.0	1.9	1.9	1.6	<1
Levofloxacin	10	2.4	2.0	1.9	1.9	1.6	<1
	30	1.9	0.5	0.4	0.4	<1	<1

[a]Data from Levasseur et al., 2003.

Table 39 In vitro activities of fluoroquinolones against *Mycoplasma* spp.

Organism and compound	*n*	MIC (μg/ml)	
		50%	90%
M. pneumoniae	31		
Garenoxacin		0.06	0.06
Gatifloxacin		0.12	0.25
Moxifloxacin		0.12	0.12
Levofloxacin		0.5	1.0
Ofloxacin		1.0	2.0
Ciprofloxacin		1.0	2.0
Trovafloxacin	11	0.25	
ABT-492	18	0.12	0.12
WCK 919	10	0.015	0.03
M. genitalium	6		
Garenoxacin		0.06–0.12[a]	
Gatifloxacin		0.12[a]	
Moxifloxacin		0.06[a]	
Levofloxacin		0.5[a]	
Ofloxacin		0.5–1.0[a]	
Ciprofloxacin		1.0–2.0[a]	
M. hominis	32		
Garenoxacin		≤0.015	≤0.015
Gatifloxacin		0.12	0.12
Moxifloxacin		0.06	0.12
Levofloxacin		0.5	1.0
Ofloxacin		0.5	1.0
Ciprofloxacin		1.0	2.0
Trovafloxacin	11	0.03	
WCK 919		0.004	0.004
Ureaplama spp.	34		
Garenoxacin		0.12	0.25
Gatifloxacin		0.25	0.5
Moxifloxacin		0.12	0.25
Levofloxacin		0.5	1.0
Ofloxacin		0.5	2.0
Ciprofloxacin		1.0	4.0
Trovafloxacin	11	0.5	
WCK 919		0.03	0.12
M. fermentans[a]	9		
Garenoxacin		≤0.015	
Gatifloxacin		0.12–0.25	
Moxifloxacin		0.06	
Levofloxacin		0.12–1.0	
Ofloxacin		0.25	
Ciprofloxacin		0.25	
M. penetrans[a]	2		
Garenoxacin		≤0.015	
Gatifloxacin		0.06	
Moxifloxacin		0.06–0.12	
Levofloxacin		0.12–0.25	
Ofloxacin		0.12–0.5	
Ciprofloxacin		0.25–1.0	

[a]MIC range, in micrograms per milliliter.

(pH 7.3) and *U. urealyticum* (pH 6.3). The activity of the fluoroquinolones depends on the pH of the culture media; the MICs are lower when the pH is high, which might explain the difference in activity of these molecules against *U. urealyticum* and *M. hominis*.

The mutation in the GyrA subunit (Ser83 → Leu) causes a loss of activity of the fluoroquinolones against *M. hominis*. The *parC* and *parE* genes of *M. hominis* have been cloned and sequenced. The ParC and ParE proteins comprise 639 and 866 amino acids, respectively, and exhibit a high degree of homology with the equivalent proteins of *S. aureus* and *S. pneumoniae*.

The incidence of mutation is 10^{-7} with ofloxacin. The fluoroquinolones would appear to be half as active against *M. pneumoniae* as against *M. hominis*, as the amino acid at position 83 of GyrA is nonpolar and does not have a hydroxyl group (methionine 83). Other *Mycoplasma* species are associated with genitourinary manifestations, such as *Mycoplasma genitalium*, *Mycoplasma fermentans*, and *Mycoplasma penetrans*. The available data are limited (Table 46). *M. penetrans* has been isolated from AIDS patients. Hayes et al. (1995) have shown that of the antibacterial agents tested, only the fluoroquinolones are bactericidal (levofloxacin and ciprofloxacin). The respective MIC_{50}s of levofloxacin and ciprofloxacin are 0.078 and 0.156 μg/ml.

Table 40 In vitro activities of fluoroquinolones against different resistance phenotypes of *N. gonorrhoeae*[a]

Phenotype[b]	No. of strains	MIC_{50} (μg/ml)		
		Ofloxacin	Ciprofloxacin	Trovafloxacin
Pen[b]	28	0.01	0.004	0.004
CMRNG	56	0.06	0.01	0.008
PPNG	67	0.03	0.01	0.008
PP/TR	15	0.01	0.004	0.004
TRNG	17	0.01	0.004	0.004

[a]Data from Knapp et al., 1995.
[b]Pen[s], MIC of ≤0.1 μg/ml; CMRNG, chromosome-mediated resistance; PPNG, penicillin G resistance (β-lactamase); TRNG, tetracycline resistance; PP/TR, penicillin G resistance/tetracycline resistance.

Table 41 In vitro activities of fluoroquinolones against *G. vaginalis*

Compound	MIC_{50} (μg/ml)
Garenoxacin	0.5
Moxifloxacin	0.5
Gatifloxacin	0.5
Ciprofloxacin	1.0
Levofloxacin	1.0
Trovafloxacin	1.0
ABT-492	0.12

Table 42 In vitro activities of fluoroquinolones against *Mobiluncus spp.*

Compound	MIC (μg/ml)		
	50%	90%	Range
Ciprofloxacin	0.5	1	0.03–1
Enoxacin	8	8	2–8
Gatifloxacin	0.2	0.2	0.1–0.2
Levofloxacin	0.78	0.78	0.39–0.78
Moxifloxacin	0.25	0.5	
Ofloxacin	1	2	0.5–2
Sitafloxacin	0.05	0.05	0.05–0.2
Sparfloxacin	0.1	0.2	0.05–0.2

Table 43 In vitro activities of fluoroquinolones against *P. bivia*

Compound	MIC (μg/ml)		
	50%	90%	Range
Levofloxacin	2	4	2–4
Trovafloxacin	1	1	0.06–4
Grepafloxacin	16	16	0.125–64
Moxifloxacin	1	2	0.25–4
Lomefloxacin	32	32	32
Gatifloxacin	4	8	4–8
Clinafloxacin	0.25	0.25	0.25–0.5
Ciprofloxacin	32	32	0.25–64
Metronidazole	2	4	0.25–8
Clindamycin	≤0.01	0.03	≤0.01–>32
Telithromycin	0.25	0.5	≤0.01–0.15
Ofloxacin	4	8	4–8
Sitafloxacin	0.5	0.5	≤0.04–1
Sparfloxacin	8	32	4–16
Clarithromycin	0.12	0.25	0.06–>32
Roxithromycin	1	1	0.12–>32
Azithromycin	0.5	1	0.25–>32

Table 44 In vitro activities of quinolones against *C. trachomatis*[a]

Compound	MIC range (μg/ml)
Ciprofloxacin	0.5–1.0
Trovafloxacin	0.06
Levofloxacin	0.12–0.5
ABT-492	0.03–0.06
Sitafloxacin	0.03–0.06
Grepafloxacin	0.03–0.125
Sparfloxacin	0.03–0.06
Tosufloxacin	0.06–0.125
Ofloxacin	0.06–0.125
Olamufloxacin	0.016–0.03
Temafloxacin	0.125
Norfloxacin	16
Gatifloxacin	0.06–0.125
Erythromycin A	0.25–0.5

[a]Data from Nilius et al., 2002; Niki et al., 1997; Kimura et al., 1993; and Miyashita et al., 1997, 2001.

Table 45 In vitro activities of fluoroquinolones against *M. hominis* and *U. urealyticum*[a]

Compound	MIC_{50} (μg/ml)	
	U. urealyticum	*M. hominis*
Ofloxacin	2	0.5
Ciprofloxacin	2	0.5
Levofloxacin	0.5	0.25
Sitafloxacin	0.12	0.06
Sparfloxacin	1	0.03
Grepafloxacin	1	0.12
Temafloxacin	2	0.25
Fleroxacin	4	2
Lomefloxacin	4	2
Norfloxacin	8	8
Pefloxacin	2	2
Enoxacin	8	8
Trovafloxacin	0.12	0.06
Gatifloxacin	1	0.12
Gemifloxacin	0.125	0.1
Nalidixic acid	64	≥256
Cinoxacin	≥128	≥128
Moxifloxacin		0.06

[a]Data from Bébéar et al. and Kenny et al.

Table 46 In vitro activities of fluoroquinolones against *Mycoplasma* species[a]

Organism	MIC (μg/ml) or MIC_{50} (μg/ml)[b]				
	OFX	LVX	SPX	MXF	GEM
M. genitalium	1	0.5	0.03	0.03	0.05
Mycoplasma fermentans	0.05	0.1	≤0.01–0.03	≤0.01–0.03	0.01
Mycoplasma penetrans	0.05	0.1	≤0.01	0.03–0.06	0.005
Mycoplasma pirum					0.01

[a]Data from Bébéar and Renaudin.
[b]Gem, gemifloxacin; for other abbreviations, see Table 9, footnote *a*.

5.10. Bacterial Agents Responsible for Infections Following Bites

Animal and human bites are common and account for thousands of medical consultations annually (Table 47).

E. corrodens is often involved in bites of human origin, while *Pasteurella* spp. and *Porphyromonas* spp. (eight species) are of animal origin, particularly Canidae or Felidae.

5.11. Antiparasitic Activity of Fluoroquinolones

In the search for new drugs, fluoroquinolones have been tested against malaria, *Pneumocystis carinii* (Brun-Pascaud et al., 1992), toxoplasmosis (Khan et al., 1996; Khan et al., 1999a, 1999b), leishmaniosis (Raether et al., 1989; Savoia et al., 1993), and, recently, trypanosomiasis (Nenortas et al., 1999). Parasites of the phylum Apicomplexa include more than 5,000 species, some being important human and veterinary pathogens such as *Plasmodium*, *Toxoplasma*, *Eimeria*, and *Cryptosporidium*. Studies have identified an additional organelle in these parasites: plastid.

Apicomplexan parasites contain three classes of DNA: (i) genome (~1 to 19 Mb), (ii) mitochordrial genome (6-kb element), and (iii) plastid (35-kb circular DNA episome). Replication of these unusual DNAs needs topoisomerase functions.

5.11.1. Trypanosomiasis

The existence of both mitochondrial and nuclear topoisomerases in trypanosomes has been demonstrated (Shapiro et al., 1989; Shapiro and Englund, 1990). Six fluoroquinolones introduced into clinical practice (norfloxacin, enoxacin, ciprofloxacin, pefloxacin, ofloxacin, and fleroxacin) and four tetracyclic investigational fluoroquinolones (Fig. 43) have been investigated for in vitro activity against the bloodstream form of *Trypanosoma brucei brucei*.

Table 47 In vitro activities of fluoroquinolones against agents responsible for infections from bites

Organism	MIC$_{50}$ (μg/ml)[a]					
	OFX	CIP	LVX	MXF	SPX	TVA
Pasteurella multocida subsp. *multocida*	0.016	0.008	0.008	0.008	0.008	0.008
Pasteurella multocida subsp. *septica*	0.03	0.004	0.008	0.01	0.004	0.008
Pasteurella canis	0.016	0.004	0.008	0.008	0.002	0.004
Actinobacillus/Haemophilus	0.016	0.016	0.008	0.01	0.004	0.016
Capnocytophaga spp.	0.06	0.06	0.03	0.03	0.01	0.016
Corynebacterium spp.	0.25	0.06	0.06	0.03	0.01	0.06
EF 4b	0.038	0.008	0.008	0.01	0.002	0.06
E. corrodens	0.016	0.008	0.008	0.01	0.01	0.06
Porphyromonas gingivalis	0.25	0.25	0.12	0.06	0.06	
Porphyromonas salivosa	0.5	1	0.5	0.12	0.5	
Neisseria weaveri	0.06	0.01	0.008	0.03	0.03	0.06
Weeksella zoohelcum	0.06	0.03	0.016	0.008	0.008	0.016

[a]See Table 19, footnote *b*.

All tested compounds had measurable activity, but the tetracyclic analogs were most potent (50% inhibitory concentration [IC$_{50}$], 1.7 to 14 μg/ml), and trypanosomes were more susceptible than L1210 leukemia cells (Table 48) (Nenortas et al., 1999).

These results, even if these compounds did not seem to be useful in the clinical setting, provide evidence that fluoroquinolone inhibition of type II DNA topoisomerases may be a novel approach for development of new antitrypanosomal drugs.

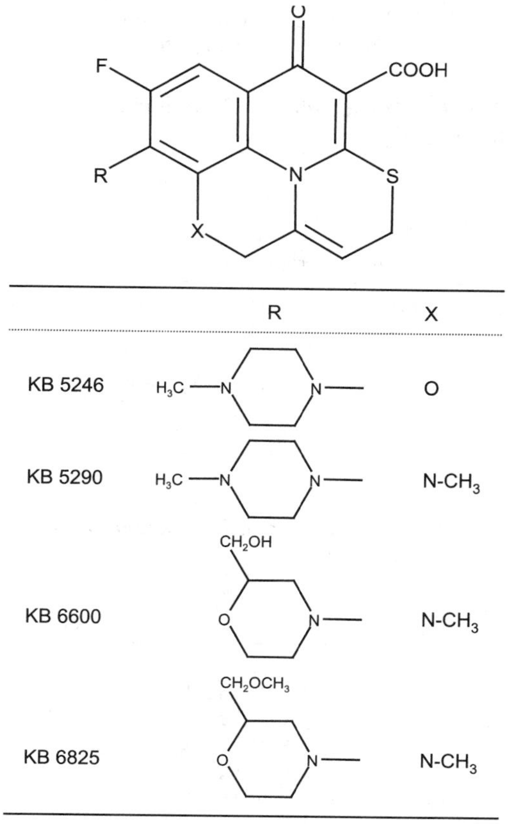

	R	X
KB 5246	H_3C—N(piperazine)N—	O
KB 5290	H_3C—N(piperazine)N—	N-CH_3
KB 6600	CH_2OH (morpholine O…N—)	N-CH_3
KB 6825	CH_2OCH_3 (morpholine O…N—)	N-CH_3

Figure 43 Antitrypanosomal quinolones

5.11.2. Toxoplasmosis

Gatifloxacin antitoxoplasmal activity was investigated in vitro and in vivo. Gatifloxacin inhibited intracellular replication of RH strain tachyzoites in vitro; the IC$_{50}$ following 48 of exposure was 0.12 μg/ml with human foreskin fibroblasts.

In RH-infected mice (outbred Swiss Webster female mice), treatment with gatifloxacin (initiated 24 h after challenge and for 10 days) alone (400 mg/kg) resulted in significant prolongation in time until death (above 3 days) and a 40% survival benefit at this dose. Combination of gatifloxacin and pyrimethamine provided a significant enhancement in survival of RH-infected mice compared with the activity of either drug alone. However, no data have been shown concerning intracerebral infection and the sterilization of mice. The clinical relevance of those data needs to be documented.

The IC$_{50}$ of trovafloxacin against *Toxoplasma gondii* is 2.93 μM. A series of 11 trovafloxacin derivatives were evaluated for their in vitro activities against *T. gondii*, and a tentative structure-activity relationship was investigated.

Different substituents have been fixed on the 7-bicyclic ring, with either a 2′,4′-difluorophenyl ring at position 1 or an N-1 cyclopropyl. All derivatives were 1.8-naphthyridone derivatives except one which was a quinoline analog. One compound also bears a 5-CH_3; it is six times more active than trovafloxacin. Replacement of 2′,4′-difluorophenyl by cyclopropyl at N-1 increased the activity twofold (IC$_{50}$, 1.68 μM). Moving the NH_2 decreased the activity (IC$_{50}$, 12.47 μM).

Table 48 In vitro activities of fluoroquinolones against *T. brucei*

Compound	IC$_{50}$ (μM)
Norfloxacin	70
Enoxacin	51
Ciprofloxacin	52
Pefloxacin	97
Fleroxacin	>100
Ofloxacin	>100
KB-5246	1.7
KB-5290	3.7
KB-6600	11
KB-6625	14

It was previously hypothesized that the 7-ring is critical for antitoxoplasmal activity. Substituted quinoline or 1,8-naphthyridone derivatives with a 7-substituted or not piperazinyl or pyrrolidinyl ring are devoid of antitoxoplasmal activities. It was shown that addition of a methyl group at C-5 of the 1,8-naphthyridone ring, at C-2′ of the azabicyclohexane ring, or on the C-6′-amino group of the bicyclic ring resulted in a four- to sixfold increase in activity. Moreover, replacement of the 2′,4′ difluorophenyl moiety by cyclopropyl at N-1 of the 1,8-naphthyridone ring decreased antitoxoplasmal activity. It was shown that ciprofloxacin could inhibit *T. gondii* growth (Fichera and Ross, 1997).

By studying structure relationships of fluoroquinolones, the following were shown: (i) 3-COOH is not essential for antitoxoplasmal activity, (ii) 6-fluorine is important for activity, (iii) activity is enhanced by the presence of the C-5 methyl group, and (iv) a nucleophilic substituent at C-8 seems to be essential for the activity of gatifloxacin and moxifloxacin (Gozalbes et al., 2000).

5.11.3. Malaria

Ciprofloxacin induces cleavage of 35-kb plastid organelle of *Plasmadium falciparum* and does not appear to target nuclear DNA.

5.11.4. Leishmaniasis

Since 1945, the treatment of leishmaniasis has remained sodium stibogluconate or meglumine antimoniate. With the emergence of the AIDS pandemic, serious problems in treating kala azar occurred; in addition, due to emergence of resistant strains, a need for new therapeutics has developed.

In vitro, it was shown that some fluoroquinolones have limited activity against *Leishmania donovani.* Pefloxacin seems to reduce significantly lesions in *Leishmania major*-infected rodents (Savoia et al., 1993). Female and male Syrian hamsters (weight, 80 to 110 g) were infected with *L. donovani* strain Calcutta; results are shown in Table 49 (Raether et al., 1989). Ciprofloxacin has been found to be effective in the treatment of one case of human cutaneous leishmaniasis due to *L. major* (Sanguigni et al., 1993). It has been shown in murine infection that the combination of pefloxacin and gamma interferon is highly effective in treating mice [BALB/c] infected with *L. major* (Zucca et al., 1996).

5.11.5. *Cryptosporidium parvum*

DNA gyrase of *C. parvum* was studied and may represent a future target for drugs (Christopher and Dyksta, 1994).

5.11.6. *Pneumocystis carinii*

The in vitro activity of six fluoroquinolones against *P. carinii* was evaluated; results are shown in Table 50. The efficacy of pefloxacin in a rat model of pneumocystis pneumonia has been determined (Brun-Pascaud et al., 1990). The reduction of *P. carinii* burden in infected immunocompromised rats was assessed for six fluoroquinolones (Brun-Pascaud et al., 1992) (Table 51). Of the tested fluoroquinolones, pefloxacin had the highest efficacy.

Table 49 **In vivo activities of fluoroquinolones against *L. donovani* infection in mice ($n = 6$)**

Compound	Dose (mg/kg per os)	No. of amastigotes/1,000 liver cell nuclei
Pentamidine	10	10–270
Ofloxacin	5	50–1,600
Norfloxacin	5	340–1,230
Ciprofloxacin	5	90–2,028
Enoxacin	5	480–2,520
Pefloxacin	5	1,320–2,970
Control		2,130–3,730

5.12. In Vitro Activity of Quinolones at the Preclinical Stage

A number of molecules are regularly described each year, and some have reached phase I. Their in vitro properties are summarized in Table 52.

5.12.1. DC-756

DC-756 is an 8-methoxy quinolone having a 7-pyrrolidinyl moiety substituted by a 3-amino group and 4(S)-fluoromethyl group (Fig. 44). DC-756 is as active as sitafloxacin (DU-6859a), one of the most active fluoroquinolones against gram-positive cocci, against *S. aureus* (MIC_{50}, 0.015 μg/ml), *S. pneumoniae* (MIC_{50}, 0.06 μg/ml), and *Streptococcus pyogenes* (MIC_{50}, 0.06 μg/ml). It is less active against *Enterococcus faecalis* (MIC_{50}, 0.25 μg/ml) and poorly active against *Enterococcus faecium* (MIC_{50}, 2 μg/ml). It shares cross-resistance with other fluoroquinolones against ofloxacin-resistant *S. aureus* isolates. It is two tubes less active than ciprofloxacin against *E. coli* (MIC_{50}, 0.03 μg/ml) and *Klebsiella pneumoniae* (MIC_{50}, 0.03 μg/ml). It is four times less active than ciprofloxacin against *P. aeruginosa* (MIC_{50}, 0.5 μg/ml, versus 0.12 μg/ml for ciprofloxacin).

In murine experimental sepsis induced with a strain of *S. pneumoniae* resistant to penicillin G, DC-756 displayed activity comparable to that of trovafloxacin (ED_{50}, 8.54 mg/kg, versus 9.05 mg/kg for trovafloxacin).

Preliminary toxicological and pharmacokinetic evaluations of DC-756 have been conducted. After a single intravenous administration of 50 mg/kg to 6-week-old male

Table 50 **In vitro activities of fluoroquinolones against *P. carinii***

Compound	IC (μg/ml)			
	50%		90%	
	Cysts	Trophozoites	Cysts	Trophozoites
Lomefloxacin	>64	>64	>64	>64
Norfloxacin	>64	>64	>64	>64
Ofloxacin	>64	>64	>64	>64
Pefloxacin	64	64	>64	>64
Rufloxacin	>64	>64	>64	>64
Pentamidine	1.0	1.0	10	10

Table 51 **In vivo efficacies of fluoroquinolones in pneumocystosis in rats**

Compound	*n*	Dose(s)	No. of cysts/g of lung tissue
Control	18		5.7×10^6
Co-trimoxazole	18	40/20 mg/kg 2 × /wk	9×10^2
Pefloxacin	10	100 mg/kg 3 × /wk	2.7×10^3
Temafloxacin	5	100 mg/kg 3 × /wk	6×10^5
Ofloxacin	5	100 mg/kg 3 × /wk	7.9×10^5
Ciprofloxacin	5	100 mg/kg 3 × /wk	2.2×10^6
Sparfloxacin	5	100 mg/kg 3 × /wk	3.8×10^6
Norfloxacin	5	100 mg/kg 3 × /wk	1.5×10^7

Table 52 In vitro activities of the new quinolones

Organism(s)	MIC$_{50}$ (μg/ml)[a]								
	GEM	GAR	OLU	DW 116	CFC 222	CAR	PAZ	PRU	MXF
S. aureus	0.01	0.01	0.03	1	0.06	0.06	0.25	0.39	0.06
S. epidermidis	≤0.008	0.01	0.5	1	0.12	0.12	0.25	0.39	0.12
S. pneumoniae	0.03	0.03	0.03	4	0.5	0.25	1.56	1.56	0.12
S. pyogenes	0.01	0.12	0.06	2	0.25	0.25	0.78	0.2	0.12
E. faecalis	0.12	0.12	0.5		2	0.5	4	1.56	4.0
E. faecium	16	4	0.12			1	6.25	1.56	8.0
N. meningitidis	0.002	0.008					0.01		0.004
N. gonorrhoeae	0.002	0.008			0.12	0.01	0.01	0.01	0.002
H. influenzae	0.008	0.008	0.008	0.06		0.008	0.01	0.02	0.03
M. catarrhalis	0.01	0.03	0.03		0.12	0.01	0.1	0.1	0.06
E. coli	0.01	0.03	0.06	8	0.25	0.03	0.1	0.02	0.06
K. pneumoniae	0.03	0.12	0.06	0.5	0.06	0.06	0.05	0.02	0.12
K. oxytoca	0.06	0.06		0.5	0.06	0.03		0.02	0.12
E. cloacae	0.03	0.12	0.03	0.5	0.06	0.03	0.1	0.02	0.06
C. freundii	0.12	0.12	0.5	0.5	0.5	0.06	0.2	0.05	0.12
S. marcescens	0.25	1	1	2	0.5	0.5	6.25	0.78	0.25
P. mirabilis	0.12	0.5	0.06	2	0.25	0.12	0.1	0.02	0.25
P. rettgeri			0.5	0.5	0.25	0.5	6.25		
P. stuartii				1	0.008	0.12	0.1	0.29	0.06
Salmonella spp.	0.01	0.03		0.25	0.008	0.03	0.1	0.05	0.06
Shigella spp.		0.03		0.12	0.25	0.01	0.1	0.01	0.03
M. morganii	0.06	0.25	0.06	0.5		0.01	0.1	0.02	0.025
Y. enterocolitica	0.01	0.06			8	0.01			0.06
P. aeruginosa	1	1	0.5	16	2	0.25	>100	0.2	2.0
S. maltophilia	1			8	1	0.25	0.78	6.25	0.5
A. baumannii	4.0	0.06	0.03	2		0.01	1.56	0.78	1.0
L. pneumophila	0.004–0.01	0.01					0.01		
C. pneumoniae	0.06–0.12								
M. pneumoniae	0.01	0.03						1.56	
C. trachomatis	0.03–0.12	0.008							
M. tuberculosis	0.12	0.03					2		
V. cholerae		0.008							0.03
B. cepacia	8.0	8.0							2.0
Flavobacterium	0.25								0.25
Acinetobacter lwoffii	0.06								0.06
Alcaligenes	8.0								2.0
Bordetella	0.06								0.06
Viridans group streptococci	0.06								0.25
S. haemolyticus	0.03								0.06
S. mitis	0.12								0.25
L. monocytogenes	0.5								0.5
Streptococcus groups C, G, and F	0.12								0.25
S. saprophyticus	0.03								0.06
S. agalactiae	0.06								0.25

[a]GEM, gemifloxacin; GAR, garenoxacin; CFC 222, ecenofloxacin; PAZ, pazufloxacin; OLU, olumafloxacin; CAR, cardifloxacin; PRU, prulifloxacin; MXF, moxifloxacin.

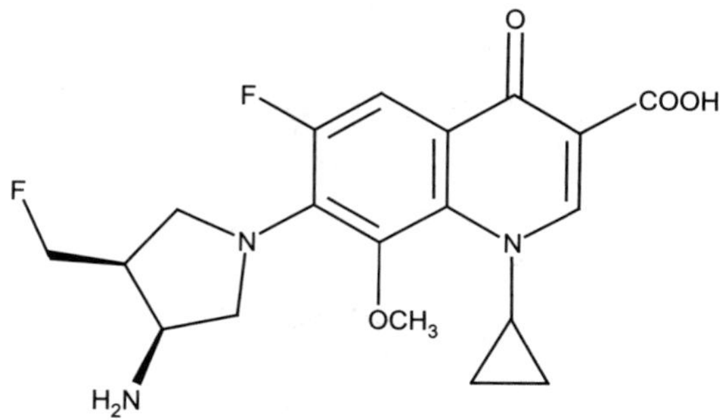

Figure 44 DC-756

S/C:ddY mice, no abnormalities were recorded. The mortality rate reached 80% of the animals at 200 mg/kg (50% lethal dose, 173 mg/kg). After oral repeated doses for 14 days, no severe alterations were noted either in rats (150 mg/kg) or in monkeys (30 mg/kg).

Using a proper model, no abnormalities in female mice (5-week-old female crj:BALB/c mice) were found after a single administration of 150 mg of DC-756 per kg, followed immediately by irradiation with UV-A for 4 (20 J/cm^{2}h). In 3-week-old ddY mice, no convulsions or mortality was recorded after a single intracisternal administration of 5 μg of DC-756 per mouse with or without oral dosing of 4-biphenylacetic acid (400 mg/kg).

Up to 30 mg/kg, no epiphysial cartilage lesions occurred in male juvenile dogs (3-month-old beagles) receiving 7 days of oral administration of DC-756. Lesions occurred at 10 mg/kg with ofloxacin. No genotoxicity has been found in vitro (Chinese hamster cell lines) or in vivo (micronuclear test, ddY mice, 6 weeks old). In rats, the bioavailability after oral and intravenous administrations of 20 mg/kg was 78% (as determined by the area under the curve [AUC]).

5.12.2. WQ-2724 and WQ-2743

Series of 6-fluoroquinolones with a 7-azetidinyl moiety substituted or not have been synthesized. They differ by the 3′ substituent on the azetidinyl moiety, i.e., 3′-hydroxyl (WQ-3034) or 3′-aminomethyl (WQ-2724 and WQ-2743), and the C-8 substituent, i.e., chlorine or bromine.

All of them bear an original N-1 substituent: a 5-amino, 2′,4-difluoropyridinyl moiety. Previous compounds of the 7-azetidinyl series bearing a 5′-amino, 2′,4′-difluorophenyl in position 1 have been synthesized (WQ-2756 and WQ-2765) but have limited oral bioavailability. New analogs were synthesized by changing the aromatic ring in N-1 in order to improve oral bioavailability. After a single oral dose of 10 mg/kg in dogs, oral bioavailability was 50.4 and 48.4% for WQ-2724 and WQ-2743, respectively. However, in dogs, WQ-2743 is highly eliminated in bile. No convulsant activity was seen after coadministration of biphenylacetic acid intravenously to mice. No phototoxicity has been demonstrated in mice (ear redness model).

WQ-2724 and WQ-2743 were 10 times more active than sparfloxacin against methicillin-susceptible *S. aureus* (MSSA) (MIC_{50} and MIC_{90}, 0.013 and 0.05 μg/ml) and 16 times more active than sparfloxacin against *S. pneumoniae* (MIC_{50} and MIC_{90}, 0.06 and 0.10 μg/ml). They showed activity similar to that of ciprofloxacin against *P. aeruginosa* (MIC_{50} and MIC_{90}, 0.20 and 1.56 μg/ml). Both compounds efficiently cured disseminated infections, chest infections, and subcutaneous infections (Amano et al., 1997).

5.12.3. WQ-3034 (ABT-492)

WQ-3034 displayed broad antibacterial activity including against methicillin-resistant *S. aureus* (MRSA) isolates which are resistant to ciprofloxacin, especially in an acidic environment (Fig. 45). Then in vitro activity of ABT-492 is reported in Table 53.

5.12.4. KRQ 10018 and Analogs

Series of 2-pyridones and fluoroquinolones bearing a bicyclic nucleus have been synthesized (Park et al., 1997). The in vitro activities of the main compounds have been compared to those of sparfloxacin and ciprofloxacin.

KRQ 10099 is an analog of ofloxacin bearing a bicyclic nucleus instead of a piperazinyl moiety. KRQ 10018 is an 8-methyl-2-pyridone derivative. Against reference strains, KRQ 10018 is extremely active against gram-positive cocci, including ciprofloxacin-resistant *S. aureus* isolates (MIC, 0.025 μg/ml) and ofloxacin-resistant *Staphylococcus epidermidis* (MIC, 0.013 μg/ml). It is more active than ciprofloxacin against *Enterobacteriaceae* and *P. aeruginosa*. The *trans* racemate KRQ 10071 displays activity comparable to that of KRQ 10018.

KRQ 10018 was the most active of all the compounds tested, even compared to KRQ 10196, a quinoline derivative which is a sparfloxacin analog with a bicyclic moiety at position 7. In ICR mice, the pharmacokinetic profile was determined after subcutaneous and oral administrations of KRQ 10018 (dose of 40 mg/kg). The bioavailability (AUC per os/AUC subcutaneously) was 57.9%.

5.12.5. WQ-3330 and WQ-2942

A series of N-1 2′,4′-difluoro-5′-aminophenyl derivatives has been synthesized, and the structure-activity relationships among the subgroup of fluoroquinolones have been reported (Fig. 46).

Irrespective of the position 7 substituents (azetidinyl or amino group), the replacement of the 2′-fluorine with a 3′-methyl on the N-1 phenyl ring decreased in vitro activity against gram-positive and gram-negative bacteria. At the C-8 position, the presence of an 8-methyl group instead of an 8-chlorine group enhanced significantly the photostability of this class of compounds in an aqueous solution under UV-irradiation.

WQ-3330 and WQ-2942 (Fig. 46) are both more active in vitro against gram-positive cocci than trovafloxacin. The difference in terms of in vitro activity against gram-positive cocci between the compounds is difficult to draw; their respective activities are strain dependent. WQ-2942 is more active than ciprofloxacin against *P. aeruginosa* and *Enterobacteriaceae* except *Serratia marcescens*. However, WQ-3330 seems to be more active than WQ-2942 against MRSA (MIC_{50}, 1.56 versus 12.5 μg/ml), and other tested fluoroquinolones are inactive (trovafloxacin MIC_{50}, 1.25 μg/ml).

In disseminated staphylococcal infections, WQ-3331 (maleic acid salt of WQ-3330) is more active than WQ-3345 (ethanolamine salt of WQ-2942) against *S. aureus* Smith (ED_{50}, 0.15 versus 0.60 mg/kg) and more active than trovafloxacin against MRSA W44 (ED_{50}, 17.5 versus 39.7 mg/kg). WQ-3345 and WQ-3331 are less active than trovafloxacin against *S. pneumoniae* infection (ED_{50}s, 10.5, 23.2, and 8.17 mg/kg for WQ-3345, WQ-3331, and trovafloxacin, respectively). WQ-3345 is more active than WQ-3331 in *P. aeruginosa* infections (ED_{50}, 4.23 versus 72.4 mg/kg), but ciprofloxacin was not tested in this model.

Five-week-old male CBA/J mice were intranasally infected with *S. pneumoniae* and then were administered compounds orally after 6, 24, and 48 h. After bacterial challenge the survival rates after treatment with both compounds were 100%, but a significant reduction in lung burden was obtained after an oral dose of 50 mg/kg, in the same magnitude as that recorded with trovafloxacin at 50 mg/kg. The reductions were over 5, 3, and over 5 $\log_{10}$ CFU/lung for WQ-3345, WQ-3331, and trovafloxacin, respectively.

The pharmacokinetics of both compounds were investigated in 5-week-old ddY male mice after an oral dose of 10 mg/kg. The levels in plasma and lungs were determined using a microbiological assay and *B. subtilis* ATCC 6633 as the test organism.

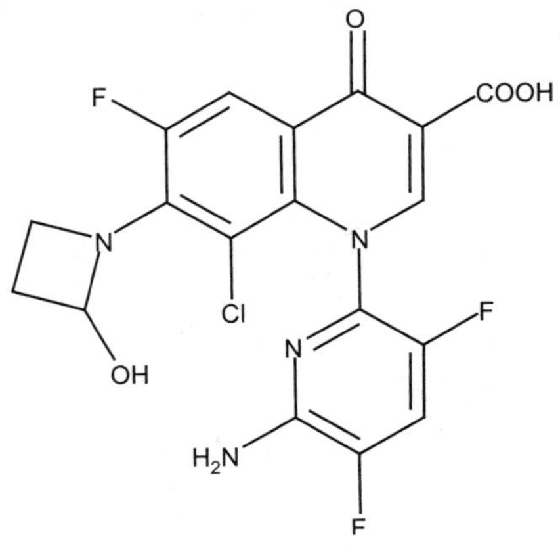

O
F
COOH
N
N
Cl
F
N
OH
H_2N
F

Figure 45 ABT-492 (WQ-3034)

Table 53 Comparative in vitro activity of ABT-492

Organism	*n*	MIC$_{50}$ (μg/ml)					
		ABT-492	GAT	MXF	CIP	LVX	GEM
MSSA	50	0.004	0.12	0.06	0.5	0.25	0.03
MRSA	25	0.5	4.0	2.0	64	16	8.0
S. epidermidis	20	0.004	0.12	0.06	0.25	0.25	0.03
S. saprophyticus	30	0.008	0.25	0.12	0.5	0.5	0.03
S. pneumoniae	91	0.008	0.25	0.25	1.0	1.0	0.03
H. influenzae	88	0.001	0.015	0.015	0.015	0.015	0.004
M. catarrhalis	44	0.008	0.06	0.06	0.03	0.06	0.015
S. milleri	30	0.015	0.5	0.25	1.0	1.0	0.03
S. pyogenes	19	0.015	0.25	0.25	1.0	1.0	0.03
S. agalactiae	17	0.015	0.25	0.12	1.0	1.0	0.03
E. faecium	90	2.0	4.0	4.0	8.0	8.0	2.0
E. faecium VanA	9	0.5–8.0	1–32	0.5–8.0	2–>128	2–64	0.06–16
E. faecium VanB	8	1–16	2–64	2–32	2–>128	2–64	1–16
E. faecalis	91	0.12	0.5	0.25	2.0	2.0	0.06
C. jeikeium	10	2.0	4.0				
N. gonorrhoeae	44	0.001	0.004	0.008	0.004	0.008	0.004
N. meningitidis	11	0.001	0.008	0.008–0.015	0.004–0.008	0.008–0.015	0.002–0.0004
C. difficile	9	0.03	0.5–16	0.06–0.5	8–16	1–4	0.5–1
C. perfringens	12	0.008	0.25–0.5	0.12–1	0.5	0.25	0.06
B. fragilis	48	0.12	0.5	0.25	2.0	1.0	0.5
Prevotella	9	0.004–4	0.25–32	0.5–8	1–32	0.5–64	1–8
Peptostreptococcus	15	0.004	0.25	0.12	1.0	0.5	0.12
B. thetaiotaomicron	18	0.25	1.0	1.0	8.0	4.0	1.0
E. coli	100	0.03	0.015	0.03	0.015	0.03	0.008
K. pneumoniae	100	0.12	0.03	0.06	0.03	0.06	0.03
P. mirabilis	50	0.06	0.12	0.25	0.03	0.06	0.12
P. vulgaris	11	0.15	0.15	0.06	0.008	0.015	0.015
P. rettgeri	6	0.03	0.03	0.06	0.015	0.06	0.03
M. morganii	12	0.06	0.03	0.06	0.008	0.015	0.03
Enterobacter sp.	50	0.12	0.06	0.06	0.03	0.06	0.03
P. aeruginosa	50	0.25	0.5	1.0	0.12	0.5	0.25

[a]GAT, gatifloxacin; MXF, moxifloxacin; CIP, ciprofloxacin; LVX, levofloxacin; GEM, gemifloxacin.

Concentrations in plasma and AUC for WQ-3345 were significantly higher than those recorded with levofloxacin, sparfloxacin, and trovafloxacin, but the values for WQ-3331 were significantly lower than those for a reference quinolone. In beagles (27 to 39 months old, male), after an oral administration of 20 mg/kg, apparent elimination half-lives were 4.0 and 5.2 h for WQ-3345 and WQ-3331, respectively. The urine elimination was low, less than 10%, in comparison with 36.9% for levofloxacin.

After coadministration in cerebral ventricles with biphenylacetic acid in ddY mice, neither compound induced convulsions or death, even after administration of the high dose of 80 μg/head. No phototoxicity in mice after UV-A irradiation (180 μw/cm^2) has been recorded at the higher dose of 80 mg/kg.

The original features of these compounds are the trisubstituted N-1 phenyl group and especially the good in vitro and in vivo activities of the 7-amino derivative, WQ-2942 (or WQ-3345) (Hayashi et al., 1999).

5.12.6. PGE-9262932, PGE-4175997, and PGE-9509924

New series of six des-6F-fluoroquinolones have been synthesized. The first series led to the development of garenoxacin (Bryskier, 1997). The aim of the new series was to obtain new quinolones active against multiresistant gram-positive cocci (Fig. 47).

A structure-activity study with compounds having an N-1 cyclopropylquinoline core has shown that the size of the position 8 substituent is important for activity against gram-positive organisms. Various substituents at position 7 demonstrated that the most potent compounds were obtained with 3′-aminoethylpyrrolidinyl and 3′-aminopiperidinyl rings (Ledoussal et al., 1999). Furthermore, it has been shown that a 6-fluorine instead of a nonsubstituted ring increased the genotoxicity in the in vitro micronucleus assay (CHO cells), whatever the substituent at position 8 (H, Cl, or OCH_3).

Three compounds were selected for further investigation: PGE-9262932, PGE-4175997, and PGE-9509926 (Fig. 1). It has been shown that these new des-6-fluorinated quinolones exhibited a less clastogenic effect than their 6-fluorinated counterparts (Hannah-Hardy et al., 1999). The acute intravenous toxicity in male Sprague-Dawley rats (8 to 12 weeks old) was explored in comparison with those of ciprofloxacin (minimal toxic dose, 300 mg/kg), trovafloxacin (minimal toxic dose, 30 mg/kg), and gatifloxacin (minimal toxic dose, 90 mg/kg). In this series, PGE-9509924 (minimal toxic dose, 240 mg/kg) was the best-tolerated compound, followed by PGE-9262932 (minimal toxic dose, 90 mg/kg) and PGE-4175997 (minimal toxic

	R_7	R_6
WQ 3330	H_5C_2—N(H)—(azetidinyl)N—	—CH_3
WQ 2942	H_2N—	—CH_3
WQ 2756	H_2N—(azetidinyl)N—	Cl
WQ 2908	H_2N—(azetidinyl)N—	—CH_3

Figure 46 **WQ-3330 and WQ-2942**

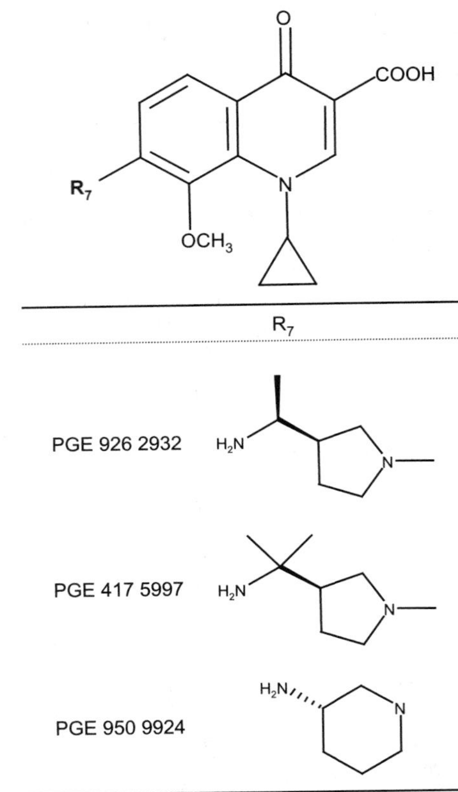

Figure 47 **Des(6F) quinolones**

dose, 60 mg/kg). Preliminary data on the affinity of these compounds in comparison with other fluoroquinolones, or in combination with 4-biphenylacetic acid for γ-aminobutyric acid (GABA) receptors, were comparable to those of comparative fluoroquinolones.

An in vitro phototoxicity study has been done, and not the in vivo reference method on ear swelling in mice, and the data are not convincing (Murphy et al., 1999).

In vitro activity has been investigated (Brown et al., 1999) in comparison with those of ciprofloxacin, trovafloxacin, and other compounds. The three derivatives could be considered inactive against *B. cepacia* (MIC_{50}, ≥8 μg/ml) and poorly active against *P. aeruginosa* (MIC_{50}, 1 to 4 μg/ml) in comparison with ciprofloxacin (MIC_{50}, 0.25 μg/ml). They are less active (10 times or more) than ciprofloxacin against *Enterobacteriaceae*. They exhibit good activity against *H. influenzae* and *M. catarrhalis*, comparable to or less than (1 test tube dilution) that of ciprofloxacin.

Among the three compounds, one, PGE-4175997, is always less active than the two others, which show differential activities depending on the bacterial species. They displayed activity comparable to that of trovafloxacin against staphylococci. They are more active against *S. pneumoniae* isolates than trovafloxacin, irrespective of their susceptibility to penicillin G.

The most active compound is PGE-9262932, with a MIC_{50} and MIC_{90} of 0.015 and 0.03 μg/ml, in comparison with a MIC_{50} and MIC_{90} of 0.12 and 0.12 μg/ml for trovafloxacin. PGE-9262932 is also very active against *S. pyogenes* (MIC_{50} and MIC_{90}, 0.015 and 0.03 μg/ml) and the viridans group streptococci (MIC_{50} and MIC_{90}, 0.03 and 0.12 μg/ml) in comparison with trovafloxacin (MIC_{50} and MIC_{90}, 0.12 and 0.50 μg/ml).

The MICs of PGE-9262932 remain low for *S. pneumoniae* isolates with a single *parC* mutation (MIC, 0.06 μg/ml), double *parC* mutations (MIC, 0.012 μg/ml), or a combination of double *parC* mutations and *gyrA* (MIC, 0.5 μg/ml) in comparison with trovafloxacin (Roychoudhury et al., 1999).

All compounds exhibit good in vitro activity against *L. pneumophila* using a medium without charcoal; the MIC_{50}s and MIC_{90}s ranged from 0.03 to 0.06 μg/ml and 0.06 μg/ml, respectively, but the compounds are less active than levofloxacin (MIC_{50}, and MIC_{90}, 0.008 and 0.015 μg/ml). For *M. pneumoniae*, the MIC_{50}s and MIC_{90}s ranged from 0.03 to 0.12 μg/ml and 0.06 to 0.25 μg/ml, respectively; however, clarithromycin and levofloxacin were more active. For *C. pneumoniae*, MICs were determined in McCoy cells treated with cycloheximide; PGE-4175997 and PGE-9262932 exhibited good antichlamydial activity (MIC and MCC, 0.03 to 0.06 μg/ml and 0.12 to 0.25 μg/ml) in comparison with PGE-9509924 (MIC and MCC, 0.25 and 0.25 to 1.0 μg/ml). The first two compounds exert in vitro activity comparable to that of clarithromycin but higher than that of levofloxacin.

The three compounds are less active than ciprofloxacin against *Enterobacteriaceae* (MIC_{50} and MIC_{90}, 0.12 and 1.0 μg/ml) and they share full cross-resistance with ciprofloxacin. They are inactive against *P. aeruginosa* (MIC_{50} and MIC_{90}, 0.12 and 1.0 μg/ml), *B. cepacia*, *S. maltophilia*, and *B. fragilis*, with a MIC_{50} and MIC_{90} of 4.0 μg/ml. They exhibit good in vitro activity against gram-positive cocci, including *Enterococcus* spp. (MIC_{50}s, ≤0.008 to 0.02 μg/ml).

S. aureus mutants were first selected at a frequency of $<5.7 \times 10^{10}$ in the presence of twice the MIC of the three compounds; in comparison, the frequencies were 9.1×10^{-8} and 5.7×10^{-9} for ciprofloxacin and trovafloxacin, respectively, and the MIC_{90}s for the resulting strains ranged from 2.0 to 4.0 μg/ml.

A unique point mutation in the His103 or Ser52 residue of *grlA* is a prerequisite for high-level resistance to these compounds in *S. aureus*.

The pharmacokinetic profiles in rats (Sprague-Dawley VAF rats, 230 to 250 g) and in dogs (male beagles, 11 to 15 kg) have been established after oral and intravenous dosing. The bioavailability in dogs was high (65 to 100%). The highest bioavailability was reached with PGE-9509924 (7-aminopiperidinyl derivative). For PGE-9262932 and PGE-4175997 the oral bioavailability was 67% ± 32% and the apparent elimination half-lives were 7.0 ± 1.4 h and 5.4 ± 0.5 h, respectively. The bioavailability was low in rats (4 to 9%), with an apparent elimination half-life of 1.5 to 2.0 h (Mallalieu et al., 1999).

5.12.7. NSFQ-105 and Derivatives

A series of benzenesulfonylamido 7-piperazinyl quinolones has been synthesized (Fig. 48). A first series had been described in 1994 (Allemandi et al., 1994) with compounds showing a good antipneumococcal activity. This series was synthesized with the aim of exploring the role of position 7 substituents in ciprofloxacin analogs in activity against *S. pneumoniae* resistant to fluoroquinolones. All of the derivatives differ from ciprofloxacin by the 4′ substituent on the 7-piperazinyl ring. Quinolones could be divided into two groups for *S. pneumoniae*, those acting against *gyrA* (sparfloxacin and gatifloxacin) and those acting as a first step against *parC* (ciprofloxacin, norfloxacin, levofloxacin, and trovafloxacin).

It was clearly demonstrated that the C-7 substituent is important for governing target selection. The piperazinyl ring of ciprofloxacin was replaced with benzosulfonamide groups. With this substituent, the primary target on *S. pneumoniae* became *gyrA* instead of *parC*. More studies are needed to explore in detail the putative role of the C-7 substituent on *S. pneumoniae* intracellular targets and the possibility to overcome cross-resistance (Alovero et al., 2000).

5.12.8. 7-Alkylamino, N-1 5′-amino-2′,4′-difluorophenyl quinolones: WQ-2944, WQ-2942, and WQ-3199

A series of compounds having at N-1 a 5′-amino-2′,4′-difluorophenyl moiety has been synthesized. Four compounds having a novel amino side chain have been investigated for their biological potential: WQ-2942 (7-amino), WQ-2944 (7-methylamino), WQ-3188 (7-hydroxylethylamino), and WQ-3199 (7-hydroxypropylamino) (Fig. 49).

The substitution at position 8 with a methyl group yielded compounds with improved photostability and reduced cytotoxicity. All of them exhibited higher activity against gram-positive cocci than levofloxacin or ciprofloxacin. There is no significant difference among all of them. MICs ranged from 0.015 to 0.25 μg/ml, except for *E. faecium* ATCC 51559, for which MICs are above 4 μg/ml.

All of them exhibit activity comparable to that of ciprofloxacin against *E. coli* (MICs ranged from 0.015 to 0.12 μg/ml), *Citrobacter freundii* (MICs, 0.008 to 0.06 μg/ml), and *K. pneumoniae* (MICs, 0.015 to 0.12 μg/ml), but they are far less active than ciprofloxacin against *S. marcescens* (MICs, 0.25 to 8 μg/ml) and *P. aeruginosa*, against which they are poorly active (MICs ranged from 0.5 to 4.0 μg/ml). These derivatives are also weakly active against *Proteus* spp. *Providencia* spp., and *Morganella morganii*. WQ-2942 is the most active derivative; the least active is WQ-3287. They share cross-resistance with ciprofloxacin. Their in vitro activity against enterococci harboring a phenotype of resistance to vancomycin has been explored in comparison with that of linezolid. Against enterococci with a VanA phenotype, linezolid is more active (geometric MIC, 2.21 μg/ml), and the most active analogs were WQ-2944 and WQ-3287 (geometric mean MIC, 5.38 μg/ml). Against VanB enterococci, WQ-2944 (geometric mean MIC, 0.65 μg/ml) and WQ-3287 (geometric mean MIC, 1.15 μg/ml) are more active than linezolid (geometric mean MIC, 2.0 μg/ml). All of these compounds are up to 40 times more active than linezolid against VanC1 and VanC2/3 enterococcal isolates.

In murine experimental staphylococcal (MRSA strain W44) infections and oral therapy, all of them are more active than levofloxacin (ED_{50}, 59 mg/kg, but with a MIC of 12.5 μg/ml). WQ-3345 exhibits good antipseudomonal activity (*P. aeruginosa* E-2) compared with that of levofloxacin (ED_{50}, 5.5 versus 26 mg/kg).

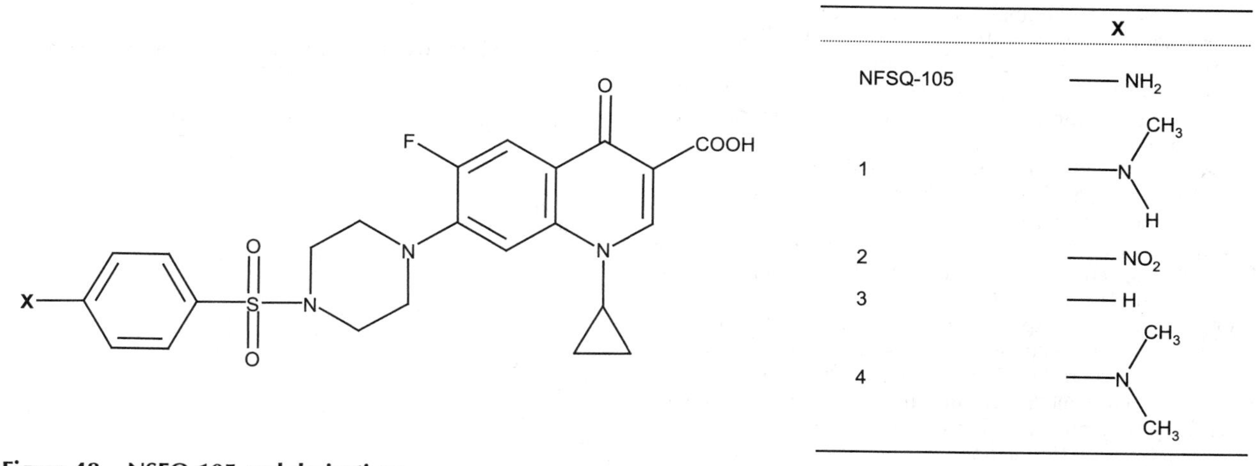

	X
NFSQ-105	$-NH_2$
1	$-N(H)CH_3$
2	$-NO_2$
3	$-H$
4	$-N(CH_3)_2$

Figure 48 NSFQ-105 and derivatives

	R
WQ 2942	H
WQ 2944	CH_3
WQ 3096	CH_2CH_3
WQ 3098	
WQ 3097	
WQ 3188	HO
WQ 3198	HO

Figure 49 7-Alkylamino, N-1 5′-amino-2′,4′-difluorophenyl quinolones

Five-week-old male CBA/J mice were challenged intranasally with *S. pneumoniae* W-28. Oral therapy with WQ-3345, WQ-3402, and levofloxacin was initiated 6, 24, and 48 h after bacterial challenge. After an oral dose of 50 mg/kg, a significant reduction of the lung burden (reduction above 3 $\log_{10}$ CFU/lung) was recorded. Pharmacokinetics after oral administration of WQ-3345, WQ-3402, WQ-3285, and WQ-3287 in mice (20 mg/kg) and dogs (10 mg/kg) in comparison with those of levofloxacin and trovafloxacin were assessed. In dogs, these derivatives are poorly eliminated in urine (≤5%, versus 36.9% for levofloxacin).

In dogs, the apparent elimination half-lives range from 2.3 to 4.9 h, compared to 6.9 and 3.6 h for levofloxacin and trovafloxacin, respectively.

In mice, the AUC from 0 to 4 h was higher for WQ-3345 (6.27 μg·h/ml) than for levofloxacin (4.16 μg·h/ml) and trovafloxacin (16.1 μg·h/ml) in lungs.

Phototoxicity was explored in 5- to 6-week-old female ICR mice after intravenous administration of WQ-3345, WQ-3402, and WQ-3287 and UV-A irradiation (320 to 400 nm to 26 J/cm^2) for 4 h immediately after intravenous administration of the different compounds. Ear redness of mice was scored at 0, 24, and 48 h postirradiation. At the dose of 80 mg/kg no abnormality was recorded.

5.12.9. WQ-2756

WQ-2756 is an 8-chlorofluoroquinolone having at N-1 appended a difluorophenyl amino group and an amino-azetidinyl ring at C-7 (Fig. 50). This molecule covers gram-positive and -negative microorganisms. It seems that addition of an amino group at the phenyl ring decreases the potential of photoxicity (Table 54) (Hayashi et al., 2002).

5.12.10. YH-6

A new tricyclic fluoroquinolone related to ofloxacin but differing by the N′4 substituent (pyridine moiety instead of a methyl group) (Fig. 51) has been disclosed. This compound was tested against *M. hominis, Mycoplasma orale, Mycoplama salivarium* and *U. urealyticum*, for which MICs of YH-6 are 0.5, 0.125, 0.125, and 0.25 μg/ml, respectively. YH-6 is active against *U. urealyticum* resistant to tetracycline (MIC, 0.25 μg/ml).

5.12.11. 6-Nitroquinolone

In the recent patent literature (JP2000256329) a 6-nitroquinolone (Fig. 52) has been shown, but no in vitro activity has been disclosed.

5.12.12. DQ-113

DQ-113 is a new investigational fluoroquinolone from Daichi which is characterized by a 5-amino group, an 8-methyl

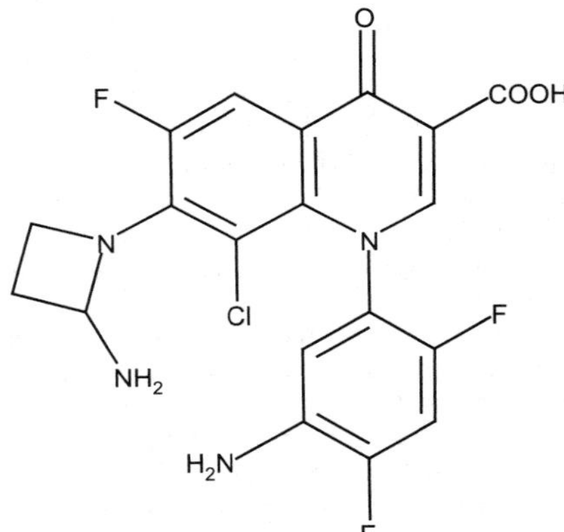

Figure 50 WQ-2756

Table 54 Phototoxicity potential of fluoroquinolones

Compound	No. of mice irradiated	No. of mice with ear redness		
		0 h	24 h	48 h
Norfloxacin	3	0	0	0
Levofloxacin	3	0	0	0
Ciprofloxacin	3	1	0	0
Lomefloxacin	6	6	6	6
Sparfloxacin	5	5	5	5
BAY y 3118	6	6	6	6
Clinafloxacin	6	6	6	6
WQ-2756	4	0	0	0
Desamino WQ-2756	6	6	6	6
Moxifloxacin	4	0	0	0
Gatifloxacin	4	0	0	0

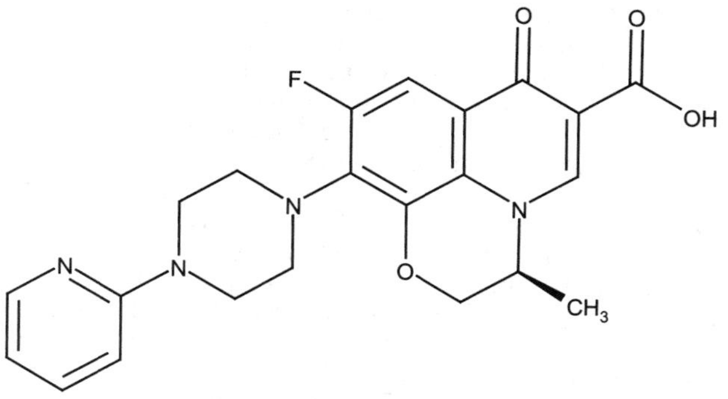

Figure 51 YH-6

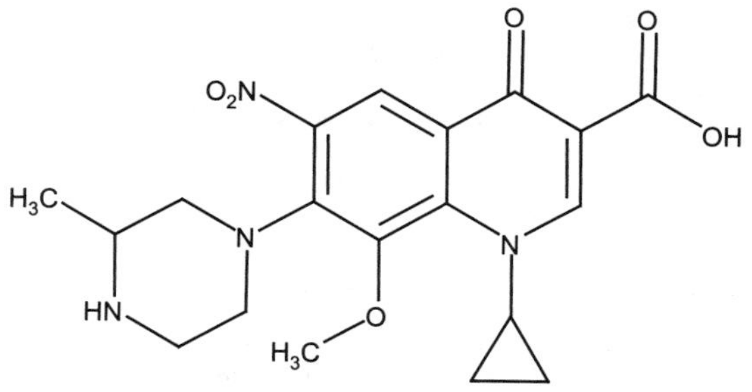

Figure 52 6-Nitroquinolone

group, an N-1 fluorocyclopropyl, and a complex 3′-fluoro-amino, 4′-aminocyclopropyl pyrrolininyl moiety at position 7 of the quinoline ring (Fig. 53).

This compound is extremely active against gram-positive cocci, including *E. faecalis*, and *Enterobacteriaceae*. DQ-113 is more active than ciprofloxacin and trovafloxacin against *Enterobacteriaceae* and gram-positive cocci, respectively, but it is less active against *P. aeruginosa* (MIC_{50}, 0.5 μg/ml, versus 0.12 μg/ml for ciprofloxacin).

It is one of the most active available fluoroquinolones against gram-positive cocci. However, no in vitro data on activity against anaerobes and intracellular or atypical microorganisms have been released. D-61-1113 seems to be active against *S. aureus* isolates resistant to ofloxacin, with a MIC_{50} and MIC_{90} of 0.06 and 0.25 μg/ml, respectively (Table 55).

In vivo activities in induced staphylococcal endocarditis and mouse enterococcal septicemia were promising. The apparent elimination half-lives in monkeys (10 mg/kg), rats (20 mg/kg), and mice (20 mg/kg) when the compound is administered intravenously are 4.3, 1.1, and 0.8 h respectively. Human protein binding is 74.9%; in comparison, trovafloxacin binds for 76.4% to serum protein in humans.

No convulsive effect after a single intracisternal administration in mice (5 μg/mouse) was recorded. No phototoxicity was induced in the mouse ear model, after a dose of 100 mg/kg and irradition for 4 h with UV-A (20 J/cm²). The cardiotoxicity in the model of isolated guinea pig myocardium at a concentration of 100 μM was comparable to that of levofloxacin and ciprofloxacin.

5.12.13. DK-507k

DK-507k is an 8-methoxy fluoroquinolone with an N-1 fluorocyclopropyl and a 3′-amino, 4′-cyclopropylpyrrolidinyl (Fig. 54) DK-507k has kept the same nucleus in position 1 as sitafloxacin: a fluorocyclopropyl. The second part, the 3′-aminopyridyl at position 7, is substituted with a 4′-cyclopropyl.

An important point, this compound seems to be soluble in water: 491 μg/ml (a parenteral solution could be done). However, lipophilicity (8.7) is high.

This compound seems to be as active as sitafloxacin against gram-positive bacteria and 1 dilution more active than moxifloxacin. It is inactive against MRSA resistant to ciprofloxacin (MIC_{90}, 4.0 μg/ml). It is also inactive against *E. faecium* (MIC_{90}, 8.0 μg/ml) even if DK-507k exhibits a higher activity than moxifloxacin but the MIC_{90} is at the limit of activity.

Concerning gram-negative bacteria, except *H. influenzae* and *M. catarrhalis*, the in vitro activity against *Enterobacteriaceae* is lower than those of sitafloxacin (four to eight

Table 55 In vitro activity of DQ-113

Organism[a]	*n*	MIC_{50} (μg/ml)
MSSA	48	0.008
MRSA	24	0.008
MRSA CIP^r	99	1.0
S. pneumoniae Pen^r	60	0.06
S. pyogenes	49	0.008
E. faecalis	50	0.03
E. faecium	47	0.50
E. coli	48	0.03
K. pneumoniae	49	0.06
H. influenzae β^+	21	≤0.004
H. influenzae β^- BLNAR	25	≤0.004
M. catarrhalis	46	0.015
P. aeruginosa	51	0.5

[a]CIP, ciprofloxacin; β^+, β-lactamase producing; β^-, non-β-lactamase producing.

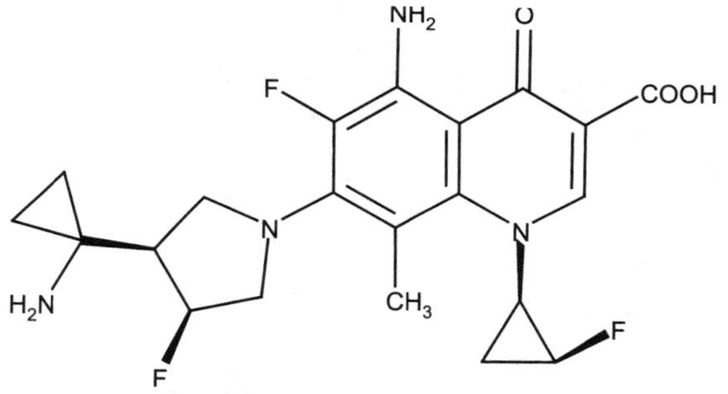

Figure 53 DQ-113

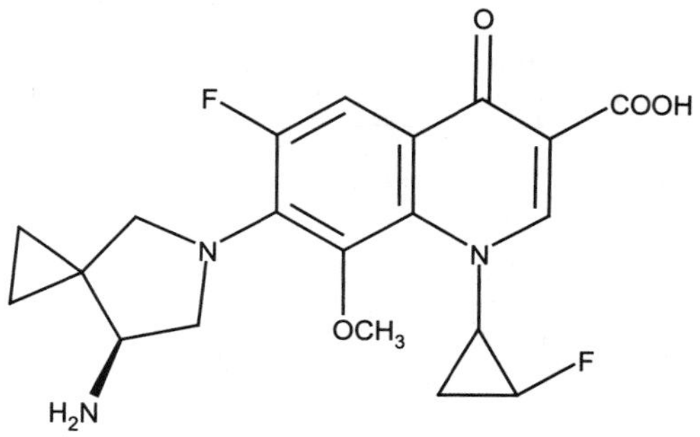

Figure 54 DK-507k

times) and ciprofloxacin (equally as active or two times less active). It is not very active against *N. gonorrhoeae* resistant to ciprofloxacin (MIC_{90}, 1 μg/ml).

Ciprofloxacin and sitafloxacin are two times more active than DK-507k against *P. aeruginosa*. For anaerobic organisms, only reference strains (ATCC) have been tested, and DK-507k is more active than moxifloxacin but less active than sitafloxacin (Table 56).

DK-507k retains activity against *S. pneumoniae* resistant to fluoroquinolones. The frequency of selecting resistant mutants is close to those observed with levofloxacin, gatifloxacin, and moxifloxacin.

Intravenous and oral treatments have been given to mice challenged with MSSA and penicillin-susceptible *S. pneumoniae* (PSSP). The ED_{50}s were quite lower than those of comparative fluoroquinolones (Table 57). In mice, DK-507k is more active than gatifloxacin, moxifloxacin, and levofloxacin against staphylococcal infections due to MSSA (ED_{50}, 9.70 mg/kg) and MRSA (ED_{50}, 97.5 mg/kg), and against pneumococcal infections irrespective of susceptibility to benzylpenicillin (ED_{50}s, 15 and 9.52 mg/kg for PSSP and penicillin-resistant *S. Pneumoniae* respectively).

DK-507k was administered to rats at the dose of 5 mg/kg (radiolabeled ^{14}C compound). Data are reported in Table 58 for rats and in Table 59 for monkeys. After 48 h, cumulative excretion of radioactivity was as follows: bile, 39.0% ± 4.6%; urine, 35.4% ±4.0%; and feces, 20.3% ± 2.6%. The apparent elimination half-life in monkeys seems to be extremely long (89 h). The cumulative excretions of radiolabeled DK-507k were as follows: urine, 41.0% ± 4.4% (168 h); feces, 56% ± 3.4% (168 h).

Protein binding in rats, monkeys, and humans is reported in Table 60. ^{14}C radiolabeled DK-507k is highly concentrated in lungs (up to 8 h), in the liver (up to 168 h), in the kidneys (up to 8 h), and in the skin (up to 8 h). Except for the first 0.5 h, the level in the brain is low.

The 50% lethal doses were assessed in mice (ddY mice, 6 weeks) and rats (IGS BR rats, 6 weeks) intravenous and orally; results are shown in Table 61.

Four-week repeated doses in rats and monkeys were assessed. For rats, doses up to 600 mg/kg were orally administered; NOAEL was considered to be 150 mg/kg. In monkeys (cynomolgus, 20 to 28 weeks), doses up to 100 mg/kg were orally administered; NOAEL was considered

Table 56 Comparative in vitro activity of DK-507k

Organism[a]	n	MIC_{90} (μg/ml)[b]					
		DK-507k	GAT	MXF	LVX	CIP	SIT
MSSA	25	0.12	0.25	0.12	0.5	1.0	0.12
MRSA CIP[s]	24	0.06	0.25	0.12	0.5	1.0	0.06
MRSA CIP[r]	25	4.0	16	8.0	64	>128	4.0
MSCoNS	36	0.5	4.0	4.0	16	64	0.5
PSSP	25	0.12	0.5	0.5	2.0	4.0	0.12
PRSP (I)	17	0.12	0.5	0.5	2.0	4.0	0.12
S. pyogenes	25	0.12	0.5	0.5	0.5	1.0	0.06
E. faecalis	25	2.0	16	8.0	32	32	2.0
E. faecium	23	8.0	32	16	128	64	8.0
E. coli	22	0.25	0.25	1.0	0.5	0.5	0.06
K. pneumoniae	25	1.0	1.0	1.0	1.0	0.5	0.25
S. marcescens	22	1.0	2.0	2.0	2.0	1.0	0.25
P. aeruginosa	24	1.0	2.0	4.0	2.0	0.25	0.25
Acinetobacter	24	0.5	0.5	1.0	1.0	2.0	0.25
H. influenzae	14	0.008	0.008	0.03	0.015	0.015	≤0.004
N. gonorrhoeae CPFX[s]	12	0.12	0.12	0.25	0.5	0.5	0.03
N. gonorrhoeae CIP[r]	23	1.0	4.0	8.0	16	32	0.25

[a]MSCoNs, methicillin-susceptible coagulose-negative staphylococci; PRSP, penicillin-resistant *S. pneumoniae*.
[b]GAT, gatifloxacin; MXF, moxifloxacin; LVX, levofloxacin; CIP, ciprofloxacin; SIT, sitafloxacin.

Table 57 Therapeutic efficacy of DK-507k in murine systemic infections

Route	Compound[a]	MSSA		PSSP	
		MIC (μg/ml)	ED_{50} (mg/kg)	MIC (μg/ml)	ED_{50} (mg/kg)
Oral	DK-507k	0.06	9.70	0.06	15.0
	GAT	0.12	15.91	0.25	32.4
	MXF	0.06	15.27	0.25	25.8
	LVX	0.25	24.65	1.0	72.49
Intravenous	DK-507k		0.76		3.11
	GAT		2.47		>20.0
	MXF		2.73		>20.0
	LVX		5.96		>80.0

[a]See Table 56, footnote *b*.

Table 58 Pharmacokinetics of DK-507k in rats (5 mg/kg)[a]

Parameter	Oral	Intravenous
C_{max} (μg/ml)	0.34 ± 0.04	
T_{max} (h)	0.7 ± 0.3	
$AUC_{0-\infty}$ (μg·h/ml)	1.01 ± 0.05	3.87 ± 0.16
$t_{1/2}$ (h)	2.2 ± 0.1	1.6 ± 0.1

[a]Data from Kawakami et al. and Tanaka et al.

Table 59 Pharmacokinetics of DK-507k in male monkeys (5 mg/kg)

Parameter	Value
C_{max} (μg/ml)	1.27 ± 0.24
T_{max} (h)	2.3 ± 1.5
$AUC_{0-\infty}$ (μg·h/ml)	14.5 ± 2.7
$t_{1/2}$ (h)	89 ± 14

Table 60 Protein binding of DK-507k

Concn (μg/ml)	Ratio of binding to protein (%)		
	Rat	Monkey	Human
0.1	39.3 ± 3.2	38.3 ± 4.1	43.7 ± 1.6
1.0	40.8 ± 1.1	38.5 ± 0.7	41.8 ± 0.8
10	40.5 ± 3.5	37.7 ± 0.7	40.5 ± 0.5

to be 30 mg/kg. Apparently, there is no phototoxicity up to 1,000 mg/kg orally and 100 mg/kg intravenously. The classical test was performed in comparison with ciprofloxacin and no convulsion or death was recorded in SIC:ddY male mice (coadministration of DK-507k and biphenylacetic acid). Juvenile beagles (4 months) received 7.5 to 30 mg/kg orally or 40 mg/kg intravenously for 8 days. No changes in chondrocyte levels were detected. In this experiment, it seems that histamine release syndrome has been recorded. Two studies have been carried out. The first, in comparison with sparfloxacin, was on cardiac repolarization; no effect was shown. The second experiment was an analysis of electrocardiogram on conscious cynomolgus monkeys in comparison with gatifloxacin and moxifloxacin. The three compounds were administered at a daily dose of 100 mg/kg. No effect was recorded for DK-507k, but I am not sure that it is the most reliable and suitable experimental model.

5.12.14. DW-286

DW-286 is a fluoro-1,8-naphthyridone derivative (Fig. 55). It is substituted at the N-1 position with a cyclopropyl moiety and at C-7 with a pyrrolidinyl moiety (Yun et al., 2002). The in vitro activity of DW-286 is reported in Table 62. The in vivo activity in murine infections was assessed and is shown in Table 63.

5.12.15. DW-224a

DW-224a is a fluoroquinolone with an N-1 cyclopropyl and a 7-pyrrolidinyl moiety substituted with an azetidinyl substituent and an alkyl side chain (Fig. 56).

DW-224a covers gram-positive and gram-negative bacteria. For *S. pneumoniae* resistant to fluoroquinolone, the MIC_{50} was 0.12 μg/ml. It is active in vitro against *M. pneumoniae* and *M. hominis* (MIC_{50}s and MIC_{90}s, 0.12 and 0.25 μg/ml and 0.03 and 0.06 μg/ml, respectively) and *C. pneumoniae* (MIC_{50}, 0.004 μg/ml).

5.12.16. DX-619

DX-619 is a des-(6F) fluoroquinolone having an 8-OCH_3 group, a fluorocyclopropyl at N-1, and an aminocyclopropyl-pyrrolidinyl moiety at C-7 (Inagaki et al., 2003) (Fig. 57). It is active against gram-positive and gram-negative bacteria; it is more active than moxifloxacin and exhibits activity similar to that of ciprofloxacin (Table 64). It displays good in vitro activity against vancomycin-resistant *S. aureus* (MIC, 0.25 μg/ml) (Hoellman et al., 2003).

5.12.17. AM-1939

AM-1939 is a tricyclic fluoroquinolone having a 3′-cyclopropylaminomethyl-pyrrolidinyl moiety at position 10 of the core ring (Fig. 58).

In vitro, AM-1939 exhibits good activity against staphylococci, including against isolates harboring a *norA* gene, and against enterococci, including VanA enterococci (Takei et al., 2003) (Table 65).

In murine staphylococcal infection (*S. aureus* KYR-5), AM-1939 is more active (ED_{50}s, 5.9 and 24 mg/kg subtaneously and orally, respectively) than levofloxacin (ED_{50}, >100 mg/kg), gatifloxacin, and clinafloxacin.

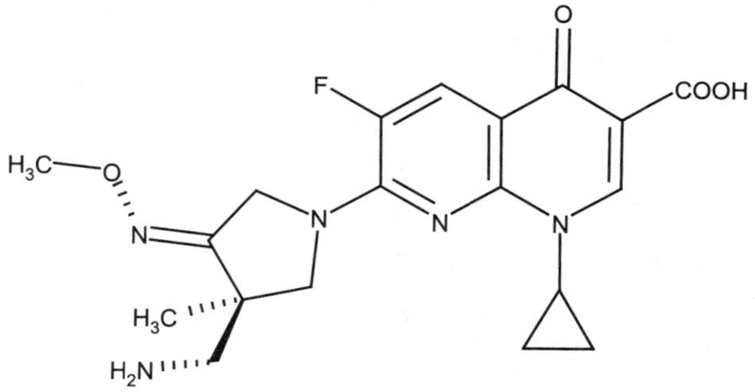

Figure 55 DW-286

Table 61 Single-dose toxicity in rats and mice

Route	No. of animals	LD_{50} (mg/kg)[a]			
		Mice		Rats	
		F	M	F	M
Oral	5	>2,000	>2,000	>2,000	>2,000
Intravenous	5	134	167	153	153

[a]LD_{50}, 50% lethal dose; F, female; M, male.

Table 62 In vitro activity of DW-286

Organism(s)[a]	*n*	MIC (μg/ml)			
		DW-286		Ciprofloxacin	
		50%	90%	50%	90%
QSSA	112	0.008	0.016	0.25	0.5
QRSA	128	0.5	8.0	64	>64
S. epidermidis	63	0.03	0.25	0.25	16
S. pyogenes	34	0.016	0.03	1.0	2.0
E. faecalis	62	1.0	4.0	4.0	>64
E. faecium	54	4.0	8.0	16	>64
S. pneumoniae	30	0.016	0.0125	1.0	4.0
E. coli	97	0.06	0.5	0.03	0.5
K. pneumoniae	78	0.06	0.05	0.06	0.5
K. oxytoca	50	0.016	0.125	0.03	0.125
C. freundii	45	1.0	2.0	0.125	0.5
E. cloacae	65	0.031	0.5	0.06	0.5
E. aerogenes	30	0.125	0.25	0.06	0.5
P. mirabilis	45	0.25	2.0	0.016	4.0
P. vulgaris	13	0.25	1.0	0.06	2.0
P. rettgeri	11	0.03	0.125	0.016	0.03
P. stuartii	17	0.25	1.0	0.25	1.0
M. morganii	28	0.25	0.5	0.016	0.5
Salmonella enterica serovar Typhimurium	41	0.125	0.25	0.03	0.06
S. enterica serovar Enteritidis	20	0.0125	0.25	0.03	0.06
Shigella spp.	60	0.01	0.125	0.06	0.03
S. maltophilia	35	1.0	4.0	2.0	8.0
Acinelobactoe calcoaceticus	35	0.25	2.0	0.5	1.0
H. influenzae	20	0.004	0.008	0.004	0.016
P. aeruginosa	70	4.0	32	0.25	2.0

[a]QSSA, QRSA, quinolone-susceptible or -resistant *S. aureus*.

Table 63 In vivo efficacies of DW-286

Organism	PD_{50} (mg/kg)	
	DW-286	Ciprofloxacin
S. aureus Smith	0.12	3.43
MRSA	0.12	3.99
QRSA[a]	0.25	32
S. pyogenes	0.12	15
S. pneumoniae	0.19	10.05
E. coli	0.37	0.32
P. aeruginosa	6.29	0.94
K. pneumoniae	0.5	0.19

[a]QRSA, quinolone-resistant *S. aureus*.

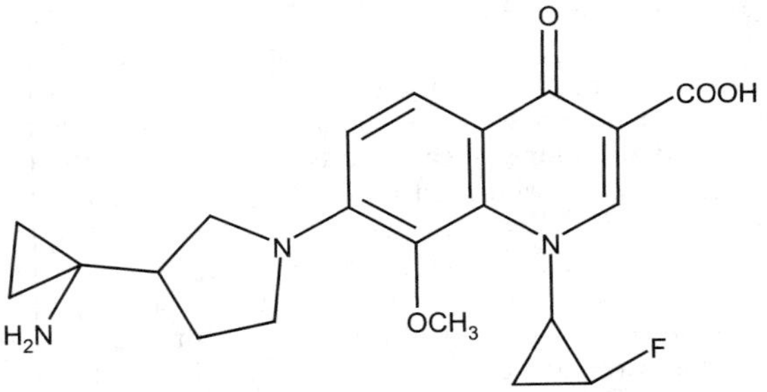

Figure 57 DX-619

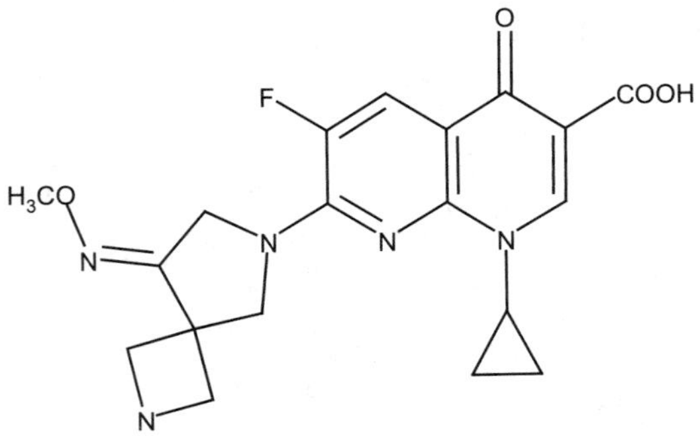

Figure 56 DW-224

5.12.18. Pradifloxacin

Pradifloxacin is an 8-cyano fluoroquinolone having a bicyclic moiety at C-7 and an N-1 cyclopropyl (Fig. 59). It seems mainly directed for veterinary use.

The pradifloxacin melting point is 241.9.°C, with a pK_a1 of 5.5 and a pK_a2 of 8.8. The water solubility is 33.5 g/liter at 20°C.

Pradifloxacin was tested comparatively with other veterinary fluoroquinolones against gram-negative bacilli of feline origin (Table 66).

Pradifloxacin displays good activity against anaerobes from cats and dogs (Table 67). The pharmacokinetics in dogs have been assessed after single and multiple doses; results are shown in Table 68.

Table 64 In vitro activity of DX-619

Organism[a]	n	MIC_{50} (μg/ml)
MSSA	48	0.008
MRSA	24	0.015
MRSA CIP[r]	99	1.0
S. pneumoniae Pen[r]	60	0.06
S. pyogenes	49	0.008
E. faecalis	50	0.06
E. faecium	47	1.0
E. coli	48	0.03
K. pneumoniae	49	0.06
H. influenzae β^+	21	≤0.004
H. influenzae β^- BLNAR	25	≤0.004
M. catarrhalis	46	0.015
P. aeruginosa	51	1.0

[a]CIP, ciprofloxacin; β^+, β-lactamase producing; β^-, non-β-lactamase producing.

5.12.19. Piperazinyl-linked Fluoroquinolones

It was shown that some piperazinyl-linked fluoroquinolone dimmers are able to overcome efflux-mediated resistance in gram-positive organisms. Some of them exhibited good in vitro activity against *S. aureus* (MIC, ≤0.03 to 9.125 μg/ml) (Fig. 60) (Kerns et al., 2001).

5.12.20. WQ-0835

WQ-0835 is a tricyclic fluoroquinolone (Fig. 61). In vitro, WQ-0835 is less active than temafloxacin against gram-positive cocci but more active than ciprofloxacin. It is inactive against *E. faecium* and showed activity against *Enterobacteriaceae* equivalent to that of ciprofloxacin. It is less active than ciprofloxacin against *P. aeruginosa* (Table 69).

5.13. Combinations of 4-Quinolones and Other Antibiotics

The treatment of severe infections, whether of nosocomial origin or occurring in deficiency states, often requires the combination of two antibacterial agents. In the case of the

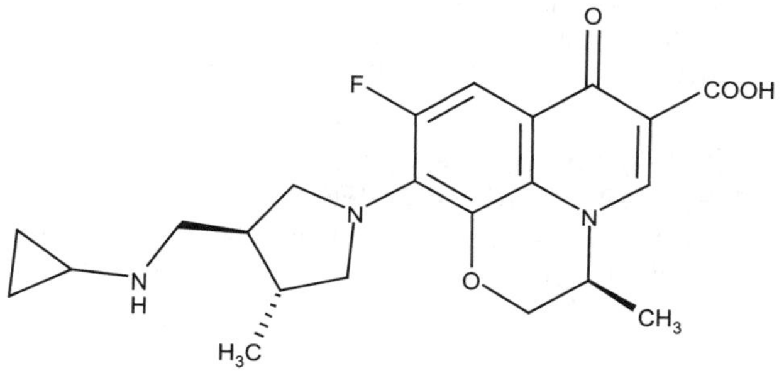

Figure 58 AM-1939

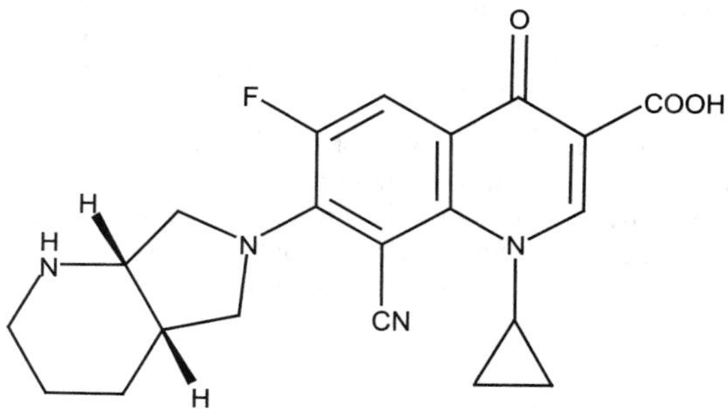

Figure 59 Pradofloxacin

Table 65 In vitro activity of AM-1939 against gram-positive cocci

Organism	MIC (μg/ml)		
	AM-1939	Levofloxacin	Ciprofloxacin
S. aureus SA 113	0.008	0.06	0.06
S. aureus SA 113 NY 12 (*norA*)	0.03	1.0	4.0
E. faecalis KU 1856 (VanA)	0.5	16	32
E. faecalis 1857 (VanB)	1.0	32	64
S. epidermidis	1.0	128	32
S. pneumoniae	0.5	32	64

Table 66 In vitro activity of veterinary fluoroquinolone against gram-negative bacilli from Felidae

Organism	n	MIC_{50} (μg/ml)				
		Pradofloxacin	Difloxacin	Enrofloxacin	Marbofloxacin	Orbifloxacin
B. bronchiseptica	113	0.12	4.0	0.5	0.5	2.0
E. coli	1,065	0.008	0.06	0.015	0.03	0.06
K. pneumoniae	31	0.015	0.12	0.03	0.03	0.12
P. multocida	47	0.002	0.015	0.008	0.015	0.015
P. mirabilis	98	0.12	1.0	0.12	0.06	1.0
P. aeruginosa	400	0.5	1.0	1.0	0.5	4.0
Salmonella	58	0.008	0.06	0.03	0.03	0.06
S. intermedius	1,420	0.03	0.25	0.12	0.25	0.5
S. aureus	232	0.03	0.25	0.12	0.25	0.25

Table 67 Pradofloxacin activity against anaerobes from cats and dogs

Organism	n	MIC (μg/ml)	
		Pradofloxacin	Metronidazole
Sporomusa	9	0.25–2.0	0.125–4.0
Porphyromonas	8	0.03–0.25	0.06–4.0
Eubacterium	7	0.06–8.0	0.25–2.0
Propionibacterium	6	0.25–2.0	0.125–256
Actinomyces	4	0.125–8.0	0.25–8
Peptostreptococcus	4	0.06–8.0	0.25–16
Ruminococcus	3	0.25–4.0	0.06–0.5
Desulfomonile	2	0.125–4.0	1.0–256
Megamonas	2	0.5–1.0	0.5
Sebaldella	2	0.06–0.125	0.5–4.0
Selenomonas	2	0.5–1.0	1.0–16

fluoroquinolones, it is recommended that these be combined against strains of *Enterobacteriaceae* of reduced susceptibility and in the case of *S. aureus* and *P. aeruginosa* infections.

Against difficult-to-treat *Enterobacteriaceae* (*S. marcescens, C. freundii, Enterobacter* spp., and certain strains of *K. pneumoniae*), the combination of a fluoroquinolone and an aminoglycoside is additive and rarely synergistic or antagonistic.

For *P. aeruginosa*, this type of combination is synergistic for about 30% of strains. The combination of ciprofloxacin and tobramycin has been shown to be synergistic against *Acinetobacter baumannii*. Against MRSA strains, the combination of a fluoroquinolone and an aminoglycoside is usually additive.

The combination of a fluoroquinolone and a β-lactam is additive but is sometimes synergistic (≤5%) or antagonistic (~1%).

The combination of ciprofloxacin and vancomycin is not synergistic against MRSA strains. In some cases, this combination may be indifferent or even antagonistic. Likewise, the combination of ofloxacin and phosphomycin is indifferent or sometimes synergistic.

The combination of ciprofloxacin and clindamycin is synergistic against 20 to 30% of the strains of *B. fragilis* tested. The combination of ciprofloxacin and metronidazole is indifferent. The combination of levofloxacin and metronidazole against *B. fragilis* is additive.

5.14. Breakpoints in France

Table 70 lists the breakpoints proposed by the French Antibiotic Sensitivity Test Committee in 1998. All of the disks of fluoroquinolones are loaded with 5 μg of drug substance, except trovafloxacin (10 μg).

5.15. Intracellular Concentrations

A number of pathogenic agents are localized inside phagocytic cells. The molecules must not only penetrate but also accumulate in those areas where the bacteria are found. Some fluoroquinolones concentrate in the cytoplasm of phagocytic cells, but few do so in phagolysosomes (Table 71).

6. MECHANISMS OF ACTION OF FLUOROQUINOLONES

The mechanisms of action and resistance have only partially been elucidated. The mode of action of the 4-quinolones is

Table 68 Pharmacokinetics of pradofloxacin in dogs after oral dosing

Treatment days	Parameter	Dose (mg/kg)			
		1	3	6	9
1	C_{max} (μg/ml)	0.47	1.44	3.15	4.17
	T_{max} (h)	1.5	2.1	1.5	1.9
	AUC (μg·h/ml)	3.82	12.69	23.39	32.78
5	C_{max} (μg/ml)	0.62	1.60	3.63	5.15
	T_{max} (h)	1.4	1.5	1.1	1.8
	AUC (μg·h/ml)	4.65	13.11	25.71	35.85
28	C_{max} (μg/ml)	0.56	1.66	3.83	5.57
	T_{max} (h)	1.4	1.6	1.3	1.6
	AUC (μg·h/ml)	3.32	9.87	19.56	29.52
	$t_{1/2}$ (h)	5.6	7.2	6.8	6.1
	Ratio	1.1	1.1	1.1	1.1

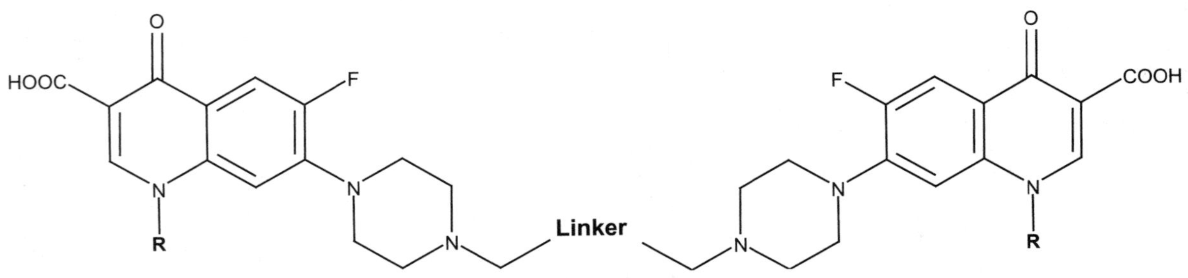

Figure 60 Piperazinyl-linked fluoroquinolones

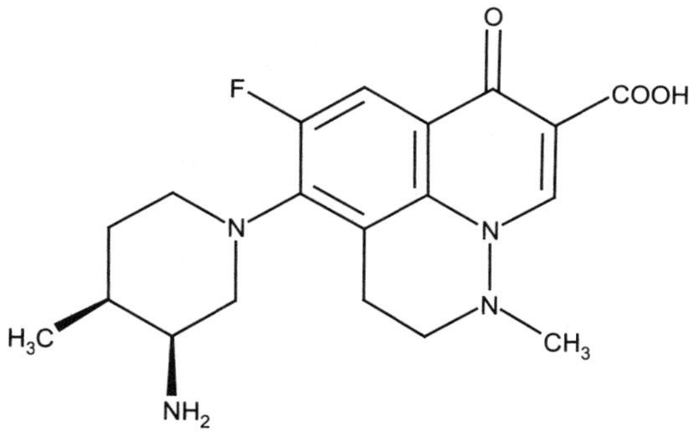

Figure 61 WQ-0835

Table 69 In vitro activity of WQ-0835

Organism	MIC_{50} (μg/ml)	
	WQ-0835	Ciprofloxacin
MSSA	0.39	0.78
MRSA	0.78	3.13
S. epidermidis	0.10	0.39
S. pneumoniae	0.39	0.78
S. pyogenes	0.39	0.78
E. faecalis	0.78	1.56
E. faecium	3.13	6.25
K. pneumoniae	0.05	0.05
C. freundii	0.20	0.10
E. cloacae	0.05	0.05
S. marcescens	0.20	0.20
M. morganii	0.05	0.05
P. rettgeri	0.20	0.05
P. aeruginosa	0.78	0.39

based on the capacity of the molecules to cross the bacterial membranes and to inhibit DNA synthesis, associated with one or more other mechanisms that induce cell death. The intrabacterial concentration is the result of an equilibrium between the accumulation of the molecules and their efflux through the cytoplasmic membrane (active efflux). The quinolones have a common mechanism of action, but because of their specific structures they have additional mechanisms that explain the difference in their in vitro activities. The mechanism of action is dependent on their physicochemical properties.

6.1. Transmembrane Transport

Transmembrane penetration is more complex for gram-negative bacilli than for gram-positive cocci.

In gram-negative bacteria, there are several routes of penetration for antibacterial agents, especially the porins and the auto-induced pathway for cationic molecules. Transport via porin or nonporin pathways is dependent on the hydrophobicity of the molecules.

6.1.1. Gram-Positive Bacteria

In gram-positive cocci, the cell wall is composed mainly of peptidoglycan, which does not obstruct the penetration of antibacterial agents. The cell wall contains teichoic acid, a polymer consisting of glycerol and ribitol phosphate and which is negatively charged, facilitating the passage of positively charged molecules and inhibiting that of anions. The most hydrophobic molecules penetrate best.

Table 70 Breakpoints of fluoroquinolones (French Antibiotic Sensitivity Test Committee, 1998)

Compound	MIC (μg/ml)		Zone diam (mm)	
	Susceptible	Resistant	Susceptible	Resistant
Ofloxacin	≤1	>4	≥22	<16
Ciprofloxacin	≤1	>2	≥22	<19
Norfloxacin	≤1	>2	≥22	<19
Pefloxacin	≤1	>4	≥22	<16
Lomefloxacin	≤1	>2	≥22	<19
Sparfloxacin	≤1	>2	≥20	<16
Trovafloxacin	≤1	>2	≥20	<17
Grepafloxacin	≤1	>2	≥20	<17
Levofloxacin[a]	≤2	>4	≥17	<15
Levofloxacin[b]	≤1	>4	≥20	<15

[a]*S. pneumoniae*.
[b]Other bacteria.

6.1.2. Gram-Negative Bacteria

The wall is complex and constitutes an important barrier to the penetration of anti-infective agents. The bacterial wall consists of two main elements: lipopolysaccharide (LPS) and porin proteins. Before reaching the cytoplasm, the 4-quinolones must cross the LPS, the bacterial outer membrane, and the cytoplasmic membrane.

6.1.2.1. LPS

LPS is composed of lipid A, a polysaccharide core, and external polysaccharide chains. The whole arrangement is maintained by the presence of bivalent metal ions such as Mg^{2+}, which allows the formation of bridges between the different LPS chains. LPS is linked covalently to peptidoglycan. The 4-quinolones are capable of crossing LPS by chelating magnesium ions, disorganizing this structure and causing the appearance of hydrophobic zones (auto-induced pathway) (Fig. 62). The polysaccharide chain exhibits no barrier effect to derivatives with a partition coefficient (*n*-octanol–0.1 M phosphate buffer) equal to or less than 0.1. When the partition coefficient is between 0.1 and 2.0, the activity against rough strains is increased, demonstrating indirectly that LPS is a potential barrier to certain 4-quinolones. When the partition coefficient is between 2.0 and 13.0, the MICs for rough strains are 4 to 16 times weaker than against smooth strains.

6.1.2.2. Porins

The outer membrane of gram-negative bacilli comprises numerous proteins, including the porins OmpC, OmpF, PhoE, and LamB. The bacterial outer membrane contains up to 10^5 copies of the different porins per cell. The majority of porins are in the form of trimers. The outer membrane of *E. coli* K-12 contains two porins, OmpC and OmpF, which possess porin channels of 1.2 and 2.9 nm, respectively, and which are coregulated, particularly in relation to the osmolarity of the culture medium. The importance in quantitative terms of each of the two porins is related to the supercoiling of DNA.

The porins allow the transparietal passage of hydrophilic molecules. The majority of fluoroquinolones use the porin pathway, as has been demonstrated with porin-deficient strains of *E. coli* or *Salmonella enterica* serovar Typhimurium as a result of mutation of the *ompF* gene. They principally use the OmpF porin and, more secondarily, the OmpC and PhoE porins. Intrabacterial accumulation is reduced in the absence of the three proteins, but it has been shown with norfloxacin that there was still 40% accumulation of the

Table 71 Intracellular concentration and efflux of fluoroquinolones[a]

Compound	Method	Cells	Intracellular/ extracellular ratio (time)	Intracellular location	Efflux (%) time	Bactericide
Pefloxacin	R	PMN	4 (0.5 h)			*S. aureus* + *K. pneumoniae*
	R	J774	8 (0.5 h)	Cytosol		
	R	PMPH			80 (5 min)	
	R	GR	0.07 (0.5 h)			
	R	MPH	9.6 (0.5 h)			
Ciprofloxacin	M	MPH	2.7 (0.5 h)			
	HPLC	PMN	8 (5 min)			*S. aureus*
	HPLC	PMN	4 (0.5–2 h)			
	F	PMN	4.7 (0.3 h)			
	F	PMN	8.6 (0.5 h)		30 (5 min)	
	F	J774	4.4 (5 min)			*P. aeruginosa* + *S. aureus*
Ofloxacin	F	PMN	4.6 (0.3 h)			
	F	PMN	4.9 (5 min)		88 (5 min)	
	F	PMN	6.7 (0.3 h)		65 (5 min)	
	F	PMN	6.0 (5 min)			*P. aeruginosa*
	F	PMN	7.6 (0.5 h)		70 (5 min)	*S. aureus*
	HPLC	WI-38	8.6 (0.5 h)			
	F	HEp-2	2.8 (10 min)			
	F	McCoy	4.7 (10 min)			*Salmonella* serovar Enteritidis
	F	Vero	2.4 (10 min)			
	F	MDCK	1.9 (10 min)			
	F	J774	5.3 (5 min)			
Levofloxacin	F	PMN	6.1 (20 min)			
	F	PMN	8.3 (10 min)			*S. aureus*
	F	PMN	7.9 (0.5 h)			
	F	HEp-2	2.1 (10 min)			
	F	McCoy	3.9 (10 min)			
	F	Vero	2.1 (10 min)			
	F	MDCK	3.4 (10 min)			
	R	PMN	6.0 (5 min)	Cytosol	80 (5 min)	
Sparfloxacin	F	PMN	6.9 (20 min)			
	F	PMN	13.2 (5 min)			
	F	PMN	6.5 (20 min)		60 (5 min)	
	F	HEp-2	7.0 (20 min)			
	F	McCoy	10 (20 min)			*S. aureus*
	F	J774	6.4 (20 min)			
Trovafloxacin	R	PMN	11 (20 min)		80 (5 min)	
	R	PMPH (H)	10 (20 min)		65 (5 min)	*S. aureus*
	R	McCoy	9.6 (20 min)			*S. aureus*
Gatifloxacin	F	PMN	6.2 (0.5 h)		80 (5 min)	
	F	J774	6.9 (0.5 h)		100 (5 min)	
Grepafloxacin	R	THP-1		Cytosol	80 (60 min)	
	F	PMN	66 (0.5 h)		54 (5 min)	*S. aureus*
Prulifloxacin	F	PMN	12 (1 h)		43 (20 min)	
Fleroxacin	R	PMN	2 (0.5 h)	Cytosol		
	R	GR	0.14 (0.5 h)			*P. aeruginosa*
	R	J774	2 (0.5 h)			
Lomefloxacin	R	PMN	3.8 (0.5 h)	Cytosol		
	R	GR	0.7 (0.5 h)			
	R	J774	3.8 (0.5 h)			
Moxifloxacin	F	PMN	10.9 (20 min)		60 (1 h)	
	F	PMN			80 (5 h)	
	F	McCoy	8.7		80 (5 min)	*S. aureus*
Olamufloxacin	M	PMN	35.4	Cytosol	67 (2 min)	
Gemifloxacin	R	MPH	28 (5 min)		30 (60 min)	
Pazufloxacin		MPH	7 (0.5 min)			*S. aureus* + *Salmonella* serovar Typhimurium
						L. pneumophila
						P. aeruginosa + *Salmonella* serovar Enteritidis

[a]Data from Labro et al., 1988. PMN, polymorphonuclear neutrophils; GR, erythrocytes; MPH, macrophages; PMPH, peritoneal macrophages; F, Fluorimeter; M, microbiology; HPLC, high-performance liquid chromatography; R, radioisotopy.

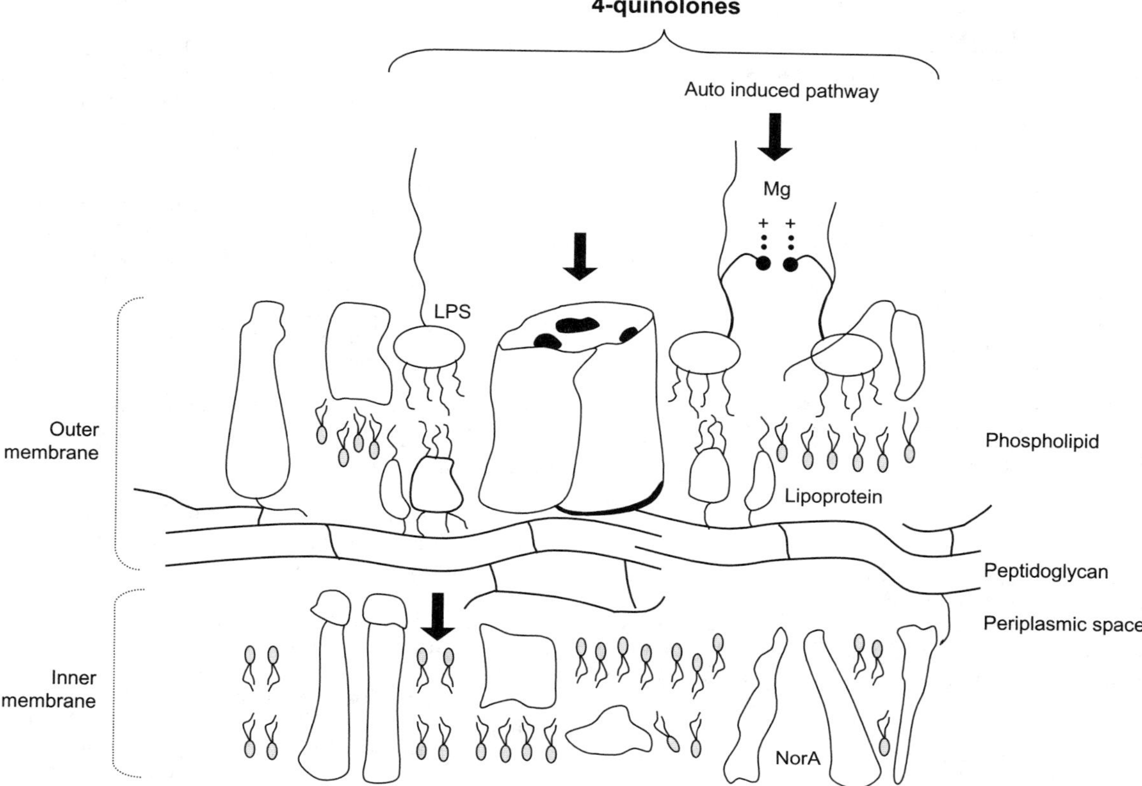

Figure 62 Transmembrane passage of fluoroquinolones

molecule in *E. coli*, suggesting other mechanisms of penetration of the bacterial outer membrane.

This mechanism is not specific, since it involves other chemical entities, such as tetracyclines, cephalosporins, or chloramphenicol.

K. pneumoniae possesses a 39-kDa wall protein, the functions of which are similar to that of the OmpF protein of *E. coli*. In *S. marcescens*, the 40- and 41-kDa wall proteins appear to be similar to the OmpF protein of *E. coli*. In *K. pneumoniae* and *S. marcescens*, the absence of the 39- and 41-kDa proteins produces resistance to norfloxacin, but also to other antibiotics such as cefoxitin, the tetracyclines, and chloramphenicol.

In *C. freundii* 791, resistance to ciprofloxacin is associated with the absence of a 45-kDa outer membrane protein and the increased presence of another 37-kDa protein. In *P. aeruginosa*, transparietal passage of the fluoroquinolones appears to be the same as for imipenem via the $OprD_2$ wall protein.

In *Alcaligenes faecalis*, ciprofloxacin does not accumulate within the bacterial cell because of the small porin diameter, whereas there is a strong affinity for DNA gyrase (IC_{50}, 0.015 μg/ml).

6.1.2.3. Inner Membrane

The precise mechanism by which fluoroquinolones pass through the inner membrane is poorly elucidated. It might involve either an energy-independent passive process or an energy-dependent active transport process. It would seem, however, that passage through this membrane occurs by means of a transporter and is controlled by a pH gradient.

6.2. Intrabacterial Concentration

The intrabacterial concentrations are the result of the equilibrium obtained between the quantity of fluoroquinolones penetrating the bacterial cell and that eliminated by active efflux.

6.2.1. Intrabacterial Accumulation

Intrabacterial accumulation varies according to the molecule and the bacterial species. However, the antibacterial activity appears to be independent of the intracellular concentration.

In *E. coli* and *S. aureus*, transparietal penetration is rapid, about 10 to 20 s, and a plateau is reached in 60 to 80s for a concentration of 27 to 45 μM (10 μg/ml). This phase is followed by a slower period of accumulation, lasting about 30 min.

In *P. aeruginosa* and *K. pneumoniae*, the fluoroquinolones accumulate more slowly, reaching a plateau in about 6 min. Penetration is nonsaturable in *E. coli* and *P. aeruginosa*, which appears to indicate that transparietal diffusion is a passive phenomenon. However, accumulation within the same bacterial species may vary and depends on the method of determination (Table 72).

6.2.2. Efflux

The existence of an active efflux has been demonstrated in *E. coli, P. aeruginosa, S. pneumoniae, E. faecalis, B. fragilis*, and *V. parahaemolyticus*. The efflux pump unit is a complex composed of several proteins: EmrAB and TolC. The EmrAB unit protects *E. coli* from oxidative phosphorylation. In particular, it causes the extrusion of the fluoroquinolones and thiolactomycin, an antibacterial agent that inhibits fatty

Table 72 Intracellular accumulation of fluoroquinolones in *E. coli*

Compound	*E. coli* strain	I/E[a] ratio	Method
Ofloxacin	NIHJ-JC2	11.6	HPLC[b]
Ciprofloxacin	NIHJ-JC2	19.5	^{14}C
	KL-16	20	^{14}C
	NCTC 10358	6	Fluorimeter
Pefloxacin	KL-12	16.2	^{14}C
Norfloxacin	KL-16	16	^{14}C
	KL-16	20	^{14}C
Fleroﬂoxacin	JF 568	4	Fluorimeter
Lomefloxacin	KL-16	3.7	^{14}C
Enofloxacin	SA 1306	9	^{14}C
	KL-16	80	^{14}C
Amifloxacin	KL-16	2.6	^{14}C
Sparfloxacin	NCTC 10538	5.3	^{14}C

[a]I/E, intracellular/extracellular.
[b]HPLC, high-performance liquid chromatography.

acid synthesis. The TolC protein is localized in the outer membrane. It is one of the components of the EmrAB pump. The EmrA protein acts with the TolC protein, which possesses porin properties. The EmrAB/TolC efflux pump is very common in gram-negative bacilli. The *emrAB* operon is regulated by the *emrR* gene. Several molecules induce this pump.

Another molecule belongs to the RND (resistance modulation cell division) family.

6.2.2.1. AcrAB/TolC Efflux Pump in *E. coli*

See Fig. 63.

The AcrAB pump protects the bacterial cell from the toxic effects of a large number of agents. AcrA is equivalent to EmrA with an association with the TolC protein. The AcrB protein is a 1,000-kDa translocase.

The *emr* operon is localized at 57.5 min on the *E. coli* chromosome and codes for two proteins, EmrA and EmrB. EmrA is a hydrophilic protein attached to the cytoplasmic membrane via a hydrophobic domain. EmrB is a membrane protein of the 14-TMS family. Hyperproduction of the *erm* gene (multiple plasmid copies) causes reduced susceptibility of *E. coli* to nalidixic acid, but not to the hydrophilic fluoroquinolones. The Erm system of *E. coli* differs from that of *S. aureus* or *P. aeruginosa*, as it only exports hydrophobic molecules.

The efflux of norfloxacin is subject to the AcrB system, which is expressed as a phenotype of the MAR system (multiple antibiotic resistance).

6.2.2.2. MexAB/Opr Pump of *P. aeruginosa*

In *P. aeruginosa*, resistance to the fluoroquinolones reflects the hyperexpression of one or more efflux systems capable of exporting fluoroquinolones, tetracyclines, chloramphenicol, and β-lactams, including carbapenems. The mechanism of this multiple resistance appears to be related to an OprK protein. The *oprK* gene belongs to an operon composed of three genes coding for two cytoplasmic membrane proteins of 40 and 108 kDa and for OprK. It has been shown that the OprM protein plays an important role in this system. The *mexAB-oprK* operon has been renamed

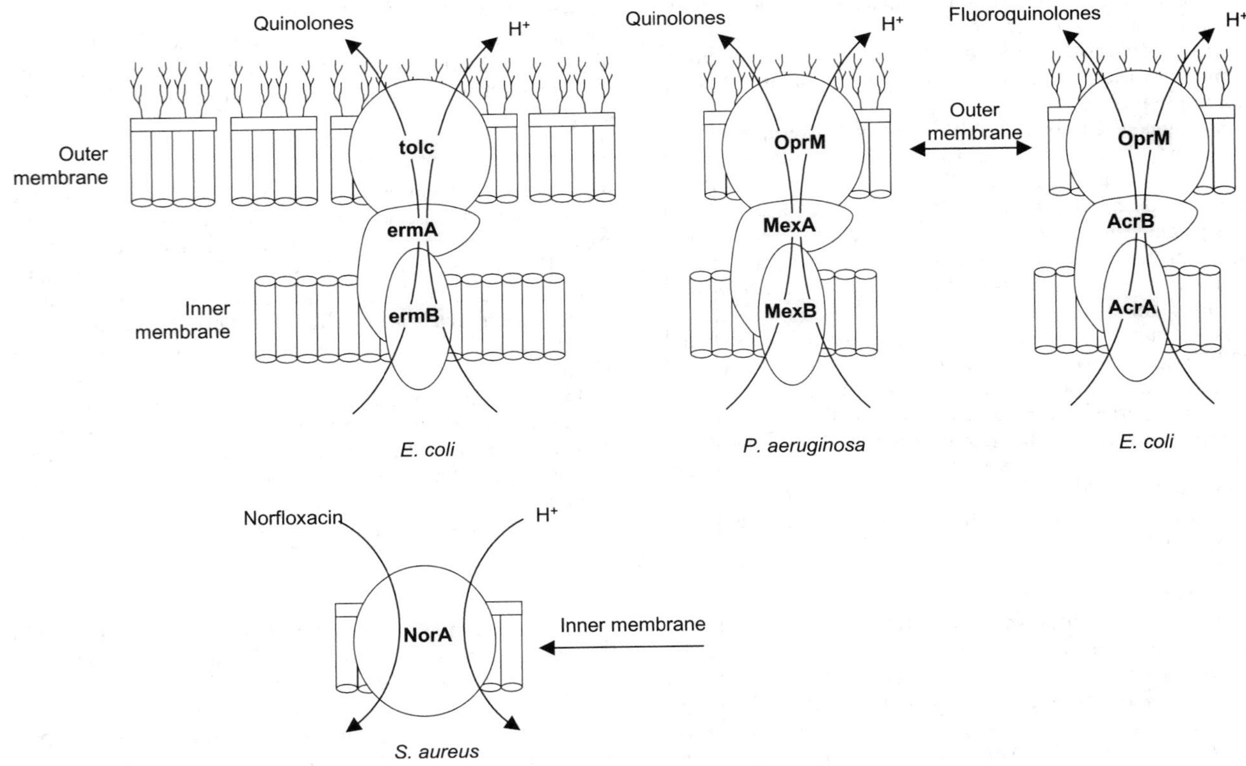

Figure 63 Efflux pump of fluoroquinolones

mexAB-oprM. The natural function of this operon is to allow the exportation of pyoverdin and its degradation products. However, it is a nonspecific transport system. The expression of this operon is under the control of the *mexR* regulatory gene. A mutation in this gene (*nalB*: Arg60→Trp) causes activation of the operon and hyperproduction of the OprM protein. In *P. aeruginosa*, there is at least one efflux system. A mutation in the *nfxB* regulatory gene (as distinct from *nalB*) yields mutants that remain susceptible to meropenem and that hyperproduce a 54-kDa wall protein, OprJ. Intrabacterial accumulation of norfloxacin in these mutants is greatly reduced. The *nfxC* mutants (46 min) are resistant to fluoroquinolones, imipenem, and chloramphenicol, but they become hypersensitive to the other β-lactams and aminoglycosides. They have a smaller quantity of OprD and an increase in OprN (50 kDa).

Loss of the OprF protein in mutant strains is accompanied by hyperproduction of an OprH protein. The strains are hypersusceptible to the majority of fluoroquinolones.

6.2.2.3. Efflux System in Gram-Positive Bacilli and Cocci

The reduction in the susceptibility of *S. aureus* to fluoroquinolones due to an efflux phenomenon was described in 1990. As opposed to the gram-negative bacilli, gram-positive bacteria do not have an outer membrane. The efflux pumps belong to three families: MFS, SMR, and ABC.

In the MFS protein family, the proteins concerned are as follows: for *B. subtilis*, Bmr and Blt; for *S. aureus*, NorA, QacA, and QacB; for *Lactococcus lactis*, LmrP; for *Streptomyces pristinespiralis*, Ptr; and for *M. smegmatis*, LfrA. They belong to the 12- and 14-TMS family (Fig. 64).

6.2.2.3.1. NorA protein. The NorA protein is a 43-kDa polypeptide localized on the cytoplasmic membrane of *S. aureus* and *S. epidermidis*. The NorA protein of *S. aureus* is a polypeptide composed of 388 amino acids and containing 12 hydrophobic regions, 9 of which have proline residues. The *norA* gene is localized on the D fragment of the *S. aureus* chromosome. These residues are associated with the presence of transmembrane transport molecules; they allow the reversible conformational changes necessary for the opening or closing of the pores.

This involves an energy-dependent pump that allows the efflux of the 4-quinolones. In the event of a mutation (aspartic acid 27→alanine of the C-terminal region) the rate of efflux is increased for the most hydrophilic molecules.

Efflux is an active phenomenon that is inhibited by carbonyl cyanide-*m*-chlorophenylhydrazone (protonophore). The natural function of the NorA protein has not been elucidated. By analogy with the Bmr protein, it is assumed that it allows the elimination of a number of toxic agents, such as chloramphenicol, fluoroquinolones, and ethidium bromide.

The increase in efflux is due to hyperproduction of the NorA protein. Ng et al. (1994) have shown that hyperexpression of the *norA* gene in an *flqB* mutant is due to the replacement of a single nucleotide in the promoter of the *norA* gene. It differs from the *bmr* gene, whose hyperexpression is due to genetic amplification. Resistance due to hyperexpression of the *norA* gene is inducible. For the hydrophilic quinolones, a mutation in the *norA* gene is responsible for a 32-fold increase in the MIC. However, the hydrophobicity of the quinolones is not the sole factor allowing the NorA protein to be used. The steric hindrance of the substituents at positions 7 and 8 of the quinoline and 1,8-naphthyridine nucleus also plays a part.

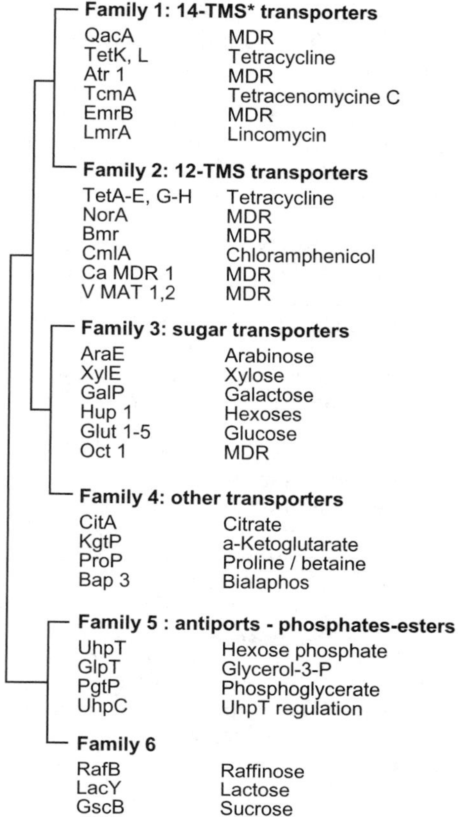

Figure 64 Phylogenetic tree of the evolution of six transporter families (TMS, tansmembrane segments)

A NorA-type polypeptide has also been detected in *E. coli*. In *B. subtilis*, the polypeptide Brm plays a role similar to that of the NorA protein in relation to the fluoroquinolones. The TetA to -E and TetG and H proteins belong to this family. The *norA* gene is of chromosomal origin. It is present in *S. aureus* and *S. epidermidis* but has not been detected in *E. faecalis*.

6.3. Cell Targets: DNA Gyrase and/or Topoisomerase IV

Inhibition of DNA synthesis is the first biochemical event to occur, within a few minutes, in the presence of low concentrations of 4-quinolone. This stage is bacteriostatic. The bactericidal activity is related to other mechanisms.

6.3.1. Bacterial Chromosome and DNA Gyrase

The *E. coli* chromosome is composed of a helicoidal, circular, two-chain DNA measuring 1,300 μm in length. A bacterium measures, on average, 1 to 2 μm in length. An intracellular DNA "condensation" mechanism is therefore required. The DNA is supercoiled by means of two enzymes: DNA gyrase (topoisomerase II) and topoisomerase I. DNA gyrase is responsible for topological changes, supercoiling, and relaxation. Topoisomerase I modulates the DNA gyrase-induced supercoiling phenomenon by increasing the relaxation component.

The tertiary structure of a circular, double-stranded DNA is defined by three parameters: *LK* (linking), *T* (twisting), and *W* (supercoiling or writhing). *T* is the number of times the double chain winds around itself. It depends on the length and thread of the helix, which is determined by the geometry of the molecule, itself dependent on the medium in which it is located.

LK is the number of times that one of the chains of the molecule crosses over the other chain in space. It is an algebraic whole number. This parameter represents a topological property of DNA and remains constant in all deformations of the double chain not involving a cut.

When the axis of the double helix can be maintained in one plane, the two numbers *LK* and *T* are equal and correspond to the relaxed state.

If the axis is out of plane, the molecule is said to be supercoiled with a supercoiling number equal to *W*. The parameter is therefore defined as follows: $W = LK - T$. The writhing number is a geometric value and cannot be an integer.

The replication of DNA is a highly controlled, complex phenomenon that is coordinated with cell growth. In *E. coli*, replication begins in a specific zone of the chromosome known as oriC. It occurs in two directions along the chromosome at the replication fork until it meets an end sequence. The joint action of two enzymes, DNA helicase and DNA polymerase, introduces positive supercoiling into the DNA, which allows the progression of the replication fork. DNA gyrase regulates this fork by introducing negative supercoiling, and topoisomerase IV allows the separation of the daughter DNA strands. Because of the rapid multiplication of bacteria, there are several simultaneous replication forks, hence the need for coordination and effective control. The roles of DNA gyrase and topoisomerase IV are therefore essential for bacterial survival.

6.3.2. Topoisomerases

There are four topoisomerases in bacteria. They catalyze the passage of a DNA strand through a DNA nick. Two types of enzymes have been described: type I, which catalyzes the passage of a single strand, and type II, which catalyzes the passage of two strands of DNA. These two enzymes then allow the DNA to reseal. The characteristics of the four topoisomerases are summarized in Table 73.

6.3.2.1. Topoisomerase I

Topoisomerase I was isolated in 1969 from *E. coli*. It is a 110-kDa monomer encoded by the *topA* gene in *E. coli*. Topoisomerase I or protein ω intervenes in the regulation of negative supercoiling by preventing excessive supercoiling of the DNA. It acts in the absence of ATP. It is an essential enzyme, as it equilibrates DNA gyrase activity.

6.3.2.2. Topoisomerase III

Topoisomerase III also enables negative supercoiling of DNA to be undone; it acts at the moment of decatenation.

6.3.3. Topoisomerase II, or DNA Gyrase

DNA gyrase is composed of four subunits: two A subunits and two B subunits, which are the products of the chromosomal genes *gyrA* and *gyrB*. The characteristics of the two subunits are summarized in Table 74.

DNA gyrase has two essential activities: supercoiling (involved in the replication of the chromosome) and decatenation (involved in the division of the chromosome).

DNA gyrase is necessary and essential for the survival of the bacterium, as it is involved in the replication, repair, genetic transcription, and recombination of DNA. DNA gyrase allows the temporary cleavage of the two DNA strands and then reseals them and supercoils them.

From a two-chain, circular, and relaxed DNA, DNA gyrase transiently cuts the two strands between a thymidine and a guanine, forming a covalent and temporary bond with an O^4 phosphate of DNA. To change the topography of the supercoiled DNA, DNA gyrase uses the hydroxyl of tyrosine 122 of the A subunit as a nucleophil to allow the hydrolysis of the phosphodiester bond between two base pairs, so that one base releases its 3′-OH and the enzyme remains temporarily attached to the 5′-OH of the adjacent base. Similar hydrolysis occurs four residues further along on the other strand.

6.3.4. DNA Gyrase and 4-Quinolones

It appears to be accepted that DNA gyrase is one of the principal targets of the 4-quinolones.

6.3.4.1. Inhibition of Supercoiling Activity

The GyrA subunit, the target of the quinolones, is cleaved in two domains by trypsin: on the one hand, a 64-kDa functional N-terminal domain containing the active

Table 74 Molecular weights of the two DNA gyrase subunits of different bacterial species

Organism	Mol wt	
	Subunit A	Subunit B
E. coli	97	90
C. freundii	107	96
P. aeruginosa	92	108
S. aureus	72	99.7
E. faecalis	100	85
B. subtilis	100	85
Micrococcus luteus	115	87
C. jejuni	95	90
K. pneumoniae	97	
H. pylori	92.5	
N. gonorrhoeae	86	
Aeromonas salmonicida	101	
S. pneumoniae		72
M. pneumoniae		72
M. hominis		73
Clostridium acetobutylicum	92.5	72

Table 73 Properties of bacterial topoisomerases

Topoisomerase	Gene(s)	Localization (min)	Other name	Property
I	*topA*	28	Protein ω	Negative relaxation of supercoiled DNA
II	*gyrA, gyrB*	48.83	DNA gyrase	DNA negative supercoiling
III	*topB*	39		Decatenation
IV	*parC, parE*	66, 66		Chromosome partition

site of DNA gyrase (tyrosine 122, the site of cutting/resealing of DNA gyrase) and the mutation site associated with resistance to the quinolones, and on the other hand, a 33-kDa structural C-terminal domain providing the stability of the DNA-DNA gyrase complex. Subunit B also comprises two domains: a functional N-terminal domain, which includes the site of hydrolysis of ATP, and a structural C-terminal domain, responsible for the interaction with the GyrA subunit and with DNA.

DNA gyrase causes relaxation of the DNA by means of DNA gyrase subunit A (a 64-kDa fragment of the N-terminal region) and a 47-kDa fragment of the C-terminal region of the B subunit.

The DNA coils around the A_2B_2 tetramer, forming a loop of 140 bp (Fig. 65). Each end of the DNA molecule remains attached to one of the A subunits by a covalent bond between the phosphorus atom at 5′ of a nucleotide and an oxygen atom of tyrosine 122 (*E. coli*) of the active site. After passage of the second DNA segment through this cut, it is sealed by a second transesterification reaction between the hydroxyl groups of the DNA and the phosphorus-tyrosine bridges. Finally, the DNA gyrase detaches itself from the DNA, to which two negative supercoil turns have been added. The reaction requires Mg^{2+}, and two ATP molecules are hydrolyzed at each cycle.

On the basis of crystallographic studies of topoisomerase II in yeasts and *E. coli*, a so-called two-gate mechanism has been proposed.

In the absence of a bond with DNA, the enzyme is in the shape of an open pincer. An open gate of GyrB allows the passage of a two-chain DNA fragment known as G and causes an initial conformational change of the enzyme. The attachment of an ATP molecule to the ATPase domains of each GyrB subunit induces a series of conformational changes with dimerization of the ATPase domains.

A second DNA fragment (known as T for transport) is then captured by the central cavity of the enzyme and passes through the temporary cut in the G segment. Fragment T is then released by the opening of a second gate in GyrA, while the cut in fragment G is repaired. Finally, hydrolysis of ATP allows the reversion to the initial conformation (open pincer), releasing segment G (Fig. 66).

DNA gyrase cleaves the two strands of DNA at the catalytic site, the cleavage sites being separated from one another by 4 bp. The cleavage site in the presence of quinolone is probably different from the spontaneous site. It occurs in a region composed of 20 bp between a thymine and a guanine. The presence of Mg^{2+} is important, and the presence of Ca^{2+} inhibits cleavage by ciprofloxacin and oxolinic acid. The negative supercoiling phase requires the presence of ATP, but the DNA relaxation phase does not (Fig. 67).

The molecular mechanism is poorly elucidated and remains disputed. It has not been definitively determined whether the 4-quinolones act directly on DNA gyrase or indirectly by binding to the bacterial DNA, given that this action is probably dependent on the chemical structure of the different molecules. DNA gyrase might recognize the 4-quinolones. The 4-quinolones could bind either to the DNA or to the DNA-DNA gyrase complex. The 4-quinolones appear to inhibit DNA gyrase activity by a specific bond at a site of the DNA revealed during the binding of DNA gyrase. At high concentrations, the 4-quinolones bind nonspecifically to DNA without the participation of the enzyme. Norfloxacin binds to pure DNA and not to DNA gyrase.

The 4-quinolones inhibit DNA synthesis biphasically. There is an early and rapid phase with induction of the SOS response proportional to the 4-quinolone concentration, followed by a slow phase.

The fluoroquinolones bind to the different purine and pyrimidine bases by hydrogen bonds via the 3-carboxyl group and the 4-carbonyl of the pyridone β-carboxylic acid nucleus (Fig. 68). Analysis of the nalidixic acid crystal shows that two molecules are attached opposite one another in the same plane by a bond at their N-1 hydrophobic groups. An aggregate composed of two, four, or more molecules of 4-quinolone is attached by hydrogen bonds between the 3-carboxyl and 4-carbonyl groups of the quinoline or 1,8-naphthyridine nuclei and the purine and pyrimidine

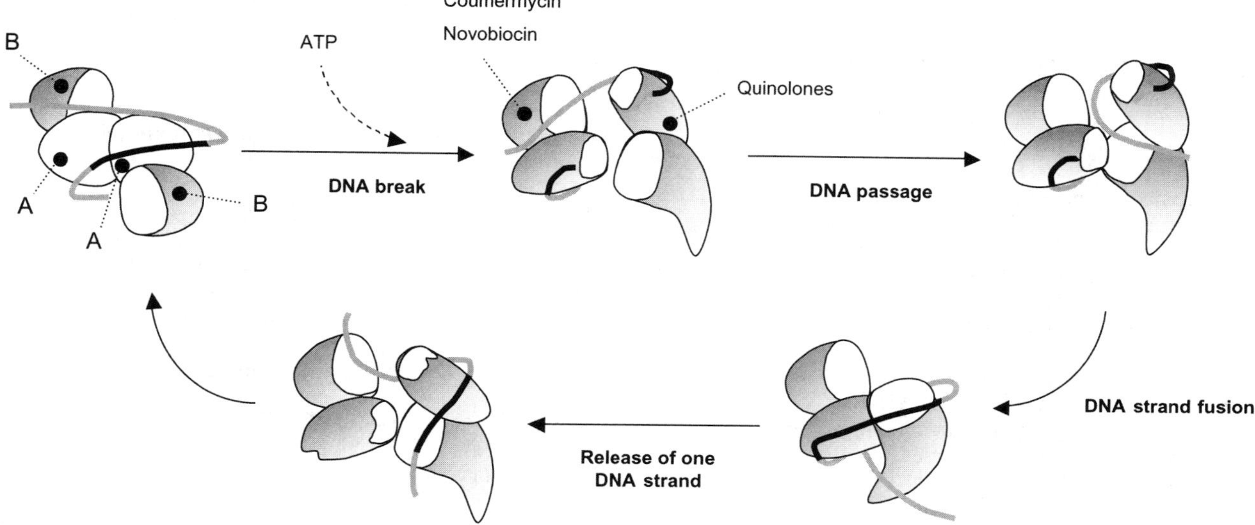

Figure 65 Model of the mode of action of DNA gyrase

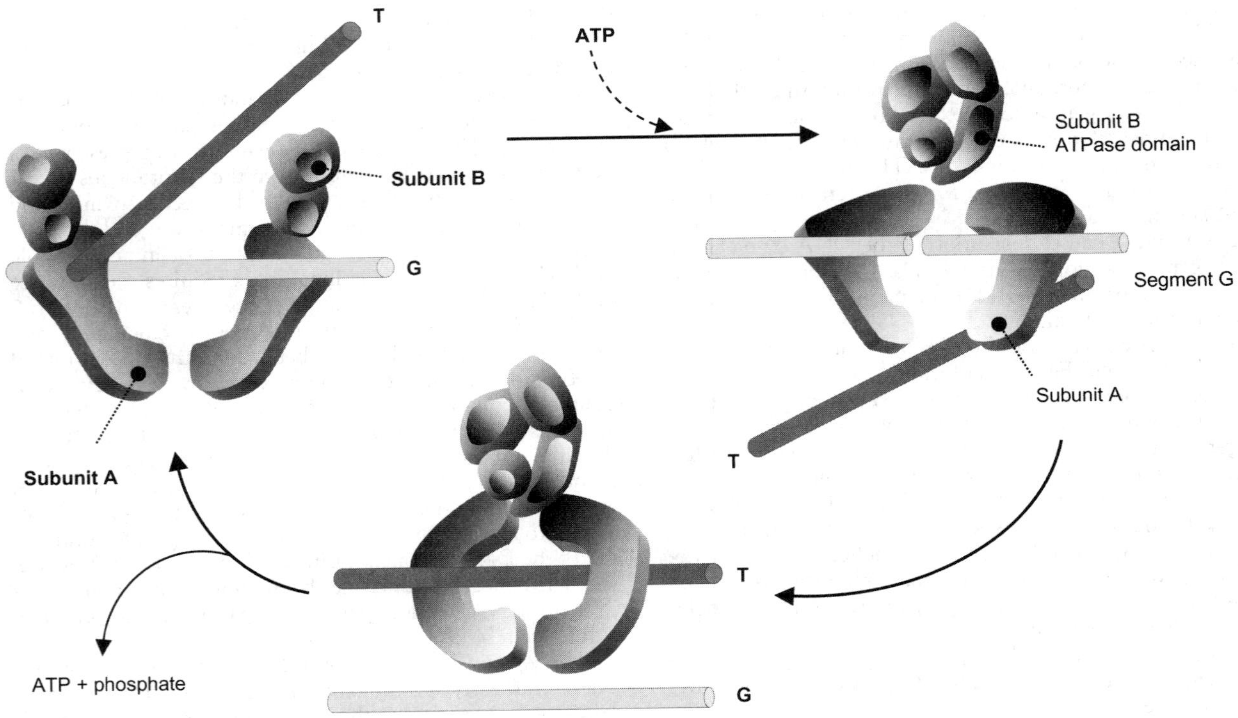

Figure 66 Two-door model

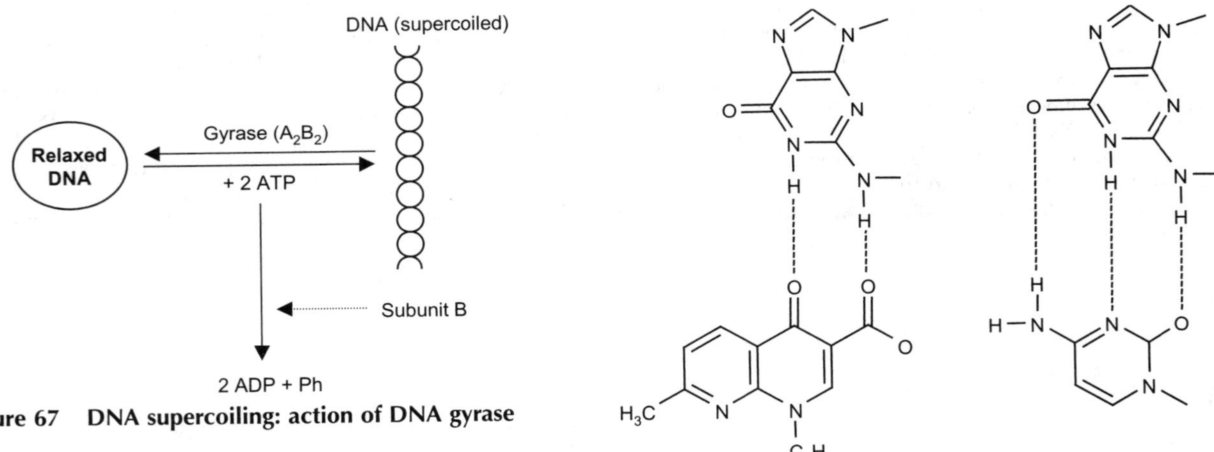

Figure 67 DNA supercoiling: action of DNA gyrase

Figure 68 Fixation of quinolone to DNA strand

bases inside the opening of the DNA strand. Binding to thymidine occurs via both groups, whereas for cytosine, guanine, and adenine it occurs via the 3-carboxyl group.

The 7-piperazine nucleus acts on DNA gyrase, not on DNA. There appears to be an electrostatic bond between this heterocycle and the B subunit, increasing the stability of the DNA gyrase–4-quinolone complex.

6.3.4.2. Quinolone Binding Models

Different models of quinolone binding to the DNA-DNA gyrase complex have been proposed, none of which are currently accepted.

In the models proposed by Shen et al. (1989) and Palumbo et al. (1993), the quinolones bind to the DNA at the free extremities of a 4-bp DNA strand released on cutting. The quinolones are bound either directly to the DNA via hydrogen bonds or via magnesium ions that form a bridge between the DNA phosphates and the quinolones (Fig. 69). In these models, cutting of the DNA is an essential precondition for binding of the quinolones. However, Critchlow et al. (1996) showed that the quinolones might bind to the DNA-DNA gyrase complex if the DNA is not opened.

In the models proposed by Maxwell et al. (1992) and Yoshida et al. (1993), the quinolones interact with the DNA-DNA gyrase complex at a specific site on the enzyme. This binding site forms a sort of pocket that appears at the time of the DNA cutting/sealing reaction and involves the GyrA and GyrB proteins.

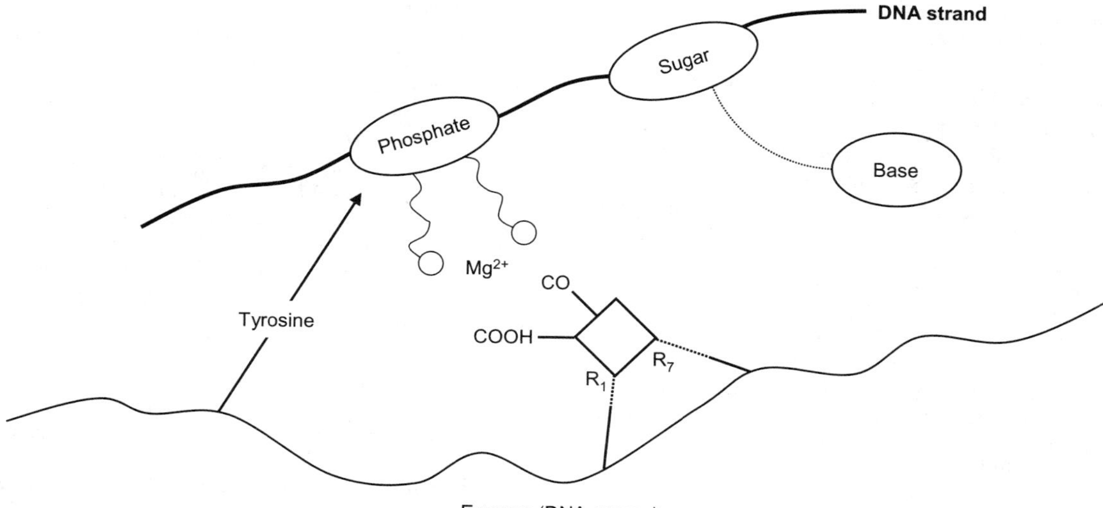

Figure 69 Model of DNA gyrase interaction in quinolones

6.3.5. Topoisomerase IV

Topoisomerase IV is a tetrameric protein composed of two A subunits (ParC) and two B subunits (ParE). These proteins are the products of the *par*C and *parE* genes. In *E. coli*, the *par*C gene has 30% homology with *gyrA* and the products have 60% amino acid homology. The *parE* gene shares 42% identity with *gyrB* and the products have 62% similarity in terms of their amino acids. The catalytic site of topoisomerase IV is located in the ParC subunit (Tyr420 in *E. coli*), whereas the ParE subunit contains the ATPase site. The molecular weights of the topoisomerase IV subunits differ with the bacterial species (Table 75).

Topoisomerase IV is necessary for bacterial survival. It is involved in the process of decatenation of DNA. It also plays a role in the sequencing of chromosomes during cell division and in addition is capable of relaxing DNA.

Division of the chromosome involves topological changes (decatenation of replicated chromosomes) and topographic segregation (positioning) of the daughter chromosome. This division is under the control of the *par*C gene. The 4-quinolones modify chromosomal division at subinhibitory concentrations.

The decatenation activity of *E. coli* topoisomerase IV is four times greater than the relaxation activity. It does not permit DNA supercoiling. Topoisomerase IV appears to be associated with the bacterial membrane. A protein has been described for *Salmonella* serovar Typhimurium, ParF, that might play a part in the binding of the tetramer to the membrane.

Topoisomerase IV is the primary target of gram-positive bacteria and *H. influenzae*.

Analysis of the *H. pylori* genome has shown that there is no topoisomerase IV in this bacterial species.

There are few studies on the interaction of the quinolones and topoisomerase IV. The molecules appear to bind to the tetramer before cleavage of the DNA. The quinolones would then act by promoting the distortion of DNA within the topoisomerase IV-DNA complex and intervene before the cleavage of DNA.

Table 75 Molecular weights of the topoisomerase IV subunits of different bacterial species

Organism	Mol wt[a]	
	GrlA	GrlB
E. coli	84 (752 aa)	70 (630 aa)
S. aureus	91 (800 aa)	74 (663 aa)
S. pneumoniae	93 (823 aa)	72 (647 aa)
M. hominis	92.2 (866 aa)	71.7 (639 aa)
B. subtilis	91.3 (806 aa)	69.8 (627 aa)
Salmonella serovar Typhimurium	85 (757 aa)	630 aa
N. gonorrhoeae	768 aa	
H. influenzae	747 aa	632 aa
P. aeruginosa	83 (754 aa)	69 (629 aa)
M. pneumoniae	789 aa	635 aa
M. genitalium	781 aa	633 aa

[a]GrlA is encoded by *parC*; GrlB is encoded by *parE*. aa, amino acids.

6.4. Genetic Regulation

6.4.1. DNA Gyrase Genes

6.4.1.1. GyrB Gene

The *gyrB* gene product (DNA gyrase subunit B) allows the production of the ATP necessary for DNA gyrase activity. The studies conducted with *E. coli* have shown that a mutation in the *gyrB* gene (58 min) induces low-level resistance to nalidixic acid due to a modification of cell wall permeability. An isolated mutation in the *gyrB* gene does not cause resistance to the fluoroquinolones.

This mutation in the *gyrB* gene is due to the replacement of the amino acids at position 447 (lysine → glutamic acid) or 426 (aspartic acid → asparagine); these are located in the C-terminal part (between amino acids 394 to 804) of the B subunit known as *v*. The region responsible for resistance to nalidixic acid is located at the binding site of the protein produced by the *gyrA* gene.

6.4.1.2. GyrA Gene

6.4.1.2.1. *E. coli.* The *gyrA* structural gene allows the production of DNA gyrase subunit A polypeptides. A mutation in the *gyrA* gene causes high-level resistance to nalidixic acid in *Enterobacteriaceae* but only a moderate increase in the MICs for fluoroquinolones. The level of resistance appears to be related to the mutation site and the replacement amino acid. Thus, at position 83 (nucleotide 318), the serine may be replaced by a leucine, a tryptophan, or another amino acid. Only the presence of a leucine or a tryptophan generates high-level resistance. This mutation causes a localized modification of the conformation of the A subunit and a change in the hydrophobicity of this region, due specifically to the hindrance produced by the leucine or tryptophan. This indicates that the site of this mutation lies on the surface of the A subunit. In *E. coli*, a mutation in the *gyrA* gene may also occur at other nucleotides.

6.4.1.2.2. *S. aureus.* The fluoroquinolones also exert activity on *S. aureus* DNA gyrase. The sequence of amino acids of the A subunit of *S. aureus* is homologous with that of *E. coli.* A mutation in the *gyrA* gene at codon 84 (serine → leucine) and/or codon 85 (serine → proline) causes resistance of *S. aureus* to 4-quinolones. Proline and leucine, hydrophobic amino acids, disorganize the DNA gyrase–4-quinolone interaction. The *gyrA* and *gyrB* genes are close to one another on the G fragment of the *S. aureus* chromosome.

6.4.1.2.3. Other bacteria. A mutation in the *gyrA* gene has been demonstrated in other bacterial species, such as *H. influenzae*, *P. aeruginosa*, *C. freundii*, *S. marcescens*, *B. subtilis*, and *E. faecalis*.

6.4.1.3. *flq* Gene

S. aureus also has another resistance gene, *flq*, localized on fragment A of the chromosome, which also contains the *cfxB* and *ofxC* genes.

6.4.1.4. *nfxC* Gene

An *nfxC* resistance gene localized on the chromosome of *P. aeruginosa* PAO in the *catA* gene (46 min) causes a reduction in the OprD protein, with the appearance of a 50-kDa protein in the bacterial wall. These strains possess cross-resistance with chloramphenicol and imipenem, but not with the other β-lactams. Strains of this kind have been isolated clinically.

6.4.1.5. Other Mutations

Other mutations in the *nfxB*, *cfxB*, *norB*, and *norC* genes are also responsible for low-level resistance to the 4-quinolones.

In *P. aeruginosa*, mutations in the *nfxB* and *nalB* genes are the source of abnormalities of membrane permeability. This type of resistance is accompanied by the appearance of new 54-kDa (*nfxB*) and 49-kDa (*nalB*) membrane proteins. Mutant strains of the *nfxB* type exhibit hypersensitivity to aminoglycosides and β-lactams.

Table 76 summarizes the genes involved in the activity of the fluoroquinolones.

Other mutations acquired by mutagenesis in *E. coli* have caused a reduction in the activity of nalidixic acid. These are genes implicated in bacterial metabolism, such as the *icd* (isocitrate dehydrogenase) or *purB* (adenosuccinate lyase) gene.

6.4.2. Topoisomerase IV Genes

The ParC and ParE proteins are coded for, respectively, by the *parC* and *parE* genes, with a chromosomal localization. The complete sequences of the topoisomerase IV genes are known for few bacterial species.

Table 76 Genes involved in the activity of fluoroquinolones[a]

Locus	Position (min)	Gene function	MIC (μg/ml)	
			NAL	CIP
gyrA	48	DNA gyrase A	>128	0.5–64
gyrB	83	DNA gyrase B	>32	0.06
ompF	21	Porin	16	0.12
marR	34	*mar* operon control protein	16	0.25
soxR	92	Stress oxidant protein regulation		0.5
emr	57.5	Efflux pump protein	8	
nalB	58	*ompF* gene	8	
norC	8	Unknown	1	0.06
nalD	89	OM/lipid content	32	
nfxB	19	*ompF* gene	16	0.5
cya	85	Adenyl cyclase: cAMP synthesis	>8	
crp	74	cAMP protein receptor	>8	
recA	58	Induction of SOS response	16	0.03
lexA	92	Protein of regulation: SOS response	16	0.016
sfiA	22	Dividing-cell regulation	8	0.03
ftsZ	2	Cellular division	32	0.03
hipA	34	OM metabolism	10	
hipQ	2	OM metabolism		0.12
icd	25	Isocitrate dehydrogenase	>10	
purB	25	Adenosuccinate lyase	>10	
Control			4	0.03

[a]Data from Piddock et al., 1998. NAL, nalidixic acid; CIP, ciprofloxacin; OM, outer membrane.

Bacterial topoisomerase IV genes are usually contiguous or close to one another, the *parC* gene being located at the 3′ extremity of the *parE* gene. It seems that when the gyrase genes are contiguous, so are those of topoisomerase IV (*B. subtilis, S. aureus, Mycobacterium genitalium, M. pneumoniae, B. burgdorferi, Chlamydia*).

6.5. "Distress" Response

The majority of the *E. coli* genes are arranged in a functional unit known as a regulon, which includes unrelated genes coordinated by a regulatory gene.

The "distress" response is under the control of three stress systems: the heat shock response, oxidant stress and the SOS response, and a regulatory system. These systems are related, as they respond to the same environmental stimuli, they share a certain number of genes, and some of their proteins interact between the various systems. Within 30 min the 4-quinolones induce a phenomenon of filamentation often associated with the onset of bacterial lysis, persisting for a minimum of 2 h, and modifications of the nucleoid. This filamentation is the result of several factors: the SOS response, the intervention of the heat shock system, an interaction with penicillin-binding protein 3 (PBP 3), and probably the generation of oxidant stress. At high concentrations, the 4-quinolones inhibit bacterial growth without filamentation.

6.5.1. SOS Response

The 4-quinolones induce an SOS response (Fig. 70) in gram-negative bacilli, which is a defensive response to a DNA insult. The organization and regulation of this system are only partially known.

Any break in a DNA fragment is a signal for induction of the synthesis of exonucleases, which hydrolyze the cut strand from the 5′ position with the formation of oligonucleotides, thereby inducing the SOS response. This allows the exonuclease activity to be inhibited and the damaged DNA to be repaired. This phenomenon is under the control of two proteins: LexA and RecA. These proteins govern the transcription of a set of genes, referred to as the SOS response. The LexA protein plays the part of repressor of the SOS response by inhibiting the transcription of the other genes. The RecA protein is induced by a modification of the DNA.

The RecA protein acts by cleaving the LexA protein. There is then derepression of the SOS response genes.

It is accepted that if the SOS response is not modulated, it becomes fatal to the bacterial cell. If the induction of the SOS response persists, a large quantity of SfiA protein is produced. This protein is an inhibitor of cell division that causes excessive filamentation and cell death. The SfiA protein acts on another protein, FtsZ, and forms a stable complex that produces increased filamentation. The target of this complex is the *hipA* gene product, which is toxic in large quantities to the bacterial cell. The excess SfiA protein is degraded by the LonA protein, which belongs to the heat shock system. The LonA protein is a protease requiring ATP for its activity.

A consequence of the induction of the SOS response is the inhibition of cell division and the activation of autolysins that contribute to the bactericidal activity of the fluoroquinolones. The final stage in the action of the fluoroquinolones is similar to that of the β-lactams.

6.5.2. Chaperonins (Heat Shock Proteins)

The heat shock-type reaction is a preservative, immediate, and transient response of the cell to an increase in tempera-

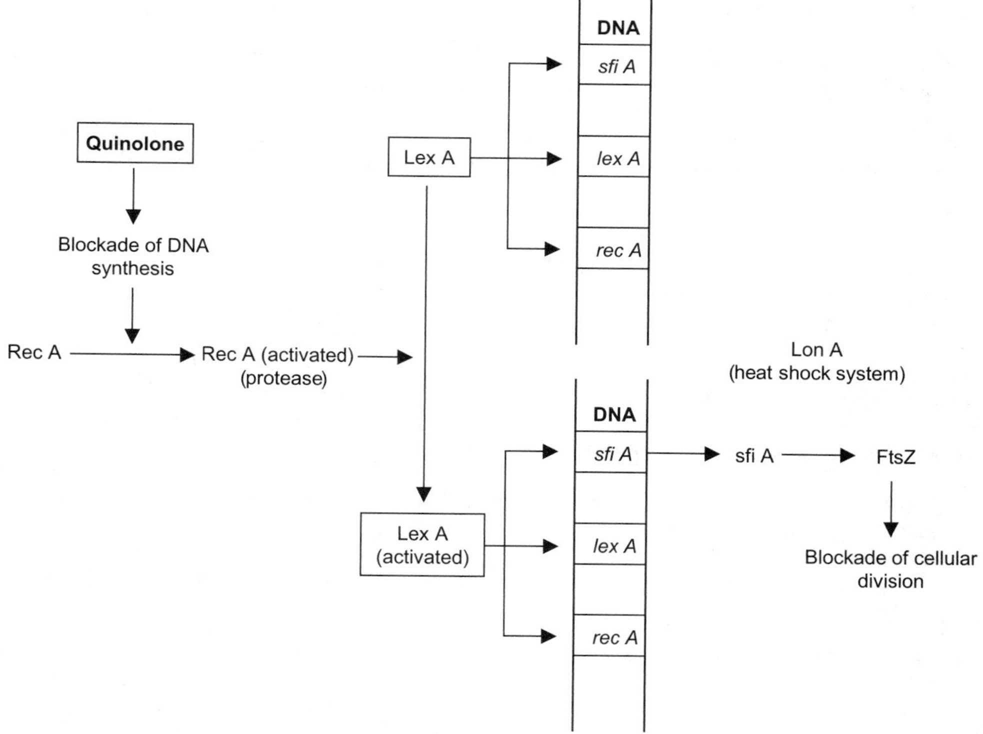

Figure 70 SOS response

ture, anoxia, heavy metals, H_2O_2, RNA and DNA viruses, ethanol, and 4-quinolones that takes the form of the synthesis of new proteins.

The inhibition of DNA gyrase activity by the 4-quinolones is reflected in the expression of the SOS response regulon but also in the increased expression of heat shock system genes. This response consists of the induction of the synthesis of 17 proteins in *E. coli*, including two major ones, GroeL and Dnak. These proteins are also known as chaperonins. The heat shock system plays a part in regulating the SOS response system.

6.5.3. Generation of Oxidant Stress

Paraquat and UV light, the bactericidal mechanism of which is based on the generation of oxidant stress, cause an SOS response. A strain of *P. aeruginosa* resistant to the bactericidal effect of fluoroquinolones and exhibiting increased resistance to acellular oxidant systems such as H_2O_2 or xanthine-xanthine oxidase has been described.

6.5.4. PBP 3

The bacterial filamentation induced by the 4-quinolones appears to increase the production of PBP 3, a protein involved in bacterial septation and which is inhibited by a large number of β-lactams.

6.6. Modification of Peptidoglycan

Weak concentrations of 4-quinolones profoundly alter the structure of peptidoglycan. The mechanisms of bactericidal activity against dividing cells appear to be similar for 4-quinolones and β-lactams. This hypothesis is strengthened by the isolation of mutants of *E. coli hipA* which are partially tolerant of ampicillin but also of nalidixic acid, ofloxacin, and norfloxacin.

6.7. Role of Oxygen

If the size of the bacterial inoculum is increased, the MICs are little affected, if at all, in contrast to the MBCs. At bacterial inocula of up to 10^6 to 10^7 CFU/ml, ofloxacin, ciprofloxacin, and norfloxacin have marked bactericidal activity against *E. coli* KL-16 and *S. aureus* ET3. If the inoculum size is increased to 10^8 CFU/ml, the bactericidal activity decreases. Beyond 10^{10} CFU/ml the molecules are only bacteriostatic. This inoculum effect is independent of pH and magnesium ion content but is dependent on the O_2 content of the medium. If the oxygen content of the environment is increased, the molecules revert to being bactericidal in the presence of an inoculum of 10^{10} CFU/ml. Under anaerobic conditions, ofloxacin and ciprofloxacin are simply bacteriostatic, irrespective of the inoculum size. This bacteriostatic activity of the fluoroquinolones in an anaerobic medium may inhibit their efficacy at poorly oxygenated infectious sites. However, this property may be an interesting feature in the oral administration of these derivatives, preventing the destruction of fecal flora. This weak activity of ciprofloxacin and ofloxacin against anaerobic bacteria is probably associated with several mechanisms, such as a reduction in or absence of transmembrane penetration, as with the aminoglycosides, and/or a modification of DNA gyrase.

6.8. Interaction of 4-Quinolones with Bacterial RNA

Several mechanisms are implicated in the antibacterial activity of the quinolones.

Weak concentrations of quinolones cause reversible blockade of DNA synthesis and are responsible for bacteriostatic activity.

Stabilization of the DNA gyrase by the quinolones on DNA would prevent the progression of the replication fork and that of RNA polymerase, causing a stoppage of replication and RNA synthesis, and indirectly of protein synthesis. The activity is bacteriostatic.

The bactericidal activity of the quinolones would appear to be due to the release of DNA fragments from the DNA-DNA gyrase complex.

6.8.1. Bactericidal Mechanisms

In *E. coli* KL-16, the bactericidal mechanism is paradoxically reduced when the 4-quinolone concentrations are increased beyond a certain threshold. The bactericidal activities of the 4-quinolones differ with the molecules. The addition of a protein synthesis inhibitor such as rifampin highlights a number of different mechanisms of action.

For Mechanism A, the bactericidal activity is abolished and only bacteriostatic activity remains. This mode of action requires the presence of proteins and RNA synthesis. Mechanism A is common to all 4-quinolones and acts on bacteria in the process of division. It would appear to involve an unidentified protein factor, culminating in the dissociation of DNA from the quinolone-gyrase complex without any repair of the break.

For Mechanism B, the addition of rifampin to the culture medium only partially inhibits the bactericidal activity. The 4-quinolones act on *E. coli* in the growth phase. Mechanism B does not require the presence of proteins or RNA synthesis and is concentration independent. It has been demonstrated in *E. coli* KL-16 with ciprofloxacin and ofloxacin, but only ofloxacin possesses this second mechanism in *S. aureus* ET3 and *Staphylococcus warneri* (Fig. 71 and 72).

For Mechanism C, norfloxacin is incapable of exerting lytic activity in the absence of protein and RNA synthesis. Norfloxacin is bactericidal against *E. coli* KL-16 in the stationary phase (in phosphate buffer), which suggests a mechanism different from those described previously. Norfloxacin might act extrinsically to the DNA-DNA gyrase binding. This mechanism has also been demonstrated with enoxacin, levofloxcin, ofloxacin, and ciprofloxacin (Fig. 73).

This bactericidal activity against bacteria irrespective of whether they are in the process of division would explain the therapeutic successes obtained with the fluoroquinolones in immunodepressed and infected patients.

6.8.2. Paradoxical Effect

See Fig. 74.

When the concentrations of the 4-quinolones are increased, a paradoxical effect is observed. The bactericidal activity against different strains of *E. coli* is proportional to the concentration of nalidixic acid. Beyond an optimum bactericidal concentration (OBC) (50 to100 μg/ml), the bactericidal activity progressively declines and is replaced by bacteriostasis (from 300 μg/ml).

Ofloxacin and ciprofloxacin are more rapidly bactericidal, as their OBCs are 0.15 and 0.90 μg/ml. They kill 90% of *E. coli* KL-16 organisms in 19 min, whereas norfloxacin achieves this result in 52 min (OBC, 1.5 μg/ml). The biphasic response of the paradoxical effect is due to the inhibition of RNA synthesis by the 4-quinolones when the concentration is below the OBC. This would appear to be due to the fact that negatively supercoiled DNA is a better substrate for DNA polymerase-dependent RNA than relaxed DNA. It would appear that at concentrations above the OBC, DNA gyrase inhibition causes relaxation of DNA so that it is no longer transcribed to RNA.

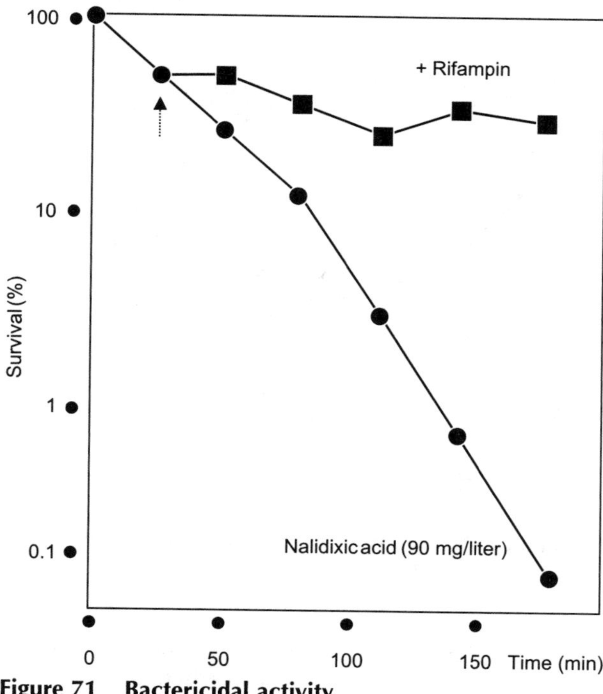

Figure 71 **Bactericidal activity**

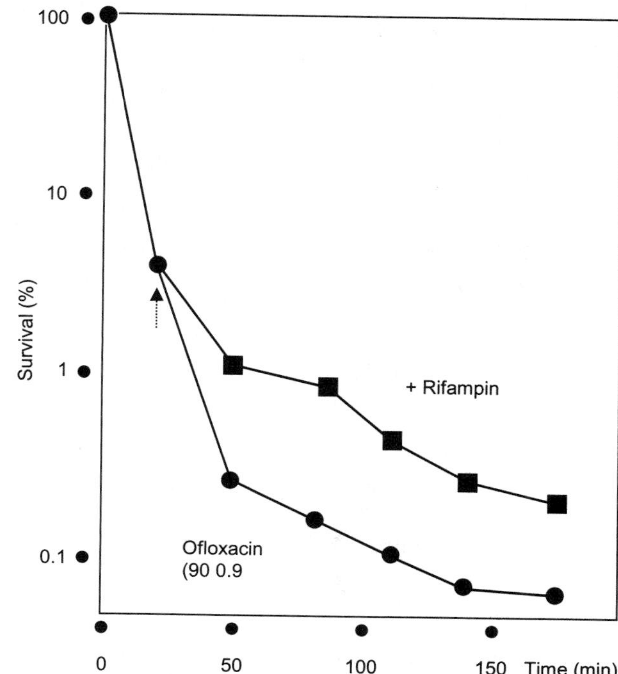

Figure 72 **Bactericidal activity**

Clinically, the biphasic response does not appear to be significant as long as the peak concentration in serum is greater than the OBC for the microorganism responsible for the infection.

In the case of *P. aeruginosa* there does not appear to be a paradoxical phenomenon with ofloxacin, pefloxacin, fleroxacin, ciprofloxacin, nalidixic acid, or oxolinic acid; the other molecules have not been tested.

6.9. Conclusion

The mechanism of action of the fluoroquinolones is complex and not unequivocal. Their synthesis has resulted in a better investigation of these mechanisms, which are based on the possibility of penetrating the bacterial wall and reaching the cell target, and on the equilibrium that exists between intrabacterial accumulation and active efflux in the cytoplasmic membrane, the whole arrangement being under the control of a very complex genetic system.

7. RESISTANCE MECHANISMS OF FLUOROQUINOLONES

The mechanisms that induce so-called low-level or high-level resistance to fluoroquinolones are complex and still

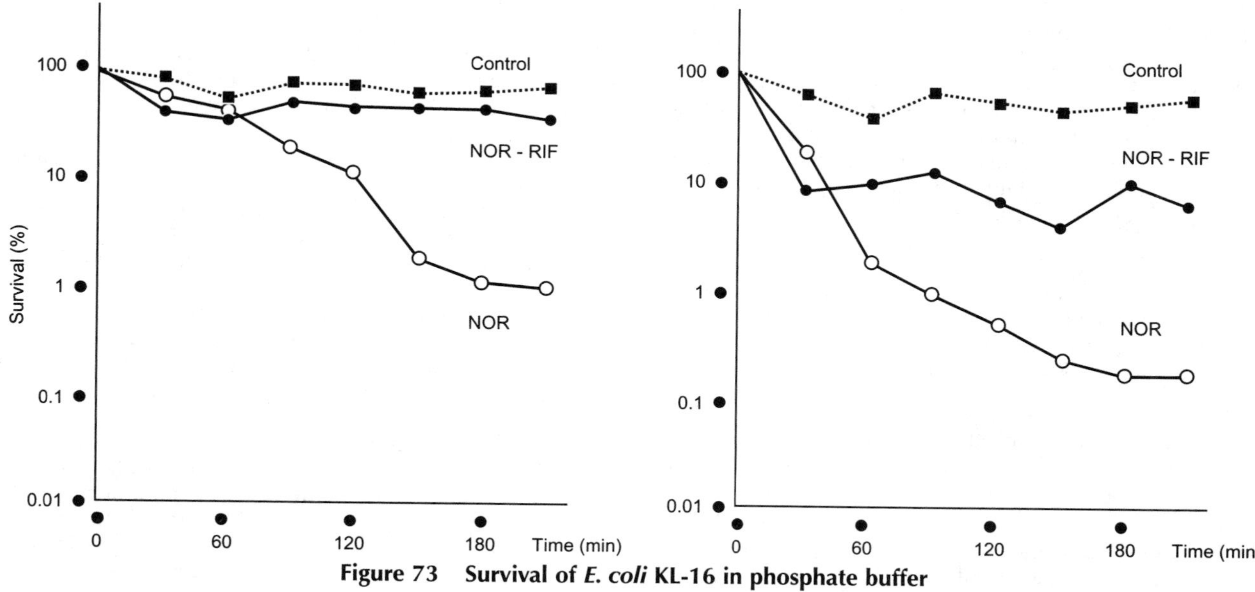

Figure 73 **Survival of *E. coli* KL-16 in phosphate buffer**

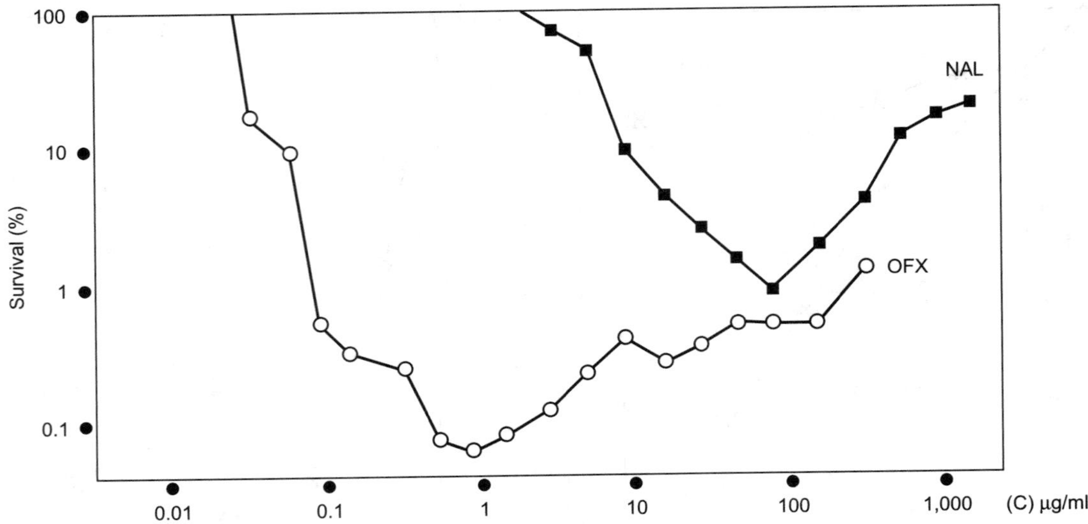

Figure 74 Biphasic killing curves in *E. coli* KL-16 at different concentrations of ofloxacin and nalidixic acid

incompletely elucidated. However, it appears to be accepted that the resistant strains possess one or more resistance mechanisms. Bacterial resistance may be acquired or intrinsic. It may be related to a defect of accumulation in the bacterial cell and/or a modification of the intracellular target or targets.

7.1. Acquired Resistance

The source of resistance to quinolones is a chromosomal mutation. Until recently, no strain with a plasmid-mediated mechanism of resistance had been described.

7.1.1. Mutation Frequency

In vitro studies conducted to determine the frequency of spontaneous mutation in the presence of fluoroquinolones have shown that this is lower than for nalidixic acid and oxolinic acid. However, it varies with the bacterial species, being higher with *S. aureus* and *P. aeruginosa* than with *Enterobacteriaceae*.

When a strain is resistant to nalidixic acid, it is generally less susceptible to the fluoroquinolones, but the MICs are very much below the therapeutic concentrations. These strains are at high risk of mutation. Consequently, in severe infections the fluoroquinolones must be combined with another antibacterial agent. The systematic testing of nalidixic acid as a "sentry" cannot be recommended highly enough. So-called low-level-resistant strains may be detected with a pefloxacin disk and high-level-resistant strains may be detected with a ciprofloxacin or sparfloxacin disk.

7.1.2. *S. pneumoniae*

It is possible with all the fluoroquinolones to select mutant strains when an appropriate methodology is used.

Against *S. pneumoniae*, the fluoroquinolones are distinguished by the following parameters (Table 77):

- The frequency of mutation
- The MICs attained with the different molecules
- The different resistance phenotypes according to the selection agents and the mechanism of resistance (GyrA or ParC)
- When the concentrations in serum are more than four times the MIC, the probability of selecting mutants is low.

When the strain is already resistant through a modification of the target (e.g., ParC), the selection of resistant mutants is obtained with very high MICs, sometimes up to 120 times the MIC. For this reason caution is required when using fluoroquinolones against which the organism has a resistance mechanism (Table 78).

- Bacterial clones with different resistance levels are obtained for each antibacterial agent.
- The ParC mutation is difficult to detect in routine laboratory tests. Pefloxacin might enable this type of mutation to be detected.

7.1.3. GyrA Mutation in *B. fragilis*

The role of *gyrA* mutations in *B. fragilis* has been explored. In vitro with ciprofloxacin as a selector, two steps were needed to obtain ciprofloxacin- and trovafloxacin-resistant mutants, and 50% of them harbored a *gyrA* mutation (Ser83 → Phe). By contrast, with trovafloxacin as a selector, first-step mutants harbored a new *gyrA* mutation (Asp82 → Asn and Ala119 → Val). These mutations resulted in an 8- to 16-fold decrease of trovafloxacin activity, but only a 4-fold decrease of ciprofloxacin activity (Bachoual et al., 1999).

7.1.4. Risk Factors

A number of risk factors have been proposed, particularly subinhibitory concentrations of the antibacterial agent.

Weak elimination in sweat might be a predisposing factor (Table 79).

To be able to act on the skin, the antibacterial agents must be eliminated through sudoriferous glands, whether these are eccrine (arms, legs, and the majority of the anatomical regions) or apocrine (axillary, inguinal, and perineal regions).

Quantifiable levels are detected 8.5 h after a single oral dose of 750 mg of ciprofloxacin. The peak concentration attained in the axillary region is 1.11 µg/ml, and the peak concentration in the forearm is 0.42 µg/ml. Subinhibitory concentrations of ciprofloxacin may promote the selection of fluoroquinolone-resistant strains of *S. epidermidis*.

Table 77 Frequency of selection of mutants from *S. pneumoniae* R 6[a]

Compound	Concn (μg/ml)	No. of times the MIC	Mutation frequency	Clone	No. of times the MIC at indicated concn (μg/ml)							
					PEN 0.015	TET 0.25	MXF 0.25	LVX 2	CIP 4	SPX 0.5	TVA 0.25	PEF 128
MXF	0.25	2	High density	A	1	1	1	1	1	2	1	1
	0.5	4	$<7 \times 10^{-9}$	B	1	1	2	1	2	8	1	1
LVX	2.0	2	$<7 \times 10^{-9}$			1						
CIP	1.0	1	High density	A	1	1	1		16	1	1	1
				B	1	1	1	1	2	1–2	1–2	4–8
SPX	2.0	2	5.7×10^{-7}	A	1	1	1	1–2	2–4	2	2	8
		2		B	1	1	2	2	2–4	1–2	1	1
TVA	0.5	4	3.6×10^{-8}	A	1	1–2	1	1	1–2		1	1
	0.5		7×10^{-8}	B	1	1–2	1	1	2	4	1	1
				C	1	1–2	1	1–2	2	1	1	4–8
				D	1	1–2	4	2	4	2	2	8
								2	4	4–8	2	8
								4	4	2	4	

[a]PEN, penicillin; TET, tetracycline; MXF, moxifloxacin; LVX, levofloxacin; CIP, ciprofloxacin; SPX, sparfloxacin; TVA, trovafloxacin; PEF, pefloxacin.

Table 78 Frequency of selection of mutants from *S. pneumoniae* R 6 t LLR6P16[a]

Compound	Mutation agent			No. of times the MIC at indicated concn (μg/ml)							
	Concn (μg/ml)	No. of times the MIC	Mutation frequency	PEN 0.015	TET 0.25	MXF 0.25	LVX 2	CIP 4	SPX 0.5	TVA 0.25	PEF 128
MXF	4	16	5×10^{-8}	1	1	16	8–16	16	32–64	32	ND
LVX	32	16	10^{-7}	1	1	16	16	8–16	32–64	32	ND
CIP	16	4	1.6×10^{-8}	1	1	16	16	16	32–64	16–32	ND
	32	8	1.2×10^{-8}								
SPX	8	16	10^{-7}	1	1	16	16	16	32–128	16–32	ND
	16	32	2×10^{-8}								
TVA	4	16	10^{-7}	1	1	16	16	16	32–128	32	ND
	8	32	2×10^{-8}	1	1						

[a]ND, not determined. For other abbreviations, see Table 77, footnote *a*.

7.1.5. MPC

The mutation prevention concentration (MPC) is defined as the concentration (in micrograms per milliliter) of antibacterial agents which prevent the emergence of mutants resistant to the compounds tested (Dong et al., 1999). MPC testing was performed by agar dilution using an inoculum size of the tested organisms of 10^{10} CFU/ml. By comparison, MICs are determined with 10^5 CFU of the organisms tested per ml.

Blondeau et al. (1999) showed that the MPC, irrespective of the susceptibility to penicillin G of 96 *S. pneumoniae* isolates, ranged from 0.5 to 4, 0.5 to 4, 1 to 4, ≤0.06 to 4, and 0.25 to 4 μg/ml for 90% of the isolates for gatifloxacin, grepafloxacin, levofloxacin, moxifloxacin, and trovafloxacin, respectively.

This parameter is an addition in the risk assessment of selection of mutants, but this parameter has to be compared with concentrations in plasma and tissue.

Table 79 Elimination of fluoroquinolones in the sudoriferous glands

Compound	Dose (μg/ml)[a]	C_{max} (μg/ml)	AUC (μg·h/ml)
Ciprofloxacin	200 i.v.	0.05	0.47
Enoxacin	400 p.o.	0.39	3.2
Fleroxacin	400 p.o.	1.4	21.5
Lomefloxacin	400 p.o.	0.9	10.9
Ofloxacin	200 i.v.	0.45	5.3
Sparfloxacin	400 p.o.	1	19.2
Temafloxacin	400 p.o.	0.71	9.9

[a]i.v., intravenously; p.o., per os.

7.1.6. Epidemiology of Resistance to Fluoroquinolones

In terms of the appearance of fluoroquinolone-resistant strains, the problem differs with the bacterial genera and species.

Since the introduction of the fluoroquinolones into therapeutic practice, the proportion of fluoroquinolone-resistant *Enterobacteriaceae* has varied with the country, with a very slow progression in the number of resistant strains for reputedly difficult species such as *Enterobacter cloacae*, *S. marcescens*, and *C. freundii*. The incidence of ciprofloxacin-resistant strains of *E. coli* is considerable in certain regions such as France, Spain, and Germany, in some cases exceeding 10% of the bacterial population. A reduction in the activity of fluoroquinolones has been reported in Vietnam for *Salmonella* serovar Typhi. The incidence of resistance of *Shigella* spp. is high in China, whereas it is ≤5% in the other parts of the world. The incidence of resistance in *Enterobacteriaceae*, however, needs to be modulated according to the nature of the infections; for example, the incidence of ciprofloxacin-resistant strains is higher when nosocomial or urinary tract infections are involved (e.g., *K. pneumoniae*, a species for which 40% resistant strains have been reported in France).

P. aeruginosa belongs to the bacteria against which the fluoroquinolones, including ciprofloxacin (MIC between 0.5 and 2 μg/ml), have borderline activity. The number of resistant strains varies with the author, as the definitions of breakpoints are not always the same. However, the incidence ranges from 5% to more than 50% (Table 80).

It seems that the emergence of resistant strains following the treatment of urinary tract infections is related to the accumulation of certain predisposing factors. Resistance development appears to be independent of the administered dose.

It has also been shown that the number of fluoroquinolone-resistant strains of *A. baumannii* is constantly increasing.

The incidence of strains of *S. aureus* that have become fluoroquinolone resistant is greater for methicillin-resistant than for methicillin-susceptible strains. In some centers it is very high, raising the problem of the administration of fluoroquinolones in the treatment of staphylococcal infections (Table 81).

The incidence of ofloxacin-resistant strains of *S. pneumoniae* in France and Spain is currently on the order of 1%. Rare strains of fluoroquinolone-resistant *H. influenzae* have been reported, particularly in Spain and France, usually for subjects with particular predispositions such as cystic fibrosis. The same applies to *M. catarrhalis* and *Mycoplasma* spp.

Ofloxacin-resistant strains of *M. tuberculosis* and *Mycobacterium leprae* have been reported, hence the need to avoid the administration of these drugs alone.

The incidence of resistant strains of *C. jejuni* and *C. coli* is high in certain regions, such as the Netherlands, affecting up to 30 to 50% of isolates.

Since 1993 to 1994, there has been a progressive loss of activity of fluoroquinolones against *N. gonorrhoeae* in certain parts of the world, particularly Southeast Asia (Thailand, the Philippines, and Hong Kong), Australia, Japan, the United Kingdom, Spain, the Canary Islands, the United States, Canada, the Caribbean, and eastern Europe, including Baltic countries (Fig. 75 and 76). This loss of activity may be accompanied by an increase in MICs for ceftriaxone. Strains of intermediate susceptibility to the fluoroquinolones may account for 50% of the bacterial population, particularly in Southeast Asia. In the United States, the incidence on these strains is on the order of 16 to 20%, depending on the region.

There is increased concern worldwide about bacterial resistance and the rapid potential decrease of activity of new drugs introduced into clinical practice. Mainly, these studies investigated the profile of resistance of respiratory pathogens: *S pneumoniae, H. influenzae*, and, to a lesser extent, *M. catarrhalis*.

A total of 15,458 fresh clinical isolates of *S. pneumoniae, H. influenzae*, and *M. catarrhalis* were collected in 377 hospitals in the United States from 1997 to 1998. Using NCCLS-recommended breakpoints, 13.7 and 22.5% of 5,640 *S. pneumoniae* isolates were resistant and intermediately susceptible respectively, to penicillin G; 4.1 and 11.2% were resistant and intermediately susceptible to ceftriaxone; 24% were resistant to erythromycin A; and less than 0.2% were resistant to fluoroquinolones (levofloxacin, moxifloxacin, trovafloxacin, sparfloxacin, and grepafloxacin).

No fluoroquinolone-resistant isolates of *H. influenzae* or *M. catarrhalis* have been identified. A total of 33.3% of *H. influenzae* isolates produced β-lactamase (2,195 of 6,588), and 92.6% (3,349) of *M. catarrhalis* isolates produced β-lactamase (Critchley et al., 1999b).

During the 1997–1998 cold season, 27 centers spread geographically throughout Great Britain (21 centers) and Northern Ireland (2 centers) and Ireland (4 centers) collected isolates of *S. pneumoniae* from patients with lower respiratory tract infections. MICs were determined using

Table 81 Incidence of resistance of methicillin-resistant strains of *S. aureus* to ciprofloxacin[a]

Country	% of strains	
	Met[r]	CIP[r]
France	33.6	96
Italy	34.4	83.8
Spain	30.3	84.7
Belgium	25.1	91.7
Austria	21.6	82.9
Germany	5.5	93
Switzerland	1.8	52.9
The Netherlands	1.5	55.5
Sweden	0.3	
Denmark	0.1	

[a]Data from Goldstein et al., 1997. CIP, ciprofloxacin.

Table 80 Epidemiology of resistance to fluoroquinolones in 1992 to 1993[a]

Organism(s)	Susceptibility (%)			
	France	Germany	Italy	Japan
S. aureus	46	94	85	87
Coagulase-negative staphylococci	71	92	86	91
E. coli	100	100	87	98.8
Enterobacter spp.		100		96.6
Salmonella spp.	100	100	100	100
S. marcescens	79.2	95.5	31.5	89.9
K. pneumoniae	90	99.6	94.9	97.3
P. aeruginosa	66	88.5	54.5	77.5

[a]Data from Jones et al., 1993.

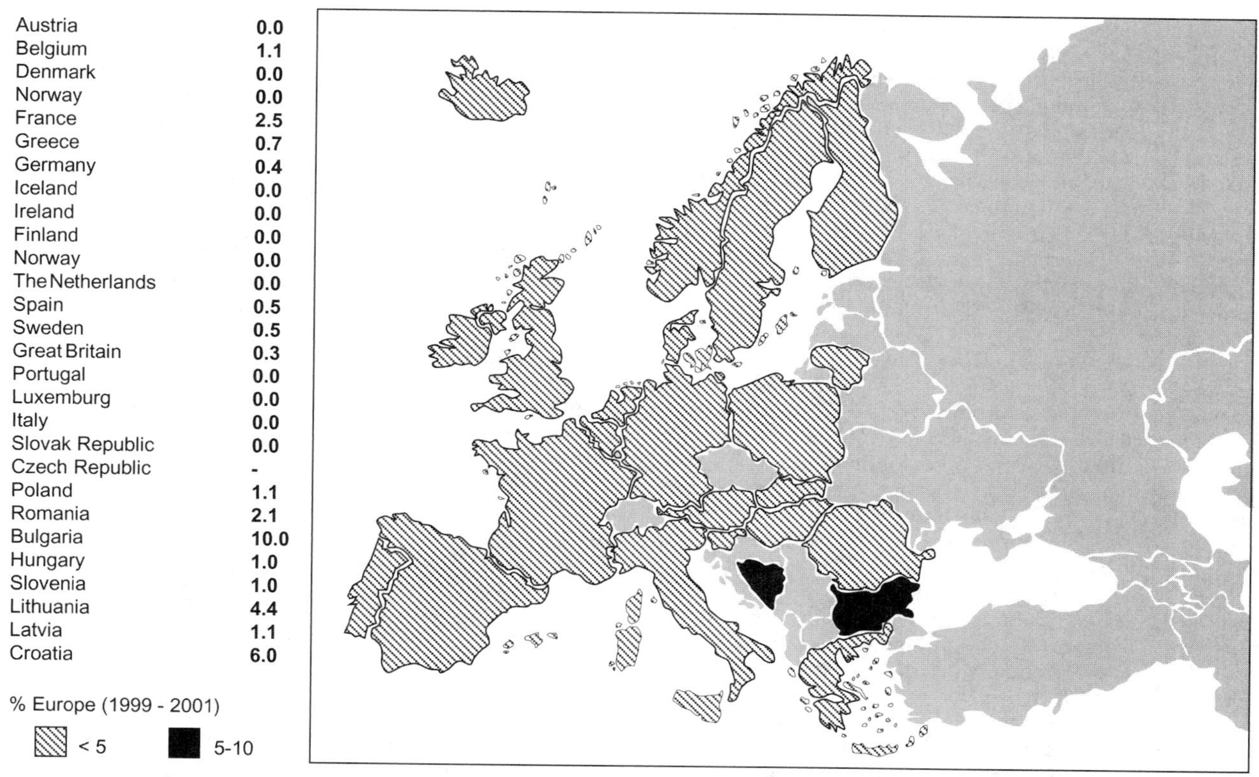

Figure 75 Epidemiology of the activity of levofloxacin and other fluoroquinolones against *S. pneumoniae* in Europe

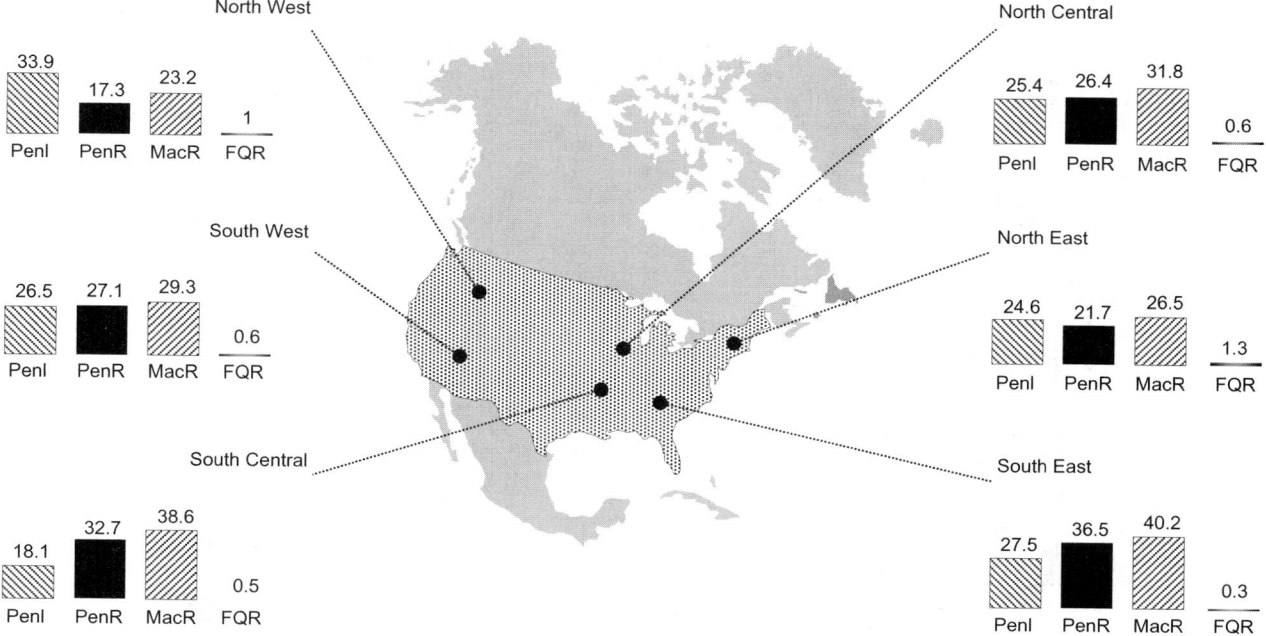

Figure 76 Epidemiology of the activity of levofloxacin and other fluoroquinolones against *S. pneumoniae* in the United States

NCCLS recommendations and recommended NCCLS breakpoints. The resistance rates throughout Great Britain (England, Wales, and Scotland) for *S. pneumoniae* were 9.1, 5.7, 5.3, 10.7, and 0.3% for penicillin G (intermediate plus resistant), amoxicillin-clavulanic acid, cefotaxime, clarithromycin, and levofloxacin, respectively.

The incidence of penicillin G resistance is higher in Northern Ireland and Ireland, at 27.5; 24.7% of strains were resistant to amoxicillin-clavulanic acid, 7.1% of *S. pneumoniae* isolates were resistant to clarithromycin, and no strains were resistant to levofloxacin (Felmingham et al., 1999).

A centralized, multicenter study with recent clinical isolates from lower respiratory tract infections from 31 sites in Austria, France, Germany, Italy, and Switzerland was conducted. The rates of *S. pneumoniae* penicillin G resistance were 5%, 45% (26% intermediate and 19% resistant), 6%, 8%, and 23% (13% intermediate and 10% resistant) for Austria, France, Germany, Italy, and Switzerland, respectively. The rate of erythromycin A resistance was 20.8% for the 31 sites and ranged from 0 to 0.6% for fluoroquinolones. No strains of *H. influenzae* or *M. catarrhalis* resistant to fluoroquinolones were isolated (Critchley et al., 1999a).

The emergence of resistance in the province of Quebec, Canada, was investigated from 1996 to 1998 in 26 centers. Pneumococcal isolates were collected from blood cultures or cerebrospinal fluid (CSF) or other sterile sites. Among the 13,545 *S. pneumoniae* isolates, the rates of resistance were as follows: penicillin G, 9.8% in 1996 to 13.6% in 1998; ceftriaxone, 7.7%; chloramphenicol, 2.7%; erythromycin A, 8.1%; rifampin, 0.1%; co-trimoxazole, 20.2%; and ofloxacin, 1.9%; no strains resistant to vancomycin were collected (Jetté et al., 1999). Prior to the early 1990s, penicillin G resistance remained uncommon among clinical isolates of *S. pneumoniae* in Germany. Resistance to penicillin G increased from 1.8% in 1992 to 5.2% in 1998 and 6.8% in 1999. A more dramatic increase in resistance was observed with erythromycin A (3.6 to 10.5%). In 1999, resistance rates of 13.4 and 0.2% were recorded for tetracycline and levofloxacin, respectively (Reinert, 1999).

7.1.7. Genetic Mutations

Bacteria may develop resistance to the 4-quinolones by at least two mechanisms: (i) a defect of intrabacterial accumulation and (ii) modification of the cell target. The different mechanisms and their targets are summarized schematically in Table 82.

7.1.7.1. Defect of Intrabacterial Accumulation

Schematically, the reduction in intracellular accumulation comes down to a decrease in, or even an absence of, transparietal permeation in gram-negative bacilli, or in an increase in efflux (Table 83).

Quinolone-resistant mutant strains obtained in the laboratory or from pathological specimens have a total or partial loss of OmpF. Passage via this porin canal is shared with the tetracyclines, imipenem, certain cephalosporins, and chloramphenicol. Thus, the loss of the OmpF protein results in resistance to all of these molecules. Mutations may interfere with the regulatory complex of the *ompF* gene, such as mutations of the cyclic AMP (cAMP) receptor protein (*crp*) or adenyl cyclase (*cya*) genes that affect cAMP-controlled regulatory genes. Other mutations in *E. coli* (*nfxC*, *cfxB*, *and norB*) are alleles at the *mar* operon (multiple resistance).

7.1.7.2. Efflux and the *mar* Operon

It now appears certain that microorganisms possess an intrinsic protective system against a wide range of toxic substances, including fluoroquinolones. The multiple antibiotic resistance (MAR) in *E. coli* is the result of a series of mutations at the *mar* locus localized at 34 min on the *E. coli* chromosome. A number of studies suggest that this system exists in all *Enterobacteriaceae* and other bacterial species.

In *E. coli*, the *mar* locus consists of two operons that are localized on either side of the *marR* gene: *marC* and *marAB*. These genes are essential for expression of the MAR phenotype. The *marA*, *marB*, and *marC* genes are under the control of Mar, which is a DNA-bound protein.

A mutation that alters *mar* causes hyperproduction of the MarA, MarB, and MarC proteins. This results in an increase in resistance to tetracyclines, chloramphenicol, rifampin, ampicillin, and nalidixic acid.

The MarA protein itself regulates transcription by activating the expression of numerous operons, including *micF*, *inhA*, and *acrAB*, all of which contribute to the MAR phenotype.

The *micF* gene codes for a small supplementary RNA at position 5′ of the mRNA of OmpF. Activation of MarA inhibits the production of OmpF. The function of the *inhA* gene is unknown. The *acrAB* gene codes for an efflux pump.

The functions of the MarB and MarC proteins are unknown.

The MAR phenotype may be induced by certain antibiotics, such as tetracyclines, and chloramphenicol (weak acids), and by other substances such as salicylates. This induction causes multiple resistance to antibacterial agents, including nalidixic acid (Fig. 77).

Table 82 Mechanisms of resistance of the fluoroquinolones[a]

Microorganism	Primary target	Secondary target(s)	Efflux
E. coli	*gyrA*	*gyrB*, *parC*, *parE*	AcrAB
Salmonella serovar Typhimurium	*gyrA*	*gyrB*	
Klebsiella	*gyrA*	*gyrB*	RamA
P. aeruginosa	*gyrA*	*gyrB*	MexAB-OprM MexCD-OprJ
N. gonorrhoeae	*gyrA*	*parC*	MexEF-OprN
Campylobacter	*gyrA*		
H. pylori	*gyrA*		Unnamed
Mycobacterium	*gyrA*	*gyrB*	
S. aureus	*gyrA*	*gyrA*, *gyrB*	LfrA
E. faecalis	*gyrA*		NorA
S. pneumoniae	*parC* (CIP) or *gyrA* (SPX)	*gyrA*, *gyrB* (CIP), *parC* (SPX)	Unnamed Unnamed

[a]Data from Köhler et al., 1998. CIP, ciprofloxacin; SPX, sparfloxacin.

Table 83 Mutations responsible for a reduction in intracellular accumulation[a]

Organism	Gene(s)	Location (min)	Compound(s)	Mechanism
E. coli	*nalB*	58	NAL	?
	nalD	89	NAL	?
	crp	74	NAL	?
	cya	86	NAL	?
	icd	26	NAL	?
	purB	25	NAL	?
	ctr	?	NAL	?
	norB	34	NOR	OmpF↓
	norC	8	Q hydrophiles	OmpF↓, LSP
	nfxB	19	NOR	OmpF↓, MicF↑
	nfxC	34	NOR	OmpF↓, MicF↑
	cfxB (*marB*)	34	MDR	OmpF↓, MicF↑, Q efflux↑
	marAB (*soxQ*)	34	MDR	OmpF↓, MicF↑, Q efflux↑ genetic activation
	marC (*soxR*)	92	MDR	OmpF↓, MicF↑, Q efflux↑
	soxRS	92	MDR	OmpF↓, MicF↑, Q efflux↑ genetic activation
	soxQ (*marA*)	34	MDR	OmpF↓, MicF↑, Q efflux↑ genetic activation
	emrAB	57.5	MDR	NAL efflux↑
	mcb		SPX	SPX efflux↑
	rob	?	MDR	OmpF↓, MicF↑ genetic activation
P. aeruginosa	*nalB* (*mexR*), *cfxB*	30	Q	OprM↑, Q efflux↑
	nfxB	4–8	Q	OprJ↑, Q efflux↑
	nfxC	46	Q + carbapenems	OprN↑, OprD↓, Q efflux↑
P. vulgaris	*pqr*			
C. jejuni	?			
S. aureus	*norA* (*flqB*)			Q efflux↑ (hydrophilicity)
S. epidermidis	*norA*			Q efflux↑ (hydrophilicity)
B. subtilis	*bmr*			
M. smegmatis	*ifr*			

[a]Data from Nakamura, 1997. NAL, nalidixic acid; SPX, sparfloxacin; NOR, norfloxacin; MDR, multidrug resistance; Q, quinolones.

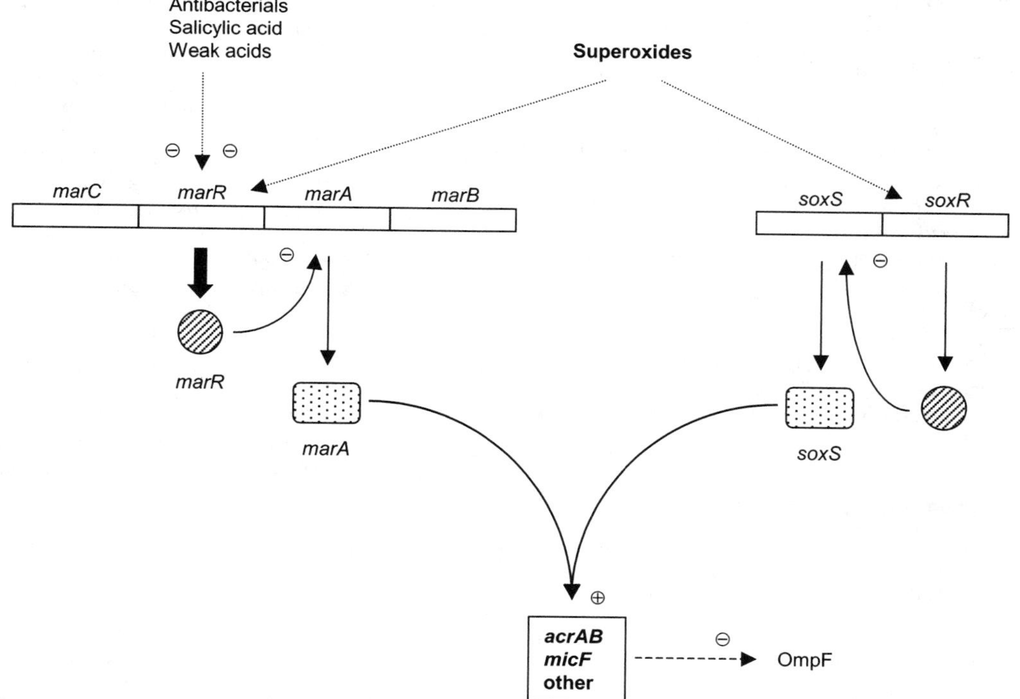

Figure 77 Regulation of the *mar* and *sox* genes of MAR

The MAR phenotype, whether acquired by induction or by mutation, protects the bacterial cell from the action of the fluoroquinolones.

7.1.8. Modifications of Cell Targets

Bacterial resistance due to a modification of the cell targets is a complex event. The main characteristics of this event are as follows:

- Resistance usually results from a single point mutation.
- A double or triple mutation is less common and usually associated with high-level resistance.
- The point mutations usually involve a single DNA gyrase or topoisomerase IV subunit.
- The mutations in *gyrA* are at a variable site along the polypeptide chain; this zone is situated in a region containing 55 nucleotides.
- The strains mutated in *gyrB* are either hypersensitive or resistant to the action of quinolones.

7.1.8.1. DNA Gyrase

7.1.8.1.1. DNA gyrase subunit B. Mutations in the *gyrB* gene of bacteria may be responsible for the inactivity of the fluoroquinolones. This phenomenon was described by Yamagoushi et al. (1982), who isolated two fluoroquinolone-resistant strains of *E. coli*. They named the genes implicated in this mechanism of resistance *nalC* (nal-31 mn) and *nalB* (nal-24 mn).

The molecular structure concerned is the substitution of an asparagine by an aspartic acid (position 426) and a glutamine by a lysine (position 447).

Mutations in *gyrB* are events that occur more rarely than in the *gyrA* gene among the microorganisms isolated in pathological specimens. They are very important for an understanding of the mechanisms of resistance involving modification of the cell target.

A mutation at lysine 447 (*nalC*) and its replacement by a glutamic acid are responsible for resistance to the quinolones of the weak acid type (nalidixic acid, oxolinic acid, etc.) but for hypersensitivity to amphoteric fluoroquinolones when they possess a basic group (piperazinyl nucleus, pyrrolidinyl, etc.) at position C-7. Lysine 447 competes with the basic groups of the fluoroquinolones at the ion bond formed with aspartic acid at position 426. Replacement of the lysine by an aspartic acid at position 447 promotes the natural ionic interaction at the expense of those that might be established with the fluoroquinolones, thus explaining the hypersensitivity of these mutant strains to amphoteric fluoroquinolones. These mutations are borne by recessive genes.

This type of mutation has been reported to date for several bacterial species, such as *E. coli*, *Salmonella* serovar Typhimurium, *S. aureus*, *N. gonorrhoeae*, and *P. aeruginosa* (Table 84).

Table 84 Mutations in *gyrB* in *E. coli*

Microorganism	Mutation
E. coli	Asp426 → Asn
	Lys447 → Gly
N. gonorrhoeae	Asp437 → Asn
S. aureus	Asp437 → Asn
	Arg458 → Glu
Salmonella serovar Typhimurium	Ser464 → Tyr

No cross-resistance between the coumarin derivatives (coumermycin and novobiocin) and the fluoroquinolones has been reported to date. This shows that the sites of action in the B subunit polypeptide of DNA gyrase differ for the two families of antibacterial agents. The coumarins interact at the N-terminal part, and the fluoroquinolones interact at the C-terminal part.

In mycobacteria, the presence of an arginine at position 447 that is more hindering than lysine (*E. coli*) and that possesses a supplementary charge and an asparagine at position 464 that is not hydroxylated and is less hindering than the serine of *E. coli* causes a weaker interaction with the DNA-DNA gyrase complex, partly explaining the weaker activity of the fluoroquinolones against mycobacteria.

7.1.8.1.2. DNA gyrase subunit A. A number of mutations have been described for the GyrA polypeptide and for numerous bacterial species. Table 85 provides a nonexhaustive list of the literature data.

The mutation points are generally located between amino acids 67 and 106 of the N-terminal region of the GyrA polypeptide. This region is known as the quinolone resistance determining region. All of the mutations are localized in a relatively hydrophobic zone which is close to the tyrosine at position 122, considered to be the site of covalent binding of DNA-DNA gyrase.

In *E. coli*, a number of mutations occur at serine 83. This is replaced by a more hydrophobic amino acid, resulting in an increase in the MIC of ciprofloxacin (from 0.03 to 0.5 μg/ml). It has been shown that two mutation points are necessary (MIC of ciprofloxacin, ≥8 μg/ml; as, for example, the combination of the following mutations: Ser83 → Leu plus Asp87 → Gly). This is a phenomenon that has been observed clinically with the administration of ciprofloxacin or another fluoroquinolone. Likewise, the level of resistance appears to be correlated with the mutation site (Table 86).

In the amino acid at position 87 (aspartic acid), resistance would appear to be due to the loss of the negative charge present in aspartic acid.

For the other bacterial species, comparable mutations at the equivalent of serine 83 have been described. In *S. aureus*, this involves serine 84, while in *P. aeruginosa* and *C. jejuni* the serine residue is replaced by a threonine residue at positions 83 and 86, respectively. Threonine comprises a hydroxyl group, giving rise to the hypothesis that the hydroxyl group is important for binding fluoroquinolones.

In *M. tuberculosis* and other mycobacteria, the majority of mutations occur at alanine 90, which is equivalent to serine 83 of *E. coli*. Mutations have also been described to occur at the amino acid at position 91.

S. aureus and *E. faecalis* possess a glutamic acid residue at position 87, which corresponds to the aspartic acid of *E. coli* and the other *Enterobacteriaceae*.

The binding of fluoroquinolones at polypeptide A differs for gram-negative bacilli and gram-positive cocci.

In a number of microorganisms, the mutation at serine 83 is responsible for a loss of the *HinfI* restriction zone (*E. coli*, *S. aureus*, *Salmonella* serovar Typhimurium, and *S. epidermidis*).

7.1.8.2. Topoisomerase IV

In gram-negative bacilli such as *E. coli*, the level of resistance to fluoroquinolones depends on an additional mutation in the *parC* gene. Topoisomerase IV is a secondary target for the fluoroquinolones in these bacterial species. The *S. aureus* and *B. subtilis* topoisomerase IV genes have been cloned and sequenced. They have been termed *grlA* (gyrase A like) and

Table 85 Mutations in GyrA of different bacterial species

Microorganism	Mutation point	Microorganism	Mutation point
A. baumannii	Gly81→Val	*E. faecalis*	Ser83→Ile
	Ser83→Ile		Gln106→His, Arg
A. salmonicida	Ser83→Ile	*H. pylori*	Asn87→Lys
	Ala67→Gly		Ala88→Val
C. burnetti	Glu87→Gly		Asp91→Gly, Asn, Tyr, Val
C. jejuni	Ala70→Thr	*C. trachomatis*	Ser83→Ile
Campylobacter lari	Thr86→Ile	*M. avium*	Ala90→Val
	Asp90→Ala, Asn	*M. smegmatis*	Ala90→Val
	Ser83→Arg		Ala94→Gly
	Glu87→Lys, Gly	*M. tuberculosis*	Gly88→Cys
	Thr86→Ile		Ala90→Val
	Pro104→Ser		Ser91→Pro
E. cloacae	Ser83→Leu, Tyr, Phe, Ile, Thr		Asp94→Asn, His, Gly, Tyr, Ala
E. coli	Asp87→His, Gly, Val, Ala, Asn	*N. gonorrhoeae*	Ser83→Phe
	Ala67→Ser	*P. aeruginosa*	Asp87→Asn
	Gly81→Cys, Asp		Thr83→Ile
	Ser83→Leu, Trp, Ala	*S. dysenteriae*	Asp87→Tyr, Asn, Gly, His
C. freundii	Ala84→Pro	*Salmonella* serovar Typhi	Ser83→Leu
E. aerogenes	Asp87→Asn, Val, Thr, Gly, His, Asp	*Salmonella* serovar Typhimurium	Ser83→Phe
K. pneumoniae	Thr83→Ile		Asp87→Gly, Tyr, Asn
	Asp87→Gly		Ser83→Phe, Tyr
K. oxytoca	Thr83→Ile		Ala119→Glu
P. stuartii	Ser83→Phe, Tyr		Ala67→Pro
S. marcescens	Asp87→Gly, Asn		Gly81→Ser
	Thr83→Ile		Ser83→Ala
	Ser83→Arg, Ile	*S. aureus*	Asp87→Asn
	Gly81→Cys		Ser 84→Leu, Ala, Phe
H. influenzae	Ser83→Ile, Arg		Ser85→Pro
	Asp87→Asn		Gly106→Asp
	Ser84→Leu, Tyr	*S. epidermidis*	Glu88→Lys, Gly
	Asp88→Asn, Tyr		Ser84→Phe

Table 86 Activities of ciprofloxacin and nalidixic acid in terms of the mutation points in *E. coli* GyrA

Amino acid location	GyrA mutation	No. of times the MIC[a]	
		NAL	CIP
67	Ala→Ser	8	4
81	Gly→Cys	16	8
83	Ser→Leu	128	32
83	Ser→Trp	128	32
84	Ala→Pro	8	8
87	Asp→Asn	64	16
106	Glu→His	4	4

[a]NAL, nalidixic acid; CIP, ciprofloxacin.

grlB. These genes have been described for other bacterial species. In gram-positive cocci, topoisomerase IV is considered to be the primary target of the fluoroquinolones. However, the primary target is dependent on the molecule. For example, the primary target of sparfloxacin in *S. pneumoniae* is GyrA.

Mutations in ParC have been described for numerous bacterial species (Table 87).

Several studies have shown that the high-level resistance to ciprofloxacin in *S. aureus* (MIC, ≥8 μg/ml) was due to a double mutation in ParC (Ser80→Tyr or Phe), associated with a mutation in GyrA (Ser84→Leu).

It has been shown that strains of *S. aureus* with high-level resistance to trovafloxacin (MIC, ≥8 μg/ml) and ciprofloxacin (MIC, 128 μg/ml) exhibited a mutation in GyrA (Ser84→Leu) and a double mutation in ParC (Ser80→Tyr or Phe plus Glu84→Lys or Gly).

It would appear that ciprofloxacin-resistant strains of *S. aureus* and those with reduced susceptibility to trovafloxacin (MIC, 0.75 μg/ml, versus 0.03 μg/ml for a wild strain) only have a mutation point at position 80 of GrlA (ParC). It has been shown that the *nfxD*-type mutation in *E. coli* responsible for its resistance to norfloxacin is in fact a mutation in the *parE* gene. The *nfxD*-type mutation is responsible for the replacement of the leucine at position 445 by a histidine that causes only a moderate increase in the MIC for a GyrA mutant strain, but not if the strain is of the *gyrA*$^+$ type. Leucine 445 corresponds to leucine 451 of GyrB, replacement of which is responsible for resistance to nalidixic acid.

Two mutations in GrlA (ParC) in *S. aureus* at the amino acids at positions 80 and 84 or two mutations on GyrA at amino acids 84 and 88 are clearly associated with high-level resistance to ciprofloxacin (MIC, ≥8 μg/ml).

Replacement of aspartic acid 435 by an asparagine in ParE in a strain of *S. pneumoniae* is responsible for low-level resistance to fluoroquinolones.

Modification of polypeptide A of DNA gyrase is an essential feature in the resistance of *N. gonorrhoeae* to fluoroquinolones. However, a modification of ParC is an additional

Table 87 Mutations in topoisomerase IV

Microorganism	Mutation point	
	parC	*parE*
E. coli	Ser80→Leu, Arg, Ile	Leu445→His
	Glu84→Leu, Arg, Ile	
K. pneumoniae	Ser80→Ile, Gly	
	Glu84→Gly, Lys	
E. cloacae	Ser80→Ile	
	Asp87→Gin, Lys	
N. gonorrhoeae	Ser88→Pro	
	Glu91→Glu, Lys	
S. aureus	Ser80→Phe, Tyr	Glu422→Asp
	Glu84→Lys, Val	Asp432→Gly
	Ala116→Glu, Pro	Pro45→Ser
	Ala48→Thr	Leu445→His
	Ile45→Met	
	Val41→Gly	
	Pro→Ser	
S. pneumoniae	Ser79→Tyr, Phe	Asp435→Asn
	Asp83→Thr, His, Tyr	
	Lys93→Glu, Cys	
	Ser95→Cys	
H. influenzae	Ser84→Leu, Tyr	
	Glu88→Lys	
M. hominis	Ser91→Ile	Asp426→Asn
	Ser92→Pro	
	Glu95→Lys, Gly	

feature. The combination of several mutations in GyrA associated with a mutation in ParC yields high-level resistance to ciprofloxacin (Table 88).

7.1.8.2.1. Clinical incidence of resistance. The level of resistance may be low and have no apparent effect on the clinical activity of these molecules. However, the fluoroquinolones should be combined with another antibacterial agent in severe infections. In fact, a mutation in the *gyrA* gene causes high-level resistance to nalidixic acid but produces only a reduction in the activity of the fluoroquinolones, with an increase of 1 or 2 dilutions of the MIC. A possible delay in the killing pharmacokinetics should be noted, as has recently been described with *Salmonella* serovar Typhi in Vietnam.

Table 88 Activity of ciprofloxacin against mutant strains of *N. gonorrhoeae* in cell targets

GyrA and/or *parC* subunits	Mutation point(s)	Ciprofloxacin MIC (μg/ml)
GyrA	Ser91→Phe	0.06–0.5
	Ser→Tyr	0.12
	Asp95→Asn	0.125
	Ser91→Phe + Asp95→Asn	0.25–0.5
GyrA	Ser91→Phe	0.5
+*parC*	Ser87→Ile	
GyrA	Ser91→Phe + Asp95→Asn	2
+ *parC*	Ser88→Pro	
GyrA	Ser91→Tyr/Asp95→Gly	8
+ *parC*	Glu91→Gly	

A mutation in the *gyrB* gene is responsible for a fivefold increase in the MIC of nalidixic acid (80 to 100 μg/ml), but concentrations of the molecule in the urinary apparatus are markedly higher (>200 μg/ml).

Ofloxacin-resistant strains of *S. aureus* that have lost their coagulase have been described; likewise, a fluoroquinolone-resistant strain of *E. coli* that has lost the capacity to produce type I pili has been reported.

These results indicate that these mutants may grow in vivo in the presence of 4-quinolones but lose some of their pathogenicity.

Studies have shown that certain ciprofloxacin-resistant strains of *S. aureus* have two distinct forms of resistance: (i) resistance in aerobic and anaerobic media and (ii) resistance in aerobic media but susceptibility under anaerobic conditions.

7.2. Intrinsic Resistance

Certain microorganisms are intrinsically resistant to the available 4-quinolones at therapeutic concentrations, particularly certain species of nonfermenting gram-negative bacilli, such as *Burkholderia mallei*, *B. pseudomallei*, fungi, and yeasts.

The mechanism of resistance for these microorganisms has not been determined exactly and probably involves the combination of membrane impermeability and a weak affinity for the intracellular targets such as DNA gyrase or topoisomerase IV.

In the case of yeasts, it has been shown that nalidixic acid and oxolinic acid do not inhibit *Saccharomyces cerevisiae* topoisomerase II activity, but molecules that have the capacity to inhibit DNA gyrase activity in yeasts have been described.

7.3. 4-Quinolones and Plasmids

A number of authors have demonstrated the elimination of plasmids to various degrees following bacterial exposure to 4-quinolones.

The bacterial genotype is important for plasmid maintenance and replication. Elimination of a plasmid by fluoroquinolones is the result of interference with *polA*-type chromosomal genes.

Plasmid-mediated resistance in *Shigella dysenteriae* was reported in 1983; the plasmid was a 20-kb transmissible plasmid associated with an increase in the phenomenon of resistance to nalidixic acid by mutation in a strain of *S. dysenteriae* type I. However, this observation has never been confirmed. In 1991, Fouet et al. demonstrated that the vector plasmid for the virulence of *B. anthracis* also carried genes coding for topoisomerase type 1. Gomez-Gomez et al. (1997) showed that it was possible to transfer fluoroquinolone resistance in *E. coli* via a plasmid. These laboratory data were confirmed in a strain of *K. pneumoniae* isolated from a pathological specimen.

8. PHARMACODYNAMICS

Determination of the in vitro activity by the MIC method enables the intrinsic activity of the molecules to be established, but it does not reveal the fate of the molecules in the patient. Other parameters are necessary to determine the dosage rate according to whether the activity is dependent on the total administered dose (maximum concentration of durg in serum/MIC or AUC/MIC) or whether it depends on the contact time between two administrations.

The pharmacodynamic profile of a molecule can be defined on the basis of various parameters:

- The bactericidal activity of the molecule
- The bactericidal potency of the serum
- Animal models for determining the pharmacodynamic profile
- The pharmacokinetics in humans
- The pharmacodynamic studies in the patient

The pharmacodynamics are the relationship between the pharmacotoxicological effects and the concentrations in plasma. For antibacterial agents, the therapeutic efficacy is the result of the intrinsic activity of the molecule and the concentrations of the drug in plasma and tissue. The interrelation between the pharmacokinetics and pharmacodynamics of the molecule is the expression of this activity.

8.1. Bactericidal Activity

The determination of the intrinsic activity is based on the determination of the MICs for a given bacterial population, and particularly the distribution of this population within a given genus, as illustrated by the following figure of the distribution of the population of *S. pneumoniae* strains with respect to levofloxacin.

This essential, quantitative analysis is necessary but insufficient; other parameters also need to be considered.

The bactericidal activity is determined in vitro by killing pharmacokinetics at two and four or even eight times the MIC. These studies have shown that the fluoroquinolones are highly bactericidal antibacterial agents. However, it is essential to perform these studies with inocula of different sizes, which more faithfully reflect the clinical situation. For example, levofloxacin remains bactericidal against *S. pneumoniae* at inocula of 10^5 and 10^6 CFU/ml, whereas at an inoculum of 10^6 CFU/ml sparfloxacin is only bacteriostatic.

The bactericidal activity must also be determined on the basis of the plasma pharmacokinetics, either by a method simulating the pharmacokinetics, or by killing pharmacokinetics as a function of the concentrations in plasma.

Animal models may help to assess this bactericidal activity, such as the models of experimental endocarditis in the rabbit in which human plasma pharmacokinetics are simulated. This model has shown levofloxacin to have a curative effect in experimental endocarditis due to viridans group streptococci, whereas at the proposed doses of trovafloxacin the results were poor.

Depending on the bacterial species, some of the fluoroquinolones exert bactericidal activity against bacteria in the stationary phase (ciprofloxacin, levofloxacin, and ofloxacin), but others, such as norfloxacin, do not possess this property.

8.2. Postantibiotic Effects

The postantibiotic effect may be determined in vitro and in vivo, but it is difficult to demonstrate in vitro for the fluoroquinolones which are highly bactericidal.

In vivo in the nonneutropenic mouse, the postantibiotic effect of the fluoroquinolones is twice as long as in the neutropenic mouse.

8.3. Serum Bactericidal Activity

The determination of the presence and duration of bactericidal activity in the serum or CSF is an excellent indicator of the potential therapeutic properties of a molecule. This can enable the unit dose and the dosage rate to be adjusted. One example is the bactericidal potency of serum determined in healthy volunteers with respect to *S. pneumoniae* and levofloxacin.

8.4. Pharmacodynamic and Pharmacokinetic Parameters and Efficacy

Shah et al. (1976) were the first to show that the bactericidal activity of the different molecules was either independent of the dose but dependent on the exposure time (β-lactams, vancomycin, clindamycin, erythromycin A, clarithromycin, and roxithromycin) or concentration dependent (aminoglycosides, fluoroquinolones, azithromycin, telithromycin, and metronidazole).

The fluoroquinolones have concentration-dependent pharmacodynamics. The AUC/MIC and maximum concentration of drug in serum/MIC ratios are the parameters that provide a better correlation between the efficacy and the intrinsic activity of the molecules (Fig. 78).

For the majority of fluoroquinolones, it is the AUC/MIC ratio that is the most appropriate parameter. It is therefore the total dose rather than the dosage that determines the activity of the fluoroquinolones.

The optimum ratio in experimental infections (murine infections localized in the thigh) is ≥35, which implies that the AUC from 0 to 24 h is 1.5 times the MIC ($1.5 \times 24\,h = 36$). This value is independent of the interval between two drug administrations and of the infection site. It has been shown in experimental infections with treatments lasting more than 2 days that there is more than 50% mortality when the ratio is less than 30, whereas if the ratio is ≥100 there is almost no mortality. Consequently, concentrations in plasma must be ≥4 times the MIC to obtain 100% survival ($4 \times 24 = 96$) in rodents. However, the activity of the fluoroquinolones disappears (paradoxical effect) beyond a certain concentration (OBC), which varies from one molecule to another (Table 89). Although difficult to interpret, this parameter must be taken into account when analyzing the pharmacodynamics of the fluoroquinolones.

However, this analysis is sometimes more complex, particularly in very severe infections where allowance must be made for the exposure time, as has been shown in experimental endocarditis models. A maximum concentration of drug in serum/MIC ratio of between 8 and 10 (in vitro and in vivo) appears to prevent the selection of resistant mutants during treatment with fluoroquinolones.

8.5. Pharmacodynamics and Therapeutic Efficacy in Humans

Forrest et al. (1993) have shown that the AUC/MIC ratio in patients treated with ciprofloxacin must be ≥125 to obtain a satisfactory therapeutic result. Below this value, satisfactory clinical and microbiological results are obtained only in ≤50% of patients. Another study conducted with levofloxacin has shown that the maximum concentration of drug in serum/MIC ratio must be ≥12 and the AUC/MIC ratio must be 100.

9. PHARMACOKINETICS

The principal characteristic of the fluoroquinolones is that they are absorbed orally and in some cases can be administered parenterally. They are eliminated via the kidneys or in the bile, but some of them undergo extensive hepatic metabolism. Their absorption varies, which partly explains the difference in unit dose between the various molecules.

The lowest oral unit doses are those of ofloxacin (200 mg), as it is very active in vitro and not metabolized

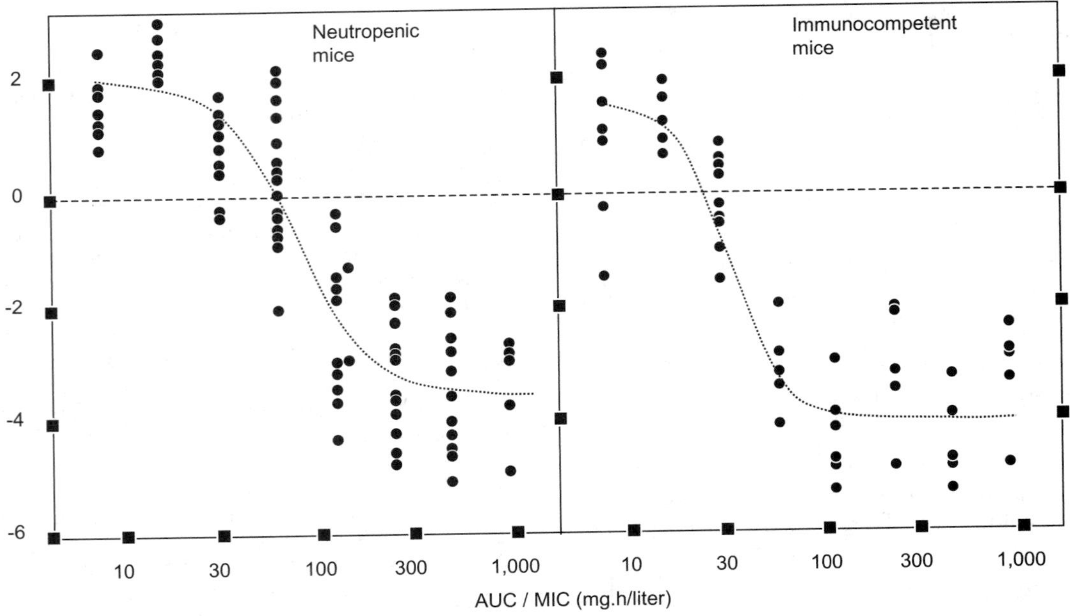

Figure 78 Pharmacodynamics (murine model)

Table 89 OBCs of quinolones (*E. coli* KL-16)[a]

Compound	MIC (μg/ml)	OBC (mg/liter)	T_{90}[b]
Ciprofloxacin	0.004	0.15	19
Ofloxacin	0.03	0.9	19
Norfloxacin	0.04	1.5	52
Oxolinic acid	0.2	9	58
Pipemidic acid	0.75	50	59
Nalidixic acid	3	90	62
Flumequine	0.4	15	53
Piromidic acid	7.5	300	92

[a]Data from Smith, 1984.
[b]T90, time to kill 90% of bacteria.

(≤5%), and trovafloxacin (200 mg). The majority of molecules are administered orally at a unit dose of 400 mg: pefloxacin, norfloxacin, lomefloxacin, enoxacin, fleroxacin, and temafloxacin. The unit dose of ciprofloxacin is 500 or 750 mg, and that of levofloxacin is 500 mg.

The daily dosage of sparfloxacin is 200 mg in a single dose following a loading dose of 400 mg on the first day.

9.1. Oral Pharmacokinetics in Volunteers

See Table 90.

Absorption of the various molecules is rapid. The peak concentration in serum for a unit dose of 400 mg is between 1.5 and 5.8 μg/ml and is reached between 0.7 and 1.5 h after administration of the drug. Ciprofloxacin is absorbed in the duodenum and jejunum. The AUCs from 0 h to infinity are between 9.9 μg·h/ml (ciprofloxacin, 500 mg) and 54.5 μg·h/ml (pefloxacin, 400 mg). The apparent elimination half-life is between 3.3 and 12.0 h. For sparfloxacin and HSR-903 it is about 18 h. For molecules with a half-life at β phase of ≥6.0 h, a single daily dose in moderately severe infections may be proposed.

Absorption occurs principally passively in the digestive tract. It has been shown that a certain proportion is actively absorbed by dipeptide transporters (enoxacin, ofloxacin, and sparfloxacin).

Elimination occurs principally via the kidneys, but the parent molecule may only be eliminated in small quantities. For example, 9 to 10% of the ingested dose of pefloxacin is eliminated, the remainder being found in the form of metabolites, including an active metabolite, demethylpefloxacin (= norfloxacin).

Ofloxacin and fleroxacin are filtered by the glomerulus and are not secreted or reabsorbed by the tubules.

Pefloxacin, but not demethylpefloxacin, is filtered by the glomerulus and then reabsorbed by the tubules. Ciprofloxacin, lomefloxacin, temafloxacin, and enoxacin are filtered by the glomerulus and secreted by the tubules.

Ten percent of the administered dose of ciprofloxacin is secreted by the cells of the duodenojejunal mucosa and is then eliminated in the feces. The same applies to ofloxacin, fleroxacin, and moxifloxacin.

The peak concentration in serum of gemifloxacin (SB 265805) after a single oral dose (0.2 to 1.5 μg/ml) is reached in 1 h (dose of 40 to 320 mg), with a dose-dependent AUC (1.3 to 9.8 μg·h/ml). The apparent elimination half-life is on the order of 6 to 9 h. About 30% of the administered dose is eliminated in the urine. The absorption of gemifloxacin is delayed and reduced (~60%) by a fatty meal.

9.2. Parenteral Pharmacokinetics

All of the fluoroquinolones can be administered orally. A number of them are also administrable parenterally: ofloxacin, levofloxacin, pefloxacin, ciprofloxacin, fleroxacin, temafloxacin, lomefloxacin, gatifloxacin, and alatrofloxacin. Norfloxacin cannot be administered intravenously. Tosufloxacin hydrochloride and tosylate are slightly soluble in water. It is difficult to obtain a formulation for parenteral use. A prodrug, 3-formyltosufloxacin, has been synthesized (A-71497).

The parenteral formulations are of considerable interest in the treatment of very severe infections, in which the

Table 90 Oral pharmacokinetics of fluoroquinolones

Compound	Dose per os (mg)	C_{max} (μg/ml)	T_{max} (h)	$t_{1/2\beta}$ (h)	$AUC_{0-\infty}$ (μg·h/ml)	Metabolites (%)	Urine (%)	Feces (%)
Ofloxacin	100	1.33	0.7	6.74	7.75	2–<5	69.6	5
	200	2.64	0.8	6.96	15.6		87	
	400	5.64	0.7	7.4	35.4		80.8	
Ciprofloxacin	400	1.5	1	3.3	5.76	3–19	29	30
	500	2.3	1.3	3.9	9.9		30.6	
	750	2.65	1.2	4.75	12.2		33	
Pefloxacin	200	1.5	1.8	11.7	25.7	5–60	11.8	40
	400	3.6	2.6	10.5	54.5		11.1	
	600	5.4	1.16	11	87.9		14	
	800	6	1.61	12.6	105		17	
Norfloxacin	400	1.5	1.5	3.3	5.4	6–23	27	29
Lomefloxacin	200	2.23	0.73	7.34	11.9	1–8	60	9
	400	2.74	1.27	7.8	24.8		59	9
Enoxacin	400	3.09	1.4	4.9	18.5	1–15	44	15
	600	4.18	1.7	4.7	27.3			
	800	3.70	1.5	5.4	27			
Temafloxacin	100	0.98	1.2	7.1	7.51		59.4	30
	200	1.61	1.9	7.9	15.02	1–8	60.9	
	300	3.1	2	8.4	28.3	1–5	70	
	400	2.43	2.5	7.9	29.7		59.2	
	600	3.87	2.6	7.8	49.5		46.8	
Sparfloxacin	100	0.44	2.6	16.8	8.9	1–27.3	12.3	56
	200	0.7	4	20.8	18.7	1–22.5	10.3	
	400	1.18	5	18.2	32.7	1–21.3	9.5	
Tosufloxacin	150	0.37	1.9	3.77	2.73	4–≥5	25	54
	300	1.19	3.06	6.93	8.32		32.7	
	600	1.86	2.19	5.60	7.42		32.8	
	900	2.83	3.13	6.33	8.53		31	
Fleroxacin	200	2.33	1.1	8.9	20.9	2–8	64.6	10
	400	4.36	1.3	9.2	48.3	2–9.2	49.8	
	800	7.04	1.9	10.3	106.1	2–11.5	50.1	
Rufloxacin	300	2.8	4.2	39.5	46.3	−4	ND[a]	25
	400	3.6	4	36	58.5		ND	
	400	4.4	1.9	28.2			26.2	
Grepafloxacin	100	0.44	1.5	11.6	4.42	4–8.5	10.2	35
	200	0.68	2.1	11.1	8.78		11.9	
	300	0.94	2.9	12.4	14.15		12.2	
	400	1.79	2.2	10.4	21.1		11.4	
	200	0.47	2.1	10.7	5.19	ND	ND	
	400	0.92	2.7	11.6	13	ND	ND	
	600	1.33	3.1	16.3	20.1	ND	ND	
	800	2.08	2.3	14.1	28.1	ND	ND	
	1,200	3.17	3	14.7	44.3	ND	ND	
Clinafloxacin	25	0.22	1.31	4.6	1.16		43.6	ND
	50	0.63	0.67	4.9	2.39		52.2	
	100	0.89	0.69	5	4.17	ND	65	
	200	2.5	0.69	6.1	10.2		50.9	
	400	2.4	1.6	6.1	18.5		63	
Gatifloxacin	100	0.87	1.6	6.9	7	10	90	6
	200	1.71	1.4	7.1	14.5			
	400	3.35	2	8.4	32.4			
	600	5.41	2.3	8.1	53.5			
Prulifloxacin	100	0.68	1.25	7.7	3.99	7	49	53 + 4.2 (ester)
	200	1.09	0.67	8.9	6.41			
	400	1.88	0.67	7.9	9.72			
	300	1.3	10.6	3.9				23
	450	1.4	12.1	5.6				19.5
	600	1.6	10.7	6.2				16.7
BAY y 3118	50	0.26	0.69	7.95	2.49	ND	9	ND
	100	0.51	0.36	13.4	4.65			

(*Continued on next page*)

Table 90 Oral pharmacokinetics of fluoroquinolones (*Continued*)

Compound	Dose per os (mg)	C_{max} (μg/ml)	T_{max} (h)	$t_{1/2\beta}$ (h)	$AUC_{0-\infty}$ (μg·h/ml)	Metabolites (%)	Urine (%)	Feces (%)
Balofloxacin	100	1	1	7	7.4	2–5	77	5.9
	200	2.2	1.1	7.8	17.1		80	
	400	3.7	1.2	8.3	32.5		72	
Pazufloxacin	100	0.94	0.93	2	3.85	ND	81	ND
	200	2.97	0.57	2.27	7.87			
	400	4.51	0.87	2.48	18.36			
Levofloxacin	50	0.57	2.41	4.34	4.70	<5	85–92	
	100	1.22	0.92	3.96	7.46			5
	200	2.04	1.48	5.97	19.9			
	250	2.8	1.57	7.27	27.2		79	
	500	5.09	1.33	6.33	47.9		75	
	750	7.13	1.90	7.70	82		73	
	100	8.85	1.70	7.90	111			
DR-3354	200	1.23	1.93	8.11	3.16			
Y-26611	100	0.72	0.8	5.2	2.89	ND	34.4–43.2	29.6
	200	1.18	1.3	5.4	4.46			
	400	2.50	1.3	5.1	9.66			
DV-7751	100	0.27	1.1	8.75	2.41	ND	26.6	12
	200	0.62	1.1	10	5.46		25.6	
	400	1.05	1.3	9.46	9.95		26.8	
	800	1.98	1	9.11	20		22	
Sitafloxacin	25	0.29	1.3	4.4	1.52	ND	69	3
	50	0.51	1.2	4.6	2.62			
	100	1	1.2	5	5.55			
	200	1.86	1	4.6	12.02			
CI-990	100	0.31	1.17	7.37	2.92	ND	46.2	
	300	1.09	1.35	8.08	10.3		58.2	
Olamufloxacin	50	0.18	1.3	17.6	2.71	ND	15	ND
	100	0.45	1.9	17.7	6.7		15	
	200	0.86	1.8	18	12.82		15	
	400	1.75	2.4	17.9	28.54		15	
Moxifloxacin	50	0.29	1.75	11.4	3.88	15.9	20.4	45
	100	0.59	2	12.2	8.51		18.9	
	200	1.15	2.5	14	15.4		19.8	
	400	2.5	1.5	13.1	26.9		20.1	
	600	3.19	2.5	12.5	39.9		17.5	
	800	4.73	3	12.3	59.9		18.7	
Trovafloxacin	30	0.3	0.7			20	7.4	60
	100	1.4	0.7	7.1	9.6		10.5	
	200	2.9	1.2	10.1	26.2			
	300	4.3	0.7	9.6	40.6		7	
	600	6.5	1.1	9.7	70.6		6.6	
	1,000	10.1	3.3	12.4	168.6		6.9	
DW-116	100	1.19	2.33	18.72	18.54	ND	43.3	ND
	200	2.44	2	14.92	46.41		45.2	
	300	3.57	3.57	15.1	67.14		44	
	800	8.73	8.73	14.83	186.5		43.1	
Ecenofloxacin (CFC 222)	25	0.13	1.5	18	2.28	<10	15	ND
	50	0.29	1	15	4.56		20	
	100	0.55	1.5	18.7	9.33		20	
	200	1.35	2.5	17	27.21		20	
	400	2.91	1.8	13.8	53.73		20	
Gemifloxacin	20	0.12	0.5	4.75	0.65		31.7	
	40	0.20	1.0	7.58	1.28		25.9	
	80	0.44	1.0	5.88	2.54		25.9	
	160	1.27	1.0	8.77	5.48		28.8	
	320	1.48	1.0	6.65	9.82		27.5	
	600	3.86	1.0	8.23	24.4		32	
	800	4.33	1.8	8.02	31.4		39.4	
ABT-492	250	3.6	1.5	8.3	13.6			

[a]ND, not determined.

intravenous form is superior to the oral route, particularly in patients who are unable to swallow or have major transit disorders.

The pharmacokinetic profile is identical to that of the oral forms. What changes is the unit dose, which either is identical to that of the oral formulation (ofloxacin and pefloxacin) or varies with the severity of the infection (ciprofloxacin) (Table 91).

The elimination pathways of the principal group IV fluoroquinolones are summarized in Fig. 79.

9.3. Repeat-Dose Pharmacokinetics

Administration of 500, 750, and 1,000 mg of levofloxacin for 10 days revealed no accumulation of this molecule (Table 92).

After repeated oral doses of 100 and 200 mg of trovafloxacin, the accumulation indices were 1.42 and 1.35 in healthy volunteers. After repeated doses of moxifloxacin the accumulation index was on the order of 1.2.

9.4. Ciprofloxacin Extended-Release Tablets

Ciprofloxacin extended-release tablets are made of a bilayer matrix composed of two different salts of ciprofloxacin. The outer part (35% of the tablet) is made of ciprofloxacin hydrochloride and is released immediately. The remaining part (inner part, 65% of the tablet) is made of ciprofloxacin betaine and is released more slowly. When the formulations are compared (same daily dose but different rhythms of administration), the AUCs from 0 to 24 h and the maximum concentrations of drug in serum are found to be similar (Table 93) (Baker et al., 1999).

9.5. Bioavailability

The absolute bioavailability of the different quinolones is not always known because of the impossibility of obtaining an intravenous formulation, as with norfloxacin and sparfloxacin. The bioavailability ranges from 40 to 100% (Table 94).

	Urine	Bile
Levofloxacin	+++	(+)
Trovafloxacin	+	+++
Grepafloxacin	+	+++
Sparfloxacin	+	++
Moxifloxacin	+	++
Gatifloxacin	+++	(+)

Figure 79 Elimination pathway of fluoroquinolones

Table 91 Intravenous pharmacokinetics of fluoroquinolones

Compound	Dose (mg)	C_{max} (μg/ml)[a]	t_{perf} (min)[b]	$AUC_{0-\infty}$ (μg·h/ml)	$t_{1/2\beta}$ (h)	CL_P (ml/min)	CL_R (ml/min)	Urinary elimination (%)
Ofloxacin	100	2.8	30	7.7	8.8	228	179	78.6
	200	5.1	30	15.6	13.3	231	187	81.3
Ciprofloxacin	100	0.8	30	2.6	4.8	701	409	58.5
	200	3.9	30	5.4	3.3	670	374	56
	200	2.31	60	23.4	9.7	156.4	19.6	13.7
Pefloxacin	400	4.37	60	54.3	10.4	123.1		12.7
	600	5.83	60	82.2	11.8	127.2	15.2	12.7
	800	8.67	60	130.9	13.8	104.8	12	10.8
	200	1.83	60	5.35	3.3	648	347	53
Enoxacin	400	5.5	60	17.8	5.1			
	800	6.58	60	29.8	4.7	479	257	51
Fleroxacin	100	2.85	20	12	9.5	122.1	88.9	72.9
Levofloxacin	500	5.7	60	44	6.7	19	95.5	100
	750	8.12	90	61.1	6.91	186		
Alatrofloxacin	30	0.4	60				9.7	<10
	100	1.8	60	16.4	10.4	85.4	7	<10
	200	2.3	60	31.2	12.3	76.3	9.7	<10
	300	4.3	60	43.4	10.8	96.9	11.2	<10
	400	5.9	60			83		
Temafloxacin	100	1.26	60		6.2	247	178	
	200	2.82	60		6.6	209	148	69
	400	5.59	60		7	199	134	
	600	8.4	60		7.3	183	121	
	800	8.95	60		7.4	195	145	
Clinafloxacin	25	0.24	60	0.89	4.6	372	206	55.4
	50	0.38	60	1.52	4.9	468	342	73.7
	100	0.9	60	4.1	5.6	399	270	67.4
	200	1.61	60	8.3	6	381	262	68.8
	400	3.52	60	20.8	5.8	319	235	74.8
Moxifloxacin	100	1.17	30	8.9	13	187	37	19.5
	200	2.07	30	17.9	12.7	186	37	19.7
	400	4.60	30	36.9	13.4	181	37	25.7
Gatifloxacin	200	2.2	60	15.9	11.1	214	155	71.7
	400	5.5	60	35.1	7.4	196	124	62.3

[a]End of infusion.
[b]Infusion duration.

Table 92 Fluoroquinolones: repeated-dose oral pharmacokinetics

Compound	Days	Dose (mg)	C_{max} (μg/ml)	T_{max} (h)	AUC (μg·h/ml)	$t_{1/2}$ (h)	CL/F (ml/min)	CL_R (ml/min)	Urinary elimination (%)
Levofloxacin	1	500	5.19	1.3	47.7	7.4			64
	10	500	5.72	1.1	47.5	7.6			67
	1	750	7.13	1.9	82 ± 14	7.7 ± 1.3	157 ± 28	118	75
	10	750	8.6	1.4	91 ± 18	8.8 ± 1.5	143 ± 29	116	79
	1	1,000	8.9	1.7	111 ± 21	7.9 ± 1.5	156 ± 34	113	73
	10	1,000	11.8	1.7	118 ± 19	8.9 ± 2.5	143 ± 29	106	71
Grepafloxacin	1	400	0.92	2.7	11.6	13			7.8
	14	400	1.23		15.6	7.96			12.7
	1	800	2.08	2.3	28.1	14.7			14.3
	14	800	3.06		34.7	8.73			12.7
Moxifloxacin	1	400	3.36	1.49	30.24	9.3	ND[a]	ND	ND
	10		4.52	1.24	47.97	11.95	ND	ND	ND
	1	600	4.21	1	50.3	9.11		40	23
	10	600	5.67	1.5	60.3	13.7		55	24.2
Prulifloxacin	1	400	1.26	1.83	6.89				46.2
	7	400	1.41	2.17	9.67	8.34			48.6
Trovafloxacin	1	100	1	0.9	9.4	9.2		66.6	20.3
	17	100	1.1	1	11.8	10.5		78	22
	1	300	2.9	1.2	26.2	10.5		58.3	28.3
	17	300	3.3	1.3	34.6	12.2		70.1	23.8
Pefloxacin	1	400	4.3	1.3	29.5	12.3	115		
	4	400	10	1.4	83.7	12.5		6.6	
Enoxacin	1	400	3.09	1.4	18.5	4.9	348	216	
	5	400	4.5	1.1	25.8	5.7	252	144	
	1	600	4.18	1.7	27.3	4.7	360	228	
	5	600	5.9	2	37.3	5.9	264	168	
	1	800	3.7	1.5	26.9	5.4	576	324	
	5	800	6.9	2.5	47.4	6.3	294	144	
Ciprofloxacin	1	500	3.2		9.9	3.2			
	5	500	3.7		11.3	3.1			
Fleroxacin	1	400	5	1.3	65.6	11.2	104.1	53.2	50.3
	5	400	6.7	1.1	71.3	12.5	95.97	53.5	74.9
	1	800	8.2	1.6	144.4	13.5	98.8	46.7	46.5
	5	800	14.3	1.4	182.9	15.6	77.7	38.8	75.3
Ofloxacin	1	400	3.2	2	33	3.8			
	5	400	5	1.7	61	5.2			
Garenoxacin	1	100	1.2	1.25	15.1			56.1	37.3
	7		1.5	1.13				55.2	50.7
	14		1.6	1.13		17.8		55.7	52
	1	200	2.4	1.75	29.6			40.6	28
	7		2.9	1.5				48.4	44.4
	14		3.0	1.75		15.5		46.9	44.3
	1	400	4.6	1.75	55.2			34.9	23.2
	7		5.2	1.25				44.6	37.6
	14		5.6	1.5		13.3		50.4	33.1
	1	800	9.5	1.75	130.3			27	21.1
	7		12.6	1.5				33.3	36.6
	14		14.4	2.5		15.5		25.6	33.1
	1	1,200	16.3	2.5	230			29.4	25.4
	7		21.5	2.5				28	36.5
	14		24	2.0		15.4		27.5	4.0.9
ABT-492	1	100	1.4	1.1	4.1	3.2			
	10		1.3	1.1	4.5	4.2			
	1	200	3.2	1.0	11.2	3.8			
	10		3.1	1.8	11.5	7.4			
	1	400	4.5	1.1	14.8	4.1			
	10		5.0	1.1	17.8	8.4			
	1	800	8.2	1.1	28	4.3			
	10		8.2	1.1	31.4	8.5			
	1	1,200	11.5	1.7	50.7	4.5			
	10		11.5	1.4	54.3	7.6			

[a]ND, not determined.

Table 93 Pharmacokinetics of ciprofloxacin extended-release tablets

Compound[a]	Dose[b]	C_{max} (μg/ml)	T_{max} (h)	AUC_{0-24} (μg·h/ml)	$t_{1/2}$ (h)
CIP ER	500 mg q.d.	1.59	1.5	7.97	6.6
CIP	250 mg b.i.d.	1.14	1.0	8.25	4.8
CIP ER	1,000 mg q.d.	3.11	2.0	16.83	6.31
CIP	500 mg b.i.d.	2.06	2.0	17.04	5.66

[a]CIP, ciprofloxacin; ER, extended release.
[b]q.d., once a day; b.i.d., twice a day.

9.6. Effects of Food

The process of absorption has been fully studied with ciprofloxacin throughout the digestive tract. Ciprofloxacin is predominantly absorbed in the duodenum and to a lesser extent in the jejunum (relative bioavailability, 37%). Absorption in the colon is much weaker (5 to 7%). In the more distal part of the digestive tract, ciprofloxacin is actively secreted from the blood circulation by the enterocytes. This phenomenon has been demonstrated with other fluoroquinolones, such as ofloxacin, fleroxacin, and levofloxacin. However, it is probably a class phenomenon.

The presence of nondairy food in the digestive tract delays the time to peak concentration in serum but does not significantly alter the bioavailability of the products, except perhaps for prulifloxacin, which is an ester, and rufloxacin. The peak concentration in serum is reduced with certain fluoroquinolones, such as ciprofloxacin, norfloxacin, ofloxacin, and rufloxacin; this effects appears to be less pronounced with the other molecules. Nevertheless, these minor modifications have no major effect in terms of the time of administration of the fluoroquinolones.

The effect produced by dairy products varies with the molecule. Simultaneous absorption of ciprofloxacin and 300 ml of milk or 300 ml of yogurt reduces the bioavailability of ciprofloxacin by 30 or 36%, respectively. In the case of norfloxacin with the same protocol, the reduction in bioavailability is 50%. No major reduction in bioavailability has been noted with ofloxacin after 300 ml of milk or yogurt (6 or 9%), and the same applies with sparfloxacin and enoxacin. The effect of milk is probably related to the presence of calcium. The bioavailability of enoxacin does not appear to be affected by the ingestion of milk. As a general rule, it is preferable to avoid the simultaneous administration of a fluoroquinolone and dairy products, even if with some of them there does not appear to be any interference (Tables 95 and 96).

Table 94 Bioavailability and protein binding of quinolones

Compound	Protein binding (%)	Bioavailability (%)
Ofloxacin	25	100
Ciprofloxacin	20–30	60–80
Pefloxacin	30	83–100
Norfloxacin	15	35–45
Lomefloxacin	10	95–100
Fleroxacin	23	99
Enoxacin	43	80–90
Rufloxacin	60–80	50
Clinafloxacin	50–60	80–98
Sitafloxacin	50	>70
Levofloxacin	24–38	100
Grepafloxacin	50	72
Trovafloxacin	76	70–90
Moxifloxacin	30–45	86
Pazufloxacin	23	
Balofloxacin	15.5	
DV-7751	35	85
Gatifloxacin	20	85
Nalidixic acid	90	
Sparfloxacin	45	40–60
Gemifloxacin	60	ND[a]

[a]ND, not determined.

9.7. Pharmacokinetics in Elderly Subjects

Elderly subjects are a heterogeneous group of patients often receiving multiple medications and for this reason more often subject to adverse effects. The dosages usually need to be modulated according to the patient's age and renal function, if the drug is eliminated renally, added to which there are disorders of digestive absorption that may be related to an underlying condition.

The studies undertaken with the various fluoroquinolones show no significant difference in terms of the time to reach the peak concentration in plasma, but the peak concentration in serum and the AUC are higher than in young subjects. The volume of distribution is often reduced in elderly subjects.

For fluoroquinolones that are eliminated unchanged via the kidneys, the reduction in glomerular filtration, as well as secretion or tubular reabsorption, may affect certain parameters. Renal clearance is reduced and the apparent elimination half-life is prolonged (Table 97).

9.8. Pharmacokinetics in Patients with Renal Insufficiency

For products eliminated predominantly or almost exclusively renally, a reduction in the daily dosage is often recommended when the creatinine clearance is less than 50 ml/min.

The majority of fluoroquinolones are eliminated principally renally and/or biliarly. Some are eliminated predominantly via the kidney (ofloxacin), and others, such as pefloxacin, grepafloxacin, trovafloxacin, and moxifloxacin, are eliminated in the bile.

In patients with renal insufficiency, it is important to know the pharmacokinetic fate of these molecules as a function of the creatinine clearance (Table 98).

In patients undergoing hemodialysis, the dialysis of the different fluoroquinolones is on the order of 10 to 15% of the administered dose.

Peritoneal infections are one of the major complications of ambulatory peritoneal dialysis. *S. aureus* and *S. epidermidis* are the bacterial agents most often implicated. The fluoroquinolones may be an oral therapeutic alternative, as has been shown by clinical studies with ciprofloxacin and ofloxacin. Because of

Table 95 Pharmacokinetics of fluoroquinolones: effect of food

Compound	Food	Dose (mg p.o.)	C_{max} (μg/ml)	T_{max} (h)	AUC (μg·h/ml)	$t_{1/2}$ (h)
Ciprofloxacin	Fasting	250	1.35	1.3	5.6	3.97
	Fed	250	1.02	1.9	5.4	4.32
Ofloxacin	Fasting	200	2.6	1.0	1.46	
	Fed	200	1.8	2.0	13.3	
Enoxacin	Fasting	400	2.39	1.38	14.75	5.71
	Fed	400	2.16	2.33	16.03	5.66
Norfloxacin	Fasting	200	0.46			
	Fed	200	0.32			
Levofloxacin	Fasting	200	1.36	0.82	10.42	5.12
	Fed	100	1.22	0.92	7.46	3.96
	Fasting	500	5.9		50.5	6.2
	Fed	500	5.1		45.6	6.5
Lomefloxacin	Fasting	200	1.78	0.86	13.33	8.47
	Fed	200	1.35	3.14	12.9	7.77
Fleroxacin	Fasting	200	2.92	1.8	36.6	9.9
	Fed	200	2.73	1.8	28.7	10.6
Sparfloxacin	Fasting	200	0.65	3.83	15.6	16.28
	Fed	200	0.74	5.17	17.78	15.38
Temafloxacin	Fasting	400	2.77	2.33	33.98	7.71
	Fed	400	3.21	2.92	35.14	7.46
Rufloxacin	Fasting	800	10.2	3.2	48.4	54.6
	Fed	800	8.5	3.4	32.3	49.6
Moxifloxacin	Fasting	200	1.24	1.5	15	13.9
	Fed	200	1	3.5	15	13.3
Sitafloxacin	Fasting	100	1	1.2	5.6	5.0
	Fed	100	0.9	2.0	5.8	6.4
Trovafloxacin	Fasting	200	2	2.1	24.8	12.3
	Fed	200	1.9	3.4	25.6	12.4
Grepafloxacin	Fasting	200	0.68	2.1	8.8	11.1
	Fed	200	0.64	3.3	7.9	10.7
Gatifloxacin	Fasting	200	1.71	1.4	14.5	7.1
	Fed	200	1.65	1.9	12.7	6.5
	Fasting	400	3.44	0.75	32.2	7.25
	Fed	400	3.10	2.0	29.8	7.19
Pazufloxacin	Fasting	200	2.96	0.85	8.65	1.91
	Fed	200	1.67	1.61	7.15	1.79
Prulifloxacin	Fasting	200	1.1	0.7	6.4	8.9
	Fed	200	0.8	2.1	6.1	7.4
Ecenofloxacin	Fasting	200	1.2	1.5	24.1	20.7
	Fed	200	1.1	3.5	22.9	21.0
DX-116	Fasting	300	3.9	1.6	50.4	14.2
	Fed	300	5.5	2.9	82.2	18.3
	Fasting	400	5.4	1.9	69.7	15.1
	Fed	400	7.4	2.3	107.4	17.2
Pefloxacin	Fasting	400	4.36	1.65	54.6	11.0
	Fed	400	3.99	1.27	55.8	11.7
Balofloxacin	Fasting	200	2.17	1.1	17.11	7.83
	Fed	200	1.68	2.5	10.81	8.34

their low molecular weight and relatively low protein binding, the mean peritoneal clearance of the different fluoroquinolones is 3 to 4 ml/min. The concentrations obtained in the peritoneal dialysis fluid vary with the patient.

9.9. Hepatic Insufficiency

Severe hepatic impairment moderately increases the apparent elimination half-life and concentrations in plasma of ciprofloxacin, lomefloxacin, and norfloxacin. The apparent elimination half-life of ofloxacin increases in severe hepatic impairment, but this probably affects cirrhotic patients with abnormal tubular secretion. Severe impairment may increase the elimination half-life of pefloxacin up to 15 to 16 h. The problem is exacerbated if there is accompanying renal insufficiency. However, these changes may be related to the changes in renal function associated with the picture of hepatic insufficiency in a number of patients.

On the basis of a study undertaken with cirrhotic patients with or without ascites, it is recommended that the fleroxacin regimen be reduced by half.

About 30 to 35% of temafloxacin is eliminated extrarenally. However, there are no changes due to hepatic

Table 96 Effects of dairy products on the pharmacokinetics of fluoroquinolones

Compound	Dose (mg)	C_{max} (μg/ml)	T_{max} (h)	$AUC_{0-\infty}$ (μg·h/ml)
Ofloxacin alone	300	3.04	1.3	23.6
Ofloxacin + milk	200	1.6	1.4	12.3
	300	2.95	1.4	22.9
Lomefloxacin	200	1.6	1.4	11.6
Lomefloxacin + milk	400	4.7	1	42.4
Ciprofloxacin	400	5.1	1.3	44.4
Ciprofloxacin + milk	500	2.9	1.2	15.1
Norfloxacin	500	1.9	1.3	10.1
Norfloxacin + milk	200	0.7	1.1	3.5
Olamufloxacin	200	0.3	1.4	1.8
Olamufloxacin + milk	200	0.94	2.1	16.5
Enoxacin	200	0.92	1.4	14.9
Enoxacin + milk	400	2	1	14.3
Moxifloxacin	400	2.2	1.3	15.3
Moxifloxacin + milk	400	2.4	0.9	31.8
	400	2.9	2.8	33.9

Table 97 Pharmacokinetics of fluoroquinolones in elderly subjects

Compound	Dose (mg)[a]	C_{max} (μg/ml)	T_{max} (h)	$AUC_{0-\infty}$ (μg·h/ml)	CL_R (ml/min)	CL_P (ml/min)	$t_{1/2}$ (h)
Ofloxacin	200	3.6	2	47.1		8.2	13.3
Levofloxacin	100	1.77	3.6	20.7			4.54
	500	7	1.4	74.7	91	121	7.6
Ciprofloxacin	500	3.24	1.1	20.9	152	394	6.8
	750	6.58	1.8	41.9	150	401	4.9
Pefloxacin	400	10.7		151.4		48	12.6
Norfloxacin	400	1.36	2	9.37	ND[b]	ND	5.18
Enoxacin	400	3.55	2.3	37.6	82	177.3	7.3
Lomefloxacin	400	4.48	1.3	49.2	84.3	143	8.75
Fleroxacin	800	15.6	2.7	39.8	43	16.9	16
Temafloxacin	600	5.2	2.4	55.5	106.6	185.5	8.7
Tosufloxacin	150	0.37	1.63	6.14			4.73
Sparfloxacin	400	1.69		22.72	19.5	193.3	19.9
Grepafloxacin	600	1.56	3.7	17.4	34.5		15.2
Pazufloxacin	200	3.85	1.2	27.97	96.85		3.16
Prulifloxacin	200	1.15	2.35	14.54			11.77
Trovafloxacin	300	2.8	1.8	30.6			
Rufloxacin	400	6.46	4.8	103		35	28.7
Moxifloxacin	200	1.6		19.9			

[a]Single dose.
[b]ND, not determined.

insufficiency. Ruhnke et al. showed that the elimination of ciprofloxacin is delayed in patients with hepatic insufficiency (Child-Pugh score, B or C); urinary elimination of ciprofloxacin is increased, but urinary elimination of the metabolites is reduced.

Trovafloxacin is partly eliminated in the bile, and about 30% is eliminated renally. In patients with hepatic insufficiency (Child-Pugh score, A or B), the product is accumulated in a ratio of 1.18 to 1.95 in type A and B patients with hepatic insufficiency after 14 days of treatment (Child-Pugh score B), but a third group of patients of Child-Pugh index C would be necessary to be investigated (Table 99).

Grepafloxacin is mainly eliminated by the hepatobiliary route. Renal elimination accounts for less than 10% of the administered dose. The pharmacokinetics are altered in patients with hepatic insufficiency (Table 100).

The peak concentration in serum of grepafloxacin is increased by 36 and 48%, respectively, in group A and B patients, whereas plasma clearance is reduced by 33 and 55%.

Eight patients suffering from hepatic insufficiency (indices B and C of the Child-Pugh classification) received a single dose of 400 mg of gatifloxacin. In patients with hepatic insufficiency, the geometric mean of the peak concentrations in serum was greater than 32% (5.14 versus 3.91 μg/ml) and the AUC was 23% (45.2 versus 36.9 μg·h/ml). The plasma clearance was 18% lower ($P = 0.03$) in the group of patients with hepatic insufficiency (105.8 versus 183.3 ml/min). The other parameters were comparable: half-life at β phase (8.9 versus 9.3 h), urinary elimination (69.8 versus 66.0%), and renal clearance (105.4 versus 123.6 ml/min).

As the product is eliminated predominantly renally, it does not appear to be necessary to modify the dosage or

Table 98 Pharmacokinetics of fluoroquinolones in patients with renal insufficiency

Compound	Dose (mg)	Elimination half-life (h) at indicated CL_{CR} (ml/min)			
		120–80	80–40	40–20	20–5
Ofloxacin	200	7.9 ± 1.8	15 ± 4.4	25.4 ± 8.6	34.8 ± 15.5
Ciprofloxacin	200	4.27 ± 0.84	6.12 ± 1.61	7.7 ± 1.22	8.55 ± 3.27
Pefloxacin	400	11.7 ± 1.61	14.74 ± 4.33	15.22 ± 5.6	16.8 ± 5.6
Norfloxacin	400	2.3 ± 0.56	4.4 ± 1.6	6.64 ± 1.7	12.23 ± 6.29
Lomefloxacin	400	7.5 ± 0.7	18.2 ± 3.7	20.3 ± 5.7	26.9 ± 3.7
Enoxacin	200	3.2 ± 0.78	9.43 ± 3.17	9.53 ± 4.66	6.91 ± 1.91
Fleroxacin	400	13.5 ± 7.1	25.2 ± 8.9	34 ± 7.5	42.6 ± 6.9
Temafloxacin	400	10.6 ± 2.4	15 ± 2.9	19.3 ± 4.8	24.6 ± 7.3
Tosufloxacin	150	3.85	4	9.8	10.5
Gatifloxacin	100	6.9	8.9	16.4	29.6
	400		11.2	17.2	30.7
Grepafloxacin	600	12.8	15.6	18	17.3
Levofloxacin	100	3.96	6.44	11.06	28.22
	500	7.6	9.1	26.57	34.83
Moxifloxacin	400	14.9	15.1	16.2	14.5
Sparfloxacin	200	20.8	17.5	20.3	17.3
	400	19.1		34.9	38.5
Clinafloxacin	200			7.5–18.1	14.6
Prulifloxacin	200		9.53	13.4	33.72

Table 99 Trovafloxacin pharmacokinetics in patients with hepatic insufficiency

Subjects	Dose (mg)	AUC_{0-24} (μg·h/ml)	C_{max} (μg/ml)	T_{max} (h)	k_{el} (h^{-1})	CL_R (ml/min)	$t_{1/2}$ (h)	Urinary elimination (%)	R[a]
Group A 1	100	8	1.1	1.1	0.11	8.8	6.3	30.4	
Controls 14	100	11.3	1.6	0.7	0.09	9.8	7.8	31.7	1.42
Patients 1	100	14.3	1.5	1.1	0.06	8.6	10.8	30.6	
Patients 14	100	16.4	1.7	1	0.07	10.3	10.2	33	1.18
Group B 1	200	17	2.1	1.5	0.08	12	8.7	25.2	
Controls 14	200	22.6	3.1	0.9	0.07	10	10.1	26.4	1.35
Patients 1	200	18.2	1.7	1.9	0.06	8.6	12.3	31.7	
Patients 14	200	34.1	3.3	2.7	0.06	7.9	12.6	30.6	1.95

[a]R, accumulation ratio.

Table 100 Grepafloxacin (400 mg every 24 h for 7 days) pharmacokinetics in patients with hepatic insufficiency

Subject[a]	n	C_{max} (μg/ml)	T_{max} (h)	AUC (μg·h/ml)	$t_{1/2\beta}$ (h)	CL_P/F (ml/min)	CL_R (ml/min)	Urinary elimination (%)
Control	14	1.16	2.25	13.1	12.2	597.5	36	6.3
A	10	1.52	2.55	20.1	13	386.6	34.5	9.8
B	12	1.65	1.83	28.6	19.5	249.4	33.5	13.1

[a]A and B, score on Child-Pugh scale.

dosage rate of gatifloxacin. For gemifloxacin, parameters are listed in Table 101.

9.10. Obesity

The increased content in fat tissue may result in altered pharmacokinetics, especially for a lipophilic compound like alatrofloxacin. In 21 subjects, alatrofloxacin pharmacokinetics were assessed after an intravenous dose of 300 mg; results are shown in Table 102.

9.11. Metabolism

All of the fluoroquinolones are metabolized to various degrees in the liver. Two sites on the molecule are subject to this metabolism: the aromatic nucleus attached at position 7 and the carboxyl group at position 3.

A number of fluoroquinolones are glucuroconjugated to various degrees at position 3: pefloxacin, difloxacin, lomefloxacin, temafloxacin, sparfloxacin, ofloxacin, balofloxacin, gatifloxacin, prulifloxacin (NM 394), tosufloxacin, moxifloxacin, and rufloxacin (Table 103).

Table 101 Gemifloxacin pharmacokinetics in hepatically impaired patients (320 mg single dose once a day)

Subjects	n	C_{max} (μg/ml)	T_{max} (h)	$AUC_{0-\infty}$ (μg·h/ml)
Volunteers	45	1.16	1.0	6.89
Child-Pugh A	9	1.42	1.0	9.05
Child-Pugh B	11	1.40	1.0	10

Table 102 Pharmacokinetics of alatrofloxacin in obese patients[a]

Subjects	n	C_{max} (μg/ml)	$AUC_{0-\infty}$ (μg·h/ml)	CL_P (ml/h/kg)	$t_{1/2}$ (h)
Obese persons	6	3.6	37	53.5	12.1
Controls	15	4.3	43.4	96.9	10.8

[a]Data from Pai et al., 2001.

Table 103 Fluoroquinolones: metabolism

Compound	Dose (mg)	Route[a]	% of administered dose: Parent compound, Urine	Parent compound, Feces	Metabolites, Urine	Metabolites, Feces
Ciprofloxacin	200	i.v.	61.5	15.2	9.5	2.6
Ofloxacin	200	i.v.	90		5	
Pefloxacin	400	i.v.	10		60	
Norfloxacin	400	p.o.	20–40		10	
Lomefloxacin	400	i.v.	71.8		10	
Fleroxacin	100	i.v.	61	15	15	
Levofloxacin	500	p.o.	88	12	<5	<5
Gatifloxacin	400	p.o.	85		≤1	
Grepafloxacin	400	p.o.	9.8	31.4	6.8	7
Trovafloxacin	200	p.o.	23.1	63.3	15.1	13.1
Moxifloxacin	400	p.o.	24.2		15.9	
Enoxacin	400	i.v.	53.6		12.5	
Prulifloxacin	400	p.o.	46.6	52.9	7	
Balofloxacin	200	p.o.	90.4	5.9	4.5	

[a]i.v., intravenous; p.o., per os.

The 7-piperazinyl nucleus is extensively metabolized (Fig. 80):

- The N-4′-methylated derivatives may be N-oxidated or N-demethylated.
- The N-4′-demethylated derivatives are converted to 4′-oxo metabolites.
- There are other more minor metabolic pathways: N acetylation, N formylation, N sulfatation, rupture of the piperazine ring: 7-(aminoethylamino), 7-amino derivatives.

The 7-(3′-aminopyrrolidine) nucleus of tosufloxacin is metabolized to two main metabolites, as follows. (i) Trovafloxacin has a bicyclic nucleus at position 7 of the 1,8-naphthyridine nucleus, which may be metabolized (Fig. 81 and 82). Conversely, that of moxifloxacin is relatively little metabolized (~10%) (sulfatation). (ii) The piperidine nucleus of balofloxacin (Q-35) is demethylated and accounts for 0.2% of the quantity of product eliminated in the urine (Table 104).

Prulifloxacin is esterified. The parent molecule is released by hydrolysis of the ester bond under the control of paraoxanase, a type A esterase.

The esterases are classified into three groups, A, B, and C, according to their reactivities with organophosphorous compounds (Table 105).

The esterases play a major role in the hydrolysis of prodrugs in humans and laboratory animals. However, there are major variations within the esterases, particularly with carbonic anhydrase, butylcholinesterase, carboxylesterase, and paraoxanase (arylesterase and *S*-formylglutathione hydrolase).

Pazufloxacin is a tricyclic fluoroquinolone that has an aminocyclopropyl instead of a heterocycle. This may be metabolized either by opening of the cyclopropyl ring (metabolite M_2), by attachment of an alkyl chain to the amino group (metabolite M_1), or, finally, by opening of the propyl ring and elimination of the amino group (metabolite M_3) (Fig. 83).

The metabolization of the group II and III fluoroquinolones is summarized in Fig. 84.

Two major metabolites of garenoxacin are recovered in urine and bile: the *N*-sulfonic acid (~37%) and the glucuronide derivative (~17%).

For gemifloxacin, all metabolites represented less than 10% of the administered dose: *N*-acetyl gemifloxacin, E-isomer of gemifloxacin, and carbamoyl glucuronide gemifloxacin.

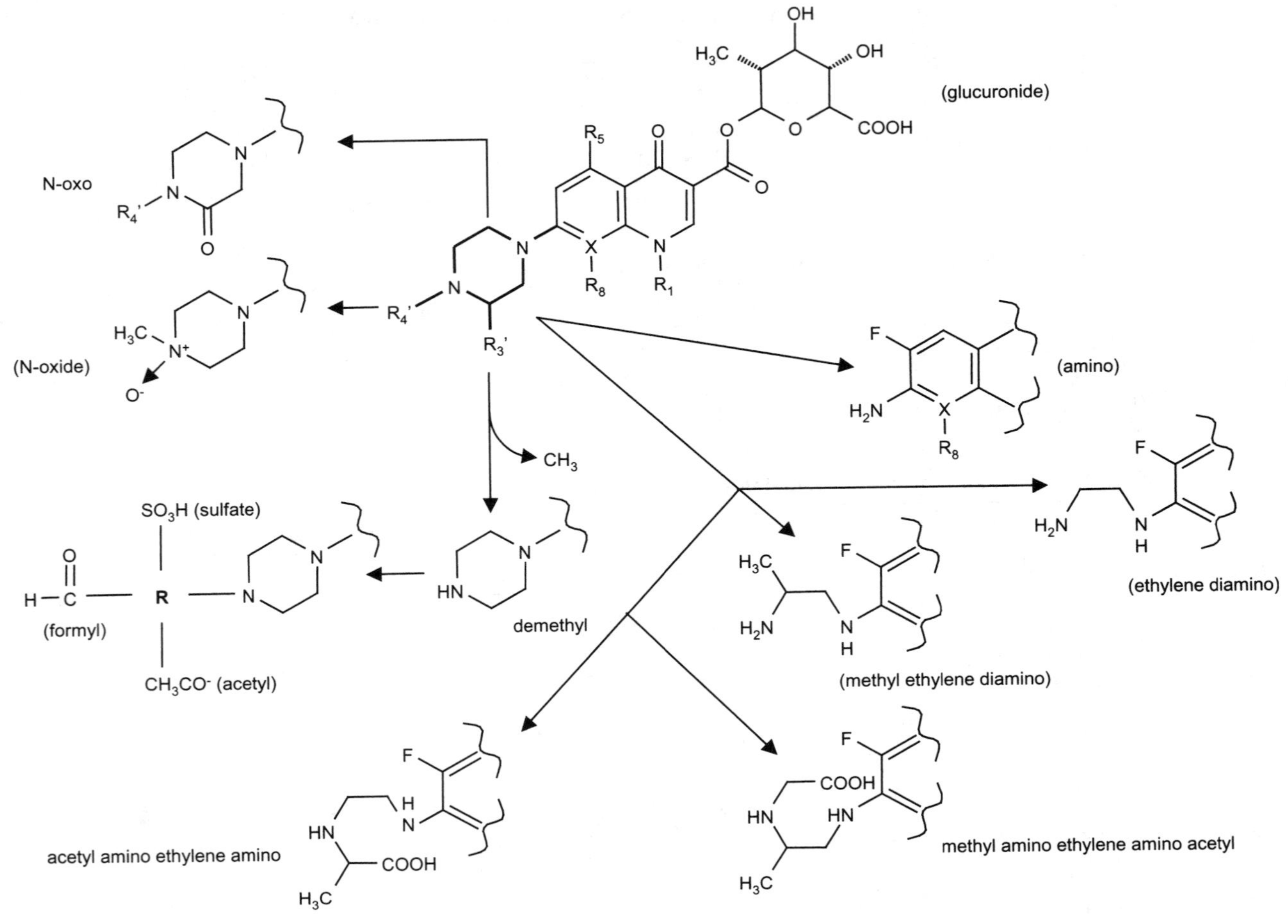

Figure 80 Metabolism of the 7-piperazinyl nucleus

9.12. Pharmacokinetics in Burn Patients

The pharmacokinetics of pefloxacin in burn patients have been studied by Galizia et al. Two groups of patients were included: those with more than 40% of the body surface area burned and those with burns on between 20 and 30% of the body surface area. The pharmacokinetic study was undertaken during two periods: the initial period (P-1) and the hypermetabolism period (P-2) (Table 106).

When the burns are very extensive, the plasma half-life is extended but the concentrations in serum are lower. When the burns are less extensive, the pharmacokinetics of pefloxacin are practically superimposable on those in subjects without burns, but elimination increases during the P-2 phase. It therefore appears to be important to monitor concentrations in serum in burn patients.

9.13. Pharmacokinetics in Pregnant or Lactating Women

Sixty parturients were included in a study of fluoroinolone pharmackinetics in pregnant women. The gestational age was between 19 and 25 weeks, and the fetuses were suffering from β-thalassemia major (Table 107).

The amniotic fluid drug concentrations are summarized in Table 108.

The concentrations of ciprofloxacin in plasma measured in pregnant women are very much lower than those obtained in women in a nongestational state. Those of pefloxacin are comparable to those obtained in nonpregnant women. These three molecules extensively penetrate the amniotic fluid (Table 108). In the rat, [^{14}C]-moxifloxacin crosses the placental barrier and is excreted in the colostrum.

9.14. Pharmacokinetics in AIDS Patients

It has been shown that the absorption of drugs in AIDS patients is abnormal. As a consequence, there is a potential reduction in efficacy of the drug.

Twelve AIDS patients received 200 mg of trovafloxacin orally or an infusion of alatrofloxacin (Table 109). The absolute bioavailability in these patients was 88%. The results are comparable to those obtained in healthy volunteers after a dose of 200 mg of trovafloxacin; the peak concentration in serum was 2 μg/ml, the AUC was 26.6 μg·h/ml, and the plasma clearance was 93 ml/min, with an absolute bioavailability of 87%.

Twenty-three human immunodeficiency virus (HIV)-positive patients received one or more doses of levofloxacin orally (750 mg) in comparison with healthy volunteers; pharmacokinetics are shown in Table 110.

10. TISSUE DISTRIBUTION

10.1. Respiratory Tissue

The fluoroquinolones are extensively distributed in all bronchorespiratory tissues. The concentrations in the pulmonary

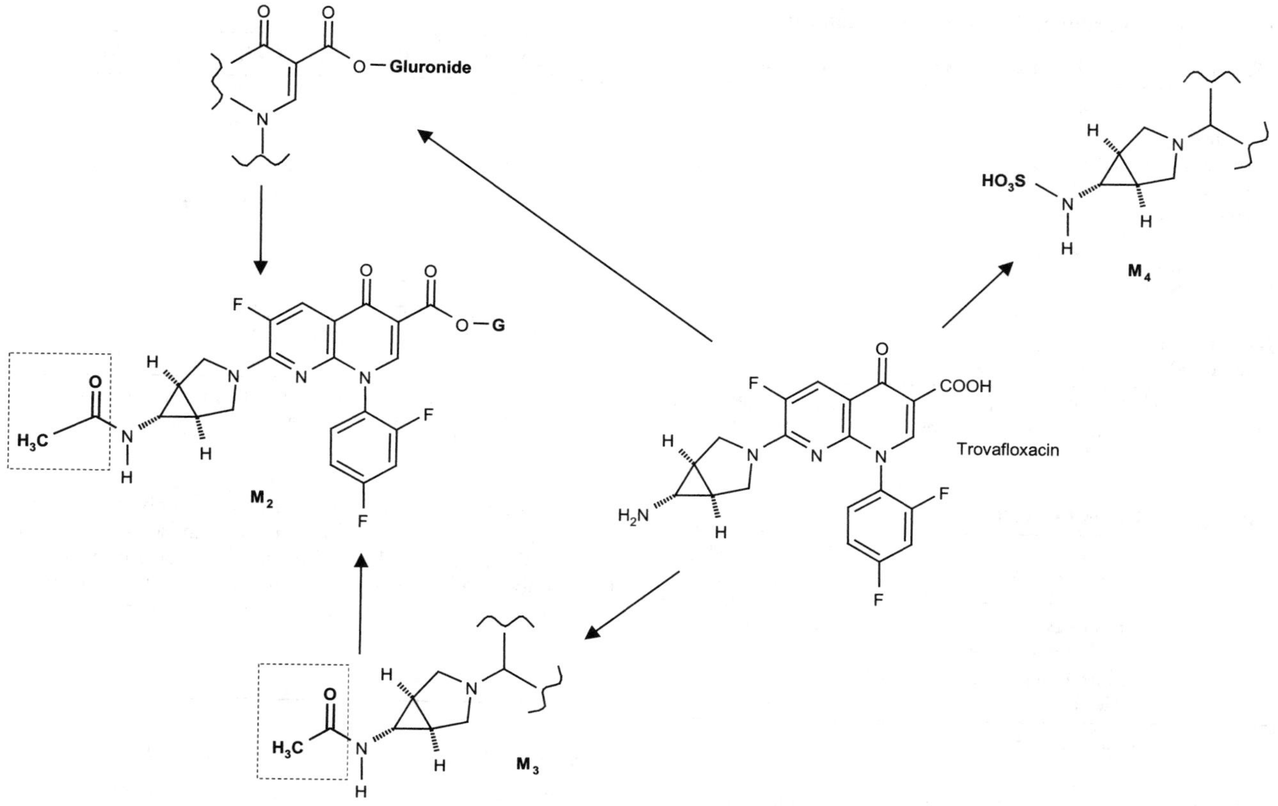

Figure 81 Metabolism of trovafloxacin

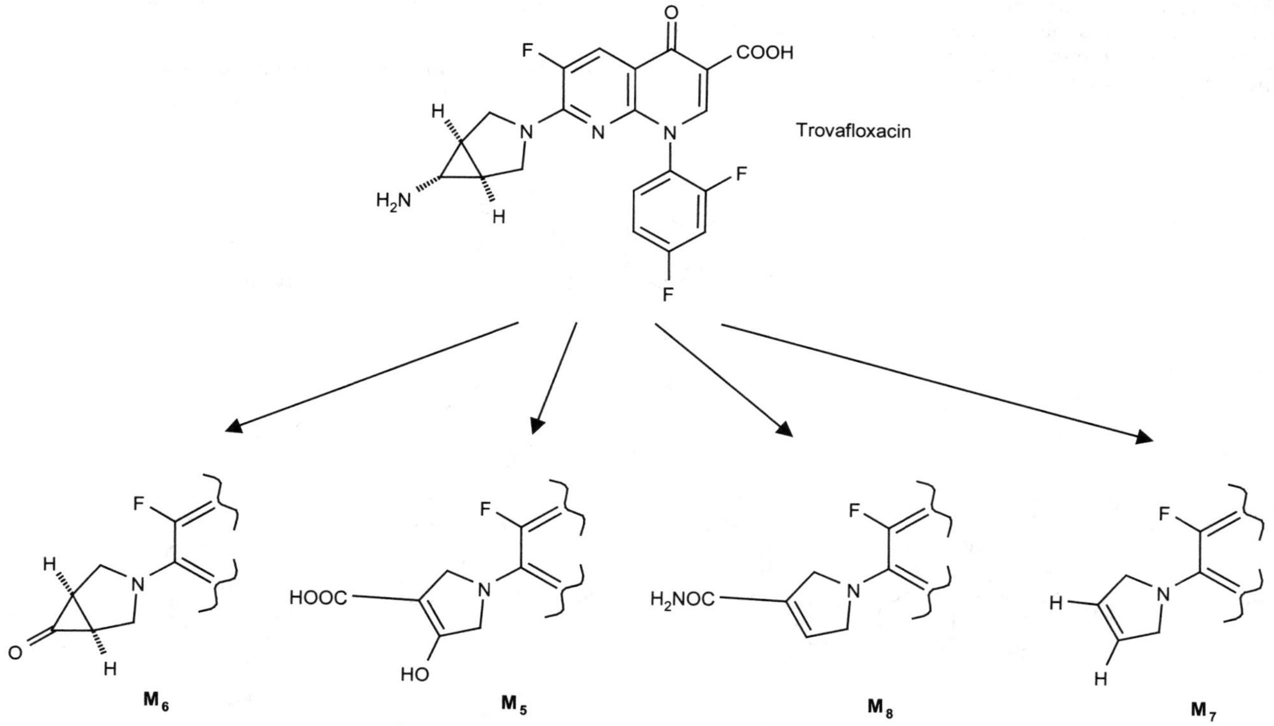

Figure 82 Metabolites (others) of trovafloxacin

Table 104 Fluoroquinolones: main metabolites[a]

Metabolite	CIP	DIF	ENX	FLE	LVX	SPX	LOM	NOR	OFX	PEF	GRX	PRU	GAT	TVA	BAL	MXF
Oxo	+		+	+				+		+		+				
N-Formyl	+		+	+				+		+						
N-Sulfonyl	+										+					
N-Oxide		+		+					+	+						
N-Acetyl								+		+				+		
N-Sulfate														+		+
Acetylamino											+					
Ethylenediamino	+	+	+				+	+		+	+	+	+			
Amino		+	+					+		+	+		+			
N-Demethyl		+	+	+					+	+			+		+	
Glucuronide	+				+	+	+	+		+	+	+		+	+	+

[a]CIP, ciprofloxacin; DIF, difloxacin; ENX, enoxacin; FLE, fleroxacin; LVX, levofloxacin; SPX, sparfloxacin; LOM, lomefloxacin; NOR, norfloxacin; OFX, ofloxacin; PEF, pefloxacin; GRX, grepafloxacin; PRU, prulifloxacin; GAT, gatifloxacin; TVA, trovafloxacin; BAL, balofloxacin; MXF, moxifloxacin.

Table 105 Classes of esterases

Group	Enzyme(s)	Organophosphate interaction
A	Arylesterases	Hydrolysis
B	Acetylcholinesterases, carboxylesterases (nonspecific)	Inhibition (DFP[a])
C	Acetylesterase	No interaction

[a]DFP, diisopropylfluorophosphate.

parenchyma and the bronchial mucosa are between 1.0 and 25.0 mg/kg (Table 111).

In bronchial infections, such as bacterial superinfections occurring during acute episodes of chronic bronchitis, the bacteria are found on the surface of the bronchial epithelium or in the wall of the bronchi. In parenchymatous infections the bacteria are localized in the bronchial wall but also in the alveolar fluid and in alveolar macrophages. The respiratory quinolones are present at therapeutic concentrations in these three localizations (Table 112).

The concentrations obtained in the bronchial secretions are on the order of 2 to 5 μg/ml, and those in the bronchoalveolar film are 1.4 to 8.5 μg/ml. Distribution in pleural fluid is about 40 to 80% of that in plasma. The concentrations of ciprofloxacin remain constant between 2 and 8 h

Group II (%)		Group III (%)	
• Pefloxacin	60	• Levofloxacin	< 5
• Norfloxacin	23	• Grepafloxacin	8
• Ciprofloxacin	19	• Gatifloxacin	10
• Enoxacin	15	• Moxifloxacin	16
• Fleroxacin	10	• Trovafloxacin	20
• Lomefloxacin	8	• Sparfloxacin	25
• Ofloxacin	5		

Figure 84 Metabolism of fluoroquinolones

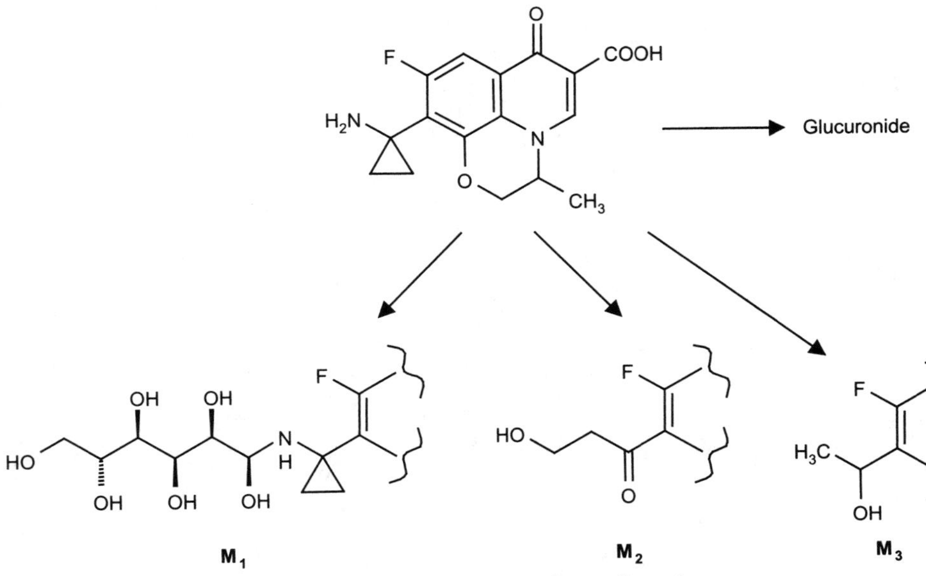

Figure 83 Metabolism of pazufloxacin

Table 106 Pharmacokinetics of pefloxacin in burn patients

% of body surface burned	Phase	C_0 (μg/ml)	C_{12} (μg/ml)	$t_{1/2\beta}$ (h)	AUC (μg·h/ml)	CL_P (ml/min)	V (liters/kg)
>40	P-1	22.1	5.8	20.1	268.6	83.5	1.6
	P-2	12.4	3.9	12.3	195.6	122	2.6
20–30	P-1	32	3.4	12.3	144.1	135.8	2
	P-2	35	3.4	8.3	107	181.5	1.7

Table 107 Fluoroquinolones: concentrations in serum in pregnant women

Drug	n	Dose (mg)	Route	T_{max} (h)	Concn (μg/ml) at:			
					4 h	6 h	8 h	12 h
Ciprofloxacin	20	200 every 12 h for 2 days	i.v.[a]	0.5	0.18	0.1	0.04	0.01
Pefloxacin	20	400 every 12 h	i.v.	0.5	3.8	3.8	3.3	2.9
Ofloxacin	20	400 every 12 h	i.v.	0.5	0.8	0.4	0.2	0.05

[a]i.v., intravenously.

Table 108 Concentrations of fluoroquinolones in amniotic fluid

Compound	n	Sampling time (h)	Concn (μg/ml)	
			Mother blood	Amniotic fluid
Ciprofloxacin	7	2–4	0.28	0.12
	7	6–8	0.09	0.13
	6	10–12	0.01	0.10
Pefloxacin	8	3–6	4.31	2.06
	5	6.5–8	3.87	2.74
	7	9.5–12.5	2.65	1.97
Ofloxacin	6	3–6	0.68	0.25
	8	6–10	0.21	0.15
	6	11–12	0.07	0.13

Table 109 Pharmacokinetics of trovafloxacin in AIDS patients

Compound	Dose (mg)	C_{max} (μg/ml)	$AUC_{0-\infty}$ (mg·h/liter)	$t_{1/2}$ (h)	CL_P (ml/min)
Trovafloxacin	200	2.1	14.1	9.4	
Alatrofloxacin	200	2.8	29.7	9.6	99

after its administration. These results are dose (single or repeated) and sampling time dependent.

10.2. ENT Tissues

Penetration by the fluoroquinolones into ear, nose, and throat (ENT) tissues is excellent. All of the quinolones attain concentrations in tissue two to three times those obtained in plasma. Because of their broad antibacterial spectrum, they are used in the treatment of chronic infections, but also in certain pathological conditions, such as Chandler's malignant otitis due to *P. aeruginosa*.

Concentrations in the tonsils are between 1.0 and 3.0 mg/kg, and those in the sinus mucosa are between 0.5 and 3.0 mg/kg. In nasal secretions, the concentrations are between 0.7 and 3.0 μg/ml. The concentration of enoxacin was tested in inflammatory middle ear fluid in 19 patients after a single dose of 400 mg of enoxacin. Its penetration is rapid, but its elimination is slow. The peak concentration achieved (after 4 h) is 0.9 μg/ml, followed by a plateau of 0.6 μg/ml for a few hours. After oral administration of 200 or 400 mg of fleroxacin, the concentration in chronic otorrhea fluid was 0.28 to 2.95 μg/ml at 2 h and 0.95 to 3.78 μg/ml at 6 h.

The mean concentrations of ciprofloxacin and enoxacin in the nasal secretions are higher than those observed in

Table 110 Pharmacokinetics of levofloxacin in HIV-positive patients

Subjects	Day	C_{max} (μg/ml)	T_{max} (h)	$t_{1/2}$ (h)	CL/F (ml/min)	CL_R (ml/min)
HIV-positive persons	1	8.79	1.4	7.17	184	125
	3	10.7	1.4	8.10	175	130
Volunteers	1	7.13	1.9	7.7	157	117
	3	8.6	1.4	8.8	143	136

Table 111 Distribution of fluoroquinolones in the bronchial mucosa

Compound	Dose (mg)a	No. of subjects	Concn (μg/ml)	
			Bronchial mucosa	Serum
Ciprofloxacin	250 p.o.		2.02	0.39
	750 p.o.		4.86	2.01
	200 i.v.		4.05	0.88
	500 p.o. every 12 h for 8 days		1.17–17.32	1–9.2
	250 p.o. every 12 h for 4 days		3.85–29	0.3–1.4
	250 p.o. every 12 h		1.8	1.1
Ofloxacin	200 p.o. SD 14	14	1.3–15.5	0.1–5
	200 p.o. every 12 h for 14 days		1.7–21	1.6

[a]p.o., per os; i.v., intravenously; SD, single dose.

Table 112 Concentrations of fluoroquinolones in respiratory tissue

Compound	Dose (mg)	n	Time (h)	Concn (μg/ml or mg/kg)[a]			
				Serum	BM	ELF	AM
Ciprofloxacin		5	2.5	2.3		2.1	5.4
		5	5	1.13		ND	7.6
		5	12–24	0.43		ND	3.8
Temafloxacin	600 b.i.d. for 3 days	14	2–16	9.6	14.9	26.5	83
Grepafloxacin	400 o.d. for 4 days	7	0.5	0.41	1.39	5	87.3
		6	2.5	1.7	4.9	17.8	170
		5	4.5	1.8	5.3	27.1	278.4
		6	12.5	1.2	3.5	9.2	322.4
Moxifloxacin	400 SD		3	3.3	5.5	24.4	61.8
			12	1.3	2.2	8.4	113.6
			24	0.5	1	3.5	38.6
Trovafloxacin	200 o.d., SD		6	1.42	1.52	3.01	19.06
			12	0.85	1.01	4.81	16.22
			24	0.37	ND	0.93	10.23
Levofloxacin	500 SD		0.5	4.73	4.3	4.74	19.1
			1	6.6	8.3	10.8	32.5
			2	4.9	6.5	9	41.9
			4	4.1	6	10.9	27.7
			6–8	4	4	10.1	38.4
			12–24	1.2			13.9
Sparfloxacin	400 SD		2.2	0.8	2.4	10.3	34.1
			13.1	1.2	2.6	9.8	61.3
			24.6	0.6	1.6	10.2	36.3
			49.4	0.3	1.1	4.8	37.9
	400 SD + 200 o.d. for 2 days		3–50	1.2	4.4	15	53.7
Clinafloxacin	200 SD	15	1–2	1.5	15.6 ± 11.8	2.7 ± 5.1	2.7 ± 1.5
Rufloxacin	400SD				3.3	11.9	41.9

[a]b.i.d. twice daily; SD, single dose; BM, bronchial mucosa; ELF, epithelial lining fluid; AM, alveolar macrophages; ND, not determined; o.d., every day.

plasma, being on the order of 1.4 ± 0.4 μg/ml. Thirty-three patients suffering from chronic suppurative sinusitis received 400 mg of pefloxacin every 12 h. After the second dose, the concentration in the nasal secretions was, on average, 6.9 μg/ml, compared with a mean concentration in plasma of 5.0 μg/ml.

Tolsdorff detected high concentrations of ofloxacin in the mastoid process, aural mucosa, and ossicles after administration of 400 mg/day in single or repeated doses (Table 113).

Seventy-five patients received 400 mg of ofloxacin preoperatively, and the mean concentration in plasma at 2 h was 2.6 μg/ml. The concentration in bone was 1.1 mg/kg, that in the cartilage of the nasal septum was 3.4 mg/kg, and that in the nasal mucosa was 3.5 mg/kg.

10.3. Cardiac Tissue

A number of studies of experimental endocarditis have been undertaken with the majority of fluoroquinolones. These have shown activity similar to that of vancomycin. There are few published cases of the therapeutic use of fluoroquinolones in the treatment of endocarditis.

The concentrations in cardiac tissue, aortic or mitral valves, mediastinal fat, and sternum were measured at different times

Table 113 Distribution of ofloxacin in the ear bones

Site	Concn of ofloxacin (mg/kg)		
	400-mg single dose (18 h)	400-mg 2nd dose (90–150 min)	400-mg 5th dose (90–150 min)
Serum	0.73	2.79	3.6
Mastoid bone			
Cortical	0.11		36
Spongy	0.17	1.34	1.18
Median ear mucosa	0.7	6.77	9.14
Auditory ossicles	0.16	0.92	1.03
Conchal cartilage	0.82	2.66	3.8
Choleasteatoma	0.93	2.9	2.8

after intravenous administration of pefloxacin (800 mg), ofloxacin (400 mg), and ciprofloxacin (200 mg).

In the myocardium and valves, the concentrations were high, on the order of 3 to 20 mg/kg, but concentrations were lower in the mediastinal tissue (1 to 5 mg/kg) and sternum (0.5 to 6 mg/kg).

10.4. Urinary Tissues

10.4.1. Kidney

The concentrations of the various quinolones in renal tissue are 5 to 10 times those in plasma. These ratios are the same in the renal medulla and cortex. In bladder tissue, the concentration of norfloxacin is on the order of 3.0 mg/kg.

10.4.2. Prostatic Tissue

Penetration into prostatic tissue is good and higher than for the majority of tissues. Concentrations are one to six times those in plasma for ciprofloxacin, ofloxacin, and norfloxacin and twice those for enoxacin.

10.4.3. Prostatic and Seminal Fluids

The different fluoroquinolones are extensively concentrated in seminal fluid. The concentrations are between 0.7 and 7.0 μg/ml, depending on the molecules and their isoelectric points. The concentration of ofloxacin is one to two times that in plasma.

The concentration is four to five times that in plasma for norfloxacin, and higher in the case of ciprofloxacin and sparfloxacin. The concentration in prostatic fluid is 40% of that in plasma for enoxacin, while in seminal fluid it is two to three times that in plasma.

Penetration into prostatic fluid is more difficult to interpret because of the risk of contamination with urine. The concentrations of the different products are 2 to 10 times those in plasma. There is a relationship between the degree of ionization of the molecule and the penetration of prostatic fluid. In fact, the pH of prostatic fluid is between 6.38 and 7.7 and that of seminal fluid is between 7.18 and 8.23.

10.4.4. Epididymal Tissue

Acute epididymitis is a common infection among sexually transmitted diseases. It is usually due to *C. trachomatis* and *N. gonorrhoeae*. Blondin et al. studied the penetration of norfloxacin into epididymal tissue in 10 patients due to undergo prostatectomy. Norfloxacin was administered at a dosage of 400 mg every 12 h for 3 days. The tissue concentration was 3.42 ± 1.98 mg/kg, and the concentration in plasma was 3.74 ± 2.11 μg/ml. Ten patients due to undergo prostatectomy received 400 mg of pefloxacin orally every 12 h for 3 days. Two hours after the last administration (a dose of 400 mg of pefloxacin intravenously), the concentrations in the epididymis were between 8.15 and 21.8 mg/kg (mean of 13.44 mg/kg).

A single dose of 300 mg of fleroxacin was administered to four volunteers 4 h prior to orchidectomy. Concentrations in the serum, testicular tissue, and epididymis were 4.36 ± 0.28 mg/kg, 7.59 ± 1.13 mg/kg, and 6.71 ± 1.51 mg/kg at 4 h and 2.94 mg/kg, 13.6 ± 3.39 mg/kg, and 12.3 ± 1.63 mg/kg at 6 h.

10.5. Gynecological Tissue

The concentrations of the different quinolones were measured in uterovaginal and ovarian tissues. The tissue concentrations decreased with time and in parallel to those in plasma. After a single dose of the various molecules, the mean concentration was between 1.0 and 4.0 mg/kg.

The concentrations of sparfloxacin in the vaginal secretions were high between 4 and 12 h after oral administration of 400 mg (3.7 and 8.9 μg/ml).

10.6. Cutaneous and Subcutaneous Tissues

Penetration of fluoroquinolones into skin and adipose tissue was less than that into the other tissues. Concentrations in the skin were dose dependent and similar to those in plasma (0.23 to 4.0 mg/kg) and slightly higher in muscle (0.5 to 8 mg/kg) (Table 114). In necrotic tissues, the concentrations of ofloxacin were between 1.6 and 6.4 mg/kg and those in plasma were between 2.3 and 5.9 μg/ml 2 h after the fifth dose of 200 mg orally.

The concentrations of ofloxacin in the colonic wall were very high, ranging from 2.7 to 10.2 mg/kg (Table 115).

10.7. Central Nervous System

The fluoroquinolones exhibit good activity against the majority of species responsible for central nervous system infections, including *S. pneumoniae* but excluding *L. monocytogenes*. In meningeal infections of nosocomial origin, they are a good therapeutic alternative to conventional treatments. The fluoroquinolones readily penetrate the CSF because of their physicochemical properties and their weak protein binding. They also penetrate noninflammatory CSF at not insignificant levels (Table 116).

In inflammatory CSF, the concentrations of the different molecules tested are compatible with treatment (Table 117).

Penetration of pefloxacin was determined in 15 patients suffering from brain tumors. The patients were given six doses of 400 mg every 12 h. The mean cerebral concentration

Table 114 Distribution of fluoroquinolones in cutaneous and subcutaneous tissues

Compound	Dose (mg)[a]	Time (h)	Concn in:			
			Serum (μg/ml)	Muscle (mg/kg)	Skin (mg/kg)	Fat (mg/kg)
Ciprofloxacin	500 p.o.	4	1.32	7.9	2.4	1.4
	500 p.o.	8	0.47	3.5	2.8	0.3
	750 p.o.	1	2.3		4	
	750 p.o.	11	0.6		1.3	
	750 p.o. every 12 h for 2 days	1	2.1		3.3	
	750 p.o. every 12 h for 2 days	11	1.3		1.9	
	100 i.v.	4	0.25	0.75	0.2	0.2
Ofloxacin	400 p.o. for 2 days		3.3	4.6	1.3	0.8
Pefloxacin	400 p.o. every 12 h for 3 days	12	3.3	5.6	7.6	2.2
Enoxacin	200 p.o. every 12 h for 3 days		2.5	3.5	2.2	0.9

[a]p.o., per os; i.v., intravenously.

Table 115 Concentrations of ofloxacin in cutaneous tissue and the colonic wall[a]

Dose (mg)[b]	Time (h)	Concn (mg/kg)	
		Skin	Colon tissue
200 i.v.	0–1	4.6	10.2
	1–2	4.1	5.6
200 p.o.	2	1.4	2.7
400 p.o.	2	2.3	7.4
200 p.o.	3	1.6	2.8
400 p.o.	3	2.4	5.3
400 p.o.	4–5		6.9

[a]Data from Wenzel et al., 1994.
[b]i.v., intravenously; p.o., per os.

was 8.2 μg/ml, with very major variations: 1.2 to 33.3 μg/ml. Branger et al. administered a single dose of 800 mg of pefloxacin intravenously (30-min infusion) to 10 patients. The concentrations in cerebral tissue were 10.22 ± 10.9, 8.30 ± 6.58, 11.14 ± 4.9, and 8.85 ± 0.02 mg/kg 1.5, 2.5, 3.5, and 4.5 h after administration.

10.8. Hepatobiliary Tissues

Although the renal pathway is the preponderant mode of elimination, the fluoroquinolones are eliminated in the bile and are concentrated in the wall of the gallbladder and in hepatic tissue (Table 118).

After a single dose of 300 mg of ciprofloxacin intravenously, biliary elimination is 4.45 ± 2.14 μg/ml and concentrations in the gallbladder mucosa are 9.52 ± 1.31, 14.80 ± 4.51, and 10.27 ± 4.08 mg/kg 0.5, 1.0, and 2.0 h after administration.

10.9. Bone Tissues

The fluoroquinolones are a therapeutic alternative in certain forms of acute osteomyelitis in adults and in chronic infections. The data concerning the penetration of the fluoroquinolones into bone are contradictory and often difficult to interpret. After administration of a dose of 400 mg orally followed by a dose of 200 mg 12 h later, the concentrations of ofloxacin were, on average, 0.4 ± 0.15 mg/kg in cartilage, 1.13 ± 0.5 mg/kg in compact bone, and 1.03 ± 0.32 mg/kg in spongy bone. The assays were performed from 1.5 to 10.5 h after administration. In cortical bone, the concentration of enoxacin was 5.9 ± 0.8 mg/kg, and in spongy bone it was 3.95 ± 1.01 mg/kg. In the serum, the concentration was 2.88 ± 0.9 μg/ml 2 h after the last of four doses of 400 mg given every 12 h. After a single oral dose of 400 mg of lomefloxacin, the peak concentration in plasma was reached after 3 h (3.57 ± 3.1 μg/ml), and at 24 h the concentration was 0.45 ± 0.2 μg/ml. In spongy tissue, the peak was the same, but at 24 h the concentration was higher: 1.83 ± 1.3 mg/kg.

Table 116 Distribution of fluoroquinolones in noninflammatory CSF

Compound	Dose (mg)	No. of patients	Concn in:	
			CSF (μg/ml)	Plasma (μg/ml)
Ofloxacin	200	15	0.36	2.4
Ciprofloxacin	200	17	0.06	0.8
Norfloxacin	200	11	0.05	0.8
Enofloxacin	200	12	0.11	1.4
Fleroxacin	200	11	0.4	2.5
Sparfloxacin	300	12	0.15	0.6
Alatrofloxacin	300	12	0.14–0.91	0.8–6.6

Table 117 Distribution of fluoroquinolones in inflammatory CSF

Compound	Dose (mg)[a]	Time (h)	Concn in: CSF (μg/ml)	Concn in: Plasma (μg/ml)
Ofloxacin	200 every 12 h p.o., multiple		0.2–9.5	0.5–13.9
Ciprofloxacin	200 i.v. every 12 h	5	0.15–0.56	5.5
Pefloxacin	7.5 mg/kg every 12 h i.v., multiple		4.8	10.3
	15 mg/kg every 12 h p.o., multiple		8.3	20.1
	7.5 mg/kg every 12 h p.o., multiple		3.8	8.2
	15 mg/kg every 12 h p.o., multiple		10.2	21.4
	800 mg i.v., single	1.5	5.13 ± 2.01	13.37 ± 4.24
		2.5	5.7 ± 2.66	12.08 ± 4.03
		3.5	5.99 ± 2.17	10.04 ± 2.66
	180 mg/m^2	4.5	4.3	8.5 ± 0.14
Alatrofloxacin		1	0.5–1.4	
		2	0.99–1.22	

[a]p.o., per os; i.v., intravenously.

Table 118 Distribution of fluoroquinolones in hepatobiliary tissues

Compound	Dose (mg)[a]	No. of patients	Time (h)	Concn in: Bile (μg/ml)	Concn in: Gallbladder (mg/kg)	Concn in: Liver (mg/kg)
Ofloxacin	200 every 8 h for 4 days			2.7–36.6	2.8–9.9	
	200 SD			7.3		
	400 SD		10	11.9 ± 4.7	4.6 ± 2.7	4.6 ± 3.5
	200 every 12 h for 7 days	6	6	24.6	5.3	
	400 SD	10		0.6–1.56	0.1–7.5	
Norfloxacin	200 every 12 h for 6 days	14			1.24 ± 0.4	
	200 every 12 h for 12 days	14		15.8 ± 7.6	1.72 ± 0.4	
	200 SD	2	2		1.7–3.4	
Pefloxacin	400 SD		12	8		
	500 SD p.o.	12	1–2	7.5 ± 2.8		
	500 SD p.o.	12	12–24	1.1 ± 0.4		
Ciprofloxacin	400 SD p.o.	8	12	12		
	300 SD i.v.	12	0.5		6.23 ± 1.1	
	300 SD i.v.	12	1		5.43 ± 2.58	
	300 SD i.v.	12	2		6.08 ± 2.71	
	750 SD p.o.	1	3			9.8
Enoxacin	400 SD	12	4.5	17.7		
	400 SD	16	5.5		3.6	
Lomefloxacin	200 SD			20–33	1.1–4.6	
Levofloxacin	100 SD	9	2	2.03 ± 1.03	1.25 ± 0.24	
	100 SD	9	2–3	1.96	2.47	
Fleroxacin	800 every 24 h for 5 days	12	24	5.9–73.3	2.9–10.6	
Sparfloxacin	400 SD	4	24	9.7 ± 2		
			48	12.2 ± 3	9.6	
Grepafloxacin	30 every 24 h for 3 days	6	0–72	−5		

[a]SD, single dose; p.o., per os; i.v., intravenously.

In cortical bone, the concentration at 24 h was 0.38 ± 0.8 mg/kg. After repeated doses of pefloxacin (400 mg intravenously every 12 h for 4 days and then 400 mg every 12 h for 7 days orally), bone concentrations were between 3.7 and 21 mg/kg. After a single dose of 400 mg of pefloxacin, the peak concentration of 1.22 μg/ml was reached in 4.5 h. The concentrations of ciprofloxacin after repeated doses of 500 and 750 mg were on the order of 1.4 ± 1.0 mg/kg.

10.10. Pancreas

Infections secondary to acute pancreatitis are associated with extensive morbidity and mortality. *S. aureus* is the bacterial agent most commonly involved.

Five patients received a single dose of 500 mg of ciprofloxacin orally. The concentration of ciprofloxacin in the pancreatic fluid remained high for more than 12 h, with a ratio to plasma on the order of 6 to 12. Penetration of pefloxacin into pancreatic fluid was studied with five patients due to undergo pancreatic transplantation. A single dose of 400 mg was administered orally. The mean concentration of pefloxacin in the pancreatic fluid was 4.6 ± 0.9 μg/ml and occurred after 2.5 h. The apparent elimination half-life was 5.0 h, and the AUC was 40.4 ± 2.2 μg·h/ml. The mean pancreatic fluid/plasma ratio ranged from 0.8 to 1.3. The penetration of ofloxacin and pefloxacin into pancreatic fluid was better than that of ciprofloxacin. The mean concentration of ofloxacin after oral administration of 400 mg was 2.7 ± 0.7 μg/ml, with an apparent elimination half-life of 11.4 h and an AUC of 65.9 ± 2.41 μg·h/ml, the mean ratio being 0.92.

After administration of 500 mg of ciprofloxacin orally, the mean peak concentration in the pancreatic fluid was 0.5 μg/ml, with an apparent elimination half-life of 5.0 h and an AUC of 3.94 ± 0.65 μg·h/ml. The mean ratio was 0.36. Concentrations of ciprofloxacin in the head, body, and tail of the pancreas were 0.02, 2.13, and 0.4 to 1.3 μg/g, respectively.

10.11. Eye

In the aqueous humor, the concentrations of ofloxacin, pefloxacin, and ciprofloxacin were between 0.6 and 1.5 μg/ml. The concentrations in the tear fluid obtained after oral or intravenous administration were between 0.2 and 0.6 μg/ml. After local application of a 0.3% suspension of ofloxacin, the concentrations in tears were between 1.2 and 22.2 μg/ml. The fluoroquinolones penetrate the vitreous humor weakly. After a single intravenous administration of 400 mg of ciprofloxacin, the concentrations in the vitreous humor were 0.05 μg/ml (1.0 h), 0.10 μg/ml (4.0 h), and 0.14 μg/ml (6.0 h) (Table 119). The concentrations of the different fluoroquinolones have been determined in tears. After a dose of 320 mg of gemifloxacin, the level in tears was 0.51 μg/ml after 1.22 h and the level in nasal secretions was 1.36 μg/g after 2.0 h. Table 120 shows the pharmacokinetics of fluoroquinolones in tears.

10.12. Saliva and Dental Tissues

See Table 121.

Ciprofloxacin levels in saliva are constant and on the order of 40% of those in plasma. Those of ofloxacin and

Table 119 Concentrations of fluoroquinolones in the eye

Compound	Dose (mg)[a]	No. of patients	Sampling time (h)	Concn (mg/kg)		
				Serum	Aqueous humor	Vitreous
Pefloxacin	400 i.v.	20	2	4.4	0.8	0.09
			6	3.5	1.5	0.2
			12	2.5	1	0.26
			24	1.2	0.9	0.43
Ofloxacin		20	2	5	1	0.04
			6	3.2	1	0.04
	400 p.o.		12	2	1	0.02
			24	0.5	0.3	<0.01
	200 p.o.	30	2	3	0.3	
			6	2.6	0.6	
Ciprofloxacin	200 i.v.	16	1	1.8	0.2	
			3	0.9	0.1	

[a]i.v., intravenously; p.o., per os.

Table 120 Pharmacokinetics of fluoroquinolones in tears

Compound	Dose (mg)	C_{max} (μg/ml)	T_{max} (h)	AUC (μg·h/ml)	$t_{1/2}$ (h)
Ofloxacin	200	1.36	2		
Ciprofloxacin	200	0.51	1	1.54	1.03
Enoxacin	200	0.81	0.6	3.59	4.03
Lomefloxacin	200	1.02	1.5	12.7	9.2
Fleroxacin	200	1.05	2	20	14.9
Levofloxacin	100	0.61	1.2	5.6	3.41
Sparfloxacin	200	0.62	4	18.9	18

Table 121 Penetration of fluoroquinolones into saliva

Compound	Dose (mg)	C_{max} (μg/ml)	T_{max} (h)	$t_{1/2}$ (h)
Gatifloxacin	200 p.o.[a]	1.55	2–3	9.28
	400 p.o.	3.05	2–3	7.06
Prulifloxacin	200 p.o.	0.28	1.5	
	400 p.o.	0.51	1.5	
Pazufloxacin	200 p.o.	0.84	1	
Grepafloxacin	200 p.o.	0.3	1.5	
Pefloxacin	400 p.o.	1.64	9	

[a]p.o., per os.

pefloxacin are similar to those in plasma. Enoxacin levels are 80% of those in plasma, but there is major interindividual variability. The concentration of ofloxacin in the gingival mucosa was determined in 12 patients receiving a single dose of ofloxacin of 300 mg and was between 3.0 and 7.0 mg/kg. After a single oral dose of 320 mg of gemifloxacin, a level of 0.78 μg/ml was achieved in 2.2 h.

10.13. Colostrum

The excretion of fleroxacin into colostrum was determined in seven lactating women after administration of a single dose of 400 mg. The plasma and colostrum were collected for 48 h.

A lactating patient received treatment with ofloxacin at a dose of 200 mg every 12 h for 10 days. Colostrum was withdrawn 44, 61, and 75 h after the last dose of ofloxacin to determine at what time she might start breast-feeding again. The elimination half-life in colostrum, 12.4 h, was greater than that in plasma. The residual concentrations at 44, 61, and 75 h were 0.03, 0.01, and 0.006 μg/ml, respectively. The pharmacokinetics of temafloxacin and fleroxacin in colostrum were comparable (Table 122).

Ciprofloxacin, pefloxacin, and ofloxacin diffuse into colostrum, and peak concentrations are reached after 2 h. The concentrations are still high at 12 h and even at 24 h (Table 123).

10.14. Skin Blister Fluid

The fluoroquinolones are well distributed in extravascular fluids (Table 124).

10.15. Elimination in the Hair

Elimination of fluoroquinolones in the hair may allow therapeutic monitoring. In fact, elimination at this level not only allows early monitoring but also makes it possible to detect drug administration many months after the last dose (hair growth of 1 cm per month). For ofloxacin, there is a linear relationship between the total dose administered per kilogram of weight and the concentration in milligrams per kilogram of hair. Ofloxacin has a high affinity for melanin.

11. INTERACTIONS

11.1. Interactions During the Absorption Process

The pharmacokinetic interactions of the fluoroquinolones potentially interfere in the enteral processes of absorption, metabolism, and urinary excretion. Protein binding is generally between 20 and 60%, and for this reason a drug interaction by displacement from protein binding is unlikely. Pharmacodynamic interactions may be due to a comparable affinity for a receptor or to an antagonistic effect (Table 125).

11.2. Antacids and Antiulcer Agents

See Fig. 85.

Aluminum- or magnesium hydroxide-based antacids reduce the absorption of the majority of fluoroquinolones. A complex appears to form between the Al^{3+} and Mg^{2+} ions and the fluoroquinolone molecule between the carboxyl group at position 3 and the keto at position 4. The other ions are less complexed by the fluoroquinolones. Anti-H_2 inhibitors (cimetidine and ranitidine) delay, but do not reduce, the absorption of fluoroquinolones. Sucralfate, which contains Al^{3+} ions, reduces the absorption of quinolones. Drugs that delay gastric emptying reduce the quantity of quinolones absorbed. Metoclopramide, an intestinal transit accelerator, causes ciprofloxacin and the other fluoroquinolones to be absorbed more rapidly, but without altering the pharmacokinetic parameters. N oxidation and N demethylation of pefloxacin constitute one of the first stages of the hepatic metabolization of the molecules. This stage may be partially inhibited by cimetidine. In

Table 122 Pharmacokinetics of fleroxacin and temafloxacin in plasma and colostrum

Compound	Plasma				Colostrum			
	C_{max} (μg/ml)	T_{max} (h)	AUC (μg·h/ml)	$t_{1/2}$ (h)	C_{max} (μg/ml)	T_{max} (h)	AUC (μg·h/ml)	$t_{1/2}$ (h)
Fleroxacin	5.6	2.4	6.7	8.0	3.7	2.0	43.8	8.0
Temafloxacin	5.6	2.8	5.1	6.3	4.5	4.5	41.6	7.7

Table 123 Concentrations of fluoroquinolones in colostrum

Sampling time (h)	Concn (μg/ml) in[a]:					
	Serum			Colostrum		
	CIP	PEF	OFX	CIP	PEF	OFX
2	2.06	4.75	2.45	3.79	3.54	2.41
4	1.06	3.63	1.47	2.26	3.43	1.91
6	0.54	2.82	0.90	0.86	2.93	1.25
9	0.30	2.24	0.51	0.51	2.24	0.64
12	0.12	1.82	0.26	0.20	1.79	0.29
24	0.02	0.88	0.03	0.02	0.59	0.05

[a]CIP, ciprofloxacin; PEF, pefloxacin; OFX, ofloxacin.

Table 124 Concentrations of fluoroquinolones in skin blister fluid

Compound	Dose (mg)	Route[a]	C_{max} (μg/ml)	T_{max} (h)	$t_{1/2}$ (h)	AUC (μg·h/ml)	Penetration (%)
Ciprofloxacin	500	p.o.	1.4	2.6	5.6	11.6	21
	100	i.v.	0.6	1.3	4.4	3.4	117
Norfloxacin	400	p.o.	1	2.3	3.5	5.7	105
Ofloxacin	600	p.o.	5.2	5.3	8	71.8	125
Enoxacin	400	p.o.	2.9	3.7	7.2	32.8	114
	400	i.v.	2.2	0.5	6.5	23.1	133
Fleroxacin	400	p.o.	3.8	4	12.7	70.4	89.7
Pefloxacin	400	p.o.	3.9	2.4	12.7	62.5	99.3
	400	i.v.	3.3	1.8	11.7	38.8	70
Lomefloxacin	400	i.v.	3.5	2.7	6	32.4	100
Temafloxacin	400	p.o.	1.9	4.7	8.3	29.4	104.5
Clinafloxacin	200	p.o.	1.1	3.8	4.6	9.22	93
Grepafloxacin	400	p.o.	1.1	4.8	13	22	183
Levofloxacin	500	p.o.	4.3	3.7	8	54	100
Trovafloxacin	200	p.o.	1.2	4.2	7.1	15	62.5
Sparfloxacin	400	p.o.	3.5	1.3	20	37	116

[a]p.o., per os; i.v., intravenously.

Table 125 Interactions of fluoroquinolones with other medicinal products

Interaction	Product(s)
Absorption interaction	Food and dairy
	Al^{3+}, Ca^{2+}, Mg^{2+} (antacids)
	Sucralfate
	Didanoside
	Anticancer agents
Metabolism interaction	Activated charcoal
	Other ions
	Theophylline, caffeine, and derivatives
	Antipyrine
	Anti-H_2 (cimetidine, ranitidine, etc.)
	Inhibitors K^+/Na^+-ATPase
Renal elimination alteration	Warfarin
Pharmacodynamic interaction	Cyclosporine
	Contraceptives (steroid, oral)
	Benzodiazepines (diazepam, temazepam)
	Probenecid
	β-Lactams
	Anti-inflammatory drugs
	Metronidazole

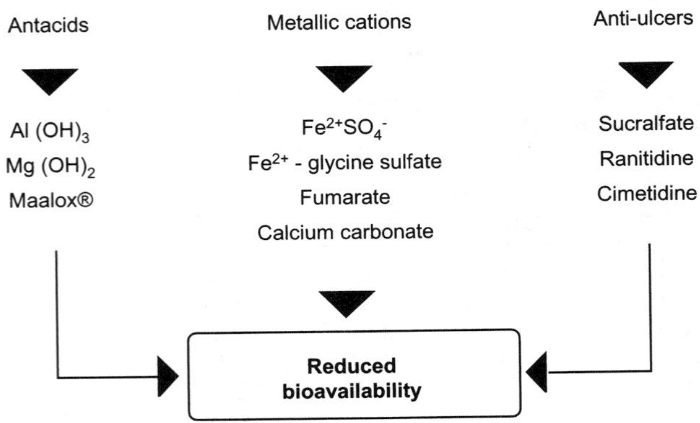

Figure 85 Interactions of cations, antacids, and antiulcer agents

the presence of cimetidine, the AUC of pefloxacin is increased, the apparent elimination half-life is prolonged (10.3 versus 15.6 h), and renal and plasma clearance is decreased (Tables 126 and 127).

The complexes formed are not absorbable and reduce the bioavailability of the fluoroquinolones. The complex is formed in a ratio of up to 1:3 (metal ions/fluoroquinolones). Simultaneous administration of Maalox [10 doses of 600 mg of $Mg(OH)_2$ and 600 mg of $Al(OH)_3$] substantially reduces the bioavailability of the different fluoroquinolones.

However, the time between administration of the fluoroquinolone and that of Maalox plays an important role. Administration of 30 ml of Maalox [17 mmol of $Al(OH)_3$ and 20.6 mmol of $Mg(OH)_2$] has shown that the bioavailability of ciprofloxacin is only affected if the antacid is administered 6 h before or 2 h after ingestion of ciprofloxacin (Table 128).

Table 126 Quinolones and antiulcer agents

Quinolone	Antiulcer agent or patient status	C_{max} (μg/ml)	T_{max} (h)	AUC (μg·h/ml)
Ofloxacin (200 mg)	Ranitidine	2.3	62	14.5
	Pirenzepine	2.4	78	16
	Maalox	0.7	72	4.5
	Fasting	1.6	57	5.6
Ofloxacin (200 mg)	None	3.1	1.6	29.5
	Sucralfate	0.9	2.9	11.5
	Sucralfate (24 h before)	3.3	1.3	27.3
Ciprofloxacin (500 mg)	Ranitidine	1.9	70	8.2
	Pirenzepine	1.8	95	8
	Maalox	0.13	60	0.7
Trovafloxacin (300 mg)	Maalox (0.5 h before)	1.12	2	14.2
	Placebo	2.8	2.4	42.1
	Maalox (2 h after)	2.5	1.9	30.2
	Omeprazole	1.9	2.9	34.7
Trovafloxacin (200 mg)	Cimetidine	2.8	1.4	27.8
	Placebo	2.5	1.5	27.1
	Calcium carbonate	1.5		22.1
	Sucralfate	0.4		8.3
	Ferrous sulfate	1		16
	Placebo	1.9		26.5
Lomefloxacin (400 mg)	Calcium carbonate (500 mg)	5.1	1.3	44.4
	Ferrous sulfate (100 mg)	3.4	1.8	36.4
	Sucralfate (1 g)	1.6	1.9	20.6
	Placebo	4.7	1.0	42.4
Prulifloxacin (200 mg)	$Al(OH)_3$	1.52	1.17	6.89
	$Mg(OH)_2$	0.1	1.75	1.02
	Calcium carbonate	0.6	1.17	2.95
	Ferrous sulfate	0.66	1.7	3.25
		0.24	0.75	1.83
	None	0.55	2	4.16
Pazufloxacin (200 mg)	$Al(OH)_3$	4.28	0.88	8.85
	Cimetidine	1.77	1.17	6.24
	None	2.75	0.76	8.93
Balofloxacin (200 mg)	$Al(OH)_3$	1.95	1.75	18.02
	Cimetidine	0.41	4.5	6.02
	None	0.68	2.83	11.42
Gatifloxacin (400 mg)	Maalox	3.8	1.4	33.5
	Maalox (2 h before)	1.2		19.4
	Maalox (2 h after)	2.1		11.9
	None (gatifloxacin orally)			25.9
Clinafloxacin (200 mg)	Cimetidine	1.3	2.1	9.3
	None (clinafloxacin i.v.[a])	1.5	1.6	13.4
	Cimetidine	1.9		9.6
	None	1.8		12.4
Norfloxacin (400 mg)	Sucralfate	1.3	1.6	7.4
	Sucralfate (2 h before)	0.1	1.8	0.6
	None (100 mg of norfloxacin)	1.4	1.3	7
Levofloxacin	$Mg(OH)_2$ (500 mg)	1.8	0.8	10
	$Al(OH)_3$ (1 g)	1.1	0.8	7.8
	None (100 mg of levofloxacin)	0.6	1.5	5.6
	Calcium carbonate (500 mg)	1.5	1.1	8.4
	Ferrous sulfate (160 g)	1.1	1.3	8.1
	None (100 mg of levofloxacin)	0.8	1.3	6.8
	Ranitidine (150 mg)	1.6	1.0	9.8
	None (100 mg of levofloxacin)	1.7	0.9	9.5
	Cimetidine (400 mg every 12 h)	7.3	1.1	53.2
	Probenecid (500 mg every 6 h)	6.9	1.1	67.6
	None (500 mg of levofloxacin alone)	7.1	1.0	73.5
	Sucralfate	5.9	1.04	49.4
	None	6.7	1.0	46.9
Moxifloxacin	None (400 mg of moxifloxacin alone)	7.3	1.1	53.2
	Ferrous sulfate	2.9		34
		1.2		20.8

[a]i.v., intravenously.

Table 127 Modifications of the pharmacokinetic parameters of fluoroquinolones after ingestion of aluminum hydroxide [$Al(OH)_3$][a]

Compound	Dose (mg)	C_{max} (μg/ml)			T_{max} (h)			AUC (μg·h/ml)		
		S	Al	%	S	Al	%	S	Al	%
Pazufloxacin	200	4.28	1.77	−59	0.9	1.2	+33	8.9	6.2	−30
Temafloxacin	200	2.33	0.81	−65	1.8	3.3	+83	22.9	9.8	−57
Sparfloxacin	200	0.87	0.68	−22	5.3	4	−25	22.1	13.7	−35
Fleroxacin	200	2.37	1.81	−24	0.8	1.3	+63	32.6	27	−17
Ofloxacin	200	2.05	0.79	−61	1.2	3	+150	10.4	4.9	−53
Lomefloxacin	200	2.03	0.60	−70	1.3	1.8	+38	9.1	3.4	−63
Enoxacin	200	2.26	0.46	−80	0.8	1.6	+100	11.4	1.8	−84
Norfloxacin	200	1.45	<0.1	−100	1.2	?	NA[b]	6.7	0.2	−97

[a]Data from Shiba et al., 1995. %, percent variation; S, without $Al(OH)_3$; Al, with $Al(OH)_3$.
[b]NA, not available.

Table 128 Interactions of Maalox and ciprofloxacin

Treatment with ciprofloxacin (750 mg)	Timing of Maalox administration	C_{max} (μg/ml)	T_{max} (h)	AUC (μg·h/ml)	Urinary elimination (%)	Bioavailability (%)
Alone		3.42	1.25	16.1	36.4	0
With Maalox	10 min before	0.68	0.66	2.4	5.5	85
	2 h before	0.88	1.50	3.7	9.2	77
	4 h before	2.62	1.25	10.3	22.6	30
	6 h before	2.64	1.5	12.8	40.9	0
	2 h after	3.96	1.25	15.8	35.8	0

Simultaneous oral administration of 400 mg of gatifloxacin and Maalox reduces the bioavailability of gatifloxacin by 64% and the peak concentration in serum by 68%. If Maalox is administered 2 h before gatifloxacin, the peak concentration in serum is reduced by 45% and the AUC is reduced by 42%. Conversely, if it is given 2 h after administration of gatifloxacin, the AUC is reduced by 18%. If it is administered 4 h afterwards, there is no further change in the pharmacokinetics of gatifloxacin.

Cimetidine and probenecid alter the elimination of levofloxacin. Coadministration with cimetidine is responsible for a 23% reduction in renal clearance (90.6 versus 119.2 ml/min). Extrarenal clearance was constant (plasma clearance/bioavailability − renal clearance) in the three arms of the study, which shows that the reduction in plasma clearance is compensated for (plasma clearance/bioavailability, 158.5 ml/min; + cimetidine, 124.8 ml/min; + probenecid, 114.5 ml/min).

11.3. Interactions with Ca^{2+}, Mg^{2+}, and Fe^{2+} Ions

See Fig. 86.

Calcium carbonate is used in the treatment of osteoporosis and in various “calcium deficiencies.” Reductions of more than 50% in the peak concentrations in serum and AUCs have been observed after administration of calcium carbonate and various fluoroquinolones.

However, contradictory studies have been published regarding the interaction between calcium and ciprofloxacin. These differences probably arise from the method of administration of the calcium (liquid or solid) and the quantity of calcium carbonate provided.

Theophylline is commonly prescribed to patients suffering from obstructive bronchitis. The bronchodilator effect of theophylline is dependent on its levels in plasma; it is optimal when the concentrations are between 10 and 20 μg/ml. The therapeutic index is low, and regular monitoring of serum theophylline levels is required. Adverse effects of the digestive, neurologic, or circulatory type are associated with high circulating levels. Fluoroquinolones of the 7-piperazinyl type are metabolized, with a few exceptions, such as ofloxacin, lomefloxacin, levofloxacin, and sparfloxacin. The presence of a 3′-oxopiperazinylquinolone metabolite, such as is found with enoxacin, ciprofloxacin, pefloxacin, and norfloxacin, causes an interaction with the metabolism of theophylline. In fact, this 3′-oxopiperazine nucleus has a structure similar to that of the N-1–N-3 part of the methylxanthine structure of theophylline. It is possible that this nucleus competes with theophylline for the isoenzymes of cytochrome P450. Theophylline is metabolized (85 to 90% by the cytochrome P450 system in the liver), and the major metabolites, 1,3-methyluric acid, 3-methylxanthine, and 1-methyluric acid, are eliminated in the urine. The major system is CYP1A2 (Fig. 87), the activity of which may be inhibited by the fluoroquinolones. Simultaneous administration of theophylline

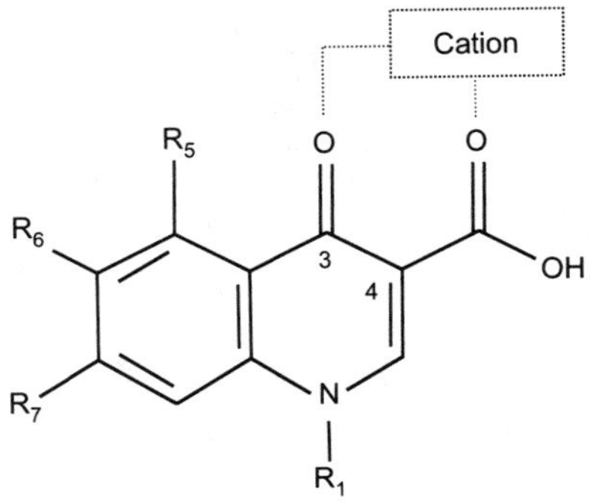

Figure 86 Al^{2+}, Mg^{2+}, Ca^{2+}, Fe^{2+}, and other cations form complexes with fluoroquinolones

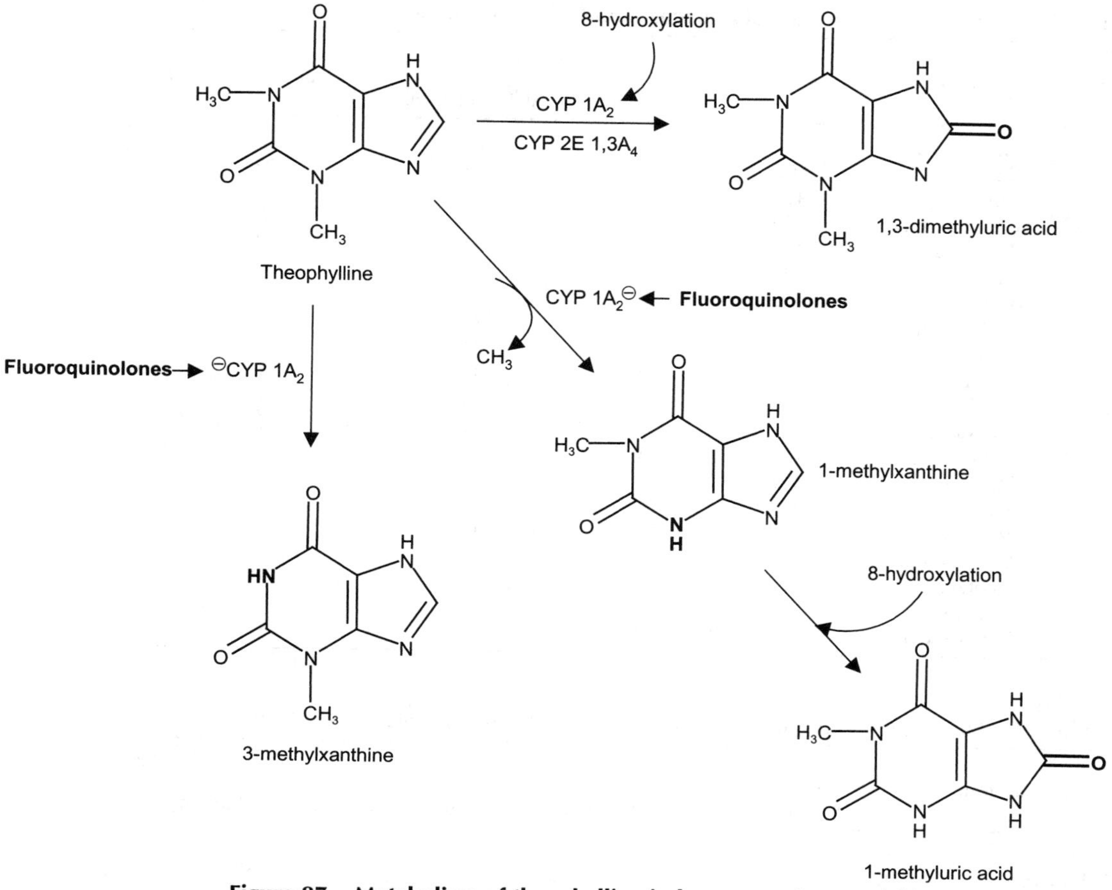

Figure 87 Metabolism of theophylline in humans and potential interaction with fluoroquinolones

Table 129 Fluoroquinolones and pharmacokinetics of theophylline

Drug(s)	C_{max} (μg/ml)	C_{min} (μg/ml)	AUC (μg·h/ml)	$t_{1/2}$ (h)	CL_P (ml/min)
Theophylline					
Alone	9.2	6.3	146	5.9	85.9
+ Enoxacin	19.4	16.6	537	15.3	31.3
+ Pefloxacin	11	8.6	224	8.6	60.9
+ Ciprofloxacin	11.3	8.8	222	8.4	59.8
+ Ofloxacin	8.5	6.3	147	6	81.5
+ Trovafloxacin	10.1		107.3	9	
+ Placebo	10.8		113.7	8.3	
+ Sitafloxacin	9.4		98.4		
+ Placebo	8.9		93.5		
+ Pazufloxacin	7.8		74.3		
+ Placebo	8.1		71.5		
+ Balofloxacin	7.8		68.9		
+ Olamufloxacin	9.7		104.6		
+ Levofloxacin	11.3		126	8.1	48.6
+ Gemifloxacin	12.6	9.4	12.9		

and a fluoroquinolone in some cases requires regular monitoring of blood theophylline levels throughout the duration of treatment with the fluoroquinolones.

The quinolones may be classified schematically into three groups according to their interference with the pharmacokinetics of theophylline (Tables 129 and 130).

11.4. Nonsteroidal Anti-Inflammatory Drugs

Simultaneous administration of fenbufen and enoxacin may cause seizures. It would appear that some quinolones have a high affinity for the GABA receptors, and combination with certain nonsteroidal anti-inflammatory drugs seems to promote convulsive episodes (Table 131).

Table 130 Interference with the pharmacokinetics of theophylline

Group	Quinolone	Dose (mg)	% of theophylline at day 5		Adverse events (%)
			C_{max} (μg/ml)	AUC (μg·h/ml)	
I	Pipemidic acid	1,500	71	79	20
	Enoxacin	600	74	84	40
II	Pefloxacin	400	17	19	0
	Ciprofloxacin	600	17	22	0
	Tosufloxacin	450	23	24	0
	Grepafloxacin	200	28	33	20
	Y-26611	400	20	24	0
	Prulifloxacin	400	24	21	0
	Olamufloxacin	200	23	24	0
	Pazufloxacin	1,000	29	32	0
III	Norfloxacin	600	4	4	0
	Ofloxacin	600	9	11	0
	Lomefloxacin	600	−8	−13	0
	Fleroxacin	400	−4	−4	0
	Sparfloxacin	300	0	0	0
	Temafloxacin	600	−12	−10	0
	Levofloxacin	300	3	3	0
	Balofloxacin	300	0.3	−1.3	0
	Pazufloxacin	600	−3	3.9	0
	Gatifloxacin	400	9	3	0

Table 131 Fluoroquinolones and nonsteroidal anti-inflammatory drugs (NSAIDs)

Fluoroquinolone	IC_{50}					
	Control	Aspirin	Fenbufen	Indomethacin	Flurbiprofen	Acetate-4-biphenyl[a]
Norfloxacin	1.4	1.4	12	190	1,400	<1,000
Ofloxacin	0.01	0.76	3.6	0.12	30	830
Enoxacin	0.14	8.3	13	530	3,300	1,100
Ciprofloxacin	7.6	0.1	13	0.1	100	3,000
Tosufloxacin	0.57	>0.01	>0.01	>0.01	NT[b]	0.12
Fleroxacin	0.76	0.76	0.58	0.58	0.25	0.1
Sparfloxacin	0.91	0.01	0.4	0.28	0.16	5.2
Levofloxacin	0.01				NT	3.5

[a]Main metabolite of fenbufen, IC_{50} (10^{-5} M) of fluoroquinolones with NSAIDs (10^{-4} M).
[b]NT, not tested.

11.5. Anticoagulants

Antibacterial agents may interfere with anticoagulant medications by destroying the fecal flora and thus modifying the cycle of vitamin K synthesis or by interacting with the metabolism of the anticoagulants. Enoxacin inhibits hydroxylation at positions 6, 7, and 8 of *R*-warfarin and at position 8 of *S*-warfarin. However, this pharmacological effect is of minor importance, as *R*-warfarin has weaker therapeutic activity than *S*-warfarin. The quinolones do not modify the various coagulation parameters.

The combination of 500 mg of levofloxacin in 16 volunteers with 30 mg of warfarin sodium did not modify the pharmacokinetics of warfarin (Table 132) or the parameters of hemostasis.

Studies conducted with temafloxacin (600 mg every 12 h), ciprofloxacin (500 mg every 12 h for 10 days), and norfloxacin (400 mg) have not revealed any pharmacodynamic changes.

Ofloxacin (200 mg every 24 h for 7 days) does not alter the anticoagulant effect of phenprocoumon.

11.6. Didanosine

Didanosine (2′,3′-dideoxyinosine) is an antiretroviral agent. It is used in the treatment of HIV-infected patients. As this molecule is extremely labile at a pH of less than 3, it was necessary to introduce dihydroxyaluminum sodium, magnesium hydroxide, and sodium citrate into its pharmaceutical formulation to reduce the effect of gastric acidity. Simultaneous administration of didanosine and ciprofloxacin in 12 volunteers substantially reduced the absorption of ciprofloxacin (Table 133).

11.7. Caffeine

The fluoroquinolones do not appear to affect the metabolism of cyclosporine, oral steroidal contraceptives, or glyburide.

Ofloxacin does not interfere with the metabolism of caffeine. Ciprofloxacin interferes moderately with the pharmacokinetics of caffeine by increasing the elimination half-life by about 15%. Conversely, simultaneous administration of enoxacin and caffeine significantly increases the elimination half-life of caffeine (3.3 to 11.8 h), with an increase in

Table 132 Pharmacokinetics of warfarin alone or in combination with levofloxacin

Compound	C_{max} (μg/ml)	T_{max} (h)	AUC (μg·h/ml)	$t_{1/2}$ (h)	CL/F (ml/min)
Warfarin *R*(+)					
Alone	1.64	1.5	86.1	43.6	2.9
+ Levofloxacin	1.6	1.3	87	46	2.9
Warfarin *R*(−)					
Alone	1.7	1.3	52.1	31.7	3
+ Levofloxacin	1.6	1.3	54.2	47.2	4.6

Table 133 Pharmacokinetics of ciprofloxacin and didanosine

Compound	C_{max} (μg/ml)	T_{max} (h)	AUC (μg·h/ml)	$t_{1/2}$ (h)
Ciprofloxacin				
Alone	3.38	1.56	15.5	4.3
+ Didanosine	0.25	0.75	0.26	Not evaluated

the peak concentration in plasma on the order of 41% (3.9 to 5.5 μg/ml) and a reduction in plasma clearance of 78%.

Twelve volunteers received 200 mg of caffeine monohydrate (183 mg of caffeine) for 6 days. One group of volunteers at the same time received either 200 mg of trovafloxacin or placebo from days 1 to 3. From days 4 to 6, the volunteers who had received trovafloxacin took placebo and the others took trovafloxacin. The pharmacokinetics of caffeine were determined on days 3 and 6 (Table 134). In this study, the pharmacokinetics of caffeine were unaffected.

11.8. Interaction with Ethanol

Twelve volunteers received ciprofloxacin (500 mg every 12 h) and a single dose of 3 g of ethanol for 3 days; pharmacokinetics are shown in Table 135.

Ethanol is a central nervous system depressant. At a concentration of 15 to 100 mM, it significantly reduces the fluidity of the lipid membranes, which appears to be correlated with the sedative effect in animal models.

On the basis of psychomotor tests, no changes have been demonstrated that would appear to be due to an interaction between ingestion of ethanol and absorption of ciprofloxacin.

11.9. Interaction with Digoxin

The therapeutic index of digoxin is low, and the risk of toxicity is high. The interaction of levofloxacin with the metabolism of digoxin after repeated doses was studied in 16 male volunteers (Table 136). There was no modification of the pharmacokinetics of digoxin in combination with levofloxacin.

11.10. Interactions of Fluoroquinolones with Other Antibacterial Agents

A number of bacterial infections require treatment with combinations of antibacterial agents, whether staphylococcal infections; infections caused by *P. aeruginosa*, mycobacteria (tuberculosis, leprosy, and atypical mycobacteriosis), *Enterobacteriaceae*, or nonfermenting gram-negative bacilli; or multibacterial infections involving anaerobic bacteria.

A number of combinations involving a fluoroquinolone have been tested pharmacokinetically, particularly with agents against anaerobic bacteria (metronidazole and clindamycin), antistaphylococcal or antimycobacterial agents (rifampin), and agents against gram-negative bacteria (β-lactams).

11.10.1. Metronidazole and Clindamycin

The new fluoroquinolones have good in vitro activity against anaerobic bacteria.

Ciprofloxacin, ofloxacin, and the other group II derivatives are relatively inactive against these bacterial species. It is therefore logical to combine them with an antibacterial agent that is active against anaerobic bacteria, such as metronidazole or clindamycin.

11.10.1.1. In Vitro Activity

Several studies have been conducted to determine the activity of the combinations of ciprofloxacin and clindamycin or metronidazole against anaerobic bacteria.

The combination of ciprofloxacin and metronidazole would appear to be more active than the products alone against *C. perfringens* and *C. difficile*.

The combination of ciprofloxacin and clindamycin is synergistic against gram-negative bacilli, except for the genus *Fusobacterium*.

Table 134 Pharmacokinetics of caffeine with trovafloxacin

Compound	C_{max} (μg/ml)	T_{max} (h)	AUC_{0-24h} (μg·h/ml)	$t_{1/2}$ (h)
Trovafloxacin (200 mg)	7.03 ± 1.31	0.9	45.77 ± 9.1	4.6
Placebo	6.12 ± 1.23	1	39.19 ± 5.8	4.5

Table 135 Pharmacokinetics of ethanol in the presence of ciprofloxacin

Compound	C_{max} (μg/ml)	AUC_{0-24h} (μg·h/ml)	T_{max} (h)	Elimination rate (μg/ml/h)
Ciprofloxacin	483	734	0.5	133
Placebo	466	736	0.6	134

Table 136 Pharmacokinetics of digoxin in the presence of levofloxacin

Compound	C_{max} (μg/ml)	C_{min} (μg/ml)	T_{max} (h)	AUC (μg·h/ml)
Levofloxacin	2.0	0.4	1.2	16.5
Placebo	1.9	0.4	1.1	15.4
Levofloxacin	2.2	0.4	0.8	15.6
Placebo	1.6	0.3	1.1	13.2

No synergy was detected for the combination ciprofloxacin-metronidazole against *B. fragilis*. The activity is additive or neutral. The same effect has been shown with levofloxacin.

The combinations of trovafloxacin and metronidazole or clindamycin are additive or neutral by the killing pharmacokinetic method against the *Bacteroides* group, *Prevotella* spp., *Peptostreptococcus* spp., *Fusobacterium* spp., and *Clostridium* spp.

11.10.1.2. Pharmacokinetics

Ciprofloxacin and ofloxacin were administered simultaneously with metronidazole or clindamycin to 10 healthy volunteers. The pharmacokinetics of ofloxacin and cipro-floxacin were not significantly affected, except for the concentrations in serum at the end of infusion for ofloxacin and the apparent elimination half-life. Likewise, the plasma pharmacokinetics of clindamycin and metronidazole were unchanged (Table 137).

Ofloxacin and fleroxacin were administered orally in combination with clindamycin, metronidazole, or ornidazole. No changes in the pharmacokinetics of these two fluoroquinolones (Table 138) or in those of the agents against anaerobic bacteria were observed.

11.10.1.3. Side Effects

Neurologic disorders in the form of seizures have been described for a patient receiving ciprofloxacin (500 mg per os every 12 h), metronidazole (250 mg every 8 h), and theophylline. Cerebellar disorders have been described for a patient receiving metronidazole and pefloxacin simultaneously.

11.10.2. Rifampin

Rifampin is a hepatic enzyme inducer that may alter the pharmacokinetics of drugs present concurrently.

Chandler et al. (1990) showed that a combination of 750 mg of ciprofloxacin every 12 h and 300 mg of rifampin every 12 h for 14 days did not significantly modify the pharmacokinetics of ciprofloxacin.

Humbert et al. (1991) showed that in the presence of rifampin the plasma clearance of pefloxacin (administration of 400 mg every 12 h for 3 days) was reduced by 35%.

Fleroxacin, administered simultaneously with 600 mg of rifampin for 7 days, had a 27% increase in the plasma clearance, a 12% reduction in the apparent elimination half-life, and a 14% reduction in the AUC. Simultaneous administration of enoxacin and rifampin did not significantly alter the pharmacokinetics of enoxacin after 10 days.

11.10.3. β-Lactams

The combination of ciprofloxacin and azlocillin has been used in the treatment of severe infections due to *P. aeruginosa*. These two compounds are organic acids and are eliminated renally and hepatically.

Table 137 Pharmacokinetics of fluoroquinolones with clindamycin or metronidazole

Compound	Additional agent	Dose (mg)	C_{max} (μg/ml)	T_{max} (h)	AUC (μg·h/ml)	$t_{1/2}$ (h)	CL_P (ml/min)	CL_R (ml/min)	Urinary elimination (%)
Ciprofloxacin	None	200 i.v.[a]	5.8	0.5	5	6.9	660	411	62.7
	Metronidazole	500 i.v.	10.5	0.5	5.6	6.2	577	346	60.5
	Clindamycin	600 i.v.	12	0.5	5.8	7.1	570	332	59.3
Ofloxacin	None	200 i.v.	8.4	0.5	16.3	15.6	199	178	87.4
	Metronidazole	500 i.v.	6.7	0.5	16	11	203	182	88.9
	Clindamycin	600 i.v.	6.4	0.5	15.1	7.6	212	177	82.3
Enoxacin	None	800 i.v.	1.8	1.4	11.1	7.3	599	337	55.5
	Metronidazole	400 i.v.	1.8	1.3	10.5	5.4	686	375	58.6
	Clindamycin	300 i.v.	1.6	1.5	10	6.1	668	380	58
Fleroxacin	None	400 i.v.	4.2	2.1	61.5	10.5	107	68	63.1
	Metronidazole	400 i.v.	4.6	1.9	60.5	10.3	107	69	63.5
	Clindamycin	300 i.v.	4.5	1.9	66.7	10.7	98	66	66.4
	Omeprazole	500 i.v.	4.9	1.6	63.6	10.3	100	67	65.7

[a]i.v., intravenously.

Table 138 Plasma pharmacokinetics of metronidazole and clindamycin alone or in combination with fluoroquinolones

Compound	Dose (mg)[a]	Concn (μg/ml)					
		0.5 h	1 h	2 h	6 h	12 h	24 h
Metronidazole	500 i.v.	16.4			7.3	3.3	1.3
	400 p.o.		7.9	7.7	6.3	2.7	
Ornidazole	500 p.o.		7.4	8.1	7.2	4.4	2.2
Clindamycin	600 i.v.	17.1			3.6	0.4	
	300 p.o.		2.6	2.2	1	0.1	

[a]i.v., intravenously; p.o., per os.

Six volunteers received ciprofloxacin or azlocillin alone or in combination intravenously. The pharmacokinetics of azlocillin were unchanged. Conversely, renal and extrarenal clearance of ciprofloxacin and the volume of distribution at steady-state were reduced by 35, 39, and 31%, respectively.

The combination of ofloxacin (400 mg) and amoxicillin (3 g) did not modify the pharmacokinetic parameters of the two drugs.

11.11. Zidovudine

In addition to its antiviral activity, zidovudine possesses a certain antibacterial activity against *Enterobacteriaceae* through its action on bacterial DNA (Table 139). As a result of its activity on DNA, zidovudine might modify the activity of the fluoroquinolones.

No antagonistic activity has been found between the fluoroquinolones tested (lomefloxacin, ciprofloxacin, levofloxacin, ofloxacin, and enoxacin) and zidovudine. The activity against *Enterobacteriaceae* is additive or neutral. The pharmacokinetics of levofloxacin are unchanged in the presence of zidovudine.

11.12. Morphine

Morphine reduces gastric acid secretion, prolongs gastric emptying time, and delays the passage of the gastric contents into the duodenum by up to 12 h, which might therefore delay the absorption of orally administrable drugs. In addition, it reduces pancreatic, intestinal, and biliary secretions.

Morphine is commonly coadministered during the surgical phase. An interaction may either reduce the efficacy of the antibacterial agent or increase the toxicity of morphine.

Table 139 In vitro activity of zidovudine

Microorganism	MIC (μg/ml)	
	Zidovudine	Levofloxacin
E. coli KL-16	0.15	0.01
E. coli 9b346	1.5	0.01
S. typhimurium NCTC 5710	1.0	0.03
Salmonella group B	1.0	0.03
Salmonella group C_1	1.5	0.02
Salmonella group D	1.5	0.03
Salmonella group E	1.5	0.05
S. aureus E3T	>500	0.07
P. aeruginosa CP	>500	0.20

Nineteen healthy volunteers received trovafloxacin (200 mg) orally with or without morphine (0.15 mg/kg intravenously).

The concentrations in plasma of trovafloxacin, morphine, and its main metabolite, 6-β-glucuronide, are summarized in Table 140.

The pharmacokinetics of morphine and its main metabolite were not affected by simultaneous administration with trovafloxacin.

The AUC of trovafloxacin was reduced by 46%, the peak concentration in serum was reduced by 36%, and the time to the peak concentration in serum was reduced by 4 h. The results are comparable to those obtained with ciprofloxacin.

11.13. Cyclosporine

In the presence of levofloxacin, the pharmacokinetics of cyclosporine are unchanged (Table 141).

11.14. Terfenadine

Sparfloxacin and terfenadine are responsible for the electrocardiographic lengthening of the QTc interval. There is an additive effect from the combination of these two drugs. The pharmacokinetics of sparfloxacin are unaffected by terfenadine.

12. CLINICAL INDICATIONS

12.1. Genitourinary Infections

A number of drugs can be used in the treatment of urinary tract infections, but the fluoroquinolones have a privileged place in complicated urinary tract infections and chronic prostatitis.

The antibacterial spectrum of the fluoroquinolones includes the majority of pathogenic agents responsible for urinary tract infections. Urinary tract infections are common in women; about 10 to 20% of women will suffer a urinary tract infection at some time during their lives. Among nosocomial infections, 40% are urinary tract infections, due in particular to the presence of an indwelling urinary catheter.

Fluoroquinolone concentrations in tissue and urine are very high. According to Wolfson et al., the basic precondition for sterilization of the urine is that the concentration in the urine should be equal to at least five times the MIC necessary to inhibit the growth of the causative pathogenic agent.

Table 140 Pharmacokinetics of morphine in combination with trovafloxacin

Compound	Additional agent	C_{max} (μg/ml)	T_{max} (h)	AUC (μg·h/ml)	k_{el} (h^{-1})	$t_{1/2}$ (h)
Morphine	Trovafloxacin	159.5	0.17	104.2	0.3	2.2
	None	148.3	0.17	106.7	0.3	2.4
β-Glucuronide	Trovafloxacin	29.5	0.9	122	0.3	2.4
	Morphine	26.1	1.0	117	0.3	2.4
Trovafloxacin	None	2.0	1.7	28.5	0.07	10.4
	Morphine	1.1	5.8	17.7	0.07	9.0

Table 141 Pharmacokinetics of cyclosporine in the presence of levofloxacin

Compound	C_{max} (μg/ml)	T_{max} (h)	$AUC_{0-\infty}$ (μg·h/ml)	$t_{1/2}$ (h)	CL_P/F (ml/min)
Placebo	1.1	1.8	7.24	6.4	25.9
Levofloxacin (500 mg)	1.1	2.4	7.62	8.8	23.6

12.1.1. Noncomplicated Urinary Tract Infections

Noncomplicated urinary tract infections may be treated by short courses of potent antibacterial agents whose urinary concentrations remain high for a long period. This is the case with co-trimoxazole, trimethoprim, and certain fluoroquinolones. The fluoroquinolones are very often used in this indication because of their potent bactericidal activity and because they are active against strains resistant to other antibacterial agents. The main bacterial causative agents are *E. coli*, *Staphylococcus saprophyticus*, and *K. pneumoniae*.

The bactericidal activity in the urine varies with the bacterial genera and the molecules (Table 142).

The evaluation of antibacterial agents in the treatment of noncomplicated urinary tract infections, including the fluoroquinolones, is difficult. In fact, it is possible to obtain sterilization of the urine in a large proportion (71%) of patients after treatment for 1 month with placebo, and 80% of these will have sterile urine 5 months after the end of treatment. In order to demonstrate improvement with an antibacterial therapeutic agent, the therapeutic efficacy rate must be at least 70 to 80%.

In a comparative, nonrandomized study, Garlando et al. compared the therapeutic efficacy of ciprofloxacin administered in a single dose at doses of 100 and 250 mg. The therapeutic efficacies among the 38 patients studied were 84 and 89%, respectively, on day 5. Identical results were obtained after single doses of amoxicillin (3 g) and co-trimoxazole (480 and 2,400 mg), with efficacy rates of 74 and 79%. In a comparative, randomized, double-blind study, ciprofloxacin (250 mg every 12 h) and co-trimoxazole (160 and 800 mg every 12 h) were administered for 10 days to 65 patients. A clinical cure and sterilization of the urine were obtained with ciprofloxacin in 100% of patients, whereas in the co-trimoxazole group the respective rates were 94 and 91%. In the fourth week after the end of treatment, 18% of patients in the co-trimoxazole group had relapsed, compared with 6.5% in the ciprofloxacin group. In the treatment of acute cystitis in young women, single doses of pefloxacin, ofloxacin, lomefloxacin, enoxacin, rufloxacin and others yielded good therapeutic results. Enthusiasm regarding these results must be tempered by the knowledge of the emergence of fluoroquinolone-resistant strains of *E. coli*, *K. pneumoniae*, and *S. saprophyticus*. In addition, various precautions should be taken with these patients, as treatment is given on an outpatient basis and certain fluoroquinolones are responsible for light intolerance at the least (lomefloxacin).

12.1.2. Complicated Urinary Tract Infections

The fluoroquinolones represent the reference treatment for complicated urinary tract infections, particularly those due to *P. aeruginosa* and multiresistant bacteria. Complicated urinary tract infections occur during pregnancy and in patients with anatomical abnormalities or with an underlying condition, such as diabetes. The difficulties associated with the treatment of complicated urinary tract infections are the need for prolonged treatment to prevent relapses, the presence of multiresistant bacteria, and the selection of resistant bacteria.

Until the introduction of the fluoroquinolones into the therapeutic arsenal, there was no oral treatment of urinary tract infections due to *P. aeruginosa*. In the various studies published, ciprofloxacin was shown to have 35 to 84% efficacy. All of the fluoroquinolones have the same activity. In a study comparing ciprofloxacin and ofloxacin over a 7-day period, the responses were identical: 61% clinical success with ofloxacin and 59% with ciprofloxacin, the microbiological efficacy being better with ofloxacin (66%) than with ciprofloxacin (50%). Leigh et al. showed that norfloxacin and ciprofloxacin have the same activity.

Table 142 Duration of bactericidal activity of fluoroquinolones in the urine

Organism	Duration (h) of activity			
	Ciprofloxacin		Ofloxacin	
	Day 1	Day 3	Day 1	Day 3
E. coli	6.0	4.0	6.0	6.0
K. pneumoniae	8.0	6.0	12.0	12.0
S. saprophyticus	NB[a]	4.0	8.0	12.0

[a]NB, nonbactericidal.

12.1.3. Chronic Prostatitis

Chronic prostatitis of bacterial origin is an infection that is difficult to treat. The standard treatment used to be co-trimoxazole, but the results were disappointing. Relapses following treatment were common, the principal reason being the absence of an inflammatory state, which usually encourages the diffusion of antibacterial agents.

The pH of prostatic fluid in patients suffering from chronic prostatitis has been shown to be alkaline, whereas it is acidic in healthy subjects or in canine experimental models. The fluoroquinolones are zwitterions that are extensively concentrated in acidic or alkaline liquids. Naber undertook an analysis of 23 studies. As a general rule, the therapeutic results are good in infections due to *E. coli* or other *Enterobacteriaceae* but disappointing in the case of *P. aeruginosa* and enterococci. *E. coli* infections require a minimum treatment period of 1 month, but this period is less than that for co-trimoxazole, which requires a minimum of 3 months. A number of studies of the efficacy of fluoroquinolones in the treatment of complicated and noncomplicated upper and lower urinary tract infections have been performed. Studies comparing the efficacies of ciprofloxacin (250 mg for 2 days), norfloxacin (400 mg for 2 days), ofloxacin (200 mg for 2 days), and co-trimoxazole have demonstrated greater therapeutic efficacy for the fluoroquinolones. The fluoroquinolones produce satisfactory results in the treatment of chronic prostatitis, but treatment must be continued for several weeks.

12.1.4. Noncomplicated Pyelonephritis

Noncomplicated pyelonephritis is responsible for about 8% of urinary tract infections. On the basis of their antibacterial spectrum and their pharmacokinetic properties, the fluoroquinolones represent a therapeutic alternative. Blomer et al. compared the activity of ofloxacin (200 mg every 12 h) with that of co-trimoxazole (160 or 800 mg every 12 h) administered for 7 days to patients suffering from pyelonephritis. Bacterial eradication was obtained in 82 and 80% of patients, respectively. Guibert et al. treated 18 patients with ciprofloxacin (500 mg every 12 h) for 10 to 84 days. Bacterial eradication without relapse was obtained (4 to 6 weeks) in 10 patients. Norfloxacin (400 mg every 12 h) achieved bacterial eradication in 92% of patients.

12.2. Sexually Transmitted Diseases

Sexually transmitted diseases are due to a wide variety of pathogenic agents: *N. gonorrhoeae*, *C. trachomatis*, *U. urealyticum*, *M. hominis*, *H. ducreyi*, *Treponema pallidum*, etc.

The fluoroquinolones are a good therapeutic alternative in the treatment of complicated or noncomplicated acute gonorrhea. They provide an answer to certain problems: strains resistant to standard treatment (spectinomycin or β-lactams), reduction in the duration of treatment, and oral administration. A cure of noncomplicated acute gonococcal infection may be obtained after a single dose of ciprofloxacin (250 mg), enoxacin (600 mg), norfloxacin (800 mg), ofloxacin (400 mg), pefloxacin (800 mg), or trovafloxacin (100 mg).

Gonorrhea is accompanied in 30 to 35% of patients by a *C. trachomatis* infection, treatment of which requires at least 10 days.

Strains of *N. gonorrhoeae* of reduced susceptibility or resistant to ciprofloxacin have been described more or less everywhere in the world and pose a problem for the future, as they are often accompanied by reduced susceptibility to third-generation (extended-spectrum) cephalosporins.

Nongonococcal urethritis due to *C. trachomatis* may be treated with a fluoroquinolone. Likewise, soft chancre due to *H. ducreyi* may be treated with a quinolone. The administration of ciprofloxacin in a single dose (1,000 mg) or for 3 days (500 mg every 12 h) or co-trimoxazole every 12 h for 3 days in 122 patients obtained the eradication of genital ulceration in 93% of patients; however, failures have been noted after a single dose. Fleroxacin in a single dose has achieved the same results in HIV-seronegative African patients but has proved less active in HIV-seropositive patients.

These molecules are ineffective in the treatment of syphilis. The fluoroquinolones are not active in *U. urealyticum* urethritis. The therapeutic results are contradictory regarding the efficacy of the fluoroquinolones in the treatment of bacterial vaginosis due to *G. vaginalis* and *Mobiluncus*. The fluoroquinolones are inactive against *P. bivia* responsible for vaginosis.

12.3. Gastrointestinal Infections

Gastrointestinal infections are usually due to gram-negative bacilli from food or water or manually transmitted. The majority are noninvasive and are cured spontaneously. Some bacterial species may be invasive, such as *Salmonella* spp., or, more rarely, *Shigella* or *Campylobacter* spp. Others are noninvasive but produce toxic syndromes: *E. coli, Shigella* spp., and *V. cholerae*. There are asymptomatic carriers of *Salmonella* spp. or *V. cholerae*.

The fluoroquinolones are very active against the pathogenic agents responsible for bacterial diarrhea, such as *E. coli, Shigella* spp., and *Salmonella* spp.

High concentrations have been observed in the stools with norfloxacin after a single dose of 400 mg: 600 mg/kg in 24 h. Similar results have been obtained with ciprofloxacin, for which the fecal concentration is between 185 and 2,200 mg/kg after administration of 500 mg every 12 h for 7 days. After 4 days of ofloxacin (400 mg/day) the concentration in the stools is 327 ± 274 mg/kg. Ten volunteers ingested 800 mg of pefloxacin daily for 8 days; the fecal concentration was, on average, 645 mg/kg (Table 143).

12.3.1. Traveler's Diarrhea

The risk of acquiring infectious diarrhea varies from one country to another, with a high incidence on the African continent, particularly North Africa, in Latin America, and in Southeast Asia. In countries in which hygiene is defective, traveler's infectious diarrhea is usually due to enteropathogenic *E. coli* and *Shigella* spp. However, other bacterial species or genera are not excluded: *Salmonella* spp., *C. jejuni* (15% of traveler's diarrhea in Bangladesh), *V. parahaemolyticus, A. hydrophila,* and *P. shigelloides*. Because of the high number of strains resistant to ampicillin and/or co-trimoxazole, the fluoroquinolones are a good therapeutic alternative. Norfloxacin was administered for 3 days versus placebo in a double-blind study. Treatment with norfloxacin achieved bacterial eradication in 74% of patients, versus 38% for placebo, and a reduction in the duration of treatment. Norfloxacin and ciprofloxacin were administered prophylactically versus a placebo. The prevention obtained was 68 to 92% with norfloxacin, depending on the studies, and 94% with ciprofloxacin. There is no consensus on the prevention of traveler's diarrhea, a pragmatic approach prevailing totally. Table 144 shows the activity of fluoroquinolones against bacteria causing traveler's diarrhea.

12.3.2. Other Etiologies of Diarrhea

In a double-blind, placebo-controlled study, norfloxacin was administered to patients with diarrhea due to *P. shigelloides*. The pathogenic agent was eradicated in 97% of cases versus 40%, but the durations of the signs and symptoms were identical. In diarrhea due to *Salmonella* spp., several studies have been undertaken with ciprofloxacin versus co-trimoxazole or placebo. In one of them, treatment produced an improvement

Table 143 Fecal concentrations of fluoroquinolones

Compound	No. of patients	Dose (mg/day) per os	No. of days	Concn in feces (mg/kg)
Ciprofloxacin	12	1,000	7	185–2,220
	21	1,500	1	<0.1–858
Ofloxacin	5	400	5	327 ± 274
Norfloxacin	12	400	1	207–2,716
	6	400	5	2,271 ± 859
	10	400	7	3,030 ± 1,906
	10	400	7	72–960
Pefloxacin	10	800	7	645 ± 67
Enofloxacin	10	800	7	100–500
Lomefloxacin	10	400	7	203
Fleroxacin	30	800	7	159 ± 64
Sparfloxacin	5	200	5	177–535

Table 144 Activities of fluoroquinolones against bacterial species responsible for traveler's diarrhea

Compound	MIC$_{50}$ (μg/ml)				
	Shigella spp.	*P. shigelloides*	*C. jejuni*	*Aeromonas* spp.	*V. parahaemolyticus*
Ofloxacin	0.06	0.01	0.05		0.25
Pefloxacin	0.125		2.0	0.12	
Ciprofloxacin	0.01	0.008	0.12	0.008	0.06
Fleroxacin	0.06		0.25		0.12
Sparfloxacin	0.01	≤0.008	0.03	0.06	0.25
Levofloxacin	0.03	0.01	0.12	0.01	0.12
Trovafloxacin	0.01	0.01		0.03	
Clinafloxacin	0.008	≤0.004	0.03	≤0.004	
Lomefloxacin	0.12			≤0.06	
Grepafloxacin	≤0.03		0.06		
Trovafloxacin	40.01			0.004	
Moxifloxacin	0.01		0.05	0.01	
Gatifloxacin	0.01			0.01	

in the signs and symptoms in 1.9 days, compared to 3.4 days. In 25% of patients receiving ciprofloxacin a bacteriological relapse was noted from the third week. Some limited studies have shown the efficacy of ciprofloxacin in diarrhea due to *Y. enterocolitica*.

C. jejuni is a gram-negative bacillus that is among the most common agents of infectious diarrhea, particularly in the United States. The picture of infection lasts, on average, 3 to 5 days but may persist for up to 2 weeks. *C. jejuni* is susceptible to the action of the fluoroquinolones. The administration of fluoroquinolones to AIDS patients with diarrheal infections due to *Salmonella, Shigella,* or *Campylobacter* spp. produces a marked improvement in the clinical picture.

12.3.3. Cholera

The fluoroquinolones have good in vitro activity against *V. cholerae* (Table 145).

Infections due to *V. cholerae* have been treated successfully with norfloxacin, lomefloxacin, fleroxacin, ciprofloxacin, and ofloxacin. Antibacterial treatment reduces the duration of the signs and symptoms (reduction in the daily number of stools) and breaks the epidemiological chain. The standard duration of treatment is a minimum of 3 days; administration of a fluoroquinolone produces sterile stools in 1 day, whereas 3 days are required to obtain the same results with cyclines.

12.3.4. Carriage of *Salmonella*

The treatment of healthy carriers of *Salmonella* spp. with fluoroquinolones appears to be slightly more disappointing, but the dosage and optimum duration of treatment remain to be determined.

Carriage of *Salmonella* spp. is often refractory to standard treatments. Norfloxacin, ciprofloxacin, and ofloxacin produce bacterial eradication, but treatment must be sufficiently long. In a comparative, double-blind study conducted in Peru, norfloxacin (400 mg every 12 h) was administered versus placebo for 28 days to two groups of 12 patients. In the group treated with norfloxacin, 11 patients out of 12 were negative for elimination of *Salmonella* serovar Typhi, in contrast to the control group. In the control group, 11 patients were then treated with norfloxacin and 7 showed bacterial eradication. In a study conducted in Chile, ciprofloxacin was administered at a dosage of 750 mg every 12 h for 28 days to 12 serovar Typhi carriers. Bacterial eradication was obtained in all 12.

Table 145 In vitro activities of fluoroquinolones against *V. cholerae*

Compound	MIC (μg/ml)	
	50%	90%
Ofloxacin	0.008	0.008
Ciprofloxacin	0.002	0.002
Fleroxacin	0.015	0.015
Sparfloxacin	0.002	0.002
Levofloxacin	0.004	0.004
Trovafloxacin	0.08	0.03
Sitafloxacin	0.002	0.002

12.3.5. Prevention of Infections in Cirrhotic Patients

Bacterial infections are one of the most common complications in cirrhotic patients and are said to be responsible for 25% of deaths among these patients. Infections due to gram-negative bacilli are more common in patients with gastrointestinal hemorrhage. Norfloxacin used in association with selective digestive decontamination has significantly reduced the incidence of gram-negative bacillary infections in neutropenic patients. Norfloxacin has also significantly reduced the incidence of infections due to gram-negative bacilli in cirrhotic patients with digestive hemorrhage.

12.4. Typhoid Fever

Epidemics of typhoid fever in developing countries pose therapeutic problems when the strains are multiresistant to standard treatment, chloramphenicol or ampicillin, and to a lesser extent to co-trimoxazole. The first epidemic was described in 1972, and since then about 1 to 35% of strains isolated have been multiresistant. Since 1990, the use of fluoroquinolones has arrested an epidemic of typhoid fever due to multiresistant strains on the Indian subcontinent. The fluoroquinolones are very active against *Salmonella* serovar Typhi and *S. enterica* serovar Paratyphi, whether the strains are susceptible or resistant to the commonly used antibacterial agents such as ampicillin, chloramphenicol, or co-trimoxazole (Table 146).

A marked reduction in the duration of treatment is possible. Studies with ciprofloxacin and pefloxacin have shown that a 10-day course of treatment produces a relapse-free recovery. Ofloxacin was administered at a dose of 400 mg daily to about 200 patients for 5 days, with good clinical results. Smith et al. (1994) demonstrated that ofloxacin at a dose of 400 mg/day was more effective than ceftriaxone administered at a dose of 3 g/day. Patients receiving ofloxacin were apyretic within 3 to 4 days, with a marked improvement in their general status, whereas patients receiving ceftriaxone remained febrile, with a poor general status after 1 week of treatment.

Nearly a thousand patients were treated for 3 days in Vietnam with an increased daily dosage (15 mg/kg instead of 10 mg/kg), taking into account the dose-dependent pharmacodynamics of the fluoroquinolones. The therapeutic results were excellent (100% eradication, versus 96% in the two published studies), with no bacterial relapses in the third month after the end of treatment. Strains of serovar Typhi resistant to nalidixic acid and of reduced susceptibility to ofloxacin have recently been described in Vietnam. The bactericidal activity is markedly reduced, with MICs of ofloxacin of up to 1 μg/ml. An increase in the daily doses has been tried.

Administration of fluoroquinolones to AIDS patients with a *Salmonella* infection produces a marked improvement in the clinical picture.

12.5. Crohn's Disease

The etiology of Crohn's disease remains a subject of dispute, but a series of arguments militates in favor of the involvement of *Mycobacterium paratuberculosis* in the etiopathogenesis of this condition. These arguments are based on the isolation of this bacterium from tissue samples or detection of the bacterium by PCR. *M. paratuberculosis* is a specific agent of enteric infections that can develop in a number of animal species, including primates. Epidemiological studies have shown that transmission to humans might occur via pasteurized milk. *M. paratuberculosis* belongs to the same genomic group as *M. avium*. Few in vitro studies have been conducted to determine the susceptibility of *M. paratuberculosis*. Rastogi et al. (1996), using a radiometric method in Middlebrook's 7 H12 medium at pH 6.8, showed moderate activity for sparfloxacin (MIC_{50}, 1.0 μg/ml) and no activity for ciprofloxacin (MIC_{50}, 5.0 μg/ml) or ofloxacin (MIC_{50}, >5.0 μg/ml). In this study, the most active molecule was clarithromycin (MIC_{50}, 0.25 μg/ml). Antituberculosis agents such as ethambutol and rifampin are weakly active, if at all.

Table 146 In vitro activities of fluoroquinolones against *Salmonella* serovar Typhi

Compound	MIC (μg/ml)	
	50%	90%
Ofloxacin	0.06	0.12
Ciprofloxacin	0.03	0.03
Pefloxacin	0.25	0.25
Norfloxacin	0.25	0.50
Sparfloxacin	0.06	0.12
Levofloxacin	0.03	0.06
Lomefloxacin	0.25	0.50
Trovafloxacin	0.03	0.03
Gatifloxacin	0.06	0.25
Grepafloxacin	0.06	0.12
Sitafloxacin	0.015	0.015
Fleroxacin	0.12	0.25
Clinafloxacin	≤0.008	0.05

12.6. Respiratory Tract Infections

12.6.1. Nonparenchymatous Lower Respiratory Tract Infections

Acute episodes in chronic obstructive bronchitis are among the most common infections. The presence of extensive bacterial flora and purulent secretions points to an infectious origin of the acute episode. These infections are generally confined to the bronchial mucosa, and spontaneous resolution of the clinical signs is commonly observed. Anthonisen et al. have shown that in patients with at least two episodes a year, antibiotic therapy produces a rapid improvement in the clinical signs and symptoms. A meta-analysis conducted on nine clinical studies showed the advantage of antibiotic therapy in these acute episodes of infectious origin.

Three groups of patients suffering from chronic bronchitis have recently been described in terms of their respiratory vital capacity. The bacteria implicated in the infectious processes in acute episodes differ according to the group (Table 147).

When antibiotic treatment proves necessary, the medication will differ according to the group. The choice of antibiotic therapy and the need for it remain the subject of dispute in the treatment of superinfections of chronic bronchitis. The activity of the fluoroquinolones is good against all bacterial species responsible for these superinfections, including *S. pneumoniae* for the new molecules (levofloxacin, trovafloxacin, grepafloxacin, sparfloxacin, etc.).

In infectious episodes in acute exacerbations of chronic bronchitis, ofloxacin, ciprofloxacin, sparfloxacin, trovafloxacin, grepafloxacin, and levofloxacin are more active than cefaclor, cefixime, cefuroxime axetil, and amoxicillin-clavulanic acid, with an improvement in the clinical signs and symptoms and a bacteriological response of between 85 and 90% for all molecules; enoxacin is the least active molecule.

12.6.2. Parenchymatous Lower Respiratory Tract Infections

Lower respiratory tract infections of parenchymatous origin are among the most common infections in humans and represent about 45 and 25% of community- and hospital-acquired infections, respectively.

12.6.2.1. Community-Acquired Pneumonia

Community-acquired pneumonia remains one of the most common infections and is accompanied by a mortality rate of between 2 and 21% depending on the pathogenic agent responsible for the infection and the patient's predisposition (age or underlying condition).

Table 147 Bacteriology of superinfections of chronic bronchitis

Group 1	Group 2	Group 3
>1.5 liters	0.75–1.5 liters	≤0.75 liter
S. pneumoniae	*H. influenzae*	*P. aeruginosa*, *Enterobacteriaceae*
Gram-positive cocci	*H. parainfluenzae* *M. catarrhalis*	

The bacterial etiology is distributed as shown in Table 148.

The use of fluoroquinolones in the treatment of parenchymatous respiratory tract infections is now well documented clinically with the new fluoroquinolones. Their use in community-acquired pneumonia has opened a debate, the crux of which remains the predominant incidence of *S. pneumoniae*.

The combination of penicillin G (12 MU/day) and ofloxacin (400 mg/day) was administered as first-line treatment to 38 patients suffering from a parenchymatous respiratory tract infection followed by secondary treatment with ofloxacin alone. The therapeutic result was good in 84.9% of patients. Fragmentary but excellent results have been obtained in the treatment of atypical pneumonia (Table 149).

Several retrospective studies have demonstrated the activity of the fluoroquinolones in the treatment of pneumonia due to intracellular bacteria or *M. pneumoniae*.

The efficacy of ciprofloxacin in the treatment of community-acquired pneumonia has been studied extensively. However, publications of therapeutic failures in pneumococcal pneumonia limited the use of ciprofloxacin in this indication, as well as that of the other fluoroquinolones.

This trend, however, has been reversed with the demonstration of the good efficacy of temafloxacin in this indication, rapidly followed by that of sparfloxacin (loading dose of 400 mg, followed by 200 mg daily) in 1,137 episodes of pneumonia, divided between a group of 560 patients treated with sparfloxacin and 577 treated with a comparator. The clinical efficacies were, respectively, 88 and 84% for sparfloxacin and the comparator drugs. Various studies have demonstrated efficacy with a single daily dose of 500 mg of levofloxacin in this indication, including against penicillin G-resistant strains of *S. pneumoniae*. About a thousand patients received either levofloxacin or a reference molecule (cefuroxime axetil, ceftriaxone, amoxicillin-clavulanic acid, or amoxicillin—including at a dosage of 3.0 g daily). The clinical and microbiological efficacy was between 94 and 96%, and that obtained with the comparator drugs was between 74 and 79% (microbiological) and 90% (clinical), including in bacteremic patients. Similar studies have been conducted with grepafloxacin (600 mg/day) and trovafloxacin (300 and 400 mg daily). The results were comparable to those obtained with sparfloxacin and levofloxacin.

Table 148 Causative agents of community-acquired pneumonia[a]

Organism	Incidence (%)
S. pneumoniae	8–76
H. influenzae	0–12
M. catarrhalis	0.5–1
C. pneumoniae	6–34
M. pneumoniae	0–18
L. pneumophila	1–15
S. aureus	1–9
C. psittaci	0–6
C. burnetii	0.8–3

[a]Data from Goldstein et al., 1998.

12.6.2.2. Nosocomial Infections

Pneumonia is one of the most common nosocomial infections (47 to 60%), followed by urinary tract infections (17 to 20%) and septicemic states (10 to 20%), particularly in intensive care units. Analysis of the literature shows that mortality is high and may attain 60% depending on the bacterial etiology.

The prevalence of nosocomial infections ranges from 3 to 20%, depending on the studies, and is much greater in patients admitted to intensive care units or at risk (Table 150).

The bacterial etiology is variable. Gram-negative bacilli are responsible for about 60% of cases of nosocomial pneumonia, followed by *S. aureus* (10 to 28%), coagulase-negative staphylococci (up to 19%), enterococci (up to 11%), *S. pneumoniae* (2 to 10%), and, in certain units, yeasts (up to 17%). *P. aeruginosa* and *S. aureus* are the bacterial agents most commonly isolated in intensive care units. However, there appears to be a "bacteriological sequence" in an intensive care unit, depending on the duration of ventilation (Fig. 88). It is not rare for the flora to be polymicrobial.

Initial antibiotic therapy is usually empirical, depending on the local ecology, and is administered with a broad-spectrum antibacterial agent.

A number of studies have shown the activity of fluoroquinolones, whether ofloxacin, ciprofloxacin, or trovafloxacin.

12.6.3. Cystic Fibrosis

The etiology of acute episodes of cystic fibrosis is still poorly elucidated, but the presence of bacteria is a standard feature. The pathogenic agents most commonly identified are *P. aeruginosa*, *S. aureus*, *H. influenzae*, and *B. cepacia*. These are present either alone or jointly, depending on the stage of development of the disease. In patients suffering from cystic fibrosis, bacterial eradication is unlikely, but antibiotic ther-

Table 149 Fluoroquinolones and atypical pneumonia

Compound	Dose (mg/day)	No. of cases cured/total				
		C. pneumoniae	*M. pneumoniae*	*L. pneumophila*	*C. psittaci*	*C. burnetii*
Ofloxacin	400–600		7/7	10/10	13/13	5/5
	600					1/1
	800	4/4				
Ciprofloxacin	1,500		1/1	2/5	5/5	
	500–1,000		33/33		17/17	
	?		4/4	5/5	2/2	
Pefloxacin	800					2/2
Temafloxacin	1,200		2/2	3/3	2/2	
Grepafloxacin	600		112/118	25/28		
Levofloxacin	500	27/28	85/85	24/26		

Table 150 Prevalence of nosocomial infections in Europe in 1992[a]

Country	No. of ICUs[b]	No. of patients	Prevalence of infections (%)		Mortality (%) in ICUs
			Hospitals	ICUs	
Austria	75	420	9.3	20	15.3
Belgium	72	669	9.9	17.2	14.9
Ireland	15	91	9.9	18.7	11.8
France	264	2,359	11.8	24.2	18.7
Germany	268	2,010	8.1	17.3	14.9
Greece	37	200	15.5	30.5	28.5
Italy	110	617	7.8	31.6	20.3
Luxembourg	5	29	3.5	17.2	13
The Netherlands	78	472	8.9	15.7	13.8
Spain	137	1,233	7.8	27	19.4
Scandinavia	94	649	11	10.5	9.8
Switzerland	49	329	10.5	9.7	8.4
Great Britain	194	840	12	16	19.9
Portugal	19	120	9.2	23.3	33.9

[a]Data from Vincent et al., 1993.
[b]ICUs, intensive care units.

apy produces a reduction in the bacterial burden and a marked improvement in the patient's general status.

The possibility of arthropathy due to fluoroquinolones is often difficult to detect, as reversible arthropathies are present in 7 to 14% of patients in the period of an acute exacerbation of the disease. It has even been suggested that almost 40% of patients have an asymptomatic articular effusion.

In 1987, Scully et al. reported the therapeutic activity of ciprofloxacin in an 8-year-old child in the terminal phase of the disease.

Superinfections of the respiratory tree in patients suffering from cystic fibrosis are sometimes amenable to treatment with fluoroquinolones. These are administered orally, or intravenously and then orally, and often used in combination with a cephalosporin with antipseudomonal activity, or even alone.

The pharmacokinetics of a number of molecules are modified in patients suffering from cystic fibrosis; these modifications involve an increase in the volume of distribution and an increase in plasma clearance, causing a reduction in concentrations in plasma. The various pharmacokinetic studies conducted with ciprofloxacin have not shown any modifications in the pharmacokinetic parameters (Table 151).

Conversely, it has been shown that the pharmacokinetics of fleroxacin are modified in subjects suffering from cystic fibrosis; with pefloxacin, the apparent volume of distribution is slightly increased.

Several studies have enabled the therapeutic efficacy and safety of ciprofloxacin to be evaluated in acute episodes of bronchial or parenchymatous superinfections in patients suffering from cystic fibrosis. The therapeutic response is similar to that obtained with combinations of β-lactams and aminoglycosides. At a roundtable devoted to the use of ciprofloxacin in patients suffering from cystic fibrosis, it was proposed that ciprofloxacin only be administered to patients over the age of 18 years and for a period of 2 to 4 weeks. No consensus was obtained regarding its preventive use.

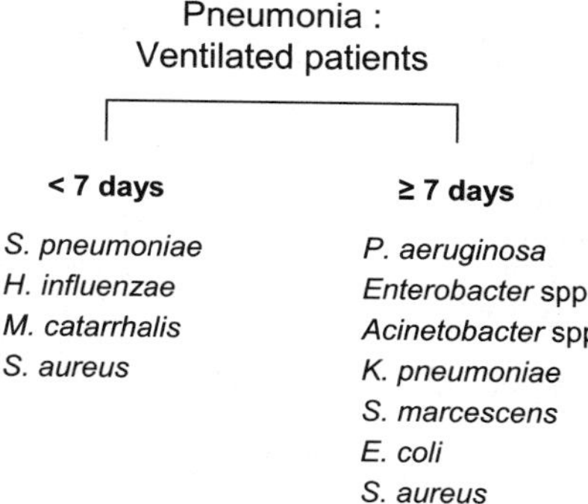

Figure 88 Nosocomial infection: microbiology

12.7. Infections of the ENT Sphere

The treatment of acute infections of the upper respiratory tract is based on β-lactams, co-trimoxazole, and macrolides. The antibacterial spectrum of the fluoroquinolones suggests

Table 151 Pharmacokinetics of fluoroquinolones in patients with cystic fibrosis

Compound	Subject group	C_{max} (μg/ml)	T_{max} (h)	$t_{1/2}$ (h)	CL/F (ml/min)	CL_R (ml/min)	V_{ss} (liters/kg)
Ciprofloxacin	Cystic fibrosis	2.8	1.6	2.6	49.7	28.4	2.1
	Control	2.3	1.3	3.9	54.5	23.8	3.8
Ofloxacin	Cystic fibrosis	3.3	1.7	4.2	126		1.7
	Control	2.6	0.8	5.6	116		1.8
Pefloxacin	Cystic fibrosis	3.2	1.3	11.3			1.5
	Control	2.6	1.6	10.7			1.7
Fleroxacin	Cystic fibrosis	9.9	2.4	10.5	80.9	38.5	1.5
	Control	8.2	1.6	13.5	98.8	46.7	1.9

that their use in the treatment of acute infections of the ENT sphere, such as tonsillitis, acute otitis, and pharyngitis, is not recommended. Studies in this area have been carried out with ciprofloxacin, ofloxacin, and sparfloxacin.

12.7.1. Chronic Otitis

Middle ear suppuration without cholesteatoma is characterized by otorrhea from a perforated tympanic membrane for more than 6 weeks. The standard treatment is based on systemic antibiotic therapy and local treatment. These measures are disappointing and ineffective, and a surgical procedure of the tympanomastoidectomy type is often necessary. The bacterial agents most commonly found in chronic otitis without cholesteatoma are *P. aeruginosa*, *S. aureus*, *S. pneumoniae*, *E. coli*, and *Proteus* spp.; in chronic otorrhea with cholesteatoma, the microorganisms most commonly isolated are, in descending order, *P. aeruginosa*, *Proteus* spp., *S. aureus*, *S. pyogenes*, and *E. coli*.

Chronic otorrhea of the middle ear is difficult to treat, possibly because of the weak penetration of antibacterial agents and the presence of bacteria that are different to treat, such as *P. aeruginosa*, *S. aureus*, and *Proteus* spp. The fluoroquinolones diffuse well at this level, and the concentrations obtained are usually above the MIC or MBC necessary to eradicate the causative pathogenic agents.

Gehanno et al. treated 21 children suffering from chronic otitis with ciprofloxacin at a dosage of 30 mg/kg/day for 14 to 21 days in two daily doses, combined with local treatment with ciprofloxacin. In 18 of the children, the suppuration was eliminated. After an average follow-up of 15.4 months, 6 of the 18 children had not relapsed. Esposito et al. showed that oral treatment with ciprofloxacin alone was insufficient to obtain definitive resolution of the ear discharge. By contrast, the combination of local instillation of ciprofloxacin drops every 12 h (250 μg/ml) and oral administration yielded satisfactory results.

The value of fluoroquinolones in chronic otorrhea is either to produce a resolution of the discharge in inoperable subjects so as to prevent the not-infrequent and dangerous meningoencephalic complications or to prepare for a surgical procedure; in this context, peri- and postsurgical antibiotic therapy is required.

12.7.2. Malignant External Otitis

Malignant external otitis is infrequent and occurs principally in elderly and diabetic subjects. *P. aeruginosa* is responsible for this severe infection. Treatment is based on a local surgical procedure in combination with a bactericidal antibiotic therapy. Chandler's malignant otitis in diabetic patients may be treated successfully with fluoroquinolones. The mean duration of treatment is about 2 months.

12.7.3. Sinusitis

Sinusitis may be divided into three types:

- Acute sinusitis follows a trivial purulent rhinitis. It is usually maxillary and is characterized by local pain and purulent discharge. The signs and symptoms rapidly regress with antibiotic therapy, in the absence of which spontaneous resolution is obtained, on average, in 2 weeks in 80% of patients. Van Buchen et al. (1997) disputed the value of antibiotic therapy. The difficult task is to be able to distinguish acute rhinitis from acute maxillary sinusitis. The most common bacterial etiology is *S. pneumoniae* (20 to 41%), followed by *H. influenzae* (6 to 50%) and a combination of the two bacterial genera (1 to 9%). *M. catarrhalis* is responsible for only 2 to 4% of episodes.
- Recurrent sinusitis is an acute sinusitis that recurs three or four times a year, with the absence of clinical, endoscopic, or radiological signs between episodes.
- Chronic sinusitis is defined as suppuration lasting for at least 3 months and often accompanied by nasal obstruction and even olfactory disorders; it is usually painless.

Chronic maxillary sinusitis may be the cause of irreversible lesions of the mucosae with replacement of the ciliated epithelium by a stratified epithelium, entailing the loss of bacterial elimination. The concentrations obtained with the different fluoroquinolones and their antibacterial spectrum point to their use in this indication. The most common causative bacterial agents are gram-negative bacilli and anaerobes (~25%), but also *S. pneumoniae* and *H. influenzae*. In chronic sinusitis, the level of moxifloxacin in sinus tissues was assessed after 5 days of once-a-day oral dosing of 400 mg; results are shown in Table 152.

12.7.4. Nasopharyngeal Carriage of *N. meningitidis*

The drug currently recommended for eradication of nasopharyngeal carriage of *N. meningitidis* is rifampin. In a placebo-controlled, double-blind, randomized study with ciprofloxacin (250 mg every 12 h for 2 days) conducted in Finland in a military setting, it was shown that carriage of *N. meningitidis* was eliminated in 96% of subjects, compared with 13% in the placebo group.

Eradication of the nasopharyngeal carriage of *N. meningitidis* is important in controlling meningococcal infections. Experiments restricted to the administration of a single dose of ciprofloxacin in children obtained the eradication of carriage in 90% of children and produced results comparable to those obtained with 2 days of rifampin or those of an intramuscular injection of ceftriaxone.

Table 152 Moxifloxacin concentrations in sinus tissues

Sampling time (h)	Concn (μg/ml or μg/g)			
	Plasma	Maxillary sinus mucosa	Anterior ethmoidal mucosa	Nasal polyps
1	2.76	4.56	4.98	5.10
3	3.58	7.48	8.19	9.09
4	3.37	6.50	7.05	6.19
6	2.62	5.73	4.09	3.97
12	1.13	2.81	4.75	2.52
24	0.68	1.47	1.20	1.57
36	0.38	1.25	0.77	0.93

12.8. Osteoarticular Infections

Because of the complexity of the concept of osteomyelitis, several classifications have been proposed that are not incompatible with one another but that are the source of difficulty as regards analysis of the published results. Waldwogel and Medloff proposed an etiopathogenic classification in three groups: (i) hematogenic, (ii) related to an adjacent infectious focus, and (iii) related to a peripheral vascular disorder. The clinical classification is the one most commonly used and distinguishes acute and chronic osteomyelitis. The former has a favorable prognosis if treated early; the latter is often recurrent, and treatment is long and complex. Cierny and Mader (1981) proposed an anatomical classification based on the localization of the infection (medullary or superficial—"cortical") and its localized or diffuse nature.

Rissing (1997) reviewed the literature on bone infections treated with fluoroquinolones. Noncomparative and comparative studies have been undertaken with ciprofloxacin, pefloxacin, and ofloxacin, and a single study has been undertaken with fleroxacin. These drugs were administered alone or in combination with rifampin or a β-lactam. The difficulty in interpreting the data stems from the patient populations, which are not homogeneous in terms of infections (infections in diabetic patients and infections of prostheses). However, the combination of a fluoroquinolone with a surgical procedure has shown that the fluoroquinolones are drugs of choice in this category of infections. In these studies, however, it is apparent that the fluoroquinolones tested have insufficient activity against gram-positive cocci.

Hematogenic osteomyelitis due to *S. aureus* is not uncommon in adults, particularly in elderly subjects, but gram-negative infections are more frequent and are often associated with an underlying disease. They are often difficult to treat.

Septic arthritis due to *E. coli* or other *Enterobacteriaceae* is a major problem in drug addicts (intravenous inoculation) or in patients with a joint prosthesis, a hemoglobinopathy, or a neoplasia.

Treatment of osteoarticular infections with fluoroquinolones represents a major therapeutic advance. Infections of prostheses may be amenable to treatment with fluoroquinolones. Bone infections of staphylococcal origin or due to *Salmonella* serovar Typhi in patients with sickle cell anemia can be treated successfully with fluoroquinolones.

12.9. Soft Tissue Infections

12.9.1. Miscellaneous Skin Infections

Primary infections occurring in normal skin may be divided into three groups: epidermal, follicular, and dermal. Epidermal infections are due principally to *S. aureus* and group A beta-hemolytic streptococci. Follicular infections have a wider etiopathogenesis: gram-negative bacilli, *S. aureus*, and *Propionibacterium acnes*. Primary dermal infections are due to group A beta-hemolytic streptococci (erysipelas and cellulitis) and, less commonly, to *S. aureus*, *H. influenzae*, *Pseudomonas* spp., and anaerobic bacteria. Secondary infections in abnormal skin may also be due to *S. aureus* (lesions of the face), group A beta-hemolytic streptococci, or gram-negative bacilli. In primary infections, the choice of antibacterial agent is easier, with the exception of *S. aureus* infections. In secondary infections, the problem is complicated by the multiplicity of pathogenic agents and the emergence in this condition of new bacterial entities such as *S. marcescens*, *Providencia stuartii*, and *S. epidermidis*. For all these reasons, the fluoroquinolones offer an important therapeutic alternative.

The fluoroquinolones have been tested in the treatment of superinfections of varicose ulcers, eschars, subcutaneous abscesses, and wounds.

Ciprofloxacin (750 mg every 12 h for 9.3 days on average) was compared with cefotaxime in 461 patients in a large, comparative, double-blind, multicenter study. The majority of bacteria were gram-negative bacilli, 8% of which were strains of *P. aeruginosa*; 25% of isolates involved a strain of *S. aureus*. A clinical cure was obtained in 81% of patients, and bacteriological eradication was obtained in 87% of the group treated with ciprofloxacin. Identical results were obtained with ofloxacin. One hundred five patients, including 30% diabetics, were treated with ofloxacin at a dosage of 400 mg every 12 h for skin infections refractory to another conventional antibiotic therapy. A satisfactory result was obtained in 87% of patients.

12.9.2. Foot Infections in Diabetic Patients

Foot infections in diabetic patients are one of the major complications of the disease. Foot infections may be divided into those that involve only the skin and subcutaneous tissue and those that also affect the bone. Bone infections are found in about 13% of patients with an ulceration. Infections at this site are usually multimicrobial and usually involve gram-positive cocci, *Enterobacteriaceae*, and anaerobic flora. For this reason a combination of a fluoroquinolone and metronidazole or clindamycin is an interesting therapeutic alternative. Two studies with ciprofloxacin have shown that treatment must last at least 3 weeks, and 3 months in the case of bone lesions. Comparable results have been obtained with ofloxacin. In infections of the extremities in diabetic patients, a successful therapeutic outcome was obtained in only 50% of cases, with the appearance of numerous resistant strains. Landon et al. (1994) have shown that administration of ofloxacin intravenously (400 mg every 12 h) followed by oral treatment yielded results comparable to those obtained with the combinations amoxicillin-clavulanic acid (500 and 125 mg every 8 h) and ampicillin-sulbactam. In this study, the predominant bacterial agent was *S. aureus*. Twenty-two percent of patients had osteomyelitis concurrently. In the ofloxacin group, an improvement or cure was obtained in 83% of patients, compared with 77% in the amoxicillin-clavulanic acid group.

12.9.3. Nadifloxacin

Nadifloxacin is a tricyclic fluoroquinolone with a 7-hydroxy pepridinyl moiety (OPC-7251) (Fig. 89). Nadifloxacin is prepared for topical use (1% [wt/vol]).

In acnes vulgaris, the gram-positive organisms are important in the maintenance of inflammation in acne. Early treatment with antibacterials helps to reduce inflammation and prevent scarring. Four groups of bacteria frequently colonize acne vulgaris lesions: *P. acnes*, *Propionibacterium granulosum*, *S. aureus*, and coagulase-negative staphylococci. It seems that the development of acne is associated with colonization of the pileo sebaceous follicle by *P. acnes*. Infections or skin diseases such as folliculitis, sycosis vulgaris, impetigo, or secondarily infected wounds are mainly caused by *S. aureus* and *S. pyogenes*. The in vitro activity of nadifloxacin is shown in Table 153.

12.9.4. T-3912

T-3912 is a non-6-fluorinated quinolone having a 7-methylaminopyrido moiety and a C-8 methyl group (Fig. 89) (Yamakawa et al., 2002). The in vitro activity of T-3912 was compared to that of nadifloxacin; results are shown in Table 154.

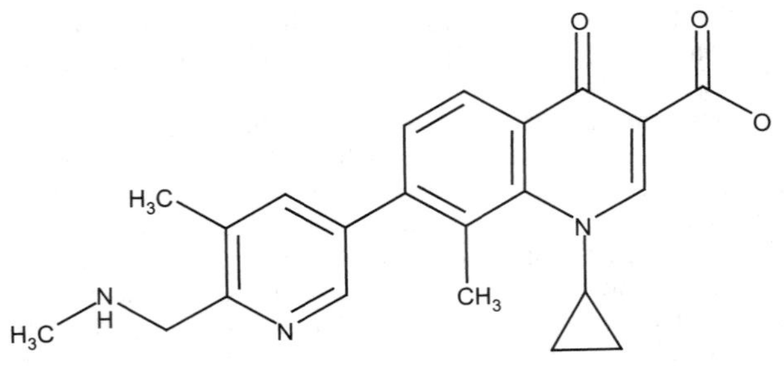

T-3912

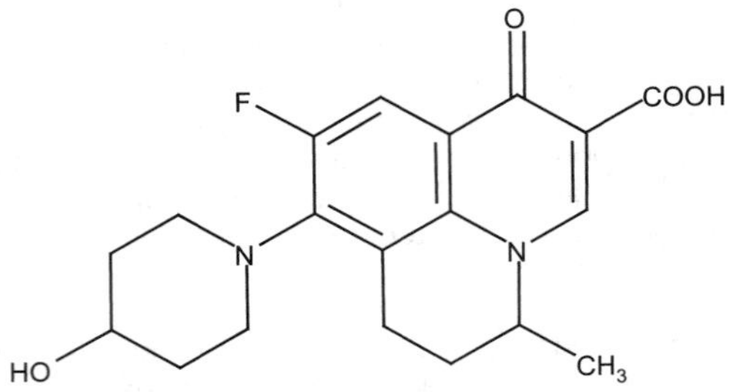

Nadifloxacin

Figure 89 Nadifloxacin and T-3912

12.10. Gynecological Infections

Several studies have been conducted to determine the concentrations of various fluoroquinolones in gynecological tissues.

The fluoroquinolones possess good activity against *C. trachomatis* and *N. gonorrhoeae*. The activity of the fluoroquinolones is well established in upper genital tract infections. In endometritis, in which there is a marked involvement of anaerobes, combination with a 5-nitroimidazole derivative (metronidazole, ornidazole, etc.) is recommended.

Peixoto et al. undertook a prospective, randomized, comparative study of pefloxacin and ampicillin combined with gentamicin. Pefloxacin was administered at a dosage of 400 mg every 8 h. The indication was salpingitis, due principally to *E. coli*, *Klebsiella* spp., and *N. gonorrhoeae*. All of the bacterial agents were eradicated in the pefloxacin group, in contrast to the control group, in which a good bacteriological result was obtained in only 61% of cases.

Table 153 In vitro activity of nadifloxacin

Organism(s)	*n*	MIC (μg/ml)	
		50%	90%
P. acnes	50	0.25	1.0
P. granulosum	5	0.125	
S. aureus	50	0.03	0.06
CoNS[a]	50	0.06	4.0

[a]CoNS, coagulase-negative staphylococci.

Table 154 In vitro comparative activity of T-3912

Organism[a]	*n*	$MIC_{50/90}$ (μg/ml)	
		T-3912	Nadifloxacin
MSSA	25	0.06/0.06	0.025/0.05
MRSA OFX[r]	23	0.2/0.2	1.56/1.56
S. epidermidis	27	0.06/0.12	0.05/0.05
S. epidermidis OFX[r]	26	0.1/0.2	0.78/1.56
PSSP	20	0.05/0.1	0.78/1.56
S. pneumoniae Pen[r]	22	0.05/0.05	0.78/1.56
S. pyogenes	26	0.02/0.05	0.39/0.78
P. aeruginosa	27	1.56/6.25	3.13/12.5
P. acnes	27	0.02/0.05	0.39/0.39

[a]OFX, ofloxacin.

12.11. Miscellaneous Infections

12.11.1. Endocarditis

A number of studies of experimental endocarditis have been conducted with the majority of fluoroquinolones. Sullam et al. compared the activities of pefloxacin and cephalothin in a model of experimental endocarditis due to MSSA and found them to be identical. Pefloxacin proved to have activity similar to that of vancomycin in reducing animal mortality and the number of bacteria in the vegetations in a model of MRSA infection. In an identical model in the rat, Thauvin et al. found an incidence of 4% pefloxacin-resistant strains during treatment, but this resistance did not appear if pefloxacin was combined with another antibacterial agent. The majority of fluoroquinolones have proved to have activity identical to that of pefloxacin. However, the appearance of strains resistant to the test molecule following treatment is not uncommon and may be as much as 8% with fleroxacin.

Ciprofloxacin in combination with rifampin (4 weeks) produced bacterial eradication and a cure of right-sided endocarditis in drug-addicted patients. However, therapeutic failures were noted for patients suffering from endocarditis due to *S. aureus* or *P. aeruginosa*. Levofloxacin showed good activity in experimental staphylococcal or viridans group streptococcal endocarditis in the rabbit, in which human plasma pharmacokinetics were simulated by means of a system of pumps, and in contrast to ciprofloxacin, levofloxacin did not select resistant mutants.

12.11.2. Central Nervous System

The fluoroquinolones possess good activity against the majority of bacterial species responsible for infections of the central nervous system, except for *L. monocytogenes*. The concentrations attained in the CSF in meningitis are high.

The fluoroquinolones represent a good therapeutic alternative in meningeal infections of nosocomial origin, particularly against gram-negative bacteria and *S. aureus*, in combination with other antibacterial agents. Although their activity against *N. meningitidis* is excellent, with MIC_{50}s on the order of 0.015 μg/ml for the majority of molecules, they are not the treatment of choice because of the excellent activity of the β-lactams and their contraindication in children. However, they might be a therapeutic alternative in pneumococcal meningitis due to a multiresistant strain of *S. pneumoniae*.

They are in particular a good therapeutic alternative against gram-negative bacilli, whether cephalosporin-resistant strains of *Enterobacteriaceae*, *P. aeruginosa*, or *Acinetobacter*. Some therapeutic successes have been described with ofloxacin, pefloxacin, and ciprofloxacin. One patient was treated successfully for *P. aeruginosa* meningitis with ciprofloxacin (200 mg every 12 h intravenously) in combination with tobramycin (120 mg every 8 h intravenously) for 14 days. The current question concerns the place of the new fluoroquinolones (trovafloxacin, moxifloxacin, etc.) in the treatment of *S. pneumoniae* meningitis, with some studies showing good activity for trovafloxacin.

The fluoroquinolones have good penetration of the CSF. There are some articles that report good activity for the fluoroquinolones in ventriculitis due to gram-negative bacilli.

Because of its lack of dependence on a state of meningeal inflammation for penetration of the CSF and its good efficacy in animals, trovafloxacin (3 mg/kg intravenously or per os) proved as effective and well tolerated as ceftriaxone (100 mg/kg intramuscularly or intravenously) for 5 days in a study conducted in Nigeria.

12.11.3. Ophthalmological Infections

Penetration of the fluoroquinolones into the aqueous humor and tears is good.

There is weak penetration of the vitreous humor. Concentrations were determined after a single dose, but it is possible that repeated administrations would yield higher levels. Ocular infections may be divided into three categories: conjunctivitis, keratitis, and endophthalmitis. The first two usually only require external treatment, while the third requires local and systemic treatment. The causative bacteria are usually *S. pneumoniae, H. influenzae, S. aureus, S. epidermidis* and, less commonly, *N. gonorrhoeae, Proteusvulgaris, N. meningitidis, Haemophilus aegyptius, Moraxella lacunata, C. diphtheriae*, and *Francisella tularensis*. *C. trachomatis* is an important cause of conjunctivitis. *P. aeruginosa* is a frequent cause of endophthalmitis.

Topical application of norfloxacin was compared to that of tobramycin in the treatment of purulent conjunctivitis in a randomized prospective study comprising 30 patients in each group. A clinical cure was obtained in 79%, compared to 90% with tobramycin, and bacterial eradication was obtained in 70% with norfloxacin and 63% with tobramycin. An ophthalmological suspension of 0.3% ofloxacin has proved to be active in the treatment of purulent conjunctivitis.

The visual prognosis is poor and uncertain in endophthalmitis. Systemic treatments are usually insufficient. Direct injection into the vitreous humor or vitrectomy with the continuous infusion of antibiotics has been recommended. In albino rabbits a dose of 50 μg of ofloxacin has been shown to be necessary to obtain a bactericidal and curative effect.

12.11.4. Peritoneal Infections

The bacteria responsible for peritoneal infections vary with the pathogenesis of the peritonitis: ascites in decompensated cirrhosis, peritoneal dialysis, or other. Distribution of the various molecules in the ascites fluid is excellent. In a multicenter study, Schacht et al. treated 54 patients suffering from peritoneal infections. All exhibited an improvement with ciprofloxacin. Flemming et al. treated peritoneal dialysis patients suffering from peritonitis with oral ciprofloxacin at a dosage of 250 to 500 mg every 6 h for 10 to 15 days. Some patients responded well from day 5. Some cases of intraperitoneal abscesses have been treated with ciprofloxacin alone, with variable results. Better results were obtained when ciprofloxacin was combined with metronidazole. This combination is as active as the combination amoxicillin-clavulanic acid. Because of the presence of a mixed flora, a 5-nitroimidazole derivative (metronidazole or ornidazole) must be combined with a fluoroquinolone in the treatment of intraperitoneal abscesses. A number of new fluoroquinolones exhibit good activity against anaerobic gram-negative bacilli. Studies are in progress to determine their place in the therapeutic arsenal for these peritoneal infections.

A study comparing the therapeutic activity of alatrofloxacin (300 mg) and imipenem-cilastatin or co-amoxiclav or trovafloxacin (200 mg) has been reported by Duke et al. (1998) for intra-abdominal infections. Three hundred eight patients were included in this study. The activity of trovafloxacin was comparable to that of the molecules used as reference therapy.

12.11.5. Miscellaneous

The antibacterial activity of the quinolones allows them to be used in the treatment of yersiniosis, rickettsiosis, coxiellosis, and pasteurellosis.

12.11.5.1. Tularemia

Tularemia is due to *F. tularensis* biovar B. Although not fatal, tularemia is a cause of infirmity if treatment is poorly managed. Conventional anti-infective therapy involves streptomycin and cyclines. Two studies have shown the efficacy of ciprofloxacin and norfloxacin.

12.11.5.2. Leprosy

In 1981, the World Health Organization recommended the use of the triple combination dapsone-rifampin-clofazimine in the treatment of leprosy to prevent the spread of resistant strains. However, the high incidence of dapsone-resistant strains (reported since 1964) and the emergence of rifampin-resistant strains (from 1976) have necessitated the search for new medications. In a murine model, pefloxacin (150 mg/kg) and ofloxacin (50 mg/kg), but not ciprofloxacin, were shown to possess bactericidal activity against *M. leprae*. The combination of ofloxacin and dapsone was synergistic, but that of ofloxacin and rifampin was additive. A marked clinical improvement was observed in lepromatous patients treated with ofloxacin (200 mg every 12 h) or pefloxacin (400 mg every 12 h); as with rifampin, the size of the bacterial inoculum was reduced by 4 $\log_{10}$ on the 22nd day. Studies conducted with moxifloxacin demonstrated its excellent activity in murine experimental models. Clinafloxacin appears to possess better activity than sparfloxacin against *M. leprae*.

An ofloxacin-resistant strain has been reported (multiresistant strain, dapsone-rifampin and ofloxacin). This resistance is due to a mutation in the *gyrA* gene with the replacement of the alanine by a valine at position 91.

On their first visit, almost 50% of patients present with only an isolated skin lesion. The lesions have a natural tendency to heal spontaneously and the bacillary population is small, usually at the limit of detection by conventional methods. Grosset (1998) proposed the so-called ROM treatment (rifampin, ofloxacin, and minocycline). A single dose of each antibacterial agent is administered to the patient.

12.11.5.3. Tuberculosis

The standard treatment of tuberculosis is a combination of two bactericidal antituberculosis agents, such as isoniazid, rifampin, ethambutol, and/or pyrazinamide. The increase in the number of resistant strains of *M. tuberculosis* and in the incidence of tuberculosis has necessitated the search for new medications.

The incidence of resistance of *M. tuberculosis* to the various antituberculosis agents varies from one country to another, reflecting the health structures of the countries concerned. In western Europe, the incidence of multiresistant strains (two major antituberculosis agents) remains low (on average, 1 to 2%), except in Berlin, Germany, where it has reached almost 5.4% because of the extensive emigration from central and eastern European countries. Conversely, there is a high incidence of isolation of multiresistant strains in central Europe; eastern Europe; the countries of the former Soviet Union, Asia, Africa, and Latin America; and certain towns in the United States.

The fluoroquinolones are useful in the management of tuberculosis, as they are easy to administer (once or twice daily), are relatively well tolerated, exhibit good tissue distribution, and are bactericidal against M. *tuberculosis*. Their use in this area is still under study. Ofloxacin and ciprofloxacin have been used successfully in the treatment of pulmonary tuberculosis where the causative strains are resistant to standard antituberculosis agents. Sparfloxacin, levofloxacin, moxifloxacin, and trofloxacin, as well as certain molecules under development, such as sitafloxacin, have good experimental activity (Table 155).

Ofloxacin-resistant strains of M. *tuberculosis* have been described, particularly in monotherapy. This resistance is due to a mutation in the *gyrA* gene.

Caution must be exercised in interpreting the in vitro results, which can vary with the medium used, whether for the radiometric method in a liquid medium (Middlebrook 7 H12 medium) or for the method of proportions a solid medium (Middlebrook 7 H10 medium), or even egg-containing media (Löwenstein-Jensen or Ogawa). The MIC is also affected by the growth conditions.

Yew et al. (1994) showed that the in vitro activities of the fluoroquinolones were comparable irrespective of whether the strain of M. *tuberculosis* was susceptible or resistant to one or more of the major antituberculosis agents (streptomycin, isoniazid, and rifampin). Conversely, the activity of the fluoroquinolones against a small number of multiresistant strains, i.e., resistant to five antituberculosis agents (streptomycin, isoniazid, rifampin, pyrazinamide, and ethambutol), decreased 8- to 10-fold, as a result of which the strains were capable of becoming resistant or of intermediate susceptibility.

Table 155 In vitro activities of fluoroquinolones against *M. tuberculosis*

Compound	MIC (μg/ml)		
	Range	50%	90%
Ofloxacin	0.25–1	0.5	0.5
Fleroxacin		2	4
Pefloxacin		4	8
Ciprofloxacin	0.12–0.5	0.25	0.25
Levofloxacin	0.12–0.5	0.25	0.25
Sparfloxacin	0.03–0.25	0.06	0.06
Temafloxacin	0.25–2	1	2
Tosufloxacin	4–>8	>8	>8
Clinafloxacin	0.03–0.25	0.12	0.25
Trovafloxacin	3–64	16	32
Moxifloxacin	0.12–0.25	0.125	0.25
Gatifloxacin	0.06–0.5	0.12	0.25
Sitafloxacin		0.25	0.25
Norfloxacin		4	8
Nalidixic acid	16–128	64	128

12.11.5.4. Other Mycobacteria

The fluoroquinolones are weakly active in vitro against M. *avium*, but they may have good activity against other so-called atypical mycobacteria. Ofloxacin and ciprofloxacin have been used successfully in the treatment of pulmonary parenchymatous infections due to M. *fortuitum* (Table 156).

Interpretation of the in vitro results is difficult. In fact, the activity varies with the methodology used and the source of the strains. The activity might be less good if the strains were collected from chronic bronchitic patients already receiving fluoroquinolones, which might have selected less susceptible strains.

Ciprofloxacin and gatifloxacin were tested against rapidly growing mycobacteria; results are shown in Table 157.

12.12. Prevention of Postsurgical Infections

The factors involved in selecting an antibacterial agent for the prevention of postsurgical infections are its activity, antibacterial spectrum, distribution in the infectious focus, safety, and cost. The antibacterial spectrum of the fluoroquinolones, their tissue pharmacokinetics, and their good tolerance mean that they may be administered preventively for postsurgical infections in bone, cardiothoracic, and neurologic surgery. They would appear to be less indicated in abdominal surgery because of the marked presence of anaerobic flora. However, after a dose of 200 mg, the concentration of ciprofloxacin in the jejunal mucosa is greater than 5 mg/kg; after repeated doses of ciprofloxacin (750 mg every 12 h on the day before surgery and 400 mg intravenously on anesthesia induction), the concentration found in the colonic mucosa was 2.7 to 37.8 mg/kg and the fecal concentration was 858 mg/kg. In colorectal surgery, Offer et al. compared the preventive activity of ciprofloxacin (200 mg every 12 h for 2 days) with that of intravenous metronidazole

Table 156 In vitro activities of fluoroquinolones against atypical mycobacteria

Organism	MIC_{50} (μg/ml)[a]							
	OFX	LVX	SPX	CIP	CLX	SIT	MXF	PEF
M. *kansasii*	4	2	1	4	8	0.39	0.06	2
Mycobacterium marinum	12.5		6.25			0.78	0.5	
Mycobacterium scrofulaceum	2	1	0.5	1	2	0.78		
M. *avium*	>8	8	4	8	>8	1.56	2	16
Mycobacterium intracellulare	>8	8	4	8	>8	3.13	2	16
Mycobacterium abscessus	>8	>8	>8	8	>8	3.13		
Mycobacterium chelonae	>8	>8	>8	>8	>8	0.39	>2	
M. *fortuitum*	2	2	0.5	0.5	1	0.2	0.12	1

[a]OFX, ofloxacin; LVX, levofloxacin; SPX, sparfloxacin; CIP, ciprofloxacin; SIT, sitafloxacin; CLX, clinafloxaxin; MXF, moxifloxacin; PEF, pefloxacin.

Table 157 In vitro comparative activities of ciprofloxacin and gatifloxacin against rapidly growing mycobacteria

Mycobacterium species	*n*	MIC (μg/ml)			
		Ciprofloxacin		Gatifloxacin	
		50%	90%	50%	90%
M. abscessus	20	16	16	16	
M. chelonae	27	4	>16	1.0	
M. fortuitum group	26	0.25	1.0	≤0.12	≤0.12
M. immunogenum	1	8[a]		8[a]	
M. smegmatis	1	0.5[a]		≤0.12[a]	
M. wolinskyi	1	0.5[a]		≤0.12[a]	
M. goodii	1	≤0.12[a]		≤0.12[a]	

[a]MIC, in micrograms per milliliter.

(500 mg every 8 h for 3 days) and cefazolin (2.0 g every 8 h for 3 days). The results showed preventive activity in 31 patients out of 34 treated with ciprofloxacin and 31 out of 36 treated with cefazolin. A comparative study of pefloxacin and cefuroxime yielded identical results. Failures are due principally to superinfections with *Candida albicans* or enterococci.

Administration of an antibacterial agent in cardiac surgery may reduce the incidence of postsurgical infections. This prevention must be directed against *S. aureus* and gram-negative bacilli. Penetration of the fluoroquinolones into the different cardiac tissues is high. There are few studies: Auger et al. compared the activity of pefloxacin (400 mg intravenously every 12 h before surgery) and cefazolin (1.0 g every 6 h for 2 days) in a randomized study involving 110 patients. The results showed colonization in 14 patients receiving pefloxacin and 11 patients receiving cefazolin; one patient receiving cefazolin developed mediastinitis due to a cefazolin-resistant strain of *S. epidermidis*. The results for the two medicinal products were comparable.

In the prevention of postsurgical infections in urology, the antibacterial agents must be eliminated in the urine and be active against *Enterobacteriaceae* and enterococci, the bacterial agents most commonly found in such infections. Use in transurethral surgery remains a matter of dispute. Several randomized studies show the value of ciprofloxacin, enoxacins, or norfloxacin versus placebo or co-trimoxazole.

12.13. Hepatobiliary Infections

The majority of fluoroquinolones are eliminated to only a limited extent in the bile, but at sufficient concentrations to allow their use in hepatobiliary infections. Few specific studies have been carried out. The majority of hepatobiliary infections that have been treated were so in conjunction with the treatment of various severe infections. Administration of ofloxacin for 4 to 7 days cured 23 patients with biliary tract infections due to *Enterobacteriaceae* and *P. aeruginosa*. Several teams have shown that the administration of ciprofloxacin yields good results in cholecystitis (~100% success) and to a lesser extent in cholangitis (~85% success). The same results have been found with other fluoroquinolones. A comparative study of the combination pefloxacin-metronidazole versus ampicillin-gentamicin in 59 patients with biliary tract infections revealed equivalent therapeutic activities.

12.14. Infections in Neutropenic Patients

Infection is one of the major problems in severe neutropenia induced by anticancer chemotherapy and one of the main causes of death in affected patients. The incidence of deaths may be as high as 55 to 75% of infected patients. In the absence of preventive measures, 50 to 90% of these patients will develop an infection during this phase. Although rigorous hygiene measures have significantly reduced mortality, they have still not abolished infectious morbidity. The endogenous flora is responsible for the majority of infections occurring in these patients. Ciprofloxacin, norfloxacin, and ofloxacin have been administered from the beginning of chemotherapy until the end of the neutropenic period. The results are difficult to interpret, but a reduction in the incidence of infections due to gram-negative bacilli has been reported by some authors. In one study, 3% of patients receiving a fluoroquinolone developed an infection, as opposed to 19% among patients receiving another antibacterial cover (co-trimoxazole). The failures were due to carriage or an infection of the upper airways, principally by gram-positive cocci, or to fungal superinfections (Table 158).

Infections occurring in neutropenic and immunodepressed patients must be treated with a bactericidal antibacterial agent. Usually the pathogenic agent is unknown, hence the need to use broad-spectrum, bactericidal agents. During long-term treatments, the possibility of switching from a parenteral formulation to an oral form is a useful attribute. These infections are often due to *S. aureus* and *P. aeruginosa*, and a combination of antibiotics is essential. Smith et al. reported good efficacy in 64% of febrile neutropenic patients with ciprofloxacin alone; however, better results were obtained with the combination of ciprofloxacin and vancomycin (77% good results). Daniels-Bosman et al. treated 32 febrile episodes in 20 neutropenic patients with a mean age of 57 years with pefloxacin, administered intravenously at a dosage of 400 mg every 8 h for 9 days. The results were satisfactory in 72% of cases.

A meta-analysis of the efficacy of fluoroquinolones (ofloxacin, ciprofloxacin, norfloxacin, and enoxacin) versus co-trimoxazole or placebo in the prevention of infections in 1,408 neutropenic patients was performed on 18 studies. This meta-analysis demonstrated the superiority of the fluoroquinolones over co-trimoxazole or placebo in terms of the relative risk of infections due to gram-negative bacilli and the occurrence of fever. Norfloxacin had activity significantly inferior to that of ofloxacin and ciprofloxacin. They significantly reduced the incidence of infections and septicemic states due to gram-negative bacilli, the incidence of infections in general, and the occurrence of fever. However, mortality during infections was not significantly modified. None of the studies showed any advantage in terms of the

Table 158 Efficacies of fluoroquinolones in the prevention of infections in neutropenic patients

Drug(s)	No. of patients	No. of infections	No. of documented infections	No. of pathogens			
				Gram negative	Gram positive	Anaerobes	Fungi
Ciprofloxacin	15	9	5	0	4	1	0
Ciprofloxacin	28	18	5	0	4	1	0
Co-trimoxazole + colistin	28	21	14	7	7	0	0
Norfloxacin	36		17	13	13	0	4
Vancomycin + polymyxin	30		18	6	6	0	6
Norfloxacin	35	35		4	16	1	10
Placebo	33	33		13	13	0	8
Norfloxacin	31		9	0	9	0	0
Co-trimoxazole	32		8	4	2	0	3
Norfloxacin ± vancomycin	48	27	7	1	6	0	0
Vancomycin + polymyxin + neomycin	48	31	7	2	5	0	0

occurrence of infections due to gram-positive cocci or fungal agents. The mean duration of the neutropenic state was 7 to 32 days. With the fluoroquinolones, the incidence of infections was the same irrespective of the duration of the neutropenia. The relative risk of emergence of resistant bacteria is difficult to define because of the absence of a sufficient number of placebo-controlled studies that consider this parameter. The incidence of emergence of resistant strains of gram-negative bacilli or gram-positive cocci is 3 or 9.4%, respectively. The emergence of gram-positive bacteria in the course of neutropenic states requires a study of the activity of the new fluoroquinolones that provide better cover against these pathogenic agents.

The fluoroquinolones are important products in the therapeutic arsenal for the prevention of infections in this type of patient and also in the treatment of infections, as these molecules have a broad antibacterial spectrum, are bactericidal, and attain high tissue concentrations. Another important parameter is the possibility of oral and parenteral administration.

12.15. Postsurgical Infections

The use of antibacterial agents in the treatment of postsurgical infections has contributed substantially to improving the prognosis. Postoperative wound infections remain a major cause of morbidity in surgical departments. In American hospitals these occur in about 5% of patients. A number of factors play a part in the patient's resistance to developing an infection: age, nutritional status, underlying diseases, etc.

The microorganisms most often isolated are *Enterobacteriaceae*, staphylococci, and *P. aeruginosa*. The in situ concentrations of the fluoroquinolones are greater than the MICs for the main pathogenic agents responsible for these superinfections.

Postsurgical intra-abdominal infections are a major cause of mortality, in some studies attaining 50%. Treatment of these infections is based principally on good surgical drainage, elimination of the source of infection, and well-managed antibiotic therapy. The fluoroquinolones might be a therapeutic alternative, but there are few studies in this area.

In the few studies undertaken with pefloxacin and ciprofloxacin, these products were combined with metronidazole or clindamycin.

12.16. Pediatric Patients

The use of fluoroquinolones in children remains a subject of dispute because of the cartilaginous lesions observed in young animals. A review on the risk for pediatric patients has been conducted recently (Gendrel et al., 2003).

12.16.1. Cartilage Problems

The quinolones cause abnormalities of the cartilage of weight-bearing bones. Abnormalities have been detected in all laboratory animals: mice, rats, dogs, marmosets, guinea pigs, rabbits, and ferrets. These abnormalities are only found in immature animals, except in the case of pefloxacin, when they can be induced in mature dogs. Young dogs are the animals most susceptible to articular disorders among the animal species tested.

Inflammation of the synovial membranes is inconsistent and dependent on the molecule.

In the dog, rabbit, and rat, the lesions are not totally reversible.

In the young dog, the cartilaginous changes are localized in the epiphysial cartilage complex.

The initial modifications involve vacuolization and mitochondrial dilatation in the chondrocytes. Fissures are then formed in the extracellular matrix, with the loss of collagen and glucosaminoglycans. In the rat, magnesium deficiency produces similar lesions.

The mechanism would appear to be chelation of the magnesium ions, which modify the functions of the chondrocyte integrin receptors. The transduction signal through the integrins appears to play a role in maintaining the integrity of the cartilaginous matrix.

12.16.2. Clinical Indications

The fluoroquinolones are contraindicated in children until the completion of bone growth. The use of fluoroquinolones in infants is contraindicated because of the risk of metabolic acidosis; this risk appears to be greater with fluoroquinolones with a hepatic metabolism, such as pefloxacin or ciprofloxacin, because of the hepatic immaturity. The two other risks are adverse effects on the central nervous system and arthralgia. In two retrospective studies it was shown that administration of nalidixic acid to children had not caused arthropathy. Schaad et al. (1995) failed to show any abnormalities by nuclear magnetic resonance in 18 children, 13 of whom were prepubertal, after 3 months of treatment with ciprofloxacin. For two patients, histological examinations of the knee showed no lesions after prolonged treatment with ciprofloxacin. The fluoroquinolones were administered to children suffering from cystic fibrosis or severe life-threatening infections.

It should be pointed out that they are used in some countries in the treatment of infectious diarrhea requiring antibiotic therapy.

The indications might be cystic fibrosis, chronic ENT infections such as chronic otitis due to *P. aeruginosa*, osteomyelitis due to microorganisms resistant to other antibacterial agents, the prevention of infections in children in the neutropenic period, certain complicated urinary tract infections, meningitis due to *Enterobacteriaceae* and superinfections resulting from their spread to the central nervous system, life-threatening infections due to multiresistant bacteria, the treatment of salmonellosis (including typhoid and paratyphoid fever), and multiresistant *Shigella* infections.

Dagan et al. treated children aged 4 months to 7 years suffering from severe infections, meningitis, or generalized infections due to *Acinetobacter* or *P. aeruginosa* with pefloxacin (200 mg/kg every 12 h) or ciprofloxacin.

Ciprofloxacin was administered orally (20 mg/kg) or intravenously (3.2 to 11.5 mg/kg) to 634 children. The infections treated were for the most part respiratory tract infections. In this population, 122 adverse effects were noted for 80 children (12.6%). In most cases the disorders were gastrointestinal (31%), cutaneous (21%), and central nervous system (14%—hallucinations, anxiety, migraine, dizziness, etc.), but also arthralgia in 10 small girls (1.6%), which resolved.

Three hundred seventeen patients aged over 5 years but under 15 years were treated with norfloxacin at a daily dose of 8 to 12 mg/kg for respiratory tract and intestinal infections; the incidence of adverse effects was 1.5%.

Schaad's recommendations in 1993 are summarized in Table 159.

12.16.3. Pharmacokinetics

Peltola et al. studied the pharmacokinetic profile of ciprofloxacin in six children aged 13 months to 5 years. The children received a single dose of 15 mg of ciprofloxacin per kg. The peak concentration in serum was between 0.5 and 5.3 μg/ml and was reached between 0.5 and 1.5 h after drug administration. The mean apparent elimination half-life was 1.42 ± 0.44 h. The concentration in plasma at 6 h in three children was 0.25 μg/ml. The apparent volume of distribution was between 5.5 and 7.9 liters/kg.

Peltola et al. studied the pharmacokinetics of ciprofloxacin in children carrying *Salmonella* after administration of 15 mg/kg orally. In infants, the apparent elimination half-life was prolonged and the AUC was greater (Table 160).

Fujii et al. studied the pharmacokinetics of norfloxacin in children; results are shown in Table 161.

The use of ciprofloxacin, ofloxacin, norfloxacin, and nalidixic acid in children has been reported in more than 30 publications. More than 7,000 children have been treated, and no articular abnormality has been detected. None of these drugs has had an adverse effect on the children's growth.

Two studies were conducted with premature patients. In one study, ciprofloxacin (10 mg/kg every 12 h) was administered to six premature infants. The mean peak concentration in serum was 0.31 μg/ml. There was 60 to 70% penetration of the CSF.

In another study, two children were treated with ciprofloxacin and five were treated with pefloxacin. Monitoring up to the age of 30 to 42 months (for a 6-month period) failed to reveal any joint or growth abnormalities.

In two studies, one including 406 children (aged 2 to 11 years) and the other (conducted in China) including 433 children with diarrhea administered norfloxacin, no adverse effect was noted.

One exception to these studies was pefloxacin administered to 63 children suffering from cystic fibrosis, among whom 9 developed synovial effusion in the knees, reversible on discontinuation of treatment. Another study conducted by Reinert demonstrated the same phenomenon in 5 of 50 patients receiving pefloxacin. Treatment with ofloxacin was well tolerated.

Table 160 Pharmacokinetics of ciprofloxacin in pediatric subjects

Subjects	Age	$t_{1/2}$ (h)	$AUC_{0-\infty}$ (μg·h/ml)	MRT[a] (h)
Neonates	5–14 wk	2.73	16	4.6
Infants	1–5 yr	1.28	5.31	2.4

[a]MRT, mean response time.

Table 159 Recommended treatment duration according to Schaad

Infection[a]	Underlying disease or feature	Pathogens	Proposed treatment duration
Parenchymal RTI	Cystic fibrosis	*P. aeruginosa*, *S. aureus*	2–8 wk
Complicated UTI	Urinary tract abnormalities	*P. aeruginosa*, *S. aureus*	2–3 wk
Otitis media	>6 wk	*P. aeruginosa*, *S. aureus*	2–4 wk
Shigellosis	Countries under development	*Shigella* spp.	5–7 days
Invasive salmonellosis		*Salmonella* spp.	
Fever prophylaxis	Neutropenia	Miscellaneous	?
Meningitis prophylaxis	ENT carrier	*N. meningitidis*, *H. influenzae* type b	2 days
Osteomyelitis	Subacute and localized forms	*P. aeruginosa*, *S. aureus*	3–12 wk

[a]RTI, respiratory tract infection; UTI, urinary tract infection.

Table 161 Pharmacokinetics of norfloxacin in children

Dose (mg/kg)	n	C_{max} (μg/ml)	T_{max} (h)	AUC (μg·h/ml)	$t_{1/2}$ (h)	Urinary elimination (%)
1.0–2.9	35	0.37	1.8	1.76	2.5	25.3
3.0–4.9	26	0.56	2.1	2.52	2.6	25.3
5.0–6.9	15	0.92	2.0	4.17	2.6	27.1

However, these results must be interpreted with caution because of the spontaneous features of cystic fibrosis.

The pharmacokinetics of alatrofloxacin were determined in 14 children and 6 infants at a dose of 4 mg/kg by infusion for 60 min (Table 162).

After a 7-mg/kg single intravenous dose of levofloxacin, the pharmacokinetics were determined; results are shown in Table 163.

For gatifloxacin, it was shown that exposure of children following a 10-mg/kg dose intravenously is comparable to the exposure in adults following a 400-mg oral tablet (Table 164).

12.17. Parasitic Infections

The emergence and spread of drug resistance to chloroquine in *P. falciparum* and *Plasmodium vivax* have produced a resurgence of interest in the antibacterial agents. Norfloxacin yielded the eradication of *P. falciparum* in semi-immune subjects in India. However, various publications have reported only weak activity for pefloxacin and ciprofloxacin in nonmalarial subjects. The currently available fluoroquinolones are not treatments for acute forms of malaria, but they may abolish a pauciparasitic form if administered simultaneously for another disease. Norfloxacin was tested against chloroquine-resistant strains of

Table 162 Pharmacokinetics of alatrofloxacin in pediatric subjects

Subjects	n	Age (yrs)	$t_{1/2}$ (h)	CL_P (liters/h/kg)	C (μg/ml)	$AUC_{0-\infty}$ (μg·h/ml)
Infants	14	7.2	9.42	0.14	4.1	34.3
Neonates	6	0.59	8.25	0.16	4.6	28.8

Table 163 Pharmacokinetics of levofloxacin in pediatric subjects

Group (age, yr[a])	n	C_{max} (μg/ml)	$AUC_{0-\infty}$ (μg·h/ml)	$t_{1/2}$ (h)	CL_P (liters/h/kg)	CL_R (liters/h/kg)
0.5–2	6	5.19	21.5	4.1	0.35	NA[b]
2–5	7	6.02	2.7	4.0	0.32	NA
5–10	9	6.11	29.2	4.8	0.25	0.18
10–12	7	6.12	39.8	5.4	0.19	0.15
12–16	11	6.15	40.5	6.0	0.18	0.11
Adults (500 mg)	23	6.18	48.3	6.0	0.15	NA

[a]Children up to 16 years of age were given 7 mg/kg.
[b]NA, not available.

Table 164 Pharmacokinetics of intravenous gatifloxacin in children

Dose (mg/kg)[a]	Age	n	C_{max} (μg/ml)	AUC (μg·h/ml)	$t_{1/2}$ (h)
2–5	3 mo–2 yr	6	2.9	9.9	4.9
	2–12 yr	6	1.6	6.4	4.4
	12–16 yr	6	2.7	9.9	5.6
5	3 mo–2 yr	3	3.2	14.9	4.4
	2–12 yr	5	2.9	12.9	4.1
7.5	2–12 yr	6	5.5	21.2	3.9
10	2–12 yr	3	8.2	34.9	4.4
12.5	2–12 yr	3	13.2	43.6	4.3
400-mg tablet	Adults	30	5.5	35.1	7.4
5, oral	0.5–2 yr	22	2.1	14.4	4.8
10	2–6 yr	31	4.1	36	5.4
10	6–12 yr	14	5.4	44.7	7.0
15	12–16 yr	23	5.4	48.7	4.9

[a]Doses are intravenous unless otherwise noted.

P. vivax and exhibited weak activity. The fluoroquinolones have shown no activity against *T. gondii*. Pefloxacin has interesting activity in the treatment of experimental pneumocystosis in the rat, but the other quinolones tested appear to be less active.

13. SAFETY

The currently available fluoroquinolones are relatively well tolerated. The frequency of adverse effects does not appear to be greater than that observed with other classes of antibacterial agents (1 to 20%). In clinical trials, the incidence is on the order of 4 to 8%. The adverse effects of the quinolones were first described with nalidixic acid and oxolinic acid, the latter being held responsible for insomnia. The principal incidents are of a digestive, neurologic, metabolic, neuropsychiatric, phototoxic, and cardiologic nature.

The fluoroquinolones share the same adverse effects, but they vary in degree according to the molecule.

13.1. Adverse Effects Noted During Preregistration Clinical Studies

The side effects may be divided into digestive disorders (3.2 to 11.4%), skin disorders (0.6 to 5.1%), neuropsychiatric disorders (0.9 to >20%), musculoarticular disorders (0.9%), and miscellaneous phenomena, such as bitterness (~1%) (Table 165).

During this phase a number of side effects were not detected, such as torsade de pointes (sparfloxacin), hematologic disorders, metabolic disorders (such as severe hypoglycemia [temafloxacin]), or hepatic disorders (trovafloxacin).

13.1.1. Skin Disorders

Although conventional adverse effects, such as pruritus, skin rash, and urticaria, have been reported with all fluoroquinolones, the incidence remains small (<1%). The major problem is phototoxicity, which has been detected with lomefloxacin, pefloxacin (1.3%), fleroxacin (0.6%), and sparfloxacin (2%). One molecule currently under development, clinafloxacin, also exhibits this property. However, these effects have not been detected with the other products of this class. A few cases of phototoxicity have been reported retrospectively with enoxacin.

13.1.2. Effects on the Central Nervous System

The most common effects are insomnia (0.1 to 1.3%), which has been described and studied with oxolinic acid, and headache (~0.3%). The most disruptive is dizziness, which is uncommon with the majority of quinolones (0.1 to 2%) but which rises to 18% (200 mg orally) or more with trovafloxacin, depending on the dose.

13.1.3. Phototoxicity

Phototoxicity reactions were first described with nalidixic acid by Brauner. They appear to be more frequent in women, affecting the dorsal aspect of the hands, feet, and legs but sparing the face. The minimum clinical signs are erythema, possibly followed by pigmentation that may progress to a second- or even third-degree burn. Some cases of onycholysis have been reported.

13.1.3.1. Mechanism of Phototoxicity

The mechanism of phototoxicity is complex and remains incompletely elucidated.

The skin is composed of several cell types. A number of factors may contribute to cutaneous toxicity, particularly the distribution of fluoroquinolones in the skin. The accumulation of sparfloxacin in rat skin is greater than for the majority of fluoroquinolones, with a long apparent elimination half-life; the same phenomenon has been described with lomefloxacin.

Other properties of the fluoroquinolones play a part, such as their stability to light or the duration of the triplet excitation stage. Following exposure to light, fluoroquinolones produce $^1O_2$ and O_2^-. The OH° radicals are also responsible for these lesions. The reactive species of oxygen such as $^1O_2$ damage DNA.

Phototoxicity is induced by exposure to UV-A at a wavelength of 320 nm.

The phototoxicity is dependent on the dose of fluoroquinolone administered.

13.1.3.2. Structure-Activity Relationship

A certain number of structure-activity studies have shown that the nature of the substituents at position 8 of the quinoline nucleus is responsible for the occurrence of phototoxicity. Molecules with a halogen (F, Cl, or Br) at C-8, particularly a fluorine, have a greater phototoxic potential than the other molecules. Domagala et al. proposed the following hierarchy among the substituents at C-8: CF ≥ C-Cl > N > CH > CF_3 > C-OR (particularly OCH_3). Marutani et al. (1993) clearly showed the effect of the substituent at C-8 using balofloxacin, which possesses an OCH_3 at C-8, and nonsubstituted or fluorine-substituted derivatives as a model. The fluorine compound is responsible for an inflammatory phenomenon in mice exposed to UV-A (5.6 m W/cm²) at the low dose of 12.5 mg/kg; the same result was obtained with the nonsubstituted derivative but at a high dose (200 mg/kg). No inflammatory effect was noted when the substituent was a methoxy, even at a dose of 800 mg/kg (Fig. 90).

13.1.3.3. Photodegradation

The quinolones require a metabolic or physicochemical transformation before becoming photoactive.

Table 165 Adverse effects recorded during phase II and III clinical trials[a]

Parameter	NOR	CIP	PEF	FLE	OFX	ENX	SPX	LVX	TVA	GRX
Patient no.	1,540	1,690	781	4,234	4,785	2,530	1,040	3,292	875	1,069
Gastrointestinal (%)	1.08	5	4.2	11	3.2	3.8	11.4	5.1	11	11
Skin (%)	0.6	1.4	2.4	3	0.7	0.6	5.1	1.1	<1	<1
CNS[b] (%)	1.4	1.6	1.1	9	0.9	1.2	4.2	1.7	20	1
Bone and joints (%)			0.9					0.3		
Others (%)	0.2			1				<1		

[a]NOR, nonfloxacin; CIP, ciprofloxacin; PEF, perfloxacin; FLE, fleroxacin; OFX, ofloxacin; ENX, enoxacin; SPX, sparfloxacin; LVX, levofloxacin; TVA, trovafloxacin; GRX, grepafloxacin.

[b]CNS, central nervous system.

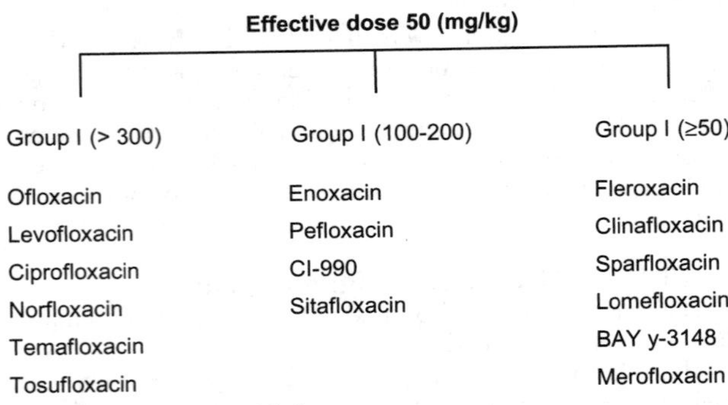

Figure 90 Phototoxicity

When a quinolone is exposed to UV-A, it may do one of the following:

- Not be degraded
- Decompose slowly
- Be transformed into a photoactive molecule

13.1.3.4. Exploratory Mode of Phototoxicity

The preventive exploration of phototoxicity may be done by in vitro and in vivo studies during the preclinical development phase of the molecule.

One of the best predictive tests is that described by Wagai et al. (1990). This allows the potential phototoxicity of a molecule to be predicted by using the exposure to UV-A (21.6 J/cm^2) of a group of BALB/c mice given different doses of quinolones as an experimental model. The ears of the mice are examined 0, 24, and 48 h after exposure. A phototoxic reaction is characterized clinically by an edematous and inflammatory reaction. It is manifested histologically in inflammatory edema (neutrophils) localized in the connective tissue surrounding the cartilage. Three groups of quinolones may be described on the basis of the 50% dose causing lesions in the mouse (Fig. 91).

In group 1, in which the ED_{50} is greater than 300 mg/kg, the potential risk of phototoxicity is rare and has been confirmed by the prescription of certain fluoroquinolones, such as ofloxacin and ciprofloxacin, to millions of patients. Conversely, the greatest risk of phototoxicity exists in group 3, in which the ED_{50} is $\leq$50 mg/kg, as has been demonstrated with sparfloxacin, lomefloxacin, and clinafloxacin. The interpretation of the phototoxic potential of the molecules belonging to group 2, in which the ED_{50} is between 100 and 200 mg/kg, is more complex. This is the case with enoxacin and pefloxacin, for which some cases of phototoxicity have been reported.

Another in vivo method involves the use of guinea pigs. The quinolones are administered in a single dose to guinea pigs, which are then exposed to UV-A (30 J/cm^2). The results are inconsistent with the clinical tolerance, and it is a poor predictive model.

Studies have been carried out with healthy volunteers with type 1 or 2 skin (sensitive to UV-A) according to Fitzpatrick's classification (1988). The phototoxic potential is simulated in terms of day and night.

13.1.3.5. Phototoxic Potential of Quinolones

Nalidixic acid, sparfloxacin, lomefloxacin, and clinafloxacin have a strong phototoxic potential. Other compounds, such as pefloxacin, enoxacin, and fleroxacin, exhibit a weaker potential.

Postmarketing drug surveillance in France has shown that the occurrence of a phototoxic phenomenon varies with the different quinolones commercially available (Table 166).

Sparfloxacin is associated with signs of severe phototoxicity, accompanied by second-degree (15.6%) and even third-degree burns (necessitating hospitalization in 8.6% of patients with sequelae).

The phototoxicity is dose dependent. In a double-blind study with fleroxacin in patients treated for *C. trachomatis* urethritis, photointolerance was reported in 0, 11, and 19% of patients taking 400, 600, and 800 mg of fleroxacin, respectively.

F, COOH, O, N, N, 8, X, CH_3

X	Dose (mg/kg)	Number of irradiated mice	Time after irradiation 0.5	24	48	72	Inflammation incidence
8-OCH$_3$	200	6	0	0	0	0	0/6
	800	6	0	0	0	0	0/6
8-F	3.1	6	0	0	0	0	0/6
	12.5	6	3	3	0	0	3/6
	50.0	6	6	6	6	6	6/6
8-H	50	6	0	0	0	0	0/6
	200	6	6	6	6	4	6/6
	800	6	6	6	6	6	6/6

from Maratuni

Figure 91 Phototoxic potential of fluoroquinolones (murine model)

Table 166 Incidence of phototoxicity in patients of fluoroquinolones

Compound	No./total cases
Sparfloxacin	1/4,000
Pefloxacin	1/18,200
Ciprofloxacin	1/387,000
Norfloxacin	1/403,000
Ofloxacin	1/1,640,000

13.1.3.6. Photocarcinogenicity and Photomutagenicity

A photocarcinogenicity study of certain fluoroquinolones was undertaken with SKH-1 mice (hairless albino mice). The reference molecule was 8-methoxypsoralen. Treatment was given for 78 weeks. After each drug administration, the animals were exposed for 1.5 h to a dose of 25 J of UV-A per cm^2. Tumor development varied with the molecule (Table 167).

The nature and number of tumors also differed with the molecule.

In this study, lomefloxacin caused 29 carcinomatous tumors, compared with 12 with 8-methoxypsoralen (positive control) and 1 with fleroxacin. In the case of ofloxacin, ciprofloxacin, and nalidixic acid, the tumors were benign and of the kind found after prolonged exposure to UV-A.

13.2. Adverse Effects on the Central Nervous System

The second type of adverse effect following administration of quinolones is neurologic or psychiatric. The incidence is between 0.4 and 4.0%, with a mean of 1.0%. Severe reactions of the type of hallucinations, mania, psychosis, depression, convulsions, and nightmares have been reported for ≤0.5% of patients. These effects on the central nervous system may be divided into two groups: mental disorders and neurologic disorders (Table 168).

Convulsions are rare and appear to affect elderly or epileptic patients, subjects with head injuries or who are alcoholic or suffering from a cerebrovascular disease, drug addicts, and patients with renal insufficiency. The route of administration is important. Convulsive episodes have been reported with nalidixic acid, norfloxacin, enoxacin, and ciprofloxacin. Studies with DBA/2 mice (strains genetically susceptible to noise-induced seizures) have enabled the convulsant activity of the fluoroquinolones to be determined.

A review of the literature has revealed a correlation between the incidence of side effects on the central nervous system and the number of prescriptions of a given fluoroquinolone (Table 169).

The effect of the fluoroquinolones would appear to result from a dose-dependent interaction with GABA.

Table 167 Photocarcinogenicity of quinolones

Compound	t_{50} (% wks)
8-Methoxypsoralen	4
Lomefloxacin	16
Fleroxacin	38
Ofloxacin	>50
Ciprofloxacin	>50
Nalidixic acid	>50

Table 168 Neuropsychiatric disorders due to quinolones

Psychiatric troubles
- Delirium
- Psychosis
- Mania, schizophrenia, paranoia
- Depression
- Anxiety
- Insomnia, nightmares

Neurologic troubles
- Seizures
- Ataxia
- Paresthesia
- Dizziness
- Headache
- Tremor

Table 169 Occurrence of adverse effects on the central nervous system with fluoroquinolones

Compound	Incidence of adverse effects (%)
Fleroxacin	1.86
Enoxacin	0.99
Lomefloxacin	0.86
Sparfloxacin	0.61
Ofloxacin	0.56
Ciprofloxacin	0.43
Tosufloxacin	0.43
Norfloxacin	0.22

Combination with certain nonsteroidal anti-inflammatory drugs increases the inhibition of the GABA receptor by the fluoroquinolones and is the source of a convulsive syndrome, particularly with the combination of fenbufen and enoxacin. The affinity for GABA varies with the molecule (Table 170).

The convulsant activity of the fluoroquinolones has been attributed to inhibition of the binding of GABA to its receptor site. However, other authors have assumed that the dopaminergic, glutaminergic, or opioid receptors are involved in the effects of the fluoroquinolones on the central nervous system. It seems therefore that inhibition of the GABA system is necessary but not sufficient and that binding to a specific ligand does not fully explain the complex mechanism that causes excitation of the central nervous system by the quinolones. Quinolones with the 8-methoxy group have stronger convulsant activity, but no interaction with anti-inflammatory drugs has been noted. It has been hypothesized that fluoroquinolone

Table 170 Concentrations of fluoroquinolones required to inhibit binding to the GABA receptor by 50%

Compound	IC_{50} (M, 10^{-5})
Enoxacin	1.4
Norfloxacin	0.14
Ofloxacin	0.01
Ciprofloxacin	7.6
Fleroxacin	0.76
Tosufloxacin	0.57
Sparfloxacin	0.91

derivatives with an 8-methoxy group and a free piperazinyl moiety might have stronger convulsant activity.

In order to analyze the excitatory potential of the fluoroquinolones better, an in vitro model of analysis of the electrical waves in the C_{A1} region of the rat hippocampus was used. This model provides a classification of the fluoroquinolones. There is a good correlation between the preclinical and the clinical data.

The majority of fluoroquinolones have a relatively low, dose-dependent excitatory effect. Trovafloxacin, clinafloxacin and enoxacin have the greatest excitatory potential (Table 171).

These results suggest that trovafloxacin and clinafloxacin have potentially high convulsant activity.

13.3. Rheumatological Adverse Effects

Lesions of articular cartilage are observed when the fluoroquinolones are administered to young animals (dogs, rats, and rabbits), whereas connecting cartilage is unaffected. Mice are insensitive to the action of fluoroquinolones. All of the quinolones accumulate in cartilage and are eliminated slowly. The lesions appear to be dose independent; they are not inflammatory in nature and are reversible.

The incidence of toxicity to the cartilage varies with the publications. Table 172 shows the incidence of toxicity, to the cartilage when 100 to 500 mg of a fluoroquinolones per kg is administered to juvenile rats.

Other adverse effects such as vasculitis, hypercalcemia, and hyperuricemia are exceptional.

13.4. Tendinopathies

Myalgia (predominantly in the morning), arthralgia, and tendinitis, possibly accompanied by rupture of the Achilles tendon, have been described. They appear to be more common in male subjects over 60 years of age.

Tendinitis of the Achilles tendon may occur after short-term treatment (2 to 13 days). It may be unilateral or bilateral and may be accompanied in 20 to 30% of cases by rupture of the tendon. It takes 30 to 60 days for the clinical signs to regress.

The fluoroquinolones are involved to various degrees in this phenomenon. In a retrospective study conducted in France over the period between 1985 and 1992, 75% of cases of tendinitis were due to administration of pefloxacin. However, although it is a serious event, the frequency should not be exaggerated. The pathogenesis is poorly elucidated, and predictive models are not truly validated.

An in vitro predictive model using rabbit tenocytes isolated from the Achilles tendon has been proposed. Using this model, Rat et al. (1998) showed that pefloxacin and norfloxacin were markedly cytotoxic but ofloxacin and nalidixic acid were only weakly so.

There are numerous reports in the literature about an association between the use of fluoroquinolones and oral corticosteroids and possible increased incidence of tendon injuries. In some reviews (Khaliq and Zhanel, 2003), it was suggested that males (~59 years old) are more likely to experience tendon injuries. However, young women (28 to 29 years old) may be affected.

The predominance of Achilles tendon injuries was noted. The drugs most commonly implicated were pefloxacin and ciprofloxacin. In a retrospective study in France the incidences of drug-related injuries among 421 cases were as follows: pefloxacin, 68%; ofloxacin, 18%; norfloxacin, 8%; and ciprofloxacin, 5%. This reflects the local habits of prescription. The mean age of patients was 62 years, the mean duration of treatment was 13 days, the mean onset was 9.3 days, and patient recovery was 15 to 30 days.

In the Netherlands, of 1,841 patients, 7 had a history of tendinopathies due to fluoroquinolones; the calculated incidence was 7.74 cases per 10^5 days. In comparison, for other antibacterials the incidence was 3.27 cases per 10^5 days. In Switzerland from 1986 to 1999, the Swiss Drug Monitoring Center received a total of 460 reports of adverse events for fluoroquinolones. Tendinopathies were reported in 19 of the 460 (4.1%).

13.5. Hematologic Disorders

Nalidixic acid can cause thrombocytopenia. Identical disorders have been described with norfloxacin and pefloxacin. Leukopenia has been reported with nalidixic acid, ciprofloxacin, and norfloxacin. An episode of hemolytic anemia has been described with nalidixic acid. A few cases of hemolytic anemia have been noted for patients with glyceraldehyde-6-phosphate dehydrogenase deficiency taking quinolones.

Dose-dependent thrombocytopenia has been described with pefloxacin.

13.6. Metabolic Disorders

A case of lactic acidosis has been reported for a 16-year-old patient with hepatic insufficiency taking 2 g of nalidixic acid every 12 h.

In 1991 attention was drawn to the induction of severe hypoglycemia following administration of enoxacin. Severe hypoglycemia has been described with other fluoroquinolones, such as temafloxacin, lomefloxacin, and sparfloxacin. Studies of insulin release in the rat have given rise to the hypothesis that the increase in circulating insulin levels is

Table 171 Increase in wave amplitude: excitatory potential of fluoroquinolones on the central nervous system

Compound	Concn used (μmol)	% Waves
Ciprofloxacin	0.25	39.2 ± 3.0
	2.0	155 ± 12.1
Enoxacin	0.25	76.2 ± 49
	2.0	192 ± 13.8
Norfloxacin	0.25	52.6 ± 4.4
Ofloxacin	0.25	52.7 ± 3.6
Pefloxacin	0.25	60.4 ± 4.5
Clinafloxacin	2.0	233 ± 12.6
Trovafloxacin	2.0	27 ± 9.0
Moxifloxacin	2.0	170 ± 4.7
Nalidixic acid	0.25	68.2 ± 3.9
	2.0	165 ± 1.7

Table 172 Incidence of cartilaginous toxicity in juvenile rats

Compound	Toxicity incidence (%)
Ciprofloxacin	0–5
Norfloxacin	25–45
Ofloxacin	0–5
Pefloxacin	0–5
Nalidixic acid	25–45

due to a blockade of ATPase-sensitive potassium channels. Sparfloxacin (1 mM glucose), lomefloxacin (3 mM glucose), and pipemidic acid (0.1 to 1 mM glucose) stimulate insulin release in the nonstimulated state, in contrast to enoxacin and tosufloxacin. In the stimulated state, all of the quinolones cause a dose-dependent release of insulin.

13.7. Renal Tolerance

There have been anecdotal reports of reversible renal insufficiency with norfloxacin and ciprofloxacin in patients over 65 years.

Crystalluria, with or without hematuria, has been noted with ciprofloxacin, tosufloxacin, and norfloxacin, but not with ofloxacin. Crystalluria is observed when the administered doses are high and the urine is alkaline. The poor solubility in water increases the probability of crystalluria.

13.8. Gastrointestinal Disorders

The incidence of gastrointestinal disorders is on the order of 3 to 7%. They are moderate and involve nausea, vomiting, epigastric burning, and abdominal cramping. There are rare reports of pseudomembranous colitis.

13.9. Ocular Toxicity

Pefloxacin and rosoxacin induce cataracts in animals. Ophthalmological surveillance of 800 patients treated with ciprofloxacin failed to reveal any ocular lesions.

13.10. Hepatic Toxicity

A case of fulminant hepatitis following administration of ciprofloxacin has been reported. Cytolysis and hepatic cholestasis have been described with trovafloxacin.

13.11. Cardiotoxicity

Following rapid intravenous administration of fluoroquinolones to dogs or cats, the majority are responsible for systolic or diastolic hypertension. These effects would appear to be due to a marked and dose-dependent release of histamine. When a fluoroquinolone has to be administered intravenously, it is recommended that it be given in the form of a slow infusion. Other adverse effects in the form of torsade de pointes have been reported, particularly with sparfloxacin. In beagles, sparfloxacin caused lengthening of the QT interval on the electrocardiogram following oral ingestion of a dosage of 45 mg/kg/day for 4 weeks. Grepafloxacin caused dose-dependent abnormalities of cardiac rhythm in anesthetized rabbits. This transient effect was observed in one of four rabbits at a dose of 10 mg/kg and in all rabbits at a dose of 30 mg/kg intravenously. In volunteers receiving the recommended dose of sparfloxacin (400 mg followed by 200 mg daily), a lengthening of the QT interval of ≥19 ms on the electrocardiogram was observed. Among 813 patients receiving sparfloxacin during phase III studies, 3% had a significant lengthening of the QT interval, and in 1.2% of cases the QT interval was greater than 500 ms (0.3% of patients with a prolongation of 100 ms compared to the normal value). This adverse effect is manifested in some patients in cardiac rhythm disorders accompanied by torsade de pointes.

This quinolone-induced abnormality may be studied during the development phase of a molecule using an in vitro model in rabbit Purkinje cells. One study has shown that, in contrast to sparfloxacin, levofloxacin and ofloxacin do not induce repolarization disorders in rabbit Purkinje cells.

Grepafloxacin and moxifloxacin have been associated with tachycardia in animals and humans.

13.12. Abnormal Laboratory Test Results

As with all antibacterial agents, treatments with fluoroquinolones may affect certain laboratory parameters, but the incidence of this is low (Table 173).

Results obtained with certain tests for the presence of opiate derivatives (codeine, morphine, hydrocodone, hydromorphone, oxycodone, oxymorphone, methadone, and meperidine) in urine may be affected by the concomitant administration of fluoroquinolones.

With the EMIT II opiate kit, ofloxacin (200 μg/ml) produces false-positive responses (apparent morphine level of >300 μg/ml), with a cross-reaction in 0.16% of cases. Ciprofloxacin and norfloxacin do not appear to produce false-positive responses with the EMIT II kit.

The risk of a cross-reaction with ofloxacin with the Abbott TDx kit is on the order of 0.03%. There are no data for the other kits, such as the Roche KIMS and CEDIA.

It is therefore advisable to inquire about potential treatments with fluoroquinolones in the event of a positive reponse for opiates and possibly to undertake a urinary assay for fluoroquinolones.

13.13. Effect on Fecal Flora

The fluoroquinolones substantially reduce the *Enterobacteriaceae* in the fecal flora and have a moderate effect on anaerobic flora, with the exception of trovafloxacin, and a variable effect on enterococci (Table 174).

Two studies have shown that administration of ciprofloxacin fosters intestinal colonization by yeasts, in con-

Table 173 Frequency of abnormal laboratory test results

Compound	Frequency of result (%)				
	Transaminase increase	Alkaline phosphatase	Creatinine	Leukopenia	Eosinophilia
Norfloxacin	2.6	0.3	0.1	0.1	0.5
Ofloxacin	2.2	0.07	0.5	0.7	2.2
Ciprofloxacin	4.3		0.2	0.2	2.1
Enoxacin	0.9		0.5	0.2	0.7
Lomefloxacin	1.8	0.4	0.4	0.2	0.5
Fleroxacin	0.6	0.1	0.7		0.3
Sparfloxacin	3.2	0.4	0.1	0.4	1.2
Levofloxacin	0.6	3.5	0		

Table 174 Effect of fluoroquinolones on fecal flora

Compound	*Enterobacteriaceae*	*Enterococcus*	Anaerobes	Yeasts
Ofloxacin	+++	++	(−)	(−)
Ciprofloxacin	+++	++	(−)	(+)
Pefloxacin	+++	+++	++	−
Lomefloxacin	+++	+	−	−
Fleroxacin	+++	+	−	−
Norfloxacin	+++	+	−	−
Enoxacin	+++	+	−	−
Levofloxacin	+++	+	(−)	(−)
Sparfloxacin	+++	++	ND[a]	ND

[a]ND, not determined.

Table 175 Toxicity of fluoroquinolones

Compound	Cardiotoxicity	Phototoxicity	CNS[a]	Metabolism
Levofloxacin	−	−	−	−
Trovafloxacin	−	−	+	−
Sparfloxacin	+	+	−	(+)
Gatifloxacin	(+)	−	−	−
Moxifloxacin	(+)	−	−	−
Grepafloxacin	(+)	−	−	−
Clinafloxacin	−	+	−	(+)
Garenoxacin	−	−	−	−

[a]CNS, central nervous system.

trast to ofloxacin and norfloxacin. Pefloxacin may occasion the selection of resistant strains of *B. fragilis* and a slight reduction in anaerobes. Pefloxacin and fleroxacin cause a reduction in *E. faecalis*, but not *E. faecium*.

13.14. Risks of Intolerance of Group III Quinolones

The risks of intolerance of group III quinolones are summarized in Table 175.

REFERENCES

Allemandi DA, Alovero FL, Manzo H, 1994, In vitro activity of new suphanilil fluoroquinolones against *Staphylococcus aureus*, J Antimicrob Chemother, 34, 261–265.

Alovero FL, Pan XS, Morris JE, Manzo H, Fisher LM, 2000, Engineering the specificity of antibacterial fluoroquinolones: benzenesulfonamide modifications at C-7 of ciprofloxacin change its primary target in *Streptococcus pneumoniae* from topoisomerase IV to gyrase, Antimicrob Agents Chemother, 44, 320–325.

Amano H, Hayashi N, Oshita Y, Nino Y, Yazaki A, 1997, WQ 2724 and WQ 2743, novel fluoroquinolones, in vitro and in vivo activities, pharmacokinetics and toxicity, 37th Intersci Conf Antimicrob Agents Chemother, abstract F-163, p 173.

Avila-Aguero M, Blumer J, Bradley J, Saez-Lorens X, O'Ryan M, Grasela D, Lacreta F, Swingle M, McCracken G, Jafri H, 2002, Single dose safety and pharmacokinetics of intravenous gatifloxacin in pediatric patients, 42nd Intersci Conf Antimicrob Agents Chemother, p 39.

Bachoual R, Tankovic J, Dubreuil L, Soussy CJ, 1999, Role of a gyrA mutation in fluoroquinolone resistance of Bacteroides fragilis, 39th Intersci Conf Antimicrob Agents Chemother, abstract 1385, p 122.

Baker KE, Wooton M, Rogers CA, 1999, Comparison of in-vitro pharmacodynamics of once and twice daily ciprofloxacin, J Antimicrob Chemother, 44, 661-667.

Blondeau JM, Borsos S, Drlica K, 1999, Mutation prevention concentration of moxifloxacin and levofloxacin against clinical isolates of S. pneumoniae and S. aureus, 39th Intersci Conf Antimicrob Agents Chemother, abstract 363, p 251.

Brown SD, Barry AL, Fuchs PC, 1999, In vitro antibacterial activity of a series of novel nonfluoroquinolones (NFQs) against bacterial pathogens, 39th Intersci Conf Antimicrob Agents Chemother, abstract 549, p 305.

Brun-Pascaud M, Fay M, Zhong M, Guyot A, Pocidalo JJ, 1990, 30th Intersci Conf Antimicrob Agents Chemother, abstract 862.

Bryskier A, 1997, Novelties in the field of fluoroquinolones, Exp Opin Investing Drugs, 6, 1227–1245.

Bryskier A, 2002, Bacillus anthracis and antibacterial agents, Clin Microb Infect, 8, 467–478.

Bryskier A, Labro MT, 1990, Quinolones and malaria, an avenue for the future, Quinolones Bull, 6, 1.

Chien S, Abels R, Blumer J, Chow A, Goldstein H, Kearns G, Maldonado S, Noel G, Well T, Spielberg S, 2002, Single dose pharmacokinetics and tolerability of levofloxacin in pediatric patients, 42nd Intersci Conf Antimicrob Agents Chemother.

Christopher LJ, Dyksta CC, 1994, Identification of a type II topoisomerase gene from Cryptosporidium parvum, J Eukaryot Microbiol, 41, 28S.

Critchley A, Mayfield D, Thornsberry C, Piazza G, Vaughan D, Sahm DF, 1999a, Benchmarking the activity of moxifloxacin against recent isolates of Streptococcus pneumoniae (SP), Haemophilus influenzae (HI), and Moraxella catarrhalis (MC) in Europe, 39th Intersci Conf Antimicrob Agents Chemother, abstract 370, p 253.

Critchley A, Thornsberry C, Piazza G, Vaughan D, Sahm DF, 1999b, Activity of moxifloxacin (MXF) against resistant and susceptible populations of Streptococcus pneumoniae (SP) and Haemophilus influenzae (HI) and Moraxella catarrhalis (MC) isolated in the United States, 39th Intersci Conf Antimicrob Agents Chemother, abstract 369, p 253.

Dhople AM, Namba K, 2002, In vitro activity of sitafloxacin (Du 6859a) alone or in combination with rifampicin, J Antimicrob Chemother, 50, 727–729.

Dong Y, Zhao X, Drlica K, 1999, Effect of fluoroquinolone concentration on selection of resistant mutants of *Mycobacterium bovis* (BCG) and *Staphylococcus aureus*, Antimicrob Agents Chemother, 43, 1756–1758.

Felmingham D, Tesfaslasie Y, Dencer C, Robbins MJ, 1999, The in vitro activity of moxifloxacin against 817 isolates of S. pneumoniae collected from 27 centers throughout the UK and Ireland during the 1997-98 cold season, 39th Intersci Conf Antimicrob Agents Chemother, abstract 379, p 256.

Fichera ME, Ross DS, 1997, A plastid organelle as a drug target in apicomplexan parasites, Nature, 390, 407–409.

Fung-Tomc JC, Minassian B, Kolek B, Huczko E, Aleksunes L, Stickle T, Washo T, Gradelski E, Valera L, Bonner DP, 2000, Antibacterial spectrum of a novel desfluoro (6) quinolone, BMS 284756, Antimicrob Agents Chemother, 44, 3351–3356.

Gendrel D, Chalumeau M, Moulin F, Raymond J, 2003, Fluoroquinolones in pediatrics, a risk for the patient or for the community, Lancet Infect Dis, 3, 537–546.

Gozalbes R, Brun-Pascaud M, Garcia-Domenechi R, Galvez J, Girard P-M, Doucet JP, Derouin F, 2000, Antitoxoplasma activities of 24 quinolones and fluoroquinolones in vitro, prediction of activity by molecular topology and virtual computational techniques, Antimicrob Agents Chemother, 44, 2771–2776.

Hannah-Hardy J, Murphy V, Kuzmak B, Murli H, Curry P, Ledoussal B, Gray J, Flaim S, Kim N, Young P, Swing E, Nikolaides N, Mundla S, Reilly M, Schunk T, 1999, Acute IV toxicity and clastogenicity of novel 8-methoxy-nonfluoroquinolones compared with 8-methoxy-fluoroquinolones, 39th Intersci Conf Antimicrob Agents Chemother, abstract 553, p 306.

Hayashi N, Hashimoto K, Yazaki A, 2002, A novel substituent at 1-position markedly decreased the phototoxicity of an 8-chloro fluoroquinolone WQ-2756 in vitro, in vivo, 42nd Intersci Conf Antimicrob Agents Chemother, abstract F-556.

Hayashi N, Oshita Y, Amano H, Hirao Y, Nino Y, Yazaki A, 1999, WQ 3330 and WQ 2942, structure activity relationships of novel 8-methyl quinolones containing an aminophenyl group at the N-1 position, 39th Intersci Conf Antimicrob Agents Chemother, abstract 557, p 307.

Higa F, Araki N, Tateyama M, Koida M, Shinzato T, Kawakani K, Saito A, 2003, In vitro and in vivo activity of olamufloxacin against Legionella sp., J Antimicrob Chemother, 52, 920–924.

Hoellman DB, Kelly LH, Smith KA, Bozdogan B, Jacob MR, Appelbaum PC, 2003, Antistaphylococcal activity of DX-619 (including a VRSA strain) compared to eleven other agents, 43rd Intersci Conf Antimicrob Agents Chemother, abstract F-1056.

Inagaki H, Miyauchi RN, Itoh M, Kimura K, Chiba M, Tanaka M, Takahashi H, Takemura M, Hayakawa I, 2003, DX-619, a novel des-F(6) quinolone, synthesis and in vitro antibacterial activity against multidrug resistant gram-positive bacteria, 43rd Intersci Conf Antimicrob Agents Chemother, abstract F-1054.

Jetté LP, Ringuette L, Delaye G, The Pneumococcus Study Group, 1999, Surveillance program of invasive Streptococcus pneumoniae strains in the province of Quebec from 1996 to 1998, 39th Intersci Conf Antimicrobial Agents Chemother, abstract 1048, p 152.

Kerns RJ, Vaka F, Grucz RG, Kaatz GW, Tyback MJ, Cha R, Diwardka V, 2001, Synthesis and antibacterial activity of novel piperazinyl-linked fluoroquinolones, 41st Intersci Conf Antimicrob Agents Chemother, abstract F-565.

Khaliq Y, Zhanel G, 2003, Fluoroquinolone-associated tendinopathy, a critical review of the literature, Clin Infect Dis, 36, 1401–1410.

Khan AA, Slifer T, Araujo FG, et al, 1996, Trovafloxacin is active against *Toxoplasma gondii*, Antimicrob Agents Chemother, 40, 1855–1859.

Khan AA, Araujo FG, Brighty KE, Gootz TD, Remington JS, 1999a, Anti-*Toxoplasma gondii* activity and structure-activity relationships of novel fluoroquinolones related to trovafloxacin, Antimicrob Agents Chemother, 43, 1783–1787.

Khan AA, Araujo FG, Remington JS, 1999b, Gatifloxacin is active against Toxoplasma gondii, 39th Intersci Conf Antimicrob Agents Chemother, abstract 1848, p 728.

Kimura M, Kishimoto T, Niki Y, Soejima R, 1993, In vitro and in vivo antichlamydial activities of newly developed quinolone antimicrobial agents, Antimicrob Agents Chemother, 37, 801–803.

Klopman G, Wang S, Jacobs MR, et al, 1993, Anti-*Mycobacterium avium* activity of quinolones, in vitro activities, Antimicrob Agents Chemother, 37, 1799–1806.

Ledoussal B, Almstead JK, Flaim SM, Gallagher CP, Gray JL, Hu XE, Kim NK, Mckeever HD, Miley CJ, Twinem TL, Zheng SX, 1999, Novel nonfluoroquinolones (NFQs), structure-activity, and design of new potent and safe agents, 39th Intersci Conf Antimicrob Agents Chemother, abstract 544, p 3031.

Levasseur P, Lowther J, Bryskier A, Hsia C, Lemaitre O, Hodgson J, Patel MV, de Souza NJ, Khorakiwala HF, 2003, Efficacy of WCK 1152, a novel fluoroquinolone, against Legionella pneumophila serogroup 1 in experimental guinea pig infection model, 43rd Intersci Conf Antimicrob Agents Chemother, abstract 1504.

Mallalieu NL, Ellis DH, Zoutendam PH, Gavin M, Dirr MK, Martin MJ, Ledoussal B, 1999, Preclinical pharmacokinetics of a series of nonfluoroquinolones (NFQs), 39th Intersci Conf Antimicrob Agents Chemother, abstract 550, p 305.

Miyashita N, Fukano H, Yoshida K, Niki Y, Matsushima T, 2002, In vitro activity of moxifloxacin and other fluoroquinolones against Chlamydia species, J Infect Chemother, 8, 115–117.

Miyashita N, Niki Y, Kishimoto T, Nakajima M, Matsushima T, 1997, In vitro and in vivo activities of AM-1155, a new fluoroquinolone, against *Chlamydia* spp., Antimicrob Agents Chemother, 41, 1331–1334.

Miyashita N, Niki Y, Matsushima T, 2001, In vitro and in vivo activities of sitafloxacin against *Chlamydia* spp., Antimicrob Agents Chemother, 45, 3270–3272.

Murphy V, Hannah-Hardy J, Murli H, Raabe H, Douds G, Sealover K, Young P, Swing E, Nikolaides N, Mundla S, Reilly M, Schunk T, 1999, Preliminary toxicology of a series of nonfluoroquinolones (NFQs), 39th Intersci Conf Antimicrob Agents Chemother, abstract 554, p 306.

Nenortas E, Burri C, Shapiro TA, 1999, Antitrypanosomal activity of fluoroquinolones, Antimicrob Agents Chemother, 43, 2066–2068.

Niki Y, Miyashita N, Kubota Y, Nakajima M, Matsushima T, 1997, In vitro and in vivo antichlamydial activities of HSR-903, a new fluoroquinolone antibiotic, Antimicrob Agents Chemother, 41, 857–859.

Nilius A, Hensey-Rudloff D, Almer I, Beyer J, Flamm RK, 2002, Comparative in vitro activity of the new quinolone ABT 492, trovafloxacin, levofloxacin and ciprofloxacin, 42nd Intersci Conf Antimicrob Agents Chemother, abstract 546.

Pai MP, Bordley J, Amsden GW, 2001, Plasma pharmacokinetics and tissue penetration of alatrovafloxacin in morbidly obese individuals, Clin Drug Investing, 21, 219–224.

Park TH, Nam KS, Ha YH, Choi YK, Choi YJ, Kong JY, Kim YH, 1997, Synthesis and antibacterial activity of KRQ 10018 and its analogues, potent DNA gyrase inhibitors, 37th Intersci Conf Antimicrob Agents Chemother, abstract F-173, p 175.

Raether N, Seidenath H, Hofmann J, 1989, Potent antibacterial fluoroquinolones with marked activity against Leishmania donovani in vivo, Parasitol Res, 75, 412–413.

Reinert RR, 1999, Antimicrobial resistance of Streptococcus pneumoniae recovered from respiratory tract infections (RTI) of outpatients in Germany, 1998–1999, results of a 20 center national surveillance study, 39th Intersci Conf Antimicrob Agents Chemother, abstract 1041, p 150.

Roblin PM, Reznik T, Kutlin A, Hammerschlag M, 1999, In vitro activities of gemifloxacin against recent clinical isolates of *Chlamydia pneumoniae*, Antimicrob Agents Chemother, 43, 2806-2807.

Roychoudhury S, Makin KM, McIntosh EJ, Mckeever HD, Twinem TL, Koenigs PM, Catrenich CE, 1999, In vitro antibacterial activity of a series of nonfluoroquinolones (NFQs) against penicillin- and quinolone-resistant strains of Streptococcus pneumoniae, 39th Intersci Conf Antimicrob Agents Chemother, abstract 548, p 304.

Sanguigni S, Marangi M, Gramiccia M, Orsini S, Paparo BS, Nicodermo G, Gradoni L, 1993, Ciprofloxacin in the treatment of leishmaniosis, Gio Malatt Infet Paras, 45, 447–449.

Savoia D, Biglino S, Cestaro A, Zucca M, 1993, In vitro and in vivo activity of some fluoroquinolones on two Leishmania species, Eur Bull Drug Res, 2, suppl 1, 135–138.

Shapiro TA, Englund PT, 1990, Selective cleavage of kinetoplast DNA minicircles promoted by antitrypanosomal drugs, Proc Natl Acad Sci USA, 87, 950–954.

Shapiro TA, Klein VA, Englund PT, 1989, Drug-promoted cleavage of kinetoplast DNA minicircles, evidence for type II topoisomerase activity in trypanosome mitochondria, J Biol Chem, 264, 4173–4178.

Takei M, Asahima Y, Gomorii H, Fukada Y, Fukada H, 2003, Antibacterial activity of Am-1939, a novel fluoroquinolone, having potent activity against gram positive bacteria including quinolone-resistant strains, 43rd Intersci Conf Antimicrob Agents Chemother, abstract F-425.

Thangaraj HS, Adjei O, Allen BW, Portaels F, Evans MRW, Banerjee K, Wansbrough-Jones MH, 2000, In vitro activity of ciprofloxacin, sparfloxacin, ofloxacin, amikacin, and rifampin against Ghanaian isolates of Mycobacterium ulcerans, J Antimicrob Chemother, 45, 231–233.

Trujillano-Martin I, Garcia-Sanchez E, Montes-Martinez I, Fresnadillo MJ, Garcia-Sanchez JE, Garcia-Rodriguez JA, 1999, In vitro activities of six new fluoroquinolones against *Brucella melitensis*, Antimicrob Agents Chemother, 43, 194–195.

Visalli MA, Bajaksouzian S, Jacobs MR, Appelbaum PC, 1997, Comparative activity of trovafloxacin, alone and in combination with other agents, against gram-negative nonfermentative rods, Antimicrob Agents Chemother, 41, 1475–1481.

Yamakawa T, Mitsuyama J, Hayashi K, 2002, In vitro and in vivo antibacterial activity of T-3912, a novel non-fluorinated topical quinolone, J Antimicrob Chemother, 49, 455–465.

Yun HJ, Min YH, Lim JA, Kang JW, Kim SY, Kim MJ, Jeong JH, Choi YJ, Kwon HJ, Jung YH, Shim MJ, Choi EC, 2002, In vitro and in vivo antibacterial activities of DW 286, a new fluoronaphthyridone antibiotic, Antimicrob Agents Chemother, 46, 3071–3074.

Zucca M, Millesimo M, Giovarelli M, Diverio D, Musso T, Savoia D, 1996, Protective role of the pefloxacin-INFγ association in Leishmania major-infected mice, New Microbiol, 19, 39–46.

DNA Gyrase Inhibitors Other Than Fluoroquinolones

A. BRYSKIER

27

1. INTRODUCTION

Conventional DNA gyrase inhibitors belong to two major families of antibacterial agents, the fluoroquinolones and the coumarin derivatives.

A number of other antibacterial agents possess DNA gyrase-inhibitory activity, directed against either the A subunit or the B subunit of DNA gyrase. These are principally cinodine, coumadin, the pyrimido[1,6-*a*]benzimidazoles, cyclothialidine, clerocidin, or 2-pyridinecarboxyl derivatives. The potential point of interest of these molecules is that they have a mode of action similar to that of the fluoroquinolones or coumarin derivatives, but the molecular target is different, suggesting partial cross-resistance.

2. CINODINES

The cinodines are glycocinnamoylspermidines (Fig. 1). They are produced by *Nocardia* spp. The cinodines comprise three molecules: cinodines β, γ_1, and γ_2 (Tresner et al., 1978). The structure is original and consists of a combination of a trisaccharide with a *p*-hydroxycinnamoylspermidine chain. The cinodines differ from one another by the structure of the pentose attached to the terminal part of the trisaccharide. They are basic molecules, soluble in water.

The antibacterial activities of these molecules are similar to those of aminoglycosides (Table 1). They are active against *Enterobacteriaceae*, *Acinetobacter* spp., *Pseudomonas aeruginosa*, and *Staphylococcus aureus*. However, they are weakly active against enterococci and anaerobes. Cinodine γ is rapidly bactericidal against gram-negative bacteria.

In vivo in murine models of experimental infections (CD-1 mouse), cinodine γ is very active against *Enterobacteriaceae* and *S. aureus*, with 50% effective doses of between 0.04 and 0.9 mg/kg of body weight. However, it is less active against *P. aeruginosa* (50% effective dose, ~9 mg/kg). It is more active than gentamicin in this model. The cinodines bind to DNA and irreversibly inhibit DNA synthesis. They inhibit *Micrococcus luteus* DNA gyrase but do not affect topoisomerase I

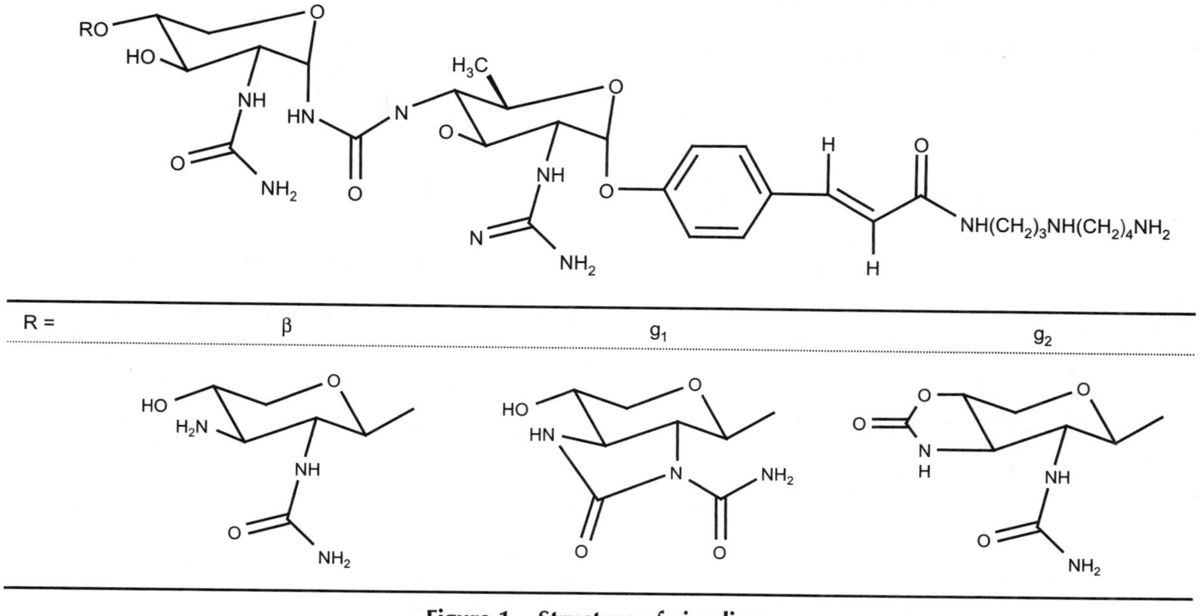

Figure 1 Structure of cinodines

Table 1 In vitro activity of cinodine γ

Organism(s)	MIC (μg/ml)			
	Cinodine	Gentamicin	Tobramycin	Amikacin
E. coli	1–2	2–4	2–4	4–8
Enterobacter	0.25–4	0.5–16	1–4	2–8
Acinetobacter	0.015–16	0.06–8	2–16	1–16
P. aeruginosa	0.25–64	1–>128	0.06–16	0.12–4
S. aureus	0.12–0.25	0.06–0.12	<0.06–0.12	1–64
Enterococcus	8–32	16		0.25–1
Bacteroides spp.	>128	>128		
Fusobacterium spp.	>128	>128		

or *Bam*HI restriction endonuclease. They inhibit DNA gyrase supercoiling at concentrations of between 0.5 and 1 mg/liter.

3. COUMAMIDINE

Coumadins are synthetic molecules of the dienoyl tetramic acid type. A number of derivatives, including molecule A, possess in vitro activity against certain bacterial genera (Table 2), and they possess activity similar to that of clindamycin against anaerobes. They are bactericidal against *S. aureus* and *Bacteroides fragilis*.

They moderately inhibit DNA gyrase activity. They apparently do possess cross-resistance with norfloxacin and coumermycin A_1 against *S. aureus*.

The most active derivative possesses a nonsubstituted 2-naphthyl nucleus attached to the terminal part of the diene (Fig. 2). The presence of a methyl group on the adjacent carbon of the terminal part of the diene increases the antibacterial activity through a spatial effect.

4. PYRIMIDO[1,6-*a*]BENZIMIDAZOLES

The β-keto group of the fluoroquinolones is attached by hydrogen bonds to the purine and pyrimidine bases of DNA, with the exception of the cytosine. Studies by Hubschwerlen et al. involved replacing this β-keto group by complementary structural analogs of these purine and pyrimidine bases. Only the derivatives with an additional structure of the thymidine type possess antibacterial activity and inhibit DNA gyrase activity at the A subunit level (Fig. 3). However, the antibacterial activity of the best compound, Ro-42-6890, is weaker than those of fleroxacin and norfloxacin (Table 3).

Table 2 In vitro activity of the 2-naphthyl derivative, molecule A

Organism	MIC (μg/ml)
S. aureus	1.56
S. epidermidis	1.56
M. luteus	1.56
Streptococcus bovis	200
S. pyogenes	50
E. coli	200
P. aeruginosa	200

Figure 2 Coumamidine derivative

Ro 42-6890

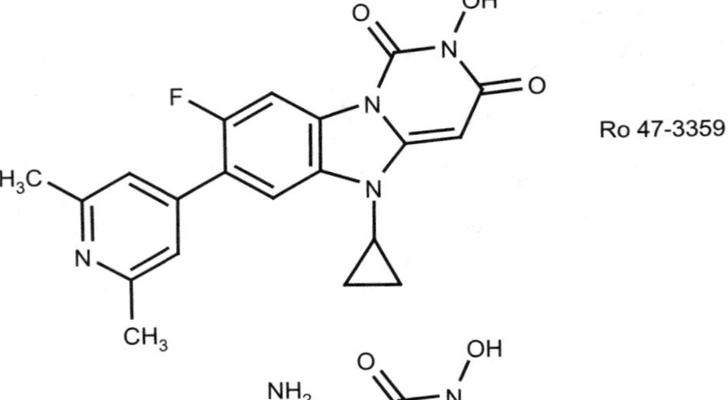

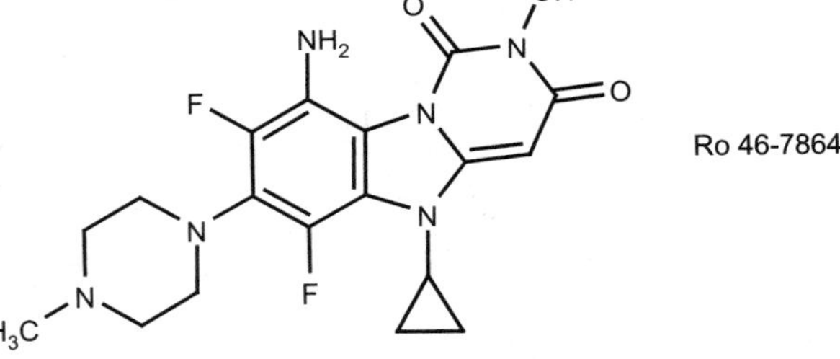

Figure 3 Pyrimido[1,6-*a*]-benzimidazoles

Table 3 In vitro activity of Ro-42-6890

Organism	MIC (μg/ml)		
	Ro-42-6890	Norfloxacin	Fleroxacin
E. coli	0.25	0.12	0.06
K. oxytoca	8.0	0.25	0.12
E. cloacae	8.0	0.25	0.12
P. aeruginosa	32	1.0	0.5
S. aureus	32	4.0	2.0
Staphylococcus haemolyticus FQ-R	>32	>64	32

They possess cross-resistance with the fluoroquinolones against *Escherichia coli* and *S. aureus*. They have a different binding site on the DNA gyrase A subunit.

5. CYCLOTHIALIDINE (Ro-09-1437)

Cyclothialidine is produced by *Streptomyces filipinensis* NR 0484. Cyclothialidine (Fig. 4) is an amphoteric molecule with a molecular mass of 641 Da. It is composed of a 12-membered lactone nucleus fused with a benzene nucleus and incorporated in a pentapeptide chain, of which the five amino acids are in the L configuration: two serines, a *cis*-3-hydroxy-L-proline, an alanine, and a cysteine.

Cyclothialidine acts by inhibiting ATPase activity at the DNA gyrase B subunit of *E. coli*. Cyclothialidine is active against novobiocin-resistant DNA gyrase, suggesting that the binding site is different from that of novobiocin. Its inhibitory activity is twice that of novobiocin or coumermycin A_1. It has little affinity for topoisomerases I and II of mammalian cells. It is inferior to the coumarin antibacterial agents or fluoroquinolones.

This molecule is active against *Eubacterium*, *Streptococcus pyogenes*, *Neisseria meningitidis*, *Moraxella catarrhalis*, and *M. luteus*, but it is inactive against *Bacillus subtilis*, *S. aureus*, and *E. coli*, which would be related to weak penetration of the cytoplasmic membrane.

This molecule has served as the lead compound for structural modifications. It has been shown that the two hydroxy phenol groups at positions 12 and 14 are essential for the DNA gyrase-inhibitory activity, and in fact 12,14-dideoxycyclothialidine is inactive. The hydroxyl group at position 14 must not be substituted, while that at position 12 may receive a methyl group. The lactone is essential for the expression of antibacterial activity but may undergo chemical alterations. The chain at position 4 must be in the *R* configuration to exert enzyme-inhibitory activity. This configuration appears to control the spatial conformation of the lactone. The substituents at position 7 of the lactone nucleus may be equally well in the *R* or *S* configuration. A derivative, Ro-46-9288, possesses a methoxy group at position 12, an ethyl carboxy group at position 4, and a thioacetyl at position 7 (Fig. 5). This molecule is four times less active than vancomycin against *S. aureus* and is very markedly more active against streptococci and enterococci (Table 4). Ro-46-9288 is bacteriostatic, like novobiocin.

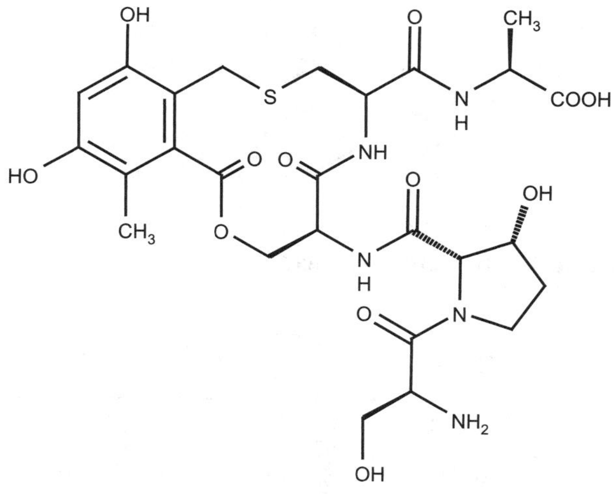

Figure 4 Structure of cyclothialidine

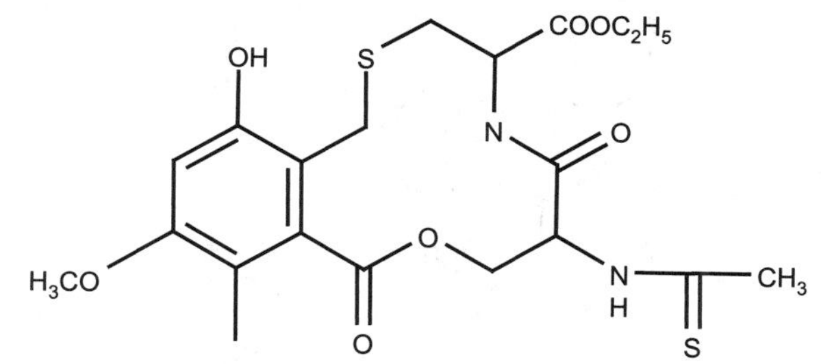

Figure 5 Ro-46-9288

Table 4 In vitro activity of Ro-46-9288

Organism(s)	MIC (μg/ml)		
	Ro-46-9288	Vancomycin	Novobiocin
MSSA	4.0	1.0	<0.25
S. aureus Met[r]	8.0	1.0	<0.25
S. epidermidis	2.0	2.0	<0.25
S. pyogenes	16	0.5	4.0
S. agalactiae	32	0.5	2.0
Viridans group streptococci	8.0	0.5	1.0
E. faecalis	16	4.0	16
Enterococcus faecium	16	2.0	16

GR-122222X (Fig. 6) was isolated from the fermentation of a strain of *Streptomyces*. It differs from cyclothialidine by the presence at the N-terminal chain of an alanine instead of a serine. It is similar to cyclothialidine D. The side chains are composed of the following amino acids: methionine and alanine, serine, proline, and alanine, to which is attached a resorcinol nucleus substituted by a methyl group. GR-122222X acts by inhibiting the ATPase activity of DNA gyrase by competing with ATP at the B subunit of this bacterial enzyme.

Yamaji et al. (1997) isolated a new series of natural cyclothialidines from the fermentation of different strains of *Streptomyces* (NR 0660, NR 0661, and NR 0662). These were called cyclothialidines B to E. Cyclothialidine A was the first molecule in this class to be described (Fig. 7). These derivatives possess greater *E. coli* DNA gyrase-inhibitory activity than novobiocin (50% inhibitory concentration [IC_{50}], 1.2 μM) and coumermycin A_1 (IC_{50}, 1.8 μM). They are inactive against intact microorganisms, as they do not cross the bacterial wall. Their physicochemical properties are summarized in Table 5.

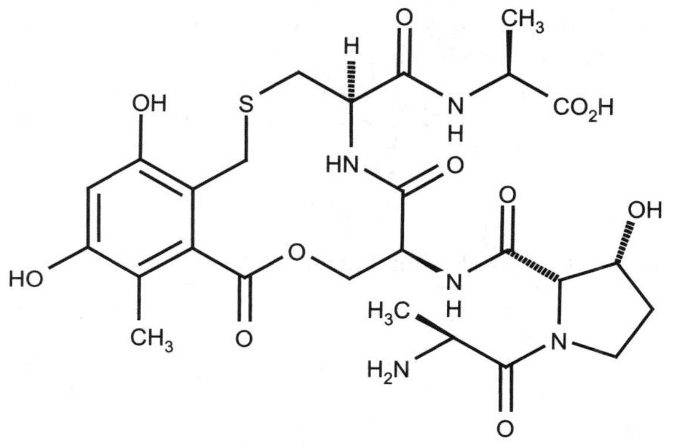

Figure 6 Structure of GR-22222X

	R_1	R_2
Cyclothialidine	NH_2, OH	CH_3
Cyclothialidine B	NH_2, OH	H
Cyclothialidine C	H_3C, NH_2	CH_3
Cyclothialidine D	H_3C, NH_2	H
Cyclothialidine E	NH_2, HOOC	CH_3

Figure 7 Derivatives of cyclothialidine

6. CLEROCIDIN

Clerocidin was isolated from *Oidiodendron truncatum* and *Fusidium viride*. It is a biterpenoid derivative of the clerodan type (Fig. 8). Intraperitoneally, the median lethal dose in the mouse is 250 mg/kg.

Clerocidin exhibits cross-resistance with the fluoroquinolones against gram-negative bacilli, but this is only partial against *S. aureus*.

It has moderate activity against *Enterobacteriaceae*. It is active against *P. aeruginosa* (MIC, 0.8 μg/ml) and inactive against *Burkholderia cepacia* (MIC, 25 μg/ml). Conversely, it has good activity against gram-positive cocci and anaerobes (Table 6). It is inactive in vitro against microscopic fungi and yeasts (MIC, >100 μg/ml). It exhibits cytotoxic activity against cells of the leukemic lymphocyte line P-388.

7. 2-PYRIDONE CARBOXYLIC ACID DERIVATIVES

A-86719.1 was preselected from a series of 2-pyridine carboxylic acid compounds. It is a bicyclic 4-*H*-4-oxo-quinolizine-3-carboxyl acid derivative (Fig. 9). A-86719.1 is characterized by the presence of a fluorine atom at position 7, a 3(*S*)-aminopyrrolidinyl ring at position 8, a cyclopropyl group at position 1, and a methyl group at position 9.

Synthesis requires 14 steps. The other molecules in this series vary in the nature of the substituents on the pyrrolidinyl ring and the groups attached at position 9 or 8.

Other derivatives have been synthesized (Fig. 10 and 11).

7.1. Physicochemical Properties

A-86719.1 has good solubility in water (Table 7) and a hydrophilic partition coefficient (Table 8).

7.2. In Vitro Activity

A-86719.1 has a broad antibacterial spectrum and is more active than ciprofloxacin in models of experimental infections due to *S. aureus* NCTC 10649, *Streptococcus pneumoniae* 6303, and *E. coli* Juhl. Its activity is similar to that of ciprofloxacin in *P. aeruginosa* infections.

7.2.1. Factors Affecting In Vitro Activity

The MICs are not affected by the nature of the culture medium; the addition of human, murine, or guinea pig serum; or the size of the inoculum (10^5 to 10^6 CFU/ml). The MIC depends on the pH of the culture medium. With *S. aureus*, the MICs are increased two- to four-fold when the pH of the medium is 5.5, compared to a pH of 7.5. Conversely, for *Enterobacteriaceae* (*E. coli, Klebsiella pneumoniae*, and *Enterobacter cloacae*), the MICs are 32 times higher at pH 5.5 than at pH 7.5. The Mg^{2+} content interferes with the in vitro activity. If the culture medium contains 9 mM Mg^{2+}, the MICs and minimum bactericidal concentrations increase 2- to 4-fold, whereas those of the fluoroquinolones increase 16-fold.

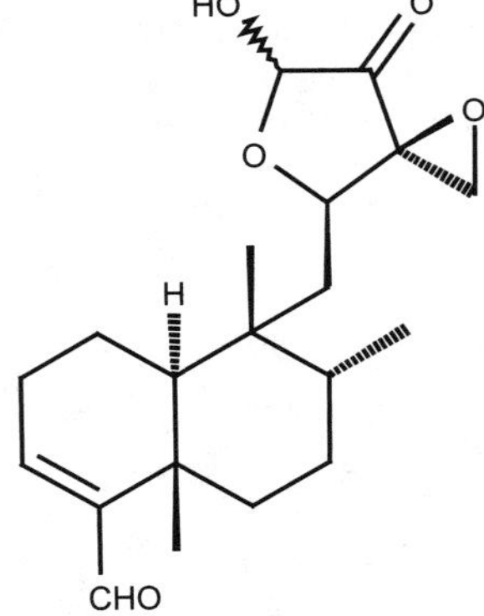

Figure 8 Structure of clerocidin

Table 5 Physicochemical properties of cyclothialidines

Property	A	B	C	D	E
Empirical formula	$C_{26}H_{36}N_5O_{12}S$	$C_{25}H_{33}N_5O_{11}S$	$C_{26}H_{35}N_5O_{11}S$	$C_{24}H_{31}N_5O_{11}S$	$C_{25}H_{33}N_5O_{11}S$
Molecular weight	641	611	625	597	611
$[\alpha]^{21}$ (c = H_2O)	−13° (1.0)	−36° (0.25)	−15° (0.25)	−26° (0.10)	11° (0.28)
IC_{50} (μM) of DNA gyrase	0.3	0.7	0.3	0.5	1.0

Table 6 In vitro activity of clerocidin

Organism	MIC (μg/ml)	
	Clerocidin	Ciprofloxacin
S. aureus 1276	0.1	0.2
E. faecalis 9011	0.1	1.6
S. agalactiae 9287	0.1	0.8
S. pneumoniae 8900	0.8	3.1
Viridans group streptococcus 11382	0.8	3.1
B. subtilis 3777	0.1	<0.05
M. luteus 2495	<0.05	1.6
B. fragilis 9844	<0.05	3.1
Clostridium perfringens 11256	0.2	0.4
Clostridium difficile 11251	0.2	12.5
Bifidobacterium dentium	0.4	1.6
Peptostreptococcus viriabilis	<0.05	0.2
Propionibacterium acnes 4020	<0.05	1.6
Mycobacterium fortuitum	0.4	0.4
Nocardia autotrophica	0.4	100

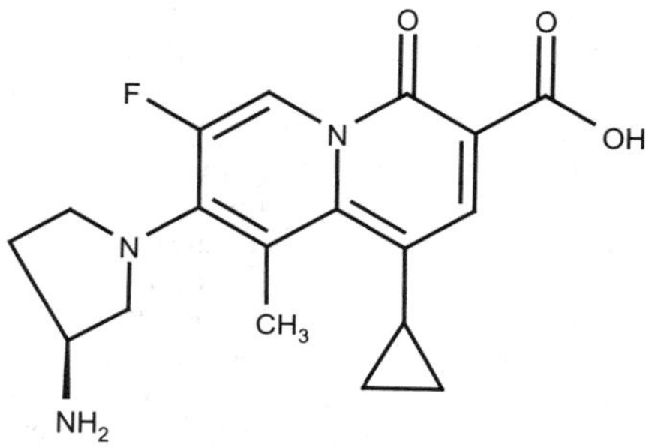

Figure 9 A-86719.1

7.2.2. In Vitro Activity against Gram-Positive Cocci

A-86719.1 is twice as active as clinafloxacin against all gram-positive cocci (Table 9). Against methicillin-susceptible strains of *S. aureus* (MSSA), it is twice as active as sparfloxacin. Killing-kinetic studies have shown that A-86719.1 is bactericidal against ciprofloxacin-resistant MSSA strains and against *Enterococcus faecalis*.

7.2.3. In Vitro Activity against Gram-Negative Bacilli

In vitro, A-86719.1 has the same activity or is twice as active as clinafloxacin. It is four to eight times more active than sparfloxacin or ciprofloxacin.

Against nonfermentative gram-negative bacilli, its activity is identical to that of clinafloxacin, but A-86719.1 is four to eight times more active than ciprofloxacin against *B. cepacia* and *Stenotrophomonas maltophilia* (Table 10). A-86719.1 has good activity against ceftazidime-resistant strains of *P. aeruginosa*. It has good activity against *Neisseria gonorrhoeae* (MIC at which 50% of isolates tested are inhibited [MIC_{50}], 0.004 μg/ml), *M. catarrhalis* (MIC_{50}, 0.06 μg/ml), and *Haemophilus influenzae* (MIC_{50}, 0.004 μg/ml).

7.2.4. Other Bacterial Genera

A-86719.1 is less active than clinafloxacin against *Legionella* spp. (MIC_{50}, 0.25 versus 0.06 μg/ml). It is inactive against *Mycobacterium avium* complex (MIC_{50}, 8 μg/ml).

It is very active against anaerobes, like clinafloxacin.

8. CJ-12371 AND CJ-12372

CJ-12371 and CJ-12372 were isolated from the fermentation products of a taxonomically unidentified fungal strain referenced N 983-46. Chemically, they are related to atrovenetinone. These derivatives have a naphthalene and decaline nucleus attached by a spiroketal nucleus (Fig. 12). The two derivatives principally have good activity against gram-positive bacteria, including ciprofloxacin-resistant strains. The MICs for *S. aureus*, *Staphylococcus epidermidis*, *S. pyogenes*, *Streptococcus agalactiae*, and *E. faecalis* are between 25 and 100 μg/ml. CJ-12372 has better DNA gyrase-inhibitory activity than CJ-12371 (Table 11).

Six derivatives have been prepared by modification of the substituents at positions 8 and 15, and some of these possess excellent inhibitory activity against DNA gyrase, but also against topoisomerase II (Fig. 13).

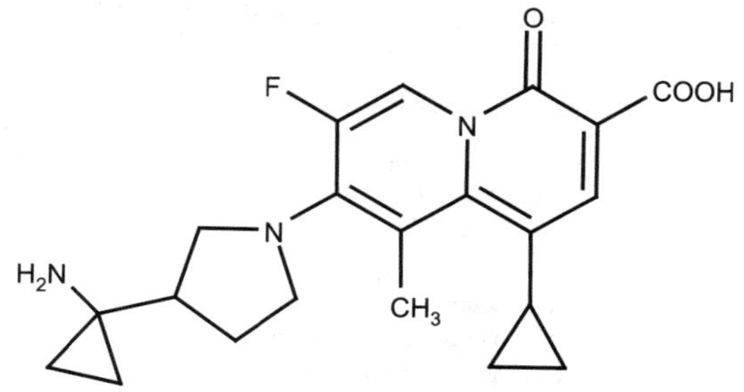

Figure 11 A-101211

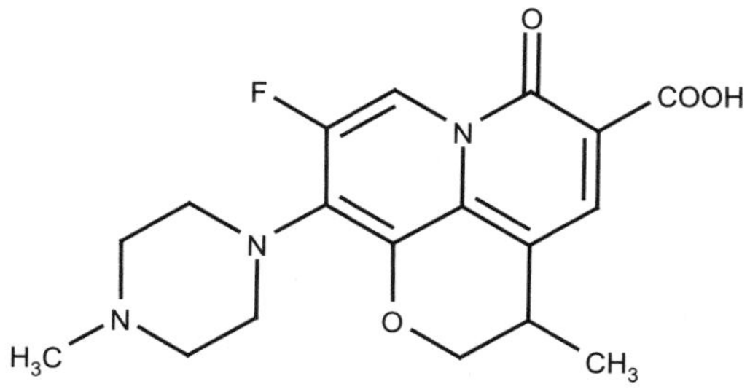

A-84066

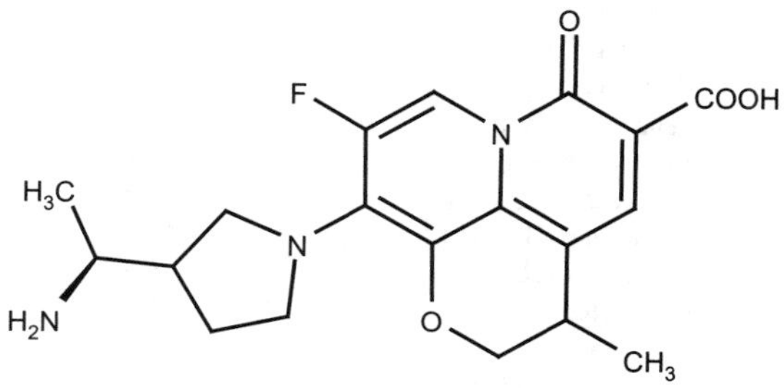

A-104954

Figure 10 2-Pyridones

Table 7 Solubility in water

Drug	Solubility (mg/ml)		
	Water	Buffer (pH 7.4)	Human urine (pH 7.4, 37°C)
A-86719.1	>20.17	0.252	0.289
Temafloxacin	5.13	0.523	1.2
Difloxacin	2.25	0.094	0.32
Sarafloxacin	0.71	0.312	20.82

Table 8 Lipophilicity of A-86719.1

Drug	LogP (*n*-octanol/water)
Difloxacin	0.523
Oxolinic acid	0.323
Pefloxacin	0.156
A-86719.1	−0.009
Temafloxacin	−0.334
Ofloxacin	−0.422
Ciprofloxacin	−1.156
Norfloxacin	−1.170

9. MICROCIN B17

In the search for living space to allow them to multiply and feed, bacteria synthesize polypeptides (bacteriocins) that selectively kill microorganisms that compete with them.

The bacteriocins are characterized by important posttranscriptional changes that endow them with specific chemical and toxic properties that would otherwise be impossible to obtain. In addition, they must only be activated in the external medium in order to allow the producer bacteria to protect themselves against their own bacteriocins. Once released into the environment, these bacteriocins have the property of binding to a specific host and not destroying any other host.

Four groups of bacteriocins have been described: colicins, microcins, lantibiotics, and nonlantibiotic bacteriocins (Table 12).

Microcin B17 is produced by certain strains of *E. coli* and possesses the property of inhibiting DNA gyrase activity.

The microcins are low-molecular-weight bacteriocins that enable producer *E. coli* strains to compete for living space in the intestines of mammals with other nonproducing strains of *E. coli*. Synthesis occurs during the stationary phase of bacterial growth and requires the involvement of numerous genes. The *mcb* genes are specific to the synthesis of microcin B17. The *mcbA* to -*G* genes form a single posttranscriptional genetic unit that controls the stationary phase of bacterial growth. Microcin B17 is produced from a precursor, promicrocin, which is a polypeptide of 69 amino acids. This precursor is the product of the *mcbA* gene. The products of the *mcbB* to -*D* genes allow the conversion of the glycyl-cysteine and glycyl-serine residues to 2-aminomethylthiazolyl-4-carboxylic acid and 2-aminomethyloxazolyl-4-carboxylic acid, respectively, which are essential for the activity of microcin B17. Conversion of the precursor to microcin B17 occurs through the detachment of a chain of 26 amino acids from the N-terminal part by a microcin B17 synthetase (Li et al., 1996), which appears to be the product of the *pmbA* gene, and the remaining unit is exported to the external medium by the McbE and McbF proteins. This bacteriocin recognizes the OmpF porin on the surfaces of the outer membrane of

Table 9 In vitro activity of A-86719.1 against gram-positive bacteria

Organism(s)	MIC_{50} (μg/ml)			
	A-86719.1	Ciprofloxacin	Clinafloxacin	Sparfloxacin
S. aureus OXA^{s}	0.03	0.5	0.06	0.03
S. aureus OXA^{r}	0.25	16	0.5	4.0
S. pyogenes	0.06	1.0	0.12	0.25
S. agalactiae	0.06	2.0	0.12	0.5
Viridans group streptococci Pen^{s}	0.06	1.0	0.12	0.25
Viridans group streptococci Pen^{r}	0.06	2.0	0.12	
S. pneumoniae Pen^{s}	0.06	2.0	0.12	0.25
S. pneumoniae Pen^{r}	0.12	2.0	0.12	0.25
Listeria monocytogenes	0.12	1.0	0.25	0.5
Corynebacterium jeikeium	1.0	32	1.0	0.125
Lactobacillus spp.	0.06	2.0	0.12	
Pediococcus spp.	0.25	16	0.5	
Leuconostoc spp.	0.12	2.0	0.25	
Erysipelothrix spp.	0.03	0.5	0.03	
E. faecalis	0.12	1.0	0.25	
E. faecalis HLGR[a] BLA^{+}	0.06	0.5	0.12	
E. faecalis HLGR	0.12	1.0	0.25	
E. faecalis Van^{r}	0.06	1.0	0.12	
E. faecium	0.25	4.0	0.5	0.5
E. faecium HLGR	0.25	4.0	0.5	0.5
E. faecium Van^{r}	0.25	4.0	1.0	0.5

[a]HLGR, high-level gentamicin resistant.

Table 10 In vitro activity of A-86719.1 against gram-negative bacilli

Organism(s)	MIC_{50} (μg/ml)			
	A-86719.1	Ciprofloxacin	Clinafloxacin	Sparfloxacin
E. coli	0.008	0.03	0.008	0.016
Enterobacter aerogenes	0.016	0.06	0.06	
E. cloacae	0.016	0.06	0.016	0.06
K. pneumoniae	0.016	0.06	0.03	0.06
Citrobacter freundii	0.06	0.06	0.06	0.03
Serratia marcescens	0.12	0.12	0.12	0.5
Proteus mirabilis	0.06	0.12	0.06	0.25
Morganella morganii	0.03	0.06	0.06	0.12
Salmonella spp.	0.016	0.06	0.03	0.03
Providencia spp.	0.03	0.03	0.008	0.12
Aeromonas hydrophila	0.08	0.016	0.008	0.06
P. aeruginosa	0.12	0.25	0.25	0.5
B. cepacia	0.06	0.25	0.06	4.0
S. maltophilia	0.25	4.0	0.25	0.5
Acinetobacter spp.	0.03	1.0	0.12	0.03

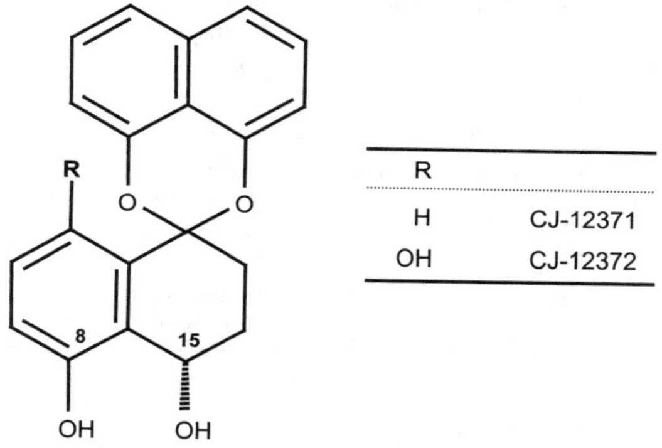

Figure 12 CJ-12371 and CJ-12372

Table 11 Activities against DNA gyrase

Drug	DNA gyrase IC_{50} (μg/ml)		
	Supercoiling	Relaxation	Eukaryotic topoisomerase II
CJ-12371	100	200	140
CJ-12372	12.5	12.5	75
Novobiocin	0.62	300	400

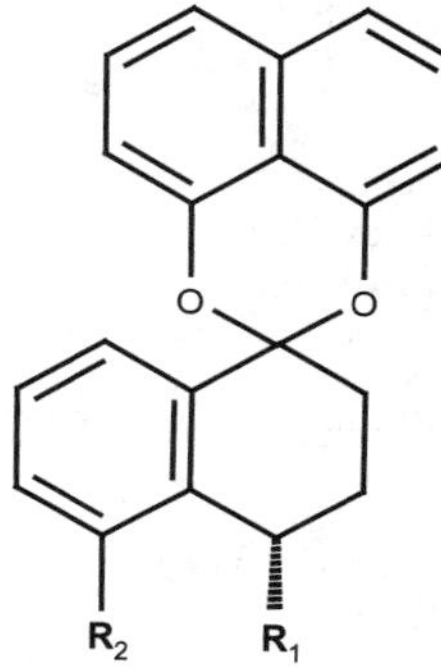

	R_1	R_2	DNA gyrase	Topoisomerase II
CJ-12371	-OH	-OH	100	144
Compound A	$-OC_2H_5$	-OH	6	13
B	$-OCH_3$	-OH	19	34
C	-OH	$-OCH_3$	38	13
D	$-OCOCH_3$	$-OCOCH_3$	13	13

Figure 13 Activity of CJ-12371 and derivatives

the host and the producer bacterium. The *mcbG* gene protects the producing bacterium, giving it immunity to microcin B17. Microcin B17 then crosses the cytoplasmic membrane of the host via the Sbma protein.

Microcin B17 is a polypeptide composed of 43 amino acids with a molecular mass of 3,200 Da (Fig. 14). This peptide antibiotic, which is bactericidal against *E. coli*, acts by inhibiting DNA replication and induces an SOS-type response. At the molecular level it binds to the B subunit of bacterial DNA gyrase, as evidenced by the mutants with changes to the *gyrB* gene (position 2251, tryptophan 751).

The *mprA* (*emrR*) gene of *E. coli* has a dual function: repressing the synthesis of microcin B17 and repressing the *emr* operon. This operon is induced by numerous molecules, including the fluoroquinolones. Its product is the efflux pump EmrAB, which causes multiresistance through efflux. The McbEFG proteins have been shown to provide protection against the action of sparfloxacin (Lomovskaya et al., 1996).

Table 12 Characteristics of bacteriocins

Group	Bacteriocins	Size[a]	Targeted bacteria	Bacterial host	Mode of action
Colicins	Pores	25–80 kDa	$Gram^-$	*E. coli*	Porin
	Nuclease E9	583	$Gram^-$	*E. coli*	Nuclease
	M	271	$Gram^-$	*E. coli*	Inhibition of lipid transport
Microcins	C7	7	*Enterobacteriaceae*	*Enterobacteriaceae*	Protein synthesis inhibitor
	B17	43	$Gram^-$	*E. coli*	DNA gyrase
	25	20	$Gram^-$	*E. coli* AY 25	Inhibition of cellular division
	Colicin V	103	*Enterobacteriaceae*	*E. coli*	Porin
	Trifolitoxin	11	*Rhizobium leguminosarum*	*Rhizobium* spp.	Nodulation inhibition
Lantibiotics	Nisin	34	$Gram^+$	*Lactobacillus lactis*	Porin
	Subtilin	32	$Gram^+$	*B. subtilis*	Porin
	Pep5	34	$Gram^+$	*S. epidermidis*	Porin
	Galidermin	21	*P. acnes*	*Streptococcus gallinarum*	Porin
	Epidermin	21	$Gram^+$	*S. epidermidis*	Porin
	Cinnamycin	19	$Gram^+$	*Streptomyces*	Phospholipase A_2 inhibition
	Cytolysin LL/LS	38/21	Streptococci	*E. faecalis*	Porin/hemolysis
	Carnocin U148	4,635 Da	Lactic bacilli	*Carnobacterium piscicola*	Porin
	Lactocin S	37	$Gram^+$	$Gram^+$	Porin
	Lactacin F	48/57	*E. faecalis*, *Lactobacillus*	*Lactobacillus johnsonsii*	Porin
Nonlantibiotic bacteriocins	Sakacin A	41	*Listeria*	*Lactobacillus sakei*	Porin
	Pediocin PA-1	44	*Listeria*	*Pediococcus acidilactici*	Porin
	Lactococcin A	68	$Gram^+$	*L. lactis*	Potassium channels
	Lactococcin Gα/β	35/29	$Gram^+$	*L. lactis*	Porin
	AS-48	70	$Gram^+$ + $Gram^-$	*E. faecalis*	Porin
	Lysostaphin	22 kDa	Staphylococci	*Staphylococcus simulans*	Endoprotease glycylglycine

[a]Values are numbers of amino acids unless otherwise noted.

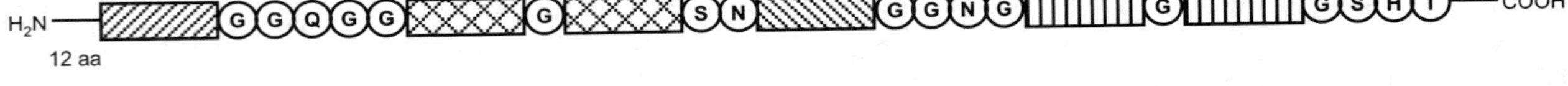

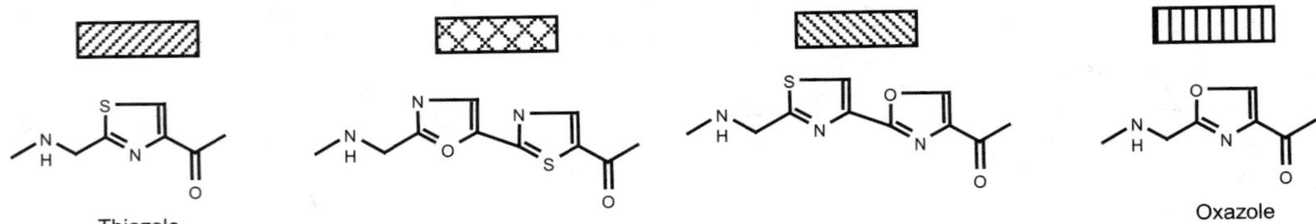

Figure 14 Microcin B17. aa, amino acid; G, glycyl; S, serine; I, isoleucine; H, histidine; N, norvaline. From Baba et al., 1998.

REFERENCES

Alder J, Clement J, Meulbroek J, Shipkowitz N, Mitten M, Jarvis K, Oleksijew A, Hutch T Sr, Paige L, Flamm B, Chu D, Tanaka K, 1995, Efficacies of ABT-719 and related 2-pyridones, members of a new class of antibacterial agents, against experimental bacterial infections, Antimicrob Agents Chemother, 39, 971–975.

Andersen NR, Lorck HOB, Rasmussen PR, 1983, Fermentation, isolation and characterization of antibiotic, PR 1350, J Antibiot, 36, 753–760.

Andersen NR, Rasmussen PR, 1984, The constitution of clerocidin, a new antibiotic isolated from Oidiodendron truncatum, Tetrahedron Lett, 25, 465–468.

Arasawa H, Watanabe J, Kamiyama T, Nakada N, Shimada H, Shimma N, Sawairi S, Yokose S, 1992, Cyclothialidine (Ro-09-1437), a new DNA gyrase inhibitor: isolation, structure and biological characterization, 32nd Intersci Conf Antimicrob Agents Chemother, abstract 493.

Baba T, Schneewind O, 1998, Instruments of bacterial warfare: bacteriocin synthesis, toxicity and immunity, Trends Microbiol, 3, 66–70.

Bayer A, Freund S, Jung G, 1995, Post-translational heterocyclic backbone modifications in the 43-peptide antibiotic microcin B17. Structure, elucidation and NMR study of the ^{13}C, ^{15}N-labelled gyrase inhibitor, Eur J Biochem, 234, 414–426.

Eliopoulos GM, Wennersten CB, Cole G, Chu D, Pizzuti D, Moellering RC Jr, 1995, In vitro activity of A-86719.1, a novel 2-pyridone antimicrobial agent, Antimicrob Agents Chemother, 39, 850–853.

Ellestad GA, Cosulich DB, Broschard RW, Martin JH, Kunstmann MP, Morton GO, Lancaster JE, Fulmor W, Lovell FM, 1978, Glycocinnamoylspermidines, a new class of antibiotics. III. Structure of LL-BM 123 β, τ_1, and τ_2, J Am Chem Soc, 100, 2515–2524.

Gmünder H, Kuratli K, Keck W, 1995, Effect of pyrimido[1,6-*a*]benzimidazoles, quinolones, and Ca^{2+} on the DNA gyrase-mediated cleavage reaction, Antimicrob Agents Chemother, 39, 163–169.

Goetschi E, Angehrn P, Gmünder H, Hebeisen P, Link H, Masciadri R, Nielsen J, 1993, Cyclothialidine and its congeners: a new class of DNA gyrase inhibitors, Pharmacol Ther, 60, 367–380.

Greenstein M, Speth JL, Maiese WM, 1981, Mechanism of action of cinodine, a glycocinnamoylspermidine antibiotic, Antimicrob Agents Chemother, 20, 425–432.

Hubschwerlen CP, Pflieger P, Specklin JL, Gubernator K, Gmünder H, Angehrn P, Kompis I, 1992, Pyrimido[1,6-*a*]benzimidazoles: a new class of DNA gyrase inhibitors, J Med Chem, 35, 1385–1392.

Kamiyama T, Shimma N, Ohtsuka T, Nakayama N, Itezono Y, Nakada N, Watanabe J, Yokose K, 1994, Cyclothialidine, a novel gyrase inhibitor. II. Isolation, characterization and structure elucidation, J Antibiot, 47, 37–44.

Kaneda K, Iwata E, Sugie Y, Inagaki T, Yamauchi T, Sakakibara T, Norcia M, Wondrack LM, Sutcliffe JA, Kojima N, 1993, Atrovenetinone-related compounds inhibit procaryotic and eucaryotic type II topoisomerase, 3rd Int Conf Biotech Microb Products, p 26.

Kawada S, Yamashita Y, Fujii N, Nakano H, 1991, Induction of a heat-stable topoisomerase II-DNA cleavable complex by nonintercalative terpenoids, terpentecin and clerocidin, Cancer Res, 51, 2922–2925.

Kuck NA, Redin GS, 1978, Glycocinnamoylspermidines, a new class of antibiotics. V. Antibacterial evaluation of the isopropyl derivative of LL-BM 123γ, J Antibiot, 31, 405–409.

Li YM, Milne JC, Madison LL, Kolter R, Walsh CT, 1996, From peptide precursors to oxazole and thiazole-containing peptide antibiotics: microcin B17 synthase, Science, 274, 1188–1193.

Lomovskaya O, Kawai F, Matin A, 1996, Differential regulation of the *mcb* and *emr* operons of *Escherichia coli*: role of *mcb* in multidrug resistance, Antimicrob Agents Chemother, 40, 1050–1052.

Martin JH, Kunstmann MP, Barbatschi F, Hertz M, Ellestad GA, Dann M, Redin GS, Dornbusch AC, Kuck NA, 1978, Glycocinnamoylspermidines, a new class of antibiotics. II. Isolation, physicochemical and biological properties of LL-BM 123 β, γ_1, and γ_2, J Antibiot, 31, 398–404.

McCullough JE, Muller MT, Howells AJ, Maxwell A, O'Sullivan J, Summerill RS, Parker WL, Wells JS, Bonner D, Fernandes PB, 1993, Clerocidin, a terpenoid antibiotic, inhibits bacterial DNA gyrase, J Antibiot, 46, 526–530.

Nakada N, Gmünder H, Hirata T, Arisawa M, 1994, Mechanism of inhibition of DNA gyrase by cyclothialidine, a novel gyrase inhibitor, Antimicrob Agents Chemother, 38, 1966–1973.

Oram M, Dosanjh B, Gormley NA, Smith CV, et al, 1996, Mode of action of GR 122222X, a novel inhibitor of bacterial DNA gyrase, Antimicrob Agents Chemother, 40, 473–476.

Osburne MS, Maiese WM, Greenstein M, 1990, In vitro inhibition of bacterial DNA gyrase by cinodine, a glycocinnamoylspermidine antibiotic, Antimicrob Agents Chemother, 34, 1450–1452.

Rosen T, Fernandes PB, Marovich MA, Shen L, Meo J, Pernet AG, 1989, Aromatic dienoyl tetramic acids: novel antibacterial agents with activity against anaerobes and staphylococci, J Med Chem, 32, 1062–1069.

Sakemi S, Inagaki T, Kaneda K, Hirai H, Iwata E, Sakakibara T, Yamauchi Y, Norcia M, Wondrack LM, Sutcliffe JA, Kojima N, 1995, CJ-12371 and CJ-12372, two novel DNA gyrase inhibitors: fermentation, isolation, structural elucidation and biological activities, J Antibiot, 48, 134–142.

Tresner HD, Korshalla JH, Fantini AA, Korshella JD, Kirby JP, Goodman JJ, Kele RA, Shay AJ, Borders DB, 1978, Glycocinnamoylspermidines, a new class of isopropyl derivatives. I. Description and fermentation of the organism producing the LL-BM 123 antibiotics, J Antibiot, 31, 394–404.

Vizan J, Hernandez-Chico C, Castillo I, Moreno F, 1991, The peptide antibiotic microcin B 17 induces double-strand cleavage of DNA mediated by E. coli DNA gyrase, EMBO J, 10, 467–476.

Watanabe J, Nakada N, Sawarai S, Shimada H, Ohshima S, Kamaiyama T, Arasiwa M, 1994, Cyclothialidine, a novel gyrase inhibitor. I. Screening, taxonomy, fermentation and biological activity, J Antibiot, 47, 32–36.

Yamaji K, Masubuchi M, Kawahara F, Nakamura Y, Nishio A, et al, 1997, Cyclothialidine analogs, novel DNA gyrase inhibitors, J Antibiot, 50, 402–411.

Codrugs

A. BRYSKIER

28

1. INTRODUCTION

Humans and bacteria have embarked on a race to destroy or neutralize the most modern antibacterial agents (bacteria) or to discover new molecules (humans). The bacteria produce β-lactamases to inactivate β-lactams, modifying the intracellular targets and protecting them from DNA gyrase or topoisomerase IV inhibitors. They prevent intrabacterial penetration by modifying the penetration pathways, particularly in the porin channels. The difficulties that confront chemists in developing new chemical entities will in the long run engender therapeutic difficulties in the area of infectious diseases.

The development of new molecules in the β-lactam family that are stable against hydrolysis by the new β-lactamases (extended-broad-spectrum enzymes) or the combination of a β-lactam with enzyme inhibitors (broad-spectrum β-lactamases), such as clavulanic acid, sulbactam, tazobactam, brobactam, the halopenams, or penems, has already produced solutions to a number of therapeutic problems, or will do so in the future.

Following this line of reasoning, O'Callaghan's team in 1975 tested a third route using a cephem as a vehicle for a molecule that was active in itself. This type of study was resumed 10 years later by Mobashery's team (1986). Since then, a number of studies have resulted in the synthesis of molecules releasing entities possessing activity different from that of the β-lactams, such as the fluoroquinolones.

2. RATIONALE OF CODRUGS

The studies are based on the fact that hydrolysis of the lactam carbonyl bond of the cephem nucleus is accompanied by expulsion of the chain attached to the methylene group at C-3′, particularly if this residue is capable of accepting an electron, such as a pyridine, azide, or acetoxy nucleus (Fig. 1).

In 1976, O'Callaghan et al. described a cephalosporin possessing dual antibacterial activity. Like cefamandole, this molecule had a D-mandeloyl chain at position 7 and a mercaptopyridine-*N*-oxide (omidine) residue at position 3 (Fig. 2). In the form of the zinc pyrithione salt, this omidine chain possesses antiseptic activity. This molecule is more active than cephalothin against gram-negative bacteria (Table 1).

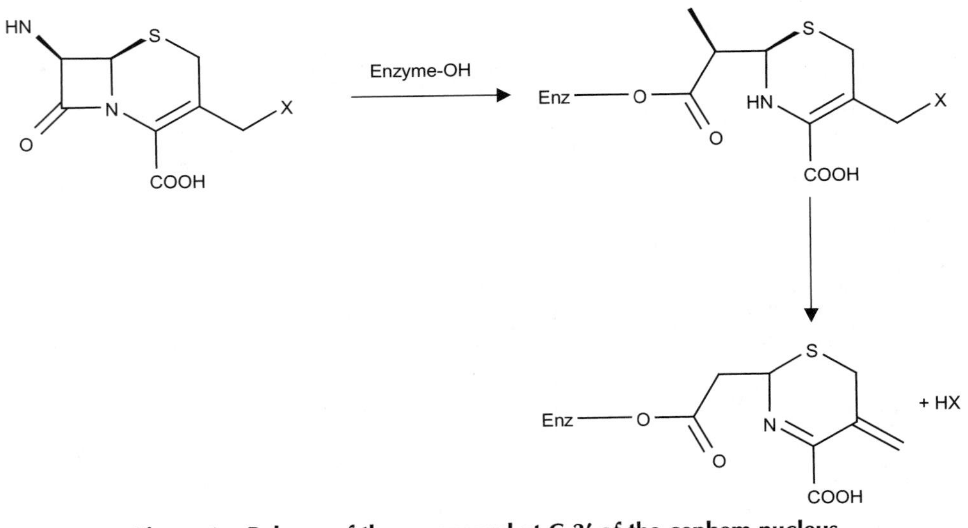

Figure 1 Release of the compound at C-3′ of the cephem nucleus

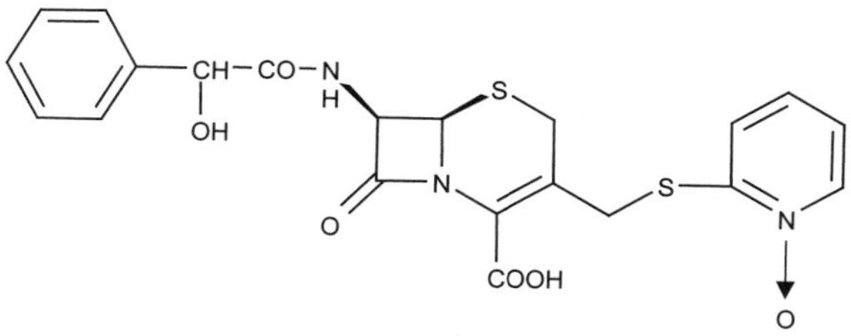

Figure 2 Cephem: C-3′-omidine derivative mercaptopyridine-*N*-oxide (MCO)

Table 1 In vitro activity of mercaptopyridine-*N*-oxide

Organism	MIC (μg/ml)	
	MCO[a]	Omidine ring
S. aureus	8	2
E. coli	2	2
C. freundii	64	2
E. cloacae	1	2
Hafnia alvei	16	2
Klebsiella aerogenes	1	2
Providencia rettgeri	0.5	8
Morganella morganii	2	8

[a]MCO, mercaptopyridine-*N*-oxide.

The molecule with the omidine nucleus has also has been shown to be active against β-lactamase-producing *Enterobacteriaceae* (Table 2).

Other entities have been prepared using a cephem as a transporter for another molecule possessing antibacterial activity attached to C-3′ by a carbamate or ether bond or a haloalanyl (Mobashery et al., 1986) (Fig. 3).

The presence of a mandeloyl residue and a hydroxyl group increases stability against hydrolysis by class 1 enzymes. However, it has been shown that the *N*-methylthiotetrazole nucleus is bacteriologically inactive.

3. DEFINITION

A codrug is a hybrid antibacterial agent resulting from the combination of a β-lactam and another antibacterial agent (fluoroquinolones, nitrofuran, etc.). It permits both components to exert their specific antibacterial activities.

This combination achieves the following:

- It increases the antibacterial activity of the cephems.
- the fluoroquinolones are poorly soluble in water under physiological conditions. This combination increases their solubility.

Table 2 Activity of the omidine nucleus against β-lactamase-producing strains

Organism[a]	MIC (μg/ml)	
	MCO[b]	Omidine nucleus
E. coli TEM$^+$	8	2
E. coli TEM$^-$	2	2
E. cloacae P99$^+$	64	2
E. cloacae P99$^-$	1	2
K. aerogenes BLA$^+$	16	2
K. aerogenes BLA$^-$	1	2
M. morganii NCTC 235	0.5	8
P. mirabilis 431	2	8

[a]BLA, β-lactamase.
[b]MCO, mercaptopyridine-*N*-oxide.

- the mechanisms of action of the two combined molecules are compatible and not antagonistic.
- The potential toxicity of certain molecules might be reduced (e.g., fluoroquinolones and carbapenems).

New codrugs without β-lactams have been synthesized, combining a fluoroquinolone and an oxazolidinone.

4. CLASSIFICATION

4.1. Combined Molecules

The most widely studied combinations are those combining a β-lactam and a fluoroquinolone. The important factor is not only the molecules constituting the codrug but also the point of attachment on the fluoroquinolone and the type of bond.

All of the different types of β-lactams have been proposed as constituents of a codrug: cephalosporins, oxacephems, cephamycins, isocephems, penams, carbapenams, penicillins, monocyclic β-lactams, nocarcidins, methylenepenams, 2,3-methylenecarbapenems, γ-lactams, lactivicins, and pyrazolidinones (Fig. 4).

The molecules combined with the β-lactams may be quinolones, 1,8-naphthyridones, pyridobenzoxazinones, isothiazoloquinolones, or other derivatives.

4.2. β-Lactam–Fluoroquinolone Bond

The bond between the β-lactam and the fluoroquinolone molecules may occur at the heterocycle attached to position 7 of the fluoroquinolone, whether this is a piperazinyl or a 3′-aminopyrrolidine nucleus (Fig. 5), via its amino chain.

The most widely studied is the linkage between the carboxyl group at position 3 of the β-pyridone nucleus and a β-lactam, the prototype for which is Ro-23-9424 (Fig. 6).

4.3. β-Lactam Bond

The majority of codrugs studied possess either a cephalosporin, a penem, or a carbapenem. The linkage for

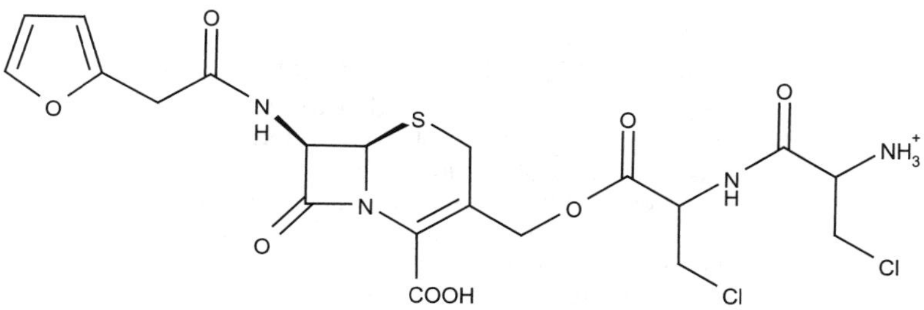

Figure 3 Haloalanyl cephalosporin

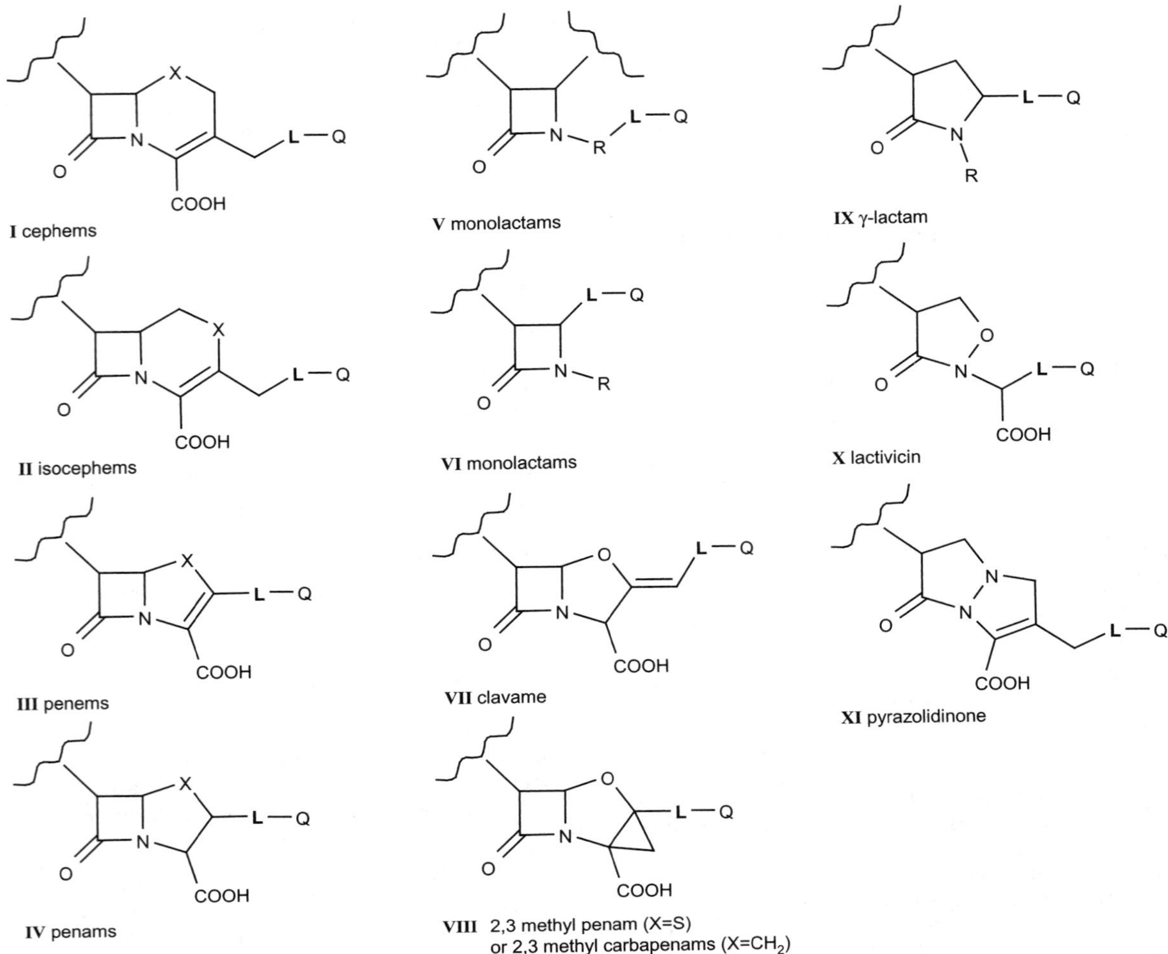

Figure 4 Classification of combined molecules

the penems and carbapenems occurs via the chain attached to position 2.

In the case of the cephalosporins, the bond occurs through the methylene chain attached to position 3 of the cephem nucleus. Two molecules have recently been described with molecules of enrofloxacin (CQ-397) and norfloxacin (CQ-414). The bond occurs in the chain at position 7 of the cephem nucleus (Fig. 7).

4.4. Intermolecular Bonds

The bonds between the β-lactam and fluoroquinolone molecules are of different types: 3′-esters, carbamate, quaternary ammonium, thiocarbamate, tertiary or secondary amine, thioethylcarbamate, urea, thiourea, pyridinium, guanidinium, amide, dithiocarbamate, etc.

5. MECHANISMS OF ACTION

The β-lactams act by acylating the serine residues of the transpeptidases responsible for the formation of the cross-linked network of peptidoglycan.

Opening of the β-lactam ring is accompanied by elimination of the group attached to C-3′ of the cephem nucleus. The β-lactam acts as a "prodrug" for the second molecule, releasing it near its site of action.

Piperazinyl nucleus

Pyrrolidinyl nucleus

Figure 5 β-Lactam–fluoroquinolone bond

Cefotaxime

Ro-23-9424

Desacetyl-cefotaxime

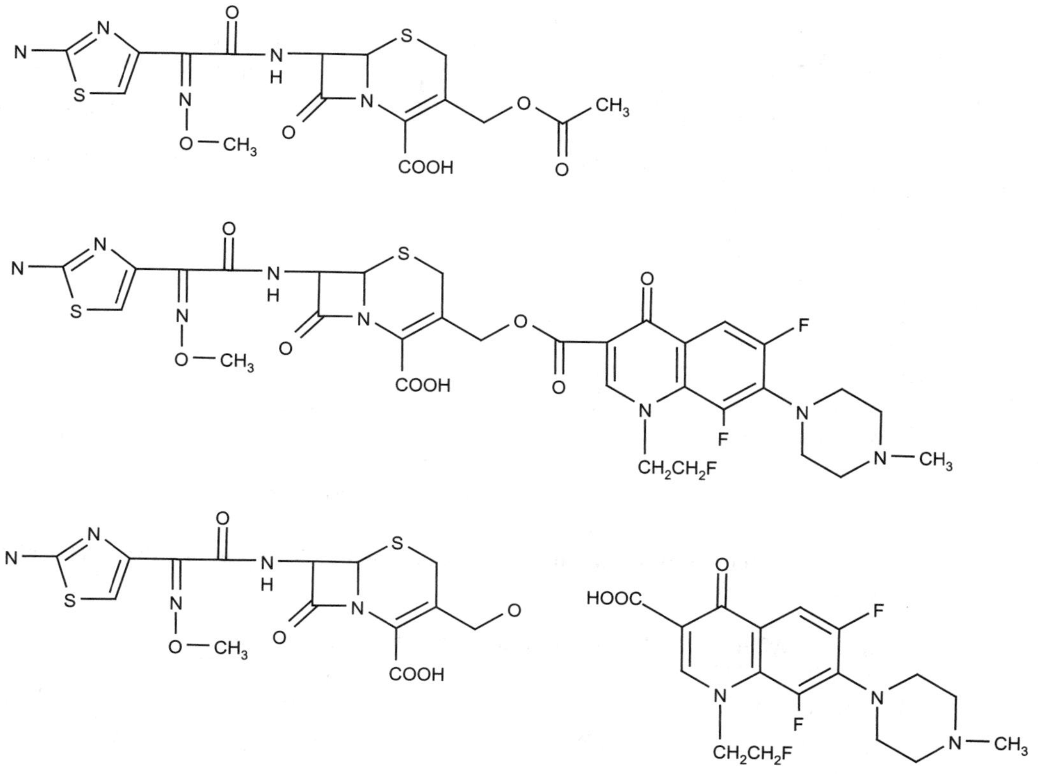

Fleroxacin

Figure 6 Structures of cefotaxime, Ro-23-9424, desacetylcefotaxime, and fleroxacin

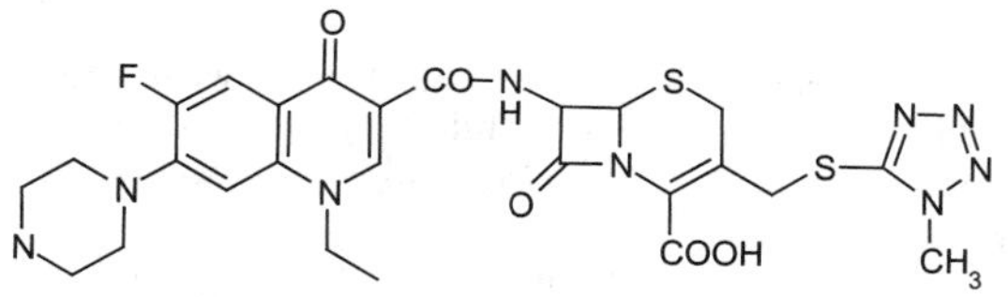

CQ-414

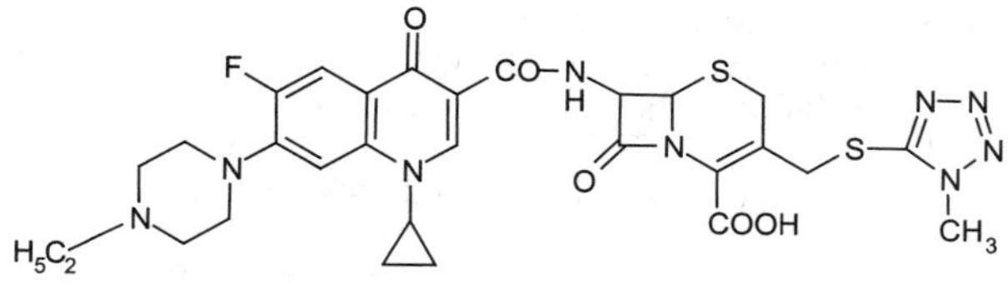

CQ-397

Figure 7 CQ-414 and CQ-397

Studies of the mechanisms of action of codrugs have been conducted principally with Ro-23-9424 (3′-ester), Ro-24-4384 (carbamate), and Ro-24-8138 (tertiary amine).

The activity of the fluoroquinolones is evaluated in vitro in terms of the inhibition of DNA gyrase activity and in vivo in the bacterium in terms of its action on the nucleoid (topoisomerase IV) using 4′,6′-diamidino-2-phenylindole. This compound allows the activity of the fluoroquinolones on the division of the nucleoid in the exponential growth phase of *Escherichia coli* to be assessed (Georgopapadakou and Bertasso, 1993).

The activity of the β-lactams is analyzed with reference to the binding to penicillin-binding proteins (PBP), the stability against hydrolysis by the different β-lactamases, and the rate of penetration of the outer membrane of gram-negative bacilli (*E. coli* wall mutants $OmpF^-$ and $OmpC^-$). Several molecules have been the subject of an analysis of their mechanism of action (Fig. 8).

5.1. β-Lactam-Type Activity

All of the molecules induce filaments at a concentration equal to the MIC.

5.1.1. Binding to PBP

Ro-23-9424 (3′-ester-type derivative) binds principally to PBP 3 of *E. coli, Enterobacter cloacae, Streptococcus pneumoniae, Proteus mirabilis*, and *Proteus vulgaris* (Georgopapadakou et al., 1989).

The molecule binds to *Pseudomonas aeruginosa* PBP 1 and 3, *Haemophilus influenzae* PBP 5, *Enterococcus faecalis* PBP 6, and *S. pneumoniae* PBP 1, 2b, and 3.

In *Staphylococcus aureus* ATCC 25923, Ro-23-9424 binds to PBP 1, 2, and 3 with greater affinity than cefotaxime and ceftriaxone. The affinity of desacetylcefotaxime for *S. aureus* PBP is very weak (Table 3).

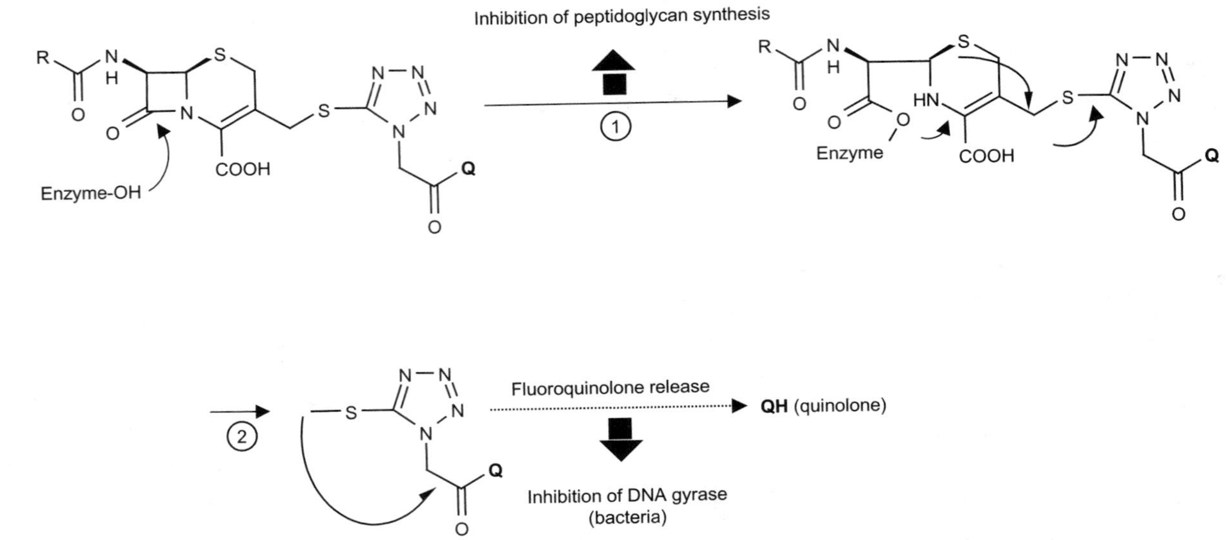

Figure 8 Mechanism of action of β-lactams–fluoroquinolones (adapted from Dax et al., 1993)

Table 3 Affinities of β-lactams for *S. aureus* ATCC 25923 PBP

Compound	IC_{50} (μg/ml) with PBP:				MIC (μg/ml)
	1	2	3	4	
Ro-23-9424	0.1	0.1	0.1	30	1
Cefotaxime	0.1	0.5	100	100	1
Ceftriaxone	0.5	2	0.5	>100	1
Desacetylcefotaxime	100	>100	30	>100	4
Ro-25-0534	0.6	1	7.6	31	4

Georgopapadakou and Bertasso (1993) showed that in *E. coli*, the carbamate and tertiary amine derivatives bind to PBP 3. The affinity for PBP 1a is weak in the case of desacetylcefotaxime (50% inhibitory concentration [IC_{50}], 2 μg/ml) and the tertiary amine derivative. Likewise, cefotaxime, ceftriaxone, desacetylcefotaxime, and Ro-24-8138 (tertiary amine derivative) have a weak affinity for PBP 1b, in contrast to the 3′-ester (Ro-23-9424 and Ro-24-6392) and carbamate (Ro-24-4383) derivatives. Cefotaxime and ceftriaxone have moderate affinity for PBP 2 (IC_{50}s of 1.4 and 1.5 μg/ml, respectively), whereas the other molecules have no affinity, with an IC_{50} of ≥30 μg/ml. The two 3′-ester derivatives (Ro-23-9424 and Ro-24-6392) have good affinity for PBP 4 (IC_{50}, ~1.5 μg/ml), as do cefotaxime (IC_{50}, 1.6 μg/ml) and ceftriaxone (IC_{50}, 2 μg/ml). The IC_{50}s of the other molecules are ≥13 μg/ml. A tertiary amine derivative of the cephalosporin-catechol type, Ro-25-0534 (Georgopapadakou and Bertasso, 1993), forms filaments with *E. coli* UB 1005 and binds to PBP 3 (IC_{50}, <0.1 μg/ml) and PBP 4 (IC_{50}, 0.5 μg/ml). It has little affinity for the other PBP (IC_{50}, ≥20 μg/ml). In *S. aureus* ATCC 25923 (MIC, 4 μg/ml), it binds principally to PBP 1 and 2.

5.1.2. Interaction with β-Lactamases

Enzymatic activity against the codrugs was studied by Georgopapadakou and McCaffrey (1994) with Ro-23-9424 (3′-ester), Ro-25-0534 (tertiary amine-catechol), and Ro-25-4825 (carbamate).

The 3′-ester derivative (Ro-23-9424) is weakly hydrolyzed by TEM-1 (V_{max}, 0.03 nmol/min/mg), but with good affinity for the enzyme (K_m, 113 μM), and is also weakly hydrolyzed by TEM-3.

The tertiary amine-catechol derivative (Ro-25-0534) is weakly hydrolyzed by TEM-1 (V_{max}, 0.002 nmol/min/mg), but its affinity for the enzyme is greater than that of cefotaxime. There is a low hydrolysis rate and weak affinity for TEM-3.

The carbamate derivatives (Ro-25-2016 and Ro-25-4835) (Fig. 9) have different affinities and hydrolysis rates. The Ro-24-2016 derivative is more hydrolyzed and has greater affinity for TEM-1 than cephalothin but, paradoxically, is weakly hydrolyzed by TEM-3. The second derivative, Ro-25-4835, is more weakly hydrolyzed than cephacetrile and has a weak affinity for the enzyme.

Class 1 enzymes have a low hydrolysis rate with Ro-23-9424. Conversely, despite a high hydrolysis rate (V_{max}, 276 nmol/min/mg), the affinity of Ro-25-2016 is weak (K_m, 11 μM). The same applies to the other compounds.

5.2. Fluoroquinolone-Type Activity

5.2.1. Activity against DNA Gyrase

Derivatives of the 3′-ester type (Ro-23-9424) weakly inhibit DNA supercoiling, as do molecules of the carbamate and tertiary amine types.

DNA synthesis is weakly inhibited by Ro-23-9424. Ro-24-6392 appears to be slightly more active. DNA biosyn-

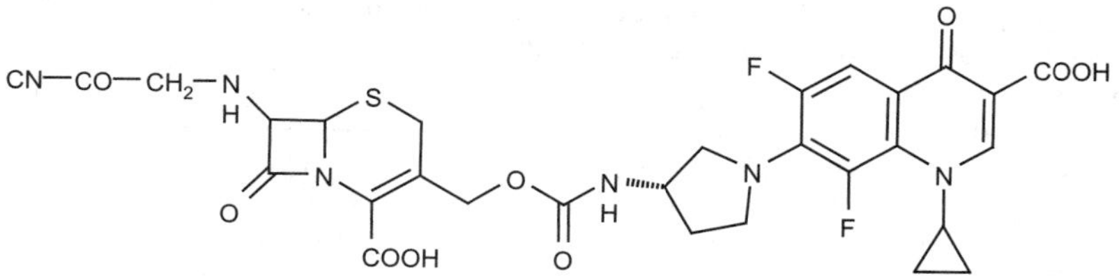

Ro-25-4835

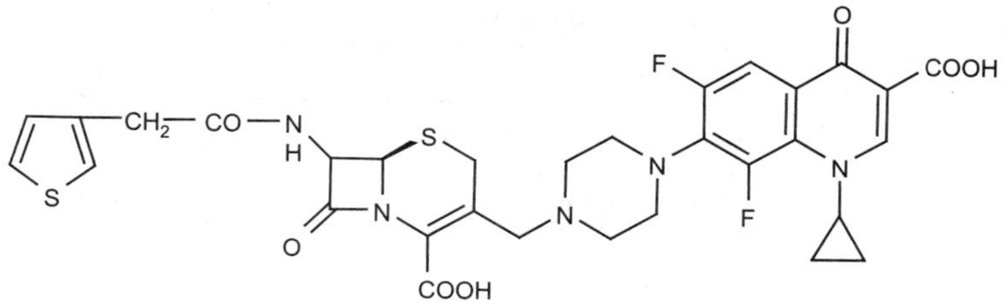

Ro-25-2016

Figure 9 Carbamate derivatives

thesis is weakly inhibited by the carbamate derivative (Ro-24-4383) and the tertiary amine derivative (Ro-24-8138) compared to the parent molecules, ciprofloxacin and fleroxacin (Table 4).

5.2.2. Action against the Nucleoid (Topoisomerase IV)

In *E. coli* ATCC 25922 (fluoroquinolone susceptible), the 3′-esters cause a modification of the nucleoid in 2 h, whereas the carbamate (Ro-24-4383) and the tertiary amine (Ro-24-2126) cause the same modification in 1 h. The response to the cephalosporins appears in 1 h.

For *E. coli* EN-225 (fluoroquinolone resistant), the carbamate derivative (Ro-24-4383) has a MIC of 20 μg/ml and the tertiary amine derivative has a MIC of 5 μg/ml, causing a cephalosporin-like response after incubation for 1 to 2 h.

5.3. Analysis of Mechanism of Action

The 3′-ester derivatives (Ro-23-9424 and Ro-24-6392) act as fluoroquinolone and cephalosporin prodrugs, as the carboxyl group at position 3 of the β-pyridone nucleus is essential for the antibacterial activity of the fluoroquinolones. The cephalosporins bind to PBP 1a, 1b, and 3, produce filaments, and do not modify the bacterial nucleoids.

The lack of cell lysis indicates binding to bacterial cell PBP 3, a weak concentration in the periplasmic space, and weak transparietal penetration (Georgopapadakou et al., 1989). As prodrugs, the fluoroquinolones act on DNA synthesis and topoisomerase IV.

In the molecules of the carbamate and tertiary amine types, the carboxyl group at position 3 of the β-pyridone nucleus is free. The bond occurs via the piperazine ring. The molecules act as intact molecules. They inhibit DNA synthesis at concentrations greater than those necessary for the parent fluoroquinolones and act on topoisomerase IV. They act like cephalosporins by binding to PBP 3. However, in bacterial cells in the growth phase, the cephalosporin activity appears only in the absence of that of the fluoroquinolones.

This has been also demonstrated with Ro-25-0534 (tertiary amine-catechol), which inhibits the DNA synthesis of *E. coli* H 560 and EN-225 less well than ciprofloxacin (36 times less) (Georgopapadakou and Bertasso, 1993).

Table 4 Activities of codrugs against DNA

Compound	IC_{50} (μg/ml)		
	DNA supercoiling (*E. coli* MK47)	*E. coli*: DNA biosynthesis	
		ATCC 25922	EN 225
Ro-23-9424	20	17	140
Ro-24-6392	5	5	35
Ro-24-4383	2	3.6	38
Ro-24-8138	2	5.2	72
Fleroxacin	0.05	0.3	5.5
Ciprofloxacin	0.02	0.05	1.4

6. MECHANISMS OF RESISTANCE

Studies have been conducted on *E. coli* TE-18, which is a strain derived from *E. coli* K-12. It hyperproduces class 1 enzymes (Pace et al., 1991).

This strain is susceptible to Ro-23-9424 (MIC, 0.2 μg/ml), but is resistant to desacetylcefotaxime (MIC, 50 μg/ml). In addition, it possesses a reduced number of OmpF-type porins, which helps reduce its susceptibility to cephalosporins.

The affinity of Ro-23-9424 for the β-lactamase produced by *E. coli* TE-18 is weak (K_m, 0.035 μM) compared to those of desacetylcefotaxime (K_m, 0.04 μM) and cefotaxime (K_m,

0.28 μM). However, the V_{max} is greater than that of cefotaxime (1.21 versus 0.4 nmol/min/mg) although considerably lower than that of desacetylcefotaxime (V_{max}, 36 nmol/min/mg). With this strain, the transparietal penetration rate is lower than that of desacetylcefotaxime (0.08×10^{-5} versus 0.02×10^{-5} cm/s) and cefotaxime (2.26×10^{-5} cm/s).

The selection of fleroxacin-resistant mutants from this strain is greater than that observed with fleroxacin alone or from another strain, such as *E. coli* JF 568.

The mutants observed in the first stage have cross-resistance with all the fluoroquinolones. Conversely, after two steps the mutants do not have cross-resistance with the other fluoroquinolones and are resistant only to fleroxacin and ofloxacin. In these mutants the level of OmpF porins is still lower than that of *E. coli* TE-18. The inhibitory activity of DNA replication is weaker with Ro-23-9424 (IC_{50}, 0.8 μg/ml) in *E. coli* TE-18. Ro-23-9424 penetrates the *E. coli* TE-18 wall less well because of its high molecular mass (732 Da) and the steric hindrance due to the 2-amino-5-thiazolyloxyimino side chain.

The activity of Ro-23-9424 against class 1 β-lactamase-producing strains is probably due to its weak affinity for the enzyme, enabling it to cross the periplasmic space and bind to PBP.

Four mutants of *E. coli* K-12 possessing low-level resistance to Ro-23-9424 have been reported with a frequency of 10^{-10} to 10^{-11} CFU. These strains are resistant to fleroxacin and ciprofloxacin.

Strains resistant to ceftriaxone but not to fleroxacin do not have cross-resistance with Ro-23-9424.

The four resistant strains have a modification of their porins, either OmpF alone or the combination of OmpF and OmpC. For these four strains, DNA replication is not inhibited by fleroxacin or, in the case of two of them, by norfloxacin. The inhibitory activity of ciprofloxacin is unaffected. There are no modifications of the PBP and no increase in β-lactamase production.

7. PHYSICOCHEMICAL PROPERTIES

The 3′-esters are much less chemically stable than the other derivatives.

The degradation half-life of Ro-23-9424 varies with the biological medium used (Table 5).

In the case of plasma, this must be collected on heparin and separated immediately by centrifugation in an equal volume of acetonitrile. The protein sediment is removed by centrifugation and the supernatant is stored at −70°C.

Ro-23-9424 is slightly soluble in water, but the solubility increases at alkaline pH. At alkaline pH the molecule is unstable due to the lability of the ester bond. The alkaline solution is obtained with L-arginine sodium benzoate (Nickerson et al., 1995).

The degradation half-lives of other derivatives are shown in Table 6.

8. CEPHALOSPORIN-TYPE DERIVATIVES

The first molecule in which a cephalosporin and a quinolone were combined was Ro-23-5068 (Fig. 10). This involved a cephem of the 7-phenoxyacetylamino type and oxolinic acid (Albrecht et al., 1990). It was a molecule obtained by a 3′-ester-type bond. The degradation half-life of this product is 6 h.

Mice treated with oxolinic acid have been shown to exhibit more locomotor disorders than those treated with Ro-23-5068.

Table 5 Degradation half-lives of Ro-23-9424 according to the biological medium

Medium	Degradation $t_{1/2}$ (h)
Buffer phosphate, pH 7.4, 37°C	2.7
Mueller-Hinton	3.4
Rat serum CD-1 (37°C)	4.5
Beagle serum (37°C)	3.9
Baboon serum (37°C)	5.6
Human serum (37°C)	6.3
Whole rat blood CD-1	5.8
Whole beagle blood	3.4

Table 6 Degradation half-lives of codrugs

Derivatives	Degradation $t_{1/2}$
Carbamates	10 h
Tertiary amines	12 h
Quaternary ammonium	12.5 days

These good results directed the research towards other molecules, such as Ro-23-9424. Because of its modest chemical stability, and in order to increase the antibacterial activity and its solubility in water and to improve the synthesis process and the pharmacokinetic profile, other molecules with different bonds or different components were synthesized.

8.1. 3′-Ester Derivatives

The most widely studied molecule has been Ro-23-9424, but Ro-24-6392 has also been widely studied in vitro and in terms of the mechanism of action.

Ro-23-9424 is a codrug combining desacetylcefotaxime and fleroxacin. The two components are linked by an ester bond between the carboxyl group at position 3 of the β-pyridone nucleus and the acetoxymethyl chain at C-3 of the cephem nucleus.

8.1.1. In Vitro Antibacterial Activity

A number of in vitro studies with Ro-23-9424 have been published (Beskid et al., 1989; Gu and Neu, 1990; Jones and Barry, 1989; Qadri et al., 1993; Rolston et al., 1992; Spangler et al., 1993).

This molecule possesses a broad antibacterial spectrum, including gram-positive and gram-negative bacteria (Table 7).

Among gram-negative bacilli, Ro-23-9424 possesses good activity against class 1 β-lactamase-producing *Enterobacteriaceae*, in contrast to desacetylcefotaxime and cefotaxime. In this case it is more active than fleroxacin (Table 8).

It manifests little activity against *P. aeruginosa*, *Burkholderia cepacia*, and *Stenotrophomonas maltophilia*.

Ro-23-9424 is active against fleroxacin-resistant strains of *Enterobacteriaceae*.

Ro-23-9424 possesses excellent activity against *S. pneumoniae* irrespective of the profile of susceptibility to penicillin G, in contrast to fleroxacin, which is inactive (MICs, 4 and

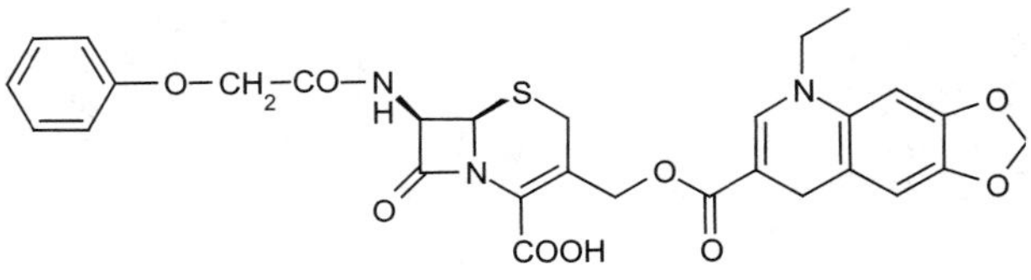

Figure 10 Ro-23-5068

Table 7 Activity of Ro-23-9424 against gram-negative bacilli

Organism(s)	MIC (μg/ml) 50%	MIC (μg/ml) 90%
E. coli	0.13	0.25
K. pneumoniae	0.25	0.50
P. mirabilis	0.13	0.25
P. vulgaris	0.25	0.25
P. rettgeri	0.06	0.50
Providencia stuartii	0.25	1
Providencia alcalifaciens	0.03	0.06
E. cloacae	0.25	2
E. aerogenes	0.25	0.25
Enterobacter agglomerans	0.12	0.25
C. freundii	0.25	1
Citrobacter diversus	0.13	0.13
S. marcescens	0.50	16
M. morganii	0.06	0.12
Salmonella spp.	0.12	0.12
Shigella spp.	0.06	0.12
Klebsiella oxytoca	0.12	0.5
Yersinia enterocolitica	0.12	0.12
Acinetobacter baumannii	1	2
Alcaligenes denitrificans	16	16
S. maltophilia	8	16
B. cepacia	4	>16
Aeromonas hydrophila	<0.03	0.12
P. aeruginosa	4	16
M. catarrhalis	0.12	0.25
Neisseria gonorrhoeae	0.12	0.25
H. influenzae ($\beta^+/\beta^-/S$)[a]	0.25	0.25

[a]β^+, β-lactamase producing; β^-, non-β-lactamase producing; S, susceptible.

Table 8 In vitro activity of Ro-23-9424 against cephalosporinase-producing *Enterobacteriaceae*

Drug	MIC (μg/ml) *S. marcescens* 50%	*S. marcescens* 90%	*C. freundii* 50%	*C. freundii* 90%
Ro-23-9424	0.06	0.12	0.12	0.125
Fleroxacin	0.5	>4	0.12	0.25
Cefotaxime	10	>16	0.25	0.50

8 μg/ml) (Table 9). Ro-23-9424 is more active than desacetylcefotaxime and is more active than a combination of the two separate components in a ratio of 1:1 (Spangler et al., 1993).

Ro-23-9424 possesses good activity against gram-positive cocci, except for *Enterococcus* spp. and coagulase-negative staphylococci, against which its activity is moderate. It is inactive against *Listeria monocytogenes* and weakly active against *Corynebacterium jeikeium* (Table 10). There is cross-resistance between Ro-23-9424 and ciprofloxacin in ciprofloxacin-resistant strains of *S. aureus* (Aldridge et al., 1992).

The in vitro activity of Ro-23-9424 against *Brucella melitensis* is moderate (MICs at which 50 and 90% of isolates tested are inhibited [$MIC_{50/90}$], 1.0/4.0 μg/ml) compared to that of rifampin ($MIC_{50/90}$, 0.25/1.0 μg/ml) and fleroxacin ($MIC_{50/90}$, 0.25/0.5 μg/ml). However, strains resistant to ciprofloxacin and fleroxacin are susceptible to Ro-23-9424 (Qadri et al., 1993).

Ro-23-9424 is inactive against *Bacteroides fragilis* (MIC_{50}, >32 μg/ml) and moderately active against *Clostridium perfringens* ($MIC_{50/90}$, 1/2 μg/ml).

Ro 23-9424 possesses activity identical to that of erythromycin A against *Legionella* spp. The $MIC_{50/90}$s are 0.08 μg/ml in buffered charcoal-yeast extract medium supplemented with α-ketoglutarate and 0.64 μg/ml in nonsupplemented buffered charcoal-yeast extract medium (Edelstein and Edelstein, 1992).

The selection of resistant mutants after a series of passages is similar to that of fleroxacin (Table 11) (Gu and Neu, 1990).

The proposed breakpoint is ≤8 μg/ml (Pfaller et al., 1993).

Table 9 In vitro activity of Ro-23-9424 against *S. pneumoniae*

S. pneumoniae phenotype	*n*	MIC (μg/ml) 50%	MIC (μg/ml) 90%
Pen[s]	49	<0.06	0.125
Pen[i]	38	<0.06	0.25
Pen[r]	83	0.125	0.50

Table 10 In vitro activity of Ro-23-9424 against gram positive bacteria

Organism(s)	MIC (μg/ml) 50%	MIC (μg/ml) 90%
S. aureus Met[s]	2	2
S. aureus Met[r]	2	2
Staphylococcus hominis	2	4
Staphylococcus saprophyticus	4	4
Staphylococcus haemolyticus Met[r]	2	16
Staphylococcus epidermidis Met[s]	1	2
S. epidermidis Met[r]	1	2
S. pyogenes	≤0.03	≤0.03
Streptococcus. agalactiae	0.13	0.13
Streptococcus group C	≤0.03	≤0.03
Streptococcus group G	≤0.03	≤0.03
Viridans group streptococci	0.5	4
E. faecalis	16	32
Enterococcus faecium	32	32
L. monocytogenes	16	16
C. jeikeium	2	2
Bacillus cereus	1	2

8.1.2. In Vivo Activity

See Beskid et al., 1990.

Ro-23-9424 is four times less active than fleroxacin in systemic infections due to methicillin-susceptible or -resistant *S. aureus*. Its activity is similar to that of cefotaxime (50% effective dose [ED_{50}], 5.6 versus 5.4 mg/kg of body weight) in

Table 11 Selection of mutants of Ro-23-9424

Microorganism	MIC (μg/ml) after no. of passages		
	0	5	14
E. coli	0.06	4	32
K. pneumoniae	0.25	4	64
S. marcescens	0.5	2	32
E. cloacae	0.5	16	128
C. freundii	0.25	4	16
P. aeruginosa	4	64	128
S. aureus	1	8	16

methicillin-susceptible *S. aureus* infections; cefotaxime is inactive in methicillin-resistant *S. aureus* infections.

Fleroxacin is inactive in *S. pneumoniae* infections. Ro-23-9424 and cefotaxime possess similar activities (ED_{50}, <1.0 mg/kg), while in infections due to *Streptococcus pyogenes* Ro-23-9424 is half as active as cefotaxime (ED_{50}, 8.8 versus 5.2 mg/kg). Fleroxacin is three to five times more active, depending on the species of enterobacteria, than Ro-23-9424, which is seven times more active than cefotaxime against class 1 β-lactamase-producing strains. Ro-23-9424 is weakly active against *P. aeruginosa* (ED_{50}, 60 mg/kg), in contrast to fleroxacin (ED_{50}, 8.9 mg/kg).

In *S. pneumoniae* pneumonia, Ro-23-9424 has activity similar to that of cefotaxime (ED_{50}, 12 mg/kg), whereas fleroxacin is inactive (ED_{50}, >100 mg/kg). In *Klebsiella pneumoniae* pneumonia, fleroxacin is more active than Ro-23-9424 (ED_{50}, 1.5 versus 41 mg/kg). In the immunodepressed mouse infected with *P. aeruginosa*, Ro-23-9424 is five times less active than fleroxacin (ED_{50}, 1.58 versus 32 mg/kg). In the nonimmunodepressed mouse, Ro-23-9424 is 10 times less active than fleroxacin (ED_{50}, 6.0 versus 6 mg/kg).

8.1.3. Pharmacokinetics in Animals

The plasma pharmacokinetics were determined in the mouse, rat, dog, and baboon. The pharmacokinetics of cefotaxime were used for comparison (Table 12).

In the baboon and mouse, Ro-23-9424 was shown to be the principal component of urinary elimination, but fleroxacin could represent between 20 and 30% of the product eliminated in the urine.

Slight accumulation has been found in the baboon. Some Ro-23-9424 is eliminated in the bile and hydrolyzed in the digestive tract. The fleroxacin released is then absorbed.

8.1.4. Pharmacokinetics in Humans

The pharmacokinetics were determined in humans after infusions of 250 and 500 mg for 1 h. At the end of infusion, levels in plasma were 6.2 and 9.1 μg/ml, with an apparent elimination half-life of between 0.7 and 1.7 h (Table 13) (Mould et al., 1991).

8.2. Carbamates

8.2.1. Ro-24-4383

Among the series prepared by Albrecht et al. (1991), the reference cephalosporin is that with the 7-(phenoxyacetyl)amino chain. This molecule has good activity against streptococci (MIC, ~0.125 μg/ml) but is devoid of activity against gram-negative bacilli, *S. aureus*, and *Enterococcus* spp. (MIC, ≥32 μg/ml). A number of other substituents have been attached to position 7. 2-Amino-5-thiazolyloxyimino derivatives with various substituents on the oxime residue and derivatives with a dioxopiperazine nucleus have been synthesized.

The best derivative in this series has excellent activity against *Enterobacteriaceae* but much weaker activity against *P. aeruginosa* (MIC, 1 μg/ml), *S. aureus* (MIC, 2 μg/ml), and *E. faecalis* (MIC, 4 μg/ml). The in vitro activity against streptococci and pneumococci is greater than that of ciprofloxacin, which conversely is more active against gram-negative bacilli.

The molecules are active against strains of *Enterobacteriaceae* which are cefotaxime resistant as a result of cephalosporinase production (*E. cloacae* P99, *Serratia marcescens* 1071, *P. vulgaris* 1082BC, and *Citrobacter freundii* BS-16, for which the MIC of cefotaxime is greater than or equal to 32 μg/ml).

In vivo, the molecule Ro-24-4383 is more active than cefotaxime in staphylococcal infections but less active than ciprofloxacin; it is more active in pneumococcal infections than the two reference molecules. It is 11 times less active than ciprofloxacin in *P. aeruginosa* infections (Table 14).

The molecules principally inhibit PBP, in some cases to a level similar to that of cefotaxime (IC_{50}, ≤0.1 μg/ml). They have little affinity for PBP 1a, 1b, and 2 of *E. coli* UB 1005 (DCO). They inhibit DNA replication, but to a lesser extent than ciprofloxacin, which can have 10 to 30 times greater inhibitory activity than that exerted by the codrugs. Ro-24-4383 penetrates the wall of *E. coli* as a single chemical entity.

Table 13 Plasma pharmacokinetics of Ro-23-9424 in humans

Dose (mg)	C_0 (μg/ml)	$t_{1/2}$ (h)	V(h)	CL_P (liters/h)
250	6.2	1.7	49	54
500	9.1	0.7	41	29

Table 12 Plasma pharmacokinetics of Ro-23-9424 (20 mg/kg intravenously) in animals

Animal	Compound	$AUC_{0-\infty}$ (μg·h/ml)	$t_{1/2}$ (min)	CL_P (ml/h/kg)
Mouse, CD-1	Ro-23-9424	7.4	13	2,796
	Cefotaxime	NA[a]	18	NA
Rat, CD-1	Ro-23-9424	19	17	1,063
	Cefotaxime	14	15	1,481
Beagle	Ro-23-9424	45	36	449
	Cefotaxime	41	43	488
Baboon	Ro-23-9424	75	75	268

[a]NA, not applicable.

Table 14 In vivo activity of Ro-24-4383

Organism	LD_{50}[a] (mg/kg) of Ro-24-4383	ED_{50} (mg/kg) subcutaneously		
		Ro-24-4383	Cefotaxime	Ciprofloxacin
S. aureus 753 Met[r]	6	28	>100	2
S. pneumoniae 6301	5,623	10	15	>50
P. aeruginosa 8780	240	33	>100	3

[a]LD_{50}, 50% lethal dose.

8.2.2. Ro-24-6392

The components of Ro-24-6392 are desacetylcefotaxime and ciprofloxacin, linked by a carbamate bond on the carboxyl group at position 3 of the β-pyridone nucleus (Fig. 11).

The molecule is more active than desacetylcefotaxime but less so than ciprofloxacin. It is active against strains of enterobacteria which are cefotaxime resistant as a result of class 1 β-lactamase production (Jones, 1990).

8.2.3. Oral Codrugs

Three series of derivatives have been synthesized (Sanchez et al., 1995; Vander Roest et al., 1995) (Fig. 12) with the aim of permitting oral absorption.

Three cephalosporins were selected: cefuroxime, cephaloglycin, and cephacetrile. They are linked to the quinolones by a carbamate bond. These molecules were esterified on the carboxyl group at position 4 of the cephem. The C-7 chain of the quinolone nucleus is either a piperazinyl nucleus or a 3′-aminopyrrolidinyl nucleus.

The in vitro activity is greater when the components are not esterified.

The most active molecules in vivo are those that possess an esterified cephacetrile nucleus.

Oral-bioavailability studies have shown that only one derivative of the cephacetrile type esterified by a pivaloyloxymethyl chain (PD-152915) (Fig. 13) remains intact after oral absorption in the rat, but not in the mouse (Table 15) (Saunders et al., 1995).

8.3. Secondary Amine Bond-Type Derivatives

Gray et al. (1995) synthesized a series of β-lactam–quinolones linked by a secondary amine bond (3′-aminopyrrolidinyl nucleus). The various compounds (Fig. 14) have good activity against gram-positive cocci and gram-negative bacilli. One derivative with a phenoxy nucleus on the C-7 chain of the cephem nucleus has good activity against *P. aeruginosa* ($MIC_{50/90}$, 0.5/2 μg/ml) but is inactive against *B. fragilis* ($MIC_{50/90}$, 60/32 μg/ml). The antipneumococcal activity is moderate, particularly against penicillin G-resistant strains ($MIC_{50/90}$, 1/2 μg/ml).

8.4. Tertiary Amine Bond-Type Derivatives

A series of derivatives with a tertiary amine bond was synthesized by Albrecht et al. (1991). These are chemically more stable than Ro-23-9424 but less active than the carbamate-type molecules.

Ro-25-0534 (Fig. 15) is a combination of a catechol-type cephalosporin and ciprofloxacin, linked by a tertiary amine bond. This molecule is active against strains of *Enterobacteriaceae* which are cefotaxime resistant as a result of cephalosporinase production. However, Ro-25-0534 is less

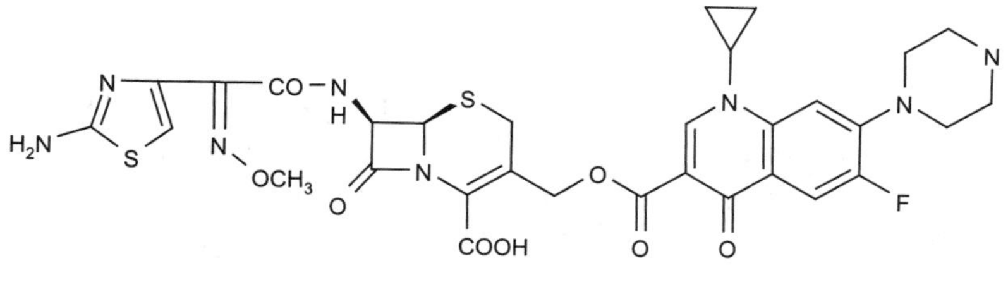

Figure 11 Ro-24-6392

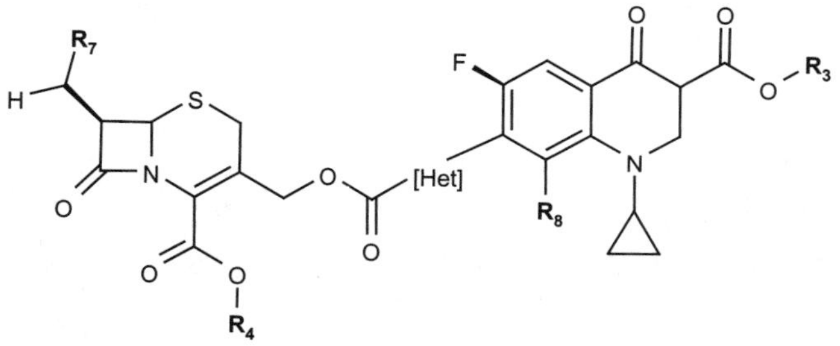

R_4 = H, ester
R_7 = Cefuroxime, cephaloglycin, cephacetrile
[Het] = piperazinyl, pyrrolidinyl
R_8 = H, F, Cl
R_3 = H, C_2H_5

Figure 12 Oral codrugs

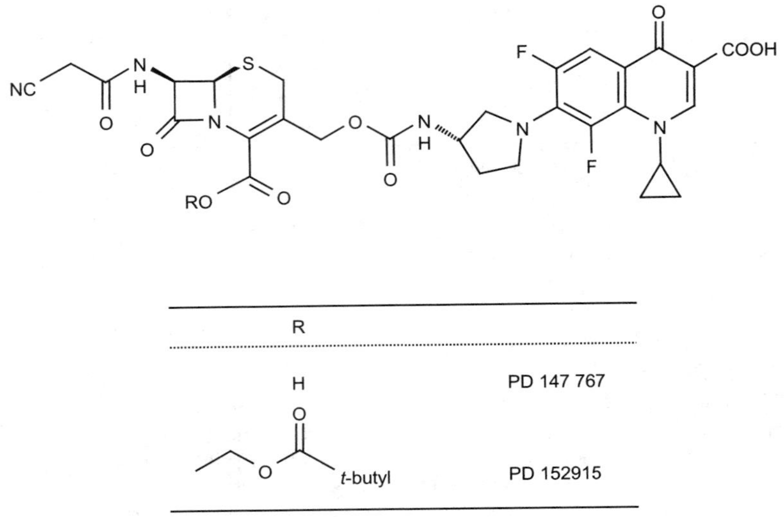

R	
H	PD 147 767
(ethoxy-carbonyl-t-butyl) t-butyl	PD 152915

Figure 13 PD-147767 and PD-152915

Table 15 Plasma pharmacokinetics kinetics of PD-152915 and PD-147767 orally (50 mg/kg) in the rat

Sampling time (h)	Concn in plasma (μg/ml)
0.5	0.14
1	0.09
2	0.04
3	0.14
6	0.22
24	ND[a]

[a]ND, not determined.

active than the most active component of the codrug. It is active against the extended-broad-spectrum-β-lactamase-producing strains of *Enterobacteriaceae*. Overall, it is less active than Ro-23-9424 (Jones and Sanchez, 1994).

Ma et al. (1996) synthesized a series of codrugs linked by a tertiary amine bond via a 3′-aminopyrrolidinyl nucleus. All the molecules prepared are inactive against *P. aeruginosa* and methicillin, and ciprofloxacin-resistant strains of *S. aureus*. They are generally less active than Ro-93-9424.

8.5. Thioester-Type Derivatives

A derivative of Ro-23-9424 has been synthesized with a thioester bond (Fig. 16). The bond is stable. At pH 10, it is four times more stable than the 3′-ester bond of Ro-23-9424 (degradation half-life is 200 versus 55 min). Its activity is similar to that of Ro-23-9424, but it is weakly active against β-lactam-resistant strains of *Enterobacteriaceae* (Keith et al., 1993).

8.6. Quaternary Ammonium-Type Derivatives

The fluoroquinolones have a reactive group on the carboxyl group at position 3 of the β-pyridone nucleus, but also on the primary, secondary, or tertiary amine, which may allow stable bonds to be established. For this reason, the cephalosporins are linked at position C-3′ to the fluoroquinolones via ammonium groups (piperazinyls and 3′-aminopyrrolidines) (Albrecht et al., 1991).

Six molecules comprising either pefloxacin (Ro-24-8138) or fleroxacin have been synthesized. These molecules differ in the chain attached to position 7 (Fig. 17).

The most active molecule is the combination of a 2-amino-5-thiazolylmethoxyimine chain and fleroxacin (compound 3). It is more active in vivo against *S. pneumoniae* and

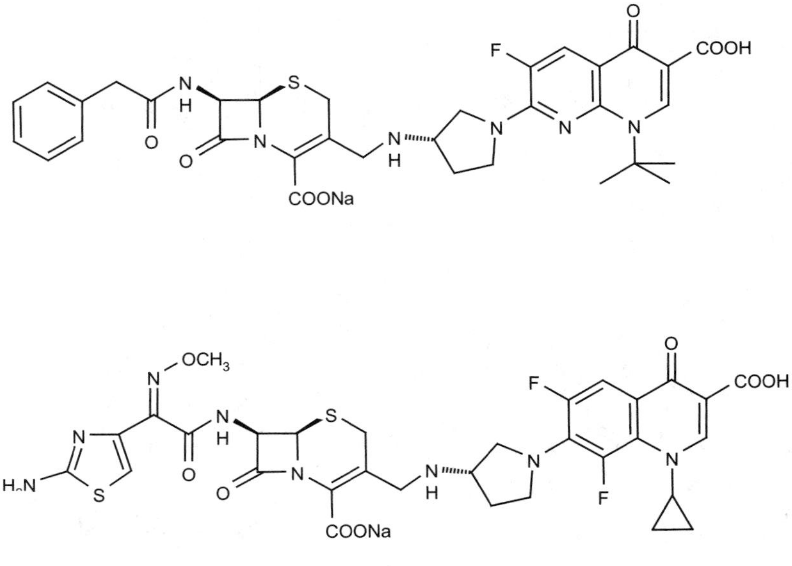

Figure 14 Quinolonyl-cephem secondary amines

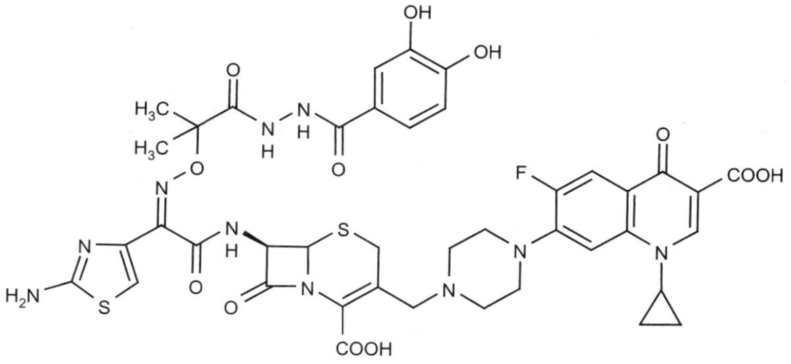

Figure 15 Ro-25-0534

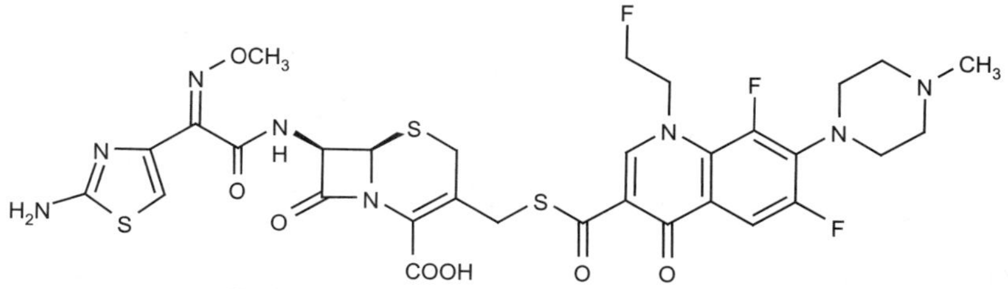

Figure 16 Thioester derivative of Ro-23-9424

S. pyogenes than is cefotaxime. It is inactive against *P. aeruginosa*, is more active than cefotaxime against *S. marcescens* SM, and possesses similar activity against *E. coli* 257. It binds to PBP 3 (IC_{90}, 0.1 μg/ml) but does not bind to the other PBP. It induces filaments. The MIC for *E. coli* is 0.2 μg/ml.

Derivative 2 is weakly active, as the 7-formylamino chain engenders weak antibacterial activity. The 7-phenoxyacetylamino derivative is moderately active, except against gram-positive cocci (streptococci) and *Enterobacteriaceae*. The other molecules are active against cephalosporinase-producing strains of *Enterobacteriaceae* (*C. freundii* BS-16 and *E. cloacae* P99).

Overall, they are less active than Ro-23-9424.

8.7. Dithiocarbamate Derivatives

Two series of compounds have been synthesized: those linked by a piperazinyl nucleus and those linked by a 3′-aminopyrrolidinyl nucleus (Demuth et al., 1993).

The cephalosporins either contain a thiophene nucleus and a 2-amino-5-thiazolylmethoxyimine chain, or the oxime

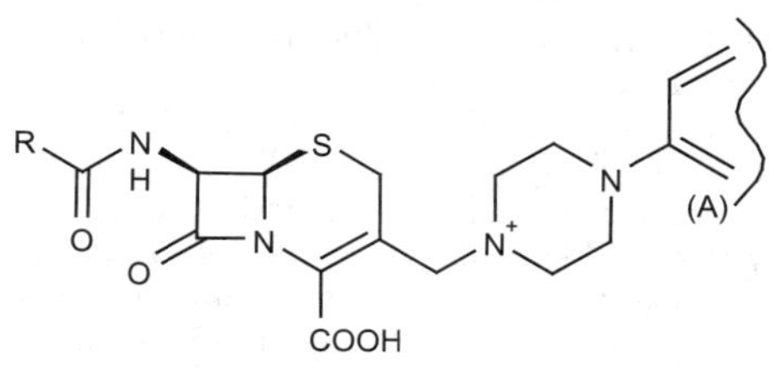

Compound	R	(A)
1	H	Fleroxacin
2	2-amino 5-thiazolyl	Fleroxacin
3	$PhOCH_2$	Fleroxacin
4	ATIBA	Fleroxacin
5	2-amino 5-thiazolyl	Pefloxacin

Figure 17 Quaternary ammonium codrugs

residue is substituted by an isobutyl chain. The quinolones vary according to the substituent at N-1: cyclopropyl or 2′,4′-difluorophenyl.

The piperazinyl compound (Fig. 18) has a 2-amino-5-thiazolylmethoxyimine cephalosporin. This compound is moderately active against *S. aureus* (MIC, ~1 μg/ml), weakly active against *E. faecalis* (MIC, ~8 μg/ml), very active against *S. pneumoniae* and *S. pyogenes* (MIC, ~0.008 μg/ml), moderately active against enterobacteria, and inactive against *P. aeruginosa* (MIC, ~16 μg/ml).

The other molecules containing a 3′-aminopyrrolidinyl nucleus are more active than ciprofloxacin against gram-positive cocci, including methicillin-resistant strains of *S. aureus*. They exhibit partial cross-resistance with ciprofloxacin against strains of ciprofloxacin-resistant *S. aureus*. They are inactive against *P. aeruginosa* and active against cephalosporinase-producing strains of *Enterobacteriaceae*.

The frequency of mutation of PGE-8335534 is low, on the order of 10^{-11} for *S. aureus* and 10^{-9} for *E. coli*. The bactericidal activity of this derivative against *S. pneumoniae* 9163 is good, equivalent to two, four, and eight times the MIC. It is moderate with *E. coli* ATCC 25922 and absent for *S. aureus* ATCC 29213 (Kraft et al., 1996).

8.8. Carboxamide Derivatives

See Johnson et al., 1996.

Two molecules have been prepared, the fluoroquinolone being enrofloxacin (CQ-397) or norfloxacin (CQ-414). They are attached to position 7 of the cephem nucleus (Fig. 7). The cephalosporin is a derivative with an *N*-methylthiotetrazole at position 3.

They are more active than cefamandole against *Enterobacteriaceae*, but less so than enrofloxacin (Table 16).

9. PENEM-QUINOLONE COMBINATIONS

Combinations of penems and fluoroquinolones have been synthesized with the various bonds described for the cephalosporins.

The chemical stability of the esters or carbamates of the penem-type derivatives is much greater than that observed

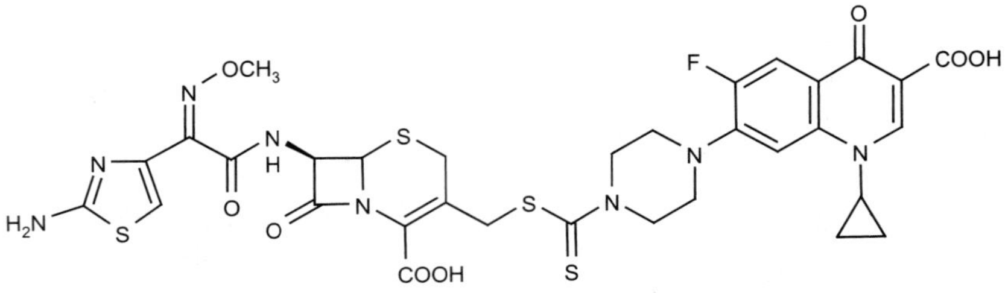

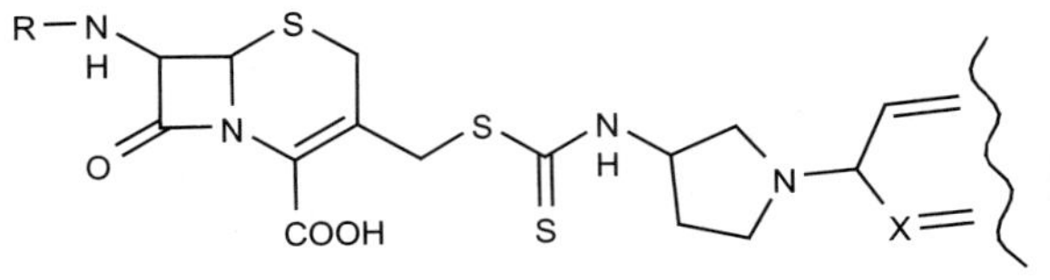

Figure 18 PGE-8335534

Table 16 In vitro activities of CQ-397 and CQ-414

Organism	MIC (μg/ml)			
	CQ-397	CQ-414	Enrofloxacin	Cefamandole
C. freundii	0.25	0.12	0.03	>32
E. cloacae	0.06	0.06	0.001	1
S. marcescens	0.5	0.5	0.12	>32
K. pneumoniae	0.12	0.06	0.03	1
P. aeruginosa	1	1	0.5	>32
S. aureus Met^s	0.25	0.25	0.056	0.5
S. aureus Met^r	32	32	4	32
S. pneumoniae Pen^s	2	1	1	0.06
S. pneumoniae Pen^r	1	1	0.5	2

with the cephalosporins. Their apparent degradation half-life is 64 to 81 h, which is similar to that of ritipenem, suggesting that the penem is hydrolyzed first of all. It has been shown that the C-2′ side chain is eliminated after attachment of the β-lactam to the enzyme.

The first molecule in this series was produced by attachment of an imine bond to a nitrofuran. Other derivatives in this series have been synthesized with different nuclei and ester-, ether-, carbamate-, and thioester-type bonds (Perronne et al., 1992).

In addition, the penems are stable against hydrolysis by class 1 β-lactamases and have the potential to be administered orally.

Compared with the reference molecules, there is increased activity against gram-negative bacilli but a loss of activity relative to that of fleroxacin or ciprofloxacin.

9.1. Ro-25-0447

A series of compounds was published by Corraz et al. (1992). This series comprises two types of penems: one without a chain at C-6 and the other with a standard penem chain. One of the series is of the carbamate type and the other is of the ester type. Ro-25-0447 and Ro-24-8705 are two molecules of the ester type (Fig. 19). Both are linked to a fleroxacin molecule by a 2′-ester bond with the carboxyl group at C-3 of the β-pyridone nucleus.

Ro-25-0695 is a penem attached to C-2′ by a carbamate bond to the piperazine nucleus of ciprofloxacin.

The codrugs are more active than the penem alone (Ro-25-1132) but less active than fleroxacin. They are inactive against *P. aeruginosa*, except perhaps the carbamate derivative (Ro-25-0695) (Fig. 20). Their activity against anaerobic bacteria is good, including against *Clostridium difficile* (Table 17).

Ro-24-8705, Ro-25-0447, and Ro-25-0695 are very stable at pH 7.4 in phosphate buffer at 37°C. Their degradation half-lives are, respectively, 16, 52, and 44 h.

They induce filaments in *E. coli* UB 1005. They bind principally to PBP 1a (IC_{50}, 2 μg/ml) and, more weakly, to PBP 2 (IC_{50}s of 30 and 10 μg/ml for Ro-25-0695 and Ro-25-0447, respectively). The affinity for the other PBP is weak.

Ro-25-0447 has very strong affinity for *S. aureus* ATCC 29213 PBP, but Ro-25-0695 has weaker affinity (Table 18).

The inhibitory activity of the three penems-quinolones against *E. coli* H560 DNA biosynthesis is weaker than that of ciprofloxacin or fleroxacin. For the derivative comprising ciprofloxacin, the inhibitory activity is 10 times weaker than that of ciprofloxacin (IC_{50}s of Ro-25-0695, 3 μg/ml, versus 0.3 μg/ml). It is only two or three times weaker when the constituent is fleroxacin (IC_{50}s, 1 and 2 μg/ml for Ro-24-8705 and 3 μg/ml for Ro-25-0447).

Ro-25-1132 (FCE 22056)

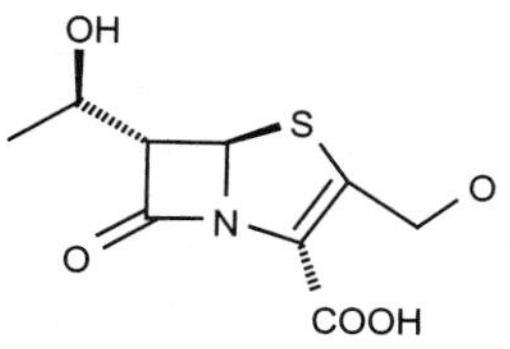

Ro-25-0447

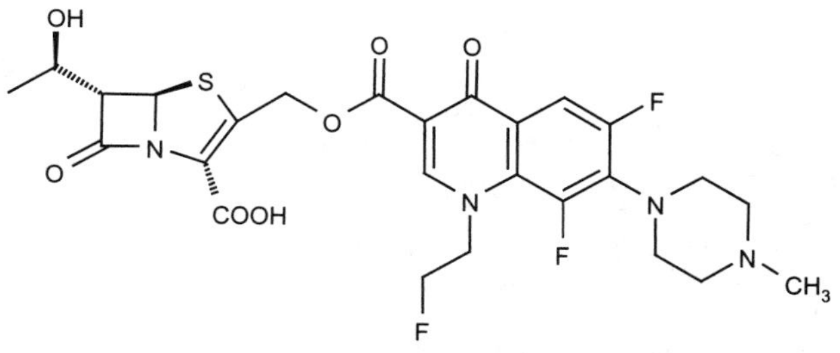

Ro-24-8705

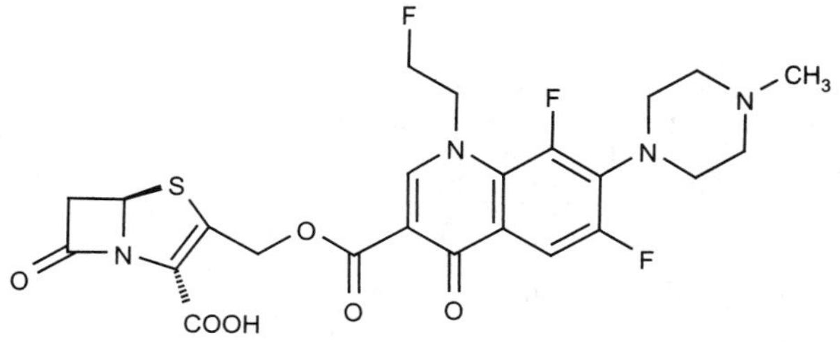

Figure 19 Penem-quinolone codrugs

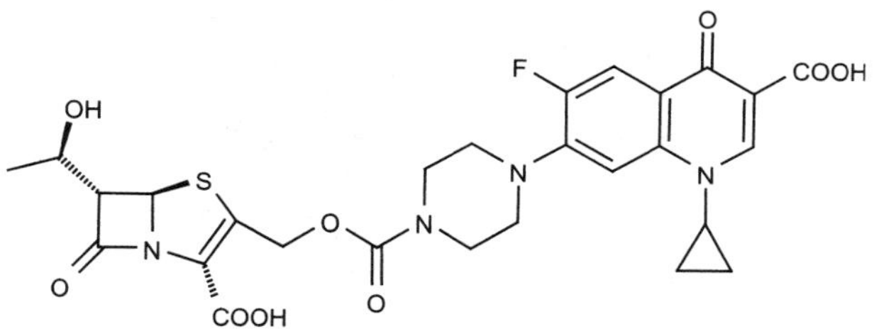

Figure 20 Ro-25-0695

The penems are hydrolyzed by renal dehydropeptidase, resulting in a loss of activity. Ro-25-0447 is less stable than imipenem against hydrolysis by porcine renal dehydropeptidase I (DHP-I). The hydrolysis rate is 2.3 nmol/min, and that of imipenem is 1.0 nmol/min.

9.2. Farmitalia Series

See Perronne et al., 1992.

A series of molecules comprising FCE-22056 (Ro-25-1132) as the penem combined with various fluoroquinolones has been synthesized with three types of bonds: ether, carbamate, and ester.

Table 17 In vitro activities of penem-quinolone codrugs

Organism	MIC (μg/ml)			
	Ro-24-8705	Ro-25-0447	Ro-05-0695	Ro-25-1132
E. coli 257	0.235	0.25	0.06	4
C. freundii BS-16	0.25	0.5	0.125	4
E. cloacae P99	0.125	0.5	0.06	8
S. marcescens SM	0.25	0.5	0.25	8
P. aeruginosa 8780[a]	16	16	2	64
S. aureus Smith	1	0.125	0.125	0.25
S. aureus Met[r]	2	2	4	1
S. pneumoniae	0.125	≤0.01	0.03	0.125
S. pyogenes 4	0.125	≤0.01	0.03	0.125
B. fragilis 52	ND[b]	≤0.125	16	≤0.125
C. difficile	ND	1	8	2

[a]Constitutive β-lactamase.
[b]ND, not determined.

Table 18 Affinities of penem-quinolone prodrugs for *S. aureus* ATCC 29213 PBP

Compound	MIC (μg/ml)				MIC (μg/ml)
	PBP 1	PBP 2	PBP 3	PBP 4	
Ro-25-0695	0.5	0.5	0.5	>100	0.125
Ro-25-0447	2	2	2	2	0.25
Ro-25-1132	30	>100	10	>100	0.25

As a general rule there is little or no activity against *P. aeruginosa*, except in the case of one derivative, and they are inactive against *E. faecalis*. There is moderate or no activity against *B. fragilis*. The activity against methicillin-resistant strains of *S. aureus* is moderate and varies with the molecule. The activity of all of the molecules against gram-positive cocci and *S. pyogenes* is good, as is that against enterobacteria, including cephalosporinase producers.

As a rule, it seems that the weaker the activity of the fluoroquinolone component against gram-negative bacilli, the weaker the activity of the codrug.

One derivative, FCE-26600 (ester-type combination with ciprofloxacin), has good in vivo activity in infections due to staphylococci (ED_{50}, 1.99 mg/kg), *E. coli* TEM-1 (ED_{50}, 0.66 mg/kg), and even *P. aeruginosa* ATCC 2598 (ED_{50}, 3.27 mg/kg).

9.3. Norwich Series (Procter & Gamble)

A number of derivatives have been synthesized. A first series contains penems linked by a carbamate bond to sparfloxacin or derivatives with a 3′-aminopyrrolidinyl at C-7. These molecules (Fig. 21) are more active than ciprofloxacin against oxacillin-susceptible strains of *S. aureus* and are also active against ciprofloxacin-resistant strains of *S. aureus*. Their activity is more moderate against methicillin-resistant strains of *S. aureus*. Overall they have excellent activity against *Enterobacteriaceae*, although the activity is inferior to that of ciprofloxacin. The activity against *P. aeruginosa* is good (MIC_{50}, 0.5 to 2 μg/ml), but they have cross-resistance with ciprofloxacin. The activity against *B. fragilis* is moderate. The activity of these molecules is not affected by the presence of broad-spectrum β-lactamases (TEM-1, SHV-1, etc.) and cephalosporinases (Rourke et al., 1993).

A second series of the secondary and tertiary amine types has been synthesized (Ma et al., 1996). The tertiary amine derivatives have good activity against gram-positive cocci, and some of them are active against methicillin- and ciprofloxacin-resistant strains of *S. aureus* (PGE-120208 and PGE-9565671; PGE-3941527). Some molecules are active against *P. aeruginosa* ATCC 25922 but have cross-resistance with ciprofloxacin (*P. aeruginosa* and *K. pneumoniae*). The activity against *B. fragilis* is moderate.

Hu et al. (1996) showed that some penem-fluoroquinolone codrugs with a carbamate bond possessed the same kind of antibacterial activity as that of the tertiary amines.

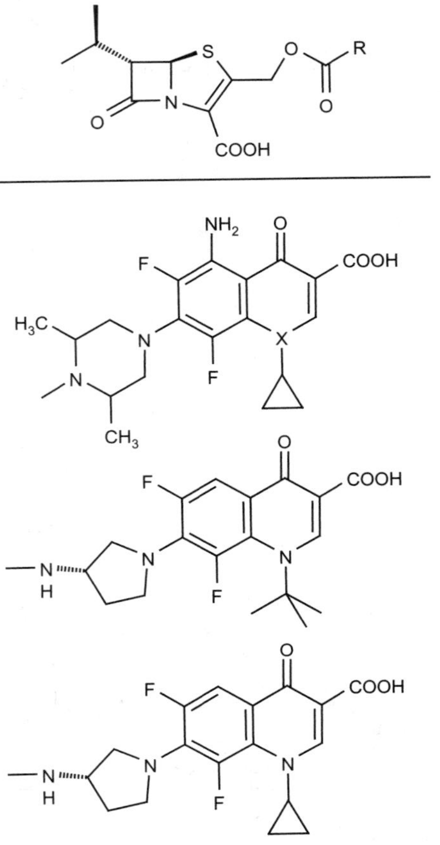

Figure 21 Procter & Gamble molecules (1993)

The pharmacokinetics of PGE-4924490 (ciprofloxacin plus penem linked by a secondary amine bond) in the dog and rat are summarized in Table 19.

10. CARBAPENEMS-FLUOROQUINOLONES

10.1. Series Synthesized by Hoffmann La Roche

See Corraz et al., 1992.

There are two types of carbapenems, 1-β-methyl carbapenems (Ro-25-0993) and those without a β-methyl

Table 19 Plasma pharmacokinetics (20 mg/kg intravenously) of PGE-4924490

Animal	$AUC_{0-\infty}$ (μg·h/ml)	$t_{1/2\beta}$ (h)	V (liters/kg)	CL (ml/min/kg)
Sprague-Dawley rat	27.7	0.29	0.37	16.23
Dog	51.4	1.50	0.78	6.77

(Ro-24-7341) (Fig. 22). Ro-25-0993 has a carbamate bond, and Ro-24-7341 has an ester bond.

Ro-25-0993 is the most active molecule against gram-positive cocci. It possesses excellent activity against *Enterobacteriaceae* and *P. aeruginosa* (Table 20).

It is weakly hydrolyzed by DHP-I (0.27 nmol/min) compared to imipenem. This activity is based on the presence of a 1-β-methyl group. It is less stable than the penems, with a degradation half-life of 5 h. The Ro-24-7341 derivative, which does not possess a 1-β-methyl, is slightly more stable, with a degradation half-life of 11 h, but is unstable against hydrolysis by DHP-I, with a hydrolysis rate of 37.5 nmol/min.

10.2. Carbapenems-Quinolones (Procter & Gamble)

A series of derivatives with a 2-thioether bond has been synthesized (Herschberger et al., 1996).

These molecules are weakly active against *P. aeruginosa* and cephalosporinase-producing *Enterobacteriaceae*. They exhibit cross-resistance with ciprofloxacin.

Analysis of the action of PGE-5428060 against the NorA protein of *S. aureus* shows that, unlike ciprofloxacin, this molecule is not expelled.

11. PENICILLINS-QUINOLONES

A series of penicillins linked by their C-3-carboxyl group to the piperazine nucleus of norfloxacin through a carbamate bond was prepared by Alex and Kulkarni (1995). These are cloxacillin or ampicillin (Fig. 23). These molecules would appear to have good activity against *S. aureus* and *E. coli* and variable activity against *Salmonella* spp.

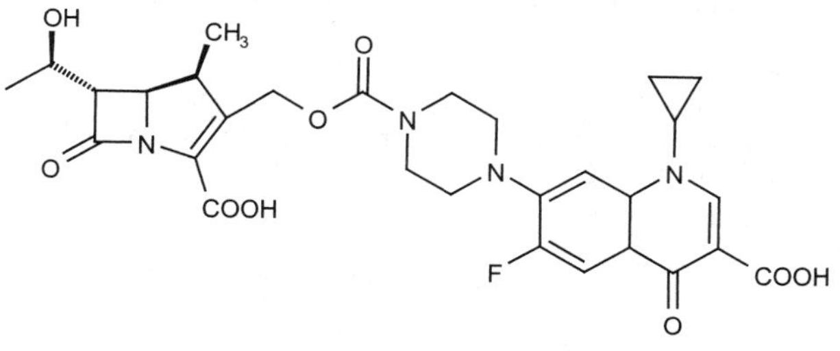

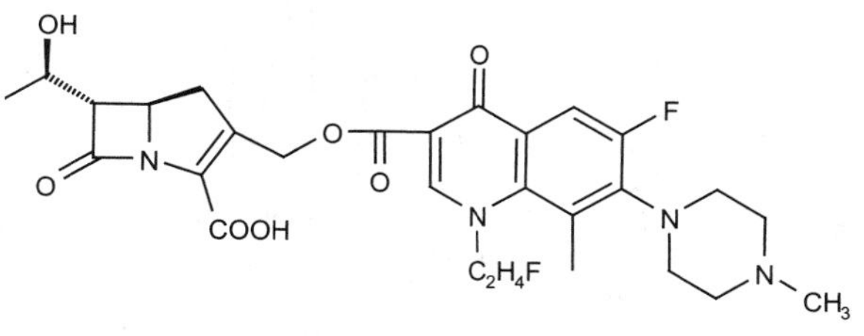

Figure 22 Carbapenems synthesized by Hoffmann-La Roche

12. MONOCYCLIC β-LACTAMS/QUINOLONES

A series of derivatives combining a monocyclic β-lactam and a fluoroquinolone (Fig. 24) has been synthesized (Zhang and Gao, 1996). Four molecules have been selected, but none

Table 20 In vitro activities of carbapenem-quinolone codrugs

Organism	MIC (μg/ml)		
	Ro-25-0993	Ro-24-7341	Ro-carbapenem
E. coli 257	≤0.01	0.125	0.5
C. freundii BS-16	0.06	0.25	0.5
E. cloacae P99	0.03	0.125	0.5
S. marcescens SM	0.06	0.25	1
P. aeruginosa 8780	0.5	4	32
S. aureus Smith	0.125	0.125	0.125
S. aureus Met^r	0.5	1	32
S. pneumoniae	0.03	0.01	0.06
S. pyogenes 4	0.03	0.01	0.06
B. fragilis 52	1	≤0.125	ND
C. difficile	4	ND[a]	ND

[a]ND, not determined.

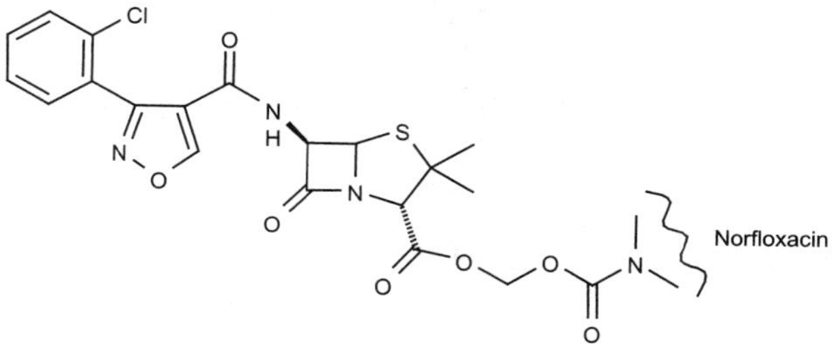

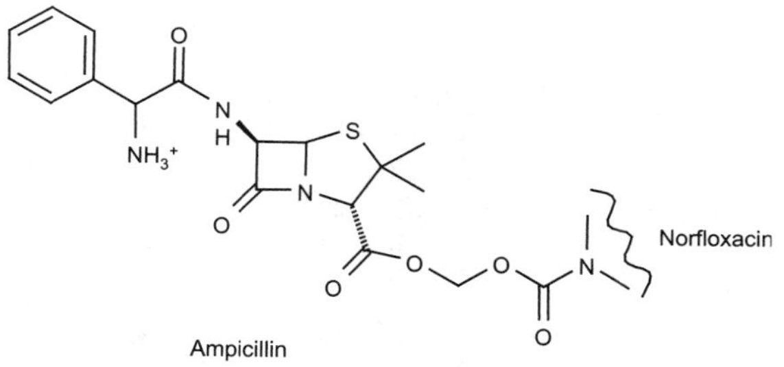

Figure 23 Penicillin-norfloxacin codrugs

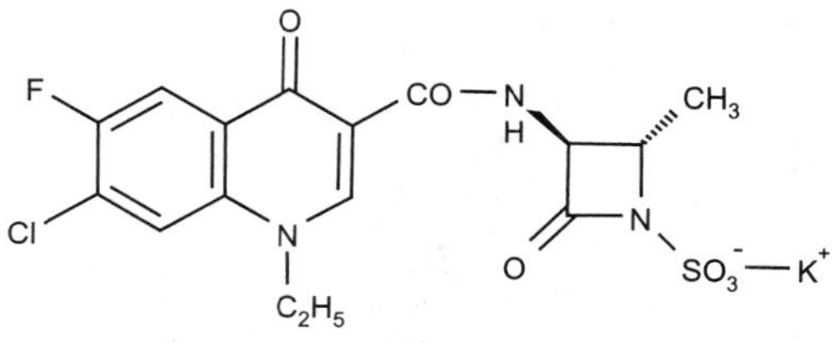

Figure 24 Monobactam-quinolone

possess activity against *S. aureus* 209 P, *B. subtilis* ATCC 6633, *E. coli*, *K. pneumoniae*, *S. marcescens*, or *P. vulgaris*.

13. OXAZOLIDINONES-QUINOLONES

A series of oxazolidinones with a spacer containing an amino residue was synthesized (Fig. 25).

MCB 1033, with 3-aminopyrrolidine as a linker, has a strong quinolone type of activity. It is more potent against gram-positive cocci than ciprofloxacin. It does not inhibit protein synthesis.

MCB 116 and MCB 2038, with a piperazinyl spacer, act primarily as inhibitors of protein synthesis, similar to linezolid. They display weak activity against DNA gyrase and topoisomerase IV. MCB 2038 shows an activity against *H. influenzae* and *Moraxella catarrhalis* (Table 21).

	Q	X
MCB 116	N N (piperazinyl)	CH
MCB 2038	N N (piperazinyl)	N
MCB 2038	NH (3-aminopyrrolidinyl)	CH

Figure 25 MCB 116, MCB 2038, and MCB 1033

Table 21 Antibacterial activities of oxazolidinones-quinolones

Strain (no. of isolates)[a]	Compound	MIC (μg/ml) 50%	MIC (μg/ml) 90%
MRSA (20)	MCB 2038	0.25	0.5
	MCB 116	0.25	0.5
	MCB 1033	2	2
MSSA (12)	MCB 2038	0.25	0.25
	MCB 116	0.25	0.5
	MCB 1033	≤0.03	≤0.03
MRSE (20)	MCB 2038	0.125	0.25
	MCB 116	0.125	0.5
	MCB 1033	0.5	2
MSSE (10)	MCB 2038	0.125	0.125
	MCB 116	0.125	0.25
	MCB 1033	≤0.03	≤0.03
E. faecalis (16)	MCB 2038	0.125	0.125
	MCB 116	0.25	0.25
	MCB 1033	0.5	1
E. faecium (20)	MCB 2038	0.125	0.125
	MCB 116	0.25	0.25
	MCB 1033	1	8
S. pneumoniae (23)	MCB 2038	0.06	0.125
	MCB 116	0.125	0.25
	MCB 1033	0.06	0.25
S. agalactiae (12)	MCB 2038	0.06	0.125
	MCB 116	0.125	0.125
	MCB 1033	0.5	0.5
S. pyogenes (11)	MCB 2038	0.06	0.06
	MCB 116	0.125	0.125
	MCB 1033	0.125	0.25
M. catarrhalis (12)	MCB 2038	0.25	0.5
	MCB 116	1	2
	MCB 1033	0.06	0.125
H. influenzae (10)	MCB 2038	0.5	2
	MCB 116	2	4
	MCB 1033	≤0.03	≤0.03
E. coli (14)	MCB 2038	32	64
	MCB 116	32	32
	MCB 1033	0.5	0.5

[a]MRSA, methicillin-resistant *S. aureus;* MSSA, methicillin-susceptible *S. aureus;* MRSE, methicillin-resistant *S. epidermidis;* MSSE, methicillin-susceptible *S. epidermidis.*

REFERENCES

Albrecht HA, Beskid G, Chan KK, et al, 1990, Cephalosporin 3′-quinolone esters with a dual mode of action, J Med Chem, 33, 77–86.

Albrecht HA, Beskid G, Christenson JG, 1991, Dual-action cephalosporins: cephalosporin 3′-quaternary ammonium quinolones, J Med Chem, 34, 669–675.

Albrecht HA, Beskid G, Christenson JC, et al, 1991, Dual-action cephalosporins: cephalosporin-3′-quinolone carbamates, J Med Chem, 34, 2857–2864.

Albrecht HA, Beskid G, Christenson JC, et al, 1994, Dual-action cephalosporins incorporating a 3′-tertiary-amine linked quinolone, J Med Chem, 37, 400–407.

Aldridge KE, Jones RN, Barry AL, Gelfand MS, 1992, In vitro activity of various antimicrobial agents against S. aureus isolates including fluoroquinolone- and oxacillin-resistant strains, Diagn Microbiol Infect Dis, 15, 517–521.

Alex RR, Kulkarni VM, 1995, Design and synthesis of penicilloyloxymethyl quinolone carbamates as a new class of dual-activity antibacterials, Eur J Med Chem, 30, 815–818.

Beskid G, Fallat V, Lipschitz ER, et al, 1989, In vitro activities of a dual-action antibacterial agent, Ro-23-9424, and comparative agents, Antimicrob Agents Chemother, 33, 1072–1077.

Beskid G, Siebelis J, McGarry CM, Cleeland R, Chan K, Keith DD, 1990, In vivo evaluation of a dual-action antibacterial, Ro 23-9424, compared to cefotaxime and fleroxacin, Chemotherapy, 36, 106–109.

Christenson JG, Chan KK, Cleeland R, et al, 1990, Pharmacokinetics of Ro 23-9424, a dual-action cephalosporin, in animals, Antimicrob Agents Chemother, 34, 1895–1900.

Corraz AJ, Dax SL, Dunlap NK, et al, 1992, Dual-action penems and carbapenems, J Med Chem, 35, 1828–1839.

Craig W, Andes D, Walker R, Urban A, Ebert S, 1994, Pharmacodynamic activities of a quinolonyl-penem carbamate (QD) in an animal infection model, 34th Intersci Conf Antimicrob Agents Chemother, abstract F-157, p 204.

Demuth TP Jr, White RE, Tietjen RA, et al, 1991, Synthesis and antibacterial activity of new C-10 quinolonyl-cephem esters, J Antibiot, 44, 200–209.

Demuth TP Jr, White RE, Tietjen RA, et al, 1993, Synthesis and antimicrobial activity of new, high potency C-10 quinolonyl-cephem dithiocarbamates, 33rd Intersci Conf Antimicrob Agents Chemother, abstract 1490, p 392.

Edelstein P, Edelstein MAC, 1992, In vitro activity of Ro 23-9424 against clinical isolates of *Legionella* species, Antimicrob Agents Chemother, 36, 2559–2561.

Georgopapadakou N, Bertasso A, Chan KK, et al, 1989, Mode of action of the dual-action cephalosporin Ro 23-9424, Antimicrob Agents Chemother, 33, 1067–1071.

Georgopapadakou N, McCaffrey C, 1994, β-Lactamase hydrolysis of cephalosporin 3′-quinolone esters, carbamates, and tertiary amines, Antimicrob Agents Chemother, 38, 959–962.

Georgopapadakou NH, Bertasso A, 1993, Mechanisms of action of cephalosporin 3′-quinolone esters, carbamates, and tertiary amines in *Escherichia coli*, Antimicrob Agents Chemother, 37, 559–565.

Gray JL, Shram GP, Gasparski CM, Wang AM, Ramberger NR, Davis BW, McKeever HD, Koenigs PM, Paule PM, Twinem TL, Kraft WG, Rourke FJ, Demuth TP Jr, 1995, Antibacterial activity of multifunctional quinolonyl-cephem 2° amines, 35th Intersci Conf Antimicrob Agents Chemother, abstract F-27.

Gu JW, Neu HC, 1990, In vitro activity of Ro 23-9424, a dual-action cephalosporin, compared with activities of other antibiotics, Antimicrob Agents Chemother, 34, 189–195.

Herschberger PM, Switzer AG, Yelm KE, et al, 1996, Synthesis and biological evaluation of 2-thioether-linked quinolonyl-carbapenems, 36th Intersci Conf Antimicrob Agents Chemother, abstract F-170.

Hu XE, Morgan JD, Herschberger PM, et al, 1996, Multifunctional quinolonyl-penem carbamates and their antibacterial activities, 36th Intersci Conf Antimicrob Agents Chemother, abstract F-168.

Johnson D, Erwin M, Jones RN, 1996, Antimicrobial activity and spectrum of novel cephalosporin-fluoroquinolone dual action compounds (DAC), CQEPCTM-397 and CQEPCTM-414, 36th Intersci Conf Antimicrob Agents Chemother.

Jones RN, 1990, In vitro activity of Ro 24-6392, a novel ester-linked co-drug combining ciprofloxacin and desacetylcefotaxime, Eur J Clin Microbiol Infect Dis, 9, 435–438.

Jones RN, Barry AL, 1989, In vitro activity of Ro 23-9424, ceftazidime, and eight other newer beta-lactams against 100 Gram-positive blood culture isolates, Diagn Microbiol Infect Dis, 12, 143–147.

Jones RN, Barry AL, Thornsberry C, 1989, Antimicrobial activity of Ro 23-9424, a novel ester-linked codrug of fleroxacin and desacetylcefotaxime, Antimicrob Agents Chemother, 33, 944–950.

Jones RN, Sanchez ML, 1994, Antimicrobial activity of a new antipseudomonal dual-action drug, Ro 25-0534, Diagn Microbiol Infect Dis, 18, 61–68.

Keith DM, Albrecht HA, Beskid G, et al, 1993, Mechanism-based dual-action cephalosporins, p 79–92, in Bentley PH, Ponsford R, ed, Recent Advances in the Chemistry of Anti-Infective Agents, The Royal Society of Chemistry.

Kraft WG, Rowke FS, Demuth TP Jr, Swift RA, Davis BW, White RE, 1996, In vitro activity of quinolonyl-cephem dithiocarbamates, 36th Intersci Conf Antimicrob Agents Chemother, abstract F-165.

Ma X, Davis BW, O'Hara TL, et al, 1994, Synthesis and multifunctional antibacterial activity of new quinolonyl-cephem 3°-amines, in 34th Intersci Conf Antimicrob Agents Chemother, abstract F-159, p 204.

Ma X, Hu XE, Davis BN, et al, 1996, Synthesis and multifunctional antibacterial activity of amine-linked quinolonyl-penems, 36th Intersci Conf Antimicrob Agents Chemother, abstract F-167.

Mobashery S, Lerner SA, Johnston M, 1986, Conscripting β-lactamase for use in drug delivery: synthesis and biological activity of a cephalosporin C_{10}-ester of an antibiotic dipeptide, J Am Chem Soc, 108, 1685–1686.

Mould D, Patel I, Ginsberg R, et al, 1991, The pharmacokinetics of Ro 23-9424, a novel antimicrobial agent, Pharm Res, 8, Suppl PPDM 8326R, p S-307.

Nickerson B, Cunningham B, Scypinski S, 1995, The use of capillary electrophoresis to monitor the stability of a dual-action cephalosporin in solution, J Pharm Biomed Anal, 14, 73–83.

O'Callaghan C, Sykes RB, Stanforth SE, 1976, A new cephalosporin with a dual mode of action, Antimicrob Agents Chemother, 10, 245–248.

Pace J, Bertasso A, Georgopapadakou N, 1991, *Escherichia coli* resistant to cephalosporins and quinolones is still susceptible to the cephalosporin-quinolone ester Ro 23-9424, Antimicrob Agents Chemother, 35, 910–915.

Perronne E, Jabes D, Alpegiani M, et al, 1992, Dual-action penems, J Antibiot, 45, 589–594.

Pfaller MA, Barry AL, Fuchs PC, 1993, Ro 23-9424, a new cephalosporin 3′-quinolone: in vitro antimicrobial activity and tentative disk diffusion interpretive criteria, J Antimicrob Chemother, 31, 81–88.

Qadri SMH, Ueno Y, Ayub A, 1993, Anti-Brucella activity of Ro 23-9424, a dual action antibacterial, Chemotherapy, 39, 386–389.

Qadri SMH, Ueno Y, Saldin H, Cunha BA, 1993, In vitro activity of Ro 23-9424, a dual-acting cephalosporin-quinolone antimicrobial agent, J Clin Pharmacol, 33, 923–928.

Rolston KVI, Nguyen HT, Ho DH, Le Blanc B, Bodey GP, 1992, In vitro activity of Ro 23-9424, a dual-action antibacterial agent, against bacterial isolates from cancer patients compared with those of other agents, Antimicrob Agents Chemother, 36, 879–882.

Rourke FJ, Davis BW, Kraft WC, et al, 1993, In vitro activity of two new quinolonyl-penem carbamates, 33rd Intersci Conf Antimicrob Agents Chemother, abstract 1489, p 391.

Sanchez J, Gogliotti R, Dax S, Albrecht H, Vander Roest S, Saunders J, 1995, Synthesis and antimicrobial activity of a series of dual-action cephalosporins (DACs) as potential oral agents, 35th Intersci Conf Antimicrob Agents Chemother, abstract F-24.

Saunders J, Bradford L, Guttendorf R, Gogliotti R, Sanchez J, Vander Roest S, 1995, Oral bioavailability of a series of new dual-action cephalosporins (DACs), 35th Intersci Conf Antimicrob Agents Chemother, abstract F-26.

Spangler SK, Jacobs MR, Pankuch GA, Appelbaum PA, 1993, Susceptibility of 170 penicillin-susceptible and penicillin-resistant pneumococci to six oral cephalosporins, four quinolones, desacetylcefotaxime, Ro 23-9424 and RP 67829, J Antimicrob Chemother, 31, 273–280.

Vander Roest S, Gogliotti R, Sanchez J, Saunders J, 1995, Synthesis and antimicrobial activity of new dual-action cephalosporins (DACs) as potential oral agents, 35th Intersci Conf Antimicrob Agents Chemother, abstract F-25.

Walling MA, White RE, Swift RA, et al, 1996, Pharmacokinetics and in vivo efficacy of quinolyl-lactam antibacterials, 36th Intersci Conf Antimicrob Agents Chemother, abstract F-169.

White RE, Demuth TP Jr, Berk JD, et al, 1993, Preparation and comparative antibacterial activity of quinolonyl-cephem amines and carbamates, 33rd Intersci Conf Antimicrob Agents Chemother, abstract 1491, p 392.

Zhang Q, Gao J, 1996, Synthesis of monobactam-quinolone amide derivative, Chinese J Med Chem 6, 262–268.

Coumarin Antibiotics: Novobiocin, Coumermycin, and Clorobiocin

A. BRYSKIER AND M. KLICH

29

1. INTRODUCTION

Antibacterial agents containing a coumarin nucleus might experience a resurgence of interest for two reasons: (i) their activity against methicillin-resistant strains of *Staphylococcus aureus* and (ii) their mechanism of action against bacterial topoisomerase II (DNA gyrase).

Novobiocin was the first antibacterial agent of this chemical class to be described. It was discovered simultaneously by three teams and for this reason bears several names. It was decided that the generic name would be novobiocin and the other names under which it has been published would be proprietary names: Cathomycin, Streptonivicin, Albamycin, and Cardelmycin.

Two other chemical entities have been described: the coumermycin complex and clorobiocin. The rubradirin complex constitutes a separate group within the coumarin-type derivatives. A semisynthetic derivative was described, RU-79115.

2. STRUCTURE AND PHYSICOCHEMICAL PROPERTIES

All of the derivatives have a coumarin nucleus (Table 1). They differ in the other molecular constituents.

2.1. Novobiocin

Novobiocin (Fig. 1) is an acidic substance consisting of three parts, A, B, and C: a central coumarin nucleus (B) (4,7-dihydroxy-3-amino-8-methylcoumarin), a benzene residue (C) (3-[3-methylbutenyl-2]-4-hydroxybenzoic acid), and a monosaccharide residue (A) (carbamoylnoviose).

Novobiocin was extracted from the fermentation products of *Streptomyces spheroides* and *Streptomyces niveus*.

Novobiocin is soluble in methanol, ethanol, butanol, acetic acid, and dioxane. It is insoluble in ether, benzene, and chloroform.

The acid form is insoluble in water, whereas the monosodium form is soluble.

2.2. Clorobiocin

Clorobiocin (Fig. 2) was isolated in 1972 from culture broths of several strains of *Streptomyces* from different species: *Streptomyces hygroscopicus* 9571, *Streptomyces roseochromogenes* subsp. *oscitans* 12976, and *Streptomyces albocinerescens* 21647.

Clorobiocin dissolves in dimethyl sulfoxide, dioxane, and acetone. It is moderately soluble in methanol and ethanol. It is insoluble in water.

Clorobiocin is composed of an 8-amino chlorocoumarin nucleus, a sugar (L-noviose substituted with a 5-methyl-1H-pyrrole-2-carboxylic moiety), and a benzoic chain identical to that of novobiocin.

2.3. Coumermycin

Coumermycin (antibiotic B4 620) (Fig. 3) is a series of five bacteriologically active derivatives extracted from the fermentation products of *Streptomyces rishiriensis* in 1956. The fermentation medium contains equal quantities of compounds A_1 and A_2 and small quantities of products B, C, and D.

Berger et al. isolated a complex of six antibiotics from *Streptomyces hazeliensis* subsp. *hazeliensis* called sugordomycins. Two products are identical to coumermycin A_1 (sugordomycin D-1a and sugordomycin D-1d). The other derivatives are sugordomycins D-A_b, D-1c, and D3.

Coumermycin A_1 is a molecule that contains two hydroxycoumarin nuclei linked by a 5-methylpyrroline nucleus. The two sugars are coumeroses (5-methylpyrrolenoviose). Coumermycin A_2 differs from coumermycin A_1 by the absence of methyl groups on the pyrrole nuclei.

Coumermycin A_1 is soluble in an alkaline but not an acidic medium. It is soluble in dioxane and acetone but is moderately soluble in ethanol, benzene, and chloroform. The mono- and disodium salts are soluble in ethanol.

Table 1 Physicochemical properties of coumarinic antibacterials

Compound	Empirical formula	Mol wt	pK 1	pK 2	Specific rotation	Melting point (°C)	LogP
Novobiocin	$C_{30}H_{36}O_11N_2$	612.63	4.3	9.1	$[\alpha]^{25}$-62	174–178	5.6
Clorobiocin	$C_{35}H_{37}ClN_2O_{11}$	697.14			$[\alpha]^{25}$-68	204–206	8.03
Coumermycin A_1	$C_{35}H_{59}N_5O_{20}$	1,110.09	6.0	>11	$[\alpha]^{25}$-141	258–260	7.88

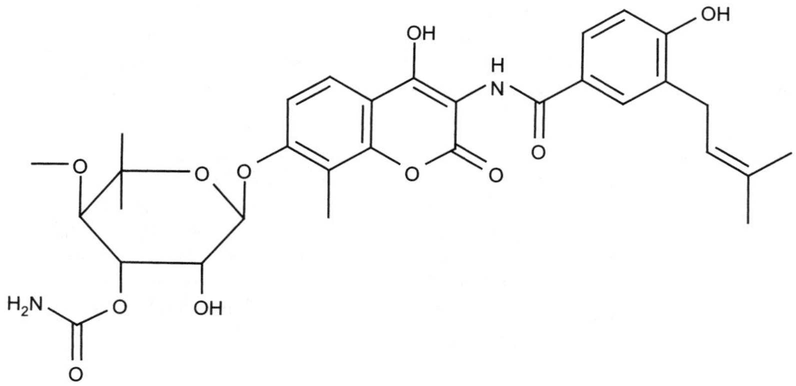

Figure 1 Novobiocin

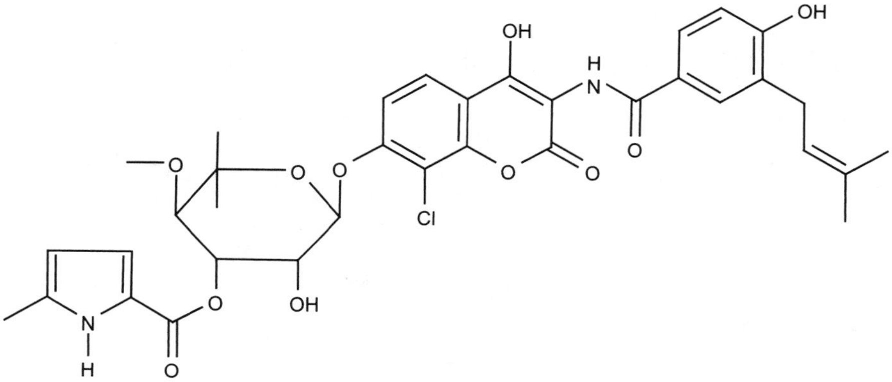

Figure 2 Clorobiocin

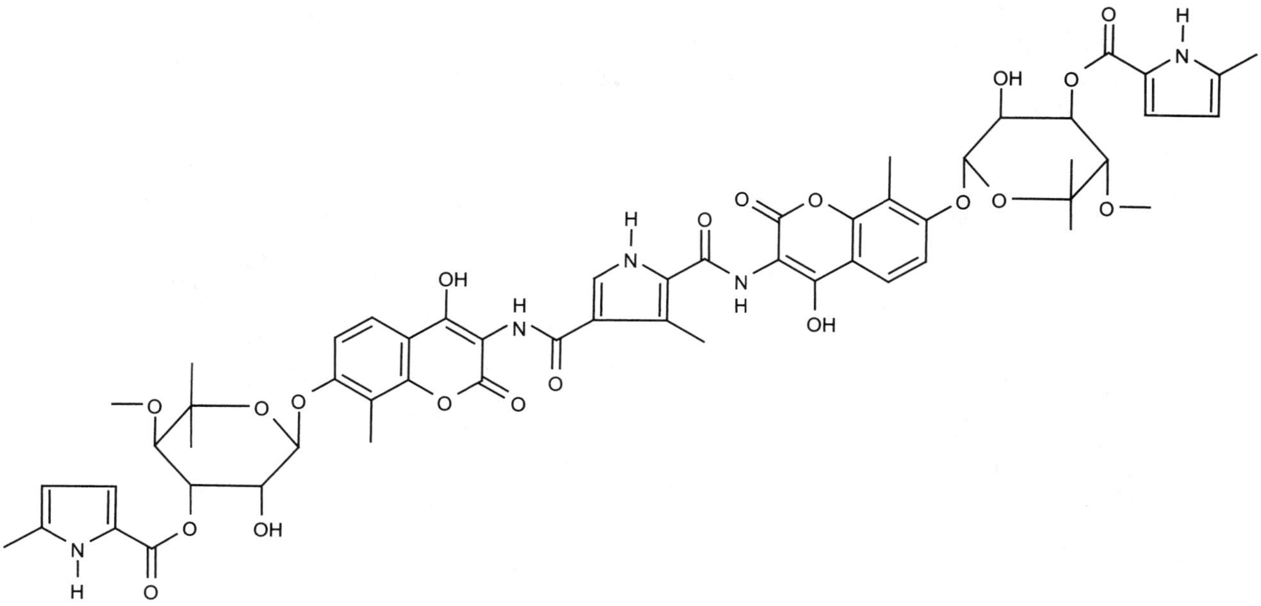

Figure 3 Coumermycin (*S*)

A number of chemical modifications have been made (Fig. 4).

2.4. Rubradirin

The rubradirin complex was isolated from the fermentation of *Streptomyces achromogenes*. The central nucleus of the molecule is a dipicolinic nucleus to which a large ansa is attached. The carboxyl group at position 6 forms an amide bond with a 3-aminocoumarin nucleus, substituted at position 4 by a nitro sugar, L-rubaniriose, the epimer of everniriose found in the everninomicins.

Four derivatives have been described, A, B, C, and D. Rubradirins B and C do not have sugars.

2.5. BL-C43

BL-C43 is a derivative of coumermycin A_1 obtained by semisynthesis and which has undergone partial development. It differs from coumermycin A_1 in the isobutyric chain attached to the coumarin nucleus (Fig. 5).

2.5.1. In Vitro Antibacterial Activity

BL-C43 is active against gram-positive cocci and bacilli and against certain fastidious gram-negative bacilli, such as *Haemophilus influenzae, Moraxella catarrhalis, Pasteurella multocida,* and gram-negative cocci such as *Neisseria gonorrhoeae*. It is inactive against *Enterobacteriaceae* and nonfermentative gram-negative bacilli.

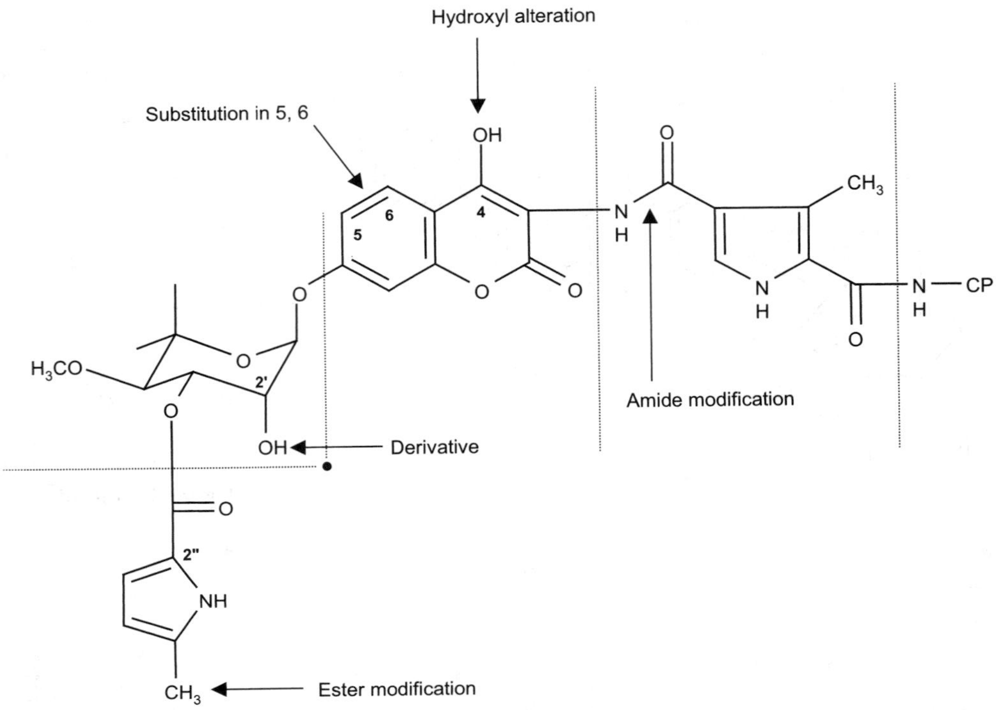

Hydroxyl alteration

Substitution in 5, 6

Amide modification

Derivative

Ester modification

Figure 4 Chemical modifications of coumermycin

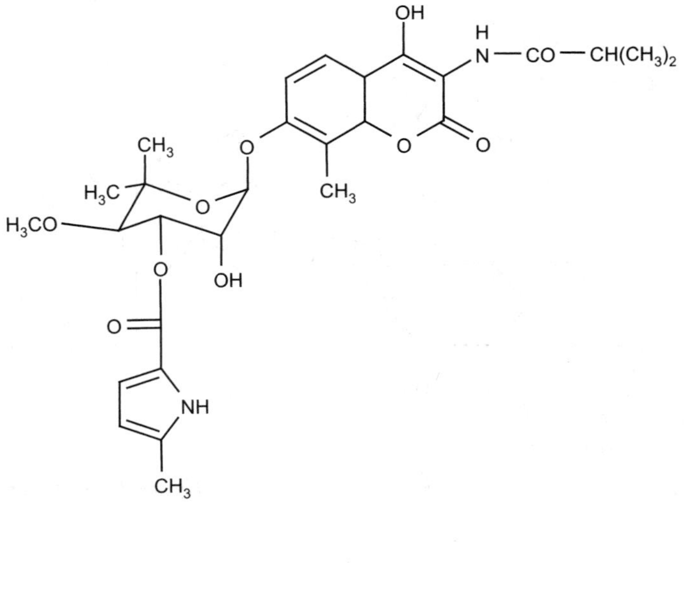

Figure 5 BL-C43

This molecule appears to be slightly less active in vitro than novobiocin, but it is more active than lincomycin or erythromycin A. These in vitro properties are summarized in Table 2.

The selection of resistant mutants of *S. aureus* A 9497 occurs more rapidly than with novobiocin. In the fourth passage, the MICs are 32 μg/ml (starting at 0.6 μg/ml) for BL-C43 and 8 μg/ml (starting at 0.6 μg/ml) for novobiocin.

2.5.2. In vivo Antibacterial Activity

In vivo in murine models of disseminated infections, BL-C43 is 3 to 10 times more active than novobiocin. The median protective doses (PD_{50}) against *S. aureus* infections are between 4 and 10 mg/kg of body weight.

The in vitro activities against *Streptococcus pyogenes* and *Streptococcus pneumoniae* are weaker, with PD_{50} of between 140 and 196 mg/kg. These are six times lower than those obtained with novobiocin. The in vivo activity against *P. multocida* is moderate (PD_{50}, 96 mg/kg).

2.5.3. Pharmacokinetics in the Mouse

After intramuscular administration of 25 mg of BL-C43 and novobiocin (sodium salt) per kg, the peak concentrations in serum were reached after 1 h. That of BL-C43 was double that of novobiocin (30 versus 15 μg/ml). The residual concentration of BL-C43 was 5 μg/ml at 7.5 h.

After oral administration of 25 mg of BL-C43 and novobiocin (sodium salt) per kg, the peak concentrations in serum were reached after 1 h and were, respectively, 11 and 9 μg/ml. The residual concentration at 12 h was 3 μg/ml for BL-C43, whereas novobiocin was no longer detectable after 9 h.

Doses of 6.25 to 200 mg/kg were administered orally to mice. The maximum concentrations in serum were proportional to the administered dose.

After an intravenous dose of 10 mg/kg in mice, the concentration was 6.5 μg/ml; after 4 h it was 4 μg/ml.

BL-C43 is weakly eliminated in the urine (<10%) in the mouse. The bile is the main route of elimination.

BL-C43 accumulates principally in the liver and very slightly in the lung tissues.

2.6. RU-79115

Intensive research was directed against coumarinic acid antibacterials by altering their chemical structure. In a series with various 5,5′-dialkyl noviose compounds (Fig. 6), a compound was selected for further investigation: RU-79115. The aim was to enhance the antibacterial activity of coumarinic analogs, but also to overcome hepatic toxicity of novobiocin and to improve physicochemical properties.

RU-79115 does not inhibit the UDP glucuronyltransferase which is responsible for the conjugation of bilirubin in the liver. No anti-vitamin K was recorded after oral administration of 30 or 100 mg of RU-79115 per kg.

RU-79115 is the 5,5′-spirocyclopentylnoviose analog (Fig. 7).

It was shown by analysis of gyrase B amino acid sequences from 12 gram-positive bacteria that enterococcal and streptococcal gyrase B activity could be influenced by 5,5′-dialkyl group of noviose in comparison to that of *Escherichia coli*. Their hydrophobic pockets consist of Val94 and Phe95, which is slightly larger than that of *E. coli* (Table 3).

RU-79115 has good activity against gram-positive bacteria irrespective of their susceptibilities to other antibacterials.

Table 2 In vitro activity of BL-C43

Microorganism[a]	MIC (μg/ml)
S. aureus OXA[s]	0.04
S. aureus OXA[r]	0.08
S. epidermidis OXA[r]	0.04
S. pyogenes	0.6
S. pneumoniae	0.16
E. faecium	2.0
E. faecalis	4.0
Listeria monocytogenes	2.0
H. influenzae	2.0
N. gonorrhoeae	2.0
P. multocida	0.25
E. coli	>128

[a]OXA, oxacillin.

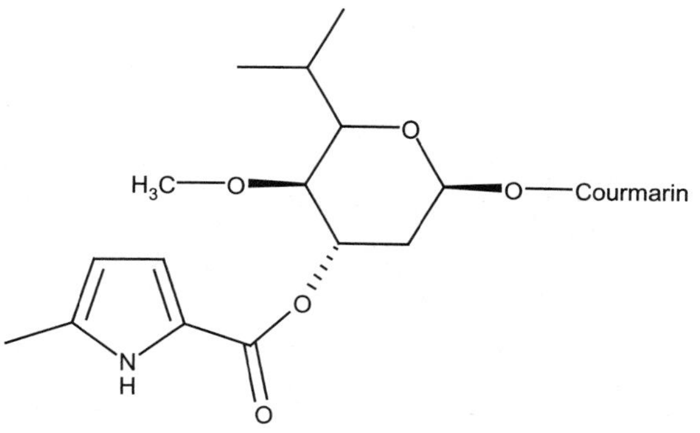

Figure 6 5,5′-Substituted L-noviose

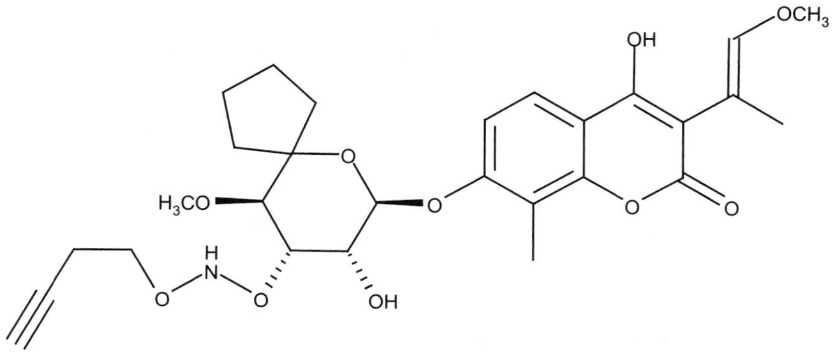

Figure 7 RU-79115

It is about 10 times more active than eperezolid, an oxazolidinone derivative, but it seems to be less active than vancomycin and teicoplanin against susceptible *Streptococcus* isolates (Tables 4 and 5).

RU-79115 is more active than eperezolid and vancomycin against *Streptococcus* species (geometric mean MICs, 0.06, 1.15, and 0.6 μg/ml, respectively).

RU-79115 is bactericidal against *Enterococcus faecium* Van^r, with a 3-$\log_{10}$ reduction at 24 h; bactericidal activity against susceptible *S. aureus* is reached after 12 h of contact.

Table 3 Amino acids at position 94 and 95 in the hydrophobic pocket from various bacteria

Position	Amino acid in:		
	E. coli	Staphylococci	Enterococci, streptococci
94	Ile	Ile	Phe
95	Met	Leu	Phe

Table 4 In vitro activity of RU-79115 against well-defined gram-positive cocci

Microorganism	Susceptibility[a]	MIC (μg/ml)
S. aureus O11HT3		0.04
S. aureus O11GO64	OFX^r, OXA^r, Ery^r	0.04
S. aureus O11HT1	Nov^r	1.2
S. epidermidis O12GOO42	OXA^r	0.04
S. pyogenes O2A1UC1		0.15
E. faecium O2D31P2	Van/TEC, Ery^r	0.15

[a]OFX, ofloxacin; OXA, oxacillin; TEC, teicoplanin.

Table 5 In vitro activities of RU-79115 against gram-positive cocci

Microorganism(s)[a]	*n*	MIC (μg/ml)[b]	
		50%	90%
S. aureus	91	0.08	0.15
S. aureus OFX^r	59	0.08	0.15
S. aureus OXA^r	66	0.08	0.15
S. aureus OXA^r OFX^r	47	0.08	0.15
Viridans group streptococci	25	0.04	2.5
S. pneumoniae	29	0.15	0.3
Enterococcus Van^r/TEC^r	17	0.15	0.3
Enterococcus Van^r	65	0.3	0.6

[a]OFX, ofloxacin; OXA, oxacillin; TEC, teicoplanin.
[b]50% and 90%, MICs at which 50 and 90% of isolates are inhibited, respectively.

Table 6 Pharmacokinetics of RU-79115 in the mouse

Route	C_{max} (μg/ml)	T_{max} (h)	$t_{1/2}$ (h)	*P* (%)
Intravenous			2.5	
Oral	5.4	0.5		62

In animal models, RU-79115 is more active than vancomycin and eperezolid against *S. aureus* (PD_{50}, 1 to 5.6 mg/kg) but less active against *S. pneumoniae* and *S. pyogenes* (PD_{50}, 30 to 40 mg/kg) and against *Enterococcus faecalis* and *E. faecium* (PD_{50}, <15 mg/kg).

Table 6 shows the pharmacokinetics of RU-79115 in mice at a dose of 10 mg/kg.

A metabolite has been detected in serum (Fig. 8).

The protein binding in mice is 75 to 90%.

3. STRUCTURE-ACTIVITY RELATIONSHIP

Novobiocin can be divided into two entities according to the presence or absence of noviose on the benzene chain (Table 7). Novenamine, which does not have the benzoic chain, inhibits DNA gyrase activity in the same way as novobiocin. However, novenamine is bacteriologically inactive, suggesting that it cannot penetrate the bacterial cell wall. Novobiocic acid has little affinity for DNA gyrase. This fraction appears to allow novobiocin to be transported inside the bacterial cell.

The substituent of noviose is an important factor in the affinity for DNA gyrase. The absence of the carbamoyl group suppresses any affinity. Coumermycin A_1 exhibits greater affinity for DNA gyrase than novobiocin. It differs in the presence of a 5-methylpyrrole nucleus instead of a carbamoyl group. The absence of the 5-methyl group reduces the activity fourfold compared to the activity of coumermycin A_1.

A number of semisynthetic derivatives have been prepared. The derivatives obtained by semisynthesis of coumermycin A_1 meet a dual need: an increase in the antibacterial activity and in the solubility in water and oral absorption. In fact, the weak hydrosolubility is probably partly responsible for its poor absorption and gastrointestinal irritability. It has been postulated that the large size of coumermycin and the lack of polar groups are responsible for this poor hydrosolubility.

4. IN VITRO ANTIBACTERIAL ACTIVITY

The coumarin derivatives include gram-positive cocci and bacilli in their antibacterial spectrum. They are inactive against fermentative gram-negative bacilli. The MICs are between 1.6 and 6.3 μg/ml.

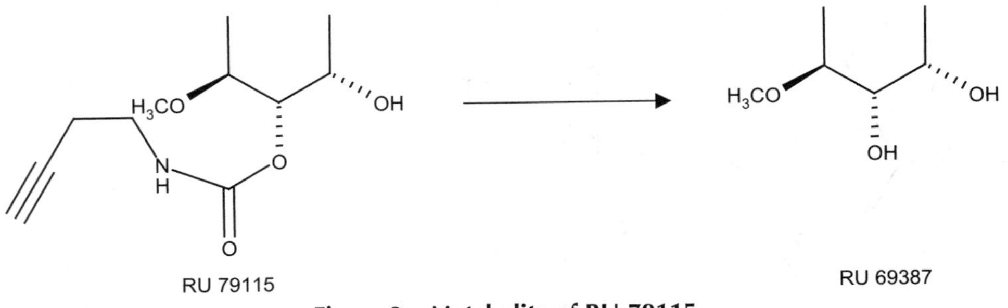

H_3CO OH N H O O — RU 79115 → H_3CO OH OH — RU 69387

Figure 8 Metabolite of RU-79115

Table 7 Structure of natural coumaric acid derivatives

Derivative	Noviose	Coumarinic moiety	Benzoic chain
Novobiocin	+	+	+
Novenamine	+	+	−
Novobiocic acid	−	+	+

Coumermycin A_1 is active in vitro against certain species of mycobacteria. Against *Mycobacterium tuberculosis*, coumermycin A_1 is active in vitro, with MICs of between 0.3 and 2.5 μg/ml, but it does not exhibit in vivo activity.

The antibacterial activity is summarized in Table 8.

The activity of coumermycin A_1 and novobiocin is affected by the pH of the medium, the size of the bacterial inoculum, and the presence of serum (Table 9).

The activity decreases in the presence of serum and in an alkaline medium.

Against *S. aureus*, coumermycin A_1 acts synergistically with fluoroquinolones, such as ofloxacin, enoxacin, and norfloxacin, but combinations with rifampin, nafcillin, and vancomycin are indifferent. Against *Staphylococcus epidermidis*, combinations with fluoroquinolones are indifferent. Coumermycin A_1 is more active than coumermycin A_2 (Table 10).

Table 10 In vitro activity of coumermycin complex

Microorganism	MIC (μg/ml)	
	Coumermycin A_1	Coumermycin A_2
S. aureus Smith	0.004	0.25
S. aureus Smith+serum	1.6	50
S. pyogenes	0.062	0.5
Bacillus subtilis	6.2	12.5
E. coli	12.5	>100

5. NOVOBIOCIN: LABORATORY TESTS

Coagulase-negative staphylococci may be divided into novobiocin-susceptible species (MIC, <1 μg/ml) and novobiocin-resistant species. The distribution in terms of human or animal origin and susceptibility to novobiocin is summarized in Table 11. For novobiocin-resistant strains, the activity is summarized in Table 12.

The determination of susceptibility by the antibiotic sensitivity test method involves disks with a dose of 5 μg. The diameters of zones of inhibition are between 16 and 36 mm for susceptible strains and less than 13 mm for resistant strains.

With disks containing 30 μg, strains are susceptible if the diameter is greater than or equal to 22 mm on Mueller-Hinton medium and 26 mm on Iso-Sensitest medium (Oxoid).

Table 8 Antibacterial activities of natural coumarinic acid derivatives[a]

Microorganism	Novobiocin			Coumermycin			Clorobiocin
	MIC	MIC_{50}	MIC_{90}	MIC	MIC_{50}	MIC_{90}	MIC
S. aureus Met[s]	0.05			<0.003–0.2	≤0.003	0.025	0.005
S. aureus Met[r]	≤0.03–1.0	0.12	0.25	0.001–0.08	0.0125	0.05	<0.04–0.3
S. epidermidis Met[s]	<0.04			0.006–0.8	0.0125	0.05	0.08
S. epidermidis Met[r]	<0.04			0.006–0.12	0.006	0.006	0.08
S. pneumoniae	1.6			0.5–6.3	0.2	1.6	0.03
S. pyogenes	1.6			0.8–3.1	1.6	3.1	0.3
Streptococcus agalactiae				1.6–3.1	1.6	3.1	
E. faecalis	2.5–5.0			3.1–12.5	6.3	6.3	2.5–5.0
L. monocytogenes				0.05–0.8	0.2	0.8	
Bacillus cereus	6.2			6.2			
Corynebacterium jeikeium				0.4–1.6	1.6	1.6	
M. catarrhalis							0.005
H. influenzae	1.0			0.04–3.12			
E. faecium	0.6			1.95	3.9		
Bacillus anthracis	2.0			3.9			2.5–2.0
Clostridium perfringens	1.0			0.1			
N. gonorrhoeae	1.0–4.0			0.0004			0.4
Neisseria meningitidis							0.05

Table 9 Factors affecting in vitro activity against *S. aureus* 209P

Compound	MIC (μg/ml)					
	Medium		Inoculum size (CFU/ml)		Serum	
	pH 6	pH 8	5×10^5	5×10^6	0%	50%
Novobiocin	0.0125	0.4	0.1	0.4	0.05	3.2
Coumermycin A_1	0.00015	0.16	0.005	0.1	0.0025	0.16

Table 11 Distribution of species of coagulase-negative staphylococci

Novobiocin resistance phenotype	Staphylococci in:		
	Humans	Humans and animals	Animals
Susceptible (MIC, <1.0 μg/ml)	*Staphylococcus auricularis* *Staphylococcus capitis* *Staphylococcus hominis* *Staphylococcus saccharolyticus*	*S. epidermidis* *Staphylococcus haemolyticus* *Staphylococcus simulans* *Staphylococcus warneri*	*Staphylococcus caprae* *Staphylococcus carnosus* *Staphylococcus caseolyticus* *S. hyicus* subsp. *chromogenes* and *Staphylococcus hyicus* subsp. *hyicus*
Resistant (MIC, >1.0 μg/ml)	*Staphylococcus cohnii* *Staphylococcus saprophyticus* *Staphylococcus xylosus* *Staphylococcus kloosii* *Staphylococcus lentus* *Staphylococcus sciuri*	*Staphylococcus arlettae* *Staphylococcus equorum* *Staphylococcus gallinarum*	

Table 12 Activity of novobiocin against coagulase-negative staphylococci

Microorganism	MIC (μg/ml)
S. arlettae	8.0
S. cohnii	3.1–12.5
S. equorum	16.0
S. gallinarum	4.0–32
S. kloosii	16–64
S. lentus	1.6–12.5
S. saprophyticus	3.16–12.5
S. sciuri	1.6–12.5
S. xylosus	1.6–12.5

6. MECHANISM OF ACTION

The coumarin derivatives act on DNA gyrase subunit B after penetrating the bacterial cell wall.

DNA gyrase is an enzyme that catalyzes negative DNA supercoiling of prokaryotic cells.

The *E. coli* enzyme is a tetramer composed of two A subunits of 97 kDa and two B subunits of 90 kDa, as for all prokaryotes.

Novobiocin binds to a 24-kDa protein fraction of the B subunit.

6.1. 43-kDa Protein Fragment

The 43-kDa fragment comprises two distinct crystallographic domains. This fragment is between amino acids 2 and 393.

Domain 1 is between amino acid residues 2 and 220 and contains the ATP binding site (24-kDa fragment). Domain 2 is between amino acid residues 221 and 393. This protein contains a number of arginine residues, particularly in the C-terminal part.

The 43-kDa fragment is a dimer. The majority of contacts between the molecules constituting the dimer occur from the N-terminal part (amino acids 2 to 15), which projects from the surface of the monomer and coils around domain 1 of the other subunit.

6.2. ATP Binding Site

ATP binds to lysine 102 via a β-phosphate. Magnesium plays an important role in this bond through asparagine 46. There is also an interaction between an ATP γ-phosphate and lysine 337 and glutamic acid 335 of domain 2. This contact between ATP and the domain is necessary for the hydrolysis of ATP. ATP binds to tyrosine 109 and N-3 of the adenine nucleus. The DNA strand crosses through this protein in a tunnel with a 20-Å diameter (the diameter of the DNA helix is 20 Å). The arginine-rich C-terminal part forms the floor of the canal. These residues form a binding site for DNA within the tunnel. The N-terminal part contains ATP and the binding sites of the coumarin derivatives.

6.3. Interactions Between the A and B Subunits

The first step is the binding of the enzyme to DNA, forming a complex that coils around 120 DNA base pairs. The second step is the cleavage of DNA into two strands with the formation of covalent bridges between the 5′-phosphate group and tyrosine 122 of the A subunit. The following step causes a structural modification, allowing the passage of a DNA strand through the protein. This stage requires the presence of ATP, which stabilizes the interactions between the domains of the N-terminal part of the β subunit.

Novobiocin binds to the 24-kDa protein fragment and stabilizes the structure so as to prevent the binding of triphosphate nucleosides. This reduces the pool of available enzymes and inhibits the hydrolysis of ATP.

A mutation point on arginine 136 (Arg136→His) causes resistance to the coumarin derivatives. The same applies to a mutation on glycine 164. This glycine-rich region is similar to that of the ATP binding site.

In summary, the DNA gyrase A subunit binds and temporarily cleaves the two DNA strands, while the B subunit, which is attached to the A subunit and to the DNA, allows supercoiling by hydrolyzing ATP (Fig. 9). The catalytic site of the hydrolysis of ATP is functional only if the B subunit is in a dimerized form. In fact, each B subunit of this dimer provides a tyrosine located on the N-terminal part, allowing the hydrolysis of ATP. The coumarin derivatives entirely occupy the site of this tyrosine and partially the neighboring ATP site. They prevent ATP from penetrating and the two subunits from dimerizing. The attachment of novobiocin to the receptor site is illustrated in Fig. 10.

The DNA gyrase-inhibitory activity of the dicoumarin derivatives is summarized in Table 13.

6.4. Binding Site of the Coumarin Derivatives

The binding sites of ATP and the coumarin derivatives are similar and overlap. It has been shown that all of the

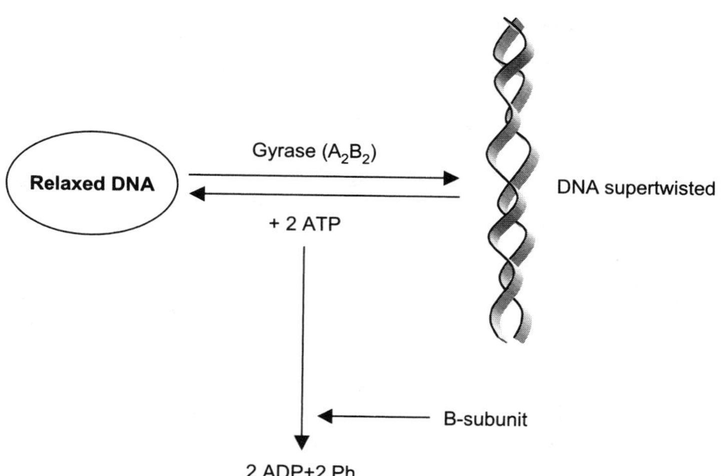

Figure 9 DNA supercoiling: action of DNA gyrase

Figure 10 Attachment of novobiocin and others to the 24-kDa fragment of gyrase B

Table 13 DNA gyrase-inhibitory activity

Compound	IC_{50}[a] (μg/ml)
Novobiocin	1.0
Noveamine	
Novobiocic acid	>77
Decarbamoyl novobiocin	>210
Coumermycin A_1	0.17–0.28
Clorobiocin	0.44

[a]IC_{50}, 50% inhibitory concentration.

mutation points on the B subunit cause resistance to novobiocin when they are located on the 24-kDa fragment of gyrase B. Binding to a loop of 98 to 120 amino acids on the 24-kDa fragment occurs. Noviose and the pyrrole nucleus of clorobiocin are superimposed, respectively, on the adenine and ribose of ATP, whereas coumarin and the isopentenyl chain are close to the terminal nucleotide bond. They are also close to proline 79, thus reducing the hydrophobic surface area of the molecule and allowing hydrophobic bonds with the protein. The most important interactions are the hydrogen bond between arginine 136 and the oxygen of the 2-carbonyl of the coumarin nucleus (2.9 Å). The other important hydrogen bonds are those linking the 2′-hydroxyl group of the noviose and the oxygen of the carbonyl of asparagine 46 (2.7 Å) and those existing between the amino group of the pyrrole nucleus and asparagine 73 (2.8 Å). The hydrophobic pocket is composed of valines 43, 71, and 167 and isoleucine 78, located between alanine 47 and tyrosine 165.

There are other hydrophobic bonds between the coumarin nucleus and the isopentanyl group of clorobiocin, such as Arg76, Ile78, and Ile94 (Fig. 11).

6.5. Novobiocin Binds to Chaperonin Hsp90

Hsp90 is a chaperonin responsible for conformational maturation of nascent polypeptides into biologically active three-dimensional structures. ATP is bound in an unusual bent conformation like Hsp90. Novobiocin binds to a similarly shaped ATP binding site in DNA gyrase and has cytotoxicity

Figure 11 Interactions with the hydrophobic pocket of DNA gyrase B

in cancer cell lines. It was shown that novobiocin binds to Hsp90—not to the N-terminal region but to an unrecognized portion of the C-terminal region.

7. TOXICOLOGY

The lethal doses are summarized in Table 14.

Novobiocin is responsible for unconjugated-bilirubin jaundice. The main characteristics of the jaundice caused by bilirubin are as follows. The jaundice is due to a predominant or exclusive increase in unconjugated bilirubin. It is not accompanied by signs of hepatic insufficiency, and there is no hyperhemolysis. The jaundice disappears within 4 days of the discontinuation of treatment.

Novobiocin acts by temporary inhibition of hepatic bilirubin glucuronyltransferase.

8. PHARMACOKINETICS

8.1. Pharmacokinetics of Novobiocin

Novobiocin is well absorbed by the gastrointestinal tract. After a dose of 500 mg, the peak concentration in serum, on average 10 to 20 μg/ml, is reached in 1 to 4 h. Therapeutic levels are present at 24 h. Following a dose of 500 mg, Drusano et al. obtained a peak concentration in serum of 62.5 ± 13.4 μg/ml (mean ± standard deviation) in 2.0 ± 1.0 h, with an apparent elimination half-life of 5.85 ± 1.2 h. The area under the curve is 407 ± 102 μg·h/ml and the elimination rate constant is 0.123 ± 0.023 h^{-1}. Novobiocin is 90% albumin bound. Less than 3% of the administered dose is eliminated in the urine; the drug is mainly eliminated in the bile. Concentrations in the feces are high.

Table 14 Acute toxicities of coumarin derivatives

Compound	Route of administration[a]	50% Lethal dose for mice (mg/kg)
Coumermycin A_1	p.o.	2,500
	s.c.	250–380
	i.p.	150–183
	i.m.	500
	i.v.	25
Clorobiocin	p.o.	2,200
	s.c.	1,700

[a]p.o., per os; s.c., subcutaneously; i.p., intraperitoneally; i.m., intramuscularly; i.v., intravenously.

8.2. Pharmacokinetics of Coumermycin A_1

Absorption of coumermycin A_1 is weak but may be increased by administration with a mixture of *N*-methylglucosamine in a ratio of 1:4 (20 mol of *N*-methylglucosamine to 1 mol of antibiotic). The peak concentration in serum is on the order of 1 μg/ml following a dose of 4 to 5 mg/kg. Concentrations are undetectable at 4 to 6 h. The apparent elimination half-life is on the order of 8 to 10 h.

8.3. Tissue Concentration

Novobiocin is distributed in a number of tissues, but not the cerebrospinal fluid. After administration of 2.0 g, novobiocin levels in pleural fluid are 1.6 to 12.8 μg/ml and those in ascites fluid are 0.4 to 51.2 μg/ml.

Novobiocin is eliminated in the bile. After administration of 500 mg, biliary levels are 3.2 and 9.6 μg/ml at 2 and 4 h, respectively.

ADDITIONAL BIBLIOGRAPHY

Drusano GL, Townsend RJ, Walsh TJ, Forrest A, Antal EJ, Standiford HC, 1986, Steady-state serum pharmacokinetics of novobiocin and rifampin alone and in combination, Antimicrob Agents Chemother, 30, 42–45.

Ferroud D, Collard J, Klich M, Dupuis-Hamelin C, Mauvais P, Lassaigne P, Bonnefoy A, Musicki B, 1999, Synthesis and biological evaluation of coumarin carboxylic acids as inhibitors of gyrase B: L-rhamnose as an effective substitute for L-noviose, Bioorg Med Chem Lett, 9, 2881–2886.

Galm U, Heller S, Shapiro S, Page M, Li S-M, Heide L, 2004, Antimicrobial and DNA gyrase-inhibitory activities of novel clorobiocin derivatives produced by mutasynthesis, Antimicrob Agents Chemother, 48, 1307–1312.

Laurin P, Ferroud D, Klich M, Dupuis-Hamelin C, Mauvais P, Lassaigne P, Bonnefoy A, Musicki B, 1999, Synthesis and in vitro evaluation of novel highly potent coumarin inhibitors of gyrase B, Bioorg Med Chem Lett, 9, 2079–2084.

Laurin P, Ferroud D, Schio L, Klich M, Dupuis-Hamelin C, Mauvais P, Lassaigne P, Bonnefoy A, Musicki B, 1999, Structure activity relationship in two series of aminoalkyl substituted coumarin inhibitors of gyrase B, Bioorg Med Chem Lett, 9, 2875–2880.

Meyer CE, 1964, Rubradirin, a new antibiotic. II. Isolation and characterization, Antimicrob Agents Chemother, 10, 97–99.

Musicki B, Periers A-M, Laurin P, Ferroud D, Benedetti Y, Lachaud S, et al, 2000, Improved antibacterial activities of coumarinic antibiotics bearing 5,5′-dialkylnoviose: biological activity of RU 79115, Bioorg Med Chem Lett, 10, 1695–1699.

Periers A-M, Laurin P, Ferroud D, Haesslein J-L, Klich M, Dupuis-Hamelin C, Mauvais P, Lassaigne P, Bonnefoy A, Musicki B, 2000, Coumarin inhibitors of gyrase B with N-propargyloxy-carbamate as an effective pyrrole bioisostere, Bioorg Med Chem Lett, 10, 161–165.

Shen G, Yu XM, Blagg SJ, 2000, Syntheses of photolabile novobiocin analogues, Bioorg Med Chem Lett, 14, 5903–5906.

Yun B-G, Huang W, Hartson SD, Matts RL, 2004, Novobiocin induces a distinct conformation of Hsp90 and alters Hsp90-cochaperone-client interactions, Biochemistry, 43, 8217–8229.

Peptide Antibiotics

A. BRYSKIER

30

1. INTRODUCTION

The family of peptide antibiotics comprises more than 400 molecules. It is an extremely complex class, the limits of which are somewhat vague. Among these molecules, the most important chemical family in therapeutic terms is that of the β-lactams. However, in this chapter I present the antibiotics belonging to two other classes: homopeptide antibiotics and heteropeptide antibiotics. Homopeptide antibiotics consist solely of amino acids, which may be linear or cyclic. Heteropeptide antibiotics, in addition to the chain of linear or cyclic amino acids, comprise other constituents such as pyrimidine bases, amino sugars, fatty acids, variable acids, and sulfurated aromatic nuclei. Bacteria produce peptide antibiotics (*Streptomyces, Erwinia*, etc.). Fungi, molds, amphibians, arthropods, and mammals (which produce molecules such as magainins, defensins, etc.) are less involved. Peptolides are a class of antibiotic that include streptogramins and are described in chapter 20.

Peptide antibiotics differ structurally from conventional peptides in that they are cyclic and contain ester bonds and D-configured or unusual amino acids, unusual nuclei (such as saturated or unsaturated fatty acids), and heterocycles or amino or nonamino sugars.

The peptide antibiotics can be divided into seven groups: I, linear peptides; II, cyclic peptides; III, glycopeptides; IV, lipoglycopeptides; V, lipopeptides; VI, thiazolopeptides; and VII, thiopeptides and chromopeptides.

Each group can be divided into subgroups according to their chemical structures, as in group V (linear lipopeptides and cyclic lipopeptides), or their antibacterial activities, as in group V_2 (anti-gram-positive organisms, anti-gram-negative organisms, and antifungal).

Within the same group of peptides the mechanism of action may differ and/or the nature of the cell target may be different. The mechanism of synthesis may be of ribosomal or nonribosomal origin. Because of the complexity of the molecules, antibacterial agents of miscellaneous origin that fall outside the classification are presented in a special section.

2. ANTIBIOTICS OF MISCELLANEOUS ORIGIN

Peptides of ribosomal origin are large and are composed of more than 100 amino acids (Fig. 1).

2.1. Antineoplastic Agents

Peptide antineoplastic agents are large proteins, such as neocarzinostatin, macromomycin, and actinoxanthin, that have antineoplastic action. The polypeptides comprise 20 proteins containing chromophoric nuclei. They bind covalently to tumor cell DNA. Other peptides in this class have been described, such as esperamicin and calichemicin, isolated from *Actinomadura verrucosospora* and *Micromonospora echinospora*, respectively.

2.2. Hormonal Peptides and Neuropeptides

Polypeptide antibiotics induced during an infection in insects, such as cecropins or attacins, have been described in this class. Likewise, peptides that act through phagocytic cells have been described for vertebrates: defensins. The skin of amphibians contains peptides, magainins and caeruleins, which have a certain similarity to peptide hormones and neurotransmitters.

2.2.1. CAPs

To avoid opportunistic infections, plants and animals have developed antimicrobial peptides in their epithelia that form pores in the inner membranes of microorganisms (Hancock, 1998).

The cationic antimicrobial peptides (CAPs) are produced by bacteria, fungi, plants, insects, amphibians, crustaceans, fish, and mammals.

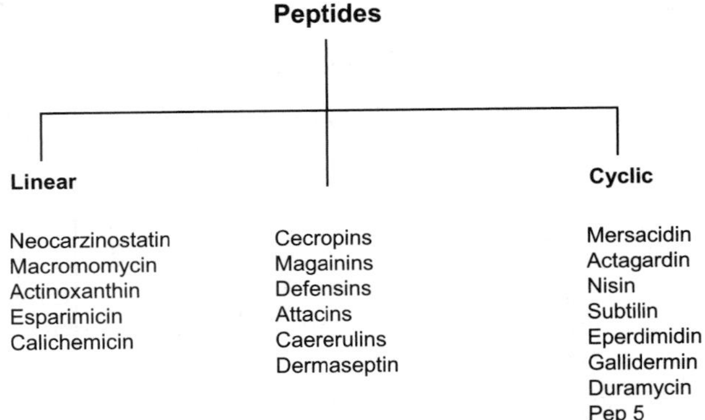

Figure 1 Classification of ribosomal peptides

In plants and insects, CAPs are under the control of a conserved complex regulatory system, involving the transcription nuclear factor NF-κB.

In higher animals, CAPs are mainly induced locally (in the skin of amphibians, fish, and humans) at mucosal sites. In humans and cows, they are produced in granules of neutrophils attracted to infection sites.

CAPs are small peptides, consisting of 12 to 50 amino acid residues, and positively charged (at +2) due to the presence of excess basic residues, lysine or arginine. They are amphiphatic molecules.

In cystic fibrosis, epithelial cells produce CAPs such as β-defensins which normally kill *Pseudomonas aeruginosa*, but in the high-salt environment of cystic fibrosis they are ineffective.

CAPs are apparently inactive against *Burkholderia cepacia*.

CAPs may be classified into three groups:

- Helical linear peptides with two prototypes: cecropins and magainins
- Peptides with one or more disulfide bridge. This group is composed of 2- to 5-kDa peptides. Main representatives are mammal defensins α and β and insect and plant defensins. Protegrin and heliomycin (ETD-15) are prototypes for humans and insects, respectively.
- Peptides composed of amino acids other than lysine and arginine

Table 1 shows peptides identified in the frog.

2.2.2. Magainins

See Zasloff, 1987.

A number of peptides possess antibacterial and, in some cases, hemolytic activities and have been isolated from the skin of various amphibian species. They have been detected in *Bombina variegata* and *Bombina orientalis* (Discoglossidae family), *Xenopus laevis* (Pipidae family), *Phyllomedusa sauvagii* (Hylidae family), and *Rana esculenta* and *Rana brevipoda porosa* (Ranidae family).

Table 1 Peptides from frogs

Compound	Species of frog	Family of frogs
Magainins	*X. laevis*	Pipidae
Bombesin-like	*B. variegata*	Discoglossidae
	B. orientalis	Discoglossidae
Dermaseptin	*P. sauvagii*	Hylidae
Brevinins	*R. brevipoda porosa*	Ranidae
Esculentin	*R. esculenta*	Ranidae
Rugosins A, B, and C	*Rana rugosa*	Ranidae
Gaegurin 4	*R. rugosa*	Ranidae
Dermaseptin	*Phyllomedusa bicolor*	Hylidae

Most of the structures of these peptides have been elucidated. Magainins have been the subject of extensive research, and some derivatives have been selected for development for topical use in human therapy.

Magainins possess a broad antibacterial spectrum. They are extracted from the skin of a toad of African origin, *X. laevis*.

There are two peptides containing 23 amino acids and which differ with respect to 2 of these. Amino acid 10 is a glycine in one (magainin 1) and a lysine in the other (magainin 2), and amino acid 22 is a lysine in one and an asparagine in the other (Fig. 2).

They possess a broad antimicrobial spectrum, including bacteria, fungi, and protozoa. Magainins are membrane-active peptides. They interact electrostatically with negatively charged moieties of the bacterial surface, such as lipopolysaccharide.

They have also been reported to be cytotoxic for tumor cells, but they are not hemolytic and are noncytotoxic against nontumor cells.

Magainin 2 possesses antibacterial (Table 2) and antiprotozoal activities, particularly against *Acanthamoeba polyphaga*, which is responsible for eye infections. More than 200 magainin derivatives have been prepared, and some MSI derivatives are in the process of clinical development for treatment of skin and eye infections. A number of derivatives manifest antifungal activity. The antibacterial activity is increased by lengthening the peptide chain and adding charged amino acids.

Magainin analogs called magainin mimetics have been synthesized (Attendo-Genco et al., 2003). Two compounds of this series were shown to exert antibacterial activity against pathogens involved in periodontal disease: MSI-751 (*N*-amidino-phenylalanyl-dioctylamide) and MSI-754 (1, 12-[di-(N-amidino-arginino-phenylalanyl)] diamino dodecan (Table 3).

Magainin-like analogs have been isolated from human submandibular and labial salivary glands.

2.2.3. Other Derivatives

Table 4 lists other peptide derivatives.

Table 2 Antibacterial activity of magainin 2[a]

Organism	MIC (μg/ml)
S. epidermidis	10
S. aureus	50
E. faecalis	>100
E. coli	5
K. pneumoniae	10
Citrobacter freundii	30
Enterobacter cloacae	50
P. aeruginosa	100
Pseudomonas putida	10

[a]Data from Zasloff, 1987.

Magainin 1

Gly— Ile — Gly— Lys— Phe(5)— Leu— His— Ser— Ala— <u>Gly</u>(10)— Lys— Phe— Gly— Lys— Ala(15)—

Phe— Val— Gly— Glu— Ile(20) — Met— <u>Lys</u>— Ser

Magainin 2

Replacement at: 10 = Lys
22 = Asn

Figure 2 Magainins 1 and 2

Table 3 In vitro activities of MSI-751 and MSI-754

Microorganism	MIC (μg/ml)	
	MSI-751	MSI-754
P. gingivalis	20	80
Fusobacterium nucleatum	20	40
Prevotella intermedia	5	10
Actinobacillus actinomycetemcomitans	40	20
Eikenella corrodens	40	40
Prevotella loescheii	10	10
E. coli	40	5
S. aureus	1.25	1.25
Y-4	40	20

2.2.3.1. Dermaseptin

Dermaseptins are CAPs (28 to 34 amino acid residues) expressed in amphibian skin. They are probably too toxic for systemic treatment. Three synthetic analogs were obtained by replacement of the C-terminal 12 residues by a carboxamide. They are bactericidal against *Staphylococcus aureus* (Navon-Venezia et al., 2001).

2.2.3.2. Cecropins

There are other molecules, such as cecropins, that are amphiphilic, nonhemolytic peptides containing 37 amino acids. They act as defense proteins in insects. Cecropins were initially isolated from the hemolymph of *Hyalophora cecropia*. They represent the primary system of defense in invertebrates that do not possess a lymphocytic system or immunoglobulins. Six cecropins have been described (A to F). Cecropins A, B, and D have been sequenced. Cecropins have been isolated from pig intestine (P1 and Shiva-1) (Lee et al., 1989).

Cecropin A is a polypeptide containing 37 nonsulfurated amino acids and a C-terminal part with an amide function.

Cecropins would appear to act on the lipids of the cytoplasmic membrane to form ion channels (Christensen et al., 1988). The N-terminal part is basic, and the C-terminal part is hydrophobic; they are connected by a flexible Gly-Pro loop.

The amino acids of the N-terminal part (amino acids 1 to 11) are important for the antibacterial activity of the cecropins. The C-terminal part is important for the activity against gram-positive bacteria. Gram-negative bacteria are more susceptible to cecropin B than gram-positive bacteria.

2.2.3.3. Defensins

Defensins are cysteine rich cationic and structural polypeptides with three or four disulfide bridges. Lehrer (1993) describes them as polypeptides composed of 29 to 35 amino acids that have three disulfide bonds essential for their antibacterial activity and no amide function in the C-terminal part. The most active defensins have eight or nine arginine residues. They possess an amphiphilic structure able to invade the lipid part of the cytoplasmic membranes.

They have been isolated from neutrophils and alveolar macrophages in humans, mammals (epithelial cells and intestinal epithelia), insects (hemolymph), and plants.

Mammalian defensins are made of two distinct subfamilies (α and β) of cationic trisulfide peptides (Raju et al., 2002).

In terms of higher-vertebrate epithelial antimicrobial peptides, phagocytes have the capability of killing ingested microorganisms through oxygen-dependent and oxygen-independent mechanisms. Leukocytes are a rich source of endogenous antimicrobial peptides called α-defensins. Neutrophils of cattle and birds do not seem to produce α-defensins, but only β-defensins. In bovines, there are 13 β-defensins of about 4 kDa constituted of 38 to 42 amino acids.

Table 4 Other peptide derivatives

Peptide	Location	No. of peptides	Peptide name(s)	Activity
Mammals				
Human	Neutrophils	4	Defensins: HNP-1 to HNP-4	Gram$^+$, gram$^-$, fungi, enveloped virus
Rabbit	Alveolar macrophages	2	Defensins: MCP-1, MCP-2	Gram$^+$, fungi, virus
	Neutrophils	6	Defensins: NP-1, NP-2, NP-3a, NP-3b, NP-4, NP-5	Gram$^+$, gram$^-$, fungi, virus
Bovine	Seminal fluid	1	Plasmin	Gram$^+$, gram$^-$
	Neutrophils	1	Bactenecins: Bac-5, Bac-7	Gram$^+$, gram$^-$
Arthropods				
Hyalophora cecropia	Lymph	6	Cecropins A to F	Gram$^+$, gram$^-$
Sarcophaga peregrina	Lymph	4	Sarcotoxins I and II	Gram$^+$
Phormia terranovae	Lymph	5	Sapecins A, B, C	Gram$^-$
	Lymph	2	Defensins A and B	Gram$^-$
Apis mellifera	Lymph	3	Ia, Ib, II	Gram$^+$
	Lymph	1	Bactenecins	Gram$^+$
	Lymph	1		Gram$^+$
Tachypleus tridentatus	Lymph	1	Tacheplysin	Gram$^+$, gram$^-$
Bombyx mori	Lymph	3	Lepidopteran A, B, C	Gram$^-$
Amphibians				
X. laevis	Skin	6	Magainins 1 and 2, CPF, XPF, LPF, PLGa	Gram$^+$, gram$^-$, yeast, virus
P. sauvagii	Skin	1	Dermaseptin	Gram$^+$, gram$^-$
R. brevipoda porosa	Skin	2	Brevenins 1 and 2	Gram$^+$, gram$^-$
R. esculenta	Skin	5	Brevenins 1-E, 2-E, A_1, B_9, esculentin	Gram$^+$, gram$^-$
B. variegata	Skin	1	Bombinin	Gram$^+$, gram$^-$
B. orientalis	Skin	1	Bombinin	Gram$^+$, gram$^-$

2.2.3.3.1. α-Defensins and β-defensins. α-Defensins are found in neutrophils of humans, rabbits, guinea pigs, rats, macaques, and hamsters, as well as in rabbit alveolar macrophages and in rodent and human small intestine Paneth cells. They consist of 29 to 35 amino acids.

β-Defensins were reported to be expressed in skin, pancreas, kidney, salivary glands, prostate, placenta, endocervix, and urinary and gingival epithelial cells of vertebrates. They consist of 38 to 42 amino acids.

2.2.3.3.1.1. HUMAN. Human β-defensin 1 (HBD-1) and HBD-2 are found in skin, plasma, saliva, and the urogenital tract. HBD-1 is a 3.9-kDa basic peptide consisting of 36 amino acids. There is strong evidence for a role of HBD-1 in cystic fibrosis lung pathogenesis. With both HBD-1 and HBD-2, skin and soft tissue infections due to gram-negative bacteria are less frequent. HBD-2 is a 42-amino-acid peptide of 4 kDa. It is highly effective against gram-negative bacilli like *Escherichia coli* and *P. aeruginosa*, whereas gram-positive cocci, such as *S. aureus*, are poorly inhibited. *Candida albicans* is killed efficiently by HBD-2.

HBD-3 has been identified in adult heart, skeletal muscle, placenta, skin, esophagus, gingival keratinocytes, and trachea and in fetal thymus.

HBD-4 has been shown in testis, uterus, thyroid gland, lung, and kidney.

Other antimicrobial peptides besides defensins have been isolated, such as ALP, found in skin and mucosal surfaces. It is active against *E. coli* and *S. aureus*. It is fungicidal against *Aspergillus fumigatus* and *C. albicans*. Cathelin derivatives are produced by granulocytes in bone marrow and testis.

2.2.3.3.1.2. PLECTASIN. Plectasin is a natural peptide isolated from a black mushroom growing in pine forest in Scandinavian countries (*Pseudoplectania nigerella*). Plectasin contains 40 amino acids. It is mainly active against streptococci (MICs range from 0.5 to 8.0 μg/ml) and less active against staphylococci (MICs from 2.0 to 32 μg/ml), *Corynebacterium* sp., and *Bacillus* sp. Two interesting features of plectasin are that it is not hemolytic and it is stable in serum. Plectasin is apparently well tolerated in mice after intravenous administration. In mice, plectasin is eliminated via the kidney.

2.2.3.3.1.3. BOVINE. The bovine tracheal mucosa is free of infections, which led to the discovery of TAP. TAP is active against *Enterobacteriaceae*, *P. aeruginosa*, and *S. aureus* (MICs, 12 to 50 μg/ml) as well as against *C. albicans* (MICs, 6 to 12 μg/ml).

It was demonstrated that LAP helps in the rapid healing of the bovine tongue after abrasions.

The distal small intestine and colon of cows express epithelial β-defensin.

2.2.3.4. Cathelicidins

The most widely used defense system against microorganisms involves membrane active protein.

The antimicrobial peptides found in mammals belong to the defensin (α- and β-defensins) and cathelicidin families. They are expressed in human keratocytes after induction by inflammatory stimuli.

Cathelicidins are found in the secondary granule of neutrophils and are expressed early in myeloid differentiation.

Cathelicidins share a highly conserved X-terminal domain, identical to a cathelin protein, but are structurally diverse at the C terminus, which also determines the antibacterial activity.

Table 5 Cathelicidins: in vitro activity

Peptide	Activity
CAP-18	Rabbit leukocytes
P15	Rabbit leukocytes
Bac-5	Bovine neutrophils
Indolicidin	Bovine neutrophils
Cyclic dodecapeptide	Bovine neutrophils
C-12	Porcine bone marrow
Trytrypsin	Phages
SMAP-29	Sheep
Novispirin G10	Sheep
CATH-1, -2, -3	Horse

The expression of the human cathelicidin FALL 39 (hCAP18) has been shown in keratinocytes and in nonsquamous epithelia of the mouth and tongue in humans.

Cathelicidins are present in saliva and expressed in gingival tissue.

CAP-18 has been described to occur in rabbit neutrophils; SMAP-29 has been described to occur in sheep.

Table 5 shows the cathelicidin peptides that have been reported.

2.2.3.5. Dermacidin

Dermacidin is expressed in the sweat glands (Schittek et al., 2001). Dermacidin is a 47-amino-acid peptide produced and exported by sweat to the epidermal surface in response to a variety of pathogenic microorganisms.

2.2.3.5.1. Bactericidal permeability-increasing protein. Polymorphonuclear leukocytes contain a number of proteins and peptides having antimicrobial activity:

- Bactericidal permeability-increasing protein
- Defensins
- Azurocidins (CAP-37)
- Cathelicidins (CAP-18)

Antimicrobial peptides are widely distributed in nature and represent an ancient mechanism of host defense.

In the innate immune system, chemical substances are produced that control microbial growth on the surface of human epithelial cells.

In plants the main innate immune system consists of thionins. Thionins comprise a family of cysteine-rich antimicrobial peptides containing 45 to 47 amino acids. They are divided into two subgroups (Table 6).

Thionins are abundant in plant epidermal cells (Schröder, 1999).

For insects, many peptides have been described (Table 7).

2.2.3.6. Mellitin

Mellitin is a polypeptide isolated from bee venom. It is an antibacterial agent that also manifests antirheumatic and hemolytic properties. It is composed of 26 amino acids, divided into two α-helices with a free segment. The N-terminal part is hydrophobic, and the C-terminal part is basic. They contain only a single tryptophan residue. Semisynthetic derivatives have been prepared, and the central part of mellitin—particularly lysine 7—has been shown to be responsible for the hemolytic activity. The replacement of Lys7 by an alanine or a glutamic acid has shown that the hemolytic activity is independent of the charge of the amino acid. However, the activity against *P. aeruginosa* is reduced

Table 6 Plant innate immune system: in vitro activity

Peptides	Amino acids	Activity		
		Gram positive	Gram negative	Fungi
Thionins	6 cysteines	+++	+++	++
	8 cysteines	+++	+++	++
Plant defensins		(+)	(+)	+++
Hevein-type peptides		++	(−)	++
Knottin-type peptides		++	(−)	+++

Table 7 Insect innate immune system: in vitro activity

Peptide(s)	Activity		
	Gram positive	Gram negative	Fungi
Cecropins	(+)	+++	−
Drosocin	(+)	+++	−
Apidaecin	(+)	+++	−
Diptericin	(+)	+++	−
Metchnikowin	+++	+++	+++
Thanatin	+++	+++	+++
Defensins	+++	(+)	−
Drosomycin	−	−	+++
Heliomycin	−	−	+++

sevenfold and that against *S. aureus* is reduced fourfold (Wade et al., 1992). The antibacterial and hemolytic activities may be dissociated.

2.2.3.7. Sarcotoxins

Sarcotoxins have been isolated from *Sarcophaga peregrina* and possess antibacterial activity.

2.2.3.8. Bacteriocins

Bacteriocins are protein ribosomally synthesized. Their production in gram-positive bacteria has been documented extensively, and they can be divided into four distinct classes.

Class 1 comprises lantibiotics. Class 2 contains bacteriocins without modified residues: at least 14 derivatives have been reported (e.g., pediocin PA-1, leucocin A, mesentericin Y 105, sakacins A and P, and curvacin).

The initial definition of bacteriocins was as follow: bacteriocins inhibit activity against closely related bacteria. However, this definition needs to be extended.

Bacteriocin has been isolated from *Enterococcus faecalis* AS-48; it is a cyclic peptide active against gram-positive and gram-negative bacteria. It is composed of 70 amino acid residues, for a molecular mass of 7,149.25 Da (Samyn et al., 1999).

Pediocin-like antibiotics exhibit high anti-*Listeria* activity. They are characterized by a YGNGV motif and a disulfide bridge in the C-terminal region, such as in pediocin PA-1. Analogs of pediocin PA-1 which possess a methionine in position 31 were synthesized, and antibacterial activity was investigated; results are shown in Table 8.

Bacteriocins produced by lactic bacilli have been the subject of intensive investigation.

Brevibacterium linens is one of the most important surface bacteria in the cheese-making process due to its role in colonizing the surface and its flavoring activity. It is an average cheese coryneform bacterium (Ryser et al., 1994).

Due to the industrial process of making cheese, there is a risk of contamination, and there is a considerable interest in developing starter which inhibits undesired microorganisms. Today, only nisin has been approved by the Food and Drug Administration. Nisin was shown to reduce the level of *Listeria monocytogenes* in cheese.

Table 8 Pediocin-like antibiotics: in vitro activity

Microorganism	MIC (μg/ml) of pediocin:				
	A1	31A[a]	31I[b]	31L[c]	31D[d]
Lactobacillus sakei	0.2	0.1	0.1	0.1	20
Lactobacillus coryniformis	0.1	0.1	0.1	0.1	10
E. faecalis	0.2	0.2	0.2	0.2	30
Carnobacterium piscicola	0.5	0.5	0.5	0.6	60
Pediococcus pentosaceus	0.1	0.4	0.5	0.2	NT[e]
Pediococcus acidilactici	2.0	1.0	10	6	NT
L. mesenteroides	4.0	4.0	4.0	10	NT

[a]Alanine.
[b]Isoleucine.
[c]Leucine.
[d]Aspartate.
[e]NT, not tested.

B. linens produces a bacteriocin inhibiting the growth of *L. monocytogenes*.

Other bacteriocins from *B. linens* have been described, such as linencin OC_2 from the surface of Gruyère cheese and linencin A. They are bactericidal against *L. monocytogenes* and *S. aureus* but are inactive against gram-negative bacteria and yeasts.

Due to an increase tolerance of *L. monocytogenes* to nisin and pediocin (Rasch and Knochel, 1998; van Schaik et al., 1999), an intensive search for new bacteriocins has been undertaken.

2.2.3.8.1. Kappacin. The caseins are the most abundant bovine milk proteins, and there are a few major types: α_{S1}-, α_{S2}-, β-, and κ-casein. The terminal polypeptide κ-casein is known as the caseinomacropeptide. It is a heterogenous C-terminal fragment (residues 106 to 169) composed of glycosylated and phosphorylated forms of different genetic variants. Caseinomacropeptide has growth-inhibitory activity against *Streptococcus mutans*, *Porphyromonas gingivalis*, and *E. coli*. This inhibition has been proposed to be the mechanism of anticariogenicity of milk protein fraction in animal caries models.

2.2.3.8.2. Carnocin H. Carnocin H is a bacteriocin belonging to class 2 of bacteriocins, with 75 amino acids with a highly cationic N terminus (six consecutive lysines). Carnocin H is produced by *Carnobacterium sp. strain* 377 and inhibits lactic acid bacilli, clostridia, enterococci, some *S. aureus* strains, *Listeria*, and *Pediococcus*.

2.2.3.9. Pleurocidins

Pleurocidins have a broad antibacterial spectrum covering gram-positive and gram-negative bacteria. They were isolated from the winter flounder *Pleuronectes americanus* in 1997 (Cole et al., 2000). Other cationic antimicrobial peptides have been isolated from flatfish by amplification of genomic DNA. Some of them, like NCR-12 and NCR-13, displayed activity against both gram-positive and gram-negative bacteria (MICs, 2.0 to 4.0 μg/ml) (Patrzykat et al., 2003).

2.2.3.10. Bombesin-Like Peptides (GRP)

Bombesin was first discovered in frog skin, and later bombesin-like peptides were discovered in mammalian brain, gut, and lung. Bombesin-like peptides were found as a larger form and identified as GRP, a 27-amino-acid peptide (Table 9) (Hernanz, 1990).

2.2.3.11. Protegrins (IB-367) (Iseganan)

Protegrins are derived from porcine leukocytes. IB-367 is under investigation for the treatment of lung infections in cystic fibrosis patients (Fujii et al., 2001). Forty cystic fibrosis patients were treated by aerosol and the flora found was tested for antibacterial susceptibility in vitro; results are shown in Table 10.

The prevalence of pathogens in 40 patients enrolled at Washington University is shown in Table 11.

The microflora of the mouth is complex: viridans group streptococci are dominant on the surface of the buccal mucosa (Loesch, 1994). The microflora can be modified in patients having an oral cancer with dominance of gram-negative bacteria and yeasts (Table 12) (Mosca et al., 2000).

Table 9 Localization of GRP

Animal	Gastric tissue	Brain	Lung cancer	Intestine
Pig	+	–		
Guinea pig		+		+
Rat		+		+
Human			+	
Dog				+

Table 10 Protegrins are also active against anaerobes involved in oral infections

Microorganism	*n*	MIC (μg/ml)	
		50%	90%
P. aeruginosa	222	4	8
S. aureus	48	2	4
Alcaligenes xylosoxidans	10	8	32
Stenotrophomonas maltophilia	9[a]	2–16	
B. cepacia	2[a]	>64	

[a]Range.

Table 11 Prevalence of pathogens in cystic fibrosis patients at Washington University

Organism	Prevalence (%)
P. aeruginosa	89
Mucoid only	31
Nonmucoid	8
Both patterns	50
S. aureus	59
MRSA	3
S. maltophilia	10
A. xylosoxidans	10
B. cepacia	3

Table 12 Prevalence of pathogens in oral microflora and iseganan in vitro activity

Microorganism(s)	*n*	MIC (μg/ml)	Prevalence (%)
MRSA ATCC 33591		4	
P. aeruginosa ATCC 9027			
Viridans group streptococci			93–99
S. salivarius	12	0.25–5.0	50–75
S. sanguinis	14	4.0–64	25–75
S. mitis	15	2.0–43	25–75
S. mutans	3	0.7–1.3	25–75
Gram-positive bacteria			
Group D streptococci	6	0.25–4	90–100
Streptococcus	16	1.3–16	1–5
Corynebacterium	5	0.13–0.25	15–90
Propionibacterium		NT[a]	11–12
Staphylococcus	35	0.13–4	3–70
Lactobacillus		NT	1–37
Gram-negative bacilli			
Moraxella	12	0.2–0.8	81–97
Neisseria	1	8.0	5–97
Haemophilus	15	1.0–8.0	5–35
Acinetobacter	4	0.06–2.0	5–30
K. pneumoniae	4	1.0–5.0	5
P. aeruginosa	18	1.0–8.0	5
E. coli	5	0.25–1.0	
S. marcescens	16	16–>256	
Yeasts			
C. albicans	6	4.0–16	3–6

[a]NT, not tested.

3. LANTIBIOTICS

See Jung, 1991.

3.1. Classification

Lantibiotics are synthesized ribosomally from gene-encoded peptide precursors, which are extensively modified by complex translational processes.

Peptide derivatives containing thioether amino acids, such as *meso*-lanthionine and 3-methyl-lanthionine, and α,β-unsaturated amino acids are known as lantibiotics.

These molecules may be divided into two groups, A and B, according to their structures (Fig. 3).

Group A molecules are cationic antimicrobial peptides that have two to seven positive charges and, with the exception of mersacidin and actagardin, molecular masses of more than 2,100 Da. They have in common the N-terminal amino acid, which is a thioether in the D configuration, and

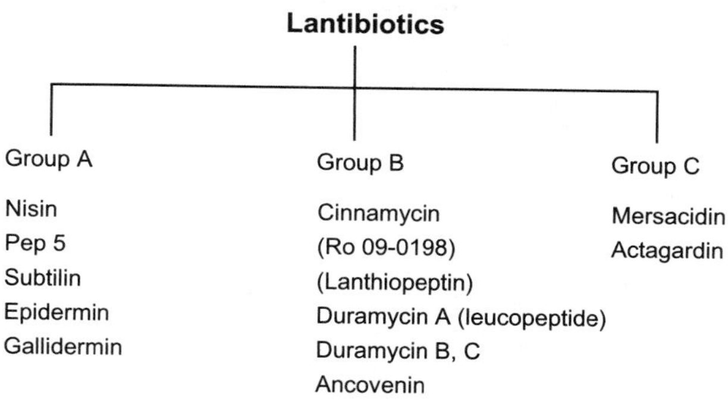

Figure 3 Lantibiotic classification

the C-terminal amino acid in the L configuration, except for mersacidin and actagardin. Group A lantibiotic-producing strains are staphylococci, streptococci, or *Bacillus* organisms.

Group B lantibiotics are produced by *Streptomyces*. They are mainly of globular aspect. The prototype is duramycin, an inhibitor of phospholipase A_2. These molecules also have a positive charge. These peptides contain α,β-dehydroamino acids and sulfurated rings of various sizes.

The following molecules belong to this group: subtilin (produced by *Bacillus subtilis*); epidermin (produced by *Staphylococcus epidermidis*), which is active against *Propionibacterium acnes*; and nisin (produced by *Lactococcus lactis*), which is used as a food additive in animals but which has been proposed in the local treatment of *Helicobacter pylori*.

Two antibiotics have recently been included in this group, mersacidin and actagardin.

3.2. Mersacidin

Mersacidin (Fig. 4) is an oligopeptide produced by *Bacillus* sp. strain Y-85 (Ganguli et al., 1989). Its antibacterial spectrum includes gram-positive cocci (Table 13), and the molecule is bactericidal (Niu and Neu, 1991).

It is presented as a white, amorphous powder, slightly soluble in water, which decomposes at 240°C. The specific rotation is $[\alpha]^{20}_{D} - 9.4°$ (c = 0.3, methanol). It has a molecular mass of 1,825 Da.

It is composed of 20 amino acids, including four methyllanthionines and one dehydroamino acid. It contains cysteines.

Table 13 In vitro activity of mersacidin[a]

Microorganism(s)	MIC_{50} (μg/ml)	
	Mersacidin	Vancomycin
MSSA	4	1
MRSA	4	1
S. epidermidis Met[s]	4	1
S. epidermidis Met[r]	4	1
S. pyogenes	1	0.25
S. agalactiae	8	0.5
S. bovis	4	1
E. faecalis	64	2
S. pneumoniae	2	0.25
C. jeikeium	4	0.5
L. monocytogenes	16	1
Clostridium perfringens	2	0.25
Peptostreptococcus spp.	2	2
P. acnes	8	0.25

[a]Data from Niu and Neu, 1991.

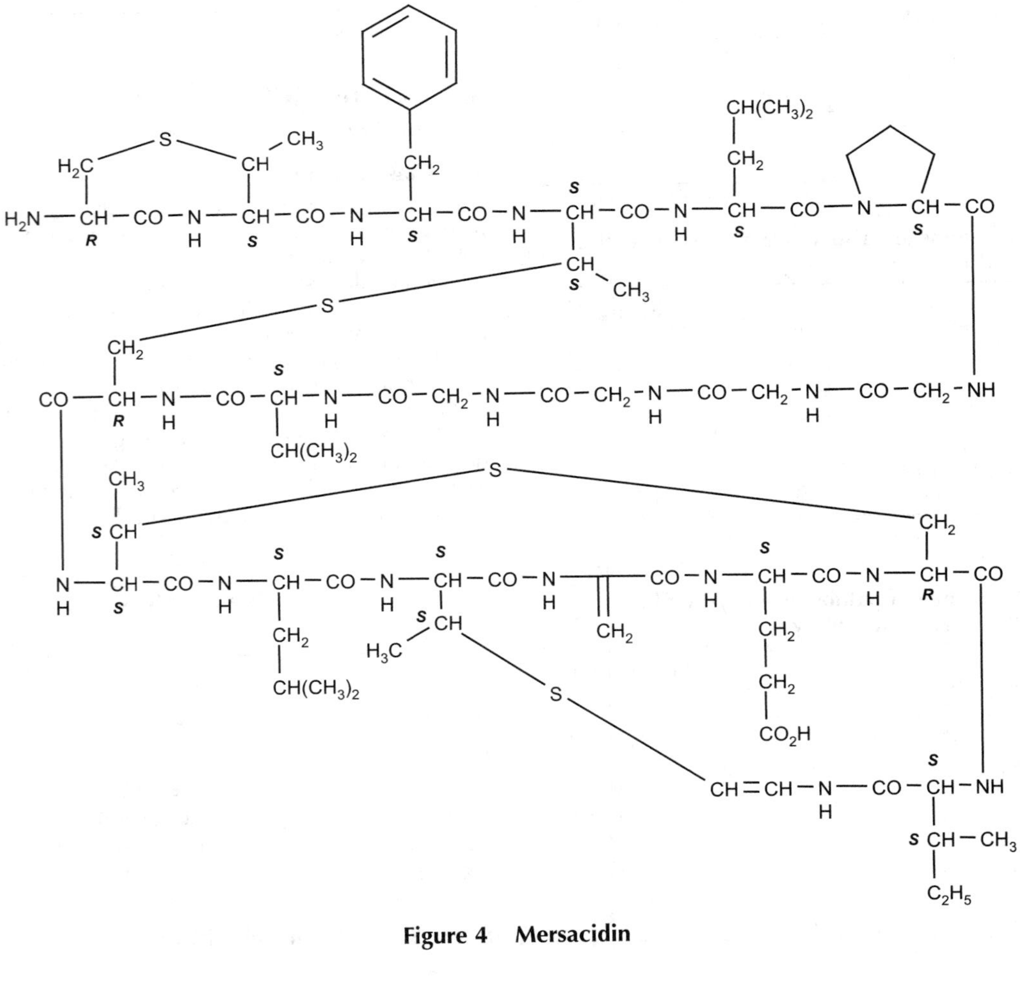

Figure 4 Mersacidin

3.3. Actagardin

Actagardin (Fig. 5) is a derivative obtained by fermentation of *Actinoplanes* sp. strain ATCC 31048, which has a molecular weight of 1,890 and is composed of 19 amino acids, including a lanthionine, 3-methyl-lanthionine, and an aromatic amino acid, tryptophan, with four thioether bonds. The acid function is due to aspartic acid (γ-COOH). The NH_2 terminus and the COOH terminus are those of the alanine contained in the two β-methyl-lanthionines.

Actagardin and its derivative compound D are active in vitro against gram-positive cocci, particularly streptococci and anaerobic bacteria. They inhibit peptidoglycan biosynthesis.

Semisynthetic derivatives of actagardin have been prepared. One derivative, 3,3-dimethylamino-1-propylamide actagardin hydrochloride, is more soluble in water than the parent molecule and more active and bactericidal. However, these derivatives are active against streptococci such as *Streptococcus pyogenes* and *Streptococcus mitis* but weakly active against *Streptococcus pneumoniae* and the other species of streptococci belonging to the viridans group and inactive against *S. aureus*.

3.4. Gallidermin

Gallidermin was isolated from *Staphylococcus gallinarum* Tu 3928. It has a molecular mass of 2,164 Da. It is composed of 22 amino acids, of which 2 are lanthionines and 1 is methyllanthionine. It is active against *P. acnes* (MIC, <0.12 μg/ml) and staphylococci.

3.5. Ruminococcin A

Ruminococcin A is produced by an anaerobic bacterium, *Ruminococcus gnavus*, from the human gut. Ruminococcin A is a 2,675-Da peptide harboring a lanthionine structure with 21 amino acid residues. It is active against *Clostridium* spp. except *Clostridium sporogenes*. *Bacillus cereus* is resistant to ruminococcin A (Dabard et al., 2001).

3.6. API 17444

Lantibiotic AK-127-1744 (API 17444) was isolated from the fermentation broth of *Actinomyces* sp. strain AD 1744. It is a 23-amino-acid peptide including lanthionine and methyllanthionine. The antibacterial spectrum covers gram-positive cocci, such as staphylococci (MIC at which 50% of isolates tested are inhibited [MIC_{50}] and MIC_{90}, 4.0 and 8.0 μg/ml), *S. pneumoniae*, and *S. pyogenes* (MIC_{50} and MIC_{90}, 0.25 and 0.25 μg/ml), but it is inactive against *Enterococcus* spp. (MIC, >32 μg/ml) (Toriya et al., 2004).

4. GROUP I: LINEAR PEPTIDES

4.1. Group IA: Dipeptides

The intention was to cause antibacterial agents to penetrate the bacterial wall by means of peptide transporters, the active part being released within the bacterial cell by peptidases (Fig. 6). To be most effective, this active part must not

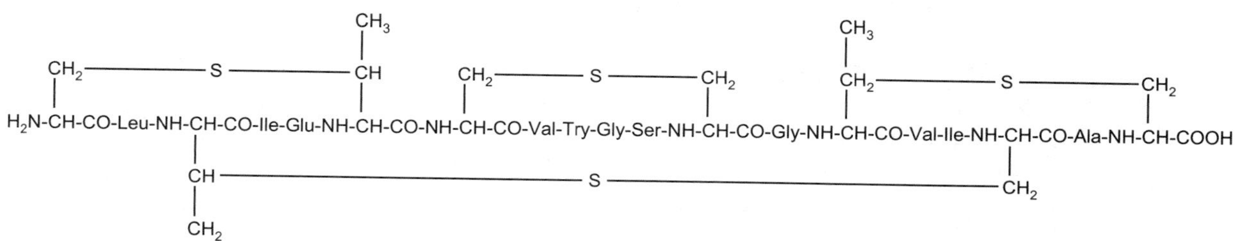

Figure 5 Actagardin

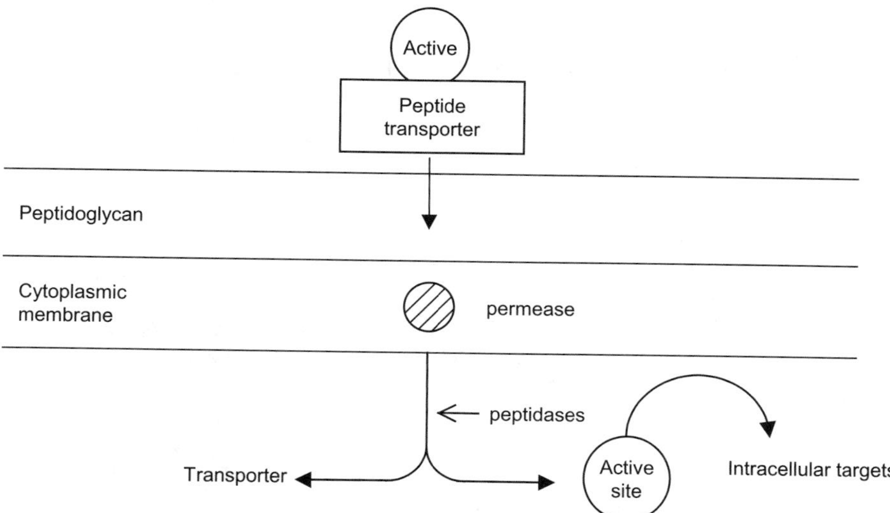

Figure 6 Intracellular dipeptide transport

be capable of crossing the wall by itself, thus enabling it to accumulate within the cell since it cannot be eliminated by the efflux system.

4.1.1. Peptidoglycan Synthesis

See Walsh, 1989.

Peptidoglycan synthesis (Fig. 7) is a complex process, from the elaboration of the precursors of the elementary disaccharide in the cytoplasm to the formation in the membrane of the elementary disaccharide bearing the peptide chains and the constitution in the wall of a cross-linkage through a transpeptidation reaction. Inhibitors can disrupt peptidoglycan synthesis throughout the whole length of this chain. The first stage, which is the constitution of UDP-*N*-acetylglucosamine, may be blocked by bacilysin, thus inhibiting the start of the synthesis chain.

A number of derivatives act on the transpeptidation that produces the cross-linking of peptidoglycan. However, the formation of the pentapeptide requires the provision of a D-Ala–D-Ala dipeptide. This dipeptide comes from two sources: either direct formation from two D-alanines by means of D-alanine ligase, which may be inhibited by a number of synthetic dipeptides, or from L-alanine and transformation to D-alanine, which requires a D-alanine racemase that can be inhibited by dipeptides such as alafosfalin.

4.1.2. Natural Peptides

4.1.2.1. Bacilysin

Bacilysin (I) (Fig. 8) is an L,L-dipeptide produced by a strain of *B. subtilis* that causes partial lysis of *S. aureus* cultures. Its structure includes an unusual amino acid. Bacilysin penetrates the bacterial wall, and the active part, anticapsin, is released by means of a peptidase into the bacterial cells.

Bacilysin inhibits L-glutamine-D-fructose-6-phosphate aminotransferase. It acts prior to the stage inhibited by fosfomycin.

4.1.2.2. Lindenbein

Lindenbein is a dipeptide isolated from *Streptomyces collinus*, the active part of which is fumarylcarboxyamido-L-2,3-diaminopropionyl-L-alanine. Its mechanism of action has been poorly elucidated.

4.1.2.3. Phosphinothricyl-Alanyl-Alanine

Phosphinothricyl-alanyl-alanine (II) is a homo-L-tripeptide, the active part of which is in the N-terminal position. It was isolated from *Streptomyces viridochromogenes*. It is active against gram-negative and gram-positive bacteria. The active part is phosphinothricin, which is a γ-phosphinate analog of glutamic acid. It is a potent inhibitor of *E. coli* glutamine synthetase.

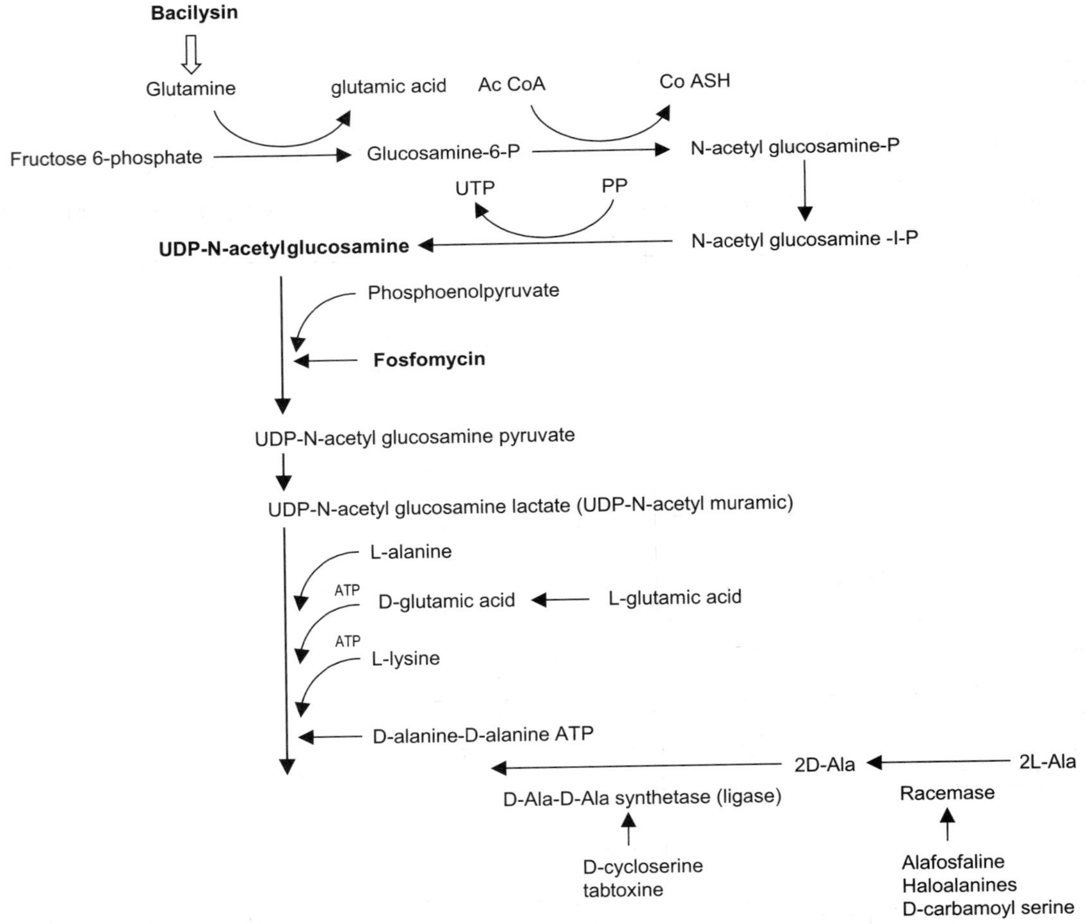

Figure 7 Peptidoglycan synthesis and sites of action of antibacterial agents

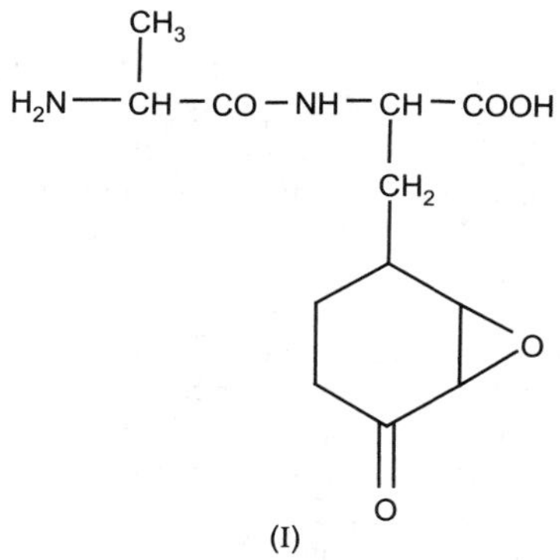

(I)

Bacilysin (tetaine, bacillin)

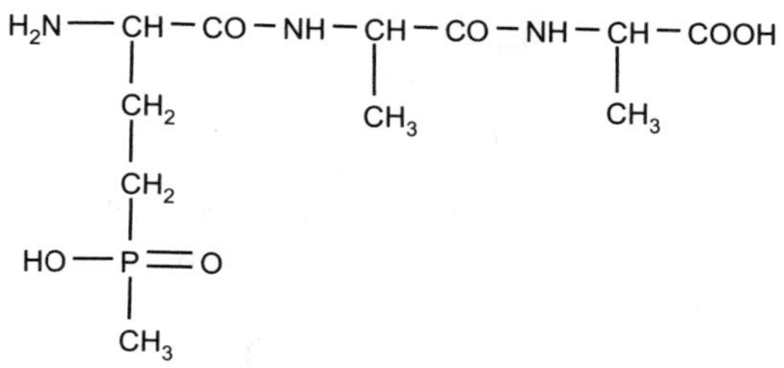

(II)

L-Phosphinothricyl alanylalanine

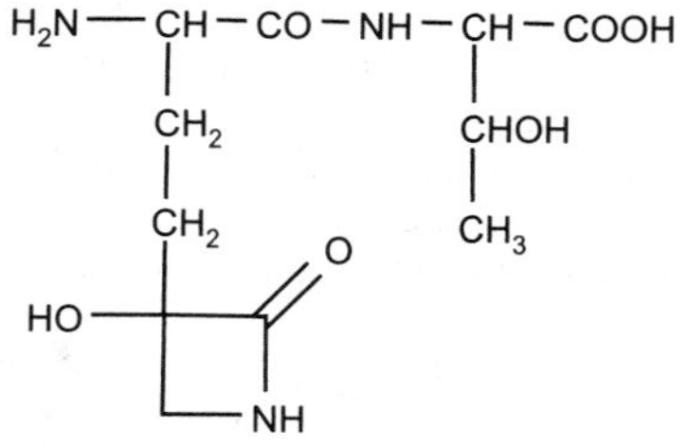

(III)

Tabtoxin

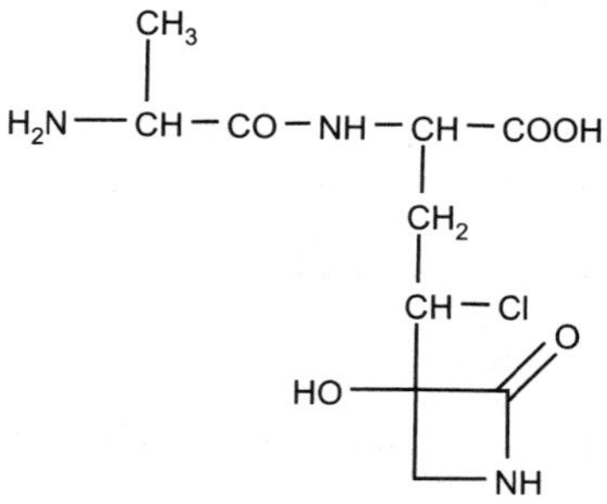

(IV)

Figure 8 Bacilysin, tabtoxin, and L-phosphinothricyl-alanyl-alanine

4.1.2.4. Analogs of Phosphinothricyl-Alanyl-Alanine

Analogs of phosphinothricyl-alanyl-alanine, L-N^5-phosphonomethionine-sulfoximinyl-alanylalanine and L-methionine-*S*-dioxydialanylalanine, have an active part that inhibits glutamine synthetase. Two transport systems may be used: oligopeptide permease for the tripeptide and methionine permease for the active part.

A number of other peptides have been described, such as alazopeptin and duazomycin B, tripeptides transporting a 6-diazo-5-oxo-L-norleucine antimetabolite that inhibits glutamine synthetase.

Two dipeptides with a β-lactam ring have been described and act on glutamine synthetase: tabtoxin (III) and (*S*)-alanyl-3-[α-(*S*)-chloro-3-(*S*)-hydroxy-2-oxo-3-azetidinyl-methyl]-(*S*)-alanine (IV).

The C-terminal part of tabtoxin may be a threonine, but also a serine. Dipeptide IV has the active β-lactam part in the C-terminal part and the L-alanine serving as a transporter. In addition, the active part contains a chlorine atom in the γ position.

Other peptides do not act on glutamine synthetase, such as stravidin (V) and valyl-1-hydroxy-2-amino-1-cyclobutane acetic acid (VI).

4.1.2.5. Stravidin

Stravidin (MSD 235 S_3) (Fig. 9) comprises a C-terminal part transporting an *N*-methyl isoleucine. The active part is amiclenomycin. The valylcyclobutane peptide (VI) is only active against gram-positive bacteria, and its activity is reversed by L-cysteine or L-methionine, the γ-C-terminal part serving as an active moiety.

4.1.2.6. Feldamycin

Feldamycin (VII) is a dipeptide containing *N*-methyl-histidine in the N-terminal part. It acts on DNA synthesis. Phaseolotoxin (*N*-phosphosulfamyl-ornithylalanylhomoarginine) is produced by *Pseudomonas phaseolicola*.

Other peptides act as antifungal agents: polyoxins and nikkomycins, which are peptide nucleoside complexes. They are active against a large number of fungi and yeasts, including *C. albicans*. The peptide transports the nucleoside fragment inside the fungal cell, where it acts by inhibiting chitin synthetase.

4.1.3. Synthetic Peptides

Based on observations made with natural peptides, a number of synthetic compounds have been prepared.

The first peptides were synthesized in 1947, such as glycylleucine and derivatives like β-2-thienylalanine. Their activities were limited and depended on the presence of a growth factor in the culture medium containing phenylalanine.

Peptides containing ethionine or norleucine showed some activity as transporters; preliminary studies demonstrated that transporter peptides had optimal activity when the active part was localized in the C-terminal part. Some amino acids have the property of inhibiting bacterial growth, such as valine, or of being bactericidal, such as glycine. However, these properties are dependent on the bacterial

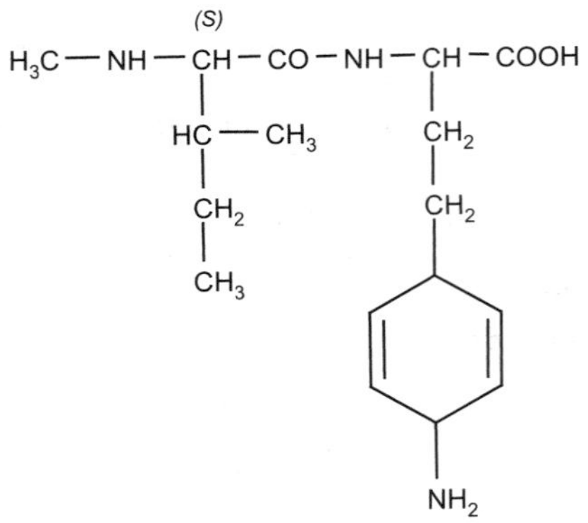

Stravidine (V)
(N-methyl isoleucine-amiclenomycin)

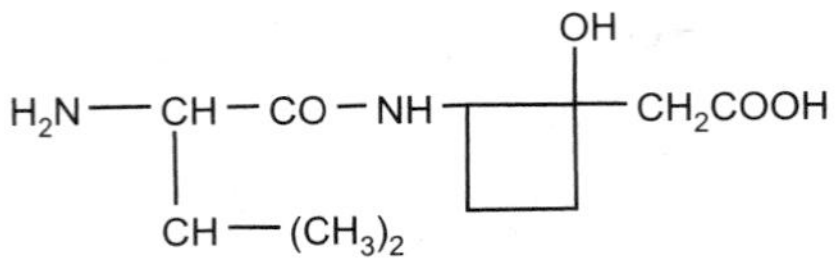

1-(S)-hydroxy-2-(S,S)-valyl amido-cyclobutane-1-acetic (VI)

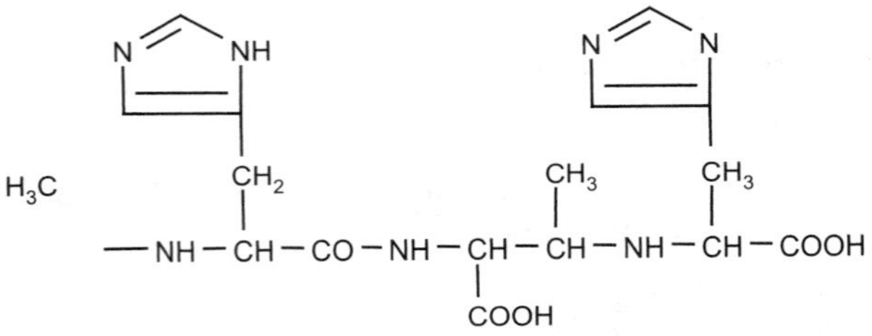

Feldamycin (VII)

Figure 9 Feldamycin and analogs

species; the activity of valine, for example, is limited to *E. coli*.

A subsequent development was the application of the principle of dual inhibition, with a dually active substance transported by a dipeptide containing a cyclopentane-glycine (an isoleucine analog) and a β-2-phenylalanine (a phenylalanine analog).

Other synthetic peptides containing ethionine, norvaline, norleucine, dioxydemethionine, azaadenylaminohexanoic acid, cysteine sulfamide, or fluorophenylalanine have been synthesized as antibacterial or antifungal agents.

The majority of peptides of natural or synthetic origin cannot be used as therapeutic agents, as they are unstable in biological liquids, they are toxic, their antibacterial spectrum is limited, and they manifest only weak activity.

Another approach was to replace the C-terminal carboxyl function by other acid functions such as phosphonates, phosphinates, sulfonates, sulfonamides, hydroxamates, tetrazoles, and others.

4.1.3.1. Alafosfalin

In a series of 300 phosphopeptides (Allen et al., 1978) comprising different α-aminoalkylphosphonic acids and in which the structural modifications related to the length of the chain, the stereochemistry, and the amino acid sequence, alafosfalin (Ro-03-7008) (Fig. 10) was selected as the most active derivative.

Alafosfalin has a broad antibacterial spectrum including gram-positive and gram-negative bacteria (Table 14).

The antibacterial activity is limited when the culture medium contains peptones or casein, or when the pH is greater than or equal to 7.5. The optimum pH is 5.5. There is a marked inoculum effect, the MICs increasing when the size of the inoculum is increased from 10^4 to 10^7 CFU/ml. It is bactericidal. There is synergy of action between alafosfalin and D-cycloserine or β-lactams.

In contrast to the natural peptides, alafosfalin is active in experimental infections because of its absorption and its stability against peptidases.

Alafosfalin acts as the transporter via bacterial peptide permeases, followed by cleavage by intracellular peptidases with the release of the active part: L-1-aminomethylphosphonic acid. Because the active part cannot penetrate by itself or be expelled (efflux) by the bacteria, it reaches very high concentrations inside the bacterium. The target is alanine racemase and, to a minor extent, UDP-*N*-acetylmuramyl-L-alanine ligase.

Inhibition of peptidoglycan synthesis occurs rapidly, and cell lysis is visible after 20 to 40 min, depending on the bacterial species. In some gram-negative bacteria, alafosfalin is metabolized inside the bacterial cell to yield muramyl-1-aminoethylphosphonic acid.

In humans, alafosfalin is well absorbed orally (Allen and Lees, 1980). The oral bioavailability is on the order of 50%, whereas intramuscularly it is practically 100% compared to that intravenously (intramuscular area under the curve

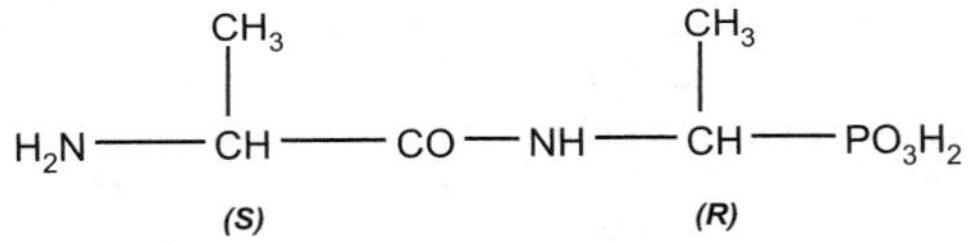

Figure 10 Alafosfalin

Table 14 In vitro activity of alafosfalin[a]

Microorganism	MIC_{50} (μg/ml)	
	Alafosfalin	Ampicillin
S. aureus	32	0.06
E. faecalis	1	0.5
N. gonorrhoeae	32	
E. coli	0.06	1
Enterobacter	1	8
S. marcescens	4	8
Salmonella serovar Typhimurium	4	0.5
Klebsiella	0.5	32
Citrobacter	0.12	4
Shigella	0.25	32
H. influenzae	8	0.25
V. cholerae	4	

[a]Data from Allen et al., 1994.

[AUC], 2.47 μg · h/ml, and intravenous AUC, 2.09 μg · h/ml, for a dose of 500 mg). Orally, alafosfalin is rapidly absorbed. The compound is detectable after 20 min and reaches a peak concentration is serum in 1 to 2 h. The apparent elimination half-life is on the order of 1.0 h. The AUCs increase linearly with the dose. Urinary elimination of the unchanged drug is complete after 8 h and is on the order of 15 to 17%, depending on the administered dose. The concentrations in plasma are at the limit of detection after 3 h (Table 15).

Alafosfalin is metabolized to L-Ala (P), and high concentrations are found in the systemic circulation and urine (Allen et al., 1979b).

Alafosfalin is probably absorbed by an active mechanism in the intestinal mucosa and is partially hydrolyzed by intestinal peptidases.

The increase in chain length among phosphonodipeptides by the addition of L-alanine to the C-terminal part of the L-1-aminoethylphosphonic fragment produces an increase in activity against *E. faecalis* and *Haemophilus influenzae* between the tripeptide and the hexapeptide $(\text{L-Ala})_5$–L-Ala (P). In the case of enterobacteria, the increase in chain length does not significantly modify the activity beyond a pentapeptide, $(\text{L-Ala})_4$–L-Ala (P). However, *Enterobacter* spp. and *Salmonella enterica* serovar Typhimurium are susceptible only to dipeptides or even tripeptides, $(\text{L-Ala})_2$–L-Ala (P).

The stereochemistry is important, and peptides with L-configured amino acids are more active than those in a D configuration. Only L-amino acids can be transported inside the bacterial cell.

Replacement of the L-alanine at the active site by other amino acids causes a reduction or loss of activity, with the exception of Gly (P). This is due to the difference in the rate of penetration inside the bacterial cell and intracellular hydrolysis.

4.1.3.2. Peptides with Other Acid Functions

Other acid functions have been attached. The tetrazole group has a charge identical and a size similar to those of the carboxyl group. However, peptides with a C-terminal aminotetrazole group have weak antibacterial activity, with differences between the peptides: phenyl-Pro[Ile-tetrazole] is more active than Ile-tetrazole. Peptides with a sulfonate are weakly active. The activities of those with an arylsulfonamide differ according to the bacterial species.

4.1.4. Other Peptides

It has been shown that alanine racemase activity can be inhibited by alafosfalin but also by other derivatives, such as peptides of the chloroalanine type (haloalanines), *O*-carbamoylserines, and D-fluoroalanine. β-β-β-Trifluoroalanine is a potent racemase inhibitor.

O-Carbamoylserine has weak antibacterial activity since its transport by D-alanineglycine permease is poor. β-Chloro-D-alanine is an excellent inhibitor of bacterial growth, but it is also the substrate of the renal enzyme D-amino acid oxidase, causing the formation of a β-chloropyruvate that is inactivated by a number of enzymes (Cheung et al., 1983).

Some 3-halovinylglycine derivatives inhibit alanine transferase activity and possess good activity (L-Nva-L-chlorovinylglycine) against gram-positive cocci (MICs, ~2 to 8 μg/ml depending on the inoculum).

However, the stage in which the D-ala–D-ala dipeptide is formed, which is under the control of a ligase, may be inhibited by numerous peptides, such as tabtoxinine and its semisynthetic derivatives, by aminophosphinic acids, or by phosphoamidic acids.

The ligase requires ATP to exert its activity and possesses two binding sites, one for ADP and the second for the dipeptide (Fig. 11).

The carboxyl group of the alanine binds to the donor site, which is activated by ATP. During or after the process, an attack is launched by the amino group of the second alanine attached to the acceptor site, causing the formation of a dipeptide and ADP. The precise mechanism has yet to be fully elucidated, but it is likely that a D-alanine-phosphate intermediate is formed. This would occur during the conversion of glutamic acid to glutamine by glutamine synthetase (Fig. 12). It is at this level that a number of inhibitors might act, such as tabtoxin or its derivatives.

Phosphonic dipeptides have been synthesized, including (1*S*)-aminoethyl-[2-carboxy-2-(*R*)-methylthio-1-ethyl] phosphonic acid, which possesses moderate antibacterial activity, with MICs of between 4 and 128 μg/ml (Fig. 13).

D-Norvaline–D-alanine inhibits the growth of *E. coli* K-12 by replacing D-Ala–D-Ala as the substrate in the synthesis of UDP-*N*-acetylmuramylpentapeptide.

Other peptides act on bacterial metabolism: peptides containing proparglycines act by blocking cystathionine-γ-synthetase, a bacterial enzyme essential for the metabolism of methionine.

4.1.5. Phosphonic Dipeptides

A series of 4-amino-4-phosphonobutyric dipeptides has been synthesized (Zboinska et al., 1993). The C-terminal part is an aminoalkane phosphonic acid, and the N-terminal part is constituted by L-alanine, L-leucine, etc. The majority of these derivatives are active against *E. coli* and *Serratia marcescens*, but inactive against *B. subtilis*, *Micrococcus luteus*, and *Pseudomonas fluorescens*. Peptides that contain an alanine, a leucine, a valine, or a phenylalanine are more active than those containing a methionine, a lysine, an isoleucine, or a proline.

4.2. Group IB: Linear Oligopeptides

Some dipeptides have been described.

Table 15 Pharmacokinetics of alafosfalin orally (tablets)

Dose (mg)	No. of subjects	C_{max} (μg/ml)		Alafosfalin AUC (μg·h/ml)
		Alafosfalin	Metabolite	
500	9	7.1 ± 0.6	NM[a]	0.86 ± 0.07
1,000	5	17.1 ± 3.1	9.2 ± 1.6	1.92 ± 0.23
1,500	5	19.9 ± 1.8	10.3 ± 1	3.12 ± 0.18
2,000	5	32 ± 2.2	14 ± 0.8	4.92 ± 0.57
2,500	4	39.1 ± 3.5	18.5 ± 1.6	6.18 ± 0.57

[a]NM, not measured.

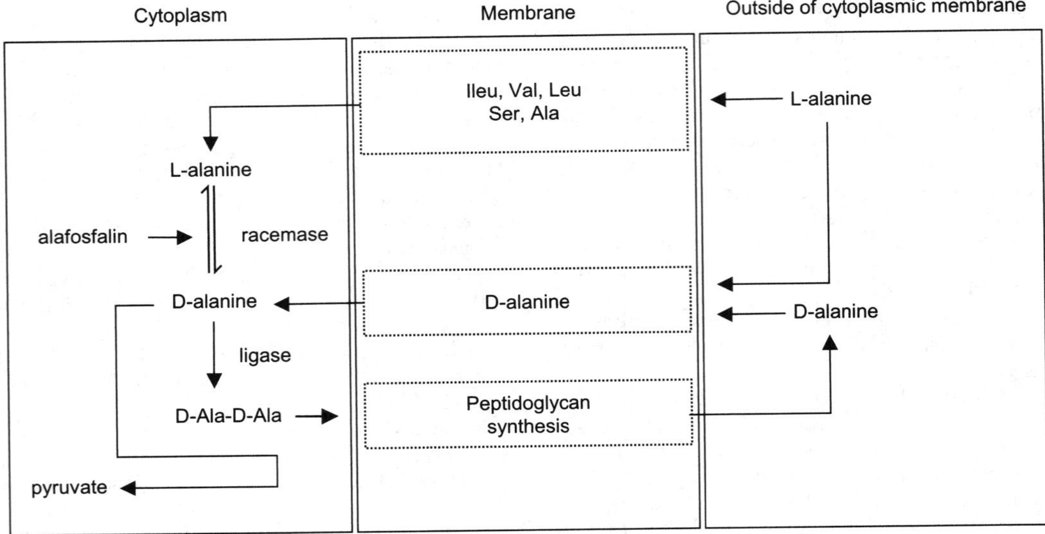

Figure 11 Alafosfalin mode of action

Figure 12 Formation of glutamine (adapted from Greenlee et al., 1989)

$H_2N—CH(CH_3)—P(=O)(OH)—CH_2—CH(SCH_3)—COOH$

Figure 13 (1 (*S*)-aminoethyl-[2-carboxy-2-(*R*)-methylthio]-1-ethyl)phosphonic acid

4.2.1. Negamycin

Negamycin (I) (Fig. 14) is a δ-hydroxylysine attached to methylhydrazinoacetic acid and is produced by a strain of *Streptomyces purpeofuscus*. It is active against gram-negative bacterial species, including *P. aeruginosa*. It acts by inhibiting protein synthesis through inhibition of the terminal chain. Derivatives obtained by semisynthesis have shown that the (*R*) configuration of the amino group on the β carbon is important for the antibacterial activity, that the δ-hydroxyl groups are not essential, and that acylation of the ε-amino group causes a loss of activity. Few synthetic analogs have been synthesized, such as VRC-4334, which exerts a weak activity against *E. coli* (MIC, 4 to 16 μg/ml) (Raju et al., 2002).

4.2.2. Linatine

Linatine acts by interacting with pyridoxal phosphate.

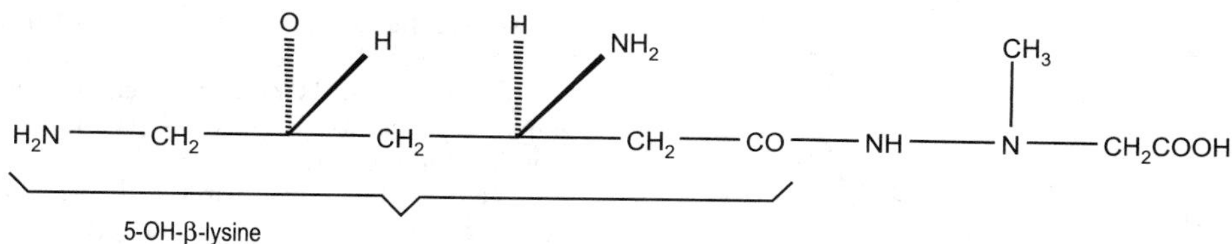

Figure 14 Negamycin (I)

4.2.3. Gramicidin A

Gramicidin A (II) (Fig. 15) is the most widely studied peptide among the linear antibiotic peptides.

Gramicidins A, B, C, and D are linear pentapeptides produced by *Bacillus brevis* ATCC 8185, at the same time as gramicidin S and the tyrocidines. The tyrothricin complex was isolated by Dubos in 1939; it is a mixture of gramicidins and tyrocidines. Gramicidin is the most active part of the complex, but it is too toxic (hemolysis) for systemic use. Its antibacterial spectrum primarily includes gram-positive bacteria (Table 16).

Gramicidins A, B, C, and D have the same amino acid composition. In gramicidins B and C, the tryptophan (amino acid 1) is replaced by a phenylglycine and a tyrosine, respectively.

Argicillin is hydroxymethylgramicidin A. It is less toxic than gramicidin.

Gramicidin A is composed of 15 amino acids, arranged in alternating L and D configurations, with a tryptophan as the amino acid in the C-terminal position and which is included in the ethanolamine. Gramicidin is present in the cytoplasmic membrane as a dimeric helix, forming a canal to allow H^+ and K^+ exchanges.

The formyl group (N-terminal part) is necessary for the antibacterial activity of gramicidin A but may be reduced by an acetyl group. The ethanolamine group is responsible for the hemolytic activity of the molecule. The four indole nuclei of the tryptophans are necessary for the antibacterial activity.

Other antibacterial agents have been described, such as edeines A and B, distamycin A, congocidine, anthelvecin A, and kikumycin A. With the exception of edeine, these molecules are characterized by the presence of a pyrrole nucleus. Edeines A and B are basic pentapeptides similar to spermidine. Bestatin inhibits the action of peptidases.

5. GROUP II: CYCLIC PEPTIDES

The cyclic peptides are among the best-studied peptide antibiotics.

Their structures provide a high degree of resistance to enzymatic degradation. They do not in general have free α-amino or α-carboxyl groups. The amino acids are often in the D configuration. The bonds inside the peptide are of the ether, β-peptide, or γ-peptide type, in addition to the normal α-peptide bond. The majority of cyclic peptides form sheets that are stabilized by intermolecular hydrogen bonds.

5.1. Amino Acids

5.1.1. D-Cycloserine

The smallest cyclic peptide is D-cycloserine (Fig. 16). The amino acid component is aminooxy-D-alanine (D-amino-S-isoxazolidone). It inhibits D-Ala–D-Ala synthetase (ligase) and alanine racemase. The rigid plane of the structure of D-cycloserine is important for its activity. It crosses the bacterial wall via the D-alanine pathway.

This molecule was isolated from the fermentation of *Streptomyces orchidaceus* and *Streptomyces garyphalus*. This molecule is a crystalline substance with a low molecular weight.

It is active against *Mycobacterium tuberculosis*, including multiresistant strains, and also possesses good activity against atypical mycobacteria. It has not insignificant activity against certain species of enterobacteria.

Cycloserine is well absorbed after oral administration. After ingestion of 250 mg, the peak concentration in serum of 10 μg/ml is reached in 3 to 4 h. There is slight accumulation following repeated doses. Thirty-five percent of the administered dose of cycloserine is metabolized, but the metabolites have not been identified. Sixty to seventy percent of the administered dose of cycloserine is eliminated by glomerular filtration. It penetrates the cerebrospinal fluid well.

Table 16 In vitro activities of gramicidin A and tyrocidine A

Microorganism	MIC (μg/ml)	
	Gramicidin A	Tyrocidine A
S. pneumoniae	0.5–1	40
S. pyogenes	5–20	100
S. mitis	10–60	80–120
E. faecalis	20–60	160–320
S. aureus	100	140–300

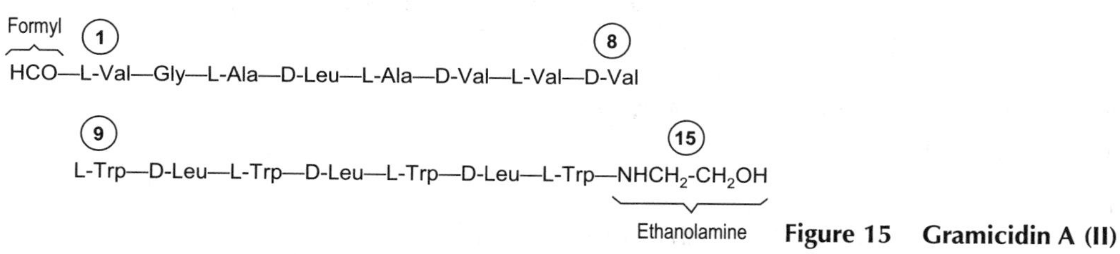

Figure 15 Gramicidin A (II)

D-cycloserine D-alanine

Figure 16 D-Cycloserine

D-Cycloserine is a minor antituberculosis agent that has more or less been abandoned because of the neuropsychiatric side effects in the form of psychosis.

5.1.2. Amino Acid Derivatives

Amino acid derivatives such as RI-331 and cispentacin have antifungal activity.

5.1.2.1. RI-331

RI-331 is (*S*)-2-amino-4-oxo-hydroxypentanoic acid (Fig. 17). It acts by inhibition of protein synthesis. This mechanism has been studied in *Saccharomyces cerevisiae*. The molecule inhibits the synthesis of amino acids derived from aspartic acid, such as methionine, isoleucine, and threonine. This inhibition occurs in the absence of biosynthesis of a precursor, homoserine, by blockade of homoserine dehydrogenase (Fig. 18). RI-331 is extracted from the fermentation of *Streptomyces* spp. It is active against yeasts such as *C. albicans* and *Cryptococcus neoformans* (Yamaguchi et al., 1989).

5.1.2.2. Cispentacin

Cispentacin, or (1*R*, 2*S*)-2-aminocyclopentane-1-carboxylic acid (Fig. 19), was isolated from *B. subtilis* L-450-B2. It possesses moderate in vitro activity against *C. albicans* (Oki et al., 1989) (50% inhibitory concentration [IC_{50}], 6.3 to ~12.5 μg/ml) and *Candida krusei*, but it is inactive in vitro against *C. tropicalis* (IC_{50}, >100 μg/ml) as determined by a turbidimetric method.

In vivo in the mouse (oral and intravenous administrations of cispentacin), the median protective dose (PD_{50}) is between 10 and 30 mg/kg of body weight (amphotericin B PD_{50}s, 0.4 and >4.0 mg/kg, respectively). In vivo it is not active orally in *C. tropicalis* infections (50% effective dose [ED_{50}], 81 mg/kg) or intravenously against *A. fumigatus* (PD_{50}, >100 mg/kg) (amphotericin B PD_{50}, ~0.3 mg/kg). It has good activity in experimental murine pulmonary and vaginal infections due to *C. albicans* but is inactive in infections due to *C. neoformans*.

5.1.2.3. 2-Amino-4-Oxo-5-Chloropentanoate

See Hirth et al., 1975.

2-Amino-4-oxo-5-chloropentanoate, a synthetic molecule, inhibits *E. coli* K-12 homoserine dehydrogenase.

Other amino acids act as antibacterial agents by inhibiting the synthesis of amino acids derived from aspartic acid. Their target is aspartate kinase, aspartate semialdehyde dehydrogenase, or homoserine dehydrogenase. The derivatives concerned are β-hydroxynorvaline, *O*-methylthreonine, and *O*-methylserine (Fowden et al., 1967).

5.1.2.4. Derivatives of Glycine-Betaine (Osmoregulation Inhibitors)

See Abdel-Ghany et al., 1993.

Bacterial cells must have a system for regulating intracellular osmolarity to prevent them from bursting. Extracellular osmolarity is greater than intracellular osmolarity. The osmolarity of enteric bacteria is controlled by osmoregulation genes. Osmolarity is maintained through certain osmolytes, such as potassium ions, proline, glutamate, and

Figure 17 RI-331

Figure 19 Cispentacin

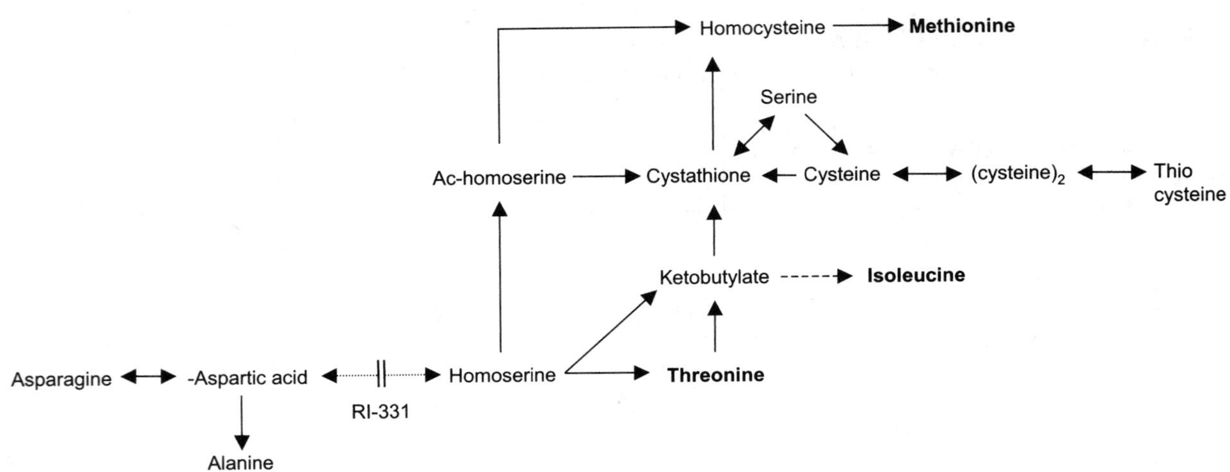

Figure 18 Activity of RI-331

trehalose. Osmoregulation is also under the control of certain compounds acquired by the bacterium. Betaine-glycine is a major osmoprotector. Because of its bipolar nature, it forms a sort of shield around the proteins that eliminates intracellular ions. When the osmolarity changes, the bacterium takes up betaine-glycine from the environment or synthesizes it from choline. The penetration of betaine-glycine and choline occurs by means of active transporters (Fig. 20).

The use of analogs that are toxic to the cell and that employ the same penetration pathways has led to the synthesis of derivatives with a sulfone, a phosphonic acid, or an arylsulfonyl nucleus instead of the terminal carboxyl group.

The bioisosteric replacement of the carboxyl group by a sulfonic acid yields molecules with osmoprotective activity identical to that of the original molecule; conversely, this effect is lost with a phosphonic acid.

The arylsulfonyl derivatives, such as the *N*-benzenesulfonylamide analogs, have only a moderate osmoprotective effect.

Replacement of the trimethylammonium part by a methylpyridinium, methylpiperidium, or methylmorpholinium inhibits the osmoprotective activity.

5.2. Cyclic Peptides

5.2.1. Capreomycin

Capreomycin is a cyclic polypeptide antibiotic (Fig. 21) isolated in 1960 from the fermentation of *Streptomyces capreolus*. It is composed of a complex of four components, IA, IB, IIA, and IIB. Capreomycin II differs from capreomycin I by the absence of a β-lysine.

Capreomycin is active only against *M. tuberculosis*. The MIC for the H_{37RV} strain of *M. tuberculosis* is 10 μg/ml. Multiresistant strains may be susceptible to capreomycin.

Capreomycin is not absorbed orally but is well absorbed intramuscularly. After an intramuscular injection of 1.0 g, the peak concentration in serum of 30 to 35 μg/ml is reached in 1 to 2 h. The concentration in serum is 10 μg/ml

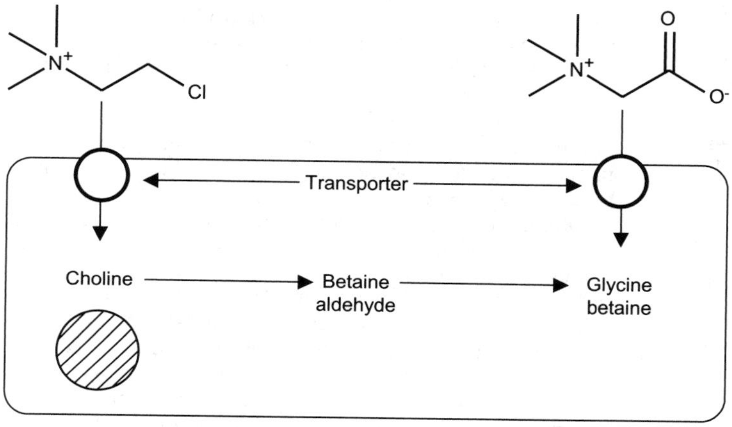

Figure 20 Transport structure of choline and glycine-betaine in gram-negative bacteria (adapted from Abdel-Ghany et al., 1993)

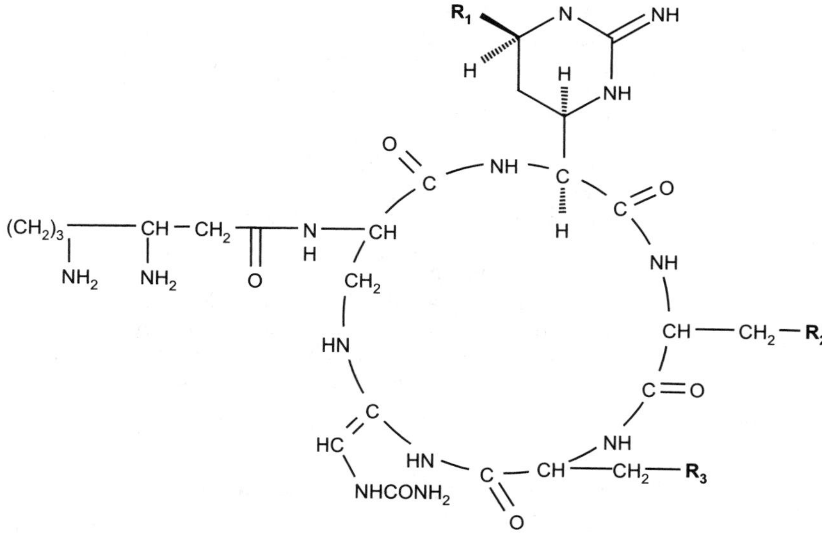

	R_1	R_2	R_3
Viomycin (II)	OH	OH	OH
Capreomycin I_A (I)	H	OH	NH_2

Figure 21 Viomycin and capreomycin

at 6 h and 1 μg/ml at 24 h. It does not accumulate after repeated doses. About 50 to 60% is eliminated in the urine in 12 h. It does not penetrate the cerebrospinal fluid well. It is nephrotoxic and ototoxic.

5.2.2. Viomycin (Tuberactinomycin B)

Viomycin (II) is a basic cyclic polypeptide antibiotic similar to capreomycin (Fig. 20) isolated from *Streptomyces floridae*. The sulfate or hydrochloride salts are soluble in water. It is active against *M. tuberculosis* but exhibits cross-resistance with capreomycin. It can be administered intramuscularly. It is ototoxic and nephrotoxic.

5.2.3. Tyrocidin

Tyrocidin (Fig. 22) is the second component of tyrothricin. The tyrocidin complex consists of five molecules, A, B, C, D, and E. Tyrocidin A (Fig. 21) is a cyclic decapeptide. Part of the molecule possesses five amino acids in common with gramicidin S.

Tyrocidin B has an L-trytophan instead of an L-phenylalanine. Its antibacterial activity is five times weaker than that of gramicidin A.

Tyrocidin is inactive against *E. coli* (MIC, >64 μg/ml) and moderately active against *H. influenzae*, but it exhibits good activity against *S. aureus* (MIC_{50} and MIC_{90}, 2.0 and 2.0 μg/ml) and *S. epidermidis* (MIC_{50} and MIC_{90}, 0.25 and 0.5 μg/ml) (Table 17). Tyrocidin acts by disrupting cellular membrane.

5.2.4. Gramicidin S

Gramicidin S (Fig. 23) is a cyclic decapeptide produced by *B. brevis* ATCC 9999. It is composed of repetitive pentapeptide sequences (Val–Orn–Leu–D–Phe–Pro). Numerous derivatives have been synthesized, and modification of the amino acids does not significantly alter its activity. It possesses moderate antibacterial activity (Table 18). It is used as a local antiseptic. Two minor derivatives of gramicidin S have been described. The minor derivative I contains a γ-aminobutyric acid in place of the valine (amino acid 1), and compound II possesses a γ-aminobutyric acid at amino acid 1′ instead of a valine. Gramicidin S is active against gram-positive cocci, such as *S. pyogenes, S. pneumoniae, E. faecalis, Enterococcus faecium* (MIC_{50}, and MIC_{90}, 0.125 μg/ml), *S. aureus* (MIC_{50}, and MIC_{90}, 1.0 and 2.0 μg/ml), and *Neisseria meningitidis* (MIC_{50}, and MIC_{90}, 0.25 and 1.0 μg/ml), but it is poorly active against *H. influenzae* (MIC_{50}, and MIC_{90}, 2.0 and 8.0 μg/ml) and inactive against *E. coli* (MIC, >64 μg/ml).

	1	2	3	4	5
	L-val —	L-Orm —	L-Leu —	D-Phe —	L-Pro
	L-aa10 —	L-Gln —	L-Asn —	D-aa7 —	L-aa6

	aa6	D-aa7	aa10
Tyrocidin	Phe	Phe	Tyr
"	Trp	Phe	Tyr
"	Trp	Trp	Tyr
"	Trp	Trp	Trp
"	Phe	Phe	Phe

Figure 22 Tyrocidins

Table 17 Tyrocidin in vitro activity

Microorganism	MIC (μg/ml) 50%	90%
E. faecalis	≤0.125	0.25
E. faecium	≤0.125	0.25
S. pneumoniae Pen^s/Pen^r	≤0.125	≤0.125
S. pyogenes	≤0.125	0.5
Streptococcus dysgalactiae	≤0.125	≤0.25
M. catarrhalis	1.0	2.0
N. meningitidis	4.0	8.0

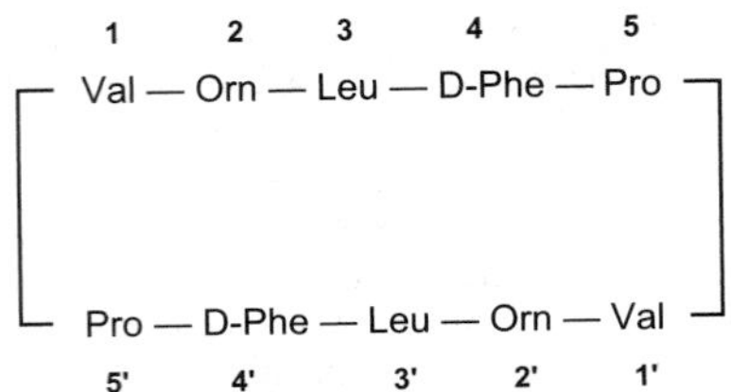

Figure 23 Gramicidin S

5.2.5. Other Derivatives

Antamanide is a cyclic decapeptide composed of amino acids in the L configuration that acts as an antidote to *Amanita phalloides*, which contains a potent poison, phalloidin.

Cyclic hexapeptides, such as monamycin and enniatins A and B, acting as ionophores have been described. Monamycin contains two unusual amino acids, L-hydroxypiperidiazine carboxylic acid and D-piperidiazine carboxylic acid. Enniatin B has alternating L- and D-amino acids and an ester-amide sequence (L-Met–Val–D-hydroxyisovalerate). Monomycin is a membrane-lytic agent. Ostreogrycin B, globomycin, evoldin, partricin, and ilamycin may also be mentioned, the last three being cyclic heptapeptides.

5.2.6. LL-A0341

Streptomyces candidus produces a complex of cyclic peptide antibiotics. This complex is a decadepsipeptide (Fig. 24), the major component of which is LL-A0341 β_1 (Lee et al., 1992). LL-A0341 β_1 is inactive against gram-negative bacteria. It is active against glycopeptide-resistant strains of enterococci (MIC_{90}, 2.0 μg/ml). It is bactericidal within 2 h against *S. aureus* Smith, whereas vancomycin is only bactericidal after 6 h (Petersen et al., 1992).

5.2.7. Janthinomycins

Janthinomycins A and B are cyclic decapeptide lactones isolated from *Janthinobacterium lividum*. They show good activity against aerobic and anaerobic gram-positive bacteria except for *Clostridium difficile* (MIC, ≥50 μg/ml).

Table 18 In vitro activity of gramicidin S

Organism	MIC (μg/ml)
S. aureus	10–25
S. pyogenes	12–25
Bacillus anthracis	25
Corynebacterium diphtheriae	50
C. perfringens	7–10

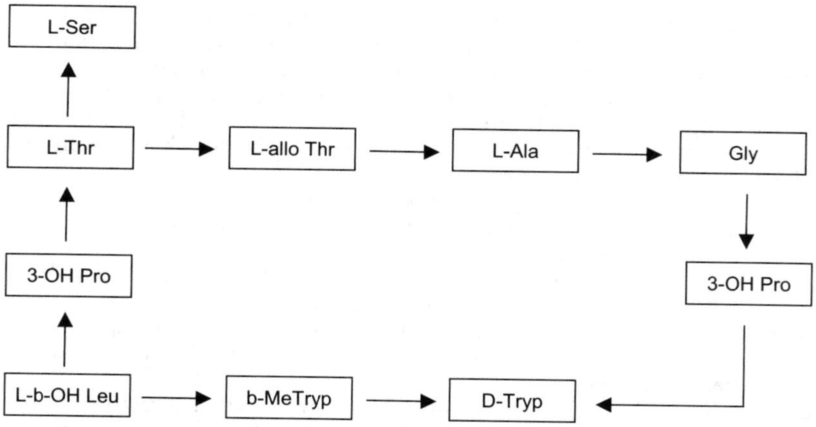

L-Ser ↑ L-Thr → L-allo Thr → L-Ala → Gly ↓ 3-OH Pro → D-Tryp ← b-MeTryp ← L-b-OH Leu → 3-OH Pro → L-Thr

Figure 24 LL-A034 β_1

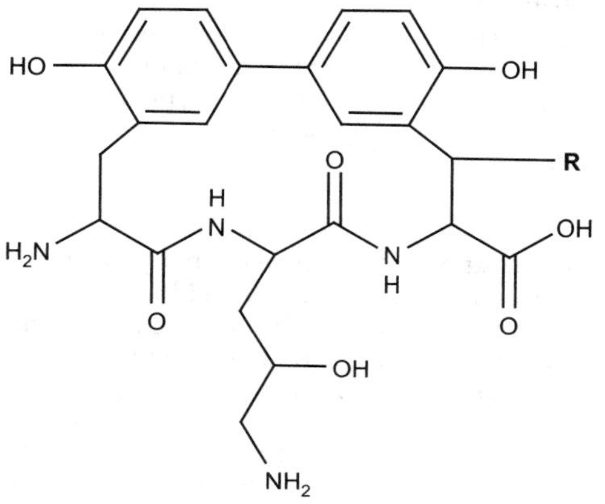

	R
WS 43708 A	OH
WS 43708 B	H

Figure 25 Structures of WS-43708

5.2.8. Chlorazicomycin

Chlorazicomycin is a depsipeptide isolated from a strain of *Streptomyces*. It has moderate activity against gram-positive bacteria. It is inactive against gram-negative bacteria and fungi.

5.2.9. WS-43708 A and B

WS-43708 A and B (Fig. 25) were isolated from a culture filtrate of *Streptomyces griseorubinosus* 43708. They are cyclic peptide antibiotics with a biphenyl nucleus. They are active against gram-positive bacteria but relatively inactive against gram-negative bacteria. WS-43708 A has good in vivo activity (Umehara et al., 1984).

5.2.10. Histatins

Histatins are naturally occurring peptides secreted by the salivary glands of humans. Histatin 5 has 24 amino acid residues. P-113 is a 12-amino-acid peptide derived from the 24-amino-acid histatin 5, being amidated at its C terminus.

P-113 exhibits in vivo activity in the prevention of gingivitis. It exerts anti-*C. albicans* activity. The D isomer of P-113 retains activity against the main pathogens isolated from bronchial secretions of patients with cystic fibrosis (Sajjan et al., 2001).

6. GROUP III: GLYCOPEPTIDES

6.1. Introduction

The nomenclature is relatively confusing because it covers a number of molecules that differ in structure. The name dalbaheptide was proposed by Cavalleri in 1990 and is derived from "dal" (D-alanine–D-alanine) "b" (binding), "a" (antibiotics), and "h" (heptapeptide).

In the last decade the class of glycopeptides has experienced a resurgence of interest because of the spread of methicillin-resistant *S. aureus* (MRSA) strains, the identification of *C. difficile* responsible for pseudomembranous colitis, and the emergence of penicillin G-resistant strains of *S. pneumoniae*. Vancomycin and teicoplanin are currently extensively used in therapy.

Ristocetin was described in 1953; it was obtained by fermentation of *Amycolatopsis orientalis* subsp. *lurida*. Vancomycin was isolated in 1956 from the fermentation of *Amycolatopsis orientalis*.

The chemical structure of vancomycin was elucidated in 1981 (Pfeiffer). The demonstration that part of the toxicity of vancomycin was related to the impurities and the purification of the molecule produced a revival of interest in its therapeutic use.

The therapeutic use of ristocetin was abandoned because it caused platelet aggregation disorders. It is currently used as a diagnostic test in von Willebrand's disease.

Teicoplanin was discovered by an analysis of the inhibitory activity against *S. aureus* of molecules resulting from the fermentation of *Actinoplanes teichomyceticus*. The izupeptins were isolated in the same way.

The subsequent molecules were isolated for their inhibitory action on wall fragments or on D-Ala–D-Ala synthetic peptides. This led to the discovery of A-40296, kibdelin, parvodicin, and A-42867.

The antibiotic A-82846 was discovered using polyclonal antibodies directed against vancomycin.

6.1.1. Oritavancin

Oritavancin is the chlorinated biphenyl derivative of orienticin C (A-82846C). The chain is attached to *epi*-vancosamine (Fig. 26). This molecule has the characteristic of being active against MRSA strains and against the different species of enterococci, whether these are susceptible or resistant to vancomycin or teicoplanin. In addition, it is bactericidal against MRSA strains, in contrast to vancomycin. In vivo it is 30 times more active than vancomycin in experimental murine infections with *E. faecalis* and *E. faecium*. It is also 20 times more active than vancomycin against *S. pneumoniae* in vivo (ED_{50}, 1.7 mg/kg) and *S. pyogenes* (ED_{50}, 0.8 mg/kg) and 3 to 4 times more active against *S. aureus* (ED_{50}, 1.2 mg/kg).

All glycopeptide antibiotics are active only against gram-positive bacteria. However, they are not active against *Leuconostoc, Pediococcus*, or *Nocardia*. They inhibit peptidoglycan synthesis by acting on transglycosylation and/or transpeptidation (Fig. 27).

6.2. Structure

About 50 molecules have been described. Structurally, they are fairly similar.

The glycopeptides are linear heptapeptides. Five amino acids are aromatic compounds. They are connected to one another to form a triphenyl ether nucleus and a diphenyl nucleus. The aromatic nuclei may be substituted by hydroxyl or methyl groups, sugars, or chlorine atoms. Five amino acids are common to all glycopeptides: the first (C terminal) is a *meta*-dihydroxyphenylglycine; the second and sixth are substituted β-hydroxytyrosines. The fourth and fifth are *para*-hydroxyphenylglycines.

The hydroxyl groups may form acetal bonds with a large variety of sugars: neutral or basic sugars; mono- or polysaccharidic acids such as glucose, mannose, or glucosamine; and atypical sugars specific to these molecules, such as vancosamine and ristosamine.

In molecules A-47934 and UK-68597 (group III), the hydroxyl of the phenyl nucleus is esterified by a monosulfate ester.

A methyl group may esterify the terminal carboxyl group, as can the terminal NH_2. UK-68597 also has a carbonyl group instead of a terminal amino group.

6.3. Classification

The glycopeptides may be divided into five groups on the basis of their chemical structures (Fig. 28). Teicoplanin, being a lipoglycopeptide, does not belong to the glycopeptide groups.

The classification is based on the structure of the heptapeptide (Fig. 29).

6.3.1. Group I

Group I is characterized by the presence of an asparagine at position 3, and the NH_2-terminal amino acid is a leucine that may be methylated. In some molecules the asparagine may be replaced by an aspartic acid or a glutamine.

The sugars are glucose, vancosamine, or 4-epivancosamine, with a few exceptions, such as olivose (orienticin B) and eremosamine (eremomycin). The majority of molecules have two chlorine atoms on the triphenyl ether nucleus. Chloroorienticin B (S-3362) is in the preclinical

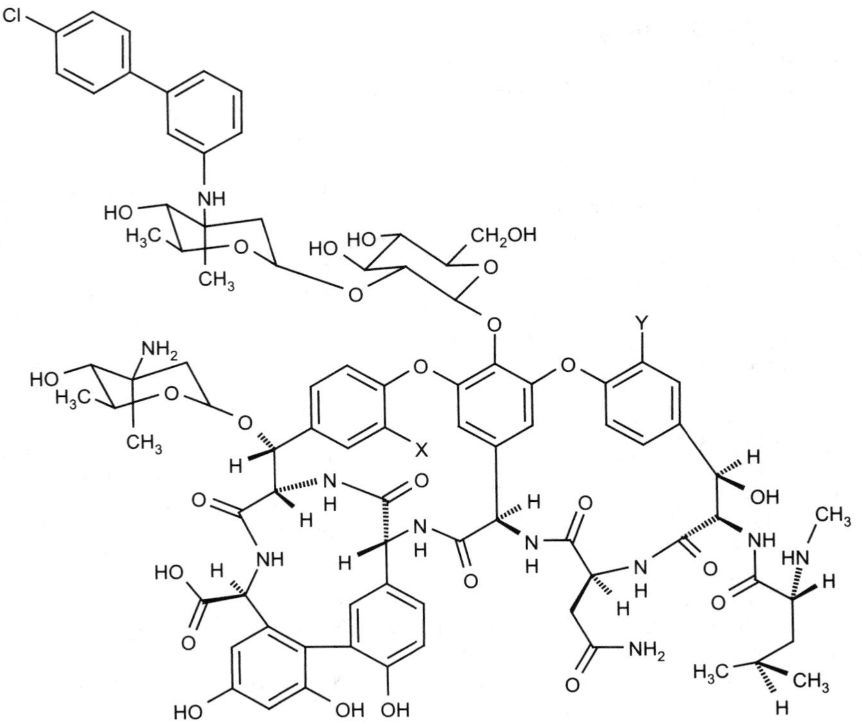

Figure 26 Oritavancin

Outer membrane peptide

Amino acids 1, 2, 3 and 4 glycopeptides (N-terminal)

Link of N-terminal amino acids with D-alanine-D-alanine

Figure 27 Mechanism of action of glycopeptides

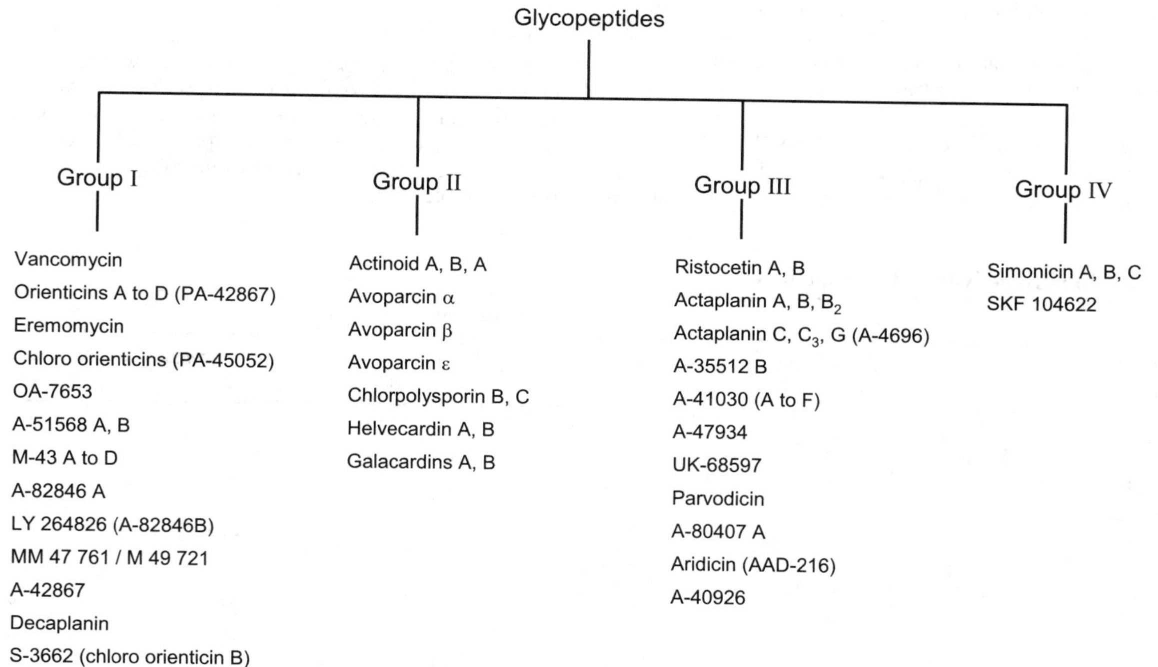

Figure 28 Classification of glycopeptides

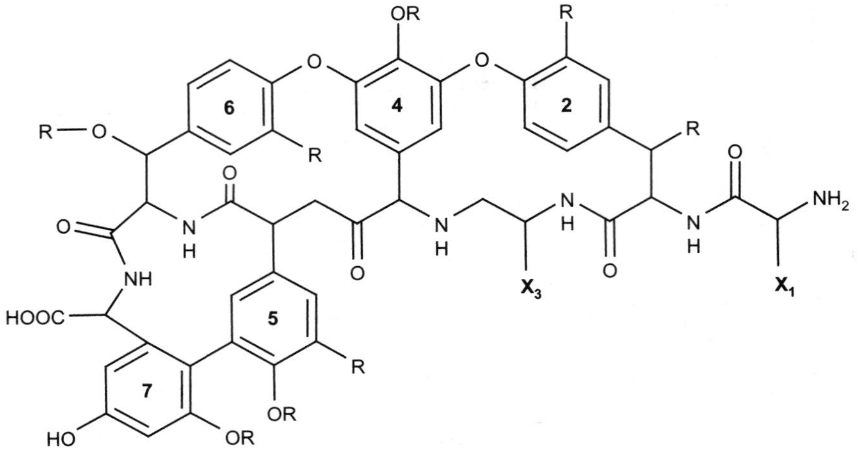

	HOOC—X7	X_6	X_5	X_4	X_3	X_2	X_1—NH_2
Vancomycin	m, m'-OH-Phg	β-OH-Tyr	β-OH-Phg	β-OH-Phg	Asn	β-OH-Tyr	Leucine
Ristocetin	m, m'-OH-Phg	β-OH-Tyr	β-OH-Phg	β-OH-Phg	m, m''-OH-Phg	β-OH-Tyr	β-OH-Phg
Avoparcin	m, m'-OH-Phg	β-OH-Tyr	β-OH-Phg	β-OH-Phg	p-OH-Phg	β-OH-Tyr	β-OH-Phg
Synmonicin	m, m'-OH-Phg	β-OH-Tyr	β-OH-Phg	β-OH-Phg	Met	β-OH-Tyr	β-OH-Phg

Tyr = tyrosine (β-OH Tyr = β-hydroxytyrosine)
Leu = leucine
M,m''-OH-Phg = metadihydroxy phenylglycine
Asn = asparagine

Figure 29 Glycopeptide structures

development phase (Komatsu et al., 1991) and exhibits partial cross-resistance with vancomycin.

6.3.2. Group II (Actinoidin)

The molecules belonging to group II possess a *para*-hydroxyphenylglycine as amino acids 3, 4, and 5 and as the NH_2-terminal amino acid. The sugars vary: acosamine, actinosamine, ristosamine, mannose, and rhamnose.

6.3.3. Group III (Ristocetin-Type Derivatives)

Group III consists of molecules with a *meta*-hydroxyphenylglycine as the amino acid at position 3, the N-terminal amino acid being a β-hydroxylphenylglycine. The aromatic moiety of these two amino acids are linked by an ether bond. Ristocetin does not have a chlorine atom and possesses a tetrasaccharide sugar, ristosamine.

6.3.4. Group IV

Currently group IV consists of synmonicin, which is characterized by a *para*-hydroxyphenylglycine as the N-terminal amino acid; the third amino acid is a thioamine aliphatic acid, methionine. One molecule is under development (SKF-104662).

The antibacterial activities of glycopeptides are summarized in Tables 19 and 20.

Table 19 In vitro activities of glycopeptides[a]

Compound	MIC (μg/ml)					
	MSSA	*S. epidermidis* ATCC 1228	*S. pyogenes* C203	*E. faecalis* ATCC 7080	*C. perfringens* ISS 30543	*N. gonorrhoeae* ISM 681126
Ristocetin	4	2	0.25	1	2	64
Vancomycin	0.25	0.5	0.13	0.5	0.13	32
Avoparcin	2	2	0.25	0.25	0.5	128
Actaplanin	1	2	0.13	0.5	1	128
Teicoplanin	0.13	0.13	0.06	0.13	0.003	32
A-35512B	1	0.5	0.13	0.5	2	64
A-41030	0.03	0.008	0.13	0.13		64
A-47934	0.06	0.03	0.13	0.13	0.25	8
Aridicin	1	4	0.13	2	0.06	64
A-40926	0.06	0.06	0.06	0.06	0.004	2

[a]Data from Parenti et al., 1990.

Table 20 In vitro activities of glycopeptides[a]

Microorganism	MIC$_{50}$ (μg/ml)				
	Vancomycin	Teicoplanin	Decaplanin	LY-264826	SKF 104662
MSSA	1	0.5	0.5	0.25	1
MRSA	2	0.5	0.5	0.25	1
S. epidermidis	2	0.5	1	0.25	2
S. haemolyticus	4	16	4	1	
E. faecalis	1	<0.03	1	0.25	0.5
E. faecium	1	0.25	0.5	0.12	0.5
Enterococcus avium	0.5	0.125			0.25
S. pyogenes	0.25	<0.03	0.25	<0.03	
S. pneumoniae	0.5	<0.03	0.12	0.06	<0.06
B. cereus	2	0.25	0.4	0.12	
C. jeikeium	0.5	0.25	0.25	0.06	0.25
L. monocytogenes	0.5	0.06	2	0.12	0.5
Viridans group streptococcus Pen[s]	0.5	0.125			0.25
Viridans group streptococcus Pen[r]	0.5	0.125			0.25

[a]Data from Yao et al., 1989.

6.3.5. AC-98 Complex

AC-98 complex was isolated in 1958 from the fermentation broth of *Streptomyces hygroscopicus*. This complex is exclusively directed against gram-positive organisms.

AC-98 is composed of five components: α, β, γ, δ, and ε, or 1 to 5. These components are glycosylated cyclic hexapeptides containing two stereoisomers of an unusual amino acid: α-amino-3[4′-(2′-imidazolidinyl)]-β-hydroxy propionic acid. This hexapeptide is made of alternating L- and D-amino acids that include β-methyl phenylalanine. A D-tyrosine residue is O glycosylated with a 1→4 α-linked mannose disaccharide.

Mannopeptimycins γ, δ, and ε have an isovaleryl group at the C-2, C-3, and C-4 positions on the terminal mannose ring, respectively. Mannopeptimycin ε is the most active component against MRSA. On the other hand, both α and β components are inactive against MRSA. All components except β exerted an in vivo efficacy against disseminated murine staphylococcal infections.

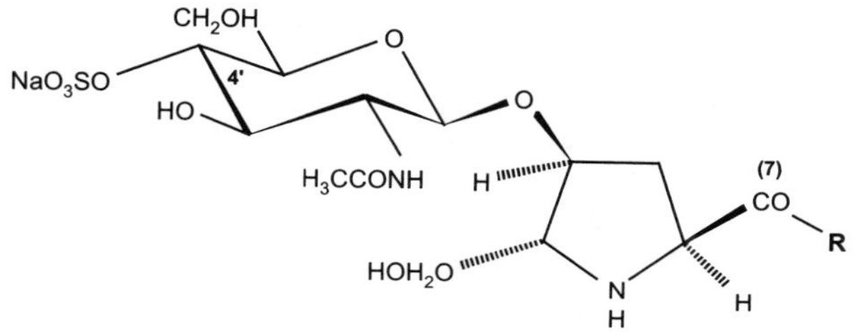

6.3.6. Bulgecins

Pseudomonas acidophila G 6302 and *Pseudomonas mesoacidophila* SB 72310 produce sulfazecin and isosulfazecin, but also bulgecins, which are small glycopeptides. Three molecules, A, B, and C, have been isolated (Fig. 30). They are composed of a specific amino acid, 4-hydroxy-5-hydroxymethylproline (iminocyclic acid), and a sugar, substituted 4-hydroxysulfonyl-β-D-glucopyranose. They are water soluble. Their lytic activities are potentiated in combination with β-lactams.

6.3.6.1. Biological Properties

The physicochemical properties vary with the substituents of the molecules, particularly the isoelectric point and lipophilicity.

It has been shown that if the isoelectric point increases, the clearance and volume of distribution decrease, while the apparent elimination half-life increases. When the isoelectric point remains the same, the clearance decreases and the apparent elimination half-life is prolonged if the lipophilicity is increased. Plasma protein binding (albumin) increases with the lipophilicity, while the free fraction decreases.

	R
Bulgecin A	NH-CH$_2$-CH$_2$-SO$_3$H
Bulgecin B	NH-CH$_2$-CH$_2$-COOH
Bulgecin C	OH

Figure 30 Bulgecins

These molecules share the same antibacterial spectrum, but their antibacterial activities differ.

6.3.6.2. Structure-Activity Relationship

The antibacterial activity stems essentially from the peptide. For vancomycin, it is based on amino acids 2, 3, and 4 from the N-terminal acid. The spatial configuration of the amino acids is important in terms of the bond with the D-alanine–D-alanine. The position requiring the least binding energy is the configuration *R*, *R*, *S*, and *R* (amino acids 1, 2, 3, and 4 from the N-terminal acid). This results in repulsive forms at positions 1 and 3, causing rotation of the N-terminal part. However, the oxygen of the carbonyl group is in an unfavorable steric position in relation to the amino group of amino acid 4. The amide bond is then rotated by 180°. This conformation with the target is the same for all of the glycopeptide antibiotics of the vancomycin type.

Amino acids 2 and 4 are in the same plane with a bond between their side chains. In the ristocetin family, the side chains of amino acids 1 and 3 are bound covalently.

Glycopeptide binding to the substrate occurs through five hydrogen bonds. The molecule binds to the carboxylate anions of the C-terminal part of the wall peptide (Cristofaro et al., 1995). For vancomycin, the hydrophobic part of the

Figure 31 Interaction between D-alanyl–D-alanine and the glycopeptide aglycon

cavity is formed by residue 1 (*N*-methyl-D-leucine) and the nonpolar parts of residues 2 and 3, whereas the N-H amide groups of these three residues form hydrogen bonds with the wall peptide carboxylates.

Sugars such as vancosamine are involved in the binding to the target. The 6-methyl group of vancosamine blocks the interaction between H_2O and H_2 of the C-terminal alanine residue, causing an increase in hydrophobicity at this point. The positively charged NH^{3+} group of vancosamine is important, as its absence reduces peptide binding threefold (Fig. 31).

The C-terminal amino acid must be a glycine or a D-amino acid. Semisynthetic derivatives of vancomycin have been prepared. About 80 *N*-alkylvancomycin derivatives have been obtained by reductive alkylation of vancomycin in the presence of aldehyde. Some *N*-alkylvancomycin derivatives have greater antibacterial activity than that of the corresponding *N*-acyl derivatives or vancomycin (Nagarajan et al., 1988a and 1988b). Alkylation occurs on the amino group of vancosamine and/or the *N*-methyl-leucine. The *N*-decanoyl derivatives of vancomycin are more active than the *N*-deacyl derivatives, and the C-10 alkyl derivatives are more active than the corresponding molecules in the alkanoyl series. The monoalkyl derivatives are more active than the di-*N*-alkyl derivatives.

7. GROUP IV: LIPOGLYCOPEPTIDES

The lipoglycopeptide group comprises a number of molecules (Fig. 32): teicoplanin, ramoplanin, aradacin, kibdelin,

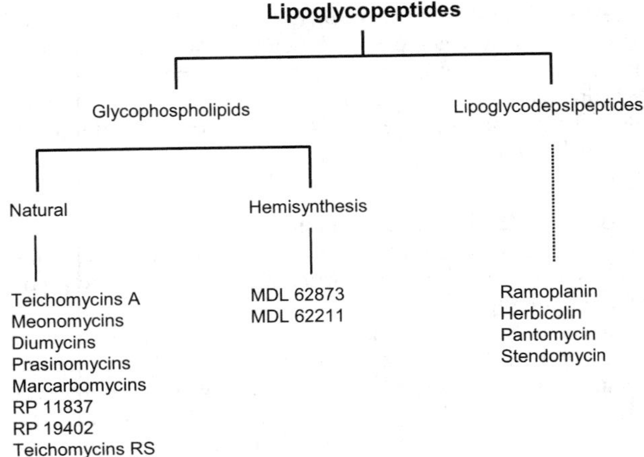

Figure 32 Classification of lipoglycopeptides

parvodicin, and A-40926. The lipoglycopeptides are characterized by a glycopeptide nucleus of the ristocetin type (glycopeptide group III) and a lipid chain attached to the amino group of the amino sugar. This chain may be linear or branched (iso or anteiso) and may be unsaturated. It contains 10 to 12 atoms of carbon.

The mechanism of action of the lipoglycopeptides is the same as that of vancomycin. The antibacterial spectrum coincides with that of vancomycin, but the antibacterial activity differs. One molecule, teicoplanin, is used therapeutically, and two are under development, ramoplanin and a semisynthetic derivative of teicoplanin, MDL-62873 (mideplanin).

7.1. Group VA: Glycophospholipid Derivatives

7.1.1. Teicoplanin

The teichomycins are lipoglycopeptide antibiotics obtained from fermentation of an actinomycete, *A. teichomyceticus*. The teichomycins are constituted by two major compounds, teichomycin A_1 and the teichomycin A_2 complex, or teicoplanin (Fig. 33), and a minor component, teichomycin A_3 (this compound does not possess *N*-acyl-β-glucosamine). Teichomycin A_1 is a phosphoglycolipid antibiotic. Teichomycin A_1 belongs to the group of glycophospholipid antibiotics, which include the moenomycins, diumycins, prasinomycins, marcarbomycins, RP-11837, RP-8036, and RP-19402.

Teichomycin A_1 is active against gram-positive cocci (MICs, 0.05 to 0.5 μg/ml) and has not insignificant activity against enterobacteria. It is inactive against the L forms of *S. aureus* and against mycoplasmas. It has a high molecular mass (3,255 Da).

The teicoplanin complex comprises five major components, TA-1, -2, -3, -4, and -5, and four minor components, RS-1, RS-2, RS-3, and RS-4.

The minor components contain the following fatty chains: RS-1 and RS-2 have 10-methylundecanoic acid and *n*-dodecanoic acid and RS-3 and RS-4 have 6-methyloctanoic acid and *n*-nonanoic acid, respectively. The fatty chains attached to the D-glucosamine present on the fourth amino acid have 10 or 11 carbons (Fig. 34).

The teicoplanin sugars are D-glucosamine and D-mannose.

The five components have the same in vitro activity. The in vivo activity and the median lethal dose differ (Table 21).

It has been shown that the two chlorine atoms at positions 22 and 55 on the aglycon are important for the antibacterial activity, as they stabilize the binding of the molecule to the binding site by preventing the mobility of the aromatic rings, in addition to that obtained with the diphenylether group. The chlorine atom at position 55 plays a major role in the antistreptococcal activity.

7.1.2. Mideplanin (MDL-62873)

Mideplanin is a semisynthetic derivative of teicoplanin A_2 obtained by binding a 3,3-dimethylamino-1-propylamine chain attached at N^{63} to the carbonyl at position 38 of the aglycon (Fig. 35 and 36).

This molecule is more active in vitro and in vivo than vancomycin. Its activity against *S. aureus*, *S. pyogenes*, and *S. pneumoniae* is similar to that of teicoplanin. It is characterized by good activity against *S. epidermidis* (MIC_{50}, 0.25 μg/ml) and *Staphylococcus haemolyticus* (MIC_{50}, 1.0 μg/ml).

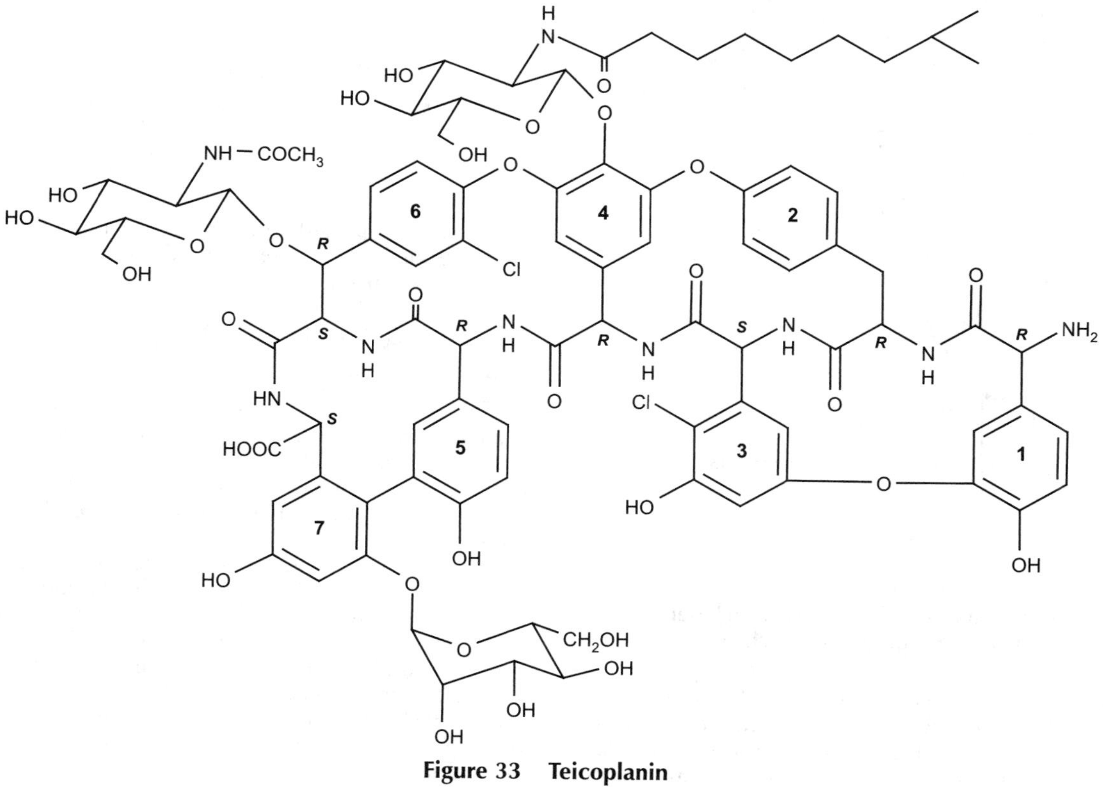

Figure 33 Teicoplanin

T-A2-1

R =

$C_{88}H_{95}Cl_2N_9O_{33}$

T-A2-2

R =

$C_{88}H_{97}Cl_2N_9O_{33}$

T-A2-3

R =

$C_{88}H_{97}Cl_2N_9O_{33}$

Figure 34 Teichomycin complex

Table 21 In vivo activity of teicoplanin A_2[a]

Teicoplanin A_2	ED_{50} (mg/kg)		Lethal dose (mice, i.p.[b]) (mg/kg)
	S. pneumoniae L44	*S. pyogenes* L49	
1	0.47	0.31	−2,000
2	0.28	0.15	−2,000
3	0.27	0.13	−1,500
4	0.12	0.098	−1,000
5	0.13	0.1	−1,000

[a]Data from Borghi et al., 1984.
[b]i.p., intraperitoneally.

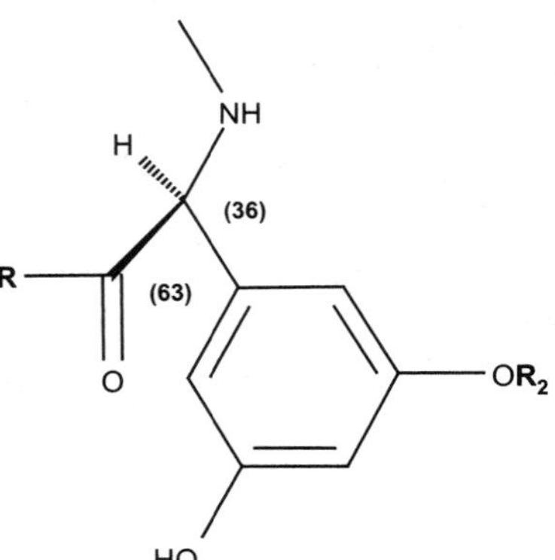

Figure 35 Derivatives of teicoplanin: attachment of a 3,3-dimethylamino-1-propylamine chain

MDL-62211 is a semisynthetic amide derivative of teicoplanin A_2 possessing good activity against methicillin-susceptible *S. aureus* (MSSA) (MICs, ≃0.5 to 1 μg/ml) and MRSA (MICs, 0.5 to 1 μg/ml), against enterococci (MICs, 0.5 to 1 μg/ml), and against *C. difficile* (MICs, 0.12 to 0.25 μg/ml). It is more active than teicoplanin, ramoplanin, and vancomycin.

7.1.3. A-40926 and MDL-63246

7.1.3.1. A-40926

The A-40926 series stems from lipopeptide derivatives related to teicoplanin. These come from natural products discovered simultaneously by two teams, one from the fermentation of *Actinomadura* sp. strain ATCC 39727 (A-40926) and the other from the fermentation of *Actinomadura parvosala* (parvodicin).

A-40926 is a complex of four molecules, A, B, PA, and PB. Compounds A and B differ in the lipid chain attached to the aminoglucuronic acid: factor A has an *n*-undecanoic acid chain, and factor B has a 10-methylundecanoic chain. The PA and PB factors are transformed rapidly to A and B. They differ from factors A and B in the presence of an acetate chain at position 6 of the D-mannose. A-40926 has two carboxyl groups, conferring on it two negative charges at neutral pH.

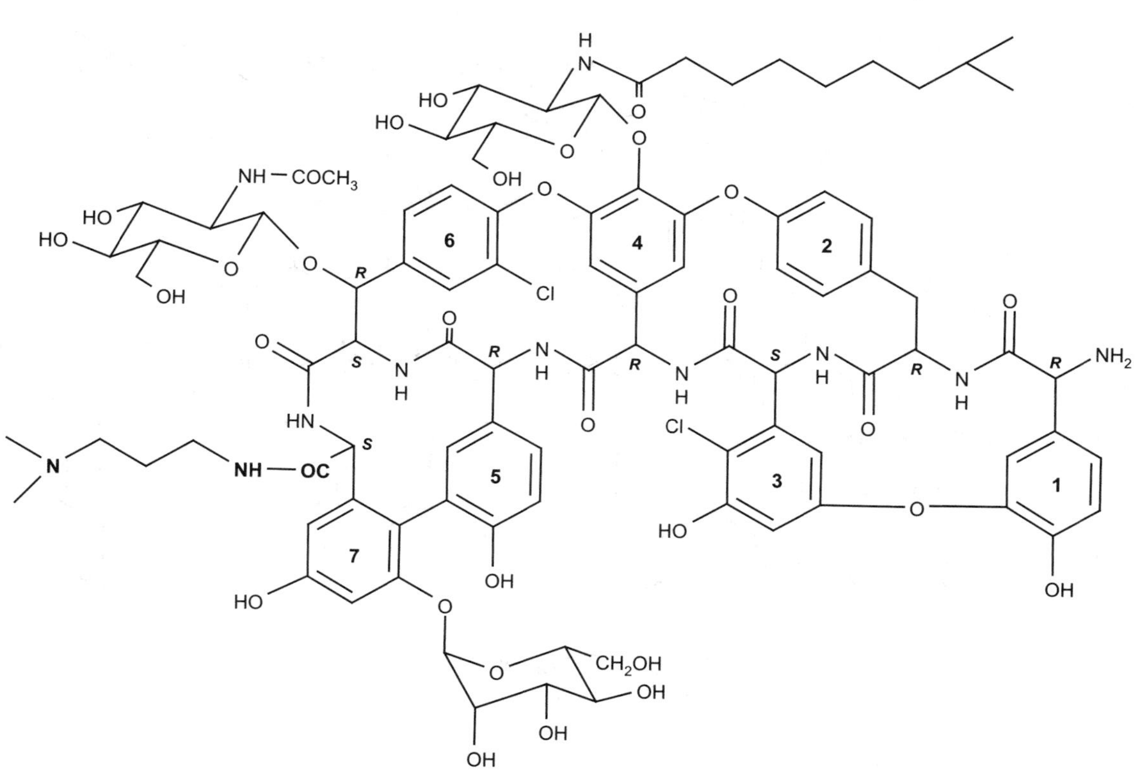

Figure 36 Mideplanin

Factors A and B have good antibacterial activity. The aglycon and the *N*-acylaminoglucuronyl aglycons have better in vitro activity against coagulase-negative staphylococci than the parent molecules (Selva et al., 1988). Factor B is slightly superior against gram-positive anaerobic bacteria. One of the characteristics of A and B is that, in contrast to teicoplanin, they are active against *Neisseria gonorrhoeae*.

7.1.3.2. MDL-63246

MDL-63246 is a semisynthetic derivative of A-40926 produced by attachment of a 3,3-dimethylaminopropylamine chain at position 38 of the aglycon (Fig. 37). Structure-activity studies have shown that in the group of teicoplanin and its derivatives the activity against enterococci is related to the absence of a 34-acetylglucosamine chain, as was demonstrated with the amide derivative of A-40926 and with 34-deacetylglucosaminyl teicoplanin, which has not inconsiderable activity against enterococci. The presence of mannose interferes little with the antienterococcal activity, whereas the presence of *N*-acylglucosamine or *N*-acylglucuronic acid or methylester derivatives of these two sugars is essential for activity against strains of enterococci of the VanA phenotype (Malabarba et al., 1995). Two in vitro studies versus vancomycin, teicoplanin, and mideplanin showed that MDL-63246 is the most active molecule. All of the molecules tested were active against *S. aureus*, whether the strains were susceptible or resistant to oxacillin. Compared to teicoplanin and vancomycin, MDL-63246 has good activity against *S. epidermidis* (MIC_{50}, 0.125 μg/ml) and *S. haemolyticus* (MIC_{50}, 0.5 μg/ml, versus 16 μg/ml for teicoplanin). The activity of MDL-63246 against *S. pyogenes, Streptococcus agalactiae, S. pneumoniae*, and beta-hemolytic or viridans group streptococci is excellent (MIC_{50}, ≤0.03 μg/ml). Its activity against enterococci is variable. Against vancomycin-susceptible *E. faecalis* it has the same activity as teicoplanin (MIC_{50}, ~0.25 μg/ml). However, while it is active against vancomycin-susceptible strains of *E. faecium* (MIC_{50}, ~0.25 μg/ml), it is moderately active against VanA strains (MICs, 8 to 32 μg/ml), although it is active against VanB strains (MIC_{50}, ~0.25 μg/ml) and VanC strains (MIC_{50}, ~0.06 μg/ml). It is also active against *Enterococcus durans* (MIC_{50}, ~0.13 μg/ml). Against VanA strains the molecule is weakly active, but markedly more than vancomycin (Malabarba et al., 1995).

Its activity against gram-negative bacilli is variable. It is good against *Corynebacterium* spp. (MIC_{50}, ~0.13 μg/ml), *L. monocytogenes* (MIC_{50}, ~0.06 μg/ml), *Bacillus* spp. (MIC_{50}, 0.06 μg/ml), *Micrococcus* spp. (MIC_{50}, ~0.13 μg/ml), *Lactobacillus garviae* (MIC, 0.25 μg/ml), and vancomycin-susceptible *Lactobacillus* (MICs, 0.03 to 0.1 μg/ml). Conversely, it is inactive against *Leuconostoc mesenteroides* (MIC, >128 μg/ml), *Pediococcus* spp. (MIC_{50}, 128 μg/ml), and vancomycin-resistant strains of *Lactobacillus* (Goldstein et al., 1995; Kenny et al., 1995).

Against *S. aureus*, MDL-63246 has slow and time-dependent bactericidal activity.

7.1.4. Telavancin (TD-6424)

Telavancin is a semisynthetic lipoglycopeptide obtained by substitution of the amino group of vancosamine by a fatty acid side chain.

The antibacterial properties of these analogs depends on the length of the hydrophobic side chain. The optimum side chain was reached for antienterococcal activity with a 13-methylene length.

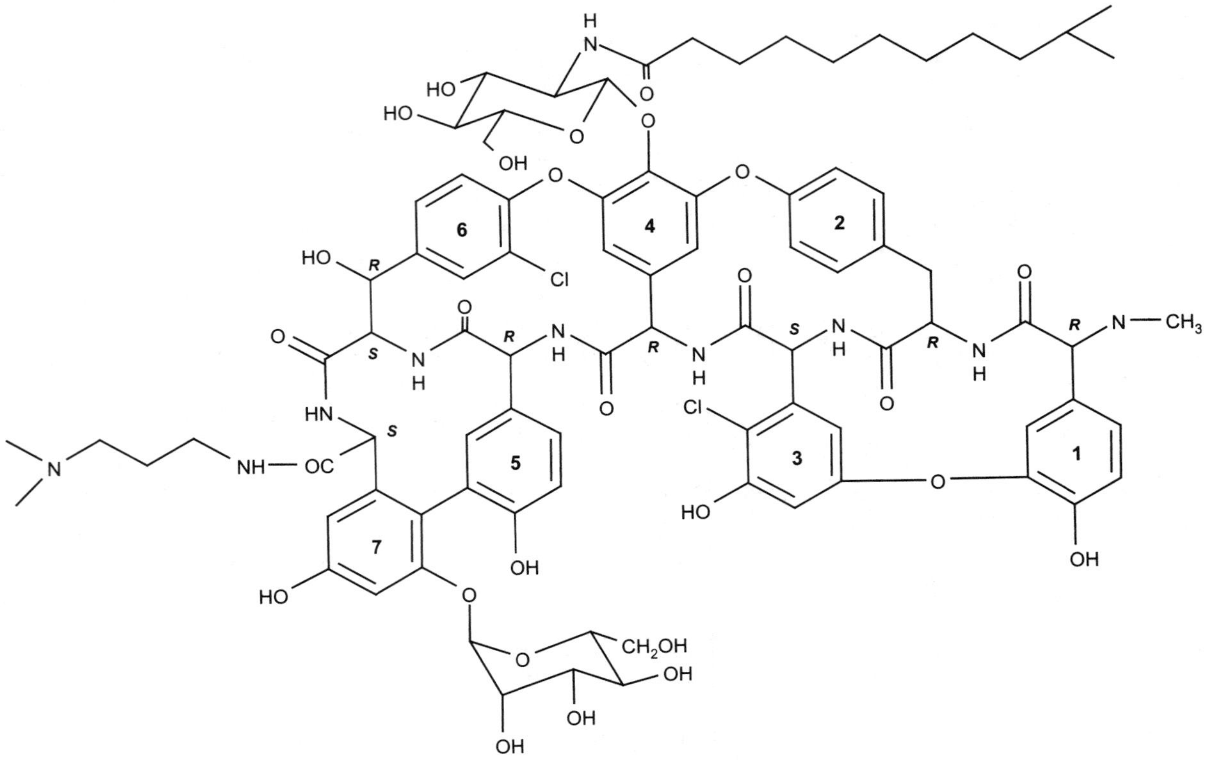

Figure 37 MDL-63246

Telavancin is more active than vancomycin but less active than oritavancin. Telavancin is more active against *S. aureus* but less active against *S. pneumoniae* and *Enterococcus* spp. than dalbavancin. Against glycopeptide-intermediate *S. aureus* (GISA) HIP 5836 strains, telavancin (MIC, 2 μg/ml) is more active than vancomycin and teicoplanin (MICs, 8 μg/ml).

Telavancin, unlike vancomycin, is bactericidal against *S. aureus*. For a concentration of 4 μg/ml, the initial inoculum was reduced from $6.22 \pm 0.08 \log_{10}$ CFU/ml mean ± standard deviation to $2.36 \pm 0.18 \log_{10}$ CFU/ml for MSSA after 4 h of contact. For MRSA, after 4 h of contact with concentrations of 8 and 32 μg/ml, the initial inoculum was reduced from $6.05 \pm 0.008 \log_{10}$ CFU/ml to $4.87 \pm 0.5 \log_{10}$ CFU/ml and $1.26 \pm 0.26 \log_{10}$ CFU/ml, respectively. For GISA strains, the contact concentrations were 8 and 32 μg/ml to obtain a reduction of the inoculum after 4 h from $5.76 \pm 0.07 \log_{10}$ CFU/ml to $2.73 \pm 0.08 \log_{10}$ CFU/ml (Pace et al., 2003).

Telavancin is active in staphylococcal infections irrespective of the resistance pattern and the mouse immune system status (Judice and Pace, 2003).

In human volunteers after a dose of 5 mg/kg of body weight intravenously, 45 and 5 μg/ml were determined to be the maximum and minimum plasma concentrations. The apparent elimination half-life is about 7 h.

7.2. Group VB: Lipoglycodepsipeptides

The lipoglycodepsipeptide group of antibiotics comprises few molecules: ramoplanin, herbicolin, and pantomycin and a similar compound, stendomycin. Herbicolin is a complex composed of two molecules isolated from the fermentation of *Erwinia herbicola*. It has antifungal activity.

Pantomycin is an antimicrobial agent isolated from the fermentation of *S. hygroscopicus*. It possesses antibacterial and antifungal activities.

Stendomycin is an antibacterial agent produced by fermentation from a strain of *Streptomyces antimycoticus*. It is a complex comprising two compounds, A and B. This molecule possesses good antifungal activity, but it is weakly active or even inactive against bacteria.

7.2.1. Ramoplanin

Ramoplanin is a complex composed of three molecules, A_1, A_2, and A_3, isolated from the fermentation of *Actinoplanes* sp. strain ATCC 33076 (Fig. 38). The components are in the ratio 12, 74, and 14%. Mutant strains have enabled the proportion of A_2 to be increased so as to represent more than 85% of production. Ramoplanin is an amphoteric molecule (pK, ~8 to 10) with a high molecular weight. It is presented in the form of a white powder that decomposes at 210 to 230°C. The specific rotation, $[\alpha]^{20}_D$, is equal to +78.3° ($c = 1.0$, H_2O). It is a basic molecule with an isoelectric point of 9.25.

The physicochemical properties of components A_1, A_2, and A_3 are summarized in Table 22.

Ramoplanin consists of three parts: a peptide part, a carbohydrate part, and a lipid part.

The peptide part is composed of 17 amino acids. An ester bond between the carboxyl group of the terminal amino acid (amino acid 17) and the hydroxyl group of amino acid 2 (β-hydroxyaspartic acid) creates a depsipeptide of 16 amino acids, leaving a free amino acid at the NH_2-terminal part.

The presence of two ornithines (amino acids 4 and 10) gives the molecule its basic character.

The saccharide part is composed of an α-D-mannosyl-α-D-mannose unit; the mannoside unit is attached by a hemiacetyl bond to the 4-hydroxyphenylglycine (amino acid 11).

The lipid part is attached to the aspartic acid (amino acid 1) by its NH_2 part and forms an amide bond. This aspartic acid is carried by an asparagine (amino acid 2), bound to the

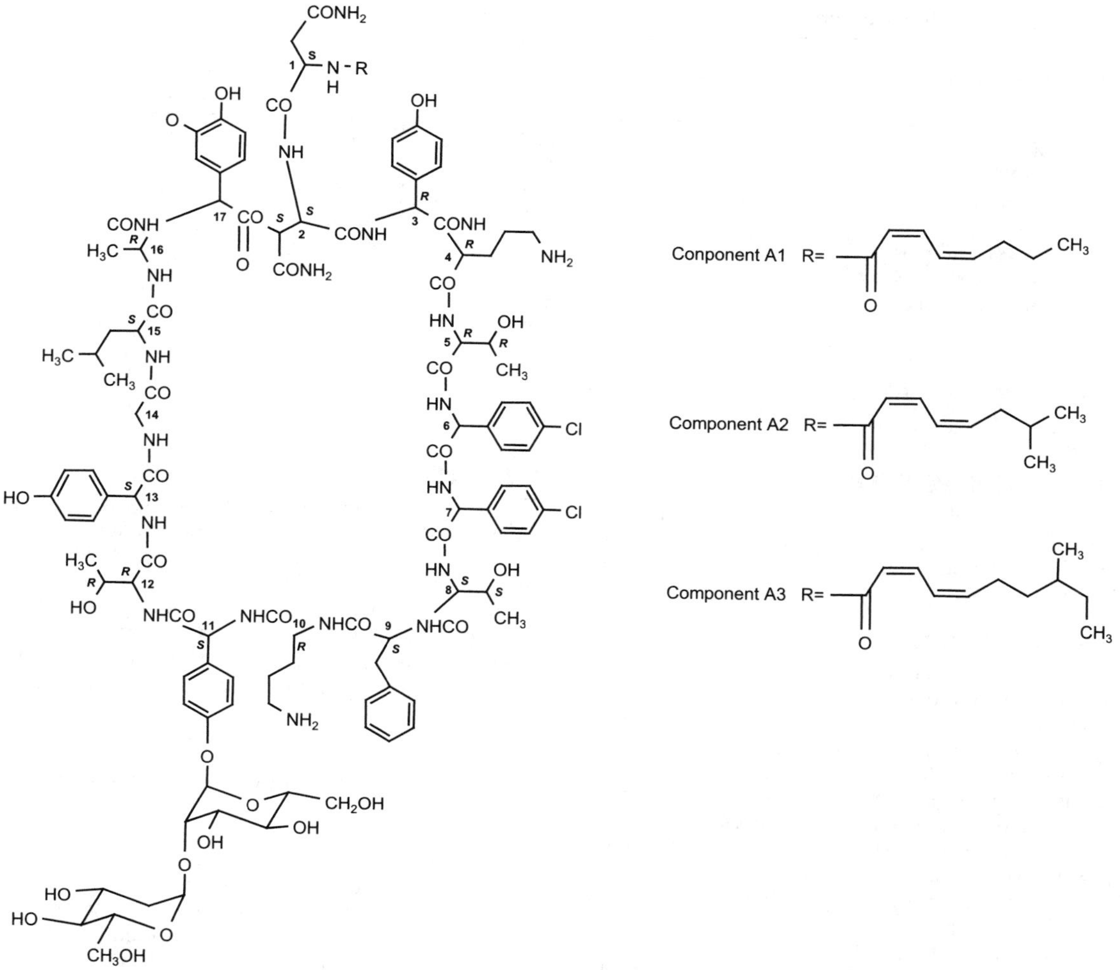

Figure 38 Structure of ramoplanin

Table 22 Physicochemical properties of the ramoplanin complex

Component	Mol mass (Da)	Empirical formula	Specific rotation $[\alpha]^{20}_D$
A_1	2,540.07	$C_{118}H_{152}ClN_{21}O_{40}$	$+57° \pm 4°$ (c = 0.5 H_2O)
A_2	2,554.09	$C_{119}H_{154}ClN_{21}O_{40}$	$+73° \pm 4°$ (c = 0.5 H_2O)
A_3	2,568.12	$C_{120}H_{156}ClN_{21}O_{40}$	$+50° \pm 4°$ (c = 0.5, 0.01 NHCl)

C-terminal amino acid (amino acid 17), 3-chloro-4-hydroxyphenylglycine acid, by a lactone bond.

The three compounds differ in their unsaturated lipid chains: octadienoic acid (A_1), 7-methyloctadienoic acid (A_2), and 8-methylnonadienic acid (A_3).

7.2.2. Antibacterial Activity

Ramoplanin is much more active than vancomycin and teicoplanin against strains of *S. aureus* and against the different species of coagulase-negative staphylococci (Francis et al., 1990), with a MIC_{50} of 0.5 μg/ml. This molecule is active against *P. acnes*. Table 23 shows the in vitro activity of ramoplanin.

Ramoplanin inhibits peptidoglycan synthesis after the formation of the cytoplasmic precursors. It does not inhibit peptidoglycan synthesis by complexing the acyl–D-Ala–D-Ala unit like the glycopeptides. The number of molecules binding to the *S. aureus* cell is lower (4×10^4 molecules) than with vancomycin (10^7 molecules).

In fact, the glycopeptides bind to the growth zone of peptidoglycan and to specific amino acids. The primary target of ramoplanin appears to be *N*-acetylglucosaminyl transferase, which catalyzes the conversion of lipid intermediate I to lipid intermediate II. It blocks the transfer of one or two precursors.

For this reason, there would appear to be no cross-resistance between ramoplanin and the glycoprotein antibiotics.

Because of its poor systemic tolerance, ramoplanin is currently under development for topical use, like mupirocin.

Table 23 In vitro activities of ramoplanin and mideplanin[a]

Microorganism(s)[b]	MIC_{50} (μg/ml)			
	Teicoplanin	Ramoplanin	Mideplanin	Vancomycin
MSSA	0.37	1.85	0.69	1.50
MRSA	0.62	2.0	0.72	1.45
MSSE	1.60	0.71	0.35	1.47
MRSE	2.15	0.77	0.44	1.43
S. haemolyticus Met[s]	2.19	<1.0	0.82	1.35
S. haemolyticus Met[r]	2.80	1.3	1.52	<2.0
Enterococcus spp.	0.20	4.35	0.33	2.25
C. difficile	0.19	0.39	0.09	0.85

[a]Data from Bartolini et al., 1990.
[b]MSSE, methicillin-susceptible *S. epidermidis*; MRSE, methicillin-resistant *S. epidermidis*.

8. GROUP V: LIPOPEPTIDES

The lipopeptides are characterized by a peptide chain to which is attached a fatty acid side chain. The lipopeptides may be divided into linear lipopeptides and cyclic lipopeptides (Fig. 39).

8.1. Linear Lipopeptides (Group V-1)

Cerexin is a linear decapeptide with a fatty acid at C-11 and a preponderance of amino acids in the D configuration.

Amphomycin (Fig. 40) was described by Heinemann et al. (1953). Its structure is that of a linear undecapeptide with a branched, unsaturated fatty acid chain at C-13. It is active against gram-positive microorganisms. The MIC_{50}s are between 2 and 4 μg/ml for staphylococci, whether the strains are susceptible or resistant to methicillin or fluoroquinolones. For the group of enterococci and streptococci, the MIC_{50} is between 0.5 and 1 μg/ml. It inhibits peptidoglycan synthesis in terms of the formation of the lipid PP, N-acetylmuramylpentapeptide. The median lethal doses in the mouse are 177.8 mg/kg (sodium salt) and 120.2 mg/kg (calcium salt) intravenously. It is used as a topical antibiotic in veterinary medicine.

Viscosin is a hexapeptide with activity against *M. tuberculosis*.

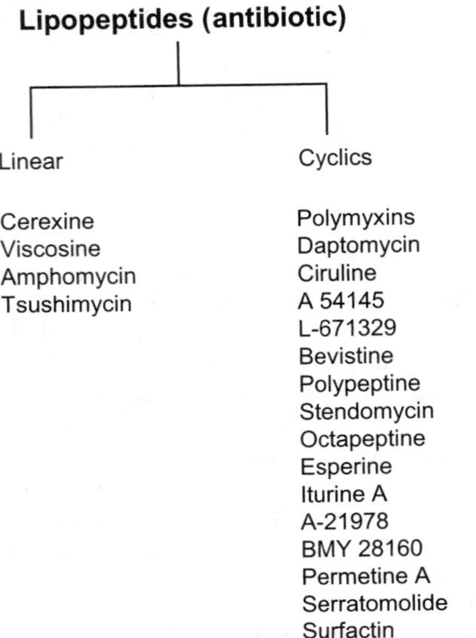

Figure 39 Classification of lipopeptide antibiotics

8.2. Cyclic Lipopeptides (Group V-2)

The cyclic lipopeptides comprise a large number of molecules, some of which are used therapeutically (polymyxin), while others are undergoing clinical development (daptomycin).

These molecules are divided schematically according to their biological activities into four groups: those active against gram-negative bacteria, those active against gram-positive bacteria, antifungal agents, and antimycobacterial agents.

8.2.1. Lipopeptides Active against Gram-Negative Bacteria

8.2.1.1. Polymyxin Complex

The main molecule of lipopeptides active against gram-negative bacteria is the polymyxin complex. Polymyxin is a decapeptide whose fatty chain is attached to the peptide nucleus. They were isolated in 1947 from the fermentation of *Bacillus polymyxa*. The polymyxins are basic decapeptides containing a heptapeptide ring and a fatty chain in the N-terminal position comprising eight or nine carbon atoms. They contain five or six γ-diaminobutyric acid residues.

The heptapeptide ring is attached by the α-amino and carboxyl groups of γ-aminobutyric acid to the fatty acid chain. Eight different polymyxins have been characterized: A(M), B_1, B_2, D_1, E_1, E_2, S, and T_1 (Table 24). Circulin produced by *Bacillus circulans* is included in this group. It is divided into subgroups 1, 2, 3, and 4 according to the fatty acid chain (Table 25).

Only polymyxins B (B_1 and B_2), E (E_1 or colistin A, and E_2 or colistin), and M in Russia (polymyxin A) are used therapeutically.

8.2.1.1.1. Physicochemical properties. The polymyxins have a high molecular mass, on the order of 1,150 Da. They are water-soluble bases that are unstable in an alkaline medium. Polymyxin B and E sulfates are salts obtained after protonation of the five L-Dab amino groups that bind sulfate ions in the presence of sulfuric acid.

They are white, crystalline, odorless, bitter, hygroscopic powders stable for several years in the dry state. Certain divalent ions (cobalt, magnesium, manganese, and calcium), strong acids, and strong bases inactivate polymyxin B sulfate.

Protonation of polymyxins in an aqueous solution causes these molecules to behave like cationic detergents, which partly explains the essential features of their toxicity.

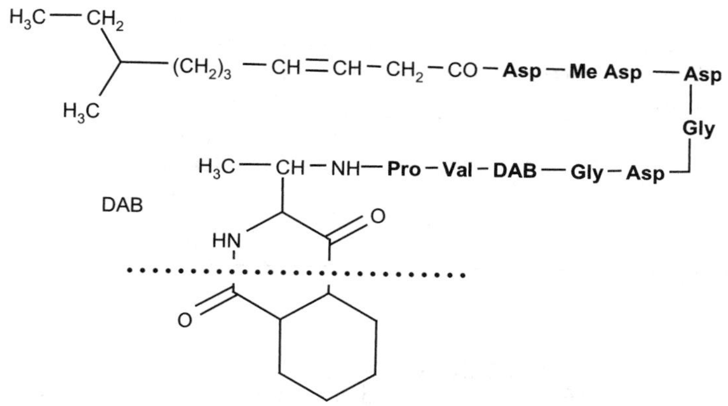

H_3C-CH_2
$(CH_2)_3-CH=CH-CH_2-CO-$**Asp**$-$**Me Asp**$-$**Asp**
H_3C
Gly
$H_3C-CH-NH-$**Pro**$-$**Val**$-$**DAB**$-$**Gly**$-$**Asp**
DAB
HN
O
O

Figure 40 Amphomycin

Table 24 Classification of polymyxins[a]

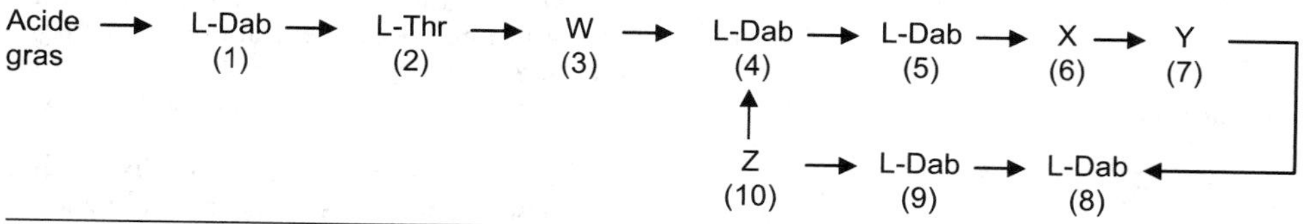

Acide gras → L-Dab (1) → L-Thr (2) → W (3) → L-Dab (4) → L-Dab (5) → X (6) → Y (7) → L-Dab (8) → L-Dab (9) → Z (10) → L-Dab (4)

Molecule(s)	W (3)	X (6)	Y (7)	Z (10)	Mol wt
Circulins A and B	L-Dab	D-Leu	L-Ile	L-Thr	1,169.47/1,155.45
Polymyxin A (M)	L-Dab	D-Leu	L-Thr	L-Thr	1,157.42
Polymyxins B1 and B2	L-Dab	D-Phe	L-Leu	L-Thr	1,198.45/1,184.42
Polymyxin (or P)	L-Dab	D-Leu	L-Thr	L-Thr	
Polymyxin D1/D2	D-Ser	D-Leu	L-Thr	L-Thr	1,144.38/1,130.35
Polymyxin E1 (colistin A)	L-Dab	D-Leu	L-Leu	L-Thr	1,169.47
Polymyxin S1	D-Ser	D-Phe	L-Thr	L-Thr	1,178.39
Polymyxin T1	L-Dab	D-Phe	L-Leu	L-Leu	1,215.54

[a]Acide gras, fatty acid.

Table 25 Classification of polymyxins by fatty acids

Polymyxin	Fatty acid
1	(+)-6-Methyloctanoyl (MOA)
2	6-Methyl heptanoyl (iso-octanoyl) (IOA)
3	Octanoyl (OA)
4	Heptanoyl, Dab-acid α-γ-aminobutyric (HA)

Polymyxin E sodium methanesulfonate has been prepared from colistin sulfate by sulfamethylation of the amino groups in the presence of formaldehyde and sodium bisulfite.

8.2.1.1.2. International and weight units. Table 26 defines the value by weight (in micrograms) of the three international standards deposited in London, England (World Health Organization, 1977).

The sulfate unit of polymyxin B corresponds to 2 IU of polymyxin sulfate and 1.25 IU of sodium methanesulfonate.

One milligram of colistin base is equal to 1.5 mg of colistin sulfate and 2.4 mg of colistin sodium methanesulfonate.

8.2.1.1.3. Physicochemical incompatibilities. Colistin is stable in solution at a pH of between 5.5 and 8 and polymyxin B is stable at neutral pH.

There is incompatibility in solution with a number of antibiotics (β-lactams, chloramphenicol, novobiocin, kanamycin, and nitrofurantoin) and other drugs: cyanocobalamin, heparin, hydrocortisone hemisuccinate, prednisone, and phenobarbital.

8.2.1.1.4. Antibacterial activity. All of the polymyxins exhibit the same antibacterial spectrum, but their activities are different. They are inactive against gram-positive bacteria. They are active against *Enterobacteriaceae* such as *E. coli*, *Klebsiella pneumoniae*, *Enterobacter*, *Salmonella* spp., and *Shigella* spp. (MIC_{50} and MIC_{90}, 0.5 and 1.0 μg/ml) but are inactive against *Proteus* spp. and *S. marcescens* (MIC, >32 μg/ml). They have good activity against *P. aeruginosa* (MIC_{50} and MIC_{90}, 2.0 and 2.0 μg/ml), *Acinetobacter* (MIC_{50} and MIC_{90}, 0.5 and 1.0 μg/ml), *H. influenzae* (MIC_{50} and MIC_{90}, 0.25 and 1.0 μg/ml), *Moraxella catarrhalis* (MIC_{50} and MIC_{90}, 2.0 and 4.0 μg/ml), and *Bordetella pertussis*, but they are inactive against *Neisseria*. *Vibrio* is conventionally susceptible, but *Vibrio cholerae* El Tor (seventh pandemic) is resistant. *Bacteroides fragilis* is resistant. Polymyxin B is the most active molecule (Table 27).

8.2.1.1.5. Mechanism of action. Polymyxins penetrate the cell wall of gram-negative bacilli by a self-induced

Table 26 Polymyxins—international units

Compound	Wt for 1 IU/μg	Accepted wt for 1 IU/μg	Concn (IU/μg)	Wt for 10^6 IU
Polymyxin B base		0.1	10	100 mg
Polymyxin B sulfate	0.119	0.1	10	100 mg
Colistin base		0.033	30	33.3 mg
Colistin methane sulfonate sodium	0.07874	0.08	12.5	80 mg
Colistin sulfate	0.04878	0.045	20	50 mg

Table 27 In vitro activity of polymyxins

Microorganism(s)	MIC (μg/ml)	
	Polymyxin B	Colistin A
E. coli	0.06–4	0.01–4
K. pneumoniae	0.06–1	0.01–8
S. marcescens	>128	>128
Enterobacter spp.	1–2	0.25–4
Proteus spp.	>128	>128
Salmonella serovar Typhimurium	0.06–2	0.01–4
Shigella sonnei	0.06–2	0.12–16
P. aeruginosa	0.03–4	0.12–8
Yersinia spp.		0.25–16
Acinetobacter spp.		0.5–4
H. influenzae	0.25–4	0.5–2
B. pertussis	0.5–4	0.01–4
C. freundii		0.5–2

mechanism. By chelating divalent cations, they destabilize the wall and can insinuate themselves into it. They act on the phosphatidylethanolamine-rich cytoplasmic membrane of gram-negative bacilli. They are inactive against gram-positive bacilli, which are poor in phosphatidylethanolamine. Methylation of the phospholipids yields lecithin, which has a weak affinity for polymyxins. The bactericidal activity of polymyxins derives from their interaction with the cytoplasmic membrane, causing the disorganization of this structure and the release of intracellular constituents into the extracellular medium.

8.2.1.1.6. Resistance. Resistance to polymyxins is of chromosomal origin and is uncommon. The origin of this resistance is a modification of the bacterial wall and, in particular, an increase in the quantity of H_1 membrane protein, which causes a reduction in the quantity of divalent cations necessary for the bacterial wall. The initial stage of the penetration of polymyxin through the bacterial wall is its binding to divalent cations, and the H_1 protein plays the role of a divalent cation; the polymyxins lose their anchorage point in the bacterial wall. A modification of the phospholipids of the cytoplasmic membrane also appears to play a part.

8.2.1.1.7. Pharmacokinetics. Some studies have been published and are based on microbiological assays using *Bordetella bronchiseptica* ATCC 4617 as the test strain, but because of the physicochemical characteristics of the polymyxins they are nonspecific. A study has been conducted with colistin methanesulfonate, and the assays were performed by a chromatographic method.

8.2.1.2. Polymyxin B

After intramuscular administration of 50 mg of polymyxin B, the peak concentration in serum is reached after about 2 h. The peak concentration ranges from 1 to 8 μg/ml. Levels in serum decline slowly, and polymyxin B is still detectable at 12 h. The apparent elimination half-life is about 6 h. After repeated doses, accumulation of polymyxin B occurs. After intravenous administration of 50 mg in 500 ml of isotonic glucose solution, the concentrations are 4.1 μg/ml at the end of the infusion (60 min), 1.1 to 3.5 μg/ml at the end of the first hour, 0.6 to 2 μg/ml at 3 h, and 0.6 to 1.3 μg/ml at 4 h.

8.2.1.3. Polymyxin E (Colistin Methanesulfonate)

Colistin sulfate is used for oral and topical application, and colisitin methanesulfonate is used for parenteral and aerosol applications. Colistin methanesulfonate is less active than colistin sodium. In aqueous solution, colistin methanesulfonate is hydrolyzed; colistin is freed and the salt methanesulfonate is transformed into a sulfomethyl complex. Colistin alone is more active in vitro than colistin methanesulfonate. Colistin methanesulfonate hydrolyzes to colistin via its partial derivatives when stored in plasma at 37°C.

Colistin was relegated to a second-line antibiotic because of its potential systemic toxicity, including neurotoxicity and nephrotoxicity.

After intramuscular administration of 80 mg, the peak concentration in serum of 5.3 μg/ml is reached in 1 to 2 h, the AUC from 0 h to infinity is 25 to 70 μg·h/ml, the apparent elimination half-life is about 3.5 h, the apparent volume of distribution is 15.8 liters, and the plasma clearance is 5.3 liters/kg. The residual concentration at 12 h is 0.35 μg/ml. Polymyxins are eliminated principally renally by glomerular filtration, and there is no tubular secretion or reabsorption. Renal clearance of polymyxins is about 63 ml/min. Colistin methanesulfonate is eliminated more rapidly than polymyxin B. Between 40 and 60% of the administered dose is found in the urine. Elimination may be prolonged for up to 3 days after the end of administration.

Biotransformation is moderate (15 to 20%), and metabolites have been detected in the urine. Biliary elimination is very weak.

In patients with renal insufficiency, the apparent elimination half-life may be 2 to 3 days, with major interindividual variations (Table 28). Polymyxins are weakly dialyzable, probably because of their size and high molecular weight. Plasma protein binding is on the order of 15 to 20%.

In animals, polymyxins bind persistently in the liver, kidneys, brain, myocardial tissue, and lungs. High concentrations are found 72 h after a single dose and after up to 5 days following repeated dosing. Colistin methanesulfonate is more strongly concentrated than polymyxin B in the kidneys, lungs, and liver, but polymyxin B is more concentrated in the brain than colistin.

Table 28 Pharmacokinetics of polymyxin B sulfate in renally impaired patients

Compound	Apparent elimination half-life (days) at indicated creatinine clearance (ml/min)			
	>80	80–30	<30	<5
Polymyxin B sulfate				
Day 1	2.5–3	2.5	2.5	2.5
Following days	2.5–3	1–1.5	1–1.5 (2–3 days)	1 (5–7 days)
Colistin methanesulfonate				
Day 1	3–5	3	3	2.5
Following days	1.5–2.5	1.5–2.5	1.5 (2–3 days)	(5–7 days)

In humans, concentrations in serous effusion or inflammatory fluids are weak. Polymyxins do not diffuse into the cerebrospinal fluid.

In children, particularly neonates and premature infants, there is not inconsiderable oral absorption. This feature contraindicates their gastrointestinal use in children in these age ranges. Parenterally, the kinetics are identical to those in adults.

In elderly subjects, renal elimination is delayed. In pregnant women, mother-fetus transmission occurs after intravenous administration. The polymyxin concentration in the cord blood ranges from 1.2 to 1.9 μg/ml 8 h after administration of the product to the mother.

The antibiotic has not been detected in amniotic fluid. Excretion in colostrum is slight.

The polymyxins are not absorbed in the intestinal mucosa. They are for this reason poor antibiotics for the treatment of enteroinvasive intestinal infections.

Following local application to wounds, burns, and mucous membranes (ears and conjunctiva) and after bladder lavage, absorption is nonexistent. Conversely, when colistin is applied to hairless areas the absorption is not insignificant.

Administered in aerosol form, polymyxins cross the bronchopulmonary barrier and concentrations in plasma are similar to those obtained after parenteral administration. Concentrations in plasma following irrigation in the peritoneal cavity may be high. Colistin can be incorporated in acrylic cements.

The pharmacokinetics in 12 cystic fibrosis patients after a 30-min infusion are shown in Table 29.

Polymyxins are never prescribed to patients receiving curarizing agents or muscle relaxants, which they potentiate because of their action on neuromuscular transmission.

Combination with antibiotics with a nephrotoxic potential, such as aminoglycosides, is not recommended.

A patient was treated with intravenous colistin methanesulfonate sodium (5 mg/kg/day) for 5 days. On day 4, culture of cerebrospinal fluid was negative. Colistin levels in cerebrospinal fluid reached 1.25 μg/ml (Jimenez-Mejias et al., 2000).

8.2.1.3.1. Nonantibiotic action. Polymyxins have nonantibiotic effects: they interact with bacterial endotoxins, the complement system, coagulation, and histamine. In the presence of calcium, polymyxin B experimentally induces mastocyte degranulation and histamine release.

8.2.1.3.2. Tolerance. Polymyxins, particularly polymyxin B, are responsible for nephrotoxicity and neurologic incidents.

8.2.1.3.3. Therapeutic indications. The therapeutic indications are theoretically those of their antibacterial spectrum. In practice, because of their side effects they are used only when other antibacterial agents are ineffective.

The local uses of polymyxins are principally infections due to *P. aeruginosa*, such as superinfected wounds and ulcers, otitis externa, ocular infections, pleurisy, arthritis, and Kehr's drains. They are used alone or, more often, in combination with another antibacterial agent.

In aerosol form, polymyxins are used in the treatment of respiratory tract infections due to *P. aeruginosa* in patients suffering from cystic fibrosis or bronchial dilatation. In severe or systemic infections, polymyxins are second-line antibiotics.

8.2.2. Lipopeptides Active against Gram-Positive Bacteria

8.2.2.1. A-21978C Complex

The A-21978 complex was obtained by fermentation of *Streptomyces roseoporus*.

Five groups of compounds have been isolated by thin-layer chromatography (Table 30). The C compounds are the most important. Three major C compounds have been

Table 29 Pharmacokinetics of colistin methanesulfonate in cystic fibrosis patients

Parameter	Colistin methanesulfonate	Colistin
C_{max} (μg/ml)	3.6–13.2	1.2–3.1
C_{min} (μg/ml)	0.1–62.0	0.14–1.3
AUC (μg·h/ml)		
CL_P (ml/min/kg)	2.01 ± 0.46	
V (ml/kg)	340 ± 95	
$t_{1/2}$ (min)	124 ± 52	251 ± 79

Table 30 R_f of complex A-21978 by thin-layer chromatography

A-21978	R_f
A	0.65
B	0.57
C (complex)	0.31
D	0.51
E	0.48

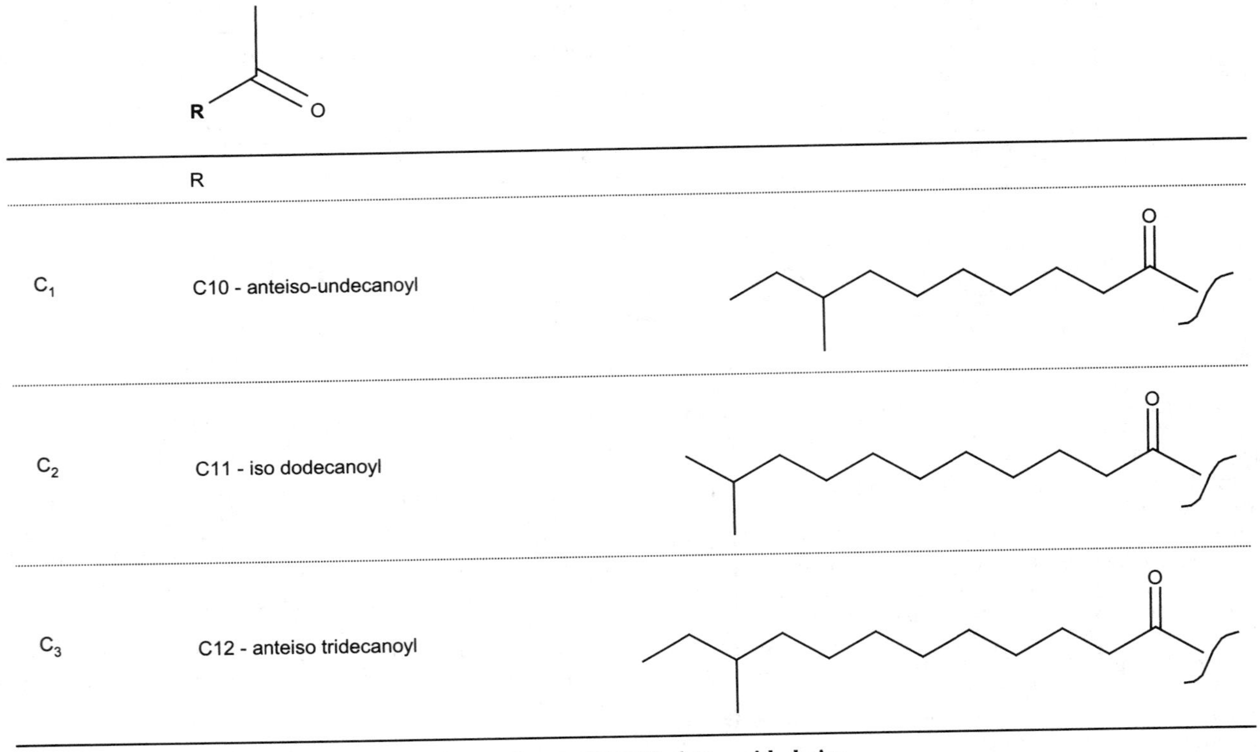

	R
C_1	C10 - anteiso-undecanoyl
C_2	C11 - iso dodecanoyl
C_3	C12 - anteiso tridecanoyl

Figure 41 A-21978C: fatty acid chains

described, 1, 2, and 3, and three minor compounds have been described, C_0, C_4, and C_5.

All of the compounds of the A-21978C complex have the same peptide nucleus, obtained by fermentation of the A-21978C complex in the presence of *Actinoplanes utahensis* NRRL 12052, which eliminates the terminal *N*-acyl chain. The peptide chain is composed of 13 amino acids: L-kynurenine, L-threo-3-methylglutamic acid, L-asparagine, three L-aspartic residues, two glycine residues, L-tryptophan, L-ornithine, D-alanine, D-serine, and L-threonine.

The various compounds differ in their *N*-acyl chains. The C_1 compound has a chain composed of 10 carbons (anteisoundecanoyl), the C_2 compound has an 11-carbon chain (isododecanoyl), and for the C_3 compound the chain length is 12 carbons (anteisotridecanoyl) (Fig. 41). In vitro, the C complex is more active than the others (Table 31).

The C_1 compound is the most active molecule in vivo as well as the least toxic, with a median intravenous lethal dose greater than 600 mg/kg (Table 32). More than 60 semisynthetic derivatives have been prepared, including daptomycin.

Table 32 Comparative biological activities of the three major components of the A-21978C complex

A-21978C	ED_{50} (mg/kg, 2 doses s.c.[a])		LD_{50} (mg/kg i.v.)[b]
	S. aureus	*S. pyogenes*	
C_1	0.2	0.064	>600
C_2	0.18	0.03	175
C_3	0.8	0.32	175

[a]S.C., subcutaneously.
[b]LD_{50}, 50% lethal dose; i.v., intravenously.

Table 31 In vitro activity of the A-21978 complex

Compound	MIC (μg/ml)			ED_{50} (mg/kg)		LD_{50} (mg/kg i.v.)[a]
	S. aureus	*S. epidermidis*	*E. faecalis*	*S. aureus*	*S. pyogenes*	
A-21978						
C_1	1	1	8	0.22	0.064	>600
C	0.25	0.25	2	0.27	0.03	450
D	0.5	0.25	8	0.99	>0.06	600
E	0.5	0.5	4	4.12	0.15	450
Daptomycin	0.5	0.5	16	0.11	0.03	600

[a]LD_{50}, 50% lethal dose; i.v., intravenously.

8.2.2.2. Daptomycin (Ly-146032)

Daptomycin is a semisynthetic derivative obtained from the compound A-21978C_1. Daptomycin is a 13-amino-acid cyclic lipopeptide isolated from *S. roseoporus*. It differs from A-21978C in the fatty acid chain attached to the tryptophan (Fig. 42).

8.2.2.2.1. Physicochemical properties. Daptomycin is a lipophilic polar molecule with a high molecular mass (about 1,639 Da). It is stable in Mueller-Hinton liquid medium supplemented with calcium or human serum.

8.2.2.2.2. Structure-activity relationship. Daptomycin was chosen from among 60 derivatives of the A-21978C nucleus comprising different N_{Trypt}-acyl chains.

In the series of chains containing a phenylalanine, the length of the *N*-acyl chain varies from 8 to 14 carbon atoms, the greatest activity being found with the C-10 chain.

Chains of 9 to 11 carbon atoms have the weakest toxicity, and the addition of an amino acid does not increase the activity.

In the *N*-acyl series, there is an increase in activity until the chain reaches 12 to 13 carbon atoms. Beyond a chain of 11 carbon atoms, the toxicity increases. The presence of an unsaturated fatty chain does not increase the antibacterial activity.

N-acylated-ornithine analogs of daptomycin were synthesized (Hill et al., 2003). Some of them expressed good activity against gram-positive bacteria in vitro and in vivo (PD_{50} for MRSA, 0.17 to 21 mg/kg), with prolonged half-lives in mice (>6 h) due probably to high protein binding.

It was shown that increasing the length of the acyl tail improved in vitro activity against a number of bacteria. A new series of compounds with introduction of a benzyl ring on the ornithine moiety has been prepared. Ornithine amine might be a secondary location for membrane interaction. Compounds having polar functionality, such as sulfonamides and amides, or polar spacers, such as piperazine, exhibited good activity against gram-positive bacteria (MICs, 0.78 to 3.13 μg/ml) (Siedlecki et al., 2003).

The toxicity is dependent on the nature of the fatty acids (Table 33).

8.2.2.2.3. Antibacterial activity. Daptomycin is active against gram-positive bacteria but is inactive against gram-negative bacteria (MIC, >64 μg/ml). The antibacterial activity depends on the calcium ion content of the culture medium (Table 34). The activity increases when the calcium content of the medium is increased. Conversely, the CO_2 content of the atmosphere has no effect. The activity of daptomycin is dependent on the inoculum size and the serum content.

Daptomycin is active against MRSA strains. It exhibits good activity against *S. haemolyticus*. It is more active than vancomycin and ramoplanin. It possesses activity identical to that of teicoplanin against *S. epidermidis*. It is active against penicillin G-resistant strains of *S. pneumoniae* (MIC_{90},

Table 33 Acute toxicity of the semisynthetic derivatives of A-21978C

Fatty acid side chain	No. of mice surviving/ total (1.000 mg/kg i.v.[a])
A-21978C	7/10
n-Decamoyl (daptomycin)	2/10
α-*N*(*n*-Decanoyl)-L-phenylalanine	10/10
N-(*n*-Decanoyl)-*p*-aminophenylacetyl	9/10
N-(*n*-Decanoyl)-*n*-undecanoyl	10/10

[a]i.v., intravenously.

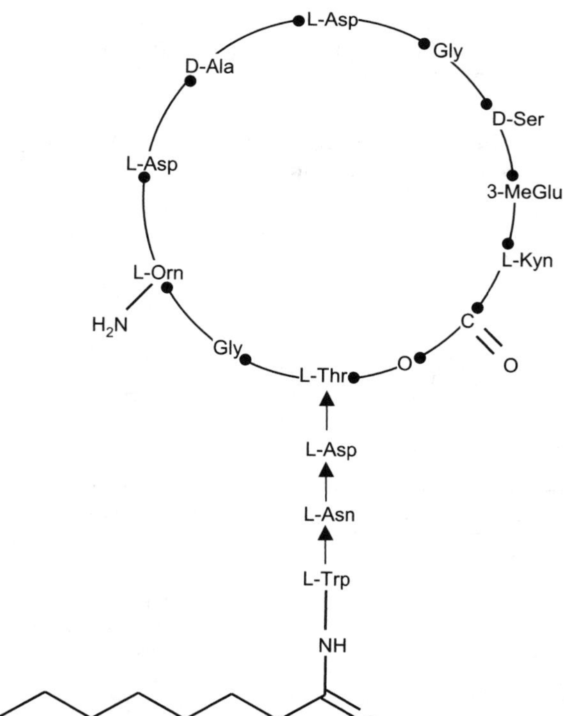

Figure 42 Daptomycin (LY-146032)

Table 34 In vitro activity of daptomycin

Microorganism(s)	MIC (μg/ml)	
	50%	90%
MSSA	0.5	1
MRSA	1	1
Coagulase-negative staphylococci, Met[s]	1	1
Coagulase-negative staphylococci, Met[s]	1	2
S. pyogenes	0.12	0.25
Group C and G streptococci	0.25	0.5
S. agalactiae	0.25	0.5
S. milleri	0.25	0.5
S. bovis	0.25	0.5
S. pneumoniae Pen[s], Pen[i], Pen[r]	0.125	0.125
E. faecalis	0.5	0.5
E. faecium	0.5	1
C. jeikeium	0.25	0.5
L. monocytogenes	0.25	0.5
E. rhusiopathiae	2	16
Leuconostoc spp.	0.25	0.25
Pediococcus spp.	0.25	0.25
Lactobacillus spp.	0.25	0.25
Bacillus spp.	6.2	6.2

~0.125 μg/ml). It is bactericidal against *E. faecalis* and *E. faecium* and possesses good activity against viridans group streptococci (for *S. milleri*, the MIC_{50} is ~0.25 μg/ml; for *S. bovis*, the MIC_{50} is ~0.25 μg/ml). For *S. pyogenes*, *S. agalactiae*, and group C and G streptococci, the MIC_{50}s are 0.25 μg/ml.

Daptomycin is moderately active against *L. monocytogenes*, *Corynebacterium jeikeium*, and *Bacillus* spp. (MIC_{90}s, 0.5 to 6.2 μg/ml) and *Erysipelothrix rhusiopathiae* (MIC_{50}, ~2 μg/ml). Conversely, in contrast to vancomycin, it has good activity against *Leuconostoc*, *Pediococcus*, and *Lactobacillus* spp. (MIC_{50}s, ~0.25 μg/ml). Daptomycin has excellent activity against anaerobic gram-positive cocci (MIC, <2 μg/ml), *Clostridium* spp. (including *C. difficile*), *Propionibacterium* spp., and *Actinomyces* spp. It is inactive against anaerobic gram-negative cocci and against anaerobic gram-negative bacteria, such as *Bacteroides* and *Fusobacterium* spp. (MIC_{90}, >64 μg/ml).

Daptomycin is rapidly bactericidal, in contrast to the glycopeptides; the bactericidal activity is concentration dependent. Daptomycin is active against strains of *E. faecalis* resistant to glycopeptides and gentamicin, and/or β-lactamase producers. It is bactericidal in vitro and in vivo. It is bactericidal against MSSA strains. Its bactericidal activity against MRSA strains is slower since their growth is slow.

Daptomycin produces a greater postantibiotic effect than vancomycin against *S. aureus*, *S. epidermidis*, and *E. faecalis*. This postantibiotic effect is concentration dependent. For *S. aureus* it is 0.7 to 7.9 h and for *E. faecalis* it is 0.5 to 7 h when determined with a concentration equal to the MIC or to 32 times the MIC.

The combination of daptomycin with imipenem or fosfomycin is usually synergistic. Conversely, the combination with vancomycin is more often neutral.

The criteria of susceptibility determined in accordance with the NCCLS recommendations with a disk containing 30 μg are as follows: bacterial strains are considered susceptible if the diameter is greater than 16 mm (MIC, 2.0 μg/ml) and resistant if the diameter is less than or equal to 12 mm (MIC, 8.0 μg/ml).

8.2.2.2.4. Mechanism of action. Daptomycin is inactive against gram-negative bacilli, as the bacterial wall is impermeable to it. Daptomycin does not penetrate the cytoplasm of gram-positive bacteria. It acts on the cytoplasmic membrane. Calcium binds to a specific site of the peptide moiety of daptomycin. It is essential for the activity of the molecule. Daptomycin causes a modification of the membrane potential without affecting the proton gradient, resulting in rupture of the membrane and death of the bacterial cell.

8.2.2.2.5. Resistance development. There is a low incidence of selection of resistant mutants ($<10^{-6}$ to 10^{-10}), and the MICs for these mutants are two to four times greater than those for wild strains. The highest incidence occurs with *S. pneumoniae* (1.2×10^{-6}), for which the MIC is more than 16 times the original MIC, followed by coagulase-negative staphylococci (3.3×10^{-7}), *Enterococcus* spp. (2×10^{-8} to 6.6×10^{-8}), and *S. aureus* (7×10^{-10}).

8.2.2.2.6. Pharmacokinetics. Daptomycin is highly bound to albumin (90 to 96%) and to α_1-glycoprotein (25 to 45%).

The pharmacokinetics are summarized in Tables 35 and 36.

After doses of 0.5 to 6 mg/kg intravenously, the pharmacokinetics are linear, with a plasma clearance of between 0.13

Table 36 Pharmacokinetics of daptomycin in patients with renal insufficiency

Parameter	Creatinine clearance (ml/min)		
	130	<30	<5
C_{max} (μg/ml)	14.6	14.5	13
$t_{1/2}$ (h)	8.8	16.4	27.3
CL_P (liters/h)	0.6	0.27	0.2
CL_R (liters/h)	0.268	0.215	0.230

Table 35 Pharmacokinetics of daptomycin

Dose (mg/kg)	C_{max} (μg/ml)	$t_{1/2}$ (h)	AUC (μg·h/ml)	CL_P (ml/min/kg)	CL_R (ml/min/kg)
0.5	6.37	5.78	41.8	0.201	0.091
1.0	13.02	6.42	93.4	0.183	0.009
1.5	17.43	9.37	139	0.183	0.078
2.0	23.02	8.25	162	0.210	0.099
3.0	41.55	8.35	329	0.155	0.052
4.0	52.25	8.56	382	0.179	0.066
6.0	82.0	8.06	598	0.171	0.064

and 0.21 ml/min/kg and a volume of distribution of 0.10 to 0.15 liters/kg. The apparent elimination half-life is about 8 h.

Plasma clearance of the free fraction is greater than that of the bound fraction (about 2.4 ml/min) (Table 35).

No accumulation has been observed in patients after repeated doses. In patients with renal insufficiency, the apparent elimination half-life is increased. If the creatinine clearance is less than 30 ml/min, the apparent elimination half-life is about 16 h, and that in hemodialyzed patients is 27 h when the creatinine clearance is <5 ml/min (Table 36).

Therapeutic failures at dosages of 2 mg/kg and greater than or equal to 12 mg/kg have resulted in the abandonment of clinical development and the occurrence of adverse events.

One of the explanations for these failures is an insufficient dose due to the high plasma protein binding. In addition, daptomycin is only bactericidal against strains of *S. aureus* in the exponential growth phase. *S. aureus*, in endocarditis vegetations, is in the stationary state and therefore less susceptible to daptomycin.

8.2.2.3. A-54145 Complex

The A-54145 complex was extracted by fermentation from *Streptomyces fradiae*. It is composed of eight molecules, A, A_1, B, B_1, C, D, E, and F. These molecules are cyclic peptides comprising 13 amino acids (Fig. 43 and 44).

The C-terminal part (amino acid 13) is an isoleucine or a valine attached by an ester bond to the threonine at position 4 to form a ring. The N-terminal part (tryptophan) is acylated by a fatty acid chain. Unusual amino acids, such as a 3-hydroxyasparagine (amino acid 3), a sarcosine (amino acid 5), or a 4-methoxyaspartic acid (amino acid 9), form part of the peptide ring.

Four peptide nuclei may be described according to amino acids 12 and 13 (Table 37).

On the basis of these four nuclei, eight molecules can be distinguished with respect to three fatty acid chains at C-10 or C-11 (8-methylnonanoic acid, *n*-decanoyl acid, and 3-methyldecanoyl acid) (Fig. 43).

The molecules of the A-54145 complex are active against gram-positive bacteria (Table 38). As with daptomycin, the

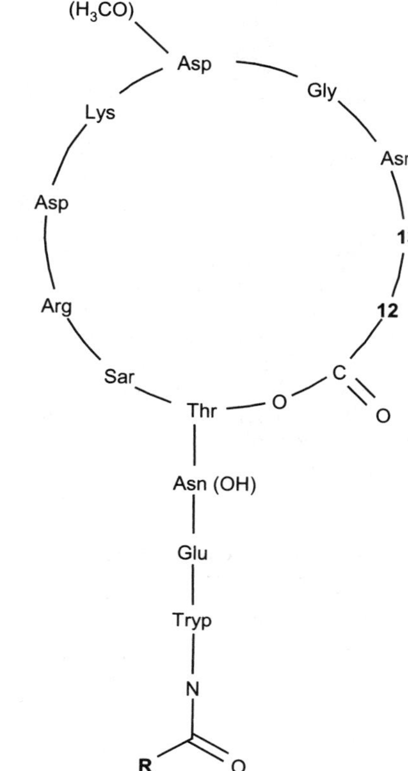

Figure 44 A-54145 complex

Acyl chains	Peptidic rings			
	A	B	C	F
C10 : 8-methyl onanoic	A	B	-	F
C10 : n-decanoyl	A_1	B_1	-	-
C11 : 3-methyl decanoyl	D	E	C	-

Figure 43 A-54145 complex: fatty acid chains

Table 37 A-54145 complex: peptide core

Component (peptide)	Amino acid at position	
	12	13
A	Glu	Ile
B	3-Methyl-Glu	Ile
C	3-Methyl-Glu	Val
D	Glu	Val

in vitro activity depends on the calcium content of the culture medium.

Semisynthetic products have been obtained after elimination of the acylated chain by fermentation of the complex in the presence of *A. utahensis*. The length of the N_{Tryp} chain on the A-54145 nucleus is an important factor in the antibacterial activity. The nucleus is devoid of antibacterial activity. The activity increases with the length of the acyl chain. For compound A, the maximum is reached with an *n*-tetradecanoyl chain. When comparing the molecules in terms of the nuclei A, B, C, and F with identical acylated chains, the most active molecule is that with a B nucleus, but this molecule is also the most toxic.

8.2.2.4. Laspartomycin

Laspartomycin was originally described in 1957 by Umezawa. Laspartomycin is a lipopeptide related to amphomycin. The natural product is a cyclic peptide core and has an aspartic acid external to the core linking the core at a C-15 αβ-unsaturated fatty acid side chain. Many analogs have been synthesized using the *A. utahensis* deacylase (Curran et al., 2002). The C component is the major element of the complex.

8.2.3. Lipopeptides with Antifungal Activity

The lipopeptides have a broad anti-infective spectrum, including molecules with antibacterial activity (daptomycin) and antifungal and antiparasitic agents (cilofungin, etc.).

Schematically, the antifungal lipopeptides may be divided into three groups (Fig. 45): cyclic or acyclic lipopeptides containing a high percentage of hydrophobic amino acids, lipopeptides that are more hydrophilic but possessing a fatty acid chain, and a third group that contains various molecules. The lipophilicity of the molecules is an important parameter, as it determines the transparietal penetration of the molecules.

The antifungal lipopeptides act as inhibitors of β-1,3-glucan synthetase.

Table 38 In vitro activities of the components of the A-54145 complex

A-54145 component	MIC (μg/ml)				
	S. aureus	*S. epidermidis*	*S. pyogenes*	*K. pneumoniae*	*Enterococcus* sp.
A	8.0	4.0	2.0	8.0	16
A_1	8.0	4.0	1.0	4.0	16
B	2.0	2.0	0.5	2.0	4.0
B_1	2.0	1.0	0.5	2.0	8.0
C	2.0	1.0	0.5	2.0	4.0
D	4.0	2.0	0.5	4.0	4.0
E	2.0	1.0	0.25	1.0	2.0
F	16	8.0	4.0	8.0	16

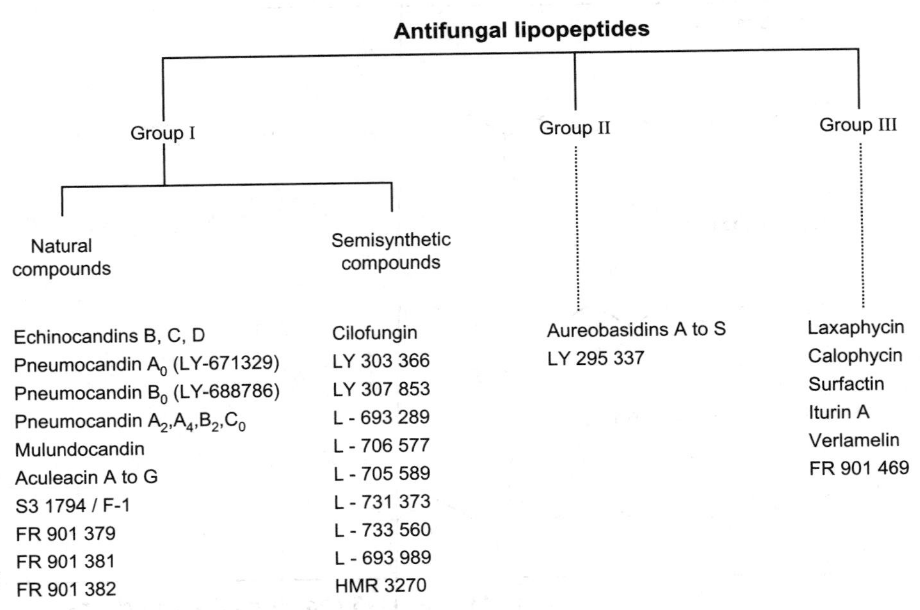

Figure 45 Classification of antifungal lipopeptides

8.2.3.1. Hydrophilic Lipopeptides

Five groups of antifungal agents are currently described in this class:

- Echinocandin and aculeacins
- Pneumocandin
- Mulundocandins
- Sporiofungins
- Lipopeptides isolated from *Coleophoma*

8.2.3.1.1. General characteristics. Hydrophilic lipopeptides are cyclic hexapeptides with a fatty acid chain. As a general rule, these molecules have poor bioavailability. The lipopeptides extracted from *Coleophoma* are slightly soluble in water.

The aims of the semisynthesis performed with these derivatives have been to increase oral bioavailability, to obtain hydrosoluble molecules, and to prepare formulations for intravenous administration. All of the molecules have a different fatty acid chain, which is important for the antifungal activity. All of the active molecules possess a homotyrosine residue that is or is not hydroxylated at position C-3 or C-4. Two amino acids with a β-hydroxyl residue are present on either side of a proline residue.

8.2.3.2. Echinocandins and Aculeacins

Echinocandin is a molecular complex obtained in 1974 from the fermentation of *Aspergillus nidulans* var. *echinulatus* or *Aspergillus rugulosis*. Echinocandin B was described by Ciba-Geigy (A-32204), and echinocandins C and D were described by Sandoz (SL 7810) and Eli Lilly (A-30912). Aculeacin was described by Toyo Jozo.

8.2.3.2.1. Structures. See Fig. 46.

Echinocandins B, C, and D are cyclic hexapeptides that have a linoleoyl chain. They differ with respect to the hydroxylation in the peptide ring.

The hexapeptide contains threonine and a 4-hydroxyproline, as well as three unconventional amino acids: 3,4-dihydroxyhomotyrosine, 4,5-dihydroxyornithine, and 3-hydroxy-5-methylproline.

The sixth amino acid may be either a threonine (echinocandin and aculeacin), a serine (mulundocandin), or a 3-hydroxyglutamine (pneumocandin A_0).

The aculeacins (Aα, γ, Dα, and γ) are also composed of a cyclic hexapeptide and differ from echinocandin with respect to the fatty acid chains, which are either a myristoyl (α derivatives) or a palmitoyl (γ derivatives). For each derivative, there are seven subgroups (A to G). They differ from one another in the nature of the amino acids that constitute the hexapeptides.

Echinocandins B, C, and D have similar antifungal activities. These derivatives are active against *C. albicans*, *C. tropicalis*, *C. krusei*, *Candida glabrata*, *Aspergillus fumigatus*, and *Trichophyton*. No natural derivative is active against *C. neoformans*.

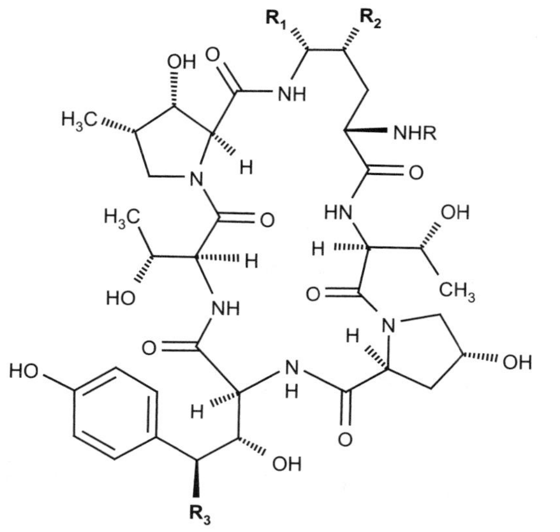

	R	R_1	R_2	R_3
Echinocandin B	linoleoyl	OH	OH	OH
Echinocandin C	linoleoyl	OH	OH	H
Echinocandin D	linoleoyl	H	H	H
Aculeacin Aa	myristoyl	OH	OH	OH
Aculeacin Ag	palmitoyl	OH	OH	OH
Aculeacin Aa	myristoyl	OH	OH	H
Aculeacin Ag	palmitoyl	OH	OH	H

Figure 46 Natural echinocandins and aculeacins

8.2.3.2.2. Semisynthetic derivatives. The first molecule to be selected was cilofungin. This molecule is active against *C. albicans* and *A. fumigatus*. These molecules also manifest activity against *Pneumocystis carinii* through the prevention of cyst formation in the rat.

The synthesized molecules are illustrated in Fig. 47.

8.2.3.3. Cilofungin (LY-121019)

Echinocandin B is a cyclic lipopeptide produced by *A. nidulans* var. *echinulatus*. In the same class of antifungal agents, aculein A is produced by *Aspergillus aculeatus*, and papulacandin is produced by *Papularia sphaerosperma*. These molecules act on yeasts by inhibiting glucan synthesis. Cilofungin is a derivative obtained by semisynthesis from echinocandin B by replacement of the fatty acid chain with 4-*n*-octyloxybenzoic acid. It is a molecule with a high molecular mass (1,030.14 Da), presented in the form of a water-insoluble white powder.

It has a narrow spectrum. It is active against yeasts, more specifically, *C. albicans* (MIC_{50} and MIC_{90}, 0.27 and 0.63 μg/ml). The activities against other species of *Candida* vary.

Structure-activity relationship studies have shown that 3-hydroxy-4-methylproline acid increases antifungal activity, but the absence of L-homotyrosine prevents the inhibition of β-1,3-glucan synthetase.

Cilofungin is very active against *C. albicans* and *C. tropicalis*, moderately active against *C. glabrata* and *C. krusei*, and inactive against *Candida parapsilosis* and *C. neoformans*. The real advantage of cilofungin over echinocandin B is its property of inducing less hemolysis. Cilofungin is moderately active against *P. carinii* and is insoluble in water. The product was discontinued after a reported case of fulminant hepatitis, although its relationship to the medication appears to be uncertain because of the use of polyethylene glycol as a solvent.

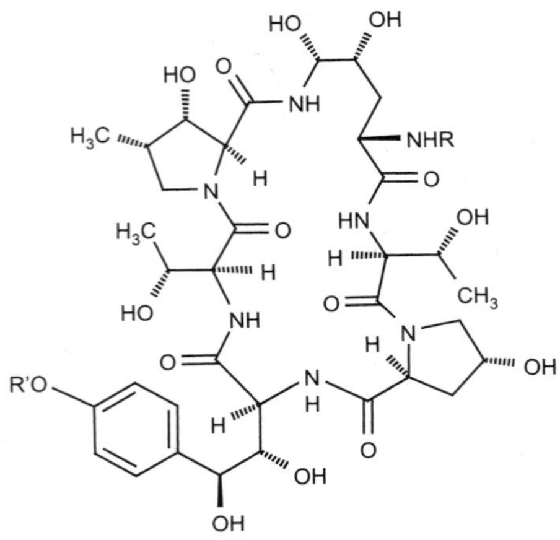

	(R)	OR'
Cilofungin (LY 121019)	C(=O)—Ph—OC_8H_{17}	OH
LY 303366	C(=O)—Ph—Ph—Ph—OC_5H_{11}	OH
LY 307853	C(=O)—Ph—Ph—Ph—OC_5H_{11}	O—P(=O)(OH)—ONa

Figure 47 Semisynthetic derivatives of echinocandin B

8.2.3.4. Polyphenyl Derivatives

The analysis of the structure-activity relationships showed that optimal activity is obtained when the lipid chain is linear, when it has a $\log_P$ of between 4.5 and 7, and when it is composed of a rigid proximal and flexible distal structure.

LY-303366 is a terphenyl derivative of echinocandin B that is a potent inhibitor of β-1,3-glucan synthetase of *C. albicans* (IC_{50}, 0.72 μg/ml) and *A. fumigatus* (IC_{50}, 0.17 μg/ml). It manifests good in vitro and in vivo activities against *Candida* spp., *Histoplasma capsulatum*, and *P. carinii*. Its activity against *Blastomyces dermatitidis* and *A. fumigatus* is moderate. It is inactive against *C. neoformans*.

8.2.3.5. Mulundocandins

The mulundocandin complex (Fig. 48) was isolated by Hoechst AG from the fermentation of *Aspergillus sydowii* var. *mulundensis* in 1980.

They differ from the echinocandins in the presence of a serine residue instead of the threonine, and the lipid chain is composed of a 12-methylmyristoyl (Fig. 49).

They are active against *C. albicans* and *Aspergillus niger* and relatively inactive against other fungal genera and species.

The semisynthetic derivative aminocandin (HRM 3270) is fungicidal against *Candida* species as well as against *Aspergillus fumigatus*. The pharmacokinetics of aminocandin were investigated in 12 healthy volunteers after intravenous administration of single ascending doses (75 to 600 mg). Concentrations assayed at the end of infusion ranged from 4.9 μg/ml (75 mg) to 16.12 μg/ml (600 mg). The AUC was 238.6 (75 mg) to 848.6 (300 mg) μg·h/ml, and the apparent elimination half-life was about 53 h (Sandage et al., 2005).

8.2.3.6. Sporiofungins

Sporiofungins A, B, and C (Fig. 50) were isolated from *Cryptosporiopsis* spp. They are structurally similar to the pneumocandins. They differ from them in the presence of a serine instead of a threonine in the constitution of the hexapeptide. The fatty acid chain is composed of 10,12-dimethylmyristoyl.

Sporiofungin A is the principal derivative. Sporiofungins are active against yeasts and filamentous fungi.

8.2.3.7. Pneumocandins

The pneumocandins differ from the echinocandins in the structure of the hexapeptide (Fig. 51). The threonine situated between the homotyrosine and the 3-hydroxy-4-methylproline is replaced by a 3-hydroxyglutamate. They differ in the lipid chain, which is a 10,12-dimethylmyristoyl.

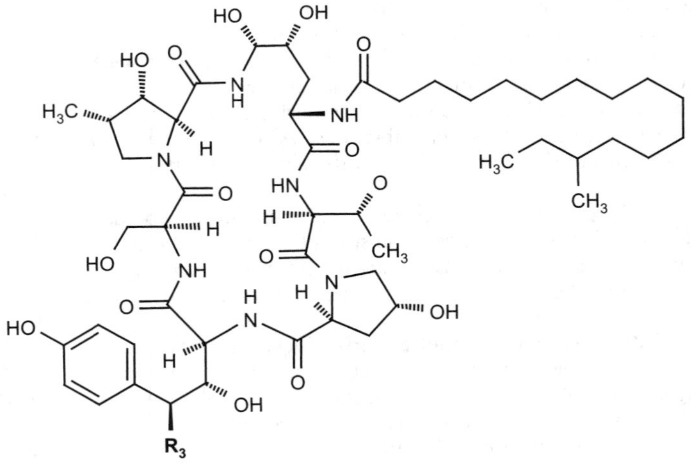

	R_3
Mulundocandin	OH
Deoxymulundocandin	H

Figure 48 Natural mulundocandins

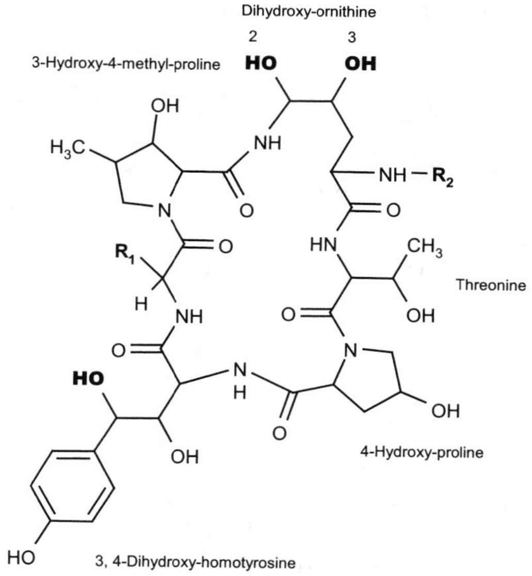

	R_1
Mulundocandin	Serine 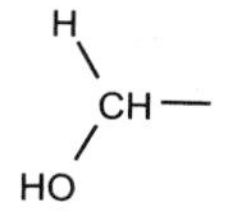
Echinocandin & aculeacin	Threonine 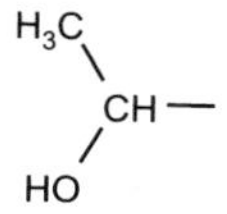
L 671 329 & S 31 794 / F1 (pneumocandin Ao)	Hydroxyglutamine 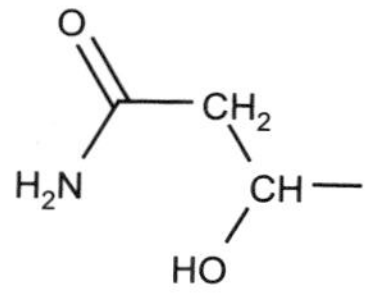

Figure 49 Lipopeptide antifungals

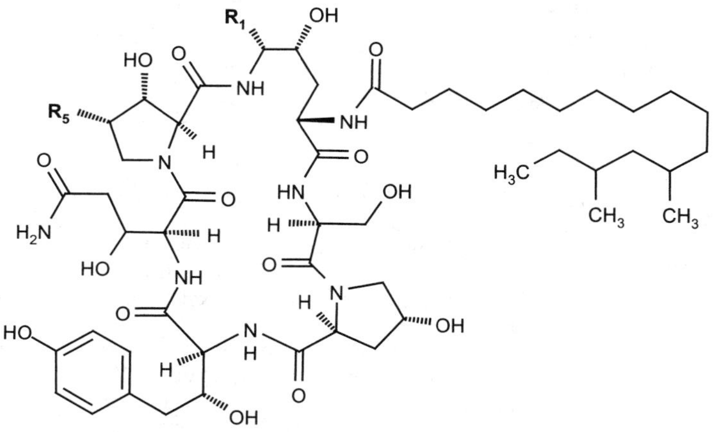

	R_3	R_5
Sporiofungin A	OH	CH_3
Sporiofungin B	OH	H
Sporiofungin C	OCH_3	CH_3

Figure 50 Natural sporiofungins

A similar derivative, S.317941F-1, discovered by Sandoz, may be classified as a pneumocandin.

The pneumocandins are extracted from *Zalerion arboricola*. This is a molecular complex, classified A to C, with subgroups. Groups B and C correspond to the presence of a 3-hydroxy-4-methylproline, a 3-hydroxyproline, and a 4-hydroxyproline situated beside the 3-hydroxyglutamine residue.

The natural pneumocandins are less active than aculeacin but are eight times more hemolytic. Pneumocandin B_0 is a more potent inhibitor (IC_{50}, 70 nM) of β-1,3-glucan synthetase than pneumocandin C_0 (IC_{50}, 500 nM). In order of inhibitory activity, the pneumocandins may be classified as follows: $B_0 > A_0$, $A_4 > A_2$, $B_2 > C_0$. They have good activity against *C. albicans* and are inactive against *C. neoformans* (Table 39).

8.2.3.7.1. Semisynthetic pneumocandins. The derivatives L-705589, L-731373, and L-733560 (Fig. 52) are aminoethylether derivatives obtained by reduction of the glutamic residue. These compounds are water soluble and manifest good activity against *C. albicans*, *A fumigatus*, and *P. carinii*.

The introduction of an amino function in the form of an aminoethylether group or by reduction of the 3-hydroxyglutamine to 3-hydroxyornithine has yielded derivatives that

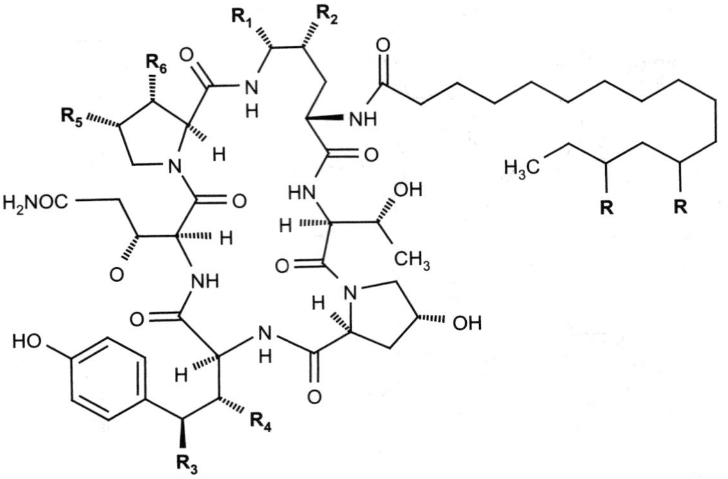

	R	R_1	R_2	R_3	R_4	R_5	R_6
S 31794/F-1	H	OH	OH	OH	OH	CH_3	OH
Pneumocandin A_0	CH_3	OH	OH	OH	OH	CH_3	OH
Pneumocandin A_2	CH_3	H	H	OH	OH	CH_3	OH
Pneumocandin A_4	CH_3	H	H	H	H	CH_3	OH
Pneumocandin B_0	CH_3	OH	OH	OH	OH	H	OH
Pneumocandin B_0	CH_3	H	H	OH	OH	H	OH
mocandin C_0	CH_3	OH	OH	OH	OH	OH	H

Figure 51 Natural pneumocandins

Table 39 In vitro activities of pneumocandins against yeasts

Yeast	MIC (μg/ml)	
	Pneumocandin A_0 (L-671329)	Pneumocandin B_0 (L-688786)
C. albicans	0.12–2.0	0.25
C. tropicalis	0.12	0.5
C. parapsilosis	4.0–8.0	4.0
C. glabrata		2.0
C. lusitaniae		2.0
C. krusei		4.0
C. guilliermondii		>64
C. neoformans		>64

are seven times more potent in terms of enzymatic inhibition than pneumocandin B_0.

L-733560 is a fungicidal derivative. It is active against *C. albicans* (minimum fungicidal concentration at which 90% of isolates tested are inhibited [MFC_{90}], 0.5 μg/ml), *C. tropicalis* (MFC_{90}, 0.25 μg/ml), *C. parapsilosis* (MFC_{90}, 0.5 μg/ml), *Candida lusitaniae* (MFC_{90}, 0.5 μg/ml), *C. glabrata* (MFC_{90}, 0.5 μg/ml), and *C. guilliermondii* (MFC_{90}, 2 μg/ml). It is inactive against *C. neoformans* (MFC_{90}, 32 μg/ml) and *Aspergillus* spp. (MFC_{90}, ≥128 μg/ml). It is active against strains of *C. albicans* resistant to azole derivatives. This molecule does not induce erythrocyte hemolysis at concentrations of up to 400 μg/ml.

8.2.3.8. Lipopeptides from *Coleophoma*

See Fig. 53.

Lipopeptides from *coleophoma*, which are water soluble, were isolated by Fujisawa (1991). They possess a palmitoyl chain and a catechol sulfate nucleus on the homotyrosine residue. The increased solubility in water might be due to the presence of the sulfate group, since its absence yields a water-insoluble catechol molecule. The three derivatives described differ in the number of hydroxyl groups present on the hexapeptide ring.

FR-901379 inhibits β-1,3-glucan synthetase to a greater extent than echinocandin B or cilofungin; the IC_{50}s are 0.8, 2.6, and 2.9 μg/ml for FR-901379, echinocandin B, and cilofungin, respectively. This molecule is active against *C. albicans*, *C. tropicalis*, and *C. krusei* (IC_{50}s, 0.003 to 0.16 μg/ml) and *A. fumigatus* and *A. niger* (IC_{50}s, 0.02 to 1.9 μg/ml). It is inactive against *C. neoformans* (IC_{50}, >2.5 μg/ml). The molecule is more active in vivo in murine candidosis than aculeacin A and fluconazole. It is active against *P. carinii*.

Semisynthetic derivatives have been prepared with the attachment of lipid chains of the γ-octyloxybenzoyl or 6-octyloxynaphthyl type to FR-901379.

8.2.3.9. Hydrophobic Lipopeptides: Aureobasidins

8.2.3.9.1. Aureobasidin complex. The second group of antifungal lipopeptide molecules has a large number of hydrophobic amino acids.

The aureobasidins form a molecular complex extracted from the fermentation medium of *Aureobasidium pullulans* no. R106, a species of black yeasts. Eighteen different molecular structures have been isolated.

The molecules are fungicidal in vitro against *C. albicans* (MICs, <0.05 to 1.56 μg/ml) and *C. neoformans* (MICs, 0.78 to 3.12 μg/ml). They are inactive against *A. fumigatus*. Aureobasidin A (Fig. 54) (LY-295337, R-106-1) is active against *C. albicans*, *C. tropicalis*, *C. parapsilosis*, *C. krusei*,

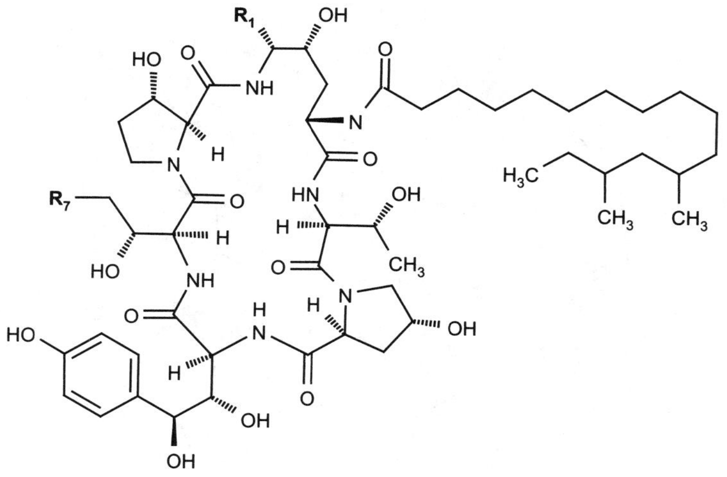

Pneumocandin B_0	R_1	R_2	Glucan IC_{50} (nM)[a]
L-705,589	$OCH_2CH_2NH_2$	$CONH_2$	11
L-731,373	OH	CH_2NH_2	11
L-733,560	$OCH_2CH_2NH_2$	CH_2NH_2	1

[a] Glucan synthase IC_{50} for *C. albicans* MY 1208

Figure 52 Amino derivatives of pneumocandin B_0

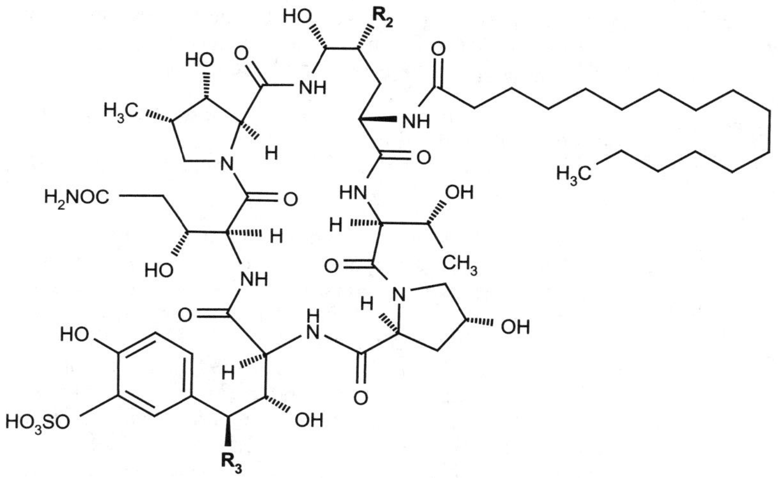

	R_2	R_3
FR 901379	OH	OH
FR 901381	OH	H
FR 901382	H	H

Figure 53 Natural lipopeptides from *Coleophoma*

C. glabrata, *C. guilliermondii*, *C. neoformans*, *H. capsulatum*, and *B. dermatitidis*. It has good oral bioavailability. LY-295337 is more active than amphotericin B. It was not possible to induce resistance after 12 passages.

8.2.3.9.2. LY-295337. LY-295337 is aureobasidin A, a cyclic depsipeptide composed of eight L-amino acids linked by 2-hydroxy-3-methylpentanoic acid. The product has a molecular mass of 1,101 Da and is insoluble in water.

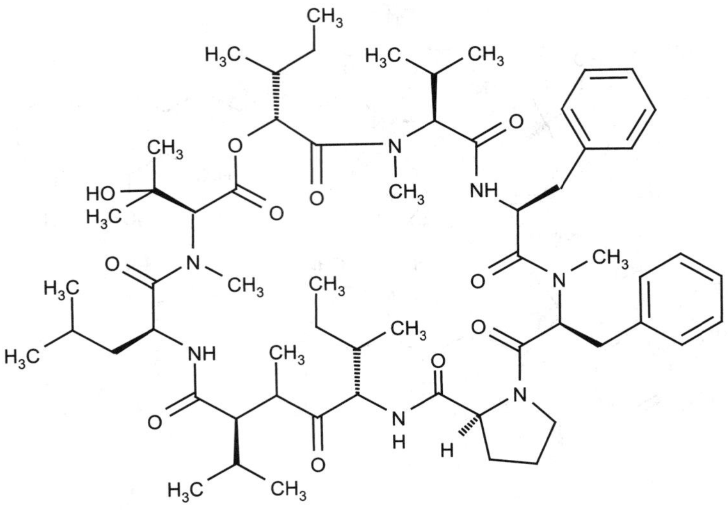

Figure 54 Aureobasidin A (R 106-1, LY-295337)

LY-295337 is fungicidal against *C. albicans* (MIC, <0.05 μg/ml) (including azole-resistant strains), *C. glabrata* (MIC, ~0.05 μg/ml), *C. krusei, C. parapsilosis, C. guilliermondii, C. neoformans, Histoplasma* spp., and *Paracoccidioides brasiliensis*. Conversely, it is inactive against *Sporothrix schenckii* and has variable and moderate activity against dermatophytes (*Trichophyton, Microsporum*, and *Epidermophyton*). It has some activity against molds (*Cladosporium*). Table 40 shows the in vitro activity of LY-295337 against various fungi.

In vivo studies of generalized murine candidosis have shown that the ED_{50} is 5.1 mg/kg orally (repeat doses twice a day for 8 days). In immunodepressed mice, the ED_{50} is 8.8 mg/kg.

An oral dose of 10 mg/kg causes a reduction of more than 99.9% of fungal cells in the kidneys and lungs.

Orally, the ED_{50}s for *B. dermatitidis, C. neoformans*, and *H. capsulatum* are, respectively, 7.4, 33.4, and 15.2 mg/kg.

LY-295337 shows no benefit in experimental *Aspergillus* lung infections (~200 mg/kg orally). In a model of experimental *C. neoformans* meningitis, a moderate prolongation of survival (29 versus 23 days) and a moderate reduction in cerebral colonization are obtained.

The acute toxicology was evaluated in female mice aged 5 to 6 weeks. The median lethal doses were greater than 1,000 mg/kg orally and subcutaneously, 1,000 mg/kg intraperitoneally, and 231 mg/kg intravenously.

Table 40 In vitro activity of LY-295337

Yeast or fungus	MIC (μg/ml)	
	Aureobasidin A (LY-295337)	Amphotericin B
C. albicans	0.04	2.5
C. tropicalis	0.08	2.5
C. parapsilosis	0.16	5.0
C. krusei	0.04	2.5
C. guilliermondii	0.08	1.25
C. glabrata	0.04	2.5
C. neoformans	0.63	2.5
A. fumigatus	20	5.0
H. capsulatum	0.16	2.5
P. brasiliensis	0.31–60	2.5–20
B. dermatitidis	0.04	0.31

In the Fischer rat, the median lethal dose was greater than 1,750 mg/kg. In the beagle, it was greater than 600 mg/kg. After repeated doses for 30 days to mice (doses of 12.5, 50, and 200 mg/kg), an increase in cholesterol and unsaturated fatty acid levels to 200 mg/kg was noted.

After repeated doses in rats, dose-dependent changes in lipid metabolism have been noted (reduction in plasma triglyceride levels).

Induction of a hepatic enzyme, benzophetamine *N*-demethylase, has been demonstrated in the beagle after repeated doses, probably related to the metabolism of the molecule. Vacuolization of the centrilobular hepatocytic cells was noted at doses of 50 and 150 mg/kg.

8.2.3.9.2.1. PHARMACOKINETICS. Unidentified metabolites have been found in animals.

Elimination is less than 5% in the urine and occurs principally in the feces.

8.2.3.9.2.2. HUMAN PHARMACOKINETICS. Two studies have been conducted; an incremental-dose study (5 to 980 mg) with 12 volunteers, and a low-dose (40, 80, and 160 mg) and high-dose (320, 640, and 980 mg) study.

The mean peak concentrations in serum were, respectively, 0.62 and 3.12 μg/ml after doses of 80 and 980 mg. The AUCs were, respectively, 2.4 and 29.2 μg·h/ml for doses of 80 and 980 mg. The apparent elimination half-lives were, respectively, 1.9, 1.9, 4.5, 9.3, and 10.5 h for doses of 80, 160, 320, 640, and 980 mg. There was, however, major interindividual variability. The pharmacokinetics are not linear. The effect of food is variable and requires further study.

LY-295337 has a number of interesting properties:

- There is good in vitro fungicidal activity against the main fungal genera, with the exception of *Aspergillus* spp.
- LY-295337 is fungicidal against *C. albicans*, which might enable the rapid emergence of resistant strains to be avoided.
- It appears to be well tolerated toxicologically (acute and 1-month chronic toxicology).
- It is effective in vivo in the murine model of generalized candidosis (immunocompetent or nonimmunocompetent mice).
- It has oral bioavailability, in contrast to the other lipopeptides.

8.2.3.10. Iturins

Iturin is a cyclic lipopeptide found in the soil of Ituri (Zaire) in 1957, by extraction from *B. subtilis*. Iturin A is the active component of the complex (composed of iturins A, B, and C). Iturin A is an antifungal compound. Iturin A-8 was found to be produced by *Bacillus amyloliquefaciens* strain RC-2; this compound is active against anthranose of the leaves of the mulberry tree, which is widely cultivated as a feed food for silkworms. The pathogen involved, *Colletotrichum dematium*, is inhibited by iturin A-8, which prevents conidial germination of the fungus. This compound is also active against *Agrobacterium tumefaciens*, and *Xanthomonas campestris* subsp. *camprestris* (Hiradate et al., 2002).

Other lipopeptide antifungals were extracted from *B. subtilis*, such as mycosubtilin and bacillomycins L, D, and F. These lipopeptides are characterized by the presence of β-amino fatty acid (C-14–C-17), a lipid moiety. The Cβ was found to be in the *R* absolute configuration. The peptide chain contains seven α-amino acid residues.

8.2.4. Other Lipopeptides

Other lipopeptides with a different cyclic structure have been isolated and have antifungal activity. These are laxaphycins produced by a blue algae, *Anabaena laxa*; calophycin, which is a cyclic decapeptide produced by *Calothrix fusca*; surfactin and iturin A, coproduced by *B. subtilis*; and verlamelin, which is active against phytopathogens.

8.2.5. Lipopeptides with Activity against Mycobacteria

Dihydromycoplanecin A (DHMPA) was discovered as an active metabolite in the urine of mice receiving mycoplanecin A, a compound that possesses activity against mycobacteria; this molecule is produced by *Actinoplanes awajinensis* subsp. *mycoplanecinus* subsp. nov. DHMPA has a cyclic peptide structure consisting of 10 amino acids, including three prolines, and a N-terminal chain comprising an α-hydroxybutyryl group (Fig. 55).

DHMPA is inactive against common gram-positive and gram-negative pyogens but has good activity against mycobacteria (Haneishi et al., 1985). This molecule is active against atypical mycobacteria and *M. tuberculosis*, whether the strains are susceptible or multiresistant (Table 41).

Toxicologically, the median lethal dose after oral administration is greater than 6,000 mg/kg and that intraperitoneally is 1,500 mg/kg in mice. In the rat, the median lethal dose orally is identical to that in the mouse, but intraperitoneally it is 760 to 1,200 mg/kg.

The combination of DHMPA and isoniazid is synergistic; combinations with streptomycin, rifampin, and ethambutol are neutral but not antagonistic. This has been confirmed in vivo (Takahashi et al., 1995).

Studies of intravenous kinetics in the mouse and dog have shown apparent elimination half-lives of 0.5 and 5.5 h, respectively. Twenty and thirty-seven percent of the

Table 41 In vitro activity of DHMPA against mycobacteria[a]

Mycobacterium sp.[b]	MIC (μg/ml)
M. tuberculosis H_{37RV}	0.78
M. tuberculosis STR[r]	0.39
M. tuberculosis INH[r]	0.39
M. tuberculosis VAN[r]	0.78
M. tuberculosis RIF[r]	0.39
M. smegmatis ATCC 607	0.39
M. phlei IFM 2952	0.10
M. avium 19075	6.25
M. avium Kirchberg	12.5
M. intracellulare ATCC 15984	0.39
M. kansasii P8	0.39
M. scrofulaceum P6	0.39
M. bovis BCG France	0.78
M. chelonae[c]	>50
M. marinum[c]	3.13

[a]Kirchner semiliquid medium with 10% calf serum (inoculum, 10^3 CFU/ml).
[b]STR, streptomycin; INH, isoniazid; VAN, vancomycin; RIF, rifampin.
[c]Ogawa medium supplemented with 2% glycerol.

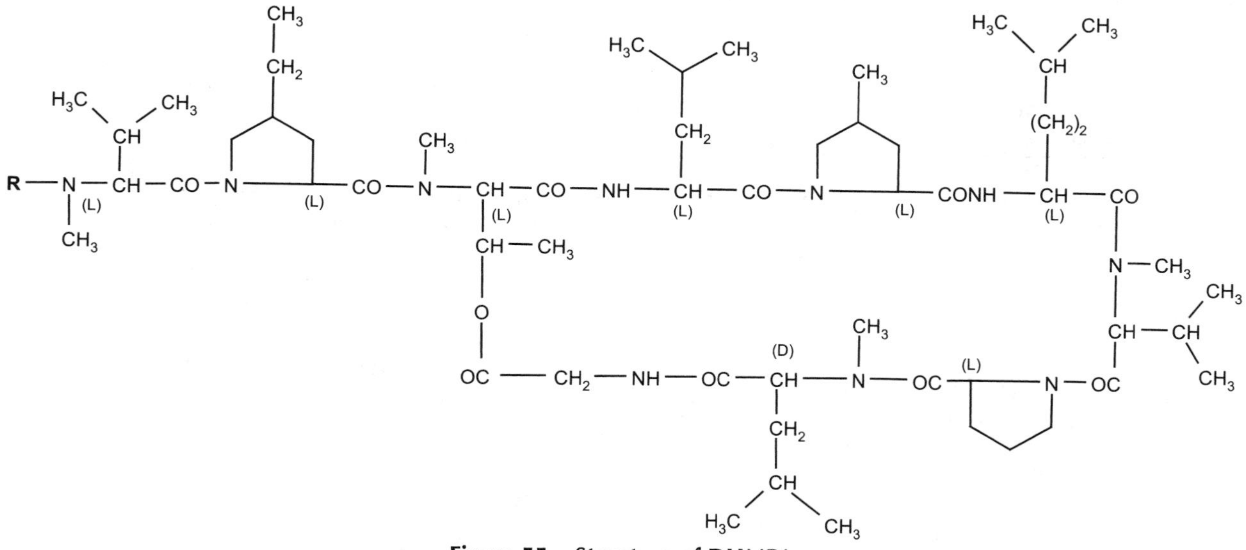

Figure 55 Structure of DHMPA

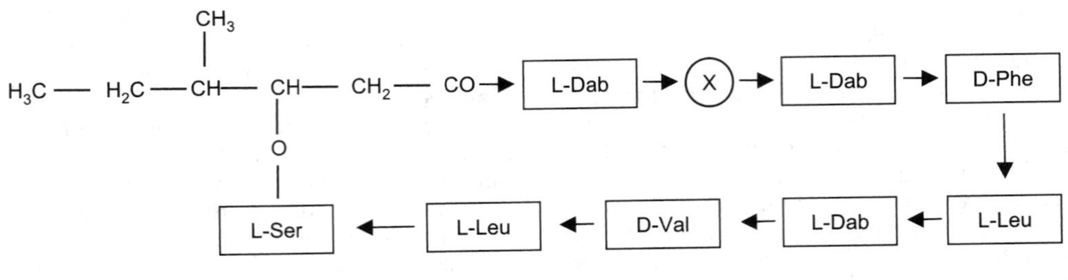

Figure 56 BMY-28160

product, respectively, is eliminated via the kidneys in the mouse and dog.

8.2.6. BMY-28160, Permeatin, and Polypeptin

Three molecules belong to a subgroup within the lipopeptides: they are the cyclic lipodepsipeptides permeatin A, polypeptin, and BMY-28160.

BMY-28160 (Sugarawa et al., 1984) is a fermentation product of *B. circulans* H 913-B4 (Fig. 56). Its biological spectrum includes gram-positive and gram-negative bacteria, together with dermatophytes and yeasts (Tables 42 and 43).

Other molecules belong to these subgroups, such as serratomolide, which is a cyclic dimer of L-serine-β-hydroxydecanoic acid produced by *S. marcescens* and which exhibits weak antibacterial activity.

The polypeptide is a cyclic nonapeptide with a fatty chain of seven carbons incorporated in the ring.

8.2.7. Cyclic Lipopeptides: Miscellaneous

Brevistin, polypeptin, and stendomycin are cyclic peptides that differ in the number and sequence of amino acids and in the nature of the fatty acids.

Stendomycin is a heptapeptide lactone attached to an acyl heptapeptide chain, whereas brevistin is a lactone decapeptide attached to a fatty acid chain at C-9.

The octapeptins constitute a group of cyclic heptapeptides possessing a D-Dab group with a fatty acid chain. The mechanisms of action of octapeptins A and B (EM-49) have been studied in detail.

The octapeptins act on the cytoplasmic membrane by interfering with oxidative phosphorylation.

Octapeptin C_1 (antibiotic 333-25) and other derivatives are not well characterized.

Esperin is a cyclic lipopeptide with a fatty chain included in the ring.

Surfactin contains seven amino acids and a lipid chain at C-15 incorporated in the ring. It acts as an anionic detergent agent and ruptures the bacterial membranes.

Table 42 In vitro activity of BMY-28160 against gram-positive bacteria

Organism(s)	MIC (μg/ml)	
	50%	90%
MSSA	0.25	0.5
MRSA	0.25	0.5
S. epidermidis	0.5	0.5
S. pyogenes	≤0.06	≤0.06
S. agalactiae	0.25	0.25
Viridans group streptococci Pen[s]	≤0.06–4.0	
Viridans group streptococci Pen[r]	0.25	0.25
Group G streptococci	≤0.06	≤0.06
S. pneumoniae	≤0.06–0.125	
E. faecalis	0.5	1.0
E. faecium	2.0	2.0
L. monocytogenes	8.0	16

Table 43 In vitro activity of BMY-28160

Microorganism	MIC (μg/ml)
S. aureus 209 P	12.5
S. aureus Smith	25
S. pyogenes	3.1
E. coli NIH-JC2	6.3
K. pneumoniae	25
Proteus vulgaris	>100
P. aeruginosa	25
B. fragilis	>100
C. difficile	12.5
P. acnes	2.5
C. albicans	50
C. neoformans	50
Trichophyton mentagrophytes	12.5

8.2.8. M-1396

M-1396 is a semisynthetic derivative of amphomycin. It is active in vitro against *S. aureus* irrespective of methicillin susceptibility, coagulase-negative staphylococci; *Enterococcus* spp. irrespective of their phenotypes of resistance to vancomycin, linezolid, or quinupristin-dalfopristin; and viridans group oral streptococci.

9. GROUP VI: THIAZOLOPEPTIDES

The thiazolopeptides comprise a few molecules, such as bacitracin, GE 2270A, the amythiamicins (Berdy, 1980), and thioxamycin (Matsumoto et al., 1989).

9.1. Bacitracin

The bacitracin group consists of hexapeptide antibiotics with a substituted thiazolidine nucleus. It was isolated from the fermentation of *Bacillus licheniformis*. Six compounds have been detected, A, B, C, D, E, and F. Compound A represents about 70% of the complex.

Bacitracin A (Fig. 57) differs from bacitracin B by the presence of an isoleucine instead of a valine. The majority of amino acids are in the L configuration, except for phenylalanine, glutamic acid, ornithine, and aspartic acid, which are D configured.

Bacitracin is a yellowish-white powder, soluble in water and alcohol and insoluble in ether, chloroform, benzene, and acetone. The molecular weight of bacitracin A is about 1,450.

Bacitracin displays good activity against gram-positive cocci. Its spectrum includes *Treponema pallidum*. The antibacterial activity is sometimes expressed in international units (1 IU = 18.2 mg of the standard preparation). Cariogenic *S. mutans* is known to be resistant to bacitracin.

Resistance is infrequent and chromosomally mediated. Other mechanisms of resistance are efflux, due to an ABC-type system which consists of the BcrA, BcrB, and BcrC proteins of *B. licheniformis*. The lack of oligosaccharide led to reduced sensitivity to bacitracin due to a reduced isoprenyl phosphate at position C-55 (Table 44).

Bacitracin acts by inhibiting peptidoglycan biosynthesis. During peptidoglycan synthesis, C-55 soprenyl phosphate

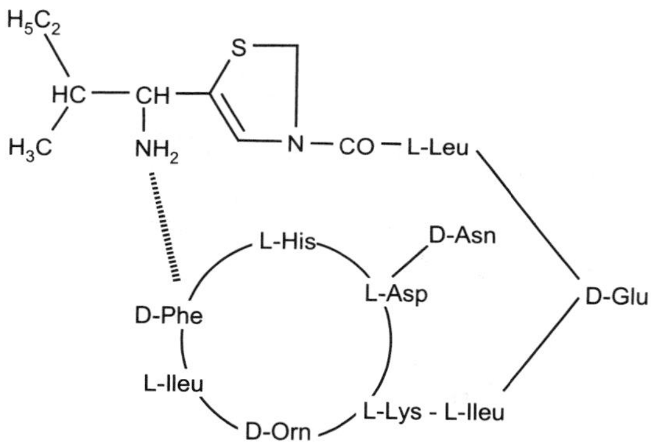

Figure 57 Bacitracin A

Table 44 Activity of bacitracin A

Microorganism(s)[a]	MIC (μg/ml)	
	50%	90%
E. coli	>64	>64
H. influenzae β^-	>64	>64
H. influenzae β^+	>64	>64
MSSA	16	32
MRSA	16	32
MSSE	32	64
MRSE	32	64
E. faecalis	32	>64
E. faecium	32	>64
S. pneumoniae Pen[s]	0.25	1
S. pneumoniae Pen[r]	0.5	1
S. pyogenes	0.25	0.25
Group C and G streptococci	8	16
N. meningitidis	32	64
M. catarrhalis	1	1

[a]β^-, non-β-lactamase producing; β^+, β-lactamase producing; MSSE, methicillin-susceptible *S. epidemidis*; MRSE, methicillin-resistant *S. epidermidis*.

serves as a lipid carrier after the translocation of sugar-peptide units to the ends of the linear peptidoglycan strands. The C-55 isoprenyl pyrophosphate is detached and dephosphorylated to C-55 isoprenyl phosphate by a membrane-bound pyrophosphatase, the recycling C-55 isoprenyl phosphate for subsequent peptidoglycan synthesis. Bacitracin inhibits this stage specifically by binding tightly to the C-55 isoprenyl pyrophosphate, forming a tertiary complex in the presence of bivalent ions which prevents pyrophosphatase from interacting with C-55 isoprenyl pyrophosphate, thus reducing the amount of C-55 isoprenyl phosphate that is available for carrying sugar-peptide units. The nitrogen atoms of the terminal amino group of the thiazole nucleus and the histidine ring are involved in this process (Fig. 58).

In *E. coli*, phosphorylation of C-55 isoprenyl phosphate due to elevated intracellular levels of the lipid kinase encoded by *bacA* appeared to confer resistance to bacitracin (Cain et al., 1993).

Bacitracin is not orally absorbed. It is degraded in the intestinal lumen. Applied locally (to the skin or mucous membrane), it is weakly absorbed. After intramuscular administration of 200 to 300 IU/kg, concentrations in serum are on the order of 0.2 to 3 IU/kg. Elimination occurs in the urine by glomerular filtration.

Bacitracin is not used parenterally, as it is nephrotoxic.

9.2. GE 2270A (MDL-62879)

GE 2270A (MDL-62879) is a thiazolide-type polypeptide isolated from *Planobispora rosea* ATCC 53773 (Fig. 59). It is a 1,289-Da molecule.

This polypeptide antibiotic is related to kirromycin and pulvomycin in terms of its mechanism of action.

This molecule inhibits protein synthesis by inhibiting elongation factor Tu (EF-Tu) (Selva et al., 1990; Goldstein et al., 1990).

It has good activity against gram-positive cocci, including MRSA strains. It possesses not insignificant activity against *P. acnes*, *B. fragilis*, and *M. tuberculosis* (Table 45). It has good activity against highly aminoglycoside-resistant strains of *E. faecalis* (MIC_{50} and MIC_{90}, 0.005 and 0.009 μg/ml). It is moderately bactericidal.

Likewise, it has good in vivo activity against *S. aureus* (ED_{50}, 1.54 mg/kg), moderate activity against *S. pyogenes* (ED_{50}, 9.12 mg/kg), and weaker activity against *S. pneumoniae* (ED_{50}, 15.2 mg/kg).

9.3. MDL-63908

GE 2270A is slightly soluble in water. Chemical modifications have enabled a hydrosoluble derivative to be obtained, while still retaining the antibacterial activity of GE 2270A. The last two amino acids are eliminated from this compound by hydrolysis of the terminal part of GE 2270A. Attachment of a 6-aminocaproic acid yields MDL-63908, which has good solubility in water (100 mg/ml). The sodium salt of MDL-63908 has been used in experimental infections.

9.4. Amythiamicins

The amythiamicin complex comprises four molecules, A, B, C, and D (Fig. 60). These were isolated from the fermentation of *Amycolatopsis* sp. strain M-1481-42 F′ (Shimanaka et al., 1994a, 1994b). They differ from GE 2270A by the presence of a methyl group on carbon 15 of the aminothiazolyl ring instead of a methoxymethyl group. They differ from one another in the substituent of carbon 41 of the aminothiazolyl nucleus. The serine propyl residues of moleules A, B, and C are attached to the aminothiazolyl

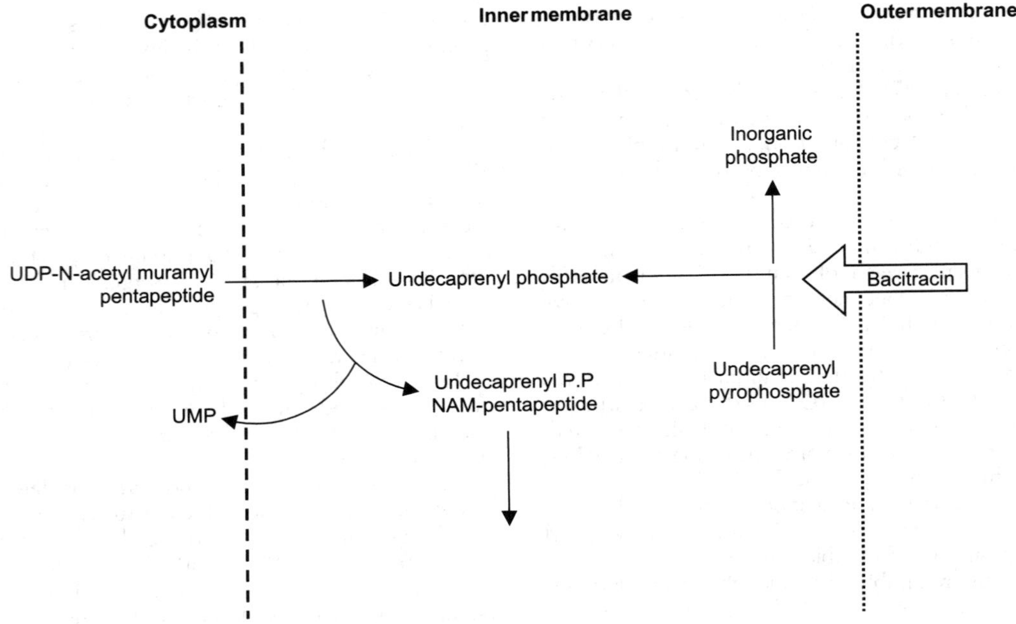

Figure 58 Mechanism of action of bacitracin

Figure 59 GE 2270A (MDL-62879)

nucleus by an oxazoline nucleus (A) or an amide (B) or ester (C) bond. Molecule D has a methoxycarbonyl chain.

Components A and D are active against gram-positive cocci, including oxacillin-resistant strains of *S. aureus*. Components D and B are weakly active or inactive.

EF-Tu is essential in the protein synthesis process and is controlled by the *tuf* gene. The sequence of amino acids of *E. coli* has been divided functionally into three domains: domain I (1 to ~200) is responsible for the GTP/GDP bond and the tRNA amino acid, and domain II (210 to ~295) and domain III (301 to ~393) are responsible for EF-TS (Clark et al., 1990). Amythiamicin acts on domain II, and GE 2270A acts on domain I (Shimanaka et al., 1995; Landini et al., 1993).

9.5. Thioxamycin

Thioxamycin was isolated from the culture filtrate of *Streptomyces* sp. strain PA-46025. It is a lipophilic and acidic molecule (Egawa et al., 1969) related to the sulfomycins (Abe et al., 1988).

Thioxamycin is a peptide molecule containing thiazolide and oxazole nuclei. This molecule is active against anaerobic gram-positive bacteria but weakly active against gram-negative

Table 45 In vitro activity of GE 2270A (MDL-62879)[a]

Microorganism(s)	MIC (μg/ml)		
	50%	90%	Range
MSSA	0.06	0.06	0.03–0.06
MRSA	0.03	0.03	0.03–0.06
S. epidermidis	0.06	0.125	0.06–0.125
Staphylococcus saprophyticus	0.125	0.25	0.06–0.125
S. haemolyticus	0.06	0.125	0.06–0.5
S. pyogenes	0.25	0.5	0.06–0.125
S. pneumoniae	0.25	0.25	0.125–0.5
S. agalactiae	1.0	1.0	0.25–1.0
Viridans group streptococci	0.25	1.0	0.06–2.0
Group C and G streptococci	0.5	0.5	0.125–0.5
E. faecalis	0.03	0.03	0.008–0.03
E. faecium Van[s]			0.004–0.03
E. faecium Van[r]			0.03
Enterococcus Van[s]	0.016	0.06	0.008–1.0
Enterococcus Van[r]	0.016	0.03	0.008–0.03
P. acnes			≤0.008
Peptostreptococcus spp.	0.016	0.03	0.001–0.03
Clostridium sp.	0.06	2.0	0.016–>64
Mobiluncus spp.	0.001	0.016	0.001–0.03
Prevotella spp.	1.0	>64	0.004–>64
Peptostreptococcus asaccharolyticus			0.03–>64
Bacteroides spp.	>64	>64	0.5–<64
Fusobacterium spp.	>64	>64	2.0–>64
C. difficile ATCC 9889			0.03
N. gonorrhoeae			32
M. tuberculosis	4.0	8.0	1.0–8.0
M. avium complex			>128
H. influenzae			128
M. catarrhalis			1.0

[a]Data from Goldstein et al., 1993; King et al., 1993; and Selva et al., 1991.

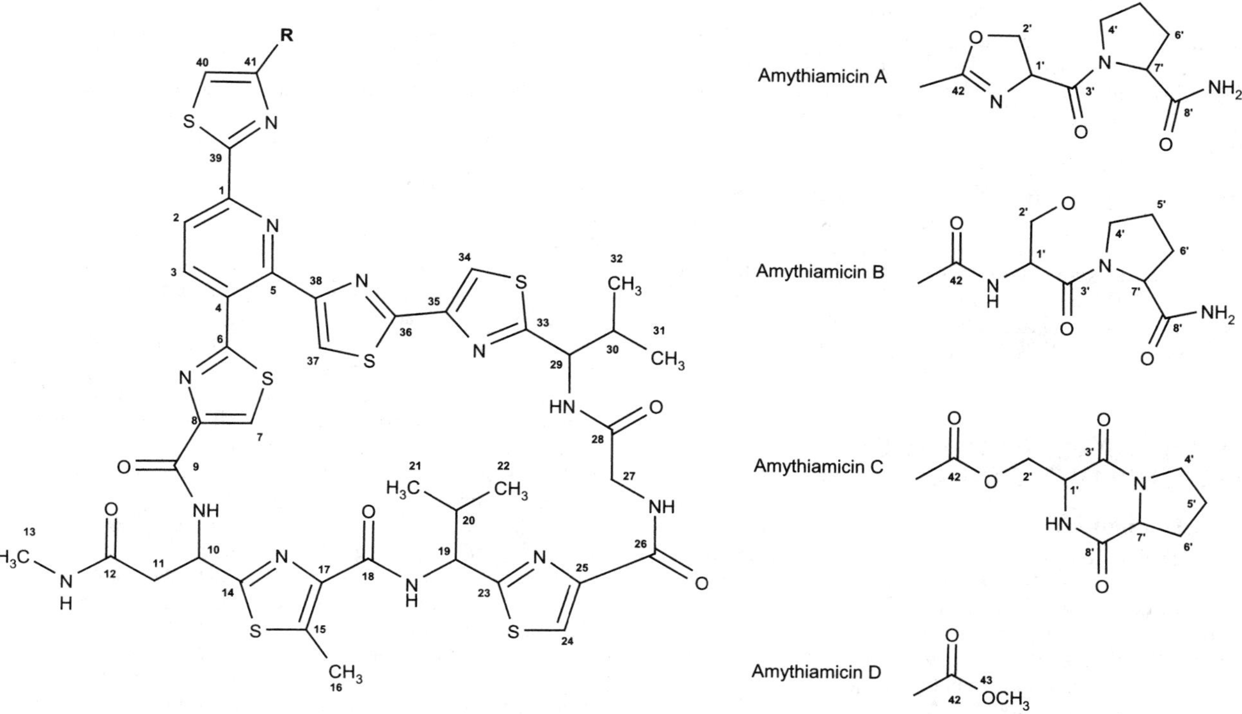

Figure 60 Structures of amythiamicins A, B, C, and D

bacteria (MIC, >25 μg/ml). It has moderate activity against gram-positive cocci, such as *S. aureus* 209 P JC-1 (MIC, 3.13 μg/ml). It is more active against *S. pneumoniae* type 1 (MIC, 0.78 μg/ml) and *S. pyogenes* C-203 (MIC, 0.39 μg/ml). It is inactive against enterobacteria and *P. aeruginosa* (MIC, >128 μg/ml). It acts by inhibiting protein synthesis.

9.6. Nocathiacins

Nocathiancins I and II are tricyclic peptide antibiotics. They were isolated from the fermentation broth of *Nocardia* and *Amycolatopsis* spp.

They inhibit the elongation process during protein synthesis (Porse et al., 1998). Chemical alterations of nocathiacins were performed with the aim of increasing their water solubility while maintaining biological activity.

The presence of several hydroxyl functionalities in nocathiacins presents an opportunity for the introduction of water-soluble substituents. The semisynthesis of bis- and mono-*O*-alkyl *n*-derivatives has been done. Some analogs exhibited high antipneumococcal activity (MICs, 0.002 to 0.5 μg/ml) and antistaphylococcal activity (MICs, 0.07 to 1.0 μg/ml), as well as antienterococcal activity (MICs, 0.03 to 4.0 μg/ml).

In vivo antistaphylococcal efficacy has been demonstrated (PD_{50}s, 0.3 to 4.0 mg/kg).

In general, the introduction of neutral or basic polar moieties improved aqueous solubility at acidic pH (pH > 1) (Regueiro-Ren et al., 2004).

9.7. Other Molecules

Other antibacterial agents of this class have been described: thiostrepton, nosiheptide, micrococcin, thiocillin, sulfomycin (Egawa et al., 1969), berninamycin, thiopeptide, sporangiomycin, and siomycin.

Common to all of these molecules are thiazole nuclei and a pyridine nucleus included in a peptide chain. Some molecules, such as thiostrepton and nosiheptide, also have a lipid chain. Micrococcin and thiocillin, like GE 2270A, have a chromophoric center composed of four thiazole nuclei. GE 2270A, like the other peptides, does not have a threonine or a dehydroalanine. GE 2270A is characteristic in that it has a methyl and a methoxymethylene at C-5 (Selva et al., 1991).

GE 37468A (Fig. 61) was obtained by fermentation of *Streptomyces* sp. strain ATCC 55365. Its chromophore differs from that of GE 2270A by the presence of a methyloxazole nucleus instead of a thiazole nucleus. This molecule has an α-hydroxyproline residue. In general, it is less active than GE 2270A against common pathogens and has cross-resistance with the latter. Its mechanism of action is identical to that of GE2270A (Stella et al., 1995).

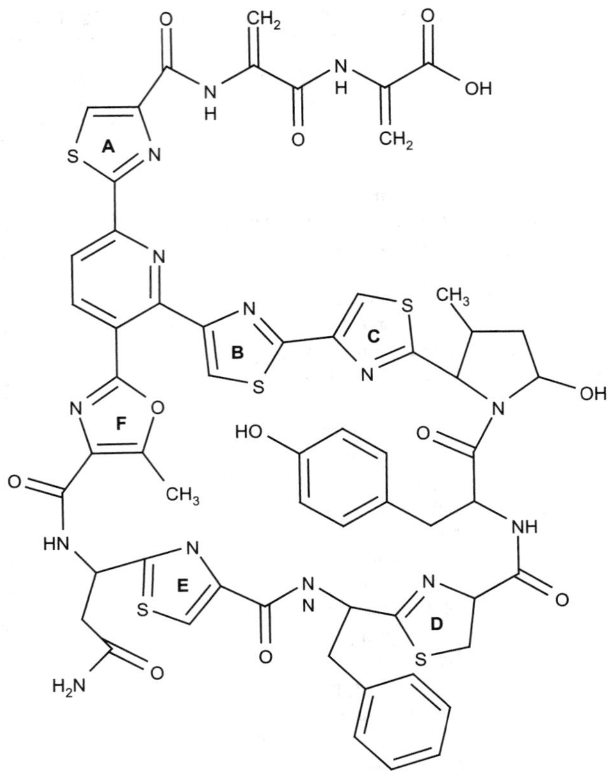

Figure 61 **GE 37468A**

10. GROUP VII: THIOPEPTIDES AND CHROMOPEPTIDES

10.1. Thiopeptides

A molecular complex, A-10255, has been isolated from *Streptomyces gardneri* NRRL 15537. It comprises seven molecules containing a sulfur residue: B, C, E, F, G, H, and J. Factors B and G are the major components (Fig. 62). A-10255 is a complex that is insoluble in water and soluble in polar solvents. The molecular mass is between 1,022 Da (compound J) and 1,255 Da (compound E). After intraperitoneal administration to mice, the median lethal doses are greater than 600 mg/kg (compounds B, C, and F) and 476 mg/kg (compound E) (Michel et al., 1989; Boeck et al., 1992).

A-10255 is a cyclic heptapeptide comprising thiazole and oxazole residues and with a side chain made up of dehydroalanine residues.

The antibacterial spectrum includes gram-positive bacteria and anaerobic bacteria (Counter et al., 1989). These molecules are for agroveterinary use (poultry industry).

10.2. Chromopeptides

10.2.1. Actinomycins

Chromopeptides derived from the fermentation of a strain of *Streptomyces* have been progressively isolated. These molecules contain a heterotricyclic chromophoric nucleus known as an actinocin (phenoxazone), responsible for their red color, connected to two lactone pentapeptides responsible for its solubility. All of the actinomycins have the same chromophoric nucleus. They differ in one or two amino acids at position 2′ or 3′. Actinomycin is not symmetrical. There are numerous actinomycins, C, D, E, F, S, X, and Z, with subgroups C_1, C_2, C_3, etc. Actinomycin D (Fig. 63) is the most well-known molecule of the group. These molecules have antibacterial but also, and above all, antineoplastic activities.

Actinomycin inhibits DNA-dependent RNA polymerase by binding to DNA in guanine-cytosine-rich regions via the phenoxazone nucleus. The two peptide nuclei are necessary for the formation of this complex via hydrogen bonds between the deoxyguanosine residues and the phosphate sugars. The main intrapeptide hydrogen bonds are those between the two D-valines above and below the plane of the chromophore, and likewise the hydrogen bond between the threonines and the deoxyguanosine.

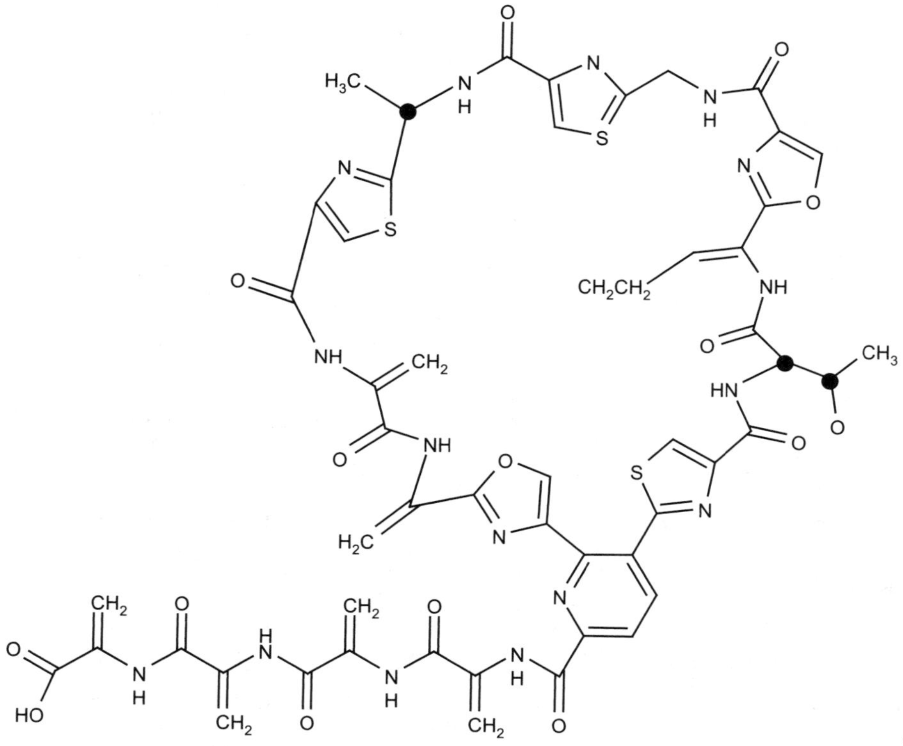

Figure 62 Thiopeptides: A-10255B

Table 46 In vitro activity of peptide 4, a cyclic D, L-α peptide

Organism	MIC (μg/ml)
B. subtilis	3
B. cereus	2
S. aureus	3
L. monocytogenes	20
E. faecalis	10
S. pneumoniae	10
Salmonella sp.	>70

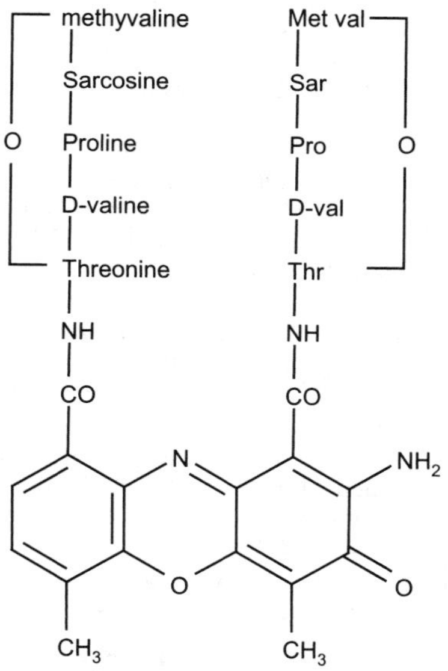

Figure 63 Actinomycin D

10.2.2. Echinomycin

Echinomycin is a cyclic octapeptide containing two chromophores: quinoxaline carboxylic acid. It binds to DNA. Its mechanism of action appears to be similar to that of actinomycin.

10.2.3. Kedarcidin

Kedarcidin is a chromophoric peptide isolated from *Streptoalloteichus* spp. which is active against gram-positive bacteria but inactive against gram-negative bacteria. It has excellent activity against *S. aureus* (MIC, ~0.008 μg/ml) and *E. faecalis* (MIC, ~0.016 μg/ml).

11. MISCELLANEOUS PEPTIDES

11.1. Peptide Dendrimers

Dendrimers are highly ordered, hyperbranched polymers. It was hypothesized that multicharged dendrimers may have high affinity for the bacterial membrane.

Series of dendrimeric peptides were synthesized and their antistaphylococcal activity was investigated (Janiszewska et al., 2003). It was shown that basic amino acids (lysine) or guanido groups and aromatic components exert antistaphylococcal activity.

The minimal dipeptide, LysPhen NH_2, expresses weak antibacterial activity. The presence of a substituted benzyl oxycarbonyl group enhanced the antistaphylococcal activity

(MIC, 16 μg/ml). The location of the aromatic groups significantly changes the in vitro activity.

11.2. Cyclic D,L-α Peptides

Cyclic D,L-α peptides with an even number of alternating D- and L-α amino acids can adopt flat ring-shaped conformations in which the backbone amide functionalities are oriented perpendicular to the side chain and the plane of the ring structure.

By interaction with the bacterial membrane, they increase the membrane permeability.

Some of them, like peptide 4 (KQRWLWLWLW), exhibit antibacterial activity (Table 46) (Fernandez-Lopez et al., 2001).

REFERENCES

Abdel-Ghany YS, Ihnat MA, Miller DD, Kunin CM, Tang HH, 1993, Structure-activity relationship of glycine-betaine analogs on osmotolerance of enteric bacteria, J Med Chem, 36, 784–789.

Abe H, Kushida K, Shiobara Y, Kodama M, 1988, The structures of sulfomycin I and berninamycin A, Tetrahedron Lett, 29, 1401–1404.

Allen JG, Atherton FR, Hall MJ, Hassall CH, Holmes SW, Lambert RW, Nisbet LJ, Ringrose PS, 1978, Phosphonopeptides, a new class of synthetic antibacterial agents, Nature, 272, 56–58.

Allen JG, Atherton FR, Hall MJ, Hassall CH, Holmes SW, Lambert RW, Nisbet LJ, Ringrose PS, 1979a, Phosphonopeptides as antibacterial agents: alaphosphin and related phosphopeptides, Antimicrob Agents Chemother, 15, 684–695.

Allen JG, Havas L, Leicht E, Lenox-Smith L, Nisbet LJ, 1979b, Phosphonopeptides as antibacterial agents: metabolism and pharmacokinetics of alafosfalin in animals and humans, Antimicrob Agents Chemother, 16, 306–313.

Allen JG, Lees LJ, 1980, Pharmacokinetics of alafosfalin, alone and in combination with cephalexin, in humans, Antimicrob Agents Chemother, 17, 973–979.

Andres E, Dimarcq JL, 2001, Les peptides antimicrobiens cationiques et leurs perspectives d'applications thérapeutiques, Antibiotique, 3, 201–205.

Aronof GR, Sloan RS, Luft FC, 1988, LY 146032 kinetics in normal subjects and patients with renal insufficiency, 28th Intersci Conf Antimicrob Agents Chemother, 125.

Atherthon FR, Hall MJ, Hassall CH, Lambert RW, Ringrose PS, 1979, Phosphonopeptides as antibacterial agents, rationale, chemistry, and structure-activity relationships, Antimicrob Agents Chemother, 15, 677–683.

Attendo-Genco C, Maloy WL, Kari UP, Motley M, 2003, Antimicrobial activity of magainin analogues against anaerobic oral pathogens, Int J Antimicrob Agents, 21, 75–78.

Balkovec JM, 1994, Lipopeptide antifungal agents, Expert Opin Investig Drugs, 3, 65–82.

Bartoloni A, Colao MG, Orsi A, Dei R, Giganti E, Parenti F, 1990, In vitro activity of vancomycin, teicoplanin, ramoplanin, MDL 62873 and other agents against staphylococci, enterococci and Clostridium difficile, J Antimicrob Chemother, 26, 627–633.

Berdy J, 1980, Thiazolyl peptides, p 389–417, in Berdy J, ed, Handbook of Antibiotic Compounds, vol IV/1, CRC Press.

Bessalle R, Haas H, Goria A, Shalit L, Fridkin M, 1992, Augmentation of the antibacterial activity of magainin by positive-charge chain extension, Antimicrob Agents Chemother, 36, 313–317.

Bloom H, Katla T, Nissen H, Holo H, 2001, Characterization, production, and purification of carnocin H, a bacteriocin produced by Carnobacterium 377, Curr Microbiol, 43, 227–231.

Boeck LD, Berry DM, Mertz FP, Wetzel RW, 1992, A 10255, a complex of novel growth-promoting thiopeptide antibiotics produced by a strain of Streptomyces gardneri: taxonomy and fermentation studies, J Antibiot, 45, 1222–1230.

Borghi A, Coronelli C, Faniuolo L, Allievi G, Pallanza R, Gallo GG, 1984, Teichomycins, news antibiotics from Actinoplanes teichomyceticus nov sp. IV. Separation and characterization of the components of teichomycin (teicoplanin), J Antibiot, 37, 615–620.

Bourlioux P, 1989, Biochimie fonctionnelle des structures bactériennes, p 22–51, in Le Minor L, Veron M, ed, Bactériologie médicale, 2nd ed, Flammarion.

Cain BD, Norton PJ, Eubanks W, Nick NS, Allen CM, 1993, Amplification of the *bcaA* gene confers bacitracin resistance in *Escherichia coli*, J Bacteriol, 175, 3784–3789.

Cheung KS, Wasserman SA, Dudek E, Lerner SA, Johsnton M, 1983, Chloroalanyl and propargylglycine dipeptides: suicide substrate containing antibacterials, J Med Chem, 26, 1733–1741.

Christensen B, Fink J, Merrifield RB, Mauzerall D, 1988, Channel-forming properties of cecropins and related model compounds incorporated into planar lipid membranes, Proc Natl Acad Sci USA, 85, 5072–5076.

Clark BFC, Kjeldgaard M, Lacour TFM, Thirup S, Nyoborg J, 1990, Structural determination of the functional sites of E. coli elongation factor Tu, Biochim Biophys Acta, 1050, 203–208.

Cole A, Deronich MRO, Legarda D, Connell N, Diamond G, 2000, Characterization of a fish antimicrobial peptide: gene expression, subcellular localization, and spectrum of activity, Antimicrob Agents Chemother, 44, 2039–2045.

Counter FT, Ensminger PW, Wu CEY, 1989, A10255, a new thiopeptide antibiotic complex, produced by Streptomyces gardneri. 3. Microbiological evaluation, 29th Intersci Conf Antimicrob Agents Chemother, abstract 411.

Cristofaro MF, Beauregard DA, Yan H, Osbrn NJ, Williams DH, 1995, Cooperativity between non-polar and ionic forces in the binding of bacteria cell wall analogues by vancomycin in aqueous solution, J Antibiot, 48, 805–810.

Curran WV, Leese RA, Borders DB, Koontz MZ, Liu H, Simon RJ, 2002, Semisynthetic approaches to laspartomycin analogs, 42nd Intersci Conf Antimicrob Agents Chemother, abstract 1175.

Dabard J, Bridonneau C, Phillipe C, Anglade P, Molle D, Nardi M, Ladiré M, Girardin H, Marcille F, Gomez A, Fons M, 2001, Ruminococcin A, a new lantibiotic produced by a *Ruminococcus gnavus* strain isolated from human feces, Appl Environ Microbiol, 67, 4111–4118.

Egawa Y, Umino K, Tamura Y, Shimizu M, Kaneko K, Sukurazawa M, Awataguchi S, Okuda T, 1969, Sulfomycins, a series of new sulfur-containing antibiotics. I. Isolation, purification and properties, J Antibiot, 22, 12–17.

Fernandez-Lopez S, Kim HS, Choi EC, Delgado M, Granja JR, Khasanov A, Kraehenbuehl K, Long G, Weinberger DA, Wilcoxen KM, Ghadiri MR, 2001, Antibacterial agents based on the cyclic D,L-α peptide architecture, Nature, 412, 452–456.

Fowden L, Lewis D, Tristam H, 1967, Toxic amino acids: their action as antimetabolites, Adv Enzymol, 1967, 89.

Francis J, Webster H, Newsom SWB, 1990, In vitro activity of ramoplanin on Staphylococci, Drugs Exptl Clin Res, 16, 457–460.

Fujii CA, Boggs A, Stapp J, Burns JL, Redman R, 2001, In vitro activity of isogenan (IB-367) against bacterial isolates obtained from cystic fibrosis enrolled in a phase I trial, 41st Intersci Conf Antimicrob Agents Chemother.

Ganguli BN, Chatterjee S, Jani GP, Pai GP, Chatterjee DK, Blumbach J, Kogler H, Fehlhaber HW, Teetz V, Klesel N, Seibert G, 1989, Mersacidin, a novel peptide antibiotic: discovery and antimicrobial evaluation, 29th Intersci Conf Antimicrob Agents Chemother, abstract 478.

Goldstein BP, Berti M, Ripamonti F, Candiani GP, Romano G, Bellini S, Denaro M, 1990, Antimicrobial activity of GE 2270A, a new peptide antibiotic which inhibits protein synthesis elongation factor EF-tu, 30th Intersci Conf Antimicrob Agents Chemother, abstract 800.

Goldstein BP, Berti M, Ripamonti F, Resconi A, Scotti R, Denaro M, 1993, In vitro antimicrobial activity of a new antibiotic, MDL 62879 (GE 2270 A), Antimicrob Agents Chemother, 37, 741–745.

Goldstein BP, Candiani G, Arain TM, Romano G, Ciciliato I, Berti M, Abbondi M, et al, 1995, Antimicrobial activity of MDL 63,246, a new semisynthetic glycopeptide antibiotic, Antimicrob Agents Chemother, 39, 1580–1588.

Gordee R, Farmer J, Zeckner D, 1992, LY 295337, a novel cyclic depsipeptide antifungal antibiotic. I. In vitro antifungal activity, 32nd Intersci Conf Antimicrob Agents Chemother, abstract 496.

Greenlee WJ, Springer JP, Patchett AA, 1989, Synthesis of an analogue of Tabtoxinine as a potential inhibitor of D-alanine-D-alanine ligase (ADP forming), J Med Chem, 32, 165–170.

Hancock REW, 1998, The therapeutic potential of cationic peptides, Expert Opin Investig Drugs, 7, 167–174.

Haneishi T, Nakajima M, Shiraishi A, Katayama T, et al, 1985, A new antimycobacterial antibiotic, dihydromycoplanecin A. I. In vitro activities and pharmacokinetics in mice and dogs, Recent Adv Chemother, 3, 2544–2545.

Heinemann B, Kaplan MA, Muir RD, Hooper IR, 1953, Amphomycin—a new antibiotic, Antib Chemother, 3, 239.

Hernanz A, 1990, Characterization and distribution of bombesin-like peptide in the rat brain and gastrointestinal tract, Biochem Cell Biol, 68, 1142–1145.

Hill J, Siedlecki J, Parr I, Morytko M, Yu X, Zhang Y, Silverman J, Controneo Y, Laganas V, Li T, Lai J-J, Keith D, Shimer G, Finn J, 2003, Synthesis and biological activity of N-acylated ornithine analogues of daptomycin, Bioorg Med Chem Lett, 13, 4187–4191.

Hiradate S, Yoshida S, Sugie H, Yada H, Fujii Y, 2002, Mulberry anthracnose antagonists (iturins) produced by Bacillus amyloliquefaciens RC-2, Phytochem, 61, 693–698.

Hirth GG, Veron M, Villar-Parasi C, Hurion N, Cohen GN, 1975, The threonine-sensitive homoserine dehydrogenase and aspartokinase activities of Escherichia coli K-12, Eur J Biochem, 50, 425.

Janiszewska J, Swieton J, Lipkowski AW, Urbanczyk-Lipkowska Z, 2003, Low molecular mass peptide dendrimers that express antimicrobial properties, Bioorg Med Chem Lett, 13, 3711–3713.

Jimenez-Mejias ME, Becerril B, Marquez-Rivas FJ, Pichardo C, Cuberos L, Pachon J, 2000, Successful treatment of multidrug-resistant Acinetobacter baumannii meningitis with intravenous colisitin sulfomethane sodium, Eur J Clin Microbiol Infect Dis, 19, 970–971.

Judice JK, Pace JL, 2003, Semisynthetic glycopeptide antibacterials, Bioorg Med Chem Lett, 13, 4165–4168.

Jung G, 1991, Lantibiotics—ribosomally synthesized biologically active polypeptides containing sulfide bridge and α,β-didehydroamino acids, Angew Chem, 30, 1051–1192.

Kellner R, Jung G, Horner T, Zahner H, Schnell N, Entian KD, Götz F, 1988, Gallidermin, a new lanthionine containing polypeptide antibiotic, Eur J Biochem, 177, 53–59.

Kenny MT, Brackman MA, Dulworth JK, 1995, In vitro activity of the semisynthetic glycopeptide amide MDL 63,246, Antimicrob Agents Chemother, 39, 1589–1590.

King A, Bethune L, Phillips L, 1993, In vitro activity of MDL 62879 (GE 2270 A) against aerobic gram-positive and anaerobic bacteria, Antimicrob Agents Chemother, 37, 746–749.

Komatsu Y, Miwa H, Matsumoto K, et al, 1991, S-3662, a new glycopeptide antibiotic for parenteral use, laboratory evaluation, 31st Intersci Conf Antimicrob Agents Chemother, abstract 413.

Landini P, Bandera M, Soffientini A, Goldstein BP, 1993, Sensitivity of elongation factor Tu (RfTu) from different bacterial species to the antibiotics efrotomycin, pulvomycin and MDL 62,879, J Gen Microbiol, 139, 769–774.

Lee JY, Boman A, Chuanxin S, Anderson M, Jornvall H, Mutt V, Boman H, 1989, Antibacterial peptides from pig intestine, isolation of a mammalian cecropin, Proc Natl Acad Sci USA, 86, 9159–9162.

Lee MD, Roll DM, Williams F, Ashcroft J, Siegel M, Chang CC, Manning JK, Pinho F, Borders DB, 1992, LL-A0341 antibiotics. I. Isolation and chemical structure of LL-A0341 β, γ_1, γ_2, δ_1, and α, 32nd Intersci Conf Antimicrob Agents Chemother, abstract 508.

Lehrer RI, 1993, Defensins, antimicrobial and cytotoxic peptides of mammalian cells, Annu Rev Immunol, 11, 105–128.

Loesch WJ, 1994, Normal microflora of the human body, p 120–128, in Nissengard RJ, Neuman MG, ed, Oral Microbiology and Immunology, The WB Saunders Co, Philadelphia, Pa.

Malabarba A, Ciabatti R, Scotti R, Goldstein BP, Ferrari P, Kurz M, Andreini BP, Denaro M, 1995, New semisynthetic glycopeptide MDL 63,246 and MDL 63,042, and other amide derivatives of antibiotic A-40,926 active against highly glycopeptide-resistant Van A enterococci, J Antibiot, 48, 869–883.

Malabarba A, Pallanza R, Berti M, Cavalleri B, 1990, Synthesis and biological activity of some amide derivatives of the lantibiotic actagardin, J Antibiot, 43, 1089–1100.

Malkoski M, Dasper S, O'Brien-Simpson NM, Talbo GH, Macris M, Cross KJ, Reynolds EC, 2001, Kappacin, a novel antibacterial peptide from bovine milk, Antimicrob Agents Chemother, 45, 2309–2315.

Matsumoto M, Kawamura Y, Yassuda Y, Tanimoto T, Matsumoto K, Yoshida T, Shoji JI, 1989, Isolation and characterization of thioxamycin, J Antibiot, 42, 1465–1469.

Michel KH, Hoehn MM, Boeck LD, Martin JW, Abbott MA, Godfrey OW, Meitz FP, 1989, A10255, a new thiopeptide complex. I. Discovery, fermentation, isolation and characterization, 29th Intersci Conf Antimicrob Agents Chemother, abstract 409.

Mosca DA, Hurst MA, So W, Viajar BSC, Fujii CA, Falla TJ, 2000, IB-367, a protegrin peptide with in vitro and in vivo activities against microflora associated with oral mucositis, Antimicrob Agents Chemother, 44, 1803–1808.

Nagarajan R, Schabel AA, Occolowitz JL, Counter FT, Ott JL, 1988a, Synthesis and antibacterial activity of N-acyl vancomycins, J Antibiot, 42, 1430–1438.

Nagarajan R, Schabel AA, Occolowitz JL, Counter FT, Ott JL, Felty-Duckworth AM, 1988b, Synthesis and antibacterial evaluation of N-alkyl vancomycins, J Antibiot, 42, 63–72.

Navon-Venezia S, Fedor R, Gaidukov I, Carmeli Y, Mor A, 2001, Antibacterial dermaseptin S4 derivatives, 41st Intersci Conf Antimicrob Agents Chemother, abstract F-348.

Niu WW, Neu HC, 1991, Activity of mersacidin, a novel peptide, compared with that of vancomycin, teicoplanin, and daptomycin, Antimicrob Agents Chemother, 35, 998–1000.

Oki T, Hirano M, Tomatsu K, Numata KI, Kamei H, 1989, Cispentacin, a new antifungal antibiotic. II. In vitro and in vivo antifungal activities, J Antibiot, 42, 1756–1762.

Pace JL, Krause K, Johnston D, Debabov D, Wu T, Farrington L, Lane C, Higgins DL, Christensen B, Judice JK, Koniga K, 2003, In vitro activity of TD 6424 against *Staphylococccus aureus*, Antimicrob Agents Chemother, 47, 3602–3604.

Parenti F, Cavalleri B, 1990, Novel glycopeptide antibiotics of the dalbaheptide group, Drugs Future, 15, 57–72.

Parenti F, Ciabatti R, Cavalleri B, Kettenring J, 1990, Ramoplanin, a review of its discovery and its chemistry, Drugs Exp Clin Res, 16, 451–455.

Patchett AA, Taub P, Weissberger B, Valiant ME, Gadebusch H, Thornberry NA, Bull HG, 1988, Antibacterial activities of fluorovinyl- and chlorovinylglycine and several derived dipeptides, Antimicrob Agents Chemother, 32, 319–333.

Patrzykat A, Gallant JW, Seo J-K, Pytyck J, Douglas SE, 2003, Novel antimicrobial peptides derived from flatfish genes, Antimicrob Agents Chemother, 47, 2464–2470.

Petersen PJ, Weiss WJ, Jacobus NV, Testa RT, 1992, Comparative in vitro and in vivo activity of LL-A0341 β_1, a cyclic depsipeptide antibiotic, 32nd Intersci Conf Antimicrob Agents Chemother, abstract 502.

Pfeiffer RR, 1981, Structural features of vancomycin, Rev Infect Dis, 3, suppl, S205–S209.

Porse BT, Leviev J, Mankin A, Garrett RA, 1998, The antibiotic thiostrepton inhibits a functional transition within protein 11α at the ribosome GTPase center, J Mol Biol, 276, 391–404.

Raj PA, Deutino AR, 2002, Current status of defensins and their role in innate and adaptative immunity, FEMS Microbiol Lett, 206, 9–18.

Raju B, Mortell K, O'Dowd H, Gao H, Kumar AS, Gomez M, Hackbarth C, Wu C, Wang W, Yuan Z, White R, Trias J, Patel DW, 2002, N- and C-terminal modifications of negamycin, 42nd Intersci Conf Antimicrob Agents Chemother, abstract F-1685.

Rasch M, Knochel S, 1998, Variations in tolerance of Listeria monocytogenes to nisin, pediocin PA-1 and bavaricin A, Lett Appl Microbiol, 27, 275–278.

Regueiro-Ren A, Naidu BN, Zheng X, Hudyma T, Connolly TP, Matiskella J, Zhang Y, Kim OK, Sorensen ME, Pucci M, Clark J, Bronson JJ, Ueda Y, 2004, Novel semisynthetic nocathiacin antibiotics: synthesis and antibacterial activity of bis- and mono-O-alkylated derivatives, Bioorg Med Chem Lett, 14, 171–175.

Ringrose PS, 1980, Peptides as antimicrobial agents, p 641-692, in Payne JW, ed, Microorganisms and Nitrogen Source, John Wiley and Sons Ltd.

Rolston KVI, Nguyen H, Messer M, 1990, In vitro activity of LY 264826, a new glycopeptide antibiotic, against gram-positive bacteria isolated from patients with cancer, Antimicrob Agents Chemother, 34, 2137–2141.

Ryser ET, Maisnier-Patin S, Gratadoux JJ, Richard J, 1994, Isolation and identification of cheese smear bacteria inhibitory to Listeria spp., Int J Food Microbiol, 21, 237–246.

Sajjan US, Tran LT, Sole N, Rovaldi C, Akiyama A, Friden PM, Forstner JF, Rothstein DM, 2001, P-113D, an antimicrobial peptide active against *Pseudomonas aeruginosa*, retains activity in the presence of sputum from cystic fibrosis patients, Antimicrob Agents Chemother, 45, 3437–3444.

Samyn B, Martinez-Bueno M, Devreese B, Maquela M, Galvez A, Valdivia E, Coyette J, van Beenmen J, 1999, The cyclic structure of the enterococcal peptide antibiotic AS-48, FEBS Lett, 352, 87–90.

Sanchez ML, Wenzel RP, Jones RN, 1992, In vitro activity of decaplanin (M86-1410), a new glycopeptide antibiotic, Antimicrob Agents Chemother, 36, 873–875.

Sandage B, Cooper G, Najarian N, Lowther J, Girard AM, 2005, Pharmacokinetics and fungicidal activity of aminocandin (HMR 3270), a novel echinocandin, in healthy volunteers, 15th Eur Cong of Chemother, Microbiol and Infect Dis, Copenhagen.

Schittek B, Hipfel R, Sauer B, Bauer J, Kalbacher H, Stevanovic S, Schirle M, Schroeder K, Blin N, Meier F, Rassner G, Garbe C, 2001, Dermacidin: a novel human antibiotic peptide secreted by sweat glands, Nat Immunol, 2, 1133–1137.

Schröder JM, 1999, Epithelial peptide antibiotics, Biochem Pharmacol, 57, 121–134.

Schwartz SN, Warren MR, Barkley FA, Landis L, 1959, Microbiological and pharmacological studies of colistin sulfate and sodium colistin methane sulfonate, Antib Annu 1959, p 41.

Selva E, Beretta G, Montanini N, Gastaido L, Lorenzetti R, Landini P, Montanaro L, Parmoggiani A, Goldstein BP, Denaro M, 1990, Antibiotic GE 2270 A, a novel inhibitor of bacterial protein synthesis. I. Discovery, isolation, characterization, 30th Intersci Conf Antimicrob Agents Chemother, abstract 798.

Selva E, Beretta G, Montanini N, Saddler GS, et al, 1991, Antibiotic GE 2270 A, a novel inhibitor of bacterial protein synthesis. I. Isolation and characterization, J Antibiot, 44, 693–701.

Selva E, Goldstein BP, Ferrari P, Pallanza R, Riva E, Berti M, Borghi A, et al, 1988, A 40926 aglycone and pseudoaglycones, preparation and biological activity, J Antibiot, 41, 1243–1252.

Shimanaka K, Iinuma H, Hamada M, Ikeno S, Tsuchiya S, Arita M, Hori M, 1995, Novel antibiotics, amythiamicins. IV. A mutation in the elongation factor Tu gene in a resistant mutant of Bacillus subtilis, J Antibiot, 48, 182–184.

Shimanaka K, Takahashi Y, Iinuma H, Naganawa H, Takeuchi T, 1994a, Novel antibiotics, amythiamicins. II. Structure elucidation of amythiamicin D, J Antibiot, 47, 1145–1152.

Shimanaka K, Takahashi Y, Iinumura H, Naganawa H, Takeuchi T, 1994b, Novel antibiotics, amythiamicins. III. Structure elucidation of amythiamicin A, B, C, J Antibiot, 47, 1153–1159.

Shinagawa S, Kasahara F, Wada Y, Harada S, Asai M, 1984, Structures of bulgecins, bacterial metabolites with bulge-inducing activity, Tetrahedron, 40, 3465–3470.

Siedlecki J, Hill J, Parr I, Yu X, Moryto M, Zhang Y, Silverman J, Controneo Y, Leganas V, Li T, Li J, Keith D, Shimer G, Finn J, 2003, Array synthesis of novel lipodepsipeptide, Bioorg Med Chem Lett, 13, 4245–4249.

Stella S, Montanini N, Le Monnier F, Ferrari P, Colombo L, Landini P, Ciciliato I, Goldstein BP, Selva E, Denaro M, 1995, Antibiotic GE 37468 A, a new inhibitor of bacterial synthesis. I. Isolation and characterization, J Antibiot, 48, 780–786.

Sugawara K, Konishi M, Kawaguchi H, 1984, BMY 28160, a new peptide antibiotic, J Antibiot, 37, 1257–1259.

Takahashi H, Kondo E, Koseki Y, Haneishi T, Arai M, Tokunoga T, 1995, A new antimycobacterial antibiotic, dihydromycoplanecin A. II. In vivo activities of dihydromycoplanecin A in combination with isoniazid on the experimental mycobacteriosis in mice, Recent Adv Chemother 3, 2546–2547.

Tavecchia P, Lociuro S, Ripamonti F, Berti M, Bellini S, Selva E, Ciabatti R, Goldenstein BP, Denaro M, 1992, Synthesis and antibacterial activity of MDL 63,908, a water-soluble analog of MDL 62,879 (GE 2270 A), 32nd Intersci Conf Antimicrob Agents Chemother, abstract 1354.

Toriya M, Shizuki Ishiquro M, Ogawa K, 2004, In vitro and in vivo antibacterial activity of a novel lantibiotic API 17444, 44th Intersci Conf Antimicrob Agents Chemother, abstract F-1932.

Tsuda H, Yamashita Y, Shibata Y, Nakawa Y, Koga T, 2002, Genes involved in bacitracin resistance in Streptococcus mutans, Antimicrob Agents Chemother, 46, 3756–3764.

Umehara K, Ezaki M, Iwami M, Yamashita M, et al, 1984, Novel peptide antibiotics, WS43708A and B, 24th Intersci Conf Antimicrob Agents Chemother.

van Schaik W, Gahan CG, Hill C, 1999, Acid-adapted Listeria monocytogenes displays enhanced tolerance against the lantibiotics nisin and lacticin 3147, J Food Protect, 62, 536–539.

Wade D, Andreu D, Mitchell SA, Silveira AMY, Boman A, Boman HG, Merrifield RB, 1992, Antibacterial peptides designed as analogs or hybrids of cecropins and mellitin, Int J Peptide Protein Res, 40, 429–436.

Walsh CT, 1989, Enzymes in the D-alanine branch of bacterial cell wall peptidoglycan assembly, J Biol Chem, 264, 2393–2396.

Wang CLJ, 1992, Antifungal agents: recent patent activity, Curr Opin Therap Patent, 247–252.

Williams AH, Grüneberg RN, 1984, Teicoplanin, J Antimicrob Chemother 14, 441.

Woodworth JR, Nyhart EH Jr, Brier GL, Wolny JD, Black HR, 1992, Single-dose pharmacokinetics and antibacterial activity for daptomycin, a new lipopeptide antibiotic, in healthy volunteers, Antimicrob Agents Chemother, 36, 318–325.

Yamaguchi H, Uchida K, Hiratani T, Nagase T, Watanabe N, Omura S, 1989, RI-331, a new antifungal antibiotic, Ann N Y Acad Sci, 544, 188–189.

Yao JDC, Elioupoulos GM, Moellering RC Jr, 1989, In vitro activity of SKF 104662, a new glycopeptide antibiotic, Antimicrob Agents Chemother, 33, 965–967.

Zasloff M, 1987, Magainins, a class of antimicrobial peptides from Xenopus skin, isolation, characterization of two active forms and partial C-DNA sequence and precursors, Proc Natl Acad Sci USA, 84, 5449–5453.

Zboinska E, Lejczak B, Kafarski P, 1993, Antibacterial activity of phosphonopeptides based on 4-amino-4-phosphono butyric acid, FEMS Microbiol Lett, 108, 225–230.

Glycopeptides and Lipoglycopeptides

A. BRYSKIER AND P. VEYSSIER

31

1. INTRODUCTION

The glycopeptide and lipoglycopeptide antibiotics are natural antibiotics obtained from cultures of certain microorganisms. These are complex molecules with high molecular masses (1,500 to 2,000 Da). One glycopeptide and one lipoglycopeptide are currently used in clinical practice: vancomycin, discovered in 1956, and teicoplanin, discovered in 1978. These antibiotics inhibit bacterial cell wall peptidoglycan synthesis but cannot cross the cell wall of gram-negative bacteria. Their antibacterial spectrum includes aerobic and anaerobic gram-positive bacteria.

Because of impurities (cofermentation products) responsible to a large extent for its poor tolerance and toxicity, the discovery of antistaphylococcal β-lactams, and the emerging problem of β-lactam-resistant gram-positive cocci, vancomycin was for a quarter of a century a second-line weapon that was difficult to use. However, since the beginning of the 1980s it has experienced a major resurgence of interest due to several factors:

- Increase in nosocomial infections due to gram-positive cocci accompanying therapeutic progress
- Emergence of resistance to first-line antibiotics (resistance to β-lactams and other antistaphylococcals, rifampin, 14- and 15-membered-ring macrolides, aminoglycosides, and fluoroquinolones), but also among streptococci, enterococci, and pneumococci
- Processes of purification of vancomycin and the description of its chemical structure and its pharmacokinetics

Vancomycin, however, remains difficult to use, and the emergence of infections due to resistant strains of gram-positive cocci resulted in the search for new glycopeptides. More than 50 glycopeptide molecules have been identified from cultures of potentially productive microorganisms, and their antibacterial and pharmacokinetic properties have been evaluated.

2. CLASSIFICATION

The glycopeptides may be divided into at least five groups on the basis of their chemical structures. Teicoplanin, being a lipoglycopeptide, does not belong to the glycopeptide groups. Since Lancini (1989) subdivided the glycopeptide family into four subgroups, on variation of amino acids 1 and 3, many new compounds, even unclassified, have arisen.

The classification is based on the structure of the heptapeptide.

2.1. Group I (Vancomycin Type)

Group I is characterized by the presence of an asparagine at position 3, and the NH_2-terminal amino acid is a leucine that may be methylated. In some molecules the asparagine may be replaced by an aspartic acid or a glutamine. They have aliphatic amino acids at positions 1 and 3.

The sugars are glucose, vancosamine, and 4-epivancosamine, with a few exceptions, such as olivose (orienticin B) or eremosamine (eremomycin). The majority of molecules have two chlorine atoms on the triphenyl ether nucleus. Chloroorienticin B (S-3362) is in the preclinical development phase and exhibits partial cross-resistance with vancomycin.

The following compounds belong to group I: vancomycin, oritavancin, chloroorienticin, orienticin, decaplanin, eremomycin, A-82846, *N*-desmethylvancomycin, and UK-72051.

2.2. Group II (Avoparcin Type)

The molecules belonging to group II possess a *para*-hydroxyphenylglycine as amino acids 3, 4, and 5 and the NH_2-terminal amino acids. The sugars vary: acosamine, actinosamine, ristosamine, mannose, and rhamnose. The molecules belonging to group II are mainly actinodin, avoparcin, chloropolysporin, galacardin, helvecardin, and synmonicin.

Synmonicin is characterized by a *para*-hydroxyphenylglycine as the N-terminal amino acid, and the third amino acid is a thioamine aliphatic acid, methionine. One molecule is under development (SKF-104662). Other derivatives belong to group II, such as actaplanin and UK-68597. The antibiotics in group II differ from those in group I in having aromatic amino acids at positions 1 and 3.

2.3. Group III (Ristocetin-Type Derivatives)

Group III consists of molecules with a *meta*-hydroxyphenylglycine as the amino acid at position 3, the N-terminal amino acid being a β-hydroxylphenylglycine. The aromatic nuclei of these two amino acids are linked by an ether bond. Ristocetin does not have a chlorine atom and possesses a tetrasaccharide sugar, ristosamine.

2.4. Group IV (Teicoplanin-Like)

The arrangement of the amino acids in the peptide core is the same. They have fatty acid residues attached to the amino sugar. Group IV is composed at least of teicoplanin, dalbavancin, televancin, ardacin, kibdelin, and parvocidin.

3. VANCOMYCIN

The basic structure of vancomycin is a peptide skeleton of seven amino acids known as an aglycone. The five amino acids at positions 2, 4, 5, 6, and 7 are aromatic (phenyl nucleus) and more or less constant for all of the glycopeptides: three phenylglycines and two β-hydroxychlorotyrosines.

The differences between the glycopeptides relate to the nature of amino acids 1 and 3; the number, situation, and nature of the sugar residues (monosaccharides and disaccharides) substituted on this heptapeptide skeleton; and the existence or otherwise of an acyl residue (fatty acid), which constitutes the originality of teicoplanin. The spatial configuration of the glycopeptides is that of a pocket or "baseball glove," and their attachment to the preferential target, the terminal D-alanyl–D-alanine group of the disaccharide pentapeptide, produces steric hindrance, blocking the synthesis of peptidoglycans.

Vancomycin, which has a molecular mass of 1,450 Da, is produced by fermentation of *Streptomyces orientalis*. Originally nicknamed "Mississippi mud" because of impurities (cofermentation and degradation products), it currently benefits from modern purification techniques, including liquid chromatography, that yield an active substance of more than 92% purity. However, the degree of purification varies with the commercial specialties. Amino acids 1 and 3 of vancomycin are two aliphatic amino acids, *N*-methyl-leucine and an amino aspartic acid, giving it a tricyclic structure. The sugar bearing the phenylglycine at position 4 is an amino disaccharide: glucose and vancosamine.

3.1. Physicochemical Properties of Vancomycin

Vancomycin hydrochloride is a white, odorless powder, soluble in water at acid or neutral pH and unstable in alkaline solution. It is a basic molecule with an isoelectric point of 8 possessing vein irritant properties. The intramuscular route is painful and cannot be used in humans. It is physically incompatible (precipitation and inactivation) in the same intravenous infusion with barbiturates, sodium bicarbonate, high concentrations of heparin or hydrocortisone succinate, chloramphenicol, and methicillin. The recommended solvents are 0.9% sodium chloride (physiological saline) or 5% (isotonic) glucose solution.

3.2. Assays

Vancomycin may be assayed in biological media by three methods:

- Microbiological method using a reference strain of *Staphylococcus aureus* or *Bacillus subtilis*
- Immunological methods: radioimmunoassay or fluorescence polarization (Merieux EMIT-SYVA and Abbott TDX kits)
- High-performance liquid chromatography (HPLC)

3.3. Mechanism of Action

The main mechanism of action of the glycopeptides occurs on the internal part of the bacterial cell wall (peptidoglycan) in the periplasmic space, a region between the cytoplasmic membrane and the cell wall in which peptidoglycan synthesis occurs. Because of their large mass, glycopeptides cannot cross the lipoprotein cell wall of gram-negative bacteria and are therefore totally inactive against them.

In gram-positive bacteria, glycopeptides cross the bacterial cell wall and bind specifically inside to the terminal D-alanyl–D-alanine dipeptide (D-Ala–D-Ala) of the disaccharide pentapeptide chain, the base unit and precursor of peptidoglycan synthesis.

As a result of the steric hindrance that it causes, this binding blocks two of the main enzymatic reactions necessary for peptidoglycan synthesis, transglycosylation and transpeptidation, causing inhibition of growth and the subsequent death of the bacterium. However, the bactericidal activity of the glycopeptides is slow: nonspecific binding of glycopeptides also occurs within the already mature peptidoglycan, and this nonspecific binding appears to affect the action of autolysins involved in the physiological hydrolysis of peptidoglycan.

In addition to this mechanism common to all glycopeptides, vancomycin appears also to have specific activity on RNA synthesis and on the permeability of the cytoplasmic membrane in *S. aureus* (Fig. 1).

3.4. Pharmacokinetics of Vancomycin

3.4.1. Modes of Administration of Vancomycin

3.4.1.1. Oral Route

The oral bioavailability of vancomycin is practically nonexistent in an intact gastrointestinal tract. Concentrations in plasma as high as 5 μg/ml have been observed after oral administration in patients suffering from extensive gastrointestinal lesions. The concentrations in the stools are about 350 μg/g after a 125 mg dose of vancomycin and 3,100 μg/g after a 500-mg dose. Concentration as high as 24,000 μg/g of stool have been observed (Cooper and Given, 1986). The oral route is reserved for the treatment of *Clostridium difficile* pseudomembranous colitis and digestive decontamination in oncology-hematology patients.

Different types of research are ongoing to improve oral absorption, such as liposomes, multiple emulsion, and using glycocholate as an absorption promoter or Labrasol, a surfactant obtained from coconut oil.

3.4.1.2. Intramuscular

Although the bioavailability of intramuscular vancomycin is satisfactory, this route of administration is very painful and necrotizing and cannot be used in humans.

3.4.1.3. Intravenous

The sole route for parenteral administration is therefore the intravenous route. Intravenous bolus injection is dangerous because of the risk of an abrupt and extensive release of histamine with red man syndrome and an anaphylactoid reaction. Vancomycin is administered by slow intravenous infusion. A flow rate of ≥500 mg/h reduces the risk of histamine release. The usual dosage in adults with normal renal function is 30 mg/kg of body weight/24 h, corresponding to infusions of about 1 g over 2 h every 12 h or 500 mg over 1 h every 6 h. The peripheral venous route can be used, but it is then recommended that vancomycin be diluted in a large volume (500 mg/125 or 250 ml) of isotonic saline or glucose solution to attenuate the local causticity. To optimize vancomycin therapy, it was recommended that adjustments in dose and dosage interval be guided by trough (5 to 10 μg/ml) and peak (30 to 40 μg/ml) levels in serum (Rotschafer et al., 1982; Zimmermann et al., 1995).

3.4.1.4. Peritoneal

Continuous infusion is possible. It is accompanied by better tissue distribution and has specific indications, such as the treatment of neuromeningeal infections. The drawbacks

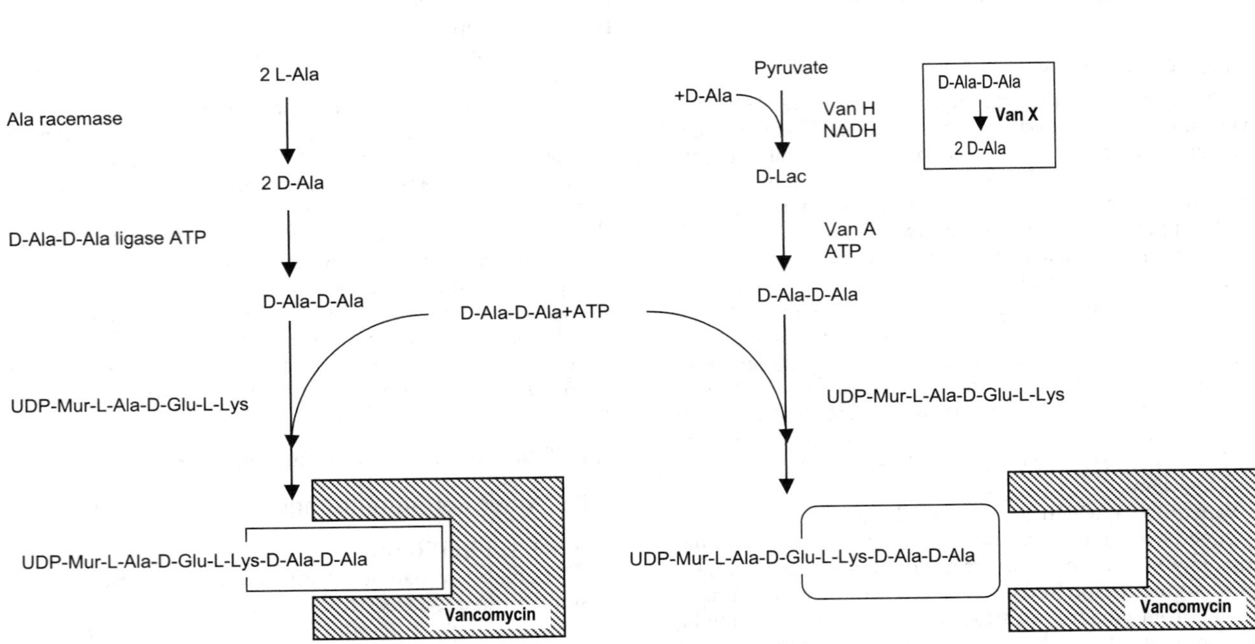

Figure 1 Vancomycin mode of action

are related to possible drug incompatibilities and perhaps slightly increased renal toxicity.

The intraperitoneal route is of interest for patients on peritoneal dialysis. There is in fact a preferential transfer of vancomycin from the peritoneal fluid to the vascular sector, enabling high intraperitoneal concentrations and effective concentrations in serum to be obtained at the same time. After an injection of 30 mg/kg in 2 liters of dialysis solution left in contact for 6 h, a peak concentration in serum of 30 ± 7 μg/ml (mean ± standard deviation) is reached after 6 h and residual concentrations of 21 ± 2 μg/ml and 7 ± 1 μg/ml are reached at 24 h and on day 7, respectively.

Vancomycin and teicoplanin can be stably incorporated into polymethylmethacrylate and are eluted well. The combination is often loaded into cement spacers. In vivo, incorporation of teicoplanin in cement was shown to be beneficial in bone infections in rabbits (Ismael et al., 2003).

3.4.1.5. Other Sites

The use of vancomycin intrathecally or intraventricularly via an Ommaya reservoir is possible at a dose of 3 to 5 mg per administration in order to obtain concentrations in the cerebrospinal fluid (CSF) of about 25 μg/ml. Dosages ranging up to 20 mg/24 h have been used.

3.4.2. Protein Binding, Distribution, Pharmacokinetic Characteristics, and Elimination

Vancomycin is bound to serum albumin. At concentrations in serum of between 10 and 100 μg/ml, this binding is 30 to 60%.

In adults with normal renal function, the concentrations in serum obtained are about 30 μg/ml at the end of an intravenous infusion of 500 mg in 1 h, 50 to 70 μg/ml after infusion of 1 g in 1 h, and about 40 μg/ml after an infusion of 1 g in 2 h. There are major interindividual variations. The mathematical model used to describe the pharmacokinetics of vancomycin is a two- or three-compartment model. The apparent elimination half-life ($t_{1/2\beta}$) is 6 to 8 h. The apparent volume of distribution is 0.4 to 0.9 liter/kg.

Vancomycin is eliminated in the nonmetabolized active form almost entirely via the kidneys (80 to 90% of the administered dose is found in the urine in 24 h), essentially by glomerular filtration. There are tubular secretion and reabsorption phenomena that may be affected by other compounds: furosemide and anti-inflammatory nonsteroidal drugs. A close correlation, however, exists between creatinine clearance (CL_{CR}) and plasma and renal clearance of vancomycin. Hepatobiliary elimination of vancomycin is very weak. The residual concentration in serum appears to be the parameter most correlated with clinical efficacy, and residual concentrations of 10 to 20 μg/ml are currently considered satisfactory, depending on the clinical severity of the infection. In the indications requiring continuous infusion, the usual initial dosage is 30 mg/kg/24 h, the aim being a mean concentration in serum of about 20 μg/ml.

3.4.3. Pharmacodynamics

Vancomycin exhibits time-dependent killing that is maximized at four times the MIC for a given microorganism. In animal models, the most predictive parameter for vancomycin efficacy is the area under the concentration-time curve/MIC ratio.

3.4.4. Specific Pharmacokinetics

There are major variations in the pharmacokinetic characteristics of vancomycin according to age, renal function, and certain pathological conditions, reflected in major variations in its ($t_{1/2\beta}$) necessitating regular monitoring of the levels in order to adapt the unit dose and the dosage interval to each clinical situation.

3.4.4.1. Pediatric Patients

In premature neonates weighing <1,000 g, the $t_{1/2\beta}$ is prolonged (10 h). It is reduced in premature infants weighing more than 1,000 g and in full-term neonates ($t_{1/2\beta}$, 5 to 6 h), and even more so in infants and children up to 10 years ($t_{1/2\beta}$, 2.5 to 3 h). The usual recommended dosage in children is therefore higher than in adults (40 mg/kg/day).

3.4.4.2. Elderly Patients

In elderly subjects, the $t_{1/2\beta}$ may be prolonged (12.1 versus 7.2 h), although this cannot entirely be explained by an impairment of renal function, but the volume of distribution was increased (Cutler et al., 1984).

3.4.4.3. Renally Impaired Patients

The pharmacokinetics of vancomycin, which is eliminated almost entirely by the kidneys, are deeply affected by renal insufficiency.

The $t_{1/2\beta}$ are about 11 h in subjects with mild renal insufficiency (CL_{CR}), (>40 ml/min for 1.73 m^2), 20 h in subjects with moderately severe renal insufficiency (CL_{CR}, 10 to 40 ml/min for 1.73 m^2), and 7 to 9 days in totally anuric patients. Adaptation of the vancomycin dosage in patients with renal insufficiency can be done in "stable" patients by using formulae involving the CL_{CR} (measured in milliliters per minute): Moellering's or Matzke's normograms, where the daily dose (in milligram per day) is determined by the equation ($CL_{CR} \times 15$) +150 mg. However, there are major interindividual variations in the pharmacokinetics of vancomycin for a given CL_{CR}, probably related to a number of different factors (tubular secretion-reabsorption phenomenon, protein binding, variations in hemodynamic status and renal function, and combined therapeutic agents) that make these adaptations very approximate. The pharmacokinetics of vancomycin were characterized in 56 patients with different degrees of renal function after an intravenous dose of 18.4 ± 4.7 mg/kg; results are shown in Table 1.

In practice, after an initial dose of 15 to 20 mg/kg in adults, the dosages must be adapted on the basis of regular measurements of the residual concentration with administration of 15 to 20 mg/kg when the residual concentration is between 10 and 20 μg/ml. In anuric patients, the interval between injections may thus vary from 3 to 7 days.

It appears that the dialysance of vancomycin, which is negligible by conventional hemodialysis using cuprophan membranes, must be taken into account with modern polyacrylonitrile membranes. It is weak by peritoneal dialysis. Following accidental overdosing, vancomycin has been eliminated satisfactorily by hemoperfusion on a resin or charcoal column. Between 1.5 and 21.2% of the administered vancomycin was eliminated during hemodialysis. The dialysis clearance of vancomycin ranged from 50.6 to 76.8 ml/min (average, 62.4 ± 10.4 ml/min). Table 2 shows the pharmacokinetics after administration of 1.0 g of vancomycin.

Table 1 Vancomycin pharmacokinetics in renally impaired patients[a]

CL_{CR} (ml/min)	n	CL_P (ml/min)	$t_{1/2\beta}$ (h)	C_{max} (μg/ml)
Group I, >60	7	62.7	9.1	1.49
Group II, 60–10	13	28.3	32.3	1.15
Group III, <10	36	4.87	146.7	1.16

[a]Data from Matzke et al., 1984.

Table 2 Vancomycin (1g) pharmacokinetics in anuric patients[a]

Parameter	Value
C_0 (μg/ml)	64.9 ± 21.7
C_{168h} (μg/ml)	6.55 ± 2.8
$t_{1/2\gamma}$ (h)	131 ± 46.7
V (liters/kg)	0.158 ± 0.121
V_{ss} (liters/kg)	0.92 ± 0.24
CL_P (liters/kg)	0.10 ± 0.0049

[a]Data from Gonzalez-Martin et al., 1996.

In patients on peritoneal dialysis, a bidirectional flow is observed between the vascular sector and the peritoneal fluid, although preferentially from the peritoneum to the circulating blood. After intravenous infusion of 15 mg of vancomycin per kg, a peak concentration in the peritoneal fluid of about 6 μg/ml is observed at 6 h. After injection of 30 mg of vancomycin per kg into the peritoneal dialysis solution, a peak concentration in serum of about 30 μg/ml is observed at 6 h, and the concentration in serum is 20 μg/ml at 24 h and 7 μg/ml at 48 h. The $t_{1/2\beta}$ in dialysis patients on continuous ambulatory peritoneal dialysis (CAPD) is about 4 days. This has two benefits: local administration of vancomycin allows local treatment of infections of the peritoneal fluid caused by susceptible bacteria, and it also represents a possible means of systemic treatment in this type of patient.

The pharmacokinetics of vancomycin were studied in four patients on CAPD. After a single intravenous infusion of 10 mg/kg, blood and dialysate samples were collected during the 72-h evaluation period. The peritoneal dialysate vancomycin concentration reached 2.2 ± 0.7 μg/ml throughout the observation period (Table 3).

In patients with end-stage renal disease (CL_{CR}, <10 ml/min), the $t_{1/2\beta}$ of vancomycin is significantly prolonged (90.2 ± 24.2 h) in comparison with that in subjects with normal renal function (4.7 to 11.2 h).

After a single 1-g intraperitoneal dose was administered to four patients, approximately 54% of the dose was absorbed into the systemic circulation, and a peak concentration in serum of, on average, 24 μg/ml was reached. The mean apparent elimination half-life was 66.9 h, and the peritoneal dialysis clearance was 2.4 ml/min (Pancorbo and Comty, 1982).

Table 3 Vancomycin pharmacokinetics in CAPD patients[a]

Dose (mg)	$t_{1/2\alpha}$ (h)	$t_{1/2\beta}$ (h)	CL_P (ml/min)	CL_R (ml/min)	CL_{CAPD} (ml/min)
600	0.75	59.4	7.37	0.65	1.83
700	0.80	84.3	6.94		1.02
750	1.50	101.8	6.50	0.65	1.37
650	2.07	115.4	4.85		1.17

[a]Data from Blevins et al., 1984.

3.4.4.4. Other Pathological Situations

The $t_{1/2\beta}$ is reduced (about 3 h) in burn patients, highly obese subjects, neutropenic subjects, and pregnant women, necessitating shorter dosage intervals at a higher daily dose. The dosage must be adapted on the basis of measurements of residual concentrations in serum.

Vancomycin was shown in dogs not to be concentrated in bile (Lee et al., 1957). In humans, vancomycin pharmacokinetics are affected by hepatic function (Brown et al., 1983) (Table 4).

3.4.5. Distribution into Biological Fluids and Tissues

The diffusion of vancomycin into pleural fluid, ascitic fluid (3.6 μg/ml at 1.5 to 5.2 h after 500 mg), pericardial fluid (0.6 to 5.5 μg/ml at 1.5 to 5.5 h after 500 mg), and synovial fluid (5.7 μg/ml at 1 h after 500 mg) is relatively good. The concentrations obtained are, on average, between 40 and 70% of the concentration in serum, i.e., on the order of 3 to 10 μg/ml.

Table 5 shows vancomycin levels in pleural fluid of 16 patients receiving vancomycin either at 15 mg/kg twice a day as a 60 min infusion (8 patients) or at 30 mg/kg as a continuous infusion after administration of a loading dose of 500 mg over 30 min (8 patients).

The continuous infusion allowed the concentration in pleural exudates to be more sustained (Byl et al., 2003).

It was shown that the serum vancomycin concentration drops during cardiopulmonary bypass (Ortega et al., 2003).

Concentrations in the bile (3.1 μg/ml 1 h after 500 mg) and aqueous humor, however, are very weak. Aqueous and vitreous vancomycin was assayed in 14 patients with endophthalmitis. Nine patients received 2 mg of vancomycin, and another five received 1.0 mg of vancomycin. In six patients, the intravitreous injection was repeated at 48 h and in seven it was repeated at 72 h. The aqueous vancomycin levels varied from 8.4 to 170 μg/ml, and the vitreous vancomycin levels ranged from 21.2 to 220 μg/ml (Haider et al., 2001).

Diffusion into the CSF varies with the state of inflammation of the meninges and is better in children than adults. With inflamed meninges, the concentrations of vancomycin found in the CSF may attain 10 to 20% of the concentrations in serum, i.e., 1 to 5 μg/ml.

In general, diffusion of vancomycin is improved by continuous infusion, and this property may be used in the treatment of neuromeningeal infections in particular.

Urinary concentrations obtained after infusion of 500 mg of vancomycin are on the order of 100 to 300 μg/ml.

Concentrations close to levels in serum may be reached in abscess fluids.

The parenchymatous concentrations found in the kidneys, liver, myocardium, and lungs, are very much higher than the concentrations in serum. Conversely, diffusion in bone is poor (about 1 to 3 mg/kg).

3.5. Adverse Effects and Toxicity of Vancomycin

The improvement in the manufacturing of vancomycin (currently very purified active substance) and the better control of its method of administration (slow infusion) have contributed to a marked improvement in its tolerance.

The most spectacular side effect of vancomycin, known as red man or red neck syndrome, is related to histamine release. The frequency of occurrence of this reaction is estimated as about 20% following infusion of 1 g over 1 h in infected patients and up to 80% in healthy volunteers. In its minor form, red man syndrome combines pruritus and an erythematous rash of the face, neck, and trunk. In the most severe forms, this flushing may be associated with other anaphylactoid reactions: angioedema, collapse, and digestive disorders. This histamine release reaction is related not to an immunological mechanism but to direct activation of mastocytes and basophils. The principal determinant of the occurrence of this syndrome is the rate of infusion of vancomycin. Infusion of vancomycin at a rate greater than or equal to 500 mg/h (1 g over at least 2 h) has been shown to reduce the

Table 4 Vancomycin pharmacokinetics in hepatically impaired patients

Hepatic function	n	C_0 (μg/ml)	C_6 (μg/ml)	$t_{1/2\beta}$ (h)	AUC (μg·h/ml)	CL_P (ml/min)
Volunteers	6	26	2.1	2.6	59	162
Impaired	9	59	19	37	3,434	48

Table 5 Vancomycin levels in pleural fluid after continuous and discontinuous infusions

Time after administration (h)	Concn (μg/ml)			
	Intermittent infusion		Continuous infusion	
	Blood	Pleural fluid	Blood	Pleural fluid
0	4.1	5.5	14.0	11.8
0.5		5.8		
1.0	48.3	9.4		
1.5		15.3		
2.0	22.4	19		
4.0	14.4	16	14.0	12.1
6.0	10.3	13		
8.0	8.6	9.8	14.7	13.0
12	5.6	6.6	16.0	13.7
AUC_{0-12h} (μg·h/ml)	172	145	178	152
AUC_{0-12h}/AUC_{blood}		0.88		0.86

frequency and severity of this reaction, and likewise premedication with an antihistamine such as hydroxyzine (Atarax).

The nephrotoxicity of vancomycin has become virtually negligible with the current preparations when used as monotherapy. However, it potentiates the nephrotoxicity of any other combined compounds, particularly aminoglycosides, amphotericin B, cyclosporine, etc. An underlying predisposition (elderly subject, septic state, hypovolemia, and impaired hemodynamic status) and, likewise, excessively high concentrations (residual concentrations in serum of >30 μg/ml) may also potentiate this nephrotoxicity. It involves a reversible tubulopathy. Regular monitoring of serum vancomycin concentrations and renal function remains justified, particularly in the presence of associated risk factors.

The ototoxicity of vancomycin remains a fact. It involves cochlear toxicity (VIIIth cranial nerve) that is predominantly, if not totally, irreversible and may take the form of tinnitus and hypoacusia, initially at high frequencies. It appears to be related to the total administered dose (treatment duration and high concentration in serum, particularly peak concentrations in serum greater than 80 μg/ml).

Local venous causticity (chemical thrombophlebitis) is reduced with the current preparations and correct handling of the drug (sufficient dilution, long infusion time, and absence of an incompatible combined medication).

Hypersensitivity reactions such as generalized skin rash, fever, and hypereosinophilia may occur in 5% of patients, generally from the seventh day of treatment onwards. They are more common (10 to 20%) in subjects allergic to β-lactams. This is not a matter of cross-resistance but probably a bias associated with selection of an atopic subpopulation.

Neutropenia may be observed. It appears to depend on the total administered dose, generally occurring during treatment lasting more than 2 weeks, and is reversible.

Finally, vancomycin has exceptionally been implicated in *C. difficile* pseudomembranous colitis (during treatment with intravenous vancomycin) and against a background of vasculitis.

4. TEICOPLANIN

4.1. Structure of Teicoplanin

Teicoplanin is a mixture of five major components designated A2-1 to A2-5 and a more polar component designated A3-1 (molecular weight, 1,562). Minor components are also present (Fig. 2).

This complex was obtained from the fermentation broth of *Actinoplanes teichomyceticus*. All teicoplanin components are lipoglycopeptide analogs with molecular weights that range from 1,564.3 to 1,907.7. The A3-1 component possesses the core glycopeptide that is common to teicoplanin components. The structure includes a bisphenylether moiety identical to vancomycin and contains three sugars (α-D-mannose, acetyl α-D-glucosamine, and acyl-β-D-glucosamine) and an acyl-aliphatic side chain. All of the components of the A2 group contain an additional *N*-acyl-β-D-glucosamine and differ only in the nature of the acyl-aliphatic side chain (Barna et al., 1984).

Teicoplanin (Fig. 3), a heptapeptide structure, is amphoteric, containing six ionizable groups: a terminal carboxylic group, a terminal amino group, and four weakly acid phenolic groups.

Teicoplanin sodium is stable for 48 h at room temperature and for 7 days at 4°C. It is highly soluble in water at pH >7.0. At its isoelectric point (pI 5.1) the logP in *n*-octanol/buffer was −1.1 (hydrophilic nature), the vancomycin logP was 2.5.

4.2. Physicochemical Properties of Teicoplanin

The lyophilisate of teicoplanin is a whitish, colorless powder. It is a weak acid with an isoelectric point of 5.1, well tolerated intravenously or intramuscularly, and highly lipophilic (50 to 100 times more than vancomycin). These global physicochemical characteristics of the teicoplanin complex, however, differ for each of the components. The gently reconstituted solution (foam) may be diluted in physiological saline or glucose solution. The molecular mass is 1,993 Da. The pK_as are 5.0 (carboxyl group), 7.1

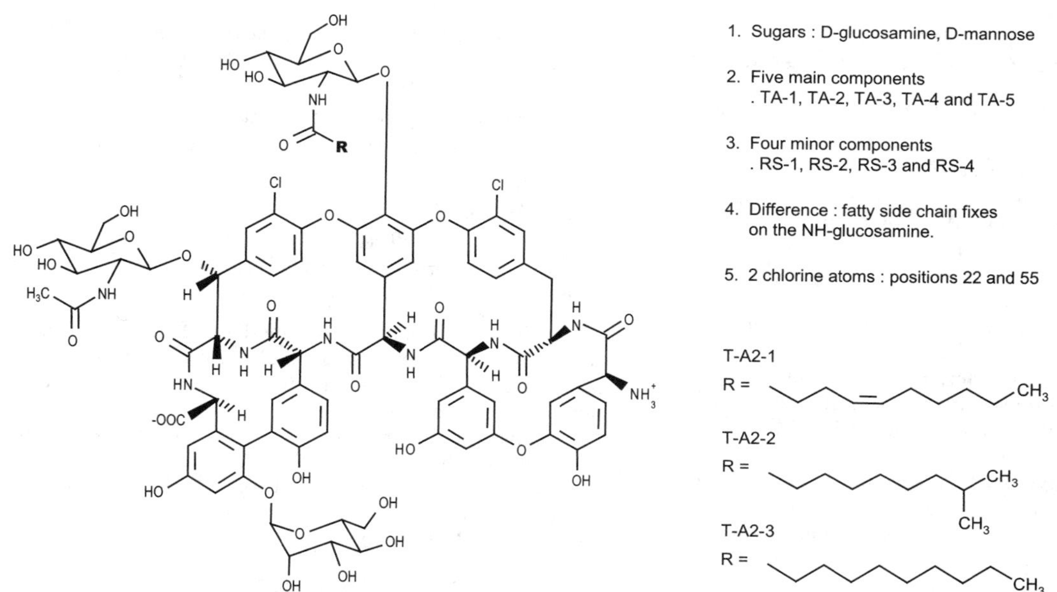

Figure 2 Teicoplanin complex

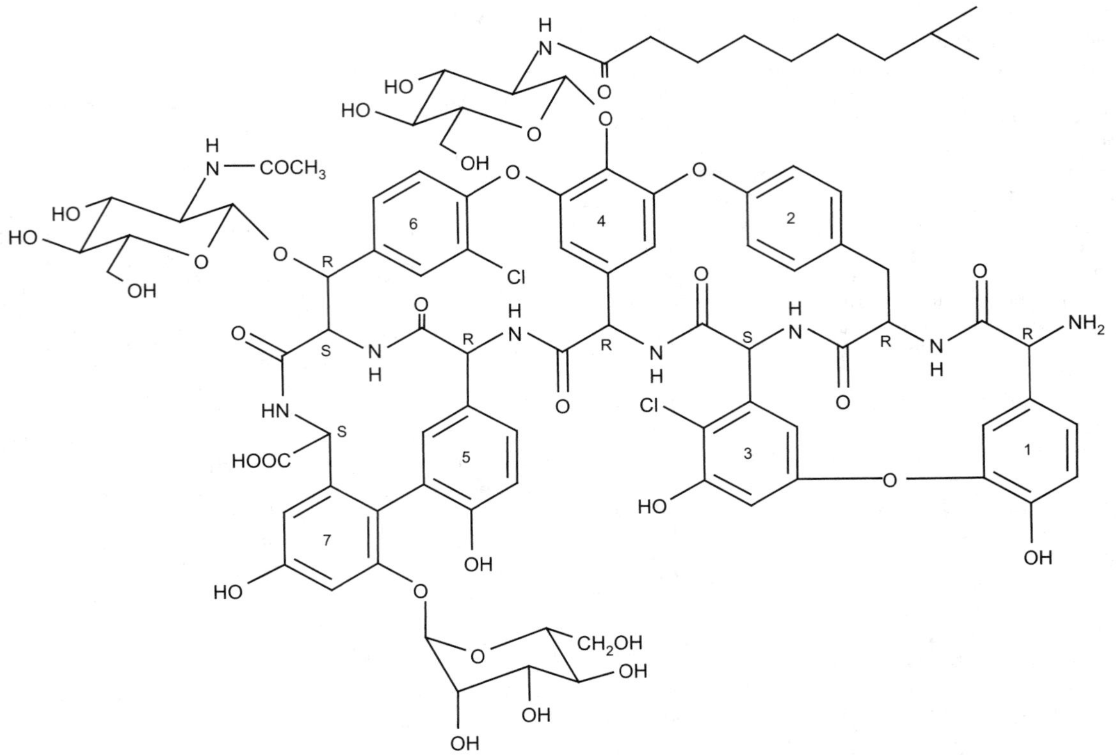

Figure 3 Structure of teicoplanin

(amino group), and 9 to 12.5 (phenol groups). The partition coefficient (logP [n-octanol/water]) ranges from 1.9 (pH 1.0) to 2.1 (pH 9.0) (Table 6). Four hundred milligrams of teicoplanin must be dissolved in at least 3 ml of liquid to prevent the formation of a gel.

4.3. Assay of Teicoplanin

Teicoplanin may be assayed by a microbiological method, by recently developed immunological methods (Abbott TDX kit), or by HPLC (not usable routinely, but enabling each of the components to be assayed specifically).

4.4. In Vitro Antibacterial Activity and Resistance

4.4.1. Antibacterial Spectrum and Antibacterial Activity

The in vitro antibacterial activity of the glycopeptides is currently determined by using the following breakpoints in broth (NCCLS): susceptible, MIC of $\leq$4 μg/ml; intermediate, MIC of 8 to 16 μg/ml; and resistant, MIC of $\geq$32 μg/ml.

Teicoplanin and vancomycin are inactive against aerobic or anaerobic gram-negative bacteria, mycobacteria, fungi, *Chlamydia*, *Mycoplasma*, and *Rickettsia*.

Disk diffusion will not differentiate staphylococcal strains with reduced susceptibility to vancomycin or teicoplanin (MICs of 4 to 8 μg/ml) for susceptible strains (MICs from 0.5 to 2.0 μg/ml).

Some gram-positive bacterial species are naturally resistant to vancomyin and teicoplanin: *Leuconostoc, Pediococcus, Nocardia, Lactobacillus,* and *Erysipelothrix rhusiopathiae*.

In general, the following are susceptible to teicoplanin:

- Staphylococci (*S. aureus* and coagulase-negative staphylococci [CoNS]), whether methicillin susceptible or resistant
- Streptococci: *S. pyogenes,* Lancefield group C, F, and G streptococci; *S. agalactiae* (group B); *S. pneumoniae*; and viridans group streptococci
- Enterococci: *E. faecalis* and *E. faecium*
- Corynebacteria: *C. diphtheriae*, *C. jeikeium*, and *C. urealyticum*
- *Listeria monocytogenes* (in vitro)
- *Bacillus* spp.
- Clostridia (*C. difficile* and *C. perfringens*) and all gram-positive anaerobic bacteria: *Peptostreptococcus, Propionibacterium,* and *Eubacterium* (Table 7)

Table 6 Physicochemical properties of teicoplanin

Property	Value
Molecular mass	1,993 Da
Empirical formula	$C_{89}H_{108}N_9O_{35}Cl_2$
Melting point	Amorphous
Isoelectric point	5.1
LogP	1.9–2.1
pK	5.0 (COOH), 7.1 (amino group), 9–12.5 (phenol)

Against glycopeptide-intermediate *S. aureus* (GISA) strains (vancomycin intermediately susceptible), teicoplanin is inactive, as is oritavancin; linezolid and dalfopristin-quinupristin remain active (Table 8).

Against the majority of strains of *S. aureus* and streptococci tested, the in vitro activity of teicoplanin is slightly greater than that of vancomycin (half the MIC). The activity of teicoplanin against enterococci is greater than that of vancomycin (MIC, three to eight times lower).

4.4.2. Resistance of Staphylococci

In the mid-1950s, Gerani was able to induce vancomycin resistance in two initially vancomycin-susceptible *S. aureus*

Table 7 In vitro activities of teicoplanin and vancomycin

Microorganism(s)[a]	*n*	MIC (μg/ml)[b]			
		Teicoplanin		Vancomycin	
		50%	90%	50%	90%
MSSA	31	0.5	2.0	1.0	2.0
MRSA	50	2.0	2.0	1.0	2.0
MSSE	28	0.5	2.0	1.0	2.0
MRSE	46	2.0	64	2.0	2.0
S. pneumoniae Pen[s]	19	≤0.01	≤0.01	0.25	0.25
S. pneumoniae Pen[i]	27	≤0.01	≤0.01	0.25	0.25
S. pneumoniae Pen[r]	45	≤0.01	≤0.01	0.25	0.5
S. pyogenes	34	≤0.01	0.25	0.25	0.25
S. agalactiae	18	≤0.01	0.12	0.5	1.0
Group C, F, and G streptococci	104	0.06	0.125	0.5	1.0
Streptococcus anginosus	7	0.06		1.0	
Streptococcus bovis	13	0.12	0.12	0.5	0.5
Streptococcus mitis	27	0.06	0.6	0.75	1.5
Streptococcus oralis	6	0.06		1.0	
Streptococcus salivarius	4	0.03		1.0	
Streptococcus sanguinis	16	0.03		1.0	
Listeria spp.	35	0.25	0.5	1.0	1.0
Rhodococcus equi	16	0.25	0.25	0.5	8.0
E. rhusiopathiae	6	16		2.0	
C. urealyticum	27	0.25	0.5	0.5	0.5
Corynebacterium jeikieum	34	1.0	1.0	0.5	0.5
Corynebacterium striatum	25	0.25	0.25	0.25	0.25
Arcanobacterium haemolyticus	25	0.06	1.0	1.0	2.0
E. faecalis	27	0.25	0.5	0.5	2.0
E. faecium	51	≤0.25	0.5	2.0	2.0
E. casseliflavus	67	≤0.25	0.5	2.0	2.0
E. gallinarum	29		32		8
S. haemolyticus	11		1		1
Staphylococcus simulans	8	4		2	
Staphylococcus saprophyticus	21		4		2
Other CoNS[c]	12	32		8.0	
C. difficile	18	0.5	0.5	1.0	1.0
C. perfringens	11	≤0.06	0.125	0.5	0.5
Pasteurella multocida	30	>32	>32	>32	>32
Actinobacillus spp.	4	4		8	
M. catarrhalis	11	8	8	4	32
Neisseria spp.	10	8	16	4	32
Eikenella corrodens	20	32	32	32	32
Bacteroides spp.	17	64	128	64	128
Fusobacterium spp.	15	>256	>256	>256	>256
Peptostreptococcus spp.	13	0125	0.25	05	1.0
Porphyromonas spp.	10	≤1.0	2.0	2.0	4.0
Prevotella spp.	12	0.5	4.0	>16	>16

[a]MSSE, methicillin-susceptible *S. epidermidis*; MRSE, methicillin-resistant *S. epidermidis*.
[b]50% and 90%, MICs at which 50 and 90% of isolates tested are inhibited, respectively.
[c]*S. cohnii* (6 isolates), *S. hominis* (5) *S. xylosus* (4) *S. capitis* (12) *S. sciuri* (2) and *S. warneri* (2).

strains by daily subcultures in increasing concentrations of vancomycin for 28 days.

The in vitro study of resistance to vancomycin and teicoplanin by successive subcultures at subinhibitory concentrations shows a much more marked induction for teicoplanin (four to eight times the MIC or more for 75% of strains) than for vancomycin (four times the MIC for 5 to 10% of strains) in both CoNS and *S. aureus*.

Acquired resistance to vancomycin or teicoplanin has appeared recently in clinical practice among CoNS and enterococci. The first *S. aureus* isolates resistant or of reduced susceptibility to vancomycin were described in Japan in 1997. An *S. aureus* isolate resistant to vancomycin was reported by the Centers for Disease Control in 2002 (Centers for Disease Control, 2002).

The vancomycin MIC for *S. aureus* HMC3 was 32 μg/ml, though this strain remains susceptible to teicoplanin (MIC, 4 μg/ml). Dalbavancin and oritavancin MICs ranged from 0.125 to 0.5 μg/ml. Teicoplanin, dalbavancin, and oritavancin retain bactericidal activity against this isolate at one to two times the MIC. However, regrowth was observed at the MIC after 24 h with dalbavancin (Bozdogan et al., 2003). The presence of the *vanA* gene suggests that the resistance determinant was acquired through exchange of

Table 8 In vitro activities of teicoplanin and vancomycin against GISA strains

Strain	MIC (μg/ml)				
	Teicoplanin	Vancomycin	Oritavancin	Linezolid	Q-D
Mu50 (Japan)	8.0	8.0	4.0	2.0	0.5
Mu3 (Japan)	16	2.0	4.0	2.0	1.0
966 (Michigan)	16	4.0	4.0	2.0	1.0
N20 (Japan)	1.0	4.0	4.0	2.0	0.5

genetic material from enterococci, as was demonstrated in vitro (Noble et al., 1992).

4.4.3. Resistance of CoNS

Strains of *Staphylococcus haemolyticus* responsible for urinary tract infections have been reported as being of intermediate susceptibility to vancomycin and resistant to teicoplanin.

Ten to twenty percent of strains of methicillin-resistant and vancomycin-susceptible *Staphylococcus epidermidis* are resistant to teicoplanin. Detection of this resistance to teicoplanin in the standard antibiotic sensitivity test (agar disk method) is not very reliable, and in practice teicoplanin should only be used in a CoNS infection after the MIC has been determined precisely in a liquid medium. The mechanism of this resistance has not been elucidated.

In addition, the production of a biofilm ("slime") by certain strains of CoNS might explain certain therapeutic failures.

4.4.4. Resistance of Enterococci

Resistance to vancomycin and teicoplanin is due to synthesis of modified precursors that display decreased affinity for both compounds.

Six types of resistance have been reported to date: VanA, VanB, VanC, VanD, VanE, and VanG (Table 9).

VanF resistance was described for *Paenibacillus popilliae* (Patel et al., 2000).

The first glycopeptide-resistant strains of enterococci were isolated in France in 1988. This type of clinical isolate has been reported in France, Spain, Germany, and the United Kingdom. In a survey in 1986, less than 1% of the isolates were resistant to vancomycin. In 1996, 16% of enterococci throughout the United States had become resistant to vancomycin (Moellering, 1998). In the United States, the emergence of nosocomial *E. faecium* was characterized by increasing resistance to ampicillin in the 1980s and a more rapid increase in vancomycin resistance in the 1990s.

4.4.4.1. VanA, VanB, and VanD

4.4.4.1.1. VanA. High-level resistance to vancomycin (MIC, 1,024 μg/ml) and teicoplanin (MIC, 512 μg/ml) is usually observed in *E. faecium* and sometimes in *E. faecalis*. It was shown that vancomycin resistance arises when bacteria acquire the ability to replace D-Ala–D-Ala with D-Ala–D-Lac. This structural change results in the loss of a critical hydrogen bond between the binding pocket of vancomycin and the peptide substrate.

In *E. faecium* (strain BM 4147), the resistance genes are carried by transposon Tn*1546*. Transposon Tn*1546* encodes seven polypeptides that act cooperatively to confer high-level vancomycin resistance. Two of them, VanR and VanS, are involved in the regulation of resistance gene expression. Three of them, VanH, VanA, and VanX, confer resistance to vancomycin and teicoplanin; the other two, VanY and VanZ, are accessory proteins that are apparently not essential for expression of resistance to vancomycin and teicoplanin. VanA is homologous to bacterial ligases which are chromosally encoded. VanA catalyzes the formation of an ester bond between D-alanine and D-lactate to produce a dipeptide, D-Ala–D-Lac. VanA cooperates with VanH, a deshydrogenase which reduces pyruvate in D-lactate, the substrate of VanA. To be fully resistant, VanX, a D,D-dipeptidase, is needed, which hydrolyzes D-Ala–D-Ala but not D-Ala–D-Lac and thus prevents synthesis of precursors ending in D-alanine. VanY, a D,D-carboxypeptidase, contributes to resistance by cleaving the terminal D-Ala of late peptidoglycan precursors that escaped hydrolysis by VanX. VanZ confers low-level resistance to vancomycin and teicoplanin by an unknown mechanism.

Expression of the resistance genes of the VanA and VanB clusters is regulated by the VanRS and VanR$_B$S$_B$ two-component regulatory systems, each composed of a membrane-associated sensor-kinase (VanS and VanS$_B$) and a cytoplasmic response regulator (VanR and VanR$_B$) that acts as a transcriptional activator. The regulatory and resistance

Table 9 Vancomycin and teicoplanin resistance in enterococci

Resistance	Acquired					Intrinsic
Phenotype	VanA	VanB	VanD	VanG	VanE	VanC
MIC (μg/ml)						
Vancomycin	64–1,000	4–1,000	64–128	8–16	16	2–32
Teicoplanin	16–512	0.5–1	4–64	0.5	0.5	0.5–1
Expression	Inducible		Constitutive	Inducible		Constitutive Inducible
Location	Plasmid Chromosome		Chromosome	Chromosome		Chromosome
Genetic elements	Tn*1546*	Tn*1547* Tn*1549*				
Modified target		D-Ala–D-Lac			D-Ala–D-Ser	

genes are transcribed from distinct promoters that appear to be coordinately regulated.

The VanRS regulatory system controls transcription of the *vanRS* and *vanHXYZ* operons at the P_R and P_H promoters.

The $VanR_BS_B$ regulatory system controls transcription of the *vanR*$_B$*S*$_B$ and *vanH*$_B$*X*$_B$*Y*$_B$*W* operons at the P_{rB} and P_{YB} promoters.

VanS consists of a putative membrane-associated N-terminal sensor domain and a C-terminal cytoplasmic histidine protein kinase domain (Arthur et al., 1992). VanS was found to catalyze ATP-dependent autophosphorylation of a histidine residue. Upon addition of VanR, the phosphoryl group was transferred from the phospho histidine residue of VanS to an aspartate residue of the response regulator. The membrane-associated domains of VanS and $VanS_B$ are thought to sense the presence of vancomycin and teicoplanin in the culture medium; the mechanism is unknown.

Phospho VanS was also shown to transfer its phosphoryl group to the PhoB response regulator of the *Escherichia coli* Pho regulon.

VanR is structurally related to response regulators of the OmpR subclass and is required for transcription initiation at the P_H promoter.

Phospho VanR binds upstream from the transcription initiation site of P_H and P_R located upstream from VanR. Phosphorylation increases the affinity of VanR for both promoters.

This high-level resistance is inducible by vancomycin. It is plasmid mediated and transferable by conjugation.

4.4.4.1.2. Van B. Low-level resistance to vancomycin (MIC, 32 μg/ml) with continuing susceptibility to teicoplanin (MIC, 0.5 μg/ml) is observed in certain strains of *E. faecium* (Van B-type resistance).

Mutations responsible for constitutive expression of the VanB cluster led to amino acid substitution at two specific positions located at position 233. Constitutive expression of vancomycin or teicoplanin resistance is most probably due to impaired dephosphorylation of $VanR_B$ by $VanS_B$.

In the inducible phenotype, teicoplanin resistance is introduced by amino acid substitutions in the sensor domain of $VanS_B$.

Teicoplanin resistance is acquired in two steps: vancomycin resistance due to mutation in the D-Ala–D-Ala ligase gene and mutation in the *vanS*$_B$ gene (Arthur and Quintiliani, 2001).

4.4.4.1.3. Van D. VanD is constitutively expressed and is not transferable by conjugation to other enterococci.

It should be stressed that the first vancomycin-resistant strains of *S. aureus* have recently been reported. The emergence of resistance to teicoplanin has been observed in the treatment of *S. aureus* endocarditis by teicoplanin monotherapy.

In a surveillance study carried out in the European Union between April 2001 and January 2003 in 39 centers, 454 *E. faecium* isolates were collected; if the global prevalence of teicoplanin resistance was 10.8%, there was great variability (Table 10).

In the United States, the incidence of all nosocomial infections attributable to vancomycin-resistant enterococci increased from 0.3% in 1989 to 7.9% in 1993. In a transcontinental survey in the United States in 1997, it was shown that the prevalence of vancomycin-resistant *E. faecium* isolates varied from one center to another: 80% in Chicago, Ill., and 0% in Wilmington, Del. In all other centers in which vancomycin-resistant *E. faecalis* strains were detected, the prevalence of vancomycin resistance ranged from 21 to 80%. In another study, the prevalence of *E. faecalis* vancomycin resistance was low (0 to 4%) (ASCP, 1997). In Argentina, the prevalence of methicillin-resistant *S. aureus* (MRSA) was 14.41%, but no vancomycin-intermediate *S. aureus* strains were detected (Bantar et al., 2000). Table 11 shows the results of a 1995 epidemiological survey of teicoplanin and vancomycin resistance carried out in nine countries.

Table 10 Prevalence of *E. faecium* resistance in Europe among patients

Country(ies)	% Resistance
Scandinavian countries[a]	0
The Netherlands	0
Italy	32.8
Greece	8.3
United Kingdom/Ireland	21.4
Belgium	0
France	1.8
Germany	11.9
Portugal	15.2
Spain	3.2
Luxembourg	0

[a]Denmark, Sweden, Iceland, Norway, and Finland.

4.4.4.2. VanC, VanE, and Van G

Enterococci belonging to the species *E. gallinarum*, *E. casseliflavus*, and *E. flavescens* are intrinsically resistant to low levels of vancomycin but retain susceptibility to teicoplanin. Resistance results from the production of peptidoglycan precursors ending in D-serine.

For VanC, three *van* genes have been described: *vanC-1* (*E. gallinarum*), *van-C2* (*E. casseliflavus*), and *vanC* (*E. flavescens*).

VanC is chromosomally encoded and generally constitutively expressed, but it is inducible for some strains.

The *vanC* operon is composed of three genes, *vanT*, *vanC*, and *vanXY*$_C$. VanT encodes a membrane-bound serine racemase, and VantT produces D-serine by converting L-serine.

$VanY_CX$ has both D,D-dipeptidase and D,D-carboxypeptidase activities, resulting in hydrolysis of D-Ala–D-Ala and removal of the ultimate D-Ala from the pentapeptide. A two-component regulatory system, $VanR_C$-$VanS_C$, is also present (Leclercq and Courvalin, 1997; Arthur et al., 1996) (Table 12).

Table 11 European survey of teicoplanin and vancomycin susceptibility among gram-positive cocci[a]

Microorganism(s)	*n*	% Resistance	
		Vancomycin	Teicoplanin
S. haemolyticus	91	0	3.3
E. faecium	183	9.5	9.3
E. faecalis	1,237	0.8	0.7
Viridans group streptococci	165	0.6	0.6
Other CoNS	1,353		0.3

[a]Data from Felmingham et al., 1998.

Table 12 Distribution of *van* genes in bacterial species

Microorganism(s)	*van* gene					
	A	B	C	D	E	G
E. faecalis	+	+		+	+	+
E. faecium	+	+				
Enterococcus durans	+					
E. flavescens			+			
Enterococcus mundtii	+					
Enterococcus avium						
E. gallinarum			+			
E. casseliflavus			+			
Streptococcus gallolyticus	+	+				
Arcanobacterium	+					
Lactococci	+					
S. bovis		+				

4.4.5. Factors Affecting Teicoplanin Activity

MICs of teicoplanin depend mainly on the methods used for determination. MICs for teicoplanin have been shown to vary according to the medium used. MICs of vancomycin were always ≤4.0 µg/ml whatever the method and medium used (Table 13).

Felmingham et al. (1987) demonstrated that the presence of 10% saponin-lysed horse blood can increase the MICs of teicoplanin but not vancomycin for CoNS.

There is an inoculum effect (increase in MIC with the size of the inoculum) with teicoplanin (Table 14).

A four- to eightfold rise in MICs as the bacterial inoculum was raised from 10^3 to 10^7 CFU/ml has been reported.

The addition of serum or blood to the medium causes an increase in the MIC, particularly with teicoplanin. When 50% human serum was added to Mueller-Hinton broth, the MICs of teicoplanin for several strains of staphylococci fell by a factor of 2 to 8.

In addition, glycopeptides diffuse poorly in agar medium, and the regression line between the diameters of the zones of inhibition in agar and the MIC in a liquid medium are not good. The current recommendations of the Antibiotic Sensitivity Test Committee of the French Microbiology Society are as follows: a CoNS strain may be considered susceptible if the zone of inhibition for teicoplanin is greater than or equal to 17 mm. If the zone of inhibition is less than 17 mm, it is recommended that the MIC be determined in a broth medium.

Small variations in MICs over pH 5.5 to 8.7 were observed, with greater activity at pH 7.4.

Table 13 Effect of media on MICs of teicoplanin and vancomycin

Microorganism (no. of isolates)	Medium	$MIC_{50/90}$ (µg/ml)[a]	
		Teicoplanin	Vancomycin
S. aureus (37)	Difco Mueller-Hinton agar	4.0/4.0	2.0/2.0
	Bio-Rad Mueller-Hinton agar	8.0/8.0	4.0/4.0
	Difco Mueller-Hinton broth	2.0/4.0	1.0/2.0
S. epidermidis (34)	Difco Mueller-Hinton agar	4.0/8.0	2.0/2.0
	Bio-Rad Mueller-Hinton agar	8.0/16	2.0/4.0
	Difco Mueller-Hinton broth	4.0/8.0	2.0/2.0
S. haemolyticus (39)	Difco Mueller-Hinton agar	4.0/16	2.0/2.0
	Bio-Rad Mueller-Hinton agar	16/32	2.0/4.0
	Difco Mueller-Hinton broth	4.0/16	1.0/2.0

[a]$MIC_{50/90}$, MICs at which 50 and 90% of isolates tested are inhibited, respectively.

Table 14 MICs of teicoplanin and vancomycin according to medium and inoculum size

Microorganism (no. of isolates)	Medium	MIC (µg/ml) at indicated inoculum size (CFU/ml)			
		Teicoplanin		Vancomycin	
		10^4	10^6	10^4	10^6
S. epidermidis (18)	Iso-Sensitest agar	0.7	2.9	0.9	1.5
	Mueller-Hinton agar	1.0	2.6	1.0	1.8
	DST agar	2.1	4.5	1.4	1.9
S. haemolyticus (14)	Iso-Sensitest agar	2.6	5.4	1.0	1.2
	Mueller-Hinton agar	3.8	5.9	1.0	1.6
	DST agar	8.3	17.7	1.9	2.2

4.4.6. Combination with Other Antibacterials

The combination of a glycopeptide with an aminoglycoside is synergistic against the majority of strains of staphylococci and enterococci. Glycopeptide-aminoglycoside combination is essential to obtain bactericidal activity against enterococci. However, there is no synergy in the case of enterococci or streptococci with high-level resistance to aminoglycosides. A recent study has shown that the combination vancomycin-penicillin-gentamicin could nevertheless be effective against a strain of *E. faecium* resistant to the three molecules alone.

Combination of a glycopeptide with rifampin in vitro yields contradictory results according to the teams and the strains of *S. aureus*: synergy, neutrality, or antagonism.

Combination with fosfomycin is usually synergistic.

Combination with fusidic acid produces variable results in vitro: usually indifferent but sometimes synergistic or antagonistic.

Interestingly synergy against strains of *E. faecium* with high-level resistance to glycopeptides has been observed with combinations of glycopeptides with various penicillins: penicillin G, amoxicillin, piperacillin, and imipenem. This synergy is potentiated still further in the triple combination glycopeptide-penicillin-gentamicin.

However, the glycopeptide-penicillin synergy is only observed for glycopeptide-resistant strains of enterococci, whereas antagonism is observed between the two molecules for glycopeptide-susceptible strains.

Combinations with fluoroquinolones are usually indifferent.

In vitro, vancomycin and cefpirome are synergistic against strains of homogeneously methicillin-resistant *S. aureus*. Vancomycin and teicoplanin, combined with cefotaxime or cefpirome or even with levofloxacin, have synergistic and bactericidal activity against penicillin G-resistant strains of *S. pneumoniae*.

4.4.7. Postantibiotic Effect Pharmacodynamics

A postantibiotic effect has been demonstrated with vancomycin against *S. aureus*.

The glycopeptides behave like time-dependent antibiotics: rather than a high peak, it is the maintenance of serum or tissue concentrations above the MIC for a maximum period or permanently that appears to be important. The measurement of residual concentrations in serum before a new administration is therefore of greater interest than the determination of the peak concentration in serum in assessing the efficacy of a therapeutic regimen.

4.4.8. Intracellular Concentrations

It was shown that teicoplanin accumulates in polymorphonuclear leukocytes and vancomycin weakly. The intracellular/extracellular ratio for teicoplanin was 65 to 82% for an extracellular concentration of 5 to 20 μg/ml (Van der Auwera et al., 1988).

4.5. Pharmacokinetics of Teicoplanin

4.5.1. Modes of Administration of Teicoplanin

The oral bioavailability of teicoplanin is negligible. This route can only be used in the treatment of *C. difficile* pseudomembranous colitis at a dosage of 200 mg two to four times daily.

Teicoplanin can be used intramuscularly with satisfactory local tolerance and 90% bioavailability.

An intramuscular injection of 3 mg/kg yields a peak concentration in serum of 7.1 μg/ml after 2 h. This dosage, which is insufficient for treatment of a severe infection, must be at least double (6 mg/kg, concentration of 400 mg in 3 ml) and the interval between injections possibly reduced in order to obtain residual concentrations that are currently considered satisfactory, i.e., between 10 and 20 μg/ml. This route is useful in subjects with a depleted venous stock (infection in drug addicts) or those who are debilitated or on prolonged ambulatory treatment (chronic bone infection).

The peripheral intravenous route may be used in the form of either a slow bolus (1 to 5 min) or a short infusion (30 min). Where possible, the potential benefit of a longer infusion with respect to tissue diffusion might be considered by analogy with vancomycin, but there is insufficient information on this point.

The dosages of 3 mg/kg every 12 h and every 24 h studied initially (usually as monotherapy) have been shown to be ineffective in the treatment of severe infections, often in several studies. The dosages currently recommended in the initial treatment of severe infections are 6 mg/kg every 12 h for 1 to 5 days to obtain residual concentrations of between 10 and 20 μg/ml rapidly. Doses of 10 to 12 mg/kg have been used in specific situations (endocarditis). After steady state is attained with clinically effective residual concentrations, injections of 6 to 12 mg/kg may be administered once daily.

Due to the long $t_{1/2\beta}$, an alternate mode of administration was investigated in order to reduce the number of injections to patients for long-term treatment. At day 11 the trough levels are similar in both groups (13.5 μg/ml) (Rouveix et al., 2002).

The intraperitoneal route may be used as a method of systemic administration in patients on peritoneal dialysis. In fact, as with vancomycin, there is a preferential flow from the peritoneal dialysis fluid towards the vascular sector. The systemic bioavailability of teicoplanin by this route is about 80%. After injection of 6 mg of teicoplanin per kg with the peritoneal dialysis solution, a peak concentration in serum of 8 μg/ml is observed after 6 h and residual concentrations in serum of 2 to 3 μg/ml are observed at 24 h. The storage of peritoneal dialysis fluid is of importance, especially for a combination of ceftazidime and teicoplanin.

After subcutaneous administration of 6 mg of teicoplanin per kg, the bioavailability relative to the intravenous dose was 82% ± 5%. Absorption occurs slowly from the subcutaneous site, with a peak appearing at 8 ± 3 h. Trough concentrations in serum of teicoplanin were always >10 μg/ml in all investigated patients (Amrein et al., 1982).

4.5.2. Pharmacokinetics of Teicoplanin by Intravenous Route in Healthy Volunteers

After an intravenous administrations of 2 or 3 mg/kg to volunteers, concentrations in serum and urine were determined by agar diffusion using a multiresistant isolate of *B. subtilis* as the test organism. The limit of quantification was fixed at 0.2 μg/ml (Table 15).

Fifty-two percent of the administered dose was eliminated by urine.

The pharmacokinetics after administration of single ascending doses of teicoplanin to five healthy adults are listed in Table 16.

Teicoplanin pharmacokinetics were investigated after multiple-dose intravenous administration of 3, 6, 9, 12, and 30 mg/kg in healthy volunteers using a two-period randomized crossover design (Table 17).

Table 15 Pharmacokinetics of teicoplanin after 2 to 3 mg/kg intravenously as a single dose[a]

Dose (mg/kg)	n	C_0 (μg/ml)	AUC (μg·h/ml)	CL_P (ml/h/kg)	CL_R (ml/h/kg)	$t_{1/2}$ (h)
2	5	15.7	123.58	16.21	9.52	46.49
3	5	22.4	189.72	15.89	10.35	45.30

[a]Data from Traina et al., 1984.

Table 16 Teicoplanin pharmacokinetics after 30-mininfusion of single ascending doses[a]

Dose (mg/kg)	n	C_{max} (μg/ml)	AUC (μg·h/ml)	$t_{1/2}$ (h)	CL_P (ml/h/kg)	CL_R (ml/h/kg)	U_{0-13} (%)[b]
15	5	194.11	1,444	88.14	10.86	8.12	70.82
20	5	196.56	1,756	82.98	11.0	8.92	77.87
25	5	252.98	2,379	91.75	11.34	8.82	73.99

[a]Data from Del Favero et al., 1991.
[b]U_{0-13}, urinary elimination from 0 to 13 days.

Table 17 Teicoplanin pharmacokinetics after intravenous multiple doses

Dose (mg/kg)	n	C_{min} (μg/ml)	V_{ss} (liters/kg)	CL_P (ml/h/kg)	CL_R (ml/h/kg)	$t_{1/2\gamma}$ (h)
6	10		1.4	11.1	12.2	159
12	10		1.2	14	10.3	155
3	6	8.3	1.12	10.4	14.8	176
3	10	7.2	0.9	12.1	11.8	139
9	12	27.7		11.9	11.0	151
30	4	58.1	0.7	12.0	12.6	92.3

Five healthy volunteers received a 1-min intravenous bolus of 400 mg of teicoplanin labeled with 41 μCi of ^{14}C. The $t_{1/2\beta}$ was 77 h, the body clearance was 7.8 ml/h/kg, the concentration in serum in 5 min was 71.7 ± 3.3 μg/ml, the level at 24 h was 4.0 ± 0.4 μg/ml, and the residual concentration at 10 days was 0.4 ± 0.1 μg/ml. Teicoplanin is eliminated in urine for 80% of the administered doses in 16 days and 2.7% in feces (Buniva et al., 1988).

4.5.3. Protein Binding, Distribution, Pharmacokinetic Characteristics, and Elimination

Teicoplanin is more than 90% protein bound (albumin).

In adults with normal renal function, the concentrations in serum obtained after intravenous administration of 6 mg/kg are 53 μg/ml at the end of the infusion (0.5 h) and 4 to 10 μg/ml at 24 h. There are major interindividual variations. The mathematical models used to describe the pharmacokinetics of teicoplanin are two- or three-compartment or noncompartmental models. The $t_{1/2\beta}$ of teicoplanin is 30 to 70 h, and its apparent volume of distribution is 0.3 to 1 liter/kg. Steady state is not reached until after 5 to 10 days, justifying the use of initial loading doses (unit doses of 6 mg/kg every 12 h for 1 to 5 days). The elimination of teicoplanin is slow and almost exclusively urinary (40 to 60% of the administered dose is found in the urine in 5 days). There is tissue storage so that once steady state is reached, renal clearance represents 100% of the total clearance of teicoplanin (12 ml/h/kg). This renal elimination occurs essentially by glomerular filtration, but there are also tubular secretion-reabsorption phenomena. The areas under the curve are, respectively, 256 and 512 μg · h/ml after single doses of 3 and 6 mg/kg.

The hepatobiliary elimination of teicoplanin is negligible. Biliary concentrations do not exceed 1 μg/ml. The residual concentrations in serum targeted are 10 μg/ml or even 20 μg/ml (because of the small free fraction).

After infusion of 12 mg/kg, the concentration in plasma is on the order of 112 μg/ml, declining to 15 to 20 μg/ml at 12 h and 10 μg/ml at 24 h. Twenty-four hours after doses of 15 and 25 mg/kg, the residual concentrations are, respectively, 19.8 and 10.5 μg/ml, and at 48 h they are 10 and 6 μg/ml.

4.5.4. Metabolism

In urine collected over 0 to 24 h after [^{14}C]teicoplanin administration in rats, more than 3 to 5% of the administered dose was found to be metabolized.

In humans, teicoplanin components seems to be metabolized in A3-1 by detachment of *N*-acylglucosamine.

Two metabolites representing 1 to 2% of total teicoplanin were isolated after intravenous administration of [^{14}C]teicoplanin. They are two teicoplanin-like compounds, bearing an 8-hydroxy decanoic (metabolite 1) or 9-hydroxy decanoic (metabolite 2) acyl moiety. The metabolic transformation is likely due to hydroxylation in the Ω2 and Ω1 positions for metabolites 1 and 2, respectively, of the C-10 linear side chain of component A2-3.

4.5.5. Pharmacokinetics in Specific Populations

4.5.5.1. Pediatric Patients

In neonates and children, the $t_{1/2\beta}$ of teicoplanin is reduced (from 20 to 30 h) and the recommended unit dosage is 10 mg/kg (Table 18).

A low renal clearance in some children may be due to incomplete urine completion.

Table 18 Pharmacokinetics of teicoplanin in neonates and children

Parameter	Value in:		
	Neonates ($n = 4$)	Adults	Children ($n = 6$)[a]
V_c (liters/kg)	0.30	0.09	0.13
V_{ss} (liters/kg)	0.77	0.76	0.90
CL_P (liters/h/kg)	0.0158	0.098	0.028
$t_{1/2}$ (h)	40	77	20.5
CL_R (liters/h/kg)			0.045

[a]Four to twelve years old.

Table 19 shows the Pharmacokinetics after repeated doses in 12 children (2.4 to 11 years old) of 6 mg/kg given intravenously over a 30-min infusion once daily for 5 consecutive days.

Twenty-one critically ill children (7 days to 12 years old) were treated with teicoplanin after three loading doses of 10 mg/kg at 12-h intervals followed by a maintenance dose of 10 mg/kg; the Pharmacokinetics are shown in Table 20.

4.5.5.2. Elderly Patients

The pharmacokinetics of teicoplanin were investigated in 10 elderly patients suffering from mild renal impairment (CL_{CR} of 51.3 ml/min) after an intravenous bolus (3 to 5 min) of 6 mg/kg. Teicoplanin was assayed by a microbiological method (Table 21) (Rosina et al., 1988).

In elderly patients, the $t_{1/2\beta}$ is prolonged (114 h), probably due in part to impairment of renal function and also the different tissue distribution (more extensive adipose tissue in elderly subjects).

The decrease with age in body clearance and increase of half-life with age are predictable: approximately 1% annual decrease in glomerular filtration rate in adults beyond 25 years.

The loading dose remains the same, but the maintenance dose varies according to age. After the ages of 65 and 95 years, 60 and 30% of the adult dose, respectively, have to be administered.

Table 19 Teicoplanin pharmacokinetics after multiple doses in children

Parameter	Value	
	Day 1	Day 5
C_0 (μg/ml)	39.3 ± 7.6	40.8 ± 7.4
C_{24} (μg/ml)	1.8 ± 0.6	3.1 ± 1.2
$t_{1/2\gamma}$ (h)	11.3	16.1
CL_P (ml/min/kg)	39.7	36.5
CL_R (ml/min/kg)	18.2	
U_{0-24} (%)[a]	48.6	

[a]U_{0-24}, urinary elimination from 0 to 24 h.

Table 20 Teicoplanin pharmacokinetics in children after a loading dose of 10mg/kg

Parameter	Value
C_{max} (μg/ml)	26.2
C_{min} (μg/ml)	5.8
$t_{1/2\beta}$ (h)	17.41
AUC (μg·h/ml)	224.5
CL_P (liters/kg/h)	45

Table 21 Teicoplanin pharmacokinetics in the elderly

Parameter	Value
C_0 (μg/ml)	71.76 ± 7.05
AUC (μg·h/ml)	606.86 ± 37.15
$t_{1/2}$ (h)	114.32 ± 8.62
CL_P (ml/h/kg)	10.21 ± 0.62
CL_R (ml/h/kg)	3.84 ± 0.36
Urinary elimination (%) (0–8 h)	28.38 ± 0.36

4.5.5.3. Renally Impaired Patients

In patients with stable chronic renal insufficiency, there is a close correlation between CL_{CR} and renal clearance of teicoplanin, and the $t_{1/2\beta}$ is increased to 111 h in patients with severe renal insufficiency (CL_{CR}, ≈ 10 ml/min). However, in intensive care patients with various degrees of acute renal insufficiency suffering from severe infections and/or hemodynamic disorders, the correlation is less good, and major interindividual variations are observed in teicoplanin clearance for equivalent CL_{CR}s, so, a regular assay of the residual concentrations is essential to adapt the unit dosage and/or the interval between two doses (Table 22).

Table 22 Pharmacokinetics of teicoplanin in renally impaired patients[a]

Group (CL_{CR})	AUC (μg·h/ml)	CL_R (ml/mn)	CL_P (ml/mn)	$t_{1/2\gamma}$ (h)
I (>80 ml/min)	193 ± 25	11.8 ± 1.3	18.1 ± 3.4	41
II (30–80 ml/min)	325 ± 51	2.5 ± 1.6	10.3 ± 2.1	77
III (10–29 ml/min)	388 ± 83	1.1 ± 0.2	10.2 ± 2.3	102
IV (3–9 ml/min)	509 ± 96	0.4 ± 0.05	6.3 ± 1.8	125
V (<2 ml/min), CAPD	609 ± 130		5.6 ± 2.0	149
VI (<2 ml/min), hemodialysis				163

[a]Data from Bonati et al., 1987.

In practice, the initial treatment procedures (loading doses of 6 to 12 mg/kg every 12 h for 2 to 4 days) may be identical in patients with renal insufficiency and subjects with normal renal function. The subsequent doses of 6 to 12 mg/kg should be administered every 24 to 72 h or longer in order to maintain residual concentrations in serum of between 10 and 20 μg/ml, depending on the severity of the infection and the clinical response.

Teicoplanin is practically undialyzable by hemodialysis. Flow in the vascular sector-peritoneal fluid direction is very weak. Conversely, a marked flow from the peritoneal dialysis fluid to the vascular sector is observed with vancomycin so that, in addition to local treatment of an infection of the dialysis fluid with a susceptible bacterium, this might allow systemic treatment, based constantly on serum assays. The dosage and rate of administration to be used are not defined, but a dosage of 6 mg/kg once daily is certainly too low (residual concentration in serum, less than 5 μg/ml at 24 h).

In 1976, Popovich et al. described the technique of CAPD for the treatment of end-stage renal disease (Oreopoulos et al., 1979). Many investigations with teicoplanin in CAPD patients have been undertaken.

Teicoplanin may be added to CAPD fluid. The half-life of absorption from the peritoneal cavity is approximately 2 h, producing a peak concentration in serum of 2.8 to 5.5 μg/ml after an intraperitoneal dose of teicoplanin of 3 mg/kg, with approximately 77% of the dose absorbed during a dwell time of 5 h (Brouard et al., 1989).

Five patients with end-stage renal disease maintained on CAPD received 22 mg of lyophilized teicoplanin. Teicoplanin was recovered in the peritoneal fluid for 6.8% ± 1.2% of the administered dose. The body clearance was 4.6 to 7.38 ml/h/kg, for a peritoneal clearance of 0.31 to 0.37 ml/h/kg (Traina et al., 1986).

A single 3-mg/kg dose was given intraperitoneally in dialysate during a 6-h dwell time. Teicoplanin was detected in plasma within 15 min at 0.70 ± 0.45 μg/ml in all five patients, and peak concentrations in serum ranged from 5.53 to 2.80 μg/ml (4.84 ± 1.43 μg/ml) at 6 h.

The rate constant for peritoneal transfer averaged $0.38\ h^{-1}$, and the half-life of the rate constant was 2.18 h (Bonati et al., 1988).

4.5.5.3.1. Components of teicoplanin. Falcoz et al. (1987), using an HPLC method, monitored the six main components of teicoplanin over 120 h after administration of a dose of 3 mg of teicoplanin per kg to healthy volunteers and to noninfected patients with various degrees of renal dysfunction. All components of teicoplanin were equally affected by renal impairment. The renal clearance decreased 10-fold. All components are eliminated by glomerular filtration (Table 23).

4.5.6. Diffusion in Biological Fluids and Tissues

Like vancomycin, teicoplanin is handicapped by its high molecular weight. In addition, it is highly bound to serum proteins. Conversely, its lipophilicity is a theoretical advantage. After an injection of radioactive teicoplanin in the rat, the highest concentrations are found in the kidneys, lungs, liver, tracheal mucosa, and adrenal glands. The concentrations in the eyes, brain, muscles, soft tissues, adipose tissue, bile, and bone are low. Likewise, the autoradiographic study of labeled teicoplanin in an experimental endocarditis model shows poor diffusion in the vegetations.

In humans, the concentration in the exudate fluid reaches 50 to 75% of levels in serum. Levels equivalent to those in serum or higher may be reached in the kidneys, liver, myocardium, mucosae, and tonsils. The diffusion is satisfactory in spongy bone (bone marrow) but poor in cortical bone. It is poor in the CSF, but there are no data on different modes of administration (continuous infusion) that might be advantageous. In contrast to vancomycin, teicoplanin is concentrated in phagocytic cells.

4.6. Adverse Effects and Toxicity

A few cases of red man syndrome have also been reported with teicoplanin, some of them occurring in patients already exhibiting intolerance to vancomycin. Other observations, however, reflect good tolerance of teicoplanin in subjects suffering from red man syndrome with vancomycin. These might be reactions related to the methods of administration rather than a vancomycin-teicoplanin cross-reaction.

The nephrotoxicity of teicoplanin is minor, and studies comparing the combinations vancomycin-aminoglycoside and teicoplanin-aminoglycoside favor the latter combination. The ototoxicity of teicoplanin has the same characteristics as that of vancomycin but appears to be less commonly observed.

Hypersensitivity reactions may be observed: rash, fever, bronchospasm, and hypereosinophilia. The existence of cross-resistance with vancomycin is disputed.

Local venous tolerance is better than that of vancomycin, with 1 to 3% of patients suffering chemical thrombophlebitis or pain or local induration on intramuscular injection.

Reversible neutropenia and thrombocytopenia have been reported, together with a transient elevation of transaminases.

In general, the tolerance of teicoplanin appears to be better than that of vancomycin, but with two reservations: first, the still relatively short track record of teicoplanin and, second, the fact that the current tendency for higher dosages

Table 23 Disposition pharmacokinetics of components of teicoplanin in healthy volunteers after a 5-mg/kg dose[a]

Parameter	Value for component					Value for complex
	A2-1	A2-2	A2-3	A2-4	A2-5	
% of complex	4.4	37.5	12.5	11.7	10.7	100
$t_{1/2}$ (h)	48	54	49	58	67	54
CL_P (liters/h/kg)	0.0193	0.0148	0.011	0.0088	0.0054	0.0121
CL_R (liters/h/kg)	0.0161	0.0112	0.0064	0.0046	0.0028	0.0084

[a]Data from Bernareggi et al., 1990.

(6 to 12 mg/kg once or twice daily) than those initially studied should encourage vigilance with respect to the occurrence of these adverse effects.

5. ORITAVANCIN

5.1. Structure

Oritavancin is a semisynthetic derivative of a natural compound, A-82846 (LY-264826). The parent compound has the same peptide backbone as vancomycin but differs in that 4-epivancosamine replaces the vancosamine sugar and an additional epivancosamine is present on the molecule. A side chain is attached by reductive alkylation to the amine group of the epivancosamine that is linked to the glucose (Nicas et al., 1997) (Fig. 4).

The rationale for adding alkyl and aryl-linked groups to vancomycin at an analogous site was to lengthen the $t_{1/2/\beta}$s. After chemical alterations of LY-264826, the best analog had an *N-p*-chlorobenzyl side chain on the disaccharide amino sugar of LY-264826.

Further modifications of the alkyl group, including biphenyl and chlorobiphenyl side chains, led to the discovery of oritavancin (Fig. 5). Oritavancin ($C_{86}H_{97}Cl_3N_{10}O_{26}$) has a molecular weight of 1,793.12.

5.2. Antibacterial Activity

The antibacterial activity of oritavancin is summarized in Table 24.

Gene clusters related to the *vanA* confer high-level resistance to vancomycin and teicoplanin. In contrast, enterococci harboring the *vanB* gene remain susceptible to teicoplanin because the *vanS*$_B$ sensor kinase does not trigger induction of the resistance gene in response to this antibiotic.

In one study, it was shown that enterococci may acquire moderate-level resistance to oritavancin (MIC, ≥16 μg/ml) in a single step by various mechanisms.

Oritavancin accumulates in macrophages (J774 cell line), especially in vacuoles. The accumulation ratio was 150 to 250% over 24 h. Oritavancin efflux is slow: 30% release in 6 h. In THP-1 (myelomonoblastic line), accumulation was 50 times over 5 h. Bacteriostatic activity was demonstrated against *L. monocytogenes*.

It seems that oritavancin acts on lipid II formation and especially on transglycosylation in peptidoglycan biosynthesis.

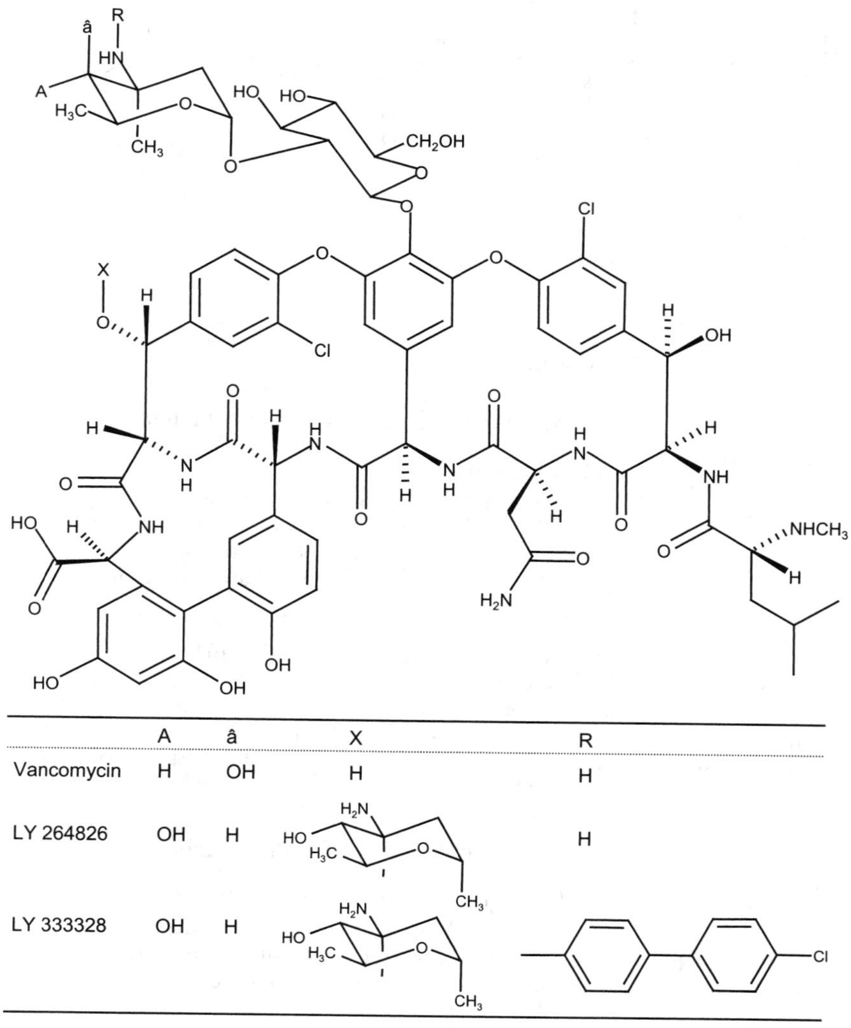

	A	â	X	R
Vancomycin	H	OH	H	H
LY 264826	OH	H		H
LY 333328	OH	H		

Figure 4 LY-264826

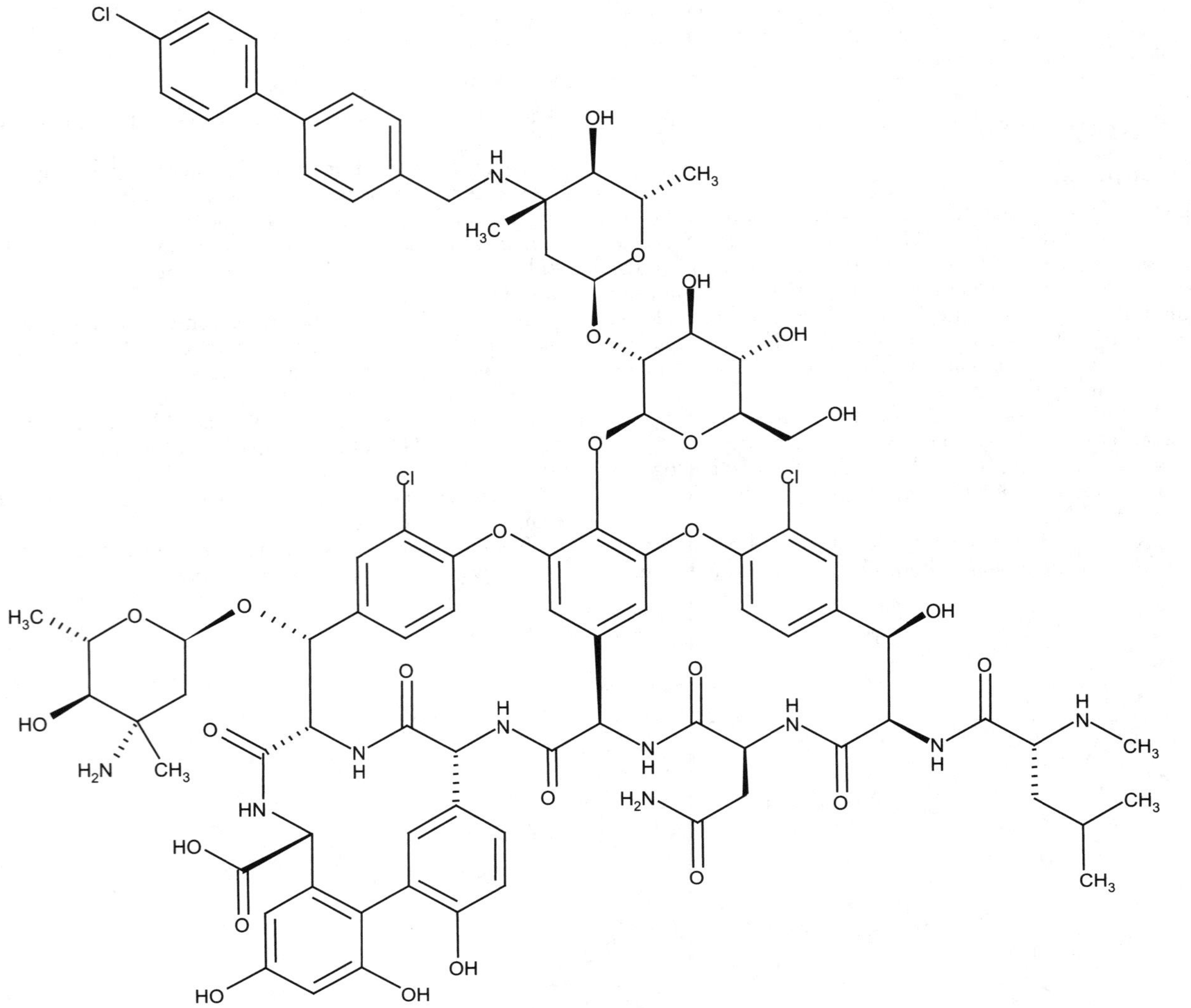

Figure 5 Oritavancin

5.3. Pharmacokinetics of Oritavancin

A pharmacokinetic study of oritavancin after intravenous administration of ascending doses was carried out on volunteers, after infusions for 0.5 h (1.5 to 3.0 mg/kg), 1.0 h (6 mg/kg), and 1.5 h (9 mg/kg). The $t_{1/2\beta}$s ranged from 8 to 10 days (Table 25).

The levels of human protein binding of [^{14}C]oritavancin at 1.0, 10, and 91 μg/ml were determined to be 85.7% ± 0.7%, 88.8% ± 0.4%, and 89.9% ± 0.4%, respectively.

6. DALBAVANCIN

Dalbavancin (BI 397, MDL-62476) is a semisynthetic derivative of a teicoplanin-like naturally occurring compound (A-409269).

6.1. Structure

Dalbavancin has an acyl chain attached to the amino sugar. This side chain is longer than that of teicoplanin and seems to be responsible for the long $t_{1/2\beta}$.

The polyamine substituent is in part responsible for its activity against gram-positive bacteria (aerobes and anaerobes) (Fig. 6).

6.2. Antibacterial Activity of Dalbavancin

6.2.1. In Vitro Activity

The in vitro activity of dalbavancin was investigated by following NCCLS-recommended methods and comparatively with vancomycin, linezolid, and quinuprisitin-dalfoprisitin (Q-D) (Table 26) (Jones et al., 2001; Goldstein and Citron, 2002).

6.2.2. Factors Influencing In Vitro Activity

MICs are not affected by various pHs (pH 6.0, 7.2, and 8.0). MICs increased significantly, from 0.12 μg/ml in brain-heart infusion or Brucella blood agar to 2.0 μg/ml in chocolate Mueller-Hinton agar. The inoculum size does not alter MICs (10^2 to 10^5 CFU/spot), nor does the atmosphere of incubation (ambient air, 5 to 6% CO_2, or anaerobic).

6.3. Pharmacokinetics of Dalbavancin

6.3.1. Single Dose in Healthy Volunteers

Dalbavancin pharmacokinetics were investigated in 55 healthy volunteers after single intravenous and ascending doses of 140, 500, and 1,120 mg; results are shown in Table 27.

Table 24 In vitro activities of oritavancin[a]

Microorganism(s)[b]	*n*	MIC (μg/ml)[c]					
		Oritavancin		Vancomycin		Teicoplanin	
		50%	90%	50%	90%	50%	90%
MSSA	172	2.0	2.0	1.0	1.0	0.5	1.0
MRSA	128	2.0	2.0	1.0	1.0	0.5	1.0
MSSE	13	2.0	4.0	1.0	2.0	2.0	8.0
MRSE	19	2.0	4.0	1.0	2.0	4.0	8.0
S. pneumoniae Pen[s]	209	≤0.015	≤0.015	0.5	0.5		
S. pneumoniae Pen[i]	40	≤0.015	≤0.015	0.5	0.5		
S. pneumoniae Pen[r]	53	≤0.015	≤0.015	0.5	0.5		
S. haemolyticus OXA[s]	11	2.0	4.0	1.0	2.0	2.0	8.0
S. haemolyticus OXA[r]	10	2.0	4.0	2.0	2.0	4.0	4.0
S. pyogenes	23	0.125	0.25	0.25	0.25	≤0.03	0.06
Listeria spp.	22	≤0.03	0.06	0.5	1.0	0.125	0.25
C. jeikeium	12	0.06	0.125	0.25	0.25	0.25	0.25
C. difficile	24	0.25	1.0	0.5	1.0	0.125	0.25
Lactobacillus spp.	12	16	32	>256	>256	>256	>256
Leuconostoc spp.	5	1-8	–	>256	–	>256	–
Pediococcus spp.	3	2-8	–	>256	–	>256	–
E. rhusiopathiae	11	2.0	4.0	64	64	2.0	8.0
E. faecalis vanA	4	2.0	–	512	–	64	–
E. faecalis vanB	1	0.6	–	32	–	2.0	–
E. faecium vanA	13	0.12	0.25	256	512	32	64
E. faecium vanB	14	0.06	0.12	16	32	0.25	2.0
E. durans	7	0.06	–	512	–	64	–
Peptostreptococcus spp.	48	0.03	0.5	0.25	2.0	0.06	0.5
Propionibacterium acnes	31	0.03	0.03	0.25	0.5	0.25	4.0
C. perfringens	49	0.25	1.0	0.25	4.0	0.25	–

[a]Data from Sillerström et al., 1999; Fraise et al., 1997; and Biavasco et al., 1997.
[b]MSSE, methicillin-susceptible *S. epidermidis*; MRSE, methicillin-resistant *S. epidermidis*; OXA, oxacillin.
[c]50% and 90%, MICs at which 50 and 90% of isolates tested are inhibited, respectively.

Table 25 Pharmacokinetics of oritavancin after ascending doses (intravenous route)[a]

Dose (mg/kg)	*n*	CL_P (liters/h)	V_c (liters)	AUC_{24} (μg·h/ml)	$t_{1/2\beta}$ (h)
1.5	4	0.55	7.3	71.8	192
2.0	5	0.49	7.5	143	209
3.0	4	0.43	7.8	211	223
3.0	4	0.57	9.5	175	182
3.0	4	0.40	8.6	186	233
6.0	4	0.44	8.1	375	220
9.0	4	0.54	8.3	465	186

[a]Data from Braun et al., 2001.

In another study, the pharmacokinetics of dalbavancin were assessed in an open-label, noncomparative study in six healthy volunteers after a single dose of 1,000 mg intravenously. Dalbavancin was assayed using a validated liquid chromatography-mass spectrometry method. Results are shown in Table 28.

Dalbavancin has a long $t_{1/2\beta}$, 9 to 12 days, and is eliminated by both renal and nonrenal routes. The plasma clearance was about 0.042 ± 0.0074 liter/h. The estimated fraction of dalbavancin eliminated unchanged into urine was 40% of the administered dose, and renal clearance was estimated as 0.018 liter/h.

6.3.2. Multiple Doses in Healthy Volunteers

A loading dose was administered as two equal doses given 12 h apart, followed by a maintenance dose for 6 days. Pharmacokinetics are shown in Table 29. After infusion of 300 and 30 mg, steady state was reached at about 48 h (day 3) following the loading dose.

No unexpected accumulation occurred throughout the multiple-dose regimen. On day 7, serum samples from volunteers receiving a single dose of 630 mg showed bactericidal activity at 4 to 16 times the MIC.

6.3.3. Hepatically Impaired Patients

The pharmacokinetics of dalbavancin were assessed in hepatically impaired patients after an intravenous loading dose of 1,000 mg on day 1 followed by 500 mg on day 8. Patients suffered from mild to moderate hepatic impairment (Child-Pugh class A and class B). The study included five or six patients with each of the above-mentioned

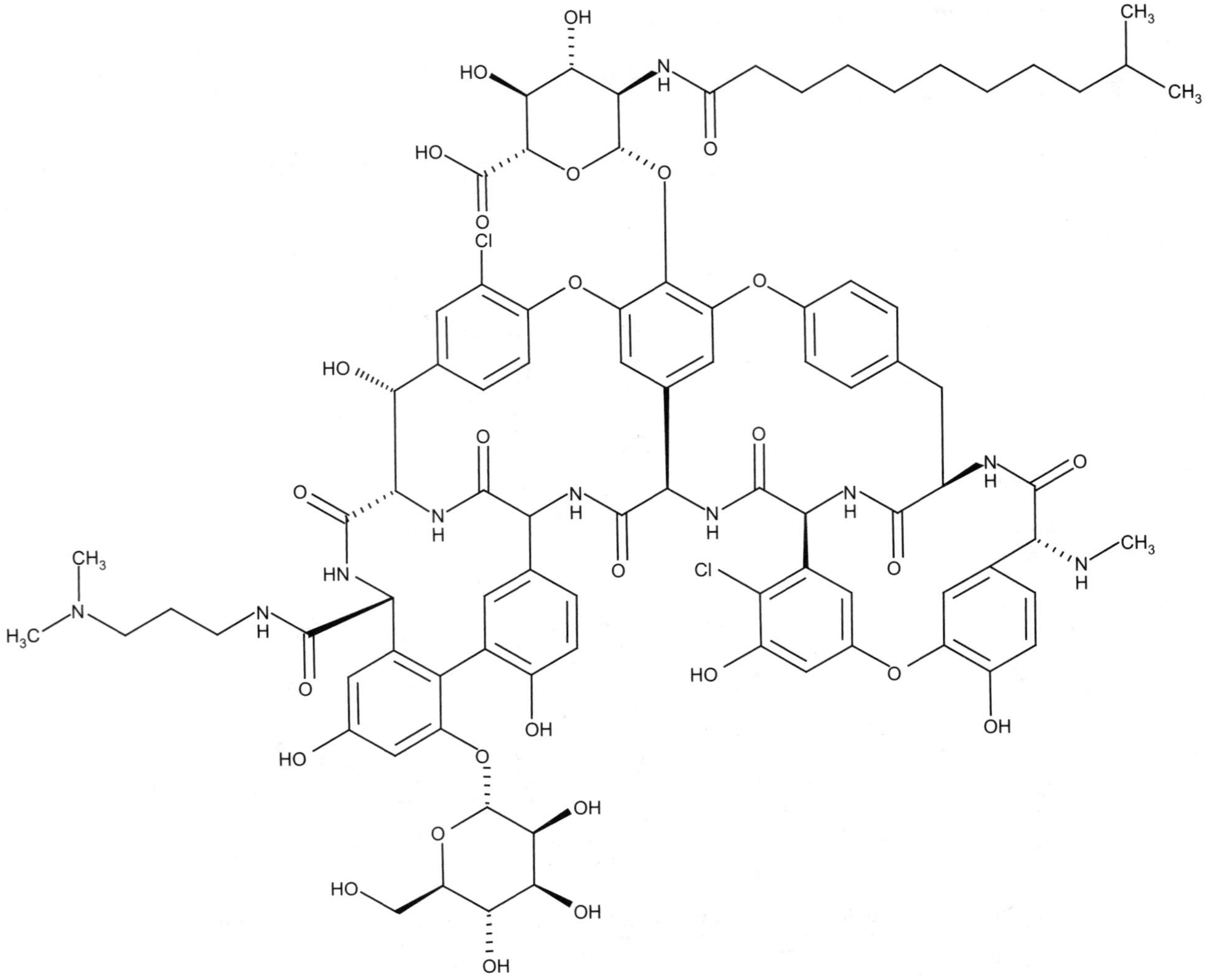

Figure 6 Dalbavancin

Child-Pugh scores; pharmacokinetics are shown in Table 30.

6.3.4. Protein Binding

Dalbavancin is practically insoluble at physiological pH. The protein binding levels are summarized in Table 31.

7. AC 98-6646

7.1. AC-98

AC-98 is a complex of antibacterial agents which was obtained from the fermentation broth of *Streptomyces hygroscopicus* in 1958. The nature of the complex was elucidated, and the complex was found to contain five naturally occurring esterified derivatives designated AC-1 to AC-5 (Fig. 7). The in vitro activities of the different components were evaluated (Petersen et al., 2002a, 2002b, 2002c); results are shown in Table 32.

The complex belongs to the mannopeptimycin group, which contains a cyclic hexapeptide core composed of alternating L- and D-amino acids that include a β-methylphenylalanine and two epimeric residues of unknown amino acids containing a cyclic guanidine moiety. One of the residues is N glycosylated with mannopyranose, while the D-tyrosine residue is D-glycosylated with a 1,4α-linked mannose disaccharides.

In mannopeptimycin α, a mannose disaccharide unit is attached to the tyrosine phenolic group; in mannopeptimycins γ, δ, and ϵ, an isovaleryl group is attached to the terminal mannose at various positions.

Mannopeptimycin α is bactericidal and inhibits cell wall synthesis, probably via inhibition of lipid II and peptidoglycan production.

Mannopeptimycins γ, δ, and ε are more active than mannopeptimycin α, indicating that substitution at the terminal mannose could enhance the antibacterial activity.

7.2. Structure of AC 98-6646

AC 98-6646 is a semisynthetic derivative from mannopeptimycin α, with an adamantly ketal side chain (Fig. 8) and a cyclohexyl alanine instead of β-methylphenyl alanine (Dushin et al., 2002).

Table 26 In vitro activity of dalbavancin

Microorganism(s)	n	MIC (μg/ml)[a]							
		Dalbavancin		Vancomycin		Linezolid		Q-D	
		50%	90%	50%	90%	50%	90%	50%	90%
MSSA	1,815	0.06	0.06						
MRSA	1,177	0.06	0.06						
E. faecalis Van[s]	586	0.03	0.06						
E. faecalis Van[r]	20	4.0	32						
E. faecium Van[s]	77	0.06	0.12						
E. faecium Van[r]	51	8.0	0.03						
S. pneumoniae Pen[s]	1,396	≤0.015	0.03						
S. pneumoniae Pen[r]	400	≤0.015	0.03						
Viridans group streptococci, Pen[s]	104	≤0.015	0.03						
Viridans group streptococci, Pen[r]	30	≤0.015	0.03						
Beta-hemolytic streptococci	234	≤0.015	0.03						
Actinomyces israelii	11	0.25	0.25	0.5	1.0	0.5	16	0.12	0.25
Actinomyces spp.	38	0.25	0.5	4.0	16	0.5	1.0	0.12	0.25
Clostridium clostridioforme	19	4.0	8.0	0.5	1.0	4.0	8.0	0.5	8.0
C. difficile	26	0.25	0.25	1.0	2.0	2.0	8.0	0.5	4.0
Clostridium innocuum	15	0.25	0.25	16	16	2.0	4.0	0.5	1.0
C. perfringens	10	0.06	0.12	0.5	0.5	2.0	2.0	0.5	0.5
Clostridium ramosum	15	1.0	1.0	4.0	4.0	8.0	8.0	0.5	4.0
Eubacterium	25	0.25	1.0	0.5	2.0	2.0	4.0	2.0	4.0
Lactobacillus spp.	23	0.5	>32	0.5	2.0	4.0	8.0	0.5	2.0
Propionibacterium spp.	15	0.25	0.5	1.0	>32	0.5	1.0	0.06	0.25
Peptostreptococcus spp.	30	0.12	0.25	0.5	1.0	0.5	1.0	0.25	0.5
Corynebacterium spp.	20	0.25	0.5	0.5	1.0	0.5	1.0	0.25	1.0
Corynebacterium amycolatum	14	0.25	0.5	0.25	0.5	0.5	2.0	0.25	0.5
C. jeikeium	12	0.5	0.5	0.5	0.5	0.5	0.5	0.25	0.5
Bacillus spp.	12	0.12	0.25						
Haemophilus influenzae	97	32	64						

[a]50% and 90%, MICs at which 50 and 90% of isolates tested are inhibited, respectively.

Table 27 Pharmacokinetics of dalbavancin after a single intravenous dose

Dose (mg)	C_{max} (μg/ml)	T_{max} (h)	AUC (μg·h/ml)	$t_{1/2}$ (h)	CL_P (liters/h)
140	39.7	0.667	3,251	189	0.043
500	153	0.5	12,451	159	0.0408
1,120	325	0.5	25,790	149	0.0437

Table 28 Pharmacokinetics of dalbavancin after a single intravenous dose of 1,000mg[a]

Parameter	Value
C_0 (μg/ml)	301 ± 65
$t_{1/2}$ (h)	257 ± 21
AUC (μg · h/ml)	23,843 ± 4,526
CL_P (liters/h)	0.0431 ± 0.0074
CL_R (liters/h)	0.0181 ± 0.0036
Urinary elimination (%)	41.9 ± 2.7

[a]Data from Dowell et al., 2002.

7.3. In Vitro Activity of AC 98-6646

The antibacterial activity of AC 98-6646 is reported in Table 33.

7.4. In Vivo Activity of AC 98-6646

Female CD-1 mice (Charles River, 20 to 22 g) were challenged with either *S. aureus*, *S. pneumoniae*, or *E. faecalis* by the intraperitoneal route and were treated 30 min postinfection with a single intravenous dose (0.2 ml/mouse) of vancomycin or AC 98-6646; results are shown in Table 34.

AC 98-6646 exhibits bactericidal activity in an *E. faecalis* endocarditis model in the rat, with a reduction from control of 3.84 $\log_{10}$ CFU/ml after a dosage of 10 mg/kg/day (Vans) or 5.92 $\log_{10}$ CFU/ml for a Van[r] strain.

7.5. Animal Pharmacokinetics

The pharmacokinetics of AC 98-6646 were assessed in different animals after administration by the intravenous route at different doses; results are shown in Table 35 (Murphy et al., 2002).

Table 29 Pharmacokinetics of dalbavancin after intravenous multiple doses[a]

Day	Repeated dose/dose (mg)	C_{max} (μg/ml)	C_{min} (μg/ml)	CL_P (liters/h)	$t_{1/2}$ (h)
1	300/30	57.3	14.4		
7	300/30	29.6	22.7	0.0508	191
1	600/60	115	30.2		
7	600/60	63.7	47.1	0.0493	98
1	1,000/100				
7	1,000/100	98.9	77.7	0.0508	89

[a]Data from Leighton et al., 2001.

Table 30 Pharmacokinetics of dalbavancin in hepatically impaired patients

Day	Hepatic function	Dose (mg)	*n*	C_{max} (μg/ml)	AUC (μg·h/ml)
1	Normal	1,000	2	252	10,420
	Class A	1,000	6	253	10,639
	Class B	1,000	5	220	8,005
8	Normal	500	2	159	10,242
	Class A	500	6	169	9,612
	Class B	500	5	130	7,391

[a]Data from Dowell et al., 2002.

Table 31 Protein binding of dalbavancin and teicoplanin

Protein and antibiotic concn (μg/ml)	Protein binding (%)	
	Dalbavancin	Teicoplanin
Human albumin		
1	98.8	98.3
100	98.8	98.3
165	98.7	98.0
200	98.5	ND[a]
500	98.0	ND
α_1-Glycoprotein		
1	73.0	9.6
10	68.2	9.1
100	26.2	6.0
165	16.9	ND
250	11.4	ND
500	5.9	ND

[a]ND, not determined.

8. TELEVANCIN

Televancin is a semisynthetic lipoglycopeptide obtained by replacement of the amino group of vancosamine by a fatty acid side chain. It is more active than vancomycin but less active than oritavancin. Televancin is more active against *S. aureus* but less active against *S. pneumoniae* and *Enteroccocus* spp. than dalbavancin. Against GISA HIP 5836 strains, televancin (MIC, 2 μg/ml) is more active than vancomycin and teicoplanin (MICs, 8 μg/ml).

Televancin is bactericidal against *S. aureus*. For a concentration of 4 μg/ml, the initial inoculum was reduced by about 4 $\log_{10}$ CFU/ml for methicillin-susceptible *S. aureus* (MSSA) after 4 h of contact. For MRSA, after 4 h of contact with concentrations of 8 and 32 μg/ml, the initial inoculum was reduced by 2 and 5 $\log_{10}$ CFU/ml, respectively. For GISA strains, the contact concentrations were 8 and 32 μg/ml to obtain a reduction of the inoculum size above 3 $\log_{10}$ CFU/ml after 4 h of contact.

Televancin inhibits both fatty acid and phospholipid biosynthesis. Televancin does not inhibit transglycolase activity.

Televancin is active in disseminated staphylococcal infections irrespective of the resistance phenotype and the mouse immune system status.

In human volunteers after a 5-mg/kg dose intravenously, maximum and minimum concentrations in plasma of 45 and 5 μg/ml were assayed, respectively. The $t_{1/2\beta}$ is about 7 h.

Televancin and comparators were tested against *Bacillus anthracis*; results are shown in Table 36 (Kaniga et al., 2004).

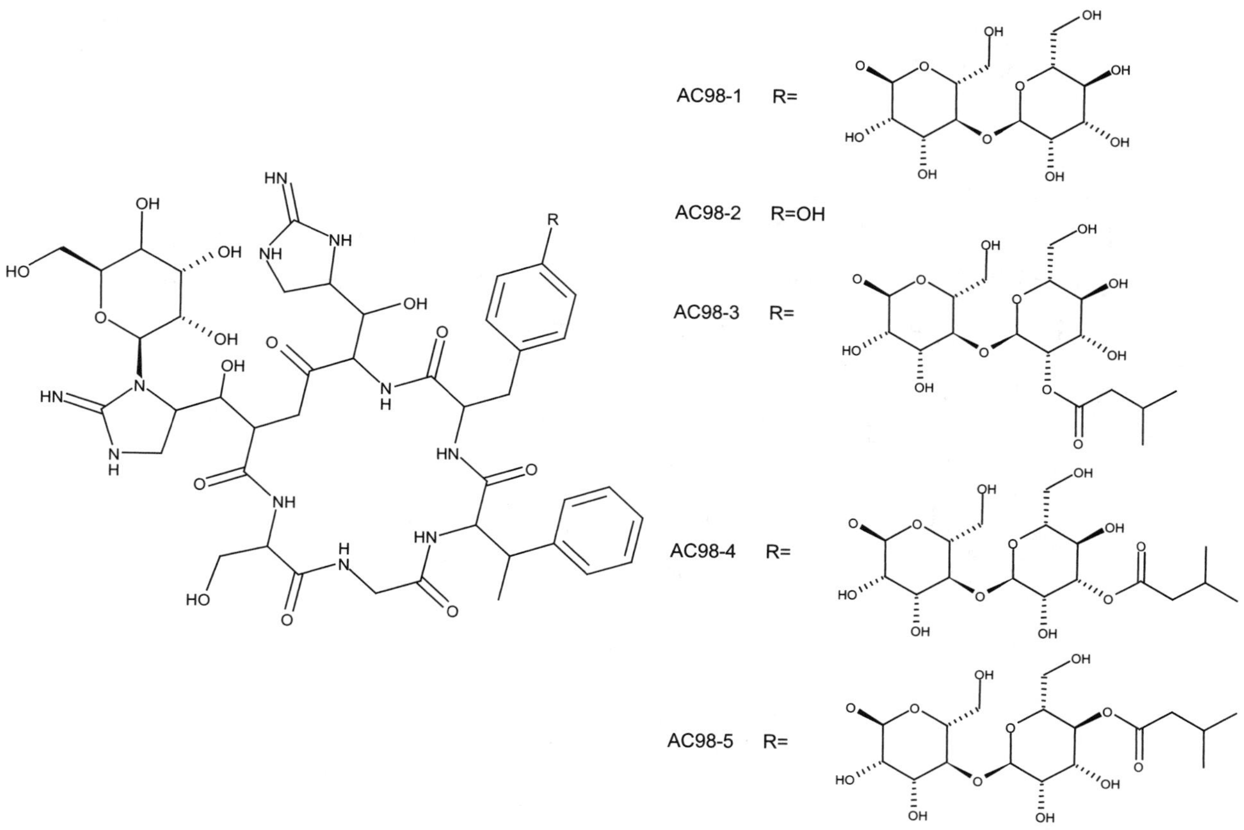

Figure 7 AC-98 complex

Table 32 In vitro activity of AC-98 complex

Microorganism(s)	*n*	MIC (μg/ml)						
		AC-1	AC-2	AC-3	AC-4	AC-5	Complex	Vancomycin
MSSA	3	>128	128	8	8	4	16	0.5–1
MRSA	4	128	64	8	4–8	4	8–16	0.5–1
CoNS Met^s	4	128	64	8	8	4–8	8–16	0.5–1
CoNS Met^r	3	64–>128	32–128	4–8	2–8	2–4	4–16	0.5–1
E. faecalis	5	>128	128	64–128	32–64	16–32	64	0.5–128
E. faecium	3	>128	128	64	8–64	8–64	16–64	0.5–128
Streptococcus spp.	8	>32	64	8	8	4–8	4–8	0.25–0.5
S. agalactiae	10			16	8			0.5
S. pyogenes	10			16	8			0.5
S. pneumoniae Pen^s	10			8	4			0.5
S. pneumoniae Pen^i	10			4	4			0.5
S. pneumoniae Pen^s	10			4	4			0.5

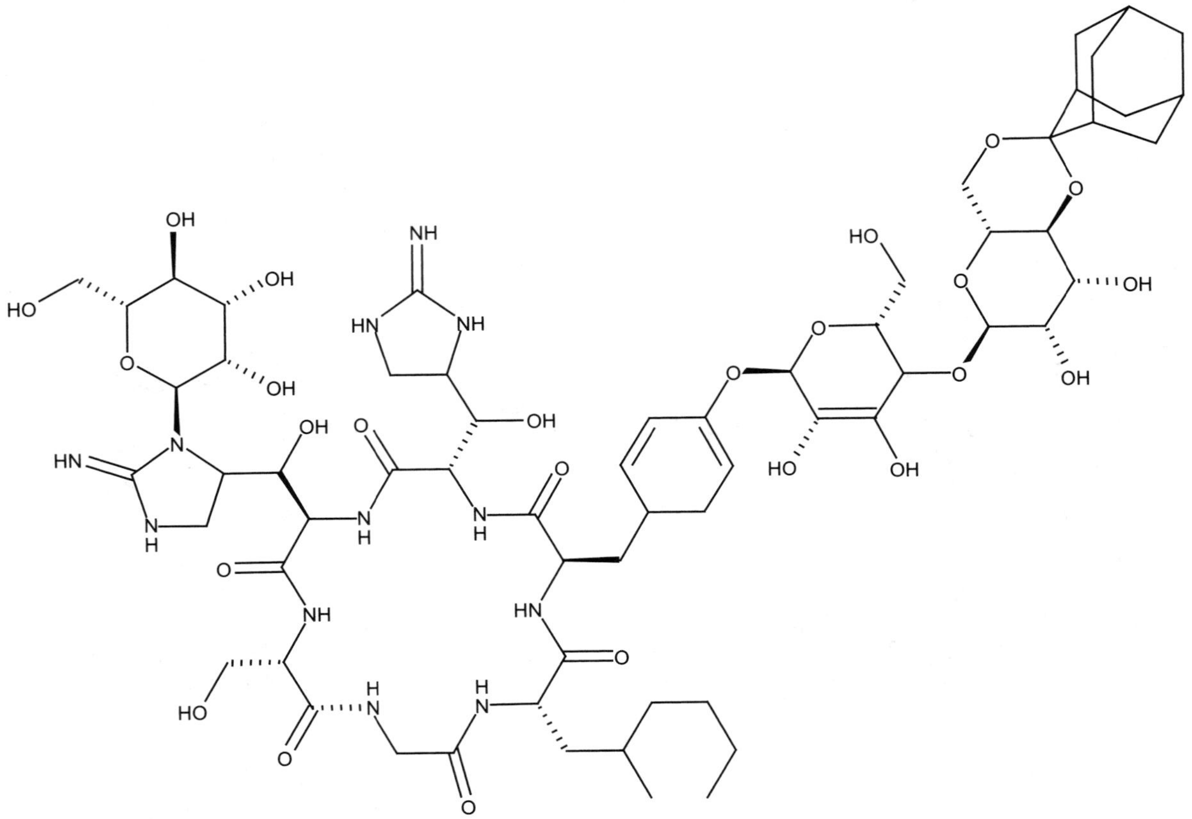

Figure 8 AC 98-6646

Table 33 In vitro activity of AC 98-6646[a]

Microorganism(s)	*n*	MIC (μg/ml)[b]					
		AC 98-6646		Vancomycin		Teicoplanin	
		50%	90%	50%	90%	50%	90%
MSSA	10	0.03	0.03	0.03	1.0	1.0	1.0
MRSA	10	0.03	0.06	0.06	1.0	1.0	1.0
VISA[c]	17	0.03	0.06	0.06	4.0	4.0	8.0
S. pneumoniae Pen^{s}	10	≤0.008	≤0.008	0.25	0.25	≤0.008	0.015
S. pneumoniae Pen^{i}	10	≤0.008	≤0.008	0.25	0.25	≤0.008	≤0.008
S. pneumoniae Pen^{r}	11	≤0.008	≤0.008	0.5	0.5	0.015	0.03
S. pyogenes	10	0.015	0.03	0.25	0.25	≤0.008	≤0.008
S. agalactiae	10	0.015	0.03	0.25	0.5	0.03	0.06
S. epidermidis	53	0.25	0.5	2.0	4.0	2.0	8.0
E. faecalis	10	0.12	0.25	0.25	2.0	0.25	0.25
E. faecalis Van^{r}	10	0.12	0.12	0.12	>8.0	>8.0	>8.0
E. faecium	10	0.12	0.12	0.12	1.0	0.5	1.0
E. faecium Van^{r}	10	0.12	0.12	0.12	>8.0	>8.0	>8.0
Clostridium spp.	10	0.06	0.12	1.0	16		
Peptostreptococcus spp.	10	0.06	>128	0.5	1.0		
Bacteroides spp.	10	>128	>128	64	128		
Prevotella spp.	10	>128	>128	128	>128		

[a]Data from Labthavikul et al., 2002, and Petersen et al., 2002a, 2002b, 2002c.
[b]50% and 90%, MICs at which 50 and 90% of isolates tested are inhibited, respectively.
[c]VISA, vancomycin-intermediate *S. aureus*.

Table 34 In vivo activity of AC 98-6646

Microorganism	ED_{50} (mg/kg)[a]	
	AC 98-6646	Vancomycin
S. aureus Smith	0.08	0.69
S. aureus NEMC-89-4 Met[r]	0.27	2.89
E. faecalis GC 6169 Van[r]	0.39	20
S. pneumoniae CG 1894 Pen[r]	0.05	0.40
S. pneumoniae ATCC 6301 Pen[s]	0.07	1.55

[a] ED_{50}, 50% effective dose.

Table 36 In vitro activity of televancin against *B. anthracis*

Compound	MIC (μg/ml)
Televancin	≤0.03–0.5
Daptomycin	0.06–4.0
Vancomycin	0.5–1.0
Teicoplanin	0.06–0.12
Ceftriaxone	0.25–>8.0
Penicillin G	≤0.06
Ciprofloxacin	0.015–0.03
Doxycycline	≤0.008

Table 35 Pharmacokinetics of AC 98-6646 in animals

Animals	Dose (mg/kg)	C_{max} (μg/ml)	AUC (μg·h/ml)	$t_{1/2}$ (h)	CL_P (ml/h/kg)
Mice	1.0	3.9	10.1	1.5	99
	10	18.2	10.2	3.3	97.9
	20	31.6	16.4	3.3	121
	60	14.8	23.9	5.4	250
Rats	2	16.3	22.6	1.2	88.7
	20	231	240	1.5	83.1
Monkeys	2	17.9	279	14.9	7.2
	20	187.9	3,241	10.2	6.2
Dogs	2	19	252	9.5	7.9
	20	201	1,247	11	16

REFERENCES

Amrein C, Hilaire-Buys D, Guillemin R, Taburet AM, Valser C, Despaux E, Singlas E, 1982, Teicoplanin can be administered by subcutaneous route, 32nd Intersci Conf Antimicrob Agents Chemother, abstract 221.

Arthur M, Molinas C, Courvalin P, 1992, The VanS-VanR two-component regulatory system controls synthesis of depsipeptide peptidoglycan precursors in *Enterococcus faecium* BM4147, J Bacteriol, 174, 2582–2591.

Arthur M, Quintiliani R Jr, 2001, Regulation of VanA- and VanB-type glycopeptide resistance in enterococci, Antimicrob Agents Chemother, 45, 375–381.

Arthur M, Reynolds P, Courvalin P, 1996, Glycopeptide resistance in enterococci, Trends Microbiol, 4, 401–407.

ASCP, 1997, Susceptibility testing group 1999, United States geographic bacteria: susceptibility pattern, Diagn Microbiol Infect Dis, 35, 143–151.

Bantar C, Famiglietti A, Goldberg M, 2000, Three year surveillance study of nosocomial resistance in Argentina, Int J Infect Dis, 4, 85–90.

Barna JCJ, Williams DH, Stone DJM, Leung C, Dodrell DM, 1984, Structure elucidation of teicoplanin antibiotics, J Am Chem Soc, 106, 4895–4902.

Bernareggi A, Danese A, Cometti A, Buniva G, Rowland M, 1990, Pharmacokinetics of individual components of teicoplanin in man, J Pharmacokinet Biopharm, 18, 525–543.

Biavasco F, Vignarolli C, Lupidi R, Manso E, Facinelli B, Varaldo PE, 1997, In vitro antibacterial activity of LY 333328, a new semisynthetic glycopeptide, Antimicrob Agents Chemother, 41, 2165–2172.

Blevins RD, Halstenson CE, Salem NG, Matzke GR, 1984, Pharmacokinetics of vancomycin in patients undergoing continuous ambulatory peritoneal dialysis, Antimicrob Agents Chemother, 25, 603–606.

Bonati M, Traina GL, Gentile MG, Fellen G, Rosina R, Cavenaghi L, Buniva G, 1988, Pharmacokinetics of peritoneal teicoplanin in patients with chronic renal failure on continuous ambulatory peritoneal dialysis, Br J Clin Pharmacol, 25, 761–765.

Bonati M, Traina GL, Villa G, Salvadeo A, Gentile MG, Fellin G, Rosina R, Cavenagh L, Buniva G, 1987, Teicoplanin pharmacokinetics in patients with chronic renal failure, Clin Pharmacokinet, 12, 292–301.

Bozdogan B, Esel D, Whitener C, Browne FA, Appelbaum PC, 2003, Antibacterial susceptibility of a vancomycin-resistant *Staphylococcus aureus* strain isolated at the Hershey Medical Center, J Antimicrob Chemother, 53, 864–868.

Braun DK, Chien JY, Farlow DS, Phillips DL, Wasilewski M, Zeckel ML, 2001, Oritavacin LY333328, a dose-escalation safety and pharmacokinetics study in patients, Eur Congr Chemother Infect Dis, Istanbul, Turkey, abstract P 434.

Brouard RJ, Kapusnik TE, Gambertoglio JG, Schoenfeld PY, Sachdeva M, Freel K, Tozer TN, 1989, Teicoplanin pharmacokinetics and bioavailability during peritoneal dialysis, Clin Pharmacol Ther, 45, 674–681.

Brown N, Ho DHW, Fang KLL, Bogard L, Maksymiuk A, Bolivar R, Fainstein V, Bodey GP, 1983, Effect of hepatic function on vancomycin clinical pharmacology, Antimicrob Agents Chemother, 23, 603–606.

Buniva G, Del Favero A, Bernareggi A, Patioa L, Palumbo R, 1988, Pharmacokinetics of ^{14}C teicoplanin in healthy volunteers, J Antimicrob Chemother, 21, suppl A, 23–28.

Byl B, Jacobs F, Wallemacq P, Rossi C, de Fraequen P, Cappelo M, Leal T, Thys JP, 2003, Vancomycin penetration of uninfected pleural fluid exudate after continuous or intermittent infusion, Antimicrob Agents Chemother, 47, 2015–2017.

Calain P, Krause KH, Vaudaux P, et al, 1987, Early termination of a prospective randomized trial comparing teicoplanin and flucloxacillin for treating severe staphylococcal infections, J Infect Dis, 155, 187–191.

Campoli-Richards DM, Brogden RN, Faulds D, 1990, Teicoplanin: a review of its antibacterial activity, pharmacokinetic properties and therapeutic potential, Drugs, 40(3), 449–486.

Cavalieri M, Cooper A, Nutley MA, Stogniew M, 2002, Protein binding of dalbavancin using intrathermal titration microcalorimetry, 42nd Intersci Conf Antimicrob Agents Chemother, abstract A-1385.

Centers for Disease Control, 2002, *Staphylococcus aureus* resistant to vancomycin—United States, Morb Mortal Wkly Rep, 51, 565–567.

Cooper GL, Given DB, 1986, Vancomycin: a comprehensive review of 30 years of clinical experience, p 81, Wiley & Sons.

Cutler NR, Narang PK, Lesko LJ, 1984, Vancomycin disposition, the importance of age, Clin Pharmacol Ther, 36, 803–810.

Del Favero A, Patoia L, Rosina R, Buniva G, Danese A, Bernareggi A, Molini E, Cavenaghi L, 1991, Pharmacokinetics and tolerability of teicoplanin in healthy volunteers after single increasing doses, Antimicrob Agents Chemother, 35, 2551–2557.

Domart Y, Pierre C, Clair B, et al, 1987, Pharmacokinetics of teicoplanin in critically ill patients with various degrees of renal impairment, Antimicrob Agents Chemother, 31, 1600–1604.

Dowell JA, Gottlieb AB, Van Saders C, Dorr MB, Leighton A, Cavalieri M, Guanci M, Colombo L, 2002, The pharmacokinetics and renal excretion of dalbavancin in healthy subjects, 42nd Intersci Conf Antimicrob Agents Chemother, abstract A-1386.

Dowell JA, Pu F, Seltzer E, Stagniew M, Dorr MB, Fayocavitz S, Krause D, Henkel T, 2003, Dalbavancin pharmacokinetics in subjects with mild or moderate hepatic impairment, 43rd Intersci Conf Antimicrob Agents Chemother, abstract A-19.

Drusano GL, 1988, Role of pharmacokinetics in the outcome of infections, Antimicrob Agents Chemother, 32, 289–297.

Dushin RG, Wang T-Z, Fortier G, Iera S, Papamichalakis M, Richard L, Sellstedt J, Shah S, 2002, Synthesis of AC 98-6646, a semisynthetic mannopeptimycin derivative, 42nd Intersci Conf Antimicrob Agents Chemother, abstract F-352.

European Organization for Research and Treatment of Cancer (EORTC) International Antimicrobial Therapy Cooperative Group and the National Cancer Institute of Canada—Clinical Trials Group, 1991, Vancomycin added to empirical combination antibiotic therapy for fever in granulocytopenic cancer patients, J Infect Dis, 163, 951–958.

Falcoz C, Ferry N, Pozet N, Cuisinaud G, Zech PY, 1987, Pharmacokinetics of teicoplanin in renal failure, Antimicrob Agents Chemother, 31, 1255–1262.

Felmingham D, Brown DFG, Soussy CJ, 1998, European glycopeptide susceptibility survey of gram-positive bacteria for 1995, Diagn Microbiol Infect Dis, 31, 563–571.

Fraise AP, Andrews J, Wise R, 1997, In vitro activity of a new glycopeptide antibiotic, LY 333328, against enterococci and other resistant gram-positive organisms, J Antimicrob Chemother, 40, 423–425.

Gilbert DN, Wood CA, Kimbrough RC, and the Infectious Diseases Consortium of Oregon, 1991, Failure of treatment with teicoplanin at 6 milligrams/kilogram/day in patients with *Staphylococcus aureus* intravascular infection, Antimicrob Agents Chemother, 35, 79–87.

Goldstein E, Citron D, 2002, In vitro activities of dalbavancin and nine comparator agents against anaerobic gram-positive species and corynebacteria, 42nd Intersci Conf Antimicrob Agents Chemother, abstract E-1454.

Goldstein F, Coutrot A, Sieffert A, Acar JF, 1990, Percentages and distributions of teicoplanin and vancomycin-resistant strains among coagulase-negative staphylococci, Antimicrob Agents Chemother, 34, 899–900.

Gonzalez-Martin G, Acuna V, Perez C, Labarca J, Guevara A, Tagle R, 1996, Pharmacokinetics of vancomycin in patients with severely impaired renal function, Int J Clin Pharmacol Ther, 34, 71–75.

Guau DR, Awni WM, Halstenson CE, et al, 1989, Teicoplanin pharmacokinetics in patients undergoing continuous ambulatory peritoneal dialysis after intravenous and intraperitoneal dosing, Antimicrob Agents Chemother, 33, 2012–2015.

Haider SA, Hassett P, Bron AJ, 2001, Intraocular vancomycin levels after intravitreal injection in post cataract extraction endophthalmitis, Retina, 21, 210–213.

Healy DP, Sahai JV, Fuller SH, Polk RE, 1990, Vancomycin-induced histamine release and red man syndrome, comparison of 1- and 2-hour infusions, Antimicrob Agents Chemother, 34, 550–554.

Ismael F, Bléton R, Saleh-Mghir A, Dautrey S, Massias L, Cremieux AC, 2003, Teicoplanin-containing cement spacers for treatment of experimental *Staphylococcus aureus* joint prosthesis infection, Antimicrob Agents Chemother, 47, 3365–3367.

Jones RN, Biedenbach DJ, Johnson DM, Pfaller MA, 2001, In vitro evaluation of BI 397, a novel glycopeptide antimicrobial agent, J Chemother, 13, 244–254.

Kaniga K, Blosser RS, Karlowsky JA, Sahm DF, 2004, In vitro activity of televancin against Bacillus anthracis, 44th Intersci Conf Antimicrob Agents Chemother, abstract E-2010.

Kureishi A, Jewesson P, Rubinger M, et al, 1991, Double-blind comparison of teicoplanin versus vancomycin in febrile neutropenic patients receiving concomitant tobramycin and piperacillin, effect on cyclosporin A-associated nephrotoxicity, Antimicrob Agents Chemother, 35, 2246–2252.

Lancini GC, 1989, Fermentation and biosynthesis of glycopeptide antibiotics, in Bushell ME, Graefe V, ed, Bioactive Metabolites from Microorganisms, Elsevier, Amsterdam, Pub Prog Ind Microbiol, 27, 283–287.

Leclercq R, Courvalin P, 1997, Resistance to glycopeptides in enterococci, Clin Infect Dis, 24, 545–556.

Leclercq R, Derlot E, Weber M, Duval J, Courvalin P, 1989, Transferable vancomycin and teicoplanin resistance in *Enterococcus faecium*, Antimicrob Agents Chemother, 33, 10–15.

Lee CC, Andreson RC, Chen KK, 1957, Vancomycin, a new antibiotic. V. Distribution, excretion and renal clearance, Antibiot Annu, 1956-1957, 82–89.

Leighton A, Mroszczak E, White R, Romano G, Gottlieb AB, Baylor M, Perry M, Henkol T, 2001, Dalbavancin, phase I single and multiple doses placebo controlled intravenous safety: pharmacokinetics study in healthy volunteers, 41st Intersci Conf Antimicrob Agents Chemother, abstract 951.

Leport C, Perronne C, Massip P, et al, 1989, Evaluation of teicoplanin for treatment of endocarditis caused by gram-positive cocci in 20 patients, Antimicrob Agents Chemother, 33, 871–876.

Matzke GR, McGory RW, Halstenson CE, Keane WF, 1984, Pharmacokinetics of vancomycin in patients with various degrees of renal function, Antimicrob Agents Chemother, 25, 433–437.

Matzke GR, Zhanel GG, Guay DR, 1986, Clinical pharmacokinetics of vancomycin, Clin Pharm, 11, 257–282.

Moellering RC Jr, 1998, The specter of glycopeptide resistance, current trends and future considerations, Am J Med, 104, suppl 5A, 3S-6S.

Morse GD, Farolino DF, Apicella M, Walshe JJ, 1987, Comparative study of intraperitoneal and intravenous vancomycin pharmacokinetics during continuous ambulatory peritoneal dialysis, Antimicrob Agents Chemother, 31, 173–177.

Murphy TM, Lenoy EB, Young M, Weiss WJ, 2002, In vivo efficacy and pharmacokinetics of AC-98-6646, a novel glycopeptide, in experimental models of infection, in 42nd Intersci Conf Antimicrob Agents Chemother, abstract F-356.

Nagarajan R, 1991, Antibacterial activities and modes of action of vancomycin and related glycopeptides, Antimicrob Agents Chemother, 35, 605–609.

Nicas TI, Zeckel ML, Braun DK, 1997, Beyond vancomycin, new therapies to the challenge of glycopeptide resistance, Trends Microbiol, 5, 240–249.

Noble WC, Virani Z, Cree RG, 1992, Co-transfer of vancomycin and other resistance genes from *Enterococcus faecalis* NCTC 12201 to *Staphylococcus aureus*, FEMS Microbiol Lett, 93, 195–198.

Oreopoulos DG, Robson M, Faller B, Ogiluine R, Rapoport A, de Veber GA, 1979, Continuous ambulatory peritoneal dialysis, a new era in the treatment of chronic renal failure, Clin Nephrol, 11, 125–128.

Ortega GM, Marti-Bonmatti E, Guevara SJ, Gomez IG, 2003, Alteration of vancomycin pharmacokinetics during cardiopulmonary bypass in patients undergoing cardiac surgery, Am J Health Syst Pharm, 60, 260–265.

Pancorbo S, Comty C, 1982, Peritoneal transport of vancomycin in 4 patients undergoing continuous ambulatory peritoneal dialysis, Nephron, 31, 37–39.

Patel R, Piper K, Cockerill FR III, Steckelberg JM, Yousten AA, 2000, The biopesticide *Paenibacillus popilliae* has a vancomycin resistance gene cluster homologous to the enterococcal VanA vancomycin resistance gene cluster, Antimicrob Agents Chemother, 44, 705–709.

Petersen PJ, Hartman HE, Wang TZ, Dushin RG, Bradford PA, 2002a, Time kill kinetics and post-antibiotic effects of AC 98-6646 novel semisynthetic glycopeptide antibiotic derivative, in 42nd Intersci Conf Antimicrob Agents Chemother, abstract F-354.

Petersen PJ, Labthavikul P, Wang TZ, Dushin RG, Bradford PA, 2002b, In vitro comparative activity of AC 98-6646, a novel semisynthetic cyclic glycopeptide derivative of the natural product mannopeptimycin αAC98-1, in 42nd Intersci Conf Antimicrob Agents Chemother, abstract F-353.

Petersen PJ, Weiss WJ, Lenoy EB, He H, Testa RT, Bradford PA, 2002c, In vitro activity of a novel cyclic glycopeptide natural product antibiotic, AC 98, and comparative antibiotics against gram-positive bacteria, in 42nd Intersci Conf Antimicrob Agents Chemother, abstract 1148.

Rodvold KA, Blum RA, Fischer JH, et al, 1988, Vancomycin pharmacokinetics in patients with various degrees of renal function, Antimicrob Agents Chemother, 32, 848–852.

Rosina R, Villa G, Danese A, Cavenaghi L, Picardi L, Salvadeo A, 1988, Pharmacokinetics of teicoplanin in the elderly, J Antimicrob Chemother, 21, suppl A, 39–45.

Rotschafer JC, Crossley K, Zaske DE, Mead K, Sawchuk RJ, Solem LD, 1982, Pharmacokinetics of vancomycin: observations in 28 patients and dosage recommendations, Antimicrob Agents Chemother, 22, 391–394.

Rouveix B, Garnier M, Pinta P, Kreutz C, 2002, Residual serum concentrations and safety of teicoplanin administered intravenously to healthy volunteers at 15 mg/kg dose on alternate days, compared with 6 mg/kg, in 42nd Intersci Conf Antimicrob Agents Chemother, abstract P-949.

Sillerström E, Wahlund E, Nord CE, 1999, In vitro activity of LY 333328 against anaerobic gram positive bacteria, J Chemother, 11, 90–92.

Torras J, Cao C, Rivas MC, et al, 1991, Pharmacokinetics of vancomycin in patients undergoing hemodialysis with polyacrylonitrile, Clin Nephr, 36, 35–41.

Traina GL, Bonati M, 1984, Pharmacokinetics of teicoplanin in man after intravenous administration, J Pharmakinet Biopharm, 12, 119–128.

Traina GL, Gentile G, Fellin G, Rosina R, Cavenghi L, Buniva G, Bonati M, 1986, Pharmacokinetics of teicoplanin in patients on continuous ambulatory peritoneal dialysis, Eur J Clin Pharmacol, 31, 501–504.

Van der Auwera P, Aoun M, Meunier F, 1991, Randomized study of vancomycin versus teicoplanin for the treatment of gram-positive bacterial infections in immunocompromised hosts, Antimicrob Agents Chemother, 35, 451–457.

Van der Auwera P, Matsumoto T, Husson M, 1988, Intraphagocytic penetration of antibiotics, J Antimicrob Chemother, 185–192.

Watanakunakorn C, 1988, In vitro induction of resistance in coagulase-negative staphylococci to vancomycin and teicoplanin, J Antimicrob Chemother, 22, 321–324.

Watanakunakorn C, 1990, In vitro selection of resistance of Staphylococcus aureus to teicoplanin and vancomycin, J Antimicrob Chemother, 25, 69–72.

Zimmermann AE, Katona BG, Plaisance KL, 1995, Association of vancomycin serum concentrations with outcomes in patients with gram-positive bacteria, Pharmacotherapy, 15, 85–91.

Ansamycins

A. BRYSKIER

32

1. INTRODUCTION

Ansamycin is the name given by Prelog and Oppolzer in 1973 to a series of derivatives possessing a chromophore (aromatic nucleus) and an aliphatic chain spanning an aromatic nucleus (ansa). The term "ansa" had been proposed in 1942 by Luttringhaus and Grahler to describe molecules with an aliphatic chain attached at the *meta* and *para* positions of a benzene nucleus. The rifamycins were isolated in 1957 by Sensi et al. from the fermentation broth of *Nocardia mediterranei* (then known under the name of *Amycolatopsis mediterranei*), isolated from the soil of a pine forest in the region of Saint Raphael in France. This strain produces a complex of five components that have been isolated chromatographically. Other derivatives of rifamycin have been described: rifamycins Y, L, W, and P and a number of biosynthetic intermediates.

The principal derivative, rifamycin B, is converted into two bacteriologically active components, rifamycins O and S. The presence of diethylbarbituric acid in the fermentation broth yields large quantities of rifamycin B. The reduction of rifamycin S to rifamycin SV produced the first drug of this chemical class to be introduced into clinical practice. The second derivative to have been prepared by semisynthesis was rifamycin B diethylaminide, or rifamide. Rifamycin SV was introduced into clinical practice in 1962 for the treatment of staphylococcal infections, infections due to gram-positive cocci, hepatobiliary infections, and tuberculosis. Rifamycin SV and rifamide are parenteral antibiotics. In fact, after oral administration, they are characterized by erratic digestive absorption, are concentrated in the liver, and are rapidly eliminated in the bile; levels in serum are low and inconsistent.

Rifampin was obtained by semisynthesis from the 3-formylrifamycin derivative. The aim of research was to obtain a molecule that was well absorbed orally and that had potent activity against *Mycobacterium tuberculosis* and gram-positive bacteria.

The research continued with changes of the substituents at position 3. A dual aim was pursued: an improvement in the pharmacokinetics and the production of molecules having only partial cross-resistance with rifampin. Three molecules that partly fulfill this expectation are under development or already introduced into clinical practice: rifabutin, rifapentine, and rifalazil. Rifaximin, a nonabsorbable molecule used in the treatment of gastrointestinal infections, is a separate entity.

Current research is directed towards the semisynthesis of molecules that are active against *Mycobacterium avium*.

2. CLASSIFICATION

It is possible to separate two groups of molecules within the ansamycin family according to the aromatic nucleus: ansamycins of the naphthalene type and ansamycins of the benzene type.

This structural difference is also accompanied by a difference in terms of biological activity. The molecules of the first group are antibacterial or antiviral agents, whereas those in the second group are mainly anticancer molecules, although some of them also have antiprotozoal or antifungal activity (Fig. 1).

2.1. Molecules Other than Rifamycins

2.1.1. Halomicin

Halomicin is transformed fairly readily to rifamycin S. Four molecules, A to D, have been isolated from the fermentation of *Micromonospora halophytica*.

2.1.2. Streptovaricins

Streptovaricins, a molecular complex comprising ten components (A to J), are difficult to separate by chromatography. These molecules exert activity against HeLa cells. The most active is streptovaricin D. The whole complex was isolated from the fermentation of *Streptomyces spectabilis*. Streptovaricin C was introduced into clinical practice under the name of Dalacin (Upjohn Company) as an antituberculosis agent, but because of its toxicity and low therapeutic index, it has been abandoned.

2.1.3. Tolypomycins

Tolypomycins are the metabolic product of *Streptomyces tolypophorus*. The principal molecules are tolypomycin Y and its derivative, tolypomycin R. Tolypomycin has good activity against gram-positive bacteria but has not been developed because of its chemical instability.

2.1.4. Naphthomycins

Naphthomycins are a molecular complex comprising eight compounds (A to H). Naphthomycin A was extracted from *Streptomyces collinus*, naphthomycin B was extracted from

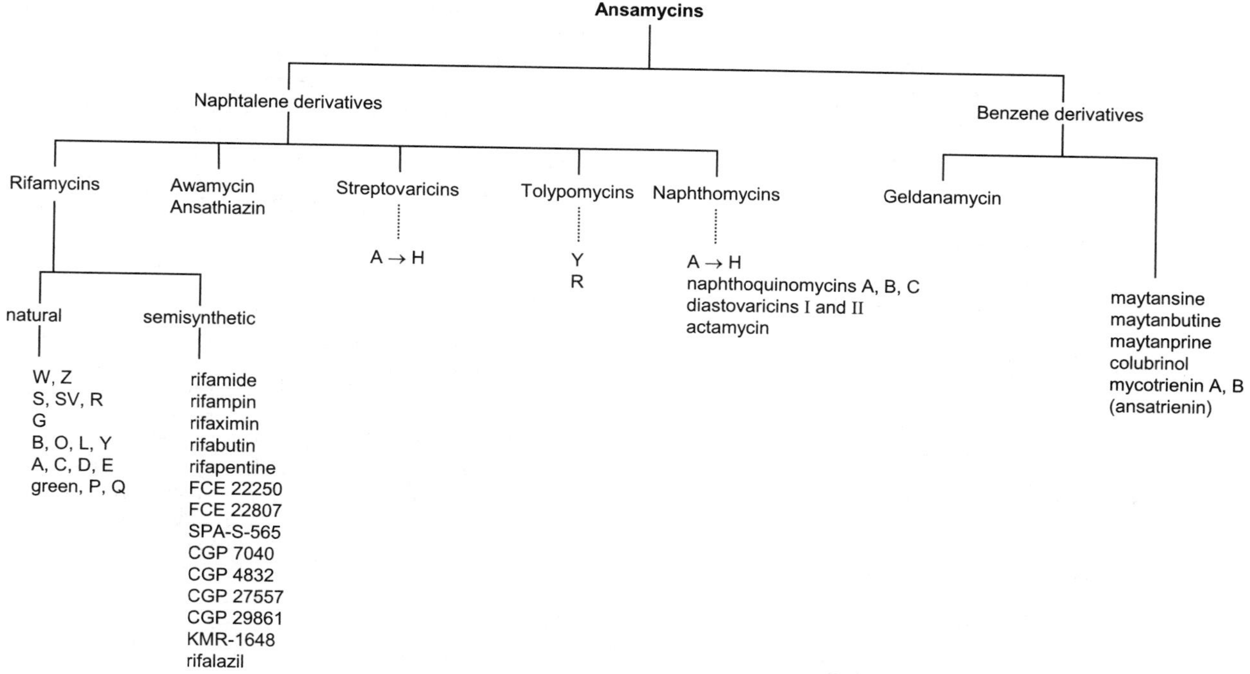

Figure 1 Classification of ansamycins

Streptomyces galbus, and naphthomycin C, the nonchlorinated derivative of naphthomycin B, was extracted from *Streptomyces diastatochromogenes*. Naphthomycins A, B, and C are *Escherichia coli* fatty acid biosynthesis inhibitors and are extracted from *Streptomyces* spp.

2.1.5. Awamycin and Ansathiazin

Awamycin and ansathiazin have been extracted from *Streptomyces albolongus* and have a sulfur atom.

2.2. Benzene Derivatives

The molecules that make up the benzene derivatives have been extracted either from plants, such as the maytansinoid derivatives (maytansine, maytanbutine, and maytanprine) that come from *Maytenus buchananii*; colubrinol, which comes from *Colubrina texensis*; or geldanamycin, which comes from the fermentation of *Streptomyces hygroscopicus* (Fig. 2). The last derivative is also active against protozoa, particularly *Crithidia fasciculata* and *Tetrahymena pyriformis*.

Figure 2 Ansamycins: naphthalene derivatives

3. CHEMICAL STRUCTURE

The rifamycins are characterized by an aliphatic chain attached to position 2 of the naphthalene nucleus and to position 12 of the same nucleus.

The nucleus is composed of 17 atoms. The carboxyl group is attached by means of an amide bond. This ensures the stability of the geometric configuration of the molecules. The molecule contains a naphthohydroquinone nucleus, and a pentaatomic nucleus is attached above it.

The double bonds at C-16 and C-17 and at C-18 and C-19 are in the *cis* and *trans* positions, respectively. The chain forms an angle of 71° with the plane of the naphthoquinone nucleus. The closest zone between the ansa and the naphthoquinone nucleus is the carbon at position 26, to which is attached a methyl group (C-34) located 3.5 Å from the plane of the nucleus. The molecule contains eight centers of asymmetry: 20*S*, 21*S*, 22*R*, 23*R*, 24*R*, 25*S*, 26*R*, and 27*S* (Fig. 3).

Figure 4 shows ansamycins with antibacterial activity.

The molecules obtained by semisynthesis differ mainly in the chain attached to position 3 of the naphthalene nucleus (Figs. 5 and 6) and the presence of a hydroxyl group or its quinone form at position 4.

4. STRUCTURE-ACTIVITY RELATIONSHIP

Chemical modifications of the ansa in general cause a reduction or even complete abolition of antibacterial activity.

Deacetylation of the acetoxy group at position 25 and demethylation of the group attached to position C-27 constitute an exception. The derivatives obtained have better activity against gram-negative bacteria but reduced activity against gram-positive bacteria.

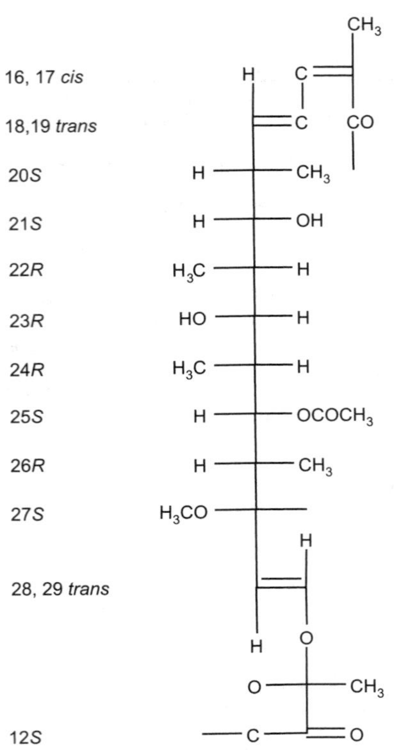

Figure 3 Absolute configuration of rifamycin S (data from Brufani, 1977)

On the naphthalene nucleus, hydroxyl groups 1 and 2 (attached to positions 1 and 8) and 9 and 11 (attached to C-23 and C-21) must not be modified, as they are essential to the antibacterial activity of the rifamycins on the aliphatic chain. The most suitable positions on the naphthalene nucleus for modification are the carbonylquinone groups at position 4, and position 3 of the quinone nucleus.

The starting point for the semisynthesis of the rifamycins was the preparation of 3-formylrifamycin SV by oxidation of the Männich bases of rifamycin SV.

A large number of derivatives have thus been obtained, including rifampin.

By condensing 3-formylrifamycin SV with different reagents, it has been possible to prepare derivatives of the imine type (CH=N-R′), hydrazones [CH=N-N (R_1R_2)], oximes (CH=N-OR), and hydrazine-hydrazones (CH=NH-C-R_1).

Derivatives of the imino type are more active against *M. tuberculosis* but do not provide a substantial improvement against gram-positive and gram-negative bacteria. The hydrazine-hydrazone derivatives are weakly active. A general increase in antibacterial activity can be obtained with the hydrazone derivatives. Among derivatives of the oxime type, some possess partial cross-resistance with rifampin, probably associated with their lipophilicity. Among the hydrazone derivatives, the most active molecule was that having an *N*-amino-*N′*-methylpiperazine chain: rifampin. Other molecules with this chain have been synthesized since then: SPA-S-565, FCE-22807, FCE-22250, rifapentine, R-76-1, rifalazil, etc.

Rifamycin B is inactive because of the presence of an acetoxy group at position 3, the carboxyl group preventing

	Position 4	Position 3	N° code
Rifamycin SV	OH	H	
Rifampin	OH	—C(H)=N–N N–CH3	
Rifabutin	-	NH, N, N, CH, CH3	LM 427
Rifaxime	4, N, N, CH3		L-105
Rifapentine	OH	N, N, N	MDL 473
SPA-S-565	OH	–CH–N–N=C(CH3)–N	
FCE 22807	=OH	—C(H)=NN·CH·N	
FCE 22250	OH	—C(H)=NN·CH·N	

Figure 4 Ansamycins with antibacterial activity

	Position 4	Position 3
CGP 4832		—N O
AF/103	-O	—$CH{=}N{-}O(CH_2)_7CH_3$
Rifamazine	-O	$R{-}CH{=}N{-}N{=}CH{-}R$
CGP 40/469A (SPA-S-565)	-O	$CH{=}N{-}N{=}C(CH_3){=}N(C_2H_5)_2$
CGP 7040	-O	—N N—CH_2— (H_3C, CH_3, CH_3)
Rifamide	$-OCH_2CO\text{-}N\text{-}(C_2H_5)_2$	H
R-76-1	-O	$CH{=}N{-}N$ N—$CH_2-CH_2\text{-}CH(CH_3)_2$

Figure 5 Ansamycin derivatives

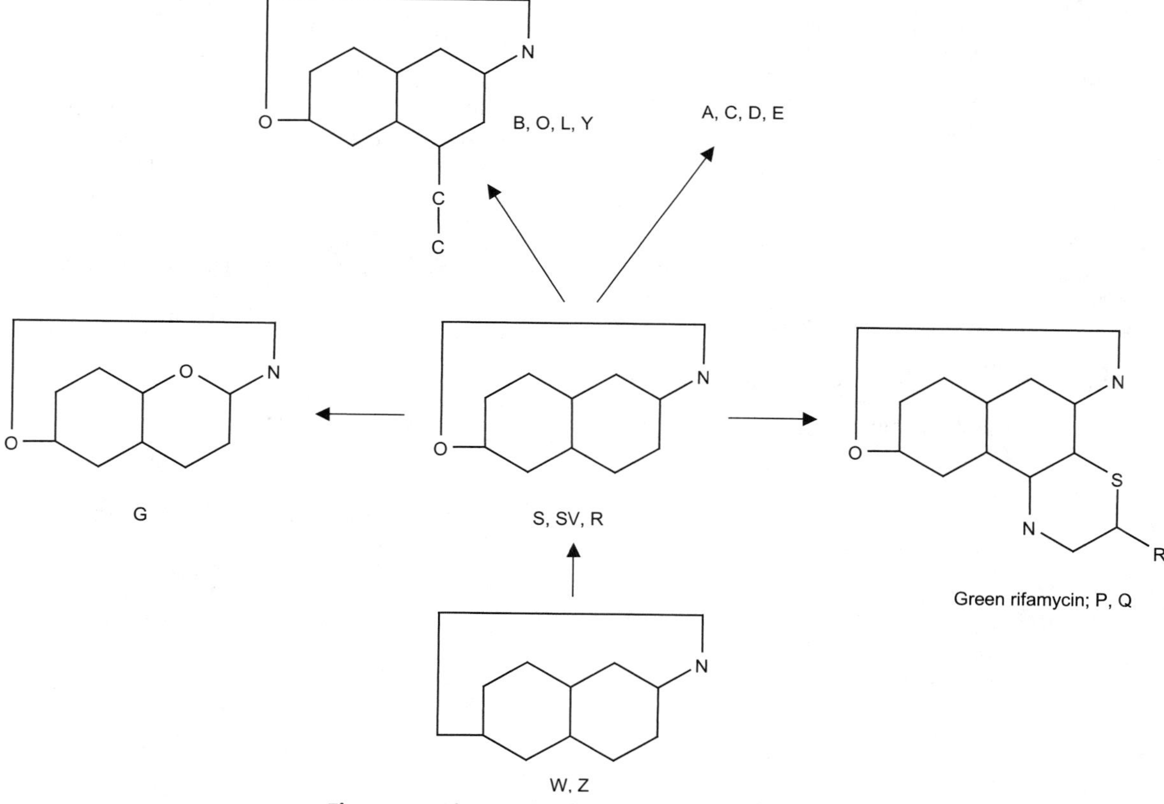

Figure 6 Biogenetic classification of rifamycins

transmembrane passage. Derivatives with an amide group, hydrazines, or an ester at position 3 have good antibacterial activity, but this activity depends on the amides or hydrazines attached. Di- or trisubstituted amides are the most active; the antibacterial activity is dependent on the lipophilicity of the molecule. In vivo, the dialkylamide derivatives of rifamycin B have better activity than rifamycin SV, the most active being rifamide.

Derivatives have been synthesized with an aromatic nucleus attached directly to the carbon at position 3 of the naphthalene nucleus, such as CGP-7040.

A new series of benzoxazinorifamycins has been synthesized. These molecules possess a 3′-hydroxy-5-(4-alkylpiperazine) chain. Various groups have been attached to the piperazine nucleus: isobutyl (rifalazil), propyl (KRM-1657), *sec*-butyl (KRM-1668), *sec*-butyl (*R*) (KRM-1686), and *sec*-butyl (*S*) (KRM-1687).

A new series of compounds has recently been semisynthesized: ABI-1131, which differs from rifalazil by the C-3 methyl group instead of a isobutyl, and ABI-1649, which has an azetidinyl ring instead of a piperazinyl ring. They display in vitro activity against rifampin-resistant isolates.

The activity of these molecules has been tested against different species of mycobacteria and is superior to that of rifampin against slow-growing mycobacteria. Likewise, they have better intramacrophagic activity against *M. tuberculosis*.

5. PHYSICOCHEMICAL PROPERTIES OF RIFAMYCINS

See Table 1.

5.1. Rifamycin SV

Rifamycin SV is a crystalline, yellow-orange substance with a poorly defined melting point; it starts to decompose at 140°C and does not melt below 300°C. It is a levogyre substance, $[\alpha]^{20}_{D}$, −4° (methanol, c = 1). Rifamycin SV is a strong acid (pK 2.7). It is poorly soluble in water, soluble in ether and bicarbonate, and slightly soluble in methanol, ethanol, and acetone.

5.2. Rifampin

Rifampin crystallizes in acetone in the form of red-orange crystals. It is poorly soluble in water when the pH is greater than 6 but more soluble when the pH is less than 6. It is soluble in the majority of organic solvents but is poorly soluble in acetone.

It is a zwitterionic molecule with an acid pK of 1.7 and an alkaline pK of 7.9. It is stable in solution, but under very acidic conditions it degrades to 3-formylrifamycin SV.

5.3. Rifamide

Rifamide is the diethylamide derivative of rifamycin B. It is a yellow-orange crystalline substance with a melting point of more than 140°C. The specific rotation in methanol (c = 0.4) is −48.7°.

5.4. Rifabutin

Rifabutin is a spiropiperidyl derivative (2-spiro-*N*-isobutyl-1-4-piperidylrifamycin S). Rifabutin is a violet-red crystalline powder; the pK is 6.9. It is soluble in chloroform, slightly soluble in ethanol, and insoluble in water.

5.5. FCE-22250

FCE-22250 is a 3-azinomethylrifamycin derivative that crystallizes in solution in methanol or acetone to red-orange crystals. The melting point is between 270 and 277°C.

FCE-22250 is a zwitterionic molecule with an acid pK (hydroxyl at C-8) of 1.7 and a pK of 5.1 corresponding to the nitrogen atom of the piperidine nucleus. FCE-22807 is the quinone form of FCE-22250.

5.6. Rifaximin

Rifaximin is a non-water-soluble compound which differs from rifamycin SV by having a 4′-methylpyridoimidazolyl nucleus at position 4 of the ansamycin ring.

5.7. CGP-27557 and CGP-29861

CGP-27557 and CGP-29861 belong to a series of 3-hydrazone products with a diazabicycloalkyl side chain. Both compounds are red-orange and insoluble in water.

5.8. CGP-7040

CGP-7040 is a derivative of rifamycin SV that differs from it in the presence of a piperazine nucleus at position 3. It is soluble in water. The crystals are yellow-orange.

5.9. Rifapentine

Rifapentine (DL-473) is a semisynthetic derivative of rifamycin SV belonging to the class of 3-piperazinylhydrazone derivatives. It has a 3-cyclopentylpiperazinylamino chain. This molecule is insoluble in water.

Table 1 Physicochemical properties of ansamycins

Compound	Empirical formula	MW	pK 1	pK 2	Color of the powder	Trade name
Rifamycin SV	$C_{37}H_{47}NO_{12}$	69.77	1.8		Yellow-orange	Rifocin
Rifamide	$C_{43}H_{58}N_2O_{13}$	810.95	3.7		Yellow-orange	
Rifampin	$C_{43}H_{58}N_4O_{12}$	822.95	1.7	7.9	Red-orange	Rifadine, Rimactan
Rifabutin	$C_{46}H_{62}N_4O_{11}$	847.12	1.6	6.9	Red-purple	Mycobutin, Ansatipine
Rifapentine	$C_{47}H_{64}N_4O_{12}$	877.04	2.4	6.5	Red-orange	Priftin
Rifalazil	$C_{51}H_{61}N_4O_{18}$					
Rifaximin	$C_{43}H_{51}N_3O_{11}$	785.89			Red-orange	Normix
FCE-22250	$C_{44}H_{51}N_4O_{11}$	811.33	1.7	5.1	Red-orange	
SPA-S-565	$C_{43}H_{58}N_4O_{12}$	822.31				
R-76-1	$C_{45}H_{63}N_3O_{12}$	837.33				
CGP-7040	$C_{51}H_{75}N_3O_{12}$	914.10			Yellow-orange	
CGP-27557	$C_{45}H_{63}N_4O_{12}$	851.33			Red-orange	
CGP-29861	$C_{47}H_{67}N_4O_{12}$	879.35			Red-orange	
CGP-4832	$C_{49}H_{65}N_3O_{15}$	935.34			Red-purple	

5.10. Rifalazil

Rifalazil (KRM-1648) is a 3′-piperazinyl analog which is a benzoxazinorifamycin.

6. PRODUCTION OF RIFAMYCINS

More than 20 biosynthetic intermediates have been isolated from the fermentation of *N. mediterranei*. Rifamycin S represents the focal point of the biogenesis of the rifamycins. On the basis of this compound, six families of rifamycins may be described (Fig. 6):

- Combination of the whole series produces rifamycin W or Z.
- Structural modifications to rifamycin give rise to rifamycins S, SV, and R.
- Introduction of a sulfur atom at position 3 gives rise to the green rifamycins P and Q.
- Replacement of the carbon atom at position 1 by an oxygen atom gives rise to rifamycin G.
- The last group is that of the complex of molecules A, C, D, and E.

The origin of the carbon skeleton of the rifamycins is the condensation of eight propionate units and two acetate units. The biosynthesis of the polyketide chain is initiated from 3-amino-5-hydroxybenzoic acid, which derives in part from shikimic acid, a unit comprising seven carbon atoms that is the starting point of the synthesis of the aliphatic chain through the provision of propionate and acetate units followed by cyclization, yielding a bicyclic nucleus characteristic of the naphthalene type of ansamycins. The nitrogen is supplied from 3-amino-5-hydroxybenzoic acid, while the methoxy groups originate from the methionines. The methyl groups, with the exception of the acetic groups, derive from the propionic units.

7. ASSAYS OF RIFAMPIN

Microbiological, spectrophotometric, and chromatographic methods have been described.

The microbiological method uses either *Sarcina lutea* ATCC 9341 or *Bacillus subtilis* ATCC 6633 as the test strain for urinary assays.

The sample size is 100 μl, and the limit of sensitivity is 0.2 μg/ml. However, these methods do not detect the metabolites and do not allow an assay to be performed in the case of a combination of drugs (Table 2).

The high-performance liquid chromatography method can be used to assay rifampin and the two metabolites, 25-diacetylrifampin and 3-formylrifampin. A sample of 50 μl is sufficient, and the limit of detection is on the order of 0.5 μg/ml.

Table 2 Microbiological assay: test strains

Compound	Test strain
Rifamide	*S. aureus* 209 P
Rifamycin SV	*S. lutea* ATCC 9341
Rifampin	*S. lutea* ATCC 9341
Rifabutin	*S. lutea* ATCC 9341
Rifapentine	*S. lutea* ATCC 9341
Rifalazil	*S. lutea* ATCC 9341
SPA-S-565	*S. aureus* ATCC 6538 P
CGP-7040	*S. aureus* K 1098
CGP-27557	*B. subtilis* ATCC 6633

8. STABILITY OF ANSAMYCINS IN CULTURE MEDIA

The activity of the ansamycins decreases in parallel over time in phosphate-buffered saline (PBS) medium or in 7 H10 medium with or without Tween 80. They are less stable in a medium without Tween 80. The detection varies with the molecules (Table 3).

9. MECHANISMS OF ACTION

See Fig. 7.

The majority of rifamycins inhibit the transcription of DNA to RNA. Their differential activity derives from their capacity to cross the bacterial cell wall.

9.1. Bacterial Cell Wall

Rifamycin B has weak bacteriological activity. Its poor in vitro activity is due to its inability to cross the bacterial cell wall; in fact, it has good inhibitory activity against isolated DNA polymerase. This inability to cross the bacterial cell wall is related to the presence of the carboxyl group of the chain attached to position 4 of the naphthalene nucleus. The derivatives with an amide, hydrazine, or ester group at position 4 have good antibacterial activity.

9.2. DNA-Dependent RNA Polymerase

Rifampin binds to and specifically inhibits bacterial DNA-dependent RNA polymerase (transcriptase). It is inactive against prokaryotic cells.

Synthesis of RNA from DNA is the first stage in genetic transcription. RNA polymerase catalyzes transcription by binding to a specific sequence of a DNA strand. *E. coli* RNA polymerase is a 950-kDa enzyme composed of a core and a σ subunit. The core is a tetramer comprising two α subunits (371 kDa, 329 amino acids), a β subunit (151 kDa, 1,342 amino acids), and a β' subunit (155 kDa, 1,470 amino acids), which are the products of the *rpoA* (73 min), *rpoB*, and *rpoC* genes. *rpoB* and *ropC* are located contiguously at 90 min in a polycistronic operon that codes for the ribosomal proteins L10, L7, and L12. *rpoD* is located at 67 min.

The σ subunit (110 kDa, 90 amino acids) is the product of the *rpoZ* gene.

The whole unit constitutes a holoenzyme of the metalloenzyme type containing two Zn^{2+} atoms. A Zn^{2+} atom is

Table 3 Stability of ansamycins in 7 H10 medium with or without Tween 80[a]

Compound	Medium	Ansamycin concn (μg/ml)		
		Day 0	Day 2	Day 7
Rifampin	+Tween 80	0.80	0.88	0.22
	−Tween 80	0.80	0.70	0.44
	PBS	0.80	0.82	0.42
FCE-22807	+Tween 80	0.68	0.03	0
	−Tween 80	0.69	0.35	0.16
	PBS	0.85	0.34	0.21
FCE-22250	+Tween 80	0.80	0.06	0
	−Tween 80	0.84	0.40	0.18
	PBS	0.94	0.61	0.19
SPA-S-565	+Tween 80	0.70	0	0
	−Tween 80	0.90	0.46	0.13
	PBS	0.80	0.45	0.07

[a]Tween 80 was at 0.5% (vol/vol) and 37°C in solution at 1 μg/ml.

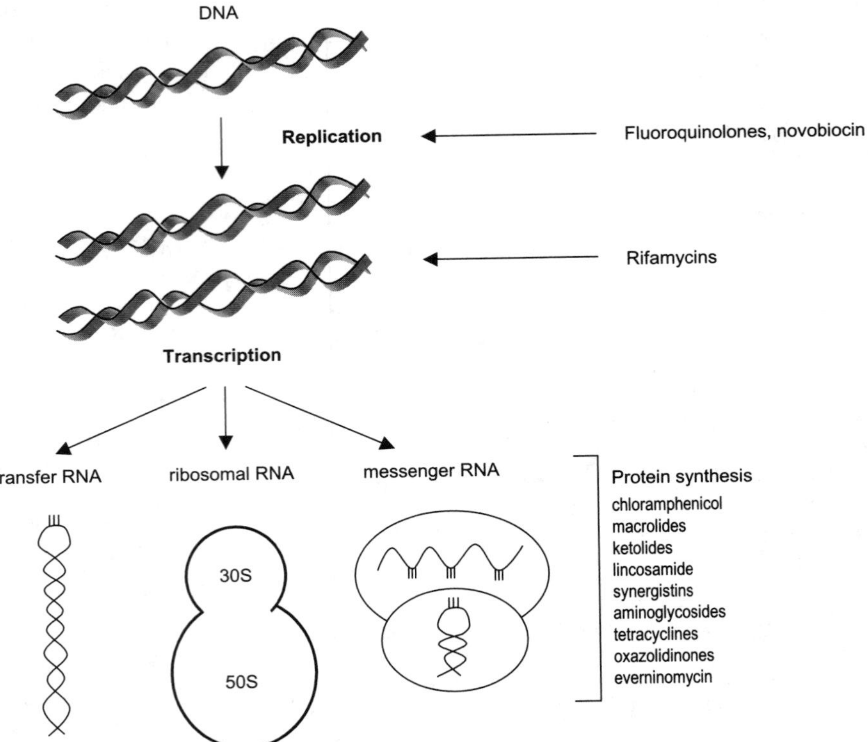

Figure 7 Mechanism of action of rifamycins

attached to both the β and the β′ subunits. The β subunit allows the formation of the phosphodiester bonds. The β′ subunit binds to DNA.

The holoenzyme is involved in the selection of promoter sites on the DNA and the initiation of RNA synthesis, while the core participates in the phenomenon of elongation.

A single rifampin molecule inhibits the activity of a transcriptase molecule. The enzyme-rifampin combination can be readily dissociated by 6 M guanidine chloride. The activity produced is of the bacteriostatic type. Rifampin binds to the β subunit and prevents the holoenzyme from initiating RNA synthesis.

The holoenzyme-rifamycin combination is obtained by a π-π type interaction between the naphthoquinone nucleus and the aromatic acids of the enzyme, principally the tyrosine residues. In the β subunit, the rifamycins bind to the basic amino acids in a cavity of 1.4 to 1.9 nm by means of hydroxyl groups at positions 1 and 2. At the same time, the aliphatic chain of the antibiotic inserts itself inside the enzyme and allows the hydroxyl fragments at positions 9 and 10 to enter into allosteric competition for the binding site of the enzyme on the RNA chain in the process of formation, the hydroxyl group at position 9 playing a more important role than the hydroxyl at position 10. The tertiary complex of DNA, RNA, and holoenzyme is thus destabilized.

Analysis of the structure-activity relationships has revealed that the hydroxyl groups at positions 1, 2, 9, and 10 are essential for the antibacterial activity of the rifamycins. Groups 1 (which may be in a quinone form) and 2 are phenols; the groups at positions 9 (C-23) and 10 (C-21) are alcohols. In order to be active, the molecule must have the four phenol hydroxyl groups binding to the enzyme by means of hydrogen bonds.

In support of this hypothesis, esterification of the hydroxyl groups at positions 9 and 10 abolishes any antibacterial activity.

The substituents introduced at position 3 of the antibiotic alter the inhibitory activity of the antibiotic against transcriptase by modifying the π-π interaction. The substituents may in particular modify the polarity of hydroxyls 1 and 2 by controlling the acidity of the O(1)-O(2) system. The reduction of the double bonds of the aliphatic chain suppresses the antibacterial activity, as it decreases the rigidity of the tertiary structure and modifies the oxidative stress interaction of the hydroxyl groups with RNA polymerase.

9.2.1. Oxidative Stress

The bactericidal activity is probably based on the combination of two mechanisms: stability of the holoenzyme-rifamycin bond and superoxide anion formation. The quinone ring of the rifamycins may be in either the hydroquinone (reduced) or quinone (oxidized) form, corresponding to rifamycins SV and S, respectively.

Oxidation of rifamycin SV in the presence of oxygen and Mn^{2+} causes the production of superoxide anion O_2^- and hydrogen peroxide (H_2O_2). The release of OH° hydroxyl radicals contributes to the bactericidal activity (Fig. 8).

9.3. Other Proteins

Apart from specific binding to the β subunit of bacterial RNA polymerase, the rifamycins bind to other bacterial proteins whose exact role remains poorly elucidated.

10. RESISTANCE

Enteric gram-negative bacilli and *Pseudomonas* spp. are resistant to rifampin because of its poor outer membrane penetration. In fact, *E. coli* RNA polymerase is highly

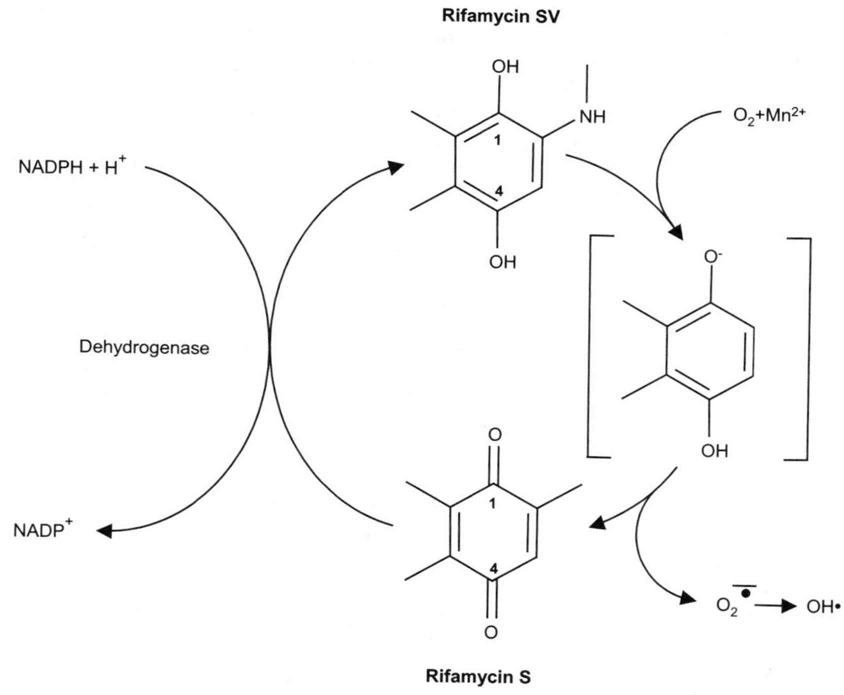

Figure 8 Production of free radicals

susceptible to the action of rifampin. A number of strains of gram-positive bacteria become resistant by chromosomal mutation. In *E. coli*, the antibiotic no longer binds to the enzyme, in particular because of the fact that the β subunit is modified by isolated mutations of amino acids.

Rifampin-resistant mutants may be obtained in vitro and in vivo with the majority of bacterial species. Resistance appears in a single stage.

The appearance of resistant mutants among strains of *M. tuberculosis* is rare, on the order of 10^{-10}.

The use of rifampin as monotherapy is associated with the rapid appearance of resistant mutants among common pathogens, particularly *Staphylococcus aureus*, *Streptococcus pyogenes*, *Streptococcus pneumoniae*, and *Neisseria meningitidis* (10^{-7}). Combination of rifampin with another antibacterial agent delays the emergence of resistant strains but does not prevent it, as has been demonstrated with *S. aureus*.

A number of semisynthetic molecules have been prepared to overcome the resistance to rifampin, particularly with so-called lipophilic rifamycins characterized by a hindering and lipophilic aromatic nucleus at position 3 of the naphthalene nucleus. Some of these molecules have good activity against rifampin-resistant strains of *S. aureus*. However, they have the drawback that they inhibit the action of a number of polymerases of eukaryotic cells. One compound, AF/103, has been tested. Another approach has been to prepare dimeric molecules such as rifamazine, obtained by condensation of two molecules of 3-formylrifamycin SV.

10.1. *S. pneumoniae*

In South Africa, for patients having an *S. pneumoniae* strain resistant to rifampin, the isolate was shown to be due to missense mutations within the *ropB* gene. Sequence analysis of 24 rifampin-resitant isolates revealed the presence of mutations within cluster I as well as novel mutations in an area designated cluster III.

Rifampin is widely used for treatment of tubercle bacilli, especially in children. The majority of children have colonization with rifampin-resistant pneumococci in the nasopharynx, a fact which results in the bacteria being indirectly exposed to the selective pressure of rifampin.

The mutations within the *ropB* gene appear to cluster into three distinct areas and are generally numbered according to the *E. coli* protein coordinates: cluster I, amino acids 505 to 532, and cluster II, amino acids 560 to 572. For *S. pneumoniae*, cluster I is amino acids 406 to 434 and cluster II is amino acids 523 to 600. These clusters are part of the rifampin binding site.

It was observed that 75% of rifampin-resistant isolates contained cluster I mutations (both Asp512→Asn and His425→Asn [*E. coli* His526]). The substitution Asp425→Asn has been reported to confer low-level resistance to rifampin (MIC, 8 μg/ml) on *S. pneumoniae* and *M. tuberculosis*. The mutation His425→Asn has been reported for *S. pneumoniae*, *N. meningitidis*, and *M. tuberculosis*. *S. pneumoniae* and *M. tuberculosis* isolates resistant to rifampin that did not contain mutations in cluster I or cluster II have been noticed. Eight mutations have been described: Arg523→Lys, Glu526→Ala, Iso534→Val, Asn549→Ser, Asn595→Glu, Ile550→Ser, Gln597→Lys, and Tyr600→Phe. Cluster II was renamed cluster III in *S. pneumoniae*, but it is different from cluster III of *E. coli*.

In a Spanish hospital study from 1979 to 1990, it was found that only 0.1% of *S. pneumoniae* isolates were resistant to rifampin. A similar low prevalence of rifampin resistance was found in the United States (0.5%) and in Brazil (3.1%).

Rifampin is not routinely used in the treatment of pneumococcal infections, although it is an alternative in combination with vancomycin or cefotaxime or ceftriaxone in the treatment of multidrug-resistant pneumococcal infections.

10.2. *S. aureus*

Two mutational changes, His526→Asn in cluster I and Ser574→Leu in cluster II, are responsible for high-level rifampin resistance.

10.3. *S. pyogenes*

Rifampin may be an alternative therapy in penicillin V failures, including pharyngeal carriage. Rifampin-resistant strains represent 0.31% of clinical *S. pyogenes* isolates in Spain (MIC, 32 μg/ml). Mutations occur at His425→Asp (*E. coli* His526). Other mutations leading to rifampin resistance have been reported, such as Ser421→Leu. Two base pair changes in the *ropB* gene resulted in amino acid substitutions in cluster I at position 522 (Ser522→Leu) leading to rifampin resistance.

10.4. *Treponema pallidum*

Rifampin resistance is due to a mutation in the *ropB* gene in cluster I (amino acids 507 to 533): S532→N.

10.5. *Rickettsia conorii*

R. conorii belongs to the spotted fever group of *Rickettsia*. Rifampin resistance is due to mutation in the *ropB* gene: Phe973→Leu. The MIC for *R. conorii* is below 1 μg/ml, and the Typhi group (*Rickettsia typhi* and *Rickettsia prowazekii*) is susceptible to rifampin; however the spotted-fever group *rickettsiae* (*R. montanensis, R. massiliae, R. aeschlimannii*, and *R. rhipicephali*) are resistant to rifampin, with MICs of 2 to 4 μg/ml.

10.6. *Rhodococcus equi*

R. equi is highly susceptible to rifampin, with a MIC at which 50% of isolates tested are inhibited (MIC_{50} and MIC_{90} of 0.06 and 64 to 128 μg/ml).

The first reported *R. equi* infection in a human occurred in 1967 in an immunosuppressed patient. A combination of erythromycin and rifampin is considered to be effective for treating *R. equi* infection.

Resistance to rifampin is still rare but has been reported. High-level resistance to rifampin involved a Ser531→Trp mutation or a His526→Tyr mutation in the *ropB* gene. Low-level rifampin resistance involved a Ser 509→Pro mutation. Resistance of *R. equi* to erythromycin is still rare. Most human patients who have developed *R. equi* infections are known to have been in contact with herbivores, their manure, or soil. On the other hand, many AIDS patients are treated with rifampin for tuberculosis.

11. IN VITRO ACTIVITY

The natural spectrum of the ansamycins covers mycobacteria, gram-positive and gram-negative cocci, intracellular bacteria, and fastidious gram-negative bacilli, such as *Haemophilus* and *Moraxella* spp. The ansamycins have weak activity against enteric gram-negative bacilli and nonfermenting gram-negative bacteria (*Pseudomonas* and *Acinetobacter* spp., *Stenotrophomonas maltophilia*, etc.). Rifampin is inactive against *Yersinia pestis* (MIC_{50} and MIC_{90}, 8.0 and 16 μg/ml).

Rifapentine is less active against gram-positive and gram-negative cocci than rifampin, but it is more active against *M. tuberculosis, M. avium* complex, *Mycobacterium leprae*, and *Chlamydia trachomatis* (Tables 4 and 5). Rifabutin is 2.5 times more active than rifampin against *M. tuberculosis* (Table 6). CGP-27557 and rifapentine have fourfold greater activity than rifampin against rifampin-susceptible strains. CGP-7040 and CGP-29861 have eightfold greater activity than rifampin against *M. tuberculosis*. Rifabutin is active only against 31% of rifampin-resistant strains, but the MICs are higher (Table 7).

CGP-4832 is the 3-morpholine derivative of rifamycin SV. This molecule is up to 400 times more active than rifampin against enterobacteria. Its activity not only is linked to inhibition of DNA polymerase but also is associated with improved parietal penetration that seems to be related to a transporter.

The benzoxazinorifamycin derivatives, rifalazil, etc. (Fig. 9), are more active than rifampin against mycobacteria. However, they are inactive against *Mycobacterium chelonae* and *Mycobacterium fortuitum* (Table 8). Some derivatives have moderate activity against rifampin-resistant strains of *M. tuberculosis*. Two metabolites have been identified, the desacetyl (KRM-1671) and the hydroxy (KRM-1690).

Rifalazil exhibits high activity against *Helicobacter pylori* irrespective of the pH of the medium (pH 7.4, MIC = 0.004 μg/ml; pH 5.4, MIC = 0.002 μg/ml). Rifalazil also exerts good activity against *Chlamydia pneumoniae*, with a MIC of 0.0006 μg/ml (HeLa cell line), and *C. trachomatis* (MIC, 0.0025 μg/ml).

A new semisynthetic derivative of rifamycin SV has recently been described: T-9. This is 3(4-cinnamyl-1-piperazinyl)iminomethyl (Fig. 10).

T-9 is four times more active than rifampin against the H_{RV37} strain of *M. tuberculosis* (MIC, 0.03 versus 0.25 μg/ml), but it exhibits cross-resistance with rifampin. It is active against strains resistant to ethambutol (MIC, ≤0.06 μg/ml) and isoniazid (MIC, 0.03 μg/ml) and strains that are multiresistant to drugs other than rifampin (MIC, 0.06 μg/ml). In animals, it is 3 log units more active than rifampin (5 versus 20 mg/kg) (Geeta et al., 1995). Against strains of *M. leprae*, T-9 is twice as active as rifampin and rifabutin (MIC, ~0.1 μg/ml). Like rifabutin but unlike rifampin, T-9 acts synergistically with ofloxacin (Dhople, 1995).

12. PLASMA PHARMACOKINETICS

12.1. Rifabutin

Rifabutin is weakly absorbed orally. About 10 to 20% of the administered dose is absorbed. After oral administration, the peak concentrations in plasma are obtained in 2.0 to 3.0 h. They are low, on the order of 0.5 to 1.0 μg/ml depending on the administered dose (300 to 1,200 mg). After intravenous administration, plasma clearance is 10 to 18 liters/h and renal clearance is on the order of 1.5 liters/h. Nonrenal clearance is 8.8 liters/h (147 ml/min). The volume of distribution is 8 to 9 liters/kg. About 10% of the administered dose is eliminated unchanged in the urine, and 20% is eliminated in the form of active or inactive metabolites. Protein binding is on the order of 71%. The apparent elimination half-life is on the order of 38 h (Table 9). After administration of a single dose of 600 mg orally, the peak concentration of rifabutin in serum is 0.6 μg/ml and that of the principal metabolite is 0.05 μg/ml. After administration of rifabutin labeled with ^{14}C on the 9′ carbon, about 70% of the radioactivity is recovered in the urine in 4 days and 30% is recovered in the feces, a small proportion being eliminated in the expired air. Five to ten percent of the administered dose is eliminated in the form of rifabutin. A very small proportion (<1%) is eliminated in the form of glucuroconjugated rifabutin. About 20 metabolites have been detected. Rifabutin undergoes either deacetylation at position 25 of the aliphatic chain or oxidation, particularly at positions 30, 31, and 32 of the chain on the piperidine nucleus

Table 4 In vitro activity of ansamycins

Microorganism	MIC$_{50}$ (μg/ml)					
	Rifamycin SV	Rifamide	Rifampin	Rifabutin	Rifapentine	Rifaximin
S. aureus	0.01	0.01	0.002	0.002	0.05	0.01–1.5
Staphylococcus epidermidis			0.01		0.05	
S. pyogenes	0.002	0.01	0.02		0.05	
S. pneumoniae	0.1	0.02	0.01		0.05	
S. agalactiae	0.1	0.05	0.03–0.5		0.1	
Enterococcus faecalis	0.8	0.1	0.25	0.5	0.05	
N. gonorrhoeae	0.1–1	0.05	0.03–16	0.39	0.03	
N. meningitidis	0.1–10	0.05	0.03–128	0.09	0.5	
Moraxella catarrhalis	≤1–10	0.02	0.001		0.06	
Haemophilus influenzae	≤1	0.02	0.2–0.4	0.6	0.5	
Bacillus anthracis	0.1–1	0.2	0.01		0.01	
Corynebacterium diphtheriae	0.01–0.1		0.1–5.0			
H. ducreyi			<0.002–0.1			
E. coli	25	10	10	10	10	
Pseudomonas aeruginosa	50	50	8–32	5	50	
C. meningosepticum			0.25–2			
L. monocytogenes			0.04		0.01	
Brucella melitensis	>1–10	2.0	0.8–12			
Brucella abortus	>10	10	0.125			
Bordetella pertussis	1–10		0.05		0.5	
Pasteurella multocida		0.5	>100			
Nocardia asteroides	>10	>100	0.012		8.0	
M. tuberculosis	0.05	0.2	0.2	0.006	0.01	
M. avium		10	4	1	2	
C. trachomatis		1	0.007		0.06	
C. pneumoniae			0.01		0.06	
C. psittaci			0.32		0.32	
B. fragilis			<0.12	<0.12	<0.12	
Clostridium perfringens			<0.12	<0.12	<0.12	
L. pneumophila			0.018	0.078	0.008	
R. prowazekii			0.01			
H. pylori			1.0		1.0	
C. burnetii			0.08			
Mycoplasma pneumoniae			64		≥128	
Mycoplasma genitalium			32		≥128	
Erysipelothrix rhusiopathiae			>10			
C. difficile			<0.006–1		0.08	<0.01–1
Vibrio cholerae			>0.01–1		2	
Campylobacter jejuni			0.1–1			0.1–1

Table 5 In vitro activity of ansamycins

Microorganism[a]	MIC$_{50}$ (μg/ml)				
	CGP-7040	CGP-27557	CGP-29861	SPA-S-565	CGP-4832
S. aureus	0.02	0.002	0.005	0.01	0.01
S. pyogenes	0.05	0.01	0.01	0.06	0.001
E. faecalis	16	1.0	4.0		1.0
E. coli	>128	4.0	16	32	8.0
P. aeruginosa	16	4.0	8.0		4.0
M. tuberculosis H_{37RV} RIF^s	0.03	0.03	0.03	0.016	
M. tuberculosis H_{37RV} RIF^r	>32	>32	>32		
M. avium	0.03–0.25	0.25–4.0	0.25–1.0		

[a]RIF, rifampin.

Table 6 Activities of rifapentine, rifampin, and R-76-1 against mycobacteria

Microorganism	MIC (μg/ml)		
	Rifapentine	Rifampin	R-76-1
M. tuberculosis H_{37RV}	1.56	6.25	0.39
M. bovis	1.56	6.25	0.20
M. avium	3.13	12.5	0.78
M. intracellulare	1.56	0.78	0.39

Table 7 Comparative in vitro activities of ansamycins against mycobacteria

Compound	MIC (μg/ml)		
	M. tuberculosis	*M. microti*	Macrophages
Rifampin	0.02	0.02	0.10
Rifabutin	0.02	0.007	0.02
Rifapentine	0.017	0.01	0.23
FCE-22807	0.008	0.01	0.15

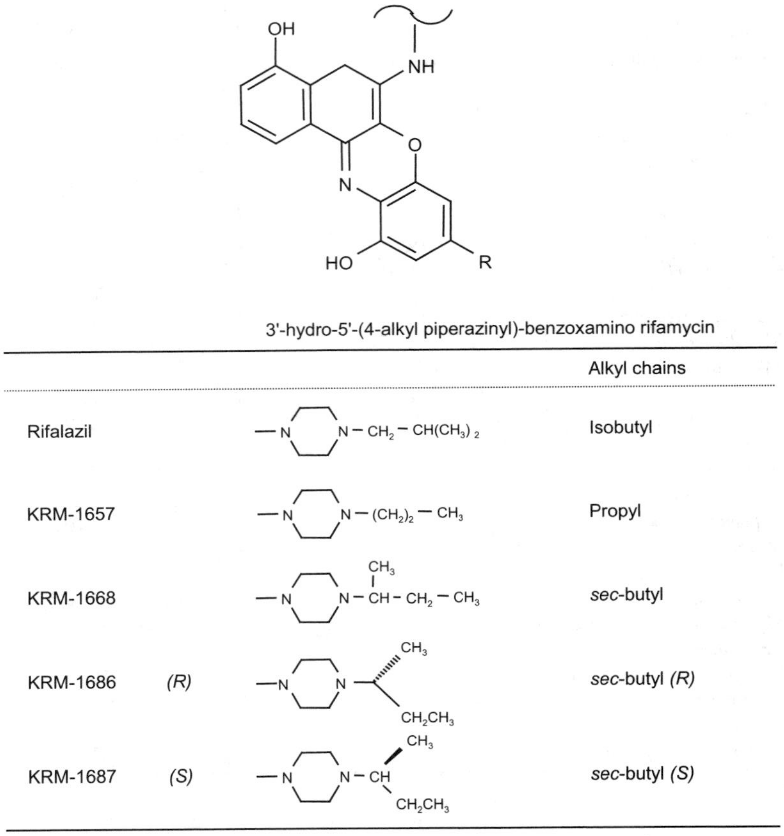

3'-hydro-5'-(4-alkyl piperazinyl)-benzoxamino rifamycin

		R	Alkyl chains
Rifalazil		$-N(C_4H_8)N-CH_2-CH(CH_3)_2$	Isobutyl
KRM-1657		$-N(C_4H_8)N-(CH_2)_2-CH_3$	Propyl
KRM-1668		$-N(C_4H_8)N-CH(CH_3)-CH_2-CH_3$	*sec*-butyl
KRM-1686	*(R)*	$-N(C_4H_8)N-CH(CH_3)CH_2CH_3$	*sec*-butyl *(R)*
KRM-1687	*(S)*	$-N(C_4H_8)N-CH(CH_3)CH_2CH_3$	*sec*-butyl *(S)*

Figure 9 Benzoxazinorifamycin series

Table 8 In vitro activities of benzoxazinorifamycin derivatives against mycobacteria

Microorganism	MIC (μg/ml)					
	KRM-1648	KRM-16657	KRM-1668	KRM-1686	KRM-1687	Rifampin
M. tuberculosis RIF[s][a]	<0.01	<0.01	<0.01	<0.01	<0.01	0.2
M. tuberculosis RIF[r]	12.5	1.56	3.13	1.56	1.56	>100
M. avium	0.05	0.1	0.1	0.1	0.1	1.56
M. fortuitum	>100	25	25	6.25	25	>100
M. marinum	≤0.01	0.02	0.05	0.02	0.05	1.56
M. kansasii	≤0.01	≤0.01	0.02	≤0.01	0.02	0.4
M. chelonae subsp. *abscessus*, *M. chelonae* subsp. *chelonae*	>100	>100	>100	>100	>100	>100

[a]RIF, rifampin.

Rifamycin SV

CH=N—N N—N—C_6H_5—CH=CH—CH_2

Figure 10 T9

Table 9 Comparative pharmacokinetics of the ansamycins orally

Compound	Dose (mg)	C_{max} (µg/ml)	T_{max} (h)	AUC (µg·h/ml)	$t_{1/2}$ (h)	Protein binding (%)	Urinary elimination (%)
Rifampin	600	8.52	3.19	73.95	2.2		
	900	14.91	2.84	117.93	2.5	70–80	~10
	1,200	21.45	2.58	195.54	4.0		
Rifabutin	150	0.19	3.0	2.51			
	300	0.49	4.0	1.8	38	71	<10
	600	0.60	4.0	1.7	38		
	900		4.0	1.7	32		
	1,200	0.9	4.0	1.7	38		
Rifapentine	300	11.1	4.8	276	14.1		
	450	13.1	6.1	378	17.8	97	
	600	14.5	5.0	542	24.5		
CGP-7040	150	1.25	7.0	106.8	42.5	<10	
	300	1.99	8.0	61.4	45.7	<10	
	600	5.58	8.0	301.3	35.9		<10
CGP-27557	150	0.17	3.0	5.0		<10	
	300	0.59	3.0	8.5	4.9	<10	
	600	3.17	3.0	17.4	7.1	<10	
CGP-29861	600	6.8	3.0	367.6	40		<10

(*N*-oxide). The main metabolite is 25-*O*-desacetylrifabutin, accounting for 1.7% of the administered dose, the other derivatives being 31-hydroxyrifabutin, 30-hydroxyrifabutin, 32-hydroxydesacetylrifabutin, and 25-*O*-desacetyl-*N*-oxide rifabutin. All of the other metabolites account for about 17% of the administered dose (Fig. 11). Food does not significantly affect the absorption of rifabutin.

12.2. Rifamide

Oral absorption of rifamide is erratic. Some volunteers have good absorption with relatively high peak concentrations in plasma after a dose of 0.5 or 1.0 g, but the majority of volunteers absorb part of rifamide tablets.

After administration of 100, 150, 250, or 500 mg intramuscularly, the peak concentration in serum (1.04 to 3.97 µg/ml) is reached in 1.0 h. Residual concentrations are 0.1 µg/ml at 6 h; only after injection of 0.5 g is it possible to measure 0.3 µg of rifamide per ml at 8 h.

After administration of 150 mg intravenously, the levels after 1 h are 1.0 µg/ml and those after 8 h are 0.01 µg/ml. Urinary elimination is 4 to 7% of the administered dose. Eight percent of the elimination occurs in the bile.

12.3. Rifamycin SV

In order to prevent the oxidation of rifamycin SV to rifamycin S, a reducing agent such as ascorbic acid or sodium bisulfate must be added to the solution. It is difficult to reconstitute rifamycin SV in an aqueous solution, as the long-term local tolerance is poor due to traces of rifamycin S.

After oral administration of a dose of 500 mg of rifamycin SV, levels in plasma are less than 0.1 µg/ml. They are higher in cirrhotic patients, rising 2 µg/ml 1 h after administration. Peak concentrations in plasma after intramuscular administration are variable.

After a dose of 500 mg, the mean peak concentration in plasma is about 4.0 µg/ml at 1 h, with a residual concentration of 0.3 µg/ml at 6 h.

In children, a peak concentration in plasma of 0.9 to 1.0 µg/ml is reached within 30 min after administration of 4 mg/kg but no rifamycin SV is detectable after 5 h.

Levels of 15 to 20 µg/ml and of 132 µg/ml are observed after intravenous infusion of 250 and 500 mg of rifamycin SV, respectively. At the end of the first hour, the levels are 0.5 and 28.6 µg/ml for doses of 250 and 500 mg, respectively. The apparent elimination half-life is 1.46 h.

Rifamycin SV is extensively distributed in cerebrospinal fluid, pleural fluid, and ascites fluid.

12.4. Rifapentine

After administration of single doses of 300, 450, and 600 mg of rifapentine, levels in plasma can be measured from the first hour (0.4, 2.3, and 3.7 µg/ml, respectively). The peak concentrations in plasma are high (11.1, 13.1, and 14.5 µg/ml) and late to appear, occurring after between 4.8 and 6.1 h. There is no linearity after administration of ascending doses (Table 9). Food increases the absorption of rifapentine. As rifapentine is insoluble in water, it is possible that only a fraction dissolves in the digestive tract, thus explaining the incomplete absorption of the drug.

The apparent elimination half-life increases with the administered dose (14.4 to 24.5 h), as has been shown with rifampin. Only 6 to 18% of the administered dose is eliminated in the urine in 72 h.

The salivary concentration is rarely greater than 0.5 µg/ml, probably related to the high plasma protein binding (>90%) and its lipophilic nature.

Rifapentine has a principal metabolite, 25-desacetylrifapentine.

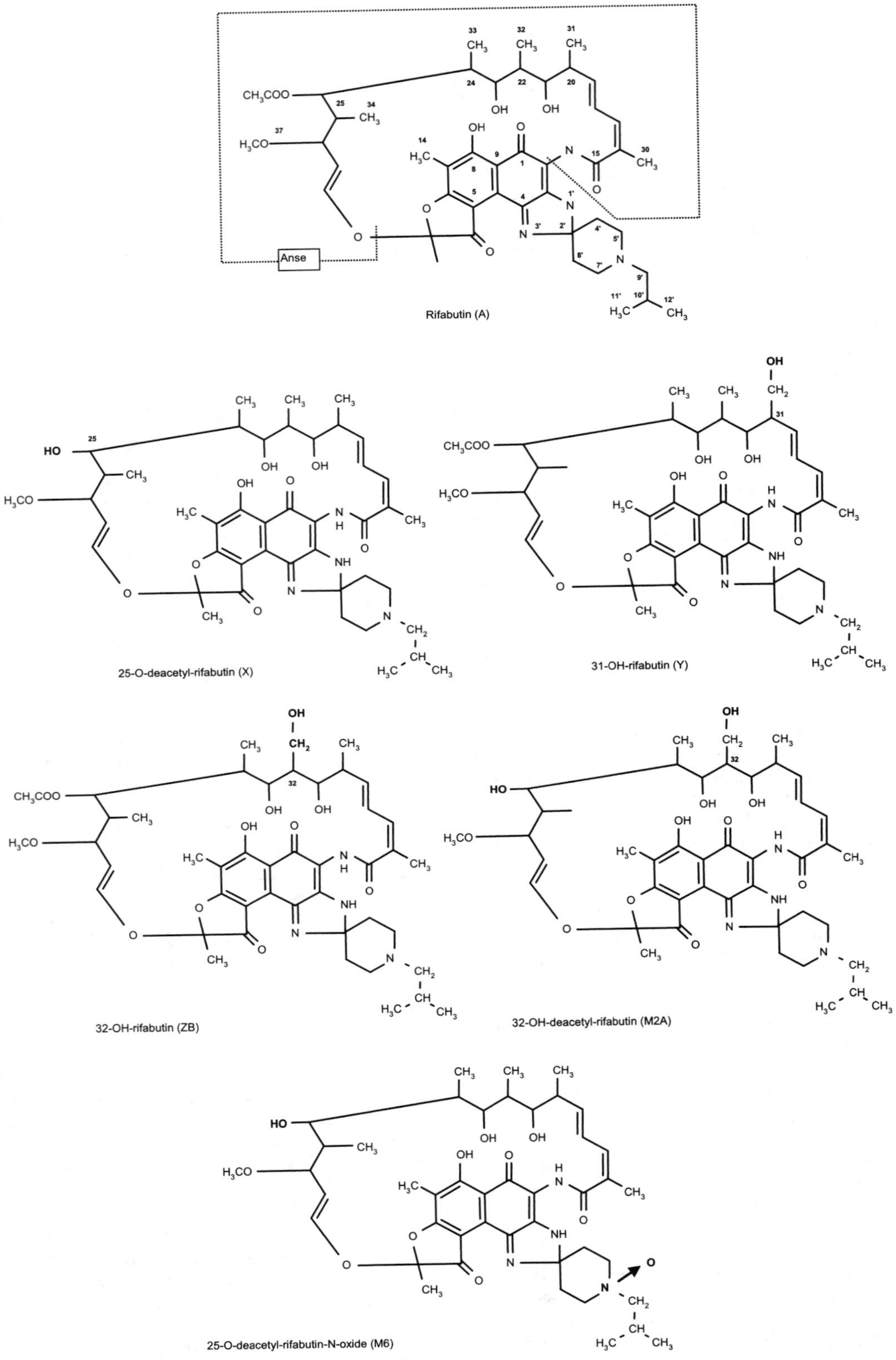

Rifabutin (A)

25-O-deacetyl-rifabutin (X)

31-OH-rifabutin (Y)

32-OH-rifabutin (ZB)

32-OH-deacetyl-rifabutin (M2A)

25-O-deacetyl-rifabutin-N-oxide (M6)

Figure 11 Metabolism of rifabutin

12.5. Derivatives CGP-7040, CGP-27557, and CGP-29861

After administration of single oral doses of 150, 300, and 600 mg of CGP-7040, CGP-27557, and CGP-29861, the concentrations in plasma increase in a dose-dependent manner. CGP-27557 has the shortest apparent elimination half-life (7 to 9 h), whereas those of CGP-7040 and CGP-27557 are 30 and 40 h, respectively. Peak concentrations in plasma are between 3 and 6 μg/ml (capsules), with a long time to maximum concentration. Absorption of CGP-29861 increases with food. Urinary elimination is weak, on the order of 2% (Table 9).

12.6. Rifampin

12.6.1. Absorption

The solubility of rifampin in water increases as the pH decreases. At acid pH (gastric secretion, pH ~2), the solubility is 10 g/100 ml. Absorption of rifampin varies with the gastric acidity. If the gastric pH is reduced by administration of histamine to volunteers (15 min before administration of rifampin), the peak concentration in serum is 9.7 ± 1.7 μg/ml (mean ± standard deviation) (time to maximum concentration, about 2 h) and the area under the curve from 0 to 24 h (AUC_{0-24h}) is 48.2 μg·h/ml. If the gastric pH is increased by administering 2.0 g of $NaHCO_3$ to volunteers, the quantity of rifampin absorbed is reduced by half but the absorption rate is unchanged; the peak concentration in serum is 4.1 ± 1.0 μg/ml, with an AUC_{0-12h} of 23.5 μg·h/ml (Table 10).

There is a delay in the absorption of rifampin in fasting subjects who have undergone total or subtotal gastrectomy or who are suffering from celiac disease or diverticulosis of the small intestine, but the quantity of product absorbed is identical (Table 11).

Food reduces the quantity of rifampin absorbed and delays absorption; the peak concentration in plasma is reduced by about 30%.

12.6.2. Pharmacokinetics

After single doses of 600, 900, and 1,200 mg of rifampin, the peak concentrations in plasma are 8.5, 14.9, and 21.4 μg/ml, respectively, and are reached in about 3 h. The apparent elimination half-life is 2 to 4.0 h.

After intravenous administration in the form of a 3-h infusion of a dose of 600 mg of rifampin, the apparent elimination half-life is 2.9 h, with an AUC_{0-12} of 64.1 μg·h/ml.

12.6.3. Elimination

Rifampin is metabolized hepatically by deacetylation at C-25. This metabolite is not a polar molecule, which increases its possibility of being eliminated in the bile. Hydrolysis in the urine yields 3-formylrifampin (Fig. 12).

The peak biliary concentration is reached in 2 to 3 h. An increase in the dose of rifampin does not increase biliary elimination of the product, suggesting that there is a phenomenon of saturation of the capacity for hepatic elimination. In the bile, 50 to 79% is 25-desacetylrifampin 3 to 4 h after administration of rifampin, and 88% is 25-desacetylrifampin at 5 h.

Gastrointestinal absorption of 25-desacetylrifampin is weak. There is, however, an enterohepatic cycle, as concentrations of 4.0 and 0.8 μg of each rifampin per ml are detected in the portal vein and in the general circulation after administration of 300 mg of rifampin.

Renal clearance is 12% of that by glomerular filtration. If biliary clearance of rifampin is overwhelmed, the quantity of rifampin eliminated in the urine increases.

The quantity of 25-desacetylrifampin eliminated in the urine decreases after repeated doses; the total quantity of product eliminated in 12 h may be reduced by 50% after administration of rifampin for 7 days. A glucuroconjugated derivative of rifampin has also been detected in the urine.

About 7% of rifampin is hydrolyzed to 3-formylrifampin, and an uncertain quantity is oxidized to quinone.

12.6.4. Repeated-Dose Pharmacokinetics

Oral or parenteral administration of repeated doses of rifampin causes reductions in the concentrations in serum and apparent elimination half-life and an increase in the plasma clearance within a few days; the volume of distribution remains unchanged. This effect is apparent from the

Table 10 Pharmacokinetics of rifampin as a function of gastric pH

Condition	Dose (mg)	C_{max} (μg/ml)	T_{max} (h)	AUC (μg·h/ml)
+ Histamine (pH acid)	300	9.7 ± 1.7	2.0	48.2
+ $NaHCO_3$, fasting	300	4.1 ± 1.0	2.0	23.5
	450	9.5	2.0	45.2
+ $NaHCO_3$, fed	450	5.8	4.0	22.9
Food effect				
Fasting	600	8.6	2.0	45.5
Fed	600	6.6	4.0	35.1

Table 11 Pharmacokinetics of rifampin with underlying gastrointestinal diseases

Subjects	*n*	Dose (mg)	T_{max} (h)	AUC (μg·h/ml)
Healthy volunteers	6	450	1.7	30.7
Patients undergoing gastrectomy (subtotal)	6	450	2.7	29.5
Healthy volunteers	10	300	1.5	21.6
Patients with:				
Celiac disease	9	300	3.0	22.1
Diverticulosis	9	300	3.0	21.7
Crohn's disease	5	300	1.5	21.9

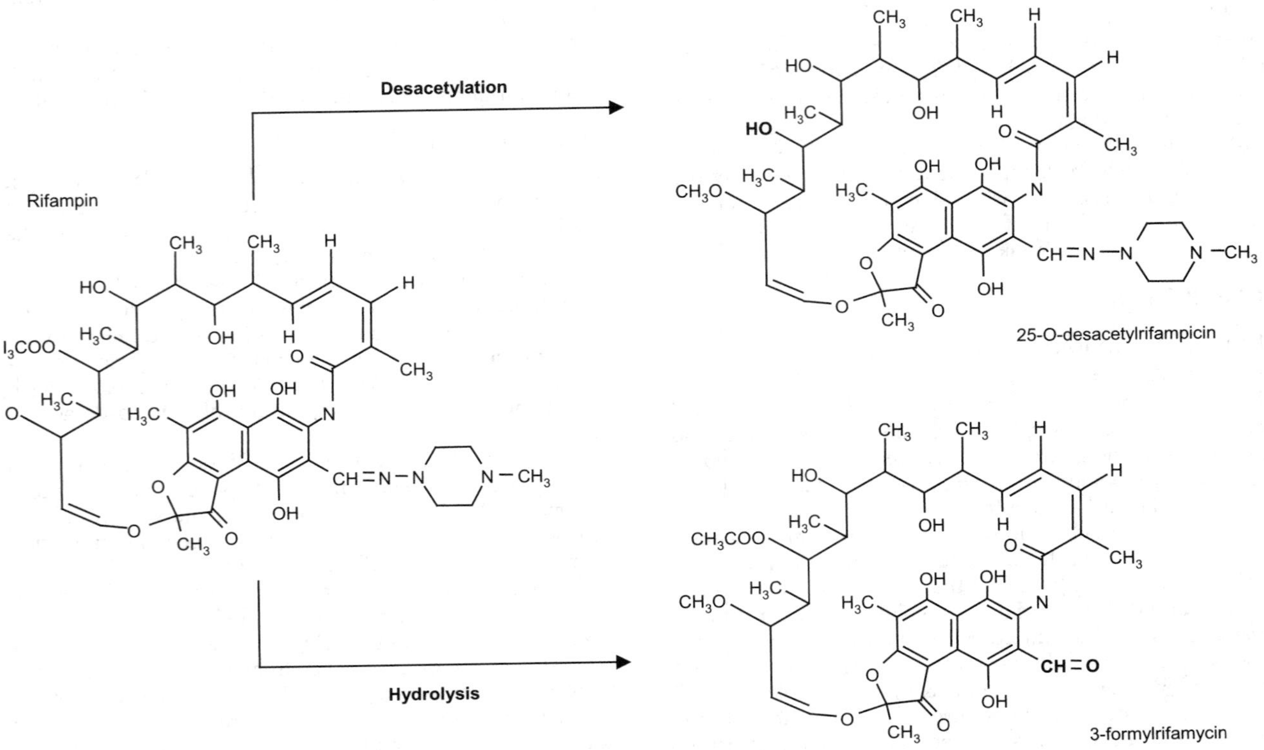

Rifampin

Desacetylation

25-O-desacetylrifampicin

Hydrolysis

3-formylrifamycin

Figure 12 Principal metabolites of rifampin

sixth day. The phenomenon is due to an increase in metabolic autoinduction. A return to normal occurs 30 days after the discontinuation of treatment. Table 12 shows the pharmacokinetics of rifampin after repeated doses.

The bioavailability of the oral form is 93%, decreasing to 68% after the third week of administration.

After multiple doses, the AUCs of the two metabolites, 25-desacetylrifampin and 3-formylrifampin, decrease. It is, however, difficult to assess accurately the apparent volume of distribution and the plasma clearance, as it is difficult to determine the exact quantities of these products in the body.

12.6.5. Pharmacokinetics in Children

The concentrations of rifampin in the umbilical cord are 12 to 33% of those in the maternal plasma.

There are few pharmacokinetic studies for children.

McCracken et al. studied the pharmacokinetics of rifampin in children aged 6 to 58 months. After administration of 10 mg of a suspension of rifampin per kg of body weight, the peak concentration was 10.7 μg/ml and was reached in 1 h; the apparent elimination half-life was about 2.9 h, with an AUC of 56 μg·h/ml. These values are similar to those obtained after a dose of 600 mg in adults (Table 13).

Table 12 Pharmacokinetics of rifampin (600 mg) after repeated doses

Route	Days	AUC (μg·h/ml)	$t_{1/2}$ (h)	CL_P (liters/h)	V (liters)	Bioavailability (%)
Intravenous	2	108.7 ± 31.4	2.8	5.9 ± 1.69	25 ± 7.4	
	9	87.4 ± 17.4	1.8	7.1 ± 1.59	21.9 ± 9.9	
	23	69.9 ± 28.5	1.51	10 ± 4.65	18.7 ± 3.5	
Oral	2	116 ± 29.2	3.14	5.48 ± 1.46	25.3 ± 6.8	94.8 ± 17.4
	9	70.2 ± 17.1	2.09	9.02 ± 2.37	27.3 ± 6.7	86.3 ± 37.3
	23	81.3 ± 24.3	2.07	8.03 ± 2.71	23.6 ± 4.7	70.5 ± 27

Table 13 Pharmacokinetics of rifampin in children

Subjects	Dose	C_{max} (μg/ml)	C_{24} (μg/ml)	T_{max} (h)	AUC (μg·h/ml)
Adults	600 mg	9.0	0.78	2	45–65
Infants and children	10 mg/kg	10.7		1	56
Neonates	10 mg/kg	6.0		8	

In neonates, the pharmacokinetics are different from those in children and infants.

Administration of a dose of 10 mg of rifampin per kg yields a peak concentration in plasma of 6 μg/ml reached after 8 h, with a delay in urinary elimination. After multiple doses, the maximum concentration in serum is higher (12 μg/ml) and the time to maximum concentration is 2 h, with an increase in the AUC and urinary elimination. These data suggest the possibility of accumulation of rifampin in neonates. This is probably due to hepatic immaturity.

12.6.6. Pharmacokinetics in Patients with Hepatic and Renal Insufficiency

Hepatic conditions modify the metabolism of rifampin. In cirrhotic patients (with a portacaval shunt), the quantity of rifampin that does not pass through the liver increases. The amount of 25-desacetylrifampin decreases in parenchymatous lesions (hepatitis). Biliary atresia causes a important reduction in the biliary elimination of rifampin and its metabolites. The result is an increase in the concentration in plasma of rifampin and an increase in its apparent elimination half-life (Table 14).

Renal clearance of rifampin is reduced in patients with renal insufficiency, but there is no significant accumulation of rifampin in plasma (Table 15).

It does not appear to be necessary to modify the doses of rifampin in patients undergoing hemodialysis or patients on peritoneal dialysis.

12.6.7. Protein Binding

The plasma protein binding of rifampin has been determined by all of the known methods: ultracentrifugation, ultrafiltration, dialysis, spectrophotometry, radioisotopes, etc.

The published values show major variability: 57 to 80% after ultracentrifugation, 79 to 90% after ultrafiltration, and 4 to 92% after dialysis.

Rifampin binds principally to albumin, and a small proportion binds to gamma globulins and fibrinogen.

12.6.8. Pharmacokinetics in Malnourished Subjects

Rifampin is one of the pivotal drugs in the treatment of tuberculosis. Tuberculosis is one of the scourges of poor countries. Polasa et al. (1984) investigated the pharmacokinetics of rifampin in tuberculous and malnourished patients. Patients received a single oral 10-mg/kg dose of rifampin. In malnourished patients the AUC was significantly reduced and the peak concentration in plasma was half that in healthy subjects. The quantity of protein-bound rifampin was lower, but there was a correlation with plasma protein levels, which were significantly reduced. The outcome was a higher level of circulating free rifampin, which might partially offset the lower bioavailability. Table 16 shows the pharmacokinetics of rifampin in malnourished patients.

12.6.9. Tissue Distribution of Rifampin

The tissue distribution of rifampin is affected by the fact that only 25% of the molecule is ionized at physiological pH (negative charge) and that it is highly liposoluble. High concentrations of rifampin, greater than those in plasma, have been measured in the bile (300 to 400 μg/ml at 6 h after a dose of 600 mg), in the urine (>450 μg/ml at 6 h after 450 mg), and in hepatic tissue (36 mg/kg after 450 mg). Likewise, high concentrations have been detected in the pulmonary parenchyma, in the gallbladder wall, in the wall of the stomach, and in the extracellular fluid.

Levels of 12 μg/ml have been measured in the bronchial secretions after a dosage of 900 mg daily in tuberculous patients.

The salivary concentration is high: 1.7 μg/ml (0.54 to 7.2 μg/ml) 2 h after administration of 10 mg/kg. The peak concentration in tears is on the order of 7.2 μg/ml, identical to that in serum. After a single dose of 600 mg of rifampin the concentration in bone is 3.35 ± 0.75 mg/kg.

There is extensive passage into the cerebrospinal fluid in the presence of inflamed meninges. The concentration in the cerebrospinal fluid of patients suffering from tuberculous meningitis after administration of 600 mg of rifampin daily is 0.18 to 1.37 μg/ml.

12.6.10. Intracellular Concentrations

The ansamycins are extensively concentrated in phagocytic cells (Table 17).

Table 18 shows the pharmacokinetics of rifalazil after a single oral dose.

13. THERAPEUTIC INDICATIONS

Rifampin, rifabutin, and rifapentine are primarily antituberculosis and antileprosy agents. Their use is reviewed in other chapters. Staphylococcal infections are one of the indications of rifampin.

However, because of its antibacterial spectrum, rifampin may be used in other infectious indications, such as *Legionella pneumophila* infections.

13.1. Tuberculosis and Leprosy

Rifampin combined with isoniazid and ethambutol or pyrazinamide is the standard treatment for pulmonary and extrapulmonary tuberculosis.

Table 15 Pharmacokinetics of rifampin in patients with renal insufficiency

Creatinine clearance (ml/min)	AUC_{0-24h} (μg·h/ml)	$t_{1/2}$ (h)
>80	89.1	3.6
50–30	127	5.0
<30	147.3	7.3
<5	173.3	11.0

Table 14 Pharmacokinetics of rifampin in patients with chronic hepatic insufficiency

Subjects	Days	AUC_{0-12h} (μg·h/ml)	$t_{1/2}$ (h)	Urinary elimination (%)
Healthy volunteers	1	83.1	2.9	20.5
	7	55.1	1.8	12.6
Hepatically impaired patients	1	87.3	4.7	9.9
	7	15.2	3.2	11.1

Table 16 Pharmacokinetics of rifampin in malnourished patients

Subjects	C_{max} (μg/ml)	AUC (μg·h/ml)	$t_{1/2}$ (h)	Protein binding (%)
Malnourished patients	5.6 ± 0.5	42.2 ± 4.2	4.6 ± 0.5	65.4 ± 1.7
Healthy volunteers	11.1 ± 1.3	59.1 ± 4.9	4.6 ± 0.6	77.8 ± 2.4

Table 17 Intracellular concentration of rifampin

Compound	Concn (μg/ml) in:	
	PMN[a]	Macrophages
Rifampin	8	5
Rifabutin		14.6
Rifapentine	87.6 ± 3.9	61.4 ± 5.8

[a]PMN, polymorphonuclear leukocytes.

Table 18 Pharmacokinetics of rifalazil

Dose (mg)	C_{max} (ng/ml)	T_{max} (h)	$t_{1/2}$ (h)	AUC (ng·h/ml)
30	17.8	3.1	48.7	504.9
100	58.8	4.0	43.1	1,543
300	115.7	3.0	206.6	5,045

Rifampin is bactericidal against *M. leprae* and belongs to the standard treatment of leprosy.

13.2. Staphylococcal Infections

Staphylococcal endocarditis may be treated with a combination of vancomycin and rifampin or rifampin and oxacillin when treatment with vancomycin or with a β-lactam alone does not produce a rapid therapeutic response. These combinations are particularly useful in vascular prosthesis infections, in endocarditis complicated by a myocardial or peripheral abscess, or when the strain of *S. aureus* is relatively nonsusceptible to vancomycin and/or oxacillin.

Chronic staphylococcal osteomyelitis may be treated with a combination of rifampin and other antistaphylococcal agents.

The combination rifampin-vancomycin has been shown to produce a rapid response in infections of central nervous system shunts due to a coagulase-negative staphylococcal species.

Nasal carriage of *S. aureus* can be reduced by rifampin.

13.3. Infections Due to Gram-Positive Bacteria

13.3.1. Gram-Positive Bacilli

Listeria monocytogenes is responsible for severe infections, particularly meningeal, septicemic, and endocarditic infections. The in vitro results are contradictory, and rifampin generally exhibits only bacteriostatic activity against *L. monocytogenes*. Animal studies have shown good activity.

Infections due to *R. equi* and *Rhodococcus rubropertinctus* respond well to rifampin.

Against *Corynebacterium jeikeium* and *Corynebacterium urealyticum*, rifampin has very variable activity.

13.3.2. Gram-Positive Cocci

Rifampin may be a therapeutic alternative in infections due to *S. pyogenes*. The activity against *Streptococcus agalactiae*, and likewise against enterococci, is only bacteriostatic, while infections due to multiresistant strains of *S. pneumoniae* may respond to treatment with rifampin.

13.4. Infections Due to Gram-Negative Bacteria

13.4.1. Gram-Negative Cocci

Rifampin is recommended in the prevention of infections due to *N. meningitidis*. However, rifampin-resistant strains resulting in a failure of prevention have been described. The combination rifampin-erythromycin has been used successfully in the treatment of acute infections due to *Neisseria gonorrhoeae*.

13.4.2. Gram-Negative Bacilli

The antibacterial spectrum of rifampin does not include enteric gram-negative bacilli, and for this reason it is not indicated in the treatment of these infections.

Several publications have reported therapeutic activity for rifampin in infections due to *Chryseobacterium (Flavobacterium) meningosepticum*.

The combination rifampin-trimethoprim has been used successfully in the treatment of chancroid (*Haemophilus ducreyi*).

The combinations rifampin-doxycycline and rifampin–co-trimoxazole have proved very effective in the treatment of brucellosis.

Rifampin is one of the treatments of *L. pneumophila* pneumonia.

13.4.3. Anaerobic Bacteria

It has been shown that *Clostridium difficile* infections may be treated with the combination rifampin-vancomycin. Experimental murine peritoneal infections with *Bacteroides fragilis* have been treated successfully with rifampin.

13.5. Chlamydiosis

In vitro, *C. trachomatis* is highly susceptible to rifampin, but resistant strains appear rapidly in tissue cultures whether rifampin is used alone or in combination. Clinical studies have shown good activity for rifampin in nongonococcal urethritis or in ocular infections involving topical treatment.

Some publications report good activity for rifampin in *Chlamydia psittaci* infections or in venereal lymphogranulomatosis.

13.6. Other Infections

One publication has reported good activity for rifampin combined with tetracycline in a case of endocarditis due to *Coxiella burnetii*. Some publications report therapeutic activity for rifampin in pneumonia due to actinomycetes.

13.7. Antiviral Activities

At high doses (100 μg/ml), rifampin has been shown to have activity against a number of viruses in mammals. The activity against poxviruses has been most extensively studied.

A number of derivatives of the ansamycin type inhibit retroviral reverse transcriptase.

13.8. Antiparasitic Activities

Antiplasmodial and antileishmaniasis activities have been described for rifampin.

13.9. Rifaximin

Rifaximin is not absorbed by the digestive tract. After oral administration, rifaximin is not detected in the plasma in assays performed by high-performance liquid chromatography with a limit of sensitivity of 25 ng/ml. Small quantities of product are found dose dependently in the urine. A small proportion is eliminated in the bile.

The indications for the therapeutic use of rifaximin appear to be diarrhea of infectious origin, selective digestive decontamination, and hepatic encephalopathy.

14. DRUG INTERACTIONS

Rifampin is an antituberculosis or antileprosy agent administered over a period of 4 to 12 months. It may interfere with the metabolism of drugs used in combination for antituberculosis treatment or in parallel treatments for other infections or conditions.

Rifampin is a potent but selective inducer of drug metabolism, as not all of the drugs metabolized by oxidation are affected. Rifampin also induces its own metabolism by increasing its plasma clearance and reducing its apparent elimination half-life. The maximum level of induction is reached on day 7 of treatment.

Coadministration of rifampin and anticoagulants requires a progressive increase in the doses of anticoagulants because of the increase in warfarin metabolism.

Elimination of digoxin is principally renal. Rifampin administered simultaneously with digoxin in patients undergoing hemodialysis reduces plasma digoxin concentrations and may be responsible for heart failure. Digoxin is eliminated by the hepatobiliary route, and a reduction in levels in plasma has been demonstrated if rifampin is administered simultaneously. A decrease in concentrations of quinidine, β-blockers (metoprolol and propanolol), verapamil, lorcainide, mexiletine, pirmenol, and propafenone in plasma after simultaneous administration of rifampin has been described.

Rifampin increases the elimination of steroidal contraceptives, cortisol, and prednisolone. The activity of oral antidiabetic agents is reduced likewise: tolbutamide, chlorpropamide, glucodiazine, etc. Plasma methadone levels are decreased when the drug is administered simultaneously with rifampin.

Cyclosporine is a cyclical endecapeptide with potent immunosuppressant properties and is metabolized by the liver (cytochrome P450). Simultaneous administration of rifampin reduces the efficacy of cyclosporine.

Simultaneous administration of rifampin and theophylline alters the metabolism of the latter. Theophylline clearance is increased by 20 to 80%, and the plasma half-life is reduced by 20 to 30%. The pharmacokinetics of theophylline return to normal about 2 weeks after the end of rifampin administration.

In epileptic patients receiving phenytoin, rifampin may be the cause of epileptic seizures as a result of a reduction in plasma phenytoin levels.

Rifampin reduces plasma thyroxine levels and increases those of triiodothyroxine; however, the clinical significance of these changes has not been clearly established.

Rifampin and isoniazid significantly reduce circulating 25-hydroxycholecalciferol levels but do not affect those of 1,25-dihydroxycholecalficerol or calcitonin. It is possible that administration of rifampin over a period of 1 year does not cause any major modifications of bone metabolism, except in childhood and pregnancy.

Rifampin does not modify the metabolism of pyrazinamide. The combination isoniazid-rifampin is sometimes hepatotoxic. Rifampin reduces the apparent elimination half-life of dapsone by half, as well as concentrations in the skin and nerves. However, the concentrations of dapsone remain sufficiently high to be therapeutic. Absorption of clofazimine is not affected by administration of rifampin. The incidence of side effects appears to be abnormally high in lepromatous patients receiving rifampin and ethionamide or protionamide simultaneously.

Levels of chloramphenicol, novobiocin, trimethoprim, and barbiturates in plasma are reduced when these drugs are administered simultaneously with rifampin.

15. ADVERSE EFFECTS

The adverse effects of rifampin are dependent on treatment duration and dose. Treatments based on high doses of rifampin (once or twice weekly) are associated with more severe side effects, particularly with doses greater than or equal to 1,200 mg.

Cutaneous reactions are seen in fewer than 5% of patients, are transient, and do not require the discontinuation of treatment. Following an overdose, a reddish-orange color of the skin occurs, giving rise to the red man syndrome.

Gastrointestinal effects occur in fewer than 2% of patients in the form of anorexia, nausea, abdominal pain, and, more rarely, diarrhea or vomiting.

Disorders of hepatic metabolism (raised enzymes), hepatitis, and fulminant hepatitis are rare, and the relationship with treatment is often difficult to establish, as patients are multimedicated (isoniazid, ethambutol, etc.).

Minor disorders of the central nervous system have been described, but these are rare.

Severe hematologic side effects have been described with intermittent doses of rifampin due to the formation of rifampin-dependent antibodies, such as hemolytic anemia and thrombocytopenic purpura. Branched-chain proteinuria may be associated with administration of rifampin. Intermittent administration of rifampin has been held to be responsible for acute renal failure.

An influenza-like syndrome occurring between 1 and 2 h after each dose of rifampin has been described. This syndrome is of immunological origin and is associated with the presence of antirifampin antibodies. Women and elderly subjects are most often affected.

Rifampin intoxication as a result of overdose is characterized by an abnormal coloring of the integument and a red color of the urine, stools, sweat, and plasma. These signs are accompanied by digestive disorders, pruritus, and edema.

The combination of rifabutin and fluconazole has been held to be responsible for uveitis in AIDS patients. Likewise, the combination of rifabutin and clarithromycin reduces clarithromycin concentrations in plasma.

Rifabutin has been considered to be responsible for arthralgic and neurologic syndromes in AIDS patients.

REFERENCES

Bergamini N, Fowst G, 1965, Rifamycin SV, Arzneim Forsch, 15, 951–1002.

Binda G, Domenichini E, Gottardi A, Orlandi B, Ortelli E, Pacini B, Fowst G, 1971, Rifampicin, a general review, Arzneim Forsch, 21, 1907–1977.

Dhople AM, 1995, In vitro and in vivo activities of T9, a new rifampicin derivative, against *Mycobacterium leprae*, 35th Intersci Conf Antimicrob Agents Chemother, abstract F-10.

Dickinson JM, Mitchison DA, 1970, In vitro activities against mycobacteria of two long-acting rifamycins, FCE 22807 and CGP 1469 A (SPA-S-565), Tubercle, 71, 109–115.

Geeta B, Reddy MV, Dimova V, Gangadharam PRJ, 1995, In vitro and intracellular antimycobacterial activity of new rifampicin analogue 3-(4-cinnamyl-piperazimyl-iminomethyl-) rifampicin-SV, 19th Int Congr Chemother, abstract 1152.

Gurgoc A, Bridges S, Green M, 1982, Rifamycins, p 519–555, in Came PE, Caliguiri LA, ed, Chemotherapy of Viral Infections, Springer-Verlag.

Loos U, Musch E, Jensen JC, Mikus G, Sehwabe HR, Eichelbaum M, 1985, Pharmacokinetics of oral and intravenous rifampicin during chronic administration, Klin Wochenschr, 63, 1205–1211.

Morris AB, Brown RB, Sands M, 1993, Use of rifampin in non-staphylococcal, nonmycobacterial disease, Antimicrob Agents Chemother, 37, 1–7.

Pallanza R, Füre'sz S, Timbal MT, Carniti G, 1963, In vitro bacteriological studies on rifamycin B diethylamide (rifamide), Arzneim Forsch, 13, 800–802.

Pascual A, Tsukayama D, Kovarik J, Gekker G, Peterson P, 1987, Uptake and activity of rifapentine in human peritoneal macrophages and polymorphonuclear leukocytes, Eur J Clin Microbiol, 6, 152–157.

Shalit I, 1988, Rifampin, p 373–403, in Koren G, Prober CG, Gold R, ed, Antimicrobial Therapy in Infants and Children, Marcel Dekker.

Venkatesan K, 1992, Pharmacokinetic drug interaction with rifampicin, Clin Pharmacokinet, 22, 47–65.

Williams JD, Phillips I, 1984, Rifampicin as an anti-staphylococcal agent, J Antimicrob Chemother, 13, suppl C.

Phenicols

A. FISCH AND A. BRYSKIER

33

1. INTRODUCTION

Chloramphenicol was the first broad-spectrum antibiotic to be used both systemically and orally. It was first isolated in 1947 from a soil actinomycete found in a field close to Caracas, Venezuela (*Streptomyces venezuelae*). It is now produced industrially by chemical synthesis.

The number of human lives that this antibiotic has saved is incalculable. However, the hematologic toxicity of chloramphenicol and the risk of unpredictable fatal accidents rapidly came to light. Despite extensive research with the aim of synthesizing less dangerous derivatives, only thiamphenicol (1952) has been adopted.

This hematologic risk, combined with the commercial availability of other, more effective antibiotics, means that phenicols only exceptionally retain any indications in industrialized countries. On the other hand, they are still of some interest in developing countries, particularly for the treatment of meningitis.

In the veterinary field a fluoro derivative is commonly used, florfenicol.

2. CHEMICAL STRUCTURES AND PHYSICOCHEMICAL PROPERTIES

The phenicols have one of the simplest chemical structures of all antibiotics.

All phenicols are derived from dichloroacetic acid, with two other parts: an aromatic nucleus with an alkyl group in the *para* position and an aminopropanediol chain (Fig. 1). There are two asymmetrical carbon atoms and hence four stereoisomers; only the D(−)-threo isomer (the natural antibiotic) is active. The possibilities of substitution offered by this structure are numerous, but although many derivatives have been synthesized, only two molecules, characterized by the R_1 group, are used in humans as antibiotics: chloramphenicol and thiamphenicol. The R_2 group varies according to the ester (succinate, palmitate, and glycinate).

Figure 1 Basic structure of the phenicols

2.1. Chloramphenicol

See Fig. 2.

The R_1 group is NO_2-$C_{11}H_{12}C_{12}N_2O_5$. The molecular weight is 323.1. 2,2-Dichloro-*N*-((*R*,*R*)-2-hydroxy-1-hydroxymethyl-4-nitrophenethyl)acetamide is the basic substance, produced originally from *S. venezuelae* but now prepared by synthesis. The white, whitish, grayish, or yellowish powder is composed of elongated and sharp crystals. It is soluble in water (1:400), alcohol (1/2.5), and propylene glycol (1/7); it is freely soluble in acetone and ethyl acetate and slightly soluble in ether. It has a bitter taste. It must be stored under vacuum and away from light, like all of its derivatives.

Two esters are usable: chloramphenicol succinate and palmitate.

2.1.1. Chloramphenicol Succinate

The molecular weight of chloramphenicol succinate is 445.2. A 1.4-g amount of chloramphenicol succinate is equivalent to about 1 g of chloramphenicol. It is presented in the form of a white or yellowish powder. It is soluble in water

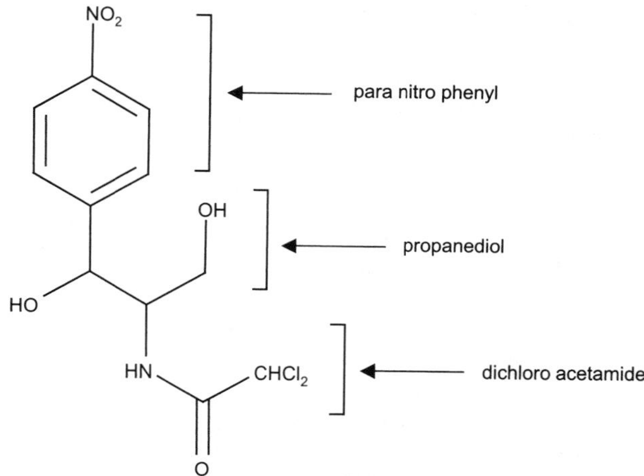

Figure 2 Structure of chloramphenicol

(approximately 1/1) and alcohol (1/1) and insoluble in ether. It has a slightly bitter taste. It must be stored away from air and light.

2.1.2. Chloramphenicol Palmitate

The molecular weight is 561.5. A 1.7-g amount of sodium palmitate is equivalent to about 1 g of chloramphenicol. It is presented in the form of a white powder. It is in practice insoluble in water, soluble in alcohol (1/45) and ether (1/14), and freely soluble in acetone. It is practically tasteless. It must be stored away from air and light.

2.2. Thiamphenicol

See Fig. 3.

The R_1 group is CH_2-SO_2-$C_{12}H_{15}C_{12}NO_5S$. The molecular weight is 356.2. 2,2-Dichloro-*N*-((*R*,*R*)-2-hydroxy-1-hydroxymethyl-4-methylsulfonylphenylethyl)acetamide is the basic substance. It has been produced solely by synthesis since its discovery in 1952. It is presented in the form of a fine white or yellowish powder. It is slightly soluble in water, ether, and ethyl acetate; soluble in dehydrated alcohol and acetone; and very soluble in dimethylacetamide. It has a slightly bitter taste. It must be stored away from light and humidity.

2.2.1. Thiamphenicol Glycinate

Thiamphenicol glycinate is the only ester used. The molecular weight is 449.7. A 1.26-g amount of thiamphenicol glycinate is equivalent to about 1 g of thiamphenicol. It has a slightly bitter taste. It must be stored away from light and air.

2.3. Florfenicol

Florfenicol has the same chemical structure as thiamphenicol but it possesses a fluorine atom instead of a hydroxyl group (Fig. 4). Having a hydroxyl group, florfenicol is less affected by enzymatic modifications.

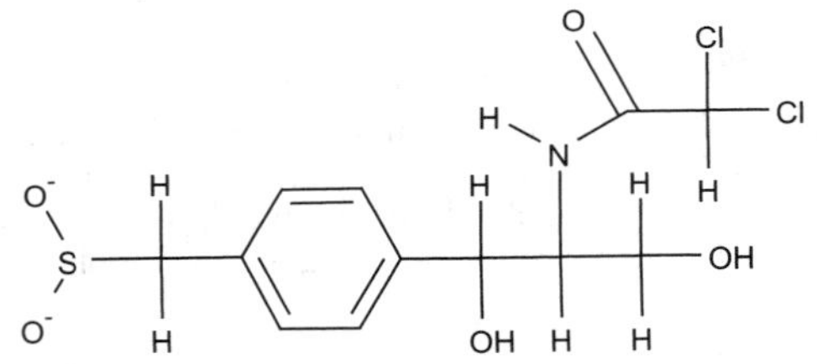

Figure 3 Structure of thiamphenicol

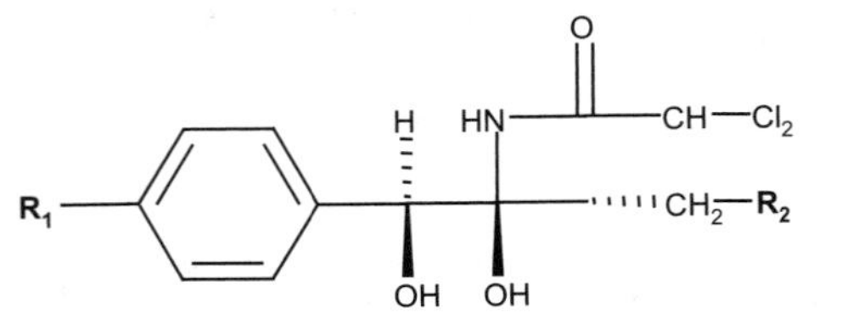

	R_1	R_2
Chloramphenicol	$-NO_2$	O, H
Thiamphenicol	$-SO_2CH_3$	OH
Fluorinated chloramphenicol analog	$-NO_2$	F
Florfenicol	$-SO_2CH_3$	F

Figure 4 Phenicol derivatives

3. IN VITRO PROPERTIES

The palmitate and succinate esters have no antibacterial activity in vitro; they only acquire antibacterial activity in vivo through the action of the body's enzymes (esterases and lipases of pancreatic origin).

The phenicols are broad-spectrum antibiotics. Table 1 lists the MICs for the main bacterial species. The phenicols

Table 1 MICs of phenicols

Organism(s)	MIC (μg/ml)
S. aureus	1–4
S. aureus Met^r	1–4
Staphylococcus epidermidis	1–4
Group A streptococci	1–4
Group B streptococci	2–4
Enterococci	4–>8
S. pneumoniae	0.5–2
Neisseria gonorrhoeae	0.25–1
N. meningitidis	0.25–1
Pasteurella multocida	0.5
H. influenzae	0.5
Haemophilus ducreyi	0.12–1.6
Gardnerella vaginalis	0.5–2.0
Brucella spp.	1.0–8.0
Bordetella pertussis	0.5–1.0
Erysipelothrix rhusiopathiae	0.1–25
Listeria monocytogenes	2–8
Corynebacterium diphtheriae	1.5–4
E. coli	1–8
Klebsiella pneumoniae	1–8
Salmonella enterica serovar Typhi	1–4
Proteus spp.	6–64
Enterobacter spp.	4–16
P. aeruginosa	16–32
Acinetobacter spp.	16–64
Salmonella spp.	1–4
Yersinia pseudotuberculosis	1–8
Yersinia enterocolitica	1–4
Serratia marcescens	1–8
Shigella spp.	1–8
Vibrio cholerae	1–4
Campylobacter jejuni	1–4
A. butzleri	16–64
A. cryaerophilus	8–64
Helicobacter pylori	4
Legionella pneumophila	0.5–1
B. fragilis	4–8
Prevotella melaninogenica	0.5–1
Fusobacterium spp.	0.12–1
Clostridium spp.	1–4
Clostridium perfringens	0.5–4
Eubacterium	2–4
Bifidobacterium spp.	2–4
Propionibacterium acnes	0.5–2
Actinobacillus actinomycetemcomitans	0.5–1
Eikenella corrodens	≤2
Actinomyces israelii	0.5–2
Veillonella parvula	0.5–2
Peptostreptococcus spp.	0.5–2
Mycobacterium smegmatis	4
Leptospira spp.	0.39–3.13
Coxiella burnetii	≥8
Tropheryma whipplei	1.0–2.0

are commonly known as bacteriostatic antibiotics. They indeed have bacteriostatic activity against the majority of gram-negative bacilli, *Enterobacteriaceae* (particularly *Escherichia coli, Klebsiella,* and *Proteus*), and *Staphylococcus aureus*, but the term "bacteriostatic" is relatively incorrect for its activity against the majority of other bacterial species, particularly those responsible for meningitis (*Neisseria meningitidis, Streptococcus pneumoniae,* and *Haemophilus influenzae*) and *Bacteroides fragilis*. They are also active against brucellae, spirochetes, rickettsiae, and *Chlamydia, Mycoplasma,* and *Vibrio* spp. *Pseudomon aeruginosa* is usually resistant.

The 1997 Antibiotic Sensitivity Test Committee (France) considers the MICs for susceptible bacteria to be less than or equal to 8 μg/ml; resistant strains are those for which the MIC is greater than 16 μg/ml.

In a recent survey, no resistance to chloramphenicol, metronidazole, piperacillin-tazobactam, cefoxitin, or imipenem had been detected among gram-positive anaerobic cocci.

Among the five species of *Arcobacter*, only two, *Arcobacter butzleri* and *Arcobacter cryaerophilus*, have been associated with enteric infections in humans. Other *Arcobacter* spp. are environmental isolates.

Aeromonas spp. have been isolated as a cause of traveler's diarrhea in 2% of patients. The strains are resistant to ampicillin and exhibit variable susceptibilities to chloramphenicol.

Burkholderia pseudomallei is intrinsically resistant to many antibiotics. Generally it is susceptible to chloramphenicol, the tetracyclines, co-trimoxazole, ureidopenicillins, aminothiazolyl cephalosporins, carbapenems, and co-amoxiclav.

Chloramphenicol is active against *Francisella tularensis*.

4. MECHANISM OF ACTION

In bacteria, the phenicols inhibit protein synthesis, but not that of peptidoglycan, polysaccharides, or nucleic acids. This inhibition is selective: it does not exist in the majority of eukaryotic organisms.

Binding of phenicols to the 50S ribosomal subunit inhibits the peptidation reaction, as chloramphenicol reduces the catalytic activity of peptidyltransferase; the translation of bacterial mRNA is therefore inhibited.

The existence of (weak) schizonticidal antiplasmodial activity—at least for chloramphenicol—should also be noted, although the molecular mechanism of this has not been clearly elucidated.

5. MECHANISMS OF RESISTANCE

5.1. Natural Resistance

Only a few bacterial species have natural resistance: *P. aeruginosa*, mycobacteria, *Acinetobacter* spp., and *Nocardia*.

5.2. Acquired Resistance

Resistance to chloramphenicol generally occurs rapidly. It is usually crossed with resistance to thiamphenicol.

This resistance is primarily due to production of chloramphenicol acetyltransferases, several isolated variants of which are known, particularly for gram-negative bacilli. Acetylation of the two hydroxyls of the aminopropanediol chain results in an inactive derivative.

Sometimes another, more contingent mechanism of resistance is involved: acquired reduction in permeability of the bacterial outer membrane to phenicols.

Resistance by enzymatic inactivation is related to the presence of a plasmid and is usually transferable. A single plasmid may transfer resistance to several antibiotics (tetracyclines, aminoglycosides, and sulfonamides), particularly as was noted in the typhoid fever epidemic in Mexico in 1973.

Plasmid-mediated resistance to florfenicol by efflux of the compound was first described for a fish pathogen, *Photobacterium damselae* subsp. *piscicida* (formerly *Pasteurella piscicida*). The resistance gene is *floR*. The gene is carried on a transposon.

6. PLASMA PHARMACOKINETICS

The phenicols may be administered as follows:

- Orally: chloramphenicol base and palmitate
- Intravenously (or intramuscularly): chloramphenicol succinate and thiamphenicol glycinate
- Intrathecally (this route is no longer used)
- Locally: in ophthalmology and otorhinolaryngology, for example

The esters of chloramphenicol are in fact inactive prodrugs from which the active molecule is released into the body under the action of endogenous esterases.

6.1. Pharmacokinetics in Healthy Volunteers

Oral absorption is rapid and virtually complete, varying between 80 and 95% according to the size of the crystals. The peak concentration in serum is reached about 2 h after absorption, approximating to 10 μg/ml for an oral dose of 1 g of chloramphenicol. A dose of 500 mg every 6 h usually yields levels in blood of more than 4 μg/ml. The oral pharmacokinetics of chloramphenicol are not affected by food.

When Chloramphenicol is given intravenously, the peak concentration in serum can be reached after between 15 min and 3 h, depending on the ester and the infusion rate.

About 50% of plasma chloramphenicol circulates in the protein-bound form. The protein binding coefficient of thiamphenicol is lower, on the order of 10 to 20%.

The half-life of chloramphenicol in healthy subjects ranges from 1.5 to 5 h depending on the study. That of thiamphenicol is comparable, on the order of 2 h.

In the liver, chloramphenicol undergoes glucuroconjugation, in contrast to thiamphenicol, which is eliminated in the active form, principally in the urine (more than 75%). About 2 to 3% of the administered dose of chloramphenicol is eliminated in the bile in the inactive form, and 1% is eliminated in the feces in the inactive form.

6.2. Pharmacokinetics in Specific Subjects

6.2.1. Subjects with Renal Insufficiency

The apparent elimination half-life of chloramphenicol is only slightly prolonged in the case of terminal renal insufficiency. Conversely, under these circumstances the half-life of thiamphenicol may be prolonged more than fourfold. In patients on hemodialysis, the half-life may be prolonged two to three times compared to the half-life in those with normal renal function. The dosage of thiamphenicol must therefore be adapted according to the creatinine clearance.

6.2.2. Patients with Hepatic Insufficiency

In cirrhotic patients with edematous and ascitic decompensation, the apparent elimination half-life of chloramphenicol may be prolonged up to 13 h. This increase is correlated with that of bilirubin and inversely correlated with that of serum albumin. The kinetics of thiamphenicol are not affected by hepatic disorders.

6.2.3. Pharmacokinetics in Pediatric Patients

The pharmacokinetics of chloramphenicol are modified in neonates (even more so if they are premature) and also in infants, with a prolongation of the half-life. However, this prolongation is not systematic because there are so many factors that are involved: hepatic maturity, enzyme maturity (pancreatic esterases), plasma proteins, etc., to the extent that the dosages must be adapted on the basis of the levels in plasma. In 24 children (aged 2 weeks up to 7 years) the pharmacokinetic profile of chloramphenicol succinate was investigated. The apparent elimination half-life was 0.4 h, the average body clearance was 0.72 liter/kg/h, and 35% of the administered dose was eliminated in urine.

6.2.4. Pharmacokinetics in Elderly Subjects

There are no data available for elderly subjects.

6.2.5. Other Pathological Conditions

6.2.5.1. Malnutrition

Pharmacokinetic studies with malnourished subjects are rare, although the phenicols are widely used in the most disadvantaged countries. Oral absorption appears to be erratic. Studies following parenteral administration have yielded divergent results.

6.2.5.2. Cardiac Insufficiency

A few studies appear to show a risk of accumulation in subjects with decompensated heart failure and in patients in a state of cardiovascular shock.

7. TISSUE DISTRIBUTION

The distribution of chloramphenicol in body tissues and fluids is very extensive, partly as a result of its marked lipophilicity. The volume of distribution is generally greater than 1 liter/kg. It crosses the blood-brain barrier even in the absence of meningeal inflammation, resulting in concentrations in the cerebrospinal fluid equal to about half the concentrations in blood. It diffuses well in the aqueous humor and the vitreous body. Diffusion is considered good in sputum, whether mucous or purulent.

It crosses the fetoplacental barrier and is excreted in breast milk. Chloramphenicol is also distributed in a number of body compartments: pleural, ascites, synovial, and lymphatic fluids and the central nervous system (intracerebral concentrations are more than five times the levels in serum).

Finally, chloramphenicol accumulates in cells and exerts its antibiotic action within phagocytic cells (neutrophils and alveolar macrophages). The cellular/extracellular concentration ratios are between 2.6 and 10.

8. DRUG INTERFERENCE

Chloramphenicol may interfere with a number of drugs, chiefly because of its hepatic metabolism. This interference has not been described with thiamphenicol.

By inhibiting hepatic microsomal enzymes, chloramphenicol is capable of increasing the half-life of hypoglycemic sulfonamides, vitamin K antagonists, and hydantoins.

Pretreatment with chloramphenicol delays the waking of animals anesthetized with pentobarbital. It is responsible for a slower response in episodes of anemia to treatment with iron, folic acid, and vitamin B_{12} (in Biermer's disease). Chloramphenicol inhibits the action of cyclophosphamide.

Other interactions with methotrexate, dexamethasone, and paracetamol have been described, but these appear to require no more than straightforward monitoring.

Finally, in some subjects it appears that chloramphenicol may have an antabuse effect.

9. TOLERANCE

The principal problem of tolerance relates to chloramphenicol and the possibility of induction of hematologic accidents that are often irreversible and fatal.

9.1. Severe Bone Marrow Aplasia

The risk of occurrence of bone marrow aplasia is the main limitation of the use of chloramphenicol. It is rare (estimated as 1 case in 20,000 to 60,000 subjects treated) but serious, with a fatality rate of more than 50%. This accident is not dose dependent and has been observed with all routes of administration, even local; its mechanism is unknown. Pancytopenia appears within a period that varies considerably, from 3 weeks up to 4 months.

The later the onset, the more serious the outcome. It is generally irreversible. In some patients the subsequent occurrence of myeloblastic leukemia has been observed.

Although this risk also theoretically hangs over thiamphenicol, no case of fatal aplasia has been reported with this antibiotic, which means that it is preferred to chloramphenicol even if its overall antibiotic activity is weaker.

9.2. Late, Reversible, Dissociated Bone Marrow Hyperplasia

Late, reversible, dissociated bone marrow hyperplasia is the direct opposite of the aplasia described above. It is observed with thiamphenicol as well as with chloramphenicol, is usually dose dependent, and occurs early. The bone marrow lesion is not general. This accident occurs more frequently in subjects with previous bone marrow deficiency or renal insufficiency or who have taken an accidental overdose. No fatal outcome has ever been reported.

9.3. Other Hematologic Accidents

Very rare cases of hemolytic anemia have been reported for subjects suffering from extensive glucose-6-phosphate dehydrogenase deficiency.

9.4. Gray Syndrome

Gray syndrome refers to the occurrence in a neonate (particularly a premature one) of a syndrome involving abdominal distension, vomiting, hyperthermia, and cardiovascular collapse associated with a grayish color of the integument and culminating in death. It is related to the accumulation of chloramphenicol associated with enzymatic immaturity.

9.5. Allergic Reactions

Essentially local (cutaneous and ocular), allergic reactions take the form of dermatitis and conjunctivitis. Phenicols are only exceptionally associated with general allergic reactions.

9.6. Other Incidents and Accidents

9.6.1. Digestive

Digestive incidents include nausea, vomiting, and diarrhea in the event of an overdose; possible but rare intestinal superinfections associated with disequilibrium of the intestinal flora; and pseudomembranous colitis.

9.6.2. Neurologic and Psychiatric

Optic neuritis, central deafness, and various mental disorders have been noted exceptionally with high and prolonged dosages.

9.6.3. Herxheimer's Reaction

Herxheimer's reaction is a state of shock occurring at the beginning of treatment with excessively high dosages for advanced typhoid fever with a high toxin burden, the antibiotic therapy causing a sometimes fatal increase in the toxins released.

10. CLINICAL INDICATIONS

The clinical indications are nowadays very limited, at least in industrialized countries; this is partly due to the potential hematologic toxicity, but also to the ever greater availability of increasingly more potent and increasingly less toxic alternative antibiotics, to the extent that chloramphenicol and even the less toxic thiamphenicol are currently very little prescribed in industrialized countries.

The only legitimate indication perhaps remains a cerebral abscess or subdural empyema because of the excellent cerebral parenchymatous diffusion of the phenicols. However, even in this rare indication the phenicol is usually combined with other antibiotics that usefully supplement its spectrum.

Despite the regular occurrence of resistance or reduced susceptibility to β-lactams of the bacteria responsible for meningitis, the phenicols have little place in this indication any longer, as it can be controlled by dosage increases and possibly combinations (penicillin A, 2-amino-5-thiazolyl cephalosporin or C3′-quaternary ammonium cephalosporins, and possibly fosfomycin).

Typhoid fever, a classic indication, has now become rapidly curable with fluoroquinolones.

The remaining indications for phenicols currently are represented by exceptional, severe infectious conditions for which no other antibiotic therapy can be used because of multiple or unusual resistance.

The phenicols, however, retain a certain place in developing countries, particularly in the treatment of bacterial meningitis. Prolonged-release chloramphenicol (oily suspension) prescribed in a dose of two intramuscular injections (one injection of 3 g every 24 to 48 h) has exhibited efficacy comparable to that of an infusion of ampicillin for 1 week (Pecoul et al., 1991). After a single administration of 3 g intramuscularly, concentrations in the cerebrospinal fluid are 2.1 and 0.6 μg/ml at 24 and 48 h, respectively (Wali et al., 1979). The hematologic risk appears to be very minor compared to the very marked mortality of this condition and is to a large extent offset by the feasibility of effective treatment, the availability of chloramphenicol on-site, and chloramphenicol's low relative cost.

On the basis of these tropical public health data, the indications for phenicols very definitely remain much more extensive than in the industrialized countries.

REFERENCES

Ambrose PJ, 1984, Clinical pharmacokinetics of chloramphenicol and chloramphenicol succinate, Clin Pharmacokinet, 9, 222–238.

Bertrand A, 1988, Chloramphenicol et thiamphenicol, Rev Prat, 38, 486–492.

Gale EF, Cundliffe E, Reynolds PE, 1981, The Molecular Basis of Antibiotic Action, J Wiley and Son, London.

Glecksman RA, 1975, Warning: chloramphenicol can be good for your health, Arch Intern Med, 135, 1125–1126.

Hahn FE, 1983, Chloramphenicol, p 34–35, in Hahn FE, ed, Antibiotics, vol IV, Springer Verlag, New York.

Najean Y, Tognoni G, Yunis AA, 1981, Safety Problems Related to Chloramphenicol and Thiamphenicol Therapy, Raven Press, New York.

Pecoul B, Varaine F, Keita M, Soga G, Djibo A, Soula G, Abdou A, Etienne J, Rey M, 1991, Long-acting chloramphenicol versus intravenous ampicillin for treatment of bacterial meningitis, Lancet, 338, 862–866.

Philippon A, Paul G, Giroud JP, 1988, Phénicolés: chloramphenicol et thiamphenicol, p 1421–1431, in Giroud JP et al, ed, Pharmacologie clinique, Bases de la therapeutique, Expansion Scientifique Francaise, Paris.

Rahal JJ Jr, Simberkoff MS, 1977, Bactericidal and bacteriostatic action of chloramphenicol against meningeal pathogens, Antimicrob Agents Chemother, 16, 13–18.

Standiford HC, 1990, Tetracyclines and chloramphenicol, p 284–295, in Mandell GL, et al, ed, Principles and Practice of Infectious Diseases, 3rd ed, Churchill Livingstone, New York.

Wali SS, MacFarlane JT, Weir WRC, et al, 1979, Single injection treatment of meningococcal meningitis. 2. Long-acting chloramphenicol, Trans R Soc Trop Med Hyg, 73, 698–702.

World Health Organization, 1990, Meningococcal meningitis in Africa, Wkly Epidemiol Rec, 16, 120–122.

5-Nitroimidazoles

L. DUBREUIL

34

1. INTRODUCTION

Used orally in the treatment of trichomoniasis, amoebiasis, giardiasis, and vaginitis caused by *Gardnerella vaginalis* (formerly *Haemophilus vaginalis*), metronidazole and ornidazole are currently indicated in the treatment of anaerobic bacterial infections. In this chapter, the information summarized relates mainly to the antibacterial activity of the 5-nitroimidazoles. Three 5-nitroimidazoles have been selected: metronidazole, ornidazole, and tinidazole. Metronidazole is the prototype and is therefore used most often as the representative molecule of the class; tinidazole is principally used as an antiprotozoal agent.

2. STRUCTURE

Metronidazole is 1-(2-hydroxyethyl)-2-methyl-5-nitroimidazole ($C_6H_9N_3O_3$), ornidazole is 1-(3 chloro-2-hydroxypropyl)-2-methyl-5-nitroimidazole ($C_7H_{10}N_3O_3Cl$), and tinidazole is 1-[2-(ethylsulfonyl)ethyl]-2-methyl-5-nitroimidazole ($C_8H_{13}N_3O_4S$).

The chemical structure of the three compounds is detailed in Fig. 1.

3. PHYSICOCHEMICAL PROPERTIES

5-Nitroimidazoles are slightly soluble in water and nonionized at physiological pH. They are soluble in alcohol and slightly liposoluble.

3.1. Metronidazole

The molecular mass is 171.16 Da; the melting point is 159 to 163°C. The pK_a is 2.62.

Figure 1 Chemical structure of the 5-nitroimidazoles

The aqueous solution for intravenous infusion is adjusted to pH 5 with a citric acid solution. The sodium content is 13.5 mmol.

3.2. Ornidazole

The molecular mass is 219.6 Da; the melting point is 87 to 92°C.

The solubilities for 100 ml of solvent are as follows: water, 1.5 g; ethanol (96%), 30 g; and phosphate buffer (pH 7), 1.5 g. In a 1% aqueous solution, the pH is between 4.5 and 7.5. The pK_a is about 2.3. It is slightly soluble in dimethylformamide but soluble in dilute acids.

3.3. Tinidazole

The molecular mass is 247.26 Da; the melting point is 127 to 128°C.

Solutions of 5-nitroimidazoles must be stored away from light.

4. ANTIBACTERIAL ACTIVITY

4.1. Methodological Problems

Without entering into the technical details, it should be pointed out that the 5-nitroimidazoles only act in vitro if the anaerobic conditions are correct. Divergent results are obtained when the different techniques used are compared, depending on whether an anaerobic chamber, oxygen replacement jars, or gas-generating envelopes are employed. As regards antibiotic susceptibility tests, there is at present no fully standardized agar diffusion method. The MICs are measured for anaerobes by an agar dilution method. Replacement methods (microdilution, elution of disks in broth, E-test, etc.) have been proposed, but none of these techniques provides a totally satisfactory solution.

4.2. Breakpoints

In the anaerobic area, and irrespective of the antibiotic considered, the NCCLS recommends only one breakpoint, separating the strains into susceptible and resistant groups. A strain is said to be resistant to metronidazole if the measured MIC is greater than 8 μg/ml. The French Antibiotic Sensitivity Test Committee has adopted a breakpoint of 4 μg/ml.

4.3. Spectrum

4.3.1. Obligate Anaerobes

See Table 1.

The 5-nitroimidazoles are very active against the majority of gram-negative anaerobic bacteria and *Clostridium*. Rare resistant strains, however, have been described among members of the *Bacteroides fragilis* group and *Clostridium*. Metronidazole is active against 73% of strains of *Bacteroides gracilis*. Anaerobic gram-positive cocci are more often susceptible to 5-nitroimidazoles, even if in the majority of studies 2 to 10% resistant strains are observed. Their action against nonsporulating gram-positive bacilli needs to be defined: three-fourths of strains of *Eubacterium* and two-thirds of strains of bifidus are susceptible to imidazole, while the majority of *Actinomyces* strains (80%) and all propionibacteria are resistant to the 5-nitroimidazoles. *Anaerobiospirillum succiniciproducens* is always resistant. Taking all obligate anaerobes isolated in human pathological specimens together, metronidazole is active against 96% of the strains studied (99% of gram-negative bacilli, 98% of gram-positive cocci, 99% of *Clostridium* isolates). The 5-nitroimidazoles may therefore be considered excellent antibacterial agents acting on the majority of anaerobes, with the exception of *Actinomyces* and propionibacteria.

The MIC of metronidazole for *B. fragilis* was 2 to 4 times higher in 25% horse plasma and 8 to 16 times higher in pure plasma.

Table 1 Activity of metronidazole against obligate anaerobes

Organism	MIC (μg/ml)	
	50%	90%
Gram-negative bacteria		
B. fragilis[a]	0.5–1	1–2
Bacteroides distasonis[a]	0.5	1
B. thetaiotaomicron	1	2–4
B. fragilis group	0.5–1	1–4
P. bivia[a]	1–62	2–4
Prevotella disiens	1	4
Prevotella oralis	1	4
Prevotella melaninogenica[a]	0.5	1–4
Prevotella intermedia[a]	0.5–1	1–4
Prevotella spp.[a]	1	2–4
Porphyromonas gingivalis	0.015	0.03
Porphyromonas asaccharolytica[a]	1	2
Fusobacterium nucleatum	0.25	0.5–4
Fusobacterium mortiferum	0.25	1
Fusobacterium necrophorum	0.25	0.5
Fusobacterium varium[a]	0.5	2
Bacteroides splanchnicus	0.06	0.12
Bacteroides stercoris	4	4
Bacteroides tectus	0.5	0.5
Bacteroides forsythus	<0.06	<0.06
Bacteroides ureolyticus	1	2–4
Other *Bacteroides* spp.[a]	0.5	2
Anaerorhabdus furcos[a]	2	4
Bilophila wadsworthia	0.125	0.25
Sutterella wadsworthensis	2	64
Campylobacter gracilis	1	8
Campylobacter rectus[a]	1	4
Anaerobiospirillum spp.	4	8
Veillonella spp.	1	2
Selenomonas spp.	<0.25	<0.25
Gram-positive bacteria		
Mobiluncus spp.	64	>128
C. perfringens	0.25–0.5	1–8
C. difficile[a]	0.125–0.25	0.25–4
Other clostridia[a]	0.25–0.5	0.5–4
Eubacterium spp.	0.5	2–32
Actinomyces spp.	32	>128
Bifidobacterium spp.	0.25	8
P. acnes	128	128
Micromonas micros	0.125	1
Finegoldia magna	0.06	0.25
Peptostreptococcus and *Peptoniphilus* spp.	0.5–1	2–8

[a]Resistance for a MIC of >8 μg/ml.

4.3.2. Activity against Other Bacteria (Excluding Anaerobes)

Metronidazole is theoretically inactive against *G. vaginalis*, as the usual MICs are 64 to 128 μg/ml. However, this antibiotic yields excellent results in the treatment of vaginosis (a specific vaginitis). This is an additional argument advanced by proponents of the involvement of anaerobes in this type of vaginitis. The strains of *Mobiluncus* (obligate anaerobes) often associated with *Gardnerella* are also resistant in vitro to 5-nitroimidazoles.

Under anaerobic conditions, metronidazole inhibits the growth of *Escherichia coli*, and it is therefore possible that the 5-nitroimidazoles might act in situ on certain strains of *E. coli* when adequate anaerobiosis is obtained at the infection site. However, the simultaneous presence of *B. fragilis* suppresses this effect.

The action of 5-nitroimidazoles on *Campylobacter* isolates varies with the species concerned: the measured MICs for *C. fetus* and *C. jejuni* are usually 12 and 32 μg/ml, respectively; *Helicobacter pylori* appears to be more susceptible in vitro (MIC at which 50% of isolates tested are inhibited [MIC_{50}], <0.12 μg/ml; MIC_{90}, 2 to 4 μg/ml), but in the majority of studies 8 to 12% of the strains studied are resistant to 5-nitroimidazoles (MIC, 64 μg/ml). Metronidazole has been used successfully against susceptible strains, alone or in combination with amoxicillin and/or bismuth salts. The failures or recurrences observed preclude any definitive conclusion about the value of 5-nitroimidazoles in the treatment of *H. pylori* gastritis.

Metronidazole inhibits 25% of strains of *Arachnia* and about 50 and 90% of strains of *Capnocytophaga ochracea* at concentrations of 4 and 16 μg/ml, respectively.

The antibacterial spectrum of metronidazole also includes oral spirochetes and *Treponema pallidum*. Metronidazole, however, is not used in the treatment of syphilis.

4.3.3. Activity against Bacteria in Mixed Culture

Enterococcus faecalis is capable of inactivating metronidazole in vitro and thus allowing the coculture of *B. fragilis* (MIC, 0.5 μg/ml) in the presence of 4 μg of metronidazole per ml. Likewise, when *Bacteroides thetaiotaomicron* and *E. coli* in mixed culture are treated with metronidazole the *Bacteroides* strain decreases, whereas if *E. faecalis* is added regrowth of *B. thetaiotaomicron* is observed. The practical significance of these observations has not been established.

4.4. Bactericidal Activity

The minimum bactericidal concentrations of the 5-nitroimidazoles for obligate anaerobes are equal or very close to the MICs. It should be pointed out that the bactericidal activity of metronidazole (reduction of 3 to 4 logarithms in the initial population) against *B. fragilis* is obtained in vitro after between 3 and 5 h if the correct anaerobic conditions are met during the experiments. The growth phase and the size of the inoculum have no effect on the killing rate. Within the limit of variations in pH from 5.5 to 8, the bactericidal effects are not affected.

In vitro, metronidazole exhibits rapid concentration-dependent bactericidal activity over a broad range of clinically achieved concentrations against *Bacteroides* and demonstrates a prolonged postantibiotic effect (>3 h). In an anaerobic infection model in which human pharmacokinetics were simulated, Lewis et al. demonstrated a bactericidal activity within a 12-h period for all strains (MICs, 0.25 to 4 μg/ml). Using metronidazole (500 mg every 8 h or 750 mg every 12 h) the percentage of the dosing interval during which the metronidazole concentration was above the MIC was 100%. The area under the inhibitory concentration curve (AUIC) was 650 to 670 μg·h/ml for most strains (MIC, 0.5 μg/ml). When the isolate demonstrated decreased susceptibility to metronidazole (MIC, 4 μg/ml), the AUIC decreased to 60 μg·h/ml, but the bactericidal activity was still present.

4.5. Combination with Other Antibiotics

Metronidazole does not interfere at all with the activity of antibiotics active against *Staphylococcus aureus, E. coli*, or *Proteus mirabilis*. The only antagonism described involves the combination with chloramphenicol, which may be antagonistic, neutral, or synergistic depending on the strains of *B. fragilis* concerned. The combination of metronidazole with other antibiotics does not, to my knowledge, cause antagonism in the majority of obligate anaerobes susceptible to 5-nitroimidazoles. Thus, studies conducted with *B. fragilis* have shown a lack of antagonism between metronidazole on the one hand and clindamycin, erythromycin A, carbenicillin, cefoxitin, spectinomycin, spiramycin, and benzylpenicillin on the other. The most widely studied combinations have been those involving spiramycin, where synergy against strains of *Bacteroides, Prevotella*, and *Propionibacterium* is observed and an additive effect against *Actinomyces* is observed. This synergy has been utilized in the treatment of periodontal infections. Partial synergy has been demonstrated between metronidazole and rifampin versus *Clostridium difficile*. More recently, combinations with new fluoroquinolones (ciprofloxacin, ofloxacin, and levofloxacin) have proved neutral or synergistic.

4.6. Mode of Action

Metronidazole is a compound with a low molecular weight that diffuses equally well inside the cells of aerobic and obligate anaerobic bacteria. The feature common to susceptible strains is the presence of an electron transport system with a low redox potential (ferredoxin-like or flavodoxin-like). These proteins are capable of reducing the nitro group by a nonenzymatic chemical reaction. This reduction plays a dual role. It reduces the intracellular concentration of unchanged metronidazole and hence maintains a penetration gradient, and it produces intermediate compounds that are toxic to the bacterial cell; this toxicity is due not to the final reduction product but to the unstable intermediates generated and/or the free radicals produced. These reduction intermediates bind to DNA and subsequently inhibit its synthesis, resulting in bacterial cell death. Inhibition of growth or protein synthesis by chloramphenicol does not interfere with the action of metronidazole against *B. fragilis*.

Returning to certain aspects of the mechanism of action in greater detail, it is possible to explain both the loss of activity of 5-nitroimidazoles under aerobic conditions and their selective toxicity against obligate anaerobes. Thus, the intracellular reduction of metronidazole ($R-NO_2$) occurs through an electron donor: $e + R-NO_2 \rightarrow R-NO_2^-$.

Oxygen antagonizes this reduction, either by competing with metronidazole in the capture of electrons or by oxidizing the reduced compound ($R-NO_2^-$), resulting in the regeneration of the original molecule with the production of a superoxide anion: $R-NO_2^- + O_2 \rightarrow R-NO_2 + O_2^-$.

In the absence of metronidazole in the bacterial cell, the electron acceptor is a hydrogen proton, itself reduced to molecular hydrogen under the action of a dehydrogenase: $2e + 2H^+ \rightarrow H_2$.

The 5-nitroimidazoles compete to capture the electrons and thus block the production of hydrogen in *Trichomonas vaginalis* and obligate anaerobes. However, as hydrogen production resumes once metronidazole is reduced, irreversible inhibition of the dehydrogenase does not constitute the mechanism of action. This enzyme therefore serves to reduce metronidazole without an adverse effect on the bacteria, while generating electrons with a low redox potential. A second nonenzymatic reaction is then essential, the electrons generated having to find an electron transporter (ferredoxin) between the enzyme and metronidazole.

In the reduction of metronidazole, the source of electrons is pyruvate-ferredoxin oxidoreductase, the role of which is to decarboxylate pyruvate with the production of acetate and carbon dioxide. The redox reaction potentials of the different systems, pyruvate-acetate + CO_2 (−700 mV), $H_2/2H^+$ (−420 mV), and ferredoxin$^-$/ferredoxin (−420 mV), are more negative than or identical to those of the metronidazole$^-$/metronidazole pair, while the ubiquitous NADH/NAD^+ system is much more positive (>100 mV). These thermodynamic considerations partly explain the mechanism of action; the selective toxicity of anaerobes is due to the fact that a redox potential of −430 to −460 mV is necessary to reduce the nitro group of the 5-nitroimidazoles. The lowest potential that can be obtained with aerobes is −350 mV. Strains of *H. pylori* are capable of having potentials of less than −430 mV under anaerobic conditions. Metronidazole-resistant strains have lost this faculty.

4.7. Mechanisms of Resistance

The natural resistance of aerobic and microaerophilic bacteria is associated with insufficient nitroreductase activity, preventing the formation of reduced intermediate compounds generating DNA breaks in the adenine- and thymidine-rich regions.

Acquired resistance is rare, once the many technical errors have been excluded. Metronidazole is cross-resistant with other 5-nitroimidazoles.

There are few data on the acquisition of resistance to metronidazole by anaerobic bacteria. In a laboratory study involving six strains of *B. fragilis*, no resistance was detected after 20 serial passages in metronidazole-containing medium; however, acquisition of resistance was recorded for a strain of *B. fragilis* isolated from a patient receiving long-term treatment (3.5 years) for Crohn's disease.

The mechanism of resistance appears related either to

- Impermeability of the outer membrane or the inability to concentrate the antibiotic
- A reduction in nitroreductase activity
- The loss of activity of the pyruvate-dehydrogenase system (essential in *Clostridium perfringens* and *B. fragilis*)

The combination of two mechanisms (impermeability and reduced nitroreductase activity) has been described for a strain of *B. fragilis*. Compared with those in a metronidazole-susceptible strain of *B. fragilis*, it was shown that the penetration of metronidazole was weaker in a metronidazole-resistant strain and that the rate of reduction of metronidazole was four times less, again reflecting a reduction in nitroreductase activity.

Several teams have shown that metronidazole-resistant strains of *T. vaginalis, C. perfringens*, and *B. fragilis* had lost the pyruvate-ferredoxin oxidoreductase generating the electrons necessary to reduce metronidazole.

4.8. Metronidazole Resistance of the *B. fragilis* Group

Metronidazole penetrates within the cells of *B. fragilis* strains by a single diffusion, and a linear relationship is established between intracellular accumulation and the extracellular concentration of metronidazole. Metronidazole was not reduced in resistant cells metabolically active and with their entire genetic material throughout the experiment. On other hand, susceptible strains presented chromosomal breakage, a rapid consumption of dissolved metronidazole, and a lethality of the bacterial population during the first 30 min of exposure.

Under strict anaerobic conditions, a 5-nitroimidazole such as dimetridazole is metabolized without major ring cleavage or nitrate formation. Two distinct metabolic pathways are involved depending on the susceptibility of the strains. In a *B. fragilis* strain the classical reduction pathway of nitroaromatic compounds is followed at least as far as the nitroso-radical anion, with further formation of the azo-dimer, 5,5′-azobis-(1,2-dimethylimidazole). In the resistant strain containing the *nimA* gene, dimetridazole is reduced to the amine derivative, namely, 5-amino-1,2-dimethylimidazole, preventing the formation of the toxic form of the compound that causes DNA breakage. It was suggested that *nimA* and related genes may encode a 5-nitroimidazole reductase.

Members of the *B. fragilis* group were classified in three groups according to susceptibility to 5-nitroimidazoles (Dublanchet, 1990): (i) susceptible strains (S), MIC of 5-nitroimidazoles of <2 μg/ml; (ii) strains of reduced susceptibility (RS), MIC of metronidazole of 2 to 4 μg/ml and MIC of tinidazole of 4 to 8 μg/ml; and (iii) resistant strains (R), MIC of 5-nitroimidazoles of 16 to 64 μg/ml.

By measuring the diameter of the zone of inhibition observed around a disk of tinidazole or metronidazole applied to Wilkins-Chalgren agar seeded with the test strain, the strain can be assigned to one of the proposed three groups: no inhibition around the disk, R. strain; zones of inhibition of 14 mm (tinidazole) and 21 mm (metronidazole), RS strain; and zones of inhibition of >46 mm (tinidazole) and >43 mm (metronidazole), S strain.

Strains of reduced susceptibility and metronidazole-resistant strains (MIC, >16 μg/ml) have frequently been found in vitro in French studies. This reduced susceptibility to the 5-nitroimidazoles does not have a clinical expression.

In France, two clinical isolates were reported in 1988; one of the strains was also resistant to imipenem.

A specific transmissible genetic determinant conferring a low level of resistance on *B. fragilis* was shown in 1989 (Breuil et al., 1989b).

Two resistance determinants (*nimA* and *nimC*) were shown to be located on small mobilizable plasmids designated pIP 417 (7.7 kb) and pIP 419 (10 kb) from *Bacteroides vulgatus* BV17 and *B. thetaioataomicron* BT13, respectively.

Another determinant (*nimB*) was found to be located on the chromosome of *B. fragilis* BF8.

The 5-nitroimidazole resistance genes of *B. fragilis* BF8 (*nimA*) and *B. thetaioataomicron* BT13 (*nimB*) have been sequenced; they are closely related (70% identity). Morever, an identical insertion sequence (IS*1186*) was shown to activate the gene *cfiA*, which encodes a carbapenemase for *B. fragilis* and is present immediately upstream of *cfiA*.

The transcription of the *cfiA* gene was found to be driven from a promoter identified on the right end of the insertion sequence. The same promoter could be efficient in the transcription of the *nimA* and *nimB* genes. Thus, resistance to both 5-nitroimidazoles and β-lactams may be encountered on rare occasions only among the *Bacteroides* species.

The *nimC* gene was described from a *B. thetaiotaomicron* plasmid (pIP 419) and the *nimD* gene was described from a *B. fragilis* plasmid (pIP 421). An insertion sequence element (IS*1170*) was identified upstream of the *nimC* gene. IS*1170* is 1,604 bp in length and is flanked by imperfect inverted repeats (15 bp). IS*1170* is similar to *Bacteroides* IS942, which serves as a promoter for the *ccrA* gene, which also encodes a carbapenemase, resulting in possible coresistance between 5-nitroimidazoles and β-lactams.

Detection by PCR of the *nim* genes using primer pair NIM-3 and NIM-5 has been described. Plasmid-borne genes have higher copy numbers (10 to 20 copies per cell) than chromosomal genes (1 or 2 copies per cell). Recently the *nimA* and *nimC* genes were found on the chromosome of *B. fragilis* strains from Morocco. The low MICs (0.2 to 2.0 μg/ml) indicated that the *nim* genes were not efficiently expressed in these clinical isolates.

Schematic comparison of the nucleotide sequences of the inverted repeat right and the outward-oriented promoter carried in the right ends of the two insertion sequence families was performed (Table 2).

DNA sequencing confirmed the presence of *nimA* genes in propionibacteria, *Actinomyces odontolyticus, Clostridium bifermentans*, and *Prevotella bivia* and of the *nimB* genes from *B. fragilis*. These authors demonstrated the presence of *nim* genes in 20 of 22 metronidazole-resistant strains (MIC, >16 μg/ml). Reduced susceptibility to metronidazole for 5 of

Table 2 The genes *nim, cfiA*, and *ccrA*

Location of 5-nitroimidazole resistance	Promoter on IS–distance between the 2 regions–gene *nim*
Plasmid pIP 417	IS*1168* (1,320 bp)–14 bp–*nimA* (528 bp)
Chromosomal	IS*1168* (1,320 bp)–12 bp *nimB* (492 bp)
Plasmid pIP 421	IS*1169* (1,325 bp)–*nimD* (8 bp)
	IS*1169* (1,325 bp)–*cfiA* (8 bp)[a]
Plasmid pIP 419	IS*1170* (1,604 bp)–*nimC* (24 bp)
	IS942 (1,604 bp)–*ccrA* (19 bp)[a]

[a]The *cfiA* and *ccrA* genes encode *B. fragilis* metallo-β-lactamases.

6 strains was associated with the presence of a *nim* gene. A *nimE* gene was reported for 5 *B. fragilis* isolates.

The lack of *nim* genes was associated with susceptibility (MIC, <2.0 μg/ml) to metronidazole. Three groups of *B. fragilis* strains classified according to the presence of *nim* genes were described: (i) absence of the *nim* genes if the MIC of metronidazole is <1.0 μg/ml, (ii) presence of the *nim* genes for a MIC of >4 μg/ml, and (iii) heterogeneity for MICs between 1 and 2 μg/ml.

Among 39 *B. fragilis* isolates, the *nim* genes were not found within 33 of 33 metronidazole-susceptible strains (MICs, 0.25 to 1.0 μg/ml). The *nimB*, *nimD*, and *nimE* genes were detected by PCR in 6 of 6 strains with decreased susceptibility to metronidazole (MICs, 4 to 8 μg/ml). In a highly resistant *B. fragilis* isolate (MIC, 64 μg/ml), the *nimA* gene was found on the chromosome, and the *nimE* gene was found in a *Veillonella* isolate (MIC, 12 μg/ml).

Bacteroides species highly resistant to metronidazole (MIC, >16 μg/ml) were associated with clinical failure.

4.9. Resistance to Metronidazole in *H. pylori*

Anaerobes and *H. pylori* share the same metronidazole mode of action: the antibacterial activity of metronidazole is dependent on reductive activation of the redox system in the target cell. In theory, any redox system possessing a reductive potential more negative than that of metronidazole in the cell will give its electrons preferentially to metronidazole and result in reductive inactivation.

In *H. pylori* strains, the oxygen-insensitive nitroreductase RdxA is likely to inactivate metronidazole by reduction and formation of cytotoxic intermediates.

Mutations in the *rdxA* gene have been associated with metronidazole resistance. DNA sequence analysis of the *rdxA* alleles of susceptible (MICs, 0.25 to 1.0 μg/ml) or resistant (MICs, 16 to 256 μg/ml) isolates showed that six of nine resistant isolates contained insertion or deletion mutations. One isolate harbored a substitution at codon 148 introducing a premature stop codon.

A second metronidazole nitroreductase responsible for resistance is encoded by the gene *frxA* (NADPH flavin oxidoreductase). Several groups of *H. pylori*, based on susceptibility to metronidazole, have been proposed after comparison of the amino acid sequences for both proteins, RdxA and FrxA, including highly metronidazole-resistant isolates (MIC, 128 μg/ml) harboring premature truncation of and/or altered RdxA and FrxA due to nonsense, framshift, and unique missense mutations and low-level resistant strains (MIC, 8 μg/ml) containing unique missense mutations in FrxA but no specific changes in RdxA.

4.10. Parasite Resistance to Metronidazole

The metronidazole-resistant *T. vaginalis* isolates are more sensitive to oxygen than susceptible isolates. In resistant trichomonads, the intracellular oxygen concentration is higher and interacts with metronidazole to prevent its reduction.

Increased activity of superoxide dismutase in resistant trichomonads may be beneficial for the parasite if it is coupled to a system removing hydrogen peroxide.

T. vaginalis and *Entamoeba* lack catalase and a gluthatione-based antioxidant system. In resistant *T. vaginalis* and *Entamoeba* a high activity of superoxide dismutase with increased expression of this enzyme have been found.

4.11. Role of 5-Nitroimidazoles among Antibiotics Active against Obligate Anaerobes

The profiles of susceptibility to 5-nitroimidazoles of obligate anaerobes other than *B. fragilis* are shown in Tables 3 and 4.

In orofacial and lung infections, the bacteria commonly involved belong to the genera *Fusobacterium*, *Prevotella*, and *Peptostreptococcus*. Forty-two percent of the strains of *Fusobacterium* and *Prevotella* are producers of β-lactamases, the result of which is that penicillin G and the α-aminopenicillins cannot be used alone; they should therefore be combined with either a 5-nitroimidazole or a β-lactamase inhibitor. *B. fragilis* strains have a predominant place among the bacteria involved in abdominal infections. The percentages of *B. fragilis* isolates susceptible to metronidazole reported in 2001 in France are summarized in Table 5.

5. PHARMACOKINETICS OF METRONIDAZOLE

See Tables 6 and 7.

5.1. Absorption

Metronidazole is rapidly absorbed after oral administration (at least 80% of the dose 1 h after ingestion) so that, for equal dosages, the same peak concentrations are obtained as those that occur intravenously within a period of 1 to 3 h.

The bioavailabilities of the oral and rectal forms are close to 100 and 70%, respectively. Although the peak concentrations are the same whether metronidazole is administered on an empty stomach or with food, food consumption prolongs the time to the peak concentration in plasma.

5.2. Concentrations in Plasma

Oral administration of 500 mg of metronidazole yields concentrations in blood of 13 μg/ml at 3 h. The same levels in blood are obtained at the end of a 20-min infusion. The apparent elimination half-life is 8 to 10 h in both of these cases.

Repeated administration of 500 mg intravenously every 8 h results in a steady state in which the peak and trough concentrations are, respectively, 26 and 12 μg/ml.

Table 3 Susceptibility profiles of gram-negative anaerobes other than members of the *B. fragilis* group[a]

Microorganisms	AMX	AMC	TIC + PIP	FOX	CTT	CTX	IMP	MOL	CLI
Prevotella spp. (*P. bivia*, *P. oralis*, *P. disiens*) and pigmented *Prevotella* spp.	+	++++	++	++++	+++	+	++++	+++	+++
Porphyromonas spp.	+++	++++	++++	++++	++++	++++	++++	+++	++++
Fusobacterium spp.	++	++++	++	+++	+++	+/++	+++	++++	++++
Other gram-negative bacilli	+	++++	+++	++	++	+/++	++++	++	++
Veillonella spp.	++	++++	+++	++++	++++	++	++++	+++	++++

[a]AMX, amoxicillin; AMC, co-amoxiclav; TIC, ticarcillin; PIP, piperacillin; FOX, cefoxitin; CTT, cefotetan; CTX, cefotaxime; IMP, imipenem; MOL, metronidazole; CLI, clindamycin.

Table 4 In vitro activities of antibacterials against gram-positive anaerobes[a]

Microorganism(s)	PEN G	TIC + PIP	AMC	C_1G	FOX	CTT	CTX	IMP	MOL	CLI	VAN	CMP
C. perfringens	++++	+++	++++	+++	++++	++++	+++	++++	+++	+++	++++	+++
C. difficile	++++	+++	++++	R	R	16–32 μg/ml	R	4–16 μg/ml	+++	+/R	+++	+
Clostridium spp.	+++	+++	+++	+	+	+	+	++++	+++	+	+++	++
Eubacterium spp.	++++	++++	++++	++	++	++	+	++++	+	++	++++	+++
Propionibacterium spp.	++++	++++	++++	++	++++	++++	++++	++++	R	+/++	++++	+++
Other nonsporulated rods	+++	++++	++++	++	++	+++	+++	++++	+	+++	++++	+++
Gram-positive anaerobic cocci	+++	+++	+++	+	+++	+++	++	++++	+/++	+	++++	+++

[a]PEN G, penicillin G; TIC, ticarcillin; PIP, piperacillin; C_1G, first-generation cephalosporin; FOX, cefoxitin; CTT, cefotetan; CTX, cefotaxime; IMP, imipenem; MOL, metronidazole; CLI, clindamycin; VAN, vancomycin; CMP, chloramphenicol. ++++, ≥95% S; +++, ≥95% of rare strain are resistant; ++, 90 to 95% S; +, 70 to 90% S.

Table 5 Antibiotic resistance of *Bacteroides* isolates in 2001

Microorganism(s) (*n*)	% of strains resistant to compound[a]												
	AMC (≥32/2)	TIC (≥128)	TCC (≥128/2)	FOX (≥64)	CTT (≥64)	CTX (≥16)	IMP (≥16)	MOL (≥32)	CLI (≥8)	CIP (≥4)	LVX (≥8)	MFX (≥4)	GAT (≥4)
B. fragilis (189)	4.8	28.6	1.6	11	19	27	1.6	0.5	21				
Other *Bacteroides* spp. (170)	6.5	39.4	2.9	15.2	72	52	0	0	45.3				
B. fragilis group (359)	5.6	33.7	2.2	13	44	38.7	0.8	0.3	32.6	73	25	11	16

[a]AMC, co-amoxiclav; TIC, ticarcillin; TCC, ticarcillin plus clavulanic acid; FOX, cefoxitin; CTT, cefotetan; IMP, imipenem; MOL, metronidazole; CLI, clindamycin; CIP, ciprofloxacin; MFX, moxifloxacin; LVX, levofloxacin; GAT, gatifloxacin; LZD, linezolid. Values in parentheses after the abbreviations are breakpoints in micrograms per milliliter.

Table 6 Dose pharmacokinetics of metronidazole and ornidazole

Route	Dose (mg)[a]	Period (h)	Concn in plasma (μg/ml)				
			Metronidazole		Ornidazole		
			C_{max}	C_{24}	C_{max}	C_1	C_{24}
Oral	SD						
	200		5.5				
	500		9.8				
	750				11		
	1,000		11.8				
	2,000		40				
	MD or SD						
	200	12	13–21				
	500	8	13–21				
Rectal	500 SD		7				
	1,000 SD		7–11				
	20,000 SD		14				
Intravenous	500 SD		9.2			8	2
	1,000 SD		23			17.7	4.9
	2,000 SD		71				
	500 MD	8	14–60	5–21			
		8	26	14			
		12	21	6.6		15	3–4
		24	16	1.6			

[a]SD, single dose; MD, multiple doses.

Table 7 Principal pharmacokinetics of the 5-nitroimidazoles

Parameter	Metronidazole	Ornidazole
$t_{1/2}$ (h)	8.2	12–14
V (liters/kg)	0.6–0.85	1
<15% Protein binding (%)	1–20	<15
Dialysis ($t_{1/2}$, h)	Yes (2.6 h)	Yes (3 h)
Peritoneal dialysis	Yes	
Colostrum (%)	50–100	
Metabolism (%)	85	95
CL_P (ml/min, 1.73 m^2)	72 ± 16	82
CL_R (ml/min, 1.73 m^2)	10	4
Elimination		
Renal (%) unchanged	8–15	
Metabolites (%)	70	63
Biliary (%)	14	22

When metronidazole is administered by infusion every 12 h, a mean peak concentration of 13 μg/ml is reached.

5.3. Diffusion

Diffusion of metronidazole is rapid and extensive in the lungs, kidneys, liver, skin, alveolar bone, brain, bile, cerebrospinal fluid (CSF), amniotic fluid, cord blood, saliva, seminal fluid, vaginal secretions, hepatic abscesses, and pelvic tissue (the concentrations in the myometrium and fallopian tubes are close to levels in plasma). It crosses the fetoplacental barrier and is excreted in breast milk. Peak concentrations in plasma obtained in pregnant women are identical to those found in the fetus. In the aqueous humor, the concentrations are equivalent to between 33 and 50% of the concentrations in plasma. Concentrations measured in bile and CSF are similar to levels in plasma. It is concentrated in urine and is inactivated in the feces by the saprophytic bacterial flora.

5.4. Metabolism

Metronidazole is metabolized to five main compounds, more than 70% in the liver. The two side chains of metronidazole may be oxidized, probably in the liver, resulting in the two main "alcohol" and "acid" metabolites (Fig. 2). The first metabolite has activity against anaerobes estimated as 65% of that of the parent molecule, whereas the acid metabolite has negligible activity, 5%. After a single dose of 500 mg, peak concentrations in plasma of the alcohol metabolite range from 1 to 2 μg/ml, and the concentration in plasma of the acid metabolite is 0.2 μg/ml.

Protein binding is weak (<10%).

5.5. Elimination

Although high hepatic and biliary concentrations are observed, the colonic concentration is low; the same applies

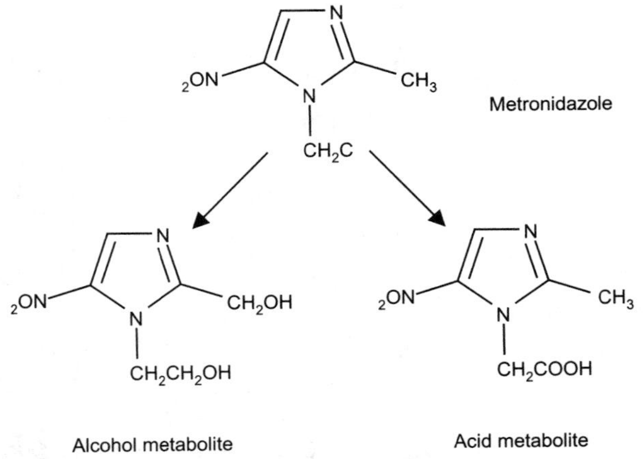

Metronidazole

Alcohol metabolite

Acid metabolite

Figure 2 Metabolism of metronidazole: principal alcohol and acid metabolites

to fecal elimination. Excretion is essentially urinary (40 to 70%, of which about 20% is in the unchanged form), causing a reddish-brown color of the urine. It is eliminated by hemodialysis (the half-life is reduced to 2.5 h); peritoneal dialysis is slight.

5.6. Effect of Age

Metronidazole may be used in premature infants, neonates, infants, and children. In infants aged 28 to 40 weeks, the apparent elimination half-life is inversely proportional to the age, on average 21.6 ± 12.4 h (mean $\pm$ standard deviation). The recommended dosage in the first week of life is 7.5 mg/kg of body weight every 12 h. Plasma metronidazole levels in subjects over 70 years of age are 50% higher than those in young adults for the same doses, and the volume of distribution is reduced by 33%. It is recommended that the dosage be reduced by 30 to 40% in patients over the age of 70 years.

5.7. Pathological Disorders

The apparent elimination half-life of metronidazole is prolonged in patients with hepatic insufficiency; however, a permanent continuous monitoring needs to be undertaken. The dosage should be reduced by 30 to 50%.

It does not accumulate in patients with renal insufficiency, although accumulation is possible if administration is prolonged. It is also eliminated with its metabolites by hemodialysis. It is contraindicated in pregnant women during the embryonic period (except in the event of need) and during lactation (the concentrations in milk are between 50% and more than 100% of the levels in plasma; the half-life of metronidazole in milk is close to that in plasma). Allergy to 5-nitroimidazoles constitutes a strict contraindication. In patients with an ileostomy, metronidazole is absorbed more rapidly and peak concentrations in plasma are higher than in controls. The bioavailability is reduced in patients with Crohn's disease.

5.8. Toxicology

The median lethal doses (metronidazole) in the rat and mouse are very high (1 to 5 g/kg). Chronic toxicity assumes the form of neurologic disorders in the dog (from 75 mg/kg daily) and testicular dystrophy in the rat (300 mg/kg daily). Because of the nitro moiety of the 5-nitroimidazoles, experimental studies have been conducted to test for a potential mutagenic or carcinogenic effect of these compounds, particularly the older metronidazole. These studies have shown the mutation rate of bacteria (*Salmonella enterica* serovar Typhimurium) to be increased in vitro. In animals, contradictory results have been obtained: in the mouse, one study reports an increase in the incidence of pulmonary tumors and lymphomas. In other studies, these phenomena have not been observed in the mouse, hamster, or rat.

In humans, abnormalities of circulating lymphocytes have been observed in patients receiving long-term treatment for Crohn's disease. However, a retrospective epidemiological study conducted at the Mayo Clinic revealed no abnormal incidence of malignant tumors in women treated for *Trichomonas* infections between 1960 and 1969.

No embryofetal or teratogenic effect has been observed in animals. No increased teratogenic risk was noted in the offspring of women receiving metronidazole during their pregnancy, even in the first trimester.

6. PHARMACOKINETICS OF ORNIDAZOLE

See Tables 6 and 7.

After oral administration of a single dose of 500 mg of ornidazole, the peak concentration in plasma of 8 μg/ml is reached after between 2 and 4 h.

It is 95% metabolized in the liver. Five free, glucuroconjugated, or sulfoconjugated metabolites are known. The two main metabolites are M1 and M4 (Fig. 3). Ornidazole is principally eliminated via the urine (65%) and bile (22%). Urinary elimination occurs in the unchanged (30%) or conjugated (70%) form.

Ornidazole levels measured in the CSF and brain represent at least 80% of levels in plasma; the same applies to concentrations in appendiceal fluid. In amniotic fluid, about half the concentration in plasma is found.

The apparent elimination half-life and plasma clearance of ornidazole in nondialyzed subjects with renal insufficiency are similar to those in subjects with normal renal function. Peritoneal elimination of ornidazole is weak: in 48 h only 6% of the administered dose is found in the dialysis fluids. Elimination by hemodialysis is extensive: 42% of the administered dose is eliminated after 4 h of dialysis. During the dialysis session, the plasma half-life of ornidazole is 3 h. No dose adjustment is needed in patients with renal impairment (even if severe), in nondialyzed patients, or in those treated by continuous ambulatory peritoneal dialysis. However, in

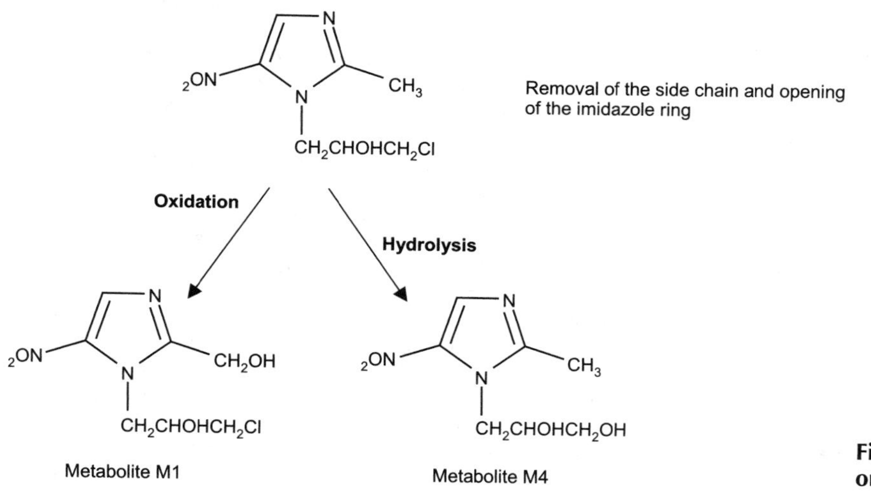

Figure 3 Metabolism of ornidazole

hemodialyzed patients it is recommended that a new dose of ornidazole be administered.

In patients with hepatic insufficiency, the peak concentrations in plasma occur later and the apparent elimination half-lives are prolonged. In order to prevent accumulation of ornidazole, the interval between doses should be doubled.

Toxic concentrations of more than 30 μg/ml are obtained after an oral dose of 3 g.

7. PHARMACOKINETICS OF TINIDAZOLE

Administration of a single dose of 2 g of tinidazole orally yields peak concentrations in plasma of 40 to 51 μg/ml within 2 h and levels in plasma of 11 to 20 μg/ml at 24 h. The bioavailability of the oral form is 90%. Absorption is not affected by food. The apparent elimination half-life is 12 to 14 h. Plasma protein binding is weak, 8 to 20%. Tissue distribution is similar to that of the other 5-nitroimidazoles. Tinidazole crosses the meningeal and placental barriers and is excreted in breast milk. The levels in the vaginal secretions, CSF, saliva, and bile are similar to those assayed in plasma. It is eliminated mainly in the urine and to a minor extent in the bile. Twenty to twenty-five percent of the administered dose is found in the urine in the unchanged form, 2 to 3% is found in the form of a metabolite (hydroxymethyltinidazole), and 10% is found in the form of unidentified compounds. In northern Europe, tinidazole has been extensively used in the injectable form. Intravenous administration of 800 and 1600 mg yields peak concentrations in plasma of 15 and 32 μg/ml, respectively. Tinidazole may affect vigilance, and drivers of vehicles and users of machines should be warned accordingly.

8. ADVERSE EFFECTS OF THE 5-NITROIMIDAZOLES

The 5-nitroimidazoles are generally well tolerated. The adverse effects are classified as frequently (f) or occasionally (o) reported, while the other effects are rarely mentioned:

- Gastrointestinal disorders: epigastric pain, nausea (f), vomiting (o), diarrhea (o), metallic taste (f), dry mouth (f), and pseudomembranous colitis (rare)
- Hematologic disorders: transient neutropenia (rare)
- Skin disorders: rash, pruritus, and urticaria
- Hepatic disorders
- Neurologic disorders: polyneuritis, seizures in the case of long-term, high-dose treatment
- Miscellaneous disorders: insomnia (o), stomatitis (o), urethral burning (o), phlebitis at the injection site (o), paresthesia (o)

It is on the neurologic level that the most serious adverse effects are observed during high-dose and/or prolonged treatments. Metronidazole should be used with caution in patients with tremors prior to treatment. Although metronidazole is used in the treatment of pseudomembranous colitis, it may itself be responsible for this condition in exceptional cases.

Metronidazole turns the urine a brownish red color, which ornidazole does not.

In healthy subjects, metronidazole does not affect the intestinal flora. Under conditions of intestinal anaerobiosis it is difficult to explain the lack of impact on the bacteria capable of reducing it. However, a reduction in the anaerobic flora is observed in the presence of high concentrations of metronidazole and in the case of diarrhea or during simultaneous treatment with other antibacterial agents; imidazole-aminoglycoside combinations have been used prophylactically for abdominal surgery.

The teratogenic effect of metronidazole remains disputed. There is no suspected carcinogenicity in humans, but the product has proved carcinogenic in a species of mouse, although not in the rat or hamster.

The solvent of ornidazole, propylene glycol, may exceptionally be responsible for serious complications, particularly in children: hemolysis, neurologic disorders, hyperosmolarity, metabolic acidosis, heart rhythm disorders, hypotension, and respiratory depression.

9. CHANGES IN BIOCHEMICAL CONSTANTS

Metronidazole interferes in the assay of transaminases (serum glutamic oxalacetic transaminase) and procainamide. It produces a false-positive reading in Nelson's treponema immobilization test.

10. DRUG INTERACTIONS

Because of the disulfiram-like effect, the consumption of alcoholic beverages and alcohol-containing drugs should be avoided. Combination with disulfiram is not recommended because it can cause delusional episodes or a confusional state.

As metronidazole potentiates the oral anticoagulant effects (warfarin), the prothombin time should be monitored more often and if necessary the dosage of these anticoagulants should be adjusted during treatment with metronidazole and for up to 8 days after its discontinuation.

An increase in the toxicity of 5-fluorouracil is observed as a result of a reduction in its clearance, and also potentiation of the curarizing effect of vecuronium.

Phenobarbital reduces the half-life of metronidazole. The dosage of metronidazole should therefore be increased in patients receiving phenobarbital.

11. THERAPEUTIC INDICATIONS

The excellent distribution of metronidazole in all organs and its intense bactericidal activity, including against quiescent bacteria, make it the antibiotic of choice in infections in which anaerobes are implicated. It acts either as curative treatment for medicosurgical infections or as prophylaxis for postoperative infections due to susceptible anaerobic bacteria. The main situations in which anaerobes are involved are digestive and genital infections (sigmoiditis, hepatic abscess, peritonitis, Douglas abscess), pleuropulmonary infections, brain abscess, endocarditis, and septicemia.

Actinomycosis and rare infections due to *Propionibacterium acnes* (brain abscess) are excluded. In mixed infections in which the antibiotic therapy instituted is ineffective against obligate anaerobes (particularly β-lactamase-producing *Bacteroides*, *Prevotella*, and *Fusobacterium*), metronidazole is generally used in combination to have an effect on these anaerobes. Metronidazole should not be combined with antibiotics that show excellent activity against the *B. fragilis* group or *Prevotella*, such as β-lactam–β-lactamase inhibitor combinations (amoxicillin or ticarcillin plus clavulanic acid and piperacillin plus tazobactam), cephamycins (cefoxitin and cefotetan), and carbapenems (imipenem and meropenem).

Its penetration of the central nervous system means that it is extensively used in brain abscesses and other infections of the central nervous system; it is used in anaerobic endocarditis, severe infections in immunodepressed patients, and lower respiratory tract infections (pleural empyema, lung abscess, and suppurative pneumonia) in combination with a penicillin or a macrolide. These antibacterial agents have also demonstrated their efficacy in a number of infections: bacteremia; bone and joint infections; tooth and orofacial infections; infection of the head, face, and neck; soft tissue infections (cellulitis and diabetic foot); obstetric and gynecological infections (pelvic or vaginal cellulitis); chronic sinusitis and otitis; and Vincent's angina. Significant results have been obtained in the treatment of vaginosis in which anaerobes, *G. vaginalis*, and other pathogenic agents have been implicated. In abdominal infections, the 5-nitroimidazoles are frequently combined with aminoglycosides, supplemented with a penicillin or a cephalosporin depending on the protocol. Like vancomycin, metronidazole is also used orally in the treatment of *C. difficile* pseudomembranous colitis. In specific subjects unable to tolerate oral antibiotic therapy, the colitis has been treated intravenously.

It is used prophylactically in patients at high risk of infection (immunodepressed patients and subjects having undergone prolonged intensive care or repeated surgical procedures or having received multiple antibiotic therapy) in the following circumstances: major gastrointestinal, septic gynecological, thoracoabdominal, vascular, or bone surgery involving a threat of gas gangrene; in multiple open traumas; or following the discovery of gangrenous, necrotic, or perforated lesions during surgery. Some antibiotic protocols are selective for gram-negative anaerobes (combination of aminoglycosides with α-aminopenicillins or cephalosporins or aztreonam).

The combination metronidazole-spiramycin is widely used in the treatment of orodental infections.

12. PHYSICOCHEMICAL INCOMPATIBILITIES

The 5-nitroimidazoles are administered in the form of an infusion in an isotonic saline or glucose solution. The main incompatibilities in solution in the same infusion bottle are penicillin G, cefamandole, cefoxitin, 10% amino acid solutions, and dopamine hydrochloride. A pink color appears when metronidazole and aztreonam solutions are mixed; similarly, β-lactams with a 2-amino-5-thiazolyl nucleus react chemically with metronidazole in an acidic medium (diazotization reaction).

Table 8 shows the presentation of the 5-nitroimidazoles.

Ornidazole needs to be administered as a slow infusion. Ampoules of 125 mg (1 ml), 500 mg (3 ml), and 1 g (6 ml) are diluted in 10 to 20, 50 to 125, and 100 to 250 ml, respectively, of injectable isotonic glucose or in saline.

A dosage of 1 g in adults may be administered in a single slow infusion.

The intravenous slow infusion administration of 500 mg of metronidazole is realized in a period of 30 to 60 min (100-ml bottle or plastic bag).

13. DOSAGE

When the patient's condition allows, the 5-nitroimidazoles are preferably administered orally.

13.1. In the Treatment of Anaerobic Infections

See Table 9.

13.1.1. Metronidazole

Metronidazole is administered in two or three daily doses according to the daily dosage adopted. A specific vaginitis requires 1 g daily in two doses for 7 days. Prevention of postoperative infections due to anaerobic bacteria is achieved by administration of an infusion of 500 mg 1 h before surgery, followed by two other infusions 8 and 16 h later. The same procedure is followed in children with a dosage of 20 mg/kg. In surgical chemoprophylaxis in combination with an antibiotic active against enteric gram-negative bacilli, metronidazole has been used orally at a dosage of 500 mg three times daily, beginning 48 h before the surgery. In children, the same protocol is used at a dose of 20 to 30 mg/kg/day.

The usual maximum dose of metronidazole is 4 g in adults.

Table 8 Presentation of the 5-nitroimidazoles

Generic name	Trade name	Route of administration
Metronidazole	Flagyl	Vial of 500 mg for i.v.[a] infusion Tablets, 250 mg Suspension, 4%
Metronidazole + spiramycin	Rodogyl	Tablets: metronidazole, 125 mg; spiramycin, 75,000 IU
Ornidazole	Tiberal	Tablets, 500 mg Vials of 125 and 500 mg
Tinidazole	Fasigyn	Tablets, 500 mg

[a]i.v., intravenous.

Table 9 Dosages of 5-nitroimidazoles used in treatment of anaerobic infections

Use	Patients	Metronidazole	Ornidazole
Treatment	Adults	1–1.5 g	1–1.5 g
	Children	25–30 mg/kg	20–30 mg/kg
	Infants		20 mg/kg
	Neonates		
Prophylaxis	Adults		1 g/day
	Children		20 mg/kg/day
Pseudomembranous colitis		250 mg every 6 h	

13.1.2. Ornidazole

Prevention of postoperative infections due to anaerobic bacteria in adults is achieved by administration of an infusion of 1 g at the time of induction; in children 20 mg/kg is administered in two infusions. In curative treatment, ornidazole is generally administered in two daily doses.

13.1.3. Tinidazole

Prevention of postoperative infections due to anaerobic bacteria in adults is achieved by administration of 2 g in a single dose 4 to 8 h before the operation.

13.2. Monitoring of Treatment

Alcohol is not recommended. Neurologic and hematologic functions should be monitored. Leukocyte counts should be performed if there is a history of blood abnormalities or in the case of high-dose and/or prolonged treatment. In the presence of leukopenia, the advisability of continuing treatment depends on the severity of the infection.

In patients with renal insufficiency, the interval between doses is unchanged.

14. CONCLUSION

The three 5-nitroimidazole derivatives have very similar antibacterial properties; the pharmacokinetics are very similar, with a longer apparent elimination half-life for ornidazole than for metronidazole, possibly allowing the number of doses of ornidazole to be reduced. These imidazole derivatives have excellent in vitro activity and well-established clinical efficacy in the treatment of anaerobic infections or in mixed infections when combined with antibiotics effective against aerobes. Once again it should be pointed out that this activity does not extend to all obligate anaerobes, since nonsporulating gram-positive bacilli appear to be partially or totally resistant to the 5-nitroimidazoles, depending on the species.

REFERENCES

Breuil J, Burnat C, Patey O, Dublanchet A, 1989a, Survey of Bacteroides fragilis patterns in France, J Antimicrob Chemother, 24, 69–75.

Breuil J, Dublanchet A, Truffaut N, Sebald M, 1989b, Transferable 5-nitroimidazole resistance in the Bacteroides fragilis group, Plasmid, 21, 151–154.

Dublanchet A, 1990, Bacteroides de sensibilité reduite au metronidazole. Une expression phenotypique inhabituelle, Med Malad Infect, 20, Hors serie, 113–116.

ADDITIONAL BIBLIOGRAPHY

Cederbrant G, Kahlmeter G, Ljungh A, 1992, Proposed mechanism for metronidazole resistance in Helicobacter pylori, J Antimicrob Chemother, 29, 115–120.

Cuchural GJ, Tally FP, Jacobus NV, Aldridge K, Cleary T, Finegold SM, Hill G, Laninni J, O' Keefe JP, Pierson C, Crook D, Russo T, Hecht D, 1988, Susceptibility of the Bacteroides fragilis group in the United States, analysis by site of isolation, Antimicrob Agents Chemother, 32, 717–722.

Dubreuil L, Derriennic M, Sedallian A, Romond C, Courtieu AL, 1989, Evolution in antibiotic susceptibility of Bacteroides fragilis group strains in France based on periodic surveys, Infection, 17, 197–200.

Duerden BL, Drasar BS, 1991, Anaerobes in humans, Arnold E., London.

Finegold SM, Baron EJ, Wexler HM, 1992, A Clinical Guide to Anaerobic Infections. Wadsworth Anaerobe Laboratory, Los Angeles, California. Star Publishing Company, Belmont, Calif.

Finegold SM, Mathisen GE, 1985, Metronidazole, in Mandell GL, Douglas RG, Bennett JE, ed, Principles and Practice of Infectious Diseases, Churchill Livingstone, New York.

Finegold SM, Wexler HM, 1988, Therapeutic implications of bacteriologic findings in mixed aerobic-anaerobic infections, Antimicrob Agents Chemother, 32, 611–626.

Kernbaum S, 1988, 5 nitro-imidazole et infections A anaerobies, p 1512–1519, in Giroux JP, Mathé G, Meyniel G, ed, Pharmacologie clinique, Edts Expansion scientifique française, Paris.

Knapp CC, Ludwig ML, Washington JA, 1991, In vitro activity of metronidazole against *Helicobacter pylori* as determined by agar dilution and agar diffusion, Antimicrob Agents Chemother, 35, 1230–1231.

Lockerby DL, Rabin HR, Bryan LE, Laishley EJ, 1984, Ferrodoxin-linked reduction of metronidazole in *Clostridium pasteurianum*, Antimicrob Agents Chemother, 26, 665–669.

Nagy E, Földes J, 1991, Inactivation of metronidazole by Enterococcus faecalis, J Antimicrob Ther, 27, 63–70.

National Committee for Clinical Laboratory Standards, 1990, Reference dilution procedure for antimicrobial testing of anaerobic bacteria. Approved standard M11-A2. NCCLS, Villanova, Pa.

Oldenburg B, Speck WT, 1983, Metronidazole, Pediatr Clin N Am, 30, 7175.

Scully BE, 1988, Metronidazole, Med Clin North Am, 72, 613–621.

Wexler HM, 1991, Susceptibility testing of anaerobic bacteria: myth, magic, or method? Clin Microbiol Rev, 4, 470–484.

Whiting JL, Cheng N, Chow AW, 1987, Interactions of ciprofloxacin with clindamycin, metronidazole, cefoxitin, cefotaxime, and mezlocillin against gram-positive and gram-negative anaerobic bacteria, Antimicrob Agents Chemother, 31, 1379–1382.

Dihydrofolate Reductase Inhibitors, Nitroheterocycles (Furans), and 8-Hydroxyquinolines

P. VEYSSIER AND A. BRYSKIER

35

1. SULFONAMIDES AND COMBINATIONS

The sulfonamides were the forerunner of the modern era of antibacterial chemotherapy after the discovery of sulfamidochrysoidine (Prontosil) in 1935 by Dogmagk. A number of drugs have been synthesized, not only antibacterial agents but also hypoglycemic agents and diuretics. Adverse effects resulted in an important reduction of sulfonamide usage in anti-infective therapy. Furthermore, the combination of bacterial resistance and the usage of other antibacterial agents also led to a dramatic decrease in sulfonamide prescriptions. The interest in sulfonamides was revived because of their potential against parasitic infections, particularly in immunodepressed patients or in combination with erythromycin in the treatment of otitis media in children. Since 1968 sulfonamides have been one of the components in combinations with dihydrofolate reductase (DHFR) inhibitors, such as trimethoprim (co-trimoxazole).

1.1. Sulfonamides

1.1.1. Structure

The sulfonamides are derived from sulfanilamide (*para*-aminobenzenesulfonamide), which has a structure similar to that of *para*-aminobenzoic acid, a factor required by bacteria to synthesize folic acid. An amino group at position 4 is associated with increased antibacterial activity. An increase in the inhibition of *para*-aminobenzenesulfonamide acid is obtained by substitution of the SO_2 attached at C-1, as in sulfadiazine, sulfisoxazole, and sulfamethizole, all of which are more active than sulfanilamide. Substituents are invoved in pharmacological modifications (absorption, solubility, and digestive tolerance). Reduced gastrointestinal absorption has been obtained following substitution on the amino group at C-4.

1.1.2. Classification

1.1.2.1. Short- or Intermediate-Acting Sulfonamides

Sulfisoxazole and sulfamethoxazole are still used in urinary tract infections. Sulfadiazine alone is prescribed in a limited number of countries.

These sulfonamides can also be used in combination: sulfadiazine and trimethoprim, sulfamoxole and trimethoprim, sulfamethoxazole plus trimethoprim, and N^1-acetylsulfisoxazole plus erythromycin (Fig. 1).

1.1.2.2. Long-Acting Sulfonamides

Few long-acting sulfonamides are currently prescribed, such as sulfadoxine and sulfamethoxine. Their elimination half-lives range from 100 to 230 h. A peak concentration in plasma of 50 to 75 μg/ml is reached 2.5 to 6 h after administration of an oral dose of 300 mg. In combination with pyrimethamine (25 mg), it may be used in malaria due to chloroquine-resistant *Plasmodium falciparum*.

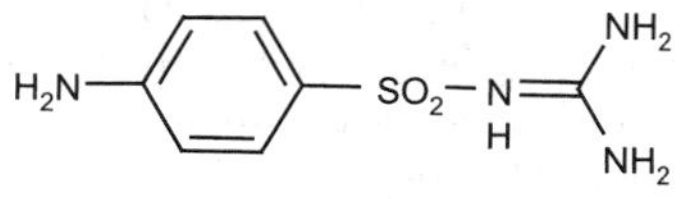

$H_2N-C_6H_4-SO_2-NH-C(=NH_2)NH_2$ Sulfaguanidine

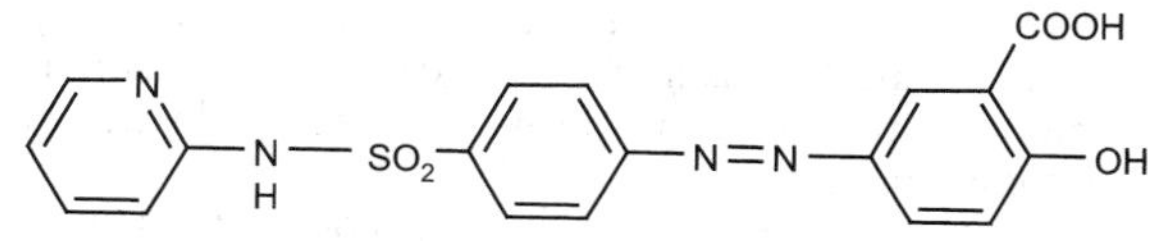

Sulfasalazine

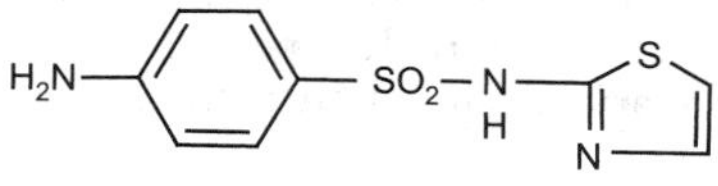

Sulfathiazole

Figure 1 Sulfonamides for systemic use

1.1.2.3. Intestinal Sulfonamides

Sulfaguanidine (*N*′-amidinosulfanilamide), succinylsulfathiazole, and phthalylsulfathiazole (Sulfathalidine) are poorly absorbed by the gastrointestinal tract. Salicylazosulfapyridine (sulfasalazine) is transformed in sulfapyridine and is used in ulcerative colitis (Fig. 2).

1.1.3. Mechanism of Action

The sulfonamides are bacteriostatic agents. Sulfonamides and sulfones inhibit the dihydropteroate synthase (DHPS) enzyme of the folate pathway.

Sulfonamide antimicrobial agents inhibit the formation of dihydropteroic acid by competing with *para*-aminobenzoic acid for condensation with 7,8-pterin pyrophosphate, a reaction catalyzed by DHPS. Inhibition results in the cells becoming depleted of tetrahydrofolate.

1.1.4. In Vitro Antibacterial Activity

The antibacterial spectrum of sulfonamides includes the following:

- Gram-positive bacteria: *Staphylococcus aureus, Streptococcus pyogenes, Streptococcus pneumoniae*, viridans group streptococci, *Bacillus anthracis, Clostridium perfringens, Actinomyces*, and *Nocardia; Enterococcus faecalis* is resistant.
- Gram-negative enteric bacteria and *Neisseria* spp., *Bordetella pertussis, Haemophilus influenzae*, and some *Pseudomonas* spp. and *Legionella* spp., as well as *Chlamydia*

Mycobacteria, *Treponema, Coxiella, Mycoplasma*, and *Leptospira* are resistant to sulfonamides. The susceptibility of *Mycobacterium leprae* to sulfonamides is comparable to that to dapsone.

Combination with trimethoprim (co-trimoxazole) potentiates the activity of sulfonamides against a large number of

H_2N—C₆H₄—SO_2—NH—**R**

	R
Sulfadiazine	
Sulfadimethoxine	
Sulfamethoxazole	
Sulfamoxole	
Sulfisoxazole (sulfafurazole)	

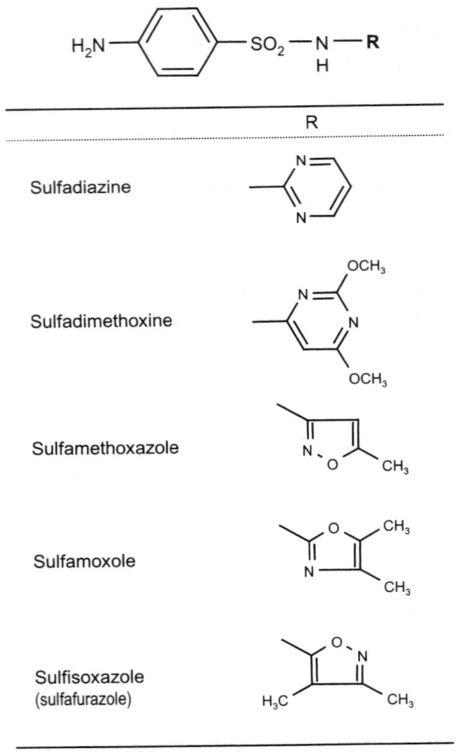

Figure 2 Sulfonamides for intestinal use

bacteria. Combinations of proguanil and certain sulfonamides (sulfisoxazole) are used in malaria due to *P. falciparum*.

1.1.5. Resistance

Mutations in the primary sequence of the *dhp* gene are associated with sulfonamide resistance. Emergence of resistance is not uncommon in streptococci during therapy. Resistant strains of gram-negative bacilli are now very common. The emergence of such strains involves plasmid-mediated resistance. *Neisseria gonorrhoeae* is often resistant, as is *Neisseria meningitidis* (25 to 80%). Sulfonamide resistance is commonly mediated by alternative, drug-resistant forms of DHPS. In enteric bacteria two plasmid-borne genes, *sul1* (or *sulI*) and *sul2* (or *sulII*), encode resistant enzymes. *sul1* forms part of the conserved region at the 3′ end of most class 1 integrons. *sul2* was originally found to be carried predominantly on small nonconjugative plasmids or on larger plasmids; *sul2* is usually linked to the streptomycin resistance genes *strA* and *strB*. By contrast, sulfonamide resistance in a number of other species, including *S. pneumoniae* and *N. meningitidis*, is mediated by mutation of the chromosomal gene encoding DHPS. The gene encoding DHPS is also named *folP*. Proline 64 is highly conserved among DHPSs, and changes around this position are involved in mutation to resistance. Various duplications of one or two amino acids in this region of the protein can mediate resistance in *S. pneumoniae*. In *N. meningitidis* a change of proline 68 (equivalent to proline 64 in *H. influenzae*) to serine or leucine has been found to influence the level of sulfonamide resistance, although other changes were also required for resistance. In a laboratory mutant of *Escherichia coli*, a Pro64→Ser substitution resulted in the development of sulfathiazole resistance. The crystal structures of DHPSs from *E. coli* and *S. aureus* have shown that the polypeptide is folded into an eight-stranded αβ TIM barrel (i.e., a structure with the same fold configuration as triosephosphate isomerase). In *E. coli*, residues 58 to 71 form an interconnecting loop between β-strand 5 and α-helix E. Within this loop, threonine 62 is involved in the binding site for 7,8-pterin pyrophosphate and arginine 63 is involved in the binding site for sulfonamide and *para*-aminobenzoic acid. A large insertion in this region could significantly alter binding specificity.

1.1.6. Pharmacokinetics

The sulfonamides are administered orally or intravenously (sulfadiazine). They are well absorbed by the gastrointestinal tract (Table 1). Their tissue distribution is good. They diffuse well into cerebrospinal fluid (CSF) and pleural and peritoneal fluid and cross the placental barrier. Tissue and serum levels depend on their protein binding and their solubility in lipids (Table 2).

The sulfonamides are metabolized in the liver. The biotransformation of sulfamethoxazole is well known in humans. After oral administration of 1 g of sulfamethoxazole, 86.5% of the parent molecule and the metabolites is found in the urine. The main metabolite is an *N*-acetyl derivative which accounts for 61% of the quantity eliminated, while 15% is in the form of the glucuroconjugate. A minor metabolite has also been detected: hydroxymethyl-3-sulfanilamidoisoxazole.

Sulfadiazine is also metabolized, and six to eight metabolites have been reported depending on the animal species. After metabolism, they are then eliminated (free and conjugated) in the urine by glomerular filtration and a slight tubular reabsorption. Urinary elimination is pK dependent and is greater for a low pK. Urinary alkalinization increases this elimination (Fig. 3 and 4).

Table 1 Pharmacokinetics of sulfonamides

Compound	$t_{1/2}$ (h)	Protein binding (%)	CL_R (ml/min)	pK	Lipophilicity (%)	Metabolism (%)		Urinary elimination (%)
						OH	N_4	
Sulfamethoxazole	10	65	5.0	6.9	20.5	30	50	10
Sulfadiazine	10–12	50	6–18	6.52	26.4	20	19/14	25
Sulfadimethoxine	40	98	0.25	7.4	78.7	75	16	5
Sulfadoxine	110	98	0.20				1	10
Sulfafurazole	6–18	85	10	5.2	48	10	88	60
Sulfamerazine	12–24	87	5	6.98	62		35/14	30
Sulfamethomidine	25	97	0.5				16	10
Sulfamethoxypyridazine	38	96	0.8	7.2	70.4		16	50
Sulfametrole	9	75	1–8	4.8			40	10
Sulfamoxole	4	75	4	7.17	41	50	33	10
Sulfapyridine	5–10	60	10			50	60/32	15
Sulfathiazole	5	82	0.5–1				30	50
Sulfatroxazole	26	85	1	7.0		70	5	10
Sulfamethoxine	150	95		6.1	5			

Table 2 Solubilities of sulfonamides at 25°C

Compound	Solubility at 25°C (μg/ml)	
	pH 5.5	pH 7.0
Sulfadiazine	265	950
N[4]-Acetylsulfadiazine	411	1,620
Sulfadoxine	186	2,387
N[4]-Acetylsulfadoxine	221	3,420
Sulfafurazole	1,533	4,724
N[4]-Acetylsulfafurazole	250	6,893
N[4]-Diacetylsulfafurazole	12	5
Sulfamerazine	378	658
N[4]-Acetylsulfamerazine	300	800
Sulfamethomidine	430	605
N[4]-Acetylsulfamethomidine	356	547
Sulfamethoxazole	300	1,900
N[4]-Acetylsulfamethoxazole	115	1,000
N[1]-Acetylsulfamethoxazole	66	66

N_4-acetyl transferase (Acetyl CoA)

Figure 3 N_4-acetylation of sulfonamides. Acetyl CoA, acetyl coenzyme A

Acetyl sulfafurazole is deacetylated intestinally and absorbed in the form of sulfafurazole. Its apparent elimination half-life is 6 h. It is 90% plasma protein bound. For peak concentrations in serum of 100 μg/ml, the concentrations in the middle ear fluid are 20 μg/ml. After a few hours the product is found in the free and metabolized forms. Its elimination is essentially urinary.

The pharmacokinetics in children are summarized in Table 3.

Among all sulfonamides, many have been selected for combination with trimethoprim. The products that have been chosen have an apparent half-life of 11 h (sulfamethoxazole and sulfamoxole) or 9 h (sulfadiazine). Table 4 shows the tissue diffusion of trimethoprim, sulfamethoxazole, and sulfadiazine.

Metabolism and elimination of sulfonamides are summarized in Table 5.

1.1.7. Drug Interactions

Hypoglycemia has been reported to occur in diabetic patients receiving tolbutamide and another sulfonamide at the same time, the latter interfering in the metabolism and elimination of tolbutamide.

The microsomal hepatic metabolism of drugs such as phenytoin and warfarin is inhibited by the usual dosages of sulfadiazine and sulfamethizole, and likewise sulfamethoxazole (in combination with co-trimoxazole).

However, sulfadimethoxine does not modify the metabolism of phenytoin. Thus, in the case of concomitant treatment with sulfonamides and vitamin K inhibitors or phenytoin, coagulation or phenytoin levels must be monitored, particularly in patients with hypoalbuminemia, as sulfonamides may also displace drugs from their protein binding sites.

The combination of sulfonamides with phenytoin is not recommended because of the increase in concentrations in plasma of this product up to toxic levels as a result of inhibition of its metabolism. Likewise, there is a risk of potentiation of oral anticoagulants, particularly warfarin.

An interaction with the sulfonamide-erythromycin combination is therefore particularly to be avoided with vitamin K inhibitors.

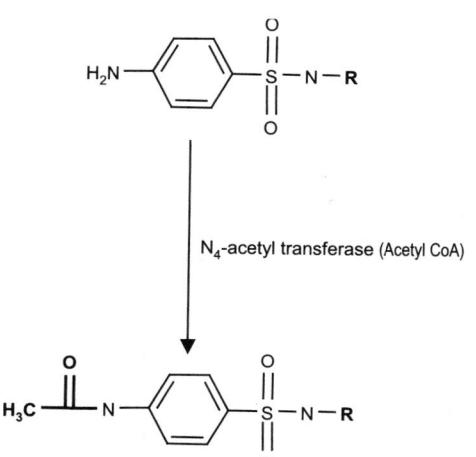

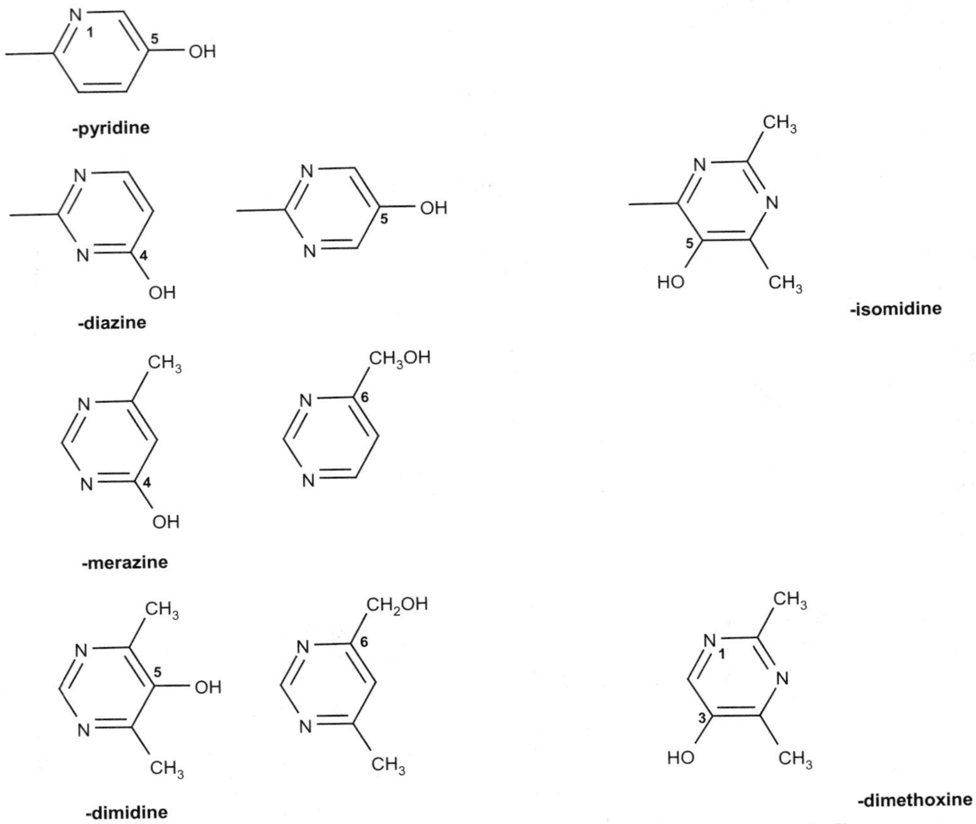

-pyridine

-diazine

-isomidine

-merazine

-dimidine

-dimethoxine

Figure 4 Pyrimidine and pyridine sulfonamides: structures of hydroxy metabolites

Table 3 Half-lives of sulfonamides in children

Compound	$t_{1/2}$ (h)					
	Days 1–7	1–4 wk	1–12 mo	2–7 yr	7–15 yr	Adults
Sulfathiazole					10	4
Sulfamoxole	19.5	11.5	7.4–10.5			8
Sulfafurazole	18	12	8	8	8	6–9
Sulfadiazine	10–40		10			10–15
Sulfamerazine			24–60	10	18	11–24
Sulfadimethoxine	120	88	20–40			30–40
Sulfadoxine	14 days	70–140				110

Table 4 Tissue diffusion of sulfonamides and trimethoprim

Fluid or tissue	Concn (μg/ml or μg/g)		
	Trimethoprim	Sulfamethoxazole	Sulfadiazine
Plasma	1	1	1
Bronchial secretions	2	<0.05	0.25
Lung tissues	3	0.5	0.50
CSF	1	0.25	0.70
Bile	1	0.5	0.50
Prostate	1.5	0.25	0.10
Bone	0.4	0.20	0.20
Tonsils	0.9	0.20	

Table 5 Percentage of the sulfonamide administered dose eliminated unchanged or as metabolites in urine

Sulfonamide	% of dose eliminated unchanged			
	Sulfonamide + N^4-acetyl	Hydroxysulfonamides	N^4-Acetyl	N_4OH
Sulfachloropyridazine			10	
Sulfaclomide	60		30	
Sulfacytine	85		10	
Sulfadiazine	25	20	25	10
Sulfadimethoxine	5	75	10	
Sulfadimidine	10		80	
Sulfadoxine	10		5	
Sulfaethidole	80			
Sulfaethylpyrazole	20		20	
Sulfaphenazole	60		10	
Sulfafurazole	60	10	20	
Sulfaguanidine	60		25	
Sulfiodizole	40		40	
Sulfisomidine	80		15	
Sulfalene	5		35	
Sulfamerazine	30		55	
Sulfamethioxaole	80	30	5	
Sulfamethomidine	10		10	
Sulfamethoxazole	10		50	
Sulfamethoxypyridazine	50		15	
Sulfametrole	10		60	
Sulfamethylthiazole	5		60	
Sulfamoxole	10	50	15	
Sulfanilamide	70		20	
Sulfapyridine	15	50	15	20
Sulfaquinoxaline				
Sulfasymazine	60		10	
Sulfasomizole	40			
Sulfathiazole	50		10	
Sulfatroxazole	10	70	20	

1.2. Trimethoprim and Sulfonamides

Trimethoprim, sulfonamides, and their combinations have well-established therapeutic activity in respiratory, digestive, and urinary infections, particularly in short-term treatments and as prophylaxis.

There are new indications for the combination in the prophylaxis of granulocytopenic cancer patients, for the curative treatment and prophylaxis of pneumocystosis in human immunodeficiency virus (HIV)-infected patients. However, a very high incidence of side effects has been observed in patients suffering from AIDS. Trimethoprim is usually combined with sulfamethoxazole but may be combined with sulfadiazine or sulfamoxole in a ratio of 1 to 5.

1.2.1. Trimethoprim

Trimethoprim is a 2,4-diamino-5-(3,4,5-trimethoxybenzyl) pyrimidine. It is a DHFR inhibitor that potentiates the activity of sulfonamides by sequential inhibition of folic acid synthesis. It may be used alone or in combination with sulfonamides.

1.2.1.1. Classification of DHFR Inhibitors

DHFR inhibitors belong to three major therapeutic classes: anticancer agents, antiparasitic agents, and antibacterial agents. These compounds may be divided into three clinical groups, including the benzylpyrimidines, to which trimethoprim and its derivatives belong (Fig. 5).

These compounds have good antibacterial activity and are devoid of inhibitory activity against epithelial cell DHFR. Three structures determine their antibacterial activity: a pyrimidine heterocycle, a benzene ring, and an intercyclic chain. The activity is based on the presence of amino groups at positions 2 and 4 and the absence of a pyrimidine heterocycle, a methylene bridge, and a benzene ring substituted at 3′4′5′. The various components differ in the substituent at position 4′.

1.2.2. Mode of Action of Trimethoprim and Its Derivatives

After penetrating the bacterial cell wall, the derivatives inhibit DHFR.

1.2.2.1. Uptake of Trimethoprim and Brodimoprim

A hydrophobic pathway is responsible for drug passage through either the outer or inner membrane.

Trimethoprim and brodimoprim contain two nitrogen atoms on the pyrimidine ring which are easily protonable according to the pH of environment (Fig. 6).

Brodimoprim is more hydrophobic than trimethoprim. Both drugs present a hydrophilic character at low pH values, where the molecules are protonated and are unable to cross the lipophilic outer membrane. With an increase in the pH,

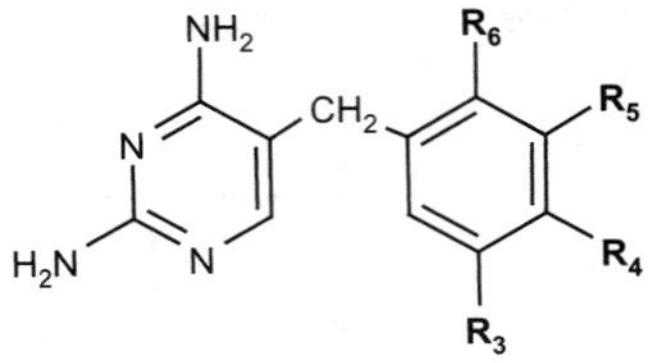

	R_3	R_4	R_5	R_6
Trimethoprim	OCH_3	OCH_3	OCH_3	H
Tetroxoprim	OCH_3	$O(CH_2)_2OCH_3$	OCH_3	H
Brodimoprim	OCH_3	Br	OCH_3	H
Aditoprim	OCH_3	$N(CH_3)_2$	OCH_3	H
Epiroprim	OC_2H_5	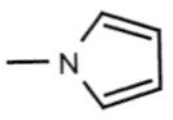 —N	OC_2H_5	H
Baquiloprim	CH_3	$N(CH_3)_2$		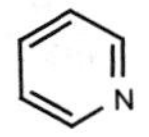 N
Ormetoprim	OCH_3	OCH_3	CH_3	H
Diaverdin	OCH_3	OCH_3	H	H
Metioprime	OCH_3	SCH_3	OCH_3	H

Figure 5 **2,5-Diaminopyrimidine derivatives**

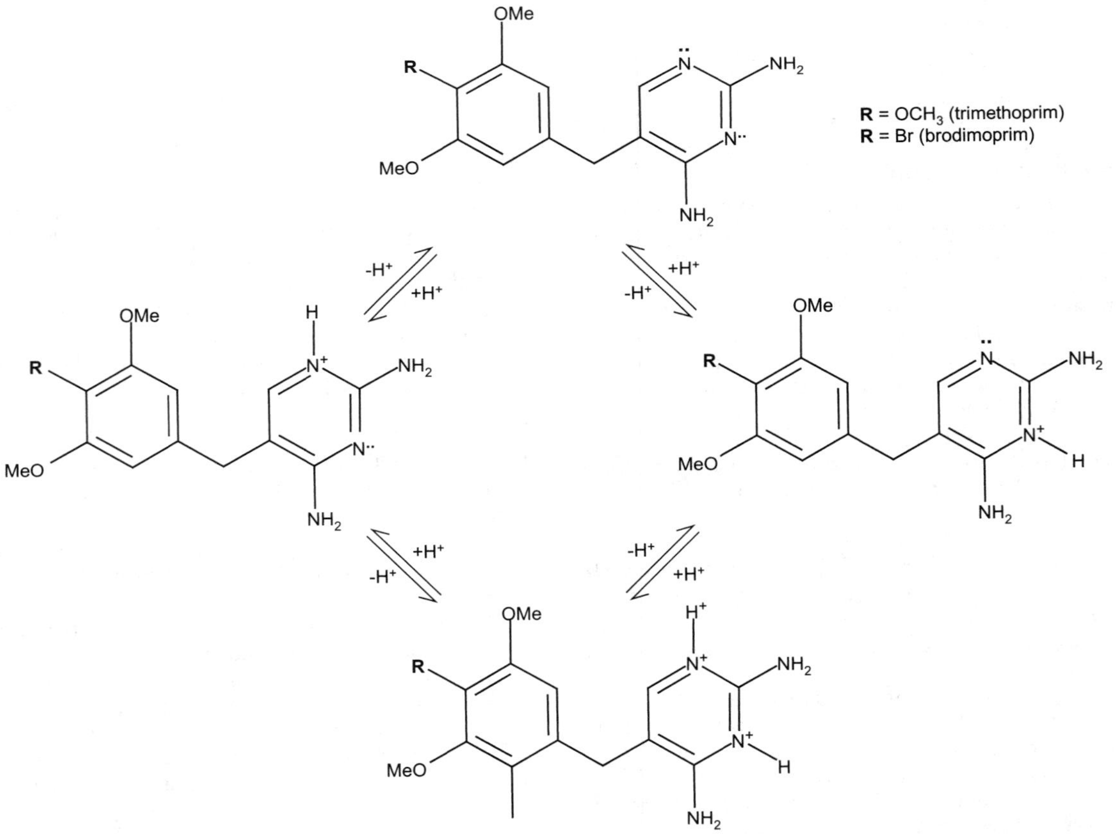

R = OCH_3 (trimethoprim)
R = Br (brodimoprim)

Figure 6 **Protonation and deprotonation of trimethoprim**

compound protonation decreases, and the hydrophobic character increases up to pH ~7.

1.2.2.2. DHFR

The enzyme DHFR catalyzes the NADPH-dependent reduction of the dihydrofolate (Fig. 7) to tetrahydrofolate.

DHFR is required for the de novo synthesis of purines, thymidylate, and certain amino acids, such as methionine.

Tetrahydrofolic acid acts as a coenzyme for a number of biochemical reactions, such as the synthesis of purine and pyrimidine bases, and intervenes in the metabolism of serine and methionine (Fig. 8).

Microorganisms are unable to use exogenous tetrahydrofolic acid and must synthesize it. This synthesis occurs schematically in two stages: synthesis of dihydrofolates, which are then converted to tetrahydrofolates by DHFR. The first stage may be inhibited by sulfonamides and the second may be inhibited by competitive inhibitors of DHFR (Fig. 9).

The active sites of all of these enzymes contain an anionic residue, which in *E. coli* is an aspartic acid (aspartic acid 27). The NH atoms of the pyrimidine ring form hydrogen bonds in *E. coli*. The protons of the nitrogen at position 1 and of the amino group at position 2 also form hydrogen bonds with the aspartic acid at position 27. NH_2 also forms a bond with the tryptophan at position 30 and the hydroxyl group of threonine at position 113.

The affinities of various compounds for DHFRs of several bacterial species are summarized in Table 6.

1.2.2.3. Thymidylate

A key nucleotide component of DNA is thymidylate (deoxythymidine 5′-monophosphate). The de novo synthesis of thymidylate is regulated by thymidylate synthase ThyA, an enzyme methylating dUMP. The reaction for a biological reaction is linked to formation of H_2 folate (dihydrofolate), because ThyA uses methylenetetrahydrofolate (CH_2H_4 folate) as both a carbon source and reductant. H_2 folate formed by ThyA is rapidly reduced by FolA (specifically inhibited by trimethoprim). However, in some bacterial species, ThyA is lacking in the genome and another gene was characterized, *thyX* (also known as *thy1*), which encodes a protein belonging to a flavin-dependent thymidylate synthase (Table 7 and Fig. 10).

ThyX-containing organisms do not require FolA for their folate metabolism. *E. coli* strains carrying inactive FolA and having an alternate pathway, being resistant to trimethoprim, remain viable. Both ThyA and ThyX are CH_2H_4 folate-dependent enzymes, but the two thymidylate synthases differ by their reductive mechanisms. ThyX uses CH_2H_4 folate as only a one-carbon donor, whereas the electrons required for formation of a methyl group are transferred from reduced pyridine nucleotides via an enzyme-bound flavin cofactor to thymidylate.

S. pneumoniae is poorly susceptible to trimethoprim. Position 30 of *S. pneumoniae* is occupied by a glutamic acid instead of the conserved aspartic acid. Except in *Lactococcus lactis*, a Glu residue is normally associated with enzymes which are resistant to trimethoprim. The amino acid at position 30 forms strong hydrogen bonds with trimethoprim and DHFR of sensitive strains (Fig. 11).

1.2.3. Physicochemical Properties of Benzylpyrimidines

The physicochemical properties of the benzylpyrimidines are summarized in Table 8.

Tetroxoprim is a molecule that is more soluble in water at 30°C (2.65 mg/ml) than trimethoprim (0.64 mg/ml), and also in chloroform (69 versus 26 mg/ml). Trimethoprim is degradated in solution; the main degradation products are listed in Fig. 12.

1.2.4. Antibacterial Spectrum of Trimethoprim

Trimethoprim has a broad antibacterial spectrum. The antibacterial activities of the 2,4-diaminopyrimidines vary according to the thymidine content in the culture medium. The optimum concentration of thymidine appears to be 0.05 μg/ml of medium.

1.2.4.1. Gram-Positive Bacteria

Trimethoprim is active against *S. aureus* (including methicillin-resistant [MRSA] strains) streptococci (*S. pyogenes*, *S. pneumoniae*, and viridans group streptococci), *E. faecalis*, and *Corynebacterium diphtheriae*. For *Nocardia* spp., the MICs are between 10 and 50 μg/ml. The MICs at which 50 and 90% of isolates tested are inhibited (MIC_{50} and MIC_{90}, respectively) *Rhodococcus equi* are 3.2 and

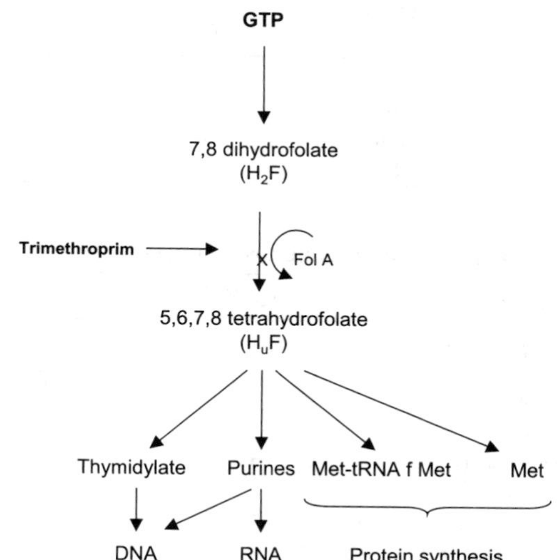

Figure 8 Mode of action of trimethoprim

NADPH NADP+

Figure 7 Reduction to tetrahydrofolate

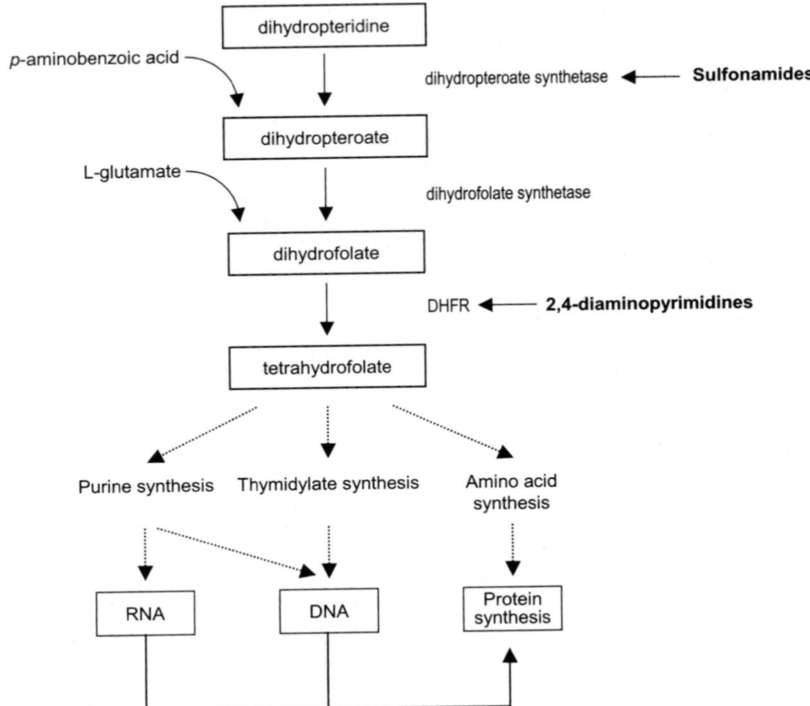

Figure 9 Role of tetrahydrofolates and sites of action of sulfonamides and benzylpyrimidines

Table 6 Affinity for DHFR

Compound	IC_{50} (μM)			
	E. coli	*S. aureus*	*Proteus mirabilis*	Rat hepatocytes
Trimethoprim	0.092	0.125	0.007	549
Brodimoprim	0.43	0.012	0.002	95
Epiroprim	0.025	0.020	0.002	170
Metioprim	0.038	0.031	0.003	576

Table 7 ThyX and FolA gene distribution

Microorganism(s)	ThyX	ThyX + FolA
Rickettsia prowazekii	+	–
C. jejuni	+	–
Helicobacter pylori	+	–
Borrelia burgdorferi	+	–
Treponema pallidum	+	–
Rickettsia conorii	+	–
Clostridium spp.	+	+
Chlamydia spp.	+	+

12.8 μg/ml, respectively. Table 9 shows the in vitro activities of trimethoprim and brodimoprim against gram-positive cocci.

Co-trimoxazole is poorly active against *Brevibacterium otitidis* (MIC, 1 to 2 μg/ml) and is inactive against coryneforms (MIC, ≥32 μg/ml), *Brevibacterium* (MIC, >256 μg/ml), and *Arthrobacter* (MIC, 4 to 16 μg/ml). It is inactive against *Actinomyces* (MIC, ≥ 64 μg/ml).

Trimethoprim is inactive against *Arcobacter butzleri* (MIC_{50} and MIC_{90}, 64 to 128 μg/ml) and *Arcobacter cryaerophilus* (MIC_{50} and MIC_{90}, 4 to 128 μg/ml).

1.2.4.2. Gram-Negative Bacteria

The majority of enteric gram-negative bacilli are susceptible to trimethoprim, as are *Yersinia enterocolitica* and *Yersinia pestis*. Co-trimoxazole is active against *Yersinia pseudotuberculosis* and against ampicillin-resistant shigellae. *H. influenzae, Pasteurella*, and *Vibrio cholerae* are usually susceptible (Table 10).

Melioidosis is due to *Burkholderia pseudomallei* and is endemic in southern Asia and northern Australia and has been prevalent in tropical and subtropical areas between latitudes 20° north and 20° south of the equator. *B. pseudomallei* is resistant to major aminoglycosides, polymyxins, and many β-lactams but is susceptible to tetracyclines, chloramphenicol, sulfonamides, novobiocin, carbapenems, and ceftazidime. Co-trimoxazole is part of the treatment of the conventional acute form of melioidosis. It is combined with ceftazidime or meropenem. However, the co-trimoxazole susceptibility of *B. pseudomallei* in vitro is often considered ambiguous; interpretation of the disk diffusion method is difficult due to many factors, such the inoculum size and the disk load, which may be inappropriate for *B. pseudomallei*. Antagonism with Mueller-Hinton agar has been described. Furthermore, there are discrepancies between the agar method, the MicroScan device, and E-test strips. The ratios of the two components are different for these methods: 1:5, 1:19, and 1:19, respectively.

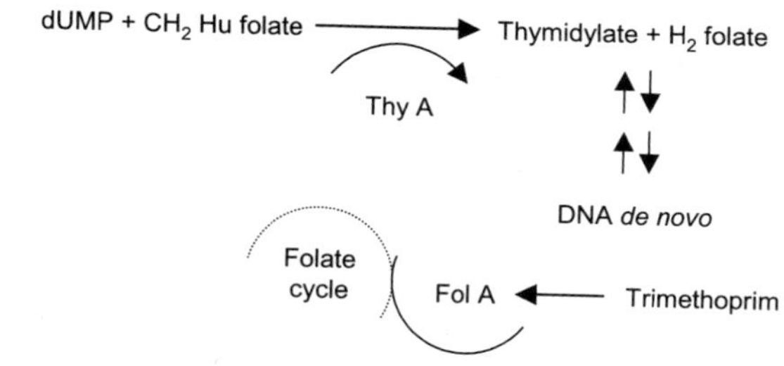

Figure 10 Mode of action of 2,4-diaminopyrimidines

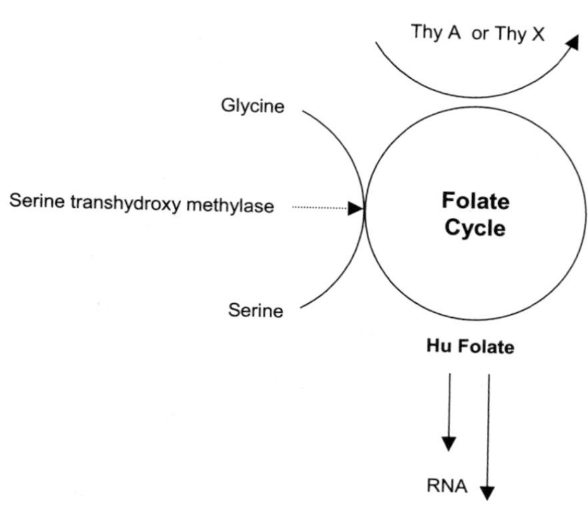

Figure 11 Thymidylate activity

Stenotrophomonas maltophilia has become an important nosocomial pathogen. It is often resistant to multiple antibiotics, including β-lactams (class B β-lactamase) and aminoglycosides. Fluoroquinolone activity is structure dependent. Activity against this organism is summarized in Table 11.

1.2.4.3. Anaerobic Gram-Negative Bacteria

Bacteroides, Fusobacterium, and *Clostridium* are resistant to trimethoprim and co-trimoxazole. However, *Bacteroides fragilis* may be susceptible to sulfamethoxazole or co-trimoxazole if trimethoprim concentrations are increased.

1.2.4.4. Breakpoints

Trimethoprim disks contain 1.5 μg. The breakpoints and the diameters of the zones of inhibition are reported in Table 12.

1.2.5. Resistance to Trimethoprim

Resistance to 2,5-diaminopyrimidines may be natural or acquired. Acquired resistance may occur following mutation or may be plasmid mediated. A bacterial strain is considered resistant to trimethoprim when the MIC is greater than 8 μg/ml.

1.2.5.1. Natural Resistance

A number of bacterial species and genera exhibit natural resistance to trimethoprim and other available 2,5-diaminopyrimidines: *Pseudomonas aeruginosa, Acinetobacter, Moraxella, Neisseria, Brucella, Campylobacter, Nocardia, Actinomyces,* mycobacteria, *Bacteroides, Clostridium,* and

Compound	R_1	R_2	R_3	X
A	$-NH_2$	$-NH_2$	$-CH_3$	-CH
B	$-NH_2$	$-NH_2$	$-CH_3$	-C=O
C	-OH	-OH	$-CH_3$	$-CH_2$
D	-OH	$-NH_2$	$-CH_3$	$-CH_2$
E	$-NH_2$	-OH	$-CH_3$	$-CH_2$
F	$-NH_2$	-OH	-H	$-CH_2$
G	$-NH_2$	$-NH_2$	-H	$-CH_2$

Figure 12 Degradation products of trimethoprim

Table 8 Physicochemical properties of 2,4-diaminopyrimidines

Compound	Mol wt	Melting point (°C)	pK	LogP (*n*-octanol/ phosphate buffer, pH 7.4)	Water solubility (log/s)
Trimethoprim	290.3	199	7.15	0.89	−2.62
Brodimoprim	339.2	225–228	7.15	1.82	−3.99
Metioprim	306.4	224–230	7.15	1.38	−3.44
Tetroxoprim	334.4	160	8.25	0.25–0.54	
Epiroprim	353.4	173–175	7.15	1.74	−4.30
Iclaprim	450.2	204	7.2		3 mg/ml

Table 9 In vitro activities of trimethoprim and brodimoprim against gram-positive cocci

Microorganism(s)	MIC_{50} (μg/ml)	
	Trimethoprim	Brodimoprim
MSSA	0.5	0.5
MRSA	0.5	0.5
S. pneumoniae	1.0	0.5
S. pneumoniae Pen[i]/Pen[r]	>128	>128
Beta-hemolytic streptococci (A, B, and G)	1.0	1.0
Enterococcus spp.	0.06	0.125
H. pylori	64	64
Legionella pneumophila	1.0	0.25
Nocardia spp.	64	8.0

Table 10 In vitro activities of benzylpyrimidines against gram-negative bacilli

Microorganism(s)	MIC_{50} (μg/ml)	
	Trimethoprim	Brodimoprim
E. coli	0.1	0.1
Klebsiella pneumoniae	0.5	1.0
K. pneumoniae (ESBL[a])	>256	>256
Proteus spp.	0.5	0.5
Salmonella spp.	0.05	0.1
P. aeruginosa	128	>256
Acinetobacter baumannii	16	16
H. influenzae	0.25	1.0
M. catarrhalis	16	32
V. cholerae	0.05	0.01

[a]ESBL, extended-spectrum β-lactamase.

Table 11 In vitro activity against S. *maltophilia*

Compound	MIC (μg/ml)	
	50%	90%
Fluoroquinolones		
Ciprofloxacin	1.0	4.0
Clinafloxacin	0.06	0.25
Levofloxacin	0.5	2.0
Sparfloxacin	0.125	1.0
Pefloxacin	2.0	8.0
Sitafloxacin	0.125	0.5
Aminoglycosides		
Amikacin	>128	
Tobramycin	>128	
β-Lactams		
Ceftazidime	16	128
Cefotaxime	32	128
Piperacillin	16	128
Piperacillin-tazobactam	16	128
Ticarcillin-clavulanic acid	32	64
Others		
Co-trimoxazole	0.25/1.25	0.25/1.25
Chloramphenicol	32	>64
Doxycycline	2.0	8.0

Table 12 Breakpoints (French Committee for Antibiotic Susceptibility Testing)

Phenotype	MIC (μg/ml)	Zone diam (mm)
Susceptible	<2	>16
Resistant	>8	<10

Treponema. With respect to the recent compounds—2,5-diaminopyrimidine derivatives—some appear to be active against *B. fragilis*.

1.2.5.2. Acquired Resistance

Two mutation mechanisms have been described: some microorganisms reduce their thymidine requirement, while others qualitatively or quantitatively reduce their DHFR.

Plasmid-mediated resistance always results in high MICs, usually above 1,000 μg/ml. The plasmids involved belong to the following incompatibility groups: W, I, C, M, N, FII, B, S, O, P, H2, and X.

Plasmids have been isolated in *E. coli, Salmonella, Shigella, Citrobacter, Klebsiella, Enterobacter, Serratia, Proteus, Providencia, V. cholerae,* and *Acinetobacter*. Two transposons carrying resistance to trimethoprim have been identified in several plasmids: Tn*7*, which is associated with resistance to streptomycin, and Tn*402*. This resistance may be transferable, and the mechanism of resistance appears to be the production of a highly resistant or nontransferable additional DHFR.

1.2.5.3. Epidemiology of Resistance

Acquired resistance to trimethoprim was very rare before 1983; only 1 to 6% of clinical isolates were reported to be trimethoprim resistant.

The first report of widespread trimethoprim resistance among staphylococci came from Australia and the United States from 1983 to 1986. From 1992 to 1995 two studies were carried out and showed that at least one-third of MRSA strains are resistant to trimethoprim and to sulfamethoxazole. In one study, the prevalence of co-trimoxazole-resistant *S. aureus* and *Enterobacteriaceae* isolated from all hospitalized patients increased significantly, from <5.5% of isolates before 1986 to 20% in 1995, during which time co-trimoxazole prophylaxis was increasing in HIV-infected patients. In addition, the rise in resistant organisms was significantly more prominent in samples obtained from HIV-infected patients, in whom resistant isolates increased from 6.3% in 1988 to 53% in 1995. Another study found that significantly more co-trimoxazole-resistant organisms were isolated from HIV-infected patients who had received co-trimoxazole than from patients who had not received co-trimoxazole.

For coagulase-negative staphylococci, such as *Staphylococcus epidermidis* resistant to methicillin, two-thirds of the strains are resistant to co-trimoxazole.

In Russia, 300 clinical isolates of *H. influenzae* have been collected. Twenty-one percent are resistant to co-trimoxazole (MICs, 0.016 to 32 μg/ml) and only 2.3% are resistant to ampicillin (MICs, 0.016 to 128 μg/ml). These strains were collected from children.

The nasopharyngeal carriage rate of resistant strains from day care centers in France was 43%, that in Switzerland was 39.4%, and that in Russia was 44%. In centers in Pakistan and Costa Rica, the carriage rates were 28.6 and 27.9%, respectively. In Malawi, 46% of the pneumococcal isolates were resistant to co-trimoxazole and 21% were resistant to penicillin G. A Protekt surveillance study had demonstrated resistance of *S. pneumoniae* to co-trimoxazole worldwide (Table 13).

Co-trimoxazole is one of the main antibacterial agents for the treatment of uncomplicated cystitis. In a survey carried out from 1992 to 1999 of the incidence of *E. coli* resistant to drugs used in lower urinary tract infections, the rate was around 16% for co-trimoxazole resistance (Table 14).

1.2.6. Co-trimoxazole

There is a synergistic effect in terms of antibacterial activity between trimethoprim and other benzylpyrimidines and sulfonamides when the bacteria are susceptible to both compounds, particularly when the two components are used globally in the ratio of their MICs. However, with sulfonamide-resistant and trimethoprim-susceptible bacteria there is no potentiation of the effect of trimethoprim (Table 15). This action is observed against a number of bacteria and certain protozoa. Some authors have evoked the potential interest of this combination in certain enterococcal infections.

1.2.7. Mechanisms of Resistance to Trimethoprim

1.2.7.1. Additional DHFR

Production of additional DHFR enzymes which are less sensitive to trimethoprim inhibition was described. Sixteen of these enzymes have been characterized and are mainly prevalent in enteric gram-negative bacilli. They are encoded by gene cassettes with plasmids or transposons.

1.2.7.2. Mutations

In staphylococci, plasmid-mediated high-level trimethoprim resistance is dominated by the ubiquitous Tn*4003*-mediated S1 DHFR. The enzyme may be mutated from the original *S. epidermidis* chromosomal DHFR. S2 DHFR has been isolated from *Staphylococcus haemolyticus* (Phe98 → Tyr).

1.2.7.3. Alteration of DHFR

In some clinical isolates of *E. coli* and *H. influenzae*, trimethoprim resistance has been shown to result from alterations in the host chromosomal DHFR. These changes include regulatory mutations resulting in overexpression of DHFR and mutations to the host chromosomal DHFR which result in a decreased affinity of trimethoprim for DHFR. In *E. coli* the most significant changes in the structural gene are from Gly30 (active site) to a tryptophan and from Gln158 to

Table 13 Prevalence of co-trimoxazole resistance

Country	% Resistance
South Korea	70.7
Hong Kong	62.85
Japan	10.7
France	41.3
Germany	8.3
The Netherlands	5.88
Belgium	17.55
Portugal	21.7
Italy	23.53
Sweden	7.81
United Kingdom	7.69
Austria	10.52
Switzerland	5.4
Spain	38.28
Poland	44
Hungary	26.47
Turkey	35.06
Mexico	47.29
Argentina	36.36
Brazil	46.15
Canada	18
United States	20.2
Australia	16.66

Table 15 In vitro activities of trimethoprim and co-trimoxazole

Microorganism(s)	MIC (μg/ml)	
Gram positive		
S. aureus	0.15–2	0.04–1.6
S. epidermidis	0.02	
S. pneumoniae	0.004–5	0.05–1.5
S. pyogenes	0.02–1	0.015–0.4
E. faecalis	0.15–0.5	0.015–0.4
C. diphtheriae	0.015–0.5	0.05–0.15
L. monocytogenes	0.05–1.5	0.015–0.15
C. perfringens	2–50	
Propionibacterium acnes	0.07	
Gram negative		
E. coli	0.01–>5	0.005–>5
Klebsiella spp.	0.15–5	0.05–3.1
P. mirabilis	0.15–1.5	0.05–0.15
Serratia marcescens	0.8–50	0.4–50
Salmonella spp.	0.01–0.4	0.05–0.15
Shigella spp.	0.04–0.8	0.02–0.5
C. freundii	0.2	
V. cholerae	0.2	
H. influenzae	0.1–12.5	0.04–50
N. gonorrhoeae	0.2–128	0.15–3.1
N. meningitidis	3.1–50	0.01–1.6
P. aeruginosa	50–1,000	3.1–100
Burkholderia cepacia	1–2	
S. maltophilia	>32	>32
B. fragilis	24	
Other		
Nocardia asteroides	3–100	1.5
Chlamydia trachomatis	20	

Table 14 Prevalence of resistance of *E. coli* in urinary tract infections in France

Yrs	*n*	% Resistance			
		Ampicillin	Ciprofloxacin	Co-trimoxazole	Nitrofurantoin
1992–1993	123	34.1	0	8.1	0
1994–1995	107	29.0	0	6.5	0
1996–1997	206	25.7	0	11.6	1.5
1998–1999	165	30.9	0	15.8	2.9

glutamic acid. In *H. influenzae*, the alterations in either the C terminus or the middle section of DHFR may cause resistance, probably as a result of a change in the secondary structure and the subsequent loss of trimethoprim binding.

1.2.7.4. The dfr Genes

In 1972, 4 years after the introduction of co-trimoxazole into clinical practice in the United Kingdom, transferable resistance to trimethoprim was reported. Since 1972, more than 20 different trimethoprim-resistant *dhfr* genes have been characterized. The most prevalent of these genes is *dhfrI* and variants. The gene *dhfrII* mediates high-level trimethoprim resistance (MIC, >1,000 μg/ml). These genes are mostly found in enteric gram-negative bacilli.

The *dfr* genes occur in streptococci and *S. pneumoniae*. *S. pneumoniae* is moderately susceptible to trimethoprim. In *S. pneumoniae* only the mutation Ile100→Leu seems to be involved in trimethoprim resistance (mutation occurring in binding site) (homologous to Ile94 of *E. coli* DHFR), as Ile100 makes van der Waals contact with the pyrimidine moiety of trimethoprim.

The *dfrD* gene has been found in *Listeria monocytogenes*.

In *E. faecalis* the genes conferring resistance to trimethoprim are called *dfrE* and *dfrF*. The trimethoprim resistance is due to the presence of an additional DHFR.

Two genes, *drfA* and *drfC*, are carried by staphylococci. The *drfC* gene results in a single mutation, Phe98→Tyr, and in a high level of trimethoprim resistance. The *drfA* gene evolved from the *S. epidermidis* chromosome.

In *Campylobacter jejuni* the genes *dfr1* and *dfr9* are responsible for trimethoprim resistance. They are located on transposon Tn*5393*.

1.2.8. Tetroxoprim and Brodimoprim

Trimethoprim is 5 to 50 times more active in vitro than tetroxoprim against gram-positive cocci and gram-negative bacilli (Table 16). Brodimoprim is slightly less active than trimethoprim.

1.2.9. Antimalarial and Other Antiparasitic Activities

The first-line treatment of malaria in areas of endemicity may be pyrimethamine-sulfadoxine, especially for chloroquine-resistant *P. falciparum* isolates. It has been demonstrated in children that *S. pneumoniae* isolates colonizing the oropharynx 3 and 4 weeks after pyrimethamine-sulfadoxine administration may be resistant to co-trimoxazole (increase in incidence from 38.1% at the initial visit to 44% at week 4).

In the co-trimoxazole-treated children, the proportion colonized with non-co-trimoxazole-susceptible *S. pneumoniae* increased from 4.5% at the initial visit to 52% at week 1 and decreased to 41.7% at week 4.

DHFR of *P. falciparum* is a bifunctional enzyme linked to thymidylate synthase. Resistance of *P. falciparum* to pyrimethamine has been shown to be due to mutations of DHFR, mainly Ser108→Asn, which may accompanied by other mutations, mostly at residues 51, 59, and 64. A single point mutation causes moderate pyrimethamine resistance, and the addition of an Asn→Ile51 or Cys59→Arg mutation confers a higher level of pyrimethamine resistance.

Trimethoprim is cross-resistant with pyrimethamine in vitro. Trimetrexate and piritrexim are used in the treatment of *Pneumocystis carinii* and *Toxoplasma gondii* infections in AIDS patients (Fig. 13). These compounds were originally developed as anticancer agents and bind very tightly to mammalian DHFR. They can be used without sulfonamides, being more potent than trimethoprim (Table 17).

Table 16 Comparative in vitro activities of trimethoprim and tetroxoprim

Microorganism	MIC (μg/ml)	
	Trimethoprim	Tetroxoprim
S. aureus CN 491	0.1	1.0
S. pyogenes CN 10	0.5	5.0
E. faecalis CN 478	0.1	0.5
Pasteurella multocida ATCC 6587	0.1	5.0
Salmonella enterica serovar Typhi CN 512	0.05	1.0
Shigella flexneri CN 6007	0.1	5.0
E. coli CN 314	0.1	1.0
S. marcescens UNC 18	0.5	10
K. pneumoniae CN 3632	0.5	5.0
Enterobacter aerogenes 2200/86	0.5	5.0
C. freundii 2200/77	0.5	5.0
Proteus vulgaris CN 329	1.0	50

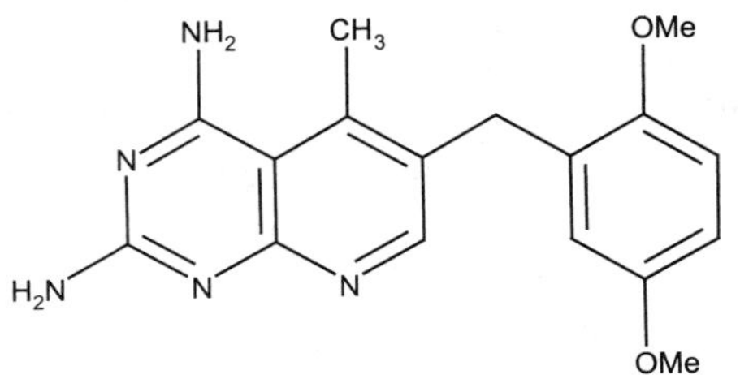

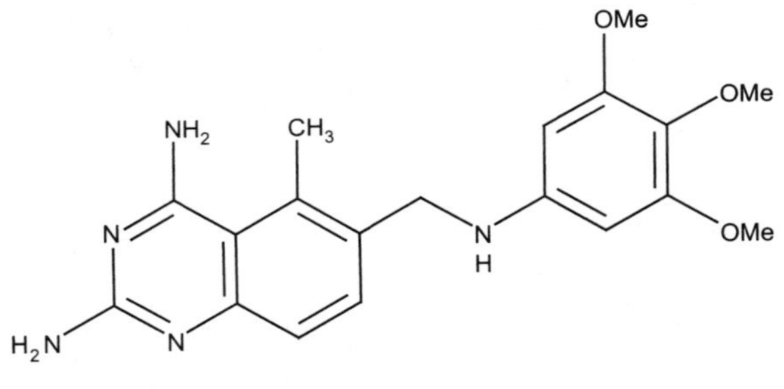

Piritrexim

Trimetrexate

Figure 13 2,4-Diaminobenzylpyrimidines with antiparasitic activities

Table 17 Affinities for DHFR of trimethoprim and piritrexin

Organism	IC_{50} (μM)	
	Trimethoprim	Piritrexim
P. carinii	13	0.013
T. gondii	2.8	0.0043
M. avium	0.3	0.00061
Rat	180	0.0038

Table 18 Pharmacokinetic characteristics of the different benzylpyrimidine derivatives

Parameter	Trimethoprim (160 mg)	Metioprim (80 mg)	Brodimoprim (200 mg)	Tetroxoprim (200 mg)
C_{max} (μg/ml)	1.2–2.1	0.89 ± 0.12	2.0 ± 0.4	2.9
T_{max} (h)	2–4	1.84 ± 0.32	4.0 ± 3.0	1.4
AUC (μg·h/ml)			94 ± 23	28.6
CL_P (ml/min)	148 ± 51	8 ± 13.1	37	120
CL_R (ml/min)	92.9 ± 47	9.0 ± 1.6	2.3	67
V (liters/kg)	1.39 ± 0.35	1.1 ± 0.11	1.5 ± 0.2	1.03 ± 0.21
Protein binding (%)	40–60	80	89	10–14
$t_{1/2\beta}$ (h)	7.4 ± 1.9	10.1 ± 1.8	34 ± 7	6.1
Urinary elimination (%)	41.4 ± 8.3	20–27	7	60.9 ± 4.5
Bioavailability (%)	85	86.8 ± 5.9		

P. carinii infections are treated with pentamidine, trimethoprim-dapsone, co-trimoxazole, and trimetrexate. Pyrimethamine plus sulfonamide is used for the treatment of *T. gondii* infections. The host tissues can be selectively protected by coadministration of leucovorin (5-formyl tetrahydrofolate), which is taken up by mammalian cells, and reverse toxicity associated with DHFR inhibitors. These drugs do not need an active carrier for their cellular uptake, in contrast classical antifolate, which needs a polar glutamate side chain.

1.2.10. Pharmacokinetics and Metabolism

Trimethoprim is metabolized to various bacteriologically inactive metabolites. The pharmacokinetic characteristics of the different derivatives are listed in Table 18.

1.2.11. Iclaprim

Iclaprim (AR-100) is a racemate of 2,4-diaminopyrimidine (Figs. 14 and 15) with a molecular weight of 354.4.

It is administered as a methanesulfonate salt. It is a benzopyranyl substituted with 7,8-dimethoxy groups and a 2-cyclopropyl moiety. The water solubility is 3 mg/ml, and in propylene glycol the solubility is >20 mg/ml. The molecular weight is 450.52, and the melting point is 204°C.

Iclaprim is 10 times more active than trimethoprim against staphylococci and 20 to 40 times more active against streptococci, including *S. pneumoniae* resistant to penicillin G. It is as active as trimethoprim against *H. influenzae* and *Moraxella catarrhalis*. Iclaprim is less active than trimethoprim against *Enterobacteriaceae*. It displays good in vitro activity against gram-negative anaerobes; trimethoprim is inactive (Table 19).

The affinity for DHFR of gram-positive organisms, including those of trimethoprim-resistant isolates, is high (Table 20).

Iclaprim is more active than vancomycin against MRSA and methicillin-susceptible *S. aureus* (MSSA) (MICs, 0.06 to 0.12 mg/ml, versus 1.0 μg/ml for vancomycin) and more active than linezolid (MIC, 1.0 μg/ml).

1.2.12. Human Pharmacokinetics

Preliminary pharmacokinetics are summarized in Table 21. Iclaprim possesses an elimination half-life of about 2 h, with a peak concentration in plasma at the end of intravenous administration ranging from 0.6 to 8.3 μg/ml depending on the administered dose. Different combinations may be used (Table 22).

1.2.12.1. Pharmacokinetics of Combinations

1.2.12.1.1. Oral administration. When trimethoprim and a sulfonamide are administered simultaneously, the levels in plasma obtained for each of the constituents are similar to those observed when the two products are administered separately. A standard dose of co-trimoxazole (ratio, 1/5)

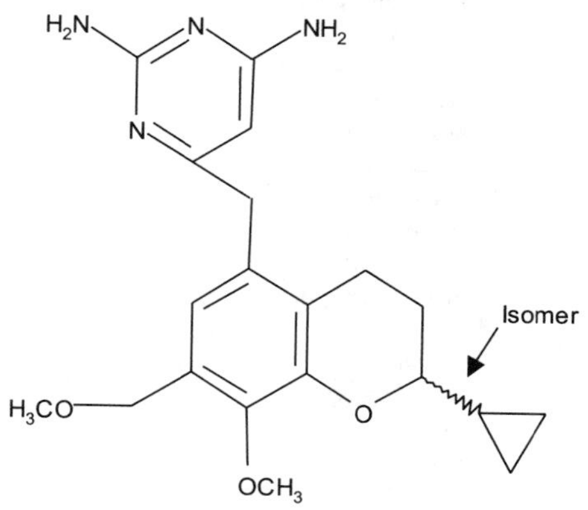

H_2N, N, NH_2, N, Isomer, H_3CO, O, OCH_3

Figure 14 Iclaprim

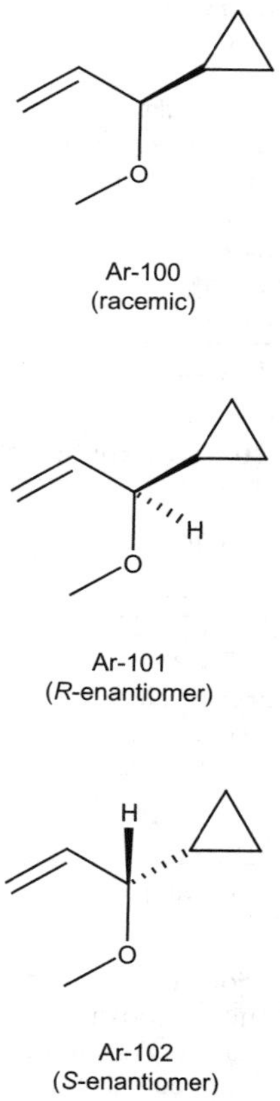

Ar-100 (racemic)

Ar-101 (*R*-enantiomer)

Ar-102 (*S*-enantiomer)

Figure 15 Enantiomers of AR-101

Table 19 In vitro activity of iclaprim

Microorganism(s)[a]	*n*	MIC (μg/ml)			
		Iclaprim		Trimethoprim	
		50%	90%	50%	90%
MSSA	24	≤0.03	0.03	0.5	0.5
MRSA	34	≤0.03	0.03	0.5	1.0
S. aureus TMP[r] (MIC, 8–128 μg/ml)	45	1.0	4.0	32	64
S. aureus TMP[r] (MIC, ≥512 μg/ml)	11	32	32	512	≥512
S. pneumoniae	18	0.06	1.0	4.0	64
Streptococcus agalactiae	18	0.5	1.0	8.0	128
S. pyogenes	20	0.25	128	8.0	256
Viridans group streptococci	15	0.5	16	8.0	128
E. faecalis	24	≤0.03	4.0	0.25	64
Enterococcus faecium	16	≤0.03	16	0.5	256
L. monocytogenes	10	0.06	0.06	0.25	0.25
MAC	7	32		>128	>128
H. influenzae	24	0.25	1.0	0.25	1.0
Haemophilus parainfluenzae	13	1.0	4.0	0.25	0.25
M. catarrhalis	17	2.0	8.0	64	64
N. meningitidis	10	2.0	4.0	64	128
Acinetobacter spp.	17	8.0	32	4.0	16
E. coli	19	4.0	>128	0.5	>128
S. flexneri	6	>128	>128	>128	>128
Burkholderia spp.	13	0.5	>128	0.125	>128
K. pneumoniae	19	2.0	4.0	0.5	1.0
P. vulgaris	19	8.0	32	2.0	8.0
P. mirabilis	19	32	>128	2.0	>256
C. freundii	18	0.5	>128	0.25	>256
Morganella morganii	19	4.0	>128	2.0	>256
Enterobacter cloacae	20	1.0	2.0	0.5	1.0
S. marcescens	18	8.0	>128	4.0	>256
P. aeruginosa	19	>128	>128	128	>256
B. fragilis		0.25		≥8.0	
Bacteroides thetaiotaomicron		1.0		16	
Fusobacterium necrophorum		1.0		16	
Gemella morbillorum		2.0		32	
P. acnes		2.0		>32	
C. difficile		>32		>32	
Peptostreptococcus		2.0		>32	
Chlamydia spp.		0.5	0.5		

[a]TMP, trimethoprim; MAC, *M. avium* complex.

Table 20 Affinity for DHFR of gram-positive cocci

Organism	IC_{50} (μM)		MIC (μg/ml)	
	Iclaprim	Trimethoprim	Iclaprim	Trimethoprim
S. aureus ATCC 25925	0.0034	0.008	0.06	2.0
S. aureus TMP[ra]	1.1	16	2.0	>128
S. pneumoniae TMP[s]	0.008	0.075	0.06	2.0
S. pneumoniae TMP[r]	0.043	3.0	2.0	64
E. coli ATCC 25922	0.0029	0.08		
P. carinii	2.0–4.0	43		
Human	>300	>300		

[a]TMP, trimethoprim.

yields peak concentrations in serum of 1 μg of trimethoprim per ml and 20 μg of sulfamethoxazole per ml between 2 and 4 h after oral administration. This ratio (1:20) is that at which the greatest synergy has been demonstrated for the largest number of bacterial species. The percent absorption of trimethoprim is greater than 90%. That of the sulfonamides (sulfamethoxazole, sulfadiazine, sulfamoxole, and sulfametrole) ranges from 85 to 95%.

1.2.12.1.2. Distribution. Protein binding of trimethoprim is not reduced when sulfonamides are added to plasma; the protein binding of the sulfonamides is not modified by

Table 21 Preliminary pharmacokinetics of iclaprim

Dose (mg/kg)	C_{max} (μg/ml)	T_{max} (h)	$AUC_{0-\infty}$ (μg·h/ml)	$t_{1/2}$ (h)	CL_P (ml/min)
0.25	0.686	0.008	0.598	1.9	495
0.50	1.912	0.008	0.988	1.3	561.6
1.0	4.726	0.008	2.574	2.0	429.9
2.0	8.3057	0.008	4.280	2.0	429.9

Table 22 Proprietary names of combinations

Combination	Proportion (mg/mg) of drug in combination				
	Trimethoprim	Sulfametrole	Sulfamethoxazole	Sulfamoxole	Sulfadiazine
Bactrim					
Oral	80		400		
Oral	160		800		
Children's	40		200		
Suspension	80		400		
Intramuscular	160		400		
Intravenous	80		400		
Eusaprim	80		400		
Bactekod	80				
Supristol	80			400	
Antrima	80				400
Quam	80	400			

trimethoprim, and the highly ionized and less liposoluble sulfonamides are more diffusible than trimethoprim (Table 23).

Sulfonamide is found in serum in the free and conjugated forms and in the form of metabolites. Trimethoprim is found free, protein bound, and in the form of metabolites. The serum ratio of 1/20 is in fact 1/10 with respect to the active forms.

Penetration is excellent for trimethoprim in bronchial secretions (Table 24), CSF, the prostate, and peritoneal fluid. Tissue penetration varies because of the differing chemical natures and liposolubilities. The most interesting sulfonamide appears to be sulfamoxole, the pK_a and partition coefficient of which are similar to those of trimethoprim. It should be noted that almost all of the tissues are the site of higher trimethoprim concentrations than serum, whereas tissue sulfonamide levels are lower than levels in serum. There is no appreciable difference when trimethoprim and sulfonamides are administered simultaneously. The meningeal penetration of trimethoprim is 18%, and that of sulfamethoxazole is 12%. In healthy subjects, after intravenous and oral administration of tetroxoprim and sulfadiazine, the concentrations attained in the CSF are greater than the MICs for the majority of bacteria. In blister fluid the level of trimethoprim was 2.21 ± 1.08 μg/ml (mean ± standard deviation) after 6 h (plasma, 3.95 ± 1.06 μg/ml). The time to maximum concentration of drug in plasma was 2.0 h (Table 25).

Trimethoprim absolute recoveries were 92.0% ± 9% and 91% ± 8% for sputum and saliva, respectively.

Table 23 Plasma protein binding

Compound	Protein binding (%)	V (liters/kg)
Trimethoprim	45	1.5–2
Sulfamethoxazole	65–70	0.25–1.2
Sulfadiazine	40	0.50
Sulfamoxole	80	0.30

1.2.12.1.3. Metabolism and elimination. Sixty to seventy percent of trimethoprim is eliminated in the unmetabolized form, the remainder being eliminated in the glucuroconjugated form. Twenty to sixty percent of the sulfonamide is eliminated in the metabolized form; 40 to 70% is eliminated in the acetylated or conjugated form. The dissociation constants are 7.3 for trimethoprim and 5.7 for sulfamethoxazole (similar to those for the others) in relation to their renal elimination levels. An acid load increases unmetabolized trimethoprim levels in the urine. An alkaline load increases unmetabolized sulfamethoxazole levels. The ratios of their concentrations in serum may therefore vary from 1:1 to 1:5 depending on these modifications, but with no appreciable modification of antibacterial activity.

The combination is eliminated renally by glomerular filtration and tubular secretion. Sulfonamide levels are three times higher than levels in serum; trimethoprim levels are up to 100 times the levels in serum. In patients with renal insufficiency in the absence of any dosage adjustment, there is essentially a risk of accumulation of the sulfonamide. The various sulfonamides obey the same rule, and the different combinations do not behave markedly differently. The apparent elimination half-lives of the different molecules are similar, 10 to 12 h for trimethoprim, 9 to 11 h for sulfamethoxazole, 10 h for sulfadiazine, 11 h for sulfamoxole, and about 6 h for sulfametrole.

At 72 h, 65% of trimethoprim and 85% of the sulfonamide are eliminated in the urine. Overall, the pharmacological behaviors of the combinations are very similar. Sulfadiazine is eliminated essentially in the unmetabolized form, and this fact is important in the treatment of urinary tract infections. In addition, there is less accumulation in renal insufficiency, making the combination co-trimoxazole more manageable in risk patients.

Pharmacokinetic studies have been conducted with malnourished subjects. In these patients, the elimination half-life is prolonged for sulfamethoxazole, with an increase in

Table 24 Penetration in bronchial secretions

Compound	Sampling time (h)	Concn (μg/ml) in:	
		Bronchial secretions	Serum
Trimethoprim (160 mg, per os)	8–12	1.97 ± 0.33	1.93 ± 0.21
Sulfamethoxazole (800 mg/day per os)	8–12	7.9 ± 0.95	59.4 ± 7.05

Table 25 Trimethoprim distribution in blister fluid

Parameter	Plasma	Skin blister fluid
C_{max} (μg/ml)	3.95 ± 1.08	2.21 ± 0.62
T_{max} (h)	2.0 ± 1.0	6.0 ± 1.0
AUC (μg·h/ml)	52.5 ± 13.4	43.9 ± 13.2
$t_{1/2}$ (h)	7.18 ± 2.40	10.23 ± 4.42
CL_P (liters/h)	7.49 ± 1.82	

the area under the curve. In patients suffering from AIDS, the high frequency of side effects of the co-trimoxazole combination appears to be correlated with a modification of the pharmacokinetic data. The doses of co-trimoxazole are higher in these patients, but sulfamethoxazole concentrations are higher than in healthy subjects, with a trimethoprim/ sulfamethoxazole ratio of 1:32, versus 1:20 in non-AIDS subjects.

1.2.12.1.4. Parenteral route. After intramuscular administration, the concentrations in plasma are higher than after oral administration, by 10% for trimethoprim and 5% for the sulfonamide.

Following intravenous injection, concentrations in serum 15 min after the end of the infusion are identical to those obtained after an injection of 400 mg of sulfamethoxazole or 80 mg of trimethoprim separately: 38 μg of free sulfamethoxazole per ml and 1.1 μg of trimethoprim per ml. The ratios of the serum and tissue concentrations and the apparent elimination half-life differ very little from the parameters observed after oral administration. If the duration of infusion is greater than 1.5 h, the peak concentrations are lower and occur with a delay. In patients suffering from renal insufficiency, prolongation of the apparent elimination half-life of trimethoprim and sulfamethoxazole is also observed after intravenous infusion, that of trimethoprim exceeding that of sulfamethoxazole for creatinine clearances of less than 30 ml/min. Infusions should therefore be given at intervals to avoid the risk of accumulation of sulfamethoxazole metabolites.

In cystic fibrosis, there is increased clearance of sulfamethoxazole (induction and/or activation of the metabolism-mediating enzymes) and trimethoprim (increase in renal clearance).

After intraperitoneal administration, rapid absorption is observed (80% compared to the systemic route for sulfamethoxazole). It is possible to use continuous administration in dialysis.

Pharmacology studies show that the combination of compounds does not modify their behavior and that if co-trimoxazole is compared with the other combinations an advantage may be found for trimethoprim-sulfadiazine in urinary tract infections and renal insufficiency. However, a number of authors consider there to be insufficient clinical arguments to assume that another combination is superior to co-trimoxazole.

In patients with renal insufficiency, the serum trimethoprim/sulfamethoxazole ratio remains 20/1 since trimethoprim, which accumulates less in serum than sulfamethoxazole, is less well eliminated by the kidneys. Despite this consideration, monitoring of levels in serum might be useful in the event of prolonged administration.

The pharmacology of co-trimoxazole is thus well known. Dosage adjustments in patients with renal insufficiency are needed. If the creatinine clearance is greater than 30 ml/min, the dosage need not be adjusted. For more severe cases of renal insufficiency, Siber's rule may be applied with unit dosages of 4 mg/20 mg/kg of body weight. The concentrations of trimethoprim then need to be checked.

In the case of hemodialysis, an infusion should be given after each session. In the case of peritoneal dialysis, an infusion of 2 ampoules daily is sufficient, with concentrations in serum being monitored twice weekly.

2. NEW EXPLORATORY DERIVATIVES

2.1. Antibacterial Agents

The continued development of this class of antibacterials has been directed to solve many problems, e.g., the need for improved activity against *S. aureus* and *S. pneumoniae*.

A series of 2,4-diaminopyrimidine derivatives incorporating basic N-disubstituted aminomethyl residues at position 5 have been synthesized with the aim of increasing the water solubility of trimethoprim. One, compound A (Fig. 16), showed an appreciable inhibitory activity against trimethoprim-resistant DHFR from *S. pneumoniae*, but it is less active against *S. aureus*.

2.2. Antiparasitic Agents

AIDS patients and those suffering from other immune disorders are often infected with opportunistic parasites such as *P. carinii*, *T. gondii*, *Cryptosporidium parvum*, and *Mycobacterium avium* complex. New inhibitors of DHFR are needed, eventually hybrids of trimethoprim and piritrexim. Trimethoprim is not potent enough to achieve significant reduction of parasitemia, and piritrexim is potent enough but not selective, and coadministration of leucovorin is required to protect mammalian cells from hematopoietic toxicity.

2.2.1. *T. gondii* and *P. carinii*

Series of 2,4-diamino-substituted pyrimidines have been synthesized. Some analogs displayed affinity for DHFR with an S108N mutation. The most interesting compounds are the unsubstituted 5-phenyl analogs of 2,4-diaminopyrimidine giving low to no toxicity in mammalian cells. Many 6-6 fused rings have been prepared with the aim of increasing the selectivity for *T. gondii* and *P. carinii* DHFR. These

	IC_{50} (μM)		MIC (μg/ml)	
	S. aureus TMP-R	*S. pneumoniae* TMP-R	*S. aureus*	*S. pneumoniae*
Trimethoprim	19	34.00	> 32	2.0
Compound A	> 100	0.21	> 32	0.5

Figure 16 Compound A. TMP, trimethoprim

include cyclopentyl[*d*] pyrimidine, pyrrolo[2,3-*d*] pyrimidine, furo[2,3-*d*] pyrimidine, and pyrrolo[3,2] pyrimidine (Table 26). However, all of them possess a glutamate side chain which is not suitable for *P. carinii* and *T. gondii* lacking the reduced folate carrier.

A series of hybrids was synthesized. The 5′ substituents were either a long chain with an alkoxy group, water-soluble, or ω-carboxyalkoxy, ω-carboxyalkynyl, ω-carboxyallyl, carboxybenzoxy, or carboxyphenoxypropenyl groups. Within this series one analog was 500-fold more potent than trimethoprim against *P. carinii* and *T. gondii* and displayed an excellent selectivity. The 50% inhibitory concentration (IC_{50}) was 3.7 nM for *M. avium* complex.

2.2.2. *C. parvum*

Cryptosporidiosis is acquired from unsterilized drinking water and is usually self-limiting except in immunocompromised patients.

Some therapeutic successes have been reported with pyrimethamine and co-trimoxazole in patients infected with *Isospora belli*. The *C. parvum* DHFR is a bifunctional enzyme which was sequenced.

Table 26 2,4-Diaminopyrimidine systems for parasites

System
5/6 system
Thieno[2,3-*d*] pyrimidine
Furo[2,3-*d*] pyrimidine
Pyrrolo[2,3-*d*] pyrimidine
Pyrazolo[2,3-*d*] pyrimidine
Cyclopenta[*d*] pyrimidine
6/6 system
Quinazoline
Pyrido[2,3-*d*] pyrimidine
Pyrido[4,3-*c*] pyrimidine
Pyrido[3,2-*d*] pyrimidine
Tricyclic and other systems
Indenopyrido[2,3-*d*] pyrimidine
Benzopyrido[2,3-*d*] quinazolines
Pyrimido[4,5-*c*] isoquinoline
Benzo[3,4]cyclohepto[1,2-*d*] pyrimidine
Pyrimido[4,5-*c*] naphthyridine
Pyrido[4′,3′:4,5]furo[2,3-*d*] pyrimidine
5,6 (Bicycloalkano) tetrahydro quinazolines

By screening of 93 lipophilic antifolates of the chemical library, Nelson et al. (2001) found that trimethoprim is >100 times more potent against *C. parvum* enzyme than against human enzyme. Three compounds out of the 93 were more potent than trimethoprim. However, trimethoprim seems to be more selective.

The trimethoprim IC_{50}s were 4.0 and 3.8 μM for cpI and cpII, respectively (IC_{50} for human DHFR, 890 μM). In this series 25 out of 93 compounds exhibit for at least one of the cp enzymes an IC_{50} of 10 μM. The best compound had an IC_{50} of 0.065 μM for cpI enzyme.

2.3. Epiroprim (Ro-11-8958)

Epiroprim was design to be more active against *S. pneumoniae* than trimethoprim.

The antibacterial activity of epiroprim is reported in Table 27.

Epiroprim is more active than trimethoprim against gram-positive cocci but is poorly active against enteric gram-negative bacilli. Epiroprim displays some activity against nontuberculous bacteria (Table 28).

Epiroprim is inactive against *Clostridium difficile* (MIC, >32 μg/ml).

The in vitro activity of epiroprim translated well to in vivo activities (Table 29). Epiroprim is more active than trimethoprim against *P. carinii*. The combination of epiroprim and dapsone is highly effective against *P. carinii* pneumonia in rats and *T. gondii* infection in mice.

3. SULFONES

Sulfones are primarily used in the treatment of leprosy. Sulfones are also used in other therapeutic areas. They are used in dermatology (dermatitis herpetiformis, bullous pemphigoid, and ulcers due to brown recluse spider bites), rheumatology, and certain inflammatory infections of the digestive tract. They also possess antiplasmodial activity and have recently been proposed in the preventive treatment of malaria. New indications are under evaluation, in particular in certain opportunistic infections during an HIV infection as curative treatment and as primary and secondary prophylaxis, particularly of pneumocystosis.

Adverse effects have been reported, such as methemoglobinemia, hemolysis, and neurologic disorders, limiting its usefulness.

The sulfones are derived from bis(4-aminophenyl)sulfone or dapsone and are usually symmetrical disubstituted diaminophenyl sulfones (Fig. 17).

Table 27 In vitro activity of epiroprim

Microorganism(s)[a]	*n*	MIC (μg/ml)			
		Epiroprim		Trimethoprim	
		50%	90%	50%	90%
MSSA TMP[s]	24	0.06	0125	0.5	0.5
MRSA TMP[r]	34	0.06	0.125	0.5	1.0
S. aureus TMP[r] (MIC, 8–128 μg/ml)	45	8.0	32	32	64
S. aureus TMP[r] (MIC, ≥256 μg/ml)	11	256	256	512	>512
CoNS TMP[s]	36	0.125	0.25	0.25	4.0
CoNS TMP[r]	70	32	64	64	128
S. pneumoniae Pen[s]	19	0.125	1.0	4.0	64
S. pneumoniae Pen[r]	55	16	32	128	>128
S. agalactiae	18	2.0	64	8.0	128
S. pyogenes	20	1.0	128	8.0	256
Viridans group streptococci	15	1.0	64	0.06	128
E. faecalis	24	≤0.03	16	0.5	64
E. faecium	16	≤0.03	64	0.25	256
L. monocytogenes	10	≤0.03	0.06	0.25	0.25
H. influenzae	24	2.0	8.0	0.25	1.0
M. catarrhalis	17	8.0	8.0	64	64
Acinetobacter spp.	17	64	128	4.0	16
N. meningitidis	10	16	16	64	128
E. coli	19	4.0	>128	0.	>128
S. flexneri	6	>128		>256	
Salmonella spp.	13	1.0	>128	0.12	>128
K. pneumoniae	19	8.0	16	0.5	1.0
P. vulgaris	19	32	128	2.0	8.0
P. mirabilis	19	32	128	2.0	>256
C. freundii	18	4.0	>128	0.25	>256
M. morganii	19	16	>128	2.0	>256
E. cloacae	20	4.0	8.0	0.5	1.0
S. marcescens	18	>128	>129	4.0	>256
P. aeruginosa	19	>128	>128	128	>256
Bacteroides spp.	12	4.0	4.0	16	32

[a]TMP, trimethoprim; CoNS, coagulase-negative staphylococci.

Table 28 In vitro activity of epiroprim against mycobacteria

Microorganism	MIC (μg/ml)			
	Epiroprim	Epiroprim + dapsone (1:19)	Trimethoprim	Trimethoprim + sulfamethoxazole (1:19)
M. fortuitum ZH5	32	0.25	>128	0.06
M. chelonae ZH9	>128	8.0	>128	>16
M. smegmatis 607	2.0	≤0.06	4.0	0.125
M. marinum ZH 11	8.0	≤0.03	16	≤0.03
M. kansasii ZH1	4.0	≤0.03	64	≤0.03
MAC[a] 158-0	64	1.0	>128	1.0

[a]MAC, *M. avium* complex.

3.1. Physicochemical Properties

The physicochemical properties are summarized in Table 30.

3.2. Structure-Activity Relationship

The reference molecule is dapsone with a sulfonyl group disubstituted symmetrically by a *para*-aminophenyl group. As this product has moderate activity and definite toxicity, studies have been conducted to synthesize molecules with greater antibacterial and antiplasmodial activities and weaker toxicity.

Among the monosubstituted sulfones, *p*-propylamino-*p*′-aminodiphenyl sulfone and *p*-ethylamino-*p*′-aminodiphenyl sulfone have good antiplasmodial activity.

Among the disubstituted sulfones, the following may be distinguished:

- Derivatives with symmetrical substituents, including glucosulfone (Promin), metabolized to dapsone in the body, and diformyldapsone and diacetyldapsone, which have identical activities but differing pharmacokinetics

Table 29 In vivo efficacy of epiroprim

Microorganism	Drug[a]	ED_{50}[b] (mg/kg)
S. aureus Smith	Epiroprim	11.7
	Trimethoprim	16.8
	EPM + DDS	<0.35
	DDS	>25
S. aureus Schoch	Epiroprim	3.5
	Trimethoprim	7.2
	EPM + DDS	0.77
	DDS	14.2

[a]EPM, epiroprim; DDS, dapsone.
[b]ED_{50}, 50% effective dose.

- Derivatives with asymmetrical substituents and variable activities (value of the morpholine nucleus at R_2 and the pentylamine at R_1)
- Derivatives with nonamino substituents and modifications of the sulfonyl or phenyl nucleus, associated with the search for sustained-release sulfones that may be of value in combination with cycloguanil, particularly by alkylation of the amino functions, the most effective molecule in this respect being acedapsone

3.3. Different Sulfones

3.3.1. Dapsone

Dapsone was the first sulfone studied. It is 4,4′-diaminodiphenyl sulfone with a molecular weight of 218.3. It is presented in the form of colorless lamellar crystals melting at 128°C. The solubility in water at 25°C is 14 mg/100 ml.

3.3.2. Glucosulfone

Glucosulfone is 4,4′-diaminodiphenylsulfone-*N*,*N*′-galactose sodium sulfonate. Its molecular weight is 572.58. It is highly soluble in water, and its melting point is 268°C. It may be administered intravenously.

3.3.3. Diacetyldapsone (Acedapsone)

Acedapsone is 4,4′-diacetylaminodiphenyl sulfone with a molecular weight of 332.4. It is a white powder, almost insoluble in water and with a melting point of between 282 and 292°C. Its essential value lies in its slow elimination. It has good efficacy in the curative and/or preventive treatment of *P. falciparum* malaria.

3.3.4. Diformyldapsone

Diformyldapsone is 4,4′-diformylaminodiphenyl sulfone. It has a molecular weight of 340.3. Its solubility is similar to that of dapsone. Its melting point is between 267 and 271°C.

3.4. Activity of Sulfones

3.4.1. Antibacterial Activity

The activity against bacteria such as streptococci or *E. coli* is anecdotal. The essential value of dapsone and acedapsone is their activities against M. *leprae*. Concentrations of 0.03 μg/ml inhibit Hansen's bacillus in animals. In humans, more than 90% of bacilli are destroyed after 4 months of treatment, but persistent bacilli are observed, and the emergence of secondary resistance, particularly in lepromatous subjects, is observed in 2 to 7% of cases.

3.4.2. Antiparasitic Activity

Dapsone and its derivatives are active against ankylostomas and promastigote forms of *Leishmania*.

The antiplasmodial activity of the sulfones has been studied. All of the sulfones have the same qualitative activity against the different plasmodial species in animals. They are active against the asexual blood forms and inactive against the tissue forms. They are inactive against gametocytes.

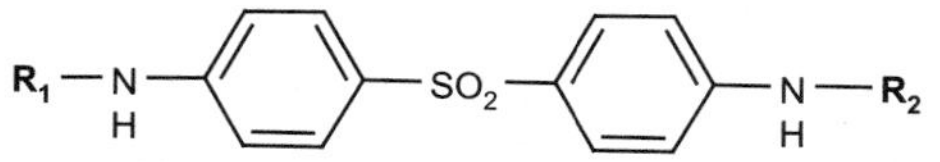

$R_1-NH-C_6H_4-SO_2-C_6H_4-NH-R_2$

		R_1	R_2
Diphenylsulfone	Dapsone ®	-H	-H
Diformyldapsone	-	-CHO	-CHO
Acedapsone	-	$-COCH_3$	$-COCH_3$
Glucosulfone	Promin ®	SO_3-Galactose	SO_3-Galactose
Acediasulfone	-	-	$-CH_2COOH$

Figure 17 Sulfones

Table 30 Physicochemical properties of sulfones

Compound	Mol wt	Melting point (°C)	pK	Lipophilicity (%)	Water solubility (mg/100 ml at 25°C)
Diphenyl sulfone	218.3	128–129	13	13	14
Acedapsone	332.37	289–292			0.3
Diformyldapsone	340.3	267–270			
Acediasulfone	306.35	194			
Glucosulfone	572.58	268			

They are active against *Plasmodium berghei* and *Plasmodium cynomolgi*. They are active against *P. falciparum* and ineffective against *Plasmodium vivax* and *Plasmodium malariae*. Dapsone has slow schizonticidal activity against *P. falciparum*, whether or not it is susceptible to chloroquine, and no sporonticidal or gametocidal activity. Acedapsone has good activity against *P. falciparum*, but slower than the combination acedapsone-cycloguanil. It also has good preventive activity (Bryskier and Labro, 1989).

In vitro, the sulfones are active against *T. gondii*, particularly dapsone.

In murine *P. carinii* pneumocystosis, dapsone is effective in treatment and prevention. In humans, the combination trimethoprim-dapsone in curative treatment and dapsone alone in preventive treatment are effective.

Sulfones are also used in rheumatology and dermatology.

3.5. Mode of Action of Sulfones

Like the sulfonamides, the sulfones interfere with folate synthesis. They also have a potent antioxidant action. Lastly, dapsone inhibits the transport of adenosine through the erythrocyte wall and prevents its incorporation in the nucleic acid of plasmodia and probably toxoplasmas and *P. carinii*.

3.6. Pharmacokinetics

Orally administered dapsone is almost entirely absorbed. The peak concentration in serum is obtained 1 to 3 h after administration and reaches 2 μg/ml for a dose of 100 mg. Dapsone is mainly metabolized by N acetylation. A proportion of dapsone is acetylated by an *N*-acetyltransferase to monoacetyldapsone. This metabolite can also be deacetylated by another enzyme back to dapsone. Dapsone acetylation exhibits a polymorphic distribution with ethnic variation (slow and fast acetylators). The main route of metallic elimination is N hydroxylation (dapsone hydroxylamine and monoacetyldapsone hydroxylamine). It accounts for between 30 and 40% of orally administered dapsone. It is mediated by cytochrome P450, 3A4, 2E1, and 2C9. The metabolites are one cause of hematologic toxicities, in constrast to monoacetyldapsone, which is not toxic to red blood cells. The apparent elimination half-life is, on average, 28 h (10 to 50 h). Metabolism is very extensive. Dapsone and its acetylated metabolite (4-amino-4′-acetamidodimethyl sulfone) are 60 to 70% serum protein bound. The metabolite represents a larger fraction of the sum of dapsone plus metabolite in rapid acetylators than slow acetylators (Table 31).

Table 31 Dapsone slow and rapid acetylators (100-mg single oral dose to nine patients)

Parameter	Value for phenotype	
	Slow	Rapid
Acetylation ratio		
First dose	0.26	0.73
Steady state	0.19	0.63
Dapsone recovery ratio (hydroxylation)		
First dose	0.60	0.42
Steady state	0.58	0.41
Dapsone (level in plasma, μg/ml)		
First dose	0.31	0.33
Steady state	1.57	1.63
Monoacetyldapsone (level in plasma, μg/ml)		
First dose	0.08	0.24
Steady state	0.30	1.06

Diffusion in biological fluids and tissues, including the placenta, is good, reaching 2 μg/ml after a dose of 100 mg. The concentrations are higher in soft tissue, liver, and kidneys. There is an enterohepatic cycle.

Elimination is essentially urinary (60 to 80% in 120 h). A large fraction of the dose is probably excreted by various routes of metabolism and elimination, as demonstrated by the differences between animals and humans. Biliary concentrations of dapsone are minor.

4. NITROHETEROCYCLES: FURANS

The search for molecules possessing antibacterial activity in the furan series initially met with only limited success with furfural, furoic acid, and the furylmercuric compounds.

In 1944, Dood and Stillman in a study involving 40 mono- or disubstituted furan derivatives demonstrated that the introduction of a nitro group at position 5 caused the appearance or increase of antibacterial activity.

The results of the various studies showed that only 5-nitro-2-furfural semicarbazone manifested appreciable in vitro activity.

The compound was tested clinically and has been selected for use as a local antiseptic, while a derivative, nitrofurantoin, is used as an antiseptic of the urinary tract.

4.1. Structure-Activity Relationship

4.1.1. Nitro Derivatives

Nitration at position 5 of the 2-substituted derivatives of furan causes a very marked increase in in vitro bactericidal activity, with a few exceptions (5-nitrofuroic acid).

This improvement is not observed if another group such as a halogen, methyl, carbonyl, or chloromethyl is introduced at position 5. With an amino substituent, it is relatively minor. Similarly, the reduction of the nitro group suppresses antibacterial activity.

The position of the nitro group appears to be the determinant. The furans nitrated at position 3 or 5 have only weak activity, if any.

4.1.2. Azomethine Group (–CH=N–)

The results observed in vivo in the treatment of various experimental infections show narrow structural specificity based on the skeleton of the molecule.

Acid hydrolysis of the azomethine group abolishes the antibacterial activity of the nitrofurans.

Exploitation of this group resulted in the synthesis of antibacterial and antiprotozoal compounds: nitrofurantoin, furazolidone, and nitrofuraldezone (Fig. 18).

Other modifications of the R chain yielded (5-nitro-8-furyl)ethylene derivatives possessing schistosomicidal activity.

At position 2, vinyl (–CH=CH–) groups and substitution directly by heterocycles have been described and have given rise to two compounds, nifurpirinol and nifurthiazole, without further clinical development.

4.1.3. Other Nitro Derivatives

Based on the concept of isosterism, the furan heterocycle was replaced by other pentagonal heterocycles: nitrothiophene, nitrothiazole, nitroimidazole, and nitropyrrole.

These compounds are antibacterial, antiprotozoal, and antifungal agents used in human and veterinary medicine.

After defining the structure-activity relationships of the furans, we consider their mechanism of action, the

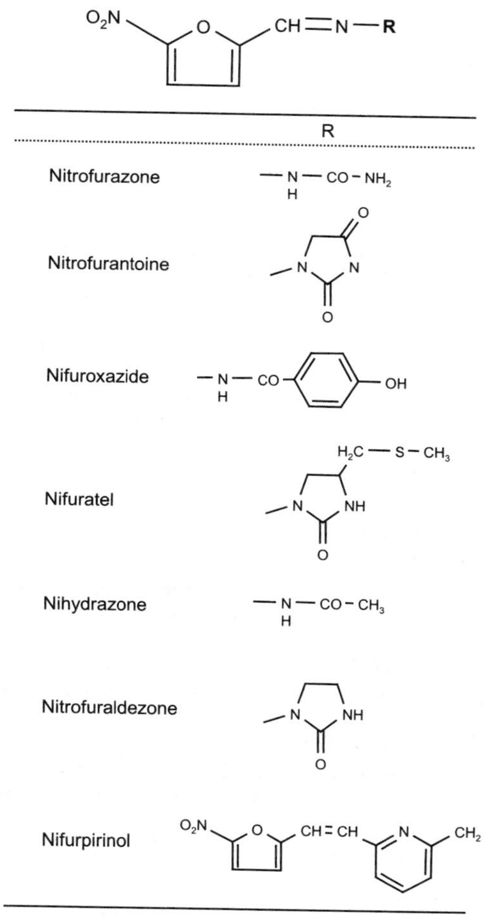

	R
Nitrofurazone	—NH—CO—NH_2
Nitrofurantoine	
Nifuroxazide	
Nifuratel	
Nihydrazone	—NH—CO—CH_3
Nitrofuraldezone	
Nifurpirinol	

Figure 18 Nitroheterocycle furans

antibacterial activity of nitrofurantoin, its pharmacology, its metabolism, its clinical indications, and its side effects.

The other derivatives are mentioned briefly, highlighting their specific features.

4.2. Mechanism of Action, Resistance, and Antibacterial Activity

4.2.1. Mechanism of Action and Resistance

The nitro groups of the nitrofurans must be reduced by nitrofuran reductases present in bacteria to amino or hydroxylamino derivatives, which are themselves reduced by opening of the ring to nitrile derivatives.

It has been shown that the furans act on the Krebs cycle by exerting a threefold inhibitory action on acetyl coenzyme A, citric acid, and oxaloacetic acid. The result of this triple inhibition is to reduce the production of energy necessary for bacterial multiplication and survival, with bacterial DNA and RNA synthesis being blocked beyond a certain concentration.

Bacterial resistance to furans appears to be related to membrane impermeability and in particular to a chromosomally or plasmid-mediated functional deficiency of nitrofuran reductase.

4.2.2. Antibacterial Activity

Furans are active against enterobacteria, except *Serratia, Proteus,* and *Providencia*. They are inactive against *P. aeruginosa* and *Acinetobacter*. They are active against gram-positive cocci such as staphylococci and streptococci.

The mean MIC for strains deemed to be susceptible is on the order of 8 to 16 μg/ml. A strain is considered resistant when the MIC is greater than 32 μg/ml.

4.2.3. Pharmacokinetics

Nitrofurantoin has different physicochemical properties according to whether it is presented in the form of an amorphous powder or in the crystalline form.

After intravenous administration at the recommended therapeutic dosage, concentrations in serum are 1 to 5 μg/ml, with an apparent elimination half-life of 30 min.

After oral administration, absorption in the small intestine yields a peak of 1 μg/ml at 30 min in animals and in humans treated for several days; concentrations in serum remain low.

Protein binding of nitrofurantoin ranges between 50 and 75%, and the apparent volume of distribution is 0.7 liter/kg. Administration of nitrofurantoin yields substantial tissue levels. There is weak transplacental passage and passage into the arachnoid spaces. Elimination in milk is disputed.

After parenteral administration of nitrofurantoin, 40 to 60% of the dose is found in the urine; elimination of the microcrystalline form (Furadantin) is weaker and slower in the first few hours than that of the micronized form, but after 24 h the quantities of product found in the urine are identical.

Nitrofurantoin is a weak acid, and its renal clearance is affected by pH. In an acidic medium, the activity is greater. Tubular reabsorption is greater and renal tissue concentrations are higher. The opposite is observed in an alkaline medium. There is little modification of renal elimination by phenobarbital, diuretics, and probenecid.

After administration of nitrofurantoin to dogs, 20% is found in the bile. A certain amount is reabsorbed and recycled in the enterohepatic circulation. The quantity of product eliminated in the bile is lower after oral administration.

The metabolism of nitrofurantoin has been the subject of several studies. The product may be eliminated in the intact form and in the form of metabolites with enzymatic degradation, essentially by hydroxylation of the furan ring.

In animals, the first stages of metabolism of the nitrofuran heterocycle take place in the cytoplasmic membrane and involve a reduction of the nitro group to a hydroxylamine.

Amino reductions occur in the following stages with the opening of the furan ring and fragmentation. The nitrofurans are converted to β-ketoglutaramic and ketoglutamic acids, which reintegrate the metabolic pool.

Acid hydrolysis of the azomethine group may also occur followed by oxidation, yielding 5-nitrofuroic acid, which can be detected in certain animals.

Overall, nitrofurantoin is rapidly absorbed and distributed in the majority of tissues. It is eliminated essentially in the urine with complex secretion-reabsorption phenomena in the kidneys. It has a short elimination half-life. It is eliminated in the intact form and in different metabolites after enzymatic degradation.

5. 8-HYDROXYQUINOLINE DERIVATIVES

5.1. Nitroxoline

Nitroxoline is an antibacterial agent related to the oxyquinoline derivatives by its chemical structure. Nitroxoline is used exclusively in urinary tract infections (Fig. 19).

	R_5	R_6	R_7	Trade name
Nitroxoline	H	H	NO_2	Nibiol ®
Diodohydroxyquinoline	I	H	I	Direxiode ®
Methyl-5-bromo-7-quinoline	Br	H	CH_3	Intetrix ®

Figure 19 8-Hydroxyquinoline derivatives

5.1.1. Antibacterial Activity

Nitroxoline is active against bacteria and yeasts. Usually susceptible species include *E. coli*, *Ureaplasma urealyticum*, and *Mycoplasma hominis*. Yeasts such as *Candida albicans*, *Candida tropicalis*, and *Candida krusei* are usually susceptible, and likewise *Candida glabrata*. Species of inconsistent susceptibility include staphylococci. Species that are usually resistant are *Pseudomonas*, *Providencia*, *Klebsiella*, *Enterobacter*, and *Serratia*. Nitroxoline has no activity against anaerobic bacteria.

5.1.2. Pharmacokinetics

Nitroxoline is administered orally. It is rapidly absorbed, whether in the form of an oral suspension or as unscored coated tablets. Absorption is on the order of 90%.

For a dose of 200 mg, the peak concentration in serum is 4 to 4.8 μg/ml and is reached 1.5 to 2 h after administration. The elimination half-life is about 2 h. For the same dose, this half-life and the peak concentrations in serum of the tablet form and the oral solution form are identical.

Plasma protein binding of nitroxoline is 10%.

Nitroxoline is eliminated in the bacteriologically active form with a free form and a conjugated form. Fifty percent of nitroxoline is found in the urine, and 10% is found in the stools. Nitroxoline is 5% eliminated in the free form and 95% eliminated in the conjugated form, the active derivatives being the sulfoconjugated derivatives.

Renal elimination occurs by glomerular filtration. The urinary concentrations observed after administration of a dose of 200 mg are 200 μg/ml for up to 4 h and greater than 30 μg/ml for 12 h. The dosage must be reduced in patients with renal insufficiency, and likewise in patients with hepatic insufficiency.

5.2. Derivatives for Intestinal Use

The 8-hydroxyquinoline derivatives have yielded drugs for urinary use (nitroxoline) and for intestinal antisepsis (Intetrix and Direxiole). Halogenation of the quinoline nucleus (bromine, iodine, and chlorine) and introduction of a methyl group at position 2, 5, or 6 of the quinoline nucleus increase the intrinsic activity of the 8-hydroxyquinoline nucleus.

5.2.1. Antibacterial Spectrum

These drugs are active against *E. coli*, *Salmonella*, *Shigella*, *Proteus*, and *V. cholerae*, as well as against staphylococci and streptococci. They possess antiprotozoal activity: *Lamblia*, *Trichomonas*, *Entamoeba histolytica* (vegetative and cystic forms), and *C. albicans*.

5.2.2. Mechanism of Action of 8-Hydroxyquinolines

These drugs appear to act through a metal-chelating effect, causing inhibition of a number of enzyme complexes.

5.2.3. Pharmacokinetics

These drugs are not absorbed by the intestinal mucosa.

5.3. Other Derivatives

Derivatives for external use, particularly gynecological, such as chlorquinaldol, are used in nongonococcal leukorrhea, particularly due to *Trichomonas vaginalis*.

REFERENCES

SULFAMIDES

Bryskier A, 1983, Les inhibiteurs de la dihydrofolate réductase—classification et relation structure activité, p 19-36, in Modai J, ed, Triméthoprime et sulfamides, Soc Pathol Infect Langue Fse.

Chauvin P, Cnudde F, Leynadier F, Halpern GM, Dry J, 1991, Aspects physiopathologiques des réactions d'intolérance aux sulfamides au cours du SIDA, Med Hyg 49, 1013–1024.

Fegueux S, de Truchis P, Balloul H, Maslo C, Matheron S, Coulaud JP, 1990, Réintroduction de la sulfadiazine au cours du SIDA, Presse Med 19, 1947.

Fischl MA, Dickinson GM, La Voie L, 1988, Safety and efficacy of sulfamethoxazole and trimethoprim chemoprophylaxis for Pneumocystis carinii pneumonia in AIDS, JAMA, 259, 1185–1189.

Fox BC, Sollinger HW, Belzer FO, Maki DG, 1990, A prospective randomized double blind study of TS for prophylaxis of infection in renal transplantation: clinical efficacy, absorption of TS, effects on the microflora and the cost benefits of prophylaxis, Am J Med, 89, 255–274.

Glatt AE, Chirgwin K, Landesman SH, 1988, Current concepts: treatment of infections associated with human immunodeficiency virus, N Engl J Med, 319, 1439–1448.

Hughes WT, 1988, Trimethoprim and sulfonamides, p 229–237, in Peterson PK, Verhoef J, ed, Antimicrobial Agents Annual III, Elsevier Science Publishers BV.

Hughes WT, Killmar JT, 1991, Synergistic anti-pneumocystis carinii effects of erythromycin and sulfisoxazole, J Acquir Immune Defic Syndr, 4, 532–537.

Hutabarat RM, Unadkat JD, Sahajwalla C, McNamara S, Ramsey B, Smith AL, 1991, Disposition of drugs in cystic fibrosis. Sulfamethoxazole and trimethoprim, Clin Pharmacol Ther, 49, 402–409.

Kucers A, Bennet N, 1979, Trimethoprim sulfamethoxazole, p 687–729, in Use of Antibiotics, W Heinemann, London.

La pneumocystose au cours de l'infection HIV, 1990, Conference de consensus 1990, Med Mal Infect, 20 (n° special), 320–324.

Masur H, Kovacs JA, 1988, Treatment and prophylaxis of pneumocystis carinii pneumoniae, p 181–191, in Sande MA, Volberding PA, ed, Medical Management of AIDS, WB Saunders Co, Philadelphia.

Pang LW, Limsomwong N, Snigharaj P, Canfield CJ, 1989, Malaria prophylaxis with proguanil and sulfisoxazole in children living in a malaria endemic area, 671, 51–58.

Remington JS, Luft BJ, 1988, Drugs used in the treatment of toxoplasmosis, p 327–336, in Peterson PK, Verhoef J, ed, Antimicrob Agents Annual III, Elsevier Science Publishers BV.

Saimot AG, Girard PM, 1990 Interactions des traitements antiviraux et antiparasitaires, p 141–152, in Journees de reanimation de l'hopital Claude Bernard, Arnette, Paris.

White MW, Haddad ZH, Brunner E, Sainz C, 1989, Desensitization to TS in patients with acquired deficiency and pneumocystis carinii pneumonia, Ann Allergy, 62, 177–179.

Wolff M, 1990, Posologie des médicaments antiparasitaires chez l'adulte en insuffisance rénale, p 153–161, in Journees de reanimation de l'hopital Claude Bernard, Arnette, Paris.

SULFONES

Biggs JT, Uher AK, Levy L, Gordon GR, Peters JH, 1975, Renal and biliary dispositions of dapsone in the dog, Antimicrob Agents Chemother, 7, 816–824.

Bryskier A, Labro MT, 1989, Les antifolates—classification, relation structure-activité, propriétés biologiques, p 69–100, in Paludisme et Medicaments, Arnette, Paris.

Medina L, Mills J, Leoung G, Hopewell PC, Lee B, Modin G, Benowitz N, Wofsy CB, 1990, Oral therapy for Pneumocystis carinii pneumonia in the acquired immunodeficiency syndrome: a controlled trial of trimethoprim-sulfamethoxazole versus trimethoprim-dapsone, N Engl J Med, 323, 776–782.

Stone OJ, 1990, Sulfapyridine and sulfones decrease glycosaminoglycans viscosity in dermatitis herpetiformis, ulcerative colitis, and pyoderma gangrenosum, Med Hypotheses, 31, 99–103.

Wordell CJ, Hauptman SP, 1988, Treatment of pneumocystis pneumonia in patients with AIDS, Clin Pharm, 7, 514–527.

Wozel G, 1989, The story of sulfones in tropical medicine and dermatology, Int J Dermatol, 28, 17–21.

FURANES

Conklin JD, 1978, The pharmacokinetics of nitrofurantoin and its related bioavailability, Antibiot Chemother, 25, 233–252.

Holmberg L, Boman G, Bottiger LE, Eriksson B, Spross R, Wessling A, 1980, Adverse reactions to nitrofurantoin, analysis of 921 reports, Am J Med, 69, 5, 733–738.

Veyssier P, Bryskier A, 1985, Agents antibactériens de synthèse, Enc Med Chir Thérapeutique, 25016 D-10.

NITROXOLINE

Hannedouche T, Godin M, Fillastre JP, 1983, Les effets secondaires des medicaments utilisés pour le traitement des infections urinaires, Therapie, 38, 281–293.

Lambert Zechovsky N, Leveque B, Bingen E, Pillion G, Chapelle J, Mathieu H, 1987, Activité clinique et effet de la nitroxoline sur la flore fécale chez l'enfant, Pathol Biol, 35, 669–672.

Mupirocin

A. BRYSKIER

36

1. INTRODUCTION

Pseudomonas aeruginosa and other *Pseudomonas* spp. produce a number of substances that possess antibacterial activity, such as pyocyanin, chlororaphin, pyoluteorin, pyrrolnitrin, pyolipic acid, pyoklastin, viscosin, magnesidin, and fluopsin C.

In 1887, Garré had noted the presence of a substance possessing antibacterial activity produced by *Pseudomonas fluorescens*. This substance, which was diffusible in agar medium, proved capable of inhibiting the growth of *Staphylococcus aureus*, *Salmonella enterica* serovar Typhi, and *Klebsiella pneumoniae* and partially preventing the growth of *Vibrio cholerae* and *Bacillus anthracis*. In the following years a number of studies confirmed this observation and resulted in the identification of a dialyzable and thermostable substance possessing antibacterial activity. However, it was not until the 1960s that the team under E. Chain attempted to isolate, purify, and characterize this substance for use as a medicinal product. By using a strain of *P. fluorescens* (NCIB10586) with a high fermentation yield, these studies resulted in the isolation of a molecular complex known as pseudomonic acid. Recently, seven derivatives have been obtained from the fermentation of a strain of *Alteromonas* isolated from a marine sponge, *Darwinella rosacea*.

2. STRUCTURE OF PSEUDOMONIC ACID

Following the initial description by Fuller et al. (1971), the precise structure was not determined until 1977.

Pseudomonic acid is a complex containing four molecules, A, B, C, and D. The pseudomonic acids have been synthesized.

2.1. Pseudomonic Acid A

Pseudomonic acid A, or mupirocin, is a molecule that is decomposed into two parts: a fatty acid chain and monic acid (Fig. 1). The fatty acid chain, 9-hydroxynonanoic acid, is attached to the remainder of the molecule by an α, β-unsaturated ester bond.

2.2. Pseudomonic Acids B, C, and D

Pseudomonic acid B has a additional hydroxyl group on the ring. The epoxy is replaced by a double bond for pseudomonic acid C, while pseudomonic acid D has an unsaturated fatty acid chain (Fig. 2).

3. PHYSICOCHEMICAL PROPERTIES

Pseudomonic acid is unstable at a pH of less than 4 or greater than 11, causing the formation of inactive products. These products are poorly soluble in water (3 mg/ml at 20°C) (Table 1).

4. ANTIBACTERIAL PROPERTIES

4.1. Activity and Antibacterial Spectrum

See Tables 2 and 3.

Mupirocin is active against gram-positive cocci: it has moderate activity against gram-positive bacilli such as *Listeria monocytogenes* (MIC, ~8.0 μg/ml) and *Erysipelothrix rhusiopathiae* (MIC, ~8.0 μg/ml); it is inactive against corynebacteria and *B. anthracis* (MIC, ≥64 μg/ml). It has good activity against *Haemophilus influenzae*, *Moraxella catarrhalis*, *Bordetella pertussis*, and *Pasteurella multocida*. It is inactive against anaerobes, *Enterobacteriaceae*, and *Pseudomonas* spp. It is active against *Neisseria meningitidis* and *Neisseria gonorrhoeae*.

Mupirocin possesses good activity against beta-hemolytic streptococci of Lancefield groups A, C, and G (MICs, ~0.05 and 0.25 μg/ml). Group B streptococci are less susceptible

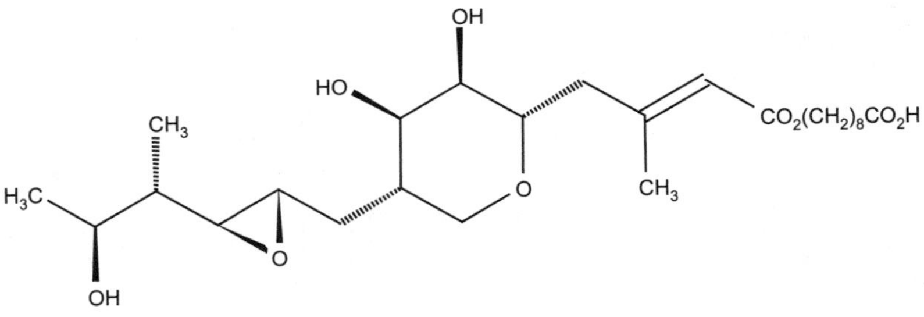

OH
HO
$CO_2(CH_2)_8CO_2H$
CH_3
CH_3
H_3C
O
O
OH

Figure 1 Mupirocin (pseudomonic acid A)

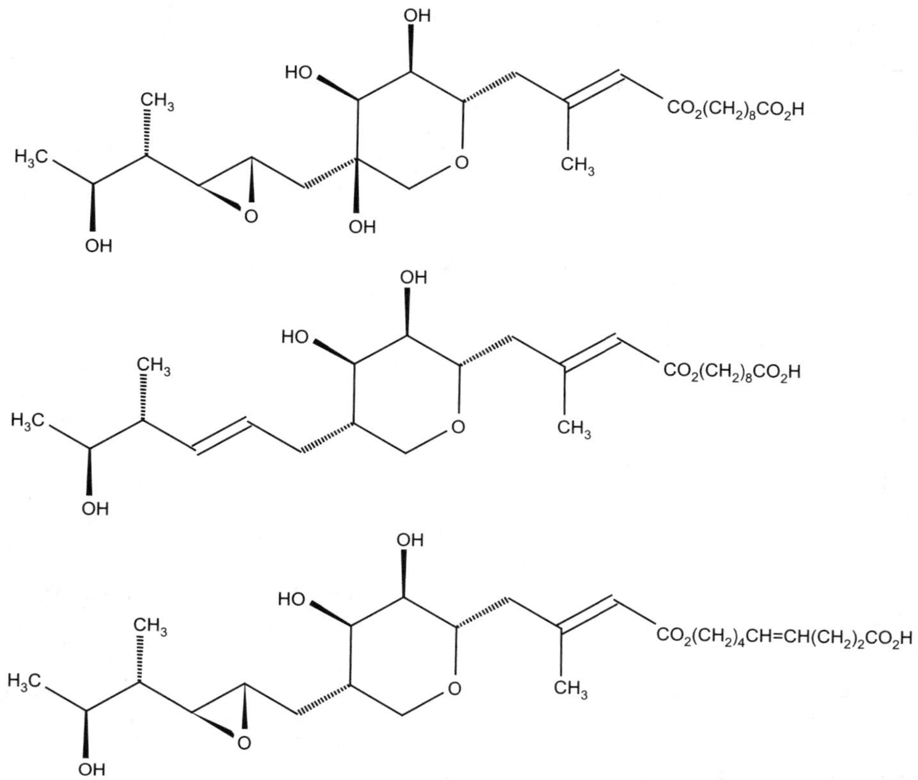

Figure 2 Pseudomonic acids B, C, and D

Table 1 Physicochemical properties of pseudomonic acids

Pseudomonic acid	Empirical formula	Molecular mass (Da)	Melting point (°C)	pK
A	$C_{26}H_{44}O_9$	500.63	77–78	4.9
B	$C_{26}H_{44}O_{10}$	516.63		
C	$C_{26}H_{44}O_8$	484.63	47–49	
D	$C_{26}H_{42}O_9$	498.61		

(MICs, 0.5 to 1.0 μg/ml). Viridans group streptococci have variable activity, depending on the species (MICs, 0.25 to 1 μg/ml). Enterococci, whether *Enterococcus faecalis* or *Enterococcus faecium*, are relatively nonsusceptible (MIC, ≥64 μg/ml). *Streptococcus pneumoniae* is susceptible to mupirocin (MIC, ~0.12 μg/ml) (Table 4). Mupirocin is inactive against *Chlamydia* spp. It is active against *S. aureus*, whether the strains are susceptible or resistant to penicillin G, tetracyclines, erythromycin A, fusidic acid, lincomycin, chloramphenicol, or methicillin. These strains are inhibited by a concentration ≤0.5 μg of mupirocin per ml. Mupirocin also manifests good activity against coagulase-negative staphylococci.

It should be noted that bacterial species or genera responsible for skin and skin structure infections, such as *Propionibacterium acnes* and *Corynebacterium* spp., are not susceptible to mupirocin.

Mupirocin has good activity against human and animal mycoplasmas (Table 5).

4.2. Factors Influencing the In Vitro Activity of Mupirocin

The antibacterial activity of mupirocin is not affected by the culture medium, although the addition of blood in the presence of isoleucine may modify the MIC. The activity, however, is affected by the pH of the culture medium, as mupirocin is more active in an acidic medium than in a neutral or alkaline medium (Table 6). It is twice as active at pH 6 as at pH 7.4 and is less active at pH 8.

Regarding the activity of mupirocin against *S. aureus*, the inoculum size does not appear to exert an effect at 5×10^5 CFU/ml. However, above 10^6 CFU/ml the activity decreases fourfold. As mupirocin is highly serum protein bound (~95%), the in vitro activity is reduced in the presence of human serum. MICs are 10 to 25 times higher in a medium containing 50% human serum (MICs, 2.5 to 5.0 μg/ml) than in a serum-free medium (MICs, 0.1 to 0.5 μg/ml) (Table 7).

4.3. Bacteriostatic Activities

Mupirocin is a bacteriostatic antibiotic.

Killing kinetics show that growth is inhibited during the initial period, accompanied by a reduction in the number of CFU per milliliter. A marked reduction in the number of bacteria is observed after 6 h of contact, depending on the concentration of the antibiotic (Fig. 3).

4.4. Mechanism of Action

Mupirocin alters protein synthesis by blocking the incorporation of isoleucine into the peptide during synthesis.

Table 2 Activity of mupirocin against gram-positive bacteria

Organism(s)	MIC_{50}[a] (μg/ml)
S. aureus	0.25
Staphylococcus epidermidis	0.5
Staphylococcus saprophyticus	0.12
Staphylococcus haemolyticus	0.5
Staphylococcus hominis	0.5
Micrococcus luteus	>128
Streptococcus pyogenes	0.12
Streptococcus agalactiae	0.5
E. faecalis	64
S. pneumoniae	0.12
E. rhusiopathiae	8.0
Corynebacterium hofmannii	64
Corynebacterium xerosis	>128
Corynebacterium jeikeium	>128
L. monocytogenes	8.0
B. anthracis	64
Bacillus subtilis	0.12
Peptostreptococcus spp.	32
Clostridium difficile	32
Clostridium sporogenes	32
Peptococcus spp.	>128
P. acnes	>128

[a]MIC_{50}, MIC at which 50% of isolates tested are inhibited.

Table 3 Activity of mupirocin against gram-negative bacteria

Organism	MIC_{50} (μg/ml)
H. influenzae	0.12
N. gonorrhoeae	0.05
N. meningitidis	0.05
M. catarrhalis	0.2
B. pertussis	0.02
P. multocida	0.25
E. coli	128
K. pneumoniae	128
Proteus mirabilis	128
Proteus vulgaris	64
Morganella morganii	>64
Enterobacter cloacae	64
Enterobacter aerogenes	128
Citrobacter freundii	128
Serratia marcescens	>128
P. aeruginosa	>128
Bacteroides fragilis	>128

Table 4 Activity of mupirocin against streptococci

Organism	MIC_{50} (μg/ml)
S. pyogenes	0.12
S. agalactiae	0.5
Streptococcus mitis	0.5
Streptococcus mutans	0.5
Streptococcus anginosus (milleri)	1.0
Streptococcus sanguinis	1.0
Streptococcus salivarius	0.5
S. pneumoniae	0.12
E. faecalis	32
E. faecium	64

Table 5 Activity of mupirocin against mycoplasmas

Organism	MIC_{50} (μg/ml)
Mycoplasma pneumoniae	2.5
Mycoplasma hyorhinis	0.156
Mycoplasma bovis	0.039
Mycoplasma dispar	0.625

Table 6 Effect of pH on antibacterial activity of mupirocin

Organism	MIC (μg/ml)		
	pH 6.0	pH 7.4	pH 8.0
S. aureus NCTC 6571	0.12	0.5	2.0
S. aureus NCTC 11561	0.5	1.0	2.0
S. pyogenes CN10	0.01	0.25	0.5
E. faecalis	64	128	>128

Table 7 In vitro activity in the presence of serum

Organism	MIC (μg/ml)	
	Agar medium	Agar medium+ 50% human serum
S. aureus NCTC 6571	0.25	2.5
S. aureus NCTC 11561	0.5	5.0
S. pyogenes 421	0.10	2.5
S. pneumoniae CN33	0.10	2.5

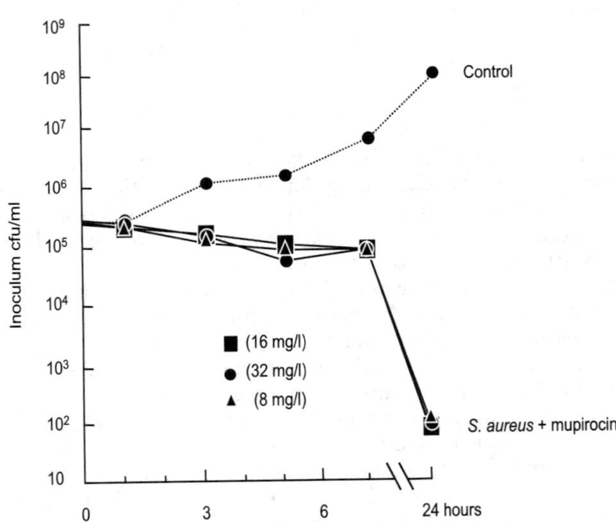

Figure 3 Bactericidal activity of mupirocin against *S. aureus*

It exerts its action through mimicking the epoxy moiety of monic acid and isoleucine tRNA synthetase (Fig. 4).

In fact, mupirocin competes at the isoleucine binding site on the enzyme via the hydrophobic domains: the methyl and ethyl groups of isoleucine.

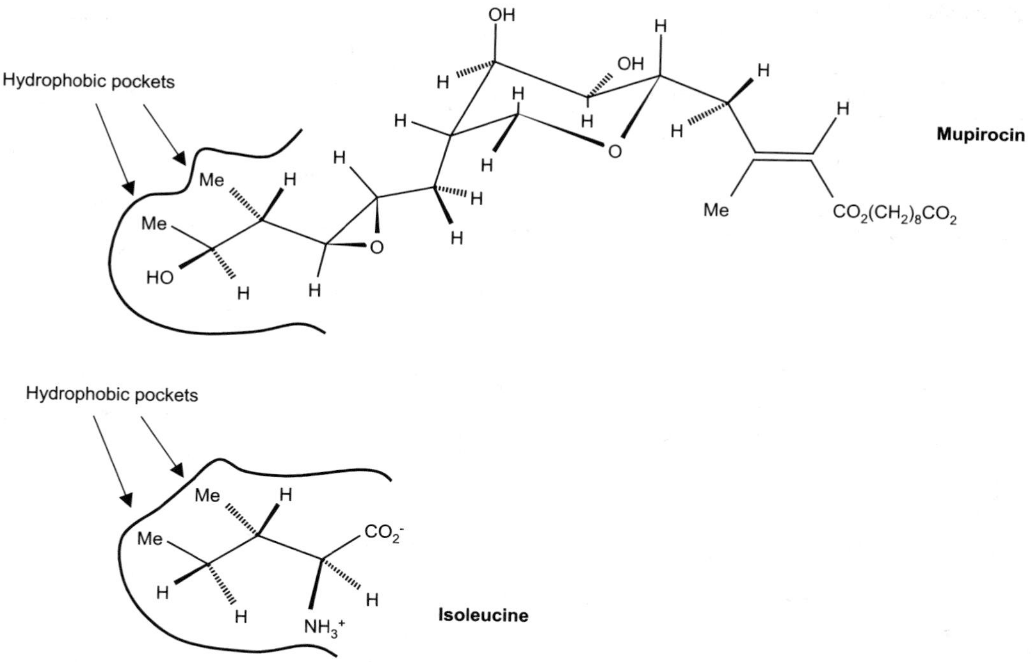

Figure 4 Mechanism of action of mupirocin

Pseudomonic acid is inactive against gram-negative bacilli because of the lack of cell wall penetration, as has been shown with lipopolysaccharide-deficient cell wall mutants of *Escherichia coli* and *P. aeruginosa* K799/61.

4.5. Mechanism of Resistance

Since 1985, when mupirocin was introduced into clinical practice, two types of resistant strains have been described: those for which the MICs are between 8 and 256 μg/ml and those for which the MICs are ≥512 μg/ml.

This resistance is of stable chromosomal origin as a result of a modification in isoleucine tRNA synthetase (50% inhibitory concentration of about 19 to 43 ng/ml, versus 0.7 to 3 ng/ml for susceptible strains).

This type of mutant, however, is uncommon, and its incidence varies with the use of mupirocin: between 1 and 2% depending on the centers. In an epidemiological study conducted in 1990 on 7,137 strains of *S. aureus*, 0.3% were resistant, including 4 strains (0.06%) with high-level resistance (MIC, ≥512 μg/ml). The level of resistance among coagulase-negative staphylococci was higher (about 3%), but no strain had high-level resistance.

High-level resistance appears to be due to a gene localized on a transposon. For the strains of *S. aureus* with high-level resistance to mupirocin, two isoleucine synthetases coexist: one normal and one plasmid mediated, with a 50% inhibitory concentration of 7,000 to 10,000 ng/ml. The question is whether the intensive use of mupirocin will cause the rapid emergence of resistant strains and thus restrict its use. However, it would appear that the selection of the resistant clone occurs gradually. Extensive use of mupirocin has resulted in the emergence of resistant strains of *S. aureus* (MIC, >8 μg/ml) in the United Kingdom. The incidence of resistant strains was 0.3% in 1990 and 8.3% in 1991 (19 of 228 strains).

4.6. Quality Control Strains

A strain is considered susceptible to mupirocin when the MIC is less than 4 μg/ml (≥18 mm). The strain is moderately resistant when the MIC is between 4 and 8 μg/ml (≤17 mm) and highly resistant when the MIC is above 512 μg/ml. The diameters of the zones of inhibition with *S. aureus* ATCC 25933 are between 22 and 27 mm.

5. PHARMACOKINETICS AND METABOLISM

5.1. Percutaneous Pharmacokinetics

Occlusive dressings containing 0.5 g of radiolabeled 2% mupirocin were applied locally to six volunteers.

No radioactivity was detected in the 24-h urine or in the stools. It has been calculated that the probability of penetration of the systemic general circulation is less than 0.24%. However, penetration via pathological or damaged skin is certainly greater. Local application of mupirocin yields in situ concentrations of 20,000 mg/kg.

5.2. Plasma Pharmacokinetics

Intravenous administration of mupirocin sodium (equivalent doses of 31.3 to 252 mg) showed that in the case of low doses, about 90% of the administered dose was eliminated in the urine in 6 to 12 h, whereas only 56% of the dose was eliminated by this route at high doses.

Unchanged mupirocin is detected in the urine (4.6%) only at doses of 125 mg and above. This appears to indicate that enzymatic transformation to monic acid is close to saturation at these doses. The apparent elimination half-life is between 19 and 35 min after doses of 125 and 252 mg, respectively. When the plasma mupirocin concentration declines, that of monic acid increases. For the latter, the half-life at β phase is about 60 min (Table 8).

Table 8 Pharmacokinetics of mupirocin intravenously

Dose (base) (mg)	n	Peak concn in plasma (μg/ml)		$t_{1/2}$ (min)		Urinary elimination (%)	
		Mupirocin	Monic acid	Mupirocin	Monic acid	Mupirocin	Monic acid
31.3	1	1.87	0.46			0	95.2
61.2	1	1.94	0.82			0	92.6
125	2	7.12	2.6	18.9	76.6	0.5	72.4
252	3	14.1	3.22	35.5	32.2–73.1	4.59	57.7

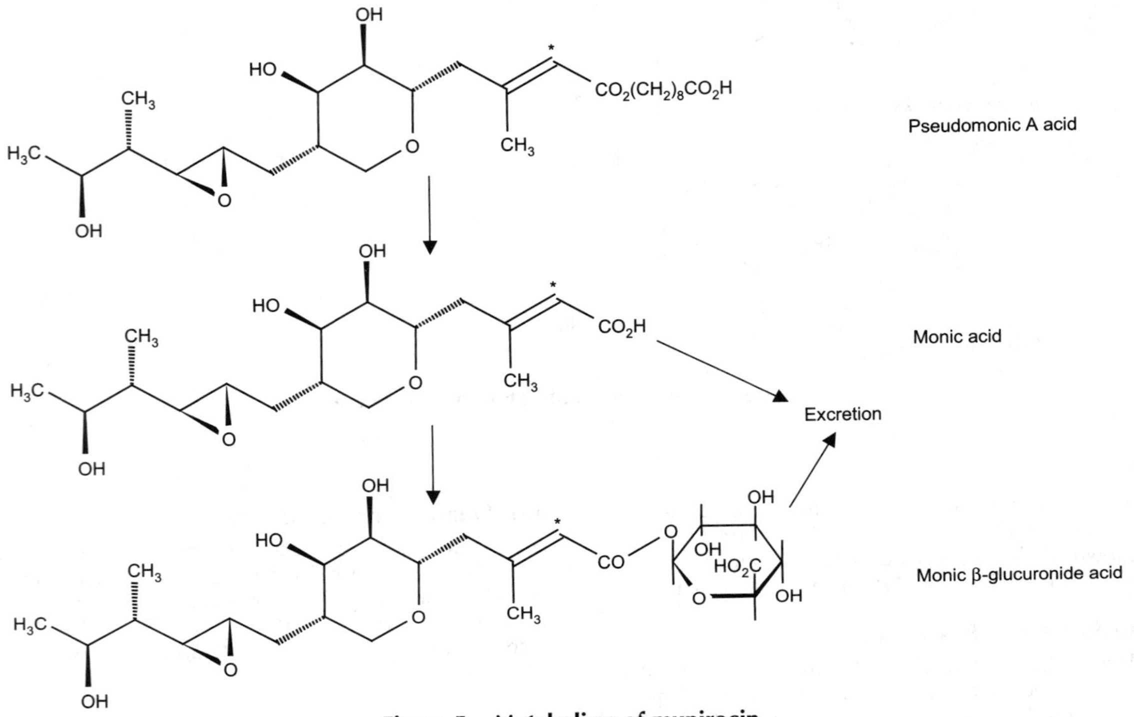

Figure 5 Metabolism of mupirocin

After a dose of 125 mg, the peak concentration in serum is 2.6 μg/ml and is reached after 1 h. At 5 h, the concentration in plasma is 0.29 μg/ml.

5.3. Metabolism

See Fig. 5.

Mupirocin is used as a topical antibiotic. Following systemic administration, it is rapidly metabolized to monic acid. After subcutaneous administration of 10 mg of ^{14}C-radiolabeled pseudomonic acid per kg of body weight in the rat, rabbit, and dog, the radioactivity was eliminated rapidly in the urine and feces. In the rat, about 36% of the intramuscularly administered dose is eliminated in the bile in 10 h.

Transformation of labeled mupirocin to monic acid is weaker in human, rat, and rabbit skin homogenates: 2.7, 11, and 27%, respectively, in 48 h. In the dog, some of the monic acid is eliminated in a glucuroconjugated form.

6. SEMISYNTHETIC DERIVATIVES

A number of chemical modifications of pseudomonic acid A have been undertaken with the following goals:

- Reducing protein binding
- Improving the pharmacokinetics
- Increasing the antibacterial spectrum

One of the main concerns is the hydrolysis of pseudomonic acid A to release monic acid and the fatty acid chain. Monic acid does not possess antibacterial activity.

Monic acid ethyl ether (ethylmonate A) has antibacterial activity similar to that of pseudomonic acid A, with the exception of streptococci, against which its activity is 5 to 20 times inferior to that of pseudomonic acid A. Ethylmonate A is more active against mycoplasmas.

Ethylmonate A is only 30% bound to human plasma proteins. In humans, levels in plasma are higher. The peak concentration of ethylmonate A (about 2 μg/ml) orally in humans is lower than that of pseudomonic acid A. Nothing is detectable after 2 h.

Klein et al. (1989) prepared a series of semisynthetic derivatives of pseudomonic acid A with the aim of preventing metabolic inactivation. They modified the structures and functions of the fragment from C-1 to C-3 by preparing 2-halo or 2-alkylated derivatives and by the formation of amides at C-1 (Fig. 6).

Inhibition of isoleucine tRNA synthetase is possible without the presence of the carbonyl group at position 1. In fact,

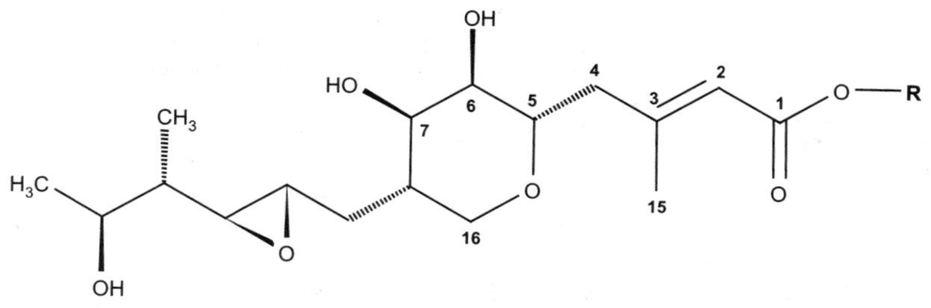

Figure 6 Modifications of pseudomonic acid A

a 20-fold increase in inhibition is possible with ether and thioether derivatives. A nine-carbon side chain produces better inhibition than a butyl chain. However, the antibacterial activity is weaker than that of pseudomonic acid A.

Derivatives of the ketoester, butenolide, or furan type have weak inhibitory and antibacterial activities.

7. THERAPEUTIC ACTIVITY

7.1. Topical Antibiotic Therapy

Skin and skin structure infections are very common, but the use of topical antibiotics or other antibacterial agents is limited by a number of factors: the complexity of the anatomy of the skin, the bacterial ecology of the skin, and the nature of the microorganisms involved in these infections. The skin is composed of different layers that form a physical barrier to infection and produce substances that inhibit the invasive potential of a number of microorganisms. In addition, the stratum corneum is constantly desquamating and renewing itself, and for this reason the relationship with bacterial colonization and bacterial products is complex.

The nature of the infection of the skin lining is dependent on the causative pathogen: staphylococcal infections are more localized because of the production of a coagulase, whereas streptococcal infections are more widespread because of the production of a hyaluronidase.

The site of infection is in fact important since dermal infections are less susceptible to topical antibiotics than superficial infections. Topical antibiotics are more often used in acute infections such as impetigo and ecthyma in which staphylococci and beta-hemolytic streptococci invade the dermis and epidermis, in superficial infections of the pilosebaceous follicles, or in secondary infections due to epidermal detachment.

Topical antibiotics are infrequently used in dermal infections such as erysipelas, cellulitis, or deep lesions of the pilosebaceous follicles, such as furunculosis.

The results are disappointing in infections such as anthrax, chancroid, syphilitic lesions, or mycobacterial lesions, since the causative bacteria are present in other tissues. Likewise, wound infections respond poorly to topical antibiotics in the case of opportunistic microorganisms such as *P. aeruginosa*.

Not only must local antibiotics have an antibacterial spectrum compatible with the bacteria responsible for skin infections, but also the pharmaceutical formulation must not be toxic, irritant, or allergenic.

Penicillin G has been used in some countries as a local antibiotic but is responsible for hypersensitivity disorders.

Fusidic acid may be used in cutaneous staphylococcal infections. Erythromycin and clindamycin act slowly, and resistance is not infrequent.

Chloramphenicol, although active, is not widely recommended because of the risks of hypersensitivity and above all hematotoxicity. Cyclines are used particularly in acne. Aminoglycosides, alone or in combination with gramicidin, are used in dressings or ointments. Neomycin B is allergenic.

7.2. Skin Infections

Mupirocin eradicates methicillin-resistant strains of *S. aureus* colonizing the skin (Denning and Haiduven-Griffiths, 1988) and produces an improvement in the healing of skin wounds (Watcher and Wheeland, 1989). The use of mupirocin before a surgical procedure for skin cancer results in decolonization of the infectious sites and a reduction in the number of skin infections. The combination of mupirocin and iodine solution reduces the number of central-catheter infections due to cutaneous microorganisms (Czarnecki et al., 1991).

Mupirocin has been used successfully in the treatment of various skin infections (Breneman, 1990), as well as eczematiform superinfections (Leyden, 1990), impetigo (Rice et al., 1992), and vulvovaginal infections (Coll-Foley et al., 1991). In hemodialyzed patients, the incidence of skin infections is decreased by reducing nasal carriage of *S. aureus* (Yu et al., 1986).

7.3. S. aureus Carriage

7.3.1. Carriage—Antibiotics

About a third of adults permanently carry *S. aureus* in their nostrils, and about half are intermittent carriers. Permanent *S. aureus* carriers (Casewell and Hill, 1986; Williams, 1963) are at increased risk of recurrent furunculosis, exfoliative lesions, and superinfections of surgical wounds. There are certain predisposing factors, such as the use of intravenous medications, terminal renal failure (hemodialysis and peritoneal dialysis), respiratory tract infections, or long periods of hospitalization.

The oropharynx is the second site of recolonization after the nostrils. Half of healthy nasal carriers of *S. aureus* are also oropharyngeal carriers.

There is, however, a variation in carriage within the population according to geographical location and population analyzed. For example, health care personnel have a higher rate of carriage than the general population. Eradication of *S. aureus* nasal carriage in hemodialyzed patients requires a reduction or even eradication of hand carriage at the same time.

A number of studies have been conducted with different antibiotics to reduce or try to eradicate nasal carriage.

Local use of penicillin G, vancomycin, or bacitracin for periods of 1 to 3 months produces bacterial eradication (Bryan et al., 1980; Gould, 1955).

Topical gentamicin has good activity, but its action is short-lived. Oral administration of rifampin has been tested but rapidly selects rifampin-resistant strains of *S. aureus*. Combinations of rifampin with cloxacillin or co-trimoxazole have also been tried: 10 days of rifampin in a single daily dose with or without cloxacillin every 6 h. Immediate eradication was obtained in 95 to 100% of subjects, persisting in 60 to 65% at 3 months and 59% at 12 months.

The combination of rifampin and cloxacillin in dialyzed patients proved effective in 90% at 3 months and 60% at 1 year.

Ciprofloxacin, with or without rifampin, has proved effective in eradicating carriage of methicillin-resistant strains of S. *aureus*. However, an increase in the MICs of mupirocin has been observed in a third of patients.

Clindamycin has been used successfully in some patients.

The benefit of topical antibiotics is that they avoid the administration of major systemic antibiotics and the selection of resistant strains. These local preparations are responsible for fewer side effects.

7.3.2. Mupirocin

Mupirocin in solution in polyethylene glycol is irritant to the nasal mucosa in about 3 to 5% of patients. A new pharmaceutical formulation combining mupirocin calcium and paraffin base appears to be less irritant.

A workshop organized by the British Society for Antimicrobial Chemotherapy and the Society of Hospital Infection (1986) recommended the local use of mupirocin in the form of three daily applications to the anterior part of the nostril for 5 days.

Mupirocin eradicates S. *aureus* nasal carriage, in most cases permanently, representing a major therapeutic breakthrough in that this eradication is only temporary with other antibacterial agents (Wheat et al., 1981).

Casewell and Hill (1986) showed that S. *aureus* is eliminated 48 h after local application of mupirocin. This eradication still persists in 50% of subjects after 5 months. Reagan et al. (1991) showed that nasal application of mupirocin calcium for 5 days significantly reduced nasal and hand carriage. Boelaert et al. (1989) showed that the local application of mupirocin calcium three times weekly significantly reduced nasal S. *aureus* carriage in hemodialyzed patients over a period of 9 months. They also noticed a lower incidence of S. *aureus* infections in these patients.

Frank et al. (1989) treated 31 patients carrying S. *aureus*. Three of them had an intolerance reaction, but 22 patients out of 24 with evaluable dossiers no longer had S. *aureus* after 4 days of treatment.

REFERENCES

Alexander RG, Clayton JP, Luk K, Rogers NH, King TJ, 1978, The absolute configuration of pseudomonic acid, J Chem Soc Perkins Trans, 1, 561–565.

Ayliffe GAJ, Sanderson PJ, Meers PD, 1986, Guidelines of the control of epidemic methicillin-resistant staphylococcus aureus: report of a combined working party of the Hospital Infection Society and British Society for Antimicrobial Chemotherapy, J Hosp Infect 7, 193–201.

Baader A, Garre C, 1887, Ueber antagonisten unter den Bacterien, Corresp Bl Schweitz Aertze, 17, 385–392.

Basker HJ, Comber KR, Clayton JP, Hannan PCT, Mizen LN, Rogers NH, Slocombe B, Sutherland R, 1980, Ethylmonate A, a semisynthetic antibiotic derived from pseudomonic acid A, Curr Chemother Infect Dis 1, 471–473.

Boelaert JR, De Smedt RA, De Baere YA, Godard CA, Matthys EG, et al, 1989, The influence of calcium mupirocin nasal ointment on the incidence of Staphylococcus aureus infections in haemodialysis patients, Nephrol Dial Transplant, 4, 278–281.

Breneman DL, 1990, Use of mupirocin ointment in the treatment of secondarily infected dermatoses, J Am Acad Dermatol, 22, 886–892.

Bryan CS, Wilson RS, Meade P, Stille LG, 1980, Topical antibiotic ointments for staphylococcal nasal carriers, survey of current practices and comparison of bacitracin and vancomycin ointments, Infect Control, 1, 153–156.

Casewell HW, Hill RLR, 1986, The carrier-state, methicillin-resistant S. aureus, J Antimicrob Chemother, 18, suppl A, 1–12.

Chain EB, Mellow G, 1974, Structure of pseudomonic acid, an antibiotic from Pseudomonas fluorescens, J Chem Soc Chem Comm, 847–848.

Chain EB, Mellow G, 1977, Pseudomonic acid. Part I. The structure of pseudomonic acid A, a novel antibiotic produced by Pseudomonas fluorescens, J Chem Soc Perkins Trans, 1, 294–309.

Clayton JP, Luk K, Rogers NH, 1979, The conversion of pseudomonic acid A into monic acid A and its esters, J Chem Soc Perkins Trans, 308.

Coll-Foley AA, Nathan C, O'Donovan C III, Simon D, 1991, Eradication of methicillin-resistant S. aureus vaginitis with mupirocin, Am Pharmacother, 25, 1331–1333.

Czarnecki DB, Nash CG, Bohl TG, 1991, The use of mupirocin before skin surgery, Int J Dermatol, 30, 218–219.

Denning DW, Haiduven-Griffiths D, 1988, Eradication of low level methicillin-resistant Staphylococcus aureus skin colonization with topical mupirocin, Infect Control Hosp Epidemiol, 9, 261–263.

Florey HW, Chain EB, Heatley NG, Jennings MA, Saunders AG, Abraham EP, Florey ME, 1949, Antibiotics, vol 1, p 554–555, Oxford University Press, Oxford.

Frank U, Lenz W, Damrath E, Kappstein I, Daschner FD, 1989, Nasal carriage of Staphylococcus aureus treated with topical mupirocin (pseudomonic acid) in a children's hospital, J Hosp Infect, 13, 117–120.

Fuller AT, Mellows G, Woodford M, Banks GT, Barrow KD, Chain EB, 1971, Pseudomonic acid, an antibiotic produced by Pseudomonas fluorescens, Nature, 234, 416–417.

Gould JC, 1955, The effect of local antibiotic on nasal carriage of Staphylococcus pyogenes, J Hyg, 53, 379–385.

Hill RL, Fisher AP, Ware RJ, Wilson S, Casewell MW, 1990, Mupirocin for the reduction of colonization of internal jugular cannulae, a randomised controlled trial, J Hosp Infect, 15, 311–321.

Hudson L, 1992, Mupirocin resistance, Lancet, 339, 56.

Jackson D, Tasker TCG, Sutherland R, Mellows G, Cooper DL, 1985, Clinical pharmacology of Bactroban®, pharmacokinetics, tolerance and efficacy studies, p 54–67, in Bactroban® (Mupirocin), Proc Int Symp, Excerpta Medica.

Klein LL, Yeung CM, Kurath P, Mao JC, Fernandez PB, Lartey PA, Pernet AG, 1989, Synthesis and activity of nonhydrolyzable pseudomonic acid analogues, J Med Chem, 32, 151–160.

Lewis JM, 1929, Bacterial antagonism with special reference to the effect of *Pseudomonas fluorescens* on spore-forming bacteria of soils, J Bacteriol, 17, 89–103.

Leyden JJ, 1990, Mupirocin, a new topical antibiotic, J Am Acad Dermatol, 22, 879-883.

Mellows G, 1985, Pseudomonic acid, its chemistry and metabolism, p 3–10, in Bactroban® (mupirocin), Proc Int Symp, Excerpta Medica.

Reagan DR, Doebbeling BN, Pfaller MA, Sheetz CT, Houston AK, Hollis RJ, Wenzel RP, 1991, Elimination of coincident Staphylococcus aureus nasal and hand carriage with intranasal application of mupirocin calcium ointment, Ann Intern Med, 114, 101–106.

Rice TD, Duggan AK, De Angelis C, 1992, Cost-effectiveness of erythromycin versus mupirocin for the treatment of impetigo in children, Pediatrics, 89, 210–214.

Slocombe B, Perry C, 1991, The antimicrobial activity of mupirocin—an update on resistance, J Hosp Infect, 19 (suppl B), 19–25.

Snider BB, Phillips GB, Cordova R, 1983, Formal total synthesis of (±) pseudomonic acid A and C. The quasi-intramolecular Lewis acid catalyzed Diels-Alder reaction, J Org Chem, 26, 3003–3010.

Stierle DB, Stierle AA, 1992, Pseudomonic acid derivatives from a marine bacterium, Experientia, 48, 1165–1169.

Watcher MA, Wheeland RG, 1989, The role of topical agents in the healing of full-thickness wounds, J Dermatol Surg Oncol, 15, 1188–1195.

Wheat LJ, Kohler RB, White A, 1981, Treatment of nasal carriers of coagulase-positive staphylococci, p 50–58, in Maibach HI, Aly R, ed, Skin Microbiology: Relevance to Clinical Infections, Springer-Verlag, New York.

Williams DR, Moore JL, Yamada M, 1986, The total synthesis of (+) pseudomonic acid C, J Org Chem, 51, 3916–3918.

Williams RED, 1963, Healthy carriage of *Staphylococcus aureus*, its prevalence and importance, Bacteriol Rev, 27, 56–71.

Yu VL, Goetz A, Wagener M, Smith PB, Rihs JD, Hanchett J, Zuravleff JJ, 1986, Staphylococcus aureus nasal carriage and infection in patients on hemodialysis. Efficacy of antibiotic prophylaxis, N Engl J Med, 315, 91–96.

Fosfomycin and Derivatives

E. BERGOGNE-BÉRÉZIN

37

1. INTRODUCTION

Fosfomycin belongs to the class of phosphonic antibiotics possessing a broad spectrum and exhibiting bactericidal activity against bacteria that fall within that spectrum. The bacterial target of fosfomycin is wall mucopeptide synthesis, and fosfomycin acts at an early stage in this synthesis by inhibiting phosphoenolpyruvate transferase, the first enzyme involved in the synthesis of peptidoglycan. Extracted initially by screening from several strains of *Streptomyces* (*Streptomyces fradiae*, *Streptomyces viridochromogenes*, and *Streptomyces wedmorensis*), fosfomycin was isolated in 1969. Fosfomycin is currently a synthetic antibiotic that has no structural relationship with the other known classes of antibiotics. There is no cross-resistance, and fosfomycin may be administered in combination with a number of other antibiotics.

2. CHEMICAL STRUCTURE

Fosfomycin is a small molecule, the sodium salt of L-*cis*-1,2-epoxypropylphosphonic acid, the epoxide of which is the determining feature in its antibacterial activity. Fosfomycin possesses a phosphorus atom attached directly to a carbon atom without the intermediate of an oxygen bond usually present in organophosphorous compounds. The chemical formula of an oral form of fosfomycin, fosfomycin trometamol, is that of a mono(2-ammonium-2-hydroxymethyl-1,3-propanediol) (2*R*-*cis*) (3-methoxyoxiranyl) phosphate. Its synthesis is obtained by treating bis(2-ammonium-2-hydroxymethyl-1,3-propanediol) (2*R*-*cis*) (3-methyl-2-oxiranyl) phosphonate with *p*-toluenesulfonic acid in hot ethanol, as illustrated in Fig. 1. A calcium salt of fosfomycin was prepared for oral administration but abandoned because of its poor bioavailability. The chemical formulae of fosfomycin, fosfomycin trometamol (oral form), and fosmidomycin are illustrated in Fig. 2.

3. CLASSIFICATION

Fosfomycin belongs to the class of phosphonic antibiotics. Three phosphonic antibiotics for parenteral use are known: fosfomycin, fosmidomycin, and alafosfalin (this one has been abandoned). In addition, fosfomycin has recently been developed in an oral form, fosfomycin trometamol, which is a monobasic hydrosoluble fosfomycin salt.

The description that follows is confined to fosfomycin and its trometamol salt because of the very limited data about the other products belonging to the class of phosphonic antibiotics.

4. PHYSICOCHEMICAL PROPERTIES

Fosfomycin disodium salt occurs in the form of a fine, white, insipid powder that is hygroscopic above a relative humidity of 30%. It is freely soluble in water. A 20% aqueous solution is clear and has a pH of 7.6 ± 0.4. The drug substance is stable under normal storage conditions (2 to 3 years). Fosfomycin is a small molecule, the smallest existing antibiotic molecule, with a low molecular mass (138 Da) which ensures extensive diffusibility. Fosfomycin is also a very polar and hence very soluble molecule. The product is unstable in an acidic medium, which is reflected in vivo in its decomposition in the acidic gastric medium and accounts for its poor oral bioavailability in the form of the disodium salt, which is reserved for the parenteral route. Conversely, fosfomycin trometamol, which displays the main features of fosfomycin, from which it is derived, is a hydrosoluble product, and trometamol is present in the molecule as an anion to form a monobasic salt with fosfomycin, allowing its oral administration. After absorption, fosfomycin trometamol releases fosfomycin by hydrolysis. The molecular weight of fosfomycin trometamol is 259.2, and the product is presented in the form of a white crystalline powder.

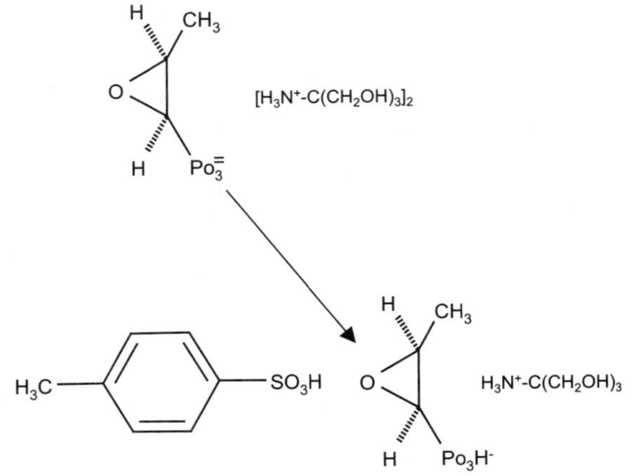

Figure 1 Synthesis of fosfomycin trometamol

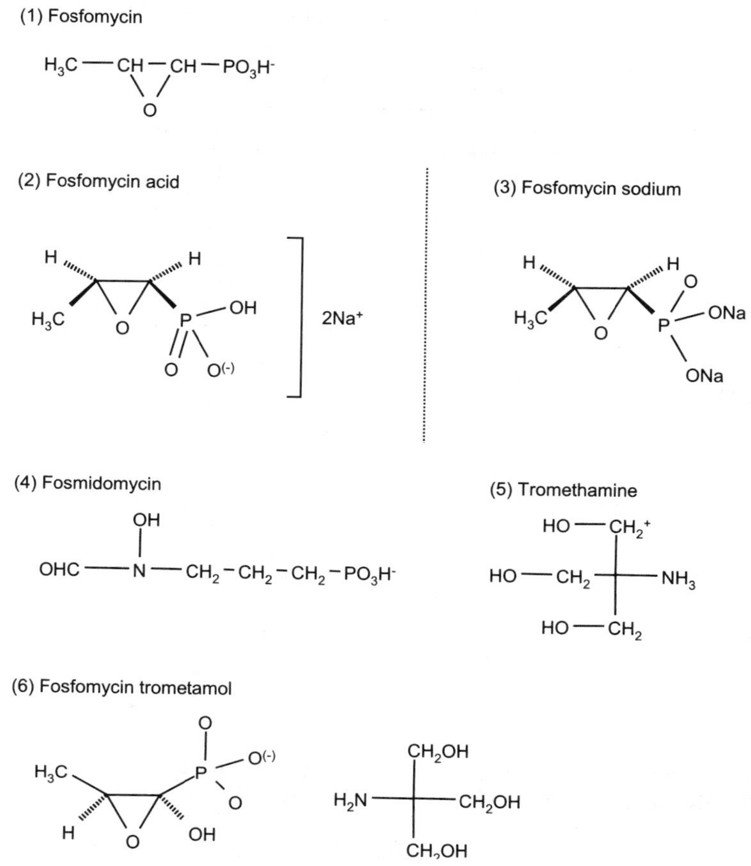

(1) Fosfomycin

(2) Fosfomycin acid

(3) Fosfomycin sodium

(4) Fosmidomycin

(5) Tromethamine

(6) Fosfomycin trometamol

Figure 2 Chemical formulae of fosfomycin, fosmidomycin, tromethamine, and fosfomycin trometamol

5. IN VITRO PROPERTIES

5.1. Antibacterial Activity

5.1.1. Fosfomycin

Fosfomycin is a broad-spectrum antibiotic which has moderate activity against numerous bacterial species (Table 1). Its activity depends on transport into the bacterial cell by L-α-glycerophosphate and hexose monophosphate systems involving the presence of glucose-6-phosphate (G-6-P). For this reason the antibacterial activity of fosfomycin in vitro requires the addition of G-6-P to the medium to determine the MIC. The MICs of fosfomycin are higher in the absence of G-6-P, particularly for enteric gram-negative bacteria. As shown by the data in Table 1, the MICs can vary considerably within the same study for species belonging to the antibacterial spectrum of fosfomycin. The MICs also vary fairly markedly from one study to another, probably due to the technical factors mentioned above. In addition, the bacterial populations contain fosfomycin-resistant variants that may contribute to the variations in the MICs for the populations tested. The antibacterial spectrum of fosfomycin includes staphylococci, *Haemophilus* spp., and the majority of enteric gram-negative bacteria, but with considerably higher MICs for the *Klebsiella-Enterobacter-Serratia* group. Fosfomycin is moderately active against *Pseudomonas aeruginosa*, with variable MICs ranging from 4 to >512 μg/ml but often below the in vivo concentrations of the antibiotic. *Acinetobacter* spp. are not susceptible to fosfomycin (MIC from 16 to 128 μg/ml), nor are gram-positive bacteria (Table 1).

Gram-negative anaerobes are not part of its antibacterial spectrum. Streptococci, *Staphylococcus saprophyticus*, corynebacteria, *Chlamydia*, and mycoplasmas are also resistant. The breakpoints adopted for fosfomycin correspond to a MIC of ≤32 μg/ml (in Mueller-Hinton agar supplemented with G-6-P) or ≤8 μg/ml (in nutrient agar supplemented with G-6-P). Strains for which the MICs of fosfomycin are >32 μg/ml in Mueller-Hinton agar or >8 μg/ml in nutrient agar (supplemented with G-6-P) are resistant (Salhi, 1978).

5.1.2. Fosfomycin Trometamol

Designed for the treatment of uncomplicated lower urinary tract infections, the oral form of fosfomycin, fosfomycin trometamol, has been tested principally in vitro against agents of community-acquired urinary tract infections. Two studies are reported in the literature; in one a broth medium (Difco) was used to determine the MICs (Gismondo et al., 1986), while in the other the MICs in Mueller-Hinton agar were investigated (Lerner et al., 1988). The results of these studies are presented in Tables 2 and 3. The in vitro activity of fosfomycin trometamol was better then that of pipemidic acid against *Staphylococcus aureus* and *Enterococcus faecalis* and better than that of amoxicillin against *Escherichia coli* and *Klebsiella pneumoniae*. In both studies, co-trimoxazole and norfloxacin appeared to be more active against bacteria involved in urinary tract infections.

5.2. Bactericidal Activity

Fosfomycin is a bactericidal antibiotic whose molecular target is the bacterial cell wall and which, like all antibiotics that inhibit cell wall mucopeptide synthesis, is only active

Table 1 In vitro activity of fosfomycin in Mueller-Hinton medium supplemented with G-6-P at 50 μg/ml[a]

Microorganism(s)	MIC (μg/ml)[b]			
	Range (Study 1)	Range (Study 2)	50%	90%
S. aureus	1–64	2–16	3	13
S. epidermidis	1–64		2	38
Streptococcus pneumoniae	4–32	8–64	5	10
E. faecalis	64–128	16–32	14	41
Streptococcus pyogenes	2–64	4–16	28	53
Streptococcus agalactiae	2–64		13	45
E. coli	1–32	0.12–1	0.4	8
Klebsiella spp.	4–>1,024	0.5–2	1.0	31
Enterobacter spp.	1–>1,024	0.12–16	1.0	11
S. marcescens	1–1,024	4–128	0.8	6
P. mirabilis	2–32	4–128	0.4	2
Proteus, indole+	0.5–128	0.12–2	24	115
P. aeruginosa	1–>1,024	8–128	5	14
Salmonella spp.	6–>512	1–16	0.45	2.6
Shigella spp.	1–8		<0.125	0.3
Vibrio cholerae	64–>1,024			
Bacteroides fragilis	>1,024			
Haemophilus influenzae	1–128	0.5–2	0.7	3

[a]Data from Forsgren and Walder, 1983; Fosfomycin International Symposium, 1977; Lorian, 1991; Maur, 1990; Neu and Williams, 1988; and Salhi, 1978.

[b]50% and 90%, MICs at which 50 and 90% of isolates tested are inhibited, respectively.

Table 2 In vitro activity of fosfomycin trometamol in nutrient broth and in the presence of urine comparison with fosfomycin calcium, pipemidic acid, and co-trimoxazole[a]

Organism(s)	Antibacterial[b]	*n*	MIC (μg/ml)			
			Nutrient broth		Urine	
			50%	90%	50%	90%
E. coli	FT	45	12.5	50	25	200
	F		12.5	50	25	200
	PIP		1.56	6.25	100	>200
	COT		6.25	12.5	100	>200
Enterobacter spp.	FT	30	12.5	50	50	200
	F		12.5	50	50	200
	PIP		25	50	100	>200
	COT		3.12	200	50	>200
Providencia rettgeri	FT	28	100	>200	200	>200
	F		100	>200	200	>200
	PIP		50	200	50	>200
	COT		100	>200	>200	>200
P. mirabilis	FT	34	12.5	50	50	200
	F		12.5	50	50	200
	PIP		1.56	100	50	>200
	COT		6.25	12.5	50	200
Pseudomonas spp.	FT	40	50	200	50	>200
	F		50	200	50	>200
	PIP		25	>200	25	>200
	COT		>200	>200	>200	>200
S. aureus	FT	93	6.25	12.5	25	50
	F		6.25	12.5	25	50
	PIP		25	100	100	>200
	COT		3.12	200	50	>200
E. faecalis	FT	30	3.12	50	25	200
	F		3.12	50	25	200
	PIP		50	>200	200	>200
	COT		3.12	>200	50	>200

[a]Data from Gismondo et al., 1986.

[b]FT, fosfomycin trometamol; F, fosfomycin calcium; PIP, pipemidic acid; COT, co-trimoxazole.

Table 3 Susceptibility of *E. coli* and other agents of urinary tract infections to fosfomycin trometamol compared with four other antibiotics (urinary)[a]

Microorganism	Findings[b]	n	MIC (μg/ml)[c]				
			FT	NFL	PIP	COT	AMX
E. coli	Chicago University	45					
	MIC_{50}		1	0.0156	2	0.08/1.6	4
	MIC_{90}		16	0.0156	4	0.16/3.2	>128
	Range		0.5–>256				
	Wayne State University	32					
	MIC_{50}		4	0.0156	2	0.08/1.6	4
	MIC_{90}		31	0.0312	4	0.32/6.4	>128
	Range		0.5–64				
K. pneumoniae		13					
	MIC_{50}		32	0.0312	4	0.08/1.6	>128
	MIC_{90}		64	0.250	32	0.28/25.6	>128
	Range		1–256				
P. mirabilis		9					
	MIC_{50}		4	0.0078	2	0.08/1.6	2
	MIC_{90}		64	0.0156	4	0.32/6.4	4
	Range		0.5–64				
Proteus vulgaris		1	32	0.0156	4	0.16/3.2	>128

[a]Data from Lerner et al., 1988.
[b]MIC_{50} and MIC_{90}, MICs at which 50 and 90% of isolates tested are inhibited, respectively.
[c]FT, fosfomycin trometamol; NFL, norfloxacin; PIP, pipemidic acid; COT, co-trimoxazole; AMX, amoxicillin.

against bacteria in the log phase (the exponential growth phase). The in vitro bactericidal effect of fosfomycin trometamol was studied by means of killing curves against *E. coli*, *K. pneumoniae*, and *Proteus mirabilis* (Lerner et al., 1988). Fosfomycin exhibits identical bactericidal activities against the three enteric gram-negative bacilli tested, and these bactericidal activities occurred rapidly, since the bacterial count declines by 3 $\log_{10}$ at 1 or 2 h even in the presence of the lowest concentration of antibiotic (the MIC). However, regrowth is observed after 5 h for *E. coli* at this concentration. When using a weak concentration of fosfomycin trometamol (half the MIC) against *S. aureus* (Gismondo et al., 1986), a bacterial decline from 10^5 to 3×10^2 CFU/ml was obtained in 4 h, but a resistant population developed, giving rise to regrowth that culminated in the initial inoculum after 24 h. It should be noted that the majority of bactericidal studies of fosfomycin have been undertaken using antibiotic combinations because of this phenomenon of rapid emergence of resistant mutants.

5.3. Effects of Variations in Experimental Conditions on In Vitro Activity of Fosfomycin

The initial in vitro work on fosfomycin and the studies with fosfomycin trometamol (Albini et al., 1986; Gismondo et al., 1986; Lerner et al., 1988) compared the results obtained by varying (i) the nature of the medium used for the tests, showing that nutrient agar is more favorable than Mueller-Hinton agar to the expression of in vitro activity against susceptible bacteria; (ii) the presence or absence of G-6-P, addition of which to the medium has been seen to be essential for intrabacterial transport of the antibiotic; (iii) the size of the bacterial inoculum, for which it has been shown that an increase from 10^5 to 10^7 CFU/ml causes an approximately twofold increase in the MIC and a retardation of bactericidal activity against *E. coli* or a reduction of this activity by 2 $\log_{10}$, although it should be noted that this size of inoculum was observed for only 10% of the strains studied (Greenwood et al., 1986); and (iv) the pH of the medium, showing that a reduction in pH from 7 to 5.5 causes an increase in bactericidal activity that is maximal at pH 5.5 and that appears to be correlated with the results of the tests performed in urine producing acidic pH conditions (Albini et al., 1986; Greenwood et al., 1986). However, other studies indicate a tendency to bactericidal curves with a greater decline in nutrient broth than in urine (Gismondo et al., 1986).

5.4. In Vitro Combinations of Fosfomycin with Other Antibiotics

The risk of the rapid development of resistant strains was revealed by the very early in vitro studies (Fosfomycin International Symposium, 1977; Gevaudan et al., 1978). The search for synergistic combinations revealed a synergistic effect for fosfomycin in combination with β-lactams or vancomycin against staphylococci and with aminoglycosides against *Enterobacteriaceae* and *Pseudomonas* spp. Fosfomycin is often synergistic with bacteriostatic antibiotics such as tetracycline or chloramphenicol; fosfomycin combined with rifampin is neutral in terms of bacteriostasis and antagonistic in terms of bactericidal activity (Drugeon and Kazmierczak, 1987). Conversely, with fluoroquinolones such as pefloxacin, fosfomycin is additive or synergistic (Drugeon and Kazmierczak, 1987). The synergy of the combinations is tested either by the checkerboard method, involving the calculation of the fractional inhibitory concentration index, or by killing kinetics (Figueredo and Neu, 1988). Against *P. aeruginosa*, the combinations of fosfomycin with ciprofloxacin and ofloxacin have shown synergy against 63% of strains and an additive effect against 100% of strains tested. Synergy of the combination of ciprofloxacin (8 μg/ml) and fosfomycin (32 μg/ml) in terms of killing kinetics was obtained in 24 h, with a decline from 10^7 to 10^3 CFU in 8 h. (These values chosen for the killing kinetics study correspond to the minimum bactericidal concentrations of these antibiotics for the strain studied.) In the same study fosmidomycin, reputedly more active than fosfomycin against *P. aeruginosa*, was not found to be synergistic with ciprofloxacin (Figueredo and Neu, 1988).

6. MECHANISMS OF ACTION OF FOSFOMYCIN

6.1. Molecular Target of Fosfomycin

Fosfomycin inhibits bacterial cell wall biosynthesis by acting on the initial stage in the synthesis of peptidoglycan precursors. It thus exerts a bactericidal action by disrupting the integrity of the cell wall, accompanied by the formation of protoplasts in *S. aureus* followed by bacterial lysis and of spheroplasts in *E. coli* or, depending on the antibiotic concentrations, rapid direct lysis of the bacteria. Fosfomycin inhibits the conversion of UDP-*N*-acetylglucosamine to UDP-*N*-acetylmuramic acid in the presence of phosphoenolpyruvate. The enzyme that catalyzes this reaction is an enolpyruvyl transferase, the target of fosfomycin, and concerns *N*-acetylglucosamine-3-*O*-enolpyruvyl transferase, an enzyme that activates fosfomycin and is thereby destroyed by the formation of a covalent bond with the product. In fact, fosfomycin offers a certain homology of structure with phosphoenolpyruvate and therefore binds stably to the enzyme, which has the effect of inactivating the synthesis of UDP-*N*-acetylmuramic acid. *N*-Acetylglucosamine-3-*O*-enolpyruvyl transferase is essential for any bacterium possessing muramic acid in its cell wall structure, which accounts for the broad spectrum of antibacterial activity of fosfomycin since numerous gram-positive or -negative species possess muramic acid that constitutes cell wall peptidoglycan. Finally, fosfomycin has no detectable activity in mammals, particularly in reactions involving other enzymes using phosphoenolpyruvate; it thus possesses a narrow specificity for pyruvyl transferase.

6.2. Penetration of Fosfomycin into the Bacterial Cell

Fosfomycin should theoretically inhibit any bacterium containing muramic acid in its cell wall on the condition that the antibiotic can reach the target enzyme inside the cell. Penetration of the antibiotic within the bacterium occurs by active transport and uses one of the following two transport systems (Kahan et al., 1974; Kanimoto and Greenwood, 1987): one, constitutive, is the L-α-glycerophosphate system; the other, inducible and predominant, is the hexose monophosphate route, operating only in the presence of an inducer, G-6-P. The antibacterial activity is therefore dependent on the presence in the medium of G-6-P. Fructose-6-phosphate and glucose-1-phosphate perform the same function in the cell, but to a lesser extent. An understanding of these mechanisms of active transport necessary for the entry of fosfomycin into the cell explains various specific features of this antibiotic: glucose acts as a repressor of the transport system and reduces the antibacterial activity of fosfomycin; glycerol, on the other hand, enhances the efficacy of the transport system and increases the susceptibility of the bacteria to fosfomycin. Bacteria possessing the dual transport system of fosfomycin are highly susceptible to the antibiotic. Reversion to susceptibility on the part of mutants through the loss of the L-α-glycerophosphate system occurs via the inducible system on the condition that there is induction in the presence of G-6-P.

6.3. Other Phosphonic Antibiotics

Fosfomycin trometamol does not appear to exhibit differences from fosfomycin in terms of its mode of antibacterial action, although no precise study of the mechanism of action of this fosfomycin salt on the bacterial wall is found in the literature. The bacterial permeability to fosfomycin in its trometamol form appears to involve the same mechanisms as those of fosfomycin, the addition of G-6-P also significantly affecting the MICs of the product for staphylococci, enterococci, and *Enterobacteriaceae*. The effect of G-6-P, which acts by reducing MICs and which is marked in nutrient broth, is moderate, nonexistent, or even inverted in other media (Mueller-Hinton, Iso-Sensitest, Eugonbroth) (Greenwood et al., 1986).

For fosmidomycin, the principal intracellular target has not been identified (Kanimoto and Greenwood, 1987). It would appear that fosfomycin and fosmidomycin have different targets in *E. coli* and/or that, in the absence of the hexose phosphate transport route, these two products are transported into the bacterial cell by different mechanisms. The literature data in this respect are very limited and often divergent (Kanimoto and Greenwood, 1987).

6.4. Mechanisms of Action of Fosfomycin Combined with β-Lactams

The results of studies of combinations of fosfomycin with other antibiotics, particularly β-lactams, are described above. Two bacterial species in particular have been studied in terms of the synergistic or antagonistic mechanism of action of these combinations in view of the difficulties encountered clinically in eradicating these bacteria. Against methicillin-resistant *S. aureus* (MRSA) fosfomycin, which is capable of reducing penicillin-binding protein (PBP) 2 and 4 levels in *S. aureus*, appears to act in the same way against MRSA-specific PBP 2′, which would account for the efficacy of fosfomycin in combination with oxacillin or cephalosporins (Utsui et al., 1986). Against *P. aeruginosa* fosfomycin, which is active against this bacterium, is often combined with α-carboxypenicillins, ureidopenicillins, or 2-amino-5-thiazolyl cephalosporins, and the synergy of these combinations and those of fosfomycin with aminoglycosides has been demonstrated (Takahashi and Kanno, 1984). Antagonistic effects have, however, been reported (Reguera et al., 1990), suggesting (i) β-lactamase induction by fosfomycin; (ii) reduced expression of *P. aeruginosa* PBP 3, which is the primary target of β-lactams in this species; and (iii) reduced affinity of PBP 3 under the effect of fosfomycin. These mechanisms, combined with the fosfomycin–β-lactam antagonism, may emerge in vivo and result in therapeutic failure.

7. MECHANISMS OF RESISTANCE

The permeability of the bacterial outer membrane to intrabacterial penetration of fosfomycin is the sine qua non for the expression of its antibacterial activity, nonpenetration of fosfomycin being expressed by resistance on the part of the bacterium.

7.1. Natural Resistance

Natural resistance to fosfomycin in certain bacterial species appears to result from the absence of the L-α-glycerophosphate transport system in the bacteria. Natural resistance may also be related to the absence of outer membrane in certain bacterial species, such as *Chlamydia* and mycoplasmas, the target of fosfomycin being an early stage of peptidoglycan synthesis. The activity of fosfomycin against these bacteria is comparable to that of the β-lactams, whose target is also wall synthesis but at a later stage (transpeptidase closing the polyglycine bonds of parietal mucopeptide).

7.2. Acquired Resistance

Acquired resistance may be related to the loss of the inducible transport system of G-6-P. In vitro studies of fosfomycin and fosfomycin trometamol (Albini et al., 1986; Forsgren and Walder, 1983; Fosfomycin International Symposium, 1977; Greenwood et al., 1986; Kanimoto and Greenwood, 1987) have shown the importance of the size of the inoculum, particularly in a broth medium. This effect is related to the rapid emergence of resistant mutants. Clinically, the selection of resistant mutants with high-level resistance was observed at an early stage when fosfomycin first started to be used as monotherapy.

7.3. Chromosomal Resistance

Chromosomal resistance is due essentially to disruption of the mechanisms of active transport of fosfomycin into the bacterial cell. The frequency of occurrence of this resistance is on the order of 10^{-6} to 10^{-7} for staphylococci, *E. coli*, and *Enterobacter* spp. and higher for *Klebsiella* and *Serratia* spp. (Fosfomycin International Symposium, 1977). In resistant mutants, incorporation of fosfomycin is 10 times lower than that normally obtained for the susceptible strain. The chromosomal mutation may be carried either on the gene governing the transport of L-α-glycerophosphate (*glpT* locus) (Kahan et al., 1974), but in this case the hexose phosphate system may be induced by addition of G-6-P and the bacterium reverts to being susceptible, or on genes governing the two transport systems, in which case the strains are totally resistant, as they are incapable of transporting the antibiotic as a result of impairment of both the L-α-glycerophosphate system and the hexose phosphate pathway.

7.4. Plasmid-Mediated Resistance

Recognized since 1980 in strains of *Serratia marcescens* and subsequently in other species of *Enterobacteriaceae*, the plasmids governing resistance to fosfomycin are of high molecular weight, are conjugative, and carry genes for resistance to other antibiotics (Llaneza et al., 1985). This mechanism confers a high level of resistance to fosfomycin, greater than 1,024 μg of fosfomycin per ml. This is a mechanism of enzymatic resistance, and the enzyme produced is a cytoplasmic polypeptide of 16,000 to 18,000 Da, synthesis of which is constitutive (Arca et al., 1988). This plasmid-mediated enzymatic resistance degrades the fosfomycin molecule to an inactive derivative that persists inside the bacterial cell. This derivative appears to be 1-(S-glutathionyl)-2-hydroxypropylphosphonic acid. Catalyzed by a cytoplasmic glutathione S-transferase, a glutathionyl residue is incorporated in the fosfomycin molecule by means of the sulfur atom of the cysteine of the tripeptide, resulting in the opening of the epoxide moiety of fosfomycin (Fig. 3). Glutathione S-transferases are enzymes known to occur in eukaryotes and described for the first time for bacteria in relation to enzymatic resistance to fosfomycin (Arca et al., 1988).

8. PLASMA PHARMACOKINETICS

8.1. Pharmacokinetics of Fosfomycin in Healthy Volunteers

A small and very soluble molecule, fosfomycin as the disodium salt for parenteral administration attains high concentrations in serum, i.e., a maximum value of 123 ± 16 μg/ml at the recommended dosages and by the recommended methods of administration (intravenous administration of 4 g by infusion over 4 h). The pharmacokinetic parameters are presented in Table 4. The pharmacokinetics of fosfomycin correspond to a two-compartment model. The apparent elimination half-life in plasma is about 2 h, and the volume of distribution is 20 to 25 liters (0.32 to 0.38 liter/kg). Binding of fosfomycin to plasma proteins is weak (less than 10%). Elimination is principally by glomerular filtration. Renal clearance of fosfomycin is similar to that of creatinine (100 to 120 ml/min); more than 85% of the product is eliminated in 12 h and urinary concentrations are high, reaching 3,000 μg/ml during an infusion of 4 g of fosfomycin in 4 h and 3,800 μg/ml between 4 and 8 h after the end of the infusion. In addition, fosfomycin is not metabolized and does not undergo an enterohepatic cycle, but a small quantity of product (0.075%) is found in the feces.

8.2. Pharmacokinetics of Fosfomycin in Subjects Other Than Adult Volunteers

8.2.1. Neonates

In neonates, the apparent elimination half-life is longer and may reach 7 h, while renal elimination is slow. The dosage in children is reduced to, on average, 100 to 200 mg/kg per 24 h by infusion.

8.2.2. Patients with Renal Insufficiency

In patients with renal insufficiency, depending on the reduction in glomerular filtration, fosfomycin accumulates in the blood proportionately to the variations in creatinine clearance and serum creatinine (Table 5). The apparent elimination half-life is prolonged, reaching 6 h when creatinine clearance is about 50 ml/min/1.73 m^2 and 11 to 12 h for a clearance of 5 to 10 ml/min/1.73 m^2. In patients with moderate renal insufficiency (creatinine clearance greater than or equal to 60 ml/min), the dosage and rhythm of infusions do not need to be modified. Conversely, for a creatinine clearance of less than 60 ml/min, the dosage must be adapted, retaining the unit dose of 4 g per infusion but modifying the interval between infusions.

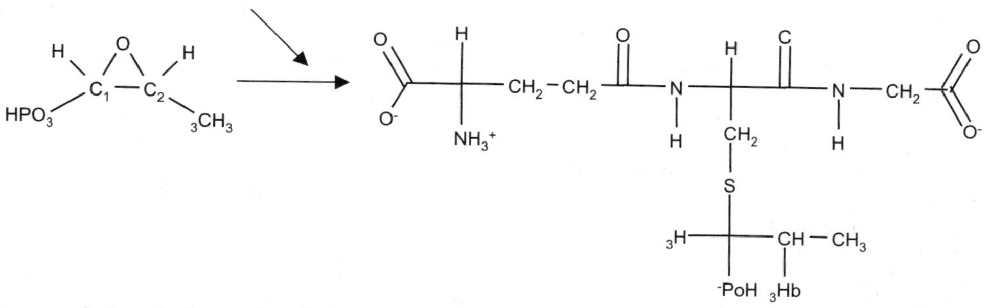

Figure 3 Proposed chemical reaction during the enzymatic inactivation of fosfomycin in the presence of glutathione

Table 4 Pharmacokinetic parameters of fosfomycin, fosmidomycin, fosfomycin trometamol, and fosfomycin calcium[a]

Antibacterial[b]	Dose (mg/kg)[c]	n	C_{max} (μg/ml)	C_{min} (μg/ml)	T_{max} (h)	$t_{1/2}$ (h)	V_{ss} (liters/kg)	$AUC_{0-\infty}$ (μg·h/ml)	CL_R (ml/min/kg)	CL_P (ml/min/kg)
F	20 i.v.	7	132	4.1		2.25	0.32	167.9	1.74	
	40 i.v.	7	259	6.8		2.22	0.36	290.8	1.91	2.08
F	50 i.v.	8	281			3.08		30.234[d]		2.31
	50 i.v.	13	297			2.79		29.721[d]		
FD	30 i.v.	10	157			1.65		210[d]		2.38
FT	25 p.o.	13	12.3		2.5	4.11		6.72[d]		
	25 p.o.	13	22		2.26	3.84		10.887[d]		
FC	50 p.o.	8	5.8		2.85	5.51		3.567[d]		
FT	50 p.o.	10	22.55		2.5	7.31		227.86		
			12.74		3.89	10.29		168.54		

[a]Data for fosfomycin, fosmidomycin, and fosfomycin trometamol are from Goto et al., 1981; Murakawa et al., 1982; and Wilson et al., 1988, respectively.
[b]F, fosfomycin; FD, fosmidomycin; FT, fosfomycin trometamol; FC, fosfomycin calcium.
[c]i.v., intravenously; p.o., per os.
[d]In micrograms per minute per milliliter.

Table 5 Concentrations of fosfomycin in plasma in patients with renal insufficiency

Patient no.	Dose (g/24 h)	Plasma creatinine (μl/liter)	Concn of drug in plasma (μg/ml)		
			End of infusion	4 h	24 h
1	8	92	186.6	35.4	15.8
2	8	212	240	155	
3	4	566	654	535	
4	4	778	617.5	154.3	

8.2.3. Patients Undergoing Hemodialysis

In hemodialyzed patients, 80% of the administered dose is eliminated in 6 h. After administration of 2 g of fosfomycin (direct intravenous line) 15 min before the beginning of hemodialysis, the plasma drug concentration reaches more than 100 μg/ml and is 32.3 μg/ml at the end of dialysis. This level still persists 4 h after the end of dialysis. The elimination half-life (mean ± standard deviation) is 4.2 ± 0.27 h during the hemodialysis session, while outside of hemodialysis the half-life is between 30 and 70 h. The dosage must be adapted to take account of these parameters, and administration of 2 g by infusion after each dialysis session is the recommended frequency.

8.3. Pharmacokinetics of Fosmidomycin and Alafosfalin

After a single dose of 30 mg/kg of body weight intravenously, or about 2 g of fosmidomycin, in healthy volunteers, a peak concentration in serum of 157 μg/ml is reached in 0.25 h and the residual concentration at 4 h is 9.2 μg/ml. The pharmacokinetics of this compound correspond to a two-compartment model (Murakawa et al., 1982) with a half-life in plasma of 1.65 h and urinary elimination of 85.5% of the unchanged product in 24 h. A repeat-dose study of 29 infusions (30 min) of 2 g every 6 h failed to reveal accumulation in the serum or urine, and the pharmacokinetic parameters were unchanged. In addition, binding of fosmidomycin to plasma proteins was estimated as 1% or less. The intramuscular and oral routes have also been studied for fosmidomycin, revealing bioavailability of 80.3 and 30%, respectively, and lower urinary elimination of only 26% after administration of 500 mg orally (Murakawa et al., 1982). The apparent elimination half-lives were 1.87 and 1.5 h after oral and intramuscular administration, respectively. Regarding the pharmacokinetic characteristics of alafosfalin, a phosphonic antibiotic, a good absorption was reached after oral and intramuscular administration, but this compound is unstable in humans, as only 4% of the compound is found in the urine, whereas a metabolite was found at levels of 51%.

8.4. Pharmacokinetics of Fosfomycin Trometamol

The pharmacokinetic parameters of fosfomycin trometamol are reported in Table 4. The concentrations in serum are higher (about 22 μg/ml) when the compound is administered before food (Bergogne-Berezin et al., 1987; Muller-Serieys et al., 1987) and the apparent elimination half-life varies with the study, from 2.5 h (Wilson et at., 1988) to about 7 h (Muller-Serieys et al., 1987). Obtained during fasting and after food in the same subjects (Bergogne-Berezin et al., 1987; Muller-Serieys et al., 1987), the pharmacokinetic parameters indicate that absorption is significantly reduced after food. Serial assays of levels in serum indicate the existence of secondary peaks corresponding to enterohepatic recirculation, and fosfomycin is found in the bile. Elimination of the product is essentially renal, and 58% of the administered dose is found in the urine in 24 h (Bergan, 1990). Urinary concentrations, which are dose dependent, are very high and may exceed 2,000 μg/ml 4 h after administration of a single dose. Urinary levels remain high for a prolonged period (over 24 h), constituting an argument in favor of the use of fosfomycin trometamol in the treatment of common urinary tract infections (Naber and Thyroff-Friesinger, 1990). The pharmacokinetic properties of fosfomycin calcium (Wilson et al., 1988) studied versus those of fosfomycin trometamol (Table 4) clearly indicate better bioavailability for the latter.

9. TISSUE DISTRIBUTION

Fosfomycin diffuses readily into various tissues and biological fluids in humans because of the small size of the molecule. A fairly large number of studies have enabled the extravascular concentrations of the product to be measured, the data for which are reported in Table 6. The tissue distribution of fosfomycin varies according to the presentation of the product, and the oral form of fosfomycin trometamol, which yields levels in serum about 10 times lower than those of fosfomycin intravenously, has given rise to a small number of studies of tissue concentrations in view also of the fact of its limited indications, which are confined to lower urinary tract infections only.

9.1. Membrane Transfer of Fosfomycin

Recent studies (Ishizawa et al., 1990, 1991) using a rat small intestine model to analyze the mechanisms of diffusion of fosfomycin have shown that the product is transported by an active transport system common to fosfomycin and the phosphate ion, using in particular the Na^+ ion and proton gradients (H^+) as vectors. Demonstrated intestinally, this mechanism of active transport may possibly not be transposable to other membrane systems.

9.2. CSF and Ventricular Fluid

Fosfomycin concentrations in the cerebrospinal fluid (CSF) of patients with meningitis have been extensively studied at

Table 6 Tissue distribution of fosfomycin[a]

Fluid or tissue	Dose (mg/kg)	*n*	Sampling time (h)	Concn (μg/ml or μg/g) in:	
				Plasma	Tissue
CSF	200 (2 days)	16	0.15	84	10.8
			1	63	13.4
			2	45	16
			4		
	200		3		38.9
	12,000 (days 1–11)	4	End of infusion		25
Respiratory tissues					
Lung	2,000 i.m.	12	1–2	22–52	8–22
	2,000 i.v.	14	1–2	24–64	6.4–25
	5,000 by infusion	13	1	172–209	114–140
			2	77–86	45–64
			3	48–54	18.5–43
			4	24–60	5.5–49
Pleural fluid	30 mg/kg	6	0.25	195.2	42.6
			3.7		
Bronchial secretions	4,000 by infusion (4 h)	11	0.15	120	13.1
			2	52.5	7.05
Burn wound	50 mg/kg	21	0.5	191.1	
			1	141	77
			2	92.5	71.6
			4	42.4	43.2
Blister fluid			1		75.4
			2		69.7
			4		49.9
Wound (exudate fluid)			1		70.5
			2		46.2
			4		22.4
Lochia	2,000 i.v.	3			14.1
	6,000/6 h/day	13			10.3
Prostate	4,000 i.v.	10		80–410	3.2–74
					13.6–128
Colostrum		2		30	6
Amniotic fluid		3		46	45.3
Miscellaneous					
Aqueous humor		4		65	4
Bile		4		30	6
Bone					
Medulla	4,000 by infusion (4 h)	10	1	56.9	12.8
			1	79.5	20.1
			2	56.9	5.1
			2	79.5	15.8
Cortex	4,000 by infusion (4 h)	10	1	42–107	6.4
			1		18.1
			2	75.9	6.8–53.5
			2		16.4

[a]Data from Dominguez-Gil et al., 1983; Fosfomycin International Symposium, 1977; Kafe et al., 1983; Quentin et al., 1983; and Stahl et al., 1982, 1983.
[b]i.m., intramuscularly; i.v., intravenously.

various dosages and under various experimental conditions. CSF fosfomycin concentrations are higher after administration of repeated doses than after a single dose, but studies have shown lower levels on day 5 than on day 2, probably related to the reduction in the inflammatory state of the meninges (Stahl et al., 1983), which promoted meningeal diffusion of fosfomycin in the initial stage of the meningitis. Overall, concentrations range from 7 to 30 μg/ml and are in a ratio of 13 to 38% of the levels in serum measured at the end of the infusion. Combination of systemic treatment (12 g daily in three infusions of 4 g) with an intraventricular injection of 10 mg/day produces an increase in local levels to 352 μg of fosfomycin per ml 2 h after the end of the infusion and the maintenance of high levels (51.8 and 32.6 μg/ml) at 4 and 6 h. These diffusion characteristics have important implications in the treatment of meningitis and acute ventriculitis due to staphylococci or gram-negative bacilli.

9.3. Respiratory Tissues

As indicated in Table 6, several studies have enabled fosfomycin concentrations to be established in the lung parenchyma (on the order of between 8 and >50 μg/g and even 100 μg/g of tissue), pleural fluid (42.6 ± 16 μg/ml), and bronchial secretions (~13 μg/ml). These local concentrations are in a ratio of 13 to >80% of simultaneous levels in serum, although the concentrations in bronchial secretions are lower than in tissue because of the dilution factor associated with this study model (Kafe et al., 1983).

9.4. Other Tissues and Biological Fluids

Fosfomycin diffuses well into interstitial fluids, where it reaches levels close to the simultaneous concentration in serum. In the genital apparatus, particularly in the lochia of patients with a puerperal infection (endometritis with sepsis), fosfomycin concentrations are variable but attain values of up to 26 or 27 μg/ml, while concentrations in prostatic tissue are 13 to 80% of simultaneous levels in serum. In breast milk, low levels, on the order of 3.6 μg per ml, of fosfomycin have been measured, equivalent to 7% of levels in serum. Fosfomycin concentrations are lower in bone tissue, but the coefficient of penetration into bone remains on the order of 20 to 27%, indicating good diffusion in bone (Quentin et al., 1983). In the tonsils and sinus mucosa, fosfomycin concentrations are, respectively, 50 and 30% of levels in serum.

9.5. Renal Tissue

Fosfomycin trometamol is concentrated in renal tissue, where, after administration of 50 mg of compound (orally), per kg, it reaches early levels (2 h) of 155.75 ± 39.94 μg/g. These levels then decline progressively but are still 78.00 ± 4.72 μg/g at 12 h. These tissue concentrations are consistent with the renal elimination of fosfomycin trometamol, the characteristics of which are described above.

10. DRUG INTERFERENCE

10.1. Electrolytes

10.1.1. Sodium

Administered intravenously in the form of the disodium salt, fosfomycin represents a high sodium intake, 14.5 mEq of Na per g of compound, i.e., 0.33 g of sodium. A daily dosage of 12 g therefore provides 4 g of sodium. This sodium content must be taken into account when calculating the electrolytes to be infused, particularly in cardiac patients.

10.1.2. Potassium

Fosfomycin is a weak acid that may induce increased urinary K^+ excretion in the distal tubule (a passive process induced by the increase in potential difference between the tubular lumen and the cell). An increase in urinary flow in the distal tubule is also possible with a greater quantity of Na^+/K^+ exchanged for (through an active process under the control of aldosterone). Repeated infusions may therefore be accompanied by a loss of potassium with hypokalemia. Potentiation of hypokalemia may occur with the simultaneous use of other hypokalemic agents, such as diuretics, amphotericin B, digitalis derivatives, other weak acids acting as nonabsorbable anions, aminoglycosides, and β-lactams at high doses (α-carboxypenicillins and *N*-acylpenicillins).

The interactions with electrolytes necessitate regular monitoring of the water and electrolyte constants throughout the treatment period and the intake of potassium if necessary.

10.2. Favorable Interactions: Synergy of Combinations

As fosfomycin is liable to cause rapid selection of a resistant mutant when used alone, it must be combined with different classes of antibiotics with which it exerts a "favorable," i.e., synergistic, interaction. It has been seen above that in vitro studies, confirmed by clinical studies (Baron et al., 1981; Drugeon and Kazmierczak, 1987; Dureux et al., 1981; Figueredo and Neu, 1988), indicate that combinations of fosfomycin with β-lactams (particularly 2-amino-5-thiazolyl cephalosporins), aminoglycosides, and fluoroquinolones are favorable. However, in the choice of a companion drug for fosfomycin, account must be taken of the nature of the bacterium involved and the site of infection for good local diffusion of the two antibiotics combined. Combinations of fosfomycin and fluoroquinolones meet this criterion. The above-mentioned drugs are used in combination with fosfomycin for the following reasons:

- Fluoroquinolones are active against infections due to staphylococci, enteric gram-negative bacteria, and *P. aeruginosa*.
- Vancomycin and fusidic acid are active against staphylococci.
- 2-Amino-5 thiazolyl cephalosporins are active in meningitis and ventriculitis due to *Enterobacteriaceae* or staphylococci.
- Imipenem is active in severe infections due to staphylococci and *P. aeruginosa*.

10.3. Other Interactions

Experimentally in the rat, concomitant administration of fosfomycin and aminoglycosides is accompanied by a decrease in aminoglycoside nephrotoxicity through a reduction in alanine aminopeptidase activity and reduced impairment of lysosomal permeability, toxic phenomena associated with the aminoglycoside (Neuman, 1983). A decrease in the renal toxicity of vancomycin and cisplatin is apparently also obtained when they are combined with fosfomycin.

10.4. Fosfomycin Trometamol

Simultaneous administration with metoclopramide delays the gastrodigestive absorption of the oral form of fosfomycin and alters the rates of urinary elimination.

11. TOLERANCE

Fosfomycin is considered atoxic. Repeated doses, however, may be accompanied by adverse effects, as follows.

Administration of fosfomycin by infusion may be accompanied by venous irritation phenomena necessitating a change of infusion site. These reactions are reduced with slow discontinuous infusion (4 h) or continuous infusion (by pump).

Metabolic effects associated with sodium intake and urinary potassium wastage have been observed.

Rare allergic phenomena have been mentioned in the literature, particularly from the combination of fosfomycin with a penicillin, involving the occurrence of a morbilliform rash or conjunctivitis (with elevated eosinophil levels) and rare cases of diarrhea. No cross-allergy has been reported with other antibiotics.

The precautions for use already reported are principally monitoring of blood electrolytes and dosage adjustment in renal insufficiency when creatinine clearance is less than 60 ml/min. Use of fosfomycin should be avoided in breast-feeding women because of the presence of high fosfomycin levels in breast milk, which may exert an ecological impact on the digestive flora in infants.

The ecological impact of the administration of fosfomycin has been studied only for the oral trometamol form. The product has been shown to cause a considerable reduction in coliforms in the fecal flora, with a significant increase in gram-positive aerobic species. The total number of anaerobes increases as the result of an elevation of levels of *Bacteroides* spp., whereas clostridia, lactobacilli, *Bifidobacterium* spp., and *Veillonella* spp. show a relative reduction.

The adverse effects of fosfomycin trometamol associated with oral administration of the product are essentially gastrointestinal disorders, such as nausea and diarrhea, and rare skin rashes. These signs disappear spontaneously and rapidly on discontinuation of treatment, which is always very short, although they can appear even with a single dose.

12. CLINICAL INDICATIONS

The main indications for fosfomycin are severe hospital-acquired infections, and fosfomycin is always used in combination with an antibiotic belonging to one of the following classes: β-lactams, aminoglycosides, fluoroquinolones, glycopeptides and glycolipopeptides.

12.1. Purulent Meningitis

A number of studies have shown the efficacy of fosfomycin combined with an aminoglycoside or cefotaxime in the treatment of purulent meningitis due to gram-negative bacilli, *S. aureus*, and, recently, pneumococci of reduced susceptibility to penicillin (MIC, >0.1 μg/ml).

12.2. Severe Pulmonary Infections

In the treatment of severe pulmonary infections (nosocomial pneumonia), particularly when the bacteria concerned are *P. aeruginosa* and *S. aureus*, combinations of fosfomycin with a ureidopenicillin or ceftazidime in the first case and vancomycin in the second have proved highly active.

12.3. Severe Urinary Tract Infections

Severe urinary tract infections have been treated with fosfomycin monotherapy in view of the excellent urinary elimination of this product: it is eliminated in the unchanged form at very high levels in the urine. Favorable results have been obtained in severe pyelonephritis, with sterilization of the urine obtained in 79% of cases at the end of treatment (7 days). The lack of nephrotoxicity of fosfomycin in patients suffering from parenchymatous renal infection, together with the antibacterial spectrum of this compound (enteric gram-negative bacilli), is an argument in favor of this indication (Fries et al., 1981).

12.4. Infectious Endocarditis and Septicemia

In infectious endocarditis and septicemic states, fosfomycin has important indications when staphylococci are involved. In *Staphylococcus epidermidis* infections the limited number of active antibacterial agents endows fosfomycin with a position of choice as long as it is combined with vancomycin or teicoplanin, an aminoglycoside, or a fluoroquinolone after previously testing these combinations in vitro for their bactericidal activities. The combination fosfomycin-aminoglycoside has been found to be most consistently bactericidal (95%) (Drugeon and Kazmierczak, 1987) and remarkably effective in staphylococcal septicemia (Baron et al., 1981; Dureux et al., 1981). In endocarditis (Dureux et al., 1981), the results of the use of fosfomycin vary: poor in the case of streptococci (which are not part of the antibacterial spectrum of fosfomycin) but more favorable in staphylococcal endocarditis, where the combination of fosfomycin with an aminoglycoside for *S. aureus* or with a fluoroquinolone for methicillin-resistant staphylococci represents a good therapeutic choice and has demonstrated efficacy.

12.5. Other Indications

Because of its good diffusion into bone, fosfomycin has been recommended in the treatment of staphylococcal bone and joint infections (osteomyelitis) or those due to *Pseudomonas*. In this indication, fosfomycin must always be combined with oxacillin in chronic osteomyelitis or with an aminoglycoside or pefloxacin in septicemia with an osteoarticular localization. The place of fosfomycin in the treatment of *P. aeruginosa* infections is still poorly established, and contradictory results, particularly the notion of antagonistic combinations of fosfomycin in vitro (Reguera et al., 1990), urge caution. However, favorable results for combinations of fosfomycin with an aminoglycoside have been reported in cases of cystic fibrosis in children with episodes of superinfection involving *P. aeruginosa*. In *P. aeruginosa* septicemia, cure rates on the order of 83% have been reported (Wolf, 1987), and it has been seen that nosocomial pneumonia and osteomyelitis involving *P. aeruginosa* also constitute indications for fosfomycin.

REFERENCES

Albini E, Belluco G, Marca G, 1986, Influence of pH, inoculum and media on the in vitro bactericidal activity of fosfomycin-trometamol, norfloxacin and cotrimoxazole, Chemioterapia, v, 268–272.

Arca P, Rico M, Brana AF, Villar CJ, Hardisson C, Suarez JE, 1988, Formation of an adduct between fosfomycin and glutathione: a new mechanism of antibiotic resistance in bacteria, Antimicrob Agents Chemother, 32, 1552–1556.

Baron D, Drugeon H, Courtieu AL, Nicolas F, 1981, Septicémies et infections graves à germes multiresistants. Résultats du traitement par la fosfomycine, Med Mal Infect, 11, 255–261.

Bergan T, 1990, Degree of absorption, pharmacokinetics of fosfomycin trometamol and duration of urinary antibacterial activity, Infection, 18, Suppl 2, S65–S69.

Bergogne-Bérézin E, Muller-Serieys C, Joly-Guillou ML, Dronne N, 1987, Trometamol-fosfomycin (Monuril). Bioavailability and food-drug interaction, Eur Urol, 13, Suppl 1, 64–68.

Dominguez-Gil A, de Portugal Alvarez J, Fernandez Lastra C, Marino EL, Barrueco M, Gomez Gomez F, Santiago Gervos M, 1983, Pharmacokinetics of phosphomycin in patients with pleural effusion, part 37, p 20–23, Proc 13th Int Congr Chemother.

Drugeon HB, Kazmierczak A, 1987, Les associations avec la fosfomycine sur Staphylococcus: les partenaires les plus intéréssants, Sem Hop Paris, 63, 3549–3552.

Dureux JB, Canton PH, Weber M, Toussain P, Roche G, 1981, La fosfomycine dans le traitement des états septicémiques et des endocardites bactériennes, Med Mal Infect, 11, 524–532.

Figueredo VM, Neu HC, 1988, Synergy of ciprofloxacin with fosfomycin in vitro against Pseudomonas isolates from patients with cystic fibrosis, J Antimicrob Chemother, 22, 41–50.

Forsgren A, Walder M, 1983, Antimicrobial activity of fosfomycin in vitro, J Antimicrob Chemother, 11, 467–471.

Fosfomycin International Symposium, Madrid, July 1975, 1977, Chemotherapy, 23, 1–447, S Karger AG, Basel.

Fries D, Jacques L, Mathieu D, Hardy N, 1981, Intérêt de la fosfomycine dans le traitement des formes sévères de pyélonéphrites, Med Mal Infect, 11, 425–429.

Gevaudan MJ, Mallet MN, Gulian C, Dalmas N, Gevaudan P, 1978, Recherche de synergie entre la fosfomycine et divers autres antibiotiques, Med Mal Infect, 8, 657–665.

Gismondo MR, Romeo MA, Lo Bue AM, Chisari G, Nicoletti G, 1986, Microbiological basis for the use of fosfomycin trometamol as single-dose therapy for simple cystitis, Chemioterapia, 5, 278–282.

Goto M, Sugiyama M, Nakajima S, Yamashina H, 1981, Fosfomycin kinetics after intravenous and oral administration to human volunteers, Antimicrob Agents Chemother, 20, 393–397.

Greenwood D, Jones A, Eley A, 1986, Factors influencing the activity of the trometamol salt of fosfomycin, Eur J Clin Microbiol, 5, 29–34.

Ishizawa T, Tsuji A, Tamai I, Terasaki T, Hosoi K, Fukatsu S, 1990, Sodium and pH dependent carrier-mediated transport of antibiotic, fosfomycin, in the rat intestinal brush-border membrane, J Pharmacobio-Dyn, 13, 292–300.

Ishizawa T, Yayashi H, Awazu S, 1991, Effect of carrier-mediated transport system on intestinal fosfomycin absorption in situ and in vivo, J Pharmacobio-Dyn, 14, 82–86.

Kafe H, Berthelot G, Daumal M, Gillon JC, Bergogne-Bérézin E, 1983, A study of the penetration of fosfomycin into respiratory secretions, part 37, p 37–139, Proc 13th Int Congr Chemother, Vienna, Austria.

Kahan FM, Kahan JS, Cassidy PJ, Kropp H, 1974, The mechanism of action of fosfomycin (phosphonomycin), Ann N Y Acad Sci, 235, 364–386.

Kanimoto Y, Greenwood D, 1987, Comparison of the response of Escherichia coli to fosfomycin and fosmidomycin, Eur J Clin Microbiol, 6, 386–391.

Lerner SA, Price S, Kulkarni S, 1988, Microbiological studies of fosfomycin trometamol against urinary isolates in vitro, p 121–129, in Neu H, Williams JD, ed, New Trends in Urinary Tract Infections, Int Symp Rome, 1987, Karger, Basel.

Llaneza J, Villar CJ, Salas JA, Suarez JE, Mendoza MC, Hardisson C, 1985, Plasmid-mediated fosfomycin resistance is due to enzymatic modification of the antibiotic, Antimicrob Agents Chemother, 28, 163–164.

Lorian V, ed, 1991, Antibiotics in Laboratory Medicine, 3rd ed, Williams and Wilkins Publishers, Baltimore.

Maur N, ed, 1990, Vade-mecum des antibiotiques et agents chimiothérapiques anti-infectieux, 5th ed, Editions Maloine, Paris.

Muller-Serieys C, Bergogne-Bérézin E, Joly-Guillou ML, 1987, La fosfomycine-trométamol (Monuril): pharmacocinétique et interaction aliment-médicament, Pathol Biol, 35, 753–756.

Murakawa T, Sakamoto H, Fukada S, Konishi T, Nishida M, 1982, Pharmacokinetics of fosmidomycin, a new phosphonic acid antibiotic, Antimicrob Agents Chemother, 21, 224–230.

Naber KG, Thyroff-Friesinger U, 1990, Fosfomycin-trometamol versus ofloxacin/co-trimoxazole as single dose therapy of acute uncomplicated urinary tract infection in females: a multicentre study, Infection, 18, Suppl 2, S70–S76.

Neu HC, Williams JD, ed, 1988, New trends in urinary tract infections, S Karger AG, Basel.

Neuman M, 1983, Protective effect of fosfomycin on the nephrotoxicity of anukacin, part 37, p 14–19, Proc 13th Int Congr Chemother.

Quentin C, Besnard R, Pinaquy C, Cruette D, Le Rebeller A, Bébéar C, 1983, Fosfomycin penetration into non-infected human bone, part 37, p 32–36, Proc 13th Int Congr Chemother.

Reguera JA, Baquero F, Berenguer J, Martinez-Ferrer M, Martinez JL, 1990, β-Lactam-fosfomycin antagonism involving modification of penicillin-binding protein 3 in *Pseudomonas aeruginosa*, Antimicrob Agents Chemother, 34, 2093–2096.

Salhi A, 1978, Activité bactériostatique in vitro de la fosfomycine. Etude préliminaire multicentre avant tout usage thérapeutique en France, Med Mal Infect, 8, 677–684.

Stahl JP, Croise J, Bru JP, Girard-Blanc MF, Franqois P, Gaillat J, Micoud M, 1983, Fosfomycin diffusion into cerebrospinal fluid of human bacterial meningitis, part 37, p 5–7, Proc 13th Int Congr Chemother.

Stahl JP, Gaillat J, Marcel JP, Salhi A, Micoud M, 1982, Diffusion expérimentale de la fosfomycine dans le liquide céphalo-rachidien du chien. Premiers résultats, Med Mal Infect, 12, 370–373.

Takahashi K, Kanno H, 1984, Synergistic activities of combinations of beta-lactams, fosfomycin, and tobramycin against *Pseudomonas aeruginosa*, Antimicrob Agents Chemother, 26, 789–791.

Utsui Y, Ohya S, Magaribuchi T, Tajima M, Yokota T, 1986, Antibacterial activity of cefmetazole alone and in combination with fosfomycin against methicillin- and cephem-resistant *Staphylococcus aureus*, Antimicrob Agents Chemother, 30, 917–922.

Wilson P, Williams JD, Rolandi E, 1988, Comparative pharmacokinetics of fosfomycin trometamol, sodium fosfomycin and calcium fosfomycin in humans, p 136–142, in Neu H, Williams JD, ed, New trends in urinary tract infections, Int Symp Rome, 1987, Karger, Basel.

Wolf M, 1987, Place de la fosfomycine dans le traitement des infections à Pseudomonas aeruginosa, Sem Hop Paris, 63, 3570–3572.

Orthosomycins

A. BRYSKIER

38

1. SUMMARY

The family of orthosomycins includes the everninomicins, which are oligosaccharide antibiotics containing two orthodiester bonds and a dichloroeverninic acid residue. Evernimicin, or SCH 27899, has been selected for development as a medicinal product (Ziracin) and is characterized by an antibacterial spectrum that principally includes gram-positive bacteria. It is inactive against enteric gram-negative bacilli and nonfermentative gram-negative bacilli. Its relatively long apparent elimination half-life (about 13 h) and its pharmacodynamic profile allow daily administration in the form of an intravenous infusion over 1 h.

2. BACKGROUND

The everninomicin complex, which includes at least 10 components, was described in 1965 and obtained from the fermentation of *Micromonospora carbonacea* subsp. *africana* (isolated from the bank of the Nyiro River in Kenya).

The major component was termed everninomicin D and has good in vitro activity against gram-positive cocci, but it has proved to be nephrotoxic and neurotoxic (ataxia) in animals.

Other components of the everninomicin complex have been obtained from the fermentation of *M. carbonacea*, particularly components 13-384-1 (evernimicin) and 13-384-5 (Sch-27900) and three other derivatives belonging to this subgroup. Since then, another molecule has been described, everninomicin-6.

Component 13-384-1 (evernimicin) has been selected for development. Unfortunately, development was stopped for safety concerns.

Five other derivatives have been isolated from the fermentation broth: Sch-58769, Sch-58771, Sch-58773, Sch-58775, and Sch-58777. All of them except Sch-58777 are equipotent to evernimicin against *Staphylococcus aureus*. This highlights the fact that the left side of the molecule, including a nitro sugar A ring as well as the chlorine-containing benzyl ester functionality, plays an important role in the antibacterial activity (Fig. 1).

3. CLASSIFICATION

3.1. Orthosomycins

The everninomicins are original antibiotics that belong structurally to the oligosaccharide antibacterial agents. They are characterized by an oligosaccharide structure with the presence of one or more orthodiester-type bonds. This type of bond is unusual in nature but has been described for a series of molecules grouped together in a family known as orthosomycins.

Within this group of molecules, two subgroups may be defined asccording to their chemical structures (Fig. 2). Subgroup I comprises the everninomicins; flambamycin; the avilamycins (A, B, C, and 13 other components); a food additive for veterinary use, curamycin; and sporocuracins A and B. These molecules are characterized by the presence of a dichloroeverninic acid (Fig. 3). Subgroup II contains molecules possessing residues of the aminocyclic type. It comprises principally hygromycin B; destomycins A, B, and C; and the antibiotics A-396-1, SS-56C, and AB-74.

3.2. Everninomicins

The everninomicin complex comprises at least 10 molecules. These are oligosaccharides that in structural terms include eight sugars, two orthodiester bonds in positions 16 and 49, a nitro sugar (evernitrose), and a dichloroeverninic acid residue (Fig. 4).

The structures of everninomicins B, C, and D are illustrated in Fig. 5. The structures of the various everninomicins differ in the substituents at positions 52 and 23.

3.3. Evernimicin

Evernimicin (SCH 27899) is component 13-384-1, the structure of which has been described in detail (Fig. 6).

The stereoisomerism at the C-16 orthodiester bond is important, as there are three stereoisomers. Only SCH 27899 is active; the second stereoisomer is weakly active and the third is inactive.

Cycles A, B, and C are identical to those of everninomicin D. SCH 27899 has an additional hydroxyl group at position 23 (E ring) and a hydroxyl in place of the methoxy group at position 45 (H ring). The substituent at position 52 is 4-dihydroxy-6-methylbenzoyloxyl.

Structures of everninimicin and analogues 1-4

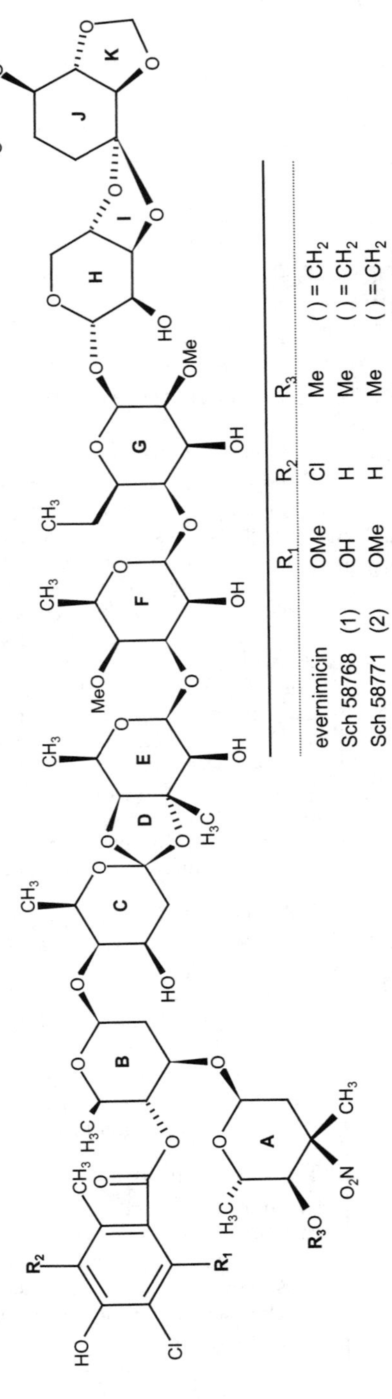

		R_1	R_2	R_3	
everninimicin		OMe	Cl	Me	( ) = CH_2
Sch 58768	(1)	OH	H	Me	( ) = CH_2
Sch 58771	(2)	OMe	H	Me	( ) = CH_2
Sch 58773	(3)	OMe	Cl	H	( ) = CH_2
Sch 58775	(4)	OMe	Cl	Me	( ) = OCOH, H

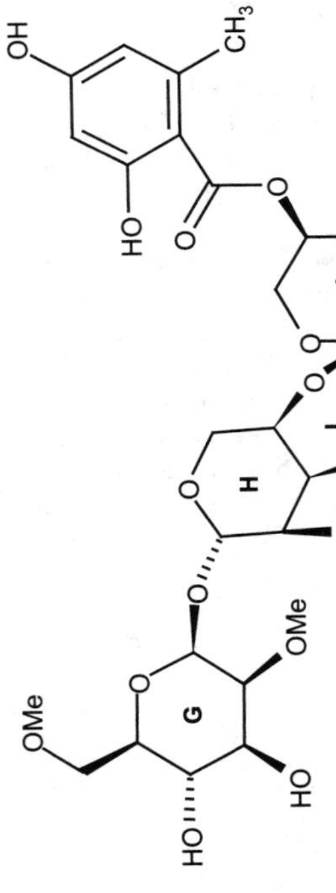

Structure of Sch 58777

Figure 1 Everninomicin analogs

Orthosomycins

Group I (dichloroevernininc acid)	Group II (aminocyclitols)
Everninomicin C, D	Hygromycin B
Everninomicin 2,3,7	Destomycins A,B,C
Everninomicin –B *(B)*	A-396-1
Everninomicin 13-314 (2,3,4)	SS-56 C
Everninomicin (Sch 27699)	AB-74
Sch 27800	
Avilamycin(s) A,B,C,D1,D2,E,A'	
Avilamycins F to N	
Curamycin	
Sporocuracin(s) A,B	
55-56 A,B	

Figure 2 Classification of orthosomycins

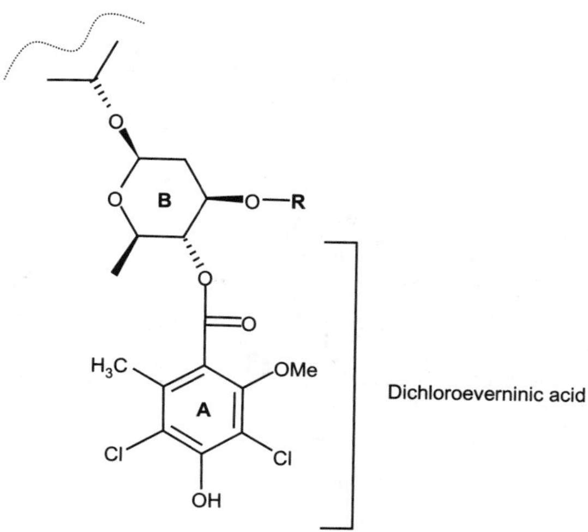

Figure 3 Dichloroevernininc acid

Dichloroevernininc acid

Oethoester links

Evernitrose

Figure 4 Everninomicin complex

Everninomicins	R_1	R_2	MW (daltons)
B	$CH(OCH_3)_2$ (drawn)	OH	1553.4
C	H	H	1479.3
D	$H_3CCH(OCH_3)$	H	1537.4

Figure 5 Everninomicins

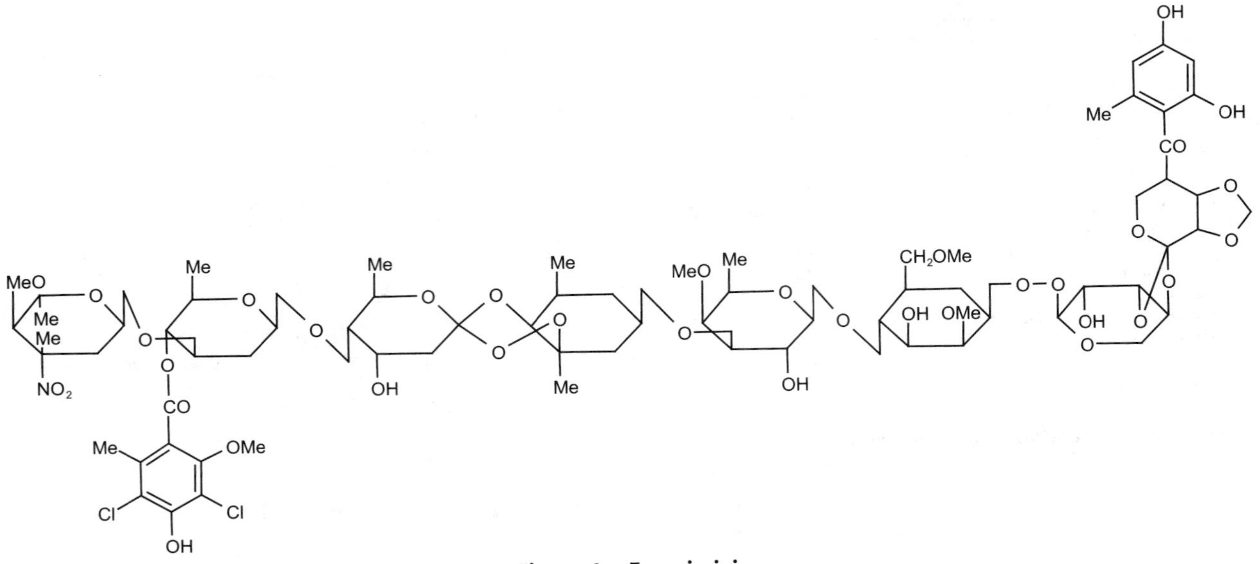

Figure 6 Evernimicin

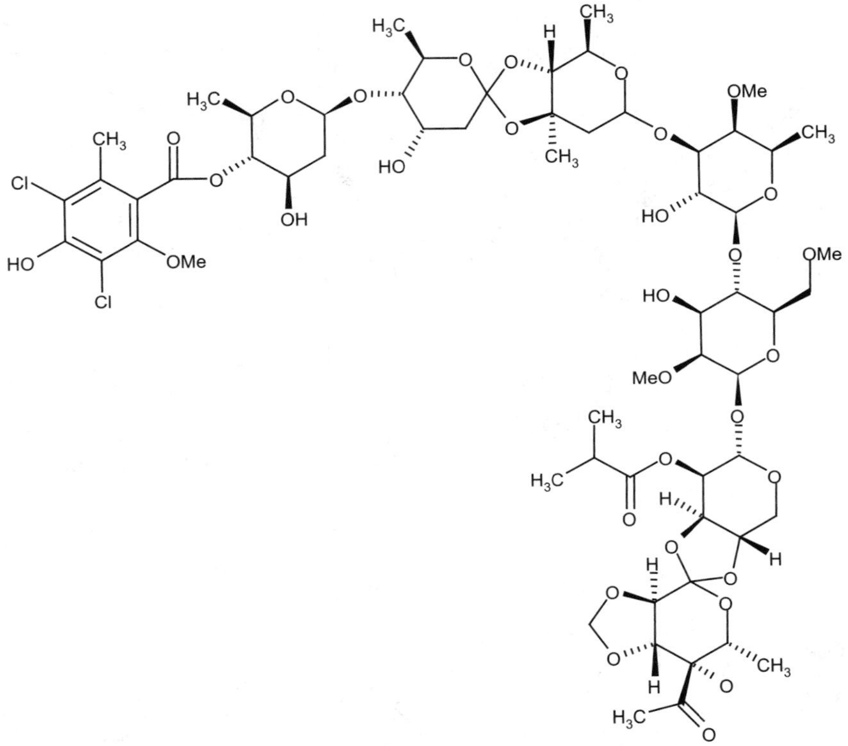

Figure 7 Avilamycin A

3.4. Avilamycin

Avilamycin is an orthosomycin complex extracted from *Streptomyces viridochromogenes* Tü 57 in 1965. It is a mixture of several major and minor components (avilamycins A to N); avilamycins A is the main component (Fig. 7).

Avilamycin is used as a growth promoter in the veterinary field.

Its mechanism of action is similar to that of everninomicin. Avilamycin is active against gram-positive bacteria.

The physicochemical properties of avilamycin A are summarized in Table 1.

Avilamycin at 60 ppm is eliminated through feces, and only small residues are found in tissues of swine and rats.

4. PHYSICOCHEMICAL PROPERTIES OF EVERNIMICIN

The physicochemical properties of SCH 27899 are summarized in Table 2. It is an amorphous powder, unlike everninomicin D, with a high molecular weight. Evernimicin has three ionizable phenol groups with a pK_a of 7.9 and greater than about 11.

Table 1 Physicochemical properties of avilamycin A

Parameter	Value(s)
Empirical formula	$C_{63}H_{94}O_{35}Cl_2$
Melting point (°C)	188–189
λ_{max}	214 and 288 nm
Mol wt	1,324

Table 2 Physicochemical properties of evernimicin (SCH 27899)

Parameter	Value
Empirical formula	$C_{70}H_{97}NO_{38}Cl_2$
Mol wt	1,631.43
ν_{max}	1,540 cm^{-1}
$[\alpha]^{26}_D$	−47.2° (1% methanol)
Solubility	
Water	<0.001 mg/ml
Ethanol	>300 mg/ml
Methanol	>300 mg/ml
pH	4.5–7.0 (solution 1%)
pK_a	7 (monophenol),
	9 (diphenol),
	>11 (3rd phenol)
Lipophilicity	octanol (pH 3)/0.1 M citrate
	buffer, $\log K_{o/w} \geq 2.96$
	octanol/water, $\log K_{o/w} \geq 3.03$
CAS no.	109545-84-8

5. STRUCTURE-ACTIVITY RELATIONSHIP

An approach to the structure and activity of everninomicins has been undertaken by means of chemical modifications, particularly of evernimicin.

The configuration of the two orthoester bonds at C-49 and C-16 is important for the antibacterial activity.

The nitro group of the evernitrose sugar has been reduced by adding nitroso, hydroxyamino, amino, or alkylamino groups; all of these derivatives retain good antibacterial activity. The pharmacokinetic properties in animals may be modulated at this level, depending on the substituents.

The sugars that make up the structure of this oligosaccharide have five hydroxyl groups (positions 18, 23, 30, 38, and 45) that may be substituted. Their substitution may modify the solubility and kinetic properties. Polar and non-polar groups have been attached to the hydroxyl groups.

Monosubstitution of 45-OH by an ethanol does not affect the antibacterial activity; conversely, attachment of hydrophobic groups to one or more hydroxyl groups is responsible for a reduction in antibacterial activity. Modification of the phenol groups at positions 57 and 59 causes a marked reduction in antibacterial activity.

6. ANTIBACTERIAL ACTIVITY OF EVERNIMICIN

See Table 3.

Evernimicin is an antibiotic that has good in vitro and in vivo activities against gram-positive bacteria but is inactive against gram-negative bacteria. Some in vitro activity has been demonstrated against other bacterial species, such as *Legionella pneumophila* and *Borrelia* spp.

Evernimicin possesses good activity against different species of enterococci, whether susceptible or resistant to vancomycin, with MICs at which 50% of isolates tested are inhibited (MIC_{50}) of between 0.125 and 0.50 μg/ml. Its activity against *S. aureus*, *Staphylococcus epidermidis*, and *Staphylococcus haemolyticus* is the same

Table 3 In vitro activity of evernimicin

Microorganism(s)	*n*	MIC (μg/ml)	
		50%	90%
S. aureus Met[r]	341	0.5	1.0
S. aureus Met[s]	448	0.25	0.5
S. epidermidis Met[r]	202	0.5	1.0
S. epidermidis Met[s]	186	0.25	1.0
S. haemolyticus Met[r]	44	0.5	2.0
S. haemolyticus Met[s]	59	1.0	1.0
Staphylococcus cohnii	11	1.0	4.0
Staphylococcus hominis	23	1.0	2.0
Staphylococcus intermedius	5	0.2	
Staphylococcus lugdunensis	5	16	
Staphylococcus saprophyticus	16	2.0	4.0
Staphylococcus simulans	20	1.0	2.0
Staphylococcus warneri	10	1.0	
Staphylococcus xylosus	3	0.5	
S. pneumoniae Pen[r]	40	0.06	0.5
S. pneumoniae Pen[s]	176	0.13	0.5
Streptococcus pyogenes	149	0.13	0.25
Streptococcus agalactiae	151	0.13	0.50
Group C streptococci	38	0.25	0.50
Group G streptococcci	39	0.25	0.5
Group F streptococci	4	0.13	
Viridans group streptococci	7	≤0.125	
E. faecalis Van[s]	802	0.5	1.0
E. faecalis Van[r]	36	0.25	1.0
E. faecium Van[s]	243	0.25	1.0
E. faecium Van[r]	233	0.25	1.0
Enterococcus gallinarum	204	0.25	0.5
Enterococcus avium	43	0.13	0.5
Enterococcus casseliflavus	37	0.25	0.50
Bacillus spp.	10	0.06	0.12
Corynebacterium jeikeium	4	≤0.125	
Listeria monocytogenes	10	0.25	0.5
Corynebacterium diphtheriae	2	0.78	
L. pneumophila	50	0.03	0.06
Legionella spp.	52	0.03	0.06
Borrelia spp.	15	0.25	0.5
Neisseria meningitidis	122	≤0.06	0.125
Neisseria gonorrhoeae	120	≤0.06	0.125
Haemophilus influenzae[a]	118	2.0	4.0
Moraxella catarrhalis	119	0.5	1.0
M. fortuitum	25	4	>16
M. chelonae	20	0.25	0.5
M. abscessus	22	>16	>16
M. smegmatis	4	2	
M. mucogenicum	5	0.25	
Micrococcus luteus	1	0.05	
Bacillus subtilis	1	0.78	
Bacillus anthracis	1	0.78	
Bacillus cereus	7	0.12	
P. acnes	10	1.0	4.0
Peptostreptococcus	2	0.06	
Bacteroides spp.		>32	
C. difficile	44	0.1	0.2
Clostridium perfringens	13	0.1	0.5

[a]β-Lactamase producing and non-β-lactamase producing.

whether the strains are methicillin susceptible or resistant (MIC_{50} and MIC_{90}, 0.25 to 1.0 and 0.5 to 2.0 μg/ml). Likewise, the activity against Lancefield group A, B, C, F, and G streptococci and against *Streptococcus pneumoniae* is good whether the strains are susceptible or resistant to penicillin G.

Evernimicin is active against *L. pneumophila* and other *Legionella* spp., with a MIC_{50} and MIC_{90} of 0.03 and 0.06 μg/ml, respectively, in buffered yeast extract α medium. The intracellular activity of evernimicin has not been determined, as the molecule is inactivated by cell cultures.

The activity of evernimicin has been tested against five species of *Borrelia*: those responsible for different syndromes in Lyme's disease (*B. burgdorferi, B. afzeliim,* and *B. garinii*) and those responsible for recurrent fevers (*B. hermsii* and *B. turicatae*). The MICs ranged between 0.06 and 0.25 μg/ml. Evernimicin exhibits bacteriostatic activity against *Borrelia* spp. at twice the MIC and bactericidal activity at four times the MIC.

Evernimicin is inactive against *Chlamydia pneumoniae* and *Chlamydia trachomatis*, with MICs greater than or equal to 8 μg/ml.

The activity against rapidly growing mycobacteria is variable. Evernimicin is inactive against *M. abscessus* (MIC_{50}, >16 μg/ml) and weakly active against *M. fortuitum* (MIC_{50} and MIC_{90}, 4 and 16 μg/ml) and *M. smegmatis* (MIC_{50} and MIC_{90}, 2 and 4 μg/ml), but its activity is better against *M. chelonae* (MIC_{50} and MIC_{90}, 0.5 and 1 μg/ml) and *M. mucogenicum* (MIC_{50} and MIC_{90}, 0.25 and 1 μg/ml).

The activity of evernimicin against two strains of *M. tuberculosis* is moderate (MIC, 16 μg/ml), and evernimicin is inactive against *M. avium* complex (MIC, >64 μg/ml).

Evernimicin exhibits good in vitro activity against gram-positive anaerobes, including *Clostridium difficile*, with MIC_{50}s ranging from ≤0.0015 to 0.12 μg/ml. It is inactive against *Bacteroides fragilis, Bacteroides thetaiotaomicron, Fusobacterium nucleatum,* and *Veillonella* spp. (MIC, >16 μg/ml) and moderately active against *Porphyromonas* spp. (MIC_{50}, 0.25 μg/ml) and *Prevotella bivia* (MIC, 2 μg/ml). Among gram-positive bacteria, evernimicin is inactive against *Propionibacterium acnes* (MIC_{50}, >16 μg/ml).

7. MECHANISM OF ACTION

Using evernimicin-resistant mutants of *S. pneumoniae*, it has been shown that evernimicin can act on domain V of 23S rRNA of the 50S ribosomal subunit, but at a site different from that of the macrolides, lincosamides, streptogramin B, and oxazolidinones. Mutations occur mainly at the adenine (A→C) at position 2469 and the cytosine (C→U) at position 2480, which interact with the ribosomal protein L16. This part also interacts with the 3′ end of tRNA and forms part of site A. The binding of tRNA has also been described as a function of protein L16.

Evernimicin inhibits protein synthesis by interfering with the (3′) tRNA binding site at site A of the ribosome (Fig. 8).

Evernimicin acts by inhibiting protein synthesis. However, its action is exerted on the ribosomal protein L16, which is at the interface of the two ribosomal subunits.

Protein L16 appears to be involved in the fixation of the aminoacyl stem of the tRNA to the ribosome at its A-site.

Evernimicin occupies the same ribosome site that is required for initiation factor 2 (IF-2) and aminoacyl-tRNA interactions. Evernimicin inhibits the early step of translation by interfering with aminoacyl-tRNA binding. Evernimicin inhibits the stimulating activity of IF-2 during initiation complex formation. The site is immediately adjacent to the nucleotide methylated by AviRb (see below).

It was shown that evernimicin is able to block the synthesis of the 50S ribosomal subunit.

8. MECHANISMS OF RESISTANCE

Mechanisms of resistance to evernimicin are complex phenomena which include mainly mutations, methylation, and efflux. Recently it was shown that avilamycin A and evernimicin share common mechanisms of resistance.

8.1. Mutations

In *Enterococcus faecalis, Enterococcus faecium, S. pneumoniae,* and *S. aureus*, mutations in the *rplP* gene, which encodes ribosomal protein L16, confer resistance to avilamycin A and evernimicin.

Mutations occur mainly on domain V of the 23S rRNA at positions 2469 (A→C) and 2480 (C→U). Other mutations have been reported at positions 2535 (G→A) and 2536 (G→C).

The mutations occur both in the *rplP* gene (protein L16) in *S. pneumoniae* and *S. aureus* and in domain V of the 23S rRNA of *S. pneumoniae* and *Halobacterium halobium*. The *rplP* gene mutations have been also reported for enterococcal isolates resistant to avilamycin A.

In protein L16, an Arg51→His mutation has been detected for an *E. faecalis* strain, and this mutation could be associated with high MICs for evernimicin (8 to 16 μg/ml). By chemical mutagenesis, Arg51→His and Cys changes have been obtained in *S. aureus*; these mutations cause a marked increase in the MIC of evernimicin (30 to 60 times). The Arg51→His change has been also reported for *S. pneumoniae* mutants obtained by site-directed mutagenesis. Other mutations in *E. faecium* have been reported at positions 52 (Ile→Thr) and 56 (Arg→His) (Fig. 8).

8.2. Methylations

Apparently three methylated sites have been reported.

Avilamycin A producer *S. viridochromogenes* Tü 57 possesses three resistance factors that protect the organism from its own metabolites. Two of these factors (AviRa and AviRb) are methyltransferases, whereas the third factor is an ATP-binding cassette-type efflux pump.

Expression of AviRb in *Streptomyces lividans* renders the bacterium highly resistant to avilamycin A, whereas AviRa expression confers low-level resistance to avilamycin A. AviRb targets the 2′ position of nucleotide U2479 ribose, in which AviRb adds a single methyl group. AviRa adds a

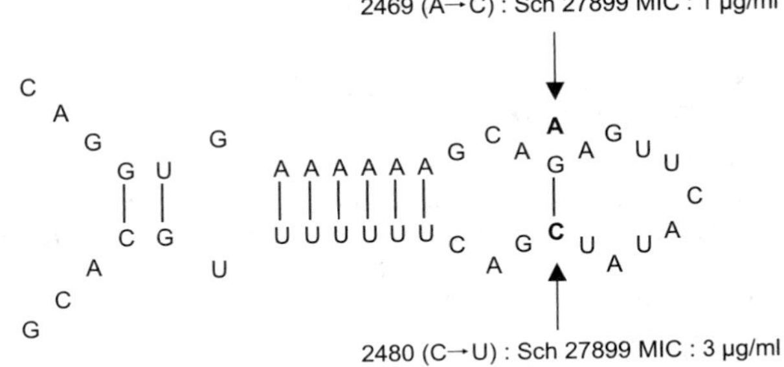

Figure 8 Mutation sites of evernimicin (SCH 27899)

single methyl group to the base of 23S rRNA nucleotide G2585 (helix 91).

The third methyltransferase was described for an *E. faecium* strain and is encoded on a transposon. This methyltransferase, EmtA, is able to add a methyl group on nucleotide G2470 of 23S rRNA, at position N-1 of the base (helix 89).

The methylations and the mutations are all located close to the IF-2 site, indicating that the IF-2 binding site overlaps that of orthosomycin compounds.

9. PHARMACODYNAMICS

In a model of infection of the thigh in neutropenic mice infected with strains of *S. pneumoniae*, *S. aureus*, and *E. faecalis* exhibiting different phenotypes of resistance to antibiotics, it has been shown that the best predictive parameter of the pharmacodynamics of evernimicin is the area under the curve (AUC)/MIC ratio, the pharmacodynamics of evernimicin being concentration dependent.

10. PHARMACOKINETICS

10.1. Plasma Pharmacokinetics

10.1.1. Healthy Young Volunteers

At the end of a 1-h infusion of 6 mg/kg of body weight in 16 volunteers, the concentration in plasma was between 49.1 and 55.2 μg/ml, with an AUC of 47 to 48.5 μg·h/ml. The plasma clearance was 34.3 to 29.7 ml/h/kg, with a mean apparent elimination half-life of 13 h.

The steady-state apparent volume of distribution is on the order of 22 liters, indicating that evernimicin is distributed in the extravascular media. The concentrations in plasma and pharmacokinetic parameters are 15% higher in women. Ascending doses of evernimicin were administered to Japanese volunteers in the form of a 1-h infusion. The pharmacokinetics were linear between 1 and 9 mg/kg, and the plasma clearance was between 31 and 46 ml/h/kg, with an AUC that increased proportionally to the dose (Table 4).

Sixty volunteers received ascending doses of evernimicin in the form of a 60-min infusion once daily for 13 days. The subjects were divided into groups of 6 subjects (doses of 1, 3, 6, 9, and 12 mg/kg). The pharmacokinetics are shown in Table 5. There was little plasma accumulation on day 13, with a ratio of between 1.2 and 1.5. The pharmacokinetics were linear at doses up to 9 mg/kg, but not above, as shown by the nonproportionality of the AUCs between 9 and 12 mg/kg.

Five groups of four patients, distributed according to their creatinine clearance, received a 30-min infusion of 3 mg of evernimicin per kg. Because of the weak elimination of evernimicin in the urine (about 5% of the administered dose), the dosage or rhythm of administration did not need to be adjusted in renally impaired patients.

Evernimicin is not dialyzable. In animals, evernimicin is eliminated principally by the hepatobiliary route.

10.1.2. Intracellular Accumulation

Evernimicin rapidly penetrates THP-1 monocytes, where it reaches a plateau in 20 min. The ratio of cellular to extracellular concentrations is 16.7 ± 2.1 (mean ± standard deviation).

10.1.3. Metabolism

Less than 2% of the product was metabolized after a 1-h infusion of [^{14}C]evernimicin (437 mg/72 μCi). The main metabolites are di- or monoglucuronides, di- or monosulfates, or hydrolysis products of the orthoester structures.

10.1.4. Passage into the Cerebrospinal Fluid

An experimental study of induced pneumococcal meningitis in the rabbit appeared to show weak penetration of evernimicin into the cerebrospinal fluid.

Table 4 Pharmacokinetics of evernimicin at ascending doses

Dose (mg/kg)	C_{max} (μg/ml)	$t_{1/2}$ (h)	$AUC_{0-\infty}$ (μg·h/ml)	CL_P (ml/h/kg)
1	8.5 ± 0.7	15.1 ± 2.3	22.5 ± 6.1	46 ± 11
3	29.7 ± 5.2	14.2 ± 1.2	88.0 ± 19.6	37 ± 7
6	55.7 ± 5.3	17.4 ± 0.6	202 ± 15	31 ± 3
9	84.3 ± 6.1	18.4 ± 2.0	283 ± 23	34 ± 3

Table 5 Pharmacokinetics of evernimicin at repeated ascending doses

Parameter	Day	Value at dose (mg/kg):				
		1	3	6	9	12
C_0 (μg/ml)	1	11.4	34.6	63.9	98.8	109
	13	11.8	37.4	69.7	104	129
AUC_{0-24} (μg·h/ml)	1	22.5	73.4	187	304	320
	13	27.1	92.2	252	443	481
$t_{1/2\beta}$ (h)	1	6.8	13	14	16	16
	13	7.0	14	18	24	19
CL_P (ml/h/kg)	1	42	36	28	24	30
	13	38	33	24	21	25
Accumulation (%)	13	1.22	1.27	1.42	1.46	1.50

11. CLINICAL INDICATIONS

In a phase II study, 55 patients suffering from pneumococcal respiratory tract infections rated as nonsevere received either 3 or 6 mg of evernimicin per kg or 2 g of ceftriaxone daily for 3 days, followed by oral treatment with amoxicillin for 7 days. For 40 of the 53 patients a strain of *S. pneumoniae* was isolated from the purulent sputum, and for 6 of them it was isolated from blood cultures as well.

A favorable clinical response was obtained in 94% of patients on day 4 of treatment in all groups of patients.

12. CONCLUSION

Evernimicin (SCH 27899) was expected to add to the existing therapeutic arsenal for the treatment of infections due to gram-positive bacteria, particularly those due to methicillin-resistant strains of staphylococci. The lack of cross-resistance with vancomycin and teicoplanin might also provide an additional therapeutic weapon against so-called GISA strains (strains of reduced susceptibility, if not resistant, to vancomycin, as described in Guatemala in 1999). Likewise, its activity against vancomycin-resistant strains of *E. faecium* would provide an adjunct to drugs such as Synercid (dalfopristin-quinipristin). However, its in vitro activity against the various species of coagulase-negative staphylococci, with the exception of *S. epidermidis*, is one of the weak features of this molecule.

Evernimicin was thought to be an alternative in severe pneumococcal infections for which no other treatment is possible because of a multiresistant strain (β-lactams and macrolide-lincosamide-streptogram compounds, including linezolid).

Unfortunately the development process was given up for obvious reasons.

REFERENCES

Banfield CR, Glue P, Affrime MB, et al, 1997, Multiple-dose safety, tolerance, and pharmacokinetics of Ziracin® (Sch 27899): a new novel oligosaccharide antibiotic, 37th Intersci Conf Antimicrob Agents Chemother, abstract A-114.

Bauernfeind A, Jungwirth R, 1993, The in vitro activity of everninomicin in comparison with vancomycin and teicoplanin, 33rd Intersci Conf Antimicrob Agents Chemother, abstract 458.

Black J, Calesnick B, Falco FG, Weinstein MJ, 1965, Pharmacological properties of everninomicin D, Antimicrob Agents Chemother, p 38–46.

Boyce JM, Medeiros AA, 1993, In vitro activity of Sch 27899 against multi-drug resistant gram-positive cocci, 33rd Intersci Conf Antimicrob Agents Chemother, abstract 466.

Chin NX, Neu HC, 1993, In vitro activity of Sch 27899 against aerobic and anaerobic gram-positive Haemophilus influenzae and Moraxella, 33rd Intersci Conf Antimicrob Agents Chemother, abstract 465.

Cormican MG, Marshall SA, Jones RN, 1995, Preliminary interpretative criteria for disk diffusion susceptibility testing of everninomicin, 35th Intersci Conf Antimicrob Agents Chemother.

Ganguly AK, Pramanik B, Chan TM, Sarre O, Liu YT, Morton J, Girijavallabban V, 1989, The structure of new oligosaccharide antibiotics 13-384 components 1 and 5, Heterocycles, 28, 83–88.

Luedemann GM, Brodsky BC, 1965, Micromonospora carbonacea sp n, an everninomicin-producing organism, Antimicrob Agents Chemother, 5, 47–52.

Menon S, Pai S, Banfield CR, Cayen M, Affrime MB, Batra V, 1997, Effect of gender on the pharmacokinetics of Ziracin® (Sch 27899) in healthy volunteers, 37th Intersci Conf Antimicrob Agents Chemother, abstract A-113.

Nakashio S, Iwasawa H, Dun FY, Kanemitsu K, Shimada J, 1995, Everninomicin, a new oligosaccharide antibiotic: its antimicrobial activity, post-antibiotic effect and synergistic bactericidal activity, Drugs Exptl Clin Res, 21, 7–16.

Nishino T, Sakurai M, 1993, In vitro activity of everninomicin (Sch 27899), 33rd Intersci Conf Antimicrob Agents Chemother, abstract 462.

Schlaes DM, Schlaes H, Etter L, Hare RS, Miller GH, 1993, Sch 27899, an everninomicin active against multiply-resistant enterococci and staphylococci, 33rd Intersci Conf Antimicrob Agents Chemother, abstract 460.

Urban C, Mariano N, Mosinka-Snipas K, Wadee C, Chahrour T, Rahal JJ, 1993, Comparative in vitro activity of Sch 27899, a novel everninomicin, 33rd Intersci Conf Antimicrob Agents Chemother, abstract 463.

Vesga O, Craig WA, 1997, In vivo pharmacodynamic activity of Sch 27899 (Ziracin®), an everninomicin antibiotic, 37th Intersci Conf Antimicrob Agents Chemother, abstract A-32.

Weinstein MJ, Luedemann GM, Oden EM, Wagman GH, 1965, Everninomicin, a new antibiotic complex from Micromonospora carbonacea, Antimicrob Agents Chemother, p 24–32.

Peptidyl Deformylase Inhibitors

ANDRÉ BRYSKIER AND JOHN LOWTHER

39

1. INTRODUCTION

The spread of resistance among gram-positive and gram-negative bacteria and parasites resulted in an intensive research for novel compounds acting on unexploited bacterial targets. One of them is a protein: peptidyl deformylase (PDF).

2. PDF

PDF is a prokyarotic metalloprotease essential for bacterial growth which was described in the 1960s (Adams, 1968; Marker and Sanger, 1964). The enzyme was not characterized until 1993, when the deformylase gene, *def,* was cloned and PDF was overexpressed in *Escherichia coli* (Rajagopalan et al., 1997).

An exhaustive review was issued recently on deformylase and inhibitors (Yuan et al., 2001).

2.1. Classification

Metallohydrolases may be classified in at least four subfamilies.

2.1.1. PDF

Bacterial PDF belongs to subfamily 3, with at least two other members: thermolysin and matrix metalloproteases (MMPs), namely, matricins and/or metzincins. MMPs are a major group of enzymes that regulate cell matrix composition. The MMPs are time-dependent endopeptidases known for their ability to cleave one or several extracellular matrix constituents as well as nonmatrix proteins.

All have a histidine and a glutamate as the third metalloligand. PDF has a hydrophobic "cork" blocking one end of the active crevice. This extremity is open in thermolysin and MMPs, allowing these enzymes to act as endoproteases. The cork is believed to play an important role in restricting the selectivity of PDF as an aminopeptidase. This subfamily also contains the HEXXH motif.

PDFs can be subdivided into three classes. Class I consists of *E. coli* PDFs, class II is composed of PDFs from gram-positive bacteria and some fastidious gram-negative bacteria, and class III may be constituted by sequences from kinetoplastid protists.

Perhaps a fourth class may be proposed: two adjacent PDF-like genes have been identified in *Drosophila melanogaster.*

There are partially expressed sequence tags encoding PDF homologs in mice and humans. The genomic fragment is known, but the intracellular location and exact function of these PDF-like sequences are unknown.

Class I and class II PDFs have two sequence insertions at the N-terminal end just upstream from the α-helix and the β_1-strand of motif 1, which is located at the entrance of the active site of PDF.

The C-terminal domains of class II PDFs contain many hydrophobic amino acids, whereas those of class I PDFs do not. This suggests that the C-terminal domains of class II PDFs may not fold into α-helices.

In *E. coli,* two forms can be distinguished. Form I retains a zinc ion which is poorly active. In this form the HEXXH motif is present, as for thermolysin and metzincins. Form II corresponds to an apoenzyme with a ferrous ion. It is believed to be the physiologically active protein.

More than 80 bacterial PDF sequences have been identified. Similar sequences were also identified in higher plants: the small mustard plant *Arabidopsis thaliana,* tomato, corn, rice, turnip, lotus, alfalfa, and wheat. Deformylases have been shown to occur in some alga chloroplasts and in various plant mitochondria and chloroplasts. PDF is not present in the organelles of animals or fungal cells. The protein synthesis in mammalian mitochondria retains the *N*-formyl group. PDFs have been reported for *Plasmodium falciparum, Trypanosoma cruzi, and Leishmania* spp.

Def homologs have been identified in all eubacteria, but not in *Archaea, Saccharomyces cerevisiae,* or the nematode *Caenorhabditis elegans.*

Bacillus subtilis contains an additional deformylase-like gene called *ykrB* whose product is similar to the class II deformylase from *Bacillus stearothermophilus* (Haas et al., 2001).

In plants such as *A. thaliana* and *Lycopersicon esculentum,* there are two PDFs: PDF1A and PDF1B. (Table 1). The amino acid sequences of these two PDFs display less than 25% similarity (Giglione et al., 2000b; Sereno et al., 2001).

Table 1 Structure of PDFs of two higher plants

Plant	PDF	No. of amino acids	Mol wt
A. thaliana	PDF1A	192	21.6
	PDF1B	193	21.9
L. esculentum	PDF1A	190	21.0
	PDF1B	197	2.3

The characteristics of PDF1A include the following:

- Zinc ion
- Differs significantly from eubacterial PDFs except that of *Streptomyces coelicolor*
- Is found only in mitochondria
- Is present in most vertebrate insects and in humans

The characteristics of PDF1B include the following:

- Closely related to cyanobacterial PDFs
- Found in the two organelles (chloroplasts and mitochondria)
- Ferrous ion
- Found in plants and *P. falciparum*

They have distinct localization in the plant cells.

These proteins are composed of two domains: an N-terminal presequence attaching the protein to the organelle and a C-terminal catalytic domain.

PDFs 1A and 1B display deformylase activity similar to that of *E. coli*, *Thermus thermophilus*, and *Bacillus stearothermophilus*.

2.1.2. MAP

Two classes of aminopeptidases have been described: MAP-1 and MAP-2. MAP-1 and MAP-2 have similar specificities, with methionine cleavage depending on the nature of the second amino acid.

MAP-2 is inhibited by fumagillin and TNP-470 (Fig. 1).

Yeast and mammalian cells also possess a MAP-1 protein which exhibits a catalytic core, as does bacterial MAP-1.

MAP-1 and MAP-2 are located in the cytoplasm of eukaryotic cells.

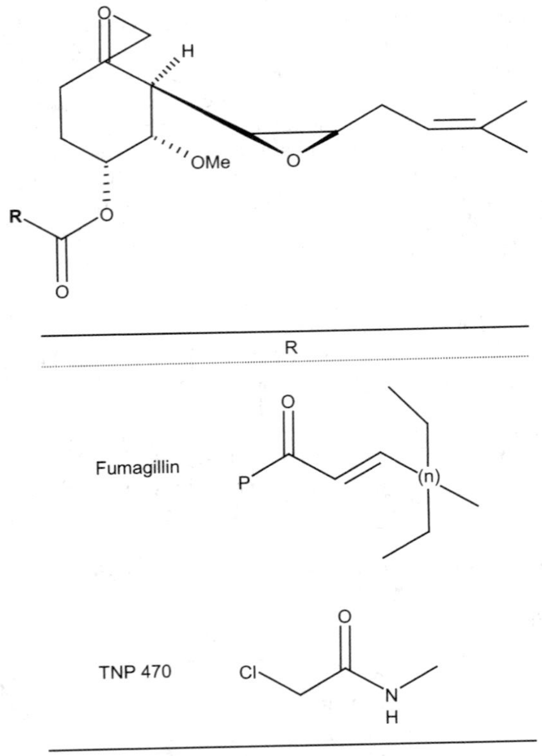

Figure 1 Fumagillin and TNP-470

2.2. Genetics

The *def* gene encodes PDF and is present in all sequenced bacterial genomes. It is not possible to construct null mutants of the *def* gene in wild-type *E. coli*, suggesting that the gene is essential for growth. Many gram-negative organisms, including *E. coli*, have one chromosomal copy of the *def* gene; however, most of the gram-positive bacteria have two homologs. The wild type of *E. coli* is naturally resistant to actinonin.

The *fmt* gene itself is not essential for *E. coli*, *Staphylococcus aureus*, or *Pseudomonas aeruginosa*.

Mutants of *fmt* have been described and have an impaired growth phenotype. All *fmt* genes are essential for *Streptococcus pneumoniae*.

All gram-positive bacteria and a few gram-negative bacteria (e.g., *Vibrio cholerae*) which have been examined have two homologs: *defA* and *defB*. The *defB* gene has the conserved domains associated with the active site, whereas the *defA* gene does not encode a functional PDF. Its product is a deformylase paralog. The *def* gene has no mammalian counterpart. It was shown that the deformylase gene, *def*, could not be inactivated unless the transformylase gene, *fmt*, was also inactivated. Often, but not systematically, the *def* gene is expressed as the first cistron of a biscistronic unit with the *fmt* gene. The *fmt* gene encodes methionyl-tRNA formyl transferase, the enzyme responsible for addition of the formyl group onto the first methionine.

2.3. Structure

Bacterial PDFs are small monomers composed of about 160 to 200 amino acids with few variations in the lengths of their N- and C-terminal extremities. Full-length PDF is about a 19-kDa protein.

2.3.1. Amino Acids

The active site of the enzyme is composed of three motifs of amino acids: motif I (GϕGϕAAXQ), motif 2 (EGCϕS), and motif 3 (HEϕDH), where ϕ is a hydrophobic amino acid and X is any amino acid. The three motifs are from the three sides of the active-site crevice. The metal ion is liganded by two histidine residues, a cysteine residue, and a water molecule.

Some amino acids are essential, such as Gln50 in motif 1 and Glu133 in motif 2, which are involved in formyl group recognition, as well as the carboxylate of glutamate in motif 2.

The link between the amino acids of the different motifs is complex. The cysteine of motif 2 and the two histidines of motif 3 are involved in metal cation binding. The hydrogen of the serine side chain of motif 2 bonds with the glutamine side chain of motif 1. The carboxylates of the glutamate of motif 2 and the aspartate of motif 3 hydrogen bond with the arginine located between motifs 2 and 3. Without these links PDF is unstable.

An asparagine located between motifs 1 and 2 is hydrogen bonded with the backbone of an amino acid located at the N terminus of the protein. Glycine and alanine side chains in motif 1 are essential for catalysis. The alternate hydrophobic and hydrophilic residues in motif 1 are involved in the formation of the β_1-strand. It has been shown that the PDF of *E. coli* is an α/β-type protein where a central helix is wrapped by a five-stranded anti-parallel β-sheet and by a two-stranded anti-parallel β-sheet.

The side chains thought to participate in the catalytic process are strictly conserved in the PDF family. Most of them belong to the three signatures sequences: GXGLAAXQ, ECGCLS, and QHEXDH. In addition, two carboxylic groups of the last two motifs make salt bridges with the guanidium groups of an isolated but strictly conserved arginine. The NH group at R2 is crucial for catalysis and for substrate recognition. Peptides with acidic groups at R3 or R4 display significantly reduced deformylation efficacies compared to the wild type and less acidic peptides.

2.3.2. Metal Ion Center

The liability of PDF was shown to be due to sensitivity of the catalytic ferrous ion to environmental oxygen. The ferrous ion in PDF is unstable and can be quickly and irreversibly oxidized to the ferric ion, resulting in an inactive enzyme. Several laboratories have replaced the ferrous ion (Fe^{2+}) with Zn^{2+}, Mg^{2+}, Ni^{2+}, and Co^{2+}, or cadmium through reconstitution or overexpression in defined medium. The metal ion allows two lobes of the protein to be linked. Zinc enzyme has weak PDF activity even if *E. coli* PDF can bind a zinc cation (Meinnel et al., 1995).

2.3.3. Active Center

The three-dimensional structure of PDF shows a large hydrophobic active site. The only ionizable groups are the metal-bound water and the side chain of Cys90, Glu133, His132, and His137. Glu133 may help ionize the metal-bound water by abstracting one of the water protons and/or facilitate the leaving NH-R group by protonation. Glu133 must be required as donating a proton to the leaving amide ion.

The catalytic metal ion of PDF is tetrahedrally coordinated with two histidines (HEXXH motif) and a serine from the EGCLS motif. A water molecule that presumably hydrolyzes the amide bond occupies the fourth position in the tetrahedron (Fig. 2).

2.3.4. Function

2.3.4.1. Mode of Action of the Enzyme Sequence

Deformylation is part of the methionine cycle involved in the protein synthesis of at least five enzymes:

- Methionyl-tRNA synthetase
- Methionyl-tRNA^{FMet} formyl transferase
- Deformylase (PDF)

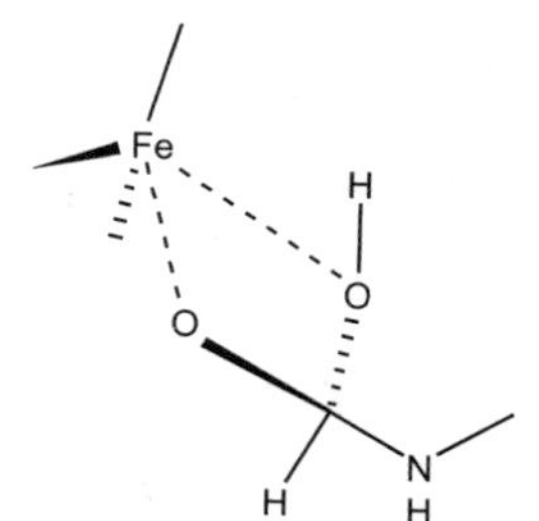

Figure 2 Ferrous ion binding

- Methionine aminopeptidase
- Peptidytl-tRNA hydrolase

A methionyl-tRNA-synthetase adds a methionine to the 3′CCA end (terminal adenine in tRNA^{Met}). Before forming the ternary complex with an mRNA and the 30S ribosomal subunit, methionyl-tRNA must be modified by a tRNA^{fMet} transformylase.

A formyl group from N^{10}-formyltetrahydrofolate is transferred by the formyl transferase to the amino goup of tRNA^{Met}. In eubacteria, this step is believed to be essential for interaction with initiation factor 2. The N-terminal sequence has a transient function, and most proteins are synthesized as precursor proteins. The N-terminal sequence of a polypeptide chain appears to be a major determinant of its fate. It can act as a signal sequence.

Following translation initiation, the PDF cleaves the formyl group from the nascent polypeptide. The *N*-formylmethionine is removed by the sequential action of PDF and aminopeptidase. Then the methionyl aminopeptidase removes the N-terminal methionine from certain deformylated peptides to produce mature proteins depending on the identity of the penultimate residue (Fig. 3 and 4).

2.3.4.2. PDF and MAP Activities

In the prokaryotic cell (bacteria mainly), unlike in mammalian cells, protein synthesis starts with a formylated

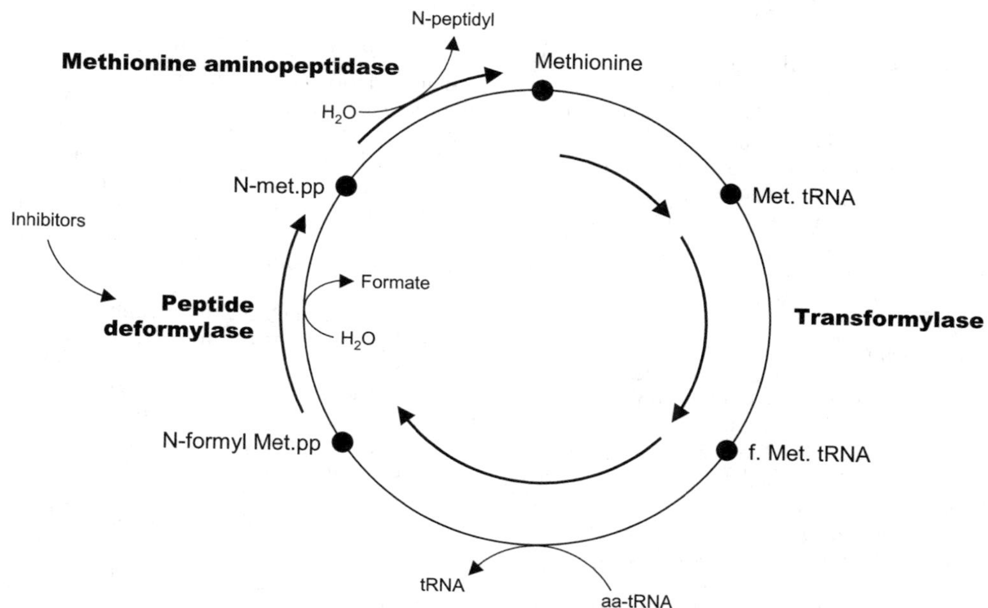

Figure 3 Formylation-deformylation cycle

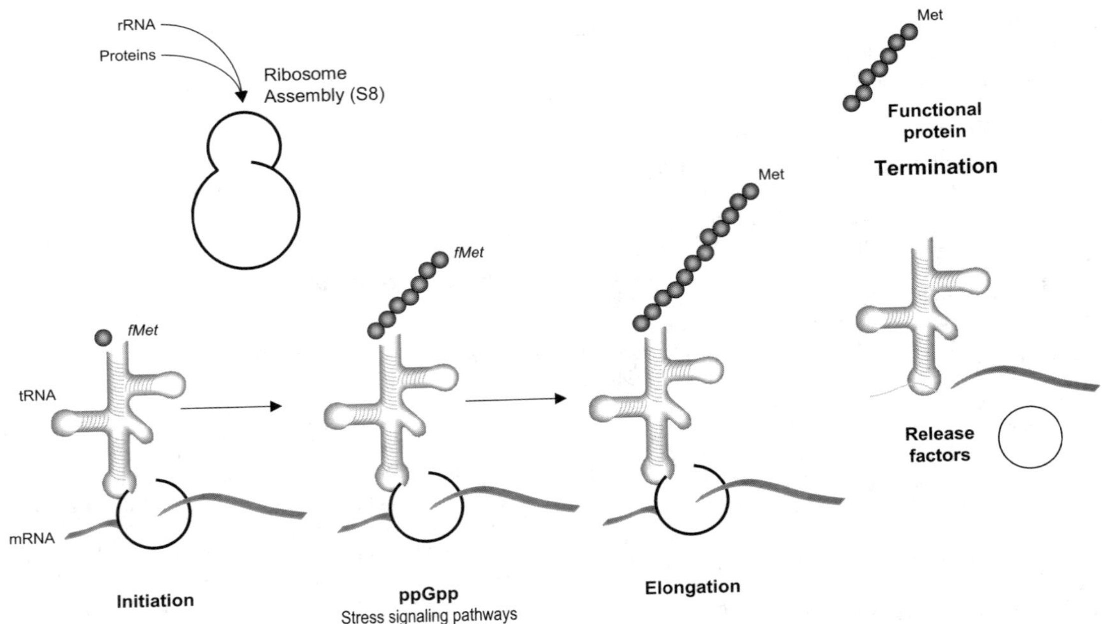

Figure 4 Protein synthesis process

methionine residue. It was recently reported that not all bacteria require the formylation pathway. Although N-formylation is not strictly essential for the survival of the bacteria, it can stimulate protein synthesis by facilitating the use of Met-tRNA in translation initiation and preventing its recognition by the elongation apparatus. The removal or maintenance of the methionine depends on the nature of the second amino acid of the polypeptide chain.

PDF specificity is more uniform because only a minority (four) of the sequences escape deformylation. The nature of the second residue seems to have little effect, whatever the characteristic of the side chains: hydrophilic (Asn and Thr), hydrophobic (Leu), positively charged (Arg), or negatively charged (Glu).

MAP cleavage seems to depend on the length of the side chain of the second amino acid. This rule is well respected for Ala, Gly, Pro, Ser, Val, Cys, and Thr. If the side chain is large (Arg, Asn, Glu, Ile, Leu, and Lys), the initiator methionine at the N terminus of the mature protein is retained.

In *E. coli* and plant organelles, many proteins have cleaved and uncleaved methionine according to the presence of Val as a second amino acid. Valine appears to be an amino acid whose side chain is intermediate for the specificity of MAP.

However, certain membrane proteins are known to retain their *N*-formyl group, such as leader peptidase, aspartate chemoreceptor, ATPase component, and H subunit of the photosynthetase reaction center.

Deformylation is a prerequisite. Methionine aminopeptidase is unable to hydrolyze *N*-blocked methionine polypeptides. PDF exhibits strict substrate specificity for *N*-formyl peptides, being weakly active against N-acetylated peptides or having no endopeptidase activity. N-formylated methionine di- or tripeptides are PDF substrates, including the chemotactic peptide *N*-formyl-Met-Leu-Phe, but *N*-formyl methionine itself is poorly hydrolyzed by PDF. PDF has a preference for *N*-formyl methionine peptide over formylated peptides, except for *N*-formyl-L-norleucine peptide.

PDF also shows a strict stereoselectivity for N-formyl-L-methionine peptide substrate over the D-amino acid. The specificity of *N*-formyl group recognition is strong, with the conserved glutamine of motif 1 playing a crucial role in this process.

Two amino acids are necessary for efficient catalysis.

The deformylation is a requirement for activity of MAP. It is probably an essential process in eubacteria.

It has been suggested that in bacteria, proteins can escape PDF action if their N termini are located at the exoplasmic surface of the membrane.

2.3.5. Resistance to PDF and MAP

If deformylation is blocked, resistance might occur due to mutations, inactivating the *fmt* gene. However, the *fmt*-containing mutants grow very poorly, and such resistance is not believed to be a major obstacle. Nevertheless, fast-growing *fmt*-containing mutants have been isolated. Resistance to PDF inhibitors has been reported for *S. aureus*, *E. coli*, and *S. pneumoniae*. The mechanism of resistance is based on the loss of transformylase activity. However, the biological cost for *S. aureus* is a reduction of growth, and virulence is attenuated. Resistant mutants of *S. pneumoniae* harbor mutations in the *defB* gene but not in the *fmt* gene. Resistant strains possessed a single missense mutation in *defB* (Q172K). This position lies immediately upstream of the $_{173}$HEXXH$_{177}$ motif. A nonconservative substitution (Q131A) at the equivalent position in the *E. coli* enzyme has been shown to decrease enzyme activity. Mutation at A133D was observed. The mutation introduces a charge amino acid five residues upstream of the $_{128}$EGCLS$_{132}$ motif, which has been shown to be involved in binding the metal ion. The frequencies of mutation are 10^{-8} and 10^{-6} for *S. pneumoniae* ATCC 49619 and *S. aureus* ATCC 25923, respectively (Margolis et al., 2000, 2001).

3. DEFORMYLASE INHIBITORS

PDF is a bacterial target for the discovery of new antibacterials (Giglione et al., 2000a).

To date most of all of the synthetic compounds are derived from the natural compound actinonin. All of the published PDFs share the same link with the ferrous ion (Fig. 5). X represents a chelating pharmacophore (hydroxomate or *N*-formyl hydroxamic acid) that is the major component in providing binding energy. The *n*-butyl group mimics the methionine side chain and fills the deep S1′ hydrophobic pocket in the PDF active site. R2 and R3 are regions of the inhibitors that can provide additional binding energy, selectivity, and favorable pharmacokinetic properties. Deformylase inhibitors can be classified in three groups: natural compounds, hydroxamate derivatives, and miscellaneous compounds (Fig. 6).

3.1. Actinonin

Actinonin is a natural hydroxamic acid pseudopeptide (Fig. 7) which was isolated in 1962 but was only tested for antibacterial activity in the 1970s. Actinonin is produced by actinomycetes (Gordon et al., 1962). The PDF-inhibitory activity was discovered (Chen et al., 2000) after screening of a chemical library of compounds having a hydroxamic moiety chelating with a 50% inhibitory concentration (IC_{50}) of $<10^{-5}$M. The hydroxamic moiety is crucial for the antibacterial activity, but the pseudopeptide backbone can be altered, such as the methionine-like structure.

In addition to the antibacterial activity, it was shown that actinonin inhibits several aminopeptidases, such as human seminal alanyl aminopeptidase, as well as tumor growth.

Depending on the metal ion, the IC_{50}s vary (Table 2). The affinity is less important when the metal ion is zinc and the strongest with a ferrous ion.

The antibacterial activity of actinonin is summarized in Table 3. Actinonin is bacteriostatic even at 10 times the MIC. At 24 h after exposure the reduction of viable cells is $\leq$1.0 $\log_{10}$ CFU/ml for *S. aureus*.

Actinonin is a tight-binding inhibitor of PDF, with a K_i of 0.28 nM.

All inhibitors favor a four-carbon side chain with various substituents. The compounds with other metal binding groups are much weaker inhibitors of PDF. IC_{50}s are listed in Table 4.

The proline moiety of actinonin may be removed and changed, but the pseudopeptide backbone needs to be retained.

The K_i varies according to the residue (Table 5).

The different groups interacting with the PDF active site have been studied. The average oxygen-nickel

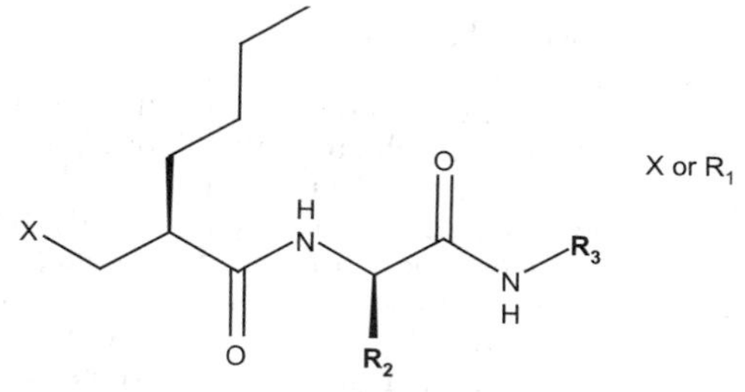

Figure 5 Basic structure of hydroxamic acid

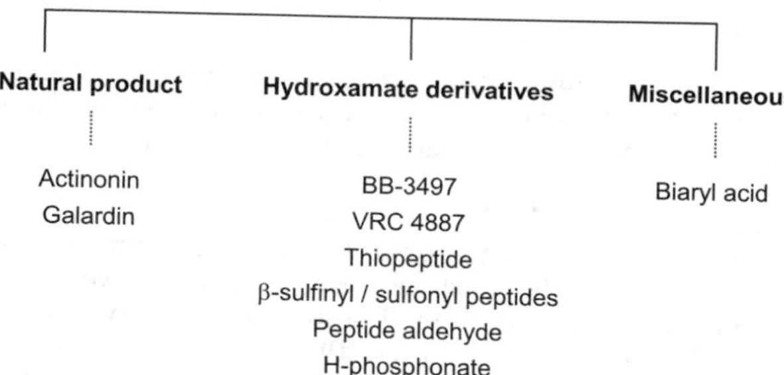

Figure 6 Classification of inhibitors of PDF

Figure 7 Actinonin

Table 2 PDF versus metal ions

PDF source	Ion	IC_{50} (μM)
E. coli	Zn^{2+}	90
	Ni^{2+}	3
	Fe^{2+}	0.8
S. aureus	Ni^{2+}	11

Table 3 In vitro activity of actinonin

Microorganism	*n*	MIC (mg/liter)
S. aureus	4	8–16
S. epidermidis	2	2–4
E. faecium	2	32–64
S. pneumoniae	1	8
S. pyogenes	1	8
E. coli acr	1	0.25
E. coli	1	>64
H. influenzae	3	1–8
Haemophilus parainfluenzae	1	0.13
M. catarrhalis	1	0.5
N. gonorrhoeae	3	1–4
B. fragilis	1	0.25
P. aeruginosa	1	128

Table 4 Inhibition of various metalloproteases by actinonin

Protein[a]	IC_{50} (nM)
Ni-PDF	10
MMP-1	1,000
MMP-2	3,000
MMP-3	6,000
MMP-7	60%[b]
Encephalokinase	7,000
ACE-1	$>10^5$

[a]ACE, angiotensin-converting enzyme; MMP-7, matrilysin.
[b]Percent inhibition at 100 μM.

Table 5 K_i **values for various groups**

Groups	K_i (μM)
Hydroxamic methionine-like	0.28
Phosphonate	37
Sulfhydroxyl	2.5
Formaldehyde	9.5

distance is 2.1Å (to the carbonyl oxygen atom of the *N*-formylhydroxylamine or the nitrogen-bound oxygen atom of the *N*-formylhydroxylamine). Hydrogen bonds are made to the hydroxamate or R1 formylhydroxylamine by the side chain of Gln133 and Gln50 and the main-chain NH of Leu91.

There is hydrogen bound between the main-chain NH of Ile44 and R1 carbonyl and Gly89 and R2.

The hydrophobic pocket is delineated by residues Ile44, Ile86, Glu88, Leu125, Ile129, and His132 and is occupied by the *n*-pentyl side chain of actinonin. The pyrrolidine ring interacts with Glu87. The isopropyl side chain does not make interactions, especially with Arg97 (Fig. 8).

Actinonin was not further developed due to the poor bioavailability and the lack of in vivo efficacies. For instance, in rats no actinonin was detected in blood following an oral dose of 50 mg/kg of body weight.

3.2. Galardin

Following a screening in a chemical library it was shown that a natural product, galardin, exhibited anti-PDF activity. Galardin is a peptide hydroxamic inhibitor (Fig. 9). It belongs to the MMP family. It is a competitive inhibitor of PDF, with a K_i of 1.9 ± 0.1 μM (mean ± standard deviation). It may serve, like actinonin, as a substrate for drug discovery.

3.3. Alteration of the Hydroxamic Acid Scaffold

Numerous teams are working on the original hydroxamic acid core in order to improve the antibacterial activity and especially to obtain a bactericidal compound, to enlarge the antibacterial spectrum, and to improve the toxicological

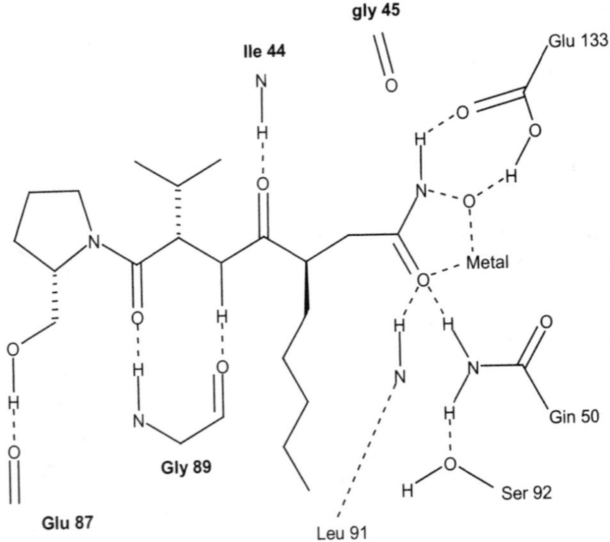

Figure 8 **Actinonin interactions in PDF active site**

Figure 9 **Galardin**

profile (no cytotoxicity) and the oral pharmacokinetics. For the antibacterial activity, it was needed not only to get or improve the overall affinity for the targeted enzyme but also to obtain a compound active against the whole bacterium. Within hydroxamate analogs, potent inhibitors are not always active antibacterial agents due to either poor membrane permeability, efflux pump, or intracellular metabolism.

The agents have to be selective for bacteria and to not interfere with mammalian systems.

N-Formyl-D-methionyl peptides are not PDF substrates. The identity of the R1 side chain is critical for high-affinity binding to the PDF active site. Truncation of the *n*-butyl side chain to a methyl group caused nearly a 10^3 reduction in affinity for the *E. coli* enzyme (15.7 μM). Shortening the R1 side chain by one and two methylene groups also decreased the potency about 40- and 750-fold, respectively. Even a minor change from an *n*-butyl group to isobutyl resulted in a 20-fold decrease in affinity. PDF is known to strongly prefer a methionine or norleucine and to a lesser extent a phenylalanine at the R1 position of a substrate.

3.3.1. Versicor Series

The design of inhibitors consists of having a nonspecific chelating pharmacophore that binds to the catalytic metal ion and is combined with a moiety that binds to the active site.

3.3.1.1. VRC-4232

The urea pharmacophore was tested as a constained carbonyl isostere of the alkyl succinate backbone. Two compounds were optimized by iterative parallel synthesis, VRC-3324 and VRC-3852 (Fig. 10).

In a series of *N*-alkyl urea hydroxamic acids (Hackbarth et al., 2002) several compounds achieved MICs of ≤4.0 μg/ml for gram-positive (*S. aureus* and *S. pneumoniae*) and gram-negative rods. This new series of compounds displays bacteriostatic activity against *S. pneumoniae* and *Haemophilus influenzae*. Two compounds have been selected for being less cytotoxic than those of previous series: VRC-4232 and VRC-4307 (Fig. 11). They do not exhibit any activity against *E. coli*, like actinonin (MIC, >64 μg/ml), and they are poorly active against *Enterococcus faecium* (MIC, 2 to 4 μg/ml) as well as against *S. pneumoniae* (MIC, 1.0 to 4.0 μg/ml) and *H. influenzae* (MIC, 2.0 to 4.0 μg/ml), but both have good antistaphylococcal activity (MIC, 0.25 to 1.0 μg/ml). Both show cross-resistance with other hydroxamic acid derivatives.

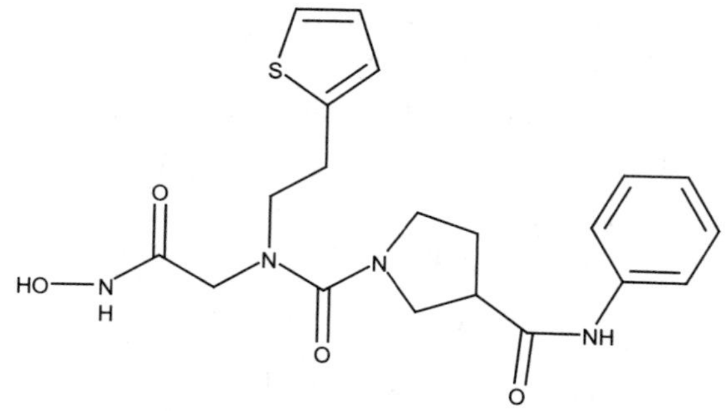

Figure 10 VRC-3324 and VRC-3852

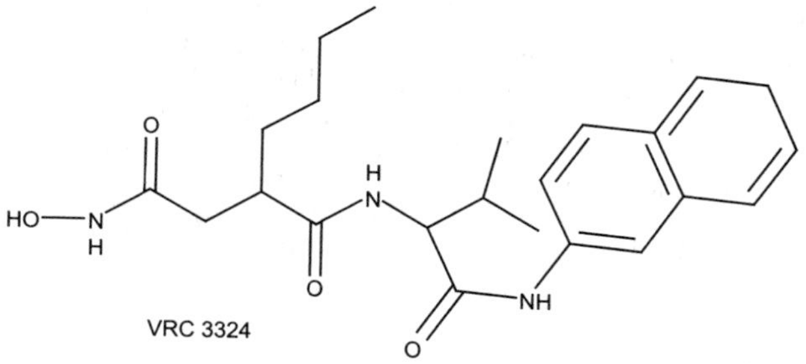

The pharmacokinetics have been studied in mice and are listed in Table 6. Both compounds are rapidly metabolized in vivo by mice and in vitro by rat microsomes (Fig. 12).

By the subcutaneous route the 50% effective doses (ED_{50}) are 30.8 and 17.9 mg/kg for VRC-4232 and VRC-4307, respectively.

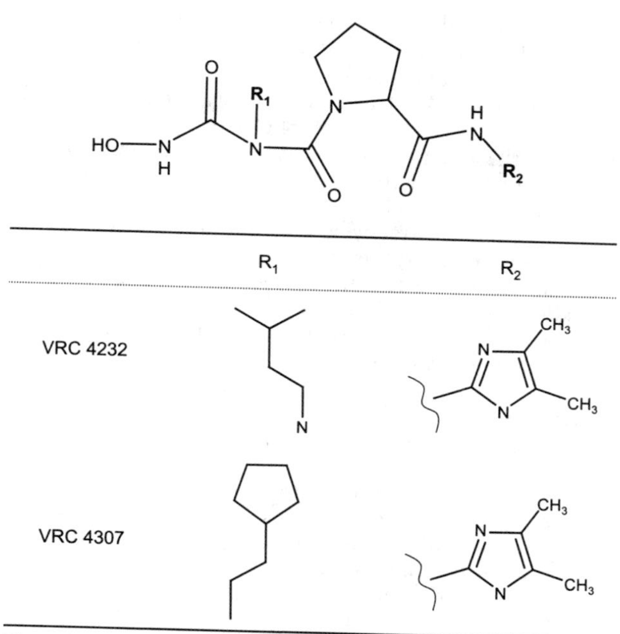

Figure 11 VRC-4232 and VRC-4307

VRC-4307 is a potent Ni-PDF inhibitor.

A series of 22 compounds has been synthesized to analyze the structure-activity relationships that could lead to the discovery of potent PDF inhibitors but with less cytotoxicity.

Only proline at R2 provides antibacterial activity with a minimum of cytotoxicity. Compounds with *p*-chlorobenzyl, cyclopentyl, or isopropyl at the R3 position are more likely to be associated with cytotoxicity.

3.3.1.2. VRC-3375

VRC-3375, with proline at R2 and *ter*-butyl ester at R3, was selected for further investigation (Fig. 13). (Chen et al.,

Table 6 Pharmacokinetics of VRC-4232 and VRC-4307 in mice

Compound	Dose (mg/kg)	Route[a]	C_{max} (ng/ml)	T_{max} (h)	AUC (ng·h/ml)	$t_{1/2}$ (h)	Bioavailability (%)
VRC-4232	13	i.v.	5.58	0.08	1.12	1.1	
		p.o.	0.167	0.08	0.035	ND[b]	3.2
VRC-4307	3.7	i.v.	1.72	0.08	0.413	0.1	
		p.o.	0.015	0.25	0.003	ND	0.1

[a]i.v., intravenous; p.o., per os.
[b]ND, not determined.

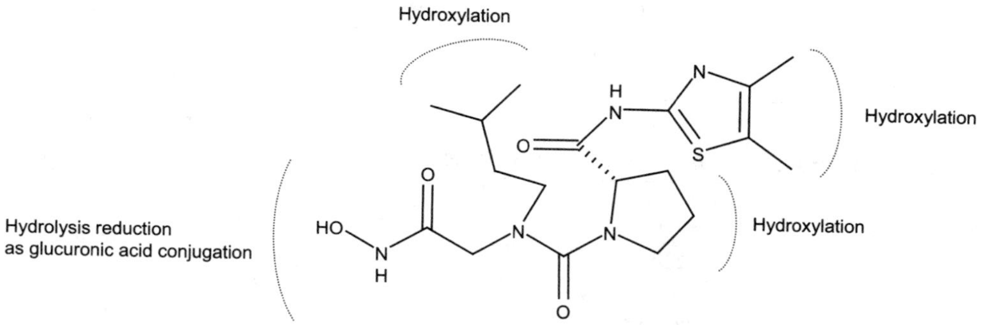

Figure 12 Metabolism of VRC-4232

2004; Jain et al., 2003). Optimization of VRC-3375 was carried out. In the succinate series VRC-3375 and VRC-4462 (*N*-formylhydroxolamine analogs) are the most potent agents. An IC_{50} of 4 nM for VRC-3375 against *E. coli* Ni-PDF was noted. Increasing the hydrophobicity at the R3 position improved the antibacterial activity of the PDF inhibitor.

Comparative in vitro activities of VRC-3375 and actinonin are listed in Table 7.

In disseminated staphylococcal murine infection, VRC-3375 was administered by the intravenous, subcutaneous, and oral routes to mice. The ED_{50} were 32, 7, and 21 mg/kg, respectively (vancomycin ED_{50}, 1.0 mg/kg).

Table 8 shows the pharmacokinetics in mice after 100 mg/kg as a single dose.

3.3.1.3. VRC-4237

VRC-4237 interacts at the active site of the enzyme (Fig. 14).

In another series it has been demonstrated that the α-position (R1) can tolerate only very small noncharged groups such as hydroxy or fluoro groups. Large substituents such as methoxy or methyl groups result in a loss of antibacterial activity. Compounds with charged groups are inactive.

In the α-fluoro series, the best configuration is *S* (VRC-4071), while no special preference was observed in the α-hydroxy series. At R3, linear alkyl chains improve antibacterial activity, but an increased cytotoxicity was noted. The cyclic amine substitutions reduced the cytotoxicity and MMP-7 inhibition. A piperidinyl ring leads to improved antipneumococal and antistaphylococal activities but reduced in vitro activity against *H. influenzae*. In the α-hydroxy series, aryl and heteroaryl substituents improved antibacterial activity but unfortunately also increased cytotoxicity. An increase of the hydrophobicity increases the overall activities against gram-negative bacteria. The best well-balanced analog bears a pyrrolidinyl moiety at the R3 position and an α-fluoro atom (VRC-4415). The α-hydroxy counterpart is less active in vitro, but the compounds exhibit similar in vivo activities in murine infections (ED_{50} by the intravenous route, 1.7 versus 1.2 mg/kg), suggesting better pharmacokinetics of the α-hydroxy series. However, the oral bioavailability is less than 15%. The *S*-configuration in the α-fluoro series exerts higher in vitro activity against *S. pneumoniae*, *S. aureus*, and *H. influenzae* (Table 9). However, some derivatives in the α-fluoro series exert improved antibacterial activity, such as VRC-4249 and VRC-4299 (Fig. 15).

They differ by the aryl moiety at the 3 position: a dichlorophenyl for VRC-4299 and a dimethyl thiazolyl for VRC-4249. For VRC-4299 an α-fluoro atom is fixed, compared to an α-hydroxy group for the remaining compounds.

Figure 13 VRC-3375

Table 7 In vitro activity of VRC-3375

Microorganism	*n*	MIC (μg/ml)	
		Actinonin	VRC-3375
S. aureus	3	8–16	1.0–4.0
S. epidermidis	1	4.0	1.0
E. faecalis	3	32–64	32–64
S. pneumoniae	3	8–32	8.0–32
S. pyogenes	1	8.0	64
H. influenzae	3	1.0–2.0	2.0–4.0
H. influenzae acr	1	0.13	0.13
M. catarrhalis	1	0.5	0.25
E. coli	1	>64	>64
E. coli acr	1	0.25	0.25
B. fragilis	1	0.25	1.0

Table 8 Pharmacokinetics of VRC-3375 in mice

Route[a]	C_{max} (ng/ml)	T_{max} (min)	AUC (ng·h/ml)	$t_{1/2}$ (min)
i.v.	147		2,456	16
s.c.	65.7	20	2,794	15
p.o.	43	10	1,568	15

[a]i.v., intravenous; s.c., subcutaneous; p.o., per os.

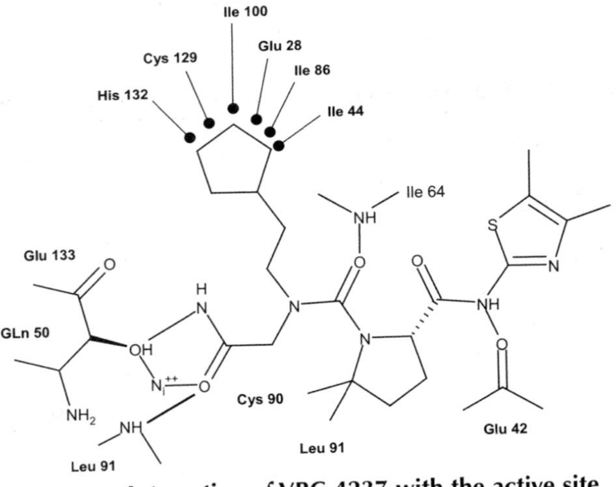

Figure 14 Interaction of VRC-4237 with the active site

Table 9 In vitro activity of the α-fluoro succinate hydroxamate

Compound	α-Fluoro	MIC (mg/liter)		
		S. pneumoniae	*S. aureus*	*H. influenzae*
VRC-4102	Racemate	16–32	>64	>64
VRC-4071	*S*-configuration	2.0–4.0	0.25–1.0	1.0–2.0
VRC-4088	*R*-configuration	16–32	2.0–8.0	16–32

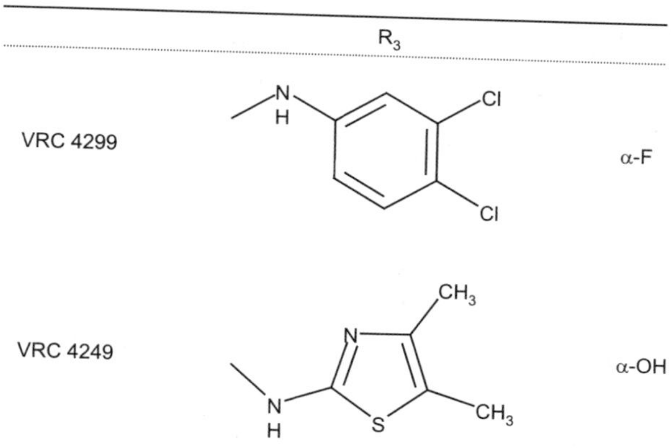

	R_3	
VRC 4299	(N-methyl-3,4-dichloroanilino: NH, Cl, Cl)	α-F
VRC 4249	(N-methyl-4,5-dimethylthiazol-2-ylamino: N, H, S, CH_3, CH_3)	α-OH

Figure 15 VRC-4249 and VRC-4299

3.3.2. VRC-4887 (NVP-PDF386)

The compound VRC-4887 (NVP-PDF386) is currently under investigation. The antibacterial spectrum and the antibacterial activity are reported in Table 10. VRC-4887 is as active as vancomycin against *S. aureus*, but it is less active than macrolides and penicillin G against *S. pneumoniae*, *Streptococcus pyogenes*, and *Streptococcus agalactiae*. It is less active than linezolid against *Enterococcus* species. It has the same MIC range as ampicillin against *H. influenzae* and as macrolides against *Moraxella catarrhalis*. It is more active than metronidazole but less active than clarithromycin and amoxicillin against *Helicobacter pylori*. VRC-4887 seems to retain activity against methicillin-resistant *S. aureus* (MRSA) and penicillin G-resistant *S. pneumoniae*, as well as vancomycin-resistant enterococci (Table 11). VRC-4887 displays good activity against *Mycoplasma pneumoniae*, but not against mycobacteria, and potent activity against *Chlamydia pneumoniae* (MICs at which 50 and 90% of isolates tested are inhibited [MIC_{50} and MIC_{90}], 0.008 and 0.008 μg/ml) (Roblin and Hammerschlag, 2003) (Table 12).

VRC-4887 has no affinity against human cell lines, such as the K562 cell line (>100 μg/ml) and the P-388 cell line (>100 μg/ml).

VRC-4887 is slowly bactericidal; killing occurs after about 12 h of contact for *H. influenzae* and *S. pneumoniae* at four and eight times the MIC, respectively. Spontaneous resistant mutants were obtained on agar plates containing ≥10 times the MIC. *S. pneumoniae* resistant mutants were obtained at a frequency of 10^{-9}, and *H. influenzae* resistant mutants were obtained at a frequency of 10^{-7}. For *S. aureus* the frequency of selection was 10^{-6}.

The in vivo efficacy of VRC-4887 in NMRI mice (21 to 25 g) is reported in Table 13.

VRC-4887 is more active than linezolid but shows activity similar to that of vancomycin against staphylococcal infections in mice. Orally, telithromycin is more active against pneumococcal infections due to penicillin G-susceptible strains but displays similar activity for penicillin G-resistant strains.

Relative efficacies in murine pneumococcal pneumonia established in female BALB/c mice (19 to 22 g) by intranasal inoculation of 50 μl of *S. pneumoniae* ATCC 6303 (10^4 to 10^5 CFU/mouse) are reported in Table 14.

Table 10 In vitro activity of VRC-4887

Microorganism	*n*	MIC (μg/ml)
S. aureus	56	0.12–4.0
S. pneumoniae	43	0.12–2.0
S. agalactiae	11	0.5–1.0
E. faecalis	23	1.0–8.0
H. influenzae	31	1.0–4.0
M. catarrhalis	22	0.06–32
H. pylori	19	0.5–2.0

Table 11 In vitro activity of VRC-4887 against resistant isolates

Microorganism(s)	*n*	Geometric mean MIC (μg/ml)
MRSA	24	0.77
S. pneumoniae Pen^r	17	0.69
Enterococcus spp., Van^r	23	2.0
H. pylori CLR^{r}[a]	5	0.87

[a]CLR, clarithromycin.

Table 12 In vitro activity against mycobacteria and intracellular and atypical pathogens

Microorganism	Strain	MIC (μg/ml)
M. pneumoniae	ATCC 15531	0.002
M. hominis	ATCC 23114	128
C. pneumoniae	ATCC VR 1355	≤0.002
C. trachomatis	ATCC VR 902B	0.008
M. smegmatis	ATCC 700084	4.0
M. fortuitum	ATCC 6841	16
M. abscessus	ATCC 19977	>64
M. aurum		0.13
M. peregrinum	ATCC 700686	16
B. fragilis		0.125

Table 13 In vivo efficacy of VRC-4887

Microorganism	Strain	CFU/mouse	Route[a]	Schedule (h)	ED_{50} (mg/kg)
S. aureus	ATCC 49951	1.7×10^7–2.2×10^7	s.c.	1–5	1.0
			p.o.		2.5
S. pneumoniae	ATCC 13709	5.4×10^7–7.5×10^7	p.o.	1–5	13.1
	ATCC 01021	2.7×10^7–3.1×10^7	p.o.	4	2.3
	ATCC 6301	1.6×10^2–2.1×10^2	p.o.	t.i.d.,[b] 4 days	5.3
	ATCC 700677	2.6×10^7–5.7×10^6	p.o.	t.i.d., 4 days	<6.0

[a]s.c., subcutaneous; p.o., per os.
[b]t.i.d., three times per day.

Table 14 Antipneumococcal activity of VRC-4887 (administered orally)

Infectious inoculum (CFU/ml)	Treatment duration	Compound	Dose (mg/kg)	No./total	ED_{50} (mg/kg)	$\log_{10}$ CFU/g
1.6×10^4–4.1×10^4	4 times a day for 3 days	Control		10/14		7.07 ± 2.0
		VRC-4887	1.56	11/14	7.4	6.1 ± 1.6
			3.12	8/12		5.9 ± 2.6
			6.25	12/12		4.0 ± 1.8
			12.5	12/12		<1.7
1.4×10^5–1.7×10^5	2–3 days	Control		4/6		8.0 ± 1.9
		VRC-4887	12.5	6/6	22.5	5.7 ± 2.2
			25	6/6		2.4 ± 1.1
			50	6/6		3.6 ± 2.5
		Telithromycin	0.83	4/6	5.6	7.6 ± 1.7
			2.5	6/6		5.4 ± 0.3
			7.5	5/5		3.6 ± 1.1
		Moxifloxacin	11.1	6/6	14.3	4.9 ± 0.6
			33.3	6/6		1.9 ± 0.5
			100	6/6		2.6 ± 1.0

VRC-4887 is less active in induced pneumococcal pneumonia in mice than telithromycin and moxifloxacin, which were administered at lower doses than VRC-4887.

The pharmacokinetic profile of VRC-4887 has been determined in CD-1 female mice after oral and intravenous administration. After dosing, the compound is recovered in urine in low quantities (2.4% of the administered intravenous dose). The main plasma parameters are summarized in Table 15.

In mice, 46% of the compound is bound to plasma proteins. VRC-4887 is rapidly distributed in lung tissues, the liver, the kidneys, and fatty tissues but not in the brain.

VRC-4887 is slowly metabolized in vitro in rodent microsomes, but in humans the compound seems to be less metabolized.

Apparently no genotoxicity by the micronucleus assay with Chinese hamster lung fibroblasts was detected, and no toxicity was detected in CD-1 mice after a single dose of 55 mg/kg and with subchronic administration for 5 days.

3.4. LBM-415 (NVP-PDF713, VIC-04959)

LBM-415 is a new hydroxamate derivative (Fig. 16). Its in vitro activity is summarized in Table 16.

LBM-415 was shown to exhibit a MIC_{50} and MIC_{90} of 0.5 and 1.0 μg/ml for and *S. pneumoniae* irrespective of the susceptibility of the clinical isolates to penicillin G (Ednie et al., 2004).

LBM-415 exhibited good in vitro activity against *M. pneumoniae* (MIC_{50} and MIC_{90}, 0.0005 and 0.001 μg/ml) and weak activity against *Ureaplasma* spp. (MIC_{50} and MIC_{90}, 2.0 and 8.0 μg/ml) and is inactive against *Mycoplasma hominis* and *Mycoplasma fermentans* (MICs, ≥256 μg/ml) (Reddy et al., 2004).

LBM-415 was evaluated in murine pneumonia due to *M. pneumoniae* ATCC 29342 after intranasal inoculation (8-week-old female BALB/c mice). Twenty-four hours after

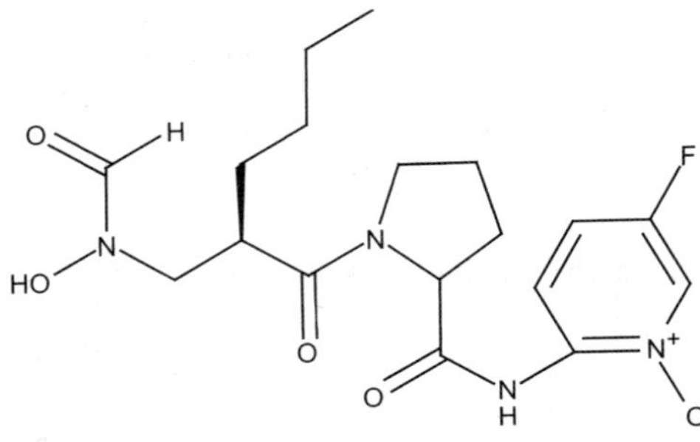

Figure 16 LBM-415

Table 16 In vitro activity of LBM-415 against common pathogens[a]

Microorganism	*n*	MIC_{90} (μg/ml)
S. aureus	56	2.0
S. pneumoniae	43	1.0
S. pyogenes	16	4.0
S. agalactiae	11	0.5
E. faecalis	23	8.0
E. faecium	31	4.0
H. influenzae	33	4.0
M. catarrhalis	22	0.5
H. pylori	19	0.5
MRSA	24	0.71[b]
MSSA[c]	32	1.0[b]
H. pylori clarithromycin[r]	5	0.16[b]
H. pylori clarithromycin[s]	14	0.20[b]
N. meningitidis	13	2.0

[a]Data from Ryder et al., 2004.
[b]Geometric mean.
[c]MSSA, methicillin-susceptible *S. aureus*.

Table 15 Pharmacokinetics of VRC-4887 in mice

Dose (mg/kg)	Route[a]	C_{max} (μg/ml)	T_{max} (h)	AUC_{0-4} (ng·h/ml)	$t_{1/2}$ (h)	Bioavailability (%)
5.4	i.v.	2.15	0.083	983	0.7	
14.4	p.o.	1.64	0.25	1,662	1.3	63.1

[a]i.v., intravenous; p.o., per os.

Table 17 Pharmacokinetics of LBM-415 in rodents

Animals	Route[a]	Dose (mg)	C_{max} (µg/ml)	T_{max} (h)	$t_{1/2}$ (h)	AUC (µg·h/ml)	CL/F (liters/h/kg)	F (%)
Mice (CD-1)	i.v.	4.9	2.06		0.43		0.919	
	p.o.	14.9	0.76	0.5	1.8		1.746	64.4
Rats (Sprague-Dawley)	i.v.	3.6	5.89		2.2	2.797		
	p.o.	11.9	0.58	0.25	2.35	2.028		21.9
	p.o.	44.2	3.47	0.5	2.10	10.22		29.8
	p.o.	124.2	20.27	0.5	3.45	45.11		46.8
	p.o.	436.2	128.3	0.5	3.29	341.7		100.8

[a]i.v., intravenous; p.o., per os.

bacterial challenge, mice were treated with 50 mg of LBM-415 per kg for 13 days (Fonsera-Aten et al., 2004). In vitro, LBM-415 was shown to be weakly active against *Neisseria gonorrhoeae* (MIC_{50} and MIC_{90}, 1.0 and 16 µg/ml) and *Neisseria meningitidis* (MIC_{50} and MIC_{90}, 1.0 and 2.0 µg/ml).

In another in vitro study it was shown that LBM-415 exhibited good antichlamydial activity, with a MIC of 0.004 µg/ml for *Chlamydia trachomatis*, and variable in vitro activity against atypical mycobacteria, with MICs of 0.5, 1.0, >64, 8.0, and 0.12 µg/ml for *M. smegmatis*, *M. fortuitum*, *M. abscessus*, *M. peregrinum*, and *M. avium*, respectively.

The pharmacokinetics in rodents were investigated and are reported in Table 17. After intravenous doses of 4.9 and 3.6 mg/kg, the urinary elimination, levels at 24 h were 19.33 and 47.64%, respectively; elimination in bile was 22.4% for rats.

Protein binding in mice ranged from 27 to 63.7% for concentrations in plasma of 5.0 to 0.1 µg/ml (Chen et al., 2004).

3.5. BB-3497 Series

3.5.1. BB-3497

BB-3497 is a hydroxamate derivative (Fig. 17) with an IC_{50} of 7 nM for Ni-PDF of *E. coli*. Many alterations of BB-3497 were done (Davies et al., 2001, 2003; Smith et al., 2002).

A *ter*-butyl analog is currently under development, and the in vitro activity against common respiratory pathogens (Wise et al., 2002) is listed in Table 18. Figure 18 shows BB-3497 in the PDF active site.

BB-3497 is active against gram-negative bacteria, poorly active against *S. pneumoniae*, and weakly active against *C. pneumoniae* (Table 19).

BB-3497 retains activity against *S. pneumoniae* strains which are resistant to fluoroquinolones, erythromycin A, and penicillin G and also against multidrug-resistant strains.

These PDF inhibitors are bacteriostatic agents. An improved in vitro activity has been reached with a series of keto compounds at R3.

Figure 17 BB-3497

Table 18 In vitro activity of BB-3497 against common pathogens causing respiratory tract infections

Compound	MIC (µg/ml)		
	S. pneumoniae (*n* = 40)	*M. catarrhalis* (*n* = 29)	*H. influenzae* (*n* = 35)
BB-3497	8	0.06	0.25
BB-83698	0.25	0.06	8
BB-83815	0.50	0.06	8
BB-83857	0.50	0.06	8
BB-84416	1.0	0.12	8
BB-84518	1.0	0.06	1
Ciprofloxacin	1.0	0.03	0.008
Amoxicillin	0.015	0.03	0.5

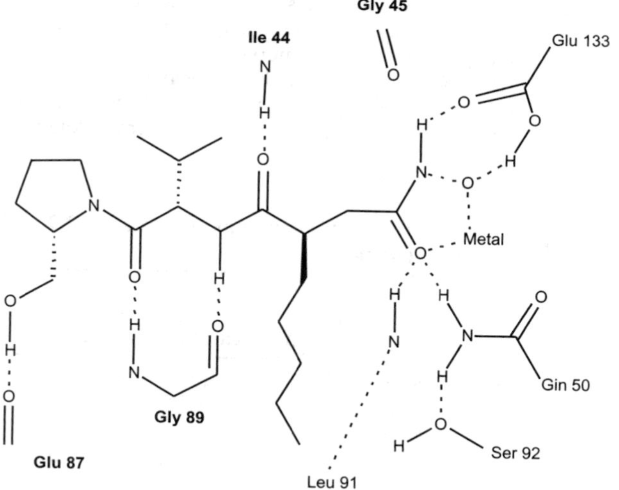

Figure 18 BB-3497 in the PDF active site

Table 19 In vitro activities against *Chlamydia* spp.

Compound	MIC (µg/ml)	
	C. pneumoniae TW-183	*C. trachomatis* CT 815
BB-3497	2.0	0.25
BB-83698	2.0	0.25
BB-83815	0.5	1.0
BB-83857	1.0	1.0
BB-84416	0.5	2.0
Ciprofloxacin	2.0	2.0

A series of compounds has an amino ketone group at R3 and c-pentylmethyl at R1 which result in an improved, broad antibacterial spectrum. Aminoaryl analogs have enhanced in vitro activity against *H. influenzae*. Some derivatives of the keto series have improved activity against intracellular and atypical respiratory pathogens (Table 20).

3.5.2. BB-83698

Figure 19 shows the structure of BB-83698, a keto analog whose in vitro activity has been explored (Table 21). BB-883698 is less active than telithromycin against *M. catarrhalis* (MIC_{50} and MIC_{90}, 0.06 and 0.12 μg/ml), *H. influenzae* (MIC_{50} and MIC_{90}, 16 and 64 μg/ml), *S. aureus* (MIC_{50} and MIC_{90}, 4 to 8 μg/ml), and *S. pyogenes* (MIC_{50} and MIC_{90}, 0.06 and 0.12 mg/ml).

BB-2948, BB-85377, and BB-85384 are bactericidal against *S. aureus* ATCC 29213 in about 6 h of contact without regrowth. They are less active than linezolid and vancomycin, with MICs of 2.0 to 4.0 μg/ml for *Enterobacter* species, 1.0 to 8.0 μg/ml for *S. aureus*, and 1.0 to 4.0 μg/ml for *Staphylococcus epidermidis*. The frequency of spontaneous mutation was estimated at $<10^{-8}$ in gram-positive bacteria.

Another series of analogs was investigated comprising nine compounds: BB-85318, BB-84888, BB-83698, BB-85128, BB-84879, BB-84880, BB-64885, BB-84887, and BB-85035 (Bowker et al., 2003).

BB-83698 was shown to exert antituberculosis activity, with a MIC (geometric) of 0.25 μg/ml (Cynamon et al., 2004).

BB-83698 efficacy was demonstrated in a murine model of experimental pneumococcal pneumonia after intratracheal administration of virulent strains and treatment with either 80 mg/kg/12 h or 160 mg/kg/34 h (Azoulay-Dupuis et al., 2004).

A dose-dependent central nervous system effect was observed only in dogs, apparently linked to high maximum concentrations in serum (tremors, unsteady gait, and convulsions). An ascending-dose study of intravenous pharmacokinetics (long infusion [1 to 2 h]) was conducted (Ramanathan-Girish et al., 2004); results are shown in Table 22.

3.6. Calpeptin and Aldehyde PDF Inhibitors

Peptide aldehydes are not specific for metalloproteases such as PDF, they also act as inhibitors of serine, cysteine, and aspartyl proteases. These inhibitors seem to bind to metalloproteases as their hydrates. Such complexes are similar in structure to the proposed tetrahedral intermediate formed during peptide hydrolysis. It was found that calpeptin (*N*-benzyloxycarbonyl-L-leucyl-norleucinal) is a potent inhibitor of both *E. coli* and *B. subtilis* PDFs. This peptide inhibits PDF at 0.5 mM. It was also shown that charged functional groups of peptide analogs do not inhibit PDF activity. Calpeptin and other analogs are more active

Table 21 In vitro activity of BB-83698[a]

Microorganism(s)[b]	*n*	MIC (μg/ml)	
		50%	90%
S. pneumoniae Pen-S	91	0.25	0.5
S. pneumoniae Pen-I	47	0.25	0.5
S. pneumoniae Pen-R	75	0.25	0.25
S. pyogenes	21	0.06	0.12
S. agalactiae	21	0.06	0.12
Viridans group streptococci	26	0.12	0.5
S. aureus oxa-S	74	4.0	8.0
S. aureus oxa-R	80	4.0	8.0
H. influenzae β −ve	60	8.0	32
H. influenzae β +ve	50	16	64
M. catarrhalis β −ve	25	0.06	0.12
M. catarrhalis β +ve	25	0.12	0.12

[a]Data from Lofland et al., 2004.
[b]S, susceptible; I, intermediate; R, resistant; β −ve, non-β-lactamase producing; β +ve, β-lactamase producing.

Table 20 In vitro activities of keto PDF inhibitors against intracellular and atypical pathogens

Compound	MIC (μg/ml)		
	M. pneumoniae (*n* = 12)	*Legionella pneumophila* (*n* = 50)	*C. pneumoniae* (*n* = 5)
BB-83698	0.002	1.0	0.25–0.5
BB-84887	0.001	0.25	
BB-84888	0.0001	1.0	4.0
BB-85035	0.00025		2.0
BB-3497		1.0	1.0–2.0
Clarithromycin	0.002	0.004	0.03
Levofloxacin	8.0	1.0	1.0

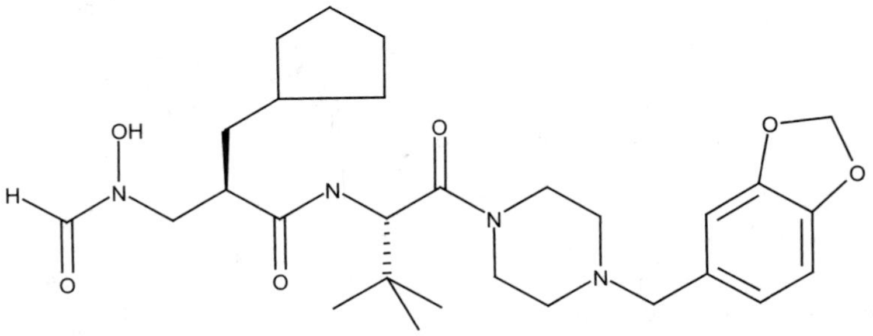

Figure 19 BB-83698

Table 22 Pharmacokinetics of BB-83698 in humans after intravenous administration

Dose (mg)	C_0 (μg/ml)	$AUC_{0-\infty}$ (μg·h/ml)	$t_{1/2}$ (h)	CL_P (ml/min)
10	0.5	0.4	4.8	520.6
25	1.2	1.3	5.0	335.1
50	2.7	3.7	6.0	233.5
100	5.3	10.3	10.1	173.3
200	9.6	26.6	15.4	135.4
325	15.6	41.3	16.7	141.5
400	18.5	39.2	8.7	175.9
475	19.3	45.8	8.5	188.5

against cobalt-containing PDFs than against those containing zinc. The 1,10-phenanthroline metalloprotease inhibitor displayed anti-PDF activity, with a K_is for cobalt and zinc PDFs of 0.60 ± 0.06 nM and 0.38 ± 0.02 nM, respectively.

Calpeptin is a competitive inhibitor of PDFs. It forms a 1:1 complex with Co(II)-substituted *E. coli* and *B. subtilis* deformylase.

These aldehyde PDF inhibitors form covalent complexes with the active-site cysteine residue. They bind to the PDF N terminus, where the formyl group is located.

3.7. PCLNA

PCLNA is the (*S*)-2-*O*-(H-phosphonoxy-L-caproyl-L-leucyl-*p*-nitroanilide (Fig. 20). L-Caproyl is used instead of L-methionine to facilitate protein synthesis. The H-phosphonate group mimics the tetrahedral intermediate implicated during formyl hydrolysis.

PCLNA acts as a competitive inhibitor of both the zinc and iron forms of PDF, with K_i values of 76 and 37 μM, respectively.

Three hydrogen bonds are formed between the main-chain atoms of the inhibitor and β-strand IV of the protein. The *p*-nitroanilide group is crucial for binding; removal of the moiety significantly reduced the enzyme affinity for the substrate. L-Leucine forms a van der Waals interaction with Leu91 and with Glu42 and Gly43. The L-caproyl group is close to the metal ion and close to Gly43, Ile44, Gly45, Glu88, Cys129, His132, and Glu133. It is bound via a hydrogen to the nitrogen of Ile44 (Fig. 21).

The proposed mechanism involves a nucleophilic attack on the formyl group by a metal-bound hydroxide ion (or water molecule) to generate a tetrahedral intermediate which is stabilized by the metal ion and the side chain of the PDF active-site residue. The phosphonate derivative which has the P1′ residue in the L-form exhibits K_i values of

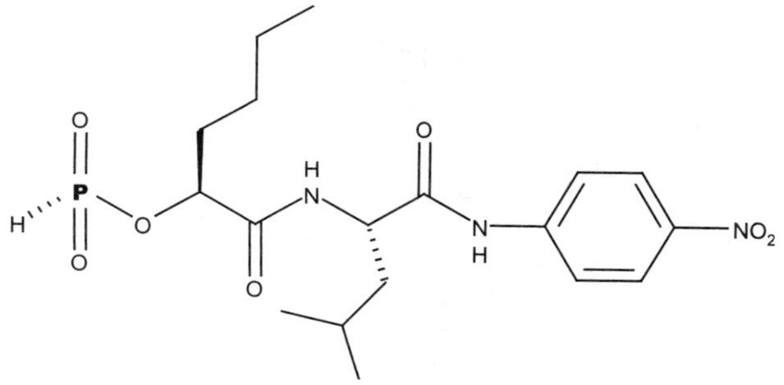

Figure 20 Phosphonate derivatives

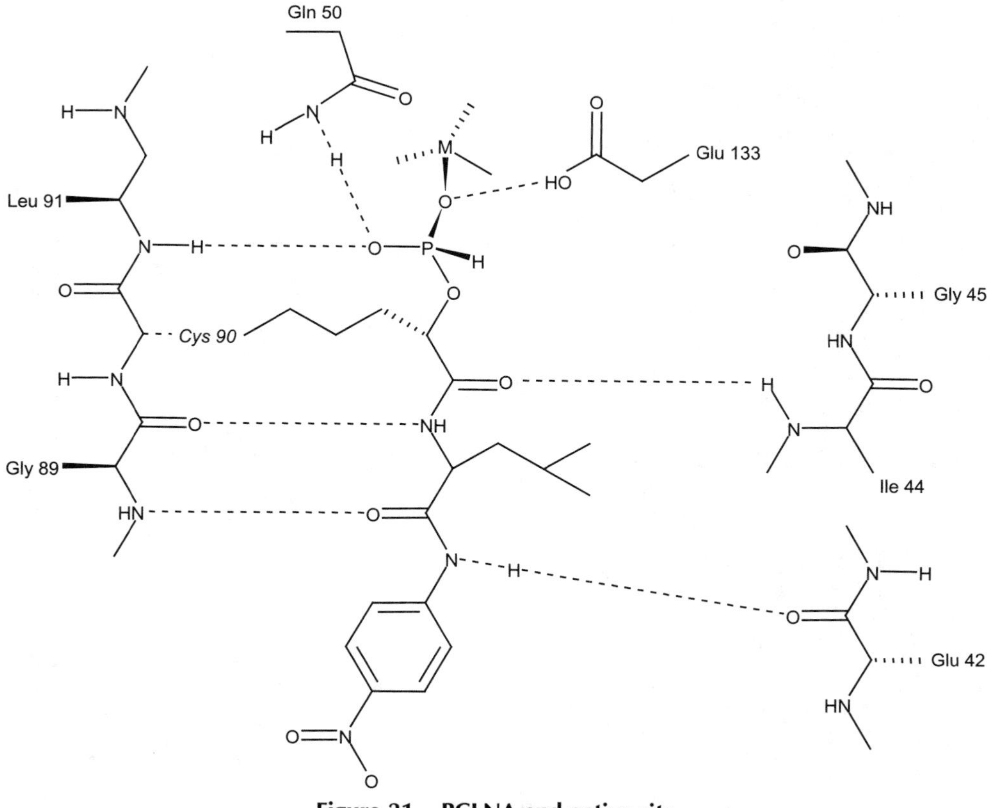

Figure 21 PCLNA and active site

37 and 76 μM for the Fe^{2+} and Zn^{2+} enzymes, respectively. The D-form is less potent, with a K_i value of 125 μM (Hue et al., 1998).

3.8. Hydroxamate Derivatives from Pharmacia

Screening of the library of Pharmacia (Thorarensen et al., 2001) against *S. aureus* PDF identified potent inhibitors (Fig. 22) exhibiting IC_{50}s in the low nanomolar range, but unfortunately these inhibitors are inactive against whole cells. Many compounds with a hydroxamic moiety have no antibacterial activity even if the affinity for the enzyme is high (IC_{50}, >50 μM). Several α-hetero-substituted amides have been prepared. The urea analog was found to have PDF activity, with an IC_{50} of 2.2 μM, and antibacterial activity. The original compound was probably inactive due to efflux pump or outer membrane impermeability.

3.9. NB Series

A series of compounds with various toxophores and a linker between the toxophore and the recognition site has been synthesized. Two of them were explored for their activities and their pharmacokinetics: NB 3057 and NB 3068 (Fig. 23). NB 3057 is poorly stable in human plasma (Table 23). The stability varies according to the linker (Fig. 24).

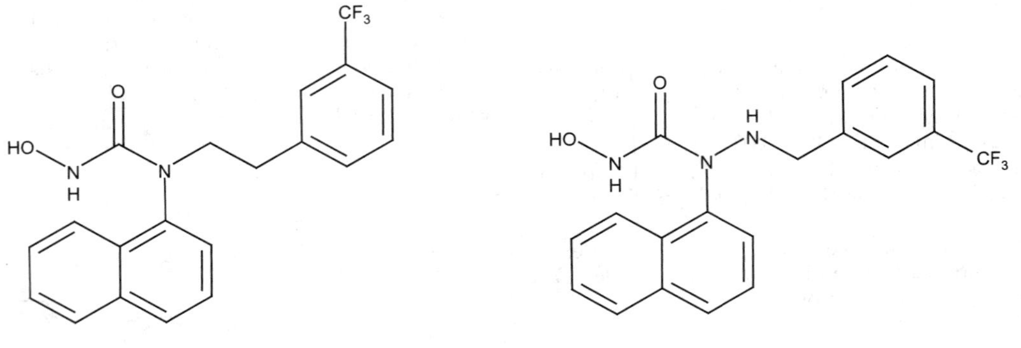

IC_{50} : 2.2 μM
MIC : 32 mg/ml
S. aureus

IC_{50} : 5 nM
MIC : >128 mg/ml
S. aureus

Figure 22 Derivatives from Pharmacia

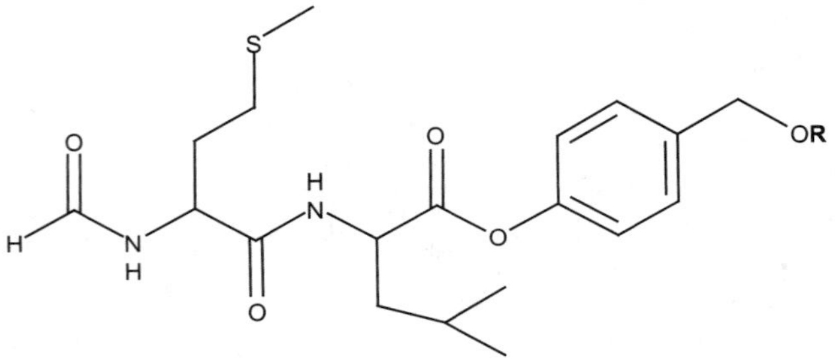

		T ½ (h)			
	R	PBPs	Broth	Mouse plasma	Human plasma
NB 3057	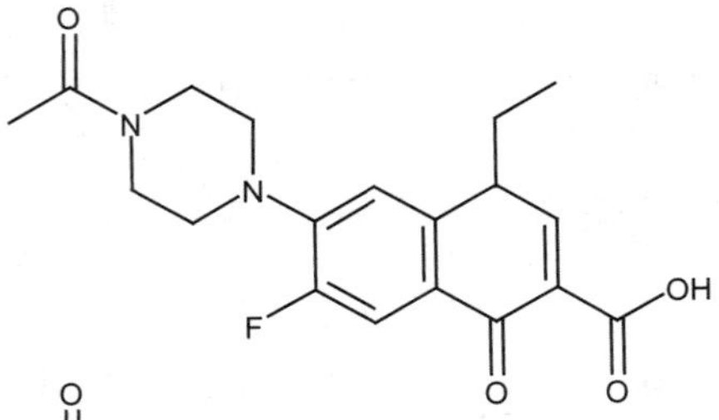	20	10	1.4	0.6
NB 3068	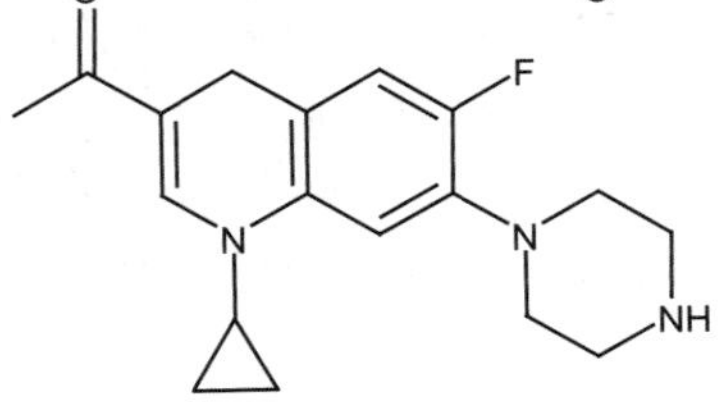	18	13	< 0.5	4.1

Figure 23 NB series of anti-PDF

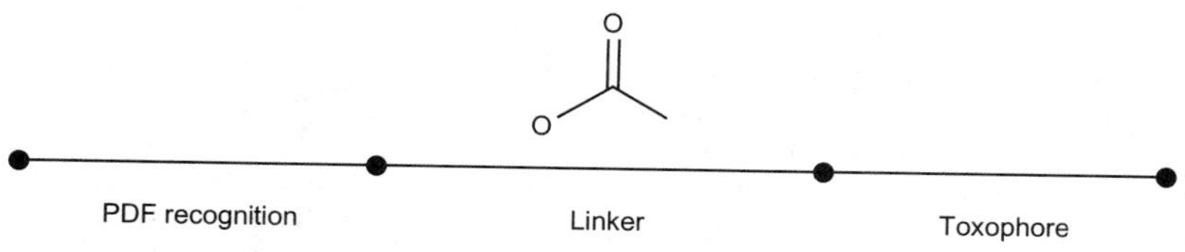

PDF recognition Linker Toxophore

Figure 24 Structure of PDF inhibitors

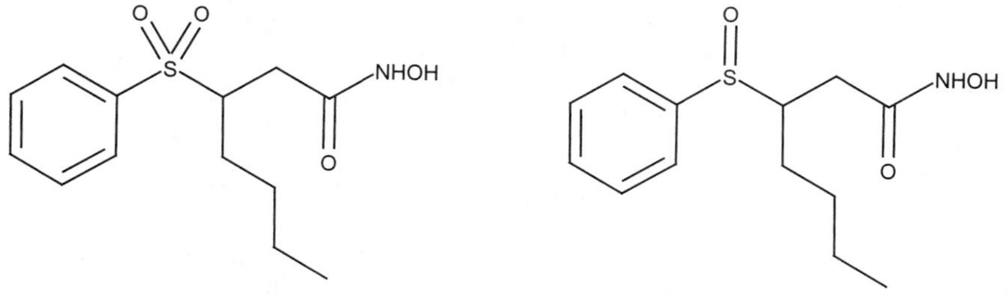

Ro 66-0376 Ro 66-.976

Figure 25 β-Sulfonyl and β-sulfinyl hydroxamate derivatives

3.10. β-Sulfonyl and β-Sulfinyl Hydroxamate Derivatives

A series of β-sulfonyl and β-sulfinyl hydroxamic acid derivatives (Fig. 25) has been shown to be potent PDF inhibitors with in vitro antibacterial activity. In this series the activity of PDF inhibitors is strongly influenced by the nature of the substituent which occupies the same position as the methionine side chain. Stronger inhibition is obtained with unsubstituted aromatic rings or linear aliphatic chains (propyl or pentyl). The activity of the inhibitors is also largely dependent on the stereochemistry at the carbon in the β position to the hydroxamic acid (Apfel et al., 2000; Gupta et al., 2002).

Trimethoprim inhibits dihydrofolate reductase and thereby promotes the depletion of the tetrahydrofolate pool. It was shown by Magel et al. in 1994 that an *E. coli* strain with an inactivated *pdf* gene can grow slowly in a rich medium containing trimethoprim and thymidine. These artificial conditions mimic a mutation in the *fmt* gene; the lack of available folate forces protein synthesis to initiate with methionine not formylated.

Resistant colonies of *E. coli* XL_2-blue appeared after 3 days at a frequency of 10^{-7}. In the mutant isolate a Tn*10* insertion in the *fmt* gene was found. All isolated mutants exhibited lower growth rates than the wild type, with doubling times of 1.2 to 2.0 h, instead of 0.44 h in the wild type.

Table 23 Stability of anti-PDF analogs in various media

Compound	$t_{1/2}$ (h)			
	PBS[a]	Broth	Mouse plasma	Human plasma
NB 3057	20	10	1.4	0.6
NB 3068	18	13	<0.5	4.1

[a]PBS, phosphate-buffered saline.

In this series good antibacterial activity against the outer membrane mutant *E. coli* strain DC2 and *M. catarrhalis* was observed, with a good correlation with the PDF-inhibitory activity. The β-sulfinyl hydroxamic acid derivatives are more potent than the corresponding β-sulfonyl acid derivatives (Table 24).

3.11. Nonpeptidic PDF Inhibitors

Several groups of workers have reported hydroxamate derivatives but only a few nonpeptidic inhibitors of PDFs.

Table 24 In vitro activities of Ro-66-0376 and Ro-66-6976

Microorganism	Strain	MIC (μg/ml)		
		N = 1 sulfonyl Ro-66-6976	N = 2 sulfinyl Ro-66-0376	Erythromycin A
E. coli	ATCC 25922	128	32	>64
Stenotrophomonas maltophilia	1 AC 739	<0.25	4.0	32
M. catarrhalis	RA 21	0.06	<0.25	<0.125
H. influenzae	11	0.25	1.0	2.0
M. pneumoniae	ATCC 29342	16	256	<0.06
C. pneumoniae	AR 39	0.25	0.5	0.06
S. aureus	ATCC 25923	16	256	0.25
B. subtilis	ATCC 585969	0.25	1.0	<0.125
S. pneumoniae	ATCC 49619	32	128	<0.125

3.11.1. Thiol Derivatives

Thiophan (3-mercapto-2-benzyl propanoyl glycine) is a competitive inhibitor of bacterial PDFs showing moderate activity.

The sulfur group was shown to bind to free valence of the methyl group and the benzyl group to enter the S′1 cavity of the enzyme. Thiophan equally inhibits PDF1A and PDF1B.

It was shown that for the thiol derivative N-Leu-Arg-OCH_3 the inhibition constant was higher for PDF1A than for PDF1B and bacterial PDFs.

The phenyl-arginine-β-naphthylamine (FRN) peptide is a specific inhibitor of bacterial PDFs. It binds to PDF1B and poorly to PDF1A (Table 25).

It was shown that monothiol compounds weakly inhibited deformylase activity, whereas dithiol derivatives, which are also known as inhibitors of a zinc metallopeptidase (Van X) of *E. faecium*, are potent inhibitors of PDF. Ethanediol, 1,3-propanedithiol, and 2,3-mercapto-1-propanol exhibit time-dependent kinetics. The first two compounds are the more potent inhibitors, with K_i values of 29 and 4.0 μM, respectively. The inhibition is irreversible. Other dithiol inhibitors have been tested, but they are less potent (Table 26).

3.11.2. Thyropropic Analogs

Thyropropic analogs (Fig. 26) increased the K_i twofold. The addition of an iodine group at R3 does not increase the inhibitory activity.

Table 25 Binding affinity for PDFs

Compound	K_i (μM)	
	E. coli Ni-PDF	*Arabidopsis thaliana* Ni-PDF
Actinonin	0.0018 ± 0.003	0.025 ± 0.003
Thiophan	189 ± 20	900 ± 200
FRN	95 ± 10	52 ± 5

Table 26 Kinetic parameters of dithiol compounds as time-dependent inhibitors

Compound	K_i (μM)
1,2-Ethanedithiol	4.0 ± 0.8
1,3-Propane dithiol	2.9 ± 0.7
2,3-Dimercapto-1-propanol	10.4 ± 2.0
2,3-Dimercapto-1-propanesulfonic acid	40.2 ± 8.8
1,5-Pentanedithiol	38.0 ± 5.0

Compound	R_1	R_2	R_3	R_4	n	R_5	IC_{50} (μM)
A	H	H	H	I	1	OH	0.94 ± 0.05
B	H	H	I	I	1	OH	2.81 ± 0.8

Figure 26 Thyropropic analogs

3.11.3. Biaryl Derivatives

Members of a series of biaryl (Fig. 27) analogs (Green et al., 2000) were identified as inhibitors of PDF by screening of a chemical library.

Each compound is composed of a fused heterocyclic aromatic ring, a biaryl group, and an acidic group such as a tetrazole ring on the biaryl ring. The biphenyl acyl sulfonamide derivative (compound 1) and the tetrazole derivative (compound 2) inhibit PDF activity, with IC_{50}s of 3.9 ± 0.2 μM and 15.0 ± 1.7 μM, respectively. Both are competitive inhibitors of deformylase, with K_i values of 1.2 ± 0.1 μM and 6.0 ± 0.2 μM, respectively. The R2 substituent is important for anti-PDF activity; a methyl or a diaminomethyl is deleterious for activity. A variety of fused heterocyclic aromatic ring systems were found to be acceptable head groups for the biaryl acid analog inhibitors of deformylase (Fig. 28).

Compound 1 was reported to be a potent competitive inhibitor of recombinant metallo-β-lactamase Ccra of *Bacteroides fragilis* (K_i value, 1.5 ± 0.1 μM). Some compounds of this series were potent Ccra inhibitors, especially those having a biphenyl tetrazole moiety. The original activity of these biaryl analogs was as angiotensin II receptor antagonists. Their acid groups, such as tetrazole, acylsulfonamide, carboxyl, and carboxamide, are important pharmacophores for activity (Fig. 29).

These anions bind in the receptor to a lysine residue. In Ccra of *B. fragilis* β-lactamase, the biphenyl tetrazole anion ligates to one of the active-site zinc ions.

In this series the development of resistance is relatively rapid.

3.12. Thiopeptide Derivatives

The carbonyl group is important for catalysis. A replacement of the oxygen atom of the carbonyl group by a sulfur atom yields a molecule with a thiol, which is not a substrate for PDF (Meinnel et al., 1999) (Fig. 30 and 31).

A series of thiopeptides with anti-PDF activity has been synthesized (Huntington et al., 2000). They act as reversible inhibitors of PDF from *E. coli* and *B. subtilis*. The most potent inhibitor has a K_i value of 11 nM for the *B. subtilis* enzyme. Some of the derivatives display activity against *B. subtilis* but not against *E. coli*. These compounds are

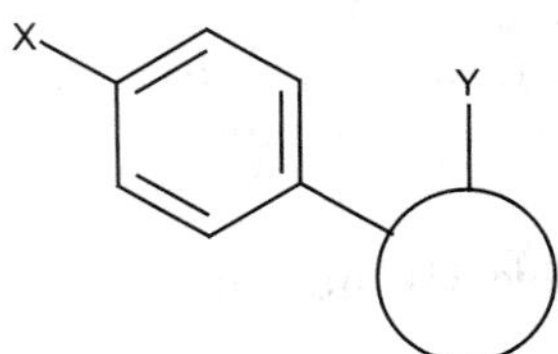

Figure 27 General structure of biaryl analogs

Figure 28 Biaryl acid

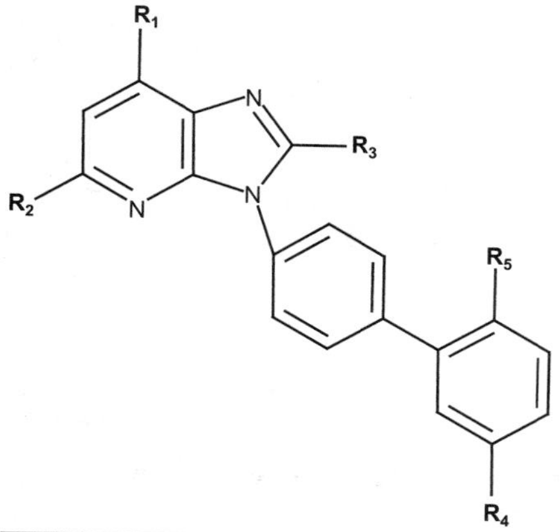

Compounds	R_1	R_2	R_3	R_4	R_5	IC_{50} (μM)
1	-H	-Cl	n-propyl	H	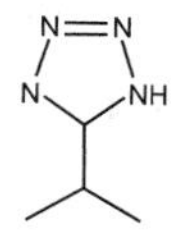	3.9±0.2
2	-H	$-CH_3$	n-propyl	H		> 50
3	-H	$-N(CH_3)_2$	n-propyl	H		> 50
4	$-CH_3$	$-CH_3$	$-C_2H_5$	Benzyl		> 50
5	$-CH_3$	$-CH_3$	$-C_2H_5$	-		34.2 ± 4.1
6	$-CH_3$	$-CH_3$	$-C_2H_5$	-	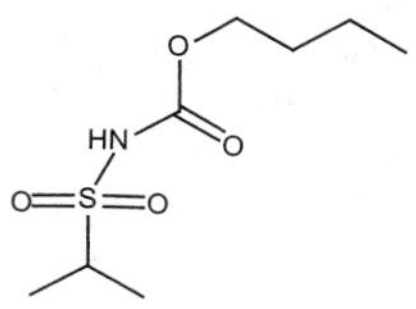	15.0 ± 1.7
7	$-CH_3$	$-CH_3$	$-C_2H_5$	-	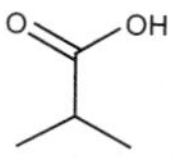	> 50
8	$-CH_3$	$-CH_3$	$-C_2H_5$	-	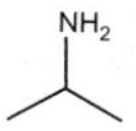	> 50

Figure 29 Biaryl derivatives

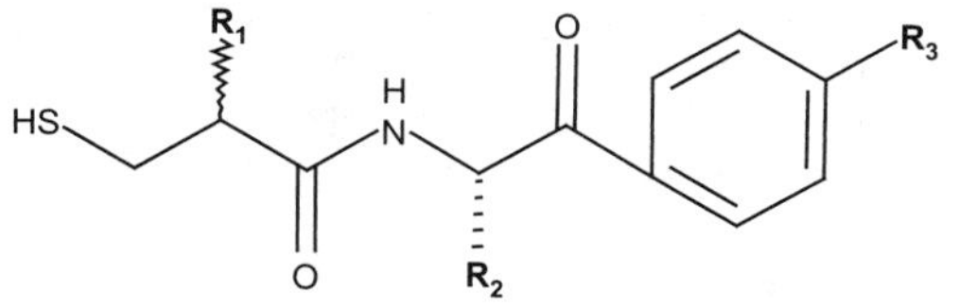

R_1	R_2	R_3
CH_2-$(CH_2)_2CH_3$	CH_2-$(CH_2)_2NH_2$	NO_2

Figure 30 Thiopeptides (1)

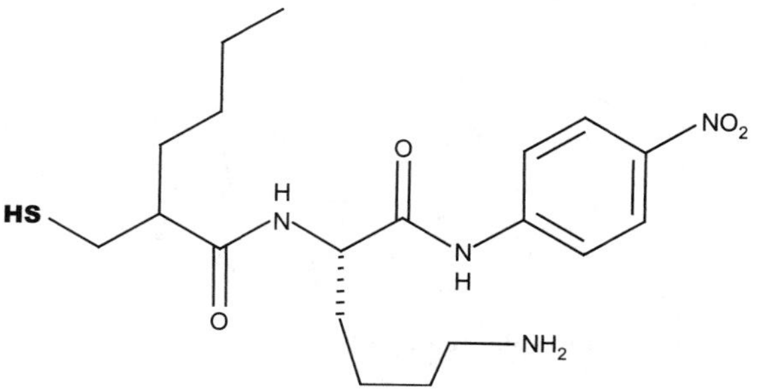

Figure 31 Thiopeptides (2)

bactericidal against *S. epidermidis*, *Enterococcus faecalis*, and *B. subtilis*. The frequency for selection of resistant mutants of *B. subtilis* is $>10^9$. It was shown in the phosphonate series that the phosphonate oxygen is directly ligated to the catabolic metal ion, replacing the metallo-bound water. It was hypothesized that the replacement of the phosphonate group by a thiol group should increase the inhibitory potency because sulfur is a stronger ligand for a transition metal such as Fe^{2+} than is oxygen. Among the PDF inhibitors of this series, one compound was the most potent, with a K_i of 19 nM for *E. coli* PDF. It is an L-diastereoisomer; the D-diastereoisomer is less potent, with a K_i of 170 nM. This compound has a polar lysine group which may enhance the water solubility and therefore reduce the nonspecific binding to lipophilic targets. In addition, this amino group might improve the membrane permeability.

3.13. Isoxazole Derivatives

A series of PDF nonpeptide inhibitors was synthesized in order to avoid metabolic instability. The central core of this series is an isoxazole-3-hydroxamic acid (Fig. 32). The inhibitory activity of these molecules against PDFs of *E. coli* and *S. aureus* ranged from 0.8 to 42 μM (*S. aureus*) and 3.4 to 62 μM (*E. coli*). In comparison, actinonin IC_{50}s were 0.0007 and 0.002 μM for *E. coli* and *S. aureus*, respectively. They are inactive in vitro (MIC, >64 μg/ml) (Cali et al., 2004).

3.14. Benzothiazole Derivatives

A series of benzothiazolylidene hydroxamic acids as PDF inhibitors was investigated (Fig. 33).

Affinity for PDF is strongly influenced by the nature of the *N*-alkyl substituent R. The affinity was enhanced as the length of the *N*-alkyl chain was increased from ethyl (IC_{50}, >100 μM) to *n*-propyl (IC_{50}, 8.39 μM) or *n*-butyl (IC_{50}, 1.04 μM). However, the affinity decreased with an *n*-pentyl (IC_{50}, 9.91 μM). Compounds with *n*-butyl and *n*-propyl exerted antistaphylococcal activity (MICs of 10 and 30 μg/ml, respectively).

3.15. Quinazoline Derivatives

A series of derivatives having a quinazoline feature was synthesized. Among them two compounds displayed good affinity for Fe-PDF of *E. coli* but exhibited poor antibacterial activity (Apfel et al., 2000b) (Fig. 34).

Compounds having a CO instead of SO_2 displayed lower affinity for PDF (IC_{50}, 0.310 versus 0.120 μM).

3.16. Bicyclic Peptides

Series of PDF inhibitors have been synthesized as bicyclic peptides. The lead compound (Fig. 35) with a metal-chelating hydroxamic acid attached to a benzothiazone core displayed good affinity for Ni-PDF (IC_{50}, <5 nM) and is soluble in water (>500 μM). This compound is unable to permeate the *E. coli* cell membrane, explaining the lack of activity (Molteni et al., 2004). Optimization of the moiety with either a bromine atom or an *n*-pentyl group improved the antibacterial activity, with a MIC of 2.0 μg/ml for *M. catarrhalis*.

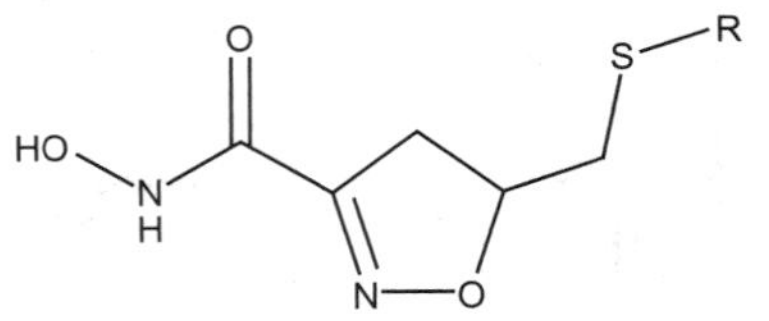

Figure 32 Isoxazole hydroxamates

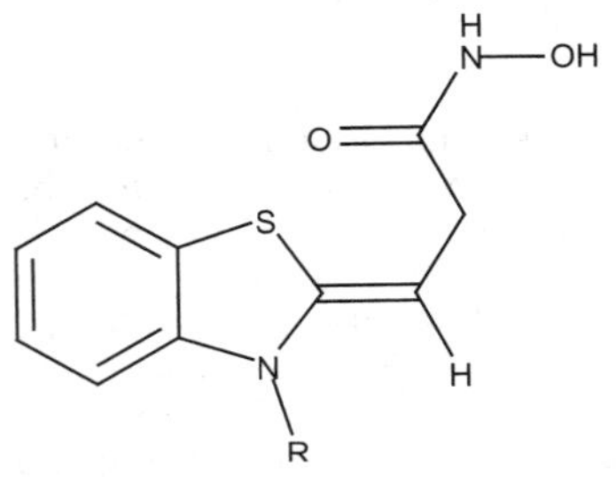

Figure 33 Benzothiazole hydroxamic acid derivatives

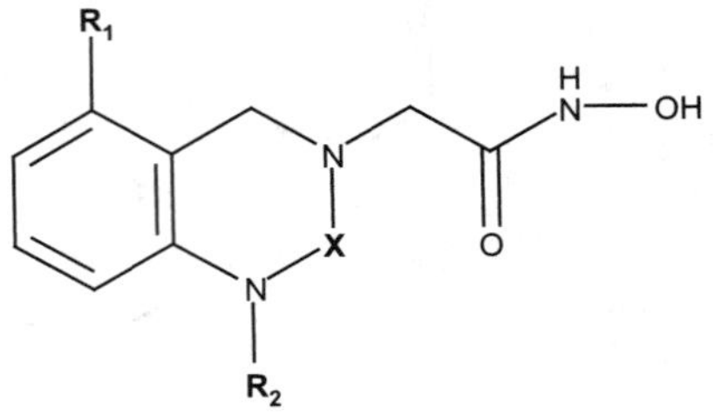

X = CO or SO_2
R_1 = H, F, Br, CF_3
R_2 = H, allyl, benzyl etc...

Figure 34 Quinazoline derivatives

3.17. Sch-382583

Sch-382583 (Fig. 36) was obtained from the fermentation broth of *Streptomyces* (Chu et al., 2001; Coats et al., 2004). This pseudopeptide contains a piperazinic acid and a succinamide side chain substituted by a 3-methylbutyl group.

Sch-382583 has a strong affinity for PDF, with a K_i of 60 nM.

The piperazinic acid ring, which is a hydrazine amino acid found in many biologically active natural products (Ciufolini and Xi, 1998), imparts the conformational rigidity.

3.18. Thioxo-4-Thiazolidinone

In a series of 2-thioxo-4-thiazolidinones discovered through screening of a chemical library, some analogs with *N*-hexanoic acid exhibited potent inhibitory activity against PDF of plants (IC_{50}, 4.6 μM). Following this previous series, a new series of molecules was synthesized with a variety of heteroarylidene groups at position 5 (Fig. 37). They showed low levels of inhibition. Analogs having shorter side chain at R2 such as acetic acid or propionic acid had no affinity for PDF.

The most potent 2-thioxo-4-thiazolidinone bears at the C-5 position a furan. The IC_{50} was 0.85 μM for PDF of soybean (Howard et al., 2004).

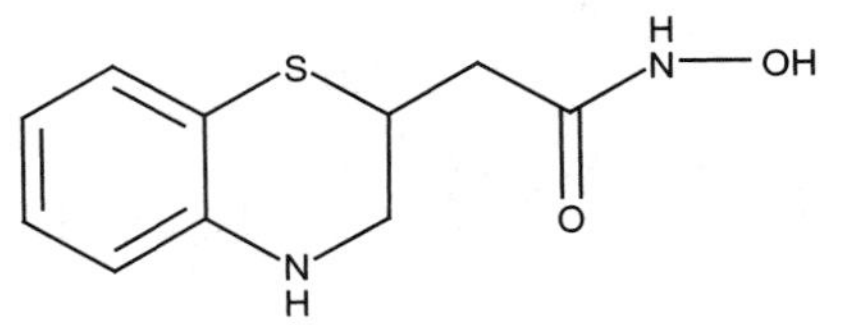

Compound A

Figure 35 Bicyclic peptide PDF inhibitors

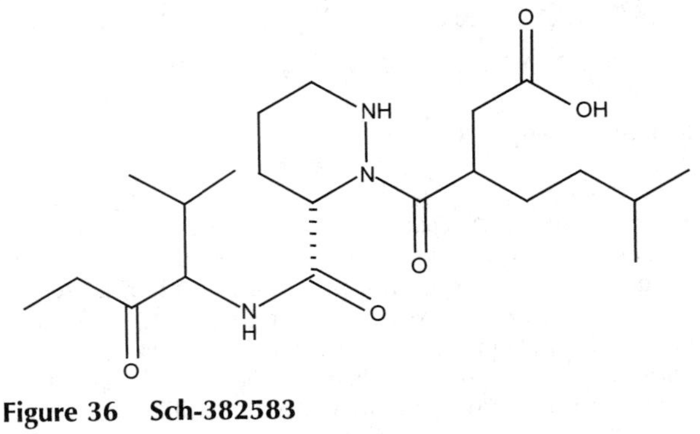

Figure 36 Sch-382583

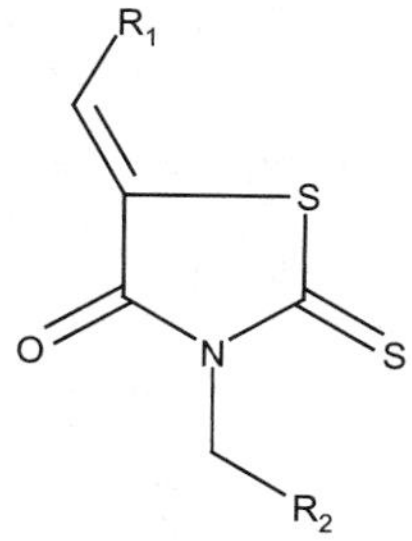

Figure 37 Thioxo-4-thiazolidinone

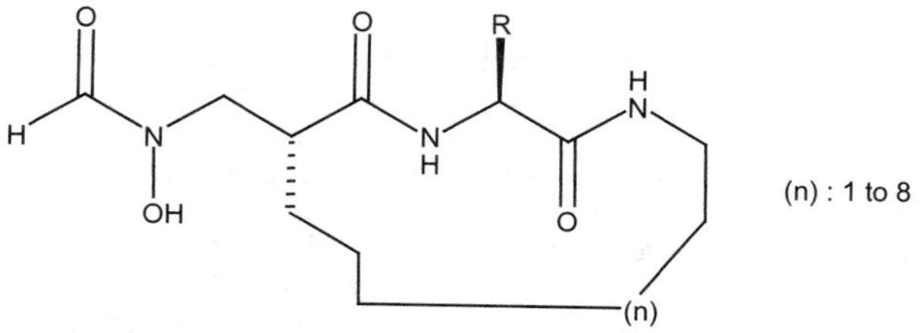

Figure 38 Macrocyclic peptide PDF inhibitors

3.19. Macrocyclic Peptides

In order to improve stability (proteolysis) and selectivity of these pseudopeptide inhibitors, it was proposed to form cyclic peptides or depsipeptides (Guilloteau et al., 2002).

A macrocyclic deformylase peptide inhibitor was reported (Hu et al., 2003). In this peptide the P1′ and P3′ side chains are covalently cross-linked (K_i, 0.67 nM) (Fig. 38).

The improved affinity for PDF is probably due to the rigidity introduced by cyclization. Some compounds exhibited good activity against *B. subtilis* (MIC, 0.7 to 1.4 μg/ml), *H. influenzae* (MIC, 0.5 μg/ml), and *M. catarrhalis* (MIC, 0.6 μg/ml) but weak activity against *S. pneumoniae* (MIC, 2.0 to 4.0 μg/ml); they were inactive against *S. aureus* (MIC, 16 μg/ml).

REFERENCES

Adams JM, 1968, On the release of the formyl group from nascent protein, J Mol Biol, 33, 571–589.

Apfel C, Banner DW, Bur D, Dietz M, Hirata T, Hubschwerlen C, Locher H, Page MGP, Pirson W, Rossé G, Specklin JL, 2000, Hydroxamic acid derivatives as potent peptide deformylase inhibitors and antibacterial agents, J Med Chem, 43, 2324–2331.

Apfel C, Banner DW, Bur D, Dietz M, Hubschwerlen C, Locher H, Marlin F, Masciadri R, Pirson W, Stalder H, 2001, 2-(2-Oxo-1,4-dihydro-2H-quinazolin-3-yl)- and 2-(2,2-dioxo-1,4-dihydro-2H-2λ^6-benzo[1,2,6]thiadiazin-3-yl)-N-hydroxy-acetamides as potent and selective peptide deformylase inhibitors, J Med Chem, 44, 1847-1852.

Azoulay-Dupuis E, Mohler J, Bédos JP, 2004, Efficacy of BB-83698, a novel peptide deformylase inhibitor, in a mouse model of pneumococcal pneumonia, Antimicrob Agents Chemother, 48, 80–85.

Bowker KE, Noel AR, MacGowan AP, 2003, In vitro activities of nine peptide deformylase inhibitors and five comparators against respiratory and skin pathogens, Int J Antimicrob Agents, 22, 557–561.

Cali P, Naerum L, Mukhija S, Hjelmencrantz A, 2004, Isoxazole-3-hydroxamic acid derivatives as peptide deformylase inhibitors and potential antibacterial agents, Bioorg Med Chem Lett, 14, 5997–6000.

Chen D, Hackbarth C, Ni ZJ, Wu C, Wang W, Jain R, He Y, Bracken K, Weidman B, Patel DV, Trias J, White RJ, Yuan Z, 2004, Peptide deformylase inhibitors as antibacterial agents, identification of VRC 3375, a proline-alkyl succinyl hydroxamate derivative, by using an integrated combinatorial and medicinal chemistry approach, Antimicrob Agents Chemother, 48, 250–261.

Chen D, Patel DV, Hackbarth CJ, Wang W, Dreyer G, Youg DC, Margolis PS, Wu C, Ni Z-J, Trias J, White RJ, Yuan Z, 2000, Actinonin, a naturally occurring antibacterial agent, is a potent deformylase inhibitor, Biochemistry, 39, 1256–1262.

Chu M, Mierzwa R, He L, Xu L, Gentile F, Terracciano J, Patel M, Miesel L, Bohanon S, Kravec C, Gramer C, et al, 2001, Isolation and structure elucidation of two novel deformylase inhibitors produced by Streptomyces sp., Tetrahedron Lett, 42, 3549–3551.

Ciufolini MA, Xi N, 1998, Synthesis, chemistry and conformational properties of piperazic acids, Chem Soc Rev, 27, 437–445.

Coats RA, Lee SL, Davis KA, Patel KM, Rhoads EK, Howard MH, 2004, Stereochemical definition and chirospecific synthesis of the peptide deformylase inhibitor Sch 382583, Bioorg Med Chem Lett, 69, 1734–1737.

Cynamon MH, Alvarez-Freites Z, Yeo AET, 2004, BB-3497, a peptide deformylase inhibitor, is active against Mycobacterium tuberculosis, J Antimicrob Chemother, 53, 403–405.

Davies SJ, Ayscough AP, Beckett P, Bragg RA, Clements JM, Doel S, et al, 2003, Structure-activity relationships of the peptide deformylase inhibitor BB-3497, modification of the methylene spacer and the P′ side chain, Bioorg Med Chem Lett, 13, 2709–2713.

Davies SJ, Ayscough AP, Beckett P, Clements JM, Doel S, Pratt LM, Spavold ZM, Thomas SW, Whittaker M, 2001, Structure-activity relationships of the peptide deformylase inhibitor BB 3497, modification of P2′ and P3′ side chain BB-3497, Bioorg Med Chem Lett, 13, 2715–2718.

Ednie LM, Pankuch G, Appelbaum PCL, 2004, Antipneumococcal activity of LBM415, a new peptide deformylase inhibitor, compared with those of other agents, Antimicrob Agents Chemother, 48, 4027–4032.

Fonsera-Aten N, Rios AM, Mejias A, Chavez-Bueno S, Katz K, Gomez AM, McCracken GH, Hardy RD, 2004, Evaluation of NVP-PDF 713 for the treatment of experimental Mycoplasma pneumoniae. I. Pneumonia, 44th Intersci Conf Antimicrob Agents Chemother, abstract F-1966.

Giglione C, Pierre M, Meinnel T, 2000a, Peptide deformylase as a target for new generation broad spectrum antimicrobial agents, Mol Microbiol, 36, 1197–1205.

Giglione C, Sereno A, Pierre M, Boisson B, Meinnel T, 2000b, Identification of eukaryotic peptide deformylase reveals universality of N-terminal protein processing mechanisms, EMBO J, 19, 5616–5629.

Gordon JJ, Kelly BK, Miller GH, 1962, Actinonin, an antibiotic substance produced by an actinomycete, Nature, 195, 701–702.

Green BG, Toney JH, Kozarich JW, Grant SK, 2000, Inhibition of bacterial peptide deformylase by biaryl acid analogs, Arch Biochem Biophys, 375, 355–358.

Guilloteau JP, Mathieu M, Giglione G, Blanc V, Dupuy A, Chevrier M, Gil P, Famechon A, Meinnel T, Mikol V, 2002, The crystal structures of four peptide deformylases bound to the antibiotic actinonin reveal two distinct types: a platform for the structure-based designed antibacterial agents, J Mol Biol, 320, 951–962.

Gupta MK, Mishra P, Prathipati P, Saxena AK, 2002, 2D-QSAR in hydroxamic acid derivatives as peptide deformylase inhibitors and antibacterial agents, Bioorg Med Chem Lett, 10, 3713–3716.

Haas M, Beyer D, Gahlmann R, Freiberg C, 2001, YkrB is the main peptide deformylase in Bacillus subtilis, a eubacterium containing two functional peptide deformylases, Microbiology, 147, 1783–1791.

Hackbarth CJ, Chen DZ, Lewis JG, Clark K, Mangold JB, Cramer JA, Margolis PS, et al, 2002, N-Alkyl urea hydroxamic acids are a new class of peptide deformylase inhibitors with antibacterial activities, Antimicrob Agents Chemother, 46, 2752–2764.

Howard MH, Cenizel T, Gutteridge S, Hanna WS, Tao Y, Totrov M, Wittenbach VA, Zheng YG, 2004, A novel class of inhibitors of peptide deformylase discovered through high-throughput screening and virtual ligand screening, J Med Chem, 47, 6669–6672.

Hu X, Nguyen KT, Verlinde CLM, Hol WG, Pei D, 2003, Structure-based design of a macrocyclic inhibitor for peptide deformylase, J Med Chem, 46, 3771–3774.

Hue Y-J, Rajagopalan PTR, Pei D, 1998, H-phosphonate derivatives as novel peptide deformylase inhibitors, Bioorg Med Chem Lett, 8, 2479–2482.

Huntington KM, Yi T, Wei Y, Pei D, 2000, Synthesis and antibacterial activity of peptide deformylase inhibitor, Biochemistry, 39, 4543–4551.

Jain R, Sundram A, Lopez S, Neckermann G, Wu G, Hackbarth C, Chen D, Wang W, Ryder NS, Weidmann B, Patel D, Trias J, White R, Yuan Z, 2003, α-Substituted hydroxamic acids as novel bacterial deformylase inhibitor-based antibacterial agents, Bioorg Med Chem Lett, 13, 4223–4228.

Jayasekera MMK, Kendall A, Shammas R, Dermeyer M, Tomala M, Shapiro MA, Holler JP, 2000, Novel nonpeptidic inhibitor of peptide deformylase, Arch Biochem Biophys, 381, 313–316.

Lofland D, Difuntorum S, Waller A, Clements JM, Weaver MK, Karlowsky JA, Johnson K, 2004, In vitro antibacterial activity of the peptide deformylase inhibitor BB-83698, J Antimicrob Chemother, 53, 664–668.

Margolis PS, Hackbarth CJ, Lopez S, Maniar M, Wang W, Yuan Z, White R, Trias J, 2001, Resistance of *Streptococcus pneumoniae* to deformylase inhibitors is due to mutations in *defB*, Antimicrob Agents Chemother, 45, 2432–2435.

Margolis PS, Hackbarth CJ, Young DC, Wang W, Chen D, Yuan Z, White R, Trias J, 2000, Peptide deformylase in *Staphylococcus aureus*: resistance to inhibition is mediated by mutations in the formyl transferase gene, Antimicrob Agents Chemother, 44, 1825–1831.

Marker K, Sanger F, 1964, N-Formyl methionyl 6S-RNA, J Mol Biol, 8, 835–840.

Meinnel T, Lazennec C, Blanquet S, 1995, Mapping of the active site zinc ligands of peptide deformylase, J Mol Biol, 254, 175–183.

Meinnel T, Patiny L, Ragusa S, Blanquet S, 1999, Design and synthesis of substrate analogue inhibitors of peptide deformylase, Biochemistry, 38, 4287–4295.

Molteni V, He X, Nabakka J, Yang K, Kreusch A, Gordon P, Bursulaya B, Warner I, Shin T, Biorac T, Ryder NS, Goldberg R, Doughty J, He Y, 2004, Identification of novel potent bicyclic peptide deformylase inhibitor, Bioorg Med Chem Lett, 14, 1477–1481.

Rajagopalan PTR, Datta A, Pei D, 1997, Purification, characterization and inhibition of peptide deformylase from Escherichia coli, Biochemistry, 36, 13910–13918.

Ramanathan-Girish S, McColm J, Clements JM, Taupin P, Barrowcliffe S, Hevizi J, Safrin S, Moore C, Patou G, Moser H, Gadd A, Hoch U, Jiang V, Lofland D, Johnson KW, 2004, Pharmacokinetics in animals and humans of a first-in-class peptide deformylase inhibitor, Antimicrob Agents Chemother, 48, 4835–4842.

Reddy NB, Crabb DM, Duffy LB, Waites KB, 2004, Comparative in vitro activity of an investigational peptide deformylase inhibitor LBM 415 and other agents against human mycoplasmas and ureaplasma, 44th Intersci Conf Antimicrob Agents Chemother, abstract E-2050.

Roblin PM, Hammerschlag MR, 2003, In vitro activity of a new antibiotic, NVP-PDF386 (VRC4887), against *Chlamydia pneumoniae*, Antimicrob Agents Chemother, 47, 1447–1448.

Ryder NS, Dziuk-Fox J, Kubik B, Mlineritsch W, Alvaraz S, Bracken K, Dean K, Jain R, Sundaram A, Weidmann B, Yuan Z, 2004, LBM 415, a new peptide deformylase inhibitor with potent in vitro activity against drug resistant bacteria, 44th Intersci Conf Antimicrob Agents Chemother, abstract F-1959.

Serero A, Giglione G, Meinnel T, 2001, Distinctive features of the two classes of eukaryotic peptide deformylase, J Mol Biol, 314, 695–708.

Smith HK, Beckett RP, Clements JM, Doel S, East SP, Launchbury SB, Pratt LM, Spavold ZM, Tmas W, Todd RS, Wittaker M, 2002, Structure-activity relationships of the peptide deformylase inhibitor BB 3497, modification of the metal binding group, Bioorg Med Chem Lett, 12, 3595–3599.

Thorarensen A, Deibel MR Jr, Rohrer DC, Vosters AF, Yem AW, Marshall VD, Lynn JC, et al, 2001, Identification of novel potent hydroxamic acid inhibitors of peptidyl deformylase and the importance of the hydroxamic acid functionality on inhibition, Bioorg Med Chem Lett, 11, 1355–1358.

Wise R, Andrews JM, Ashby J, 2002, In vitro activities of peptide deformylase inhibitors against gram-positive pathogens, Antimicrob Agents Chemother, 46, 1117–1118.

Yuan Z, Trias J, White RJ, 2001, Deformylase as novel antibacterial target, Drug Discovery Today, 6, 954–961.

Helicobacter pylori and Antibacterial Agents

ANDRÉ BRYSKIER, JOHN LOWTHER, AND CATHERINE COUTURIER

40

1. INTRODUCTION

Spiral bacteria have been observed in studies including known patients since 1889 (Kidd and Modlin, 1998). The first well-known report of gastric *Helicobacter* was done by Bizzazero in Turin, Italy, in 1893. He observed gram-negative "spirochetes" inhabiting the glands in the gastric mucosa of dogs. Salomon (1896) was able to induce colonization with these spirochetal organisms in mouse stomachs after feeding ground-up gastric mucosa from rats and dogs.

In the early 20th century, spiral organisms in the human mucosa were reported occasionally, initially adjacent to carcinomas (Kriewitz, 1906).

Almost 40% of resected gastric specimens were found to have spirochetal organisms (Freedberg and Baron, 1940). In 1967, an enlarged spirochete within a parietal cell gland was published in anatomical photography of the gastric corpus (Ito, 1967).

In 1975, it was shown that in 80% of gastric ulcer specimens, spiral bacteria were present (Steer and Colin-Jones, 1975). Unfortunately, the authors were unable to culture the microorganism. In 1979, Warren, a pathologist of the Perth Hospital in Australia, and coworkers observed from gastric biopsies the presence of curved bacilli in the mucus layer overlying the gastric mucosa; they were able to isolate and culture *Helicobacter pylori* from patients with abnormal abdominal complaints (Marshall and Warren, 1983). Since then, a tremendous number of studies of human gastritis have been carried out and have demonstrated the involvement of *H. pylori* in the pathogenesis of gastric diseases (Enroth and Engstrand, 2001).

The recognition of *H. pylori* as an etiological agent of gastric peptic ulcer, gastric adenocarcinoma, and mucosa-associated lymphoid tissue lymphoma is one of the most important advances made in gastroenterology in the past 50 years. In 1994, the World Health Organization and International Agency of Research and Cancer Consensus considered that there was sufficient epidemiological and histological evidence to classify *H. pylori* as a group 1 carcinogen (Huang et al., 1998; World Health Organization, 1994).

In the United States, around 80 million people are infected with *H. pylori*, and a significant portion of those infected patients will have symptoms of gastric disease (Copeland et al., 2000). Worldwide, the rate of *H. pylori* infection varies from 25 to above 75% of the population, depending on sanitation levels and other socioeconomic factors.

The relative uneffectiveness of singly administered antibiotics has empirically led to the use of dual therapies or, better, triple therapies including a proton pump inhibitor and two antibiotics. The search for optimal *H. pylori* treatment was mainly and empirically based on the results of a great number of clinical trials.

The development of new anti-*H. pylori* agents is needed in order to overcome some threats: adverse events such as vomiting, diarrhea, nausea, or disulfiram-like syndrome resulting in noncompliance with therapy; the emergence of *H. pylori* isolates resistant to clarithromycin, metronidazole, and, as recently described, amoxicillin; and the broad antibacterial spectrum of the standard antibacterial therapy, which may be a problem in disturbing the normal flora, which can result in selecting resistant bacteria of other species.

It has been argued whether all *H. pylori* infections should be treated. Nonulcer dyspeptic patients with *H. pylori* infections constitute a large patient group, and according to recommendations made by the National Institutes of Health in 1994, the patients should not be treated.

However, in the Maastricht Consensus report made by the European *H. pylori* study group in 1997, this patient group is suggested for treatment especially if a patient has a family history of gastric cancer. The recommended regimen is a combination of a proton pump inhibitor with antibacterial agents.

Eradication therapy is recommended for infected persons who develop peptic ulcer disease or gastric lymphoma or who are beginning long-term treatment with nonsteroidal anti-inflammatory drugs. However, it is claimed that therapy against *H. pylori* may worsen gastroesophageal efflux disease and increase the risk of esophageal cancer.

2. *H. PYLORI*: TAXONOMY

H. pylori is a fastidious, gram-negative, microaerophilic spiral bacillus (Dunn et al., 1997). It is the only microorganism that regularly colonizes the stomach.

H. pylori belongs to the family *Campylobacteraceae*, which was proposed in 1991 (Vandamme et al., 1991).

Taxonomic studies divided the genus *Campylobacter* into three genera (i) *Campylobacter* species, including *Bacteroides gracilis*; (ii) *Helicobacter* species, including *Flexispiras*; and (iii) *Arcobacter, Wolinella, Thiovulum*, and *Anaerobiospirillum*.

Table 1 Main *Helicobacter* species and their hosts[a]

Helicobacter species	Natural hosts	Experimental hosts
H. pylori	Human, rhesus monkeys, cats	Mice, piglets, monkeys, cats, gerbils, guinea pigs
H. felis	Cats, dogs	Mice, rats, dogs
H. heilmannii	Birds, cats, dogs, ferrets, monkeys	Humans, mice
H. mustelae	Ferrets	Ferrets
H. pullorum	Chickens, humans	ND[b]
H. canis	Dogs, cats	ND
H. bilis	Mice, rats	Mice
H. hepaticus	Mice	Mice
H. rappini	Sheep, dogs, mice, humans	Guinea pigs
H. fennelliae	Humans	Macaques
H. cinaedi	Humans, hamsters	Macaques
H. acinonychis	Cheetahs	Mice
H. cholecystus	Syrian hamsters	
H. rodentium	Mice	
H. survius	Musk shrews	
H. aurati	Syrian hamsters	
H. mesocricetorum	Syrian hamsters	

[a]Data from Ferrero et al., 2001.
[b]ND, not described.

The genus *Helicobacter* was established in 1989 (Goodwin et al., 1989), and now more than 20 species belong to this genus (On, 2001) (Table 1).

H. pylori was the first bacterial species for which the determination of the complete genome sequences of two strains was accomplished.

3. EPIDEMIOLOGY OF *H. PYLORI* INFECTION

The majority of *Helicobacter* species are found in the stomach and intestines of different animals, as well as in humans.

H. pylori is unique among bacterial species in its ability to colonize the stomachs of more than half of all populations worldwide, and it is able to persist for years once it has become established (Taylor and Blaser, 1991).

H. pylori is associated with chronic active gastritis B, and eradication of *H. pylori* is always followed by resolution of the gastritis.

The vast majority of persons carrying *H. pylori* do not report any related clinical symptoms. However, persons carrying *H. pylori* also have an increased risk of developing both intestinal-type and diffuse-type noncardiagastric adenocarcinoma.

H. pylori is most frequently found in the central part of the human gastric mucosa in untreated patients. In patients treated with acid-suppressing drugs (proton pump inhibitors and H_2 antagonists), *H. pylori* may be present in the body of the stomach. Thus, it is always important to obtain antral biopsy samples, as well as corpus biopsy samples, from patients recently treated with acid-suppressive drugs.

Although our understanding of H. pylori has advanced, many questions are unsolved, such as how *H. pylori* is transmitted (Parsonneet et al., 1999). A part from *H. pylori*, *Helicobacter heilmannii* is the most common bacterium in the human gastric mucosa, with a prevalence of up to 0.5% in dyspeptic patients in Western Europe (Holck et al., 1997). *H. heilmannii* is usually found in the foveolae associated with mild chronic gastritis, whereas *H. pylori* is usually found on the surface epithelium associated with severe gastritis. Occasionally, *H. pylori* and *H. heilmannii* are found simultaneously (Dent et al., 1987).

An improved socioeconomic situation has resulted in the disappearance of *H. pylori* in industrialized countries (Blaser and Berg, 2001) and declining prevalence in some developing countries.

4. VIRULENCE OF *H. PYLORI*

Several virulence factors for gastric colonization, tissue damage, and survival have been identified in *H. pylori* (Andersen and Wadström, 2001) (Table 2).

H. pylori persists on the surfaces of gastric epithelial cells, in the overlying mucin, and it seems to enter certain epithelial cells (Noach et al., 1994). Around 80% of *H. pylori* isolates live free in gastric mucus; some attach to the gastric mucosa via adherence pedestals.

Table 2 Virulence factors of *H. pylori*

Function	Virulence factor(s)
Colonization	Flagella
	Urease
	Adhesins
Tissue damage	Proteolytic enzymes
	GacA (cytotoxins)
	VacA (vacuolating cytotoxins)
	Urease
	Phospholipase A
	Alcohol dehydrogenase
Survival	Intracellular
	Superoxide dismutase
	Catalase
	Coccoid forms
	Heat shock proteins
	Urease
Other	LPS
	Lewis factors (X/Y)

H. pylori multiplies despite important host defenses, including gastric acidity, peristalsis, epithelial cell turnover, and immune and inflammatory responses.

Significant advances have been made in recent years with regard to the virulence determinants expressed by *H. pylori*. However, the exact mechanisms of pathogenesis and immune evasion remain unclear. The putative pathogenic determinants of *H. pylori* can be divided into two major groups: maintenance factors, which allow colonization, and virulence factors, which contribute to pathogenicity. Urease and adherence to epithelial cells are maintenance factors.

One-half to two-thirds of U.S. and European strains carry the *cag* pathogenicity island (PAI). A 40-kb DNA segment in many of these genes seems to help induce interleukin 8 and thereby a strong and potentially damaging inflammatory response. Such strains are recovered preferentially from patients with overt disease.

All East Asian *H. pylori* strains carry the *cag* PAI independent of disease status. More than half of U.S. and European isolates carry toxigenic alleles (*vacAs* 1) of the vacuolating cytoxin gene, with other strains carrying nontoxigenic alleles (*vacAs* 2). In general, *vac*As 1 strains carry the *caf* PAI.

All East Asian strains carry *vacAs* 1 alleles. The East Asian and Western *H. pylori* strains differ markedly in DNA sequence motifs in the *vacA* and *cagA* genes.

H. pylori strains can be classified into two types with regard to the presence of a PAI (Xiang et al., 1995) within the bacterial genome, which is associated with an increased virulence of *H. pylori* (Rappuoli et al., 1998).

Type 1 *H. pylori* strains express a highly immunogenic protein of unknown function called CagA, which is encoded within the PAI, and the VacA cytotoxin, which induces vacuole formation in epithelial cells (de Bernard et al., 1997). Other genes encode a putative type IV secretion protein.

Type 2 *H. pylori* strains do not possess the PAI and therefore do not express CagA. They also exhibit no cytotoxic activity in vitro, despite the fact that the *vacA* gene is present (Ghiara et al., 1995).

It has been shown that type 1 *H. pylori* isolates are associated with more severe gastritis and a higher risk of developing disease (Covacci et al., 1999). However, one-half of the world's population is infected with CagA-positive strains, yet only a minority will develop clinical disease.

Recent studies demonstrated that gastric epithelial cells in *H. pylori*-infected patients exhibit an increased rate of apoptosis, in addition to necrosis, contributing to the increased loss of gastric epithelial cells (Ahmed et al., 2000) and leading in the medium term to fibrosis.

It has been shown that *H. pylori* inhibits the synthesis and secretion of mucin through cell wall lipopolysaccharide (LPS) (Slomiany et al., 1997). *H. pylori* LPS induces the mucosal inflammatory process due to enhancement of proinflammatory properties of cytokine expression, nitric oxide generation, and massive epithelial cell apoptosis triggered by the mucosal rise of insoluble tumor necrosis factor alpha. Release of tumor necrosis factor alpha occurs mainly through selective activation of p38 and extracellular signal-regulated kinase (ERK) mitogen-activated protein kinase pathways. Activation of the p38 kinase cascade appears to be coupled with apoptosis, and ERK activation is associated with cell survival. The detrimental influence of *H. pylori* LPS on gastric mucin synthesis is closely linked to caspase 3 activation and apoptosis. The inhibition of caspase 3 blocks *H. pylori*-induced apoptosis but also results in an increase in mucus synthesis. Inhibition of ERK with PD-98059 potentiated the LPS-induced caspase 3 activity. Inhibition of p38 kinase with SB 203580 blocked caspase 3 activation, the kinase having a proapoptotic activity.

The mobility of *H. pylori* is considered a virulence factor, being a colonization factor (O'Toole et al., 2000).

Urease is one of the key enzymes in *H. pylori* pathogenesis. Urease is necessary for *H. pylori* to maintain a pH-neutral microenvironment around the bacteria, compulsory for survival in the acidic stomach. Superoxide dismutase breaks down superoxide production by polymorphonuclear neutrophils and macrophages and thereby prevents the killing of these organisms. Catalase protects *H. pylori* against the damaging effect of hydrogen peroxide released from phagocytes.

The *H. pylori* outer membrane contains at least five porins, which are part of the 32-member family of outer membrane proteins. These porins are expressed weakly in comparison with those in other bacteria. However, the main porin, HopE, formed a large channel, of 1.5 nS. There are approximately 2,000 copies of HopE. Among the few conserved families of efflux systems associated with bacterial resistance to antibacterial agents, one is widespread among gram-negative bacilli: the RND family. The presence of three gene fragments encoding components of a putative RND efflux system in *H. pylori* 11637 was reported. Apparently, *H. pylori* lacks an effective RND efflux system for antibiotics. It was shown that tetracycline, chloramphenicol, and metronidazole are not pumped out by *H. pylori* in an energy-dependent fashion. Of the three putative efflux systems identified in *H. pylori*, only one, HefABC, showed any homology to the RND efflux system involved in multidrug resistance in other bacteria. It was apparently expressed under laboratory conditions, as was HefDEF but not HefGHI, a relative of the cation efflux subfamily of the RND system.

H. pylori transforms into coccoid forms under certain conditions, such as nutrient starvation, and in media containing growth inhibitors: bismuth, proton pump inhibitors, and certain antibiotics. The virulence of *H. pylori* decreases when the bacterium is in the coccoid form, but no deletion exists in amplification fragments of the *ureA*, *ureB*, *hpaA*, *vacA*, and *cagA* genes, suggesting that coccoid *H. pylori* may have pathogenicity.

Lactoferrin is a multifunctional glycoprotein with antibiotic, anti-inflammatory, and immunomodulation properties. It is found in neutrophils and in human exocrine secretions such as breast milk, tears, saliva, bile, and pancreatic juice, where it is associated with mucosal defense. Lactoferrin seems to be able to block or displace bacterial attachment. Recombinant human lactoferrin was tested in a *Helicobacter felis* murine model. Treatment for 2 weeks with lactoferrin partially reverses both infection-induced gastritis and the infection rate.

5. TREATMENT OF *H. PYLORI* INFECTIONS

H. pylori can colonize the stomach during childhood and cause lifelong chronic gastritis. Curing *H. pylori* infection cures ulcer disease, and reinfection seems to be of rare occurrence. *H. pylori* is difficult to eradicate, and successful treatment requires the concurrent administration of two or more antibacterials. None of the drug regimens currently used to treat *H. pylori* cures the infection in 100% of patients (Wood, 1995).

Over the past decade many different therapies were promoted and recommendations changed rapidly.

Empirical therapies with bismuth compounds were used in ancient times. Since the 19th century, bismuth compounds have been advocated in the form of bismuth subnitrate, subcarbonate, and subcitrate for the treatment of nonspecific gastrointestinal symptoms.

A triple therapy combining bismuth salts or acid-suppressive drugs and two antibacterial agents was promoted. These antibacterial agents comprised amoxicillin, tetracycline, metronidazole, and clarithromycin.

A quadruple therapy is currently being promoted. In meta-analysis the quadruple regimen had the highest cure rate. Antibacterial therapy for ulcers has been recommended since 1994, following a Consensus Development Conference of the National Institutes of Health (NIH Consensus Development Panel, 1994).

6. IN VITRO STUDIES

6.1. E-Test

The E-test is recommended by the British Society for Antimicrobial Chemotherapy (BSAC) for determination of the MICs of antibacterials for *H. pylori*.

In a multicenter European study, the correlation between E-test and agar dilution for testing metronidazole was not as good as those obtained with amoxicillin and clarithromycin. There was a large proportion of discrepancies, 22%, in metronidazole testing. The E-test method led to higher MICs, and more strains were categorized as resistant. The degree of agreement within ±1 dilution was 57%, and that within ±2 dilutions was 76%.

In another study metronidazole resistance was 39% by E-test and 21.6% by agar dilution ($P < 0.001$). For clarithromycin, the proportions of *H. pylori* resistant strains were 12 and 10.6% by the E-test method and agar dilution, respectively. Forty-two percent of the metronidazole MICs differed by 2 log units or more and resulted in a difference in susceptibility pattern in 17.6%. In contrast, the difference in susceptibility pattern was only 3% with clarithromycin.

There were not only discrepancies between E-test and agar dilution for metronidazole but also a lack of reproducibility for some isolates.

The European *H. pylori* study group proposed a standardized method for use of E-test (Table 3).

Three days of incubation seems more accurate, as 5 days gave greater variability. With E-test, susceptibility results were similar with inoculum sizes of 10^6 and 10^8 CFU/ml, and correlation with agar dilution was good with either inoculum when read at 3 days.

6.2. MIC Determination in Agar

The NCCLS subcommittee for antibiotic susceptibility testing has published guidance on susceptibility testing by agar dilution (NCCLS document M-100, A7). The European consensus in Maastricht has made recommendations on susceptibility testing, and the BSAC has made recommendations on susceptibility testing using E-test. There are no published internationally agreed-upon methods for susceptibility testing by disk diffusion for *H. pylori*.

6.2.1. Factors Influencing Susceptibility Testing

6.2.1.1. Influence of pH of the Medium

It has been shown that the pH of the medium influences greatly the MICs of all antibacterial agents (Table 4).

6.2.1.2. Media

In published studies, several culture media have been used: Brucella agar, Wilkins-Chalgren agar, yeast charcoal agar anaerobic medium, GAB-camp agar, Columbia agar, and Mueller-Hinton agar. A false high rate of metronidazole resistance can be attributed to media and growth factors, such as Columbia blood agar supplemented with factors X and Y and menadione. The X-factor and menadione used as growth factors inhibit metronidazole activity. Mueller-Hinton agar supplemented with 5 to 10% sheep blood can be used.

6.2.1.3. Age of Culture

It was shown that with *H. pylori* isolates recovered after more than 4 days of incubation, the correlation between E-test and zone diameter was only 0.742. In contrast, for isolates recovered within 4 days of primary incubation, the correlation between both methods was 0.937.

Coccoid strains are not inhibited in vitro by amoxicillin, although they remain susceptible to metronidazole.

Bacteria should be harvested for susceptibility testing during the active phase of growth, and the colonies recovered from the primary plates beyond 4 days should be recultured to produce younger isolates for susceptibility testing.

6.2.1.4. Size of Inoculum

The sizes of the inocula used in the different studies varied from McFarland 0.5 to 4 to 6. However, the most common

Table 4 Influence of pH on anti-*H. pylori* activities of various antibacterials[a]

Compound	MIC (μg/ml)	
	pH 7.0–7.4	pH 5.0–5.7
Ampicillin	<0.06	0.06
Erythromycin A	0.12	4.0
Clarithromycin	<0.01–0.03	0.5–0.75
Azithromycin	0.094–0.25	1.5–2.0
Roxithromycin		
Clindamycin	0.75	16
Metronidazole	2.0–12	1.0–32
Ciprofloxacin	0.12	2.0

[a]Data from Debets-Ossenkop et al., 1995; Malonoski et al., 1993; and Rubinstein et al., 1994.

Table 3 E-test methods for *H. pylori*

Method	Inoculation method	Size of inoculum	Medium	Incubation
European group	Flooding	McFarland 4	Mueller-Hinton + 10% horse blood	37°C, microaerophilic, 3 days
BSAC	Swabbing	McFarland 3	Mueller-Hinton or Wilkins-Chalgren + 5–10% horse blood	37°C, microaerophilic, 3–5 days

Table 5 Zone size for metronidazole against *H. pylori*

Medium	Zone diam (mm)		
	Susceptible	Resistant	Intermediate
Mueller-Hinton + 7–10% blood	>21	<16	16–21
Columbia agar + 7–10% blood	≥16	<16	

inoculum size used is McFarland 4 (10^8CFU/ml). It was suggested that an inoculum size of 10^8CFU/ml (equivalent of McFarland 4) be used to allow results to be read by 3 days.

6.2.1.5. Zone Diameters

McNulty et al. (2001) recommended the following for disk susceptibility testing for *H. pylori*.

- For clarithromycin, the medium to be used is either Mueller-Hinton supplemented with 7 to 10% blood or Columbia agar plus 7 to 10% blood. When the organism is resistant, no zone is visible; the presence of any zone indicates susceptibility. Disks contain 2 μg of clarithromycin.
- For metronidazole, it is more complex:
  - Avoid high (≥50 μg) or low (1 μg) metronidazole disk content. Disks loaded with 5 μg of metronidazole are recommended.
  - Mueller-Hinton or Columbia agar supplemented with 5 to 10% horse blood
  - Use cultures less than 4 days old for setting up susceptibility testing.
  - Inoculum size of 10^8CFU/ml (McFarland 4)
  - Include a metronidazole-susceptible strain as a control (e.g., NCTC 12822).
  - Zone sizes for metronidazole are given in Table 5.
  - Follow-up testing of strains exhibiting a metronidazole-intermediate zone by another quantitative method may be required.
  - Overall discordant results for 5 to 10% of patients due to coinfection with multiple strains may be expected.

7. ANIMAL STUDIES

Initial attempts to establish *H. pylori* infection models in laboratory animals (mice, rats, and rabbits) were unsuccessful. Alternative *Helicobacter* models were developed using animals that were already naturally infected with *Helicobacter* species (ferrets) and nonhuman primates, or those that could be experimentally infected with *H. pylori*, including dogs and gnobiotic piglets.

The first report of experimental *H. pylori* infections in immunocompetent mice was published in 1995 (Marchetti et al., 1995). Using fresh clinical *H. pylori* isolates that had been cultured extensively in vitro, it was possible to establish transient infection in mice.

A mouse model permitting the establishment of a long-term, high-bacterial-density *H. pylori* colonization was also reported (Lee et al., 1997).

Experimental *H. pylori* models have also been developed in Mongolian gerbils (Matsumoto et al., 1997; Yokota et al., 1991) and in guinea pigs (Shomer et al., 1998), cats (Fox et al., 1995), and macaques (Dubois et al., 1996, 1999).

An optimization of Lee's mouse model (C57BL/6-H mice) using *H. pylori* strain SS1 with 1-day dosing was proposed. The aim was to be able to test at an early stage a promising lead compound in vivo.

8. EPIDEMIOLOGY OF RESISTANCE TO *H. PYLORI*

The true figure of resistance to *H. pylori* in one country is difficult to assess. Until recently, most studies aiming to assess the prevalence of resistance to *H. pylori* have been single-centered and have included a fairly limited number of clinical isolates originating from the same geographical area. In addition, comparison between centers is difficult due to the lack of standardization of susceptibility testing methods.

However, a tentative summary of published data is reported here by geographical area.

With the currently available data, results need to be taken with caution due to the following:

- Technical limitations for metronidazole MIC determination with the E-test method
- Low number of clinical isolates tested, which leads to very large confidence intervals
- The limited representativeness of the isolates tested, sometime including posttreatment strains (failures) and strains from patients having received multiple eradication therapies
- Reports usually available are from a single center or, in the best case, from two centers for one country.
- Studies are carried out irrespective of patient age.
- Breakpoints for the current antibacterials for *H. pylori* are not yet available.

Anti-*H. pylori* activities of four main antibacterials are usually investigated. These antibacterials are companion drugs in triple or quadruple therapy for eradication of *H. pylori*. These antibacterials are clarithromycin, metronidazole, tetracycline, and amoxicillin.

The prevalence of resistance worldwide for clarithromycin, with few exceptions, ranges from 0 to 20% of the isolates. For metronidazole there is a clear-cut difference between countries using metronidazole in large scale for gastrointestinal infections (amoebiasis and gardiasis) and gynecological infections (mainly trichomoniasis) and other parts of the world. In the former, metronidazole resistance can reach up to 80%, and in the latter, the metronidazole resistance rate is less than 60% depending on the population tested. The tetracycline resistance rate is low, with few exceptions, as is the amoxicillin resistance rate.

The first report of an *H. pylori* strain resistant to metronidazole was in 1988, and the first tetracycline-resistant strain was reported in 1996. Amoxicillin resistance was not considered a problem until it was described in the United States, Canada, and Italy.

Few studies have analyzed the rate of secondary resistance observed after treatment failures.

8.1. Resistance Rate in Europe

8.1.1. Adult Patients

Reports have been made from individual countries, and a study involving 17 European countries has been reported.

In France, a program of active surveillance was set up to study the susceptibility of *H. pylori* to antibacterials. Gastroenterologists throughout the country were asked to enroll patients randomly. Among 500 *H. pylori* strains, the level of primary resistance to clarithromycin was 14.1%.

In 2001, the rate of resistance to clarithromycin reached 17%. It is of interest that the resistance rate among strains isolated from ulcer patients (2%) was significantly lower than those from other gastric pathology. The resistance rate for metronidazole was 23.9% for the same period. In France, in 1991, the prevalence of clarithromycin-resistant *H. pylori* strains was 11%; it has been stable since then, at 10, 12, and 14% in 1992, 1994, and 1996, respectively. In this study MICs were determined by E-test.

The resistance rate in the southern part of Switzerland was investigated. One hundred forty-two *H. pylori* isolates were collected in 1996 and 1997. Of these isolates, none were found to be resistant to amoxicillin (MIC, ≥2.0 μg/ml), 12% were resistant to clarithromycin (MIC, ≥8.0 μg/ml), and 29% were resistant to metronidazole (MIC, ≥8.0 μg/ml). In Basel, Switzerland, *H. pylori* resistance to antibacterials was investigated in isolates from 153 patients who had undergone an antral gastric biopsy. Metronidazole resistance (MIC, >8.0 μg/ml) was found in 38% of the isolates (47 of 153 patients). No strains were resistant to amoxicillin, and 3% were resistant to clarithromycin.

In the Netherlands, a total of 231 *H. pylori* isolates were collected throughout the country over a period of 6 months during 1997 and 1998. The overall rates of resistance to clarithromycin and metronidazole were 1.7 and 21.1%, respectively. None of the strains were resistant to tetracycline or amoxicillin. The prevalence of primary resistance to trovafloxacin was 4.7%. There is a 3% increase in metronidazole resistance in comparison with a survey carried out in 1994 and 1995. However, the pattern of resistance to metronidazole was determined by the disk diffusion method in 1993 and the E-test method between 1994 and 1996. Metronidazole resistance rose from 7% (18 of 245 patients) in 1993 to 32% (161 of 509 patients) in 1996. More patients with nonulcer dyspepsia and more non-Western European patients were enrolled in 1996 than in 1993, but age and sex differences were not observed.

Between January 1990 and December 1999, a total of 473 clinical isolates of *H. pylori* were collected from dyspeptic patients in one center in Lisbon, Portugal. MICs were determined by E-test. The overall rates of resistance to amoxicillin, tetracycline, metronidazole, clarithromycin, and ciprofloxacin were 0, 0, 30.6, 19, and 9.6%, respectively. The prevalence of resistance to metronidazole was stable during this period, but for clarithromycin and ciprofloxacin a significant rise of resistant isolates was noted (Table 6).

H. pylori isolates were collected from 166 Portuguese patients by gastric biopsy, and rates of clarithomycin and metronidazole resistance of 5.8 and 60%, respectively, were obtained.

Consecutive patients with *H. pylori*-positive antral gastric biopsy samples were studied from 1994 to 1999 in the United Kingdom in a single center. A total of 1,064 patients were enrolled; the overall rate of metronidazole resistance was 40.3%, decreasing with age. Clarithromycin resistance was associated with metronidazole resistance. No isolates were resistant to amoxicillin. The overall rates of resistance to tetracycline and clarithromycin were 0.5 and 4.4%, respectively (Table 7).

Table 6 Prevalence of *H. pylori* resistance in Lisbon, Portugal

Years	% of resistance		
	Metronidazole	Clarithromycin	Ciprofloxacin
1990–1993	28.5	4.6	0
1994–1997	33.8	12.2	8.6
1998–1999	32.3	14.6	11.1

In another study, 1,215 *H. pylori* isolates were tested for susceptibility to antibacterials using the disk diffusion method in England; data are reported in Table 8.

In Croatia, the rate of *H. pylori* resistance to azithromycin was 4.87%. In Tartu, Estonia, 56 patients suffering from *H. pylori* infections were enrolled for testing of the susceptibility of *H. pylori* clinical isolates to antibacterial agents. MICs were determined by E-test. The metronidazole resistance rate was 46% (MIC, ≥8 μg/ml). All of the *H. pylori* strains were inhibited by ≤2.0 μg of clarithromycin per ml.

In Norway, the resistance rate was similar to that in Estonia.

Eighty *H. pylori* isolates from antral biopsy specimens obtained from dyspeptic patients were tested using E-test in Naples, Italy. All *H. pylori* isolates were inhibited by less than 4.0 μg of amoxicillin per ml and by less than 2.0 μg of tetracycline per ml. Seventy-nine strains (98.7%) were inhibited by less than 8 μg of ofloxacin per ml, but for one isolate, the ofloxacin MIC was above 64 μg/ml. Seventy percent of isolates (56 of 80 patients) were resistant to metronidazole (MIC, ≥8.0 μg/ml). The clarithromycin MIC was above 1.0 μg/ml for 12.0% of *H. pylori* strains (10 of 80 patients). In Turin, Italy, from 1997 to 1998, 49 previously untreated patients suffering from gastric or duodenal ulcers underwent biopsies of the gastric mucosa, and *H. pylori* strains were tested for susceptibility to antibiotics. MICs were determined by agar diffusion and E-test. All clinical isolates were susceptible to amoxicillin (MIC, <0.06 to 0.12 μg/ml). The prevalence of clarithromycin resistance was 5 to 7%. Coexistence of clarithromycin-susceptible and -resistant pretreatment strains was found in two patients. Pretreatment strain resistance to metronidazole was 6% in another study in Italy.

In Seville, Spain, *H. pylori* isolates were cultured from gastric biopsy samples from 58 patients. MICs were determined by E-test. The rates of resistance were 41, 22, and 12% for metronidazole, clarithromycin, and both compounds,

Table 7 Prevalence of *H. pylori* isolates resistant to antibacterials in the United Kingdom

Years	No. of patients	% of resistance		
		Clarithromycin	Tetracycline	Metronidazole
1994–1995	96		0.0	20.8
1995–1996	167		0.0	46.7
1996–1997	228	2.7	0.0	39
1997–1998	313	4.8	0.6	41.9
1998–1999	260	5.8	1.2	42.7

Table 8 Prevalence of *H. pylori* isolates resistant to antibacterials in England

Year	% of resistance	
	Metronidazole	Clarithromycin
1992	18	
1993	22	1
1994	33	2
1995	32	4
1996	37	6
1997	37	8

respectively. Of the metronidazole- and clarithromycin-resistant isolates, 2% were also resistant to tetracycline. None of them were resistant to amoxicillin.

The prevalence of resistance of *H. pylori* in the area of Magdeburg, Germany, during the period from 1996 to 1997 was studied using isolates from 271 gastric biopsy specimens. MICs were determined by E-test. The prevalence of metronidazole resistance was 32.1%; the resistance rate was higher in women (38.5%) than in men (24.4%). The rate of clarithromycin resistance was 3.3%. Eight of nine strains resistant to clarithromycin were resistant to metronidazole. All of the isolates were susceptible to amoxicillin or tetracycline. High-level resistance to metronidazole was also reported in another part of Germany.

In Ireland, of 50 *H. pylori* isolates, 26% were resistant to clarithromycin due to an A2143G mutation. In a previous study, the clarithromycin resistance rate was 5%.

In Malmö, Sweden, the rate of resistance to metronidazole was 29 to 40%. From 1994 to 1999, clarithromycin resistance increased in prevalence from 1.0 to 7.0%. In Göteborg, Sweden, in 109 patients from whom *H. pylori* was collected by antral gastric biopsy, the resistance rates were 40.3% for metronidazole and 2.8% for clarithromycin. No isolates resistant to tetracycline or amoxicillin were recovered. A study was designed to investigate the development of resistance in Swedish *H. pylori* isolates from 1990 to 1996. A total of 415 clinical isolates were collected from 10 clinical microbiological laboratories. None of the isolates were resistant to ampicillin or tetracycline, but 30% were resistant to metronidazole. In 1996, 9% of *H. pylori* isolates were resistant to clarithromycin.

Primary resistance in *H. pylori* was investigated using isolates from 192 patients suffering from peptic ulcer or chronic gastritis in Sofia, Bulgaria, collected from three hospitals from 1993 to 1999. Susceptibilities were assessed by the disk diffusion method. The rates of resistance were 28.6, 9.7, 3.9, and 1.9% for metronidazole, clarithromycin, ciprofloxacin, and tetracycline, respectively. The rates of combined resistance to dual and triple antibacterials were 2.8 and 2.3%, respectively. The metronidazole resistance rate was stable, being 28.1% from 1993 to 1996 and 27.3% from 1998 to 1999. The rates of clarithromycin resistance were 8.2% from 1993 to 1996 and 11.5% from 1997 to 1999. For ciprofloxacin, resistance rates were 2.1% from 1993 to 1996 and 9.1% from 1997 to 1999. Tetracycline resistance was detected only in 1999.

In Poland, the rates of metronidazole resistance were stable between 1993 and 1996: 38, 60, 59, and 35% in 1993, 1994, 1995, and 1996, respectively. In 1996, the resistance rates for ciprofloxacin and clarithromycin were 0.8 and 16.9% respectively. No strains resistant to tetracycline or amoxicillin were reported.

8.1.2. Pediatric Patients

From 1989 through 2000, in Belgium, *H. pylori* gastritis was diagnosed in 569 children, and antibiotic susceptibility was investigated for 555 patients. Data are reported in Table 9. All strains were found to be susceptible to amoxicillin. For 238 patients the antibiotic susceptibilities were compared among the strains isolated from the antrum and gastric body in the same patient. Discrepant results were found in five samples (2%): for clarithromycin susceptibility in two patients and for metronidazole susceptibility for the three remaining patients.

In a French series, 64 of 150 (43%) *H. pylori* isolates from children were resistant to metronidazole, 21% (32 of 150) were resistant to clarithromycin, and 9% (14 of 150) were resistant to both metronidazole and clarithromycin. The overall prevalence of resistance to metronidazole and clarithromycin did not change significantly between 1994 and 1999. In another series resistance rates varied from 1 of 23 (4%) to 3 of 38 (7%) for clarithromycin and from 6 of 23 (26%) to 15 of 38 (40%) for metronidazole.

In a study carried out in Greece, 5% of *H. pylori* isolates were resistant to clarithromycin, a rate similar to that reported for adult patients in the same geographical area, and 27% were resistant to metronidazole or tinidazole (one-half the rate in adults).

In a survey carried out in Germany, the prevalence of *H. pylori* resistance in children was high: 16 and 32% for clarithromycin and metronidazole, respectively.

Table 9 *H. pylori* resistance in children in Belgium

Year	*n*	% of resistance		
		Metronidazole	Clarithromycin	Clarithromycin + metronidazole
1989	31	0	19	0
1990	30	10	17	0
1991	42	5	7	3
1992	51	4	24	2
1993	31	3	16	0
1994	33	6	9	3
1995	44	16	20	5
1996	61	23	10	0
1997	79	13	15	1
1998	51	10	22	0
1999	53	4	19	6
2000	49	18	14	6

In Spain, a survey carried out between 1991 and 1999 with 246 children allowed the pattern of resistance of *H. pylori* to antibacterials to be profiled. No strain resistant to amoxicillin was detected. Rates of resistance to metronidazole and clarithromycin are reported in Table 10.

The prevalence of primary resistance was assessed in 98 pediatric patients from 1998 to 2000 in the Children's Health Institute in Warsaw, Poland. Twenty-three of 98 (23.5%) *H. pylori* isolates were categorized as resistant to clarithromycin by agar dilution and E-test (MIC, >1.0 μg/ml). An A2142G mutation was detected in 70% (16 of 23 patients) of clarithromycin-resistant strains. Four resistant isolates harbored an A2143G mutation. Sequence analysis revealed that two of them contained an A2142G transversion and one contained a T2812C mutation. One isolate with an A2142T transversion also had a C1953T mutation.

8.1.3. Secondary Resistance

The impact of resistance in clinical and bacteriological outcome on resistance to metronidazole is dramatic. Up to a 50% decrease in the success of the metronidazole-containing triple therapy was observed in the case of resistance to this drug. The impact of resistance to clarithromycin on eradication was even higher. Data on the epidemiology of resistance after therapeutic failure are scarce.

A comparison of prevalence of *H. pylori* resistance to antibacterials during a 3-year period was carried out in Germany in two geographically distinct centers: Regensburg and Freiburg. Results are shown in the Table 11. These strains were collected from patients in whom one or two therapies failed to eradicate *H. pylori* (Heep et al., 2000).

In France, the rate of secondary resistance to clarithromycin reached 60% in one study. In a study by Bomtems et al. (2001), eradication of *H. pylori* failed in 128 of 451 children treated (28.4%). After eradication failure, antibiotic susceptibility determination was carried out for 87 of 128 strains.

Table 10 Epidemiological survey in Spain for *H. pylori* susceptibility in children

Compound	Years	*n*	% of resistance
Clarithromycin			
(MIC, ≥1.0 μg/ml)	1991–1993	45	1
	1994–1996	81	17
	1997–1999	120	34
Metronidazole			
(MIC, ≥8.0 μg/ml)	1991–1993	42	3
	1994–1996	79	16
	1997–1999	118	36

Table 11 Prevalence (secondary) of *H. pylori* resistant strains in two geographical areas in Germany

Compound	% of resistance in:	
	Regensburg (*n* = 302)	Freiburg (*n* = 252)
Metronidazole	75	66
Clarithromycin	58	49
Amoxicillin	0	0
Ciprofloxacin	9	9
Doxycycline	0	0
Rifampin	0	0

Secondary resistance developed in 57 of 87 strains (65.1%). All but 5 strains isolated from different gastric locations showed identical susceptibilities. Acquired resistance to the last antibiotic used was recorded for 39 of 87 strains (44.8%).

8.1.4. Pan-European Surveys

The first European multicenter survey was carried out to investigate metronidazole resistance in *H. pylori* in 12 hospitals in 11 European countries. MICs were determined by E-test. In this prospective study, 443 *H. pylori* strains were collected. The frequency of resistance to metronidazole (MIC, >8.0 μg/ml) varied among centers from 7% in Madrid, Spain, to 49% in Athens, Greece (Table 12).

The overall rate of resistance to metronidazole was higher in women than in men (34.7 versus 23.9%).

Another multicenter in vitro survey of resistance of *H. pylori* to antibiotics was carried out in 1998 in 22 European centers. MICs were determined by E-test. Data are reported in Table 13.

Resistance rates ranged from 18.8% in Brussels, Belgium, to 61% in Helsinki, Finland. For clarithromycin the rate varied from 0% in Frederikstad, Norway, to 27.2% in Chieti, Italy.

Overall, metronidazole-resistant strains were isolated more frequently from women than from men (38.5 versus 28.4%; $P = 0.001$).

In this study, the mean resistance rate was of the same magnitude as those reported in another six European countries and in the MACH2 study.

8.2. Resistance in North America

There are few data regarding the *H. pylori* resistance rate in the United States. The frequency of primary clarithromycin and metronidazole resistance among patients enrolled in different geographical areas in the U.S.-based clinical trials between 1993 and 1999 was assessed by MIC determinations using E-test.

The rate of resistance to clarithromycin varied from 6.1% in 1993 to 9% in 1999, with a peak of 14.5% in 1997 (Table 14).

The rate of resistance to amoxicillin and tetracycline in this study among *H. pylori* isolates was low: 0.04% (three strains; MICs of amoxicillin, >16 μg/ml). The rates of resistance to metronidazole were 39% (690 of 1,768) and 25.2% (367 of 1,454) using E-test and agar dilution, respectively. Marked regional differences were noted. The highest level of metronidazole resistance occurred in the southeast (22.1% [91 of 412]). The highest rate of clarithromycin resistance (13% [67 of 156]) occurred in the northeast, while the lowest rate of clarithromycin resistance (8.3% [44 of 533]) was found in the West.

Table 12 Prevalence of *H. pylori* resistance to metronidazole in Europe from 1990 to 1991

Country	% of resistance
France	20
The Netherlands	37.5
United Kingdom	38.5
Belgium	18.2
Ireland	22.9
Greece	49
Sweden	10
Finland	30
Portugal	20
Spain	7.0

Table 13 Prevalence of *H. pylori* resistance to antibacterials in Europe in 1998

Country	Center	*n*	% of resistance		
			Metronidazole	Clarithromycin	Amoxicillin
Austria	Vienna	49	44.9	23.4	0.0
Belgium	Yvoir	81	25.6	23.1	0.0
	Brussels	86	18.9	10.5	0.0
Denmark	Copenhagen	25	32	4.0	0.0
Finland	Helsinki	73	61.6	6.7	0.0
France	Bordeaux	48	25	8.8	0.0
	Nancy	22	19.7	4.7	0.0
Germany	Freiburg	115	24.6	2.7	0.9
Greece	Athens	59	44.1	10.2	1.7
Ireland	Dublin	51	27.4	3.9	0.0
Italy	Chieti	61	49	27.2	8.2
The Netherlands	Hoogeven	72	23.4	1.3	0.0
Norway	Frederikstad	23	21.7	0.0	0.0
Poland	Wrocław	47	44.6	12.6	0.0
Portugal	Lisbon	63	33.3	20.7	0.0
United Kingdom	Gloucester	83	28.9	1.3	1.2
Spain	Madrid	78	37.2	15.2	0.0
Sweden	Lund	23	38.9	5.1	0.0
Switzerland	Lausanne	42	38.1	16.6	0.0

Table 14 Rate of resistance of *H. pylori* to clarithromycin (MIC, >1.0 μg/ml) in the United States

Year	*n*	% of resistance
1993	66	6.1
1994	521	8.1
1995	141	12.1
1996	1,099	12.1
1997	317	14.1
1998	1,050	11.1
1999	211	9.0

Analysis of 11 studies carried out in Canada between 1980 and 1999 showed that resistance rates for metronidazole and clarithromycin varied from 11 to 48% and 0 to 12%, respectively.

In 1999, the prevalence in Canada of primary resistance in *H. pylori* appeared to be 18 to 22% for metronidazole and less than 4% for clarithromycin. These rates appeared to be consistent across the regions, but in many regions the prevalence was not investigated. In the province of Alberta, the rates of resistance to metronidazole were 12 and 14% when MICs were determined by agar dilution and E-test, respectively. One of the 31 strains was considered resistant to clarithromycin (MIC, 8.0 μg/ml). No strain was resistant to tetracycline or metronidazole. In another report it was shown that the prevalence of resistance ranged from 33% in 1993 to 42% in 1998. In this survey, clarithromycin resistance was 8% in 1996.

8.3. Resistance in Asia

In Japan from December 1999 to March 2001, a total of 51 H. pylori isolates were collected from gastric antrum or body biopsy samples from 48 pediatric patients. The rates of *H. pylori* resistance were 29, 24, and 0% for clarithromycin, metronidazole, and amoxicillin, respectively. In clarithromycin-resistant isolates, the main mutation was A2144G for 92% of the strains.

The prevalence of *H. pylori* isolates resistant to metronidazole was assessed in two areas of Japan from 1996 to 1999; results are shown in Table 15.

No strain was resistant to amoxicillin or tetracycline.

The prevalence of *H. pylori* isolates resistant to metronidazole was investigated from 1993 to 1996 to Singapore. The overall resistance rate was 62.7%. There was a significant rise in resistance, from 50.5% in 1993 to 72.7% in 1996.

In another report, the rates of metronidazole resistance were 20, 50, and 62% in 1995, 1996, and 1997, respectively.

In a study using the disk method with incubation under a CO_2 atmosphere, it was found that 25% (50 of 199) *H. pylori* isolates were resistant to metronidazole.

In Hong Kong, 57% of patients carried *H. pylori* isolates resistant to metronidazole. Among them, 77% carried a mixture of susceptible and resistant strains nonuniformly distributed in the gastric mucosa. The prevalence of clarithromycin resistance was 11%.

More than 50% of the *H. pylori* isolates in Malaysia are resistant to metronidazole.

The prevalence of *H. pylori* isolates resistant to clarithromycin in Taiwan was 18% among 245 children. The dominant mutation was A2144G (83%), while in adults the dominant mutation was reported to be A2143G in another study. Nine percent of the isolates were resistant to metronidazole.

Table 15 Prevalence of metronidazole and clarithromycin resistance of *H. pylori* in two areas in Japan

Year(s)	% of resistance			
	Metronidazole		Clarithromycin	
	Sapporo	Kyoto	Sapporo	Kyoto
1996	5.7	17	5.7	11.3
1997	5.9	40	9.6	13.3
1998–1999	11.6	18.2	17	27.3

For Korea, Kim et al. (2001) summarized the prevalence of *H. pylori* resistance to six antibacterial agents from 1994 to 1999. The rate of *H. pylori* infection ranged from 22% in children to 75% in adults in 1999 (Table 16).

Song et al. (1999) reported that for 169 *H. pylori* isolates, the rates of resistance were 34.3, 31.9, 20.7, 12.4, 10.1, 0.0, and 0.0% for clarithromycin, metronidazole, amoxicillin, erythromycin A, josamycin, ciprofloxacin, and tetracycline, respectively. Dual and triple resistances were detected in 9.6 and 3.9%, respectively.

In one survey it was found that 6.7% (7 of 105 isolates) and 4.9% (22 of 460 isolates) of *H. pylori* isolates were resistant to tetracycline in Japan and Korea, respectively. Rates of resistance to metronidazole were 40.4 and 23.8% for Korea and Japan, respectively. For clarithromycin, 15.2 and 5.3% of *H. pylori* isolates in Japan and Korea, respectively, were resistant. No isolate was resistant to amoxicillin. All 29 *H. pylori* isolates resistant to tetracycline were resistant to metronidazole (coresistance) but not vice versa. This fact was observed by other workers.

In Shanghai, China, between January 1998 and February 1999, it was shown that the rates of *H. pylori* resistance were 77.8, 71.9, and 58.8% for metronidazole, amoxicillin, and tetracycline, respectively. In a 3-year period, the prevalence of metronidazole resistance climbed from 37.3 to 77.8%. Metronidazole resistance was more frequent in women than in men, probably due to the large use of metronidazole in gynecological infections. In 2000, the prevalence of *H. pylori* isolates in Beijing, China, was 16.5%. All strains resistant to clarithromycin were characterized by an A2143G mutation. The prevalence of clarithromycin-resistant *H. pylori* strains in Shanghai and Guangzhou, China, was 5% in 1995. The mutation on the 23S rRNA was at A2143G. Clarithromycin MICs ranged from 2.0 to 4.0 μg/ml. In another area of China, of 50 *H. pylori* isolates collected between 1996 and 1999, 50% were resistant to metronidazole, 8.0% were resistant to clarithromycin, and all were susceptible to tetracycline.

In Calcutta, India, in 2000, about 90% of *H. pylori* isolates were resistant to metronidazole.

In Dhaka, Bangladesh, in 1996, 86% of *H. pylori* isolates were resistant to metronidazole.

8.4. Resistance in Australia

In a prospective study, the prevalence of *H. pylori* isolates resistant to antibiotics was assessed in 732 patients undergoing a gastric biopsy for dyspeptic syndrome in the area of Sydney, Australia, from 1996 to 1997. From 340 infected patients, only 237 *H. pylori* strains were tested for their susceptibility to antibacterials by E-test. The overall metronidazole resistance rate was 59.1%. In Melbourne, metronidazole resistance was present in 32% of the 37 patients. In Perth, the metronidazole resistance rate was 64% in 58 patients enrolled in the survey. In outer Western Sydney, the metronidazole resistance rate was 64%. In another prospective study carried out between July 1998 and July 1999 in western Australia, *H. pylori* was cultured from gastric biopsy samples from 108 patients. Rates of resistance to metronidazole and clarithromycin were 36 and 11%, respectively. No isolates were resistant to tetracycline or amoxicillin.

8.5. Resistance in Latin America

In Brazil, the number of *H. pylori* strains resistant to clarithromycin has increased significantly since 1996 (Table 17).

In 2000, of 107 *H. pylori* isolates, 52.97% were resistant to metronidazole. A positive correlation has been found between metronidazole and female gender which may be explained by the use of metronidazole for the treatment of gynecological infections. Combined resistance was found in 7.43% of *H. pylori* isolates. Among clarithromycin-resistant *H. pylori* strains, 90% harbored a 23S rRNA mutation of A2142G (16.7%), A2143G (66.7%), or both (16.6%). In another part of Brazil, the rates of *H. pylori* resistance were 42, 29, 7.0, 7.0, and 4.0% for metronidazole, amoxicillin, clarithromycin, tetracycline, and furazolidone, respectively.

One hundred ninety-five *H. pylori* strains were isolated during the period from 1995 to 1997 in Mexico City, Mexico. The rates of resistance were 76.9, 24, and 18.5% for metronidazole, clarithromycin, and amoxicillin, respectively. Among resistant *H. pylori* isolates, 30.7% were multidrug resistant, 17.9% were resistant to metronidazole and clarithromycin, and 12.8% were resistant to metronidazole and amoxicillin. The rate of resistance for the three antibiotics was 8.7%. Rates of resistance to metronidazole were similar from 1995 to 1997. In contrast, resistance to amoxicillin and clarithromycin increased significantly during this period. Resistance to clarithromycin increased from 10% in 1995 to 27% in 1997, and the prevalence of resistance to amoxicillin increased from 13% in 1995 to 26% in 1997.

Ninety-one *H. pylori* isolates were collected between August 1997 and August 2000 in Chile. All strains were susceptible to amoxicillin, 42% were resistant to metronidazole, and two strains were resistant to clarithromycin. In another study in Chile, the prevalence of metronidazole resistance reached 25% of isolates.

Table 17 Clarithromycin resistance of *H. pylori* in Brazil

Year	% of resistance
1996	4.48
1997	7.69
1998	10.0
1999	12.19
2000	19.05

Table 16 Prevalence of *H. pylori* isolates resistant to antibacterials in Korea

Compound	Breakpoint (μg/ml)	% of resistance				
		1994 (*n* = 63)	1995 (*n* = 130)	1996 (*n* = 129)	1997 (*n* = 69)	1998–1999 (*n* = 65)
Metronidazole	>8.0	33.3	38.5	42.6	40.6	47.7
Clarithromycin	≥1.0	4.8	4.6	3.9	11.6	7.7
Tetracycline	>2.0	3.0	6.9	4.7	2.9	7.7
Amoxicillin	>8.0	0.0	0.0	0.0	0.0	0.0
Furazolidone	>2.0	1.6	0.0	3.9	0.0	1.5
Nitrofurantoin	>2.0	1.6	0.0	3.9	0.0	1.5

In Peru, the prevalence of *H. pylori* resistance to metronidazole was reported to be 61%. In Lima from 1993 to 1994, 70.8% of the strains were resistant to metronidazole. For 76.5% of patients, both metronidazole-susceptible and -resistant isolates were isolated. Clarithromycin resistance was detected in 4.2% of isolates.

8.6. Resistance in the Middle and Near East

In Israel from 2000 to 2001, the rates of resistance of 138 *H. pylori* isolates were 8.2, 38.2, 1.87, 0.9, and 0.0% for clarithromycin, metronidazole, cefixime, amoxicillin, and tetracycline, respectively.

In Lebanon, the E-test method was used determine resistance among 44 *H. pylori* isolates; results are summarized in Table 18.

In Bahrain, the susceptibilities of *H. pylori* isolates from 150 patients to metronidazole, clarithromycin, and amoxicillin were investigated using the E-test method from 1998 to 1999. The rates of resistance were 57 and 32.5% for metronidazole and clarithromycin, respectively. No isolates were resistant to tetracycline or amoxicillin.

In Saudi Arabia, the prevalence of *H. pylori* resistance to antibacterials was assessed by the disk diffusion method from 1987 to 1998. Results are summarized in Table 19.

In Saudi Arabia, tetracycline and metronidazole are commonly used for the treatment of *H. pylori* infection. An increase in metronidazole resistance, from 35.2 to 78.5%, was reported in the period from 1990 to 1996. No isolates were resistant to tetracycline in this period.

In the United Arab Emirates, the prevalence of *H. pylori* resistance to metronidazole was 62.5%, but no strains were resistant to tetracycline.

In Iran, prevalence of metronidazole resistance was 42% (47 of 112 patients undergoing biopsy for duodenal ulcer). Susceptibility was determined by disk diffusion.

8.7. Resistance in Africa

Epidemiological surveys on *H. pylori* resistance to antibiotics in Africa are not numerous. In African countries such as Zaire or Malawi, the prevalence of resistance to metronidazole is high. Most patients in sub-Saharan Africa received metronidazole or derivatives for gastrointestinal parasites. In Malawi, in 1991, of 141 *H. pylori* isolates collected, 74% were resistant to metronidazole but none were resistant to amoxicillin or tetracycline.

Fifty-five *H. pylori* isolates were cultured from adult patients in Nigeria between November 1997 and October 1998. All isolates were susceptible to amoxicillin. The rates of resistance to tetracycline, clarithromycin, and metronidazole were 11, 12.7, and 60%, respectively. In Zaire, the rate of resistance to metronidazole reached 87%.

Table 18 Prevalence of *H. pylori* resistance in Lebanon

Compound	Breakpoint (μg/ml)	% of resistance
Metronidazole	>8.0	31.5
Clarithromycin	>1.0	4.0
Tetracycline	>2.0	2.0
Amoxicillin	>1.0	0.0

Table 19 Prevalence of *H. pylori* resistance in Saudi Arabia

Compound	*n*	% of resistance
Tetracycline	52	1.9
Metronidazole	54	35.2
Erythromycin A	42	2.4
Nalidixic acid	54	90.8
Gentamicin	41	0.0
Chloramphenicol	40	0.0
Ampicillin	43	0.0
Penicillin G	42	0.0

8.8. Resistance in the Caribbean

In Barbados, resistance to metronidazole was found in 39% of *H. pylori* isolates. In Guyana, 11% of *H. pylori* isolates are resistant to metronidazole.

9. NONANTIBACTERIAL AGENTS

Luminal acidity influences the effectiveness of some drugs against *H. pylori*. Raising the gastric pH from 3.5 to 5.6 increases the in vitro effectiveness of amoxicillin and erythromycin more than 10-fold (Grayson et al., 1989). This increased activity at higher pH values may explain the effectiveness of regimens that combine acid-suppressing drugs and antibacterial agents.

The following drugs are combined with antibacterial agents: bismuth salts, H_2-antagonists, and proton pump inhibitors. Cytoprotective agents have been tried.

9.1. Bismuth Salts

Bismuth salts are topical antibacterial drugs that disrupt the integrity of bacterial cell walls (Van Caekenberghe and Breyssens, 1987). Bismuth lyses *H. pylori* near the gastric surface and prevents the adhesion of *H. pylori* to the gastric epithelium. Bismuth salts inhibit urease, phospholipase, and proteolytic activities of *H. pylori*.

In the United States, only bismuth subsalicylate is available; elsewhere in many parts of the world tripotassium dicitrate bismutate (De-Nol) is available.

Due to the high incidence of adverse events, bismuth salts have been banned in many countries. The side effects of bismuth in high doses include central nervous system toxicity, especially for a level in plasma above 50 to 100 μg/ml (Gorbach, 1990).

In vitro activities of the various bismuth salts are listed in Table 20. Bismuth salts exhibit moderate in vitro activity against *H. pylori*.

H. pylori possesses alcohol dehydrogenase activity which results in acetaldehyde formation, production of which could be partly responsible for *H. pylori*-associated gastric injury; *H. pylori* is unable to effectively remove acetaldehyde due to the lack of aldehyde dehydrogenase. Alcohol dehydrogenase activity of *H. pylori* is significantly inhibited by colloidal bismuth subcitrate at 0.01 mM, as well as omeprazole at 0.5 mM. The inhibitory effect of ranitidine was comparable to that of omeprazole (0.25 mM), whereas

Table 20 In vitro anti-*H. pylori* activity of bismuth salts ($n = 16$)[a]

Salt	MIC (μg/ml)		
	50%	90%	Range
Bismuth nitrate	4.0	4.0	2.0–4.0
Tripotassium diacetate bismuth	8.0	16	4.0–32
Bismuth sodium nitrate	8.0	16	2.0–32

[a]Data from MacNulty et al., 1985.

famotidine decreases alcohol dehydrogenase activity only slightly at high concentrations.

Acetaldehyde is known to be a highly reactive and toxic compound; it readily forms adducts with different cellular proteins and may also induce lipid peroxidation, both of which can lead to tissue injuries (Roine et al., 1992).

Ciprofloxacin possesses two ionic sites and could be protonated at the ring carbonyl oxygen (C-4 position of the pyrridone ring) and the N-4′ position of the 7-piperazinyl moiety. A combination of ciprofloxacin with bismuth (III) was proposed. The bismuth ions are coordinated by chloride ions forming a dinuclear centrosymmetric $(Bi_2Cl_{10})^{4-}$ anion. The ionic compound consists of a positively charged quinolone molecule and negatively charged chlorobismuthated (III) anions. This molecule is dissolved in dimethyl sufoxide bismuth salts being prone to hydrolysis. This complex exhibits in vitro activity against *H. pylori*. MICs are above 0.3 μg/ml, irrespective of the ratio of ciprofloxacin and bismuth (1:1 or 1:2).

9.2. Proton Pump Inhibitors

Proton pump inhibitors are substituted 2-pyridylmethyl sulfinyl benzimidazoles with the same core structure (Fig. 1). These agents are protonable weak bases with pK values of about 4, except for rabeprazole (pK of 5). These compounds accumulate selectively in the secretory canaliculus of the gastric parietal cell, where the pH is below 4. In this environment the nitrogen atoms of the pyridyl and benzoimidazolyl rings are protonated and form a metabolite with antibacterial activity, a tetracyclic sulfenamide. This structure binds covalently to the cysteine residue of the α subunit of the H^+/K^+ ATPase, thus inhibiting the activity of the pump of the canalicular membrane of the parietal cell (Horn, 2000; Fellenius et al., 1981).

9.2.1. In Vitro Activity

It was demonstrated that lansoprazole inhibits the growth of *H. pylori* (Iwahi et al., 1991). Proton pump inhibitors inhibit the growth of *H. pylori* at concentrations similar to those that inhibit gastric H^+/K^+ ATPase. A P-ATPase has been cloned and sequenced for *H. pylori* (Melchers et al., 1996).

In vitro activity was investigated for the proton pump inhibitors and is summarized in Table 21. It was hypothesized that the growth-inhibitory effects of proton pump inhibitors may be sufficient to achieve eradication of *H. pylori* by coadministered antibacterials.

Omeprazole and lansoprazole exhibit some in vitro activity against *H. pylori*, but in vivo they only suppress the organism without eradicating it.

9.2.2. Mode of Action

The mode of action of proton pump inhibitors against *H. pylori* is complex and is not completely understood.

9.2.2.1. Urease

The proton pump inhibitors inhibit *H. pylori* urease activity by binding to the active site of the enzyme. The affinities for *H. pylori* urease vary among these compounds (Nagata et al., 1993).

H. pylori possesses several putative colonizing factors, including urease. Urease accounts for about 5% of *H. pylori* protein. It is present in all *H. pylori* isolates. Genetically engineered urease-deficient *H. pylori* is unable to colonize germfree piglets, ferrets, or mice (Eaton et al., 1991).

H. pylori urease is a potent stimulus of mononuclear phagocyte activation and inflammatory cytokine production (Harris et al., 1996). In vitro, urease activity is toxic to human gastric epithelial cells. Both activities promote colonization and pathogenesis of gastric mucosa damage.

Table 21 Anti-*Helicobacter* activities of proton pump inhibitors

Inhibitor	*n*	MIC (μg/ml)		
		50%	90%	Range
Omeprazole	30	16	32	8–32
	4			2.0–16
	17	25	25	12.5–50
	18	64	128	16–256
Pantoprazole	30	48	128	8–128
Lansoprazole	4			0.25–1.0
	17	6.25	6.25	3.13–12.5
B-8203-010				8–32
Rabeprazole	4			0.01–0.5
	8	1.54		1.56–3.3

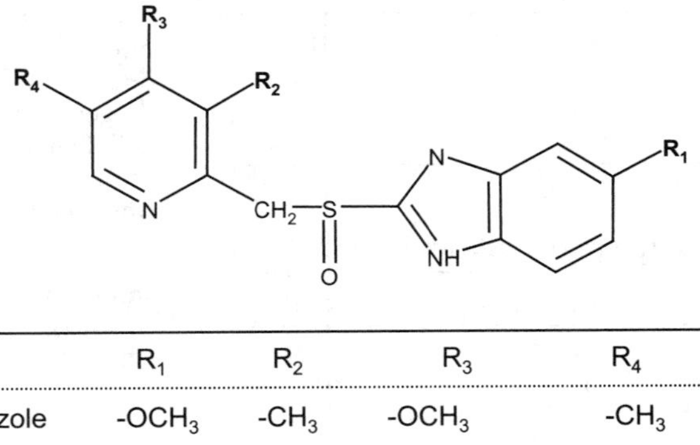

	R_1	R_2	R_3	R_4	Molecular weight
Omeprazole	$-OCH_3$	$-CH_3$	$-OCH_3$	$-CH_3$	345.42
Lansoprazole	-H	$-CH_3$	$-OCH_2CF_3$	-H	369.37
Pantoprazole	$-OCHF_2$	$-OCH_3$	$-OCH_3$	-H	432.40
Rabeprazole	-H	$-CH_3$	$O(CH_2)_3OCH_3$	-H	381.43

Figure 1 Proton pump inhibitors

H. pylori urease is a nickel-containing hexameric molecule with molecular mass of 540 kDa, consisting of two subunits, UreA and UreB, in a molar ratio of 1:1. The transition metal nickel is an essential trace element of at least five biological processes: hydrolysis of urea, oxidation and evolution of molecular hydrogen, carbon monoxide dehydrogenase-mediated acetate metabolism under anaerobic conditions, reduction of methyl coenzyme M to methane, and detoxification of superoxide dismutase radicals.

Uptake of nickel is a prerequisite for those organisms which catalyze nickel-dependent reactions.

Two types of nickel-specific uptake systems have been identified: a multiple-component ATP-binding cassette system called NIK (*Escharichia coli, Brucella suis*, and *Vibrio parahaemolyticus*) and the nickel-cobalt transporters family, comprising homologous single polypeptides in a variety of microorganisms, including *H. pylori*.

H. pylori strains have a high-affinity nickel transport protein, NixA. NixA scavenges the low levels of nickel from the human body, which are estimated to be in the range of 2 to 11 mM.

Urease converts urea monochloramine and carbamate, the latter decomposing spontaneously to carbon dioxide and ammonia. Monochloramine and neutrophil-derived hypochlorous acid have been suggested to play an important role in gastric mucosa injury. Urease catalyzes the hydrolysis of urea to ammonia and carbon dioxide.

Synthesis of active urease by *H. pylori* requires the presence of the structural genes *ureA* and *ureB* and the accessory genes *ureIEFGH*, which are needed for the full expression of urease activity (Cussac et al., 1992) as well as nickel transport enzymes such as NixA. The hydrolysis of urea by cytoplasmic urease results in energy generation in the form of proton motive force which drives flagellar rotation, allowing bacterial motility in the mucus layer of the stomach.

Some urease activity has been observed within the cytoplasm of *H. pylori*, suggesting a role in assimilation of organic nitrogen. The association between urease and the bacterial surface is apparently stabilized by divalent cations such as Ca^{2+} and Mg^{2+}, although other cations can inhibit the activity of the enzyme (Perez-Perez et al., 1994). Acid-suppressive activity of proton pump inhibitors is followed by elevation of intragastric pH, which improves the protection of many antibiotics from acid degradation (Van Zeneca et al., 1992).

The in vitro activities of rabeprazole, omeprazole, and lansoprazole against urease were assessed in cell-free and cellular environments at various pHs (Table 22) (Tsuchiya et al., 1995).

It was clearly shown that 50% inhibitory concentrations (IC_{50}s) are pH dependent except in the case of AG-2000, which is a lansoprazole analog; rabeprazole, lansoprazole, and AG-2000 inhibited both cellular and cell-free urease equipotently.

Table 22 Activity against urease (measured by the indophenol method)

Compound	Environment	IC_{50} (μM)		
		pH 5.0	pH 7.0	pH 8.1
Rabeprazole	Cellular	0.24	4.2	40
	Cell free	0.29	7.6	55
Omeprazole	Cellular	8.0	72	170
	Cell free	5.4	5.6	29
Lansoprazole	Cellular	14	20	590
	Cell free	9.3	10	500
AG-2000	Cellular	1.2	2.5	1.2
	Cell free	0.3	1.0	1.3

Rabeprazole thioether, one of the main metabolites of rabeprazole, did not inhibit urease activity despite being a more potent inhibitor of *H. pylori* growth than the parent compound.

Omeprazole was also shown to inhibit *H. pylori* via a urease-independent mechanism, with inhibition of growth seen at a low pH in the absence of urea and in a urea-deficient strain of *H. pylori*. This phenomenon highlights the fact that other potential mechanisms are involved.

9.2.2.2. H^+/K^+ ATPase

Another target of proton pump inhibitors in *H. pylori* may be a membrane-bound H^+/K^+ ATPase, similar to that found in human parietal cells. By this mechanism, the bacterium is able to maintain a proton gradient in an acidic environment (Mauch et al., 1993).

9.2.2.3. Chemotactic Mobility

The velocity of *H. pylori* increases when the viscosity of the mucus increases. The high viscosity enhances bacterial contact with epithelial cells. Most populations of *H. pylori* are located within the mucus layer, but about 2% are associated with the gastric epithelia. Due to the high turnover of the mucus, *H. pylori* must move towards the epithelial cell surface. This chemotaxis needs urea and sodium carbonate (Yoshigama et al., 2000).

It has been shown that proton pump inhibitors are able to inhibit the chemotactic mobility of *H. pylori* in a highly viscous environment at concentrations similar to those inhibiting urease activities (Yoshiyama and Nakazawa, 2000).

9.2.2.4. Respiratory Inhibition

H. pylori is a microaerophilic bacterium exhibiting a strict respiratory form of metabolism and oxidizing organic acids as an energy source. It has been suggested that lansoprazole inhibits the respiratory pathway of *H. pylori*. Lansoprazole concentrations required for 50% inhibition of respiration in H. pylori were close to MICs (Nagata et al., 2001).

9.2.2.5. Metabolic Pathway

Omeprazole inhibits alcohol deshydrogenase activity of *H. pylori* (Roine et al., 1992).

9.3. H_2-Antagonists

9.3.1. Standard H_2-Antagonists

Since Black et al. (1972) first defined the histamine H_2 receptor and its involvement in gastric acid secretion, cimetidine, ranitidine, roxatidine, and nizatidine have been developed and used clinically as anti-acid secretagogues. *H. pylori* is intrinsically resistant to all available H_2-receptor blockers (Piotrowski et al., 1991) (Table 23).

Table 23 In vitro activities of H_2-antagonists against *H. pylori*

Compound	MIC (μg/ml)
Cimetidine	400–1,600
Ranitidine	>1,600
Roxatidine	>1,600
Famotidine	800–1,600
Nizatidine	>1,600

H_2-antagonists increase the gastric concentrations of antibiotics (Peterson, 1997). Westblom and Duriiex (1991) assayed concentrations of clindamycin in serum and tissue of guinea pigs premedicated with cimetidine. They found that the mucosal concentration of clindamycin was fivefold higher at an alkaline pH of 5.9 than the concentration at a physiological pH of 2.0.

Amoxicillin uptake into the gastric mucosa was reduced by acid pH in volunteers. It has been demonstrated that amoxicillin and cimetidine clear *H. pylori* infection from the antrum, but not from the gastric fundus or body. It was shown that omeprazole alone resulted in low oral flora alterations in comparison with those induced by the combination of omeprazole and amoxicillin. Triple therapy caused the most important disturbances in the oral microflora. In the intestinal microflora, very few alterations were seen during treatment with omeprazole-placebo or omeprazole-amoxicillin in comparison with the triple therapy.

It has been shown that NADH dehydrogenase and NADH cytochrome *c* reductase are absent or weakly active in *H. pylori*, indicating that the pathway from fumarate reductase to complex II-IV is the main electron transport chain in *H. pylori*. Fumarate reductase is an essential component of the energy metabolism of *H. pylori*. Fumarate reductase catalyzes the reduction of fumarate to succinate. Succinate might be the primary electron donor for the respiratory chain of *H. pylori*.

It was demonstrated that nizatidine exerts a concentration-dependent inhibitory effect (10 to 100 μg/ml of protein) on fumarate reductase of the respiratory chain of *H. pylori* and inhibits SCC reductase (complex II-III) at a high concentration (1,000 μg/ml of protein) but had no effect on succinate dehydrogenase. Omeprazole did not inhibit fumarate reductase.

9.3.2. Ebrotidine

Ebrotidine is an H_2-antagonist (Fig. 2). This compound exhibits antisecretory activity comparable to that of ranitidine and displays gastroprotective effects.

Ebrotidine inhibits the effect of the cytotoxin protease and lipase of *H. pylori*. Ebrotidine also inhibits urease activity of *H. pylori*. The effect was shown to be concentration dependent and reached a maximum of 77% inhibition at 2.1 μM. In comparison, ranitidine gave a maximum inhibition of 73% at a concentration of 6.4 μM. Omeprazole and lanzoprazole inhibit urease activity of *H. pylori* at concentrations three to five times higher than ebrotidine (Piotrowski et al., 1995).

Using agar dilution methods, the in vitro activity of ebrotidine against *H. pylori* was determined. The MIC was 150 μg/ml (Table 24).

Structurally, ebrotidine shares many features with ranitidine and cimetidine. It contains the *N*-sulfonylformamidine group instead of the cyanoguanidine group of cimetidine and the 2-nitro ether diamino group of ranitidine, whereas the imidazolyl ring of cimetidine is replaced by guanidothiazole (Anglada et al., 1988).

These modifications endow ebrotidine with diminished cytochrome P450 binding and eliminate the potential for mutagenic nitrosamine formation.

Ebrotidine enhances the anti-*H. pylori* activities of amoxicillin, tetracycline, and erythromycin A (Piotrowski et al., 1995).

Due to liver toxicity, clinical use of ebrotidine was stopped (Torello et al., 1998).

9.3.3. Benzyloxyisoquinoline Derivatives

The screening of the Fujisawa chemical library, in a random program of various nonantimicrobial agents, resulted in 5-hydroxyquinoline (Fig. 3), which displays weak anti-*H. pylori* activity (MIC, 25 to 50 μg/ml).

In order to enhance the anti-*H. pylori* activity of the lead compound, a series of derivatives was prepared and one compound was selected: FR-180102 (Fig. 4). It was shown that other isomers of the lead compounds are devoid of any anti-*H. pylori* activity and that introduction of lipophilic

Table 24 Comparative anti-*H. pylori* activity of ebrotidine

Compound	MIC (μg/ml)
Ebrotidine	150
Erythromycin A	0.10
Amoxicillin	0.12
Tetracycline	0.15
Metronidazole	14
Ranitidine	1,600

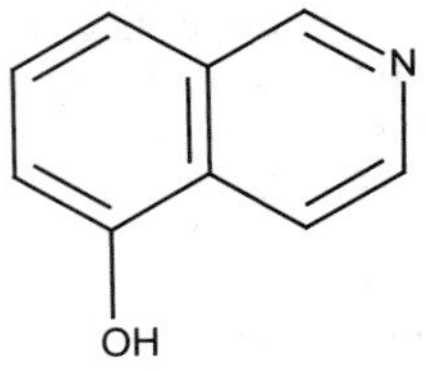

Figure 3 5-Hydroxyquinoline

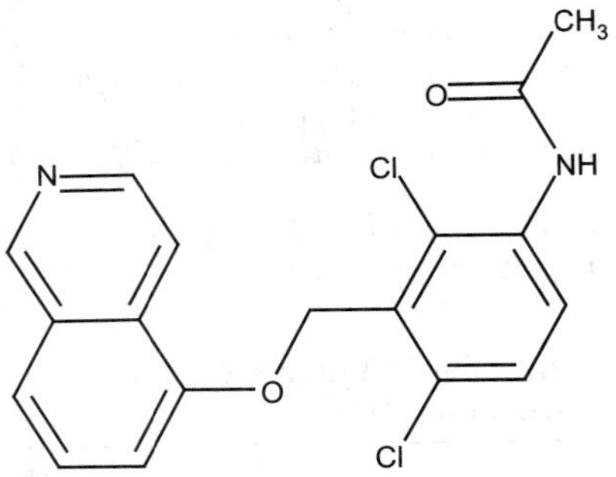

Figure 4 FR-180102

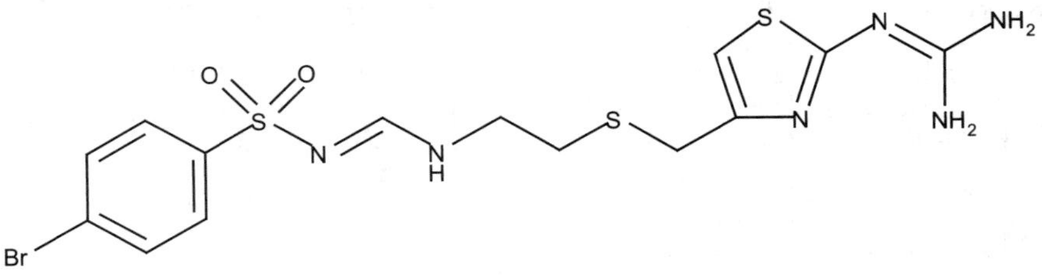

Figure 2 Ebrotidine

substituents improved the anti-*H. pylori* activity. Benzyl derivatives of the lead compound showed about 20-fold-enhanced in vitro activity. It was shown that a combination of amino and chloro groups enhanced the anti-*H. pylori* activity. FR-180102 is devoid of any activity against gram-negative and gram-positive bacteria tested (MICs, >100 μg/ml). MICs are listed in Table 25.

FR-180102 is poorly bactericidal after 6 h of contact even at 16 times the MIC (decrease of 1 $\log_{10}$CFU/ml), similar to other benzyloxyisoquinolines. The lack of in vivo activity of FR-180102 may be due to the lack of early bactericidal activity combined with the rapid peeling of the mucosa in the stomach leading to an absence of contact, which may explain this phenomenon (Yoshida et al., 1999).

9.3.4. Piperidyl Derivatives

A series of piperidyl derivatives has been prepared and one compound displayed improved anti-*H. pylori* activity (MIC, 1.56 μg/ml) and good H_2-antagonist activity (Fig. 5 and Table 26).

Table 25 Comparative anti-*H. pylori* activity of FR-180102

Compound	MIC (μg/ml) for *H. pylori* strain:			
	8007	9005	13001	FP1757
FR-180102	0.025	0.05	0.025	0.0125
Ampicillin	0.10	0.10	0.02	0.02
Clarithromycin	0.05	0.1	0.05	0.05

Figure 5 Piperidyl derivatives

Table 26 Anti-*H. pylori* activity of piperidyl derivative[a]

Compound	MIC (μg/ml) for *H. pylori* 9470	H_2-antagonist activity (IC_{50} [μg/m])
Cimetidine	>100	3.7
Ranitidine	>100	1.05
Roxatidine acetate	>100	1.43
Compound 12e	1.56	0.43

[a]Data from Kajima et al., 1996.

9.3.5. Guanidino Derivatives

9.3.5.1. Guanidino Analogs

In the course of searching for a novel class of H_2-antagonists with anti-*H pylori* activity, many series of compounds have been prepared.

Among them is a lead compound (Fig. 6), structurally related to classical anti-H_2 compounds, which demonstrated anti-*H. pylori* activity close to that of bismuth subcitrate (MICs, 27 versus 18 μg/ml).

The lead compound was intensively chemically modified, and one compound was selected for further investigation: FR-145745. The compounds were modified around a central core: thiazolylguanidine.

It was shown first that the guanidino moiety is essential for anti-*H. pylori* activity. In the side chain fixes on the guanidino moiety, flexibility is required for activity. The alkyl side chain length enhances the activity against *H. pylori*. However, gastric and antisecretory activities are not related to the length of the side chain. Ethyl and *n*-propyl derivatives showed strong activities, higher than that of cimetidine. The *n*-butyl and *n*-hexyl derivatives exhibited marginal activity. The methyl and isopropyl derivatives showed weak activities on both gastric secretion and H_2-antagonist assays (Table 27).

In a series of furothiazolyl compounds (Katsura et al., 1998), substituents such as cyclic alkyls, unsaturated alkyls, and hetero atoms containing alkyl have been introduced on the guadinino moiety. Among them, ethoxyethyl and cyclohexylmethyl compounds were the most active (Table 28).

A third series of compounds has been prepared in which the alicyclic part was replaced with an aromatic group (Katsura et al., 1999). In a fourth and fifth series, the furyl moiety was replaced by other aryl moieties (Katsura et al., 2000, 2002).

Keeping the *n*-butyl and 2(2-methoxy phenyl) ethyl moieties on the guanidino residue, which are favorable substituents, it was shown that pyridyl, thienyl, and thiazolyl derivatives displayed anti-*H. pylori* activity. However, pyrimidyl,

Table 27 Anti-H_2 activities of guanidino derivatives

Carbon length or compound	Inhibition (%)	
	Gastric secretion (rats given 1 mg/kg i.v.[a])	H_2 antagonist (10^{-6} g/ml)
H	68	85
Methyl	24	25
Ethyl	79	51
n-Propyl	97	81
n-Butyl	45	78
n-Hexyl	44	79
Isopropyl	32	27
Bismuth subcitrate	9	0
Cimetidine	53	43

[a]i.v., intravenously.

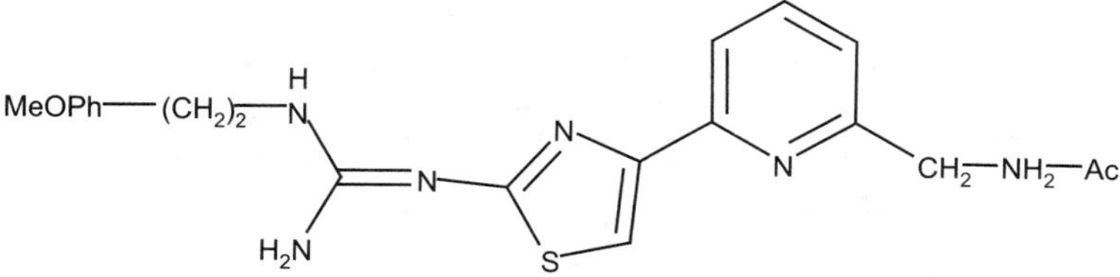

Figure 6 Guanidine analogs

Table 28 Anti-*H. pylori* activities and anti-H2-receptors of furothiazolyl derivatives

Derivative	MIC (μg/ml)	% Inhibition		
		Gastric secretion[a]		H_2-antagonist (10^{-6} g/ml)
		Rat	Dog	
Cyclohexylmethyl	0.025–0.1	60	38	33
Ethoxyethyl	0.2–0.78	64	71	85
Cimetidine		53	22	43

[a]Rats were given 1 mg/kg intravenously; dogs were given 1 mg/kg per os.

isoxazolyl, imidazolyl, and oxazodiazolyl derivatives did not have attractive in vitro activity.

Here also, in the pyridylthiazolyl series, it was shown that introduction on the guadinino moiety of bulky substituents tended to increase the in vitro activity; the incorporation of a hetero atom, a basic function, or an ionizable hydrogen was deleterious.

The pyridyl derivative showed potent anti-H_2 activity, comparable to those of reference compounds. Thienyl, thiazolyl, and oxazolyl analog possessed weak or no H_2-antagonist activities.

The most active agent against *H. pylori* is the 4-thienyl thiazolyl derivative with a 2(2-methoxy phenyl) ethyl substituent on the guanidino moiety. MICs ranged from 0.005 to 0.025 μg/ml, but it was devoid of H_2-antagonist activity.

The pyridyl counterpart exhibited good anti-*H. pylori* activity (MIC, 0.025 to 1.0 μg/ml) and H_2-antagonist activities (Table 29).

9.3.5.2. FR-145175

FR-145175 is a thiazolyl phenylguanidino derivative (Fig. 7). It displayed good in vitro activity against *H. pylori*, comparable to that of clarithromycin and superior to that of metronidazole (Table 30).

In experimental *H. pylori* infections in piglets, FR-145175 significantly inhibited the growth of *H. pylori* in all parts of the gastric mucosa (Table 31).

In isolated guinea pig atrium studies, FR-145175 antagonized histamine-induced positive chronotropic response, with approximately three times more potent action than ranitidine.

Table 29 Anti-H_2 activity of a pyridyl derivative

Compound	Inhibition (%)	
	Gastric secretion (rats given 1 mg/kg i.v. periods[a])	H_2-antagonist (10^{-6} g/ml)
Compound A	65	78
Cimetidine	53	43
Ranitidine	72	44

[a]i.v., intravenously.

In histamine-stimulated acid secretion in Schild's rats, FR-145175 was approximately 6 and 16 times less potent than ranitidine when administered intravenously and intraduodenally, respectively.

FR-145175 significantly inhibited gastric lesions induced by aspirin in the presence of 200 mM HCl at doses of 10 and 32 mg/kg, while ranitidine and cimetidine failed to prevent gastric lesions at identical doses.

10. ANTIBACTERIAL AGENTS

10.1. β-Lactam Antibiotics

β-Lactam antibiotics are a large class of antibacterial agents composed of four groups: penams, cephems, β-lactam monocyclic agents, and penems.

The in vitro activities of the different compounds against *H. pylori* have been assessed.

Amoxicillin is one of the companion drugs in triple or quadruple therapy. Other antibacterials are not commonly used in therapy.

10.1.1. Amoxicillin

10.1.1.1. Resistance to Amoxicillin

Amoxicillin-resistant isolates of *H. pylori* have been identified in many countries, such as Italy, the United States, and Canada (Dore et al., 1998). The presence of amoxicillin resistance was associated with a marked reduction in efficacy of treatment (Dore et al., 1998).

During attempts to confirm and characterize *H. pylori* isolates resistant to amoxicillin, it was observed that freezing

Table 30 Anti-*H. pylori* activity of FR-145715

Compound	MIC (μg/ml) range
FR-145715	0.20–0.39
Amoxicillin	<0.1
Clarithromycin	0.025–0.1
Metronidazole	1.56–25

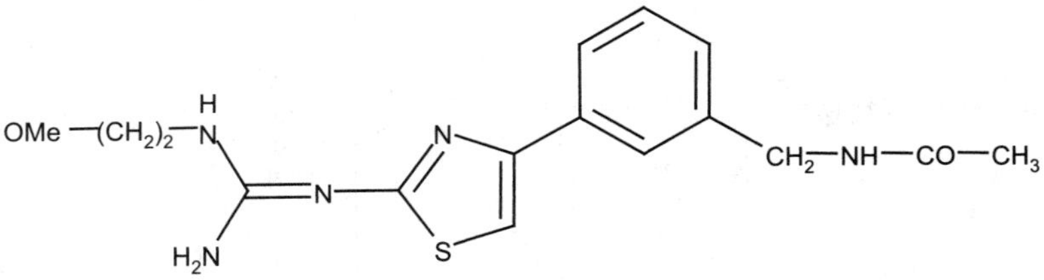

Figure 7 FR-145175

Table 31 Eradication of *H. pylori* in gnobiotic piglets with FR-145715

Compound	Piglet no.	CFU/g (10^8) in gastric mucosa	Strains in section			
			Cardia	Fundus	Antrum	Pylorus
Control	1	1.61	+	+	+	+
	2	0.89	+	+	+	+
	3	0.66	+	−	+	−
FR-145715	1	0	−	−	−	−
(16 mg/kg)	2	0	−	−	−	−
	3	0	−	−	−	−

H. pylori strains at −80°C resulted in a loss of the amoxicillin resistance phenotype (Dore et al., 1999). This phenomenon was observed in other bacteria with β-lactams. Of 17 *H. pylori* isolates highly resistant to amoxicillin (MIC, ≥256 μg/ml), no β-lactamase activity was detected in any strain by the nitrocefin assay.

The genomes of *H. pylori* strains 26695 and J 99 have been completely sequenced, and the open reading frames (ORFs) were grouped into 95 protein families. For about two-thirds of all ORFs, a function was assigned by sequence comparisons. A group of seven ORFs that were unique to *H. pylori* were identified. This group was named family 12, but a functional assignment was not possible. The product of gene *hp0160* was identified and is able to bind penicillin derivatives. This product, a cysteine-rich protein A (30 kDa) named HcpA, seems to belong to a new class of β-lactamases designated class E, which is able to hydrolyze β-lactams. The presence of β-lactamases in significant amounts could not be detected in vivo, which can be explained by the moderate catalytic activity of HcpA in vitro.

All *H. pylori* isolates irrespective of their susceptibilities to amoxicillin were resistant to nafcillin and oxacillin.

10.1.1.2. PBPs

Penicillin-resistant *H. pylori* bacteria lack a penicillin-binding protein (PBP) with a molecular mass of 30 to 32 kDa named PBPD (Dore et al., 1998).

Many workers have investigated PBPs of *H. pylori*, but the number of PBPs remains debatable.

Four PBPs were reported for *H. pylori* ATCC 43479, with molecular masses of 66, 63, 60, and 47 kDa. The first three PBPs were named PBP 1, PBP 2, and PBP 3. The last one is considered a putative PBP of *H. pylori*.

However, another team identified three high-molecular-mass PBPs named PBP 1, PBP 2, and PBP 3 from *H. pylori* 84-183, with a molecular masses range of 66 to 55 kDa, and they pointed out that these corresponded to PBPA, -B, and -C reported by Ikeda et al.

Dore et al. and Krishnamurthy et al. identified a small PBP with a molecular mass of 30 to 32 kDa under the name of PBPD or PBP 4.

Other PBPs in *H. pylori* were recently identified by Harris et al. at 72, 62, 54, 50, 44, 33.5, and 28 kDa.

Dehoney et al. (2000) showed in their PBP system that there is a decreased affinity for PBP 1 and PBP 2 in amoxicillin-resistant strains. During exposure of *H. pylori* to amoxicillin, microscopy showed spheroplasts after 21 h of contact, which is a concentration-dependent induction that occurs after 2 h.

10.1.1.3. Other Mechanisms

A decrease in intracellular ATP levels was noticed during exposure of *H. pylori* to high concentrations of amoxicillin.

A bactericidal effect of amoxicillin was noted against *H. pylori* associated with cells (HEp-2 cells) or free, sessile, or planktonic bacteria, at 10, 1, and 0.1 μg of amoxicillin per ml at 24 h of contact (inoculum size, 2×10^5 CFU/ml). The combination of amoxicillin and metronidazole was additive.

Chromosomal DNA from an amoxicillin-resistant *H. pylori* strain was isolated and introduced into an amoxicillin-susceptible *H. pylori* strain by natural transformation. This resulted in the occurrence of amoxicillin-resistant colonies at a frequency of 10^{-5}. The MIC for the resistant mutant colonies was increased more than 400-fold compared with that for the susceptible strain. Repetitive subculture of the resistant mutant proved also that this acquired resistance was stable.

An amoxicillin-resistant strain exhibited *pbp1* and *pbp2* mutations. Mutations in *pbp1* contribute to amoxicillin resistance in *H. pylori*. This mutation rendered *H. pylori* moderately resistant (MIC, 0.5 to 1.0 μg/ml). Transformation within the *pbp2* gene does not cause amoxicillin resistance. Amino acids changes resulting from *pbp1* mutation are presented in Table 32. All of those mutations were located in the putative transpeptidase domains of the proteins. In the Hardenberg *H. pylori* strain, mutation in the *pbp1A* gene resulted in a single Ser 144-to-Arg substitution, resulting in a high amoxicillin MIC for *H. pylori*.

10.1.1.4. Gastric Tissue Concentrations

After oral absorption of [^{35}S)pivampicillin and [^{35}S]bacampicillin, 10 to 20% of the radiolabeled compound was taken up by the stomach. Absorption in the duodenum is important, and cumulative uptake for both compounds averages 65%. In the proximal jejunum the cumulative uptake levels were 83 and 71% of the dose for [^{35}S]pivampicillin and [^{35}S]bacampicillin, respectively. The corresponding values for [^{35}S]ampicillin are 24 to 45%. Ampicillin esters are absorbed unchanged and are hydrolyzed not only in the blood but also in the intestinal wall and the liver.

It has been reported that the viscosity of the gastric mucus decreases due to the increase of intragastric pH when omeprazole is administered to healthy volunteers. A change in the viscosity of gastric mucus may be one factor that explains the increased uptake of [^{14}C]amoxicillin into gastric

Table 32 Amino acid changes in strain 69A (amoxicillin resistant)

MIC (μg/ml)	Gene	Amino acid change
0.5	*pbp1*	S414 → R
		Y484 → C
		T541 → I
		P600 → T

Table 33 Concentrations of amoxicillin and ampicillin in gastric tissue

Compound	No. of subjects	Sampling time (h)	Concn in: Serum (μg/ml)	Gastric tissue (mg/kg)
Amoxicillin	3	0.75–1.15	<1.0–24	20–>155
	4	1.25–2.0	10.8–26	15–>153
Pivampicillin	4	0.5–1.0	>1.0–21	>120–209
	1	2.0	16.2	107

tissue in vivo. It was shown that lansoprazole influences the penetration of [^{14}C]amoxicillin in gastric tissue of rats. Gastric amoxicillin and ampicillin (pivampicillin) concentrations were determined in 20 patients undergoing endoscopy. The dose of both antibiotics was 500 mg (Table 33).

Amoxicillin is an amphoteric compound, containing both a basic (-NH_2) and an acidic (-COOH) group (pK_1, 2.4; pK_2, 7.2) A greater proportion of the molecule is in the nonionized form at alkaline pH, and at very acidic pH, and the lipid solubility of amoxicillin may be enhanced.

The passive diffusion across the gastric mucosa partially depends on the pK, lipophilicity, and protein binding of the compounds and on the pH gradient according to the Henderson-Hasselbach equation. In human gastric juice the mean degradation half-lives at pH 2.0 are as summarized in Table 34, whereas the half-lives of degradation at pH 7.0 are above 68 h.

The mucous gel that adheres to the surface of the gastric epithelium represents a barrier which may retard hydrogen ion back-diffusion. A significant pH gradient has been documented from the gastric lumen through the gastric mucus to the surface of the mucosa, with no significant differences between healthy subjects and patients with nonulcer dyspepsia and *H. pylori* gastritis (Table 35).

In controls, luminal and juxtaluminal pHs (mean ± standard error of the mean) of 3.29 ± 0.3 and 4.48 ± 0.25, respectively, were noted in distal esophagus. pHs of 2.57 ± 0.15, 7.16 ± 0.13, and 6.84 ± 0.1 were recorded in the duodenal cap, and a pH of 7.03 ± 0.19 was recorded in the proximal duodenal loop. In the duodenal loop and cap and in the gastric corpus and fundus, the mucosal pH is relatively unaffected by marked variations in luminal pH. In the distal esophagus and antrum, mucosal pH values are influenced to a greater extent, particularly by luminal pH values under 3.0, suggesting that these regions are less able to maintain a pH gradient. In duodenal ulcers, the mean luminal pH is lower at all sites.

Levels of amoxicillin in the gastric mucosa are controversial. In one study, after an oral dose of 0.5 g of amoxicillin as a syrup administered to 15 healthy volunteers (receiving or not 150 or 2,300 mg of ranitidine), the concentrations of amoxicillin in the gastric mucosa and in the gastric juice were higher than those assayed in the serum. After administration of a 1.0-g tablet or water-dissolved tablets of amoxicillin, the levels in the gastric mucosa were up to 40 times higher than those assayed in the serum (Table 36).

Table 34 Half-lives of degradation of antibacterials at pH 2.0

Compound	$t_{1/2}$ of degradation (h)	pK	logP
Amoxicillin	19	2.4, 7.2	
Clarithromycin	1.3		3.24
Metronidazole	2,200	2.52	

10.1.2. Cephems

Cephems are believed to display poor anti-*H. pylori* activity. They are fundamentally stable under acidic conditions, and they are less susceptible to degradation in the stomach than is ampicillin. However, among oral cephems, cefixime and cefuroxime exhibit good in vitro activity, whereas cefetamet and cefteram are weakly active. In an in vitro study carried out by Loo et al. (1992), the MICs at which 50 and 90% of isolates tested are inhibited (MIC_{50} and MIC_{90}) by cefixime were 0.06 and 0.5 μg/ml, and only one strain was considered resistant to this cephem (MIC, ≥4.0 μg/ml).

Among parenteral cephems, the 2-amino-5-thiazolyl cephems also exhibit good in vitro activity against *H. pylori*, with MIC_{50} ranges from 0.12 to 0.5 μg/ml. Cefoperazone is less active, with a MIC_{50} and MIC_{90} of 1.0 and 2.0 μg/ml.

Screening from the Fujisawa cephem library resulted in a compound having a 1,2,4-triazolyl moiety at position 3 of the cephem nucleus which displayed good anti-*H. pylori* activity. MICs ranged from 0.006 to 0.1 μg/ml (Fig. 8).

The anti-*H. pylori* activity of this compound was compared to those of cefdinir and FK-041, which also displays anti-*H. pylori* activity (Fig. 9).

The trifluorocitrate salt of the 4'-pyridyl thiazolyl cephem (Fig. 10) was claimed to exhibit in vitro activity against *H. pylori* NCTC 11637 and TN2, with MICs of ≤0.006 μg/ml, compared to MIC of 0.05 μg/ml for clarithromycin.

FR-182024 (Fig. 11), which has phenyl and thienyl acetamido groups at position 7, showed excellent anti-*H. pylori* activity. However, the presence of an oxime moiety results in decreased activity.

FR-182024 exhibited excellent in vivo activity in eradicating *H. pylori* from mice after oral administration (Table 37).

Table 35 Intragastric pH gradient in humans[a]

Subject condition	*n*	Mean intraluminal pH: Fundus	Corpus	Antrum	Mean juxtamucosal pH: Fundus	Corpus	Antrum
Healthy	21	2.01 ± 0.17	1.82 ± 0.12	3.52 ± 0.34	4.84 ± 0.37	5.50 ± 0.15	5.42 ± 0.29
Duodenal ulcers	9	1.38 ± 0.27	1.50	1.89 ± 0.22	3.80	3.38 ± 0.6	4.19 ± 0.4

[a]Data from Quigley et al., 1987.

Table 36 Amoxicillin concentrations in serum and gastric tissues[a]

Dose (g) and form	n	Sampling time (h)	Concn (μg/ml or mg/kg)					
			Serum	Gastric mucosa			Duodenum	Gastric juice
				Antrum	Fundus	Corpus		
0.5 (syrup)	5	1.5	2.57	3,600	2,000	ND[b]	2,500	2,122
	5	1.5[c]	2.35	1,650	1,200	ND	1,100	1,700
	5	1.5[d]	2.38	1,300	900	ND	1,350	333
1.0 (tablets)	6	0.5	3.0	0.20	0.14	0.14	ND	ND
	6	1.0	7.2	0.08	0.06	0.06	ND	ND
	6	1.5	7.0	0.08	0.06	0.04	ND	ND
1.0 (water dissolved tablets)	6	0.5	1.5	0.63	0.13	0.16	ND	ND
	6	1.0	4.2	0.09	0.06	0.07	ND	ND
	6	1.5	3.5	0.04	0.03	0.04	ND	ND

[a]Data from Cooreman et al., 1993.
[b]ND, not determined.
[c]Plus ranitidine at 150 mg.
[d]Plus ranitidine at 300 mg.

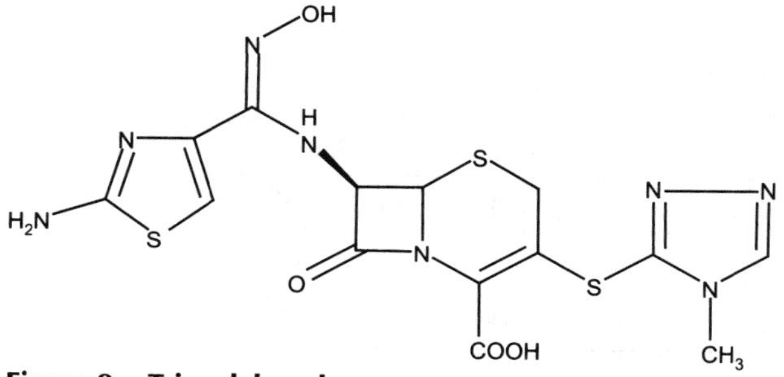

Figure 8 Triazolyl cephems

It exhibits good in vitro activity against *H. pylori* 16021 isolates (clarithromycin resistant) (Yoshida et al., 1999).

10.1.3. Other β-Lactam Antibiotics

Tigemonam, a monocyclic β-lactam, exhibits moderate in vitro activity, with a MIC_{50} and MIC_{90} of 0.25 and 0.5 μg/ml. Aztreonam is poorly active (MIC_{50} and MIC_{90} of 1.0 and 4.0 μg/ml). The in vitro activities of tigemonam and other β-lactam antibiotics are listed in Table 38.

Fropenem (or faropenem), a penem derivative, also displays good in vitro activity against *H. pylori* (Sanofi-Aventis, data on file) and is more active in vitro than amoxicillin (Table 39).

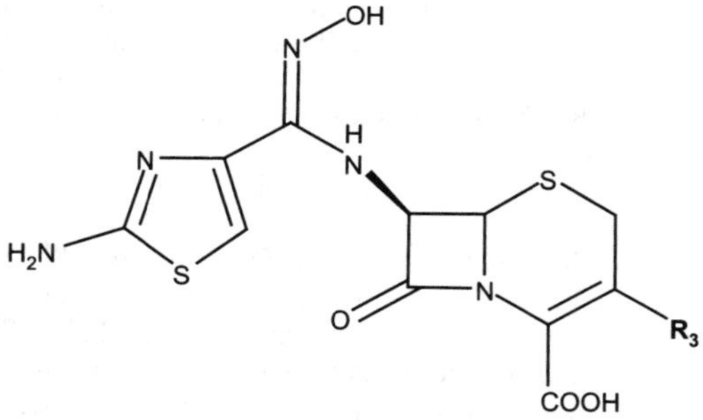

MIC (μg/ml) for *H. pylori* strain:

	R_3	9005	13001	FR 1757
Compound A	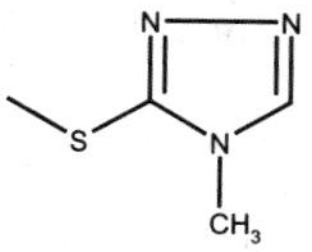	0.10	0.006	0.006
Cefdinir	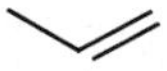	0.20	0.39	0.20
FK 041	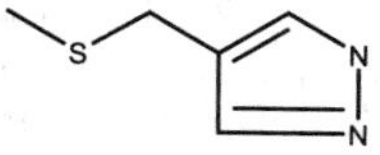	0.20	0.10	0.10

Figure 9 Anti-*H. pylori* action of cephems

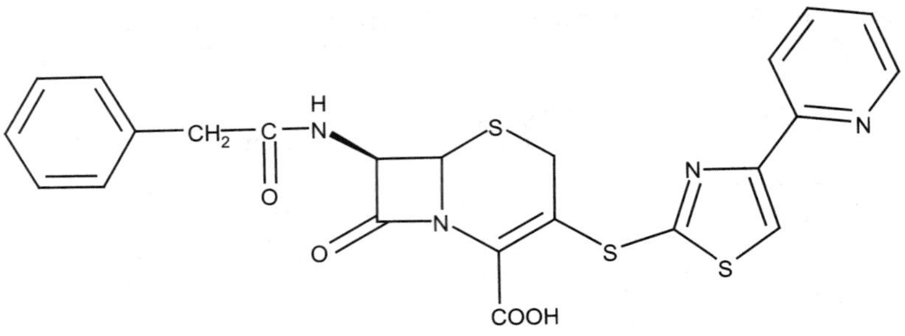

Figure 10 Thiazolyl cephems

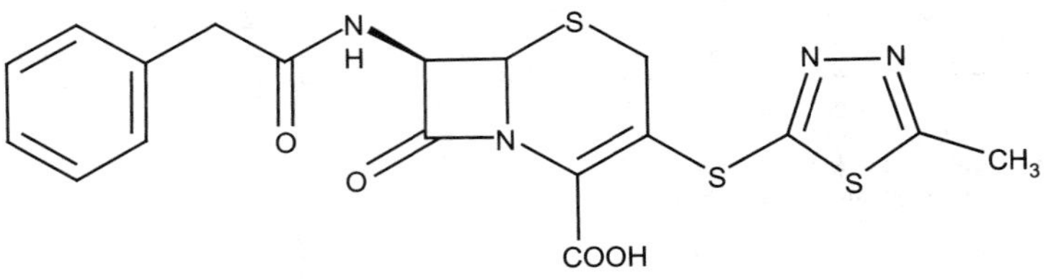

Figure 11 FR-182024

Table 37 In vitro activity of FR-182024 against *H. pylori* isolates

Compound	MIC (μg/ml) for *H. pylori* strain:				Eradication ratio at dose (mg/kg):			
	9005	13000	FP 1757	16021	0.1	0.32	1.0	32
FR-182024	0.006	0.0007	0.001	0.0001	5/8	8/8	ND[a]	ND
Amoxicillin	0.05	0.025	0.01	0.01	0/8	1/8	3/8	7/8
Clarithromycin	0.2	0.05	0.1	5.0	ND	0/8	0/8	0/8

[a]ND, not determined.

10.2. Macrolides

Macrolides constitute an important family of antibiotics and can be divided into three main groups according to the size of the lactone ring. A macrolide is one of the components of triple or quadruple therapy for *H. pylori* infections.

14-Membered-ring macrolides are the most active in vitro and in therapies against *H. pylori*. The most common macrolide used in triple or quadruple therapy is clarithromycin. Azithromycin is less active than the 14-membered-ring macrolides, and 16-membered-ring macrolides are weakly active against *H. pylori* (Table 40).

10.2.1. PAE

A long postantibiotic effect (PAE) of clarithromycin, approximately 15 h, was demonstrated for *H. pylori* after exposure to 10 times the MIC for 5 h.

The PAE of flurithromycin on 10 *H. pylori* strains was studied by exposure of the bacteria to flurithromycin at 5 and 10 times the MIC for 1 or 2 h. The mean durations of PAE varied between 1.5 and 6.0 h.

10.2.2. Bactericidal Activity of Macrolides against *H. pylori*

Clarithromycin exhibited bactericidal activity, with a reduction of 3 $\log_{10}$CFU/ml within 2 to 8 h. Erythromycin A and azithromycin exhibited a reduction of >3 $\log_{10}$CFU/ml after 24 h of contact. Clarithromycin in combination with the 14-OH metabolite and amoxicillin demonstrated an additive effect against 32% of *H. pylori* isolates tested.

10.2.3. Mode of Action of Macrolides

14- and 15-membered-ring macrolides inhibit protein synthesis. They block the exit of the nascent polypeptide. They interact with domain V of the peptidyltransferase loop (23S rRNA). It was shown that clarithromycin has a high affinity for the *H. pylori* ribosome. The half-life of dissociation ranged from 7 to 16 h (Table 41).

10.2.4. In Vitro Intracellular Activity of Macrolides

Observations both in vitro and in vivo have shown that *H. pylori* is able to invade epithelial cells. Some electron microscopic studies have also shown that *H. pylori* is often at the intercellular junctions between gastric epithelial cells or within intercellular spaces and the gastric mucosa.

It has been shown that *H. pylori* can survive intracellularly for at least 48 h in vitro and can be killed by clarithromycin.

H. pylori penetrates rapidly into HEp-2 cells, but it is not able to replicate inside the cells and no intracellular bacteria were viable after 72 h. Only a subpopulation of *H. pylori* has the capacity to "switch on" virulence determinant-associated genes that allow intracellular penetration. Clarithromycin exhibited early bactericidal activity within the cell, with complete killing at four times the MIC (2 μg/ml). Azithromycin is active against a clinical isolate of *H. pylori* internalized by HEp-2 cells. However, extracellular concentrations of 200 times the minimum bactericidal concentration (100 μg/ml) were necessary to achieve intracellular killing.

Table 38 In vitro activities of β-lactam antibiotics against *H. pylori*

Compound	*n*	MIC (μg/ml)		
		50%	90%	Range
Penicillin G	18	0.06	0.125	<0.03–1.0
	70	0.01	0.03	0.002–0.06
Ampicillin	18	0.06	0.125	<0.03–1.0
	16	0.01	0.03	0.008–0.03
Amoxicillin	30	<0.008	0.06	<0.008–0.06
	18	0.06	0.125	0.06–0.5
Carbenicillin	26	0.0	0.8	0.025–1.6
Cephalothin	18	4.0	16	1.0–16
Cefazolin	18	1.0	2.0	0.06–2.0
Cephradine	25	1.6	3.1	0.2–6.2
Cefuroxime	30	0.125	0.25	0.01–0.25
	18	0.125	0.25	<0.03–0.25
	23	0.125	0.125	0.06–2.0
	16	1.0	4.0	0.25–8.0
Cefaclor	24	8.0	128	0.25–128
	16	1.0	2.0	0.12–2.0
Loracarbef	16	0.5	2.0	0.25–2.0
Cefadroxil	16	8.0	16	0.5–16
Cefetamet	30	2.0	4.0	1.0–8.0
	16	16	16	4.0–16
Cefteram	30	0.5	2.0	0.03–2.0
Cefixime	30	0.06	0.25	0.008–0.25
	18	0.125	0.125	0.06–1.0
	16	1.0	4.0	0.5–8.0
Ceftibuten	16	4.0	8.0	2.0–8.0
	30	2.0	8.0	0.25–8.0
Cefpodoxime	16	1.0	4.0	0.5–4.0
	30	0.5	4.0	0.12–4.0
Cefdinir	16	0.5	2.0	0.5–2.0
Cefprozil	16	2.0	8.0	0.25–8.0
Bay 3522	16	2.0	4.0	0.06–4.0
Moxalactam	23	0.25	0.25	0.06–0.5
Cefoperazone	18	1.0	2.0	<0.03–2.0
	23	1.0	1.0	0.25–1.0
Ceftriaxone	18	0.12	0.5	<0.03–0.5
	23	0.12	0.5	0.06–0.5
Ceftazidime	23	0.5	2.0	0.06–2.0
Ceftizoxime	23	0.5	0.25	0.06–0.5
	25	0.4	1.6	0.1–1.6
Cefoxitin	70	0.12	0.12	0.01–0.5
	23	0.06	0.12	0.06–>2.0
Cefsulodin	18	4.0	16	0.06–16
	23	64	>64	8.0–>64
Tigemonam	30	0.25	0.5	0.01–0.5
Aztreonam	18	1.0	4.0	<0.03–16

Table 39 In vitro comparative activities of fropenem and other antibacterials against *H. pylori* (*n* = 100)

Compound	MIC (μg/ml)		
	50%	90%	Range
Fropenem	0.008	0.015	≤0.008–0.125
Roxithromycin	0.06	0.125	≤0.03–8.0
Clarithromycin	0.03	0.06	≤0.03–32
Metronidazole	1.0	<32	0.12–32
Tetracycline	0.06	0.25	0.015–0.5
Amoxicillin	0.015	0.03	≤0.008–0.25

Rifabutin in this study showed good intracellular activity against *H. pylori*, as did lansoprazole. Metronidazole and amoxicillin exhibited poor intracellular activity against *H. pylori*.

10.2.5. Macrolide Resistance

The importance of de novo mutation in developing resistance was reported for the first time in 1943. The frequency of spontaneous resistance to erythromycin A ranges from 10^{-5} to 10^{-9}.

After serial passages, 26.9% of *H. pylori* isolates became resistant to azithromycin. The frequency of spontaneous

Table 40 In vitro activities of macrolides against *H. pylori*

Compound	*n*	MIC (μg/ml)		
		50%	90%	Range
Erythromycin A	70	0.06	0.12	0.01–0.5
	18	0.125	0.25	<0.03–0.25
	13	0.12	0.25	0.12–0.25
	30	0.01	0.03	0.01–0.12
	16	0.12	0.5	0.12–0.5
	10	0.12	0.25	0.06–0.25
	18	0.03	0.06	0.008–012
Clarithromycin	13	0.03	0.03	0.03–0.06
	100	0.03	0.06	≤0.03–32
14-OH clarithromycin	13	0.06	0.06	0.06–0.12
Roxithromycin	13	0.12	0.25	0.12–0.25
	30	<0.008	0.01	<0.008–0.03
	10	0.25	0.25	0.12–0.25
	100	0.06	0.12	≤0.03–32
Dirithromycin	13	0.5	0.01	0.25–0.5
	30	0.25	0.5	0.125–0.25
Erythromycylamine	13	0.5	0.25	0.25–1.0
Flurithromycin	13	0.12	0.5	0.06–0.25
Davercin	16	0.5	2.0	NI[a]
Azithromycin	13	0.25	0.12	0.25
	18	≤0.25	≤0.25	≤0.25
	10	0.25	0.25	0.12–0.5
	16	0.5	2.0	NI
Josamycin	13	1.0	0.25	0.5–2.0
Spiramycin	13	0.5	1.0	0.25–2.0
Miokamycin	13	0.5	1.0	0.25–1.0
Rokitamycin	13	0.5	0.5	0.5–1.0

[a]NI, not indicated.

Table 41 Kinetics of macrolide interaction with *H. pylori* 70S ribosomes

Compound	k_{-1} ($M^{-1}min^{-1}$)	k_1 (min^{-1})	k_d (M)
Erythromycin A	6.83×10^{-4}	3.3×10^{6}	2.07×10^{-10}
Clarithromycin	7.07×10^{-4}	305×10^{6}	2.32×10^{-10}
14-OH clarithromycin	16.6×10^{-4}	8.47×10^{6}	1.96×10^{-10}

mutations in *H. pylori* conferring antibiotic resistance was determined for clarithromycin, metronidazole, rifampin, and ciprofloxacin. Data are reported in Table 42.

Xia et al. (1996) found that 9 of the 20 (45%) clarithromycin-resistant *H. pylori* isolates tested reverted to susceptibility after two to five subcultures on clarithromycin-free agar. Hulten et al. (1997) were unable to reproduce those data.

In a third investigation it was shown that clarithromycin resistance was unstable in 3 out of 30 (10%) *H. pylori* isolates. The investigators found that resistance was not stable after 10, 13, and 18 subcultures. Two isolates had an A216G mutation and one had an A21426 mutation.

In a fourth study, Debets-Ossenkopp et al. (1998) found that after 21 passages in clarithromycin-free medium all strains remained resistant.

10.2.6. Mechanisms of Resistance to Macrolides

A point mutation is associated with macrolide resistance in *H. pylori*, and this mutation (adenine to guanine) could be in either of two positions (Table 43).

Table 42 Frequency of spontaneous mutation in *H. pylori*

Selective antibiotic (concn, μg/ml)	No. of subcultures	Frequency of mutants	Mutation rate/ cell division
Rifampin (20)	15–30	3.8×10^{-8}–6.6×10^{-8}	1.1×10^{-8}–1.6×10^{-8}
Ciprofloxacin (1)	15	3.8×10^{-8}	1.1×10^{-8}
Clarithromycin (0.5)	12	3.0×10^{-9}	8×10^{-10}
Metronidazole (8)	15	5.1×10^{-9}	6.9×10^{-10}

Table 43 Correlation between *E. coli* and *H. pylori* numeration

H. pylori	*E. coli*
2142	2058
2143	2059

No methylation process (*erm*) has been shown to date in *H. pylori*.

The two main transition mutations are A2142G and A2143G. Another mutation has been described in the transversion A2142G that is of rare occurrence. In vitro, other unstable mutations have been reported: A2143C, A2142T, and A2143T. Two mutations, A2115G and G2141A, reported by Hulten et al. have never been found again.

Two identical copies of the 23S rRNA have been sequenced, and the transcription start site of the gene from a clarithromycin-susceptible strain was determined. A-to-G mutations at position 2142 or 2143 were predominantly observed in clarithromycin-resistant *H. pylori* clinical isolates. Very few cases of A-to-C and A-to-T mutations were reported. The A-to-G mutation resulted in competitive growth advantages compared with the A-to-C or A-to-T mutation. It is possible that A-to-C and A-to-T mutations impair ribosome function in protein synthesis, but not A-to-G mutations. Two major types of macrolide-lincosamide-streptogramin (MLS_B) resistance were identified and correlated with specific point mutations in the 23S rRNA.

The A2142G mutation was linked with high-level cross-resistance to all MLS_B antibiotics (type I), and the A2143G mutation gave rise to an intermediate level of resistance to clarithromycin and clindamycin but no resistance to streptogramin B (type II).

In addition, streptogramins A and B were demonstrated to have a synergistic effect on both MLS_B-susceptible and -resistant *H. pylori* isolates.

Infection by a mixed population of clarithromycin-susceptible and clarithromycin-resistant *H. pylori* has been reported.

The A2142G mutations was consistently associated with clarithromycin MICs >256 μg/ml, whereas mutants carrying A2143G had MICs ranging from ≤0.01 to >256 μg/ml. There is a dissociation between susceptibility to clarithromycin and resistance to erythromycin A.

Clarithromycin resistance carries a biological cost, as measured by a decreased competitive ability caused by *H. pylori* resistance in mice.

10.2.6.1. Gastric Tissue Levels

The roxithromycin level in the gastric mucosa was assayed after four oral doses of 150 mg. Higher concentrations in tissue were achieved 8 and 12 h after the last administration. Data are reported in Table 44.

Twenty-three healthy *H. pylori*-negative volunteers received 500 mg of clarithromycin three times per day for 5 days, and biopsy samples were taken from the gastric mucosa for clarithromycin level determinations. Clarithromycin is more concentrated in the fundus of the stomach than in the antrum. The level of clarithromycin is low in mucus. In the presence of omeprazole the level of clarithromycin increased up to 2 times in the fundus and antrum and up to 40 times in mucus (at 2 h the mucus clarithomycin level in combination with omeprazole is 39.3 ± 32.8 mg/kg of body weight, with high interindividual variation). Data are reported in Table 45.

Azithromycin distribution in gastric tissues was studied for 32 patients with proven gastric cancer due to be resectioned. The azithromycin concentrations in gastric tissue, mucus, and gastric juice (Table 46) were in sharp contrast with levels in plasma, which were undetectable 24 h after dosing. The mean azithromycin concentration in the gastric mucosa following a single 500-mg oral dose were similar to those attained in lung tissue.

Seven patients suffering from gastritis received a combination of azithromycin (500 mg on day 1 and 250 mg on days 2 to 5), pantoprazole once daily, and 800 mg of metronidazole daily. The median concentrations of azithromycin in gastric tissue amounted to 7.5 mg/kg on day 2 and 9.7 mg/kg on day 5. Four days after the end of treatment, median concentrations were still at 3.9 mg/kg.

Gastric mucosal concentrations of erythromycin after an oral dose of 500 mg of erythromycin ethyl succinate or stearate were determined for 18 patients undergoing endoscopies (Table 47).

Table 44 Gastric mucosa tissue concentration of roxithromycin

Time of sampling (h)	Concn (μg/ml or mg/kg)	
	Serum	Gastric mucosa
4.0	11.85 ± 9.64	13.14 ± 3.71
8.0	7.81 ± 5.48	12.31 ± 7.43
12	2.54 ± 2.87	8.8 ± 2.03

Table 45 Gastric tissue level of clarithromycin and the main metabolite

Compound	Time of sampling (h)	Concn (μg/ml or mg/kg)			
			Gastric tissue		
		Plasma	Antrum	Fundus	Mucus
Clarithromycin	0	1.7 ± 0.6	5.3 ± 2.1	9.8 ± 1.5	0.7 ± 0.9
	2	3.8 ± 1.1	10.5 ± 2.0	20.8 ± 7.6	4.2 ± 7.7
	4	3.7 ± 0.8	7.5 ± 1.8	16.5 ± 3.6	0.8 ± 1.1
	6	2.5 ± 1.0	5.2 ± 2.9	13.6 ± 11.0	1.0 ± 0.9
14-OH clarithromycin	0	0.7 ± 0.9	0.6 ± 1.5	2.9 ± 0.6	0.3 ± 0.3
	2	1.0 ± 0.1	2.2 ± 1.4	4.8 ± 0.7	0
	4	0.8 ± 0.3	1.3 ± 0.9	2.8 ± 2.1	0
	6	0.7 ± 0.2	0.4 ± 0.8	3.6 ± 2.0	0

Table 46 Azithromycin concentrations in gastric juice and tissue

Location	Concn in μg/ml or mg/kg (range) at time:			
	24–48 h	49–72 h	73–96 h	97–120 h
Gastric juice	0.02 (0–0.59)	0.15 (0–0.16)	0.20 (0–0.37)	0.0 (0–0.38)
Gastric mucosa	0.48 (0–0.49)	0.52 (0.23–0.80)	0.47 (0–0.83)	0.44 (0–1.6)
Gastric tissue	3.97 (1.6–13.4)	4.07 (1.7–10.8)	4.61 (4.3–5.3)	2.27 (0–5.8)

Table 47 Gastric tissue concentration of erythromycin

Erythromycin	*n*	Sampling time (h)	Gastric tissue (mg/kg)	Serum (μg/ml)
Stearate	5	0.75–1.0	1.9–36.7	<0.2–1.0
	5	1.5–2.25	2.5–5.2	0.4–1.8
Ethyl succinate	3	0.6–1.0	2.0–40.9	0.3–1.45
	5	1.5–2.5	1.8–21.7	0.2–1.35

10.2.7. A-69334 and A-70310

A series of erythromycin A derivatives having an amino group at C-9 were prepared and tested against *H. pylori*. Two compounds, A-69334 and A-70310 (Fig. 12), in comparison with other antibacterials were shown to display good anti-*H. pylori* activity, but less than that of clarithromycin (Table 48).

A-69334 is equipotent to erythromycin A against *H. pylori*; A-70310 is far less active than azithromycin, clarithromycin, and erythromycin A against *H. pylori*.

10.3. Ketolides

10.3.1. Telithromycin

Ketolides are new semisynthetic derivatives of erythromycin A which differ in having a 3-keto group instead of an L-cladinose on the erythronolide A ring. One compound reached clinical practice in 2001: telithromycin (Fig. 13).

Telithromycin in vitro activity has been tested against 136 *H. pylori* isolates (Table 49). In vitro, telithromycin shows good activity against *H. pylori*, higher than that of erythromycin A and azithromycin but less than that of clarithromycin.

In another study, the in vitro activity of telithromycin was tested against 100 isolates of *H. pylori* either susceptible ($n = 50$) or resistant ($n = 50$) to clarithromycin. In each group half of the strains were either susceptible or resistant to metronidazole. MIC determinations were done by agar dilution using a Wilkins-Chalgren agar supplemented with 10% sheep blood. Incubation was carried out for 48 h at 37°C in a microaerophilic atmosphere (Sanofi-Aventis, data on file). Results are shown in Table 50.

In another study, the in vitro activities were determined using Mueller-Hinton agar supplemented with 10% horse whole blood. The inoculum size was 10^8 to 10^9 CFU/ml. Incubation was carried out for 72 h in a microaerophilic atmosphere. MIC determinations were done at pH 7.4, 6.5, and 5.9; results are shown in Table 51.

The in vitro activities of telithromycin and clarithromycin are influenced by pH. Full cross-resistance has been shown between clarithromycin and telithromycin when a mutation in the 23S rRNA (A2144G or A2143G) is present. A2142, A2143, and A2144 are included in the *H. pylori* peptidyltransferase loop.

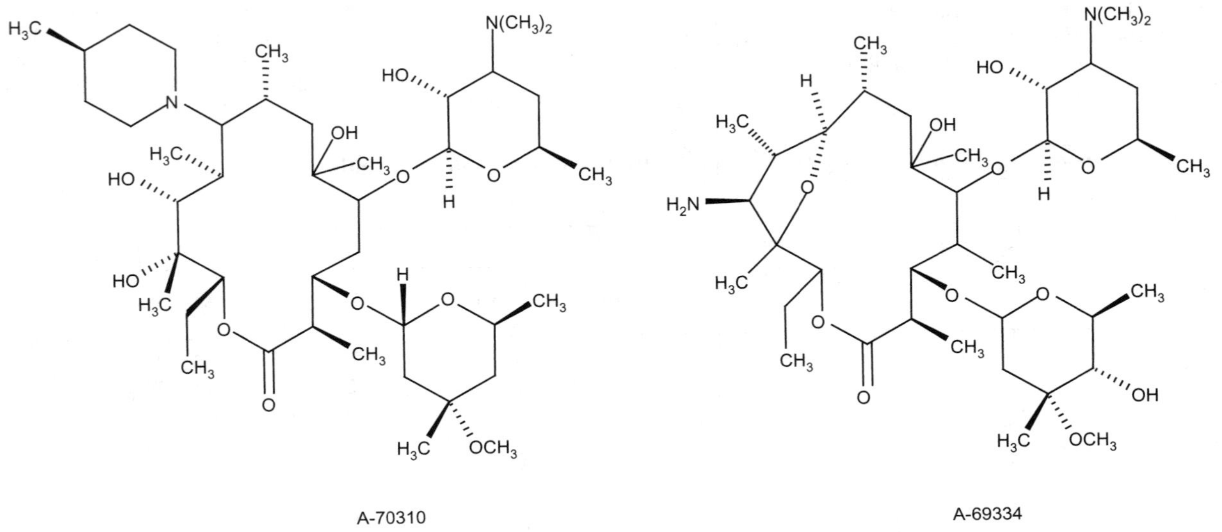

Figure 12 Macrolides with anti-*H. pylori* activity

Table 48 In vitro activities of A-69334 and A-70310 against *H. pylori*

Strain	MIC (μg/ml)				
	A-69334	A-70310	Azithromycin	Clarithromycin	Erythromycin
NCTC 11637	0.12	1.0	0.06	≤0.06	0.12
ATCC 43526	0.12	0.25	≤0.06	≤0.06	0.06
ATCC 43579	0.12	0.5	0.12	≤0.06	0.12
ATCC 43629	0.12	0.5	0.06	≤0.06	0.12
AC 2758	0.06	0.5	0.12	≤0.06	0.12
AC 2759	0.12	0.5	0.12	≤0.06	0.12
A 2761	0.12	1.0	0.12	≤0.06	0.12
A 2764	0.12	1.0	≤0.06	≤0.06	0.12

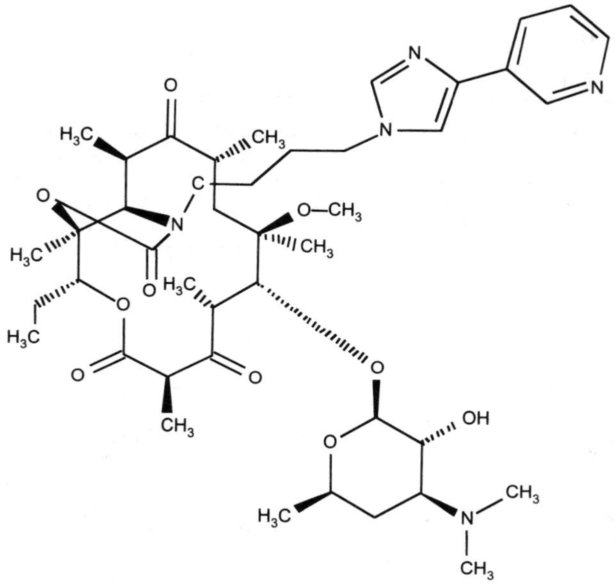

Figure 13 Telithromycin

Telithromycin exhibits bactericidal activity against *H. pylori* NCTC 11637, with a 3-$\log_{10}$CFU/ml reduction, 3 h after contact at 50 times the MIC; within 6 h for 10 times the MIC and for 12 h only 2 times the MIC are needed.

The PAE was 6 h (5 to 33 h). Within HEp-2 cells, telithromycin exhibited a 1.8 to 2.0-$\log_{10}$ reduction of intracellular bacteria within 8 h.

The in vitro activity of HMR 3004 against *H. pylori* was investigated. For 100 *H. pylori* isolates, the MIC_{50} and MIC_{90} were 0.06 and 0.25 μg/ml (range, ≤0.03 to 8.0 μg/ml). HMR 3004 was as active as telithromycin. The bactericidal effect of HMR 3004 was achieved at 6.0 h for 50 times the MIC, and at 12 h for 10 times the MIC. At 5 and 2 times the MIC only a 2-$\log_{10}$CFU/ml reduction was achieved at 24 h. The PAE was reached at 13 h (8 to 22 h). In HEp-2 cells, a reduction of 1.8 to 2.0 $\log_{10}$ bacteria within 8 h was shown.

10.3.2. Cethromycin (ABT-773)

In a study, the MIC of cethromycin (ABT-773) (Fig. 14) for *H. pylori* was determined using a modified NCCLS method. Ten percent defibrinated horse blood was used as a blood supplement instead of 5% aged sheep blood. Plates were incubated in a 10% CO_2 incubator rather than under microaerophilic conditions (5% oxygen, 10% CO_2, and 85% N_2) used for *Campylobacter*. Supplementation with horse blood resulted in better growth than supplementation with sheep blood. Data are reported in Table 52.

There was full cross-resistance between ABT-773 and clarithromycin against *H. pylori* (Table 53).

The combination of cethromycin and metronidazole demonstrated additive effects against 69% of *H. pylori* isolates. The combination of cethromycin and tetracycline showed a 100% additive effect. Fractional inhibitory concentrations (FICs) of ≤0.75 were seen in 93% of *H. pylori* isolates. The combination of ABT-773 and amoxicillin demonstrated an additive effect against 43% of *H. pylori* isolates.

10.4. Tetracyclines

Tetracycline belongs to a family of broad-spectrum antibiotics that have been widely used for the treatment of bacterial infections since the late 1950s. Resistance to tetracycline has been reported for almost all bacterial species. The in vitro activities of tetracycline and analogs are reported in Table 54.

Table 49 In vitro activity of telithromycin against *H. pylori*

Compound	*n*	MIC (μg/ml)		
		50%	90%	Range
Telithromycin	21	0.25	0.25	0.00–0.25
	15	0.06	0.125	0.008–0.5
	100	0.06	0.125	0.03–8.0
Clarithromycin	21	0.015	0.06	0.008–0.12
	15	≤0.002	≤0.002	≤0.002
	100	0.03	0.06	≤0.03–16
Erythromycin A	21	0.25	0.5	0.25–0.5
Azithromycin	21	0.25	0.5	0.03–0.5

Table 50 In vitro activity of telithromycin against clarithromycin-resistant *H. pylori*

Compound	Phenotype[a]	MIC (μg/ml)		
		50%	90%	Range
Telithromycin	CLR^{s}	0.125	0.5	0.06–2.0
	CLR^{r}	16	128	0.5–128
Clarithromycin	CLR^{s}	0.03	0.125	0.007–0.2
	CLR^{r}	32	>128	4–>128
Azithromycin	CLR^{s}	0.12	0.25	0.03–128
	CLR^{r}	>128	>128	64–>128

[a]CLR, clarithromycin. Susceptibility corresponds to a MIC of <1.0 μg/ml.

Table 51 Influence of pH on determination of MICs for *H. pylori*

Compound	MIC (μg/ml)								
	pH 7.4			pH 6.5			pH 5.9		
	50%	90%	Range	50%	90%	Range	50%	90%	Range
Telithromycin	0.12	0.12	0.03–0.25	0.25	0.5	0.06–1.0	0.5	1.0	0.25–2.0
Clarithromycin	0.03	0.03	≤0.008–0.06	0.06	0.25	0.06–0.25	0.25	0.5	0.12–1.0

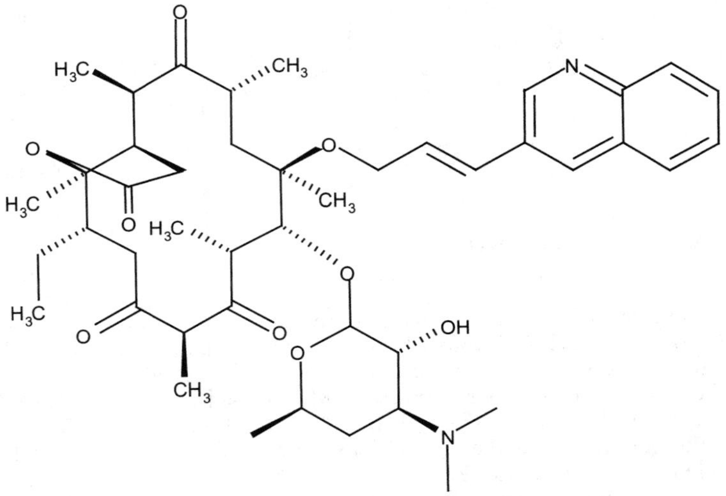

Figure 14 Cethromycin

Table 52 In vitro activity of ABT-773 against *H. pylori*

Compound	MIC (mg/ml)[a]			
	10% CO_2 atmosphere		Microaerophilic condition	
	10% HB	5% ASB	10% HB	5% ASB
ABT-773	0.25	0.25	0.125	0.125
Amoxicillin	0.015	0.015	0.015	0.015
Clarithromycin	0.03	0.06	0.03	0.03
Metronidazole	128	128	128	128
Tetracycline	0.125	0.25	0.25	0.5

[a]HB, horse blood; ASB, aged sheep blood.

Table 53 In vitro activity of ABT-773 against *H. pylori* isolates resistant to clarithromycin (*n* = 15)

Compound	Phenotype[a]	MIC (μg/ml)		
		50%	90%	Range
ABT-773	CLR[s]	0.03	0.06	0.008–0.06
	CLR[r]	32	64	4–64
Clarithromycin	CLR[s]	0.008	0.01	0.008–0.06
	CLR[r]	32	128	4–128
Azithromycin	CLR[s]	0.25	0.5	0.06–0.5
	CLR[r]	>128	>128	128–>128
Erythromycin A	CLR[s]	0.12	0.25	0.06–0.25
	CLR[r]	128	>128	64–>128

[a]CLR, clarithromycin.

Tetracycline-resistant *H. pylori* strains were isolated in 1996 in Australia. Tetracycline-resistant strains are uncommon in the United States and the European Union. However, the prevalence of tetracycline resistance is high and increasing in Brazil, Korea, Japan, Lebanon, Estonia, and India. In China it was reported that 59% of the clinical isolates are resistant to tetracycline.

Tetracycline binds to the 30S ribosomal subunit and blocks the binding of aminoacyl-tRNA, thus stalling the synthesis of nascent polypeptide. In the crystal structure of the 30S ribosomal subunit, two to six binding sites for tetracycline have been identified. It has been shown that protein S7 and 16S rRNA bases G693, A892, U1052, C1054, G1300, and G1338 all contribute to tetracycline binding.

Tetracycline resistance in *H. pylori* is relatively low, with an average incidence of 5 to 7% of the isolates. There is cross-resistance between tetracycline and metronidazole, but not vice versa. Furthermore, this resistance was transferred to susceptible strains by transformation with the genomic DNA of the resistant organisms.

When *H. pylori* is subjected to serial passages with increasing concentrations of tetracycline, resistant *H. pylori* strains for which the tetracycline MIC is 32 μg/ml can be easily obtained. However, this resistance is unstable and is lost when *H. pylori* is subcultured in tetracycline-free medium.

It was shown that mutations found in the 16S rRNA genes are responsible for the resistance of tetracyclines by affecting the binding site of tetracyclines.

The $AGA_{965-967}TTC$ (h31 loop) mutation and 6-942 deletions are located in domain III.

Several nucleotides in this region interact with tRNA molecules. In particular, base G966 directly contacts the anticodon loop of the tRNA in the P-site. These mutations are located at the primary tetracycline-binding site.

Triple mutations are responsible for high-level resistance; single or double mutations are responsible for low-level resistance. However, resistance to tetracycline is due in 50% of the cases to involvement of membrane permeability (efflux).

The finding that all characterized tetracycline-resistant *H. pylori* strains are also resistant to metronidazole suggests that there may be a progressive acquisition of resistance where metronidazole resistance may be required before tetracycline resistance can develop. Metronidazole in *H. pylori* is converted into an active mutagenic form that could increase mutations in the 16S rRNA genes.

Table 54 In vitro activities of cyclines against *H. pylori*

Compound	*n*	MIC (μg/ml)		
		50%	90%	Range
Doxycycline	18	0.5	2.0	0.25–8.0
	16	1.0	1.0	
Tetracycline	100	0.06	0.25	0.015–0.5
Minocycline	16	0.5	0.5	
	24	0.5	2.0	0.12–2.0
	30	0.25	0.5	0.06–0.5
DMAM[a]	16	0.25	0.5	

[a]DMAM, *N*,*N*-dimethylaminidominocycline.

10.5. 5-Nitroimidazole Derivatives

10.5.1. Metronidazole

10.5.1.1. Clinical Use

Metronidazole is a 5-nitroimidazole derivative which was introduced in to clinical practice at the end of the 1950s for the treatment of *Trichomonas vaginalis* and used later for the treatment of intestinal protozoa: *Giardia lamblia* and *Entamoeba histolytica*. In the early 1970s, it was demonstrated that metronidazole is an excellent antianaerobic drug. It was shown that *H. pylori*, a microaerophilic bacterium, is highly susceptible to metronidazole. Metronidazole is actively secreted into the gastric juice, and its bactericidal activity is weakly affected by a decrease of pH.

Metronidazole is the companion drug in triple and quadruple therapy for *H. pylori* infections.

In different studies, it was shown that up to 76% of patients infected with metronidazole-resistant isolates were cured. However, in the MACH2 study the eradication rates for metronidazole-susceptible and -resistant *H. pylori* isolates were 95 and 76%, respectively. In another study, triple therapy was successful in 93 and 69% of cases when susceptible and resistant *H. pylori* isolates were involved.

Coinfections located in different parts of the stomach due to *H. pylori* strains resistant and susceptible to metronidazole have been identified.

Smith et al. discovered differences in susceptibility in isolates obtained from both the corpus and antrum. The discrepancies may be due to coinfection with two different strains of distinct lineages. This was confirmed by DNA fingerprinting.

Metronidazole is metabolized to a hydroxy metabolite that also has activity against *H. pylori*. Addition of the metronidazole hydroxy metabolite to the parent compound resulted in enhanced activity when combined with paromomycin against *H. pylori*.

The in vitro activities of metronidazole and tinidazole are reported in Table 55.

10.5.1.2. Mode of Action

Metronidazole exerts its antibacterial activity via one-electron reduction of the nitro group, which leads to the production of radical species that can cause DNA damage. Metronidazole has a low reduction potential and is normally effective in organisms with a low intracellular redox state. *H. pylori* belongs to these organisms, which grow better at low oxygen tensions than under anaerobic conditions. *H. pylori* has a pyruvate-flavodoxin oxidoreductase complex and is sensitive to metronidazole. In addition, *H. pylori* possesses a number of genes encoding a putative ferredoxin-like (*fdxB* gene) electron carrier protein which may be involved in the activation of metronidazole under microaerophilic conditions. Other nitroreductase-encoding genes, including *frxA*, which encodes NADPH flavinoxidoreductase, have been described for *H. pylori*. Oxygen has a higher reduction potential than metronidazole (~486 mV); the molecule of oxygen outcompetes metronidazole as an acceptor in redox reductions. Consequently, anaerobic or anoxic conditions are required for metronidazole to be reduced.

Oxygen-insensitive NADPH nitroreductase activity has been associated with susceptibility to metronidazole in *H. pylori*.

This nitroreductase, encoded by *rdxA*, reduces nitroaromatic compounds through sequential two-electron reductions to generate nitroso intermediate and hydroxylamine end products.

This enzyme reduces the nitro group of metronidazole to active metabolites that are directly toxic to the bacteria, and in *H. pylori*, the bactericidal activity of metronidazole is largely due to the induction of DNA single-strand breakage.

The selective toxicity of metronidazole for anaerobic bacteria and protozoa is due to the redox potential of the components of their electron transport chains, which are sufficiently negative to reduce the nitro group of metronidazole. Within these organisms, electrons produced by the pyruvate oxidoreductase complex from the decarboxylation of pyruvate are passed on to ferredoxin or flavodoxin.

This low-redox electron carrier protein then reduces another component, usually a proton, which acts as the terminal electron acceptor. Accepting electrons from reduced ferrodoxin or flavodoxin activates metronidazole, which has a very low redox potential. The ongoing reduction of metronidazole maintains a favorable transmembrane metronidazole concentration gradient.

Table 55 In vitro activity of metronidazole against *H. pylori*

Compound	*n*	MIC (μg/ml)		
		50%	90%	Range
Metronidazole	59	2.0	64	0.5–>128
	16	2.0	2.0	2–64
	70	1.0	8.0	0.5–8.0
	100	1.0	>32	0.12–>32
	30	0.25	0.5	0.06–0.5
Tinidazole		1.0	2.0	0.25–2.0

An alternative mechanism of action, named "futile cycling," has been proposed, for when metronidazole is exposed to aerobic atmospheric conditions.

Molecular oxygen may oxidize the nitroso radicals generated from the reduction of metronidazole generated by a one-electron transfer stepback to the parent compound. Under normal circumstances, superoxide ions are converted by superoxide dismutase to hydrogen peroxide, which is further reduced by the action of catalase.

10.5.1.3. Mechanism of Resistance

The widespread use of metronidazole in the treatment of amoebiasis and giardiasis in developing countries is thought to account for the high prevalence of metronidazole-resistant *H. pylori* in these countries. The slightly higher prevalence of metronidazole-resistant strains in women than in men in developed countries may be attributed to the use of metronidazole in the treatment of gynecological infections (*T. vaginalis*, *Gardnerella vaginalis*, and *Prevotella bivia*, agents of vaginosis).

Several mechanisms of resistance to metronidazole have been proposed based upon the effects on metronidazole enzyme activity and gene expression, but the full nature of the resistance remains unclear. There is a relationship between the intracellular oxygen-cavenging ability of *H. pylori* and the susceptibility of *H. pylori* to metronidazole. Metronidazole-resistant *H. pylori* isolates possess lower soluble cytosolic NADH oxidase activity than metronidazole-susceptible *H. pylori* strains.

In strains resistant to metronidazole, oxygen outcompetes metronidazole for the electrons from the flavodoxin, resulting in no metronidazole activation, or metronidazole is reduced by the flavodoxin but is oxidized back to the inactive parent compound by a futile-cycling mechanism. This hypothesis was named "scavenging of oxygen." Short exposure of metronidazole-resistant cultures of *H. pylori* to anaerobic conditions causes them to become sensitive to metronidazole.

The majority of resistance is associated with mutational inactivation of the *rdxA* gene, which codes for a putative oxygen-insensitive NADPH nitroreductase. Inactivation of other nitroreductase-encoding genes, including *frxA* and *frxB*, is also associated with resistance and seems to be involved in the transition to high-level resistance. The relative importance of the *rdxA* and *frxA* nitroreductase genes in metronidazole resistance in *H. pylori* remains controversial. Jeong et al. (2000) have proposed dividing metronidazole resistant *H. pylori* isolates into two groups: type I, in which there is only inactivation of *rdxA* for resistance, and type II, requiring inactivation of both genes. Inactivation of *frxA* by itself was not sufficient to confer resistance. On the other hand, Kwon et al. (2001) showed that metronidazole resistance could occur from inactivation of either *frxA* or *rdxA*. In an additional study, Jeong et al. (2001) showed that *frxA* mRNA and, perhaps, *rdxA* mRNA were more abundant in type II than in type I strains. They confirmed their previous results. Metronidazole-susceptible *H. pylori* isolates which highly express *frxA* genes are uncommon (less than 10% of *H. pylori* metronidazole-susceptible isolates) except in Lithuania, where half of the isolates were of this type.

There is a heterogeneity of resistance to metronidazole which can be explained by *rdxA* mutations. Resistance to metronidazole is due to extensive deletions in the *rdxA* ORF but also to a single amino acid change.

It was shown that two alterations of the RdxA protein, C19Y and T49K, have the same effect on the phenotype of *H. pylori* as RdxA multimutations. The same is true for deletion of the C-terminal 14 amino acids of RdxA. RdxA protein is not produced by the majority (90%) of metronidazole-resistant *H. pylori* strains. Some strains produce RdxA protein which is functionally inactive by having missense mutations resulting in a P51L amino acid substitution or having an additional mutation, Y47H. This nonfunctional protein is subsequently degraded. A mutation within the promoter region of *rdxA* is associated with a metronidazole resistance phenotype.

Although several genes in *H. pylori* were found to be associated with metronidazole resistance, the nature of the exact mechanism of cause and spread of metronidazole-resistant strains remains unclear.

Horizontal gene transfer can occur via conjugation, transduction, or transformation, and most *H. pylori* strains are naturally competent for transformation. The possibility that a natural transformation process could be involved in the mutation of *rdxA*, due to the replacement of a short patch of DNA sequence, 26 to 124 bp, was shown. In one study, 80.2% of *H. pylori* clinical isolates were naturally competent, while the remainder were not competent, and natural competence was associated with high MICs for metronidazole (Table 56).

Part of the resistance to metronidazole may be due not to an alteration of the scavenging of oxygen but to modification of NAD(P)H oxidase activity. NAD(P)H oxidase activity may interact with alkyl chains, reducing them in their alcohol counterparts through an alkyl peroxide reductase. Alkyl peroxide reductase consists of two subunits, AhpC and AhpF. NAD(P)H is used to reduce FAD bound to AhpF, which in turn is used to reduce a disulfide bound in this subunit.

The reduced disulfide reduces a disulfide bound in AphC, which then supplies the reducing power for the conversion of an alkyl compound to its corresponding alcohol.

The oxidase activity exhibited by the enzyme is due to leakage of electrons from the reduced $FADH_2$ cofactor. A number of flavoenzymes, such as thioredoxin reductase and glutathione reductase, with disulfide reductase activity possess NAD(P)H oxidation and dehydrogenation.

AhpC was found in *H. pylori*, and thioredoxin was found instead of AphF. No gene encoding a typical AhpF subunit is present in the full *H. pylori* genome.

This activity is absent in metronidazole-resistant *H. pylori* isolates (Fig. 15).

10.5.2. Other Nitroimidazole Derivatives

Nitroimidazole derivatives are a wide class of synthetic antimicrobial agents, the nitro group being fixed in either position 5, 2, or 4. The in vitro activities of the different analogs against *H. pylori* were assessed using the disk diffusion method. Each disk contained a 0.58 μM concentration of each compound. Data are summarized in Table 57.

10.5.2.1. Gastric Tissue Concentration of Metronidazole

In volunteers receiving intravenous infusion (30 min) of 500 mg of metronidazole either alone or after 7 days of 20 mg of omeprazole per day orally, the level of metronidazole in gastric juice was assayed by a high-performance liquid chromatography method. Results are reported in Table 58. The marked decrease of metronidazole in gastric juice after repeated administration of omeprazole is explained by the elevation of gastric pH induced by omeprazole. For the weak acid salt of metronidazole (metronidazole HCl), a shift occurs in the ratio of nonionized to ionized compound at pHs near its pK, which is 2.0. The proportion of nonionized compound is less than 20% below pH 2.0, while at a pH above 4.0 all of the compound is in the nonionized form (>95%). The ionized form is less soluble in lipids and does not cross the mucosal membrane. At low pH, most of the compound diffuses in gastric juice and is immediately ionized, and then it is no longer available to diffuse back through the gastric membrane into the serum. In contrast, at a higher pH, only a small part is ionized and the nonionized form could shuttle back to the serum, lowering the concentration of metronidazole in the gastric juice. No data are available today on the levels of metronidazole attainable in the gastric mucosa.

Table 56 In vitro activity of metronidazole against competent and noncompetent *H. pylori* strains[a]

Strain	n	MIC (μg/ml)			
		50%	90%	Range	% Resistance (MIC, ≥8 μg/ml)
Naturally competent	65	>32	>32	0.004–>32	61.5
Noncompetent	16	2.0	8.0	0.025–>32	25

[a]Data from Yeh et al., 2002.

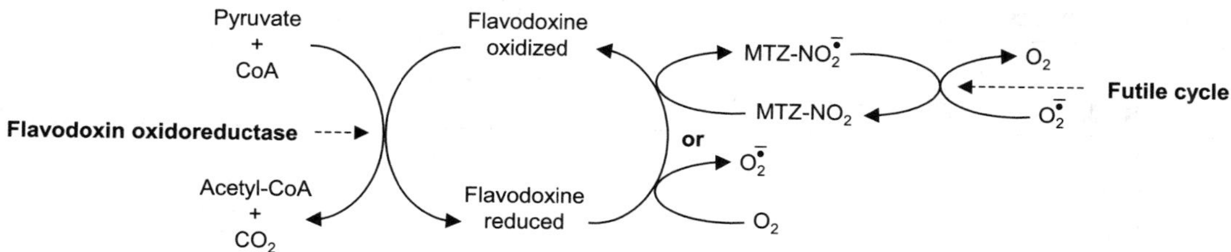

Figure 15 NADH oxidase in metronidazole-resistant *H. pylori*

Table 57 In vitro activities of nitroimidazole analogs against *H. pylori*[a]

Compound	Zone of inhibition (mm)	
	UC744 Res	UC946 Sus
5-Nitroimidazole		
Metronidazole	0	20
Dimetronidazole	0	26
MSD L-595	0	13
MSD L-594	3	11
Flunidazole	7	18
Ipronidazole	0	30
Ornidazole	0	23
Ronidazole	20	30
SC-28905	0	12
SC-29027	4	27
Tinidazole	0	26
2-Nitroimidazole		
Azomycin	7	22
Benznidazole	8	13
Desmethyl misonidazole	22	25
Misonidazole	20	25
4-Nitroimidazole		
4-Imidazole	0	13

[a]Data from Moore et al., 1995.

10.6. Quinolones

10.6.1. Fluoroquinolones

In vitro, ciprofloxacin has relatively low MICs for *H. pylori*. In patients, ciprofloxacin failed to eradicate *H. pylori*. Fluoroquinolones with a 7-piperazinyl ring have shown decreased antibacterial activity at low pH. Ofloxacin and ciprofloxacin combined with the proton pump inhibitor omeprazole resulted in a higher *H. pylori* eradication rate; ciprofloxacin in combination with omeprazole yielded a 76% eradication rate, versus 26% when ciprofloxacin was administered alone.

Using ciprofloxacin alone to treat patients with *H. pylori* infections results in poor clearance of the organism and rapid conversion to ciprofloxacin resistance.

The in vitro activity of fluoroquinolones against *H. pylori* is summarized in Table 59.

10.6.2. Mechanism of Resistance

The *gyrA* gene of *H. pylori* was cloned and sequenced. An ORF of 2,478 nucleotides encodes a polypeptide of 826 amino acids with a molecular mass of 92.51 kDa. The amino acid sequence showed 76.5% identity with the *gyrA* subunit of *Campylobacter jejuni*.

In ciprofloxacin-resistant *H. pylori*, four classes of mutations were shown, with substitutions at amino acid 87 (Asn → Lys), amino acid 88 (Ala → Val), and amino acid 91 (Asp → Gly, → Asn, or → Tyr) and a double mutation at amino acids 91 and 97 (Ala → Val). One isolate did not have alteration within the quinolone resistance determining region.

Regardless of the type of substitution, the MICs of ciprofloxacin for all of the resistant isolates were similar, ranging from 4 to 8 μg/ml.

The synergistic effect of fluoroquinolones, sitafloxacin, and levofloxacin in comparison with amoxicillin or clarithromycin was assessed using the checkerboard method for 17 *H. pylori* strains. A synergistic effect was observed for the combinations of pantoprazole and sitafloxacin, pantoprazole and levofloxacin, omeprazole and levofloxacin, and lansoprazole and sitafloxacin (FIC index, <0.29).

When clarithromycin was combined with proton pump inhibitors, mainly an additive effect was observed (FIC index, 0.54 to 0.89). With amoxicillin, the FIC indices were >1.467.

10.6.3. Fluoroquinolone Concentrations in Gastric Tissue

Westblom and Duriiex (1991) assayed the ciprofloxacin level in gastric tissue of guinea pigs, which is a good model mimicking humans, with a physiological pH of 2.0. The ciprofloxacin concentration was lower than the MIC_{90} for *H. pylori*.

Ciprofloxacin was administered as a single dose of 500 mg in 15 patients undergoing biopsies. Ciprofloxacin levels ranged from 1.5 to 1,762 mg/kg. Optimal concentrations were obtained after 1 h of dosing and reached 500 mg/kg. A residual concentration of 35 mg/kg was detected in one patient at 8 h.

After an intravenous infusion of 200 mg of ciprofloxacin, tissue concentrations were 0.9 and 1.36 mg/kg at 90 and 180 min, respectively, after dosing.

The enoxacin level is nine times higher in gastric tissue than in plasma.

Nineteen patients who underwent gastrectomy received a single oral dose of 400 mg of ofloxacin 2 h before surgery. In the gastric mucosa, the ofloxacin concentration was, on average, 5.0 mg/kg (0.1 to 11.7 mg/kg), with large interindividual variations. Sampling was done between 2 and 8 h.

10.6.4. 7-Bicyclic Derivatives

A series of quinoline and 1,8-naphthyridone derivaties having a 7-bicyclic (Fig. 16) moiety was reported to have anti-*H. pylori* activity, with a MIC of 0.125 μg/ml (Matzke et al., 1998).

10.6.5. 7-Morpholino Quinolone

In the course of optimization of 7-morpholino derivatives, it was shown that Y-26611 (Fig. 17) possessed good anti-*H. pylori* activity. However, the compound has poor oral efficacy in

Table 58 Pharmacokinetics of metronidazole in gastric juice with and without omeprazole

Subject	T_{max} (h)		C_{max} (μg/ml)		$AUC_{0-\infty}$ (μg·h/ml)	
	MTR[a] alone	+Omeprazole	MTR alone	+Omeprazole	MTR alone	+Omeprazole
1	2.0	1.0	107.7	14.6	498.7	69.3
2	3.0	5.0	100.8	17.3	510.8	97
3	1.0	6.0	95	19.7	534.2	122.7
4	3.0	1.0	22.1	8.6	122.7	41.3

[a]MTR, metronidazole.

Table 59 In vitro activities of quinolones against *H. pylori*

Compound	*n*	MIC (μg/ml)		
		50%	90%	Range
Nalidixic acid	30	>128	>128	16–>128
Oxalinic acid	30	4.0	4.0	2.0–4.0
Ciprofloxacin	16	0.25	0.25	0.12–0.25
	30	0.03	0.125	0.008–0.25
	26	0.25	0.5	0.13–1.0
	57	0.25	2.0	0.03–4.0
Ofloxacin	16	1.0	1.0	1.0
	30	1.0	2.0	0.25–2.0
Pefloxacin	16	4.0	4.0	4.0
	30	4.0	4.0	0.5–8.0
Norfloxacin	16	2.0	2.0	1.0–2.0
	30	1.0	2.0	0.5–2.0
Enoxacin	16	8.0	8.0	4.0–8.0
	30	8.0	8.0	1.0–32
Lomefloxacin	16	2.0	2.0	2.0–4.0
Fleroxacin	16	2.0	2.0	2.0–4.0
	30	1.0	2.0	1.0–4.0
Tosufloxacin	16	0.25	0.5	0.25–0.5
Levofloxacin	26	0.25	0.5	0.13–2.0
Moxifloxacin	26	0.25	0.5	0.13–2.0
	57	0.12	2.0	0.06–4.0
Gatifloxacin	21	0.01	0.03	0.004–0.06
Gemifloxacin	26	0.06	0.13	0.03–1.0
Garenoxacin	21	0.004	0.008	≤0.002–0.03
Sitafloxacin	57	≤0.008	≤0.008	≤0.008–0.03
Clinafloxacin	57	≤0.008	≤0.008	≤0.008–0.12
Temafloxacin	16	1.0	1.0	0.5–1.0
	30	1.0	1.0	0.12–4.0
Irloxacin	30	2.0	2.0	1.0–16
Trovafloxacin	21	0.01	0.01	0.004–0.12
CI-934	30	0.06	0.06	0.01–0.5
E-3846	30	0.008	0.008	0.008–0.03
Olamufloxacin	19	0.20	0.13	0.05–3.13
Sparfloxacin	19	0.78	12.5	0.25–25
Difloxacin	16	2.0	2.0	2.0–4.0

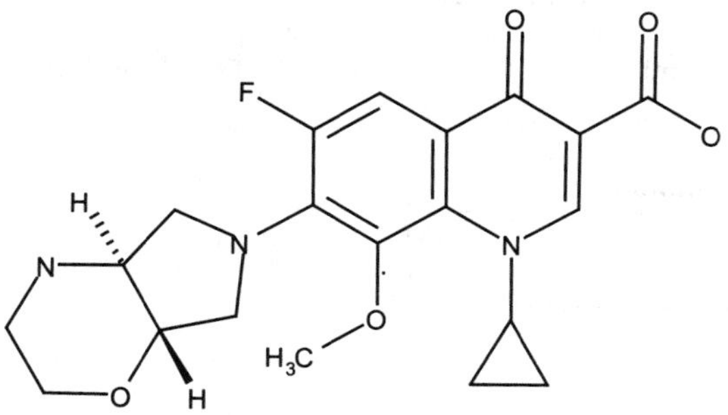

Figure 16 Bicyclic fluoroquinolone with anti-*H. pylori* activity

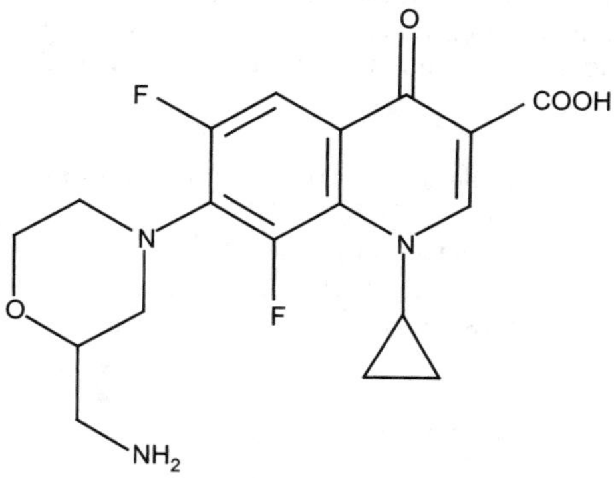

Figure 17 Y-26611

experimentally *H. pylori*-infected Mongolian gerbils (Hirayama et al., 1996).

Another series was set up to optimize the anti-*H. pylori* activity. Modification of the primary amine of Y-26611 with bulky groups decreased anti-*H. pylori* activities (propylamino and acetylamino analogs). Compounds having a dimethyl aminomethyl group exhibited enhanced anti-*H. pylori* activity. The photostability was improved by incorporating an 8-methoxy group instead of 8-fluorine. The (*S*-)-isomer was 30 times more potent than the (*R*-)-isomer. In Mongolian gerbils infected with *H. pylori*, Y-34867 (Fig. 18) exhibited a higher therapeutic efficacy than Y-26611, levofloxacin, tosufloxacin, sparfloxacin, amoxicillin, and clarithromycin (Table 60).

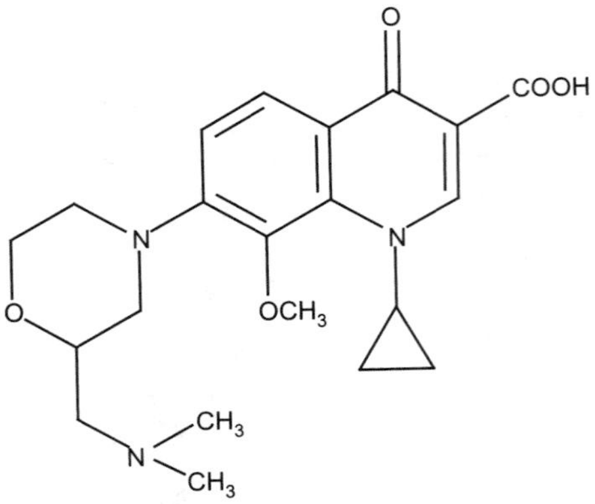

Figure 18 Y-34867

10.6.6. Quinolones Extracted from *Evodia rutaecarpa*

In the quinolone class, a series of natural quinolones isolated from the fermentation broth of *E. rutaecarpa* has been described.

The fruit of *E. rutaecarpa* (Rutaceae), which is a traditional Chinese drug (wu-chu-yu), has long been used in the treatment of abdominal pain, dysentery, amenorrhea, migraine, and nausea. Gosyuyu, which is a crude extract of the fruit of *E. rutaecarpa*, exhibits marked anti-*H. pylori* activity. Purification yielded the active part, which is composed of two components. They are two quinolone derivatives which are characterized by an N-1 methyl and no substituent at position 3 (no methyl group such as in a natural quinolone, or β-carboxylic group for synthetic derivatives) and a C-2 long alkyl chain: a 8-tridecenyl and 7-tridecenyl for compound A (evocarpin) and compound B, respectively, in a ratio of 10:1, which could not be separated from each other.

MICs obtained by agar dilution ranged from 0.02 to 0.05 μg/ml (albumin agar after 3 days under microaerobic conditions), and MICs of 2 μg/ml were recorded for *H. pylori* reference strains NCTC 11916, NCTC 11637, and ATCC 43504. These compounds are poorly active against *C. jejuni*, *V. parahaemolyticus*, *Salmonella enterica* serovar Enteritidis, *E. coli*, and *Pseudomonas aeruginosa* (Hamasaki et al., 2000).

In a clinical trial, the combination of omeprazole, amoxicillin, and gosyuyu (gosyuyu, jujube, ginger, and ginseng) yielded in 31 patients an 87% eradication rate for *H. pylori* (Higuchi et al., 1999).

10.6.7. Anti-*H. pylori* Quinolones from *Pseudonocardia* spp.

In a screening program to discover anti-*H. pylori* compounds from microbial products, a series of quinolones displaying such in vitro activity was discovered. These compounds were obtained from fermentation of *Pseudonocardia* sp. strain CL 38489 (Dekker et al., 1998).

Eight compounds were isolated having a 5-methyl group and a 2-substituted side chain on the pyridine ring. In vitro activities were assessed by the disk (loaded with 0.5 μg of drug substance) inhibition zone. The most potent compound was the epoxy derivative CJ-13564. Modifications of the terpene unit, such as a double bond in place of the epoxide (CJ-13217) and addition to a hydroxy group at C-1′ (CJ-13567) or C-3′ (CJ-13568), reduced the anti-*H. pylori* activity. Quinolones with an *N*-methyl group seem to be more active than those without an *N*-methyl group (CJ-13,136 versus CJ-13565 and CJ-13212 versus CJ-13566).

These compounds did not show any activity against gram-positive bacteria or *Pasteurella haemolytica*. The MIC of CJ-13136 for *H. pylori* is 0.1 μg/ml, and the minimum bactericidal concentraton is 10 μg/ml (Fig. 19).

10.7. Ansamycin

10.7.1. In Vitro Activity

Ansamycins belong to a complex family. One group is composed of antibacterial agents derived from rifamycin SV, such as rifampin, rifabutin, rifapentine, and rifalazil.

The in vitro activities of ansamycin derivatives are listed in Table 61. The in vitro activities of rifalazil and KRM-1657 were shown to not vary significantly when MICs were determined at pH 7.4 and 5.4 for two isolates of *H. pylori* (Table 62) (Akada et al., 1999).

Kill kinetics were determined to assess the potential bactericidal activities of rifalazil, rifampin, and KRM-1657. *H. pylori* HPK5 was the test isolate. The kill kinetics of the three compounds were assessed at the MIC and 10 times the MIC (inoculum size, 3×10^6 CFU/ml); results are shown in Table 63.

Morphological studies revealed that all *H. pylori* cells are lysed after incubation with rifalazil (concentration of 0.04 μg/ml) or KRM-1657 (concentration of 0.001 μg/ml).

Table 60 Anti-*H. pylori* activities of 7-morpholinoquinolones

Compound	Dose (mg/kg)[a]	Clearance (%)[b]	MIC (μg/ml) for *H. pylori* ATCC 43504
Y-26611	10	80	0.05
Y-34867	1	100	0.012
	0.3	0	
Levofloxacin	10	60	0.20
	3	0	
Tosufloxacin	10	0	0.39
Sparfloxacin	10	0	0.20
Amoxicillin	10	100	0.025
	3	0	
Clarithromycin	30	100	0.025
	10	0	

[a]Administered per .5 twice a day for 7 days (n = 5).
[b]Determined 3 days after final administration.

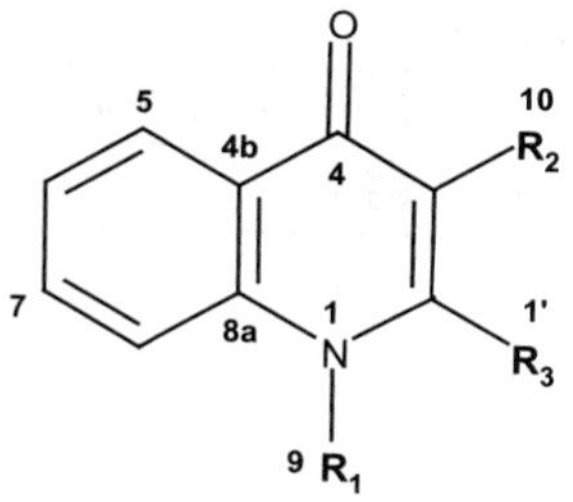

	R_1	R_2	R_3	Inhibition zone (mm) At 0.5 μg/disk
CJ-13,136	H	Me	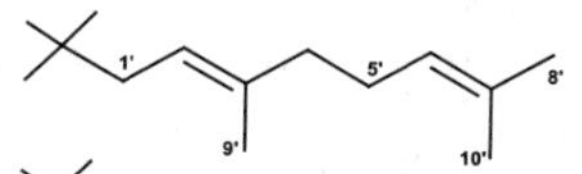	23
CJ-13.217	Me	Me	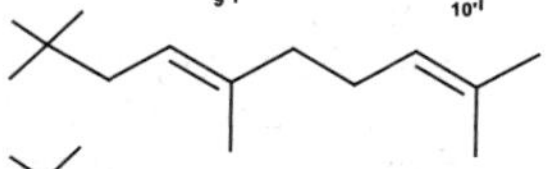	24
CJ-13.536	-CH_2SMe	Me	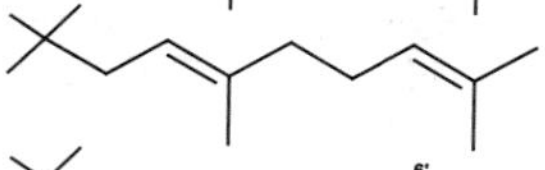	12
CJ-13,564	Me	Me	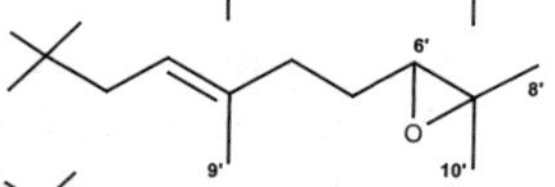	29
CJ-13,565	H	H	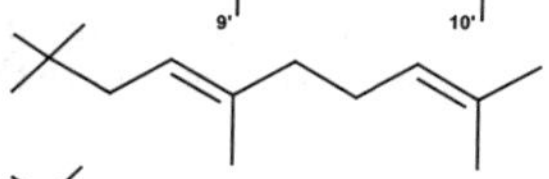	17
CJ-13,566	Me	H	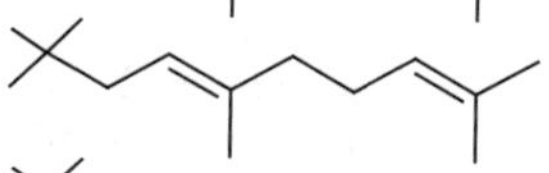	16
CJ-13.567	Me	H	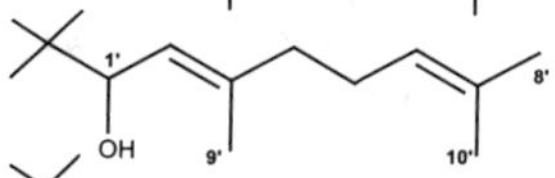	8
CJ-13,568	Me	H	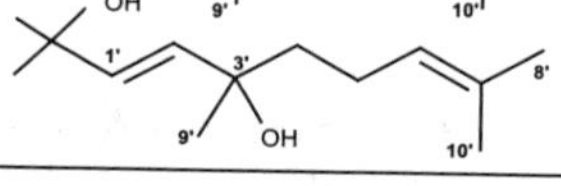	20

Figure 19 Structure and activity of natural quinolones against *H. pylori*

Table 61 In vitro activities of ansamycin derivatives

Compound	*n*	MIC (μg/ml) 50%	90%	Range
Rifampin	81	0.25	1.0	0.03–2.0
	44	1.0	4.0	0.06–8.0
	25	0.12	0.12	0.12–0.75
	10	1.0	1.0	<0.06–1.0
Rifapentine	20	1.0	2.0	1.0–2.0
Rifabutin	81	0.008	0.008	0.004–0.016
Rifalazil	44	0.004	0.008	0.005–0.008
Rifaximin	40	4.0	8.0	4.0–16
KRM-1657	44	0.001	0.002	0.0002–0.002

Table 62 In vitro activities of rifalazil and KRM-1657

Compound	MIC (μg/ml) Strain NCTC 11637 pH 7.4	Strain NCTC 11637 pH 5.4	Strain CPY 3281 pH 7.4	Strain CPY 3281 pH 5.4
Rifalazil	0.004	0.002	0.008	0.004
KRM-1657	0.001	0.001	0.001	0.002
Clarithromycin	0.06	0.5	0.03	0.5

In contrast, amoxicillin contact yields coccoid forms (Akada et al., 1999).

10.7.2. Mechanism of Resistance

The Frequency of occurrence of spontaneous mutations was assessed for six *H. pylori* isolates (Table 64). In serial passages, it was shown that the MICs of rifampin for the resistant mutants ranged from 32 to 64 μg/ml in the agar dilution assay and were higher with the E-test method. While all of the mutants were resistant to rifampin, the MICs of rifabutin ranged from 0.06 to 64 μg/ml, suggesting different mutations.

The target of all rifamycins is the β subunit of the DNA-dependent RNA polymerase encoded by the *rpoB* gene. Resistant mutants of *H. pylori* ATCC 43504 selected in vitro by serial passages in the presence of rifampin showed mutations in codons 525 to 545 or codon 586 (Heep et al., 1999).

rpoB random mutations at codon 149 were generated and induced different levels of resistance, depending on the replacement amino acids (Table 65).

Parts of the *rpoB* gene product deduced from the published *H. pylori* genome sequence exhibit amino acid similarity to homologous resistance-determining regions in *E. coli* and *Mycobacterium tuberculosis*.

The four residues (codons 527, 530, 540, 545) were the most frequent mutations found in serial passages performed (Heep et al., 1999).

Table 63 Bactericidal activities of ansamycins against *H. pylori*

Compound	MIC (μg/ml)	No. of times the MIC	Kill kinetics (log_{10} CFU/ml)	
			3 h	24 h
Rifalazil	0.004	1		
		10		−4.5
KRM-1657	0.001	1	−1	−3
		10		−4.5
Rifampin	0.25	10		−2
Amoxicillin	0.03	1		−1
		10		−1

Table 64 Frequency of mutation induced with ansamycins against *H. pylori*

Compound	Frequency of mutation (range)
Rifampin	1.2×10^{-6}–2.1×10^{-8}
Rifalazil	1.5×10^{-6}–7.1×10^{-8}
KRM-1657	2.3×10^{-7}–7.1×10^{-8}
Amoxicillin	$<7.1 \times 10^{-9}$

Table 65 *H. pylori*: *rpoB* mutations[a]

Mutation at V149	MIC (μg/ml)	
	Rifampin	Rifabutin
Q (glutamine)	32–64	0.5–1.0
H (histidine)	32	0.125–1.0
K (lysine)	16	2.0–8.0
E (glutamate)	32–64	2.0–8.0
D (aspartate)	32	16
F (phenylalanine)	32	16–64
W (tryptophan)	32	64
I (isoleucine)	32	2.0

[a]Data from Heep et al., 2000.

In a German survey, the rates of resistance to rifampin and rifabutin were assessed, and no isolates were considered resistant to both compounds (Heep et al., 2000).

A triple therapy composed of pantoprazole (twice daily), 1 g of amoxicillin (twice a day), and 400 mg of rifabutin (every day) yielded a success rate of 78.6% (Perri et al., 1998).

In patients treated with rifampin, the eradication rate was 23.1% (Fujimura et al., 2000).

A clinical isolate of *H. pylori* developed resistance during therapy and harbored a mutation at codon 149 (V→F) (Heep et al., 2000).

10.8. Other Antibacterial Agents

The in vitro activities of various antibacterial agents against *H. pylori* have been assessed, including linezolid, dalfopristin-quinupristin, mupirocin, aminoglycosides, and fosfomycin.

H. pylori is not susceptible to the polycationic lipopeptide polymyxin B or to antibacterial peptides. *H. pylori* isolates are resistant to trimethoprim and sulfamethoxazole (MIC, >256 μg/ml). In vitro data are summarized in Table 66.

11. MISCELLANEOUS ANTI-*H. PYLORI* AGENTS

11.1. Compounds Containing Rotenoids

Compounds containing rotenoids were claimed to be active against *H. pylori* (Takashima et al., 2002) (Fig. 20). Compounds selectively inhibit *H. pylori* but no other bacterial species. The MIC of compound II for *H. pylori* was 0.08 μg/ml.

Table 66 In vitro activities of various antibacterials against *H. pylori*

Compound(s)	*n*	MIC (μg/ml)		
		50%	90%	Range
Sulfonamides	30	128	128	128
Trimethoprim	30	64	128	64–128
Colistin	30	4.0	128	4.0–128
Clindamycin	24	4.0	16	1.0–>128
	30	2.0	4.0	1.0–8.0
Chloramphenicol	30	4.0	128	0.12–128
Fosfomycin	24	32	64	2.0–64
Linezolid	57	8.0	8.0	4.0–16
Eperezolid	57	4.0	4.0	1.0–4.0
Dalfopristin-quinupristin	57	2.0	4.0	1.0–4.0
Mupirocin	57	0.06	0.25	≤0.008–0.5
Tobramycin	18	0.5	0.5	0.06–0.5
Gentamicin	18	0.125	0.125	0.06–0.125
	70	0.125	0.25	0.06–0.5
Kanamycin	24	8.0	16	0.5–64

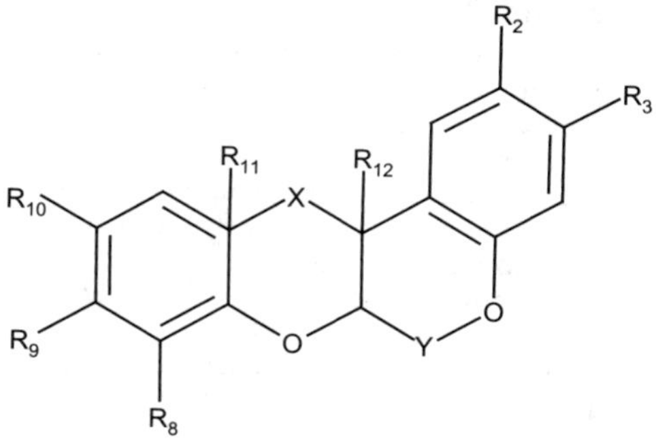

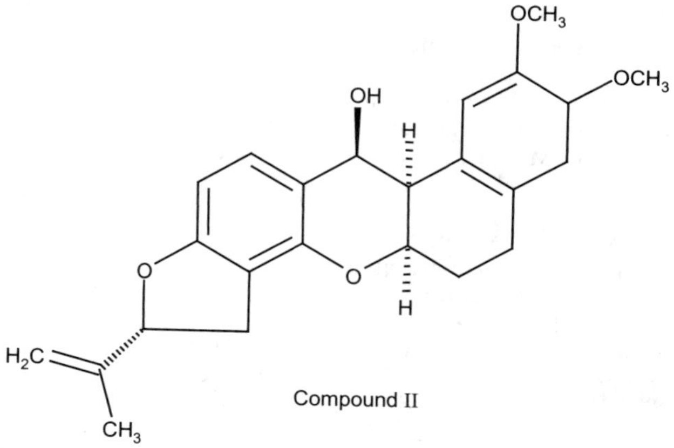

Compound I

Compound II

Figure 20 Rotenoids

11.2. TAK-083

TAK-083 (Fig. 21) was isolated from the fermentation broth of *Streptomyces* sp. strain HC-21. It is an indolmycin derivative. The mechanism of antibacterial activity of indolmycin lies in its ability to inhibit bacterial tryptophanyl-tRNA synthetase. Indolmycins are poorly active against common pathogens and were not developed as antibacterial agents. TAK-083 is highly selective for *H. pylori* (Table 67).

TAK-083 is inactive against gram-negative bacteria (MIC, ≥32 μg/ml), exhibits some activity against *C. jejuni* (MIC, 0.5 μg/ml), and is weakly active against *Staphylococcus aureus* (MIC, 2.0 μg/ml).

The MICs of TAK-08 are not affected by pH variations from 4.5 to 7.5. TAK-083 exhibits for *H. pylori* a concentration-dependent bactericidal activity which occurs at four times the MIC. Selection of mutants did not occur following 10 exposures to TAK-083. TAK-083 selectively inhibits the formation of tryptophanyl-tRNA in *H. pylori* (IC_{50}, 12.2 nM), whereas the corresponding eukaryotic system (bovine liver) was hardly affected (IC_{50}, 4.04 mM).

In Mongolian gerbils given TAK-083, in a dose-dependent fashion, a complete clearance was obtained at a dose of 10 mg/kg (Kanamuru et al., 2001).

Figure 21 TAK-083

11.3. BAS-118

BAS-118 is an *N*-methyl-3[(2-naphthyl) acetylamino] benzamide derivative (Fig. 22) (Ando et al., 2001). It is selectively active against *H. pylori* but not *C. jejuni* (MIC, 0.008 μg/ml). The in vitro activity of BAS-118 is listed in Table 68.

BAS-118 retains activity against *H. pylori* isolates resistant to clarithromycin and metronidazole.

MICs were determined on blood agar base no. 2 (Oxoid) supplemented with 5% horse blood and incubated at 35°C for 72 h under microaerophilic conditions.

No selection of mutants after 10 serial passages has been shown (Kobayashi et al., 2002).

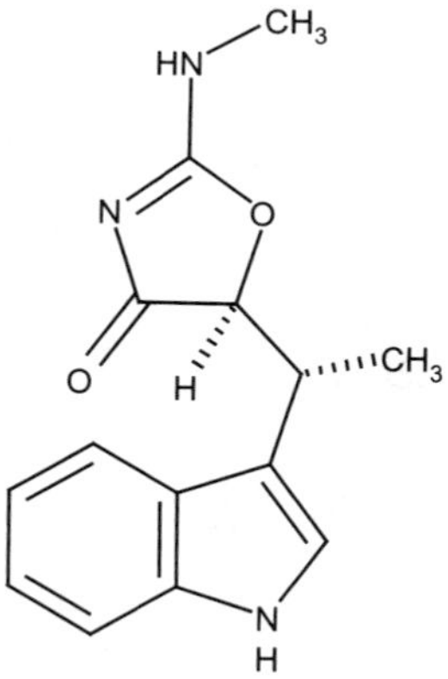

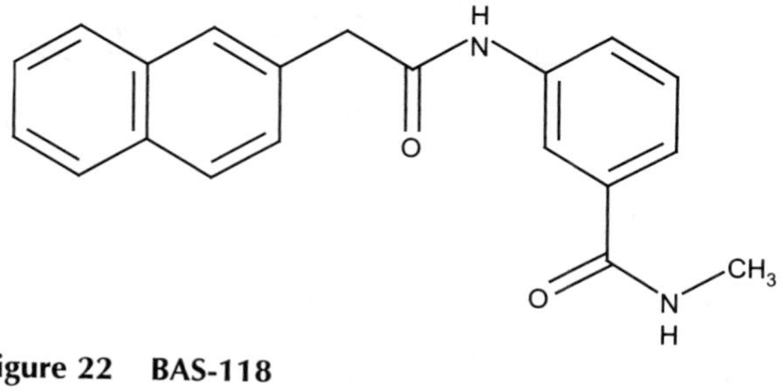

Figure 22 BAS-118

Table 67 In vitro activity of TAK-083 against *H. pylori* (*n* = 54)

Compound	MIC (μg/ml)		
	50%	90%	Range
TAK-083	0.016	0.031	≤0.008–0.031
Amoxicillin	0.031	0.125	≤0.008–0.5
Clarithromycin	0.063	64	0.016–128
Metronidazole	4.0	8.0	2.0–128

Table 68 In vitro activity of BAS-118 against *H. pylori* (*n* = 100)

Compound	MIC (μg/ml)		
	50%	90%	Range
BAS-118	≤0.003	0.013	≤0.003–0.025
Clarithromycin	≤0.025	6.25	≤0.025–25
Amoxicillin	≤0.025	0.06	≤0.025–0.39
Metronidazole	0.78	3.13	0.39–100

11.4. Moenomycin

Moenomycin belongs to the class of phosphoglycolipid antibiotics. Anti-*H. pylori* activity of moenomycin sodium or moenomycin salt was assessed against isolates susceptible or resistant to either clarithromycin or metronidazole. The MIC_{50}s and MIC_{90}s ranged from 1.0 to 4.0 and 4.0 to 16.0 μg/ml, respectively (Aventis data on file, 1997).

11.5. Catechin Derivatives

Recent studies have demonstrated a variety of biological activities for tea catechins, which constitute about 15% of the dry weight of green tea.

The different components of the tea catechins were tested against 108 *H. pylori* isolates and reference *H. pylori* strains. MICs were determined by broth microdilution with an inoculum size of 5×10^4 CFU per well (Mueller-Hinton broth supplemented with 10% heat-inactivated horse serum). Only the (−) epigallocatechin exhibited some in vitro activity with MICs ranging from 1.0 to 64 μg/ml. The in vitro activity of this compound is pH dependent; no antibacterial activity was shown at a pH of ≤5.0. This compound inhibits the urease activity of *H. pylori* and probably damages the membrane lipid bilayer, as was shown for other bacterial species (Ikagai et al., 1993).

In Mongolian gerbils, catechin was able to eradicate *H. pylori* in 10% of the animals tested, but a decrease in the burden in the stomach cell wall was recorded in comparison with the control. The pH dependence of antibacterial activity and the short gastric transit tissue may explain the weak in vivo activity (Fig. 23).

11.6. Pyloricidin Derivatives

Four pyloricidin derivatives (A, B, C, and D) were extracted from the fermentation broth of *Bacillus* sp. strain HC-70. They are composed of (2*S*, 3*R*, 4*R*, 5*S*)-5-amino-2,3,4,6-tetrahydroxyhexanone acid and several amino acids: *L*-valine, *L*-leucine and β-*D*-phenylalanine (Fig. 24).

By total synthesis, it was clearly shown that the β-*D*-phenylalanine part and the stereochemistry of the 5-amino-2,3,4,6-tetrahydroxyhexanone acid moiety are crucial for anti-*H. pylori* activity.

The four natural compounds display good anti-*H. pylori* activity, and no activity against other bacterial species has been detected (Table 69).

Pyloricidin B inhibits protein synthesis in *H. pylori*, with an IC_{50} of 0.42 μM (0.235 μg/ml).

The therapeutic effect has been assessed in Mongolian gerbils challenged with *H. pylori* TN2GF4. In control Mongolian gerbils, gastric *H. pylori* was maintained at a level of about 10^6 CFU. Pyloricidin B, administered orally twice a day for 7 days, decreased the burden of *H. pylori* in the stomach tissue in a dose-dependent manner, and clearance was attained at doses of 10 and 30 mg/kg (Table 70).

11.7. Triazole Antifungal Compounds

It was reported that antifungal azoles might have activity against gram-positive bacteria and anaerobes. It was shown that some triazolyl derivatives may have acceptable in vitro activity (Table 71).

Amphotericin B is inactive against *H. pylori* (MIC, >32 μg/ml).

	R	N strains	MIC (μg/ml) 50	90	Range
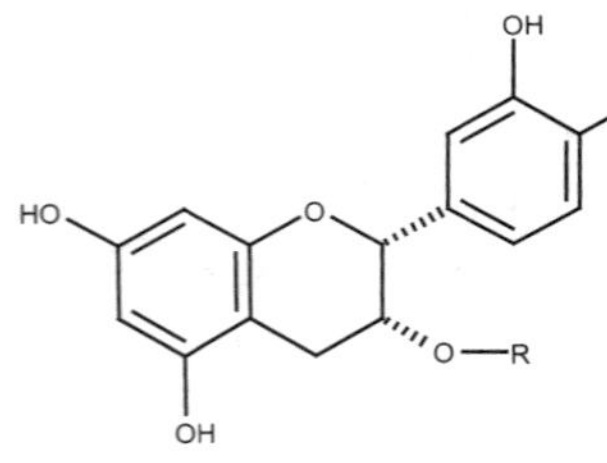	H (-) Epicatechin	55	256	512	16-1024
	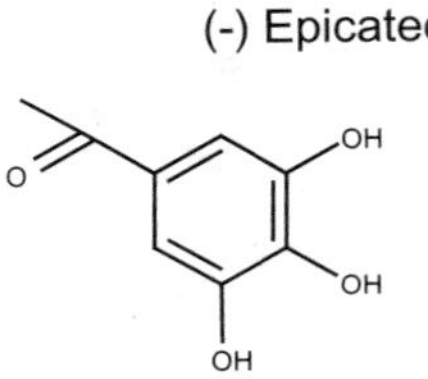 (-) Epicatechin gallate	55	16	32	1.0-256
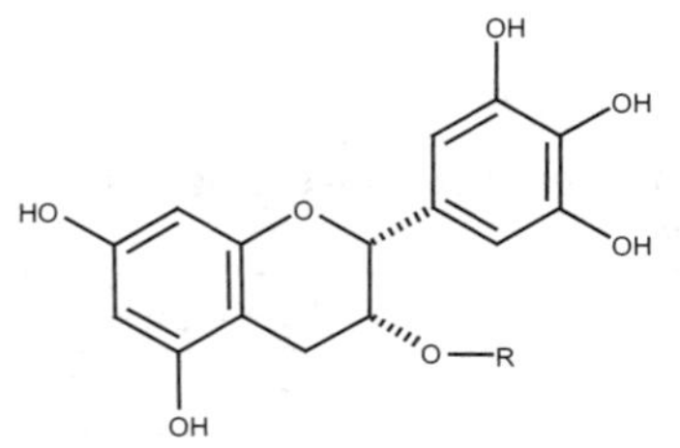	H (-) Epigallocatechin	55	64	128	16-1024
	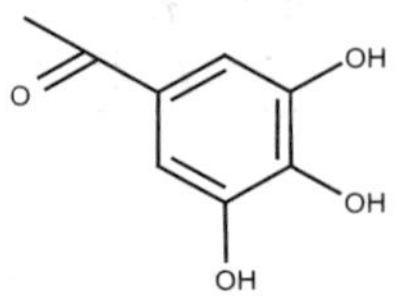 (-) Epigallocatechin gallate	110	8	32	1.0-64

Figure 23 Catechin derivatives

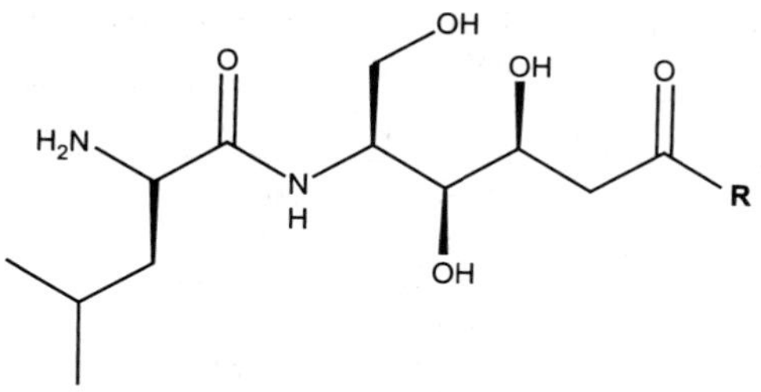

Compound	R	MIC (μg/ml) NCTC 11637	CYP 43	TN 2	TN 58
Pyloricidin	β-D-Phe-OH	0.20	3.13	0.78	1.56
A	Gly-OH	> 6.25	> 6.25	> 6.25	> 6.25
B	β-Ala-OH	> 6.25	> 6.25	> 6.25	> 6.25
C	DL Phe-OH	> 6.25	> 6.25	> 6.25	> 6.25
D	D-Phe-OH	1.56	6.25	6.25	1.56
E	β-D-Phe(4CH_3)OH	6.25	> 6.25	> 6.25	> 6.25
F	β-L-Phe-OH	12.5	> 6.25	> 6.25	> 6.25

Figure 24 Pyloricidin derivatives

Table 69 In vitro activity of pyloricidin B against *H. pylori* (*n* = 50)

Compound	MIC (μg/ml) 50%	90%	Range
Pyloricidin B	0.063	0.25	0.016–0.5
Amoxicillin	0.03	0.125	≤0.008–0.5
Clarithromycin	0.125	64	0.016–128
Metronidazole	4.0	16	2.0–128

11.8. Nitazoxanide

Nitazoxanide is a nitro thiazolamide derivative (Fig. 25). It is a nitrothiazolylsalicylamide derivative with a predictive redox potential of ~360 mV. The active compound in vivo is the main metabolite, the deacetyl derivative tizoxanide. This compound exhibits antianaerobic activity (Dubreuil et al., 1996) and displays antihelmintic activity as well as antiprotozoan activities (cryptosporidia, microsporidia, trichomonads, entamoebae, giardiae). The MICs of nitazoxanide and tizoxanide for 103 strains ranged from 0.25 to 8.0 μg/ml (the MIC_{50} and MIC_{90} were 1.0 and 4.0 μg/ml, respectively). The mode of action of nitazoxanide against *H. pylori* is its efficient activation by a pyruvate oxidoreductase, an essential enzyme of central intermediate metabolism. Nitazoxanide is activated via nitroreductase by three enzymes: pyruvate oxidoreductase (RdxA), oxygen-insensitive NADPH nitroreductase, and FrxA, another oxygen-insensitive flavin NADPH nitroreductase. *H. pylori* metronidazole- and nitrofuran-resistant isolates remain susceptible to nitazoxamide.

Table 70 In vivo activity of pyloricidin B against *H. pylori*

Compound	Dose (mg/kg)	No. showing clearance/total (%)	Log_{10}CFU in gastric wall
Vehicle control	0	0/5 (0)	6.04 ± 0.19
Pyloricidin B	1	2/5 (40)	3.05 ± 0.71
	3	3/5 (60)	1.83 ± 0.29
	10	5/5 (100)	ND[a]
	30	5/5 (100)	ND

[a]ND, not detected.

Table 71 In vitro activities of azole antifungals against *H. pylori*

Compound	*n*	MIC (μg/ml)		
		50%	90%	Range
Itraconazole	57	2.0	2.0	2.0–8.0
Miconazole	61	4.0	4.0	0.5–8.0
Clotrimazole	60	8.0	8.0	0.25–8.0
Ketoconazole	59	16	32	8.0–32
Fluconazole	61	>64	>64	>64

Figure 25 Nitazoxanide

11.9. Nitecapone

Nitecapone, 3-(3,4-dihydroxy-5-benzylidione)-2,4-pentanedione, is a catechol-O-methyltransferase inhibitor known for its gastroprotective effect.

Nitecapone inhibits protease and lipase produced by *H. pylori*. MICs were determined in Brucella agar supplemented with 7% horse blood. Nitecapone activity against 59 *H. pylori* isolates was assessed. The MIC_{50} and MIC_{90} were 64 and 128 μg/ml, respectively (range, 32 to 128 μg/ml). In comparison, for omeprazole in vitro, the MIC_{50} and MIC_{90} were 8 and 128 μg/ml, respectively (MIC ranged from 16 to >128 μg/ml) (Rautelin et al., 1992).

11.10. Inhibitors of Pyrimidine Biosynthesis: Pyrazole Derivatives

In the complete genome of *H. pylori*, metabolic pathways for purine and pyrimidine synthesis and for purine salvage are clearly identifiable. There is an apparent lack of key enzymes of the pyrimidine salvage pathway common to both prokaryotic and eukaryotic organisms (Table 72).

The lack of these enzymes makes *H. pylori* dependent on de novo pyrimidine biosynthesis for both growth and survival.

In an investigation, compounds inhibiting a key enzyme of the de novo pyrimidine biosynthetic pathway, dihydroorotate dehydrogenase (DHODase), were prepared. This enzyme catalyzes the fourth step in de novo pyrimidine biosynthesis: the oxidation of dihydroorotate to orotate (Copeland et al., 1995). DHODase of *H. pylori* belongs to family 2, which includes all known enzymes from gram-negative bacteria and the enzymes from mammalian sources.

All of these enzymes are membrane-associated flavoproteins that utilize an endogenous FMN redox cofactor and exogenous coenzyme Q_6 as an electron acceptor in the FMN oxidative half-reaction of the enzyme. The coenzyme Q binding pocket for the *H. pylori* DHODase displays distinct behavior relative to the mammalian enzyme. The *H. pylori* enzyme donates electrons to coenzymes Q_6 and Q_0. The human enzyme acts only on coenzyme Q_6. Furthermore, the *H. pylori* enzyme donates electrons to naphthoquinone (vitamine K_2) and menadione (vitamine K_3), whereas the human enzyme utilizes these cofactors very poorly.

In a series of pyrazole derivatives, one compound displayed acceptable inhibitory activity against DHODase of

Table 72 Genes of pyrimidine biosynthesis and salvage pathways[a]

Gene(s)	Presence in *H. pylori* genome
De novo synthesis	
pyrAa and *pyrAb*	+
pyrB₁	+
pyrC	+
pyrD	+
pyrE	+
pyrF	+
pyrH	+
pyrG	+
ndK	+
Salvage	
cdd	–
codA	–
codB	+
tdK	–
deoA	–
upp	–
udk	–
udp	–

[a]Data from Copeland et al., 2000.

H. pylori, with MICs from 2 to 8 μg/ml (Copeland et al., 2000) (Fig. 26).

11.11. Sulglicotide

It has been shown that sialoglycopeptide from the duodenal mucosa of swine (molecular mass, 81.0 ± 2 kDa) possesses antiulcer and anti-inflammatory properties in rats. Sulfatation of gastric mucin and polysaccharides enhances the antiulcer properties of sialoglycopeptide. The presence of sulfate groups in polysaccharide molecules gives rise to antipeptic properties.

Sulglicotide is a sulfated glycopeptide derived from pig duodenal mucus obtained by an extensive proteolysis of the glycoprotein, followed by the chemical etherification of its carbohydrate chains with sulfate groups (Psilogenis et al., 1991).

This compound exhibits gastroprotective and antiulcer properties, including the stimulation of bicarbonate secretion, inhibition of peptic erosion of mucus gel, and endogenous prostaglandin generation.

Sulglicotide has the ability to interfere with *H. pylori* mucosal attachment.

Sulglicotide possesses a structural resemblance with endogenous gastric sulfomicins, which are known to interfere with *H. pylori* colonization of the mucosa (Piotrowski et al., 1991).

11.12. Plaunotol

Plaunotol (Fig. 27), which is the most important component of a Thai medicinal plant called plau-noi, has been found to possess a broad antiulcer spectrum (Ogiso et al., 1978; Kobayashi et al., 1982). The in vitro activities of cytoprotective agents are summarized in Table 73.

Plaunotol exhibits in vitro (Table 73) and in vivo activities. Treatment of nude mice infected with *H. pylori* at a dose of 100 mg/kg/day for 9 days resulted in a significant decrease in the number of viable *H. pylori* organisms in the stomach (Koga et al., 1996).

In serial passages, it was shown that the MIC of plaunotol before passage was 10.2 μM and the MIC after five

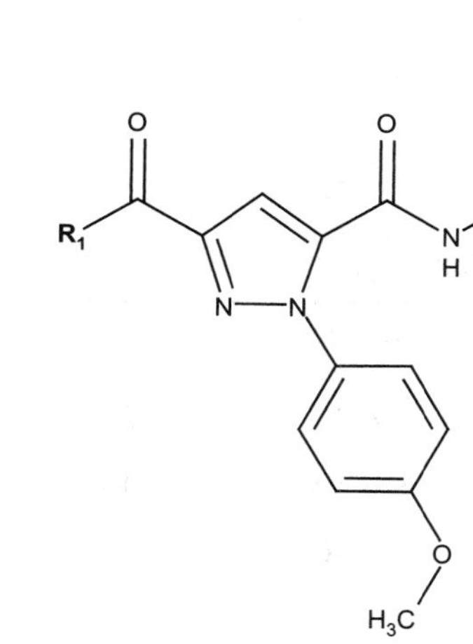

Compound	R_1	R_2	Enzyme inhibition *H. pylori*	human	*E. faecalis*
1	benzyl	N-pyrolidine	26 ± 12	> 10^5	> 10^5
2	benzyl	Phenyl	150 ± 20	> 10^5	> 10^5
3	o-hydroxyphenyl	N-pyrolidine	50 ± 4	> 10^5	> 10^5
4	p-hydroxyphenyl	N-pyrolidine	2.4 ± 10^4	> 10^5	> 10^5

Figure 26 Pyrrazolyl derivatives: inhibition of DHODase of *H. pylori*

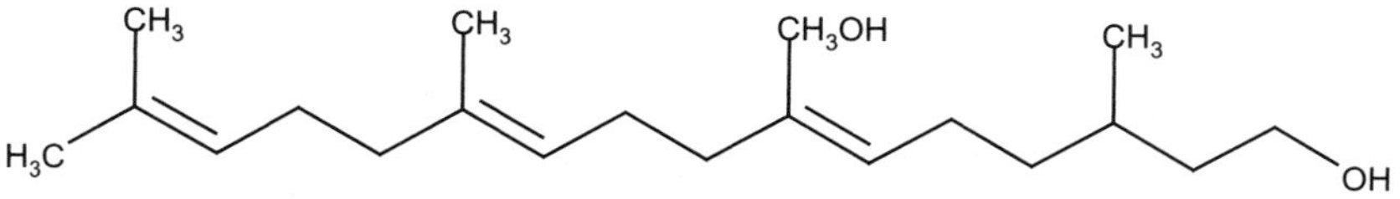

Figure 27 Plautonol

Table 73 Anti-*H. pylori* activities of cytoprotective antiulcer agents ($n = 14$)

Compound	MIC (µg/ml) 50%	90%	Range
Plaunotol	6.25	12.5	6.25–12.5
Benexate hydrochloride	50	50	25–100
Sofalcone	100	100	25–100
Teprenone	100	>100	100–>100
Cetraxate hydrochloride	>100	>100	>100
Gefarnate	>100	>100	>100

passages was 20.4 µM. In contrast, the MIC of metronidazole was 4.6 µM before passage and that after five passages was 58.2 µM. After five passages, a metronidazole-resistant strain remained susceptible to plaunotol (Koga et al., 1998).

No spontaneous resistant mutant was selected at 0.25 times the MIC of plaunotol.

The primary target of plaunotol is the cytoplasmic membrane of *H. pylori*.

Plaunotol has been obtained through a synthetic route. A series of thiourea derivatives has been prepared (Kogen et al., 1999) and displayed anti-*H. pylori* activity.

Thiourea is known to inhibit urease activity. For this reason, several aryl thiourea (1-phenylthiourea) were synthesized. Some of them exhibited potent in vitro activity against *H. pylori* (Fig. 28).

A series of diol derivatives of plaunotol has been synthesized. These analog displayed weak anti-*H. pylori* activity (MIC, 3.13 to 6.25 µg/ml) (Fig. 29).

11.13. Cabreuvin

In a search for a new lead anti-*H. pylori* compound from Brazilian medicinal plants, methanol extracts of 80 species of Brazilian medicinal plants were tested for the ability to inhibit *H. pylori* growth.

One active compound, cabreuvin (Fig. 30), was isolated in the extract of "Oles yermerbo" (trunk wood, *Myroxylon peruiferum*). The bioactive compound was identified as an isoflavone. It was shown that the isoflavone or isoflavan skeleton, as well as the position of the phenolic hydroxy groups and their alkylation, is critical for anti-*H. pylori* activity.

Cabreuvin is inactive against gram-positive and -negative bacteria, as well as against yeasts. MICs are above or equal to 625 µg/ml. The MIC of cabreuvin for *H. pylori* is 7.8 µg/ml (Ohsaki et al., 1999).

11.14. Sucralfate

Sucralfate has local cytoprotective effect for the gastric mucosa, but it is not absorbed into the systemic circulation. It was shown that sucralfate inhibits the hemagglutination, mucolytic, proteolytic, lipolytic, and urease activities of *H. pylori* (Slomiany et al., 1992, 1997). In vivo studies have confirmed that sucralfate reduces the density of *H. pylori* in the stomach. Sucralfate is also reported to enhance the anti-*H. pylori* activities of metronidazole, erythromycin A, tetracycline, and amoxicillin (Slomiany et al., 1995).

Eradication rates for sucralfate-based triple therapies have ranged from 59 to 100%, and the efficacy of sucralfate for *H. pylori* eradication seems to be questionable (Adachi et al., 2000).

Sucralfate is poorly active in vitro with MICs from 400 to 3,200 µg/ml (Table 74).

11.15. Terpene Derivatives

11.15.1. Mastic Gum from *Pistacia lentiscus*

Mastic gum is a natural resin obtained from the stem of *P. lentiscus*, an evergreen tree of the Anacardiaceae family which is cultivated in Mediterranean countries.

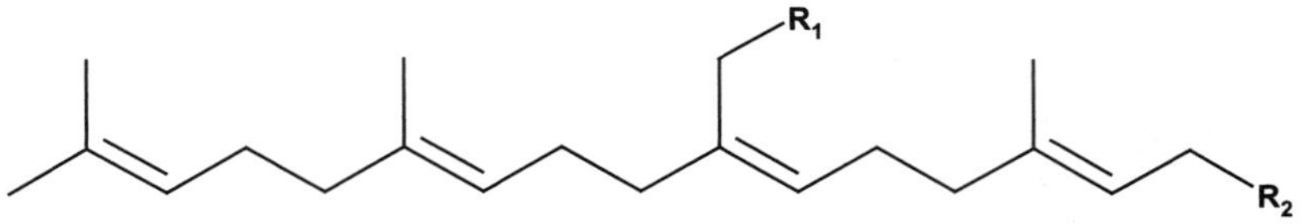

Compound	R_1	R_2	MIC (μg/ml) NCTC 11637	CPY 2052	N° 7
1	OH	OH	12.50	6.25	12.50
2	OH	$NHC(S)NH(CH_2)_2Ph$	≤ 0.10	≤ 0.10	≤ 0.10
3	$NHC(S)NH(CH_2)_2Ph$	OH	25.00	1.56	1.56
4	$NHC(S)NH(CH_2)_2Ph$	$NHC(S)NH(CH_2)_2Ph$	2.25	0.78	6.25
Amoxicillin	-	-	0.02	0.05	0.10

Figure 28 Thiourea analogs of plautonol with *H. pylori* activity

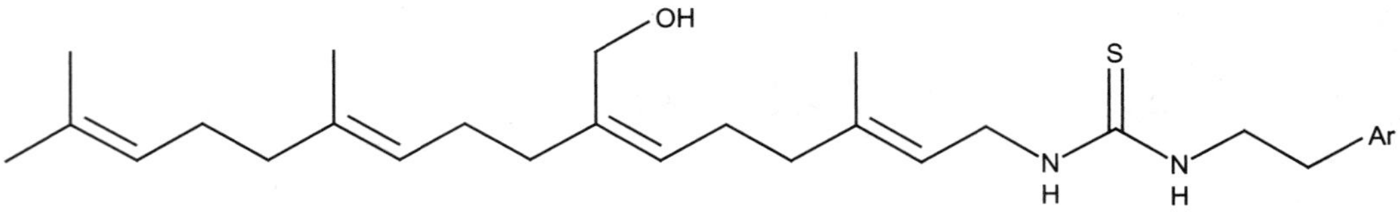

Compound	Ar	MIC (μg/ml) NCTC 11637	CYP 2052	N° 7
2c	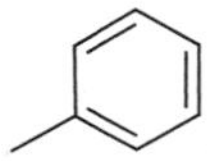 phenyl	≤ 0.10	≤ 0.10	≤ 0.10
2d	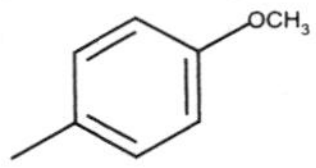 OCH_3	≤ 0.10	0.20	≤ 0.10
2e	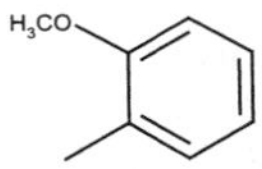 H_3CO	0.78	3.13	1.56
2f	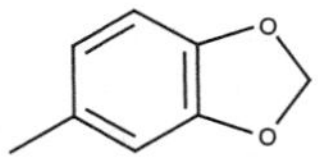 O, O	0.20	0.78	0.39
2g	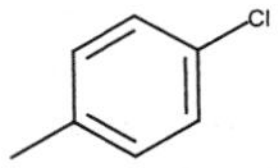 Cl	≤ 0.10	0.39	0.20

Figure 29 Diol plaunotol analogs

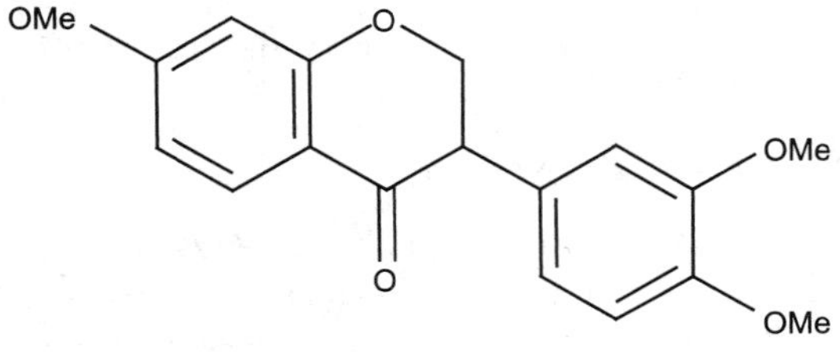

Figure 30 Cabreuvin

Table 74 In vitro activity of sucralfate

Compound	*n*	MIC (μg/ml) 50%	90%	Range
Sucralfate	27	1,600	3,200	400–3,200
Nitrofurantoin	25	0.8	1.6	0.2–5.1
Cimetidine	27	800	3,200	400–3,200

The resin is extracted from incisions made in the tree trunk. It is white-yellow and has a balsamic-like taste and smell. The substance was used in the Hellenistic time for the relief of abdominal discomfort, gastralgia, dyspepsia, and peptic ulcer.

Mastic inhibited 50% of *H. pylori* growth at a concentration of 12 μg/ml and 90% of growth at 500 μg/ml. Mastic induced ulcer ultrastructural changes in the microorganism as demonstrated by transmission electron microscopy.

The structures of 10 triterpenoid acids were tentatively identified on the basis of mass spectroscopy.

11.15.2. Capsaicin

A terpenoid constituent, capsaicin, from chile pepper shows bactericidal activity against *H. pylori*.

11.15.3. Trichorabdal

Trichorabdal A, a terpene from a Japanese herb, can directly inhibit *H. pylori*. Trichorabdal was isolated from *Rabdosia trichocarpa* (Kadota et al., 1997).

11.16. Calvatic Acid

Calvatic acid has a diazene *N*-oxide chemical structure. It is an antibiotic isolated from the culture broth of the gasteromycete *Calvatia lilacina* (Fig. 31). Many of its derivatives exhibit potent antibacterial, antifungal, and antitumor properties.

MICs have to be determined in media without cysteine, which decreases in vitro activity by interacting with the -SH groups. Calvatic acid is a strong acid, with a pK of 3.2.

The core —N(O)=NCH moiety is responsible for the in vitro activity, with a high degree of specificity against *H. pylori*.

Calvatic acid is equally potent against metronidazole-susceptible and resistant *H. pylori* isolates (Table 75).

Preliminary studies of the in vivo activity show that calvatic acid is able to eliminate 67% of *H. felis* organisms in mice at 50 mg/kg three times a day by gavage for 4 days. Metronidazole eliminated 100% at 10 and 50 mg/kg.

Synthetic derivatives of calvatic acid were obtained by combining the latidine-derived pharmacophore group and calvatic acid. These compounds displayed moderate anti-*H. pylori* activity and H_2-antagonism.

11.17. Other Plant Extracts

Many natural plant extracts have been tested against *H. pylori*.

Resveratrol, which is the 3,5,4′-trihydroxystilbene, is a phytoalexin derivative extracted from grape skin, red wine, and other foods. It was tested against 15 clinical isolates of *H. pylori*. The MIC_{50} and MIC_{90} of the red wine extract were 25 and 50 μg/ml, respectively (range, 12.5 to 50 μg/ml). The MIC_{50} and MIC_{90} of resveratrol were 12.5 and 25 μg/ml respectively (range, 6.25 to 25 μg/ml). Amoxicillin MICs ranged from 0.02 to 0.06 μg/ml. In another study, it was found that red wine exhibited bactericidal activity against *H. pylori*.

Various bioactive substances in kiwi fruit extracts were fractionated by organic solvent extractions. All fractions were inactive against *H. pylori*.

A methanol extract of dried garlic bulbs (*Allium sativum*) and alexin (3-hydroxy-5-methoxy-2-pentyl-4H-pyranone), a phenolic phytoalexin, were tested against 15 clinical *H. pylori* isolates. The garlic extract was inactive (MIC, >100 μg/ml). The MIC_{50} and MIC_{90} for alexin were 25 μg/ml (range, 12.5 to 50 μg/ml).

From the Brazilian medicinal plant pariparoba (*Pothomorphe umbellata*), four compounds were identified. One of them, *N*-benzyl mescaline, exhibits anti-*H. pylori* activity.

Protolichestirinic acid from the lichen *Cetraria islandica* was shown to be poorly active against *H. pylori*. The MIC_{50} and MIC_{90} were 32 μg/ml. The reason to investigate the anti-*H. pylori* activity of this compound is the use in Iceland of lichen extracts for the relief of gastric and duodenal ulcers. Authors speculated that the relief of abdominal pains could be due to the in vitro inhibiting activity of protochesterinic acid against 5-lipoxygenase.

One author reported that several patients suffering from ulcer disease experienced unexpectedly dramatic relief of their symptoms after consuming 3-day-old broccoli sprouts. These cruciform sprouts are rich sources of sulforaphane. Sulforaphane was originally isolated for its antibacterial activity from hoary cress (*Cardaria draba*, white top). Sulforaphane (Fig. 32) is [(−)-1-isothiocyanate-(4*R*)-(methylsulfinyl) butane].

Sulforaphane was tested against 48 *H. pylori* isolates. The MICs of sulforaphane ranged from 0.06 to 8.0 μg/ml. This activity was demonstrated irrespective of the susceptibility of the strains to clarithromycin and metronidazole. A bactericidal effect was demonstrated at five times the MIC (MIC of 2.0 μg/ml) at 24 h irrespective of pH (pH 7.4 and 5.8). Sulforaphane is rapidly concentrated in HEp-2, ARPE-19, AGS, and Hepa 1c1c cells. At 30 min, for an extracellular concentration of 5 μM, an intracellular concentration of

HOOC—C_6H_4—N(→O)=N-CN

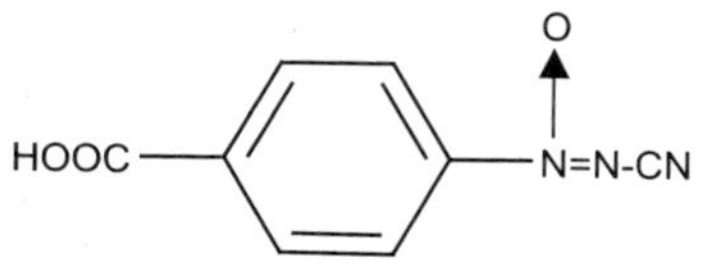

Figure 31 Calvatic acid

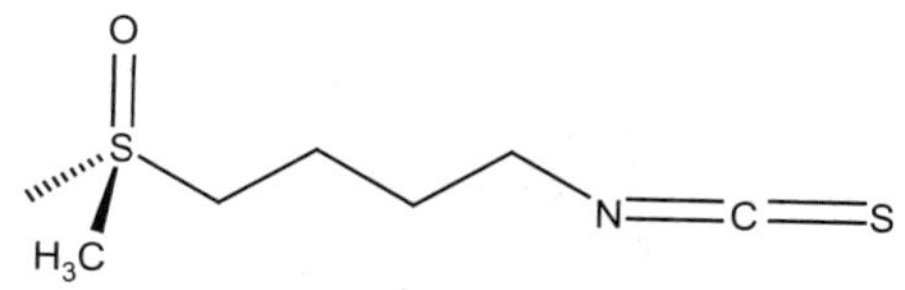

H_3C—S(=O)—$(CH_2)_4$—N=C=S

Figure 32 Sulforaphane

Table 75 In vitro activity of calvatic acid against *H. pylori*

Compound	MIC (μg/ml)			
	All strains		Metronidazole-resistant strains	
	MIC_{50}	MIC_{90}	NCTC 11637	102B
Calvatic acid	0.01	0.03	0.007	0.03
Metronidazole	0.25	8.0	16.0	8.0

500 μM was recorded. It is bactericidal within HEp-2 cells for *H. pylori*.

11.18. Hydroxamic Acid Derivatives

Ureases are ubiquitous in nature and are inhibited by a variety of agents, such as fluorides, thiols, and hydroxamic acids. In a first series of hydroxamic acid analogs substituted with amino acids and dipeptides, it was shown that some compounds diplayed good anti-*H. pylori* activity by significantly inhibiting *H. pylori* urease. A new series of 24 analog was prepared showing good affinity for *H. pylori* urease at the pocket level.

REFERENCES

Adachi K, Ishihara S, Hashimoto T, Hirakawa K, Niigaki M, Takashima T, Kaji T, et al, 2000, Efficacy of sucralfate for Helicobacter pylori eradication triple therapy in comparison with a lansoprazole-based regimen, Aliment Pharmacol Ther, 14, 919–922.

Ahmed A, Smoot D, Liyttleton G, Tackey R, Walters CS, Kashanchi P, Atten CR, Ashktorab H, 2000, Helicobacter pylori inhibits gastric cell cycle programme, Microbes Infect, 2, 1159–1169.

Akada JK, Shirai M, Faji K, Okita K, Nakazawa T, 1999, In vitro anti-*Helicobacter pylori* activities of new rifamycin derivatives, KRM-1648 and KRM-1657, Antimicrob Agents Chemother, 43, 1072–1076.

Andersen LP, Wadström T, 2001, Basic bacteriology and culture, p 27–38, in Mosley HLT, Mencz GL, Hazzell SH, ed, *Helicobacter pylori*: Physiology and Genetics, ASM Press, Washington, D.C.

Ando R, Kawamura M, Chiba N, 2001, 3-(Arylacetylamino)-N-methylbenzamides: a novel class of selective anti-Helicobacter pylori agents, J Med Chem, 44, 4468–4474.

Anglada L, Marquez M, Sacristan A, Ortiz JA, 1988, Inhibitors of gastric acid secretions, N-sulphonyl formamidines in a series of a new histamine H2 receptors antagonists, Eur J Med Chem, 23, 97–100.

Bizzazero G, 1893, Über die Schlauch formeigen Drusen des magen Darmkanals und die bezienhungen ihres Epiteloz zu dem oberflachen Epithel der Schleimhaut, Arch Mikr Anat, 42, 82.

Black JW, Owen DA, Parsons ME, 1997, An analysis of the depressor responses to histamine in the cat and dog: involvement of both H1- and H2-receptors. 1975, Br J Pharmacol, 120 (4 Suppl), 420–425.

Blaser MJ, Berg DE, 2001, Helicobacter pylori, genetic diversity and risk of human disease, J Clin Investig, 107, 767–773.

Bryskier A, Belfiglio S, 1999, Cephalosporins, p 703–748, in Yu VL, Merignan CT Jr, Barrière SL, ed, Oral Antimicrobial Therapy and Vaccines, Williams & Wilkins, Baltimore, Md.

Copeland RA, Davis JP, Dowling RL, Lombardo D, Murphy KB, Patterson TA, 1995, Recombinant human dihydroorotate dehydrogenase: expression, purification, and characterization of a catalytically functional truncated enzyme, Arch Biochem Biophys, 323, 79–86.

Copeland RA, Marcin Keviciene J, Haque TS, Kopcho LM, et al, 2000, Helicobacter pylori-selective antibacterials based on inhibition of pyrimidine biosynthesis, J Biol Chem, 275, 33373–33378.

Covacci A, Telford JL, del Giudice G, Parsonnet J, Rappuoli R, 1999, Helicobacter pylori virulence and genetic geography, Science, 284, 1329–1353.

Cussac V, Ferrero RL, Labigne A, 1992, Expression of Helicobacter pylori urease genes in *Escherichia coli* grown under nitrogen-limiting conditions, J Bacteriol, 174, 2466–2473.

de Bernard M, Arico B, Papini E, Rizzuto R, Grandi G, Rappuoli R, et al, 1997, Helicobacter pylori toxin VacA induces vacuole formation by acting in the cell cytosol, Mol Microbiol, 26, 665–674.

Dekker KA, Inagaki T, Gootz TD, Huang LH, Kojima Y, Kohlbrenner WE, Matsunaga Y, McGuirk PR, Nomura E, Sakakibara T, Sakemi S, Suzuki Y, Yamauchi Y, Kojima N, 1998, New quinolone compounds from Pseudonocardia sp. with selective and potent anti-Helicobacter pylori activity, taxonomy of producing strains, fermentation, isolation, structural elucidation and biological activation, J Antibiot, 51, 145–152.

Dent JC, McNulty CAM, Uff JC, Wilkinson SP, Gear MWL, 1987, Spiral organisms in the gastric antrum, Lancet, ii, 96.

Dore MP, Graham DY, Sepulveda AR, 1998, PBD D, a novel penicillin-binding protein, is involved in amoxicillin-resistant Helicobacter pylori, Gastroenterology, 114–A-109. (Abstract.)

Dore MP, Graham DY, Sepulveda AR, Realdi G, Osato MS, 1999, Sensitivity of amoxicillin-resistant *Helicobacter pylori* to other penicillins, Antimicrob Agents Chemother, 43, 1803–1804.

Dubois A, Berg DE, Incecik ET, Fiala N, Heman-Ackah LM, Del Valle J, Yang M, Winck HP, Perez-Perez GI, Blaser MJ, 1999, Host specificity of Helicobacter pylori strains and host responses in experimentally challenged non-human primates, Gastroenterology, 116, 90–96.

Dubois A, Berg DE, Incecik ET, Fiala N, Heman-Ackah LM, Perez-Perez GI, Blaser MJ, 1996, Transient and persistent experimental infection of nonhuman primates with *Helicobacter pylori*: implications for human disease, Infect Immun, 64, 2885–2891.

Dubreuil L, Houcke I, Mouton Y, Rossignol JF, 1996, In vitro evaluation of nitazoxanide and tizoxanide against anaerobes and aerobic organisms, Antimicrob Agents Chemother, 40, 2266–2270.

Dunn BE, Cohen H, Blaser MJ, 1997, *Helicobacter pylori*, Clin Microbiol Rev, 10, 720–741.

Eaton KA, Radin MJ, Kramer L, Wack R, Sherding R, Krakowka S, Morgan DR, 1991, Gastric spiral bacilli in captive cheetahs, Scand J Gastroenterol Suppl, 181, 38–42.

Enroth H, Engstrand L, 2001, An update on Helicobacter pylori microbiology and infection for the new millennium, Scand J Infect Dis, 33, 163–174.

Ernst PB, Gold BD, 2000, The disease sprectrum of Helicobacter pylori, the immunopathogenesis of gastroduodenal ulcers and gastric cancer, Annu Rev Microbiol, 54, 615–640.

Fellenius E, Berglindh T, Sachs G, Olbe L, Elander B, Sjostrand SE, Wallmark B, 1981, Substituted benzimidazoles inhibit gastric acid secretion by blocking (H+/K+) ATPase, Nature, 290, 159–161.

Fox JG, Batchelder M, Marini R, Yan L, Handt L, Li X, Shames B, Hayward A, Campbell J, Murphy JC, 1995, *Helicobacter pylori*-induced gastritis in the domestic cat, Infect Immun, 63, 2674–2681.

Freedberg AS, Baron LE, 1940, The presence of spirochetes in human gastric mucosa, Am J Dig Dis, 74, 443–445.

Fujimura S, Kawamura T, Asib N, Takahashi H, Watanabe A, 2000, Helicobacter pylori infection rate in patients treated with rifampicin: eradication effect of rifampicin on Helicobacter pylori, Jpn J Antibiot, 48, 839–842.

Ghiara P, Marchetti M, Blaser MJ, Tummuru MKR, Cover TL, Segal ED, et al, 1995, Role of the *Helicobacter pylori* virulence factors vacuolating cytotoxin, CagA, and urease in a mouse model of disease, Infect Immun, 63, 4154–4160.

Goodwin CS, et al, 1989, Transfer of *Campylobacter pylori* and *Campylobacter mustelae* to *Helicobacter* gen. nov. as *Helicobacter pylori* and *Helicobacter mustelae*, respectively, Int J Syst Bacteriol, 39, 397–405.

Gorbach SL, 1990, Bismuth therapy in gastrointestinal diseases, Gastroenterology, 99, 863–875.

Grayson ML, Eliopoulos GM, Ferraro MJ, Moellering RC Jr, 1989, Effect of varying pH on the susceptibility of Campylobacter pylori to antimicrobial agents, Eur J Clin Microbiol Infect Dis, 8, 888–889.

Hamasaki N, Ishi E, Tominaga K, Tezuka Y, Nagaoka T, Kadota S, Kuroki T, Yano I, 2000, Highly selective antibacterial activity of novel alkyl quinolone alkaloids from a Chinese herbal medicine, Gosyuyu (Wu-Chu-Yu), against Helicobacter pylori in vitro, Microbiol Immunol, 44, 9–15.

Hara Y, Antioxidants in tea and their physiological functions, p 49–65, in Hiramatsu M et al, ed, Food and Free Radicals, Plenum Press, New York, N.Y.

Harris PR, Mobley HL, Perez-Perez GL, Blaser MJ, Smith PD, 1996, Helicobacter pylori urease is a potent stimulus of mononuclear phagocyte activation and inflammatory production, Gastroenterology, 111, 419–425.

Heep M, Beck D, Bayerdörffer E, Lehn N, 1999, Rifampin and rifabutin resistance mechanism in *Helicobacter pylori*, Antimicrob Agents Chemother, 43, 1497–1499.

Heep M, Odenbreit S, Beck D, Decker J, Prohaska E, Rieger U, Lehn N, 2000, Mutations at four distinct regions of the *rpoB* gene can reduce the susceptibility of *Helicobacter pylori* to rifamycins, Antimicrob Agents Chemother, 44, 1713–1715.

Higuchi K, Arakawa T, Ando K, Fujiwara Y, Uchida T, Kurochi T, 1999, Eradications of Helicobacter pylori with a Chinese herbal medicine without emergence of resistant colonies, Am J Gastroenterol, 94, 1419–1420.

Hirayama F, Takagi S, Yakoyama Y, Iwao E, Ikeda Y, 1996, Establishment of gastric Helicobacter pylori infection in Mongolian gerbils, J Gastroenterol, 31, suppl 9, 24–28.

Holck S, Ingeholm P, Blom J, Norgaard A, Elsborg L, Adamsen S, Andersen LP, 1997, The histopathology of human gastric mucosa inhibited by Helicobacter heilmannii-leko (Gastrospirillum hominis) organisms including one culturable case, APMIS, 105, 746–756.

Horn J, 2000, The proton pump inhibitors, similarities and differences, Clin Ther, 22, 266–280.

Huang JQ, Sridhar S, Chen Y, Hunt RH, 1998, Meta-analysis of the relationship between Helicobacter pylori seropositivity and gastric cancer, Gastroenterology, 114, 1169–1179.

Ikagai H, Nakae T, Hara Y, Shimamura T, 1993, Bactericidal catechins damage the lipid bilayer, Biochim Biophys Acta, 1147, 132–136.

Ito S, 1967, Anatomic structure of the gastric mucosa, p 705–741, in Code CF, ed, Alimentary Canal, American Physiological Society, Washington, D.C.

Iwahi T, Satoh H, Nakao M, Iwasaki T, Yamazaki T, Kubo K, Tamura T, Imada A, 1991, Lanzoprazole, a novel benzimidazole proton pump inhibitor, and its related compounds have selective activity against *Helicobacter pylori*, Antimicrob Agents Chemother, 35, 490–496.

Kadota S, Basnet P, Ishii E, Tamura T, Namba T, 1997, Antibacterial activity of trichorabdal A from Rabdosia trichocarpa against Helicobacter pylori, Zentralbl Bakteriol, 286, 63–67.

Kajima K, Nakajuma K, Karata H, Tabata K, Utsui Y, 1996, Synthesis of a piperidinomethylthiophene derivative as H2-antagonist with inhibitory activity against Helicobacter pylori, Bioorg Med Chem Lett, 1796–1798.

Kanamuru T, Nakano Y, Toyoda Y, Miyagawa KI, Tada M, Kaisho T, Nakao M, 2001, In vitro and in vivo antibacterial activities of TAK-083, an agent for treatment of *Helicobacter pylori* infection, Antimicrob Agents Chemother, 45, 2455–2459.

Katsura Y, Nishino S, Inoue Y, Sakane K, Matsumoto Y, Morinaga C, Ishikawa H, Takasugi H, 2002, Anti-Helicobacter pylori agents. 5. 2-(substituted guanidino)-4-arylthiazoles and aryloxazole analogues, J Med Chem, 45, 143–150.

Katsura Y, Nishino S, Ohno M, Sakane K, Matsumoto Y, Morinaga C, Ishikawa H, Takasugi H, 1999, Anti-Helicobacter pylori agents. 3. 2-[(Arylalkyl)guanidino]-4-furylthiazoles, J Med Chem, 42, 2920–2926.

Katsura Y, Nishino S, Tomishi T, Sakane K, Matsumoto Y, Ishikawa H, Takasugi H, 1998, Anti-Helicobacter pylori agents. 2. Structure-activity relationship in a new series of 2-alkylguanidino-4-furylthiazoles, Bioorg Med Chem Lett, 8, 1307–1312.

Katsura Y, Tomishi T, Inoue Y, Sakane K, Matsumoto Y, Morinaga C, Ishikawa H, Takasugi H, 2000, Anti-Helicobacter pylori agents. 4. 2-(Substituted guanidino)-4-phenylthiazoles and some structurally rigid derivatives, J Med Chem, 43, 3315–3321.

Kawakami Y, Akahane T, Yamaguchi M, Oana K, Takashi Y, Okimura Y, Okabe T, Gotoh A, Katsuyama T, 2000, In vitro activities of rubeprazole, a novel proton pump inhibitor, and its thioether derivative alone and in combination with other antimicrobial agents against recent clinical isolates of *Helicobacter pylori*, Antimicrob Agents Chemother, 44, 458–461.

Kidd M, Modlin IM, 1998, A century of Helicobacter pylori: paradigms lost, paradigms regained, Digestion, 59, 1–15.

Kobayashi I, Muraoka H, Hasegawa M, Saika T, Nishida M, Kawamura M, Ando R, 2002, In vitro anti-Helicobacter pylori activity of BAS-118, a new benzamide derivative, J Antimicrob Chemother, 50, 129–132.

Kobayashi S, Ishibashi C, Morita A, Masuda H, Ogiso A, 1982, Anti-ulcer activities of (E,Z,E)-7-hydroxymethyl-3,121,15 trimethyl-2,6,10,14-hexadecatetraen-1-01 (CS 684), a new cyclic diterpene alcohol from Thai medicinal plant, on experimental acute gastric and duodenal ulcers, Pharmacometrics, 24, 599–607.

Koga T, Kawada H, Utsui Y, Domon H, Ischii C, Yasuda H, 1996, In-vitro and in-vivo antibacterial activity of plaunotol, a cytopredictive antiulcer agent, against Helicobacter pylori, J Antimicrob Chemother, 37, 919–929.

Koga T, Watanabe H, Kawada H, Takahashi K, Utsui Y, Domon H, Ishii C, Narita T, Yasuda H, 1998, Interactions of plaunotol with bacterial membranes, J Antimicrob Chemother, 42, 133–140.

Kogen H, Tago K, Arai M, Minomi E, Masuda K, Akiyama T, 1999, A highly stereoselective synthesis of plaunotol and its thiourea derivatives as potent antibacterial agents against Helicobacter pylori, Bioorg Med Chem Lett, 9, 1347–1350.

Kriewitz W, 1906, Über das Auftreten von Spirochäten verschiedene form im Magen hinhält bei Carcinoma ventriculi, Dtsch Med Wochenschr, 32, 872.

Lee A, O'Rourke J, Corazon de Ungria M, Robertson B, Daskalopoulos G, Dixon MF, 1997, A standardized mouse model of Helicobacter pylori infection, introducing the Sydney strain, Gastroenterology, 112, 1386–1397.

Loo VG, Sherman P, Matlow AG, 1992, *Helicobacter pylori* infection in a pediatric population: in vitro susceptibilities to omeprazole and eight antimicrobial agents, Antimicrob Agents Chemother, 36, 1133–1135.

The Maastricht Consensus, 1997, Current European concepts in the management of Helicobacter pylori infection, report, Gut, 41, 8–13.

Marchetti M, Arico B, Burroni D, Figura N, Rappuoli R, Ghiara P, 1995, Development of a mouse model of Helicobacter pylori infection that mimics human disease, Science, 267, 1655–1658.

Marshall BJ, Warren JR, 1983, Unidentified curved bacilli on gastric epithelium in active chronic gastritis, Lancet, i, 1273–1275.

Matsumoto SY, Washizuku Y, Matsumoto Y, Tanara S, Ikeda F, Yokota Y, Karita M, 1997, Induction of ulceration and severe gastritis in Mongolian gerbil by Helicobacter pylori infection, J Med Microbiol, 46, 391–397.

Matzke M, Peterson U, Jaetsch T, Bartel S, Schenke T, et al, 1998, Use of 7(2-oxa-5,8 diazabicyclo [430] non 8-91) quinolone and naphthyridonecarboxytic acid derivatives for the treatment of Helicobacter pylori infections and associated gastroduodenal illnesses, patent WO 98-007672-1898.

Mauch F, Bode G, Malferheiner P, 1993, Identification and characterization of an ATPase system of Helicobacter pylori and the effect of proton pump inhibitor, Am J Gastroenterol, 88, 1801–1802.

McGowan CC, Cover TH, Blaser MJ, 1994, The protein pump inhibitor omeprazole inhibits survival of Helicobacter pylori by a urease-independent mechanism, Gastroenterology, 107, 738–743.

Mégraud F, Occhialini A, Rossignol JF, 1998, Nitazoxanide, a potential drug for eradication of *Helicobacter pylori* with no cross-resistance to metronidazole, Antimicrob Agents Chemother, 42, 2836–2840.

Melchers K, Wertzenegger T, Buhmann A, Steinhilber W, Sachs G, Schafer KP, 1996, Cloning and membrane topology of a P-type ATPase from Helicobacter pylori, J Biol Chem, 271, 456–457.

Nagata K, Satoh H, Iwahi T, Shimoyama T, Tamura T, 1993, Potent inhibitory action of the gastric pump inhibitor lansoprazole against urease activity of *Helicobacter pylori*, unique action selective for *H. pylori* cells, Antimicrob Agents Chemother, 37, 769–774.

Nagata K, Sone N, Tamura T, 2001, Inhibitory activities of lansoprazole against respiration in *Helicobacter pylori*, Antimicrob Agents Chemother, 45, 1522–1527.

NIH Consensus Development Panel, 1994, Helicobacter pylori in peptic ulcer disease, JAMA, 272, 65–69.

Noach LA, Roef TM, Tytgat GNJ, 1994, Electron microscopic study of association between Helicobacter pylori and gastric and duodenal mucosa, J Clin Pathol, 47, 699–704.

Ogiso A, Kitazawa E, Karabasyashi M, Sato A, Takahashi S, Nogurhi H, et al, 1978, Isolation and structure of antipeptic ulcer diterpene from Thai medicinal plant, Chem Pharm Bull, 26, 3117–3123.

Ohsaki A, Takashima J, Chiba N, Kawamura M, 1999, Microanalysis of a selective potent anti-Helicobacter pylori compound in a Brazilian medicinal plant, Myroxylon peruiferum, and the activity of analogues, Bioorg Med Chem Lett, 9, 409–412.

On SLW, 2001, Taxonomy of Campylobacter, Arcobacter, Helicobacter and related bacteria, current status, future prospects and immediate concerns, J Appl Microbiol, 90, 1S-15S.

O'Toole PW, Lane MC, Porowollik S, 2000, Helicobacter pylori mobility, Microbes Infect, 2, 1207–1214.

Parsonnet J, Shmuely H, Haggerty T, 1999, Fecal and oral shedding of Helicobacter pylori from healthy infected adults, JAMA, 282, 2240–2245.

Perez-Perez GL, Gower CB, Blaser MJ, 1994, Effects of cations on *Helicobacter pylori* urease activity, release, and stability, Infect Immun, 62, 299–302.

Perri F, Festa V, Andricelli A, 1998, Treatment of antibiotic-resistant Helicobacter pylori infection, N Engl J Med, 339, 53.

Peterson WL, 1997, The role of antisecretory drugs in the treatment of Helicobacter pylori infection, Aliment Pharmacol Ther, 11, Suppl 1, 21–25.

Piotrowski J, Piotrowski E, Slomiany A, Slomiany BL, 1995, Susceptibility of Helicobacter pylori to antimicrobial agents: effect of ebrotidine and ranitidine, J Physiol Pharmacol, 46, 463–469.

Piotrowski J, Slomiany A, Murty VLN, Fekete Z, Slomiany BL, 1991, Inhibition of Helicobacter pylori colonization by sulfated gastric mucin, Biochem Int, 24, 749–756.

Psilogenis M, Alberico P, Bianchi G, Nazzaci M, 1991, Sulglycotide, p 232–244, in Broga PD, ed, Drugs on Gastroenterology, Raven Press, New York.

Rappuoli R, Lange C, Censini S, Covacci A, 1998, Pathogenicity island mediated Helicobacter pylori interaction with the host, Folia Microbiologia, 43, 275–278.

Rautelin H, Renkonen OV, Kosunen TU, 1992, In vitro susceptibility of Helicobacter pylori to nitecapone, Eur J Clin Microbiol Infect Dis, 11, 274–275.

Rautelin H, Vaara M, Renkonen OV, Kosanen TU, Seppäla K, 1992, In vitro activity of antifungal azoles against Helicobacter pylori, Eur J Clin Microbiol Infect Dis, 11, 273–274.

Roine RP, Salmela KS, Hook-Nikanne J, Kosunen TU, Salaspuro M, 1992, Alcohol dehydrogenase mediated acetaldehyde production by Helicobacter pylori—a possible mechanism behind gastric injury, Life Sci, 51, 1333–1337.

Shomer NH, Dangler CA, Whary MT, Fox JG, 1998, Experimental *Helicobacter pylori* infection induces antral gastritis and gastric mucosa-associated lymphoid tissue in guinea pigs, Infect Immun, 66, 2614–2618.

Slomiany BL, Piotrowski J, Majka J, Slomiany A, 1995, Sucralfate affects the susceptibility of Helicobacter pylori to antimicrobial agents, Scand J Gastroenterol, 30 (S210), 82–84.

Slomiany BL, Piotrowski J, Slomiany A, 1992, Effect of sucralfate on the degradation of human gastric mucus by Helicobacter pylori protease and lipases, Am J Gastroenterol, 87, 595–599.

Slomiany BL, Piotrowski J, Slomiany A, 1997, Suppression of Helicobacter pylori urease activity by sucralfate and sulglycotide, Biochem Mol Biol Int, 42, 155–161.

Steer HW, Colin-Jones DG, 1975, Mucosal changes in gastric ulceration and their response to carbenoxolone sodium, Gut, 16, 590–597.

Takashima J, et al, 2002, Derrisin, a new rotenoid from Derris malaccensis, plain and anti-Helicobacter pylori activity of its related constituents, J Nat Prod, 65, 611–613.

Talley N, Full-Young C, Wyatt JMA, Adam S, Lau A, Borody T, Tseng-Shing C, Daskofojoloor C, Cheung K, Talley XIA, 1998, Nizatidine in combination with amoxycillin and clarithromycin in the treatment of Helicobacter pylori infection, Alim Pharmacol Ther, 12, 527–532.

Taylor DN, Blaser JH, 1991, The epidemiology of Helicobacter infection, Epidemiol Rev, 13, 42–59.

Torello J, Castillo JR, Gonzales S, Mariguez P, Merino MN, Jimenez MC, 1998, Liver injury associated with ebrotidine, Methods Finds Exp Clin Pharmacol, 20, Suppl A, abstract 015.

Tsuchiya M, Imamura L, Park J-B, Kobashi K, 1995, Helicobacter pylori urease inhibition by rabeprazole, a proton pump inhibitor, Biol Pharm Bull, 18, 1053–1056.

Van Caekenberghe DL, Breyssens J, 1987, In vitro synergistic activity between bismuth subcitrate and various antimicrobial agents against *Campylobacter pyloridis* (*C. pylori*), Antimicrob Agents Chemother, 31, 1429–1430.

Vandamme P, Falsen E, Rossau R, Hoste B, Segers P, Tytgat R, De Ley J, 1991, Revision of *Campylobacter, Helicobacter*, and *Wolinella* taxonomy: emendation of generic descriptions and proposal of *Arcobacter* gen. nov. Int J Syst Bacteriol, 41, 88–103.

Van Zeneca SJO, Goldie J, Hollingworth J, et al, 1992, Secretion of intravenously administered antibiotics in gastric juice, implication for management of H. pylori, J Clin Pathol, 45, 225–227.

Westblom TU, Duriiex DE, 1991, Enhancement of antibiotic concentrations in gastric mucosa by H2-receptor antagonist: implications for treatment of Helicobacter pylori infections, Dig Dis Sci, 36, 25–28.

Wood AJJ, 1995, The treatment of Helicobacter pylori infection in the management of peptic ulcer disease, N Engl J Med, 333, 984–991.

World Health Organization, 1994, International Agency for Research on Cancer Monographs, 61, 177–220.

Xiang Z, Censini S, Bayeli PF, Telford JL, Figura N, Rappuoli R, Covacci A, 1995, Analysis of expression of CagA and VacA virulence factors in 43 strains of *Helicobacter pylori* reveals that clinical isolates can be divided into two major types and that CagA is not necessary for expression of the vacuolating cytotoxin, Infect Immun, 63, 94–98.

Yokota K, Kurebayashi Y, Takagawa Y, Hayashi S, Isogai H, Isogai E, Imai K, Yabana T, Yachi A, Oguma K, 1991, Colonization of Helicobacter pylori in the gastric mucosa of Mongolian gerbils, Microbiol Immunol, 35, 473–480.

Yoshida Y, Barrett D, Azami H, Morinaga C, Matsumoto S, Matsumoto Y, Takasugi H, 1999, Studies on anti-Helicobacter pylori agents. Part 1. Benzyloxoisoquinoline derivatives, Bioorg Med Chem, 7, 2647–2666.

Yoshiyama H, Nakazawa T, 2000, Unique mechanism of Helicobacter pylori for colonizing the gastric mucus, Microbes Infect, 2, 55–60.

Microbial Efflux of Antibiotics and Inhibitors of Efflux Pumps

ANDRÉ BRYSKIER

41

1. INTRODUCTION

Living microorganisms communicate with the environment in part via solute-specific transport systems. Considered clinically important only for tetracyclines up to a few years ago, antibiotic efflux pumps are now recognized as one of the components of bacterial resistance to many classes of antibacterials.

Active efflux processes have been shown to yield drug resistance in gram-negative bacteria since 1992.

The intrinsic resistance of gram-negative bacteria cannot only be attributed to the low permeability of the outer membrane, including for *Pseudomonas aeruginosa*. Narrow porin channels slow down the penetration of even small hydrophilic solutes, and the low fluidity of the lipopolysaccharide leaflet decreases the rate of transmembrane (TM) diffusion of lipophilic solutes. The equilibrium across the outer membrane is achieved very rapidly partially due to the surface-to-volume ratio being very large in a small bacterial cell.

The periplasmic concentrations of many antibacterials are expected to reach 50% of their external concentrations in 10 to 30 s in *P. aeruginosa* and in a much shorter period in *Escherichia coli*.

Antibiotic efflux could be associated with other mechanisms of resistance, such as methylase (*erm* gene) in *Streptococcus pneumoniae*, *Streptococcus pyogenes*, and other streptococci for 14- and 15-membered-ring macrolides, conferring high levels of resistance to a given antibacterial. Another example of this type of "cooperation" is penicillin efflux pumps and β-lactamases, both of which significantly decrease the cellular concentrations of the β-lactams and the target; penicillin-binding proteins are no longer saturated with penicillin. These types of synergy have been described for *P. aeruginosa*.

2. ROLE OF EFFLUX PUMPS

The early studies of transport in bacteria were focused on how substances, particularly nutrients, get into the cells. In the 1970s, investigations were focused on identifying how certain substances came out of the cells. Initially, those studies of efflux dealt with simple cations (Na^+, K^+, and Ca^{2+}), which are extruded by an energy-dependent process linked to the proton motive force.

Efflux pumps are part of a physiological process that allows the maintenance of homeostasis within the bacterial cell. Transport is the process of uptake and extrusion of drugs, chemicals (dyes), and nutrients from the cell cytoplasm and the environment to maintain a balance between the uptake of essential nutrients and elimination of toxic agents such as dyes, drugs, cationic agents, and metabolites.

Gram-negative bacteria are more resistant to lipophilic and amphiphilic inhibitors than gram-positive bacteria. Such inhibitors include dyes, detergents, free fatty acids, antibacterials, and other chemotherapeutic agents. This property is used in the selective enrichment of gram-negative bacteria (Enterobacteriaceae), for example, with MacConkey agar (containing crystal violet and bile salts), eosin-methylene blue agar (containing dyes), and deoxycholate agar (containing sodium deoxycholate). Efflux pumps remove compounds from the cytoplasm and those dissolved in the lipid phase of the membrane.

A protective function is likely attributable to the MtrCDE system, which provides for resistance to fecal lipids in rectal isolates of *Neisseria gonorrhoeae*. AcrAB, EmrAB (*E. coli*), VcAB (*Vibrio cholerae*), and CmeABC (*Campylobacter jejuni*) efflux pumps greatly contribute to resistance of the organisms to bile, which is an important factor for these organisms to survive in the intestinal tract.

Detergent-like bile salts kill bacterial cells by destroying bacterial multidrug resistance (MDR) efflux systems. These not only play an important role in antibacterial resistance but also contribute to bacterial pathogenesis.

3. POTENTIAL ROLE IN ANTIBACTERIAL RESISTANCE

In the environment, bacteria may be exposed to antibiotic-producing microorganisms during evolution. The ability of some efflux transporters to extrude a variety of chemicals is in favor of adaptability or selection of novel or mutant bacterial efflux pumps. Bacteria have inventive and versatile ways to resist antibacterials and other toxic elements. The earliest characterized mechanisms were those which inactivated the drugs or altered the target in the cell. Decreased permeability or decreased binding was initially the proposed explanation. However, it is known that active efflux is one of the primary mechanisms of resistance by decreasing the concentrations of compounds in the cells.

Direct efflux mediates increases in MIC for a given class of antibacterials (e.g., macrolides, tetracyclines, and fluoroquinolones).

Efflux can result in decreasing the concentration of a given antibacterial at the target site and results in an increase in MIC.

The reduced amount of antibacterial at the target site may allow more frequent mutations. Drug efflux decreases the load on enzyme-mediated detoxification systems, thereby avoiding their saturation, while chemical modifications by the enzyme-based system, which usually increase the amphilicity of compounds, provide drug pumps with better substrates.

4. CLASSIFICATION OF EFFLUX PUMPS

Nearly 200 families of transport proteins have been identified, and about 100 of those have been detected in bacteria.

These systems consist of integral membrane proteins that usually span the cytoplasmic membrane of the cell multiple times as α-helices. These proteins form solute-specific channel or transport pathways. Both gram-positive and -negative bacteria possess a cytoplasmic (inner) membrane, with an additional outer membrane for gram-negative bacteria.

The outer membrane of gram-negative bacteria acts as a permeability barrier and contains several classes of channel proteins (porins, facilitated-diffusion pore proteins, TonB, and other high-affinity proteins). These facilitate the transport of the precursors of energy-producing nutrients. The efflux pump proteins exist in the inner membranes of both gram-negative and -positive bacteria.

Energy coupling proteins, located on the cytoplasmic surface of the membrane, and extracytoplasmic receptors, tethered to or localized to the external surface of the membrane, may be superimposed on the transporters to provide increased pumping capacity and high-affinity solute recognition, respectively.

Efflux pump proteins are an extremely complex class of proteins. Efflux pumps can be classified by the mechanism of antibacterial extrusion, which is either TM protein gradient energy driven or H^+-ATP hydrolysis energized.

Identified transport proteins have been classified according to topology, protein family, substrate specificity, bioenergetics, and distribution of homology in other organisms.

4.1. Proton (H^+) Gradient Energy-Driven Class

The H^+ gradient energy-driven class is composed of at least four families: the major facilitator superfamily (MFS), the resistance nodulation cell division family (RND), the small MDR family (SMR), and the multidrug and toxic compound extrusion family (MATE).

4.2. ATP Hydrolysis Class

The ATP hydrolysis-driven energy class, ATP-binding cassette (ABC) transporters, are functionally related to the eukaryotic MDR P-glycoprotein.

4.3. Bacteria and Efflux Pumps

A single bacterial cell may possess a vast and complex arsenal of efflux pumps, allowing extrusion of a very wide set of antibacterials. The known and putative multidrug efflux systems of bacteria for which extensive genome analysis has been done are summarized in Table 1.

In *E. coli*, 9 of 29 putative efflux pumps have been shown to be involved in MDR. The number of efflux pumps is approximately proportional to the genome size (Table 2).

Comparison with nonpathogenic organisms such as *Bacillus subtilis* revealed that they possess similar number of multidrug efflux proteins relative to the total number of encoded transporters. The fact that pathogenic and nonpathogenic bacteria exhibit comparable numbers of chromosomally encoded MDR efflux systems argues against the tenet that those systems arose recently in pathogens as a result of extensive exposure to anti-infective drugs. They play an important physiological role in the extrusion of naturally occurring toxic substances.

Table 1 Family of transporters in some bacterial species

Transporter	No. of members				
	E. coli	*H. influenzae*	*Mycoplasma genitalium*	*B. subtilis*	*P. aeruginosa*
ABC	2	0	2	1	1
MFS	18	4	0	7	20
SMR	4	1	0	1	6
RND	5	1	0	0	12
MATE			0	0	3
Total	29		2	9	42

Table 2 Numbers of transporters in some bacterial species

Parameter	Value for[a]							
	Ec	Hi	Hp	Nme	Pa	Bsub	Mt	Mge
Potential drug efflux pumps	31	6	8	8	35	28	20	2
Total transporter systems	285	89	53	83	300	239	107	22
Genome size (Mb)	4.6	1.8	1.7	2.3	6.3	4.2	4.4	0.6
No. of efflux systems/100 kb	6.7	3.3	4.8	3.5	5.6	6.7	4.5	3.4
No. of transporter systems/100 kb	6.2	4.9	3.2	3.7	4.8	5.7	2.4	3.8

[a]Ec, *E. coli*; Hi, *H. influenzae*; Hp, *H. pylori*; Nme, *Neisseria meningitidis*; Pa, *P. aeruginosa*; Bsub, *B. subtilis*; Mt, *M. tuberculosis*; Mge, *M. genitalium*.

Expression of those pumps is controlled by regulatory proteins, and their overexpression is controlled by mutations in the regulatory elements, resulting in an MDR phenotype.

4.4. The Four-Letter-Digit Classification

Transporters can be classified on the basis of three main criteria, namely, the energy source, the phylogenetic relationship, and the substrate specificity. A four-letter nomenclature has been proposed in which the first group of digits refers to the mode of transport and energy source, the second and the third refer to the phylogeny (superfamilies and families), and the fourth refers to the substrate (Table 3).

5. MFS FAMILY

5.1. Characteristics of the Families

The MFS transporters belong to a very large family, widespread in archaebacteria and eukaryotes. Multidrug transporters occur mostly in several subfamilies. The MFS family is also known as the uniporter-symporter-antiporter family.

These transporters are composed of 400 amino acids putatively arranged into 12 or 14 membrane-spanning helices, with a large cytoplasmic loop between helices 6 and 7. In effect, the cytoplasmic loop joins the two halves of the transporters, which usually have related sequences, leading to the proposal that this structure arose by gene duplication. A few of those transporters have a putative 14-helix topology, but these transporters usually have a much smaller cytoplasmic loop.

The MFS superfamily of transporters consists of at least 18 families of transporters; some are responsible for import, others are responsible for export, and others are either transporters or antiporters.

Mainly found in the families DHA-1 to -3 and DHA-2 for 12- and 14-TM proteins, respectively, are the efflux MDR pumps.

A number of highly conserved amino acid motifs have been identified within MFS proteins which are likely to be essential for the structure and function of these transporters. These motifs could be ubiquitous or family specific.

Globally, the MFS family can be classified into two subfamilies: the 12-helix transporters, such as *E. coli* TetA, and the 14-helix transporters, such as the class K tetracycline transporter (TetACK) (Table 4).

The 12-helix arrangement varies with the different proteins. For instance, the arrangement of the antiporter NhaA couples Na^+ efflux to H^+ influx of *E. coli*. Six of the helices are arranged into a right-handed bundle, and the remainder are arranged into two layers of four and two helices.

TetA(B) of *E. coli* possesses different arrangements than NhaA. TetA(B) crystallizes as a trimer, whereas NhaA crystallizes as a dimer.

MFS transporters are thought to derive from a common ancestor. Sequence analysis suggests that a simple duplication of a gene encoding a 6-TM segment protein led to the appearance of the 12-TM segment family.

The 14-TM segment family evolved from the insertion of an increasingly hydrophobic central loop of the 12-membrane precursor into the membrane. This family displays a long intracytosolic peptide loop running between the sixth and the seventh TM segments.

Some MFS transporters are closely related to mammalian vesicular monoamine transporters that can handle a wide

Table 3 Four-letter classification of efflux pumps

Superfamily	Family	Pump(s)	Antibacterial(s)[a]
MFS	DHA-1	Tet A, B, E	CHL, NAL, TET
		Tet C	TET
		Tet H	TET
		CmlA	CHL
		Bcr	SUL
		NorA	CHL, FQ, TET
		Blr	CHL, FQ
	DHA-2	EmrB	NAL
		MdfA	TET, AG, CHL, ERY, FQ, RIF
		LfrA	FQ
		Tet K	TET
	DHA-3	MefA	14- and -15-membered-ring macrolides
		MefE	14- and -15-membered-ring macrolides
		Emr	CHL, ERY, TET
		Tet V	TET
		Tap	TET
MATE		NorM	AG, FQ
SMR	2.7.1	EmrE	ERY, SULF, TET
		Mmr	ERY
RND	HAE-1	Acr	β-LACT, CHL, ERY, FUS, NAL, RIF, TET
		Mex	AG, β-LACT inhibitors, β-LACT, CHL
		MtrD	β-LACT, CHL, ERY, FUS, TET
		AmrB	AG, ERY
ABC	Drug E-1	MsrA	ERY
		OleC	OLE
		SrmB	SPI
		TirC	TYL
	Drug E-2	LmrA	

[a]β-LACT, β-lactam; CHL, chloramphenicol; TET, tetracycline; AG, aminoglycosides; FQ, fluoroquinolones; ERY, erythromycin A; OLE, oleandomycin; TYL, tylosin; RIF, rifampin; NAL, nalidixic acid; SUL, sulfonamide; FUS, fusidic acid; SPI, spiramycin.

Table 4 MFS family of efflux pumps

Class	Organism(s)	No. of membrane-spanning domains	Substrate(s)[a]
Blt	*B. subtilis*	12	FQ, HC
Bmr	*B. subtilis*	12	FQ, HC
EmrB	*E. coli*	14	NAL, thiolactomycin
LfrA	*M. smegmatis*	14	FQ, HC
LmrP	*L. lactis*	12	HC, quinine
MdfA	*E. coli*	14	CP, DA, DX, ERY
GmlA	*E. coli*	12	NEO, NOR, PM, RIF, TET
MdrL	*Listeria monocytogenes*	12	CHL, CF
NorA	*S. aureus*	12	CHL, FQ, HC, PM
PmrA	*S. pneumoniae*		FQ
Tap	*M. fortuitum/M. smegmatis*	12	TET
Tet A	*E. coli*	12	TET
Tet K	*E. coli*	14	TET
VceB	*V. cholerae*	14	CHL, DV, ERY, NAL
Tap	*M. tuberculosis*	12	TET
QacA	*S. aureus*	14	EB, QAC, CHL, PI
MefA and MefE	*S. pneumoniae, S. pyogenes, other Streptococcus* spp., *Enterococcus faecium, M. luteus, C. jeikeium*	12	ERY
Ca MDR 1	*C. albicans*		fluconazole

[a]CHL, chloramphenicol; HC, hydrophobic cations; TET, tetracycline; FQ, fluoroquinolone; ERY, erythromycin A; NAL, nalidixic acid; NOR, norfloxacin; NEO, neomycin; DX, doxorubicin; DA, daunomycin; QAC, quaternary ammonium compounds; PM, puromycin; DV, daunorubicin; CP, cetylpyridinium chloride; EB, ethidium bromide; PI, pentamidine isothionate; CF, cefotaxime.

range of catecholamine-type neurotransmitters, such as dopamine, epinephrine, norepinephrine, and serotonin, and to vesicular acetylcholine transporters that can also pump various quaternary amine compounds.

5.2. NorA

NorA is located in the cytoplasmic membrane and is the product of the *norA* gene. The *norA* gene was first isolated from a norfloxacin-resistant clinical isolate by screening of a library of chromosomal DNA in plasmid pBR3222 for an ability to confer resistance on *E. coli* HB101, a norfloxacin-susceptible isolate. The gene encodes a 388-residue protein which exhibits 12 putative TM domains.

NorA is dependent on the proton motive force and is therefore sensitive to protonophores such as 2,4-dinitrophenol and carbonyl cyanide-*m*-chlorophenylhydrazone (CCCP).

Initial studies suggested that NorA is somehow activated by mutation in drug-resistant isolates. In one *Staphylococcus aureus* strain, resistance to fluoroquinolones was attributed to an Asp362→Ala mutation in *norA*. Other resistant isolates were shown to carry NorA promoter mutations that acted to upregulate NorA expression. The *norA* gene was cloned and the nucleotide sequence was determined.

NorA confers resistance to fluoroquinolones and to lipophilic and monocationic compounds such as chloramphenicol, cetrimide, ethidium bromide, benzalkonium chloride, oriflavine, rhodamine, puromycin, and others. In the *S. aureus* genome, it was shown that at least 10 regions encoding polypeptides and having homology with *norA* can be identified.

The structural features of a fluoroquinolone that determine whether it is affected by an efflux system are not fully defined but correlate with hydrophobicity in the NorA pump of *S. aureus*.

NorA appears to have higher affinity for more hydrophilic fluoroquinolones (ciprofloxacin, enoxacin, and norfloxacin) than more hydrophobic compounds (levofloxacin, sparfloxacin, and trovafloxacin).

The risk of acquisition of resistance may be reduced for quinolones that are poor substrates for efflux pumps, since overexpression of such pumps would be unlikely to be effective as a resistance mechanism.

NorA, Bmr, and Blt pump out organic cations in addition to fluoroquinolones. Fluoroquinolones are monocationic when the pH of the cell surface is slightly acidic, although NorA and Bmr pump out uncharged compounds, such as chloramphenicol.

Blt pumps out spermidine (a natural polyamine), and the *blt* gene is part of an operon apparently involved in detoxification of natural polyamines. Verapamil, a calcium channel blocker, was shown to decrease the effect of NorA on fluoroquinolone resistance.

Reserpine and H^+/K^+ ATPase inhibitors (omeprazole and lansoprazole) can significantly reduce MICs, increase killing activity, and prolong the postantibiotic effect of fluoroquinolones (Table 5). Levofloxacin MICs were not affected by omeprazole. The development of levofloxacin resistance did not occur in *S. aureus* 1199 and occurred in only a few colonies of *S. aureus* 1199-3. In contrast, high levels of norfloxacin and ciprofloxacin resistance occurred in both strains of *S. aureus*.

In the *S. aureus* genome there are at least 17 open reading frames (ORFs) encoding putative drug transporters. Some pumps are already encountered in the clinical setting, such as NorA, MsrA and MsrB, Tet(K), and QacA and QacB. A putative protein unrelated to NorA which demonstrated significant homology to AcrA has been identified in the *S. aureus* genome. Growth of *S. aureus* in the presence of salicylate increases intrinsic resistance to the fluoroquinolones, fusidic acid, and tea tree oil (terpene mixture). There is a reduced accumulation of ciprofloxacin. This reduction was not energy dependent, since the addition of the protonophore

Table 5 Activities of omeprazole against resistant staphylococci in combination with fluoroquinolones

S. aureus strain	Drug(s)	MIC (μg/ml)		
		Norfloxacin	Ciprofloxacin	Levofloxacin
1199	FQ[b] alone	0.5	0.25	0.12
	+Omeprazole	0.12	0.12	0.12
1199-3[a]	FQ alone	8.0	4.0	0.5
	+Omeprazole	1.0	0.5	0.12

[a]Expression of NorA was induced with 0.25 the MIC of cetrimide.
[b]FQ, fluoroquinolone.

CCCP and inhibition of ATP transporters (orthovanadate) did not affect the process.

5.3. QacA and QacB

QacA is a protein with 14 TM helices which is encoded by the gene *qacA*, which is plasmid mediated. QacB and QacA have different substrate specificities due to a single amino acid substitution at position 323 with the presence of an acidic residue in QacA (QacA, Asp323; QacB, Ala323). This amino acid is essential for a high level of resistance to diamidines and biguanidines. In QacA, an amino acid with a negative charge at position 34 in TM-1 is essential, as is an arginine at position 114 in TM-4.

Three determinants, the *qacA*, *qacB*, and *qacC* genes, have been identified which confer resistance to organic cations by means of proton motive force-dependent multidrug efflux.

The *qacA* gene confers resistance to a range of structurally disparate organic cations, including monovalent cations, such as ethidium bromide, benzalkonium, and cetrimide, and divalent cations, like chlorhexidine and pentamidine. It is located on plasmids and chromosomes.

The *qacA* gene encodes a 514-amino-acid protein with a molecular mass of 55 kDa. The *qacB* gene confers resistance primarily to monovalent organic cations and, at low levels, to some divalent compounds. It is located on several plasmids, including heavy-metal resistance plasmids, like pSK23. Sequence analysis revealed that *qacA* and *qacB* differ from each other only by seven nucleotides. The phenotypic differences between the proteins are solely due to the carriage of an acid residue: Asp323 in loop 10 in the QacA polypeptide and Ala323 in QacB.

The *qacC* gene, which is identical to the *qacD*, *ebc*, and *smr* genes, confers resistance to quaternary ammonium compounds and ethidium bromide. It is usually located on both conjugative and nonconjugative plasmids (class III) in clinical isolates of staphylococci.

The in vitro activities of antiseptics against *S. aureus* isolates harboring either *qacA*, *qacB*, or *qacC* are summarized in Table 6.

The multidrug efflux protein QacA is able to confer resistance to more than 30 cationic lipophilic antimicrobial compounds that belong to 12 distinct chemical classes. No resistance was observed for trivalent cationic substances or anionic substances.

The resistance specificity of QacA is restricted to monovalent and bivalent cationic substrates.

Expression of both *qacA* and *qacB* is regulated by a divergently encoded transcriptional repressor, QacR, a member of the TetR family of repressors.

The QacR repressor in *S. aureus* is a 23-kDa protein. The gene *qacR* (previously called *orf188*) is located on IR1. IR1 is a large inverted repeat located immediately adjacent to and downstream from the *qacA* and *qacB* promoter. IR1 is unusually large for an operator sequence bound of TetR family regulator, comprising 15-bp half-sites separated by a 6-bp spacer region. QacR is induced by binding mono- and divalent cationic lipophilic compounds. The C-terminal of QacR is involved in the binding of inducing compounds.

Table 6 Qac subfamily of efflux pumps

Compound	MIC (μg/ml)		
	qacA	*qacB*	*qacC*
Biguanidines			
Alexidine	6.0	4.0	4.0
Chlorguanide	250	250	250
Chlorhexidine	12	6.0	1.0
Diamidines			
Amicarbalide	1,200	400	200
Diamidinophenylalanine	250	50	50
Dibromopropamidine	10	1.0	1.0
Diminazene	400	200	200
Hexamidine	300	200	100
Pentamidine	350	200	100
Phenamidine	1,800	200	200
Propamidine	300	100	100
Stilbamidine	400	200	100
Guanylhydrazones			
1i 39/JC-1-134	>2,000	1,600	100
1a 62/JC-1-127	1,600	1,600	500
Methylglyoxal bisguanylhydrazone	1,200	1,200	1,200

In clinical practice, one of the important hygiene measures used to prevent spread of methicillin-resistant *S. aureus* (MRSA) is the decontamination of potentially contaminated rooms, utensils, and colonized patients. It is of concern that *S. aureus* isolates may carry antiseptic resistance genes.

Between 1997 and 1999, in 24 hospitals located in 14 European countries, 297 MRSA and methicillin-susceptible *S. aureus* (MSSA) isolates were collected. It was found that 186 of 297 (63%) MRSA isolates and 24 of 200 (12%) MSSA isolates harbored *qacA* and/or *qacB*. The gene *qacC* was found in 6.4% (19 of 297) and 5% (10 of 200) MRSA and MSSA isolates, respectively.

In Japan, in 1992, Noguchi et al. detected *qacA* and *qacB* in 10 of 71 (14%) and *qacC* in 20 of 71 (28%) MRSA isolates. The three genes have been found concomitantly in five isolates (1%), including one MSSA and four MRSA isolates.

In a follow-up study, it was shown that 42% of MRSA isolates carried *qacA* and *smr*. It was proposed that since *qacA* and *qacB* are very similar, and *smr* is identical to *qacC*, *qacD*, and *ebc*, these genes should be divided into two subclasses, *qacA* and *smr*.

In this study, the authors also demonstrated a chromosomal *norA23* gene from an MRSA strain which exhibits high-level resistance to acriflavine.

The *qacB* determinant was identified on plasmids in *S. aureus* isolates in the early 1950s, whereas *qacA* has only been detected in staphylococcal strains isolated since 1980. The *qacA* determinant may be derived from *qacB* after acquiring a high-affinity binding site for divalent ligands.

5.4. PmrA

An active efflux mechanism of resistance to ciprofloxacin in *S. pneumoniae* was first reported in 1997. *pmrA* encodes a putative efflux pump for fluoroquinolones, which mediates low-level resistance to norfloxacin, ethidium bromide, and acriflavine. PmrA is inhibited by reserpine.

Piddock et al. suggested that the normal efflux pump in wild-type bacteria and overexpression of *pmrA* do not contribute to resistance to fluoroquinolones other than norfloxacin.

In the pneumococcal genome, it is clear that several putative efflux pump genes are present.

5.5. MdfA (Cmr)

The *E. coli* multidrug transporter MdfA possesses a single acidic residue, Glu26, in its putative TM domains, which provides drug selectivity. A single membrane-embedded negative charge is critical for recognition of positively charged compounds by the *E. coli* MDR protein, MdfA. The substitution of Glu26 for a basic residue abolishes transport of positively charged ethidium bromide but not uncharged chloramphenicol. CmlA contains an aspartate as amino acid 26.

MdfA possesses a broad spectrum of drug recognition. MdfA is able to recognize as a substrate basic aromatic and lipophilic compounds and neutral nonaromatic, zwitterionic, and nonaromatic hydrophilic compounds (Table 7).

Extensive sequence alignment showed similarity between MdfA and YjiO (CmlA).

The *mdfA* gene is 1,233 bp and encodes a putative 410-amino-acid protein with a molecular mass of 44,300 Da. It is a 12-TM protein efflux pump.

The YjiO gene, located at 98.3 min on the *E. coli* chromosome, is able to confer drug resistance.

Recently MdfA homologs were identified in *Salmonella enterica* serovar Typhi (90% identity) and *Yersinia pestis* (73% identity). In a secondary-structure model it was predicted that MdfA contains 12-TM proteins with the N and C termini on the cytoplasmic side of the membrane and a single embedded charged residue.

It was shown that the entire C-terminal TM domain and the cytoplasmic C terminus are not essential for MdfA-mediated drug resistance and transport.

Table 7 Resistance of *E. coli* HB101 harboring pT 7-4 (*mdfA*) or pT 7-5

Compound	MIC (μg/ml)	
	pT 7-5	pT 7-4 (*mdfA*)
Ethidium bromide	75	750
TPP	839	2,517
Benzalkonium	50	400
Puromycin	82	217
Tetracycline	2	8
Daunomycin	70	180
Rhodamine CG	70	160
Rifampin	10	80
Chloramphenicol	2	30
Erythromycin A	50	200
Neomycin	0.6	1.5
Kanamycin	1.0	2.0
Ciprofloxacin	0.002	0.007
Norfloxacin	0.03	0.1

5.6. CmlA$_1$

In most of the strains resistant to chloramphenicol the resistance is due to an encoded chloramphenicol acetyltransferase which is plasmid mediated. However, new enzymatic resistance to chloramphenicol has been induced after exposure to subinhibitory concentrations of chloramphenicol.

The first of these chloramphenicol determinants was demonstrated in a multiresistant *P. aeruginosa* isolate on a transposon, Tn*1696*, carried on an IncP plasmid.

cmlA$_1$ encodes a 419-amino-acid polypeptide with 12 helices (molecular mass, 44.2 kDa). Regulation of CmlA$_1$ induction is posttranscriptional with chloramphenicol as an inducer.

The CmlA$_1$ protein is located in the inner membrane and confers resistance to chloramphenicol by proton motive force-driven active efflux of chloramphenicol from *E. coli* cells. Recently, genes encoding proteins that are related to CmlA$_1$ have been identified. Two of those genes are also preceded by a translational attenuator signal. CmlA$_2$ and CmlA$_4$ are 90 and 98% identical, respectively, to CmlA$_1$. A CmlA$_3$ gene (*pp-flo*, *flo-st*, or *flo-SR*) has been found in various bacterial species, and this gene confers resistance to florfenicol and chloramphenicol.

5.7. EmrE

The *emrE* gene (*mvrC*) produces EmrE protein. Overproduction of EmrE protein makes *E. coli* strains slightly more resistant to tetracycline, erythromycin A, and sulfadiazine.

The EmrE pump is a 14-TM protein which extrudes nalidixic acid and thiolactomycin.

5.8. Tet Pumps

Active efflux of tetracycline is a resistance mechanism found in both gram-positive and gram-negative bacteria. The nomenclature of tetracycline resistance determinants has recently been revised (Table 8). The distribution of

Table 8 Tetracycline resistance determinants

Tet determinant or gene	GenBank accession no.
Tet A	X00006
Tet B	J01830
Tet C	J01749
Tet D	X65876
Tet E	L06940
Tet F (?)	Unsequenced
Tet G	S52437
Tet H	U00792
Tet I (?)	Unsequenced
Tet J	AF038993
Tet K	M16217
Tet L (plasmid)	M11036
Tet L (chromosomal)	X08034
Tet P	L20800
Tet V	AF030344
Tet Y	AF070999
Tet Z	AF121000
otrB	AF079900
tcr3 (*tcrC*)	D38215
Tet 30	AF090987

Table 9 Distribution of tetracycline resistance determinants

Organisms or type of protection	One determinant	Two or more determinants
Gram-negative bacteria	*Actinobacillus* Tet B	*Edwardsiella* Tet A, D
	Moraxella Tet B	*Providencia* Tet B, E, I
	Treponema Tet B	*Plesiomonas* Tet A, B, D
	Yersinia Tet B	*Proteus* Tet A, B, C
	Alcaligenes TE	*Enterobacter* Tet B, C, D
	Pasteurella multocida Tet H	*Pseudomonas* Tet A, C, E
		Aeromonas Tet A, B, D, E
		Serratia Tet A, B, C, E
		Citrobacter Tet, A, B, C, D
		Klebsiella Tet A, B, C, D
		Shigella Tet A, B, C, D
		Salmonella Tet A, B, C, D
		E. coli Tet A, B, C, D, E, I
		Vibrio Tet A, B, C, D, E, G
Gram-positive bacteria	*Nocardia* Tet K	*Actinomyces* Tet L (M)
		Bacillus Tet L, K
		Eubacterium Tet K (M, Q)
		Clostridium Tet KLP(M)
		Listeria Tet KL (MS)
		Mycobacterium Tet KL, OtrB (OtrA)
		Staphylococcus Tet KL (M,O)
		Peptostreptococcus Tet KL (MOQ)
		Enterococcus Tet KL (MOS)
Ribosomal protection		*Streptococcus* Tet KL (MOQ)
		Streptomyces Tet KL OtrB (OtrA, OtrC)

tetracycline resistance determinants among bacteria for an efflux mechanism of resistance is summarized in Table 9.

The following genes for tetracycline resistance determinants have been identified: *tetA*, *tetB*, *tetC*, *tetD*, *tetE*, *tetG*, *tetH*, *tetK*, *tetL*, *tet*A(P), and *Otr B*.

All of these genes encode energy-dependent membrane-associated patterns which extrude tetracyclines out of the bacterial cells.

The genes in gram-positive bacteria, *tetK*, *tetL*, and *tetA* (P), and the genes in gram-negative bacteria, *tetA*, *tetC*, *tetD*, *tetE*, *tetG*, and *tetH*, encode efflux proteins which confer resistance to tetracycline but not to minocyline.

The *tetB* gene encodes an efflux protein in gram-negative bacteria which confers resistance to both tetracycline and minocycline.

None of the known efflux genes confer resistance to the glycylcycline compounds.

Each of the efflux genes encodes an approximately 46-kDa protein which possesses either 12 (gram-negative bacteria) or 14 (gram-positive bacteria) hydrophobic TM domains.

Tet proteins exist as multimers in the cell membrane.

The efflux genes in gram-negative bacteria are widely distributed on large conjugative plasmids. These plasmids often carry other antibiotic resistance genes.

Some genes are carried on transposons, such as *tet*A(B) on Tn*10* on the chromosome, the gene activated by the *marRAB* regulatory system.

5.8.1. TetA(B)

The TetA(B) protein (401 amino acids) is encoded by the *tet*A(B) gene on Tn*10* and represents class B of a set of seven related TetA tetracycline efflux pumps from gram-negative bacteria. Tetracyclines are extruded from the bacterial cell as a divalent cation cholate in exchange for a proton.

A low-level endogenous efflux system(s) that pumps tetracycline directly into the medium appears to operate in wild-type cells. Tet protein pumps tetracycline into the periplasm.

5.8.2. TetB

The TetB protein is composed of 12 TMs which are α-helices, the N- and C-terminal (alpha and beta) halves of the protein, with each six TMs joined by a large interdomain cytoplasmic loop. Both domains are required for Tet function. The alpha and beta domains of TetB interact between TM-5 and TM-8 and between TM-2 and TM-11.

Mutations can occur at various sites. Mutation of a residue near the periplasmic side of TM-8 in TetB, such as a replacement of Gly217 with Asp or Asn, resulted in loss of tetracycline resistance. The following mutations are also involved in tetracycline resistance: in TM-5, Gly132 → Asp, Ala136 → Val, and Thr146 → Leu; in TM-8, Ala262 → Thr and Gly254 → Ser; in TM-8 and TM-9 (loop), Glu274 → Lys; in TM-10, Gly320 → Glu or Lys; and in TM-1, Ser340 → Asn.

5.9. VceAB

V. cholerae, a gram-negative bacillus, is responsible for the noninvasive diarrheal disease cholera.

A putative multidrug efflux pump, VceAB, has been described (Colmer et al., 1998). The pump consists of at least two proteins which are encoded by the *vceA* and *vceB* genes.

The gene *vceA* encodes a 42.4-kDa protein which shares homology with the ErmR and ErmK proteins of *E. coli.* and *Haemophilus influenzae*. The gene *vceB* encodes a 55.8-kDa protein which shares homology with the EmrB and EmrV proteins of *E. coli* and EmrH of *H. influenzae*.

VceAB is a 14-TM protein. It is responsible for both *V. cholerae* and *E. coli* with resistance to several toxic compounds, including hydrophobic agents (such as deoxycholate), antibiotics (chloramphenicol and nalidixic acid), and the uncoupler CCCP (Table 10).

VceAB differs from both the AcrAB and EmrAB pumps in the requirement for TolC, an outer membrane protein.

Table 10 AVCE efflux pumps in *V. cholerae*

Compound	MIC (μg/ml)	
	V. cholerae 569B (wild type)	*V. cholerae* 569B (AvceB:Gm)[a]
Deoxycholate	8,800	2,000
CCCP	8.09	0.102
Phenylmercuric acetate	0.168	0.042
Pentachlorophenol	11.3	2.82
Erythromycin A	1.0	0.5
Nalidixic acid	5.0	0.625
Tetracycline	0.5	0.5

[a]Isogenic mutant.

5.10. Mef family

Mef is a membrane protein which is involved in the energy-dependent efflux of 14-and 15-membered-ring macrolides (erythromycin A, clarithromycin, roxithromycin, and azithromycin) out of the cell.

The efflux pump is less efficient on 16-membered-ring macrolides (josamycin, spiramycin, midecamycin, etc.), ketolides (telithromycin and cethromycin), lincosamides, and streptogramin type B.

The 16-membered-ring macrolides are not substrates for Mef. The ketolides are weak inducers of Mef relative to erythromycin A (50-fold versus 500- to 200-fold, respectively). (A variety of gram-positive bacteria carry mobile *mef* genes (Table 11).

MefA and MefE have been shown to be 90% identical, and it was proposed that they be referred to collectively as MefA. However, it has since been demonstrated that the genes for these proteins are genetically different. Both *mefA* and *mefE* are found in *S. pneumoniae*. The gene *mef* was found in *N. gonorrhoeae*.

5.10.1. *mefA*

The *mefA* gene encodes a 44.2-kDa hydrophobic molecule, MefA.

The *mefA* gene of *S. pyogenes* is predicted to encode a protein with 12 membrane-spanning regions which can be divided into two domains, similar to the tetracycline protein motive force transporters found in gram-negative bacteria.

The mefA gene is carried in a genetic element and is related to the Mega macrolide efflux genetic assembly named Tn*1270.1*.

Table 11 Organisms which carry *mefA* or *mefE*

Organism(s)
S. pneumoniae
S. pyogenes
S. agalactiae
Viridans group streptococci
S. milleri
S. mitis
Lancefield group C and G streptococci
M. luteus
C. jeikeium
E. faecium
L. monocytogenes
L. lactis

Tn*1270.1* is a 7,244-bp defective transposon containing *mefA* and four downstream ORFs with homology and position similar to those of the corresponding ORFs of Mega. However, the sequence 5′ of *mefA* in Tn*1270.1* contains three additional ORFs with recombinase and integrase homology.

The insertion site of the *mefA*-containing Tn*1270.1* is a transformation-specific locus of the pneumococcal locus.

In *S. pneumoniae*, Tn*1270.1* was found to be integrated at a specific site in the chromosome, downstream of the A nucleotide at position 1676 of the *cel* gene.

The integration of Tn*1270.1* caused a 1,947-bp deletion in the pneumococcal genome (nucleotides 1393 to 3339) involving the 5′ end of *celB* (nucleotides 2775 to 3339 of contig 4139) and the 5′ end of *orf436* (nucleotides 1393 to 1784 of contig 4139).

orf5, whose coding sequence starts 119 bp downstream of the *mefA* stop codon, was found to be homologous to *msrA* and *vagA*. The last two genes are putative members of the ABC transporter superfamily and mediate resistance by encoding antibiotic-specific efflux pumps.

orf6, *orf7*, and *orf8* are homologs of the pneumococcal conjugative transposon Tn*5252*. *orf8* is truncated, since its gene product is homologous to the C terminus of UmuC, a UV resistance protein encoded by Tn*5252*.

Tn1270.1 should be considered a defective transposon since it terminates with a truncated ORF at the right side. It is of nonconjugative nature.

The *mefA* gene has been demonstrated to be transferred from *S. pyogenes*, *S. pneumoniae*, *Micrococcus luteus*, and *Corynebacterium jeikeium* into their respective species or a common heterologous host (*Enterococcus faecalis* JH2-2). It has been shown in the laboratory that *mefA* is transmissible to a variety of bacterial species, such as *Acinetobacter junii*, *N. gonorrhoeae*, and a variety of gram-negative bacteria recipients.

5.10.2. *mefE*

The macrolide efflux mechanism of resistance for *S. pneumoniae* was described in 1999. A 3.7-kb pneumococcal fragment containing *mefE* was cloned in *E. coli* and was shown to encode a proton motive force-driven transporter sufficient to confer the M-phenotype.

The *mefE* gene encodes a 405-amino-acid hydrophobic protein with 12 TM-spanning regions.

The *mefE* gene was found on the 5′ end of a 5.5- or 5.4-kb insertion, designated the macrolide efflux genetic assembly (Mega), which was found in ≥4 or more distinct sites of the pneumococcal genome.

The 5′ nucleotide sequence of Mega contained a 944-bp segment (33.8% guanine-cytosine content). The 5′ end 180-bp region immediately preceding *mefE* in Mega was identical to the same sequence preceding *mefA* in Tn*1270.1* and included a putative promoter region.

The ORF, which demonstrated above 99% sequence homology to *mefE*, started at position 1125 of Mega. The sequence immediately 3′ of *mefE* contained a 1,464-bp ORF with the same orientation and was designated *mel* (for the 1-letter symbol of the first 3 amino acids). The predicted protein of the ORF showed 36.2% amino acid identity to erythromycin A resistance ATP binding MsrA of *Staphylococcus epidermidis*.

There is a 119-bp intergenic region between *mefE* and *mel*. This region contains a consensus Shine-Dalgarno sequence upstream from the predicted start codon for *mel*. *mefE* and *mel* are cotranscribed.

The 944- and 150-bp 5′ and 3′ termini including the *lexA* binding sequence are unique to Mega.

The first ORFs form an operon which contains *mefE* and *mel*.

The three other ORFs (3 to 5) of Mega share homology with ORFs 11 to 13 of Tn*5252*. The function of these ORFs is unknown, but recent evidence suggests that ORF 13 of Tn*5252* is involved in the SOS response in *S. pneumoniae*. The other potential regulatory components of Mega, a *lexA* binding domain in ORF 5 and *cin* box with *mefE*, suggest that this element might be regulated by competitive and SOS response events.

The amino acid sequence homologous between ORFs 5, 4, and 3 of Mega is related to conjugative transposons, which insert by a nonduplicative site-specific recombination mechanism.

ORF 13 of Tn*5252* and ORF 5 of Mega have homology to *umu* C. In Tn*5252*, ORF 13 is followed by ORF 14, a *umuD* homolog. The UmuC and UmuD homologs of Tn*5252* restore error-prone repair in *S. pneumoniae*, and the expression of the Tn*5252 umuCD* gene is regulated by the RecA and LexA proteins.

Although a UmuD homolog is absent in Mega, ORF 5, the Mega UmuC homolog, has a consensus LexA binding sequence.

In addition to ORFs 3 to 5, the complement of the strand containing *mefE* contains a TACGAATA sequence. It was postulated that this sequence is part of a core promoter consensus recognized by an alternative sigma factors critical for the expression of competitively induced elements. This sequence, referred to as a *cin* box, is found in nine putative competitive loci of the pneumococcal genome.

Mega may be influenced by the induction of competence and the SOS network.

Mega appears to have entered the pneumococcal genome on ≥4 occasions by site-specific recombination events but has expanded rapidly in the pneumococcal population by selection of Mega-containing clones and has spread horizontally by transformation.

5.10.3. Induction of *mef* Genes

No evidence that *mefE* is a normally silent resident in *S. pneumoniae* or *Enterococcus* spp. has been obtained, as PCR with *mef*-specific primers did not yield a PCR product for macrolide-susceptible strains of pneumococci or enterococci.

Induction of *mefE* by erythromycin A was confirmed by Northern blotting using an internal *mefE*-specific probe. After 45 min, two bands, one at 1,100 bp and one at 2,300 bp, were expressed in an inducible manner. The smaller band has a size that corresponds to the coding sequence of the MefE protein (Table 12).

In a transcription-translation experiment with wild-type pneumococcal ribosomes, both cethromycin (ABT-773, a ketolide) and erythromycin A at 1 μM efficiently inhibited protein synthesis.

In methylated ribosomes, erythromycin A lost most of its inhibitory activity, while cethromycin was able to completely block translation at a higher concentration.

In the *mef*-containing *S. pneumoniae* strains, there is a competition between the ribosome and the Mef binding sites for the intracellular compound, although the efflux pump might also intercept the compound within the membrane.

Cethromycin, which possesses tight ribosome binding kinetics, may not bind as tightly to the efflux pump, resulting in a net influx site which exceeds the capacity of the pump.

Table 12 Inducibility of *mef(A)* by MLS_B antibiotics and ketolides in *S. pneumoniae*

Compound	MIC (μg/ml)		
	Strain R6	R6 *mefE* (Ind^-)[a]	R6 *mefE* (Ind^+)[a]
Erythromycin A	0.02	12.5	12.5
Clarithromycin	0.006	12.5	12.5
Azithromycin	0.05	25	25
Spiramycin	0.10	0.10	0.10
Tylosin	0.20	0.20	0.39
Josamycin	0.05	0.02	0.02
Telithromycin	0.002	0.10	0.20
HMR 3004	0.0004	0.02	0.5
Streptogramin B	3.12	1.56	1.56
Clindamycin	0.02	0.02	0.02

[a]Growth in the presence (+) or in absence (−) of 0.05 μg of erythromycin A per ml as an inducer.

Inactivation of the Mef pump with CCCP resulted in a 2.6-fold increase in initial erythromycin A uptake but little or no change in the initial uptake of cethromycin in *S. pneumoniae* 5649 (*mef*-containing strain).

5.10.4. Other *mef* Genes

The *mef214* gene was described as part of plasmid pk 214 from an MDR *Lactobacillus lactis* strain, k 214, used in cheese manufactured by lactic fermentation. The Mef214 protein is about 36% identical at the amino acid level to MefA. The *mefA* gene does not confer macrolide resistance on *L. lactis* k 214 but does confer it on *E. coli*.

6. SMR FAMILY

6.1. General Characteristics

SMR transporters are smaller than MFS transporters and are composed of about 100 amino acids putatively arranged into four helices.

There is no known TM linker or outer membrane channel associated with transporters of this family.

SMR transporters have been found so far only in bacteria.

The putative mechanism of drug transport, as established by site-directed mutagenesis of an SMR transporter, could involve the following steps:

- Exchange between the compound and a proton fixed on a charged residue
- Translocation of the compound by a series of conformational changes driving it through a hydrophobic pathway
- Replacement of the compound by a proton in the external medium and return to the initial conformational state

The overall results of the transport are therefore an exchange between the drug and a proton (antiport).

Table 13 lists members of the SMR family.

It seems that SMR transporters exist in the membrane as homo-oligomers and are soluble in organic solvents.

The genome of *B. subtilis* reveals that it can encode six SMR homologs. The six *B. subtilis* homologs and two *E. coli* homologs were encoded from gene pairs in four distinct operons (Table 14).

Ten members of the SMR family, which is well conserved, have been sequenced to date, and all are from bacteria.

Table 13 SMR family

Protein	Organism	Antibacterial(s) extruded[a]
EmrE (= Mvrc, Ebr)	*E. coli*	Erythromycin A Sulfadiazine
Mmr	*M. tuberculosis* *Mycobacterium simiae* *Mycobacterium gordonae* *Mycobacterium marinum* *Mycobacterium bovis*	Tetracycline Erythromycin A TPP, cationic dyes
Smr/Qac	*S. aureus*	EB, CP, QA, TPP
EbrAB	*E. coli*	EB, AC, PY, SO, TPP
YkkCD	*B. subtilis*	CHL, PS, STR, TET

[a]CHL, chloramphenicol; STR, streptomycin; TET, tetracycline; EB, ethidium bromide; QA, quaternary amine compounds; AC, acriflavin; PS, phosphonomycin.

Table 14 SMR family: gene pairs

Organism	Pair
B. subtilis	*ebrA-ebrB* *yvdR-yvdS* *ykkC-ykkD*
E. coli	*b1599-b1600*

Table 15 Structure of SMR pair proteins

Protein	Organism	No. of amino acids
YkkC	*B. subtilis*	112
YkkD	*B. subtilis*	105
EbrA	*B. subtilis*	105
EbrB	*B. subtilis*	117
YvdR	*B. subtilis*	106
YvdS	*B. subtilis*	114
YvaE	*B. subtilis*	119
Ebr	*E. coli*	115
SugE	*E. coli*	105
b1599	*E. coli*	109
b1600	*E. coli*	121
EmrE	*E. coli*	110

The SMR family consists of two phylogenetic subfamilies: subfamily 1, which confers MDR and catalyzes drug efflux via a drug: H^+ antiport mechanism, and subfamily 2, for, which no drug resistance has been reported.

One member of each *B. subtilis* protein pair is shorter (Table 15). This difference proved to be due to a partially conserved C-terminal hydrophilic extension present in the latter protein.

6.2. EmrE

EmrE, a multidrug transporter from *E. coli*, functions as an oligomer (probably a trimer), suggesting that the functional complex is comparable in tertiary structure to the MFS transporters. This fact was demonstrated with tetraphenyl phosphonium ion (TPP^+). One mole of TPP^+ is bound with a K_d of 10 nM to 3 mol of EmrE.

Binding of TPP^+ is pH dependent, as was demonstrated in a mutant strain, in which the only embedded charged residue, Glu14, was substituted for Asp14. Binding occurred at a pK of <5.0 instead of 7.5, but in mutants no or little export activity was demonstrated.

It was also shown that each monomer might have different structures in the functional unit.

EmrE from *E. coli* catalyzes efflux of erythromycin A in addition to lipophilic monovalent cations and tetracycline.

Table 16 In vitro activities of *ykkC-ykkD*

Compound	MIC (μg/ml)		
	ykkC	*ykkD*	*ykkC-ykkD*
Cationic dyes			
Ethidium bromide	50	50	2,000
Proflavine	20	20	500
Tetraphenyl arsonium bromide	200	200	2,000
Crystal violet	2	2	50
Pyronine Y	5	5	500
Methyl viologen	50	50	1,000
Cetrimide	50	50	500
Neutral antibacterials			
Chloramphenicol	2	2	10
Streptomycin	2	2	100
Tetracycline	0.5	0.5	2
Anionic antibacterial			
Phosphonomycin	0.1	0.1	10

6.3. YkkCD

Expression of paired genes is required to confer resistance to a range of cationic dyes, such as ethidium bromide. This fact was demonstrated for both *ebrA* and *ebrB* in *E. coli*.

This suggests that the two protein subunits of Ykk and Ebr transporters interact with each other to produce an asymmetric dimeric functional complex.

When both the *ykkC* and *ykkD* genes were expressed in *E. coli* strain HH5α, a broad-spectrum multidrug resistance (MDR) phenotype was observed for cationic dyes and neutral and anionic antibacterials (Table 16).

6.4. *mmr*

The gene *mmr* has been cloned and sequenced in *Mycobacterium tuberculosis*. It exhibits 43% identity to EmrE and confers resistance to erythromycin A in a heterologous host, *Mycobacterium smegmatis*.

7. MATE FAMILY

7.1. General Characteristics

MATE (multidrug and toxic compounds extrusion family) is a family which contains at least 30 proteins, including proteins representative of eukaryotes, archaea, and eubacteria. They are Na^+-driven efflux pumps.

Two proteins, NorM and YdhE, are representative of MDR efflux pumps. These proteins do not share any significant sequence similarity with any member of the MFS family.

There is significant amino acid sequence similarity between NorM and other members of the family.

The proteins in this family range in size from 363 to 1,141 amino acid residues. These proteins possess 12 TM segments, and highly conserved regions are located in the vicinity of TM-5 and TM-6 and near the terminus of TM-8. Phylogenetic analysis of this family revealed the presence of three distinct clusters (Brown et al., 1999).

Table 17 Activities of aminoglycosides and erythomycin A on *B. pseudomallei*

Compound	MIC (μg/ml) for mutant strain:				
	1026b	RM101	RM102	+pRM105	D 503
Gentamicin	256	2	2	96	0.75
Kanamycin	16	<1	<1	24	ND
Neomycin	32	<4	<4	ND[a]	<4
Spectinomycin	>1,064	64	64	ND	64
Streptomycin	1,064	16	16	512	>1,024
Tobramycin	48	0.75	1.5	16	0.75
Clarithromycin	>256	12	16	192	8
Erythromycin	>256	8	16	>256	8
Clindamycin	>256	>256	>256	ND	>256

[a]ND, not determined.

The first cluster includes the bacterial multidrug efflux proteins NorM and YdhE, as well as proteins from *Haemophilus* (HmrM) (Xu et al., 2003), *Bacillus*, and *Synechocystis*.

The constituents of the second cluster are exclusively eukaryotic proteins from either fungi or plants. One member of the cluster is the yeast Erc1 protein, which confers resistance to the methionine analog ethionine.

The third cluster includes the DinF protein of *E. coli* and *S. pneumoniae*. The function of DinF is not known, but expression on both organisms has been demonstrated to be DNA damage inducible. It may be a stress-induced efflux protein. A CdeA protein has been described for *Clostridium difficile*.

7.2. NorM Protein

7.2.1. *Vibrio parahaemolyticus*

V. parahaemolyticus, a halophilic murine bacterium, is one of the major causes of food poisoning in Japan.

V. parahaemolyticus possesses an energy-dependent efflux system for norfloxacin. The NorM gene was sequenced and encodes a 12-TM protein of 456 amino acid residues, with a molecular mass of 42,422 Da. This protein is very rich in hydrophobic residues, showing that the protein is a membrane protein. This protein induces resistance to ciprofloxacin, ethidium bromide, kanamycin, and streptomycin in addition to norfloxacin.

7.2.2. *Burkholderia pseudomallei*

B. pseudomallei is the causative agent of melioidosis and is intrinsically resistant to a wide range of antibacterials. The efflux RND pump AmrAB-OprA is specific for both aminoglycosides and macrolides (Table 17).

7.3. Other Proteins

Other proteins in this family yielding MDR resistance have been described, such as YdhE. YdhE was found in *E. coli* (457 amino acids) and *H. influenzae* (HmrH, 464 amino acids). Cells of *E. coli* transformed with the cloned *ydhC* gene exhibited resistance to norfloxacin, ciprofloxacin, acriflavine, and TPP^+, but not to ethidium bromide (Table 18).

Kanamycin, minocycline, and tetracycline activities are not modified in *E. coli* harboring *ydhE*.

In *B. subtilis*, the protein YojI had an amino acid sequence that was similar to that of NorM (35% identity and 77% similarity).

BexA of *Bacteroides thetaiotaomicron* is responsible for fluoroquinolone resistance.

VcrM is a 445-amino-acid protein encoded by the *vcrM* gene of *Vibrio cholerae* non-O1 (Huda et al., 2003). PmpM is an H^+-drug antiporter of the MATE family harbored by *Pseudomonas aeruginosa* (He et al., 2004). VcmA is harbored by *Vibrio cholerae* non-O1 (Huda et al., 2001) and encoded by the chromosomal gene *vcmA*. This protein has 12 hydrophobic domains; in comparison with YdhE it has an additional amino acid at position 414 (Gln). VmrA, a 447-amino-acid polypeptide with a calculated molecular mass of 49 kDa, belongs to cluster 3 (DinF subfamily) and was isolated in *Vibrio parahaemolyticus*. In a tigecycline-resistant strain of *Staphylococcus aureus*, an efflux pump of the MATE family was isolated (MepA) (McAleese et al., 2005). CdeA is an efflux pump isolated in a strain of *Clostridium difficile* (Dridi et al., 2004).

Table 18 In vitro activities of antibacterials against *E. coli ydhE*

Compound	MIC (μg/ml)	
	Wild type	*ydhE*
Chloramphenicol	0.39	0.78
Norfloxacin	0.025	0.20
Enoxacin	0.05	0.39
Trimethoprim	3.13	12.5
Fosfomycin	1.56	3.13
Ethidium bromide	12.5	25
TPP	6.25	200
Benzalkonium	3.13	6.25
Deoxycholate	1,250	40,000

7.4. NorM I Protein

Four bacterial members, NorM and VmrA of *V. parahaemolyticus*, YdhE of *E. coli*, and BexA of *Bacteroides thetaiotaomicron*, have been reported to mediate MDR. NorM and VmrA were also reported to function by a drug:Na^+ antiport mechanism.

Among the eukaryotic members, the two only functionally characterized proteins are yeast Erc1, which confers resistance to the methionine analog ethionine, and *Arabidopsis* Alf5, conferring resistance to toxins.

Two putative efflux pumps belonging to the MATE family are encoded by the genome of *Brucella melitensis*.

The first, NorMI, is encoded by the gene BME 11585 and was identified as a potential virulence factor.

The second was named NorMII and is encoded by the gene BME 11612.

These proteins share 27.7 and 19.9% identical amino acids, respectively, with NorM protein of *V. parahaemolyticus*.

NorMI possesses 12 TM helices.

NorMII, like YdhE, confers resistance to norfloxacin, ciprofloxacin, acriflavine, berberine, and TPP^+.

NorMI confers resistance to kanamycin and streptomycin.

8. RND FAMILY

8.1. General Characteristics

The RND family contains multidrug efflux transporters of a unique type found in gram-negative bacteria. All members of the RND family are involved in secretion or excretion of multiple ligands, antibacterials, and toxic metal ions. RND transporters are larger than MFS transporters, being composed of approximately 1,000 amino acid residues.

The RND family evolved as a mean of self-defense for bacteria. An RND pump was shown in a plant pathogen, *Agrobacterium tumefaciens*, and its induction by a plant defense compound, isoflavonoid, suggests its involvement in the survival of the bacterium in its normal habitat.

RND transporters are a three-component system. This system bypasses the periplasmic space and provides efflux across both the inner membrane and the outer membrane. Such systems require three partners: an inner membrane transporter, a periplasmic membrane fusion protein (MFP), and an outer membrane channel. These pumps utilize the energy of the proton motive force to extract dyes, detergents, disinfectants, solvents, and antibiotics from the cell.

MFP has two α-helical domains which form a coiled-coil and are flanked by regions of β-structures, each of which contains a motif that resembles the lipoyl domain of enzymes involved in the transfer of a covalently attached lipoyl or biotinyl moiety between proteins. The functional role of MFP is not well understood. It was suggested that MFP (i) forms a channel between the inner and outer membranes or (ii) acts to pull inner and outer membranes together, allowing direct ligand and transfer between the inner and the outer membrane translocases. (iii) Homologous proteins have been found in gram-positive bacteria, but their function is unknown. The inner membrane transporter and the MFP are invariably encoded by the same operon.

This unusual putative topology is characteristic of this family. At the amino-terminal end of each protein, the polypeptide chain traverses the cytoplasmic membrane (inner) once from the cytoplasm to the periplasm, and this spanner is followed by a large water-soluble domain located in the periplasmic or extracytoplasmic space. The polypeptide chain then spans the membrane into the periplasmic space six more times before it again emerges into the periplasm as another water-soluble domain of the same size as the first one. The carboxy-terminal end of the permease is again embedded in the membrane with five additional spanners.

Each permease has 12 putative spanners as well as two large extracytoplasmic domains.

Phylogenetic analysis of the members of the RND family revealed that these proteins fall into three clusters: cluster 1 is specific for divalent and heavy metal ions, cluster 2 is specific for lipooligosaccharides, and cluster 3 is a single putative three-component transporter, NolFGH, which catalyzes efflux of multiple drugs.

The current drug resistance members of the RND family probably arose from a single primordial drug resistance protein as noted for the ABC-2, MFS, and SMR families. The different proteins involved in MDR are summarized in Table 19.

Homologies of the RND-MFP-type MDR systems with and without linked outer membrane genes are identifiable in the genomes of many bacteria. The genomes have been sequenced for many bacteria, such as *Rickettsia prowazekii*, *Helicobacter pylori* (the *hef*ABC operon has been identified), *Cyanobacterium*, *Synechocystis*, and *Rhodobacter capsulatus*. Unfinished genome sequences and numerous homologous genes have been found in *Salmonella enterica* serovar Typhimurium (four genes), *Bordetella pertussis* (four), *Y. pestis* (four), *C. jejuni* (one), and *V. cholerae* (one).

For each efflux pump, the substrate (antibacterial) may vary (Table 20).

8.2. *P. aeruginosa*

In *P. aeruginosa*, each of the RND pump-containing efflux operons occurs with a specific regulatory gene, but small molecules that regulate the expression of these systems are unknown.

Table 19 Proteins of RND efflux family

Microorganism	Efflux component			Regulatory gene	Expression		Substrates
	MFP	RND	OEP		Wild	Mutant	
B. cepacia	CeoA	CeoB	OpcM	*unk*	–	+	Antibiotics
E. coli	AcrA	AcrB	TolC	*ArR1*, *marA*, *robA*, *soxS*	+	*marR*++ *acrR*++	Antibiotics
	AcrE (EnvC)	AcrF (EnvD)	?	*acrS*	–	+	Antibiotics
H. influenzae	AcrA	AcrB	?	+		+	Antibiotics
N. gonorrhoeae	MtrC	MtrD	MtrE	*mtrR*	+	+	Antibiotics
P. aeruginosa	MexA	MexB	OprM	*mexR*	+	*nalB*+++ *nalC*+++	Antibiotics
	MexC	MexD	OrpJ	*nfxB*	–	++	Antibiotics
	MexE	MexF	OprN	*mexT*	–	*nfxC*++	Antibiotics
	MexX (AmrA)	MexY (AmrB)	OprM	*mexZ* (*amrR*)	+	+	Antibiotics
Salomenella serovar Typhimurium	AcrA	AcrB	?	?	+	+	Antibiotics
S. maltophilia	SmeA	SmeB	SmeC	*smeRS*	?		Antibiotics
E. aerogenes	AcrA	AcrB	TolC				
B. pseudomallei	AmrA	AmrB	OprA	*amrAB*, *oprA*			Antibiotics
Acinetobacter	AdeA	AdeB	AdeC	*adeABC*	+	+	Antibiotics

Table 20 Antibacterial substrates for RND proteins

Microorganism	Efflux pump	Antibiotic substrates
B. cepacia	CeoAB-OpcM	Chloramphenicol, trimethoprim, fluoroquinolones
E. coli	AcrAB-TolC	β-Lactams, novobiocin, erythromycin A, fusidic acid, tetracycline, chloramphenicol, fluoroquinolones, nalidixic acid, aminoglycosides
H. influenzae	AcrAB-TolC	Erythromycin A, rifampin, novobiocin
N. gonorrhoeae	MtrCDE	β-Lactams, chloramphenicol, erythromycin A, fusidic acid, rifamycin, tetracycline
B. pseudomallei	AmrAB-OprA	Erythromycin A, aminoglycosides
P. aeruginosa	MexAB-OprM	β-Lactams, novobiocin, erythromycin A, fusidic acid, tetracyclines, chloramphenicol, fluoroquinolones, β-lactamase inhibitors
	MexCD-OprJ	Chloramphenicol, fluoroquinolones, tetracycline, quaternary ammonium cephems, β-lactams, novobiocin
	MexXY	Aminoglycosides, erythromycin A, tetracyclines, fluoroquinolones
	MexEF-OprN	Chloramphenicol, fluoroquinolones, trimethoprim
	MexGHI-OrmD	Acetylated homoserine lactone?
	MexJK	Tetracyclines, erythromycin A
	EzrAB	Cadmium, zinc
S. enterica serovar Typhimurium	AcrAB-TolC	Chloramphenicol, fluoroquinolones, aminoglycosides, cyclines, β-lactams
S. maltophilia	SmeABC, SmeDEF	Fluoroquinolones, chloramphenicol, tetracyclines
E. aerogenes	AcrAB-TolC	Chloramphenicol, erythromycin A, fluoroquinolones, tetracyclines, β-lactams

The intrinsic resistance of *P. aeruginosa* to a wide range of antibacterial agents cannot be explained solely by the low permeability of its outer membrane. It has been demonstrated that efflux pumps are involved in the mechanisms of resistance to many antibacterials, such as β-lactams, tetracyclines, fluoroquinolones, and chloramphenicol in *P. aeruginosa*.

Among these efflux systems, MexAB-OprM and MexXY-OprM contribute to both intrinsic resistance and acquired resistance, while MexCD-OprJ and MexEF-OprN contribute only to acquired resistance in *P. aeruginosa*.

All three efflux systems have slight but significant differences in substrate specificity for β-lactams (Table 21).

8.2.1. MexAB-OprM

The operon *mexAB-oprM* encodes an MFP linker protein (MexA), a large transporter of about 112 kDa (MexB), and a putative outer membrane channel protein, OprM. The disruption of these genes caused hypersusceptibilities to several agents.

MexB contains 12 α-helices, but unlike other transporters of this class, it contains large periplasmic domains between helices 1 and 2 and helices 7 and 8.

The MexAB-OprM system appears to pump out a wide range of compounds and to be overexpressed in carbenicillin-resistant clinical isolates of *P. aeruginosa*. This can be caused by *nalB* mutation.

The *nalB* mutation has been located in the local repressor gene *mexR*, which occurs immediately upstream of the efflux operon and encodes a repressor of *mexAB-oprM* expression.

Table 21 Substrate specificities for β-lactams in *P. aeruginosa*

Efflux system	β-Lactam substrates
MexAB-OprM	Penicillins, cephems, and meropenem-like carbapenems-penems
MexXY-OprM and MexCD-OprJ	Penicillin but not α-carboxypenicillins (carbenicillin), and sulbenicillin Various cephems Many carbapenems

The MexAB-OprM operon is expressed constitutively in wild-type cells and contributes to intrinsic resistance to fluoroquinolones and other antibacterial agents. The MexAB-OprM system increases at the late log phase of growth.

The *nalC* mutant harbors a mutation in an unidentified regulator of the *mexAB-oprM* operon.

MexB pumps out the quorum-sensing signaling molecule dodecanoyl homoserine lactone.

Among the carbenicillin-resistant isolates of *P. aeruginosa* from British sources, almost 80% did not produce a carbenicillin-hydrolyzing β-lactamase and appeared to belong to the elevated-efflux *nalB* type.

In a French survey, about one-third of ticarcillin-resistant *P. aeruginosa* isolates exhibited a resistance problem of the *nalB* type.

OprM is a periplasmic protein which is anchored to the outer membrane through a lipid moiety.

One compound (Fig. 1) was found to potentiate levofloxacin, with an MPC_8 (see section 10 below) of $\leq$0.06 μg/ml for *P. aeruginosa* expressing MexAB-OprM; however, this combination is inactive in vivo due to the properties of this compound (high lipophilicity, high protein binding, and low water solubility).

To improve the physicochemical properties of this compound, a few analogs were synthesized, first by incorporation of polar groups to reduce the protein binding; however, this

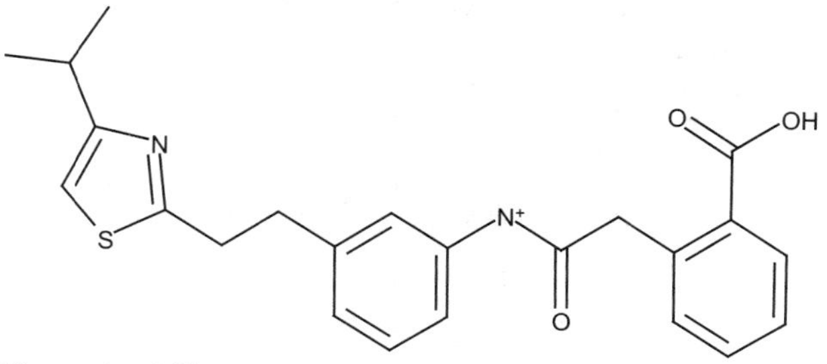

Figure 1 Efflux pump inhibitor of MexAB-OprM (*P. aeruginosa*)

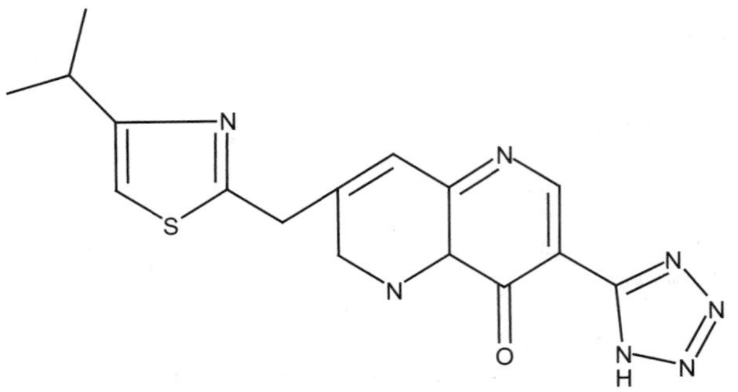

Figure 2 Pyridinopyrimidine-tetrazole (inhibitor of MexAB-OprM from *P. aeruginosa*)

modification was unsuccessful. Modifying the scaffold by introducing a pyridopyrimidine with a tetrazole moiety resulted in an analog (Fig. 2) which potentiates either levofloxacin or sitafloxacin in vitro and in vivo. The protein binding was less than 90%.

8.2.2. MexCD-OprJ

The MexCD-OprJ system does not pump out conventional cephems but pumps out C-3′ quaternary ammonium cephems (cefpirome, cefepime, etc.).

MexCD-OprJ requires that its substrate contain at least one positively charged group at its hydrophobic end.

This system is not expressed in wild-type cells. It is overexpressed in *nfxB* and *nfxC* mutants.

The *nfxB* gene is located upstream of the efflux operon and encodes a repressor of *mexCD-oprJ* expression. Two classes of *nfxB* mutants have been described: type A, which results in moderate resistance, and type B, which yields high-level resistance.

The nature of mutations in *nfxC*-containing strains has yet to be elucidated.

8.2.3. MexEF-OprN

MexEF-OprN hyperexpression is dependent upon the *mexT* gene, which is located upstream of the *mefEF-oprN* operon and encodes a positive regulator of *mefEF-oprN* expression.

The substrate range of MexEF-OprN seems to be narrow, and overexpression of this system produces resistance to only fluoroquinolones and chloramphenicol.

8.2.4. MexXY-OprM (AmrAB)

MexXY appears to use the product of the *oprM* gene as its outer membrane constituent (OprM).

MexXY-OprM-mediated resistance to fluoroquinolones has only been demonstrated with the cloned gene in *E. coli* and *P. aeruginosa*.

A gene, *mexZ* (*amrR*), has been identified upstream of *mexXY* and apparently encodes a repressor of *mexXY* (*amrAB*) expression.

An extensive survey of aminoglycoside resistance in clinical isolates has established the prevalence of the aminoglycoside impermeability-type resistance phenotype in *P. aeruginosa*. Impermeability resistance predominates (>90%) among *P. aeruginosa* isolates collected from cystic fibrosis patients.

In these strains, *mexXY-oprM* was observed to be upregulated.

8.2.5. MexGHI-OprM

Sequence data from the *P. aeruginosa* genome project predicted the existence of at least six unidentified species homologous to the MexAB-OprM RND family system, in addition to the four efflux systems already described.

Outer membrane efflux proteins such as OprM and OprJ cooperatively function not only with native inner membrane complexes such as MexAB and MexCD, respectively, but also with nonnative inner membrane complexes such as MexAB (for OprJ), MexCD (for OprM), and the MexXY (for OprM) aschimeric system.

mexGHI-opmD encodes RND efflux proteins. The proteins are composed of 105 amino acids (gene PA4205 [*mexG*]), and 370 amino acids (gene PA420 [*mexM*]) respectively. *mexI* encodes a protein close to OprN, OpmD. After the gene PA4208 cluster, and transcribed in the opposite orientation, is the gene *phZM* (PA4209), encoding an O-methyltransferase essential for the biosynthesis of pyocyanin. The mutant expressing OmpD produced less pyocyanin and pyoverdin (*mexI* mutant).

Vanadium exerts a bacteriostatic effect on *P. aeruginosa*, especially when the cells are grown under conditions of iron limitation. It was shown that vanadium is complexed by the two *P. aeruginosa* siderophores, pyoverdin and pyochelin. Vanadium could be also toxic for *S. pneumoniae*. Efflux metal systems have been described for cadmium and zinc in *P. aeruginosa* and *Pseudomonas fluorescens*. An increased resistance to ticarcillin-clavulanic acid and netilmicin as well as resistance to tetracycline was recorded when *mexGMI-opmD* was expressed. One possible explanation is that clavulanic acid (lactone) is excreted by the pump (Table 22).

Five multidrug efflux systems have been demonstrated in *P. aeruginosa* (Table 23). These systems are usually chromosally encoded, but recent identification of an RND-type efflux pump gene on a plasmid indicates that efflux-mediated MDR may be plasmid determined as well.

The *mexAB-oprM* operon (previously named *mexAB-oprK*) is expressed constitutively and contributes to intrinsic

Table 22 Activities of antibacterials against *P. aeruginosa* PAO-1 and PAO-ncr

Antibacterial	Zone diam (mm)	
	Wild type	Ncr *mexGHI-opmD*
Tobramycin	20	20
Amikacin	21	20
Netilmicin	21	13
Imipenem	27	27
Ticarcillin-clavulanic acid	21	0
Colistin	15	15
Tetracycline	10	10
Ciprofloxacin	32	29

Table 23 *P. aeruginosa* multidrug efflux proteins

Proteins	Characteristics
MexAB-OprM; MexXY-OprM	Intrinsic; MDR
MexCD-OprJ; MexEF-OprN	Not expressed in wild-type cells; acquired resistance
MexGHI-OprD	Vanadium and clavulanic acid resistance

Table 24 ***P. aeruginosa*, antibacterials, and efflux pumps**

MexAB-OprM	Antibacterial(s) invloved in efflux pump			
	MexXY-OprM (AmrAB)	MexCD-OprJ	MexEF-OprN	MexGHI-OprM?
Carbenicillin	Aminoglycosides	Macrolides	Fluoroquinolones	Clavulanic acid
Aztreonam	Tetracyclines	Chloramphenicol	Tetracyclines	Netilmicin
Meropenem	Erythromycin A	Tetracyclines	Chloramphenicol	Tetracycline
Fluoroquinolones		Novobiocin	Imipenem	
Macrolides		Trimethoprim	Trimethoprim	
Chloramphenicol		C-3′ quaternary ammonium cephems		
Trimethoprim		Ceftazidime		
Novobiocin		Cefoperazone		
Sulfonamide				

resistance to β-lactams, tetracyclines, macrolides, novobiocin, trimethoprim, and sulfonamide.

MexAB-OprM also exports a variety of dyes and detergents, inhibitors of fatty acid biosynthesis, organic solvents, and homoserine lactone (quorum sensing). There is a concern, therefore, that nonchemotherapeutic agents can promote the emergence of resistance to clinically relevant antibacterials in this organism.

Table 24 lists antibacterials involved in different efflux pumps in *P. aeruginosa*.

CCCP abolishes efflux-mediated resistance.

OprM, unlike TolC, contains N-terminal signature sequence for acylation (so-called lipoprotein box) within which is a conserved cysteine residue, the presumed site of acylation.

Acylation of OprM appears to be somewhat dispensable.

Efflux-mediated MDR attributable to MexAB-OprM and MexCD-OprJ appears to require the predicted *tonB* gene (now called *tonB1*), which encodes a protein whose *E. coli* counterpart is known to interact with the outer membrane of certain bacteria.

Outer channel-forming proteins (i.e., those involved in the uptake of ferric siderophore and vitamin B12) are located at the N terminus. In *P. aeruginosa*, outer membrane components may be TonB-dependent channel proteins.

8.3. *E. coli*

8.3.1. AcrAB-TolC

The *E. coli* AcrAB-TolC efflux system is one of the most investigated systems (AcrAB for acridine system). In *E. coli* several efflux systems seem to share the same outer membrane channel TolC.

AcrA, an MFP, has been shown to have an elongated shape with a length of 20 nm, which is enough to cross the periplasmic space.

AcrAB appears to regulate primarily by global regulators such as MarA (which responds to the presence of antibiotics or inhibitors). In addition to increasing the efflux due to elevating transcription of the *acrAB* operon, MarA (also called SoxS or Rob) downregulates the synthesis of the major porin OmpF through increasing the production of an antisense RNA, *micF*.

AcrAB and MexAB differ from EmrB in that the MFPs AcrA and MexA are linked to the inner membrane by a lipid moiety.

AcrAB interacts with TolC. TolC is composed of three proteins. This trimer forms a 140-Å protein cylinder that is open at the outer membrane end, with an internal diameter of 35 Å, but which becomes narrower at the periplasmic space. The structure can be divided into two major domains.

Of 36 *E. coli* strains resistant to ciprofloxacin at a high level, it was found that 22 accumulated lower levels of ciprofloxacin than the wild type, in addition to the *gyrA* mutations.

Excessive production of AcrA and AcrB is prevented by the dimeric repression of AcrR and SdiA (a regulatory protein involved in cell division). The intracellular level of MarA is controlled by MarR, which binds to *marO*. Mar could be inhibited by salicylates. MarA binds to *marO* and activates *marAB* transcription.

It was found that 21 of 57 high-level fluoroquinolone-resistant *E. coli* clinical isolates showed tolerance to cyclohexane, suggesting an important broad-spectrum efflux activity.

In high-level ciprofloxacin-resistant *E. coli* isolates, there is an overexpression of AcrA, at a level ≥170% of that found for a control strain, *E. coli* AG100. In addition, an outer membrane β-barrel which is composed of 12 β-strands, 4 donated by each TolC molecule, is arranged into a right-twisted barrel.

The system allows extrusion of lipophilic antibiotics (β-lactams, chloramphenicol, erythromycin A, and tetracycline), dyes, and detergents in addition to fluoroquinolones.

A periplasmic α-helical barrel, which is a 12-helix domain but with a lift twist, is 100 Å long, which is close to the level of the periplasmic space.

8.3.2. EmrAB

EmrAB is composed of EmrB, a putative 14-helix multidrug H^+ antiport, and the MFP EmrA, which has a short amino-terminal cytoplasmic domain, a single membrane helix, and a large periplasmic domain. The EmrAB proteins provide a continuous pathway across the bacterial membranes by operating in conjunction with the outer membrane TolC.

8.4. *Enterobacter aerogenes*

E. aerogenes, a gram-negative bacillus, is a commensal from the human normal flora which emerged recently as a nosocomial pathogen in some intensive care units. Some *E. aerogenes* isolates are resistant to many antibacterial agents. The *acrA-acrB-tolC* gene efflux pump was recently identified. In *E. aerogenes* ATCC 13048, resistance to norfloxacin, chloramphenicol, polymyxin, and tetracycline was induced when the strain was cultured in the presence of 0.5 to 16 μg of imipenem per ml. Imipenem may be an inducer of the efflux pump in *Enterobacteriaceae*. This efflux pump belongs to related AcrA.

8.5. *Burkholderia* spp.

8.5.1. *Burkholderia cepacia*

In *B. cepacia*, the operon *ceoAB-oprM* was first identified as a chloramphenicol resistance mechanism. A regulatory gene has been reported for this efflux system, although salicylate induction of fluoroquinolone MDR in *B. cepacia* is suggestive of a *mar* locus in this organism.

8.5.2. *Burkholderia vietnamiensis*

B. cepacia is now classified into distinct genomovars that form the *B. cepacia* complex. *B. vietnamiensis* belongs to genomovar V. NorM of *B. vietnamensis* is a protein which contains 462 amino acids with an estimated molecular mass of 47.9 kDa. NorM extrudes norfloxacin.

8.5.3. *B. pseudomallei*

In *B. pseudomallei*, an AmrAB-OprA system resulting in resistance to aminoglycosides and macrolides but not fluoroquinolones has been described.

8.6. *Stenotrophomonas maltophilia*

S. maltophilia is an aerobic, nonfermentative gram-negative bacterium which is ubiquitous in nature and is an opportunistic pathogen. Several multidrug efflux systems have been identified in *S. maltophilia*, including SmeABC and SmeDEF.

Several clinical MDR strains of *S. maltophilia* expressing homologs of MexAB-OprM efflux in *P. aeruginosa* have been reported.

This system is encoded by the *smABC* operon, yielding resistance to fluoroquinolones as well as other antibacterial agents.

S. maltophilia infections are difficult to treat due to the intrinsic resistance of this organism to many antibacterial agents.

S. maltophilia is resistant to many β-lactams, including combinations of β-lactams and inhibitors of β-lactamases, by harboring two β-lactamases, L-1 metallo and L-2 serine β-lactamases. Fluoroquinolone resistance has been increasingly reported, and aminoglycoside-inactivating enzymes have been detected. The presence of a gene encoding a phosphotransferase (gram-positive bacteria) in an *S. maltophilia* D457 R mutant has also been reported.

SmeF is close to OprM, and the molecular mass is 50 kDa. The cytoplasmic membrane protein SmeD has a molecular mass of 110 kDa.

The operon *smeDEF* is overexpressed by 33% of clinical *S. maltophilia* isolates. Overexpression might contribute to increased resistance to tetracycline, chloramphenicol, erythromycin A, and fluoroquinolones in clinical isolates of *S. maltophilia*.

8.7. *N. gonorrhoeae*

N. gonorrhoeae is a strictly human pathogen. It often infects mucosal sites bathed in fluid containing host-derived antibacterial hydrophobic agents such as free fatty acids and bile salts. Its resistance has been attributed to the *mtrCDE*-encoded efflux pump.

In *N. gonorrhoeae*, elevated expression of the MtrCDE efflux system makes mutants more resistant to various lipophilic antibiotics (azithromycin), dyes (crystal violet), and detergents. Three proteins form a channel across the inner membrane and outer membrane, through which antibacterials are extruded. Mtr is encoded by the operon *mtrCDE*, which is regulated by a transcriptional repressor, MtrR (encoded by the *mtrR* gene). MtrR binds within the 250-bp intergenic region between *mtrR* and *mtrC* that accommodates the promoter for *mtrCDE* transcription, thereby downregulating expression of the efflux operon. Mutations in *mtrR* or in the promoter region of the gene result in increased resistance of *N. gonorrhoeae* to hydrophobic antibacterials. The suppressor mutation is located in a novel gene, *mtrF*, which is downstream of *mtrR*.

MtrRC belongs to the MFS family and is presumed to link MtrD (RND transporter) located in the cytoplasmic membrane with MtrE, an outer membrane protein that serves as a channel for export of antibacterials to the extracellular fluid.

MtrF is encoded by the *mtrF* gene, which is located downstream of the *mtrR* gene. MtrF is a 56.1-kDa membrane protein containing 12 TM domains. It is important in the expression of high-level detergent resistance in *N. gonorrhoeae*.

For *N. gonorrhoeae* a second efflux pump has been described, the *far*-encoded system. This system confers resistance to long-chain fatty acids. It is composed of the FarA membrane transporter protein and the FarB cytoplasmic membrane transporter protein. Their expression is controlled by FarR, which regulates directly in a negative manner the operon *farAB*. FarR is upregulated by MtrR.

FarR belongs to the Mar family and to MFS. At the amino acid sequence level, the *farAB* system is similar to the *emrAB* efflux pump system of *E. coli*.

In a study conducted in the United States, 62 *N. gonorrhoeae* isolates resistant to erythromycin A were collected in the Seattle, Wash., area; these represented 22.7% of the clinical isolates. The mechanisms of resistance were numerous, such as *ermB*, *ermE*, *mefA*, *ermF*, and a 1-bp deletion in *mtrR*. Mutations at the level of 23S rRNA have been described. The mutations occurred at positions G2057, A2058, A2060, A2064, and C2605 (C→T). Modifications of the ribosomal target by methylases have been described for *N. gonorrhoeae*.

Rectal isolates of *N. gonorrhoeae* often harbor missense mutations in the repressor *mtrR* gene; the mutation apparently allows the bacteria to survive in an environment rich in lipophilic inhibitors by upregulation of the efflux system. *N. gonorrhoeae* mutants which overexpress the MtrCDE system sometimes have a short deletion in the promoter sequence of this operon.

8.8. *H. influenzae* (AcrAB-Like)

AcrB is a 12-TM protein. The genome of *H. influenzae* indicates that the organism does not possess a homolog of TolC but does have an outer membrane protein with 21.1% identity to OprM from *P. aeruginosa*. In addition to *acrA* (HI0894) and *acrB* (HI0895), a third gene has been identified, *acrR* (HI0893). AcrAB substrates include both positively charged (dyes and erythromycin A) and negatively charged (novobiocin) amphiphilic compounds.

H. influenzae possesses only one porin, Omp2, which produces larger, highly permeable channels. The large size of the channel allows the penetration of 1,845-Da oligosaccharides. Omp2 has a high permeability to β-lactams, chloramphenicol, tetracyclines, and fluoroquinolones. The *H. influenzae* porin channel significantly reduces the permeation by relatively bulky agents, such as erythromycin A and novobiocin, and the AcrAB-like efflux system of *H. influenzae* can produce detectable resistance to these agents.

The more rapid influx of the relatively small agents through the Omp2 porin channel of *H. influenzae* may counterbalance the relatively slow efflux, generating little resistance.

8.9. *C. jejuni* (CmeABC)

C. jejuni is one of the leading causes of human enteritis in many industrialized countries.

The sequence of the genome of *C. jejuni* NCTC 11168 has been completed, and it has such characteristics as a lack of inserted sequence elements, prophages, and transposons which often carry genes encoding drug resistance. It has been shown that several genes share significant homology with known multidrug transporters.

A CmeABC system has been described for *C. jejuni*.

The three ORFs (*cmeA*, *cmeB*, and *cmeC*) are located in the same coding strand and are tandemly positioned on the chromosome of *C. jejuni* strain 81-176.

cmeA (nucleotides 207 to 1307), *cmeB* (nucleotides 1310 to 4429), and *cmeC* (nucleotides 4425 to 5900) encode 367-, 1,040-, and 492-amino-acid proteins, respectively. Other proteins potentially regulate the *cmeABC* operon. CmeA, CmeB, and CmeC possess molecular masses of 37.9, 114, and 53 kDa, respectively.

The *cmeABC* operon is expressed in wild-type *C. jejuni* 81-176. In a *C. jejuni* mutant strain, 9B6, with a transposon insertion in *cmeB* (this transposon encodes a 360-amino-acid peptide), resulted in increased susceptibilities to many antibacterial agents. *C. jejuni* is intrinsically resistant to rifampin, which is used in selective *C. jejuni* media. This resistance can be attributed to expression of CmeABC (Table 25).

The Mre acronym came from macrolide resistance efflux. MreA protein was found in *Streptococcus agalactiae* CO H31 γ/δ. This strain was resistant to 14-, 15-, and 16-membered-ring macrolides and to clindamycin.

The gene *mreA* encodes a 310-amino-acid protein with a predicted molecular mass of 35.4 kDa. This protein is hydrophilic, with interspersed hydrophobic and amphiphatic sequences. The protein displayed homology with RibC, a flavokinase/flavin adenine dinucleotide synthetase from *B. subtilis*.

It was shown that the product of *mreA* displays a flavokinase activity and is responsible for broad-spectrum resistance to a variety of compounds when cloned in *E. coli* but not when expressed in *E. faecalis*.

The *mreA* gene is located on the chromosome. MreA seems to belong to the RND family.

Table 25 Susceptibilities of *C. jejuni* 81-176 and its *cmeB* mutant to different antibacterial agents

Compound	MIC (μg/ml)	
	Strain 81-176 (wild type)	9B6 (mutant)
Ciprofloxacin	0.312	0.039
Norfloxacin	0.078	0.039
Nalidixic acid	1.25	0.625
Erythromycin A	0.078	0.02
Ampicillin	0.312	0.01
Cefotaxime	1.60	0.006
Rifampin	100	0.78
Trimethroprim	>200	>200
Tetracycline	50	6.25
Chloramphenicol	0.850	0.425
Gentamicin	0.265	0.133
Polymyxin B	3.0	3.0
Cycloheximide	>500	>500
Protamine	25	12.5
Ethidium bromide	0.625	0.078
$CoCl_2$	312	156
$CuCl_2$	391	196
$ZnSo_4$	78	78
Sodium dodecyl sulfate	250	62.5
Cholic acid	6,250	98
Chenodeoxycholic acid	5,000	12.5
Taurocholic acid	>50,000	780
Deoxycholic acid	10,000	10

8.10. *Acinetobacter baumannii*

Acinetobacter species are ubiquitous nonfermentative, gram-negative bacteria which play a significant role in colonization and infection in patients in intensive care units. Few antibiotics are effective for the treatment of *Acinetobacter* infections due to the numerous mechanisms of resistance and the frequency of MDR strains. Resistance of *Acinetobacter* to β-lactams is partially intrinsic due to the synthesis of species-specific cephalosporinase. Mutations in *gyrA* have been associated with high-level resistance to fluoroquinolones. Aminoglycoside resistance is also common in *Acinetobacter* due to inactivating enzymes, such as acetyltransferase, phosphotransferase, and adenyltransferase. Efflux pumps have been recently reported for *A. baumannii* BM 4454. The *adeB* gene encodes an RND protein which is responsible for resistance to aminoglycoside, fluoroquinolones, tetracycline, chloramphenicol, erythromycin A, trimethoprim, cefotaxime, and ethidium bromide. The *adeB* gene is part of a cluster that includes *adeA* and *adeC*.

AdeB can apparently recognize hydrophobic, amphiphilic, and hydrophilic molecules which can be either positively charged or neutral.

Among aminoglycosides, kanamycin and amikacin appeared to be less effectively transported than other compounds by AdeABC. Kanamycin and amikacin are the most hydrophilic aminoglycosides. In the same manner, sparfloxacin and ofloxacin, which are hydrophobic fluoroquinolones, appeared to be slightly better substrates than norfloxacin and pefloxacin.

8.11. *L. lactis*

Lactococci belong to the lactic acid group of bacteria used in the dairy product industry. *L. lactis* K214, isolated from a raw milk soft cheese, has been shown to harbor a multiple antibiotic resistance 30-kb plasmid, pK214, which also carries genes for chloramphenicol (acetyltransferase), streptomycin (adenylase), and tetracycline (*tetS* gene) resistance and a putative efflux gene, *mef*214 (MdtA). Two multidrug transporters have been described for *L. lactis*: LmrA (ABC transporter) and LmrP. MdtA, encoded by the gene *mdtA*, is a plasmid-specified protein belonging to the MFS family. The *mdtA* gene confers resistance to erythromycin A, clarithromycin, azithromycin, spiramycin, clindamycin, lincomycin, and quinupristin-dalfopristin. The protein is composed of 12 putative TM-spanning domains.

8.12. *M. tuberculosis*

Pyrazinamide is transformed through a pyrazinamidase to an active metabolite, pyrazinoic acid, in mycobacteria, especially in *M. tuberculosis* and less in other mycobacteria. It was shown that an acidic pH enhances pyrazinoic acid accumulation in the bacterial cell. In mycobacterial species an efflux pump extrudes pyrazinoic acid, leading to resistance.

Other active efflux pumps have been described for tubercle bacilli (see chapter 43).

8.13. *Pseudomonas putida*

P. putida S-12 is able to transform toxic concentrations of toluene and other organic solvents. *P. putida* employs at least two mechanisms for active defense against the detrimental effects of solvents: efflux and a mechanism which prevents solvents from partitioning into cell membranes (ratio of *trans* to *cis* unsaturated fatty acids). The genes *sprABC* encode this pump (RND family): an outer membrane channel protein (SrpB), a periplasmic linker protein (SprA), and an inner membrane transporter (SrpC).

8.14. *S. enterica* Serovar Typhimurium

S. enterica serovar Typhimurium DT 104 harbors a gene cluster conferring resistance to ampicillin, chloramphenicol, florfenicol, streptomycin, sulfonamides, and tetracyclines, as well as fluoroquinolones.

Two genes, *floR* and *tetC*, encode efflux pumps belonging to the MFS family. The AcrAB-TolC multidrug efflux system is responsible for resistance to fluoroquinolones, florfenicol, chloramphenicol, and tetracyclines.

Table 26 ABC transporters

ABC transporter	Organism(s)	Antibacterial agent(s)
LmrA	*L. lactis*	DN, DR, DA, VB, VC
VgaB	*Staphylococcus* spp.	S_B
MsrA	*S. aureus*, coagulase-negative staphylococci	14-and 15-membered-ring MLs; S_B
TlC	*Streptomyces fradiae*	Tylosin
CarA	*Streptomyces thermotolerans*	Carbomycin
SrmB	*Streptomyces ambofaciens*	Spiramycin
Msr	*Streptomyces rochei*	Erythromycin complex, spiramycin
OleB	*S. antibioticus*	Oleandomycin
ErtX	*Streptomyces erythraeus*	ND
ArsAB	*E. coli*	Arseniate
RbsAC	*E. coli*	ND
LsA	*E. faecalis*	Q-D, clindamycin

[a]DN, daunorubicin; DR, doxorubicin; DA, daunomycin; VB, vinblastin; VC, vincristine; S_B, streptogramin; B ML, macrolides; ND, not defined; Q-D, quinupristin-dalfopristin.

9. ABC TRANSPORTERS

9.1. General Characteristics

ABC-type efflux transporters generally consist of an integral membrane protein with six putative TM α-helical spanners and an energy-coupling protein localized to the cytoplasmic side of the membrane.

ABC transporters are composed of at least 28 families for sugars, amino acids, ions, drugs, antibiotics, vitamins, iron complexes, peptides, proteins, complex carbohydrates, etc.

ABC transporters are multicomponent, multidomain systems. The total size is above 1,000 amino acid residues, with usually 12 spanners. More than 500 members have been sequenced. Drug efflux pumps are found in a few (three or four) of the many recognized families.

Most of the known ABC transporters that contain two ABCs but no hydrophobic domain(s) were found in antibiotic-producing microorganisms, in which they are involved in the active excretion of those molecules.

Several ABC transporters which do not have alternating hydrophobic domains have been grouped in a subfamily to distinguish them from the other members of ABC-2 transporter subfamilies, the members of which contain hydrophobic TM domains. These proteins are usually present as dimeric complexes, and the complete prototypical system therefore possesses 12 spanners.

ABC transporters responsible for resistance are listed in Table 26.

In *Leishmania, Entamoeba histolytica, Plasmodium falciparum*, and *Trypanosoma cruzi* (Chagas' disease), MDR is catalyzed by an ABC transporter.

In *P. falciparum*, Pfmrd1, a 12-TM protein, induces resistance to chloroquine, mefloquine, and artemisin. In *Candida albicans*, the protein Cdr1, a 12-TM efflux protein, induces resistance to fluconazole, ketoconazole, miconazole, and steroids.

The ABC family includes the MDR P-glycoprotein, a 1,280-amino-acid protein that confers resistance to anticancer drugs.

Related ABC transporters have been found in other fungi, such as *Aspergillus fumigatus* and *Cryptococcus neoformans*.

The ABC drug efflux has been classified extensively in families according to structural homology.

ABC domains present a high degree of homology, whereas TM domains differ between transporters and might contribute to defining their substrate specificities.

ABC transporters which contain two ABC domains derive their energy from the hydrolysis of ATP. An additional characteristic of an MRP transporter is that its activity is strictly dependent on the presence of glutathione. The role of glutathione remains unclear.

A conformational change of the ABC protein is necessary for drug extrusion and probably is triggered by drug binding and ATP hydrolysis.

The physiological transporters of phospholipids and glutathione conjugates are known as flippases.

The archetype ABC transporter has two nucleotide-binding sites (NB and 12 membrane-spanning α-helices arranged in two groups of 6). Although the α-helical model is widely accepted, an alternative β-barrel has been proposed.

Bacterial ABC transporters frequently include ATPase subunits with allosteric sites that control the ATPase activity. In this system, the transporter protein located in the cytoplasmic membrane is thought to be brought into opposition with an outer membrane channel protein such as TolC, PrtF, or CyaE through the linker protein such as HlyD, PrtE, and CyaD, which were shown to make up the MFP. Transporters of those systems are all members of the ABC family.

ABC transporters usually contain four single or joined components that are arranged into two homologous halves containing an ATP-binding domain and a membrane-spanning domain composed of several (usually six) putative α-helical TM segments.

The numbers of amino acids which compose some ABC transporters are listed in Table 27.

In the ABC-2 permease family, which is composed of four clusters, all of the functionally characterized drug resistance permeases can be found in cluster D: OleCJ is an oleandomycin pump of *Streptomyces antibioticus*, and OrrB1 and DrrC pump daunorubicin in *Mycobacterium leprae*.

9.2. MsrA and MsrB

MsrA is a protein of 488 amino acids (molecular mass, 55.9 kDa) that contains two ATP-binding domains

Table 27 ABC transporters (bacterial)

Protein	Microorganism	No. of amino acids	Molecular mass (kDa)
YjcA	*L. lactis*	513	
MsrC	*E. faecium*	493	
VgA	*S. aureus*	522	60
VgB	*S. aureus*	552	61
MsrA	*S. aureus*	488	
LmrA	*L. lactis*		
LsA	*E. faecalis*	498	498

characteristic of the ABC transporters. The two ATP-binding domains are separated by a rather long Q-linker (23Q; 1,160 amino acids).

The gene *msrA* has been sequenced for both *S. epidermidis* and *S. aureus*.

MsrA is specific for 14- and 15-membered-ring macrolides and streptogramin B.

Two TM proteins, SmpA and SmpC, were identified, but they do not seem to be essential for expressing MsrA. In MsrA, the two ATP-binding regions are fused into a single protein with internally homologous domains. In other proteins, the ATP-binding regions are monomeric and likely form dimers in vivo.

MsrB protein has been identified in *Staphylococcus xylosus*. This protein is identical to the C-terminal half of MsrA of *S. aureus*.

The first Msr protein efflux was identified in 1976 in Czechoslovakia. In a study published in 1993, 8 of 11 *Staphylococcus cohnii* strains isolated from human skin harbored the gene *msrA*. (*msrA* is the most frequently encountered erythromycin A resistance determinant in both *Staphylococcus hominis* and *S. cohnii*, and possibly in other staphylococcal species as well. *msrA* was reported in 1982 for an *S. aureus* strain isolated from Hungary.)

9.3. Lsa Protein

In the *E. faecalis* genome, 34 possible transporter homologies have been identified.

One strain harboring *lsa* (formerly called *abc*23) exhibits reduced susceptibility to quinupristin-dalfopristin and clindamycin.

The gene *lsa* encodes a protein containing 498 amino acids (Singh et al., 2002). A 45-amino-acid putative peptide was identified preceding the *lsa* start codon. The presence of this sequence seems to be important for the expression of drug resistance.

The presence of leader peptide sequences has been reported for *msrA*, *ermB*, and *ermC*. They are postulated to be involved in posttranscriptional regulation of the expression of the resistance genes.

LsA and MsrA contain no hydrophobic domains.

9.4. VgaA

The *vgaA* gene encodes a 522-amino-acid protein of 60,115 Da. VgaA has two ATP-binding domains, containing each of the A and the B motifs.

The *vgaB* gene encodes a 552-amino-acid protein, VgaB, of 61,327 Da. VgaB has two ATP-binding domains but does not include a TM hydrophobic domain. The 155-amino-acid sequence between the two ATP-binding domains of VgaB is rich in Glu compared to the remaining part of the molecule.

The *vgaB* gene was found in 21 of 52 streptogramin A-resistant strains and is carried on a plasmid of 50 to 90 kDa also harboring the *vatB* gene, which encodes an acetyltransferase inactivating streptogramin A. In all plasmids, *vgaB* and *vatB* have the same relative positions.

Several staphylococcal plasmids (26 to 45 kb) carry all three streptogramin resistance genes, *vat*, *vgb*, and *vga*. The gene *vat* encodes a streptogramin acetyltransferase, the *vga* gene encodes an ATP binding protein (efflux), and the *vgb* gene encodes a streptogramin B lactonase.

9.5. Other Proteins

ArsA is the ATPase subunit of the arsenical efflux pump, which binds antimonite and arsenate.

10. ANTIBACTERIALS AND EFFLUX

When an efflux pump inhibitor was combined with an antibacterial agent, the potentiation activity was expressed as the lowest concentration of the efflux pump inhibitor achieving an eightfold reduction in antibacterial MIC; this parameter was named MPC_8.

10.1. Aminoglycosides

Quite a few efflux pumps extrude aminoglycosides. This is probably due to the high hydrophilicity of these compounds, which enter the cells by nonspecific diffusion.

Aminoglycosides mimic polyamines, an essential substrate for many types of cells, and use their inward transport system for entering bacteria.

Aminoglycoside-producing organisms generally protect themselves not by efflux pumps but by the production of aminoglycoside-inactivating enzymes.

10.2. Glycopeptides

There are no published efflux pumps for glycopeptides. These compounds are bulky and hydrophilic and act in the outer space of gram-positive bacteria.

10.3. Fluoroquinolones

Fluoroquinolone resistance attributable to an efflux mechanism has been reported for numerous gram-negative and -positive bacteria (Table 28).

A CCCP-promoted increase in fluoroquinolone accumulation has been observed in the absence of an efflux mechanism. Demonstration of CCCP-enhanced fluoroquinolone accumulation in bacterial cells is insufficient to support the existence of a fluoroquinolone efflux mechanism.

MexCD-OprJ and MexEF-OprN hyperexpression is the predominant mechanism of fluoroquinolone resistance in strains isolated from the lungs of cystic fibrosis patients.

10.4. Macrolides

Fourteen- and 15-membered-ring macrolides are pumped out with the Mef group. A putative pump has been shown in mycobacteria. Mef pumps are found mainly in gram-positive cocci. For group B streptococci another pump has been described, MreA. For *S. pneumoniae*, it has already been reported that *mef* and *mel* are cotransmitted. Efflux of erythromycin A is abolished by arsenate and strongly inhibited by dinitrophenol.

10.5. Tetracyclines

Efflux genes encode a 46-kDa membrane-bound protein. This protein can be divided into six groups according to

Table 28 Known bacteria with fluoroquinolone resistance due to efflux mechanisms

Organism(s)
A. baumannii
B. cepacia
Bacteroides fragilis
Brucella melitensis
B. thetaiotaomicron
Citrobacter freundii
C. jejuni
E. aerogenes
E. coli
K. pneumoniae
P. aeruginosa
Proteus vulgaris
S. aureus
Shigella dysenteriae
S. enterica serovar Typhimurium
S. maltophilia
S. pneumoniae
V. parahaemolyticus
V. cholerae
Viridans group streptococci

amino acid sequence identity. The efflux pump exchanges a tetracycline cation complex (tetracycline-Mg^{2+}) against a concentration gradient.

Nine ribosomal protection proteins have been described. They are cytoplasmic proteins that protect ribosomes from the action of tetracycline and confer resistance to doxycycline and minocycline.

Resistance to cyclines has been studied for respiratory pathogens but not in detail at the gene level (Table 29).

Table 29 Resistance to tetracycline in respiratory pathogens from 1999 to 2000 (Protekt)

Organism[a]	*n*	MIC (μg/ml)[b] 50%	MIC (μg/ml)[b] 90%	% Resistance
S. pneumoniae				
Asia	515	>16	>16	81.6
Australasia	121	0.25	>16	13.4
Europe	1,521	0.6	32	24.1
Latin America	518	0.125	>16	24.9
North America	687	0.25	>16	13.8
H. influenzae β+	489	0.5	8.0	6.6
H. influenzae β−	2,459	0.5	1.0	0.7
Moraxella catarrhalis	2,948	0.5–1.0	0.5–1.0	3.3

[a]β+, β-lactamase producing; β−, non-β-lactamase producing.
[b]50% and 90%, MICs at which 50 and 90% of isolates tested are inhibited, respectively.

10.6. β-Lactams

10.6.1. Penems

It was demonstrated in AmpC-lacking *P. aeruginosa* that an efflux system extrudes penems, that MexAB-OprM pumps out penems more efficiently than it pumps out norfloxacin and tetracyclines, and that the extreme potency of MexAB-OprM for penems is higher than those of MexCD-OprJ and MexXY-OprM. Penems are extruded mainly by the MexAB-OprM efflux pump and also by a minor efflux pump, MexCD-OprJ (Table 30).

The fixed combination quinolyl-carbapenem seems to be a poor substrate for the norA-encoded quinolone efflux pump.

10.7. Antibacterial Specificities

The importance of lipophilicity is often difficult to assert in the absence of published data with homogeneous series of drug derivatives.

However, for penicillins, the following ranking has been established: cloxacillin > nafcillin > penicillin G > carbenicillin > penicillin N (the latter being almost not transported). There is a close relationship with their corresponding octanol/water partition coefficients.

Meropenem selects for a loss of specific basic amino acid/carbapenem channel protein OprD in the outer membrane of *P. aeruginosa* as well as for the overproduction of the MexAB-OprM efflux complex.

The physicochemical properties of the antibiotics transported by a given class of pumps correspond to those of the nonantibiotic compounds as well as those of the putative physiological substrates. One major discrepancy is with chloramphenicol, which is extruded by MFS despite its neutral character. Probably the recognition of this compound is mediated by interactions which differ from those observed for other antibacterials.

Table 30 Activities of penems according to phenotype of resistance[a]

P. aeruginosa strain	Phenotype[b]					MIC (μg/ml)[c]					
	AB	XY	CD	M	J	F	R	AMA	S	Sch-29482	Sch-34343
PAO-1	+	−	−	+	−	512	128	128	32	256	128
KG 5002	−	−	−	−	−	1	2	1	0.12	0.5	1
KG 5004	++	−	−	++	−	4,096	256	1,024	64	2,048	1024
KG 5006	−	++	−	++	−	4	8	8	0.5	8	8
KG 5008	−	−	++	−	++	16	4	64	2	32	32
KG 2504	+	−	−	+	−	256	32	ND	8	256	ND
KG 2504 F1	++	−	−	++	−	2,048	128	ND	64	1,024	ND
KG 2505	−	−	−	−	−	1	128	1	0.12	1	1
KG 2505 F1	−	−	++	S	++	16	2	ND	2	16	ND
KG 2505 F1 ΔD	−	−	−	S	−	1	4	ND	0.12	1	ND

[a]Data from Okamoto et al., 2002.
[b]S, lower but significant expression; −, undetectable expression; ++, overexpression; +, wild-type-level expression.
[c]F, fropenem (faropenem); R, ritipenem; AMA, AMA-3176; S, sulopenem; ND, not determined.

11. MAGNITUDE OF RESISTANCE TO EFFLUX PUMPS

The epidemiological impact of antibiotic efflux pumps on resistance in the clinical setting was only established for *S. pyogenes* and *S. pneumoniae* for 14- and 15-membered-ring macrolides and ketolides (telithromycin), allowing comparison with other mechanisms of resistance such as methylation (macrolides-lincosamides-streptogramin B [MLS_B] [*erm*]) or mutation in the L4 and L22 ribosomal proteins for *S. pneumoniae*.

11.1. Streptococcus spp.

11.1.1. *S. pyogenes*

S. pyogenes is responsible for upper respiratory tract infections and skin and soft tissue infections. Since the mid-1990s, there has been an increase in resistance to macrolides worldwide. In the United States, the main mechanism of resistance is efflux driven by the MefA protein, encoded by *mefA* (Table 31).

Another pump was recently described belonging to the ATP cassette.

11.1.2. *S. pneumoniae*

Of a total of 1,037 clinical isolates of *S. pneumoniae* collected during 1996 and 1997 from patients in the United Kingdom, 273 showed reduced susceptibility to norfloxacin and ciprofloxacin (MICs, >8 and >1 μg/ml, respectively). These isolates could be divided into two groups on the basis of the effect of reserpine: group A ($n = 149$), for which the MIC of norfloxacin was reduced only twofold or less by reserpine, and group B ($n = 124$), for which the MIC of norfloxacin was reduced fourfold or greater by reserpine. The strain with the efflux phenotype remained susceptible to the more hydrophobic compounds sparfloxacin and moxifloxacin. This suggests that hydrophobic fluoroquinolones are poor substrates for the pneumococcal efflux pump.

Table 31 ***S. pyogenes*** **resistance to erythromycin A: prevalence of the different genes in the European community from 1999 to 2000**

Country	*n*	No. of gene(s) detected				
		SR[a]	*mefA*	*ermB*	*ermA*	*ermB*+*mef*
Austria	206	20	13	2	5	
Belgium	599	92	219	33	10	
Denmark	377	11		2	2	7
Finland	133	10	3	3	4	
France	441	36	17	19		
Germany	216	17	12	1	4	
United Kingdom	994	53	16	5	28	1
Greece	161	30	21		10	
Ireland	158	3	1	2		
Italy	160	52	22	22	6	2
Luxembourg	86	9	1	3	2	3
The Netherlands	383	5		2	1	2
Norway	199	2				
Portugal	300	82	16	64	2	
Spain	202	48	40			8
Sweden	199	0				

[a]SR, strain resistant.

Table 32 MIC ranges for *S. agalactiae* containing the *mefA* gene

Compound	MIC range (μg/ml)
Erythromycin A	0.1–1.0
Clarithromycin	0.1–0.5
Azithromycin	1.0–4.0
Telithromycin	0.03–0.5

11.1.3. *S. agalactiae*

The *mef* determinants were characterized for 18 clinical *S. agalactiae* isolates from France. The MIC ranges of 14- and 15-membered-ring macrolides for *mef*-containing isolates were lower than those usually recorded for *mef*-containing *S. pyogenes* or *S. pneumoniae* isolates (Table 32).

In a multicenter study involving 10 French clinical microbiological laboratories in 1999, 126 *S. agalactiae* isolates were collected in the community from patients. Of these, 27 (21.4%) were considered resistant to erythromycin A (MIC, ≤1.0 μg/ml). The most prevalent genes were *ermB* and *ermTR*, in 40.7% (11 of 27) and 37% (10 of 27 strains), respectively. One isolate harbored both genes. The *mefA* gene alone was detected in two isolates and in combination with ermB in one isolate.

11.1.4. Viridans Group Streptococci

Viridans group streptococci form the major part of the commensal flora of the human upper respiratory tract. They may be the reservoir of erythromycin A resistance.

In the southwest of France, between 1988 and 1995, 90 viridans group streptococci were collected from patients. This set of strains was composed of 57 isolates belonging to the *Streptococcus mitis* group, 24 belonging to the *Streptococcus milleri* group, and 9 belonging to the *Streptococcus salivarius* group. Overall, 8.9% of the isolates (8 of 90 strains) harbored the M-phenotype. Six strains carried an unidentified M-phenotype.

In two other studies, the incidence of the M-phenotype in viridans group streptococci was about 20%.

12. EFFLUX PUMP INHIBITORS

Efflux pump inhibitors may be novel molecules belonging to a given new chemical family.

12.1. Chemical Families

12.1.1. Tetracycline

It has been shown that thiatetracycline, a sulfur derivative of tetracycline, the sulfur atom being at position 6, is active against plasmid-containing tetracycline-resistant bacteria, probably because of an inability of the cells to remove accumulated compound. Unfortunately, thiatetracycline is too toxic for clinical use. Tetracyclines, which are substituted with a dimethyl glycylamido side chain at C-9, are not recognized by the tetracycline pumps.

Class A to E, G, and H determinants among gram-negative bacteria and class K and L determinants among gram-positive bacteria are specifically an active-efflux mechanism for tetracycline. The class P resistance determinant from *Clostridium perfringens* contains two overlapping resistance genes, one for an active-efflux protein and one for a ribosomal protective-type cytoplasmic protein. Using everted inner membrane of *E. coli* harboring a *tet(B)* determinant, inhibitors of [^{3}H]tetracycline were assessed. The C-13 substituted thiol derivatives of methacycline had pronounced inhibitory effects on the accumulation of [^{3}H]tetracycline in everted membrane. 13-Cyclopentylthio-5-OH-TC (13-CPTC) is able to interfere with tetracycline transport by competitively binding to the *tet*-(B) antiporter but is itself transported less effectively than tetracycline.

13-CPTC possesses antibacterial activity alone, especially against isolates harboring *tet*(K) and *tet*(L) as well as *tet*(M) (Fig. 3 and 4).

12.1.2. Ketolides

The ketolides telithromycin and cethromycin have improved activity against gram-positive cocci harboring an efflux pump for erythromycin A (*mefA* and *mefE*).

To enter the cell, macrolides and ketolides are passively taken up from the outer membrane. The efflux is the result of two things: induction of the pump and affinity for the pump.

Both ketolides are poor inducers of the *mefA* and *mefE* genes and have poor affinity for the efflux pump.

Ketolides and macrolides have a high affinity for the 50S ribosomal subunit. Ketolides have a higher affinity for the ribosomal subunit than does erythromycin A, clarithromycin, or azithromycin, and they display higher affinity for ribosome than for efflux pump proteins.

Whether protonated or not, both ketolides are minimally extruded from the cell, efflux being a balance between influx and efflux.

12.1.3. Fluoroquinolones

Fluoroquinolone extrusion is more complex; depending on the lipophilicity, the pump is or is not a good substrate for efflux proteins, explaining why some new fluoroquinolones are not extruded from the bacterial cells as easily as others.

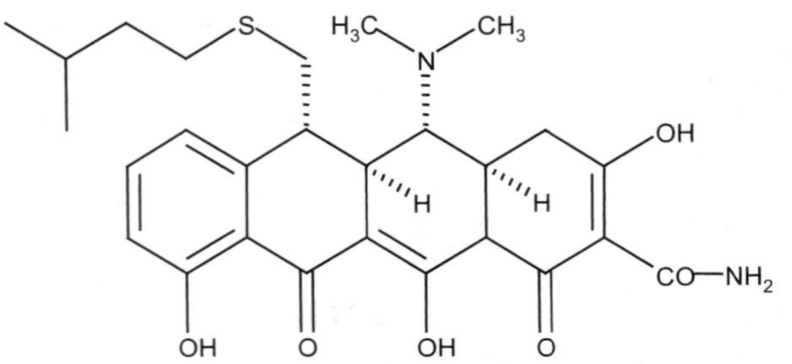

Figure 3 Inhibitor of Tet protein efflux

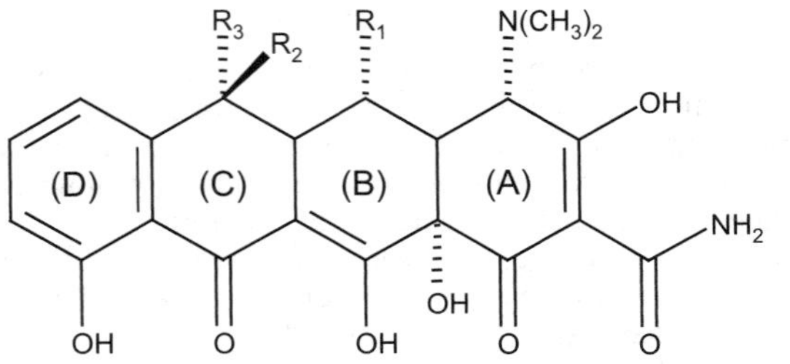

	R_1	R_2	R_3
Tetracycline	H	OH	CH_3
Doxycycline	OH	H	CH_3
13-CPTC	OH	H	CH_2-S–(cyclopentyl) 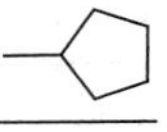

Figure 4 New tetracyclines

12.2. Inhibitors of Efflux Groups

The first flavolignan was reported in 1968 (silybin or silymarin) for fruit of the medicinal plant *Silybum marianum*.

The second flavolignam reported was hydnocarpin in 1973, isolated from *Hydnocarpus wightiana*; it was also shown to occur in *Cassia absus*. Hydnocarpins are devoid of optical activity and are scalenic isolates. The stereochemistry at C-12 and C-13 was *trans* in all flavolignans.

Americanis A. was isolated from *Phytolacca americana*.

In 1974, two minor components were recorded for *H. wightiana*, isohydnocarpin and 5′-methoxyhydnocarpin (5′-MHC).

Today, a new approach is to prepare or discover from natural screening agents devoid of antibacterial activity (or a weak one at a high concentration) which can be combined with antibacterial agents to overcome efflux pumps or to minimize them.

12.2.1. Reserpine-Like Derivatives

Quinolone resistance may be due to the combination of three mechanisms of resistance: mutations on *gyrA* and *parC* and efflux. The degree of efflux varies among fluoroquinolones.

In one study, 40% of *S. pneumoniae* isolates showed efflux of ofloxacin and trovafloxacin and 55% showed efflux of gemifloxacin; the MICs were double those for wild strains.

For fluoroquinolones and *S. pneumoniae*, the efflux pump is PmrA and has been sequenced.

Other efflux pumps have been reported, such as NorA for *S. aureus* and enterococci and Bmr for *B. subtilis*. Brm and NorA promote efflux of a variety of organic compounds, including ethidium bromide, rhodamine, acridine, TTP, puromycin, benzalkonium, cetrimide, and pentamidine.

NorA can be inhibited by the alkaloid plant product reserpine, which is an antihypertensive drug.

Fluoroquinolone resistance may arise via horizontal transfer of mutated topoisomerase genes from viridans group streptococci to *S. pneumoniae*. It has been possible to transfer both mutated *parC* and *gyrA* in a single step from *S. mitis* to *S. pneumoniae*. Given the homology among the topoisomerase genes of *S. mitis*, *Streptococcus oralis*, and *S. pneumoniae*, genetic exchanges via transformation between those species could be envisaged in a clinical setting.

In addition to being involved in the reduced susceptibility of gram-positive bacteria to fluoroquinolones, efflux pumps contribute to the acquired resistance which is selected upon exposure to the antibacterials. Inhibition of NorA may increase the bactericidal activity and the postantibiotic effect of ciprofloxacin on *S. aureus*.

In the clinic, reserpine cannot be used at the dose required for inhibition because of its neurotoxicity. Reserpine displays antibacterial activity at a concentration of 5 μg/ml. Reserpine contains an indole moiety.

Compounds from the chemical library of Diverset were screened for activity against a well-characterized *B. subtilis* strain. It has been shown that compounds having a nitro indole as well as compounds with a trichlomethyl functional group were active. Unfortunately, the group makes them toxic for human use. The compounds INF-392, INF-277, and INF-240 exhibited some activity at a concentration of ≤5 μg/ml. The most potent indole analog was INF-392, and the most potent phenylurea derivative was INF-271.

Table 33 Activities of reserpine-like compounds

Compound	EtBr[a] concn (μg/ml)	Ciprofloxacin	
		FIC index (μg/ml)	*S. aureus* 1199-B
INF-55	0.08	0.25	0.25
INF-240	0.16	0.12	0.28
INF-271	0.07	0.12	0.18
INF-277	0.09	0.5	0.28
INF-392	0.14	0.28	0.15

[a]Etbr, ethidium bromide.

The most potent inhibitor able to reverse resistance was INF-392, being able to reverse ethidium bromide and ciprofloxacin resistance, which was found by checkerboard titration (Table 33).

The reserpine inhibitory activity was discovered to reverse Bmr- and NorA-mediated drug resistance.

The large number of identified inhibitors and their broad structural diversity apparently lie in the low substrate specificity of this multidrug transporter. There is strong evidence that reserpine exerts its inhibitory effect directly by binding to the transporter that mediates the efflux. Sparfloxacin and tosufloxacin are poor substrates of NorA.

12.2.2. Berberine and Derivatives

Berberis fremontii, a berberine product used in Native American traditional medicine, synthesizes a potent MDR inhibitor: 5′-MHC (Fig. 5).

Berberine is an alkaloid, which is a common component of a variety of plant species in the family Berberidaceae. Berberine exhibits weak antibacterial activity, due to the MDR efflux in particular (MIC, ≥30 μg/ml). Berberine was found in *Berberis aquifolium*, *Berberis repens*, and *B. fremontii.*

The alkaloid protopine, allocryptopine, glaucine, isocotcyclinemethiodine, tetrahydropalmatene, a mixture of bis benzyltetrahydroquinoline, and the lignan asamarin all are inactive against *S. aureus*, and mixtures of each with subinhibitory berberine were all inactive.

Hydnocarpin was reported to have lipolipidemic, anti-inflammatory, and antineoplastic activities.

It was demonstrated that chloroform extract from leaves of *B. fremontii* inhibits growth of *S. aureus*. The content of 5′-MHC in *B. fremontii* is estimated at 0.05 to 0.10% of dry leaf weight.

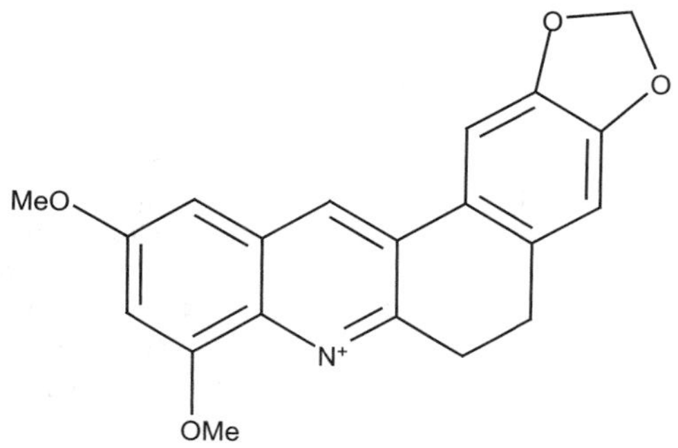

MeO
N+
OMe

Figure 5 Berberine

Any prospective microbial MDR inhibitor to be used in medicine should be devoid of activity against P-glycoprotein MDR.

5′-MHC was also reported as a minor component of *H. wightiana* in the family Flaconstaceae.

The 7-OH of 5′ MHC has a pK of 7.3. Flavonoids with alkylated 7-OH groups are active against P-glycoprotein, whereas 7-OH forms are completely inactive, probably because of acidic properties of this group. The 7-OH-containing 5′-MHC is likely to be a specific microbial MDR inhibitor. Norfloxacin in the wild type inhibits at 1 μg/ml; an addition of 5′-MHC decreases the norfloxacin MIC to 0.25 μg/ml.

Ethidium bromide binds to DNA and has a high level of fluorescence, and increase of ethidium bromide causes a decrease in fluorescence. Efflux of ethidium bromide is significant in wild bacterial cells harboring NorA MDR.

Addition of 5′-MHC completely inhibits NorA-dependent efflux of ethidium bromide in wild-type cells. Berberine is a planar catonic molecule that reassembles ethidium bromide and binds to DNA. The DNA binding apparently contributes to the antibacterial activity of berberine. 5′-MHC was reported as a minor component of chaulmoogra oil from seeds of Hydnocarpus trees.

12.2.3. Flavolignan and flavones and derivatives

It was shown that two plant-derived compounds, flavolignan and 5′-MHC, and the porphyrin pheophorbide A are potent inhibitors of NorA of *S. aureus*. Both are bacteriologically inactive but potentiate the inhibitory activities of berberine, norfloxacin, and benzalkonium chloride (Fig. 6) against resistant *S. aureus*.

Many flavolignans, such as (−)-silandrin (isolated from *Silybum marianum*) or scutellaprostin A and B (isolated from *Scutellinia prostata*), were tested in the presence of 30 μg of berberine against resistant *S. aureus*.

A series of flavolignan compounds (Fig. 7) has been synthesized. None of them display antibacterial activity, but some exhibit inhibitory activity (MIC, 125 μg/ml) (Table 34). The compounds with or without free phenolic groups at positions 5 and 7 were comparably active (compounds 6, 9, 10, 18, and 19). The most potent analog (compound 9) completely lacks A-ring OH groups.

The presence of 3-hydroxy groups resulted in markedly decreased activity (compound 11). Some changes in the D-ring played an important role. The majority of flavolignans had 3-methoxy-4-hydroxy groups.

In flavones, a relatively high potency was reduced when 4′ (D-ring) was alkylated, which can lead to various ethers of 4′-hydroflavones.

12.2.4. Pyridoquinolones

E. aerogenes is one of the most commonly encountered nosocomial respiratory pathogens. The *mar* regulon was described for *E. coli*, *Senterica* serovar Typhimurium, *Shigella*

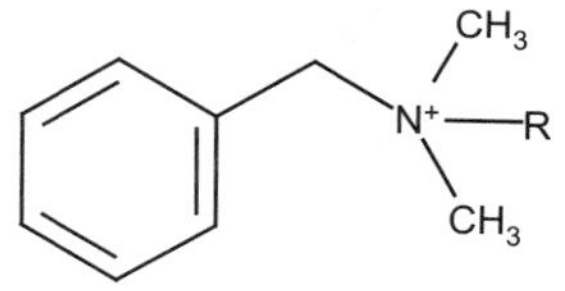

CH_3
N+—R
CH_3

Figure 6 Benzalkonium

Figure 7 5-MHC

Table 34 Antibacterial activities of flavolignan analogs

Compound(s)	MIC (μg/ml)
1	1–2
5	3.1
6	0.1
6a	0.1
8	4–8
9	0.08
10	0.8
10a	1.6
11	
12, 12a	Inactive
14	Inactive
15	3.1
15a	1.6
16	1.9
17	12.5
18	1.9
19	0.6
20	Inactive
21	Inactive

flexneri, *Klebsiella pneumoniae*, and *E. aerogenes*. The MarA activator increases the expression of the AcrAB- TolC pump and decreases porin synthesis.

The 4,6-bis(dimethylaminoethylthio)pyrido[3,2,9] quinolone and 4,6-bis (pyrrolidinoethylthio)pyrido[3,2,9] quinoline (Fig. 8) are effective in restoring fluoroquinolone accumulation in a strain expressing MarA-mediated efflux. The *mar* cascade generates a decrease in porin expression.

12.2.5. MC-02595

C-capped dipeptides (D-ornithine-DhPhe-3-aminoquinoline) potentiate the activity of levofloxacin in *P. aeruginosa*. The compounds exemplified by L-phenylalanine-L-ornithine-β-naphthylamine potentiate levofloxacin activity eightfold at a concentration of 2.5 μg/ml (Fig. 9).

The reference parameter was MPC_8, which is the value needed for the inhibitor to reduce the MIC of levofloxacin eightfold.

The compound is unstable in rat serum. The initial product of serum degradation was L-ornithine-β-naphthylamine and did not potentiate levofloxacin activity.

To overcome the instability, a series of N-methylated derivatives was prepared, and the compound obtained was as active as the nonmethylated analog. However, at pH 2 to 4, it was shown that the 5-amino group of ornithine readily cyclized to form a lactam, liberating β-naphthylamine. The amide linkage of the capping group was replaced with an ether or hydroxyethylene moiety, yielding different compounds

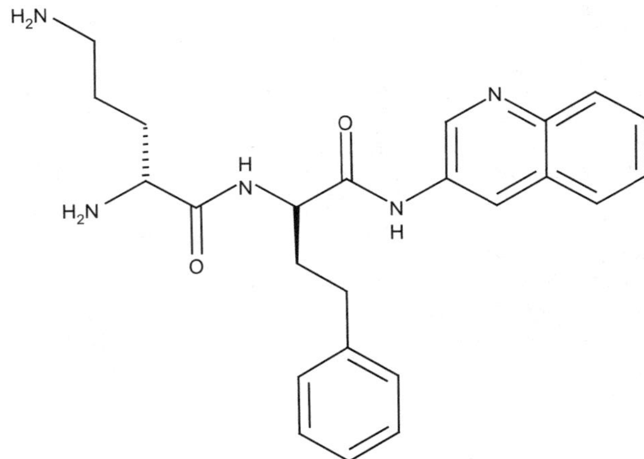

Figure 9 MC-02595

R
Diamethylamino ethyl
Diethylamino ethyl
Dimethylamino propyl
Di-isopropylamino ethyl
Piperidino ethyl
Pyrrolidino ethyl
Morpholino ethyl

Figure 8 Pyridoquinolones

such as L-ornithine-L-phenylalanine-β-naphthylamine which continue to potentiate levofloxacin, but this compound is unstable in rat serum.

Replacement of phenylalanine with homophenylalanine gave a twofold improvement in potentiation.

The replacement of β-naphthylamine with a 3-amino quinoline moiety furnishes the compound with higher potentiator activity.

The stereochemistry of the potentiation was an important parameter yielding MC-02595.

12.2.6. MC-207110

MC-207110 (L-phenylalanine-L-arginine-β-naphthylamine) (Fig. 10) is an inhibitor of the RND efflux pump family. Following the previous series, a new one was prepared. A basic amino acid is a prerequisite for activity.

L-Lysine gave a compound as active as the lead compound with an L-ornithine, but the compound with an L-histidine is devoid of activity.

However, compounds with an L-lysine or an L-ornithine are unstable when incubated with mouse, rat, or human serum at 37°C. The cleavage of the peptide linkage occurred between amino acids 1 and 2 (Fig. 11).

To circumvent the problem, an *N*-methyl compound was prepared. Among 500 analogs, it was shown that substitution of the phenylalanine moiety yields less active compounds, except replacement of phenylalanine by L-homophenylalanine gave rise to a compound twofold more active than those bearing a phenylalanine.

Compounds with a variety of groups, such as 5-aminoindan, aniline, or derivatives, were synthesized; the first was as active as those having a β-naphthylamine group. The series is poorly active or inactive.

When MC-207110 was administered with levofloxacin, a 3-$\log_{10}$ reduction in CFU/ml was recorded after 4 h of contact but was followed by regrowth. There was a significant potentiation, whereas each compound as a single agent was not active.

In studying the structure-activity relationship of toxicity, it was shown that the ornithine residue was the major contributor to toxicity. Analog bioisosters of arginine, which itself is a bioisoster of ornithine, were synthesized. One of the most active compounds was MC-04124 (proline moiety), which displays a protein binding of 68%.

12.2.7. Pheophorbide A

Pheophorbide A (Fig. 12) was isolated first from *Artemisia capillaris*, which belongs to the Compositae family of plants.

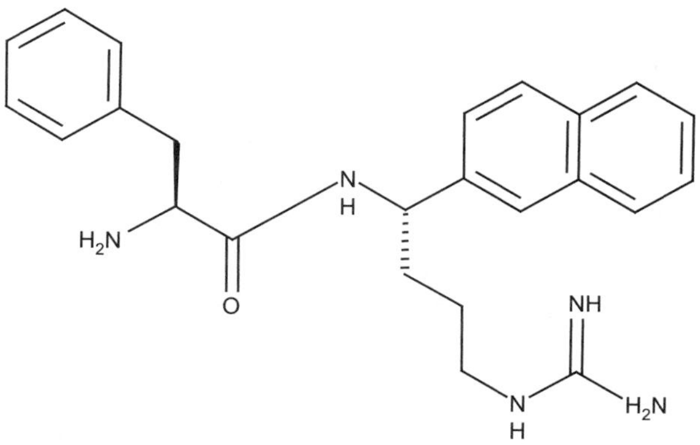

Figure 10 MC-207110

Phosphobide is an intermediate in the natural breakdown of chlorophyll in both the higher plants and algae. It has a porphyrin structure. Some porphinoid-type compounds from cyanobacteria are known anticancer MDR reversal agents that potentiate P-glycoprotein-transported compounds.

12.2.8. UK-57562

UK-57562 (Fig. 13) is a tetracycline efflux reverser. It is devoid of antibacterial activity (MIC, 50 to 100 μg/ml). UK-57562 potentiates tetracycline activity. MICs for *Pasteurella haemolytica* and *E. coli* decreased 8- to 32-fold by 0.5 times the MIC of UK-57508. The effect on gram-positive species, like streptococci and *S. aureus,* is 4-fold.

UK-57562 is able to potentiate tetracycline activity against susceptible strains. UK-57562 potentiates MICs for gram-negative bacteria four- to eightfold.

12.2.9. MC-510050

MC-510050 is a natural product obtained from *Streptomyces* fermentation. The compounds are *O*-sulfate derivatives of benastatins A and B (Fig. 14). They are able to inhibit the MexAB pump from *P. aeruginosa* and lower the MIC of levofloxacin fourfold (concentration of 0.625 μg/ml). A derivative, MC-510051, has a moderate cytotoxicity, which convinced Microcide to halt development of these compounds.

A new series of MC-04124 analogs was prepared in order to explore the physicochemical properties in relation to pharmacokinetics.

The lead compound, MC-04124 (Fig. 15), has two amine moieties and a moderate basicity (pK 9.6 and 6.9; logP, 2.2).

The in vitro activity as an efflux pump inhibitor is dependent upon both basicity and lipophilicity; the ratio of compound level in tissues versus serum did not correlate with any of the physicochemical parameters examined.

12.2.10. MC-510125 and MC-510126

MC-510125 and MC-510126 (MF-BA 1768-α and -β) were obtained in a *Microbispora* sp. isolated from the soil roots of *Arachis hypogaea* in West Java (Indonesia). The two antibiotics are small cyclic peptides (<4 kDa). MC-510125 and MC-510126 are active against gram-positive bacilli (MIC range, 2 to 32 μg/ml). They are rapidly bactericidal (2 h of contact) against *S. aureus*. They are not toxic to the human cell line K-562.

12.2.11. GG 918

GG 918 is a semisynthetic compound that was originally discovered as part of a screening program designed to identify inhibitors of mammalian P-glycoprotein (ABC transporters).

The effects of GG 918 and reserpine are equivalent.

In general, norfloxacin and ciprofloxacin had better potentiation activities. Both fluoroquinolones are quite hydrophilic compounds with small substituents at C-7 and C-8, which made them more favorable substrates for NorA. Levofloxacin and moxifloxacin are more hydrophobic compounds (Table 35).

GG 918 may have affinity for the pump MrsA and Tet K.

12.2.12. Phenothiazines and Thioxanthenes

NorA protein is able to translocate hydrophilic fluoroquinolones, monocationic dyes, and disinfectants. *S. aureus* has a genome size of 2.8 Mb and possesses approximately

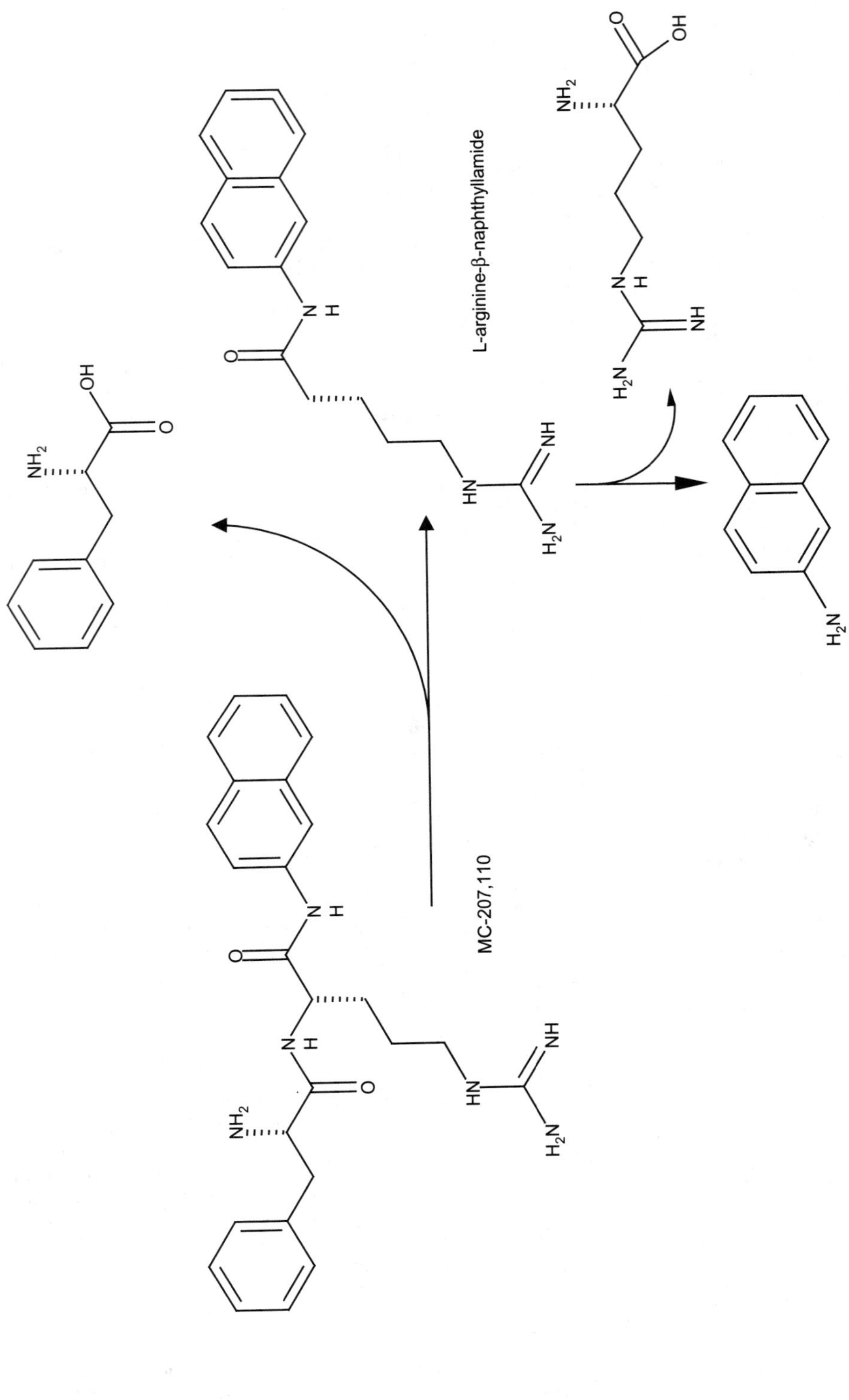

MC-207,110

L-arginine-β-naphthyllamide

β-naphthylamine

Figure 11 Cleavage of MC-207110

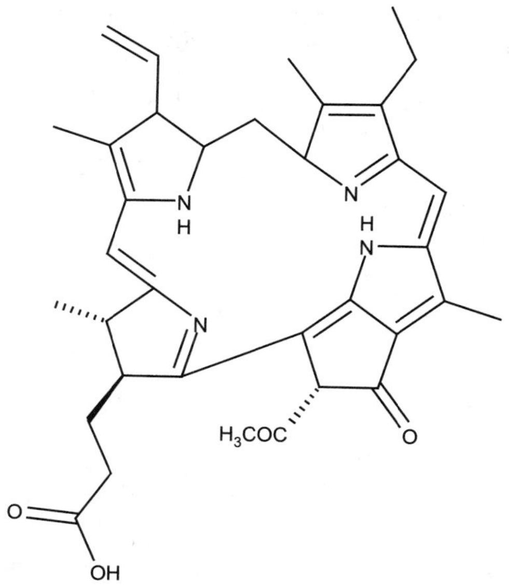

Figure 12 Pheophorbide A

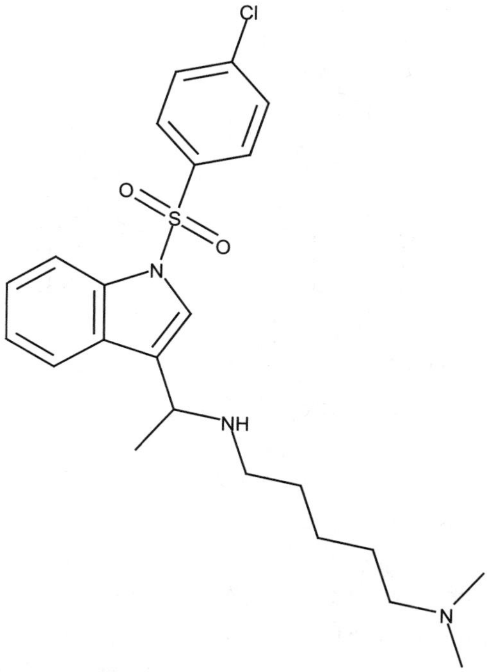

Figure 13 UK-57562

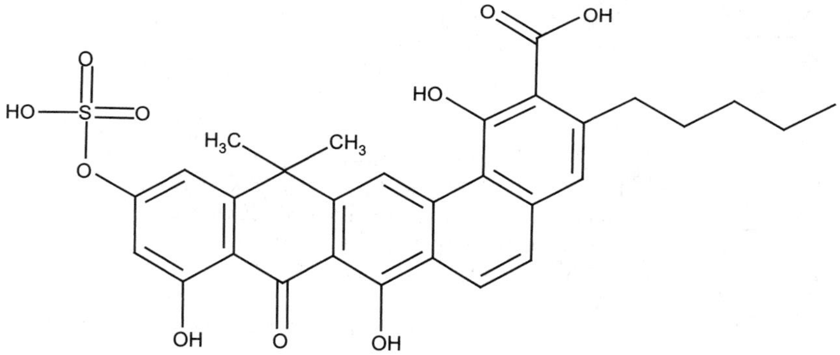

Figure 14 MC-510050

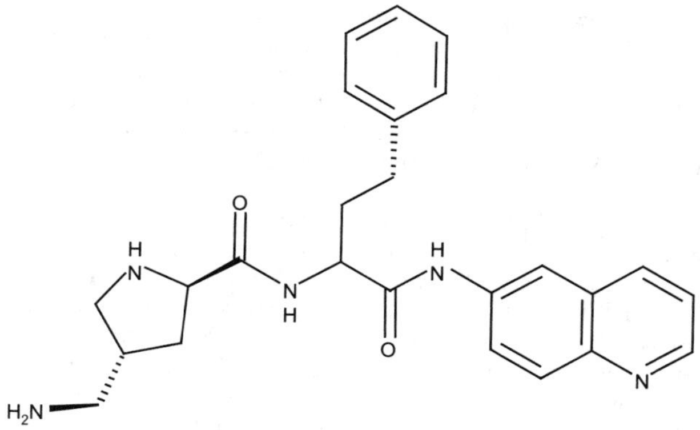

Figure 15 MC-04124

Table 35 Activity of GG 918 against *S. aureus* resistant to fluoroquinolones

Drug(s)	MIC (μg/ml) for *S. aureus* strain:	
	1199 (NorA)	K2068 (MDR)
Norfloxacin	32	8.0
+ GG 918	4.0	2.0
Ciprofloxacin	8.0	0.5
+ GG 918	1.0	1.0
Levofloxacin	1.0	0.5
+ GG 918	0.25	0.25
Moxifloxacin	0.25	0.25
+ GG 918	0.25	0.25
Erythromycin A	0.25	0.5
+ GG 918	0.12	0.5
Tetracycline	0.12	0.5
+ GG 918	0.06	0.5

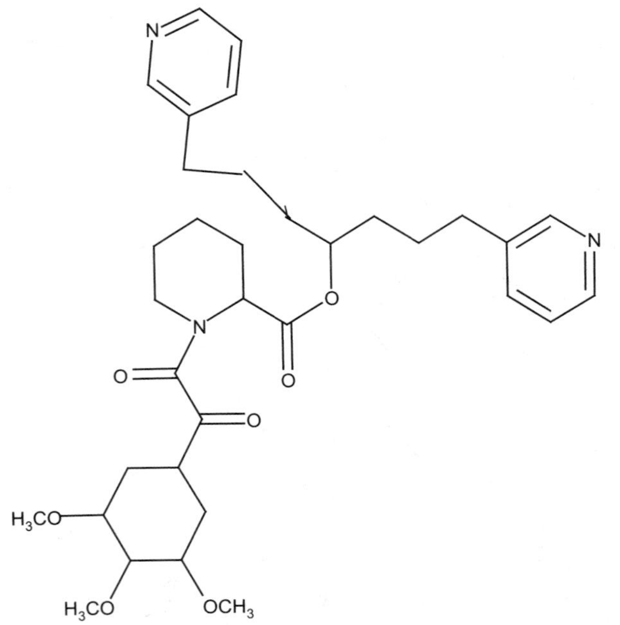

Figure 16 Biricodar

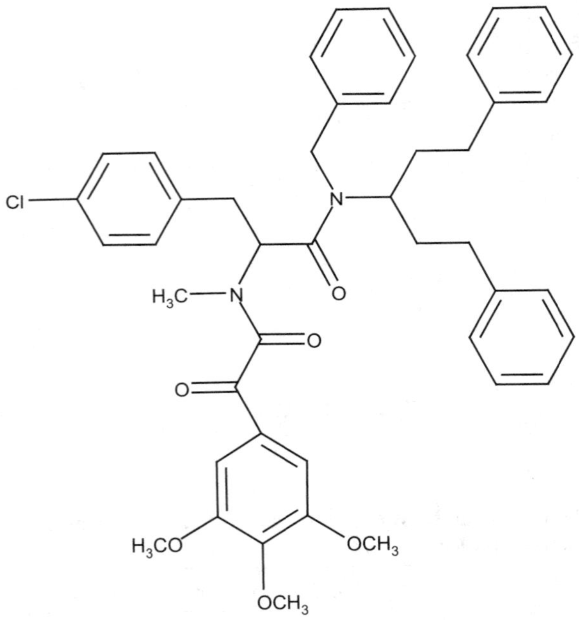

Figure 17 Timcodar

253 ORFs encoding putative transport pumps; of these, 17 may be MDR efflux pumps.

Verapamil and reserpine are able to inhibit the NorA pump, but the concentrations required are too high to be used in clinics.

Phenothiazines and thioxanthene compounds, which are dopamine receptor antagonists, and calmoduline inhibitors are administered as neuroleptics and antiemetics in clinics.

Table 36 Activities of efflux pump inhibitors in combination with antibacterial agents against *S. aureus*

Compound	MIC (μg/ml) without EPI	MIC (μg/ml) with EPI (4 × MEC)[a]		
		Reserpine	Biricodar	Timcodar
Tetracycline	0.25	0.25	0.125	0.25
Novobiocin	0.125	0.06	0.06	0.06
Levofloxacin	025	0.125	0.125	0.125
Ciprofloxacin	0.25	0.06	0.06	0.125
Norfloxacin	1.0	0.5	0.25	0.5
Gatifloxacin	0.5	0.125	0.125	0.25

[a]EPI, efflux pump inhibitor; 4 × MEC, four times the minimum effective concentration.

For thioxanthenes, the compound which is active against coagulase-negative staphylococci is the *cis* isomer, but the two isomers exhibit similar antistaphylococcal activities. However, the *trans* isomer is twofold more potent than the *cis* isomer. Among neuroleptics, possibly prochlorperazine is superior, being equipotent to at least reserpine in terms of inhibitory effect.

12.2.13. Epicatechin Gallate

Epicatechin gallate and epigallocatechin are weakly active against *S. aureus*, with MICs above 32 μg/ml. When incorporated in the growth medium at a concentration of 20 μg/ml, both compounds exhibited a fourfold potentiation of norfloxacin activity (*S. aureus* harboring NorA). Epicatechin gallate is only slightly more active than epigallocatechin.

When less than 20 μg/ml was added to the medium, both compounds paradoxically stimulated efflux.

12.2.14. Timcodar and Biricodar

Biricodar (VX-710) and timcodar (VX-853) are small molecules that inhibit mammalian MDR and confer increased drug susceptibility to cells expressing both P-glycoprotein and MRP-1 (Fig. 16 and 17; Table 36).

12.2.15. Omeprazole and Miscellaneous Compounds

NorA is present in wild-type *S. aureus* and confers a baseline low level of intrinsic resistance to fluoroquinolones and other structurally unrelated compounds. H^+ and K^+ ATPase pump inhibitors such as omeprazole and lansoprazole exert a synergistic activity with fluoroquinolones by restoring their activities. These compounds presumably affect the activity of NorA by affecting the cell proton gradient in a manner analogous to that of CCCP. Omeprazole and lansoprazole produced 4- to-16-fold decreases in the MICs of norfloxacin and ciprofloxacin and 2- to 4-fold decreases for levofloxacin. (These inhibitors were used at 1- and 10-μg/ml concentrations [Table 37].)

The time-kill curves for norfloxacin and ciprofloxacin against *S. aureus* 1199 in combination with omeprazole and lansoprazole showed significant inhibition of growth at the 4- and 8-h points compared with that achieved with norfloxacin or ciprofloxacin alone. Against *S. aureus* 1199-B, the combination of lansoprazole and norfloxacin resulted in better synergy than with other inhibitors. For *S. aureus* 1199-3, a reduction of about 1.5 to 2.5 $\log_{10}$ CFU/ml was observed at the 4- and 8-h points.

Table 37 In vitro activities of omeprazole and miscellaneous compounds against NorA-containing *S. aureus* in combination with fluoroquinolones

S. aureus strain	Compound	MIC (μg/ml)		
		Norfloxacin	Ciprofloxacin	Levofloxacin
1199 (NorA)	FQ alone	0.5	0.25	0.25
	FQ+:			
	Cyclosporine	1.0	0.25	0.125
	Reserpine	0.6	0.06	0.06
	Omeprazole	0.125	0.125	0.125
	Lansoprazole	0.125	0.06	0.125
	Verapamil	0.25	0.125	0.125
	Diltiazem	0.25	0.125	0.125
1199 (NorA inducible)	FQ alone	8.0	4.0	0.5
	FQ + :			
	Cyclosporine	16	8.0	0.5
	Reserpine	0.5	0.25	0.125
	Omeprazole	1.0	0.5	0.125
	Lansoprazole	1.0	0.5	0.125
	Verapamil	2.0	1.0	0.25
	Diltiazem	2.0	2.0	0.5
1199 (NorA constitutive + *grlA*)	FQ alone	32	4.0	1.0
	FQ +			1.0
	Cyclosporine	32	8.0	0.25
	Reserpine	2.0	0.5	0.5
	Omeprazole	4.0	1.0	0.5
	Lansoprazole	4.0	1.0	0.5
	Verapamil	8.0	2.0	0.5
	Diltiazem	16	4.0	0.5

Omeprazole and lansoprazole display moderate activities compared with that of reserpine but significantly higher activity than those of verapamil, diltiazem (channel calcium blockers), and cyclosporine.

REFERENCES

Ainsa JA, Blokpoel MC, Otal I, Young DB, De Smet KA, Martin C, 1998, Molecular cloning and characterization of Tap, a putative multidrug efflux pump present in Mycobacterium fortuitum and Mycobacterium tuberculosis, J Bacteriol, 180, 5836–5843.

Baucheron S, Tyler S, Boyd D, Mulvey MR, Chaslus-Dancla E, Cloeckaert A, 2004, AcrAB-TolC directs efflux-mediated multidrug resistance in Salmonella enterica serovar typhimurium DT104, Antimicrob Agents Chemother, 48, 3729–3735.

Brenwald NP, Appelbaum PC, 2003, Evidence for efflux pumps, other than PmrA, associated with fluoroquinolone resistance in Streptococcus pneumoniae, Clin Microbiol Infect, 9, 140–143.

Brown MH, Paulsen IT, Skurray RA, 1999, The multidrug efflux protein NorM is a prototype of a new family of transporters, Mol Microbiol, 31, 393–395.

Capobianco JO, Cao Z, Shortridge VD, Ma Z, Flamm RK, Zhong P, 2000, Studies of the novel ketolide ABT-773: transport, binding to ribosomes, and inhibition of protein synthesis in Streptococcus pneumoniae, Antimicrob Agents Chemother, 44, 1562–1567.

Chen J, Morita Y, Huda MN, Kuroda T, Mizushima T, Tsuchiya Y, 2002, VmrA, a member of a novel class of Na^+-coupled multidrug efflux pumps from Vibrio parahaemolyticus, J Bacteriol, 184, 572–576.

Chollet R, Chevalier J, Bryskier A, Pages JM, 2004, The AcrAB-TolC pump is involved in macrolide resistance but not in telithromycin efflux in Enterobacter aerogenes and Escherichia coli, Antimicrob Agents Chemother, 48, 3621–3624.

Clarebout G, Villers C, Leclercq R, 2001, Macrolide resistance gene mreA of Streptococcus agalactiae encodes a flavokinase, Antimicrob Agents Chemother, 45, 2280–2286.

Colmer JA, Fralick JA, Hamood AN, 1998, Isolation and characterization of a putative multidrug resistance pump from Vibrio cholerae, Mol Microbiol, 27, 63–72.

Dridi L, Tankovic J, Petit JC, 2004, CdeA of Clostridium difficile, a new multidrug efflux transporter of the MATE family, Microb Drug Resist, 10, 191–196.

Gibbons S, Udo EE, 2000, The effect of reserpine, a modulator of multidrug efflux pumps, on the in vitro activity of tetracycline against clinical isolates of methicillin resistant Staphylococcus aureus (MRSA) possessing the tet(K) determinant, Phytother Res, 14, 139–140.

Guz NR, Stermitz FR, Johnson JB, Beeson TD, Willen S, Hsiang J, Lewis K, 2001, Flavonolignan and flavone inhibitors of a Staphylococcus aureus multidrug resistance pump, structure-activity relationships, Med Chem, 44, 261–268.

He GX, Kuroda T, Mima T, Morita Y, Mizushima T, Tsuchiya T, 2004, An H^+-coupled multidrug efflux pump, PmpM, a member of the MATE faily of transporters, from Pseudomonas aeruginosa, J Bacteriol, 186, 262–265.

Hendricks O, Butterworth TS, Kristiansen JE, 2003, The in-vitro antimicrobial effect of non-antibiotics and putative inhibitors of efflux pumps on Pseudomonas aeruginosa and Staphylococcus aureus, Int J Antimicrob Agents, 22, 262–264.

Higgins MK, Bokma E, Koronakis E, Hughes C, Koronakis V, 2004, Structure of the periplasmic component of a bacterial drug efflux pump, Proc Natl Acad Sci USA, 101, 9994–9999.

Huda MN, Morita Y, Kuroda T, Mizushima T, Tsuchiya T, 2003, Na^+-driven multidrug efflux pump VcmA from Vibrio cholerae non-O1, a non-halophilic bacterium, FEMS Microbial Lett, 203, 235–239.

Huda N, Chen J, Morita Y, Kuroda T, Mizushima T, Tsuchiya T, 2003, Gene cloning and characterization of VcrM, a Na+-coupled multidrug efflux pump, from Vibrio cholerae non-O1, Microbiol Immunol, 47, 419–427.

Jo JT, Brinkman FS, Hancock RE, 2003, Aminoglycoside efflux in Pseudomonas aeruginosa, involvement of novel outer membrane proteins, Antimicrob Agents Chemother, 47, 1101–1111.

Jonas BM, Murray BE, Weinstock GM, 2001, Characterization of emeA, a NorA homolog and multidrug resistance efflux pump, in Enterococcus faecalis, Antimicrob Agents Chemother, 45, 3574–3579.

Kristiansen MM, Leandro C, Ordway D, Martins M, Viveiros M, Pacheco T, Kristiansen JE, Amaral L, 2003, Phenothiazines alter resistance of methicillin-resistant strains of Staphylococcus aureus (MRSA) to oxacillin in vitro, Int J Antimicrob Agents, 22, 250–253.

Lee EH, Rouquette-Loughlin C, Folster JP, Shafer WM, 2003, FarR regulates the farAB-encoded efflux pump of Neisseria gonorrhoeae via an MtrR regulatory mechanism, J Bacteriol, 185, 7145–7152.

Lee EH, Shafer WM, 1999, The farAB-encoded efflux pump mediates resistance of gonococci to long-chain antibacterial fatty acids, Mol Microbiol, 33, 839–845.

Lee EW, Huda MN, Kuroda T, Mizushima T, Tsuchiya T, 2003, EfrAB, an ABC multidrug efflux pump in Enterococcus faecalis, Antimicrob Agents Chemother, 47, 3733–3738.

Levy SB, 2002, Active efflux, a common mechanism for biocide and antibiotic resistance, Symp Ser Soc Appl Microbiol, 31, 65S–71S.

Lewis K, 2001, In search of natural substrates and inhibitors of MDR pumps, J Mol Microbiol Biotechnol, 3, 247–254.

Lin J, Michel LO, Zhang Q, 2002, CmeABC functions as a multidrug efflux system in Campylobacter jejuni, Antimicrob Agents Chemother, 46, 2124–2131.

Lomovskaya O, Warren MS, Lee A, Galazzo J, Fronko R, Lee M, Blais J, Cho D, Chamberland S, Renau T, Leger R, Hecker S, Watkins W, Hoshino K, Ishida H, Lee VJ, 2001, Identification and characterization of inhibitors of multidrug resistance efflux pumps in Pseudomonas aeruginosa: novel agents for combination therapy, Antimicrob Agents Chemother, 45, 105–116.

Lomovskaya O, Watkins W, 2001, Inhibition of efflux pumps as a novel approach to combat drug resistance in bacteria, J Mol Microbiol Biotechnol, 3, 225–236.

Lomovskaya O, Watkins WJ, 2001, Efflux pumps, their role in antibacterial drug discovery, Curr Med Chem, 8, 1699–1711.

Mallea M, Mahamoud A, Chevalier J, Alibert-Franco S, Brouant P, Barbe J, Pages JM, 2003, Alkylaminoquinolines inhibit the bacterial antibiotic efflux pump in multidrug-resistant clinical isolates, Biochem J, 376, 801–815.

McAleese F, Petersen P, Ruzin A, Dunman PM, et al, 2005, A novel MATE family efflux pump contributes to the reduced susceptibility of laboratory-derived Staphylococcus aureus mutants to tigecycline, Antimicrob Agents Chemother, 49, 1865–1871.

Miyamae S, Ueda O, Yoshimura F, Hwang J, Tanaka Y, Nikaido H, 2001, A MATE family multidrug efflux transporter pumps out fluoroquinolones in Bacteroides thetaiotaomicron, Antimicrob Agents Chemother, 45, 3341–3346.

Mullin S, Mani N, Grossman TH, 2004, Inhibition of antibiotic efflux in bacteria by the novel multidrug resistance inhibitors biricodar (VX-710) and timcodar (VX-853), Antimicrob Agents Chemother 48, 4171–4176.

Musumeci R, Speciale A, Costanzo R, Annino A, Ragusa S, Rapisarda A, Pappalardo MS, Iauk L, 2003, Berberis aetnensis C. Presl. extracts: antimicrobial properties and interaction with ciprofloxacin, Int J Antimicrob Agents, 22, 48–53.

Nakayama K, Ishida Y, Ohtsuka M, Kawato H, Yoshida K, Yokomizo Y, Hosono S, Ohta T, Hoshino K, Ishida H, Yoshida K, Renau TE, Leger R, Zhang JZ, Lee VJ, Watkins WJ, 2003a, MexAB-OprM-specific efflux pump inhibitors in Pseudomonas aeruginosa. Part 1. Discovery and early strategies for lead optimization, Bioorg Med Chem Lett, 13, 4201–4204.

Nakayama K, Ishida Y, Ohtsuka M, Kawato H, Yoshida K, Yokomizo Y, Ohta T, Hoshino K, Otani T, Kurosaka Y, Yoshida K, Ishida H, Lee VJ, Renau TE, Watkins WJ, 2003b, MexAB-OprM specific efflux pump inhibitors in Pseudomonas aeruginosa. Part 2. Achieving activity in vivo through the use of alternative scaffolds, Bioorg Med Chem Lett, 13, 4205–4208.

Nikaido H, 1998, Antibiotic resistance caused by gram-negative multidrug efflux pumps, Clin Infect Dis, 27, Suppl 1, S32–S41.

Nikaido H, Zgurskaya HI, 2001, AcrAB and related multidrug efflux pumps of Escherichia coli, J Mol Microbiol Biotechnol, 3, 15–18.

Peric M, Bozdogan B, Jacobs MR, Appelbaum PC, 2003, Effects of an efflux mechanism and ribosomal mutations on macrolide susceptibility of Haemophilus influenzae clinical isolates, Antimicrob Agents Chemother, 47, 1017–1022.

Renau TE, Leger R, Flamme EM, Sangalang J, She MW, Yen R, Gannon CL, Griffith D, Chamberland S, Lomovskaya O, Hecker SJ, Lee VJ, Ohta T, Nakayama K, 1999, Inhibitors of efflux pumps in Pseudomonas aeruginosa potentiate the activity of the fluoroquinolone antibacterial levofloxacin, J Med Chem, 42, 4928–4931.

Renau TE, Leger R, Filonova L, Flamme EM, Wang M, Yen R, Madsen D, Griffith D, Chamberland S, Dudley MN, Lee VJ, Lomovskaya O, Watkins WJ, Ohta T, Nakayama K, Ishida Y, 2003, Conformationally-restricted analogues of efflux pump inhibitors that potentiate the activity of levofloxacin in Pseudomonas aeruginosa, Bioorg Med Chem Lett, 13, 2755–2758.

Rosenberg EY, Bertenthal D, Nilles ML, Bertrand KP, Nikaido H, 2003, Bile salts and fatty acids induce the expression of Escherichia coli AcrAB multidrug efflux pump through their interaction with Rob regulatory protein, Mol Microbiol, 48, 1609–1619.

Siddiqi N, Das R, Pathak N, Banerjee S, Ahmed N, Katoch VM, Hasnain SE, 2004, Mycobacterium tuberculosis isolate with a distinct genomic identity overexpresses a tap-like efflux pump, Infection, 32, 109–111.

Singh KV, Weinstock GM, Murrary BE, 2002, An Enterococcus faecalis ABC homologue (Lsa) is required for the resistance of this species to clindamycin and quinupristin-dalfopristin, Animicrob Agents Chemother, 46, 1845–1850.

Steinfels E, Orelle C, Fantino JR, Dalmas O, Rigaud JL, Denizot F, Di Pietro A, Jault JM, 2004, Characterization of YvcC (BmrA), a multidrug ABC transporter constitutively expressed in Bacillus subtilis, Biochemistry, 43, 7491–7502.

Stermitz FR, Lorenz P, Tawara JN, Zenewicz LA, Lewis K, 2000, Synergy in a medicinal plant: antimicrobial action of berberine potentiated by 5′-methoxyhydnocarpin, a multidrug pump inhibitor, Proc Natl Acad Sci USA, 97, 1433–1437.

Sudano Roccaro A, Blanco AR, Giuliano F, Rusciano D, Enea V, 2004, Epigallocatechin-gallate enhances the activity of tetracycline in staphylococci by inhibiting its efflux from bacterial cells, Antimicrob Agents Chemother, 48, 1968–1973.

Sutcliffe J, Grebe T, Tait-Kamradt A, Wondrack L, 1996, Detection of erythromycin-resistant determinants by PCR, Antimicrob Agents Chemother, 40, 2562–2566.

Truong-Bolduc QC, Zhang X, Hooper DC, 2003, Characterization of NorR protein, a multifunctional regulator of norA expression in Staphylococcus aureus, J Bacteriol, 185, 3127–3138.

Van Bambeke F, Balzi E, Tulkens PM, 2000, Antibiotic efflux pumps, Biochem Pharmacol, 60, 457–470.

Xu XJ, Su XZ, Morita Y, Kuroda T, Mizushima T, Tsuchiya T, 2003, Molecular cloning and characterization of the HmrM multidrug efflux pump from Haemophilus influenzae Rd, Microbiol Immunol, 47, 937–943.

Yang S, Clayton SR, Zechiedrich EL, 2003, Relative contributions of the AcrAB, MdfA and NorE efflux pumps to quinolone resistance in Escherichia coli, J Antimicrob Chemother, 51, 545–556.

Paldimycin

A. BRYSKIER

1. INTRODUCTION

Paldimycin belongs to the group of antibiotics containing an isothiocyanate group. Three groups of molecules have been isolated: the proceomycins (Tsukiura et al., 1964), senfolomycins A and B (Mitsher et al., 1966) and the paulomycins (Wiley et al., 1986).

1.1. Proceomycin

Proceomycin was isolated from the fermentation broth of *Streptomyces albolongus* sp. nov. (Tsukiura et al., 1964). It is a weak acid, the powder of which has a yellow-orange color, and it inhibits the growth of a number of gram-positive cocci. It is inactive against *Enterobacteriaceae* (MIC, >25 μg/ml) and against *Pseudomonas aeruginosa* (MIC, >25 μg/ml). The MICs are ≤0.1 μg/ml for *Staphylococcus aureus* and coagulase-negative staphylococci. For *Streptococcus pneumoniae* and *Enterococcus faecalis* they are, respectively, 0.39 and 1.56 μg/ml. The median lethal doses in the mouse after subcutaneous, intravenous, and oral administration are, respectively, 180, 26.6, and 3,750 mg/kg.

The structure of proceomycin has not been well established, but it contains an isothiocyanate group. The physicochemical properties are summarized in Table 1.

1.2. Senfolomycins A and B

Senfolomycins A and B were isolated from the fermentation products of *Streptomyces ochrosporus* sp. nov. (NRRL 3146). The physicochemical properties are summarized in Table 1. They have good activity against *S. aureus* (MIC, ~0.2 μg/ml) and *E. faecalis* (MIC, ~0.78 μg/ml), but they are inactive against gram-negative bacilli (Mitsher et al., 1966).

1.3. Paulomycins

The paulomycin complex is produced by fermentation of *Streptomyces paulus* 273 (Wiley et al., 1986). It has been possible to isolate paulomycins A and B, paldimycins A and B (products 273a1α [A] and 273a1β [B]), and products 273a2α and 273a2β.

2. STRUCTURE OF THE PAULOMYCINS

See Fig. 1.

The six molecules possess an isothiocyanate group. The paulomycins differ from one another in the group at R_1, which is a 2-methylbutyryl for paulomycin A and an isobutyryl for paulomycin B. The paldimycins and the 273a2 compounds are produced by the addition of two and one *N*-acetyl-L-cysteine, respectively, to paulomycins A and B.

3. PHYSICOCHEMICAL PROPERTIES

These molecules are weak acids and have high molecular weights (Table 2).

4. IN VITRO ACTIVITY

Paldimycin exhibits optimal antibacterial activity when the pH of the culture medium is less than 7. It is much more active when tests are performed in nutrient broth than in Mueller-Hinton medium (Pohlod et al., 1987). This difference appears to be due to the greater stability of paldimycin in nutrient broth.

Paldimycin has good activity against *S. aureus* and coagulase-negative staphylococci, irrespective of whether the strains are methicillin susceptible or resistant (Table 3)

Table 1 Physicochemical properties of proceomycin and senfolomycins

Parameter	Proceomycin	Senfolomycin A	Senfolomycin B
Molecular mass (Da)	734.4	845.9	864
Melting point (°C)	100–105	122–124°C	
Specific rotation ($[\alpha]^{25}$)	−2.2° (ethanol)	−58° (methanol)	−60° (methanol)
pK	−6.73		
UV (ethanol) (nm)	235, 275, 325	236, 277, 322	236, 277, 322
Infrared (cm^{-1})	2,060	2,050	2,050

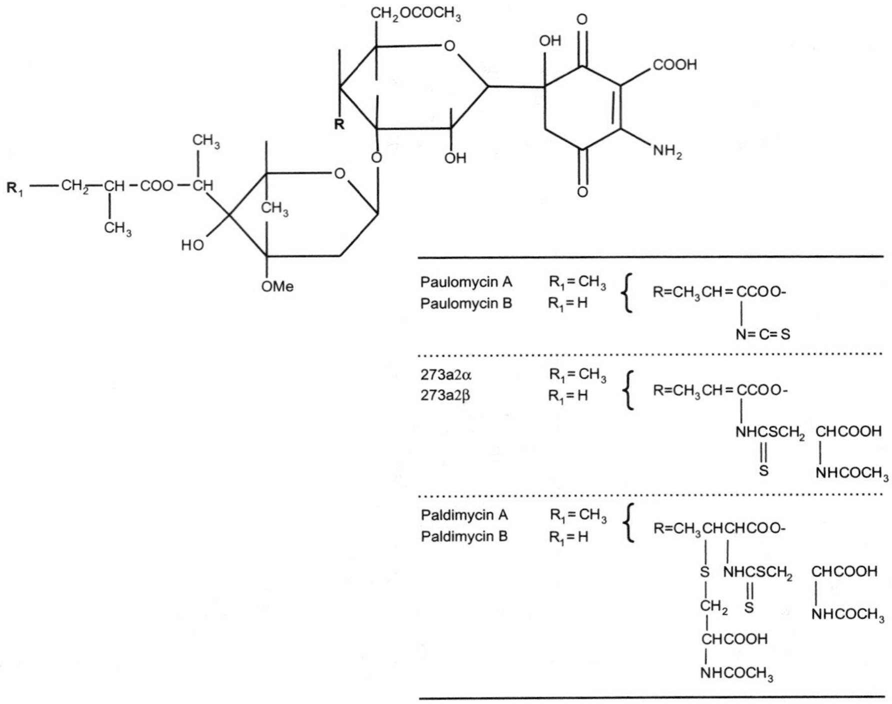

Paulomycin A	$R_1=CH_3$	R=$CH_3CH=C(N=C=S)COO-$
Paulomycin B	$R_1=H$	
273a2α	$R_1=CH_3$	R=$CH_3CH=C(NHC(=S)SCH_2CH(NHCOCH_3)COOH)COO-$
273a2β	$R_1=H$	
Paldimycin A	$R_1=CH_3$	R=$CH_3CH(SCH_2CH(NHCOCH_3)COOH)CH(NHC(=S)SCH_2CH(NHCOCH_3)COOH)COO-$
Paldimycin B	$R_1=H$	

Figure 1 Paulomycin classification

Table 2 Physicochemical properties of paulomycins

Parameter	Paulomycin A	Paulomycin B	Paldimycin A[a]	Paldimycin B[a]	273a2α	273a2β
Empirical formula	$C_{34}H_{46}N_2O_{17}S$	$C_{33}H_{44}N_2O_{17}S$	$C_{44}H_{64}N_4O_{23}S$	$C_{42}H_{62}N_4O_{23}S$	$C_{39}H_{55}N_3O_{23}S_2$	$C_{38}H_{53}N_3O_{20}S_2$
MW	786.25	772	1,112	1,098	949	935
Melting point (°C)	95–105	105–143	120	120	119–150	122
Specific rotation ($[\alpha]^{25}$)	−22°	−28°	631°	−35°	−33.6°	−34°
pK	3/7.4	3/7.4	3.8–4	3.8–4	3.8–4	3.8–4

[a]Paldimycin: U70, 138E, or 273a1.

Table 3 Activity of paldimycin against gram-positive bacteria

Organism(s)	MIC$_{50}$ (μg/ml)	
	Paldimycin	Vancomycin
S. aureus Pen[s]	0.5	1.0
S. aureus Met[s]	0.5	1.0
S. aureus Met[r]	0.5	1.0
Staphylococcus epidermidis Met[s]	0.125	2.0
S. epidermidis Met[r]	0.125	2.0
Staphylococcus haemolyticus	0.5	2.0
Staphylococcus saprophyticus	0.5	0.8
Staphylococcus hominis	0.25	1.0
Streptococcus pyogenes	0.06	0.5
Streptococcus agalactiae	0.125	0.5
S. pneumoniae	0.06	0.25
Group G streptococci	0.125	0.25
E. faecalis	1.0	1.0
C. jeikeium	≤0.03	1.0
L. monocytogenes	2.0	1.0
Bacillus cereus	2.0	1.0

(Brumfitt et al., 1987; Pfaller et al., 1987). Among the molecules that manifest good activity against methicillin-resistant strains of *S. aureus*, paldimycin is one of the most active (Table 4) (Maple et al., 1989). It is bactericidal against staphylococci (Chandrasekar and Sluchak, 1989).

It is highly active against Lancefield group A and B streptococci and against *E. faecalis*.

Paldimycin has moderate activity against *Listeria monocytogenes* (MIC at which 50% of isolates tested are inhibited

Table 4 Antistaphylococcal activity

Drug	MIC (μg/ml)	
	50%	90%
Vancomycin	1.5	2.2
Teicoplanin	0.8	1.2
Ramoplanin	0.5	1.0
Paldimycin	0.17	0.5
DUP-721	1.6	3.0
DUP-105	5.2	7.4

Table 5 Activity of paldimycin against gram-positive anaerobic bacteria

Organism	MIC$_{50}$ (μg/ml)		
	Paldimycin	Daptomycin	Vancomycin
Peptostreptococcus anaerobius	1.0	≤0.12	0.5
Peptostreptococcus magnus	8.0	≤0.12	1.0
Clostridium perfringens	8.0	0.25	1.0
Clostridium difficile	32	≤0.12	1.0
Lactobacillus	32	2.0	1.0
Eubacterium lentum	8.0	4.0	8.0
Propionibacterium acnes	8.0	0.5	1.0
Bifidobacterium	16	0.5	1.0
Actinomyces	16	0.25	0.5

[MIC$_{50}$], ~2 μg/ml), but it has good activity against *Corynebacterium jeikeium* (MIC$_{50}$, ≤0.03 μg/ml) (Rolston et al., 1987).

In comparison with daptomycin and vancomycin, paldimycin has moderate activity against anaerobic gram-positive bacilli (Table 5) (Chow and Cheng, 1988). However, the tests were performed on Wilkins-Chalgren medium at pH 6.8 and supplemented with cations, whereas it has been shown that the cation content and the nature of the medium affect the in vitro activity. Paldimycin appears to be active against *Chlamydia trachomatis* (Stamm et al., 1986).

It is inactive against anaerobic gram-negative bacilli (MIC, >64 μg/ml).

It appears to act by inhibiting protein synthesis.

REFERENCES

Argoudelis AD, Baczynskyj L, Buege JA, Marshall VP, Mizsak SA, Wiley PF, 1987, Paulomycin-related antibiotics: palimycins and antibiotic 273a$_2$. Isolation and characterization, J Antibiot, 40, 408–418.

Argoudelis AD, Baczynskyj L, Mizsak SA, Shilliday FB, Spinelli PA, Dezwaan J, 1987, Paldimycins A and B and antibiotics 273a$_{2a}$ and 273a$_{2\beta}$—synthesis and characterization, J Antibiot, 40, 419–436.

Argoudelis AD, Brinkley TA, Brodasky TF, Buege JA, Meyer HF, Mizsak SA, 1982, Paulomycins A and B—isolation and characterization, J Antibiot, 35, 285–294.

Brumfitt W, Hamilton-Miller JMT, Whiter G, 1987, Paldimycin: a novel antibiotic highly active against Gram-positive bacteria, J Antimicrob Chemother, 19, 405–406.

Carley NH, Wadsworth SJ, Starr E, Truant AL, Suh B, 1989, In vitro susceptibilities of Campylobacter pylori to quinolone and selected antibiotics, Clin Res, 37, 425A.

Chandrasekar PH, Sluchak JA, 1989, Susceptibility of staphylococci to paldimycin, and emergence of resistance, in vitro, J Antimicrob Chemother, 24, 821–824.

Chow AW, Cheng N, 1988, In vitro activities of daptomycin (LY 146032) and paldimycin (U-70138F) against anaerobic gram-positive bacteria, Antimicrob Agents Chemother, 32, 788–790.

Maple PAC, Hamilton-Milller JMT, Brumfitt W, 1989, Comparative in-vitro activity of vancomycin, teicoplanin, ramoplanin (formerly A 16686), paldimycin, DO 721 and DO 105 against methicillin and gentamicin resistant Staphylococcus aureus, J Antimicrob Chemother, 23, 517–525.

Mitsher LA, McCrae W, DeVoe SE, Shay AJ, Hausmann WK, Bohonos N, 1966, Senfolomycin A and B, new antibiotics, Antimicrob Agents Chemother, 1965, 828–831.

Pfaller MA, Bale M, Barrett M, 1987, In-vitro activity of paldimycin against methicillin-resistant and susceptible isolates of Staphylococcus aureus and S. epidermidis, J Antimicrob Chemother, 20, 286–288.

Pohlod DJ, Saravolatz LD, Somerville MM, 1987, In vitro susceptibility of gram-positive cocci to paldimycin, Antimicrob Agents Chemother, 31, 104–107.

Rolston KVI, LeBlanc B, Ho DH, Bodey GP, 1987, In vitro activity of paldimycin (U-70138F) against gram-positive bacteria isolated from patients with cancer, Antimicrob Agents Chemother, 31, 650–652.

Stamm WE, Suchland R, 1986, Antimicrobial activity of U-70138F (paldimycin), roxithromycin (RU 965), and ofloxacin (ORF 18489) against *Chlamydia trachomatis* in cell culture, Antimicrob Agents Chemother, 30, 806–807.

Tsukiura H, Okanishi M, Koshiyama H, Ohmori T, Miyaki T, Kawaguchi H, 1964, Proceomycin, a new antibiotic, J Antibiot, 17, series A, 223–229.

Wiley PF, Mizsak SA, Baczynskyj L, Argoudelis AD, Duchamp DJ, Watt W, 1986, The structure and chemistry of paulomycin, J Org Chem, 51, 2493–2499.

Antituberculosis Agents

ANDRÉ BRYSKIER AND JACQUES GROSSET

43

1. INTRODUCTION AND HISTORY OF TB

1.1. History of TB

Tuberculosis (TB) is a chronic, necrotic, and communicable infectious disease caused by a group of mycobacteria that includes *Mycobacterium tuberculosis*. It affects the lung, but any body site in the body can be involved. TB, or phthisis (from the Greek, meaning wasting away or consumption), was called the "white plague" by René Dubos in 1952, and has also been called the King of Disease or Captain of Death. TB was present at the dawn of humankind. Skeletal remains of prehistoric humans dating back to 8000 BCE found in Germany have shown evidence of the disease. Egyptian skeletons dating from 2500 to 1000 BCE, skeletons from the Nubian dynasty, and skeletons from nomadic desert-living tribes have revealed Pott disease of the spine.

Herodotus (484–425 BCE) described the exclusion of those afflicted with leprosy and scrofulous lesions. Hippocrates (460–377 BCE) gave a description and used the name phthisis. Galen and Coelius Aurelianus, as well as Arété of Cappadocia, described the illness during the Roman period.

Ancient Chinese writings have documented the presence of the disease, as did the "Luminary Surrata" from India in 500 AD. Hebrews knew the illness (Leviticus 21:16). The sickness was described in detail in the Babylonian Talmud, which was compiled in the fifth and sixth centuries AD. In the Americas, the best proof of TB came from an Inca mummy dated from 700 AD and subsequent cases in South America. Herds of bison were infected with *M. tuberculosis*. In the New World, TB appears to have predated the arrival of Christopher Columbus and other settlers. However, TB-like lesions seem to have been confined mainly in sedentary agriculturally based communities and were rare among groups of hunters, who were less exposed to crowding. The peak figure reached in New England was 1,600 per 10^5 inhabitants. With industrial development, the epidemic spread to the Midwest years later. The peak was reached in 1840 in New Orleans, La., and in the West in 1880. There were few problems among American Indians since they were gathered on reservations; the peak of the epidemic in this population was reached in 1910. The epidemic swamped the Northeast. The Alaskans and American Indians were the last populations to be involved by the TB epidemic.

TB was unknown in sub-Saharan Africa until recently; Livingstone (1857) found no TB in South Africa. The Hawaiian Islands had little or no TB in the mid-1800s. Priests who explored the Great Lakes regions in the 19th century reported rare cases of glandular infections and chronic pulmonary infections that were probably of tubercular nature. Tubercular changes in the vertebral skeleton have been found in remains in 9 of 290 persons in Ohio dated to 1275 AD.

The study of TB began during the Renaissance in the early 16th century, when Giralomo Frascator (1483–1555) recognized the contagious nature of TB.

The transmission of TB was demonstrated by Jean Antoine Villemin (1827–1892) in 1868. Airborne transmission was suspected in 1862 by Louis Pasteur but was proven by William Wells in 1934. However, transmission by expectoration was referred to in cuneiform writings. Hippocratus and Isocrates (436–338 BCE) accepted this mode of transmission.

After the school of Cos and Alexandria ceased to exist, Arabs took over. Avicenna (980–1037) studied TB, continuing the work of Izshak Seraphion (circa 820). The convincing nature of the bacterial origin of TB was put forward by Robert Koch in 1882 with the description of *M. tuberculosis*. That TB was due to a microorganism was discovered in 1722 by Benjamin Marten in London, England. The development of the acid-fast stain by Paul Ehrlich in 1885, modified by Ziehl and Neelsen, and the discovery by Roentgen in 1895 of X rays made possible and more accurate the diagnosis of the disease.

The name "tuberculosis" derived from the description by Francis Sylvius (1614–1672) of minitubercles in the lungs of patients who died from TB. The name was introduced into medicine by J. L. Schönlein (1793–1864).

The pathology of TB was described by Pierre Descaut in 1733 and Gaspard Laurent Bayle in 1810, who published a book entitled *Recherche sur la phtisie pulmonaire*. But the real clinical approach was allowed after the research of Hyacinthe Laennec (1781–1826), who published his famous treatise of medicine in 1819 and in 1826 titled *Auscultation Mediate*.

During this period, numerous well-known persons suffered from TB, such as the children of Catherine de Medici (Henri III and Charles IX, who were kings of France), and many are supposed to have died from TB infection, such as

Molière, Joseph II of Austria, the Cardinal Richelieu, John Calvin, Frederic Chopin, Friedrich Von Schiller, and Laennec.

Extrapulmonary TB was recognized gradually. Pleural effusion was described by Landouzy, and pericarditis was observed by Sénac in 1819 and Corvisart in 1806. Tuberculous meningitis was suspected by Morgagni in 1761 and Whytt in 1768; the diagnosis was made possible by Quincke's use of lumbar punction. The etiology of phthisis and scrofula was found to be the same by P. Dessault in 1733. Percival Pott (1713–1788) and Jacques Matthieu Delpech (1777–1832) described TB in bone and joints.

All of these extrapulmonary manifestations were attributed to M. *tuberculosis* for the first time in 1679 by Sylvius de la Pöe and confirmed two centuries later by H. Laennec and Louis (1885). Many controversies arose between the laboratories of Laennec and Virchow (1821–1902).

1.2. History of Therapies

1.2.1. Prechemotherapy Era

TB treatment does not solve the problem of the disease; even though numerous anti-M. *tuberculosis* agents exist, several persons die each year from TB.

In industrialized countries many efforts were made to eradicate *Mycobacterium bovis* among cattle herds. One of the oldest descriptions of therapy for TB is in the Ayurveda from India, which recommends lukewarm baths, effusion of water in the absence of fever, and massage with sesame oil. In the 10th century B.C.E., walking, high altitudes, and fresh air were recommended, along with a diet composed of meat, vegetables, and milk mixed with honey, pepper, and citrus juice. In China in the pre-Christian era, tussilago (infusions), ginseng, roots, caraway, thuja leaves, cardamom leaves, violet, jujubes, coltsfoot with opium, ground hartshorn, arsenic, and phosphate were common prescriptions.

In ancient Greece, physicians advocated baths in lukewarm water and hot ablutions, but not on the head. In the presence of fever, red and white wines as well as milk mixed with hydromel and with animal blood were recommended. Hippocrates added hydrotherapy and psychological treatments.

In ancient Rome, medical potions were brewed from mixtures of figs, hyssop, mint, common horehound, and lily seeds. Turpentine and vinegar were used as well, for coughing and pulmonary hemorrhages, respectively. Grapes, sodium carbonate, arsenic, and copper were added to concocted medicines, and cupping glasses were applied.

The ancient Hebrews followed recipes in the Babylonian Talmud which recommended a special mixture containing chopped mangold, chopped leeks, jujubes, lentils, caraway, and chabla, stuffed into a sausage skin coming from a first-born animal, all washed down with a strong beer.

Arab physicians in Salerno, Italy, added milk baths and medicines concocted from pine cones, opium, arsenic, sulfur, myrrh, oxymel, and opobalm.

In the Middle Ages, Hildegard of Bingen (1098–1179) recommended a mixture of balmony, caraway, muscat, chamomile, and sweet-scented herbs to make the potion pleasant to absorb. She proposed staying indoors if the air was damp or foggy. Throughout the Middle Ages, apothecaries ordered decoctions of lungwort for pulmonary diseases.

Scrofula, defined as TB of the lymphatic gland, has afflicted humankind for thousands of years. In the Middle Ages, the European name of the illness was "King's Evil." Miraculous cures were not uncommon incidents in the lives of emeritus and saintly kings. Clovis the First (466–511 A.D.) was the first Roman Catholic king of France to claim to cure scrofula after his baptism in 466 following his victory in the battle of Tolbiac. The "royal touch" was practiced in England from Edward the Confessor to Queen Anne in the 18th century. After being chosen by a priest and touched by the ruler, patients received a gold coin which was to protect them from subsequent scrofulous attacks. Newly crowned kings of France and England were believed to have special healing powers. Edward the Confessor washed the neck of a scrofulous and infertile woman; her scrofula disappeared and within a year she gave birth to twins. It was said that King Charles II of England touched more than 90,000 people during his rule.

Modern therapies, including the use of high altitude, were advocated for the first time by Florence Nightingale (1820–1910).

Specific establishments were set up in 1645 in the city of Reims, France, for the treatment of scrofula. The first hospital set up for the treatment of TB was opened in Italy at the end of the 18th century. Others were opened in England in 1814, in Germany in 1859, and in France by the end of the 19th century. Italy established quarantines in 1699, followed by Spain, although in northern Europe TB was not widely viewed as a public health problem.

Sea treatment became popular by the end of the 18th century. In 1839 Chopin stayed in Majorca, Spain, to seek relief from his symptoms. He was ejected from the island and stayed for a short period in Barcelona, Spain, where the local authorities requested that the bed in which he rested be burned.

In Germany, sanitorium treatment was codified by Brehmer and Dettweller in the mid-19th century. Afterwards, this method was adopted in Switzerland and France.

Many drugs were used in the Middle Ages, some strange, like crushed lung of fox by treatment analogy. Folk therapy remedies included wolf's liver boiled in wine, weasel blood, pigeon dung, and essence of skunk. Eating live snails was said to prevent the disease. In the Renaissance period, drugs containing arsenate or mercury were added as for syphilis. From the 17th century to the middle of the 19th century, treatments included diet and phlebotomy (bloodletting). Climatology therapy was predominant from the mid-1800s up to the mid-1900s but was also used in the 18th century, as for Louis the Dauphin, son of Louis XVI of France, for whom a special apartment in the castle of Meudon on the top of a hill was built. However, he died from TB in 1789.

In the 20th century physicians prescribed creosote, digitalis, opium, cod-liver oil, and Fowler's solution (a tonic rich in arsenic).

The first aggressive therapy started with Forlani (1847–1918), the "collapsotherapie." Numerous derivatives of this procedure were applied, such as artificial pneumothorax, phrenic nervous paralysis, and thoracoplasty. Surgery of the lung started to be used in 1935. Surgical resection of residual pulmonary lesions was frequently performed in the early years of chemotherapy, when physicians were unsure of the long-term benefits of chemotherapy. The surgical procedures were given up when the efficacy of medical therapy was well documented. The first surgical treatment of Pott disease occurred in 1911 and was done by the Alibe method.

1.2.2. Chemotherapy Era

In the prechemotherapy era, the mortality rate in New York Sanitorium of patients suffering from TB was high; in 1938,

69% of those with advanced disease died. The treatment of TB was revolutionized by the discovery of several antibiotics highly active against M. *tuberculosis* within the space of 25 years. In November 1944, the first patient received intravenous streptomycin. In 1952 came the first use of isoniazid in the United States. Successful use of chemotherapy for TB was launched.

In 1943, the discovery of streptomycin by S. Waksman's team provided a cure for meningitis and miliary TB and was a vital adjuvant to therapeutic pneumothorax. The discovery of the anti-TB activity of *p*-aminosalicylic acid (PAS) and isoniazid led to the standard 18-month treatment of TB with the triple combination of streptomycin, isoniazid, and PAS.

Finally, the discovery of rifampin in 1967 opened the way for the modern, "short-term" 9-month or even 6-month treatment employing rifampin combined with pyrazinamide (Table 1).

Over the course of the 20th century, improvements in hygiene and nutrition produced a steep decline in the incidence of TB in industrialized countries. The decline was accelerated by the introduction of potent chemotherapeutic agents.

Investigation of sulfonamides revealed that thiazole or thiadiazole rings exert a certain anti-M. *tuberculosis* activity. G. Domagk and Hegler in 1942 explored chemically all possibilities and discovered the anti-TB activity of thiosemicarbazone (Combentin). Domagk initiated in the mid-1940s in Germany a large clinical trial enrolling more than 20,000 patients and obtained good clinical and bacteriological outcomes.

In 1940, Bernheim observed that virulent M. *tuberculosis* growth was stimulated by respiration in the presence of small quantities of benzoic acid and salicylic acid. Lehmann looked for inhibitors and rediscovered the compound described in 1901 by Seidel, which fulfilled his expectation. The 2-hydroxy-4-aminobenzoic acid was named PAS. Schatz and coworkers in December 1943 found that the filtrate of the fermentation broth of *Streptomyces griseus* contains a substance they named streptomycin. The major drawback of monotherapy with streptomycin was the selection of mutants resistant to streptomycin. In an effort to prevent resistance, combination therapy with PAS was tried and was shown to be successful by the British Medical Society.

Table 1 Chronology of anti-TB drugs

Compound(s)	Year of discovery as anti-TB agent
Sulfones	1940
Isoniazid	1951
Rifampin	1966
Streptomycin	1943
Pyrazinamide and morphozamide	1952
Thiocarbanilide	1953
Protionamide	1963
Ethambutol	1962
Ethionamide	1956
D-Cycloserine	1952
Capreomycin	1962
Viomycin	1951
Kanamycin	1957
Amikacin	
Thiacetazone	1943–1946
PAS	1940
Fluoroquinolone (norfloxacin)	1976

In 1951, the anti-M. *tuberculosis* activity of isoniazid was discovered from a compound synthesized in 1912 by Meyer and Mally at the Charles University of Prague (Prague, Czech Republic). Isoniazid was discovered fortunately after Chorine discovered that nicotinamide exerts anti-M. *tuberculosis* activity. A search of compounds having a pyridine led to isoniazid.

Isoniazid became a major component of first-line therapy against TB. Soon after, the anti-M. *tuberculosis* activity of pyrazinamide as well as those of ethambutol and rifampin was shown.

The marked antituberculostatic activity of aliphatic polyamines and substituted ethylenediamines yielded ethambutol in the work of Wilkinson and coworkers in 1962.

A semisynthetic analog of rifamycin SV resulted in the major bactericidal anti-TB drug rifampin, which is a component of first-line therapy.

Pyrazinamide was synthesized by Dalmer and Walter in 1931 and was manufactured as an intermediate for the synthesis of 2-aminopyrazine, which was being investigated as an antibacterial. Its anti-M. *tuberculosis* activity was demonstrated in 1952 by two different teams.

Numerous other compounds called minor anti-TB drugs were isolated, such as viomycin, D-cycloserine, ethionamide and other thioamides, kanamycin, amikacin, and capreomycin. A number of rifamycin SV semisynthetic compounds with various anti-TB activities have been prepared, such as rifabutin, rifapentine, and rifalazil.

The real novelty in this therapeutic area is the introduction into clinical practice of fluoroquinolones, but only those having a quinoline ring are expected to exhibit anti-TB activity. Recently, diaryl quinoline has been reported to have anti-M. *tuberculosis* activity.

1.3. Epidemiology

In the 19th century, cancer, silicosis, and lung abscesses were confused with TB, making the accuracy of the data doubtful. In England and Wales, from the 17th to the 19th centuries more than 20% of deaths were due to TB. In 1715, TB accounted for 13% of deaths in western Europe; the epidemic probably achieved its height in the late 18th or early 19th century. The peak was delayed to the end of the 19th century (1888) in eastern Europe. In England the epidemic began in the 16th century and reached a peak in 1780 as a result of industrialization and growth of the cities, which allowed the spread of the disease from person to person.

In the United States the peak was reached in 1900. In Salem, Mass., from 1768 to 1773, pulmonary TB accounted for 18% of deaths. Between 1799 and 1808 the proportion rose to about 25%. During the first half of the 19th century, most cities on the East Coast reported a prevalence of 400 cases per 10^5 inhabitants, and 15 to 30% of all deaths were attributable to TB.

The larger Asiatic countries experienced the height of the epidemic in the late 19th century. The peak in sub-Saharan Africa is occurring now.

TB is caused by a group of mycobacteria including M. *tuberculosis*, M. *bovis* (including the BCG strains), M. *africanum*, and M. *microti*. Transmission is by the airborne route. Most individuals who become infected do not experience clinical illness but remain asymptomatic and noninfectious. The only evidence of colonization may be a reaction to a tuberculin skin test. This could persist for years; however, the person remains

Table 2 Rates of mortality due to TB

WHO region(s)	No. of deaths due to TB per 10^5 inhabitants	% of all TB deaths
Africa	100	18
Latin America	46	7
Eastern Mediterranean	43	5
Southeast Asia	72	32
Western Pacific	50	4
China	72	27
United States, Canada, Japan, Australia, New Zealand	1.4	0.2
Europe	3.9	1.0

Table 3 Prevalence of TB and deaths

Region(s)	Total no. of patients	No. of new patients	No. of deaths
Africa	171,000	1,398	656
America	117,000	564	220
Eastern Mediterranean	52,000	594	163
Southeast Asia	426,000	2,480	932
Western Pacific	574,000	2,557	894
Industrialized countries	382,000	409	42

at high risk of developing apparent disease, especially if the immune system becomes impaired.

Even in treated patients, viable organisms may cause a relapse after therapy ends. Appropriate combination therapies will reduced the risk as well as the emergence of multidrug-resistant *M. tuberculosis*. Without a suitable therapy, the mortality rate is high, reaching 50 to 60% of patients. The TB mortality rates in 1990 as reported by the World Health Organization (WHO) are listed in Table 2.

Eight million new TB cases occur every year, with an estimate of approximately three million patients who will die from TB (Table 3).

A 1998 WHO survey estimated the incidence of TB in the 22 highest-burden countries; rates are listed in Table 4.

It is important to know the prevalence of resistance to a single drug or multiple drugs in a given area before beginning anti-TB therapy. When microorganisms are resistant to both isoniazid and rifampin, the length of treatment increases from 6 months to 18 to 24 months and the cure rate decreases from nearly 100% to less than 60%. In some outbreaks occurring in the United States, *M. tuberculosis* strains resistant to seven drugs have been reported. Most of the patients were infected with human immunodeficiency virus (HIV); in these patients the mortality rate ranged from 72 to 89%, and the average interval between TB diagnosis and death was shortened from 4 to 16 weeks. The emergence of TB in New York, N.Y., in the 1980s has been closely linked to the AIDS epidemic.

In a survey in New York City, 33% of the cases involved organisms resistant to at least one drug and 19% involved organisms resistant to both isoniazid and rifampin.

It has been more than 60 years since PAS and streptomycin were discovered as anti-TB drugs and were able to provide the first pharmaceutical alternative to fresh air, diet, and exercise as the basis of TB treatment. TB was thought to be under control in the Western countries. In 1989, a target date of 2010 was set for the elimination of TB in the United States (defined as <1 case per 10^6 inhabitants).

Since then, however, the number of TB patients in the United States has risen. After years of steady decline, during which TB had become confined to definable population groups such as disadvantaged populations, immigrants from countries with a high prevalence of TB, aged people, drug addicts, persons in correctional facilities and nursing homes, and the homeless, the reported prevalence of TB in the United States plateaued in 1985 and then started to climb in 1989.

Table 4 Incidence of TB in high-burden countries

Country	Population, 10^5	Rate/10^{-5}	Cumulative incidence (%)
India	9,820	186.1	23
China	1,255	112.6	40
Indonesia	206	286.6	47
Bangladesh	124	244.7	51
Pakistan	148	181	55
Nigeria	106	243.4	58
The Philippines	73	306.7	61
South Africa	40	437.9	63
Ethiopia	60	268.6	65
Vietnam	78	189.3	66
Russia	147	105.7	68
Zaire	49	263.7	70
Brazil	166	74.7	71
Tanzania	32	308.6	73
Kenya	29	296.8	74
Thailand	60	140.9	875
Myanmar	44	181.9	76
Afghanistan	21	353.1	77
Uganda	25	332.3	78
Peru	11	265	78
Zimbabwe	11	560.1	79
Cambodia	10.8	540.5	80

Today, for many reasons, TB is reemerging as a plague worldwide. Globally, it is estimated that between 2000 and 2020 nearly 1 billion persons will be newly colonized, 200 million will be ill, and 35 million will die from TB if it is not controlled. An increased number of immunocompromised patients are at risk, and a number of multidrug-resistant *M. tuberculosis* strains have been reported, with high mortality rates. Serious economic problems such as civil war, homelessness, and fiscal constraints in government at all levels have resulted in cutbacks in many anti-TB campaigns. There have been shortages of antibacterials and inadequate resources to follow up on noncompliant patients and to bring outbreaks under control.

It is clear that TB has become a major health problem within industrialized and developing countries alike.

2. IN VITRO TESTING OF ANTI-TB DRUGS

M. tuberculosis replicates at a low rate, generally every 24 h instead of 20 to 40 min for common pathogens.

It is possible to detect mycobacteria in undiluted samples from patients if the specimen, such as sputum, is smeared on a glass slide. Detection of mycobacteria under the microscope requires either Ziehl-Neelsen or, better, a fluorochrome stain (auramine); however, the smear is positive when the specimen contains about 10^4 organisms/ml. It is important to note that a smear is not able to differentiate living or dead bacilli; for this reason, a culture of the pathological specimen is compulsory.

Specific media such as Löwenstein-Jensen or Middlebrook 7H10 or 7H11 agar should be used. Standard bacterial growth media are not suitable for *M. tuberculosis* growth.

The conventional method for susceptibility testing of *M. tuberculosis*, known as the proportion method, generally requires 3 to 8 weeks to provide susceptibility data.

Adaptations of the in vitro method have been developed for pyazinamide, because an acidic environment is required to demonstrate in vitro activity against *M. tuberculosis*. In order to offset this major drawback, a simple and rapid but indirect method of detection of resistance is based on the demonstration of pyrazinamidase, an enzyme for the activity of pyrazinamide. Unfortunately, there is no correlation between resistance to pyrazinamide and loss of pyrazinamidase. For this reason the incidence of primary and secondary resistance of *M. tuberculosis* to pyrazinamide is not well explored.

With the radiometric method (BACTEC 460), results are obtained between 1 to 6 weeks. 7H12 Middlebrook broth contains [^{14}C]palmitic acid as the carbon source to detect the $^{14}CO_2$ produced by living organisms.

Simultaneous infections with multiple strains of *M. tuberculosis* may occur in immunocompetent hosts (susceptible and resistant isolates) and may be responsible for drug susceptibility test result discrepancies.

The breakpoints were empirically established for most compounds used in therapy. Breakpoints may be different according to the medium used (Table 5).

The *M. tuberculosis* reference strain is *M. tuberculosis* $H37_{RV}$ (Table 6).

Table 5 Breakpoints of anti-TB compounds

Compound	MIC (μg/ml) on indicated medium			
	7H10	7H11	Löwenstein Jensen	BACTEC
Isoniazid	0.2	0.2	0.2	0.1
PAS	2.0	8.0	0.5	
Streptomycin	2.0	2.0	4.0	2.0
Rifampin	1.0	1.0	40.0	2.0
Ethambutol	5.0	7.5	2.0	2.5
Ethionamide	5.0	10.0	20.0	5.0
Kanamycin	5.0	6.0	20.0	5.0
D-Cycloserine	20.0	30.0	30.0	50.0
Pyrazinamide	50.0	50.0	100.0	100.0

Table 6 In vitro activities of anti-TB agents against *M. tuberculosis* $H37_{RV}$

Compound	MIC (μg/ml) range
Isoniazid	0.01–0.25
Pyrazinamide	25–150
Ethionamide/protionamide	0.6–2.0/0.4–0.8
Ethambutol	0.5–1.0
Rifampin	0.125
Rifabutin	0.016
Rifapentine	0.5
Rifalazil	0.004
Streptomycin	0.4–2.0
Kanamycin	5.0
Viomycin	2–12
Capreomycin	16–32
Thiosemicarbazone	0.5–2
PAS	0.5–1.5
D-Cycloserine	6.25–25

3. ANTI-TB ANTIBIOTICS

Depending on their antibacterial activities and their toxicities to humans, anti-TB antibiotics are classified as first-line antibiotics, administered as first-choice treatment in any new case of TB, and second-line antibiotics, reserved for the treatment of patients with *M. tuberculosis* resistant to the first-line antibiotics. In addition, new antibiotics are currently under study.

The first-line anti-TB antibiotics are streptomycin, rifampin, isoniazid, pyrazinamide, and ethambutol.

3.1. Physicochemical Characteristics

See Table 7.

Capreomycin is soluble in water, ethambutol is readily soluble in water, thiosemicarbazone is weakly soluble (88 mg/ml at 20°C); pyrazinamide and isoniazid are 1.5 and 13%, soluble, respectively; viomycin is weakly soluble (7.8 mg/ml); D-cycloserine is highly soluble in water; and tiocarlide as well as ethambutol is insoluble in water.

Rifampin is zwitterionic, with pKs of 1.7 (4-hydroxy) and 7.9 (3-piperazine nitrogen).

4. STREPTOMYCIN

The antibacterial spectrum of streptomycin (Fig. 1) includes gram-positive and gram-negative bacteria (see chapter 16). Streptomycin is very potent against mycobacteria (Table 8).

In macrophages, after 7 days of contact the cellular/extracellular ratio (C/E ratio) is about 5.

Table 9 lists concentrations of streptomycin in cerebrospinal fluid (CSF) after a 600-mg dose.

Table 7 Physicochemical characteristics of anti-TB compounds

Compound	Molecular mass (Da)	Melting point (°C)	LogP *n*-octanol/water	pK
Isoniazid	137.15	171.4	−2.54	3.8
Pyrazinamide	123.1	188–189	−2.66	0.5
Ethionamide/protionamide	166/180	166/142	−1.76/−1.28	0.36
Ethambutol	277.2	201–202	ND[a]	6.6, 9.5
Streptomycin/kanamycin	581.23/484.5	200/178–182	ND	7.2
Rifampin	822.97	183–188	3.2	1.7, 7.9
Rifabutin	870.2	148–156	3.2	1.6, 6.9
Rifapentine	877.04	179–181	3.45	2.4, 6.5
Rifalazil			4.81	
Thiacetazone	236.39	233		
Capreomycin	850.79	253–255		6.2, 8.2, 10.2, 13.3
Viomycin	685	280		8.2, 10.3, 12
D-Cycloserine	102.09	152–156		4.5, 7.4
PAS	153.13	147–240		
Tiocarlide	400.5	148–149		
Clofazimine	473.41	210–212		

[a]ND, not determined.

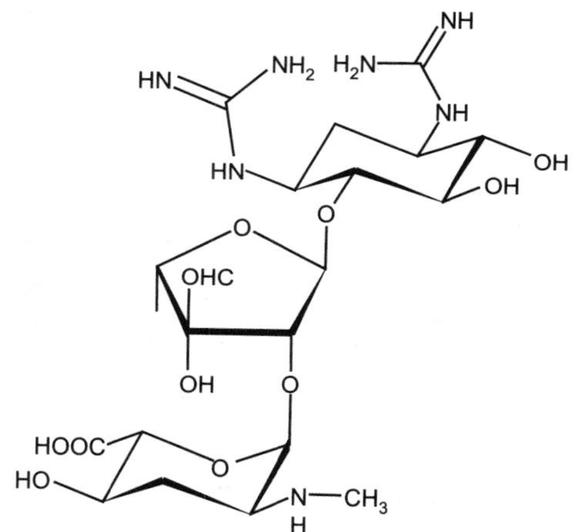

Figure 1 Streptomycin

Table 8 Streptomycin activity against mycobacteria

Organism	MIC (μg/ml) range
M. tuberculosis H37$_{RV}$	0.4–2.0
M. bovis	0.09–3.12
M. tuberculosis	0.09–11.5
M. avium	0.39–50

Table 9 Concentrations of streptomycin in the CSF

Sampling time (h)	*n*	Dose (mg/kg)	Concn (μg/ml) in: Serum	Concn (μg/ml) in: CSF
2	10	14.2	30.5	2.1
4	6	13.1	16.4	1.6
6	6	12.8	10.6	2.3

5. ANSAMYCIN DERIVATIVES

5.1. Rifampin

5.1.1. General Characteristics

Rifampin is a semisynthetic derivative of rifamycin SV belonging to the ansamycin family of antibiotics. Rifamycin SV is produced by *Nocardia mediterranei*. The structure is illustrated in Fig. 2.

5.1.2. Mechanism of Action, Antibacterial Spectrum, and Antibacterial Activity

Rifampin inhibits bacterial DNA-dependent RNA polymerase. It inhibits the extrusion of nascent RNA transcript and the elongation of full-length mRNA. Rifampin binds to the β subunit of the enzyme (DNA-dependent RNA polymerase, which is an oligomer of four different subunits).

Rifampin has no effect on human RNA polymerase. Its antibacterial spectrum is similar to that of rifamycin B (rifamycin SV). It is bactericidal against members of the *M. tuberculosis* complex: *M. tuberculosis, M. bovis, M. africanum,* and *M. microti*. In contrast to rifamycin B, it is active against *Mycobacterium kansasii* and *Mycobacterium szulgai*. Rifampin is

Figure 2 Structure of rifampin

active against the other mycobacteria, but poorly in vivo (*M. marinum*, *M. ulcerans*, *M. xenopi*, and *M. avium*).

Rifampin concentrates in phagocytes and exhibits bactericidal activity against *M. tuberculosis* irrespective of the metabolism status.

A strain of *M. tuberculosis* is considered susceptible when the MIC of rifampin is less than or equal to 0.4 μg/ml when measured in an agar medium and less than 40 μg/ml measured in Löwenstein-Jensen medium. In agar medium, MICs range from 0.005 to 1.0 μg/ml. However, in Ogawa medium, MICs range from 2.5 to 10 μg/ml.

5.1.3. Pharmacokinetics

In contrast to rifamycin B, rifampin is rapidly absorbed by the gastrointestinal tract. The enteric absorption depends not only on the quality of the pharmaceutical formulation but also on the crystallization of the molecule. After oral administration of 600 mg, the average peak concentration in serum of 8 to 10 μg/ml is reached 2 to 4 h later. Rifampin diffuses well in the tissues, and the concentrations in CSF attain 50% of concentrations in blood when the meninges are inflamed. Rifampin reaches an adequate level in the tuberculous cavitaries. The volume of distribution is 70 to 100 liters, and plasma protein binding is 80 to 90%. The apparent elimination half-life is, on average, 3 h and declines progressively during the first weeks of treatment to stabilize at 2 h. After oral administration of less than 600 mg, the fraction of antibiotic reaching the systemic circulation is reduced because of a hepatic first-pass effect and biliary excretion.

Rifampin is metabolized in the liver to a bacteriologically active derivative, 25-O-deacetylated rifampin, which is eliminated in the bile but not absorbed by the gastrointestinal tract. When the process of hepatic deacetylation is saturated, a fraction of the free rifampin taken up by the hepatocytes is eliminated in the bile and reabsorbed by the gastrointestinal tract (true enterohepatic cycle). Deacetylation diminishes intestinal reabsorption and increases fecal elimination. About 60% of the administered dose is eliminated in the feces. Because of autoinduction of the enzymes of hepatic deacetylation, biliary elimination increases during the first weeks of treatment. As a result of enzymatic induction, rifampin therefore accelerates its own metabolism and that of other drugs with a similar metabolic pathway (Table 10).

The formylrifampin metabolite exhibits 10% of the antibacterial activity of rifampin.

In patients above 65 years old, the plasma clearance and the area under the concentration-time curve (AUC) are slightly modified (Table 11). No changes in daily dose are needed.

Elimination of rifampin is mainly biliary and secondarily urinary. Concentrations in serum and urine are increased in patients with hepatic insufficiency. Administration of probenecid reduces the excretion of rifampin by blocking hepatic uptake. Elimination in the urine, saliva, tears, and sweat is reflected by a red color of these secretions.

Under fasting conditions, variability in absorption of rifampin is small (Table 12).

The absolute bioavailability of rifampin from tablets and the intravenous form in adults has not been determined.

Rifampin is not removed by peritoneal dialysis or hemodialysis. It should be administered in normal doses in renally impaired patients. Because the apparent elimination half-life is prolonged in hepatically impaired patients, the daily dose must be reduced.

The C/E ratio can reach 3 in less than 1 min in alveolar macrophages and a level of about 5 in half an hour. Rifampin is able to inhibit or kill *M. tuberculosis* in cultured monocyte-derived human macrophages (Table 13).

Table 14 lists concentrations of rifampin in the CSF after a 600-mg dose.

Table 10 Pharmacokinetics of rifampin (600-mg dose)

Parameter	Value
C_{max} (μg/ml)	8.52
T_{max} (h)	3.19
$AUC_{0-\infty}$ (μg·h/ml)	73.95
$t_{1/2\beta}$ (h)	2.2
Urinary excretion (%)	10.9
CL_R (ml/min)	103 ± 25
Protein binding (%)	80

Table 11 Rifampin pharmacokinetics in elderly patients

Parameter	Value for age	
	<65 yr ($n = 19$)	>65 yr ($n = 18$)
Dose (mg/kg)	9.9	9.2
AUC (μg·h/ml)	64.87	80.95
C_{max} (μg/ml)	10.37	12.95
T_{max} (h)	3.47	2.56
$t_{1/2}$ (h)	3.02	3.60
CL_P (ml/min/kg)	3.01	2.27

Table 12 Pharmacokinetics of rifampin after food

Condition	C_{max} (μg/ml)	T_{max} (h)	$AUC_{0-\infty}$ (μg·h/ml)
Fast 1	10.54	2.43	57.15
Fast 2	11.32	2.18	58.98
Antacid	10.89	2.36	58.37
Fed	7.27	4.43	55.20

Table 13 Rifampin in lung tissues[a]

Sample	Concn (range)
Serum (μg/ml)	8.9–23.4
ELF[b] (μg/ml)	3.3–7.5
Alveolar macrophages (μg/ml)	145.4–738.7
Bronchial mucosa (mg/kg)	6.2–16.6

[a]Single oral dose of 600 mg to 15 subjects.
[b]ELF, epithelial lining fluid.

Table 14 Rifampin concentrations in CSF[a]

Sampling time (h)	n	Dose (mg/kg)	Concn (μg/ml) in:	
			Serum	CSF
2	19	10.7	11.5	0.39
4	10	11.1	10.6	0.38
5	7	10.1	10.1	0.78
6	7	10.5	4.7	0.47

[a]Single dose of 600 mg.

5.1.4. Drug Interactions

Enzymatic induction causes an acceleration of the metabolism of a number of drugs: corticosteroids, estrogen-progestogen combinations (oral contraceptives), and vitamin K inhibitors (warfarin, phenprocoumon, and acenocoumarol), but also methadone, cyclosporine, digitoxin, quinidine and hydroquinidine, tolbutamide (and other hypoglycemic sulfonamides), theophylline, and propranolol (and other beta-blockers inactivated by the liver). This induction reaches a peak after 3 weeks. A dosage adjustment of the drug used in combination is required: an increase in dose during the prescription of rifampin and a reduction on its discontinuation.

6. DERIVATIVES OF RIFAMYCIN SV

6.1. General Characteristics

Three rifamycin analogs have been introduced into clinical practice: rifabutin, rifapentine, and rifampin. The MIC of rifabutin for *M. tuberculosis* is 10 to 20 times lower than that of rifampin. This advantage, however, is offset by 10- to 20-fold-lower concentrations in serum than those of rifampin. The MIC of rifapentine for *M. tuberculosis* is only slightly lower than that of rifampin, but its apparent elimination half-life is longer (≥15 h). Rifapentine looks like a sustained-release rifampin that is as active administered once weekly as rifampin administered daily. As there is cross-resistance among rifampin, rifabutin, rifapentine, and rifalazil, the new molecules, with few exceptions, have no therapeutic activity in patients with rifampin-resistant strains of *M. tuberculosis*.

6.2. Rifapentine

6.2.1. General Characteristics

Rifapentine is a semisynthetic derivative of rifamycin SV harboring a cyclopentyl piperazinyl side chain (Fig. 3).

The MICs for *M. tuberculosis* range from 0.02 to 0.2 μg/ml (MIC at which 50% of isolates are inhibited [MIC_{50}] and MIC_{90}, 0.1 and 0.1 μg/ml).

6.2.2. Pharmacokinetics

Rifapentine is absorbed slowly from the gastrointestinal tract, with the peak concentration in plasma occurring after 4 to 5 h. Rifapentine is extensively metabolized, with the 25-deacetyl as a main metabolite. Rifapentine was quantifiable in plasma up to 48 h after dosing for all studied subjects and up to 72 h for 12 of 15 subjects when given with food. Protein binding is as follows: albumin > lipoproteins > α_1 acid glycoprotein. Rifapentine is linked for about 97.7%, and the metabolite is linked for 93.3%. The metabolite exhibits in vitro activity.

Pharmacokinetics are listed in Table 15.

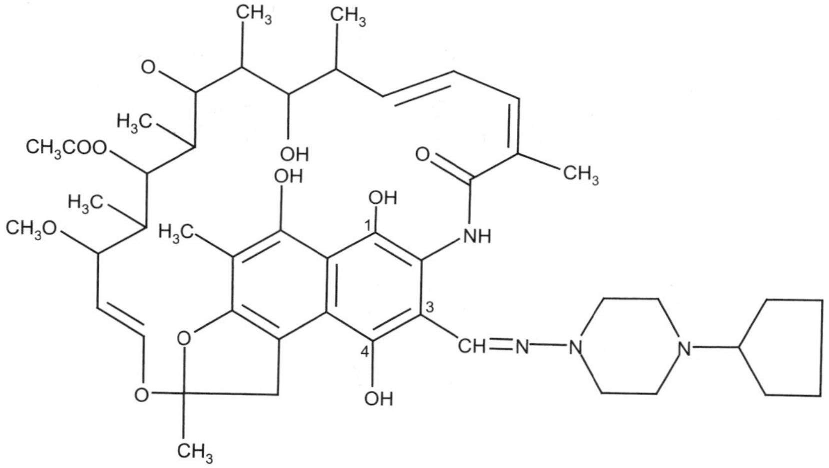

Figure 3 Rifapentine

Table 15 Pharmacokinetics of rifapentine

Compound and parameter	Value in subjects			
	Young	Fed	HIV+	Fed, HIV+
Rifapentine				
n	20	20	16	15
C_{max} (μg/ml)	11.76	17.57	9.42	14.09
T_{max} (h)	5.0	6.58	4.82	5.34
AUC (μg·h/ml)	319	499	256	374
CL_P (liters/h)	2.02	1.3	2.62	1.68
$t_{1/2}$ (h)	15.74	15.11	17.63	16.47
Protein binding (%)	97.7			
25-Deacetyl rifapentine				
C_{max} (μg/ml)	4.03	5.91	4.45	6.25
T_{max} (h)	19.25	21.68	15.64	19.61
AUC (μg·h/ml)	177	267	215	294
$t_{1/2}$ (h)	14.29	13.27	18.32	14.17
Protein binding (%)	93.3			

Table 16 Rifapentine pharmacokinetics: ascending doses

Parameter	Single dose			Steady state		
Dose (mg)	150	300	600	150	300	600
C_{max} (μg/ml)	3.6	8.6	15.8	5.3	11.2	24.3
AUC (μg·h/ml)	7.0	178	386	74	159	367
$t_{1/2}$ (h)	13.2	13.5	14.1	13.3	11.3	11.9
CL_P (liters/h)	2.19	1.8	1.69	2.08	1.98	1.72

A linear increase has been found between 150- and 600-mg oral doses of rifapentine (Table 16).

At steady state the time to maximum concentration in serum ranged from 5 to 4.6 h, and after a single dose it ranged from 4.2 to 5.1 h. Rifapentine is absorbed slowly in hepatically impaired patients. The time to maximum concentration in serum is about 30% longer. The maximum concentration in serum in patients with moderate to severe hepatic dysfunction was 8.4 μg/ml, compared with 11.8 μg/ml in healthy volunteers.

Rifapentine is well distributed in lung tissues (Table 17).

Rifapentine lacks autoinduction. However, rifapentine may induce CYP 3A4 and 2C8/9 enzymes.

In pediatric patients, the mean maximum concentration in serum and AUC for rifapentine are similar to those in adults and adolescents.

6.3. Rifabutin

Rifabutin is a semisynthetic derivative of rifamycin SV harboring an imidazolylpiperidyl side chain (Fig. 4).

It is a red-violet drug substance.

Table 17 Distribution of rifapentine in lung tissues

Parameter	Value in: Plasma	ELF[a]	Alveolar macrophages
C_{max} (μg/ml)	26.2	3.2	5.3
T_{max} (h)	5.0	5.0	7.0
AUC (μg·h/ml)	520	111	183
$t_{1/2}$ (h)	28.3	20.8	13

[a]ELF, epithelial lining fluid.

6.3.1. Pharmacokinetics

Table 18 summarizes the pharmacokinetics of rifabutin after a single oral dose of 150 mg either in tablet form or in suspension. Rifabutin is poorly absorbed by the gastrointestinal tract. The apparent elimination half-life is about 36 h. Rifabutin is mainly bound in the plasma to albumin (70%). The bioavailability is around 53%. The volume of distribution

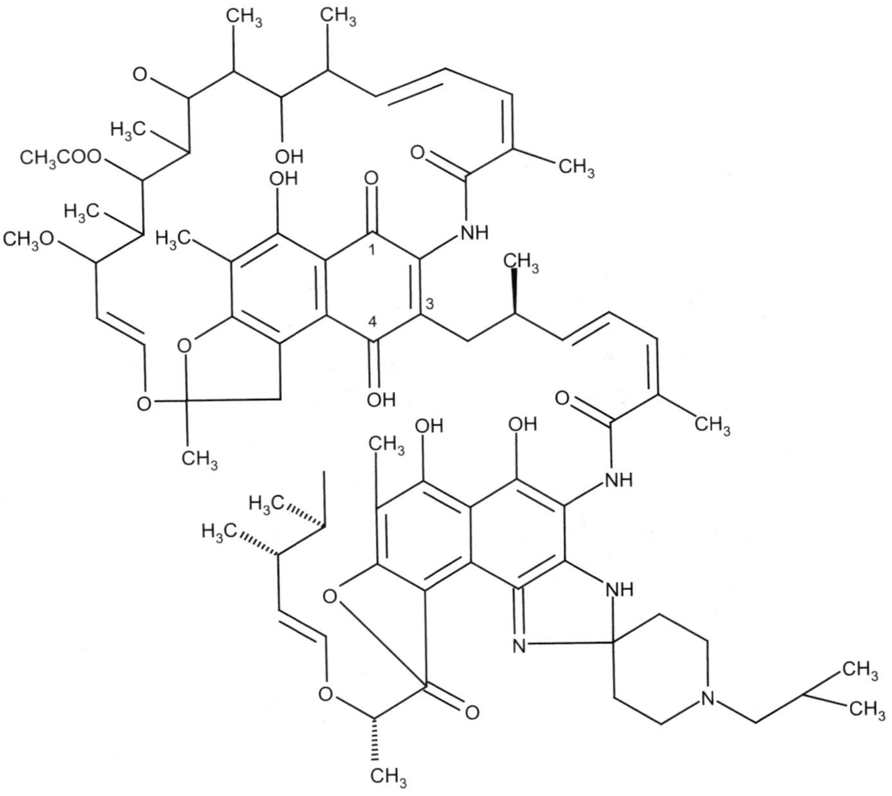

Figure 4 Rifabutin

Table 18 Pharmacokinetics of rifabutin after a single dose of 150 mg

Parameter	Value for:	
	Tablets	Suspension
C_{max} (ng/ml)	187.9	237.5
T_{max} (h)	3.0	2.5
$AUC_{0-\infty}$ (ng·h/ml)	2,271	2,715
Urinary excretion (%)	11	11

Table 19 Effect of food on pharmacokinetics of rifabutin

Parameter	Value under condition	
	Fed	Fasting
C_{max} (ng/ml)	156.2	187.9
T_{max} (h)	5.4	3.0
$AUC_{0-\infty}$ (ng·h/ml)	2,640	2,516
Urinary elimination (%)	17.1	13.6

is 9.3 liters/kg, the renal clearance is 0.03 liter/h/kg, and the plasma clearance is 320 to 370 ml/min (0.69 liter/h/kg).

There is no influence on the extent of rifabutin absorption if the drug is taken simultaneously with a fatty meal (Table 19).

Rifabutin is metabolized to six metabolites. 25-Deacetyl and 31-hydroxy rifabutin are found in animals and humans. In rats, rabbits, and monkeys, a 31-hydroxy metabolite was detected as well. In dogs, after a dose of 100 mg/kg of body weight, three metabolites were shown in urine: 25-deacetyl, hydroxy, and 25-deacetyl-30-hydroxy rifabutin.

In humans, four additional metabolites have been detected: 32-hydroxy, 30-hydroxy, 32-OH-25-deacetyl, and 25-*O*-deacetyl-*N*-oxide rifabutin. All of the metabolites eliminated in urine represent about 10% of the administered dose of rifabutin.

The pharmacokinetic profile does not change significantly in HIV patients (Table 20).

When rifabutin is combined with anti-AIDS drugs such as saquinavir, nevirapine, ritonavir, and amprenavir, the rifabutin regimen needs to be significantly modified.

The pharmacokinetics after different rhythms of administration are shown in Table 21.

6.4. Rifalazil

Rifalazil (KRM-1648) is 3′-hydroxy-5′-(4-isobutyl-1-piperazinyl) benzoxazino rifamycin (Fig. 5). This compound was synthesized in 1993.

Table 20 Pharmacokinetic profile of rifabutin in HIV patients

Patient status	Dose (mg)	C_{max} (μg/ml)	AUC (μg·h/ml)
HIV^-	300	0.375	4.298
	450	0.568	6.755
	600	0.724	8.555
HIV^+	300	0.384	5.4
	600	0.579	10.2
	900	0.877	11.7

It has the same antibacterial spectrum as rifampin but is more active against *M. tuberculosis* than rifampin.

6.4.1. Antibacterial Activity

Rifalazil is more active than rifampin against mycobacteria (Table 22).

For *Helicobacter pylori* the MICs range from 0.002 to 0.004 μg/ml; for *Chlamydia pneumoniae* the MICs are under 0.001 μg/ml.

6.4.2. Pharmacokinetics

Rifalazil is not an inducer of drug metabolism. Two main metabolites have been reported for humans: 25-deacetyl and 30-hydroxy rifalazil.

Table 23 lists the pharmacokinetics after single ascending doses to healthy volunteers.

Rifalazil is detectable in plasma for approximately 36 and 168 h after administration of 30- and 100-mg single oral doses, respectively.

Less than 2% of the administered dose is eliminated in the urine. The concentrations in plasma of the metabolites are less than 2 ng/ml.

Rifalazil is metabolized in animals and humans. Two metabolites have been detected in the urine of dogs: M-1 and M-2, which are 25-*O*-deacetyl rifalazil (KRM-1671) and 30-hydroxy rifalazil (KRM-1690), respectively. In mice M-2 is predominant and M-1 is not detected. In rats and guinea pigs neither M-1 nor M-2 was detected. In monkeys, M-2 and four unknown metabolites were detected, but not M-1. M-1 occurs in whole blood in mice and rats but not in humans. In humans M-2 formation seems to be mediated by CYP 3A3 and CYP 3A4. The main metabolites are active against *M. tuberculosis* (Table 24).

In humans, after a single oral dose of 50 mg of rifalazil, two main metabolites were found in urine: M-1 and M-4. Rates of urinary elimination at 0 to 6 h were as follows (mean ± standard deviation): rifalazil, 0.038% ± 0.015%; M-1, 0.015% ± 0.05%, and M-4, 0.01% ± 0.007%. The rates at 72 h were as follows: rifalazil, 0.194%, M-1, 0.190%;

Table 21 Rifabutin pharmacokinetics after alternative regimens

Compound	Parameter	Value for regimen	
		300 mg weekly	150 mg every 3 days
Rifabutin	C_{max} (ng/liter)	496	130
	C_{min} (ng/liter)	19.2	55
	AUC (ng·h/liter)	13.4	18.2
25-Deacetyl rifabutin	C_{max} (ng/liter)	310	103
	C_{min} (ng/liter)	27.3	52.8
	AUC (ng·h/liter)	10.5	12.1

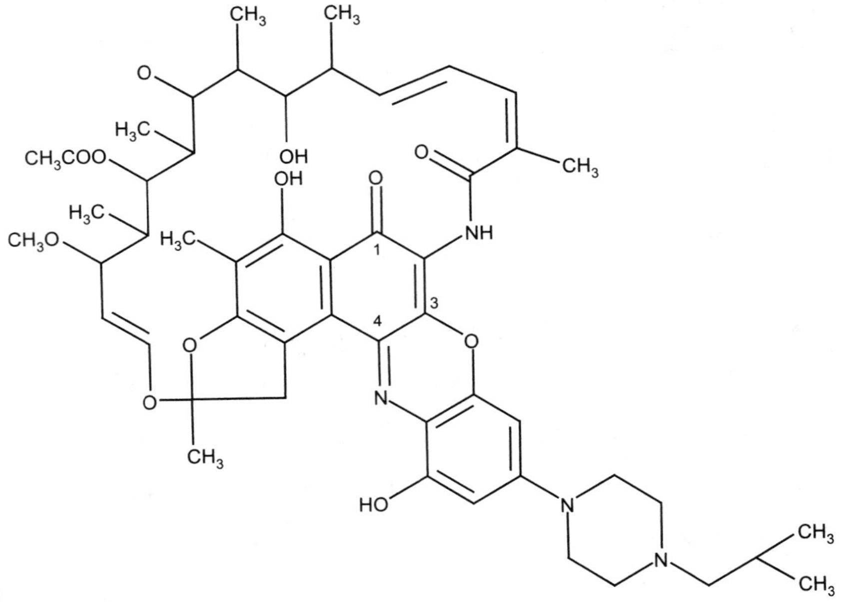

Figure 5 Rifalazil

Table 22 In vitro activities of rifamycin derivatives against TB ($n = 30$)

Compound	MIC (μg/ml)		MIC (μg/ml) for strain:	
	50%	90%	$H37_{RV}$	Kurono
Rifalazil	0.016	2.0	0.004	0.002
Rifabutin	0.016	8.0	0.016	0.016
Rifampin	4.0	>128	0.125	0.125

Table 23 Rifalazil pharmacokinetics after ascending doses

Parameter	Value for dose:		
	30 mg	100 mg	300 mg
C_{max} (ng/ml)	17.8	58.8	115.7
T_{max} (h)	3.1	4.0	3.0
$t_{1/2}$ (h)	48.7	43.1	206.6
$AUC_{0-\infty}$ (ng·h/liter)	504.9	1,543.3	5,045

Table 25 Pharmacokinetic profile of rifalazil and the main metabolites in humans after a single dose of 50 mg

Parameter	Value for:		
	Rifalazil	M-1	M-4
C_{max} (ng/ml)	50.1	3.9	2.6
T_{max} (h)	2.7	7.2	4.3
AUC (ng·h/ml)	1,250	163	94
$t_{1/2}$ (h)	34.4	23.9	26.6

Table 26 Rifalazil pharmacokinetics after repeated doses ($n = 8$)

Parameter	Value for:		
	5-mg/kg first dose	5-mg/kg last dose (day 14)	25-mg/kg first dose
C_{max} (ng/ml)	13.3	13.4	41.3
T_{max} (h)	5.25	4.57	5.6
$t_{1/2\beta}$ (h)	10.1	17.3	12.3
$AUC_{0-\infty}$ (ng·h/ml)			479
AUC_{0-24} (ng·h/ml)	137	187	688

and M-4, 0.05%. The in vitro activity of M-4 (32-hydroxy derivative) is similar to that of rifalazil against M. *tuberculosis*. The pharmacokinetics of M-1 and M-4 in plasma are shown in Table 25.

Repeated doses have been given to healthy volunteers; data are shown in Tables 26 and 27.

Rifalazil may induce a flu-like syndrome. At high doses (100 mg) a drop in neutrophil count has been observed.

Table 24 In vitro activities of rifalazil metabolites against mycobacteria

Organism	MIC_{90} (μg/ml)			
	Rifalazil	25-Deacetyl rifalazil	30-Hydroxy rifalazil	Rifampin
M. *avium*	0.25	0.25	>0.50	8.0
M. *intracellulare*	0.50	0.5	2.0	16
M. *tuberculosis*	<0.125	<0.125	<0.125	<1.0

Table 27 Rifalazil pharmacokinetics after multiple doses once a week

Parameter	Value for:			
	25 mg/kg, day 1	25 mg/kg, day 21	50 mg/wk, day 1	50 mg/wk, day 2
n	6	6	8	8
C_{max} (ng/ml)	39.3	43.9	69.8	79.1
T_{max} (h)	5.7	5.7	5.5	6.0
$t_{1/2\alpha}$ (h)	10.51	11.3	9.5	12.0
$t_{1/2\beta}$ (h)		60.9		109.1
$AUC_{0-\infty}$ (ng·h/ml)	628.7	1,347.3	1,019.1	2,840.6
AUC_{0-24} (ng·h/ml)	472.2	552.6	795.3	1,013.0

Table 28 Intracellular ratio of rifalazil

Concn in medium (μg/ml)	C/E ratio	
	Rifalazil	Rifampin
0.25	288	4.2
1.0	191	4.5
4.0	230	4.5

The concentration in human macrophages is very high for rifalazil (Table 28).

7. ISONIAZID

7.1. General Characteristics

Isoniazid, isonicotinic acid hydrazide, is a molecule which was first synthesized at the beginning of the 20th century but whose anti-TB activity was not detected until 1945. The anti-TB activity of isoniazid was demonstrated by three independent teams. Its structure is illustrated in Fig. 6.

7.2. Mechanism of Action, Antibacterial Spectrum, and Antibacterial Activity

Isoniazid is active only against the M. *tuberculosis* complex: M. *tuberculosis*, M. *bovis*, M. *africanum*, and M. *microti*. Its precise mechanism of action remains unclear. The target seems to be inhibition of mycolic acid synthesis. There is some evidence of the central role played by InhA, the product of the gene *inhA*. InhA is an enoyl reductase and interacts with another protein, KasA, which is a β-ketoacylsynthase. Both enzymes are involved in mycolic acid synthesis. Middlebrook in 1954 observed that M. *tuberculosis* strains resistant to isoniazid were devoid of catalase/peroxidase activity. For this activity another protein is involved, AphD, which is the equivalent in *Enterobacteriaceae* of AphF. AphD is thought to control the same promoter as AphC. It is an alkylhydroperoxidase. Isoniazid is a prodrug that requires cellular activation to an unknown active form. The enzyme which activates it is KatG, which is a catalase/peroxidase. KatG is a multifunctional enzyme which belongs to the hydroperoxidase I group of proteins. The KatG protein could be considered a virulence factor since it is able to detoxify the reactive oxygen generated in host macrophages. The KatG protein is able to act as a peroxynitrase and is able to enhance DNA repair when expressed in *Escherichia coli.*

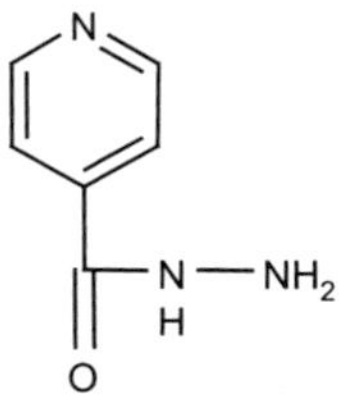

Figure 6 Structure of isoniazid

For susceptible species, the MIC of isoniazid is 0.03 to 0.05 μg/ml and varies little with the culture medium used or the incubation time. The MIC for M. *kansasii* is 0.25 to 0.50 μg/ml, but for all other mycobacterial species the MICs are very high (>5 μg/ml).

Isoniazid is unable to kill nonmultiplying M. *tuberculosis* in cultures of human macrophages.

7.3. Pharmacokinetics

Isoniazid is well absorbed by the gastrointestinal tract, exhibits good tissue diffusion, and has good concentrations in macrophages, in caseous material, and in CSF. Its apparent volume of distribution is 30 to 40 liters. It is administered orally and possibly intravenously, intramuscularly, or even locally (intrapleurally for example). After oral administration of 5 mg/kg, the recommended dose for adults and children (UICTMR-WHO), almost 90% of isoniazid is rapidly absorbed, and the peak concentration in serum, reached in 1 to 2 h, is 2.5 to 5 μg/ml. The apparent elimination half-life in plasma depends on its rate of metabolic inactivation by acetylation. In fast acetylators it is 60 to 90 min, and in slowly acetylating subjects it is 120 to 280 min. The fact of belonging to the category of fast acetylators has no therapeutic consequences for the patient, probably because of the low MIC of isoniazid for M. *tuberculosis* and the daily administration of isoniazid in combination with other bactericidal antibiotics. Isoniazid is poorly bound to plasma protein (4%).

7.3.1. Acetylation

Isoniazid is transformed to a bacteriologically inactive derivative, acetyl isoniazid, by an *N*-acetyltransferase present in the liver and small intestine as well by M. *tuberculosis*. Acetyltransferase activity is genetically determined. Slow acetylators represent 60% of the population among Caucasian and black subjects, whereas in Asians and American Indians fast acetylators account for 70% of the population (Table 29).

The acetylation of isoniazid may be delayed by hepatic insufficiency and simultaneous administration of molecules inactivated by the same metabolic pathway, such as PAS.

Table 29 Isoniazid inactivator status

Country	% of type of inactivation:		
	Rapid	Middle	Slow
Germany	36–44		56–64
Japan	38	42	20
Egypt	18		82
Finland	41		58–59
Sweden	32		68
Canada	46	10	49
United States	32		68
France	39		56–61
Czech Republic	36		61
Slovakia	45		55

In all patients, about 50% of acetylated isoniazid is metabolized to isonicotinic acid and monoacetyl hydrazine (Fig. 7). Metabolites are weakly active or inactive against *M. tuberculosis*.

Table 30 shows the formation of the metabolites after administration of 300 mg as a single oral dose to nine volunteers.

Monoacetyl hydrazine is itself metabolized by the microsomal oxidation system (cytochrome P450 in the presence of NADPH and oxygen) to an extremely toxic reactive metabolite that can cause cytolytic hepatitis. Hepatic enzyme-inducing drugs (rifampin, phenobarbital, general

Table 30 Elimination of metabolites

Compound	% Eliminated by:	
	Rapid acetylators ($n = 5$)	Slow acetylators ($n = 4$)
Acetyl isoniazid	46.3	28.9
Monoacetyl hydrazone	1.8	2.5
Diacetyl hydrazone	23	4.9
Mono- and diacetyl hydrazone	24.9	7.5

anesthetics, etc.) that are involved in the activation of the microsomal oxidation system may potentiate the hepatic toxicity of isoniazid.

Fast acetylators of isoniazid, who produce more acetylated isoniazid and hence more monoacetyl hydrazine than slow inactivators, are a priori more susceptible to toxic hepatitis than slow acetylators. However, as monoacetyl hydrazine is itself acetylated by the same *N*-acetyltransferase to a nontoxic diacetyl hydrazine, fast acetylators of isoniazid are in fact no more exposed to a risk of toxic hepatitis than slow acetylators.

7.3.2. Elimination

Elimination of isoniazid is mainly renal, 75 to 95% of administered isoniazid being eliminated in 24 h in the urine in the form of free isoniazid (25% in slow acetylators and 5% in fast

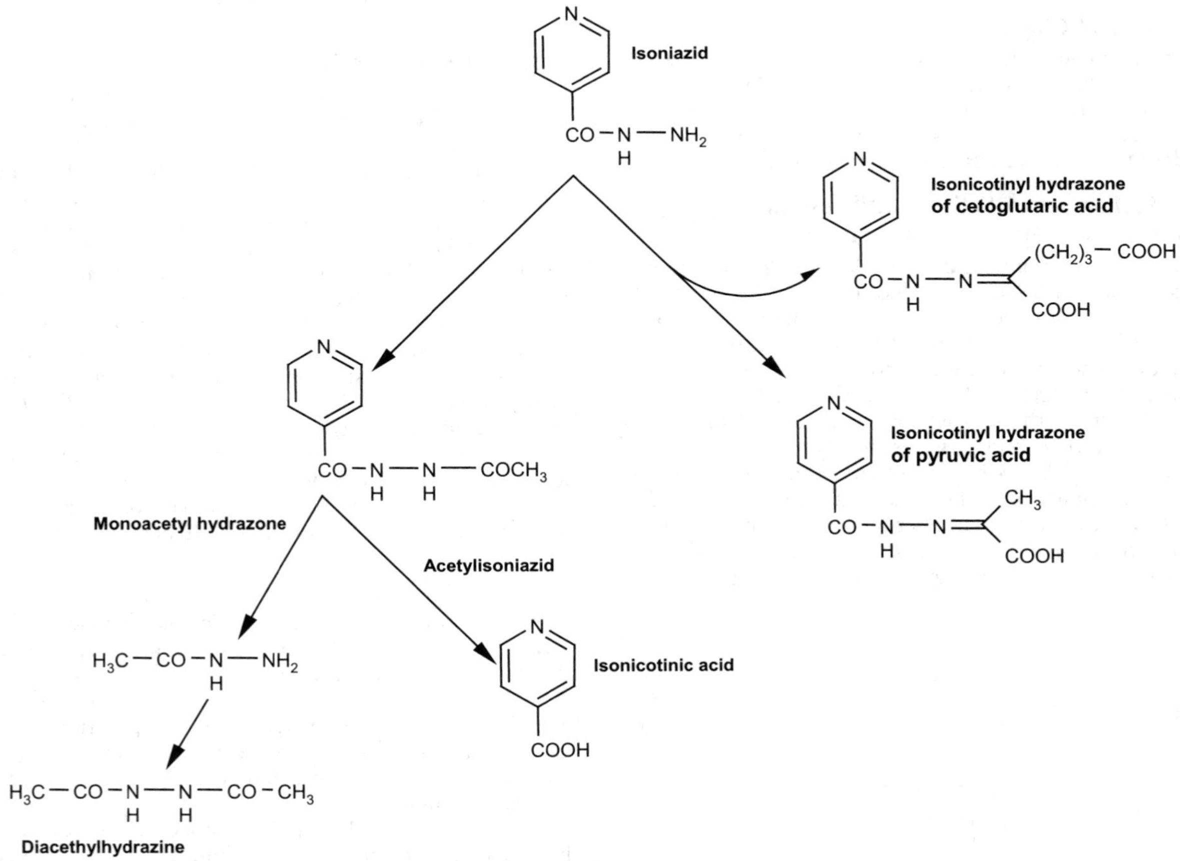

Figure 7 Metabolism of isoniazid

Table 31 Concentration of isoniazid in CSF

Time after dose (h)	n	Dose (mg/kg)	Concn (μg/ml) in: Serum	CSF
2	19	8.5 ± 0.4	4.4	1.9
4	8	9.1 ± 0.6	2.6	3.2
5	9	9.0 ± 0.8	2.1	1.8
6	8	7.5 ± 0.9	1.0	1.8

acetylators) and of isoniazid hydrazones, acetyl isoniazid, isonicotinic acid, and isonicotinuric acid. The renal clearance is around 15 ml/min.

Moderate renal insufficiency does not generally require a dosage adjustment for isoniazid, although severe renal insufficiency does. Isoniazid is eliminated in saliva.

Concentrations of isoniazid in CSF are shown in Table 31.

7.3.3. Elderly Patients

The incidence of TB in aged persons has risen in the past 20 years. The hydrazine metabolite has been implicated as a cause of isoniazid-induced liver toxicity (Fig. 8).

It has been suggested that there is a reduction in the acetylation rate with age. For this reason it seems that the risk of developing isoniazid-induced hepatitis increases with age. The pharmacokinetics in elderly patients are summarized in Table 32.

The profile of the hydrazine metabolite has been studied in young and elderly persons; data are shown in Table 33.

7.3.4. Food Effects

The absorption is delayed and the peak concentration is significantly lower with food but not with antacids (Table 34).

Gastrointestinal absorption is also delayed according to the acetylator status (Table 35).

Table 32 Isoniazid (6 mg/kg) pharmacokinetics in the elderly

Parameter	Value in: Fast acetylators		Slow acetylators	
Age (yrs)	<65	>65	<65	>65
n	17	12	2	6
C_{max} (μg/ml)	4.52	5.3	3.87	4.59
T_{max} (h)	2.32	1.92	1.5	1.17
AUC (μg·h/ml)	23.9	25.7	32.2	34.25
$t_{1/2}$ (h)	2.72	2.69	4.34	5.49
CL_P (ml/min/kg)	5.07	4.26	3.41	3.50
V (liters/kg)	1.15	1.0	1.24	1.52

Table 33 Hydrazine metabolite pharmacokinetics

Parameter	Value in: Young subjects ($n = 19$)	Elderly subjects (>65 yrs) ($n = 18$)
C_{max} (μg/ml)	0.24	0.40
T_{max} (h)	2.95	2.67
AUC (μg·h/ml)	2.0	2.5

Table 34 Isoniazid pharmacokinetics with food

Food status	C_{max} (μg/ml)	T_{max} (h)	AUC (μg·h/ml)
Fast 1	6.21	0.79	20.1
Fast 2	5.53	1.02	20.2
Antacids	5.62	0.71	20.3
Fed	2.73	1.93	17.7

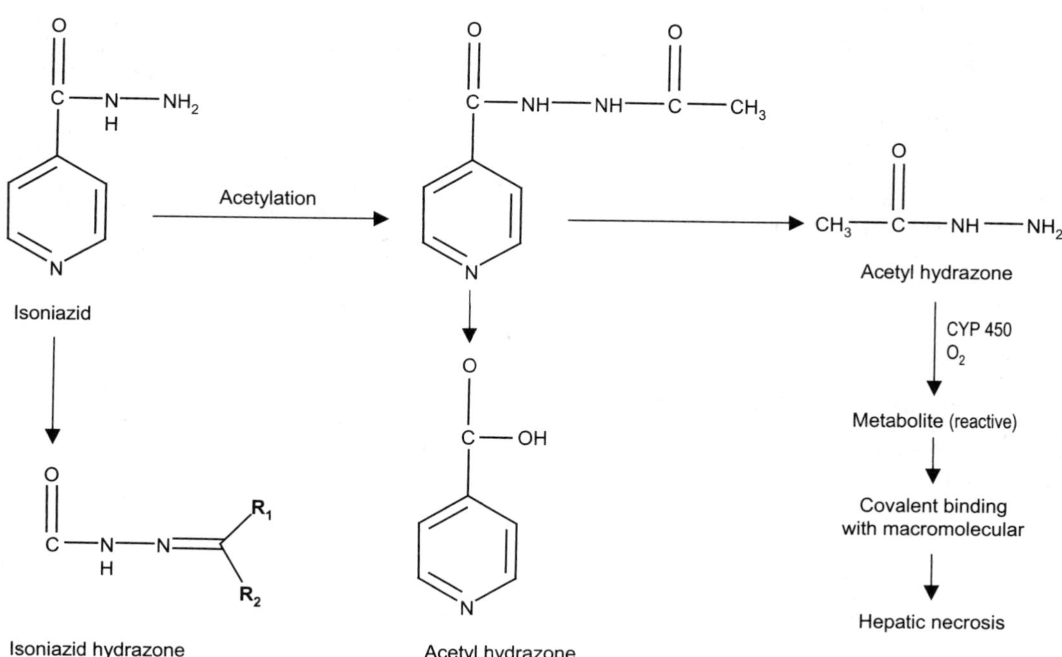

Figure 8 Isoniazid metabolism and liver toxicity

Table 35 Isoniazid pharmacokinetics with food and acetylator status

Parameter	Value in:	
	Fast acetylators	Slow acetylators
C_{max} (μg/ml)	6.20	5.26
T_{max} (h)	0.5	1.25
$AUC_{0-\infty}$ (μg·h/ml)	11.4	23.7
$t_{1/2}$ (h)	1.66	4.05
V (liters)	0.63	0.70
$t_{1/2\alpha}$ (h)	0.24	0.24
CL_R (liters/h)	3.09	
Urinary elimination (%)	10.9	

7.4. Drug Interactions

Drug interactions are rare. The risk of intoxication due to an overdose of phenytoin is increased in slow acetylators. The metabolism of other antiepileptics, carbamazepine, primidone, warfarin, and certain glucocorticosteroids might be delayed.

The combination disulfiram-isoniazid is not recommended in alcoholics. Enzyme inducers (halogenated general anesthetics, phenobarbital, and rifampin) encourage the formation of toxic metabolites. Finally, isoniazid must not be administered at the same time as niridazole because of the risk of severe psychiatric disorders.

7.5. Aconiazid

A prodrug of isoniazid was synthesized in 1960 and 1961: aconiazid (2-formylphenoxyacetic isoniazid). This prodrug was less absorbable than the parent compound, and development was stopped.

8. PYRAZINAMIDE

8.1. General Characteristics

Pyrazinamide, synthesized in 1952, is the pyrazine analog of nicotinamide (Fig. 9).

The synthesis of many nicotinamide analogs, including the pyrazine isostere pyrazinamide, followed the discovery of the effectiveness of nicotinamide in murine TB.

It was shown that nicotinamidase inside the bacterial cell hydrolyzes nicotinamide and pyrazinamide to their corresponding carboxylic acids. Pyrazinamide is active against dormant cells. It has been found that pyrazinoic acid inhibits the *fas1* gene, encoding fatty acid synthase I. In *M. tuberculosis* both systems Fas I and Fas II are present.

Pyrazinamide is soluble in water, and the pH of the solution is close to neutrality. It was shown to be effective in the treatment of experimental TB in mice in 1952 by Kushner and the same year in the treatment of human pulmonary TB by Yearge and coauthors. Pyrazinamide is stable for at least 2 months at 4 and 25°C in plastic and glass, with a loss of around 10% of the initial dose.

Figure 9 Structure of pyrazinamide

8.2. Mechanism of Action, Antibacterial Spectrum, and In Vitro and In Vivo Activities

In the cytoplasm, pyrazinamide is transformed by a deamidase, pyrazinamidase, to pyrazinoic acid, which is active against *M. tuberculosis* and *M. africanum* but inactive against *M. bovis* and other mycobacterial species. The MIC for *M. tuberculosis* ranges between 10 and 20 μg/ml in Löwenstein-Jensen agar and in broth. Pyrazinamide is active only when the pH is acidic (between 5 and 5.5) and is limited in vivo to *M. tuberculosis* in an acidic environment, i.e., within macrophages or in areas of recent caseification. Acidity promotes (or activates) it to pyrazinoic acid, the metabolite active against *M. tuberculosis*. Only mycobacteria that have the dual property of allowing pyrazinamide to penetrate their outer membrane and possessing a pyrazinamidase are therefore susceptible to pyrazinamide.

A common problem in pyrazinamide susceptibility testing is false resistance caused by large bacterial inoculum size. Large inocula (10^7 and 10^8 CFU/ml) of *M. tuberculosis* HR37ra caused significant increases in medium pH from 5.5 towards neutrality. The in vitro activity is also reduced in the presence of bovine serum albumin due to its neutralizing effect on medium pH. The age of culture can also interfere: a 3-month-old *M. tuberculosis* H37ra culture was shown to be more susceptible to pyrazinamide exposure than a 4-day log-phase culture, suggesting that pyrazinamide is more active for nongrowing bacilli.

Pyrazinoic acid is also active against *M. bovis* and *M. kansasii* even if pyrazinamide by itself is not active against these organisms. *M. bovis* has a low level of pyrazinamidase due a unique substitution, C→G, at position 169 of the enzyme.

8.3. Pharmacokinetics

Pyrazinamide is well absorbed by the gastrointestinal tract. The peak concentration in plasma of pyrazinamide, obtained after 2 h, is 30 μg/ml following a single oral dose of 20 mg/kg. The apparent elimination half-life ranges between 6 and 8 h (Table 36).

In elderly patients the apparent elimination half-life is longer and the plasma clearance is reduced (Table 37).

Pyrazinamide has good tissue distribution and concentrates in macrophages well, where it exerts bactericidal activity. It is mainly metabolized in the liver. Pyrazinoic acid is partially metabolized by a xanthine oxidase to 5-hydroxypyrazinoic acid. Pyrazinamide is almost entirely excreted renally, 3% in the unmetabolized form, 30% in the form of pyrazinoic acid, and 60 to 70% in the form of 5-hydroxypyrazinoic acid.

The urine can be colored orange. The elimination of pyrazinoic acid competes with the elimination of uric acid,

Table 36 Pharmacokinetics of pyrazinamide after a 1.0-g single oral dose

Parameter	Value
C_{max} (μg/ml)	35–45
T_{max} (h)	2.0
$t_{1/2}$ (h)	5–14
$AUC_{0-\infty}$ (μg·h/ml)	450
CL_P (liters/h)	1.5–6
V (liters)	58
CL_R (liters/h)	0.11
Urinary elimination (%)	3–4
Pyrazinoic acid in urine (%)	30
Protein binding (%)	0

Table 37 Pharmacokinetics of pyrazinamide in the elderly

Parameter	Value in subjects	
	<65 yrs ($n = 19$)	>65 yrs ($n = 18$)
C_{max} (μg/ml)	36.27	38.23
T_{max} (h)	2.97	2.11
$AUC_{0-\infty}$ (μg·h/ml)	461.22	497.53
$t_{1/2}$ (h)	5.69	9.75
CL_P (liters/h)	1.6	0.89

Table 38 Pharmacokinetics of pyrazinamide with food

Food status	C_{max} (μg/ml)	T_{max} (h)	$AUC_{0-\infty}$ (μg·h/ml)
Fast 1	33.4	1.43	656
Fast 2	52.1	1.71	652
Antacid	55.7	1.43	613
Fed	45.6	3.09	672

probably via inhibition of urate transport, and thus increases uricemia. Renal function would be expected to have a significant impact on the clearance of pyrazinamide, pyrazinoic acid, and 5-hydroxypyrazinoic acid.

Pyrazinamide is active in guinea pig TB (extracellular) but is also active in murine TB, which has an important intracellular component. Its main characteristic is to be active against dormant cells.

Food could delay the absorption of pyrazinamide (Table 38).

9. ETHAMBUTOL

9.1. General Characteristics

Discovered in 1961 by Wilkinson and coauthors among a number of synthetic molecules, ethambutol is the dextrogyre isomer of *N,N'*-bis-(1-hydroxymethylpropyl) ethylenediamine, administered in the form of the dihydrochloride salt (Fig. 10).

The *d*-isomer is 200 times more active against *M. tuberculosis* than the *l*-isomer. A series of ethambutol analogs was prepared by substitution of the two ethyl moieties at each side of the molecule, resulting in deleterious activity against *M. tuberculosis* as well as introduction of a conformational constraint, such as a prolinol, which abolishes the in vitro activity.

CH_2OH … CH_2OH

H—C—N—CH_2—CH_2—N—C—H

C_2H_5 … C_2H_5

Figure 10 Structure of ethambutol

9.2. Mechanism of Action, Antibacterial Spectrum, and In Vitro and In Vivo Activities

Ethambutol has bacteriostatic activity against *M. tuberculosis*, *M. bovis*, *M. africanum*, *M. kansasii*, and mycobacteria of the *Mycobacterium terrae* complex. The MIC for *M. tuberculosis* ranges from 0.5 to 2 μg/ml depending on whether it is measured in a liquid medium with Tween-albumin or in Löwenstein-Jensen medium.

The MICs for *M. bovis*, *M. avium*, and *M. kansasii* are 1.0 to 2.0, 1.0 to 2.4, and 1.0 to 4.0 μg/ml, respectively.

Ethambutol interacts with outer membrane synthesis, being an inhibitor of arabinosyltransferase. Ethambutol inhibits outer membrane formation by mycobacteria via the *embCAB* gene cluster. The outer membrane of mycobacteria contains mainly polysaccharides and proteins with lipid components. The carbohydrate composes most of the outer membrane. The two main components for *M. tuberculosis* are polysaccharide and glucan: arabinoglucan a neutral polysaccharide acetylated or not. It is attached to a lipid, lipoarabinomannan (β-D-arabinofuranosyl-1-monophosphodecaprenol). Ethambutol must lie between conversion of D-glucose to D-arabinose and transfers of the arabinose into arabinogalactan (activated sugar is a guanosine diphospho-D-arabinose).

9.3. Pharmacokinetics

Ethambutol is administered orally at a dose of 20 mg/kg but may also be administered intramuscularly or intravenously. Almost 75 to 80% of the administered dose is absorbed, and the peak concentration in plasma of 3 to 5 μg/ml is reached in 1 or 2 h. The apparent elimination half-life is 6 to 8 h. After intravenous infusion of 20 mg/kg over 2 h, the concentration in serum was 11.5 μg/ml, but it was 2 μg/ml 2 h later. After 25 mg/kg orally as a single dose, the maximum concentration in serum is 5.0 μg/ml and the residual concentration at 24 h is ≤1.0 μg/ml. Eight to fifteen percent of the administered dose is converted to inactive metabolites (Fig. 11).

The average pharmacokinetics after a single oral dose of 15 mg/kg are listed in Table 39.

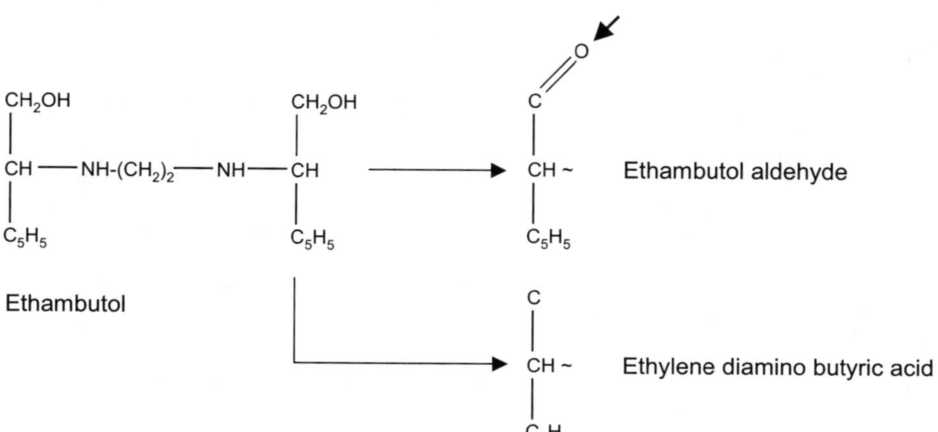

Figure 11 Metabolism of ethambutol

Table 39 Pharmacokinetics of ethambutol given as a single oral dose of 15 mg/kg

Parameter	Value
C_{max} (μg/ml)	4.0
T_{max} (h)	2.8
AUC (μg·h/ml)	28.9
$t_{1/2}$ (h)	12.4
CL_R (liters/h)	25
Urinary recovery (%)	53
Protein binding (%)	0–25
Elimination in the stool in 72 h (%)	9.1

Table 40 Pharmacokinetics of ethambutol (25 mg/kg) after food ($n = 16$)

Food status	C_{max} (μg/ml)	T_{max} (h)	$AUC_{0-\infty}$ (μg·h/ml)
Fast 1	4.52	2.46	28.9
Fast 2	4.58	2.50	30.7
Antacid	3.27	2.93	27.5
Fed	3.83	3.21	29.6

Ethambutol diffuses into the whole body, including the CSF. However, when the meninges are inflamed, the concentrations in CSF are only 10 to 20% of those in serum. Because of a storage effect, the intraerythrocyte concentrations are higher than the concentrations in serum for longer.

Almost 60% of the ingested dose is eliminated in the urine in 24 h in the unmetabolized form and 15% in the form of an aldehyde and a carboxylic acid. Elimination occurs primarily by glomerular filtration. The remaining 20 to 30% is eliminated in the feces. The dosage of ethambutol must be adapted in the event of renal insufficiency. During hemodialysis (procedure lasting 8 h), the mean half-life of ethambutol is reduced versus that in the dialysis-free period (21 versus 6 h). Ethambutol is removed by peritoneal dialysis. The apparent elimination half-life during peritoneal dialysis is 5.6 h. The circulating compound is ethambutol and not the metabolite.

The pharmacokinetics under fasting conditions and after food are summarized in Table 40. Under fasting conditions the interindividual variability is small. The maximum concentration in serum is significantly reduced in subjects taking food or antacids.

The absolute bioavailability of ethambutol tablets versus the intravenous formulation has not been published.

After intravenous administration of ethambutol, less than 1% of the administered dose is eliminated in the stool, whereas up to 20% could be eliminated by this route after oral administration of ethambutol. Erythrocytes may serve as a depot for ethambutol. Small amounts of compounds are slowly released into the circulation in the intervals between drug administration. The C/E ratio is 7 for an extracellular concentration of 5 μg/ml.

10. THIOAMIDES: ETHIONAMIDE AND PROTIONAMIDE

The second-line antibiotics are kanamycin, thioamides, PAS, D-cycloserine, capreomycin, viomycin, thiacetazone, and tiocarlide.

Ethionamide Protionamide

Figure 12 Structures of ethionamide and protionamide

Ethionamide is 3-ethylthioisonicotinamide, and protionamide is 2-propylthioisonicotinamide (Fig. 12). They exhibit anti-TB activity and similar pharmacokinetics and toxicities.

10.1. Mechanism of Action, Antibacterial Spectrum, and In Vitro and In Vivo Activities

The thioamides, derivatives of isonicotinic acid, have an antibacterial spectrum similar to that of isoniazid, essentially *M. tuberculosis* complex.

The MIC for the strains of *M. tuberculosis* vary with the pH and culture medium and the duration of incubation. They range from 0.5 to 2 μg/ml in a liquid medium and 5 to 20 μg/ml in Löwenstein-Jensen medium.

The thioamides have bactericidal activity in vitro and in vivo. In mice and humans, thioamides prevent the selection of mutants resistant to the antibiotics combined with them.

The mechanism of action seems to be similar to that of isoniazid; however, isolates resistant to isoniazid may remain susceptible to ethionamide. The *ethA* gene encodes a flavoprotein monooxygenase which activates ethionamide through thioamide oxidation. This enzyme is an NADH-dependent 2-transenoyl-ACP reductase.

10.2. Pharmacokinetics

Administered orally, the thioamides are well absorbed by the gastrointestinal tract, but their poor digestive tolerance requires them to be administered in the form of enteric coated tablets or suppositories, which produce levels in serum that vary considerably from one subject to another. The average peak concentration in plasma, obtained in 3 h, is 20 μg/ml after oral administration of 1 g. The apparent elimination half-life is about 2 h. Like isoniazid, the thioamides diffuse well into all compartments of the body and penetrate macrophages well, where they have bactericidal activity (Table 41).

They are eliminated in the urine, 1 to 3% in the active form and the remainder in the form of six metabolites. Some metabolites are active, such as the sulfoxide, the 2-ethyl isonicotinic acid, and amide, as well as the corresponding dihydropteridine derivatives (Fig. 13).

Food has a minimal effect on gastrointestinal absorption (Table 42).

There are substantial interindividual variations. Ethionamide undergoes first-pass metabolism that could explain this variability. The mean maximum concentration in serum is increased by 9% with orange juice and is slightly decreased by antacids (4%). The absorption was delayed by

Table 41 Pharmacokinetics of ethionamide and protionamide

Parameter	Value for:	
	Ethionamide	Protionamide
C_{max} (μg/ml)	55–215[a]	48–870
T_{max} (h)	1.5	0.5
$t_{1/2}$ (h)	1.85	1.78
$AUC_{0-\infty}$ (μg·h/ml)	10	
CL_P (liters/h)	51.6	
V (liters)	79	93
CL_R (liters/h)		
Urinary elimination (%)	3	3
Bioavailability	1.1	0.9
Protein binding (%)	30	60

[a]Intravenous formulation.

concomitant ingestion of orange juice by 12%, was delayed by 53% by food, and was delayed by 35% by antacids.

The pharmacokinetics of the suppository form (500 mg) are listed in Table 43.

Table 42 Pharmacokinetics of ethionamide given as a single oral dose after food

Food status	C_{max} (μg/ml)	T_{max} (h)	$AUC_{0-\infty}$ (μg·h/ml)
Fast 1	2.3	1.7	10
Fast 2	2.5	1.9	9.6
Antacid	2.3	2.6	10
Fed	2.2	2.3	10.4

Less than 1% is eliminated in the feces. Ethionamide is eliminated in the saliva at more than 1% of the administered dose, and protionamide is poorly eliminated in saliva.

11. PAS

PAS was described in 1901 and 1902 by Seidel and coworkers. During analysis of organic acids on the oxidative metabolism of *M. tuberculosis* in the 1940s by Bernheim, he discovered the effect of salicylate on oxygen consumption by *M. tuberculosis*. Based on this observation Lehmann et al. in 1946 described the anti-TB activity of PAS.

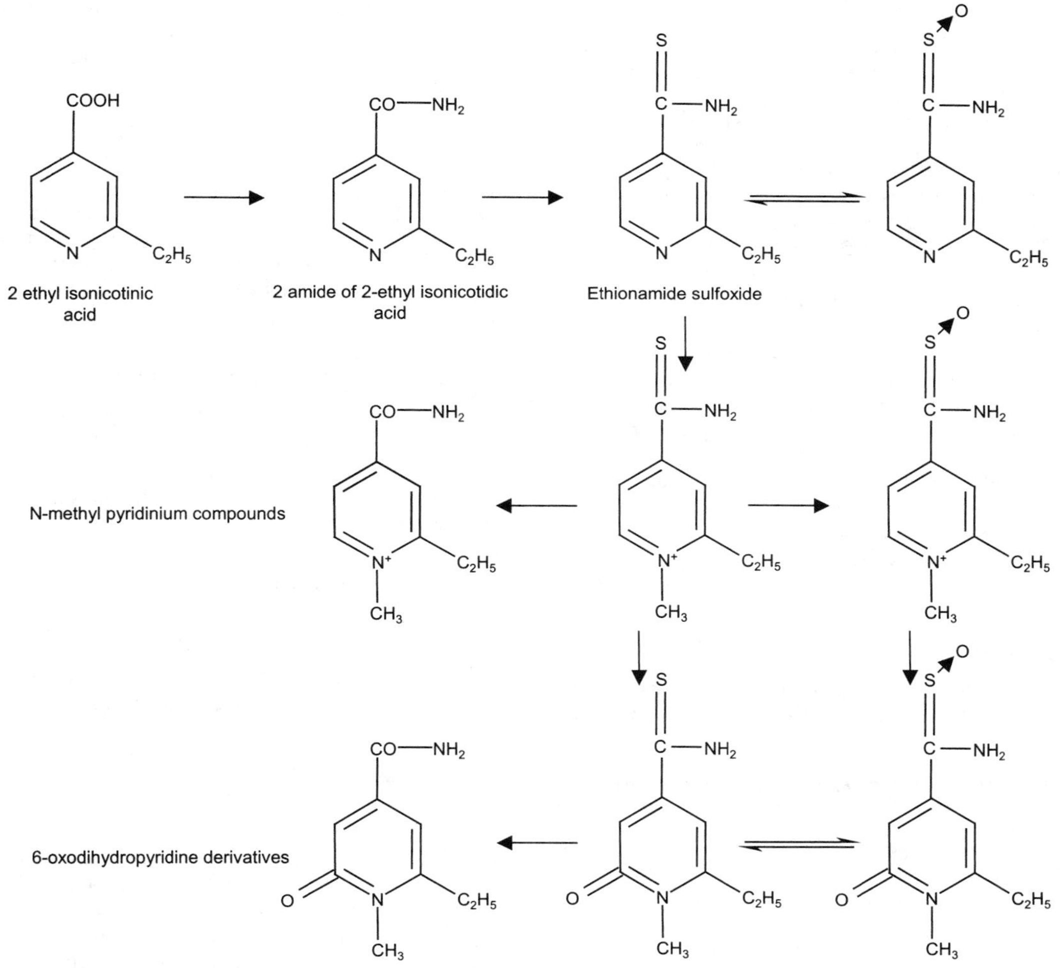

Figure 13 Metabolism of ethionamide

Table 43 Pharmacokinetics of ethionamide tablets and suppositories

Delivery route ($n = 12$)	C_{max} (μg/ml)	T_{max} (h)	AUC (μg·h/ml)	Bioavailability (%)
Oral	2.24	1.75	10.34	100
Rectal	0.74	4.42	5.34	57.28

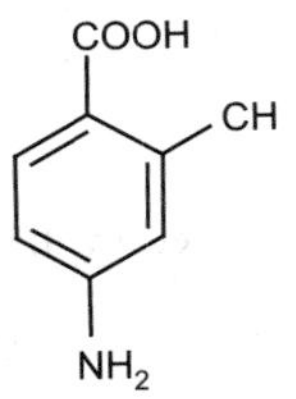

COOH
CH
NH$_2$

Figure 14 Structure of PAS

An analog of *para*-aminobenzoic acid, PAS is a synthetic antibacterial agent (Fig. 14).

11.1. Mechanism of Action, Antibacterial Spectrum, and In Vitro and In Vivo Activities

PAS is bacteriostatic against *M. tuberculosis* complex. Barring exceptions, it is inactive against mycobacterial species. PAS is inactive against common pathogens. Its MIC ranges between 1 and 10 μg/ml (Table 44).

The mechanism of action of PAS remains controversial: like that of the sulfonamides, it involves inhibition of folic acid synthesis. Some studies suggest that this compound blocks the salicylate-dependent biosynthesis of mycobactins, which are involved in iron assimilation.

PAS decomposes by decarboxylation with the release of *m*-aminophenol; this could occur under the influence of moisture, light, or air. PAS cannot be boiled or autoclaved. It is antagonized by the presence of *para*-aminobenzoic acid.

Heterogenic populations have been described. The resistance phenotype seems to be unstable and noninheritable. After a single step, the mutant is weakly resistant; high-level resistance is obtained by the second step. In this case it is a stable resistance.

PAS-resistant *M. tuberculosis* isolates are highly resistant to thiacetazone; however, isolates which are resistant to PAS at a low level remain susceptible to thiacetazone. All thiacetazone-resistant isolates remain susceptible to PAS. There is no cross-resistance with sulfonamides.

PAS, which is hydrophilic, does not accumulate in bacterial cells and probably not in macrophages.

PAS does not exert a postantibiotic effect.

Combined with isoniazid, it prevents the selection of isoniazid-resistant mutants and reduces its acetylation by a competitive effect.

11.2. Pharmacokinetics

After oral administration of 4 g, the peak concentration in plasma of 8 μg/ml is reached within 2 h. The apparent elimination half-life is on the order of 1 h. Eighty percent of the administered dose is eliminated in urine through glomerular filtration and tubular secretion. The drug has to be given in an acidic beverage to regulate the release (Table 45).

Table 44 In vitro activity of PAS against mycobacteria

Organism	MIC (μg/ml)
M. tuberculosis	0.5–1.5
M. bovis	25
M. avium	500
M. kansasii	19
M. smegmatis	125

Table 45 Pharmacokinetics of PAS

Parameter	Value
C_{max} (μg/ml)	75 (i.v.[a])
T_{max} (h)	1–2
V (liters)	7.4
$t_{1/2}$ (min)	64 (i.v.), 24.6 (oral)
CL_R (ml/min)	120–197
Protein binding (%)	
PAS	15
Acetyl	58–73
Glycine	30–35
Urinary elimination (%)	80

[a]i.v., intravenous.

PAS diffuses throughout the body, and almost 75% is metabolized in the liver to *N*-acetylaminosalicylic acid (60%) and to the glycine metabolite. The latter compound exhibits anti-TB activity, whereas the acetyl derivative is inactive.

Acetylation starts in the intestinal mucosa. After a 12-g oral dose, 45% is eliminated in feces as acetylated PAS. The esterified glycine derivative circulates in plasma. It has been reported to have up to five glucuronide derivatives, including glucuro-*p*-aminosalicyluric acid (35%). The metabolites and a small proportion of free PAS are eliminated in the urine (Fig. 15).

PAS is relatively unstable in aqueous solution in the formulation *m*-aminophenol.

Patients receiving calcium benzoyl PAS have lower concentrations in plasma than with free PAS. The AUC is smaller for all PAS salts (calcium, sodium, and potassium).

In renally impaired patients, the plasma clearance is increased by 183%.

12. D-CYCLOSERINE

D-Cycloserine was described in 1952 by Kurosawa from *Streptomyces* sp. strain K 00 under the name orientomycin. D-Cycloserine has also been isolated from *Streptomyces lavindulans* (1955), *Streptomyces garyphalus* (1955), and *Streptomyces orchidaceus* (1955).

D-Cycloserine is a cyclic derivative of serine hydroxamic acid (Fig. 16).

12.1. Microbiology

D-Cycloserine possesses a broad antibacterial spectrum, being active against the majority of mycobacteria, including *M. avium-M. intracellulare*, gram-positive bacteria such as *Staphylococcus aureus*, and gram-negative bacteria such as *E. coli*. Only the D-isomer has been developed. A structural analog of D-alanine, D-cycloserine disrupts bacterial cell

Figure 15 Metabolism of PAS

Figure 16 D-Cycloserine

wall synthesis, but its activity is inhibited in the presence of D-alanine.

The MIC of D-cycloserine for susceptible strains of *M. tuberculosis* ranges from 10 to 30 μg/ml in Löwenstein-Jensen medium.

The drug target seems to be the *alrA* gene. D-Cycloserine inhibits both D-alanine racemase and D-alanyl- D-alanine synthase (Fig. 17) in *M. tuberculosis*, resulting in accumulation of the peptidoglycan precursor UDP-glycosyl muramyl tripeptide.

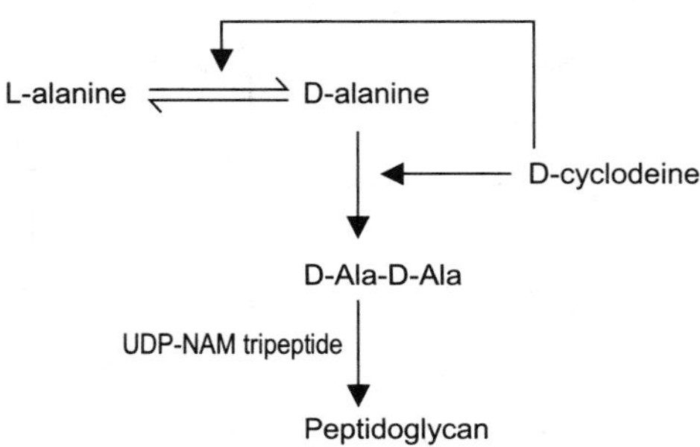

Figure 17 Mechanism of action of D-cycloserine

D-Cycloserine is transported in bacterial cells through a permease.

12.2. Pharmacokinetics

D-Cycloserine is well absorbed by the gastrointestinal tract. After oral administration of 250 mg, the peak concentration in plasma of 10 μg/ml is reached in 3 to 4 h. D-Cycloserine has good diffusion in tissue and CSF; it penetrates macrophages and crosses the blood-placenta barrier. Almost 60 to 70% of the administered dose is eliminated in the urine in the active form (47%). The renal clearance corresponds to the glomerular filtration rate. In renally impaired patients the daily dose needs to be reduced. D-Cycloserine is moderately bound to plasma proteins. Food delays or even reduces gastrointestinal absorption (Table 46).

D-Cycloserine is rapidly destroyed at acidic to neutral pH, but it is stable in alkaline solutions.

Table 46 Pharmacokinetics of D-cycloserine

Parameter	Value for:	
	D-Cycloserine	Terizidone
C_{max} (μg/ml)	14.4	16.3
T_{max} (h)	3.0	3.0
AUC (μg·h/ml)		
$t_{1/2}$ (h)	7–15	7–15
V (liters)	Unknown	Low
Protein binding (%)	47	
Urinary elimination (%)	8–17.9	

13. VIOMYCIN

Viomycin was extracted from the fermentation broth of *Streptomyces floridae* in 1951 and also from *Streptomyces puniceus*.

Viomycin is a basic peptide antibiotic (Fig. 18) whose activity against M. *tuberculosis* is four times weaker than that of streptomycin. It has been withdrawn from the market. The MIC for M. *tuberculosis* is 5 μg/ml in a liquid culture medium and 10 to 20 μg/ml in Löwenstein-Jensen medium.

There is partial inhibition of M. *tuberculosis* growth in macrophages. The in vitro activity against other mycobacteria is weak. Viomycin is weakly active against gram-positive and gram-negative bacteria.

Its pharmacokinetic profile is similar to that of capreomycin. Viomycin is administered intramuscularly at a dosage of 1 g daily. Sixty-three to one hundred percent of the administered dose is eliminated in urine. Apparently no metabolites of viomycin have been recovered. No data on plasma protein binding have been reported. After 1.0 g intramuscularly, the peak concentration in plasma of 25.6 μg/ml was reached in 1.0 to 2.0 h.

Its toxicity is mainly renal and auditory.

14. CAPREOMYCIN

Capreomycin was described in 1960 from the fermentation broth of *Streptomyces capreolus*. The capreomycin complex is composed of four components: IA, IB, IIA, and IIB. Component IA contains a serine instead of an alanine (Fig. 19).

Components IIA and IIB did not have a β-lysine in their side chains (Fig. 20). The preparation contains approximately 80% component IA and 20% component IB.

Capreomycin is an antibiotic cyclic peptide that inhibits protein synthesis. The MICs for M. *tuberculosis* strains, irrespective of their resistance to PAS, streptomycin, or ethionamide, range from 1 to 4 μg/ml. Capreomycin is poorly active against common gram-positive bacteria.

The MIC for M. *tuberculosis* is 1 to 4 μg/ml in a liquid medium and 8 to 16 μg/ml in Löwenstein-Jensen medium.

Administered intramuscularly at a dose of 1 g, capreomycin (Capastat) has a peak concentration in plasma within 1 to 2 h of 30 to 35 μg/ml. About 50 to 60% of the administered dose is eliminated in the free form in the urine.

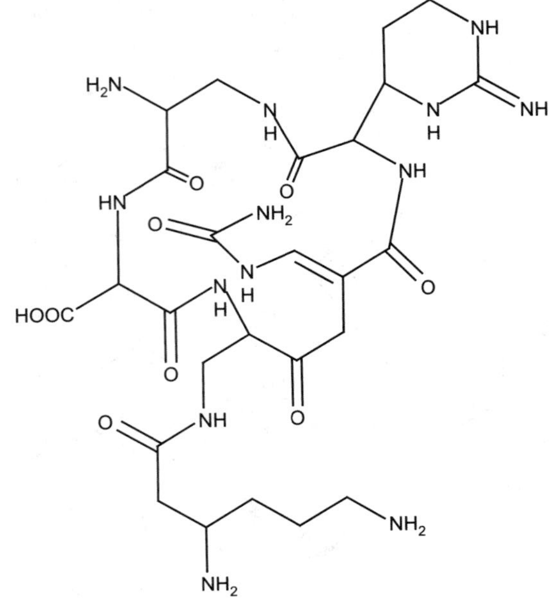

Figure 19 Capreomycin

The side effects of capreomycin are similar to those of streptomycin, particularly for the kidney and the VIIIth pair of cranial nerves.

15. THIACETAZONE

The synthesis of a series of thiosemicarbazones as intermediates in the preparation of analogs of sulfathiazole, which exhibit weak anti-TB activity, led to the discovery G. Domagk's team of thiosemicarbazone. The anti-TB activity resides in the aromatic aldehydes.

Thiacetazone is a thiosemicarbazone (Fig. 21).

The antibacterial spectrum of thiacetazone is confined to mycobacterial species and, among these, to mycobacteria of

Figure 18 Viomycin

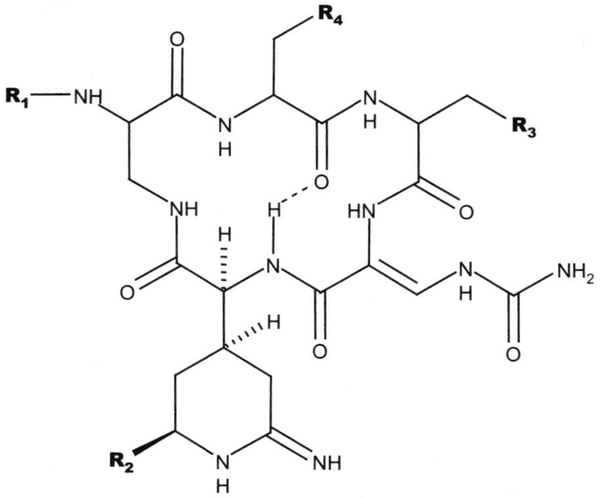

Compound	R_1	R_2	R_3	R_4
I A	H	H	NH-X	H
I B	H	H	NH-X	H
II A	H	H	NH_2	OH
II B	H	H	NH_2	H

X = H_2N–

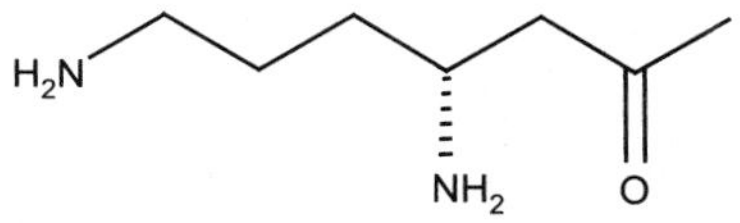

Figure 20 Capreomycin components

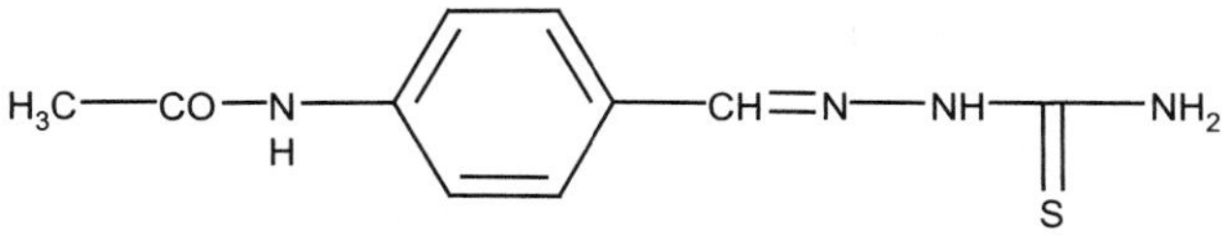

H_3C—CO—NH—C_6H_4—CH=N—NH—C(=S)—NH_2

Figure 21 Thiacetazone

the M. *tuberculosis* complex and certain atypical mycobacteria. Its MIC for M. *tuberculosis* in vitro is 1 μg/ml. Although it has bacteriostatic activity, thiacetazone is still used in a number of developing countries for first-line treatment of TB in combination with isoniazid and streptomycin.

Natural resistance of M. *africanum* to thiacetazone is common in certain regions of Africa.

After oral administration of a dose of 150 mg, the peak concentration in serum of 1 to 3 μg/ml is reached in 4 to 5 h. The apparent elimination half-life of thiacetazone is about 12 h. Thiacetazone is eliminated in the urine, 20 to 30% without transformation and the remainder metabolized. Four to twelve percent of the administered dose is recovered in the feces. The metabolites are suspected to be *para*-aminobenzaldehyde (1%) and *para*-acetylaminobenzaldehyde (5%).

16. TIOCARLIDE (ISOXYL)

Tiocarlide (Fig. 22) is 4,4′-diisoamyloxydiphenylthiourea. Tiocarlide belongs to the diaryl thiourea family and was synthesized in 1953 by Buu-Hoi et al. It is an oral drug, the drug substance being poorly soluble in water. Tiocarlide was used in TB therapy in the 1960s in combination with isoniazid, with which it exerts a synergistic activity. When the drug is used alone, the clinical outcome even after 6 months of therapy is poor. Isoxyl interacts with the biosynthesis of mycolic acid, as demonstrated in M. *bovis*, especially on the synthesis of fatty acids of free lipids. The mode of action is not totally clear. It seems that tiocarlide complexes metal ions. Tiocarlide exhibits only anti-M. *tuberculosis* activity and is active against multidrug-resistant M. *tuberculosis*. MICs determined in the presence of bovine serum range from 2.0 to 10 μg/ml and >7.5 μg/ml for other mycobacterial species. There is no cross-resistance with other anti-TB drugs except with thiosemicarbazone.

Tiocarlide is bound to the lipoprotein fraction of erythrocytes. No data on intracellular bioactivity are available.

After an oral dose of 3 g of tiocarlide, the level in blood irrespective of the pharmaceutical formulation (tablets or granules) ranged from 0.2 to 0.5 μg/ml (at 24 h). The peak concentration in plasma of 5.54 μg/ml was obtained 9 h after administration. There is considerable interindividual variation. The lag time was half an hour. Small quantities are eliminated in the urine (0 to 2%) and by the biliary route. The apparent elimination half-life and the volume of distribution were not disclosed. Metabolites with unknown structures have been detected. The daily dose is 6 to 10 g in divided doses. In rabbits it was shown to have an extrahepatic cycle.

Hypoglycemia and leukopenia in addition to skin reactions are the main side effects.

17. OTHER DRUGS

17.1. Fluoroquinolones

The therapeutic use of fluoroquinolones in the therapy of TB started in the early 1990s. Antimycobacterial activities of fluoroquinolones widely differ, depending on their structures.

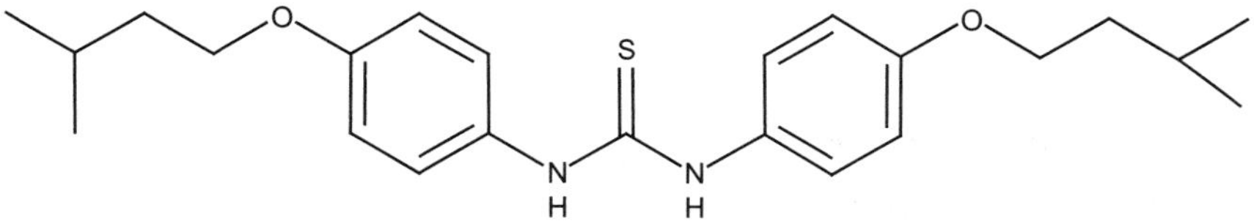

Figure 22 Tiocarlide (isoxyl)

The 1,8-naphthyridones are inactive against *M. tuberculosis*. All differences could be due to differences in fluoroquinolone penetration across the outer membrane and their affinities for DNA gyrase. Higher hydrophobicity seems to increase their penetration across the outer membrane. Mycobacterial resistance to fluoroquinolones has been associated with mutations in the quinolone resistance-determining region of subunit A at positions 90, 91, and 94. There are discrepancies between results obtained with the E-test method and genotypic analysis of ofloxacin resistance using automated sequencing.

Among the new antibacterials, only the fluoroquinolones (Fig. 23) exhibit activity against *M. tuberculosis*, even if the isolates are resistant to isoniazid and rifampin. Ofloxacin is active against *M. tuberculosis* in vitro and in vivo, but sparfloxacin and moxifloxacin are even more efficient. In vitro, its MICs are two to four times lower than those of ciprofloxacin (which is poorly active in vivo, probably for pharmacokinetic reasons) and ofloxacin. In the mouse, it is six to eight times more active than ofloxacin and appears to be almost as bactericidal as isoniazid and rifampin. Initial empirical therapy with a fluoroquinolone may be associated with a delay in the initiation of appropriate anti-TB treatment.

17.2. Clofazimine

In early experimental studies, clofazimine (Fig. 24) was found to be active in murine and hamster TB; however, the compound was poorly active in guinea pigs and monkeys. These discrepancies were attributed to inadequate absorption in certain species of animals and low levels of the compound in the plasma of these animals, in which the disease was considered extracellular. Clofazimine is one of the components of the therapy for Hansen disease. Derivatives of clofazimine were synthesized to be active against *M. tuberculosis*.

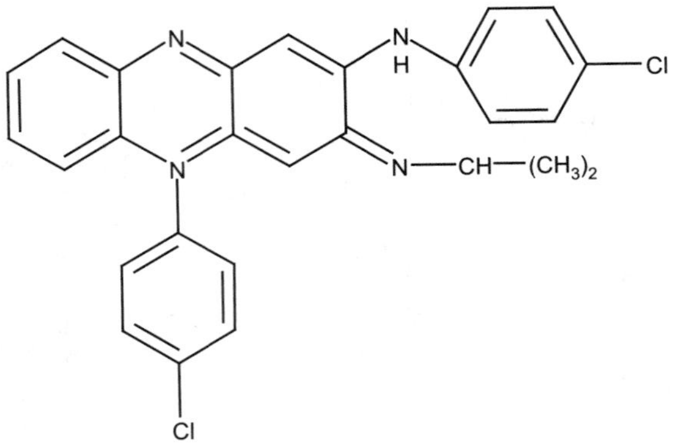

Figure 24 Clofazimine

The mechanism of action has not yet been clearly defined. Clofazimine apparently inhibits the growth of mycobacteria by potentiating the activity of phospholipase A2, leading to lysophospholipid-mediated dysfunction of membrane cation transporters. It was also proposed that clofazimine inhibits mycobacterial replication by binding to the guanine bases of DNA.

17.3. Macrolides

The macrolides available in clinical practice today lack potency against *M. tuberculosis*. Innate macrolide resistance in *M. tuberculosis* appears to be mediated by the *erm* gene (Buriankova et al., 2004).

Some macrolides and ketolides exhibit relatively low MICs against *M. tuberculosis* (MICs, 0.125–8.0 μg/ml) with low specificity, as shown by the relatively low 50% inhibitory

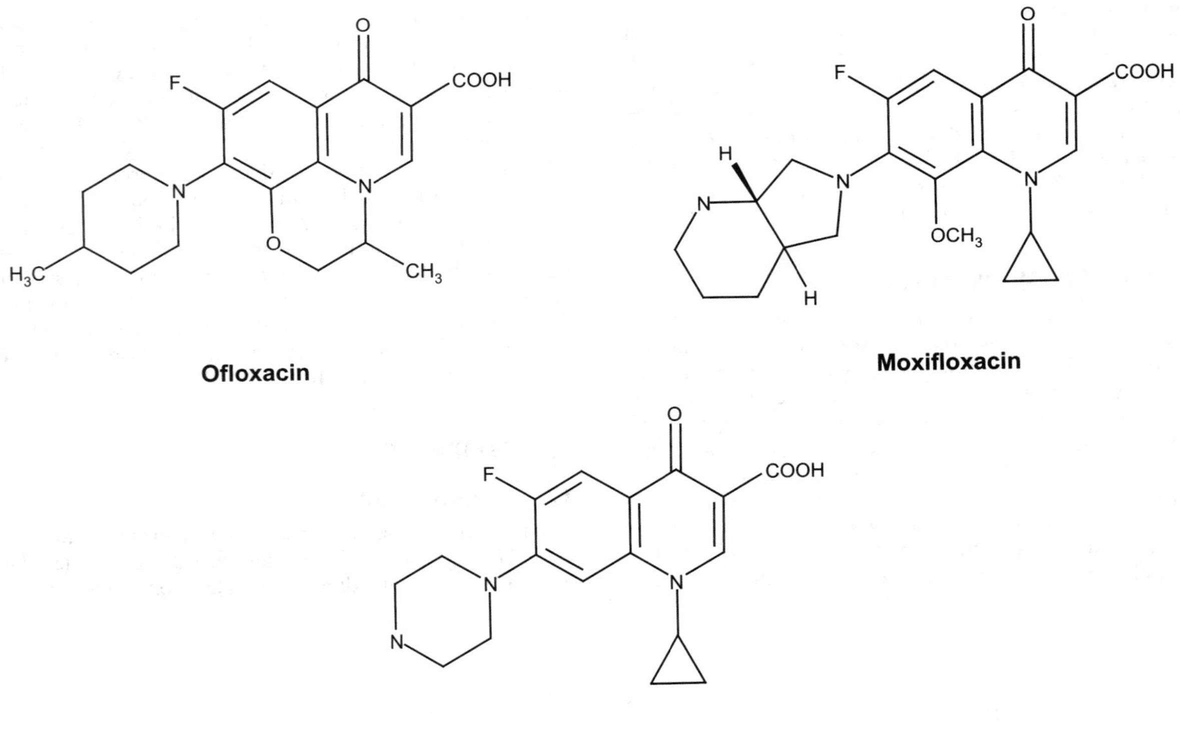

Ofloxacin

Moxifloxacin

Ciprofloxacin

Figure 23 Fluoroquinolones

concentration (IC_{50}) for Vero cells and for J 774 A.1 cells. Two macrolides, RU 60856 (having a C-11–C-12 carbamate with a quinoline butyl chain) and RU 69874 (C-11–C-12 side chain found in telithromycin), are exceptions, with MICs of 0.44 and 0.38 μM, respectively, and low cytotoxicity.

Among analogs harboring a nonsubstituted C-11–C-12 carbamate residue, the most active analog was A-323348, harboring a 2-fluorine and a 6-quinolyl isoxazolyl propyl side chain (MIC, 0.38 μM).

In macrophages, a reduction of 1 to 2 log CFU/ml in viability was recorded at 1.6 to 8.0 μM for RU 66252 (the cladinose counterpart of HMR 3004) and A-323348. The bactericidal activity was dose dependent against *M. tuberculosis* Erdman in J 774 A.1 macrophages (*M. tuberculosis* Erdman grows better in macrophages and in mice than *M. tuberculosis* $H37_{RV}$). BALB/c mice were challenged by means of an aerosol with *M. tuberculosis* Erdman and treated at the dose of 100 and 200 mg/kg with various analogs. A more pronounced inhibitory activity against *M. tuberculosis* pneumonia was obtained with RU 66252.

RU 66252 remains active against multidrug-resistant *M. tuberculosis* (MIC identical to those for wild strains: 0.25–0.50 μM) (Falzari et al., 2005).

18. RESISTANCE OF TUBERCLE BACILLI TO ANTIBACTERIALS

The different species of *M. tuberculosis* complex have natural or clinical resistance to most of the standard antibacterials, such as macrolides (specific methylase). They may also acquire resistance to antibiotics to which they are naturally susceptible. *M. tuberculosis* strains are commonly isolated in vitro in the laboratory and in vivo in experimental animals, particularly in mice and also in humans. It is important to characterize resistance patterns according to gender, age, country of origin for immigrants or pilgrims, or recent journey to areas of endemicity.

In areas where the anti-TB program was maintained, the rates of drug resistance have not increased substantially. In areas where this program was not maintained properly by the public sector, there are alarming rates of drug resistance.

Comparison of drug resistance rates among communities and countries is difficult because methods are not standardized. However, in a given country, it can be expected that serial surveys can yield comparable results and trends can be tracked.

Usually, the number of men with an *M. tuberculosis* infection is greater than that of women (ratio, 2:1). Using tuberculin tests, the prevalence of *M. tuberculosis* was higher in men than in women in China, India, and Korea, and sometimes higher after 14 years of age in males than in females. Other studies have shown that there is no difference between genders. However, it has been suggested that the tuberculin test may be less sensitive for women due to a lesser delayed-type hypersensitivity response than in men.

Unlike for many bacterial species, such as common pathogens which are able to acquire antibiotic resistance genes by transduction, conjugation, or transformation, there is no evidence of mobilization of genes between *M. tuberculosis* strains.

18.1. Incidence of Resistance

As no plasmid coding for resistance to naturally active antibiotics has been identified to date, the acquired resistance of mycobacteria of the *M. tuberculosis* complex to antibiotics is considered the result of selection of chromosomal mutants. The incidence of these mutants is on average 10^{-6} for isoniazid and streptomycin and 10^{-7} to 10^{-9} for rifampin. It is often higher for second-line antibiotics.

Table 47 Frequency and rate of mutation to resistance to first-line anti-TB drugs

Compound	Concn (μg/ml)	Mutation rate	Frequency
Isoniazid	0.2	1.84×10^{-8}	3.5×10^{-6}
	1.0	1.70×10^{-8}	3.10×10^{-6}
Streptomycin	2.0	2.90×10^{-8}	3.80×10^{-6}
Rifampin	1.0	2.20×10^{-10}	1.20×10^{-8}
Ethambutol	5.0	1.0×10^{-7}	3.10×10^{-5}

The genes responsible for the resistance of *M. tuberculosis* to isoniazid, rifampin, and ethambutol have been identified. For isoniazid, the resistance is related to loss of the catalase/peroxidase gene. The deletion of the catalase/peroxidase gene confers resistance to isoniazid, while supplementation of an isoniazid-resistant strain with the catalase/peroxidase gene restores susceptibility to isoniazid. It remains to be determined why isoniazid-resistant *M. tuberculosis* mutants have decreasing catalase activity and virulence in the guinea pig as their degree of resistance to isoniazid increases. Almost all strains of *M. tuberculosis* for which the MIC of isoniazid is 10 μg/ml or more no longer have catalase activity or pathogenic activity in guinea pigs.

M. tuberculosis mutants resistant to antibiotics of one family normally remain susceptible to antibiotics of the other families, with the exception of thioamide-resistant mutants, which are resistant to thiacetazone, and mutants that are weakly resistant to isoniazid, which sometimes exhibit marked resistance to thioamides. There is no cross-resistance between isoniazid and pyrazinamide despite the structural analogy of the two molecules.

18.2. Frequency of Resistance

Resistance to isoniazid develops at a rate of 10^{-5} to 10^{-7} in vitro, while resistance to rifampin develops less frequently, at a rate of about 10^{-9}. The rate of mutation to resistance to streptomycin, ethambutol, kanamycin, and PAS seems to be of the same magnitude as that for isoniazid. Resistance to ethionamide, capreomyin, and thiacetazone occurs approximately at a rate of 10^{-3}. The probability of developing resistance to both isoniazid and rifampin is 10^{-14} (Table 47).

18.3. Prevalence of Resistance

In Table 48 the rates of resistance to the main anti-TB drugs are listed. The incidence of therapeutic failure of anti-TB treatment has decreased considerably since the treatment has been based on the combination of several antibiotics, particularly the systematic use of rifampin. However, in occasional subjects (less than 1% of new cases of TB in France) with a relapse of TB after one or more previous treatments, *M. tuberculosis* becomes resistant to antibiotics (average of 20% of cases). Acquired or secondary resistance has serious therapeutic consequences, since half of the strains of *M. tuberculosis* with secondary resistance are resistant to isoniazid and rifampin, the two essential anti-TB antibiotics (Tables 49 and 50).

The rate of primary resistance, defined as resistance observed in patients whose TB has been recently diagnosed and not yet treated (or treated for less than 1 month), is 5 to 8% in France (Table 49). The most common forms of resistance are primary resistance to streptomycin (3 to 7%) and primary resistance to isoniazid (3 to 8%). Until recent

Table 48 Prevalence of resistant TB worldwide

Country or region	Year(s)	*n*	% of resistance[a]						
			PZA	PAS	INH	RIF	STR	EMB	MDR-TB
Africa									
Algeria	1966–1980	620			1.7		3.4		5.8
	1964–1966				3.2		3.8		
	1972–1974				2.5		2.7		
	1977–1978				3.0		3.2		
	1980				1.4		3.4		
	1980–1985				1.5		2.3		
Morocco	1997	130		3.8	34.6	33.1	26.1	9.2	27.6
	1998	510			2.7	0.2	0.6	0.0	2.2
Libya	1984–1986	598			3.0	0	4.2	5.9	
Egypt					10.4	3.0	6.0	7.0	0
Mauritania	1978	151		11.9	13.3		20	23.9	
Niger	1984	174			10.9	0.6	7.0	35.4	
Burkina Faso	1976			12.9	19.5		23.3	35.4	
	1992–1994	300			7.6	2.5	12.4	2.0	0.6
Gabon	1984				13.5	1.9	9.6	9.6	
Senegal	1987–1988	67			1.4	4.4	0	0	
Benin (Cotonou)	1990–1991	108			14.8		12.9	0	
	1991				6.5	0	4.6	0	8.3
Ghana	1985–1987	99	0	47	27	0	23	0	
Cameroon (Yaoundé)	NG	109		4.2	10		10		
	1994–1995	516			12.4	0.8	20.3	0.4	0.6
	1994–1995			3.7	6.0	0.2	15.1		0.8
	1996–1997	111			54.1	27.6	25.5	12.2	27.6
Tanzania	1982				22.3	2.2	8.0	3.0	
	1990–1994				28.1	0	0.3	2.8	1.0
Mali	1980–1982	235	24.1	0	15.5	3.5	19		
	1989–1990	498	32.7	0	6.2	1.1	7.1	3.1	
Malawi (Karonga)	1962–1963	234			8.0		4.0		
	1986	44			29.5	6.8	29.5		
	1993	119			5.04		6		1.7
	1986–1989				3.5	0.3	3.5	0	4.3
	1993								
Zaire	1983–1986	102							
Central Africa	1998	464			4.1	1.3	6.5	0.0	1.0
Guinea	1998	539			4.5	0.2	5.2	0.0	0.6
Equatorial Guinea	1999–2000	236			16.6				1.7
Ivory Coast	1989	46			20	3.0	3.0		21
Rwanda	1991–1993	298			5.4	0.7		4.7	2.4
	1991–1993				12.3	2.7		11	6.8
Uganda	1997	374			3.2	0.8	7.0	2.4	0.5
	2000	215			7.9	1.4	6.1	0.9	4.7
Kenya	1981	592			6.8	0.2	0.8		0.1
	1982	851			6.8	0.2	0.7		0.1
	1983	812			6.9	0.2	0.9		0.1
	1984	1,364			7.1	0.1	1.0		0.1
	1985	420			7.2	0.1	1.0		0.1
	1986	581			7.6	0.2	1.0		0
	1987	802			8.1	0.1	1.2		0
	1988	417			8.5	0	1.5		0
	1989	347			9.8	0.3	1.7		0
	1990	333			10.2	0	1.8		0
Nairobi	1989–1990				5.1		0.8		0.4
	1994–1997	491			12.4	0.0	2.0	0.0	0.0
	1995				12.4	0.0	2.0	0.0	0.0
Sierra Leone	1994–1997	635			21.4	4.9	28.9	4.1	4.2
	1995–1996				21.4	4.9	28.9	4.1	4.2
	1997	117			3.4	0.0	14.5	0.0	0.9
Zimbabwe	1994–1997	712			4.0	2.4	0.9	0.5	2.4
	1994–1995				4.0	2.4	0.9	0.5	2.4
	1994–1996	381							6.7

(Continued on next page)

Table 48 Prevalence of resistant TB worldwide (*Continued*)

Country or region	Year(s)	*n*	% of resistance[a]						
			PZA	PAS	INH	RIF	STR	EMB	MDR-TB
South Africa	1992–1993				10.6	4.2		0.3	4.0
	1965–1970				28.8	6.4	33.8	1.5	
	1971–1979				23.3	2.0	10.6	1.5	
	1980–1988				14.2	1.8	12.1	1.2	
	1997	661			3.5	0.2	2.3	0.0	1.5
Swaziland	1994–1995	378			3.9	0	2.4	0.3	0
Lesotho	1994–1997	383			9.3	1.2	3.9	0.2	1.2
	1994–1995				9.3	1.2	3.9	0.2	1.1
Botswana	1994–1997	521			2.4	1.7	2.2	0.5	0.8
	1995–1996				2.4	1.7	2.2	0.5	0.8
	1998	638			3.6	0.2	1.6	0.0	0.5
Ethiopia	1993				46	11	31	5	11
	1994	167			8.4	1.0	10.2	0	1.2
	1994–1995				9.6	1.9	8.3	1.4	1.9
Zambia	1993				7.4	2.5	3.2		2.2
Mozambique	NG				37	37	37	37	58
	1999	1,028			7.98	1.8	0.0	2.5	3.5
Near East									
Saudi Arabia	1991			1.2	1.8	7.2	3.3		
Gizan	1985	108			40.8	30.4			19.4
Riyadh	1989	432			19.4	9.7			8.8
	1996–2000	6,316	3.1		11	9.7	9.1		5.7
Taif	1993	678			6.5	15.0			3.8
Jeddah	1993–1995	78			10.2	5.1			5.1
Riyadh	1996	289			7.2	3.1			2.8
Jeddah	1996–1998	101			28.7	20.7			20.7
Israel	1983–1992		0	0	7.7	0	6.8	0	0
	1992				15.6	5.2	22.2	1.5	3.7
	1993				20.4	7.2	17.4	3.4	6.0
	1994				22.5	6.7	22.3	0.8	5.0
	1998	307			1.6	0.3	3.3	0.0	8.1
Iran	NG				18.1	43.6	14.9	3.2	17
	1998	666			2.7	0.9	4.2	0.3	5.0
Oman	1999	133			1.5	0.8	2.3	1.5	0.8
North America									
United States	1991	33,313	5.8		9.1	3.9	5.7	2.4	3.5
	1995				8.4	2.7	6.4	2.1	2.0
	1997	12,063			4.4	0.4	3.0	0.5	1.2
Canada	1987				5.9	1.2	4.6	1.0	1.0
Ontario	1988			0.2	6.1	2.5	5.0	2.0	2.2
	1989			2.0	8.5	2.3	4.1	2.2	2.2
	1990			2.2	7.6	2.1	4.9	1.5	2.1
	1991			1.3	11.9	2.3	3.9	1.5	2.0
	1992			1.5	9.8	2.3	5.4	0.9	2.1
	1993			1.5	10.5	2.3	5.0	1.3	1.5
	1994			2.0	10.3	1.5	4.2	0.6	1.4
	1995			1.8	10	1.5	4.8	0.9	1.2
	1996			1.6	12	2.5	4.5	0.6	2.3
	1997			2.5	10.1	1.7	6.9	1.7	1.7
	1997	1,593			4.1	0.1	2.3	0.3	1.1
	1998			2.2	11.5	1.9	6.0	2.4	1.7
Oceania									
Australia	1994–1997	705			7.5	1.1	7.5	0.3	0.7
	1996	750			9.7	0.1	2.4	0.3	2.0
	1995				7.5	1.1	7.4	0.3	6.0
New Zealand	1995–1996				4.3	0.7	0.9	0.5	0.7
	1997	179			6.7	0.0	1.1	1.1	1.1
New Caledonia	1996	93			0.0	0.0	2.2	0.0	0.0
Asia									
China	1978–1982	1,309			9.2	1.0	10	0.7	

(*Continued on next page*)

Table 48 Prevalence of resistant TB worldwide (*Continued*)

Country or region	Year(s)	*n*	% of resistance[a]						
			PZA	PAS	INH	RIF	STR	EMB	MDR-TB
	2000	392		2.8	17.6	16.6	17.3	1.3	10.7
Henan Province	1996	646			24	1.4	6.3	0.5	0.5
Guangdong Province	1997	461			9.3	0.4	2.8	0.0	1.1
Shandong Province	1997	1,009			11.3	0.6	5.4	0.1	0.6
Zheijiang Province	1999	802	6		8.9	1.6	3.7	0.2	2.2
Taiwan	1981				7.4		8.7		
	1996–2000		50.9		16	9.5		12.1	11.4
Japan	1992	946			5.2	3.93.7	5.3	0.5	2.4
Singapore	1987–1997				72		45		14
	1996	980			2.6	0.1	1.3	0.0	0.3
The Philippines	1986–1990	299	10		17	8.0	7	39	8.0
	1992–1995	299	17.1		45.2	36.1	22.1	70.2	35.8
Thailand	1991–1996	8,282			5.4	1.2	5.8	0.1	4.4
	1996–1997	131			4.6	6.9	7.6	2.3	0.8
	1997	1,137			6.2	2.0	5.6	3.0	2.1
Korea	1965				16.7		9.5		
	1970				19.6		14.1		
	1975				18.0	1.1	8.5	2.1	2.0
	1980				25		4.6	5.6	
	1985				13.7	2.5	3.7	2.7	2.5
	1990				12.6		7.1	1.6	
	1994				10	4.0	3.5	4.2	3.1
	1999	2,370			4.9	0.7	1.3	0.0	0.3
Vietnam	1996–1997	640			6.7	1.1	11.1	0.2	3
Hong Kong	1989–1999								2.1
	1996	4,424			2.6	0.0	5.3	0.0	1.4
Malaysia	1984–1987				4.2	0.95	7.59	1.44	0.1
	1997	1,001			1.0	0.4	2.4	0.4	0.1
India	1983–1986	0		13.9	0	7.4			
Delhi	1995				28.8	14	18.1	7.0	13.3
Tamil Nadu	1997	384			7.6	0.5	1.8	0.5	3.4
	2000	644			18.7	2.5			2.5
Nepal	1996								1.1
	1999	104			1.5	0.8	0.8	0.0	0.8
Pakistan	1996				1.0				
Europe									
Austria	1999	756			4.3	0.7			0.3
Malta	1994–1997								
	1999	13			0	0			0
Denmark	1993–1995	1,354			10				<1
	1998	412			1.7	0.0	7.0	0.0	0.5
	1999	416			7.4	0.3			0
Norway	1994–1997								
	1996	138			4.3	0.0	2.9	0.0	2.2
	1999	144			7.6	2.1			2.1
Sweden	1993				<3	<3	<3		
	1994–1997								
	1997	356			3.1	0.0	2.2	0.0	0.6
	1999	377			9.3	1.3			0.8
Finland	1993				1.4	0	0.2		0.2
	1997	410			4.1	0.0	0.2	0.0	0.0
	1999	450			0.5	0			0
Iceland	1999	9			0	0			0
Switzerland	1994–1997			0	3.9	0.3		0.1	0.1
	1999	428			5.6	0.9			0.7
Zurich	1991–1992				4.0	0.3			0.5
	1997	322			2.6	0.2	0.3	0.0	0.0
United Kingdom	1987–1993	358			4.5	0.3			2.8
	1999	2,138			6.2	0.5			0.5
Germany	1985				0	0	1.0	0	

(*Continued on next page*)

Table 48 Prevalence of resistant TB worldwide (*Continued*)

Country or region	Year(s)	*n*	% of resistance[a]						
			PZA	PAS	INH	RIF	STR	EMB	MDR-TB
	1986				0	0	7.0	0	
	1987				0	0	0	0	
	1988				0	0	0	0	
	1999	3,356			4.3	1.0			0.8
Frankfurt	1989–1990	3,440	3.1		5.3	1.2	3.6	1.2	<0.1
	1989				0	0	8	0	
	1990				0	0	3	0	
	1991				0	0	2	0	
	1992				0	0	4	0	
	1993				0	0	5	0	
Berlin	1993		2.0		33	0	19	1.0	5.8
	1994				0	0	5	0	
	1995				0	0	7	0	
	1995	2,579	1.4		5.5	1.6	4.7	2.0	1.3
	1998	1,458			3.2	0.3	2.4	0.2	0.9
Croatia	1999	761			1.8	0.5			0.3
Bosnia and Herzegovina	1999	1,154			0.6	0.8			0.3
Czech Republic	1999	628			1.6	0.8			0.3
	1995				2.3	1.2	1.2	1.2	1.2
	1999	311			1.0	0.3	0	0	1.6
Poland	1974–1977				4.3	0	1.2	0	0
	1997	2,976			1.5	0.1	0.8	0	0.6
Slovakia	1999	456			2.3	0			0
	1998	589			1.4	0	0.7	0	0.3
Slovenia	1999	304			2.3	0			0
	1997	290			0.3	0	1.4	0	0.7
Estonia	1993				18	21	19	17	
	1999	1,128			27.3	17.8			17.3
	1994				25.3	11.7	24	9.2	11.7
	1998	377			2.7	0.3	10.3	0.3	14.1
Latvia	1999	825			27.4	10.4			10.4
	1998	789			7.2	0	1.8	0	9.0
Lithuania	1999	819			21.7	10.1			7.8
France	1999	910			3.4	0.8			0.7
	1992	48							0.56
	1993	40							0.47
	1994	58							0.7
	1995	40							0.6
	1997	26							0.5
	1998	30							0.5
	1995–1996				4.5	1.3	7.5	0.5	0.9
	1996								0.5
	1997								0.5
	1997	787			2.3	0.1	5.3	0.3	0
Greece	1986				0.0	0.88	3.90	0.88	
	1987				2.12	0.56	2.50	0	
	1988				1.59	0.69	1.19	0.96	
	1989				2.20	0.0	1.38	0	
	1990				1.11	0	1.86	9.16	
	1991				0.8	0	1.92	0.0	
	1994				28	28	28	28	9
Spain	1999	514			3.7	0.8			0.6
Madrid	1993–1994				5.7	4.3	4.9	2.6	7.4
Galicia	1993–1994								5.0
Overall	1992–1993				5.9	5.04		1.68	1.0
Barcelona	1995–1996	218			5.4	2.7	5.8	2.3	2.3
	1998	315			1.9	0.0	2.2	0.0	0.3
Portugal	1995	776			1.8	0	6.5	0	0.2
	2000	197			7.7	1.9			1.8
Belgium	1992	1,290							1.9
	1993	1,266							2.3

(*Continued on next page*)

Table 48 Prevalence of resistant TB worldwide (*Continued*)

Country or region	Year(s)	*n*	% of resistance[a]						
			PZA	PAS	INH	RIF	STR	EMB	MDR-TB
	1997	791			8.6	0.4			2.0
The Netherlands	1995				8.6	1.2	8.7	0.4	1.1
	1996	1,042			3.8	0.3	2.1	0.4	0.6
	1999	899			5.8	0.8			0.4
England and Wales	1995				6.8	2.1	2.9	0.4	1.9
	1997	3,053			2.9	0.1	3.6	0.0	0.8
Northern Ireland	1997	41			2.4	0.0	2.4	0.0	0.0
Scotland	1997	299			3.0	0.0	2.2	0.0	0.3
Ireland	1999	260			2.0	1.0			1.O
Italy	1999	683			2.9	0.9	5.3	0.4	1.2
Albania	1999								
Hungary	1999	456			7.2	2.6			1.8
	1994				4.0	0.4	2.0		0.5
Romania	1999	2,114			9.2	5.3			3.6
	1995				9.2	4.3	4.1	1.7	5.5
Yugoslavia	1999	290			0.7	0.3			0
Turkey	1992	785			13.4	19.2	24.3	6.5	9.2
Armenia	1999	104			8.7	6.7			2.9
Russia	1999	36,217							6.7
	1995–1996				21.4	4.9	28.9	4.9	4.2
Tomsk	1999	417			2.4	0.5	7.4	0.2	6.5
Ivanov	1998	222			7.2	0.0	6.3	2.7	9.0
Archangel	1998–2000	119			73.3		31.7		25.2
Ukraine	1999	245			12.3	11.0			7.8
Moldavia	1995–1999	3,463					81.5	21.8	11.2
Georgia		215							13
Kazakhstan	1999	2,024			20.2	9.3			5.4
Kyrgyzstan	1999	141			23.4	12.8			6.4
Latin America									
Argentina	1981				1.9		6.3		
	1985–1990	76		0	1.3	0	3.9	0	1.3
	1994–1997	894			12.5	9.2	10.9	5.2	8.0
	1994				12.5	9.2	10.9	5.2	8.0
Bolivia	1985–1990	109		0	3.7	0	8.3	0	2.8
	1994–1997	605			10.3	9.2	11.1	6.6	0.8
	1996				10.3	9.2	11.1	5.6	2.1
Brazil	1985–1990	355		0	2.0	0	6.8	0	2.0
	1994–1997	2,888			6.3	1.5	3.8	0.2	1.3
	1995–1996				6.3	1.5	3.8	0.2	1.3
Chile	1981				2.4	0.4	3.5		
	1985–1990	35		0	2.9	0	5.7	0	
	1997	732			1.2	0.1	4.9	0.0	0.4
Colombia	1985–1990	105		7.6	1.9	1.0	1.9	0.0	4.8
	1999	201			3.0	0.0	5.0	0.0	0.5
Cuba	1985–1990	35		2.9	2.9	0	5.7	0.0	5.7
	1994–1997	786			2.8	1.4	9.2	0	1.0
Ecuador	1989–1996	161			14.2	11.8			8.7
Haiti	1985–1990	26		7.7	7.7	0.0	3.7	0.0	3.7
	1988–1989	381		2.0	19	1.0	5.0		1.0
	1995–1996				2.8	1.4	9.2	0.0	1.8
	1998	284			0.7	0.0	3.5	0.0	0
Dominican Republic	1994–1997	420			22.4	18.6	21.8	5.1	8.6
	1995–1996				22.4	18.6	21.8	5.1	8.6
Mexico	1985–1990	164		3.0	2.4	0.6	6.7		4.3
	1997	334			4.2	0.6	5.4	0.3	2.4
Nicaragua	1998	564			5.9	0.5	5.5	0.2	1.2
Paraguay	1985–1990	38		2.6	5.3	0	2.6	0	0
Peru	1985–1990	79		2.5	2.5	5.0	18.9	0	8.9
	1994–1997	1,958			10	7.0	10	2.3	4.5
	1995–1996				10	7	10	2.3	4.5
	1999	1,879			3.6	0.7	6.8	0.8	3.0

(*Continued on next page*)

Table 48 Prevalence of resistant TB worldwide (*Continued*)

Country or region	Year(s)	*n*	% of resistance[a]						
			PZA	PAS	INH	RIF	STR	EMB	MDR-TB
Puerto Rico	1987–1990	466	1.0		26	22	13	8.0	19
	1994–1996				7.7	3.6	4.1	2.8	4.1
	1994–1997	391			7.3	3.6	2.8	3.6	4.1
	1997	160			3.2	0.6	2.5	0.6	2.5
Uruguay	1997	484			0.4	0.4	1.4	0.8	0
Venezuela	1998	221			1.4	0.0	1.4	0.0	0.0

[a]PZA, pyrazinamide; PAS, PAS or thiacetazone; INH, isoniazid; RIF, rifampin; STR, streptomycin; EMB, ethambutol; MDR-TB, resistance to rifampin and isoniazid; NG, not given.

Table 49 Secondary resistance of *M. tuberculosis* to isoniazid and rifampin in patients from the Pitié-Salpêtrière hospital (Paris, France) relapsing after previous treatment

Phenotype[a]	1980–1987		1988–1992	
	n	%	*n*	%
INH[r]	16	8.6	8	7.7
RIF[r]	1	0.5	2	1.9
INH[r] + RIF[r]	23	12.4	13	12.5

[a]INH, isoniazid; RIF, rifampin.

Table 50 Primary resistance of *M. tuberculosis* to antibiotics in untreated patients in the Pitié-Salpêtrière hospital

Phenotype[a]	1980–1987		1988–1992	
	n	%	*n*	%
INH[r]	14	1.6	10	1.7
STR[r]	17	2.0	28	4.9
RIF[r]	1	0.1	0	0
INH[r] + STR[r]	11	1.3	12	2.1
INH[r] + RIF[r]	0	0	1	0.1
INH[r] + RIF[r] + STR[r]	0	0	4	0.7

[a]INH, isoniazid; STR, streptomycin; RIF, rifampin.

years, primary resistance to rifampin and ethambutol was of rare occurrence (0.1% or less). However, cases of primary resistance to both isoniazid and rifampin in HIV-positive patients are now being observed. Some of these cases appear to occur in clusters and might reflect nosocomial transmission.

As PAS and D-cycloserine are not often used, acquired resistance to these two antibiotics is now rare. However, primary resistance to PAS is still observed in 1 to 2% of cases. Secondary resistance to thiacetazone is rare, except in patients treated previously with a thioamide because of the cross-resistance of these two antibiotics.

Jeddah (Saudi Arabia) is an entry point for pilgrims coming to Mecca mainly from developing countries, most of which have endemic TB. Jeddah residents have considerable exposure to M. *tuberculosis*. Saudi Arabia still has a high incidence of TB despite a reduction from 135 cases per 10^5 inhabitants in 1980 to 18.6 cases per 10^5 inhabitants in 1990. In the Jeddah area, the prevalence of TB is 63.4 per 10^5 inhabitants. In 1991, 0.8% of the M. *tuberculosis* isolates were resistant to D-cycloserine.

In Africa TB is caused by either M. *tuberculosis* or M. *africanum*. In Cameroon the distribution rates were 34 and 66% for M. *africanum* and M. *tuberculosis*, respectively, with 2.0% of the strains being resistant to ethionamide and 41.4% of M. *africanum* strains resistant to thiacetazone in a survey conducted in 1993 and 1994, versus only 2.6% of M. *tuberculosis* isolates in the same period. In Ghana, among 42 (55%) of the isolates, 42 and 35% of M. *africanum* isolates were resistant to streptomycin and thiacetazone, respectively. In Ivory Coast the proportions of M. *tuberculosis*-resistant strains which were also resistant to ethionamide and capreomycin were 17 and 7.0%, respectively.

In sub-Saharan countries 447,000 cases of TB were reported in 1995 (14% of all TB cases in the world). This is likely a serious underestimate of the true burden of TB in Africa. In Israel, the highest prevalence resistance in the mid-1990s was found in immigrants coming from the former Soviet Union. From 1991 to 1994 in St. Petersburg, Russia, the prevalence of TB ranged from 25.1 to 38.6 per 10^5 inhabitants. In the northwest of Russia, the proportion of pulmonary isolates with secondary multidrug resistance increased from 21.6% from 1984 to 1995 to 33% from 1989 to 1994.

In Düsseldorf, Germany, the proportion of multidrug-resistant M. *tuberculosis* isolates ranged from 5 to 15%, with an average of 8.4%. In Germany between 1985 and 1995, no isolates were found to be resistant to protionamide.

The Indian subcontinent has the greatest burden of TB, including multidrug-resistant strains. In France the rates of TB were 11.4 and 11.1 per 10^5 inhabitants in 1996 and 1999, respectively. The rates were different between French people and immigrants (in 1997, 7.3 versus 458).

In 1997, in Colombia, the prevalence of TB ranged from 26.5 to 90.5 per 10^5 inhabitants depending on the city. In that country, 92% of patients interrupted their treatments and restarted them several times. Some did not take their medicine for at least 1 month. Other patients took suboptimal treatment instead of the recommended dose or took only part of the chemotherapy, one drug instead of three.

In the former Soviet Union, including Baltic countries, TB remains an important public health concern.

Australia has one of the lowest reported rates in the world: 5.6. For Canada, the United States, New Zealand, England and Wales, and France, reported rates are, on average, 7.0, 9.8, 10.4, 11.2, and 17.2, respectively.

The resurgence of TB in New York City from 1978 to 1982 has been closely linked to the AIDS epidemic. The immune deficit seems to allow activation of the latent form of TB. It was demonstrated that resistance to rifampin occurred after an average of 40 weeks (1 to 179%; 81% of these patients had been noncompliant before the emergence of rifampin resistance).

Table 51 Incidence of TB resistance in 2000 and 2001 in Mexico

Compound	% Resistance in subjects	
	HIV+	HIV−
Isoniazid	44	20
Rifampin	44	18
Pyrazinamide	56	20
Ethambutol	44	14
Streptomycin	67	23
Ciprofloxacin	0	3
Ethionamide	67	44

Table 52 Prevalence of TB in the former Soviet Union

Country or region	Prevalence (10^5 inhabitants)
Belarus	75.4
Moldavia	102.1
Russian Federation	62.4
Siberia	250
Ukraine	62.6
Armenia	32.1
Azerbaijan	55.3
Georgia	55.6
Kazakhstan	109.2
Kyrgyzstan	61.4
Tajikistan	87.3
Turkmenistan	72.7
Uzbekistan	77.8
Estonia	55.8
Latvia	59.6
Lithuania	65

In the United States from 1953 to 1984 the incidence of TB declined progressively, from 84,304 cases in 1953 to 22,255 cases in 1984. In 1985, the trend was reversed, resulting in 63,800 excess cases in 1993; more than 70% of cases occurred in racial and ethnic minorities, and 29% of cases occurred in persons born outside the United States. In 1991, 14.2% of reported cases were due to resistant *M. tuberculosis*. The status of the patient could be of importance in the prevalence of resistance, as was shown in Mexico (Table 51).

Surveys conducted by the WHO and other international institutions have pointed out that drug resistance is ubiquitous. Practically in more than 90% of the explored sites there was drug-resistant *M. tuberculosis* among previously treated patients (secondary resistance). Worldwide, the prevalence of resistance to at least a single drug ranged from 1.7% in Uruguay to 36.9% in Estonia.

The prevalence of multidrug-resistant *M. tuberculosis* ranged from 0 in the eighth explored site to 14.1% in Estonia. Resistance to all four compounds tested occurred in 8.5% of patients in Estonia. There is a global upward trend of prevalence of resistance to any drug. In France, Spain (Barcelona), the United States, and Switzerland, the opposite is true.

We did not find reliable data for some countries where TB is at the endemic stage.

In the former Soviet Union the prevalence of TB per 10^5 inhabitants remains high (Table 52).

The prevalence of patients suffering from TB remains high in eastern Europe, from 107.6 in Romania to 50.9 in Bulgaria. In South Korea the prevalence of TB dropped in 15 years from 580 per 10^5 inhabitants (28.6 million inhabitants) to 126 per 10^5 inhabitants (42.8 million inhabitants) in 1990.

19. MECHANISMS OF RESISTANCE OF TB

Resistance to chemically unrelated antibacterials may be due to one of four mechanisms: impermeability of the waxy outer membrane, efflux (which has not been completely explored), mutations at the level of the targets, and inactivation.

19.1. Impermeability

Treatment of mycobacterial infections is often difficult because the bacteria are intrinsically resistant to most antibacterials due to the specific outer membrane of *M. tuberculosis*.

The waxy cell wall slows down the diffusion of antibacterials into the bacterial cell but cannot completely prevent it.

19.2. Efflux

The genome sequence of *M. tuberculosis* has disclosed 20 putative genes. Transporter proteins remove toxic compounds from the bacteria by active transport after they enter the cytoplasm by diffusion.

Few efflux pumps have been reported. Such pumps include LfrA, conferring low-level resistance to fluoroquinolones and other compounds, TetV, conferring resistance to tetracycline; and Emb, conferring resistance to ethambutol in *Mycobacterium smegmatis*. The *efpA* gene encodes a putative efflux protein from *M. tuberculosis*. This protein belongs to the QacA family. Taptub confers resistance to tetracyclines but not to aminoglycosides. This pump seems to have no effect on any anti-*M. tuberculosis* drugs, chloramphenicol, lincosamides, macrolides, or vancomycin. LsrA confers resistance to hydrophobic fluoroquinolones. P55 is a membrane protein implicated in aminoglycoside and tetracycline efflux pumps.

Isoniazid may induce the synthesis of an efflux pump protein. This mechanism could occur during therapy with isoniazid. High levels of resistance to this drug can be gradually induced in isoniazid-susceptible isolates of *M. tuberculosis*. Rifampin may be pumped out by *M. tuberculosis*, conferring a low level of resistance.

The genes encoding ATP cassette transporters occupy 2.5% of the genome of *M. tuberculosis*. DrAB is a doxorubicin efflux pump which could also extrude unrelated antibacterials, such as hydrophobic compounds (tetracycline, 14-membered-ring macrolides, ethambutol, norfloxacin, streptomycin, and chloramphenicol).

19.3. Mutations

The *katG* gene encodes an 80-kDa homoprotein of 744 amino acids that has catalase and peroxidase activity. There is involvement of metal ions such as iron and manganese. There is an overexpression of this protein, with five different nucleotide alterations in the promoter region of the *aphC* gene (L48A, C54T, G551A, G74A, and C81T). For KatG there is a point mutation which results in an amino acid substitution at residue 315 (Ser→Thr). Other less frequent mutations have been reported: H108Q, T262R, A350S, and G629S. A missense mutation in *inhA* is responsible for isoniazid resistance in *M. bovis* and *M. smegmatis*. The *ndh* gene encodes an NADH dehydrogenase. A direct defect in the enzyme activity results in an increased NADH/NAD$^+$ ratio and resistance to isoniazid and ethionamide. Mutations and deletions in *ndh* occur in 9.5% of *M. tuberculosis* isolates. The mutations are mainly at positions 110 (T→A) and 268 (R→H). *M. tuberculosis* produces an acetylase which could inactivate isoniazid.

For rifampin, one or more missense mutations affecting the *rpoB* gene, which codes for DNA-dependent RNA polymerase, are responsible for resistance, as in *E. coli*. The mutation occurs in an 81-bp segment among 3,534 bp of *rpoB*. It was found that up to 15 mutations in *M. tuberculosis* involve 8 conserved amino acids clustered in a 23-amino-acid region. Amino acid substitutions were missense mutations and substitution at one or two positions (residues 521 and 531). Substitution at the codon for position 526 (CAC→TAC) leads to the replacement of a histidine by a tyrosine, and substitution at the codon for position 531 (TCG→TTG) leads to a leucine instead of a serine. Other substitutions extending the size of the core region to 27 amino acids, or 81 bp, have been described.

M. tuberculosis mutants resistant to rifampin and other antibiotics, such as streptomycin, pyrazinamide, and ethambutol, do not have reduced virulence and do not appear to have their enzyme equipment modified. There is cross-resistance between rifampin and the other derivatives of rifamycin B, such as rifapentine and rifabutin, but no cross-resistance with the other families of antibiotics. Some isolates resistant to rifampin remain susceptible to rifabutin, rifapentine, or rifalazil. It was shown that all isolates having changes of Glu513→Leu, His562→Arg, Asp, Pro, Tyr, or Gln, and Ser 531→Leu, Trp, or Tyr had high levels of cross-resistance between rifabutin and rifampin. In contrast, for isolates with Leu511→Pro or Asp516→Val or Ser changes, the rifabutin MICs were ≤ 0.5 μg/ml. All microorganisms are cross-resistant between rifapentine and rifampin, except those with an Asp516→Tyr change. Rifalazil remains active with *ropB* mutations at positions 511 and 512. The vast majority of mutations are a single nucleotide change conferring an amino acid substitution; however, deletions and insertions could occur.

Ansamycins are not active against dormant bacilli.

Acquired resistance to streptomycin in mycobacteria has been attributed to mutation in the 30S ribosomal subunit. These mutations include point mutations in the S12 ribosomal protein encoded by the gene *rpsL* and in the *rrs* operon in the 16S rRNA. It was found that pyrazinamide-resistant isolates have lost pyrazinaminidase activity due to a mutation at the *pnsA* gene level. The mutation occurs throughout the 561-bp *pncA* coding region and the −11 promoter region, including base substitutions, insertion, and deletion. The substitution of proline disrupts the α-helical structure of the enzyme, thereby accounting for the loss of enzyme activity. The mutations are frequently found at nucleotides 70, 139, 254, and 388 in the *pncA* gene.

For D-cycloserine, resistance is due to an overproduction of D-alanine racemase or D-alaninyl-D-alanine ligase.

In ethionamide-resistant organisms, mutations occurred in the gene *ethA*.

Resistance to ethambutol is due to either overexpression of the *embABC* genes or mutation at codon position 306 of the *embB* gene (methionine→valine, leucine, or isoleucine). Other mutations have been shown at codons 330 and 630 (*embA* and *embC*). It has been suggested that the lack of incorporation of D-arabinose in arabinogalactan caused by ethambutol deprives the mycolic acid molecule of its site of transfer in the cell wall, leading to an overproduction of other mycolic acid derivatives.

19.4. Inactivation

M. tuberculosis produces an acetylase which could inactivate isoniazid. Sulfonamides as well as sulfones are poorly active against *M. tuberculosis*. In *Mycobacterium fortuitum*, sulfonamide resistance was found to be conferred by an inactivating enzyme encoded on a transposon.

In 1941, Abraham and coworkers noted that the growth of *M. tuberculosis* could not be inhibited by as much as 40 U of penicillin G per ml. Mycobacteria produce β-lactamases. The β-lactamases are not metalloenzymes and are inhibited by clavulanic acid. The major enzyme belongs to class A and has some cephalosporinase activity, the predominant activity being penicillinase.

Chromosomally encoded aminoglycoside 2-*N*-acetyltransferase from *M. tuberculosis* has been overexpressed to acetylate aminoglycoside substrates in vitro. This enzyme inactivates amikacin and kanamycin, which both have a hydroxyl group.

20. RATIONAL BASES OF ANTI-TB TREATMENT

The success of treatment of TB, as with that of any other bacterial infectious disease, is based on a consideration of the main factors involved (bacteria, lesions, and antibiotics), the biological objectives to be attained, and, finally, the antibiotic treatment administered. The characteristics of *M. tuberculosis* which are important for the treatment of TB are strict aerobiosis, slow multiplication, and a high proportion of antibiotic-resistant mutants. In the infected lung, the bacillus first multiplies in the alveolar macrophages. Then, 6 weeks to 3 months later, because of the specific immunity that has become established, the infected macrophages and the pulmonary tissues surrounding them are the subject of necrosis or caseification. The necrotic or caseous lesion may liquefy, be evacuated via the bronchi, and give rise to a cavern, in which the bacilli find ideal conditions for multiplication. Anti-TB antibiotics have a certain specificity of action. Isoniazid, streptomycin, and rifampin are the most bactericidal antibiotics against *M. tuberculosis* located in the cavern wall. In the acidic environment that prevails within macrophages and in areas of recent caseification, pyrazinamide is the most active antibiotic, followed by isoniazid and rifampin. Finally, in the poorly oxygenated caseous foci and at neutral pH, where *M. tuberculosis* is in a (persistent) reduced metabolic state of life, only rifampin is active (Table 53; Fig. 25).

For antibiotic treatment of TB to be effective, it must be bactericidal for susceptible bacilli; must not select resistant mutants, which would result in therapeutic failure; and must not allow the persistence of live bacilli, which would be liable to result in a relapse of the disease after the discontinuation of treatment. Therapy length for TB differs according to the localization (Tables 54 and 55).

A 6-month regimen comprising rifampin, isoniazid, pyrazinamide, and ethambutol for the initial 2 months, followed by rifampin and isoniazid for the next 4 months, is recommended as standard treatment for adult respiratory tract infection due to *M. tuberculosis*, including isolated pleural effusion or mediastinal lymphoadenopathy, irrespective of the bacteriological status of the sputum.

Ethambutol can be omitted in patients with low risk of resistance to isoniazid. If pyrazinamide cannot be administered, a 9-month therapy is recommended.

Isoniazid, pyrazinamide, ethionamide, and protionamide penetrate into the CSF well. Rifampin penetrates less well and streptomycin and ethambutol penetrate when the

Table 53 Bactericidal activities of anti-TB drugs

Compound	Intracellular	Extracellular	C/E ratio
Isoniazid	+	+	1.5
Pyrazinamide	+++	−	
Ethionamide/protionamide			
Streptomycin/kanamycin	−	+	
Ethambutol	−	−	1.4–4.8
Capreomycin	−/+	+	
Viomycin	−	+	
Cycloserine			
PAS	−	−	<1
Rifampin	+	+	2.6–92
Rifapentine	+	+	88
Rifabutin	+	+	2.6–92
Clofazimine	++	+	1.5–17.5

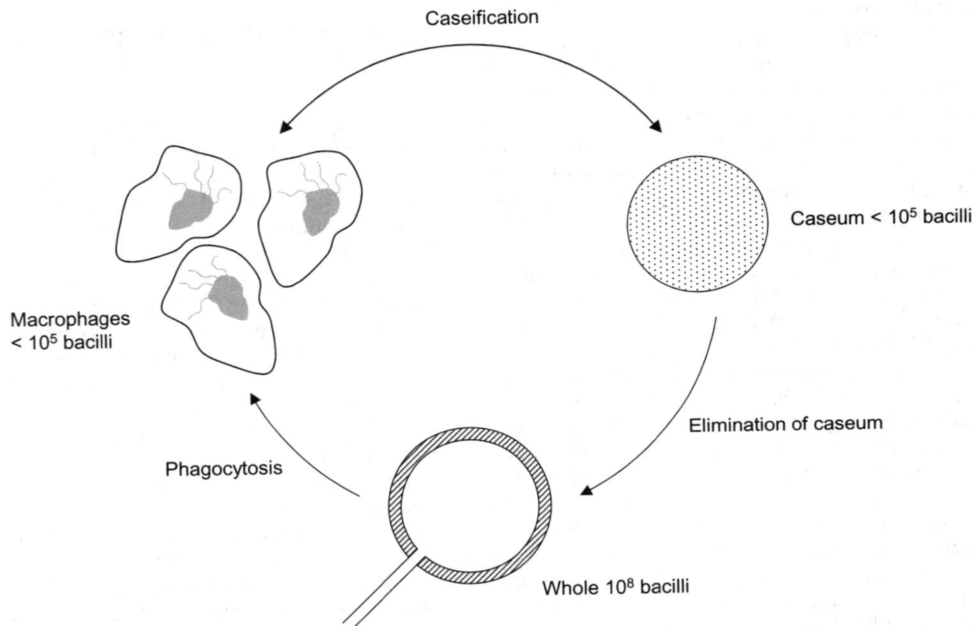

Figure 25 The three main populations of bacilli in TB and their respective prevalences

meninges are inflamed in the early stage of the treatment. Intrathechal administration of streptomycin is not useful.

Drug interactions need to be taken into consideration when anti-TB treatments are prescribed (Table 56).

21. PREVENTING SELECTION OF RESISTANT MUTANTS

To prevent the selection of resistant mutants, several antibiotics must be administered simultaneously. As the normal proportion of mutants resistant to each antibiotic is, on average, 1 in 10^6 and the tubercle cavern contains at least 10^8 bacilli, treatment with a single antibiotic, e.g., isoniazid, will select mutants resistant to this antibiotic that are already present within the susceptible population. Conversely, treatment with two antibiotics, e.g., isoniazid and rifampin, prevents selection because, as a result of the independence of mutations, the probability of there being a mutant simultaneously resistant to both the antibiotics administered is equal to the product of the individual probabilities, i.e., 1 to 10^6 + 1 to 10^6, or 1 to 10^{12}. As the tubercle cavern contains only 10^8 bacilli, the risk of selection of doubly resistant mutants is virtually nonexistent. In theory, therefore, the combination of two active antibiotics is sufficient to successfully treat a new case of TB due to susceptible bacilli. In practice, it is preferable to combine at least three antibiotics since the disease to be treated may involve a strain of *M. tuberculosis* exhibiting primary resistance to one of the antibiotics administered.

22. STERILIZING LESIONS

Simultaneous administration of several antibiotics prevents the selection of resistant mutants but considerably reduces the number of susceptible bacilli. For example, after 2 months of treatment with the triple combination isoniazid-rifampin-pyrazinamide, the number of residual bacilli in the cavern is 10^2 to 10^3. These bacilli, which are in a reduced metabolic

Table 54 Regimen of first-line anti-TB drugs

Compound	Wt (kg)	Dosage
Isoniazid		15 mg/kg 3 times/wk
Rifampin		600–900 mg 3 times/wk
Pyrazinamide	≥50	2.0 g
	≤50	2.5 g 3 times/wk
	≥50	3.0 g
	≤50	3.5 g 2 times/wk
Ethambutol		30 mg/kg 3 times/wk
		45 mg/kg 2 times/wk

Table 55 Therapy according to localization

Indication or site(s)	Length of therapy (mo)
Meningitis	12
Chemoprophylaxis	3–6
Peripheral lymph nodes	6
Bone and joints	6 (± surgery)
Pericarditis	6
Cerebral tuberculoma	12
Disseminated tuberculosis	6
Genitourinary	6
Other sites	6

Table 56 Drug interactions with first-line anti-TB drugs

Compound	Level			
	Increased by:	Decreased by:	Increase of:	Decrease of:
Isoniazid	Prednisolone		Phenytoin	Enllaranne
	Ethionamide		Carbamazepine	Azoles
			Warfarin	
			Diazepam	
Pyrazinamide			Probenecid	
Ethambutol		$Al(OH)_3$		
Rifampin		PAS		Warfarin
		Ketoconazole		Azoles
				Sulfonylureas
				Contraceptives
				Theophylline
				Diazepam
				Phenytoin
				Digitoxin
				Methadone
				Protease, isoniazid
				Cyclosporine

state, are, however, susceptible to the action of rifampin and pyrazinamide. It is for this reason that the duration of anti-TB treatment is now 6 months, whereas it was 18 to 24 months at the time that the combination isoniazid-streptomycin-PAS was used.

23. CHEMOTHERAPY OF TB: RECOMMENDED ANTIBIOTIC COMBINATIONS

The four antibiotic combinations summarized in Table 57 are currently recommended for the treatment of new cases of TB. The first, the most active, provides short-term treatment (6 months) and is recommended in all industrialized countries. The second corresponds to the conventional 9-month treatment with rifampin but without pyrazinamide. It is the most expensive and is justified only for patients who cannot tolerate pyrazinamide during the initial phase of treatment or who are carriers of pyrazinamide-resistant bacilli, such as *M. bovis*. The third combination is a compromise between the short-term treatment recommended in industralized countries (combinations 1 and 2) and the 12-month treatment recommended in developing countries because of its low cost, and it is based on the triple combination isoniazid-streptomycin-thiacetazone (combination 4). In the third and fourth combinations, thiacetazone is often replaced by ethambutol because of the risks of exfoliative dermatitis commonly observed (20%) in HIV-seropositive patients treated with thiacetazone.

24. LATENT TB

In order to eliminate TB, in the United States the Institute of Medicine set up a task force which identified the importance of latent TB. Many cases of acute TB are not due to a recent contamination but are the result of recent reactivation of latent TB. It could be important to identify individuals who are at high risk of developing TB. Developing means for directly detecting TB-specific proteins produced by *M. tuberculosis* during latency has became an important

Table 57 Anti-TB combinations

Combination	Duration of treatment (mo)	Cost (U.S. dollars in 1991 from UNICEF)
HRZE	2	52
HRE	2	60
HRZE (S)	2	18.7–7.6
HAST (E)	4	32.9
HR	4	52
HR	7	60
HT (E)	6	18.7–7.6
S2H2		32.9

research focus. HpsX, the product of the gene *hpsX*, may be a target. This is an α-crystalline protein homolog (16.2 kDa; 144 amino acids) also named Acr that is one of several proteins produced during persistent TB under low-oxygen conditions. This protein is able to reduce the production of interleukin 6. The estimated risk of a person facing a reactivation is 10% for most individuals over their lifetime to an annual risk of 10% for immunocompromised patients.

To conclude, it is important to emphasize the fact that therapeutic success depends not only on the initial susceptibility of the bacilli and the quality of the antibiotic combination prescribed but also on good treatment compliance. The HpsX protein can help M. *tuberculosis* to establish latency. It is required for growth in macrophages. It could be a new target for anti-M. *tuberculosis* treatment.

ADDITIONAL BIBLIOGRAPHY

Alangaden GJ, Kreiswirth BN, Oud A, Khetarpal M, Igno FA, Moghazeh SL, Manavathn EK, Lerner SA, 1998, Mechanism of resistance to amikacin and kanamycin in M. tuberculosis, Antimicrob Agents Chemother, 42, 1295–1297.

Albino JA, Reichman LB, 1997, Multidrug resistance in tuberculosis, Curr Opin Infect Dis, 10, 116–122.

Arioli V, Pallanza R, Füresz S, Carniti G, 1967, Rifampicin, a new rifamycin. 1. Bacteriological studies, Arzneimittel-Forsch, 17, 523–529.

Bartz QR, Ehrlich J, Mold JD, Penner MA, Smith RM, 1951, Viomycin, a new tuberculostatic antibiotic, Am Rev Tuberc, 63, 4–6.

Bernstein J, Lott WA, Steinberg BA, Yale HL, 1952, Chemotherapy of experimental tuberculosis. V. Isonicotinic acid hydrazide (Nidrazid) and related compounds, Am Rev Tuberc, 65, 357–364.

Boxenbaum HG, Riegelman S, 1974, Determination of isoniazid and metabolites in biological fluids, J Pharmacol Sci, 63, 1191–1197.

Bryskier A, Couturier C, Lowther J, 2002, Fluoroquinolones and M. tuberculosis, Exp Opinion Invest Drug.

Buriankova K, Doucet-Populaire F, Dorson D, Gondran A, Ghnassia JC, Weiser J, Perrodet JL, 2004, Molecular basis of intrinsic macrolide resistance in the M. *tuberculosis* complex, Antimicrob Agents Chemother, 48, 143–150.

Butler WR, Kilburn JO, 1983, Susceptibility of M. tuberculosis to pyrazinamide and its relationship to pyrazinamidase activity, Antimicrob Agents Chemother, 24, 600–601.

Canetti G, Gay PH, Le Lirzin M, 1972, Trends in the prevalence of primary drug resistance in pulmonary tuberculosis in France from 1962 to 1970, a national survey, Tubercle (Lond), 53, 57–83.

Canetti G, Grosset J, 1961, Teneur des souches sauvages de Mycobacterium tuberculosis en variants resistants à l'isoniazide et en variants resistants à la streptomycine sur milieu de Löwenstein-Jensen, Ann Inst Pasteur, 101, 28–46.

Canetti G, Rist N, Grosset J, 1963, Mésure de la sensibilité du bacille tuberculeux aux drogues antibacillaires par la méthode des proportions, Rev Tuberc (Paris), L7, 217–220.

Cartel JL, Naudillon Y, Artus JC, Grosset JH, 1985, Hepatotoxicity of the daily combination of 5 mg/kg protionamide + 10 mg/kg rifampicin, Int J Lepr, 51, 15–18.

Cohen SP, Levy SB, Fould J, Rosner JL, 1993, Salicylate induction of antibiotic resistance in Escherichia coli, acivation of the mar operon, an independent pathway, J Bacteriol, 175, 7856–7862.

Domagk G, Benisch R, Mietzsch F, Schmidt H, 1946, Über eine neue, gagen Tuberkelberzillen in vitro wirksame Verbindungslasse, Naturw, 22, 315.

Edlin BR, Tokars JI, Grieco MH, Crawford JT, Williams J, Sordillo EM, Ong KR, Kilburn JO, Dooley SW, Castro KG, Jarvis WR, Holmberg SD, 1992, An outbreak of multiresistant tuberculosis among hospitalized patients with the acquired immunodeficiency syndrome, N Engl J Med, 326, 1514–1521.

Ellard GA, 1984, Signification clinique potentielle du phénotype d'acétylation de l'isoniazide dans le traitement de la tuberculose pulmonaire, Rev Fr Mal Resp, 1, 207–219.

Falzari K, Zhu Z, Pan D, Liu H, Hongmanee P, Franzblau SG, 2005, The in vitro and in vivo activities of macrolide derivatives against M. *tuberculosis*, Antimicrob Agents Chemother, 49, 1447–1454.

Füresz S, Arioli V, Pallanza R, 1965, Antimicrobial properties of new derivatives of rifamycin SV, Antimicrob Agents Chemother, p 770.

Gardner TS, Wenis E, Lee J, 1954, Synthesis of compounds for chemotherapy of tuberculosis. IV. The amine function, J Org Chem, 19, 753–757.

Girling DJ, 1982, Adverse effects of antituberculosis drugs, Drugs, 23, 56–74.

Grosset J, 1989, Present status of chemotherapy for tuberculosis, Rev Inf Dis, 11, S347–S352.

Grosset J, 1990, Present and new drug regimens in chemotherapy and chemoprophylaxis of tuberculosis, Bull Int Union Against Tuberc Lung Dis, 65, 86–91.

Grosset J, 1992, Treatment of tuberculosis in HIV infection, Tubercle Lung Dis, 7, 378–383.

Grosset J, Benhassine M, 1970, La thiacétazone (Tbl), données experimentales et cliniques recentes, Adv Tuberc Res, 17, 107–153.

Grosset J, Canetti G, 1962, Teneur des souches sauvages de Mycobacterium tuberculosis en variants résistants aux antibiotiques mineurs, Ann Inst Pasteur, 103, 163–184.

Grosset J, Chauvelot-Moachon L, Giroud JP, 1988, Antituberculeux, p 1553–1573, in Giroud JP, Mathé J, Meyniel J, Advenier C, Benoist JM, Durenne-Marillaz P, Escousse A, Guidicelli JF, Imbs JL, Lapalus P, Loiseau P, Montestruc JL, Philippon A, Regoli D, Simon P, Tillement JP, ed, Pharmacologie clinique, 2nd ed, Exp Sc Fr.

Grosset J, Truffot-Pernot CH, 1988, Etat actuel de la résistance de Mycobacterium tuberculosis aux antibiotiques, La lettre de l'infectiologue, 3, 369–377.

Grunberg E, Schnitzer RJ, 1952, Studies on the activity of hydrazine derivatives of isonicotinic acid in experimental tuberculosis of mice, Quart Bull Sea View Hosp, 13, 3–11.

Harned RC, Hidy PA, Kropp La Baw EK, 1955, Cycloserine. I. A preliminary report, Antibiot Chemother, 5, 204–205.

Herr EB, Haney ME, Pittenger GE, Hyggens CE, 1960, Isolation and characterization of a new peptide antibiotic, Proc Indiana Acad Sci, 69, 134.

Heym B, Cole ST, 1992, Isolation and characterization of isoniazid-resistant mutants of Mycobacterium smegmatis and M. aurum, Res Microbiol, 143, 721–730.

Heym B, Zhang Y, Poulet S, Young D, Cole ST, 1993, Characterization of the katG gene encoding a catalase-peroxidase required for the isoniazid susceptibility of Mycobacterium tuberculosis, J Bacteriol, 175, 4255–4259.

Jenne JW, MacDonald FM, Mendoza E, 1961, A study of the renal clearances, metabolic inactivation rates, and serum fall-off interaction of isoniazid and para-aminosalicylic acid in man, Am Rev Respir Dis, 84, 371–378.

Ji B, Truffot-Pernot C, Grosset J, 1991, In vitro and in vivo activities of sparfloxacin (AT4140) against M. tuberculosis, Tubercle, 72, 181–186.

Kapur V, Li LL, Iordanescu S, Hamrick MR, Wanger A Musser JM, 1994, Characterization by automated DNA sequencing of mutations in the gene (rpoB) encoding RNA polymerase β-subunit in rifampicin-resistant M. tuberculosis from New York City, J Clin Microbiol, 32, 1095–1098.

Konno K, Feldmann FM, McDermott W, 1967, Pyrazinamide susceptibility and amidase activity of tubercle bacilli, Am Rev Respir, 25, 461–469.

Kurosawa H, 1952, Studies on the antibiotic substances from actinomyces. XXIII. The isolation of an antibiotic produced by a strain of streptomyces "K30," J Antibiot Ser B, 5, 682–688.

Kushner S, Dalalian H, Sanjurjo JL, Bach FL Jr, Safir SR, Smith VK Jr, Williams JH, 1952, Experimental chemotherapy of tuberculosis. II. The synthesis of pyrazinamide and related compounds, J Am Chem Soc, 74, 3617–3621.

Lalande V, Truffot-Pernot C, Paccaly-Moulon A, Grosset J, Ji B, 1993, Powerful bactericidal activity of sparfloxacin (AT-4140) against Mycobacterium tuberculosis in mice, Antimicrob Agents Chemother, 37, 407–413.

Lehmann J, 1946, Determination of pathogenicity of tubercle bacilli by their intermediate metabolism, Lancet, Jan 5, 114–115.

Lehmann J, 1946, Para-aminosalicylic acid in the treatment of tuberculosis, Lancet, 15–16.

Le Lirzin M, Djurovic V, 1971, Etude sur milieu de Lowenstein-Jensen de la composition des souches sauvages de Mycobacterium tuberculosis en variants résistants à la rifampicine et en variants résistants a l'ethambutol, A nn Inst Pasteur, 120, 531–548.

Lesobre R, Ruffino J, Teyssier L, Achard F, Brefort G, 1968, Les ictères au cours du traitement par la rifampicine, Rev Tuberc Pneumol, 33, 393–403.

Libermann D, Moyeux M, Rist N, Grumbach F, 1956, Sur la préparation de nouveaux thioamides pyridiniques actifs dans la tuberculose expérimentale, C R Acad Sci, 246, 2409–2412.

MacKaness GB, 1956, The intracellular activation of pyrazinamide and nicotinamide, Am Rev Tuberc, 74, 718–728.

Meier A, Kirschner P, Bange FC, Vogel U, Bottger EC, 1994, Genetic alterations in streptomycin-resistant Mycobacterium tuberculosis: mapping of mutations conferring resistance, Antimicrob Agents Chemother, 38, 228–233.

Middlebrook G, 1954, Isoniazid-resistance and catalase activity of tubercle bacilli, Am Rev Tuberc, 699, 471–472.

Moghazeh SL, Pan Y, Arain T, Stover CK, Musser JM, Kreiswirth BN, 1996, Comparative antimycobacterial activity of rifampin, rifapentine, and KRM-1648 against a collection of rifampin-resistant M. tuberculosis with known rpoB mutations, Antimicrob Agents Chemother, 40, 2655–2657.

Moulding, T, Dutt AK, Reichman LB, 1995, Fixed dose combinations of antituberculous medications to prevent drug resistance and enhance patient compliance, Ann Intern Med, 122, 951–954.

Musser JM, 1995, Antimicrobial agent resistance in mycobacteria, molecular genetic insights, Clin Microbiol Rev, 8, 496–514.

Pretet S, Lebeaut A, Parrot R, Truffot C, Grosset J, Dinh-Xuan AT, GETIM (Group for the Study and Treatment of Resistant Mycobacterial Infections), 1992, Combined chemotherapy including rifabutin for rifampicin and isoniazid-resistant pulmonary tuberculosis, Eur Respir J, 5, 680–684.

Reichman LB, 1994, Multidrug resistant tuberculosis, meeting the challenge, Hosp Pract, 29, 85–96.

Rindler H, Muskes KT, Loesher T, 2001, Hetero resistance in M. tuberculosis, Int J Tuberc Lung Dis, 5, 339–345.

Riska PF, Jacobs WR Jr, Alland D, 2000, Molecular determinants of drug resistance in tuberculosis, Int J Tuberc Lung Dis, 4, S4–S10.

Rist N, 1960, L'activité anti tuberculeuse de l'éthionamide (l'alpha-éthyl-thioisonicotinamide ou 1314 Th), étude experimentale et clinique, Adv Tuberc Res, 10, 69–126.

Roberts GD, Koneman EW, Kim YK, 1991, Mycobacterium, p 304–339, in Balows, Hausler, Hermann, Isenberg, Shadomy, ed, Manual of Clinical Microbiology, 5th ed, American Society for Microbiology, Washington, D.C.

Sachais BS, Nachamkindagger II, Mills JK, Leonard DG, 1998, Novel pncA mutations in pyrazinamide-resistant isolates of M. tuberculosis, Mol Diagn, 3, 229–231.

Schatz A, Bugle E, Waksman SA, 1944, Streptomycin, a substance exhibiting antibiotic activity against gram-positive and gram-negative bacteria, Proc Soc Exp Biol Med, 55, 66.

Scorpio A, Lindholm-Levy P, Heifets L, et al, 1997, Characterization of pncA mutation in pyrazinamide-resistant M. tuberculosis, Antimicrob Agents Chemother, 41, 540–543.

Sreevatsan S, Pan Y, Zhang Y, Kreiswirth BN, Musser JM, 1997, Mutations associated with pyrazinamide-resistance in pncA of M. tuberculosis complex organisms, Antimicrob Agents Chemother, 41, 636–640.

Sreevatsan S, Stockbauer KE, Pan Y, et al, 1997, Ethambutol resistance in Mycobacterium tuberculosis, critical role of embB mutation, Antimicrob Agents Chemother, 41, 1677–1681.

Takiff HE, Salazar L, Guerero C, et al, 1994, Cloning and nucleotide sequence of M. tuberculosis gyrA and gyrB genes and deletion of quinolone mutation, Antimicrob Agents Chemother, 38, 773–780.

Telenti A, Imboden P, Marchesi F, Lourice D, Cole S, Colston MJ, Matter L, Schopfer K, Bodner T, 1993, Detection of rifampicin-resistance mutations in Mycobacterium tuberculosis, Lancet, 341, 647–650.

Thomas JP, Baughn CO, Wilkinson RG, Shepard RG, 1961, A new synthetic compound with antituberculous activity in mice, ethambutol [dextro-2,2′-(ethylenediimino)-DI-1-butanol], Am Rev Respir Dis, 83, 891–893.

Truffot-Pernot C, Giroir AM, Maury L, Grosset J, 1988, Etude des concentrations minimales inhibitrices de rifabutine (ansamycine LM427) pour M. tuberculosis, M xenopi, M avium, Rev Mal Respir, 5, 401–406.

Truffot-Pernot C, Grosset J, Bismuth R, Lecoeur H, 1983, Activité de la rifampicine administré de manière intermittente et de la cyclopentyl rifamycine (ou DL473) sur la tuberculose expérimentale de la souris, Rev Fr Mal Resp, 11, 875–882.

Truffot-Pernot CH, Ji B, Grosset J, 1991, Activities of pefloxacin and ofloxacin against mycobacteria, in vitro and mouse experiments, Tubercle, 72, 57–64.

Tsukamura M, 1985, In vitro antituberculosis activity of a new antibacterial substance ofloxacin (DL 8280), Am Rev Respir Dis, 131, 348–351.

Tsukamura M, Nakamura E, Yoshii S, Yanase M, Yasuda Y, Amasso H, 1985, Therapeutic effect of a new antibacterial substance ofloxacin (DL 8280) on pulmonary tuberculosis, Am Rev Respir Dis, 131, 352–356.

Umezawa H, Ueda M, Maeda K, Yagishita K, Kondo S, Okami Y, Utahara R, Osato Y, Nitta K, Takenchi T, 1957, Production and isolation of a new antibiotic, kanamycin, J Antibiot Jpn Ser A, 10, 181–188.

Vivien JN, Grosset J, 1961, Le taux d'isoniazide actif dans le serum sanguin, Adv Tuberc Res, 11, 45–121.

Way EL, Smith PK, Howie PL, Weiss R, Swanson R, 1948, The absorption, distribution, excretion and fate of para-amino-salicylic acid, J Pharmacol Exp Ther, 9, 368–372.

Wayne LG, 1974, Simple pyrazinamidase and urease tests for routine identification of mycobacteria, Am Rev Respir Dis, 109, 147–151.

WHO, Guidelines for tuberculosis treatment in adults and children in national tuberculosis programmes, WHO/Tub/91161.

Wirima JJ, Harries AD, 1991, Stevens-Johnson syndrome during antituberculosis chemotherapy in HIV-seropositive patients, report on six cases, East Afr Med J, 68, 64–66.

Young DB, Cole ST, 1993, Leprosy, tuberculosis, and the new genetics, J Bacteriol, 175, 1–6.

Zhang Y, Heym B, Allen B, Young D, Cole S, 1992, The catalase-peroxydase genes and isoniazid resistance of Mycobacterium tuberculosis, Nature, 358, 591–593.

Zhang Y, Scorpio A, Nikaido H, Su Z, 1999, Role of acid pH and deficient efflux of pyrazinoic acid in unique susceptibility of M. tuberculosis to pyrazinamide, J Bacteriol, 181, 2044–2049.

Fluoroquinolones and Tuberculosis: a Review

ANDRÉ BRYSKIER AND JOHN LOWTHER

44

1. INTRODUCTION

Tuberculosis (TB) remains a major world health problem, with about one-third of humans being infected by *Mycobacterium tuberculosis*. Each year *M. tuberculosis* infection is responsible for 2 to 3 million deaths.

TB has been referred to as the "white plague" or "the King of Disease," and as a communicable infectious disease it has been a leading cause of death in Europe and North America for centuries. The first rational description of the infectious nature of TB was made by Marten in 1722, followed by autopsy studies by Laennec in 1819. Villemin in 1868 was the first to demonstrate the transmission of TB in a rabbit model.

The actual causative agent of TB was described in 1882 by Robert Koch. Subsequently Paul Ehrlich developed a staining method for tubercle bacilli based on their acid-fastness. Modification of this method by Ziehl and Neelsen produced the now widely used standard staining method. Diagnosis of TB was facilitated by this method, which opened the way for therapy.

Once the contagious nature of TB was understood, the primary treatment from the end of the 19th century up to the mid-20th century was to place the patient in specialized hospital, or sanitorium. The sanitoriums were localized at higher altitudes, where rest and fresh air constituted the main prescription for treatment.

With the advent of X-ray film, it became evident that the pulmonary cavity was pivotal in the evolution of the disease. Surgical interventions such as pneumothorax, pneumoperitoneum, extraperiosteal plombage, and thoracoplasty were aimed at elimination of the cavity.

TB only became a curable disease by means of drug therapy with the introduction in the middle of the 20th century of *p*-aminosalicylic acid (PAS), streptomycin, and isoniazid. An improvement in anti-TB chemotherapy was the discovery of rifampin. Rifampin and isoniazid as well as streptomycin eventually became the core of TB treatment.

Introduction of efficacious anti-TB therapy resulted in a dramatic decline of the prevalence of TB infections. TB ceased to be a problem not only in industrialized countries, where it was presumed to have disappeared, but also in developing countries, where mass vaccination and anti-TB chemotherapy were expected to control the disease. However, the resurgence of TB has illustrated the limits of its control.

The recent trends in TB incidence have been quite different for industrialized and developing countries. In developing countries TB incidence has changed little. In contrast, in industrialized countries the TB rate declined until the end of 1980s, after which the recorded incidence of TB began to rise again.

The cause of this resurgence of TB in industrialized countries is a combination of deteriorating public health infrastructure, inadequate institutional control of infections, urban crowding, the epidemic of human immunodeficiency virus (HIV) infection, poverty, and homelessness. Unfortunately, the resurgence of TB has coincided with the emergence of multidrug-resistant TB (defined as having resistance to rifampin and isoniazid with or without resistance to other anti-TB agents). Outbreaks have resulted in high morbidity and mortality. The underlying causes of multidrug-resistant TB have been suggested to be incorrect treatment, poor compliance and erratic drug ingestion, and frequent or prolonged storage of anti-TB drugs due to financial constraints in some developing countries.

This dramatic rise of multidrug-resistant TB resulted in an acute medical need for new anti-TB agents able to overcome this modern threat. Despite intensive research, only fluoroquinolones are able to meet this new medical challenge.

Fluoroquinolones are synthetic antibacterial agents derived from the first pyrridone-β-carboxylic derivative, nalidixic acid. They are characterized by an atom of fluorine at position 6 and an aryl substituent at position 7 of the quinoline or 1,8-naphthyridone ring. Fluoroquinolones exhibit a broad antibacterial spectrum which includes *M. tuberculosis*.

2. RATIONALE FOR USING FLUOROQUINOLONES

Ofloxacin, ciprofloxacin, and, later, sparfloxacin were shown to exhibit potent in vitro activity against *M. tuberculosis* (Tsukamura, 1985a; Collins et al., 1985; Gaya and Chadwick, 1986; Grassi, 1997). In addition, animal studies support the anti-TB activity of ofloxacin, ciprofloxacin, and sparfloxacin. On the basis of these studies, ofloxacin and ciprofloxacin have been suggested as alternate treatments for TB.

The rationale for using fluoroquinolones in the treatment of TB is the following:

- Development of shorter duration of therapy (6 months) by strengthening the regimens with powerful bactericidal drugs other than those currently used would increase the compliance of the patients.

- New drugs are needed to overcome isoniazid and/or rifampin resistance in *M. tuberculosis*.
- Fluoroquinolones are widely distributed in tissue, including within cells, where *M. tuberculosis* resides.

3. IN VITRO ACTIVITY OF FLUOROQUINOLONES

3.1. In Vitro Anti-TB Activity of Fluoroquinolones

3.1.1. Testing Methodologies

The following methods have been used to determine susceptibility: agar dilution, broth macrodilution and microdilution, disk elution (La Bombardi et al., 1993), and the BACTEC radiometric system (Trimble et al., 1987). A variety of media have been used, including Middlebrook 7H10 agar with or without enrichment with oleic acid-albumin-dextrose-catalase (OADC), glycerol, or Tween 80; Middlebrook 7H10 broth; Middlebrook 7H11 agar; Löwenstein-Jensen agar; Ogawa egg medium; the early proposed E-test method (Wanger and Mills, 1994); and luciferase (Jacobs et al., 1993; Cooksey et al., 1993).

Although a standardized method for susceptibility testing has not yet been agreed upon, the most widely used is based on either Middlebrook 7H10 or 7H11 agar with an inoculum size of 10^7 to 10^8 CFU/ml.

3.1.2. Fluoroquinolone Activities

Nonclassical fluorinated quinolones are not active against *M. tuberculosis* (Berlin et al., 1987; Garcia-Rodriguez et al., 1988, 1993; Young et al., 1987).

Many studies have been carried out to investigate the in vitro activity of available fluoroquinolones. MIC determination methodologies have varied from one team to another.

The following is a selection of 13 studies from existing literature followed by an overall summary.

3.1.2.1. Pefloxacin, Ofloxacin, and Ciprofloxacin

The in vitro activity of pefloxacin was investigated by incorporating pefloxacin drug substance into Löwenstein-Jensen medium. The final concentrations ranged from 0.25 to 16 μg/ml. The MIC at which 50% of isolates tested are inhibited (MIC_{50}) and MIC_{90} of pefloxacin were 8.0 and 16.0 μg/ml irrespective of the susceptibility of *M. tuberculosis* to isoniazid or rifampin (Truffot-Pernot et al., 1991). The MIC_{50} and MIC_{90} of pefloxacin and norfloxacin for 23 *M. tuberculosis* isolates were 4.0 and 8.0 μg/ml for both compounds. MICs were determined by broth dilution using an inoculum size of 10^4 to 10^5 CFU/ml in Youmans medium (Texier-Maugein et al., 1987). The modal MIC of pefloxacin for 15 *M. tuberculosis* isolates using a 7H10 Middlebrook OADC-enriched medium was 8.0 μg/ml (range 4.0 to 16.0 μg/ml) in comparison with ciprofloxacin and ofloxacin, for which the modal MICs were 1.0 and 2.0 μg/ml, respectively (Gevaudan et al., 1998).

Whatever the method used, the MIC_{50} and MIC_{90} of ofloxacin for *M. tuberculosis* were 0.5 to 1.0 and 1.0 to 2.0 μg/ml (Ji et al., 1991; Truffot-Pernot et al., 1991; Piersimoni et al., 1992; Fenelon and Cynamon, 1986; Banerjee et al., 1992; Tomioka et al., 1991; Rastogi and Goh, 1991; Tsukamura et al., 1985b; Texier-Maugein et al., 1987).

The MIC_{50}s and MIC_{90}s of ciprofloxacin ranged from 0.5 to 2.0 and 0.5 to 4.0 μg/ml, respectively.

3.1.2.2. Difloxacin and Fleroxacin

Using a twofold dilution in 7H11 agar medium, the MIC_{50} and MIC_{90} of fleroxacin for 25 TB isolates were 3.13 and 6.25 μg/ml, respectively (Tomioka et al., 1991).

The modal MICs of enoxacin, norfloxacin, difloxacin, A-56620, CI-934, and fleroxacin were 1.0, 2.0, 2.0, 1.0, 1.0, and 2.0 μg/ml, respectively, for 24 isolates of *M. tuberculosis* fully susceptible to standard anti-TB drugs (Young et al., 1987; Berlin et al., 1987; Gay et al., 1984) (Table 1).

As determined by the proportion method in 7H10 Middlebrook OADC-enriched medium, fleroxacin and ciprofloxacin inhibited, at 0.5 μg/ml, the growth of 11 *M. tuberculosis* isolates (Salfinger et al., 1988).

3.1.2.3. Irloxacin

Using a radiometric method with 7H12 Middlebrook medium, it was shown that irloxacin exhibited greater anti-TB activity at pH 5.0 than did other fluoroquinolones (Casal et al., 1995).

3.1.2.4. Lomefloxacin

For 79 *M. tuberculosis* isolates fully susceptible and 11 resistant to standard anti-TB drugs, lomefloxacin exhibited a MIC_{50} and MIC_{90} of 1.0 and 2.0 μg/ml (Table 2) (Piersimoni et al., 1992). A radiometric method with 7H12B Middlebrook medium was used. The MIC_{50} and MIC_{90} observed in this study were 1 tube dilution less than those in other studies.

3.1.2.5. WIN 57273

WIN 57273 is weakly active against *M. tuberculosis*, with MIC_{50}s of 2.0 and 0.5 μg/ml when tested in 7H12 broth medium at pH 6.8 and 6.0, respectively (Heifets and Lindholm-Levy, 1990) (Table 3).

Table 1 Anti-*M. tuberculosis* activities of CI-934, A-56620, irloxacin, and amifloxacin[a]

Compound	MIC (μg/ml)		
	50%	90%	Range
Ciprofloxacin	0.5	1.0	0.06–1.0
Ofloxacin	0.5	0.5	0.125–1.0
Temafloxacin	1.0	1.0	0.03–2.0
Amifloxacin	2.0	4.0	1.0–32
Difloxacin	4.0	4.0	0.5–8.0
Enoxacin	4.0	4.0	1.0–32
Irloxacin	8.0	16	2.0–32
Pefloxacin	4.0	4.0	1.0–16
CI-934	2.0	2.0	1.0–8.0
A-56620	4.0	8.0	2.0–16

[a]Data from Young et al., 1987; Berlin et al., 1987; Gay et al., 1984; and Van Caekenberghe, 1990.

Table 2 Anti-*M. tuberculosis* activity of lomefloxacin[a]

Compound	Isolate phenotype[b]	*n*	MIC (μg/ml)		
			50%	90%	Range
Ofloxacin	S	79	0.5	1.0	0.25–1.0
	R	11	0.5		0.25–4.0
Ciprofloxacin	S	79	0.25	0.5	0.12–1.0
	R	11	0.25		0.25–4.0
Lomefloxacin	S	79	1.0	2.0	0.5–2.0
	R	11	1.0		1.0–4.0

[a]Data from Piersimoni et al., 1992.
[b]S, susceptible; R, resistant.

Table 3 Anti-TB activity of WIN 57273[a]

M. *tuberculosis* strain(s)	*n*	MIC (μg/ml)					
		pH 6.8			pH 6.0		
		OFX	CIP	WIN	OFX	CIP	WIN
$H37_{RV}$[b]	1	1.0	1.0	4.0	2.0	2.0	1.0
Clinical isolates[c]	9	1.0	0.5	2.0	1.0	1.0	0.5

[a]Data from Heifets and Lindholm-Levy, 1990. OFX, ofloxacin, CIP, ciprofloxacin; WIN, WIN 57273.
[b]Values are MICs.
[c]Values are MIC_{50}s.

3.1.2.6. Clinafloxacin

For 21 M. *tuberculosis* isolates, using an inoculum size of 10^6CFU per plate on Middlebrook agar, the MIC_{90} of clinafloxacin was 1 μg/ml (range, 0.12 to 2 μg/ml) (Wise et al., 1988).

3.1.2.7. Sparfloxacin

For 25 M. *tuberculosis* isolates, the MIC_{50} and MIC_{90} of gatifloxacin were 0.1 and 0.2 μg/ml, those of sparfloxacin were 0.1 and 0.2 μg/ml, and those of ofloxacin were 0.78 and 0.78 μg/ml by agar dilution using Middlebrook 7H11 agar with an inoculum size of 5×10^3 CFU (Tomioka et al., 1993a).

3.1.2.8. BAY y 3118

Twenty-five M. *tuberculosis* isolates (10 susceptible and 15 resistant) were tested for susceptibility to BAY y 3118 on 7H10 Middlebrook agar with an inoculum size of 2×10^4 CFU. The MIC_{50} and MIC_{90} were 0.06 and 0.13 μg/ml, respectively, for a range of 0.06 to 0.13 μg/ml irrespective of the susceptibility to other antibacterial agents (Sirgel et al., 1995).

3.1.2.9. Amifloxacin

For 10 M. *tuberculosis* isolates fully susceptible to standard anti-TB compounds, the MICs of amifloxacin ranged between 0.5 and 4.0 μg/ml. MICs were determined using Middlebrook 7H10 agar (Pattyn et al., 1987). The MIC_{50} and MIC_{90} of amifloxacin for 22 M. *tuberculosis* isolates were 4.0 and 4.0 μg/ml, with a range of 2.0 to 8.0 μg/ml, using OADC-enriched 7H10 agar medium (Fenelon and Cynamon, 1986).

3.1.2.10. Levofloxacin

The in vitro activity of levofloxacin against 18 susceptible M. *tuberculosis* isolates (including $H37_{RV}$ and two ofloxacin-resistant isolates) was assessed in OADC-enriched 7H11 Middlebrook agar. For the 18 isolates the MIC_{50} and MIC_{90} of levofloxacin were 0.5 and 1.0 μg/ml. In comparison, the MIC_{50} and MIC_{90} were 0.5 and 1.0 μg/ml and 0.25 and 0.5 μg/ml for ofloxacin and sparfloxacin, respectively. For ofloxacin-resistant isolates, the MICs of levofloxacin, ofloxacin, and sparfloxacin were 8.0, 8.0, and 4.0 μg/ml, respectively (Ji et al., 1995).

In 7H12 broth medium, the MICs of levofloxacin were 0.25 to 1.0 μg/ml (Mor et al., 1994).

3.1.2.11. Enoxacin

MICs of enoxacin were investigated for 36 M. *tuberculosis* isolates using OADC-enriched 7H10 Middlebrook agar. The MIC_{50} and MIC_{90} were 2.5 and >5.0 μg/ml (range, 0.3 to >5.0 μg/ml). The MIC_{50} and MIC_{90} of norfloxacin were 2.5 and >5.0 μg/ml (range, 0.3 to >5.0 μg/ml), and the MIC_{50} and MIC_{90} of pefloxacin were 0.6 and 1.2 μg/ml (Davies et al., 1987).

The in vitro activities of four fluoroquinolones were investigated for M. *tuberculosis* isolates with various phenotypes of resistance to standard anti-TB drugs in India, using 7H10 Middlebrook agar medium (Karak and De, 1995); results are shown in Table 4.

Using a checkerboard method and combinations of ciprofloxacin with rifampin, isoniazid, streptomycin, ethambutol, and pyrazinamide against 20 fully susceptible M. *tuberculosis* isolates, an antagonism of the ciprofloxacin-rifampin combination was demonstrated independently of activity of ciprofloxacin and other anti-TB drugs (Uttley and Collins, 1988).

3.1.2.12. Y-26611

Y-26611, a 7-morpholino quinolone derivative, had a MIC_{90} of 0.4 μg/ml for 25 M. *tuberculosis* isolates (Tomioka et al., 1992).

3.1.2.13. Sitafloxacin

The MIC_{50}s and MIC_{90}s of sitafloxacin, sparfloxacin, and ofloxacin were, respectively, 0.1 and 0.2, 0.1 and 0.2, and 0.78 and 0.78 μg/ml for 25 M. *tuberculosis* isolates in 7H11 Middlebrook agar (Saito et al., 1994).

3.1.2.14. Norfloxacin

Gaya and Chadwick (1986) showed that norfloxacin, with a MIC_{50} and MIC_{90} of 4.0 and 8.0 μg/ml (range, 2.0 to 8.0 μg/ml), was less active than ciprofloxacin (MIC_{50} and MIC_{90} of 0.5 and 1.0 μg/ml [range, 0.25 to 1.0 μg/ml]) against 20 M. *tuberculosis* isolates. Tests were performed on 7H10 Middlebrook agar.

3.1.2.15. Moxifloxacin

In vitro it was shown by Ji et al. (1998) that sparfloxacin and moxifloxacin are equally active and are slightly more active than clinafloxacin against 19 M. *tuberculosis* isolates, including M. *tuberculosis* $H37_{RV}$ (Table 5). In another study, it was shown that the MICs of moxifloxacin range from 0.12 to 0.5 mg/liter (Woodcock et al., 1997).

MIC_{50}s were 1.0, 1.0, 0.25, and 0.25 μg/ml and MIC_{90}s were 4.0., 2.0, 2.0, and 2.0 μg/ml for ciprofloxacin, ofloxacin, levofloxacin, and moxifloxacin, respectively, for 50 M. *tuberculosis* isolates tested in Middlebrook 7H11 medium enriched with OADC. A MIC of ≥2.0 μg/ml was noted for 21.8% (12 of 50) for ciprofloxacin, ofloxacin, levofloxacin, and moxifloxacin. One strain was particularly resistant to ciprofloxacin, with a MIC of 128 μg/ml (Rodriguez et al., 2001).

3.1.2.16. Temafloxacin

The MICs of difloxacin, temafloxacin, and enoxacin were determined in Middlebrook 7H10 agar (inoculum size of

Table 4 Comparative in vitro activities against *M. tuberculosis* of ciprofloxacin, norfloxacin, pefloxacin, and ofloxacin[a]

M. *tuberculosis* phenotype	*n*	Drug[b]	MIC (μg/ml)		
			50%	90%	Range
Susceptible + $H37_{RV}$	25	CIP	0.3	0.6	0.3–1.2
		OFX	0.3	0.6	0.15–0.6
		PFL	1.2	2.5	1.2–2.5
		NOR	2.5	5.0	1.2–5.0
INH^r (MIC, ≥1.0 μg/ml)	16	CIP	0.6	1.2	0.6–1.2
		OFX	0.3	0.6	0.15–0.6
		PFL	1.2	2.5	1.2–2.5
		NOR	2.5	5.0	2.5–5.0
STR^r (MIC, ≥32 μg/ml)	9	CIP			0.6
		OFX			0.3–0.6
		PFL			2.5
		NOR			2.5
EMB^r (MIC, ≥8 μg/ml)	3	CIP			0.3
		OFX			0.3
		PFL			2.5
		NOR			2.5
Multi (EMB^r, INH^r, RIF^r, [MIC, 128 μg/ml], STR^r)	8	CIP			0.3–0.6
		OFX			0.3–0.6
		PFL			2.5–5.0
		NOR			2.5–5.0

[a]Data from Karak and De, 1995.
[b]CIP, ciprofloxacin; OFX, ofloxacin; PFL, pefloxacin; NOR, norfloxacin; INH, isoniazid; EMB, ethambutol; RIF, rifampin.

Table 5 Anti-*M. tuberculosis* activities of clinafloxacin and moxifloxacin[a]

Compound	MIC (μg/ml)		
	50%	90%	Range
Sparfloxacin	0.25	0.5	0.12–0.5
Moxifloxacin	0.5	0.5	0.12–0.5
Clinafloxacin	0.5	1.0	0.12–1.0

[a]Data from Woodcock et al., 1997.

Table 6 Anti-*M. tuberculosis* activities of difloxacin and temafloxacin[a]

Compound	MIC (μg/ml)		
	50%	90%	Range
Difloxacin	2.7	4.7	2.5–1.0
Temafloxacin	1.4	2.3	1.3–5.0
Enoxacin	3.0	8.3	2.5–>10
Pefloxacin	3.3	6.7	2.5–>10
Ciprofloxacin	2.0	4.3	0.6–5.0
Ofloxacin	1.3	2.4	1.3–1.0

[a]Data from Gorzynski et al., 1989.

2×10^6 CFU). Temafloxacin activity was comparable to that of ofloxacin and superior to those of difloxacin, enoxacin, and pefloxacin (Gorzynski et al., 1989) (Table 6).

The in vitro activities of 10 fluoroquinolones against 64 M. *tuberculosis* isolates were investigated. MIC determinations were carried out by an agar dilution technique using Middlebrook 7H10 agar. The inoculum size was 10^4 CFU/ml. The most active compounds were ciprofloxacin and ofloxacin, with MIC_{50}s of 0.5 μg/ml, followed by temafloxacin (MIC_{50} of 1 μg/ml) (Table 6).

3.1.2.17. Olamufloxacin

A comparison of the in vitro activities of olamufloxacin (HSR-903), sitafloxacin, gatifloxacin, and levofloxacin against 23 M. *tuberculosis* isolates fully susceptible to standard anti-TB agents and 22 multidrug-resistant M. *tuberculosis* strains was carried out using 7H11 Middlebrook agar (Tomioka et al., 1999) (Table 7).

Against strains fully susceptible to standard anti-TB agents and levofloxacin, olamufloxacin is less active than levofloxacin, sitafloxacin, and gatifloxacin. For multidrug-resistant M. *tuberculosis* a bimodal population was recorded due to the fact that some of the isolates were resistant to levofloxacin.

A cross-resistance was demonstrated between all fluoroquinolones tested, even if the MIC_{50}s of sitafloxacin and gatifloxacin remain relatively low (0.78 μg/ml) but eight times higher than that for levofloxacin-susceptible isolates (0.1 μg/ml).

3.1.2.18. Gatifloxacin

The gatifloxacin MIC_{50} and MIC_{90} for 11 M. *tuberculosis* isolates were 0.12 and 0.25 μg/ml, respectively. MICs were determined by a broth macrodilution method in 7H9 broth with 2×10^7 CFU/ml as the final inoculum size (Fung-Tomc et al., 2000).

3.1.2.19. Garenoxacin (BMS-284756, T-3811ME)

The activity of garenoxacin against 10 M. *tuberculosis* isolates was assessed using a broth macrodilution method

Table 7 Anti-*M. tuberculosis* activities of sitafloxacin, gatifloxacin, and levofloxacin[a]

M. tuberculosis phenotype	*n*	MIC (μg/ml)							
		OLF		SIT		GAT		LVX	
		50%	90%	50%	90%	50%	90%	50%	90%
Non-MDR	23	0.78	0.78	0.1	0.1	0.1	0.2	0.39	0.39
MDR	22	3.13	25	0.39	1.56	0.39	1.56	3.13	6.25
LVX[s]	27	0.78	1.56	0.1	0.1	0.1	0.2	0.39	0.78
LVX[r]	18	6.25	50	0.78	1.56	0.78	3.13	3.13	12.5

[a]Data from Tomiaka et al., 1999. SIT, sitafloxacin; GAT, gatifloxacin; LVX, levofloxacin; OLF, olamufloxacin; MDR, multidrug resistant.

with 7H9 Middlebrook broth with an inoculum size of about 10^6CFU/ml. The MIC_{50} and MIC_{90} were 1.0 and 2.0 μg/ml (range, 0.03 to 2.0 μg/ml). In comparison, the MIC_{50}s were 0.06, 0.5, 2.0, and 1.0 μg/ml and the MIC_{90}s were 0.12, 1.0, 2.0, and 4.0 μg/ml for moxifloxacin, levofloxacin, ofloxacin, and ciprofloxacin, respectively (Kolek et al., 2000).

3.1.2.20. Trovafloxacin

Twenty-three *M. tuberculosis* isolates were recovered from patients with different IS*6110* restriction fragment length polymorphism patterns and were tested for their susceptibilities to various antibacterial agents, including ciprofloxacin, levofloxacin, sparfloxacin, and trovafloxacin. MICs were determined by a radiometric method. Only two strains were susceptible to all anti-TB agents; of the other isolates, 17 were multiresistant and the remainder were considered resistant to a single agent. Data are summarized in Table 8.

Trovafloxacin could be considered to be inactive in vitro. The most active compound is sparfloxacin, followed by levofloxacin (Hoffner et al., 1997).

The weak activity of trovafloxacin against *M. tuberculosis* was confirmed by other studies. Takahata et al. (1999) demonstrated that the MIC_{50} and MIC_{90} of trovafloxacin were 1.0 μg/ml, whereas those of BMS-284756, ciprofloxacin, and levofloxacin were 0.05, 0.12, and 0.12 μg/ml, respectively. However, the methodology was unusual: MICs were determined in microtiter plates containing Dubos broth medium enriched with 5% glycerol and 10% albumin. Two hundred fifty isolates of *M. tuberculosis* were evaluated for susceptibility to trovafloxacin, grepafloxacin, gemifloxacin, levofloxacin, ofloxacin, and ciprofloxacin in Middlebrook 7H10 agar medium (Table 9). The results confirmed the poor activity of trovafloxacin and gemifloxacin against *M. tuberculosis* (Ruiz-Serrano et al., 2000). Both are 1,8-naphthyridone compounds; these structures are known to reduce the activity of pyridone-β-carboxylic acid against *M. tuberculosis* (Jacobs, 1995).

Table 8 Anti-*M. tuberculosis* activity of trovafloxacin[a] (*n* = 23)

Compound	MIC (μg/ml)		
	50%	90%	Range
Ciprofloxacin	1.0	2.0	1.0–4.0
Levofloxacin	1.0	1.0	1.0–2.0
Sparfloxacin	1.0	1.0	1.0
Trovafloxacin	>8	>8	>8

[a]Data from Hoffner et al., 1997.

Table 9 Anti-*M. tuberculosis* activities of grepafloxacin, trovafloxacin, and gemifloxacin[a]

M. tuberculosis phenotype	*n*	Compound	MIC (μg/ml)	
			50%	90%
Fully susceptible	206	Ciprofloxacin	1.0	1.0
		Ofloxacin	1.0	1.0
		Levofloxacin	0.5	1.0
		Grepafloxacin	1.0	1.0
		Trovafloxacin	32	64
		Gemifloxacin	4.0	8.0
Multidrug resistant	44	Ciprofloxacin	1.0	2.0
		Ofloxacin	1.0	2.0
		Levofloxacin	0.5	1.0
		Grepafloxacin	1.0	2.0
		Trovafloxacin	32	128
		Gemifloxacin	8.0	8.0

[a]Data from Ruiz-Serrano et al., 2000.

3.1.2.21. Grepafloxacin

Grepafloxacin exhibited in vitro activity comparable to those of ofloxacin and ciprofloxacin. Using a 7H11 Middlebrook agar medium enriched with 10% OADC, the in vitro activity of grepafloxacin against 33 *M. tuberculosis* isolates was investigated. This study confirmed the previous one, showing comparable in vitro activities of ciprofloxacin, ofloxacin, and grepafloxacin. The three compounds exhibited a MIC_{50} and MIC_{90} of 0.5 and 1.0 μg/ml (range, 0.12 to 2.0 μg/ml) (Vacher et al., 1999). These results were supported by a third study (Saito et al., 1994).

3.1.2.22. Tosufloxacin

Tosufloxacin, a 1,8-naphthyridone compound, has been shown to be inactive against 98 isolates of *M. tuberculosis* in a nonspecified agar medium (Table 10) (Yew et al., 1994). In this study, it was shown that in vitro sparfloxacin was the most active compound against all *M. tuberculosis* isolates. However, two important findings were highlighted. Against multidrug-resistant *M. tuberculosis*, all of the compounds exhibited a bimodal activity, with some isolates being probably resistant; however, these isolates were not explored. When an isolate is highly resistant to standard anti-TB drugs, fluoroquinolones could be weakly active.

3.1.2.23. Balofloxacin and Cadrofloxacin

The in vitro activities of balofloxacin, cadrofloxacin (CS-940), and other fluoroquinolones against 100 *M. tuberculosis* isolates were assessed using an egg-based Ogawa medium

Table 10 Activities of tosufloxacin and A-80556 against multidrug-resistant *M. tuberculosis* isolates ($n = 17$)[a]

Compound	MIC (μg/ml)		
	50%	90%	Range
Ciprofloxacin	2.0	4.0	0.12–4.0
Ofloxacin	4.0	8.0	0.25–8.0
Levofloxacin	2.0	4.0	0.12–4.0
Sparfloxacin	0.5	1.0	0.03–2.0
Temafloxacin	8.0	>8.0	0.5–>8.0
Clinafloxacin	1.0	2.0	0.06–4.0
Tosufloxacin	>8.0	>8.0	>8.0
A-80556	>8.0	>8.0	4.0–>8.0

[a]Data from Yew et al., 1994. Isolates were resistant to isoniazid, rifampin, streptomycin, pyrazinamide, and ethambutol.

Table 11 Anti-*M. tuberculosis* activities of WQ-3034 and olamufloxacin[a]

Compound	MIC (μg/ml)			
	Rifampin[s] ($n = 27$)		Rifampin[r] ($n = 45$)	
	50%	90%	50%	90%
Levofloxacin	0.39	1.56	3.13	6.25
Ciprofloxacin	0.78	1.56	6.25	12.5
Sparfloxacin	0.20	0.39	1.56	3.13
Gatifloxacin	0.10	0.39	0.39	1.56
Sitafloxacin	0.10	0.20	0.39	1.56
WQ-3034	0.78	1.56	1.56	6.25
Olamufloxacin	0.78	1.56	3.13	25

[a]Data from Ogasawara et al., 2000.

and 7H10 Middlebrook agar medium. The MICs determined in Ogawa medium were approximately two- to fourfold higher than those determined in Middlebrook 7H10 medium. The MIC_{50}s of cadrofloxacin and sparfloxacin were 0.25 and 0.50 μg/ml, respectively. The MIC_{50} of balofloxacin was 2.0 μg/ml (Yamane et al., 1996).

3.1.2.24. Prulifloxacin

The MIC_{50} of prulifloxacin was 0.78 μg/ml for *M. tuberculosis* in 7H11 Middlebrook agar medium (Tomioka et al., 1993b).

3.1.2.25. WQ-3034

The in vitro activities of seven fluoroquinolones, including WQ-3034 and olamufloxacin, against 37 rifampin-susceptible and 45 rifampin- and ciprofloxacin-resistant *M. tuberculosis* isolates were investigated. MICs were determined on agar dilution in 7H11 medium and for resistant strains also in Ogawa medium. No significant differences were observed in MICs between the media. Gatifloxacin and sitafloxacin retained activity against *M. tuberculosis* isolates resistant to rifampin and ciprofloxacin (Table 11) (Ogasawara et al., 2000).

Against 45 *M. tuberculosis* isolates, WQ-3034 was found to be as active as levofloxacin (MIC_{50} and MIC_{90}, 0.39 and 0.78 μg/ml) but less active than sparfloxacin (MIC_{50} and MIC_{90}, 0.20 and 0.20 μg/ml) and more active than ciprofloxacin (MIC_{50} and MIC_{90}, 0.78 and 0.78 μg/ml) against *M. tuberculosis* strains susceptible to rifampin, but these compounds were poorly active against the 22 *M. tuberculosis* isolates resistant to rifampin and ciprofloxacin (MIC_{50}, 6.25 μg/ml). MICs were determined in Middlebrook 7H11 medium (Tomioka et al., 2000).

3.1.3. Fluoroquinolone Activities against *M. tuberculosis* Complex

The in vitro activities of levofloxacin, ofloxacin, and *d*-ofloxacin against *M. tuberculosis* complex (comprising *M. tuberculosis*, *M. africanum*, *M. bovis*, and *M. bovis* BCG) were investigated using a radiometric method (BACTEC 460TB) in 7H12 Middlebrook broth (Rastogi et al., 1996).

The MICs of *d*-ofloxacin were 64 μg/ml irrespective of the component of the *M. tuberculosis* complex.

Levofloxacin was twice as active as ofloxacin. The MICs of levofloxacin were 0.5, 0.5 to 0.75, 0.5, 0.5, and 0.5 μg/ml and those of ofloxacin were 0.75 to 1.0, 0.75 to 1.0, 0.75 to 1.0, 0.75 to 1.0, and 0.75 to 1.0 μg/ml for susceptible *M. tuberculosis*, multidrug-resistant *M. tuberculosis*, *M. africanum*, *M. bovis*, and *M. bovis* BCG, respectively (Table 12).

Table 12 In vitro activity of levofloxacin against *M. tuberculosis* complex[a]

Microorganism(s)	n	MIC (μg/ml) range		
		Ofloxacin	Levofloxacin	*d*-Ofloxacin
M. tuberculosis (susceptible)				
$H37_{RV}$	1	1.0	0.5	64
Clinical isolates	5	0.75–1.0	0.5	64
MDR[b]	4	0.75–1.0	0.5–0.75	32–64
M. africanum				
ATCC 25420	1	1.0	0.5	64
Clinical isolates	2	0.75–1.0	0.5	64
M. bovis				
ATCC 19210	1	0.75	0.5	64
Clinical isolates	2	1.0	0.5	64
BCG				
BCG Pasteur	1	0.75	0.5	64
BCG Denmark	1	0.75	0.5	32
BCG Russia	1	1.0	0.5	64

[a]Data from Rastogi et al., 1996.
[b]MDR, multidrug resistant.

Table 13 In vitro activities of fluoroquinolones against *M. bovis* and *M. africanum*[a]

Microorganism	MIC (μg/ml)			
	Ofloxacin	Ciprofloxacin	Pefloxacin	Norfloxacin
M. bovis	1.0	1.0	8.0	4.0
M. bovis BCG Pasteur	0.5	1.0	2.0	1.0
M. africanum	0.5	1.0	2.0	2.0

[a]Data from Dailloux et al., 1989.

The in vitro activity of levofloxacin in combination with antimycobacterial drugs was assessed against susceptible strains and single-drug- or multidrug-resistant isolates. Combination testing of sub-MICs of levofloxacin with first-line (isoniazid, rifampin, and ethambutol) and second-line (amikacin and clofazimine) anti-TB drugs was done with two-, three-, and four-drug combinations. A synergistic activity was observed in 8 of 25, 12 of 20, and 8 of 15 tests, respectively, indicating that levofloxacin could act in synergy with standard anti-TB drugs (Rastogi et al., 1996).

Twenty-five *M. tuberculosis* isolates have been tested for susceptibility to ofloxacin, pefloxacin, norfloxacin, and ciproflaxin using 7H10 Middlebrook agar enriched with 10% of bovine calf serum (proportion method). One hundred percent of the isolates were inhibited with 1.0, 2.0, 8.0, and 4.0 μg of ofloxacin, ciprofloxacin, pefloxacin, and norfloxacin per ml, respectively. The MIC_{50}s of these four compounds were 0.5, 0.25, 4.0, and 2.0 μg/ml, respectively.

The MICs of ofloxacin, ciprofloxacin, pefloxacin, and norfloxacin were 0.25, 0.5, 2.0, and 1.0 μg/ml, respectively for *M. tuberculosis* $H37_{RA}$.

The MICs of the four quinolones for *M. bovis*, *M. bovis* BCG Pasteur, and *M. africanum* were determined; results are shown in Table 13 (Dailloux et al., 1989).

3.1.4. Summary of In Vitro Anti-TB Activities

Table 14 summarizes the in vitro activities of fluoroquinolones against *M. tuberculosis*.

Table 14 In vitro activities of fluoroquinolones against *M. tuberculosis*

Compound	MIC (μg/ml)		
	50%	90%	Range
Ciprofloxacin	0.25	0.5–1.0	0.125–4.0
Ofloxacin	0.5	0.5–1.0	0.25–4.0
Pefloxacin	4.0	4.0	1.0–1.6
Norfloxacin	4.0	8.0	2.0–4.0
Amifloxacin	2.0	4.0	1.0–32
Difloxacin	4.0	4.0	0.5–8.0
Temafloxacin	1.0	1.0	0.03–2.0
Lomefloxacin	1.0	2.0	0.5–2.0
Irloxacin	8.0	16	2.0–32
Levofloxacin	1.0	1.0	1.0–2.0
Sparfloxacin	0.25–1.0	0.5–1.0	0.12–1.0
Moxifloxacin	0.5	0.5	0.12–0.5
Gatifloxacin	0.12	0.25	0.12–0.25
Trovafloxacin	>8.0	>8.0	>8
Grepafloxacin	1.0	2.0	1.0–2.0
Sitafloxacin	0.1–0.78	0.1–1.56	0.1–1.56
Gemifloxacin	4.0	8.0	
Y-26111		0.4	
Garenoxacin	1.0	2.0	0.03–2.0
WIN 57273	1.0		1.0–4.0
WQ-3034	0.78	1.56	
Enoxacin	4.0	4.0	1.0–32
CI-934	2.0	2.0	1.0–8.0
A-80556	>8.0	>8.0	4–>8.0
Olamufloxacin	0.78	1.56	
Cadrofloxacin	0.25		
A-56620	4.0	8.0	2.0–16
Balofloxacin	2.0		
Clinafloxacin	0.5	1.0	0.12–1.0
Tosufloxacin	>8	>8	>8
Prulifloxacin	0.78		
BAY y 3118	0.06	0.13	0.06–0.13
DW 224a	0.06	0.06	0.03–0.06

3.2. Bactericidal Activity against *M. tuberculosis*

The minumum bactericidal concentrations were assessed (reduction in the viable counts by at least 99% compared with the viable counts of the initial inoculum added to the drug-containing vial) (Rastogi and Goh, 1991; Heifets and Lindholm-Levy, 1987). It was shown that ofloxacin, ciprofloxacin, and sparfloxacin exhibit bactericidal activity against *M. tuberculosis*.

3.3. Factors Affecting Susceptibility Testing

It was shown that pH affects MICs. Table 15 shows MIC_{50}s of ciprofloxacin, ofloxacin, and WIN 57273 determined in 7H12 broth at pH 6.8 and pH 6.0. The final inoculum size was 10^4 to 10^5CFU/ml.

The MICs of ofloxacin (ranges, 0.5 to 2.0 and 1.0 to 2.0 μg/ml at pH 6.8 and 6.0, respectively) were less affected by pH variation of the medium (Heifets and Lindholm-Levy, 1990).

The MICs of WIN 57273 were more pH dependent than those of ofloxacin and ciprofloxacin. *M. tuberculosis* does not grow sufficiently at pHs lower than 6.0.

Table 15 Effect of pH on in vitro activities of fluoroquinolones against TB

Compound	MIC_{50} (μg/ml)	
	pH 6.8	pH 6.0
Ofloxacin	1.0	2.0
Ciprofloxacin	1.0	2.0
WIN 57273	4.0	1.0

MICs were also determined by the radiometric method in 7H12 Middlebrook broth with an inoculum size of 10^4 to 10^5CFU/ml (Heifets and Lindholm-Levy, 1990).

In OADC-enriched 7H11 Middlebrook agar, the MICs of ofloxacin, levofloxacin, and sparfloxacin for strain $H37_{RV}$ were 1.0, 0.5, and 0.12 μg/ml, respectively (Ji et al., 1995).

3.4. In Vitro Activity against *M. tuberculosis* $H37_{RV}$

Table 16 shows the MICs of fluoroquinolones for *M. tuberculosis* $H37_{RV}$ in 7H11 agar medium (Ji et al., 1991).

Table 16 In vitro activities of fluoroquinolones against *M. tuberculosis* H37$_{RV}$

Compound	MIC (μg/ml)
Sparfloxacin	0.25
Ciprofloxacin	1.0
Ofloxacin	1.0

4. MECHANISM OF RESISTANCE

Tsukamura et al. (1985) reported prompt bacteriological conversion of sputum for 5 of 19 patients with multidrug-resistant TB treated with ofloxacin alone, and the condition of all patients improved. However, in 12 of the 19 cases, selection of ofloxacin-resistant isolates was obtained when the drug was given alone. The same results occurred in 4 of 9 patients when ofloxacin was administered with a poorly active drug (Hong-Kong Chest Service, 1992). This phenomenon was reported in New York City between 1991 and 1993 in most cases, as a result of inadequate or inappropriate treatment (Sullivan et al., 1995). The proportion of mutants resistant to fluoroquinolones among a population of susceptible *M. tuberculosis* isolates is about 10^{-6}, and the size of the bacterial population is 10^8CFU/ml in cavity pulmonary TB (Canetti and The, 1965). It is difficult to prevent the selection of fluoroquinolone-resistant mutants in patients whose organisms remain susceptible to only a few active drugs. Combination therapy is compulsory to reduce the risk of selecting a mutant.

4.1. *M. tuberculosis* DNA Gyrase

The DNA gyrase genes are located on a 480-kb *Dra*I fragment of *M. tuberculosis* H37$_{RV}$. The *gyrA* gene (2,517 bp) was found to be located 34 bp downstream of *gyrB* (2,060 bp).

The deduced GyrB protein of *M. tuberculosis* showed 79 and 63% amino acid homology with those of *Streptomyces spheroides* and *Escherichia coli* protein, respectively. The deduced GyrA protein of *M. tuberculosis* showed 69 and 68% similarity with the *E. coli* and *Staphylococcus aureus* GyrA proteins, respectively.

The *gyrA* gene is located 34 nucleotides downstream of the *gyrB* gene. Both genes seem to be transcribed from the promoter located upstream of the *gyrB* coding sequence (Madhusudan et al., 1994).

GyrB protein is composed of 714 amino acids. The GyrB sequence has been shown to be a useful phylogenetic marker for mycobacterial species identification. The internal transcribed spacer seems to be 100% identical for the four species composing the *M. tuberculosis* complex (*M. tuberculosis*, *M. bovis*, *M. africanum*, and *M. microti*) (Kasai et al., 2000). However, it has been shown that *M. africanum* subtype II and *M. tuberculosis* have an identical *gyrB* sequence that could facilitate discrimination with *M. africanum* subtype I, *M. bovis*, and *M. microti*. Pyrazinamide-resistant and -susceptible *M. bovis* strains showed specific substitution at position 756 but can be differentiated by substitution at position 1311 (Niemann et al., 2000).

The peptide sequence of the quinolone resistance-determining region (QRDR) of Gyr B were identical in all mycobacterial species, including the amino acids at the three positions known to be involved in acquired resistance to quinolones: 426 (Asp), 447 (Arg), and 464 (Asn). The last two residues could be involved in the overall low level of susceptibility of mycobacteria to quinolones, since they differ from those found in *E. coli*, which is very susceptible to fluoroquinolones (Lys447 and Ser464) (Guillemin et al., 1998, 1999).

The A-subunit of DNA gyrase of *Mycobacterium leprae*, unlike its counterpart in *M. tuberculosis*, is produced by protein splicing, as its gene, *gyrA*, harbors a 1,260-bp in-frame insertion encoding an intein, a putative homing endonuclease (Esihi et al., 1996).

It has been shown that the presence of *gyrA* inteins is a taxonomic characteristic specific for a given taxon at species or a subspecies level (Sander et al., 1998).

The gyrase of *M. tuberculosis* also exhibited considerable homology with the type IV topoisomerase of *E. coli* ParC and ParE: 62% amino acid homology between ParC and GyrB and 59% amino acid similarity between ParE and GyrA (Takiff et al., 1994). A topoisomerase IV gene was not identified in the *M. tuberculosis* genome sequence (Cole et al., 1998).

4.2. Mutations on DNA Gyrase of *M. tuberculosis*

Fluoroquinolones inhibit DNA gyrase of *M. tuberculosis* (Drlica et al., 1996; Kocagöz et al., 1996).

The nucleotide sequence corresponding to the GyrA region associated with fluoroquinolone resistance in *M. tuberculosis* was reported. The region is located at the highly conserved (interspecies) N-terminal protein region the QRDR (Takiff et al., 1994). In an extensive study, ciprofloxacin-susceptible and -resistant (MIC, >4.0 μg/ml) *M. tuberculosis* isolates were investigated by PCR for single strand conformational polymorphism (SSCP) in *gyrA* and *gyrB*.

The 320-bp *gyrA* fragment was sequenced from all strains. Two *gyrA* SSCP patterns were identified among ciprofloxacin-susceptible organisms, and eight *gyrA* SSCP patterns were found among resistant bacteria. All strains had a single *gyrB* SSCP pattern.

A total of five polymorph codons (positions 88, 90, 91, 94, and 95) were identified in *gyrA* by DNA sequencing. Codon 95 contained a naturally occurring polymorphism (AGC [Ser] or ACC [Thr]).

The four other polymorph codons contained changes unique to the ciprofloxacin-resistant strains, with position 94 being the most variable.

The *gyrA* mutations were identified in all strains for which the ciprofloxacin MIC was >2 μg/ml.

It is quite difficult to draw a general conclusion. Furthermore, numbering of codons differs among authors, rendering it difficult to compare results.

Kapur et al. (1995) sequenced a 320-bp region of *gyrA* in 17 *M. tuberculosis* isolates, including 12 strains resistant to ciprofloxacin. In all isolates, a natural mutation in codon 95 was detected (AGC→ACC [Ser→Thr]). Among ciprofloxacin-resistant isolates missense mutations have been found in codons 94 and 90.

In a strain for which the ofloxacin MIC was 32 μg/ml on the basis of results determined by the proportion method, a missense mutation (GAC→CAC [Asp→His]) was demonstrated in codon 89 (Cambau et al., 1994a, 1994b).

In another study four missense mutations were described for 15 *M. tuberculosis* isolates resistant to ciprofloxacin, in codons 88, 90, 91, and 94 (Table 17) (Takiff et al., 1994).

Analysis of the QRDRs of *gyrA* genes from fluoroquinolone-resistant strains (MIC, ≥4.0 μg/ml) showed a cross-resistance within all the fluoroquinolones tested: ofloxacin, ciprofloxacin, and sparfloxacin (Alangaden et al., 1995). Mutations resulting in a substitution of Ala83 or Asp87 were shown (Asp94 in the Takiff study). Substitution in Asp87 (codon 94) was the most common for fluoroquinolone-resistant *M. tuberculosis* isolates.

Table 17 DNA gyrase mutation in *M. tuberculosis* and ciprofloxacin in vitro activity[a]

Strain	*n*	MIC (μg/ml)	Genotype	
			SSCP	Mutation
$H37_{RA}$ mutant	1	≥3.0	E	Gly88→Cys
Ciprofloxacin[r]	3	4.0–8.0	C	Ala90→Val
	1	4.0	F	Ser91→Pro
	1	≥4.0	G	Asp94→His
	1	>8.0	D	Asp94→Asn
	5	>8.0	H	Asp94→Gly
	2	>8.0	I	Asp94→Tyr
	1	4.0	J	Asp94→Ala
	1	2.0	B	Codon 95

[a]Data from Takiff et al., 1994.

The level of fluoroquinolone activity against *M. tuberculosis* is partly related to the amino acid residue at position 90 in the QRDR. This was supported by the fact that the 50% inhibitory concentrations (IC_{50}) for the purified DNA gyrase from *Mycobacterium avium* and *Mycobacterium smegmatis*, which naturally have an alanine at position 83, were higher than those inhibiting the enzyme of *Mycobacterium fortuitum* subsp. *peregrinum*, characterized by a serine at position 83 of GyrA (Guillemin et al., 1999).

In an investigation by Onodera et al. (2001), it was shown that IC_{50} correlated well with in vitro activity of various fluoroquinolones against *M. tuberculosis* $H37_{RV}$ and mutants (Table 18).

For the two modified GyrA proteins, the IC_{50} of levofloxacin, ciprofloxacin, and sparfloxacin were above 400 μg/ml. For sitafloxacin, the IC_{50} were 22.1 μg/ml for a single mutation and 144 μg/ml for a double mutation.

4.3. Selection of Spontaneous Fluoroquinolone-Resistant Mutants

Resistance to fluoroquinolones shows a two-step pattern. Two phenotypes of resistance have been reported according to the level of MICs: a group for which the MICs of ofloxacin are equal to 5 μg/ml and a group for which the MICs of ofloxacin are above or equal to 100 μg/ml (Tsukamura et al., 1985b).

The frequency of occurrence of resistant mutants in the culture population was investigated using *M. tuberculosis* strain $H37_{RV}$ as a test organism in 7H10 Middlebrook agar containing ofloxacin, ciprofloxacin, and sparfloxacin (2.0, 4.0, and 8.0 μg of each fluoroquinolone per ml). Spontaneous mutants appeared at frequency of 2×10^{-6} to 1×10^{-8}. The highest concentration of each fluoroquinolone at which spontaneous mutants were obtained was 8.0 μg/ml for ofloxacin and ciprofloxacin an 4.0 μg/ml for sparfloxacin (Alangaden et al., 1995). Comparable frequencies have been observed by other authors (Takiff et al., 1994).

The selecting concentrations of ofloxacin are 1, 2, and 4 times the MIC, and those of ciprofloxacin are 4, 8, and 16 times the MIC; with sparfloxacin at 4 and 8 times the MIC the frequencies were 10^{-6} and 10^{-8}, and at 16 times MIC (8 μg/ml) the frequency was $<10^{-9}$. The frequencies of mutation for a given concentration were comparable for ofloxacin and ciprofloxacin. The frequency of spontaneous ciprofloxacin-resistant mutants was 10^{-6} (0.5 μg/ml) to 10^{-8} (2 μg/ml). Spontaneous ciprofloxacin-resistant mutants were selected from the avirulent strain *M. tuberculosis* $H37_{RA}$ and from the virulent strains $H37_{RV}$ and Erdman. The frequencies for a ciprofloxacin concentration of 1 μg/ml were 1×10^{-6}, 5×10^{-6}, and 2×10^{-6}, respectively. Colonies resistant to 1 μg of ciprofloxacin per ml were found 10 to 50 times more frequently than colonies resistant to 2.0 μg of ciprofloxacin per ml. No primary resistance was found for a concentration of 2 μg of ciprofloxacin per ml when an inoculum size of 10^8 CFU per plate was used (Takiff et al., 1994).

The progressive development of drug resistance in a patient while undergoing anti-TB chemotherapy is of concern.

In a 32-year-old male patient suffering from a pulmonary TB who failed to respond to standard anti-TB chemotherapy, serial isolates of *M. tuberculosis* were cultured. Each successive isolate was found to be resistant to a wider range of anti-TB drugs than its predecessors.

The initial isolate was resistant to isoniazid and rifampin; the second isolate was also resistant to ethambutol. The third was resistant to pyrazinamide and ofloxacin, and the fourth was also resistant to ciprofloxacin and sparfloxacin, which were never used in this patient. MICs increased from 0.5 to >2.0 μg/ml for ofloxacin, 0.75 to >2.0 μg/ml for ciprofloxacin, and 0.2 to >1.0 μg/ml for sparfloxacin. MICs were determined on 7H11 agar and using a BACTEC radiometric method (7H12 broth) (Table 19).

A stepwise acquisition of resistance was suggested, in the following order: ofloxacin > ciprofloxacin > sparfloxacin (Rastogi et al., 1992).

4.4. Efflux Mechanism of Resistance

It was recently shown that fluoroquinolones could be pumped out from *M. smegmatis* isolates, rendering them resistant to fluoroquinolones. In *M. smegmatis*, the LfrA protein gene is responsible for a low level of resistance to fluoroquinolones (ciprofloxacin, ofloxacin, sparfloxacin, and levofloxacin) and increases the frequency of mutation to higher-level resistance

Table 18 Affinity for DNA gyrase in mutant *M. tuberculosis* isolates of fluoroquinolones[a]

Compound	MIC (μg/ml)	IC_{50} (μg/ml)		
		Wild type	V90A[b]	V90A + V94D[c]
Sitafloxacin	0.03	1.67	22.1	144
Levofloxacin	0.5	13.9	>400	>400
Ciprofloxacin	0.5	12.2	>400	>400
Sparfloxacin	0.12	4.8	>400	>400

[a]Data from Onodera et al., 2001.
[b]V90A, Val90→Ala (GTG→GCG, Ser 83 of *E. coli*) mutant.
[c]V94D, Gly94→Asp (GCG→CAC) mutant.

Table 19 ***M. tuberculosis* stepwise acquisition of resistance to fluoroquinolones**[a]

Isolate	MIC (μg/ml)					
	Ofloxacin		Ciprofloxacin		Sparfloxacin	
	7H11	BACTEC	7H11	BACTEC	7H11	BACTEC
1	0.5	0.5	0.75	0.25	0.2	0.1
2	0.5	0.5	0.75	0.25	0.2	0.1
3	1.0	1.0	0.75	0.25	0.2	0.1
4	>3.0	>3.0	>2.0	>2.0	>1.0	0.1

[a]Data from Rastogi et al., 1992.

Table 20 **Intracellular anti-TB activities of gatifloxacin and ofloxacin**[a]

Compound	Dose (μg/ml)	CFU/100 macrophages on day:		
		0	3	5
Control		60.5 ± 3.85	179 ± 5.2	320 ± 10.7
Gatifloxacin	1.0		56.3 ± 4.6	58.3 ± 3.6
	1.0		7.4 ± 0.4	4.5 ± 0.2
Ofloxacin	1.0		175 ± 3.8	320 ± 8.9
	1.0		64 ± 1.8	47.6 ± 5.6

[a]Data from Tomioka et al., 1999.

(Takiff et al., 1996, Liu et al., 1996). These pumps belongs to the major facilitator superfamily (MFS).

A pump belonging to the small multidrug resistance family, Mmf, was described to occur in *M. tuberculosis* and pump out erythromycin A (Borges-Walmsley and Walmsley, 2001).

A putative pump which effluxes tetracycline belonging to the MFS pump family, Tap, has been reported to occur in *M. tuberculosis* and *M. smegmatis;* the substrate is tetracycline (Ainsa et al., 1998).

It can be hypothesized that in the near future, with the increased use of fluoroquinolones in the treatment of TB, low levels of resistance to these drugs will be due to an active efflux mechanism (Banerjee et al., 1996).

4.4.1. Intracellular Activity of Fluoroquinolones

In pulmonary TB, *M. tuberculosis* penetrates in alveolar macrophages and lung epithelial cells (Bermudez and Goodman, 1996). However, the precise role of lung epithelial cells is still unknown. It has been demonstrated that *M. tuberculosis* enters and vigorously multiplies within macro-phages and type II lung epithelial cells. These facts strongly suggest that the alveolar pneumocytes act as the sites of bacterial growth in lung infections caused by mycobacteria.

In most studies of intracellular activity of anti-TB compounds, the antibacterials are added directly after infection and the bactericidal effect of the compounds on the intracellular pathogens is tested only on bacilli residing in fused vacuoles. To be valid, a prolonged period of incubation is needed (3 to 4 days) in order to investigate this effect on bacteria multiplying in nonfused vacuoles.

The J-774 macrophage line was infected with the $H37_{RV}$ strain of *M. tuberculosis*. Ciprofloxacin and ofloxacin at 5 μg/ml were added 2 days after all challenge. Ofloxacin exhibited bactericidal activity intracellularly comparable to those of rifampin and isoniazid (Rastogi et al., 1987). However, ofloxacin killed *M. tuberculosis* slowly in macrophages (Crowle et al., 1988).

In murine macrophages, there is a significant reduction of *M. tuberculosis* $H37_{RV}$ after contact with 1.0 and 10 μg of gatifloxacin per ml and 10 μg of ofloxacin per ml (Table 20) (Tomioka et al., 1999).

A 2-h exposure of human monocytes to 7 μg of levofloxacin and ofloxacin per ml resulted in intracellular concentrations of 27.1 ± 0.8 μg/ml (mean ± standard deviation) (cellular/extracellular ratio [C/E ratio] of 3.9) for ofloxacin and 38.44 ± 1.1 μg/ml (C/E ratio of 5.5) for levofloxacin (Mor et al., 1994). With levofloxacin, that represents a 100-fold decrease in cell burden in comparison with ofloxacin (Mor et al., 1994).

The intracellular activity in human monocytes was less pronounced with ciprofloxacin (exposure of 5 μg/ml) than with clinafloxacin (exposure of 1.0 μg/ml) or CI-990 (exposure of 0.5 μg/ml) (Van Rensburg et al., 1995; Rastogi and Blom-Potar, 1990).

These results need to be taken cautiously. It has been highlighted that virulent *M. tuberculosis* eludes the antimicrobial mechanism of macrophages by escaping from fused phagolysosomes into nonfused vesicles or the cytoplasm. The process can take up to 4 days.

In one study, it was shown that only clinafloxacin was able to inhibit the growth of *M. tuberculosis* in nonfused vacuoles in comparison with ciprofloxacin and CI-990 (Van Rensburg et al., 1995).

Bioactivities of olamufloxacin and levofloxacin against *M. tuberculosis* strain Kurono (isoniazid and rifampin susceptible) were assessed in monocytic Mac 6 macrophages (MM6-MΦ) and in A-549 cells (human type II lung epithelial cell-like). Both compounds were added to culture medium of *M. tuberculosis*-infected cells at the maximum concentration of each compound in serum (0.86 and 2.0 μg/ml for doses of olamufloxacin and levofloxacin of 4 and 20 mg/kg of body weight, respectively). The antibacterial activities of both compounds against *M. tuberculosis* residing in A-549 cells are significantly lower than those against *M. tuberculosis* within MM6-MΦ. *M. tuberculosis* replicates in A-549 cells more vigorously than in MM6-MΦ, presumably because of the inability in A-549 cells to produce nitric oxide, and important antimycobacterial effector molecule (Bermudez et al., 1996; McDonough and Kress, 1995; Sato and Tomioka, 1999).

In A-549 cells, olamufloxacin-mediated bacterial elimination was incomplete, but with levofloxacin progressive and complete killing of *M. tuberculosis* was achieved. There was no difference between the compounds in MM6-MΦ, in which complete killing of *M. tuberculosis* was obtained. This observation was confirmed in another study (Sato et al., 2000).

This effect is concentration dependent, as demonstrated when 0.25 mg of both compounds per liter is added, which corresponds to the MICs of both against *M. tuberculosis* Kurono. At this concentration, olamufloxacin exhibited a bacteriostatic effect but levofloxacin remained bactericidal in MM6-MΦ. In A-259 cells, only a weak bacteriostatic effect at 0.25 μg/ml was recorded (Tomioka et al., 1999).

When WQ-3034 and levofloxacin were added at their MICs assayed by broth dilution (1.0 and 0.25 μg/ml, respectively), WQ-3034 exhibited a bacteriostatic activity against *M. tuberculosis* Kurono multiplying in MM6-MΦ, while levofloxacin did not exhibit such activity. Weak bacteriostatic activity effects were observed for both compounds against *M. tuberculosis* isolates within A-549 cells.

In the human monocytic cell line THP-1, *M. bovis* BCG does not grow during the first 48 h, but during days 2 and 5 the number of bacteria within the cells increases 10- to 20-fold. The activity of fluoroquinolones against *M. bovis* BCG has to be assessed during the lag phase.

PD-161148 (8-OCH_3 analog) was more efficient than PD-160793 (the 8-H counterpart) in bacterial killing.

A reduction of 1 log_{10}CFU was observed for an extracellular concentration of 2 μg/ml for the 8-OCH_3 and 8-H analogs. However, at 6 and 10 μg/ml, no growth was detected with the 8-OCH_3 analog; the effect was observed at 10 μg/ml with the 8-H analog. Against ciprofloxacin-resistant *M. bovis* BCG (strain CX1) at 2, 6, and 10 μg/ml, a survival rate of 4% was observed with the 8-OCH_3 analog and a weak effect at 10 μg/ml was observed with the 8-H analog (reduction of 24%) (Zhao et al., 1999).

In the cell line THP-1, the bactericidal activities of PD-161148, PD-160793, and ciprofloxacin against ciprofloxacin-susceptible and -resistant *M. tuberculosis* strains were assessed.

A clear reduction in numbers of bacterial cells was observed in ciprofloxacin-susceptible strains after the 1st and 15th days with PD-161148 and PD-160793, with less than 1% survival with the 8-OCH_3 analog at 2 μg/ml and with the 8-H analog at 4 μg/ml. For ciprofloxacin at day 5 at 8 μg/ml, 1.3% survival was obtained.

The strong difference was with strains with mutations at position 94, with dependency on the substitution alanine to glycine, histidine, or tyrosine. For the first type of mutant, with the 8-OCH_3 analog survival rates of 1.3 and 0.2% were obtained at day 5 for concentrations of 4 and 8 μg/ml; with the 8-H analog at 8 μg/ml, a survival rate of 20% was obtained.

For the His94 mutant, at 8 μg/ml 0.5 and 17% survival rates were obtained with the 8-OCH_3 and 8-H analogs and 42% survival was obtained with ciprofloxacin. The Tyr94 mutant is less susceptible to fluoroquinolone action. Survival rates of 6.8, 38, and 42% were obtained with the 8-OCH_3 and 8-H analogs and ciprofloxacin, respectively.

5. ANIMAL EXPERIMENTAL TB

In experimental murine TB, ofloxacin was given at a 42-μg/g dose. A significant decrease of the bacterial burden in the liver was obtained (Tsukamura, 1985a).

After TB challenge, mice received either pefloxacin or ofloxacin by the oral route (gavage, diet). Pefloxacin at a dose up to 150 mg/kg was inactive.

In terms of survival rate, the minimal effective dose of ofloxacin against *M. tuberculosis* infection was 150 mg/kg daily, but in terms of bacterial clearance, ofloxacin at a daily dose of 150 mg/kg exhibits activity comparable to that of ethambutol (100 mg/kg daily). The therapeutic efficacy of ofloxacin against *M. tuberculosis* infection is dose dependent. At 300 mg/kg daily (300 mg every day [o.d.] or 150 mg/kg twice a day [b.i.d.]), the therapeutic efficacy improved (Truffot-Pernot et al., 1991).

In 4-week-old female Swiss mice, sparfloxacin at dosages of 50 and 100 mg/kg daily six times a week for 4 weeks exhibited activity comparable to that of isoniazid at 25 mg/kg daily and superior to that of ofloxacin at 300 mg/kg daily. The efficacy of sparfloxacin was also dose dependent, with a minimal effective dosage of 12.5 mg/kg daily (Ji et al., 1991; Lalande et al., 1993).

WIN 57273 at 100 mg/kg daily was totally inactive against murine TB (Ji et al., 1991).

In a murine TB model with daily treatment six times a week for 4 weeks, in terms of CFU counts in the spleen, the ranking of anti-TB activities of the tested treatments ran in the following order: levofloxacin (300 mg/kg) = sparfloxacin (100 mg/kg) > isoniazid (25 mg/kg) > sparfloxacin (50 mg/kg) > ofloxacin (300 mg/kg) = levofloxacin (150 mg/kg) > ofloxacin (150 mg/kg) = levofloxacin (50 mg/kg) (Ji et al., 1995).

Four-week-old female outbred CD-1 mice were challenged intravenously with approximately 10^7 viable *M. tuberculosis* cells. Treatment started day 1 postinfection and was administered daily for 28 days, 5 days per week.

Levofloxacin at all doses (at 100, 200, and 400 mg/kg) reduced the organism cell counts in the spleen and lungs in comparison with control. A dose-related reduction in organ cell counts was noted with levofloxacin treatment (Klemens et al., 1994).

In a murine model of TB infection induced intravenously with 10^6CFU of *M. tuberculosis* H37$_{RV}$, the combination of ciprofloxacin and isoniazid was synergistic, and no pulmonary lesions and no *M. tuberculosis* colonies were isolated (Andriole, 1989). It was also shown that the combination of ciprofloxacin and rifampin sterilized the lungs and the spleen in infected mice faster than the combination of isoniazid and rifampin (Chadwick et al., 1989) (Table 21).

Four-week-old female Swiss mice were challenged intravenously with a suspension of 6.2×10^6CFU of *M. tuberculosis* H37$_{RV}$. One day after bacterial challenge, mice were treated orally by esophageal gavage for 4 weeks, receiving a daily dose 6 days per week. At daily doses of 25, 50, and 100 mg/kg, clinafloxacin failed to exhibit anti-TB activity in vivo. Moxifloxacin and sparfloxacin were bactericidal, but this effect was dose dependent. Furthermore, moxifloxacin at an equivalent regimen showed a higher bactericidal activity than sparfloxacin. Moxifloxacin at 100 mg/kg/day exhibited bactericidal activity comparable to that of isoniazid at 25 mg/kg/day (Ji et al., 1998).

The high efficacy of moxifloxacin was also demonstrated in another study (Miyazaki et al., 1999).

Outbred female Swiss Webster mice (5 weeks old, 18 to 20 g) were infected intravenously with a suspension of 5.9×10^5CFU of highly virulent *M. tuberculosis* strain CSU 93, which is more virulent than strain Erdman. Treatments were administered either 1 day or 1 week after bacterial challenge every day, 6 days per week, for 4 or 8 weeks. The MIC for

Table 21 In vivo activity of ciprofloxacin in a murine model of TB[a]

Compound(s)	Dose (mg/kg/day)	Organ[b]	Duration of therapy (wks)	Log_{10} CFU of viable *M. tuberculosis* organisms			
				End of therapy	1 mo	2 mo	3 mo
Rifampin	40	L	9	0.6		1.2	0.6
		S	9	NG		0.8	0.2
		L	12	0.4	0.2	0.4	
		S	12	NG	NG	NG	
		L	16	0.2	0.8	0.9	0.9
		S	16	NG	0.2	NG	NG
Isoniazid	25	L	16	1.4	0.4	0.8	0.4
		S	16	1.1	0.7	0.3	1.1
Ciprofloxacin	300	L	16	1.9	2.4	1.2	2.4
		S	16	2.1	1.0	0.8	1.1
Ciprofloxacin + rifampin		L	16	NG	NG	NG	NG
		S	16	NG	NG	NG	NG
Rifampin + isoniazid		L	9	0.7	0.5	1.3	0.8
		S	9	0.3	0.3	0.3	0.9
		L	12	0.5	0.2	0.2	NG
		S	12	NG	NG	NG	NG
		L	16	NG	0.3	NG	NG
		S	16	NG	NG	NG	NG
Control		L	9	3.7	3.6		2.9
		S	9	3.2	1.6		1.7
		L	12	3.7	2.4	3.5	3.4
		S	12	3.2	2.0	2.5	1.6
		L	16	3.3	3.0	3.5	3.6
		S	16	2.5	1.5	2.5	3.0

[a]Data from Chadwick et al., 1989. NG, no growth.
[b]L, lung; S, spleen.

Table 22 In vitro activity of moxifloxacin in murine TB[a]

Time	Treatment	Daily dose (mg/kg)	Log_{10} CFU of *M. tuberculosis*	
			Lung	Spleen
4 wks	Control		5.64 ± 0.12	4.88 ± 0.18
	Isoniazid	25	0.38 ± 0.19	1.23 ± 0.18
	Moxifloxacin	100	0.63 ± 0.22	0.51 ± 0.24
	Moxifloxacin + isoniazid	100 + 25	0.17 ± 0.11	0.66 ± 0.20
8 wks	Control		6.45 ± 0.48	4.57 ± 0.31
	Isoniazid	25	0.10 ± 0.25	0.49 ± 0.47
	Moxifloxacin	100	0 ± 0	0 ± 0
	Moxifloxacin + isoniazid	100 + 25	0 ± 0	0 ± 0

[a]Data from Miyazaki et al., 1999.

M. tuberculosis CSU 93, determined by a radiometric method, was 0.25 μg/ml.

Moxifloxacin given to mice at 100 mg/kg/day significantly reduced the bacillary population in the lungs and the spleen (Table 22).

Furthermore, at week 4, the combination of isoniazid and moxifloxacin exerted a synergistic activity. At week 8, with moxifloxacin, no bacteria were detected.

Moxifloxacin at 20 mg/kg daily allowed a 100% survival rate, in comparison with a 50% survival rate in control mice after challenge with a large inoculum of the virulent strain CSU 98 (1.0×10^7 CFU/mouse) (Miyazaki et al., 1999).

It has been shown in murine infection (outbred Swiss mice, 4 to 5 weeks old) induced by *M. tuberculosis* $H37_{RV}$ that among the fluoroquinolones (sparfloxacin, ofloxacin, and levofloxacin) and aminoglycosides (streptomycin, kanamycin, amikacin, and isepamicin), sparfloxacin at 50 mg/kg and amikacin at 200 mg/kg are the most active compounds after isoniazid (25 mg/kg) in treating TB in mice (Lounis et al., 1997).

6. STRUCTURE-ACTIVITY RELATIONSHIPS

The most active compounds against mycobacteria are the 4-fluorophenyl and 2′,4′-difluorophenyl analogs. They are also the best antibacterials of this series. None of them were more active than ciprofloxacin and sparfloxacin.

Increasing the lipophilicity by modifying the phenyl moiety did not increase the antimycobacterial activity. For example, the substitution of a methyl group between the two fluoro atoms on the phenyl group resulted in reduced activity (MIC, >16 μg/ml). Compounds having a 2′,4′-dimethyl phenyl or a 2′,4′-dichlorophenyl moiety are weakly active or inactive.

These data suggest that the lipophilicity of fluoroquinolone analogs at N-1, specifically of N-1 phenyl-substituted derivatives, is less important than the intrinsic activity against common pathogens.

Renau et al. (1996b) showed that the antimycobacterial activity imparted by the N-1 substituent was in the order *tert*-butyl ≥ cyclopropyl > 2,4-difluorophenyl > ethyl ≈ cyclobutyl > isopropyl, and substitution with either piperazinyl or pyrrolidinyl heterocycles at C-7 afforded similar activity against mycobacteria.

A series of compounds with various substitutions at C-8 has been prepared (Renau et al., 1996a). It has been shown that the contribution of the C-8 substituent is correlated with the substituent at N-1. If the N-1 substituent is a cyclopropyl, the optimal C-8 substituents are in the order methoxy > bromide, chlorine, nonsubstituted = fluorine = ethoxy > nitrogen > methyltrifluorine.

If N-1 is a 2′,4′-trifluorophenyl, the order of activity is nitrogen = nonsubstituted > fluorine, methoxy at N-1 if *tert*-butyl, N ≥ CH, and N > CH if N-1 = ethyl.

In general, analogs with a 7-piperazinyl are slightly less active against mycobacteria than those with a 7-pyrrolidinyl (Renau et al., 1996b) (Fig. 1).

The most active compound is PD-161144-like gatifloxacin, which was reported to show good antimycobacterial activity. It has an 8-methoxy group. However, in this series, the most active compound against M. *tuberculosis* is PD-161148.

It has to be noted that the in vitro activity against M. *fortuitum* does not always reflect the anti-TB activity, as was shown with PD-135661, which has a MIC of ≤0.03 μg/ml for M. *fortuitum* and a MIC of 12.5 μg/ml for M. *tuberculosis*.

Against M. *tuberculosis*, the fluoroquinolones do not exert the same activity for inhibiting the growth of resistant mutants (Xu et al., 1996). It was shown that compounds with a methoxy group attached to the C-8 position are more active against mutants than their 8-H counterparts (Dong et al., 1998; Zhao et al., 1999).

A series of Mannich bases of norfloxacin were synthetized by substituting the N4[1] hydrogen of the 7-piperazinyl moiety with various isatin derivatives (Fig. 2). Eleven compounds were prepared with various substituents, such as chlorine, bromine, or hydrogen, in R_1 and various alkyl or alkylaryl side chains in R_2. All of them exhibited anti-TB activity (M. *tuberculosis* $H37_{RV}$) for a MIC range of <6.25 to <12.5 μg/ml (Pandeya et al., 2001).

A new parameter was recently defined: the mutant prevention concentration (MPC), which is the minimal quinolone concentration that allows the mutant recovery when more than 10^{10} cells are applied to drug-containing agar (Dong et al., 1999). It was proposed that if a concentration in tissue for a given quinolone is above the MPC, selection of resistant mutants should be severely restricted. Eighteen fluoroquinolone analogs having four different substituents at C-8 (unsubstituted [8-H] or 8-OCH_3, 8-F, 8-Cl, or 8-Br) and various substituents at N-4′, C-3′, and C-2′ of the 7-piperazinyl ring have been tested. It was shown that the most active compounds against M. *smegmatis* possess an 8-OCH_3 group. It was

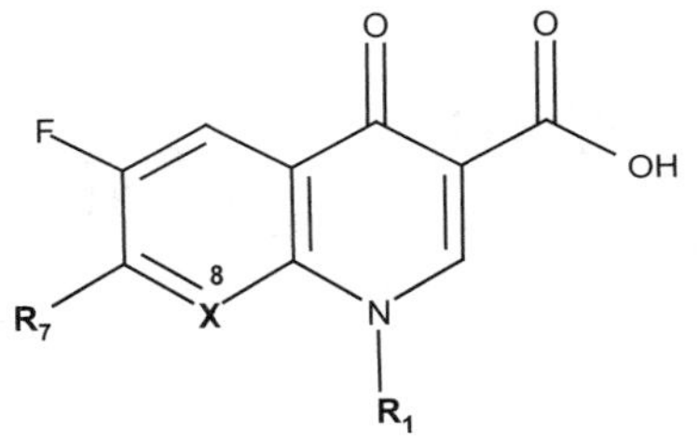

	R_1		X	R_7	*M. fortuitum*	*M. tuberculosis*
PD-163,753	Cyclopropyl	c:C_3H_5	CBr	3′ methyl-piperazinyl	≤0.03	0.78
PD-161,144		c:C_3H_5	$COOCH_3$	4′etyl	≤0.03	0.39
PD-163,048	t-butyl	$(CH_3)_3C$	N	3′ methyl-piperazinyl	0.03	0.78
PD-163,049		$(H_3)_3C$	N	3′5 dimethyl-piperazinyl	0.03	0.78
PD-161,148	Cyclopropyl		OCH_3	3′ ethyl-piperazinyl	0.03	0.10
Ciprofloxacin					0.06	0.25
Sparfloxacin					0.06	0.06

Figure 1 Structure-activity relationship of fluoroquinolones versus TB (Renau et al., 1996a, 1996b)

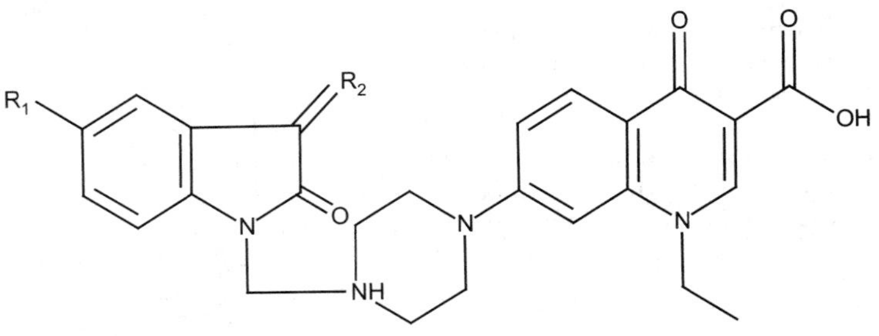

Figure 2 Isatin derivatives of norfloxacin

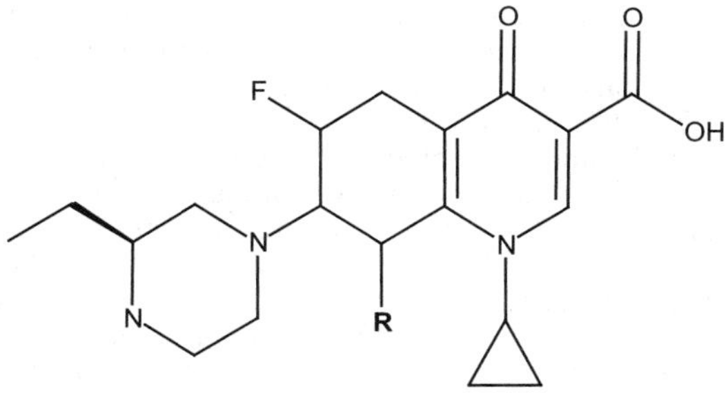

PD 161148 R = OCH_3
PD 160793 R = H

Figure 3 PD-161148 and PD-160793

shown that the MPC correlates well with the MIC for the most resistant, first-step *gyrA* mutant (Fig. 3).

Also, the MPC and MIC measurements show that there is an interaction between C-8 and C-7 substituents.

The most effective compound in preventing mutants possesses a C-3′ ethyl or monomethyl substituent on the 7-piperazinyl ring (PD-161148 or PD-135432) (Sindelar et al., 2000).

In previous studies, it was shown that adding an OCH_3 group at position C-8 of the quinoline ring enhances the bactericidal activity against *E. coli*, *S. aureus*, and *M. bovis* BCG (Dong et al., 1998), including mutant isolates moderately resistant and of the *gyrA* type or *parC* (*S. aureus*).

The comparative activities of two fluoroquinolones, PD-161148 (8-OCH_3) and PD-160793 (8-H counterpart), against *M. tuberculosis* isolates susceptible and resistant to fluoroquinolones were investigated.

PD-161148 was more bactericidal than its 8-OH counterpart and ciprofloxacin against *M. tuberculosis* TN 1626 (*gyrA*$^+$). The concentrations needed to kill 90% of the cells were 0.38, 0.80, and 1.3 μg/ml for PD-161148, PD-160793, and ciprofloxacin, respectively.

The *M. tuberculosis* TN 1625 strain, resistant to ciprofloxacin due to a substitution at position 90 of GyrA of valine for alanine, is more susceptible to the 8-OCH_3 analog (90% lethal doses were 1.5, 9.0, and 11.0 μg/ml for PD-161148, PD-160793, and ciprofloxacin, respectively).

Three other mutant isolates, which had a substitution of glycine, histidine, or tyrosine for aspartic acid at position 94 of GyrA, were killed effectively by the 8-OCH_3 analog; however, higher concentrations were needed (90% lethal doses were 3.2, 5.6, and 10 μg/ml, respectively) (Zhao et al., 1999).

N-4′ substitution of the 7-piperazinyl ring either with a methyl, an ethyl, or an isopropyl group significantly enhances the in vitro activity of ciprofloxacin. These compounds were two to four times more active than ciprofloxacin, with MIC_{50}s of 0.125, 0.125, and 0.5 μg/ml for the *N*-methyl, *N*-ethyl, and *N*-isopropyl analogs of ciprofloxacin and ciprofloxacin, respectively. N-phenylated or N-benzylated analogs were less active than ciprofloxacin (Haemers et al., 1990) (Fig. 4).

7. NEW QUINOLONES WITH ANTIMYCOBACTERIAL ACTIVITY

7.1. Nitroquinolones

A series of pyridone-β-carboxylicacid analogs has been synthesized having alkylamino substituents at C-7 and a 6-nitro group at position 6 of the quinoline nucleus. The N-1 substituents were either a cyclopropyl or a *t*-butyl.

Only one compound of this series exhibited an anti-TB activity comparable to those of ciprofloxacin and ofloxacin, with a MIC_{50} and MIC_{90} of 1.5 and 6.0 μg/ml. This compound bears at N-1 a *t*-butyl and at position C-7 an amino-*ter*-butyl (Fig. 5) (Artico et al., 1999).

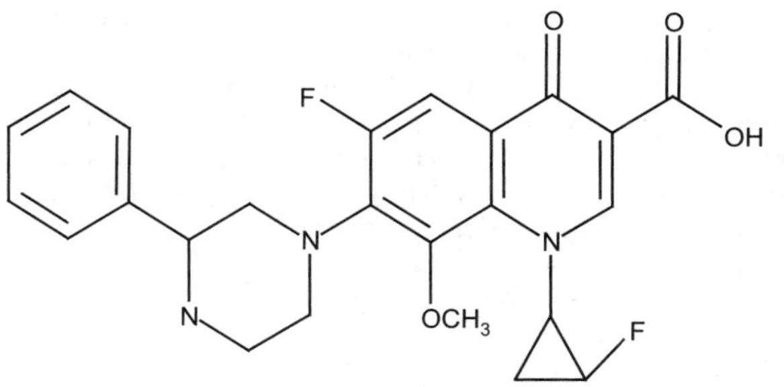

Figure 4 Antimycobacterial fluoroquinolone

7.2. Piperazinyl Substituted Quinolones

A 6-fluoroquinolone derivative having an 8-OCH_3 group, an N-1 fluorocyclopropyl substituent, and a 3′-phenyl ring substituent on the 7-piperazinyl ring directed against *M. tuberculosis* has been recently reported. The MICs of this compound range from 0.1 to 12.5 μg/ml for a panel of eight rifampin-resistant *M. tuberculosis* isolates. In all cases, it was claimed to be more active than ofloxacin (Takemura et al., 2001).

8. CLINICAL STUDIES

No clinical trials have been carried out, but anecdotal investigations have been published on single-drug therapy or on combinations with standard anti-TB drugs. Ofloxacin and ciprofloxacin have been investigated the most frequently. Few trials have been reported with levofloxacin.

However, it should be pointed out that it would not be appropriate to substitute a fluoroquinolone for any of the first-line drugs in the treatment of drug-susceptible TB.

8.1. Clinical Experiences

Favorable clinical outcomes with ofloxacin, ciprofloxacin, and levofloxacin have been seen in the treatment of pulmonary and extrapulmonary TB, as single agents or as companion drugs in susceptible or multidrug-resistant TB.

8.1.1. Disseminated TB

Miliary TB is one of the most severe clinical forms of TB, and early diagnosis and prompt therapy are essential for a favorable clinical outcome.

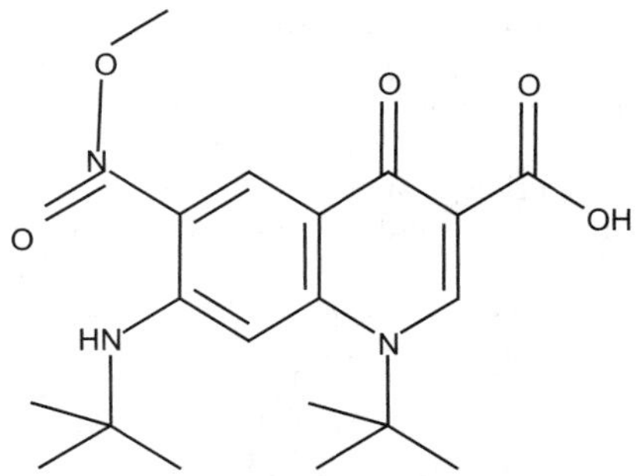

Figure 5 6-Nitro fluoroquinolone

A 27-year-old man suffering from severe miliary TB was treated successfully with a combination of ofloxacin (200 mg every 8 h) and cycloserine (250 mg every 6 h) by the oral route for 9 months. Rifampin, isoniazid, ethambutol, and streptomycin were given as first-line treatment but were discontinued due to severe adverse effects: hepatic, ocular, and vestibular toxicities (Alegre et al., 1990).

In another case, a 70-year-old male suffering from disseminated TB received after 2.5 months of isoniazid and rifampin (600 mg for 8 months) a combination of rifabutin (300 mg for 12 months) and ciprofloxacin (500 to 750 mg daily for 18 months). No relapse was reported after a follow-up of 19 months (Kahana and Spino, 1991).

8.1.2. Pulmonary TB

8.1.2.1. Ofloxacin

A total of 118 patients with intractable pulmonary TB were treated with a daily doses of 300 to 600 mg of ofloxacin for over 3 months. Within 5 months, 19.5% of the patients showed negative sputum cultures and remained culture negative for at least 6 months. However, the development of a significant resistance against ofloxacin was a serious drawback (Nakae et al., 1991). In another clinical trial, 22 patients with multidrug-resistant pulmonary TB were treated for 8 to 12 months with ofloxacin (300 or 800 mg once daily) together with second-line anti-TB agents (Yew et al., 1990).

Fifty patients with multidrug-resistant TB were given ofloxacin-containing treatment in Indonesia (Mangunnegoro and Hudoyo, 1999), a country in which the prevalence of TB is extremely high (8 per 10^3 inhabitants), representing the second leading cause of death after cardiovascular disease. Multidrug-resistant TB involving two major drugs occurred in 6.16%, involving three drugs occurred in 5.82%, and involving up to five drugs occurred in 0.16%. In total, multidrug resistance occurred in 14.24% of all patients. Ofloxacin was given at 400 mg once a day for 9 months as a companion drug of pyrazinamide (1,000 to 1,500 mg according to the patient weight) and ethambutol (750 mg daily); kanamycin or streptomycin was given selectively at a dose of 750 mg twice a week for 6 months. The follow-up after treatment completion lasted 12 to 15 months. Bacterial conversion occurred after 3 months of therapy in 46% of patients (23 of 50), in 72% at 6 months (36 of 50), and in 78% at 9 months (39 of 50). The MIC of ofloxacin ranged from 0.5 to 2 μg/ml in Ogawa medium. Those patients with isolates for which the MICs of ofloxacin were ≥2 μg/ml failed to achieve bacterial conversion. Relapses were observed at 3, 6, and 12 months in 11% of patients (4 of 36). In all relapsed patients, *M. tuberculosis* was less susceptible than at entrance to ofloxacin (MIC, ≥2.0 μg/ml).

No clinical trials have evaluated the optimal treatment of multidrug-resistant TB, and no rules regarding the regimen and duration of treatment have been recommended. However, in a retrospective study, it was shown that of immunocompetent patients with secondary multidrug-resistant TB, only 56% responded to ofloxacin-containing regimens (Yew et al., 1990). But in the same study, it was shown that clinical and bacteriological responses occurred in 50 and 80% of patients in the 300- and 800-mg/day groups, respectively.

Of 31 patients with multidrug-resistant TB, a sputum conversion occurred in 81% of those treated with an ofloxacin-containing regimen (Willcox et al., 1993). In another study, of 63 patients with multidrug-resistant TB, 51 patients were cured (81%), 9 patients showed treatment failure (14.3%), and 3 patients died (4.7%) when on ofloxacin- or levofloxacin-containing regimens (600 to 800 mg daily).

For the entire group, the mean duration of therapy was 14 months, and the mean number of companion drugs was 4.7. The mean times for sputum smear and culture conversions were 1.7 and 2.1 months, respectively (Yew et al., 2000).

For 124 patients treated with isoniazid and rifampin, ofloxacin (600 mg/day) or ethambutol was added in order to compare the two regimens. Culture conversion rates at 3 months were 98 and 94% with ofloxacin- and ethambutol-containing regimens, respectively. The MIC_{50}s for ofloxacin and ethambutol were 0.39 and 1.56 μg/ml, respectively. No relapse was recorded in either group after 24 months of treatment ended (Kohno et al., 1992).

8.1.2.2. Ciprofloxacin

Numerous studies have been published in which ciprofloxacin was a component of the anti-TB chemotherapy (Kahana and Spino, 1991; Kennedy et al., 1993a, 1993b; Mohanty and Dhamgaye, 1993; Sirgel et al., 1997).

Ciprofloxacin at 750 mg daily has been administered in combination with isoniazid, streptomycin and pyrazinamide, and rifampin in various studies.

In those studies, initial bacteriological responses occurred rapidly; however, in ciprofloxacin-containing regimens the time to response was longer, and it seems that relapses are more common than with non-ciprofloxacin-containing regimens (Mohanty and Dhamgaye, 1993; Kennedy et al., 1996).

The early bactericidal activity of ciprofloxacin at 250, 500, 1,000, and 1,500 mg in patients with pulmonary TB was assessed in the first 2 days of treatment by counting the viable tubercle bacilli in the sputum. In 80 patients, it was clearly shown that ciprofloxacin exhibited a bactericidal activity against TB which was dose dependent (Sirgel et al., 1997). Ciprofloxacin at 1,500 mg daily seems the most adequate dose in this study. However, the early bactericidal activity of ciprofloxacin was lower than that with 600 mg of rifampin and much lower than that with 300 mg of isoniazid. Another study showed an early bactericidal activity of ciprofloxacin in Tanzanian patients (Kennedy et al., 1993a). However, caution needs to be taken when analyzing these data. As pointed out by Mitchinson (1995), the methodology is extremely important. It was suggested that the rapid fall of CFU counts in sputum during the first 2 days of drug administration was due to killing of actively growing *M. tuberculosis* (Jindani et al., 1980).

Exposure to 2% NaOH for half an hour reduced the mean count of *M. tuberculosis* by 1.70 $\log_{10}$ CFU/ml when actively growing but by only 0.75 $\log_{10}$ CFU/ml when stationary. False results could be obtained for sputum specimens decontaminated with NaOH.

That results obtained with a suboptimal dose of ciprofloxacin could be disappointing was suggested by a study comparing two regimens of ciprofloxacin, 1,000 mg once daily and 500 mg every 12 h. The clinical and bacteriological outcome in the first group was superior to that in the second group. Conversion of smear and culture to negativity took longer in the group receiving 500 mg b.i.d. than in that receiving 1,000 mg o.d. (Table 23).

The tolerance of ciprofloxacin was comparable in both groups (Bergstermann et al., 1997).

8.1.2.3. Levofloxacin

Levofloxacin for treatment of pulmonary TB was given at a daily dose of 750 to 1,000 mg (Peloquin et al., 1998).

Ten patients with multidrug-resistant TB were treated with levofloxacin at a dose of 600 to 800 mg once daily. However, 7 of the 10 had bacilli susceptible to ofloxacin, and

Table 23 Bacteriological efficacy of ciprofloxacin in pulmonary TB[a]

Result	No. of days to result obtained, with indicated regimen:		P
	1,000 mg o.d.	500 mg b.i.d.	
Smear positive	84 ± 68.3	94 ± 55.9	0.19
Culture positive	60 ± 61	76 ± 60.5	0.04

[a]Data from Bergstermann and Rüchardt, 1997.

all had successful cure with the levofloxacin-containing regimen. Of the three remaining patients, two had isolates susceptible to levofloxacin (Yew et al., 2000).

A 25-year-old HIV-negative patient with multidrug-resistant pulmonary TB (isoniazid- and rifampin-resistant isolate) was treated with pyrazinamide (1,250 mg daily), isoniazid (900 mg b.i.d.), and ethambutol (1,200 mg daily) to which capreomycin and cycloserine were added. Though pulmonary function improved, the patient suffered from meningitis. Pyrazinamide, ethambutol, and cycloserine and prednisone were orally administered in combination with amikacin and levofloxacin by the intrathecal route every other day, alternating with 750 mg of levofloxacin intravenously and 1,200 mg of amikacin intravenously. Intrathecal (0.5 to 1.5 mg) administration was based on the expectation of reaching concentrations of 8 to 10 μg/ml and 40 μg/ml for levofloxacin and amikacin, respectively, given an assumed cerebrospinal fluid (CSF) volume of 120 ml. However, local tolerance was good, but the CSF levofloxacin level after 2 h reached only 1.64 μg/ml.

Marked improvement was obtained in 8 days, with CSF-negative culture, and no increase in the CSF levofloxacin level was needed (Berning et al., 2001).

8.1.2.4. Sparfloxacin

The potential role of sparfloxacin in the treatment of multidrug-resistant TB has been highlighted previously (Grosset, 1992).

The clinical experience with sparfloxacin against pulmonary TB is limited. Four studies have investigated the clinical efficacy of sparfloxacin in this area.

Used for compassionate treatment in Europe, sparfloxacin was given orally at 400 mg daily for at least 4 weeks followed by a 200-mg daily dose until sputum cultures became negative. However, some patients received 300 or 400 mg once daily for the length of the therapy course. Thirty patients received a sparfloxacin-containing regimen. The mean duration of treatment with sparfloxacin was 42.2 weeks (10 to 102 weeks). Sparfloxacin was the companion drug for mainly second-line anti-TB drugs such as kanamycin, capreomycin, amikacin, cycloserine, PAS, protionamide, and clofazimine. These drugs were combined with either pyrazinamide or ethambutol. An overall favorable clinical/bacteriological response was obtained for 19 of 30 patients (63%), and conversion of sputum was obtained for 66% (20 of 30 patients) at week 12 (Aventis Pharma, data on file).

An investigation of the clinical efficacy of sparfloxacin was carried out with 14 patients with advanced TB and who had already been treated with conventional anti-TB drugs. Sparfloxacin was given at a daily dose of 200 mg in combination with other anti-TB drugs. The short-term follow-up showed good clinical and radiological improvement and sputum conversion (Kamat, 1998).

In multidrug-resistant TB, sputum conversion was obtained after 3 months of sparfloxacin at 400 mg and in combination with four other anti-TB drugs (Dautzenberg et al., 1994).

In the fourth investigational study, conversion of sputum smears was observed after 20 weeks of administration of sparfloxacin used in combination with other anti-TB drugs in 5 of 10 patients in with multidrug-resistant TB (Schaberg et al., 1995).

Between April 1993 and April 1999, 30 patients with pulmonary TB ($n = 28$) and/or with lymph node TB ($n = 2$) were treated with a combination of sparfloxacin and at least two other anti-TB drugs. Sixteen patients were infected by one or more multidrug-resistant *M. tuberculosis* strains. The duration of sparfloxacin therapy during hospitalization ranged from 2.5 to 4 months. The daily doses ranged from 100 to 400 mg. Twenty-five patients completed therapy and were cured.

Although sparfloxacin was apparently well tolerated, five mild phototoxicity reactions and six prolongations of QT intervals (30 to 40 ms, compared to baseline of ≤450 ms) were registered by electrocardiogram without clinical symptoms (Lubasch et al., 2001)

8.1.2.5. Lomefloxacin

A total of 132 patients suffering from pulmonary TB were treated with a lomefloxacin-containing regimen at an oral daily dose of 400 mg b.i.d. They received isoniazid (5 to 6 mg/kg/day b.i.d.), pyrazinamide (30 mg/kg every other day), streptomycin (15 mg/kg o.d. intramuscularly), or ethambutol (30 mg/kg every other day per os).

The reason to combine lomefloxacin was adverse effects with other anti-TB drugs, such as hepatitis, and multidrug resistance to standard anti-TB drugs. The MICs of lomefloxacin for *M. tuberculosis* were not reported. Conversion of the sputum to negativity occurred between 1 to 3 months after the start of therapy.

The role of lomefloxacin in the anti-TB regimen was unclear. In one study, two patients suffered from phototoxicity (Mariandyshev et al., 1997; Sokolova et al., 1998; Sokolova et al., 2000; Mozhokina et al., 1998).

8.1.3. Retreatment of TB with Fluoroquinolones

Acquired resistance to isoniazid or rifampin and multidrug resistance have been reported to increase in some parts of the world.

Fluoroquinolones could be an alternative as a second-line therapy.

Fourteen patients with pulmonary TB, having serious adverse effects from standard therapy or in vitro resistance to two or more of the conventional drugs, received pefloxacin (400 mg), isoniazid (300 mg), and thiacetazone (150 mg), all in a single daily dose. The mean time taken for sputum conversion was 3 months in one patient who also received pyrazinamide, and the longest time taken was 6 months. Ten patients who completed the full duration showed good response in the form of persistently negative sputum, adequate clinical improvement, and radiological clearing (Rao, 1995).

A 25-year-old male noncompliant patient had pulmonary TB for 4 years. The last treatment he received was a combination of isoniazid (300 mg), cycloserine (500 mg), ethionamide (500 mg), and ethambutol (1,000 mg) for the last 20 months. At admission, the isolate of *M. tuberculosis* was resistant to isoniazid, streptomycin, ethambutol, rifampin, and thiacetazone. The regimen comprised amikacin (750 mg intranasally once daily), ofloxacin (600 mg o.d.), clofazimine (1,000 mg o.d.), and INAPAS (a combination of PAS [5 g] and isoniazid

[150 mg b.i.d.]). Within 1 month after initiation of the treatment, the patient was asymptomatic (Shah et al., 1993).

In a 3-year-old female suffering from multidrug-resistant pulmonary TB, a combination of three anti-TB drugs, pyrazinamide, ethionamide, and cycloserine, was given and pefloxacin (1,200 mg daily) was added for 9 months; pyrazinamide and cycloserine were stopped due to adverse effects after 2 months (Fur et al., 1987).

In a study whose aim was to investigate if rifabutin has a potential role in the retreatment of patients with chronic pulmonary TB for which standard retreatment has failed, it was shown that rifabutin does not have a useful role in this kind of patient. All patients in whom this treatment failed received an ofloxacin-containing regimen (800 mg o.d.). Seventeen patients were retreated with ofloxacin, and 5 patients received ofloxacin alone, as there were no remaining companion drugs available. In 14 patients, the M. *tuberculosis* isolate was considered susceptible to ofloxacin. Only one patient out of five responded to ofloxacin alone. In 7 of 10 patients, only a temporary response was obtained; for the 3 remaining patients smear conversion was obtained and remained negative for 12, 18, and 18 months (Girling et al., 1992). Such results have been reported by other authors (Sahoo, 1993).

8.1.4. Extrapulmonary TB

Anecdotal reports on various locations of TB treated with ofloxacin, ciprofloxacin, or pefloxacin have been published.

Ofloxacin was efficient in intracranial TB in a 38-year-old alcoholic patient (Caparros-Lefebvre et al., 1989), in combination with rifampin and ethambutol and 2 months of streptomycin. This is an infrequent pathology in western countries but has a high incidence rate in the Middle East (Jenkins et al., 1987) and the Far East (De Angelis, 1981).

One patient with peritoneal TB was treated with pefloxacin (800 mg daily) intravenously before M. *tuberculosis* was isolated by culture. The patient became apyretic after 8 days of therapy (Wesenfelder and Eugene, 1993).

Patients were treated with either pefloxacin, ciprofloxacin, or ofloxacin for TB osteoarthritis (Gagnerie et al., 1988; Hussey et al., 1992). Improvement of osteoarthritis was achieved, but after a variable period of time a relapse occurred.

The efficacy of ofloxacin in the treatment of urogenital TB was assessed and compared to that of other anti-TB drugs. At 200 mg every 12 h for 6 months, the therapeutic efficacy of ofloxacin was comparable to those of rifampin (600 mg every 24 h for 3 months) and isoniazid (300 mg every 24 h for 3 months).

9. ROLE OF FLUOROQUINOLONES IN TB

9.1. Preventive Therapy

A recent outbreak of multidrug-resistant TB in the United States prompted the Centers for Disease Control and Prevention (CDC) to implement recommendations for its prevention, as isoniazid and rifampin are ineffective against multidrug-resistant TB.

The CDC proposed a two-drug preventive regimen of pyrazinamide and a fluoroquinolone, such as ciprofloxacin (Stevens and Daniel, 1995) or ofloxacin, for 6 to 12 months in people recently exposed to and infected with multidrug-resistant M. *tuberculosis* isolates (American Thoracic Society, 1994). Combination of pyrazinamide with ofloxacin or ciprofloxacin was proposed. However, single drugs are well tolerated, although in combination ofloxacin and pyrazinamide gave rise to a higher rate of manifestations of intolerance such as nausea, rash, and asymptomatic hepatitis (Ridzon et al., 1997; Horn et al., 1994).

9.2. Role of Fluoroquinolones

Important points regarding the use of fluoroquinolones in TB can be highlighted from the literature (Berning, 2001):

- Ofloxacin, levofloxacin, and ciprofloxacin were effective as first-line therapy in TB.
- Isoniazid and rifampin are more active than the above-mentioned fluoroquinolones in first-line therapy.
- These drugs could be used in combination with two or more standard anti-TB agents to avoid rapid selection of fluoroquinolone-resistant mutants.
- The clinical response to fluoroquinolones appears to be dose related.
- As with other anti-TB agents, fluoroquinolones need to be administered for a long period. The tolerance could be a problem for some of them.
- Fluoroquinolones are second-line agents for TB (O'Brien, 1993).
- Fluoroquinolones could be an alternative therapy for TB when major side effects occur with standard anti-TB drugs, such as hepatitis (isoniazid), ocular toxicity (ethambutol), and vestibular toxicity (streptomycin).
- For ciprofloxacin (Yew et al., 1995) and ofloxacin (Yew et al., 1992; Bagnato et al., 1995), it has been shown that both drugs could be given in patients who develop significant drug-induced hepatitis (rifampin, isoniazid, and pyrazinamide) during administration of short-term therapy, which usually occurs within the first 2 months, and both drugs could be companion drugs in an "interim regimen" for treating extensive pulmonary TB during this period pending liver function recovery.

Incorporation of fluoroquinolones in second-line regimens for the management of multidrug-resistant TB has been recommended by many health authorities, including the World Health Organization (Crofton et al., 1997; Chaulet et al., 1996). However, clinical failures were reported even for a ciprofloxacin-susceptible strain.

Initial resistance to isoniazid and streptomycin has little effect on the sterilizing effect of rifampin or pyrazinamide (Mitcheson and Nunn, 1986). In contrast, initial resistance to rifampin carries a much poorer prognosis.

Randomized, controlled clinical trials on multidrug-resistant TB are difficult to conduct and have additional ethical constraints (Bhatti et al., 1990).

9.3. Choice of a Fluoroquinolone

Fluoroquinolones are not recommended in pediatric patients, even for those treated with ciprofloxacin without any noticeable adverse effects (Hussey et al., 1992), because of the potential damage to cartilage reported to occur in developing animals (Linseman et al., 1995). When fluoroquinolones have been used on a compassionate basis in children and adolescents (634 clinical cases), reversible arthropathy occurred in 1.3% of these patients (Kapila et al., 1990). Fluoroquinolones are not recommended during pregnancy. In multidrug-resistant TB during pregnancy, ofloxacin or ciprofloxacin could be a second-line therapy (Bothamley, 2001). A review of the cases of 200 pregnant women exposed to ciprofloxacin during the first trimester failed to record any musculoskeletal abnormalities, although those treated with ciprofloxacin had a higher rate of abortion (Loebstein et al., 1998). However, this information relates to short-term therapy, 5 to 7 days, at a low daily dose (250 mg b.i.d.). No published experiences are available for pregnant women undergoing long-term therapy.

Combination therapy is compulsory. However, irreversible drug interaction could occur. Combination of pyrazinamide with ofloxacin appears to increase the rates of asymptomatic hepatitis and gastrointestinal disturbances. Combination of ofloxacin with D-cycloserine has been reported to cause an increase of central nervous system adverse effects, probably due to altered γ-aminobutyric acid binding (Yew et al., 1993). Metabolism of fluoroquinolones needs to be taken into account.

In reported literature, the daily doses of ofloxacin and ciprofloxacin varied. For levofloxacin, a daily dose of 750 mg was chosen instead of 500 mg in infections due to common pathogens.

Fluoroquinolones are selected as companion drugs in chemotherapy on the basis of the results of susceptibility testing and the history of previous anti-TB chemotherapy.

A simplified rhythm of administration is needed to obtain compliance of patients. Levofloxacin (750 mg/day) and sparfloxacin (200 mg/day) could be given once daily. Ofloxacin was given at 400 mg once a day and ciprofloxacin was given at 500 to 750 mg b.i.d. A once-daily dose of 800 mg of ofloxacin and a once-daily dose of 1,000 mg of ciprofloxacin could be considered, as *M. tuberculosis* replicates only once every 24 h. These regimens were given to 103 patients, with a good clinical tolerance (Berning et al., 1995), better than with other second-line anti-TB drugs such as PAS, D-cycloserine, and ethionamide. Therapeutic drug monitoring of fluoroquinolones needs to be a standard in all institutions treating TB and especially in the HIV-infected population, in which malabsorption of drugs is a risk (Berning et al., 1992, 1995).

10. FLUOROQUINOLONES AS A DIAGNOSTIC TEST

Fluoroquinolones could be also used as a laboratory test to differentiate mycobacteria at the species level (Leysen et al., 1989; Tsukamura and Mizuno, 1986). Enoxacin could be used to differentiate between *M. gordonae*, *M. scrofulaceum*, and *M. szulgai* (Tsukamura and Mizuno, 1986).

11. CONCLUSION

TB still remains a serious public health problem worldwide, one that is particularly acute in developing countries. HIV infection, poverty, homelessness, and emergence of multidrug-resistant TB have yielded a difficult situation, and alternative or new companion drugs are compulsory. Some fluoroquinolones have been demonstrated to be effective companions in standard regimens of TB therapy, but the emergence of *M. tuberculosis* isolates resistant to fluoroquinolones, all of them having a cross-resistance, has led to discontinuation of their use in monotherapy (Gillespie and Kennedy, 1998). On the basis of in vitro studies, one of the proposed combinations includes either ofloxacin (400 mg twice daily) or ciprofloxacin (750 mg/kg/day). Another alternative regimen is the combination of fluoroquinolones with pyrazinamide and ethambutol (15 to 25 mg/kg/day) (Alangaden et al., 1997). Fluoroquinolones are administered worldwide, especially in Eastern Europe, Pakistan, India, China, and Far East countries (Chen et al., 1989; Kapur et al., 1995).

REFERENCES

Ainsa JA, Blockpoel MC, Otul I, Young DB, De Smet A, Martin C, 1998, Molecular cloning and characterization of Tap, a putative multidrug efflux pump present in Mycobacterium fortuitum and Mycobacterium tuberculosis, J Bacteriol, 180, 5836–5843.

Alangaden GJ, Lerner SA, 1997, The clinical use of fluoroquinolones for the treatment of mycobacterial diseases, Clin Infect Dis, 25, 1213–1221.

Alangaden GJ, Manavathu EK, Vakulenko SB, Zvonok NM, Lerner SA, 1995, Characterization of fluoroquinolone-resistant mutant strains of Mycobacterium tuberculosis selected in the laboratory and isolated from patients, Antimicrob Agents Chemother, 39, 1700–1703.

Alegre J, Fernandez de Sevilla T, Faka V, Martinez-Vazquez JM, 1990, Ofloxacin in miliary tuberculosis, Eur Resp J, 3, 238–239.

American Thoracic Society, 1994, Treatment of tuberculosis and tuberculosis infection in adults and children, Am J Resp Crit Care, 149, 1359–1374.

Andriole VT, 1989, An update on the efficacy of ciprofloxacin in animal models of infection, Am J Med, 87, Suppl 5A, 532–534.

Artico M, Mai A, Sbardella G, Massa S, Misiu C, Lostia S, Demontis F, La Colla P, 1999, Nitroquinolones with broad spectrum antimycobacterial activity in vitro, Bioorg Med Chem Lett, 8, 1651–1656.

Bagnato GF, Di Cesare E, Gulli S, Cucinotta D, 1995, Long-term treatment of pulmonary tuberculosis with ofloxacin in a subject with liver cirrhosis, Monaldi Arch Chest Dis, 50, 279–281.

Banerjee DK, Ford J, Makanday S, 1992, In vitro activity of lomefloxacin against pathogenic and environmental mycobacteria, J Antimicrob Chemother, 30, 236–238.

Banerjee SK, Bhatt K, Rana S, Misra P, Chakraborti PK, 1996, Involvement of an efflux system in mediating high level of fluoroquinolone resistance in Mycobacterium smegmatis, Biochem Biophys Res Commun, 226, 362–368.

Bergstermann H, Rüchardt A, 1997, Ciprofloxacin once daily versus twice daily for the treatment of pulmonary tuberculosis, Infection, 25, 227–232.

Berlin OGW, Young LS, Bruckner DA, 1987, In vitro activity of six fluorinated quinolones against Mycobacterium tuberculosis, J Antimicrob Chemother, 19, 611–615.

Bermudez LE, Goodman J, 1996, Mycobacterium tuberculosis invades and replicates within type II alveolar cells, Infect Immun, 64, 1400–1406.

Berning SE, 2001, The role of fluoroquinolones in tuberculosis today, Drugs, 61, 9–18.

Berning SE, Cherry TA, Iseman MD, 2001, Novel treatment of meningitis caused by multidrug resistant Mycobacterium tuberculosis with intrathecal levofloxacin and amikacin, case report, Clin Infect Dis, 32, 643–646.

Berning SE, Huitt GA, Iseman MD, et al, 1992, Malabsorption of antituberculous medications by patients with AIDS, New Engl J Med, 327, 1817–1818.

Berning SE, Madsen L, Iseman MD, Peloquin CA, 1995, Long-term safety of ofloxacin and ciprofloxacin in the treatment of mycobacterial infection, Am J Respir Crit Care Med, 151, 2006–2009.

Bhatti N, Chronos N, White JP, Larson E, 1990, A case of resistant tuberculosis, Tubercle, 71, 141–143.

Borges-Walmsley MI, Walmsley AR, 2001, The structure and function of drug pumps, Trends in Microbiol, 9, 1–9.

Bothamley G, 2001, Drug treatment for tuberculosis during pregnancy—safety considerations, Drug Safety, 24, 553–565.

Cambau E, Sougakoff W, Bessen M, Truffot-Pernot C, Grosset J, Jarlier V, 1994a, Selection of gyr A mutant of Mycobacterium tuberculosis resistant to fluoroquinolones during treatment with ofloxacin, J Infect Dis, 170, 479–483.

Cambau E, Sougakoff W, Jarlier V, 1994b, Amplification and nucleotide sequence of the quinolone determining region in the gyr A gene of mycobacteria, FEMS Microbiol Lett, 116, 49–54.

Canetti G, The J, 1965, Burns Ambersen Lecture, present aspects of bacterial resistance in tuberculosis, Am Rev Resp Dis, 92, 687–703.

Caparros-Lefebvre D, Salomez JL, Petit H, 1989, Tuberculomes intracrâniens multiples: aspect en imagerie par résonance magnétique nucléaire et apport thérapeutique de l'ofloxacine, Ann Med Inter, 140, 699–701.

Casal M, Gutierrez J, Ruiz P, Morena G, 1995, Preliminary study of the in vitro activity of irloxacin against mycobacteria, Chemotherapy, 41, 204–207.

Chadwick M, Nicholson G, Gaya H, 1989, Brief report, combination chemotherapy with ciprofloxacin for infection with M. tuberculosis in a mouse model, Am J Med, 87, suppl 5A, 535–536.

Chaulet P, Raviglione M, Bustero F, 1996, Epidemiology, control and treatment of multidrug resistant tuberculosis, Drugs, 52, suppl 2, 103–108.

Chen C-H, Shih J-F, Lindholm-Levy PJ, Heifets LB, 1989, Minimal inhibitory concentrations of rifabutin, ciprofloxacin, and ofloxacin against Mycobacterium tuberculosis isolates before treatment of patients in Taiwan, Am Rev Respir Dis, 140, 987–989.

Cole ST, Brosch R, Parkhill J, Garnier T, Churche C, Harris D, et al, 1998, Deciphering the biology of Mycobacterium tuberculosis from the complete genome sequence, Nature, 393, 537–544.

Collins CH, Yates MD, Uttley AMC, 1985, In vitro susceptibility of mycobacteria to ciprofloxacin, Antimicrob Chemother, 16, 575–580.

Cooksey RC, Crawford JT, Jacobs WR Jr, Shinnick TM, 1993, A rapid method for activity against a strain of M. tuberculosis expessing firefly luciferase, Antimicrob Agents Chemother, 37, 1348–1352.

Crofton J, Choculet P, Maher D, et al, 1997, Guidelines for the management of drug-resistant tuberculosis WHO/TB/96-210 (rev 1), World Health Organization, Geneva.

Crowle AJ, Elkins N, May MH, 1988, Effectiveness of ofloxacin against Mycobacterium tuberculosis and Mycobacterium avium and rifampicin against M. tuberculosis in cultured human macrophages, Am Rev Resp Dis, 137, 1141–1146.

Dailloux M, Petitpain N, Henry C, Weber M, 1989, Détermination in vitro de la sensibilité des mycobactéries aux fluoroquinolones, Path Biol, 37, 346–349.

Dautzenberg B, Truffot-Pernot C, Bakdach H, 1994, Ambulatory regimen with sparfloxacin and combined old antituberculosis drugs plus synergy for treatment of multidrug resistant tuberculosis, Tubercle Lung Dis, 75, Suppl 1, 14 AB, 47.

Davies S, Sparham PD, Spencer RC, 1987, Comparative in vitro activity of five fluoroquinolones against mycobacteria, J Antimicrob Chemother, 19, 605–609.

De Angelis CM, 1981, Intracranial tuberculoma, case report and review of the literature, Neurology, 31, 1133–1136.

Dong Y, Xu C, Zhao X, Domagala J, Drlica K, 1998, Fluoroquinolone action against mycobacteria; effects of C-8 substituents on growth, survival, and resistance, Antimicrob Agents Chemother, 42, 2978–2984.

Dong Y, Xu C, Zhao X, Domagala J, Drlica K, 1999, Effect of fluoroquinolone concentration on selection of mutants of Mycobacterium bovis BCG and Staphylococcus aureus, Antimicrob Agents Chemother, 43, 1756–1758.

Drlica K, Xu C, Wang JY, Burger RM, Malik M, 1996, Fluoroquinolone action in mycobacteria, similarity with effects in Escherichia coli and the detection by cell lysate viscosity, Antimicrob Agents Chemother, 40, 1594–1599.

Esihi H, Vincent V, Cole ST, 1996, Homing events on the gyr A gene of some mycobacterials, Proc Natl Acad Sci USA, 93, 3410–3415.

Estebanez Zarranz MJ, Martinez Sagarra JM, Alberte A, Amon Sesmero J, Rodriguez Toves A, 1992, Treatment of urogenital tuberculosis with ofloxacin, preliminary study, Actas Urol Esp, 16, 64–68, in Spanish.

Fenleon CH, Cynamon MH, 1986, Comparative in vitro activities of ciprofloxacin and other 4-quinolones against Mycobacterium tuberculosis and Mycobacterium intracellulare, Antimicrob Agents Chemother, 29, 386–388.

Fung-Tomc J, Minassian B, Kolek B, Washo T, Huczko E, Bonner D, 2000, In vitro antibacterial spectrum of a new 8-methoxyfluoroquinolone, gatifloxacin, J Antimicrob Chemother, 45, 437–446.

Fur A, Massin P, Camus A, Waldner A, Jeanin L, 1987, Traitement de sauvetage d'une tuberculose pulmonaire multirésistante: efficacité de la péfloxacine, Presse Med, 3, 128.

Gagnerie F, Taillan B, Euller-Ziegler G, 1988, Efficacité transitoire de la péfloxacine au cours d'une ostéoarthrite tuberculeuse, Med Mal Infect, 18, 201–202.

Garcia-Rodriguez JA, Garcia-Gomez AC, 1993, In vitro activities of quinolones against mycobacteria, J Antimicrob Chemother, 32, 797–808.

Garcia-Rodriguez JA, Garcia-Sanchez JF, Gomez-Garcia AC, Trujillano I, Plata AM, 1988, In vitro activity of the new quinolones, with special reference to Mycobacterium, Nocardia and Rhodococcus, Rev Infect Dis, 10, suppl 1, S53–S55.

Gay JD, De Young DR, Roberts GD, 1984, In vitro activity of norfloxacin and ciprofloxacin against Mycobacterium tuberculosis, M. avium complex, M. chelonei, M. fortuitum, and M. kansasii, Antimicrob Agents Chemother, 26, 94–96.

Gaya H, Chadwick MV, 1986, In vitro activity of ciprofloxacin against mycobacteria, Eur J Clin Microbiol, 4, 345–347.

Gevaudan MJ, Mallet MN, Gulian C, Terriou P, Lagier P, de Micco P, 1998, Etude de la sensibilité de sept espèces de mycobactéries aux nouvelles quinolones, Path Biol, 36, 477–481.

Gillespie SH, Kennedy N, 1998, Fluoroquinolones, a new treatment for tuberculosis, Int J Tuberc Lung Dis, 2, 265–271.

Girling DJ, Hong Kong Chest Service/British Medical Research Council, 1992, A controlled study of a ribafutin and an uncontrolled study of ofloxacin in the retreatment of patients with pulmonary tuberculosis resistant to isoniazid, streptomycin and rifampicin, Tubercle Lung Dis, 73, 59–67.

Gorzynski EA, Gutman SI, Allen W, 1989, Comparative antimycobacterial activities of difloxacin, temafloxacin, enoxacin, pefloxacin, reference fluoroquinolones and a new macrolide, clarithromycin, Antimicrob Agents Chemother, 33, 591–592.

Grassi C, 1997, New drugs for tuberculosis, Exp Opin Investig Drugs, 6, 1211–1226.

Grosset JH, 1992, Treatment of tuberculosis in HIV infection, Tubercle Lung Dis, 73, 378–383.

Guillemin I, Jarlier V, Cambau E, 1998, Correlation between quinolone susceptibility patterns and sequences in the A and B subunits of DNA gyrase in mycobacteria, Antimicrob Agents Chemother, 42, 2084–2088.

Guillemin I, Sougakoff W, Cambau E, Viravau VR, Moreau N, Jarlier V, 1999, Purification and inhibition by quinolones of DNA gyrase from Mycobacterium avium, Mycobacterium smegmatis and Mycobacterium fortuitum bv. peregrinum, Microbiology, 145, 2527–2532.

Haemers A, Leysen DC, Bollaert W, Zhang M, Pattyn SR, 1990, Influence of N-substitution on antimycobacterial activity of ciprofloxacin, Antimicrob Agents Chemother, 34, 496–497.

Heifets LB, Lindholm-Levy PJ, 1987, Bacteriostatic and bactericidal activity of ciprofloxacin and ofloxacin against Mycobacterium tuberculosis and Mycobacterium avium complex, Tubercle, 68, 267–276.

Heifets LB, Lindholm-Levy PJ, 1990, MICs and MBCs of WIN 57273 against Mycobacterium avium and Mycobacterium tuberculosis, Antimicrob Agents Chemother, 34, 770–774.

Hoffner SE, Gezelius L, Olsson-Liljequist B, 1997, In vitro activity of fluorinated quinolones and macrolides against drug-resistant Mycobacterium tuberculosis, J Antimicrob Chemother, 40, 885–888.

Horn DL, Hewlett D, Alfalla C, et al, 1994, Limited tolerance of ofloxacin and pyrazinamide prophylaxis against tuberculosis [letter], N Engl J Med, 330, 1241.

Hussey G, Kibel M, Parker N, 1992, Ciprofloxacin treatment of multiply drug-resistant extrapulmonary tuberculosis in a child, Pediatr Infect Dis J, 11, 408–409.

Jacobs MR, 1995, Activity of quinolones against mycobacteria, Drugs, 49, suppl 2, 67–75.

Jacobs WR Jr, Barlett RG, Udani R, et al, 1993, Rapid assessment of drug susceptibility of M. tuberculosis by means of luciferase reporter phages, Science, 260, 819–822.

Jenkins JR, Al-Kawi MZ, Bashir R, 1987, Dynamic computed tomography of cerebral parenchymal tuberculomata, Neuroradiology, 29, 523–529.

Ji B, Lounis N, Maslo C, Truffot-Pernod C, Bonnafous P, Grosset J, 1998, In vitro and in vivo activities of moxifloxacin and clinafloxacin against Mycobacterium tuberculosis, Antimicrob Agents Chemother, 42, 2066–2069.

Ji B, Lounis N, Truffot-Pernot C, Grosset J, 1995, In vitro and in vivo activities of levofloxacin against Mycobacterium tuberculosis, Antimicrob Agents Chemother, 39, 1341–1344.

Ji B, Truffot-Pernot C, Grosset J, 1991, In vitro and in vivo activity of sparfloxacin (AT 4140) against Mycobacterium tuberculosis, Tubercle, 72, 181–186.

Jindani A, Aber VR, Edwards EA, Mitchinson DA, 1980, The early bactericidal activity of drugs in patients with pulmonary tuberculosis, Am Rev Resp Dis, 121, 939–949.

Kahana LM, Spino M, 1991, Ciprofloxacin in patients with mycobacterial infections, experience in 15 patients, DICP Ann Pharmacother, 25, 919–924.

Kamat SR, 1998, Early experience with sparfloxacin in tuberculosis, J Assoc Physicians India, 46, 827–828.

Kapila K, Chysky V, Accieri G, Schacht P, Echols R, 1990, Worldwide clinical experience on safety of ciprofloxacin in children on compassionate use basis, Third Intern Symp New Quinolones, Vancouver.

Kapur V, Li LL, Hamrick MR, Plikaytis BB, Shinnick TM, Telenti A, Jacobs WR Jr, Banerjee A, Cole S, Yuen KY, Clarridge JE III, Kreiswirth BN, Mussen JM, 1995, Rapid Mycobacterium species assignment and unambiguous identification of mutations associated with antibiotic resistance in Mycobacterium tuberculosis by automated DNA sequencing, Arch Pathol Lab Med, 119, 131–138.

Karak K, De PK, 1995, Comparative in vitro activity of fluoroquinolones against Mycobacterium tuberculosis, Indian J Med Res, 101, 147–149.

Kasai H, Ezaki T, Harayama S, 2000, Differentiation of phylogenetically related slowly growing mycobacteria by their gyrB sequences, J Clin Microbiol, 38, 301–308.

Kennedy N, Berger L, Curram L, et al, 1996, Randomized controlled trial of a drug regimen that includes ciprofloxacin for the treatment of tuberculosis, Clin Infect Dis, 22, 827–833.

Kennedy NR, Fox GM, Kisyombe GM, Saruni AOS, Uiso LO, Ramsay ARC, Ngowi FI, Gillespie SH, 1993a, Early bactericidal and sterilizing activities of ciprofloxacin in pulmonary tuberculosis, Am Rev Resp Dis, 148, 1547–1551.

Kennedy NR, Fox R, Uiso L, Ngowi FI, Gillespie SH, 1993b, Safety profile of ciprofloxacin during long-term therapy for pulmonary tuberculosis, J Antimicrob Chemother, 32, 897–902.

Klemens SP, Sharpe CA, Rogge MC, Cynamon M, 1994, In vitro activity of ofloxacin against Mycobacterium tuberculosis, Antimicrob Agents Chemother, 38, 1476–1479.

Kocagöz T, Hackbarth CJ, Ünsal I, Rosenberg EY, Nikaido H, Chambers HF, 1996, Gyrase mutations in laboratory-selected fluoroquinolone-resistant mutants of Mycobacterium tuberculosis H37Ra, Antimicrob Agents Chemother, 40, 1768–1774.

Kohno SH, Koga H, Kaku M, Maesaki S, Hara K, 1992, Prospective comparative study of ofloxacin or ethambutol for the treatment of pulmonary tuberculosis, Chest, 102, 1815–1818.

Kolek B, Huczko E, Aleksunes L, Minassian B, Valera L, Stickle T, Bonner D, Fung-Tomc J, 2000, The in vitro activity of the novel des-fluoro (6) quinolone BMS-284,756 against anaerobes, Mycoplasma, Ureaplasma, Chlamydia and Mycobacterium spp., 40th Intersci Conf Antimicrob Agents Chemother.

La Bombardi VJ, Cataldo-Caputzal L, 1993, Ciprofloxacin susceptibility testing by MIC and disk elution of drug-resistant Mycobacterium tuberculosis and Mycobacterium avium complex, Antimicrob Agents Chemother, 37, 1556–1557.

Lalande V, Truffot-Pernot C, Paccaly-Moulin A, Grosset J, Ji B, 1993, Powerful bactericidal activity of sparfloxacin (AT-4140) against Mycobacterium tuberculosis in mice, Antimicrob Agents Chemother, 37, 407–411.

Leysen DC, Haemers A, Pattyn SR, 1989, Mycobacteria and the new quinolones, Antimicrob Agents Chemother, 33, 1–5.

Linseman DA, Hampton LA, Branstetter DG, 1995, Quinolone-induced arthropathy in the neonatal mouse: morphological analysis of articular lesions produced by pipemidic acid and ciprofloxacin, Appl Toxicol, 28, 59–64.

Liu J, Takiff HE, Nikaido H, 1996, Active efflux of fluoroquinolones in Mycobacterium smegmatis mediated by LfrA, a multidrug efflux pump, J Bacteriol, 178, 3791–3795.

Loebstein R, Addis A, Ho E, et al, 1998, Pregnancy outcome following gestational exposure to fluoroquinolones, a multicenter, prospective, controlled study, Antimicrob Agents Chemother, 42, 1336–1339.

Lounis N, Ji B, Truffot-Pernot C, Grosset J, 1997, Which aminoglycoside or fluoroquinolone is more active against Mycobacterium tuberculosis in mice? Antimicrob Agents Chemother, 41, 607–610.

Lubasch A, Erbes R, Mauch H, Lode H, 2001, Sparfloxacin in the treatment of drug resistant tuberculosis or intolerance of first line therapy, Eur Resp J, 17, 641–646.

Madhusudan K, Ramesh V, Nagaraja V, 1994, Molecular cloning of gyr A and gyr B genes of Mycobacterium tuberculosis, analysis of nucleotide sequence, Biochem Mol Biol Intern, 33, 651–660.

Mangunnegoro H, Hudoyo A, 1999, Efficacy of low-dose ofloxacin in the treatment of multidrug-resistant tuberculosis in Indonesia, Chemotherapy, 45, Suppl 2, 19–35.

Mariandyshev AO, Klinberg NM, Shobina AI, Moroz MI, 1997, Use of Maxaquin® in the treatment of progressive pulmonary tuberculosis occurring with standard chemotherapy regimens, Probl Tuberk, 4, 19–21.

McDonough KA, Kress Y, 1995, Cytotoxicity for lung epithelial cells is a virulence-associated phenotype of Mycobacterium tuberculosis, Infect Immun, 63, 4802–4811.

Mitchison DA, 1995, Early bactericidal activity and sterilizing activity of ciprofloxacin in pulmonary tuberculosis, Am J Resp Crit Care Med, 151, 921–922.

Mitchison DA, Nunn AJ, 1986, Influence of initial drug resistance on the response to short-course chemotherapy of pulmonary tuberculosis, Am Rev Resp Dis, 133, 423–429.

Miyazaki E, Miyazaki M, Chen JM, Chaisson RE, Bishai WR, 1999, Moxifloxacin (BAY 12-8039), a new 8-methoxy quinolone, is active in a mouse model of tuberculosis, Antimicrob Agents Chemother, 43, 85–89.

Mohanty KC, Dhamgaye TM, 1993, Controlled trial of ciprofloxacin short-term chemotherapy for pulmonary tuberculosis, Chest, 104, 1194–1198.

Mor N, Vanderkork J, Heiflets L, 1994, Inhibitory and bactericidal activities of levofloxacin against Mycobacterium tuberculosis in vitro and in human macrophages, Antimicrob Agents Chemother, 38, 1161–1164.

Mozhokina GN, Kunichan AD, Levchenko TN, Smirnova NS, 1998, Mechanism of action of lomefloxacin on Mycobacterium tuberculosis, Antibiot Khimiother, 43, 13–16.

Nakae I, Nakatoni K, Inoue S, et al, 1991, Therapeutic effects of ofloxacin on intractable pulmonary tuberculosis and ofloxacin resistance of tubercle bacilli isolated from the patients, Chest Disease Cooperative Study Unit of National Sanatorium in Kinki District, Kekkaku, 66, 299–307.

Niemann S, Harmsen D, Ruesch-Gerdes S, Richter E, 2000, Differentiation of clinical Mycobacterium tuberculosis complex isolates by gyr B DNA sequence polymorphism analysis, J Clin Microbiol, 38, 3231–3234.

O'Brien RJ, 1993, Ciprofloxacin is not a component of first-line TB, Chest, 104, 1312.

Ogasawara K, Sato K, Tamioka H, 2000, Comparative in vitro antimicrobial activity of the newly synthesized quinolones WQ-3034 and HSR-903 and other quinolones against Mycobacterium tuberculosis and Mycobacterium avium complex, Jpn J Chemother, 48, 892–897.

Onodera Y, Tanaka M, Sato K, 2001, Inhibitory activity of quinolones against DNA gyrase of Mycobacterium tuberculosis, J Antimicrob Chemother, 47, 447–450.

Pandeya SN, Sriram D, Yogeeswari P, Ananthan S, 2001, Antituberculous activity of norfloxacin Mannich bases with isatin derivatives, Chemotherapy, 47, 266–269.

Pattyn SR, Van Caekenberghe DL, Verhoeven JR, 1987, In vitro activity of five quinolones against cultivable mycobacteria, Eur J Clin Microbiol, 6, 572–573.

Peloquin CA, Beaning SE, Huitt GW, Heman MD, 1998, Levofloxacin for drug resistant Mycobacterium tuberculosis, Ann Pharmacother, 32, 268–269.

Piersimoni G, Morbiducci V, Bornigia S, De Sio G, Scalise G, 1992, In vitro activity of the new quinolone lomefloxacin against Mycobacterium tuberculosis, Am Rev Respir Dis, 146, 1445–1447.

Rao S, 1995, An uncontrolled trial of pefloxacin in the retreatment of patients with pulmonary tuberculosis, Tubercle Lung Dis, 76, 219–222.

Rastogi N, Blom-Potar MC, 1990, Intracellular bactericidal activity of ciprofloxacin and ofloxacin against Mycobacterium tuberculosis H37Ra multiplying in the J-774 macrophage cell line, Zentralbl Bakteriol, 273, 195–199.

Rastogi N, Goh KS, 1991, In vitro activity of the new difluorinated quinolone sparfloxacin (AT-4140) against Mycobacterium tuberculosis compared with activities of ofloxacin and ciprofloxacin, Antimicrob Agents Chemother, 35, 1933–1936.

Rastogi N, Goh KS, Bryskier A, Devallois A, 1996, In vitro activities of levofloxacin used alone and in combination with first and second line antituberculous drugs against Mycobacterium tuberculosis, Antimicrob Agents Chemother, 40, 1610–1616.

Rastogi N, Potar MC, David HL, 1987, Intracellular growth of pathogenic mycobacteria in the continuous murine macrophage cell line J-774, ultrastructure and drug susceptibility studies, Current Microbiol, 16, 79–92.

Rastogi N, Ross BC, Dwyer B, Goh KS, Clavel-Sérès S, Jeantils V, Gruaud P, 1992, Emergence during unsuccessful chemotherapy of multiple drug resistance in a strain of Mycobacterium tuberculosis, Eur J Clin Microbiol Infect Dis, 11, 901–907.

Renau TE, Gage JW, Dever JA, Roland GE, Joannides ET, Shapiro MA, Sanchez JP, Grachek SJ, Domagala JM, Jacobs MR, Reynolds RC, 1996a, Structure-activity relationships of quinolone agents against mycobacteria, effect of structural modifications at the 8 position, Antimicrob Agents Chemother, 40, 2363–2368.

Renau TE, Sanchez JP, Gage JW, Dever JA, Shapiro MA, Grachek SJ, Domagala JM, 1996b, Structure-activity relationships of the quinolone antibacterials against mycobacteria, effect of structural changes at N-1 and C-7, J Med Chem, 39, 729–735.

Renau TE, Sanchez JP, Shapiro MA, Dever JA, Grachek SJ, Domagala JM, 1995, Effect of lipophilicity at N-1 on activity of fluoroquinolones against mycobacteria, J Med Chem, 38, 2974–2977.

Ridzon R, Meador J, Maxwell R, et al, 1997, Asymptomatic hepatitis in persons who received alternative preventive therapy with pyrazinamide and ofloxacin, Clin Infect Dis, 24, 1264–1265.

Rodriguez JC, Ruiz M, Climent A, Royo G, 2001, In vitro activity of four fluoroquinolones against Mycobacterium tuberculosis, Inter J Antimicrob Agents, 17, 229–231.

Ruiz-Serrano MJ, Alcala L, Martinez L, Diaz M, Marin M, Gonzalez-Abad MJ, Bouza E, 2000, In vitro activities of six fluoroquinolones against 250 clinical isolates of Mycobacterium tuberculosis susceptible or resistant to first-line antituberculosis drugs, Antimicrob Agents Chemother, 44, 2567–2568.

Sahoo RC, 1993, Ofloxacin in the retreatment of patients with pulmonary tuberculosis resistance to isoniazid, streptomycin and rifampicin, a South Indian experience, Tubercle Lung Dis, 74, 140–141.

Saito H, Sato K, Tomioka H, Dekio S, 1994, In vitro and in vivo antimycobacterial activities of a new quinolone, DU-6859a, Antimicrob Agents Chemother, 38, 2877–2882.

Saito H, Tomioka H, Sato K, 1994, In vitro antimycobacterial activity of the new quinolone OPC-17116, Chemotherapy, 42, 1–5.

Salfinger M, Hohl P, Kafader FM, 1988, Comparative in vitro activity of fleroxacin and other 6-fluoroquinolones against mycobacteria, J Antimicrob Chemother, 22, suppl D, 55–63.

Sander P, Alcaide F, Richter I, Frischkosn K, Tortoli E, Springer B, Telenti A, Boettger EC, 1998, Inteins in mycobacterial gyr A are a taxonomic character, Microbiology, 144, 589–591.

Sato K, Tomioka H, 1999, Antimicrobial activities of benzoxazino rifampicin (KRM-1648) and clarithromycin against Mycobacterium avium intracellulare complex residing in murine peritoneal macrophages, human macrophage-like cells and human alveolar epithelial cells, J Antimicrob Chemother, 43, 351–357.

Sato K, Tomioka H, Akaki T, Kawahara S, 2000, Antimicrobial activities of levofloxacin, clarithromycin and KRM-1648 against Mycobacterium tuberculosis and Mycobacterium avium complex replicating within mono Mac 6 human macrophage and A-549 type II alveolar cell line, Inter J Antimicrob Agents, 16, 25–29.

Schaberg T, Specht S, Stephan H, Lode H, 1995, Use of sparfloxacin for the treatment of multidrug resistant pulmonary tuberculosis, Tubercle Lung Dis, 76, suppl 2, 091-PA 11, 86.

Shah A, Bhagat R, Panchal N, 1993, Resistant tuberculosis, successful treatment with amikacin, ofloxacin, clofazimine and PAS, Tubercle Lung Dis, 74, 64–67.

Sindelar G, Zhao X, Liew A, Dong Y, Lu T, Zhou J, Domagala J, Drlica K, 2000, Mutant prevention concentration as a measure of fluoroquinolone potency against mycobacteria, Antimicrob Agents Chemother, 44, 3337–3343.

Sirgel FA, Botha FJ, Parkin DP, Van den Wal BW, Schall R, Donald PR, Mitchison DA, 1997, The early bactericidal activity of ciprofloxacin in patients with pulmonary tuberculosis, Am J Respir Crit Care Med, 156, 901–905.

Sirgel FA, Venter A, Heilmann HD, 1995, Comparative in vitro activity of BAY y 3118, a new quinolone, and ciprofloxacin against Mycobacterium tuberculosis and Mycobacterium avium complex, J Antimicrob Chemother, 35, 349–351.

Sokolova GB, Kunichan AD, Koriakin YA, Lazareva IV, 1998, Lomefloxacin in complex treatment of acute progressive form of pulmonary tuberculosis, Antibiot Khimiother, 43, 10–12.

Sokolova GB, Mozhokina GN, Kunichan AD, Elistratova NA, Perelman ML, 2000, Maxaquin® in the combined treatment of tuberculosis, Probl Tuberk, 5, 35–39.

Stevens JP, Daniel TM, 1995, Chemoprophylaxis of multidrug-resistant tuberculosis infections in HIV-uninfected individual using ciprofloxacin and pyrazinamide, a decision analysis, Chest, 108, 712–717.

Sullivan EA, Kreiswirth BN, Palumbo L, Kapur V, Musser JH, Ebrahimazedeh A, Frieden TR, 1995, Emergence of fluoroquinolone resistant tuberculosis in New York City, Lancet, 345, 1148–1150.

Takahata M, Mitsuyama J, Yamashino Y, Yonezawa M, Araki H, Todo Y, Minami S, Watanabe Y, Naritu H, 1999, In vitro and in vivo activities of T-3811 ME, a novel des-F(6) quinolone, Antimicrob Agents Chemother, 43, 1077–1084.

Takemura M, Takahashi H, Kawakami K, Namba K, Tanaka M, Miyanchi R, 2001, Novel anti-acid-fast bacterial agents containing pyridonecarboxylic acids, WO-00158876-2001.

Takiff HE, Cimino M, Musso MC, Weisbrod T, Martinez R, Delgado MB, Salazar L, Bloom BR, Jabcos WR Jr, 1996, Efflux pump of the proton antiporter family confers low-level fluoroquinolone resistance in Mycobacterium smegmatis, Proc Natl Acad Sci USA, 93, 362–366.

Takiff HE, Salazar H, Guerrero C, Philipp W, Huang WM, Kreiswirth B, Cole ST, Jacobs WR, Telenti A, 1994, Cloning and nucleotide sequence of M. tuberculosis gyrA and gyrB genes and detection of quinolone resistance mutations, Antimicrob Agents Chemother, 38, 773–780.

Texier-Maugein J, Mormede M, Fourche J, Bébéar C, 1987, In vitro activity of fluoroquinolones against eighty-six isolates of mycobacteria, Eur J Clin Microbiol, 6, 584–586.

Tomioka H, Saito H, Sato K, 1993a, Comparative antimycobacterial activity of the newly synthesized quinolone AM-1155, sparfloxacin, and ofloxacin, Antimicrob Agents Chemother, 37, 1259–1263.

Tomioka H, Sato K, Akaki T, Kajitani H, Kawahara S, Sakatani M, 1999, Comparative in vitro antimicrobial activities of the newly synthesized quinolones HSR-903, sitafloxacin (DU 6859a), gatifloxacin (AM-1155) and levofloxacin against Mycobacterium tuberculosis and Mycobacterium avium complex, Antimicrob Agents Chemother, 43, 3001–3004.

Tomioka H, Sato K, Kajitani H, Akaki T, Shishido S, 2000, Comparative antibacterial activities of the newly synthesized quinolone WQ-3034, levofloxacin, sparfloxacin, and ciprofloxacin against Mycobacterium tuberculosis and Mycobacterium avium complex, Antimicrob Agents Chemother, 44, 283–286.

Tomioka H, Sato K, Saito H, 1991, Comparative in vitro and in vivo activity of fleroxacin and ofloxacin against various mycobacteria, Tubercle, 72, 181–186.

Tomioka H, Sato K, Saito H, 1993b, In vitro antimycobacterial activity of a new quinolone, NM 934, Kekkaku, 68, 517–520.

Tomioka H, Sato K, Saito K, Ikeda Y, 1992, Antimycobacterial activity of a newly synthesized fluoroquinolone, Y 26,611, Kekkaku, 67, 515–520.

Trimble KA, Clark RB, Sanders WE Jr, Frankel JW, Cacciatore R, Valdez H, 1987, Activity of ciprofloxacin against Mycobacterium in vitro, comparison of BACTEC and macrobroth dilution methods, J Antimicrob Chemother, 19, 617–622.

Truffot-Pernot C, Ji B, Grosset J, 1991, Activities of pefloxacin and ofloxacin against mycobacteria, in vitro and mouse experiments, Tubercle, 72, 57–64.

Tsukamura M, 1985a, Antituberculosis activity of ofloxacin (DL-8280) on experimental tuberculosis in mice, Am Rev Respir Dis, 132, 915.

Tsukamura M, 1985b, In vitro antituberculosis activity of a new antibacterial substance, ofloxacin (DL 8280), Am Rev Respir Dis, 131, 348–351.

Tsukamura M, 1986, Differentiation of Mycobacterium gordonae from Mycobacterium scrofulaceum and Mycobacterium szulgai by susceptibility to enoxacin (antimycobacterial activity of enoxacin), Microbiol Immunol, 30, 931–933.

Tsukamura M, Mizuno S, 1986, Differentiation between mycobacterial species by the susceptibility test to ciprofloxacin: comparison of antimycobacterial spectrum between ofloxacin and ciprofloxacin, Kekkaku, 61, 357–359.

Tsukamura M, Nakamura E, Yoshii S, Yanase M, Yasuda Y, Amano H, 1985, Therapeutic effect of a new antibacterial substance ofloxacin (DL 8280) on pulmonary tuberculosis, Am Rev Respir Dis, 131, 352–356.

Uttley AHC, Collins CH, 1988, In vitro activity of ciprofloxacin in combination with standard antituberculous drugs against Mycobacterium tuberculosis, Tubercle, 69, 193–195.

Vacher S, Pellegrin JL, Leblanc F, Fourche J, Mangeiro J, 1999, Comparative antimycobacterial activity of ofloxacin, ciprofloxacin and grepafloxacin, J Antimicrob Chemother, 44, 647–652.

Van Caekenberghe D, 1990, Comparative in vitro activities of ten fluoroquinolones and fusidic acid against Mycobacterium spp., J Antimicrob Chemother, 26, 381–386.

Van Rensburg CEJ, Joone GK, Anderson R, 1995, An in vitro investigation of the bioactivities of a ciprofloxacin and the new fluoroquinolone agent clinafloxacin (CI-960) and PD 131,628 against Mycobacterium tuberculosis in human macrophages, Chemotherapy, 41, 234–238.

Wanger A, Mills K, 1994, Etest for susceptibility testing of Mycobacterium tuberculosis and Mycobacterium avium-intracellulare, Diagn Microbiol Infect Dis, 19, 179–181.

Wesenfelder L, Eugene C, 1993, Tuberculose péritonéale décapitée par les fluoroquinolones chez un malade atteint de cirrhose, Gastroenterol Clin Biol, 17, 765.

Willcox PA, Groenwald PJ, Mackenzie CR, 1993, Ofloxacin-based chemotherapy in multiply drug-resistant pulmonary tuberculosis, Drugs, 45, Suppl 3, 223–224.

Wise R, Ashby JP, Andews JM, 1988, In vitro activity of PD 127,391, an enhanced-spectrum quinolone, Antimicrob Agents Chemother, 32, 1251–1256.

Woodcock JH, Andrews JM, Boswell FJ, Brenwald NP, Wise R, 1997, In vitro activity of BAY 12-8039, a new fluoroquinolone, Antimicrob Agents Chemother, 41, 101–106.

Xu C, Kreiswith BN, Sreevatsan S, Musser JM, Drlica K, 1996, Fluoroquinolone resistance associated with specific gyrase mutations in clinical isolates of multi-drug resistant Mycobacterium tuberculosis, J Infect Dis, 174, 1127–1130.

Yamane N, Chilima BZ, Okuzawa Y, Tanno K, 1996, Determination of antimycobacterial activities of fluoroquinolones against clinical isolates of Mycobacterium tuberculosis, comparative determination with egg-based Ogawa and agar-based Middlebrook 7H10 media, Kekkaku, 71, 453–458.

Yew WW, Chan CH, Wong PC, Lee J, Wong CF, Cheung SW, Chan SY, Cheng AFB, 1995, Ciprofloxacin in the management of pulmonary tuberculosis in the face of hepatic dysfunction, Drugs Exptl Clin Res, 21, 79–83.

Yew WW, Chan CK, Chan CH, Tam CM, Leung CC, Wong PC, Lee J, 2000, Outcomes of patients with multidrug-resistant pulmonary tuberculosis treated with ofloxacin/levofloxacin-containing regimens, Chest, 117, 744–751.

Yew WW, Kwan SY, Ma WK, Khin MA, Chan PY, 1990, In vitro activity of ofloxacin against Mycobacterium tuberculosis and its clinical efficacy in multiply resistant pulmonary tuberculosis, J Antimicrob Chemother, 26, 227–236.

Yew WW, Lee J, Wong PC, Kwan SYL, 1992, Tolerance of ofloxacin in the treatment of pulmonary tuberculosis in presence of hepatic dysfunction, Int J Clin Pharmacol Res, 12, 173–178.

Yew WW, Piddock LVJ, Li MSK, Lyon D, Chan CY, Cheng AFB, 1994, In vitro activity of quinolones and macrolides against mycobacteria, J Antimicrob Chemother, 34, 343–351.

Yew WW, Wong CF, Wong PC, et al, 1993, Adverse neurological reactions in patients with multidrug-resistant pulmonary tuberculosis after co-administration of cycloserine and ofloxacin, Clin Infect Dis, 17, 288–289.

Young L, Berlin OGW, Inderlied CB, 1987, Activity of ciprofloxacin and other fluorinated quinolones against mycobacteria, Am J Med, 82, suppl 4A, 23–26.

Zhao BY, Pine R, Domagala J, Drlica K, 1999, Fluoroquinolone action against clinical isolates of Mycobacterium tuberculosis, effects of a C-8 methoxy group on survival in liquid media in human macrophages, Antimicrob Agents Chemother, 43, 661–666.

Antituberculosis Compounds under Investigation

A. BRYSKIER

45

1. INTRODUCTION

New antituberculosis (anti-TB) drugs are needed due to the emerging and spreading resistance of *Mycobacterium tuberculosis* to standard treatment such as isoniazid (INH), rifampin, pyrazinamide, ethambutol, or streptomycin.

The AIDS pandemic stimulated research into and development of novel anti-TB agents; such agents have also been used to treat the opportunistic infections associated with AIDS such as *Mycobacterium avium* complex (MAC) infections, pneumocystosis, toxoplasmosis, cryptosporidiosis, and fungal infections.

Several paths are followed in search of this grail:

- Chemical modifications of existing anti-TB agents
- Investigations of existing compounds for potential anti-TB activity (oxazolidinones, fluoroquinolones, macrolides/ketolides, 5-nitroimidazoles, etc.)
- Screening for natural products with anti-TB activity
- New targets with novel chemical entities
- New pharmaceutical formulations to improve absorption or to provide a new mode of administration (e.g., aerosol).

The World Health Organization predicted a morbidity rate of TB reaching five million patients per annum in the early 21st century.

To combat this threat, implementation of existing programs, such as Directly Observed Therapy Short Course (DOTS), was proposed or encouraged.

Since the discovery of streptomycin in 1943 and a few years later of *p*-aminosalicylic acid (PAS), thiosemicarbazone, and INH, many anti-TB drugs have been discovered and developed. After the mid-1960s with the release of rifampin, only few chemical entities were clinically developed, such as fluoroquinolones and, to a lesser extent, oxazolidinones for the treatment of TB.

The current anti-TB regimen is rather long and complex. Furthermore, in immunosuppressed patients it is not satisfactory.

2. "IDEAL" PROFILE FOR NEW ANTI-TB AGENTS

New anti-TB drugs need to fulfill several requirements, such as the following:

- Activity against susceptible and multidrug-resistant (MDR) mycobacteria
- Enhancement of in vitro and in vivo activities of existing compounds
- Intracellular penetration and activity (macrophages)
- Activity against dormant cells (such as with pyrazinamide)
- Good tolerance for long-term treatment
- Synergistic activity in combination with other anti-TB agents
- Good tissue distribution (lungs, spleen, cerebrospinal fluid, etc.)
- Easy to produce in an industrial scale-up
- Stable in difficult conditions of storage (temperature, humidity, etc.)
- Easy to handle (e.g., tablets) and administer
- Cheap, to be affordable by countries under development

3. EARLY INVESTIGATIONS FOR NEW POTENTIAL ANTI-TB AGENTS

The preselection of potential anti-TB compounds needs to meet the following requirements:

- Testing of the new entity against a reference strain ($H37_{RV}$) fully susceptible to standard anti-TB agents
- Activities against isolates resistant to one or more agents
- MICs must always be determined by the same methodology (e.g., BACTEC 460) and at various pHs
- Cytotoxicity against Vero cells
- Intramacrophagic activity (murine macrophages)
- In vivo efficacy in a murine model of TB, with determination of the burden in the lungs, spleen, and liver.
- Comparison with compounds of the same class and other classes, mainly INH, rifampin, ethambutol, pyrazinamide, and streptomycin
- Bactericidal activities (comparative)

All of the above are needed in addition to the toxicological profile to initiate phase I and further development (Anonymous, 2001).

4. ALTERATIONS OF EXISTING COMPOUNDS

4.1. INH Derivatives

INH is still a primary anti-TB agent; however, its use is jeopardized by the emergence of INH-resistant TB as well as MDR TB.

Since the discovery of the antitubercular activity of INH in the 1950s, a continuous effort has been made to enhance the INH activity not only against *M. tuberculosis* but also against nontuberculosis mycobacteria (McMillon et al., 1952).

Analogs maintain the INH pharmacophore, and it was expected that appending various moieties would enhance the lipophilicity in order to increase the intrabacterial uptake of a given derivative.

4.1.1. Isonicotinoyl Isosteres

It was assumed that precursors of isosteres of isonicotinic and pyrazinoic acids could possess antimycobacterial activities (see item 4.2 below).

A new series of isonicotinoyl hydrazone derivatives aggregated in a metallo complex (copper or nickel) were synthesized and investigated by the BACTEC 400 method for in vitro activity against *M. tuberculosis* $H37_{RV}$ (Fig. 1). All tested hydrazone (compound A) and metal (B and C) complexes produced 99 to 100% growth inhibition at a screening concentration of 12.5 μg/ml. Six compounds, B1, B2, B3, C1, C2, and C3, were very active, with MICs of ≤0.2 μg/ml, while other derivatives from classes B and C had MIC from 0.39 to 12.5 μg/ml (Bottari et al., 2000).

4.1.2. Halogenated INH Analogs

Series of new INH analogs have been synthesized such as acetophenone-isonicotinylhydrazones and a 4-aryl-1-methoxy-1-(4-pyridyl)-2,3-diaza-1,3-butadiene. They were considered inactive against *M. tuberculosis*. However, some halogenated derivatives display weak activity against *M. avium* (Vigorita et al., 1992, 1994).

4.1.3. Cyanoborane Derivatives

The class of 2-substituted-4-thiazolidones issued from acidomycin or actithiazic acid thiazolidinone isolated in 1952 from *Streptomyces virginiae* were found to be selectively and highly active against TB (Brown, 1961).

Cyanoborane derivatives were obtained by appending this moiety to the N-2′ or 2′-aryl/alkyl isonicotinohydrazide (Fig. 2 to 4).

A series of analogs were synthesized starting from the cyanoborane compound by fixing various substituents at R and R′.

The MICs of compounds A, B, and E for *M. tuberculosis* $H37_{RV}$ were 0.2 μg/ml, very similar to that of rifampin (Maccari et al., 2002).

The presence of a cyanoborane moiety is detrimental for activity (Table 1).

Fluoro and trifluoromethyl (compounds B and C) substitutions on the benzene ring appeared to be the most beneficial for activity in vitro.

Higher MICs were obtained when the trifluoromethyl group was linked to an iminic carbon (compound 1P) or a 2′-methyl group (compounds 2P and 3P).

Cyanoborane analogs are more toxic to Vero cells than compounds 1 and 2. Compounds of the 2 family are the least toxic but are more toxic than INH.

Some of the analogs exert intracellular bactericidal activity against *M. tuberculosis*. Only a few of them are active against rifampin-resistant isolates, but all derivatives seem to be devoid of any activity against *M. tuberculosis* isolates resistant to INH, ethionamide, thiacetazone, aminoglycosides, and ciprofloxacin. They remain active against ethambutol-resistant isolates (MICs, 0.78 to 6.25 μg/ml). (Ottana et al., 1998).

4.1.4. Fullerene Derivatives

It was demonstrated that a 260-μg/ml concentration of water-soluble fulleropyrrolidine inhibits the growth of

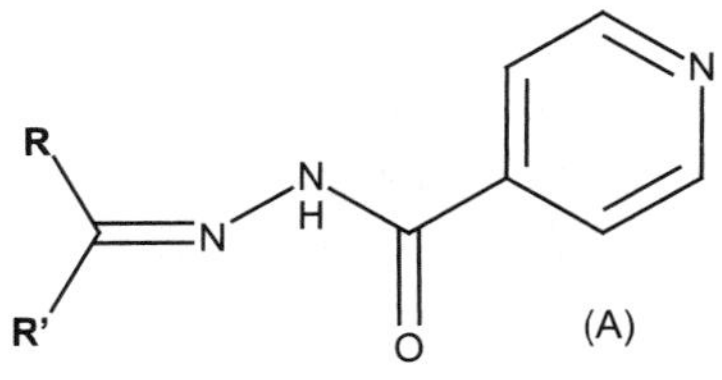

(A)

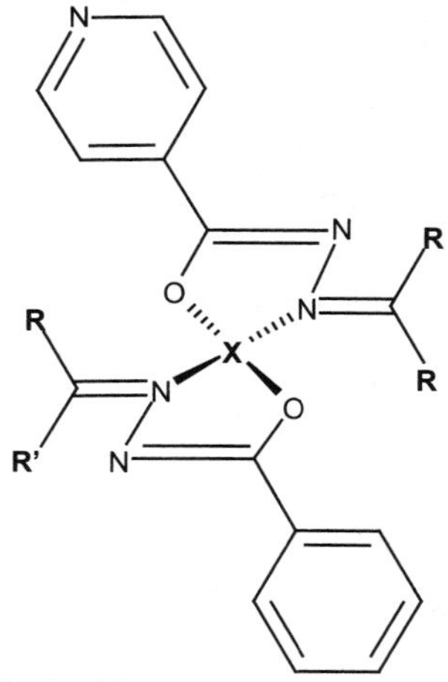

X = Cu (B)
X = NI (C)

Compound B	R	R'
1	H	2F-Ph
2	H	3F-Ph
3	H	3F,4CH_3O-Ph

Compound C	R	R'
1	H	3F_3-Ph
2	H	3CF_3-Ph
3	H	CF_3

Figure 1 New INH analogs

Isoniazid

Isonicotinoylhydrazone (ISNES) (1)

2'-alkylaryl isonicotinol hydrazides (2)

Cyanoborane derivatives (3)

Figure 2 Cyanoborane derivatives

Figure 3 Dicyanoborane analogs

M. *avium*, but it did not show any activity against M. *tuberculosis* H37$_{RV}$ or H6/99.

New series have been prepared, and two compounds, compounds B and C, exhibit good activity against M. *tuberculosis* H37$_{RV}$ and H6/99, with MICs of 5 μg/ml (Bosi et al., 2000).

4.1.5. Isonicotinoyl Hydrazones

A new series of amino hydrazone analogs structurally related to INH was described. Pyridylmethylenamino derivatives with various substituents on the phenyl ring were synthesized (Fig. 5) and investigated for their anti-M. *tuberculosis* activity. All of them were cross-resistant with INH, and within the tested compounds there are no analogs with activity comparable to that of INH (MIC, 0.06 μg/ml, versus >6.25 μg/ml for analogs).

In combination, isonicotinoyl hydrazones at subinhibitory concentrations induced significant increases in the activities of rifampin, ethambutol, and PAS with clofazimine against M. *tuberculosis* H37$_{RV}$, whereas no effects were observed (De Logu et al., 2002) in combination with clofazimine.

4.1.6. 4-Aminobenzoic Acid Hydrazones

In a series of 4-aminobenzoic acid hydrazones, one compound showed good anti-M. *tuberculosis* activity, with a MIC of 3.13 μg/ml for M. *tuberculosis* H37$_{RV}$, using BACTEC 12 B medium for the BACTEC 460 radiometric system. However, this compound is also very cytotoxic.

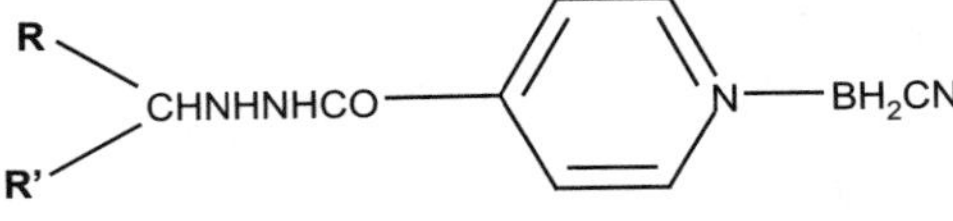

	R	R'
A	H	C_6H_5
B	H	$2F-C_6H_4$
C	H	$3F-C_6H_4$
D	H	$4F-C_6H_4$
E	H	$3,CF_3-C_6H_4$
F	H	$3,4Cl_2-C_6H_3$
G	H	$3,4(OCH_3)_2-C_6H_3$
H	CH_3	C_6H_5
I	CH_3	$2F-C_6H_4$
J	CH_3	$3F-C_6H_4$
K	CH_3	$4F-C_6H_4$
L	CH_3	$3,CF_3-C_6H_4$
M	CH_3	$3,4Cl_2-C_6H_3$
N	CH_3	$3,4Cl_2-C_6H_3$
O	CH_3	$3,4(OCH_3)_2-C_6H_3$
P	H	CF_3

Figure 4 Anti-TB INH cyanoborane derivatives

4.2. Pyrazinamide Derivatives

Pyrazinamide is an important component of short-course chemotherapy against TB because of its activity against semidormant bacilli sequestered within macrophages (Heifets and Lindholm-Levy, 1992). To be active, pyrazinamide needs to be converted to pyrazinoic acid by pyrazinamidase, which is encoded by the gene *pncA* (Scorpio and Zhang, 1996); mutation on *pncA* can render pyrazinamide inactive (Morlock et al., 2000).

Table 1 Cyanoborane derivatives of INH: in vitro activity against *M. tuberculosis* H37$_{RV}$

Compound	MIC (μg/ml)		
	ISNES[a]	2-Aryl/alkyl isonicotinohydrazides	3-Cyanoboranes
A	0.05–	0.2	0.8
B		0.2	3.13
C	0.05	0.39	0.8
D		0.39	
E	0.1	0.2	0.8
F		1.6	
G			0.39
H	0.1	6.25	12.5
I	0.2		
J	<0.05	1.6	
K	0.05	1.6	
L	0.1	1.6	
M	0.1	3.13	
N		1.6	>6.25
O		12.5	
P	0.05	0.39	0.78

[a]ISNES, isonicotinoylhydrazone; see Fig. 2.

4.2.1. Pyrazinamide Isosteres

Many cleavable isosteres have been synthesized, such as tetrazole, 4-hydroxy-7-aza-coumarin, oxadiazolones, oxadiazolothiones, and oxathiazolinones (Fig. 6).

Sulfide analogs were synthesized which could be transformed to sulfoxides by the catalase/peroxidase enzymatic system of *M. tuberculosis*. The resulting β-ketosulfoxide would be acidic enough to initiate an acid function. This sulfide could not, however, overcome drug resistance which is due to the lack of a catalase peroxidase (Gezginci et al., 2001; Wächter et al., 1998).

MICs were determined using the BACTEC 460 method. The MICs in BACTEC 6A media (pH 6) are the following: tetrazoles, 13 to 105 μg/ml; sulfoxides, 105 to 210 μg/ml; and benzyl-substituted coumarin, 210 μg/ml. In comparison, the MICs of pyrazinamide and INH were 52 and <0.02 μg/ml. The unsubstituted tetrazoles were shown to display weak in vitro activity (33 to 50% inhibition of growth relative to control) (Kushner et al., 1952).

Several other acidic heterocycles or functional groups have been used to replace the carboxyl goup or tetrazole ring itself. Only the oxathiazolinone exhibited potential anti-*M. tuberculosis* activity (MICs, 4.5 to 9.0 μg/ml). Other analogs were less active, with MICs from 13 to >256 μg/ml.

The unsubstituted isosteres of pyridine and pyrazine carboxylic acid are weakly active. These polar analogs are unable to penetrate the outer membrane of *M. tuberculosis*.

4.2.2. Pyrazinamide Esters

Pyrazinoic acid is more active in vitro than pyrazinamide against *M. tuberculosis*. Pyrazinoic acid will circumvent the need for pyrazinamide and is supposed to overcome pyrazinamide resistance.

Structural modifications of the ester side chain rather than substitutions of the pyrazine nucleus have been very

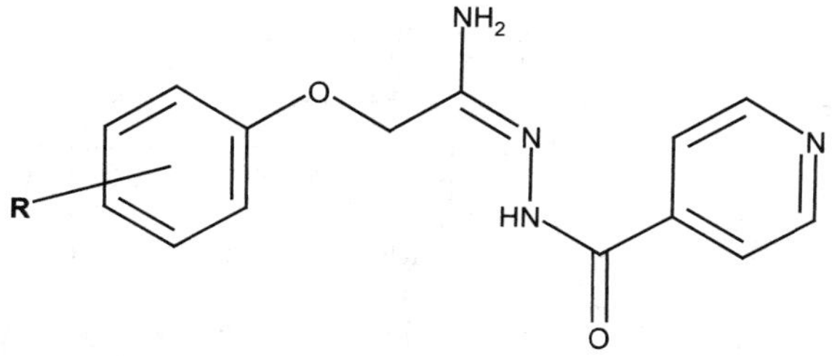

Compound	R	MIC (μg/ml) *Mycobacterium tuberculosis*					Clinical isolate n=16	
		H37 RY	INH-R	RMP-R	PZA-R	SM-R	50	90
A	2-CH_3	12.5	100	12.5	25	25	25	50
B	3-CH_3	3.12	100	1.56	3.12	6.25	12.5	12.5
C	4-CH_3	6.25	50	3.12	3.12	6.25	3.12	6.25
D	3-Cl	3.12	12.5	12.5	3.12	6.25	6.25	12.5
E	4-Cl	3.12	100	3.12	12.5	6.25	3.12	6.25
F	4-NO_2	6.25	50	12.5	12.5	3.12	12.5	12.5
Isoniazid	-	0.09	200	0.09	0.09	0.09	0.09	0.19
Rifampin	-	0.19	0.19	> 100	0.19	0.19	0.39	0.78
Ethambutol	-	6.25	3.12	6.25	3.12	6.25	3.12	3.12
PAS	-	0.39	0.19	0.19	0.9	0.19	0.39	0.78
Clofazimine	-	0.78	0.39	6.25	6.25	3.12	-	-

Figure 5 MICs of isonicotinyl hydrazones for *M. tuberculosis* isolates

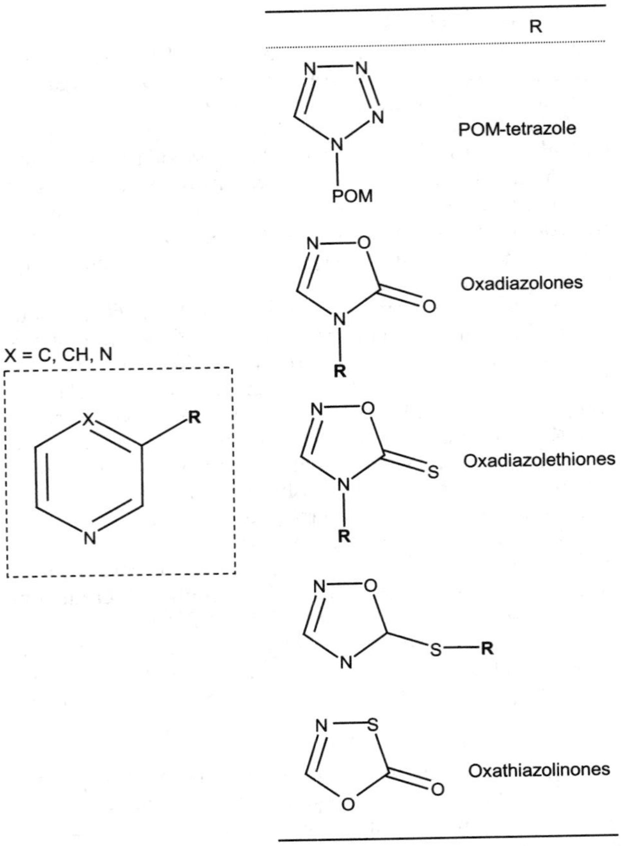

X = C, CH, N

R	
	POM-tetrazole
	Oxadiazolones
	Oxadiazolethiones
	S—R
	Oxathiazolinones

Figure 6 Pyrazinoic isostere derivatives

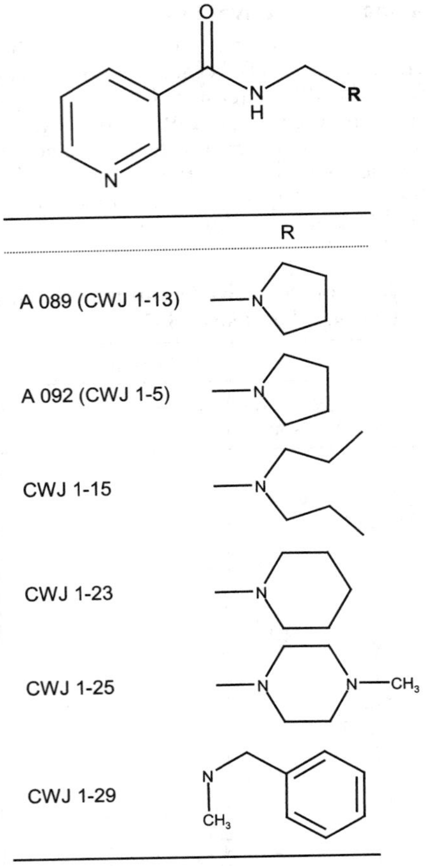

	R
A 089 (CWJ 1-13)	
A 092 (CWJ 1-5)	
CWJ 1-15	
CWJ 1-23	
CWJ 1-25	N—CH_3
CWJ 1-29	CH_3

Figure 7 Aminomethylene amido analogs of pyrazinamide

Table 2 In vitro activity of 5-chloropyrazinamide[a]

Microorganism	*n*	MIC (μg/ml)[b]			
		PZA	5-PZA	PA	5-PA
M. tuberculosis	7	32–>2,048	8–32	16–64	64–256
M. bovis	3	>2,048	8	32–64	128–256
M. kansasii	1	2,048	64	256	64
M. smegmatis	1	>2,048	32	>2,048	512
M. fortuitum	1	>2,048	32	>2,048	256
M. avium	1	>2,048	32	>2,048	>1,024

[a]Data from Cynamon et al., 1995.
[b]PZA, pyrazinamide; 5-PZA, 5-chloropyrazinamide; PA, pyrazinoic acid; 5-PA, 5-chloropyrazinoic acid.

successful in expanding the activity of pyrazinoic acid (Cynamon et al., 1995).

4.2.3. 5-Chloropyrazinamide

5-Chloropyrazinamide is poorly active, as is the metabolite (Table 2).

4.2.4. Aminomethylene Pyrazinamide

New series of aminomethylene pyrazinamide analogs (Fig. 7) have been reported. Twelve new analogs were investigated for their in vitro, in vivo, and intramacrophagic activities against *M. tuberculosis*. These compounds were tested in vitro at various pHs (pH 5.5, 6.0, and 6.8) against pyrazinamide-susceptible and -resistant *M. tuberculosis*.

These new analogs were as active as pyrazinamide against susceptible *M. tuberculosis* strains, but they also exhibit equal activity against *M. tuberculosis* isolates resistant to pyrazinamide, with a MIC of 100 μg/ml in 7H12 BACTEC broth. For two compounds, A-089 and A-092, the in vitro activity was not influenced by the pH of the medium, unlike for pyrazinamide, whose activity dropped at pH 6.8 (MIC of >300 μg/ml, instead of 12.5 μg/ml at pH 5.5).

Within J-774 macrophages, pyrazinamide does not inhibit *M. tuberculosis* growth. In contrast to pyrazinamide, the new aminomethylene analogs exhibited a bactericidal effect in a dose-dependent manner. In combination with rifampin, the A-092 analog was clearly superior to rifampin in macrophages.

In vivo in a mouse model of TB, A-092 in combination with rifalazil or rifampin was more active than pyrazinamide with the same companion drugs (Welch et al., 2000).

These new derivatives could be an alternative in the treatment of infection with *M. tuberculosis* isolates resistant to pyrazinamide.

4.3. Ethambutol Derivatives

Ethambutol was discovered and introduced into clinical practice in the 1960s (Wilkinson et al., 1962).

The rationale for expanding research on ethambutol analogs included the following:

- Improvement of antimycobacterial activity
- Easy chemical substrate to modify
- Overcoming rare but existing resistance to ethambutol

- Enhancement of water solubility
- Better pharmacokinetics
- Better tolerance (ocular toxicity)

Ethambutol inhibits the mycobacterial arabinofuranosyl transferases responsible for glycosylation steps in the biosynthesis of lipoarabinomannan and arabinogalactan, which are constituents of the mycobacterial cell wall.

The anti-*M. tuberculosis* activity is dependent upon the presence of two basic imino nitrogens and small branched alkyl groups (no larger than *sec*-butyl). The dextro derivative exerts anti-*M. tuberculosis* activity, while the levo analog is inactive (Wilkinson et al., 1962).

Analogs can be obtained by modifying the methylene linker (X) or the two side chains, such as in the cyclic analogs of ethambutol (Fig. 8) (Berthelot et al., 1983).

An iminoalditol mimics the arabinofuranosyl motif, which exhibits antimycobacterial properties in an infected-macrophage model. Other iminoalditols bearing the ethambutol partial structure were reported to be inactive.

Minor deviation from the structure of the parent compound resulted in reduced antimycobacterial activity (Häusler et al., 2001).

4.4. Ansamycin Derivatives

Recently, rifabutin and rifapentine were introduced into clinical practice; rifalazil is still under development (see chapter 32).

4.5. Clofazimine Derivatives

Clofazimine (B-663) was initially developed as an anti-TB drug (Barry et al., 1957). Clofazimine exhibits variable activities in animal models: good efficacy was demonstrated in hamsters and mice, but poor efficacy was demonstrated in monkeys and guinea pigs.

The rationale for developing new riminophenazine analogs included the following:

- Enhancement of the in vitro activity, including MDR against TB
- High in vivo activities
- High intracellular bactericidal bioactivity
- Better tolerance than with clofazimine (pigmented skin in long-term therapy)
- Activity against non-TB mycobacteria

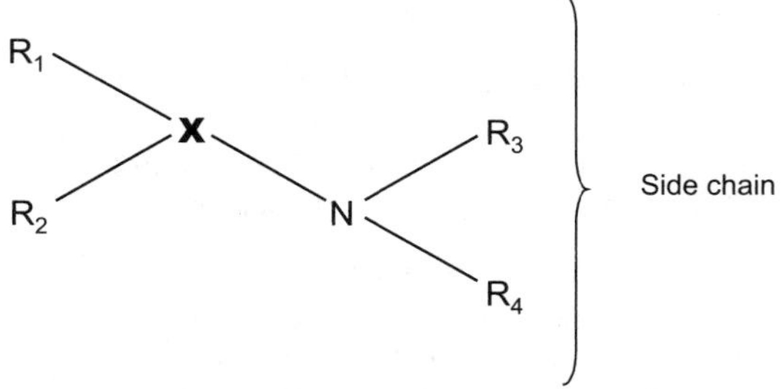

Figure 8 Diamine library with five potential points of diversity

A few series of riminophenazine analogs were synthesized. Some analogs exhibited good in vitro activity against TB, but less in macrophages and in vivo, such as B-4100 and B-4101 (Reddy et al., 1996).

Two other derivatives, B-4157 and B-4154 (Fig. 9), exhibited good activity in vitro, intracellularly, and in experimental infections (Table 3).

In vitro, B-746 (Fig. 10) is more active than B-4101 (MICs, 0.06 to 0.12 μg/ml and 0.12 to 2.0 μg/ml, respectively) and clofazimine (MICs, 0.12 to 2.0 μg/ml). B-746 markedly reduced the viable CFU counts in J-774 macrophages by day 4, and no viable bacilli could be detected by day 7, at either 0.5 or 2.0 μg/ml. The decrease in viable cells in the lungs is lower than that observed with clofazimine and similar to those in the liver and spleen (Jagannath et al., 1995).

	R	R_1
B 4154	Cl	$(CH_2)_3N(C_2H_5)_2$
B 4156	CF_3	C_2H_5

Figure 9 B-4157 and B-4154

Table 3 In vitro activities of B-4154 and B-4157

Microorganism[a]	*n*	MIC (μg/ml)		
		Clofazimine	B-4154	B-4157
M. tuberculosis	6	0.25–1.0	0.12–0.25	≤0.06–1.0
M. tuberculosis MDR	6	0.12–2.0	0.12–0.25	≤0.06–1.0
M. tuberculosis RIF^r	4	0.12–0.25	0.06–0.25	≤0.06
M. tuberculosis EMB^r	1	1.0	0.12	≤0.06
M. tuberculosis INH^r	2	0.12	0.12–0.25	≤0.06

[a]RIF, rifampin; EMB, ethambutol.

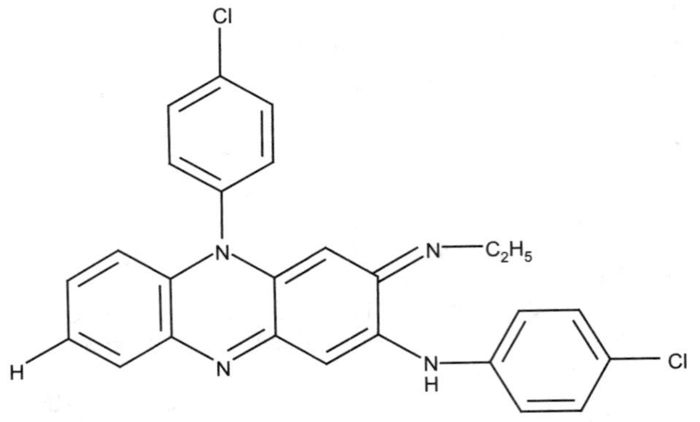

Figure 10 B-746

Table 4 In vitro activities of TMP-substituted riminophenazines against TB

Compound	MIC (μg/ml)
Clofazimine	0.06
B-4100	0.03
B-4121	0.03
B-4125	0.06
B-4128	0.03
B-4169	0.0015

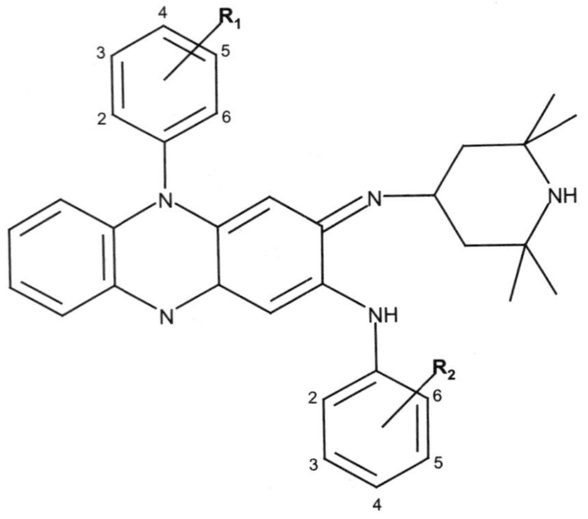

	R_1 and R_2
B 4100	3,4-di-Cl
B 4121	3,5-di-Cl
B 4125	2-Cl
B 4128	2,4-di-Cl
B 4169	3,4,5-tri-Cl

Figure 11 TMP-substituted phenazine derivatives

Tetramethyl piperidine (TMP)-substituted phenazines were tested against M. *tuberculosis* (Table 4; Fig. 11). Some derivatives were more active than clofazimine against M. *tuberculosis*. They have also been found to possess intraphagocytic activity (Reddy et al., 1996).

Table 5 In vitro activity of isoxyl against mycobacteria

Mycobacterium sp.	MIC (μg/ml)
M. *tuberculosis* H37$_{RV}$	2.5
M. *bovis* BCG	0.5
M. *avium*	2.0
M. *aurum*	2.0

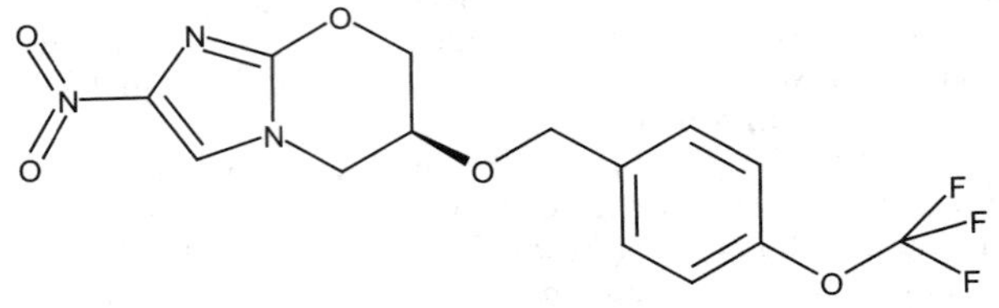

Figure 12 PA-824

Clofazimine apparently inhibits the growth of mycobacteria by potentiating the activity of microbial phospholipase A_2 (PLA_2) leading to lysophospholipid-mediated dysfunction of membrane cation transporters. B-4128 enhanced PLA_2 activity and inhibition of K^+ transport. An influx of Ca^{2+} occurred after a lag time of 2 to 3 min, possibly due to depletion of microbial ATP (Matlola et al., 2001).

4.6. Isoxyl Analogs

Isoxyl is a thiourea derivative (tiocarlide). Isoxyl inhibits the synthesis of both fatty acids and mycolic acids (α-mycolates by 91.6%, methoxymycolate by 94.3%, and ketomycolates by 91.1%). Isoxyl also inhibits the biosynthesis of short-chain fatty acids.

Isoxyl is active against all mycobacteria tested (Table 5) (Phetsuksiri et al., 1999).

5. ALTERATIONS OF EXISTING ANTIBACTERIAL AGENTS

5.1. 5-Nitroimidazole Derivatives

It was demonstrated that M. *tuberculosis* can survive in low oxygen concentrations. Metronidazole is able of killing dormant M. *tuberculosis* (Wayne and Sramek, 1994).

5.2. Nitroimidazopyran Derivatives: PA-824

PA-824 (Fig. 12) had emerged as a lead anti-TB compound (Stover et al., 2000). It exhibits good in vitro and in vivo activities. The antimycobacterial activity of nitroimidazopyran has been reported (Cynamon et al., 1997).

A series of six new nitroimidazole analogs has been tested. In vitro they display good anti-M. *tuberculosis* activity (MIC, ≤1 μg/ml). However, in vivo in mice, at 10 mg/kg of body weight, none of these derivatives was as active as INH at 25 mg/kg.

5.3. CGI 17341

CGI 17341 (Fig. 13) possesses an ethyl substituted oxazole ring fixed to the imidazole ring. In vitro it is more active than metronidazole (Table 6).

CGI 17341 did not show cross-resistance with any anti-TB agents tested. The MIC of CGI 17341 for M. *tuberculosis* H37$_{RV}$ is independent of the pH (pH 5.6 and pH 6.8) (Ashtekar et al., 1993).

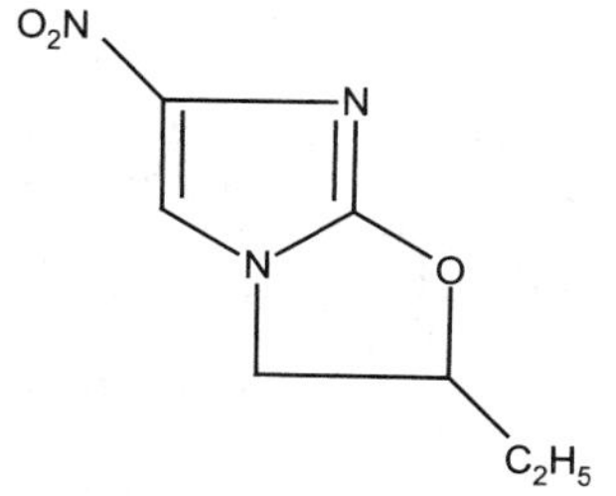

Figure 13 CGI 17341

Table 6 In vitro activity of CGI 17341

Microorganism[a]	n	MIC (μg/ml)	
		CGI 17341	Metronidazole
M. tuberculosis $H37_{RV}$	1	0.06	>256
M. tuberculosis	10	0.1–0.3	>256
M. tuberculosis RIF[r]	1	0.08	>256
M. tuberculosis INH[r]	1	0.0015	>256
M. tuberculosis MDR	1	0.2–0.4	>256
M. tuberculosis EMB[r]	1	0.08	>256

[a]RIF, rifampin; EMB, ethambutol.

5.4. Oxazolidinones

The first oxazolidinone derivatives showing anti-TB activity were DuP 105 and DuP 721. DuP 721 administered at 10 mg/kg twice a day for 30 days is lethal for rats. Three other derivatives, U-100480, U-101603, and U-101244 (active metabolites of U-100480), were extremely active against *M. tuberculosis* (Fig. 14; Table 7).

U-100480 is active in a murine model of *M. tuberculosis* infection after oral administration, with a significant reduction of the CFU in the lungs and spleen (3.1 and 4.9 $\log_{10}$ CFU/tissue). It was shown that linezolid (U-100766) and eperezolid (U-100592) also exert good anti-*M. tuberculosis* activities (Zurenko et al., 1996).

In a murine (4-week-old outbred CD-1 mice) model of *M. tuberculosis* infection, PNU-100480 was as efficient as INH (Table 8).

PNU-100480 is rapidly converted to the sulfoxide metabolite (U-101603) and, to a lesser extent, to the sulfone metabolite (U-101244) (Cynamon et al., 1999).

5.5. Inhibitors of DHFR

5.5.1. Mycobacterial DHFR

It is known that trimethoprim and available benzylpyrimidine derivatives are poor inhibitors of dihydrofolate reductase (DHFR) of *M. tuberculosis* and MAC.

Many bacteria need to synthesize folates de novo through a pathway containing at least four enzymes, such as dihydroneopterin aldolase (Escuyer et al., 2002).

5.5.2. Deazapteridines

The inhibitory activities of 2,4-diamino-5-deazapteridine analogs against DHFR of MAC were investigated (Fig. 15). Various substituents were fixed at position 5 and/or 6 of the pteridine moiety, and the resulting compounds were tested for their activities. More than 50% of the 70 analogs inhibited MAC DHFR, with a 50% inhibitory concentration (IC_{50}) of ≤10 nM. The MICs for *M. tuberculosis* varied from 1.28 to ≥128 μg/ml (Suling et al., 1999).

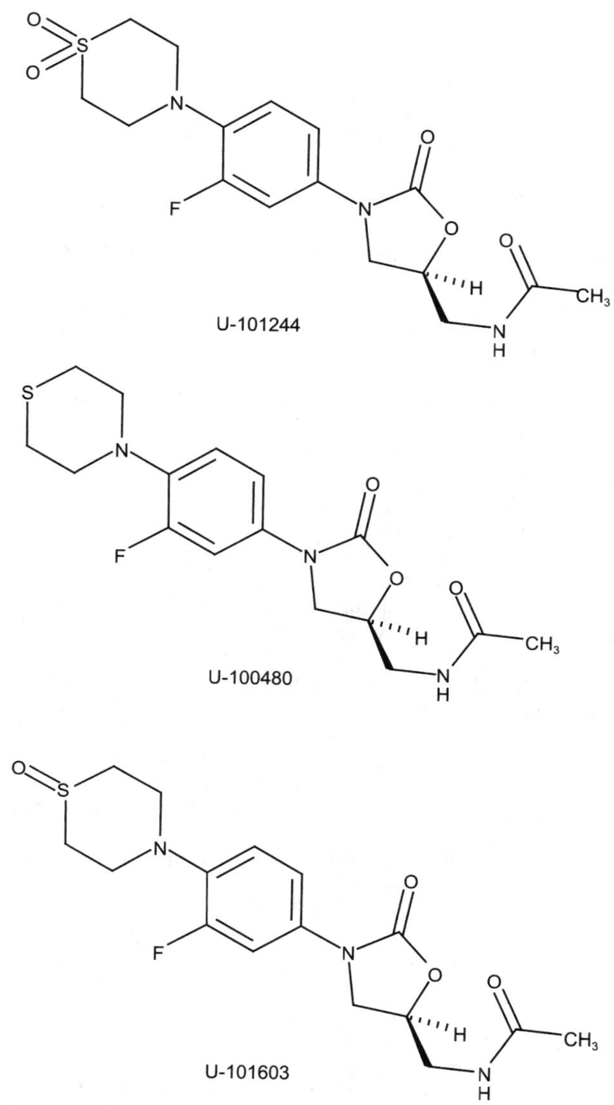

Figure 14 Oxazolidinones

Table 7 In vitro activities of oxazolidinone derivatives against *M. tuberculosis* $H37_{RV}$

Compound	n	MIC (μg/ml)
U-100480	10	0.03–2.0
U-101603	1	≤0.125
U- 101244	10	0.125–2.0
Eperezolid	10	0.125–0.5
Linezolid	10	0.5–2.0

Table 8 In vivo activities of oxazolidinones against *M. tuberculosis*

Compound	Log_{10} CFU/organ (mean ± SD)	
	Spleen	Lungs
Late control	7.63 ± 0.10	8.47 ± 0.51
INH	4.36 ± 0.31	3.81 ± 0.17
PNU-100480	4.61 ± 0.26	3.59 ± 0.33
Linezolid	5.24 ± 0.32	5.03 ± 0.65

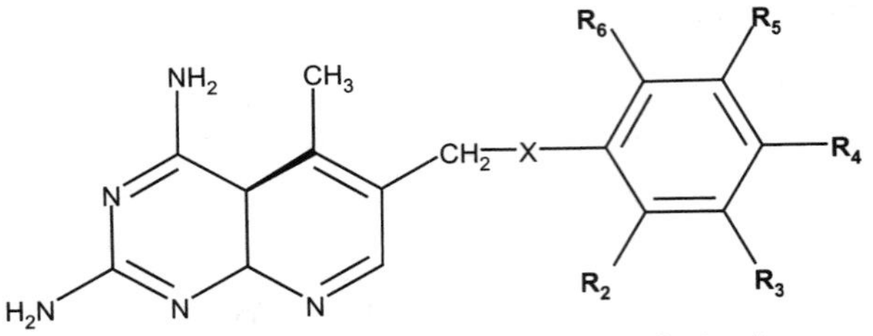

Figure 15 2,4-Diamino-5-deazapteridine derivatives

Hundreds of deazapteridine derivatives, which are inhibitors of tubulin polymerization, were prepared and screened for in vitro activity against M. *tuberculosis* using BACTEC assays. Some of them exhibited activity against M. *tuberculosis*, such as SR-1761 (MIC of 6.25 μg/ml).

Deazapteridine analogs were prepared as inhibitors of DHFR. The compounds evaluated were 2,4-diamino-5-methyl-5-deazapteridines having a structure similar to that of trimetrexate and piritrexim, which are antifolate anti-infective compounds. Follow-up research yielded 12 derivatives having antimycobacterial activities (Suling et al., 2000).

Seventy-seven compounds were synthesized and evaluated for in vitro activity against M. *avium* and MAC DHFR IC_{50}s versus those for human rDHFR. Four compounds of the 77 showed a MIC of ≤1.3 μg/ml for MAC NJ168. Twenty-one derivatives were more than 100-fold more active against MAC rDHFR than against human rDHFR. In general, selectivity was dependent on the composition of the two-atom bridge at position 6 and the attached aryl groups with substitutions at the 2′ and 5′ positions on the phenyl ring (Suling et al., 1998).

Twelve DHFR inhibitors were tested against M. *tuberculosis* H_{37RA} and three clinical MAC isolates (serovar 1, 4, or 6). They are 2-diamino-5-methyl-5-deazapteridine derivatives. The deazapteridine compounds had aryl group substitutions on position 6 of the heterocyclic moiety which were linked through a two-atom bridge [either CH_2NH, $CH_2N(CH_3)$, or CH_2S]. Six of the compounds had MICs of ≤12.8 μg/ml for M. *tuberculosis* and of ≤1.28 μg/ml for MAC. Two compounds, with the aryl group (2-methyl-5-methoxyphenyl or 2-methoxy-5-trifluoromethyl phenyl) linked to the deazapteridine moiety by a CH_2NH bridge, had MICs of ≤0.13 μg/ml for MAC strains (Suling et al., 1997).

5.6. Tetracyclines

It has been shown that minocycline is rapidly bactericidal against M. *leprae*. An investigation has been conducted with all available cycline derivatives and some other analogs to determine the structure-activity relationship of cyclines against M. *tuberculosis*. It has been suggested that a dimethylamine substitution at C-7 enhanced the anti-TB activity as well as a 6-methyl substituent or a lack of a C-5 substituent.

5.7. Fluoroquinolones

Some fluoroquinolones exhibit good activity against M. *tuberculosis* and are used in second-line therapy, because resistance mutations occur rapidly.

The activities of fluoroquinolones against atypical mycobacteria vary. The DNA gyrases from M. *avium*, *Mycobacterium smegmatis*, and *Mycobacterium fortuitum* subsp. *peregrinum* are naturally resistant, moderately susceptible, and susceptible, respectively, to available fluoroquinolones. This poor affinity of fluoroquinolones for M. *avium* and M. *smegmatis* could be due to the presence of Ala83 instead of Ser83 in the quinolone resistance-determining region of gyrase A (Guillemin et al., 1999).

Against M. *tuberculosis*, all of the fluoroquinolones do not exert the same activity for inhibiting the growth of resistant mutants (Xu et al., 1996). It was shown that compounds with a methoxy group attached to the C-8 position are more active against mutants (Dong et al., 1998; Zhao et al., 1999).

A new parameter was recently defined: the mutant prevention concentration (MPC), which is the minimal fluoroquinolone concentration that allows the mutant recovery when more than 10^{10} cells are applied to drug-containing agar (Dong et al., 1999). It was proposed that if a concentration of a given fluoroquinolone in tissue is above the MPC, selection of resistant mutants should be severely restricted. Eighteen fluoroquinolone analogs having four different substituents at C-8 (unsubstituted [8-H] or 8-OCH_3, 8-F, 8-Cl, and 8-Br) and various substituents at N-4′, C-3′, and C-2′ of the 7-piperazinyl ring have been tested. It was shown that the most active compounds against M. *smegmatis* possess an 8-OCH_3 group. It was shown that the MPC correlates well with the MIC for the most resistant, first-step *gyrA* mutant.

Also, the MPC and MIC measurements show that there is an interaction between C-8 and C-7 substituents.

The most effective compound in preventing mutation possesses a C-3′ethyl or monomethyl substituent on the 7-piperazinyl ring (PD-161148 or PD-135432) (Sindelar et al., 2000).

6. NEW TARGETS AND COMPOUNDS

Mycobacteria are relatively resistant to drying, alkali, and many chemical disinfectants, making it difficult to prevent the transmission of TB in institutions and in urban environments in general. The anatomical and the physiological structures of mycobacteria can be good targets for research of novel derivatives.

6.1. Outer Membrane of Mycobacteria

Mycobacteria belong to a large group of gram-positive eubacteria containing high-GC DNA (*Corynebacterium*, *Mycobacterium*, *Nocardia*, and *Rhodococcus*). These bacteria produce a chemotype IV cell wall containing diaminopimelic acid (peptidoglycan). In mycobacteria and *Nocardia* the muramic acid is N glycosylated and not N acylated.

The chemotype cell wall possesses a unique polysaccharide, arabinogalactan substituted by mycolic acid.

Mycolic acid contains up to 40 to 60 carbon atoms, with 70 to 90 carbon atoms for *Corybacterium*, *Nocardia*, and mycobacteria, respectively.

In addition, several other lipid species, many of them with unusual structures, belong to the mycobacterial cell wall which could be specific for a bacterial genus, such as sulfolipids for M. *tuberculosis* (Brennan and Nikaido, 1995).

6.2. Mycolic Acids

Mycolic acids are long-chain, high-molecular-weight α-alkyl, β-hydroxy fatty acids. The general structure is R-CH(OH)-CH(R′)-COOH, where R is a meromycolate chain consisting of 50 to 56 carbons and R′ is a shorter aliphatic branch consisting of 22 to 26 carbon atoms.

Mycobacteria possess both the multifunctional fatty acid synthase type I (FAS-I) system and the dissociated fatty acid synthase type II (FAS-II) system. FAS-I catalyzes de novo synthesis of C-16–C-18 or C-24–C-28 fatty acids in a bimodal fashion. FAS-II elongates palmitoyl coenzyme A following transacylation of ACP (Fig. 16). MtFabH is a critical link between the FAS-I and FAS-II systems.

Figure 16 Fatty acid and mycolic acid biosynthesis in *M. tuberculosis* (adapted from Kremer and Besra, 2002)

Mature mycolic acid is transferred to arabinoglucan from a carrier molecule, trehalose monomycolate, to trehalose to form trehalose dimycolate (cord factor). This transfer is catalyzed by the antigen 85 complex.

6.2.1. β-Sulfonyl Carboxiamides

β-Sulfonyl carboxiamides were designed to mimic the transition state of the reaction catalyzed by the β-keto acyl synthase.

N-Octanesulfonylacetamide (OSA) (Fig. 17) is an inhibitor of fatty acid and mycolic acid biosynthesis in mycobacteria. OSA inhibits the growth of *M. tuberculosis* strains irrespective of their susceptibility to anti-TB drugs (Parrish et al., 2001).

6.3. Arabinogalactan

Arabinogalactan plays a crucial role in anchoring the outer lipid layer to the peptidoglycan layer (Fig. 18). Ethambutol is an effective inhibitor of the arabinan component of arabinogalactan.

Isopentyl diphosphate is the precursor of mycobacterial polyprenyl phosphate.

6.4. Branched-Chain Amino Acids

Microorganisms and plants are able to synthesize the branched-chain amino acids isoleucine, valine, and leucine. The keto-isovalerate, an intermediate on the valine pathway, is also used for the synthesis of leucine, which is catalyzed by acetolactate synthase (ALS), keto-acid reducto-isomerase (KARI), and dihydrolase (Fig. 19).

Figure 17 OSA

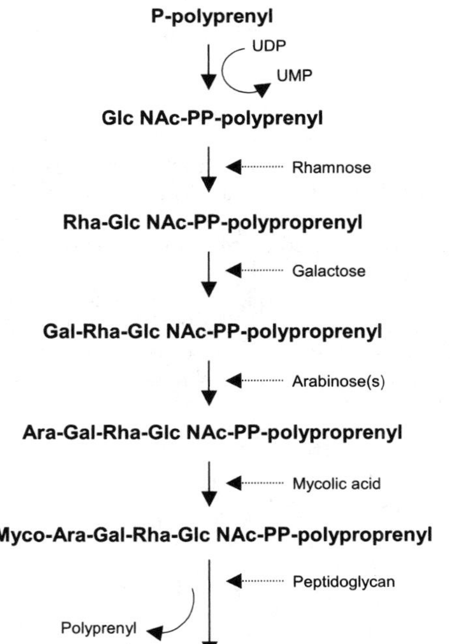

Figure 18 Proposed pathway of arabino-peptidoglycan biosynthesis (Kremer and Besra, 2002)

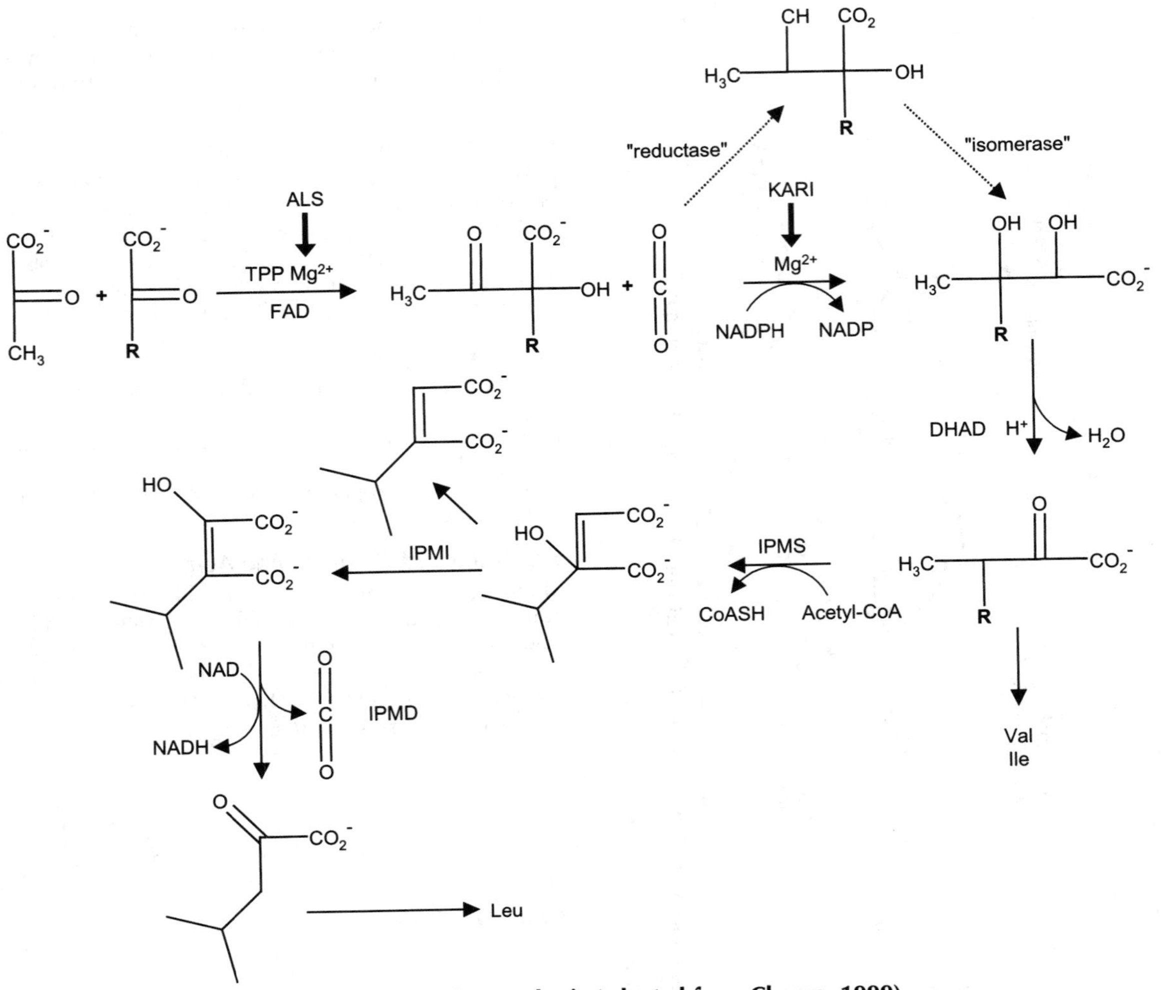

Figure 19 Leucine synthesis (adapted from Chopra, 1999)

For M. *tuberculosis*, two additional enzymes are involved in the biosynthesis of amino acids: 2,3-dihydroxy isovalerate from acetolactate, replacing the reducto-isomerase activity of KARI. Due to this alteration, inhibitors of KARI may be ineffective (Grandoni et al., 1998).

Sulfometuron methyl (Fig. 20) was discovered in 1984 as a major herbicide and inhibits ALS in bacteria. The inhibition of plant ALS is the basis for phytotoxicity of other sulfonylurea herbicides (sulfonylurea, imidazolinones, sulfonanilides, etc.).

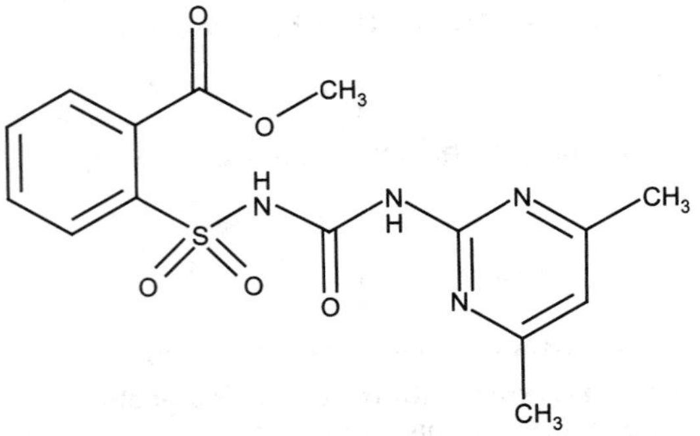

Figure 20 Sulfometuron methyl

Leucine auxotrophic strains of *Mycobacterium bovis* BCG are less effective in challenging mice. This suggests that leucine biosynthesis is required for virulence of M. *bovis* (McAdam et al., 1995). These auxotrophic isolates contained a transposon-insertion in *leuD*.

ALS inhibitor as well as KARI inhibitor activities on M. *tuberculosis* virulence were investigated. Compounds were tested for the ability to inhibit growth of M. *tuberculosis* in vitro.

Of the ALS and KARI inhibitors, sulfometuron methyl and metsulfuron methyl were the most potent inhibitors of M. *tuberculosis* ATCC 35801. In comparison, INH and rifampin were much more potent inhibitors (MIC, $<0.015\,\mu M$). At $34\,\mu M$ sulfometuron methyl and metsulfometuron methyl inhibited 85 and 97% of growth of M. *tuberculosis* $H37_{RV}$, respectively.

KARI and isopropyl malate deshydrogenase inhibitors are weakly effective in inhibiting M. *tuberculosis* growth.

In a mouse model of M. *tuberculosis* infection, after daily treatment with 500 mg/kg for 28 days, it was shown that sulfometuron methyl significantly reduced the organism burden in the lungs but had no effect on spleen burden.

M. *tuberculosis* grows in vacuoles and not in cytoplasm. This microorganism, like *Salmonella*, needs to synthesize some amino acids de novo to survive within the host cell (McAdam et al., 1995).

6.5. Other Targets

See Kremer and Besra, 2002.

6.5.1. Isocitrate lyase

Isocitrate lyase is an important enzyme in the fatty acid catabolism-associated glyoxylate shunt pathway. Mutations may render M. *tuberculosis* unable to survive (McKinney et al., 2000).

6.5.2. PcaA

PcaA is a specific cyclopropane synthase involved in cyclopropanation of the proximal double bond of mycolic acids. Inactivation of the gene for this cyclopropane synthase might alter lipid fluidity, permeability, antigenicity, and ability to neutralize exogenous free radicals (Glickman et al., 2000).

6.5.3. Phthiocerol Dimycocerostate

Disruption of genes involved in the biosynthesis or transport of phthiocerol dimycorostate restricts replication of M. *tuberculosis* in the lungs of infected mice but not in the spleen (Cox et al., 1999).

6.6. Genome

The genome of M. *tuberculosis* was elucidated. The genome contains about 4,000 genes. Today, precise or putative functions can be attributed to 52%, with the remaining 48% being conserved hypotheticals or unknown. About 8% of the genome is dedicated to lipid metabolism (Cole, 2002).

6.7. FtsZ

FtsZ is the first nonregulatory element to appear at the septum site of bacteria, and the function of the septum has been shown to depend on correct FtsZ function (Reynolds et al., 2000).

FtsZ is a cytoplasmic protein similar to bacterial tubulin.

Among 200 compounds of 2-alkoxy carbonyl aminopyridine (Fig. 21), some of them display inhibitory activity for M. *tuberculosis* FtsZ. Two of them were selected for further investigation, SRI-3072 and SRI-7614. These derivatives were shown to be active against MDR M. *tuberculosis* (MIC, 0.5 μg/ml for M. *tuberculosis* $HR37_{RA}$).

SRI-3072 inhibited the growth of M. *tuberculosis* Erdman in infected mouse marrow macrophages (90% effective concentration, 0.12 μg/ml) (White et al., 2002).

6.8. Vitamin K

Vitamin K is present in several strains of *Mycobacterium* and plays a role in the electron transport and oxidative phosphorylation of several pathogenic and nonpathogenic mycobacteria.

Coenzyme Q also stimulates the growth of M. *tuberculosis* and nonpathogenic mycobacteria.

6-Cyclo-octylamino-5,8-quinolinoquinone (CQQ) (Fig. 22) yields dual analogs of vitamin and coenzyme Q. The CQQ MIC for M. *tuberculosis* is 1.0 μg/ml, and that for MAC is 8.0 μg/ml. CQQ exerts bactericidal activity against M. *tuberculosis* (Chakraborty et al., 1981).

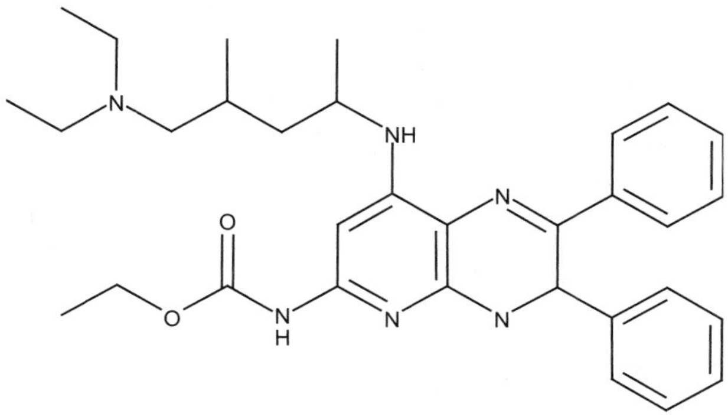

SRI-3072

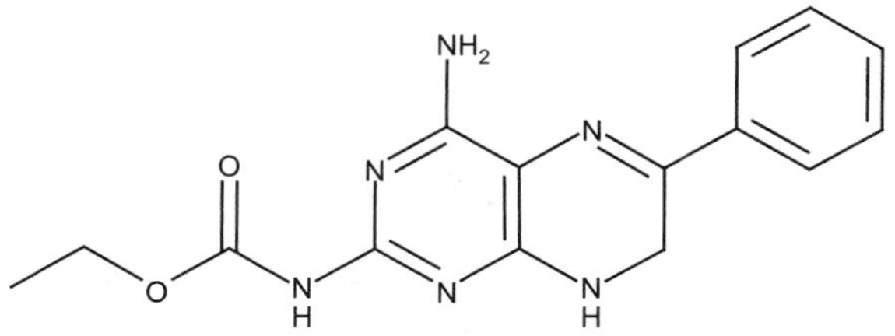

SRI-7614

Figure 21 Inhibitors of *M. tuberculosis* FtsZ

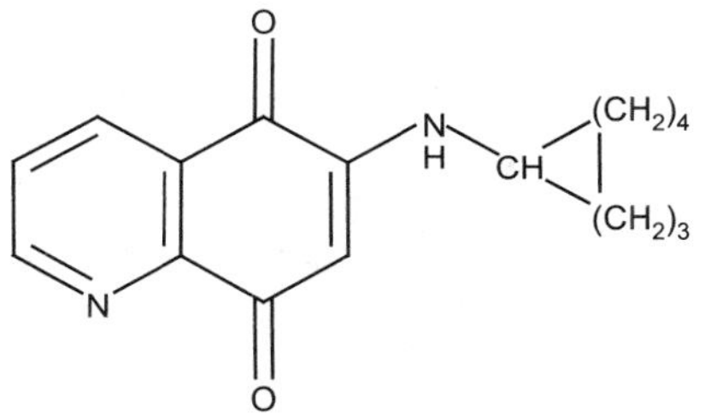

Figure 22 CQQ

7. NATURAL COMPOUNDS

7.1. Caprazamycins A to F

Novel nucleoside anti-M. *tuberculosis* caprazamycins A to F (Fig. 23) were produced by the fermentation of *Streptomyces* sp. strain MK 730-62F2.

Caprazamycin B is the major component of this complex. The MIC of caprazamycin B for M. *tuberculosis* $H37_{RV}$ is 3.13 μg/ml, and for the Kurono and Ravanel strains, the MICs were 6.25 and 12.5 μg/ml, respectively.

After nasal instillation of M. *tuberculosis* $H37_{RV}$ in mice, various doses of caprazamycin B were administered. A dose-dependent reduction of M. *tuberculosis* lung burden was observed (Igarashi et al., 2002).

7.2. Indigoferabietane

From *Indigofera longeracemosa*, a plant reported to be useful in traditional medicine, a compound was extracted and named indigoferabietone. It exhibited good anti-M. *tuberculosis* activity (MICs, 0.38 μg/ml) (Thangadurai et al., 2002).

7.3. Mycoplanecin A

Mycoplanecin A (Fig. 24) is a major component of a complex molecule produced by *Actinoplanes awajinensis* subsp. *mycoplanecinus* subsp. nov. (Torikata et al., 1983). Dihydromycoplanecin A is an active metabolite in urine of mice and dogs administered mycoplanecin A. Mycoplanecin A possesses a cyclic structure composed of 10 amino acid residues containing three kinds of proline analogs and α-ketobutyric acid, which can be differentiated from other minor components B,

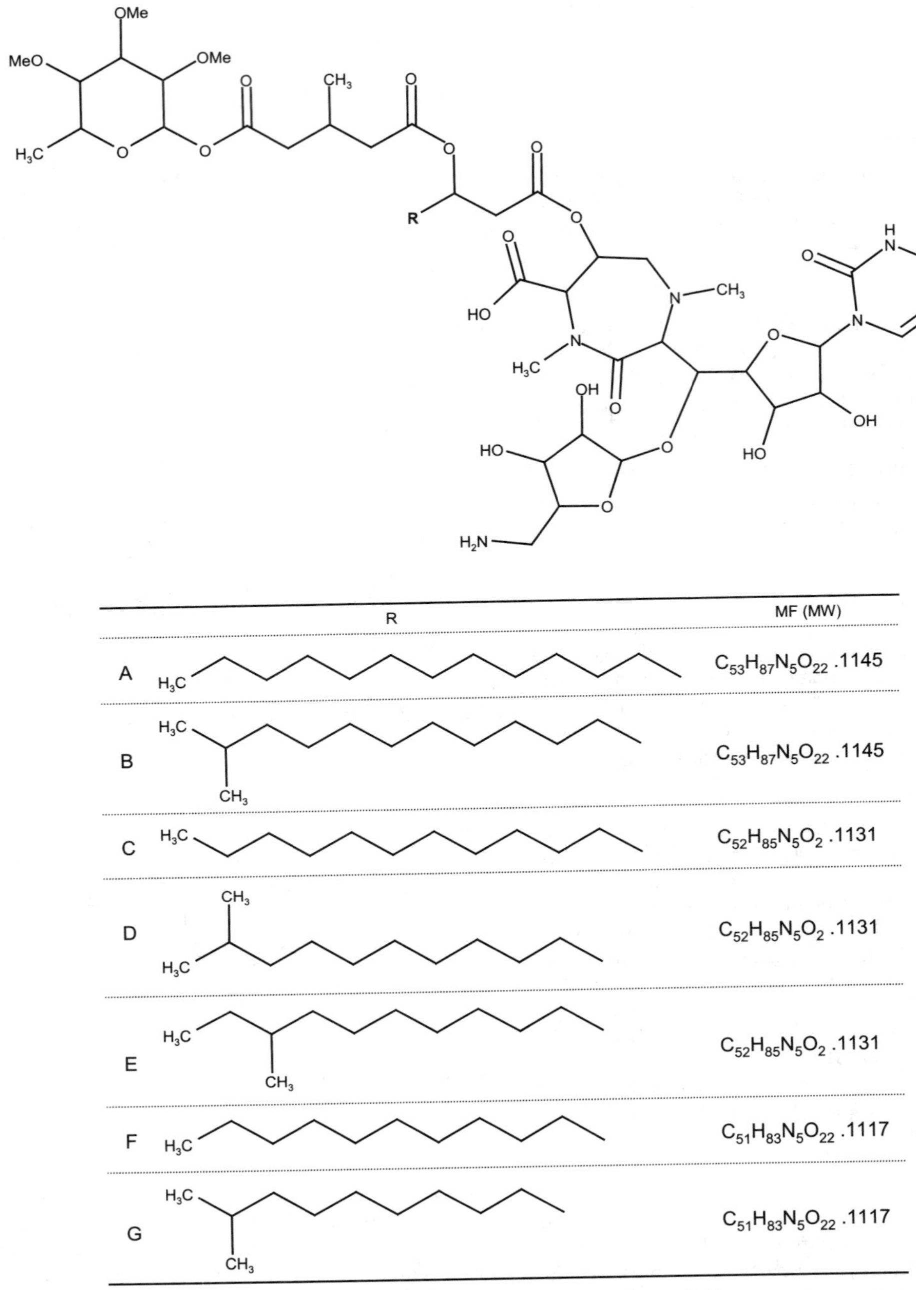

	R	MF (MW)
A		$C_{53}H_{87}N_5O_{22}$ .1145
B		$C_{53}H_{87}N_5O_{22}$ .1145
C		$C_{52}H_{85}N_5O_2$ .1131
D		$C_{52}H_{85}N_5O_2$ .1131
E		$C_{52}H_{85}N_5O_2$ .1131
F		$C_{51}H_{83}N_5O_{22}$ .1117
G		$C_{51}H_{83}N_5O_{22}$ .1117

Figure 23 Caprazamycins A through F

C, and D. Dihydromycoplanecin A has an α-hydroxybutyric acid as an *N*-acyl group. In vitro activity against mycobacteria is reported in Table 9.

After administration of 10 mg of dihydromycoplanecin A per kg to mice, the apparent elimination half-life was 0.5 h and the urinary and fecal elimination rates within 48 h were 19.6 and 78% of the administered dose, respectively.

After a single intravenous dose of 10 mg/kg to dogs, the apparent elimination half-life was 5.5 h and urinary elimination within 48 h was 37%.

7.4. Biflavonoids

Biflavonoids (Fig. 25) are a series of naturally occurring compounds that include flavone-flavone, flavonone-flavone, and flavonone-flavonone subunit linkages. More than 100 biflavonoids have been identified from plants since the isolation of gingetin in 1929.

Naturally occurring biflavonoids were isolated from seed kernels of *Rhus succedanea* and *G. multiflora*. Among all components isolated from both, few natural components are able to inhibit the growth of *M. tuberculosis* (Lin et al., 2001) (Table 10).

7.5. Rhein

Rhein is an extract of a Chinese rhubarb (*Rhei rhizoma*). Rhein belongs in traditional medicine in a mixture of five crude compounds named onpi-to (*R. rhizoma*, *Glycyrrhizae radix*, *Ginseng radix*, *Rhizoma zingiberis*, and *Aconiti tuber*). The primary

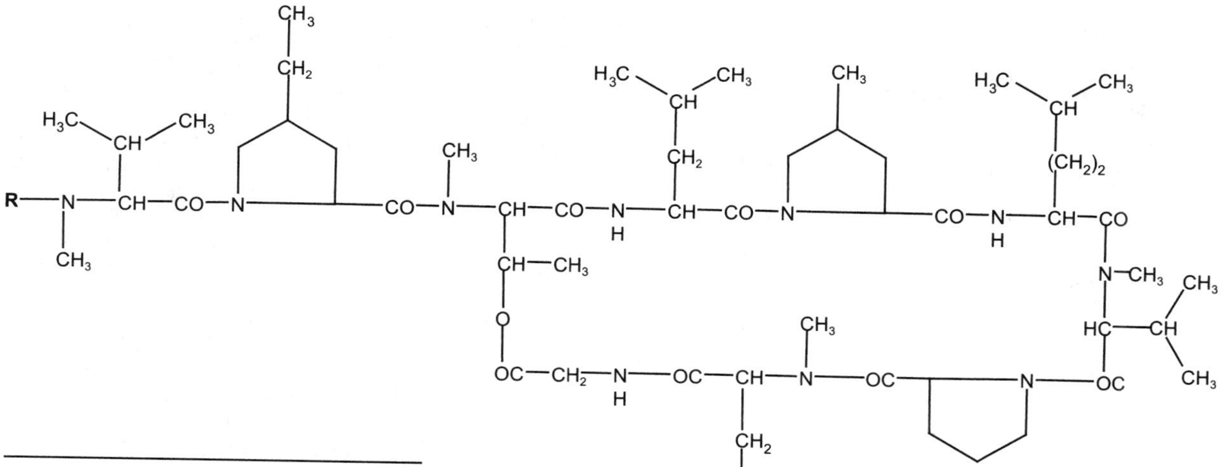

	R
Mycoplanecin A	CH_3-CH_2-CO-CO
Dihydromycoplanecin	CH_3CH_2 CH(OH)-CO

Figure 24 Mycoplanecin A

Table 9 In vitro activity of dihydromycoplanecin A

Microorganism	*n*	MIC (μg/ml) 50%	MIC (μg/ml) 90%	MIC (μg/ml) Range
M. tuberculosis	38	<0.125	0.05	
M. intracellulare	20	1.56	25	
M. kansasii	20	0.39	0.78	
M. bovis	5			0.025–0.2
M. fortuitum	4			>25
M. gordoenae	3			<0.0125–0.39
Non-chromogenes mycobacteria	3			0.39–25

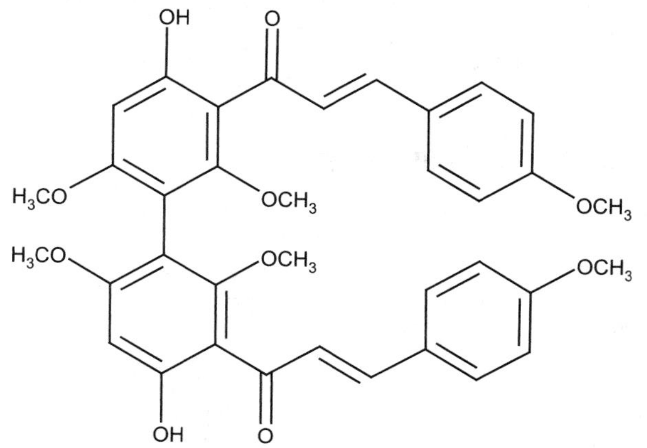

Figure 25 Anti-TB compounds: biflavonoids

constituents of *R. rhizoma* are anthranoids including sennoside A, sennoside B, rhein-8-O-glucopyranoside, and rhein. Sennosides A and B are converted to rhein by bacteria in the colon (Takizawa et al., 2003).

Table 10 In vitro activities of biflavonoids[a]

Compound	% Inhibition
6,6″-Biapigenin hexamethyl ether	96
3′-Nitro-3-O-4′-biflavone	61
Volkensiflavanone hexamethyl ether	95
3,8″-Biapigenin hexamethyl ether	87

[a]From Lin et al., 2001.

Rhein is a dried root and is derived from the outer corky layer of *R. rhizoma*. It is an anthraquinone derivative (9,10-dihydro-4,5-dihydroxy-9,10-dioxo-2-anthracene carboxylic acid (Fig. 26). Rhein is also the active metabolite of diacerein, an anti-inflammatory compound. Rhein reduces the production of superoxide anion in human neutrophils. It is either eliminated by the renal route (20%) or conjugated in the liver to rhein glucuronide and rhein sulfate (Nicolas et al., 1998). Rhein exerts antimycobacterial activity (Vittori and Collins, 1996).

7.6. Tryptanthrin

The active principle was an extract of the Taiwanese medicinal plant *Strobilanthes cusia*.

7.7. Elisapterosin B

Elisapterosin B (Fig. 27) is a diterpene compound having an elisapterane-like skeleton and possessing an antimycobacterial agent extracted from the West Indian sea whip (gorgonian coral) *Pseudopterogorgia elisabethae*. It inhibits 79% of growth of *M. tuberculosis* $H37_{RV}$ at a concentration of 12.5 μg/ml (Rodriguez et al., 2000).

7.8. *Ardisia iwahigensis*

(7)-(10-Pentadecenyl) resorcinol was extracted from leaves and twigs of *A. iwahigensis* Elmer. MICs at which 90% of isolates were inhibited (MIC_{90}s) of 2.5 to 5.0 μg/ml were found for *M. tuberculosis* $H37_{RV}$ (Onwuta et al., 1997).

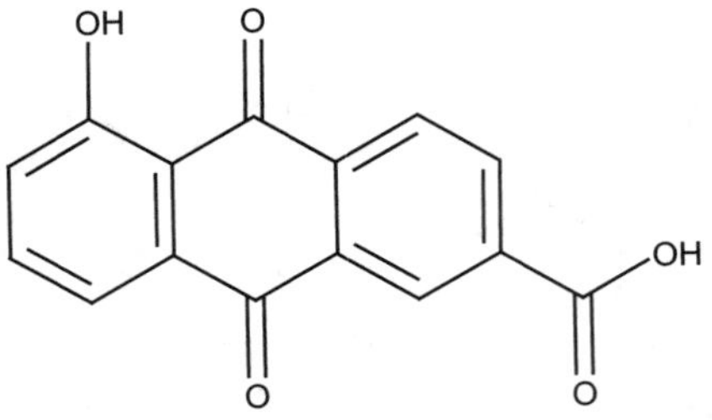

Figure 26 Rhein

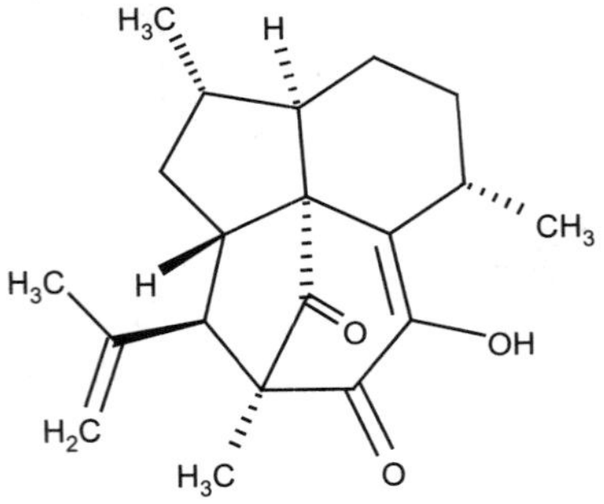

Figure 27 Elisapterosin B

7.9. Ibogaine, Texalin, and Voacangine

Natural substances were extracted from plants growing in the Caribbean island of Guadeloupe. Using the BACTEC 460 radiometric method and 7H12 Middlebrook agar medium, extracts or essential oils of nine different plants were tested against M. *tuberculosis* (Table 11; Fig. 28).

7.10. Anti-*M. tuberculosis* Agents of Marine Origin

Numerous compounds have been isolated from marine life and tested for anti-M. *tuberculosis* activity.

(+)-8-Hydroxymanzamine A is an alkaloid derivative characterized by a complex heterocycle ring system attached to a β-carboline moiety. (+)-8-Hydroxymanzamine A was first isolated from sponge (*Pachypellina* spp.) and later from Petrosiidae. The MIC for M. *tuberculosis* $H37_{RV}$ was 0.91 μg/ml. The MIC of manzamine A for M. *tuberculosis* $H37_{RV}$ was 1.56 μg/ml (Youssef et al., 2002).

Ircinol A is an alkaloid-like compound closely structurally related to (+)-8-hydroxymanzamine A.

Axisonitrole-3 is a cyano sesquiterpene isolated from a sponge, *Acanthella klethra*; its MIC for M. *tuberculosis* $H37_{RV}$ is 2.0 μg/ml (Konig et al., 2000).

Pseudopteroxazole is a benzoxazole diterpene alkaloid isolated from *P. elisabethae*. The compound induced 97% growth inhibition of M. *tuberculosis* $H37_{RV}$ at a concentration of 12.5 μg/ml (Rodriguez and Ramirez, 1999).

Ergogiaene, a serrulatane-based diterpene (or biflorane), was isolated from *P. elisabethae*. The compound induced inhibition of M. *tuberculosis* $H37_{RV}$ at a concentration of 12.5 μg/ml (Rodriguez et al., 2001).

Litosterol is a C-19 hydroxysteroid isolated from a coral, *Litophyton viridis*. The compound induced inhibition of M. *tuberculosis* $H37_{RV}$ at a concentration of 3.13 μg/ml. It is poorly water soluble (Iguchi et al., 1989).

Puupehenone induced inhibition of M. *tuberculosis* $H37_{RV}$ at a concentration of 12.5 μg/ml. The puupehenones are shikimate-sesquiterpene-derived metabolites from sponges (*Hyrtios* spp.) (Nasu et al., 1995).

8. OTHER DERIVATIVES

8.1. Purines

It was shown that the natural product agelasine F and 9-sulfonyl-6-mercaptopurines exhibited anti-TB activity (Fig. 29) (Scozzafava et al., 2001). This serendipitous discovery led to intensive research in this field. A few series of analogs were synthesized such as 9-benzyl purines (Fig. 30) (Bakkestuen et al., 2000). Some of them displayed anti-M. *tuberculosis* activity, especially those substituted at position 2 and/or 6. They inhibited 90% of M. *tuberculosis* growth at a concentration of 12.5 μg/ml. Other derivatives were more active, but only against susceptible M. *tuberculosis* isolates (Table 12) (Gundersen et al., 2002).

In a study of the structure-activity relationship, it was shown that 9-unsubstituted purines or those with small alkyl substituents (methyl) or aryl are inactive. Among the 9-aryl substituted purines, the following moieties resulted in better analogs in vitro: 2-furyl > 2-thienyl >2-phenyl substituents. 2-Chlorine also led to a high level of anti-M. *tuberculosis* activity (Fig. 31). The length of the bridge between the purine core and the phenyl group was increased from a methylene to an ethylene bridge. The thienyl purines are less active than the furyl derivatives.

Table 11 In vitro activities of compounds from Guadeloupean plants against *M. tuberculosis*[a]

Compound	Family	Plant(s)	MIC (μg/ml)	
			BACTEC 460	7H11 agar
Pilocarpine	Alkaloids	*Pilocarpus racemosa*	>100	>200
Heraclenol	Coumarin	*Amyris elemifera*	100	200
Canella	Sesquiterpene	*Canella winteriana*	100	200
Lochnerin	Indole alkaloid	*Rauwolfia biauriculata*	100	>200
Ibogaine	Indole alkaloid	*Tabernaemontana citrifolia*	50	50
Isomeranzin	Coumarin	*Triphasia trifolia*	100	200
Voacangine	Indole alkaloid	*T. citrifolia*	50	50
Texalin	Oxazole alkaloid	*A. elemifera*	25	25
Canella oil		*Canella winterana*	100	>200

[a]Data from Rastogi et al., 1998.

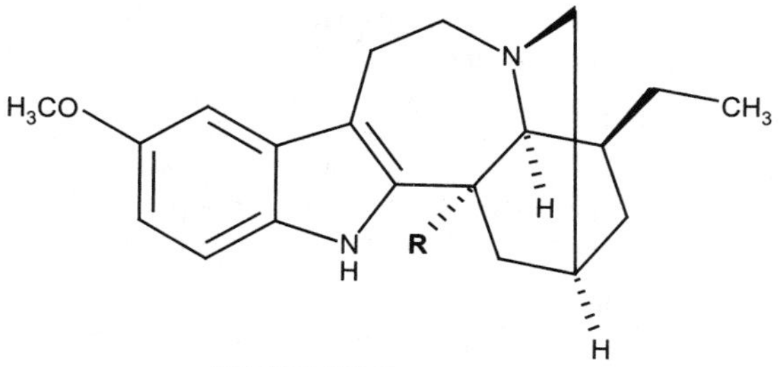

	R
Ibogaine	H
Voacangine	$COOCH_3$

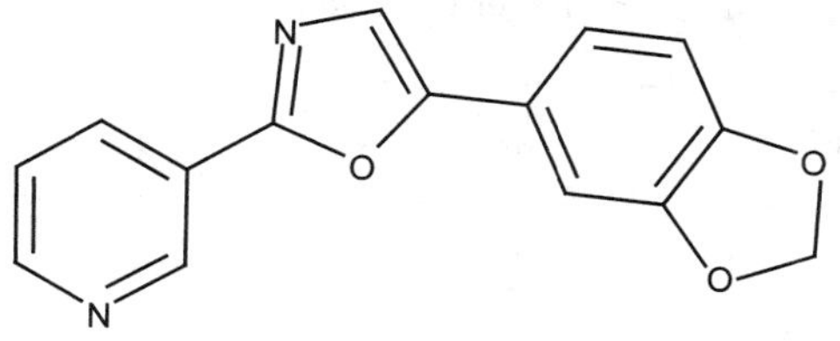

Texalin

Figure 28 Natural anti-*M. tuberculosis* products

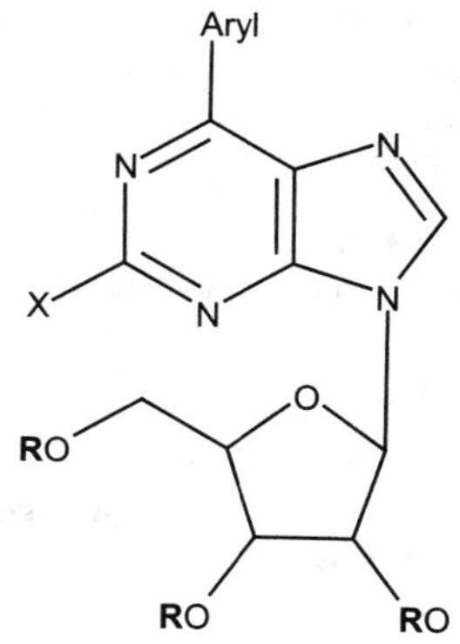

Figure 29 6-Aryl purines

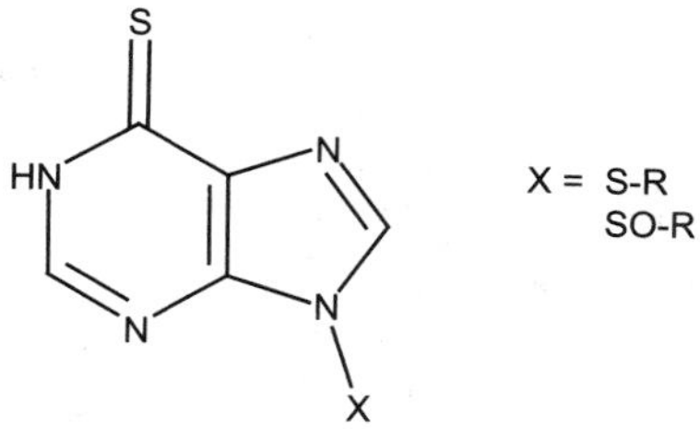

X = S-R
SO-R

Figure 31 Anti-TB compounds: 9-sulfonylated/ 9-sulfenylated 6-mercaptopurines

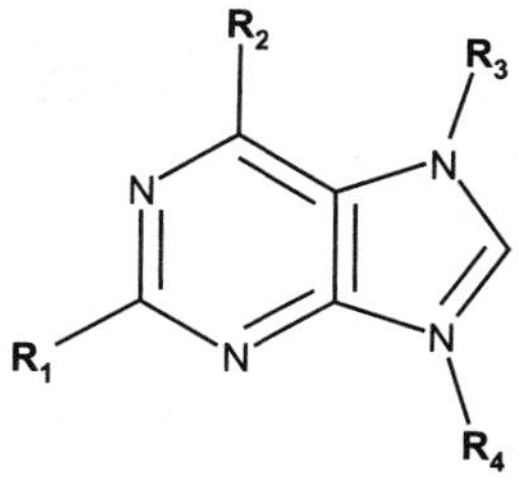

Figure 30 9-Substituted benzyl purines

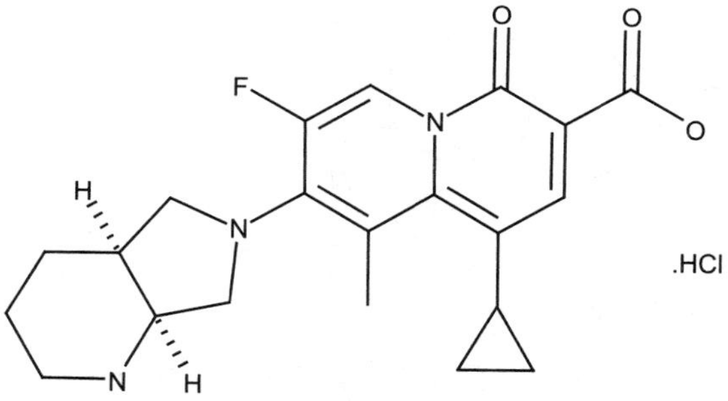

.HCl

Figure 32 ABT-255

Table 12 In vitro activities of purine derivatives against *M. tuberculosis*

Compound	R	MIC (μg/ml)
A	$4Br\text{-}C_6H_4$	0.78
B	$4\text{-}AcNHC_6H_4$	0.78
C	$2\text{-}O_2NC_6H_4$	0.78
D	$4\text{-}O_2NC_6H_4$	0.78
Rifampin		0.125

8.2. ABT-255

The MIC of AB-719, the prototype of 2-pyridones, was ≤0.4 μg/ml for susceptible and resistant M. *tuberculosis* isolates. ABT-255 (Fig. 32) is another 2-pyridone analog. Its in vitro activity is reported in Table 13.

Table 13 In vitro activity of ABT-255

Compound	MIC (μg/ml)
ABT-255	0.016–0.031
INH	0.5–0.78
Rifampin	0.016–12.5
Ethambutol	0.78–>25

ABT-255 exerts activity similar to that of INH against M. *tuberculosis* Erdman in murine M. *tuberculosis* infection (Table 14).

8.3. Pyrrole Derivatives

BM 212 (Fig. 33) is slightly less active than INH and streptomycin against M. *tuberculosis* but exhibits higher activities against non-TB mycobacteria (Table 15).

Table 14 ABT-255: in vivo efficacy in murine lung infection[a]

Compound[b]	Dose (mg/kg/day)	Log_{10} CFU/lung (mean ± SD)
ABT-255	25	1.43 ± 0.49
	12.5	3.58 ± 0.04
	6.25	5.55 ± 1.34
	3.13	7.0 ± 0.23
INH	25	1.69 ± 0.57
	12.5	2.0 ± 0.56
	6.25	1.96 ± 0.44
	3.13	2.37 ± 0.59
INH (RIF[r])	25	4.48 ± 0.25
ABT-255 (RIF[r])	25	5.24 ± 0.3
	12.5	6.58 ± 0.31
	6.25	7.46 ± 0.10
INH (EMB[r])	25	2.08 ± 0.48
ABT-255 (EMB[r])	25	4.13 ± 0.15
	12.5	5.62 ± 0.21
	6.25	6.52 ± 0.21
RIF[r]	50	7.37 ± 0.35
EMB[r]	150	7.28 ± 0.35
Controls		6.89 ± 0.23

[a]Data from Oleksijew et al., 1998.
[b]RIF, rifampin; EMB, ethambutol.

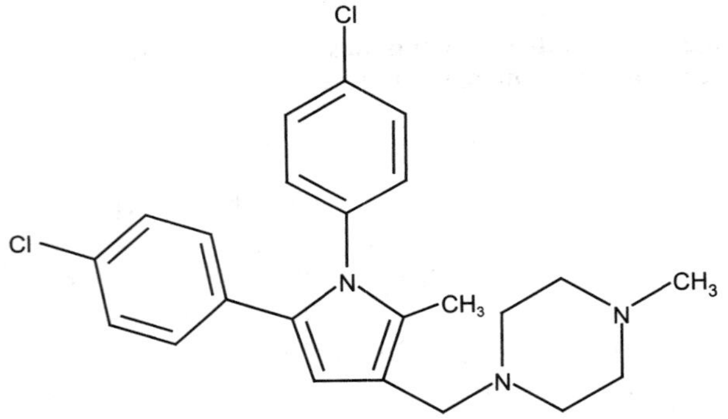

Figure 33 BM 212

M. *tuberculosis* was able to multiply in macrophages in control wells, where they increased from about 130 × 10^3 ± 77 × 10^3 per 10^6 cells (mean ± standard deviation) after infection to 380 × 10^3 ± 124 × 10^3 per 10^6 cells at the end of incubation. After 7 days of contact, BM 212 completely inhibited the intracellular mycobacteria. The effect was dose dependent, and the MIC was 0.5 μg/ml. Similar results were found for rifampin at 3.0 μg/ml (Deidda et al., 1998).

8.4. Thymidine Monophosphate Kinase Phosphatase (dTMP to dTDP)

Thymidine monophosphate kinase phosphatase is essential for DNA synthesis, and it has only 22% sequence identity with human thymidylate kinase. This enzyme acts in the synthesis of dTDP as the last enzyme of the synthesis pathway.

Between dTMP and the enzyme the links are the following:

- Pyrimidine ring and Phe70
- Hydrogen bond between O^4 of the thymine and Arg74 side chain
- Hydrogen bond between N^3 of the thymine ring and Asn100
- Hydrogen bond between 3′-hydroxyl dTMP and the terminal carboxyl of Asp9 (Mg^{2+} is responsible for positioning the phosphate oxygen of dTMP)

Hydrogen bonds and an ionic interaction occur between the 5′-*O*-phosphoryl group and Tyr39, Phe36, Arg95, and Mg^{2+}.

The presence of Tyr103 close to the 2′ position is believed to render the enzyme catalytic selective for 2′-deoxynucleotide (Vanheusden et al., 2002).

Inhibitors have been tested (Fig. 34).

8.5. Toluidine Analogs

A series of toluidine analogs was synthesized, and it was shown that the most active derivative bears an imidazole ring in the molecular structure (Fig. 35) (Biava et al., 1997).

8.6. Calmodulin-Like Compounds

Two chemical classes of calmodulin antagonists have been tested against M. *tuberculosis*: the phenothiazine and naphthalene sulfonamide classes. Among the compounds tested, only phenothiazine analogs showed in vitro activity but not in vivo, probably due to rapid liver metabolism.

8.7. Coumarin Derivatives

Coumarin analogs are important cores for drugs, anti-infectives (novobiocin) as well as DNA gyrase inhibitors, diuretics (mercumatilin), and anticoagulants (warfarin).

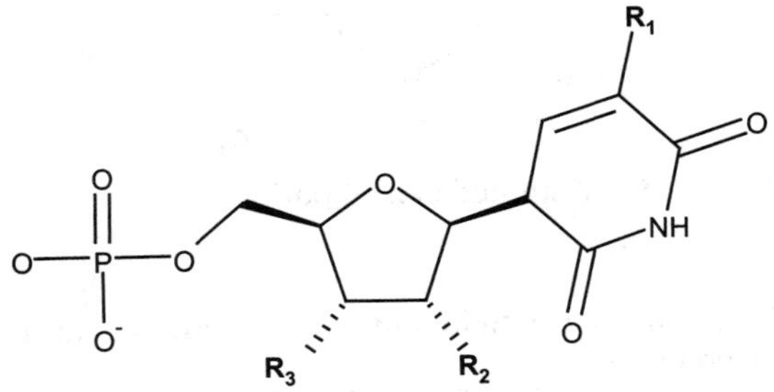

Figure 34 TMP inhibitors

Table 15 In vivo activity of BM 212

Microorganism	*n*	MIC (μg/ml)		
		BM 212	INH	Streptomycin
M. *tuberculosis*	19	0.7–6.2	0.05–0.2	0.4–6.2
M. *fortuitum*	8	3.1–12.5	12.5–50	25
M. *smegmatis*	6	3.1–25	50.6–>100	6.2–25
M. *gordonae*	6	6.2–>100	25–50	12.5–50
M. *avium*	14	0.4–3.1	25–> 100	6.2–25
M. *kansasii*	4	3.1–6.2	6.25–25	12.5–50

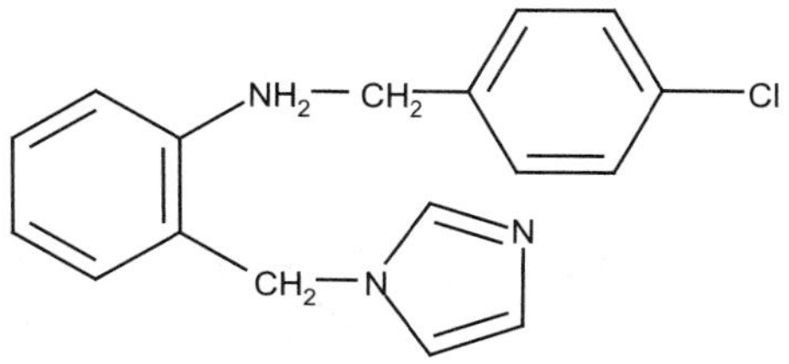

Figure 35 Toluidine derivative

Thiazolinyl hydrazones have been shown to exhibit antitubercular, antibacterial, and antifungal activities.

Within the first series of derivatives, the cyclohexyl substitution at position 3 of the thiazolidinone ring resulted in the highest antitubercular activity (Gürsoy and Karali, 2000; Karali et al., 2002).

8.8. Chaperonin Inhibitors

The molecular chaperones, or heat shock proteins, play a pivotal role in intracellular survival of *M. tuberculosis*. The chaperones play a central role in protein folding posttranslationally and are upregulated under conditions of stress.

GroEL and GroES receive unfolded polypeptides from DnaK and DnaJ posttranslationally for folding to the native state. Inhibitors of these chaperonins have been identified (Hartman, 2000) (Fig. 36).

8.9. Trifluoperazine Derivatives

It was shown that there is a correlation between *M. tuberculosis* growth and the presence of calmodulin-like protein, phospholipids, and lipids (Reddy et al., 1992). Trifluoperazine is a calmodulin antagonist and inhibits the incorporation of phospholipids into the phospholipid bilayers. It was shown that trifluoperazine inhibits the growth of *M. tuberculosis* H37$_{RV}$. In a recent study, trifluoperazine, an antipsychotic drug, displayed moderate activity against *M. tuberculosis*, even multiresistant isolates. It could be a companion drug when an MDR isolate is involved in this pathological process (Gadre and Talwar, 1999).

8.10. Phenothiazine Derivatives

Since the discovery of chlorpromazine in 1952 (Charpentier et al., 1952) the in vitro antibacterial activity of this class of drugs has been frequently demonstrated. Chlorpromazine and thioridazine have been shown to be active against MDR *M. tuberculosis* isolates and to also be highly concentrated in macrophages allowing them to display good antimycobacterial activity (Crowle et al., 1992). In a recent comparative in vitro study, the activity against 11 MDR tubercule bacilli was investigated for chlorpromazine, thioridazine, promethazine, promazine, and desipramine. It was shown that chlorpromazine and thioridazine inhibited the growth of 100% of the tubercle bacilli at a concentration of 12 μg/ml, but at 3 and 1 μg/ml the growth inhibition rates were 60 and 26%, respectively.

The peak concentration in plasma of thioridazine of 0.5 μg/ml is not sufficient to achieve antimycobacterial activity; however, thioridazine is at least 10-fold accumulated in macrophages that phagocytose mycobacteria (Crowle et al., 1992).

The antimycobacterial activity of promethazine was less pronounced than that of chlorpromazine and thioridazine. The least active compounds were promazine and desipramine (an antihistaminic drug) (Bettencourt et al., 2000).

8.11. Pyridines: Pyridinecarbothioamide Derivatives

Using a radiometric method to investigate the in vitro activity against *M. tuberculosis* and *M. avium*, it was shown that a new series of pyridinecarbothioamide derivatives of antituberculosis compounds exhibits good in vitro activity, with MICs from 1.0 to 2.0 μg/ml. The N-alkyl-1,2-dihydro-2-thioxo-3-pyridinecarbothiamide was chemically altered, and the antimycobacterial activities of the resulting compounds were investigated.

Two compounds exhibited good activity against *M. tuberculosis* H37$_{RV}$, with MICs of 0.5 μg/ml, but they were less active against *M. avium* (MIC, 4.0 μg/ml). Compound A exhibited good in vitro activity against MAC (the MICs ranged from 0.5 to 1.0 μg/ml) and against *M. tuberculosis* H37$_{RV}$ (MIC, 1 μg/ml) (Fig. 37).

Compounds B and C, having *N*-ethyl and *N*-heptyl groups, respectively, have different hydrophobicities, with logPs of 1.92 and 4.08, respectively. These compounds are poorly water

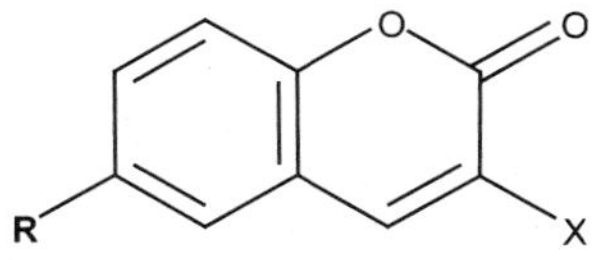

	R	X	MIC (μg/ml)
A	H	$CO\text{-}CH_2\text{-}Br$	12
B	Br		"
C	H	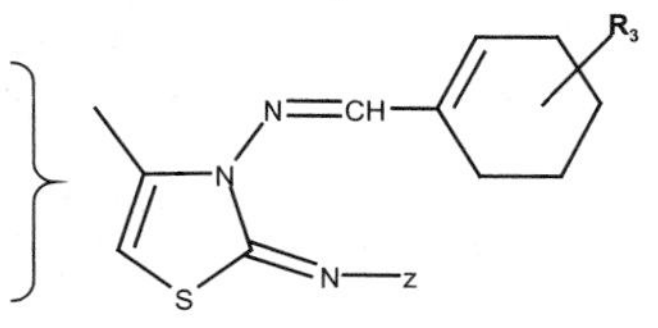	"
D	H		"
E	BH		"
F	Br		"
G			"
Rifampin			0.25

Figure 36 Chaperonin inhibitors

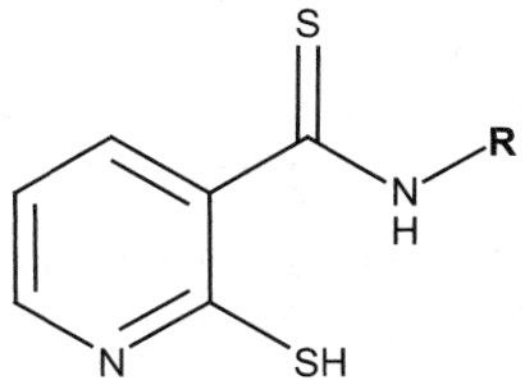

	R
A	C_2H_5
B	C_7H_{15}
C	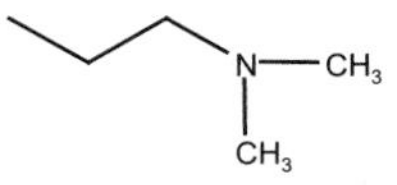
D	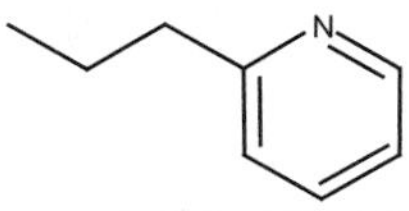

Figure 37 Pyridinecarbothioamide anti-TB agents

soluble. The 50% lethal doses after intraperitoneal administration of compounds B and C were above 200 mg/kg in mice and rats. These compounds are not absorbed orally in rats. After intravenous administration in rats, the apparent elimination half-lives were 37.2 ± 19.7 min and 28.0 ± 15.6 min for compounds B and C, respectively. They are rapidly cleared, with plasma clearances of 0.02 ± 0.007 liter/min and 0.05 ± 0.03 liter/min, respectively (Pagani et al., 2000).

It was shown that *N*-alkyl-1,2-dihydro-2-thioxo-3-pyridinecarbothioamides belong to a new class of anti-TB agents.

The pharmacokinetics of the various analogs depend on the amino substituent. When the substituent is an ethyl or a heptyl group there is a rapid elimination and poor absorption in rats.

For the *N*,*N*-dimethylaminoethyl analog) after intravenous administration, the apparent elimination half-life was 2.72 ± 0.6 h, with an area under the concentration-time curve of 6.9 ± 0.47 μg · h/ml. The hydrophilicity seems to be responsible for the pharmacokinetic improvement (Ubiali et al., 2002).

8.12. PDF Deformylase Inhibitors

BB-3497 (Fig. 38), a hydroxamate derivative with PDF deformylase-inhibitory activity, was shown to display anti-TB activity in vitro, with a MIC (geometric) of 0.25 μg/ml (Cynamon et al., 2004). However, it had been demonstrated with other hydroxamic acids that not all derivatives of this class exert anti-*M. tuberculosis* activity.

8.13. Diaryl quinolines (R-207910)

R-207910 is a diaryl quinoline derivative with anti-TB activity. R-207910 is a quinoline substituted with a methoxy group and a bromine atom and a naphthalene side chain with a dimethyl moiety (Fig. 39).

Table 16 shows the antimycobacterial activity of R-207910.

R-207910 exerts a time-dependent killing effect. A reduction of 3 $\log_{10}$ CFU/ml after 12 h at 10 times the MIC was observed (Andries et al., 2004).

The proportion of resistant mutants that emerged was 5×10^{-7} to 2×10^{-8} at four and eight times the MICs for *M. tuberculosis* and *M. smegmatis*, respectively.

The gene affected is that encoding the AtpE part of the subunit of ATPase synthase.

The point mutations identified were D32V and A63P for *M. tuberculosis* and *M. smegmatis*, respectively, which both are in the membrane-spanning domain of the protein.

Proton pump ATP synthase could be the bacterial target.

R-207910 is weakly active against *Helicobacter pylori* (MIC, 4 μg/ml).

In Swiss specific-pathogen-free mice, R-207910 is rapidly absorbed after a single dose of 6.25 or 25 mg/kg (Table 17).

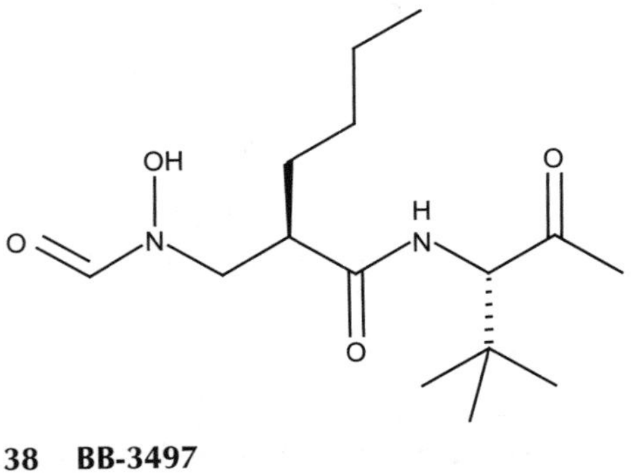

Figure 38 BB-3497

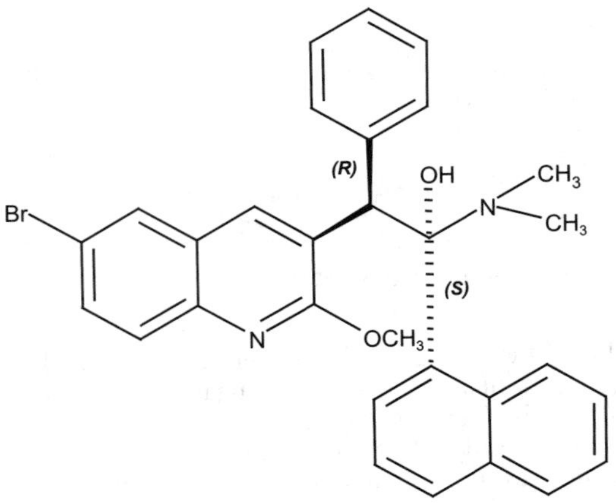

Figure 39 R-207910

Table 16 Antimycobacterial activity of R-207910

Microorganism	*n*	MIC range (μg/ml)
M. tuberculosis	6	0.03–0.12
M. tuberculosis INH^{r}	7	0.03–0.07
M. tuberculosis RIF^{r}[a]	1	0.03
M. tuberculosis, MDR	1	0.01
M. avium	7	0.007–0.01
M. kansasii	1	0.003
M. marinum	1	0.003
M. fortuitum	5	0.007–0.01
M. abscessus	1	0.25
M. ulcerans	1	0.5
M. smegmatis	7	0.003–0.01

[a]RIF, rifampin.

Table 17 Pharmacokinetics of R-207910 in mice

Dose	C_{max} (μg/ml)	T_{max} (h)	AUC (μg · h/ml)	$t_{1/2}$ (h)
6.25	0.4–0.54	1.0	5–5.9	
25	1.1–1.3	2.0–4.0	18.5–19.4	43.7–64

REFERENCES

Andries K, Verhasselt P, Guillemont J, Göhlmann HWH, Neefs JM, Winckler H, Van Gestel J, Timmerman P, et al, 2004, A diarylquinoline drug active on the ATP synthase of Mycobacterium tuberculosis, Sciences, online, 101–126.

Anonymous, 2001, Tuberculosis drug screening program—search for new drugs for treatment of tuberculosis, Antimicrob Agents Chemother, 45, 1943–1946.

Ashtekar DR, Costa-Perira R, Nagrajan K, Vishvanathan N, Bhatt AD, Rittel W, 1993, In vitro and in vivo activities of the nitro imidazole CGI 17341 against Mycobacterium tuberculosis, Antimicrob Agents Chemother, 37, 181–186.

Bakkestuen PK, Gundersen LL, Langli G, Liu F, Nolsøe JMJ, 2000, 9-Benzyl purines with inhibitory activity against Mycobacterium tuberculosis, Bioorg Med Chem Lett, 10, 1207–1210.

Barry VC, Belton JG, Conalty ML, Denneny JM, Edward DW, O'Sullivan JF, Twomey D, Winder F, 1957, A new series of phenazines (rimino-compounds) with high antituberculosis activity, Nature, 179, 1013–1015.

Berthelot P, Debaert M, Cremieux A, Baghadi N, 1983, Analogues cycliques de l'éthambutol, activité anti-mycobactérie, Il Farmaco, 38, 73–79.

Bettencourt MV, Bosne-David S, Amaral L, 2000, Comparative in vitro activity of phenothiazines against multi-drug resistant Mycobacterium tuberculosis, Intern J Antimicrob Agents, 16, 69–71.

Biava M, Fioravanti R, Porretta GC, Sleiter G, Etterre A, Deidda D, Lampia G, Pompei R, 1997, New toluidine derivatives with antimycobacterial and antifungal activities, Med Chem Res, 7, 228–250.

Bosi S, Da Ros T, Castellano S, Banfi E, Prato M, 2000, Antimycobacterial activity of ionic fullerene derivatives, Bioorg Med Chem Lett, 10, 1043–1045.

Bottari B, Maccari R, Montfort F, Ottana R, Rotondo E, Vigorita MG, 2000, Isoniazid-related copper (II) and nickel (II) complexes with antimycobacterial in vitro activity, Part 9, Bioorg Med Chem Lett, 10, 657–660.

Brennan PJ, Nikaido H, 1995, The envelope of mycobacteria, Am Rev Biochem 64, 29–63.

Brown FC, 1961, Chem Rev, 61, 463–470.

Chakraborty A, Gangdharam PR, Damle P, Pratt P, Wright P, Davidson PJ, 1981, Antituberculosis activity of 6-cyclo-octylamino-5,8 quinolinoquinone, Tubercle, 62, 37–41.

Charpentier P, Guillot P, Jacob R, Gaudechon J, Buisson P, 1952, Recherches sur les dimethylaminopropyl-N-phenothiazines, C R Acad Sci, 235, 59–60.

Cocco MT, Congiu C, Onnis V, Pusceddu MC, Schivo ML, De Logu A, 1999, Synthesis and antimycobacterial activity of some isonicotinoylhydrazones, Eur J Med Chem, 34, 1071–1076.

Cole ST, 2002, Comparative and functional genomics of M. tuberculosis complex, Microbiology, 148, 2919–2928.

Cox JS, Chen B, McNeil M, Jacobs WR, 1999, Complex lipid determines tissue-specific replication of Mycobacterium tuberculosis in mice, Nature, 402, 78–83.

Crowle AJ, Douvas GS, May MH, 1992, Chlorpromazine, a drug potentially useful for treating mycobacterial infections, Chemotherapy, 38, 410.

Cynamon M, Lang M, O'Railly T, Chmielewski A, Klemens S, 1997, In vitro and in vivo activities of new nitroimiazole derivatives against M. tuberculosis, 37th Intersci Conf Antimicrob Agents Chemother, abstract F-30, p 151.

Cynamon MH, Alvarez-Freites Z, Yeo A, et al, 2004, BB-3497, a peptide deformylase inhibitor, is active against Mycobacterium tuberculosis, J Antimicrob Chemother, 53, 403–405.

Cynamon MH, Gimi R, Guyenes T, Sharp CA, Bergmann KE, Han HJ, Grego LB, Rapoma R, Lucino G, Welch JT, 1995, Pyrazinoic acid esters with broad-spectrum in vitro antimycobacterial activity, J Med Chem, 38, 3902–3907.

Cynamon MH, Klemens SP, Sharpe CA, Chase S, 1999, Activities of several novel oxazolidinones against Mycobacterium tuberculosis in a murine model, Antimicrob Agents Chemother, 43, 1189–1191.

Deidda D, Lampis G, Fioravanti R, Biava M, Porretta GL, Zanetti S, Pompei S, 1998, Bactericidal activities of the pyrrole derivative BM 212 against multidrug-resistant and intramacrophagic Mycobacterium tuberculosis strains, Antimicrob Agents Chemother, 42, 3035–3037.

De Logu A, Onnis V, Saddi B, Congiu C, Shiva ML, Cocco M, 2002, Activity of a new class of isonicotinyl hydrazones used alone and in combination with isoniazid, rifampicin, ethambutol, para-aminosalicylic acid and clofazimine against Mycobacterium tuberculosis, J Antimicrob Chemother, 49, 275–282.

Dong Y, Xu C, Zhao X, Domagala J, Drlica K, 1998, Fluoroquinolone action against mycobacteria: effect of C-8 substituents on growth, survival, and resistance, Antimicrob Agents Chemother, 42, 2978–2984.

Dong Y, Xu C, Zhao X, Domagala J, Drlica K, 1999, Effect of fluoroquinolone concentration on selection of mutants of Mycobacterium bovis BCG and Staphylococcus aureus, Antimicrob Agents Chemother, 43,1756–1758.

Escuyer VE, White EL, Ross J, Cuningham AP, Suling WJ, 2002, A putative folate pathway gene in the Mycobacterium tuberculosis genome codes for dihydroneopterin aldolase, a potential drug target, 32nd Intersci Conf Antimicrob Agents Chemother, abstract F-753.

Gadre DV, Talwar V, 1999, In vitro susceptibility testing of Mycobacterium tuberculosis strains to trifluoperazine, J Chemother, 11, 203–206.

Gezginci MH, Martin AR, Franzblau SG, 2001, Antimycobacterial activity of substituted isosteres of pyridine and pyrazine carboxylic acid, 2, J Med Chem, 44, 1560–1563.

Glickman MS, Cox JS, Jacobs WR, 2000, A novel mycolic acid cyclopropane synthetase is required for cording, persistence, and virulence of Mycobacterium tuberculosis, Mol Cell, 5, 717–727.

Grandoni JA, Marta PT, Schloss JV, 1998, Inhibitors of branched-chain amino acid biosynthesis as potential antituberculosis agents, J Antimicrob Chemother, 42, 475–482.

Guillemin I, Sougaroff W, Cambau E, Revel-Viravau V, Moreau N, Jarlier V, 1999, Purification and inhibition by quinolones of DNA gyrases for Mycobacterium avium, Mycobacterium smegmatis and Mycobacterium fortuitum bv peregrinum, Microbiology, 154, 2527–2537.

Gundersen LL, Nissen-Meyer J, Spilberg B, 2002, Synthesis and antimycobacterial activities of 6-arylpurines, the requirements for the N-9 substituent in active antimycobacterial purines, J Med Chem, 45, 1383–1386.

Gürsoy A, Karali N, 2000, 4-(3-Coumarinyl)-4-thiazolin-2-one benzylidenehydrazones with antituberculosis activity, Arzneim Forsch, 50, 167–172.

Hartman GC, 2000, Molecular chaperonin inhibitors as novel anti-tuberculosis agents, 40th Intersci Conf Antimicrob Agents Chemother, abstract 2192, p 232.

Häusler H, Kawakami RP, Mlakor E, Severn WB, Stütz AE, 2001, Ethambutol analogue as potential antimycobacterial agent, Bioorg Med Chem Lett, 11, 161–168.

Heifets L, Lindhom-Levy P, 1992, Pyrazinamide sterilizing activity in vitro against semidormant Mycobacterium tuberculosis bacterial populations, Am Rev Resp Dis, 145, 1223–1225.

Igarashi M, Nakagara N, Hahori S, Doi N, Masuda T, Yamazaki T, Miyake T, Ishizuka M, Naganawa H, Shomura T, Omoto S, Yano I, Hamada M, Takeuchi T, 2002, Caprazamycin A–F, novel anti-TB antibiotics from Streptomyces spp, 32nd Intersci Conf Antimicrob Agents Chemother, abstract F-2031.

Iguchi K, Saitoh S, Yamada Y, 1989, Novel 19-oxygenated sterols from the Okinawa soft coral Litophyton viridis, Chem Pharm Bull, 37, 2553–2554.

Jagannath C, Reddy VM, Kailasam S, O'Sullivan JF, Pattisapu R, Gangadharam G, 1995, Chemotherapeutic activity of clofazimine and its analogs against Mycobacterium tuberculosis, in vitro, intracellular, and in vivo studies, Am J Resp Crit Care Med, 151, 1083–1086.

Karali N, Kocabalkanli A, Gürsoy A, Ates Ö, 2002, Synthesis and antitubercular activity of 4-(3-coumarinyl)-3-cyclohexyl-4-thiazolin-2-one benzylidenehydrazones, Il Farmaco, 57, 589–593.

Konig GM, Wright AD, Franzblau SC, 2000, Assessment of antimycobacterial activity of a series of mainly marine derived natural products, Planta Med, 66, 337–342.

Kremer L, Besra GS, 2002, Current status and future development of antitubercular chemotherapy, Expt Opin Invest Drugs, 11, 1033–1049.

Küçükgüzel SG, Rollas S, Küçükgüzel I, Kiraz M, 1999, Synthesis and antimycobacterial activity of some coupling products from 4-aminobenzoic acid hydrazones, Eur J Med Chem, 34, 1093–1100.

Kushner S, Dalalion H, Sanjurjo JL, Bach FL Jr, Safir SR, Smith VK Jr, Williams JH, 1952, Experimental chemotherapy of tuberculosis. II. The synthesis of pyrazinamides and related compounds, J Am Chem Soc, 74, 3617–3621.

Lin Y-M, Flavin MT, Cassidy CS, Mar A, Chen F-C, 2001, Biflavonoids as novel antituberculosis agents, Bioorg Med Chem Lett, 11, 2101–2104.

Maccari R, Ottana R, Monteforte F, Vigorita MG, 2002, In vitro antimycobacterial activities of 2′-monosubstituted isonicotinohydrazides and their cyanoborane adducts, Antimicrob Agents Chemother, 46, 294–299.

Matlola NM, Steel HC, Anderson R, 2001, Antimycobacterial action of B4128, a novel tetramethylpiperidyl-substituted phenazine, J Antimicrob Chemother, 47, 199–202.

McAdam RA, Weisbrod TR, Martin J, Scuderi JD, Brown AM, Cirillo JD, Bloom BR, Jacobs WR, 1995, In vivo growth characteristics of leucine and methionine auxotrophic mutants of Mycobacterium bovis BCG generated by transposon mutagenesis, Infect Immun, 63, 1004–1012.

McKinney JD, Honer zu Bentrup K, Munoz-Elias J, et al, 2000, Resistance of Mycobacterium tuberculosis in macrophages and mice requires the glyoxylate shunt enzyme isocitrate lyase, Nature, 406, 735–738.

McMillon FH, Leonard F, Meltzer RI, King JA, 1952, Antitubercular substances. II. Substitution products of isonicotinic hydrazide, J Am Pharm Assoc, 42, 457–464.

Morlock GP, Crawford JT, Butler RW, Brim SE, Sikes D, Mazurek GH, Woodley CL, Cooksey RC, 2000, Phenotypic characterization of pncA mutants of Mycobacterium tuberculosis, Antimicrob Agents Chemother, 44, 2291–2295.

Nasu SS, Young BKS, Hamann MT, Scheuer PI, Kelly-Borges M, Goins KD, 1995, Puupehenone-related metabolite from Hawaiian sponges, Hyrtios spp, J Org Chem, 60, 7290–7292.

Nicolas P, Tod M, Padoin C, Petitjean O, 1998, Clinical pharmacokinetics of diacerein, Clin Pharmacokinet, 35, 347–359.

Oleksijew A, Meulbroek J, Ewing P, Jarvis K, Mitten M, Paige L, Tovcimak A, Nukkula M, Chu D, Alder JD, 1998, In vivo efficacy of ABT-255 against drug-sensitive and -resistant Mycobacterium tuberculosis strains, Antimicrob Agents Chemother, 42, 2674–2677.

Onwuta US, Kanyok TP, Horgen FD, 1997, Extraction and antimycobacterial activity of an alkenyl resorcinol from Ardisia iwahigensis Elmer, 37th Interscі Conf Antimicrob Agents Chemother, abstract F-51, p 154.

Ottana R, Maccari R, Vigorita MG, Rotondo E, 1998, Synthesis of mono and di-cyanoborane adducts from isoniconoylhydrazone and cyanoborohydre, J Chem Res, S, 550–551.

Pagani G, Pregnolato M, Ubiali D, Terreni M, Piersimoni C, Scaglione F, Franschini F, Rodriguez-Gascón A, Pedraz Muñoz JL, 2000, Synthesis and in vitro antimycobacterium activity of N-alkyl-1,2-dihydro-2-thioxo-3-pyridine carbothioamides, preliminary toxicity and pharmacokinetic evaluation, J Med Chem, 43, 199–204.

Parrish NM, Houston T, Jones PB, Townsend G, Dick JD, 2001, In vitro activity of a novel antimycobacterial compound, N-octanesulfonyl acetamide and its effects on lipid and mycolic acid synthesis, Antimicrob Agents Chemother, 45, 1143–1150.

Phetsuksiri B, Baulard AA, Cooper AM, Minnikin DE, Douglas JD, Besra GS, Brennan PJ, 1999, Antimycobacterial activity of isoxyl and new derivatives through the inhibition of mycolic acid synthesis, Antimicrob Agents Chemother, 43, 1042–1051.

Rastogi N, Abaul J, Goh KS, Devallois A, Philogene E, Bourgeois P, 1998, Antimycobacterial activity of chemically defined natural substances from the Caribbean flora in Guadeloupe, FEMS Immunol Med Microbiol, 20, 267–273.

Reddy PH, Burra SS, Murphy PS, 1992, Correlation between calmodulin-like protein, phospholipids and growth in glucose grown Mycobacterium phlei, Can J Microbiol, 38, 339–342.

Reddy VM, Nadadhur G, Daneluzzi D, O'Sullivan JF, Gangadharam G, 1996, Antituberculosis activities of clofazimine and its new analogs B4154 and B4157, Antimicrob Agents Chemother, 40, 633–636.

Reynolds RC, White L, Ross LM, Seitz LE, Moore G, Leung A, 2000, Inhibitors of mycobacterial Ftsz polymerization, 40th Intersci Conf Antimicrob Agents Chemother, abstract 2030, p 226.

Rodriguez AD, Ramirez C, 2001, Serrulatane diterpenes with antimycobacterial activity isolated from the West Indian sea whip Pseudopterogorgia elisabethae, J Nat Prod, 64, 100–102.

Rodriguez AD, Ramirez C, Rodriguez GEM, 1999, Novel antimycobacterial benzoxazole alkaloid from the West Indian sea whip Pseudopterogorgia elisabethae, Org Lett, 1, 527–531.

Rodriguez AD, Ramirez C, Rodriguez I, Barnes CL, 2000, Novel terpenoids from the West Indian sea whip Pseudopterogorgia elisabethae (Bayer). Elisapterosins A and B—rearranged diterpenes possessing an unprecedented cagelike framework, J Org Chem, 65, 1390–1398.

Scorpio A, Zhang Y, 1996, Mutations in pncA gene encoding pyrazinamidase/nicotaminidase cause resistance to the antituberculosis drug pyrazinamide in tubercule bacilli, Nat Med, 2, 662–667.

Scozzafava A, Mastobrenzo A, Sapuran CT, 2001, Antimycobacterial activity of 9-sulfinylated/sulfonylated 6-mercaptopurine derivatives, Bioorg Med Chem Lett, 11, 1675–1678.

Sindelar G, Zhao X, Liew A, Dong Y, Lu T, Zhou J, Domagala J, Drlica K, 2000, Mutant prevention concentration as a measure of fluoroquinolone potency against mycobacteria, Antimicrob Agents Chemother, 44, 3337–3343.

Stover CK, Warrener PG, Sherman DR, Van Devanter NH, Langhome K, Tanaka K, Yan Y, Barry CE, Baker WR, 2000, A small molecule nitroimidazopyran drug candidate for the treatment of tuberculosis, Nature, 405, 962–966.

Suling WJ, Reynolds RC, Barrow EW, Wilson LN, Piper JR, Barrow WW, 1997, In vitro activity of lipophilic dihydrofolate reductase (DHFR) inhibitors against Mycobacterium tuberculosis and Mycobacterium avium complex, 37th Intersci Conf Antimicrob Agents Chemother, abstract F-42, p 153.

Suling WJ, Reynolds RC, Barrow EW, Wilson LN, Piper JR, Barrow WW, 1998, Susceptibilities of Mycobacterium tuberculosis and Mycobacterium avium complex to lipophilic deazapteridine derivatives, inhibitors of dihydrofolate reductase, Antimicrob Agents Chemother, 42, 811–815.

Suling WJ, Reynolds RC, Piper JR, Barrow EW, Gundy LE, Ginkel SZ, Westbrook L, Barrow WW, 1999, Vancomycin: structure activity studies of 2,4-diamino-5-deazapteridine derivatives as antimycobacterial agents and inhibitors of mycobacterial dihydrofolate reductase (DHFR), 39th Intersci Conf Antimicrob Agents Chemother, abstract 1812, p 339.

Suling WJ, Seitz LE, Pathak V, Westbrook L, Barrow EW, Zywno-Van-Ginkel S, Reynolds RC, Piper JR, Barrow WW, 2000, Antimycobacterial activities of 2,4-diamino-5-deazapteridine derivatives and effects on mycobacterial dihydrofolate reductase, Antimicrob Agents Chemother, 44, 2784–2793.

Takizawa Y, Takashi M, Takeda S, Aburada M, 2003, Pharmacokinetics of rhein from onpi-to, an oriental herbal medicine, in rats, Biol Pharm Bull, 26, 613–617.

Thangadurai D, Viswanathan MB, Ramesh N, 2002, Indigoferabietone, a novel abietane diterpenoid from Indigofera longeracemosa with potential antituberculous and antibacterial activity, Pharmazie, 57, 714–715. (Retraction, 59:336, 2004.)

Torikata A, Enokita R, Okazaki T, Nakajima M, Iwado S, Haneishi T, Arai M, 1983, Mycoplanecins, novel anti-mycobacterial antibiotics from Actinoplanes awajinensis subsp mycoplanensis subsp nov—taxonomy of producing organism and fermentation, J Antibiotics, 36, 957–960.

Ubiali D, Pagani G, Pregnolato M, Piersimoni C, Pedraz-Munoz JL, Rodriguez-Gascon A, Terreni M, 2002, New N-alkyl-1,2-dihydro-2-thioxo-3-pyridine carbothioamides as antituberculosis agents with improved pharmacokinetics, Bioorg Med Chem Lett, 12, 2541–2544.

Vanheusden V, Meunier-Lehman H, Pochet S, Herdewij P, Van Calenbergh S, 2002, Synthesis and evaluation of thymidine-5′-O-monophosphate analogues as inhibitors of Mycobacterium tuberculosis thymidylate kinase, Bioorg Med Chem Lett, 12, 2695–2698.

Van Rensburg CEJ, Jonne GK, Sirgel FA, Matlola NM, O'Sullivan JF, 2000, In vitro investigation of the antimicrobial activities of novel tetramethylpiperidine-substituted phenazines against Mycobacterium tuberculosis, Chemotherapy, 46, 43–48.

Vigorita MG, Basile M, Zappala G, Gabbrielli G, Pizzimonti F, 1992, Halogenated isoniazid derivatives as possible antitubercular and anti-neoplasic agents, Il Farmaco, 47, 893–906.

Vigorita MG, Ottana R, Zappala C, Macacari R, Pizzimonti FC, Gabbrielli G, 1994, Halogenated isoniazid derivatives as posssible antimycobacterial and anti-HIV agents—III, Il Farmaco, 49, 775–781.

Vittori N, Collins M, 1996, Production of rhein and rhein derivatives, worldwide patents WO 96/ 30034.

Wächter GA, Davis MC, Martin AR, Franzblau SG, 1998, Antimycobacterial activity of substituted isosteres of pyridine and pyrazine carboxylic acid 1, J Med Chem, 41, 2436–2438.

Wayne LG, Sramek HA, 1994, Metronidazole is bactericidal to dormant cells of Mycobacterium tuberculosis, Antimicrob Agents Chemother, 38, 2054–2058.

Welch J, Chung WJ, Kornilov A, Brodsky B, Higgins M, Sanches T, Spencer D, Heifets L, Cynamon MH, 2000, Novel aminomethylene analogs of pyrazinamide, PZA, possessing in vitro activity against M. tuberculosis in murine models of infection and intracellular activity against M. tuberculosis in infected human monocytes, 40th Intersci Conf Antimicrob Agents Chemother, abstract 2184, p 230.

White EL, Suling WJ, Ross LJ, Seitz LE, Reynold RC, 2002, 2-Alkoxy carbonyl amino pyridines, inhibitors of Mycobacterium tuberculosis FtsZ, J Antimicrob Chemother, 50, 111–114.

Wilkinson RG, Cantrall MB, Sheperd RG, 1962, Antituberculous agents III, +,-2,2-(ethylenediamine,-di-1-butanol) and some analogs, J Med Pharm Chem, 5, 835–845.

Xu C, Kreiswirth BN, Sreevatsan, S, Musser JM, Drlica K, 1996, Fluoroquinolone resistance associated with specific gyrase mutations in clinical isolates of multi-drug resistant Mycobacterium tuberculosis, J Infect Dis, 174, 1127–1130.

Youssef M, el Sayed K, Roa KU, et al, 2002, Oxamanzamines: novel biocatalytic and natural products from manzamine producing Indo-Pacific sponges, Tetrahedron, 58, 7397–7402.

Zhao BY, Pine R, Domagala J, Drlica K, 1999, Fluoroquinolone action against clinical isolates of Mycobacterium tuberculosis, effects of a C-8 methoxyl group on survival in liquid media and in human macrophages, Antimicrob Agents Chemother, 43, 661–666.

Zurenko G, Yagi BH, Schaadt RD, Al JW, Kilburn JO, Glickman SE, Hutchins DK, Barbachyn MR, Brickner SJ, 1996, In vitro activities of U-100592 and U-100766, novel oxazolidinone antibacterial agents, Antimicrob Agents Chemother, 40, 839–845.

Antibacterial Treatment of Leprosy

J. GROSSET

46

1. INTRODUCTION

Up until 1941, the year in which the antileprosy activity of the sulfones was discovered, there was no effective treatment for leprosy, although chaulmoogra oil, used for centuries in India and China, was considered to have a certain activity. Chaulmoogra oil has hydrocarpin acid for an active ingredient; it is a lipophilic compound and would be a typical substrate for broad multidrug resistance, as EmrAB or RND and ABC pumps.

Nowadays several antibiotics that are extremely active against the leprosy bacillus, *Mycobacterium leprae*, are available; they are prescribed in combination and at an early stage of the disease, with excellent results. The principles on which the combination of several antibiotics is based are now accepted by all leprologists, and multiple drug therapy of leprosy as recommended by the World Health Organization (WHO) is well established in this field.

2. AVAILABLE ANTIBIOTICS

Among the antibiotics available, four are currently in use: dapsone, rifampin, clofazimine, and a thioamide, i.e., ethionamide or protionamide. Others with weak antibacterial activity, including the sulfonamides, thiacetazone, and thiambutosine, are no longer part of the therapeutic arsenal. Finally, still others, the fluoroquinolones, 14-membered-ring macrolides, and cyclines, have only recently been shown to possess antileprosy activity and for this reason are still not part of the therapeutic regimens used in the field. Their properties are examined below in the paragraph devoted to current research in the chemotherapy of leprosy.

2.1. Sulfones

Synthesized in Germany in 1908, diaminodiphenyl sulfone or the parent sulfone (dapsone) is active against a number of bacterial infections in animals, but at effective doses it is highly toxic in humans. At the end of the 1930s, a derivative of the parent sulfone, glucosulfone sodium (or Promin), proved active against experimental tuberculosis in the guinea pig, but too toxic for use in humans. In 1941, Guy Faget administered it intravenously to lepers in Carville, La., and noted its efficacy. Shortly afterwards, Robert Cochrane tried it intramuscularly with success and launched the sustained-release form. In 1947, John Lowe replaced glucosulfone sodium with the parent sulfone orally, prescribed it at very much lower and hence much less toxic doses, and noted its marked activity. Used at low doses (100 mg daily), dapsone is cheap, well tolerated, very active, and hence very well suited to outpatient treatment.

2.1.1. Chemical Structure

All the sulfones active against *M. leprae* are derivatives of the parent sulfone, 4,4′-diaminodiphenyl sulfone, known as dapsone, the chemical structure of which is similar to that of the sulfonamides (Fig. 1). Diacetyldiphenyl sulfone, also called acedapsone or DADDS, is the sustained-release derivative most commonly used.

2.1.2. Mechanism of Action, Antibacterial Activity, and Pharmacokinetics

Like the sulfonamides, the sulfones are analogs of *p*-aminobenzoic acid, whose use in folic acid synthesis they

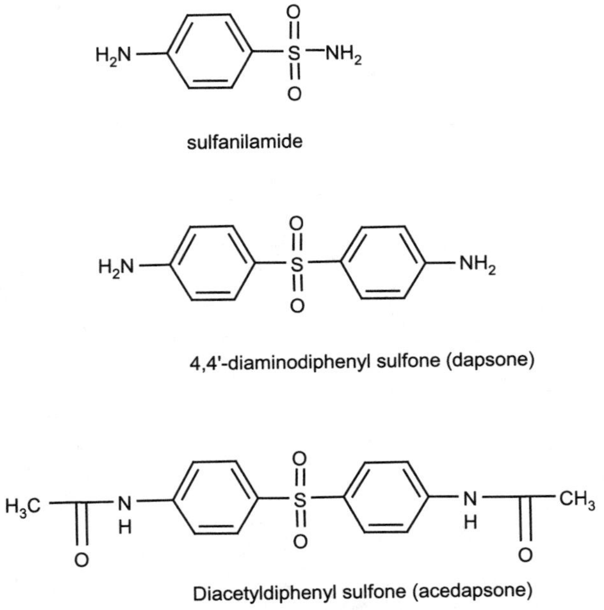

sulfanilamide

4,4'-diaminodiphenyl sulfone (dapsone)

Diacetyldiphenyl sulfone (acedapsone)

Figure 1 Comparative chemical structures of sulfanilamide, dapsone, and acedapsone

prevent by competition. More specifically, they are competitive inhibitors of dihydropteroate synthase (or dihydrofolate synthetase), an enzyme responsible for the incorporation of *p*-aminobenzoic acid in dihydropteroic acid, the immediate precursor of folic acid.

As *M. leprae* does not multiply in vitro, the antibacterial activity of antibiotics is evaluated in the mouse by inoculation in the footpad. It was shown (Shepard and Chang, 1962; Colston et al., 1978) that the MIC of dapsone for *M. leprae* is 0.003 μg/ml. Administered at a dose of 100 mg, dapsone has concentrations in serum in humans on the order of 1.5 μg/ml, i.e., 500 times the MIC (Table 1). At very much lower dosages, 10 and 1 mg/day, concentrations in serum are, respectively, 0.15 and 0.015 mg/ml and thus still above the MIC. At these dosages, the activity of dapsone is only bacteriostatic, whereas at 100 mg/day it is weakly bactericidal.

Dapsone is acetylated in the liver and excreted slowly via the kidneys. The rate of acetylation is genetically determined, so the serum elimination half-life, which is on average 24 h, differs from one subject to another; it ranges from 12 to 50 h. With daily treatment, there is an accumulation of dapsone and a risk of toxicity if the dosage is too high.

Dapsone diffuses well into the skin, adipose tissue, muscles, liver, and kidney and through the nerve sheaths. The ratio of concentrations in plasma to those in tissue is 0.6 to 1.

2.1.3. Resistance of *M. leprae*

Resistance of *M. leprae* to the sulfones emerges progressively. The first observation of sulfone resistance dates from 1964 (Pettit and Rees, 1964). It probably results from the successive selection of mutants with increasingly high levels of resistance to dapsone by a process similar to that described for the sulfonamides in bacteria culturable in vitro. The selection of low-level resistant mutants appears to have been encouraged by the low dosages used in the early years.

The progressive increase in doses used to overcome low-level resistance might in turn be responsible for the progressive increase in the level of resistance by the same process of selection of highly resistant mutants among low-resistance mutants. It is to avoid the sequential selection of high-level dapsone-resistant mutants that a daily dose of 100 mg of dapsone is recommended from the outset.

Acquired resistance to dapsone, very common in subjects suffering from multibacillary leprosy who relapse after several years of treatment with dapsone, is usually high level (Table 2). Primary resistance to dapsone, usually at a low level, is very common in regions of the world where dapsone has been extensively used. Its prevalence is close to 50% in a number of countries (Table 3).

2.1.4. Administration and Dosage

Dapsone is presented in the form of 100-mg tablets (Disulone). It is administered daily by mouth at a dose of one tablet in adults and 2 mg/kg of body weight in children. It may be administered by intramuscular injection of 600 mg once a week. The sustained-release form, DADDS, releases dapsone or its monoacetyl derivative very slowly, so the intramuscular injection of 225 mg of DADDS every 75 days has been extensively used in leprosy control programs. However, serum dapsone levels are very low, 0.02 to 0.1 μg/ml, and the antibacterial activity is much weaker than that obtained with 100 mg of dapsone per day.

Table 1 Principal pharmacokinetic parameters of the four antileprosy antibiotics

Antibacterial	MIC (μg/ml)	Dose (mg)	C_{max}/MIC ratio	$t_{1/2}$
Dapsone	0.003	100	500	24 h
Rifampin	0.3	600	30	3 h
Clofazimine	0.360.6	100	162	70 days
Thioamides	0.05	375–500	60	3–5 h

Table 2 Susceptibilities to dapsone and rifampin of strains of *M. leprae* isolated from previously treated patients (acquired resistance)

Years	*n*	Susceptible	Dapsone resistant		Rifampin[a]	
			0.0001%	0.001%	S	R
1980–1985	101	18	14	47	84	17
1986–1990	59	16	6	24	51	6

[a]S, susceptible; R, resistant.

Table 3 Susceptibilities to dapsone and rifampin of strains of *M. leprae* isolated from previously untreated patients (primary resistance)

Years	*n*	Susceptible	Dapsone resistant		Rifampin[a]	
			0.0001%	0.001%	S	R
1980–1985	133	81	37	8	133	0
1986–1990	147	110	19	4	146	1

[a]S, susceptible; R, resistant.

2.1.5. Tolerance and Toxicity

Side effects are very rare when dapsone is used at the recommended dosage of 100 mg daily in adults. At higher dosages, 200 or 300 mg/day, they are constant and comprise neuropsychiatric disorders, anemia, hypoalbuminemia, and neuropathies. Congenital NADH-dependent methemoglobin reductase deficiency may cause severe methemoglobinemia following administration of dapsone. Hemolytic disorders are observed in subjects with a congenital glucose-6-phosphate dehydrogenase deficiency. Allergic rashes, which may be accompanied by bullous skin lesions, have been described. However, the long list of complications recorded over the 30 years that dapsone has been used in the treatment of millions of lepers should not conceal its extremely good tolerance and its usual lack of toxicity.

2.2. Rifampin

Discovered in 1967, rifampin is a semisynthetic derivative of rifamycin SV, an antibiotic with a complex macrocyclic structure produced by *Streptomyces mediterranei* with potent bactericidal activity against both *Mycobacterium tuberculosis* and M. *leprae* (Fig. 2).

2.2.1. Chemical Structure

The rifamycins, rifamycin SV (Rifocine), rifampin (Rifadine and Rimactan), rifapentine (Priftin), and rifabutin (Mycobutin), all have the same central macrocyclic structure, which has led to them being referred to as ansamycins (ansa = loop). This central structure appears to be responsible for the antibacterial activity. The rifamycins differ from one another in the composition of their side chains (Fig. 2), and this difference is responsible for the pharmacokinetic properties.

2.2.2. Mechanism of Action, Antibacterial Activity, and Pharmacokinetics

Rifampin inhibits the functioning of mycobacterial RNA polymerase and that of other susceptible bacteria by binding to the β subunit of this enzyme, preventing RNA synthesis and ultimately protein synthesis. At concentrations active against M. *leprae*, it does not inhibit RNA synthesis in eukaryotic cells.

The MIC of rifampin for M. *leprae* is 0.3 μg/ml. After administration of a dose of 600 mg (10 mg/kg), the peak concentration is obtained in 2 to 4 h and on average reaches 10 μg/ml. At this concentration, rifampin is highly bactericidal to M. *leprae*. A single dose of 600 mg of rifampin renders M. *leprae* nonviable in the mouse, corresponding to bactericidal activity of between 99 and 99.99% for an initial percentage of live bacilli in humans of between 1 and 100%.

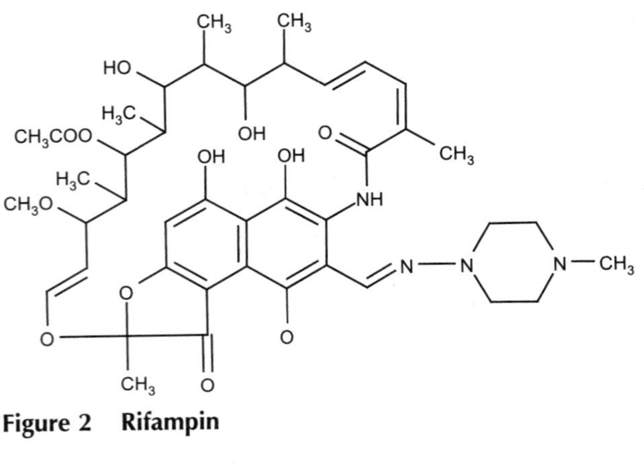

Figure 2 Rifampin

2.2.3. Resistance

Acquired or secondary rifampin resistance in M. *leprae* is rare. It was detected (Jacobson and Hastings 1976; Grosset et al., 1989) in patients relapsing after prolonged treatment with dapsone and then treated for a long period with rifampin alone (Table 2). For the time being, no confirmed case of primary resistance to rifampin has been described (Table 3). Rifampin resistance is accompanied in *Escherichia coli* by a modification of the gene coding for the β subunit (gene known as *rpoB*) of RNA polymerase. Recent studies (Honoré and Cole, 1993) have established that the same applies to M. *tuberculosis* and M. *leprae*. This discovery may lead to the development of a rapid method for measuring susceptibility to rifampin based on genetic engineering.

2.2.4. Distribution, Biotransformation, and Pharmacokinetics

Rifampin has excellent tissue diffusion, the concentrations obtained in tissue generally being equal to or greater than the concentrations in serum. The volume of distribution is high, 70 to 100 liters, and rifampin is 80 to 90% bound to plasma proteins. The liposolubility of rifampin gives it good intracellular penetration and good diffusion through the lipid-rich wall of M. *leprae*.

After oral ingestion and gastroduodenal absorption, rifampin is taken up by hepatocytes and then excreted via the bile in the form of unmetabolized native rifampin and rifampin metabolized to deacetyl rifampin, which is not liposoluble and hence not capable of being reabsorbed by the digestive tract. After several enterohepatic cycles, all of the rifampin is deacetylated and excreted in the stools. Hepatic deacetylation is microsomal and autoinducible. The peak concentration in serum of 10 μg/ml and the elimination half-life of 3 h at the beginning of treatment decrease progressively during the first few weeks of treatment to stabilize on average at 7 μg/ml and 2 h, respectively. In order to obtain high concentrations in plasma, the processes involved in the hepatic first-pass effect and in biliary excretion must be saturated. This can be achieved by administering high unit doses (10 mg/kg).

Rifampin is partially eliminated in the urine, coloring it red. The red color of the urine is good evidence of the ingestion of rifampin by the patient and of a sufficient dosage to cause high concentrations in plasma and urinary excretion. Urinary excretion, however, only plays an accessory role, and renal insufficiency in itself is not an obstacle to administration of rifampin.

2.2.5. Administration and Dosage

Rifampin is administered orally in the form of capsules containing 300 mg, or 150 mg in some countries. A syrup form is available for children. Rifampin may also be administered intravenously by infusion over 90 min, diluted in glucose solution. The standard unit dose is 10 mg/kg, or 600 mg in adults. Except in specific cases, such as severe hepatic insufficiency, the unit dose should be not less than 10 mg/kg and should be administered in a single dose to saturate the hepatic inactivation processes. Rifampin may be administered over short periods or in a single dose at 15 or 20 mg/kg, i.e., 900 to 1,200 mg in adults.

2.2.6. Drug Interference

Some medications interfere with the gastroduodenal absorption of rifampin: *p*-aminosalicylic acid, bentonite, and barbiturates. No interference with the other antileprosy antibiotics, however, has been reported.

Rifampin is a potent inducer of metabolism by hepatic microsomal enzymes. It causes acceleration of its own metabolism, but also that of drugs that are subject to the same metabolic pathway. This is the case with oral contraceptives (estrogen-progestogen combinations), orally administered anticoagulants of the coumarin type, glucocorticoids, digitoxin (Digitaline), and quinidine. The dosages of these drugs must therefore be increased during the prescription of rifampin and reduced when it is stopped. Induction by rifampin of metabolism by microsomal enzymes is marked in the case of daily treatment but negligible in the case of intermittent monthly treatment with rifampin.

2.2.7. Tolerance and Toxicity

Rifampin is usually well tolerated. In daily treatment, the most commonly observed side effect is the transient elevation of hepatic transaminases to no more than two to three times the upper limit of normal. Sometimes, and particularly in the case of preexisting hepatic impairment and the concomitant administration of hepatotoxic drugs (thioamides, for instance), the hepatic injury is severe and takes the form of anorexia, nausea, vomiting, and jaundice.

In intermittent treatment once to twice weekly, and particularly if the dosage of rifampin is greater than 10 mg/kg, immunohematologic disorders are observed in almost 20% of patients in the form of an influenza-like syndrome with fever, chills, and myalgia occurring within the first few hours of administration of rifampin. The influenza-like syndrome may be complicated by hypereosinophilia, interstitial nephritis, acute tubular necrosis, thrombocytopenia, hemolytic anemia, and shock. It necessitates the immediate discontinuation of rifampin. Rifampin is usually very well tolerated in once-monthly intermittent treatment at a dose of 600 mg.

2.3. Clofazimine

Clofazimine (B-663 or Lamprene) (Fig. 3) is a phenazine with a very pronounced orange-red color, synthesized in 1956 (Barry and Conalty, 1958) and initially proposed as an antituberculosis antibiotic. It is a crystalline substance which is insoluble in water but soluble in fats and ethanol.

2.3.1. Mechanism of Action

Clofazimine appears to bind to DNA and thus inhibit its replication (Morrison and Marley, 1976). It has an anti-inflammatory effect, which has been used to prevent and treat reactive episodes.

2.3.2. Resistance

Although one case of acquired resistance to clofazimine has been reported (Warndoff-Vandiepen, 1982), it has not been confirmed and no other cases have been identified.

2.3.3. Antibacterial Activity and Pharmacokinetics

The MIC of clofazimine for *M. tuberculosis* is 0.3 to 0.6 μg/ml (Grumbach, 1960). The MIC for *M. leprae* in the mouse has not been established because of the marked tissue binding of clofazimine and the low and variable concentrations in serum, on the order of 0.5 to 0.7 μg/ml after a daily dose of 100 mg (Banerjee et al., 1974). Its activity is weakly bactericidal. In humans, after 6 months of daily treatment with 100 mg of clofazimine, viable bacilli detected by inoculation in the mouse are still present in a third of patients (Jamet et al., 1992).

2.3.4. Administration, Dosage, and Distribution

Clofazimine, available in 50- and 100-mg capsules, is administered orally at a mean dosage of 100 mg/day. After partial absorption in the digestive tract, it is deposited in all of the tissues, but predominantly in adipose tissue and in the cells of the reticuloendothelial system. The very long apparent elimination half-life, on the order of 70 days, allows a wide variety of dosage regimens, for example, 50 mg/day supplemented by administration of 300 mg once a month, as in the therapeutic regimen recommended by the WHO, or a single dose of 1,200 mg once monthly, the efficacy and tolerability of which is virtually identical (Jamet et al., 1992). Clofazimine is sometimes administered at a daily dose of 300 mg to treat reactive episodes.

2.3.5. Tolerance and Toxicity

Clofazimine is well tolerated at the usual dosages. However, some patients have digestive disorders such as epigastric or abdominal pain and diarrhea. Others have skin disorders such as dryness of the skin or pruritus. However, the major drawback of clofazimine is the purple-reddish discoloration of the skin and conjunctiva that it causes. This discoloration, which is barely visible on black skin, is very marked in light-skinned subjects and may result in the refusal by the patient to take clofazimine. The discoloration disappears over a period of 1 to 2 years after stopping therapy.

2.4. Thioamides

The thioamides, synthesized by D. Liberman in 1956 (Rist, 1960), are represented by two molecules, ethionamide (Trecator), or α-ethylthioisonicotinamide, and protionamide (Trevintix), or α-propylthioisonicotinamide (Fig. 4). Derivatives of isonicotinic acid, like isoniazid, thioamides are second-line antituberculosis agents. Active against *M. leprae*, they may be used as a substitute for clofazimine.

2.4.1. Antibacterial Activity, Pharmacokinetics, and Distribution

The thioamides, ethionamide and protionamide, have comparable activities against *M. leprae* in both mice and humans.

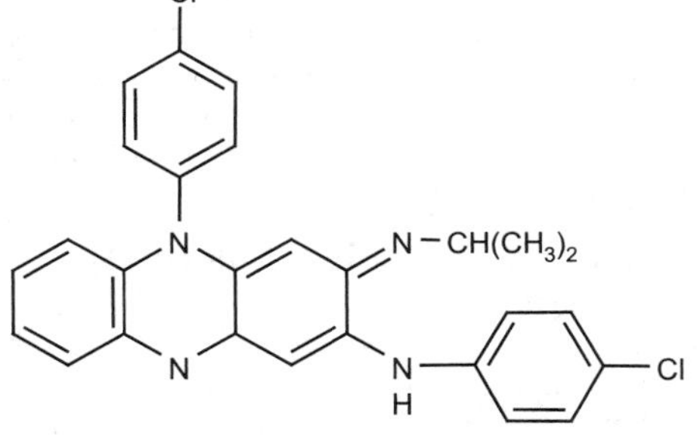

Cl
N
N
$N-CH(CH_3)_2$
N
H
Cl

Figure 3 Structure of the clofazimine molecule

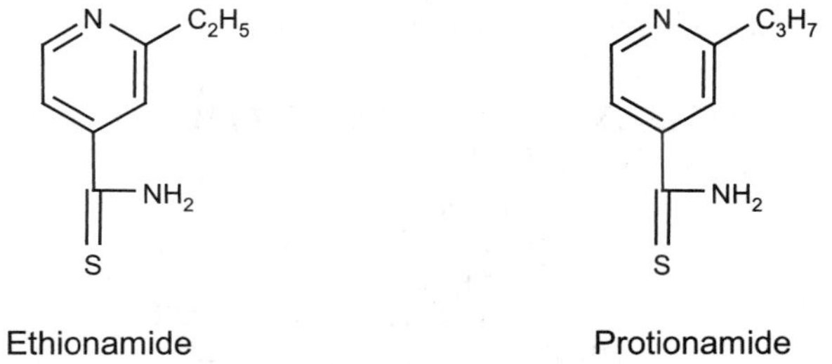

N C_2H_5 NH_2 S
N C_3H_7 NH_2 S

Ethionamide Protionamide

Figure 4 Chemical structure of ethionamide and protionamide

Their MIC is on the order of 0.05 μg/ml for M. *leprae* and, administered daily, their bactericidal activity is on the same order as or slightly superior to that of dapsone and clofazimine. The thioamides are not active by intermittent administration (WHO Study Group, 1982). After oral administration of 500 mg, the peak concentration in serum, 3 μg/ml is reached in 3 h and the apparent elimination half-life is 2 h (Ellard, 1990). Tissue distribution of the thioamides is excellent (Hamilton et al., 1962). The mechanism of action of the thioamides against M. *leprae* has not been elucidated.

2.4.2. Resistance

Acquired resistance of M. *leprae* to the thioamides has been demonstrated in patients suffering from lepromatous leprosy treated with thioamides alone (Pattyn et al., 1975).

2.4.3. Administration and Dosage

Ethionamide and protionamide are administered orally at maximum dosages of 1 g daily in adults and 15 to 25 mg/kg daily in children. A very much lower dosage (5 mg/kg) has been recommended to reduce the frequency of gastrointestinal disorders and the risks of hepatic toxicity (WHO Study Group, 1982). At this dosage, the thioamides have weakly bactericidal activity, similar to that of dapsone and clofazimine.

2.4.4. Tolerance and Toxicity

Gastrointestinal disorders—anorexia, nausea, and vomiting—are commonly observed in patients treated with thioamides. More serious conditions are hepatotoxicity, which takes the form of a marked elevation of transaminases to more than five times the upper limit of normal, and jaundice. Hepatotoxicity is observed, on average, in 5% of patients treated with the thioamides (Lesobre et al., 1968; Simon et al., 1969) and in 10 to 15% of patients treated with the combination of thioamides and rifampin (Cartel et al., 1983, 1985; Ji et al., 1984). For this reason, the use of thioamides is not recommended in leprosy control programs (WHO Expert Committee on Leprosy, 1988).

2.5. Other Antileprosy Antibiotics

The sulfonamides have long been used in place of dapsone. Having the same mechanism of action as dapsone but 100 times weaker antibacterial activity, they have no advantage over the latter and should disappear from the arsenal of antileprosy antibiotics (WHO Study Group, 1982).

The same applies to thiacetazone, an antibiotic with weak bacteriostatic activity against M. *leprae* and M. *tuberculosis*. It is active with daily administration at a dose of 150 mg but is inactive with intermittent administration. It may be responsible for serious cutaneous hypersensitivity reactions (Stevens-Johnson syndrome), the incidence of which is particularly high in subjects infected with human immunodeficiency virus (Grosset, 1992).

Isoniazid has no activity against M. *leprae*.

3. TREATMENT OF LEPROSY BEFORE MULTIDRUG THERAPY

The first antileprosy antibiotic used systematically was chaulmoogra oil (Jacobson, 1985). This is a traditional remedy of Burmese origin with limited and inconsistent activity. It was replaced at the end of the 1930s by the sulfonamides. Although undoubtedly active, they were only weakly so (Faget et al., 1942), and in their turn they were replaced by one of their derivatives, a sulfone known as glucosulfone sodium. Administered intramuscularly, it produced excellent results, but unfortunately it caused a number of side effects (Faget et al., 1943). Shortly afterwards, it was shown that the parent sulfone, dapsone (or diaminodiphenyl sulfone), was at least as active as glucosulfone sodium, but with the added advantages of being orally administrable at the low dosage of 100 mg daily in adults and of being well tolerated and cheap (Cochrane et al., 1949; Lowe and Smith, 1949; Lowe, 1950). Dapsone thus became the miracle drug for leprosy, and prolonged monotherapy with dapsone became the universal treatment for affected subjects. Early detection of the disease and its treatment with dapsone have, since the 1950s, been the basis for modern control of leprosy. In addition, the therapeutic results are excellent in countries or regions where this policy has been implemented, and the prevalence of the disease is declining.

Monotherapy with dapsone, however, has its weak points. As dapsone has limited bactericidal activity, it must be administered throughout the lifetime of subjects suffering from lepromatous leprosy and for at least 3 years in subjects suffering from tuberculoid or indeterminate leprosy. The length of treatment has commonly been the cause of poor compliance. More serious still, monotherapy is the origin of the progressive emergence of resistance of M. *leprae* to dapsone. Reported for the first time in 1964 (Pettit and Rees, 1964), dapsone-resistant strains have become increasingly common in lepromatous patients relapsing after prolonged monotherapy with dapsone (acquired resistance) and even in some patients before the beginning of their treatment (primary resistance as a result of being contaminated by patients carrying a resistant strain).

The discovery of clofazimine and subsequently of rifampin for some time offset this acquired dapsone resistance. Thus, relapsing patients with dapsone-resistant bacilli could be treated with clofazimine or rifampin. However, in its turn, monotherapy with rifampin, a highly bactericidal antibiotic (Levy et al., 1976), resulted in the selection of rifampin-resistant strains of M. *leprae* (Jacobson and Hastings, 1976; Ji, 1985; Grosset et al., 1989).

To prevent acquired resistance to antibiotics active against M. *leprae*, it was recommended (WHO Expert Committee on Leprosy, 1977) from the 1970s onward that leprosy, which like tuberculosis is a richly bacilliferous infectious disease, be treated with a combination of several antibiotics. In practice, with the failure of dapsone monotherapy, the validity of the scientific principles underlying multidrug therapy and its initial successes in the field resulted in the WHO in 1981 (WHO Study Group, 1982) recommending that all patients suffering from leprosy be treated by multidrug therapy.

4. TREATMENT OF LEPROSY BY MULTIDRUG THERAPY

Only the antibacterial treatment of leprosy, the principles on which it is based, the combinations with recommended antibiotics, and the results obtained to date in the field are discussed here. The therapeutic management of neuritis and reactive states and of the numerous other lesions of patients suffering from leprosy, albeit essential, is the subject of other chapters.

4.1. Theoretical Basis of Multidrug Therapy

Patients suffering from lepromatous or multibacillary leprosy, although in the minority in numerical terms, are the main sources of contamination by M. *leprae* and those in whom the selection of antibiotic-resistant mutant strains can most easily occur. The whole argument behind modern chemotherapy of leprosy (WHO, 1982; Grosset, 1986; Ellard, 1990, 1991) is therefore based on the treatment of these diseases, in the same way that the rationale for the chemotherapy of tuberculosis is based on the treatment of patients suffering from cavitary pulmonary tuberculosis. In both cases, it is the multibacillary nature of the mycobacterial infection that is the essential factor.

4.1.1. Different Bacterial Populations in Multibacillary Leprosy

In a patient suffering from lepromatous or multibacillary leprosy, the maximum number of bacilli may be estimated as 100 thousand million (10^{11}), of which, on average, 1% are viable, i.e., 1,000 million (10^9) viable *M. leprae* organisms (Shepard, 1974). The proportion of mutants resistant to dapsone, clofazimine, and rifampin among the 10^9 viable *M. leprae* organisms has still not yet been formally established because of the lack of an in vitro culture of *M. leprae*. However, by analogy with the known incidence of mutants resistant to antibiotics in *M. tuberculosis*, it may be estimated that there is one rifampin-resistant mutant for every 10^7 susceptible bacilli and one mutant resistant to dapsone, clofazimine, or ethionamide or protionamide for every 10^6 susceptible bacilli. If this is the case, a patient suffering from multibacillary leprosy harbors at most a population of 10^9 bacilli susceptible to all antibiotics, plus populations of 10^2 mutants resistant to rifampin and 10^3 mutants resistant to the other antibiotics (Fig. 5).

4.1.2. Objectives of Chemotherapy

To cure a patient bacteriologically, chemotherapy must be capable of preventing the selection of resistant mutants and eliminating all susceptible bacilli, or the largest possible number of them.

To prevent the selection of resistant mutants, a combination of active antibiotics must be administered until all of the resistant mutants present at the beginning of treatment are killed and the susceptible bacilli are sufficiently reduced in number not to be able to give rise to resistant mutants. The elimination of resistant mutants and that of the majority of susceptible bacilli are therefore the objectives of the initial phase of chemotherapy.

The subsequent phase, known as the continuation phase, is intended to eliminate the susceptible bacilli that have survived the initial phase. Because it is directed at a reduced number of bacilli, the risk of selecting resistant mutants has disappeared and should not necessarily be based on a combination of several antibiotics. Conversely, because it is directed at so-called persistent bacilli which are in a retarded metabolic state of life and much less accessible to antibiotic treatment, it must be based on one or more antibiotics capable of killing persistent bacilli, or be sufficiently long for the host's immune mechanisms to eliminate the majority or all of the persistent bacilli under the cover of antibiotics.

4.1.3. Initial Phase of Chemotherapy

Each antibiotic is known to be active against mutants resistant to other antibiotics as long as the antibiotics have different mechanisms of action. In principle, the combination of two antibiotics is therefore sufficient to prevent the selection of resistant mutants, since the number of live bacilli in a multibacillary leper is at most 10^9 and the incidence of mutants resistant simultaneously to two antibiotics is 1 to 10^{12} (1 to $10^6 \times 1$ to 10^6). Because of the frequency of primary and secondary resistance to dapsone (Ji, 1985; Guelpa-Lauras et al., 1987), it is, however, advisable to combine two antibiotics with dapsone. These two antibiotics are rifampin,

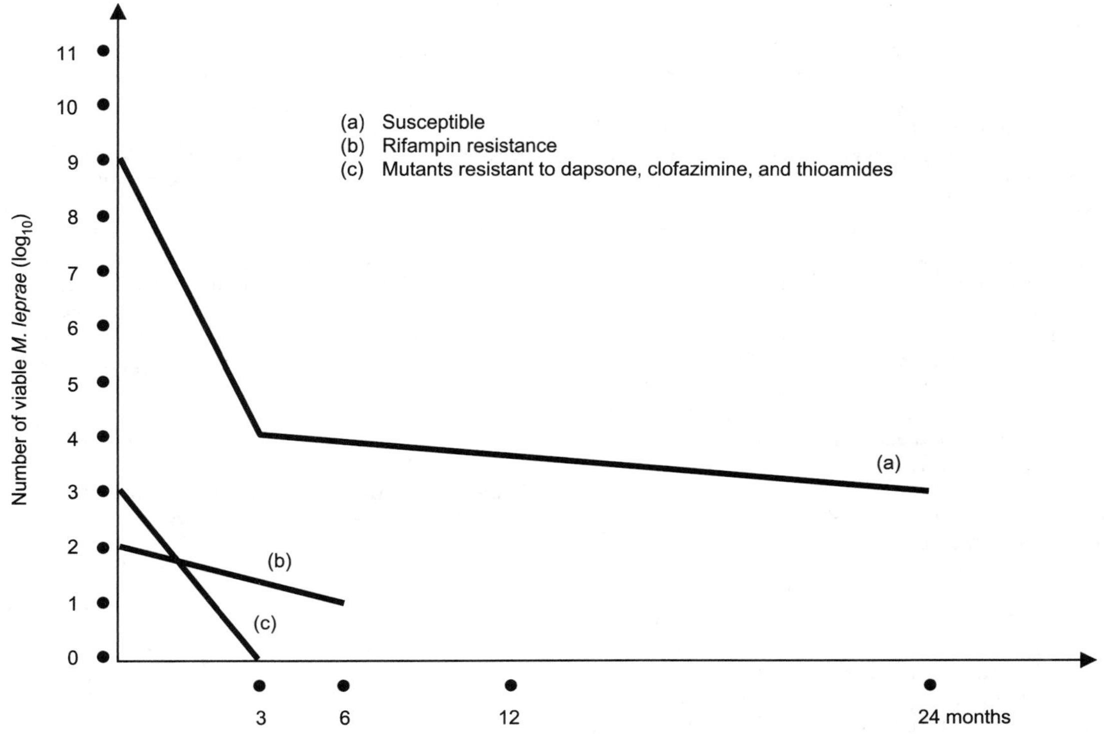

Figure 5 Principal viable microbial populations in multibacillary leprosy and their response to multidrug therapy during initial phase of treatment

because of its potent bactericidal activity, and clofazimine or one of the two thioamides. Clofazimine is perhaps slightly less bactericidal than the thioamides and causes a reddish-purple pigmentation of the skin, but its lack of hepatic toxicity means that it is preferred to the thioamides.

Dapsone, rifampin, and clofazimine therefore are automatically part of the initial phase of the chemotherapy of leprosy. The frequency and duration of administration of these antibiotics need also to be defined. In terms of the frequency of administration, dapsone must be administered daily at a dose of 100 mg in adults in order to be active. Sustained-release dapsone (acedapsone), injectable once a month, cannot be recommended, as it produces low, nonbactericidal concentrations in serum. In the case of clofazimine, studies (Jamet et al., 1992) have shown that administered once a month at a dose of 1,200 mg, it is as active as when administered daily at a dose of 50 or 100 mg. However, the custom of administering clofazimine daily in combination with dapsone has prevailed to date. Regarding rifampin, it is known that administration of a single dose of 600 mg kills more than 99% of viable bacilli, or at least as many as the daily administration of dapsone, clofazimine, or a thioamide for 3 to 6 months (Shepard et al., 1972; Levy et al., 1972). More recently (Thelep Subcommittee, 1987) it has been shown that after 3 months of daily treatment with 100 mg of dapsone and 100 mg of clofazimine combined either with 600 mg of rifampin daily, with 600 mg of rifampin weekly, or with a single dose of 1,500 mg of rifampin, the uniform outcome was 1 viable bacillus in 10^7. It may be concluded that the majority of bacilli are killed by the first dose or doses of rifampin and that it is not necessary to administer rifampin daily to obtain exceptional bactericidal activity (Ellard, 1991). Thus, in the leprosy control programs in the field, supervised monthly administration of rifampin is recommended, particularly as it often corresponds to the rate at which the medical teams pass by.

The duration of the initial phase depends finally on the rate at which the majority of susceptible bacilli and all resistant mutants are eliminated. The results of the Bamako-Chingleput study indicate that out of 10^5 viable bacilli at the beginning of treatment, only a single one remained 3 months after a single dose of 1,500 mg or the first few doses of 600 mg of rifampin. From 10^9 at the beginning of treatment, the total number of viable *M. leprae* bacilli in a patient suffering from multibacillary leprosy therefore fell to 10^4! The majority of susceptible bacilli and mutants resistant to dapsone and clofazimine, which by definition are susceptible to rifampin, were eliminated. Only 10^2 rifampin-resistant mutants are not killed by the first doses of rifampin (Fig. 5). They must be killed by the combination dapsone-clofazimine. As the length of time necessary for the combination of dapsone-clofazimine to kill rifampin-resistant mutants is not known exactly, it is advisable to administer this combination throughout the duration of treatment, particularly as the susceptibility of bacilli to dapsone may very well be reduced (Ji, 1985; Guelpa-Lauras et al., 1987).

4.1.4. Continuation Phase of Chemotherapy

After the initial phase of chemotherapy has reduced the number of viable bacilli to a level at which the risks of acquired resistance to antibiotics can be eliminated, treatment should still be continued to eliminate the 10^4 susceptible bacilli that have survived. This is the role of the so-called continuation phase. However, the major obstacle that confronts chemotherapy is that the proportion of bacilli capable of multiplying in the mouse remains constant, irrespective of the nature and frequency of administration of the antibiotics. After the rapid death of the majority of bacilli under the effect of the initial doses of rifampin, chemotherapy appears to have no effect on residual or persistent viable bacilli, even though they are totally susceptible to the antibiotics. It may therefore be wondered whether it is worthwhile continuing treatment beyond the first few doses of rifampin and, if so, for how long.

The first reason for continuing treatment beyond the first doses of rifampin is to prevent the risk of selection of rifampin-resistant bacilli. The second reason is that after very short-term multidrug therapy in patients suffering from Bamako multibacillary leprosy, it was found that the shorter the duration of antibiotic administration, the earlier relapses occurred (Table 4). Although not affecting the proportion of persistent bacilli, chemotherapy therefore appears to be active during the continuation phase. For these two reasons, chemotherapy should be continued after the first doses of rifampin, but for how long?

Three arguments may be considered. The first is that in the Bamako-Chingleput study, the bacteriological index, i.e., the number of *M. leprae* bacilli seen in the skin smears, decreased during treatment by 62% (0.62 $\log_{10}$) annually. If the regression in the number of persistent bacilli during treatment paralleled the reduction in the bacteriological index, this would require $4 \div 0.62 = 6.45$ years, or about 7 years of treatment, to eliminate all of the 10^4 persistent bacilli present in a patient suffering from very highly bacilliferous leprosy (Fig. 6). If this reasoning is correct, then the length of chemotherapy would depend on the initial bacillary burden, in practice the bacteriological index (Grosset, 1986).

One argument that supports the previous reasoning is that in patients in Bamako included in very short-term chemotherapy studies, relapses were significantly more frequent and earlier in highly bacillary subjects than in others (Table 5). In summary, there might be a relationship between the number of persistent bacilli and the risk of relapse and hence between the optimum duration of treatment and the initial bacillary burden.

The third argument is of a practical nature. In the campaigns to control leprosy in the field, it is difficult to adapt the duration of treatment to the bacillary burden of each patient. It is much more workable to standardize the durations of treatment for each of the two major categories of disease, multibacillary patients with a positive bacteriological index on the one hand and paucibacillary patients with a negative bacteriological index on the other. That is why, taking into account also the compliance of patients and health care officials with the treatments prescribed, the WHO Study Group (1982) and the WHO Expert Committee on Leprosy (1988) recommended that patients receive the standard treatments indicated below.

Table 4 Relationship between the duration of treatment with rifampin and early and late relapse rates[a]

Treatment duration	No. of relapses after treatment completion		
	Total	≤5 yr	>5 yr
≤3 mo	50	32	18
>3 mo	18	4	14
Total	68	36	32

[a]Data from Marchoux Chemotherapy Study Group, 1992.

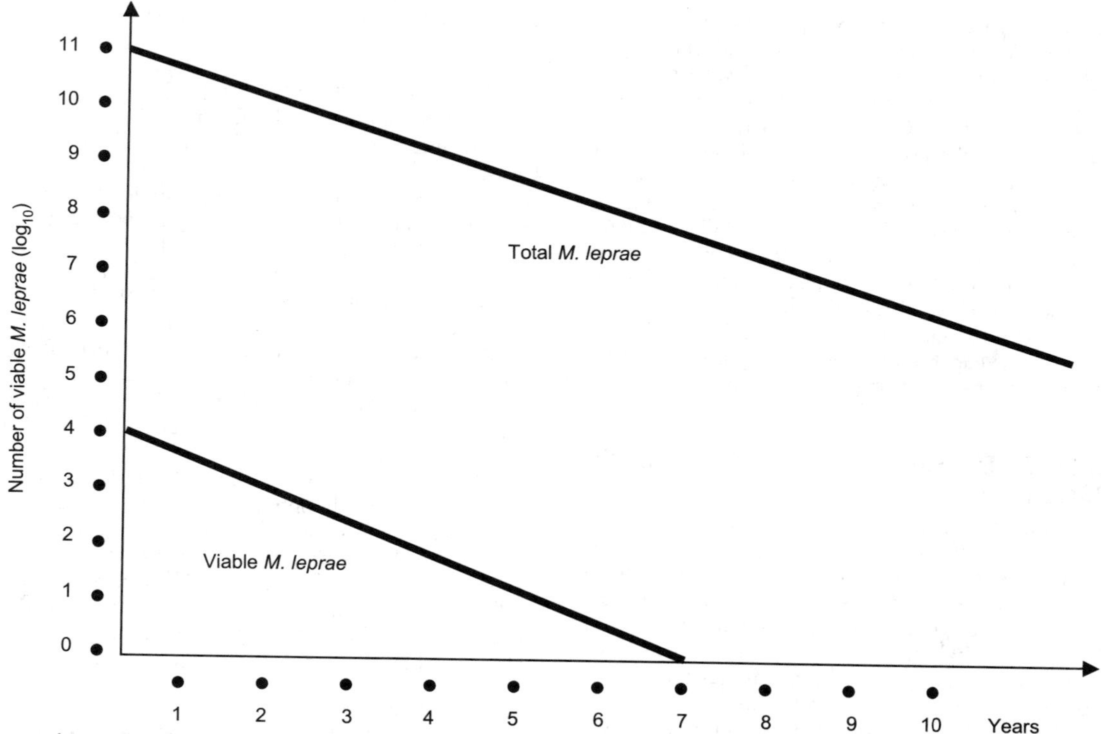

Figure 6 Regression of the total number of *M. leprae* bacilli and the probable number of viable *M. leprae* bacilli persisting on multidrug therapy in multibacillary leprosy

Table 5 Relationship between bacteriological index on discontinuation of treatment and relapse rate[a]

Bacteriological index at treatment end	No. of patients	Relapses	
		No.	%
≥5+	197	42	21.3
≤4+	184	25	13.6
Total	381	67	17.5

[a]Data from Marchoux Chemotherapy Study Group, 1992.

4.2. Therapeutic Regimens Recommended by the WHO

Patients suffering from paucibacillary leprosy, defined as a negative bacteriological index at all sampling sites, must be treated for 6 months with rifampin at 600 mg once monthly under supervision and with 100 mg daily of dapsone (1 to 2 mg/kg) by self-administration.

Patients suffering from multibacillary leprosy, defined as a positive bacteriological index at one sampling site at least, must be treated for a minimum of 2 years, and preferably until the bacteriological index is negative, with the following three antibiotics: rifampin at 600 mg, once monthly under supervision; dapsone at 100 mg (1 to 2 mg/kg) daily, self-administered; and clofazimine at 50 mg daily, self-administered, and 300 mg once monthly under supervision.

4.3. Results of WHO Standard Multidrug Therapy

Since the WHO recommendations in 1982 and 1988, multidrug therapy has been used in a number of countries around the world. At the end of 1991, almost four million patients had received or were receiving treatment with multidrug therapy. The two therapeutic regimens were well tolerated by the patients, with the exception of the discoloration caused by clofazimine, which has been a problem in light-skinned subjects (Becx-Bleuminck, 1989). The side effects have been rare and nonserious. The regimens have also been very effective. Clinical improvement has been rapid, and in leprosy control programs in the field, the relapse rates after discontinuation of treatment have been less than 0.1% per year in 85,000 paucibacillary patients and less than 0.06% in 22,000 multibacillary patients (S.K. Noordeen, personal communication). In the therapeutic trials conducted with the support of the WHO, the figures were 0.4% during the first year following discontinuation of treatment in paucibacillary patients (Boerrigter et al., 1988) and 0 in more than 8,000 patient years of follow-up in multibacillary patients (UNDP/World Bank/WHO, 1989). It is important to stress that the clinically active lesions were still present at the end of treatment in 4 to 28% of the paucibacillary patients (Boerrigter et al., 1988; Katoch et al., 1989). For patients and health care officials, these lesions were obviously considered to be still active and requiring treatment, although they could improve and even disappear after the discontinuation of treatment (Becx-Bleuminck, 1989). Opposite reactions occur in 5 to 9% of patients after the discontinuation of treatment (Boerrigter et al., 1988; Katoch et al., 1989) and may cause irreversible nerve lesions. The low relative incidence of persistent lesions and reactive episodes after 6 months argues against recommending a systematic extension of treatment of paucibacillary patients up to 12 months. Conversely, the prolongation or reintroduction of treatment in similar circumstances can very well be decided on a case-by-case basis (WHO Expert Committee on Leprosy, 1988).

In multibacillary patients, in leprosy control programs in the field, and in therapeutic trials conducted with the support of the WHO, no relapse was observed in the 5 years following the discontinuation of treatment, even in patients who received only 2 years of WHO multidrug therapy. This observation is evidence of the potent bactericidal activity of the recommended therapeutic regimen and its capacity to prevent the early resurgence of persistent bacilli. Another equally important observation is that all of the multibacillary patients who relapsed after very short-term multidrug therapy and the only patient who relapsed after 2 years of multidrug therapy (Constant-Desportes et al., 1991) had bacilli that remained susceptible to the antibiotics administered. Multidrug therapy thus appears to be capable of achieving its first objective, which is to prevent the selection of resistant mutants.

5. CURRENT RESEARCH IN CHEMOTHERAPY OF LEPROSY

Given the excellent efficacy of the therapeutic regimens recommended by the WHO, the current priority in the chemotherapy of leprosy in all countries in which it is not yet the case is to create the conditions for their implementation, to apply them on the ground, and to evaluate their results from a threefold clinical, bacteriological, and epidemiological viewpoint. At the same time, the researcher must try to improve existing regimens, at least in two areas: those of its duration and its supervision. Although the minimum 2-year treatment with WHO multidrug therapy is a considerable advance over lifetime treatment with dapsone, it still remains difficult to implement in certain regions (Ji and Grosset, 1990), and in those in which it is properly applied, it is not always regularly observed by patients (Ellard et al., 1988). Having access to shorter or totally supervised treatment or, better still, to treatment that is both short and totally supervised would therefore be of major interest.

5.1. Possible Improvements in WHO Multidrug Therapy

It is difficult to reduce the duration of the multidrug therapy recommended by the WHO. It is based on the combination of the three best-tolerated antibiotics, rifampin, dapsone, and clofazimine, of which only rifampin is highly bactericidal. It is therefore not possible to increase its antibacterial activity, particularly as the fourth antibiotic available, ethionamide or protionamide, is not more strongly bactericidal and is not recommended because of its potential hepatic toxicity. Conversely, the supervision of multidrug therapy might be improved by administering clofazimine monthly. In fact, it has been shown (Jamet et al., 1992) that monthly administration of 1,200 mg of clofazimine was as bactericidal as daily administration of 50 mg combined with a monthly administration of 300 mg. If it could be shown that a monthly dose of 900 mg was better tolerated and as bactericidal as administration of 1,200 mg, the administration of clofazimine could be totally supervised (S. K. Noordeen, personal communication).

5.2. New Antileprosy Antibiotics

New antibiotics highly bactericidal against M. *leprae* are required to shorten the duration of treatment or develop a totally supervised treatment. Ideally, these new antibiotics should have a mechanism of action different from that of the existing antibiotics, act in synergy with them, be well tolerated, and be administrable orally in a single daily dose. Currently, three antibiotics or families of antibiotics meet these requirements.

5.2.1. Fluoroquinolones

The fluoroquinolones are inhibitors of the DNA gyrase complex, the enzyme involved in the synthesis of bacterial DNA. Consequently, they have a mechanism of action different from that of the other antileprosy antibiotics. Among these, pefloxacin and ofloxacin have potent bactericidal activity against M. *leprae* in the mouse (Guelpa-Lauras et al., 1987; Grosset et al., 1988). In humans, 22 daily doses of 800 mg of pefloxacin or 400 mg of ofloxacin kill 99.99% of viable bacilli at the beginning of treatment (Ndeli et al., 1990; Grosset et al., 1990). The clinical improvement is spectacular and the side effects are minor, except in the case of one patient treated daily with 800 mg of pefloxacin, who suffered a confusional episode that resolved spontaneously on discontinuation of treatment.

Minocycline acts on ribosomal bacterial protein synthesis. A particularly lipophilic antibiotic, it is active against M. *leprae*, whereas the other cyclines are inactive. In the mouse, like the fluoroquinolones it has potent bactericidal activity (Gelber, 1987; Ji et al., 1993). In humans, it is very well tolerated when administered at a dose of 100 mg daily. It causes a rapid clinical improvement and kills more than 99% of viable bacilli in 1 month (Ji et al., 1993).

5.2.2. Clarithromycin

A derivative of erythromycin A, clarithromycin inhibits bacterial protein synthesis by a mechanism different from that of minocycline. In the mouse, it is highly bactericidal against M. *leprae* and its combination with minocycline or with minocycline plus rifampin has an additive effect (Ji et al., 1991). In humans, it is very well tolerated when administered at a dose of 500 mg daily, causes a rapid clinical improvement, and kills more than 99% of viable bacilli in 1 month. Its antibacterial activity is as bactericidal as that of minocycline. The combination of clarithromycin and minocycline is apparently no more active than each of the antibiotics used alone, perhaps because of their spectacular activity.

5.2.3. Other Antibiotics

Research is continuing with the aim of developing phenazine derivatives that do not have the adverse effects of clofazimine. So far, efforts have not been successful (Franzblau et al., 1989). Derivatives of rifamycin, particularly rifapentine, rifabutin, and R-76-1, have been tested in mice infected with M. *leprae* in parallel with rifampin. All of these derivatives are slightly more active than rifampin for equal weight, but all have cross-resistance with it (Ji and Grosset, 1990). Their potential value as a replacement for rifampin is therefore not apparent. β-Lactams, penicillins, and cephalosporins, as well as certain aminoglycosides, have bactericidal activity against M. *leprae* in the mouse. However, all have to be administered parenterally and therefore do not have a place in the new therapeutic regimens for leprosy.

5.3. Therapeutic Regimens Under Study

A new therapeutic regimen is of interest only if it is clearly more effective than the current multidrug therapy recommended by the WHO in terms of acceptability, treatment duration, and supervision, or if it can replace it in the case of proven rifampin resistance.

In the regions of the world where clofazimine is poorly accepted because of the reddish-purple color that it imparts to the skin, it might be replaced by a fluoroquinolone, clarithromycin, or minocycline, on the condition that the tolerance, cost, duration, and frequency of administration of the substitute antibiotic are acceptable. Minocycline might be an ideal candidate for this replacement were it not banned in pregnant women and young children.

As ofloxacin is capable of killing 99.99% of viable bacilli, i.e., as many as the combination of dapsone and clofazimine in 2 years, it is possible that daily treatment for 28 days with the combination rifampin-ofloxacin is as active as WHO multidrug therapy for 24 months, which comprises only 24 doses of rifampin monthly. To test this hypothesis, a multicenter therapeutic trial has just been undertaken under the aegis of the WHO.

Another line of research is that of totally supervised treatment in which the daily dose of dapsone and clofazimine is replaced by supervised monthly administration of one or more new antibiotics. For this, it must be shown that the new antibiotics, perhaps the combination minocycline-clarithromycin or the triple combination minocycline-clarithromycin-ofloxacin, are as bactericidal in a monthly dose as the combination dapsone-clofazimine in a daily dose. The promising results obtained in mice (Ji et al., 1993) must be confirmed in humans.

The new antibiotics may also be used simultaneously with dapsone and rifampin for the treatment of patients carrying resistant *M. leprae*. Although there are still few of these patients (Jacobson and Hastings, 1976; Grosset et al., 1989), they must be treated as priorities to prevent the dissemination of their bacilli. A daily treatment regimen that is definitely effective might combine ofloxacin at 400 mg plus clarithromycin at 500 mg plus minocycline at 100 mg plus clofazimine at 100 mg initially for 2 to 3 months, followed for a 6-month phase by clarithromycin at 500 mg plus minocycline at 100 mg plus clofazimine at 50 mg, and finally minocycline at 100 mg plus clofazimine at 50 mg or clofazimine at 50 mg alone until the bacteriological index was completely negative.

REFERENCES

Banerjee DK, Ellard GA, Gammon T, Waters MFR, 1974, Some observations on the pharmacology of clofazimine, Am J Trop Med Hyg, 23, 1110–1115.

Barry VC, Conalty ML, 1958, Antituberculosis activity in the phenazine series. II. N^3-substituted anilino-apo-safranines (rimino-compounds) and some derivatives, Am Rev Tuberc Pulm Dis, 78, 62–73.

Becx-Bleuminck M, 1989, Operational aspects of multidrug therapy, Int J Lepr Other Mycobact Dis, 57, 540–541.

Boerrigter G, Ponnighaus JM, Fine PEM, 1988, Preliminary appraisal of a WHO-recommended multiple drug regimen in paucibacillary leprosy patients in Malawi, Int J Lepr Other Mycobact Dis, 56, 408–417.

Cartel JL, Millan J, Guelpa-Lauras CC, Grosset JH, 1983, Hepatitis in leprosy patients treated with a daily combination of dapsone, rifampin, and a thioamide, Int J Lepr Other Mycobact Dis, 51, 461–465.

Cartel JL, Naudillon Y, Artus JC, Grosset JH, 1985, Hepatotoxicity of the daily combination of 5 mg/kg prothionamide + 10 mg/kg rifampin, Int J Lepr Other Mycobact Dis, 53, 15–18.

Cochrane RG, Ramanujam K, Paul H, Russel D, 1949, Two-and-a-half years' experimental work on the sulphone group of drugs, Lepr Rev, 20, 4–64.

Colston MJ, Hilson GRF, Banerjee DK, 1978, The proportional bactericidal test, a method for assessing bactericidal activity of drugs against Mycobacterium leprae in mice, Lepr Rev, 49, 7–15.

Constant-Desportes M, Guelpa-Lauras CC, Carolina JC, Leoture A, Grosset JH, Sansarricq H, 1991, A case of relapse with drug-susceptible M. leprae after multidrug therapy, Int J Lepr Other Mycobact Dis, 59, 242–247.

Ellard GA, 1990, The chemotherapy of leprosy. Part 1, Int J Lepr Other Mycobact Dis, 58, 704–716.

Ellard GA, 1991, The chemotherapy of leprosy. Part 2, Int J Lepr Other Mycobact Dis, 59, 82–94.

Ellard GA, Pannikar VK, Jesudasan K, Christian M, 1988, Clofazimine and dapsone compliance in leprosy, Lepr Rev, 59, 205–213.

Faget GH, Johansen FA, Ross H, 1942, Sulfanilamide in the treatment of leprosy, Public Health Rep, 57, 1892–1899.

Faget GH, Pogge RC, Johansen FA, Dinan JF, Prejean BM, Eccles CG, 1943, The promin treatment of leprosy: a progress report, Public Health Rep, 58, 1729–1741.

Franzblau SG, White KE, O'Sullivan JF, 1989, Structure-activity relationships of tetramethylpiperidine-substituted phenazines against *Mycobacterium leprae* in vitro, Antimicrob Agents Chemother, 53, 2004–2005.

Gelber RH, 1987, Activity of minocycline in Mycobacterium leprae-infected mice, J Infect Dis, 18, 236–239.

Gerald L, Mandell MA, 1990, Drugs used in the chemotherapy of tuberculosis and leprosy, p 1146–1164, in Goodman and Gilman, The Pharmacological Basis of Therapeutics. Antimicrobial Agents, 8th ed, Pergamon Press, Inc.

Grosset J, 1992, Treatment of tuberculosis in HIV infection, Tuber Lung Dis, 71, 378–383.

Grosset JH, 1986, Recent developments in the field of multidrug therapy and future research in chemotherapy of leprosy, Lepr Rev, 57, Suppl, 223–234.

Grosset JH, Guelpa-Lauras CC, Bobin P, Brucker G, Cartel JL, Constant-Desportes M, Flageul B, Frederic M, Guillaume JC, Milian J, 1989, Study of 39 documented relapses of multibacillary leprosy after treatment with rifampin, Int J Lepr Other Mycobact Dis, 57, 607–614.

Grosset JH, Guelpa-Lauras CC, Perani EG, Beoletto C, 1988, Activity of ofloxacin against Mycobacterium leprae in the mouse, Int J Lepr Other Mycobact Dis, 56, 259–264.

Grosset JH, Ji B, Guelpa-Lauras CC, Perani EG, Ndeli L, 1990, Clinical trial of pefloxacin and ofloxacin in the treatment of lepromatous leprosy, Int J Lepr Other Mycobact Dis, 58, 281–295.

Grumbach F, 1960, Activité anti tuberculeuse expérimentale de deux dérivés de phénazine pigmentée (B663 et B720) seuls et associés à d'autres antituberculeux (isoniazide et éthionamide), Ann Inst Pasteur, 98, 567–585.

Guelpa-Lauras CC, Cartel JL, Constant-Desportes M, Milian J, Bobin P, Guidi C, Brucker G, Flageul B, Guillaume JC, Pichet C, Remey JC, Grosset JH, 1987, Primary and secondary dapsone resistance to M. leprae in Martinique, Guadeloupe, New Caledonia, Tahiti, Senegal and Paris between 1980 and 1985, Int J Lepr Other Mycobact Dis, 55, 672–679.

Guelpa-Lauras CC, Perani EG, Giroir AM, Grosset JH, 1987, Activities of pefloxacin and ciprofloxacin against Mycobacterium leprae in the mouse, Int J Lepr Other Mycobact Dis, 55, 70–77.

Hamilton EJ, Eidus L, Little E, 1962, A comparative study in vivo of isoniazid and alpha-ethylthioisonicotinamide, Am Rev Respir Dis, 85, 407–412.

Hastings RC, 1985, Leprosy, Longman Group Limited.

Honoré N, Cole S, 1993, Molecular basis of rifampin resistance in *Mycobacterium leprae*, Antimicrob Agents Chemother, 37, 414–418.

Husser JA, Traore I, Daumerie D, 1994, Activity of two doses of rifampin against Mycobacterium leprae, Int J Lepr Other Mycobact Dis, 62, 359–364.

Jacobson RR, 1985, Chapter 9, in RC Hastings, ed, Treatment in Leprosy, Churchill Livingstone.

Jacobson RR, Hastings RC, 1976, Rifampin-resistant leprosy, Lancet, ii, 1304–1305.

Jamet P, Ji B, 1995, Relapse after long-term follow up of multibacillary patients treated by WHO multidrug regimen. Marchoux Chemotherapy Study Group. Int J Lepr Other Mycobact Dis, 63, 195–201.

Jamet P, Traore I, Husser JA, Ji B, 1992, Short-term trial of clofazimine in previously untreated lepromatous leprosy, Int J Lepr Other Mycobact Dis, 60, 542–548.

Jenner PJ, Ellard GA, 1981, High-performance liquid chromatographic determination of ethionamide and prothionamide in body fluids, J Chromatogr, 22, 245–251.

Jenner PJ, Ellard GA, Gruent PJK, Aber VR, 1984, Comparison of blood levels and urinary excretion of ethionamide and prothionamide in man, J Antimicrob Chemother, 12, 267–277.

Jesudassan K, Vijayakumaran P, Pannikar VK, Christian M, 1988, Impact of MDT on leprosy as measured by selective indicators, Lepr Rev, 59, 215–223.

Ji B, 1985, Drug resistance in leprosy—a review, Lepr Rev, 56, 265–278.

Ji B, Chen J, Wang C, Xia G, 1984, Hepatotoxicity of combined therapy with rifampicin and daily prothionamide for leprosy, Lepr Rev, 55, 283–289.

Ji B, Grosset J, 1990, Recent advances in the chemotherapy of leprosy, Lepr Rev, 61, 313–329.

Ji B, Jamet P, Perani EG, Bobin P, Grosset JH, 1993, Powerful bactericidal activities of clarithromycin and minocycline against M. leprae in lepromatous leprosy, J Infect Dis, 168, 188–190.

Ji B, Perani EG, Grosset JH, 1991, Effectiveness of clarithromycin and minocycline alone or in combination against *Mycobacterium leprae* infection in mice, Antimicrob Agents Chemother, 35, 579–581.

Katoch K, Ramanathan U, Natrajan M, Bagga AK, Bhatia AS, Saxena RK, Ramu G, 1989, Relapses in paucibacillary patients after treatment with three short-term regimens containing rifampicin, Int J Lepr Other Mycobact Dis, 57, 458–464.

Lesobre R, Ruffino J, Teyssier L, Achard F, Brefort G, 1968, Les icteres au cours du traitement par la rifampicine, Rev Tuberc Pneumol, 33, 393–403.

Levy L, Shepard CC, Fasal P, 1972, Clofazimine therapy of lepromatous leprosy caused by dapsone-resistant Mycobacterium leprae, Am J Trop Med Hyg, 21, 315–321.

Levy L, Shepard CC, Fasal P, 1976, The bactericidal effect of rifampicin on M. leprae in man: a) single doses of 600, 900 and 1200 mg; and b) daily doses of 300 mg, Int J Lepr Other Mycobact Dis, 44, 183–187.

Lowe J, 1950, Treatment of leprosy with diamino-diphenyl sulfone by mouth, Lancet, i, 145–150.

Lowe J, Smith M, 1949, The chemotherapy of leprosy in Nigeria; with an appendix on glandular fever and exfoliative dermatitis precipitated by sulfones, Int J Lepr, 17, 181–195.

McDermott W, 1958, Microbial persistence, Yale J Biol Med, 30, 257–329.

Mechali D, Coulaud JP, 1988, Antilépreux, p 1574–1583, in Giroud JP, Mathe G, Meyniel G, ed, Pharmacologie clinique. Bases de la therapeutique, 2nd ed.

Mitchison DA, 1988, The action of antituberculosis drugs in short-course chemotherapy, Tubercle, 68, 219–225.

Morrison NE, Marley GM, 1976, Clofazimine binding studies with deoxyribonucleic acid, Int J Lepr Other Mycobact Dis, 44, 475–481.

Ndeli L, Guelpa-Lauras CC, Perani EG, Grosset JH, 1990, Effectiveness of pefloxacin in the treatment of lepromatous leprosy, Int J Lepr Other Mycobact Dis, 58, 12–18.

Pattyn SR, Ropier MT, Rollier R, Verdoahaege G, 1975, Sensibilité envers la dapsone, la sulfaméthoxypyridazine et l'éthionamide de Mycobacterium leprae provenant de malades traités par ces substances, Int J Lepr Other Mycobact Dis, 43, 356–362.

Pettit JHS, Rees RJW, 1964, Sulphone resistance in leprosy. An experimental and clinical study, Lancet, ii, 673–674.

Rees RJW, Pearson JMH, Waters MFR, 1970, Experimental and clinical studies on rifampicin in the treatment of leprosy, Br Med J, 1, 89–92.

Rist N, 1960, L'activité antituberculeuse de l'éthionamide (l'alpha-éthylthioisonicotinamide ou 1314 Th). Etude expérimentale et clinique, Adv Tuberc Res, 10, 69–126.

Shepard CC, 1974, Recent developments in the chemotherapy and chemoprophylaxis of leprosy, Leprologia (Argentina), 19, 230–236.

Shepard CC, Chang YT, 1962, Effect of several anti-leprosy drugs on multiplication of human leprosy bacilli in footpads of mice, Proc Soc Exp Biol Med, 102, 636–638.

Shepard CC, Levy L, Fasal P, 1974, Further experience with the rapid bactericidal effect of rifampin on Mycobacterium leprae, Am J Trop Med Hyg, 23, 1120–1124.

Shepard CC, Walker LL, Van Landingham RM, Redus M, 1971, Kinetic testing of drugs against Mycobacterium leprae in mice: activity of cephaloridine, rifampin, streptovaricin, and viomycin, Am J Trop Med Hyg, 20, 616–620.

Simon E, Veres E, Banki G, 1969, Changes in SGOT activity during treatment with ethionamide, Scand J Respir Dis, 50, 314–322.

Thelep Subcommittee on Clinical Trials of the Chemotherapy of Leprosy Scientific Working Group of the UNDPI/World Bank/WHO Special Programme for Research and Training in Tropical Diseases, 1987, Persisting Mycobacterium leprae among Thelep trial patients in Bamako and Chingleput, Lepr Rev, 58, 325–337.

UNDP/World Bank/WHO Special Programme for Research and Training in Tropical Diseases, 1989, Leprosy, p 93–100, in Ninth Programme Report: Tropical Diseases, Progress in International Research, 1987–1988, WHO, Geneva.

Warndoff-Vandiepen T, 1982, Clofazimine-resistant leprosy: a case report, Int J Lepr Other Mycobact Dis, 50,139–142.

WHO Expert Committee on Leprosy, 1977, Fifth Report, Tech Rep Ser 607, World Health Organization, Geneva.

WHO Expert Committee on Leprosy, 1988, Sixth Report, Tech Rep Ser 768, World Health Organization, Geneva.

WHO Study Group, 1982, Chemotherapy of leprosy for control programmes, Tech Rep Ser 675, World Health Organization, Geneva.

Young DB, Cole ST, 1993, Leprosy, tuberculosis, and the new genetics, J Bacteriol, 175, 1–6.

Primycin

A. BRYSKIER

47

1. INTRODUCTION

Primycin, described in 1954, is a topical antibiotic developed in Hungary for the local treatment of certain superficial and deep infections of the skin and subcutaneous tissue. It is a product obtained from fermentation of *Thermomonospora galeriensis* (Szabo et al., 1976).

2. CHEMICAL STRUCTURE

Primycin is a complex of macrocyclic antibiotics comprising 20 compounds. Nine of them account for more than 90% of the total, and their structure has been elucidated. This molecular complex is stable, and the molecules are linked to one another by hydrogen bonds. The compound A_1 accounts for about 50% of the series. The three major compounds are A_1, B_2, and C_3. The other compounds are minor: A_2, A_3, B_1, B_3, C_1, and C_2. Each of them has been identified structurally (Fig. 1) and named (Table 1).

These compounds may be separated into three groups, A, B, and C, according to the substituent at R_1, and into three subgroups according to the nature of the substituent at R_2, which may be a butyl, pentyl, or hexyl group.

3. PHYSICOCHEMICAL PROPERTIES

Primycin is insoluble in water (50 μg/ml), moderately soluble in methanol (2,000 μg/ml) and 1,2-propanediol (5,000 μg/ml), and freely soluble in warm *N*-methylpyrrolidone, and it forms a stable gel that can contain up to 30% primycin (Ebrimycin). This gel forms the basis of the various pharmaceutical preparations. The topical preparation contains primycin sulfate.

The molecular mass is on the order of 1,000 Da for each of the components (Table 2), and the pK is 11. The melting point is between 160 and 170°C.

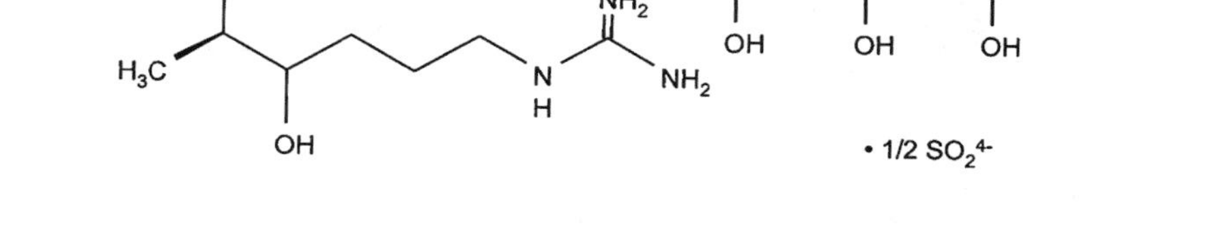

	A_1	A_2	A_3	B_1	B_2	B_3	C_1	C_2	C_3
R_1	α-D-arabofuranosyl			H	H	H	OH	OH	OH
R_2	butyl	pentyl	hexyl	butyl	pentyl	hexyl	butyl	pentyl	hexyl

Figure 1 Primycins

Table 1 Primycin derivatives

Component	Generic name
A_1	Chinopricin
A_2	Midopricin
A_3	Metipricin
B_1	Hydropricin
B_2	Hymipricin
B_3	Hymetipricin
C_1	Oxipricin
C_2	Oximipricin
C_3	Oximetipricin

Table 2 Molecular weights of the components of primycin

Component group	Molecular weight of subgroup		
	1	2	3
A	1,078	1,092	1,106
B	930	944	958
C	946	960	974

4. TOXICOLOGY

The median lethal dose in the mouse is greater than 3,000 mg/kg of body weight orally and 56 mg/kg intraperitoneally. No skin lesions have been observed after chronic cutaneous applications (90 days) in the rabbit.

5. ANTIBACTERIAL ACTIVITY

Primycin possesses good in vitro activity against *Staphylococcus aureus* and coagulase-negative staphylococci, but its activity against *Streptococcus pyogenes* and enterococci is moderate. It is active against *Micrococcus* and *Bacillus* spp. but is inactive against *Corynebacterium* spp. It is inactive against *Enterobacteriaceae* and *Pseudomonas aeruginosa*, yeasts, and dermatophytes (Table 3).

Primycin acts by modifying the membrane. At high concentrations, it inhibits membrane ATPase of gram-positive and gram-negative bacteria.

6. PHARMACOKINETICS

After oral administration of 10 mg of primycin per kg to rats, no antibacterial activity was measured in the plasma (microbiological method using *Bacillus subtilis*) between 30 and 360 min after administration. The results were the same when primycin was administered at a dosage of 5 mg/kg for 7 days.

Transdermal penetration has been studied in rats with a normal skin lining and those having suffered second-degree burns. No antibiotic activity was detected in the serum after application of 250 mg/kg.

REFERENCES

Frank J, Dékany G, Pelczer I, Apsimon JW, 1987, The composition of primycin, Tetrahedron Lett, 24, 2759–2762.

Nogradi M, 1998, Primycin (Ebrimycin®)—a new topical antibiotic, Drug To Day, 24, 563–566.

Szabo IM, Marton N, Kulcsar G, Buti I, 1976, Taxonomy of primycin-producing actinomycetes. I. Description of the type strain, Thermomonospora galeriensis, Acta Microbiol Acad Sci Hung 23, 371–376.

Table 3 In vitro activity of primycin

Organism(s)	MIC (μg/ml)				
	Primycin	Ampicillin	Erythromycin A	Tetracycline	Clindamycin
S. aureus	0.39	<0.5	>250	1.0	>250
S. aureus ATCC 25923	25	<0.5	1.0	<0.5	62.5
Staphylococcus epidermidis	0.78	<0.5	<0.5	62.5	31.3
S. pyogenes	1.56	<0.5	0.5	1.0	125
Streptococcus mitis	50	7.8	250	1.0	>250
Micrococcus	0.78	<0.5	<0.5	7.8	15.6
Coryneform(s)	50	31.3	>250	31.3	250
B. subtilis ATCC 6633	0.39	<0.5	<0.5	<0.5	15.6
Escherichia coli	50	2.0	62.5	1.0	>250
Enterobacter cloacae	50	7.8	250	2.0	>250
Propionibacterium acnes	<0.1	1.0	<0.5	<0.5	0.5

Benzonaphthyridones

A. BRYSKIER

48

The use of mupirocin and fusidic acid in topical applications is jeopardized by the emergence of resistant bacteria. New medicinal chemical entities are needed to overcome this threat. Benzonaphthyridone molecules are one of the potential alternatives.

1. RP-60556

From a new series of benzonaphthyridones, RP-60556A was selected for further preclinical investigation focused on its potential use as a topical antibacterial agent. It was shown that the most potent compound within this series of benzo[*b*]naphthyridones is RP-60556A, due to the 4-fluorophenylpiperazidinyl side chain.

1.1. Structure

RP-60556 is a 7,8-substituted benzo[*b*]naphthyridone, having a fluorine atom at position 7 and a piperazinyl moiety at position 8, bearing a fluorophenyl side chain (Fig. 1).

1.2. Physicochemical Properties

RP-60556A is a chlorinate salt. The physicochemical properties of this yellow crystalline powder are listed in Table 1. RP-60556A is unstable against intense sunlight.

1.3. In Vitro Activity

This chain allowed comparable activities against fluoroquinolone-susceptible and resistant *Staphylococcus aureus* strains (MICs, 0.25 and 0.50 μg/ml, respectively).

Table 1 Physicochemical properties of RP-60556A

Parameter	Datum
Empirical formula	$C_{24}H_{19}F_2N_4O_3$
Mol wt	553.61
Melting point (°C)	328–328°C
Chlorinate salt melting point (°C)	285–290°C
LogP	4.6
pK_a	5.8
Water solubility	>100 mg/ml

RP-60556A exhibits good antistaphylococcal activity, irrespective of the susceptibility to pefloxacin, ciprofloxacin, and sparfloxacin, with a MIC at which 50% of isolates tested are inhibited (MIC_{50}) and MIC_{90} of 0.25 μg/ml. RP-60556A is active against *S. aureus* isolates with GlrA or GyrA mutations as well as against strains harboring an efflux mechanism of resistance (NorA).

RP-60556A is inactive against *Enterobacteriaceae* (MIC, >128 μg/ml).

RP-60556A displays activity similar to those of fusidic acid and mupirocin against *S. aureus* strains susceptible to those antibacterials but remains active against mupirocin- and/or fusidic acid-resistant isolates. The compound is not affected by methicillin resistance. For Lancefield group A, B, C, and G streptococci, MICs ranged from 0.25 to 1.0 μg/ml. For *Enterococcus* species, MICs ranged from 1.0 to 2.0 μg/ml. RP-60556A is weakly active against fastidious gram-negative

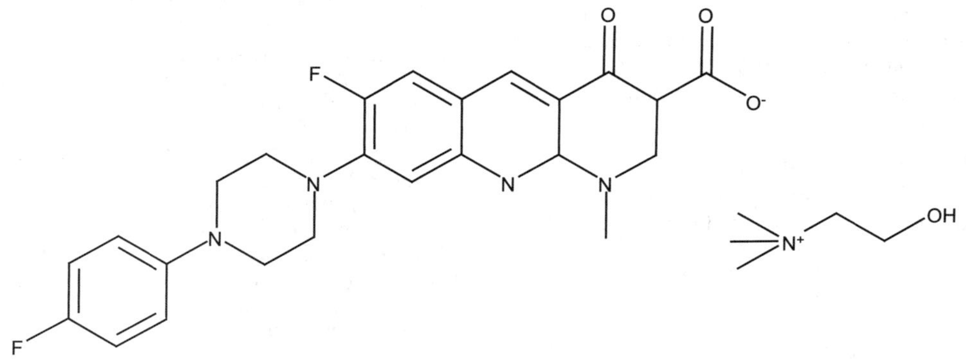

Figure 1 RP-60556A

Table 2 Pharmacokinetics of RP-60556A

Animals	Dose (mg/kg)	C_{max} (μg/ml)	T_{max} (h)	$t_{1/2}$ (h)	AUC (μg·h/ml)	F (%)
OF-1 mice	50	2.9	0.5	4.5	33.35	52
Rats	40	1.03	7.12	6.4	16.29	3.4
Dogs	40	1.646	4.5	14.6	37.04	13.3

Figure 2 RPR 203246

bacilli, with MICs of 2.0 to 8.0 μg/ml for *Moraxella catarrhalis* and 4.0 to 32 μg/ml for *Haemophilus influenzae*. RP-60556A exhibits good in vitro activity against gram-positive anaerobes (MICs, 0.12 to 0.5 μg/ml) and against *Bacteroides fragilis* (MICs, 1.0 to 2.0 μg/ml).

In vitro activity against *S. aureus* is affected by addition of 50% human serum to the culture medium (MIC, >64 μg/ml).

The bactericidal activity against *S. aureus* seems to be strain dependent, with at least above a 2-$\log_{10}$ CFU/ml reduction, mupirocin is always bacteriostatic, with a 1-$\log_{10}$ CFU/ml reduction of the bacterial burden. This slight bactericidal activity remains against mupirocin-resistant *S. aureus* isolates. RP-60556A is highly bactericidal against *Streptococcus pyogenes* (reduction of the inoculum size above 3 $\log_{10}$ CFU/ml in a 3-h period).

In vivo in a guinea pig model of cutaneous infection with *S. aureus*, a significant reduction of staphylococcal load per wound was shown in 24 h.

RP-60556A retained in vitro activity against *S. aureus* isolates resistant to fluoroquinolones due to a *gyrA* mutation (Ser80 → Phe, Glu84 → Lys, or Ser80 → Lys) or *grlA* mutation (Glu88 → Lys, Ser84 → Leu, or Ser85 → Pro) or harboring an efflux mechanism of resistance, with NorA protein. MICs ranged from 0.25 to 0.5 μg/ml.

RP-60556A exhibited a bactericidal activity at two to four times the MIC within a 3 to 6-h period of contact irrespective of the phenotype of resistance of *S. aureus* and *Staphylococcus epidermidis*. RP-60556A was bactericidal at two to four times the MIC in 3 h against beta-hemolytic streptococci.

1.4. Pharmacokinetics in Animals

In rats and guinea pigs after local application of 40 mg/kg of body weight, no compound was detected in the blood. After oral administration of 40 to 50 mg/kg to mice (OF-1) and dogs, the bioavailability ranged from 13 to 52% (Table 2). No plasma metabolites were detected.

In an ex vivo model, it was shown that in a 1% topical formulation, RP-60556A diffuses through human skin for 8 and 24 h, demonstrating activity against *S. aureus* isolates comparable to that of a 2% fusidic acid formulation.

The in vivo activity of a 2% topical formulation of RP-60556A in comparison with that of a 2% mupirocin formulation was investigated in a model of staphylococcal wound infection in guinea pigs (Hartley albinos, male). Antibacterials were applied 18 h after local bacterial challenge.

The compounds exhibited similar activities with a decrease of about 3 $\log_{10}$ CFU in comparison with control at 24 h.

2. RPR 203246

A new series of benzo[*f*]naphthyridines has been synthesized, and RPR 203246 (Fig. 2) is a representative of this series. These benzo[*f*]naphthyridines are fluorinated and substituted by various acyl side chains. RPR 203246 is slightly less active against *S. aureus* irrespective of the mechanism of resistance to pefloxacin. MICs are from 1.0 to 2.0 μg/ml.

REFERENCES

Bernard FX, Berthaud N, Desnottes JF, 2000, RP 60556A, a new topical benzonaphthyridone derivative: ex-vivo antibacterial activity through human skin samples, 40th Intersci Conf Antimicrob Agents Chemother, abstract 1516, p 212.

Berthaud N, Dutka-Malen S, Boisrobert V, Efremenko F, Gouin AM, Martin J, Rousseau J, Desnottes JF, 2000, RP 60556A, a new topical benzonaphthyridone derivative: in vitro spectrum of bacteriostatic activity, 40th Intersci Conf Antimicrob Agents Chemother, abstract 1513, p 211.

Berthaud N, Dutka-Malen S, Boisrobert V, Efremenko F, Gouin AM, Martin J, Rousseau J, Desnottes JF, 2000, RP 60556A, a new topical benzonaphthyridone derivative: in vitro spectrum of bacteriostatic activity, 40th Intersci Conf Antimicrob Agents Chemother, abstract 1514, p 211.

Berthaud N, Dutka-Malen S, Boisrobert V, Efremenko F, Gouin AM, Martin J, Rousseau J, Desnottes JF, 2000, RP 60556A, a new topical benzonaphthyridone derivative: in vitro bactericidal activity against gram-positive cocci, 40th Intersci Conf Antimicrob Agents Chemother, abstract 1515, p 212.

Berthaud N, Huet J, Bourgues A, Bussières JC, Ferreira C, Imbault F, Selingue M, Desnotttes JF, 2000, RP 60556A, a new topical benzonaphthyridone derivative: activity in a guinea-pig model of *Staphylococcus aureus* cutaneous infection, 40th Intersci Conf Antimicrob Agents Chemother, abstract 1517, p 212.

Tabart M, Picaut G, Berthaud N, Descenclois JF, 2000, Synthesis and biological evaluation of RP 60556A, a new topical antibacterial agent, 40th Intersci Conf Antimicrob Agents Chemother, abstract 1512, p 211.

Tabart M, Picaut G, Desconclois JF, Dutka-Malen S, Huet Y, Berthaud N, 2001, Synthesis and biological evaluation of benzo[b]naphthyridones, a series of new topical antibacterial agents, Bioorg Med Chem Lett, 11, 919–921.

Tabart M, Picaut G, Lavergne M, Wentzler S, Malleron JL, Dutka-Malen S, Berthaud N, 2003, Benzo[*f*]naphthyridines: a new family of topical antibacterial agents active on multiresistant gram-positive pathogens, Bioorg Med Chem Lett, 13, 1329–1331.

Agents against Methicillin-Resistant *Staphylococcus aureus*

ANDRÉ BRYSKIER

49

1. INTRODUCTION

For the last five or six decades, antibacterials have revolutionized medicine by providing cures for life-threatening infections. Infections due to methicillin-resistant *Staphylococcus aureus* (MRSA) are associated with a mortality rate of 15 to 60%. It seems from a recent meta-analysis of *S. aureus* bacteremia that there is a correlation between oxacillin susceptibility and cure rate. The mortality rate is higher with MRSA (Cosgrove et al., 2003). An epidemiological surveillance program was set up in Europe in 1999 and 2000 (Tiemersma et al., 2004). Twenty-seven countries were involved in collecting *S. aureus* from blood samples. A total of 20% of the isolates were methicillin resistant. A wide range of susceptibility was recorded, from 0.5% in Iceland to above 40% in the United Kingdom (Fig. 1). The geographical variation showed a north-south gradient with a high variation among hospitals.

From 1940 to the 1950s, *S. aureus* isolates were susceptible to benzylpenicillin, but rapidly strains producing PC-1 β-lactamase began to spread in hospital settings and then in communities. The first report of *S. aureus* resistant to penicillin occurred in 1942 (Rammelkamp, 1942). To overcome this threat, semisynthetic penams were prepared, and the resulting compounds were methicillin or oxacillin and derivatives (Deresinski, 2005). Unfortunately, MRSA rapidly

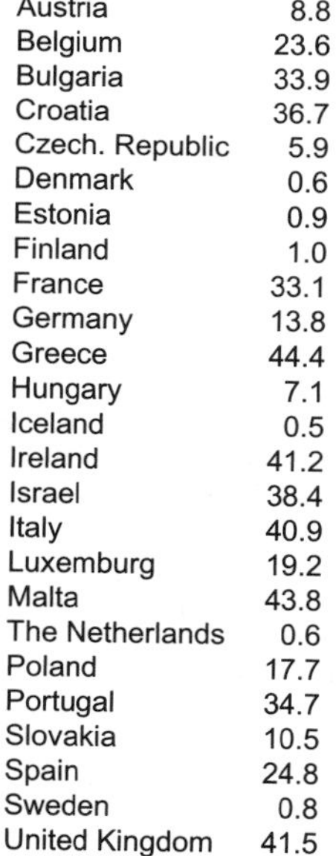

Austria 8.8
Belgium 23.6
Bulgaria 33.9
Croatia 36.7
Czech. Republic 5.9
Denmark 0.6
Estonia 0.9
Finland 1.0
France 33.1
Germany 13.8
Greece 44.4
Hungary 7.1
Iceland 0.5
Ireland 41.2
Israel 38.4
Italy 40.9
Luxemburg 19.2
Malta 43.8
The Netherlands 0.6
Poland 17.7
Portugal 34.7
Slovakia 10.5
Spain 24.8
Sweden 0.8
United Kingdom 41.5

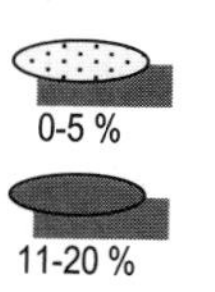

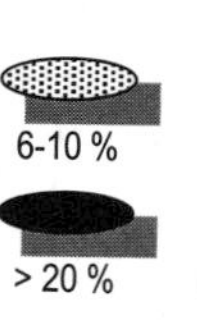

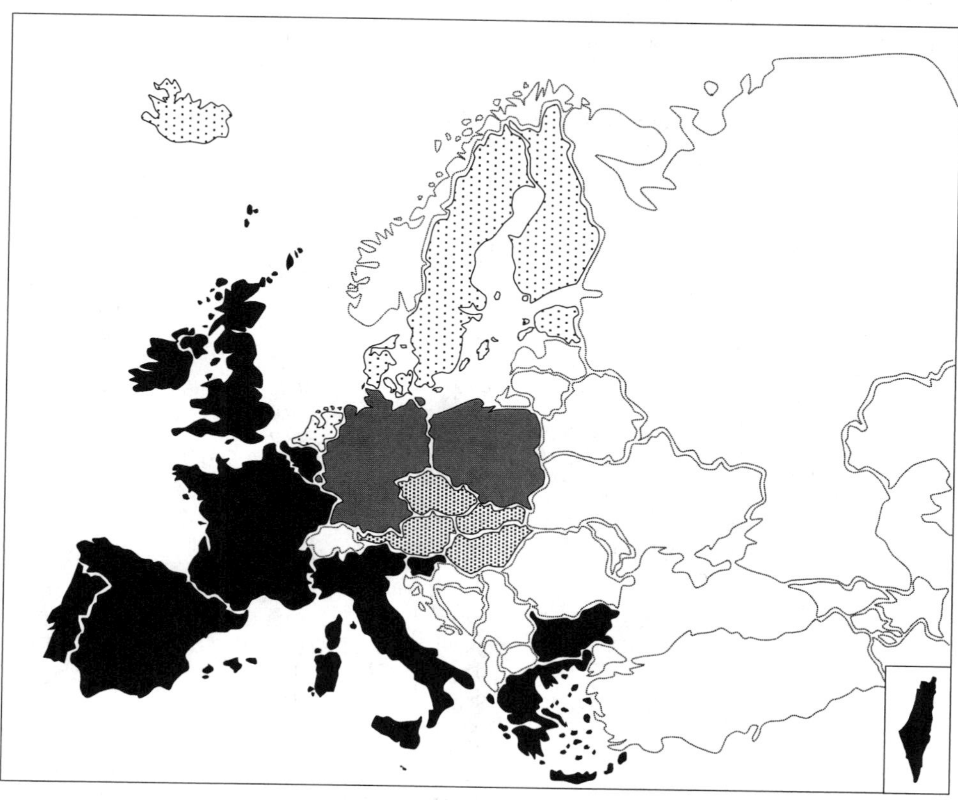

Figure 1 Prevalence of MRSA in Europe, 1999 to 2000

emerged in the early 1960s (Jevons, 1961), and vancomycin became an alternate therapy.

Since the early 1990s, hospital-acquired infections (nosocomial) shifted from gram-negative organisms to gram-positive bacteria (Rybak, 2001). MRSA isolates represent about 34, 26, 60, and 45% of clinical isolates (hospital) in the United States, Europe, Japan, and the Western Pacific region, respectively (Diekema and Jones, 2001). A surveillance program throughout the United States (SCOPE) was carried out from March 1995 to September 2002 for nosocomial bloodstream infections. Staphylococcal infections represented about 20.2% of recorded nosocomial infections, with a mortality rate of 25.4%. Of the 1,699 *S. aureus* isolates, 41% of the tested strains were resistant to methicillin (Wisplinghoff et al., 2004). In a surveillance program (SENTRY) carried out between 2000 and 2001 in Latin America, oxacillin resistance was detected in 38.6% of *S. aureus* isolates. The overall rate of resistance to mupirocin was 3.1%. The rates of resistance were 26.8 to 46.7, 22.3 to 59.5, 36.3 to 52.6, 6.1, 15.4, and 2.6% in Argentina, Brazil, Chile, Colombia, Mexico, and Venezuela, respectively (Gales et al., 2004). In western Australia, MRSA prevalence was about 12% from 1997 to 1999 (Cordova et al., 2004), and in western Africa, the prevalence of MRSA was 56.5 and 70% in Abidjan, Ivory Coast, and Dakar, Senegal, respectively (Akona-Koffi et al., 2004; Seydi et al., 2004).

The in vitro activities of 19 compounds against 3,498 *S. aureus* isolates (Fritsche et al., 2004) from hospitals and communities and susceptible or resistant to oxacillin have been investigated and are reported in (Table 1).

MRSA strains were for many years restricted to hospitals, but now community-acquired MRSA strains have started to spread. These strains mainly belong to *SSSmec* type IV.

In general, nosocomial pathogens are often multidrug resistant, and emergence of vancomycin-resistant MRSA, even if in limited areas today, is a matter of concern. This serious problem has fueled a search for novel medicinal chemical entities.

There is an effective and urgent need for new antibacterials active against MRSA with, if possible, new modes of action, for the following reasons:

- In spite of advances in medical sciences, staphylococcal infections remain a considerable cause of morbidity and mortality.
- Treatment cure rates may be variable, and treatment may even be ineffective, despite laboratory susceptibility of the microorganism to vancomycin (Moise and Schentag, 2000). Bactericidal therapy is believed to be critical in treatment of bloodstream infections; therefore, clinical failure with vancomycin may be at least partially explained by tolerance to vancomycin by some MRSA strains.
- The risk of failure of vancomycin therapy seems to be correlated with strains harboring the *agr* group II polymorphism (Moise-Brocher et al., 2004). In a recent study, it was found that 55 to 60% of glycopeptide-intermediate *S. aureus* (GISA) strains harbor the *agr* group II polymorphism, and this is an independent predictor of vancomycin treatment failure in patients with MRSA infections (Sakoulas et al., 2002). The accessory gene regulator (*agr*) operon of *S. aureus* is a global regulon that coordinately controls many critical virulence pathways in the microorganism. The *agr* gene upregulates production of secreted virulence factors (hemolysins and proteases) and downregulates production of virulence factors expressed on the staphylococcal cell surface (Arvidson and Tegmark, 2001). Four *agr* groups have been described: group II mainly contains GISA isolates, group III seems to be associated with community-acquired MRSA, and group IV is associated with exfoliatin-producing strains. Group I function is not well identified.

Table 1 Susceptibility of *S. aureus* to antibacterials in 2003 in the United States

Compound	Susceptibility (%)			
	MSSA		MRSA	
	Community (1,592)[a]	Hospital (706)	Community (652)	Hospital (548)
Tetracycline	95.9	97.2	90.8	94.7
Doxycycline	99	99	96.1	96.8
Penicillin G	17.7	17.4	0.5	0.2
Co-amoxiclav	99.4	99.2	12.1	3.5
Ceftazidime	91.2	89.9	2.0	0.5
Ceftriaxone	98.9	98.7	3.8	3.8
Imipenem	99.9	99.7	74	66.4
Erythromycin A	74.7	72.9	6.1	3.1
Clindamycin	94.5	91.6	33.7	23.5
Quinupristin-dalfopristin	99.9	100	100	100
Chloramphenicol	96.5	96.7	83.3	79.8
Ciprofloxacin	91.3	89.7	15.2	6.0
Levofloxacin	93.4	91.5	17.6	6.9
Gentamicin	98.7	97.9	89.8	86.8
Rifampin	99.8	99.7	93.1	93.1
Co-trimoxazole	96.8	96.6	92.2	92.7
Linezolid	100	100	99.8	100
Teicoplanin	100	100	100	100
Vancomycin	100	100	100	100

[a]Number of isolates.

- Starting in the mid-1990s in Japan, and rapidly thereafter elsewhere, clinical isolates intermediately susceptible to vancomycin and teicoplanin emerged (Hiramatsu et al., 1997). In 2002, the first MRSA strain resistant to vancomycin due to the *vanA* gene was reported in the United States (Liassine et al., 2004). Vancomycin-resistant *S. aureus* had been obtained in vitro by plasmid transfer (Noble et al., 1992). VanA transfer was shown in clinical isolates (Bozdogan et al., 2003).
- MRSA isolates are also resistant to many other antibacterials, such as aminoglycosides, macrolides, lincosamides, streptogramins, and fluoroquinolones. Due to its adaptability, *S. aureus* can easily develop resistance to commonly used antibiotics. The emergence of resistance is an important treatment issue (Jones et al., 1999).
- The occurrence of GISA infections has prompted recommendations that vancomycin usage be limited in order to control the emergence of vancomycin-resistant gram-positive organisms.

Many strategies are available for controlling infections: combination therapy, development of new members of existing antibiotic classes (e.g., glycopeptides, macrolides, and cephems), and introduction of novel classes of antibacterial agents.

Approximately 90% of *S. aureus* isolates produce one of 11 genotypes of capsular polysaccarides. Genotypes CP-5 and CP-8 account for 25 and 50%, respectively (Seeman et al., 2004). Resistance through reduced penetration has been shown to occur in vancomycin-intermediate resistant *S. aureus* isolates that produce a thick cell wall (Lambert, 2002).

2. GLYCOPEPTIDES

The first glycopeptide used in clinical practice was vancomycin, followed by a lipoglycopeptide, teicoplanin. In China, a desmethyl vancomycin is used.

2.1. Vancomycin and Derivatives

It has been shown that vancomycin could be selectively functionalized at position 6 of the glucose residue, allowing the synthesis of a wide variety of analogs.

Incorporation of a lipophilic side chain into vancomycin resulted in a dramatic enhancement in activity against vancomycin-resistant bacteria (Nagarajan et al., 1989).

The introduction of a hydrophilic side chain on the nitrogen of the amino sugar moiety was found to yield potent derivatives against MRSA and vancomycin-resistant enterococci (VRE) as exemplified by oritavancin and demonstrated by many teams (Kim et al., 2002). However, this side chain has an unfavorable effect on water solubility.

Vancomycin binds to the terminal D-Ala–D-Ala unit of the bacterial cell wall peptidoglycan precursor. One structural key of vancomycin for binding is the cyclic peptoid unit (Fig. 2) that incorporates several H-bond donor NH groups and one H-bond acceptor amide carbonyl group.

The cationic terminal *N*-methylamino group in vancomycin also stabilizes the bound complex through a favorable electrostatic interaction with the carboxy group of the terminal D-Ala residue of the growing cell wall.

2.1.1. Vancomycin-Like Compounds

Two natural compounds, MG3G and M43F, contain a modified residue of aspartic acid, an additional methyl, and a carboxamide side chain instead of a carboxylic group. When an L-β-cyanoalanine was used to replace a 3-L-aspartic acid, the resulting compound retained activity against MRSA (Nagarajan et al., 1994). Replacement of the carboxamide group with a nitrile group resulted in decreased activity (McAtee et al., 2002).

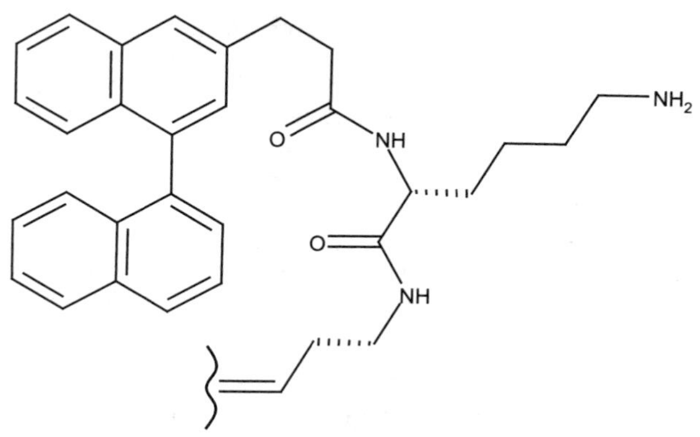

Figure 2 Cyclic peptoid

2.1.2. Disulfide Vancomycin

Over the past 20 years extensive research has been carried out on chemical modifications of vancomycin. The lipophilic modifications through alkyl-linked groups on the vancosamine sugar impart unfavorable absorption, distribution, and elimination properties. Synthesis of vancomycin derivatives bearing disulfide bonds in the lipid tail (Fig. 3) resulted in compounds with good anti-MRSA activity (MICs of 0.4 to 2.9 μg/ml), bactericidal activity, and improved pharmacokinetics. They are converted into more hydrophilic metabolites and eliminated in the urine (Mu et al., 2004).

2.2. Eremomycin and Its Semisynthetic Derivatives

2.2.1. Eremomycin

Eremomycin is a glycopeptide belonging to the dalbaheptapeptide subgroup composed of A-82846A and MM 45289.

Series of hydrophobic N′-mono and N′, N″-double alkylated derivatives of eremomycin were synthesized. The introduction of an N′-*p*-(*p*-chlorophenyl) benzyl substituent into vancomycin resulted in enhancement of vancomycin antibacterial activity against both susceptible and resistant isolates; in constrast, the same side chain resulted in decreased activity of eremomycin.

Some derivatives were more active against MRSA (MIC, 0.78 μg/ml) than the parent compound, eremomycin (MIC, 1.56 μg/ml) (Pavlov et al., 2001).

2.2.2. A-40926

A-40926 was obtained from the fermentation broth of *Actinomadura*. From A-40926 were derived many compounds,

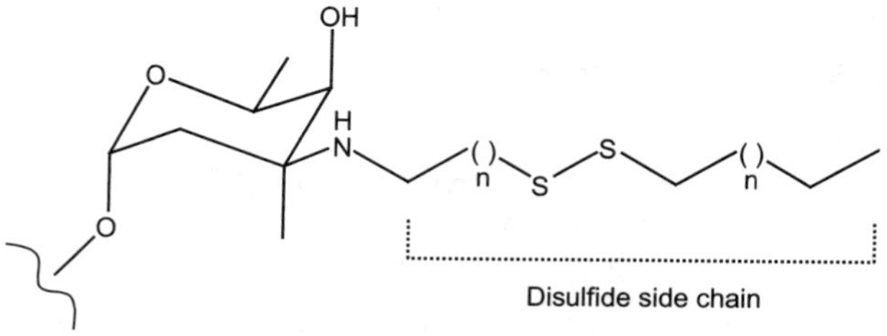

Figure 3 Lipidated vancomycin derivatives with disulfide bonds

such as MDL-63246, DA-40926, and 3-oxazolinone derivatives. The 3-oxazolinone derivatives contain the oxazolinone ring between positions C-36 and C-38. It is less active than teicoplanin against methicillin-susceptible *S. aureus* (MSSA) (MICs, 0.5 to 1.0 μg/ml) and MRSA (MIC, 16 μg/ml) (Panzone et al., 1998).

2.2.3. MDL-63246

MDL-63246 is a semisynthetic derivative of A-40926. It is an amide derivative with the amino sugar of amino acid 6 removed.

2.2.4. Oritavancin (LY-333328)

Oritavancin is a chloroeremomycin derivative. The hydrophobic substituent is a C-10–C-12 alkyl or diaryl substituent. Most of the hydrophobic derivatives are weakly effective in vivo, which may be related to their potential inactivation by serum proteins. The presence of a polar group may influence this immobilization by serum proteins and enhance the activity of hydrophobic compounds in vivo.

Oritavancin contains a chlorodiphenyl side chain. Oritavancin is bactericidal against MRSA strains, including GISA strains. It is also active against other gram-positive bacteria, including anaerobes (Sillerström et al., 1999). Oritavancin accumulates in cultured macrophages with a slow efflux (Van Bambecke et al., 2001). The mode of action of oritavancin is complex, first because oritavancin interacts with D-Ala–D-Ala and second because the hydrophobic side chain fixed on the vancosamine sugar (chlorodiphenyl) inhibits transglycosylation during peptidoglycan biosynthesis (Kim et al., 2002). In an epidemiological surveillance study, 128 MRSA clinical isolates were collected. The MIC at which 50% of isolates tested are inhibited (MIC_{50}) and MIC_{90} of oritavancin were 2.0 and 4.0 μg/ml, respectively (Critchley et al., 2002). In a prospective multicenter surveillance study carried out in 12 countries and involving 18 centers, 310 MRSA isolates were collected. Oritavancin MICs ranged from <0.06 to 4.0 μg/ml (Zeckel et al., 2000). At Hershey Medical Center, *S. aureus* HMC3 was resistant to vancomycin through the presence of the *vanA* resistance gene and also contained *mecA*, *ermB*, *tetK*, and *aac(6′)-aph(2″)* and had alterations in GyrA and GyrB. At four times the MIC a reduction of 3 $\log_{10}$ CFU/ml was recorded for dalbavancin (6 h), oritavancin (3 h), ramoplanin (3 h), daptomycin (3 h), BAL 9141 (6 h), RWJ-54428 (12 h), DK-507k and sitafloxacin (3 h), and DNA nanobinder GS-02-2 (24 h). Other comparative compounds were not bactericidal, such as PDF inhibitor NVP-PDF713, GS-02-12, tigecycline, and oxazolidinones (linezolid and ranbezolid) (Bozdogan et al., 2003). Oritavancin possesses a long elimination half-life (182 to 233 h), with a plasma clearance of 0.4 to 0.55 liter/h and an area under the concentration-time curve of 71 to 465 μg·h/ml (depending on the administered dose [1.5 to 9.0 mg/kg of body weight]) (Braun et al., 2001). After phase III, development was given up in the United States.

2.3. AC-98 (Mannopeptimycin)

2.3.1. AC-98 complex

AC-98 complex was discovered in 1958. This complex was isolated from *Streptomyces hygroscopicus*. This complex was not pursued further at that time due to its antibacterial spectrum, which consisted exclusively of gram-positive organisms.

AC-98 is composed of five components: α, β, γ, δ, and ε, or 1 to 5 (Singh et al., 2000). These components are glycosylated cyclic hexapeptides containing two stereoisomers of an unusual amino acid, α-amino-3[4′-(2′-imidazolidinyl)]-β-hydroxy propionic acid. This hexapeptide is made of alternating L- and D-amino acids that include β-methyl phenylalanine. A D-tyrosine residue is O-glycosylated with a 1→4 α-linked mannose disaccharide (Fig. 4).

The antibacterial activity seems to be correlated with the presence of a disaccharide moiety and the position of an isovaleryl substituent on the terminal mannose.

Mannopeptimycins γ, δ, and ε have an isovaleryl group at positions C-2, C-3, and C-4 on the terminal mannose ring, respectively. Mannopeptimycin ε is the most active component against MRSA. On the other hand, both the α and β components are inactive against MRSA. All components except β protect against disseminated murine staphylococcal infections (Table 2) (Petersen et al., 2002c).

After 40 serial passages, a slight increase of mannopeptomycin δ MIC was reported.

2.3.2. AC 98-6446

AC 98-6446 is a semisynthetic derivative of component α, or 1, obtained by replacement of the β-methyl phenylalanine with a cyclohexyl alanine residue and possessing an adamantyl ketal moiety across the 4-6 position of the terminal mannose of the initial disaccharide (Dushin et al., 2002).

This semisynthetic derivative is active against MSSA and MRSA, with MICs ranging from 0.01 to 0.06 μg/ml (Petersen et al., 2002b). In murine staphylococcal infections AC 98-6446 is more active than vancomycin, with 50% effective doses (ED_{50}) of 0.08 and 0.27 mg/kg for MSSA and MRSA, respectively, whereas the ED_{50} of vancomycin were 0.69 and 2.89 mg/kg, respectively. At four times the MIC, AC 98-6446 reduced the inoculum size of MRSA GC 1131 by 2 to 3 $\log_{10}$ CFU/ml after 6 h of contact (vancomycin reduced the inoculum size by 1 to 2 $\log_{10}$ CFU/ml in the same period of contact) (Petersen et al., 2002a).

After intravenous administration of AC 98-6446, the apparent elimination half-life appeared to be long whatever the animal species (mouse, rat, monkey, or dog) (Murphy et al., 2002).

2.4. Chloroorienticin B

Chloroorienticin B and its water-soluble derivatives are active against MRSA (Tsujii et al., 1988). Introduction of a hydrophobic side chain is considered to be essential for potent antibacterial activity, especially against VRE; however, these derivatives are sparingly soluble in water. To enhance water solubility, a hydrophilic side chain was added to the previous resulting compounds, such as an amino methyl of the resorcinol moiety (Yoshida et al., 2002).

2.5. Other derivatives

A series of glycopeptides was prepared at Shionogi and displayed good in vitro anti-MRSA activity, with MICs ranging from 0.20 to 6.25 μg/ml (Japan Patent 2001).

A novel thiostrepton from *Micromonospora carbonacea* with anti-MRSA activity was isolated (Puar et al., 1998).

3. LIPOGLYCOPEPTIDES

3.1. Teicoplanin Derivatives

Teicoplanin derivatives having both hydrophobic and hydrophilic substituents were synthesized. They exhibited activity against gram-positive organisms (Pavlov et al., 1998).

A new teicoplanin-like antibiotic was found from the fermentation broth of *Actinoplanes teichomyceticus* 3/w. The compounds Teico2 aglycone and teicoplanin aglycone exhibited

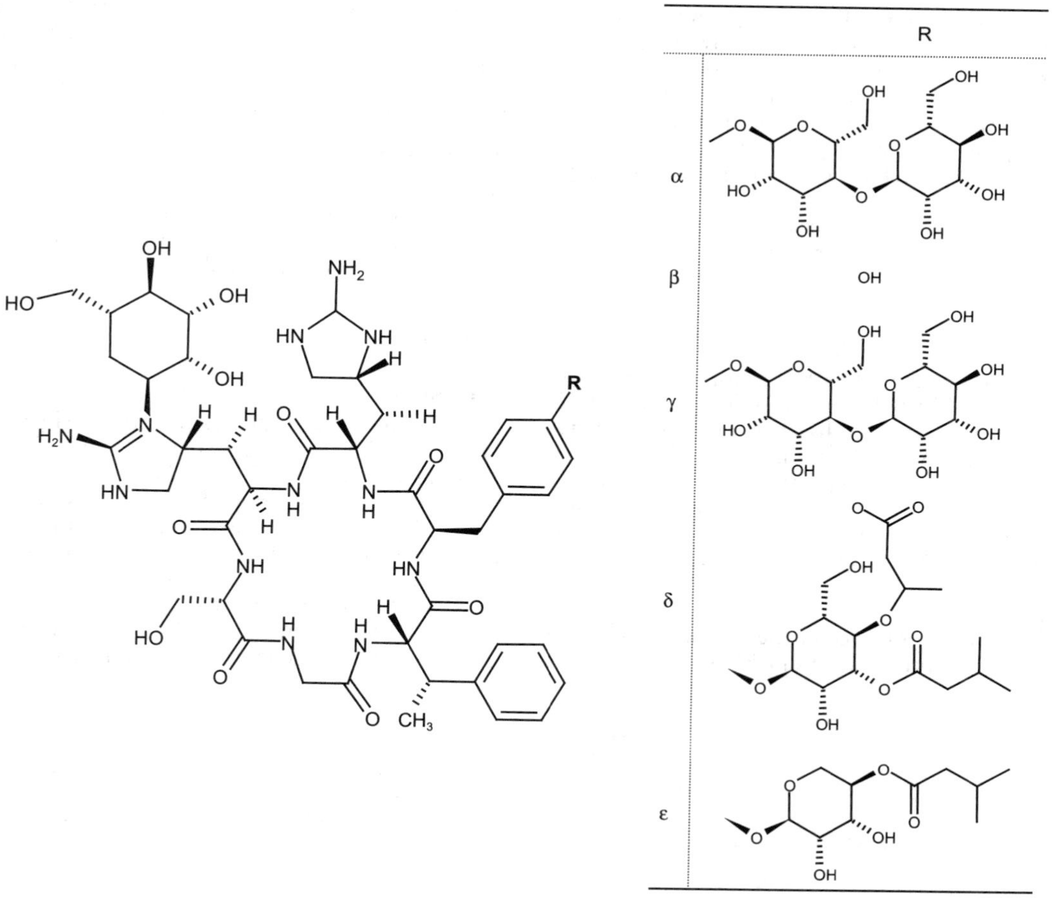

Figure 4 **AC-98 complex**

Table 2 **Antibacterial activities (in vitro and in vivo) of mannopeptimycin components**

Component or agent	MIC (μg/ml)	ED_{50} (mg/kg)
α	128	20
β	64	>32
γ	8.0	3.8
δ	8.0	2.6
	4.0	0.59
Vancomycin	1.0	0.94

MICs of 0.13 and 0.06 μg/ml, respectively, for *S. aureus* TowLI69; when 50% bovine serum was added, the MICs were 16 and 0.25 μg/ml, respectively (Quarta et al., 1996).

3.2. Dalbavancin

Dalbavancin is a semisynthetic amide derivative of MDL-62476 (A-40926). It is a complex of at least three components. For *S. aureus*, irrespective of the susceptibility to methicillin, dalbavancin MICs ranged from 0.06 to 1.0 μg/ml (MIC_{50} and MIC_{90}, 0.12 and 0.25 μg/ml).

At four and eight times the MIC dalbavancin remains bacteriostatic, with a 1- to 2-log_{10} CFU/ml reduction after 24 h of contact (Jones et al., 2001a).

After a 30-min intravenous infusion of 140 to 1,120 mg of dalbavancin to healthy volunteers, the apparent elimination half-life ranged from 145 to 193 h (mean, 1 week). At the end of infusion the concentration in plasma ranged from 3,200 to 27,000 μg/ml, and the plasma clearance was low (0.04 liter/h). Dalbavancin is highly bound to serum proteins (Leighton et al., 2004).

Dalbavancin clinical trials involving staphylococcal (MRSA) skin and soft tissue infections are expected.

3.3. Telavancin

Telavancin (TD-6424) is a semisynthetic lipoglycopeptide. It is a dimethylamino propyl amide derivative of A-40926. Telavancin is derived from a semisynthetic vancomycin analog. The decyl aminoethyl vancomycin (THRX 68-9909) via Mannich reaction yielded telavancin.

Telavancin is active against MRSA, with MICs ranging from 0.125 to 1.0 μg/ml (MIC_{50} and MIC_{90}, 0.25 and 0.5 μg/ml).

By using telavancin as a lead compound, numerous analogs were synthesized with increased sizes of the hydrophobic substituent (Judice and Pace, 2003). The antibacterial activities of the derivatives were dependent on the length of the hydrophobic substituent. Increasing the length resulted in an enhancement of in vitro activity against MRSA followed by a reduction of activity.

Telavancin does not inhibit transglycolase activity. The 50% inhibitory concentration (IC_{50}) of the transglycolase reaction decreased from 11.6 to 0.01 μg/ml for the series of glycopeptide analogs having hydrophobic substituents with sizes between 6 and 15 methylene equivalents (MIC, 16 μg/ml, except THRX 68-9909, with a MIC of 0.04 μg/ml). Telavancin inhibits both fatty acid and phospholipid biosynthesis.

After administration of 5 mg/kg intravenously to healthy volunteers, the maximum concentration of drug in serum was 45 μg/ml, and the minimum concentration in serum was 5 μg/ml. The apparent elimination half-life was 7 h.

Introduction of a hydrophobic appendage to a glycopeptide causes an increase in half-life.

The MIC_{50} and MIC_{90} of telavancin for *S. aureus* were close to those of vancomycin and teicoplanin (MIC_{50} and MIC_{90}, 1.0 and 1.0 μg/ml versus 1.0 and 2.0 μg/ml and 1.0 and 4.0 μg/ml, respectively) (Pace et al., 2003).

3.4. DA-40926

DA-40926 was obtained by microbial transformation of the parent antibiotic A-40926 through *A. teichomyceticus* ATCC 31121. DA-40926 contains two hydrophobic moieties. Fifty-nine derivatives of DA-40926 containing two hydrophobic substituents at the amino groups of the peptide backbone and glucuronic acid and their mono- and diamides and also 7-d-aminomethylated derivatives were semisynthesized and investigated (Preobrazhenskaya et al., 2002).

3.5. Tripeptins

Tripeptin is a complex of five components isolated from the culture broth of *Lysobacter* sp. strain BMK 33348F3. It is composed of eight amino acids and variable fatty acid side chains. The most active component against MRSA is the C tripeptin, with MICs ranging from 0.39 to 1.56 μg/ml. The antibacterial activity seems to be dependent on the size of the fatty acid side chain (Hashizume et al., 2001).

3.6. LY-264826

A derivative of chloroeremomycin, LY-264826 possesses lipophilic substituents on the sugar moiety and exhibits improved activity against VRE as well as against other gram-positive bacteria (Pavlov et al., 1998).

4. PEPTIDES

4.1. Nocathiacin

Nocathiacins I and II are tricyclic thiazolyl peptide antibiotics isolated from the fermentation broth of *Nocardia* and *Amycolatopsis* (Fig. 5). They inhibit protein synthesis by acting on the elongation step. They are active in vitro and in vivo against MRSA. However, they are sparingly water soluble, which a prerequisite for development as an intravenous agent (Regueiro-Ren et al., 2004).

Mono-O-alkyl nocathiacins exhibited in vitro activity superior to that of vancomycin (MIC, 0.2 to 1.0 μg/ml). Some of them displayed good in vitro and in vivo activities and

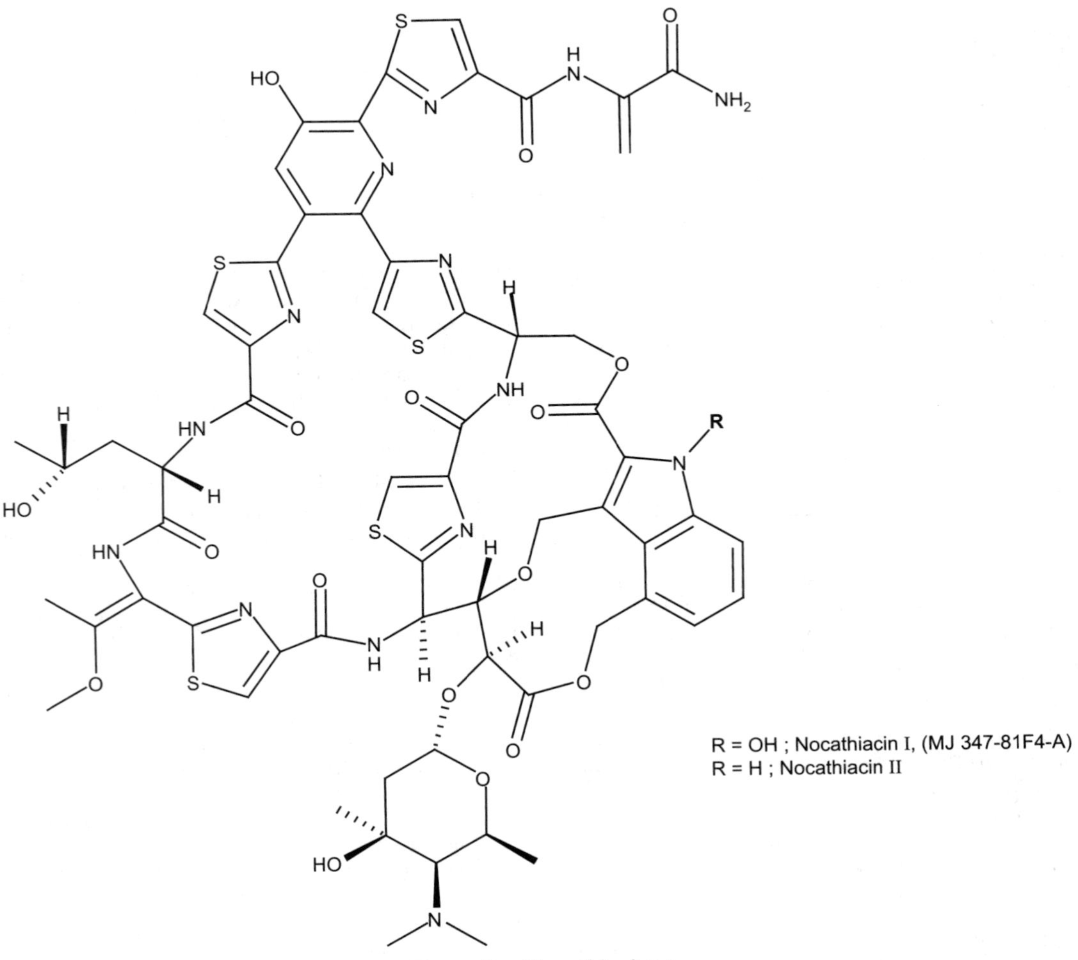

R = OH ; Nocathiacin I, (MJ 347-81F4-A)
R = H ; Nocathiacin II

Figure 5 Nocathiacin(s)

water solubility (MICs, 0.125 to 0.25 μg/ml; 50% protective dose [PD_{50}], 3.4 mg/kg). Ionic groups such as phosphate significantly improved the water solubility, to above 2 mg/ml at neutral pH.

Nocathiacin disrupts bacterial protein synthesis by interacting directly with the L11 protein and 23S rRNA regions of ribosome.

The water solubility is inadequate to produce intravenous formulations. To overcome this problem, semisynthetic compounds were prepared (Table 3).

The O-substituted analogs (A, B, and C) with polar groups (carbamate, phosphonate, and phosphates) retained potent in vitro avtivity against staphylococci as well as good in vivo activity and, for a few of them, enhanced water solubility (Naidu et al., 2004).

4.2. Methylsulfomycin

Methylsulfomycin I is a cyclic peptide isolated from the fermentation broth of *Streptomyces* sp. strain HIL-Y 9420704. It is a thiazolyl peptide containing thiazolyl and oxazolyl rings. For *S. aureus*, the MIC of methylsulfomycin I ranged from 0.06 to 0.125 μg/ml irrespective of the susceptibility to methicillin, vancomycin, or teicoplanin (Kumar et al., 1999).

4.3. Ramoplanin

Ramoplanin is a lipodepsipeptide isolated from the fermentation broth of *Actinoplanes* sp. strain ATCC 33076 in 1989. Ramoplanin is a mixture of three main components, A1, A2, and A3, with a few minor components. The three major components differ in the acyl group attached to the Asn1 N terminus and in the stereochemistry of the double bonds with the different acyl groups.

Ramoplanin belongs to a class composed of closely related antibacterials which also includes enduracibins and janiemycin.

Ramoplanin inhibits peptidoglycan biosynthesis at the level of the MurG step by binding to lipid I. Ramoplanin inhibits transglycosylases (formation of glycan chains of peptidoglycan by binding to lipid II) (Hu et al., 2003). Clinical trials were ongoing in 2004.

A ramoplanin derivative, VIC-603, was semisynthesized. Ramoplanin, which is currently under development for the treatment of diarrhea due to *Clostridium difficile* and the prevention of bacteremia due to enterococci, is limited in systemic administration by hemolytic activity and low tolerability when administered intravenously.

VIC-603 bears a 2-methylphenylacetic acid residue instead of the disubstituted fatty acid chain. MICs ranged from 0.06 to 0.25 μg/ml for MRSA, including GISA isolates (Jabes et al., 2003b). In vivo in murine staphylococcal infections (immunocompetent mice), the ED_{50} were 0.4 and 0.5 mg/kg for the intravenous and subcutaneous routes, respectively (Jabes et al., 2003a).

5. LIPOPEPTIDES

Among lipopeptides it is possible to differentiate two subgroups of compounds: those related to amphomycin, such as friulimicins, tsushimycin, zaomycin, laspartomycins, and aspartocin, and a group of lipodepsipeptides containing daptomycin and the A-21978 complex. The latter is composed of 10 amino acids with nine peptide linkages and one ester linkage within the ring.

5.1. Daptomycin

Daptomycin was isolated from *Streptomyces roseoporus*. It is a 13-amino-acid cyclic peptide with a decanoyl side chain. This side chain is responsible for the high lipophilicity and results in high protein binding in humans (>90%). Daptomycin is bactericidal against MRSA, including GISA strains, with MIC_{50}s and MIC_{90}s of 2.0 and 2.0 μg/ml and 4.0 and 16 μg/ml without calcium (50 μg/ml in the medium) and 0.25 and 0.5 μg/ml and 1.0 and 4.0 μg/ml with addition of calcium (Petersen et al., 1999). Daptomycin inhibits peptidoglycan and lipoteichoic acid biosynthesis and is responsible for inner membrane disruption. In vivo in murine staphylococcal infections, the ED_{50} were 0.07 to 0.12 mg/kg depending on the challenge inoculum size.

In an effort to enhance the antibacterial activity and the pharmacological properties of daptomycin, a series of N-acylated ornithine analogs was synthesized. It was shown previously that the ornithine amino group is not essential (Hill et al., 2001a, 2001b). Some analogs had activity against MRSA similar to that of daptomycin but possessed better pharmacokinetics (Hill et al., 2003).

Daptomycin possesses an unusual amino acid, kynurenine. Modifications of this amino acid were attempted on the ketone and anilino groups. These modifications highlighted the importance of this amino acid for antibacterial activity (Hill et al., 2001c).

Daptomycin in an intravenous formulation is now available in the United States for clinics.

5.2. HMR 1043

HMR 1043 is a cyclic lipopeptide. In calcium-adjusted Mueller-Hinton agar, MICs were 0.5 μg/ml for both MSSA and MRSA, and a MIC of 2.0 μg/ml for GISA was noted (Bemer et al., 2003).

5.3. Laspartomycin

Laspartomycin was originally reported in 1955 by Umezawa et al. It is a lipopeptide antibiotic related to amphomycin, with a C-15 αβ unsaturated fatty acid side chain (Fig. 6). Laspartomycin is produced from fermentation broth of *Streptomyces viridochromogenes* subsp. *komabensis* ATCC 29814 (Border et al., 2001).

Laspartomycin is composed of 11 amino acids and a C-15 unsaturated fatty acid side chain. C Laspartomycin is the main component. All components differ by their acyl side

Table 3 In vitro activities and water solubilities of nocathiacin and analogs

Compound	MIC (μg/ml) for MSSA	PD_{50} (mg/kg) i.v.[a]	Water solubility (mg/ml) (pH)
Nocathiacin I	0.007	0.2	0.34 (4.0)
Compound A	0.003	ND	>2.3 (3.0)
Compound B	0.125	1.6	5.6 (8.2)
Compound C	0.25	5.9	>10 (8.5)

[a]i.v., intravenously; ND, not determined.

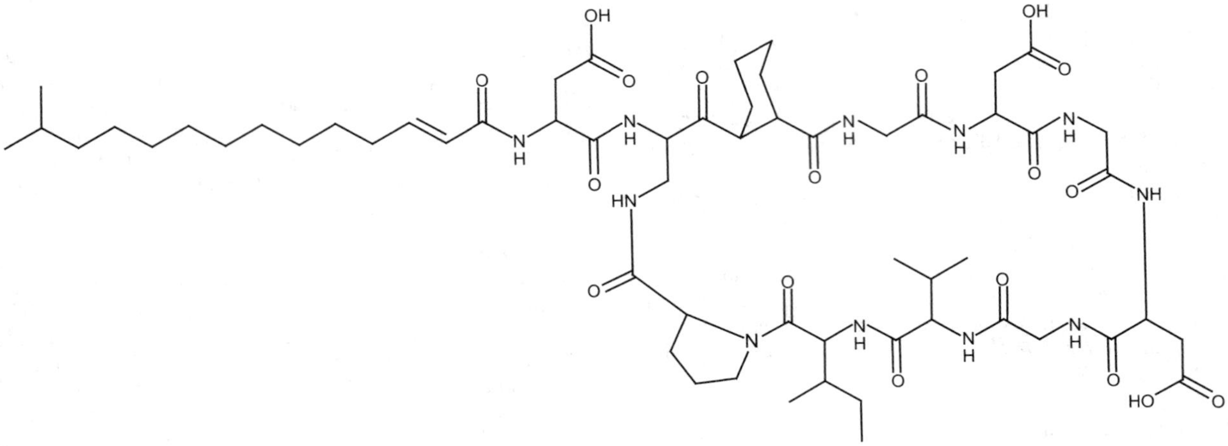

Figure 6 Laspartomycin

chains. The enzymatic cleavage of laspartomycin with a deacylase produced by *Actinoplanes utahensis* resulted in two peptides, and both have been converted by synthetic modifications to derivatives active against *S. aureus*, with MICs of 4 to >64 μg/ml) without addition of calcium and of 2.0 to >64 μg/ml with addition of calcium (4 mM calcium chloride).

The main requirement for biological activity with laspartomycin derivatives seems to be an acyl-L-aspartic acid (Simon et al., 2001).

5.4. WAP-8294A

WAP-8294A is produced by *Lysobacter* and belongs to a complex of depsipeptide antibiotics (Fig. 7). This complex is

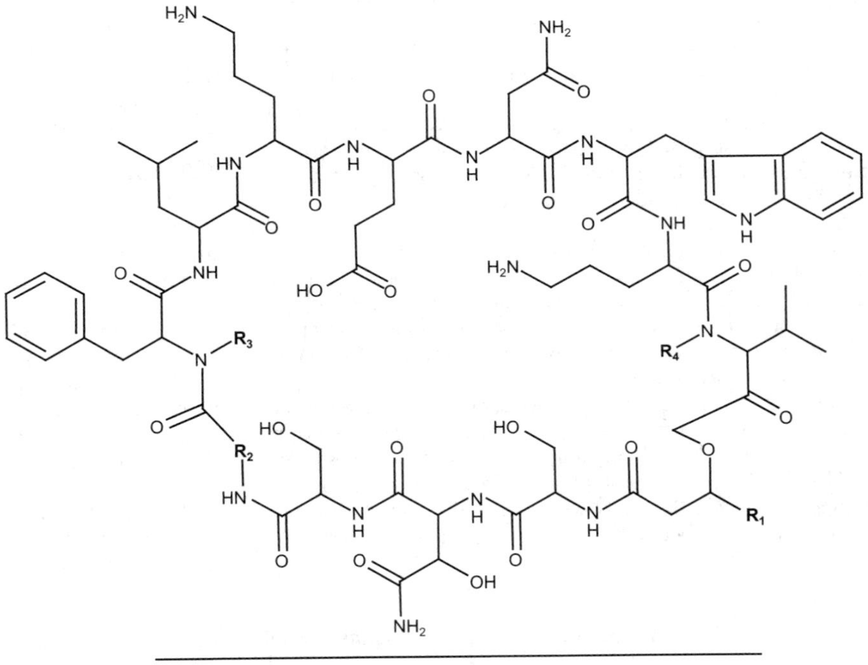

	R_1	R_2	R_3	R_4
WAP-8294 A_1	$(CH_2)_4CH_3$	CH_2	CH_3	CH_3
WAP-8294 A_2	$(CH_2)_3CH(CH_3)_2$	CH_2	CH_3	CH_3
WAP-8294 A_4	$(CH_2)_4CH(CH_3)_2$	CH_2	CH_3	CH_3
WAP-8294 Ax8	$(CH_2)_3CH(CH_3)_2$	CH_2	CH_3	CH_3
WAP-8294 Ax9	$(CH_2)_3CH(CH_3)_2$	CH_2	H	H
WAP-8294 Ax13	$(CH_2)_3CH(CH_3)_2$	$(CH_2)_2$	CH_3	CH_3

Figure 7 WAP-8294A complex

composed of 19 components. WAP-8294A is the major component, and others are considered minor components. Only six of them were isolated and their structures elucidated (Kato et al., 1997, 1998).

WAP-8294A_1, -A_2, and -A_4, with MICs of 0.39 to 0.78 μg/ml, are bactericidal, with a 5-log_{10} CFU/ml reduction after 2 h of contact at the MIC.

WAP-8294A_2 seems to interact selectively with phospholipids in the cell membrane, resulting in membrane damage. WAP-8294A is composed of 12 amino acid residues and 1 3-hydroxy fatty acid residue.

5.5. LY-301621

LY-301621 is a tripeptide composed of carbobenzoxy diphenyl alanine-proline-phenylalanine alcohol (Fig. 8). It acts synergistically with methicillin against MRSA (Eid et al., 1997).

5.6. Diperamycin

Diperamycin (Fig. 9) was isolated from the fermentation broth of *Streptomyces griseoaurantiacus*. Diperamycin is a cyclic hexadepsipeptide and is active against MRSA, with MICs of 0.1 to 0.2 μg/ml. This compound also exerted strong inhibitory activity on tumor cell lines tested (IC_{50}, 0.009 to 0.023 μg/ml) (Matsumoto et al., 1999).

5.7. TAN 1057

TAN 1057 A and B are dipeptides consisting of β-homoarginine and an amidourea heterocycle from 2, 3-diaminopropionic acid (Fig. 10) (Funabashi et al., 1993). It is a complex of four peptidic components, A to D. TAN 1057 was obtained from the fermentation broth of *Flexibacter* sp. strains PK-74 and PK-176 (Katayama et al., 1993). TAN 1057 A and D are more active against MRSA than the B and C components, probably due to their *S* configuration at C-5. TAN 1057 is more active in vivo in murine staphylococcal infections than vancomycin. Apparently there is no correlation between in vitro and in vivo activities. MICs are medium and pH dependent.

TAN 1057 seems to inhibit protein synthesis after the formation of aminoacyl-tRNA.

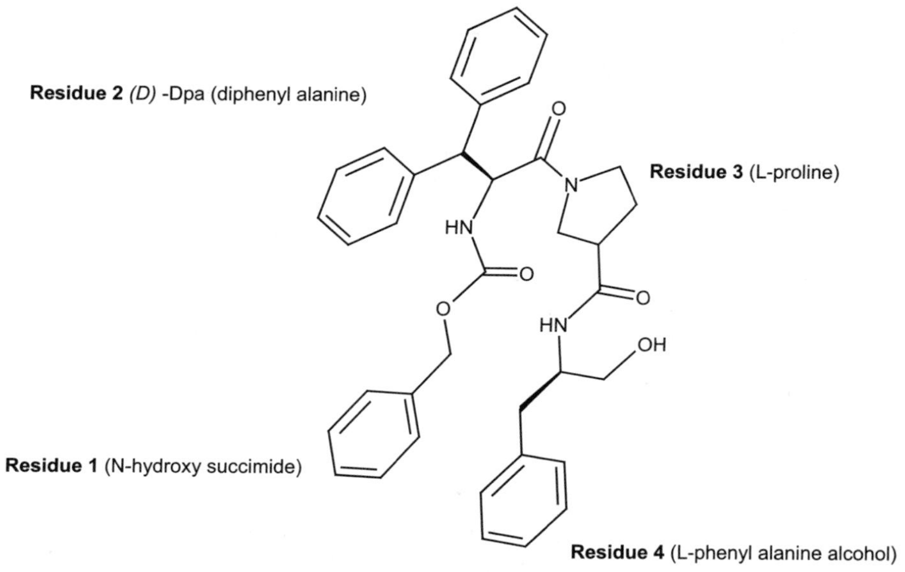

Residue 2 *(D)* -Dpa (diphenyl alanine)

Residue 3 (L-proline)

Residue 1 (N-hydroxy succimide)

Residue 4 (L-phenyl alanine alcohol)

Figure 8 LY-301621

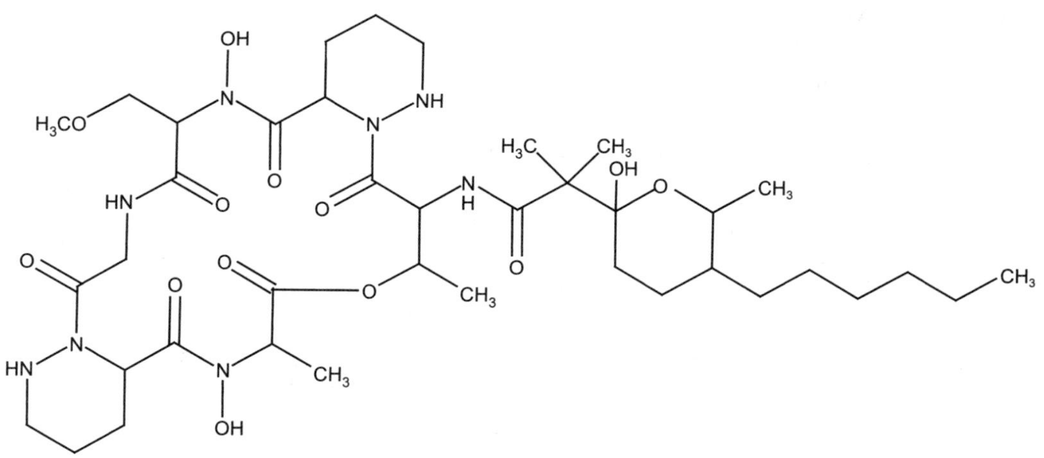

Figure 9 Diperamycin

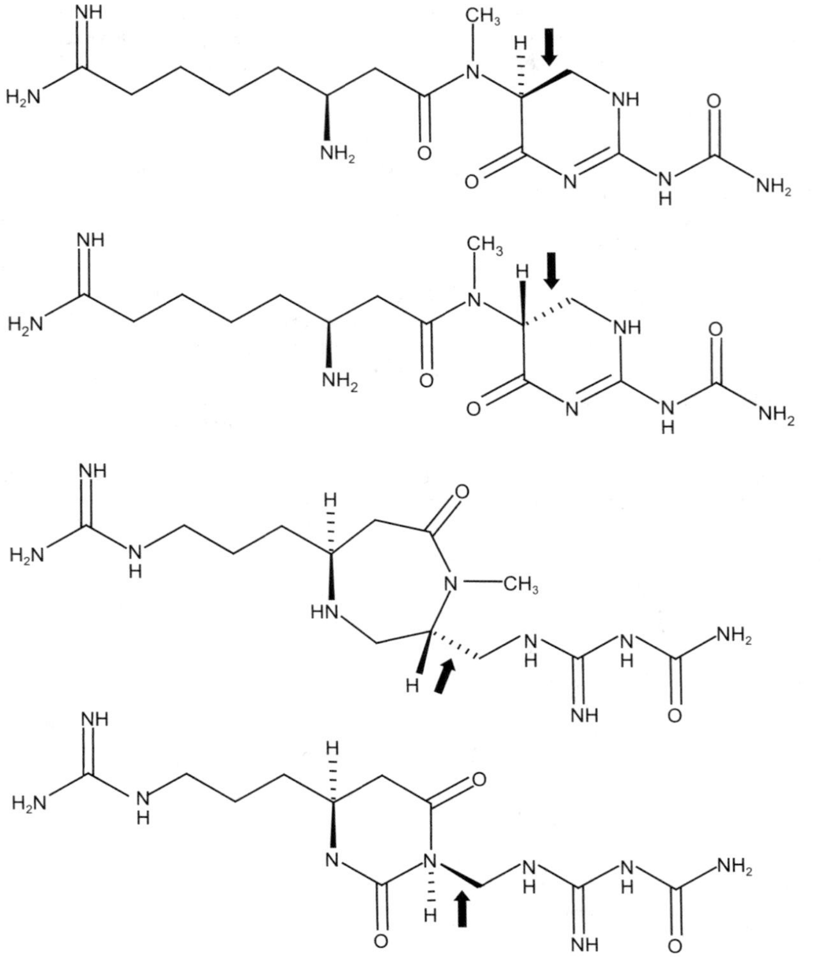

TAN 1057 A

TAN 1057 B

TAN 1057 C

TAN 1057 D

Figure 10 TAN 1057 complex

Fifty percent lethal doses (LD_{50}) are above 400, 50, and 100 mg/kg for oral, peritoneal and intravenous, and subcutaneous administrations, respectively (Table 4).

A low level of resistance might be due to the modification of the mechanism of uptake of TAN 1057 into the bacterial cell; a high level of resistance is due to *S. aureus* ribosome modifications (Limburg et al., 2002).

5.8. Sapecin B derivatives

Many insects synthesize various antibacterial proteins. They are inducible defense proteins. It was shown that an undecapeptide derived from sapecin B, an antibacterial of *Sarcophaga*, is effective against gram-positive bacteria.

Alteration of the amino acid sequence of this undecapeptide led to highly active compounds. Two peptides were obtained,

Table 4 In vitro and in vivo activities of TAN 1057[a]

S. aureus strain	Inoculum (CFU/mouse)	Compound(s)	MIC (μg/ml)	ED_{50} (mg/kg)[b]	
				s.c.	p.o.
308-A1 (MSSA)	10^8	TAN 1057	12	0.03	1.2
		Imipenem-cilastatin	0.02	0.10	
		Vancomycin	0.78	2.2	
N 133 A (MRSA)	10^8	TAN 1057	6.25	0.03	0.56
		Imipenem-cilastatin	>25	4.2	
		Vancomycin	1.56	2.3	

[a]Data from Katayama et al., 1993, and Williams et al., 1998.
[b]s.c., subcutaneously; p.o., per os.

RLKLLLLLRLK-NH_2 and KLKLLLLLKLK-NH_2. These peptides are built with two different units, basic at the terminus and hydrophobic due to five internal leucines. Cleavage sites are provided for various proteinases due to the presence of lysine and arginine residues. The D-enantiomer of KLKLLLLLKLK-NH_2 is resistant to tryptic digestion. The MICs for *S. aureus* ranged from 1.0 to 2.0 μg/ml, and the ED_{50} ranged from 0.2 to 0.3 mg/kg.

The peptides apparently interact with the phospholipid of the membrane but they are not hemolytic (Alvarez-Bravo et al., 1994); it is accepted that 20 amino acid residues are needed for inhibiting peptidoglycan biosynthesis and the lipid bilayer of the membrane.

5.9. GE 2270A

GE 2270A (Fig. 11) is a member of the cyclic thiazolyl peptide family, which inhibits protein synthesis. This family (nonribosomally synthesized) contains GE 37468, the amythiamicins, thiostrepton, nosiheptide, siomycin, and micrococcin. GE 2270A is produced by *Planobispora rosea*. GE 2270A inhibits protein biosynthesis through inhibition of elongation factor Tu (EFTu). EfTu is an essential component in the bacterial protein biosynthetic pathway. EFTu recognizes and transports noninitiator aminoacyl-tRNA to the A-site of mRNA-programmed ribosomes during the elongation cycle (Heffron and Jurnak, 2000). The IC_{50} for EFTu was 5 nM.

GE 2270A is poorly soluble in water; this fact is a limiting factor for development (water solubility <0.001 mg/ml at pH 7.4).

Series of analogs of GE 2270A were synthesized in order to enhance water solubility. Few derivatives exhibited acceptable water solubility (≥0.5 mg/ml). The MIC for MRSA was 0.12 μg/ml (Clough et al., 2003).

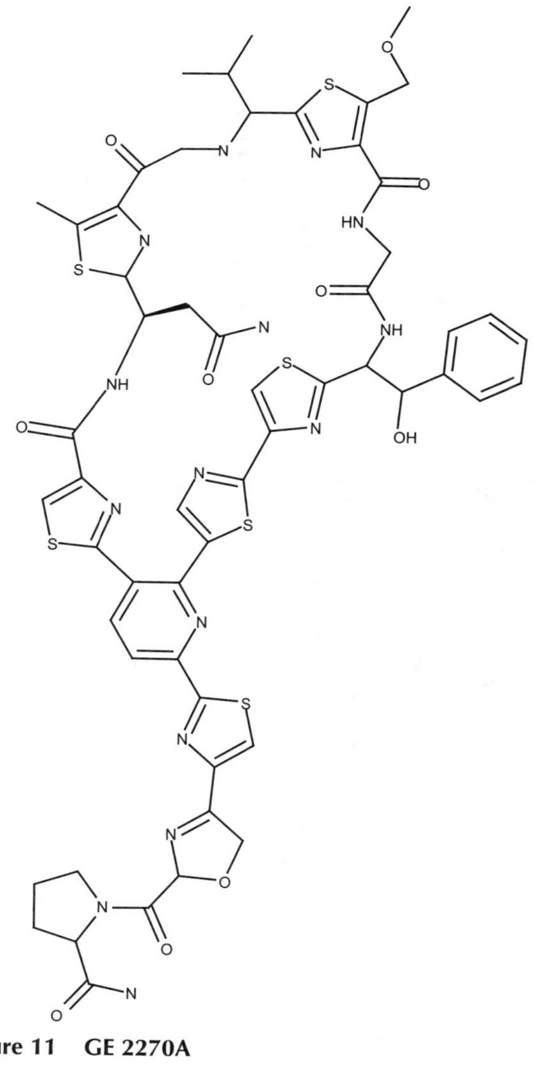

Figure 11 **GE 2270A**

5.10. M-1396

M-1396 is a semisynthetic derivative of amphomycin (Fig. 12). The MICs for MRSA ranged from 0.5 to 2.0 μg/ml irrespective of the susceptibilities of the strains to oxacillin, mupirocin, or tetracycline. For coagulase-negative staphylococci the MICs ranged from 0.5 to 4.0 μg/ml. MICs ranged from 0.5 to 2.0 μg/ml and 0.25 to 1.0 μg/ml for enterococci, irrespective of their susceptibilities to vancomycin and linezolid, and viridans group streptococci, respectively.

M-1396 seems to be rapidly bactericidal (less than 2 h of contact for *Enterococcus faecalis* at 16 times the MIC.

In murine peritonitis infections, the ED_{50} were 6.5, 0.6, and 0.8 mg/kg for *S. aureus*, *Streptococcus pneumoniae*, and *E. faecalis*, respectively.

The elimination half-lives after 10 mg/kg administered intravenously as a bolus were 481 and 275 min for Swiss CD-1 mice and Sprague-Dawley rats, respectively (Dugourd et al., 2004).

6. NATURAL PRODUCTS OF PLANT AND MARINE ORIGIN

6.1. *Camellia sinensis* (Tea Components)

The antibacterial activity of tea was recognized a century ago (McNaught, 1906).

Of all of the components extracted, one of them, epigallocatechin gallate, exerts anti-MRSA activity (MICs, 4.0 μg/ml) (Shiota et al., 1999; Yam et al., 1997). 5-Epicatechin gallate and epigallocatechin gallate (Fig. 13) are major components of Japanese green tea (*C. sinensis*). They are polyphenolic compounds. Alkyl gallates, such as acetyl gallate and dodecyl gallate, have been found to possess direct activity against MRSA (MICs, 12.5 μg/ml) (Kubo et al., 2002). The putative mode of action is prevention of production of PBP 2a by *S. aureus*. Alkyl gallates were shown to inhibit bacterial respiratory systems. They act synergistically with β-lactams to restore activity against MRSA.

6.2. Ascochital

The organic extracts of the culture filtrate of the marine ascomycete (Linder) Pleomascariaceae displayed activity against gram-positive and gram-negative bacteria, including *Pseudomonas aeruginosa*. Among these extracts, ascochital, an aromatic aldehyde, was investigated. It exhibited antibacterial activity against *Bacillus subtilis* (Kusnick et al., 2002).

6.3. MC-21 A

MC-21 A is a phenolic substance exerting anti-MRSA activity (Fig. 14). It is composed of symmetrical aromatic benzenes replaced with bromine atoms. MC-21 A was isolated from *Pseudoalteromonas phenolica* sp. nov. O-BC30(T). MC-21 A alters the permeability of the cell membrane. The MICs for MSSA and MRSA are 1.0 μg/ml. It is bactericidal at four times the MICs after 8 h of contact (Isnansetyo and Kamei, 2003).

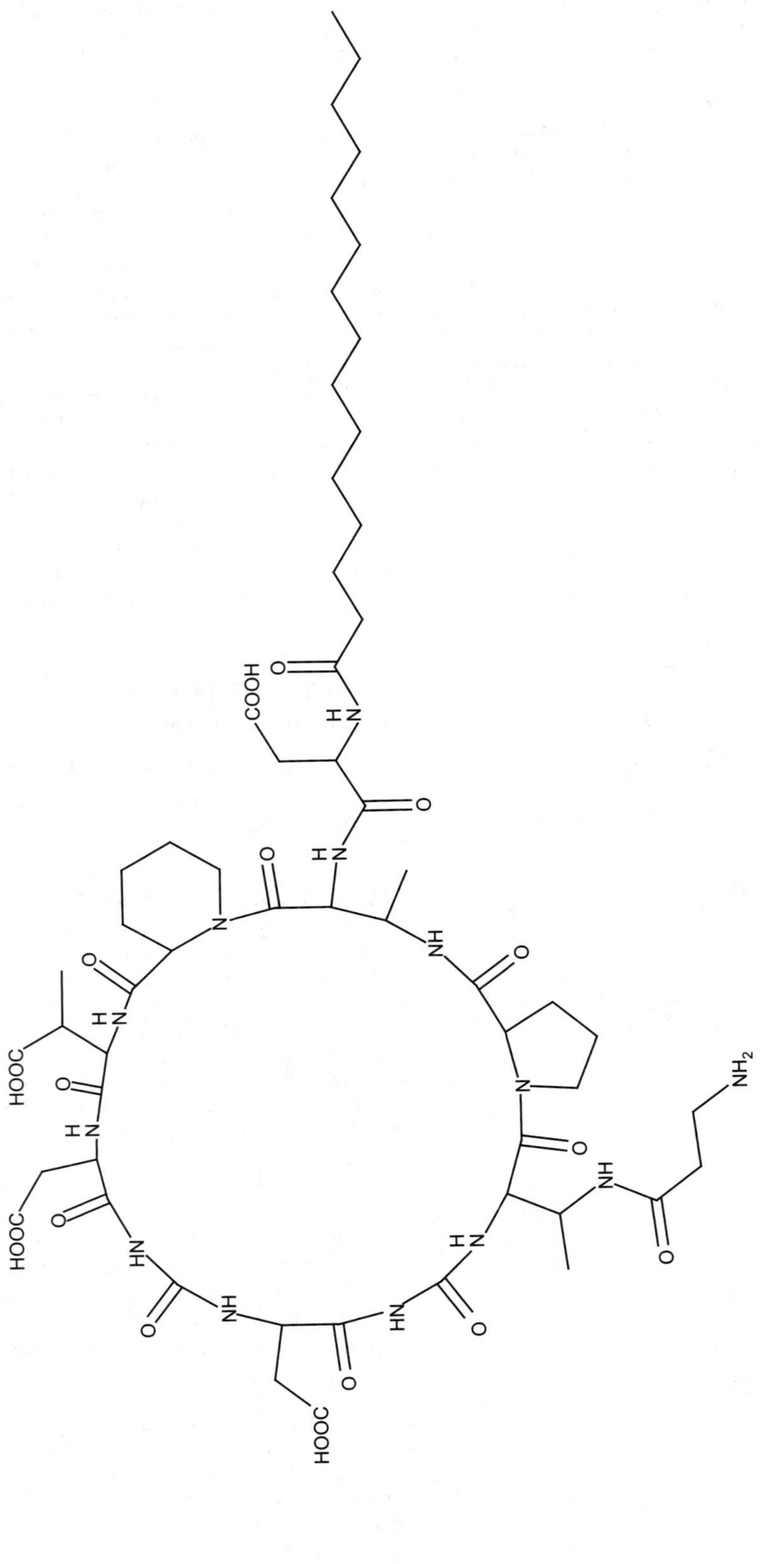

Figure 12 M-1396

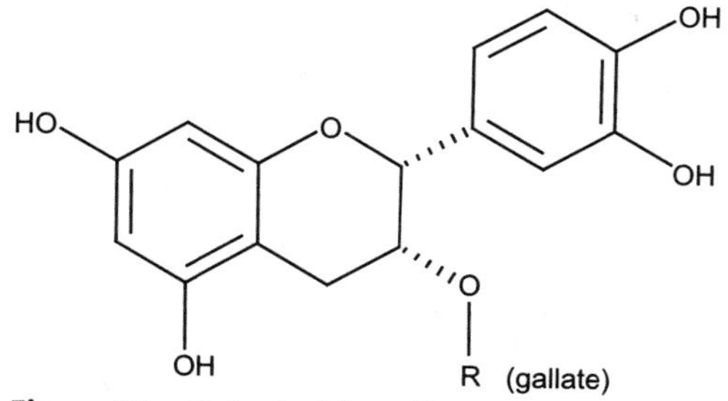

Figure 13 Epicatechin gallate

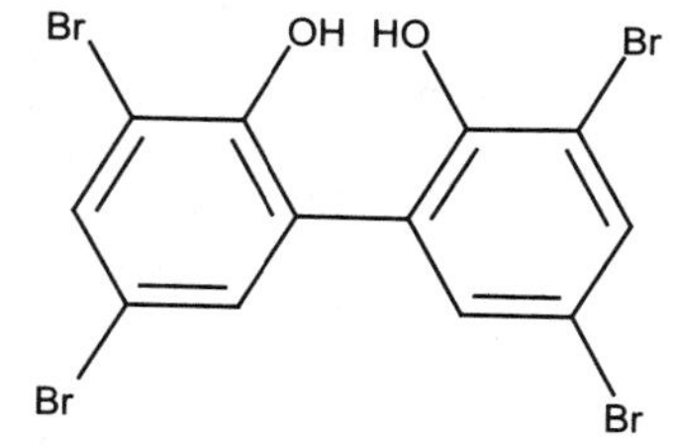

Figure 14 MC-21 A

6.4. Xanthones

Extracts of *Garcinia mangostana* (Guttiferae) possessed anti-staphylococcal activity. Some of the components exhibit anti-MRSA activity, such as a xanthone, α-mangostin, with MICs ranging from 1.56 to 12.5 μg/ml.

Rubraxanthone isolated from *Garcinia diorica*, with structural analogy to α-mangostin, exerts the highest antistaphylococcal activity (MICs, 0.3 to 1.25 μg/ml) (Iinuma et al., 1996).

6.5. Sesquiterpenoids

Artemisia gilvescens is found in some provinces of China and Japan. The sesquiterpene substance was also isolated from a marine gorgonian and *Taraxacum walchii*. It displays a MIC of 1.95 μg/ml for MRSA (Kawazoe et al., 2003) (Fig. 15).

A sesquiterpene lactone was extracted from the annual herb *Xanthium sibiricum* Patr or wild (Fig. 16). Xanthatin exhibits anti-MRSA activity (MICs, 7.8 to 15.6 μg/ml). MICs are identical whatever the susceptibility of *S. aureus* to methicillin (Sato et al., 1997).

6.6. Aaptamines

Methanol extracts of the Indonesian marine sponge *Xestospongia* were investigated for antibacterial activity. Analysis of the extracts resulted in extraction of aaptamines. One of them was identical to an aaptamine reported for the Okinawa marine sponge, *Aaptos aaptos* (Fig. 17).

One derivative displayed moderate in vitro activity against staphylococci (MIC, 6.0 μg/ml) (Calcul et al., 2003).

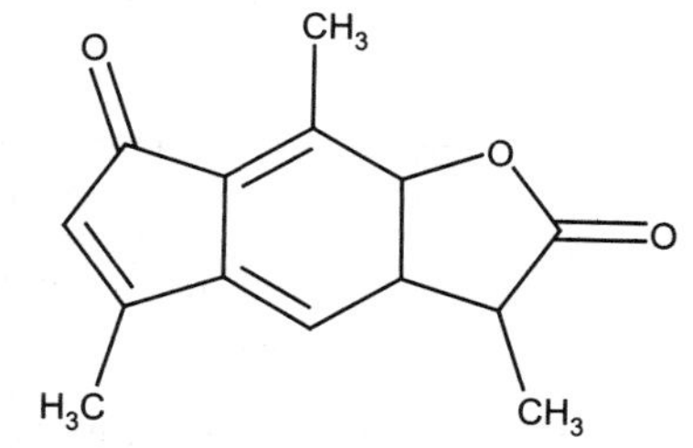

Figure 15 Sesquiterpenoids (*A. gilvescens*)

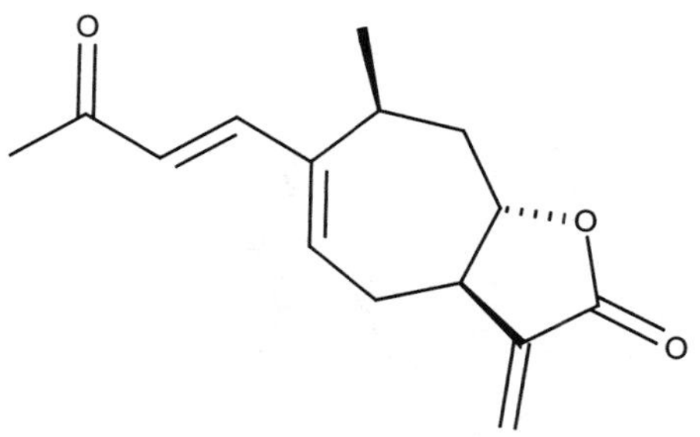

Figure 16 Xanthatin

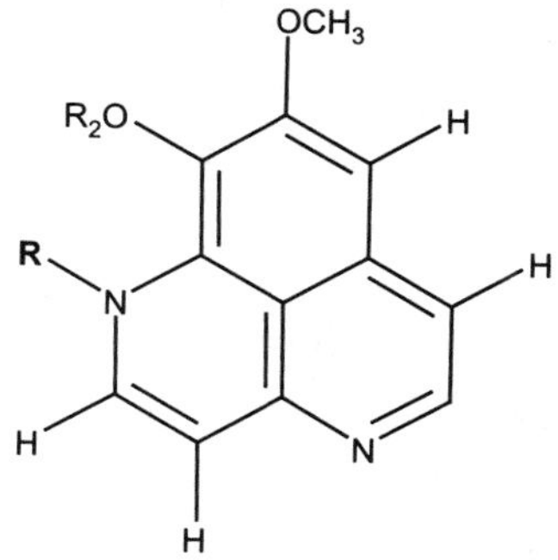

Figure 17 Aaptamines

These aaptamines are found in sponges of the orders Hadromerida (subclass Teractinomorpha) and Haplosclerimida (subclass Ceractinomorpha).

6.7. ECO-0501

ECO-0501 is a natural product obtained from *Amycolatopsis orientalis*. It is a glycosidic polyketide containing few guanidine glucuronic acid and amino-hydroxycyclopentenone groups (Fig. 18).

The MICs are 2.0 and 4.0 μg/ml for MRSA and human GISA strains, respectively. ECO-0501 is a bacteriostatic compound which acts by disrupting the inner membrane.

7. MISCELLANEOUS COMPOUNDS

7.1. Deoxyspergualin

15-Deoxyspergualin is an immunosuppressive agent used in organ transplantation. It is weakly active against *S. aureus*. It apparently acts by depleting intracellular *S. aureus* with the ubiquitous putrescine and spermidine (Hibasami et al., 1991).

7.2. Dichlorophenyl Analogs

The 6-chlorophenyl analogs (Fig. 19) displayed good anti-MRSA activity (MICs, 1.56 to 6.25 μg/ml) (Miura et al., 1994).

7.3. Rhodamine

One of the most effective antibacterial strategies is to disrupt the integrity of bacterial cell wall formation. Peptidoglycan includes four steps in which amino acid residues are ligated to uridine-diphospho-*N*-acetylmuramic acid (UDP-MurNac). MurC is encoded by the *murC* gene and catalyzes the formation of the peptide bond between UDP-MurNac and L-alanine.

Benzylidene rhodamine (Fig. 20) is an inhibitor of MurC (IC_{50}, 27 μM) and is active against MRSA (MICs, 31 μM).

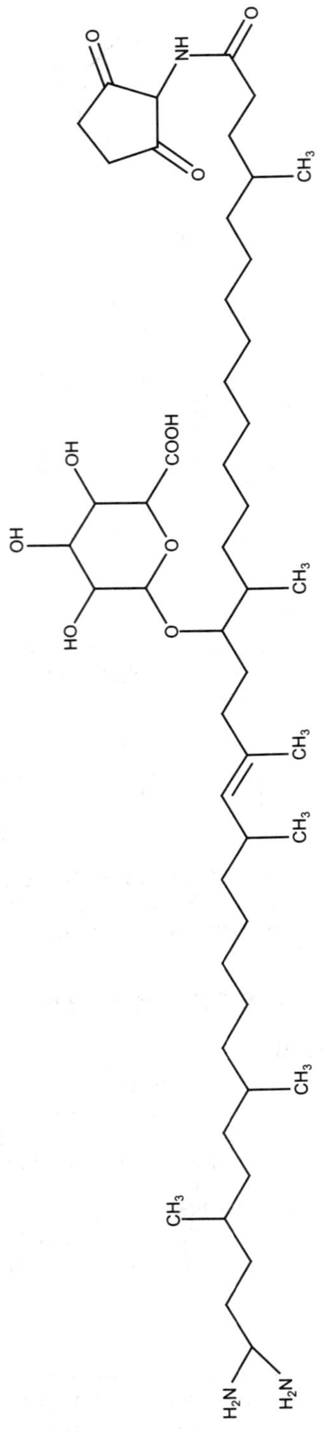

Figure 18 ECO-0501

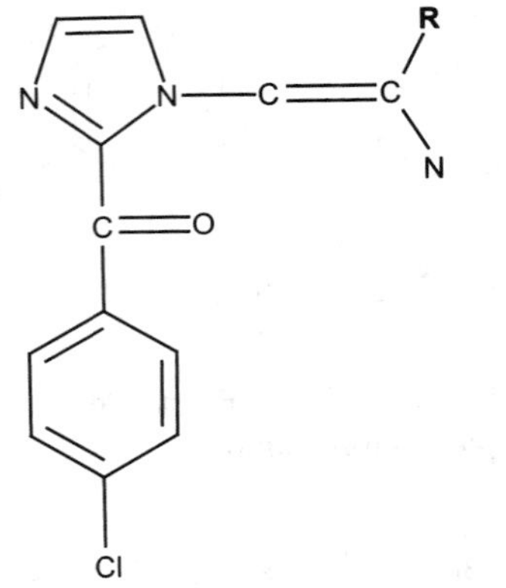

Figure 19 Dichlorophenyl analogs

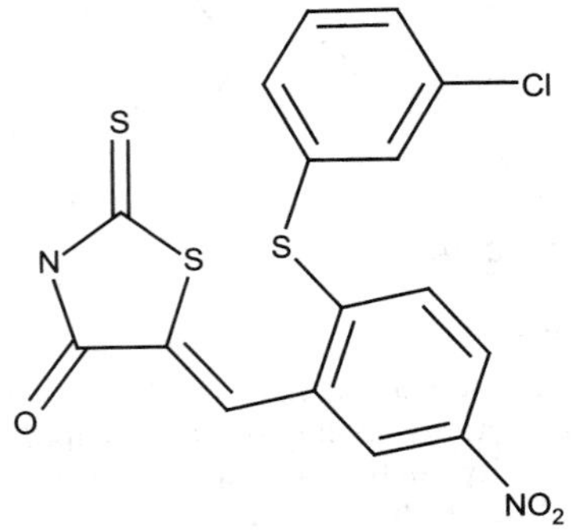

Figure 20 Benzylidene rhodamine

However, this compound is apparently toxic to Chinese hamster ovary cells (29 μM) (Sim et al., 2002).

7.4. Chorismate Synthase Inhibitors

The shikimate pathway is common to microbial eukaryotes and prokaryotes even if the sequence identity is low; the topological arrangement of secondary structure elements is almost unchanged. The biosynthesis of aromatic acids through the shikimate pathway is essential for bacteria. This pathway is absent in humans, essential amino acids being acquired through diet. The shikimate pathway is complex: five steps are needed for the conversion of 3-deoxy-D-arabinose-heptolosonuc-3-phosphate to dehydroquinate catalyzed by dehydroquinase synthetases. Using type I or II dehydroquinate synthetases encoded by the *aroB* gene followed by dehydroshikimate dehydratase, the dehydroquinate can be converted to dehydroshikimate and then to protocatechinate.

Disruption of the shikimate pathway results in attenuation for virulence of many bacteria. The coding sequence for *S. aureus* was identified as a 1,062-bp open reading frame.

Chorismate synthase is a key enzyme in the shikimate pathway, essential for the synthesis of aromatic acids in bacteria.

A series of benzofuranones inhibits chorismate synthase, with IC_{50}s ranging from 0.15 to 2.2 μM for PTX-008218 to 8 μM for PTX-110130 (Fig. 21).

By screening a series of compounds, bis-phenylsulfonamides were identified as potential inhibitors of AroB enzyme activity. The most active bis-sulfonamide inhibitor of dihydroquinate synthase was A-358 (Fig. 22), with an IC_{50} of 1.8 μM for *S. aureus* AroB. However, A-358 has a low water solubility (<100 μM) and a logP of 3 to 4 (Chana et al., 2001). The mean MIC of A-358 for *S. aureus* was 1.8 μg/ml (Stables et al., 2001). For MRSA, MICs are high (4.0 to 16 μg/ml). A-358

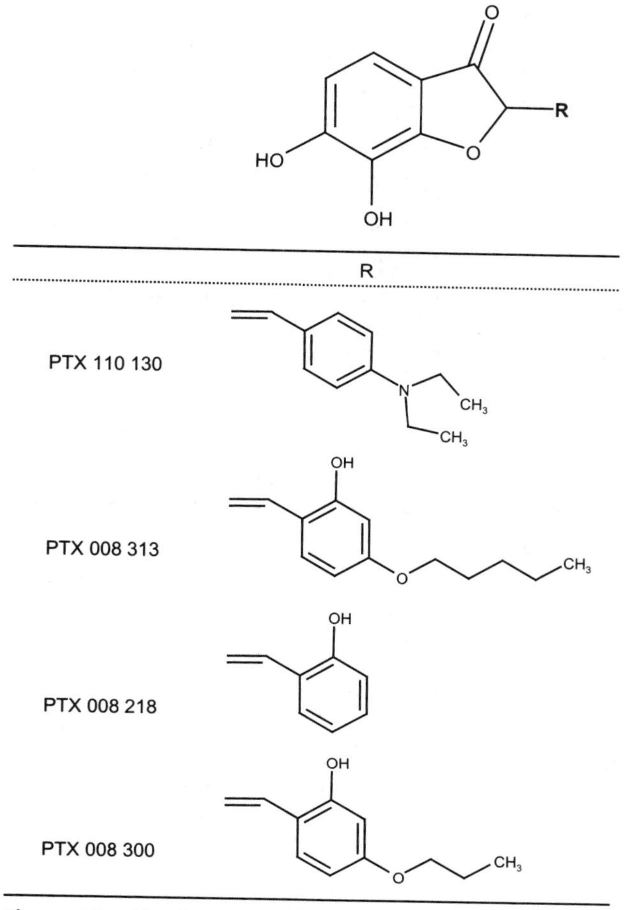

Figure 21 Chorismate synthetase inhibitors

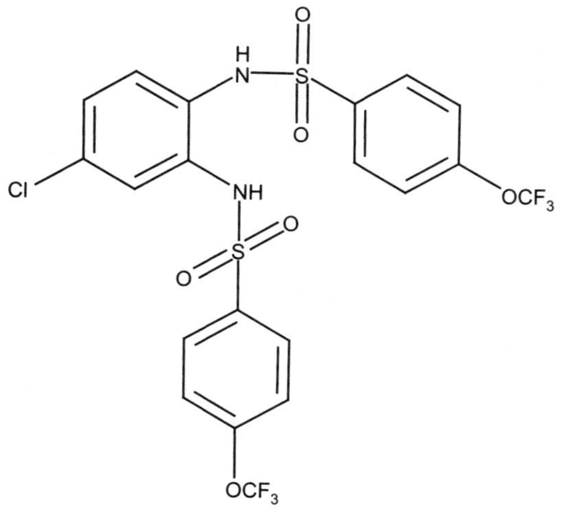

Figure 22 A-358 (shikimate dehydroquinate synthase inhibitor)

seems to be bactericidal against MSSA. No data have been disclosed for MRSA. In vivo in an experimental model of staphylococcal skin and skin structure infection in 6- to 8-week-old BALB/c mice, after topical treatment, a reduction of the bacterial burden of approximately 3 $\log_{10}$ CFU/ml was attained (Peters et al., 2001).

7.5. Methanofusidic Acid

Fusidic acid is a steroid antibacterial issued from the fermentation of *Fusidium coccineum*. The $\Delta_{17(20)}$ double bond is essential for antibacterial activity. However, it is assumed that C-17 and C-20 may be altered.

17*S*,20*S*-Dihydrofusidic acid exhibits potent antibacterial activity.

The spirocyclopropane system orients the side chain into a bioactive conformational space. 17*S*,20*S*-Methanofusidic acid (Fig. 23) exerts good antistaphylococcal activity (MIC, 0.003 μg/ml), including against MRSA (MIC, 0.01 μg/ml). However, a cross-resistance was noted with fusidic acid (Duvold et al., 2002).

7.6. Pol IIIC inhibitors

Polymerase IIIC (Pol IIIC) is an enzyme encoded by the *polC* gene. Pol IIIC is only found in gram-positive bacteria with a low G + C content, including *Staphylococcus, Enterococcus, Streptococcus, Bacillus*, and *Listeria*. This enzyme is not found in gram-positive bacteria with a high G + C content, such as *Mycobacterium* and *Corynebacterium*, or in gram-negative bacteria.

Pol IIIC is a replication-specific DNA polymerase:

- Pol IIIC is essential for bacterial DNA replication.
- Pol IIIC enzymes are highly conserved among gram-positive bacteria.
- The active site of Pol IIIC has been shown to bind specifically to the small-molecule antibiotics of the 6-anilino uracil family of inhibitors (AUs).

The potential utility of Pol III inhibitors as antibacterial agents was first described by Langley in 1962.

The AUs act through their capacity to mimic the guanine moiety of dGTP by forming base pairs with impaired cytosine of the DNA template. The aryl domain of AUs binds to Pol IIIC.

N[3]-Hydroxybutyl-6- (3′-ethyl-4′-methylamino) uracil (HBEMAU) (Fig. 24) is highly specific to Pol IIIC but does not inhibit DNA polymerase IIIE of gram-negative bacteria (Tarantino et al., 1999).

The frequency of resistance is low at eight times the MIC (Wright and Gambino, 1984): 5.9×10^{-9} for MRSA and 7.3×10^{-10} for MSSA.

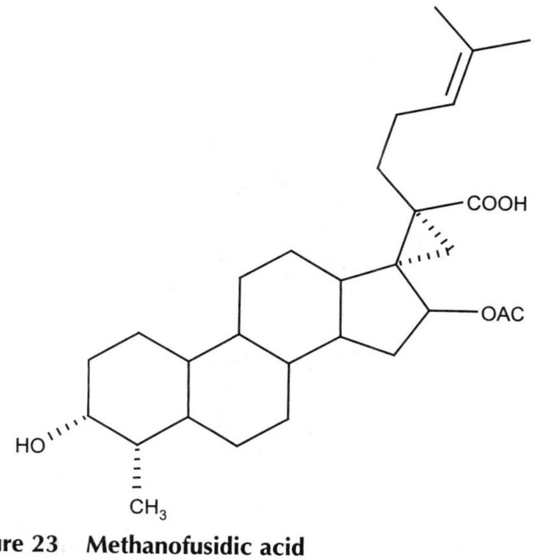

Figure 23 Methanofusidic acid

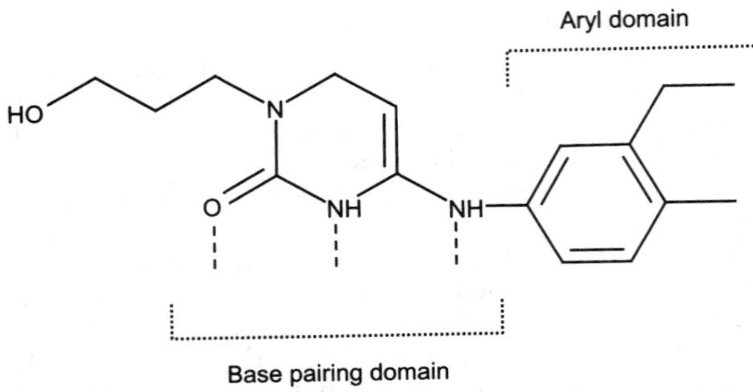

Figure 24 Pol IIIC inhibitor (HBEMAU)

By cloning the *polC* gene of HBEMAU-resistant *S. aureus*, the only mutation was a change in amino acid 1261 (Phe→Leu).

The prototype inhibitors 6-phenylhydrazino uracil, 6-benzylamino uracil, and AU were shown to inhibit a catalytically inactive ternary complex with DNA and the enzyme (Cozzarelli, 1977; Wright and Brown, 1977). These prototypes are insoluble in water (Fig. 25).

To overcome these limitations, the AU moiety was replaced with a 4-substituted-2-amino-6 (anilino) pyrimidine subunit.

The first series of 2-amino-4-chloro-6 (anilino) pyrimidine analogs was weakly active as Pol IIIC inhibitors (IC_{50}s, 50 to 120 μM). A new series of analogs with variations of the substituent at position 4 was prepared. Of these, the *p*-bromo derivative (Fig. 25) was fivefold more active than the prototype 4-chloro analog. The IC_{50} was 10 μM for Pol IIIC of *S. aureus*.

7.7. Lydicamycin

Lydicamycin was described in 1991. A new series of lydicamycins was reported as TPU A, B, C, and D. They are produced by *Streptomyces platensis* TP A 0598 (Fig. 26).

The most active component was component D, with MICs from 3.13 to 6.25 μg/ml for MRSA. Component D is the 30-demethyl-8-deoxy analog. The presence of a C-C double bound between C-14 and C-15 may diminish the antibacterial activity (Furumai et al., 2002).

7.8. Tetrahydroquinolones

In a series of 2-(1*H*-indol-3-yl) quinolines (Fig. 27) (Hoemann et al., 2000), it was shown that some derivatives were effective in vitro and in vivo against MRSA, including GISA strains, and VRE.

A series of derivatives was synthesized (Hoemann et al., 2002), with the aim of improving logP and water solubility, as well as protein binding.

Reducing the core from a quinoline to tetrahydroquinoline yielded many analogs which were active against MRSA.

7.9. Sortases-Iron

Molecular iron is an essential factor for bacterial growth, iron being used during respiration, DNA replication, and other biological processes.

Sortase (SrtA) is an enzyme that anchors surface proteins to the cell wall of gram-positive bacteria and cleaves sorting signals at the LPXTG motif. A second sortase (SrtB) in *S. aureus* is required for anchoring a surface protein with the NPQTN motif; StrB is part of an iron-regulated locus called an iron-repressive surface determinant. Deletion of the sortase gene in *S. aureus* results in severe virulence defects.

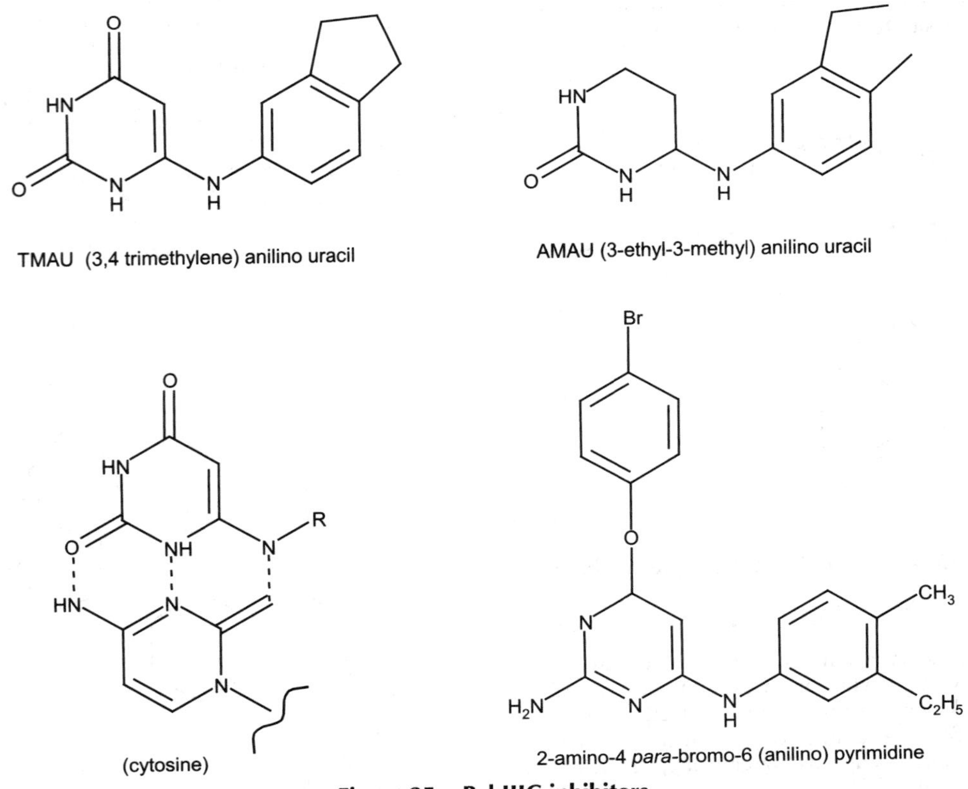

Figure 25 Pol IIIC inhibitors

$R_1 = CH_3$ = Lydicamycin $R_2 = OH$
$R_1 = H$ = TPU 0037-A $R_2 = OH$
between C14-C15 : double bond = TPU 0037-B
$R_1 = H$ = TPU 0037-C $R_2 = OH$
$R_1 = CH_3$ = TPU 0037-D $R_2 = H$

Figure 26 Lydicamycin complex

Compound	R	Isomer	MRSA MIC (μg/ml)
A	5-Br	*cis*	0.31
B	5-Cl	*cis*	0.78
C	H	*cis*	>25.00
D	6-F	*cis*	6.25
E	2-CH_3	*cis*	>25.00
F	5-Br	*trans*	3.13
G	5-Cl	*trans*	3.13
H	H	*trans*	6.25
I	6-F	*trans*	12.50

Figure 27 Tetrahydroquinoline derivatives

Inhibition of the cell wall anchoring of surface protein is a potential target for the development of novel antibacterials (Mazmanian et al., 2002).

7.10. Efflux Inhibitors

Efflux pumps are a major mechanism of resistance. The first protein characterized was NorA, but subsequently a non-NorA-related multidrug resistance phenotype was isolated.

Structural variants of certain phenylpiperidine-selective serotonin uptake inhibitors inhibited the function of multidrug resistance efflux pumps of *S. aureus* (Kaatz et al., 2003) (Fig. 28).

7.11. FabH Inhibitors

The main process in bacterial fatty acid biosynthesis is catalyzed by a set of enzymes named FAS II. This fact has led to a specific interest in this process as an antibacterial target.

Efforts to find inhibitors of FabI (isoniazid, ethionamide, and triclosan) and, more recently, of the β-ketoacyl ACP synthase-condensing enzymes (FabB, FabF, and FabH) have been undertaken.

FabH, a ubiquitous enzyme and essential for bacterial viability, has received a lot of interest.

Substituted 1,2-dethiol-3-ones are already the cores of many drugs, such as oltipraz (antiparasitic), in which a 5-halogen (chlorine or bromine) was appended; this drug exhibited both MurA and FabH inhibitors.

Some compounds exhibited moderate in vitro antistaphylococcal activity (He et al., 2004a).

7.12. Biaryl Acids

A series of biaryl acids and amides having high activity against gram-positive bacteria was discovered through a screening program. The antibacterial activity is dependent on the nature of the amino acid side chain (Fig. 29). The compounds are bactericidal, with a MIC of 20 μg/ml for MRSA for PDL 117230 and PDL 117229 (Look et al., 2004) (Fig. 30).

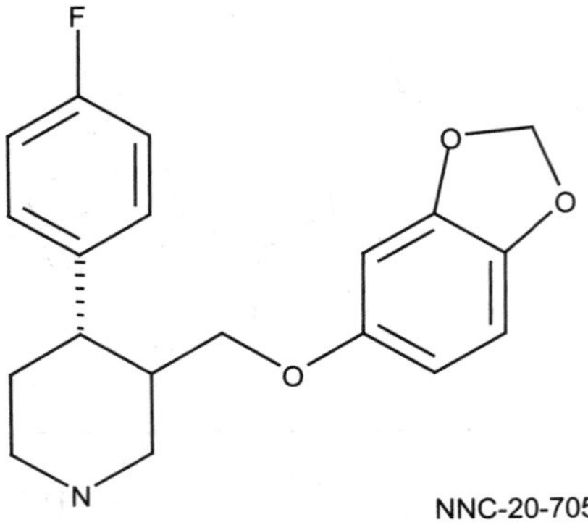

NNC-20-7052

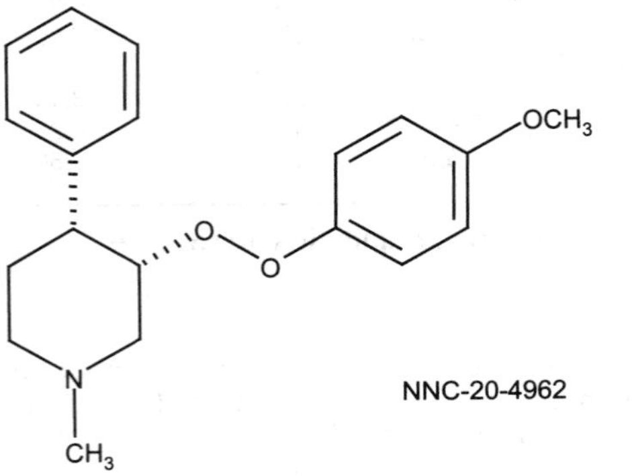

NNC-20-4962

Figure 28 Phenylpiperidine derivatives

7.13. Aminoacyl tRNA Synthase Inhibitors

Aminoacyl-tRNA synthases are essential enzymes for biological cell growth (Davis et al., 1994). One compound, mupirocin, with antistaphylococcal activity was introduced into clinical practice and inhibits isoleucyl-tRNA synthase. Aminoacyl synthases play an essential role in translation. They catalyze the formation of tRNA with its respective amino acid. The charged tRNA is then transported to the ribosome, where the amino acid is transferred to the growing peptidoglycan. This reaction is processed in two steps via the formation of an amino acid adenylate intermediate.

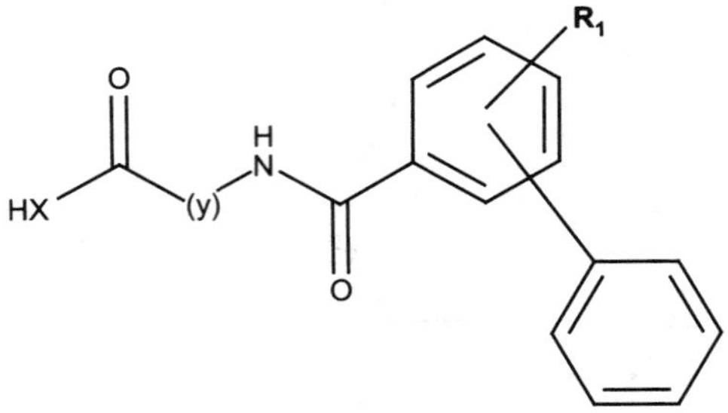

Figure 29 Biaryl acid derivative

7.13.1. Phenylalanyl-tRNA Synthase Inhibitors

A series of spirocyclic compounds was found to possess inhibitory activity against phenylalanyl-tRNA synthase through an intensive screening of a chemical library.

The IC_{50} of the lead compound (compound I) for *S. aureus* phenylalanyl-tRNA synthase was 0.38 μM, with a high selectivity over the human enzyme (IC_{50}, >100 μM). The spirocyclic furan analogs (Fig. 31) were poorly active in vitro (MIC, >50 μg/ml) due to their instability in Mueller-Hinton agar (Yu et al., 2004a).

A series of heterocyclic analogs was synthesized (Yu et al., 2004b). Some of them exhibit high inhibitory activity, with IC_{50} of 0.51 μM associated with MICs of 3.1 μg/ml (analog II), and interact with a dual mode of action. The affinity of CB 102930 for PBP 2a was 0.6 μM, with a MIC of 50 μg/ml. This compound is instable. To circumvent this problem, CB 102930 was reduced, and the resulting compounds have IC_{50}s of 0.81 and 0.51 μM, with MICs of 3.1 and 6.25 μg/ml (Hill et al., 2001d) (Fig. 32).

7.13.2. Tyrosyl-tRNA Synthase Inhibitors

Tyrosyl-tRNA synthase belongs to class I of tRNA synthases. It was shown that the tyrosyl adenylate is a potent inhibitor of tyrosyl-tRNA synthase but the polarity prevents their transport across the bacterial cell wall.

Series of substituted acyl dipeptide derivatives of tyrosine may act as *S. aureus* tyrosyl-tRNA synthase inhibitors (Fig. 33).

The tyrosyl-tyrosine had an IC_{50} of 3.8 μM, whereas IC_{50}s of 0.9 and 0.8 μM were noted for L-phenylglycine and 2-hydroxyphenylglycine, respectively (Jarvest et al., 1999).

For the tyrosyl-tyrosine analog (Fig. 33), it was shown that the N-terminal tyrosine occupies the tyrosyl binding pocket.

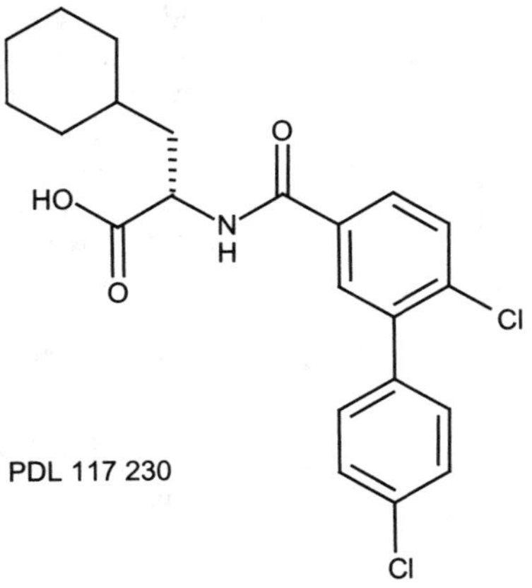

PDL 117 230

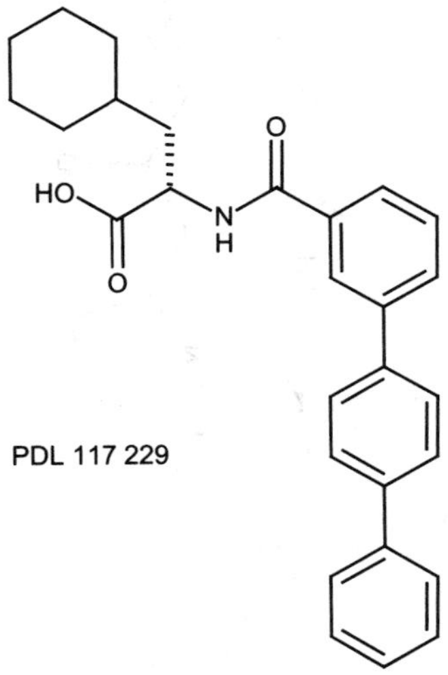

PDL 117 229

Figure 30 PDL 117230 and PDL 117229 (Biaryl derivatives)

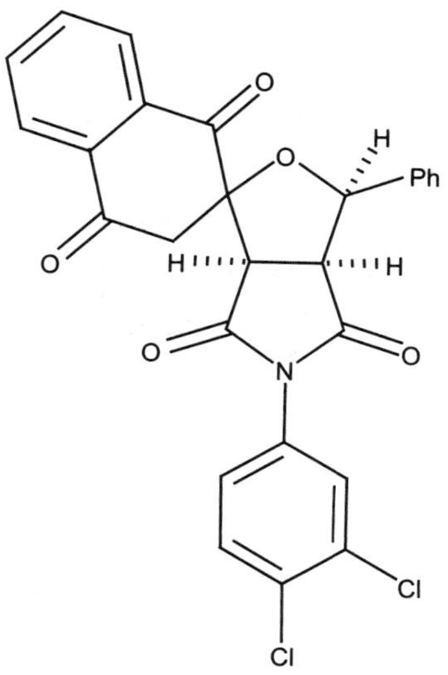

(I)

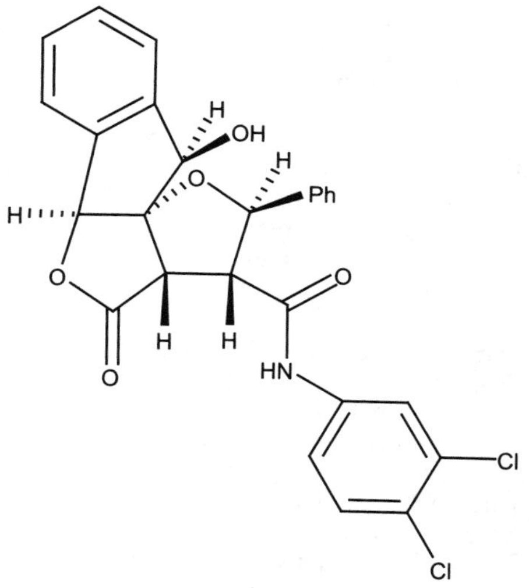

(II)

Figure 31 Phenylalanyl-tRNA synthase inhibitors (spirocyclic furan and pyrrolidine derivatives)

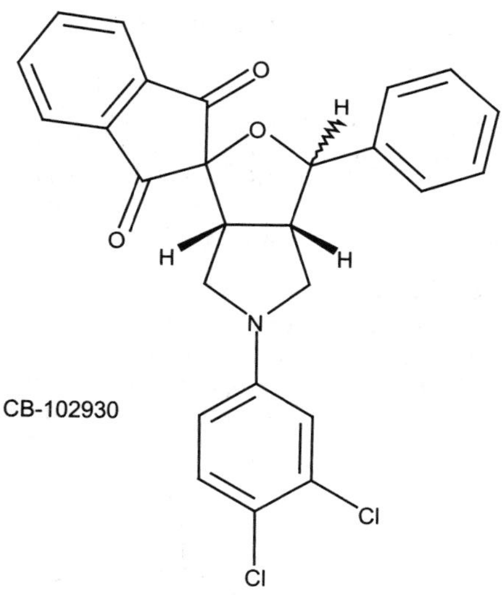

CB-102930

X = S or O

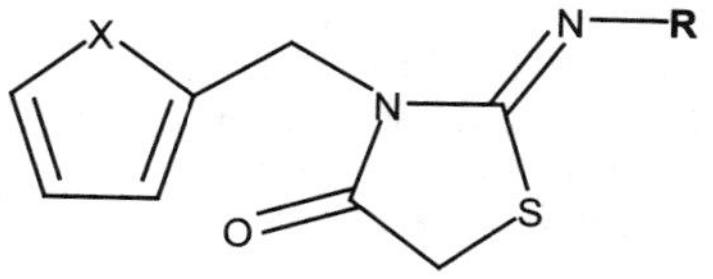

Thiazolidinones

Figure 32 CB 102930 (phenylalanyl-tRNA synthase inhibitor)

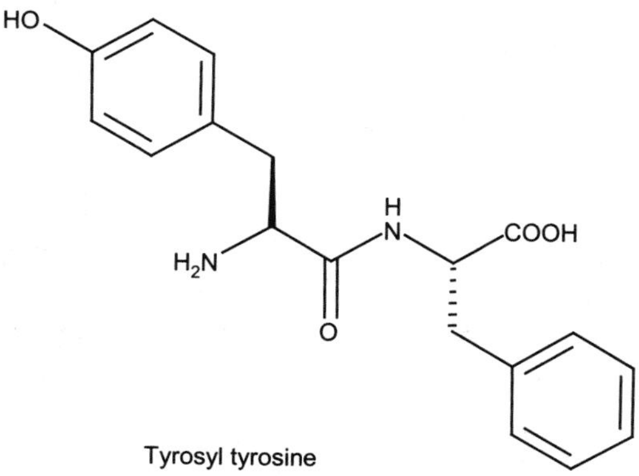

Tyrosyl tyrosine

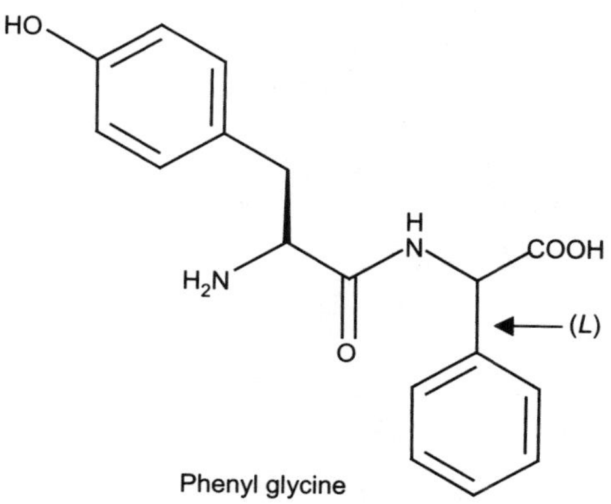

Phenyl glycine

Figure 33 Tyrosyl-tRNA synthetase inhibitor

The carbonyl group of the amide function appears to mimic the phosphoryl moiety of tyrosyl adenylate. The second tyrosine interacts with His50, and phenolic hydroxyl makes hydrogen bond to His47.

7.13.3. Methionyl-tRNA Synthase Inhibitors

A series of methionyl-tRNA synthase inhibitors has been synthesized. A 2-amino substituted quinoline exhibited antistaphylococcal activity; however, due to probably this residue it displayed a low membrane permeation (Jarvest et al., 2003a, 2003b).

One compound having an azabenzimidazole with a dibromine tetrahydroquinoline moiety (Fig. 34) exhibited an IC_{50} for *S. aureus* of 11 μM, with a MIC of ≤ 0.06 μg/ml for *S. aureus* Oxford. This compound is a racemate. The (*R*)-enantiomer was found to be the most active isomer, with an IC_{50} of 6.3 nM and a MIC of ≤0.06 μg/ml (Jarvest et al., 2004).

Two series of compounds (Fig. 35) were found to exhibit good in vitro activity against MRSA through methionyl-tRNA synthetase-inhibitory activity. Two groups of compounds were the most active: the catechol derivatives (IC_{50}, 20 nM; MIC, 3.1 μg/ml) and the proline series (IC_{50}, 210 nM; MIC, 50 μg/ml) (Finn et al., 2001).

7.13.3.1. REP 8839

Diaryl diamines have been described as inhibitors of tRNA methionyl synthase. REP 8839 is characterized by a 2-aminoquinoline pharmacophore and a bromothiophene substituted side chain (Fig. 36). REP 8839 exhibited in vitro activity against MRSA irrespective of the susceptibility to mupirocin, with MICs from ≤0.008 to 0.5 μg/ml. REP 8839 displayed a similar in vitro activity against isolates with intermediate susceptibility to vancomycin, with MICs ranging from ≤0.008 to 0.5 μg/ml, and against isolates resistant to linezolid (Critchley et al., 2004). This compound also displayed good in vitro activity against gram-positive cocci but is inactive against *Propionibacterium acnes* (Critchley et al., 2004).

7.13.4. SB 203207 and Analogs

SB 203207 was isolated from the fermentation broth of *Streptomyces* sp. strain NCIMB40513 and was shown to inhibit isoleucyl-tRNA synthetase from *S. aureus* Oxford (IC_{50}, 1.7 nM). Replacing isoleucine of SB 203207 with leucine or valine (Fig. 37) produced selective inhibitors of leucyl- and valyl-tRNA synthetases. The leucyl-tRNA synthetase and the valyl-tRNA synthetase of *S. aureus* have an IC_{50}s of 0.016 and 0.03 μM, respectively (Banwell et al., 2000).

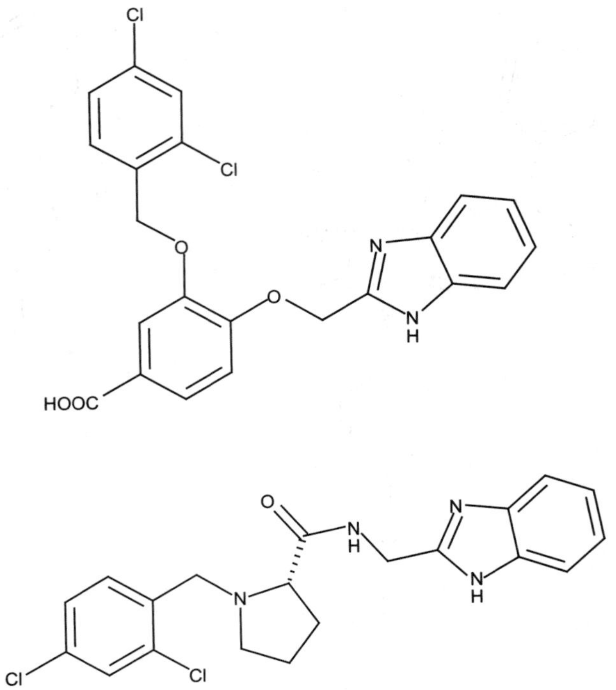

Figure 35 Methionyl-tRNA synthase inhibitors

7.14. Pantothenate Kinase Inhibitors

Coenzyme A is an essential cofactor for many enzymatic reactions. It is synthesized from pantothenic acid (vitamin B_5) in five steps. The first step is the phosphorylation of pantothenate by pantothenate kinase. The pantothenate kinase

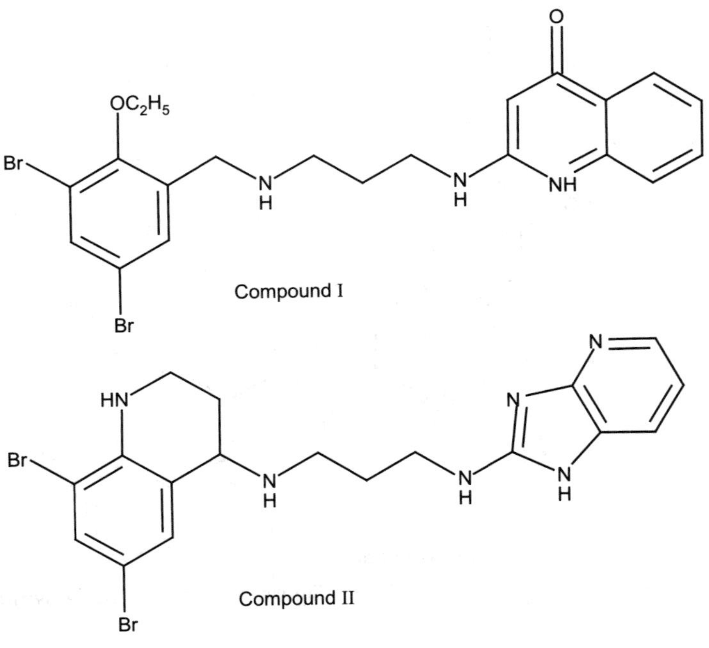

Compound I

Compound II

Figure 34 Methionyl-tRNA synthase inhibitors

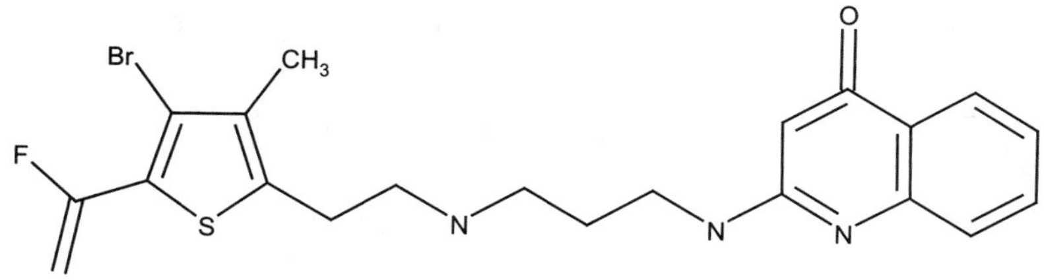

Figure 36 REP 8839

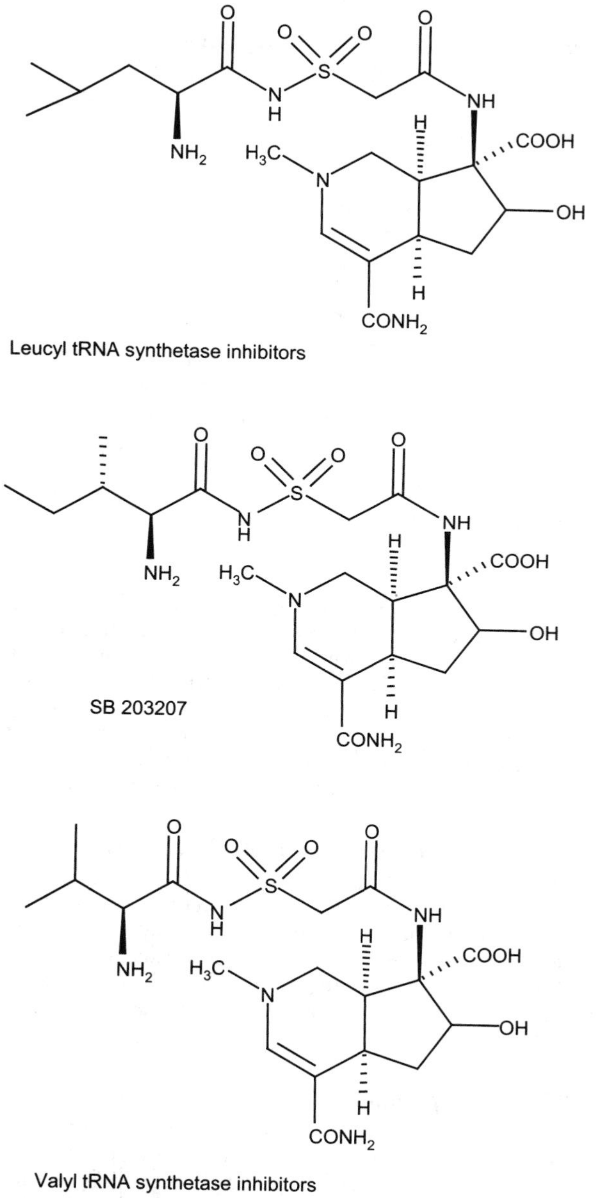

Leucyl tRNA synthetase inhibitors

SB 203207

Valyl tRNA synthetase inhibitors

Figure 37 SB 203207

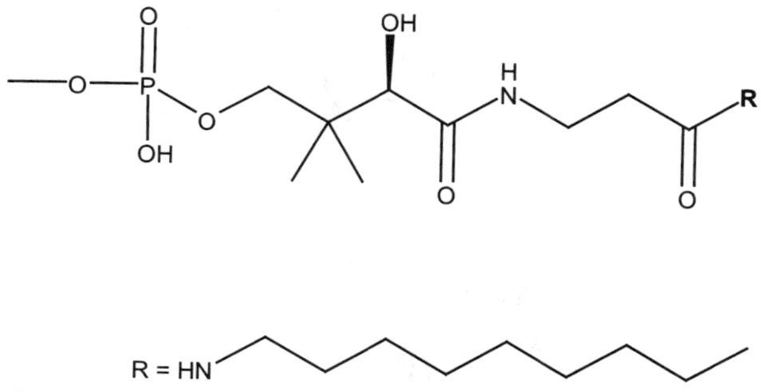

was identified and characterized. The genes for pantothenate kinase have been found in other gram-positive bacteria, including *Bacillus anthracis*.

Inhibitors of pantothenate kinase of *S. aureus* were identified (Fig. 38) having IC_{50}s of 0.4 to 2.9 μM associated with MICs from 1.0 to >64 μg/ml (Choudhry et al., 2003).

Figure 38 Pantothenate kinase inhibitors

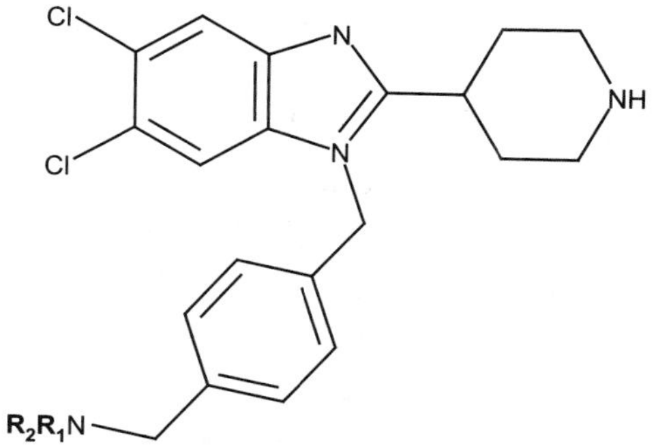

Figure 39 Benzoimidazole derivatives

7.15. Benzoimidazoles

A series of benzoimidazole derivatives (Fig. 39) was synthetized to target rRNA. Some analogs exhibited antistaphylococcal activity (He et al., 2004b).

7.16. Vancoresmycin

Vancoresmycin (Fig. 40) was isolated from *Amycolatopsis* sp. strain ST 101170. It is a tetramic acid derivative with a long oxygenated alkyl side chain. Vancoresmycin exhibits antistaphylococcal activity, with a MIC of ≤0.04 μg/ml (Hopmann et al., 2002).

7.17. Flavonoids

Flavonoids exert a variety of biological activities. The flavonoid derivatives having the highest anti-MRSA activity belong to the structural pattern of chalcone (Fig. 41). However, they are weakly active (MIC, >32 μg/ml) (Alcavaz et al., 2000).

Four components having an isoflavonoid structure were isolated from the roots of *Erythrina poeppigiana*. They are claimed to exert anti-MRSA activity; however, the reported MICs are very high, above 12.5 μg/ml (Tanaka et al., 2004).

7.18. DHFR Inhibitor

Iclaprim (AR-100) is a substituted cyclopropyl benzopyran appended to the pyrimidine ring via a methyl bridge (Fig. 42). Iclaprim is a racemate derivative of equal association with two enantiomers, AR-101 and AR-102.

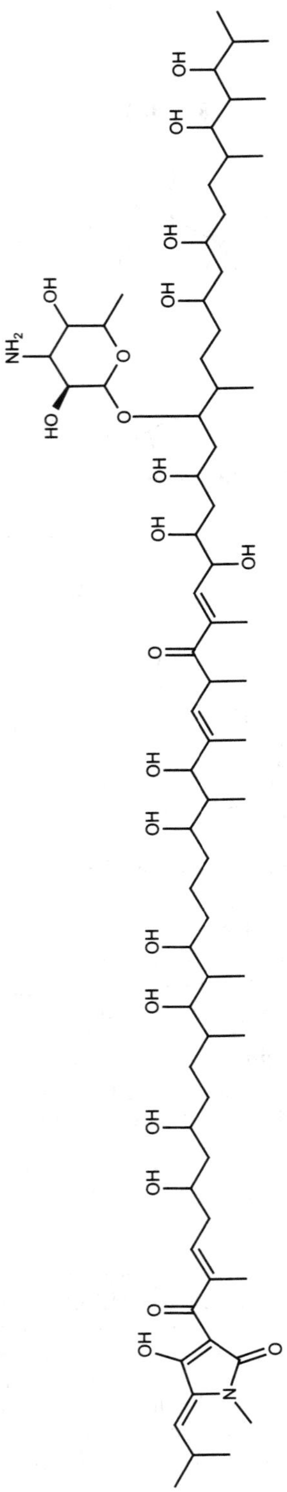

Figure 40 Vancoresmycin

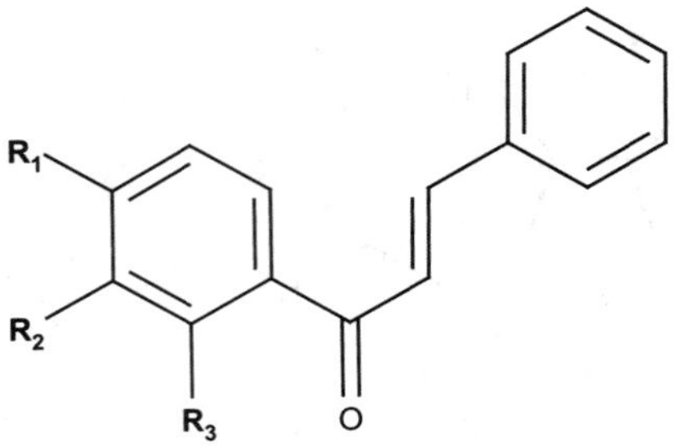

Figure 41 Flavonoid chalcone derivatives

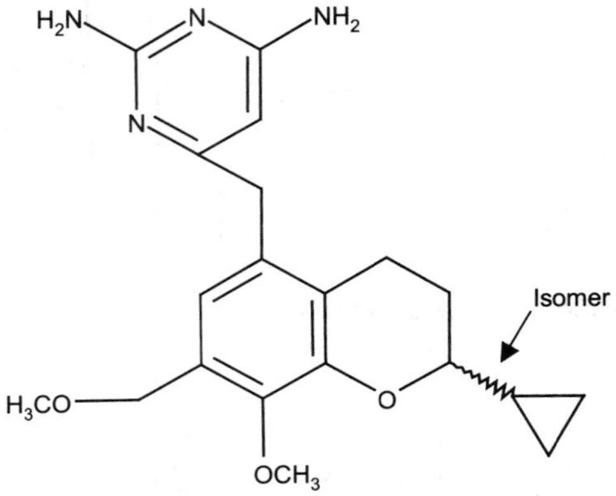

Figure 42 AR-100 (iclaprim)

Iclaprim exhibits high affinity for dihydrofolate reductase (DHFR) of *S. aureus*, with an IC_{50} of 0.007 μM (human IC_{50}, >300 μM), combined with good in vitro activity (MIC, <0.03 μg/ml). It exerts bactericidal activity against MRSA and GISA strains at four times the MIC after 6 h of contact (reduction of 3 $\log_{10}$ CFU/ml). In vivo against MRSA resistant to trimethoprim, the ED_{50} were 5.06 and 12.5 mg/kg after intravenous and oral administration (Schneider et al., 2003).

7.19. Dihydropteroate Synthase Inhibitors

Enzymes from the folate pathway are lacking in humans. Dihydropteroate synthase inhibitors have been used only through sulfonamides for at least seven decades. The sulfonamides act by competing with *p*-aminobenzoic acid.

Series of inhibitors were prepared, but none of them were potent inhibitors of dihydropteroate synthase (Dreier et al., 2001).

7.20. Streptogramins

Streptogramins in the form of pristinamycin were introduced into clinical practice in France and a few other countries. To overcome the water solubility, a semisynthetic and parenteral derivative was prepared: dalfopristin-quinupristin. Dalfopristin-quinupristin exhibits antistaphylococcal activity, with a MIC of less than 0.5 μg/ml (Jevitt et al., 2003). In order to enhance the antibacterial activity and the chemical profile, a semisynthetic oral streptogramin was synthesized, XRP 2868 (NXL103), which is made of two components: RPR 132552 (pristinamycin II derivative) and RPR 202868 (pristinamycin I derivative), in a ratio of 30:70 (Fig. 43).

The A component is a morpholino derivative, and the B component is a fluoro derivative (Bacqué et al., 2001).

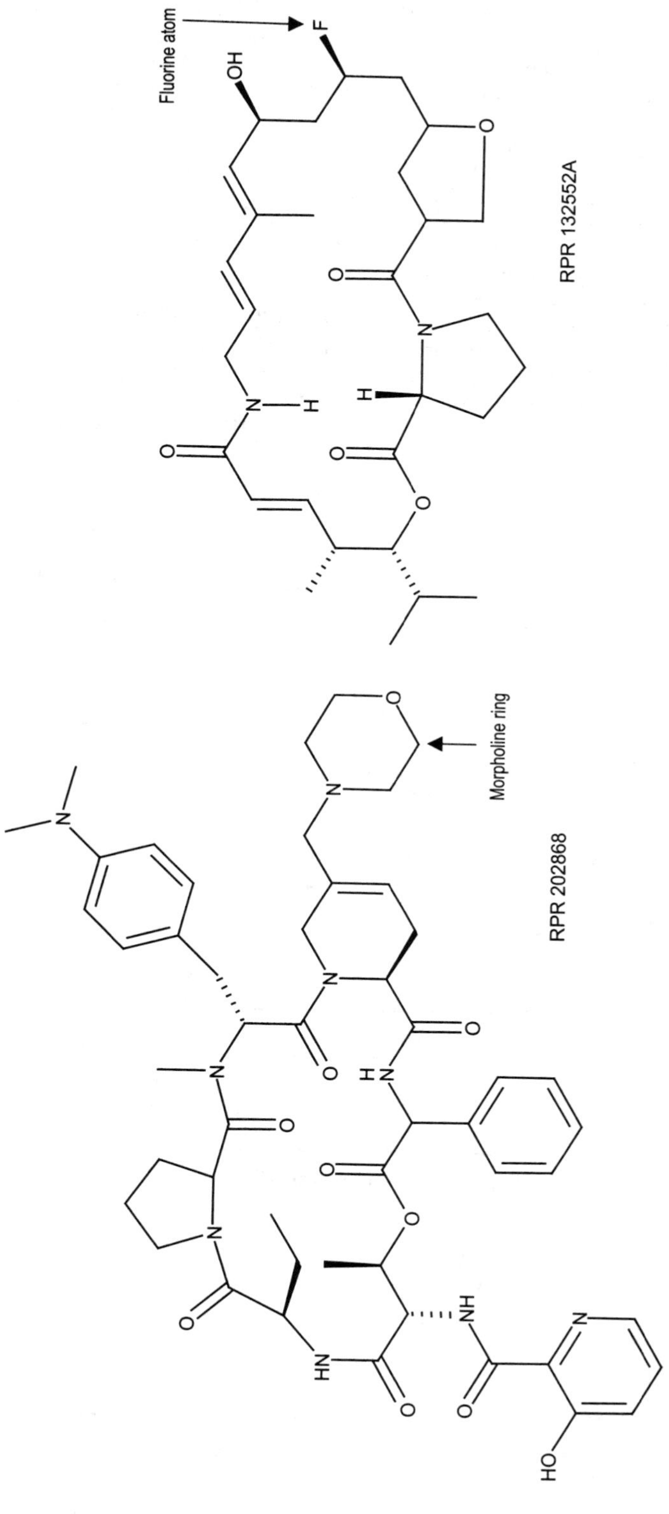

Morpholine ring

RPR 202868

Fluorine atom

RPR 132552A

Figure 43 **XRP 2868**

Resistance to the B component is mediated by methylation of the 23S rRNA (*ermB* gene). The bactericidal activity of the two components combined in a 30:70 ratio against *S. aureus* was assessed. A decrease of 3 log_{10} CFU/ml was noted after 24 h of contact (Drugeon et al., 2002). The MIC_{50} and MIC_{90} for *S. aureus* were 0.25 and 0.5 μg/ml (Felmingham et al., 2004).

Resistance to the A component is mediated by lactonases encoded by the *vgbA* and *vgbB* genes. For staphylococci, three acetyltransferase genes, *vatA*, *vatB*, and *vatC*, and two efflux genes (ABC transporter), *vgaA* and *vgaB*, have been reported.

Type B streptogramins are cyclic depsipeptides consisting of six or seven amino acids. These peptides are cyclized via an ester bond between the C-terminal carboxyl group of an invariant threonine residue at position 2. To overcome the weak point, the ester bond, an isosteric replacement was proposed via an amide cyclization (through a tyrocidine peptide). The rationale was that the amide functionality would be more thermodynamically stable, resulting in a type B streptogramin that would not provide a substrate for the lyase Vgb. This chimeric compound is poorly active in comparison to quinupristin. MICs against gram-positive cocci range from 32 to 128 μg/ml. The outer membrane is impermeable to this chimeric compound (Mukhtar et al., 2005).

7.21. Benzopyran

A series of benzopyran cyanostilbenes (Fig. 44) was synthesized and found to be active against MRSA (MIC, <50 μg/ml). A new series of benzopyrans was prepared with the aim of optimizing the in vitro activity against MRSA (Nicolaou et al., 2001). It was shown that the orientation of the stilbene moiety on the benzopyran ring system is important for biological activity. The presence of a free phenolic group on the terminal aromatic ring is essential for antibacterial activity. Compound 1 exhibited antistaphylococcal activity in general (MIC, 4 to 12 μg/ml) as well as activity against GISA strains (MIC, 6.0 μg/ml).

7.22. Topoisomerase IV Inhibitors

AVE 6971 is a disubstituted methoxyquinoline with a side chain containing a thienyl and a piperidine nucleus link with a sulfofuryl or a propyl bridge. At position 3 the side chain bears a hydroxy group (Fig. 45). In vitro, AVE 6971 exhibited

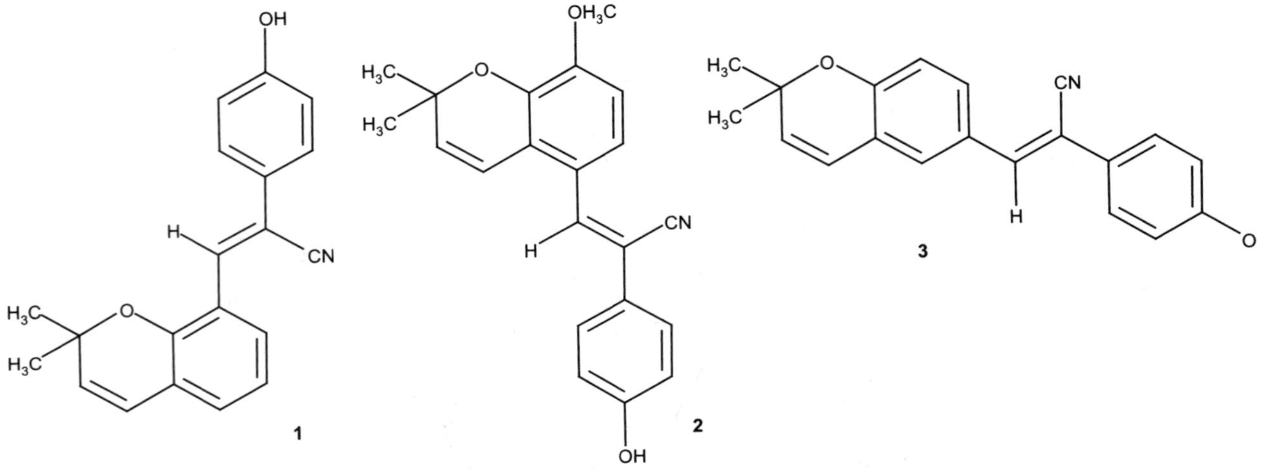

	MIC (ì g/ml)		
	MSSA	MRSA	GISA
1	4.0	4-12	6.0
2	12.0	12	12.0
3	25.0	25	12.0

Figure 44 Benzopyran stilbene

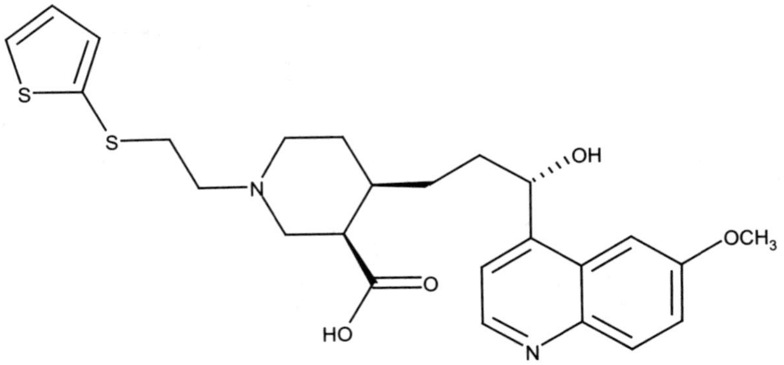

Figure 45 AVE 6971

a MIC_{50} and MIC_{90} of 5 and 0.5 μg/ml and 0.5 and 1.0 μg/ml for MSSA ($n = 41$) and MRSA ($n = 53$), respectively (Robbins et al., 2004). In a disseminated staphylococcal (MRSA) infection in mice, the ED_{50} were 3.6 and 9.5 mg/kg for subcutaneous and oral therapy, respectively.

AVE 6971 acts as a topoisomerase IV inhibitor.

Many other series of topoisomerase IV inhibitors have been synthesized by modifying the quinoline ring and/or the side chain appended on the quinoline ring.

Exploration of one compound, AVE 4221, has begun, and data have been released. AVE 4221 is the fluoro derivative of AVE 6971. It is one to two dilutions more active than AVE 6971, with a $MIC_{50/90}$ for *S. aureus* of 0.25/0.25 μg/ml. AVE 4221 is also active against *C. jeikeium* ($MIC_{50/90}$, 0.12/0.25 μg/ml) and *A. haemolyticum* ($MIC_{50/90}$, 0.25/0.25 μg/ml). AVE 4221 is bactericidal against staphylococci (Robbins et al., 2005).

7.23. FabI Inhibitor

7.23.1. 1,4-Benzodiazepine Derivatives

FabI is an enoyl carrier protein reductase that acts on fatty acid biosynthesis. It was shown that a 1,4-benzodiazepine derivative (Fig. 46) inhibits FabI of *S. aureus*, with IC_{50}s ranging from 0.15 to 15 μM.

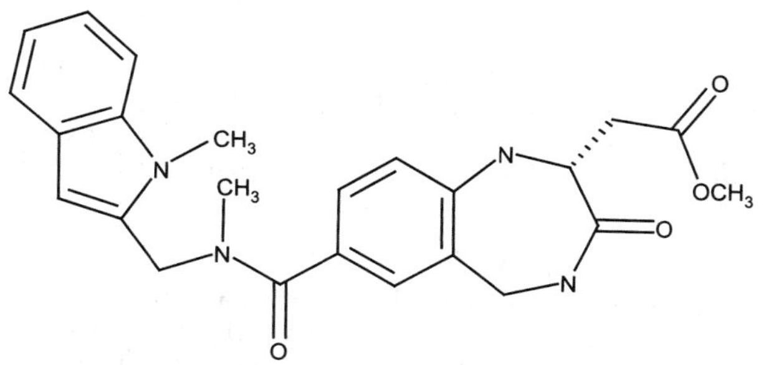

Figure 46 FabI inhibitor: 1,4-benzodiazepine derivative

7.23.2. API 1401

Naphthyridinyl enamides were recently identified as FabI-enoyl ACP reductase inhibitors. It was shown that the left side of these derivatives is set in a hydrophobic pocket of the enzyme. The right side forms a hydrogen bond with alanine 95 which needs to be retained for antibacterial activity.

A new inhibitor has recently been described, API 1401, which is a soluble pyrido-pyrimidine analog (Clarke et al., 2004; Manning et al., 2004; Bardouniotis et al., 2004).

7.24. 2-Mercaptoquinoline

In a Japanese patent it was reported that 2-mercaptoquinoline (Fig. 47) exhibited a MIC of ≤ 0.20 μg/ml for MRSA (Kato et al., 2000).

7.25. Gyrase B Inhibitors

7.25.1. Coumarins

The coumarins are DNA gyrase B inhibitors. Coumarins (Fig. 48) were synthesized with the aim of providing a compound active against MRSA.

The coumarinic moiety has been substituted at different positions. The aim was to enhance the antibacterial activity of coumarinic analogs, but also to overcome hepatic toxicity of novobiocin and to improve physicochemical properties. Novobiocin inhibits ATPase activity of DNA gyrase by competing with ATP for binding to gyrase subunit B.

One compound was selected for further investigation: RU-79115 (Fig. 49) (Musiki et al., 2000). The in vitro activity of RU-79115 against MRSA was good (MICs of 0.12 μg/ml). In disseminated staphylococcal infections, RU-79115 administered by the subcutaneous route was more active than vancomycin and linezolid.

7.25.2. Imidazolyl Derivatives

A series of imidazolyl derivatives has been synthesized; of these, one exhibited good inhibitory activity against DNA gyrase (IC_{50}, 1.0 μg/ml), combined with a MIC of 0.4 μg/ml for MRSA (Tanitame et al., 2004b).

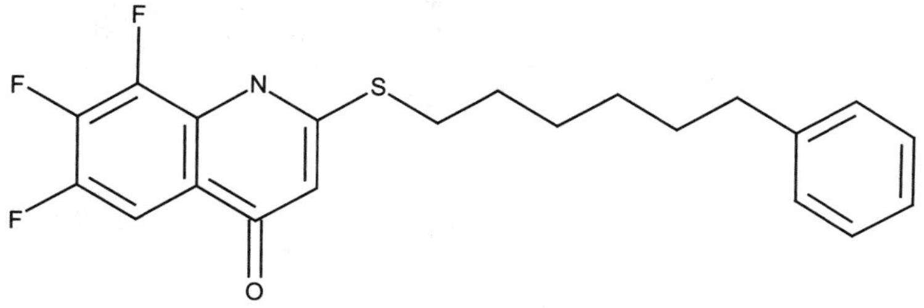

Figure 47 2-Mercaptoquinoline

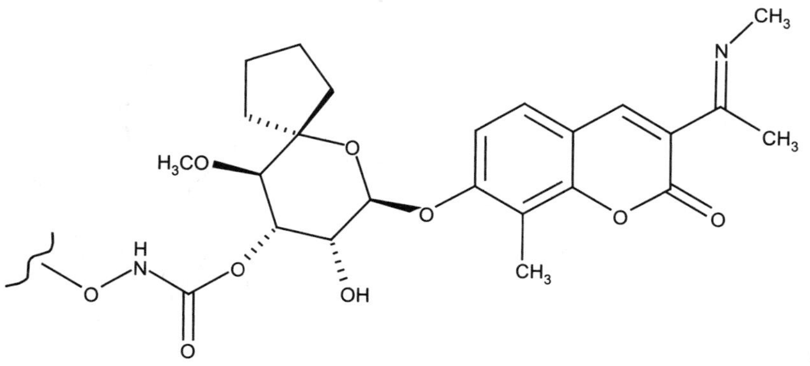

Figure 48 Coumarin derivative

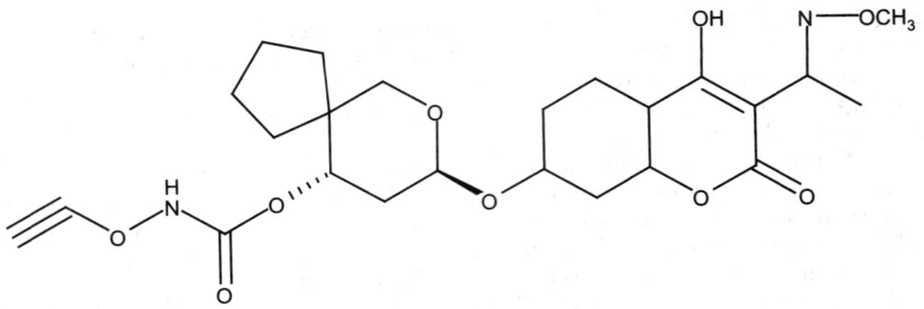

Figure 49 RU-79115

7.25.3. Pyrazolo-Pyrimidines

Series of 4-amino-pyrazolo-pyrimidines or triazines (Fig. 50) were synthesized as DNA gyrase B inhibitors. Some of them exhibit weak anti-MRSA activity, with MICs ranging between 2.0 and 8.0 μg/ml (Lübbers et al., 2000).

In a random screening of the chemical library, it was found that a pyrazole derivative exhibited weak antibacterial activity and weak inhibitory activity for topoisomerase IV. To optimize this lead compound, a series of analogs was synthesized. By modifying the lipophilicity of analogs by appending various substituents, it was found that some of them had MICs of 1 to 8 μg/ml for MRSA and IC_{50}s of 14 μg/ml for MRSA (Tanitame et al., 2004a).

7.25.4. Cyclothialidine Derivatives

Cyclothialidine (Ro-09-1437) (Fig. 51) was isolated from *Streptomyces filipinensis* NR 0484. The MIC of cyclothialidine needs to be determined on a medium supplemented with sheep blood. Cyclothialidine is not active against MRSA, due to poor membrane permeation. It is highly protein bound (96%), and the in vivo ED_{50} was above 25 mg/kg.

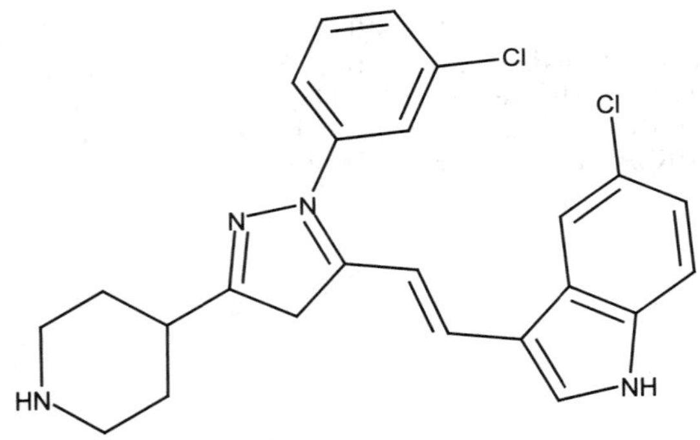

Figure 50 DNA gyrase B inhibitor: pyrazolo derivatives

In a series synthesized with the aim of investigating the structure-activity relationship, it was shown that the phenolic groups are essential, as well as the 14-hydroxyl group (H-bound with Asp75). The three-dimensional shape of the lactone is also compulsory, as is the *R*-configuration at C-7 (Angehrn et al., 2004).

To improve the pharmacokinetics, replacement of C-4 with 1,2,4-oxadiazole was found to be optimal.

One derivative exhibited activity against MRSA (MIC_{50} and MIC_{90}, 0.06 and 0.12 μg/ml). However, in a disseminated murine staphylococcal infection this analog was inactive. This poor in vivo activity may be partly explained by the pharmacokinetic behavior; this analog is highly lipophilic (logP, 3.34) and is metabolized as a glucuronic derivative.

7.25.5. TPU-0031-A and -B

TPU-0031-A and -B (Fig. 52) are produced by *Streptomyces*. The producing strain is isolated from the plant *Aucuba japonica*. These compounds are insoluble in water. The MICs of TUP-0031-A, TUP-0031-B, and novobiocin were 12.5, 3.1, and <0.2 μg/ml, respectively (Sasaki et al., 2001).

7.25.6. Indazole Analogs

It was shown that an indazole derivative interacts with the DNA gyrase B subunit of *S. aureus*. The derivative has a high affinity for the enzyme but poor in vitro activity due to low penetration through the outer membrane. Investigation in this series was given up.

However, recently a new series of analogs (Tanitame et al., 2004b) has been prepared, and one of them exhibited both high enzymatic affinity and in vitro activity (IC_{50}, 4.0 μg/ml; MICs 4 to 8 μg/ml) (Fig. 53).

7.26. Evernimicin

The everninomicins are oligosaccharide antibacterials isolated from *Micromonospora carbonacea*. Evernimicin (SCH

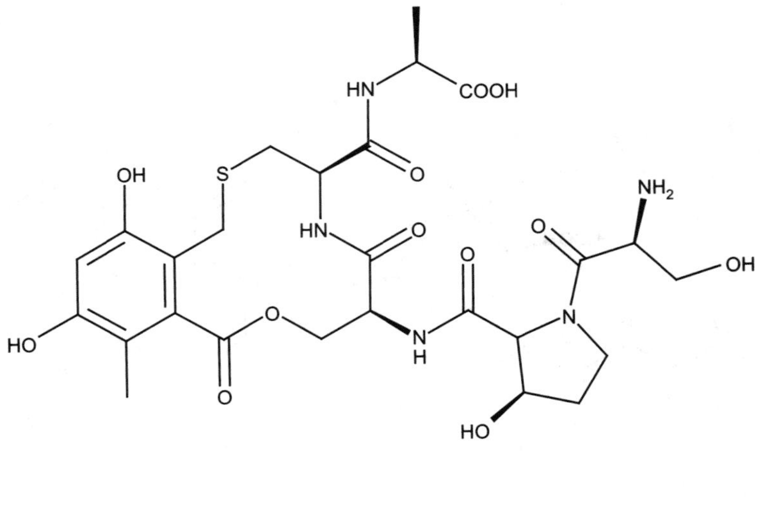

Figure 51 Cyclothialidine

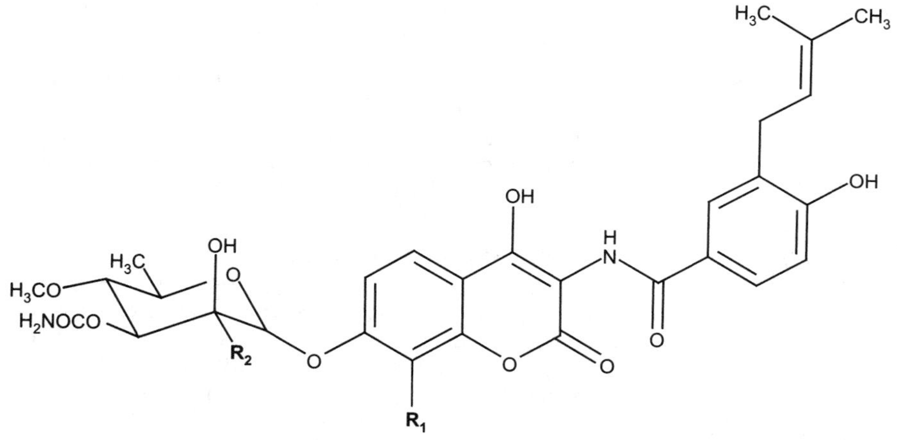

	R_1	R_2
TPU-0031 A	H	CH_3
TPU-0031 B	CH_3	H
Novobiocin	CH_3	CH_3

Figure 52 Novobiocin derivatives

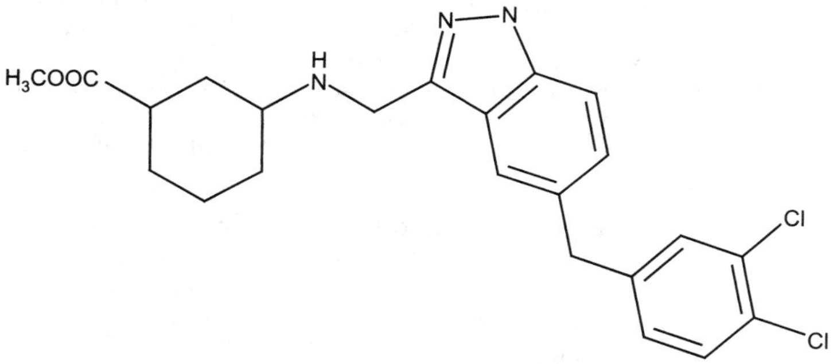

Figure 53 Indazole derivatives (DNA gyrase B inhibitor)

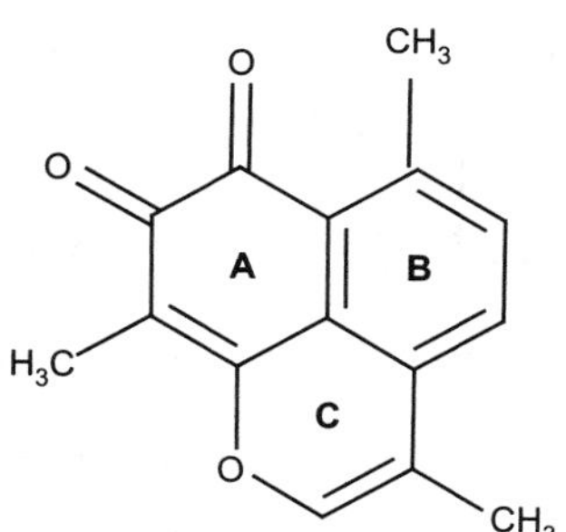

Figure 54 Mansonone F

27899) is one member of the everninomicin complex. Evernimicin activity against 763 MRSA isolates was determined by the E-test method, and the MIC_{50} and MIC_{90} were 0.25 and 0.75 μg/ml (Jones et al., 2001b). Development of evernimicin was given up due to serious adverse effects.

7.27. Mansonone F

Mansonone F is a sesquiterpenoid derivative composed of an oxaphenalene skeleton and *ortho*-naphthoquinone moiety (Fig. 54). Mansonone F was isolated from the root bark of *Ulmus davidiana*, used as a medicinal herb in traditional medicine in Korea. Mansonone F exhibited anti-MRSA activity, with a MIC_{90} of 2.0 μg/ml (Suh et al., 2000). In an effort to elucidate structure-activity relationships (Shin et al., 2004), it was shown that the *ortho*-quinone and the tricyclic skeleton are essential for the anti-MRSA activity of mansonone F.

7.28. Porphyrins

Porphyrins act as photosensitizers when irradiated. It was shown that porphyrins can be used in photodynamic antibacterial chemotherapy.

A series of 24 amino porphyrin derivatives has been semisynthesized and investigated for their antistaphylococcal activities. Some derivatives exerted good antistaphylococcal activity in vitro (MICs, 1.0 to 2.5 μg/ml) (Sol et al., 2004).

7.29. Indolquinoline

Through a screening of the chemical library, it was shown that some indolquinolines exhibited anti-MRSA activity.

A new series was synthesized in order to explore the structure-activity relationships and to enhance the antibacterial activity. Antibacterial activity is improved by the introduction of hydrophobic substituents into the quinoline ring. The dichlorinated derivative (Fig. 55) exerts good anti-MRSA activity (MIC, 0.5 to 1.0 μg/ml) as well as activity against GISA strains (MIC, 0.5 to 1.0 μg/ml) (Hoemann et al., 2000). These derivatives are only bacteriostatic. Mutants arose at a frequency of 10^{-8} for SEP 155342 (Oliva et al., 2003).

7.30. Isoquinolines

The 3-hydroxyisoquinolines were identified as possessing weak in vitro antibacterial activity (Stier et al., 2000). Further

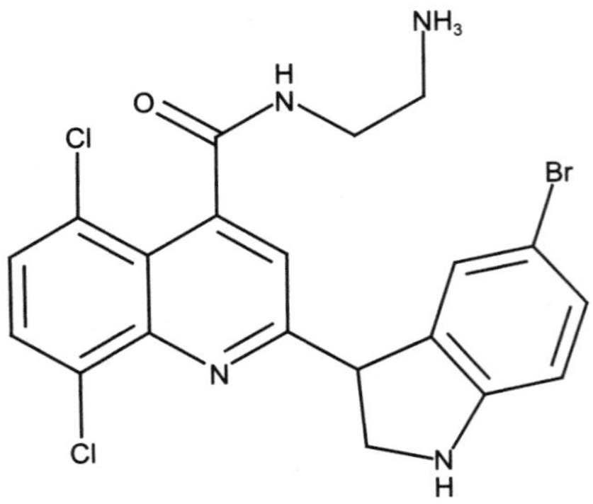

Figure 55 Indolquinoline

investigations led to the discovery of 3-hydroxyquinazolinone (Fig. 56).

The 3-hydroxy group replaces the 3-carboxylic acid moiety of fluoroquinolones. The acidity of 3-hydroxyl is similar to that of the 3-carboxylic acid functionality of fluoroquinolones (pK, 5.6 to 6.4). Many 2,4-diones inhibit bacterial DNA

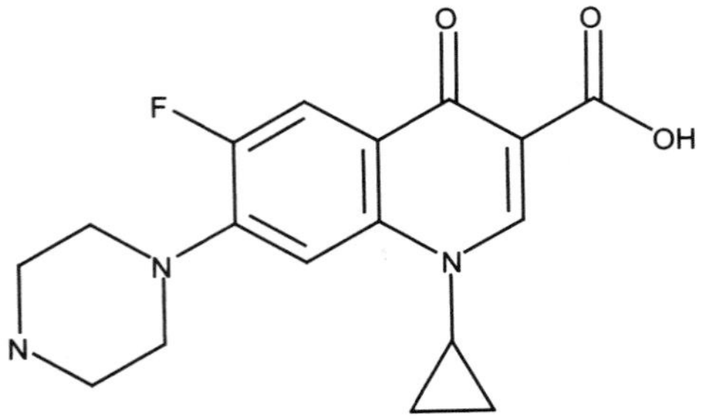

Ciprofloxacin

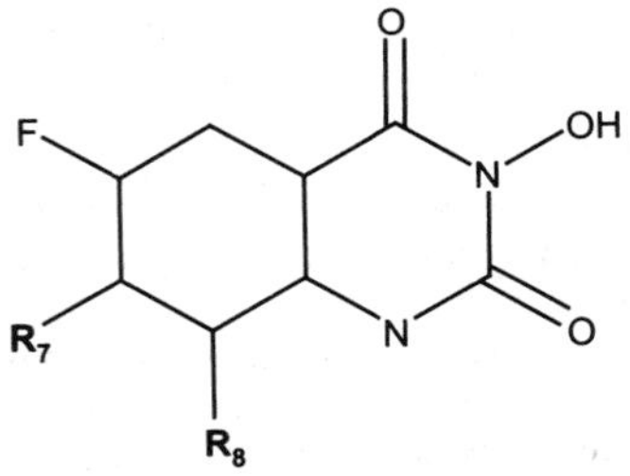

3-hydroxy isoquinoline

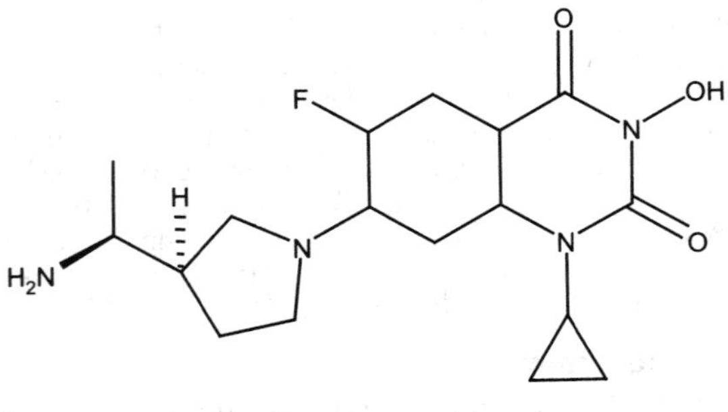

3-hydroxy quinazoline-2,4-diones

Figure 56 Isoquinoline

gyrase. Some derivatives exhibited in vitro activity against *S. aureus* (MIC, 1.0 to 4.0 μg/ml) close to that of ciprofloxacin (MIC, 2.0 μg/ml) (Tran et al., 2004).

They inhibit DNA gyrase of *Escherichia coli* H560 in correlation with MICs.

At N-1, cyclopropyl or cyclopropylmethyl substituents resulted in extremely active analogs against *S. aureus*. An amino substituent appended to position 3′ of the 7-pyrrolidinyl ring enhanced in vitro activity.

7.31. Signal Peptidase Inhibitors

After protein transport through the inner membrane, the signal sequence is cleaved by a signal peptidase. Then the mature protein is released into the outer medium or periplasm. These proteases utilize a unique catalytic serine-lysine dyad.

Series of aryl guanidines have been synthesized. Some of them inhibit signal peptidase, with IC_{50s} of 19 to 75 μM, but are inactive against the whole cell (MIC, >128 μg/ml). In a series of 5S-penems, one compound (Fig. 57) displayed high affinity for signal peptidase (IC_{50}, 5 μM) without in vitro activity (Howard et al., 2001; Grinius et al., 2001).

7.32. Isoxazolones

An approach involved searching for a bioisostere to replace the central oxazolidinone heterocycle. Already some oxazolidinone isosteres have been synthesized. Many are active, such as butenolide or isoxazoline; other analogs are inactive. Benzoisoxazolinones and pyrrole analogs have recently been prepared. Some isoxazolinones exhibited good in vitro activity against MRSA, with MICs of 1.0 μg/ml (Snyder et al., 2004) (Fig. 58).

7.33. Pyrimido-Pyrimidine Derivatives

A series of pyrimido [4,5*d*]pyrimidines was synthesized and evaluated against a panel of strains including *S. aureus* (Sharma et al., 2004). One derivative was found to have a MIC of 2.0 μg/ml for *S. aureus* ATCC 29213 (Fig. 59).

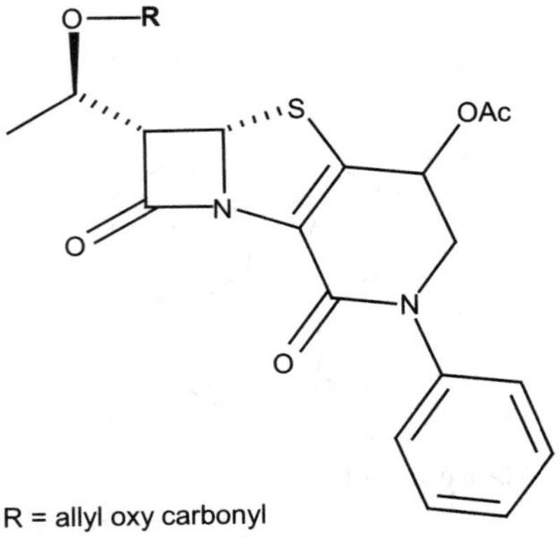

R = allyl oxy carbonyl

Figure 57 5S-penems: signal peptidase inhibitors

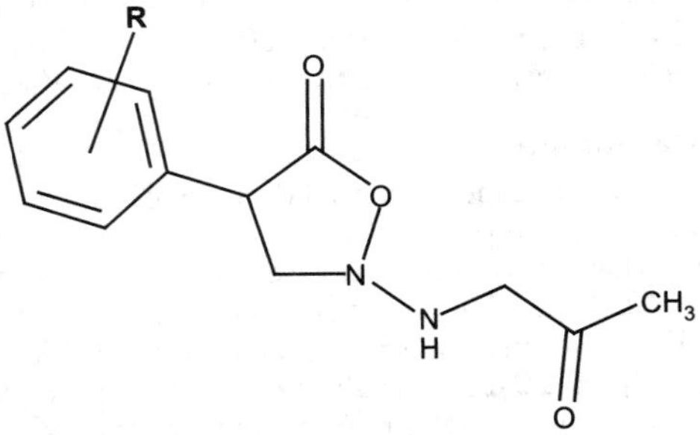

Figure 58 Isoxazolinones

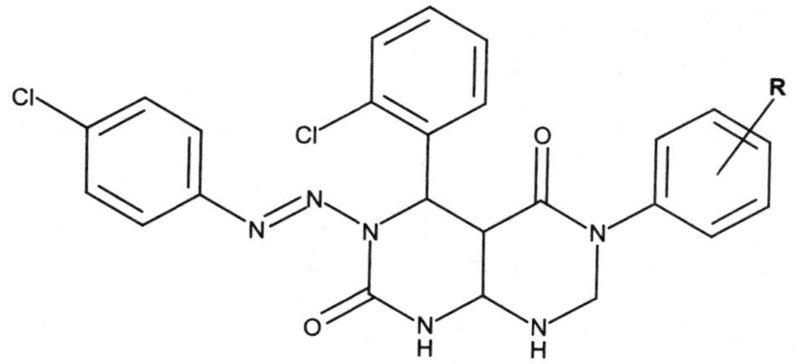

Figure 59 Pyrimido[4,5]pyrimidine derivatives

7.34. DNA Binding Agents

Netropsin and distamycin (Fig. 60) are well-characterized DNA binding agents. These antibacterials bind within the minor groove of DNA AT regions with four or five AT base pairs, respectively.

Smaller molecules were synthesized to enhance cellular uptake and pharmacokinetic properties of bis-netropsin and bis-distamycin.

A prototype structure was identified, the 3-chlorothiophene. This compound is active in vitro and in vivo against MRSA (ED_{50}, 30 mg/kg). To improve antibacterial activities an isoquinoline was synthesized; it showed an ED_{50} of 11 mg/kg for MRSA. New derivatives were prepared showing ED_{50} of 3 and 4 mg/kg (Hu et al., 2004).

A series of pyrrole tetramides analogs was prepared. Compounds with *N*-alkyl pyrrole terephthalmidea linkers exhibited good in vitro activity against MRSA, such as GL 5789225, GL 522997, GL 548043, and GL 568815 (MICs, 0.27 to 1.1 μg/ml) and good in vivo activity (Liehr et al., 2001).

7.35. HARP

HARP belongs to a small class of antibacterials acting on DNA (DNA nanobinders). One derivative was selected for investigation, GSQ 1539 (Fig. 61). This compound had a MIC_{50} and MIC_{90} of 1.0 and 4.0 μg/ml for MRSA and is active against GISA strains (MIC_{50} and MIC_{90}, 0.5 and 1.0 μg/ml). GSQ 1539 is bacteriostatic.

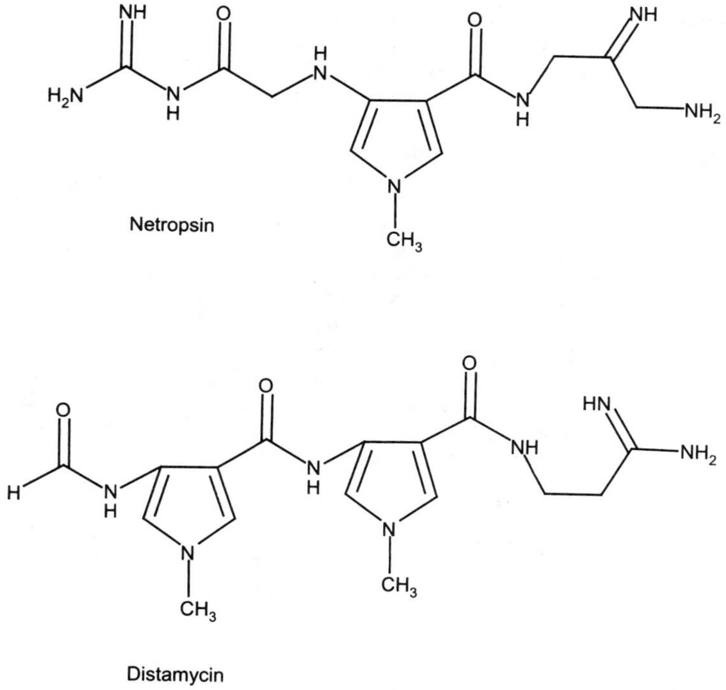

Netropsin

Distamycin

Figure 60 Netropsin and distamycin

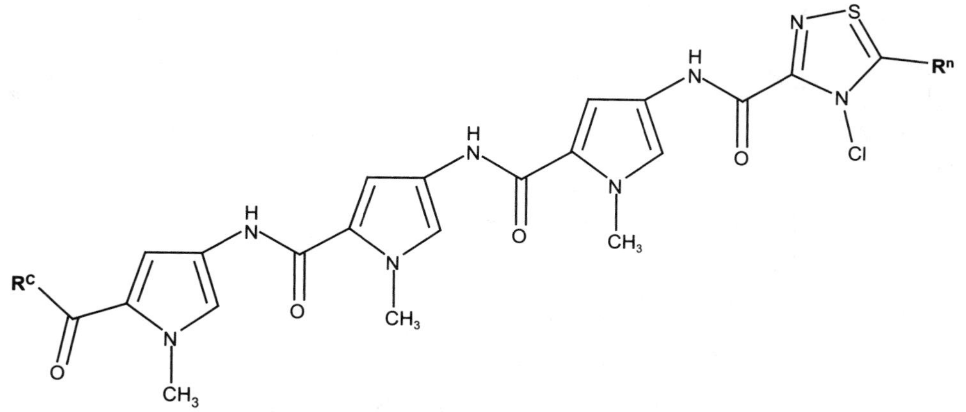

Figure 61 HARP analogs

GSQ 1539 binds to bacterial AT sequences with high affinity (IC_{50}, 2 to 30 nM). GSQ 1539 inhibits DNA synthesis and RNA transcription.

7.36. Nematophin

Nematophin was isolated from the culture broth of *Xenorhabdus nematophila* (*Enterobacteriaceae*) a bacterial symbiont of the entomopathogenic nematode *Steinernema carpocapsae*.

Nematophin (Fig. 62) was shown to be highly active against MRSA (Li et al., 1997a).

A series of nematophin analogs was synthesized, and some of them displayed antistaphylococcal activity (Li et al., 1997b; Kennedy et al., 2000). Structure-activity relationship studies were carried out (Himmler et al., 1998). It was established that replacement of the indole system with a smaller heterocycle such as pyridine or imidazole resulted in a loss of activity. The α-keto amide is required; the hydrogen on the indole ring can be replaced by either an aryl, alkyl, or benzyl group, resulting for some of them in enhancement of the antibacterial activity. Replacement at the C-3 position of the indole ring with a phenyl moiety resulted in a potent antistaphylococcal (*S. aureus* Col) derivative (MIC, 0.06 μg/ml). (Kennedy et al., 2000).

7.37. Aminoglycosides

Intensive research on aminoglycosides is ongoing in some research centers to investigate the possibility of enhancing in vitro activity without toxicity.

A series of neomycin derivatives with new sugar moieties was synthesized, and some of them exhibited MICs of 0.5 to 4.0 μg/ml for *S. aureus* ATCC 29213 (Yao et al., 2004).

In a new series of pyranmycins, some had MICs of 0.3 μg/ml for *S. aureus* ATCC 29213 (Wang et al., 2004).

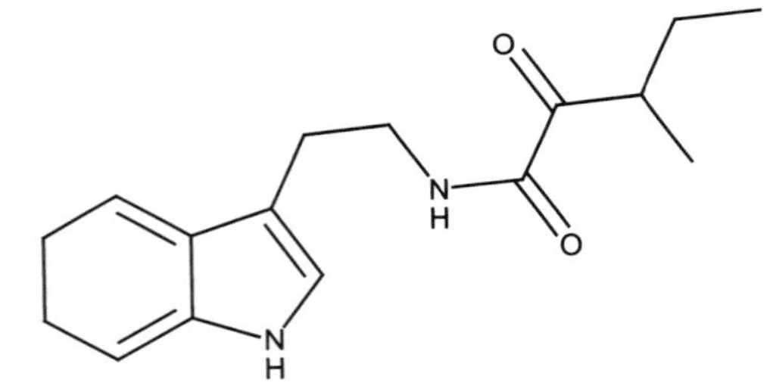

Figure 62 Nematophin

7.38. Pyrrolobenzodiazepines

The pyrrolobenzodiazepines belong to a tricyclic family of antibiotics. They bind covalently in the minor groove of double-stranded DNA, spanning 3 bp with preferential sequences. They bind selectively to Pu-G-Pu sequences. Three analogs have been investigated for their antibacterial activities: SJG-136, DRG 16, and ELB 21 (Fig. 63). They exhibited good anti-MRSA activity (MICs, 0.03 to 0.5 μg/ml) as well as activity against other gram-positive cocci, such as VRE, *Streptococcus pyogenes, Streptococcus agalactiae,* and *Listeria monocytogenes* (Hadjivassileva et al., 2004).

7.39. Cremimycin

Cremimycin is a 19-membered-ring macrocyclic lactam (Fig. 64) belonging to the same chemical family as hitachimycin and BE-14106. It was extracted from the fermentation broth of *Streptomyces* sp. strain MJ 635-86FS. Cremimycin is active against gram-positive cocci, including MRSA (MICs, 0.39 to 0.78 μg/ml), but is inactive against gram-negative bacteria and has no antitumor activity (Igarashi et al., 1998).

8. β-LACTAM ANTIBIOTICS

Considering the safety and the bactericidal properties of cephem derivatives, chemically modified cephems were expected to be active against MRSA due to high affinity for PBP 2a.

The first compounds showing potential in vitro activity against MRSA with higher affinity for PBP 2a were compounds having at C-2 (carbapenems) or C-3 (cephems) a benzothiazolyl substituent (Fig. 65). However, these compounds were inactive in vivo due to their high binding affinity for human serum albumin. These compounds were named CP0467 and LY 206763 (SM-17466); they also included an unnamed derivative from Merck Research (Tsushima et al., 1998; Ternasky et al., 1993; Sunagawa et al., 1994). Other derivatives were prepared, such as TOC-39 or isocephems (OPC-20011). Some β-lactams have been modified by introducing a hydrophobic nucleus into the C-3, C-7, and C-2 side chains for cephems and carbapenems.

8.1. Cephems

Cephems are subdivided into at least seven groups (Bryskier et al., 1994). Group VI is composed of compounds with a

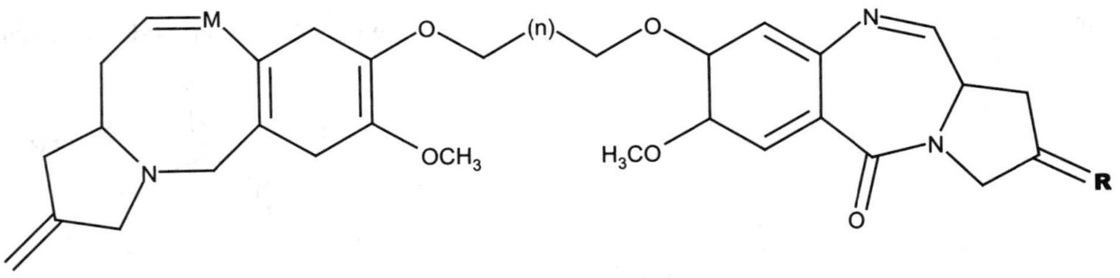

	n	R
SJG 136	1	=
DRG 16	3	=
EBL 21	3	=\

Figure 63 Pyrrolobenzodiazepines

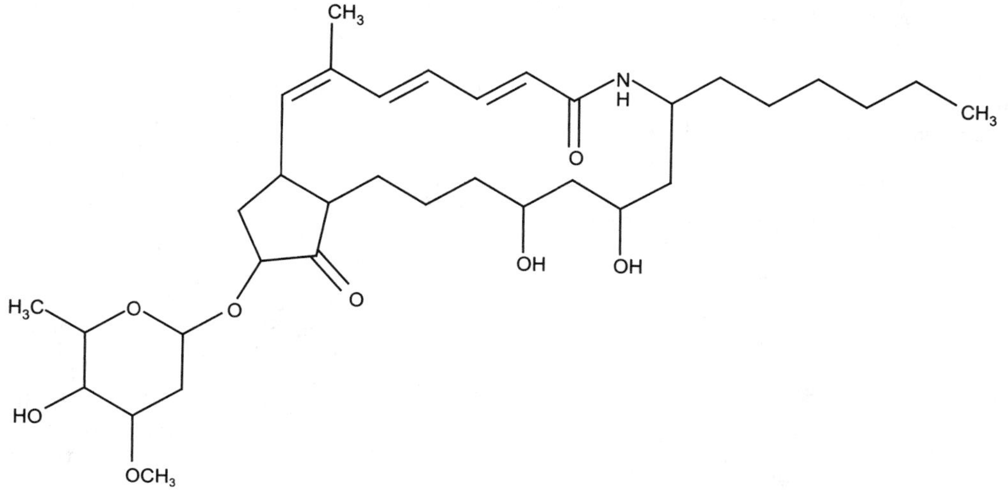

Figure 64 Cremimycin

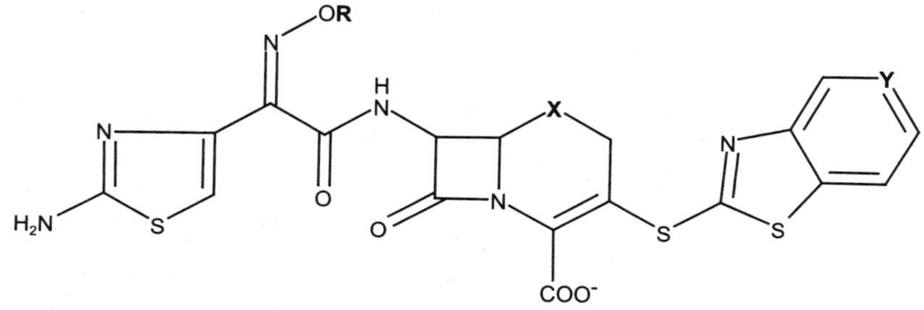

	R	X	Y
CP 0467	CH_3	S	S
LY 206763	CH_2CH_2F	CH_2	N

Figure 65 Benzothiazolyl cephems

narrow spectrum. This group can be divided into group VI_A antipseudomonal cephems like cefsulodin and group VI_B for anti-MRSA cephems (Fig. 66). One of the targets of this research was to improve water solubility, to obtain in vivo activity against MRSA, and to obtain both anti-MRSA activity and activity against gram-negative bacteria, including *P. aeruginosa*.

8.1.1. TAK-599 (PPI-0903)

In a series of derivatives, a spacer at C-3 between the core cephem and the 1-methyl pyridine group was set up. The spacer was made of thio five-membered heteroatomic rings which were expressed to adopt a conformation similar to that of the optimal parent compound.

One compound was selected, T-91825, having a thiothiazolyl as a spacer (Fig. 67). T-91825 bears an ethoxyimino group at C-7.

In order to improve the water solubility of T-91825, a prodrug, TAK-599 (Fig. 68), was prepared (Ishikawa et al., 2003). TAK-599 bears an ethoxyimino group at C-7. TAK-599 exhibits the most potent protective effect of all of the derivatives (ED_{50}, 1.74 mg/kg) and good affinity for PBP 2a.

Most of the β-lactam derivatives exhibiting anti-MRSA activity are zwitterionic compounds. Their water solubility is poor, which may be due in part to the C-3′ pharmacophore.

One strategy to improve water solubility was to synthesize prodrug. The C-7 aryl moiety (2-amino-5-thiazolyl and 5-amino-1,2 thiadiazolyl) is one possibility. Many strategies were applied: N carboxylation, N phosphorylation, N alanylation (such as with ceftizoxime [AS-924] [Kasei et al., 1999]), or *N*-phosphono and sulfo moieties (Ishikawa et al., 2001b).

The N-phosphono derivative showed protective effects comparable to that of the parent compound. The sulfo derivative showed poor in vivo activity. The *N*-phosphono derivative is transformed, in mice, in less than 5 min on parent compound. The water solubility was not too high (2 to 5 mg/ml), and the resulting pH was $1 \approx 2$. The addition of sodium bicarbonate dramatically increased the water solubility of the prodrug (<100 mg/ml).

N-Phosphono-type prodrug with a C-3 pyridinothiovinyl moiety possessed enough water solubility for intravenous administration. The resulting compound is not chemically stable for drug storage in formulation. TAK-599 is water soluble (>100 mg/ml) and stable for at least 8.0 h at pH 7. In addition, TAK-599 is a crystalline form containing an acetic

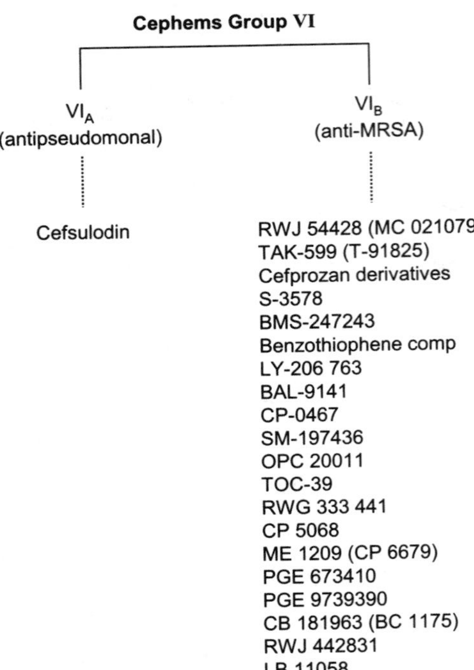

Figure 66 Classification, cephem group VI

acid solvate and is chemically stable for at least 16 weeks at 40°C in the solid state.

8.1.2. S-3578

C-3′ quaternary ammonium cephems are inactive against MRSA. An attempt was made to enhance anti-MRSA activity while retaining activity against gram-negative bacteria, including *P. aeruginosa*.

S-3578, a C-3′ quaternary ammonium cephem, is composed of an imidazolylpyridine substituted moiety (3-methylamino propyl) at the C-3 position and an ethoxyimino group and a thiadiazolyl ring at C-7 (Fig. 69). It displays anti-MRSA activity (MIC, 3.13 μg/ml) and anti-*P. aeruginosa* activity (MIC, 1.56 μg/ml). The IC_{50} for PBP 2a of MRSA was 4.5 μg/ml. S-3578 IC_{50}s for PBP 1 and PBP 2 of *S. aureus* were <0.5 μg/ml. S-3578 is bactericidal, with a reduction of 3 $\log_{10}$ CFU/ml after 6 h of contact (four times the MIC) (Fujimura et al., 2003). The compound is extremely water soluble (>50 mg/ml). In disseminated murine staphylococcal infection, the ED_{50} was 7.21 mg/kg.

8.1.3. BAL 9141 (Ceftobiprole)

BAL 9141, formerly Ro-63-9141, is a pyrrolidinone-3-ylidenenmethyl cephem (Fig. 70). It displays good in vitro activity against MRSA, with a MIC_{50} and MIC_{90} of 1.0 and 2.0 μg/ml; the MIC_{50} and MIC_{90} are 0.5 and 0.5 μg/ml for MSSA (Jones et al., 2002b). To enhance water solubility a prodrug has been synthesized, Ro-65-5788 (renamed BAL 5788) (Hebeisen et al., 2001). It is bactericidal against MRSA after 8 h of contact at five times the MIC. Only affinity for PBP 2a of methicillin-resistant Staphylococcus epidermidis was disclosed, with an IC_{50} of 0.87 μM; for MRSA, the IC_{50} was 0.31 μg/ml (Entenza et al., 2002). In experimental disseminated staphylococcal infection in mice, the ED_{50} was 2.4 mg/kg. In experimental staphylococcal (MRSA) endocarditis in rats, BAL 9141 was able to sterilize more than 90% of cardiac vegetations.

8.1.4. BMS-247243

It was shown that compounds with a lipophilic group at C-3 and a linked pyridinium moiety at C-7 exhibited anti-MRSA activity both in vitro (MIC, 0.125 μg/ml) and in vivo (PD_{50}, 1.4 mg/kg).

An aminopropyl side chain is appended to the pyridinium ring. Unfortunately, this compound (compound I) was found to be toxic to mice when administered intravenously (bolus).(Springer et al., 2001).

To overcome this toxicity, an unsubstituted ornithine side chain on the pyridinium ring was appended (compound II) (Fig. 71). This derivative exhibits good anti-MRSA activity. It is less toxic than compound I, but due to its zwitterionic nature it is poorly water soluble (Springer et al., 2003b). Compounds with a net negative charge are usually nontoxic; however, they are poorly active against MRSA.

To keep the anti-MRSA activity and to obtain a water-soluble compound, the ammonium and the carboxylate residues of the ornithine side chain at C-3 need to be separated by some distance. It was expected that the distance would attenuate the intramolecular association.

A new series of cephems was prepared in order to improve water solubility. An extra acid group improved acute toxicity and water solubility.

Some C-7 cinnamic acid derivatives were shown to display anti-MRSA activity in vitro (MIC_{90}, 3.7 μg/ml) and in vivo (PD_{50}, 3.9 mg/kg for compound III).

Figure 67 T-91825

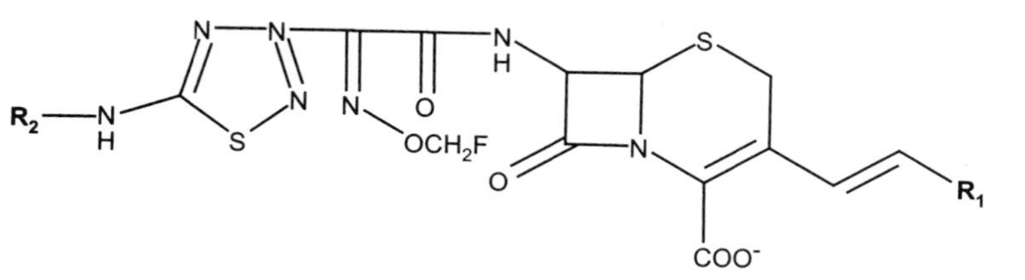

	R_2
Phosphono derivatives	$(OH)_2$-OP—
Sulfo derivatives	HO_3S—

Figure 68 TAK-599

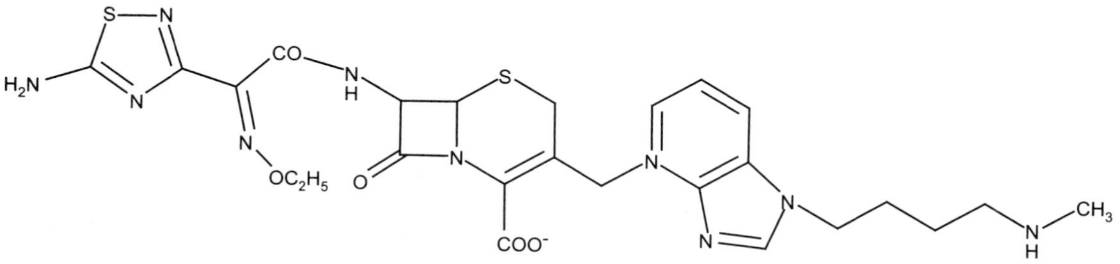

Figure 69 S-3578

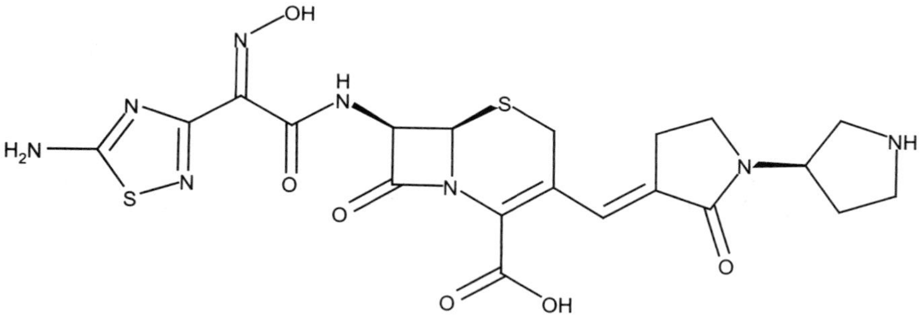

Figure 70 BAL 9141

The activity of BMS-247243 was investigated from the microbiological point of view. In vitro BMS-247243 was moderately active, with a MIC_{50} and MIC_{90} of 4.0 and 4.0 μg/ml. The affinity for PBP $_{2a}$ of MRSA is high at 0.7 μg/ml. After 6 h of contact, whatever the MRSA strains, BMS-247243 was not bactericidal; it yielded a reduction of the inoculum size of less than 2 $\log_{10}$ CFU/ml. In rabbit endocarditis due to MRSA there is a drop of 6 $\log_{10}$ CFU/ml.

The bacterial count in many vegetations treated with 30 mg/kg was $<10^2$ CFU/g (Fung-Tomc et al., 2002).

8.1.5. RWJ-54428 (MC 02,479)

RWJ-54428 is a pyridine-substituted cephem with a (2-aminoethyl)-thiomethyl side chain (Fig. 72). The pyridine ring is crucial for both antibacterial activity and water solubility. The high lipophilicity of C-3-substituents correlates with anti-MRSA activity. The pyridine ring is unprotonated at physiological pH and meets the lipophilicity criterion. At acidic pH, the pyridine moiety is positively charged, thus affording acceptable water solubility for intravenous formulation.

Replacement at C-3 by a nonbasic aromatic nucleus resulted in compounds with anti-MRSA activity and poor water solubility.

Replacement at C-7 of the 2-amino-5-thiazolyl nucleus with an aminopyridine (isostere of aminothiazole) resulted in a more soluble compound (>20 mg/ml) at pH 4.5. The aminopyridine is expected to be uncharged at physiological pH, resulting in good anti-MRSA activity (Cho et al., 2001a).

In order to obtain anti-MRSA activity in the 3-(heteroarylthio) cephem series, it is important to append electron-withdrawing substituents at positions C-7 and C-3.

The chlorine atom in the C-7 aminothiazolyl ring is beneficial to the anti-MRSA activity.

In serum, these derivatives are more or less stable due to decomposition of the C-3 unit; probably this effect is due to the electronegative C-3 substituent.

The MIC_{50} and MIC_{90} were 0.5 and 0.5 μg/ml and 1.0 and 2.0 μg/ml for MSSA and MRSA, respectively (Johnson et al., 2002). For GISA strains the MICs were 0.5 μg/ml. In a murine model of staphylococcal (MRSA) infection, the ED_{50} of RWJ-54428 was 6.1 mg/kg, for a MIC of 1.0 μg/ml (Griffith et al., 2003).

RWJ-54428 has a 4-pyridine thiol replaced with a 2-aminoethylthio methyl side chain. The pyridine moiety is unprotonated at physiological pH and met the lipophilicity criterion for antibacterial activity. By replacing the pyridine

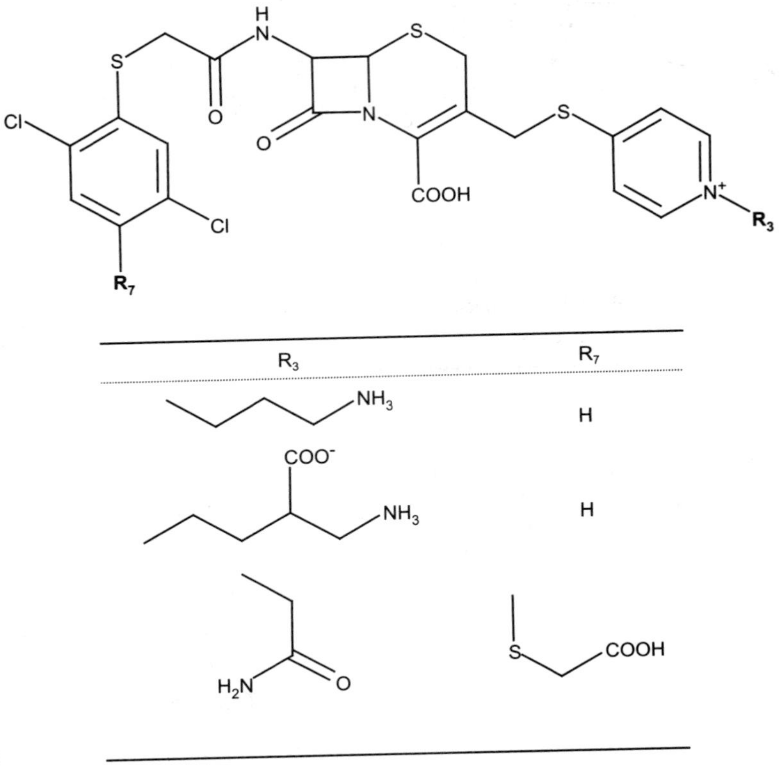

Figure 71 BMS-247243

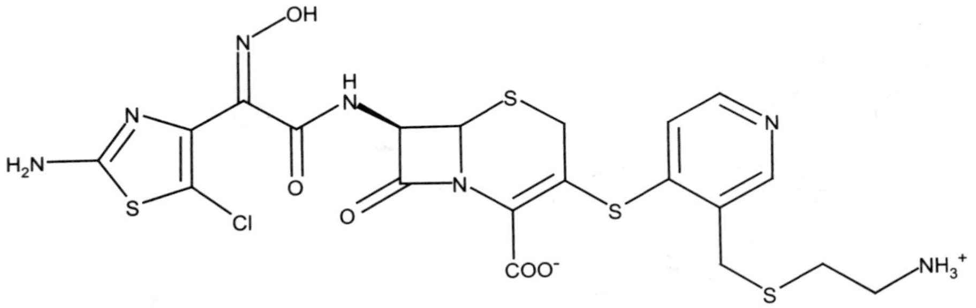

Figure 72 RWJ-54428

ring with a nonbasic aromatic ring (thiodiazolyl ring), the anti-MRSA activity remained but the water solubility was low (MIC, 1.0 μg/ml). By introducing an additional basic functionality at C-7, the desired level of water solubility was reached. Aminopyridines are isosteres of the aminothiazole ring, and analogs showed water solubility of >20 mg/ml at pH 4.5 (Cho et al., 2001a).

8.1.6. RWJ-333441 (MC-04,546)

RWJ-333441 (Fig. 73) is a zwitterionic compound with a water solubility of 4.5 mg/ml at pH 7.2, which is not enough for intravenous formulation; it possesses a low level of protein binding (Glinka et al., 2003).

RWJ-333441 exhibits antibacterial activity similar to that of RWJ-54428 but with improved pharmacokinetics.

A strategy was set up to enhance water solubility (Hecker et al., 2003). The compound is soluble at low pH due to protonation of the nitrogen of the pyridine ring. The solubility is dependent on the side chain appended: at pH 7, a valine (lipophilic; water solubility, 6.7 mg/ml), a serine (polar; water solubility, 7.8 mg/ml), or N substitution (*N*-methyl alanine water solubility, 10.3 mg/ml, alanyl-alanine water solubility, 18.1 mg/ml). Due to an additional ionizable group, the solubility of L-aspartyl is above 50 mg/ml. When an additional charge is added to a lysine, ornithine, and histidine, as well as daloxate, the water solubility is above 20 mg/ml. The ester cleavage seems to be more important with alanine derivatives or alanyl-alanine. A medium cleavage was recorded with aspartate and lysine (about 23 to 27% recovery).

The most promising compound, taking into account in vitro and in vivo activities, was the aspartate derivative RWJ-333442 (Fig. 74). The daloxate derivative is also rapidly released due to esterases (Alexander et al., 1996).

8.1.7. RWJ-442831

RWJ-442831 (Fig. 75) is an aspartic acid amide derivative of RWJ-54428 designed to enhance water solubility of RWJ-54428 at physiological pH. Against MRSA, RWJ-442831 is slightly less active than RWJ-54428 (MICs, 1.0 to 2.0 versus

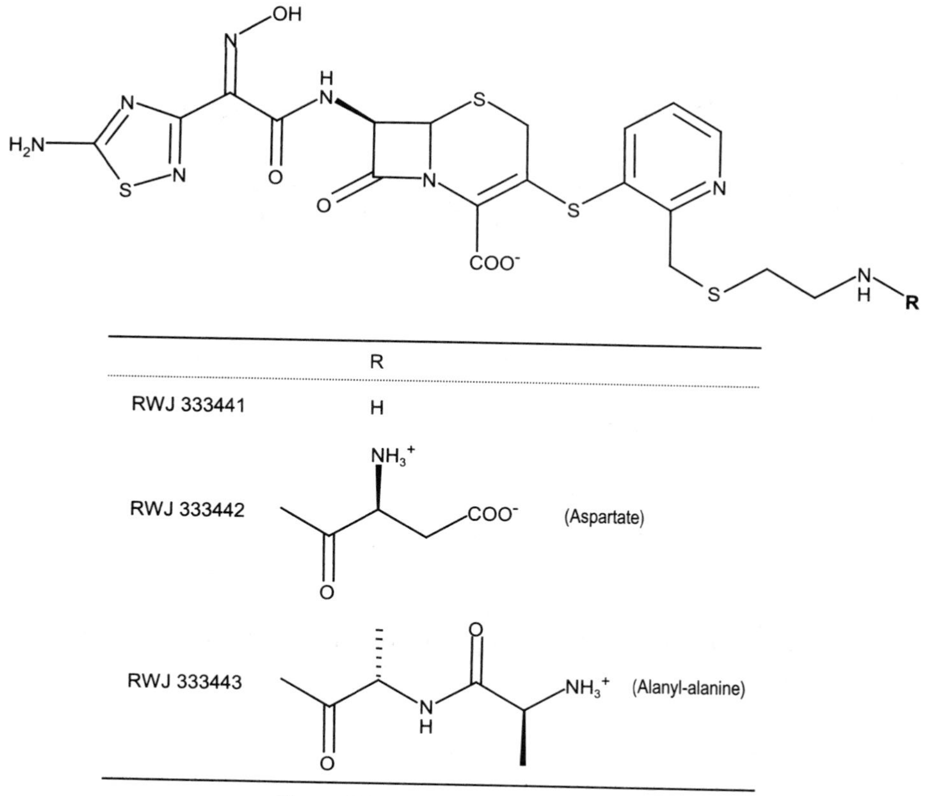

	R	
RWJ 333441	H	
RWJ 333442		(Aspartate)
RWJ 333443		(Alanyl-alanine)

Figure 73 RWJ-333441 prodrugs

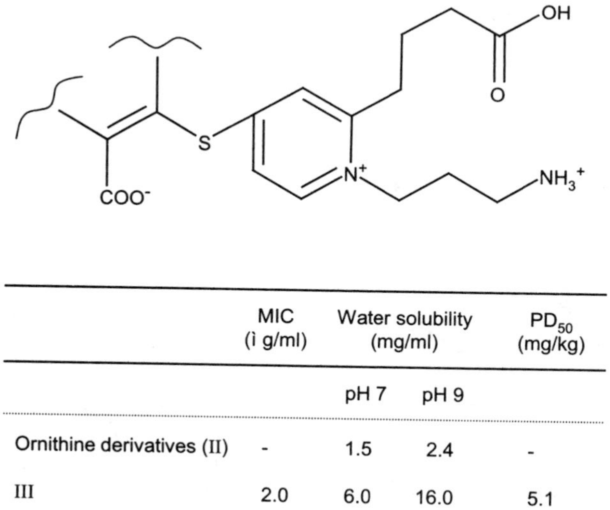

	MIC (ì g/ml)	Water solubility (mg/ml)		PD_{50} (mg/kg)
		pH 7	pH 9	
Ornithine derivatives (II)	-	1.5	2.4	-
III	2.0	6.0	16.0	5.1

Figure 74 Water solubility of anti-MRSA cephems

0.125 to 0.5 μg/ml) There is a rapid conversion (in less than 30 min) of RWJ-442831 to RWJ-54428. The two compounds displayed similar in vivo efficacies in mice challenged with MRSA (ED_{50}, 1.7 and 1.9 mg/kg, respectively) (Bush et al., 2003).

8.1.8. Other Cephems

Many other cephems were reported to display good activity against MRSA, such as ME-1209 (CP-6679) (Fig. 76), which exerts anti-MRSA activity (MICs, 4 to 16 μg/ml; IC_{50} for PBP 2a, 5.1 μg/ml; and good in vivo efficacy, with an ED_{50} of 0.37 mg/kg) as well as anti-*P. aeruginosa* activity (MICs, 0.5 to 1.0 μg/ml; ED_{50}, 0.056 to 0.015 mg/kg).

The first derivatives showing anti-MRSA activity among the cephem class were LY-206763 (IC_{50}, 2 μg/ml), TOC-39 (Hanaki et al., 1995) (IC_{50}, 0.58 μg/ml), and OPC-20011 (Matsumoto et al., 1998). These compounds were bactericidal at four times the MIC after 6 to 8 h of contact. BC 1175 (CB 181963) belongs to a group of cephems having guanylhydrazone moieties containing an additional basic substituent at N-4 (Fig. 77).

BC 1175 is soluble in water (>15%) at physiological pH in the protonated form (Ascher et al., 2003). This azomethine cephalosporin is moderately active against MRSA (MIC_{50} and MIC_{90}, 2.0 to 4.0 μg/ml) as well as against GISA strains (Draghi et al., 2003).

In a series of cephems, the C-3′ pharmacophore chosen was imidazol[1, 2*b*] pyridazinium (Fig. 78).

Introduction of a thiovinyl group or a thio group as the C-3 spacer between the C-3 position and the C-3′ pharmacophore results in improved anti-MRSA activity (Tsushima et al., 1998). One analog was selected for further investigation; MICs for MRSA ranged from 0.78 to 3.13 μg/ml, with no antipseudomonal activity (MIC, ≥6.25 μg/ml). In vivo the ED_{50} was 4.82 mg/kg and the IC_{50} for PBP 2a was 2 to 7 μg/ml (Ishikawa et al., 2001b).

Some cephems with a C-3 pyridinium moiety have anti-MRSA activity but lack appreciable water solubility. A hydroxyiminoaminothiazolyl substituent at position C-7 of 2-thioisocephem with a vinylthio linkage at position C-3 showed strong activity against MRSA, but these derivatives

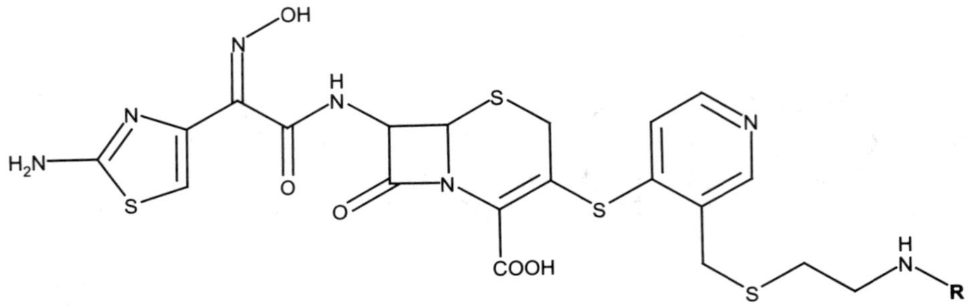

	R
RWJ 54428	H
RWJ 442831	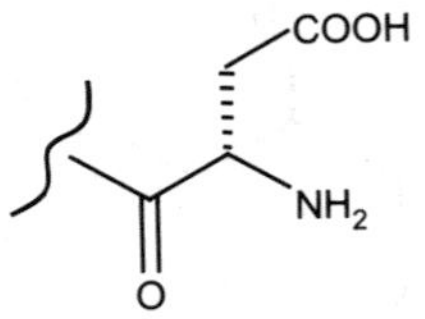 COOH, NH_2, O

Figure 75 **RWJ-442831, prodrug of RWJ-54428**

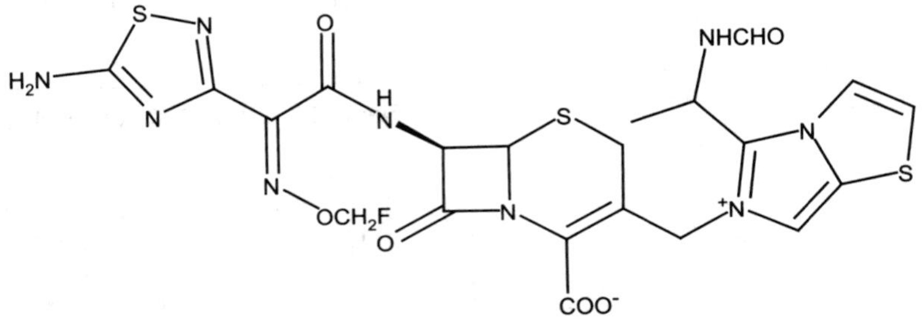

Figure 76 **ME-1209 (CP-6679)**

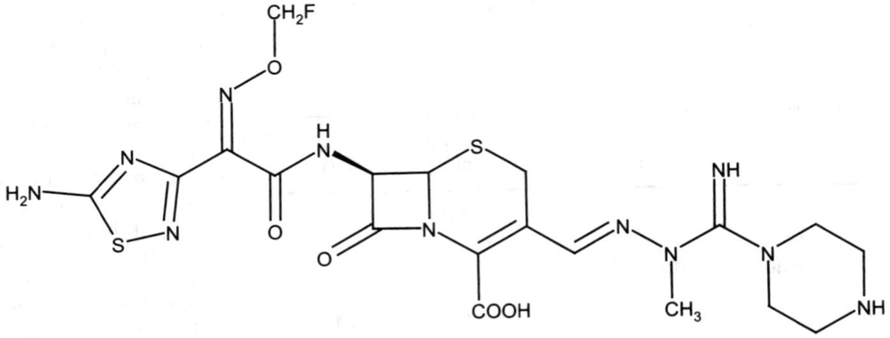

Figure 77 **BC 1175**

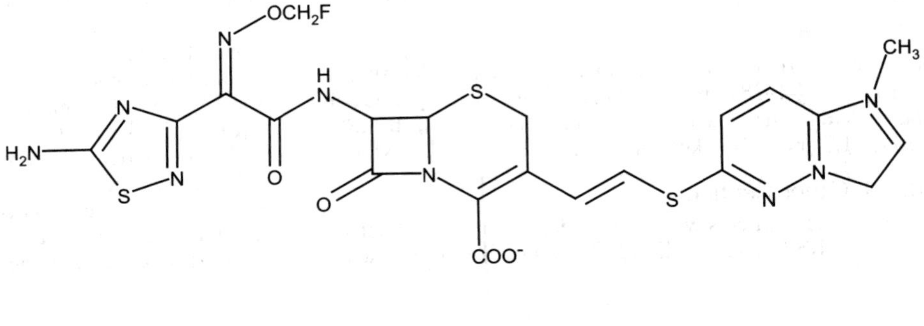

Figure 78 **Imidazolo-pyridinium cephalosporin**

have low water solubility. Series of derivatives having a C-3 thiovinyl pyridinium replaced with N-quaternary alkyl ammonium moieties and a C-7 hydroxy-imino-amino-thiazolyl side chain showed good anti-MRSA activity (MIC_{90}, 1.56 μg/ml) and acceptable water solubility (>20% at pH 7.2) (Hanaki et al., 2001).

8.1.9. LB-11058

LB-11058 (Fig. 79) displays moderate anti-MRSA activity (MIC_{50} and MIC_{90} of 1.0 and 2.0 μg/ml) even if the affinity for PBP 2a is high (0.3 μg/ml). This cephem is highly bound to human serum protein (>93%). In vivo the PD_{50} was 7.5 mg/kg for MRSA (Joo et al., 2001).

The compound seems to be bactericidal, with a reduction of 3 $\log_{10}$ CFU/ml at 12 h at four times the MIC (Cho et al., 2001b).

8.1.10. PGE-9739390

PGE-9739390 (Fig. 80) is 3-dithiocarbamoyl cephalosporin. The MIC for MRSA was 2.0 μg/ml, and the IC_{50} for PBP 2a was 0.5 μM (Chen et al., 2000).

8.1.11. Summary

Table 5 summarizes the data on various anti-MRSA cephems.

8.2. Carbapenems

Today carbapenems can be considered the most potent β-lactam family. However, they are inactive against MRSA. In recent years, it has been shown that appending some moieties at position 2 may enhance anti-MRSA activity. The moieties involved are aryl, thiazolylthio, benzothiazolylthio, aminothiocarbonylthio, and aryl-oxymethyl groups.

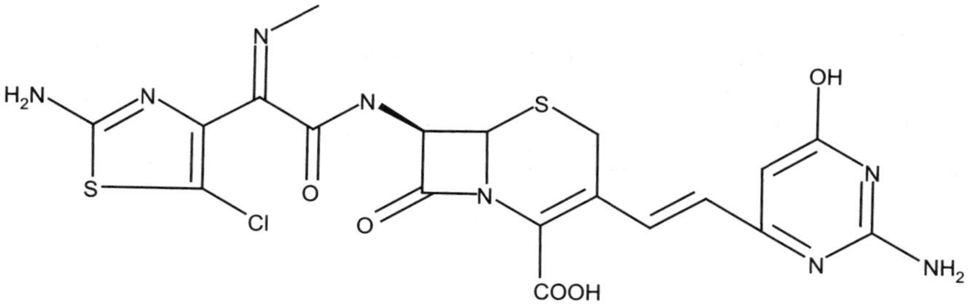

Figure 79 **LB-11058**

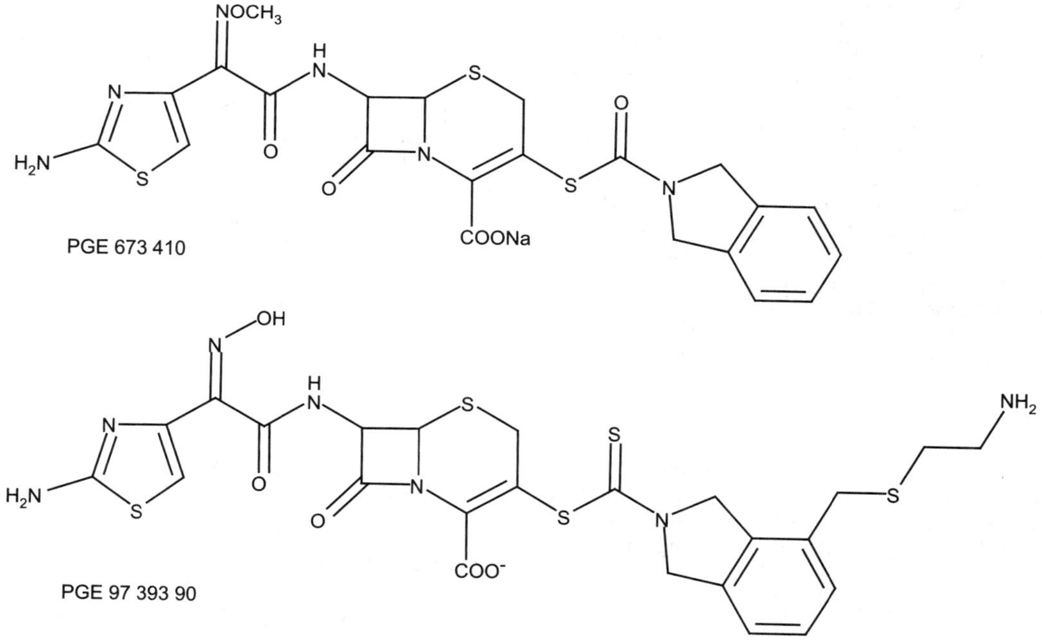

	PGE 6937410	PGE 9739390
MIC (μg/ml)	8.0	2.0
IC_{50} (μg/ml)	2.6	1.5
Solubility (pH 7.4)	2500 mg/ml	15.0

Figure 80 **PGE-69337410 and PGE-69337410**

Table 5 Profile of anti-MRSA cephems

Compound	*n*	MIC (μg/ml)			ED_{50}/PD_{50} (mg/kg)	Water solubility (mg/ml)	IC_{50} (μM or μg/ml)[a]
		50%	90%	Range			
TAK-599[b]					0.8–4.72	>100	
T-91825	81	1.0	2.0	0.25–2.0	1.74	2.3	0.9
Ceftobiprole medocaril	77	2.0	4.0	0.12–4.0	2.4	ND[d]	0.31
RWJ-54428	322	1.0	2.0	0.5–4.0	6.1		0.7
RWJ-333441[c]					1.7	14.5	
RWJ-442831[c]					1.9	20	
LB-11058	110	1.0	1.0	0.25–1.0	7.5	>20	0.3
S-3578	84	1.0	2.0	0.5–2.0	7.21–8.9	>100	4.5
TOC-39	117	1.56	3.13		23.7	<1	0.58
CP0467	25	3.13	6.25	1.56–6.25		0.49	
ME-1209				4–16	0.37		5.1
LY-206763	2			0.5–4.0	ND	ND	2.0
PGE-9739390		0.12	0.12	0.12–2.0		15	0.5
BMS-247243	67	4.0	4.0	0.5–8.0	1.4	ND	0.7
OPC-20011	33	6.25	6.25	0.78–6.25	1.0	ND	ND
BC 1175	61	2.0	4.0	1.0–8.0		>150	
CB 181963	199	2.0	4.0	0.5–4.0			
Vancomycin	67	2.0	2.0	1.0–2.0	3.37–4.80	50	

[a]Affinity for PBP 2a.
[b]PPI-0903 (prodrug of T-91825).
[c]Prodrug of RWJ-54428.
[d]ND, not disclosed.

8.2.1. L-763863

A series of amidinium 2-benzofuranyl carbapenems has been synthesized (Fig. 81), and some of them exhibited good in vitro and in vivo activities against MRSA (MIC_{50} and MIC_{90}, 1.0 and 2.0 μg/ml) and in vivo an ED_{50} of <0.096 mg/kg. The protein binding was 71% (Laub et al., 1999).

Many advanced candidates were identified but abandoned for immune-based toxicity in rhesus monkeys, such as L-763863 (benzothiazolylthio carbapenem) and L-695256 and L-742728 (2-fluoroenoyl carbapenems). Introduction in the latter two compounds of a double quaternized 1,4-diazabicyclooctane renders them sufficiently hydrophilic for high in vitro activity.

The immunotoxicity was believed to result from nonspecific acylation of lysine residues by the carbapenem, following immune recognition and response to the appended hapten. It was the lipophilic side chain which was suspected of being the main immunogenic component of the hapten.

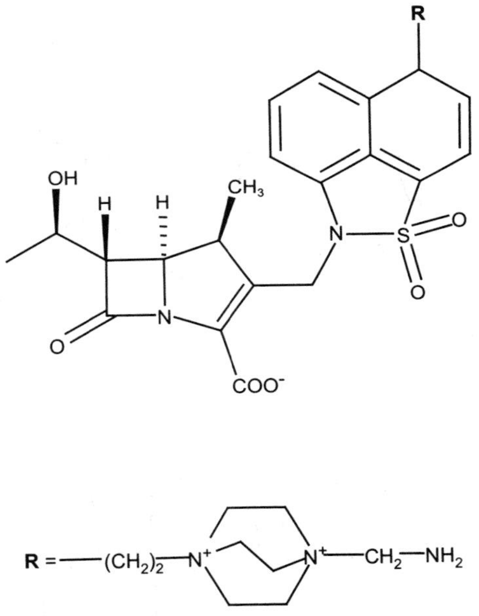

8.2.2. L-786392

Exploring the cause of immunotoxicity of previous carbapenems led to the synthesis of 2-(naphthylsultamoyl) methyl carbapenems. L-786392 (Fig. 82) exhibited a MIC of 0.7 μg/ml for MRSA and a stability of 1.77 against renal dehydropeptidase I (DHP-I), with a low toxicity profile and an IC_{50} of 8.8 μg/ml for PBP 2a (Ratcliffe et al., 1999).

Figure 81 L-763863

Figure 82 L-786392

The 1,8-naphthosultamoyl side chain was identified as a novel PBP 2a-binding anti-MRSA pharmacophore designed to be released upon opening of the β-lactam ring (Miller et al., 2000) (Fig. 83).

There is a rapid and quantitative ring opening of the β-lactam bond accompanied by simultaneous appearance of the expulsed side chain (Ratcliffe et al., 1999).

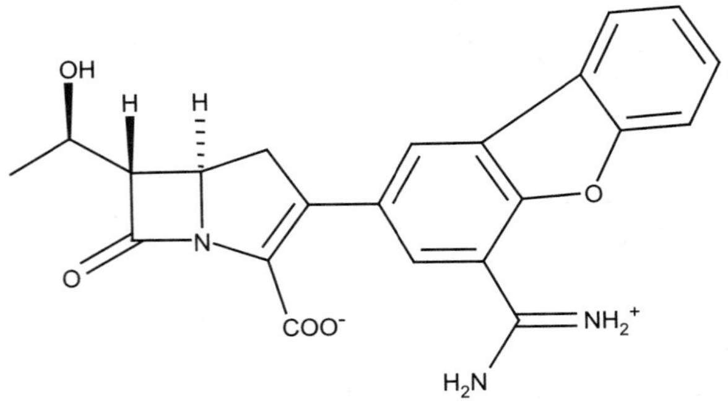

8.2.3. BO-3482: Dithiocarbamate Carbapenems

BO-3482 (Fig. 84), a dithiocarbamate analog, was selected, but in vivo efficacy and DHP-I susceptibility needed to be

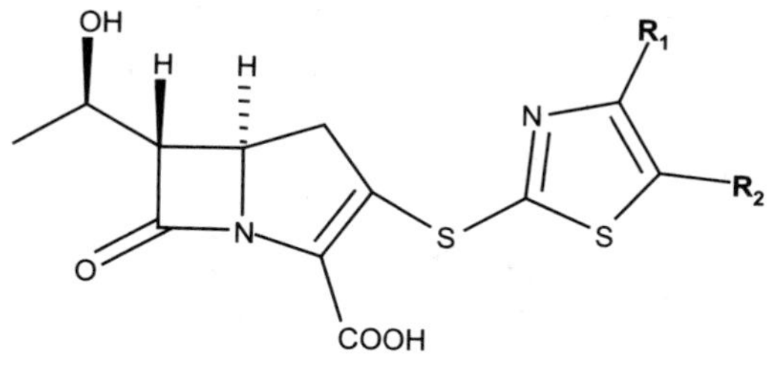

C-2 thiazolyl carbapenem

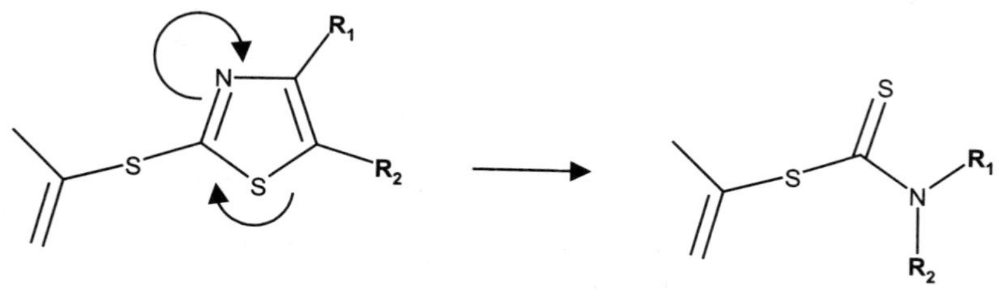

Cleavage of the thiazolyl ring

Figure 83 Cleavage of the carbapenem ring

improved (Inamura et al., 2001; Ohtake et al., 1998). Numerous points have to be taken into consideration:

- A high hydrophobicity may have a deleterious effect on the physicochemical properties.
- Introduction of a quaternary ammonium moiety into the C-2 side chain reduces the protein binding rate and improves DHP-I stability against hydrolysis. Unfortunately these analogs displayed significant epileptogenicities in an intra-cerebroventricular assay.

A series of dithiocarbamate tetrahydropyridylthio carbapenems was synthesized (Fig. 84). These dicationic derivatives exhibit anti-MRSA activity (MIC, 3.13 μg/ml) and susceptibility to DHP-I of 0.51; the IC_{50} for PBP 2a was 1.1 μg/ml. The protein binding was 55%. No epileptogenicity after administration of 200 μg/rat was noted. In murine staphylococcal (MRSA) infection the ED_{50} was 1.86 mg/kg (vancomycin ED_{50}, 5.56 mg/kg; imipenem ED_{50}, above 200 mg/kg).

8.2.4. J-111,347

The aim of other research in the field of carbapenems was to enhance the activities against both gram-positive and gram-negative bacteria, including *P. aeruginosa*.

J-111,347 is a C-2 *trans*-pyrrolidinylthio, 1-β-methyl carbapenem and was a prototype (Fig. 85) (Nagano et al., 2000).

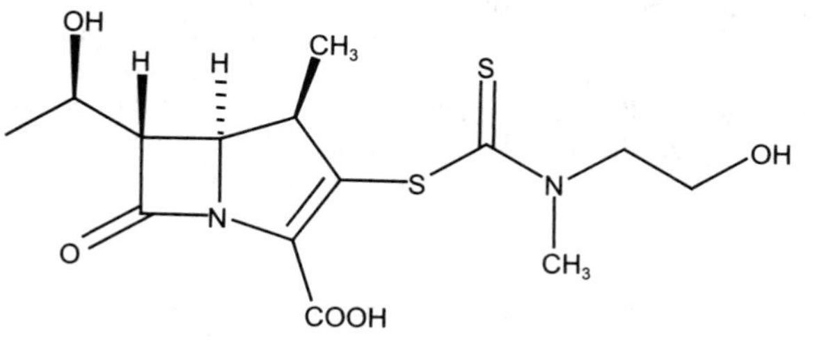

BO-3482

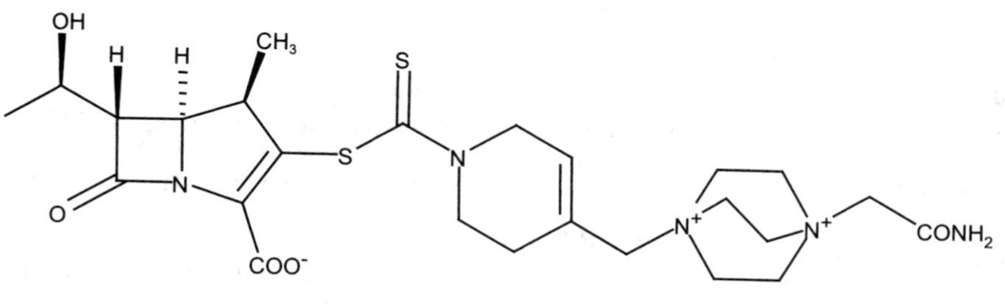

Dithiocarbamate tetrahydropyridylthio carbapenems

Figure 84 Dithiocarbamate (BO-3482)

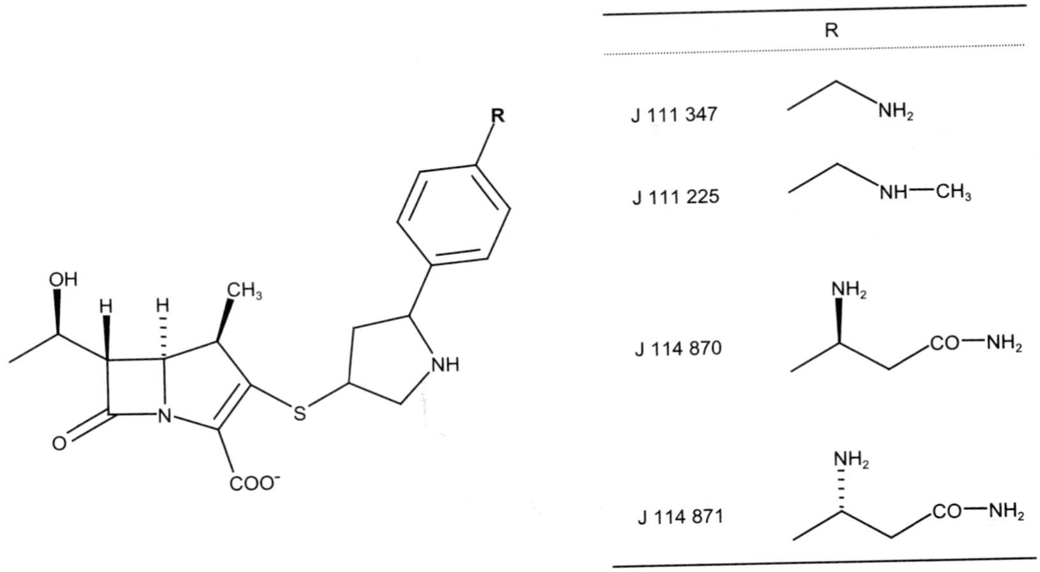

Figure 85 J-111,347 and analogs

Four compounds were investigated: J-111,347, J-111,225, J-114,870, and J-114,871. All of them displayed MIC_{50}s and MIC_{90}s of 2.0 and 4.0 μg/ml for MRSA and of 1.0 and 4.0 μg/ml for *P. aeruginosa*. They have a partial cross-resistance with imipenem-resistant *P. aeruginosa* (imipenem MIC, ≥8.0 μg/ml, versus a MIC_{50} and MIC_{90} of 4 to 8 and 16 μg/ml). They are bactericidal against *S. aureus* at four times the MIC after 6 h of contact. The IC_{50s} for PBP 2a were 2.6 and 2.5 μg/ml for J-111,347 and J-111,225 respectively (imipenem IC_{50}, 85 μg/ml).

J-111,347 investigations were given up due to epileptogenicity. This adverse effect was eliminated by N methylation (J-111,225) or introduction of a carbamoyl methyl substituent (J-114,870 and J-114,871) at the α-position of the benzylamino group.

8.2.5. Mercaptothiazolyl Carbapenems

The cleavage of the thiazolyl ring between the 1-5 bond resulted in dithiocarbamate moiety. Some derivatives exhibited anti-MRSA activity in vitro as well as favorable binding affinity for PBP 2a. MICs ranged from 0.78 to 3.13 μg/ml, the IC_{50}s were 1.8 to 5.6 μg/ml, and DHP-I susceptibility varied from 2.18 to 4.41; serum protein binding was too high (>88 to 95%). These derivatives are inactive against *P. aeruginosa*.

Introduction of a mercaptothiazolyl group at C-2 enhances anti-MRSA activity.

Human serum albumin binding and stability against DHP-I hydrolysis are correlated with the distance between the cationic amino moiety on the C-2 side chain and the carbapenem skeleton.

In a new series of mercaptothiazolyl carbapenems, some compounds remain active against MRSA (MICs, 1.56 μg/ml; IC_{50} for PBP 2a, 5.9 μg/ml) but are weakly bound to human serum albumin (15%) (Shinagawa et al., 1997).

8.2.6. Pyrrolidinyl-Substituted Carbapenems

In a series of pyrrolidinyl-substituted carbapenems, it was shown that among aminoethyl carbamoyl substituents, the most active analog bears a cyclic urea moiety (piperazinyl) (Fig. 86). MICs ranged from 0.20 to 6.25 μg/ml for MRSA.

Among the substituted carbapenems the guanidine analogs exhibited the highest anti-MRSA activity (MICs, 0.20 to 1.56 μg/ml), including antipseudomonal activity (MIC, 0.8 μg/ml) (Oh et al., 2003b).

In another study, two important points were illustrated:

- 2-Vinyl carbapenems are stable against hydrolysis by DHP-I.
- When directly linked to the carbapenem skeleton, pyrrolidinyl carbapenems are active against MRSA.

Many derivatives were active against MRSA, with MICs below 0.25 μg/ml, but some of them were weakly active (MICs, 3.13 to 6.25 μg/ml) and others were totally inactive (MICs, ≥25 μg/ml). Many of them exhibited antipseudomonal activity (MICs, 0.20 to 0.78 μg/ml) and exhibited good stability against human DHP-I hydrolysis, with urinary recovery above 40% (Hattori et al., 2002).

Introduction of an additional oxime and imine moiety on the urea form into the pyrrolidine nucleus resulted in improved activity against MRSA. KJO-16 (Fig. 87) was the most active analog, with MICs ranging from 0.03 to 3.13 μg/ml depending on the strain tested, followed by KJO-26, with MICs ranging from 0.1 to 0.78 μg/ml (Oh et al., 2003a).

8.2.7. SM-216601

SM-216601 is a β-methyl carbapenem substituted at position 2 with a thiazolyl substituted side chain (Fig. 88).

The MIC_{50} and MIC_{90} are 1.0 and 2.0 μg/ml, and the affinity for PBP 2a is 0.99 μg/ml. In disseminated murine infection the ED_{50} is 2.89 mg/kg. Apparently this carbapenem is bactericidal.

8.2.8. CS-834

CS-834 is a prodrug of R-95867 having a 2-oxopyrrolidinyl moiety. CS-834 is orally absorbed. It is inactive against MRSA in vitro (MIC_{50} and MIC_{90}, 3.13 and 12.5 μg/ml). The compound was not tested in vivo (Fukuoka et al., 1997) (Fig. 89).

8.2.9. CP-5068

CP-5068 belongs to a series of 6,7-disubstituted imidazolylthiazole carbapenem derivatives (Fig. 90) (Shitara et al., 2000).

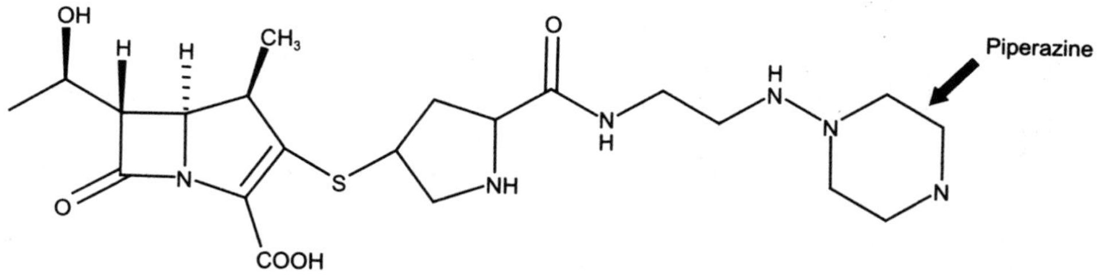

Substituted 2-pyrrolidinyl carbapenems

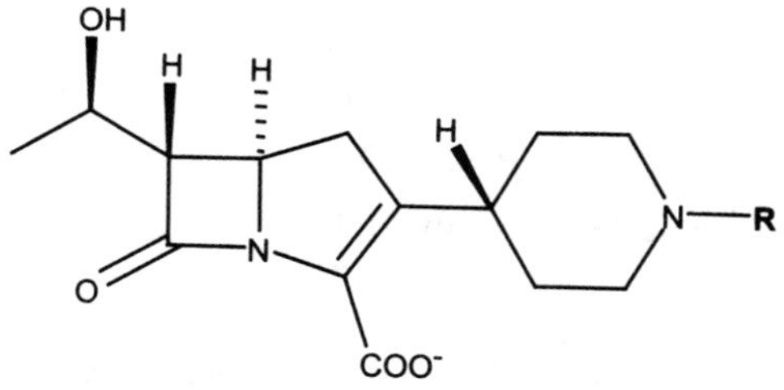

Directly 2-linked pyrrolidinyl carbapenems

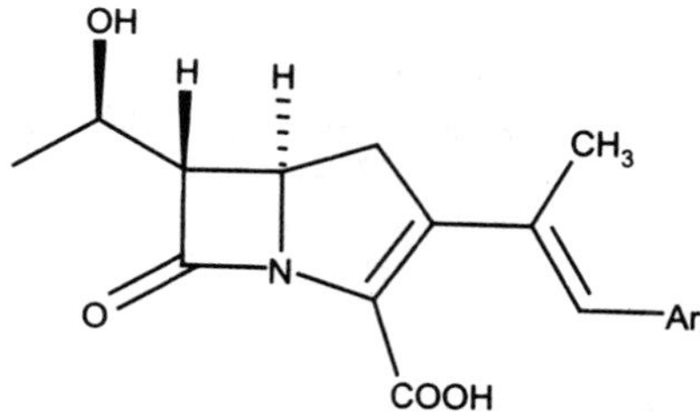

2-vinyl carbapenems

Figure 86 Pyrrolidinyl carbapenems

	R
KJO-20	
KJO-26	
KJO-8	
KJO-16	
KJO-18	

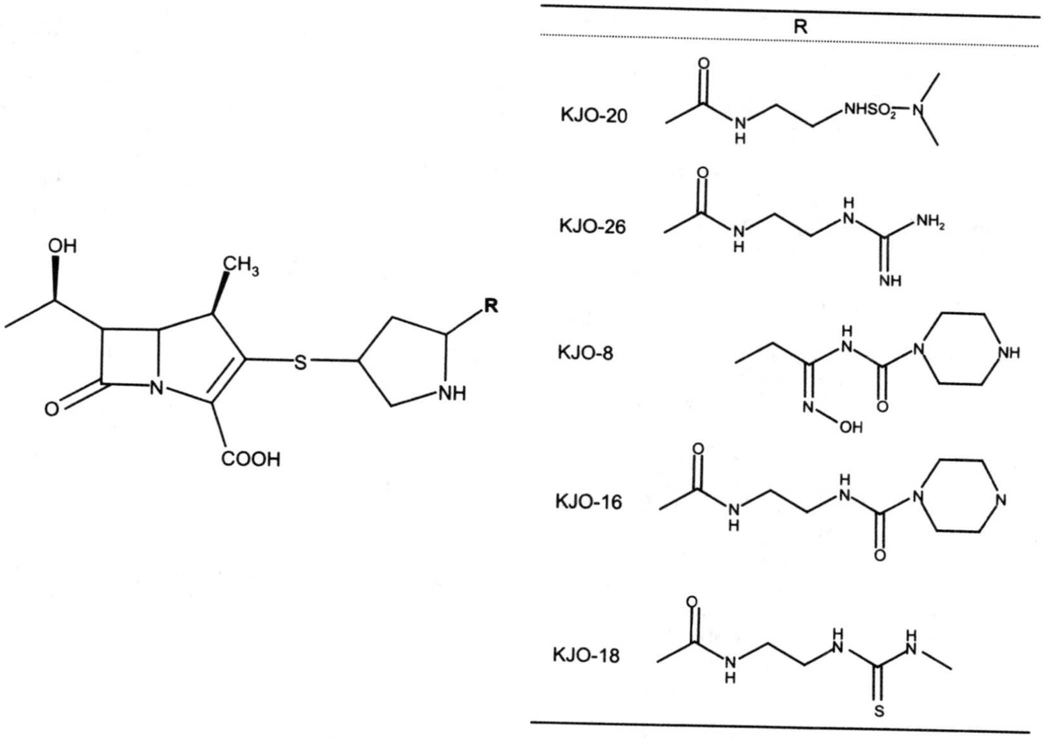

Figure 87 β-Methyl carbapenems with oxime and imino moieties

The MIC_{50} and MIC_{90} were 2.0 and 8.0 μg/ml for MRSA. In disseminated staphylococcal murine infections the PD_{50} was 5.2 mg/kg (Ida et al., 2000).

8.3. Monocyclic β-Lactams

Using purified PBP 2a, potent monocyclic-β-lactams were identified as lead compounds (IC_{50}s, 0.37 to 0.64 μg/ml) (Nieuwlandt et al., 2001).

9. TOPICAL ANTISTAPHYLOCOCCAL COMPOUNDS

S. aureus, coagulase-negative staphylococci, and *S. pyogenes* are the main pathogens involved in skin and skin structure infections. The number of antibacterials used as topical antibiotics is not large (mupirocin and fusidic acid), and strains of *S. aureus* highly resistant are not uncommon. New antibiotics for topical use are needed.

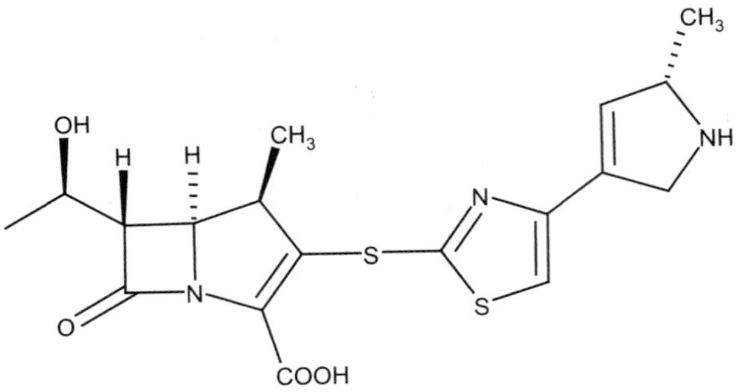

Figure 88 SM-216601

9.1. Benzo[*b*]naphthyridone—RP-60556A

The first benzo[*b*]naphthyridone was synthesized in 1967. RP-60556A (Fig. 91) and its analog RP-203246 exhibit good anti-MRSA activity (MICs, 0.5 and 1.0 to 2.0 μg/ml, respectively). They are active against mupirocin-resistant isolates (Tabart et al., 2001, 2003).

9.2. Pleuromutilins

The first pleuromutilin was isolated in 1951 from the basidiomycete *Pleurotus mutilus* (Kavanagh et al., 1951).

Pleuromutilins are composed of a tricyclic diterpenoid structure. They exert their antibacterial activity by inhibiting bacterial protein synthesis. They bind to the 50S ribosomal subunit at the level of the 23S rRNA, especially at nucleotides A2058, A2059, U2506, and U2584, as well as to ribosomal protein L3.

New synthetic derivatives with antistaphylococcal activity are currently under development.

Two semisynthetic derivatives of pleuromutilins, SB 247386 and SB 268091, were selected for further investigation.

In vitro SB 268001 is particularly active against MSSA (MIC_{90}, 0.06 μg/ml), MRSA (MIC_{90}, 0.06 μg/ml), mupirocin-resistant *S. aureus* (MIC_{90}, 0.06 μg/ml), and fusidic acid-resistant *S. aureus* (MIC_{90}, 0.03 μg/ml) as well as against *S. epidermidis* (MIC_{90}, 0.03 μg/ml) and *S. pyogenes* (MIC_{90}, ≤0.01 μg/ml). SB 247386 is less active than SB 268001 especially against isolates resistant to methicillin (MIC_{90}, 2.0 μg/ml) or resistant to mupirocin (MIC_{90}, 1.0 μg/ml) and against *S. epidermidis* (MIC_{90}, 1.0 μg/ml) (Rittenhouse et al., 1999).

Dorsal staphylococcal wound infections were induced in mice and local treatment was begun 1 h after challenge; further doses were administered at 4 and 7 h and treatment was continued thereafter three times a day for 3 days. Animals were sacrificed approximately 17 h after therapy ended. The viable bacterial cells recovered from the wounds were counted. In control mice, the number of bacterial cells was 6.4 ± 0.3 $\log_{10}$ CFU/wound (mean ± standard deviation). Treatment

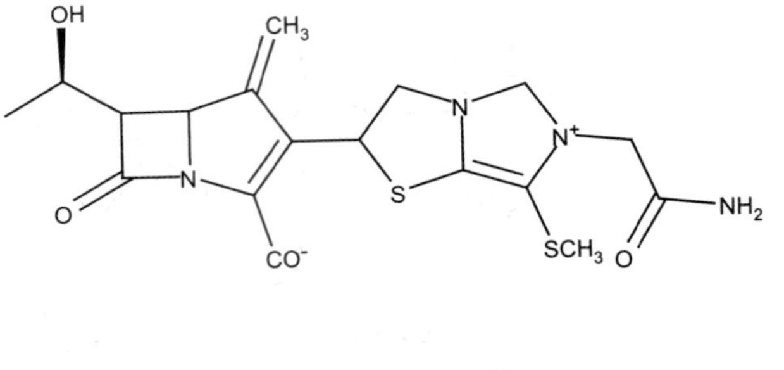

Substituted imidazole thiazolium

DHP-1 = 0.04

MIC = 1.0

PD_{50} = 0.45 - 0.08 mg/kg

Figure 90 CP-5068

with mupirocin resulted in a 2-$\log_{10}$ reduction in bacterial counts (4.4 ± 1.3 $\log_{10}$ CFU/wound). A high reduction was obtained with SB 247386 in comparison with control and mupirocin groups of mice, 1.8 ± 0.9 $\log_{10}$ CFU/wound, and no detectable bacteria were recorded for four of seven mice. The same figure was recorded with SB 247386 (1.3 ± 0.2 $\log_{10}$ CFU/wound), and four of seven mice showed sterilized wounds.

When mice were infected with *S. aureus* 1080 resistant to mupirocin (MIC, 4.0 μg/ml), mupirocin decreased the wound burden slightly (5.2 ± 1.0 $\log_{10}$ CFU/wound, versus 6.3 ± 0.3 $\log_{10}$ CFU/wound for control), but SB 247386 significantly decreased the bacterial burden (2.3 ± 0.4 $\log_{10}$ CFU/wound, versus 6.3 ± 0.3 $\log_{10}$ CFU/wound for control) and the bacterial count was under the limit of detection (<1.7 $\log_{10}$ CFU/wound) in three of seven mice (Berry et al., 1999).

9.3. Saccharomicins

Saccharomicins A and B were isolated from the culture broth of an actinomycete, *Saccharothrix espanaensis* LLC 19004 (Fig. 92). Components A and B are equipotent against gram-positive bacteria. Against MRSA, MICs ranged from <0.12 to 0.5 μg/ml. Even if an ED_{50} of 2.6 mg/kg showed good in vivo antistaphylococcal activity, the therapeutic index between the ED_{50} and LD_{50} is too low to allow parenteral administration (Singh et al., 2000).

9.4. Allicin

Allicin extracts (garlic) exhibited anti-MRSA activity in topical usage. Allicin is active against mupirocin-resistant strains (Cutler et al., 2001).

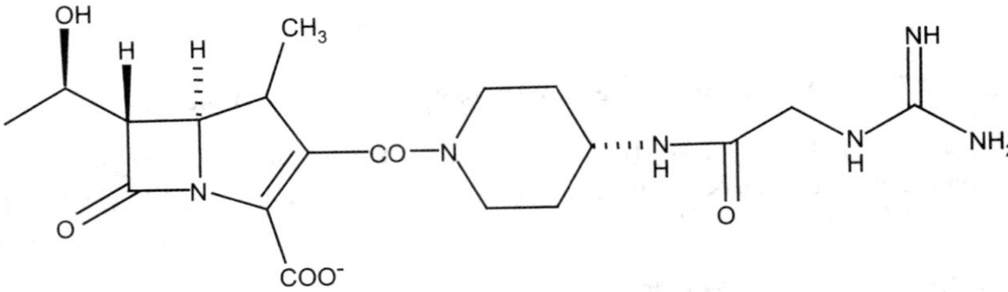

MRSA (n=52) $MIC_{50/90}$ = 4.0 / 8.0 μg/ml

ED_{50} = 7.93 mg/kg

IC_{50} PBP_{2a} ?

Figure 89 CS-834

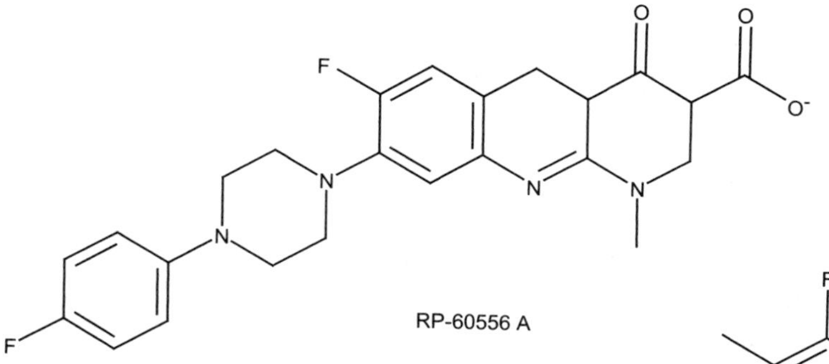

RP-60556 A

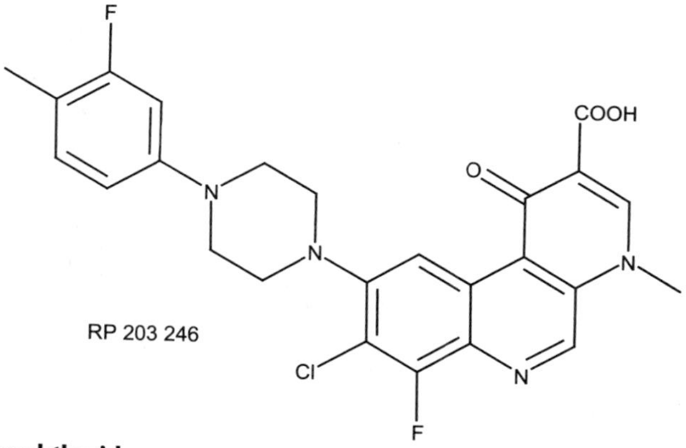

RP 203 246

Figure 91 Benzonaphthyridones

9.5. Mersacidin

Mersacidin is a 20-amino-acid peptide belonging to the lantibiotic family. Mersacidin was isolated from the fermentation broth of *Bacillus* sp. strain HIL Y-85/54728. It exhibits activity against gram-positive organisms, inhibiting bacterial cell wall biosynthesis by complexing lipid II.

It has been shown that mersacidin is able to cure disseminated staphylococcal (MRSA) murine infection and abscesses in rats after subcutaneous administration.

S. aureus can be carried asymptomatically on the nasal epithelium in healthy individuals.

Epidemiological studies have linked nasal carriage with a high risk of development of staphylococcal infection. Mersacidin administered intranasally twice daily (1.66 mg/kg twice a day) over 3 days eradicated MRSA from the nasal mucosa of colonized mice (Kruszenska et al., 2004).

10. CYCLINES

There is a renewal of interest in cycline derivatives with the semisynthesis of tigecycline and PTK 0796.

10.1. Tigecycline (GAR-936)

Tetracycline derivatives with a 9-glycylamido substituent are named glycylcyclines.

Tigecycline is a semisynthetic derivative of minocycline having a 9*t*-butyl glycylamido substitution.

Tigecycline possesses a broad antibacterial spectrum, including gram-positive, gram-negative, intracellular, and atypical microorganisms.

In vitro, the tigecycline MIC_{50} and MIC_{90} are 0.25 and 0.5 μg/ml and 0.25 and 0.5 μg/ml for MRSA and GISA strains, respectively (Petersen et al., 1999).

In a recent study, tigecycline inhibited 76.7, 93.7, and 100% of MRSA strains at concentrations of 0.12, 0.25, and 1.0 μg/ml, respectively (Stevens et al., 2004).

In murine disseminated staphylococcal infection as well as in experimental endocarditis in rats, the ED_{50} were 1.9 and 0.24 to 0.72 mg/kg for GISA and MRSA, respectively.

10.2. PTK 0796 (BAY 73-6944)

PTK 0796 is 7-dimethylamino,9-(2,2-dimethylpropyl)-aminoethylcycline (Fig. 93).

The IC_{50} and IC_{90} for MRSA are 0.25 and 0.5 μg/ml, respectively.

PTK 0796 exhibits activity against isolates harboring *tet* genes. In murine disseminated staphylococcal infection (MRSA), the ED_{50} was 5.9 mg/kg (minocycline ED_{50}, 35.2 mg/kg).

11. MACROLIDES/KETOLIDES

Today, 14- and 15-membered-ring macrolides are poorly active against MRSA. MRSA isolates often harbor a macrolide-lincosamide-streptogramin (MLS_B) mechanism of resistance.

Ketolides like telithromycin are active in vitro against MRSA having an inducible MLS_B mechanism of resistance but are inactive when the MLS_B mechanism is constitutive. The MIC_{50} and MIC_{90} are 0.12 and 0.5 μg/ml. Telithromycin inhibits superoxide anion production in a time- and concentration-dependent manner. The intracellular persistence of *S. aureus* in polymorphonuclear neutrophils has been demonstrated. Telithromycin is bactericidal against intracellular staphylococci in correlation with the MIC (Vazifeh et al., 2002).

12. LINCOSAMIDES

It was shown that 7-methyl-4′-pentyl prolamide lincosamides exhibited higher in vitro antibacterial activity against gram-positive cocci than clindamycin (Lewis et al., 2004a).

One analog was selected for further investigation, VIC-105555 (Lewis et al., 2004b) (Fig. 94).

In vitro VIC-105555 exerted activity against MRSA similar to that of clindamycin (MIC_{50} and MIC_{90}, 0.25 and 0.25 μg/ml), but VIC-105555 was more active in vivo after intravenous and subcutaneous administration (ED_{50}, 0.13 and 0.32 mg/kg, respectively) than clindamycin (ED_{50}, 1.61 and 2.27 mg/kg, respectively) (Park et al., 2004).

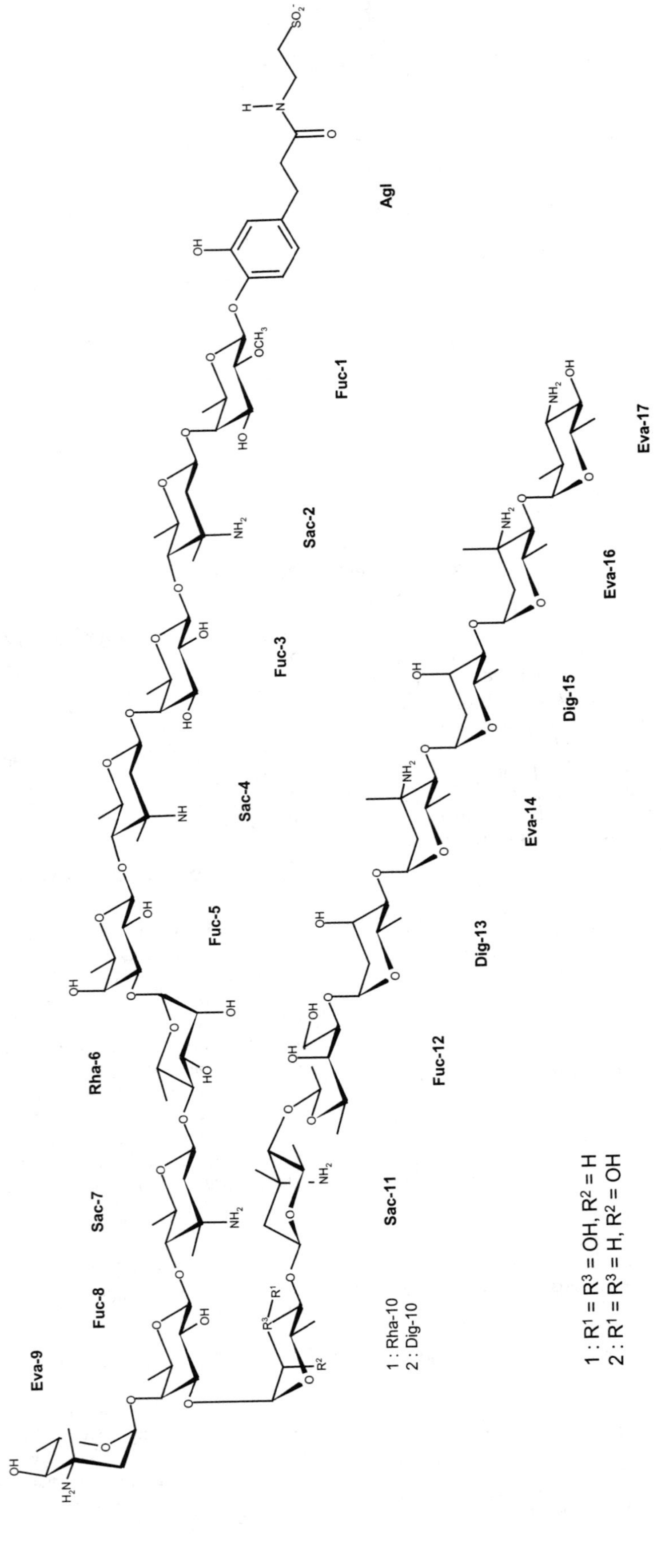

1 : Rha-10
2 : Dig-10

1 : $R^1 = R^3 = OH, R^2 = H$
2 : $R^1 = R^3 = H, R^2 = OH$

Figure 92 Saccharomicins

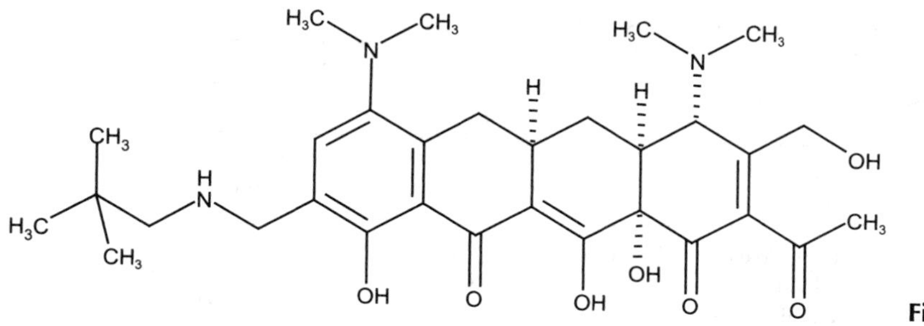

Figure 93 PTK 0796

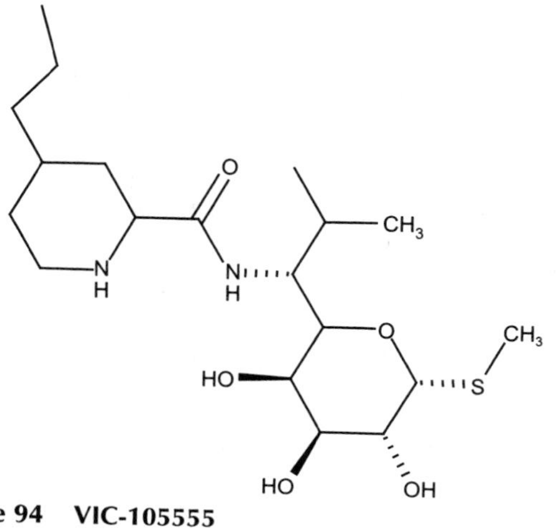

Figure 94 VIC-105555

13. FLUOROQUINOLONES

Fluoroquinolones are active against *S. aureus* strains irrespective of their susceptibilities to methicillin. Unfortunately, MRSA strains resistant to fluoroquinolones have emerged very rapidly.

To overcome this problem, intensive research on fluoroquinolones targeting gram-positive bacteria was undertaken. Although real progress in terms of in vitro and in vivo activities was made, none of the drugs reached clinics for use against MRSA. MICs are summarized in Table 6.

In murine disseminated staphylococcal infections, the ED_{50} for MRSA were 9.23, 100, 56.7, and 67.3 mg/kg for DK-507k (Fig. 95), levofloxacin, moxifloxacin, and gatifloxacin, respectively (Otani et al., 2003).

The most active molecule, including against MRSA isolates resistant to fluoroquinolones, is ABT-492. Unfortunately, for unclear reasons the development of this compound was given up during phase II.

WCK 771 is the active *S*-(−)-isomer of the racemate nadifloxacin (Fig. 96), which was developed for topical use due to its water solubility. WCK 771 is soluble in water, being an arginine salt formulation. For GISA strains the MICs of WCK 717 were 1.0 μg/ml, as were those of clinafloxacin (Jacobs et al., 2004).

DQ-113 (formerly DQ-61-113) is an 8-methyl fluoroquinolone, bearing an N-1 fluorocyclopropyl and a 5′-amino-1′-fluorocyclopropyl on the 7-pyrrolidinyl moiety (Fig. 97). In vitro its MIC_{50} and MIC_{90} for MRSA are ≤ 0.004 and 0.008 μg/ml (Tanaka et al., 2002). In murine respiratory infection induced with MRSA, DQ-113 reduced the bacterial burden after a 40-mg/kg dose by $\approx 2\ \log_{10}$ CFU/ml.

DX-619 (Fig. 98) exhibited good in vitro activity against MRSA, including strains resistant to ciprofloxacin and those showing intermediate susceptibility to vancomycin or resistant to vancomycin (Bozdogan and Appelbaum, 2004). For isolates resistant to available quinolones, the affinity of DX-619 is similar or superior to that for topoisomerase IV or GrlA of susceptible isolates (Table 7) (Ishida et al., 2004).

14. OXAZOLIDINONES

The oxazolidinones represent a relatively new class of antibacterial agents. They are synthetic compounds with activities against gram-positive bacteria.

The first oxazolidinone derivatives investigated for human use were DuP 105 and DuP 721. They were weakly active against MRSA (MIC_{50} and MIC_{90}, 8 and 16 μg/ml and 4 and 4 μg/ml, respectively) (Barry, 1988).

Linezolid was the first oxazolidinone introduced into clinical practice against MRSA, with MICs of 2.0 μg/ml; it is bacteriostatic.

Ranbezolid (RBx 7944) is a substituted (nitrofuryl) piperazinyl derivative, but it remains bacteriostatic, with a MIC_{50} and MIC_{90} of 1.0 and 2.0 μg/ml. In murine disseminated staphylococcal infections the ED_{50} were 5.2 and 1.56 mg/kg by the oral and parenteral routes, respectively (linezolid ED_{50}, 5.6 and 4.42 mg/kg, respectively).

AZD 2563 (Fig. 99) (Howe et al., 2003) is active against MRSA (MIC_{50} and MIC_{90}, 1.0 and 2.0 μg/ml) (Anderegg et al., 2002) as well as against GISA strains (MIC_{50} and MIC_{90}, 1.0 and 2.0 μg/ml). A cross-resistance was seen with linezolid-resistant strains.

The aim of efforts for new series of oxazolidinones was to improve potency and to enlarge the antibacterial spectrum as well as improve the safety of long-term linezolid treatment. Investigations were carried out to replace the morpholine ring.

Numerous exploratory oxazolidinone derivatives have been synthesized. They bear various heterocycles, such as isoxazolyltetrahydropyridine (Lee et al., 2003), thiadiazolyl (Thomasco et al., 2003), benzoazepine (Johnson et al., 2003), thiomorpholine S-oxide and S-dioxide (Singh et al., 2003b), azetidinyl, piperazinyl, imidazolyl, pyridyl, benzothiazolone (Endersmann et al., 1998), and benzoxazolone (Bartel et al., 1998) (Fig. 100).

A series of codrugs combining a fluoroquinolone and linezolid was synthesized. These molecules displayed in vitro activity against MRSA, including linezolid-resistant strains. MICs were ≤ 0.25 μg/ml (Locher et al., 2002).

15. DEFORMYLASE INHIBITORS

Deformylase is an essential bacterial metallo-enzyme responsible for the removal of the N-terminal formyl group from methionine following protein synthesis. Further, methionine aminopeptidase removes the methionine group to produce mature protein. PDF is encoded by the gene *def.*

Table 6 In vitro activities of fluoroquinolones against MRSA[a]

MRSA phenotype	Compound	MIC (μg/ml)	
		50%	90%
Fluoroquinolone susceptible	DK-507k	0.03	0.06 (24)[b]
	Sitafloxacin	0.03	0.06 (24)
	Levofloxacin	0.25	0.5 (24)
	Ciprofloxacin	0.5	1.0 (24)
	Clinafloxacin	0.015	0.03
	Gatifloxacin	0.12	0.25 (24)
	Moxifloxacin	0.12	0.12 (24)
	Garenofloxacin	0.03	0.06 (24)
	WCK 717	0.5	1.0
	WCK 919	1.0	2.0
	DQ-113	0.004	0.008 (24)
	Grepafloxacin	≤0.06	≤0.06 (62)
	Sparfloxacin	≤0.06	≤0.06 (62)
	Trovafloxacin	≤0.06	≤0.06 (62)
	DW-116	1.0	4.0 (132)
	ABT-492	0.004	0.008
	DX-619	0.008	0.008
Fluoroquinolone resistant	DK-507k	1.0	4.0 (25)
	Sitafloxacin	1.0	4.0 (25)
	Levofloxacin	16	64 (25)
	Ciprofloxacin	>128	>128 (25)
	Clinafloxacin	0.25	2.0
	Gatifloxacin	8	16 (25)
	Moxifloxacin	4	8 (25)
	Garenofloxacin	2	8 (25)
	WCK 717	0.5	1.0
	DQ-113	0.06	0.25 (25)
	Grepafloxacin	16	32 (189)
	Sparfloxacin	0.5	4 (16)
	Trovafloxacin	1.0	4 (189)
	DW-116	32	32 (107)
	ABT-492	0.12	0.25
	DX-619	0.06	0.5

[a]Data from Otani et al., 2003; Jones et al., 2002a; Tanaka et al., 2002; Choi et al., 1997; and Jacobs et al., 2004.
[b]Numbers in parentheses are numbers of isolates

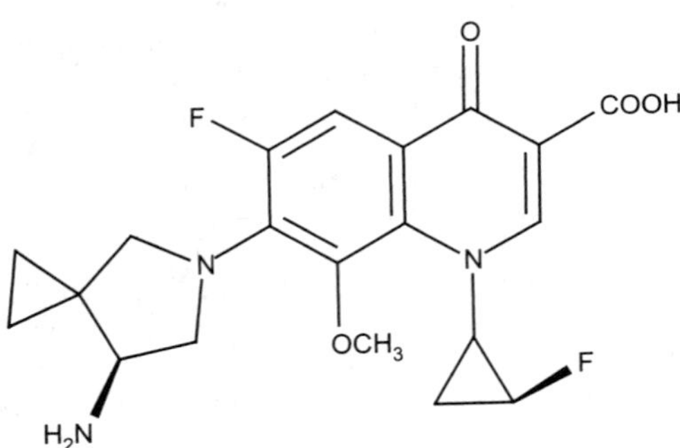

Figure 95 DK-507k

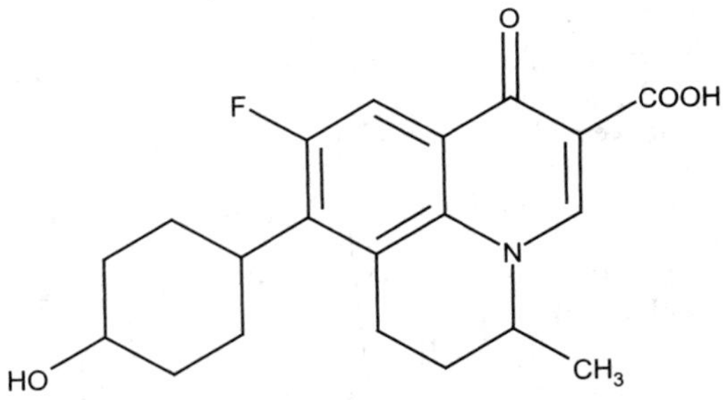

Figure 96 WCK 771

Some compounds with inhibitory activity are currently under development (Hackbarth et al., 2002). Their weakness, being pseudodipeptides, is that they are poorly metabolically stable.

Two deformylase gene homologs, *def*A and *def*B, were identified in *S. aureus*. Inhibitory activity of deformylase seems to be correlated with the *def*A gene; the function of *def*B is unknown (Margolis et al., 2000).

15.1. NVP-PDF713

NVP-PDF713 is a synthetic hydroxamic derivative (Hackbarth et al., 2002). Its MICs ranged from ≤0.06 to 4.0 μg/ml; however, for the vast majority of strains the MICs were between 0.25 and 2.0 μg/ml irrespective of their susceptibilities to oxacillin (Jones et al., 2004).

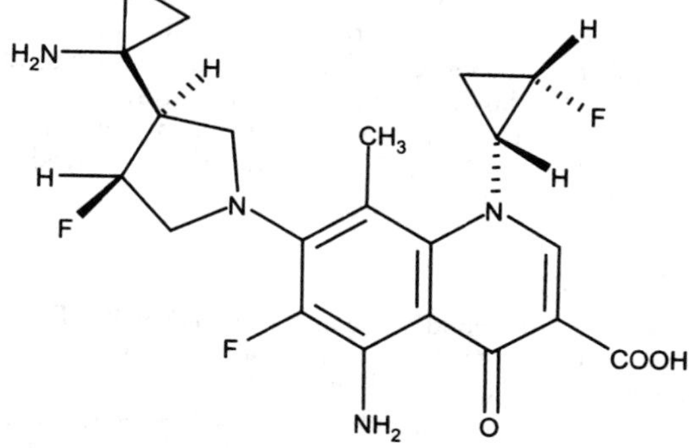

Figure 97 DQ-113

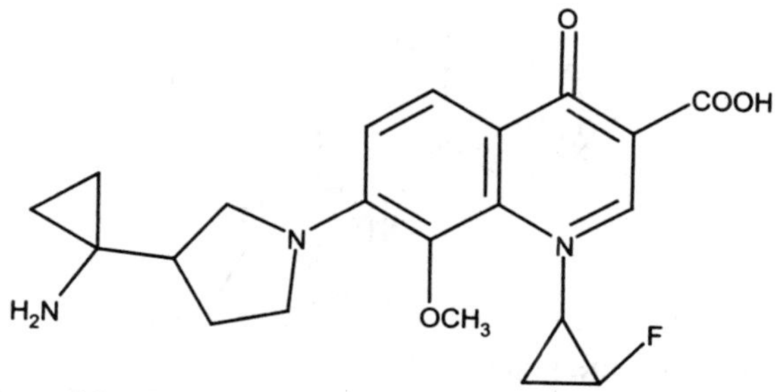

Figure 98 DX-619

Table 7 Enzymatic affinities of quinolones for topoisomerase IV and GrlA protein of *S. aureus*

Compound	IC_{50} (μg/ml)			
	Topoisomerase IV		GrlA	
	Wild type	Ser84→Leu	Wild type	Ser80→Phe
DX-619	0.8	7.81	0.309	1.76
Levofloxacin	9.41	>512	2.67	57.1
Ciprofloxacin	13.4	>256	1.24	22.4
Moxifloxacin	4.38	>512	1.36	24.2
Gatifloxacin	3.22	287	1.85	22.5

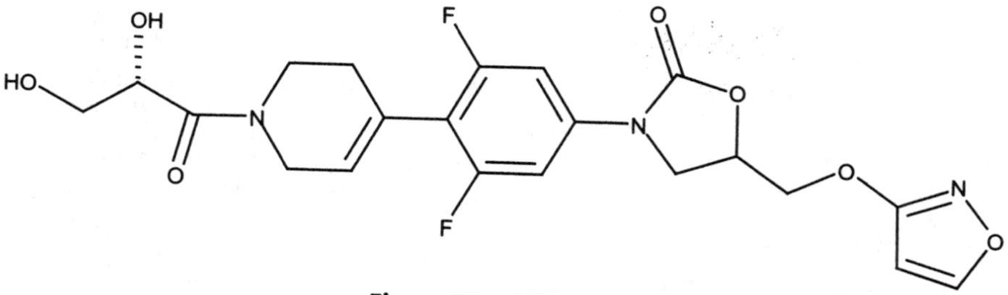

Figure 99 AZD 2563

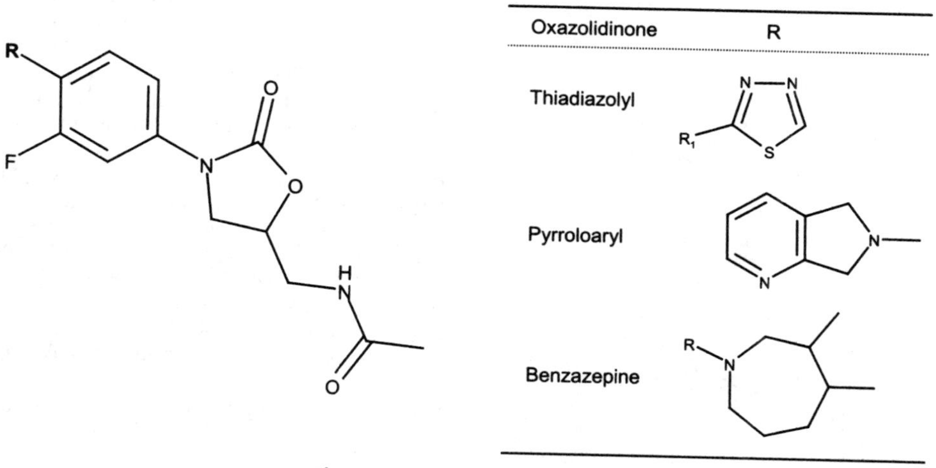

Oxazolidinone	R
Thiadiazolyl	
Pyrroloaryl	
Benzazepine	

Figure 100 Oxazolidinones

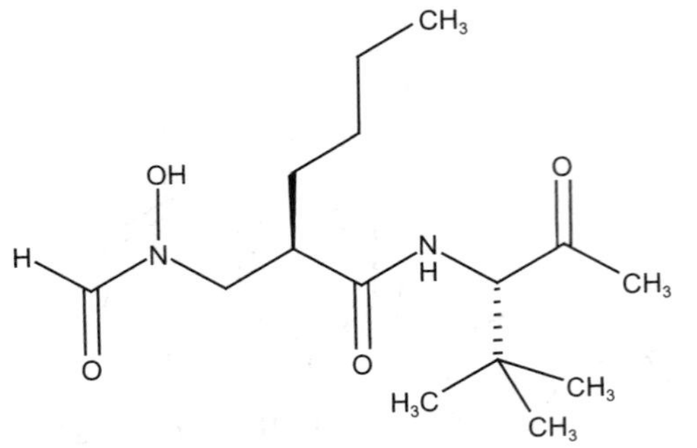

Figure 101 BB-83698

15.2. BB-83968

BB-83968 (Fig. 101) exhibited a MIC_{50} and MIC_{90} for MRSA and MSSA of 4.0 and 8.0 μg/ml, respectively (Lafland et al., 2004).

16. AMINOPEPTIDASE INHIBITORS

Methionine aminopeptidases play a pivotal role in protein biosynthesis. Methionine aminopeptidase is a metallo-enzyme, which cleaves in newly translated proteins, *N*-formyl methionine resulting in mature protein. These enzymes are divided into two classes, class I in eubacteria, mitochondria, and plastids and class II in eukaryotes and archaea.

A series of inhibitors as analogs of 5-aminomethyl-2-mercaptothiazoles (IC_{50}, 0.7 μM) was synthesized (Wademan et al., 2003) (Fig. 102).

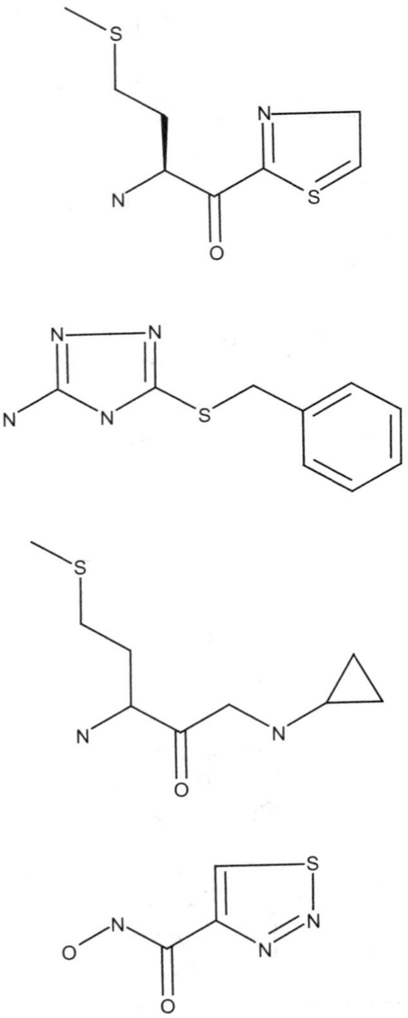

Figure 102 Methionine aminopeptidase inhibitors

REFERENCES

Akona-Koffi C, Guessennd N, Gbonon U, Faye-Ketté H, Dosso M, 2004, Methicillin-resistance of S. aureus in Abidjan (1998-2001), a new hospital problem, Med Mal Infect, 34, 132–136.

Alcavaz LE, Blanco SE, Puig ON, Thomas T, Ferretti FN, 2000, Antibacterial activity of flavonoids against methicillin-resistant S. aureus strain, J Theor Biol, 205, 231–240.

Alexander J, Binda DS, Glan JD, Holahan MA, Reyner MC, Rork GS, Sitko GR, Stanieri MT, Stupienski RF, Veerapanne H, Cook JJ, 1996, Investigation of (oxodioxolenyl) methyl carbamates as non chiral bioreversible prodrug moieties for chiral amines, J Med Chem, 39, 480–486.

Ali A, Aster SD, Graham DW, Patel GF, Taylor GE, Tolman RL, Painter RE, et al, 2001, Design and synthesis of novel antibacterial agents with inhibitory activity against DNA polymerase III, Bioorg Med Chem Lett, 11, 2185–2188.

Alvarez-Bravo J, Kurata S, Natori S, 1994, Novel synthetic antimicrobial peptides effective against methicillin-resistant S. aureus, Biochem J, 302, 535–538.

Anderegg TR, Biedenbach DJ, Jones RN, 2002, In vitro evaluation of AZD 2563, a novel oxazolidinone against 603 recent staphylococcal isolates, Antimicrob Agents Chemother, 46, 2662–2664.

Angehrn P, Buchmann S, Funk C, Goetschi E, Gmuender H, Hebeisen P, et al, 2004, New antibacterial agents derived from the DNA gyrase inhibitor cyclothialidine, J Med Chem, 47, 1487–1513.

Arvidson S, Tegmark K, 2001, Regulation of virulence determinants in S. aureus, Intern J Med Microb, 291, 159–170.

Ascher G, Heilmayer N, Hildebrandt J, Wieser J, 2003, Synthesis and SAR of novel cephalosporin-azomethines, broad spectrum antibacterial with anti-MRSA activity, 43rd Intersci Conf Antimicrob Agents Chemother, abstract F-543.

Bacqué C, Barrière JC, Berthaud N, Desmezeau F, Dutka-Mallens S, Dutuc-Rosset G, Ronan B, 2001, Design, synthesis, and in vitro evaluation of XRP 2868, a new oral streptogramin, 41st Intersci Conf Antimicrob Agents Chemother.

Banwell MG, Crasto CF, Easton CJ, Forrest AK, Karoli T, March DR, Mensah L, et al, 2000, Analogues of SB-203207 as inhibitors of tRNA synthetase, Bioorg Med Chem Lett, 10, 2263–2266.

Bardouniotis E, Thalakada R, Walsh N, Dorsey M, Schmid MB, Kaplan N, 2004, In vitro activities of novel bacterial enoyl-ACP reductase inhibitors, 44th Intersci Conf Antimicrob Agents Chemother, abstract F-316.

Barry AL, 1988, In vitro evaluation of DuP 105 and DuP 721, two new oxazolidinone antimicrobial agents, Antimicrob Agents Chemother, 32, 150–152.

Bartel S, Endermann R, Guarnieri W, Häbich D, Härber M, Kroll HP, Raddatz S, Rield B, Rosentreter U, Ruppel M, Stolle A, Wild H, 1998, Synthesis and antibacterial activity of novel hetero aryl oxazilidinones. I. Benzoxazone and benzothiazole oxazolidinones, 38th Intersci Conf Antimicrob Agents Chemother, abstract F-131.

Bemer P, Juvin ME, Bryskier A, Drugeon H, 2003, In vivo activities of a new lipopeptide HMR1043 against susceptible and resistant gram-positive isolates, Antimicrob Agents Chemother, 47, 3025–3029.

Berry V, Satterfield J, Singley C, Hunt E, Woodnutt G, 1999, In vivo efficacy of the novel topical pleuromutilins, SB-247386 and SB-268091, 39th Intersci Conf Antimicrob Agents Chemother, abstract 1804, p 337.

Blizzard TA, Kim RM, Morgan JD, Chang J, Kohler J, Kilburn R, Chapman K, Hammond ML, 2002, Antibacterial activity of G-6 quaternary ammonium derivatives of a lipophilic vancomycin analogue, Bioorg Med Chem Lett, 12, 849–852.

Border DB, Lease RA, Jarolmen H, Francis ND, Fantini AA, Falla T, Aumelas A, 2001, Laspartamycin—lipopeptide antibiotic with a unique peptide core, 41st Intersci Conf Antimicrob Agents Chemother, abstract F-1154.

Bozdogan B, Appelbaum PC, 2004, Activity of DX 619, a new quinolone against vancomycin non-susceptible staphylococci, 44th Intersci Conf Antimicrob Agents Chemother, abstract F-1940.

Bozdogan B, Esel D, Whitener C, Browne FA, Appelbaum PC, 2003, Antibacterial susceptibility of a vancomycin-resistant Staphylococcus aureus strain isolated at Hershey Medical Center, J Antimicrob Chemother, 52, 864–868.

Braun DK, Chien Y, Farlow DS, Phillips DS, Nasilewska MM, Zeckel M, 2001, Oritavancin (LY 333328), a dose escalating on safety and pharmacokinetic studies in patients, Eur Cong Chemother Microbiol Infect Dis Istambul, P 434.

Bremner JB, Coates JA, Coghlan DR, David DM, Keller PA, Pyne SG, 2002, The synthesis of a novel binaphthyl-based cyclicpeptoid with antibacterial activity, New J Chem, 26, 1549–1551.

Bryskier A, Aszodi J, Chantot J-F, 1994, Parenteral cephalosporin classification, Expert Opin Invest Drugs, 3, 145–171.

Bugg TD, Wright GD, Dutka-Mahlens S, Arthur M, Courvalin P, Walsh CT, 1991, Molecular basis for vancomycin resistance in Enterococcus faecium BM 4147, biosynthesis of a depsipeptide peptidoglycan precursor by vancomycin resistance protein Van H and Van A, Biochemistry, 30, 10408–10415.

Bürli R, Ge Y, White S, et al, 2002, DNA binding ligands with excellent antibiotic potency against drug-resistant gram-positive bacteria, Bioorg Med Chem Lett, 12, 2591–2594.

Bush K, Abbanat D, Davies T, Dudley M, Blais J, Hilliard J, Wira E, Queenan A, Foleno B, 2003, In vitro and in vivo antibacterial activity of RWJ 442831, a prodrug of the anti-MRSA cephalosporin RWJ 4428, 43rd Intersci Conf Antimicrob Agents Chemother, abstract F-548.

Calcul L, Longeon A, Al Mourabit A, Guyot M, Bourguet-Koudracki M-L, 2003, Novel alkaloids of the aaptamine class from an Indonesian marine sponge of the genus Xestospongia, Tetrahedron, 59, 6539–6544.

Chana S, Chapman S, Charles I, Cockerill S, Dolman M, Goulding E, Hawkins A, et al, 2001, Synthesis and SAR of novel inhibitors of the shikimate pathway enzyme dehydroquinate synthase, 41st Intersci Conf Antimicrob Agents Chemother, abstract F-1793.

Chen Z, White RE, Laughlin KJ, et al, 2000, Discovery of 3-dithiocarbamoylcephalosporins highly active in vitro against resistant gram-positive bacteria, 40th Intersci Conf Antimicrob Agents Chemother, abstract F-1068.

Cho A, Glinka TW, Ludnikow M, Fan AT, Wang M, Hecker SJ, 2001a, New anti-MRSA cephalosporins with a basic aminopyridine at the C-7 position, Bioorg Med Chem Lett, 11, 137–140.

Cho YR, Kim MJ, Joo HR, Kim HS, Youn H, 2001b, The in vitro activity of LB 11058, a new parenteral cephalosporin with activity against multi-resistant gram-positive bacteria, 41st Intersci Conf Antimicrob Agents Chemother, abstract F-330.

Choi KH, Hong JS, Kim SK, Lee DK, Yoon SJ, Choi EC, 1997, In vitro and in vivo activities of DW-116, a new fluoroquinolone, J Antimicrob Chemother, 39, 509–514.

Choudhry AE, Mandichak TL, Brosey JP, Egolf RW, Kingland C, Begley TP, Seefeld MA, Ku TW, Brown JR, Zulacain M, Rathman K, 2003, Inhibitors of pantothenate kinase, novel antibiotics for staphylococcal infections, Antimicrob Agents Chemother, 47, 2051–2055.

Clarke TE, Buzadzija K, Dorsey M, 2004, High resolution 3-dimension structural characterization of Staphylococcus enoyl-ACP-reductase ternary complex, 44th Intersci Conf Antimicrob Agents Chemother, abstract F-1527.

Clough J, Chen S, Gordon EM, Hackbarth C, Lam S, Trias J, White RJ, Candiani G, Donadio S, Romano G, Ciabatti R, Jacobs JW, 2003, Combinatiorial modification of natural products, synthesis and in vitro analysis of derivatives of triazolyl peptide antibiotic GE 2270 A, A-ring modifications, Bioorg Med Chem Lett, 13, 3409–3414.

Cordova SP, Heath CH, McGechie DB, Keil AD, Beers HY, Riley TV, 2004, Methicillin-resistant S. aureus bacteremia in Western Australia teaching hospital, 1997-1999: risk factors, outcomes and implications for management, J Hosp Infect, 56, 22–28.

Cosgrove SE, Sakoulas G, Perencevich EN, Schwaber MJ, Karchmer AW, Carmeli Y, 2003, Comparison of mortality associated with methicillin-resistant and methicillin-susceptible S. aureus bacteremia, a meta-analysis, Clin Infect Dis, 36, 53–59.

Cozzarelli NR, 1977, The mechanism of action of inhibitors of DNA synthesis, Annu Rev Biochem, 46, 641–668.

Critchley IA, Blosser-Middleton RS, Porter SP, Loutit JS, Jones ME, Thornsberry C, Karlowsky JA, Sahm DF, 2002, Activity of oritavancin against clinical isolates of S. aureus collected from blood specimen in the United States, 42nd Intersci Conf Antimicrob Agents Chemother, abstract E-1452.

Critchley IA, Stone K, Young C, Ochsner U, Guiles J, Tarasow T, Janjic N, 2004a, REP 8839, a novel methionyl tRNA synthetase inhibitor with potent activity against Staphylococcus aureus and Streptococcus pyogenes, 44th Intersci Conf Antimicrob Agents Chemother, abstract F-728.

Critchley IA, Young C, Stone K, Ochsner U, Dang C, Janjic N, 2004b, Spectrum of activity of REP 8839, a new antibiotic for topical use, 44th Intersci Conf Antimicrob Agents Chemother, abstract F-729.

Cutler BR, Cutler SJ, Josling PD, Wilson P, 2001, Activity of a novel, stable, allicin extract in liquid and cream formulations, against methicillin-resistant S. aureus including mupirocin-resistant MRSA, 41st Intersci Conf Antimicrob Agents Chemother, abstract 2279.

Davis MW, Buechter DD, Schimmel P, 1994, Functional dissection of a predicted class-defining motif in a class II tRNA synthetase of unknown structure, Biochemistry, 33, 9904–9911.

Deresinski S, 2005, Methicillin-resistant Staphylococcus aureus, an evolutionary, epidemiologic, and therapeutic odyssey, Clin Infect Dis, 40, 562–573.

Diekema MJ, Jones RN, 2001, Oxazolidinone antibiotics, Lancet, 358, 1975–1982.

Draghi DC, Thornsberry C, Jones ME, Flamm RK, Sahm DF, Karlowsky JA, 2003, In vitro activity of CB 181963 against 1064 gram-positive and gram-negative pathogens, 43rd Intersci Conf Antimicrob Agents Chemother, abstract F-544.

Dreier J, Ofner C, Stueber D, Danel F, Page MGP, 2001, Identifying new inhibitors of dihydropteroate synthase from S. aureus, 41th Intersci Conf Antimicrob Agents Chemother, abstract 1702.

Drugeon HB, Juvin ME, Couturier C, Bryskier A, 2002, Role of each component (RPR 202868 –PI) and RPR 132552 – PII in bactericidal synergism of XRP 2868 (a new oral semi synthetic streptogramin) against Streptococcus pneumoniae, H. influenzae and S. aureus, 42nd Intersci Conf Antimicrob Agents Chemother, abstract F-2116.

Dugourd D, Rubinchik E, Erfle DJ, Siu R, Fenn J, Patsetka C, Clement JJ, 2004, M-1396, a novel lipopeptide antimicrobial active against antibiotic resistant and sensitive gram-positive bacteria, 44th Intersci Conf Antimicrob Agents Chemother.

Dushin RG, Wang TZ, Fortier G, Tera S, Papamichelakir H, Richard L, Sellstedt J, Stahl S, 2002, Synthesis of A-98-6446, a semi-synthetic mannopeptimycin derivative, 42nd Intersci Conf Antimicrob Agents Chemother, abstract F-352.

Duvold T, Jorgensen A, Andersen NR, Henriksen AS, Sorensen MD, Björkling F, 2002, 17S,20S-Methanofusidic acid, a new potent fusidane antibiotic, Bioorg Med Chem Lett, 12, 3569–3572.

Eid CN, Nicas T, Mullen DL, Loncharich RJ, Paschal JW, 1997, Design, synthesis and potentiating activities against methicillin-resistant S. aureus of cyclic analogs of LY 301621, Bioorg Med Chem Lett, 7, 2087–2092.

Endersmann R, Bartel S, Guarnieri W, Häbich D, Härter M, Kroll HP, Raddatz S, Rield B, Rosentreter U, Ruppelt M, Stolle A, Wild H, 1998, Synthesis and antibacterial activity of novel hetero aryl oxazolidinones. III. Activities against clinically important gram-positive pathogens, 38th Intersci Conf Antimicrob Agents Chemother, abstract F-129.

Entenza JM, Hohl P, Heinze-Krauss I, Glauser MP, Moreillon P, 2002, BAL 9141, a novel extended-spectrum cephalosporin active against methicillin-resistant Staphylococcus aureus in treatment of experimental endocarditis, Antimicrob Agents Chemother, 46, 171–177.

Felmingham D, Robbin MJ, Schackcloth J, Denar C, Williams J, Bryskier A, 2004, Activity of XRP 2868 against S. pneumoniae, S. aureus, H. influenzae and 'atypical' respiratory tract pathogens, 44th Intersci Conf Antimicrob Agents Chemother.

Finn J, Hill J, Ram S, Morytko M, Yu X, Gimi R, Silverman J, Stem R, et al, 2001, Novel antibacterial agents targeting methionyl-tRNA synthetase, a cheminformatic approach to convert HTS data into quality medicinal chemistry load, 41st Intersci Conf Antimicrob Agents Chemother, abstract 2140.

Fritsche TR, Kirby J, Jones RN, 2004, Activity of tigecycline tested against 3498 Staphylococcus aureus: an assessment versus community-acquired ORSA, 44th Intersci Conf Antimicrob Agents Chemother, abstract C2-2000.

Fujimura T, Yamano Y, Yoshida I, Shimada J, Kuwahara S, 2003, In vitro activity of S-3578, a new broad-spectrum cephalosporin active against methicillin-resistant staphylococci, Antimicrob Agents Chemother, 47, 923–931.

Fukuoka T, Ohya S, Utsui Y, Domon H, Takenouchi T, Koga T, Masuda N, et al, 1997, In vitro and in vivo antibacterial activities of CS-834, a novel oral carbapenem, Antimicrob Agents Chemother, 41, 2652–2663.

Funabashi Y, Tsubotoni S, Koyama K, Katayama N, Harada S, 1993, A new anti-MRSA dipeptide TAN-1057 A, Tetrahedron, 49, 13–28.

Fung-Tomc JC, Clark J, Minassian B, Pucci M, Tsai YH, Gradelski E, Lamb L, Medina I, et al, 2002, In vitro and in vivo activities of a novel cephalosporin, BMS 247243, against methicillin-resistant and -susceptible staphylococci, Antimicrob Agents Chemother, 46, 971–976.

Furumai T, Eto K, Sasaki T, Higushi H, Onaka H, Saito N, Fujita T, Naoki N, Igarashi Y, 2002, TPU-0037 A, B, C and D, novel lydicamycin congeners with anti-MRSA activity from Streptomyces platensis TP A0598, J Antibiot, 55, 873–880.

Gales AC, Andrade SS, Sader HS, Jones RN, 2004, Activity of mupirocin and 14 additional antibiotics against staphylococci isolated from Latin American hospitals: report from the SENTRY antimicrobial surveillance program, J Chemother, 16, 323–328.

Ge Y, Touami S, Critchley I, Taylor M, Baird E, Bürli R, Pennell A, Moser H, 2001, Evaluating in vitro potency of GSQ 1530 a new class of antibiotic HARP, 41st Intersci Conf Antimicrob Agents Chemother, abstract 1687.

Ge Y, Wu J, Parekh B, White S, 2001, Mechanistic study of a novel class of antibiotic HARP, 41st Intersci Conf Antimicrob Agents Chemother, abstract 1686.

Glinka T, Huie K, Cho A, Ludwikow M, Blais J, Griffith D, Hoecker S, Dudley M, 2003, Relationships between structures, antibacterial activity, serum stability, pharmacokinetics and efficacy in 3-(heteroaryl thio) cephem: discovery of RWJ 333441 (MC 04546), Bioorg Med Chem, 11, 591–600.

Gravestock MB, Acton DG, Betts MJ, Dennis M, Hatter G, McGregor A, Swain ML, Wilson RG, Woods L, Wookey A, 2003, New classes of antibacterial oxazolidinones with C-5, methylene O-linked heterocyclic side chains, Bioorg Med Chem Lett, 13, 4179–4186.

Griffith DC, Hardford L, Williams R, Lee JL, Dudley MN, 2003, In vivo antibacterial activity of RWJ 54428, a new cephalosporin with activity against gram-positive bacteria, Antimicrob Agents Chemother, 47, 43–47.

Grinius L, Morris CM, Curnow AW, Hu EX, Canty JF, Mieling GE, Wallace CD, Zoutendam PH, Demuth TPJ, 2001, Identification and characterization of new signal peptidase inhibitors among 5S-penem, 41st Intersci Conf Antimicrob Agents Chemother, abstract 388.

Hackbarth CJ, Chen DZ, Lewis JG, Clark K, Mangold JB, et al, 2002, N-alkyl urea hydroxamic acid as a new class of peptide deformylase inhibitors with antibacterial activity, Antimicrob Agents Chemother, 46, 2752–2764.

Hadjivassileva T, Thurston DE, Taylor PW, 2004, Antibacterial activity of pyrrolobenzodiazepine dimers, a novel group of DNA-binding compounds, 44th Intersci Conf Antimicrob Agents Chemother, abstract 717.

Hanaki H, Akagi H, Masara Y, Otani T, Hyodo A, Hiramatsu K, 1995, TOC-39, a novel parenteral broad spectrum cephalosporin with excellent activity against methicillin-resistant Staphylococcus aureus, Antimicrob Agents Chemother, 39, 1120–1126.

Hanaki H, Nomura S, Akagi A, Hiramatsu K, 2001, Improvement of water-soluble cephalosporin derivatives having antibacterial activity against methicillin-resistant Staphylococcus aureus, Chemotherapy, 47, 170–176.

Hashizume H, Igarashi M, Hattori S, Hamada M, Takeuchi T, 2001, Tripropeptins, novel antimicrobial agents produced by Lysobacter sp. I. Taxonomy, isolation and biological activities, J Antibiot, 54, 1054–1059.

Hattori K, Yamada A, Kuroda S, Chiba T, Murata M, Sakane K, 2002, Synthesis and antibacterial evaluation of novel 2-[N-imidoyl pyrrolidinyl] carbapenem, Bioorg Med Chem Lett, 12, 383–386.

He X, McEtwee-Reeve A, Desai UR, Kellog GE, Reynolds KA, 2004a, 1,2-Dithiole-3-ones as potent inhibitor of the bacterial 3-ketoacyl carrier protein synthase II (FabH), Antimicrob Agents Chemother, 48, 3092–3102.

He Y, Yang J, Wu B, Risen L, Swayze EE, 2004b, Synthesis and biological evaluations of novel benzimidazoles as potential antibacterial agents, Bioorg Med Chem Lett, 14, 1217–1220.

Hebeisen P, Heinz-Krauss I, Anghern P, Hilh P, Page MGP, Then RL, 2001, In vitro and in vivo properties of Ro 63-9141, a novel broad spectrum cephalosporin with activity against methicillin-resistant Staphylococcus aureus, Antimicrob Agents Chemother, 45, 825–836.

Hecker SJ, Calkins T, Price ME, Huie K, Chen S, Glinka TW, Dudley MN, 2003, Prodrugs of cephalosporin RWJ 333341 (MC 04546) with improved aqueous solubility, Antimicrob Agents Chemother, 47, 2043–2046.

Heffron S, Jurnak F, 2000, Structure of EFTu complex with triazolyl peptide antibiotic determined at 2.35Å resolution: atomic basis for GE 2270 A inhibition of EFtu, Biochemistry, 39, 37–45.

Hibasami H, Midorikawa Y, Gasaluck P, Yoshimara H, Masuji A, Takaji S, Nakashima K, Imai M, 1991, Bactericidal effect of 15-deoxyspergualin on Staphylococcus aureus, Chemotherapy (Basel), 37, 202–205.

Hill J, Finn J, Lazarova T, Morytko M, Silverman J, Oliver N, Laganas V, Li TC, Keith D, 2001a, Novel lipopeptide. 3. Synthesis and biological activity of kynurenine modified analogs of daptomycin, 41st Intersci Conf Antimicrob Agents Chemother, abstract 1152.

Hill J, Finn J, Parr I, Silverman J, Oliver N, Laganas V, Li TC, Keith D, 2001b, Novel lipopeptide. 2. Synthesis and biological activity of aromatic amide analogs of daptomycin, 41st Intersci Conf Antimicrob Agents Chemother, abstract 1151.

Hill J, Finn J, Parr I, Yu X, Morytko M, Silverman J, Oliver N, Laganas V, Li TC, Keith D, 2001c, Novel lipopeptide. 1. Synthesis and biological activity of ornithine amino amide analogues of daptomycin, 41st Intersci Conf Antimicrob Agents Chemother, abstract 1150.

Hill J, Finn J, Yu X, Wang Z, Silverman J, Oliver N, Gallant P, Wendler P, Keith D, 2001d, Synthesis and activity of spirocyclic tetrahydrofurans as inhibitors of phenylalanine-tRNA synthase, 41st Intersci Conf Antimicrob Agents Chemother, abstract 1707.

Hill J, Siedlecki J, Parr I, Morytko M, Yu X, Zhang Y, Silverman J, et al, 2003, Synthesis and biological activity of N-acylated ornithine analogs of daptomycin, Bioorg Med Chem Lett, 13, 4187–4191.

Himmler T, Pirro F, Schmer N, 1998, Synthesis and antibacterial in vitro activity of novel analogues of nematophin, Bioorg Med Chem Lett, 8, 2045–2050.

Hiramatsu K, Hanaki H, Ito J, Yabata K, Oguri T, Tenover FC, 1997, Methicillin-resistant S. aureus clinical strain with reduced vancomycin susceptibility, J Antimicrob Chemother, 40, 135–136.

Hoemann MZ, Kumaravel G, Xie RL, Rossi RF, Meyer S, Sidhu A, Cuny GD, Hauske JR, 2000, Potent in vitro methicillin-resistant Staphylococcus aureus activity of 2-(1-H-indol-3-yl) quinoline derivative, Bioorg Med Chem Lett, 10, 2675–2678.

Hoemann MZ, Xie RL, Rossi RF, Meyer S, Sidhu A, Cuny GD, Hauske JR, 2002, Potent in vitro methicillin-resistant S. aureus activity of 2-(1-H-indol-3-yl) tetrahydroquinoline derivatives, Bioorg Med Chem Lett, 12, 129–132.

Hopmann C, Kurz M, Brönstrup M, Wink J, Le Beller D, 2002, Isolation and structure elucidation of vancoresmycin, a new antibiotic from Amycolatopsis ST 101170, Tetrahedron, 43, 435–438.

Howard JM, Moris CM, Grinius L, Renick PJ, Morris TW, Wallace CD, Koenigs PM, Li M, Neuman JF, 2001, Using membrane activity to determine the fate of signal peptidase inhibitors with antibacterial properties, 41st Intersci Conf Antimicrob Agents Chemother, abstract 1710.

Howe RA, Wootton M, Noel AR, Bowker KE, Walsh TR, MacGowan AP, 2003, Activity of AZD 2563, a novel oxazolidinone, against Staphylococcus aureus strains with reduced susceptibility to vancomycin and linezolid, Antimicrob Agents Chemother, 47, 3651–3652.

Hu W, Bürli RW, Kaizerman JA, Johnson KW, Gross MI, Iwamoto M, Jones P, Lofland D, Difuntorum S, Chen H, Bozdogan B, Appelbaum PC, Moser HE, 2004, DNA binding ligands with improved in vitro and in vivo potency against drug resistant Staphylococcus aureus, J Med Chem, 47, 4352–4355.

Hu Y, Helm JS, Chen L, Ye XY, Walker S, 2003, Ramoplanin inhibits bacterial transglycosylase by binding as a dimer to lipid II, J Am Chem Soc, 125, 8736–8737.

Ida T, Kurazono J, Nagura J, Sugano T, Takayama Y, Yoshida T, Takase Y, Takata H, Sasaki T, Komiya I, 2000, CP 5068, a new carbapenem, in vitro and in vivo activities against MRSA, 40th Intersci Conf Antimicrob Agents Chemother, abstract 1237.

Igarashi M, Tsuchida T, Kinoshita N, Kamijima M, Sawa R, Naganawa H, Hamada M, Takeuchi T, Yamaziki K, Ishizaka M, 1998, Cremimycin, a novel 19-membered lactam antibiotic from Streptomyces sp, J Antibiot, 51, 123–129.

Iinuma M, Tosa H, Tanaka T, Asai F, Kobayashi Y, Shimano R, Miyauchi K, 1996, Antibacterial activity of xanthones from guttiferaeous plants against methicillin-resistant S. aureus, J Pharm Pharmacol, 48, 861–865.

Inamura H, Ohtake N, Jona H, Shimizu Amoriya M, Sato H, Sugimoto Y, et al, 2001, Dicationic dithio carbamate carbapenems with anti-MRSA, Bioorg Med Chem Lett, 9, 1571–1578.

Ishida H, Fujikawa K, Chiba M, Tanaka M, Otani T, Sato K, 2004, DX 619, a novel des-F(6)-quinolone, mode of action against quinolone resistant MRSA, 44th Intersci Conf Antimicrob Agents Chemother, abstract F–1935.

Ishikawa T, Kamiyama K, Nakayama Y, Iizawa Y, Okonogi K, Miyake A, 2001a, Studies on anti-MRSA parenteral cephalosporins. III. Synthesis and antibacterial activity of 7β-[2-(5-amino-1,2,4-thiadiazol-3-yl)-2(Z)-alkoxyiminoacetamido]-3-[(E)-2(1-alkyl imidazo[1, 2,b](pyridazinium-6-yl)thiovinyl]-3-cephem-4-carboxylates and related compounds, J Antibiot, 54, 257–277.

Ishikawa T, Matsunaga N, Tawada H, Kuroda N, Nakayama Y, Ishibashi Y, Tomimoto M, Ikeda Y, Tagawa Y, Iizawa Y, Okonogi K, Hashiguchi S, Miyake A, 2003, TAK-599, a novel phosphono type prodrug of anti-MRSA cephalosporin T-91825, synthesis, physico-chemical and pharmacokinetic properties, Bioorg Med Chem Lett, 11, 2427–2437.

Ishikawa T, Nakayama Y, Tomimoto M, Niwa S, Kamiyama K, Hashiguchi S, Iizawa Y, Okonogi K, Miyake A, 2001b, Studies on anti-MRSA parenteral cephalosporins. IV. A novel water-soluble N-phosphono type prodrug for parenteral administration, J Antibiot, 54, 364–374.

Isnansetyo A, Kamei Y, 2003, MC21 A, a bactericidal antibiotic produced by a new marine bacterium, Pseudoalteromonas phenolica sp nov OBC 30 against methicillin-resistant S. aureus, Antimicrob Agents Chemother, 47, 480–488.

Jabes D, Candiani G, Romano G, Rivas S, Mafioli S, Cibiatti R, 2003a, Efficacy of VIC-603, a new anti-gram-positive antibiotic in experimental infection, 43rd Intersci Conf Antimicrob Agents Chemother, abstract 2113.

Jabes D, Romano G, Brunati C, Rossi R, Maffioli S, Ciabatti R, 2003b, In vitro characteristics of VIC-603, a new anti-gram-positive antibiotic, 43rd Intersci Conf Antimicrob Agents Chemother, abstract 2112.

Jacobs MR, Bajaksouzian S, Windau A, Appelbaum PC, Patel MV, Gupte SV, Bhagwat SS, De Souza Nj, Khorakiwala HF, 2004, In vitro activity of the new quinolone WCK 771 against staphylococci, Antimicrob Agents Chemother, 48, 3338–3342.

Jarraud S, Mougel C, Thioulouse J, et al, 2002, Relationships between S. aureus genetic background, virulence factors, agr groups (alleles), and human disease, Infect Immun, 70, 631–641.

Jarvest RL, Armstrong SA, Berge JM, Brown P, Elder JS, Brown MJ, et al, 2004, Definition of the heterocyclic pharmacophore of bacterial methionyl-tRNA synthase inhibitor, potent antibacterially active non-quinolone analogues, Bioorg Med Chem Lett, 14, 3937–3941.

Jarvest RL, Berge JM, Brown MJ, Brown P, Elder JS, Forrest AK, Houge-Frydrych CSV, O'Hanlon PJ, McNair DJ, Rittenhouse S, Sheppard RJ, 2003a, Optimisation of aryl substitution leading to potent methionyl-tRNA synthetase inhibitors with excellent gram-positive antibacterial activity, Bioorg Med Chem Lett, 13, 665–668.

Jarvest RL, Berge JM, Brown P, Houge-Frydrych CSV, O'Hanlon PJ, McNair DJ, Pope AJ, Rittenhouse S, 2003b, Conformational restriction of methionyl-tRNA synthetase inhibitors leading to analogues with potent inhibition and excellent gram-positive antibacterial activity, Bioorg Med Chem Lett, 13, 1265–1268.

Jarvest RL, Berge JM, Houge-Frydrych CSV, Jason C, Mensah LM, O'Hanlon PJ, Pope A, Saldanha A, Qiu X, 1999, Interaction of tyrosyl aryl dipeptide with S. aureus tyrosyl-tRNA synthetase, inhibition and crystal structure of a complex, Bioorg Med Chem Lett, 9, 2859–2862.

Jevitt LA, Smith AJ, Williams PP, Raney PM, McGowan JE Jr, Tenover F, 2003, In vitro activities of daptomycin, linezolid, and dalfopristin-quinupristin against a challenge panel of staphylococci and enterococci including vancomycin-intermediate S. aureus and vancomycin-resistant E. faecium, Microb Drug Res, 9, 389–393.

Jevons M, 1961, Celbenin resistant staphylococci, Br Med J, 1, 124–126.

Johnson AP, Warner M, Carter M, Livermoore DM, 2002, In vitro activity of a cephalosporin RWJ 54428 (MC 02479) against multidrug-resistant gram-positive cocci, Antimicrob Agents Chemother, 46, 321–326.

Johnson PD, Aristoff PA, Zurenko GE, Schaadt RD, Yagi BH, Ford CW, Hamel JC, Stapert D, Moerman JK, 2003, Synthesis and biological evaluation of benzazepine oxazolidinone antibacterials, Bioorg Med Chem Lett, 13, 4197–4200.

Jones ME, Klootwijk M, Schmitz FJ, Verhoef J, 2002a, Comparative activity of quinolone compounds moxifloxacin, grepafloxacin, trovafloxacin, levofloxacin, sparfloxacin, ofloxacin and oxazolidinone, linezolid against unrelated clinical isolates of ciprofloxacin-resistant and sensitive S. aureus, 42rd Intersci Conf Antimicrob Agents Chemother, abstract E-212.

Jones RD, Low DE, Pfaller MA, 1999, Epidemiological trends in nosocomial and community-acquired infections due to antibiotic-resistant gram-positive bacteria: the role of streptogramins and other new compounds, Diagn Microbiol Infect Dis, 33, 101–112.

Jones RN, Biedenbach DJ, Johnsen DM, Pfaller MA, 2001a, In vitro evaluation of BI 397, a novel glycopeptide antimibcrobial agent, J Chemother, 13, 244–254.

Jones RN, Despande LM, Mutnick AH, Biedenback DJ, 2002b, In vitro evaluation of BAL 9141, a novel parenteral cephalosporin against oxacillin-resistant staphylococci, J Antimicrob Chemother, 50, 915–922.

Jones RN, Fritsche TR, Sader HS, 2004, Antimicrobial spectrum and activity of NVP PDF 713, a novel peptide deformylase inhibitor, tested against 1837 recent gram-positive clinical isolates, Diagn Microbiol Infect Dis, 49, 63–65.

Jones RN, Hare RS, Sabatelli FJ, and the Ziracin Susceptibility Testing Group, 2001b, In vitro gram-positive antimicrobial activity of evernimicin (SCH 27899), a novel oligosaccharide, compared with other antimicrobials, a multicenter international trial, J Antimicrob Chemother, 47, 15–25.

Joo HY, Bu SC, Shin JE, Cho YR, Park D, Kim SH, Lee SH, Youn H, 2001, The in vivo efficacy and pharmacokinetics of LB 11058, a new parenteral cephalosporin in experimental animals, 41st Intersci Conf Antimicrob Agents Chemother, abstract F-331.

Judice JK, Pace JL, 2003, Semi synthetic glycopeptide antibacterials, Bioorg Med Chem Lett, 13, 4165–4168.

Kaatz GW, Moudgal VV, Seo SM, Hansen JB, Kristiansen JE, 2003, Phenylpiperidine selective serotonin reuptake inhibitors interfere with multidrug efflux pump activity in Staphylococcus aureus, Intern J Antimicrob Agents, 22, 254–261.

Kasai M, Hatano S, Kitagawa M, Yoshimi A, Nishimura K, Mori N, Sakai A, Sugihara T, 1999, AS-924, a novel orally active bifunctional prodrug of ceftizoxime, synthesis and relationship between physico-chemical properties and oral absorption, Chem Pharm Bull, 47, 1081–1088.

Katayama N, Fukusumi I, Funabashi Y, Iwahi T, Ono H, 1993, TAN 1057 A-D, new antibiotics with potent antibacterial activity against methicillin-resistant S. aureus: taxonomy, fermentation and biological activity, J Antibiot, 46, 606–613.

Kato A, Nakaya S, Kakubo N, Aiba Y, Ohashi Y, Hirata H, 1998, A new anti-MRSA antibiotic complex WAP-8294 A. I. Taxonomy, isolation and and biological activities, J Antibiot, 51, 929–935.

Kato A, Nakaya S, Suzuki N, Ohashi Y, Hirata H, Fujii K, Harada KI, 1997, WAP-8294 A, a novel anti-MRSA antibiotic produced by Lysobacter sp, J Am Chem Soc, 119, 6680–6681.

Kato N, Yoshida T, Nishino H, Yoshikawa Y, 2000, 2-Mercaptoquinoline derivative, Horikoriku Seyaky Patent JP 12302760.

Katz GW, Mougdal VV, Seo SM, 2002, Identification and characterization of a novel efflux-related multidrug resistance phenotype in Staphylococcus aureus, J Antimicrob Chemother, 50, 833–838.

Kavanagh F, Hervey A, Robbins WJ, 1951, Antibiotic substances from basidiomycetes. VIII. Pleurotus mutilus and Pleurotus passeckerianus Pilat, PNAS, 37, 570–574.

Kawazoe K, Tsubouchi Y, Abdullah N, Takaishi Y, Shibata H, Higati T, Hori H, Ogawa M, 2003, Sesquiterpenoids from Artemisia gilvescens, an anti-MRSA compound, J Nat Prod, 66, 538–539.

Kennedy G, Viziano M, Winders JA, Cavallini P, Gevi M, Micheli F, Rodegher P, Seneci P, Zumerle A, 2000, Studies on the novel anti-staphylococcal compound nematophin, Bioorg Med Chem Lett, 10, 1751–1754.

Kim RM, Kahne DE, Chapman KT, 2001, WO 0069-893, Chem Abstract 134, 5162.

Kim SJ, Cegelski L, Strudelska DR, O'Connor RD, Mehta AK, Schaefer J, 2002, The mode of action of vancomycin derivative LY 333328 characterized by redox, 42nd Intersci Conf Antimicrob Agents Chemother, abstract F-351.

Kruszenska D, Sahl H-G, Bierbaum G, Pag U, Hynes SO, Ljungh A, 2004, Mersacidin eradicates methicillin-resistant Staphylococcus aureus (MRSA) in a mouse rhinitis model, J Antimicrob Chemother, 54, 648–653.

Kubo I, Xiao P, Fujita K, 2002, Anti-MRSA activity of alkyl gallates, Bioorg Med Chem Lett, 12, 113–116.

Kumar V, Kenia J, Mukhopadyay T, Nadakarm SR, 1999, Methylsulfomycin I, a new cyclic peptide antibiotic from Streptomyces sp HIL-Y 9420704, J Nat Prod, 62, 1562–1564.

Kusnick C, Jansen R, Liberra K, Lindequist U, 2002, Ascochital, a new metabolite from the marine ascomycete Kirschsteiniothelia maritima, Pharmazie, 57, 510–512.

Lafland D, Di Funtorum S, Waller A, Clements JH, Weaver MK, Karlowsky JA, Johnson K, 2004, In vitro antibacterial activity of the peptide deformylase inhibitor BB-83968, J Antimicrob Chemother, 53, 664–666.

Laub J, Greenlee MC, DiNinno F, Hüber JL, Sundelof JG, 1999, The synthesis and anti-MRSA activity of amidinium-substituted 2-dibenzofuranoylcarbapenems, Bioorg Med Chem Lett, 9, 2973–2976.

Lambert A, 2002, Cellular impermeability and uptake of biocides and antibiotics in gram-positive bacteria and mycobacteria, J Appl Microbiol, 92, 46S–54S.

Lankas GR, Coleman JB, Klein HJ, Bailly Y, 1996, Species specificity of 2-aryl carbapenem-induced immunemediated hemolytic anemia in primates, Toxicology, 108, 207–215.

Lee JS, Cho YS, Chang MH, Koh HY, Chung BY, Pae AN, 2003, Synthesis and in vitro activity of novel isoxazolyl tetrahydropyridinyl oxazolidinone antibacterial agents, Bioorg Med Chem Lett, 13, 4117–4120.

Leighton A, Gottlieb AB, Dorr MP, Jakes D, Masconi G, Van Saders C, Mroszczak EJ, Campell KCM, Kelly E, 2004, Tolerability, pharmacokinetics and serum bactericidal activity of intravenous dalbavancin in healthy volunteers, Antimicrob Agents Chemother, 48, 940–945.

Lewis JG, Ategbu AE, Chen T, Kumar SA, Patel DV, Hacbarth CJ, Asano R, Wu C, Wang W, Yuan Z, Trias J, White RJ, Gordeev MF, 2004a, Novel antimicrobial 7-methyl lincosamine, prolamide analogs, 44th Intersci Conf Antimicrob Agents Chemother, abstract F-1388.

Lewis JG, Gu S, Kumar SA, Chen T, O'Dowd H, Patel DV, Blais J, Wu C, Wang W, Yuan Z, Trias J, White RJ, Gordeev MF, 2004b, Novel antimicrobial 7-methyl lincosamine, pipecolamide analogs, 44th Intersci Conf Antimicrob Agents Chemother, abstract F-1389.

Li J, Chen G, Webster JM, 1997a, Nematophin, a novel antimicrobial substance produced by Xenorhabdus nematophilus (Enterobacteriaceae), Can J Microbiol, 43, 770–773.

Li J, Chen G, Webster JM, 1997b, Synthesis and anti-staphylococcal activity of nematophin and its analogs, Bioorg Med Chem Lett, 7, 1379–1352.

Li MKW, Scheuer PJ, 1984, A guainolide pigment from a deep sea gorgonia, Tetrahedron Lett, 25, 2109–2110.

Liassine N, Auckenthaler R, Descombes MC, Bes M, Vandenesch T, Etienne J, 2004, Community-acquired methicillin-resistant Staphylococcus aureus isolated in Switzerland contains the Panton-Valentine leukocidin or exfoliative toxin genes, J Clin Microb, 42, 825–828.

Liehr S, Hansen E, Khorlin A, Roberts C, Keicher J, Zhang W, Nadherny J, et al, 2001, A new family of DNA targeting compounds have potent activity against vancomycin-resistant enterococci and methicillin-resistant S. aureus, 41st Intersci Conf Antimicrob Agents Chemother, abstract F-1699.

Limburg E, Beyer D, Gahlmann R, 2002, S. aureus resistance to TAN 1057 is mediated by modification of the bacterial ribosome, 42nd Intersci Conf Antimicrob Agents Chemother, abstract F-2032.

Locher HH, Specklin JL, Borner Y, Brohammer S, Schroeder S, Sigwalt C, Hubschwerlen C, 2002, Synthesis and antibacterial action of novel-quinolone-linked oxazolidinone, 42nd Intersci Conf Antimicrob Agents Chemother, abstract 1317.

Look FC, Vacin C, Dias TM, Ho S, Tran TN, Lee LL, Wiesner C, Fang F, et al, 2004, The discovery of baryl acids and amides exhibiting antibacterial activity against gram-positive bacteria, Bioorg Med Chem Lett, 14, 1423–1426.

Lübbers T, Angehrn P, Gmünder H, Herzig S, Kulhanek J, 2000, Design, synthesis and structure-activity relationship studies of ATP analogues as DNA gyrase inhibitors, Bioorg Med Chem Lett, 10, 821–826.

Manning DD, Xie D, Duong TN, Decornez HY, Dorsey M, Awrey DE, Kaplan N, Bardouniotis E, Clarke T, Berman J, Pauls H, 2004, Structure guided design, synthesis and in vitro characterization of aqueous soluble inhibitors of bacterial fatty acid biosynthesis, 44th Intersci Conf Antimicrob Agents Chemother, abstract F-318.

Margolis PS, Hackbarth CJ, Yong DC, Wang W, Chen D, Yuan Z, White R, Trias J, 2000, Peptide deformylase in Staphylococcus aureus, resistance to inhibition is mediated by mutations in the formyl transferase gene, Antimicrob Agents Chemother, 44, 1825–1831.

Matsumoto M, Tamaoka H, Ishigawa H, Kikuchi M, 1998, In vitro and in vivo antibacterial activity of OPC-20011, a novel parenteral broad spectrum 2-oxaisocephem antibiotic, Antimicrob Agents Chemother, 42, 2943–2949.

Matsumoto N, Momose T, Umekita M, Kinoshita N, Chino M, Iinumura H, Sawa T, Hawada M, Takeuchi T, 1999, Diperamycin, a new antimicrobial antibiotic produced by Streptomyces griseoaurantiacus MK 393AF2. I. Taxonomy, fermentation, isolation, physico-chemical properties and biological activities, J Antibiot, 51, 1087–1092.

Mazmanian SK, Thon-That H, Su K, Schneewind O, 2002, An iron-regulated sortase anchors a class surface proteins during S. aureus pathogenesis, PNAS, 99, 2293–2298.

McAtee JJ, Castle SL, Qing J, Boger DL, 2002, Synthesis and evaluation of vancomycin and vancomycin aglycone analogues that bear modifications in the residue 3 asparagine, Bioorg Med Chem Lett, 12, 1319–1322.

McNaught JG, 1906, On the action of cold and lukewarm tea on Bacillus typhosus, J Royal Army Med Corps, 7, 372–373.

Miller RA, Humphrey GR, Lieberman DR, Ceglia SS, Kennedy DJ, Grabowski EJJ, Reider PJ, 2000, A practical and efficient preparation of the releasable naphthosultam side-chain of a novel anti-MRSA carbapenem, J Org Chem, 65, 1399–1406.

Miura S, Iwasaki Y, Tatsuta K, 1994, Anti-MRSA activity of 1-(4-chlorophenyl)-3-dichlorophenyl and 3-trichlorophenyl-2-(1-H-imidazol-1-yl)-2-propen-1-one derivative, J Antibiot, 47, 1171–1172.

Moise PA, Schentag JJ, 2000, Vancomycin treatment failures in S. aureus lower respiratory tract infections, Intern J Antimicrob Agents, 16, suppl 1, S31–S34.

Moise-Brocker PA, Sakoulas G, Eliopoulos GM, Schentag J, Forrest A, Moellering RC Jr, 2004, Accessory gene regulation group II polymorphism in methicillin-resistant S. aureus is predictive of failure of vancomycin therapy, Clin Infect Dis, 38, 1700–1705.

Mu YQ, Nodwell M, Pace JL, Shaw JP, Judice JK, 2004, Vancomycin disulfide derivatives as antibacterial agents, Bioorg Med Chem Lett, 14, 735–738.

Mukhtar TA, Koteva K, Wright GD, 2005, Chimeric streptogramin-tyrocidine antibiotics that overcome streptogramin resistance, Chem Biol, 12, 229–235.

Murphy TM, Lenoy EP, Young M, Weiss WJ, 2002, In vivo efficacy and pharmacokinetics of AC-98-6446, a novel glycopeptide in experimental infections, 42nd Intersci Conf Antimicrob Agents Chemother, abstract F-356.

Musiki B, Perriers AM, Laurin P, Ferroud D, Benedetti X, Lachaud S, Chatreaux F, et al, 2000, Improved antibacterial activities of coumarin antibiotics bearing 5,5′-dialkyl noviose, biological activity of RU 79115, Bioorg Med Chem Lett, 10, 1695–1699.

Nagano R, Shibata K, Adachi Y, Imamura H, Hashizume T, Morishima H, 2000, In vitro activities of novel trans 3,5-disubstituted pyrrolidinylthio-1β methyl carbapenems with potent activities against methicillin-resistant S. aureus and P. aeruginosa, Antimicrob Agents Chemother, 44, 489–495.

Nagarajan R, et al, 1994, Glycopeptide Antibiotics, Marcel Dekker, New York.

Nagarajan R, Schabel AA, Occolowitz JL, Counter FT, Ott JL, Felty-Duckworth AM, 1989, Synthesis and antibacterial evaluation of N-alkyl vancomycin, J Antibiot, 42, 63–72.

Naidu BN, Sorenson ME, Hudyma T, Zheng X, Zhang Y, Bronson JJ, Pucci MJ, Clark JM, Ueda Y, 2004, Synthesis and antibacterial activity of O-substituted nocathiacin I derivatives, Bioorg Med Chem Lett, 14, 3743–3746.

Nicolaou KC, Roecker AJ, Barluenga S, Pfefferkorn JA, Cao CQ, 2001, Discovery of novel antibacterial agents active against methicillin-resistant S. aureus from combinatorial benzopyran libraries, Chem Biochem, 2, 460–465.

Nieuwlandt D, Kellogg E, Wecker M, Qui J, Wolk S, Tarasow T, Dewey T, Eaton B, 2001, Anti-MRSA drug leads from evolutionary chemistry, 41st Intersci Conf Antimicrob Agents Chemother, abstract F-2133.

Noble WC, Virani Z, Cree RG, 1992, Co-transfer of vancomycin and other resistance genes from Enterococcus faecalis NCTC 12201 to Staphylococcus aureus, FEMS Microb Lett, 72, 195–198.

Oh CH, Cho JH, Lee SC, 2003a, Synthesis and biological activities of 1β-methyl carbapenems having oxime and imine moieties, 43rd Intersci Conf Antimicrob Agents Chemother, abstract F-533.

Oh CH, Lee SC, Cho JH, 2003b, Synthesis and biological activity of 1-β-methyl-2-[5-(2N-substituted aminoethyl carbamoyl)pyrrolidin-3-ylthio] carbapenem, Eur Med Chem, 38, 841–850.

Ohtake N, Imamura N, Jona H, Kiyonaga H, Shimizu A, Moriya M, Sato H, Nakano M, Ushijima R, Nakagawa S, 1998, Novel dithio carbamate carbapenems with anti-MRSA activity, Bioorg Med Chem, 6, 1089–1101.

Oliva B, Miller K, Caggiano N, O'Neil AJ, Cuny GD, Hoemann MZ, Hauske JR, Chopra I, 2003, Biological properties of novel antistaphylococcal quinoline-indole agents, Antimicrob Agents Chemother, 47, 458–466.

Otani T, Tanaka M, Ito E, Kurosaka Y, Marakami Y, Onodera K, Akasaka T, Sato K, 2003, In vitro and in vivo antibacterial activity of DK-505k—a novel fluoroquinolone, Antimicrob Agents Chemother, 47, 3750–3759.

Pace JL, Krause K, Johnston D, Debabov D, Wu T, Farrington L, Lane C, Higgins DL, Christensen B, Judice K, Kaninga K, 2003, In vitro activity of TD-6424 against Staphylococcus aureus, Antimicrob Agents Chemother, 47, 3602–3604.

Paget SD, Foleno BD, Boggs CM, Goldschmidt RM, Hlasta DJ, Weidner MA, Werblood HM, Wira E, Bush K, Macielag M, 2003, Synthesis and antibacterial activity of pyrroloacyl-substituted oxazolidinones, Bioorg Med Chem Lett, 13, 4173–4177.

Panzone G, Ferrari P, Kurz M, Trani A, 1998, A novel glycopeptide carrying a 3-oxazolin-5-one ring obtained by intramolecular cyclization, J Antibiot, 51, 872–879.

Park C, Blais J, Lopez S, Gomez M, Rossi R, Candiani G, Jabes D, Kubo A, Maniar M, Margolis P, Hacbarth C, Lewis J, Gordeev M, White R, Trias J, 2004, VIC 105555, a new lincosamide with improved in vivo efficacy and good in vitro activity, 44th Intersci Conf Antimicrob Agents Chemother, abstract F-1392.

Pavlov AY, Miroshnikova OV, Printsevskaya SS, Olsufyeva EN, Preobrazhenskaya MN, Goldman RC, Branstrom AA, Baizman ER, Longley CB, 2001, Synthesis of hydrophobic N′-mono and N′, N″-double alkylated eremomycins inhibiting the transglycosylation stage of bacterial cell wall biosynthesis, J Antibiot, 54, 455–459.

Pavlov AY, Preobrazhenskaya MN, Malabarba A, Ciabatti R, Combo C, 1998, Mono and double modified teicoplanin aglycone derivatives on the amino acid 7 structure-activity relationships, J Antibiot, 51, 73–78.

Peters SE, Maskell DJ, Charles IG, Stabls JN, Powell KL, 2001, In vivo efficacy of inhibitors of the shikimate pathway enzyme dehydroquinate synthase, 41st Intersci Conf Antimicrob Agents Chemother, abstract F-1695.

Petersen PJ, Hartman HE, Wang TZ, Dushin RG, Bradford PA, 2002a, Time-kill kinetics and post-antibiotic effect of AC-98, novel semisynthetic cyclic glycopeptide antibiotic derivative AC-98-6446, 42nd Intersci Conf Antimicrob Agents Chemother, abstract F-354.

Petersen PJ, Jacobs NV, Weiss WJ, Sum PE, Testa RT, 1999, In vitro and in vivo antibacterial activity of a novel glycylcycline, the 9-t-butyl glycylamide derivative of minocycline (GAR-936), Antimicrob Agents Chemother, 43, 738–744.

Petersen PJ, Labthavikul P, Wang TZ, Dushin RC, Bradford PA, 2002b, In vitro comparative activity of A-98-6446, a novel semi-synthetic cyclic glycopeptide derivative of the natural product mannopeptimycin α (AC 98-1) and other antimicrobial agents against gram-positive clinical isolates, 42nd Intersci Conf Antimicrob Agents Chemother, abstract F-353.

Petersen PJ, Weiss WJ, Lenoy EB, He H, Testa RT, Bradford PA, 2002c, The in vitro activity of a novel cyclic glycopeptide natural product antibiotic AC-98 and comparative antibiotics, 42nd Intersci Conf Antimicrob Agents Chemother, abstract F-1148.

Preobrazhenskaya MN, Pavlov AY, Maffoli SI, Romano G, Ciabatti R, 2002, The synthesis and antibacterial activity of di-alkylated derivatives of glycopeptide DA-40926 and their amides, 42nd Intersci Conf Antimicrob Agents Chemother, abstract F-358.

Puar MS, Chan TM, Hegde V, Patel M, Bartner P, Ng KJ, Pramanik BN, MacFarlane RD, 1998, Sch 40832, a novel thiostrepton from Micromonospora carbonacea, J Antibiot, 51, 221–224.

Quarta C, Borghi A, Zerilli LF, De Pietro MT, Ferrari P, Trani A, Lancini GC, 1996, Isolation and structure determination of a novel complex of the teicoplanin family, J Antibiot, 49, 644–645.

Rammelkamp M, 1942, Resistance of Staphylococcus aureus to the action of penicillin, Proc R Soc Exp Biol Med, 51, 386–389.

Ratcliffe RW, Wilkening RR, Wildonger KJ, Waddell ST, Santorelli GM, Parker DL Jr, et al, 1999, Synthesis and properties of 2-(naphthosultamoyl) methyl carbapenems with potent anti-MRSA activity: discovery of L 786392, Bioorg Med Chem Lett, 9, 679–684.

Regueiro-Ren A, Naidu BN, Zheng X, Hudyma TW, Connolly TP, Matiskella JD, Zhang Y, Kim OK, Sorenson ME, Pucci M, Clark J, Bronson JJ, Ueda Y, 2004, Novel semi-synthetic nocathiacin antibiotics, synthesis and antibacterial activity of bis- and mono-O-alkylated derivatives, Bioorg Med Chem Lett, 14, 171–175.

Ried B, Endermann R, 1996, Recent development with oxazolidinone antibiotics, Exp Opin Ther Patents, 9, 625–633.

Rittenhouse S, Moore T, Donald B, Hunt E, Woodnutt G, 1999, In vitro activity of two novel pleuromutilin derivatives, SB-247386 and SB-268091, 39th Intersci Conf Antimicrob Agents Chemother, abstract 1805, p 337.

Robbins MJ, Shackcloth J, Dencer C, Williams L, Bryskier A, Felmingham D, 2004, Comparative in vitro activity of AVE 6971, a novel inhibitor of DNA topoisomerase IV against S. aureus, 34th Intersci Conf Antimicrob Agents Chemother.

Robbins MJ, Bryskier A, Felmingham D, 2005, Comparative in vitro activity of AVE 6971 and AVE 4221, novel inhibitors of DNA topoisomerase IV, against *Staphylococcus aureus*, 15th ECCMID, Copenhagen, abstract 1159.

Rybak MJ, 2001, Therapeutic options in gram-positive infections, J Hosp Infect, 49, suppl A, S25–S32.

Sakoulas G, Eliopoulos GM, Moellering RC Jr, et al, 2002, Accessory gene regulator (agr) locus in geographically diverse S. aureus isolates with reduced susceptibility to vancomycin, Antimicrob Agents Chemother, 46, 1492–1502.

Sasaki T, Igarashi Y, Saito N, Furumai T, 2001, TPU-0031 A and B, new antibiotics of the novobiocin group produced by Streptomyces sp TP-A0556, J Antibiot, 54, 441–447.

Sato Y, Oketani H, Yamada T, Sinyouchi KJ, Ohtsubo T, Kihara T, Shibata H, Huguchi T, 1997, A xanthanolide with potent antibacterial activity against methicillin-resistant S. aureus, J Pharm Pharmacol, 49, 1042–1044.

Schneider P, Hawser S, Islam K, 2003, Iclaprim, a novel diaminopyrimidine with potent activity on trimethoprim sensitive and resistant bacteria, Bioorg Med Chem Lett, 13, 4217–4221.

Seeman P, Day M, Russel AD, Ochs D, 2004, Susceptibility of capsular S. aureus to some antibiotics, triclosan and cationic biocides, J Antimicrob Chemother, 54, 696–697.

Seydi M, Sow AI, Soumaré M, Diallo HM, Hatim B, Tine R, Diop BM, Sow PS, 2004, S. aureus bacteremia in the Dakar Fann University hospital, Med Mal Infect, 34, 210–215.

Sharma P, Rane N, Gurram VK, 2004, Synthesis and QSAR studies of pyrimidino[4,5-d]pyrimidine-2,5-dione derivatives as potential antimicrobial agents, Bioorg Med Chem Lett, 14, 4185–4190.

Shin DY, Kim SN, Chae JH, Hyun SS, Seo SY, Lee YS, Lee KO, Kim SH, Lee YS, Jeong JM, Choi NS, Suh YG, 2004, Syntheses and anti-MRSA activities of the 3 analogs of mansonone F, a potent antibacterial sesquiterpenoid, insight into its structural requirements for anti-MRSA activity, Bioorg Med Chem Lett, 14, 4519–4523.

Shinagawa H, Yamaga H, Houchigai H, Sumita Y, Sunagawa M, 1997, Synthesis and biological properties of a new series of anti-MRSA β-lactams 2-(thiazol-2-ylthio)carbapenems, Bioorg Med Chem, 5, 607–621.

Shiota S, Shimizu M, Mizushima T, Ito M, Hatano T, Yoshida T, et al, 1999, Marked reduction in the minimum inhibitory concentration (MIC) of β-lactam in methicillin-resistant S. aureus produced by epicatechin gallate, an ingredient of green tea (Camellia sinensis), Biol Pharm Bull, 32, 1388–1390.

Shitara E, Yamamoto Y, Kano Y, et al, 2000, CP 5068, a new carbapenem, synthesis and structure activity relationships, 40th Intersci Conf Antimicrob Agents Chemother, abstract F-1236.

Sillerström E, Wahlund E, Nord CE, 1999, In vitro activity of LY 333328 against anaerobic gram-positive bacteria, J Chemother, 11, 90–92.

Sim NM, Ng SB, Buss AD, Crasla SC, Goh KL, Lee SK, 2002, Benzylidene rhodamine as novel inhibitors of UDP-N-acetyl muramic/L-alanine ligase, Bioorg Med Chem Lett, 12, 697–699.

Simon RJ, Curran WV, Leese RA, Borders DB, Koontz MZ, Liu H, 2001, Semisynthetic approaches of laspartomycin analogs, 41st Intersci Conf Antimicrob Agents Chemother, abstract F-1155.

Singh MP, Petersen PJ, Weiss WJ, Janso JE, Lucman SW, Lenoy EB, Bradford PA, Testa RT, Greenstein M, 2003a, Mannopeptimycins, new cyclic glycopeptide antibiotics produce by Streptomyces hygroscopicus LL-AC 98: antibacterial and mechanistic activities, Antimicrob Agents Chemother, 47, 62–69.

Singh MP, Petersen PJ, Weiss WJ, Kong F, Greenstein M, 2000, Saccharoamicins, novel heptadecaglycoside antibiotics produced by Saccharothrix espanaensis: antibacterial and mechanistic activities, Antimicrob Agents Chemother, 44, 2154–2159.

Singh U, Raju B, Lam S, Zhou J, Gadewood RC, Ford CW, Zurnnko GE, Schaadt RD, Morin SE, Adams WJ, Friis JM, et al, 2003b, New antibacterial tetrahydro-4 (2H)-thiopyran and thiomorpholine S-oxide and S,S-dioxide phenyloxazolidinones, Bioorg Med Chem Lett, 13, 4209–4212.

Snyder LB, Meng Z, Mate R, D'Andren SV, Marinier A, Quesnelle CA, Gill P, Denbleyker KL, Fung-Tomc JC, et al,

2004, Discovery of isoxazolinone antibacterial agents. Nitrogen as a replacement for the stereogenic center found in oxazolidinone antibacterials, Bioorg Med Chem Lett, 14, 4735–4739.

Sol V, Braland P, Chaleix V, Granet R, Guilloton M, Lamarche F, Verneuil B, Krausz P, 2004, Amino porphyrins as photo inhibitors of gram-positive and gram-negative bacteria, Bioorg Med Chem Lett, 14, 4207–4211.

Springer DM, Luh BY, Bronson JJ, 2001, Anti-MRSA cephems. Part I. C-3 substituted thiopyridinium derivatives, Bioorg Med Chem Lett, 11, 797–801.

Springer DM, Luh BY, Goodrich JT, Bronson JJ, 2003a, Anti-MRSA cephems. Part II. C-7 cinnamic acid derivatives, Bioorg Med Chem, 11, 265–279.

Springer DM, Luh BY, Goodrich JT, Bronson JJ, 2003b, Anti-MRSA cephems. Part III. Additional C-7 acid derivatives, Bioorg Med Chem, 11, 281–291.

Stables J, Chana S, Chapman S, Charles I, Cockerill S, Dolman M, Goulding E, et al, 2001, In vitro antimicrobial activity of dehydroquinate synthase inhibitors, 41st Intersci Conf Antimicrob Agents Chemother, abstract F-1694.

Stevens T, Johnson B, Johnson T, Bourchillon S, Hoban D, Gaylord C, McCarthy M, Dowazicky M, 2004, Tigecycline evaluation surveillance trial: in vitro antibacterial activity against methicillin-resistant and methicillin-susceptible Staphylococcus aureus isolates, 44th Intersci Conf Antimicrob Agents Chemother, abstract E-2061.

Stier MA, Watson BM, Domagala JM, Sanchez JP, Gracheck S, Joannides ET, Olson E, Shapiro MA, Amegadzie A, Micetich R, Singh R, Vo D, Vaiburg A, Wu K, 2000, The synthesis and SAR of a series of 2-hydroxyisoquinolones, new antibacterial gyrase inhibitors, 40th Intersci Conf Antimicrob Agents Chemother, abstract F-1503, p 209.

Suh YG, Shin DY, Min KH, Hyun SS, Jung JK, Seo SY, 2000, Facile construction of the oxaphenalene skeleton by peri ring closure: formal synthesis of mansonone F, Chem Commun, 1203–1204.

Sunagawa M, Yamaga H, Shinagawa E, Houchigai H, Sumita Y, 1994, Synthesis and biological properties of a new series of anti-MRSA β-lactams; 2-(thiazol-2-ylthio)carbapenems, Bioorg Med Chem Lett, 4, 2793–2798.

Tabart M, Picaut G, Desconclois JF, Dutka-Malens S, Huet Y, Berthaud N, 2001, Synthesis and biological evaluation of benzo[b]naphthyridones, a series of topical antibacterial agents, Bioorg Med Chem Lett, 11, 919–921.

Tabart M, Picaut G, Lavergne M, Wentzler G, Malleron JL, Dutka-Mallens S, Berthaud N, 2003, Benzo[b]naphthyridone, a new family of topical antibacterial agents active against methicillin-resistant gram-positive pathogens, Bioorg Med Chem Lett, 13, 1329–1331.

Tanaka H, Sato M, Oh-Uchi T, Yamaguchi R, Etoh H, Shimizu H, Sako M, Takeuchi H, 2004, Antibacterial properties of a new isoflavonoid from Erythrina poeppigiana against methicillin-resistant Staphylococcus aureus, Phytomed, 11, 331–337.

Tanaka M, Yamazaki E, Chiba M, Yoshihara K, Akasaka T, Takemura M, Sato K, 2002, In vitro antibacterial activities of DQ 113, a potent quinolone against clinical isolates, Antimicrob Agents Chemother, 46, 904–908.

Tanitame A, Oyamada Y, Ofuji K, Fujimoto M, Iwai N, Hiyama Y, Suzuki K, Ito H, Terauchi H, Kawasaki M, Nagai K, Wachi M, Yamagishi H, 2004a, Synthesis and antibacterial activity of a novel series of potent DNA gyrase inhibitors: pyrazole derivatives, J Med Chem, 47, 3693–3696.

Tanitame A, Oyamada Y, Ofuji K, Kyoya Y, Suzuki K, Ito H, Kawasa M, Nagai K, Wachi M, Yamagishi JI, 2004b, Design, synthesis and structure-activity relationship studies of novel indazole analogue as DNA gyrase inhibitor with gram-positive antibacterial activity, Bioorg Med Chem Lett, 14, 2857–2862.

Tarantino PM Jr, Zhi C, Wright GE, Brown NC, 1999, Inhibitors of DNA polymerase III as novel antimicrobial agents against gram-positive eubacteria, Antimicrob Agents Chemother, 43, 1982–1987.

Ternasky R, Draheim SE, Pika AJ, Bell FW, Wesh SJ, Jordan CL, Wu E, Preston D, Alborn WJ, Kasher JS, Hawkins FW, 1993, Discovery and structure-activity relationship of a series of 1-carba-1-dethiacephems exhibiting activity against methicillin-resistant Staphylococcus aureus, J Med Chem, 36, 1971–1976.

Thomasco LM, Gadwood RC, Weaver EA, Ochoada JM, Ford CW, Zurenko GE, Hamel JC, Stupert D, Moerman JK, Schaadt RD, Yagi BH, 2003, The synthesis and antibacterial activity of 1,3,4-thiadiazole phenyl oxazolidinone analogues, Bioorg Med Chem Lett, 13, 4193–4196.

Tiemersma EW, Bronzwier S, Lyytikäinen O, Degener JE, Schijnemakers P, Bruisma N, Monen J, Witte W, Grundmann H, 2004, Methicillin-resistant Staphylococcus aureus in Europe: 1999-2000, Emerg Infect Dis, 10, 1627–1634.

Tran TP, Ellsworth EL, Stier MA, Domagala JM, Showalter NDM, Gracheck SJ, Shapiro MA, Joannides TE, Singh R, 2004, Synthesis and structural activity relationships of 3-hydroxyquinazoline-2,4-dione antibacterial agents, Bioorg Med Chem Lett, 14, 4405–4409.

Tsujii N, Kamigauchi T, Kobayashi M, Terni Y, 1988 New glycopeptide antibiotics. II. The isolation and structures of chloroorienticins, J Antibiot, 41, 1506–1510.

Tsushima M, Iwamatsu JK, Tamura A, Shibahara S, 1998, Novel cephalosporin derivatives possessing a bicyclic heterocycle at the C-3 position. Part I. Synthesis and biological activities of 3-(benzothiazol-2-yl)thiocephalosporin derivatives, CP 0467 and related compounds, Bioorg Med Chem, 6, 1009–1017.

Van Bambecke F, Carryn S, Snock AS, Mingeot-Leclercq MP, Tulkens PM, 2001, LY 333328 (oritavancin) glycopeptide accumulates in cultured macrophages but only bacteriostatic towards intracellular Listeria monocytogenes, 41st Intersci Conf Antimicrob Agents Chemother, abstract E-450.

Vazifeh D, Abdelgafaffar H, Labro MT, 2002, Effect of telithromycin (HMR 3647) on polymorphonuclear neutrophil killing of S. aureus: comparison with roxithromycin, Antimicrob Agents Chemother, 46, 1364–1374.

Wademan SN, Almstetter M, Borer Y, Dalo GE, Douangamath A, D'Arcy A, Frutos-Hoener A, et al, 2003, Identification of potent inhibitors of the Staphylococcus aureus methionine aminopeptidase, 43rd Intersci Conf Antimicrob Agents Chemother, abstract F-332.

Wang J, Li J, Czyryca PG, Chang H, Kao J, Chang CWT, 2004, Synthesis of an unusual branched-chain sugar, 5-C-methyl-L-idopyranose for SAR studies of pyranmycins: implication for the future design of aminoglycoside antibiotics, Bioorg Med Chem Lett, 14, 4389–4393.

Williams KM, Yuan C, Lee VJ, Chamberland S, 1998, Synthesis and antimicrobial evaluation of TAN 1057 A analogs, J Antibiot, 51, 189–201.

Wisplinghoff H, Bischoff T, Tallet SM, Seifert H, Wenzel RP, Edmond MB, 2004, Nosocomial bloodstream infections in US hospitals, analysis of 24179 cases from a prospective nationwide surveillance study, Clin Infect Dis, 39, 309–317.

Wright GE, Brown NC, 1977, Inhibitors of Bacillus subtilis DNA polymerase. II. Structure activity relationships of 6-(phenylhydrazino) uracils, J Med Chem, 20, 1181–1185.

Wright GE, Gambino JJ, 1984, Quantitative structure-activity relationship of 6-anilinouracils, inhibitors of Bacillus subtilis DNA polymerase III, J Med Chem, 27, 181–185.

Yam TS, Shah S, Hamilton-Miller JMI, 1997, Microbiological activity of whole and fractionated crude extracts of tea (Camellia sinensis) and of tea components, FEMS Microbiol Lett, 152, 169–171.

Yao S, Sgarbi PWM, Masby KA, Rabuka D, O'Hare SM, et al, 2004, Glyco-optimization of aminoglycosides, new aminoglycosides as novel anti-infective agents, Bioorg Med Chem Lett, 14, 3733–3738.

Yoshida O, Yasukata T, Sumino Y, Manekage T, Narukawa Y, Nishitani Y, 2002, Novel semisynthetic glycopeptide antibiotics active against methicillin-resistant S. aureus and vancomycin-resistant enterococci, doubly-modified water-soluble derivative of chloroorienticin, Bioorg Med Chem Lett, 12, 3027–3031.

Yoshizawa H, Itani H, Ishikura K, Iric T, Yokoo K, Kubota T, Minami K, Iwaki T, Miwa H, Nishitami Y, 2002, S-3578, a new broad spectrum parenteral cephalosporin exhibiting potent activity against both methicillin-resistant S. aureus and P. aeruginosa: synthesis and structure activity relationships, J Antibiot, 55, 975–992.

Yu XY, Finn J, Hill JM, Wang ZG, Keith D, Silverman J, Oliver N, 2004a, A series of spirocyclic analogues as potent inhibitors of bacterial phenyl alanyl-tRNA synthetases, Bioorg Med Chem Lett, 14, 1339–1342.

Yu XY, Finn J, Hill JM, Wang ZG, Keith D, Silverman J, Oliver N, 2004b, A series of heterocyclic inhibitors of phenyl alanyl-tRNA synthetases with antibacterial activity, Bioorg Med Chem Lett, 14, 1343–1346.

Zeckel ML, Preston DA, Allen BS, 2000, In vitro activity of LY 333328 and comparative agents against nosocomial gram-positive pathogens collected in 1997: global surveillance study, Antimicrob Agents Chemother, 44, 1370–1374.

Mutilins

A. BRYSKIER

50

Pleuromutilin was discovered in 1951 from the basidiomycete *Pleurotus mutilus*, renamed *Clitopilus scyphoides*.

Some mutilins, such as tiamulin and valnemulin, were introduced into veterinary medicine for the treatment of swine infections with *Brachyspira hyodysenteriae* (diarrhea) and *Mycoplasma hyopneumoniae* (pneumonia).

In order to circumvent the issue of bacterial resistance, one approach is to reinvestigate those antibacterials known which have had so far little or no utility in human medicine.

1. STRUCTURE

Mutilins are semisynthetic derivatives having a tricyclic diterpenoid structure. They differ in their side chains (Fig. 1).

It was shown that the C-14 side chain is essential for antibacterial activity. The tricyclic diol mutilin did not inhibit protein synthesis.

Some carbamate analogs are extremely active, with MICs of 0.06, ≤0.06, 1.0, and ≤0.06 μg/ml for *Staphylococcus aureus* (methicillin resistant and susceptible), *Streptococcus pneumoniae*, *Haemophilus influenzae*, and *Moraxella catarrhalis*, respectively.

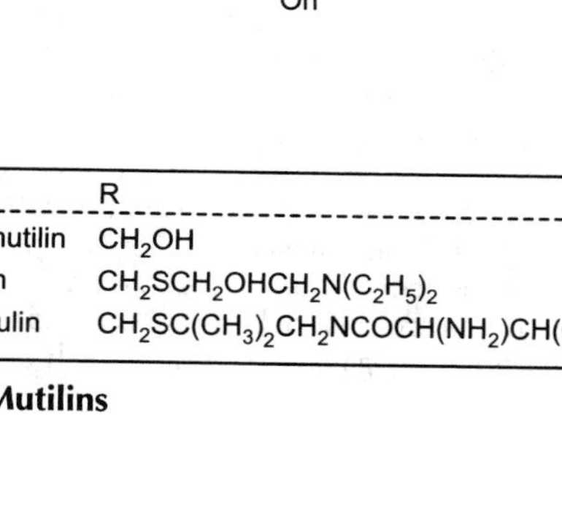

	R
Pleuromutilin	CH_2OH
Tiamulin	$CH_2SCH_2OHCH_2N(C_2H_5)_2$
Valnemulin	$CH_2SC(CH_3)_2CH_2NCOCH(NH_2)CH(CH_3)_2$

Figure 1 Mutilins

Tiamulin is a lipophilic, weak organic base with a pK_a of 7.6, for a molecular weight of 493.76 and a melting point of 147 to 148°C.

Tiamulin is a potent inducer-inhibitor of cytochrome P450 activity in the liver.

2. ANTIBACTERIAL ACTIVITY

Pleuromutilins are mainly active against gram-positive bacteria and display moderate activity against fastidious gram-negative bacilli (Table 1).

Tiamulin MICs of >32, 4.0, and 0.06 to 0.5 μg/ml are observed for *Bordetella bronchiseptica*, *Leptospira* spp., and *Mycoplasma* spp., respectively. Organisms for which the MICs are ≤4.0 μg/ml are considered susceptible, those for which the MICs are 8 to 16 μg/ml are considered moderately susceptible, and those for which the MICs are ≥32 μg/ml are considered resistant.

3. MODE OF ACTION

Tiamulin inhibits protein synthesis. It binds to domain V of 23S rRNA of the 50S ribosomal subunit.

Tiamulin and valnemulin interact with adenines 2058 and 2059 and uracils 2506, 2584, and 2585. They prevent the correct positioning of the CCA end of tRNA for peptide transfer. Tiamulin inhibits peptidyltransferase, thus inhibiting peptide bond formation. They bond to site A of peptidyltransferase centers.

4. MECHANISM OF RESISTANCE

Tiamulin resistance develops relatively slowly and in a stepwise fashion in vitro.

Protein L3 has a globular domain on the ribosome surface plus an extended domain that stretches into the ribosome interior. Protein L3 is one of the four proteins that come closest to the site of peptide bond formation through its extended domain.

It was shown that a point mutation, A445G, in protein L3 may be responsible for resistance (Asn149 → Asp).

Trp242 is located at the top of the extended domain and represents the position on protein L3 that comes closest to the catalytic center. The distance between the α-carbon of Arg144 and the phosphorus atom of nucleotide U2506 is

Table 1 In vitro activities of mutilins

Compound	MIC (μg/ml)[a]				
	MSSA	MRSA	*S. pneumoniae* Ery[r]	*H. influenzae*	*M. catarrhalis*
Pleuromutilin	0.5	0.25	2.0	1.0	0.25
Tiamulin	0.25	0.125	0.125	8.0	≤0.06
TDM 85530	0.25	0.125	0.25	4.0	0.125

[a]MSSA and MRSA, methicillin-susceptible and -resistant *S. aureus*, respectively.

approximately 10 Å. Alteration of ribosomal protein L3 at the relevant amino acid also affects the action of trichothecenes, another class of antibiotics.

Mutation Trp255 → Cys causes resistance in *Saccharomyces cerevisiae*.

5. TDM 85530

TDM 85530 (Fig. 2) is a semisynthetic compound.

5.1. Antibacterial Activity

This compound is mainly active against gram-positive bacteria (Table 2).

5.2. Pharmacokinetics

The pharmacokinetics after single oral ascending doses are listed in Table 3.

TDM 85530 is extensively metabolized:

- N-glucuronidation
- Cleavage of the S-aminotriazole bond, resulting in degradation of the side chain at C-14 to the methylsulfone via methylation
- Hydroxylation at positions 2 and 8 in which the 2β and 8α configurations seem to be preferred over the 2α and 8β configuration

6. SB 247386

A new series of semisynthetic pleuromutilins was presented and one compound was selected for further preclinical investigation, SB264128.

Two previous derivatives were explored in 1999, SB 268001 (Fig. 3) and SB 247386 (Fig. 4). SB-264128 was selected for the treatment of respiratory tract infections.

For *S. pneumoniae* isolates irrespective of their susceptibilities to penicillin G, the MIC at which 50% of isolates tested are inhibited (MIC_{50}) and MIC_{90} are 0.12 and 0.25 μg/ml. SB 264128 retains activity against *S. pneumoniae* isolates for which azithromycin MICs are above 1.0 μg/ml. SB 264128 exhibited good activity against *H. influenzae* irrespective of ampicillin resistance, with a MIC_{50} and MIC_{90} of 0.25 and 0.25 μg/ml. SB 264128 showed higher activity against *M. catarrhalis*, with a MIC_{50} and MIC_{90} of 0.03 and 0.06 μg/ml.

Respiratory infections were initiated via intratracheal inoculation (inoculum size of approximately 6.0 $\log_{10}$ CFU) in rats (100 g) with *S. pneumoniae* 1629 or *H. influenzae* H 128 (β-lactamase-producing strains). SB 264128 (50 mg/kg of body weight) and co-amoxiclav (50 and 25 mg/kg) were administered orally by gavage 1, 5, and 24 h after bacterial challenge.

Table 2 In vitro activity of TDM 85530

Microorganism	*n*	MIC (μg/ml)	
		50%	90%
S. aureus	32	0.5	1.0
Staphylococcus saprophyticus	12	2.0	4.0
S. pyogenes	30	0.12	0.12
Streptococcus agalactiae	30	0.25	0.25
Group C streptococci	14	0.25	0.25
Group G streptococci	28	0.5	4.0
Viridans group streptococci	42	4.0	128
S. pneumoniae	25	0.5	2.0
Bacillus cereus	31	64	64
Listeria monocytogenes	23	64	64
Corynebacterium spp.	6	0.06	
Corynebacterium jeikeium	17	1.0	8.0
M. catarralis	11	0.12	16
Neisseria meningitidis	13	0.5	2.0
Neisseria gonorrhoeae	56	0.25	1.0
Eikenella corrodens	15	16	32
Legionella pneumophila	10	0.5	1.0
Bordetella pertussis	6	<0.01	
Gardnerella vaginalis	16	0.03	2.0
Pasteurella multocida	12	8.0	32
Campylobacter jejuni	13	8.0	64
H. influenzae	37	1.0	2.0
Bacteroides fragilis	8	16	
Bacteroides thetaiotaomicron	8	>128	
Bacteroides distasonis	3	32	
Bacteroides bivia	10	0.25	0.5
Prevotella melaninogenica	16	0.125	0.25
Fusobacterium spp.	2	1–8	
Veillonella parvula	3	8	
Peptostreptococcus	17	0.125	1.0
Eubacterium	3	2	
Propionibacterium spp.	3	0.125	
Clostridium spp.	11	4	16

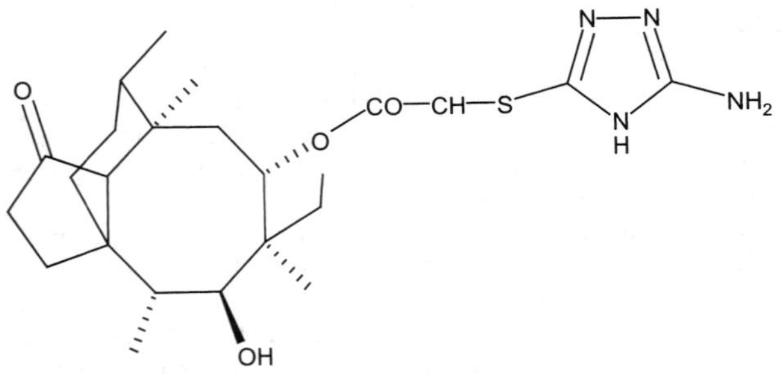

Figure 2 TDM 85530

Table 3 Pharmacokinetics of TDM 85530

Dose (mg)	C_{max} (μg/ml)	T_{max} (h)	$t_{1/2}$ (h)	$AUC_{0-\infty}$ (μg·h/ml)
250	1.88	1.35	1.29	5.22
350	2.84	1.39	2.01	10.7
500	3.90	1.27	2.64	16.8

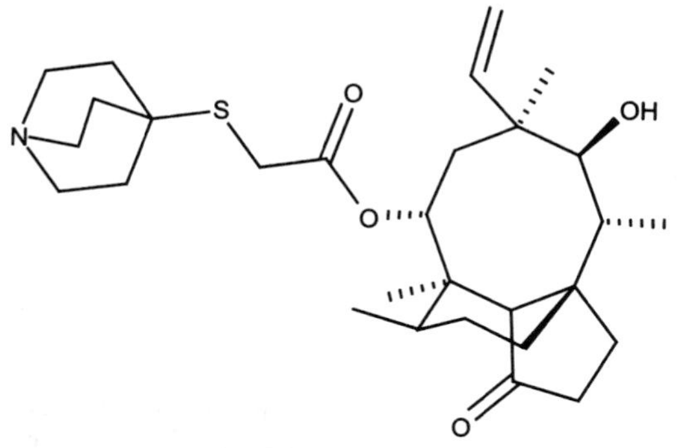

Figure 3 SB 268001

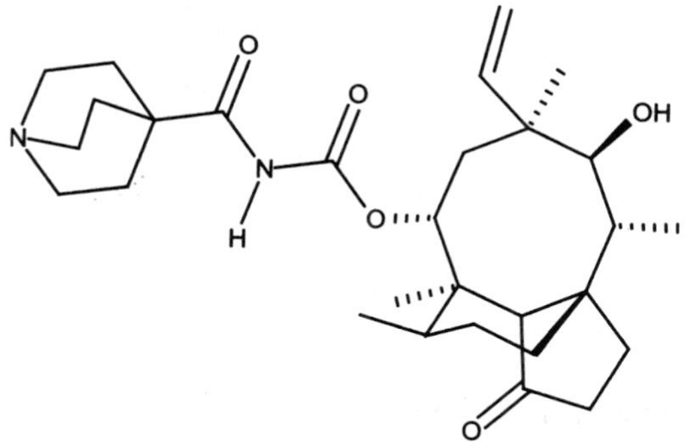

Figure 4 SB 247386

In pneumococcal infections, the burden reduction obtained with SB 264128 was significant (2.7 ± 1.0 $\log_{10}$ CFU/lung [mean ± standard deviation]). In *H. influenzae* H 128 infection, bacterial counts in untreated rats were 5.3 ± 0.7 $\log_{10}$ CFU/lung. SB 264128 exhibited a higher clearing activity (1.8 ± 0.2 $\log_{10}$ CFU/lung) than co-amoxiclav (3.5 ± 1.2 $\log_{10}$ CFU/lung).

ADDITIONAL REFERENCES

Bosling J, Poulsen SM, Vesten B, Long KS, 2003, Resistance to the peptidyl transferase inhibitor tiamulin caused by mutation of ribosomal protein L3, Antimicrob Agents Chemother, 47, 2892–2896.

Brook G, Burgess W, Colthurst D, Hinks JD, Hunt E, Pearson MJ, She B, Takle AK, Wilson JM, Woodnutt G, 2001, Pleuromutilins. Part 1.The identification of novel mutilin 14-carbamates, Bioorg Med Chem, 9, 1221–1231.

Kavanagh F, Hervey H, Robbins WJ, 1951, Antibiotic substances from Basidiomycetes. VIII. Pleurotus multilus Passecketianus Pilat, Proc Natl Acad Sci USA, 37, 570–574.

Poulsen SM, Karlson M, Johanson B, Vester B, 2001, The pleuromutilin drugs tiamulin and valnemulin bind to the RNA at the peptidyl transferase centre on the ribosome, Mol Microbiol, 41, 1091–1099.

Rittenhouse S, Moore T, Donald B., Hunt E, Woodnutt G, 1999, In vitro activity of two novel pleuromutilin derivatives, SB-247386 and SB-268091, 39th Intersci Conf Antimicrob Agents Chemother, abstract 1805, p 337.

Schlünzen F, Pyetan E, Fucini P, Yonath A, Harms JM, 2004, Inhibition of peptide bond formation by pleuromutilins, the structure of the 50S ribosomal subunit from Deinococcus radiodurans in complex with tiamulin, Mol Microbiol, 54, 1287–1294.

Springer DM, Sorensen ME, Huang S, Connolly TP, Bronson JJ, Matson JA, Hanson RL, Brzozowski DB, La Porte TL, Patel RN, 2003, Synthesis and activity of a C-8 keto pleuromutilin derivative, Bioorg Med Chem Lett, 13, 1751–1753.

In Pursuit of New Antibiotics

ANDRÉ BRYSKIER

51

1. INTRODUCTION

The question which currently faces us is whether we need new antibacterial agents. The answer is not straightforward. Bacteria that are totally resistant to all available antibacterial agents are still uncommon. However, on the basis of the growth curves of bacterial resistance, the problem of increasing numbers of multiresistant clinical strains will emerge in about 10 years' time, reaching a plateau to a greater or lesser extent in the majority of cases and rendering first-line treatment with one or more antibiotics ineffective.

As regards this last category of bacterial strains, an intensive search for new compounds for therapeutic use must be instituted rapidly to enable us to meet this challenge by 2010 to 2015. This requires the promotion of a number of different approaches in search of an appropriate response to this new threat so as to try to prevent bacterial agents from adapting too rapidly from the outset.

This observation raises a number of questions: what will be the bacterial problems of the future, and how can they be identified or how can a solution be provided, and what are the currently unresolved bacterial problems (for example, methicillin-resistant staphylococcal strains)?

1.1. Identification

The identification of future problems is very complex and involves both the assessment of bacterial sensitivity through epidemiological studies using standardized methods and the propensity of these bacteria to multiply, to retain their potential for virulence (cost to the bacterium), and, above all, to spread in the ecosystem.

1.2. Exploratory Approaches

There are a number of exploratory approaches, and some have already borne fruit.

The oldest approach is the screening of microorganism metabolites and of plant, mammal, amphibian, and insect defense proteins.

In this respect, mention may be made of defensins, which derive from the endolymph of insects, plants, and the skin coating of amphibians. Some of these have been modified chemically and are in the process of evaluation. The majority are intended initially for topical use because of their chemical instability in the body and the as-yet-unresolved difficulties of parenteral administration. This is the case with magainins, protegrins, etc.

Controlled fermentation is also one of the approaches for obtaining more active derivatives and for exploring the potential of certain microorganisms better.

The second approach, which appears to be more conventional, is the chemical modification of known molecular entities.

The third approach is the search for new targets and new compounds by means of genomics and proteomics, which as yet have not yielded any new anti-infective compounds.

1.3. Objectives of This Research

The philosophy of research in antibiotic therapy underwent a major reappraisal in the 1980s.

1.3.1. First Period

Before that time, the first stage, following the work in New York by the Frenchman Roger Dubos in 1939 on tyrocidine and covering a period of almost 20 years, was the discovery of new therapeutic entities that provided a resolution to the age-old problems of certain infections, such as typhoid fever (chloramphenicol), tuberculosis (streptomycin, isoniazid, and rifampin), and other nightmares confronting humanity. The second stage, from the 1960s onwards, was totally different, and while in principle the study of fermentation products persisted, it proved less cost-effective in terms of new medications, although not in the quantity of new molecular entities.

1.3.2. Second Period

The nature of this research changed tack and was obliged to respond to various problems and demands from the medical profession and consumers:

- To find chemical modifications by which to circumvent bacterial resistance, which gave rise to cephalosporins with an extended spectrum and antibacterial activity
- To meet the pharmacokinetic requirements of good oral absorption of existing antibiotics such as penicillin G, which gave rise to penicillin V, or erythromycin, which resulted in the semisynthesis of 14- and 15-membered-ring macrolides such as roxithromycin, clarithromycin, and azithromycin. Less obvious is the improvement in the administration regimens and daily dosages, irrespective of the patient's physiological status, which has only partially been achieved with cefotaxime. The absence of metabolites has been a line of research designed to obtain chemically

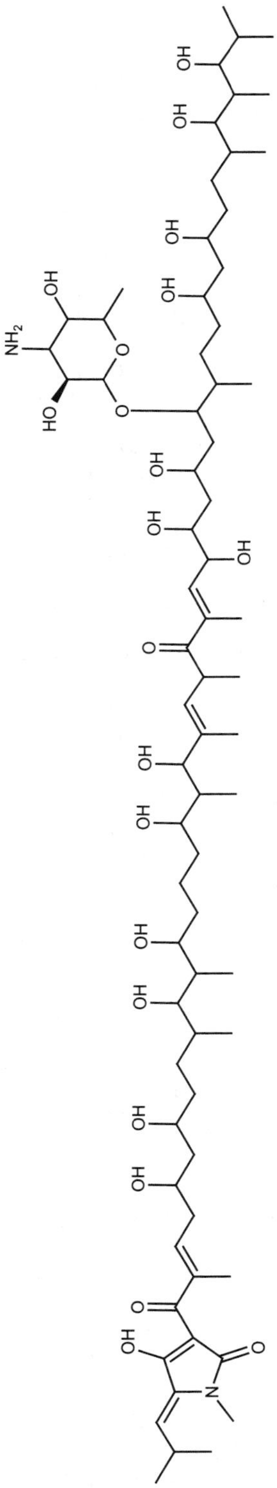

Figure 1 Vancoresmycin

and biologically stable compounds, which has been achieved by a better understanding of the chemical properties of the molecules.

In some respiratory tract infections, such as those which can be observed in cystic fibrosis, superinfections of chronic bronchitis, or bronchiectasis, the use of inhalational antibacterials in the form of aerosols has been successful. The bacteria most commonly found are gram-negative bacilli, such as *Pseudomonas aeruginosa,* and gram-positive cocci, such as *Staphylococcus aureus*. The most widely used antibacterial agents are the aminoglycosides, colistin, or β-lactams. An attempt at rationalization (dose and administration regimen) by means of appropriate pharmaceutical formulations has been undertaken with certain antibacterial agents, such as tobramycin (Cole, 2001).

In order to meet consumers' expectations, research has been conducted into improving their comfort, masking the bitterness of certain oral forms by mixtures with various salts such as josamycin propionate, reducing the number of daily administrations to a single daily dose (such as the once-daily injection of ceftriaxone) and thus increasing patients' compliance with their treatment, and reducing the duration of treatment in the community, which has been tried with certain macrolides, such as azithromycin, and certain oral cephalosporins, such as cefpodoxime proxetil.

To prolong patent life of many antibacterials, new formulations have been designed, such as extended-release clarithromycin and ciprofloxacin (a once-a-day dosing).

New chemical entities have been found, such as vancoresmycin (Fig. 1), which is a compound against gram-positive bacteria that is well tolerated in animal toxicology and has an unknown mechanism of action (Hopmann et al., 2002).

1.3.3. Third Period

With the 1980s, the objective changed since it became necessary to meet the increasingly rampant emergence of bacterial resistance which, although it had existed since the conception of antibacterial agents, was becoming a dominant factor in anti-infective therapy.

The problems associated with bacterial resistance are not new, and it very soon became obvious that bacteria were able to adapt and defend themselves. Two classic examples may be mentioned: those of antituberculosis agents and of penicillin G and *S. aureus*. In the first case, the response was therapeutic with the administration of combinations of antituberculosis agents such as streptomycin and *p*-aminosalicylic acid. This method of administration is still used now, but with more effective medications. In order to combat the production of β-lactamases by *S. aureus,* a chemical modification to the structure of the penicillins was made which resulted in methicillin and oxacillin and its derivatives. Until the middle of the 1980s, pharmaceutical research was always able to respond to the emergence of these strains, but research now is coming up against increasing difficulties, and there are a number of problems for which acceptable solutions have not been found.

The 1980s and subsequent years saw the appearance of another phenomenon associated with the improvement in knowledge through the detection of previously unknown bacterial agents such as *Helicobacter pylori, Clostridium difficile,* and *Legionella pneumophila*. Antibacterial agents were required to eradicate these microorganisms, and this objective has been achieved satisfactorily in the case of some bacterial species but not others, or intensive research has not yet resulted in one or more medications that fulfill the requirements, as for *H. pylori*.

Another unexpected phenomenon, but related to the progress of medicine and surgery, was the appearance on the infection scene of opportunistic bacteria, such as *Stenotrophomonas maltophilia*, *Burkholderia cepacia*, *Acinetobacter baumannii*, and *Alcaligenes* spp., for which often there is no satisfactory therapeutic response, and these bacterial species should in the future be included in the assessment panel for molecules produced in medicinal chemistry.

This exercise began with the modification of certain aminoglycosides by blockade of the site of action of the inactivating enzymes. This involved the restoration of antibacterial activity that had been blocked by these enzymes. This has yielded a molecule, amikacin, which remains one of the cornerstones of current antibiotic therapy.

1.3.4. Current Period

This idea has been pursued, but with a different objective: that of retaining the basic mechanism of action inherent in a given family of antibacterial agents and adding a complementary mechanism to preserve activity against strains that have become resistant. Often the addition of a supplementary mechanism has transformed a series of bacteriostatic molecules into bactericidal compounds.

Three examples of this type of modification may be mentioned, one of which has yielded a medicinal product, telithromycin.

Telithromycin is the result of a dual chemical action: removal of the L-cladinose mimicking what is found in a natural compound, narbomycin, and substitution of the lactone nucleus by a carbamate chain. This has yielded a compound possessing the mechanism of action of erythromycin A as well as another mode of interaction with 23S rRNA, the combination proving active against pneumococcal strains resistant to erythromycin A and its derivatives.

The second example is oritavencin. This is a bactericidal glycopeptide obtained by substitution of the vancosamine sugar with a biphenyl group. An active molecule is then obtained that is bactericidal against vancomycin-resistant strains of gram-positive cocci. This result is due to the addition of a supplementary mechanism of action to that of vancomycin against the synthesis of peptidoglycan (D-Ala–D-Ala), but it also acts on transglycosylation at the point of peptidoglycan synthesis so that it interacts at two levels of biosynthesis: transpeptidation and transglycosylation.

The third example is tigecycline (GAR-936). This molecule is derived from minocycline; it is active against minocycline-resistant bacterial strains, particularly those whose resistance is due to an efflux phenomenon. In addition to the conventional mechanism of tetracyclines, this compound prevents the extrusion of the molecule by steric hindrance due to the bulky substituent at position 9 of the molecule.

A less well-known avenue is the use of veterinary and agricultural antibacterial compounds as starting points. There are several examples, but one has yielded a medicinal product for human use. This concerns the oxazolidinones, which were used originally for the treatment of tomato infections due to *Agrobacterium tumefaciens*. After considerable research and disappointments with molecules derived at Dupont de Nemours (DuP 105 and DuP 721), a medicinal product has been introduced into medical practice: linezolid, which is active against gram-positive cocci such as staphylococci and enterococci. Another example is represented by the pleuromutilins, such as tiamulin, which are used in veterinary medicine and a derivative of which is undergoing investigation as a topical antibiotic in humans. Two pleuromutilin derivatives, SB 247386 and SB 268091, have been preselected (Rittenhouse et al., 1999).

Another approach is the creation of molecular hybrids or chimeras. Under the inspiration of Woodward, molecular hybrids gave rise to penems in 1976. These are a chemical hybrid between cephems (enamine function) and penams (Bryskier, 1995). After many disappointments, a molecule of this class, faropenem, was introduced into medical practice in Japan, but because of the poor pharmacokinetics, which necessitated administration every 8 h, and the large number of stages in its synthesis, it has not been developed in Europe and North America. These hybrids should not be confused with carbapenems of natural origin that were subsequently modified by semisynthesis, as was the case with thienamycin, which gave rise to imipenem. Currently, carbapenems are totally synthetic. Hybrids such as the combination of a fluoroquinolone molecule and a β-lactam (Bryskier, 1996) or oxazolidinone molecule (Hubschwerlen et al., 2003) have not undergone further development. The underlying idea was to provide the compound with a dual potential by creating a synergistic action.

During the period from the 1980s to the 1990s, at least two families of antibiotics resulting from the fermentation products of microorganisms were developed, such as mupirocin (modified pseudomonic acid) and monocyclic β-lactams from sulfazecin, giving rise to two medications, aztreonam and carumonam. However, this avenue of research proved to be a dead end because of the lack of prescription of these two medications.

The chance discovery of unknown antibacterial properties has been the starting point for intensive research. One example of this is metronidazole, which was originally an antiprotozoal agent whose activity against anaerobic bacteria was discovered towards the end of the 1970s. This "magic" compound exhibited another facet of its antibacterial activity: activity against *Mycobacterium tuberculosis* and in particular against "dormant bacterial cells," a known property of pyrazinamide. Research has been conducted in this area and has given rise to some compounds (PA-824) which have not been developed by the inventors for unspecified reasons.

No new antimycobacterial compounds have been synthesized in decades. It was shown by chance that fluoroquinolones and oxazolidinones such as PNU-100480 and derivatives displayed antimycobacterial activity.

The screening of all drug molecules, irrespective of their clinical use, is often the source of surprising discoveries. For example, chemical modifications to the skeleton of captopril permitted the synthesis of compounds capable of inhibiting class B β-lactamases (metalloenzymes). Chemical modification of proton pump inhibitors (medication for peptic ulcers) allowed the synthesis of compounds with a dual potential: antibacterial against *H. pylori* and active against gastric acidity, thereby simplifying the treatment of ulcers. For unspecified reasons, these compounds have not been developed for therapeutic use.

A new phenomenon is the rediscovery of compounds sometimes described several decades previously and resurrected from chemical libraries for a specific purpose. One example is the rediscovery of the properties of certain glycopeptides active only against gram-positive bacteria and not developed half a century ago in view of the lack of any medical need, which are being revived at the present time because of the failure to resolve the problems of methicillin-resistant staphylococcal strains.

Another approach is the study of the structure-activity relationships of compounds to find the active and nontransformable site of antibacterial activity. Along the same lines, research has been conducted into the chemical centers of toxicity of certain molecules for the purpose of eliminating these. In the first case, one example is the synthesis of an inhibitor of the B subunit of DNA gyrase by coumarin-type derivatives given all of the problems of tolerance associated with novobiocin, which binds to the B subunit of DNA gyrase in competition with a molecule of ATP. These compounds are at a very early stage of their development. RU-79115 does not inhibit UDP glycuronyl transferase, which is responsible for the conjugation of bilirubin in the liver, nor does it have any anti-vitamin K activity (Mauvais et al., 1999).

The second example is the phototoxicity induced by certain fluoroquinolones. Intensive studies conducted by research teams from Chugai in Japan have shown that the substitution of the carbon at position 8 by a fluorine atom is one of the causes of this toxicity, and this atom has now been replaced in new compounds by a methoxy group (OCH_3). The search for compounds that are better tolerated by patients is one of the current objectives, even though the new entities do not provide any major innovation in antibacterial terms.

The systematic screening of the chemical libraries of pharmaceutical companies, often very extensive as a result of several decades of research and synthesis work, without any preconceived idea about the intrabacterial target but directed against gram-positive or gram-negative test bacteria, makes it possible to discover and preselect a molecular series and to optimize it. This empirical screening method based on a chemical library is complementary to that of bacterial metabolites. One example is the demonstration of the anti-staphylococcal activity of certain heterocyclic derivatives containing a urea-type residue (Kane et al., 2003).

The limits of this research need to be understood, particularly on the industrial level: for example, an understanding of the optimized structures of cephems might in theory allow the production of an ideal cephalosporin. However, the bottleneck lies in the industrial synthesis, as demonstrated with a catechol-type cephalosporin such as RU-59863, which proved very promising in small quantities of drug substance synthesized in a research laboratory, but for which transposition to the industrial scale was impossible. Another example is the preparation of HR-790, a fluorinated monocyclic β-lactam in which the insertion of the fluorine atom in the oxime chain proved dangerous industrially; HR-790 was therefore abandoned despite all of its intrinsic antibacterial qualities (Chantot et al., 1992).

An important area is the acquisition of an absorbable and water-soluble molecule. In terms of absorbable molecules, an attempt has been made to enable the 2-amino-5-thiazolyl cephalosporins (cefotaxime, ceftriaxone, ceftizoxime, etc.) to cross the digestive barrier, unsuccessfully in the case of cefotaxime but with sufficiently acceptable bioavailability to allow oral treatment in the case of ceftizoxime. The addition of an amino acid chain to the amino group of the thiazole nucleus has allowed the oral absorption of this compound, which is currently in phase III in Japan. Cleavable esters that increase solubility have been prepared for fluoroquinolones such as tosufloxacin and more recently for an antistaphylococcal cephalosporin (RWJ-54428).

One of the most effective means of defense for enterobacteria and a certain number of nonfermentative gram-negative bacilli is the production of enzymes such as β-lactamases. Broad-spectrum enzymes such as TEM-1, TEM-2, and SHV-1 were blocked by suicide-type molecules such as clavulanic acid and sulfonated penicillins (sulbactam and tazobactam).

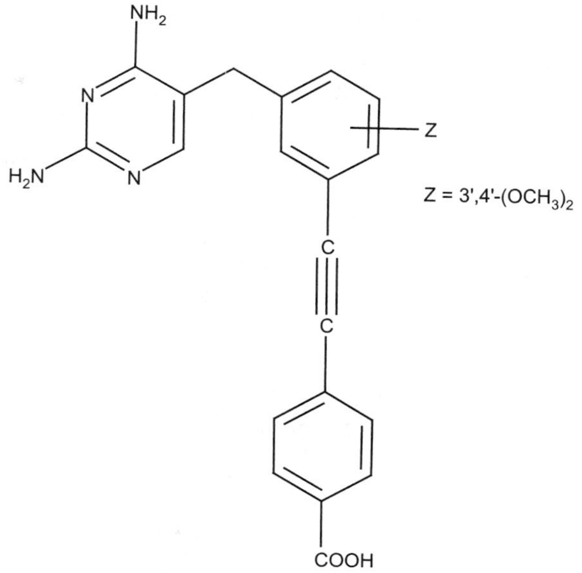

Figure 2 Inhibitors of DHFR of *M. avium* and *P. carinii*

However, the evolution of the enzyme world through mutations is now the source of an increasing number of β-lactamases. The world of these enzymes is made up of several hundred molecules divided into four classes, A, B, C, and D. The development of molecules inhibiting the activity of metalloenzymes (class B) is confronted by many difficulties and is complicated by the diversity of these enzymes. No molecule amenable to therapeutic use has been developed. Conversely, molecules with an inhibitory potential against class A and class C β-lactamases of the serine type are currently undergoing evaluation.

Among the derivatives which inhibit dihydrofolate reductase (DHFR), one, AR-100, is undergoing evaluation against *S. aureus*. Trimethoprim resistance in *S. aureus* is due to a single amino acid substitution (Phe98 → Tyr) in its DHFR. This substitution causes the loss of a hydrogen bond between the amino group at position 4 of trimethoprim and the carbonyl group of leucine 5 (Dale et al., 1997). Potent analogs of trimethoprim (Fig. 2) were synthesized with selective activity against DHFR of *Mycobacterium avium* and *Pneumocystis carinii* (Forsch et al., 2004).

2. FUTURE RESEARCH

Research in the area of anti-infective agents has developed considerably over the last half century, particularly during the last two decades.

From scientific empiricism, we have now entered upon an era of reflection and targeted research.

Previously, activity screening tests were carried out and the best compound in terms of activity, tolerance in laboratory animals, and chemical yield was selected for further development, possibly resulting in a medicinal product.

Nowadays, the requirements are more complex: compounds must be innovative, in other words, active against bacterial strains that are multiresistant to the currently available antibacterial agents, well tolerated, and with a sales price that is compatible with health care system resources in different countries, permitting their reimbursement by the welfare systems. Starting from this premise, we now find ourselves midstream, with a number of bacterial targets but no novel drugs. A better understanding of bacterial physiology is essential to better ascertain the lethal targets of bacteria.

Despite all of the efforts invested, the flexibility and adaptability of bacteria are sometimes more rapid than our research. It appears that once the phenomenon of the spread of resistance is unleashed, it is difficult to stop it or rein it in, even with the proposed therapeutic guidelines of good antibiotic prescribing practices. To escape from this vicious cycle, it is probably necessary to find other bacterial targets and perhaps new treatment formulas that have yet to be conceived.

The most dynamic approach involves research into new bacterial targets and molecules which block these, but this is a long and capricious route.

2.1. Bacterial Targets

An understanding of bacterial physiology is a prerequisite for all research into new therapeutic entities.

The marked improvements in understanding of the physioanatomy of bacteria hold out the prospect of a number of targets. We are beginning to have data banks of genome sequences of numerous bacterial species at our disposal, enabling the presence or absence of certain genes to be explored and allowing us to abandon or persevere with a particular line of research. The study of the biosynthesis of certain "organs," such as the bacterial wall, suggests new targets. These targets are numerous, but how many will be the subject of drug discoveries remains a mystery.

The most widely studied are the bacterial wall of gram-negative bacteria, that of mycobacteria (mycolic acid), and ribosomes, with respect to the inhibition not only of protein synthesis (peptidyltransferase site) but also of other ribosomal functions such as ribosomal protein assembly. Analysis of the metabolic pathways in search of vital sites for bacteria is another line of exploration. One that is less investigated is DNA, the approach to which is more difficult because of its tertiary configuration. Blockade of bacterial defense systems is also one avenue of research.

2.2. Research Methods

As a result of gaining an understanding of the bacterial genome, it is possible to see the incidence of a given target in the bacterial world.

One of the difficulties is the development of reliable, readily reproducible, validated (allowing the validity of the results to be certified), and sensitive screening tests.

The most common method is the screening in a given target of thousands of molecules contained in the chemical libraries of the different pharmaceutical companies. If one or more compounds emit even weak activity "signals," the candidate molecule or molecules can then be optimized by chemical modifications. This stage, if it proves positive, will be followed by all of the tests allowing preselection and then selection for development.

Outside chemical libraries, it is possible to turn to molecules of various origins, such as those from plants, mammals, marine products, and insects.

Difficulties have to be overcome: the screening of products of natural origin requires a synthetic process with a high yield, which is sometimes difficult to obtain. This is demonstrated by the squalamines obtained from *Squalus acanthias* (shark), which involve a long and expensive synthesis. Squalamines are multipotent molecules acting on bacteria, parasites, fungi, and cancer cells (Khabnadideh et al., 2000).

The tools currently available allow important progress to be made in medicinal chemistry. Two examples may be mentioned. The first is 14- and 15-membered-ring macrolides, some groups of which can only be obtained by genetic engineering. The second example, which involves the addition of constituents to the fermentation medium, is that of flurithromycin through the addition of a fluorine atom as an isosteric element at position 8 of the erythronolide A nucleus and of daptomycin, the lipid chain of which has been obtained by specific fermentation. The same problem is found in the structural modifications of the streptogramins by mutasynthesis.

2.3. Which Molecules?

The current research into antibacterial molecules appears to be directed along various lines:

- Towards a precise bacterial agent with specific screening: antistaphylococcal (methicillin resistant), anti-*H. pylori*, anti-*M. tuberculosis*, etc.
- Broader research without an apparent precise bacterial objective, other than finding a lethal target or a series of potential compounds inhibiting the activity of that target. The chemical structure of the molecule then has to be optimized so that it can act on the whole bacterial cell (broad antibacterial spectrum to a greater or lesser extent).

3. STATE OF PROGRESS OF RESEARCH

Several avenues of research in terms of new bacterial targets are under study, and only a few examples are mentioned here.

3.1. The Bacterial Outer Membrane

3.1.1. Peptidoglycan

Peptidoglycan (murein) is a covalent macromolecule located on the outside of the cytoplasmic membrane and specific to microorganisms.

Its main function is to maintain internal osmotic pressure so as to retain the shape of the bacterium.

Peptidoglycan biosynthesis is a complex process that has not yet been fully elucidated. Three stages are involved: intracytoplasmic (formation of monomers), transfer of the monomers through the cytoplasmic membrane, and, finally, polymerization on the surface. Each stage involves several enzyme systems.

Therapeutic compounds are known to inhibit peptidoglycan synthesis: fosfomycin, β-lactams, vancomycin and its derivatives, and D-cycloserine.

Research is currently underway to find other inhibitors acting on other enzyme systems involved in this synthesis. MraY inhibitors are compounds inhibiting lipid I biosynthesis, among which may be mentioned the tunicamycin group (tunicamycins, streptovirudins, and corynetoxins), ribosamino-uridine (liposidomycins, muramycins, caprazamycins, the FR-900493 series, and riburamycins), and, lastly, the uridylpeptides (mureidomycins, pacidamycins, and napsamycins) (see chapter 12).

3.1.2. Mycobacteria

The mycobacterial cell wall is essential for viability and virulence. The wall of mycobacteria is unique, as it comprises a large lipid component (mycolic acid) and inhibition of its biosynthesis is lethal to the microorganism (Parrish et al., 2001).

A major component of the mycobacterial cell wall is the antigen 85 complex, composed of three proteins: Ag85A, Ag85B, and Ag85C. All three molecules contribute to cell wall biosynthesis. They catalyze transfer of mycolic acid from one trehalose monomycolate to another, resulting in trehalose dimycolate and one free trehalose.

It was shown that a trehalose analog, 6-azido-6-deoxytrehalose, inhibits the mycolyl transferase activity of all three proteins. Based on this observation, series of 6,6′-bis(sulfonamido), *N,N′*-dialkyl amino trehaloses were synthesized to inhibit the Ag85 complex. Series of phosphonate inhibitors were designed to mimic the transition state of the mycolyl transferase reaction (Gobec et al., 2004).

3.1.3. Porphyrins

The activity of porphyrins is due to the capacity of the peroxidation and oxidation reactions. The absorption of photons and reactive oxygen species by the lipid component of the bacterial wall causes a lethal change in it.

Porphyrin chimeras have been synthesized by replacement of the iron atom by other elements such as gallium, manganese, indium, ruthenium, and zinc. These derivatives possess good activity against gram-negative bacteria and mycobacteria (Stojiljkovic et al., 2000).

3.2. Ribosomes

There are numerous targets in ribosomes, among which may be mentioned deformylase, ppGpp degradase, initiation factors (IF-1, IF-2, and IF-3), elongation factors (EF-Tu, EF-Ts, and EF-G), release factors (RF-1, RF-2, and RF-3), ribosomal protein assembly, and the peptidyltransferase site.

3.2.1. Ribosomal A-Site

The ribosomal A-site can be blocked by aminoglycosides. Azepane-glycoside derivatives appear to have the same action (Barluenga et al., 2004).

Benzoimidazole-type derivatives (Fig. 3) bind to the A-site at the 16S RNA level (He et al., 2004). The benzoimidazoles block the activity of bacterial translation. Some of these derivatives possess antistaphylococcal activity (MIC, 6 to 12 μg/ml), but this activity is absent in *Escherichia coli*.

Azepane-glycoside or new 2′-deoxystreptamine analogs appear to have the same site of action (Barluenga et al., 2004; Verloumis et al., 2002).

3.2.2. Aminoacyl-tRNA

Aminoacyl-tRNA synthetases are essential enzymes in the synthetic pathway of proteins, as they catalyze the binding of amino acids to tRNA prior to their uptake in the ribosome. An antibiotic acting on isoleucyl-tRNA, mupirocin, has been introduced into therapeutic use. Attachment occurs in two stages: binding to an adenylate, followed by an attack on the 2′ OH or 3′ OH group of the tRNA in the carboxyl group. It is the intermediate which can be inhibited by acyl sulfamates. tRNAs I and II react differently with aminoalkyl or acyl sulfamates. A series of spirocyclic furans with inhibitory activity against phenylalanyl-tRNA synthetase has been synthesized (Yu et al., 2004) (Fig. 4).

Tyrosyl-tRNA synthetase is a member of the class I tRNA synthetases, which are characterized by catalytically important HIGH and KMSKS sequence motifs. There are significant differences between bacterial and mammalian enzymes, so selective inhibition offers potential for new antibacterials. It was found that SB 219383 (Fig. 5) is an effective inhibitor of tyrosyl-tRNA synthetase of *S. aureus* (Jarvest et al., 1999).

Quinoline derivatives inhibiting methionyl-tRNA of *S. aureus* (50% inhibitory concentration [IC_{50}], 7.8 to 12 nM) with good antibacterial activity (MICs, <0.06 to 1.0 μg/ml) have been reported.

A natural amino acid tRNA inhibitor was reported, indolmycin, which exhibits a high affinity for tryptophan tRNA of *S. aureus* (IC_{50}, 15 ng/ml). Semisynthetic compounds from indolmycin have been synthesized. Other natural compounds have been reported, such as borrelidin (threonine tRNA), granaticin (leucyl-tRNA), furanomycin (isoleucyl-tRNA), purpuromycin (all tRNA), chuanximycin (tryptophanyl-tRNA), and ochratoxin A (phenylalanyl-tRNA).

It appears that isoleucyl-, methionyl-, phenylalanyl-, and tyrosyl-tRNA inhibitors are candidates for use as drugs.

3.2.3. Initiation Factors

There appear to be three initiation factors.

- IF-1 facilitates the association/dissociation of the ribosomal subunits and helps IF-2 to bind to the ribosomal 30S subunit.

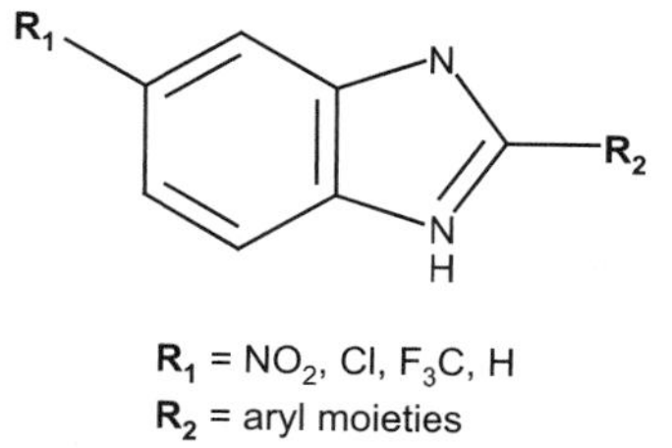

R_1 = NO_2, Cl, F_3C, H
R_2 = aryl moieties

Figure 3 Benzoimidazole derivatives: site A inhibitors

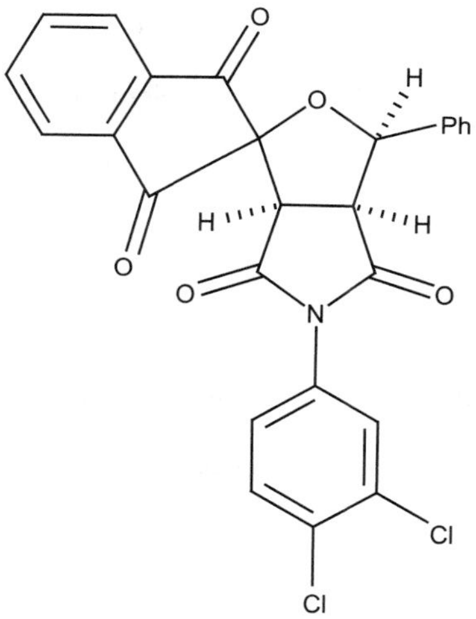

Figure 4 Phenylalanine tRNA transferase inhibitor

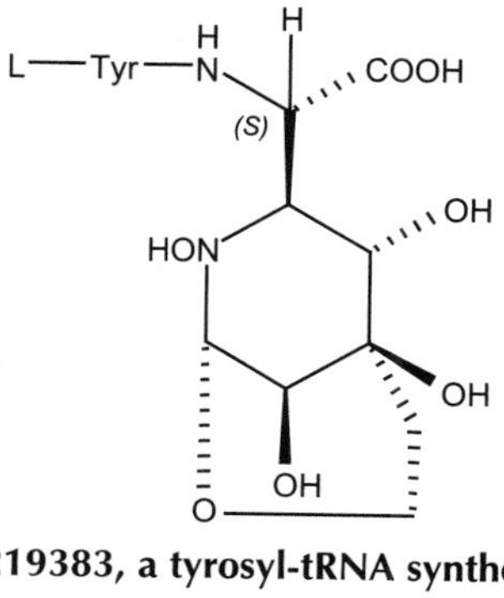

Figure 5 SB 219383, a tyrosyl-tRNA synthetase inhibitor

- IF-2 stimulates the binding of tRNA, having bound an fMet at the ribosomal P site. IF-2 specifically recognizes the formyl group of $tRNA^{fMet}$.
- IF-3 acts as a stabilization factor in the 30S subunit.

There are antibacterial agents other than aminoglycosides which are active against IF-2 (Evans et al., 2003).

3.2.4. Elongation Factors

EF-Tu is an essential component of protein synthesis. Its function is to recognize and transport (noninitiating) tRNA with its amino acid to the mRNA A-site during the elongation cycle. During this cycle, EF-Tu interacts with GTP, GDP, RF-Ts, and tRNA with a bound amino acid. Several families of antibacterial agents are known to interact with EF-Tu: thiazolyl peptides such as GE 2270A (Heffron and Jurnak, 2000), kirromycin (Fig. 6), pulvomycin, and enacyloxin IIa. The process of recognition of site A requires the presence of the EF-Tu–GTP–aminoacyl-tRNA complex. This complex penetrates at the T-site, which is adjacent to the A-site on the ribosome. Hydrolysis of a GTP molecule is essential to ensure the reading of a correct codon-anticodon unit and the rejection of any abnormal tRNA.

ET-Ts subsequently binds to EF-Tu, which promotes the release of GDP from EF-Tu after GDP hydrolysis, resulting in regeneration of the active form of EF-Tu.

Aminoglycosides appear to affect the dissociation between the ribosome and EF-G. EF-G is inhibited by fusidic acid.

EF-Tu and EF-Ts are essential and highly conserved among bacteria, and EF-Ts lacks homology with its eukaryotic counterpart.

EF-Tu has a different functionality than EF-1α from eukaryotes.

Four series of inhibitors were synthesized. Nine indole dipeptide analogs inhibit EF-Tu and EF-Ts (IC_{50}, 14 to >50 μM). The indole dipeptide shown in Fig. 7 exhibits a MIC of 2.0 μg/ml for *S. aureus*; 2-arylbenzoimidazole, N-substituted imidazole, and N-substituted guanidine had MICs of 2.0, 8.0, and 0.5 μg/ml, respectively (Jayasekera et al., 2005) (Fig. 7).

3.2.5. Peptidyltransferase Site

Macrolides, lincosamides, oxazolidinones, evernimicin, and streptogramins are known to interact in protein synthesis by blocking the P-site at different levels in 23S rRNA. Compounds such as the pleuromutilins, currently under investigation, also act at this level.

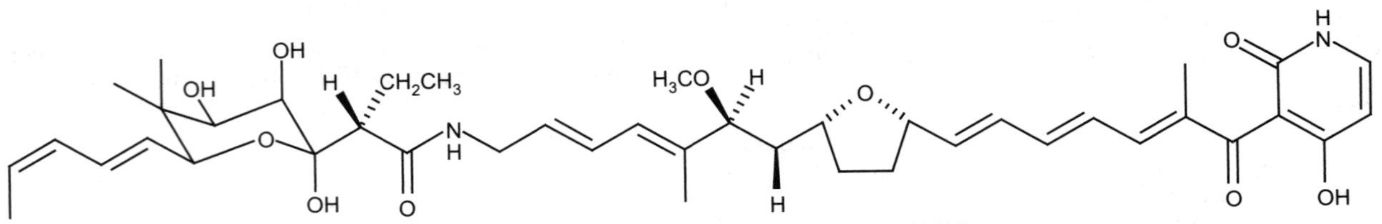

Figure 6 Kirromycin, an elongation factor inhibitor

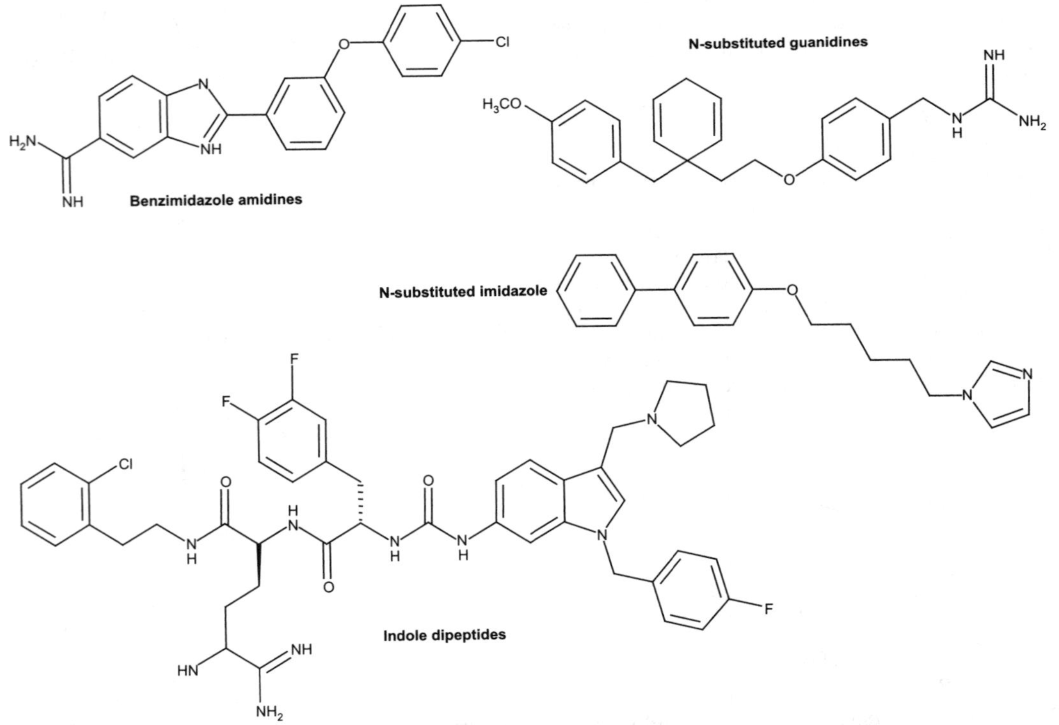

Benzimidazole amidines

N-substituted guanidines

N-substituted imidazole

Indole dipeptides

Figure 7 Structure of EF-Tu and EF-Ts inhibitors

3.2.6. Ribosomal Assembly

Ribosomal 50S subunit assembly is blocked by macrolides and related substances in gram-positive cocci and *Haemophilus influenzae*. Other antibacterial agents cause inhibition of this assembly, such as streptogramins and evernimicin (Champney, 2003).

3.2.7. Deformylases

Bacterial protein synthesis is initiated by *N*-formylmethionine. The nascent peptide is transformed to a mature protein by sequential removal of the *N*-formyl group and the methionine by a peptide deformylase and a methionine aminopeptidase (Mazel et al., 1994). This enzyme is absent in mammalian cells. It has been shown that the production of the deformylase protein is governed by two genes in gram-positive cocci (*defA* and *defB*), but only one gene appears to be involved in that of *E. coli* (*defA*). These genes are essential for bacterial growth (Margolis et al., 1999a, 1999b). The *defA* gene in *E. coli* is under the control of the *tolC* gene, which can govern the level of expression of peptide deformylase by varying the concentration of arabinose. The viability of the cells depends on the product of the *fmt* gene (gene product, tRNA-methionyl formyltransferase).

The deformylase protein is a metallohydrolase. Compounds are undergoing development.

3.2.8. GTPase

Era (*E. coli* Ras-like protein) is a GTPase which is present in gram-positive and -negative bacteria and in mycoplasmas. It is an essential enzyme. An inhibitor of this enzyme has been synthesized, but despite its good enzyme affinity, it exhibits poor penetration of the bacterial wall. A derivative of this prototype has a great affinity (IC_{50}, 0.01 to 2 μg/ml) and MICs on the order of 1.6 to 32 μg/ml (Snyder et al., 2000).

3.2.9. DnaK

Assembly of the different ribosomal proteins yields the 50S and 30S subunits. Apparent spontaneous assembly appears to occur with the participation of proteins known as chaperonins, which facilitate and accelerate assembly. The DnaK-DnaJ pair and GroEL proteins are involved in the terminal part of the ribosomal assembly of *E. coli*. DnaK accelerates the process of conversion of the 21S particles to 30S subunits and of the 32S and 45S particles to 50S subunits.

In combination with antibacterial agents, Dnak acts on bacterial ribosomal assembly and might substantially affect the activity of these compounds by accelerating the inhibition process.

3.3. DNA

3.3.1. Helicases

Helicases are present in all microorganisms. These are enzymes involved in the formation of nucleic acid strands. They are ubiquitous. Twelve helicase DNAs have been identified in *E. coli*. They act by hydrolyzing nucleoside triphosphate, causing the separation of strands of DNA-DNA, DNA-RNA, or RNA-DNA (Singleton and Wigley, 2002).

DnaA is a helicase with a great affinity for ATP and acts on DNA replication by inhibiting the binding of ATP. Inhibitors such as bis-indole derivatives have been described.

3.3.2. DNA Polymerase III

3.3.2.1. 6-Anilinouracil

In the polymerase C family, polymerase III is subdivided into C-1 (*dnaE*) and C-2 (*polC*). All bacteria possess the *dnaE* gene, but the *polC* gene is found principally in gram-positive bacteria with a low G + C content. These enzymes intervene principally in chromosomal replication. 6-Anilinouracil derivatives can block GTP purines (guanines) through their resemblance (Tarantino et al., 1999) (Fig. 8).

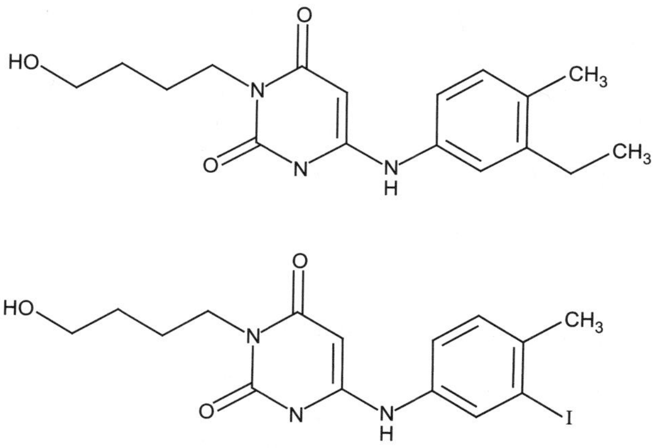

Figure 8 Polymerase III inhibitors

Anilinouracil derivatives inhibited *Bacillus anthracis*, with MICs ranging from 0.156 to 20 μg/ml and K_is of 0.006 to 0.32 μM (Butler et al., 2004).

3.3.2.2. REP 6021

DNA replication is an essential process for cells. This replication is under the control of polymerase III holoenzymes.

Thioxothiazolidinones inhibit DNA polymerases of both gram-positive and gram-negative bacteria (Fig. 9).

REP 6021 has a MIC of 0.12 μg/ml for *S. aureus*, *Enterococcus faecalis*, *Enterococcus faecium*, *H. influenzae*, *Streptococcus pneumoniae*, and *Moraxella catarrhalis*.

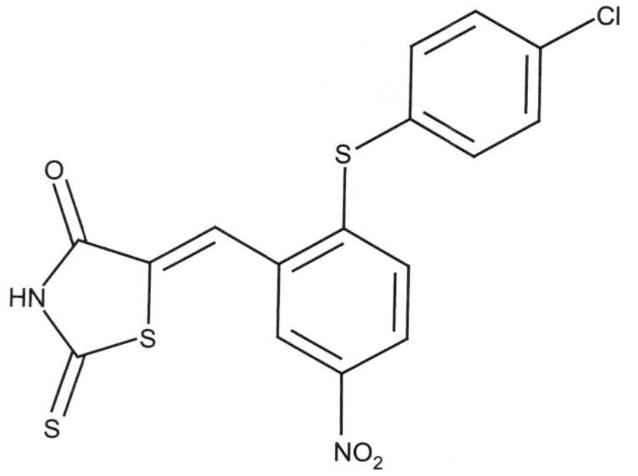

3.3.3. Thymidine Phosphatase

Thymidine phosphatase catalyzes the phosphorylation of thymidine. Hydrazine carboxamide derivatives have inhibitory potency against this enzyme in *E. coli* (McNally et al., 2003).

3.3.4. Purine Phosphatase Inhibitors

Purine nucleoside ribosyltransferase catalyzes the reversible phosphorolysis of ribo- and deoxyribonucleosides of guanine as well as adenine. Formycins A and B (Fig. 10) and analogs exhibited inhibitory activity against purine nucleoside phosphorylase of *E. coli* (Bzowska et al., 1992).

Figure 9 REP 6021

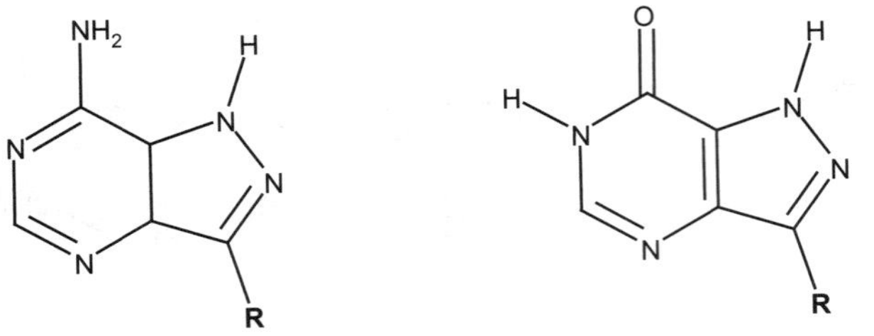

Formycin A

Formycin B

Figure 10 Formycins A and B

3.3.5. DNA Gyrase B Inhibitors

Novobiocin inhibits ATPase activity of DNA gyrase by competing with ATP for binding to gyrase subunit B. Many compounds have been synthesized as coumarin inhibitors.

It was shown that the indazole scaffold forms a hydrogen bond with Asp73 (Tanitame et al., 2004) (Fig. 11).

DNA gyrase B inhibitors from series of aminobenzoimidazoles have been shown to exhibit good in vitro and in vivo activities. Some analogs, such as V07, V08, and V09, exhibit good in vitro activities against *S. aureus* (MICs, 0.06 to 0.25 μg/ml), *Staphylococcus epidermidis* (MICs, 0.03 to 0.12 μg/ml), *E. faecalis* (MICs, 0.03 to 0.06 μg/ml), *E. faecium* (MICs, 0.06 to 0.12 μg/ml), and *S. pneumoniae* (MICs, 0.008 to 0.03 μg/ml). In rats, the apparent elimination half-life after administration of 10 mg/kg of body weight is about 1.2 h. V08 was selected for further development as VX 692. This compound is bactericidal against *Enteroccocus* spp. and *H. influenzae,* as well as against *S. aureus*. VX 692 exhibits time-dependent pharmacodynamics.

3.4. Metabolism

3.4.1. Osmotransporters

Blockade of the transport mechanisms of solutions of antibacterial agents by osmotransporters such as glycine betaine inhibitors (Fig. 12) (Cosquer et al., 2004) is one line of research. These osmotransporters prevent toxic substances from penetrating the bacterium, and their blockade indirectly causes the bacterium to become intoxicated.

3.4.2. Efflux Pumps

Efflux pumps, which have been demonstrated in a number of bacteria, are a physiological means for the bacteria to eliminate xenobiotics such as antibacterial agents. Research is currently ongoing to combine molecules that are active in expelling them from the bacterium with compounds that block their exit. Suggestions have been made to combine levofloxacin with an inhibitor for *P. aeruginosa,* and this type of molecule has been proposed for enterobacteria such as *Enterobacter aerogenes* (Chevalier et al., 2004). More complex research has shown that the mechanisms of expulsion may differ in the same family of antibiotics (macrolides in *Enterobacteriaceae*).

3.4.3. Fatty Acid Biosynthesis

Lipid metabolism is complex and represents a potential avenue for the activity of new antibiotics. Fatty acid biosynthesis is induced by one or more ubiquitous systems known as FAS. There are two systems, FAS I and FAS II.

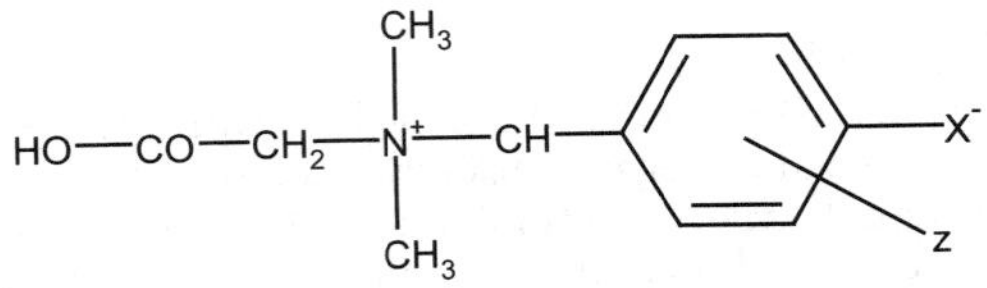

Compound	X	Z
1	Cl or Br	H
2	Br	4-NO_2

Figure 12 Osmotransporter inhibitor

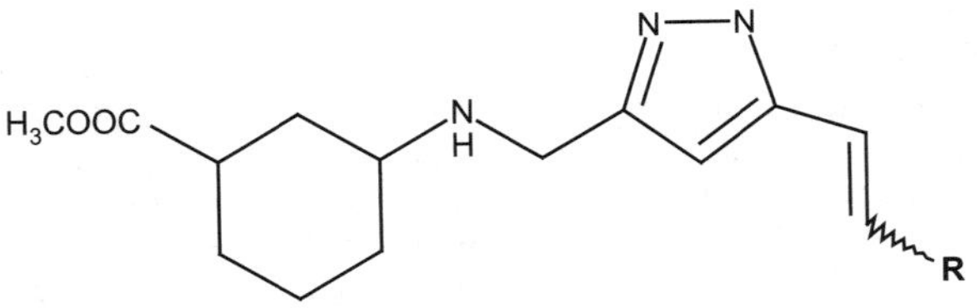

		R	MIC (μg/ml) S. aureus 209 P	MIC (μg/ml) E. faecalis ATCC 29212
Compound 1	E	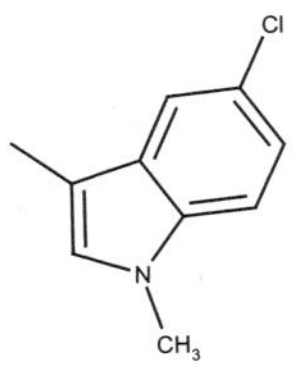	1.0	32.0
	Z		1.0	8.0

Figure 11 DNA gyrase inhibitors

Fatty acid biosynthesis is induced via several stages that are catalyzed by various enzyme systems, producing elongation of the fatty acid chain. The biosynthesis cycle is initiated by an enzyme complex known as FabH (giving the initiating step of malonyl coenzyme A) or FabD (malonyl ACP). This is followed by an enzyme cascade comprising FabG and then FabA/Z and ends with FabI, allowing the addition of two carbon atoms (Kaneda et al., 1991; Choi et al., 2000; Hoang and Schweizer, 1997; Jackowski et al., 1989). Some derivatives are known for their interaction with the different parts of the synthetic cycle, such as isoniazid, triclosan, cerulenin, and thiolactomycin (Heath et al., 2002). Investigations are in progress and have yielded exploratory derivatives such as imidazole-type molecules, diazaborines, and HR-19 and HR-12, which act on *S. aureus* FabH (He and Reynolds, 2002). FabI (ACP) reductase catalyzes the last stage of the fatty acid elongation cycle. An acrylamide derivative has been synthesized and possesses a high affinity for FabI (IC_{50}, 0.047 μM) and good anti-staphylococcal activity (MIC, 0.06 μg/ml) (Payne et al., 2002) (Fig. 13).

In a series of naphthyridinyl enamide compounds, AP-1401 was identified as the most active FabI-enoyl ACP reductase inhibitor; it is water soluble (Fig. 14).

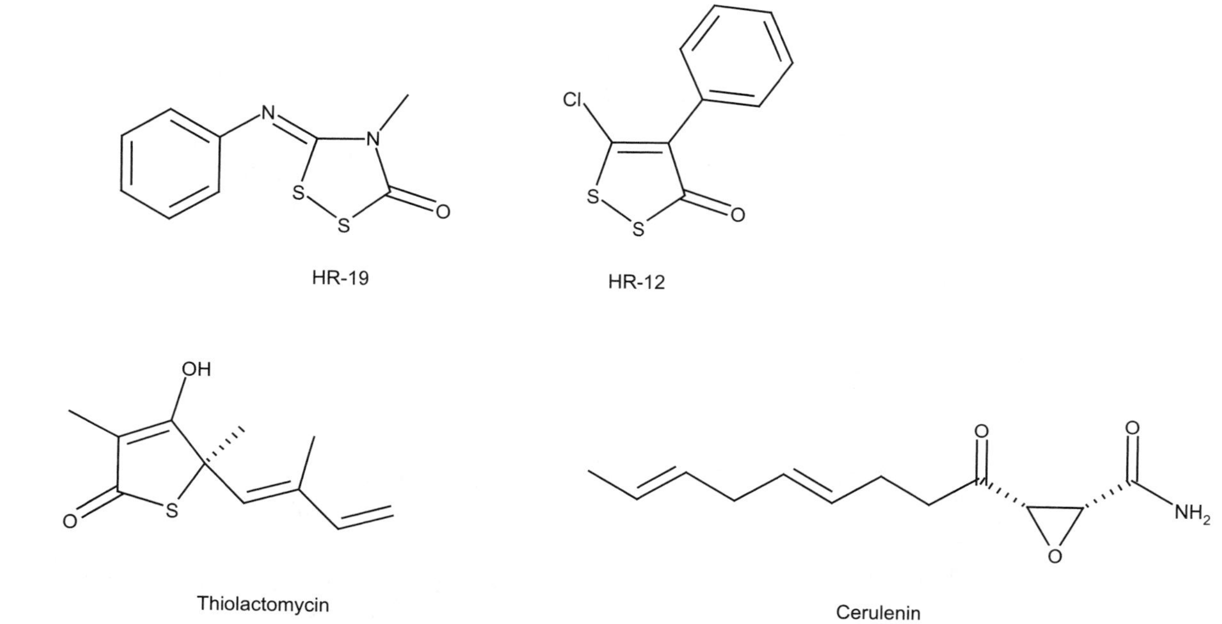

Figure 13 Fatty acid biosynthesis inhibitors

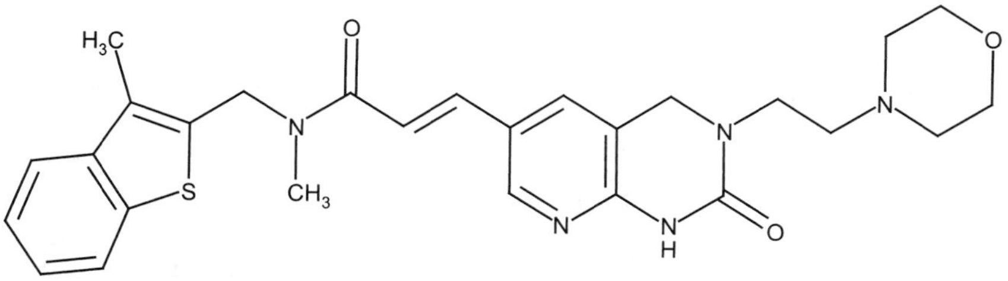

Fab I (IC_{50} - μM) (*S. aureus*)	0.02
MIC (μg/ml)	
S. aureus	≤0.06
MRSA	≤0.06
S. epidermidis	≤0.06
Water solubility (μg/ml)	
pH 7.4	8.0
pH 4.0	> 320

Figure 14 AP-1401

3.4.4. Iron Metabolism

The inability of some antibacterial agents to penetrate the bacterial wall is responsible for the resistance of the bacterium to these agents. Bacteria need the iron which is found in the external environment for their physiology, and they use siderophores to obtain it. Some antibiotics, such as cephalosporins of the catechol type, use this route as a second mechanism of action. Another solution is to allow some antibacterial agents to conjugate with a siderophore. This has been achieved by means of isocyanurate compounds with a valine as the ligand, such as the valine-5-fluorouridine derivatives (Ghosh and Miller, 1995).

3.5. Virulence

3.5.1. Adherence

The adherence of bacteria can occur through pili for gram-negative bacilli or sortases for gram-positive bacilli.

Pilicides have been synthesized and are of the β-lactam type, but they differ from the penam structure by the presence of a C-C bond instead of the C-N at position 6 of the central core and by different stereochemistry from the penams.

The sortases of all gram-positive bacilli contain the LPXTGX motif.

3.5.2. Quorum Sensing

Quorum sensing is a communication system between bacteria governed by a set of genetic components and controlled by homoserine lactones that are autoinduced in a situation of distress and which appear to be inhibited by macrolides. This phenomenon might be one of the explanations for their activity in cystic fibrosis. Quorum sensing modifies and regulates bacterial virulence, secondary-metabolite production, and biofilm formation and modulates the transition to the stationary phase of bacterial growth.

Homoserine lactone inhibitors are undergoing study, perhaps for administration in combination with known antibacterials.

3.5.3. Two-Component Systems

The two-component system is used by bacteria to detect and respond to environmental stimuli.

A histidine kinase and a regulator are used by pathogenic bacteria to regulate the virulence factors necessary for the bacterium to survive. Several series of compounds have been synthesized and inhibit the two-component KinA/Spo0F system of *Bacillus subtilis*.

A series of guanidine derivatives has led to the discovery of RWJ-49815. The IC_{50} for KinA/Spo0F is 2.0 μM, and RWJ-49815 has in vitro activity against *S. aureus* ATCC 29213 (MIC, 2.0 μg/ml), *S. aureus* OC 2089 (methicillin resistant [MIC, 1.0 μg/ml]), *E. faecalis* OC 3041 (MIC, 2 μg/ml), and *E. faecium* Van^r OC 3312 (MIC, 1 μg/ml) (Demers et al., 1997).

Members of series of benzoxazine derivatives, including RWJ-63093 and RWJ-63138, have a good IC_{50} for the KinA/Spo0F system (53 and 13 μM for RWJ-63093 and RWJ-63138, respectively), with a MIC of 4.0 μg/ml for *S. aureus* OC 2878 (Licata et al., 1997).

A series of salicylanilide derivatives has been reported. Some of these compounds possess a good inhibitory effect on the KinA/Spo0F system and good in vitro antistaphylococcal activity (Macielag et al., 1997) (Fig. 15).

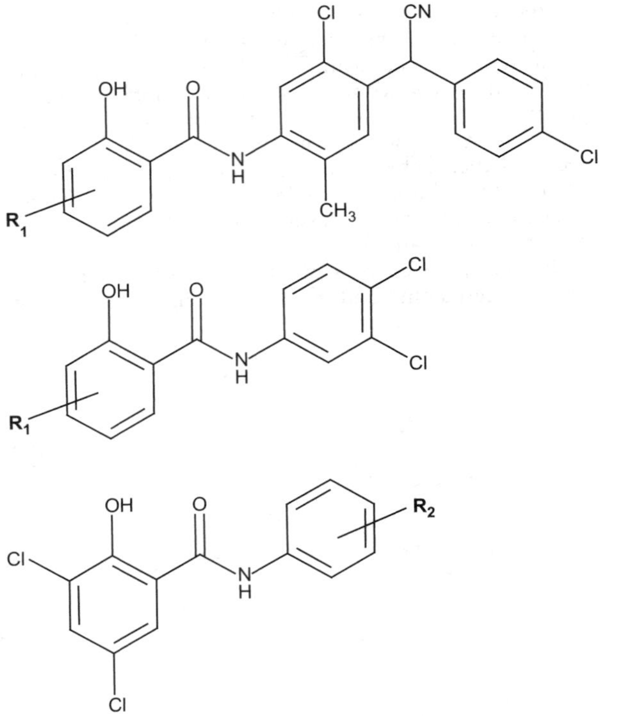

Figure 15 Two-component system inhibitors

3.5.4. Lipid A

Lipid A is a unit comprising phosphated disaccharides to which fatty acid chains are bound. It is an integral part of lipopolysaccharide, the hydrophic part of which appears to be responsible for the toxicity of lipopolysaccaride. Its biosynthesis requires the involvement of at least nine enzyme systems, of which the second stage (LpxC) appears to be the most sensitive to the action of inhibitors of its synthesis. Lipid A biosynthesis is necessary for the growth of *E. coli*. A number of derivatives are active against *E. coli* but not *P. aeruginosa*. This enzyme is a metallo(zinc)-amidase which appears to be inhibited by compounds of the types L-573655 and L-161240. These derivatives are also active in vivo in a murine model of experimental infection. Other derivatives, such as E-5532, act on the exit of tumor necrosis factor alpha.

BB-78484 and BB-78485 are derivatives of α-(R)-amino-hydroxamic acid and possess good LpxC-inhibitory activity (Clements et al., 2002) (Fig. 16 and 17).

3.5.5. TTPS

Many bacteria live in a close relationship with host organisms. This relationship is directed by proteins secreted by bacteria in the extracellular environment or by translocating them into the bacterial cell, especially for gram-negative bacteria through the type III protein secretion system (TTPS). The TTPS is composed of approximately 20 to 25 different proteins. About half of these proteins are converted in most type III systems. Effectors appear to gain entry into host cells through pores formed in host cell membrane by type III secreted proteins named translocators (Ghosh, 2004). They translocate bacterial effector proteins directly into the cytoplasm or inner membrane of target host cells and interfere with eukaryotic signal transduction.

TTPSs are virulence determinants. They are found in gram-negative bacteria.

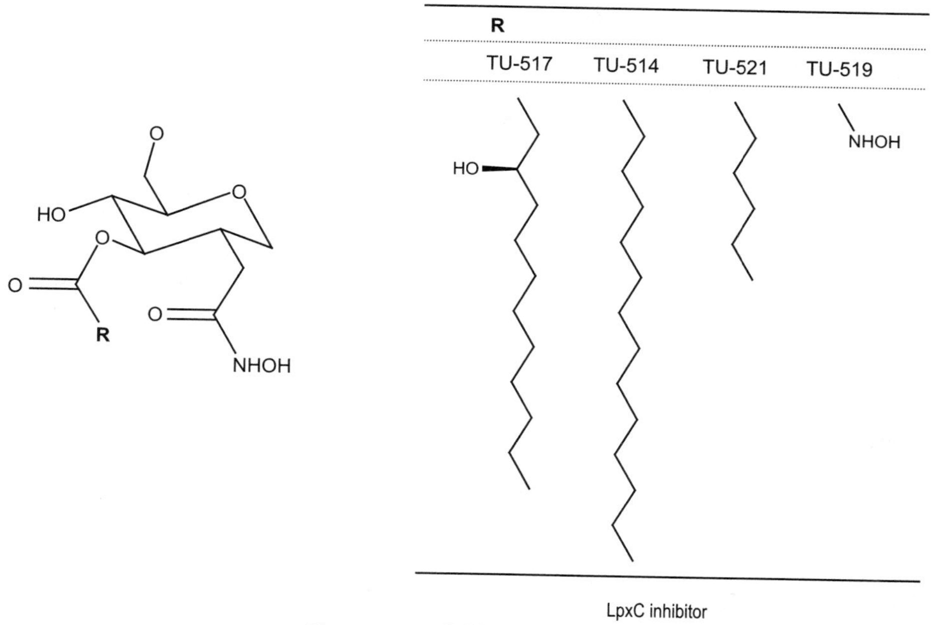

R			
TU-517	TU-514	TU-521	TU-519

LpxC inhibitor

Figure 16 Lipid A inhibitors

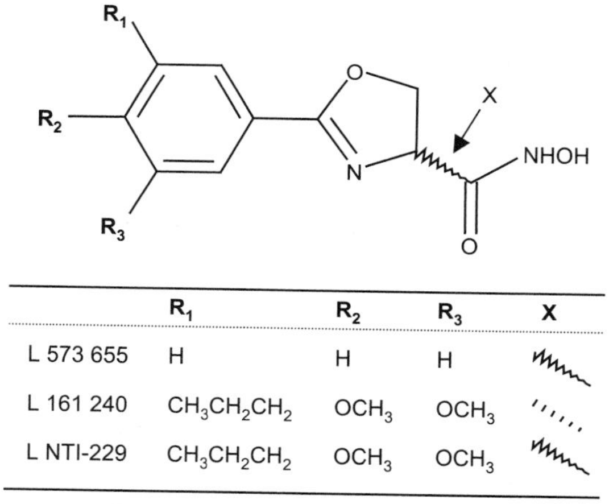

	R_1	R_2	R_3	X
L 573 655	H	H	H	
L 161 240	$CH_3CH_2CH_2$	OCH_3	OCH_3	
L NTI-229	$CH_3CH_2CH_2$	OCH_3	OCH_3	

Figure 17 Lipid A inhibitors

Several series of compounds have been synthesized containing dipeptide, oxazole, thiazole, and imidazole moieties (Fig. 18).

Compounds from the dipeptide and azole series showed broad specificity for inhibition of TTPSs from both *Salmonella* and *P. aeruginosa* (Li et al., 2004).

The carboxylic group seems to be crucial for the affinity for the pocket of the TTPS (Table 1).

MICs for *E. coli* are above 32 μg/ml.

In order to delay the growth of a strain of *P. aeruginosa*, an inhibitor of TTPS in combination with ciprofloxacin was tested in a murine experimental model (Fernandez et al., 2004).

3.5.6. ERM Methyltransferase Inhibitor

3.5.6.1. Triazine Analogs

One of the major mechanisms of resistance to macrolides, lincosamides, and streptogramin type B is the N mono- or dimethylation of base A2058, located on the peptidyltransferase loop of domain V of the 23S rRNA on the 50S subunit of the bacterial ribosomes using *S*-adenosylmethionine as a source of methyl (Denoya and Dubnan, 1989). The *erm* genes govern the production of these enzymes (Weisblum, 1995).

Using a nuclear magnetic resonance-based screen, a series of triazine derivatives was identified to bind weakly to ErmA. These initial lead compounds were optimized by synthesis of analogs, yielding compounds which were able to inhibit ErmAM. More than 400 compounds were synthesized, and analysis of the structure-activity relationships for the binding to ErmAM and ErmC′ yielded some analogs exhibiting a high inhibitory activity. Two compounds (Fig. 19) bind to ErmAM and ErmC′ via a hydrogen link with the triazine moiety and with the indan structure. ErmAM and ErmC′ interact with both compounds at I106 (L105) and D109 (Q108). These changes from aspartic acid to glutamine may explain the difference in the inhibitory activities of the two compounds. Residues I60 (L59) and S39 (T38) in ErmC′ (ErmAM) interact with the planar face of the triazine ring and with the substituent at R_2, respectively. ErmAM and ErmC′ were inhibited by compounds A and B at 8 and 75 μM and 7.5 and 12.5 μM, respectively (Hajduk et al., 1999).

3.5.6.2. *S*-Adenosyl-L-Homocysteine Analog

S-Adenosyl-L-homocysteine is a naturally occurring inhibitor of methyltransferase with a K_i of about 40 μM (Fig. 20).

Ten compounds were synthesized and tested for inhibitory activity against ErmAM and ErmC′. Two compounds exhibited IC_{50}s of 40 to 80 μM (Fig. 21) (Hanessian and Sgarbi, 2000).

3.5.7. Mar Inhibitors

To enlarge the potential of virulence factor inhibitors, the central regulatory pathway was focused to avoid the narrow spectrum obtained with antipili, antitoxins, etc.

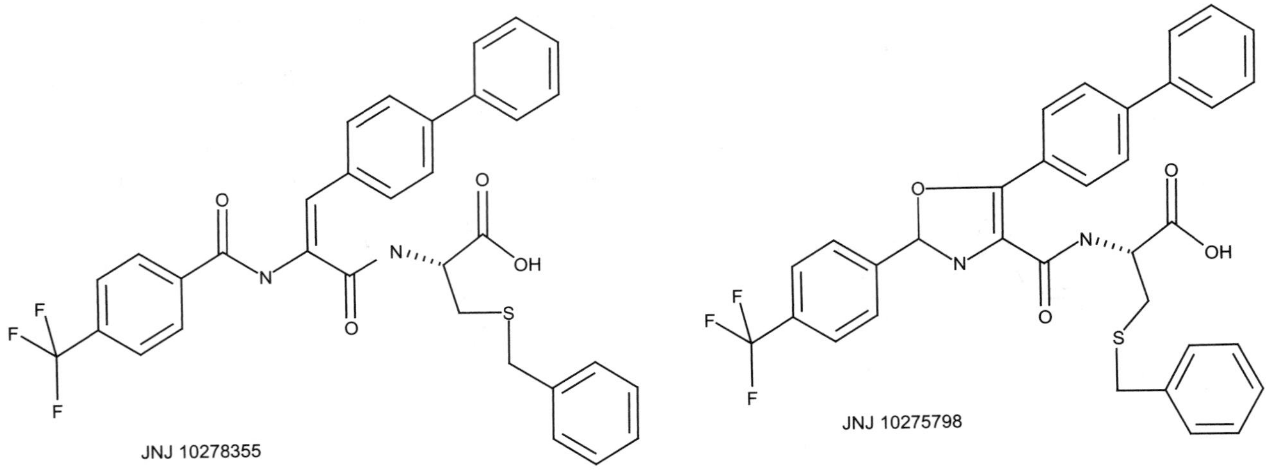

JNJ 10278355

JNJ 10275798

Figure 18 TTPS inhibitors

Table 1 Affinity for TTPS

Protein	IC_{50} (μM)	
	JNJ 10278385	JNJ 10275798
SopE	9.4	4.1
SipE	8.5	5.1
ExoU	23.5	16.8

Compounds with a benzoimidazole core were substituted (Table 2; Fig. 22) (Alekshun et al., 2004).

3.5.8. Biofilms

Biofilms are associated with many infections, both involving medical devices and not involving medical devices. Some

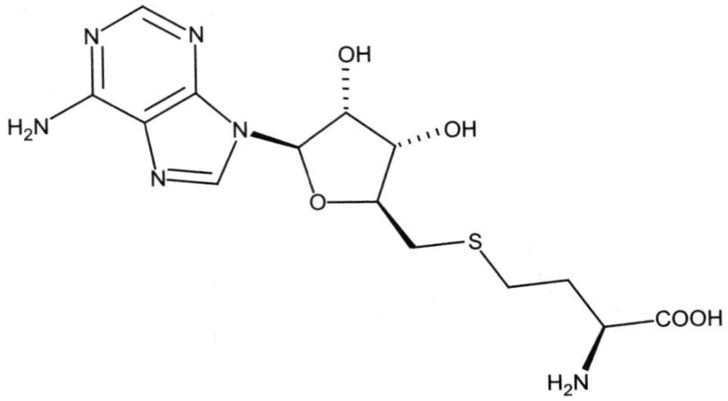

Figure 20 ERM methylase inhibitors: *S*-adenosyl-L-homocysteine

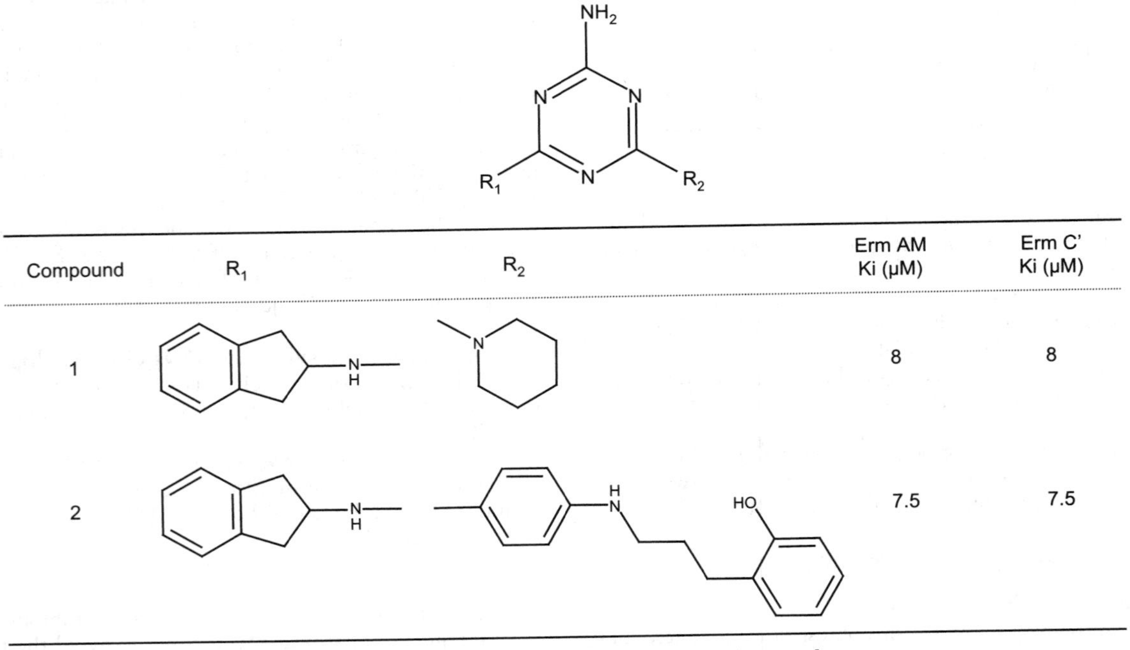

Compound	R_1	R_2	Erm AM Ki (μM)	Erm C' Ki (μM)
1			8	8
2			7.5	7.5

Figure 19 ERM methylase inhibitors: triazine analogs

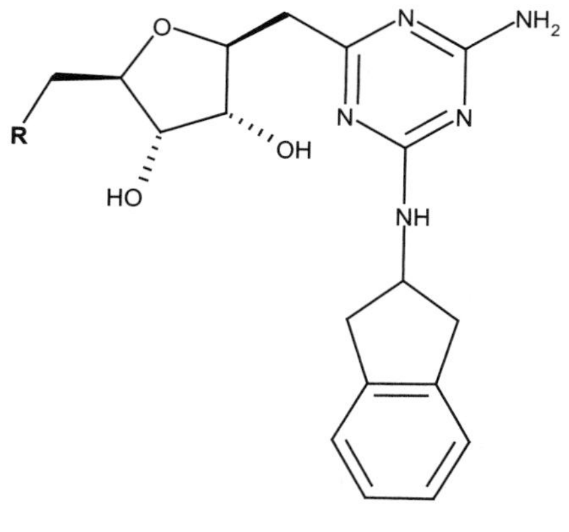

Compound	R	Ki (μM) Erm AM	Erm C'
1	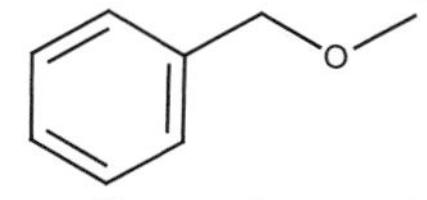	> 100	> 100
2	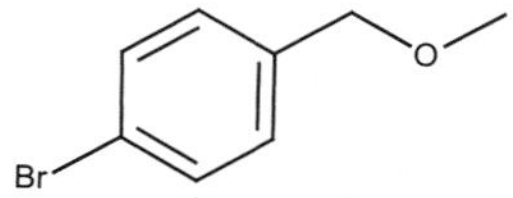 Br	-75	-40
3	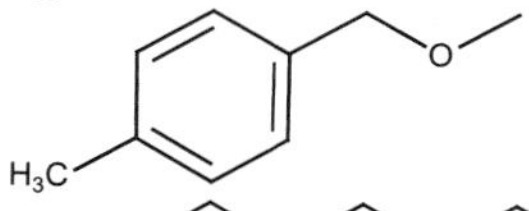 H_3C	-100	> 100
4	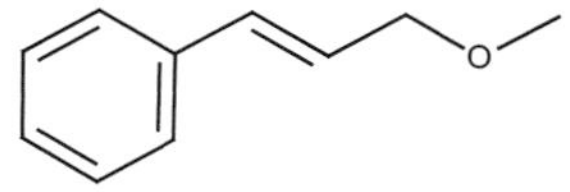	-90	-60
5	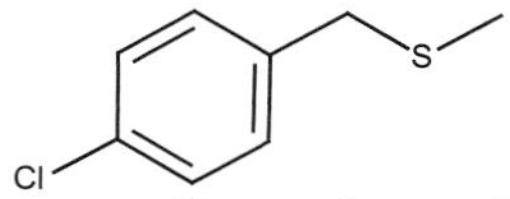 Cl	-55	-80
6	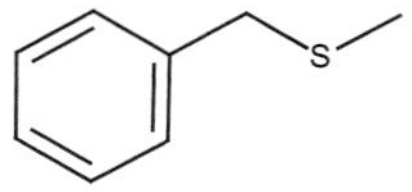	> 100	> 100

Figure 21 ERM methylase inhibitors: analogs of S-adenosyl-L-homocysteine

Table 2 Mar inhibitor activities in vitro of selected benzimidazoles[a]

Protein	IC50 (μM) of compound: 1	2	3	4	5
SoxS	8.28	3.03	4.38	0.85	2.7
MarA	11.7	ND	ND	1.2	ND
Rma	17	4.94	3.61	1.77	ND
PqrA	13.6	ND	ND	1.42	ND
Rob	28	4.73	3.45	1.34	8.01
ExsA	15.6	4.04	2.59	1.85	3.95

[a]Selected Mar inhibitors inhibited the activity of a diverse group of AraC proteins from *E. coli* (SoxC, Rob, and MarA), *Salmonella enterica* serovar Typhimurium (Rma), *Proteus mirabilis* (PqrA), and *P. aeruginosa* (ExsA). Data from Alekshun et al., 2004. IC_{50}s were determined using a dose-response analysis. ND, not determined.

compounds from Cumbre have been shown to reduce biofilms. These activities were shown to be exerted in vitro and in vivo.

3.5.9. *Clostridium histolyticum* Collagenase Inhibitor

C. histolyticum produces a collagenase which destroys the collagen that acts as a wound healer in corneal keratitis. Hydroxamates are inhibitors of these metallo(zinc)-enzymes.

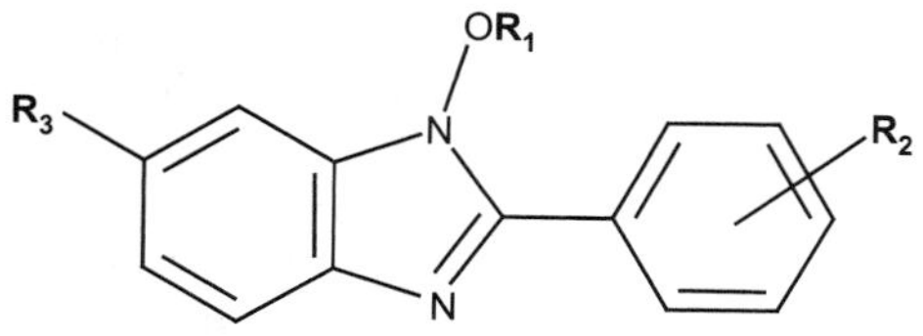

Figure 22 Mar inhibitors

The most active of the 100 derivatives prepared is a thiourea (Scozzafava and Supusan, 2000) (Fig. 23 and 24).

3.6. OPT-80

OPT-80 (Fig. 25) is an 18-membered-ring macrocyclic antibiotic, also known as tiacumicin B (Thericault et al., 1987), obtained from the fermentation broth of *Dactylosporangium aurantiacum* subsp. *handenensis*. OPT-80 is selective for *Clostridium* spp., particularly *C. difficile* and *Clostridium perfringens*. It is currently under development in the treatment of *C. difficile*-associated colitis.

Its in vitro activities (Credito and Appelbaum, 2004; Finegold et al., 2004) against some clostridia are listed in Table 3. In vitro activity against clostridia is correlated with their taxonomic clusters. The most susceptible clostridia belong to clusters I and XI.

Autism is a complex disease associated with gastrointestinal disturbances. The fecal flora of autistic patients is significantly different from that of normal subjects. There is a high incidence of *Clostridium bolteae*, often reported previously as *C. clostridioforme*. The in vitro activities of some antibacterials against *C. bolteae* are reported in Table 4.

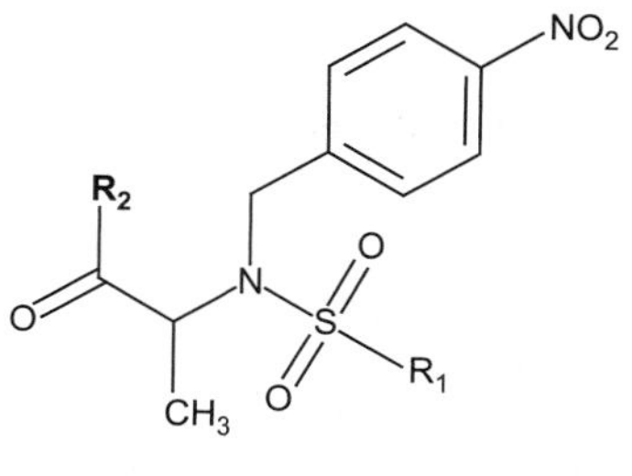

	R_2
A_1-B_{35}	OH
B_1-B_{35}	NH-OH

Figure 23 Collagenase inhibitor

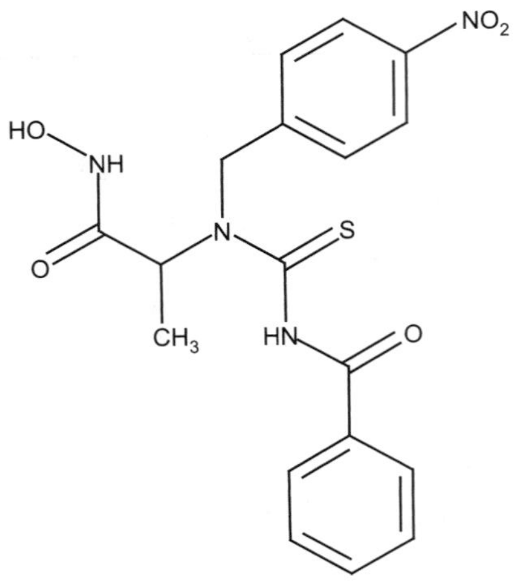

Thiourea derivative

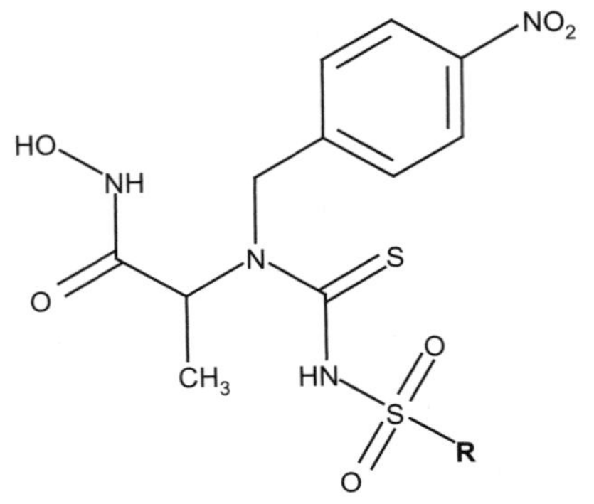

			Ki (μM)
1	4 F	C_6H_4	9
2	4 Cl	C_6H_4	7
3	4 CH_3	C_6H_4	12
4	2 CH_3	C_6H_4	8

Arylsulfonyl ureido hydroxamate derivatives

Figure 24 Collagenase inhibitor

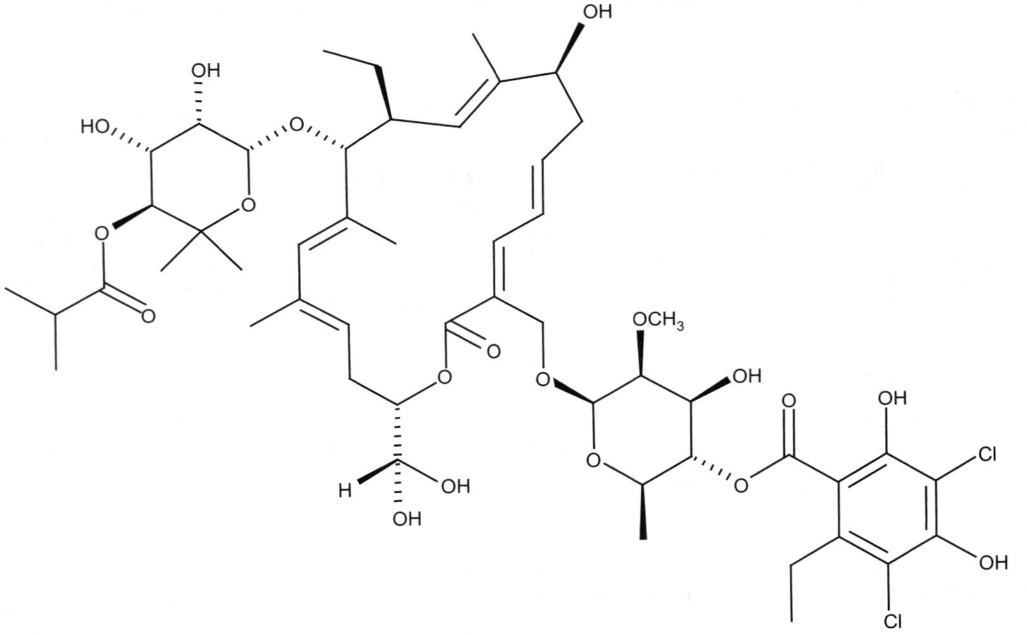

Figure 25 OPT-80

In patients, metronidazole and vancomycin (orally administered) are able to affect autistic symptoms (Finegold et al., 2002).

OPT-80 is poorly absorbed by the gastrointestinal tract: after 400 mg, a maximum concentration in serum of 26.5 ng/ml is reached after 1.5 h, and an apparent elimination half-life of 0.94 to 2.77 h was recorded. OPT-80 is unstable in urine, and 92.6% was recovered in the feces, with one metabolite, OPT-1118 (Shangle et al., 2004).

4. CONCLUSION

Anti-infective agents are not limited to antibacterial agents, and intensive research has been conducted on antifungal agents. The vast and complex world of antiprotozoal agents, however, is much more difficult to circumscribe. There is an urgent need to find agents against *Plasmodium falciparum*, but also to increase the number of agents active against *Leishmania donovani* and *Trypanosoma gambiense*, to find

Table 3 In vitro activity of OPT-80[a]

Microorganism(s)	*n*	MIC (μg/ml)[b]		
		50%	90%	Range
Bacteroides fragilis group	50	256	>1,024	
Veillonella sp.	10	32	128	
Clostridium bifermentans	9			0.25–1.0
C. bolteae	7			1.0–64
C. clostridioforme	4			0.25
C. difficile	23	0.12	0.25	
Clostridium glycolicum	9			0.06–1.0
Clostridium innocuum	9			0.25–1.0
Clostridium paraputrificum	8			0.06–8.0
C. perfringens	14	0.06	0.06	
Clostridium ramosum	10	512	512	
Clostridium sordellii	5			0.06
Other clostridia	9			0.06–>1,024
S. aureus and *S. epidermidis*	19	0.5	<1,024	
Streptococcus sp.	9			8.0–16

[a]Data from Finegold et al., 2004.
[b]50% and 90%, MICs at which 50 and 90% of isolates tested are inhibited, respectively.

Table 4 In vitro susceptibility of *C. bolteae*

Compound	MIC (μg/ml)
Co-amoxiclav	0.5–32
Ciprofloxacin	8.0–64
Clindamycin	0.5–2.0
Linezolid	4.0
Metronidazole	0.25–1.0
OPT-80	1.0–64
Tobramycin	8.0–128
Vancomycin	1.0–16

drugs active against Chagas' disease, and to produce new molecules against *Giardia lamblia*.

Less than 20% of bacterial targets are exploited as sites of action for antibacterial agents, which holds out some hope for the future, even if the discovery and exploitation of new drug entities constitute a difficult, long, and arbitrary task.

The situation as regards antibacterial agents at the moment is not yet critical but might become so if nothing is found rapidly. Difficulties are often associated with development, and the interval between synthesis, selection, and availability to the medical profession is rarely less than about 6 years.

REFERENCES

Alekshun MN, Barlett VJ, Bowser T, Verma A, Grier M, Warchol T, Ohemeng K, Levy SB, Tanaka SK, 2004, Novel anti-infective agents, small molecule transcription factor modulators, 44th Intersci Conf Antimicrob Agents Chemother, abstract F-1523.

Barluenga S, Simosen KB, Littlefeld ES, Ayida BK, Vourloumis D, Winters GC, Takahashi M, Shandrick S, Zhao Q, Han Q, Hermann T, 2004, Rational design of azepane-glycoside antibiotics targeting the bacterial ribosome, Bioorg Med Chem Lett, 14, 713–718.

Bryskier A, 1995, Penems: new oral β-lactam drugs, Expert Opin Invest Drugs, 4, 705–724.

Bryskier A, 1996, Dual β-lactam-fluoroquinolone compounds, a novel approach to antibacterial treatment, Exp Opin Invest Drugs, 6, 1479–1499.

Butler NM, Barnes MH, Zhi C, Long ZY, Xu WC, Brown NC, Leighton JJ, Wright GE, Bowlin TL, 2004, Inhibition of Bacillus anthracis DNA polymerases and cell growth by derivatives of the anilino-uracil family, 44th Intersci Conf Antimicrob Agents Chemother, abstract F-732.

Bzowska A, Kulikowska E, Sugar D, 1992, Formycins A and B and some analogues, selective inhibitors of bacterial (E. coli) purine nucleoside phosphatase, Biochim Biophys Acta, 1120, 239–247.

Champney WS, 2003, Bacterial ribosomal subunit assembly is an antibiotic target, Curr Top Med Chem, 3, 929–947.

Chantot JF, Klich M, Teutsch G, Bryskier A, Collette P, Markus A, Seibert G, 1992, Antibacterial activity of RU44790, a new N-tetrazolyl monocyclic beta-lactam, Antimicrob Agents Chemother, 36, 1756–1763.

Chevalier J, Bredin J, Mahamoud A, Mallea M, Barbe J, Pages JM, 2004, Inhibitors of antibiotic efflux in resistant Enterobacter aerogenes and Klebsiella pneumoniae strains, Antimicrob Agents Chemother, 48, 1043–1046.

Choi KH, Heath RJ, Rock CO, 2000, β-Ketoacyl-acyl carrier protein synthase III (FabH) is a determining factor in branched-chain fatty acid biosynthesis, J Bacteriol, 182, 365–370.

Clements JM, Coignard F, Johnson I, Chandler S, Palan S, Waller A, Wijkmans J, Hunter MG, 2002, Antibacterial activities and characterization of novel inhibitors of LpxC, Antimicrob Agents Chemother, 46, 1793–1799.

Cole PJ, 2001, The role of nebulized antibiotics in treating serious respiratory infections, J Chemother, 13, 354–362.

Cosquer A, Ficamos M, Jebbar M, Corbel JC, Choquet G, Fontenelle C, Uriac P, Bernard T, 2004, Antibacterial activity of glycine betaine analogues, involvement of osmotransporters, Bioorg Med Chem Lett, 14, 2061–2065.

Credito KL, Appelbaum PC, 2004, Activity of OPT 80, a novel macrocyclic, compared with those of eight other agents against selected anaerobic species, Antimicrob Agents Chemother, 48, 4430–4434.

Dale GE, Broger C, D'Arcy A, Hartman PG, DeHoogt R, Jolidon S, Kompis I, Labhardt PG, Langen H, Locher H, Page MGP, Stüber D, Then RL, Wipf B, Oefner C, 1997, Single amino acid substitution in Staphylococcus aureus dihydrofolate reductase determines trimethoprim resistance, J Mol Biol, 266, 23–30.

Demers JP, Bernstein JI, Fernandez JA, et al, 1997, The identification of RWJ 49,815, a novel inhibitor of bacterial two-component regulatory systems and a potent gram-positive antibacterial, 37th Intersci Conf Antimicrob Agents Chemother, abstract F-227, p 185.

Denoya C, Dubnan D, 1989, Mono-and dimethylating activities and kinetic studies of the ErmC 23S rRNA methyltransferase, J Biol Chem, 264, 2615–2624.

Evans JM, Turner BA, Bowen S, Ho AM, Sarver RW, Benson E, Parker CN, 2003, Inhibition of bacterial IF-2 binding to fMet-tRNA(fmet) by aminoglycosides, Bioorg Med Chem Lett, 13, 993-996.

Fernandez J, Abbanat D, Bush K, Hilliard J, Guan Q, Li X, Macielag M, Goldschmidt RM, 2004, In vivo efficacy of the bacterial type III protein secretion system (TTPS) inhibitors JNJ 10275798 and JNJ 19278385, 44th Intersci Conf Antimicrob Agents Chemother, abstract F-710.

Finegold SM, et al, 2002, Gastrointestinal microflora studies in late-onset autism, Clin Infect Dis, 35, suppl 1, S6–S16.

Finegold SM, Moletoris D, Vaisanen ML, Song Y, Liu C, Bolanos M, 2004, In vitro activities of OPT-80 and comparator drugs against intestinal bacteria, Antimicrob Agents Chemother, 48, 4898–4902.

Forsch RA, Queener SF, Rosowsky A, 2004, Preliminary in vitro studies on two potent, water-soluble trimethoprim analogues with exceptional species selectivity against dihydrofolate reductase from Pneumocystis carinii and Mycobacterium avium, Bioorg Med Chem Lett, 14, 1811–1815.

Ghosh M, Miller MJ, 1995, Design, synthesis and biological evaluation of isocyanurate-based antifungal and macrolide antibiotic conjugates, iron transport-mediated drug delivery, Bioorg Med Chem, 3, 1519–1525.

Ghosh P, 2004, Process of protein transport by the type III secretion system, Microbiol Mol Biol Rev, 68, 771–795.

Gobec S, Plantan I, Mravljak J, Wilson RA, Besra GS, Kiklj D, 2004, Phosphonate inhibitors of antigen 85 C, a crucial enzyme involved in the biosynthesis of Mycobacterium tuberculosis cell wall, Bioorg Med Chem Lett, 14, 3559–3562.

Guiles J, Janjic N, Sun X, Tregay M, Smith S, Critchley IA, Stone I, Ochsner U, Green L, Bertin J, Lin Y, Dallman HG, McHenry CS, 2004, 5-Benzylidene-2-thioxo-thiazolidin-4-ones, inhibitors of DNA polymerase III holoenzyme and potential new antibacterial agents, 44th Intersci Conf Antimicrob Agents Chemother, abstract F-731.

Hajduk PJ, Dinges J, Schkeryantz JM, Janowick D, Kaminski M, Tufano M, Augeri DJ, Petros A, Nienaber V, Zhong P, Hammond R, Coen M, Beutel B, Katz L, Fesik SW, 1999, Novel inhibitors of Erm methyltransferases from NMR and parallel synthesis, J Med Chem, 42, 3852–3859.

Hanessian S, Sgarbi PWM, 2000, Design and synthesis of mimics of S-adenosyl-L-homocysteine as potential inhibitors of erythromycin methyltransferases, Bioorg Med Chem Lett, 10, 433–437.

He X, Reynolds KA, 2002, Purification, characterization, and identification of novel inhibitors of the β-ketoacyl-acyl carrier protein synthase III (FabH) from Staphylococcus aureus, Antimicrob Agents Chemother, 46, 1310–1318.

He Y, Yang J, Wu B, Risen L, Swayze EE, 2004, Synthesis and biological evaluations of novel benzoimidazoles as potential antibacterial agents, Bioorg Med Chem Lett, 14, 1217–1220.

Heath RJ, White SW, Rock CO, 2002, Inhibitors of fatty acid synthesis as antimicrobial chemotherapeutics, Appl Microb Biotechnol, 58, 695–703.

Heffron SE, Jurnak F, 2000, Structure of an EF-Tu complex with thiazolyl peptide antibiotic determined at 3.5 Å resolution, atomic basis for GE 2270 A inhibition of EF-Tu, Biochemistry, 39, 37–45.

Hoang TT, Schweizer HP, 1997, Fatty acid biosynthesis in P. aeruginosa, cloning and characterization of the fabAB operon encoding β-hydroxyacyl-acyl carrier protein dehydratase (FabA) and β-ketoacyl-acyl carrier protein synthase I (FabB), J Bacteriol, 179, 5326–5332.

Hopmann C, Kurz M, Brönstrup M, Wink J, LeBeller D, 2002, Isolation and elucidation of vancoresmycin—a new antibiotic from Amycolatopsis sp. ST 101170, Tetrahedron Lett, 41, 435–438.

Hubschwerlen C, Specklin JL, Baeschlin DK, Borer Y, Haefeli S, Sigwalt C, Schroeder S, Locher HH, 2003, Structure-activity relationship in the oxazolidinone-quinolone hybrid series, influence of the central spacer on the antibacterial activity and the mode of action, Bioorg Med Chem Lett, 13, 4229–4233.

Jackowski S, Murphy CM, Cronan JE, Rock CO, 1989, Acetoacetyl-acyl carrier protein synthase, J Biol Chem, 264, 7624–7629.

Jarvest RL, Berge JM, Houge-Frydrych CSV, Janson C, Mensah LM, O'Hanlon PJ, Pope A, Saldanha A, Qiu X, 1999, Interaction of tyrosyl aryl dipeptides with S. aureus tyrosyl tRNA synthetase, inhibition and crystal structure of a complex, Bioorg Med Chem Lett, 9, 2859–2862.

Jayasekera MMK, Onheiher K, Keith J, Venkatesan H, Santillan A, Stocking EM, Tang L, Miller J, Gomez L, Rhead B, Delcamp T, Huang S, Walin R, Bobkova EV, Shaw KJ, 2005, Identification of novel inhibitors of bacterial translation elongation factors, Antimicrob Agents Chemother, 49, 131–136.

Kane JL Jr, Hirth BH, Liang B, Gourlie BB, Nahill S, Barsomian G, 2003, Ureas of 5-aminopyrazole and 2-aminothiazole inhibit growth of gram-positive bacteria, Bioorg Med Chem Lett, 13, 4463–4466.

Kaneda T, 1991, Iso and antiiso-fatty acids in bacteria, biosynthesis, function, and taxonomic significance, Microb Rev, 55, 288–302.

Khabnadideh S, Tan CL, Croft SL, Kendrick H, Yardley V, Gilbert IH, 2000, Squalamine analogues as potential anti-trypanosomal and anti-leishmanial compounds, Bioorg Med Chem Lett, 10, 1237–1239.

Li X, Quan Q, Macielag M, Murray W, Fernandez J, Montenegro D, Bush K, Goldschmidt R, 2004, Synthesis and SAR of inhibitors of bacterial type III protein secretion, 44th Intersci Conf Antimicrob Agents Chemother, abstract F-711.

Licata L, Melton JL, Fernandez JA, et al, 1997, In vitro characterization of a novel class of antibacterial agents that inhibit bacterial two-component systems, 37th Intersci Conf Antimicrob Agents Chemother, abstract F-226, p 184.

Macielag MJ, Bernstein J, Demers JP, et al, 1997, Antibacterial salicylamides that inhibit bacterial two-component regulatory systems, 37th Intersci Conf Antimicrob Agents Chemother, abstract F-228, p 185.

Margolis P, Hackbarth C, Lopez S, White R, Trias J, 1999a, Resistance to deformylase inhibitor VRC483 is caused by mutation in formyl transferase, 39th Intersci Conf Antimicrob Agents Chemother, abstract 1795, p 334.

Margolis P, Young D, Yuan Z, Wang W, Trias J, 1999b, Peptide deformylase as a target for discovery of novel antibacterial agents, 39th Intersci Conf Antimicrob Agents Chemother, abstract 1793, p 333.

Mauvais P, Dupuis-Hamelin C, Lassaigne P, Bonnefoy A, Shoot B, Musicki B, Haesslein J, Ferroud D, Klich M, Rowlands D, Lorenzon G, Vicat P, Julien P, Hamon G, 1999, Novel coumarin antibiotics. II. In vitro and in vivo activity of RU 79115, 39th Intersci Conf Antimicrob Agents Chemother, abstract 563, p 309.

Mazel D, Pochet S, Marliere P, 1994, Genetic characterization of polypeptide deformylase, a distinctive enzyme of eubacterial translation, EMBO J, 13, 914–923.

McNally VA, Gbaj A, Douglas KT, Stratford IJ, Jaffar M, Freeman S, Bryce RA, 2003, Identification of a novel class of inhibitor of human and E. coli thymidine phosphorylase by in silico screening, Bioorg Med Chem Lett, 13, 3705–3709.

Parrish NM, Houston T, Jones PB, Townsend C, Dick JD, 2001, In vitro activity of a novel antimycobacterial compound, N-octanesulfonylacetamide, and its effects on lipid and mycolic acid synthesis, Antimicrob Agents Chemother, 45, 1143–1150.

Payne DJ, et al, 2002, Discovery of a novel and potent class of FabI directed antibacterial agents, Antimicrob Agents Chemother, 46, 3118–3124.

Rittenhouse S, Moore T, Donald B, Hunt E, Woodnutt G, 1999, In vitro activity of two novel pleuromutilin derivatives, SB-247386 and SB-268091, 39th Intersci Conf Antimicrob Agents Chemother, abstract 1805, p 337.

Sbardella G, Mai A, Artico M, Loddo R, Setzu MG, La Colla P, 2004, Synthesis and in vitro antimycobacterial activity of novel 3-(1H-pyrrol-1-yl)-2-oxazolidinone analogues of PNU-100480, Bioorg Med Chem Lett,14, 1537–1541.

Scozzafava A, Supusan CT, 2000, Protease inhibitors, synthesis of Clostridium histolyticum collagenase inhibitors incorporating sulfonyl-L-alanine hydroxamate moieties, Bioorg Med Chem Lett, 10, 499–502.

Shangle S, Lee C, Okamu F, Walsh B, Sears P, Shue YK, Gorbach S, Preston RA, 2004, Safety and pharmacokinetics of OPT 80 in human volunteers, 44th Intersci Conf Antimicrob Agents Chemother, abstract A-5.

Singleton MR, Wigley DB, 2002, Modularity and specialization in superfamily 1 and 2 helicases, J Bacteriol, 184, 1819–1826.

Snyder NJ, Meier TL, Wu CE, Letourneau DL, Zhao G, Tabbe M, 2000, Discovery of a series of compounds that demonstrate potent broad spectrum antibacterial activity and inhibition of Era, an essential bacterial GTPase, 40th Intersci Conf Antimicrob Agents Chemother, abstract 2028, p 225.

Stojiljkovic I, Evavold BD, Kumar V, 2000, Antimicrobial properties of porphyrins, Exp Opin Invest Drugs, 10, 309–320.

Tanitame A, Oyamada Y, Ofuji K, Kyoya Y, Suzuki K, Ito H, Kawasaki M, Nagai K, Wachi M, Yamagishi JI, 2004, Design, synthesis and structure-activity relationship studies of novel indazole analogues as DNA gyrase inhibitors with Gram-positive antibacterial activity, Bioorg Med Chem Lett, 14, 2857–2862.

Tarantino PM Jr, Zhi C, Wright GE, Brown NC, 1999, Inhibitors of DNA polymerase III as novel antimicrobial agents against Gram-positive eubacteria, Antimicrob Agents Chemother, 43, 1982–1987.

Thericault RJ, Karlowski JP, Jackson M, Girolimi RL, Sunga BN, Vojtko CM, Coen LJ, 1987, Tiacumicins, a novel complex of 18-membered macrolide antibiotics. I. Taxonomy, fermentation, and antibacterial activity, J Antibiot, 40, 567–574.

Verloumis D, Takahashi M, Winters GC, Simonsen KB, Ayida BK, Barluenga S, Qamar S, Shandrick S, Zhao Q, Hermann T, 2002, Novel 2,5-dideoxystreptamine derivatives targeting the ribosomal decoding site RNA, Bioorg Med Chem Lett, 12, 3367–3372.

Weisblum B, 1995, Erythromycin resistance by ribosome modification, Antimicrob Agents Chemother, 39, 577–585.

Wright GE, Brown NC, 1999, DNA polymerase III, a new target for antibiotic development, Curr Opin Antiinfect Invest Drugs, 7, 45–48.

Yu XY, Finn J, Hill JM, Wang ZG, Keith D, Silverman J, Oliver N, 2004, A series of spirocyclic analogues as potent inhibitors of bacterial phenylalanyl tRNA synthetases, Bioorg Med Chem Lett, 14, 1339–1342.

Systemic Antifungal Agents

R. GRILLOT AND B. LEBEAU

52

1. INTRODUCTION

Antifungal therapy really developed over the past two decades; very few systemic antifungal agents had been available in the period from 1960 until then. Amphotericin B (AMB), which is very effective but toxic, for a long time remained the only truly suitable agent. This inertia was justified by the rarity of systemic mycoses, apart from certain tropical mycoses with a well-defined geographical distribution.

Three factors have totally altered this situation: the growing incidence of septicemia due to invasive yeasts and of aspergillosis as a result of the use of more effective, but also more aggressive, medical and surgical therapies, the rapid emergence of AIDS, and the appearance of new opportunistic fungi. The appearance also in the 1980s of a new class of antifungals, the azoles, then in the 1990s the targeted delivery of AMB and the development of second- and third-generation azole antifungals (see below) and subsequently new classes of antifungals, have completely changed the therapeutic panorama at the dawn of the 21st century.

In fact, the difficulties arising from the development of an antifungal compound should not be underestimated. These difficulties relate to the fungi themselves, the territory they invade, and, lastly, the antifungal agents. Some of the main limiting factors are noted here. The presence of a thick polysaccharide cell wall in micromycetes prevents the intracellular penetration of a number of molecules and implies specific physicochemical characteristics in them. The already evolved structure of the fungal cell (fungi are eukaryotes), which likens it to the mammalian cell, also explains the toxicity of a number of antifungal agents to the host organism. In addition, the majority of fungi are not parasites but usually belong to the commensal flora in humans: it is the collapse of the usual defense mechanisms that provides the basis for opportunistic disease and that explains the frequent therapeutic failures in immunodepressed patients (e.g., those treated with cancer chemotherapy or suffering from AIDS). Lastly, the majority of current antifungal agents have a fungistatic and not a fungicidal action at the usual therapeutic doses, a phenomenon that entails long-term treatments to obtain a mycological cure.

With respect to the research necessary for their development, in the case of the azole series, for example, this is confronted with difficulties associated with the in vitro screening of molecules. The evaluation of their efficacy is highly dependent on the experimental conditions, a phenomenon that requires the use of animal experimental models.

These obstacles of various kinds explain the limited number of systemic antifungals available to us today. The current development of deep mycoses therefore requires the restitution of older medications and the positioning of the most recent ones, which is the aim of this survey. Only systemic antifungals are discussed here, while products used for their local action (cutaneous or mucocutaneous, including digestive) are mentioned only for information (Table 1).

Schematically, the current systemic antifungals can be divided into two categories: that of the antifungal antibiotics, which include griseofulvin and AMB, and that of the chemical agents, which comprise all of the other molecules, flucytosine (5FC), the extremely rich series of azoles (ketoconazole, fluconazole, itraconazole, and, in the near future, voriconazole) and, more recently, the allylamines (terbinafine) and echinocandins (caspofungin). The lack of homogeneity among these different antifungals requires them to be considered separately.

2. ANTIFUNGAL ANTIBIOTICS

2.1. Griseofulvin

2.1.1. Introduction

Isolated from *Penicillium griseofulvum* in 1939, griseofulvin was not used therapeutically until 1958, thanks to Gentles, who had the idea of administering it orally in the treatment of tinea, first experimentally in the guinea pig and then in humans. This was a complete revolution in the treatment of these infections, for which at the time only epilatory radiotherapy was available. Its anti-inflammatory properties were discovered shortly afterwards.

Its excellent activity against dermatophytes explains why this antifungal still remains the major treatment of tinea of the scalp (and possibly of other extensive or refractory dermatophyte lesions).

Figure 1 shows the chemical structure of griseofulvin.

2.1.2. Physicochemical Properties

Table 2 lists the physicochemical properties of griseofulvin.

Table 1 Principal local antifungals (cutaneous and/or mucosal mycoses)[a]

Class	Active substance	Spectrum	Indications	Remarks
Antibiotics				
Polyenes	AMB	Yeasts (*Candida* spp., *M. furfur*) *Geotrichum* spp.	Gastrointestinal mycoses, cutaneous and vaginal candidosis, seborrheic dermatitis	
	Nystatin	Yeasts	Cutaneous, vaginal, and digestive candidosis	In certain dosage forms, combination of antibiotic(s) and sometimes a corticosteroid
Benzohydrofuran	Griseofulvin	Dermatophytes	Dermatophyte infections	Adjuvant for oral treatment
Sulfur derivative	Selenium sulfide	*M. furfur*	Pityriasis versicolor, seborrheic dermatitis of the scalp	Prior loosening with Mercryl Lauryle
Thiocarbamate	Tolnaftate	Dermatophytes ± *M. furfur*	Dermatophyte infections (other than tinea)	
Morpholine	Amorolfine	Dermatophytes	Dermatophyte nail infections	
Pyridone	Ciclopirox olamine	Yeasts (*Candida* spp., *M. furfur*) Dermatophytes	Cutaneous candidosis Dermatophyte infections (other than tinea) Pityriasis versicolor	Penetrates nail keratin Also bactericidal (gram-positive and -negative flora)
Imidazoles	Miconazole[b]	Yeasts (*Candida* spp., *M. furfur*) *Geotrichum* Dermatophytes	Gastrointestinal mycoses Cutaneous and vaginal candidosis Dermatophyte infections Pityriasis versicolor	
	Omoconazole[b]	See miconazole	Cutaneous and vaginal candidosis Dermatophyte infections Pityriasis versicolor	
	Oxiconazole[b]	See omoconazole	See omoconazole	
	Fenticonazole[b]	See oxiconazole	See oxiconazole	
	Tioconazole[b]	Yeasts (*Candida* spp., *M. furfur*) Dermatophytes Some moulds	See fenticonazole	
	Econazole	See tioconazole	See tioconazole	
	Isoconazole	See econazole	See econazole	
	Bifoconazole	Yeasts (*Candida* spp., *M. furfur*) Dermatophytes	Cutaneous candidosis Dermatophyte infections Pityriasis versicolor	
	Ketoconazole	See bifoconazole	Gastrointestinal mycoses Cutaneous candidosis Dermatophyte infections Pityriasis versicolor	
	Sertaconazole	*Candida* spp. Dermatophytes	Cutaneous and vaginal candidosis Dermatophyte infections	
	Butoconazole	*Candida* spp.	Vaginal yeast infections	Also bactericidal (gram-positive flora)

[a]Only systemic antifungals are discussed here, while products used for their local action (cutaneous or mucocutaneous, including digestive) are only mentioned for information.

[b]This product is also bactericidal to gram-positive bacteria. Irritation or sensitization due to active substance or excipient is rare. For tinea, adjuvant is used for systemic treatment.

2.1.3. In Vitro Properties

The spectrum of griseofulvin is limited exclusively to dermatophytes. The MICs are between 0.10 and 2.5 μg/ml depending on the genus: *Microsporum*, *Trichophyton*, or *Epidermophyton* (MIC expressed after 5 days of culture in liquid Sabouraud medium). Its in vitro and in vivo action is essentially fungistatic in nature, and clinically the appearance of resistant strains is extremely rare.

For all other agents of fungal infections, resistance is customary, whether in the case of yeasts (*Candida*, *Cryptococcus*, and *Malassezia*), moulds (*Aspergillus* and other hyaline hyphomycetes, *Dematiaceae*, and *Mucoraceae*), dimorphic

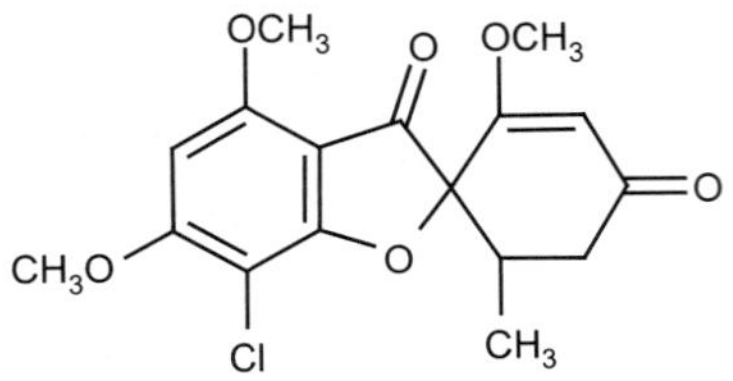

Figure 1 Griseofulvin chemical structure

fungi (*Histoplasma*, *Blastomyces*, *Coccidioides*, and *Sporothrix*), or again fungal or bacterial agents of mycetomas.

2.1.4. Mechanism of Action

As for many old molecules, the mechanism of antifungal action of griseofulvin is not fully understood. Moreover, this action is fairly surprising since it is specifically by inhibiting fungal keratolysis in the hair that its antidermatophytic action is predominantly exerted. Thus, during treatment, griseofulvin binds in the bulb and then accompanies the hair in the course of its growth. Impregnation of the hair with the antibiotic inhibits the keratolytic action of the fungus and thus causes resistance to invasion. However, this phenomenon is not indefinite, so treatment must be continued for several weeks to prevent any relapse.

This has led to an examination of the action of griseofulvin on the fungal cell. Various hypotheses have been advanced, but none in itself is entirely satisfactory and they are probably complementary, viz.

- Inhibitory action on the development of certain wall components, including chitin
- Antimitotic properties (of the colchicine type) by spindle inhibition
- An action on wall synthesis causing chemical structural modifications of the cell wall (phenomenon described under the name of "curling effect," with thickening and winding of the terminal hyphae)

Consequently, at present we can observe that griseofulvin is used successfully to treat dermatophyte infections, but without knowing exactly how it acts on the cellular and molecular levels.

The same applies to its anti-inflammatory properties: apart from its antifungal action, griseofulvin also has a noncortisone and vasotropic anti-inflammatory action at high doses, hence its indications in certain rheumatic conditions and in Raynaud syndrome.

2.1.5. Mechanism of Resistance

The explanation of the resistance of micromycetes that are nonsusceptible to griseofulvin from the outset (all fungi except dermatophytes) exhibits the same lack of precision. The following are postulated:

- The role of the wall constituents, which have a low chitin content (but it is not possible, for instance, to explain the nonsusceptibility of *Aspergillus niger*, which has a very chitin-rich wall)
- The impermeability of the fungal cell: the wall might bind the antibiotic and prevents its penetration or cause demethylation of griseofulvin and its transformation to inactive compounds through the elaboration of enzymes

2.1.6. Pharmacokinetics

Table 3 shows the pharmacokinetics of griseofulvin.

2.1.7. Tolerability, Adverse Effects, Interactions, and Contraindications

Table 4 shows the tolerability, adverse effects, interactions, and contraindications of griseofulvin.

2.1.8. Clinical Indications

Its indication is limited to dermatophyte infections. Some of these mycoses require systemic treatment and administration must be prolonged, as the growth of keratin is slow. The duration of treatment varies with the localization:

- Tinea capitis, 1 to 2 months
- Onychomycoses, several months
- Extensive dermatophyte infections of the hairless skin (*Trichophyton rubrum*), 1 to 4 months

The dosage is 500 mg or 1 g daily in adults and 10 mg/kg of body weight/day in children (administered in two doses during meals with a lipid).

Local application of an antifungal combined with systemic treatment is recommended.

2.1.9. Pharmaceutical Preparations

Griseofulvin is available as 250- and 500-mg tablets under several usp names in the United States and Grisefuline in Europe.

2.2. Polyene Antifungals

2.2.1. AMB

2.2.1.1. Introduction

The *Streptomyces* group is the source of the production of numerous polyene antibiotics possessing antifungal activity, for example, nystatin (1954), AMB (1958), natamycin (1958), and mepartricin (1975). All of these molecules are cyclic, closed by an internal ester bond, and comprise two parts: a rigid apolar part composed of conjugated double bonds (two to seven) and a polar part comprising a large number of hydroxyl groups and an amino sugar, mycosamine.

Table 2 Physicochemical properties of griseofulvin

Empirical formula	Mol wt	Solubility	Stability
$C_{17}H_{17}ClO_6$	352.8	Insoluble in water	Stable at room temperature if protected from light
		Soluble in alcohol and organic solvents	Stable against autoclaving if not in solution

Table 3 Pharmacokinetics of griseofulvin

Parameter	Description
Absorption in healthy volunteers	Intestinal, varies substantially from subject to subject Improved: By the microcrystalline form By administration during a high-fat meal 1 g per os: low levels in blood (peak concn in serum at 4 h of 1.5–2 μg/ml), plasma half-life of 10–15 h, traces after 72 h
Excretion	Majority of the product in the stools in the active free form
Metabolism	Hepatic demethylation (enzyme-inducing effect) → inactive 6-demethyl-griseofulvin, eliminated in the urine (1%) in the glucuroconjugated form
Distribution	Plasma protein binding: 80% Good skin penetration (hence therapeutic value): After 2–3 days: detectable in upper part of stratum corneum After 15 days: reaches halfway through corneal layer After 25–30 days: reaches surface of skin
Renal insufficiency	No accumulation (dosage unchanged) Nondialyzable
Hepatic insufficiency	Vigilance during long-term treatment
Children and elderly subjects	No data

Table 4 Tolerability of griseofulvin

Parameter	Description
Tolerability	Usually excellent
Adverse effects	Rarely reported in prolonged treatments: Allergic cutaneous reactions and photosensitization Transient gastrointestinal disorders (nausea, diarrhea, and dyspepsia), exceptionally entailing the discontinuation of treatment Neurotoxic disorders (headache, dizziness, asthenia, and insomnia) potentiated by alcohol Induction or exacerbation of lupus erythematosus Hematologic disorders (leukopenia, neutropenia, and anemia) Episodes of acute porphyria in subjects suffering from porphyria Teratogenic effect detected in animals, and for humans very rare cases of fetal malformations attributable to griseofulvin have been reported
Interactions	Alcohol: antabuse effect Enzyme-inducing effect of griseofulvin: reduces the efficacy of estrogen-progesterone combinations, oral anticoagulants, oral antidiabetics, cyclosporine Potentiates the hepatotoxicity of other medications with a hepatic metabolism: ketoconazole (leave an interval of 1 month) and isoniazid Absorption reduced by certain barbiturates or hypnotics
Contraindications	Allergy to griseofulvin Pregnancy Lupus erythematosus
Precautions	Monitoring: Increased in patients with hepatic insufficiency Of blood count during prolonged treatment
Changes in laboratory test results	Reduction of uricemia Leukopenia and hypochromic anemia Retention of bromosulfophthalein

This structure assimilates them to the macrolide antibiotics, but not polyenes such as erythromycin, hence the name polyene macrolides for them.

Their antifungal spectrum is very broad and is not restricted to micromycetes, since they are active against certain protozoa (*Naegleria*, *Trichomonas* and *Leishmania*) and algae (*Prothoteca*), but they possess no antibacterial or antiviral activity. However, their use in antifungal chemotherapy is limited by their toxicity when they are administered parenterally, whereas orally their tolerability is excellent since they are not reabsorbed. Of the polyene antifungals that have been used in the treatment of fungal infections, the majority are used only as oral and/or local contact antifungals. Conversely, AMB can also be used systemically. Moreover, AMB is the major first-line antifungal agent, the most effective in a number of clinical systemic mycoses. Its very broad spectrum also means that it constitutes the reference for evaluating any new molecule with antifungal activity. However, the many toxic phenomena that AMB causes when used intravenously have resulted in the last few years in research into new dosage forms designed to reduce its in vivo toxicity, while still preserving its activity against the fungal cell. This research has been the source of new formulations involving incorporation in liposomes (AMB and liposomal nystatin) or in combination with lipids (AMB lipid complex [ABLC] and colloidal dispersion [ABCD]), opening up extensive therapeutic vistas.

Consequently, in the case of the polyene macrolides, we confine our comments to the characteristics of AMB, the only commercially available systemic antifungal agent in this group (in its conventional intravenous and lipid formulations).

2.2.1.2. Chemical Structure

Resulting from the fermentation process of a soil actinomycete, *Streptomyces nodosus* (Dutcher, Squibb Laboratories, 1953), this polyene macrolide comprises seven double bonds (heptaene) responsible for the marked lipophilia of the molecule (Fig. 2).

2.2.1.3. Physicochemical Properties

AMB is a particularly insoluble yellow powder (Table 5): the presence of bile salts (sodium deoxycholate) allows the formation of mixed micelles with AMB and solubilization of the antibiotic. However, as the deoxycholate-AMB association constant is weak, below a certain critical concentration the complex dissociates and AMB is found isolated in the aqueous medium.

This instability of AMB justifies the many precautions that need to be taken during intravenous administration, since any precipitation increases the toxic phenomena: only 5% glucose serum is sufficient for producing this suspension.

2.2.1.4. In Vitro Properties and Spectrum of Activity

The antifungal spectrum of this compound is particularly broad, since the very great majority of fungi are susceptible to very low concentrations of AMB (generally at a MIC of <0.5 μg/ml), a property justifying its designation as a major antifungal agent:

- Yeasts: *Candida* spp. and *Cryptococcus neoformans*
- Filamentous fungi: *Aspergillus* spp. and *Mucorales*
- Yeast forms of dimorphic fungi: *Histoplasma*, *Blastomyces*, and *Coccidioides*

Conversely, AMB has variable activity against potential new opportunistic agents of deep mycoses: *Trichosporon cutaneum* (syn. *Trichosporon beigelii*), *Malassezia furfur* (0.3 to 2.5 μg/ml), *Fusarium*, and dematiaceous hyphomycetes such as *Bipolaris*, *Curvularia*, *Alternaria*, *Wangiella*, and *Cladosporium*.

Resistant strains are exceptional (MIC, >2 μg/ml) and principally involve *Candida lusitaniae* and the majority of strains of *Scedosporium apiospermum* (syn. *Pseudallescheria boydii*) and *Scedosporium inflatum*.

The in vitro determination of susceptibility to polyene antifungals presents no specific difficulties, as this is relatively independent of any variation in the experimental parameters (inoculum size and composition of the medium). Only the presence of sterols in the culture medium may affect the MIC determination (Casitone-type peptone medium is recommended, although there is no real standardization).

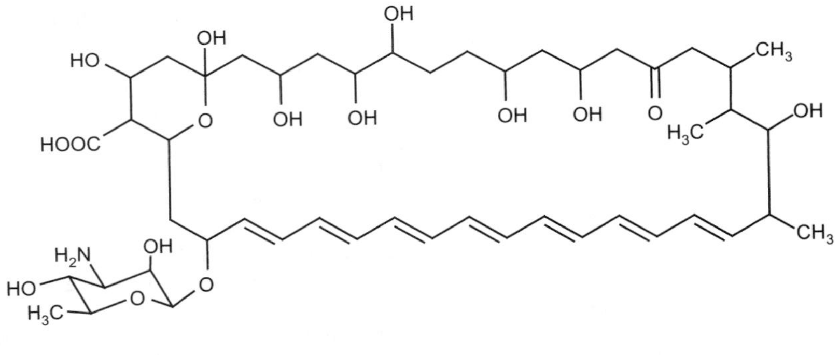

Figure 2 AMB

Table 5 Physicochemical properties of AMB

Empirical formula	Mol wt	Solubility	Stability
$C_{47}H_{73}O_{17}$	924	Yellow powder insoluble in water and in alcohol + Sodium deoxycholate and 5% glucose solution (micellar suspension) Soluble in organic solvents: DMSO[a] (30–40 mg/ml) and DMF (4 mg/ml)	Colloidal suspension Stable only at 4°C for 24 h and if concentrated Degraded by light Physical incompatibility with all solutions other than 5% glucose solution

[a]DMSO, dimethyl sulfoxide.

In vitro, AMB exerts fungicidal activity after 3 h at a concentration of 1 μg/ml, but this activity does not persist for more than 48 h. The combination AMB-5FC has proved synergistic, with a marked fungicidal effect relative to that of AMB alone. Conversely, the combination AMB-azole (irrespective of the molecule) is never synergistic, is exceptionally additive, and is usually neutral (according to the study conducted on *Candida albicans* and *Candida tropicalis* by Hennequin et al.), or even antagonistic.

2.2.1.5. Mechanisms of Action

Although AMB has been used in the treatment of deep mycoses for more than 30 years (its first use dates back to 1957), it is only in the last few years that its mechanism of action, which in any case is highly complex, has begun to be elucidated. The preparation of in vitro models in artificial membranes and whole cells has provided a better understanding of its mechanisms of action at the cellular and molecular level.

The effects of AMB on fungal or animal cells are varied, but it appears to be accepted that the initial stage of toxicity consists of an interaction with the plasma membrane sterols, in which it forms pores. This very early phenomenon immediately causes an ionic disequilibrium within the cell, particularly of the monovalent Na^+ and K^+ ions, and impairs cell permeability.

These pores (or channels) result from the aggregation of several AMB molecules within the lipid bilayer of the fungal membrane so as to form a sort of hollow cylinder through which the ions and the essential cell constituents can escape. This self-assembly phenomenon has still not been totally elucidated, but studies (Bolard, 1991; Brajtburg et al., 1990) appear to implicate the physicochemical properties of self-association of AMB.

The selectivity of AMB for the fungal cell as opposed to the host cell would appear to stem from a much greater affinity for membranes containing ergosterol, a major component of the fungal membrane, than for those containing cholesterol, which is essentially present in mammalian membranes.

This assembly process would appear to result from the steric conformation of ergosterol, which is more favorable than that of cholesterol to the creation of Van der Waals-type bonds between this sterol and the rigid chain of AMB bearing the seven conjugated double bonds.

Conversely, the hydrogen bonds that form between the carboxyl group of AMB and the OH groups of the sterols located on the flexible part of the molecule, bonds that are further strengthened by the participation of the NH_2 group of the amino sugar of AMB, involve cholesterol and ergosterol without distinction. This selectivity of action on the fungal cell is therefore not absolute, and there is also a certain lethal action on animal cells. This phenomenon is the subject of current research designed to improve its therapeutic index, in particular by incorporating AMB into liposomes, which is discussed below.

In addition to this capacity to form pores through the plasma membrane, AMB inhibits the action of membrane enzymes, such as *C. albicans* proton ATPase or erythrocyte Na^+/K^+ ATPase, and peroxidizes unsaturated fats. The hyperthermia caused in humans and animals by intravenously administered AMB would appear to result from stimulation of cell oxidation.

At subtoxic concentrations, AMB exerts stimulant effects on cell growth, as evidenced by the increased incorporation of labeled uridine or leucine; these mechanisms are not yet fully established, but they might result from the increase in intracellular free Ca^{2+} secondary to transient hyperpolarization of the membrane.

In addition, AMB might have immunostimulant effects, but the mechanisms involved and their potential clinical consequences still remain very obscure.

2.2.1.6. Resistance Mechanisms

In more than 30 years of use, the isolation of AMB-resistant fungal strains has only very rarely been reported. In fact, the true incidence is difficult to quantify and may be underestimated since susceptibility to this antifungal agent is not always determined systematically and these tests still lack standardization.

This resistance may be observed from the outset in some moulds (*Scedosporium* and *Fusarium* spp.) or yeasts (*M. furfur* and *Trichosporon* spp.), but rare cases of acquired resistance have also been reported, particularly in *C. lusitaniae*, *C. tropicalis*, *Candida parapsilosis*, and even *C. albicans*.

The majority of resistant strains have been isolated from severely immunocompromised patients previously receiving AMB empirically for prolonged periods. A significant relationship has also been found between the reduced susceptibility of strains to AMB and the clinical severity of the patients: in all cases, strains of yeasts for which the MIC of AMB is >0.8 μg/ml were associated with an unfavorable outcome (Powderly et al., 1988).

Several hypotheses have been postulated to explain the fungal resistance to AMB. These involve the following:

- The possible role of the fungal wall. Composed of chitin and β-1,3-glucans, it constitutes the first barrier that AMB has to cross to reach the cell membrane. This passage might be modified in resistant strains, but the phenomenon is still very poorly understood.
- The appearance of qualitative and quantitative changes in the lipid content of the cell membrane, particularly the depletion of ergosterol. This hypothesis is supported by the fact that resistance has appeared in patients previously receiving clotrimazole orally for prophylactic purposes. It is possible that the imidazole selects AMB-resistant strains of yeasts by decreasing the ergosterol content, reducing the possibilities for AMB-cell membrane binding.
- The reduction in the susceptibility of the fungal cell to oxidation phenomena normally induced by AMB

These observations, combined with the poor tolerability of AMB, mean that the spectrum of this antifungal agent is being substantially "eaten away" by more recent molecules. Nevertheless, AMB still remains the antifungal most often effective in the majority of clinical situations associated with the occurrence of deep fungal infections in immunodepressed patients.

2.2.1.7. Pharmacokinetics

The very poor absorption of AMB when administered orally (<5%) necessitates its intravenous use in deep mycoses: oral dosages of 1.6 to 5 g/day yield levels in serum of only 0.04 to 0.5 μg/ml.

In addition, the intramuscular route is not recommended in view of its irritant effect and its weak absorption.

The pharmacokinetic data for intravenously administered AMB are summarized in Table 6 (Gallis et al., 1990). As discussed above, our understanding of the mechanisms of action is still incomplete, particularly with respect to its metabolism.

Table 6 Pharmacokinetics of AMB

Parameter	Description
Intravenous administration in adults	Levels in serum Related to dose, frequency, and no. of infusions After infusion of 1 mg/kg in 6–8 h: At 1 h: 1.2 μg/ml At 6–8 h (end of infusion): peak serum concn of 1.5–3.5 μg/ml persisting for 6–8 h At 24 h: 1–2 μg/ml At 48 h: 0.25 μg/ml Dose dependent for dosages of 5 to 50 mg, plateau phenomenon thereafter Unmodified if daily dosage doubled and daily administration, for instance: 0.5 mg/kg/day daily 1 mg/kg one day in two May be increased by the infusion rate (45 min instead of 6–8 h), but only for levels in serum obtained 1 h after the end of the infusion. No difference at 24 and 48 h.
Distribution	Intravenous: serum lipoprotein binding (91–95%, particularly lipoproteins, erythrocytes, and cholesterol) and then tissue redistribution when AMB binds to cholesterol-rich membranes Apparent vol of distribution: 4 liters/kg Excellent tissue concn in lung, spleen, liver, and kidney Weak in fluids: pleural, peritoneal, synovial, and bronchial (less than half the levels in serum) Minimal in CSF (2–4%), but meningeal levels may be greater than those in CSF Crosses placental barrier
Excretion	Metabolism still not fully known: no metabolite has been identified Biphasic serum elimination: Initial serum half-life: 24–48 h Terminal serum half-life: 15 days Elimination partly biliary (up to 14%) and very slightly urinary (<5%), remainder unknown No accumulation after daily administration (but might increase half-life in CSF)
Renal insufficiency	Levels in blood not affected Hemodialysis does not alter levels in blood Hemodialysis in hyperlipidemic patients: decrease in levels in serum through binding of AmB-lipoprotein complex to dialysis membrane
Hepatic insufficiency	Levels in blood unaffected
In children	Still incomplete data Lower vol of distribution Peak concn in serum about half the levels obtained in adults receiving an equivalent dose Risk of accumulation; interval between infusions

2.2.1.8. Tolerability, Adverse Effects, Interactions, and Contraindications

Although AMB constitutes the treatment of first choice in deep fungal infections, its use is unfortunately considerably affected by its high level of toxicity. This includes numerous adverse effects that occur earlier or later in the course of treatment:

- Early intolerance reactions
- Thrombophlebitis
- Nephrotoxicity
- Hematotoxic effects

We report here the main toxic phenomena, describing at the same time the mechanisms potentially involved on the basis of the most recent data while mentioning only briefly the means for remedying these phenomena. In fact, all of the recommendations necessary for the management of patients treated with AMB are detailed extensively elsewhere in exhaustive reviews, which we recommend for further information (Dupont and Drouhet, 1990; Gallis et al., 1990; Denning and Stevens, 1990).

2.2.1.8.1. Immediate reactions of a general nature. The occurrence of chills, febrile reactions, digestive disorders, headache, and a sensation of malaise is common during the very first few hours of the infusion. Varying in intensity with the patient, they become attenuated as the number of administrations increases.

Although the mechanism has not really been explained, these intolerance phenomena might be related to prostaglandins, AMB being a potent inducer of prostaglandin E_2 synthesis in vitro. A double-blind placebo-controlled clinical study has shown that the frequency of occurrence of chills was halved by prior administration (30 min before the infusion) of cyclooxygenase-inhibiting nonsteroidal anti-inflammatory drugs such as ibuprofen. These reactions are conventionally countered by the preventive administration of aspirin, antihistamines, and hydrocortisone hemisuccinate and the use of a progressive dosage.

2.2.1.8.2. Thrombophlebitis. Caused by the venous irritation associated with the molecule, thrombophlebitis may be prevented by the use of a deep intravenous route, changing the duration of the infusion, and monitoring the pH of the suspension.

2.2.1.8.3. Nephrotoxicity. Renal impairment represents the major potential risk of administration of AMB: it is consistent with the characteristics of a chronic distal tubulopathy associated with the direct toxicity of the antifungal agent. AMB causes the following:

- Reduced glomerular filtration
- Reduced renal blood flow
- Impaired proximal and distal tubular reabsorption of electrolytes

The clinical and laboratory consequences occur in general after 2 or 3 weeks of treatment and reveal metabolic acidosis with hyperazotemia, oliguria, cylindruria without proteinuria, and potassium and magnesium leakage.

The principal mechanism concerned would appear to involve membrane permeability but might also relate to activation of an intrarenal mechanism known as tubuloglomerular feedback, which controls proximal and distal tubular ionic regulation and affects the vascular resistance of the afferent arteriole. This feedback is suppressed by prior sodium loading. This explains why the reduced glomerular filtration rate caused by AMB may be prevented in vivo by prior sodium loading. These are retrospective observations that still remain to be confirmed by prospective, randomized clinical studies.

The fact that nephrotoxicity involves a toxic tubulopathy implies reversibility after the discontinuation of treatment, which generally occurs if the total dose has not exceeded 4 to 5 g. However, irreversible, albeit rare, changes have been reported and might be related to individual reactions.

In practice, this risk requires close clinical and laboratory monitoring to prevent the potential metabolic consequences of renal impairment: administration of alkalinizing agents and potassium and daily assays of serum creatinine, blood urea nitrogen, and electrolytes (potassium and magnesium). If the renal impairment tends to deteriorate, the dosage may be reduced temporarily (if the patient's state allows) to permit the stabilization of renal function.

2.2.1.8.4. Hematologic effects. Normochromic and normocytic anemia may occur with a reduction of 18 to 35% in the hemoglobin concentration (up to 10 weeks after the beginning of treatment). This would appear to result from either inhibition of erythropoietin production or nephrotoxicity. This phenomenon does not appear to be dose dependent, and the hematocrit returns to normal in the months following the discontinuation of treatment.

Leukopenia is rarely associated with the administration of AMB, and no cases of bone marrow aplasia have been reported. However, in vitro and in animal models, AMB may modify lymphocyte function, increase the number of antibody-producing cells, and potentiate cell-mediated immunity and macrophage activity.

2.2.1.8.5. Other effects. The following have been reported exceptionally:

- Thrombocytopenia
- Acute allergic reaction (bronchospasm and dyspnea) in subjects with a history of asthma
- Hepatotoxicity, although the responsibility of the antifungal has not been proven

2.2.1.8.6. Drug interactions. AMB displays antagonism with a number of other medications. This is all the more significant in that the patients receiving AMB are often profoundly debilitated and are multiply medicated. Three principal types of effects are observed:

- Potentiation of drug action by the hypokalemia associated with AMB
- Cardiotonic heterosides (digitalis derivatives): reduce the dosage
- Neuromuscular relaxants: reduce the dosage
- Nonantiarrhythmic medications causing torsade de pointes: coadministration contraindicated
- Increase of potassium depletion of AMB by the following:
  - Glucocorticoids
  - Hypokalemic drugs: diuretics (ethacrynic acid and thienylic acid), stimulant laxatives, and tetracosactide (combination to be avoided; otherwise, very close monitoring of blood potassium levels)
- Synergy of the nephrotoxic effects
  - Cyclosporin and tacrolimus: require close monitoring
  - Aminoglycosides (gentamicin): combination contraindicated

Finally, there is a risk of bone marrow toxicity from an additive effect with zidovudine.

In terms of the antifungal action, a synergistic effect is observed with 5FC, but in the current state of knowledge the combination AMB-azoles is not recommended (considered in the case of 5FC and azoles). Likewise, coadministration with rifampin is not recommended, even if isolated observations of synergy in vitro have been reported, as results of clinical studies do not demonstrate any benefit from the combination.

2.2.1.9. Clinical Indications

The complexity of the dosages and durations of treatment with AMB is related not only to the different types of fungal diseases and their localization but also to the conditions specific to each patient (initial underlying disease, tolerability, etc.).

A test dose should enable the tolerability to be ascertained.

The daily dosage is reached progressively and is between 0.5 and 0.6 to 1 mg/kg/day or may be increased and administered every other day (never to exceed 1.5 mg/kg/day).

In the majority of deep fungal infections treatment is for 6 to 12 weeks, but treatment may sometimes be prolonged for several months (hepatosplenic candidosis). In very summary form, the regimens for AMB and its indications are as follows (refer to the recommendations of *Clinical Infectious Diseases,* 2000). They cover the majority of deep fungal infections due to yeasts and filamentous and dimorphic fungi, sometimes in combination with 5FC, and may be associated with a surgical procedure depending on the indications:

- Neuromeningeal cryptococcosis
- Septicemia and fungemia (if susceptible strains)
- Systemic candidosis
- Pulmonary and invasive aspergillosis and mucormycosis
- Fungal endophthalmia
- American and tropical fungal infections due to dimorphic fungi
- Empirical treatment of febrile agranulocytosis

2.2.1.10. Pharmaceutical Form

Fungizone® is the trade name for injectable powder, 50 mg (combination of AMB [25 mg] and sodium deoxycholate [25 mg]).

2.2.2. Lipid Formulations of AMB

As we have just seen in the previous section, conventional AMB, which remains the reference treatment, is associated with frequent, serious, and immediate and late adverse effects. The cumulative toxicity is principally renal and often exacerbated by the combined administration of certain types of chemotherapy, aminoglycosides, or cyclosporine. Under these conditions, research has focused on the development of molecules with the advantages of AMB, i.e., its fungicidal potency and its very broad spectrum, but without all of the adverse effects.

These new dosage forms are based on the concept of "passive delivery," which involves modifying the pharmacokinetics of a drug and increasing its concentration by targeting it to the infected organ. Phospholipid structures with or without an aqueous phase therefore readily serve as a vehicle for amphiphilic compounds such as AMB (one lipophilic pole and one hydrophilic pole).

2.2.2.1. L-AMB

Although there are several lipid formulations of AMB, there is only one Liposomal form (L-AMB). In fact, the other formulations are presented in the form of a flattened disk or ribbon and do not have the same spatial structure or the same constituents. This is the source of the very different in vivo physicochemical properties and behavior.

2.2.2.1.1. Chemical structure. L-AMB consists of unilamellar spherical vesicles with a diameter of between 60 and 80 nm. Two phospholipids are involved in their composition: hydrogenated soy phosphatidylcholine and distearoylphosphatidylglycerol. AMB, as an amphiphilic molecule, is included in the phospholipid bilayer. The presence of cholesterol incorporated into this structure is important for two reasons: it stabilizes the membrane by making the bilayer more compact, and it maintains AMB in the structure by physicochemical affinity (affinity of AMB for sterols). This thus limits the interactions of AMB with the host's cell membrane cholesterol and thereby reduces the risks of toxicity.

2.2.2.1.2. Physicochemical properties. The combined physicochemical characteristics of these liposomes make them highly stable in blood: hydrogenated soy phosphatidylcholine, the main constituent, stabilizes the liposomal structure through its alkyl chains. The reduced size of the liposomes enables them to remain for a prolonged period in the blood compartment without undergoing excessive degradation, releasing only very little AMB into the circulation.

As a lyophilisate, L-AMB is stable for at least 36 months between 2 and 27°C. Reconstituted, it is stable for 24 h at room temperature. Diluted in 5% glucose, it must be administered within 6 h.

The lyophilisate must be reconstituted in water (and not in physiological saline) and diluted in 5% glucose. Any other solution or the presence of bacteriostatic agents may cause precipitation of L-AMB. Filtration of L-AMB is essential, but the diameter may not be less than 1 μm (because of the liposomes). It is therefore not a candidate for sterile filtration.

2.2.2.1.3. In vitro properties and spectrum of activity. The spectrum of activity of L-AMB is similar to that of conventional AMB, with a tendency for its MICs and minimum fungicidal concentrations for the most frequently encountered strains to be lower (Anaissie et al., 1991).

2.2.2.1.4. Mechanisms of action. The mechanism of action of L-AMB is closely related to its liposomal nature. AMB is very strongly anchored to the liposomes and does not dissociate in an aqueous medium. This allows optimized delivery of AMB to the sites of infection where vascular permeability is increased. In addition, uptake of the liposomes by macrophages allows L-AMB to migrate towards the infected tissue. Thus, AMB interacts only weakly with human cells and serum lipoproteins but directly with the fungus in the infected tissues. The liposomes adhere to the fungal wall, where they disintegrate and release their content of AMB (see section 3.1 below).

2.2.2.1.5. Resistance mechanisms. See section 3.1 below.

2.2.2.1.6. Pharmacokinetics. Reflecting the targeted delivery, the pharmacokinetics of L-AMB differ from those of conventional AMB. After injection, the liposomes exhibit limited diffusion towards the tissues and are stable in the circulation; this is reflected in a higher peak concentration in plasma and a lower apparent volume of distribution than with conventional AMB. However, the liposomes are actively and intensively removed from the circulation by phagocytic uptake by macrophages from the reticuloendothelial system (RES), thus explaining the shorter half-life. Given that higher initial levels in serum are obtained and that the RES is saturable, the area under the curve (AUC) obtained with L-AMB is greater than that obtained with conventional AMB. Reflecting this saturation of the RES by the liposomes, there is a nonlinear increase in the peak concentration in serum and the AUC when the doses of L-AMB are increased, as well as a nonlinear reduction in apparent volume of distribution. A lower fraction of antifungal agent than with conventional AMB is found in the kidney and lung, and peak tissue concentrations are obtained in the liver and spleen.

In conclusion, liposomal delivery thus allows AMB to circulate in the vascular compartment without the diffusion to healthy organs or binding to serum lipoproteins that occurs after an injection of conventional AMB. These parameters thus indicate the sequestration of L-AMB in the circulating macrophages.

L-AMB is not eliminated by renal filtration and therefore is not dialyzable.

The effect of this formulation is prolonged (slow elimination from tissues, plasma stability, and absence of renal elimination) and allows single-daily dosing. Tissue accumulation, the metabolic pathways of elimination, and modification of the pharmacokinetics in patients with renal and hepatic insufficiency are not yet known.

The pharmacokinetics of L-AMB and the tissue concentrations are presented in Tables 7 and 8.

2.2.2.1.7. Tolerability, side effects, interactions, and contraindications. The stability of the liposomes in blood, the reduced interaction of AMB with the cell membranes, and its limited distribution in healthy tissue (particularly the kidney) constitute the major value of the liposomal formulation, characterized by excellent tolerability, particularly in terms of immediate toxicity and nephrotoxicity. The adverse events responsible for clinical reactions are significantly less common than with conventional AMB:

- Systemic tolerability (fever, chills, and cardiovascular disorders) where, according to the studies (Walsh et al., 1999; Prentice et al., 1997). L-AMB at a dosage of 3 mg/kg/day reduces immediate adverse effects by 50 to 70%. The use of premedication is therefore less common.
- Nephrotoxicity and secondary hypokalemia, which are significantly less common and later in onset. In addition, they are not dose dependent. Here again, toxicity studies show that AMB reduces renal toxicity and potassium leakage by more than 50%. In children, in whom renal tolerance of AMB is better, the gain in terms of tolerance appears to be less significant.

Hematologic tolerance, particularly anemia of central origin, which is more difficult to evaluate in patients often suffering from a blood disorder, appears to be slightly better, as does hepatic tolerance. The incubation of different lipid forms of AMB with erythrocytes shows that L-AMB causes only 15% hemolysis, whereas the other forms (ABLC and ABCD) cause, respectively, 70 and 40% hemolysis after incubation for 48 h (Jensen, 1998).

The contraindications and in particular the drug interactions are numerous and are related to the nephrotoxic, hypokalemic, and hematotoxic effects of AMB (see section 3.1 below).

2.2.2.1.8. Clinical indications. Because of its weaker toxicity, permitting higher dosages, and the contribution of targeted delivery, which allows higher concentrations to be obtained at the site of infection, greater efficacy may be expected from the liposomal form; this superiority has already been demonstrated in animals but not yet in humans (insufficient number of comparative studies).

L-AMB is indicated in the treatment of invasive aspergillosis and systemic candidosis in adults and children with impaired renal function. The recommended dosage is 3 mg/kg/day, but the excellent tolerability profile may indicate an increase in this dosage to 5 mg/kg/day or even higher in the most serious infections. It should be stressed that this product is also approved for the treatment of visceral leishmaniasis and in the United States for the treatment of febrile neutropenia.

2.2.2.1.9. Pharmaceutical form. AmBisome is the trade name for injectable powder (50 mg) of AMB.

2.2.2.2. ABLC

In a liposomal structure, when the concentration of AMB increases (between 25 and 50 mol%), the lipid structures in the liposomal form disappear in favor of lipid structures in ribbons. This is the principle of the formulation of ABLC.

2.2.2.2.1. Chemical structure. In this organization, in contrast to liposomes, there is no aqueous phase; the lipid fraction is presented in the form of a ribbon (1,600 to 6,000 nm in length) in which the AMB molecules are inserted. Two phospholipids make up this complex: dimyristoyl phosphatidylcholine and dimyristoyl phosphatidylglycerol, in a ratio of 7:3.

Table 7 Pharmacokinetics of the different forms of AMB

Parameter	Descriptions or value			
Product	AMB	L-AMB	ABLC	ABCD
Dosage form	Colloidal suspension	Liposomes	Lipid ribbon	Lipid disks
AMB (mol%)		10	33	50
Dose (mg/kg)	1	3	5	5
C_{max} (μg/ml)	1.7	14.4	1.7	3.1
AUC (μg·h/ml)	25	171	14	36
V (liters/kg)	2–4	0.4	131	18
$t_{1/2}$ (h)	26.8	13	173	27

Table 8 Tissue concentrations of AmB in rats after administration of different forms

Product	Tissue concn (μg/g) of AMB				
	Kidney	Liver	Spleen	Lung	Brain
AMB	19	93	59	13	ND[a]
AmBisome	23	176	201	17	0.56
Abelcet	7	196	290	222	1.6
Amphotec	–	++	++	–	ND

[a]ND, Not determined.

2.2.2.2.2. Physicochemical properties. ABLC is a sterile apyrogenic suspension for dilution. The ready-to-use suspension is stable for more than 24 h at 2 to 8°C and for an additional 6 h at room temperature. The compatibility of ABLC with different products has not been established. It must therefore not be diluted with saline solutions or mixed with other drugs or electrolytes. Only the 5% glucose solution may be used to obtain the final dilution, and always after filtering ABLC.

2.2.2.2.3. In vitro properties, spectrum of activity, and resistance mechanisms. The in vitro activity of ABLC against pathogenic fungal strains is similar to that of conventional AMB, as are the resistance mechanisms (see section 3.1 below).

2.2.2.2.4. Mechanisms of action. ABLC is rapidly taken up in sites with intense macrophagic activity (RES, liver, spleen, and, to a lesser extent, lungs) and by circulating mononuclear cells, hence the high product concentrations in these organs.

During an infection, the antifungal molecule is transported by the monocytic cells to the inflammatory focus or taken up directly by the macrophages at the site of infection; the increased permeability of the vascular wall also facilitates tissue diffusion in the nonendocytic free form by passage through the vascular endothelium.

Several mechanisms may contribute to the degradation of the lipid complexes: the exchange of phospholipids with cell and fungal membranes and the action of phospholipases (phagocytes and endothelial and fungal cells): this allows the progressive release of AMB inside and outside the phagocytic cells, and hence an action on both free and phagocytosed infectious agents (see section 3.1 below).

2.2.2.2.5. Pharmacokinetics. The pharmacokinetics of ABLC differ from those of AMB. The main pharmacokinetics are illustrated in Tables 7 and 8.

Compared with conventional AMB, the kinetics of ABLC are characterized by the following:

- Four- to fivefold-lower systemic concentrations
- A four- to fivefold-higher volume of distribution
- A four- to fivefold-greater total clearance
- A comparable terminal half-life
- A weaker urinary excretion

These differences are the result of more intense and more rapid tissue uptake of ABLC, principally by the RES.

For the same cumulative dose, the concentrations of ABLC are higher in the spleen, liver, and lungs and lower in the kidneys (Table 8).

2.2.2.2.6. Tolerability, side effects, interactions, and contraindications. The most common adverse effects are related directly to the infusion (fever and chills) but are less common than with conventional AMB. They can be controlled by premedication.

Renal tolerability is good in the treatment of fungal infections, even in patients suffering from preexisting renal insufficiency. Nephrotoxicity is therefore less marked and occurs later than with AMB, which has been confirmed in children.

The improvement over AMB in terms of renal tolerance may be explained by weaker renal diffusion, a more targeted action on the site of infection, and a stable structure that reduces the interactions of AMB with cell membranes and lipoproteins (low-density lipoproteins [LDL]), AMB-LDL complexes possibly being the source of toxic endocytoses for cells bearing the LDL receptor.

The hematologic and hepatic tolerance still remains to be evaluated. The tolerability profile in specific populations (pediatric and geriatric) is thus insufficiently known.

The contraindications and in particular the drug interactions are numerous and related to the nephrotoxic, hypokalemic, and hematotoxic effects of AMB (see section 3.1 below).

2.2.2.2.7. Clinical indications. ABLC at a dosage of 5 mg/kg/day is indicated in systemic candidosis and invasive aspergillosis in the event of renal impairment (preexisting or AMB induced). However, its use may be considered in the failure of conventional AMB and as first-line treatment in invasive fungal infections due to filamentous fungi other than *Aspergillus*, particularly *Fusarium* spp. and *Mucorales*, in view of the high response levels observed in these two conditions with a usually very poor prognosis.

2.2.2.2.8. Pharmaceutical form. Abelcet is the trade name for a suspension for dilution, 100 mg of AMB per 20 ml.

2.2.2.3. ABCD

ABCD is not currently commercially available in France, but it is in the United States and in other European countries. It is composed of AMB bound to cholesterol sulfate in an equimolar mixture. The particles are disk shaped, with a diameter of 120 to 140 nm and a thickness of 4 nm. Pharmacological data for this product are still limited. ABCD is rapidly taken up by the RES; hence it has a lower peak concentration than AMB and a large volume of distribution (Table 7), but while its hepatic and splenic concentrations are high, its pulmonary and cerebral concentrations are lower than with AMB. Preliminary studies of clinical efficacy are rare, but they suggest slightly greater efficacy in invasive fungal infections than that of AMB. The immediate side effects are superimposable on those of AMB, but at four- to fivefold-higher dosages. Conversely, nephrotoxicity appears to be lower.

This product is commercially available in the United States under the name of Amphotec and in Europe under the name of Amphocil.

2.2.3. Liposomal Nystatin

Liposomal nystatin, a polyene antifungal, has the same mode of action as AMB. It has been used for some 30 years in local cutaneous or mucosal treatment for its action on yeasts. Nystatin is not absorbed orally; parenteral administration causes phenomena of local intolerance and marked systemic toxicity. It is currently the subject of experimental protocols in an injectable multilamellar liposomal form that should be better tolerated. In fact, it possesses a spectrum similar to that of AMB, but extended to include certain species of opportunistic filamentous fungi. Some clinical studies show encouraging results for the use of liposomal nystatin in the treatment of disseminated aspergillosis in AIDS patients. However, its development has been stopped in France.

3. CHEMICAL ANTIFUNGALS

3.1. 5FC

3.1.1. Introduction

The synthesis of 5FC (Fig. 3), the only antifungal in the fluoropyrimidine series, was conducted in association with

Figure 3 5FC

research into an antagonist of uracil, produced in abnormal quantities by cancer cells. These studies culminated in 1957 (Heidelberg-University of Wisconsin and Duchinsky Hofmann-La Roche) in the production of 5-fluorouracil (5FU), which possesses cytostatic properties but which is toxic to the human cell, and then in 1963 (Grunberg) in the discovery of 5FC. This molecule, which is devoid of antineoplastic activity and is not metabolized in humans, possesses excellent antiyeast properties in vitro and in vivo and acts, in fact, as an antimetabolite.

This antifungal is positioned principally as an anticandidosis agent, but currently its use is restricted by the frequent occurrence of secondary resistance that precludes its administration in single-agent therapy in severe infections.

3.1.2. Physicochemical Properties

Table 9 lists the physicochemical properties of 5FC.

3.1.3. In Vitro Properties

5FC is characterized by a narrow spectrum, which distinguishes it from the outset from AMB. It has very marked and selective in vitro and in vivo activities against different species of pathogenic or potentially pathogenic yeasts, such as *C. albicans* and other species of *Candida* and *C. neoformans* (inhibition of the majority of strains at concentrations of <1 μg/ml). Its action is moderate and varies with the strains against certain filamentous fungi, such as *Aspergillus* spp. (one in three strains of *Aspergillus fumigatus* is susceptible, with a MIC of between 1 and 25 μg/ml), and against the agents of chromomycosis (*Phialophora* and *Cladosporium*: MIC of 0.2 to 12.5 μg/ml). Conversely, 5FC has no action against the other agents of deep mycoses (*Histoplasma*, *Coccidioides*, and *Blastomyces*).

However, primary resistance has been reported with *Candida* and *Cryptococcus* in certain regions, and secondary resistance is liable to occur during treatment, phenomena that may be explained by the mode of action of 5FC on the fungal cell.

We should stress that in vitro susceptibility to this antifungal agent should always be determined in a synthetic medium, since its activity is considerably affected by the composition of the culture medium.

3.1.4. Mechanisms of Action

Two initial stages are essential for 5FC to exert its action: penetration of the fungal cell, controlled by cytosine permease, and deamination to 5FU by means of a cytosine deaminase (Fig. 4). The antifungal spectrum of 5FC is essentially determined by the presence and activity of the latter enzyme. The weak toxicity of 5FC in humans may be explained by the virtual absence of cytosine deaminase in mammalian cells.

Table 9 Physicochemical properties of 5FC

Empirical formula	Mol wt	Solubility	Stability
$C_4H_4ON_3F$	129	Soluble in water at 60°C Soluble in alcohol Slightly soluble in water at 20°C (1.2%)	Solution stable at room temp

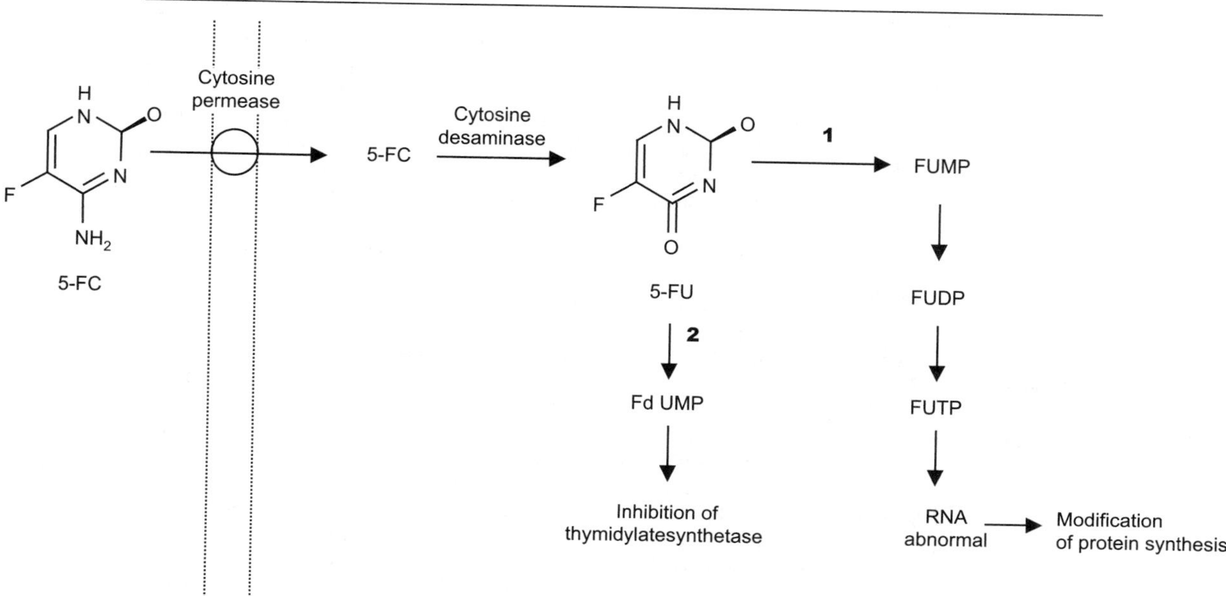

Figure 4 Mechanism of action of 5FC

Starting with the formation of 5FU, two different pathways disrupt fungal protein synthesis. After transformation to 5-fluorouridine, which is mono-, di-, and then triphosphated, 5FU is incorporated into RNA in place of uracil, resulting in the synthesis of abnormal RNA. However, the principal source of disruption stems from the formation of 5-fluorodeoxyuridine monophosphate, which acts as a potent inhibitor of thymidylate synthetase, thereby blocking DNA synthesis. Depending on the concentrations and exposure times, this type of action may be fungicidal in vitro, but it is purely fungistatic in vivo (Polak and Scholer, 1980).

Other consequences of the action of 5FC on *C. albicans* have been reported: increased volume of the fungal cell and carbohydrate content, accompanied by a change in the proportions of wall polysaccharides.

3.1.5. Resistance Mechanisms

The different biochemical transformations that 5FC undergoes in the susceptible fungal cell give rise to several types of resistance that occur through genetically stable mutations independent of one another. Resistance may involve a loss of enzymes (permease, cytosine deaminase, or UMP pyrophosphorylase) or excessive neosynthesis of pyrimidines competing with 5FC or its metabolites (six resistance phenotypes have been identified). The formation of 5FC-resistant mutants occurs permanently and spontaneously, irrespective of the presence of the substance, so there are resistant microorganisms in any susceptible population. The rate of primary resistance varies with the species and countries:

- For *C. albicans*, about 95% of isolated strains are susceptible. The great majority of these strains belong to serotype A, whereas resistant strains are primarily of serotype B, which is much more rarely isolated in France but is frequently isolated in Africa, for instance.
- For species of *Candida* other than *C. albicans*, particularly *C. tropicalis* and *C. krusei*, 25 to 50% of strains are resistant on isolation.
- Lastly, the resistance rate in *C. neoformans* is low, about 2%.

During treatment with 5FC, the selection of mutants with spontaneous resistance is likely to occur and continues until the whole population has become resistant. The appearance of this secondary resistance is all the more common if there is a large number of microorganisms, the defensive capabilities of the host are impaired, and the cellular concentrations of 5FC are reduced (less than 25 μg/ml). This major risk therefore contraindicates the use of 5FC as single-agent therapy in severe infections, particularly in cryptococcal meningitis, and its use in gastrointestinal fungal infections.

In the case of 5FC, the most significant development over the past few years has certainly been the therapeutic use of the combination 5FC-AMB in systemic fungal diseases. In fact, the synergistic or additive antifungal activity of this combination has been perfectly demonstrated in vitro and in vivo in yeastlike fungi, including *C. albicans*. Conversely, in *Aspergillus* this action is more equivocal, and the value of this combination in invasive aspergillosis still remains to be proven. As regards the triazoles, synergistic activity has also been observed in vitro in yeasts, but the clinical value of this combination is still under evaluation.

3.1.6. Pharmacokinetics

In addition to its spectrum, 5FC differs from AMB in all of its pharmacokinetic characteristics: good absorption via the gastrointestinal tract, short elimination half-life, weak protein binding, and crossing of the meningeal barrier (Table 10).

Table 10 Pharmacokinetics of 5FC

Parameter	Description
Absorption in healthy volunteers	After oral administration, rapid and almost total intestinal absorption Peak concn in serum 0.5 to 2 h after administration Half-life: 5 h After single administration: peak concn in serum in μg/ml equivalent to administered dose in mg/kg (i.e., 50 μg/ml for 50 mg/kg) After repeated administration every 6 h: accumulation and then stabilization between 25 and 40 μg/ml
Distribution	No protein binding Tissue diffusion: excellent throughout the body, including bronchial secretions, bile, and bone tissues CSF: 75% of levels in serum Aqueous humor: <30% Peritoneal fluid: variable, 10–75% according to author
Elimination	Essentially urinary (90%) in the unchanged form: glomerular filtration without reabsorption or tubular secretion
Renal insufficiency	Requires dosage adjustment according to serum creatinine levels (plasma accumulation proportional to degree of renal insufficiency) Monitoring of concns in serum (easily performed by bioassay or enzymatic assay or by HPLC[a]); residual levels must be not <25 μg/ml (risk of resistance) and never >100 μg/ml (toxic phenomena) Hemodialyzable: elimination of 65–75% of product present in body
Hepatic insufficiency	Does not contraindicate use: abnormality of hepatic function reported in 5% of cases (isolated elevation of transaminases and alkaline phosphatase)
Children and subjects >65 yrs	No formal contraindication in current state of knowledge

[a]HPLC, high-performance liquid chromatography.

Table 11 Tolerability of 5FC

Parameter	Description
Interactions	Azathioprine: increased risk of hematologic toxicity of 5FC Cytarabine: competitive inhibition of 5FC
Contraindications	No formal contraindication during: Pregnancy Postchemotherapy neutropenia
Precautions	Dosage divided into three or four daily doses Mandatory monitoring of concns in serum in the event of renal insufficiency and in any "at risk patient" (serum creatinine, blood count, differential count, transaminases, and phosphatases); never >100 μg/ml Avoid excessively low dosages (<25 μg/ml) and local use: risk of secondary resistance If using intravenous form, take account of sodium intake (2 g of NaCl per bottle) Risk of crystallization of solutions when cold: in this case, reheat on water bath without exceeding a temp of 50°C

3.1.7. Tolerability, Side Effects, Interactions, and Contraindications

5FC is a generally well-tolerated antifungal agent in the absence of major visceral impairment (Table 11).

However, in the last few years, toxic phenomena have been increasingly reported during the treatment of disseminated yeast infections in compromised patients treated with 5FC or AIDS patients treated with the combination 5FC-AMB for neuromeningeal cryptococcosis. Serum 5FC levels of >100 μg/ml are associated with a markedly higher incidence of bone marrow toxicity (leukopenia and, more rarely, thrombocytopenia) or enterocolitis. Rather than being the result of an excessive dosage, these overdoses are due to neglected or unknown renal impairment.

Among the possible mechanisms of toxicity (Fig. 5), one theory postulates the deamination of 5FC to 5FU: the 5FC secreted in the intestinal lumen (a phenomenon that occurs irrespective of the route of administration [oral or intravenous]) is deaminated by the intestinal flora to 5FU, which may cause systemic toxicity following reabsorption. The bone marrow, gastrointestinal tract, and liver are the sites most commonly affected by toxicity, both of 5FC and of 5FU.

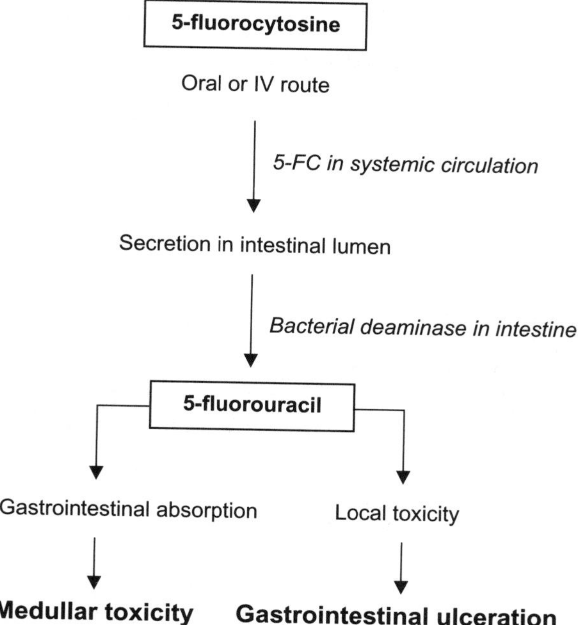

Figure 5 Toxicity of 5FC

3.1.8. Clinical Indications

5FC must be reserved for the treatment of systemic mycoses due to susceptible yeasts and in combination with AMB. Its main indication is systemic candidosis, but it is also indicated for other mycoses:

- Candidosis of the central nervous system
- *Candida* endophthalmia
- Renal and hepatosplenic candidosis
- Neuromeningeal cryptococcosis
- Possibly aspergillosis (to be considered on a case-by-case basis and only in the initial phase of treatment) in combination with AMB.

For neuromeningeal cryptococcosis, and in the absence of AIDS, the initial dosage of 5FC if renal function is normal is 150 mg/kg/day in four divided doses, in combination with AMB (0.3 mg/kg/day), with the recommendation that concentrations in serum be monitored and maintained between 50 and 75 μg/ml. The doses are then reduced as the concentrations in serum begin to increase because of the reduction in glomerular filtration induced by AMB.

For systemic candidosis, the dosages are more variable, depending on the individual predisposition: 5FC at 100 to 150 mg/kg/day combined with AMB intravenously at 0.3 to 0.7 mg/kg/day.

The duration of administration (from 2 to several weeks) is variable and related to a number of factors (type and localization of the fungal infections, underlying disease, tolerability, etc.).

3.1.9. Pharmaceutical Forms

Ancobon (European name, Ancotil) is the trade name for 500-mg tablets and 1% injectable solution in physiological saline (250-ml bottle).

3.2. Azole Derivatives

3.2.1. Introduction

The discovery of the antifungal activity of the imidazoles represents a considerable advance in the treatment of superficial and systemic fungal infections.

Their pharmacological history began some 50 years ago with the discovery of the antibacterial and antifungal properties of benzimidazole. Some of these derivatives possess excellent anthelmintic (thiabendazole [1960]) and antiprotozoal (metronidazole [1959]) activities and even immunomodulatory properties (levamisole [1974]).

Clotrimazole was the first imidazole derivative (1967) to be recognized as a potential systemic antifungal. Unfortunately, the high doses necessary to obtain sufficient concentrations in serum are poorly tolerated, and in addition the induction of microsomal hepatic enzymes responsible for its metabolism causes a reduction in levels in serum with repeated dosing. In spite of these issues, this class of imidazoles has experienced a considerable boom.

In schematic terms, three groups may be distinguished, based more on the history of their development than on a chemical structure.

The first-generation azoles include a wide variety of imidazole compounds with an antifungal action, including miconazole; like all products in this series, they act by modifying the sterol composition of the membrane by direct action on cytochrome P450. At high concentrations they can be fungicidal. These azoles are available in various pharmaceutical forms, ideally suited to the treatment of cutaneous mycoses due to yeasts or dermatophytes and of mucocutaneous mycoses (Table 1). (It should be noted that miconazole no longer has a parenteral dosage form and therefore can no longer be considered a systemic antifungal agent: its oral dosage form fails to produce sufficient levels in serum in deep mycoses.)

Ketoconazole, an orally active N-substituted imidazole, is the principal representative of the second-generation azoles. It is the first imidazole to be well absorbed orally, but its hepatotoxicity and interactions with a number of molecules restrict its conditions of use.

Finally, the third-generation azoles correspond to the triazole derivatives: fluconazole, itraconazole, and voriconazole are featured in this group. Their pharmacological properties and their generally satisfactory tolerability enable them to be used in systemic fungal infections. The former is characterized by a spectrum targeted principally to certain yeast species (*C. albicans* in particular). Itraconazole is positioned more as an anti-*Aspergillus* agent and has already undergone extensive clinical evaluation. Other triazole derivatives (voriconazole, posaconazole, and ravuconazole) are on the verge of being made commercially available or are undergoing clinical trials.

Given their value in the treatment of systemic mycoses, we discuss the three systemic azoles currently commercially available (ketoconazole, fluconazole, and itraconazole) in parallel with voriconazole, which is currently available under an authorization for compassionate use, and conclude with the most recent triazoles under development.

3.2.2. Available Azoles

3.2.2.1. Chemical structures

The only systemic imidazole available (ketoconazole) is characterized by a pentacyclic structure with two nitrogen atoms, associated with a complex chain carried by one of the nitrogen atoms (Fig. 6). The triazoles (fluconazole, itraconazole, and voriconazole) are characterized by similar structures, but the pentacycle contains three nitrogen atoms.

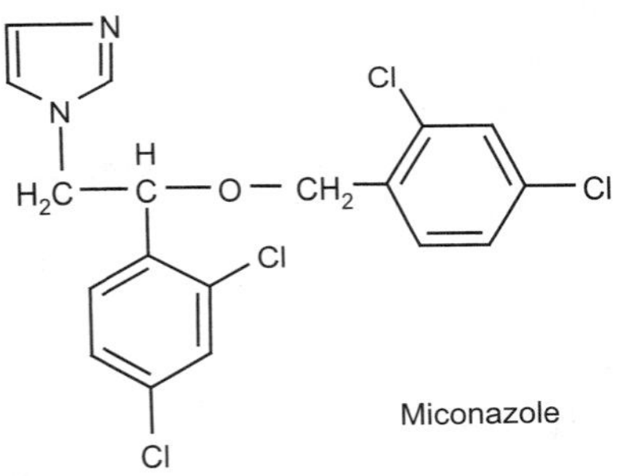

Miconazole

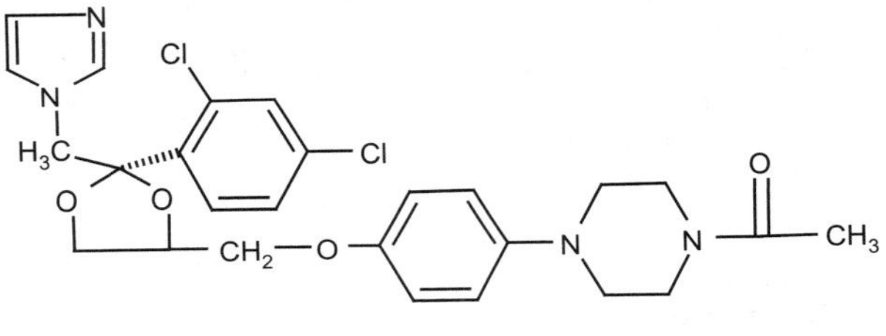

Ketoconazole

Imidazolyl derivatives

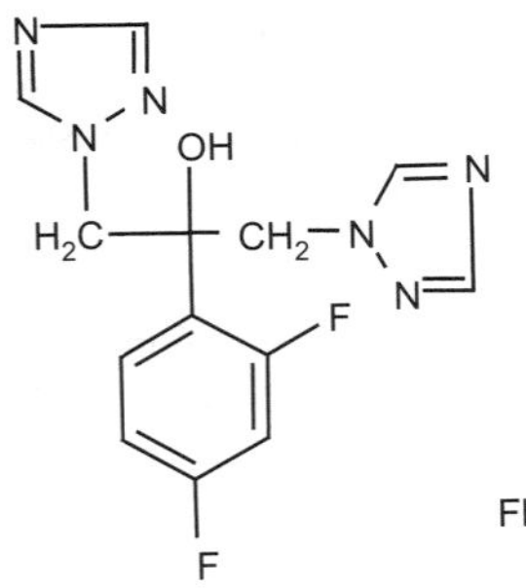

Fluconazole

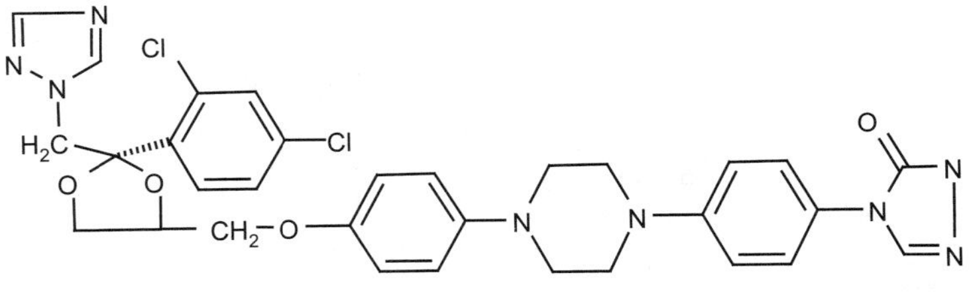

Itraconazole

Triazolyl derivatives

Figure 6 Azole antifungals

3.2.2.2. Physicochemical Properties

The great majority of antifungal azole derivatives are molecules characterized by their insolubility in an aqueous medium and their lipophilia, with the exception of fluconazole, which is original in this series in its combination of properties. Their characteristics are summarized in Table 12.

3.2.2.3. In Vitro Properties and Spectrum of Activity

The azole compounds possess a relatively broad spectrum against numerous pathogenic or opportunistic fungal species, a spectrum that is exceeded only by that of AMB.

However, although all of these derivatives share good activity against some of these fungi (such as *C. albicans*, *C. neoformans*, and dimorphic fungi), major differences have been found in vitro and subsequently confirmed in animals and in clinical trials (Table 13). For example, certain species of *Candida* are resistant from the outset to fluconazole but are not resistant in vitro to ketoconazole, itraconazole, or voriconazole (*C. krusei* and certain strains of *Candida glabrata* and *C. tropicalis* in the case of itraconazole). Itraconazole and voriconazole are the only azoles currently available therapeutically that exert genuine activity on certain filamentous fungi and specifically the different species of *Aspergillus*.

The spectrum of activity of the triazoles is presented in Table 13 on the basis of a literature review of the MICs obtained according to the recommendations of the National Committee for Clinical Laboratory Standards (NCCLS). However, considerable caution should be exercised when interpreting in vitro susceptibility. In fact, the determination of the in vitro susceptibility to these molecules is still an extremely delicate operation, given the major impact that even minimum methodological variations can have on the results: medium composition, temperature and duration of incubation, and cell phase of the fungus (spores or mycelium).

Since 1995, the NCCLS has managed to standardize the determination of the susceptibilities of yeasts and, very recently, of filamentous fungi. This work culminated in the definition of susceptibility "endpoints" for the main fungi found in respect of the principal antifungal agents and the definition of the term dose-dependent susceptible when the observed MIC points to an upwards titration of the antifungal dosage (this is particularly important for *C. glabrata* and fluconazole). However, a very complex but also essential point remains to be established: the exact correlation between in vitro resistance and clinical resistance. Vital information has been obtained from experimental animal models and randomized studies in particular during the treatment of oropharyngeal candidosis in patients suffering from AIDS, but there have also been disappointments that still necessitate the exercise of considerable caution when interpreting the MICs of this class of antifungal agents in therapeutic use.

3.2.2.4. Mechanism of Action

Essentially, the mechanism of action of the azole compounds lies in the preferential inhibition of cytochrome P450 enzymes in the fungal cell. Present in the majority of living species, bacteria, fungi, plants, protozoa, metazoa, and vertebrates, these enzymes in the eukaryote cell are an integral part of the endoplasmic reticulum and the internal membrane of mitochondria. They play a key role in metabolic phenomena and detoxification reactions and interact with a wide range of substances, including sterols.

In the fungal cell, the azoles interfere with the biosynthesis of ergosterol, a major component of the fungal membrane (this sterol is the equivalent in fungi of cholesterol in the mammalian cell) by inhibiting the enzyme responsible for the demethylation of lanosterol to ergosterol, 14α-demethylase (Fig. 7), an essential stage in the synthesis of ergosterol (in fungi) and cholesterol (in mammals). This phenomenon causes an accumulation of the precursors and conversely a depletion of ergosterol. This interference causes abnormalities of membrane permeability. More recently, it has been shown that the initial target of the azoles was the heme portion of cytochrome P450, which binds to the nitrogen located in position 1 of the triazole ring, thereby blocking the site normally occupied by oxygen.

The synthesis of cholesterol in the mammalian cell is also blocked by the azoles at the 14α-demethylation stage. However, the dose of azole necessary to obtain this inhibition is much higher than the inhibitory dose for the fungal cell. In fact, each azole has a selective affinity for the enzymes of fungal cytochrome P450 to a greater or lesser extent, thus explaining the variable tolerability and hepatotoxicity from one molecule to another.

However, this action is perhaps not alone in explaining the inhibition of fungal growth by azoles. Other phenomena have been observed:

- Direct effect on the membrane fatty acids, causing the leakage of proteins, amino acids, and other essential substances in cell metabolism
- Interference with catalase systems

Table 12 Physicochemical properties of systemic azole antifungals

Antifungal	Empirical formula	Mol wt	pK_a	LogP	Solubility
Ketoconazole	$C_{26}H_{28}O_4N_4C_{12}$	531	6.5	3.8	± insoluble in water (4 mg/100 ml) Soluble at pH <3 Soluble in organic solvents Excellent stability of solutions
Itraconazole	$C_{35}H_{38}O_4N_8C_{12}$	705	3.7	5.7	Insoluble in water Soluble in organic solvents or in acidic polyethylene glycols Highly lipophilic
Fluconazole	$C_{13}H_{12}ON_6F_2$	306			Sparingly soluble in water (8 mg/ml) and 0.1 N HCl Soluble in methanol and acetone Very slightly soluble in hexane
Voriconazole	$C_{16}H_{14}F_3N_5O$	346			Insoluble in water Soluble in organic solvents
Posaconazole	$C_{35}H_{38}F_2N_8O_4$	672			
Ravuconazole	$C_{22}H_{17}N_5OF_2S$	437			

Table 13 Antifungal spectrum of systemic azole derivatives[a]

Fungal species	Ketoconazole	Fluconazole	Itraconazole	Voriconazole
Yeasts				
C. albicans	+	+	+	(+)
C. tropicalis	–	+	(±)	(+)
C. krusei	+	–	(±)	(±)
C. glabrata	–	±	(±)	(+)
C. neoformans	–	+	+	(+)
M. furfur	+	–	+	(+)
Filamentous fungi				
Aspergillus spp.	–	–	+	+
Scedosporium spp.	+	?	?	+
Fusarium spp.	±	–	–	–
Mucor, Rhizopus	?	?	?	?
Dermatophytes	+	–	+	?
Dimorphic fungi				
C. immitis	+	+	+	(+)
B. dermatitidis	+	?	+	(+)
Histoplasma spp.	+	+	+	(+)
S. schenckii	+	?	+	(+)
Paracoccidioides brasiliensis	+	+	+	(+)

[a]Data from Chandrasekar and Manavathu, 2001, and Bodey, 1992. +, active; –, resistant; ±, uncertain action; ?, no data at present. Parentheses indicate that the data concerning the activity of itraconazole and voriconazole on *Candida* will need to be reassessed on the basis of further clinical trials.

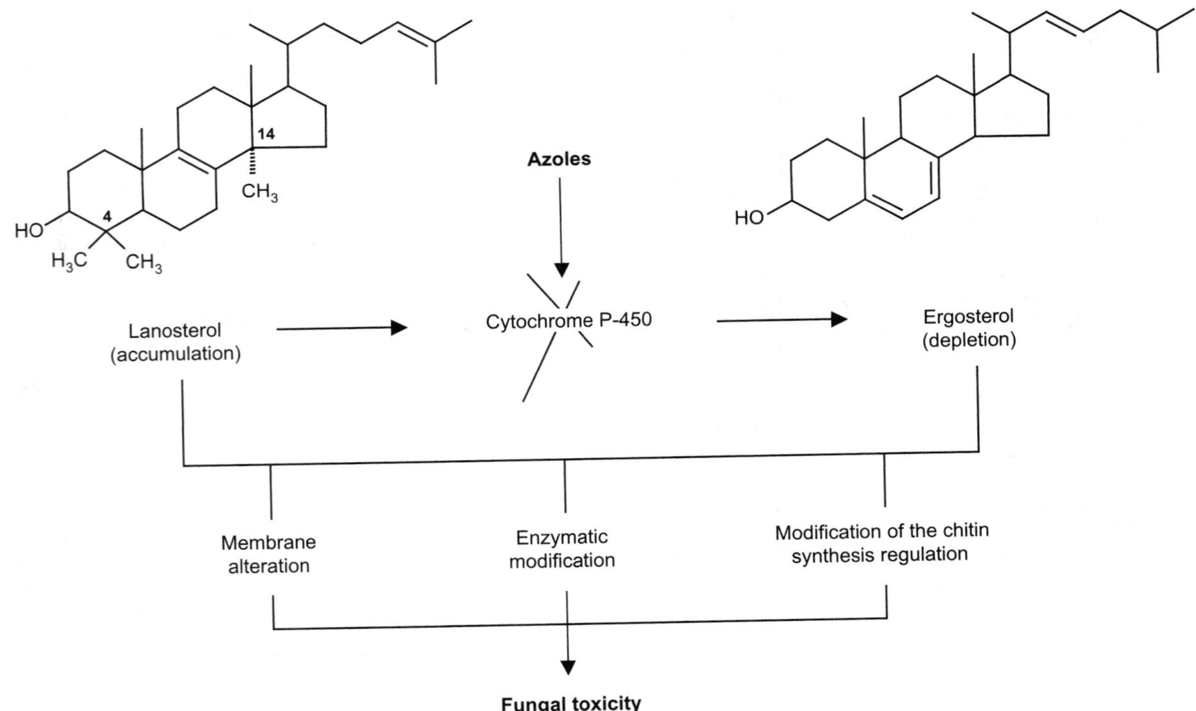

Figure 7 Mode of action of azole antifungals

- Inhibition of the formation of germ tubes and the production of mycelium
- Reduction in fungal adhesion phenomena

Generally, the azoles are considered fungistatic, but the differentiation between fungicidal and fungistatic activities is largely dependent on the laboratory techniques used.

3.2.2.5. Resistance

The emergence of strains resistant to the azoles occurred in parallel with the use of azoles (particularly fluconazole) principally in the treatment of mucocutaneous candidosis in patients suffering from AIDS.

On the basis of current data there are the following:

- Primary resistance (for example, fluconazole with *C. krusei* and certain strains of *C. glabrata* and itraconazole with *C. glabrata*)
- Secondary resistance, the extent of which varies with the species (*Candida dubliniensis*, *C. albicans*, *Candida inconspicua*, *Candida norvegensis*, etc.). For *C. albicans* it is estimated to be about 10%.

Resistance appears to involve the selection of either new pathogens during treatment or resistant mutants.

In addition, since all members of the azole family act on the same target, cross-resistance with a number of azoles is normal and regularly observed.

Three resistance mechanisms are currently postulated:

- Genetic alteration of the target of action (*ERG11* gene, coding for 14α-demethylase)
- Overproduction of the target of action by overexpression of the *ERG11* gene
- Efflux pumps through overexpression of the genes coding for the membrane transporters and chiefly involving three genes:
  - *CDR1* and *CDR2*, both encoding members of the family of ATP-binding cassette proteins and conferring comparable patterns of resistance to the azoles but also to terbinafine and cycloheximide
  - *MDR1*, exhibiting a sequence similar to major facilitator protein genes and coding principally for resistance to fluconazole

3.2.2.6. Pharmacokinetics

The principal pharmacological characteristics of the four systemic azole antifungals (ketoconazole, itraconazole, fluconazole, and voriconazole) are summarized in Table 14. Despite a common mechanism of action, the azoles differ considerably in their pharmacokinetic properties, which requires them to be discussed separately.

3.2.2.6.1. Ketoconazole. Ketoconazole, the first imidazole to be systemic after oral administration, initially constituted a considerable advance (1982), but its specific pharmacological features and its hepatotoxicity in prolonged treatment necessitated the redefinition and restriction of its conditions of use.

After oral administration, its bioavailability is markedly dependent on gastric pH, as it must be transformed to the hydrochloride to be active. After oral administration of 200 mg in healthy adults, a peak concentration in serum of 2 to 4 μg/ml is obtained 2 to 3 h after ingestion. This bioavailability is considerably modified by the administration of antacids or histamine H_2 receptor antagonists (cimetidine and ranitidine), which reduce or inhibit its absorption. Some situations also reduce gastric acidity: gastric disorders in AIDS patients, gastric surgery, and elderly status.

Conversely, the absorption of ketoconazole is enhanced if it is administered at the beginning of a meal and also by the addition of acidic substances (increase in concentrations in serum up to 5.6 μg/ml). These individual variations must be borne in mind in particular for "patients at fungal risk" receiving ketoconazole as fungal prophylaxis.

Ketoconazole is very strongly plasma protein bound (84%), with 15% of the product binding to leukocytes and only 1% remaining free in the plasma.

Study of the distribution of the product after administration of 200 mg shows good distribution, except in two compartments: cerebrospinal fluid (CSF) and urine. Penetration of the CSF is very weak (0.1 to 0.25 μg/ml when there is a meningeal inflammatory reaction, which contraindicates its use in fungal meningitis) and elimination in the urine is weak (2 to 4% of the dose).

Salivary diffusion is good (2.45 μg/ml 1 h after its administration), and the product is excreted in colostrum.

The majority of the administered dose of ketoconazole is metabolized in the liver by oxidative phenomena to inactive metabolites excreted in the bile and eliminated in the feces. The weak urinary elimination does not require modification of the dosage in patients with renal insufficiency. In the presence of hepatic insufficiency there does not appear to be accumulation of the product.

3.2.2.6.2. Itraconazole. A highly lipophilic triazole, itraconazole has been defined by Graybill as a "new and improved ketoconazole." Its activity against *Aspergillus* spp.,

Table 14 Principal pharmacokinetic characteristics of systemic antifungals[a]

Parameter	Ketoconazole	Itraconazole	Fluconazole	Voriconazole
Route of administration	Per os	Per os or I.V.[a]	Per os or I.V.	Per os or I.V.
Usual dosage	200–400 mg	100–400 mg	200–400 mg	400 mg
Peak concn in serum (μg/ml), 200 mg	3–5	1	10	1–2.5
Half-life (h)	1–4	21–37	27–37	6–24
Protein binding (%)	99	99.8	11	51–67
CSF/Concn in serum	<10	<1	50–90	50
Active product in urine (%)	2–4	<1	80	5
Visceral diffusion	++	+++	+++	+++
Absorption (%)	75	99	90	90
Metabolism	Liver	Liver	Renal elimination (80%)	Liver
Toxicity				
Renal	0	0	0	(0)
Hepatic	++	+	+	+
Endocrine	++	+/−	0	(0)
Gastrointestinal	++++	+/−	+/−	(0)
Ocular	0	0	0	+

[a]Adapted from Patterson, 1998, and Chandrasekar and Manavathu, 2001.

an important extension of its spectrum compared to ketoconazole, is of very specific interest. It is currently commercially available in an oral form (capsules and oral solution) and available in the parenteral form under an authorization for compassionate use. This has considerably altered its pharmacokinetics, particularly its absorption, a very limiting factor in its use in deep fungal infections, which generally occur in patients receiving parenteral nutrition.

In terms of absorption and bioavailability:

- The capsule form that has been commercially available since 1992 exhibits good absorption in healthy subjects as long as it is administered after meals (maximum bioavailability of 55%). However, this bioavailability may be affected in patients receiving cytotoxic drugs or radiotherapy or in AIDS patients. Levels obtained in serum after 3 to 4 h are between 0.1 and 0.5 μg/ml after a single dose of 100 to 400 mg. Repetition of the same daily dose produces a progressive improvement in the concentrations, steady state being obtained after 2 weeks (0.3 to 2 μg/ml depending on the daily dosage). The serum elimination half-life increases from 15 to 25 h after a single dose to 34 to 42 h after 2 weeks of administration. This absorption, which is related to gastric acidity, is reduced by antacids but not by anti-H2.
- The solution form (in which itraconazole is solubilized by hydroxypropyl-β-cyclodextrin) has more recently been made commercially available. It has very much better bioavailability (>30 to 60%), particularly if taken while fasting. Cyclodextrin, by contrast, is not absorbed but is transformed immediately by enzymes of the digestive flora to glucose molecules that are rapidly absorbed and metabolized. In addition, this dosage form yields high salivary levels up to 8 h after administration of a dose of itraconazole solution. This local persistence resulting in a topical effect explains the efficacy of this form in the treatment of oral mycoses.
- The intravenous form is also made from the itraconazole-cyclodextrin complex. A concentration in plasma of 0.2 to 0.5 μg/ml is obtained after infusion of 200 mg twice daily for 48 h in healthy volunteers. Cyclodextrin is rapidly eliminated by glomerular filtration, with minor accumulation in the body.

The circulating product is almost totally plasma protein bound, principally to albumin (99.8%). Concentrations in aqueous humor, CSF, saliva, and urine are negligible (<10%), but concentrations are considerably greater in sputum, bronchial secretions, and necrotic tissues. By contrast, tissue concentrations are high (kidney, liver, bone, spleen, and muscle), including tissues often affected by fungal infections (skin, nails, lungs, and genital mucosa), where the product can also persist for a very long time.

Itraconazole is metabolized entirely in the liver, the metabolites being essentially eliminated in the feces (54%) and urine (35%). One of the metabolites, hydroxyitraconazole, has antifungal activity in vitro equivalent to that of itraconazole, but weaker activity in animal models. The concentrations in plasma of hydroxyitraconazole exceed those of itraconazole, although the mean serum elimination half-life is markedly shorter (14 versus 25 h): at steady state, the concentrations of the hydroxyl metabolite are about twice those of the precursor. Therapeutically, a minimum concentration of itraconazole of at least 0.25 to 0.5 μg/ml is required, or at least 1 μg/ml if itraconazole and hydroxyitraconazole are assayed.

The pharmacokinetic characteristics of itraconazole are not altered by renal insufficiency, and the product is not eliminated by hemodialysis. Its metabolism is substantially reduced in patients with impaired hepatic function.

3.2.2.6.3. Fluconazole. Currently available in the oral and parenteral forms, fluconazole is a triazole that exhibits very original properties compared to the other systemic azoles through its very selective action on fungal cell cytochrome P450, which means that it is well tolerated and in particular possesses new pharmacological properties: hydrosolubility, metabolic stability, and low protein binding (11%).

The product is rapidly and totally absorbed gastrointestinally (>90%), peak concentrations in serum of 1.9 μg/ml being obtained 30 min after administration of a single oral dose of 100 mg and 6.7 μg/ml for a dose of 400 mg. There is a linear relationship between the concentrations in plasma of fluconazole and the administered dose. Absorption is not significantly affected by either gastric acidity or food intake. It is marginally lower in patients who have undergone bone marrow transplantation (1.75 instead of 1.9 μg/ml).

The tissue concentration-plasma concentration ratio is 0.5 to 0.8 for liver, spleen, lungs, kidney, muscle, and brain.

Repeated dosing produces steady state in 5 to 10 days with twice the concentrations, and the administration of an initial loading dose is recommended (twice the usual daily dose).

The volume of distribution is similar to that of water. The product is distributed equally between the different tissue compartments, crosses the meningeal barrier (>60%), and penetrates the vitreous humor, aqueous humor, and cornea. Salivary and peritoneal concentrations are comparable to levels in serum.

The metabolic stability of fluconazole is one of its major characteristics: 80% is eliminated in the urine in the unchanged form and 11% is eliminated in the metabolized form. The mean elimination half-life of fluconazole in healthy volunteers is 27 to 37 h. As yet preliminary results indicate that the concentration in serum may be high in elderly subjects. The half-life is shorter in children (16 to 20 h) but is considerably increased in premature infants and neonates (88 h). Dosage adaptations are therefore essential in children.

In view of its route of elimination, the dosage regimen must be adjusted in patients with renal insufficiency, as the renal clearance of fluconazole varies with glomerular filtration; with glomerular filtration of >70 ml/min, renal clearance is 1.04 liters/h; with glomerular filtration of <20 ml/min, renal clearance is 0.19 liter/h. Hemodialysis for 3 h reduces levels in serum by 48%, and the product is also eliminated by peritoneal dialysis. Its weak hepatic metabolization does not necessarily require a dosage adaptation in patients with hepatocellular insufficiency, but a significant reduction in the renal elimination of fluconazole has been observed in patients with severe hepatic impairment.

3.2.2.6.4. Voriconazole. Shortly to be available (currently available only on an authorization for compassionate use) in both the oral and intravenous forms, voriconazole (Fig. 8) is a second-generation triazole obtained by modifying the structure of fluconazole to broaden its spectrum of activity. However, their pharmacokinetic characteristics differ in a number of respects (Table 14).

Absorption after oral administration is rapid, with a time to peak concentration in serum of 1 to 2 h and bioavailability of >90%. Absorption is affected by food, being optimal if the medication is taken 1 to 2 h after food.

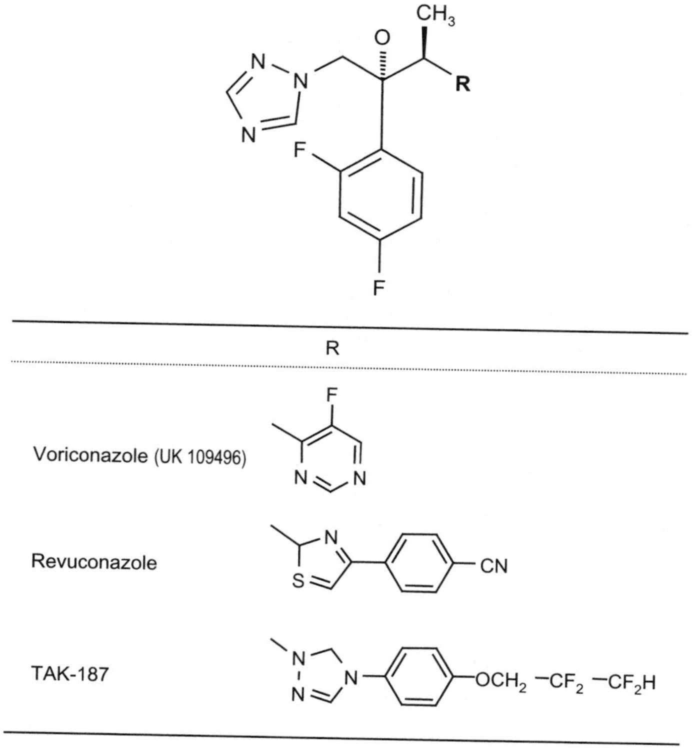

R

Voriconazole (UK 109496)

Revuconazole

TAK-187

Figure 8 Azoles under investigation

Voriconazole has a half-life of 6 h, with nonlinear pharmacokinetics, due probably to the saturable hepatic first-pass effect. It is moderately protein bound (≈55%). With a low apparent volume of distribution (2 liters/kg), voriconazole is extensively distributed in tissues and body fluids. Its plasma protein binding is moderate (≈60 to 65%).

Voriconazole is metabolized by the liver in the form of eight metabolites (three major and five minor) by the hepatic cytochrome P450 isoenzymes CYP2C9, CYP3A4, and CYP2C19. These metabolites have no antifungal action, and less than 5% of voriconazole is eliminated in the urine in the unchanged form.

3.2.2.7. Tolerability, Adverse Effects, and Drug Interference

The potential toxicity of the azole derivatives is gastrointestinal, hepatic, endocrine, metabolic, and hematologic. It varies with the following:

- The molecule: ketoconazole combines all of the drawbacks of the "standard" imidazoles, whereas the triazoles benefit from better tolerability, their affinity for fungal cell cytochrome P450 being more selective.
- The dosage: these derivatives are generally well tolerated at the standard dose, even when they are used for long periods. However, adverse effects are more common when the dosage is increased.

In addition, toxicity may also result from drug interactions, the same cytochrome P450 enzymes also being involved in the metabolism of a number of other drugs.

Generally, gastrointestinal disorders (nausea and vomiting) are moderate: they occur in 3 to 10% of patients receiving standard doses of ketoconazole (400 mg/day). They are more common (50%) if the dosage is increased (1.6 g/day). They affect less than 4% of patients receiving fluconazole (with a higher incidence in immunodepressed patients) and less than 10% of those receiving itraconazole. Headache, fever, fatigue, abdominal pain, and diarrhea are sometimes reported (particularly induced by the cyclodextrin present in the solution and intravenous forms of itraconazole).

Hypersensitivity reactions with pruritus, skin rash, and hypereosinophilia are also moderate: 2% for fluconazole, 6 to 9% for itraconazole, and 6% for voriconazole (according to the very early studies).

The principal risks associated with the azole compounds, and more specifically ketoconazole, relate to hepatotoxicity: transient elevations of transaminases and alkaline phosphatase occur during the first fortnight in about 10% of cases (15 to 20% in prolonged treatments). Cytolytic, cholestatic, or mixed types of hepatitis occur in about 1 in 10,000 to 50,000 patients but in 5% of cases during prolonged treatments. It may regress on discontinuation of the therapy, but fulminating and fatal hepatitis may occur during the first 4 to 6 weeks of treatment. It essentially affects women over 40 years of age (75%) treated for onychomycosis (70%) and who have previously exhibited allergic reactions to other treatments (50%).

This hepatotoxicity is markedly less with the triazoles (fluconazole and itraconazole): <5% transient disturbances of hepatic function (this incidence is often increased in immunodepressed patients). However, current data concerning the new forms of itraconazole (solution and intravenous) are still limited. Preliminary studies of the hepatic tolerance of voriconazole have shown a marked disturbance of liver function tests in 10 to 15% of the 1,019 patients monitored. Cases of sometimes fatal hepatitis observed with these molecules, although rare, should entail the discontinuation of treatment on the emergence of any signs or symptoms of hepatic lesions.

It should be noted that several studies have still shown only moderate toxicity of fluconazole even at high doses (≤1,200 mg/day) and/or in prolonged treatment (≥6 months).

The azoles may interfere with the conversion of lanosterol to cholesterol, the precursor of various hormones, by blockade of the enzymes 14α-demethylase, 11β-hydroxylase, and $C_{17,20}$-desmolase. In humans, ketoconazole may cause a decrease in serum testosterone levels, reduced libido, oligospermia, and gynecomastia. This phenomenon is dose dependent and regresses on discontinuation of treatment. At daily doses of >400 mg, ketoconazole can also cause a decrease in serum cortisol levels and a reduction in the response to adrenocorticotropin stimulation: a few cases of adrenocortical insufficiency have been reported.

In the case of itraconazole, results appear to suggest that at high dosages (600 mg/day) the endocrine toxicity derives from the accumulation of steroid precursors with an aldosterone-like effect, causing hypokalemia and hypertension. In very rare cases, hypokalemia has been reported in the past with fluconazole.

Again at high dosages (1.2 g/day), ketoconazole interferes with the metabolism of cholesterol: 27% reduction in levels in serum involving LDL, with high-density lipoproteins and triglycerides remaining unchanged.

The presence of dose-dependent and transient visual disorders and photophobia in 8 to 10% of patients receiving voriconazole should be noted.

Finally, the Food and Drug Administration has very recently drawn attention to several cases of congestive heart failure in patients treated with itraconazole for fungal nail disease, thereby contraindicating this antifungal agent in the treatment of onychomycoses in patients with a history of heart failure.

Azole antifungals are contraindicated during pregnancy; ketoconazole and itraconazole are teratogenic at high doses in the rat but not in the rabbit. There are no data yet for voriconazole.

Finally, one of the major questions about the azoles concerns the drug interactions associated with their interference in the enzymatic action of hepatic microsomes. These are observed in particular with ketoconazole and to a lesser extent with itraconazole and fluconazole.

These may involve the following:

- Either an interaction of the azole with various compounds:
  - Potentiation of various drugs with a hepatic metabolism (nonsedative H_1 antihistamines, cisapride, hypoglycemic sulfonamides, anti-vitamin K anticoagulants [warfarin], cyclosporine, tacrolimus, benzodiazepines, etc.)
  - Potentiation of the hepatotoxic effect of certain compounds such as griseofulvin.
- Or an antagonist effect on the azole:
  - By enzyme inducers, e.g., rifampin and phenytoin (for itraconazole and ketoconazole), which accelerate the clearance of the antifungal agent and reduce its elimination half-life
  - By drugs that inhibit or markedly reduce their gastric absorption: antacids, histamine H_2 receptor antagonists, and atropine derivatives

The main drug interactions are summarized in Table 15.

In general, the consumption of alcohol is contraindicated, as the combination of azole and ethanol causes a disulfiram effect; this abstention should continue for 48 h after the end of treatment.

Finally, no analytical interference has been observed between these azole antifungals and routine laboratory tests, particularly by autoanalyzer.

3.2.2.8. Clinical Indications

It is perhaps surprising that although the azole antifungals have been used for a number of years in the treatment of fungal infections, knowledge about their efficacy and indications is still incomplete. In fact, there are a number of reasons why clinical trials are difficult to conduct for deep mycoses: an often limited number of patients, difficulty of definitely establishing the diagnosis of infections such as candidosis and disseminated aspergillosis, often chronic infections subject to relapses after discontinuation of treatment, etc. However, there is current unanimity in recommending azoles in the following indications (some of these assessments are still in the course of being performed).

3.2.2.8.1. Miconazole. Because of its poor tolerance (related essentially to the solvent, Cremophor), the intravenous route is no longer available. The use of miconazole is therefore confined to topical mucocutaneous applications, particularly in gastrointestinal mycoses.

3.2.2.8.2. Ketoconazole. Ketoconazole has proved the treatment of choice for endemic mycoses due to dimorphic fungi: histoplasmosis, blastomycosis, paracoccidioidomycosis, and certain kinds of entomophthoromycosis:

- Recurrent infections due to superficial yeasts: oral and esophageal thrush, vaginitis, and pityriasis versicolor
- Chronic mucocutaneous candidosis and folliculitis in heroin addicts
- Extensive dermatophyte infections
- Still disputed in the prophylaxis of gastrointestinal candidosis in neutropenic patients
- To be prohibited in disseminated or localized deep infections in immunodepressed patients

The dose (200 to 400 mg) and duration of treatment (1 week to several months) vary with the indications.

3.2.2.8.3. Fluconazole. The spectrum of fluconazole, which is directed primarily against infections due to *C. albicans* and *C. neoformans*, currently justifies these indications, in which moreover the majority of clinical trials have been undertaken (evaluations still in progress):

- Oropharyngeal candidosis, esophageal candidosis (AIDS and malignant hemopathy); however, there is a risk of selection of less susceptible flora
- Systemic candidosis (urinary tract infections, candidemia, and peritonitis)
- Fundamental interest in cryptococcosis, where fluconazole constitutes an alternative to AMB and represents the treatment of choice in the prophylaxis of relapses in AIDS patients

The dose is between 100 and 400 mg, with a loading dose on the first day (intravenously or orally), for 2 to 3 weeks (mucosal infections) to several months (cryptococcosis).

3.2.2.8.4. Itraconazole. Although a number of evaluations are still in progress to determine exactly the indications and dosage (100 to 400 mg), itraconazole, which is original through its action on filamentous fungi, is of genuine interest in the treatment of the following:

Table 15 Principal drug interactions observed with systemic azole antifungals

Drugs	FLC	ITC	KTC	Adverse effects	Precautions
Action of azole on the metabolism of other drugs (potentiation of the combined drug by inhibition of its hepatic metabolism [CYP3A4 +++])					
Nonsedative antihistamines	±	+	+	Torsade de pointes, ↑QT	Contraindication (ITC and KTC)
Cisapride	+	+	+	Torsade de pointes, ↑QT	Contraindication
Cyclosporine	+	+	+	Nephrotoxicity (particularly transplant patients)	Monitoring (levels in plasma and kidney)
Tacrolimus	+	?	+	Nephrotoxicity	Monitoring (levels in plasma and kidney)
HMG-CoA reductase inhibitors	–	+	–	Rhabdomyolysis	Contraindication (ITC and KTC)
Anti-vitamin K anticoagulants (warfarin)	+	+	+	↓prothrombin time ratio, hemorrhagic risk	Monitoring (PT)
Calcium inhibitors	?	+	?	Fluctuations in hypertension and cardiac rhythm, edema	Contraindication (ITC and berepril) or monitoring
Benzodiazepines (triazolam and midazolam)	+	+	+	↑hypnotic effect	
Oral hypoglycemic agents	+	?	+	↑hypoglycemia (not FLC)	Monitoring (blood glucose)
Antiretroviral agents					
Zidovudine	+	+	+		
Ritonavir	–	+	+		
Saquinavir	–	+	+		
Indinavir	–	+	+		
Digoxin	–	+	–	Digestive and visual disorders, rhythm disorders	Monitoring (levels in plasma and ECG)
Quinidine	?	?	+	Rhythm disorders, torsade de pointes, hearing	
Prednisolone	–	–	+		
Griseofulvin	–	–	+	Hepatotoxicity	Contraindication
Antagonist effect of the combined drug on the azole by enzymatic induction					
Phenytoin	↓plasma levels	↓ITC	↓KTC	Digestive and visual disorders (FLC); failure of antifungal treatment (ITC, KTC)	Monitoring
Other enzyme-inducing anticonvulsants	–	↓ITC	–	Failure of antifungal treatment (ITC)	Monitoring
Rifampin, isoniazid	↓of both anti-infectives	↓of both anti-infectives	↓of both anti-infectives		Interval between the two doses, monitoring
Rifabutin	↑plasma levels	?	?	Ocular toxicity (FLC)	Clinical monitoring
Antagonist effect of the combined drug on the azole by inhibition of its gastric absorption					
Antacids, anti-H_2, sucralfate, proton pump inhibitors	–	↓ITC	↓KTC	Failure of antifungal treatment	Interval between the two doses (antacids) or monitoring
Didanosine (antiretroviral)	–	↓ITC	↓KTC	Presence of antacid in tablet	Interval between the two doses

[a]Adapted from Lomaestro, 1998, and Albengres et al., 1998. FLC, fluconazole; ITC, itraconazole; KTC, ketoconazole; CoA, coenzyme A; PT, prothrombin time; ECG, electrocardiogram.

- Allergic bronchopulmonary, chronic necrotizing, invasive aspergillosis and nonoperable aspergillomas, particularly in AMB-intolerant or -refractory patients
- Cutaneous dermatophyte infections and conditions due to pityriasis versicolor when local treatment is not feasible. In onychomycoses, the indication must be established extremely cautiously in view of the hepatic and cardiac toxicity in long-term treatment.
- Infections due to dimorphic fungi: coccidioidomycosis, sporotrichosis, and chromomycosis
- Keratomycosis and cryptococcosis, which appear to respond well to itraconazole

- Oral and/or esophageal candidosis in human immunodeficiency virus-positive patients (solution form only). However, its use outside the authorized indication may be an alternative to the capsule form in patients unable to feed themselves.

The dosage is between 200 and 400 mg/day, with a loading dose being required in invasive infections due to filamentous fungi of the *Aspergillus* type.

3.2.2.8.5. Voriconazole. Clinical data about its use are still limited, but voriconazole appears to be of interest in the case of resistance or problems of intolerance to conventional molecules following *Candida* or *Aspergillus* infections or those due to other susceptible microorganisms, such as *S. apiospermum*, *Fusarium* spp., or *C. neoformans*. Its use as first-line therapy in minor systemic infections or as empirical therapy remains to be determined.

The dosages currently recommended are on the order of 400 mg daily in two doses for the oral form and 3 to 6 mg/kg every 12 h for the parenteral form.

3.2.2.9. Pharmaceutical Forms

Nizoral is the trade name for ketoconazole (200-mg tablets).

Diflucan (European name, Triflucan) is the trade name for 50-, 100-, and 200-mg fluconazole capsules, as well as for powder for oral suspension (50 mg/5 ml) and injectable solution for infusion) (2 mg/ml).

Sporanox is the trade name for 100-mg itraconazole capsules, as well as oral solution (10 mg/ml) and injectable solution for infusion (10 mg/ml).

Vfend is the trade name for voriconazole.

3.2.3. Azoles under Development

Two triazoles are currently under development: posaconazole and ravuconazole.

3.2.3.1. Posaconazole

Posaconazole (Fig. 9) is a triazole with a structure similar to that of itraconazole. This substance is very slightly soluble in water (2 μg/ml) and is used only in the oral form (tablet or suspension).

Like all azoles, posaconazole acts by inhibiting cytochrome P450 14α-demethylase (CYP51), the key enzyme in ergosterol synthesis.

It has a broad spectrum of activity and exerts fungicidal activity against a number of filamentous fungi (*Aspergillus* spp., *P. boydii*, and zygomycetes). It appears to be less active against *Fusarium* spp. Posaconazole has good activity against yeasts of the *Candida* genus (particularly non-*C. albicans* species resistant to fluconazole and/or itraconazole, but for which the MIC at which 90% of isolates tested are inhibited still remain high) and *C. neoformans*, as well as dimorphic fungi such as *Histoplasma capsulatum*, *Blastomyces dermatitidis*, *Sporothrix schenckii*, and *Coccidioides immitis*.

In humans, preliminary pharmacokinetic studies show that increasing doses of posaconazole yield levels in plasma well above the MICs for the fungi most commonly found in human disease, including species of *Candida* resistant to other azoles. However, as for itraconazole, the bioavailability of the oral form (the only one studied to date) is markedly increased (fourfold) if it is administered with a fatty meal. As with itraconazole, the suspension form also has better availability than the tablet form.

Preclinical studies with animals do not show any specific toxicity at the doses used in humans.

Posaconazole is undergoing phase III clinical trials.

3.2.3.2. Ravuconazole

Ravuconazole is a triazole that is structurally similar to fluconazole and voriconazole at the beginning of testing (phase II). It has a broad spectrum of activity that includes *Candida* spp., *C. neoformans*, *A. fumigatus*, and *Dematiaceae* in vitro. Its activity appears to be more limited with respect to *S. schenckii*, *P. boydii*, *Fusarium* spp., and zygomycetes. Only an oral form is currently described.

3.3. Terbinafine

Terbinafine belongs to the class of allylamines, which are ergosterol inhibitors. Their action, therefore, as for the polyenes and azoles, occurs in the cytoplasmic membrane. Terbinafine is the only antifungal agent of this class to possess systemic action. Its indications previously were confined to superficial mycoses. However, its as yet very occasional usage recently in certain deep mycoses justifies its place in this chapter.

3.3.1. Physicochemical Properties

Table 16 lists the physicochemical properties of terbinafine.

3.3.2. In Vitro Properties and Spectrum of Activity

Terbinafine has very good in vitro activity against certain filamentous fungi (dermatophytes, *Aspergillus* spp., and

Table 16 Physicochemical properties of terbinafine

Empirical formula	Mol wt	Stability
$C_{21}H_{26}ClN$	328	Stable against heat (<50°C), moisture, and oxidizing agents Unstable against light

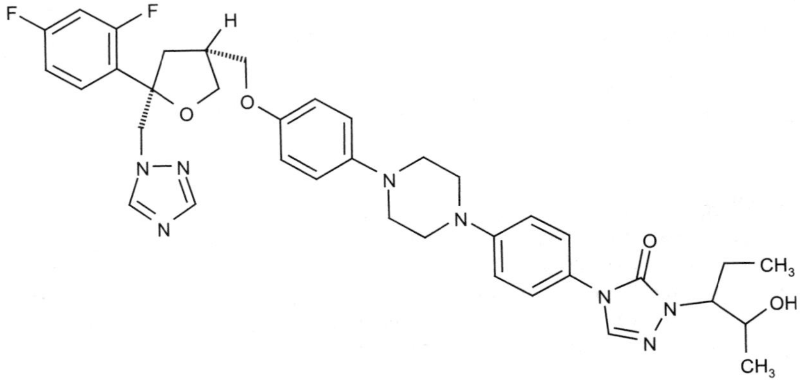

Figure 9 Posaconazole

Dematiaceae, essentially) and dimorphic fungi (*H. capsulatum, B. dermatitidis,* and *S. schenckii*), but less so against pathogenic yeasts.

3.3.3. Mechanisms of Action

Terbinafine inhibits fungal ergosterol synthesis early and specifically at the squalene epoxidation stage (Fig. 7). Inhibition of squalene epoxidase causes the following:

- A deficiency of ergosterol, causing debilitation of the fungal membrane and arrested growth, hence a fungistatic activity
- Accumulation of squalene, which causes the deposition of lipid vesicles in the cytoplasm and the fungal wall, with rupture of the cell membrane and hence fungicidal activity. However, this fungicidal action is marked to a greater or lesser extent according to the species concerned (dermatophytes and *Aspergillus*).

3.3.4. Resistance Mechanisms

Resistance to terbinafine has not been reported for dermatophytes or *Aspergillus*, although resistance has been described for *Saccharomyces cerevisiae*. However, data are still limited with respect to filamentous fungi such as *Aspergillus*.

3.3.5. Pharmacokinetics

At a dose of 250 mg, the maximum concentration in serum is 1 μg/ml and the volume of distribution is 15 liters/kg. Oral absorption is rapid and extensive (>70%). The pharmacokinetics are linear. It is markedly protein bound (>99%), but nonspecifically and hence nonsaturably. Terbinafine diffuses rapidly through the dermis and is concentrated in the stratum corneum. It also diffuses into the sebum and reaches high concentrations in the hair follicles. It is present in the nail from the first weeks of treatment. This explains the main indications of this antifungal agent in superficial mycoses. However, one study showed a two- to sevenfold-higher concentration in the lungs than in the plasma in volunteer patients treated with 500 to 750 mg of terbinafine per day prior to elective pulmonary resection. A single daily dosage, therefore, yields effective parenchymatous concentrations. These data point to the possible use of terbinafine in certain invasive mycoses.

The principal routes of metabolization are as follows:

- N dealkylation of the atom of the central nitrogen
- Oxidation of the methyl groups of the side chain
- Formation of dihydrodiols via the formation of an aromatic arene oxide

The metabolites that are formed do not possess antifungal activity. Elimination occurs in two phases, a distribution phase (half-life, 4.6 h) and an elimination phase (half-life, 17 h). Excretion is essentially urinary (70% of the administered dose is found in the urine in the form of inactive metabolites).

No difference has been observed in elderly patients and in children at steady state. In patients with hepatic insufficiency, elimination is slower because of a reduction in biotransformation and hence total clearance of the product. In patients with renal insufficiency, the total clearance of terbinafine is markedly lower, resulting in higher levels in plasma. The use of terbinafine is not recommended in children in the absence of specific studies.

3.3.6. Tolerability, Adverse Effects, Interactions, and Contraindications

The tolerability of terbinafine has been evaluated in numerous cases of onychomycosis for treatment periods of more than 6 weeks. It is relatively nontoxic, and the most commonly encountered reactions involve the gastrointestinal sphere (5%). These usually involve nausea, dyspeptic disorders, abdominal pain, and transit disorders. These reactions are moderate and transient. Minor skin reactions occur in 2% of cases. Finally, partial or total loss of taste, which may regress only after the discontinuation of treatment, has been observed. Hematologic disorders with a possible lesion of the three cell lines have been reported exceptionally.

Very recently, the Food and Drug Administration has reported 16 cases of hepatic insufficiency, including 11 deaths possibly related to terbinafine.

Few drug interactions have been described. The only known interaction is a reduction in plasma terbinafine levels with rifampin as a result of an increase in its plasma clearance.

3.3.7. Clinical Indications

The therapeutic indications for the marketing authorization are limited to superficial fungal infections: onychomycoses, dermatophyte infections, and cutaneous candidosis at dosages of 250 mg/day for several weeks or months, depending on the type of lesion and localization.

However, the in vitro activity of terbinafine against *Aspergillus* and in animal models of invasive aspergillosis has given rise to the consideration of its use in pulmonary aspergillosis. The very first clinical studies show efficacy of terbinafine in immunocompetent patients. In addition, it has been demonstrated in vitro that there is synergistic activity of the combination itraconazole-terbinafine and an additive effect of the combination AMB-terbinafine, a therapeutic avenue that might be interesting to explore in the future in invasive aspergillosis. However, the potential interactions should be carefully studied.

3.3.8. Pharmaceutical Forms

Lamisil is the trade name for terbinafine (250-mg) tablets.

3.4. Echinocandins

Whereas the previous antifungal agents act on the nucleus (5FC) or more often on the cytoplasmic membrane (polyenes, azoles, and allylamines), the new classes of antifungal agents target their action on the fungal wall. This in fact comprises three major components: β-1,3-D-glucan, chitin, and a mannoprotein, and the new agents act by inhibiting the synthesis of one of these constituents. None of these elements is present in mammalian cells, suggesting a highly targeted action by the molecules, which avoids in particular the side effects associated with a target common to mammals and fungi, as is the case with the currently available antifungals.

Among the inhibitors of β-1,3-D-glucan synthesis, the echinocandins belong to a large family of lipopeptides in which caspofungin is the first agent to have an authorization for compassionate use. Marketing authorization should follow in France very shortly.

3.4.1. Caspofungin

3.4.1.1. Chemical Structure

Caspofungin acetate is a semisynthetic lipopeptide synthesized from a fermentation product of *Glarea lozoyensis* (Fig. 10).

3.4.1.2. Physicochemical Properties

Table 17 lists the physicochemical properties of caspofungin. It is a white to whitish powder, soluble in water and

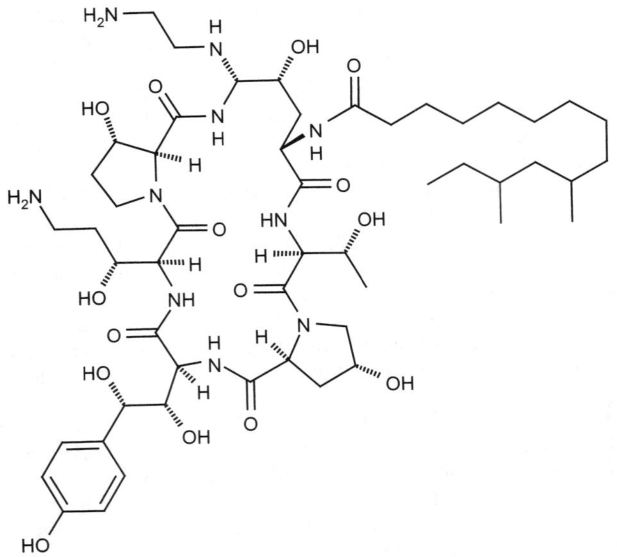

Figure 10 Caspofungin

methanol and slightly less so in ethanol. Its pH in aqueous solution is 6.6.

3.4.1.3. In Vitro Properties and Spectrum of Activity

Caspofungin appears to have a fungicidal action and is characterized by excellent in vitro activity against *Aspergillus* spp. (*A. fumigatus*, *A. flavus*, and *A. terreus*) and numerous species of *Candida*. However, this activity has been studied in accordance with the recommendations of the NCCLS in the absence of standards for inhibitors β-1,3-D-glucan synthesis. In addition, current results of in vitro susceptibility studies are not necessarily correlated with clinical results. On the other hand, there does not appear to be cross-resistance with strains resistant to AMB or azoles, particularly azole-resistant strains of *Candida* spp.

Conversely, this agent has little or no activity:

- In vitro or in vivo against *C. neoformans* (as this yeast possesses little if any β-1,3-D-glucan synthetase but does possess a β-1,6-D-glucan or 1,6-α-glucan structure)
- In vitro against filamentous fungi such as *Fusarium* and *Rhizopus* spp.

For the other fungal genera, the presence of β-1,3-D-glucan as a constituent in the wall is still insufficiently documented. Conversely, this new drug is active against *Pneumocystis carinii*.

3.4.1.4. Mechanisms of Action

Caspofungin acts by specifically inhibiting the synthesis of β-1,3-D-glucan, an essential component of the fungal wall, particularly of *Candida* and *Aspergillus* spp. This inhibition involves a noncompetitive action on β-1,3-D-glucan synthetase, leading to the formation of glucan polymers. This culminates in disruption of the wall structure and osmotic instability, resulting in cell lysis.

3.4.1.5. Resistance Mechanisms

In vitro resistance of *Aspergillus* spp. to caspofungin has not yet been observed. Results from the still limited clinical trials available to us have not shown resistance in patients treated for invasive aspergillosis.

3.4.1.6. Pharmacokinetics

The oral bioavailability is weak. Only the parenteral route is currently available.

The concentrations in plasma of caspofungin decrease multiphasically after single infusions for 1 h:

- Short α phase immediately after infusion
- β phase with a half-life of 9 to 11 h
- γ phase with a half-life of 27 h

These kinetics allow single daily administration.

Plasma clearance is slow, explained more by the distribution than by excretion or biotransformation. In fact, the last two are minor during the first 30 h following administration.

Caspofungin is strongly bound to albumin (97%) and is therefore not dialyzable. Its metabolism is slow, involving hydrolysis and N acetylation. After a single intravenous dose, the rates of excretion of caspofungin and its metabolites in humans are 35% in feces and 41% in urine. Renal clearance of the parent molecule is weak.

The pharmacokinetics are presented in Table 18. The pharmacokinetics are linear in adults and in children. The AUC increases proportionately to the dose. The half-life does not vary over time or with the clearance or volume of distribution. In the pediatric population, clearance and volume of distribution are 33 and 26% higher, respectively.

Table 17 Physicochemical properties of caspofungin

Empirical formula	Mol wt	Solubility	Stability
$C_{52}H_{88}O_{15}N_{10}2C_2H_4O_2$	1,213	Soluble in water and methanol Less soluble in ethanol	Infusion solution (undiluted) stable 24 h at ≤ 25°C

Table 18 Pharmacokinetics of caspofungin after repeated administrations in immunodepressed adults and children

Subjects and length of treatment	Dose (mg/day)	C_{max} (μg/ml)	AUC (μg·h/ml)	V (liters/kg)	$t_{1/2}$ (h)	CL (ml·h/kg)
Child (4 days)	1	20	57	0.38	17	0.28
Adult (7 days)	50	6.40	49	0.22	12.5	0.20

3.4.1.7. Tolerability, Adverse Effects, Interactions, and Contraindications

We do not currently have sufficiently large studies for this agent to evaluate its tolerability with certainty. However, according to initial studies (623 individuals), tolerability is generally good. In treated patients (287 patients), the clinical and laboratory abnormalities regarded as treatment related are mild and markedly less than with AMB:

- General (fever, headache, and pain)
- Gastrointestinal (nausea, vomiting, and diarrhea)
- Cutaneous (vasomotor flushes and pruritus)
- Vascular (complications in the infused vein)
- Hepatic (elevation of hepatic enzymes)
- Plasma (anemia)

Caspofungin has no particular affinity for cytochrome P450 as a substrate and does not exhibit any significant inhibition of this enzyme system either. It is not a substrate of P-glycoprotein.

According to the preliminary studies on drug interactions:

- Concomitant use of caspofungin and a metabolism inducer and/or inhibitor (efavirenz, nelfinavir, nevirapine, rifampin, dexamethasone, phenytoin, or carbamazepime) should entail an increase in the daily dose.
- Caspofungin does not interact with mycophenolate or tacrolimus. However, the combination of caspofungin and tacrolimus may reduce the concentrations of the latter in blood, necessitating a dosage adjustment.
- Cyclosporine causes an increase in the AUC of caspofungin, probably by reduction of its hepatic uptake. In addition, coadministration of these two drugs is not recommended because of the elevation of hepatic enzymes observed in healthy volunteers.

3.4.1.8. Clinical Indications

Caspofungin is currently indicated in the treatment of invasive aspergillosis in patients refractory or intolerant to other treatments.

The dosage is 50 mg/day, with a loading dose of 70 mg on the first day. No dosage adjustment is necessary in the case of renal insufficiency or mild hepatic insufficiency (Child-Pugh score of 5 or 6). Above that, the dosage must be adapted or treatment must be discontinued in the current absence of clinical data.

Finally, the mechanism of action of caspofungin, which is very different from that of the other families of antifungals, suggests major possibilities for the combination of caspofungin and polyenes or even caspofungin and azoles.

3.4.1.9. Pharmaceutical Forms

Cancidas (Caspofungine MSD in France) is the trade name for powder for dilution for injectable preparation for infusion (70- and 50-mg bottles).

3.4.2. Echinocandins under Development

There are two new drugs (micafungin and anidulafungin) of the class of echinochandins currently under investigation, the mechanism of action of which is based on inhibition of the synthesis of the major component of the fungal wall, 1,3-β-D-glucan. Their spectrum of activity appears to be very similar to that of caspofungin. Micafungin is active in vitro against *Candida* spp., particularly the azole-resistant strains of *C. albicans*, and against *Aspergillus* spp. It is currently in phase II clinical studies and will only be available in the intravenous form, whereas anidulafungin will have oral and intravenous forms.

4. CONCLUSIONS AND PROSPECTS

Despite the considerable advances in antifungal therapy over the last few years, we are still far from possessing the ideal antifungal and progress is still necessary. Fungal infections remain in fact a matter of concern, particularly in severe neutropenia (frequent inefficacy in disseminated mycoses) and AIDS (frequency of relapses and/or resistance in oroesophageal candidosis and cryptococcosis).

However, the therapeutic panorama has diversified and recently has allowed interesting alternatives by virtue of the following:

- New lipid forms of AMB
- A new parenteral formulation of itraconazole, a first-generation triazole
- The commercialization of voriconazole, a second-generation triazole that is very active against *Aspergillus* and *Cryptococcus*. However, it is essential to bear in mind the limits imposed by the risks of long-term toxicity of the azoles (hepatotoxicity or endocrine toxicity), none of the derivatives of this series being truly harmless when long-term treatments are involved.
- The development of totally new classes of recently discovered antifungals, enzyme inhibitors involved in the synthesis of wall components of the fungal cell (β-1,3-glucan synthetase and chitin synthetase), particularly caspofungin

In addition to the discovery of molecules with new sites of action, the consolidation of the use of previously developed molecules, and at the same time the even more precise definition of their indications and optimal dosages and extension of their potential role in prophylaxis, research in the area of antifungals is currently directed to other goals:

- Combinations of antifungals to obtain a synergistic effect or to suppress the emergence of resistance are still little used, apart from the common addition of AMB to 5FC. Although azole-polyene antagonism is conventionally assumed, the combinations of azoles or azole-5FC, AMB-echinochandin, azole-echinochandin, or again the sequential use of polyenes and azoles has as yet been little investigated.
- The incorporation of immunomodulators (interferons, interleukins, colony-stimulating factors) that might play a considerable additive role in conventional antifungal therapy of serious mycoses in immunosuppressed patients by amplifying the host's resistance to the fungal aggression
- Finally, the concept of vaccination for certain at-risk populations might, in the future, offer an alternative in terms of prevention.

REFERENCES

Albengres E, Le Louet H, Tillement JP, 1998, Systemic antifungal agents, drug interactions of clinical significance, Drug Saf, 18, 83–97.

Anaissie E, Paetznick V, Proffitt R, Adler-Moore J, Bodey GP, 1991, Comparison of the in vitro antifungal activity of free and liposome-encapsulated amphotericin B, Eur J Clin Microbiol Infect Dis, 10, 665–668.

Andrès E, Tiphine M, Letscher-Bru V, Herbrecht R, 2001, Nouvelles formes lipidiques de l'amphotéricine B, revue de la littérature, Rev Méd Interne, 22, 141–150.

Bodey GP, 1992, Azole antifungal agents, Clin Infect Dis, 14, Suppl 1, S161–S169.

Bolard J, 1986, How do the polyene macrolide antibiotics affect the cellular membrane properties? Biochim Biophys Acta, 864, 257–304.

Bolard J, 1991, Mechanism of action of an anti-Candida drug, amphotericin B and its derivatives, p 214–238, in Prasad R, ed, Candida albicans, Cellular and Molecular Biology, Springer Verlag.

Bonaly R, 1977, La griséofulvine, mode d'action et cinétique, CR Entretiens de Mycologie Fondamentale et Appliquée, CHR Hôpital Jeanne d'Arc, Dommartin les Toul, 17 Novembre 1977.

Brajtburg J, Powderly WG, Kobayashi GS, Medoff G, 1990, Amphotericin B, current understanding of mechanisms of action, Antimicrob Agents Chemother, 34, 183–188.

Chandrasekar PH, Manavathu E, 2001, Voriconazole, a second-generation triazole, Drugs of Today, 37, 135–148.

Chiller T, Stevens DA, 2000, Treatment strategies for Aspergillus infections, Drug Resistance Updates, 3, 89–97.

Dellamonica P, 1989, Réflexions sur la 5-fluorocytosine, La Lettre de l'Infectiologue, 4, 598–599.

Denning DW, Stevens DA, 1990, Antifungal and surgical treatment of invasive aspergillosis, review of 2,121 published cases, Rev Infect Dis, 12, 1147–1201.

Dodds ES, Drew RH, Perfect JR, 2000, Antifungal pharmacodynamics, review of literature and clinical applications, pharmacotherapy, 20, 1335–1355.

Drouhet E, Dupont B, 1988, Antifongiques, p 1738–1760, in Giroud JP, Mathe G, Meyniel G, ed, Pharmacologie clinique, bases de la thérapeutique, 2nd ed, Expansion Scientifique Française, Paris.

Dupont B, Drouhet E, 1990, Antifongiques, Editions Techniques Encycl Méd Chir, Maladies infectieuses, 8004 M^{10}, p 9–15.

Dykewicz C, 2001, Summary of the Guidelines for Preventing Opportunistic Infections among Hematopoietic Stem Cell Transplant Recipients, Clin Infect Dis, 33, 139–144.

Gallis HA, Drew RH, Pickard WW, 1990, Amphotericin B, 30 years of clinical experience, Rev Infect Dis, 12, 308–329.

Goa KL, Barradell LB, 1995, Fluconazole, an update of its pharmacodynamic and pharmacokinetic properties and therapeutic use in major superficial and systemic mycoses in immunocompromised patients, Drugs, 50, 658–690.

Goldman RC, Frost DJ, Capobianco JO, Kadam S, Rasmussen RR, Abad-Zapatero C, 1995, Antifungal drug targets: Candida secreted aspartyl protease and fungal wall β-glucan synthesis, Inf Agents Dis, 4, 228–247.

Grant SM, Clissold SP, 1990, Fluconazole, a review of its pharmacodynamic and pharmacokinetic properties and therapeutic potential in superficial and systemic mycoses, Drugs, 39, 877–916.

Graybill JR, 1989, New antifungal agents, Eur J Clin Microbiol Infect Dis, 8, 402–412.

Graybill JR, 1992, Future directions of antifungal chemotherapy, Clin Infect Dis, 14 (Suppl 1), S170–S181.

Hoang A, 2001, Caspofungin acetate, an antifungal agent, Am J Health-Sys Pharm, 58, 1206–1214.

Hood S, Denning DW, 1997, Treatment of fungal infection in AIDS, J Antimicrob Chemother, 37, suppl B, 71–85.

Hughes WT, Armstrong D, Bodey GP, Brown AE, Edwards JE, Feld R, Pizzo P, Rolston VI, Shenep JL, Young LS, 1997, Guidelines from the Infectious Diseases Society of America, Clin Infect Dis, 25, 551–573.

Iwata K, Vanden Bossche H, 1986, In vitro and in vivo evaluation of antifungal agents, Elsevier Science Publishers BV, Amsterdam.

Jensen GM, 1998, 38th Intersci Conf Antimicrob Agents Chemother.

Joly V, Saint-Julien L, Carbon C, Yeni P, 1990, Interactions of free and liposomal amphotericin B with renal tubular cells in primary culture, J Pharmacol Exp Ther, 255, 17–22.

Klepser ME, 2001, Antifungal resistance among Candida species, Pharmacotherapy, 21, 124S–132S.

Kobayashi GS, Odds FC, 1989, Current perspectives on antifungal susceptibility testing, focus on fluconazole, p 26, Pfizer Monograph, Scientific Therapeutic Information, Inc., New Jersey.

Kontoyiannis DP, 2001, A clinical perspective for the management of invasive fungal infections, Focus on IDSA guidelines, Pharmacotherapy, 21, 175S–187S.

Lortholary O, Dupont B, 1997, Apport des antifongiques azolés dans la prophylaxie des infections fongiques, Ann Med Interne, 3, 258–267.

Meyer RD, 1992, Current role of therapy with amphotericin B, Clin Infect Dis, 14 (Suppl 1), S154–S160.

Neely MN, Ghannoum MA, 2000, The exciting future of antifungal therapy, Eur J Clin Microbiol Infect Dis, 19, 897–914.

Odds FC, 1988, Antifungal agents and their use in Candida infections, p 279–313, in Candida and Candidosis, a Review and Bibliography, 2nd ed, Baillière Tindall, London.

Patterson BE, Coates PE, 1995, UK 109496, a novel wide-spectrum triazole derivative for the treatment of fungal infection, pharmacokinetics in man, 35th Intersci Conf Antimicrob Agents Chemother, abstract F-78.

Patterson TF, 1999, Role of newer azoles in surgical patients, J Chemother, 11, 504–512.

Polak A, 1998, The past, present and future of antimycotic combination therapy, Mycoses, 42, 355–370.

Polak A, Scholer HJ, 1980, Mode of action of 5-fluorocytosine, Rev Institut Pasteur Lyon, 13, 233–244.

Powderly WG, Kobayashi GS, Herzig GP, Medoff G, 1988, Amphotericin B-resistant yeast infection in severely immunocompromised patients, Am J Med, 84, 826–832.

Prentice HG, Hann IM, Herbrecht R, Aoun M, Kvaloy S, Catovsky D, Pinkerton CR, Schey SA, Jacobs F, Oakhill A, Stevens RF, Darbyshire PJ, Gibson BE, 1997, A randomized comparison of liposomal versus conventional amphotericin B for treatment of pyrexia of unknown origin in neutropenic patients, Br J Haematol, 98, 711–718.

Rex JH, Walsh TJ, Sobel JD, Filler SG, Pappas PG, Dismukes WE, Edwards JE, 2000, Practice guidelines for the treatment of candidiasis, Clin Infect Dis, 30, 662–678.

Rosa FW, Hernandez C, Carlo WA, 1987, Griseofulvin teratology, including two thoracopagus conjoined twins, Lancet, i, 171.

Saag MS, Graybill RJ, Larsen RA, Pappas PG, Perfect JR, Powderly WG, Sobel JD, Dismukes WE for the Mycoses Study Group Cryptococcal Subproject, 2000, Practice guidelines for the management of cryptococcal disease, Clin Infect Dis, 30, 710–718.

Smith KJ, Warnock DW, Kennedy CTC, Johnson EM, Hopwood V, Van Cutsem J, Vanden Bossche H, 1986, Azole resistance in Candida albicans, J Med Vet Mycol, 24, 133–144.

Stevens DA, Kan VL, Judson MA, Morrison VA, Dummer S, Denning DW, Bennett JE, Walsh TJ, Patterson TF, Pankey GA, 2000, Practice guidelines for diseases caused by Aspergillus, Clin Infect Dis, 30, 696–709.

Storm G, van Etten E, 1997, Biopharmaceutical aspects of lipid formulations of amphotericin B, Eur J Clin Microbiol Dis, 16, 64–73.

Vanden Bossche H, 1991, Ergosterol biosynthesis inhibitors, in Prasad R, ed, Candida albicans, Springer-Verlag, Berlin.

Vanden Bossche H, Mackenzie DW, Cauwenbergh G, Van Cutsem J, Drouhet E, Dupont B, 1990, Mycoses in AIDS patients, Plenum Press, New York.

Van Tyle HJ, 1984, Ketoconazole, mechanism of action, spectrum of activity, pharmacokinetics, drug interactions, adverse reactions and therapeutic use, Pharmacotherapy, 4, 343–373.

Walsh TJ, Finberg RW, Arndt C, Hiezmez J, Schwartz C, Bodensteiner D, et al, 1999, Liposomal amphotericin B for empirical therapy in patients with persistent fever and neutropenia, National Institute of Allergy and Infectious Diseases Mycoses Study Group, N Engl J Med, 340, 764–771.

Walsh TJ, Pizzo A, 1988, Treatment of systemic fungal infections, recent progress and current problems, Eur J Clin Microbiol Infect Dis, 7, 460–475.

Warnock DW, 1998, Fungal infections in neutropenia, current problems and chemotherapeutic control, J Antimicrob Chemother, 41, suppl D, 95–105.

White TC, Marr KA, Bowden RA, 1998, Clinical, cellular and molecular factors that contribute to antifungal drug resistance, Clin Microbiol Rev, 11, 382–402.

Antifungal Targets and Research into Antifungal Agents

A. BRYSKIER

53

1. INTRODUCTION

Systemic infections of fungal origin are an attendant feature in immunodepressed patients. This is a sector of infectious pathology that has increased rapidly over the past few years because of the increasing number of immunodepressed patients. A study conducted in the United States between 1980 and 1989 already showed that nosocomial infections of fungal origin had increased by 40%. The number of species responsible for these infections remains relatively limited: *Candida albicans* (80%), *Aspergillus fumigatus* (15%), *Candida tropicalis*, and *Cryptococcus neoformans*. Molds of the types of *Penicillium*, *Trichosporon*, and *Pseudoallescheria* are increasingly more often being isolated.

The principal opportunistic fungal agents are listed in Table 1.

The clinical emergence of strains of fluconazole-resistant *C. albicans*, particularly in AIDS patients, and the treatment-refractory nature of *Aspergillus* infections have stimulated research into new antifungal agents.

The actual incidence of *Aspergillus* infections is difficult to establish because of the lack of standardization of reliable diagnostic methods. The majority of *Aspergillus* infections occur in AIDS patients towards the end of the disease, when the immune system is very debilitated. The impairment of neutrophil and macrophage functions increases the risk of *Aspergillus* infections. The species most commonly isolated in AIDS patients are *A. fumigatus* (83%), *A. flavus* (9%), *A. niger* (5%), and *A. terreus* (3%).

C. neoformans is an opportunistic fungal agent responsible for life-threatening meningoencephalitis in 5 to 10% of AIDS patients. Mortality is high despite therapeutic efforts. The reference treatment is amphotericin B (AMB), alone or in combination with flucytosine. Patients who survive this acute phase receive fluconazole preventively throughout their lives to prevent relapses. Studies of strains of *C. neoformans* in relapsing patients have shown that the same strain was involved, indicating that treatment of the acute phase had not eradicated the fungal agent.

The genus *Paecilomyces* is composed of numerous saprophytic species of soil or atmospheric origin, but which may be isolated from food or paper. Some species are responsible for opportunistic infections ranging from nail infections to endocarditis or peritonitis occurring during peritoneal dialysis. The prognosis for these is very poor. AMB alone or in combination is the empirical treatment of such infections, with a failure rate of 40%, but the failure rate in the case of endocarditis is 100%. The species most commonly responsible are *P. variotii*, *P. lilacinus*, *P. marquandii*, *P. fumosoroseus*, and *P. javanicus*. Flucytosine is inactive, but the activities of the different azoles and AMB vary with the species. The most susceptible species is *P. variotii* (MIC [geometric mean] [MIC_{GM}] of AMB, 0.08 μg/ml; itraconazole MIC_{GM}, 0.07 μg/ml), and the most resistant is *P. lilacinus* (AMB MIC_{GM}, 10.29 μg/ml; itraconazole MIC_{GM}, 7.51 μg/ml). The activity of antifungal agents against *P. marquandii* is weak (AMB MIC_{GM}, 1.41 μg/ml; itraconazole MIC_{GM}, 5.88 μg/ml).

Table 1 Opportunistic agents of fungal infections

Agent(s)
Yeasts
C. albicans
C. krusei
Candida lusitaniae
C. parapsilosis
C. tropicalis
C. glabrata
C. neoformans
Malassezia spp.
Rhodotorula spp.
S. cerevisiae
Hyalohyphomycosis agents
Aspergillus spp.
Fusarium spp.
Scopulariopsis spp.
Zygomycosis agents
Absidia spp.
Mucor spp.
Rhizopus spp.
Phaeohyphomycosis agents
Alternaria spp.
Bipolaris spp.
Curvularia spp.
Exserohilum spp.
P. boydii
S. prolificans

2. TARGETS OF ANTIFUNGAL AGENTS

Fungal agents and mammalian cells have a common heritage in eukaryotic cells, but they differ on certain points of their structures and metabolism. Comparative physiology studies have yielded new targets for antifungal drugs and will continue to do so.

The targets of antifungal drugs are principally the cell structure—the cell wall and cytoplasmic membrane—but also the metabolism (protein synthesis) and cell division. Other metabolic pathways are undergoing study.

2.1. Cytoplasmic Membrane

The fungal cytoplasmic membrane contains a large quantity of ergosterol that plays an important physiological role. It provides membrane fluidity (barrier effect and membrane enzyme functioning), plays a regulatory role, and stabilizes the physical properties of the membrane.

Two categories of antifungal agent act on the cell membrane: polyenes, which increase membrane permeability, and ergosterol synthesis inhibitors.

2.1.1. Polyenes

The polyenes are a complex chemical class of macrocyclic agents that includes AMB (parenteral use), pimaricin, nystatin (NYT), and candicidin (Fig. 1).

AMB has a greater affinity for ergosterol than for cholesterol (a major component of mammalian cells). This affinity, even if weak, partially explains the toxicity of AMB. The first effect of AMB is to make the fungal cell more permeable by potassium ions. Cell death may be explained by the simultaneous penetration of protons that cause acidification of the intracellular medium.

2.1.1.1. Amphotericin B (AMB)

2.1.1.1.1. Chemical modifications. A number of semisynthetic derivatives of AMB have been described in the literature. One of the intentions is to reduce the nephrotoxic potential and increase the therapeutic index, while at the same time preserving the activity of AMB (Fig. 2). AMB is slightly soluble in water. The search for an improvement in the therapeutic index follows two lines of attack: chemical modifications and new pharmaceutical formulations (see chapter 52). The numerous derivatives obtained by semisynthesis have a substituent at C-16 with variable substituents at C-13 or C-14 (Fig. 3). Other chemical modifications have involved the amino group at C-3′ of the D-mycaminose.

Compound A, which is the methyl ester derivative of AMB, is less active than AMB and has greater affinity for eukaryotic cells. The product is less nephrotoxic, but during clinical trials it proved to be neurotoxic. Another modification on the carboxyl group at C-16 is the attachment of a 1-amino-4-piperazinyl (compound B). This derivative is more water soluble than AMB. Structure-activity studies have been performed by the SmithKline Beecham team.

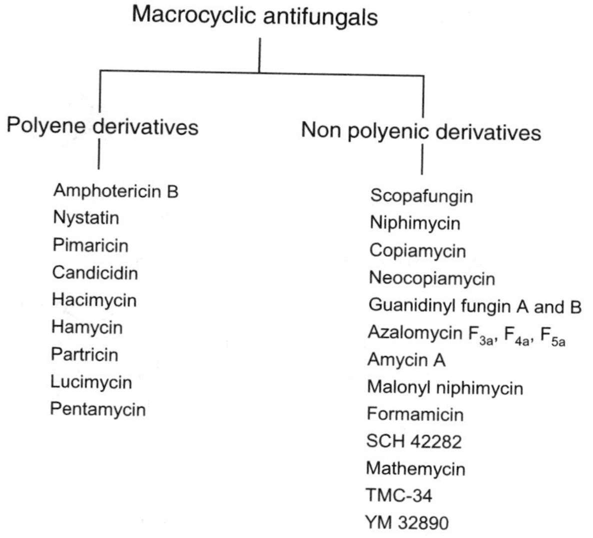

Macrocyclic antifungals

Polyene derivatives	Non polyenic derivatives
Amphotericin B	Scopafungin
Nystatin	Niphimycin
Pimaricin	Copiamycin
Candicidin	Neocopiamycin
Hacimycin	Guanidinyl fungin A and B
Hamycin	Azalomycin F_{3a}, F_{4a}, F_{5a}
Partricin	Amycin A
Lucimycin	Malonyl niphimycin
Pentamycin	Formamicin
	SCH 42282
	Mathemycin
	TMC-34
	YM 32890

Figure 1 **Classification of polyene antifungals**

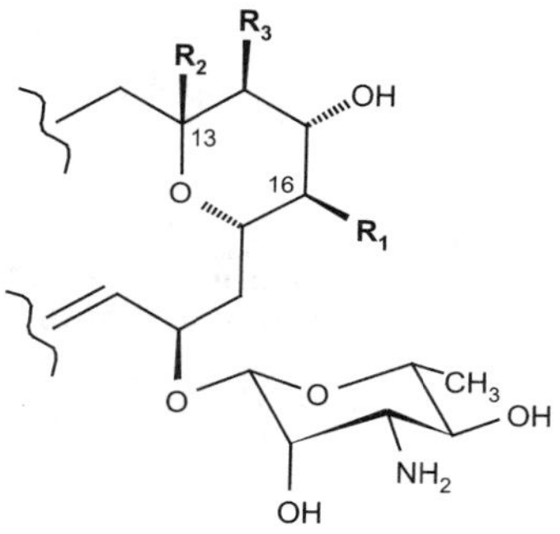

	R_1 (16)	R_2 (13)	R_3 (14)
A	CO_2CH_3	OH	H
B	CO−N−N(piperazine)NCH$_3$	OH	H
C	CH_2OH	OH	H
D	$COO\text{-}CH_3$	OH	OH
E	COOH	OCH_3	H
F	COOH	SCH_2CH_3	H
G	$COO\text{-}CH_3$	H	OH

Figure 3 **Derivatives of AMB**

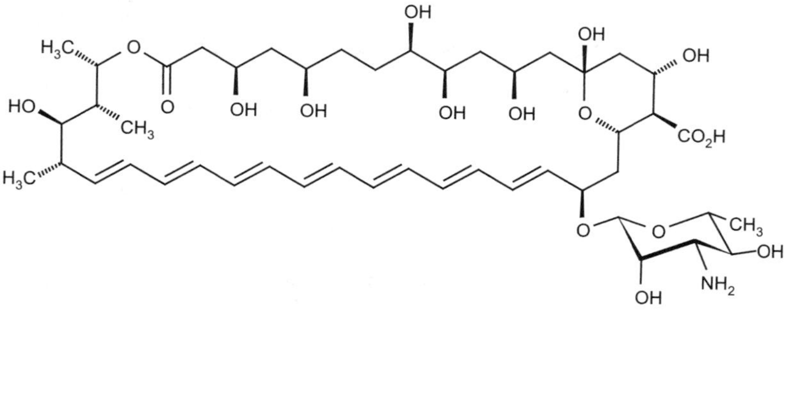

Figure 2 **Amphotericin B (AMB)**

Compound C is the result of the reduction of the carboxyl group at C-16 to a hydroxymethyl residue. It is less toxic than AMB. Other molecules have been prepared by hydroxylation (compound D) or alkoxylation at C-14 (OCH_3 [compound E]) or by a thioacetal at C-13 (compound F). Anhydro derivatives with changes at C-13 and C-14 (compound G) or a dehydroxy analog (compound H) have also been prepared (Fig. 4). All of these derivatives are less toxic but also much less active than AMB.

Modifications have been made to the sugar, combined with substituents on the carboxyl group at C-16. Substituents have been attached to the amino group of the D-mycosamine.

The most active derivative (compound I) [Fig. 5] is *N*-methyl-*N*-D-fructosyl AMB. It is less toxic than AMB (50% lethal dose, 400 versus 6 mg/kg of body weight) and appears to be more effective in the treatment of murine *C. albicans* infections (50% effective dose [ED_{50}], 2.3 mg/kg).

The V-28-3B methyl ester derivative (Fig. 6) was obtained from the fermentation of *Streptomyces aerenae*. It is less active in vitro than AMB but appears to have comparable in vivo activity. It is less toxic than AMB.

MS-8209 is a semisynthetic derivative of AMB (Fig. 7) obtained by attachment of a benzylidene-fructosyl chain.

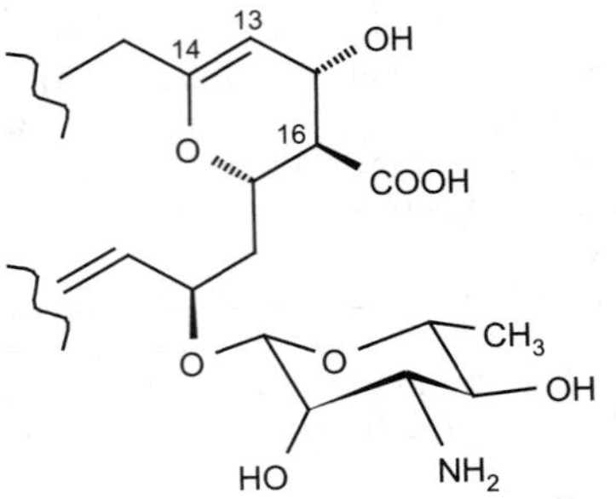

13 14 16 OH COOH O CH3 O OH HO NH2

Figure 4 C-13 dehydroxy derivative of AMB (compound H)

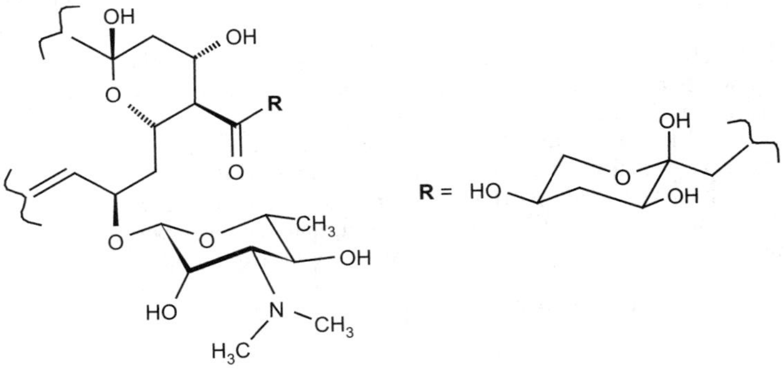

OH OH O R O O CH3 OH HO N CH3 H3C

R = HO O OH OH

Figure 5 Derivative 1: D-fructosyl AMB

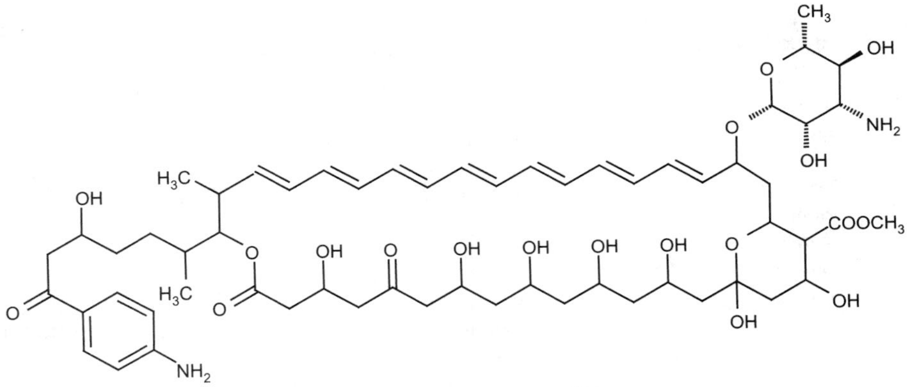

CH3 OH O NH2 OH O H3C OH COOCH3 O OH O OH OH OH OH O OH H3C O OH O NH2

Figure 6 V-28-3B methyl ester

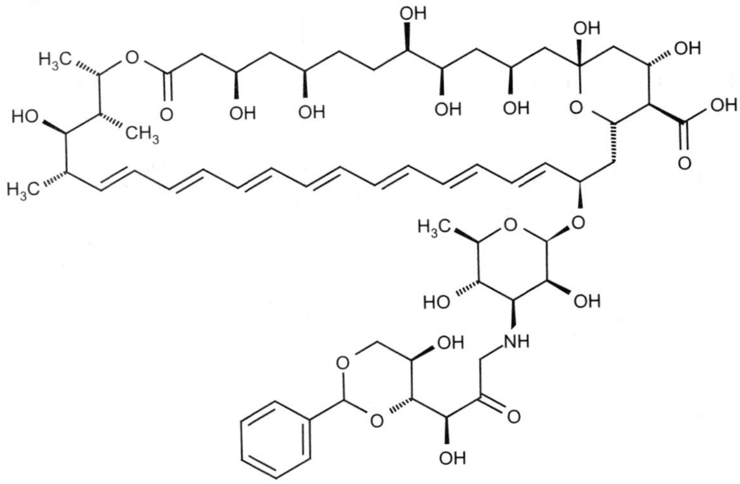

OH OH OH H3C O HO CH3 O OH OH OH OH O OH O H3C O O HO OH OH NH O O O OH

Figure 7 MS-8209

This molecule is two to five times less active than AMB. For *C. neoformans*, MS-8209 has an MIC of 0.56 μM, compared with 0.21 μM for AMB. At the maximum tolerated doses in the mouse, MS-8209 (15 mg/kg) and AMB (0.5 mg/kg) have the same efficacy in the treatment of disseminated candidosis. MS-8209 produces longer survival times in *C. neoformans* infections than AMB.

2.1.1.1.2. Pharmaceutical modifications. Despite the commercialization of a liposomal form (AmBisome) that is less toxic than AMB, new pharmaceutical formulations have been published.

A formulation combining AMB and cyclodextrin has reduced toxicity and would appear to allow enteral absorption. It appears to be slightly less active than AMB. Another formulation involves the covalent binding of AMB with a dextran amino group through an imine or amino bond. This conjugate appears to be more hydrosoluble and less toxic than AMB. A study with mice has apparently shown better efficacy in *C. albicans* infections than with nystatin.

2.1.1.2. Nystatin

NYT is a polyene antifungal agent extracted by fermentation of *Streptomyces noursei*. It is not absorbed orally, and its parenteral administration is limited by its poor local tolerance and systemic toxicity. As with AMB, a liposomal formulation has been developed (Table 2).

The antifungal spectra of NYT and AMB are different, and there is no complete cross-resistance between the two molecules. The spectrum of NYT is slightly broader and includes species, such as *Geotrichum* and *Beauvaria,* that are not included in that of AMB. NYT is active in vitro and in vivo against *Candida* spp., *C. neoformans, Coccidioides immitis, Histoplasma capsulatum, A. flavus, A. fumigatus*, and *A. terreus*. The in vitro activities of the different formulations of AMB are presented in Table 3 in comparison with those of NYT.

It would appear that the mechanisms of action of the two molecules are not identical. In fact, the resistance to AMB induced in the laboratory in *C. albicans* is not always found for NYT.

NYT and AMB, like cyclosporine, are amphiphilic and hydrophobic molecules that bind to plasma lipoproteins. Their kinetics are highly influenced by plasma high-density lipoprotein levels. Some results of clinical studies with liposomal L-NYT (Nyotran) have yielded encouraging results, particularly in immunodepressed patients suffering from disseminated aspergillosis.

2.1.1.3. Other Polyenes

Other polyene molecules have been extracted from the fermentation broths of *Streptomyces* spp. One derivative (Fig. 8) has moderate in vitro activity against *C. albicans* (MIC, 12.5 μg/ml) and *A. niger* (MIC, 3.13 μg/ml).

2.1.2. Ergosterol Inhibitors

The ergosterol skeleton derives from acetyl coenzyme A (acetyl-CoA), with the exception of the methyl group at position 24 of the side chain.The initial synthesis includes condensation of two acetyl-CoA units to form acetoacetyl-CoA, and the addition of a third acetyl-CoA unit yields β-hydroxy-3-methylglutaryl-CoA (HMG-CoA), which is reduced by NADPH to form mevalonic acid (Fig. 9). The different steps are catalyzed by cytoplasmic enzymes: acetoacetyl-CoA thiolase, HMG-CoA synthetase, and HMG-CoA reductase, a yeast mitochondrial enzyme.

Table 2 Parenteral formulations of polyene antifungal agents

Name	Formulation[a]	Molar ratio	Structure	Particle size
L-NYT[b]	DMPC-DMPC NYT	7:3:1	Multilamellar liposome	0.1–3 μm
L-AMB[c]	HSPC-cholesterol-HSPC AMb	10:5:4:2	Monolamellar liposome	80 nm
ABCD[d]	Cholesterol sulfate sodium AMb	1:1	Lipid disk	120 nm
ABLC[e]	DMPC-DMPG-AMb	7:3:10	Lipid ribbon	2–5 μm
AMB[f]	Deoxycholate sodium AMb	4:5	Colloidal suspension	

[a]HSPC, phosphatidylcholine; DSPG, diastearoylphosphatidyl glycerol; DMPC, dimyristylphosphatidylcholine.
[b]L-NYT, liposomal NYT (Nyotran).
[c]L-AMB, liposomal AMB (AmBisome).
[d]ABCD, AMB colloidal dispersion (Amphocil).
[e]ABLC, AMB liquid complex (Abelcet).
[f]Fungizone.

Table 3 In vitro activities of the different formulations of polyene antifungal agents

Microorganism	*n*	MIC (μg/ml)[a]					
		AMB	ABLC	ABCD	L-AMB	NYT	L-NYT
A. flavus	10	1	8	>8	>8	8	4
A. fumigatus	30	1	0.25	8	>8	8	2
C. albicans	40	0.25	0.12	1	4	2	1
C. glabrata	20	0.25	0.25	2	8	2	2
C. krusei	20	0.5	0.5	8	>8	4	2
C. lusitaniae	10	0.5	0.12	4	8	4	1
C. parapsilosis	20	0.25	0.12	2	8	4	2
C. tropicalis	20	0.5	0.25	4	>8	4	2
C. neoformans	20	0.25	0.06	2	8	2	1

[a]L-AMB, liposomal AMB; L-NYT, liposomal NYT. ABLC, AMB lipid complex; ABCD, AMB colloidal dispersion;

Figure 8 Polyene derivative

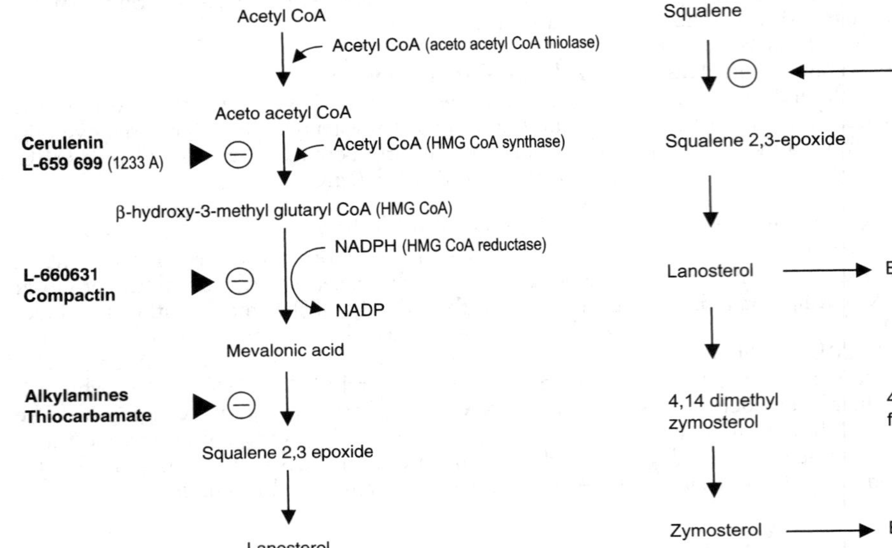

Figure 9 Inhibition of squalene-2,3-epoxide synthesis

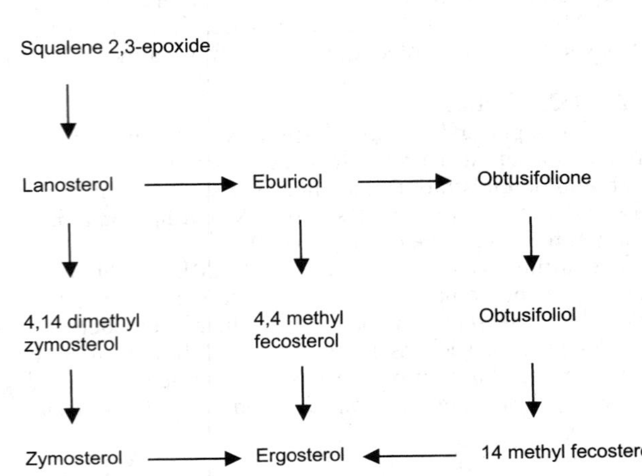

Figure 11 Biosynthetic pathway of ergosterol

Ergosterol regulates its biosynthesis through cytoplasmic enzymes. Yeast acetoacetyl-CoA thiolases may be inhibited by citrinin at a concentration of 0.2 μM, and HMG-CoA synthetase is inhibited by cerulenin and L-659699 (F-244, 1233A) (Fig. 9). The latter has in vitro activity.

The formation of mevalonate may be inhibited by L-660631, an acetyleneic fatty acid.

HMG reductase is inhibited by compactin (Fig. 10), which possesses good in vitro activity against *C. albicans* (MIC, 0.1 μg/ml).

The following stage is the formation of squalene from mevalonic acid. The epoxidation of squalene is the first step in a long biosynthesis chain that transforms the 20-carbon chain of squalene to ergosterol (Fig. 11).

The first step is the transformation of squalene to squalene-2,3-epoxide (Fig. 12) in the presence of oxygen. Alkylamines and thiocarbamates can inhibit this step (Fig. 12).

2.1.2.1. Thiocarbamates

Thiocarbamates are principally topical products, such as tolnaftate, tolciclate, and piritetrate. They are principally active against dermatophytes but not against *C. albicans*, as they cannot penetrate the wall of *C. albicans*.

2.1.2.2. Allylamines

Naftifine is used as a topical multifungal agent together with terbinafine (Fig. 13), which may also be administered

Figure 10 Squalene molecule formation inhibitors

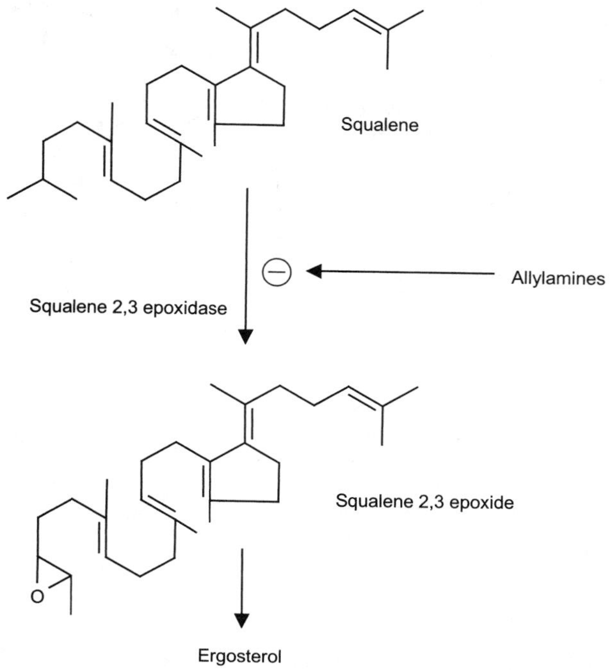

Figure 12 Mode of action of allylamines

orally. The latter possesses good in vitro activity against *Trichophyton* (MIC, 0.001 μg/ml), moderate activity against *Aspergillus* (MIC, 3.0 μg/ml), and weak activity against *C. albicans* (MIC, 12.0 μg/ml). It is inactive against *Candida (Torulopsis) glabrata* (MIC, >100 μg/ml).

Other derivatives, such as 2-aza-2,3-dihydrosqualene, inhibit squalene epoxidase.

2.1.3. 2,3-Oxidosqualene-Lanosterol Cyclase Inhibitors

2,3-Oxidosqualene-lanosterol cyclase inhibitors catalyze the cyclic rearrangement of 2,3-epoxysqualene to lanosterol (Fig. 14). Cyclization of 2,3-epoxysqualene is controlled by 2,3-oxidosqualene-lanosterol cyclase, a ubiquitous enzyme whose gene in *C. albicans* has been cloned and characterized. The enzyme induces cyclization of the 2,3-oxidosqualene derivative folded in a chair-and-boat form by protonating and opening the epoxy ring.

Several series of compounds have been synthesized. Some, such as 2,3-dihydro-2-azosqualene or *N,N*-dimethyldodecylamine (Fig. 15), interact with the acid (A) groups of the active site through nitrogen atoms.

The second approach involves interfering with the nucleophilic (N) group of the active site to block C-20 of the prosterol. Two categories of compounds may inhibit this interference: enolether derivatives and vinyl derivatives of 2,3-oxidosqualene.

A third approach involves the synthesis of derivatives with a dual action through inhibition of the A- and N-sites. The aminoketone derivatives might play this role. This dual inhibition is determined by the distance between the nitrogen atom of the tertiary amine and the carbon atom of the carbonyl electrophilic center of the benzophenone residue. The optimum distance has been estimated as 10.7 Å.

Ro-43-8212, Ro-44-4281, and Ro-44-2103 have 50% inhibitory concentrations (IC_{50}) for the *C. albicans* enzyme of 1.09, 0.32, and 0.11 μM. The optimal substituent at the *para* position of the phenyl nucleus is a halogen. The IC_{50} increase when the substituent is a CN, NO_2, or F or an alkyl chain.

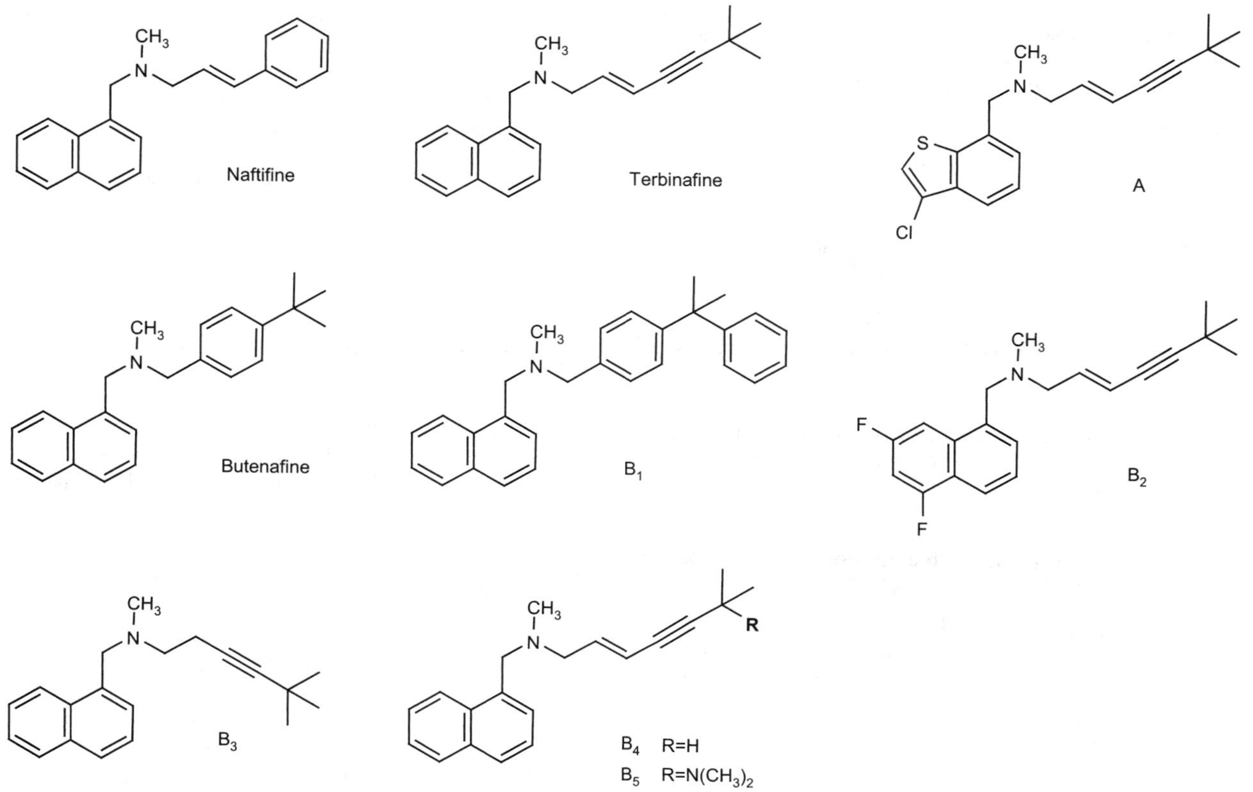

Figure 13 Allylamine derivatives

Oxidosqualene lanosterol cyclase

Inhibitor

Lanosterol

(3*S*) -2,3-oxidosqualene

Figure 14 2,3-Oxidosqualene-lanosterol cyclase inhibitors

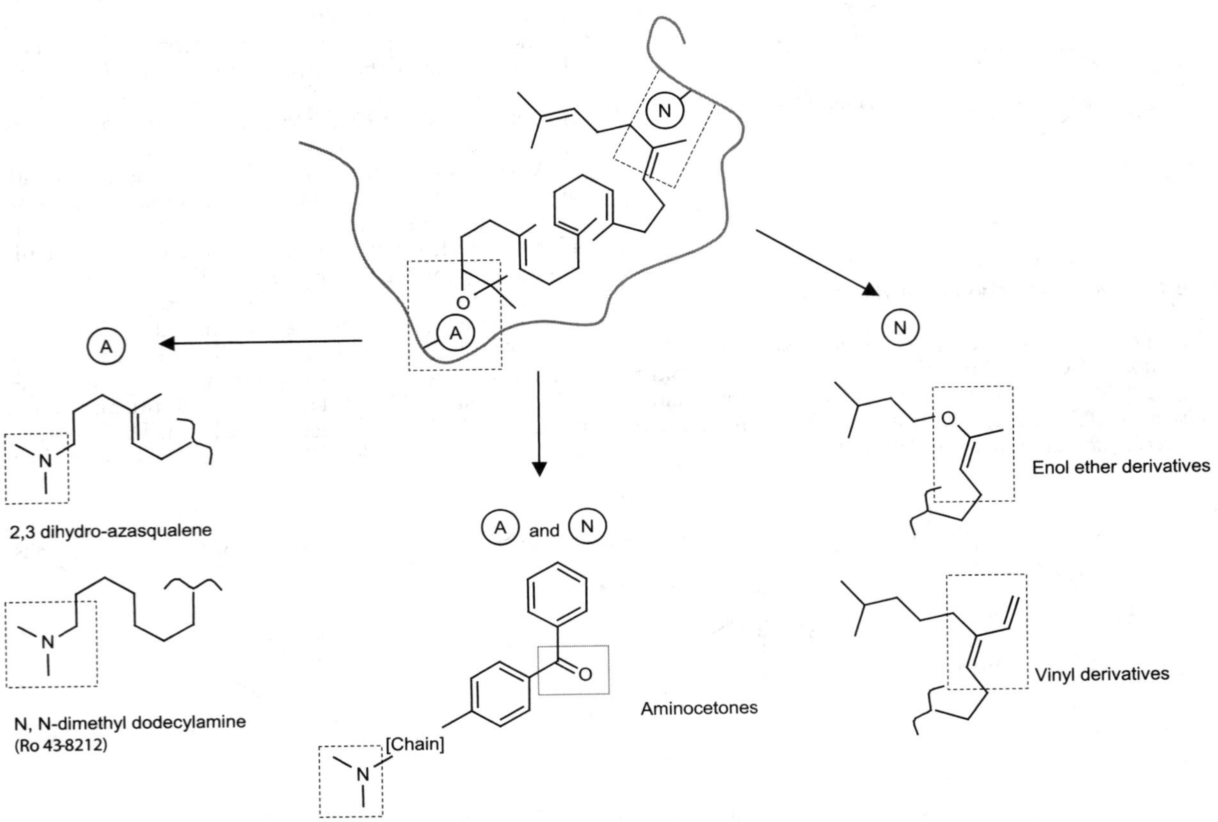

Figure 15 Different classes of 2,3-oxidosqualene-lanosterol cyclase inhibitors

Some molecules possess activity similar to that of itraconazole against yeasts but are more active against dermatophytes (Table 4).

2.1.4. C-14 Demethylation Inhibitors

One of the early stages in the biosynthetic pathway of ergosterol is demethylation at position 14. This demethylation

Table 4 In vitro activities of cyclase inhibitors[a]

Compound	IC_{50} (μM) for *C. albicans*	MIC (μg/ml)			
		C. albicans	*C. neoformans*	Dermatophytes	Dimorphs
Itraconazole		1.25	0.15	5.0	1.25
Ro-43-6913	0.66	0.60	0.35	0.30	0.30
Ro-46-6543	0.03	1.68	1.25	0.23	0.15
Ro-44-4082	0.11	1.25	3.40	1.24	0.44

[a]Data from Joridon et al., 1993.

	X	R_1	R_2	R_3	R_4
Ro 09-157	O	CH_3	H	O, O, NH_2	
Ro 09-2050	CH_2	CH_3	CH_3	N, N=N	
Ro 09-2127	CH_2	CH_3	CH_3	N, N	
A	O	CH_3	H	O, O, N, H, NH_2	

Figure 16 Derivatives of restricticin

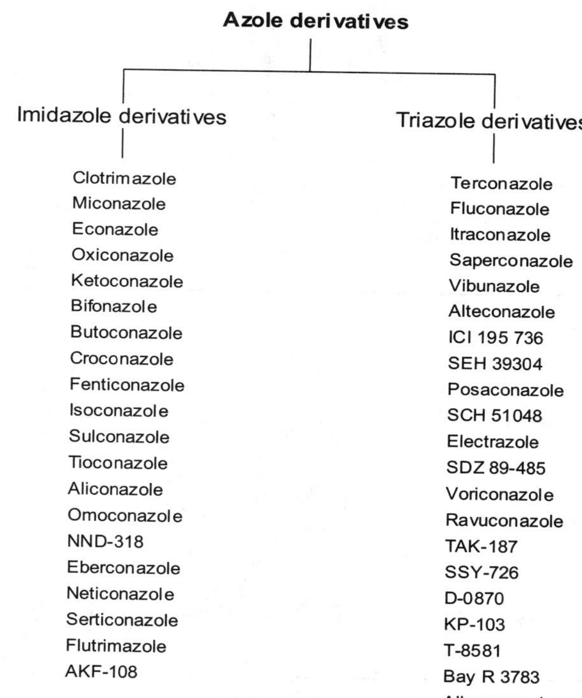

Figure 17 Classification of azoles

occurs via an enzyme, lanosterol 14α-demethylase, using cytochrome P_{450} (CYP5IA1) as a support.

The azole derivatives inhibit this stage of ergosterol synthesis. Other compounds, such as the pyrimidine, pyridine, or piperazine derivatives, also exert inhibitory activity on this enzyme.

The derivatives of restricticin (Fig. 16) are more potent inhibitors than fluconazole and itraconazole, particularly Ro-09-2127. The carbazate A derivative is active in vivo in disseminated murine *C. albicans* infections.

2.1.4.1. Azole Derivatives

Research in the field of triazole derivatives is very important, as these are topical and/or systemic drugs. The azoles are divided into two major classes: imidazoles, represented by ketoconazole and miconazole, and triazoles (Fig. 17), particularly fluconazole, saperconazole (Fig. 18), itraconazole, and SDZ 89-485 (Fig. 19).

A number of compounds either are currently undergoing clinical development, such as voriconazole (UK-109496), D-0870, posaconazole (SCH 56592), ER 30346, and SSY726, or are in the preclinical stage, such as T-8581 and U-9825.

2.1.4.1.1. Voriconazole. Voriconazole differs structurally from fluconazole through the replacement of one of the triazole nuclei by a fluorinated pyrimidine nucleus (Fig. 20). This activity is based on the *2R,3S* enantiomer. In contrast to itraconazole, this molecule possesses good activity against *C. albicans*, *C. neoformans*, and molds. Voriconazole is much more active than fluconazole against *Aspergillus* spp. There are no published clinical strains of *A. fumigatus* resistant to AMB. Strains of reduced susceptibility have been obtained by mutagenesis (irradiation). In vitro and in vivo, it has been shown that voriconazole and itraconazole have good activity against these strains.

Voriconazole is the result of an analysis of the structure-activity relationships of the azole derivatives against *Aspergillus* spp. In fact, fluconazole is only slightly active against *Aspergillus* (MIC, ~100 μg/ml), with a weak affinity for the target, 14α-demethylase (IC_{50}, 4.8 μM). The addition of a methyl group to the propanol chain increases the inhibitory activity against the target enzyme (MIC, 12.5 μg/ml; IC_{50}, 0.48 μM). Replacement of the triazole ring of fluconazole by a pyrimidine ring increases the antifungal activity. The presence of a fluorine atom at position 5 of the pyrimidine nucleus substantially increases the in vitro activity (MIC, 0.09 μg/ml) and the affinity for the target enzyme (IC_{50}, 0.053 μM), as well as the in vivo activity.

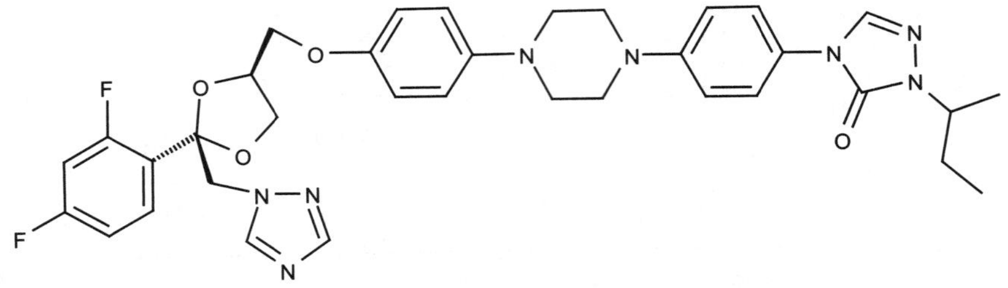

Figure 18 Saperconazole

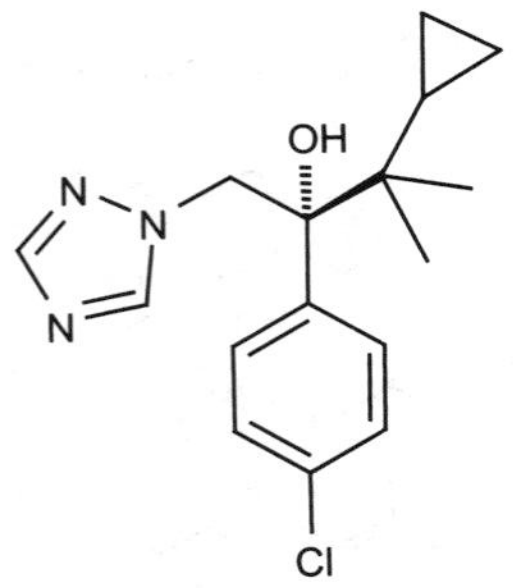

Figure 19 SDZ 89-485

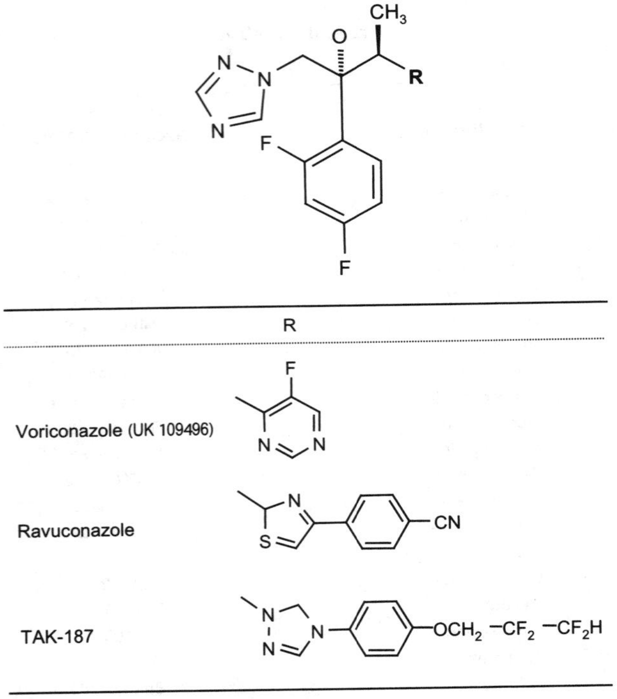

R

Voriconazole (UK 109496)

Ravuconazole

TAK-187

Figure 20 New triazole derivatives

In addition, voriconazole possesses good activity against *Fusarium, Exophiala, Bipolaris, Wangiella dermatitidis, C. immitis, Pseudallescheria boydii*, and *Sporothrix schenckii.*

The human pharmacokinetics after oral or intravenous administration of single or repeated doses have shown that absorption is rapid (time to maximum concentration in serum, <2 h) and that the apparent elimination half-life is 6 h. Voriconazole was administered orally to volunteers in single or repeated doses for 30 days. The maximum dosage was 200 mg every 12 h (5 mg/kg twice a day [b.i.d.]). Voriconazole was rapidly absorbed, the peak being reached in 1 to 2 h. Bioavailability is reduced by 22% in the presence of food. The pharmacokinetics are not linear. There is sixfold accumulation after oral administration on the basis of the areas under the curve.

After a single dose in the form of a 1-h infusion, the pharmacokinetics appear to be linear up to 4 mg/kg but not beyond (8 mg/kg). After administration of a dosage of 3 mg/kg every 12 h for 10 days, the accumulation ratio is on the order of 6. Steady-state plasma clearance is 3.7 ml/min/kg. The volume of distribution is 2 liters/kg. Plasma protein binding is 58%.

The concentration attained in the saliva is on the order of 65% of that in plasma. The absolute oral and intravenous bioavailability is on the order of 58% after a single dose and 90% after repeated doses. Elimination in the urine is less than 1% of the administered dose.

Voriconazole is metabolized and inhibits the activity of CYP2C9 and CYP3A4. Voriconazole has the potential to interfere with the metabolism of cyclosporine, phenytoin, carbamazepine, and warfarin. The comparative pharmacokinetics of the azole derivatives during development are summarized in Table 5. The plasma pharmacokinetics of ketoconazole and fluconazole are discussed in chapter 52.

The relative bioavailability is about 90%. About 1% of the administered dose is eliminated unchanged in the urine. The apparent volume of distribution is 2 liters/kg. After a dose of 200 mg of radiolabeled product, about 78 to 89% of the radioactivity is recovered in the urine and 20 to 30% is recovered in the feces, irrespective of the route of administration. Three major and five minor metabolites have been reported. The following hepatic enzymes are implicated in the metabolism process: CYP2C9, CYP2C18, and CYP3A4.

During phase I, dose-dependent visual disorders indicated the need to restrict the dosage.

Good therapeutic efficacy has been demonstrated in neutropenic patients suffering from disseminated aspergillosis, nonneutropenic patients with chronic invasive aspergillosis, and AIDS patients suffering from oropharyngeal candidosis.

2.1.4.1.2. D-0870. D-0870 (Fig. 21) is the enantiomer of ICI-195739. The development of this molecule reached phase II but was stopped. It manifests excellent activity against *C. albicans*, whether the strain is susceptible or resistant to fluconazole. It is less active than itraconazole against *Aspergillus* spp. It has activity similar to that of fluconazole against *C. neoformans*. Its activity against molds appears to be good, and likewise those against *Histoplasma* spp., *C. immitis*, and *W. dermatitidis*.

Nine healthy volunteers received a single dose of 50 mg of D-0870 followed by 10 mg once daily for 4 days. After a single dose of 50 mg, the peak concentration in serum was 0.11 μg/ml, allowing steady state to be reached from the first day. The apparent elimination half-life on day 5 was between 23 and 85 h (mean, 48.85 h).

Nine other healthy volunteers received a loading dose of 200 mg followed by four doses of 25 mg once daily (Table 5).

Table 5 Pharmacokinetics of azole derivatives

Compound	n	Dose administration[a]	Route of	C_{max} (μg/ml)	T_{max} (h) (μg·h/ml)	AUC	$t_{1/2}$ (h)
Voriconazole		3 mg/kg b.i.d.	Oral SD	1.3	1.0	3.15	5.5
		3 mg/kg b.i.d.	MD (10 days)	2.8	1.1	18.70	6.4
			i.v. SD	2.16		5.39	5.6
			MD	3.88		20.70	6.5
SCH 56592	9	50 mg	Oral SD	0.11	5.0	0.69	
	9	100 mg	MD	0.46	5.0	4.45	19.2
	9	200 mg	Oral SD	0.27	5.0	1.71	
	9	400 mg	MD	1.14	6.0	11.57	24.1
			Oral SD	0.37	5.0	2.41	
			MD	1.75	4.0	16.80	23.9
			Oral SD	0.76	5.0	5.03	
			MD	4.15	5.0	39.21	31
SSY726		10 mg	Oral	0.13		4.2	294.9
		20 mg	Oral	0.30		7.6	315.6
		40 mg	Oral	0.69		14.6	276.5
		50 mg	Oral	0.89		20.70	259.2
		60 mg	Oral	0.84		18.7	251.2
		70 mg	Oral	1.16		26.2	301.7
		80 mg	Oral	1.10		29.4	304.7
		90 mg	Oral	1.50		41.9	352.5
D-0870	9	50 mg SD	Oral	0.11		1.73	
	9	50 mg + 10 mg for 4 days	Oral	0.09		1.66	48.5
	9	50 mg SD	Oral	0.43		7.79	
	9	200 mg + 25 mg OD for 4 days	Oral	0.43		7.75	70.51
Itraconazole	6	50 mg	Oral	0.04	3.2	0.57	13
	6	100 mg	Oral	0.13	4.0	1.90	17
	6	200 mg	Oral	0.29	4.7	5.21	18
	10	100 mg SD	Oral	0.12		1.36	
	10	100 mg MD	Oral	0.67		9.42	28
Itraconazole HPC[b]		200 mg	Oral	0.31	5.0	5.8	22.1

[a]SD, single dose; MD, multiple doses; i.v., intravenous.
[b]HPC, β-hydroxycyclodextrin.

Figure 21 D-0870

The accumulation ratios were, respectively, 0.90 and 1.17 in the first and second groups. The mean apparent elimination half-life was 70.5 h (34 to 137 h) (De Wit et al., 1998) (Table 5).

In 25 patients suffering from oropharyngeal candidosis due to a fluconazole-resistant strain of *C. albicans*, the therapeutic efficacy proved satisfactory, with a favorable response in 68% of patients.

2.1.4.1.3 Posaconazole (SCH 56592). Posaconazole (Fig. 22) is a hydroxyl derivative of SCH 51048, development of which was stopped because of carcinogenicity. It is a trisubstituted tetrahydrofuran. SCH 51048 has good activity against *Aspergillus* spp. It reduced or delayed fatality in mice with disseminated aspergillosis at a dose of 5 mg/kg. However, large doses (30 mg/kg) are necessary to reduce fungal colonization of lung tissue.

Posaconazole has good in vitro and in vivo activities against *C. albicans* (MIC at which 50% of isolates tested are inhibited [MIC_{50}], 0.06 μg/ml), comparable to those of itraconazole. It also has good activity against *C. tropicalis* (MIC_{50}, 0.12 μg/ml), *Candida parapsilosis* (MIC_{50}, 0.12 μg/ml), *Candida krusei* (MIC_{50}, 0.5 μg/ml), and *C. glabrata* (MIC_{50}, 0.5 μg/ml).

Posaconazole has good activity against *A. fumigatus*, including lung infections in immunodepressed ICR mice. It is more effective than itraconazole and AMB. Good activity against *C. neoformans*, *C. immitis*, *W. dermatitidis*, and *H. capsulatum* has been demonstrated.

Yarosh-Tomain et al. (1997) showed that the activity of posaconazole and fluconazole against *C. glabrata* differs from that of itraconazole. Thus, they isolated a strain of *C. glabrata* without a lanosterol 14α-demethylase against

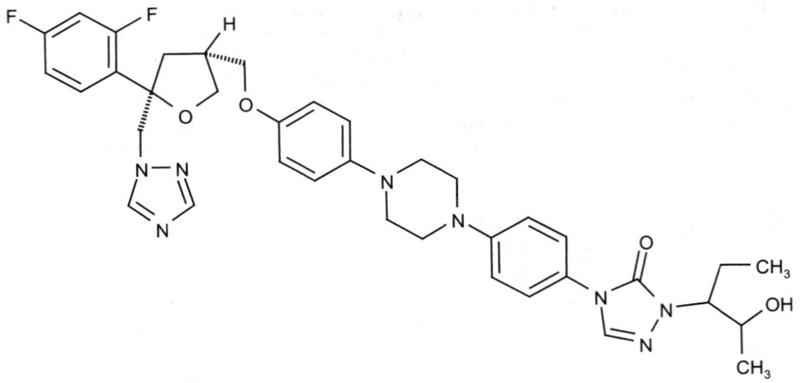

Figure 22 Posaconazole (SCH 56592)

which posaconazole and fluconazole, but not itraconazole, were active, and a strain in which the sterol was abnormal through the absence of the double bond at positions 5 and 6, against which all three molecules were inactive. It is likely that posaconazole and fluconazole have a different mechanism of action against *C. glabrata*.

The inhibitory activity of posaconazole on ergosterol synthesis by *A. flavus* and *A. fumigatus* is 10 to 100 times greater than that of itraconazole and fluconazole.

When triazole resistance in *C. albicans* involves efflux mechanisms, it would appear that there is cross-resistance between itraconazole, fluconazole, and posaconazole.

Posaconazole and voriconazole are very active against *Fusarium* spp. *Fusarium* spp. are responsible for superficial infections, particularly onychomycoses, but also for fatal disseminated infections in neutropenic patients. Medications active against this fungal genus are necessary because of the extreme severity of these infections, which are increasingly more frequently being isolated.

Three species of *Fusarium* are most often isolated: *F. solani*, *F. oxysporum*, and *F. moniliforme*.

Posaconazole has good in vitro activity against the last two species, AMB being active only against *F. oxysporum* (Table 6).

Posaconazole is inactive against *Rhizopus* spp. (MIC, 2 to 16 μg/ml). Posaconazole and itraconazole reduce the cerebral fungal load of *W. dermatitidis* at a dose of 2 mg/kg and prolong survival time in the nude mouse at a dose of more than 5 mg/kg.

Forty-eight healthy volunteers received single or repeated doses of posaconazole (50 to 800 mg) for a period of 14 days. For doses of between 50 and 800 mg, the pharmacokinetics were linear. After 14 days of administration of the product, the accumulation ratio (area under the curve from 0 to 12 h day 14/day 1) was between 6.1 (100 mg) and 8.3 (400 mg).

The apparent elimination half-life is between 19 and 31 h. Plasma clearance is between 10.3 and 13.9 liters/h, and the volume of distribution is between 343 and 486 liters (Table 5).

Table 6 Activity against *Fusarium* spp.

Compound	MIC_{GM} (μg/ml)		
	F. solani	*F. oxysporum*	*F. moniliforme*
SCH 56592	10.5	2.4	0.36
AMB	2.1	0.36	2.3

2.1.4.1.4. ER 30346. ER 30346 (BMS-207147; ravuconazole [Fig. 20]) has a 3-(4-cyanophenyl)thiazole chain at position 3 of the butan-2-ol.

This derivative has better activity than fluconazole, itraconazole, and AMB against *C. albicans*, *A. fumigatus*, and *C. neoformans*. ER 30346 is more active than itraconazole in pulmonary aspergillus infections in the mouse.

2.1.4.1.5. Other azole derivatives. A number of other azole derivatives are in the preclinical development stage. TAK-187, an azalene derivative (Fig. 20), possesses better in vivo activity than fluconazole in murine *C. albicans* and *C. neoformans* infections. Toyama has reported the activity of T-8581 (2-fluorobutamide) (Fig. 23), which is hydrosoluble at physiological pH (41.8 versus 0.02 μg/ml). It is inactive against *A. fumigatus* (71 versus 0.38 mg/ml) and weakly active against *C. neoformans* (2 versus 0.03 μg/ml). A number of morpholine derivatives have been synthesized: UR-9746 (2-hydroxymorpholine) and UR-9751 and UR-9728 (*N*-arylmorpholines). Albaconazole (UR-9825) is a triazole derivative in an enantiomeric form (Fig. 24). This molecule is more active than itraconazole against *C. albicans* (MIC_{GM}, 0.02 μg/ml), *C. glabrata* (MIC_{GM}, 0.4 μg/ml), *C. krusei*

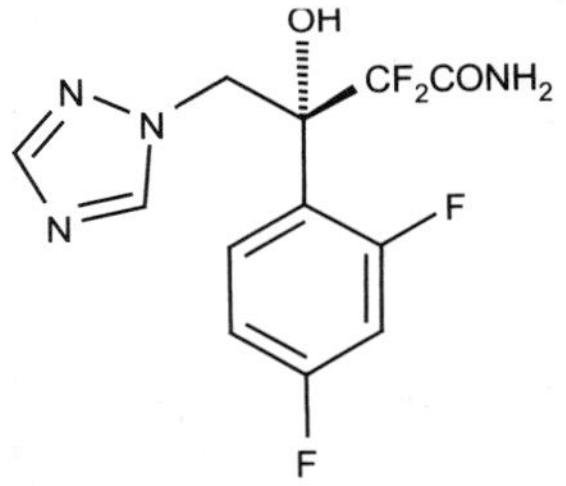

Figure 23 T-8581

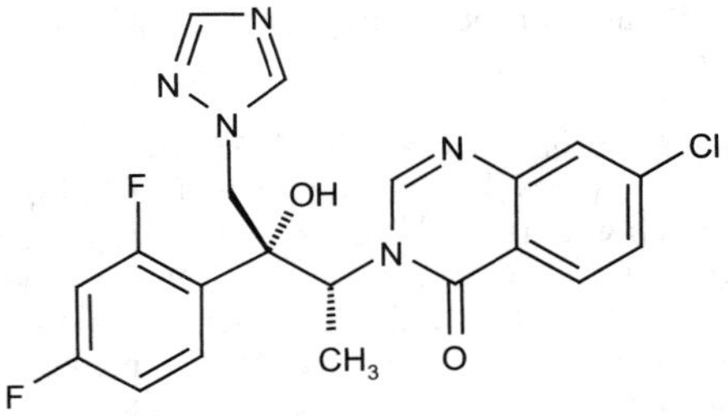

Figure 24 UR-9825

(MIC_{GM}, 0.25 μg/ml), and *C. tropicalis* (MIC_{GM}, 0.08 μg/ml). It possesses good in vivo activity in aspergillus infections, although weaker than that of AMB. SSY726 (Fig. 25) has slight in vitro activity against *C. glabrata, C. krusei,* and *C. neoformans*. It is inactive against *Aspergillus* spp. However, it seems that, as for fluconazole, its in vitro activity does not reflect its in vivo activity. The kinetics are summarized in Table 5.

2.1.5. Δ^{14}-Reductase Inhibitors

After demethylation, the sterol derivative is reduced at position 14 by a Δ^{14} reductase. This step may be inhibited by the morpholine derivatives. One derivative has been introduced into clinical practice, amorolfine (Fig. 26). It has a broad antifungal spectrum, including dermatophytes, yeasts, and molds. It is fungicidal against yeasts, dermatophytes, dimorphic fungi, and *Dematiaceae* (Table 7).

It is inactive in vitro against *Aspergillus, Fusarium,* and zygomycetes.

2.1.6. Δ^7-Δ^8 Isomerase Inhibitors

After demethylation at C-4 and C-14 and methylenation of the side chain, the following step is the production of fecosterol by isomerization of the double bond at Δ^7-Δ^8 by an isomerase. This step may be inhibited by the morpholine derivatives.

Tridemorph (Fig. 27) appears to inhibit Δ^7-Δ^8 isomerase more selectively, whereas fenpropimorph appears to inhibit both isomerases at Δ^{14} and Δ^7-Δ^8.

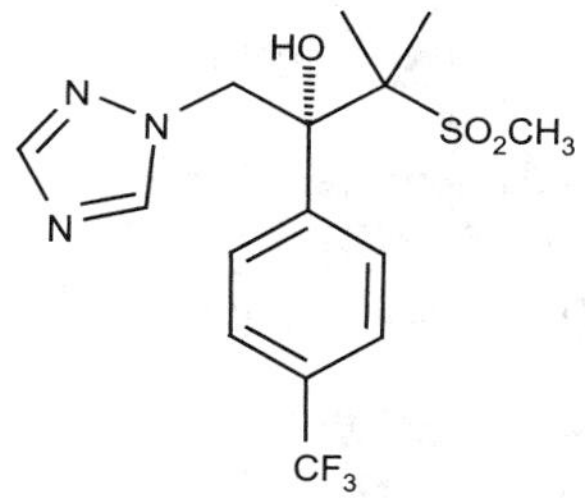

Figure 25 SSY726

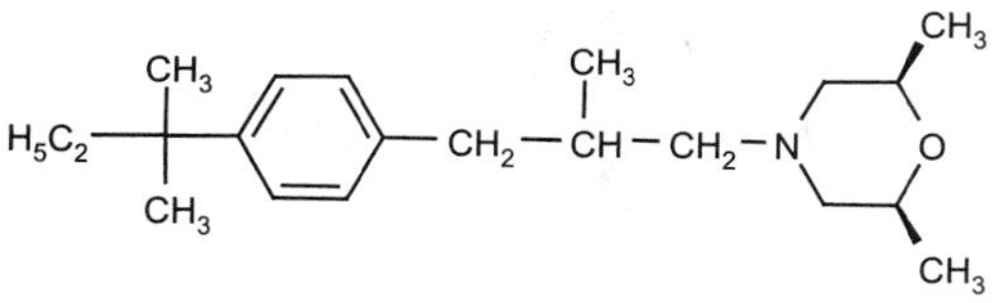

Figure 26 Amorolfine

Table 7 In vitro activity of amorolfine

Microorganism(s)	*n*	MIC_{GM} (μg/ml)
Dermatophytes	200	0.02
Pityrosporum spp.	10	0.075
C. albicans	155	0.55
Candida spp.	125	0.79
C. neoformans	55	0.033
Dimorphic fungi	70	0.08
Aspergillus spp.	65	0.12
Zycomycetes	68	100
Fusarium spp.	25	30
Alternaria spp.	8	30
Scopulariopsis	5	0.35
	3	0.8

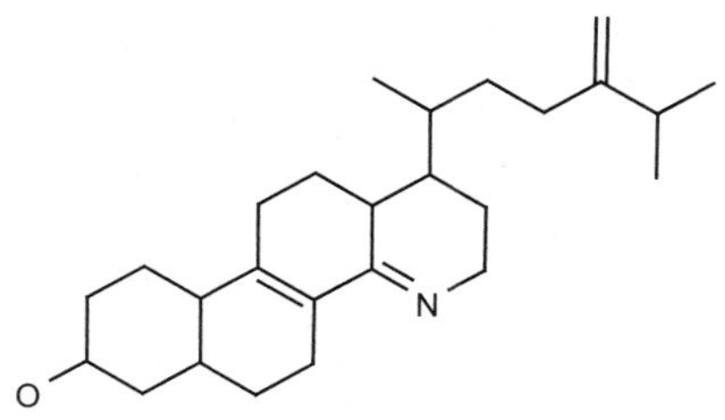

A-25228 B

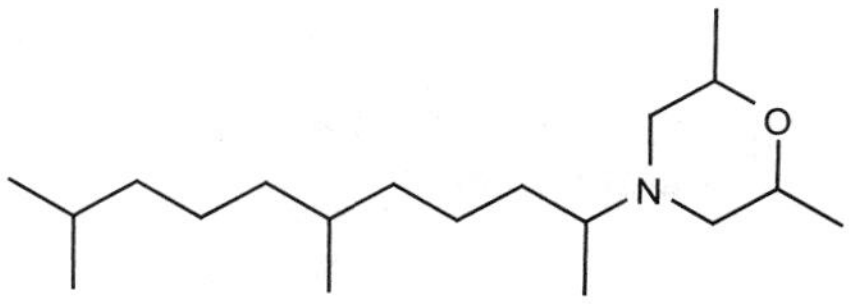

Tridemorph

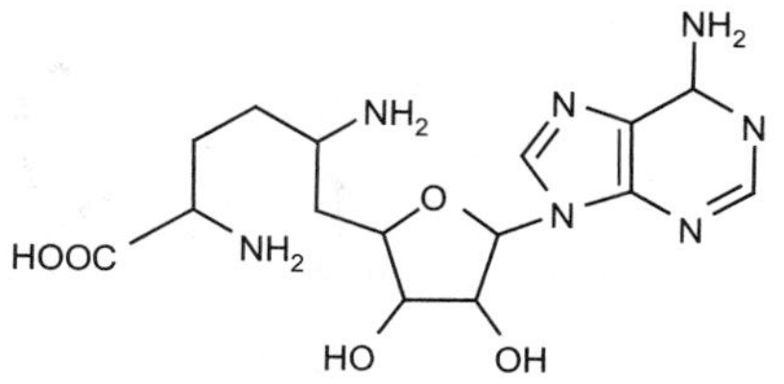

Sinefungin

Figure 27 Tridemorph

2.1.7. C-24 Methylase Inhibitors

One of the following steps is the addition of a methyl group at position 24 at the moment of production of zymosterol. This step is specific to yeasts and does not exist in mammalian cells. A number of compounds, such as tomatidine or derivatives of the ICI-62965 series (Fig. 28), inhibit this step.

2.2. Fungal Wall

The fungal wall is an important target for potential antifungal agents. This wall is in constant renewal itself, and these dynamics may allow certain key stages to be inhibited. It is complex and composed principally of three major components: 1,3-β-D-glucan, chitin (β-1,4-N-acetylglucosamine), and a mannoprotein (principally composed of α-1,6-mannose) (Fig. 29). None of these elements are found in mammalian cells.

2.2.1. Inhibition of β-1,3-D-Glucan Synthesis

In the majority of fungal agents β-1,3-D-glucan is linear, with about 3% of branches composed of β-1,6-D-glucan. The network constituted by β-1,3-D-glucan is very complex, as it contains cross-links and heteropolymers and part of the structure comprises linear polymers of the β-1,6-D-glucan-type consisting of 140 residues.

The main inhibitors of β-1,3-D-glucan synthetase are echinocandins and their derivatives and papulacandins and their derivatives. They inhibit β-1,3-D-glucan biosynthesis by preventing the incorporation of glucose in the synthetic chain (Fig. 30).

2.2.1.1. Lipopeptides

The family of lipopeptides is complex and is described in chapter 30. The lipopeptides possessing antifungal activity

R

HO

	R
Tomatidine	
ICI 62965	

CH_3 NH CH_3 H O

H_3C OH N CH_3

Figure 28 C_{24}-sterol methyltransferase inhibitors

Inhibitors of C_{24}-sterol methyl transferase

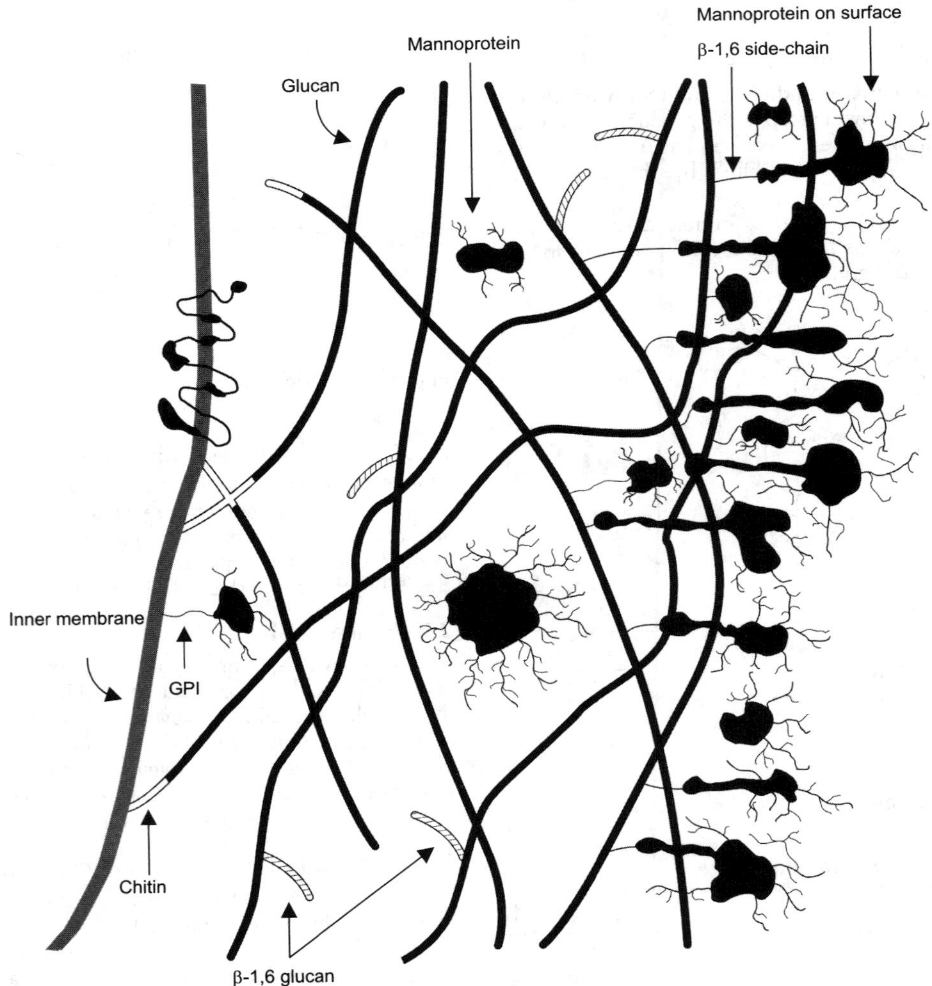

Figure 29 Constitution of the fungal wall

are divided into several subgroups: echinocandins, pneumocandins, mulundocandins, and derivatives obtained by semisynthesis.

2.2.1.1.1. Echinocandins. The lipopeptides belonging to the echinocandin family are represented by more than 20 derivatives of natural origin, divided into six subgroups. A large number of semisynthetic derivatives have been prepared from these natural products. All act by inhibiting β-1,3-D-glucan synthesis.

The first natural derivatives described were fungicidal and in some cases slightly toxic, but they possessed a narrow spectrum that included only *C. albicans*. New series have been discovered, among which some molecules are also active against *Aspergillus* spp. and *Pneumocytis carinii*. They are inactive against *C. neoformans* through the absence of a

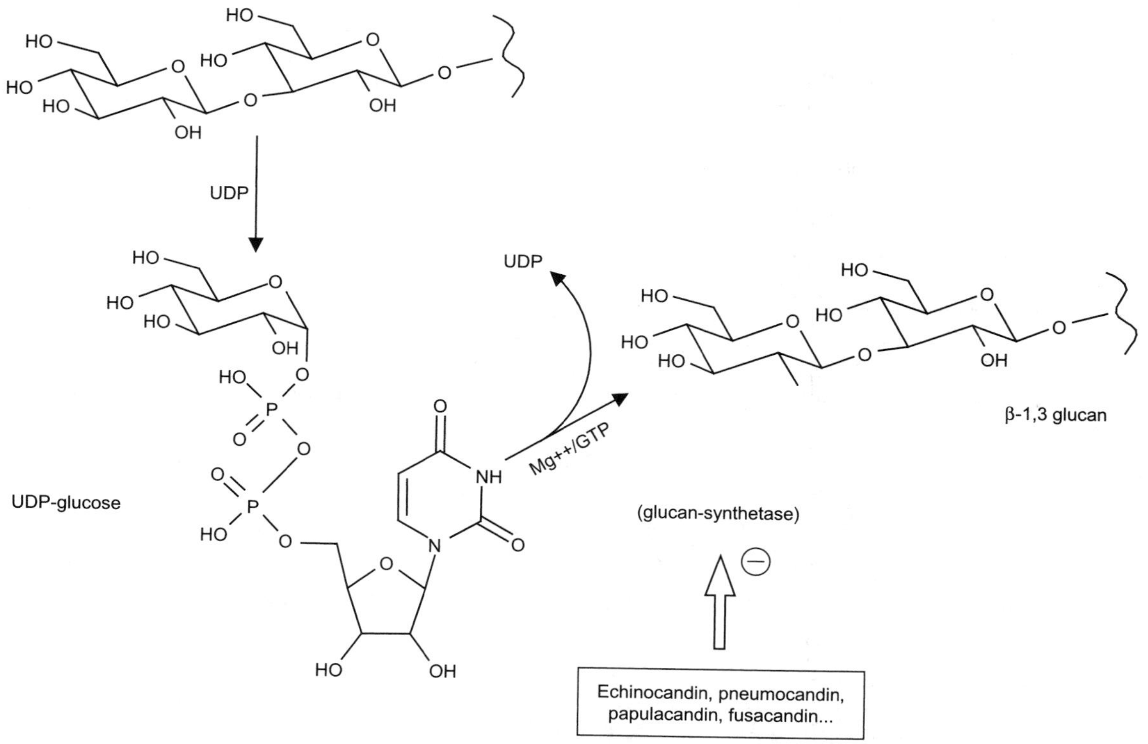

Figure 30 Echinocandin, pneumocandin, papulacandin, fusacandin, etc.

target enzyme and against *Trichosporon beigelii*. They act by noncompetitive inhibition of β-1,3-D-glucan synthetase.

The echinocandins were discovered simultaneously by three teams from E. Lilly, Sandoz, and Ciba-Geigy. They were isolated from strains of *Aspergillus nidulans* and *Aspergillus rugulosis*. Structurally, they involve hexacyclic peptides with a different fatty chain attached to the α-amino group of ornithine (Fig. 31). They contain an unusual amino acid, homotyrosine, two substituted proline residues, and a cyclized ornithine on the δ-amino group. They differ through the number of hydroxyl groups on the amino acids.

Echinocandin B is a potent anti-*Candida* agent that has not been developed because of its hemolytic potential. The antifungal and hemolytic properties are dependent on the nature of the fatty acid chain. The discovery of the possibility of removing the fatty acid chain enzymatically has allowed major progress in the chemistry of the echinocandins, particularly through the use of *Actinoplanes utahensis*. The deacylated echinocandin molecule is inactive but becomes a good substrate for the preparation of semisynthetic derivatives. It would appear that the antifungal activity and the hemolytic properties increase with the length of the unbranched fatty acid chain.

The first molecule with clinical potential was cilofungin, which has a phenyl nucleus but which had to be abandoned because of its nephrotoxicity. This was attributed to the presence of polyethylene glycol in the pharmaceutical formulation for intravenous use.

Other derivatives have been prepared and one of them, LY-280949, is also orally absorbed in animals. A number of derivatives have been prepared from this molecule to optimize the oral activity. Thus, a group of derivatives with an ED_{50} of <10 mg/kg orally has surfaced. It has been shown structurally that a linear part and a rigid part are necessary to obtain this type of activity, the lipophilia of these compounds being optimized by a flexible alkyl moiety.

2.2.1.1.2. Anidulafungin (LY-303366). Anidulafungin (Fig. 32) has good in vitro activity against the different *Candida* spp. (Table 8). It is 10 to 100 times more active than cilofungin. It also has good activity against strains of *Candida* resistant to azole derivatives.

Anidulafungin is active in vitro against *A. fumigatus*. The activity is greater than that of cilofungin (MIC, 0.12 versus 0.25 μg/ml). However, the MIC determination differs from that used conventionally. Two critical parameters may be established. The first is the time at which there is a modification of growth through the change from confluent colonies to microcolonies. This value appears to be highly correlated with the in vivo activity. The second parameter is the disappearance of the microcolonies, which is achieved at high concentrations.

The activity of anidulafungin was tested against 195 strains of filamentous fungi. The results showed that anidulafungin was active against *Paracoccidoides brasiliensis*, *H. capsulatum*, and the agents of phaeohyphomycoses, with moderate activity against *W. dermatitidis*, *Penicillium marneffei*, and *C. immitis*. Anidulafungin is inactive against *S. schenckii*, *Fusarium*, *Rhizopus*, and *Scedosporium prolificans*, the agents of chromoblastomycoses, and zygomycetes.

Anidulafungin and caspofungin are more active against *P. boydii* than AMB (Table 9).

In the murine model of disseminated candidosis, anidulafungin is 20 to 30 times more active than cilofungin intraperitoneally (ED_{50}, 0.3 versus 8.2 mg/kg) and is also active orally (ED_{50}, 7.8 mg/kg). It is as active as AMB in its capacity to reduce the aspergillus burden in the kidney. It is active in murine models of disseminated aspergillus infection at low doses (2.5 to 5.0 mg/kg).

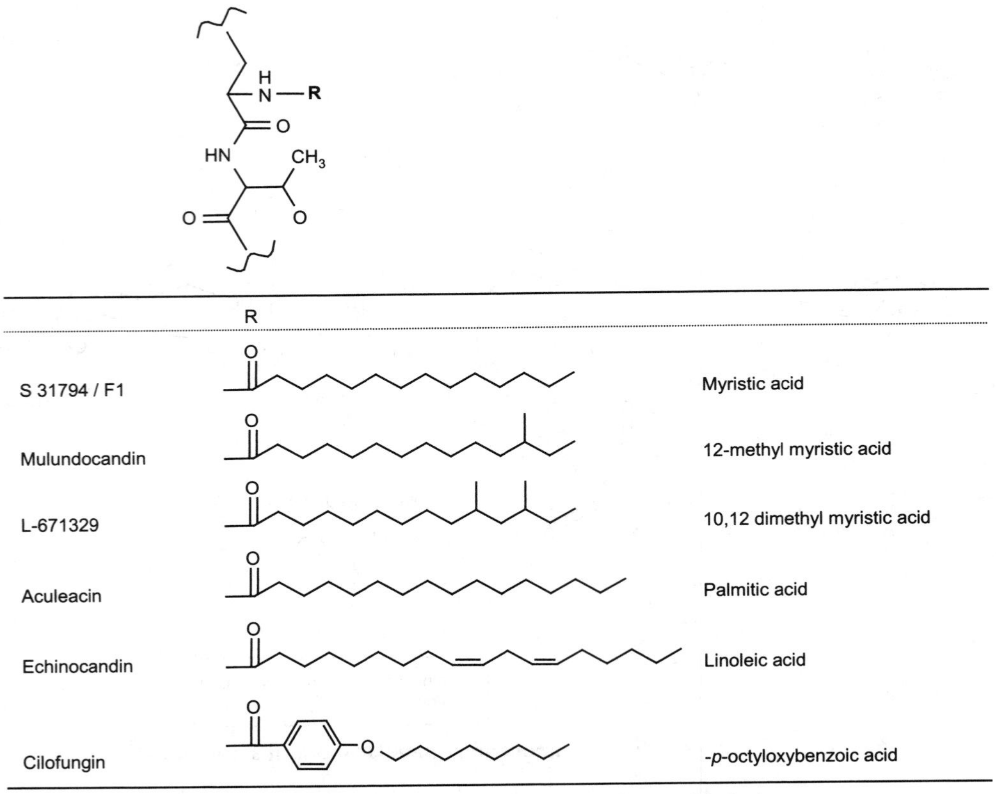

	R	
S 31794 / F1		Myristic acid
Mulundocandin		12-methyl myristic acid
L-671329		10,12 dimethyl myristic acid
Aculeacin		Palmitic acid
Echinocandin		Linoleic acid
Cilofungin		-*p*-octyloxybenzoic acid

Figure 31 Echinocandin derivatives: fatty acid chains

It is active against *P. carinii* by significantly reducing the pulmonary cyst burden in infected immunodepressed rats when given orally at a dosage of 5 mg/kg for 4 days.

It is inactive against *C. neoformans*.

The oral kinetics of anidulafungin were studied by Lucas et al. (1995), who administered increasing doses to healthy volunteers (25 to 1,000 mg). The apparent elimination half-life was long, about 32 h. The peak concentrations in serum were between 0.02 and 1.6 μg/ml, with a relatively long time to peak, on the order of 6 h (Table 10).

Food reduces the area under the curve by 40 to 50%, and similarly the peak concentration in serum, delaying its time of onset by up to 11 h.

Single increasing doses (7 to 100 mg) of anidulafungin were administered intravenously to 26 healthy volunteers in the form of an infusion. The pharmacokinetics are given in Table 11.

Comparison of the areas under the curve of the oral and intravenous doses shows that the oral bioavailability is about 45%.

A water-soluble derivative of anidulafungin has been described. This is anidulafungin phosphate (LY-307853).

2.2.1.1.3. Pneumocandins. The first molecule of the group of pneumocandins to be isolated was pneumocandin A_0, which is a less hemolytic derivative than the natural echinocandins. The activity of pneumocandin A_0 (L-6711329) is comparable to that of cilofungin. Pneumocandin B_0, which differs from A_0 by the absence of a methyl group on a proline residue, has better affinity for glucan synthetase (IC_{50}, 0.07 μM), but this enzymatic inhibition is not reflected in an increase in in vitro activity. These two derivatives are weakly soluble in water, and for this reason it is difficult to prepare a formulation for intravenous administration.

Solubilization was obtained by means of a prodrug by attaching a monoester phosphate to the hydroxyl group of the homotyrosine (L-693989). The parent product was obtained de novo by means of phosphatases.

New semisynthetic derivatives obtained from modifications on the peptide ring have given rise to caspofungin, currently undergoing clinical development.

2.2.1.1.4. Caspofungin (MK-0991, L-743872). Caspofungin (Fig. 33) is a water-soluble semisynthetic derivative of pneumocandin B_0 (L-688866). The β-1,3-D-glucan synthetase-inhibitory activity of caspofungin is 100 times greater than that of pneumocandin B_0.

Caspofungin is less active than AMB against *Candida* spp. It is inactive against *C. neoformans* (Table 12).

Caspofungin is active against fluconazole-resistant strains of *C. albicans*. This activity has been confirmed in vivo in models of generalized *C. albican* infection in neutropenic and nonneutropenic mice, but at dosages of ≥375 mg/kg every 12 h. It would appear that caspofungin is slightly more active than anidulafungin when the products are administered parenterally. However, the major advantage of anidulafungin is that it is orally active.

Caspofungin appears to possess a certain hemolytic potential.

2.2.1.1.5 Micafungin (FK 463). Micafungin is a semisynthetic lipopeptide, a derivative of FR 901379. FR 901379 is a water-soluble lipopeptide isolated from the fermentation broth of *Coleophama empedri*. It is a hexapeptide with a fatty acid side chain.

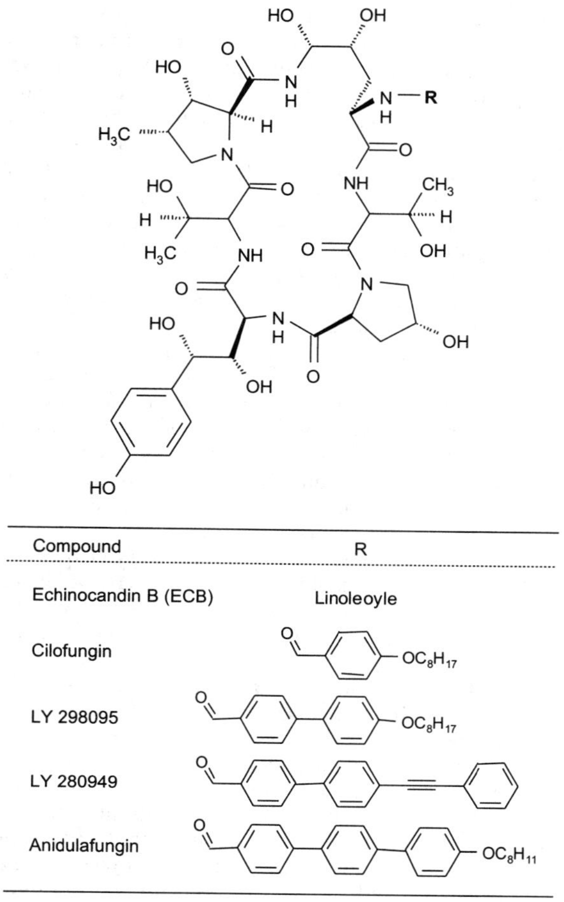

Compound	R
Echinocandin B (ECB)	Linoleoyle
Cilofungin	
LY 298095	
LY 280949	
Anidulafungin	

Figure 32 Cilofungin

Micafungin is highly active against *Candida* species (MICs, range 0.0078–0.125 μg/ml), except against *C. parapsilosis* (MIC, 1.0 μg/ml), and is fungicidal against *Candida albicans*. Against *Aspergillus* species micafungin is highly active in vitro (MICs, 0.003–0.007 μg/ml). Micafungin is only fungistatic against *Aspergillus fumigatus* (Tawara et al., 2000).

Micafungin is inactive in vitro against *Cryptococcus neoformans*, *Fusarium solanii*, zygomycetes, and dermatophytes, and the yeast form of dimorphic fungi (*Histoplasma capsulatum*, *Blastomyces dermatitidis*, *Penicillium marneffei*, *Sporothrix schenckii*, *Coccidioides immitis*). Micafungin displayed moderate activity against dematiaceous fungi (Nakai et al., 2002).

Micafungin is poorly active against some uncommon ascomycetes such as *Chaetomium* species which are responsible for skin and skin structure infections, as well as disseminated infections in immunocompromised patients, resulting in high mortality rates (Serena et al., 2003). Azole derivatives (raviconazole, albaconazole, voriconazole) exhibited MICs of ≤0.5 μg/ml.

Table 8 In vitro activity of anidulafungin against yeasts

Yeast	MIC (μg/ml)
C. albicans	0.01
C. parapsilosis	0.26
C. krusei	0.02
C. glabrata	0.01
C. tropicalis	0.02

Table 9 In vitro activities of lipopeptides[a]

Microorganism(s)	n	MIC (μg/ml)		
		Caspofungin	Anidulafungin	AMB
Acremonium spp.	1	0.03	0.5	2.0
A. flavus	10	0.03–0.5	0.015–0.03	1.0–2.0
A. fumigatus	12	0.6–0.12	0.004–0.12	1.0–2.0
Fusarium spp.	13	>8.0	>2.0	1.0–2.0
Paecilomyces spp.	1	0.5	1.0	4.0
P. boydii	5	0.25–2.0	>2.0	2.0–4.0
Rhizopus spp.	6	>8.0	0.06	1.0–2.0
Trichoderma	1	0.25		1.0

[a]Data from Pfaller et al., 1998.

Table 10 Oral pharmacokinetics of anidulafungin

Dose (mg)	C_{max} (μg/ml)	T_{max} (h)	AUC (μg·h/ml)	$t_{1/2}$ (h)	CL_P (liters/h)
25	0.02	7	0.989		
50	0.04	6.5	1.981		
50	0.009	10	0.05		
100	0.11	7	4.51	32.2	22.9
200	0.26	7	11.6	30.7	17.9
200	0.06	11	3.8	35.3	53.4
300	0.57	6.5	20.5	26.6	15
500	0.75	6.0	26.9	25.3	19
500	0.35	6.0	14.6	28.7	36.2
700	0.90	6.0	33.9	31.4	22
700	0.54	6.0	22.2	24.6	31.6
1,000	1.62	6.0	51.7	31.6	19.4

Table 11 Pharmacokinetics of anidulafungin given intravenously

Dose (mg)	C_0 (μg/ml)	T_{max} (h)	AUC (μg·h/ml)	$t_{1/2}$ (h)	CL_P (liters·h/kg)
50	0.25	0.75	51.6	39.3	0.01
70	0.29	1.0	66.7	45.4	0.01
100	0.38	1.5	101.4	42.3	0.01

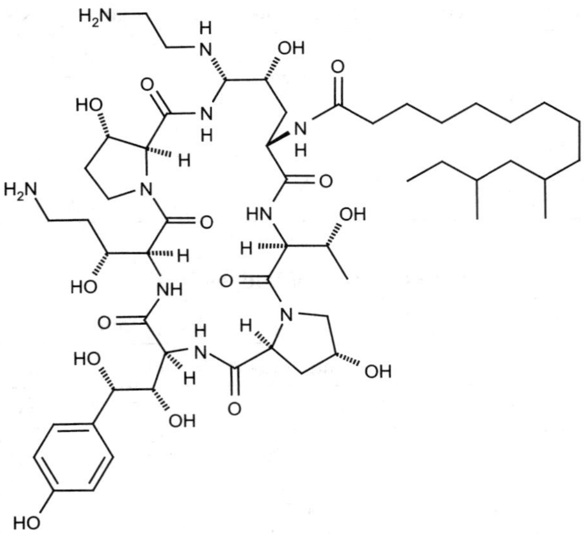

Figure 33 Caspofungin (MK-0991, L-743872)

Table 12 In vitro activity of caspofungin against yeasts

Yeast	MIC (μg/ml)	
	Caspofungin	AMB
C. albicans	0.5	0.25
C. tropicalis	0.5	0.25
C. parapsilosis	0.5	1.0
C. lusitaniae	0.25	1.0
C. guilliermondii	1.0	0.25
C. kefyr	0.25	0.25
C. glabrata	0.5	0.25
C. krusei	0.125	
C. neoformans	32	0.5

Immunocompromised patients may be infected with uncommon Basidiomycete yeasts such as *Cryptococcus laurentii*, *Sporobolomyces salmonicolor*, *Cryptococcus albidus*, *Rhodotorula glutinis*, and *Trichosporon asahii*. There is a limitation of amphotericin B therapy. Usually treatment failed to cure patients. New azole derivatives exhibited a good in vitro activity against these microorganisms (albaconazole, voriconazole, itraconazole with MICs of ≤0.5 μg/ml, except against *C. albidus*) and raviconazole exhibited poor activity against *Rhodoturula* species (Serena et al., 2004). *Paecilomyces*, a saprophytic fungus, may be responsible in immunocompetent and immunosuppressed patients for endophthalmitis and endocarditis; the current treatment is a combination of amphotericin B and an azole, but the treatment failed in 40% of patients. Micafungin displayed a good in vitro activity against *Paecilomyces variotii* (MICs, 0.06–0.5 μg/ml) but is inactive against *Paecilomyces lilacinus* (MICs, >64 μg/ml) (Ortoneda et al., 2004). Micafungin is inactive against *Pseudallescheria boydii* and *Scedosporium apiospermum* (MIC, >16 μg/ml) (Zeng et al., 2004).

In vivo in a murine (neutropenic) model of disseminated infection due to *Aspergillus* (Warn et al., 2003), mice were challenged with a lethal dose of either itraconazole-susceptible or -resistant *A. fumigatus*. Twenty-four hours after challenge they were treated for 7 days with various doses of mucafungin. All mice (100%) survived after doses of 5 or 10 mg/kg micafungin. However, no treatment regimens were able to sterilize the liver or the kidney of mice.

Micafungin when administered intravenously (1-h infusion in 100 ml of solution) exhibited a long apparent elimination half-life (~12–13 h). After repeated doses for 7 days, micafungin accumulated slightly (Table 13) (Hiemenz et al., 2005).

2.2.1.1.6. Mechanism of action of echinocandins. Echinocandins inhibit fungal cell wall synthesis by acting noncompetitively on β-1,3-D-glucan synthetase, allowing the formation of glucan polymers.

This enzyme is composed of two subunits: a catalytic subunit localized in the cytoplasmic membrane and one that binds to GTP, activating the catalytic subunit. The target gene of echinocandins is *ETG1* in *Saccharomyces cerevisiae*, which produces a 25-kDa protein possessing 16 transmembrane domains. This protein has considerable analogy with the cyclic β-1,3-glucan transporter protein. The principal function of this gene is transparietal transport.

Similar genes have been found in *C. albicans* and *Aspergillus* spp.

The echinocandins are not active against *C. neoformans*, as this fungal species has little or no β-1,3-D-glucan synthetase. *C. neoformans* has a β-1,6-D-glucan or 1,3-α- or 1,6-α-glucan structure. The echinocandins are very active against *P. carinii*, which in the cyst phase contains a large quantity of this enzyme in the cell wall.

Table 13 Human pharmacokinetics of micafungin after ascending and repeated doses

Daily dose (mg)	n	Study days	C_{max} (μg/ml)	$AUC_{0-\infty}$ (μg·h/ml)	$t_{1/2}$ (h)
12.5	8	1	0.9	11.6	11.3
	8	7	1.1	16.7	11.5
25	9	1	1.6	24.2	14.6
	8	7	4.1	34.9	12.4
50	9	1	3.6	44.6	12.5
	9	7	4.4	64.0	12.2
75	9	1	5.4	64.3	12.7
	8	7	8.3	91.1	13.4
100	9	1	7.1	81.1	13.0
	8	7	22	126.2	12.0
150	10	1	11.7	144.6	13.0
	8	7	17.6	230.3	12.9
200	8	1	13.1	164.3	14.3
	8	7	22.6	438.0	20.1

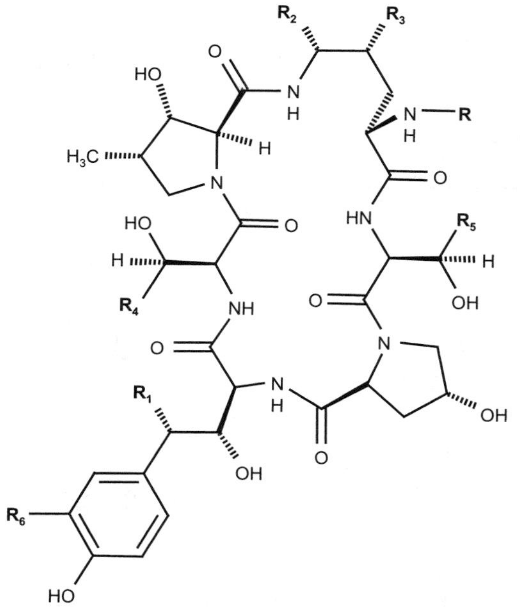

Echinocandines lipopeptide	R	R_1	R_2	R_3	R_4	R_5	R_6
Echinocandin B	Linoleoyl	OH	OH	OH	CH_3	CH_3	H
C	Linoleoyl	H	OH	OH	CH_3	CH_3	H
D	Linoleoyl	H	H	H	CH_3	CH_3	H
Aculeacin A_γ	Palmitoyl	OH	OH	OH	CH_3	CH_3	H
Mulundocandin	12-Methylmyristoyl	OH	OH	OH	H	H	H
Sporiofungin A	10,12-Dimethylmyristoyl	OH	OH	OH	CH_2CONH_2	H	H
Pneumocandin A_0	10,12-Dimethylmyristoyl	OH	OH	OH	CH_2CONH_2	CH_3	H
WF11899A	Palmitoyl	OH	OH	OH	CH_2CONH_2	CH_3	OSO_3H

Figure 34 Natural echinocandins

The presence of β-1,3-D-glucan as a constituent of the cell wall of other fungal genera is probable, although poorly documented.

2.2.1.1.7. WF 16616 and F 11899. WF 16616 was obtained by semisynthesis from pneumocandin A_0 and has good activity against *C. albicans* (MIC, 0.1 to 0.78 μg/ml) and *A. fumigatus* (MIC, 0.16 μg/ml) (Fig. 34). F-11899 is a sulfone derivative that is soluble in water. It was isolated from *Coleophoma empedri*. It has in vivo activity in the mouse against *C. albicans*, *A. fumigatus*, and *P. carinii*.

2.2.1.2. Other Peptide Derivatives

2.2.1.2.1. Cyclic depsipeptides: aureobasidin family. R-106 A (LY-295337) is the major compound obtained from the fermentation of *Aureobasidium* spp. discovered in 1989. Since then several other derivatives have been identified.

R-106 A is a octacyclic depsipeptide possessing a 2-hydroxy-3-methylpentanoic acid at *2R,3R*. The eight amino acids are in the L configuration, and four of them are N methylated. Only the hydroxyl group of *N*-methylvaline at position 8 is readily amenable to chemical modification. This highly lipophilic molecule is poorly soluble in water.

R-106A (Fig. 35) is active against *Candida* spp., *Histoplasma* spp., *W. dermatitidis*, and *C. neoformans*, but its in vivo activity is limited in the case of the last species. It is not active in vitro against *Aspergillus* spp.

A number of derivatives have been prepared by semisynthesis. The hydroxyl group in the β position on the *N*-methylvaline has been shown to be essential for activity against *C. neoformans* and even against *C. albicans*.

Structure-activity studies centered on the *N*-methylvaline residue with a β-hydroxyl group and a sarcosine residue have been conducted by researchers at Eli Lilly. It has been shown that activity against *C. albicans* is modified less with the various diastereoisomers than that against *C. neoformans*. A compound, SCH 56301, with a modification at the *N*-methylvaline site appears to possess in vivo activity comparable to that of R-106 A orally and intravenously.

2.2.1.2.2. Cyclic lipodepsipeptides: pseudomycins. A series of hydrosoluble lipodepsinonapeptides (pseudomycins) has been described. These were extracted partly from the fermentation of *Pseudomonas syringae*.

Pseudomycins are active against *C. albicans*, *C. tropicalis*, *A. fumigatus*, and *C. neoformans* (MIC, 3.12 μg/ml) (Harrison et al., 1991).

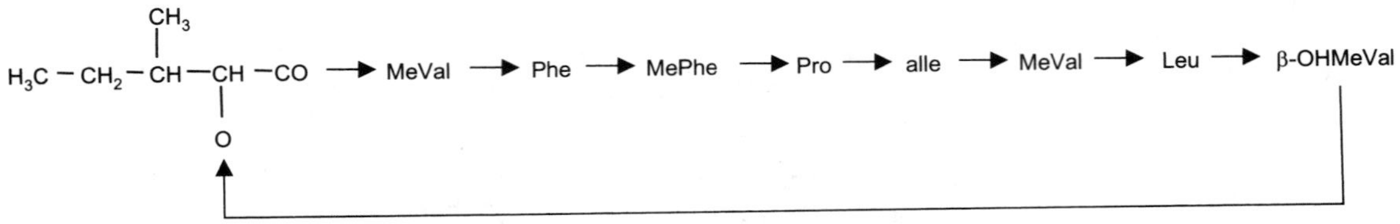

Figure 35 R-106 A (LY-295337)

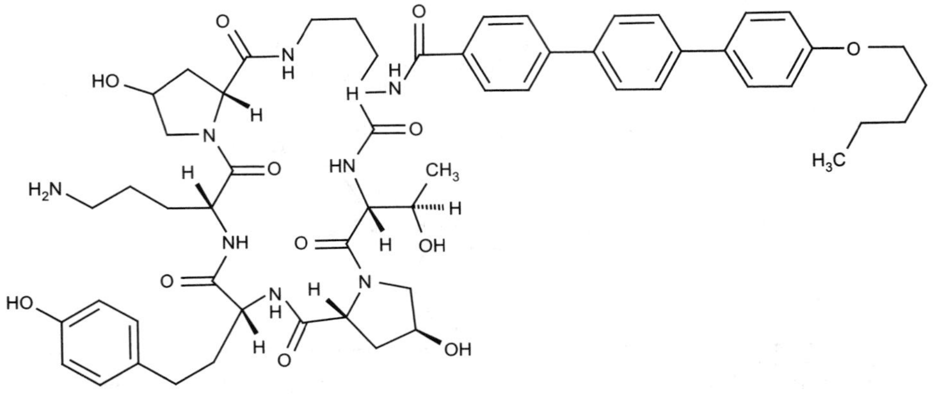

Figure 36 A-175800.0

2.2.1.2.3. Linear peptides. More than 30 derivatives have been described, and some appear to possess good activity against *C. albicans*.

2.2.1.2.4. A-175800.0. A-175800.0 is a cyclopentamine derivative (Fig. 36) that acts by inhibition of β-1,3-D-glucan synthesis. It is a hexapeptide.

In vitro A-175800.0 is two to four times more active than AMB against *C. albicans* (MIC, 0.2 to 1.56 μg/ml). It also has good activity against *C. tropicalis* and *C. glabrata*. It has bactericidal activity against *C. albicans* CCH-42 at one and four times the MIC.

2.2.1.3. Lipodisaccharide Derivatives

A number of derivatives of the papulacandin family have been described: papulacandins, BE-29602, Mer-WF 3010, saricandin, furanocandin, fusacandin A, and chaetiacandin.

2.2.1.3.1. Papulacandins. Papulacandins were described in 1988 and consist of a complex of five molecules (A to E) isolated from the fermentation of *Papularia sphaerosperma*. They are amphophilic compounds with an original structure described as being a spirocyclic oligosaccharide esterified by two unsaturated fatty acid chains (Fig. 37). They differ from one another in terms of the degree of unsaturation and the number of hydroxyl groups on the fatty acid chain. Papulacandin D is different in that it lacks a sugar and a fatty acid chain.

Each disaccharide is composed of a combination of galactosyl and glucose, the two sugars being linked to one another by a β-1,4 bond. A spirocyclic system is attached at C-1 of the glucose and at C-3 and is esterified by a fatty acid chain (*trans*-7-hydroxy-8,14-dimethyl-2,4,8,10-hexadecatetranoic acid).

L-687781 is a papulacandin extracted from *Dictyochaeta simplex*. It differs from papulacandins A and B by the fatty acid chain attached at C-6 of the galactose.

Papulacandins are very active against *C. albicans, C. tropicalis, C. krusei,* and *Candida parakrusei* (MIC, 0.1 to 0.2 μg/ml). Likewise, they possess good activity against *C. parapsilosis, C. glabrata,* and *S. cerevisiae*. *Microsporum canis* is susceptible to papulacandin B. Papulacandins A and B are inactive against *Candida guilliermondii, C. neoformans, S. schenckii, Aspergillus* spp., and *Trichophyton* spp.

Papulacandin B inhibits the enzyme that introduces the β-(1,6) branched chain during the construction of the β-(1,3)-glucan network rather than the enzyme that causes elongation of the chain.

It has been shown that the absence of a fatty acid chain on the galactose nucleus prevents the penetration of papulacandins through the wall. The fatty acid chain attached to the glucose is important, as its absence renders the molecules inactive.

The fungus *Monochaetia dimorphospora* produces chaetiacandin, which is similar to papulacandins A and B.

2.2.1.3.2. Fusocandin. Fusocandin belongs to the same family as the papulacandins. In structural terms, it differs in that is has a trisaccharide instead of a disaccharide (galactose), it possesses a C-glucoside phenol in place of the spirochetal residue of papulocandin, it is stable in the presence of acid, and it possesses unbranched side chains. Furanocandin has a galactose furanosyl residue.

It possesses activity comparable to that of AMB against *Candida* spp., *Cryptococcus* spp., and *A. niger.*

It is relatively inactive in vivo in murine *C. albicans* infections. This poor activity is based not on metabolic inactivation but on very weak protein binding due to the fatty acid moiety. Replacement of the fatty chain at position 6′ may restore activity against *C. albicans*.

Fusocandin was isolated from the fermentation of *Fusarium sambucinum*.

2.2.1.3.3. Mulundocandin and derivatives. Mulundocandin is a lipopeptide isolated from the fermentation broth of *Aspergillus sydowi* Y-30462 (Royk et al., 1987).

Mulundocandin exhibited a good in vitro activity against *C. albicans* and *C. glabrata* (MICs, range 0.5–4.0 μg/ml and 2.0–4.0 μg/ml, respectively). It is less active against *C. tropicalis*

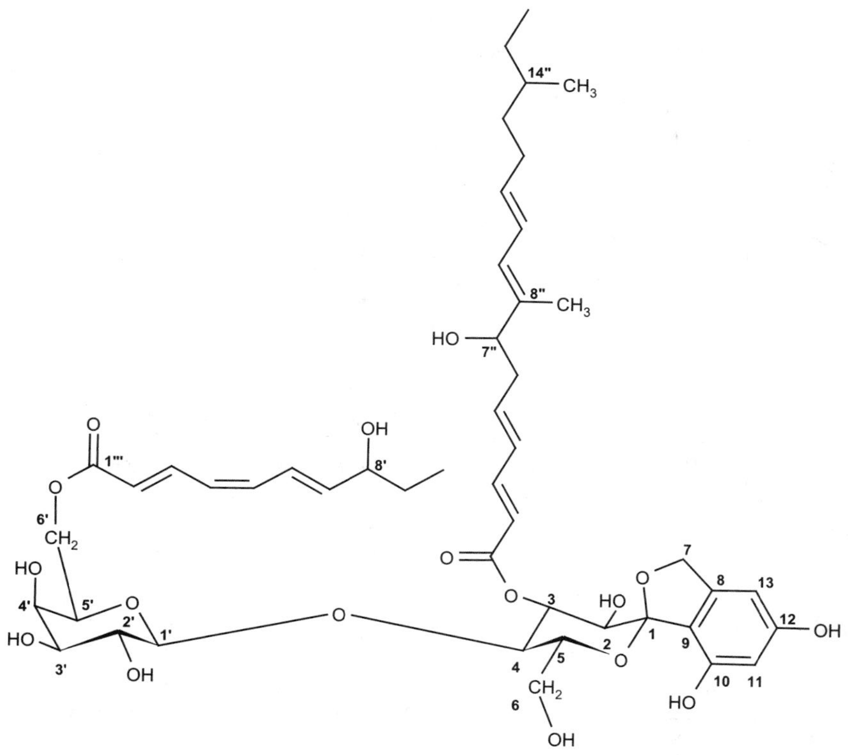

Figure 37 Structure of papulacandin B

(MICs, 1.0–8.0 μg/ml), and it is poorly active against other *Candida* species. Mulundocandin is inactive against *C. neoformans*, *Aspergillus* species, and *Trichophyton.* It is fungicidal against *C. albicans* after 8 h of contact at 4× and 8× MICs (Hawser et al., 1999; Hawser and Islam, 1999).

Many semisynthetic derivatives have been prepared in order to enhance and enlarge the antibacterial activity and spectrum. One compound, HMR 3270, was selected for further development (see chapter 30).

2.2.1.3.4. Aureothricins. Aureothricins are natural compounds obtained from the fermentation broth of *Deuteromycotinia* species. One of the three components isolated was known as FR 901469 (Fujie et al., 2000). It is considered as a threonine-rich product. All three components were subjected to chemical modifications. It is a large cyclic peptide with a molecular mass of 1,533 to 1,549 Da. In vitro this compound is active at the same level as caspofungin against *C. albicans*, *A. fumigatus*, *Fusarium solanii*, and *Scedosporium apiospermum.* In a murine model of disseminated candidiasis, ED_{50} values ranged from 0.05 to 0.4 mg/kg.

2.2.2. Inhibition of Mannoprotein Synthesis

Mannoproteins are 50% composed of carbohydrates and are a potential cell wall target of antifungal agents. They play an important role in fungal cell life, particularly at the parietal level, where they are attached to the cytoplasmic membrane by a glycosylphosphatidyl inositol chain or to the glucan or chitin network by 1,6-β-D-glucan bonds. However, the highest concentration of mannoproteins is found at the periphery of the fungal wall, where they constitute a major antigenic structure.

Benanomicins and pradimicins are two groups of antifungal agents belonging to the chemical family of benzo[α]naphthacenequinones that have a D-alanine substituting the C-15 and a mono- or disaccharide chain. Benanomicins A and B have been detected in the fermentation broth of *Actinomadura* spp. A number of components have been identified.

Pradimicins A and E (Fig. 38) are produced by a mutant strain of *Actinomadura hibisca*. Pradimicin C is identical to benanomicin N. A number of aglycone derivatives have been isolated: derivatives M, N, O, and P. The mechanism of action is poorly defined, but it would appear that these molecules have a great affinity for mannoprotein, which is calcium dependent, causing rupture of the cell wall. Benanomicins A and B (Fig. 39) exhibit moderate activity against yeasts and filamentous fungi, and likewise in vivo in disseminated murine *Candida* infections.

Pradimicins A, B, and C are less active than AMB. In vivo in a model of experimental *Candida* infection, the median intravenous protective dose is 9 mg/kg, compared to 0.2 mg/kg for AMB and 4.5 mg/kg for ketoconazole.

2.2.3. Inhibition of Chitin Synthesis

Chitin is a homopolymer composed of a β-1,4-*N*-acetylglucosamine (β-1, 4-GlcNAc) chain (Fig. 40). It was the first component of the fungal wall to have been described. It is the most abundant aminopolysaccharide in nature. Chitin is also present in the exoskeleton of insects and crustaceans. Three types of chitin have been described, α, β, and γ, according to the nature of the crystal, due to the alignment and spatial arrangement of the poly-GlcNAc chains. Chitin α is found in fungi and arthropods. The chains are antiparallel and are stabilized by means of intra- and interchain hydrogen bonds. The first bond is between the 3-OH group of each sugar and the oxygen of the pyranose ring of the following sugar, and the second is between the keto and amino groups of the acetamido residue of the adjacent chains. The stereochemistry of the repetitive units of chitin α is the

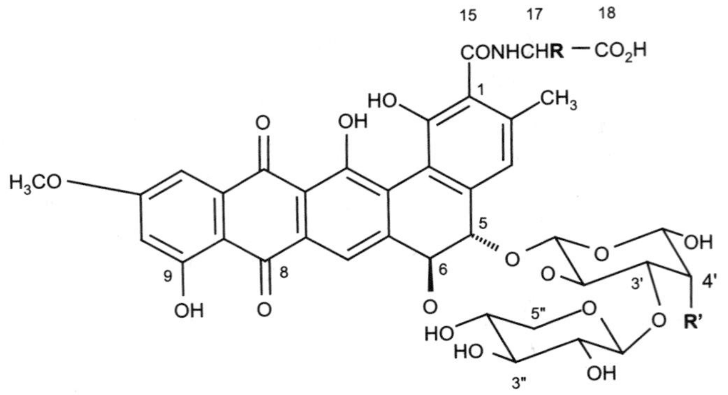

Compound	R (C17)	R (C4')	Water solubility (mg/ml)	MIC (μg/ml) *Candida albicans*	*Cryptococcus neoformans*	*Aspergillus fumigatus*
A	$-CH_3$	$-NHCH_3$	0.02	3.1	1.6	1.6
FA 1	$-CH_2OH$	$-NHCH_3$	0.26	6.3	1.6	1.6
FA 2	$-CH_2OH$	$-NH_2$	0.03	6.3	1.6	1.6
	-H	$-N(CH_3)_2$	2.00	6.3	1.6	12.5
BMY 28864	$-CH_2OH$	$-N(CH_3)_2$	> 20.00	6.3	1.6	3.1
BMS 181184	$-CH_2OH$	-OH	> 40.00	6.3	3.1	3.1

Figure 38 Pradimicin derivatives

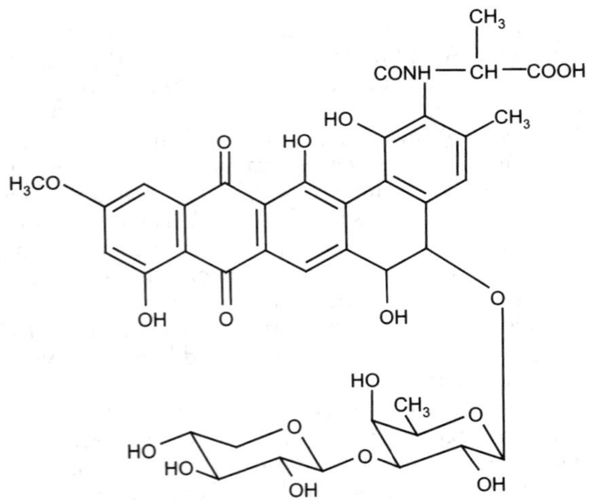

Figure 39 Structure of benanomicin A

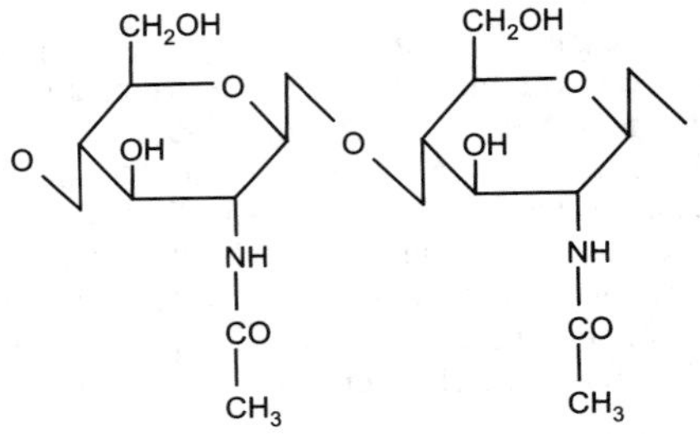

Figure 40 Structure of the β-1,4-GlcNAc unit forming chitin by repetition

dimer GlcNAc (diacetylchitobiose). In *C. albicans* and *S. cerevisiae,* chitin is a minor component (3%) localized principally in the septal region. Chitin is more abundant in the mycelial form of *C. albicans,* where is it localized in the apical region of the hypha. Chitin may also be associated with glucan.

Chitin is synthesized on the surface of the cytoplasmic membrane, where it projects perpendicularly through other components of the wall. It is in the form of microfibrils.

Noncrystallized chitin is hydrolyzed to the GlcNAc dimer under the action of a periplasmic chitinase.

2.2.3.1. Chitin Synthetase Inhibitors

Two structurally similar groups of compounds have been isolated by fermentation of different strains of *Streptomyces.* The first group is composed of polyoxins, and the second is composed of nikkomycins. They were discovered during research programs directed towards identifying insecticidal and fungicidal products for agricultural needs.

The polyoxins were discovered during the development of a research program to obtain treatment against *Pellicularia filamentosa* subsp. *sasakii,* responsible for a disease of rice plants (sheath blight). A nonpurified mixture of polyoxins has been introduced into the agricultural domain for a wide variety of indications.

The first polyoxins were isolated in 1965 from the fermentation of *Streptomyces cacaoci,* and nikkomycin was discovered in 1976 from the fermentation of *Streptomyces tendae* TU901. The latter was isolated from a soil sample from the facade of the Nikko pagoda (the five-storied pagoda) in Japan.

To date 13 natural polyoxins, A to M, have been described, as have 14 natural nikkomycin derivatives, Bx, Bz, Cx, Cz, D, E, I, J, M, N, X, Z, pseudo-J, and pseudo-Z.

Structurally, the polyoxins and nikkomycins are protein nucleosides with a great structural similarity to UDP-GlcNAc,

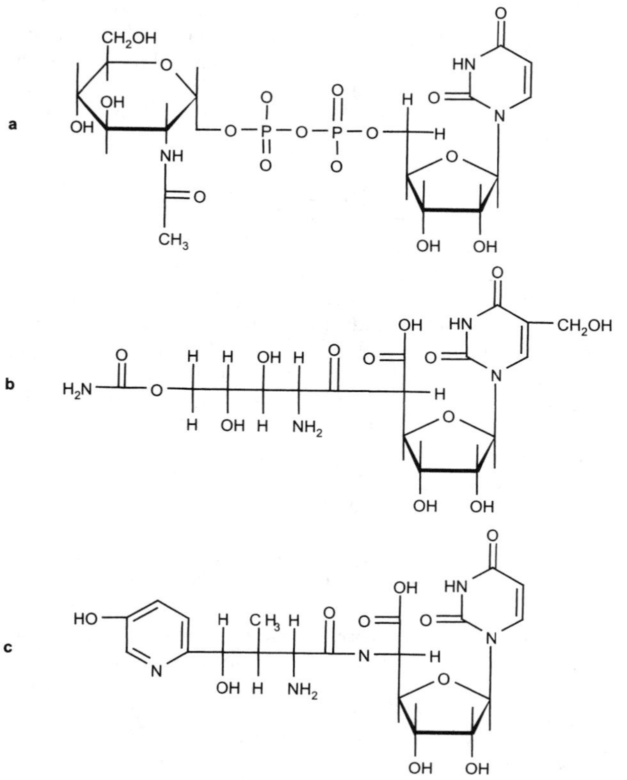

Figure 41 Structures of UDP-GlcNAc (a), polyoxin B (b), and nikkomycin Z (c)

one of the basic constituents of chitin (Fig. 41). Derivatives possessing biological activity are composed of two or three polypeptides constituted by amino acids in the α-L form and attached to a uridine or a formylimidazoline in the case of nikkomycin X.

Their mechanisms of action are unusual, as they act as chitin synthesis inhibitors by competition with GlcNAc synthetase and not as protein synthesis inhibitors, as has been demonstrated with other agents possessing this type of structure.

The polyoxins and nikkomycins have comparable affinities for the different chitin synthetases, with K_i values of between 0.6 and 3 μM, except for polyoxin B (Table 14).

This property of inhibiting chitin synthesis is not specific to fungi; it has also been demonstrated in insects. The K_is for chitin synthetase of the insect *Tribolium castaneum* are, respectively, 0.03 and 4 μM for polyoxin D and for the mixture of nikkomycins X and Z.

2.2.3.1.1. Polyoxin. The carbamoyl polyoxamic acid part of polyoxin forms a hydrogen bridge with chitin synthetase with an amino group at C-2″, the most important part

Table 14 Affinity for chitin synthetase

Compound	K_i (μM)
Polyoxin A	0.6
Nikkomycin X	0.5
Nikkomycin Z	2–3.5
Polyoxin D	0.6–3
Polyoxin B	32

for binding of the enzyme. It appears that the hydroxyl groups at C-3″ and C-4″ may also be attached by hydrogen bonds.

Polyoxins B and J have twice the affinity of UDP-GlcNAc for the enzyme.

The molecules with uridine as the nucleotide are the most effective. Replacement by thymidine reduces the activity of the derivatives by half. Other compounds with other nucleotides do not have inhibitory activity.

The polyoxins were described in 1965, but it was not until 1983 that the first studies devoted to fungi with a pathogenic potential in humans were undertaken with polyoxin D. It has been shown in yeasts that there is a ratio of 3 between chitin synthetase-inhibitory activity and activity against the whole fungal cell. The first study showed activity on the order of 1 μg/ml against *C. immitis*, particularly on the immature phase (spherules). Conversely, it is inactive during the mycelial phase and has no activity against *C. albicans* or *C. neoformans* (MIC, >200 μg/ml).

2.2.3.1.2. Nikkomycins. Substitution of the phenyl nucleus by more hydrophobic groups, such as a methyl group, yields compounds that have twice the inhibitory activity of the parent compound.

There are two transporters in *C. albicans* that allow di- or tripeptides to enter. Nikkomycin uses one of these transporters for penetration. It would appear that the polyoxins generally use these transport systems to penetrate the inside of the cell.

It has been shown with *C. albicans* that passage into the fungal cell is poor.

Various derivatives obtained by semisynthesis through modifications of the peptide chain or the nucleoside part have no greater affinity than the parent molecule.

2.2.3.1.2.1. NIKKOMYCIN X AND Z. The nikkomycins are active against dimorphic fungi such as *C. immitis* and *W. dermatitidis* and have moderate activity against *C. albicans* and *C. neoformans*, but they are inactive against *Fusarium* spp., *Aspergillus* spp., and *C. tropicalis* (MIC of 1 to 8 μg/ml).

2.2.3.1.2.2. NIKKOMYCIN Z. Nikkomycin Z is a water-soluble derivative. It possesses good activity in murine pulmonary histoplasmosis. The in vitro activity is 0.5 μg/ml. In vitro, nikkomycin Z has a MIC of >12.8 μg/ml for *W. dermatitidis*. Its activity in vivo is very moderate. Likewise, it has good activity against *C. immitis*.

Twelve healthy volunteers received incremental doses of 0.25 to 2 g of nikkomycin Z orally. Administered orally in the form of a single dose, nikkomycin Z generally appears to be well tolerated.

The peak concentrations in serum of 2.2, 4.5, and 6.1 μg/ml were reached after between 2 and 5 h for doses of 0.25, 1.0, and 1.75 g, respectively.

2.2.3.1.3. FR-900403 and FR-900848. FR-900403 differs from the polyoxin group and from nikkomycin by the fact that the nucleoside is an adenine and the peptide is attached to the nucleoside by a residue at C-3′. It is active against *C. albicans* but not against filamentous fungi.

FR-900848 is a compound composed of a nucleoside, uridine, and a monounsaturated fatty acid chain containing cyclopropyls. This derivative is active against filamentous fungi but not against yeasts.

2.2.3.1.4. Xanthofulvin. Three chitin synthetases have been identified in *S. cerevisiae* and *C. albicans*. In *S. cerevisiae*, Chs1 plays a repair role and Chs2 is partly

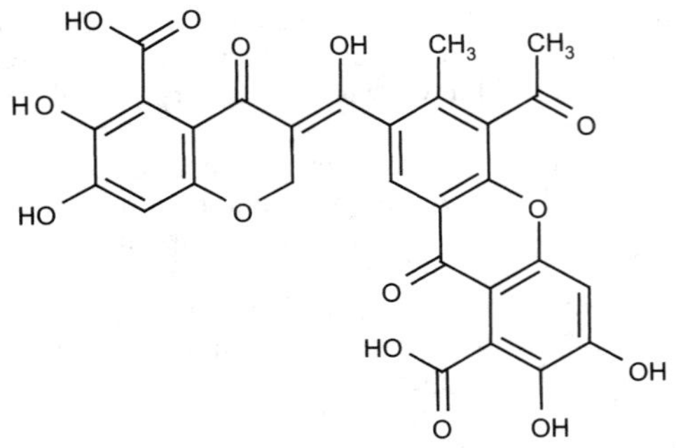

Figure 42 Xanthofulvin

responsible for maintaining cellular morphology, while Chs3 controls the production of the chitin mass. Interactions between the enzymes have not been clearly elucidated.

The polyoxins and nikkomycins principally inhibit Chs1 (IC_{50}, 0.25 μM for polyoxin D). Xanthofulvin (Fig. 42) inhibits Chs2 (IC_{50}, 2.2 mM, versus 10.3 μM for polyoxin D). Nikkomycin Z is a specific inhibitor of the isoenzyme Chs3, but it has no inhibitory activity against *S. cerevisiae* Chs2. It is probable that the moderate activity of nikkomycin Z against yeasts, or even its lack of activity, is related to the absence of activity against Chs3.

2.2.3.2. Inhibition of Chitinases

There is an equilibrium between the manufacture and destruction of chitin during the growth of the fungal cell, and likewise during reproduction and separation.

Allosamidin (Fig. 43), derived from the fermentation of a strain of *Streptomyces*, was first reported as an inhibitor of insect chitinase. It inhibits *C. albicans* chitinase (IC_{50}, 0.3 μM).

2.2.4. Other Sites of Action of Antifungal Agents

Antifungal agents have other sites of action: protein synthesis, cell division, and topoisomerases.

2.2.4.1. Cell Division

2.2.4.1.1. Flucytosine. Flucytosine penetrates the fungal cell via a cytosine permease, where it is deaminated to 5-fluorouracil by a cytosine deaminase. This enzyme is specific to the fungal cell. In fact, mammalian cells do not possess cytosine deaminase in their cytoplasm.

5-Fluorouracil is converted by a series of pyrimidine-type enzymes to 5-fluoro-UMP, which is a specific inhibitor of thymidylate synthetase, an enzyme essential for DNA synthesis, and to 5-fluoro-UTP, which is incorporated into RNA, causing the arrest of protein synthesis.

2.2.4.1.2. Griseofulvin. Griseofulvin is active against dermatophytes. It prevents nuclear division by blocking mitosis in the metaphase. It inhibits microtubule formation concentration dependently, probably by binding to the dimers of the tubules. Its action differs from that of colchicine.

2.2.4.1.3. Benzimidazole carbamate. Microtubulins are proteins of the cytoskeleton that play a major role in cell division, cell motility, and cell morphology.

The microtubulins are composed of two major proteins, α- and β-tubulins, in combination with other proteins that stabilize the assembly and dissociation complex. This unit is controlled by factors such as GTP, Mg^{2+}, and Ca^{2+}.

The benzimidazole carbamates (Fig. 44) are microtubule inhibitors acting by a rapid disintegration of microtubules and disruption of mitochondria into small bodies. Mutations in a structural gene for β-tubulin confer resistance to benzimidazole carbamates.

Benzimidazole carbamate agents have been used as anthelminthics since the 1960s.

It has been shown that *S. cerevisiae* is susceptible to the action of these molecules, and so is *C. albicans* β-tubulin.

2.2.4.1.4. Alkoxypropylamine derivatives. A series of alkoxypropylamine derivatives has been synthesized. The most active derivatives (e.g., Fig. 45) possess a four-carbon alkyl chain. The MICs for *C. albicans*, *A. flavus*, and *Trichophyton mentagrophytes* are, respectively, 0.156, 1.25, and 0.078 μg/ml. Its mechanism of action against *C. albicans* is different from that of the azoles, alkylamines, and morpholines. It does not act on membrane ergosterol, or glucan, mannan, or chitin biosynthesis, or RNA or protein synthesis, but it does act concentration dependently on DNA synthesis (Table 15).

This molecule is inactive in vivo. After intraperitoneal administration of 50 mg/kg to mice, the peak concentration in serum is 7 μg/ml and the apparent elimination half-life is 40 min. The molecule is rapidly metabolized.

Assembly and dissociation inhibitors have been identified, particularly in the field of oncology.

2.2.4.2. Topoisomerases

The fungi possess specific topoisomerases that might be inhibited.

It has been shown that *C. albicans* and *A. niger* possess topoisomerases I and II (Shen et al., 1992).

The topoisomerases are targets for antibacterial agents (fluoroquinolones and coumarin derivatives) and anticancer agents. Certain derivatives have been shown to have different

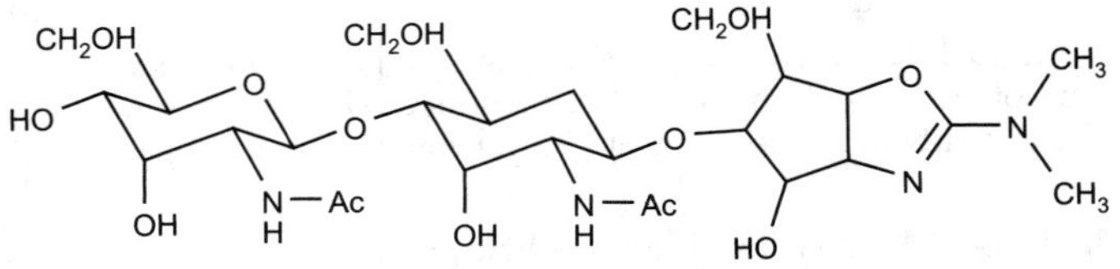

Figure 43 Allosamidin

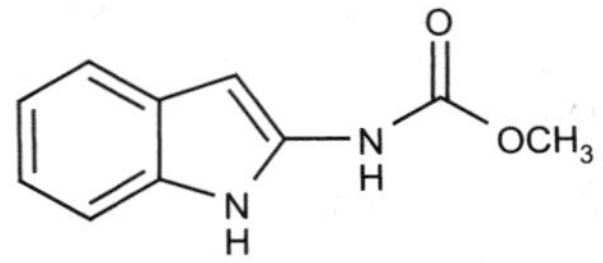

Figure 44 Methylbenzimidazole carbamate

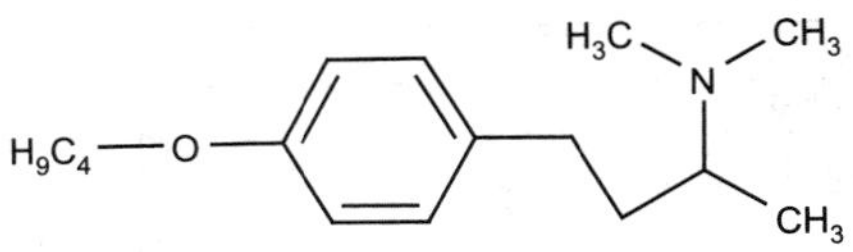

Figure 45 Alkoxyphenylpropylamine derivative

Table 15 Differential mechanisms of action of antifungal agents

Compound	Inhibition of synthesis of:				
	Ergosterol	Outer membrane	Protein	RNA	DNA
Phenylalkylamine	–	–	–	–	+
Ketoconazole	+	–	–	–	–
Fenpropimorph	+	–	–	–	–
Naftifine	++	–	–	–	–
Aculein	+	–	–	–	–
Blasticidin	+	–	+	–	–
Flucytosine	–	–	–	+	–
Actinomycin D	–	–	–	–	+

activities against mammalian cell (calf thymus) and *C. albicans* topoisomerase II, such as A-75272 (Fig. 46), suggesting that there are subtle differences between mammalian cell and fungal topoisomerase II. This phenomenon had already been demonstrated in *S. cerevisiae* by Figgitt et al. (1989) and Goto et al. (1984), who showed different inhibitory activities of relaxation by etoposide.

A. niger topoisomerase II is inhibited by podophyllotoxin derivatives (Fig. 47). These three derivatives are also active in vitro.

However, mammalian cell topoisomerase inhibitors also inhibit topoisomerase of fungal cells, which are eukaryotic cells.

P. carinii topoisomerases I and II are selectively inhibited relative to mammalian cell topoisomerases by substituted benzimidazole dication derivatives (Fig. 48). The most potent inhibitors are also active in vivo in murine *P. carinii* pneumonia. The results appear to show that these derivatives act on the first stage of action of topoisomerase at the recognition and cleavage site.

2.2.4.3. Inhibition of Protein Synthesis

2.2.4.3.1. EF-3. Fungal protein synthesis uses elongation factor 3(EF-3) (Fig. 49), which has no equivalent in other eukaryotic cells. EF-3 is essential to the fungus for life. This factor is controlled by ATPase and GTPase of ribosomal origin.

EF-3 possesses structural homology with other factors associated with translation, such as aminoacyl-tRNA synthetases and the S5 ribosomal protein of *Escherichia coli*. EF-3 appears to act at the moment of decoding of mRNA at the A-site.

A number of derivatives inhibit the action of EF-3, such as aspirochlorine (Fig. 50).

2.2.4.3.2. EF-2. EF-2 is an essential protein allowing ribosomal translocation during protein synthesis and is found in all eukaryotic cells (Fig. 49).

Sordarin (Fig. 51) blocks translocation by stabilizing the EF-2 complex in yeasts in a fashion similar to the action exerted by fusidic acid.

EF-2, although not specific to the fungal cell, may be inhibited by certain sordarin derivatives, such as GM 237354.

GM 237354 (Fig. 51) is a tetrahydrofuran derivative of sordarin obtained by semisynthesis. It inhibits protein synthesis by acting on EF-2 of *C. albicans*.

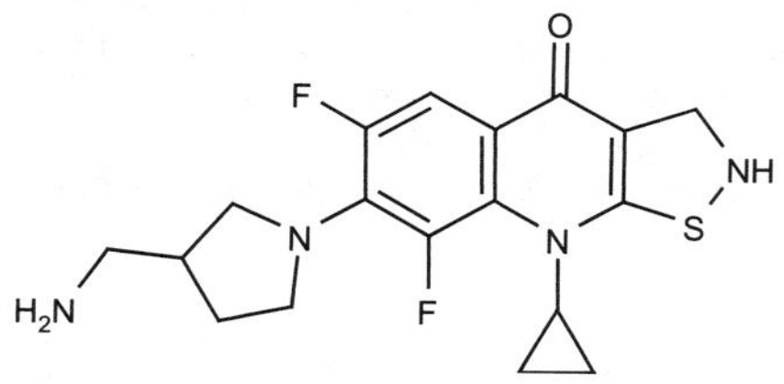

Figure 46 A-75272

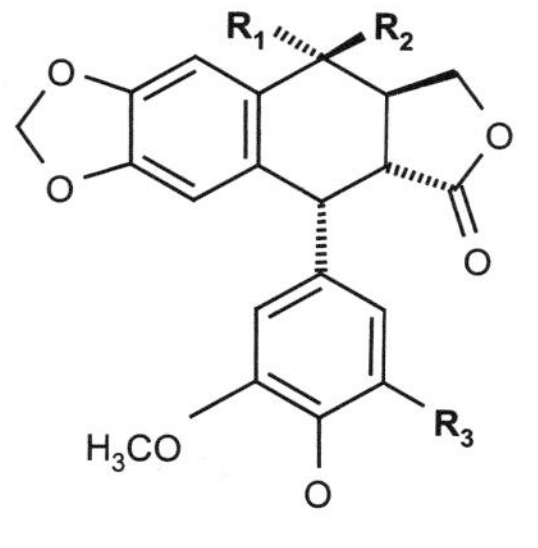

	R_1	R_2	R_3
Podophyllotoxin (P)			
4'-demethyl desoxy P	H	H	OCH_3
4'-demethyl P	=O	—	OCH_3
3',4'-didemethyl desoxy P	H	H	O

Figure 47 Podophyllotoxin derivatives

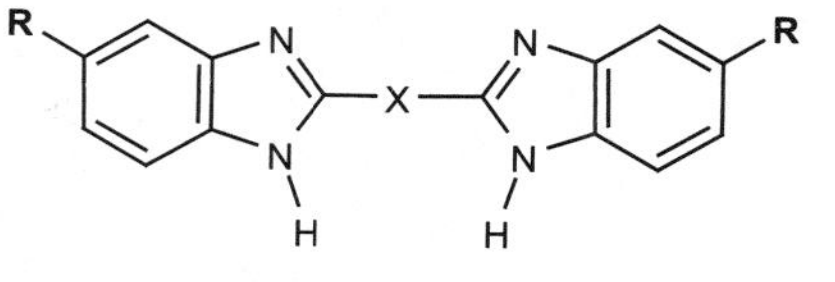

Compounds	R	X
1	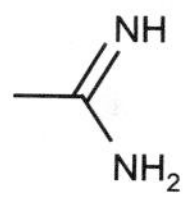 NH / NH_2	$(CH_2)_2$
2	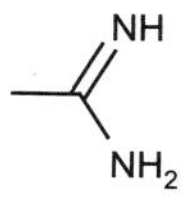 NH / NH_2	–HC=CH–

Figure 48 Bis-benzimidazole dication derivatives

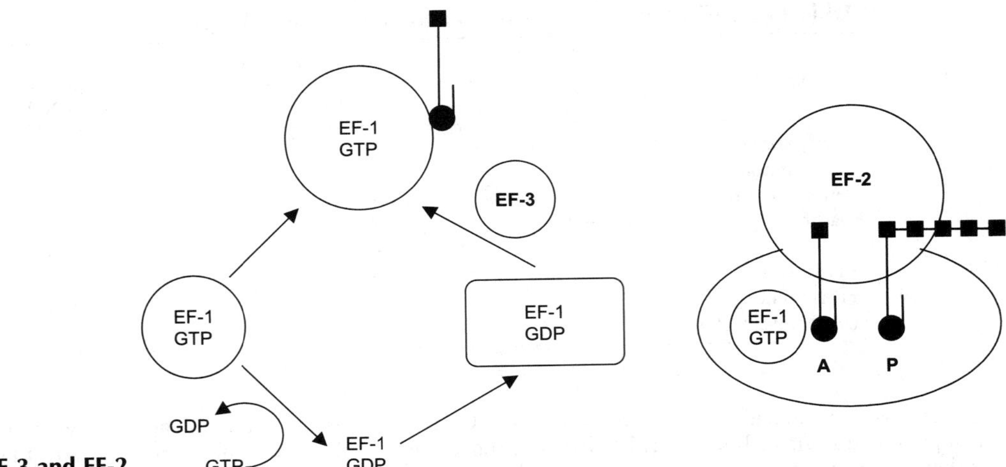

Figure 49 EF-3 and EF-2

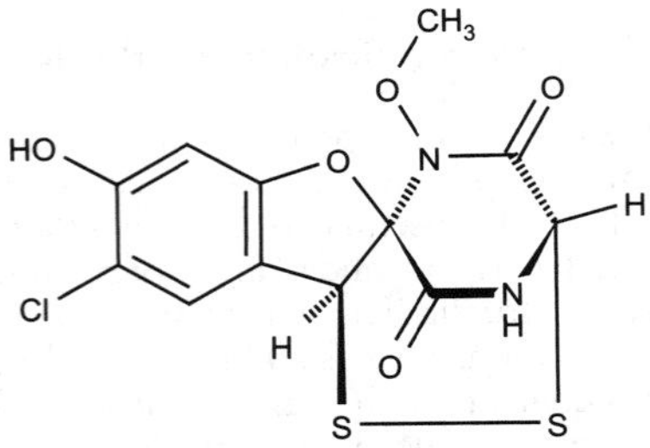

Figure 50 Aspirochlorine

GM 237354 is more active than itraconazole against *C. albicans* (MIC, 0.03 to 0.12 μg/ml), including fluconazole-resistant strains. It is active against *Candida kefyr* (MIC, 0.12 μg/ml).

Its activity against *C. glabrata* is bimodal. Seventy-five percent of strains are inhibited by 2 μg/ml. The remainder of the population is inhibited by 16 μg/ml.

C. krusei and *C. parapsilosis* are intrinsically resistant. All strains of *C. neoformans* are inhibited by ≤0.25 μg/ml. It possesses good in vivo activity in murine infections due to *C. albicans* and *H. capsulatum*. Its activity is comparable to that of fluconazole in *C. immitis* infections. It possesses good activity against *P. carinii*. In the rat, the bioavailability is 50%.

Other derivatives of the sordarin type have been isolated and characterized chemically and antifungally, but the mechanism of action has not been elucidated. The product concerned is GR-135402 (Fig. 52), which was isolated from the fermentation medium of *Graphum putredinis*. It possesses activity comparable to that of AMB against *C. albicans* (MIC, ~0.03 μg/ml). However, this molecule is inactive against *C. krusei*, *C. glabrata*, *C. tropicalis*, and *A. fumigatus*. Its

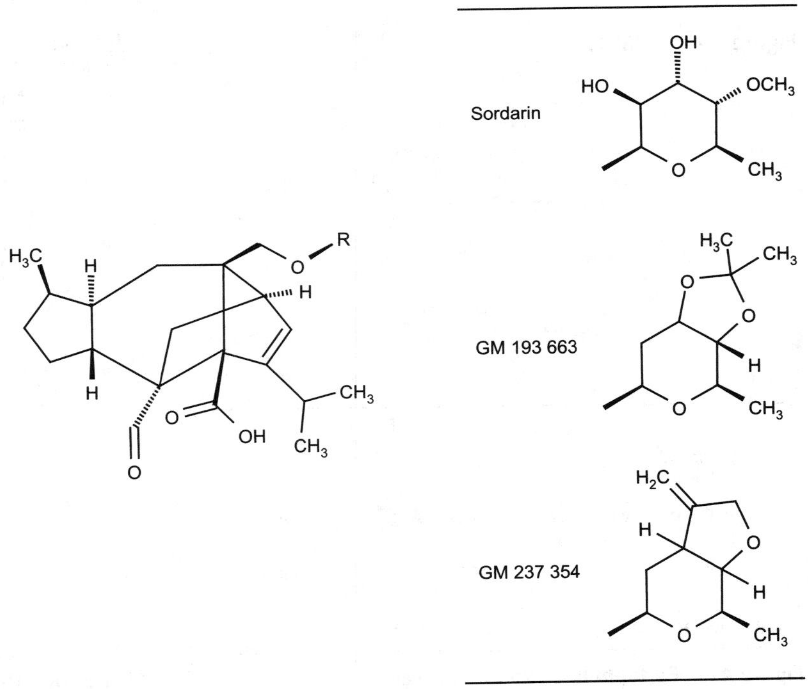

Figure 51 Sordarin derivatives

activity is moderate against *C. neoformans* (MIC, 1 μg/ml, versus 0.13 μg/ml for AMB).

A molecule related to sordarin and which is also a tetracyclic diterpene is SCH 57404 (Fig. 53), which possesses a narrow antifungal spectrum, with a MIC of ~16 μg/ml for *C. albicans* and a MIC of >128 μg/ml for dermatophytes and *Aspergillus* spp.

2.2.4.4. Other Potential Sites of Inhibition

The synthesis of sulfurated amino acids such as cysteine or methionine is essential to the fungus for life and occurs via a specific biosynthetic pathway using SO_4^{2-}, which is absent from mammalian cells. This might be a potential target.

2.2.4.4.1. RI-331. RI-331 (Fig. 54) is an antibiotic of the amino acid type (δ-hydroxy-γ-oxonorvaline) produced by *Streptomyces* spp. This antibiotic is active against *Mycobacterium tuberculosis* but also against *C. albicans*. RI-331 inhibits protein synthesis, not at the level of synthesis itself but by inhibition of amino acid synthesis.

RI-331 prevents the conversion of aspartic acid to homoserine or threonine. Likewise, it prevents the synthesis of isoleucine from threonine.

2.2.4.4.2. Azoxybacillin. Azoxybacillin is an azoxy derivative combined with amino acids (Fig. 55), isolated from the fermentation of *Bacillus* spp. It acts by preventing the binding of sulfur to methionine. This compound prevents the genetic expression of sulfite reductase (transcriptional activation of *MET4* and posttranscriptional activation of *MET10*). Its in vivo activity is moderate. A number of semisynthetic analogs, such as Ro-09-1824, have been prepared.

2.2.4.4.3. Purpuromycin and MDL-63604. Purpuromycin and its analog, MDL-63604 (Fig. 56), have activity comparable to that of AMB in vitro against *C. albicans*. They inhibit protein and RNA synthesis in fungi. However, as they are insoluble in water, it is difficult to test their activities in disseminated infections.

2.2.4.4.4. Icofungipen (Bay 10-8888, PLD-118). Icofungipen (Fig. 57) is a semisynthetic derivative of a natural product, cispentacin. It is a β-cyclic amino acid that has marked anticandidal activity.

Icofungipen accumulates to a very marked extent in cells of *S. cerevisiae* and *C. albicans*. Inside the cell, icofungipen inhibits the action of isoleucyl-tRNA synthetase, causing inhibition of protein synthesis. Intracellular accumulation is due to specific cispentacin transporters.

A study of ascending pharmacokinetics of the oral form of icofungipen was undertaken by enrolling 18 healthy

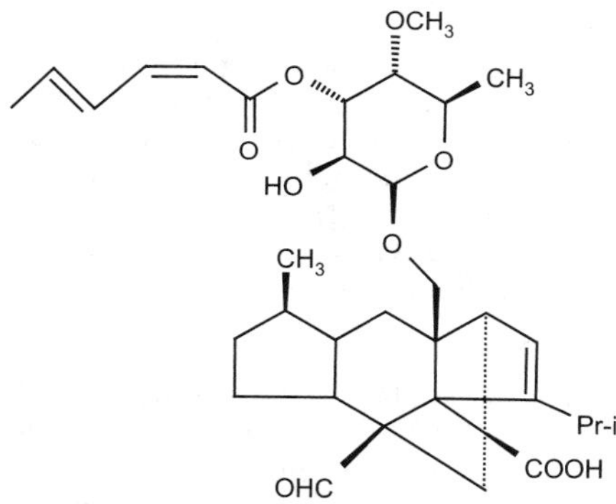

Figure 52 GR-135402

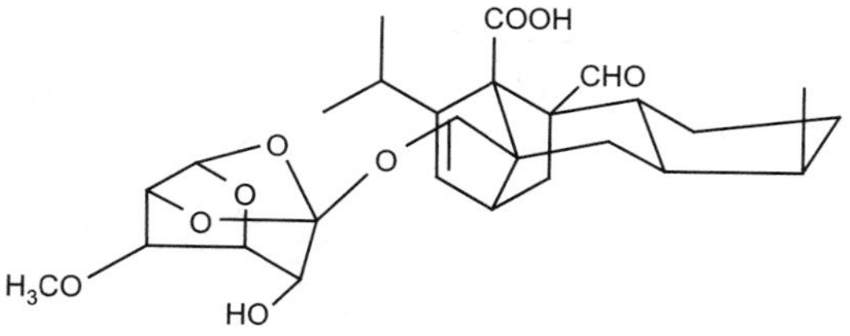

Figure 53 SCH 57404

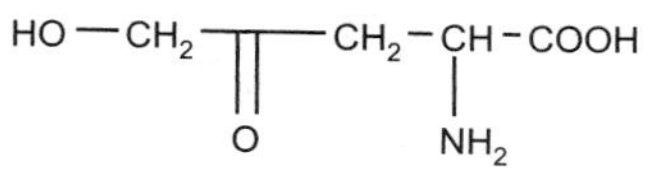

Figure 54 RI-331 (δ-hydroxy-γ-oxonorvaline)

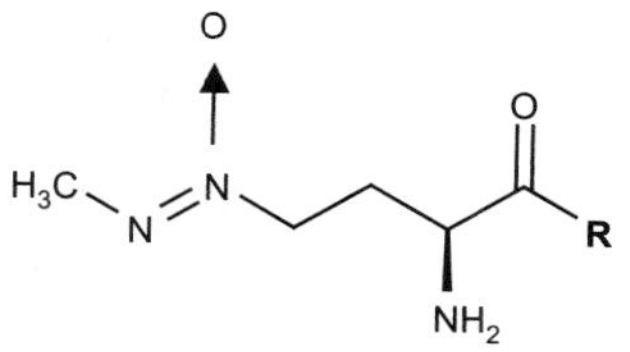

	R
Azoxybacillin	OH
Ro 09-1824	OBn

Figure 55 Azoxybacillin

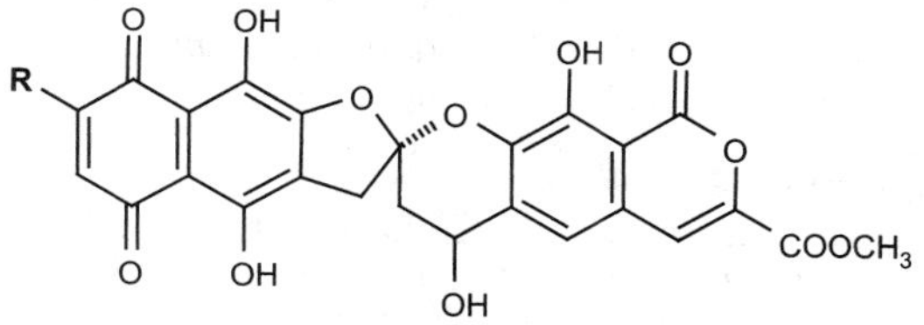

	R
Purpuromycin	OCH_3
MDL 63604	$NHCH_3$

Figure 56 MDL-63604

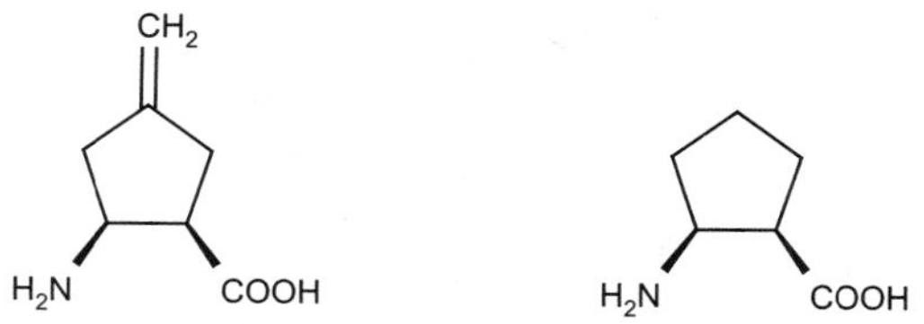

BAY 10-8888 Cispentacin

Figure 57 Icofungipen (Bay 10-8888, PLD-118)

Table 16 Pharmacokinetics of ascending doses of icofungipen

Doses (mg)	C_{max} (μg/ml)	AUC (μg · h/ml)	T_{max} (h)	$t_{1/2}$ (h)	Urinary elimination (%)
17.5	0.54	3.084	1.4	6.23	85
35	1.14	6.774	0.68	7.28	79
70	2.30	12.179	0.90	6.13	73
140	4.98	26.259	0.55	7.0	89
280	8.54	49.123	0.94	6.95	66

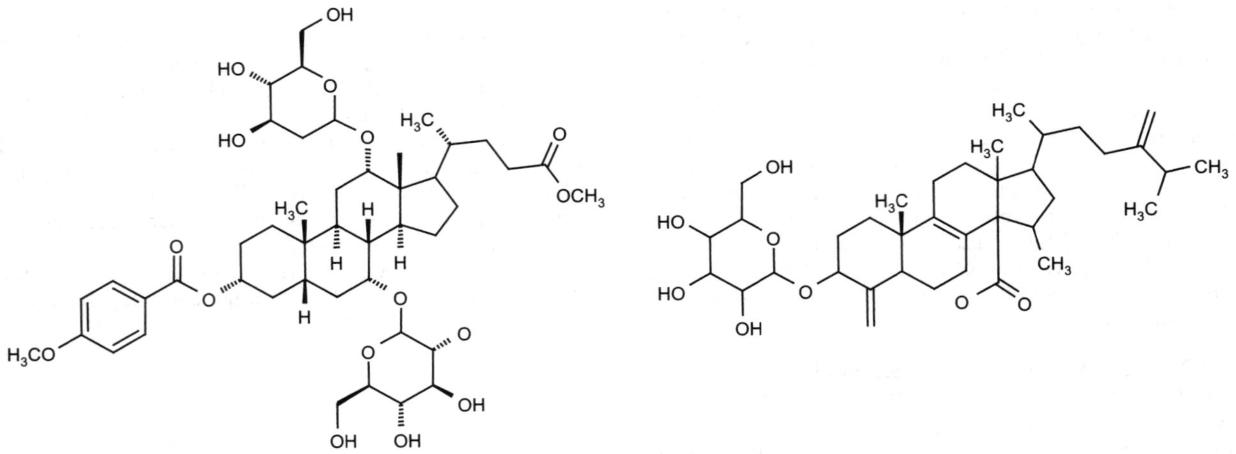

Figure 58 Steroid antifungal agents

volunteers (Oreskovic et al., 2001). Pharmacokinetic parameters are summarized in Table 16.

After food there is a delay in peak plasma concentration and a reduction above 10% of the C_{max}.

3. MISCELLANEOUS ANTIFUNGAL AGENTS

There is extensive literature on products of natural, semisynthetic, or synthetic origin possessing antifungal activity. Only a few examples are given here.

3.1. Steroid Derivatives

A series of derivatives with antifungal activity and having a steroidal structure (Fig. 58) has been extracted from the fermentation of *Mycoleptodiscus atromaculans*. One product exhibits variable activity against *Candida*, *Cryptococcus*, and *Aspergillus* (MIC, <0.03 to 64 μg/ml).

Derivatives known as ascosterosides have been isolated from the fermentation of *Ascotricha amphitricha*.

3.2. YM-47522

YM-47522 is a derivative consisting of a fatty acid chain at C-13 and a cinnamate residue, isolated from the fermentation of *Bacillus* sp. strain YL 03709B. This molecule is active against *Rhodotorula acuta* and *Pichia angusta*. It is inactive against *C. albicans* and *Aspergillus*. It possesses moderate in vitro activity against *Cryptococcus* spp. (MIC, 6.25 μg/ml) (Shibazaki et al., 1996) (Fig. 59).

3.3. SCH 2137

SCH 2137 is a polycyclic xanthone (Fig. 60) isolated from the fermentation of *Actinoplanes* sp. strain SCC 1906, belonging to the family of albofungins.

The family of albofungins also includes lysolipin, LL-D42067α and β, cervinomycins, actinoplanones (simaomicins), and everninomicins. Like albofungin, SCH 2137 has good in vitro activity (MIC, <0.125 μg/ml) against different species of *Candida*. Conversely, it is inactive against *Trichophyton* spp., like LL-D42067.

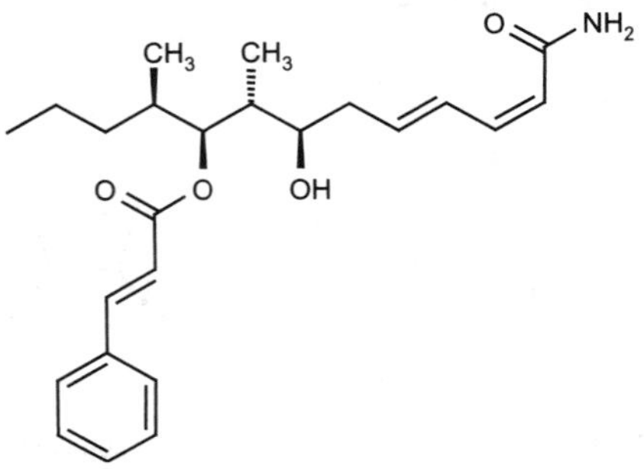

Figure 59 YM-47522

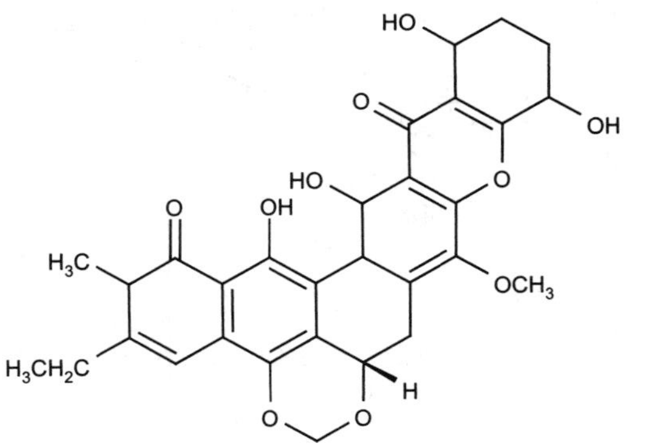

Figure 60 SCH 2137

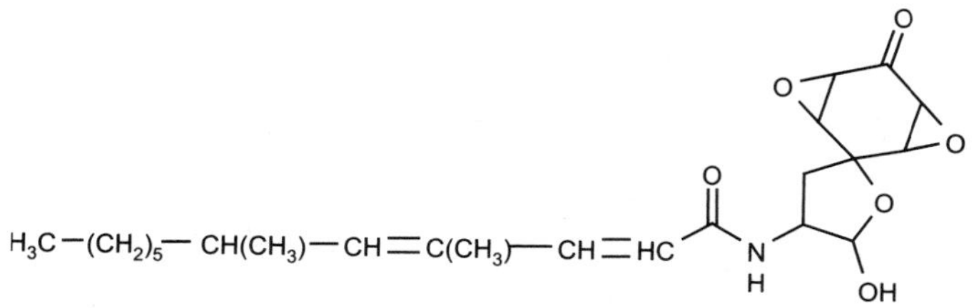

Figure 61 Aranotin

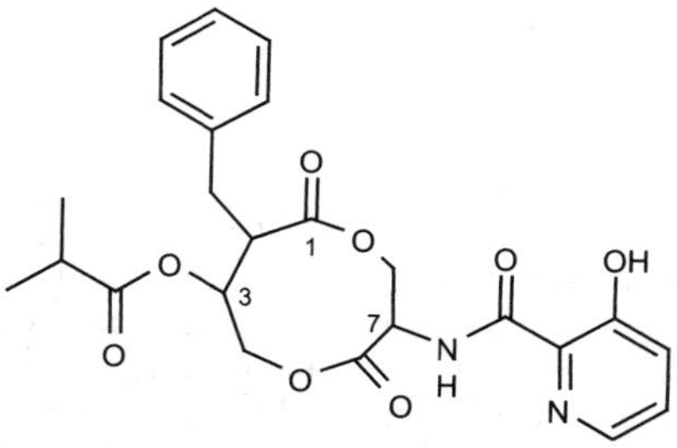

Figure 62 UK-3A

3.4. CAN-296

CAN-296 was isolated from the wall of *Mucor rouxii*. It is principally composed of multiple acetylglucosamine units (1.4, 2.4, and 4.6) and an N-terminal residue, GlcNAc (molecular mass, ~4,300 Da).

It possesses fungicidal activity against *C. albicans* dependent on the calcium concentration.

3.5. Aranotin

Aranotin (Fig. 61) was extracted from *Pseudoarachniatus roseus* HIL Y-30499. It possesses moderate activity against *C. albicans* and *A. niger*.

3.6. UK-3A

UK-3A (Fig. 62) was obtained from fermentation of *Streptomyces* sp. strain 517-02 (Ueki et al., 1997). It belongs to the family of macrocyclic dilactones, which consists of nine members, including UK-1 (benzoxazole) and UK-2A, -2B, -2C, and -2D.

UK-3A does not possess antibacterial activity. It has good activity against yeasts (*C. albicans, Rhodotorula rubra, Aspergillus, Rhizopus, Phycomyces, Neurospora,* and *Mucor*) with MICs of <1 μg/ml. It is inactive against *F. oxysporum* (MIC, 100 μg/ml). It also has cytotoxic activity.

3.7. Ambruticin and Derivatives

3.7.1. Ambruticin

Ambruticin (Fig. 63) is a cyclopropyl-polyene-pyran acid, which is the major component of a group of molecules extracted from *Polyangium cellulosum* subsp. *fulvum*. It is active in vitro against dimorphic and filamentous fungi such as *C. immitis, H. capsulatum,* and *W. dermatitidis* (MIC, ≤0.125 to 1.0 μg/ml). It is inactive in murine infections due to *C. immitis* and *H. capsulatum*. It possesses good activity in skin infections due to *T. mentagrophytes* in the guinea pig. It is not active against *P. boydii*. It is more active than AMB (MIC_{50}, 2.0 versus 32 μg/ml) against *Dematiaceae* (*Cladosporium, Phialophora,* and *Fonsecaea* spp). It is not active against *S. schenckii* (MIC_{50}, 8.0 μg/ml), but it is more so than AMB (MIC_{50}, 64 μg/ml). It possesses variable activities against *Mucor* (MIC_{50}, ≤1 μg/ml) and *Aspergillus* (MIC_{50}, 2.0 μg/ml).

Ambruticin is inactive against yeasts, with the exception of *C. parapsilosis* (MIC_{50}, ≤1.0 μg/ml). It has activity superior to that of griseofulvin against dermatophytes (*Trichophyton, Microsporum,* and *Epidermophyton* spp.).

This product has not been developed because of its inactivity against *C. albicans, C. glabrata,* and other *Candida* spp.

3.7.2. Jerangolids

Jerangolids are structurally similar derivatives of ambruticin extracted from *Sorangium cellulosum*, a myxobacterium (Gerth et al., 1996).

Their antifungal activities appear to be identical to those of ambruticin. They appear to act on the fungal wall.

3.8. Macrocyclic Antifungal Agents

A number of antifungal agents with a macrocyclic structure not belonging to the polyene family have been reported in the literature, such as the formamicins and TMC-34.

3.8.1. Formamicin

Formamicin is a macrocyclic antifungal agent with a 16-membered-ring aglycone (Fig. 64). It was isolated from the fermentation of *Saccharothrix* sp. strain MK 27-91FZ. It belongs to the family of bafilomycins-concanamycins.

It has good activity against the molds responsible for plant infections. It is inactive against *Candida, Aspergillus,* and *Trichophyton* spp. It possesses good activity against *C. neoformans* (Igarashi et al., 1997).

3.8.2. TMC-34

TMC-34 is a macrocyclic antifungal agent with a 24-membered-ring macrocycle. It was extracted by fermentation of a strain of *Streptomyces*. It belongs to the family of copiamycins and neocopiamycins. It manifests good activity in vitro against *C. albicans* ATCC 48130 (MIC, 3.1 μg/ml), *C. neoformans* 145 A (MIC, 1.6 μg/ml), *A. fumigatus* (MIC,

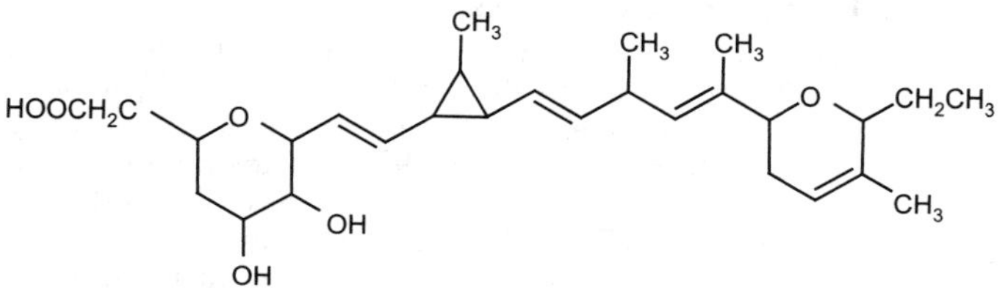

Figure 63 Ambruticin

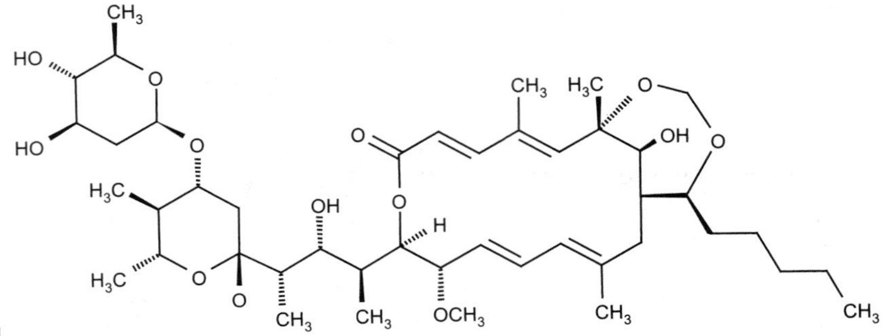

Figure 64 Formamicin

3.1 μg/ml), and *Trichophyton rubrum* (MIC, 1.6 μg/ml) (Kohno et al., 1995).

3.8.3. Mathemycin A

Mathemycin A is a macrocyclic antifungal agent extracted from the fermentation broth of *Actinomyces* sp. strain HIL Y-8620959, a soil strain from the region of Maharashta, India. The molecular mass is 1,396 Da. It is soluble in water. It is active against a certain number of molds. It is a molecule with a macrolactone composed of 40 members. There are other derivatives that belong to this group, such as desertomycins A and B, orsamycins A and B, which have 42 members, and oasamycins C and D, which have 44 members.

3.8.4. SCH 42282

SCH 42282 is a 14-membered-ring macrocyclic antifungal agent extracted from *Microtetraspora* spp. Eight monosaccharide and one disaccharide macrocyclic derivatives have been isolated from the fermentation broth. SCH 42282 is a trisaccharide macrocyclic antifungal agent.

It possesses moderate activity against *Candida* spp. (MIC_{GM}, 18 μg/ml), but it is less active than SCH 42729, a disaccharide derivative (MIC_{GM}, ≥10.7 μg/ml), and SCH 38518 (Fig. 65), a monosaccharide derivative (MIC_{GM}, 3.8 μg/ml).

The three derivatives are inactive in vitro against dermatophytes and *Aspergillus*.

3.8.5. YM-32890 A and B

YM-32890 A and B are 22-membered-ring macrocyclic derivatives extracted from the fermentation of *Cytophaga* sp. strain YL 02905 9 (Kamigiri et al., 1997). YM-32890 A possesses activity against gram-positive bacteria, including methicillin- and erythromycin A-resistant strains of *Staphylococcus aureus*, but also against yeasts.

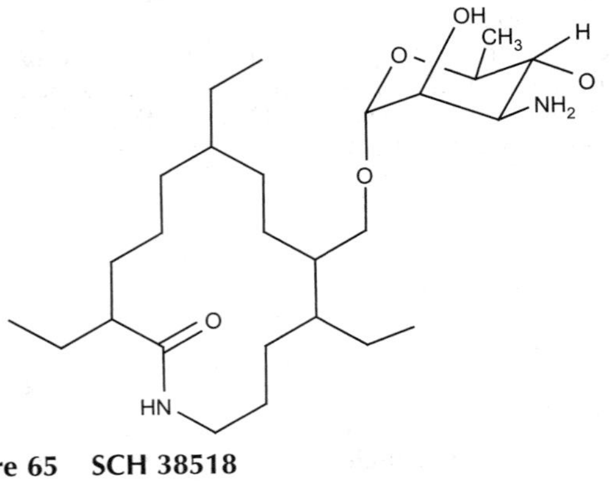

Figure 65 SCH 38518

3.8.6. Malonyl Niphimycin (AK-B7-3)

Malonyl niphimycin belongs to the same family of nonpolyene macrocyclic antifungal agents as scopafungin, niphimycin, copiamycin, neocopiamycin, guanidylfungins A and B, azalomycins (F_{3a}, F_{4a}, and F_{5a}), and amycin A. This molecule was obtained by fermentation from *Streptomyces hygroscopicus* B-7. It is a 36-membered-ring molecule derived from niphimycin A, to which a malonyl is attached at positions C-19 and C-23. It manifests activity against gram-positive bacteria, fungi, and yeasts (Ivanova et al., 1998).

3.9. Miscellaneous Antifungal Lipopeptides

Laxaphycin was extracted from the terrestrial blue-green alga *Anabaena laxa*. It is a complex of five cyclic lipopeptide compounds active against *Aspergillus*, *Candida*, *S.cerevisiae*, and *Trichophyton*.

Calophycin is a cyclic decapeptide derivative extracted from *Calothrix fusca* that has an antifungal spectrum similar to that of laxaphycin. It possesses in vitro activity against *C. albicans* and *A. fumigatus* similar to that of AMB.

Surfactin and iturin A were extracted from the fermentation of *Bacillus subtilis* and have surfactant and antifungal activities. They are active against phytopathogens, such as the lipopeptide verlamelin, which has a δ-hydroxymyristate residue.

The lipopeptide FR-901169 (Fig. 66) has good activity against *C. albicans*, *C. krusei*, and *C. tropicalis* (MIC_{50}, 0.004 to 0.16 μg/ml), with good activity in the murine model of disseminated candidosis (ED_{50}, <1 mg/kg). This derivative has good activity against *A. fumigatus* and *A. niger* (MIC_{50}, 0.63 μg/ml) but is not active against *C. neoformans* (MIC, >10 μg/ml). The activity against *P. carinii* is not known.

3.10. Other Cyclic Peptides

Chondramides (Fig. 67) are cyclic peptides isolated from *Chondromyces crocatus* that possess good activity against yeasts.

A series of cyclic peptides has been described by Mercian Corp. One derivative has good activity against *C. albicans* (MIC, 1.25 μg/ml) and *C. neoformans* (MIC, 0.63 μg/ml).

3.11. Natural Derivatives

A number of products of natural origin (Fig. 68) were reported in the literature between 1995 and 1997, including patents.

TAN 1771 is a dieneamide derivative that appears to be identical to the product YL-03709B. Activity against *C. albicans* (MIC, 25 μg/ml) and *Aspergillus* is moderate. Dorrigocins A and B are glutarimide derivatives produced by *Streptomyces platensis* subsp. *rosaceus* that manifest weak

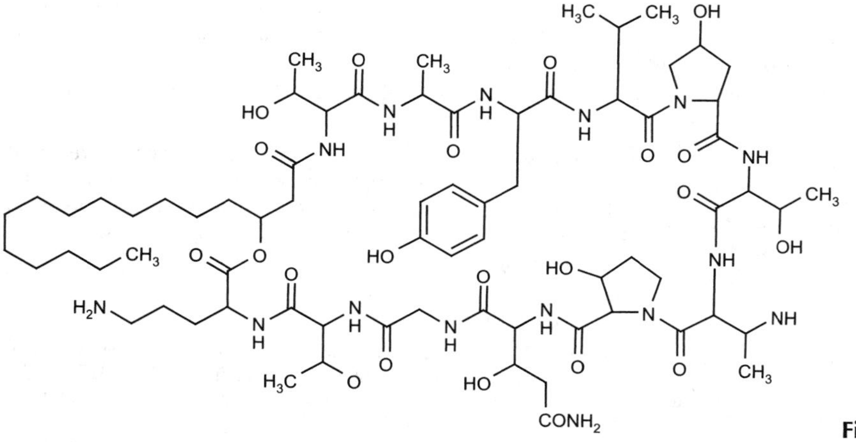

Figure 66 FR-901169

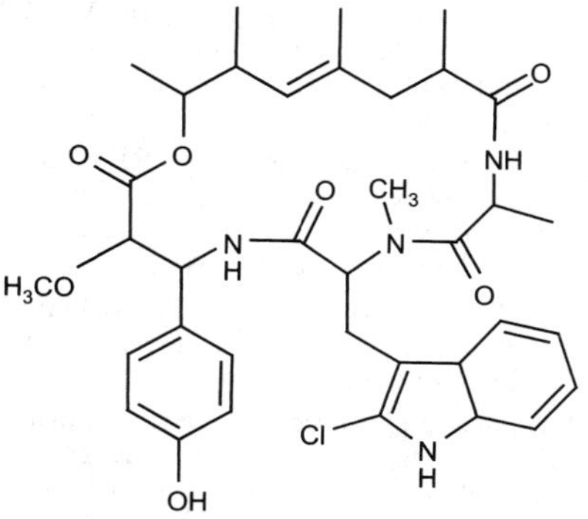

Chondramides

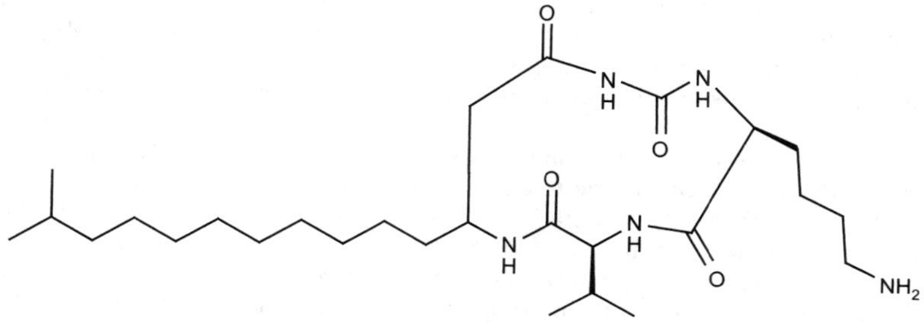

Compound Mercian Corp.

Figure 67 Peptide derivatives

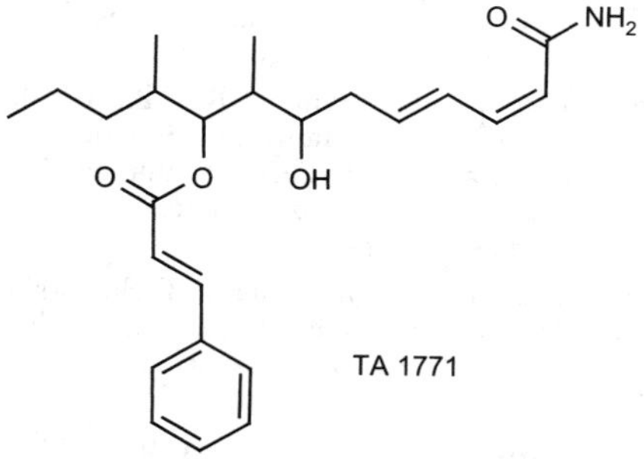

TA 1771

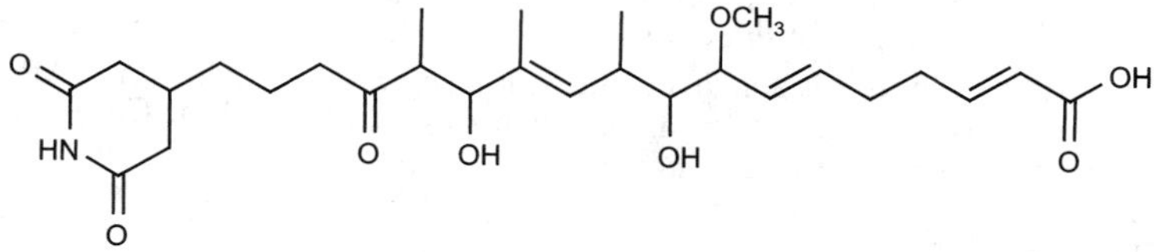

Dorrigocin A

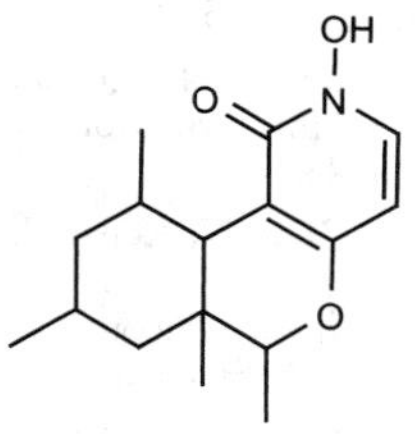

PF 1140

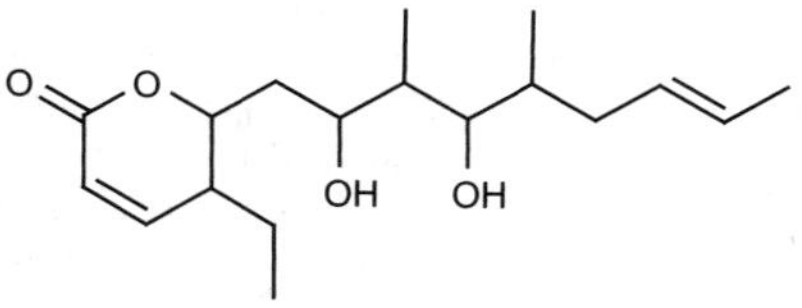

NK 10958 P

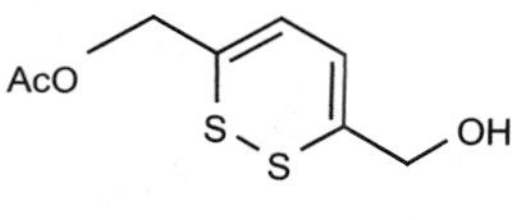

Dithricins

Figure 68 New antifungal agents

activity against *C. albicans*, *A. fumigatus*, and *A. niger* (MIC, 25 μg/ml). They appear to be inactive against the other fungi.

NK-10958P is a pyranone of natural origin with moderate activity against *C. albicans*, *C. neoformans*, and *A. fumigatus*.

PF-1140 is a product of natural origin that exerts moderate in vitro activity against *Candida* spp. (MIC, 12.5 μg/ml) and *A. fumigatus* (MIC, 12.5 μg/ml).

The melithiazols (Fig. 69) are active against *C. albicans* (MIC, 0.06 μg/ml). The dithiine derivatives cover a broad antifungal spectrum, with good activity against *C. albicans* (MIC, 0.6 to 1.25 μg/ml), *C. neoformans* (MIC, 0.31 μg/ml), and *A. fumigatus* (MIC, 0.31 μg/ml).

4. OTHER POTENTIAL SITES

Other potential sites of action of antifungal agents are under evaluation.

Myristoyl-CoA protein *N*-myristoyltransferase is a well-characterized target. Selective inhibitors of the enzyme of *C. neoformans* might be identified, as distinct from that of *C. albicans*, the former differing from the enzymes of mammalian cells.

β-1,6-Glucan might be an interesting target. A number of defective mutants of this polysaccharide have been manufactured.

Another interesting target might be cytoplasmic membrane ATPase. It is not specific to fungal cells but acts differently from that of mammalian cells, as has been demonstrated with omeprazole and ouabain.

Other studies have suggested the use of the "centrosome" as a target, which differs from that of mammalian cells, and transcription at the level of fungal mRNA.

5. RESISTANCE MECHANISMS

The majority of molecules penetrate the fungal wall readily, the first obstacle being the cytoplasmic membrane, where the molecules must use permeases to penetrate the cytoplasm. Some have been modified to active molecules (e.g., flucytosine). Resistance to antifungal agents is of several types:

- Modifications of membrane permeases. This mechanism is involved in resistance to flucytosine.
- Efflux. The mechanism is similar to the multidrug resistance mechanism of the other mammalian eukaryotic cells and has been described to occur in *C. albicans* for fluconazole.
- Modifications of activases, the enzymes allowing the transformation of flucytosine to 5-fluorouracil
- Modifications of the target, either by mutation at the enzyme or by an increase in the quantity of enzyme. This is a mechanism of resistance to azoles through the absence of inhibition of lanosterol 14α-methylase.

OCH_3 O N N S H_3CO OCH_3 S

Figure 69 Melithiazol

- Enzymes that degrade antifungal agents. Such systems might exist but have not been demonstrated for antifungal agents.
- Resistance to lipopeptides (β-1,3-D-glucan synthetase inhibitors)

It has been shown experimentally that lipopeptide-resistant strains of *C. albicans* might be obtained by reduction of the inhibitory activity of β-1,3-D-glucan synthetase. This is an extremely rare event, however, as the genome of *C. albicans* is diploid (frequency, $\sim 10^8$).

REFERENCES

Andes D, Marchillo K, Lowther J, Bryskier A, Stamstad T, Conklin R, 2003, In vivo pharmacodynamics of HMR 3270, a glucan synthase inhibitor, in a murine candidiasis model, Antimicrob Agents Chemother, 47, 1187–1192.

Castellano S, La Colla P, Musiu C, Stefancich G, 2000, Azole antifungal agents related to naftifine and butenafine, Arch Pharm (Weinheim), 333, 162-166.

Courtney R, Pai S, Laughlin M, Lim J, Batra V, 2003, Pharmacokinetics, safety, and tolerability of oral posaconazole administered in single and multiple doses in healthy adults, Antimicrob Agents Chemother, 47, 2788–2795.

De Wit S, O'Doherty E, Edwards J, Yates R, Smith RP, Clumeck AN, 1998, Pharmacokinetics of two multiple-dosing regimens of D0870 in human immunodeficiency virus-positive patients, a phase I study, Antimicrob Agents Chemother, 42, 903–906.

Figgitt DP, Denyer SP, Dewick PM, Jackson DE, Williams P, 1989, Topoisomerase II, a potential target for novel antifungal agents, Biochem Biophys Res Commun, 160, 257–262.

Fujie A, Iwamoto T, Muramatsu H, Okudaira T, Sato I, Furuta T, Tsurumi Y, Hori Y, Hino M, Hashimoto S, Okuhara M, 2000, FR901469, a novel antifungal antibiotic from an unidentified fungus No. 11243. II. In vitro and in vivo activities, J Antibiot (Tokyo), 53, 920–927.

Gerth K, Washausen P, Hofle G, Irschik H, Reichenbach H, 1996, The jerangolids, a family of new antifungal compounds from Sorangium cellulosum (Myxobacteria): production, physico-chemical and biological properties of jerangolid A, J Antibiot (Tokyo), 49, 71–75.

Greenspan MD, Yudkovitz JB, Lo CY, Chen JS, Alberts AW, Hunt VM, Chang MN, Yang SS, Thompson KL, Chiang YC, et al, 1987, Inhibition of hydroxymethylglutaryl-coenzyme A synthase by L-659,699, Proc Natl Acad Sci USA, 84, 7488–7492.

Groll AH, Mickiene D, Petraitis V, Petraitiene R, Alfaro RM, King C, Piscitelli SC, Walsh TJ, 2003, Comparative drug disposition, urinary pharmacokinetics, and renal effects of multilamellar liposomal nystatin and amphotericin B deoxycholate in rabbits, Antimicrob Agents Chemother, 47, 3917–3925.

Grzybowska J, Sowinski P, Gumieniak J, Zieniawa T, Borowski E, 1997, N-methyl-N-D-fructopyranosylamphotericin B methyl ester, new amphotericin B derivative of low toxicity, J Antibiot (Tokyo), 50, 709–711.

Hawser S, Borganovi M, Markus A, Isert D, 1999, Mulundocandin, an echinocandin-like lipopeptide antifungal agent: biological activities in vitro, J Antibiot, 52, 305–310.

Hawser S, Islam K, 1999, Comparison of the effect on fungicidal and fungistatic agents on the morphogenetic transformation of Candida albicans, J Antimicrob Chemother, 43, 411–413.

Hiemenz J, Cagnoni P, Simpson D, Devine S, Chao N, Keirns J, Lau W, Facklam D, Buell D, 2005, Pharmacokinetic and maximum tolerated dose study of micafungin in combination with fluconazole versus fluconazole alone for prophylaxis of fungal infections in adult patients undergoing a bone marrow or peripheral stem cell transplant, Antimicrob Agents Chemother, 49, 1331–1336.

Igarashi M, Kinoshita N, Ikeda T, Nakagawa E, Hamada M, Takeuchi T, 1997, Formamicin, a novel antifungal antibiotic produced by a strain of Saccharothrix sp. I. Taxonomy, production, isolation and biological properties, J Antibiot (Tokyo), 50, 926–931.

Ikeda F, Wakai Y, Matsumoto S, Maki K, Watabe E, Tawara S, Goto T, Watanabe Y, Matsumoto F, Kuwahara S, 2000, Efficacy of FK463, a new lipopeptide antifungal agent, in mouse models of disseminated candidiasis and aspergillosis, Antimicrob Agents Chemother, 44, 614–618.

Ivanova V, Schlegel R, Dornberger K, 1998, N′-methylniphimycin, a novel minor congener of niphimycin from Streptomyces sp. 57-13, J Basic Microbiol, 38, 415–419.

Kamigiri K, Tokunaga T, Sugawara T, Nagai K, Shibazaki M, Setiawan B, Rantiatmodjo RM, Morioka M, Suzuki K, 1997, YM-32890 A and B, new types of macrolide antibiotics produced by Cytophaga sp., J Antibiot (Tokyo), 50, 556–561.

Kohno J, Nishio M, Kawano K, Suzuki S, Komatsubara S, 1995, TMC-34, a new macrolide antifungal antibiotic, J Antibiot (Tokyo), 48, 1173–1175.

Krieter P, Flannery B, Musick T, Gohdes M, Martinho M, Courtney R, 2004, Disposition of posaconazole following single-dose oral administration in healthy subjects, Antimicrob Agents Chemother, 48, 3543–3551.

Kunze B, Jansen R, Sasse F, Hofle G, Reichenbach H, 1995, Chondramides A–D, new antifungal and cytostatic depsipeptides from Chondromyces crocatus (myxobacteria): production, physico-chemical and biological properties, J Antibiot (Tokyo), 48, 1262–1266.

Lucas BD Jr, Purdy CY, Scarim SK, Benjamin S, Abel SR, Hilleman DE, 1995, Terfenadine pharmacokinetics in breast milk in lactating women, Clin Pharmacol Ther, 57, 398–402.

Matsunaga T, Harada T, Hirata Z, Mitsui T, Murano H, Shibutani Y, 2000, D0870, an antifungal agent, induces reverse use-dependent QT prolongation in dogs, J Vet Med Sci, 62, 491–497.

Mehta RT, Hopfer RL, Gunner LA, Juliano RL, Lopez-Berestein G, 1987, Formulation, toxicity, and antifungal activity in vitro of liposome-encapsulated nystatin as therapeutic agent for systemic candidiasis, Antimicrob Agents Chemother, 31, 1897–1900.

Nakai T, Uno J, Otomo K, Ikeda F, Tawara S, Goto T, Nishimura K, Miyaji M, 2002, In vitro activity of FK463, a novel lipopeptide antifungal agent, against a variety of clinically important molds, Chemotherapy, 48, 78–81.

Nakai T, Uno J, Ikeda F, Tawara S, Nishimura K, Miyaji M, 2003, In vitro antifungal activity of Micafungin (FK463) against dimorphic fungi: comparison of yeast-like and mycelial forms, Antimicrob Agents Chemother, 47, 1376–1381.

Ng AW, Wasan KM, Lopez-Berestein G, 2005, Liposomal polyene antibiotics, Methods Enzymol, 391, 304–313.

Oreskovic K, Bischoff A, Schroedter A, Pavicic-Stedul H, Avdagic A, Dumic M, Kralj T, Schoenfeld W, Knoeller J, 2001, PLD-118: tolerability, safety, and pharmacokinetics following single oral dose in healthy volunteers, 41st Intersci Conf Antimicrob Agents Chemother.

Ortoneda M, Capilla J, Pastor FJ, Pujol I, Yustes C, Serena C, Guarro J, 2004, In vitro interactions of approved and novel drugs against Paecilomyces spp., Antimicrob Agents Chemother, 48, 2727–2729.

Pfaller MA, Marco F, Messer SA, Jones RN, 1998, In vitro activity of two echinocandin derivatives, LY303366 and MK-0991 (L-743,792), against clinical isolates of Aspergillus, Fusarium, Rhizopus, and other filamentous fungi, Diagn Microbiol Infect Dis, 30, 251–255.

Pfaller MA, Messer S, Jones RN, 1997, Activity of a new triazole, Sch 56592, compared with those of four other antifungal agents tested against clinical isolates of Candida spp. and Saccharomyces cerevisiae, Antimicrob Agents Chemother, 41, 233–235.

Pfaller, MA, Messer SA, Coffman S, 1997, In vitro susceptibilities of clinical yeast isolates to a new echinocandin derivative, LY303366, and other antifungal agents, Antimicrob Agents Chemother, 41, 763–766.

Roy K, Mukhopadhyay T, Reddy GC, Desikan KR, Ganguli BN, 1987, Mulundocandin, a new lipopeptide antibiotic. I. Taxonomy, fermentation, isolation and characterization. J Antibiot, 40, 275–280.

Saint-Julien L, Joly V, Seman M, Carbon C, Yeni P, 1992, Activity of MS-8209, a nonester amphotericin B derivative, in treatment of experimental systemic mycoses, Antimicrob Agents Chemother, 36, 2722–2728.

Sasse F, Bohlendorf B, Herrmann M, Kunze B, Forche E, Steinmetz H, Hofle G, Reichenbach H, 1999, Melithiazols, new beta-methoxyacrylate inhibitors of the respiratory chain isolated from myxobacteria: production, isolation, physico-chemical and biological properties, J Antibiot (Tokyo), 52, 721–729.

Serena C, Ortoneda M, Capilla J, Pastor FJ, Sutton DA, Rinaldi MG, Guarro J, 2003, In vitro activities of new antifungal agents against Chaetomium spp. and inoculum standardization, Antimicrob Agents Chemother, 47, 3161–3164.

Serena C, Pastor FJ, Ortoneda M, Capilla J, Nolard N, Guarro J, 2004, In vitro antifungal susceptibilities of uncommon basidiomycetous yeasts, Antimicrob Agents Chemother, 48, 2724–2726.

Shen LL, Baranowski J, Fostel J, Montgomery DA, Lartey PA, 1992, DNA topoisomerases from pathogenic fungi, targets for the discovery of antifungal drugs, Antimicrob Agents Chemother, 36, 2778–2784.

Shibazaki M, Sugawara T, Nagai K, Shimizu Y, Yamaguchi H, Suzuki K, 1996, YM-47522, a novel antifungal antibiotic produced by Bacillus sp. I. Taxonomy, fermentation, isolation and biological properties, J Antibiot (Tokyo), 49, 340–344.

Tawara S, Ikeda F, Maki K, Morishita Y, Otomo K, Teratani N, Goto T, Tomishima M, Ohki H, Yamada A, Kawabata K, Takasugi H, Sakane K, Tanaka H, Matsumoto F, Kuwahara S, 2000, In vitro activities of a new lipopeptide antifungal agent, FK463, against a variety of clinically important fungi, Antimicrob Agents Chemother, 44, 57–62.

Ueki M, Kusumoto A, Hanafi M, Shibata K, Tanaka T, Taniguchi M, 1997, UK-3A, a novel antifungal antibiotic from Streptomyces sp. 517-02, fermentation, isolation, structural elucidation and biological properties, J Antibiot (Tokyo), 50, 551–555.

Urbina JM, Cortes JC, Palma A, Lopez SN, Zacchino SA, Enriz RD, Ribas JC, Kouznetzov VV, 2000, Inhibitors of the fungal cell wall: synthesis of 4-aryl-4-N-arylamine-1-butenes and related compounds with inhibitory activities on beta(1-3) glucan and chitin synthases, Bioorg Med Chem, 8, 691–698.

Warn PA, Morrissey G, Morrissey J, Denning DW, 2003, Activity of micafungin (FK463) against an itraconazole-resistant strain of Aspergillus fumigatus and a strain of Aspergillus terreus demonstrating in vivo resistance to amphotericin B, J Antimicrob Chemother, 51, 913–919.

Yamada H, Tsuda T, Watanabe T, Ohashi M, Murakami K, Mochizuki H, 1993, In vitro and in vivo antifungal activities of D0870, a new triazole agent, Antimicrob Agents Chemother, 37, 2412–2417.

Zeng J, Kamei K, Zheng Y, Nishimura K, 2004, Susceptibility of Pseudallescheria boydii and Scedosporium apiospermum to new antifungal agents, Nippon Ishinkin Gakkai Zasshi, 45, 101–104.

Drug Interactions during Anti-Infective Treatments

O. PETITJEAN, P. NICOLAS, M. TOD, C. PADOIN, AND A. JACOLOT

54

1. MECHANISTIC AND METHODOLOGICAL APPROACH

Adverse drug events associated with drug-drug interactions are a well-known cause of hospital admissions. However, a large number of drug interactions could be prevented if physicians and pharmacists were trained to have a better knowledge of and to make a better evaluation of the risks associated with multidrug prescriptions. To this end, we propose a step-by-step mechanistic approach to pharmacokinetic interactions with anti-infectives, among the most commonly prescribed drugs worldwide.

It should be recalled first of all that in the last two decades this topic has been tackled either as a general review or as a focus on a single compound or antibiotic family, such as rifampin, macrolides, antifungal azoles, and fluoroquinolones. In addition, publications concerning the specific targets that subtend these interactions should also be considered: P-glycoprotein (P-gp), cytochrome P450 (CYP450) enzymes, and renal transport and metabolism.

2. INTERACTION AND DRUG ABSORPTION

The general process which an orally administered drug must undergo on its passage from the gut lumen to the systemic circulation involves two organs mounted in series: the intestine, followed by the liver. The effective oral bioavailability (F_{oral}) can thus be viewed as the product of successive events: the dissolution of the pharmaceutical form and the solubilization of the active molecule in the intestinal fluid, which determines the fraction of the dose ready to be absorbed (F_{abs}); the permeation of the molecule through the enterocyte membrane, which regulates exposure to drug-metabolizing intestinal enzymes and to absorption proteins (F_{gut}); and the fraction of the dose entering the liver via the portal route that will be lost due to hepatic first-pass metabolism and/or biliary excretion (F_{hep}). This can be described by the following equation: F_{oral} (%) $= F_{abs} \times F_{gut} \times F_{hep}$. Drug interactions can be observed at each of these steps.

2.1. Drug Interactions and F_{abs}: Solubilization of the Active Ingredient

2.1.1. Alkalinization of the Digestive Medium

The solubilization of antifungal azoles (with the exception of fluconazole), indinavir, delavirdine, or even dapsone requires an acidic pH, so acid suppressants (such as omeprazole and cimetidine) greatly reduce their bioavailability. This situation can also occur with the concomitant administration of dideoxyinosine due to the presence of a strong alkaline buffer in its pharmaceutical formulation. In the same way, it should be remembered that patients with AIDS have an almost neutral gastric pH which requires the administration of azoles with a glass of either 0.1 N HCl or a long drink of an acidic beverage such as Coca-Cola. In addition, gastric hypoacidity might be a consequence of *Helicobacter pylori* infection and thus be improved by eradication treatment.

Alkalinization of the digestive content can also significantly reduce the absorption (30 to 50% less) of some β-lactam esters with much greater solubility at pH 1 to 2, such as bacampicillin, cefuroxime axetil, and cefpodoxime proxetil. Cefotiam hexetil and cefetamet pivoxil are two major exceptions to this rule. This interaction does not appear to occur with nonesterified β-lactams.

The bioavailability of macrolides that are chemically stable at acidic pH, such as clarithromycin and azithromycin, is not significantly affected by the physiological pH gradient, unlike erythromycin free base, for which enteric-coated formulations are required for effective use in humans.

Regarding the fluoroquinolones (FQ), even with a highly variable solubility between pH 2 and 6, the bioavailability of this family is not affected by the alkalinization of the digestive contents (see Table 1).

For isoniazid, concomitant administration of aluminum antacids might delay and reduce the oral absorption.

Last, let us acknowledge the commonly admitted fact that the elderly are at risk for neutral gastric pH: studies of gastric secretion or of hydrogen ion secretion indicate a progressive fall in basal and stimulated secretion with advancing age.

2.1.2. Formation of Metal Chelates

Di- or trivalent cations (iron, zinc, aluminum, magnesium, and calcium) lead to the formation of insoluble or weakly soluble chelates with FQ (see Table 1), tetracyclines, rifampin, and ethambutol. On average, the loss of bioavailability is around 40%, but it can reach up to 90%. As a result, the use of mucosa-protective drugs such as Maalox is contraindicated and should be replaced by antisecretory drugs such as H_2-receptor antagonists or proton pump inhibitors. The use of bismuth salts does not affect the efficacy of tetracyclines, but care should be taken since Veegum, an excipient found in a commercially available liquid formulation with bismuth subsalicylate, adsorbs tetracycline and reduces its area under the concentration-time curve (AUC) by 25%. Similarly, the impairment of mycophenolate mofetil absorption by concomitant use of iron ion preparations has been described, a result that should be known since this immunosuppressive agent is administered to patients often treated with iron for anemia.

With some compounds of the above families which undergo enterohepatic recycling (biliary excretion with rifampin or transintestinal secretion with doxycycline or ciprofloxacin), the cycling can be partially interrupted, leading to a shorter elimination half-life, even after intravenous administration. Such situations have been described with the following drugs: doxycycline, ciprofloxacin, fleroxacin, sparfloxacin, temafloxacin, and ofloxacin.

With the exception of cefdinir, metal cations do not modify the oral absorption of β-lactams. The only reference found in the literature shows a 17% decrease in bioavailability of cefaclor AF when coadministered with Maalox, suggesting that divalent cations could interact with the Pep-T, H^+-coupled peptide transporters.

Finally, adsorption phenomena have already been described with cholestyramine, an anion exchange resin that can interact with sulfamethoxazole, certain oral β-lactams, vancomycin, and certain tetracyclines. Caution should also be exercised with the coprescription of activated charcoal. Last, kaolin-pectin mixture dramatically reduces oral lincomycin absorption, and the combination of guar gum with pectin usually reduces the rate of drug absorption.

2.1.3. Which Antacid Should Be Used?

When the drug interaction can be clearly explained by an elevation in gastric pH, as with ketoconazole and itraconazole and also with some β-lactam esters (see section 2.1.2), the concomitant use of antacids should be firmly discouraged.

On the other hand, when the interaction results from the formation of metal chelates (see section 2.1.1), antisecretory agents can be used. The choice should lie between proton pump inhibitors, such as lansoprazole, omeprazole, and dimethicone, but only if not associated with aluminum or magnesium, and H_2-receptor antagonists (see Table 1). Care should be exercised specifically with H_2-receptor antagonists because cimetidine is an inhibitor of hepatic CYP enzymes metabolizing fleroxacin, pefloxacin, and temafloxacin. Consequently, coprescription of cimetidine with one of these fluoroquinolones will produce a 20 to 40% increase in the AUC of the antibiotic. In the same way, it should be recalled that lansoprazole and omeprazole are inhibitors of CYP2C19 (see Table 3).

2.2. Drug Interactions and F_{gut}: Crossing the Intestinal Barrier

Although absorption is the main function of the intestinal mucosa, its metabolic capacity is now well recognized, so dual mechanical and metabolic barriers can be postulated, both of which are subject to drug interactions.

2.2.1. Mechanical Barrier

Xenobiotics cross the mechanical barrier in either of two ways, the transcellular or the paracellular pathway (Table 1). The transcellular pathway involves passage by simple diffusion or by means of transporters that are specific and saturable to a greater or lesser extent. The fact that these transporters are saturable explains the nonlinearity of the pharmacokinetics of a number of β-lactams. Transporters are localized essentially in the duodenum and jejunum, which explains for example why the SR forms of ciprofloxacin (Ciflox XR), cefaclor (Cefaclor-AF), and amoxicillin-clavulanic acid (Augmentin, Duamentin) are clinically not genuine SR forms; in fact, the dissolution of these active substances beyond the jejunum is accompanied by a substantial loss of bioavailability due to a lack of available transporters.

Alternatively, xenobiotics cross the mechanical barrier by the paracellular pathway, with a regulation that is itself possibly dependent on the intracellular concentrations produced, since high intracellular concentrations might in fact reduce the extent of access by this route.

The drug interactions described to date relate to the transporters: competition between substrates, or induction or inhibition of these transport systems. The latter are of two types, absorption promoters and efflux promoters. They are all saturable and specific to a greater or lesser extent and have a precise distribution (localization and content).

Among protein carriers promoting drug absorption is the oligopeptide transporter (Pep-T1), which transports all drugs with a structure related to di- and tripeptides such as β-lactam antibiotics, ACE inhibitors, some FQ, or L-valine esters of acyclovir or zidovudine (AZT). Pep-T1 belongs to the proton oligopeptide transporter superfamily.

The basolateral peptide transporter (BLPT) has also been described, which cooperates with Pep-T1 in the efficient transepithelial transfer of small peptides and various peptide-like drugs structurally related to small peptides (di- or tripeptides).

Besides Pep-T1, four major families of organic ion transporters have been identified which actively pump drugs into cells: organic anion transporters (OAT), organic anion transport proteins (OATP), organic cation transporters (OCT), and organic cation/carnitine transporters (OCTN/OCTP). OATP seems to be the most widely studied of all influx proteins; it is a family of transmembrane sodium and ATP-independent transporters with a wide tissue distribution. Fexofenadine is currently considered an OATP probe substrate (as well as a P-gp probe).

Lastly, a monocarboxylic acid transport system (MCT) at the blood-brain barrier (BBB) has been described, but it seems in fact to be an ubiquitously expressed transport family implicated in both the influx and efflux of acidic drugs.

Everything points to the fact that these transporters may be the subject of genetic polymorphism, as has already been described for P-gp.

Efflux promoters, of whatever kind, are designed if not to prevent, at least to limit the penetration of xenobiotics (and to facilitate their excretion), which explains their strategic localization: at the intestinal, ear, nose, and throat, bronchopulmonary, or BBB level or fetoplacentally, to prevent the influx of molecules, and in the bile canaliculi or renal tubules, to facilitate elimination.

P-gp is the most studied of the membrane efflux proteins. P-gp is a member of the ATP-binding cassette superfamily of transport proteins that utilize ATP to translocate a wide range of substrates across biological membranes, pumping drugs out of the cell into apical or basolateral extracellular fluids. P-gp is encoded by a family of genes referred to as multidrug resistance (MDR) genes.

In the case of underexpression of duodenal P-gp, which is the case with subjects homozygous for the 3435 C/T gene, the bioavailability of the substrates of this transporter is increased, as is observed in the case of coprescription of a P-gp inhibitor. This has been demonstrated for digoxin, fexofenadine, and two antiretrovirals, efavirenz and nelfinavir.

Table 1 Extent of decrease in fluoroquinolone C_{max} and AUC when coprescribed with a gastroprotective drug[a]

FQ	Maalox		Sucralfate and $Al(OH)_3$		Ferrous sulfate		Zinc		Calcium carbonate/ calcium supplements		Dairy products [yogurt]		Anti-H_2 and omeprazole		Others		Calcium-fortified orange juice	
	C_{max}	AUC	C_{max}	AUC	C_{max}	AUC	C_{max}	AUC	C_{max}	AUC	C_{max}	AUC	C_{max}	AUC	C_{max}	AUC	C_{max}	AUC
Amifloxacin	85	85																
Ciprofloxacin	80–95	85–96	72–95	84–96	33–77	48–64	37	24	38–47	41–42	36–[47]	33–[36]	0 [11]	±10–15 [13]	Pirenzepine 5	+8	40	40
Enoxacin	70	73	91	88					44–59	26–40							16	NS
Fleroxacin			25	23														
Gatifloxacin	56–69	46–63			49–54	29–35			6	10		15 (milk)	0					
Levofloxacin		56–78	65	44	45	19			23	3			0	0				
Lomefloxacin	46	41											+11 [0]	+4 [+9.5]	Benexate 0	0		
Moxifloxacin	40	45	71	60	59	39			15	3	15	6	+8	+3				
Norfloxacin	95	NP	90	98–99	75	73 55 (FU)		56 (FU)	66	63	51–[53]	48–[58]						
Ofloxacin	73	73			36	25			+3	+4	0–[18]	6–[8]			Pirenzepine 8	+10		
Pefloxacin	62	55											+8	+41	Dimethicone 11	2		
Rufloxacin	43	36																
Sparfloxacin	48	44																
Temafloxacin	59	61											+4	+22				

[a]Results are expressed as percentages of observed decrease. NS, not significant; NP, not published; FU, urinary elimination; +, an increased value.
C_{max} = peak plasma concentration
AUC = Area under the curve ± in the case of either an increased or a decreased value

In the enterocyte (and probably in the lung), the effect may be combined with that of CYPP450 (P-gp and CYP3A form a cooperative barrier against the absorption of xenobiotics). Thus, the drug is first exposed to P-gp which is expressed at the entrance to the epithelial cell, restricting its entry and thus delaying its access to the CYP. By a repeated cycle of cellular extrusion-reabsorption, drug metabolization is thus facilitated because of the lag in the saturation of the metabolic systems (repetitive recycling of drug between the intestinal lumen and CYP3A facilitates drug metabolism by preventing CYP enzymes from being overwhelmed by the high drug concentrations in the intestine). It will moreover be noted, without going as far as the idea of coexpression, that P-gp and CYP3A4 have a number of substrates in common (Table 2). Thus, evidence suggests two distinct regulatory mechanisms for the basal expression of P-gp and CYP3A4: the relatively low between-subject variability in intestinal P-gp compared to that of CYP3A, the lack of any intraindividual correlation between the two proteins, their opposite patterns of expression in humans, and their different behavior following an inductive process. For example, the response to an induction caused by St.John's wort will find a different quantitative expression, depending on the substrate concerned, as the activity of P-gp may in fact be more markedly increased than that of CYP3A4 or vice versa.

After administration of rifampin (600 mg/day for 10 days) in healthy volunteers, P-gp expression in enterocytes of duodenal biopsy samples is enhanced 3.5-fold according to Greiner et al. (1999).

Recently, the probenecid (-sensitive) transporter has been described, another efflux transporter at the BBB level involved in elimination of probenecid and a variety of other drugs, such as β-lactam compounds (penicillin, ampicillin, cefodizime, cefotaxime, and ceftriaxone), methotrexate, AZT, and dideoxyinosine. Furthermore, OATP, which is mainly an influx transporter, can work in the opposite direction at the BBB level.

Besides these efflux proteins, some other transmembrane efflux transporters have been described, such as the MRP (MDR protein) family, including cMOAT (MRP2), fatty acid binding protein (FABP) (Z-protein) ligandin (Y-protein), and MCT (see Fig. 1).

In these efflux systems, the interaction can occur by competition between substrates. Thus, moxifloxacin-digoxin coadministration induces a 33% increase in the maximum concentration in plasma (C_{max}) of digoxin without an effect on digoxin systemic clearance. The interaction can also occur directly by an increase in efficiency of the transporters following coprescription of an efflux protein inducer (this will cause a reduction in the bioavailability of the transported drug) or by reduction of the transport capacities in combination with an efflux protein inhibitor (Fig. 1).

These transporters therefore have a major role in drug metabolism and particularly here in the extent of the presystemic metabolism in its intestinal phase (intestinal first-pass effect). This mechanism explains why the same substance (e.g., dexamethasone) can be both a substrate of P-gp and an inhibitor by competition with another substrate and, independently of that, an inducer of P-gp (in the same way as any other inducer, whether or not a substrate of P-gp).

Lastly, just as metabolic autoinduction phenomena have been described with some drugs, resulting in a reduction in the elimination half-life of the inducer following repeated doses, so it has been shown that after repeated administration of rifampin, the oral bioavailability of this antituberculosis agent was reduced (without any change in its elimination half-life), in all likelihood following the induction of an efflux protein, probably P-gp (autoinduction of its own efflux from the enterocyte).

Quantitatively speaking, these interactions on enterocyte efflux proteins should not be underestimated. St. John's wort reduces the oral bioavailability of cyclosporine by 30 to 60% and has thus been the cause of a number of graft rejections. Rifampin, through a dual P-gp–CYP interaction, multiplies by 3.7 the oral clearance of cyclosporine and by induction of P-gp alone increases that of digoxin by a factor of 1.4 to 1.8, while at the same time the content of P-gp is multiplied 3.5-fold.

Dexamethasone, an inducer of both P-gp and CYP3A4, multiplies by 6 the first-pass effect of indinavir. Finally, cyclosporine increases the bioavailability of paclitaxel (Taxol) from 5 to 50% and that of docetaxel (Taxotere) from 8 to 88%. In mice, quinidine increases plasma and brain digoxin concentrations by 7%, an experimental result that could explain digoxin toxicity in clinical practice when administered with quinidine.

Table 2 Behavior of antiproteases vis-à-vis CYP3A4 and P-gp

Substrates of CYP3A4	Substrates of P-gp
Amprenavir	
Indinavir	Indinavir
Nelfinavir	Nelfinavir
Ritonavir	Ritonavir
Saquinavir	Saquinavir

2.2.1.1. Localization of Epithelial Cell Transporters

Each type of transporter often has several isoforms, the substrates of which are not always common to each, with tissue distributions that are often different and with variable directions of operation (adsorption/secretion).

- OAT, OATP: gastrointestinal (GI) tract, hepatobiliary tract, kidney, BBB
- MCT: BBB, etc. (expressed ubiquitously)
- OCT, OCTN/OCTP: GI tract, kidney
- H^+-coupled oligopeptide transporter (Pep-T1): GI tract, kidney, central nervous system (CNS) (?)
- P-gp: GI tract, liver, kidney, BBB, bronchi, nasal mucosa, placenta (this should entail the contraindication of the use of P-gp inhibitors and any other efflux protein in pregnant women to prevent any increase in exposure of the fetus to the drug substrates of these transporters)
- Testes, adrenal cortex, lymphocytes
- MRP: GI tract, liver, kidney, BBB, bronchi, heart, skeletal muscle, testes
- cMOAT (MRP2): hepatobiliary tract
- FABP (Z-protein): hepatobiliary tract (cytosolic protein).
- Ligandin (Y-protein): bile acid binding protein: hepatobiliary tract (cytosolic protein).
- OATP efflux: BBB
- MCT efflux: BBB
- Probenecid (-sensitive) transporter: BBB

Note that CYP3A4 enzyme activities as well as Pep-T1 abundance decrease gradually in a proximal to distal direction in humans (but not in rats); P-gp distribution follows the opposite pattern.

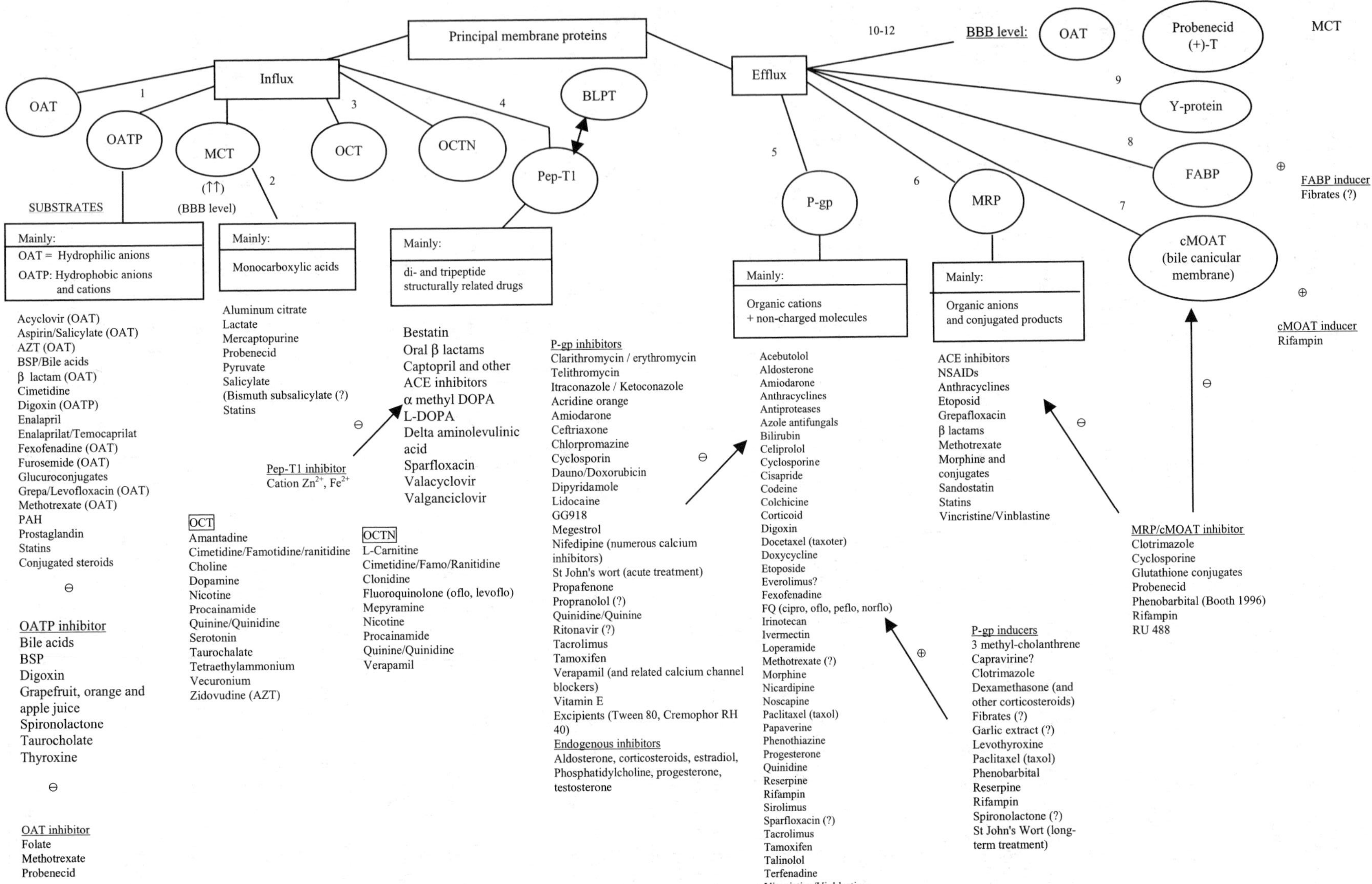

Figure 1 **Epithelial cell transporters and their main substrates, inhibitors, and inducers. *, substrates = conjugated (e.g., BSP conjugates) and unconjugated anions; cMOAT is MRP2.**

2.2.1.2. Direction of Operation of Transporters

Although it is customary to talk of absorption transporters and secretion (or efflux) transporters, it has now been clearly shown both in vitro and in vivo that these transporters, or at least some of them (P-gp and OATP), might operate in both directions.

2.2.1.3. Interindividual Variability

In intestinal biopsy samples from patients and healthy volunteers, the expression of P-gp varied 1.5- to 8-fold, with a median of 4.5-fold in men and 8-fold in women according to Schuetz et al. (1995).

The magnitude of interindividual variability in intestinal P-gp expression seems to be a lot lower than intradonor variations in CYP3A4 (>10- to 20-fold).

2.2.1.4. Sex Differences

Men have twofold-higher P-gp levels than women.

2.2.1.5. Intraindividual Variability in Intestinal P-gp Expression

Over a period of 120 days, according to Masuda et al. (2000), there was a fourfold variation in MDR1 mRNA expression level and a twofold variation in trough concentration of tacrolimus in a young patient after a small bowel transplant.

2.2.2. Metabolic Barrier

Any metabolizable drug that penetrates the enterocyte and gains access to its cytosol will be metabolized by enterocytic CYP, a new stage which may be the subject of an interaction either by competition between substrates or by modification of the metabolic capacities of the enterocyte following coprescription of an enzyme inducer or inhibitor (Table 3). The purpose is very probably to detoxify the xenobiotic agent that has been absorbed by making it more polar, thereby facilitating its elimination. Moreover, it should be remembered that oxidation by CYP and binding to liver microsomes correlate well with drug hydrophobicity.

Thus, most drugs undergo metabolic transformations in the body and are eliminated in the form of metabolites, including conjugates. A few drugs are not metabolized and are excreted unchanged. Typically, these are strongly polar compounds, e.g., strong acids (methotrexate) or bases (aminoglycocides and vancomycin).

For the same reasons, as the lungs are continually exposed to airborne environmental chemicals and to xenobiotics that enter the body through other portals, xenobiotic-metabolizing enzymes are well distributed within this organ. The main CYPs expressed in human lung are CYP1A1, -2A6, -2C9, -2E1, and -3A4. Pulmonary CYPs are induced by cigarette smoke, a means of eliminating more actively chemicals contained in the smoke.

It will be noted that all of the metabolic pathways identified in humans are the subject of genetic polymorphism, a phenomenon which contributes considerably to interindividual variability.

2.3. Crossing the Hepatocytic Barrier

The fraction of unchanged drug that leaves the enterocyte reaches the liver via the portal vein, when a new stage of metabolism is possible; only the enzyme concentration and possibly the nature of the isoforms changes. The interaction processes remain the same. This stage, which helps reduce the bioavailability of the drugs exposed to it, is known as a first-pass effect. In general, these are saturable processes and hence often dependent on the administered dose; thus, the bioavailability of propranolol is one-third lower when it is given in four doses rather than in two. For the same reasons, prolonged-release forms might tend to undergo this first-pass effect more than immediate forms. However, this reasoning ignores two major facts. First, CYP3A4 protein levels and catalytic activity are generally highest in proximal small intestine: if the tested drug is a substrate of this isoform, any modified-release formulation (extended release, sustained or slow release, etc.) will lead to a decreased intestinal metabolism. Table 4 shows substrate of CYPs. Second, P-gp expression progressively increases from proximal to distal regions of the gut, so modified-release formulations of a P-gp substrate will lead to a greater loss of bioavailability. Actually, one should consider the net result of three events (rather proximal intestinal metabolism, rather distal enterocytic extrusion, and reduced risk for saturating the presystemic liver metabolism), an assessment very difficult to draw, as well as the determination of the different risks for drug interactions at each of these three levels.

In the same way, it can be understood that interactions by competition between substrates will be more apparent if the dosage conditions (dose and dosage form) promote the saturation or prolong the presence of the inhibitor.

It may be important to note that a sodium diet appears to modulate the expression of CYP3A4 and/or intestinal P-gp, which is illustrated by the weaker bioavailability of quinidine administered with a high-salt diet (30 to 40% lower with 400 mEq of NaCl per day than with 10 mEq/day).

3. INTERACTIONS RELATING TO THE DISTRIBUTION PHASE

Interactions relating to the distribution phase may be observed at three levels:

- They may involve competitive displacement of a drug from its binding to a circulating protein; to attain clinical significance, the percent binding must then be high (>80%) and the volume of distribution of the displaced drug must be relatively low (≤0.3 to 0.5 liter/kg); in other words, the bulk of the product must not already be outside the vascular compartment.
- Modulation of active passage towards a given tissue may be involved.
- The interaction may relate to specific receptors (interactions with bacterial target proteins are not discussed here).

As regards the first point, although there are a number of antibiotics that are strongly bound to circulating proteins (isoxazolyl-penicillins, ceftriaxone, doxycycline, rifampin, teicoplanin, azole antifungals, and fusidic acid), with the exception of the sulfonamides, none is liable at present to cause or undergo an interaction of this type. The lack of interaction with circulating proteins, including antibiotics that are more than 99% bound (itraconazole is 99.8% bound to plasma albumin), shows that the binding generated is weak affinity binding. The only sulfonamide currently marketed in France, sulfamethoxazole, which is 65% bound, has only a modest effect in this area; the interactions it undergoes may be explained by an enzyme inhibitory effect. Through this mechanism, it increases the activity of warfarin, phenytoin, tolbutamide, and loperamide.

With respect to tissue penetration, seven examples may be documented.

Table 3 Distribution of substrates, enzyme inducers, and enzyme inhibitors according to the different CYPs

Parameter	CYP family						
	1	2					3
Subfamily	1A	2A	2B	2C	2D	2E	3A
Isoform(s)	1A2, 1A1 (extrahepatic)	2A6	2B6	2C8, 2C9, 2C19	2D6	2E1	3A3–3A5 (principally 3A4)
% of total hepatic CYP content (28% unidentified)	8–15%	4.0 5–12	0.09–24 1–5 0.2	10 (2C8) 15–20 (2C9) <5 (2C19)	1.5–2	6–11	30–40
Total intestinal CYP content	Very low level	0	0		40 times lower than in the whole liver	0	10–50% lower than in the liver
% of all drugs metabolized by CYPS	2 11	<0.1 3	<1 3	16 16 (2C8, 2C9) 8 (2C19)	25 19	2 4	55 36
Interindividual variability of CYP expression							10- to 100-fold in the liver (up to 30-fold in the small intestine)
Existence of polymorphism	Yes	Yes	Yes	Yes	Yes	Yes	Yes
Enzyme inducers	Altitude Bilirubin Caffeine Dioxin GH 3-Methylcholanthrene Omeprazole (in poor metabolizers) 3-Methylindole (cruciferous vegetables) Nelfinavir (?) (β-Naphthoflavone Polycyclic aromatic hydrocarbon Tobacco smoke Charcoal-broiled beef Smoked meat Pan-fried meat Polyhalogenated biphenyls	Rifampin	Efavirenz Nevirapine Phenobarbital? Pesticides?	Artemisinin (2C19) Carbamazepine (2C9) Dapsone and related compounds (in vitro) Nelfinavir Phenobarbital (2C9) Phenytoin (2C9) Rifampin (2C9, 2C19) Ritonavir Spironolactone (?)	Pregnancy	Dexamethasone Aspirin Cigarette smoke Ethanol (chronic consumption)[a] Isopropanol Isopentanol Fibrate Isoniazid Myristicin Nelfinavir (?) Organic solvent (acetone, benzene, ether, sulfide and nitrogen-containing heterocycles, trichloroethylene, toluene, xylene) Pyrazole Ritonavir St. John's wort (long-term treatment) Diabetes High-fat diet Obesity	Amprenavir Capravirine Carbamazepine (but not oxcarbazepine) Clotrimazole Dexamethasone (and related compounds) Efavirenz Ethanol? Ethosuximide Lovastatin Nevirapine Omeprazole?/ lansoprazole? Phenobarbital (barbiturates) Phenylbutazone Phenytoin Pioglitazone Pleconaril Primidone Pyrazinamide (?) Reserpine Rifabutin Rifampin

	Rifampin Ritonavir					Starvation (in rats)	Sex steroids Simvastatin Spironolactone St. John's wort Sulfinpyrazone TM 125 Troglitazone
Enzyme inhibitors	Cimetidine Ellipticine Ethanol (chronic consumption) FQ Fluvoxamine Furafylline Interleukin 2 Alpha and beta interferon Isosafrole Grapefruit juice (±) 8-Methoxypsoralene α-Naphthoflavone	Clotrimazole Grapefruit juice 8-Methoxypsoralene Miconazole Sulfamethoxazole (in vitro) Sulfadiazine (in vitro)	Orphenadrine	Amiodarone (2C9) Antiproteases (2C9, 2C19) Atovaquone (2C9) Carbamazepine (2C19) Cimetidine (weak) (2C19?) Chloramphenicol Cranberry juice Delavirdine (2C9 and 2C19) Diazepam (2C19?) Efavirenz (2C19) Fluconazole (2C9 and 2C19) Fluoxetine (2C19) Fluvoxamine (2C19) Garlic extract (2C9, 2C19?) GH (2C19) Imipramine (2C19?) Isoniazid (2C19) Ketoconazole, itraconazole, voriconazole (weak) S-Mephenytoin (2C19) Miconazole (2C9) (-naphthoflavone (2C8, 2C9) Omeprazole (2C19) Phenylbutazone (2C9) Spironolactone Sulfamethoxazole (2C9) Sulfaphenazole (2C9) Sulfinpyrazone (2C9) Tolbutamide (2C9)	Amiodarone Antiproteases Chlorpheniramine Cimetidine Encainide/Flecainide Fluoxetine Fluvoxamine Haloperidol HMG-CoA[b] reductase inhibitors Ketoconazole Moclobemide Nefazodone Orphenadrine Paroxetine Phenothiazines Quinidine Ritonavir Sertraline Somatostatin Terbinafine Telithromycin (in vitro)	2-(Allylthio)pyrazine Capsaicin CCl4 Chlormethiazole Disulfiram Ethanol (acute consumption) Garlic extract GH (?) Isoniazid Malotilate 8-Methoxypsoralene (?) Miconazole Phenylethylisothiocyanate Mustard green family vegetables Pyrazole, 4-methylpyrazole	Antiproteases (indinavir, nelfinavir, ritonavir, saquinavir) Aprepitant Bromocriptine Cimetidine Clotrimazole Cyclosporine Danazol Delavirdine Dihydroergotamine Diltiazem Ergotamine Ethinyl estradiol Fluconazole (±) FQ (±) Fluoxetine, norfluoxetine, paroxetine Fluvoxamine Furanocoumarin Gestodene Interleukin 2 Alpha and gamma interferon Grapefruit juice Ketoconazole, itraconazole, posaconazole, voriconazole Macrolides Metronidazole Mibefradil Mifepristone Vinorelbine (Navelbine)

(*Continued on next page*)

Table 3 Distribution of substrates, enzyme inducers, and enzyme inhibitors according to the different CYPs (*Continued*)

Parameter	CYP family		
	1	2	3
			Nefazodone Nicardipine, nifedipine Norfloxacin Omeprazole and analogs (±) Peppermint oil Progesterone Propoxyphene Quercetin Quinine and quinidine Sertraline Somatostatin Spironolactone Tacrolimus, tamoxifen Telithromycin (weak) Valspodar Verapamil Vinblastine, vincristine

[a]Long-term ethanol consumption increases the mutagenicity of tobacco-derived products via CYP2E1 induction; this explains why lung cancers occur primarily in heavy smokers who are also alcoholics or have CYP2E1 overexpression.
[b]CoA, coenzyme A.

Table 4 Substrates for CYP isoforms

Isoform	Substrates
1A1, 1A2	Amitriptyline; caffeine; chlorpromazine and analogues; clomipramine; clozapine; dihydralazine; imipramine; mianserin; paracetamol (high dose: hepatotoxic-reactive metabolites); phenacetin; tacrine; theophylline (1- and 3-oxidation and 8- hydroxylation); R-warfarin; zidovudine
2A6	Antipyrine; coumarins (7-hydroxylation); halothane
2B6	Bupropion; cinnarizine; cyclophosphamide (activation); ketamine; S-mephenytoin; nevirapine; propofol; tamoxifen (activation)
2C8, 2C9, 2C19[a]	Amitriptyline (2C19); antipyrine (2C9/2C19); arachidonic acid (2C8/2C9/2C19); barbiturates; carbamazepine; citalopram (2C19); coumarins (2C19); dapsone (2C9); diazepam (2C19); fluconazole (2C9); fluoxetine (2C9); fluvastatin (2C9); glibenclamide (2C9); gliclazide (2C9); glimepiride (2C9); glipizide (2C9); imipramine and analogues (2C8); indanediones (2C19); lansoprazole (2C19); loperamide; mephenytoin (2C19); methsuximide; nelfinavir (2C19); nialamide; NSAIDs (2C9) (arylacetic and arylpropionic acids); omeprazole (2C19); paclitaxel (Taxol) (2C8); papaverine; phenylbutazone; phenytoin (2C9 and 2C19) and related hydantoins; pioglitazone (2C8); pro/chloroguanil (2C19); propranolol (2C19); (oxidation of side chain); repaglinide (2C8); rosiglitazone (2C8); rosuvastatin (2C9); sartans (2C9); sulfamethoxazole (2C9); sulfinpyrazone; thienylic acid; tolbutamide (2C9) and related hypoglycemic agents; torasemide (loop diuretic and related diuretic Ag); voriconazole (2C9 and 2C19); S-warfarin (2C9)
2D6[b]	Amiflamine; amitriptyline and analogues; amphetamine; antipyrine; beta blockers (most); bufuralol; captopril; celecoxib (but not rofecoxib); chlorpromazine and analogues; cinnarizine; debrisoquine; desmethyl citalopram; dexfenfluramine; dextromethorphan/codeine; hydro/oxycodone; diphenhydramine; domperidone; ecstasy; encainide and analogues; ethylmorphine; flunarizine; fluvoxamine (?); guanoxan; haloperidol; halothane; imipramine and analogues; loratadine; methadone; methoxy amphetamine; methoxy phenamine; metoclopramide; mexiletine; mianserin; minaprine; nortriptyline; omeprazole; ondansetron; papaverine; paroxetine and analogs; perhexillin; perphenazine; phenacetin; phenformin; phenytoin; phenothiazines; propafenone; quinidine; risperidone; selegiline; sparteine; tamoxifen; thioridazine; tropisetron; yohimbine; zopiclone
2E1	Aniline; antipyrine; caffeine; chlorzoxazone; dapsone; disulfiram; environmental procarcinogens; ethanol; fatty acids (arachidonate, laurate); halothane[c] (fluranes[c]); paracetamol[c]; theophylline (8-hydroxylation), possibly activated to hepatotoxic reactive metabolites *Chemicals and xenobiotics:* alcohols; aldehydes; alkanes; alkenes; ethers; aromatics hydrocarbons (benzene, toluene, capsaicin ...); halogenated hydrocarbons; metals: chromium
3A3–5[d]	Alfentanil/fentanyl and related opioids; amiodarone; amitriptyline; antiproteases; antipyrine; astemizole; benzodiazepines (alpra/mida/triazolam/dia/broma/clonazepam); bromocriptine; busulfan; capravirine; carbamazepine; clarythro/erythromycin; cisapride; clindamycin; cocaine; cyclophosphamide; cyclosporin; dapsone; delavirdine; dextromethorphan; disopyramide; doxorubucin; ergot (alkaloids); erythromycin; ethosuximide; ethylmorphine; etoposide; everolimus; glucocorticoids-corticosteroids; granisetron, ondansetron; haloperidol; ifosfamide; imipramine and analogues; calcium inhibitors (calcium channel antagonists); irinotecan; ivermectin; keto/itraco/mico/posaco/voriconazole; lidocaine; loratadine; losartan; mibefradil; mizolastine; nefazodone/ trazadone; omeprazole; ondansetron; oral contraceptives; paclitaxel (Taxol); pentoxifylline; perphenazine; pimozide; procainamide; propafenone; quinidine; rifabutin; rifampin; risperidone; sertraline; sidenafil; statins; natural steroids; tacrolimus; tamoxifen/toremifen; telithromycin; terfenadine; valproic acid; vinblastine/vincristine; verapamil/diltiazem; warfarin; xenobiotics (aflatoxin B1, benzopyrene activations, benzphetamine, heterocyclic amines, sterigmatocystin); zonizamide; zopiclone/zolpidem

[a]The incidence of CYP 2C19 poor metabolizers is 2–6% in the Caucasian population and 18–22% in Asian populations.
[b]The incidence of CYP 2D6 poor metabolizers is 5–10% in the Caucasian population and 1–2% in Asian populations.
[c]Possibly activated to hepatotoxic reactive metabolites.
[d]40% of the total CYP 3A4 content resides in the small intestine.

(i) At the alveolar level, the concentrations of pyrazinamide in epithelial lining fluid are 20 times greater than the concentrations in serum, whereas alveolar macrophages do not concentrate the product. This therefore seems to indicate that there are efflux transporters at this level which concentrate pyrazinamide in the alveolar film. Can these proteins be induced (by rifampin or corticosteroids, for example) or inhibited? It will be noted also that OATP (absorption and efflux transporters) and P-gp are present in the lungs.

(ii) In Calu-3 cells, an airway epithelium model, accumulation of quinolones is suboptimal due to active efflux. Efflux inhibitors (P-gp/verapamil; MRP/probenecid) significantly increase cellular accumulation of quinolones and therefore may improve their activity against intracellular organisms.

(iii) Dexamethasone very significantly reduces the passage of lincomycin into the cerebrospinal fluid, the probable consequence of induction of an efflux pump rather than a change in the inflammatory situation. This is because, conversely, it does not modify the penetration of cefotaxime or ceftriaxone. By contrast, probenecid blocks organic acid transporters (MRP, OATP, and other probenecid [-sensitive] transporters) in the choroid plexus and thus delays the central elimination of β-lactams by these efflux pumps.

Everything points to the fact that high doses of β-lactams saturate these transporters, thereby promoting local accumulation. Finally, simultaneous administration of two compounds with a β-lactam structure (piperacillin plus tazobactam) prolongs the central dwell time of each of the products by competition at the same transporters.

(iv) Blockade by competition of renal megalin might reduce the renal uptake of aminoglycosides and hence their nephrotoxicity.

(v) In the same way, a negative effect of the P-gp inducers rifampin and dexamethasone on the activity of antineoplastic treatments is to be feared, whereas myocardial uptake of anthracyclines might be reduced with these products, since P-gp inhibitors (verapamil and amiodarone) enhance this uptake.

(vi) P-gp inhibitors (macrolides, azole antifungals, etc. [Fig. 1]), by promoting penetration of the BBB by its substrates, may induce neurotoxic reactions with digoxin, ivermectin, loperamide, tacrolimus, and vincristine. This is unlikely to be observed with African populations, which have an overexpression of P-gp, and this also explains why a high incidence of drug resistance to cancer treatment is observed. Conversely, no results have yet been obtained along these lines which would facilitate the central passage of antiproteases, despite hopeful results from animal studies. This could be the result of an overlapping substrate specificity between OATPs and P-gp or MRPs as has been described for many drugs, such as digoxin, fexofenadine, and opioids, the existence of alternative transport pathways reducing the opportunities of drug-drug interaction, a situation commonly encountered with CYPs when several metabolic pathways are involved.

(vii) At the ocular level, probenecid inhibits active transport across the retina of "posterior-route" drugs (penicillins, and cephalosporins), thereby forcing β-lactam drugs to escape by the anterior route with a prolonged half-life.

As a final point relating to the risks of interaction at the receptor level, attention should be drawn to the central receptors to point out that FQ displace γ-aminobutyric acid (GABA) from its central GABA-A receptors in the same way as is observed with imipenem, effects which in the case of FQ are potentiated by the coprescription of nonsterodial anti-inflammatory drugs (NSAIDs). Two aspects should be highlighted here: first, that the combination imipenem-FQ-NSAID is probably particularly at risk and, second, that the natural "antidote" to be proposed for the prevention of any epileptogenic risk is clonazepam (Rivotril) or, failing that, diazepam (Valium), substrates with a higher affinity and which mimic the effects of GABA.

In the French population, the frequency of central effects with NSAID + FQ is on the order of 5%.

Among risk factors, the presence of hepatic failure (in the case of FQ with hepatic metabolism) and the coprescription of theophylline should be mentioned.

4. INTERACTIONS RELATING TO THE ELIMINATION PHASE

4.1. Metabolic Clearance

4.1.1. General Considerations

Systemic metabolism is the culmination of a transformation process which may begin with the oral absorption phase and the purpose of which is to make drugs more polar so as to facilitate their elimination in the urine or bile. Interactions at this level are those we have described in sections 2.2.2 and 2.3 (hence Table 3).

However, the predictive application of Table 3 requires consideration of the following two points.

First, it should be borne in mind that the enzyme equipment of the intestinal cell is not qualitatively comparable to that of the hepatocyte in the same way that it is quantitatively. In particular, however, as is generally accepted, it should be realized that for the same isoform, CYP3A4 for example (a CYP that is fairly well distributed between the two sites), the comparative metabolism rate between enterocyte and hepatocyte varies substantially according to the substrate (Fig. 2).

These two aspects, the distribution of isoforms and the metabolism rate of different substrates, are probably related. In fact, for the same majority metabolic pathway—CYP3A4 as in the previous example—what will ultimately affect the (global) rate of metabolism observed will be the existence or otherwise of secondary metabolic pathways (alternative clearance pathways) and obviously therefore their extent and tissue distribution (Table 5).

Second, although theoretically for any one isoform an inducing compound, such as rifampin in the case of CYP3A4, induces the corresponding enterocyte and hepatocyte activities equally and concomitantly, it appears that in reality currently unknown regulatory mechanisms result almost systematically (at least in the example given) in the exclusive induction either of the hepatic isoform or of the intestinal isoform in a way which appears to be totally random since the substrate is not known. This is, obviously, in favor of an independent regulation of these two metabolic systems.

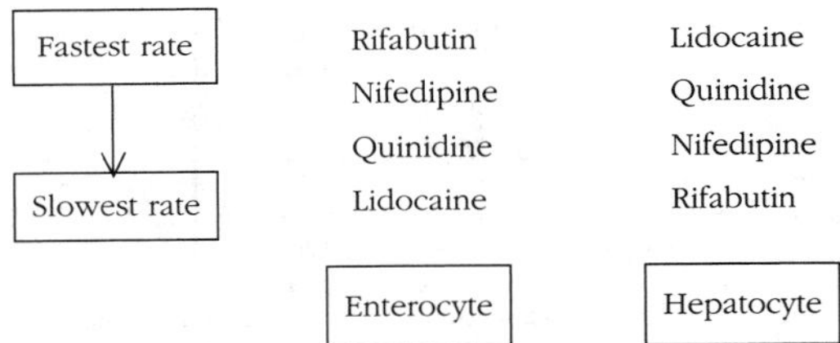

Figure 2 Metabolism rate of four substrates of CYP3A4 by rat intestinal or hepatic microsomal preparations (from Aiba et al., 2003)

Table 5 Hepatic and intestinal distributions of the isoforms CYP3A4, -2D6, and -3A9 in the rat[a]

Compound	Metabolizing isoforms	Site of metabolism	Distribution of isoform:		
			3A4	2D6	3A9
Lidocaine	CYP3A4, CYP2D6	Liver	+++	+++	0
Rifabutin	CYP3A4, CYP3A9	Intestine	+++	+	++

[a]Data from Aiba et al., 2003.

According to Greiner et al. (1999), the expression of CYP3A in duodenal samples is increased 4.4-fold after administration of a 10-day treatment with rifampin (600 mg/day).

In addition to these metabolic stages, known as phase I, which represent the majority of interactions, mention may be made under the heading of phase II reactions, in other words, conjugation, of the inhibition of glucuronidation of AZT by chloramphenicol, beta interferon, certain NSAIDs, atovaquone, valproic acid, and azole antifungals (note that morphine is conjugated by the same enzyme system both in the liver and centrally). Probenecid is also a known UDP-glucuronosyltransferase inhibitor. Conversely, rifampin, which is an inducer of glucuronyltransferase, reduces the AUC of AZT by half but does not increase the morphine glucuronide/morphine plasma AUC ratio. The following are inducers of glucuronyltransferase: carbamazepine, lamotrigine, oral contraceptive steroids, phenobarbital, phenytoin, rifampin, and ritonavir. It should be added at this point that for glucuroconjugated drugs which undergo an enterohepatic cycle (enterohepatic recycling) after biliary excretion and deconjugation by colonic bacterial glucuronidases, eradication of the colonic flora by prolonged antibiotic treatment may result in a significant reduction in the AUC of the drugs.

It might be thought that the combination of several inducers (rifampin plus dexamethasone, for example) or several inhibitors (cimetidine plus ciprofloxacin or azole antifungal plus grapefruit juice) is usually additive in its effects, as suggested by Table 6. However, this is not the rule for the simple reason that, since inducing effects as well as inhibitory effects are involved, the latter exhibit a maximum effect which, when it is achieved, can by definition no longer be exceeded either by the addition of a second effect modulator or by any increase in dosage. The outcome of the addition of another inducer or another inhibitor (as of an increase in dose) depends solely on the trio modulator-CYP-substrate and the dosage regimen used (dose as well as dosage interval). Also, the net percent increase of midazolam systemic clearance (or oral clearance) for a said group of patients and for the combination midazolam-rifampin will be that much greater than the initial value if the clearance is low.

As an example, in a "preinduced" smoking population, the magnitude of phenytoin induction of theophylline metabolism does not differ from that observed with phenytoin in nonsmoking volunteers. Similary, after long-term administration of carbamazepine, chronic dosing with St. John's wort, an effective CYP3A4 enzyme inducer, does not modify carbamazepine steady-state pharmacokinetics. These data suggest that after long-term administration of carbamazepine, CYP3A4 enzymes are already fully induced and a maximum effect is reached through an autoinduction process.

Along the same lines, it is commonly said that inducing effects are stronger in poor metabolizers than in extensive metabolizers. However, this is at present widely disputed.

As regards the induction of duodenal P-gp, this appears to be weaker in subjects homozygous for the genotype 3435C/T, in other words, in subjects with weak expression of duodenal P-gp. This is reflected during cotreatment with rifampin in this population by a twofold increase in the bioavailability of digoxin compared to that in subjects not exhibiting this genotype.

Table 6 Inhibition of the metabolism of theophylline

Drug(s)	Dose	$t_{1/2\beta}$ (h)	% Increase in inhibition
Theophylline		7.2	
+Cimetidine	400 mg b.i.d.	10.2	42
+Ciprofloxacin	500 mg b.i.d.	10.6	48
+Cimetidine	400 mg b.i.d.	12.8	78
+Ciprofloxacin	500 mg b.i.d.		

Conversely, the result of the combination of a substrate (cyclosporine) with both an inducer (rifampin) and an inhibitor (erythomycin) of its metabolism is unpredictable, particularly in the quantitative assessment of the phenomenon.

It should be added that there might be a sex-related effect, since Gorski et al. (2003) showed that the inducing effect of rifampin in relation to CYP3A4 is significantly more marked in men than in women.

Lastly, when several metabolic pathways are involved, the risk of interaction is reduced still more, at least where an interaction by competition between two substrates is involved.

Thus, while the majority of benzodiazepines are transformed by CYP3A4, as a result of which their clearance is reduced by the many inhibitors of this isoform, zolpidem, a benzodiazepine-like product, is admittedly metabolized by CYP3A4 but also by CYP1A2, -2C9, -2C19, and -2D6, which are supplementary pathways, so that this hypnotic does not undergo any significant interaction.

Likewise, among the tricyclic antidepressants, those possessing a tertiary amine (imipramine, clomipramine, and amitiptyline) have a lower risk of interaction than those with a secondary amine (nortriptyline and desipramine), the former in fact being metabolized by five different isoforms, whereas the latter are metabolized solely by CYP2D6.

Again, posaconazole, a CYP3A4 inhibitor, inhibits rifabutin, for which it is the only metabolism pathway, but not phenytoin, which can employ CYP2C9, -2C19, -2D6, and −3A4.

In fact, CYP isoforms usually exhibit distinct but overlapping substrate specificities, and only a few drugs are exclusively metabolized by a single enzyme. Otherwise drug-drug interactions would be considerably more frequent.

Based on a mathematical approach, Rowland and Matin (1973) concluded that a significant drug-drug interaction should occur only when the relative contribution of the metabolic fraction of a particular pathway that is being inhibited is greater than 50% of total clearance.

4.1.2. Enzyme Induction

4.1.2.1. Rifampin and Antibiotic Combinations

Rifampin is one of the most potent enzyme inducers in the pharmacopoeia and therefore the source of a number of drug interactions.

Often combined with FQ or novobiocin in the treatment of staphylococcal infections, rifampin reduces the elimination half-life of the latter by 30 to 60% and that of the quinolones with marked hepatic metabolism, pefloxacin and fleroxacin, to a similar extent. In the case of such combinations, the use of a nonmetabolized quinolone (ofloxacin) or one with a mixed elimination (ciprofloxacin) is preferable.

It should, however, be borne in mind that the combination FQ-rifampin may become antagonistic if the FQ is administered during the postantibiotic effect of rifampin, in other words, if administration of the two antibiotics is nonsynchronous.

A similar interaction, although often even more marked, is found with the azole antifungals with marked metabolic elimination. Rifampin, like the inducing antiepileptics (carbamazepine, phenytoin, and phenobarbital), reduces the C_{max} of ketoconazole or itraconazole by a factor of 3 to 4.

A 10-fold greater reduction has even been reported for the combination itraconazole-phenytoin. More surprisingly, rifampin itself has proved undetectable during combination with ketoconazole. Such combinations should be avoided, particularly if the necessary facilities are not available for proper therapeutic monitoring of the two partners in the combination.

The interaction rifampin-fluconazole is less marked, being at the limit of clinical significance (20 to 25% reduction in the plasma AUC of fluconazole). Rifabutin, for its part, a compound that is structurally similar to rifampin but with weaker inducing properties, does not modify the kinetics of fluconazole.

Lastly, with respect to dapsone-trimethoprim combinations as an alternative to co-trimoxazole in *Pneumocystis carinii* infections, it may be useful to know that rifampin can reduce the elimination half-life of dapsone by more than half.

4.1.2.2. Interactions of Rifampin with Nonantibiotic Compounds

Rifampin is a potent broad-spectrum enzyme inducer which induces the 1A2, 2A6, 2C9, 2C19, and 3A4 isoforms of CYP and consequently markedly reduces the concentrations in plasma of a number of drugs with metabolic clearance.

Thus, during treatment with rifampin, the half-life of quinidine is divided by 3 and its plasma AUC is divided by 4 to 6. An interaction of the same order is found with quinine, verapamil, diltiazem, and probably also with the other calcium inhibitors that undergo a major hepatic first-pass effect. The bioavailability of midazolam is even reduced by 96% with rifampin.

Under the same conditions, the plasma clearance of theophylline is practically doubled, as is that of other drugs, particularly oral anticoagulants, glycodiazine, tolbutamide, cortisol, digitoxin, oral contraceptives, methadone, ethosuximide, phenytoin, diazepam, haloperidol, tocainide, lorcainide, bunazosin, disopyramide, benzodiazepines and related substances, and losartan.

The same observation is made with the antiproteases delavirdine and efavirenz. Rifabutin, an inducer of CYP3A4 alone, in this respect has a considerably less marked effect than rifampin.

The combination rifampin-cyclosporine has resulted in graft rejections following the dramatic fall in circulating cyclosporine concentrations. If this combination is found to be necessary, the initial dose of cyclosporine should be increased by 50% and therapeutic monitoring should be undertaken daily. Recent studies by Hebert et al. (1991, 1992) and Gomez et al. (1994) seem to indicate that, rather than induction of hepatic CYP, this apparently involves either a reduction of oral absorption by induction of an efflux protein which metabolizes cyclosporine (e.g., P-gp), induction of its digestive presystemic metabolism, or, more probably, a combination of the two. In fact, in the first place the kinetics of intravenous cyclosporine are not modified by rifampin (Hebert et al., 1992), and in the second place ex vivo studies have shown that the digestive mucosa possesses the enzyme equipment necessary to metabolize cyclosporine.

Finally, it should be noted that when erythromycin, a potent inhibitor of the CYP involved in the transformation of cyclosporine, is added to previous combination rifampin-cyclosporine, it is the effect of rifampin which takes precedence, necessitating an increase in the dose of the immunosuppressant.

Conversely, the combination of fluconazole or clarithromycin (both of which are inhibitors) plus rifabutin results in an increase of 50 to 80% in rifabutin: the inhibitor here is dominant.

Some authors have proposed replacing rifampin with pyrazinamide in transplantations; however, pyrazinamide itself appears to be capable of reducing circulating concentrations of cyclosporine.

Finally, while still on the subject of antituberculosis agents, it should be pointed out that isoniazid is a specific inducer of the isoenzyme CYP2E1, involved in the biotransformation of paracetamol. This combination might therefore result in a quantitative increase in the formation of paracetamol metabolites, with the risk of attaining the toxic zone and causing the depletion of glutathione and ultimately a serious hepatocytic lesion.

4.1.3. Enzyme Inhibition

There are two major types of CYP enzyme inhibition. The first is rapidly reversible and competitive inhibition. Inhibitors (the drug itself and/or its metabolite[s]) tend to bind effectively to the catalytic site of the enzyme and compete with other substrates for that binding according to their respective K_is. Many of these inhibitors are nitrogen-containing drugs, including imidazoles, pyridines, and quinolines. Obviously the potentially implicated nitrogen must not be sterically hindered, and, in addition, in order to be good inhibitors, drugs need to have sufficient lipophilicity (Lin and Lu, 1998).

The second is irreversible or semi-irreversible and noncompetitive inhibition with the corresponding two subtypes of inhibition. The first subtype is the so-called "mechanism-based" inhibition, where the inhibitor (suicide inhibitor) is oxidized by CYPs to a reactive intermediate that subsequently causes irreversible inactivation of the enzyme. This may result from irreversible alteration of prosthetic heme through the production of radical intermediates (e.g., ethinyl estradiol, gestodene, and mifepristone) or apoproteins (chloramphenicol, thienylic acid, diallyl sulfide [a component of garlic], etc.) or both (spironolactone). The second subtype is CYP inhibition with the formation of a metabolite-intermediate complex (MI complex): such inhibitors have been shown to undergo successive oxidation to a nitrosoalkane species which in vitro forms a slowly reversible inactive complex with the prosthetic heme of the CYP. However, in vivo the MI complex is very stable and de novo biosynthesis of new enzymes is the only means by which activity can be restored. These compounds include several macrolide antibiotics; some antidepressants, such as fluoxetine, paroxetine, nortriptyline, desipramine, and imipramine; and amiodarone, diltiazem, lidocaine, tamoxifen, tiamulin, and SKF-525A.

Lastly, allosteric inhibition, a third type of inhibition, has been described; it is both reversible and noncompetitive. An allosteric change caused by the binding of a ligand may affect the binding of a second molecule. For example, quinidine acts as an allosteric noncompetitive inhibitor of CYP3A4, oxidation of nifedipine resulting in an enzymatically ineffective ternary complex.

In the case of a mixed effect, competitive, and noncompetitive inhibition, one of the two mechanisms will outweigh the other, without any possibility of knowing a priori which will gain precedence. Two contrasting examples follow:

- The inhibitory effect of erythromycin is the result of MI complex formation rather than rapidly reversible binding to the enzyme.
- In the case of diltiazem, the two metabolites desmethyl- and didesmethyldiltiazem are highly potent reversible

inhibitors of CYP3A4, so reversible in vivo inhibition by such metabolites, as they accumulate in the body, may be a more potent mechanism than MI complex formation.

As regards the degree of inactivation, this depends on the dose, and duration as well as the frequency of administration. In other respects, it might be thought that poor metabolizers are more susceptible because of a low quantity of target CYP enzyme to be inhibited. In fact, however, it is necessary to think in terms of the amount of activity inhibited rather than of the percent variation of the remaining uncomplexed CYPs, so the reverse is observed: extensive metabolizers are more susceptible to enzyme inhibitors.

The three major antibiotic families responsible for interaction by inhibition of CYP are the FQ, the macrolides, and the azole antifungals.

4.1.3.1. FQ

The inhibitory activity of the FQ essentially involves CYP1A2 and, to a lesser extent, CYP3A4, so even if therapeutic monitoring is recommended as a precaution during treatment combining an FQ with cyclosporine, this potential interaction is only exceptionally observed, the metabolism of cyclosporine being under the control of CYP3A4.

In fact, the only clinically significant interaction involves theophylline, the half-life of which may in fact be significantly prolonged (Table 7).

4.1.3.2. Macrolides, and Ketolides

Macrolides, particularly triacetyloleandomycin and erythromycin, are potent CYP3A inducers, an induction which is followed immediately by a second stage during which a metallic complex forms between the ferric ion of the heme and a nitrosoalkane intermediate which ultimately causes inactivation of the CYP3A activated initially (= formation of MI complexes).

Macrolides thus inhibit the oxidative metabolism of a number of drugs, including theophylline, cyclosporine, carbamazepine, warfarin, terfenadine (Table 8), zopiclone, midazolam, triazolam, bromocriptine, lansoprazole, methylprednisolone, disopyramide, felodipine, glyburide, and valproic acid, all drugs metabolized by CYP3A4.

On the other hand, telithromycin does not form stable CYP Fe(II)-nitrosoalkane complexes (mechanism-based inhibition) in vitro in the way that macrolides do. However, this ketolide could be a weak competitive inhibitor for CYP3A4 substrates owing to the fact that it weakly impairs cisapride elimination (registration dossier). In fact, the risks of interaction with telithromycin are much less marked than with the macrolides (registration dossier), and the increases in AUC never exceed 30%, except for digoxin (+37%) (inhibition of intestinal P-gp).

Table 7 Multiplication factor of the half-life of theophylline in combination with an FQ

Compound(s) combined	Multiplication factor
Enoxacin	2
Pipemidic acid	2
Pefloxacin	1.5–2
Ciprofloxacin	1.5
Tosufloxacin	1.5
Norfloxacin	1.2
Lomefloxacin, sparfloxacin	1.0
Gatifloxacin, levofloxacin, ofloxacin	1.0
Rufloxacin	1.0

Table 8 Drug interaction involving macrolides and ketolides[a]

Drug combined	Azithromycin	Clarithromycin	Dirithromycin	Erythromycin	Josamycin	Midecamycin, myocamycin	Roxithromycin	Spiramycin	TAO	Telithromycin
Theophylline	0	0 (two doses of 250 mg/day)	0	++	+	ND	0/+	0	+++	0/+
Cyclosporine	0	+++	ND	+++	+++	+++	+	0	ND	ND
Carbamazepine	ND	0 (two doses of 250 mg/day) + (two doses of 500 mg/day)	ND	+++	+	+	0/+	0/+	+++	ND
Midazolam	0	++	ND	++	ND	ND	+	ND	ND	ND
Warfarin	0	ND	ND	+	ND	ND	0	ND	ND	0
Terfenadine	0	++	ND	+++	0/+	ND	0	ND	ND	ND

[a]The extent of the interaction is graded from 0 (no interaction) to +++ (major interaction) (0/+, clinically nonsignificant). TAO, triacetyl oleandomycin; ND, not documented.

Interactions have also been recorded with substances metabolized by pathways other than that of CYP3A4. In fact, the induction of CYP3A4 is often associated with a relative reduction in the expression of the other CYPs, particularly CYP2C or even CYP2D, as indicated by the reduction in metabolic clearance of amitriptyline or nortriptyline observed with josamycin.

Very often, because the interaction with theophylline is at a low level, an increased incidence of nausea and vomiting can be avoided by giving theophylline 1 h before the macrolide or ketolide.

4.1.3.3. Azole Antifungals

Systemic azole antifungals behave like CYP inhibitors. However, the spectrum of inhibition varies from one compound to another. Ketoconazole has a particular affinity for the isoenzymes of the CYP2C subfamily and a weak affinity for the isoenzymes of CYP3A (particularly CYP3A4); ketoconazole, itraconazole, and voriconazole have exactly the opposite profile of affinity for CYP2C and CYP3A4 from that of fluconazole. Posaconazole appears to be similar to the ketoconazole-itraconazole group.

Fluconazole will therefore tend to inhibit metabolization of the drug substrates of CYP2C, such as phenytoin and tolbutamide, and to a considerably lesser extent those whose metabolism is effected by CYP3A4, as is the case with atevirdine and theophylline, the elimination half-life of which increases by only 9 to 10% with fluconazole. In fact, theophylline is little affected by the azoles in general, as only 8-hydroxylation is controlled by the isoenzyme CYP3A4 and demethylation is dependent on CYP1A2.

Conversely, ketoconazole, itraconazole, and voriconazole inhibit the metabolism of the substrates of the isoenzyme CYP3A4, particularly terfenadine, cyclosporine, benzodiazepines, granisetron, and probably ondansetron, as well as the antiproteases used in the treatment of AIDS, especially saquinavir, the bioavailability of which increases by 230% with ketoconazole, and likewise quinidine, corticosteroids, methylprednisolone, and budesonide. In this last case, consideration may be given to administering the two drugs at an interval of 12 h in order to minimize the interaction: one in the morning and the other in the evening.

In a normal situation, terfenadine, an oral antihistamine, undergoes a virtually total hepatic first-pass effect (99%), resulting in an active acid metabolite, M1, which is subsequently oxidized to a second inactive metabolite, M2. The first stage is under the control of the isoenzyme CYP3A4 and may be inhibited both by ketoconazole and by itraconazole, resulting subsequently in the appearance of measurable circulating concentrations of terfenadine, the cardiotoxicity of which can then be expressed. Cases of torsade de pointes with prolongation of the QT interval have thus been reported with ketoconazole as well as itraconazole (but not with fluconazole) and with erythromycin, likewise a potent inhibitor of CYP3A4. A case of torsade de pointes and cardiac arrest with the combination terfenadine-itraconazole is also found in the literature. Among associated risk factors, mention should be made of the coprescription of erythromycin, the presence of liver insufficiency, an underlying cardiovascular disease, hypokalemia (treatment with diuretics, laxatives, or amphotericin B; cirrhotic patient, etc.), and the ingestion of grapefruit juice, the CYP3A4-inhibitory nature of which is now well established. By contrast, cimetidine, an inhibitor of CYP1A, -2C, -2D and-3A, does not block the metabolism of terfenadine any more than ranitidine. Any other therapeutic agent likely per se to prolong the QT interval will also constitute a predisposing factor.

The interaction between ketoconazole and terfenadine has been the subject of in vitro modeling in human hepatic microsomes, which appears to predict the extent of the interaction during therapeutic use. QT interval prolongation can also be observed with erythromycin.

Finally, it should be noted that ketoconazole itself causes prolongation of the QT interval, which should probably be attributed to blockade of the cardiac potassium currents.

Proposed for economic reasons to reduce the dosage of cyclosporine, ketoconazole, of the three azoles studied, is the one which most inhibits the metabolism of this immunosuppressant (voriconazole and posaconazole have not been the subject of this type of study). From this aspect, ketoconazole is recommended at a dosage of 200 mg/day, which then enables the dosage of cyclosporine to be reduced by 75% during the first month of treatment, and almost 85% after 12 months (reommended dose at 1 month, 24% of the usual standard dose; 24% at 3 months; 18% at 6 months; and 16% at 12 months). Enzyme inhibition, which involves presystemic intestinal metabolization, increases in fact over the course of treatment.

An interaction with itraconazole does exist but appears to be less marked, although in a series of seven heart or heart-lung graft patients, the dose of cyclosporine had to be reduced by 33 to 84% (mean, 56%). In terms of the interaction between cyclosporine and fluconazole, its extent appears to depend on the dose of fluconazole used. At all events, it is essential to monitor the course of blood cyclosporine levels closely.

This inhibitory effect may be enhanced by the presence of hepatic failure or by the coprescription of erythromycin, calcium inhibitors, metoclopramide, or, again, grapefruit juice.

Lastly, like itraconazole, ketoconazole inhibits the metabolism of alprazolam, midazolam, and triazolam, three benzodiazepines metabolized by the isoenzyme CYP3A4. The C_{maxs} are multiplied by a factor of 3 to 4, and the plasma AUCs are multiplied by a factor of 5 to 7. Such combinations should be avoided. The risks are also increased by the presence of hepatic insufficiency or the consumption of grapefruit juice.

Among the list of interactions, that between fluconazole and AZT should also be highlighted, resulting after 7 days of treatment with 400 mg of fluconazole in an increase of almost 75% in the area under the AZT curve by inhibition of the formation of the glucuroconjugated derivative. The same type of interaction with ketoconazole is likely.

4.1.3.4. Co-trimoxazole

Sulfamethoxazole, a sulfonamide combined with trimethoprim, inhibits the metabolism of warfarin, phenytoin, and loperamide, probably by acting on CYP2C.

4.1.3.5. Enzyme Inhibition and Therapeutic Contribution

We reported above (section 4.1. 3.3) that the ketoconazole-cyclosporine interaction was proposed in order to reduce the costs of treatment of the immunosuppressant. The contribution here is strictly economic. Conversely, the combination of cimetidine with dapsone, by blocking the CYP3A4 responsible for N hydroxylation of the anti-infective agent, thus reduces the risks of methemoglobinemia associated with the production of hematotoxic derivatives: dapsone hydroxylamine and nitrosodapsone.

Lastly, the CYP3A4-inhibitory properties of ritonavir are used to boost the circulating concentrations of the other protease inhibitors, all metabolized by this isoform.

4.1.4. Variation Factors and Risk Factors

Variation and risk factors include the following:

- The existence of genetic polymorphism (see above)
- The combination of several enzyme inducers and/or inhibitors for the same substrate (see above)
- The presence of severe hepatic impairment, given that in this case the isoforms are not all affected in the same way, depending on the Child-Pugh severity score (Table 9) and whether or not cholestasis is also present, as highlighted in the study by George et al. (1995, Table 10). Cholestasis affects the CYP system, possibly through bile salt retention since bile salts inhibit CYPs in vitro. It should be noted that all of the conjugation processes may also be affected, even if this possibility remains disputed in the case of glucuroconjugation.
- Congestive heart failure. Thomson et al. (1973) first reported that lidocaine clearance was nearly halved in patients with heart failure because hepatic blood flow is modified.
- Malnutrition phenomena, probably as the result of a lack of hepatic protein synthesis and/or reduction in hepatic blood flow. However, this problem is mainly encountered in kwashiorkor patients and would not be the case in malnourished patients with global malnutrition.
- A number of serious diseases may be accompanied by a reduction in hepatic and/or extrahepatic capacities. It has thus been noted during bacterial and viral pulmonary infections that there is a significant reduction in the metabolism of nitrendipine, theophylline, and antipyrine. This might involve a direct effect by modification of the expression of pulmonary CYP (the lung is in fact a tissue with a high metabolism capacity) or again a reduction in the capacities of certain enzyme systems associated with interferon release during the infectious process. Alpha-2b interferon in fact reduces the clearance of theophylline and of antipyrine but does not affect the metabolism of hexobarbital.
- Intensive care patients also very frequently have impaired hepatic function which might affect the biotransformation of drugs administered to them. The same is observed early in sepsis despite fluid resuscitation.
- Surgery patients. It should also be realized in this respect that acute hypoxia does not significantly modify the activity of CYP (Jürgens et al., 2002), in contrast to the assessment proposed by Park (1996).
- The administration of cytokines: alpha, beta, or gamma interferon or interleukin 2 may be the cause of inhibition of CYP1A2 and-3A4 (Table 3).
- Patients with end-stage renal disease who have 30% lower baseline erythromycin breath test values than controls but an enzyme induction capacity after rifampin that is not different from that in healthy subjects. Interisoform differences are not excluded. Besides CYP3A4 modification, CYP2C9 is decreased. The same is observed during surgery- and drug-induced renal dysfunction in animals.
- Human immunodeficiency virus patient
- In celiac disease, the expression of intestinal CYP3A is markedly decreased.
- Burn patients
- Due to the difficulty in obtaining liver and other tissue material from children, limited data are available on the ontogeny of the individual CYPs, while sparse data are available on transport proteins. However, because of their global physiological immaturity, the following is observed in neonates and infants up to 1 month old:
    - An inefficient hepatic excretory function because of immaturity of carrier-mediated hepatocellular uptake and biliary efflux transport systems. If we consider the ontogeny of P-gp in the CNS and GI tract as an example, it is clear that P-gp maturity is not achieved at birth (Table 11).
    - Reduced CYP activity, both by measurements of microsomal activity and by values for plasma clearance of CYP probe substrates (Table 12). Global CYP reaches 30 to 40% of adult levels from 3 to 12 months of age, which is not very different from that observed in neonates. Consistent with this metabolic pattern, only the 4 primary metabolites of caffeine were detected by Cazeneuve et al. (1994) using liver microsomes, while 14 metabolites were recovered in vivo in the urine of adult subjects.
    - As regards the development of phase II reactions, if glucuronidation activity is about one-fourth to one-sixth of adult activity during the first month of life, sulfatation activity is more developed, even if the activity with different substrates develops fully in the postnatal period. The median ratio of glucuronidation to sulfatation activity is 0.3 at 4 weeks, compared to 1.8 in

Table 9 Decrease in CYP activity according to Child-Pugh score

Child-Pugh score	Decrease in CYP activity (% of control)			
	1A2	2C9	2D6	2E1
≥6–7	41	70–80	40–50	35
5	NS[a]	30–40	NS	NS

[a]NS, not significant.

Table 10 Decrease in CYP activity according to the presence or absence of cholestasis

Cholestasis	Decrease in CYP activity (% of control)			
	1A2	2C	2E1	3A
Absence ($n = 32$)	71[a]	43	19	75[a]
Presence ($n = 18$)	82[a]	66[a]	51[a]	59

[a]$P < 0.05$.

Table 11 Relative levels of P-gp in CNS and GI tract on Western immunoblot of FVB mouse from days 0 to 21 of life

Location	Level of P-gp[a]		
	Day 0	Day 7	Day 21
CNS	22	34	97
GI tract	17	11	89

[a]Data are expressed as percentage of adult levels. (Note that 21 days in mice is probably equivalent to 3 to 6 months in humans.)

Table 12 CYP enzyme activity in infants (1 to 28 days) as a fraction of adult activity

Activity type	Fraction of adult activity of CYP isoform(s)				
	1A2	2C9, 2C10	2D6	2E1	3A4 + 3A7
Hepatic microsomal activity	1/10–1/100	1/2–1/50	1/3–1/10	1/3	1/2
Clearance of enzyme-specific probe substrates	1/4	ND[a]	ND	ND	1/3–1/5

[a]ND, no data.

adults. Thus, sulfation can be a replacement pathway for some drugs, such as paracetamol (Table 13). The reduced capacity for glucuronidation is a well-known cause of accumulation of bilirubin in premature infants, responsible for kernicterus, and of chloramphemical, causing fatal gray baby syndrome. However, in the case of hyperbilirubinemic encephalopathy, several studies suggest that BBB P-gp may play a major role in protecting the CNS from bilirubin neurotoxicity by reducing brain bilirubin influx, a step which may be very lacking at birth.

  - Lastly, there is some evidence that both CYP3A and glucuronidation activities can be induced during fetal life as well as after birth. In the same way, antenatal dexam-ethasone treatment increases brain P-gp expression twofold in suckling mouse pups. Protein immaturity in the neonate is therefore global and affects metabolism systems, membrane transporters, receptors, and the bactericidal/permeability-increasing protein of neutrophils, which could partly explain the increased incidence of gram-negative sepsis among newborns. This leads us to postulate the hypothesis of a possible immaturity in children of megalin, a renal aminoglycoside transport protein, as the explanation for the better tolerability of these antibiotics during the first months of life.

- The elderly subject. All evidence appears to indicate that metabolic capacities decrease with age, as demonstrated by the large number of pharmacokinetic changes observed in elderly subjects in association with drugs with a high metabolic clearance. Although the reason is not yet fully understood and although there is no predictive test, it may be noted that the following are jointly present in elderly subjects:
  - A decrease in liver weight over the age of 50 to 60 years. Liver weight as a percentage of body weight in subjects in their 20s or 30s was found to average 2.5%; in subjects in their 90s, liver weight was only 1.6% of body weight. At the same time, galactose clearance, which is said to reflect functioning cell mass, decreases commensurately with hepatic volume (around 1% per year after age 40), as well as clearance of drugs such as aminopyrine, antipyrine, imipramine, caffeine, and theophylline. However, the evaluation of drug clearance is not easy, particularly in patients with cirrhosis, as it is dependent on other drugs they ingest to control edema, ascites, depression, and other mental disorders, all drugs that can cause enzyme induction or inhibition. Blood flow to and from the liver shows a corresponding decline as the relative liver mass decreases (hepatic blood flow falls by 40 to 50% between the ages of 20 and 65 to 70 years). However, this fall in hepatic blood flow is consistent with diminishing cardiac output of 1% per year after the age of 30. (This should alter the level of first-pass through the liver.)
  - A decrease of 1% annually in hepatic CYP450 content
  - A decrease in bromosulfophthalein excretion, which suggests a somewhat reduced capacity for transport and storage of organic anions, but not for active secretion in the bile
  - Phenotypical changes appear with age and enhance the phenomena of variability.
  - In addition, elderly surgical patients with marasmic protein energy malnutrition may rapidly become hypalbuminemic, and then are probably at high risk of global protein synthesis deficiency, including metabolizing enzymes, particularly if sepsis is associated.
  - Lastly, it has been suggested that induction of drug metabolism by environmental factors and other drugs is decreased in elderly humans, but this has been disputed by Gorski et al. (2003). Moreover, inhibition of drug-metabolizing enzymes appears to be similar in young and elderly subjects.
- During pregnancy, CYP1A2 and *N*-acetyltransferase 2 activities are decreased, probably because hormonal factors play a role in the regulation of hepatic metabolism in humans. Moreover, CYP activity is inducible during pregnancy (see information on newborn patients above).
- Hypothermia
- Treatment duration, since the status of a slow or rapid acetylator appears to be capable of modification during the course of treatment with isoniazid
- P-gp and/or CYP enzyme overexpression in disease states:
  - Intestinal and hepatic human P-gp, but not CYP3A4, is strongly upregulated during tissue regeneration following acute rejection of an allograft. In the event of rejection, all P-gp substrates, including tacrolimus, sirolimus, and cyclosporine, will have to be administered intravenously to avoid extremely low levels in plasma. In this situation, the intestinal MDR1 mRNA level is a good probe for predicting inter-, and intraindividual variations in P-gp substrate oral pharmacokinetics, and optimal strategy in drug dosing.

Table 13 Urinary excretion of glucuronidation and sulfatation activities for paracetamol

Subject	Urinary excretion (% of administered dose)[a]	
	G	S
Newborn (0–2 days)	17	51
Child (3–9 yrs)	30	42
Adult	46	26

[a]G, glucuronidation; S, sulfatation.

- Such mRNA overexpressions have been described to occur with diabetes and obesity for CYP2E1.

4.2. Influence of Environmental Chemicals, Social Drugs, and Life Habits

Whittaker first began to demonstrate the important role played by the environment in interindividual variability in family studies in 1970.

The measurement of clearance (or of the elimination half-life) of antipyrine (phenazone) in various population groups (Table 14) made us aware as early as the 1970s of the importance of certain variation factors related to the environment or lifestyle. Antipyrine is a substrate for CYP1A2, -2A6, -2C9, -2C19, and -3A, in other words, a nonspecific CYP probe substrate, but a global one.

This highlights the problem of population sampling when studying drug-drug interactions, and questions what is a healthy subject. Thus, Vestal et al. (1975), studying the effect of age on antipyrine disposition, showed that some of the effects observed (metabolism was slower in elderly subjects and faster in women than in men) could be explained by cigarette smoking, and possibly coffee consumption, both of which were significantly greater in young men.

Since the 1970s, a large amount of data has been published on herbal products, beverages, supplements, social drugs, and dietary products, all of which are involved in documented interactions with commonly marketed drugs. Most often induction or inhibition of drug metabolism and/or membrane transport is postulated (Table 15).

Naturally, the extent of the interaction depends in all cases on the substrate tested, but only the interactions for which significant results were obtained are mentioned in Table 15. For further information, please consult futher references available from this author and the recent review from Harris et al. (2003).

In this area, the two most extensively studied products are St. John's wort and grapefruit juice. St. John's wort (*Hypericum perforatum*) is a minor antidepressant herbal product with very efficient intestinal and/or hepatic CYP3A4- and CYP2E1-inducing activity, particularly after long-term consumption, having a paradoxical effect on P-gp activity, since it is an inhibitor at the first dose and an inducer of this efflux protein after long-term administration. Some of the constituents of St. John's wort could be P-gp substrates and act as competitors before the progressive increase in activity as P-gp induction develops. St. John's wort induces the metabolism of amitryptiline, cyclosporine, indinavir, midazolam, simvastatin, saquinavir, theophylline, and oral contraceptives. Other data indicate that St. John's wort is not the only botanical supplement involved in herb-drug interactions (Table 15). This interaction currently constitutes a genuine problem in the United States, with as many as 16% of prescription drug users consuming herbal dietary supplements.

Grapefruit juice is first of all a potent inhibitor of intestinal CYP3A4: it causes an increase in the bioavailability of the substrates of this isoform only after oral administration and is without effect if the isoform is administered intravenously. An inhibitory effect has been demonstrated in particular on dihydropyridine-type calcium channel antagonists (felodipine, nicardipine, nifedipine, nimodipine nisoldipine, and nitrendipine, but not amlopidine), verapamil, astemizole, terfenadine, cisapride, statins, benzodiazepines, buspirone, carbamazepine, cyclosporine, tacrolimus, saquinavir (but not amprenavir), sildenafil, and ethinyl estradiol.

Grapefruit juice and the related 6′,7′-dihydroxybergamottin act as "suicide inhibitors" with selective targets (intestinal CYP enzyme). However, contrary to what is generally believed, the CYP3A4 enzyme is probably not the only target for grapefruit juice, based on the fact that it inhibits the metabolism of caffeine, which is a CYP1A2 probe, and the 7-hydroxylation of coumarins, which is a CYP2A6 pathway.

Lastly, grapefruit juice is a very weak inhibitor of intestinal P-gp and most probably an inhibitor of intestinal OATP.

Of course the magnitude of the interaction is dependent upon the commercial brand and batch of grapefruit juice used, as is a general rule with natural products.

Table 14 Antipyrine half-life in different populations

Population	Antipyrine half-life (h)
Contraceptive pill users ($n = 8$)	17.3
Vegetarian Asian females ($n = 11$)	16.7
Office workers ($n = 33$)	13.1[a]
Anesthesiologists exposed (≥3 wks) to anesthetic agents ($n = 8$)	10.7[b]
Barbecue consumers ($n = 8$)	10.7
Chronic ethanol consumers ($n = 9$)	9.0
London factory workers ($n = 31$)	9.1[c]
Insecticide factory workers ($n = 26$ males)	7.7
Barbiturate addicts ($n = 8$)	5.3

[a]With a seven-fold range, probably due to cigarette smoking.
[b]The antipyrine half-life was 13.1 h when the same anesthesiologists were not exposed to anesthetic agents (crossover study, $P < 0.05$).
[c]All of them chronically exposed to high levels of cigarette smoke.

4.3. Renal and Biliary Excretion

Like the renal tubular cell, the hepatocyte is equipped with influx transporters that allow passage through the basolateral membrane (an effect which is additional to the processes of simple diffusion). These are proteins related to OATP and OCTP found in the enterocyte; they are saturable and are probably subject to inhibition and activation in the same way as the efflux proteins (including P-gp) found at the luminal pole, and which allow extraction in the bile and urine. The enterocytic model applies fully here. It is in full accordance with a finalistic point of view: in the enterocyte, OATP and P-gp are thought to transport drug in opposite directions because fundamentally OATP serve as modulators for absorption of nutriments or otherwise essential life compounds, whereas P-gp acts protectively by limiting the systemic entry of xenobiotics. In the hepatocyte or in the renal tubular cell, the two membrane transporters act in the same direction in order to facilitate xenobiotic compound or endogenous toxic metabolite uptake by the sinusoidal cells (or the tubular cells), a step followed by bile (or tubular) secretion (cooperative effect).

Clarithromycin blocks the tubular secretion of digoxin by inhibition of renal P-gp, while cimetidine blocks the extraction of cations and probenecid blocks that of anions. Zwitterions at physiological pH, such as ofloxacin, levofloxacin, cefepime, cefpirome, and imipenem, therefore undergo an increase in their AUC on administration of cimetidine and probenecid. Inducers of the type of phenobarbital, spironolactone, and clofibrate promote the biliary excretion of cholephilic anions such as rifampin.

In the same way, dual inhibition of OATP and P-gp is encountered in some cases because of an overlapping

Table 15 Influence of environmental chemicals, social drugs, and life habits on epithelial cell transporter capacity and CYP enzyme activity

Substance	Transporters		CYPs				Other modifications
	OAT, OATP, OCTP	P-gp	1A2	2C9, 2C19	2E1	3A4[a]	
Induction							
Herbal products							
St. John's wort		⇑ (long term only)	⇑ (?)		⇑ (long term)	⇑ (acute and long term) [I + H]	⇑ 2D6 (?)
Ginkgo biloba				⇑			
Echinacea						⇑ (H)	
Beverages and supplements							
Jufeng grape juice			⇑				
Red wine							Dose dumping (with extended-release felodipine)
Boost-plus nutrition formulae							⇑ F% of posaconazole (C_{max} and AUC)
Chemicals and social drugs							
Organic solvents (acetone, benzene, pyridine, etc.)					⇑		
Halogenated insecticides (DDT, lindane, aldrin, Dieldrin)							⇑ Cl antipyrine
Cigarette smoke, cannabis smoke, and polycyclic aromatic procarcinogens			⇑		⇑		
Ethanol consumption (chronic)					⇑		⇑ Cl antipyrine
Alimentary products							
Cruciferous vegetables (all kind of cabbages) and alfalfa meals			⇑				
Garlic						⇑	
Myristicin[b]					⇑		
Pan-fried meat			⇑				
Charcoal-broiled meat			⇑				
Smoked meat			⇑				
Diverse							
Physical activity (chronic exercise, athletics)			⇑				⇑ Cl antipyrine
Oral contraceptives							⇑ UDP-glucuronyltransferase
Cedar chips for the bedding of laboratory animals							⇑ Cl antipyrine
Inhibition							
Herbal products							
Echinacea						⇓(I)	
Ginkgo biloba						⇓	
Ginseng						⇓	
Sho-saiko-to			⇓				⇓ xanthine oxidase

Beverages and supplements							
Grapefruit juice	⇓ (OATP)	⇓ (very weak)	⇓ (weak)	⇓		⇓ (I)	⇓ CYP 2A6 (coumarin)
Seville orange juice						⇓ (I)	
Lime juice						⇓ (weak)	
Orange or apple juice	⇓ (OATP)	⇓					
Calcium-fortified orange juice[c]	⇓ (OATP, Pep-T)	⇓					FQ-ion complexes
Cranberry juice				⇓ (↑ warfarin effect)			
Red wine (but not white wine)						⇓	
Ensure nutrition formula							⇓ AUC gatifloxacin
Vitamin C (1–3 g/day)		⇓ (indinavir)					⇓ Acetaminophen sulfatation
Water-soluble vitamin E		⇓					
Social drugs							
Ethanol consumption (acute)					⇓		
Tetrahydrocannabinol							⇓ Cl antipyrine
Alimentary products							
Apiaceous vegetables: dill weed, celery, parsley, parsnip, carrot			⇓				
Mustard green family vegetables : kale, collard greens, kohlrabi, brussels sprouts, broccoli, watercress, mustard					⇓ (↑ isoniazid concns)		
Phenylethylisothiocyanate[d]					⇓		
Garlic oil (due to diallyl sulfide)					⇓		
Peppermint oil						⇓	
Diverse							
Oral contraceptive[e]			⇓	⇓		⇓	⇓ CYP2B6
Hormone replacement therapy[f]			⇓			0	⇓ CYP 2B6
Inert excipient: Cremophor RH 40		⇓					

[a]I, at the intestinal level; H, at the hepatic level.
[b]Myristicin is a naturally occurring benzodioxole compound found in nutmeg, carrots, and flavoring agents.
[c]Calcium-fortified orange juice decreases FQ bioavailability through three potential mechanisms: (i) formation of nonabsorbable FQ-ion complexes (with a magnitude of effect which could look like the one observed after milk consumption considering the low calcium dosing), (ii) inhibitory effect of the divalent cation on Pep-T1-mediated intestinal transport, and (iii) inhibitory effect of orange juice on OATP or eventually on OCTN (this hypothesis has never been studied, but ofloxacin and levofloxacin are substrates for OCTN). The magnitude of the global effect will probably be more important for FQ which are carried by one or more of the influx proteins (Pep-T1 and OATP).
[d]A dietary compound derived from cruciferous vegetables.
[e]Ethinyl estradiol plus desogestrel.
[f]Estradiol plus levonorgestrel.

substrate specificity between transport proteins. For example, when fexofenadine and verapamil are coadministered, the bioavailability and the K_a of fexofenadine are increased likely because of a dual decreasing of OATP-mediated sinusoidal uptake, and P-gp-mediated canalicular secretion.

Other major interactions with the efflux proteins of anions (probably of the MRP type) have been reported:

- Inhibition of the hepatobiliary excretion of cyclosporine by ceftriaxone
- Inhibition of hepatic uptake and/or tubular secretion of methotrexate by mezlocillin, amoxicillin, or probenecid

In both cases, cyclosporine and methotrexate, the concentrations in serum rapidly attain toxic values, requiring caution to be exercised with any combination of cyclosporine or methotrexate and one of the three products mentioned above, as well as with weak organic acids with pronounced biliary elimination, such as piperacillin, azlocillin, ceftriaxone, and rifampin, and with β-lactams with marked tubular secretion. This type of combination requires regular therapeutic monitoring. It should be added that the toxicity of methotrexate is itself enhanced by combination with cyclosporine, NSAIDs, and co-trimoxazole.

It should be noted under the heading of beneficial interactions that the measurement of the glomerular filtration rate by means of creatinine clearance can be improved by the administration of cimetidine: this compound in fact significantly reduces the proportion of tubular secretion of creatinine and thus corrects the excess values commonly observed, particularly when glomerular clearance is low. This interaction may be assimilated with the reduction in the secretion of creatinine during treatment with trimethoprim.

In addition, it is still the case that by promoting the dissociation of weak organic acids, alkalinization of the urine blocks their passive reabsorption and thus increases their renal elimination rate, and that the opposite is observed with weak bases. Matters become more complicated when the drug is a combination of a weak organic acid and a weak organic base, which is the case with co-trimoxazole, since here any change in pH, by promoting the urinary elimination of one of the two combined compounds, modifies the concentration ratio of these two active substances in the plasma and tissues and possibly, in the case of co-trimoxazole, the level of synergy.

Regarding active tubular reabsorption, it can be said that even now matters are not clear. Lastly, a cocktail of markers to measure simultaneously the individual renal handling pathways has recently been developed and could be used to evaluate risk factors for drug-drug interactions at this level.

4.4. Transintestinal Secretion

The possibility of transintestinal elimination of antibiotic compounds in the unchanged form in humans was demonstrated for the first time with doxycycline in 1974. Since then it has been shown that clarithromycin and certain FQ, particularly ciprofloxacin, also exhibited mixed plasma clearance involving renal, hepatic, and transintestinal elimination. This transintestinal elimination is also found with paclitaxel (Taxol) and docetaxel (Taxotere) as well as with digoxin, talinolol, and irinotecan. The transporter most commonly involved in transintestinal secretion is P-gp, owing to the fact that digoxin and talinolol are considered pure P-gp probes in humans. However, some other transport proteins could be involved.

Using in vivo segmental intestinal perfusion with a specific multiluminal perfusion catheter and inflatable polypropylene balloons, Drescher et al. (2003) demonstrated that digoxin transintestinal secretion could both be significantly induced by rifampin, a P-gp inducer (jejunal elimination increased by 170%), and inhibited by quinidine, a P-gp inhibitor (jejunal elimination halved). In the same way, doxycycline, which is not known to be extensively metabolized, has a half-life that is a third of the usual after 10 days of barbiturates, and its concentrations are halved after rifampin pretreatment. This drug-drug interaction might explain the treatment failures during brucellosis therapy despite the constantly high and uniform tetracycline sensitivity of *Brucella* spp. Lastly, Westphal et al. (2000) demonstrated 35 and 21% decreases in oral and intravenous AUCs of talinolol, respectively, after 6 days of rifampin administration and simultaneously a fourfold increase in duodenal P-gp content.

At the same time, it should be noted that segmental analysis of the intestinal absorption of ciprofloxacin shows that the extent of this absorption, like transintestinal secretion, decreases from the jejunum to the colon; in other words, it is directly dependent on the number of enterocyte transporters. It is not currently possible to determine whether these are the same transporters operating in both directions, from the apical pole to the basolateral pole and vice versa, or whether these are two different types of transporters.

5. STUDY OF CLINICAL INTERACTION PROFILES

The function of the efflux system may be to prevent uptake of toxic substrates and to facilitate the excretion of these substrates across the mucosa of the intestinal tract. This is the reason why enterocytes as well as hepatocytes have been characterized as polarized cells.

In light of all the data presented previously, it is possible to define theoretical profiles of variation according to the example in Fig. 3, taken in part from Benet et al. (2003), given that evidence for dual inhibition (enzyme plus transporter) as well as cooperative effect (enzyme plus transporter) has been produced to date only for P-gp–CYP3A4, although this does not exclude other processes of the same kind.

From the point of view of strict kinetic macroconstants, the changes shown in Fig 3 should result in the changes illustrated in Fig. 4. Often a simple decision tree might be applied to the model we have just seen, as in the example of the interaction between grapefruit juice and CYP3A4 substrates.

The initial question is, by what mechanism(s) does grapefruit juice modify the oral clearance of the substrates of CYP3A4? This entails answering the following questions in turn:

1. Is the presystemic enzyme inhibition hepatic and/or intestinal?

Data. Grapefruit juice alters the oral clearance of the principal substrates of CYP3A4, without altering their elimination half-lives. Grapefruit juice does not alter the kinetics of the same drugs (felodipine, nifedipine, nicardipine, midazolam, and cyclosporine) when they are administered intravenously.

Answer. Grapefruit juice does not affect hepatic metabolism. The interaction occurs strictly in the enterocyte.

2. In view of the frequent P-gp–CYP3A4 cooperation, is P-gp involved in this interaction or is the OATP influx protein also often associated with CYP3A4?

	Intestine			Liver		Kidney	BBB and other tissues
	Efflux apical	Absorption apical	Efflux basolateral	Efflux apical/basolateral	Absorption basolateral	Efflux	Efflux (luminal membrane)
INHIBIT							
Transporter	⇓	⇓	⇑	⇑	⇓		
Enzyme	⇓	⇓	⇓	⇓	⇓	⇓	⇓
Enzyme + transporter	⇓⇓	⇓⇓	⇔⇑⇓	⇔⇑⇓	⇓⇓		
INDUCE							
Transporter	⇑	⇑	⇓	⇓	⇑		
Enzyme	⇑	⇑	⇑	⇑	⇑	⇑	⇑
Enzyme + transporter	⇑⇑	⇑⇑	⇔⇑⇓	⇔⇑⇓	⇑⇑		

Figure 3 Postulated changes in substrate metabolism as a function of enzyme and transporter inhibition and induction (adapted from Benet et al., 2003)

VS control		F %	Cmax	t1/2β	Cl_R	Cl_{NR}	Cl_R/Cl_{NR}
INDUCERS							
CYP inducer	• Intestinal level	⇓	⇓	0	0	0	0
	• Hepatic level	⇓	⇓	⇓	0	⇓	⇑
	• Both	⇓	⇓	⇓	0	⇓	⇑
Efflux transport inducer		⇓	⇓	⇓ (4) 0 (5)	⇑ (1)	⇓ (2)	⇑ (3)
CYP + efflux transport inducer		⇓	⇓	⇓	⇑ (1)	⇓	⇑
INHIBITORS							
CYP inhibitor	• Intestinal level	⇑	⇑	0	0	0	0
	• Hepatic level	⇑	⇑	⇑	0	⇑	⇓
	• Both	⇑	⇑	⇑	0	⇑	⇓
Efflux transport inhibitor		⇑	⇑	⇑ 0 (5)	⇓	⇓	⇓⇑
CYP + efflux transport inhibitor		⇑	⇑	⇑	⇓	⇑	⇓

Figure 4 Theoretical pharmacokinetic modifications in an induction or inhibition process

- If tubular transporters are involved
- If canalicular transporters and/or transintestinal secretion are involved
- Indicates the system most strongly induced clinically
- If tubular/canalicular and/or transintestinal secretion is involved
- Only intestinal efflux transporters are involved

Note that the possible induction and inhibition of the absorption transport process are not included

Data. Grapefruit juice has virtually no effect on the pharmacokinetics of oral digoxin, which is a specific P-gp probe substrate (C_{max} is increased only 21% [not significant]). When fexofenadine, both a P-gp and an OATP inhibitor, is administered with grapefruit juice, both the rate (C_{max}) and extent (AUC_t [experimental AUC]) of this H_2 receptor antagonist are reduced by 35%.

Answer. Inhibition of intestinal OATP (but not P-gp) is responsible for some of the effects observed on coadministration of fexofenadine and grapefruit juice.

Conclusion. In the event of dual participation of CYP3A4 and intestinal OATP in the metabolism of a substrate, both will be inhibited by grapefruit juice. Conversely, if only P-gp is involved in the presystemic metabolism of a drug, no drug interaction is to be expected with grapefruit juice.

Nevertheless, however logical it may be, Fig. 4 provides no quantitative information, nor does it take account of associated factors, such as environment and disease. However, the example of digoxin might give us an idea of the natural complexity of affairs in a theoretically simple situation since digoxin is only a simple substrate of P-gp not metabolized by CYPs. The effects of pretreatment with a P-gp inducer, rifampin, may be compared with that of a P-gp inhibitor, itraconazole (Fig. 5).

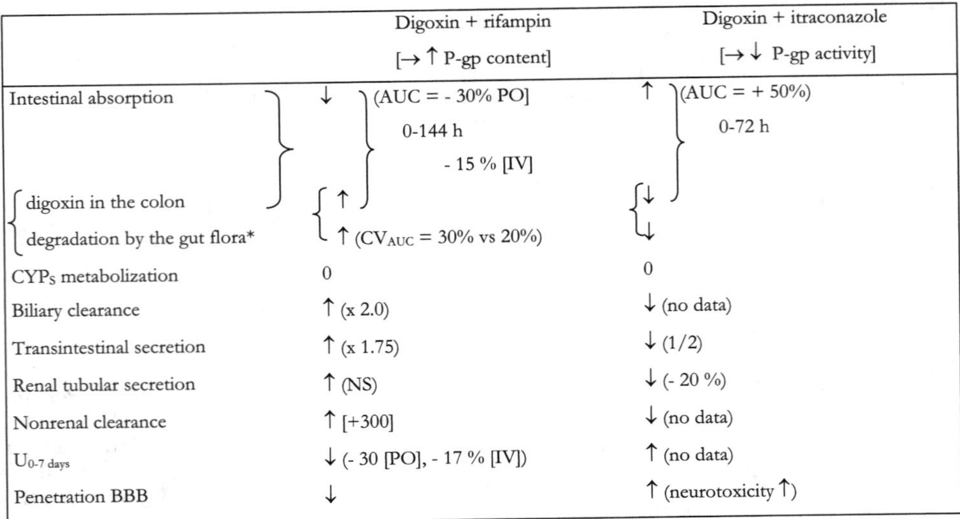

	Digoxin + rifampin [→ ↑ P-gp content]	Digoxin + itraconazole [→ ↓ P-gp activity]
Intestinal absorption	↓ (AUC = - 30% PO] 0-144 h; - 15 % [IV]	↑ (AUC = + 50%) 0-72 h
digoxin in the colon	↑	↓
degradation by the gut flora*	↑ (CV_{AUC} = 30% vs 20%)	↓
CYPs metabolization	0	0
Biliary clearance	↑ (x 2.0)	↓ (no data)
Transintestinal secretion	↑ (x 1.75)	↓ (1/2)
Renal tubular secretion	↑ (NS)	↓ (- 20 %)
Nonrenal clearance	↑ [+300]	↓ (no data)
$U_{0\text{-}7\ days}$	↓ (- 30 [PO], - 17 % [IV])	↑ (no data)
Penetration BBB	↓	↑ (neurotoxicity ↑)

Figure 5 Illustration of the digoxin-drug interaction case

Note in Fig. 5 that digoxin is inactivated via enzymatic reduction by the gut flora. Up to 40% of the administered dose can be reduced by *Eubacterium lentum*. Furthermore, it has been shown that there can be interethnic variations in the occurrence of this phenomenon. Thus, using a macrolide as a P-gp inhibitor leads quantitatively to results different from those obtained with itraconazole because antibiotic therapy reverses this bacterial process.

These results reveal three things:

- The highly inducible nature of intestinal P-gp, possibly enhanced by bacterial metabolism
- The equal in vivo effect (but how much?) of induction or inhibition of intestinal P-gp, again both possibly enhanced by the effect of colonic bacteria
- Finally, the lesser part played by tubular P-gp compared to biliary or intestinal extrarenal P-gp (or other efflux transporters) (nonrenal efflux transporters) (CL_R not modified by rifampin pretreatment)

It will be understood that under these conditions quantification becomes extremely difficult if the co-administered substrates are also the subject of hepatic and/or intestinal metabolism. The confusion will obviously be even greater if the inducer or inhibitor induces or inhibits its own metabolism, which is the case with the autoinhibition of clarithromycin, for instance, or the conventional autoinductions of carbamazepine or phenytoin. In the case of high risk, only a plasma assay of the different drugs will elucidate the levels of interaction.

6. PROSPECTS

In the near future, pharmacogenetic information may refine the appraisal of drug-drug interactions. The term pharmacogenetic information is used here to mean patient-specific information about the sequence or expression of genes involved in drug kinetics or effects. Genetic variability arises from gene deletion, single nucleotide polymorphism, or gene duplication. Any protein may be prone to such variability, especially drug-metabolizing enzymes, transporters, and receptors. To date, pharmacokinetic variability due to metabolizing enzymes has been studied most. As a result, patients may be classified as poor, extensive, or ultraextensive metabolizers for a given metabolizing isoenzyme. Examples of polymorphisms affecting CYP450 are given in Table 3. Other important examples of polymorphic enzymes are NAT2 (*N*-acetyltransferase) and GST M1 (glutathione transferase), which affect isoniazid metabolism, and UDP-glucuronyltransferases, which are involved in the glucuronidation of many drugs.

Pharmacogenetic information may be obtained by genotyping or phenotyping. Genotyping is performed using blood, saliva, hair roots, or buccal swabs and involves DNA extraction and sequencing. Phenotyping requires either (i) administration of a drug probe, repeated blood or urine collection, measurement of drug and metabolite, and calculation of a metabolic index or (ii) direct assessment of enzyme activity if the enzyme is in plasma or in blood cells. In the latter case, enzyme activity in blood may not be well correlated with that in other tissues such as liver. Consequently, genotyping is more practical than phenotyping. However, it must be stressed that not all genetic alterations result in a clinically relevant modification of drug kinetics or effect and that results can vary according to the substrate and site, while many environmental, physiological, and pathological factors add to the genetically induced variability. In other words, the genotype of an individual does not vary, but the phenotype may. Furthermore, whenever alternative clearance pathways can compensate for underdeveloped (in the case of neonates) or deficient elimination pathways, it becomes difficult to know the exact contribution of those alternative pathways. Thus, the relevance of pharmacogenetic information for drug prescription will have to be established by prospective studies case by case.

With these limits and warnings in mind, pharmacogenetic information may have a significant impact on a number of drug-drug interactions (for usual CYP probe subtrates, see Table 16).

Poor metabolizers of isoniazid have increased isoniazid concentrations in plasma, which may result in a stronger inducing effect of CYP2E1 and inhibiting effect of CYP2C19 and CYP3A.

Poor CYP2C19 metabolizers may have (i) increased voriconazole levels, enhancing its inhibition of CYP3A4,

Table 16 Substrates usually used as specific CYP probes

CYP family	Substrate(s)
1A2	Caffeine
2A6	Coumarin
2B6	Bupropion
2C9	Diclofenac, phenytoin, tolbutamide, warfarin
2C19	S-Mephenytoin
2D6	Debrisoquin, dextromethorphan, sparteine
2E1	Chlorzoxazone
3A4	Dapsone, erythromycin, midazolam, nifedipine

and (ii) increased omeprazole concentrations, resulting in higher gastric pH and stronger inhibition of CYP1A2.

Poor CYP2C9 metabolizers have (i) increased phenytoin levels, which may have a greater inducing effect on CYP2C and CYP3A isoenzymes, and (ii) a lower clearance of warfarin, resulting presumably in an increased interaction with sulfamethoxazole.

These examples show that some patients with specific genetic alterations of metabolizing enzymes may be more severely affected by drug-drug interactions. Other kinds of alteration (P-gp, etc.) probably have a similar impact on individual susceptibility to interactions, but data are still lacking.

7. EVALUATION OF POTENTIAL DRUG-DRUG INTERACTIONS

Nowadays, evaluation of potential drug-drug interactions is mandatory for the registration of new drugs by regulatory agencies. This is why the methodological aspect of such evaluation has been particularly studied in the past few years. The two main points to consider are

- The problem of in vitro/in vivo, and animal/human extrapolation
- The methodology to apply in association with an interaction study conducted with humans

The two basic questions to be answered are (i) does the new drug influence the metabolism of other compounds, and (ii) is the metabolism of the candidate drug altered by other compounds that could be administered concomitantly in clinical practice?

Over and above that, this methodological approach should allow a more critical reading of the literature by the nonspecialist.

7.1. In Vitro and In Vivo Data and Animal and Human Extrapolation

Prediction of in vivo metabolic clearance from in vitro data is still difficult, and controversial. Despite well-documented examples showing a good in vitro and in vivo correlation in humans and other animal species, no general consensus has been reached about the parameters and experimental strategies to be used.

If in vitro and/or animal screening is opted for in order to establish an initial risk profile, it is then essential when in vitro models are used to study separately (i) the risks of interaction involving transporters (models expressing OATP, OCTP, P-gp, MRT, etc.) and (ii) the risks involving a metabolic interaction.

There are two reasons for this. First, the dissociations in the behavior of P-gp and CYP are nowadays sufficiently documented for it no longer to be acceptable simply to extrapolate from data observed with CYP alone. Second, there are transporters other than P-gp that behave totally independently of CYP.

7.1.1. Preliminary Stage: Study of the Structure-Activity Relationships

At both levels, intestinal (and/or hepatic) membrane transporter and CYP enzymes, a quantitative two-dimensional (2D) or 3D structure-property relationship or structure-activity relationship (QSAR) can be used to predict whether a certain drug will be a potent substrate for the transporter or the enzyme acceptor site tested.

For transporters, two cases can be distinguished, (i) carrier-mediated transport and (ii) efflux mechanisms.

Carrier-mediated transport is a natural means for nutrients to gain access to intracellular sites. Thus, we can broadly assume that all drugs that structurally mimic the corresponding natural substrates of a given carrier will be effectively taken up by this transporter. This has been applied with success to the description of Pep-T1 substrates and has allowed a better understanding of drug-drug interactions at this level (e.g., L-3,4-dihydroxyphenylalanine β-lactam antibiotics or ACE [agonist converting enzyme] β-lactam antibiotics), as well as the prodrug design of the L-valine esters of acyclovir and related substances (valacyclovir and valganciclovir) and AZT (L-valyl-AZT) so as to make them readily transportable substrates for Pep-T1 and thus improve their bioavailability. Recently, a 3D substrate template has been developed using molecular modeling. This new model can discriminate between substrates that will be transported with high, medium, or low efficiency and thus probably give a better insight into drug-drug interactions at this level.

However, an increasing number of active transporters are being discovered, often without a clear natural substrate specificity, which complicates the identification of a substrate recognition pattern. This is the problem encountered with efflux proteins which per se are relatively "substrate aspecific" because of their role of limiting the penetration of all xenobiotics. However, consistent patterns have been proposed to characterize P-gp substrates as well as P-gp inducers, so a more comprehensive use and molecular choice of compounds within a large structurally related family is becoming possible in specific clinical fields. Thus, by using glucocorticoids data and 3D QSAR techniques, Yates et al. (2003) developed a model able to reveal molecular regions that contribute to rendering a molecule a P-gp substrate, a model in accordance with previous reports on vinblastine transport. In turn, their approach could be used to specifically design compounds with lower or, at the opposite, higher P-gp affinity in order to, respectively, increase or decrease intracellular concentration and/or tissue penetration (e.g., brain access and oral bioavailability). Right now it explains why a very high dose of intravenous methylprednisolone is needed in spinal cord injury patients in order to compensate for poor spinal cord access, and as a whole, this may lead to treatment with a glucocorticoid while being not a good substrate for P-gp, as with dexamethasone.

Some advances have been made in QSAR model development to enable drug-CYP3A4 interaction to be predicted with reasonable accuracy. Actually, the great difficulty can be how drug designers can combine the QSAR proposals leading to maximal pharmacological effect with those maximizing P-gp (or any other protein transporter) activity without omitting the possibility of a dual effect of P-gp and CYP.

7.1.2. P-gp and Other Transport Proteins

A fairly large number of in vitro tests have been developed for the purpose of screening new molecules. These tests sometimes lack specificity and may pose problems of interpretation insofar as they do not always meet the requirements:

- The cell line chosen must be able to express all of the transporters responsible for taking up the drug or drugs tested.
- The model must allow the study of phenomena of both inhibition and induction: Cao-2 is not suitable for induction studies.
- The saturability of the transporters should be evaluated in relation to the expected concentrations (always very high in the lumen of the digestive tract, for example).
- The measurement of efflux should only be global, but a distinction must be drawn between absorption efflux at the apical pole and secretion efflux at the basolateral pole: this at least avoids the fear of an interaction in the absorption phase for drugs with transintestinal secretion and essentially paracellular penetration (doxycycline).

However, all of these precautions do not totally prevent in vitro and in vivo dissociations, which may be explained to some extent by the following:

- Either, since excretory organs (kidney and liver) or tissues such as BBB are involved, by the in vivo existence of endogenous inhibitors (see Fig. 1)
- Or, in the case of oral absorption, by the failure to allow for local pH, which varies throughout the gut (from 6.4 to 8.0) and which helps modify the ionized fraction and hence the transport capacities. Finally, it has also been shown that cellular models function only over a certain range of coefficients of influx.

Consequently, it can be seen that in the best-case scenario, only the qualitative objective can be achieved. This involves screening tests, which may be supplemented by the use of an isolated organ or the whole animal. However, even with the latter it must be realized that, firstly, transporter activities vary from one species to another (and P-gp is not the only one that needs to be considered), and, secondly, animals reflect the polymorphism observed in humans to only a limited extent.

7.1.3. CYP

Nowadays, it is easy to know which CYPs are involved in the metabolism of a drug, and the first metabolic studies undertaken with humans rapidly provide us with information about the different metabolic pathways adopted and their relative importance.

From this, it is possible to establish the list of candidate drugs likely to act as inducers or inhibitors of these molecules.

In the same way, it is possible to determine whether the drug can itself behave as a metabolic inducer or inhibitor in suitable cell lines expressing the CYP to be studied.

This prerequisite makes it possible to identify fairly clearly the risks of interaction with a given product. However, it does not enable this risk to be quantified. In vitro studies provide only qualitative information. Moreover, on this subject, there are as many examples of in vitro studies that are predictive as there are of such studies that are nonpredictive of what will be observed in humans.

7.1.3.1. Major Causes of Discrepancies between In Vitro and In Vivo Data

Discrepancies between in vitro and in vivo data can be caused by a number of factors.

The first factor is the in vitro experimental design, including in vitro enzyme instability, relative abundance of CYPs, linearity of the assay, microsomal protein concentrations, clinically nonrelevant drug concentrations, inappropriate choice of test concentrations (e.g., circulating free concentration, whereas binding is permissive), nonspecific protein binding, and experimental conditions which preclude the development of an inducer effect (time problem, cell line problem, etc.).

Second, discrepancies between in vitro and in vivo data might reflect involvement of extrahepatic metabolism, including drug metabolism by intestinal microorganisms (e.g., digoxin and other drugs) with a possibility in this case of ethnic variability due to different diets.

Discrepancies might also be due to active transport by the liver. This problem of active transport raises in a different form that of the choice of the experimental concentration to be used: total concentration or free fraction. The "free drug" hypothesis does not work when plasma drug binding is permissive (or essentially permissive) rather than restrictive; it all depends on the ratio of the plasma association constant of the drug to its cellular (or tissue) association constant. Essentially, it is this ratio which governs the fraction of compound available for tissue extraction (capillary transit time also plays a role to a certain extent). Thus, in summary, it may be said that the generally accepted free-drug hypothesis cannot work when the drug penetrates hepatocytes by an active process and concentrates in the cells. This has been described for cimetidine and itraconazole inhibition of midazolam, a CYP3A4 substrate, in rat liver: the in vitro K_i of itraconazole for midazolam CYP3A4 inhibition is far higher than its steady-state free fraction in plasma (270 versus 5.3 nM). Although no systemic interaction would have been predicted, itraconazole has been shown to be a potent inhibitor of systemic clearance of midazolam because part (or all) of the total steady-state concentration of the antifungal (2.7 μM for 200 mg twice a day) is available for intrahepatic CYP3A4 inhibition.

Further, discrepancies between in vitro and in vivo data might reflect the failure to consider the inhibition of an enterocytic efflux transporter which enhances the inhibitory effect observed on CYP alone in the case of dual P-gp/CYP3A substrates (e.g., ritonavir increases the AUC of saquinavir 15 to 20 times more than was expected from metabolic studies). The same remark applies to the interactions with an inducer of both P-gp and CYP3A4.

In general, we raise here the problem of cooperation (and/or synergy) of intestinal transporters and the two successive stages of metabolization, intestinal followed by hepatocytic, which the hepatocyte model alone cannot predict (microsomes, cell culture, etc.), even if an attempt is made in the modeling used to include intestinal enzyme activity by measuring enterocytic microsomal activity, for example.

This is complicated further still if it is considered that there is a sex effect over and above these data; by way of example, the level of P-gp is twice as high in men as in women, while CYP3A activity is the same. The fact that P-gp activity is greater in men also results in a higher first-pass effect (by a specific P-gp effect and also by a cooperative effect) and hence a lower AUC in men than in women and a likewise lower oral clearance. This result, generally obtained in vivo with CYP3A substrates, is obviously not consistent with the in vitro measurements of simple metabolism since at this level there is no sex effect.

The analysis of the possible risk of a sex effect should take account of the behavior of each of the proteins, transport proteins as well as metabolism enzymes, involved in the kinetics of all of the partners combined (Table 17).

Table 17 Suggested gender differences in selected drug transporters and metabolizing enzymes

Protein function	Protein(s)	Sex effect[a]
Drug transporters		
Efflux	P-gp	M > F
	MRP	M = F
Absorption	OATP	M = F
	OCTP	M > F
Phase I metabolizing enzymes	CYP1A2	M > F
	CYP2C9, CYP2C19	M = F
	CYP2D6	F > M
	CYP2E1	M ≥ F
	CYP3A4	M = F
Phase II metabolizing enzymes	UDP-G[b]	M > F
	Sulfotransferase	M > F
	N-Acetyltransferases	M = F
	Methyltransferases	M > F

[a]M, male; F, female.
[b]UDP-G, UDP-glucuronyltransferases.

From Table 17 we can see that sex differences in the metabolism of CYP3A4 substrates are actually due to sex differences in P-gp and will only occur for substrates of both CYP3A4 and P-gp. In addition, it is interesting that the work of Gurley et al. (2002) hardly suggests a sexual dimorphism in CYP3A4 inducibility by St. John's wort and that the CYP3A4-inducing effect of rifampin (midazolam being the substrate) seems to be greater in men in the case of presystemic metabolism but greater in women for systemic metabolism. However, no such sex difference was noted in CYP2E1-induced activity.

Another possible factor in discrepancies in in vitro and in vivo data is the combination of both an enzyme inducer and inhibitor (see section 4.1.2.1).

An interaction dependent on the modes of administration might also contribute to discrepancies. For example, St. John's wort is first of all an inhibitor of P-gp in short-term administration and then an inducer after prolonged administration.

The participation of substrate metabolites in drug-drug interactions at both levels, drug transport proteins (absorptive proteins as well as efflux proteins) and CYP enzymes, could also lead to discrepancies. Preliminary results for tacrolimus and sirolimus suggest that their metabolites formed in the small intestinal mucosa and secreted back on the luminal side of the enterocyte could compete with the parent drug for the different transporters available. In the same way, when it is considered that the half-life of pefloxacin increases substantially over time from 10 to 12 h at day 1 to 20 h at day 10, it may be postulated that pefloxacin metabolites (most probably norfloxacin, which is an inhibitor of CYP3A4) compete with the parent drug for CYP metabolism.

A further factor in discrepancies between in vitro and in vivo data is dissociation of effect between the intestinal cell and the hepatic cell. Echinacea, an herbal remedy CYP3A4 modulator, induces midazolam metabolism hepatically and inhibits it intestinally.

Despite an in vitro K_i (50 to 75 μM) for CYP3A4 well above the usual steady-state concentrations in plasma (total, 339 nM; unbound, 75 nM), diltiazem is an effective inhibitor of the oral clearance of a number of CYP3A4 substrates (cyclosporine, quinidine, and numerous benzodiazepines). In fact, diltiazem is oxidized by CYP3A4 to a second metabolite which is a considerably more potent CYP3A4 inhibitor than the parent drug (didesmethyl diltiazem; $K_i = 100$ nM).

The existence of interindividual variability (polymorphism, sex, environmental factors, dietary habits, etc.) and nonlinear pharmacokinetics can lead to discrepancies.

One of the major pitfalls leading to discrepancies is the existence of a mechanism-based enzyme inactivation which is irreversible and extremely difficult to quantify despite sophisticated modeling processes.

It remains to be determined on the basis of what criteria other than measurements of circulating concentrations might it be possible to predict the highly variable level of interaction observed between grapefruit juice and the 13 drugs listed in Table 18, a variability which is not altered when they are grouped by chemical family (see the four statin studies presented in Table 18).

These are all potential reasons for resorting to the isolated organ or preferably the whole animal.

However, before using animals for drug-drug interaction studies, comparative studies using liver microsomes or cells from animals and humans will be of great value in the justifiable selection of animals, not only because of different CYPs expressed in humans and other species but also because of their relative abundance, the predominant isoform usually differing from one species to another. In the particular field of antibiotic therapy, the example of the metabolism of pefloxacin perfectly illustrates our proposition and shows that no animal species is suitable for conducting a complete interaction study with this compound (Table 19).

This is a very well-known difficulty for toxicologists. There are many examples of species-dependent toxic reactions, and some are shown in Table 20. In fact, many cases of species differences in response to toxic substances arise from metabolic differences, particularly in the metabolic pathways. In this case, one or more of the following are involved:

- Competing reactions (the most common occurrence and the most unpredictable event): the same metabolites are formed, but the relative amounts vary with the species. This kind of problem is typically illustrated by the pefloxacin example. The existence of a predominant isoform that is different from the human one, as well as probable interspecies differences in the geometry of the active sites, can:
  - Lead to the observation of a drug-drug interaction with this specific isoform which will not be relevant for humans

Table 18 AUC increases over baseline of 13 different drugs when administered with grapefruit juice

Compound	% AUC increase over baseline
Pravastatin	<50
Cyclosporine	50
Nimodipine	150
Midazolam, triazolam	150
Saquinavir	150
Atorvastatin	200
Felodipine	200
Terfenadine	250
Nisoldipine	500
Buspirone	900
Lovastatin	1,500
Simvastatin	1,600

Table 19 Mean urinary recovery of pefloxacin and main metabolites after oral administration of a single dose of pefloxacin[a]

Species	Unchanged pefloxacin	Norfloxacin	Oxoflacin-norfloxacin	Pefloxacin–*N*-oxide	Pefloxacin-glucuronide	Norfloxacin/pefloxacin ratio
Mouse	++++	0	0	+	+++	0
Rat	++	++	0	+++	++++	1
Dog	+	+	0	+++	++++	1
Monkey	++	+++	(+)	+	(+)	1.6
Human	+++	++++	+	++++	0	2.3

[a]Results are expressed as a fraction of the administered dose on the following scale: ++++, 14 to 23%; +++, 9 to 12%; ++, 6 to 7%; and (+), 2 to 3% (adapted from Montay et al., 1984).

Table 20 Species-dependent toxic effects of chemicals

Compound	Toxicity	Reactive species	Nonreactive species
Phenylthiourea	Pulmonary edema	Rat	Rhesus monkey
Norbormide	Respiratory failure	Rat	Cat, dog, mouse
DDT	Weak carcinogen	Mouse	Hamster
3-Methylcholanthrene	Carcinogen	Mouse and rat	Rhesus monkey
Thalidomide	Teratogen	Rabbit	Hamster

- Mask an interaction involving a different CYP in humans
- Species defects in common metabolic reactions: some species appear to lack the capacity to carry out certain metablic reactions (Table 21). For example, the rat does not form 14-OH clarithromycin, so this species cannot be used to predict a possible interaction involving the metabolism of clarithromycin, such as inhibition of the formation of 14-OH clarithromycin with ritonavir.
- Occurrence of uncommon reactions: more unusually, a number of metabolic reactions appear to be largely restricted to humans and other primate species, e.g., the metabolic conjugation of phenylacetic acid. In humans and in monkey species, this compound is largely conjugated with glutamine, whereas in subprimates glycine is utilized.

The same applies to induction capacities, which vary from species to species for the same product. For example, rifampin is a potent inducer in humans and rabbits but a poor inducer in rats; in contrast, pregnenolone-16α-carbonitrile, a potent inducer of CYP3A in rats, is not an inducer in either rabbits or humans.

The phenomena of enzyme inhibition are no exception either, as 8-methoxypsoralen is a suicide inactivator of the rat CYP3A4 isoform, but in humans it appears to be selective for CYP2A6. In addition, quinidine is a more potent inhibitor of CYP2D activity in human liver microsomes than in rat liver microsomes, while the reverse is observed for quinine.

Table 21 Species defects in common metabolic reactions

Defective reaction	Species
N-Hydroxylation of aliphatic amines	Rat
Glucuronide formation	Cat, Gunn rat
Sulfate formation	Pig, opossum
Arylamine acetylation	Dog, fox
Mercapturic acid formation	Guinea pig
Glycine conjugation	Fruit bat

These interspecies differences in behavior involve all of the protein binding phenomena: plasma proteins, transport proteins, membrane proteins, metabolism enzymes, and target proteins. For example, in the rat intestinal mucosa, P-gp abundance decreases gradually in the proximal to distal direction, whereas in humans, P-gp distribution follows the opposite pattern.

One final example: whereas in rabbits, *N*-acetylsulfamethazine, the normal metabolite of sulfamethazine, displaces the latter from its binding to albumin, multiplying the free fraction of this sulfonamide by 2 to 3, this interaction is not observed in humans.

All of these data raise the question of the place of animal studies in a context where the potential risks have already been identified in the in vitro phase and where the use of animals does not enable the risks to be quantified even after an allometric scaling approach.

Even if the most common interactions are of the competitive type and can usually be reasonably predicted simply by comparing K_is and from the knowledge of the expected concentrations, clinical studies are now essential, whatever the circumstances. The recent work by Skarke et al. (2003) on quinidine-morphine interactions indicates clearly the inconsistency of animal models: in vitro data and the animal model agreed in suggesting that quinidine P-gp inhibition would result in elevated plasma and CNS morphine concentrations and hence an increase in its pharmacodynamic effect. However, both the pharmacokinetics and the pharmacodynamics were similar after quinidine and placebo treatment in healthy volunteers.

We raise a major question here because it is generally assumed in regulatory guidelines that negative results in in vitro studies can eliminate the need for further clinical investigation, as is pointed out by Christians et al. (2002) in the discussion of major discrepancies between the in vitro and in vivo evaluations of tacrolimus with false-negative in vitro results. This kind of recommendation has the potential to overlook clinically significant drug interactions.

7.2. Clinical Evaluation: Methodological Problems

In light of the general issues and numerous examples that have been presented above, it is easy to understand why drug interaction studies in humans must be designed on the basis of up-to-date knowledge. Several major questions, among others, need to be addressed before planning a study:

- What is known about the presumed drug-drug interaction from in vitro studies, preclinical studies, and/or clinical studies with related drugs?
- What is the primary goal of the clinical study? A pure research strategy, aiming to characterize better the mechanism(s) of the interaction, or a more regulatory approach, aiming to evaluate the clinical relevance of the interaction?
- What are the doses and dosage schedules that are most appropriate to the primary goal of the study?
- Should the study be conducted with healthy volunteers or with patients?
- Should the results of the study be readily transposable to different subgroups, such as young people, elderly people, young women, patients with renal and/or hepatic insufficiency, or other subgroups?

It would be beyond the scope of this chapter to debate each of these questions, but the interested reader can find valuable information in a recent work published by Nix and Gallicano (2001). Here, our objective is to present what seems to be the "gold standard" approach for handling drug interaction data.

7.2.1. Drug-Drug Interaction as an Equivalence Situation

In drug-drug interaction studies, the general purpose is to establish whether the pharmacokinetics or the pharmacodynamics of one drug, when given alone, can be modified by the concomitant administration of a second drug. Immediately, two questions arise: are the experimental data indicative of a true interaction? If so, what is the clinical relevance of this interaction? Biostatisticians are familiar with such questions, but clinicians are probably less so because the statistical approach required to answer them remains somewhat sophisticated.

7.2.1.1. Pharmacokinetic Interaction

In 1991, Steinijans et al. were the first to apply the methodology of bioequivalence assessment to the drug interaction situation, introducing the expression "lack of pharmacokinetic interaction." It may be recalled that bioequivalence studies focus on bioavailability outcomes and are of major importance in the field of generic drugs. To be convinced, it is necessary only to look at the extensive literature on the subject or to consider the large number of scientific meetings and symposia held all around the world during the last three decades in search of regulatory harmonization. It may be noted that the latest guidelines on bioequivalence testing were issued in 2002 by the Food and Drug Administration (FDA) (http://www.fda.gov/cder; see text 4964dft.doc, 10 July 2002) and in 2001 by the European Community (http://www.emea.eu.int; see text CPMP/EWP/QWP/1401/98, 26 July 2001).

Briefly, two medicinal products are bioequivalent if they are pharmaceutically equivalent (the same amount of the same active substance) and if their bioavailabilities after administration in the same molar dose are similar to such a degree in terms of rate and extent of systemic exposure that both efficacy and safety will be essentially the same. Translated into statistical language, bioequivalence testing is based on two null hypotheses (H01 and H02) of inequivalence and one alternative hypothesis (H1) of equivalence, defined by a specific equivalence criterion and limits. Different inequalities can be postulated, where μ_{Ref} and μ_{Test} are population average means of bioavailability and $\theta 1$ and $\theta 2$ are bioequivalence limits for the population criterion, such that:

- Null hypothesis H01: $(\mu_{Test} / \mu_{Ref}) < \theta 1$, with a P value of $H01 \leq \alpha$
- Null hypothesis H02: $(\mu_{Test} / \mu_{Ref}) > \theta 2$, with a P value of $H02 \leq \alpha$
- Alternative hypothesis H1: $\theta 1 \leq (\mu_{Test} / \mu_{Ref}) \leq \theta 2$, with a P value of $H1 \geqslant (1 - \beta)$

In this situation, the nominal α risk, or type I error, is the risk of falsely rejecting inequivalence (i.e., incorrectly accepting equivalence), and it represents the so-called consumer risk. The β risk, or type II error, is the risk of falsely rejecting equivalence (i.e., incorrectly accepting inequivalence), and it represents the so-called producer risk. The best decision-making rule that minimizes the consumer risk without being too conservative is based on the two one-tailed tests procedure, for either normally distributed variables or distribution-free variables. When the α risk is set at 0.05, this procedure is conveniently replaced by the 90% confidence interval (CI), an approach which offers a much easier interpretation. Here, bioequivalence is assumed to exist when the 90% CI for the ratio (μ_{Test}/μ_{Ref}) is entirely within a predefined equivalence range (usually ±20%, setting the lower limit, $\theta 1$, at 80% and the upper limit, $\theta 2$, at 120% for raw data or 125% for log-transformed data).

Thus, for drug-drug pharmacokinetic interactions, Steinijans et al. (1991) proposed retaining the bioequivalence statistical approach, while replacing the expression "bioequivalence" by the expression "lack of pharmacokinetic interaction." By so doing, the type I error becomes the risk of falsely rejecting the presence of interaction (i.e., incorrectly accepting the lack of interaction), while the type II error become the risk of falsely rejecting the lack of interaction (i.e., incorrectly accepting the interaction). In other words, assuming a correct study design, with a sample size large enough to give sufficient power and with properly defined interaction limits, the equivalence approach would be able, firstly, to detect an interaction and, secondly, to evaluate its importance in terms of clinical practice. The consumer risk (type I error) becomes the patient risk of receiving a probably harmful multiple drug prescription, while the producer risk (type II error) becomes a second patient risk, that of not receiving a useful multiple drug prescription. Here again, the advantage of the equivalence approach lies in its ability to control the patient risk at the chosen α level.

7.2.1.1.1. Choice of pharmacokinetic metrics. The construction of the plasma or serum concentration time curve is generally the first step in pharmacokinetic data analysis. However, there is no single statistical test comparing the shapes of two curves and allowing a simultaneous evaluation of the rate and extent of bioavailability. As a result, there are different methods of obtaining various metrics, ranging from direct graphic constants to complicated model-based estimates with underlying assumptions about the absorption process. In order to remain within the framework of usual drug-drug interaction studies, only metrics based on noncompartmental methods are presented here.

7.2.1.1.1.1. PRESYSTEMIC DRUG-DRUG INTERACTION. Whatever the mechanism and localizations involved (intestine and/or liver), presystemic drug interactions are likely to affect both the rate and extent of absorption. The most common method for assessing the rate of absorption remains the graphical presentation of C_{max}, together with the corresponding time of occurrence of C_{max} (T_{max}). By definition, both C_{max} and T_{max} are highly dependent on the discrete sampling scheme, and sometimes the number of experimental points in the first portion of the curve is much too small to provide a reliable measurement. C_{max} is also rather insensitive to changes in the rate of absorption. For this reason, several metrics have been proposed and evaluated for their performance in assessing bioequivalence. Among these, metrics such as the ratio (C_{max}/AUC) and partial AUC up to T_{max} (AUC_p), while never used, could probably be of particular interest in presystemic drug interactions, although this is not to underestimate the difficulty of defining the interaction limits.

The extent of absorption is comparatively much easier to characterize by the unchallenged metric AUC, calculated by means of various trapezoidal rules. Obviously, measuring circulating concentrations for at least four or five apparent half-lives is crucial in obtaining an accurate metric, especially when the interaction results in a prolonged elimination process. The recent concept of exposure (i.e., peak and total exposure), presumed to have a better clinical relevance than the rate of absorption for approval and regulatory needs, could also find an application in drug interaction. It is based on three metrics: one for early exposure that could be the partial area up to a cutoff point not necessarily being t_{max}, a second one for peak exposure, readily assessed by C_{max}, and a third one for total exposure, logically measured by AUC_{∞} or AUC_{lqc} (up to the last quantifiable concentration).

7.2.1.1.1.2. POSTSYSTEMIC DRUG-DRUG INTERACTION By postsystemic interactions are meant interactions affecting either the distribution phase (competition at protein binding sites), the metabolism phase (enzymatic induction or inhibition), or the elimination phase (renal and biliary routes). Accordingly, the determination of drug bound and free fractions, C_{max}, AUC_{∞}, systemic and renal clearances, terminal elimination half-life, and ratio of AUC_{∞} to terminal half-life can serve as characteristic measurement metrics. When the interaction is related to drug-metabolizing enzymes, quantification of one or more metabolites in addition to the parent drug should be required in order to calculate metabolic (phenotype) ratios, whenever an optimized blood sampling schedule has been anticipated in the study protocol.

7.2.1.2. Pharmacodynamic Interaction

Clinical studies involving a pharmacodynamic approach to evaluate drug-drug interactions are very rare in comparison to those involving the pharmacokinetic approach. However, a pharmacodynamic interaction could also be viewed as an equivalence situation or, more precisely, as a noninferiority situation. A noninferiority trial is a trial where the main goal is to show that an experimental treatment is clinically and statistically not inferior to an active control. For this, the major issues relate to the selection of the active control (or reference treatment), the quantification of its efficacy (from previous placebo-controlled trials), and the determination of the noninferiority margin of clinical relevance. The design and the statistical analysis of such trials are also a great source of discussion. In a special issue of *Statistics in Medicine* devoted entirely to this topic, Laster and Johnson (2003) proposed a reappraisal of Blackwelder's general approach by extending one-tailed equivalence testing to a ratio definition of the percentage of effectiveness, R_{True}, based on mean values μ_{Test} (for the tested drug) and μ_{Ref} (for the reference drug) of a continuous response variate, such that

- $R_{True} = (\mu_{Test} / \mu_{Ref})$
- Null hypothesis H0: $R_{True} < R_{Lower\ Bound}$, with a P value of H0 $\leq \alpha$
- Alternative H1: $R_{True} > R_{Lower\ Bound}$, with a P value of H1 $\geq (1 - \beta)$ and where $R_{Lower\ Bound}$ is a selected lower bound based on a percentage of R_{True} indicating an allowance for clinical tolerance

Again, the rejection of H0 (with a type I error of falsely rejecting noninferiority, i.e., incorrectly accepting clinical tolerance) means the acceptance of H1 (with a type II error of falsely rejecting the clinical tolerance, i.e., incorrectly accepting noninferiority). Unfortunately here, however, the construction of one-tailed or even two-tailed CIs comes up against a dissuasively complicated calculation, so they cannot be proposed as an alternative to hypothesis testing, unlike bioequivalence testing. Nevertheless, this ratio-based approach offers a useful tool when the objective is to prove that a new drug can produce an acceptably high percentage of the standard therapy's effect because there is no need to select an absolute value for the noninferiority margin.

Thus, the transposition to pharmacodynamic interactions is straightforward whenever the primary objective is to prove that the concomitant prescription of drug Y (the interacting drug) with drug X (the drug of interest) can produce an acceptable percentage of the effect of drug X when given alone. Obviously, this may appear to be more suited to interactions where lesser efficacy is expected, rather than cases where greater efficacy is expected. Indeed, the use of nonsuperiority would probably be more difficult to defend, not so much statistically (the hypothesis would be reversed and the limit would become $R_{Upper\ Bound}$) as clinically on the basis of safety concerns.

By way of illustration, we have selected two recent studies. In the first one, the effect of rifampin (600 mg once a day for 6 days) on the pharmacokinetics and pharmacodymics of glicazide (80-mg single dose on day 7) was investigated with nine healthy Korean subjects in a randomized two-way crossover study. The expected interaction was based on the potential induction of CYP2C9 by rifampin since glicazide is extensively metabolized by this CYP isoform. The dynamic endpoint was the glucose response after an oral intake of 75 g of glucose (as orange juice) 30 min after the administration of glicazide. Blood glucose and insulin concentrations were monitored in the following 4 h. The sample size of nine subjects was not justified, and the statistical analysis was the standard null hypothesis testing with a two-tailed paired t test. The pharmacokinetic interaction was confirmed with a decrease in glicazide AUC_{∞} and terminal half-life by 70 and 61%, respectively. The pharmacodynamic response was significantly modified in terms of the glucose parameters (10% increase in glucose AUC from 0.5 to 4 h and 17.5% increase in glucose C_{max}) but not with insulin. This study has numerous methodological shortcomings, but our intention is just to say that a noninferiority approach would probably be a better way of addressing this dynamic interaction study by defining, a priori, $R_{Lower\ Bound}$ for insulin parameters and $R_{Upper\ Bound}$ for glucose parameters together with the sample size required for sufficient power.

In the second study, the effect of quinidine (800-mg single dose) on various dynamic parameters of morphine (7.5 mg,

3-h infusion, starting 1 h after quinidine intake) was investigated with 12 healthy volunteers in a randomized, double-blind, two-way crossover design. The expected interaction was based on P-gp blockade by quinidine with kinetic and dynamic implications for morphine, known to be a substrate of P-gp. The main dynamic endpoint was the morphine-induced miotic effect, assessed by pupil diameter, and results of a previous study were used to estimate the study sample size. Statistics were based on standard null hypothesis testing with multivariate repeated-measure analysis of variance. As expected, morphine produced miosis (smaller pupil diameter at the end of the infusion compared with baseline value), but coadministration of quinidine failed to produce an increased effect (with no significant quinidine-by-morphine interaction in the analysis). Here, the methodology of the study is of very good quality, but again we feel that a noninferiority approach should replace the standard approach, particularly in this case where the "reference" effect was not predicted accurately. Indeed, a percent lower (upper) bound can always be used for hypothesis testing, regardless of the magnitude of the observed reference response.

The reader interested in this approach could find other examples of pharmacokinetic-pharmacodynamic studies where the standard null hypothesis testing could be adequately replaced by equivalence hypothesis testing, such as the interaction between grapefruit juice and midazolam, the effects of enteric-coated methylnaltrexone in preventing opioid-induced delay in oral-cecal transit time, or the physostigmine reversal of midazolam-induced electroencephalographic changes in healthy subjects.

7.2.2. Design of In Vivo Interaction Studies

As described all through this chapter, great advances have been made in the mechanistic understanding of drug-drug interactions. This should allow more specific in vivo studies, reaching conclusions with greater evidence and thereby providing greater utility to clinicians. To allow this, the design of interaction studies must be carefully planned, which remains a difficult task because the diversity of the objectives is so great that a single design to fit all situations is meaningless. Thus, a case-by-case design should be the rule, even if some common recommendations must be followed to avoid insoluble difficulties in interpretating the data. (Examples of regulatory guidelines can be found at http://www.fda.gov/cber) [search for "In vivo drug metabolism/drug interaction studies," November 1999], and at http://www.emea.eu.int [search for "Note for guidance on the investigation of drug interactions," CPMP/EWP/560/95, 17 December 1997].)

7.2.2.1 Main Objective of the Trial: Mechanistic Exploration or Therapeutic-Like Conditions?

The question of the main objective must receive a clear answer prior to the design since mechanistic exploration and therapeutic-like conditions are quite different. On the one hand, a trial intended to understand the mechanism of a metabolic drug-drug interaction should maximize the chance of observing specific effects, possibly but not necessarily leading to a better estimation of the maximum risk of the interaction. Most of the time, and for statistical purposes, subjects included are young healthy volunteers or even a very narrow subgroup of subjects (gender, no tobacco, no alcohol, special dietary factors, phenotyping, etc.) in order to reduce interindividual variability so as to achieve sufficient power with a minimum sample size. Doses, pharmaceutical forms, routes of administration, and treatment durations are often far removed from therapeutic conditions, so observed results might not be generalizable to broader populations. For example, by combining a simultaneous intravenous dose of midazolam with an oral liquid form of $^{15}N_3$-midazolam (stable isotope), the relative contribution of intestinal and hepatic CYP3A inhibition by clarithromycin was assessed in 28 young male and female healthy volunteers. In addition, a two-way open-label crossover study with 21 healthy young subjects was performed to study the coordinated induction of both CYP3A and MDR1 (P-gp) by St. John's wort, using midazolam, fexofenadine, and cyclosporine as selected in vivo probes for CYP3A, MDR1, and both proteins, respectively.

On the other hand, the objective of a trial conducted under therapeutic-like conditions is to detect "clinically relevant" drug-drug interactions, i.e., large enough to require a dosage adjustment or any other additional therapeutic monitoring. Here, inclusion and exclusion criteria should be relaxed as far as possible to mirror the target population of patients, which implies a much greater sample size. Safety considerations and/or reasons for believing that the pathology may influence the magnitude of the interaction are situations where the recruitment of healthy volunteers can be ethically questionable. A review investigating the quality and quantity of 89 drug-drug interaction studies included in 14 new drug applications submitted to the FDA in 1996 revealed that 75% of the studies used healthy male subjects and 25% used patients for whom the new drugs were intended. The search for pharmacodynamic interaction studies in various databases confirms the rarity of studies conducted with patients, except for cancer therapy. For example, the pharmacodynamics of etoposide, based on a sigmoid E_{max} model using the percent decrease in white blood cell count, have been evaluated with leukemic patients receiving high-dose cyclosporine as therapy designed to reverse or modulate P-gp-mediated MDR.

7.2.2.2 Design Configuration

By definition, within-subject designs appear to be rather well suited to interaction studies since subjects act as their own control by receiving the different treatments in either fixed or random order. Thus, simple 2×2 randomized crossover designs with healthy volunteers, for example, enable the impact to be studied on the pharmacokinetics of object substrates following reversible inhibition of CYP1A2 by enoxacin, that of CYP3A4 by ritonavir, or that of CYP2C19 by ketoconazole. However, when studying interactions based on noncompetitive inhibition (e.g., CYP3A and macrolides or CYP2C and delavirdine) as well as situations involving inducing drugs (e.g., P-gp and CYP with rifampin or St. John's wort), randomized allocation of treatments may be a source of difficulty in interpreting data in the case of uncontrolled carryover. Here, a sequential crossover design with fixed-order drug administration or even a factorial design for evaluating combination therapies is probably a better solution. For example, the pharmacokinetic interaction between rifampin and AZT was evaluated in eight human immunodeficiency virus-infected patients using a two-treatment, three-period, single sequence (AZT alone, AZT plus rifampin, and AZT alone) with a 14-day duration in each period.

From a purely statistical point of view, parallel-group designs offer less advantage in evaluating drug interactions since they require larger sample sizes on the assumption that there is greater variability between subjects than within subjects. For example, the effect of growth hormone on various hepatic CYP activities was evaluated in 30 healthy elderly men enrolled in a randomized, double-blind, placebo-controlled, parallel-group study. A parallel-group design could also be an interesting solution to the study of drug interactions in patients using a population approach when curative treatments and unstable diseases preclude the use of healthy volunteers.

When analyzing data from a trial, it is good statistical practice to obtain an unbiased estimate of the treatment effect devoid of any carryover effect. In fact, the treatment of the carryover effect has been extensively discussed, with diametrically opposing statements ranging from a simple and deliberate practice of ignoring it to the use of complex statistical models. Drug interaction studies should receive particular attention in this respect since, by definition, a carryover effect is expected because of the precipitating drug. In addition, other parameters such as individual psychological factors, food intake, and/or time events are likely to affect the treatments within each period differently. Thus, potential period effects can be merged with treatment effects in a longitudinal design, while carryover and sequence effects can be combined in a randomized crossover design.

The usual way to prevent residual effects from the previous treatment is to plan an adequate washout period in the design, but this is not always sufficient to remove all of the constituents of the carryover. The prime issue here therefore remains the sample size calculation in a particular situation where the assumption of no interaction cannot hold true, remembering that testing for carryover has less power than testing for treatment effect.

To detect a reasonable target interaction effect, the trial should have adequate power, something rarely calculated in practice. Indeed, the assessment of the 89 drug interaction studies submitted to the FDA in 1996 yielded a median number of 14 subjects per study, a sample size which allows the detection of a large interaction effect only. By way of illustration, the risk of interactions between botanical supplements and commonly prescribed medications has been recently studied with 12 healthy volunteers. Four different plant chemicals (garlic oil, Ginkgo biloba, Panax ginseng, and St. John's wort) were administered three or four times daily for 28 days and expected to interact with single administrations of specific CYP probes (midazolam for CYP3A4, caffeine for CYP1A2, chlorzoxazone for CYP2E1, and debrisoquin for CYP2D6). The chosen design was an open-label study, randomized for supplementation sequence with each period followed by a 30-day washout interval. Our purpose here is not to comment on the results of this study but to point out several methodological problems: the sample size was not justified, although both inhibiting and inducing effects were expected; with four different herbal supplements, 24 possible sequences were needed for a complete carryover-balanced design, but with 12 subjects only an obvious selection has been made, which is not specified. It took almost 7 months to complete the four periods of the study, and each volunteer was asked to abstain from tobacco, alcohol, caffeine, fruit juices, cruciferous vegetables, and charbroiled meat throughout the study, conditions which are actually very difficult to control and sources of evident within-period time events. Multiple *P* values were used to determine the significance of herb-drug interactions instead of the equivalence approach with a 90% CI. Thus, while such a study offers some advantages for screening large CYP-mediated interactions, it should be considered an "intent-to-see" study rather than an "evidence-based" study, particularly when a lack of interaction is concluded.

7.2.2.3. The Washout Period in Metabolic Drug Interaction: Is It Correctly Fulfilling Its Function?

The importance of the washout period has been underlined above, and its duration should be carefully determined to ascertain that it will correctly fulfill its function. This is all the more true with metabolic drug interactions, for which a simple reasoning on the basis of elimination half-lives of the tested drugs is far from sufficient. Ideally, the mechanism responsible for the interaction, the time course of both onset and offset of interaction, and strict control of dietary intake by subjects entering the study should be known prior to the definition of the washout period. In practice, some information is still missing, but intensive research on CYPs and transport proteins during the last decade has greatly improved our understanding and should help in planning a study or in exercising a critical faculty when reading a study report.

It is now well established that the glucocorticoid pathway regulates the induction of several genes within CYP subfamilies through a complex process involving the expression of various nuclear receptors, such as PXR (pregnane X receptor), RXRα (retinoid X receptor), and CAR (constitutive androstane receptor). Experimental work on human hepatocytes prepared from lobectomy segments has shown that CYP inducibility mediated by rifampin, phenobarbital, phenytoin, and St. John's wort was actually linked to the glucocorticoid receptor network (reviewed by Pascussi et al. [2000]). Interestingly, P-gp is also regulated by the same process, since hyperforin, the active substance present in St. John's wort, is one of the most potent in vitro inducers of PXR. Dexamethasone has been shown to induce the MDR1 gene in various species, so common molecular mechanisms appear to regulate at least CYP2B6, CYP3A4, and P-gp activities.

In the vast literature dedicated to metabolic drug interactions, CYP3A4 has received the greatest attention. Depending on the precipitating drug and the experimental conditions used in clinical trials, full induction can be achieved in 4 to 5 days with phenytoin but not until 10 to 14 days with phenobarbital, a difference probably due to the long half-life of the latter drug. In addition, the induction observed with phenytoin occurs more rapidly in pericentral and midzonal areas than in the periportal region of hepatocytes obtained from posttransplant liver biopsy samples. Among rifamycin antibacterials, rifampin has the greatest potency for CYP3A induction, followed by rifapentine and then rifabutin. Assuming the half-life of CYP3A turnover to be around 2 days, maximum induction is attained in about 1 week. This result has been confirmed subsequently, since full induction has been observed in roughly 8 days following rifampin given at 600 mg daily for 12 days. In all cases, CYP3A4 activity returned to baseline within about 2 weeks after drug discontinuation. Very recently, the potency of pleconaril (an oral agent active against picornavirus) for CYP3A4 induction was evaluated with 18 healthy volunteers, using midazolam as a biomarker. Again, the pleconaril-midazolam interaction was reversible with a duration of approximately 2 weeks.

The time course of recovery of CYP3A function after single doses of grapefruit juice has been studied with 25 healthy volunteers. Grapefruit juice contains two furanocoumarin derivatives, bergamottin and DHB (6′, −7′-dihydroxybergamottin), known to inhibit or inactivate CYP3A function. The volunteers received a single oral dose of midazolam either 26, 50 or 74 h after grapefruit juice. Maximum inhibition was probably not reached, but the time required for the inhibition to resolve was around 5 days, a duration consistent with the time course of enzyme regeneration after irreversible inhibition.

Time course data from other CYPs were reported in a large study assessing the risk of drug interactions related to treatment with rhGH (0.5 to 1.5 IU per day, subcutaneous injection for 12 weeks) in 30 elderly subjects with specific CYP probes. No attempt was made to standardize diet, smoking, or drinking habits during the study. The main result was an increase in the metabolic ratio of caffeine after 12 weeks of GH administration, indicative of CYP1A2 induction with a return to baseline 4 weeks after GH discontinuation. Also, slight inhibition of CYP2C19 was observed, indicated by the ratio of *S*-mephenytoin to *R*-mephenytoin, and interestingly, this ratio continued to be increased 4 weeks after GH discontinuation. This suggests that factors other than GH could be responsible for the inhibition, without excluding a long-lasting GH metabolic effect.

No time course data with human P-gp have been retrieved. However, data are available for rats receiving cyclosporine subcutaneously (10 mg/kg of body weight per day for 5, 10, or 15 days). After 10 days of treatment, a maximum increase of P-gp levels was reached in various tissues such as liver, intestine, kidney, and lungs. In humans, using allometric extrapolations with caution, it has been estimated that full induction would be reached in roughly 1 month following repeated cyclosporine doses. However, this remains to be confirmed with real experimental data.

To summarize, onset and offset of enzyme interactions due to compounds with short elimination half-lives are not necessarily confined to the period of drug administration, whenever enzyme turnover is the rate-limiting factor. This is particularly true in the case of enzyme induction, a process which is much more complicated than enzyme inhibition. When planning a metabolic drug interaction, all of the available information should be considered so as to define the most appropriate washout period. This has been recently emphasized by the FDA in a proposal of what could be stated in a protocol example linked to various situations such as drug-drug, drug-dietary supplement, or drug-juice interactions: "For at least 2 weeks prior to the start of the study until its conclusion, volunteers will not be allowed to eat any food or drink any beverage containing alcohol, grapefruit or grapefruit juice, apple or orange juice, vegetables from the mustard green family (e.g., kale, broccoli, watercress, collard greens, kohlrabi, brussels sprouts, mustard) and charbroiled meats ..." (Huang, 2003). The rationale for this proposal appears to be well-founded, but it could lead to great difficulties in the recruitment of volunteers and in the supervision of the study. As an extreme example, if CYP inhibition were to be studied by means of common antidepressants in healthy volunteers, it would require at least 2 weeks of dosing to achieve a true steady-state condition as in clinical practice. The simple comparison of two antidepressant drugs in a randomized crossover fashion adopting the FDA proposal for subject eligibility would probably encounter some suspicion from any institutional review board because of its problems of feasibility. Once again, the primary objective of a drug interaction study, whether a mechanistic approach or a clinical approach, must be clearly presented, as this greatly influences the complexity or simplicity of the protocol.

7.2.2.4. Equivalence Margins

Setting equivalence margins or acceptance criteria in drug interaction studies is a difficult exercise. For pharmacokinetic interactions, it sounds fairly logical to follow the approach prompted by the broad experience gained with generic drugs and bioequivalence studies. Thus, if the 90% CI for the geometric mean ratio [(object drug + interacting drug)/object drug] of properly defined pharmacokinetic metrics is entirely included within the regular interval (80 to 125%), then the absence of a clinically relevant interaction may be claimed (see section 7.2.1.1.1). In the same way, different intervals can be proposed for three categories of drugs: highly variable drugs (HVD), drugs with narrow therapeutic range (NTR), and critical-dose drugs (CDD). HVD are drugs that exhibit large intraindividual variability in pharmacokinetic constants but are very safe. Most of the time, high variability is associated with a high first-pass effect (intestinal and/or hepatic) and nonlinear pharmacokinetics. Thus, the usual (80 to 125%) criterion is often judged too conservative to establish bioequivalence, so wider intervals, such as 75 to 133% or even 70 to 143%, are proposed in various regulatory guidelines. To improve the definition of the bioequivalence limits under such conditions, a procedure known as scaled average bioequivalence has recently been described, and it could be used for interaction studies with HVD, provided there is a sample size of at least 24 subjects. The term NTR applies to drugs for which there is less than a twofold difference in the minimum toxic and minimum effective systemic concentrations, thus requiring careful titration and patient monitoring for safe and effective use. The term CDD applies to the same categories of drugs but, in addition, serious clinical consequences of overdosing (toxicity) or underdosing (lack of effect) are considered. Whatever the name, examples of such drugs are found in many categories, such as immunosuppressive drugs (cyclosporine), anticancer drugs (methotrexate), cardiovascular drugs (digoxin and quinidine), anticoagulant drugs (warfarin), hormones (levothyroxine), and CNS drugs (lithium). Metabolic drug interactions with NTR or CDD are likely to happen, and in this particular case, narrower limits could be proposed to assess the risk of interaction, such as 0.90 to 1.12. This is really an open question that is still subject to extensive discussion.

For pharmacodynamic interactions, setting the decision rule is even more difficult because experience in the field is rather limited. Thus, a mixture of scarce evidence-based data and solid rule of thumb means that 10% may be proposed as a maximum relative variation for toxicity and 20% may be proposed as a maximum relative variation for efficacy. As for pharmacokinetic interactions, different margins can be justified on a case-by-case basis. For example, morphine is not considered to belong to HVD, but it exhibits highly variable pharmacodynamics. In a pivotal study comparing a modified-release form of morphine with the reference immediate-release form, interindividual variability of pharmacokinetic parameters was around 35%, while a five-fold range was observed in the antinociceptive response measured by a visual analog scale in a cancer patient (Moscotin LP, study F002-B, registration file, 1990). In a study evaluating ethnic differences in morphine pharmacokinetics and pharmacodynamics, Latinos and Colombian Indians had similar pharmacokinetics, different from those of Caucasians, but Native Americans exhibited a blunted ventilatory response to CO_2, while Latinos and Caucasians had equivalent ventilatory responses. So, when evaluating pharmacodynamic interactions with morphine (and generally speaking, with drugs showing high pharmacodynamic variability), specific margins for the decision rule could be accepted.

The question of a fixed margin versus a varying margin in noninferiority trials has been addressed statistically for anti-infective treatments, taking into account the variable underlying clinical success rate of the reference treatment. Instead of forming a CI of the difference in the treatment rates, it is proposed that a CI should be formed on the difference in the test rate and the equivalent margin. Attempts to validate this approach in pharmacodynamic drug interaction studies could be interesting, but it requires large sample sizes (at least 75 subjects per group), a condition that is still unrealistic today.

[A further list of more than 700 references may be obtained from the authors.]

REFERENCES

Aiba T, Takehara Y, Okuno M, Hashimoto Y, 2003, Poor correlation between intestinal and hepatic metabolic rates of CYP3A4 substrates in rats, Pharm Res, 20, 745–748.

Benet LZ, Cummins CL, Lau YY, Wu CY, 2003, New discoveries in enzymes and transporters (OATP, P-gp) that affect systemic exposure: what does it mean for biopharmaceutics and clinical pharmacology? Bio-International 2003: Towards harmonisation in bioavailability and bioequivalence, London, UK, 8–10 October 2003.

Cazeneuve C, Pons G, Rey E, Treluyer JM, Cresteil T, Thiroux G, d'Athis P, Oliver G, 1994, Biotransformation of caffeine in human liver microsomes from foetus, neonates, infants and adults, Br J Clin Pharmacol, 37, 405–412.

Christians U, Jacobsen W, Benet LZ, Lampen A, 2002, Mechanisms of clinically relevant drug interactions associated with tacrolimus, Clin Pharmacokinet, 41, 813–851.

Drescher S, Glaeser H, Mürdter T, Hitzl M, Eichelbaum M, Fromm MF, 2003, P-glycoprotein mediated intestinal and biliary digoxin transport in humans, Clin Pharmacol Ther, 73, 223–231.

George J, Murray M, Byth K, Farrell GC, 1995, Differential alterations of cytochrome P450 proteins in livers from patients with severe chronic liver disease, Hepatology, 21, 120–128.

Gomez D, Hebert M, Benet LZ, 1994, The effect of ketoconazole on the intestinal metabolism and bioavailability of cyclosporin, Clin Pharmacol Ther, 55, 209.

Gorski JC, Vannaprasaht S, Hamman MA, Ambrosius WT, Bruce MA, Haehner-Daniels B, Hall SD, 2003, The effect of age, sex and rifampicin administration on intestinal and hepatic cytochrome P450 3A activity, Clin Pharmacol Ther, 74, 275–287.

Greiner B, Eichelbaum M, Fritz P, Kreichgauer HP, von Richter O, Zundler J, Kroemer HK, 1999, The role of intestinal P-glycoprotein in the interaction of digoxin and rifampin, J Clin Invest, 104, 147–153.

Gurley BJ, Gardner SJ, Hubbard MA, Williams DK, Gentry WB, Cui Y, Ang CYW, 2002, Cytochrome P450 phenotypic ratios for predicting herb-drug interactions in humans, Clin Pharmacol Ther, 72, 276–287.

Harris RZ, Jang GR, Tsunoda S, 2003, Dietary effects on drug metabolism and transport, Clin Pharmacokinet, 42, 1071–1088.

Hebert MF, Roberts JP, Gambertoglio JG, Benet LZ, 1991, The effects of rifampin on cyclosporin pharmacokinetics, Clin Pharmacol Ther, 49, 129.

Hebert MF, Roberts JP, Prueksaritanont T, Benet LZ, 1992, Bioavailability of cyclosporin with concomitant rifampin administration is markedly less than predicted by hepatic enzyme induction, Clin Pharmacol Ther, 52, 453–457.

Huang, S-M, 2003, Drug interactions or lack of drug interactions: what should we care about in terms of BA, BE and PK? Lecture handouts, Bio-International, October 9, 2003, London.

Jürgens G, Christensen HR, Brosen K, Sonne J, Loft S, Olsen NV, 2002, Acute hypoxia and cytochrome P450 mediated hepatic drug metabolism in humans, Clin Pharmacol Ther, 11, 214–220.

Laster L, Johnson M, 2003, Non-inferiority trials, the "at least as good as" criterion, Statist Med, 22, 187–200.

Lin JH, Lu AYH, 1998, Inhibition and induction of cytochrome P450 and the clinical implications, Clin Pharmacokinet, 35, 361–390.

Masuda S, Uemoto S, Hashida T, Inomata Y, Tanaka K, Inui KI, 2000, Effect of intestinal P-glycoprotein on daily tacrolimus trough level in a living-donor small bowel recipient, Clin Pharmacol Ther, 68, 98–103.

Montay G, Goueffon Y, Roquet F, 1984, Absorption, distribution, metabolic fate, and elimination of profloxacin mesylate in mice, rats, dogs, monkeys, and humans, Antimicrob Agents Chemothes, 25, 463–472.

Nix D, Gallicano K, 2001, Design and data analysis in drug interaction studies, p 333–351, in Piscitelli SC, Rodvold KA, ed, Drug Interactions in Infectious Diseases, Humana Press, Totowa, N.J.

Park GR, 1996, Molecular mechanisms of drug metabolism in the critically ill, Br J Anaesth, 77, 32–49.

Pascussi JM, Gerbal-Chaloin S, Fabre JM, Maurel P, Vilarem MJ, 2000, Dexamethasone enhances constitutive androstane receptor expression in human hepatocytes, consequences on cytochrome P450 gene regulation, Mol Pharmacol, 58, 1441–1450.

Rowland M, Matin SB, 1973, Kinetic of drug-drug interactions, J Pharmacokinet Biopharm, 1, 553–567.

Schuetz EG, Furuya KN, Shuetz JD, 1995, Interindividual variation in expression of P-glycoprotein in normal human liver and secondary hepatic neoplasms, J Pharmacol Exp Ther, 275, 1011–1018.

Skarke C, Jarrar M, Erb K, Schmidt H, Geisslinger G, Lötsch J, 2003, Respiratory and miotic effects of morphine in healthy volunteers when P-glycoprotein is blocked by quinidine, Clin Pharmacol Ther, 74, 303–311.

Steinijans VW, Hartmann M, Huber R, Radtke H, 1991, Lack of pharmacokinetic interaction as an equivalence problem, Int J Clin Pharmacol Ther Toxicol, 29, 323–328.

Thomson PD, Melmon KL, Richardson JA, Cohn K, Steinbrunn W, Cudihee R, Rowland M, 1973, Lidocain pharmacokinetics in advanced heart failure, liver disease, and renal failure in humans, Ann Intern Med, 78, 499–508.

Vestal RE, Norris AH, Tobin JD, Cohen BH, Shock NW, Andres R, 1975, Antipyrine metabolism in man, influence of age, alcohol, caffeine, and smoking, Clin Pharmacol Ther, 18, 425–432.

Westphal K, Weinbrenner A, Giessmann T, Sturh M, Franke G, Zschiesche M, Oertel R, Terhaag B, Kroemer HK, Siegmund W, 2000, Oral bioavailability of digoxin is enhanced by talinolol, evidence for involvement of intestinal P-glycoprotein, Clin Pharmacol Ther, 68, 6–12.

Whittaker JA, 1970, Genetic control of phenylbutazone metabolism in man, Br Med J, 4, 323–328.

Yates CR, Chang C, Kearbey JD, Yasuda K, Schuetz EG, Miller DD, Dalton JT, Swaan PW, 2003, Structural determinants of P-glycoprotein-mediated transport of glucocorticoids, Pharm Res, 20, 1794–1803.

Antibiotic Treatments and the Intestinal Ecosystem

A. ANDREMONT

55

1. WHY THIS CHAPTER?

Antibacterial agents probably belong to the therapeutic class whose use over the last few decades has most transformed human health and the prognosis for numerous systemic or localized infectious diseases. Historically, community-acquired infections were the first to benefit from this contribution. Currently, at least in industrialized countries, nosocomial infections represent the most substantial challenge to antibiotic therapy. For both community-acquired and hospital-acquired infections, the target of antibiotic therapy varies. It may be localized in one or more organs, or it may be more diffuse in generalized infections. It is only fairly exceptionally that it is intestinal.

In that case, why devote a chapter to the effect of antibacterial agents on the intestinal flora?

There is a straightforward response to this which relates to the fact that our digestive tract, and in particular its lower colonic part, contains a considerable number of bacteria.

It is from these bacteria in the digestive tract that a number of systemic, opportunistic, and nosocomial infections arise (Tancrède and Andremont, 1985). It is also within this intestinal ecosystem that favorable conditions exist for genetic exchanges between bacteria, exchanges which when they are fruitful may be the source of dissemination of the trait of resistance.

It should be understood that because of the massive use of antibiotics in human therapy, this enormous bacterial mass has been confronted with a particularly marked selection pressure in each patient treated (Finland, 1979; McGowan, 1983). In fact, whatever the indication for which it is prescribed, antibiotic treatment, whether oral or parenteral, will culminate in the majority of cases in a large quantity of active molecules being discharged into the colon.

After oral treatment there is an unabsorbed and unmetabolized ingested fraction, to which is added the fraction excreted by the bile (and possibly for some antibiotics by the intestinal mucosa itself). After parenteral treatment, only biliary and intestinal excretion is involved, but this is often extensive.

2. COMPOSITION OF THE COLONIC FLORA

What are the bacteria that make up this colonic flora and on which this selection pressure is exerted?

The colonic flora represents almost all of the bacteria found in the human gastrointestinal tract (Bernasconi, 1984; Hentges, 1983). It is a substantial bacterial population composed of several tens—or even hundreds—of different species. It is estimated that about 10^{13} bacteria are found in the colon of a healthy adult. This is almost 100 times more than on the skin of the same individual, and 10 times more even than there are eukaryotic cells in the entire body. The contact area between the host containing them and these very large numbers of intestinal bacteria is also large, since if the colonic mucosa were to be spread out by unfolding all the villi, it would produce a surface area of several tens of square meters. It will therefore be realized that a priori there are considerable possibilities for exchange and interaction between the colonic flora and the intestinal mucosa of the host. In fact, a very large number of studies have shown a variety of actions by the intestinal flora on the immune system, bile salt metabolism, and fermentation of certain nutrients (Hentges, 1983).

3. SPECIFICITY AND STABILITY

I should like at this point to stress two essential concepts that need to be understood when attention is devoted to the human colonic flora: first of all, the host specificity of the bacterial species that make up the flora and, second, the stability of the composition within the same species and over time in the same individual.

Host specificity has been demonstrated by studies of the composition of the colonic flora in hosts belonging to different species. It has been shown that the human flora is significantly different from that in laboratory rodents or in herbivores. In contrast to the genetic code, in terms of the fecal flora what is true for the mouse is not true for the elephant.

4. DOMINANT AND SUBDOMINANT FLORA

The colonic flora in humans comprises essentially obligate anaerobic bacteria that are always present in large numbers (more than 10^9 per g of feces). They make up what is known as the dominant flora. Numerous species may be distinguished among these obligate anaerobic bacteria (several tens at least), which are often fairly difficult to classify in terms of traditional taxonomy but which may be grouped together in a small number of major bacterial genera, such as

Clostridium, Bacteroides, Eubacterium, and *Fusobacterium.* A number of other bacterial species are also always present in the colonic flora of healthy subjects. Conversely, these are always in very much smaller numbers (1,000 to 1,000,000 times less numerous) and make up what it is conventionally referred to as the subdominant flora. The combination of dominant flora and subdominant flora constitutes the resident flora in humans. This subdominant flora includes again a number of obligate anaerobic bacterial species, but also two bacterial species that grow in both the absence and presence of oxygen (hence known as facultative aerobes-anaerobes) and that are much more well known to the whole of the medical profession: *Enterobacteriaceae* and enterococci.

5. INFECTIONS DUE TO BACTERIA OF THE INTESTINAL FLORA

The reputation of the *Enterobacteriaceae* and enterococci derives obviously to some extent from the ease with which they have been cultured on the usual—and therefore widely studied—media since the very beginning of microbiology, but also and in particular from the importance that they assume in human diseases. The infections that they cause originate either from retrograde colonization of the urinary tract from the perineum (particularly in women), resulting in cystitis or pyelonephritis, or from their passage through the intestinal mucosa, resulting in bacteremia or even septicemia. This passage through the intestinal mucosa is known as translocation and occurs above all in immunodepressed subjects, particularly after major chemotherapy (Tancrède and Andremont, 1985), and probably in very profoundly malnourished children.

Diseases due to anaerobic bacteria in the intestinal flora are much less common, but these too involve opportunistic types of disease. Transparietal passage of obligate anaerobic bacteria occurs essentially when the intestinal mucosa is physically damaged, as in the case of a perforation or colonic surgery.

6. RESIDENT, TRANSIENT, AND PATHOGENIC FLORA

In addition to the resident flora, certain bacteria of exogenous origin are sometimes found in the human digestive tract, introduced for instance in the diet, and which in healthy subjects only transit (hence the name sometimes adopted of transient flora) without establishing themselves and colonizing the intestine. Sometimes, this resistance to colonization is reduced after certain antibiotic treatments, but probably also in other less well-identified circumstances, and a strain of *Pseudomonas,* staphylococcus, or yeast becomes established in and colonizes the intestine in greater or lesser concentrations. This colonization is asymptomatic and requires no treatment except, once again, during periods of profound immunodepression, where it may constitute the portal of entry for a systemic infection.

Beside these bacteria of the resident and transient flora, it is also possible to find pathogenic bacteria in the digestive tract, such as enteropathogenic salmonellae, shigellae, vibrios, *Campylobacter, Yersinia,* and *Escherichia coli.* It is rare (except for salmonellae, for which healthy and prolonged carriage is fairly often the result of an acute episode) for these bacteria to be isolated in healthy subjects. Most of the time their presence is associated with diarrheal or dysenteric disorders, or even with systemic infections in the case of salmonellae. These infections, as everyone knows, may occur even in nonimmunodepressed subjects. This therefore is not an opportunistic condition. However, it should be pointed out that some of these disorders are more common or more serious in certain situations (AIDS, gastric achlorhydria, and previous administration of antibiotics).

7. RESISTANCE TO COLONIZATION, BARRIER EFFECTS, AND MICROBIAL ANTAGONISM

Many bacterial species may also be found in the human colonic flora. In fact, this apparent diversity masks great stability within the resident flora under normal conditions. In a group of healthy volunteers, the same species will be found in the dominant flora and the same species will be found in the subdominant flora. Tests conducted at regular intervals would, barring intercurrent events, show the same results.

This stability is only comprehensible if the majority of bacteria extrinsic to the intestinal flora with which we are in contact and which we inhale or ingest with food in particular do not find the means of establishing themselves for a sustained period in the digestive tract. The majority of them are destroyed by gastric acid on passage through the stomach, but it is known that a small proportion of them (1 in 1,000 to 1 in 10,000) do reach the lower part of the digestive tract, where necessarily they can proliferate and multiply. It is this multiplication that is prevented by the resident flora and particularly the anaerobic species of the dominant flora. This phenomenon was observed 15 to 20 years ago independently by various authors, each of whom gave it a different name: colonization resistance (van der Waaij et al., 1971), barrier effect (Prevot et al., 1986), or more simply, microbial antagonism (Dutos and Schaedler, 1964).

In fact, certain details about the intimate mechanism of this phenomenon have only fairly recently been discovered, although it may be reproduced relatively easily in experimental models. A small number of bacteria are necessary for its complete expression, a single species apparently never being sufficient, but the biochemical mechanism(s) is not understood with certainty. It has also been shown that there are individual variations in the susceptibility of the strains to these antagonistic effects and that this susceptibility might be due to the presence or absence of a specific plasmid (Andremont et al., 1985a). Here again, the gene or genes responsible for this susceptibility to microbial antagonism are not known precisely.

It can thus be seen that the intestinal flora represents a formidable reservoir of microorganisms with which we generally coexist happily. It is likely that this flora has profound importance for our state of health and constitutes a genuine organ with multiple physiological functions. The study of these functions, however, remains very primitive compared with those of the other major systems of the body.

8. METHODS OF STUDYING THE EFFECT OF ANTIBIOTICS ON COLONIZATION RESISTANCE

The deleterious effect of antibiotic treatments on colonization resistance has been observed on very many occasions. Virtually all antibiotics affect it to a greater or lesser extent. It is, however, very difficult to quantify this impact. Descriptions of changes in the composition of the intestinal flora are always difficult to interpret because of the multiplicity of species and the vagueness of the taxonomy. That is why a classification of the dominant flora in major bacterial groups has been proposed in which strict anaerobes are distinguished simply between spore-forming and non-spore-forming gram-positive bacilli, gram-negative bacilli, cocci, and highly oxygen-sensitive bacteria (Pecquet et al., 1986).

The changes in the relative proportions of these various groups provide an indication of the extent of the change in the dominant flora (Pecquet et al., 1986, 1991).

The limitation of this technique, albeit simplified, of describing the intestinal flora derives from its technical complexity, which requires the study to be restricted to a small number of healthy volunteers.

A more dynamic and more functional aspect of the reports of colonization resistance may be obtained experimentally, particularly by using axenic mice kept in isolators. In fact, these animals can be associated with human intestinal flora, and it is then possible to reproduce in their digestive tract the bacterial equilibrium observed in that of the human donor. The mice can be treated with antibiotic doses that reproduce in their feces the concentrations obtained in humans (Andremont et al., 1985b).

The resultant quantitative changes can be observed, and in particular a specific microorganism can be introduced into the animals' intestine before, during, or after treatment to assess the possibilities of its establishment, or rather, the resistance to colonization with which it will be confronted from the intestinal flora (Andremont et al., 1983; Leonard et al., 1985; Pecquet et al., 1986, 1991).

The limit of this technique, which is complex but attractive, is that in practice the flora of a only one subject will be tested. The inferences that can be drawn about the general effect of an antibiotic on the intestinal flora in large-scale prescriptions are therefore at the very least limited.

At present I believe that we must look to study techniques that are similar to epidemiology, either by treating a relatively large number of healthy volunteers (several tens) or by observing the colonization of patients treated in efficacy studies of the product, particularly during phase III clinical trials.

It is also possible to study very specific aspects, as has been done for the interaction between β-lactams and intestinal β-lactamases (Chachaty et al., 1992) in short-term series of very closely monitored volunteers.

9. EFFECT OF ANTIBIOTICS ON THE RESIDENT FLORA AND DECONTAMINATION

It is now clearly demonstrated that antibiotics which thus reach the lumen of the digestive tract are capable of destroying all or some of the resident flora. It is this activity that is used in so-called "decontamination" treatments, whether this decontamination is total, in other words, intended to eliminate all the intestinal flora, or selective, i.e., intended to eliminate only a fraction of the flora, that represents a potential risk of infection for a given category of patients (for example, facultative aerobic-anaerobic gram-negative bacteria in aplastic or intensive care subjects or anaerobic bacteria in subjects due to undergo submesocolic surgery).

We are far from being certain at present whether, despite its logic, selective decontamination applied indiscriminately provides true benefit to hospitalized patients, particularly in intensive care units (Consensus, 1992; Hammond et al., 1992, Winter et al., 1992). Conversely, it seems that it can help restrict the diffusion of certain epidemic species, such as extended-spectrum β-lactamase-producing *Enterobacteriaceae* (Brun-Buisson et al., 1989).

10. RISKS OF DECONTAMINATION

The risk of decontamination is that resistant mutants present prior to the arrival of the antibiotic are selected during the treatment and to some extent assume the place of susceptible bacteria destroyed by the antibiotics. It has been clearly demonstrated that there is a significant relationship between administration of an antibiotic and intestinal carriage of bacteria resistant to it from the time that a fraction of the ingested dose arrives in the active form in the colonic lumen (Andremont et al., 1986; Raibaud et al., 1977). The culmination of this process is the excretion of resistant bacteria into the outside environment in large numbers, and their transmission to other patients, particularly in hospitals, may be the source of episodes of epidemics of nosocomial infections.

It is also under these circumstances—the arrival of active antibiotics in the colon—that resistant bacteria will multiply in the digestive tract by mechanisms involving a plasmid genetic medium. These constitute a twofold risk: the risk of dissemination into the environment of a large quantity of these bacteria (as in the case of mutants), but also an additional risk of transmission of the resistance traits by homo- or heterologous transfer in vivo to other bacteria resident in the digestive tract. It is also known that it is possible for such transfers to occur with bacteria not only of the resident flora but also of the transient flora (Doucet-Populaire et al., 1991, 1992).

11. CONCLUSION

The digestive tract is thus the preferential site of multiplication and dissemination of resistance traits during antibiotic treatment. This effect must certainly be evaluated for the new molecules brought to the market versus those that are already used. This is a genuine risk and may raise major problems of public health, as has been the case with the rapid dissemination of broad-spectrum β-lactamases (Jacoby and Medeiros, 1991; Philippon et al., 1989). Awareness of this risk means that patients carrying potentially epidemic-resistant strains can be treated appropriately, particularly by well-codified measures of enteral isolation and intestinal decontamination (Brun-Buisson et al., 1989). The proven efficacy of these measures when applied strictly and in carefully considered indications should ensure that the adverse effects of antibiotics in terms of the emergence of resistant bacteria and the dissemination of resistance traits do not prevent the prescription of molecules whose direct benefit in the treatment of bacterial infections is so important.

REFERENCES

Andremont A, Gerbaud G, Tancrède C, Courvalin P, 1985a, Plasmid mediated susceptibility to intestinal microbial antagonisms in Escherichia coli, Infect Immun, 49, 751–755.

Andremont A, Raibaud P, Tancrède C, 1983, Effect of erythromycin on microbial antagonisms, a study in gnotobiotic mice associated with a human fecal flora, J Infect Dis, 148, 579–587.

Andremont A, Raibaud P, Tancrède C, Duval-Iflah Y, Ducluzeau R, 1985b, The use of germ-free mice associated with human fecal flora as an animal model to study enteric bacterial interactions, p 219–228, in Takeda Y, Miwatami T, ed, Bacterial Diarrheal Diseases, KTX Scientific Publishers, Tokyo.

Andremont A, Sancho-Garnier H, Tancrède C, 1986, Epidemiology of intestinal colonization by members of the family Enterobacteriaceae highly resistant to erythromycin in a hematology-oncology unit, Antimicrob Agents Chemother, 29, 1104–1107.

Bernasconi P, 1984, Flore et ecosystème intestinal, Editions Scientifiques des Laboratoires Biocodex Montrouge.

Brun-Buisson C, Legrand P, Rauss A, Richard C, Montravers F, Besbes M, Meakins JL, Soussy CJ, Lemaire F, 1989, Intestinal decontamination for control of nosocomial multiresistant gram-negative bacilli, Ann Intern Med, 110, 873–881.

Chachaty E, Depitre C, Mario N, Bourneix C, Saulnier P, Corthier G, Andremont A, 1992, Presence of Clostridium difficile and of antibiotic and beta-lactamase activity in the feces of volunteers treated with oral cefixime, oral cefpodoxime (RU51807), or placebo, Antimicrob Agents Chemother, 36, 2009–2013.

Consensus, 1992, Decontamination digestive selective chez les malades de reanimation, La Lettre de l'Infectiologue, 7, 364–366.

Doucet-Populaire F, Trieu-Cuot P, Andremont A, Courvalin P, 1992, Conjugal transfer of plasmid DNA from Enterococcus faecalis to Escherichia coli in the digestive tract of gnotobiotic mice, Antimicrob Agents Chemother, 36, 502–504.

Doucet-Populaire F, Trieu-Cuot P, Dosbaa I, Andremont A, Courvalin P, 1991, Inducible transfer of conjugative transposon Tn1545 from Enterococcus faecalis to Listeria monocytogenes in the digestive tracts of gnotobiotic mice, Antimicrob Agents Chemother, 35, 185–187.

Dutos R, Schaedler RW, 1964, The digestive tract as an ecosystem, Am J Med Sci, 248, 49/267–53/271.

Finland MW, 1979, Emergence of antibiotic resistance in hospitals 1935–1975, Rev Infect Dis, 1, 4–21.

Hammond JMJ, Potgieter PD, Saunders GL, Forder AA, 1992, Double-blind study of selective decontamination of the digestive tract in intensive care, Lancet, 340, 5-9.

Hentges DJ, 1983, Human Intestinal Microflora in Health and Disease, Academic Press, New York.

Jacoby GA, Medeiros AA, 1991, More extended spectrum β-lactamases, Antimicrob Agents Chemother, 35, 1697–1704.

Leonard F, Andremont A, Tancrède C, 1985, In vivo activity of nifurzide and nifuroxazide in intestinal bacteria in man and gnotobiotic mice, J Appl Bacteriol, 58, 545–553.

McGowan JE, 1983, Antimicrobial resistance in hospital organisms and its relation to antibiotic use, Rev Infect Dis, 5, 1033–1045.

Pecquet S, Andremont A, Tancrède C, 1986, Selective antimicrobial modulation of the intestinal tract by norloxacin in human volunteers and in gnotobiotic mice associated with a human fecal flora, Antimicrob Agents Chemother, 29, 1047–1052.

Pecquet S, Andremont A, Tancrède C, 1987, Effect of oral ofloxacin on fecal bacteria in human volunteers, Antimicrob Agents Chemother, 31, 124–125.

Pecquet S, Chachaty E, Tancrède C, Andremont A, 1991, Effect of roxithromycin on fecal bacteria in human volunteers and resistance to colonization in gnotobiotic mice, Antimicrob Agents Chemother, 35, 548–552.

Philippon A, Labia R, Jacoby G, 1989, Extended spectrum β-lactamases, Antimicrob Agents Chemother, 33, 1131–1136.

Prevot MH, Andremont A, Sancho-Garnier H, Tancrède C, 1986, Epidemiology of intestinal colonization by members of the family Enterobacteriaceae resistant to cefotaxime in a hematology-oncology unit, Antimicrob Agents Chemother, 30, 945–947.

Raibaud P, Ducluzeau R, Tancrède C, 1977, L'effet de barrière microbien dans le tube digestif, moyen de defense de l'hôte contre les bactéries exogenes, Med Mal Infect, 1, 130–134.

Tancrède C, Andremont A, 1985, Bactériémies d'origine intestinale chez les leucémiques en aplasie, Med Mal Infect, 5, 214–219.

van der Waaij D, Berghuis-de-Vriies JM, van der Weese, L, 1971, Colonization resistance of the digestive tract in conventional and antibiotic treated mice, J Hyg (Lond), 69, 405–407.

Winter R, Humphreys H, Pick A, MacGovan AP, Willatts SM, Speller DCE, 1992, A controlled trial of selective decontamination of the digestive tract in intensive care and its effect on nosocomial infection, J Antimicrob Chemother, 30, 73–87.

Interaction between Antimicrobial Agents and the Oropharyngeal and Intestinal Normal Microflora

ÅSA SULLIVAN, CHARLOTTA EDLUND, AND CARL ERIK NORD

56

1. BACKGROUND

Human skin and mucous surfaces are colonized with microorganisms, and each ecological habitat harbors a specific microflora often referred as the normal microflora. These ecosystems are relatively stable in health, but variations in diet or hygiene habits give rise to large interindividual differences. The normal microflora is important in its function as a barrier against colonization by potentially pathogenic microorganisms and against overgrowth of already present microorganisms. The control of growth of opportunistic microorganisms that is accomplished by the normal microflora is termed colonization resistance (132, 137). Severe disease and administration of antibacterial agents are the major causes for decreased colonization resistance. Antibacterial agents cause disturbances in the ecological balance between the host and the normal microflora. Disturbances are dependent on the characteristics of the agents as well as of individual variations in pharmacokinetics, composition, and susceptibility of the normal microflora. The majority of studies on the ecological impact of antibacterial agents have been performed on the intestinal microflora in healthy subjects and to some extent also on the oropharyngeal microflora. The intestines harbor a dense microbial population and are a common source of pathogens. Resistant strains frequently emerge, and transmission of resistance genes between microorganisms can contribute to increased numbers of resistant, potentially pathogenic microorganisms (121). The present knowledge of the impact of antimicrobial agents on the oropharyngeal and intestinal microflora and the optimal performance of such studies are discussed in this chapter.

2. THE NORMAL OROPHARYNGEAL MICROFLORA

Microorganisms in saliva derive from all mucous surfaces in the oropharynx and from dental plaques (90, 141). Saliva comprises approximately 10^8 to 10^9 CFU/ml, and more than 300 different species have been isolated (36). Anaerobic microorganisms predominate in saliva; the relative proportion between anaerobic and aerobic microorganisms is 100:1. Major genera are streptococci, aerobic and anaerobic, belonging to the mitis, salivarius, and anginosus groups of viridans streptococci (140), and anaerobic gram-negative cocci and rods like veillonellae, fusobacteria, and prevotellae. Disturbances in the oropharyngeal microflora are caused by administration of antimicrobial agents that reach high concentrations in oral tissues. Agents that are excreted through the mucous membranes or are excreted in saliva are found in microbiologically active concentrations. Reduced numbers of streptococci and anaerobic microorganisms allow for overgrowth of organisms normally isolated only in low numbers, i.e., *Candida* species and enterobacteria. Emergence of resistant streptococci is a common consequence of a disturbed normal oropharyngeal microflora (124).

3. THE NORMAL INTESTINAL MICROFLORA

The intestinal tract harbors the largest numbers and the most diverse collection of microorganisms (128). The concentration of microorganisms in the lower intestinal tract is at least 10^{13} CFU/g, with a diversity of more than 600 different species (90). Anaerobic microorganisms outnumber aerobic bacteria by a factor of 1,000:1. Enterobacteria, mainly *Escherichia coli* and enterococci, dominate in the aerobic flora, while *Bacteroides,* bifidobacteria, anaerobic cocci, eubacteria, and clostridia are dominant anaerobic microorganisms (36).

Orally administered antimicrobial agents that are incompletely absorbed, excreted via salivary glands and bile, or excreted transluminally frequently result in a decreased colonization resistance. Enzymes produced by intestinal microorganisms inactivate antimicrobial agents to various degrees, and binding to intestinal material can also cause inactivation of the agents (41). Disturbances most often seen are changed numbers of enterococci, enterobacteria, and anaerobic microorganisms. Overgrowth of microorganisms normally present in low numbers and with natural resistance can occur, with serious clinical consequences. Overgrowth of yeasts can cause systemic infection in immunocompromised patients, and overgrowth of *Clostridium difficile* can lead to diarrhea and life-threatening colitis (6, 37). Emergence of resistant enterococci, enterobacteria, and *Bacteroides* species is observed in connection with administration of some groups of antimicrobial agents (124).

4. PERFORMANCE OF STUDIES ON THE INTERACTION BETWEEN ANTIMICROBIAL AGENTS AND THE NORMAL MICROFLORA

4.1. Study Design, Subjects, and Drug Administration

Studies on the impact of antimicrobial agents on the normal microflora should be performed as comparative double-blind studies. The subjects should be randomized for treatment and stratified for gender (44). In phase I studies that include healthy volunteers, and more rarely phase II studies, when a defined group of patients are included, it is important that the subjects have an ecologically well-balanced microflora at the start of the study. The study groups should include at least 12 subjects, and the dosing of the antimicrobial agents should be clinically relevant (39). If possible, it is favorable when pharmacokinetic and pharmacodynamic analyses as well as microbiological assays can be performed simultaneously. Not only can correlation analyses between the microflora and the concentrations of antimicrobial agents in body fluids be performed, but also it is an advantage from an economical point of view. Sampling of saliva and feces for pharmacokinetic analyses should always be performed together with sampling for microbiological analyses.

4.2. Sampling Procedures

Saliva samples are thought to reflect the total oropharyngeal microflora shed from epithelial cells and from the teeth. Saliva should be transported in special transport medium and be immediately cultured or frozen at −70°C. Fecal samples are thought to roughly reflect the colonic microflora and are most often used for determination of the intestinal microflora. The samples should be collected in sterile containers and be frozen at −70°C, ideally within 2 h.

At least two samples each before the start, during, and after the administration period should be collected. The last sampling should not be carried out until 2 to 4 weeks after the end of administration to allow for normalization of the microflora.

4.3. Assay of Concentrations of Antimicrobial Agents

The salivary and fecal concentrations of antimicrobial agents should be determined microbiologically by the agar plate diffusion method in order to determine the amount of active drug. Undiluted saliva is used for measurements of salivary concentrations. Fecal samples are diluted in phosphate buffer and centrifuged. The supernatant is used for the determinations. Standard series with known concentrations of the agent are prepared in pooled supernatants of saliva or feces. A susceptible microorganism is inoculated in a uniform layer on the agar. Wells are punched in the medium and defined volumes of test solutions are applied. All samples should be run in triplicate, and on each agar plate a concomitant standard series should be included. The drug concentrations are determined in relation to the diameters of the inhibition zones caused by the known concentrations from the linear standard series. Linear regression is used to confirm linearity of standard series. Divergence of precision determined for the analyses is regarded as acceptable if less than 10% (39).

4.4. Microbiological Procedures

For microbiological analyses of saliva, the samples are further diluted 10-fold in reduced medium to 10^{-5} and inoculated on selective and nonselective agar media (89). Fecal samples are diluted up to 10^{-7} and are inoculated on a number of selective and nonselective agar media (31). After incubation of the agar plates at 37°C, different colony types are counted, isolated in pure culture, and identified to the genus level. All isolates are analyzed according to Gram stain reaction and colony morphology, followed by biochemical tests (98). Anaerobic microorgansims are identified by gas-liquid chromatography of metabolites from glucose (126). Molecular identification of microorganisms is of great value in some instances. Methods that have been used are PCR analyses of 16S rRNA sequences, fingerprinting methods like pulsed-field gel electrophoresis, restriction fraction length polymorphism, arbitrarily primed PCR, and ribotyping (127).

4.5. Antimicrobial Susceptibility Tests

Throughout the study period, dominant species from the respective habitat should be collected to monitor emergence of resistance. From the oropharyngeal and intestinal microflora, three to five representative colonies of alpha-hemolytic streptococci as well as enterobacteria, enterococci, and *Bacteroides* species are generally collected. The colonies should be selected from samples collected before and on the last day of administration and at the end of the study period of the examined antimicrobial agent. New species that appear in connection with the administration or overgrowth of species that are normally present in low numbers should also be tested for susceptibility. The MIC for the studied agent should be determined with established methods such as the agar or broth dilution methods or the E-test (AB Biodisk, Solna, Sweden) according to NCCLS or corresponding standards (45, 100, 101).

4.6. Statistical Analysis

Logarithmic values of the microbiological counts are used in the calculations. Salivary counts are expressed as CFU per milliliter of saliva, and fecal counts are expressed as CFU per gram of feces. The median count for each species is calculated for each sampling occasion. To compare quantitative changes in counts of microorganisms within treatment groups, analysis of variance may be used. The nonparametric Wilcoxon signed-ranked test can be used to compare pretreatment versus end-of-treatment data or end-of-study-period data. To compare quantitative data between groups the Mann-Whitney U test can be performed. The Mann-Whitney U test can also be used for statistical analyses of MICs for each species within groups, between pretreatment and end of treatment, and between pretreatment and end of study. *P* values should be adjusted for the multiple analyses. *P* values of ≤ 0.05 for culture data and of ≤ 0.05 or ≤ 0.01 for MICs are considered relevant (39).

4.7. Informed Consent and Data on Safety of Drugs

All subjects should give consent to participate before taking part in the study and sign a paper to confirm that he or she is aware of the nature of the study and possible consequences.

Safety variables that ought to be included are adverse-event questioning, clinical laboratory data, blood pressure and heart rate measurements, electrocardiogram recordings, and physical examination findings. Adverse events that occur should be judged to determine the possibility of a connection with the administered drug and whether treatment is needed. Adequate documentation is mandatory.

5. IMPACT OF PENICILLINS ON THE HUMAN MICROFLORA

5.1. Oropharyngeal Microflora

Data on the impact of penicillins on the oropharyngeal microflora are summarized in Table 1. Phenoxymethylpenicillin is not excreted in saliva, and only moderate disturbances occur in the oropharyngeal microflora. Minor reductions in numbers of viridans group streptococci and in total numbers of anaerobic microorganisms have been observed. Ampicillin in combination with sulbactam has been shown to markedly reduce both the aerobic and anaerobic microflora and also lead to colonization with enterobacteria and fungi. Administration of amoxicillin, a broad-spectrum penicillin, reduces to a minor extent the numbers of some strains of streptococci, while the effect on the anaerobic microflora has been shown to be dose dependent (doses of ≥2,000 mg daily decrease the anaerobic microflora). In patients, but not in healthy volunteers, increased numbers of enterobacteria have been observed during amoxicillin administration. When analyzed, the concentration of amoxicillin in saliva has been shown to be below the detection limit. Combinations of amoxicillin and clavulanic acid reduce the numbers of *Streptococcus salivarius* and *Veillonella* organisms, while the total numbers of streptococci and of anaerobic microorganisms are unaffected. Bacampicillin is not excreted in saliva, and only minor reductions in the numbers of *S. salivarius* organisms and of fusobacteria have been detected. Likewise, only low concentrations of amdinocillin have been detected in saliva after pivmecillinam administration, and no major ecological disturbances have been observed.

5.2. Gastrointestinal Microflora

Data on the impact of penicillins on the intestinal microflora are shown in Table 2. No significant changes have been noticed in the total numbers of aerobic or anaerobic intestinal microflora during administration of phenoxymethylpenicillin. Some subjects have been colonized with new species of enterobacteria during treatment. Penicillins are mainly excreted renally, and fecal concentrations of phenoxymethylpenicillin are generally below the detection limit. Penicillinase produced by the intestinal microorganisms inactivates penicillin that reaches the intestines. Ampicillin, a penicillin with effect on both gram-positive and gram-negative microorganisms, induces moderate changes in the intestinal microflora. Increased numbers of ampicillin-resistant enterobacteria are common, and overgrowth of *Candida* species has been seen occasionally. More marked reductions in the numbers of aerobic microorganisms and moderate reduction in the anaerobic microflora have been observed with increasing doses. Combination of ampicillin and a β-lactamase inhibitor, sulbactam, is more favorable from an ecological point of view, and in particular the aerobic microflora is less disturbed. Amoxicillin, an agent that is acid stable and better absorbed than ampicillin, increases the numbers of enterobacteria, and emergence of resistant new enterobacterial strains has been observed in connection with its administration. Overgrowth of *Candida* has been found in some individuals. Resistant enterobacteria in the normal intestinal microflora have frequently been observed also in connection with administration of amoxicillin combined with clavulanic acid (β-lactamase inhibitor). Esters of ampicillin like bacampicillin, pivampicillin, and talampicillin are ecologically more favorable than ampicillin, since they are better absorbed and are found in the large intestine only in low concentrations. Azlocillin and piperacillin are excreted in bile, and both the aerobic and anaerobic microflora are effected. A combination of piperacillin and a β-lactamase inhibitor, tazobactam, reduces the effect mainly on the intestinal anaerobic microflora. Pivmecillinam has a spectrum including in particular gram-negative aerobic rods, and the main impact of this agent is also seen as reduced numbers of enterobacteria. Increased numbers of aerobic cocci and reduced numbers of anaerobic microorganisms are connected with increased doses. No measurable fecal concentrations of ticarcillin-clavulanic acid have been found, and only minor changes in the numbers of aerobic cocci and enterobacteria are associated with its administration.

6. IMPACT OF CEPHALOSPORINS ON THE HUMAN MICROFLORA

6.1. Oropharyngeal Microflora

The ecological impact of cephalosporins on the oropharyngeal microflora is summarized in Table 3. Cephalosporins are soluble in water, and therefore only minor amounts can be detected in saliva. Both parenterally and perorally administered cephalosporins disturb the normal microflora to a minor degree. Parenteral administration of ceftriaxone and peroral administration of cefadroxil and cefuroxime axetil lead to moderate suppression of the numbers of streptococci. Moxalactam suppresses the gram-negative aerobic and anaerobic microorganisms and promotes colonization with *Candida albicans*. Overgrowth of enterobacteria and enterococci is connected with the intake of cefaclor.

6.2. Gastrointestinal Microflora

The effect on the intestinal microflora of parenteral administration of cephalosporins is shown in Table 4, and that of

Table 1 Impact of penicillins on the oropharyngeal microflora[a]

Agent	Impact on: Streptococci	Impact on: Anaerobic bacteria	Resistant streptococci	Overgrowth of enterobacteria or *Candida*	Reference(s)
Phenoxymethyl penicillin	↓	↓	–	–	2, 52
Ampicillin-sulbactam	↓	↓	–	+	51
Amoxicillin	↓	↓	–	+	17, 22, 123
Amoxicillin-clavulanic acid	–	–	–	–	89
Bacampicillin	–	–	–	–	57
Pivmecillinam	–	–	–	–	125

[a]↓, mild to moderate suppression (2 to 4 $\log_{10}$ CFU/ml of saliva); –, no significant changes.

Table 2 Impact of penicillins on the oropharyngeal microflora[a]

Agent	Impact on: Aerobic Gr⁺cocci	Entero-bacteria	Anaerobic bacteria	Resistant microorganisms	Overgrowth of *C. difficile* or *Candida*	Reference(s)
Phenoxymethyl penicillin	–	–	–	+	–	2, 52
Ampicillin	↓↓	↓↓	↓	+	+	12, 77, 82
Ampicillin-sulbactam	↓	↓	↓	+	+	67, 72
Amoxicillin	–	↑	–	+	+	1, 17, 22, 41, 47, 48, 82, 94, 123
Amoxicillin-clavulanic acid	–	↑	–	+	+	18, 80, 87, 94, 95, 142
Bacampicillin	–	–	↓	–	–	49, 57
Pivampicillinam	–	↑	–	+	+	75
Talampicillin	–	↑	–	+	–	82
Azlocillin	↓	↓	↓	+	–	104
Piperacillin	↓	↓	↓	–	–	70
Piperacillin-tazobactam	↓	↓	–	+	–	106
Pivmecillinam	–	↓	–	–	–	73, 125
Ticarcillin-clavulanic acid	↑	↓	–	–	–	105

[a]↓, mild to moderate suppression (2 to 4 $\log_{10}$ CFU/g of feces); ↓↓, strong suppression (>4 $\log_{10}$ CFU/g of feces); ↑, increase of microorganisms during treatment; –, no significant changes. Gr⁺, gram positive.

Table 3 Impact of cephalosporins on the oropharyngeal microflora[a]

Agent	Impact on: Streptococci	Anaerobic bacteria	Resistant streptococci	Overgrowth of enterobacteria or Candida	Reference(s)
Parenterally administered					
Cefpirome	–	–	–	–	176
Ceftriaxone	↓	–	–	–	21, 24
Moxolactam	–	↓	–	+	51
Perorally administered					
Cefaclor	–	–	–	+	22, 109
Cefadroxil	↓	–	–	–	2
Cefpodoxime proxetil	–	–	–	–	17
Cefuroxime axetil	↓	–	–	–	89
Loracarbef	–	–	–	–	108

[a]↓, mild to moderate suppression (2 to 4 $\log_{10}$ CFU/ml of saliva); –, no significant changes.

peroral administration of cephalosporins is shown in Table 5. Cephalosporins are excreted mainly via the kidneys, but some agents, like ceftriaxone, cefoperazone, and moxalactam, are excreted in the bile. With the exception of loracarbef, the absorption of perorally administered cephalosporins is low and the outcome is high fecal concentrations that cause extensive disturbances of the microflora. The extent of disturbances is modified by the amount of β-lactamases produced by the intestinal microorganisms (41). Cephalosporins exhibit a broader antimicrobial spectrum than do the penicillins. Enterococci are intrinsically resistant to cephalosporins, and overgrowth of resistant enterococci is common during both parenteral and peroral administration. Parenteral administration of cephalosporins causes moderate to strong suppression of the number of enterobacteria, while the suppression is milder in connection with peroral administration. Colonization with new resistant enterobacterial strains is common, and overgrowth of *C. difficile* and yeasts has frequently been observed. Several of the parenterally administered agents, perorally administered cefixime, and high doses of cefpodoxime proxetil also reduce the numbers of anaerobic microorganisms.

Table 4 Impact of parenterally administered cephalosporins on the instestinal microflora[a]

Agent	Impact on:			Resistant microorganisms	Overgrowth of *C. difficile* or *Candida*	Reference(s)
	Aerobic Gr⁺cocci	Entero-bacteria	Anaerobic bacteria			
Cefazolin	–	–	—[b]	+	–	135
Cefbuperazone	↓	↓	↓	–	–	64
Cefepime	–	↓	–	–	–	5
Cefmenoxime	–	↓	–	–	+	74
Cefoperazone	↓↑	↓↓	↓	+	+	4, 50, 81
Cefotaxime	↑	↓	–	+	–	50, 79, 135
Cefotiam	–	↓	–	+	+	74
Cefoxitin	↑	↓	↓	+	+	69, 97
Cefpirome	–	↓↓	–	–	–	76
Ceftazidime	–	↓	–	–	–	74
Ceftizoxime	–	↓	–	+	–	74
Ceftriaxone	↑	↓↓	↓	+	+	21, 24, 50, 102, 136, 139
Ceftriaxone-loracarbef	↑	↓	↓	–	+	136
Moxolactam	↑	↓	↓	–	–	71

[a]↓, suppression (2 to 4 $\log_{10}$ CFU/g of feces); ↓↓, strong suppression (>4 $\log_{10}$ CFU/g of feces); ↑, increase of microorganisms during treatment; –, no significant changes. Gr⁺, gram positive.
[b]—, no data available.

Table 5 Impact of perorally administered cephalosporins on the instestinal microflora[a]

Agent	Impact on:			Resistant microorganisms	Overgrowth of *C. difficile* or *Candida*	Reference(s)
	Aerobic Gr⁺cocci	Entero-bacteria	Anaerobic bacteria			
Cefaclor	–	–	–	–	+	22, 46, 109
Cefadroxil	–	–	–	+	–	2
Cefetamet pivoxil	–	–	–	–	–	112
Cefixime	↑	↓	↓	–	+	46, 111, 112
Cefpodoxime proxetil	↑	↓	↓	+	+	17, 114
Cefprozil	–	↓	–	–	+	86
Ceftibuten	↑	↓	–	–	+	16
Cefuroxime axetil	↑	↓	–	+	+	29, 33, 84, 112, 142
Cephradine	–	–	–	–	–	18
Loracarbef	↑	–	–	+	–	47, 108

[a]↓, suppression (2 to 4 $\log_{10}$ CFU/g of feces); ↑, increase of microorganisms during treatment; –, no significant changes. Gr⁺, gram positive.

7. IMPACT OF MONOBACTAMS, CARBAPENEMS, AND GLYCOPEPTIDES ON THE HUMAN MICROFLORA

7.1. Oropharyngeal Microflora

The impact of monobactam on the normal oral microflora is shown in Table 6. Aztreonam is the only agent in this class of β-lactam antimicrobial agents. Aztreonam is stable against β-lactamases and has been shown to induce only minor changes in the oropharyngeal microflora, although superinfection with staphylococci has been observed.

There are no studies performed on the interaction between carbapenems or glycopeptides and the oropharyngeal microflora.

7.2. Gastrointestinal Microflora

The influence of monobactams, carbapenems, and glycopeptides on the intestinal microflora is shown in Table 7. The spectrum of aztreonam includes mainly aerobic gram-negative rods, and that is also clear from the results of studies on the effect on the intestinal microflora where strong reductions of enterobacteria have been seen. Aztreonam has no impact on gram-positive or anaerobic microorganisms. As in the oropharyngeal microflora, a significant increase in the number of staphylococci is connected with its administration. Of the β-lactam antibiotics, imipenem and meropenem have the broadest antimicrobial spectrum. Both agents suppress the enterobacterial and anaerobic microorganisms. Imipenem induces reductions in the numbers of gram-positive aerobic

Table 6 Impact of monobactam, macrolides, ketolide, and lincosamide on the oropharyngeal microflora[a]

Agent	Impact on:		Resistant streptococci	Overgrowth of enterobacteria or *Candida*	Reference(s)
	Streptococci	Anaerobic bacteria			
Monobactam					
Aztreonam	–	–	–	–	51, 62
Macrolides					
Clarithromycin	–	–	+	+	11, 28
Dirithromycin	–	–	–	–	27
Erythromycin	↓	–	–	+	53, 54
Ketolide					
Telithromycin	–	–	–	+	28
Lincosamide					
Clindamycin	–	↓↓	–	+	52, 53

[a]↓, mild to moderate suppression (2 to 4 $\log_{10}$ CFU/ml of saliva); ↓↓, strong suppression (>4 $\log_{10}$ CFU/g of feces); –, no significant changes.

Table 7 Impact of monobactam, carbapenems, and glycopeptides on the instestinal microflora[a]

Agent	Impact on:			Resistant microorganisms	Overgrowth of *C. difficile* or *Candida*	Reference(s)
	Aerobic Gr^+cocci	Entero-bacteria	Anaerobic bacteria			
Monobactam						
Aztreonam	↑	↓↓	–	–	+	25, 62, 63, 131
Carbapenems						
Imipenem-cilastin	↓	↓	↓	–	–	65, 110
Meropenem	↑	↓	↓	–	–	10
Lenapenem	↓	–	–	–	–	99
Glycopeptides						
Vancomycin	↓↑	–	↓	+	–	29, 88, 129
Teicoplanim	↓↑	↑	–	+	–	129

[a]↓, suppression (2 to 4 $\log_{10}$ CFU/g of feces); ↓↓, strong suppression (>4 $\log_{10}$ CFU/g of feces); ↑, increase of microorganisms during treatment; –, no significant changes. Gr^+, gram positive.

cocci, while the numbers of enterococci increase during meropenem administration. The mean total counts of aerobic and anaerobic microorganisms were not influenced by lenapenem, although the numbers of streptococci and *Veillonella* organisms decreased during administration.

Vancomycin and teicoplanin are glycopeptide antimicrobial agents, which inhibit the biosynthesis of the bacterial cell wall at an earlier stage than the penicillins. Both agents are administered intravenously, except for oral administration of vancomycin in the treatment of *C. difficile* diarrhea or colitis. Studies on the effect on the normal microflora have been performed with orally administered drugs, and since the agents are poorly absorbed high intraluminal concentrations are achieved. The numbers of enterococci decreased rapidly during administration, and isolation of vancomycin-resistant enterococci has been reported from a study performed in Belgium. Motile enterococci, pediococci, lactobacilli, and enterobacteria are intrinsically resistant to glycopeptides and increase in number during administration. The numbers of *Bacteroides* organisms are also suppressed during the administration even though gram-negative microorganisms are not susceptible in vitro to glycopeptides.

8. IMPACT OF MACROLIDES, KETOLIDES, LINCOSAMIDES, AND STREPTOGRAMINS ON THE HUMAN MICROFLORA

8.1. Oropharyngeal Microflora

The interaction between macrolides, ketolides, and lincosamides and the oropharyngeal microflora is shown in Table 6. Macrolides inhibit the bacterial synthesis of proteins and are active mainly against gram-positive microorganisms. Administration of clarithromycin is not connected with any major disturbances of the oropharyngeal microflora, but isolation of highly resistant alpha-hemolytic streptococci and overgrowth of enterobacterial species have been registered. No major impact of administration of dirithromycin on the oropharyngeal microflora has been shown. In spite of rather high concentrations of erythromycin in saliva, the impact of administration has been shown mainly on the aerobic microflora, where the numbers of streptococci are reduced. No changes have been shown in the anaerobic microflora. Overgrowth of enterobacteria is common.

Telithromycin belongs to a new class of macrolides, ketolides, and has a broad antimicrobial spectrum.

Telithromycin is also found in high concentrations in saliva, but no major ecological disturbances occur. Transient colonization with low numbers of enterobacteria has been reported.

The lincosamide clindamycin has a broad antimicrobial spectrum including anaerobic and gram-positive aerobic microorganisms. Clindamycin is secreted into saliva and exerts an influence on the anaerobic microflora that is strongly suppressed. Some of the streptococcal species are affected but to a lesser extent. The changed conditions during treatment allow for overgrowth of both aerobic and anaerobic microorganisms, including yeasts.

There are no available studies on the effect of streptogramins on the oropharyngeal microflora.

8.2. Gastrointestinal Microflora

Table 8 shows the impact of macrolides, ketolides, lincosamides, and streptogramins on the intestinal microflora. High fecal concentrations have been attained for both the macrolides and the ketolides. The macrolides are incompletely absorbed, mainly metabolized in the liver, and, like the ketolides, eliminated through bile. Clarithromycin evokes changes in the aerobic intestinal microflora mainly in reduced numbers of streptococci and *E. coli* organisms and selects for resistant enterobacteria. In the anaerobic microflora, reductions in the numbers of lactobacilli, bifidobacteria, and *Bacteroides* organisms have been seen. Highly resistant *Bacteroides* strains have been isolated in some studies. Administration of dirithromycin increases the numbers of streptococci and staphylococci and suppresses the numbers of enterobacteria, with a concomitant colonization with resistant enterobacterial species. Several anaerobic species are reduced in number during treatment. Very high fecal concentrations of erythromycin affect the intestinal flora strongly, with suppressed numbers of both enterobacteria and anaerobic microorganisms. Enterococci and staphylococci are also reduced and new colonization with resistant staphylococci, enterobacteria, and yeasts occurs. *C. difficile* has been isolated in a few subjects. Roxithromycin has been reported to induce less strong changes in the intestinal microflora, with reductions only in the numbers of enterobacteria.

The ketolide telithromycin induces moderate quantitative ecological disturbances in spite of very high fecal concentrations of the drug. Isolation of *Bacteroides* organisms for which the MICs of telithromycin are increased has been associated with its administration.

Clindamycin is well absorbed but is excreted mainly through bile, and therefore the fecal concentrations reach high levels. Naturally resistant bacteria are enterococci and enterobacteria. The numbers of enterococci and enterobacteria other than *E. coli* increase during administration, and the anaerobic microflora is strongly suppressed. Resistant enterococci and *C. difficile* are frequently isolated.

Quinopristin-dalfopristin is an injectable streptogramin that is mainly eliminated through feces. Administration increases the numbers of enterococci and enterobacteria, while anaerobic gram-negative microorganisms decrease. Isolation of *C. difficile* has not been documented, but increased numbers of resistant enterococci and gram-negative anaerobes have been reported.

9. IMPACT OF TETRACYCLINES, AMINOGLYCOSIDES, NITROFURANTOIN, OXAZOLIDINONE, NITROIMIDAZOLES, AND FOLIC ACID ANTAGONISTS ON THE HUMAN MICROFLORA

9.1. Oropharyngeal Microflora

The impact of tetracyclines and nitroimidazoles on the oropharyngeal microflora is summarized in Table 9. Tetracyclines are broad-spectrum antimicrobial agents and act by inhibiting the protein synthesis of the microorganisms. Tetracyclines are detected in mixed saliva in concentrations equivalent to those in plasma. In spite of the high salivary concentrations, only minor quantitative changes occur during administration, depending on a marked increase in the numbers of both aerobic and anaerobic tetracycline-resistant microorganisms.

Nitroimidazoles are active against anaerobic microorganisms by interfering with the synthesis of DNA. Salivary concentrations of nitroimidazoles follow the concentrations in serum, and high levels are achieved during treatment. Administration of tinidazole has no impact on the aerobic microflora, but the anaerobic microorganisms decrease in number, in particular fusobacteria. Combinations of

Table 8 Impact of macrolides, ketolide, lincosamide, and streptogramin on the instestinal microflora[a]

Agent	Impact on:			Resistant microorganisms	Overgrowth of *C. difficile* or *Candida*	Reference(s)
	Aerobic Gr^+ cocci	Entero-bacteria	Anaerobic bacteria			
Macrolides						
Clarithromycin	↓	↓↓	↓	+	–	15, 28, 31
Dirithromycin	↑	↓	↓	+	–	27
Erythromycin	↓	↓↓	↓↓	+	+	15, 53, 54
Roxithromycin	–	↓	–	–	–	117
Ketolide						
Telithromycin	↓↑	↓	–	+	–	28
Lincosamide						
Clindamycin	↑	↑	↓↓	+	+	52, 53, 66, 113
Streptogramin						
Quinupristin-dalfopristin	↑	↑	↓	+	–	122

[a]↓, suppression (2 to 4 $\log_{10}$ CFU/g of feces); ↓↓, strong suppression (>4 $\log_{10}$ CFU/g of feces); ↑, increase of microorganisms during treatment; –, no significant changes. Gr^+, gram positive.

Table 9 Impact of tetracyclines, nitroimidazoles, combination of metronidazole and penicillin or macrolides, and quinolones on the oropharyngeal microflora[a]

Agent	Impact on: Streptococci	Impact on: Anaerobic bacteria	Resistant streptococci	Overgrowth of enterobacteria or *Candida*	Reference(s)
Tetracyclines					
Doxycycline	↓	↓	+	–	55
Nitroimidazoles					
Tinidazole	–	↓	–	–	56, 58
Metronidazole-amoxicillin	↓	↓	–	+	3
Metronidazole-clarithromycin	↓	↓	+	+	3
Quinolones					
Ciprofloxacin	–	–	–	–	9
Levofloxacin	–	–	–	–	40
Lomefloxacin	–	–	–	–	32
Moxifloxacin	↓	↑	–	–	11
Norfloxacin	–	–	–	–	30
Ofloxacin	–	–	–	–	34, 40
Rufloxacin	–	–	+	+	23

[a]↓, mild to moderate suppression (2 to 4 $\log_{10}$ CFU/ml of saliva); ↑, increase of microorganisms during treatment; –, no significant changes.

metronidazole and amoxicillin or clarithromycin decrease the numbers of streptococci and anaerobic microorganisms and gives rise to overgrowth of enterobacteria and *Candida* species in some subjects. Resistant streptoccocci have been isolated in connection with combination of metronidazole and clarithromycin.

There are no studies available on the interaction between aminoglycosides, nitrofurantoin, linezolid, or folic acid antagonists and the oropharyngeal microflora.

9.2. Gastrointestinal Microflora

The influence of tetracyclines, aminoglycosides, nitrofurantoin, oxazolidinone, nitroimidazoles, and folic acid antagonists on the gastrointestinal microflora is shown in Table 10.

Extensive use of tetracyclines has led to emergence of resistance in several pathogens, such as β-hemolytic streptococci, staphylococci, and *Bacteroides fragilis*. Tetracyclines are excreted in the bile and are reabsorbed in the small intestine, which leads to high fecal concentrations. Tetracyclines do not give rise to any major changes of total numbers of intestinal microorganisms during administration, but administration is followed by a marked selection of tetracycline-resistant strains and overgrowth of both aerobic and anaerobic microorganisms. Overgrowth of *C. albicans* has been seen occasionally.

Aminoglycosides are mainly active against gram-negative aerobic microorganisms, and during administration the numbers of enterobacteria in feces decrease. β-Lactam antimicrobial agents act synergistically with aminoglycosides, and thereby the antibacterial spectrum increases.

Nitrofurantoin has an antibacterial spectrum similar to that of the aminoglycosides and is mainly used in the treatment of urinary tract infections. It acts by inhibiting the protein synthesis of the bacterial cell. Administration of nitrofurantoin does not have any major effect on the normal aerobic microflora, and no data are available for the anaerobic microflora.

Linezolid belongs to a new class of synthetic antimicrobial agents, oxazolidinones, and inhibits the initiation of bacterial protein synthesis. Administration causes reduced numbers of enterococci and increased numbers of resistant enterobacteria. Linezolid also has been shown to markedly reduce the anaerobic microflora.

Low concentrations of nitroimidazoles are detected in feces during administration since the agents are excreted via liver metabolism. Consequently, no changes in the intestinal microflora have been observed during metronidazole administration. However, proliferation of enterococci and staphylococci and decreased numbers of anaerobic microorganisms have been observed during administration of tinidazole. Combination of metronidazole and amoxicillin induces larger changes in increased numbers of enterococci, emergence of resistant new enterobacteria, and overgrowth of yeasts. Increased numbers of enterococci are also seen when combinations of metronidazole and clarithromycin are administered. Furthermore, the combination suppresses the numbers of *E. coli* and anaerobic microorganisms. Increased resistance to clarithromycin has been detected during treatment in strains of enterococci, enterobacteria, and *Bacteroides*. In one study *C. difficile* was detected in a few subjects.

The folic acid antagonist co-trimoxazole (trimethoprim-sulfamethoxazole) is excreted via the kidneys and has been shown to strongly suppress the numbers of enterobacteria during administration. The effect on the anaerobic normal microflora has not been investigated.

10. IMPACT OF QUINOLONES ON THE HUMAN MICROFLORA

10.1. Oropharyngeal Microflora

The effect of quinolones on the oropharyngeal microflora is shown in Table 9. The quinolones are well distributed in all body tissues and secretions. Salivary concentrations of the newer quinolones, like moxifloxacin, have been shown to be similar to those in serum. However, low levels of the older agents have been detected in saliva, and the proportion of the disturbances on the normal oropharyngeal microflora is also smaller than that induced by moxifloxacin. The activity

Table 10 Impact of tetracyclines, aminoglycoside, nitrofurantoin, oxazolidinone, nitroimidazoles, combinations of metronidazole and penicillin or macrolide, and folic acid antagonists on the intestinal microflora[a]

Agent	Impact on: Aerobic Gr⁺ cocci	Entero-bacteria	Anaerobic bacteria	Resistant microorganisms	Overgrowth of *C. difficile* or *Candida*	Reference(s)
Tetracyclines						
Tetracycline	–	–	–	+	+	8
Doxycycline	↓↑	↓	–	+	+	8, 55
Aminoglycosides						
Tobramycin	–	↓	–	+	–	96
Nitrofurantoin	–	–	*[b]	–	–	92
Oxazolidinone						
Linezolid	↓	↑	↓↓	+	–	87
Nitroimidazoles						
Metronidazole	–	–	–	–	–	103
Tinidazole	↑	–	↓	–	–	56, 68
Metronidazole-amoxicillin	↑	–	–	+	+	3
Metronidazole-clarithromycin	↑	↓	↓	+	+	3, 20
Folic acid antagonist						
Co-trimoxazole	–	↓↓	*	–	–	92

[a]↓, suppression (2 to 4 $\log_{10}$ CFU/g of feces); ↓↓, strong suppression (>4 $\log_{10}$ CFU/g of feces); ↑, increase of microorganisms during treatment; –, no significant changes. Gr⁺, gram positive.
[b]*, no data available.

of the first quinolones was restricted to gram-negative aerobic microorganisms, while later agents have increased activity against streptococci, staphylococci, and anaerobic microorganisms. The older agents have an impact mainly on gram-negative aerobic cocci, while moxifloxacin also reduces the numbers of alpha-hemolytic streptococci and gives rise to markedly increased numbers of gram-negative anaerobic bacteria. In connection with administration of rufloxacin, increased resistance to this agent has been observed in viridans group streptococci and coagulase-negative staphylococci.

10.2. Gastrointestinal Microflora

The interactions between the normal intestinal microflora and quinolones are described in Table 11. Fluoroquinolones act by inhibiting DNA gyrases, which are essential enzymes for DNA supercoiling. The agents are well absorbed after oral administration, and several mechanisms are involved in

TABLE 11 Impact of quinolones on the intestinal microflora[a]

Agent	Impact on: Aerobic Gr⁺ cocci	Entero-bacteria	Anaerobic bacteria	Resistant microorganisms	Overgrowth of *C. difficile* or *Candida*	Reference(s)
Ciprofloxacin	↓	↓↓	–	+	–	9, 13, 14, 19, 42, 43, 59, 78, 85, 118, 120, 130, 134, 143
Enoxacin	–	↓↓	–	–	–	35
Gatifloxacin	↓↑	↓↓	–	–	–	38
Gemifloxacin	↓	↓	–	–	–	7, 48
Levofloxacin	↓	↓↓	–	–	–	40, 60
Lomefloxacin	–	↓↓	–	–	–	32
Moxifloxacin	↓	↓↓	–	–	–	31
Norfloxacin	–	↓↓	–	–	–	26, 30, 83, 91–93, 115
Ofloxacin	↓	↓↓	–	–	–	34, 40, 116
Pefloxacin	↓	↓↓	–	–	–	134, 138
Rufloxacin	–	↓↓	↓	–	–	23, 91
Sitafloxacin	↓↓	↓↓	↓	+	+	61
Sparfoxacin	↓	↓↓	–	–	–	119
Trovafloxacin	↓	↓↓	↓	+	–	48, 133
BMS-284756	↓	↓	↓↓	+	+	107

[a]↓, suppression (2 to 4 $\log_{10}$ CFU/g feces); ↓↓, strong suppression (>4 $\log_{10}$ CFU/g feces); ↑, increase of microorganisms during treatment; –, no significant changes. Gr⁺, gram positive.

their elimination. Generally, very high fecal concentrations are achieved, but the quinolones are bound to fecal material and the major part is thereby biologically inactive. The unbound fractions are still above the MICs for enterobacteria since their numbers are strongly suppressed during administration. Ciprofloxacin, enoxacin, lomefloxacin, and norfloxacin usually do not affect other intestinal microbial groups, but in some studies on the impact of ciprofloxacin, decreased numbers of enterococci have been observed. The numbers of gram-positive cocci are partly suppressed during treatment with the remaining quinolones, as shown in Table 11. Administration of rufloxacin decreases the numbers not only of enterobacteria but also of anaerobic microorganisms. Quinolones like sitafloxacin, trovafloxacin, and BMS-284756 disturb both the aerobic and anaerobic microflora. Emergence of resistant strains has been detected during treatment with these agents. Overgrowth of *C. difficile* or yeasts is uncommon in connection with the use of quinolones.

11. CONCLUSIONS

Knowledge about the interaction between antimicrobial agents and the normal microflora gives the clinician the possibility to choose agents associated with lesser degrees of ecological disturbances. Consequently, the risk of development of resistant strains and transfer of resistance elements between microorganisms is reduced. Further, consideration of the ecological consequences is also an important step to prevent distribution of resistant strains between patients in hospital settings.

The dimension of disturbances not only is dependent on the spectrum of the agents but also is influenced by the degree of absorption of the agent, the route of elimination, and the enzymatic activity of the microflora. Individual pharmacokinetic variations as well as the character of composition and susceptibility of the normal microflora are variables that further influence the interactions.

REFERENCES

1. **Adamsson, I., C. Edlund, R. Seensalu, S. Sjöstedt, and C.E.** Nord. 1998. The normal gastric microflora and *Helicobacter pylori;* before, during and after treatment with omeprazole and amoxycillin. Clin. Microbiol. Infect. **4:**308–315.
2. **Adamsson, I., C. Edlund, S. Sjöstedt, and C.E. Nord.** 1997. Comparative effects of cefadroxil and phenoxymethylpenicillin on the normal oropharyngeal and intestinal microflora. Infection **25:**154–158.
3. **Adamsson, I., C.E. Nord, P. Lundquist, S. Sjöstedt, and C. Edlund.** 1999. Comparative effects of omeprazole, amoxycillin plus metronidazole versus omeprazole, clarithromycin plus metronidazole on the oral, gastric and intestinal microflora in *Helicobacter pylori*-infected patients. J. Antimicrob. Chemother. **44:**629–640.
4. **Alestig, K., H. Carlberg, C.E. Nord, and B. Trollfors.** 1983. Effect of cefoperazone on faecal flora. J. Antimicrob. Chemother. **12:**163–167.
5. **Bächer, K., M. Schaeffer, H. Lode, C.E. Nord, K. Borner, and P. Koeppe.** 1992. Multiple dose pharmacokinetics, safety, and effects on faecal microflora of cefepime in healthy volunteers. J. Antimicrob. Chemother. **30:**365–375.
6. **Barbut, F., and J.C. Petit.** 2001. Epidemiology of *Clostridium difficile*-associated infections. Clin. Microbiol. Infect. **7:**405–410.
7. **Barker, P.J., R. Sheehan, M. Teillol-Foo, A.C. Palmgren, and C.E. Nord.** 2001. Impact of gemifloxacin on the normal human intestinal microflora. J. Chemother. **13:**47–51.
8. **Bartlett, J.G., L.A. Bustetter, S.L. Gorbach, and A.B. Onderdonk.** 1975. Comparative effect of tetracycline and doxycycline on the occurrence of resistant Escherichia coli in the fecal flora. Antimicrob. Agents Chemother. **7:**55–57.
9. **Bergan, T., C. Delin, S. Johansen, I.M. Kolstad, C.E. Nord, and S.B. Thorsteinsson.** 1986. Pharmacokinetics of ciprofloxacin and effect of repeated dosage on salivary and fecal microflora. Antimicrob. Agents Chemother. **29:**298–302.
10. **Bergan, T., C.E. Nord, and S.B. Thorsteinsson.** 1991. Effect of meropenem on the intestinal microflora. Eur. J. Clin. Microbiol. Infect. Dis. **10:**524–527.
11. **Beyer, G., M. Hiemer-Bau, S. Ziege, C. Edlund, H. Lode, and C.E. Nord.** 2000. Impact of moxifloxacin versus clarithromycin on normal oropharyngeal microflora. Eur. J. Clin. Microbiol. Infect. Dis. **19:**548–550.
12. **Black, F, K. Einarsson, A. Lidbeck, K. Orrhage, and C.E. Nord.** 1991. Effect of lactic acid producing bacteria on the human intestinal microflora during ampicillin treatment. Scand. J. Infect. Dis. **23:**247–254.
13. **Borzio, M., F. Salerno, M. Saudelli, D. Galvagno, L. Piantoni, and L. Fragiacomo.** 1997. Efficacy of oral ciprofloxacin as selective intestinal decontaminant in cirrhosis. Ital. J. Gastroenterol. Hepatol. **29:**262–266.
14. **Brismar, B., C. Edlund, A.S. Malmborg, and C.E. Nord.** 1990. Ciprofloxacin concentrations and impact of the colon microflora in patients undergoing colorectal surgery. Antimicrob. Agents Chemother. **34:**481–483.
15. **Brismar, B., C. Edlund, and C.E. Nord.** 1991. Comparative effects of clarithromycin and erythromycin on the normal intestinal microflora. Scand. J. Infect. Dis. **23:**635–642.
16. **Brismar, B., C. Edlund, and C.E. Nord.** 1993. Effect of ceftibuten on the normal intestinal microflora. Infection **21:**373–375.
17. **Brismar, B., C. Edlund, and C.E. Nord.** 1993. Impact of cefpodoxime proxetil and amoxicillin on the normal oral and intestinal microflora. Eur. J. Clin. Microbiol. Infect. Dis. **12:**714–719.
18. **Brumfitt, W., I. Franklin, D. Grady, and J.M. Hamilton-Miller.** 1986. Effect of amoxicillin-clavulanate and cephradine on the fecal flora of healthy volunteers not exposed to a hospital environment. Antimicrob. Agents Chemother. **30:**335–337.
19. **Brumfitt, W., I. Franklin, D. Grady, J.M. Hamilton-Miller, and A. Iliffe.** 1984. Changes in the pharmacokinetics of ciprofloxacin and fecal flora during administration of a 7-day course to human volunteers. Antimicrob. Agents Chemother. **26:**757–761.
20. **Bühling, A., D. Radun, W.A. Müller, and P. Malfertheiner.** 2001. Influence of anti-Helicobacter triple-therapy with metronidazole, omeprazole and clarithromycin on intestinal microflora. Aliement. Pharmacol. Ther. **15:**1445–1452.
21. **Cavallaro, V., V. Catania, R. Bonaccorso, S. Mazzone, A. Speciale, R. di Marco, G. Blandino, and F. Caccamo.** 1992. Effect of a broad-spectrum cephalosporin on the oral and intestinal microflora in patients undergoing colorectal surgery. J. Chemother. **4:**82–87.
22. **Christensson, B., I. Nilsson-Ehle, B. Ljungberg, I. Nömm, G. Oscarsson, L. Nordström G. Goscinsky, E. Löwdin, T. Linglöf, B. Nordström, I. Denstedt-Stigzelius, K. Lindhagen, C. Edlund, and C.E. Nord.** 1991. A randomized multicenter trial to compare the influence of cefaclor and amoxycillin on the colonization resistance of the digestive tract in patients with lower respiratory tract infection. Infection **19:**208–215.
23. **D'Antonio, D., E. Pizzigallo, A. Iacone, B. Violante, A.D. Marzio, M. Lombardo, G. Fioritoni, T. Staniscia, and F. Romano.** 1996. The impact of rufloxacin given as prophylaxis to patients with cancer on their oral and faecal microflora. J. Antimicrob. Chemother. **39:**839–847.
24. **de Vries-Hospers, H.G., R.H.J. Tonk, and D. van der Waaij.** 1991. Effect of intramuscular ceftriaxone on aerobic oral and faecal flora of 11 healthy volunteers. Scand. J. Infect. Dis. **23:**652–633.
25. **de Vries-Hospers, H.G., G.W. Welling, E.A. Swabb, and D. van der Waaij.** 1984. Selective decontamination of the digestive tract with aztreonam. A study of 10 healthy volunteers. J. Infect. Dis. **150:**636–642.

26. **de Vries-Hospers, H.G., G.W. Welling, E.A. Swabb, and D. van der Waaij.** 1985. Norfloxacin for selective decontamination: a study in human volunteers. Prog. Clin. Biol. Res. **181:** 259–262.
27. **Eckernäs, S.Å., A. Grahnén, and C.E. Nord.** 1991. Impact of dirithromycin on the normal oral and intestinal microflora. Eur. J. Clin. Microbiol. Infect. Dis. **10:**688–692.
28. **Edlund, C., G. Alván, L. Barkholt, F. Vacheron, and C.E. Nord.** 2000. Pharmacokinetics and comparative effects of telithromycin (HMR 3647) and clarithromycin on the oropharyngeal and intestinal microoflora. J. Antimicrob. Chemother. **46:**741–749.
29. **Edlund, C., L. Barkholt, B. Olsson-Liljequist, and C.E. Nord.** 1997. Effect of vancomycin on intestinal flora of patients who previously received antimicrobial therapy. Clin. Infect. Dis. **25:**729–732.
30. **Edlund, C., T. Bergan, K. Josefssson, R. Solberg, and C.E. Nord.** 1987. Effect of norfloxacin on human oropharyngeal and colonic microflora and multiple-dose pharmacokinetics. Scand. J. Infect. Dis. **19:**113–121.
31. **Edlund, C., G. Beyer, M. Hiemer-Bau, S. Ziege, H. Lode, and C.E. Nord.** 2000. Comparative effects of moxifloxacin and clarithromycin on the normal intestinal microflora. Scand. J. Infect. Dis. **32:**81–85.
32. **Edlund, C., B. Brismar, and C.E. Nord.** 1990. Effect of lomefloxacin on the normal oral and intestinal microflora. Eur. J. Clin. Microbiol. Infect. Dis. **1:**35–39.
33. **Edlund, C., B. Brismar, H. Sakamoto, and C.E. Nord.** 1993. Impact of cefuroxime-axetil on the normal intestinal microflora. Microb. Ecol. Health Dis. **6:**185–189.
34. **Edlund, C., L. Kager, A.S. Malmborg, S. Sjöstedt, and C.E. Nord.** 1988. Effect of ofloxacin on oral and gastrointestinal microflora in patients undergoing colorectal surgery. Eur. J. Clin. Microbiol. Infect. Dis. **7:**135–143.
35. **Edlund, C., A. Lidbeck, L. Kager, and C.E. Nord.** 1987. Effect of enoxacin on colonic microflora of healthy volunteers. Eur. J. Clin. Microbiol. **6:**298–300.
36. **Edlund, C., and C.E. Nord.** 1991. A model of bacterial-antimicrobial interactions: the case of oropharyngeal and gastrointestinal microflora. J. Chemother. **3**(Suppl. 1)**:**196–200.
37. **Edlund, C., and C.E. Nord.** 1993. Ecological impact of antimicrobial agents on human intestinal microflora. Alpe Adria Microbiol. J. **3:**137–164.
38. **Edlund, C., and C.E. Nord.** 1999. Ecological effect of gatifloxacin on the normal human intestinal microflora. J. Chemother. **11:**50–53.
39. **Edlund, C., and C.E. Nord.** 2001. The evaluation and prediction of the ecological impact by antibiotics in human phases I and II trials. Clin. Microbiol. Infect. **7** (Suppl. 5)**:**37–41.
40. **Edlund, C., S. Sjöstedt, and C.E. Nord.** 1997. Comparative effects of levofloxacin and ofloxacin on the normal oral and intestinal microflora. Scand. J. Infect. Dis. **29:**383–386.
41. **Edlund, C., C. Stark, and C.E. Nord.** 1994. The relationship between an increase in β-lactamase activity after oral administration of three new cephalosporins and protection against intestinal ecological disturbances. J. Antimicrob. Chemother. **34:**127–138.
42. **Enzenberger, R., P.M. Shah, and H. Knothe.** 1985. Impact of ciprofloxacin on the faecal flora of healthy volunteers. Infection **13:**273–275.
43. **Esposito, S., D. Barba, D. Galante, G.B. Gaeta, and O. Laghezza.** 1987. Intestinal microflora changes induced by ciprofloxacin and treatment of portal-systematic encephalopathy. Drugs Exptl. Clin. Res. **10:**641–646.
44. **The European Agency for the Evaluation of Medicinal Products (EMEA).** 2000. Points to consider on pharmacokinetics and pharmacodynamics in the development of antibacterial medicinal products. Document CPMP/EWP/2655/99. Committee for proprietary medicinal products (CPMP), London. http://www.eudra.org/ emea.html.
45. **European Committee for Antimicrobial Susceptibility Testing (EUCAST) Definitive Document E.DEF 2.1.** 2000. Determination of antimicrobial susceptibility test breakpoints. EUCAST discussion Document, European Society of Clinical Microbiology and Infectious Diseases (ESCMID). Clin. Microbiol. Infect. **6:**570–572.
46. **Finegold, S.M., L. Ingram-Drake, R. Gee, J. Reinhardt, M.A. Edelstein, K. MacDonald, and H. Wexler.** 1987. Bowel flora changes in humans receiving cefixime (CL 284,635) or cefaclor. Antimicrob. Agents Chemother. **31:**443–446.
47. **Floor, M., F. van Akkeren, M. Rozenberg-Arska, M. Visser, A. Kolsters, H. Beumer, and J. Verhoef.** 1994. Effect of loracarbef and amoxicillin on the oropharyngeal and intestinal microflora of patients with bronchitis. Scand. J. Infect. Dis. **26:**191–197.
48. **Garcia-Calvo, G., A. Molleja, M.J. Giménez, A. Parra, E. Nieto, C. Ponte, L. Aguilar, and F. Soriano.** 2001. Effects of single oral doses of gemifloxacin (320 milligrams) versus trovafloxacin (200 milligrams) on fecal flora in healthy volunteers. Antimicrob. Agents Chemother. **45:**608–611.
49. **Gipponi, M., C. Sciutto, L. Accornero, S. Bonassi, C. Raso, C. Vignolo, and F. Cafiero.** 1985. Assessing modifications of the intestinal bacterial flora in patients on long-term oral treatment with bacampicillin or amoxycillin: a random study. Chemioterapia **4:**214–217.
50. **Guggenbichler, J.P., and J. Kofler.** 1984. Influence of third-generation cephalosporins on aerobic intestinal microflora. J. Antimicrob. Chemother. **14**(Suppl. B)**:**67–70.
51. **Heimdahl, A., L. Kager, and C.E. Nord.** 1986. Alterations in the human oropharyngeal microflora related to therapy with aztreonam, moxalactam and ampicillin plus sulbactam. Scand. J. Infect. Dis. **18:**49–52.
52. **Heimdahl, A., and C.E. Nord.** 1979. Effect of phenoxymethylpenicillin and clindamycin on the oral, throat and faecal microflora of man. Scand. J. Infect. Dis. **11:**233–242.
53. **Heimdahl, A., and C.E. Nord.** 1982. Effect of erythromycin and clindamycin on the indigenous human anaerobic flora and new colonization of the gastrointestinal tract. Eur. J. Clin. Microbiol. **1:**34–48.
54. **Heimdahl, A., and C.E. Nord.** 1982. Influence of erythromycin on the normal human flora and colonization of the oral cavity, throat and colon. Scand. J. Infect. Dis. **14:**49–56.
55. **Heimdahl, A., and C.E. Nord.** 1983. Influence of doxycycline on the normal human flora and colonization of the oral cavity and colon. Scand. J. Infect. Dis. **15:**293–302.
56. **Heimdahl, A., C.E. Nord, and K. Okuda.** 1980. Effect of tinidazole on the oral, throat, and colon microflora of man. Med. Microbiol. Immunol. **168:**1–10.
57. **Heimdahl, A., C.E. Nord, and K. Weilander.** 1979. Effect of bacampicillin on human mouth, throat and colon flora. Infection **7**(Suppl. 5)**:**446–451.
58. **Heimdahl, A., L. von Konow, and C.E. Nord.** 1982. Effect of tinidazole on the human oral microflora: a comparison between high single and low repeated doses. J. Antimicrob. Chemother. **10**(Suppl. A)**:**157–164.
59. **Holt, H.A., D.A. Lewis, L.O. White, S.Y. Bastable, and D.S. Reeves.** 1986. Effect of oral ciprofloxacin on the faecal flora of healthy volunteers. Eur. J. Clin. Microbiol. **5:**201–205.
60. **Inagaki, Y., R. Nakaya, T. Chida, and S. Hashimoto.** 1992. The effect of levofloxacin, an optically-active isomer of ofloxacin, on fecal microflora in human volunteers. Jpn. J. Antibiot. **45:**241–252.
61. **Inagaki, Y., N. Yamamoto, T. Chida, N. Okamura, and M. Tanaka.** 1995. The effect of DU-6859a, a new potent fluoroquinolone, on fecal microflora in human volunteers. Jpn. J. Antibiot. **48:**368–379.
62. **Jones, P.G., G.P. Bodey, E.A. Swabb, and B. Rosenbaum.** 1984. Effect of aztreonam on throat and stool flora of cancer patients. Antimicrob. Agents Chemother. **26:**941–943.
63. **Kager, L., B. Brismar, A.S. Malmborg, and C.E. Nord.** 1985. Effect of aztreonam on the colon microflora in patients undergoing colorectal surgery. Infection **13:**111–114.
64. **Kager, L., B. Brismar, A.S. Malmborg, and C.E. Nord.** 1986. Impact of cefbuperazone on the colonic microflora in patients undergoing colorectal surgery. Drugs Exptl. Clin. Res. **12:**983–986.

65. **Kager, L., B. Brismar, A.S. Malmborg, and C.E. Nord.** 1989. Imipenem concentrations in colorectal surgery and impact on the colonic microflora. Antimicrob. Agents Chemother. **33**:204–208.
66. **Kager, L., L. Liljeqvist, A.S. Malmborg, and C.E. Nord.** 1981. Effect of clindamycin prophylaxis on the colonic microflora in patients undergoing colorectal surgery. Antimicrob. Agents Chemother. **20**:736–740.
67. **Kager, L., L. Liljeqvist, A.S. Malmborg, C.E. Nord, and R. Pieper.** 1982. Effects of ampicillin plus sulbactam on bowel flora in patients undergoing colorectal surgery. Antimicrob. Agents Chemother. **22**:208–212.
68. **Kager, L., I. Ljungdahl, A.S. Malmborg, and C.E. Nord.** 1981. Effect of tinidazole prophylaxis on the normal microflora in patients undergoing colorectal surgery. Scand. J. Infect. Dis. **26**(Suppl):84–91.
69. **Kager, L., I. Ljungdahl, A.S. Malmborg, C.E. Nord, R. Pieper, and P. Dahlgren.** 1981. Antibiotic prophylaxis with cefoxitin in colorectal surgery. Ann. Surg. **193**:277–282.
70. **Kager, L., A.S. Malmborg, C.E. Nord, and S. Sjöstedt.** 1983. The effect of piperacillin prophylaxis on the colonic microflora in patients undergoing colorectal surgery. Infection **11**:251–254.
71. **Kager, L., A.S. Malmborg, C.E. Nord, and S. Sjöstedt.** 1984. Impact of single dose as compared to three dose prophylaxis with latamoxef (moxalactam) on the colonic microflora in patients undergoing colorectal surgery. J. Antimicrob. Chemother. **14**:171–177.
72. **Kager, L., A.S. Malmborg, S. Sjöstedt, and C.E. Nord.** 1983. Concentrations of ampicillin plus sulbactam in serum and intestinal mucosa and effects on the colonic microflora in patients undergoing colorectal surgery. Eur. J. Clin. Microbiol. **2**:559–563.
73. **Knothe H.** 1976. The effect of pivmecillinam on the human gut flora. Arzneimittel Forschung (Drug Reg.) **26**:427–430.
74. **Knothe, H., G.A. Dette, and P.M. Shah.** 1985. Impact of injectable cephalosporins on the gastrointestinal microflora. Observations in healthy volunteers and hospitalized patients. Infection **13**(Suppl. 1):129–133.
75. **Knothe, H., and U. Lembke.** 1973. The effect of ampicillin and pivampicillin on the intestinal flora of man. Zentralbl. Bakteriol. Hyg. I Abt. **223**:324–332.
76. **Knothe, H., V. Schäfer, A. Sammann, M. Badian, and P.M. Shah.** 1992. Influence of cefpirome on pharyngeal and faecal flora after single and multiple intravenous administrations of cefpirome to healthy volunteers. J. Antimicrob. Chemother. **29**(Suppl. A):81–86.
77. **Knothe, H., and B. Wiedemann.** 1965. Die Wirkung von Ampicillin auf die Darmflora des gesunden Menschen. Zentralbl. Bakteriol. Hyg. I Abt. **197**:234–243.
78. **Krueger, W.A., G. Rucksdeschel, and K. Unertl.** 1997. Influence of intravenously administered ciprofloxacin on aerobic intestinal microflora and fecal drug levels when administered simultaneously with sucralfate. Antimicrob. Agents Chemother. **41**:1725–1730.
79. **Lambert-Zechovsky, N., E. Bingen, Y. Aujard, and H. Mathieu.** 1985. Impact of cefotaxime on the fecal flora in children. Infection **13**(Suppl. 1):140–144.
80. **Lambert-Zechovsky, N., E. Bingen, M.C. Proux, Y. Aujard, and H. Mathieu.** 1984. Effect of amoxycillin combined with clavulanic acid on the fecal flora of children. Pathol. Biol. **32**:436–442.
81. **Lambert-Zechovsky, N., E. Bingen, M.C. Proux, Y. Aujard, and H. Mathieu.** 1984. Effects of cefoperazone on children's fecal flora. Pathol. Biol. **32**:439–442.
82. **Leigh, D.A.** 1979. Pharmacology and toxological studies with amoxycillin, talampicillin and ampicillin and a clinical trial of parenteral amoxycillin in serious hospital infections. Drugs Exptl. Clin. Res. **5**:129–139.
83. **Leigh, D.A., F.X.S. Emmanuel, C. Tighe, P. Hancock, and S. Boddy.** 1985. Pharmacokinetic studies of norfloxacin in healthy volunteers and effect on the faecal microflora. Proc. 14th Int. Cong. Chemother., Kyoto, p. 1835–1836.
84. **Leigh, D.A., B. Walsh, A. Leung, S. Tait, K. Peatey, and P. Hancock.** 1990. The effect of cefuroxime axetil on the faecal flora of healthy volunteers. J. Antimicrob. Chemother. **26**:261–268.
85. **Ljungberg, B., I. Nielsen-Ehle, C. Edlund, and C.E. Nord.** 1990. Influence of ciprofloxacin on the colonic microflora in young and elderly volunteers: no impact of the altered drug absorption. Scand. J. Infect. Dis. **22**:205–208.
86. **Lode, H., C. Müller, K. Borner, C.E. Nord, and P. Koeppe.** 1992. Multiple-dose pharmacokinetics of cefprozil and its impact on intestinal flora of volunteers. Antimicrob. Agents Chemother. **36**:144–149.
87. **Lode, H., N. von der Höh, S. Ziege, K. Borner, and C.E. Nord.** 2001. Ecological effects of linezolid versus amoxicillin/clavulanic acid on the normal intestinal microflora. Scand. J. Infect. Dis. **33**:899–903.
88. **Lund, B., C. Edlund, L. Barkholt, C.E. Nord, M. Tvede, and R.L. Poulsen.** 2000. Impact on human intestinal microflora of an Enterococcus faecium probiotic and vancomycin. Scand. J. Infect. Dis. **32**:627–632.
89. **Lund, B, C. Edlund, B. Rynnel-Dagöö, Y. Lundgren, J. Sterner, and C.E. Nord.** 2001. Ecological effects on the oro- and nasopharyngeal microflora in children after treatment of acute otitis media with cefuroxime axetil or amoxycillin-clavulanate as suspensions. Clin. Microbiol. Infect. **7**:230–237.
90. **Mackowiak, P.** 1982. The normal microbial flora. N. Engl. J. Med. **307**:83–93.
91. **Marco, F., M.J. Giménez, M.T. Jiménez de Anta, M.A. Marcos, P. Salvá, and L. Aguilar.** 1995. Comparison of rufloxacin and norfloxacin effects on faecal flora. J. Antimicrob. Chemother. **35**:895–901.
92. **Mavromanolakis, E., S. Maraki, G. Samonis, Y. Tselentis, and A. Cranidis.** 1997. Effect of norfloxacin, trimethoprim-sulfamethoxazole and nitrofurantoin on fecal flora of women with recurrent urinary tract infections. J. Chemother. **9**:203–207.
93. **Meckenstock, R., E. Haralambie, G. Linzenmeier, and F. Wendt.** 1985. Die Beeinflussung der Darmflora durch Norfloxacin bei gesunden Menschen. Z. Antimikr. Antineoplast. Chemother. **1**:27–34.
94. **Mittermayer, H.W.** 1983. The effect of amoxycillin and amoxycillin plus clavulanic acid on human bowel flora, p. 125–133. *In* E.A.P. Croydon and M.F. Michael (ed.), Augmentin: Clavulanate-Potentiated Amoxycillin.
95. **Motohiro, T., K. Tanaka, T. Koga, Y. Shimada, N. Tomita, Y. Sakato, T. Fujimoto, T. Nishiyama, N. Kuda, and K. Ishimoto.** 1985. Effect of BRL 25000 (clavulanic acid-amoxicillin) on bacterial flora in human feces. Jpn. J. Antibiot. **38**:441–450.
96. **Mulder, J.G., W.E. Wiersma, G.W. Welling, and D. van der Waaij.** 1984. Low dose oral tobramycin treatment for selective decontamination of the digestive tract: a study in human volunteers. J. Antimicrob. Chemother. **13**:495–504.
97. **Mulligan, M.E., D. Citron, E. Gabay, B.D. Kirby, W.L. George, and S.M. Finegold.** 1984. Alterations in human fecal flora, including ingrowth of *Clostridium difficile*, related to cefoxitin therapy. Antimicrob. Agents Chemother. **26**:343–346.
98. **Murray, P.R., E.J. Baron, M.A. Pfaller, F.C. Tenover, and R.H. Yolken (ed.).** 1999. Manual of Clinical Microbiology, 7th ed., p. 246–726. ASM Press, Washington, D.C.
99. **Nakashima, M., T. Uematsu, K. Kosuge, S. Nakagawa, S. Hata, and M. Sanada.** 1994. Pharmacokinetics and safety of BO-2727, a new injectable 1-β-methyl carbapenem antibiotic, and its effect on the faecal microflora in healthy male volunteers. J. Antimicrob. Chemother. **33**:987–998.
100. **National Committee for Clinical Laboratory Standards.** 2000. Methods for dilution antimicrobial susceptibility tests for bacteria that grow aerobically. Approved standard, 5th ed., M7-A5, p. 1–25. NCCLS, Wayne, Pa.
101. **National Committee for Clinical Laboratory Standards.** 2001. Methods for antimicrobial susceptibility testing of anaerobic bacteria. Approved standard, 5th ed., M11–A5, p. 1–34. NCCLS, Wayne, Pa.

102. **Nilsson-Ehle, I., C.E. Nord, and B. Ursing.** 1985. Ceftriaxone: pharmacokinetics and effect on the intestinal microflora in patients with acute bacterial infections. Scand. J. Infect. Dis. **17:**77–82.
103. **Nord, C.E.** 1993. Ecological impact of narrow spectrum antimicrobial agents compared to broad spectrum agents on the human intestinal microflora, p. 8–19. *In* C.E. Nord, P.J. Heidt, V.C. Rusch, and D. van der Waaij (ed.), Old Herborn University Seminar Monograph: Consequences of Antimicrobial Therapy for the Composition of the Microflora of the Digestive Tract. Herborn, Institute for Microbiology and Biochemistry.
104. **Nord, C.E., T. Bergan, and S. Aase.** 1986. Impact of azlocillin on the colon microflora. Scand. J. Infect. Dis. **18:**163–166.
105. **Nord, C.E., T. Bergan, and S.B. Thorsteinsson.** 1989. Impact of ticarcillin/clavulanate on the intestinal microflora. J. Antimicrob. Chemother. **24**(Suppl. B)**:**221–226.
106. **Nord, C.E., B. Brismar, B. Kasholm-Tengve, and G. Tunevall.** 1993. Effect of piperacillin/tazobactam treatment on human bowel microflora. J. Antimicrob. Chemother. **31**(Suppl. A)**:**61–65.
107. **Nord, C.E., D.A. Gajjar, and D.M. Grasela.** 2002. Ecological impact of the des-F(6)-guinolone, BMS-284756, on the normal intestinal microflora. Clin. Microbiol. Infect. **8:**229–239.
108. **Nord, C.E., A. Grahnen, and S.Å. Eckernäs.** 1991. Effect of loracarbef on the normal oropharyngeal and intestinal microflora. Scand. J. Infect. Dis. **23:**255–260.
109. **Nord, C.E., A. Heimdahl, C. Lundberg, and G. Marklund.** 1987. Impact of cefaclor on the normal human oropharyngeal and intestinal microflora. Scand. J. Infect. Dis. **19:**681–685.
110. **Nord, C.E., L. Kager, A. Philipson, and G. Stiernstedt.** 1984. Impact of imipenem/cilastin therapy on faecal flora. Eur. J. Microbiol. **3:**475–477.
111. **Nord, C.E., G. Movin, and D. Stålberg.** 1988. Impact of cefixime on the normal intestinal microflora. Scand. J. Infect. Dis. **20:**547–552.
112. **Novelli, A., T. Mazzei, S. Fallani, R. Dei, M.I. Cassetta, and S. Conti.** 1995. Betalactam therapy and intestinal flora. J. Chemother. **7**(Suppl. 1)**:**25–32.
113. **Orrhage, K., B. Brismar, and C.E. Nord.** 1994. Effect of supplements with *Bifidobacterium longum* and *Lactobacillus acidophilus* on the intestinal microbiota during administration of clindamycin. Microb. Ecol. Health Dis. **7:**17–25.
114. **Orrhage, K., S. Sjöstedt, and C.E. Nord.** 2000. Effect of supplements with lactic acid bacteria and oligofructose on the intestinal microflora during administration of cefpodoxime proxetil. J. Antimicrob. Chemother. **46:**603–611.
115. **Pecquet, S., A. Andremont, and C. Tancrède.** 1986. Selective antimicrobial modulation of the intestinal tract by norfloxacin in human volunteers and in gnotobiotic mice associated with human faecal microflora. Anrimcrob. Agents Chemother. **29:**1047–1052.
116. **Pecquet, S., A. Andremont, and C. Tancrède.** 1987. Effect of ofloxacin on fecal bacteria in human volunteers. Antimicrob. Agents Chemother. **31:**124–125.
117. **Pecquet, S., E. Chachaty, C. Tancrède, and A. Andremont.** 1991. Effects of roxithromycin on fecal bacteria in human volunteers and resistance to colonization in gnotobiotic mice. Antimicrob. Agents Chemother. **35:**548–552.
118. **Pecquet, S., S. Ravoire, and A. Andremont.** 1990. Faecal excretion of ciprofloxacin after a single oral dose and its effect on faecal bacteria in healthy volunteers. J. Antimicrob. Chemother. **26:**125–129.
119. **Ritz, M., H. Lode, M. Fassbender, K. Borner, P. Koeppe, and C.E. Nord.** 1994. Multiple-dose pharmacokinetics of sparfloxacin and its influence on fecal flora. Antimicrob. Agents Chemother. **38:**455–459.
120. **Rozenberg-Arska, M., A.W. Dekker, and J. Verhoef.** 1985. Ciprofloxacin for selective decontamination of the alimentary tract in patients with acute leukemia during remission induction treatment: the effect on the fecal flora. J. Infect. Dis. **152:**104–107.
121. **Salyers, A.A., and C.F. Amábile-Cuevas.** 1997. Why are antibiotic resistance genes so resistant to elimination. Minireview. Antimicrob. Agents Chemother. **41:**2321–2325.
122. **Scanvic-Hameg, A., E. Chachaty, J. Rey, C. Pousson, M.L. Ozoux, E. Brunel, and A. Andremont.** 2001. Impact of quinupristin/dalfopristin (RP59500) on the fecal microflora in healthy volunteers. J. Antimicrob. Chemother. **49:**135–139.
123. **Stark, C.A., I. Adamsson, C. Edlund, S. Sjöstedt, R. Seensalu, B. Wikström, and C.E. Nord.** 1996. Effects of omeprazole and amoxycillin on the human oral and gastrointestinal microflora in patients with *Helicobacter pylori* infection. J. Antimicrob. Chemother. **38:**927–939.
124. **Sullivan, Å., C. Edlund, and C.E. Nord.** 2001. Effect of antimicrobial agents on the ecological balance of human microflora. Lancet Infect. Dis. **1:**101–114.
125. **Sullivan, Å., C. Edlund, B. Svenungsson, L. Emtestam, and C.E. Nord.** 2001. Effect of perorally administered pivmecillinam on the normal oropharyngeal, intestinal and skin microflora. J. Chemother. **13:**299–308.
126. **Summanen, P., E. Baron, D. Citron, C. Stong, H. Wexler, and S. Finegold.** 1993. Wadsworth Anaerobic Bacteriology Manual, 5th ed., p. 1–159. Veterans Administration, Wadsworth Medical Center, Los Angeles, Calif.
127. **Tang, Y.W., and D.H. Persing.** 1999. Molecular detection and identification of microorganisms, p. 215–244. *In* P.R. Murray, E.J. Baron, M.A. Pfaller, F.C. Tenover, and R.H. Yolken (ed.), Manual of Clinical Microbiology, 7th ed. ASM Press, Washington, D.C.
128. **Tannock, G.W.** 1999. The normal microflora: an introduction, p. 1–23. *In* G.W. Tannock (ed.), Medical Importance of Normal Microflora. Kluwer Academic Publishers, London.
129. **Van der Auwera, P., N. Pensart, V. Korten, B.E. Murray, and R. Leclercq.** 1996. Influence of oral glycopeptides on the fecal flora of human volunteers: selection of highly glycopeptide-resistant enterococci. J. Infect. Dis. **173:**1129–1136.
130. **van der Leur, J.J.J.P.M., E.J. Vollaard, A.J.H.M. Janssen, and A.S.M. Dofferhoff.** 1997. Influence of low dose ciprofloxacin on microbial colonization of the digestive tract in healthy volunteers during normal and during impaired colonization resistance. Scand. J. Infect. Dis. **29:**297–300.
131. **van der Waaij, D.** 1985. Selective decontamination of the digestive tract with oral aztreonam and temocillin. Rev. Infect. Dis. **7**(Suppl. 4)**:**628–634.
132. **van der Waaij, D., and C.E. Nord.** 2000. Development and persistence of multiresistance to antibiotics in bacteria; an analysis and a new approach to this urgent problem. Int. J. Antimicrob. Agents **16:**191–197.
133. **van Nispen, C.H.M., A.I.M. Hoepelman, M. Rozenberg-Arska, J. Verhoef, L. Purkins, and S.A. Willavize.** 1998. A double-blind, placebo-controlled, parallel group study of oral trovafloxacin on bowel microflora in healthy male volunteers. Am. J. Surg. **176**(Suppl. 6A)**:**27–31.
134. **Van Saene, J.J., H.K. Van Saene, J.N. Geitz, N.J. Tarko-Smit, and C.F. Lerk.** 1986. Quinolones and colonization resistance in human volunteers. Pharm. Weekbl. Sci. **8:**67–71.
135. **Vogel, F., and H. Knothe.** 1985. Changes in aerobic faecal bacterial flora of severely ill patients during antibiotic treatment. Klin. Wochenschr. **63:**1174–1179.
136. **Vogel, F., H.R. Ochs, K. Wettich, S. Kalich, I. Nilsson-Ehle, I. Odenholt, and C.E. Nord.** 2001. Effect of step-down therapy of ceftriaxone plus loracarbef versus parenteral therapy of ceftriaxone on the intestinal microflora in patients with community-acquired pneumonia. Clin. Microbiol. Infect. **7:**376–379.
137. **Vollaard, E.J., and H.A.L. Clasener.** 1994. Colonization resistance. Minireview. Antimicrob. Agents Chemother. **38:**409–414.
138. **Vollaard, E.J., H.A.L. Clasener, and A.J.H.M. Janssen.** 1992. Influence of pefloxacin on microbial colonization resistance in healthy volunteers. Eur. J. Clin. Microbiol. Infect. Dis. **11:**257–260.
139. **Welling, G.W., G.J. Meijer-Severs, G. Helmus, E. van Santen, R.H.J. Tonk, H.G. de Vries-Hospers, and D. van der Waaij.** 1991. The effect of ceftriaxone on the anaerobic bacterial flora

and the bacterial enzymatic activity in the intestinal tract. Infection **19:**313–316.

140. **Whiley, R.A., and D. Beighton.** 1998. Current classification of the oral streptococci. Oral Microbiol. Immunol. **13:**195–216.
141. **Whittaker, C.J., C.M. Klier, and P.E. Kolenbrander.** 1996. Mechanisms of adhesion by oral bacteria. Annu. Rev. Microbiol. 50:513–552.
142. **Wise, R., S.A. Bennet, and J. Dent.** 1984. The pharmacokinetics of orally absorbed cefuroxime compared with amoxycillin/ clavulanic acid. J. Antimicrob. Chemother. **13:**603–610.
143. **Wistrom, J., L.O. Gentry, A.C. Palmgren, M. Price, C.E. Nord, A. Ljungh, and S.R. Norrby.** 1992. Ecological effects of short-term ciprofloxacin treatment of travellers diarrhoea. J. Antimicrob. Chemother. **30:**693–706.

Clinical Quality Assurance and the International Development of New Anti-Infective Agents

J. M. HUSSON, C. LIM, AND A. BRYSKIER

57

1. INTRODUCTION

Any industrial company (aeronautical, electronic, or other) must fulfill regulatory requirements and the demands of its clients, irrespective of the product manufactured or the service rendered.

The industrialist must think in terms of "total quality," since only optimal quality applied to each of the stages of manufacture of the "product" and to each of the tasks performed in each of the areas of activity will enable him to meet fully the specifications imposed by his client.

The pharmaceutical industry does not escape this rule. At all stages of development of a new pharmaceutical product, it must meet the demands of its potential clients in terms of quality. It must therefore meet predefined standards of efficacy and safety from the outset.

The clinical part of development is essential, but it is only one of the stages in the pursuit of this total quality. Chemists, pharmacologists, toxicologists, development pharmacists, and clinicians participate in this chain of quality, at the same time as their partners or clients represented by the registration authorities and ultimately the patients.

2. QA OF CLINICAL TRIALS ON MEDICINAL PRODUCTS

It is easy to accept that a new medicinal product must be produced according to "good manufacturing practice" (GMP) or undergo animal toxicology studies in accordance with "good laboratory practice" (GLP). It is more difficult to understand that any clinical drug trial, particularly if it is intended for the registration of a new medicinal product, must follow "good clinical practice" (GCP) procedures. Would "poor clinical quality" be conceivable in clinical drug trials?

The existence of a strict regulatory framework does not guarantee this quality. The interest of the healthy subject or patient from the point of view of protection, and that of the sponsor (industrial or otherwise) in terms of optimal quality and authenticity of the clinical data, make the introduction of GCP essential, and hence a clinical quality assurance system (QAS) specific to the pharmaceutical industry or any other sponsor wishing to bring a quality product to the market. A medicinal product that can be used in human healthcare must first of all be accepted by all the regulatory authorities.

The total quality so long sought after and obtained in the aeronautical industry is all the more necessary in clinical drug trials in that there is a chain of human factors (patient, investigator, pharmacist, sponsor, etc.) specific to this type of research. Quality in clinical research in fact obeys the same requirements as in other areas.

In this chapter we attempt to analyze the specific features of the clinical development of anti-infective agents (AIA) (antibacterials, antivirals, and antifungals) and to identify the general or specific rules for obtaining optimal quality.

2.1. Principles of a QAS

2.1.1. General Principles

Three basic principles underlie clinical research on medicinal products in the context of GCP: (i) protection of the subject undergoing biomedical research, (ii) the search for optimal quality for clinical data, and (iii) minimization of the risk of deviations from preestablished specifications, whatever their origin, and consequently the search for possible fraud.

Four basic concepts underlie the search for total quality. This occurs in well-defined stages, summarized by some authors in the concept of plan, do, check, and act:

1. The design or definition of the project, which comes down to defining the aims and objectives and detailing the means and methods necessary to achieve it—plan
2. The training and education of the participants and implementation of the project—do
3. Conformity with preestablished specifications: this is quality control—check
4. Performance in relation to the project and the plan: measurement of the level of results by audits. This leads to the necessary corrective measures being taken depending on the abnormalities observed—act

International standards of the ISO 9000 series define the general principles for obtaining quality, which may be applied to any area of production and enable a quality system to be established for a defined and limited activity. These standards applied by the industrialist wishing to satisfy his client are fully applicable to pharmacy and clinical research into drugs.

2.1.2. Specific Problems

The clinical development of AIA is specific in that, more than the other therapeutic classes, it involves the three types of good practice (Table 1), each corresponding to one of the components of the study: clinical trial proper, drug samples, and clinical microbiology.

2.1.2.1. Clinical Trial Proper

GCP acts as a regulatory framework in terms of quality for the clinical part of a pharmacokinetic study or a therapeutic trial.

GLP guarantees the quality of the samples and assays of biological specimens.

2.1.2.2. Drug Samples

GMP is the framework for the quality system, allowing the manufacture of batches of active substance and pharmaceutical batches for clinical trials. The pharmaceutical form of the new medicinal product must from the beginning of clinical development be as close as possible to that which will be brought onto the market, hence the importance of QA.

2.1.2.3. Clinical Microbiology

GLP should be applied and systematically incorporated into the conduct of the bacteriological studies associated with therapeutic trials on antibacterials. Paradoxically, no bacteriology laboratory of any kind (clinical or fundamental) and no country in which they are established has set up a genuine QAS based on GLP and, indirectly, GCP, which would allow in particular intercenter comparisons through the introduction of normal values and reference standards. A considerable distance remains to be covered before an international consensus is obtained on this matter and standardized common "rules" are established.

2.2. Regulatory Provisions: GCP

2.2.1. Definition of GCP

GCPs are defined as a series of "legal or regulatory texts" ensuring the quality and authenticity of clinical data, while protecting the subject undergoing clinical research.

Although strictly speaking extrinsic to scientific questions and ethics, GCP cannot in fact be dissociated from them.

GCP in general involves "technical notes" or "guidelines" whose aim is to specify standards of good practice for clinical trials on medicinal products. They must be read and interpreted in light of the pharmaceutical legislation and regulation specific to each country.

Table 1 Treatment by AIA: characteristics in relation to other medicinal products in therapeutic and quality terms

Practice	Characteristic
GCP, GLP	Activity against causal pathogens
GLP	Pathogens isolated and identified
GLP?	Predictive in vitro activity (laboratory)
GCP, GLP	Levels of AIA
GCP, GLP	Microbiological eradication rate during therapy
GCP, GLP	Microflora interactions
GLP	Resistance development
	Resistance transfer
	Hemostasis AIs[a] due to AIA

[a]AIs, adverse incidents.

2.2.2. Different GCP Texts

In the United States, the Food and Drug Administration (FDA) in 1977 published a series of regulatory texts in the *Federal Register* on the conduct of clinical trials, introducing the concept of GCP for the first time in the world; these texts were supplemented in the 1980s by several other texts defining the regulation of clinical trials on medicinal products (Table 2).

In Europe, following the publication by a number of European countries of national texts on GCP, a guideline on GCP prepared by the Committee on Proprietary Medicinal Products was published by the European Community in June 1990. This text, published in a regulatory and in part legislative form (Directive 92/318 EEC), will only be legally binding if the GCPs are included in the future directive on clinical trials in preparation and are incorporated in the national law of those member states who have not included GCPs in a legal text.

Japan published its own GCP procedures in 1990, and in September 1992 the World Health Organization published its draft guidelines.

Harmonization of the GCP texts of different countries began in 1989 at the International Conference on Harmonization between the European Community, Japan, and the United States (ICH1—Brussels, Belgium, November 1991). A parallel study of the texts from the European community, Japan, and the United States taking the "European explanatory note" as a point of reference showed that there were differences between the texts but that, in principle, a clinical trial conducted in one of these three regions was mutually acceptable from the GCP aspect. The "ICH concept" on GCP enabled certain proposals to be put forward at ICH2 (Orlando, Fla., October 1993) concerning the essential points to be included in a harmonized tripartite text.

Among the texts adopted and published in the form of an appendix for consultation, the following may be mentioned: the list of documents essential for recognition of the GCP standard (Table 3) and the plan for the "investigator's brochure."

The mutual and tripartite acceptance of clinical trials undertaken within the legal and/or regulatory framework of GCP is a necessary, but not sufficient, condition for acceptance abroad within the context of a registration dossier. There are at present, particularly between Europe, Japan, and the United States, major differences in terms of ethical factors, medical practice, therapeutic customs, and study methodology that make mutual recognition, and hence the acceptance of clinical trials for registration purposes, difficult.

Some of these points today represent some of the subjects approached within the framework of the ICH. Harmonization in this area, which is certainly achievable, will require a fundamental change of attitude and approach

Table 2 Development by the FDA of GCP

Legal	Date of Proposal	Applications
GLP	November 1976	June 1979
Informed consent	August 1979	July 1981
	August 1978	July 1981
IRB	September 1977	
Sponsor monitoring	August 1978	
Clinician investigations	October 1982	May 1985
NDA rewrite	June 1983	June 1987
IND rewrite		January 1988

Table 3 List of essential documents for clinical trials conducted in accordance with GCP (proposal)

Document(s)	Retrieval	
	Investigator	Sponsor
Standard operating procedures	?	+
Investigator brochure (up-to-date)	+	+
Protocols: signed	+	+
Protocol amendments	+	+
Contracts	+	+
Insurance	+	+
Ethics committees: protocols	+	+
Ethics committees: amendments	+	+
Authority authorizations	+	+
Investigators: addresses, curricula vitae, etc.	+	+
Clinical labs: standards	+	+
Drugs		
Technical documents		±
Distribution		±
Count	+	+
Investigator in charge	?	±
Enrollment figures	±	
Random list		±
Opening	+	+
Monitoring forms		
Telephone, fax		±
On-site visit		±
Document of origin	±	
Consent form: documentation	+	+
Adverse-event reports	+	+
Study book signed, including amendments	+	+
Clinical report signed	+	+
Audit certificate		±

by the authorities, investigators, and industrialists in countries concerned with the development of new medicinal products.

2.2.3. Scope and Applications of GCP

The scope and applications of GCP relate to the following areas (see European GCP for further details):

- The protection of subjects included in clinical studies
- Investigational review boards (IRB) or their equivalents, such as the ethics committee in France
- Informed consent
- The responsibilities of the sponsor, monitor, and investigator
- The experimental study plan, the preparation of samples, and randomization
- Data management and statistical analysis
- The clinical study report
- Data retrieval
- QA proper

2.3. QAS of the Clinical Trial of an AIA

2.3.1. Standard Operating Procedures

International pharmaceutical companies have been obliged progressively to include GCP in their daily practice and in clinical trials on their products, not only to meet the requirements of the regulatory authorities around the world but also to improve the intrinsic quality of these trials.

These companies have thus progressively instituted their own quality standards, compiled in the form of standard operating procedures. The different components of these regulatory texts are transcribed by the sponsor, but also by the pharmacist and investigator involved in the trial, in the form of standard operating procedures applicable to each of the stages of a clinical trial on a medicinal product.

2.3.2. Clinical Research on Medicinal Products and QA

For a given clinical research project, the QAS instituted by a pharmaceutical company is based on the different sectors of activity involved in the study and on several operational levels.

Four (line) management levels are involved in the implementation and conduct of studies in terms of quality.

(i) Management (medical or equivalent) ratifies the principle and the implementation of a QAS, assumes responsibility for the financing, and takes any corrective measures necessary after audit.

(ii) The study director and QA director constitute the next level down. The former decides on the principle of the clinical trial and supervises its implementation, and the second, his counterpart, supervises the audits intended to check the intrinsic quality of the study.

(iii) The project leader is responsible for conducting the study and, together with the statistician, analyzing the results. He may obtain the cooperation of a contract research organization charged with completing the study.

(iv) The QA auditor(s) checks the quality "performance" following the project.

The concept of total quality for any clinical project requires the employment of personnel whose qualifications and performance are based on up-to-date education and training, sufficient experience, suitable material and financial resources, and sufficient time to complete the study.

The team must work in accordance with the standardized operating procedures already mentioned. Each person involved is responsible for ensuring an optimum quality level, thereby guaranteeing the safety of the patient and fulfilling the requirements of the legal and/or regulatory texts.

There is one major prerequisite for the organization of the QAS, which is the need to have a complete hierarchical and operational separation between those people carrying out the clinical projects and those responsible for quality audits (Fig. 1). This restriction is related to the fact that QA personnel cannot be the judge in their own case; they must work in a neutral, open, and independent manner, free from any pressure.

The ultimate aim of QA is to include data of sufficiently high quality in the clinical study report and more generally in the clinical documentation to allow firm decisions to be taken about the risk/benefit ratio. The concept of total quality assumes that everyone involved in the project must attempt to achieve the highest level of professionalism in ensuring the patient's safety and the integrity of the clinical data. This requirement concerns both the sponsor and/or his representatives (contract research organization) and the other protagonists in the clinical study: investigator, pharmacist, IRB, etc. The healthy volunteer or patient must be provided with complete information and explanations in order to benefit as much as possible from his inclusion in the study, while at the same time guaranteeing the hoped-for level of quality.

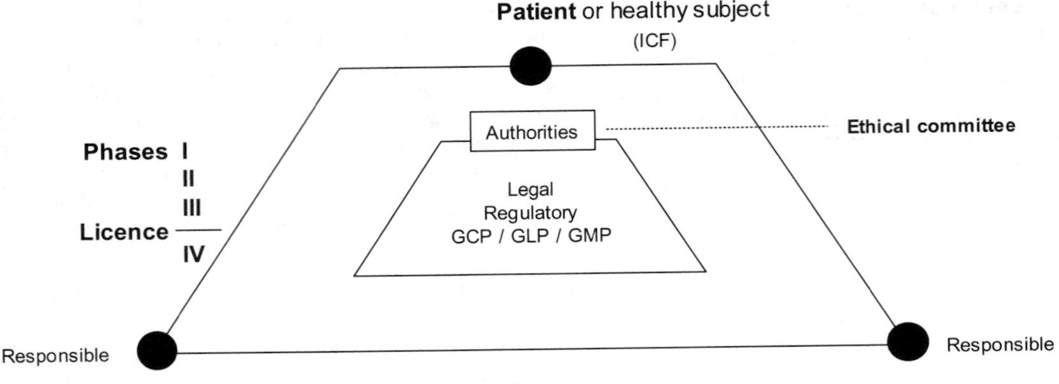

Figure 1 The different partners involved in a clinical trial. Authorities: FDA, Koseisho, national agencies (France, Sweden, United Kingdom, Germany). ICF, informed-consent form; SOP, standard operating procedures; EMEA, European Agency for the Evaluation of Medicinal Products.

2.4. Audits and Inspections

The audit, whether conducted by the sponsor or by the regulatory authorities, involves a performance evaluation undertaken during the clinical study, including the statistical part. The audit measures the quality of the study and sees whether it meets the total-quality standard.

For the sponsor, the audit is performed by a QA department independent of the clinical research unit responsible for the clinical trial proper. The site audits (investigator or sponsor) check systematically the availability of certain general documents (e.g., IRB documentation and follow-up visit by monitors) or arbitrarily and in a randomized manner a certain percentage of individual data (cross-checking of case report forms against source data, availability of consent forms, etc.).

The problem of the audit/inspection by the authorities has been raised in the majority of European countries. In France, such inspections required by the law on biomedical research of December 1988 have not yet been systematized, despite certain attempts.

This inspection, however, is one of the key elements in the mutual recognition of clinical data by the authorities of the main countries, as is the case preclinically for certain countries (e.g., Pharmaceutical Inspection Convention, established by the countries of the European Free Trade Area and today involving 16 countries, including many countries of the European community, or the convention governing toxicology [GLP] and involving the United States, Japan, and certain European countries).

Since 1980, as was pointed out at ICH2 by Frances Kelsey, the FDA has undertaken inspections abroad, including Europe (Table 4), that initially resulted in a rejection or a reanalysis of the trials in 45% of cases. The deficiencies most commonly encountered are listed in Table 5.

2.5. Scientific Quality of the Trial and GCP

Although theoretically absent from the concept of GCP, the scientific quality of the trial, based on the study protocol, cannot be dissociated from the QA defined by GCP texts. The EEC text devotes a chapter to the protocol and to its different aspects (study plan and statistical approach).

The concept of simple notification or authorization of a clinical trial varies from country to country (Table 6), which means that the verification of the scientific quality

Table 4 Routine FDA inspections—the most common deficiencies[a]

Deficiency	%		
	United States	Other countries	European Union
Consent forms incorrect	56	50	17
Protocol violations	27	77	72
Incorrect count (drugs)	23	41	28
Clinical data incorrect	21	80	78
Amendments without notification	10		
Combined treatment nonlicensed in the United States	4		
No agreement of IRB	3		
Registered data not available	3		
Other investigators not mentioned			
No. of Health Agency visits 1 June 1977 to 1 July 1991	2,592	66	18

[a]From Kelsey, ICH1, 1991.

Table 5 Comparison of site audits undertaken in France and the United Kingdom[a]

Parameter	Score	
	France	United Kingdom
Investigator performance	+++	+++
Center organization	+++	++
Responsibility: transfer	+++	+++
Documentation: retrieval	+	+
Patient protection		
Ethics committee	+++	+++
Consent forms	+++	++
Drug count	++	++
Study monitoring	++	++
Adverse-event report	++	++

[a]The audits were undertaken in France ($n = 11$) and the United Kingtom ($n = 4$) in 1991 to 1992 as part of a multicenter study on an antidepressant, the study monitoring being performed by two contract research organizations.

of the study is different within the European Union, making it difficult to draw any comparisons on a purely scientific level.

3. PROBLEMS POSED BY THE CLINICAL EVALUATION OF AIA

3.1. Specificity of the Clinical Trial of an AIA

3.1.1. Disparity or Nonhomogeneity of Study Populations

Infectious disorders assume a wide variety of different presentations for the same microorganism, depending in particular on the portal of entry, the only actual and apparent common feature of which, apart from the infectious syndrome, is the discovery of the causative agent. This fact, which often makes the diagnosis difficult and the grouping of patients in clinical trials complicated, distinguishes infectious diseases from others.

3.1.2. Evaluation of Efficacy Based on Microbiological Criteria

Infectious diseases raise problems in therapeutic trials that are specific to them.

The evaluation of the efficacy of AIA is based on clinical criteria (fever and systemic and local signs of infection), but above all on the microbiological criteria obtained in the laboratory. The efficacy of the product is tested against strains of microorganisms of defined susceptibility.

3.2. Differences between AIA and other Medicinal Products

Differences between AIA and other medicinal products are summarized by Beam et al. in the "General Guidelines for the Clinical Evaluation of Anti-Infective Drug Products." In the introduction the authors summarize the characteristics of AIA in relation to other medicinal products.

The specific profile of these products affects the prerequisites and the standards in terms of QA.

For B. Regnier there are two specific problems relating to the quality of clinical trials on antimicrobial agents. The first problem concerns the validity of the microbiological data. The absence of true QA and of standardization of the different tests makes any interpretation and comparison of the results difficult, if not impossible. It would therefore be beneficial to set up a system of accreditation of contract bacteriology laboratories with a genuine QAS. This is essential in view of the importance of the microbiological results in interpreting the results of clinical trials on an AIA (efficacy).

The ideal would be to have the microbiological tests centralized, as is the case in Japan, which would avoid any bias in the interpretation of the results. The credibility of the therapeutic evaluation of the drug product depends on the credibility of the microbiological results.

The second problem in terms of quality is the high frequency of patients placed in the improved or unevaluable category. This is related to the implementation of a poor protocol with poor evaluation criteria on a clinical and microbiological level.

Table 6 Background documentation required for clinical trials of a new medicinal product and registration

Text	Australia	Canada	European Union	Japan	Scandinavian countries	United States
Global						
GLP	+		+	+	+	+
GCP	+	+	+	+	+	+
GMP	+	Industry	+	+	+	+
Clinical authorization	CTX	IND	-	Announced	IND	IND
Registration						
Full file		PL	EMEA[a]		EMEA	NDA
File summary			+		+	+
Other documents						
Statistics				+		+
Pharmacokinetics			+	+	+	+
Bioequivalence	+	+	+		+	+
Specifics						
Elderly			+	+	+	+
Children	+		+	+	+	+
Pregnancy			+			
Compounds						
Antibacterials			+	+	+	+
Antifungals			+	+	+	+

[a]EMEA, European Agency for the Evaluation of Medicinal Products.

4. CURRENT STATE OF ACCEPTANCE OF CLINICAL TRIALS ABROAD FOR THE INTERNATIONAL REGISTRATION OF AN AIA

4.1. Intrinsic Quality of a Clinical Study

Is the quality of clinical trials of AIA the same in all countries with a drug industry? Is there a difference in quality between clinical trials conducted in France and those undertaken in the main European countries? The "gold standard" remains acceptance by the FDA, such as "pivotal studies," clinical trials undertaken abroad and in this case usually without an IND (IND = investigational new drug application, the administrative stage by which the FDA [United States] authorizes clinical development following prior consultation [phase I]).

Let us take a clinical trial in France as an example. In terms of evaluation of the dossier of an AIA and hence of the quality of its contents, the French authorities are probably the most demanding in Europe, alongside the Swedish authorities. Does this mean that the quality of clinical trials conducted in France is sufficient and that they will be accepted throughout the world? In terms of quality, have they achieved total quality, and is it possible for them to be incorporated in a registration dossier in the United States (NDA) (NDA = new drug application) (marketing authorization) that is acceptable to the FDA or in the documentation of other countries whose standard of registration dossiers is very high (e.g., Australia and Canada)?

4.2. Acceptance in Europe (European Union and European Free Trade Area) of French Studies

French clinical trials are increasingly incorporated into the clinical documentation for registration, irrespective of whether the marketing authorization (or its equivalent) is applied for nationally or by an EEC procedure. Acceptance and hence recognition of these studies in terms of quality vary from one area to another, studies of AIA together with those of antihypertensive agents and gastric antisecretory agents being among the most readily accepted. The quality of such a study measured by an audit shows that there is not necessarily nowadays a major difference between a clinical trial conducted in France and one conducted in the United Kingdom.

4.3. Japan

For various reasons, clinical trials conducted abroad are not included in the documentation submitted to the Japanese authorities (Koseisho, or Ministry of Health and Welfare).

Various factors have led the Japanese not to accept studies conducted in Caucasians except as supplementary data, including for the evaluation of drug tolerance.

There are many reasons for this rejection, including ethnic differences; environmental differences; differences of medical, legal, and regulatory practice; and differences of methodology. Whatever the origin of the dossier (United States or Europe or both), almost all clinical trials must be repeated in Japan in Japanese subjects.

4.4. United States

To be accepted by the FDA, particularly as the (sole) basis for an NDA, studies conducted abroad must meet specified standards. The scientific and regulatory level required by the FDA is not inaccessible to the French investigator, particularly if he is working in the context of an IND. The investigator and the sponsor are in this case obliged to achieve total quality, related in particular to the intensity of the monitoring performed by the sponsor or a contract research organization and the horizon represented by the FDA inspection.

One restriction specific to the United States and Canada deserves to be mentioned, which is the need to have for each of the claimed therapeutic indications in the NDA (or its equivalent, the NDS) microorganisms susceptible to the antibiotic and hence a minimum of clinical cases for each of them (some 10 or so for the rarest species).

Despite its constraints, the law on biomedical research, known as the Huriet Law, should allow clinical trials conducted in France to achieve sufficient quality to be accepted in the most demanding countries. The only means of evaluating and improving the quality of French clinical trials will be (i) the official institution of inspections (medical and pharmaceutical inspectors) by the French authorities and (ii) the possible inspection by the FDA, the ideal in the future being the mutual recognition by the United States, Europe, and Japan of clinical trials after inspection by local authorities; this would require the prior institution of a system of inspection within the framework of the European Union.

5. CONCLUSIONS

Total quality is an aim to be achieved in clinical research for any pharmaceutical company that respects human dignity and is active on an international scale.

Europe, Japan, and the United States represent the "golden triangle" in terms of the discovery of new molecules. There is, however, a discrepancy between the United States and the rest of the world in terms of the quality of clinical trials required for registration. QASs are one of the necessary conditions but are insufficient to achieve the level required by the most demanding registration authorities (e.g., Australia, Canada, Sweden, the United Kingdom, and the United States). The quality of a clinical trial may also be measured in terms of scientific quality and hence methodology, even if the quality of the clinical research does not differ fundamentally between the major industrialized countries. Apart from ethnic factors, everything divides Japan from Europe and the United States in this respect. The ICH is currently attempting to bridge this gap, which throws up differences of medical practice and therapeutic approach.

As the time factor is difficult to negotiate, only an increase in human and material resources will allow optimal clinical quality to be obtained in a minimum of time. The increase in the quality of clinical trials acceptable in the United States is reflected in Europe by an increase of about 30 to 40% in financial costs. This is the price to be paid by the European industry if it wishes to have some of its studies accepted by the FDA.

Total quality must be instituted in relation to clinical trials of AIA. The quality required for the clinical part is that applicable to all clinical research on medicinal products. This is not the case with clinical bacteriology or research into other microorganisms, which is a specific feature of the infectious disease and which is essential for the diagnosis and monitoring of an infectious syndrome, particularly during trials of AIA. The absence of standards in clinical bacteriology makes the systematic introduction of GLP and a clinical QAS within a short period a matter of necessity. Only a stricter methodological approach will allow the efficacy of AIA to be correctly evaluated but will also allow an intercenter comparison in the main countries of the world.

We will take the opportunity to define the prerequisites in another publication.

REFERENCES

Beam TR, David NG, Kunin CI, 1992, General guidelines for the clinical evaluation of anti-infective drug products, Clin Infect Dis, 15 (Suppl 1), S5-S33.

D'Arcy PF, Harron DWG, ed, 1991, International Conference on Harmonization of Technical Requirements for Registration of Pharmaceuticals for Human Use, Proceedings of the 1st International Conference on Harmonization, Brussels, vol. I.

Regnier B, 1990, Good clinical practice, Eur J Clin Microbiol Inf Dis, 9, 519-522.

GUIDELINES

Germany

The Principles for Proper Performance of the Clinical Investigation of Drugs, Bonn, 1987.

European Community

Note for Guidance. Good Clinical Practice for Trials on Medicinal Products in the European Community, July 1990.

European Guidelines for the Clinical Evaluation of Anti-Infective Drug Products, 1993, Publ. European Society for Clinical Microbiology and Infectious Diseases.

United States

Guidelines for the Evaluation of Anti-Infective Drug Products, Clin Infect Dis, 15, S1-S339, 1992.

Protection of Human Subjects, Food and Drug Administration, CFR 21: Food and Drug, Parts 50, 56, 312, 314, 600 + 5/1980-6/1987.

France

Bonnes Pratiques Cliniques, Ministère de la Sante, Bulletin Officiel, Paris, 1987.

Japan

Good Clinical Practice for Trials on Drugs, Ministry of Health and Welfare Pharmaceutical Affairs Bureau, December 1990.

Scandinavia

Nordic Council, Good Clinical Practice, NLN publication no. 28, Nordiska Läkemedelsnamnden, Uppsala, 1983.

United Kingdom

Association of the British Pharmaceutical Industry: Guidelines on Good Clinical Research Practice, PJB Publications, London, 1988.

World Health Organization

Guidelines for Good Clinical Practice (GCP) for Trials on Pharmaceutical Products (draft), Division of Drug Management and Policies, World Health Organization.

Index